a LANGE medical book

CURRENT

Medical Diagnosis & Treatment 1998

37th Edition

D0226282

Edited by

Lawrence M. Tierney, Jr., MD
Professor of Medicine
University of California, San Francisco
Assistant Chief of Medical Services
Veterans Affairs Medical Center, San Francisco

Stephen J. McPhee, MD
Professor of Medicine
Division of General Internal Medicine
Department of Medicine
University of California, San Francisco

Maxine A. Papadakis, MD
Professor of Clinical Medicine
Director of Student Programs, Medicine
University of California, San Francisco

With Associate Authors

APPLETON & LANGE
Stamford, CT

Notice: The authors and the publisher of this volume have taken care to make certain that the doses of drugs and schedules of treatment are correct and compatible with the standards generally accepted at the time of publication. Nevertheless, as new information becomes available, changes in treatment and in the use of drugs become necessary. The reader is advised to carefully consult the instruction and information material included in the package insert of each drug or therapeutic agent before administration. This advice is especially important when using new or infrequently used drugs. The publisher disclaims any liability, loss, injury, or damage incurred as a consequence, directly or indirectly, of the use and application of any of the contents of the volume.

97 98 99 00 / 10 9 8 7 6 5 4 3 2 1

Prentice Hall International (UK) Limited, *London*
Prentice Hall of Australia Pty. Limited, *Sydney*
Prentice Hall Canada, Inc., *Toronto*
Prentice Hall Hispanoamericana, S.A., *Mexico*
Prentice Hall of India Private Limited, *New Delhi*
Prentice Hall of Japan, Inc., *Tokyo*
Simon & Schuster Asia Pte. Ltd., *Singapore*
Editora Prentice Hall do Brasil Ltda., *Rio de Janeiro*
Prentice Hall, *Upper Saddle River, New Jersey*

ISSN: 0092-8682

Acquisitions Editor: Shelley Reinhardt
Development Editor: Jim Ransom
Production Editor: Jeanmarie Roche
Designer: Mary Skudlarek
Illustrator: Linda F. Harris
Associate Art Manager: Maggie Belis Darrow
Art Coordinator: Becky Hainz-Baxter

PRINTED IN THE UNITED STATES OF AMERICA

ISBN: 0-8385-1524-X
90000

9 780838 515242

Contents

Preface

Current Medical Diagnosis & Treatment 1998 is the 37th annual volume of a general medical text designed as a single-source reference for practitioners in both hospital and ambulatory settings. CMDT covers all fields of internal medicine plus important other topics of concern to primary care physicians and to all specialists who provide generalist care. It emphasizes the practical features of diagnosis and patient management.

OUTSTANDING FEATURES

- Reissued annually in January to incorporate current advances.
- Coverage of all aspects of primary care, including gynecology, obstetrics, dermatology, ophthalmology, otolaryngology, psychiatry, neurology, urology, and other topics relevant to generalist care.
- Concise, readable format, facilitating efficient use in various practice settings.
- More than 1000 diseases and disorders.
- Only book of its kind to include an annual update on HIV infection.
- Brevity, conciseness, and easy accessibility of key information.
- Emphasis on prevention and cost-consciousness.
- Handy access to drug dosages and prices.
- Inexpensively priced.

INTENDED AUDIENCE

House officers and medical students will find the concise, up-to-date descriptions of diagnostic and therapeutic procedures, with citations to the current literature, of daily usefulness in the immediate management of patients.

Internists, family physicians, and other specialists who provide generalist care will appreciate *CMDT* as a useful ready reference and refresher text.

Physicians in other specialties, surgeons, and dentists will find the book useful as a basic internal medicine reference.

Nurses, nurse practitioners, physician's assistants, and other health practitioners will welcome the concise format and broad scope of the book as a means of enhancing their understanding of diagnostic principles and therapeutic procedures.

ORGANIZATION

CMDT is developed and organized chiefly by organ system. Chapter 1 presents general information on patient care, including health maintenance and disease prevention and management of pain and other common symptoms. Chapter 2 presents information on preoperative assessment and perioperative management. Chapter 3 addresses special problems of the older patient. Chapter 4 discusses medical management of cancer. Chapter 5 addresses care at the end of life. Chapters 6–28 describe diseases and disorders of various organ systems and their treatment. Chapter 29 sets forth the basic concepts of nutrition in modern medical practice. Chapters 30–37 cover infectious diseases and antimicrobial therapy. Chapters 38 and 39 cover disorders due to physical agents and poisoning. Chapter 40 discusses the principles of genetics as applied to medical disorders. Chapter 41 discusses laboratory tests and the diagnostic process. The Appendix provides information about therapeutic drug levels and reference ranges for the commonly used laboratory tests.

NEW TO THIS EDITION

- A new chapter on care at the end of life.
- Drug information and bibliographies updated through June 1997.
- An up-to-date chapter on HIV infection and approach to multidrug antiretroviral therapy. Information on AIDS in other chapters.
- An update on antibiotics.
- New table on ophthalmic medications.
- Major revision of chapters on bacterial and chlamydial infection, the alimentary tract, and lipid abnormalities.
- Updated drug costs, including costs per unit dose and costs for 30 days' treatment.
- Cutting edge information on new developments in the treatment of diabetes mellitus, asthma, HIV infection, homocysteinemia, prophylaxis of bacterial endocarditis, and testing for and treatment of *Helicobacter pylori* infection.
- Reflects latest clinical practice guidelines from the Agency for Health Care Policy and Research of the United States Public Health Service.
- Listing of key Internet addresses for peer-reviewed, current medical information, including traveler's and immunization information from the Centers for Disease Control and Prevention, Consensus Statements from the National Institutes of Health, and Clinical Guidelines from the Agency for Health Care Policy and Research of the United States Public Health Service.
- Drug trade names included in index.
- Complete listing of USA Poison Control Centers with telephone numbers.

ANNOUNCING *CMDT 1998* ON CD-ROM

In December 1997, a new CD-ROM version of *CMDT 1998* will be available. Besides the *CMDT* text, the CD-ROM will incorporate diagnostic test information from the *Pocket Guide to Diagnostic Tests,* second edition, and drug information from the *Pocket Guide to Commonly Prescribed Drugs,* second edition. Photographs of pills and capsules will also be included. The *CMDT 1998* CD-ROM will incorporate a wide variety of multimedia illustrations, including color photographs, photomicrographs, electrocardiograms, echocardiograms, x-rays, and other diagnostic imaging procedures; graphs, algorithms, and nomograms; video footage of cardiac catheterizations, IUD insertions, and other procedures; heart sounds and lung sounds; and an extensive listing of Internet addresses for each chapter. Finally, Medline abstracts will be provided for all journal references in *CMDT 1998,* in addition to the last five years of all Medline abstracts for the 25 medical journals considered most useful for generalists.

ANNOUNCING ANNUAL SUBSCRIPTIONS TO *CMDT*

You can now subscribe to the only annually updated textbook of medicine simply by returning the enclosed postcard to Appleton & Lange. You will receive each annual edition automatically upon publication, and you will be billed when you are mailed the text.

ACKNOWLEDGMENTS

We wish to thank our associate authors for participating once again in the annual updating of this important book. In particular, we wish to thank Dr Ralph Gonzales of the University of Colorado Health Sciences Center for his editorial supervision of the CD-ROM project. Many students and physicians have contributed useful suggestions to this and previous editions, and we are grateful. We continue to welcome comments and recommendations for future editions in writing or via electronic mail. The editors' and authors' institutional and Internet e-mail addresses are given in the Authors section that follows.

Lawrence M. Tierney, Jr., MD
Stephen J. McPhee, MD
Maxine A. Papadakis, MD

San Francisco, California
September 1997

Authors

Daniel C. Adelman, MD
Associate Adjunct Professor of Medicine, University of California, San Francisco.
Internet: adelman.daniel@gene.com
Allergic & Immunologic Disorders

Joshua S. Adler, MD
Assistant Clinical Professor, Department of Medicine, University of California, San Francisco; Director of Medical Consultation, Veterans Affairs Medical Center, San Francisco.
Internet: jadler@itsa.ucsf.edu
Preoperative Evaluation

Thomas M. Amidon, MD
Clinical Instructor, University of Washington, Seattle; Cardiologist, Overlake Hospital Medical Center, Bellevue, Washington.
Heart

Michael J. Aminoff, MD, FRCP
Professor of Neurology, University of California, San Francisco.
Nervous System

Robert B. Baron, MD, MS
Professor of Clinical Medicine; Vice Chief, Division of General Internal Medicine; Director, Primary Care Internal Medicine Residency Program; Director, Continuing Medical Education, Department of Medicine, University of California, San Francisco.
Internet: baron@dgim.ucsf.edu
Nutrition; Lipid Abnormalities

Timothy G. Berger, MD
Associate Clinical Professor, Department of Dermatology, University of California, San Francisco.
Skin & Appendages

Robert V. Brody, MD
Clinical Professor of Medicine and Family & Community Medicine, University of California, San Francisco; Chair, Ethics Committee, and Chief, Pain Consultation Clinic, San Francisco General Hospital; Medical Director, Hospice & AIDS Programs, Visiting Nurses & Hospice of San Francisco.
Internet: brody@itsa.ucsf.edu
Care at the End of Life

Warren S. Browner, MD, MPH
Associate Professor of Medicine, Epidemiology, Biostatistics, and Anesthesia, University of California, San Francisco; Chief, General Internal Medicine Section, Veterans Affairs Medical Center, San Francisco.
Internet: WSBMD@ITSA.UCSF.EDU
Lipid Disorders

Maria E. Carlini, MD
Fellow in Infectious Diseases, Baylor College of Medicine, Houston.
Infectious Diseases: Viral & Rickettsial

Peter R. Carroll, MD
Professor and Chair, Department of Urology, University of California, San Francisco.
Internet: peter_carroll@quickmail.ucsf.edu
Urology

Henry F. Chambers, MD
Professor of Medicine, University of California, San Francisco; Chief, Division of Infectious Diseases, San Francisco General Hospital.
Internet: chipc@itsa.ucsf.edu
Infectious Diseases: Bacterial & Chlamydial

Richard Cohen, MD, MPH
Associate Clinical Professor, Division of Occupational and Environmental Medicine, University of California, San Francisco.
Internet: Richard.Cohen@corp.varian.com
Disorders Due to Physical Agents

William R. Crombleholme, MD
Professor and Vice Chair, Department of Obstetrics, Gynecology and Reproductive Sciences, University of Pittsburgh School of Medicine, Magee-Women's Hospital.
Obstetrics

William M. Detmer, MD, MSc
Clinical Assistant Professor of Medicine, Department of Health Evaluation Sciences, University of Virginia, Charlottesville.
Internet: bdetmer@virginia.edu
Diagnostic Testing & Medical Decision Making

Stuart J. Eisendrath, MD
Professor of Clinical Psychiatry; Director, Psychiatric Consultation and Brief Intervention Clinics, Langley Porter Psychiatric Institute, University of California, San Francisco.
Internet: Eisen@itsa.ucsf.edu
Psychiatric Disorders

R. Ron Finley, RPh
Lecturer, Division of Clinical Pharmacy, School of Pharmacy, University of California, San Francisco.
Internet: rrf@itsa.ucsf.edu
Drug Information

Paul A. Fitzgerald, MD
Associate Clinical Professor of Medicine, Department of Medicine and Metabolic Research Unit, University of California, San Francisco.
Internet: pf@fitzgeraldmd.com
Endocrine Disorders

Scott A. Flanders, MD
Chief Medical Resident, University of California, San Francisco; Assistant Chief of the Medical Service, Moffitt-Long Hospital, San Francisco.
Internet: flandrz@itsa.ucsf.edu
References

Lawrence S. Friedman, MD
Associate Professor of Medicine, Harvard Medical School; Associate Physician, Gastrointestinal Unit, Massachusetts General Hospital, Boston.
Internet: Friedman.Lawrence@mgh.harvard.edu
Liver, Biliary Tract, & Pancreas

Armando E. Giuliano, MD
Clinical Professor of Surgery, University of California, Los Angeles, School of Medicine; Chief of Surgical Oncology and Director, Joyce Eisenberg Keefer Breast Center, John Wayne Cancer Institute, Saint John's Hospital and Health Center, Santa Monica, California.
Internet: Giuliano@jwci.org
Breast

Lee Goldman, MD, MPH
Julius R. Krevans Distinguished Professor and Chairman, Department of Medicine; Associate Dean of Clinical Affairs, School of Medicine, University of California, San Francisco.
Internet: Lee_goldman@ucsfdom.ucsf.edu
Preoperative Evaluation

Robert S. Goldsmith, MD, MPH, DTM&H
Professor Emeritus of Tropical Medicine and Epidemiology, Department of Epidemiology and Biostatistics, University of California, San Francisco.
Internet: rg645@itsa.ucsf.edu
Infectious Diseases: Protozoal & Helminthic

B. Joseph Guglielmo, PharmD
Professor and Vice Chair, Department of Clinical Pharmacy, School of Pharmacy, University of California, San Francisco.
Internet: bjg@itsa.ucsf.edu
Anti-infective Chemotherapeutic & Antibiotic Agents

Richard J. Hamill, MD
Associate Professor of Medicine, Baylor College of Medicine; Staff Physician, Infectious Disease Section, Veterans Affairs Medical Center, Houston.
Internet: hamill.richard_j@houston.va.gov
Infectious Diseases: Mycotic

David B. Hellmann, MD
Mary Betty Stevens Professor of Medicine and Executive Vice Chair, Department of Medicine, Johns Hopkins University School of Medicine, Baltimore.
Internet: hellmdb1@welchlink.welch.jhu.edu
Arthritis & Musculoskeletal Disorders

Harry Hollander, MD
Professor of Clinical Medicine and Director, Categorical Medicine Residency Program, University of California, San Francisco.
Internet: drwine@itsa.ucsf.edu
HIV Infection

Robert K. Jackler, MD
Professor of Otolaryngology and Neurological Surgery, University of California, San Francisco.
Internet: rkj@itsa.ucsf.edu
Ear, Nose, & Throat

Richard A. Jacobs, MD, PhD
Clinical Professor of Medicine and Clinical Pharmacy, University of California, San Francisco.
Internet: dick_jacobs@quickmail.ucsf.edu
General Problems in Infectious Diseases; Infectious Diseases: Spirochetal; Anti-infective Chemotherapeutic & Antibiotic Agents

Michael J. Kaplan, MD
Associate Professor, Department of Otolaryngology-Head and Neck Surgery and Department of Neurologic Surgery, University of California, San Francisco.
Internet: mjkaplan@orca.ucsf.edu
Ear, Nose, & Throat

John H. Karam, MD
Professor of Medicine, Emeritus, Metabolic Research Unit and Diabetes Center, University of California, San Francisco.
Internet: BEM969KAR@AOL.COM
Diabetes Mellitus & Hypoglycemia

Mitchell H. Katz, MD
Director, Community Health and Safety, San Francisco Department of Health.
Internet: Mitch_Katz@dph.sf.ca.us
HIV Infection

Kiyoshi Kurokawa, MD, MACP
Dean and Professor of Medicine, Tokai University School of Medicine, Kanagawa, Japan
Internet: kurokawa@is.icc.u-tokai.ac.jp
Fluid & Electrolyte Disorders

Charles A. Linker, MD
Clinical Professor of Medicine and Director, Adult Leukemia and Bone Marrow Transplant Program, University of California, San Francisco.
Internet: Charles_Linker@quickmail.ucsf.edu
Blood

H. Trent MacKay, MD, MPH
Associate Clinical Professor, Department of Obstetrics and Gynecology, University of California, Davis.
Internet: txm3@cdc.gov
Gynecology

Barry M. Massie, MD
Professor of Medicine, University of California, San Francisco; Associate Staff Member, CVRI; Director, Coronary Care Unit, and Chief, Hypertension Program, Veterans Affairs Medical Center, San Francisco.
Internet: Massie.Barry@SanFrancisco.va.gov
Heart; Systemic Hypertension

Stephen J. McPhee, MD
Professor of Medicine, Department of Medicine University of California, San Francisco.
Internet: Steve_McPhee@UCSFDGIM.ucsf.edu
General Approach to the Patient; Health Maintenance & Disease Prevention; & Common Symptoms

Kenneth R. McQuaid, MD
Associate Professor of Clinical Medicine, University of California, San Francisco; Director, Endoscopy, Veterans Affairs Medical Center, San Francisco.
Internet: mcquaid.kenneth_r@sanfrancisco.va.gov
Alimentary Tract

Louis M. Messina, MD
Professor and Chief, Division of Vascular Surgery, Department of Surgery, University of California, San Francisco.
Internet: messina@itsa.ucsf.edu
Blood Vessels & Lymphatics

Brent R.W. Moelleken, MD
Clinical Instructor, Division of Plastic and Reconstructive Surgery, University of California, Los Angeles, School of Medicine.
Internet: rijuv@aol.com
Disorders Due to Physical Agents

Gail Morrison, MD
Vice Dean for Education, Director of Academic Programs, and Professor of Medicine, University of Pennsylvania School of Medicine, Philadelphia.
Internet: morrisog@mail.med.upenn.edu
Kidney

C. Diana Nicoll, MD, PhD
Clinical Professor and Vice Chair, Department of Laboratory Medicine; Associate Dean, University of California, San Francisco; Chief of Staff and Chief, Laboratory Medicine Service, Veterans Affairs Medical Center, San Francisco.
Internet: nicoll.diana@sanfrancisco.va.gov
Diagnostic Testing & Medical Decision Making; Therapeutic Drug Monitoring & Laboratory Reference Ranges

Toshihiro Okuda, MD, PhD
Staff Nephrologist, Division of Internal Medicine, Health Service Center, University of Tokyo, Japan.
Internet: okuda-tky@u-min.ac.jp
Fluid & Electrolyte Disorders

Kent R. Olson, MD, FACEP
Clinical Professor of Medicine, Pediatrics, and Pharmacy, University of California, San Francisco.
Internet: olson@itsa.ucsf.edu
Poisoning

Maxine A. Papadakis, MD
Professor of Clinical Medicine and Director of Student Programs, Department of Medicine, University of California, San Francisco.
Internet: Maxine_Papadakis@UCSFdom.ucsf.edu
Fluid & Electrolyte Disorders

Joseph C. Presti Jr., MD
Assistant Professor, Department of Urology, University of California, San Francisco; Chief of Urology, Veterans Affairs Medical Center, San Francisco.
Internet: Joe_Presti.URO@quickmail.ucsf.edu
Urology

Reed E. Pyeritz, MD, PhD
Professor and Chair, Department of Human Genetics; Professor of Medicine and Pediatrics, Allegheny University of the Health Sciences, Pittsburgh and Philadelphia.
Internet: Pyeritz@pgh.auhs.edu
Medical Genetics

Michael W. Rabow, MD
Assistant Clinical Professor of Medicine, Division of General Internal Medicine, University of California, San Francisco.
michael_rabow@ucsfdgim.ucsf.edu
Care at the End of Life

Neil M. Resnick, MD
Chief of Geriatrics, Brigham & Women's Hospital; Associate Professor, Harvard Medical School, Boston.
Internet: NMResnick@Bics.Bwh.Harvard.edu
Geriatric Medicine

Paul Riordan-Eva, FRCOphth
Honorary Senior Lecturer, Institute of Neurology, London; Consultant Ophthalmologist, Bromley Hospitals NHS Trust, England; Honorary Consultant Neuro-Ophthalmologist, National Hospital for Neurology and Neurosurgery, London.
Eye

Hope S. Rugo, MD
Assistant Clinical Professor of Medicine, Division of Hematology and Oncology, Adult Leukemia and Bone Marrow Transplant Program, University of California, San Francisco.
Internet: Hope_Rugo@quickmail.ucsf.edu
Cancer

Steven A. Schroeder, MD
President, The Robert Wood Johnson Foundation, Princeton, New Jersey; Clinical Professor of Medicine, University of Medicine and Dentistry of New Jersey, Robert Wood Johnson Medical School, New Brunswick.
Internet: ss@rwjf.org
General Approach to the Patient; Health Maintenance & Disease Prevention; & Common Symptoms

Wayne X. Shandera, MD
Assistant Professor of Internal Medicine, Baylor College of Medicine, Houston.
Internet: shandera@bcm.tmc.edu
Infectious Diseases: Viral & Rickettsial

John L. Stauffer, MD
Professor of Medicine, The Pennsylvania State University College of Medicine; Attending Physician, The Milton S. Hershey Medical Center of the Pennsylvania State Geisinger Health System, Hershey.
Internet: jstauffe@med.hmc.psu.edu
Lung

Marshall L. Stoller, MD
Associate Professor of Urology, University of California, San Francisco.
Internet: mls@itsa.ucsf.edu
Urology

Abba I. Terr, MD
Clinical Professor of Medicine, Stanford University Medical School, Stanford.
Allergic & Immunologic Disorders

Lawrence M. Tierney, Jr., MD
Professor of Medicine, University of California, San Francisco; Assistant Chief of Medical Services, Veterans Affairs Medical Center, San Francisco.
Internet: vaspa@itsa.ucsf.edu
Blood Vessels & Lymphatics

Daniel G. Vaughan, MD
Clinical Professor of Ophthalmology, University of California, San Francisco; Governor, Francis I. Proctor Foundation for Research in Ophthalmology, San Francisco.
Eye

From inability to let alone; from too much zeal for the new and contempt for what is old; from putting knowledge before wisdom, and science before art and cleverness before common sense; from treating patients as cases; and from making the cure of the disease more grievous than the endurance of the same, Good Lord, deliver us.

—Sir Robert Hutchison

General Approach to the Patient; Health Maintenance & Disease Prevention; & Common Symptoms

1

Stephen J. McPhee, MD, & Steven A. Schroeder, MD

GENERAL APPROACH TO THE PATIENT

Successful diagnosis and treatment demand consideration of the often complex personal, family, and economic circumstances of the patient as well as a supportive and open relationship.

The approach to diagnosis begins with the history and pertinent physical examination, each of which is susceptible to errors of omission and commission. The medical interview should accomplish three important functions: to collect information, to respond appropriately to the patient's emotional state, and to educate the patient and beneficially influence patient behavior. Patient satisfaction may be increased by discussing psychosocial issues and by forgoing physician dominance of the encounter. Any diagnostic procedures must be based on principles of diagnostic test selection, which in turn depend upon the test characteristics (sensitivity and specificity), disease incidence and prevalence, potential risk to the patient, and cost-benefit profile of the test determined by reference to its indications (see Chapter 41). Successful treatment—particularly management of patients with chronic illnesses—must be tailored to the circumstances of the individual patient and reinforced by a well-established doctor-patient relationship.

Patient Compliance

For many illnesses, treatment depends on fundamental behavioral changes—including alterations in diet, exercise, smoking, and drinking—that are difficult even for motivated patients. Compliance with prescribed drug regimens is a problem in every practice, with up to 50% of patients failing to achieve full compliance and a third never taking their medicines at all. Compliance rates for short-term, self-adminis-

tered therapies are higher (about 75% initially) than long-term therapies (< 25% for completion of antibiotic therapy for acute infection). Compliance rates are inversely correlated with the number of interventions prescribed, their complexity, and their cost. Thus, medication regimens should be as simple as possible (eg, once daily rather than multiple doses), and convenience devices such as MediPaks or MediSets should be used for complex regimens.

In general, patients seem better able to recall instructions to take prescribed medications than to comply with recommendations to follow a diet, exercise regularly, or perform various self-care activities (such as monitoring blood glucose levels at home). Even when the physician's instructions are kept in mind, adherence may vary markedly. Writing out advice to patients, including changes in medication, may be helpful. But in public hospitals, functional health illiteracy is endemic, with over 40% of patients unable to read and understand basic written medical instructions.

Patient compliance is improved when strong and trusting doctor-patient relationships have been established. Physicians can improve patient compliance by inquiring specifically about the behaviors in question and by reinforcement through key family members. When confronted directly, many patients will admit to noncompliance with medication regimens or with advice about giving up cigarettes or engaging only in "safe sex" practices. The productivity constraints imposed by recent market pressures limit the time for individual patient encounters, yet the importance of allocating sufficient time for health messages is paramount. Other direct ways of detecting noncompliance include pill counts; comparing dates on prescription labels with the number of pills remaining; monitoring serum, urine, or saliva levels of drugs or metabolites; or assessing predictable drug side effects such as bradycardia from beta-blockers. Indirect measures of compliance include monitoring appointment keeping, evaluating therapeutic responses, and examining pharmacy records. In general, noncompliance is associated with a poorer prognosis. In many instances, such as drug treatment of hypertension and diabetes mellitus, even partial compliance improves outcomes compared with noncompliance.

Guiding Principles

Fundamental ethical principles are intrinsic to a successful approach to diagnosis and treatment: honesty, beneficence, justice, avoidance of conflict of interest, and the pledge to do no harm. Increasingly, Western medicine involves patients in important decisions about medical care, including how far to proceed with treatment of patients with terminal illnesses (see Chapter 5).

Finally, the physician's role does not end with diagnosis and the prescribing of a treatment regimen. The importance of the empathic physician in helping patients and their families bear the burden of serious illness and death cannot be overemphasized. "To cure sometimes, to relieve often, and to comfort always" is a French saying as apt today as it was five centuries ago—as is Francis Peabody's admonition: "The secret of the care of the patient is in caring for the patient."

Butler C, Rollnick S, Stott N: The practitioner, the patient and resistance to change: Recent ideas on compliance. Can Med Assoc J 1996;154:1357. (Patients' resistance to change may stem partly from the way clinicians talk to them. An advice-giving approach is usually inadequate to motivate major lifestyle changes. Instead, the authors propose a patient-centered, negotiation-based framework that harnesses patients' intrinsic motivation to make their own decisions and promotes clinicians' acceptance of those decisions—even if they run counter to current medical wisdom.)

Cramer JA: Optimizing long-term patient compliance. Neurology 1995;45(2 Suppl 1):S25. (Key elements in prescribing include minimizing the number of daily doses, scheduling when doses are to be taken, and helping the patient to select a reminder "cue.")

Kravitz RL et al: Recall of recommendations and adherence to advice among patients with chronic medical conditions. Arch Intern Med 1993;153:1869. (The majority of 1751 patients with diabetes, hypertension, and heart disease failed to recall important advice and did not always adhere to the recommendations even when recalled.)

Wechsler H et al: The physician's role in health promotion revisited: A survey of primary care practitioners. N Engl J Med 1996;334:996. (Compared with a 1981 survey, more physicians now value and assume responsibility for important health-promoting behaviors. Notable exceptions are dietary counseling and available community resources.)

Williams MV et al: Inadequate functional health literacy among patients at two public hospitals. JAMA 1995;274:1677. (High proportions of patients were unable to read and understand basic written instructions. Illiteracy was especially high among patients over 60 years of age [80%] and for Spanish-speaking patients [60%].)

HEALTH MAINTENANCE & DISEASE PREVENTION

Preventing disease is more important than treating it. Preventive medicine is categorized as primary, secondary, or tertiary. Primary prevention aims to remove or reduce disease risk factors (eg, immunization, giving up or not starting smoking). Secondary prevention techniques promote early detection of disease or precursor states (eg, routine cervical Papanicolaou screening to detect carcinoma of the cervix, or tuberculin skin testing to identify candidates for chemoprophylaxis of tuberculosis). Tertiary prevention measures are aimed at limiting the impact of established disease (eg, partial mastectomy and radiation therapy to remove and control localized breast cancer). Primary prevention is by far the most effective and economical of all methods of disease control, but most physicians are deficient in their counseling practices concerning preventable conditions.

Table 1–1 lists deaths from preventable causes in the USA, which in 1990 accounted for 50% of all fatalities. Physicians can have a major role in reducing almost all of these risk factors.

Health maintenance and disease prevention usually begin with the office or clinic encounter. Table 1–2 compares and contrasts recommendations for periodic health examinations as developed by the United States Preventive Services Task Force, the American College

Table 1–1. Deaths from preventable causes in the United States in 1990.[1]

Cause	Estimated Number of Deaths	Percentage of Total Deaths
Tobacco	400,000	19
Dietary factors and activity patterns	300,000	14
Alcohol	100,000	5
Microbial agents	90,000	4
Toxic agents	60,000	3
Firearms	35,000	2
High-risk sexual behavior	30,000	1
Motor vehicle injuries	25,000	1
Illicit use of drugs	20,000	<1
TOTAL	1,060,000	≈50

[1]Reproduced, with permission, from McGinnis JM, Foege WH: Actual causes of death in the United States. JAMA 1993;270:2707.

Table 1–2. Expert recommendations for preventive care for asymptomatic, low-risk adults.

Preventive Service	United States Preventive Services Task Force			American College of Physicians			Canadian Task Force on the Periodic Health Examination		
	Sex	Age	Minimum Frequency	Sex	Age	Minimum Frequency	Sex	Age	Minimum Frequency
Physical examination									
Blood pressure	MF	18+	q 2 yrs[1]	MF	18+	q 2 yrs	MF	25–64	q 5 yrs
							MF	65+	q 2 yrs
Clinical breast examination	F	50–69[2]	Annually[3]	F	40+	Annually	F	50–69	Annually
Laboratory tests									
Papanicolaou smear	F	18[4]–65	q 3 yrs	F	20[4]–65	q 3 yrs	F	18[4]–69	q 3 yrs[5]
Stool for occult blood	MF	50+	Annually	MF	50–70/80	Annually[6]	NR	NR	NR
Sigmoidoscopy	MF	50+	q ? yrs[1]	MF	50–70	q 10 yrs	NR	NR	NR
Mammography	F	50–69[2]	q 1–2 yrs	F	50–75	q 2 yrs	F	50–69	Annually
Cholesterol	M	35–65	q 5+ yrs[1]	M	35–65	Once[1]	M	30–59	q ? yrs[1]
	F	45–65		F	45–65				
Immunizations									
Tetanus-diphtheria booster	MF	18+	q 15–30 yrs	MF	18+	q 10 yrs or once at age 50	MF	18+	q 10 yrs
Influenza vaccination	MF	65+	Annually	MF	65+	Annually	MF	65+	Annually
Pneumococcal vaccination	MF	65+	Once[7]	MF	65+	Once[7]	NR	NR	NR
Counseling[8]	MF	18+	At routine visits	MF	18+	At routine visits	MF	18+	At routine visits

NR = no recommendation; ? = "periodic."
[1]Owing to lack of evidence, the appropriate interval is left to clinical discretion.
[2]The benefits of clinical breast examination and mammography in women age 70 and older have not been determined. Screening decisions in older women should take into account comorbid conditions and life expectancy of each patient.
[3]Studies have also generally employed periodic mammography; the benefit of clinical breast examination alone in women of any age has not been determined.
[4]Or following onset of sexual activity.
[5]After two normal annual smears.
[6]For persons who decline screening sigmoidoscopy, barium enema or colonoscopy.
[7]Reimmunize at age 65 those high-risk individuals who are 6 years or more after primary dose.
[8]Regarding tobacco use, nutrition, exercise, sexual behavior, substance abuse, injury prevention, and dental care.

of Physicians, and the Canadian Task Force on the Periodic Health Examination. Although there is emerging consensus on many of the preventive services recommended, controversy persists for many others. Recently, there has been a shift away from recommendations based solely on patients' age and sex to recommendations based on their additional risk factors.

[*Guide to Clinical Preventive Services,* 2nd ed.]
   http://text.nlm.nih.gov/ftrs/pick?collect
     =cps&ftrsK=55784
Sox HC: Preventive health services in adults. N Engl J Med 1994;330:1589.

INFECTIOUS DISEASES

Accomplishments in immunization and antibiotic therapy notwithstanding, much of the decline in the incidence and fatality rates of infectious diseases is attributable to improved public health measures—especially improved sanitation, better nutrition, and greater prosperity.

Immunization remains the best means of preventing many infectious diseases. In the USA, immunization has contributed to an estimated 90% decline in measles, mumps, rubella, poliomyelitis, diphtheria, pertussis, and tetanus since 1900. *Haemophilus influenzae* type b invasive disease has been reduced by more than 95% in the 5 years since introduction of the first conjugate vaccines. Opportunities still exist for reducing morbidity and mortality from vaccine-preventable diseases. For example, in adults in the USA, there are an estimated 50,000–70,000 deaths annually from influenza, hepatitis B, and invasive pneumococcal disease. Among targeted adult groups, only about 40% have had influenza vaccination, only 10% hepatitis B vaccination, and only 20% pneumococcal vaccination. The American College of Physicians recommends that physicians "mainstream" immunizations into adult medical care. It recommends that physicians should review each adult's immunization status at age 50; review risk factors that would indicate need for pneumococcal vaccination and annual influenza immunizations; reimmunize at age 65 those who received an immunization against pneumococcus more than 6 years before; ensure that all adults have completed a primary diphtheria-tetanus immunization series, and administer a single booster at age 50; and assess the serologic response to hepatitis B vaccination in all recipients older than age 30.

Varicella virus causes an estimated 3.7 million cases of chickenpox and 9000 hospitalizations in the USA annually. A vaccine against varicella was released by the FDA in 1995. It is expected to be 70–90% effective in preventing this highly communicable disease. A single injection is recommended for children 12 months to 12 years of age, and two injections four weeks apart for those age 13 and older. The vaccine can be given at the same time as the measles, mumps, and rubella (MMR) immunization. It is unnecessary for those who have had chickenpox, since the disease confers lifelong immunity.

Hepatitis A accounts for about half of all hepatitis cases each year in the United States. In 1996, 29,000 cases of hepatitis A were reported in the USA; the actual incidence is probably considerably higher, perhaps 75,000–143,000 cases per year. While most patients recover, about 100 persons die of fulminant hepatitis A each year. Hepatitis A is more severe and more likely to be fatal in adults, particularly those age 50 and older. In 1995, a vaccine against hepatitis A was licensed by the FDA. Its efficacy in various trials has ranged between 94% and 97% in preventing acute hepatitis A infection. For children 2–18 years of age, the primary injections of 0.5 mL are given once and four weeks later, with a single booster injection given 6–12 months later; for adults, the primary injection of 1 mL is given once and the booster 6–12 months later.

Recent trials of trivalent and multivalent acellular pertussis vaccines have found efficacy rates that equal or exceed those of the most widely used whole cell vaccine in the United States while having substantially better safety profiles. The Advisory Committee on Immunization Practices now recommends the use of DTaP vaccine for the first four doses of the routine series of vaccinations against diphtheria, tetanus, and pertussis among children.

Recommended immunization schedules for children and adults are set forth in Table 30–4. Persons traveling to countries where infections are endemic should take special precautions, as described in Chapter 30.

Skin testing for tuberculosis and then treating selected skin-positive patients with prophylactic isoniazid reduces the risk of reactivation tuberculosis (see Table 9–10). Attention to technique is particularly important for measurements close to the cutoff point separating negative from positive results. Patients with HIV infection are at an especially high risk for reactivation of tuberculosis. The prophylaxis and treatment of tuberculosis in HIV-infected patients are discussed in Chapter 31, as is the emerging concern about multidrug-resistant tuberculosis.

AIDS is now the major infectious disease problem in the Western world. Since sexual contact is the usual mode of transmission, prevention must rely on safe sexual practices, although increasingly cases of HIV infection are transmitted by use of illicit intravenous drugs. If consistently and appropriately used, condoms can reduce the rate of HIV transmission. Retrospective data from studies of partners of HIV-infected persons suggest that consistent use of condoms may reduce the risk of HIV transmission by an estimated 69%. Among those couples who used condoms inconsistently, there was a considerable risk of infection: the rate of seroconversion was 4.8 per 100 persons per year, leading to an estimated cumulative incidence of 12.7% after 24 months of exposure. No seroconversions were noted among the couples who used condoms consistently. Other approaches to prevention of HIV infection include programs aimed at sexually transmitted diseases, behavioral interventions, development of vaginal microbicides, and vaccine development. For patients abusing intravenous drugs, HIV prevention activities should include provision of sterile injection equipment.

Although live virus vaccines (such as MMR) are not generally recommended for immunocompromised patients, *asymptomatic* HIV-infected patients have generally not shown adverse consequences when given them. Thus, these individuals should receive MMR and influenza vaccinations as well as tetanus, hepatitis B, *H influenzae* type b, and pneumococcal vaccinations. However, if poliomyelitis immunization is required, the inactivated poliomyelitis vaccine should be used. *Symptomatic* HIV-infected patients should be given annual influenza vaccinations, but live virus vaccines such as MMR should generally be avoided.

The last year for new reports of poliomyelitis cases in the Western Hemisphere was 1991. A goal has been established of worldwide eradication of poliomyelitis and dracunculiasis (dracontiasis; guinea worm disease) by the year 2000; if successful, their eradication will follow that of smallpox (1978).

[Technical recommendations and answers to common clinician questions regarding immunizations from the National Immunization Program]
http://www.cdc.gov/nip/clinical.htm

American College of Physicians Task Force on Adult Immunization, Infectious Diseases Society of America: *Guide for Adult Immunization*, 3rd ed. American College of Physicians, 1994.

Des Jarlais DC et al: Maintaining low HIV seroprevalence in populations of injecting drug users. JAMA 1995;274:1226. (In low seroprevalence areas, transmission of HIV among intravenous drug users can be limited by early action, providing sterile injection equipment, and reaching out to drug users.)

de Vicenzi I: A longitudinal study of human immunodeficiency virus transmission by heterosexual partners. N Engl J Med 1994;331:341.

Edwards KM, Decker MD: Acellular pertussis vaccines for infants. (Editorial.) N Engl J Med 1996;334:391.

Fedson DS: Adult immunization: Summary of the National Vaccine Advisory Committee report. JAMA 1994;272:1133.

Foege WH: Polio eradication—how near? (Editorial.) JAMA 1996;275:1682. (The Pacific countries are now polio-free. In a single day, China vaccinated 83 million children and India 88 million children. However, in more than 40 African countries, polio is still a public health problem.)

Gardner P et al: Adult immunizations. Ann Intern Med 1996;12(1 Part 1):35. (Reviews new vaccines for hepatitis A, varicella, and typhoid and reemphasizes pneumococcal and influenza vaccinations.)

Makadon HJ, Silin JG: Prevention of HIV infection in primary care: Current practices, future possibilities. Ann Intern Med 1995;123:715. (Barriers to prevention include narrow conceptions of medical care and the physician's role; physicians' discomfort in discussing sexuality, illicit drug use, and HIV; constraints on time and resources; and ambiguity of messages about HIV prevention.)

Pouchot J et al: Reliability of tuberculin skin test measurement. Ann Intern Med 1997;126:210. (Ballpoint pen technique more reliable than palpation. Generally good interobserver reliability, but readings close to cutoff point for positivity should be confirmed.)

Zimmerman RK, Clover RD: Adult immunizations—a practical approach for clinicians: Part I, Part II. Am Fam Physician 1995;51:859, 1139.

CARDIOVASCULAR & CEREBROVASCULAR DISEASES

Impressive declines in age-specific mortality rates from heart disease and stroke have been achieved in all age groups in North America during the past 2 decades. The chief reason for this favorable trend appears to be a modification of risk factors, especially cigarette smoking and hypercholesterolemia, plus more aggressive detection and treatment of hypertension and heart disease.

Cigarette Smoking

Cigarette smoking remains the most important cause of preventable morbidity and early demise in developed countries. It is estimated that in 1997, smoking will account for 419,000 deaths in the USA. Cigarettes are now responsible for one in every five deaths in the USA. It is likely that even these striking figures underestimate the full hazards of tobacco. Recently, pipe and cigar smoking have increased; there is also continued use of smokeless tobacco (chewing tobacco and snuff), particularly among young people. Tobacco dependence may have a genetic component. Smokers have twice the risk of fatal heart disease, ten times the risk of lung cancer, and several times the risk of cancers of the mouth, throat, esophagus,

pancreas, kidney, bladder, and cervix; a two- to threefold higher incidence of stroke and peptic ulcers (which heal less well than in nonsmokers); a two- to fourfold greater risk of fractures of the hip, wrist, and vertebrae; and a twofold increase in the risk of developing cataracts. Each year brings new discoveries of other risks from smoking. Most recently, smoking has been associated with increased risks of leukemia, of colon and prostate cancers, of breast cancer among postmenopausal women who are slow acetylators of N-acetyltransferase 2 enzymes, and of osteoporosis. In cancers of the head and neck, lung, esophagus, and bladder, smoking is linked to mutations of the *p53* gene, the most common genetic change in human cancer. Olfaction and taste are impaired in smokers, and facial wrinkles are increased. Diabetic patients who smoke may have an increased risk of proteinuria. Patients with head and neck cancer who continue to smoke during radiation therapy have lower rates of response than those who do not smoke. Those who smoke more than one pack per day have a 2.5 greater risk of developing age-related macular degeneration. Smokers die 5–8 years earlier than never smokers.

Smoking cessation lessens the risks of death and of myocardial infarction in both men and women with coronary artery disease; lessens the risk of stroke; slows the rate of progression of carotid atherosclerosis; and is associated with reversal of chronic bronchitis and improved pulmonary function. It is estimated that women smokers who quit smoking by age 35 add about 3 years to their life expectancy, and men more than 2 years to theirs. Smoking cessation can increase life expectancy even for those who stop after the age of 65.

The children of patients who smoke have lower birth weights, are more likely to be mentally retarded, have more frequent respiratory infections, less efficient pulmonary function, and a higher incidence of chronic ear infections than children of nonsmokers and are more likely to become smokers themselves. In addition, passive smoking by adults has been shown to increase the risk of cervical cancer, lung cancer, and heart disease, to promote endothelial damage and platelet aggregation, and to increase urinary excretion of tobacco-specific lung carcinogens.

There has recently been an encouraging national trend away from smoking. According to the most recent (1996) data, 28.5% of adults in the USA are smokers. Smoking is slightly more common in men than women (28% versus 23%). One-fourth of United States adults are former smokers. From 1965 through 1985, smoking prevalence declined by 0.5% per year, and from 1987 through 1990 by 1.1% per year—but since 1990, the decline has leveled off.

Despite the fact that tobacco use constitutes the most serious common medical problem, access to effective treatment remains limited for most Americans. Over 70% of smokers see a physician each year, but only about a third of them receive any medical quitting advice or assistance. (Those whom physicians advise to quit are 1.6 times as likely to attempt quitting.) Clinicians can contribute to the decline in smoking prevalence by helping smokers break the addiction to nicotine and by persuading young people not to start smoking.

Consensus guidelines for smoking cessation have recently been published. The five steps for helping smokers quit are summarized in Table 1–3. Common elements of supportive smoking cessation treatments are reviewed in Table 1–4. Most smokers who quit do so without recourse to nicotine replacement therapy. However, guidelines for nicotine replacement are summarized in Table 1–5. Suggestions for use of the nicotine patch are listed in Table 1–6 and for the nicotine gum in Table 1–7. Both the patch and the gum are now available over-the-counter. Nicotine nasal spray is now available by prescription.

Weight gain occurs in most patients (79%) following smoking cessation. For most patients, weight gain is minor, averaging 5 lb, but for some (10–14%) major weight gain—over 29 lb—may occur.

Clinicians should avoid appearing to disapprove of patients who cannot stop smoking. Thoughtful admonition, family or social pressures, or the opportunity presented by an intercurrent illness such as acute bronchitis or acute myocardial infarction may enable even the most addicted chronic smoker to quit or at least to cut back. Even under the most pessimistic assumptions, such counseling is more cost-effective than treating hypertension. The physician's role in smoking cessation is summarized in Table 1–4.

[AHCPR guideline on smoking cessation]
  http://text.nlm.nih.gov/ftrs/pick?dbName=smkc&ftrsK=
    46004&cp=1&1=858442446&collect=ahcpr
[CDC's Tobacco Information and Prevention Sourcepage]
  http://www.cdc.gov/nccdphp/osh/tobacco.htm
Christen WG et al: A prospective study of cigarette smoking and risk of age-related macular degeneration in men. JAMA 1996;276:1147. (Prospective cohort study shows 2.5-fold risk for current smokers of one pack per day or more.)
Doll R et al: Mortality in relation to smoking: 40 years' observations on male British doctors. BMJ 1994;309:901. (In a cohort of 35-year-old male physicians who smoked, half the deaths during the subsequent 35 years were attributed to smoking.)
Henningfield JE: Nicotine medications for smoking cessation. N Engl J Med 1995;333:1196. (Terse, comprehensive review of nicotine dependence and treatment.)
Joseph AM et al: The safety of transdermal nicotine as an aid to smoking cessation in patients with cardiac disease. N Engl J Med 1996;335:1792. (No evidence of increased cardiac events, but its effect in promoting abstinence attenuates by 24 weeks.)
Law M et al: An analysis of interventions intended to help people stop smoking. Arch Intern Med 1995;155:1933. (Review of 188 randomized controlled trials shows small but positive benefit from physician advice and 13% effectiveness from nicotine replacement therapy.)
Smoking Cessation Clinical Practice Guidelines Panel and Staff: The Agency for Health Care Policy and Research Smoking Cessation Guidelines. JAMA 1996;275:1270. (Best single resource about smoking cessation.)

Hypercholesterolemia

Serum cholesterol levels in the United States have declined impressively during the past 3 decades. Lowering elevated LDL cholesterol concentrations and raising low HDL levels reduce the risk from coronary heart disease, particularly in middle-aged men. Elevated plasma lipoprotein(a) is an independent risk factor for premature coronary heart disease in men but is not yet available as a routine test. Calculated gain in life expectancy from modest decreases in blood cholesterol is low, especially in patients without other risk factors such as cigarette smoking and hypertension. A recent article has questioned whether the "fibrate" and "statin" classes of lipid-lowering drugs might increase cancer risk. However, for high-risk patients, such as those who have had a myocardial infarction or men with definite hypercholesterolemia, benefits from lowering cholesterol levels may be great. Compliance with "statin"-type drugs appears to be significantly greater than for the other classes of lipid-lowering agents. Despite cardiac benefits, lowering serum cholesterol does not seem to reduce the morbidity or mortality from stroke in middle-aged men. Screening and treatment for hypercholesterolemia may not be appropriate for elderly patients unless there is clinical evidence of atherosclerosis or other risk factors for death due to coronary heart disease. Elevated plasma homocysteine may be an independent factor for coronary artery disease.

Specific guidelines for therapy, which include diet, weight reduction, exercise, and drugs, are discussed in Chapter 29.

American College of Physicians: Guidelines for using serum cholesterol, high density lipoprotein cholesterol, and triglyceride levels as screening tests for preventing coronary heart disease in adults. Ann Intern Med 1996;124:515. (Relatively conservative screening recommendations for primary prevention.)
Andrade SE et al: Discontinuation of anti-hyperlipidemic drugs: Do rates reported in clinical trials reflect rates in primary care settings? N Engl J Med 1995;332:1125. (One-year drug discontinuation rates in two HMO settings ranged from a low of 15% for lovastatin to 37% for gemfibrozil, 41% for bile acid sequestrants, and 46% for niacin.)
Boushey CJ et al: A quantitative assessment of plasma homocysteine as a risk factor for vascular disease. JAMA 1995;274:1049. (Folic acid supplementation, given concurrently with cyanocobalamin, might be used to decrease plasma homocysteine levels.)
Gillman MW et al: Protective effect of fruits and vegetables on development of stroke in men. JAMA

Table 1–3. Actions and strategies for the primary care clinician to help patients quit smoking.[1]

Action	Strategies for Implementation
Step 1. Ask—Systematically Identify All Tobacco Users at Every Visit	
Implement an officewide system that ensures that for *every* patient at *every* clinic visit, tobacco-use status is queried and documented[2]	Expand the vital signs to include tobacco use. 　Data should be collected by the health care team. 　The action should be implemented using preprinted progress note paper that includes the expanded vital signs, a vital signs stamp, or, for computerized records, an item assessing tobacco-use status. Alternatives to the vital signs stamp are to place tobacco-use status stickers on all patients' charts or to indicate smoking status using computerized reminder systems.
Step 2. Advise—Strongly Urge All Smokers to Quit	
In a *clear, strong,* and *personalized* manner, urge every smoker to quit	Advice should be 　*Clear:* "I think it is important for you to quit smoking now, and I will help you. Cutting down while you are ill is not enough." 　*Strong:* "As your clinician, I need you to know that quitting smoking is the most important thing you can do to protect your current and future health." 　*Personalized:* Tie smoking to current health or illness and/or the social and economic costs of tobacco use, motivational level/readiness to quit, and the impact of smoking on children and others in the household. Encourage clinic staff to reinforce the cessation message and support the patient's quit attempt.
Step 3. Attempt—Identify Smokers Willing to Make a Quit Attempt	
Ask every smoker if he or she is willing to make a quit attempt at this time	If the patient is willing to make a quit attempt at this time, provide assistance (see step 4). If the patient prefers a more intensive treatment or the clinician believes more intensive treatment is appropriate, refer the patient to interventions administered by a smoking cessation specialist and follow up with him or her regarding quitting (see step 5). If the patient clearly states he or she is not willing to make a quit attempt at this time, provide a motivational intervention.
Step 4. Assist—Aid the Patient in Quitting	
A. Help the patient with a quit plan	*Set a quit date.* Ideally, the quit date should be within 2 weeks, taking patient preference into account. *Help the patient prepare for quitting:* The patient must 　*Inform* family, friends, and coworkers of quitting and request understanding and support. 　*Prepare the environment* by removing cigarettes from it. Prior to quitting, the patient should avoid smoking in places where he or she spends a lot of time (eg, home, car). 　*Review* previous quit attempts. What helped? What led to relapse? 　*Anticipate* challenges to the planned quit attempt, particularly during the critical first few weeks.
B. Encourage nicotine replacement therapy except in special circumstances	Encourage the use of the nicotine patch or nicotine gum therapy for smoking cessation (see Tables 1–5 to 1–7 for specific instructions and precautions).
C. Give key advice on successful quitting	*Abstinence:* Total abstinence is essential. Not even a single puff after the quit date. *Alcohol:* Drinking alcohol is highly associated with relapse. Those who stop smoking should review their alcohol use during the quit process. *Other smokers in the household:* The presence of other smokers in the household, particularly a spouse, is associated with lower success rates. Patients should consider quitting with their significant others and/or developing specific plans to maintain abstinence in a household where others still smoke.
D. Provide supplementary materials	*Source:* Federal agencies, including the National Cancer Institute and the Agency for Health Care Policy and Research; nonprofit agencies (American Cancer Society, American Lung Association, American Heart Association); or local or state health departments. *Selection concerns:* The material must be culturally, racially, educationally, and age appropriate for the patient. *Location:* Readily available in every clinic office.
Step 5. Arrange—Schedule Follow-Up Contact	
Schedule follow-up contact, either in person or via telephone	*Timing:* Follow-up contact should occur soon after the quit date, preferably during the first week. A second follow-up contact is recommended within the first month. Schedule further follow-up contacts as indicated. *Actions during follow-up:* Congratulate success. If smoking occurred, review the circumstances and elicit recommitment to total abstinence. Remind the patient that a lapse can be used as a learning experience and is not a sign of failure. Identify the problems already encountered and anticipate challenges in the immediate future. Assess nicotine replacement therapy use and problems. Consider referral to a more intense or specialized program.

[1]Modified and reproduced, with permission, from: The Agency for Health Care Policy and Research *Smoking Cessation. Clinical Practice Guideline. JAMA* 1996;275:1270.
[2]Repeated assessment is not necessary in the case of the adult who has never smoked or not smoked for many years and for whom the information is clearly documented in the medical record.

Table 1–4. Common elements of supportive smoking treatments.[1]

Component	Examples
Encouragement of the patient in the quit attempt	Note that effective cessation treatments are now available. Note that half the people who have *ever* smoked have now quit. Communicate belief in the patient's ability to quit.
Communication of caring and concern	Ask how the patient feels about quitting. Directly express concern and a willingness to help. Be open to the patient's expression of fears of quitting, difficulties experienced, and ambivalent feelings.
Encouragement of the patient to talk about the quitting process	Ask about Reasons that the patient wants to quit. Difficulties encountered while quitting. Success the patient has achieved. Concerns or worries about quitting.
Provision of basic information about smoking and successful quitting	Inform the patient about The nature and time course of withdrawal. The addictive nature of smoking. The fact that any smoking (even a single puff) increases the likelihood of full relapse.

[1]Modified, with permission, from: The Agency for Health Care Policy and Research. *Smoking Cessation Clinical Practice Guideline.* JAMA 1996;275:1270.

Table 1–5. Clinical guidelines for prescribing nicotine replacement products.[1]

1. Who should receive nicotine replacement therapy?

Available research shows that nicotine replacement therapy generally increases rates of smoking cessation. Therefore, except in special circumstances, the clinician should encourage the use of nicotine replacement with patients who smoke. Little research is available on the use of nicotine replacement with light smokers (ie, those smoking ≤ 10–15 cigarettes/d). If nicotine replacement is to be used with light smokers, a lower starting dose of the nicotine patch or nicotine gum should be considered.

2. Should nicotine replacement therapy be tailored to the individual smoker?

Research does not support the tailoring of nicotine patch therapy (except with light smokers as noted above). Patients should be prescribed the patch dosages outlined in Table 1–6.

Research supports tailoring nicotine gum treatment. Specifically, research suggests that 4-mg gum rather than 2-mg gum be used with patients who are highly dependent on nicotine (eg, those smoking >20 cigarettes/d, those who smoke immediately upon awakening, and those who report histories of severe nicotine withdrawal symptoms). Clinicians may also recommend the higher gum dose if patients request it or have failed to quit using the 2-mg gum.

3. Should patients be encouraged to use the nicotine patch or nicotine gum?

While both pharmacotherapies are efficacious, panel opinion is that nicotine patch therapy is preferable for routine clinical use. This preference is based on the following comparisons with nicotine gum therapy:

Nicotine patch therapy is associated with fewer compliance problems that interfere with effective use.

Nicotine patch therapy requires less clinician time and effort to train patients in its effective use.

The following factors would support the use of nicotine gum:

Patient preference.

Previous failure with the nicotine patch.

Contraindications specific to nicotine patch use (eg, severe skin reactions).

[1]Reproduced, with permission, from: The Agency for Health Care Policy and Research. *Smoking Cessation Clinical Practice Guideline.* JAMA 1996;275:1270.

1995;273:1113. (Men in the highest quintile of fruit and vegetable intake—an average of almost ten servings daily—had an almost threefold reduction in stroke compared with those in the lowest quintile.)

La Rosa JC: Cholesterol agonistes. Ann Intern Med 1996;124:505. (Criticizes the ACP lipid screening guidelines [see above reference] as missing important treatment opportunities.)

Newman TB et al: Carcinogenicity of lipid lowering drugs. JAMA 1996;275:55. (All members of the fibrate and statin classes of lipid-lowering drugs show much greater rodent carcinogenicity than drugs used to treat hypertension. The authors argue that physicians should restrict the use of such drugs to obvious high-risk patients.)

Shepherd J et al: Prevention of coronary heart disease in men with hypercholesterolemia. N Engl J Med 1995;333:1302. (Middle-aged men with a mean cholesterol of 272 mg/dL were assigned either to pravastatin treatment or control and followed for 5 years. The treatment group had a 20% decline in total cholesterol and 26% decline in LDL levels. Coronary events, including fatal and nonfatal acute myocardial infarctions, were significantly less in the treatment group, and noncardiovascular deaths were not increased. Reductions in deaths from all causes achieved borderline statistical significance for the treatment group.)

Hypertension

Over 50 million adults in the USA have hypertension. In every adult age group—including those over 70 years old—higher values of systolic and diastolic blood pressure carry greater risks of stroke and congestive heart failure. Even so, clinicians must be able to apply specific blood pressure criteria as a means of deciding at what levels treatment should be considered in individual cases. Table 11–1 presents a classification of hypertension based on blood pressures that was proposed in 1993. Primary prevention of hypertension can be accomplished by intervention strategies aimed at both the general population and special, high-risk populations. The latter include persons with high-normal blood pressure or a family history of hypertension, blacks, and individuals with various behavioral risk factors such as physical inactivity, excessive consumption of salt, alcohol, or

Table 1–6. Suggestions for the clinical use of the nicotine patch.[1]

Parameter of Clinical Use	Suggestions		
Patient selection	Appropriate as a primary pharmacotherapy for smoking cessation.		
Precautions	*Pregnancy:* Pregnant smokers should first be encouraged to attempt cessation without pharmacologic treatment. The nicotine patch should be used during pregnancy only if the increased likelihood of smoking cessation, with its potential benefits, outweighs the risk of nicotine replacement and potential concomitant smoking. Similar factors should be considered in lactating women. *Cardiovascular diseases:* While not an independent risk factor for acute myocardial events, the nicotine patch should be used only after consideration of risks and benefits among particular cardiovascular patient groups: those in the immediate (within 4 weeks) post-myocardial infarction period, those with serious arrhythmias, and those with severe or worsening angina pectoris. *Skin reactions:* Up to 50% of patients using the nicotine patch will have a local skin reaction. Skin reactions are usually mild and self-limiting but may worsen over the course of therapy. Local treatment with hydrocortisone cream (5%) or triamcinolone cream (0.5%) and rotating patch sites may ameliorate such local reactions. In fewer than 5% of patients do such reactions require the discontinuation of nicotine patch treatment.		
Dosage[2]	Treatment of 8 weeks or less has been shown to be **as** efficacious as longer treatment periods. Based on this finding, we suggest the following treatment schedules as reasonable for most smokers. Clinicians should consult the package insert for other treatment suggestions. Finally, clinicians should consider individualizing treatment based on specific patient characteristics such as previous experience with the patch, number of cigarettes smoked, and degree of addiction.		
	Brand	Duration (weeks)	Dosage (mg/h)
	Nicoderm and Habitrol	4 then 2 then 2	21/24 14/24 7/24
	Prostep	4 then 4	22/24 11/24
	Nicotrol	4 then 2 then 2	15/16 10/16 5/16
Prescribing instructions	Abstinence from smoking: The patient should refrain from smoking while using the patch. Location: At the start of each day, the patient should place a new patch on a relatively hairless location between the neck and the waist. Activities: There are no restrictions while using the patch. Time: Patches should be applied as soon as patients awaken on their quit day.		

[1]Reproduced, with permission, from: The Agency for Health Care Policy and Research. *Smoking Cessation Clinical Practice Guideline.* JAMA 1996;275:1270.
[2]These dosage recommendations are based on a review of the published research literature and do not necessarily conform to package insert information.

calories, and deficient intake of potassium. Interventions of documented efficacy for primary prevention of hypertension include reduced sodium and alcohol consumption, weight loss, and regular exercise. Interventions of limited or unproved efficacy include pill supplementation of potassium, calcium, magnesium, fish oil, or fiber; macronutrient alteration; and stress management. A major cause of the recent impressive decline in stroke deaths has been improved diagnosis and treatment of hypertension. Diets rich in fruits and vegetables may also protect against stroke. Pharmacologic management of hypertension is discussed in Chapter 11.

Gillman MW et al: Protective effects of fruits and vegetables on development of stroke in men. JAMA 1995;273:1113. (Framingham study 20 year follow-up of middle-aged men showed age-adjusted risk ratio of 0.78 for stroke for each increase of three servings per day of fruits and vegetables.)

Littenberg B: A practice guideline revisited: Screening for hypertension. Ann Intern Med 1995;122:937.

Stockwell DH et al: The determinants of hypertension awareness, treatment, and control in an insured population. Am J Public Health 1994;84:1768. (Of employees with hypertension, only 71% were aware of their condition, only 49% were on treatment, and only 12% had achieved adequate blood pressure control.)

Table 1–7. Suggestions for the clinical use of nicotine gum.[1]

Parameter of Clinical Use	Suggestions
Patient selection	Appropriate as a primary pharmacotherapy for smoking cessation.
Precautions	*Pregnancy:* Pregnant smokers should first be encouraged to attempt cessation without pharmacologic treatment. Nicotine gum should be used during pregnancy only if the increased likelihood of smoking cessation, with its potential benefits, outweighs the risk of nicotine replacement and potential concomitant smoking. *Cardiovascular diseases:* Although not an independent risk factor for acute myocardial events, nicotine gum should be used only after consideration of risks and benefits among particular cardiovascular patient groups: those in the immediate (within 4 weeks) post-myocardial infarction period, those with serious arrhythmias, and those with serious or worsening angina pectoris. *Adverse effects:* Common adverse effects of nicotine chewing gum include mouth soreness, hiccups, dyspepsia, and jaw ache. These effects are generally mild and transient and can often be alleviated by correcting the patient's chewing technique (see "Prescribing instructions" below).
Dosage	*Dosage:* Nicotine gum is available in doses of 2 mg and 4 mg per piece. Patients should be prescribed the 2-mg gum initially. The 4-mg gum should be prescribed to patients who express a preference for it, have failed with the 2-mg gum but remain motivated to quit, and/or are highly dependent on nicotine. The gum is most commonly prescribed for the first few months of a quit attempt. Clinicians should tailor the duration of therapy to fit the needs of each patient. Patients using the 2-mg strength should use not more than 30 pieces per day, whereas those using the 4-mg strength should not exceed 20 pieces per day.
Prescribing instructions	*Abstinence from smoking:* The patient should refrain from smoking while using the gum. *Chewing technique:* The gum should be chewed slowly until a "peppery" taste emerges, then "parked" between cheek and gum to facilitate nicotine absorption through the oral mucosa. Gum should be slowly and intermittently chewed and parked for about 30 minutes. *Absorption:* Acidic beverages (eg, coffee, juices, soft drinks) interfere with the buccal absorption of nicotine, so eating and drinking anything except water should be avoided for 15 minutes before and during chewing. *Scheduling of dose:* A common problem is that patients do not use enough gum to get the maximum benefit: they chew too few pieces per day and do not use the gum for a sufficient number of weeks. Instructions to chew the gum on a fixed schedule (at least 1 piece every 1 to 2 hours) for at least 1 to 3 months may be more beneficial than ad lib use.

[1]Reproduced, with permission, from: The Agency for Health Care Policy and Research. *Smoking Cessation Clinical Practice Guideline.* JAMA 1996;275:1270.

Chemoprevention

As discussed in Chapters 10 and 24, aspirin is useful for the primary and secondary prevention of acute myocardial infarction and stroke.

PHYSICAL INACTIVITY & SEDENTARY LIFESTYLE

A sedentary lifestyle has been linked to 28% of deaths from leading chronic diseases. For example, the American Heart Association in 1992 declared physical inactivity to be a major risk factor for heart disease.

In 1995, the Centers for Disease Control and Prevention recommended that every adult in the United States should accumulate 30 minutes or more of moderate-intensity physical activity on most—preferably all—days of the week. The new guideline is intended to complement, not replace, previous advice urging at least 20–30 minutes of more vigorous, continuous aerobic exercise three to five times a week.

Regular moderate to vigorous exercise has been shown to lower the risk of myocardial infarction, stroke, hypertension, non-insulin-dependent diabetes mellitus, diverticular disease, and osteoporosis. In general, the benefits of exercise appear to be dose-dependent, with a major difference in benefit between no and mild to moderate exercise and a smaller difference in benefit between moderate and vigorous exercise. In recent studies, the relative risk of stroke was found to be less than one-sixth in men who exercised vigorously compared with those who were inactive; the risk of non-insulin-dependent diabetes mellitus was about half among men who exercised five or more times weekly compared with those who exercised once a week. Glucose control is improved in diabetics who exercise regularly, even at a modest level. Regular exercise is associated with a lower long-term risk of coronary events, including fatal myocardial infarctions, with elevated HDL cholesterol concentrations in both men and women and with decreased risk of hypertension. Physical activity reduces the risk of colon cancer (though not rectal cancer) in men and women and of breast and reproductive organ cancer in women. Finally, weight-bearing exercise has been shown to increase bone mineral content and retard development of osteoporosis in women.

Exercise may also confer benefits on those with chronic illness. For example, men and women with chronic symptomatic osteoarthritis of one or both knees benefited from a supervised walking program. Benefits included improvement in self-reported functional status and decreased pain medication usage. Exercise has been shown to produce sustained lowering of both systolic and diastolic blood pressure in patients with mild hypertension. In addition, it can help patients maintain ideal body weight, and the risk of myocardial infarction is estimated to be 35–55% lower for individuals who maintain ideal body weight compared with those who are obese. Physical activity has been shown to reduce depression and anxiety, to improve adaptation to stress, to improve sleep quality, and to enhance mood, self-esteem, and performance.

However, physical exertion can also trigger the onset of acute myocardial infarction, particularly in persons who are habitually sedentary. The risk of infarction is considerably less among those reporting regular (at least five times per week), heavy (six MET or more) physical exertion. Other potential complications of exercise include angina pectoris, arrhythmias, sudden death, and asthma. In insulin-requiring diabetics who undertake vigorous exercise, blood glucose levels should be carefully monitored to prevent hypoglycemia.

Recent surveys indicate that only about 22% of adults in the USA are active at the moderate level, and only 8% currently exercise at the more vigorous level recommended for health benefits. Instead, 58% report irregular or no leisure time physical activity. Generally, men are more active than women. Activity levels seem to increase with income and education and to decrease with age.

Physicians should advise patients about the benefits and risks of exercise, prescribe an exercise program appropriate for each patient, and provide advice that will help to prevent injuries or complications. Prior to prescribing exercise, physicians should perform a history and physical examination and laboratory studies directed by findings. The value of routine electrocardiography or exercise electrocardiography remains controversial. In general, healthy individuals can exercise without supervision, but patients with ischemic heart disease or other cardiovascular disease require medically supervised, graded exercise programs. Exercise should not be prescribed for patients with decompensated congestive heart failure, complex ventricular arrhythmias, unstable angina pectoris, hemodynamically significant aortic stenosis, aortic aneurysm, or uncontrolled diabetes mellitus. Five- to 10-minute warm-up and cool-down periods, stretching exercises, and gradual increases in exercise intensity help to prevent musculoskeletal and cardiovascular complications.

Most people believe that they do not have time to be physically active. Physicians must therefore educate their patients to understand that physical activity is something that can be incorporated into the daily routine—not necessarily something to be added to an already busy schedule. For example, the physician can advise the patient to take the stairs instead of the elevator, to walk or bike instead of driving, to do housework or yardwork, to get off the bus one or two stops earlier and walk the rest of the way, to park at the far end of the parking lot and walk, or to walk during the lunch hour. Table 29–2 shows energy expenditures of selected physical activities. Physicians need to emphasize that such physical activity will result in real health benefits. The basic message must be: the more the better, and anything is better than nothing.

[Physical Activity and Health: A Report of the Surgeon General]
  http://www.cdc.gov/nccdphp/sgr/sgr.htm
[Summary of recommendations for physical activity and health from various organizations]
  http://www.pitt.edu/~pahnet/pahnet/recommend.html
Blair SN et al: Influences of cardiorespiratory fitness and other precursors on cardiovascular disease and all-cause mortality in men and women. JAMA 1996;276:205. (Low fitness was an important predictor of mortality among both men [RR 1.52, 95% CI 1.28–1.82] and women [RR 2.10, 95% CI 1.36–3.21]. Highly and moderately fit persons had lower adjusted mortality rates than those with low fitness regardless of smoking status, systolic blood pressure, serum cholesterol, and general health.)
Ettinger WH et al: A randomized trial comparing aerobic exercise and resistance training to a health education program on physical disability in older adults with knee osteoarthritis. JAMA 1997;277:25. (Exercise has beneficial—but modest—effect on pain, physical performance, and disability.)
King AC et al: Moderate intensity exercise and self-related quality of sleep in older adults with osteoarthritis: A randomized controlled trial. JAMA 1997;277:32. (Exercise caused impressive improvements in sleep quality—15 minute reduction in sleep onset latency and 45 minute increase in sleep duration.)
Lakka TA et al: Relation of leisure-time physical activity and cardiorespiratory fitness to the risk of acute myocardial infarction in men. N Engl J Med 1994;330:1549. (Higher levels of both leisure time physical activity and cardiorespiratory fitness had a strong, graded inverse association with the risk of myocardial infarction.)
Lemaitre RN et al: Leisure-time physical activity and the risk of nonfatal myocardial infarction in postmenopausal women. Arch Intern Med 1995;155:2302. (Risk of myocardial infarction is decreased by 50% with modest levels of exercise, equivalent to 30–45 minutes of walking three times weekly.)

CANCER

Primary Prevention

Cigarette smoking is the most important preventable cause of cancer. Primary prevention of skin cancer consists of restricting exposure to ultraviolet light by wearing appropriate clothing and use of sunscreens. In the past 2 decades, there has been a threefold increase in the incidence of squamous cell carcinoma and a fourfold increase in melanoma in the United States. Regular physical exercise has been associated with a significant reduction in breast and colon cancer risk. Prevention of occupationally induced cancers involves minimizing exposure to carcinogenic substances such as asbestos, ionizing radiation, and benzene compounds. There is increasing evidence that chemoprevention may be an important part of primary cancer prevention (see Chapter 4).

For example, aspirin (in a dose as small as 325 mg four times weekly) and other NSAIDs may reduce the risk of colon cancer.

Secondary Prevention

Generally accepted techniques exist for secondary prevention of cancers of the breast, colon, and cervix through cancer screening procedures. Note that Table 1–8, derived from American Cancer Society guidelines, differs in many instances from the recommendations of other authorities as shown previously in Table 1–2, which take a more conservative view of the efficacy of cancer screening maneuvers. For example, there is continuing controversy regarding the value of screening mammography for women aged 40–49, serum PSA testing for men, or fecal occult blood testing for men or women older than age 50. A federal consensus panel in 1997 was unable to agree

Table 1–8. Screening for cancer: American Cancer Society (1993) guidelines for the early detection of cancer in people without symptoms.[1]

Test or Procedure	Sex	Age	Frequency
Sigmoidoscopy, preferably flexible	MF	50 and over	Every 3–5 years
Stool test for occult blood	MF	50 and over	Every year
Digital rectal examination	MF	40 and over	Every year
Prostate examination[2]	M	50 and over	Every year
Papanicolaou test	F	Women who are or have been sexually active or have reached age 18 years	Annually until at least 3 consecutive satisfactory normal examinations, then less often at discretion of physician
Pelvic examination	F	18–40	Every 1–3 years with Papanicolaou test. Not indicated if cervix has been removed for a nonmalignant condition
		Over 40	Every year
Endometrial tissue sample	F	At menopause; women at high risk[3]	At menopause and thereafter at the discretion of the physician
Breast self-examination	F	20 and over	Every month
Breast physical examination	F	20–40 Over 40	Every 3 years Every year
Mammography[4]	F	40–50 Over 50	Every year Every year
Health counseling and cancer checkup[5]	MF	Over 20 Over 40	Every 3 years Every year
Chest x-ray		Not recommended	
Sputum cytologic examination		Not recommended	

[1]From Update January 1992: The American Cancer Society Guidelines for the Cancer-Related Check-Up. CA Cancer J Clin 1992;42:44; from Mettlin C et al: Defining and updating the American Cancer Society's Guidelines for the cancer-related checkup: Prostate and endometrial cancers. CA Cancer J Clin 1993;43:42; and from the American Cancer Society 1997 update.
[2]Digital rectal examination and serum prostate-specific antigen; if either is abnormal, further evaluation by transrectal ultrasound and biopsy as indicated.
[3]History of infertility, obesity, failure of ovulation, abnormal uterine bleeding, or unopposed estrogen or tamoxifen therapy.
[4]American Cancer Society 1997 update.
[5]To include examination for cancers of the thyroid, testicles, ovaries, lymph nodes, oral region, and skin.

on the advisability of routine mammography for women aged 40–49, leaving the decision instead to the discretion of individual patients and their physicians. Even more recently, based on recommendation from an expert advisory panel which cited evidence that breast cancers may grow more quickly in younger women, the American Cancer Society mammography screening guidelines were changed to include annual mammograms for women in their 40s.

Single serum PSA measurements appear to offer relatively high sensitivity and specificity to detect prostate cancer. The sensitivity is about 67%, the specificity about 82%, and the positive predictive value for prostate cancer is about 43%. When both the digital rectal examination and serum PSA are abnormal, PSA specificity increases, but sensitivity falls (to 33%), and predictive value rises only slightly (to 49%). Whether early detection and treatment alters the natural course of the disease remains to be seen. There are still no data on the morbidity and mortality benefits of such screening. Unlike the American College of Physicians, the American Cancer Society recommends annual PSA testing for men over age 50. Many physicians remain ambivalent about recommending its routine use.

In two separate studies, the risk of death from colon cancer among patients undergoing at least one sigmoidoscopic examination was reduced by 60–80% compared with that among those not having sigmoidoscopy. A recent finding of a 33% reduction in mortality rate from colorectal carcinoma in persons undertaking annual fecal occult blood testing (FOBT) has been more controversial. The predictive value of a positive FOBT was only 2.2%, and 38% of all patients screened underwent at least one follow-up colonoscopy during the 13-year study.

Screening for vaginal cancer with a Papanicolaou smear is not indicated in women who have undergone hysterectomies for benign disease with removal of the cervix.

Screening for other cancers in normal asymptomatic or even high-risk segments of the population is not recommended because adequate screening tests are not available.

[National Cancer Institute screening recommendations] gopher://gopher.nih.gov:70/11/clin/cancernet/pdqinfo/screening

American College of Physicians: Screening for prostate cancer. Ann Intern Med 1997;126:480. (Instead of routine screening, the ACP recommends that physicians describe the potential benefits and known harms of screening, diagnosis, and treatment, listen to the patient's concerns, and then individualize the decision to screen.)

Bernstein L et al: Physical exercise and reduced risk of breast cancer in young women. J Natl Cancer Inst 1994;86:1403.

Collins MM, Barry MJ: Controversies in prostate cancer screening: Analogies to the early lung cancer screening debate. JAMA 1996;276:1976. (Cautions regarding widespread dissemination of prostate cancer screening without experimental evidence that such screening does more good than harm.)

Gabriel H, Wilson TE, Helvie MA: Breast cancer in women 65–74 years old: Earlier detection by mammographic screening. AJR Am J Roentgenol 1997;168:23. (Screening mammography revealed significantly smaller and earlier stage tumors in 65- to 74-year-old women.)

Gann PH et al: A prospective evaluation of plasma prostate-specific antigen for detection of prostatic cancer. JAMA 1995;273:289. (Single PSA had relatively high sensitivity and specificity to detect prostate cancers that arose within a 4-year period. PSA values greater than the usual cutoff of 4 ng/mL were associated with a 5.5-fold increased risk compared with levels less than 1 ng/mL.)

Giovannucci E et al: Physical activity, obesity, and risk for colon cancer and adenoma in men. Ann Intern Med 1995;122:327. (Both physical inactivity and obesity independently increased the risk for colon cancer and adenomas greater than 1 cm in size.)

Hostetler RM, Mandel IG, Marshburn J: Prostate cancer screening. Med Clin North Am 1996;80:83. (Prostate cancer is potentially detectable at early, possibly curative stages. However, the effectiveness of prostate cancer treatment is still unproved. In addition, prostate cancer may actually be multiple entities with different natural histories, needing different treatments and, consequently, different screening strategies.)

Kerlikowske K et al: Likelihood ratios for modern screening mammography: Risk of breast cancer based on age and mammographic interpretation. JAMA 1996;276:39. (The sensitivity of first screening mammography increased with age, but specificity was similar for all ages. Based on the risk of breast cancer before mammography, which increases with age, the risk of breast cancer after mammography rose from 0.01 for ages 30–39 years to 0.05 for ages 50–59 years and to 0.07 for ages 70 years and older.)

McPhee SJ: Screening for cancer: Useful despite its limitations. West J Med 1995;163:169.

Muller AD, Sonnenberg A: Prevention of colorectal cancer by flexible endoscopy and polypectomy: A case-control study of 32,702 veterans. Ann Intern Med 1995;123:904. (Evidence that endoscopic polypectomies may reduce the risk for colorectal cancer by 50% for periods lasting up to 6 years.)

Swedish Cancer Society and the Swedish National Board of Health and Welfare: Breast-cancer screening with mammography in women aged 40–49 years. Int J Cancer 1996;68:693. (The relative mortality associated with invitation to screening was 0.77 [95% CI 0.59–1.01]. Detailed analysis suggested faster tumor progression in the age group 40–49 compared with groups aged 50 or more.)

Trends in cancer screening—United States, 1987 and 1992. MMWR Morb Mortal Wkly Rep 1996;45:57. (While the findings indicate an increase in use of all cancer screening tests except Pap smear from 1987 to 1992, the rates are substantially lower than national health objectives.)

Van Dijck JA et al: Mammographic screening after the age of 65 years: Evidence for a reduction in breast cancer mortality. Int J Cancer 1996;66:727. (Regular mammographic screening of women older than age 65 [at least up to age 75] appeared to reduce breast cancer mortality by approximately 45%.)

Woolf SH: Screening for prostate cancer with the prostate-specific antigen: An examination of the evidence. N Engl J Med 1995;333:1401. (Excellent review of issues behind current controversy.)

ACCIDENTS & VIOLENCE

Accidents remain the most important cause of loss of potential years of life before age 65. Although seat belt use protects against serious injury and death in motor vehicle accidents, at least one-fourth of adults do not use seat belts routinely. In 1991, only 62% of motorcyclists and 18% of bicyclists used safety helmets. Physicians should try to educate their patients about seat belts, safety helmets, using cellular telephones while driving, drinking (or using other intoxicants) and driving, and the risks of having guns in the home. Recently, studies have documented that chronic alcohol abuse adversely affects outcome from trauma and increases the risk of readmission for new trauma. Males aged 16–35 are at especially high risk for serious injury and death from accidents and violence, with blacks and Latinos at greatest risk. Deaths from firearms have reached epidemic levels in the United States and will soon surpass in numbers deaths from motor vehicle accidents. Cocaine use is often involved. Having a gun in the home increases the likelihood of homicide by 2.7-fold and of suicide by fivefold. Finally, physicians have a critical role in detection, prevention, and management of physical or sexual abuse—in particular, routine assessment of women for risk of domestic violence. In one study, inclusion of a single question about domestic violence in the medical history—"At any time, has a partner ever hit you, kicked you, or otherwise physically hurt you?"—increased identification of this common problem from nil to 11.6%.

[National Center for Injury Prevention and Control information on prevention of unintentional injuries and violence]
http://www.cdc.gov/ncipc/ncipchm.htm
Abbott J et al: Domestic violence against women: Incidence and prevalence in an emergency department population. JAMA 1995;273:1763. (The incidence of acute domestic violence among 418 women with a current male partner was 11.7%; the cumulative lifetime prevalence of exposure to such violence was 54.2%.)
Adler KP et al: Firearm violence and public health. Limiting the availability of guns. JAMA 1994;271:1281. (Firearms now account for one-fifth of all injury deaths in the USA, and for every fatal injury an estimated seven nonfatal injuries occur.)
Annest JL et al: National estimates of nonfatal firearm-related injuries: Beyond the tip of the iceberg. JAMA 1995;273:1749. (Firearm-related nonfatal injuries treated in hospital emergency rooms outnumber fatalities by an estimated ratio of 2.6:1.)
Brookoff D et al: Testing reckless drivers for cocaine and marijuana. N Engl J Med 1994;331:518. (Over half of reckless drivers who were not intoxicated with alcohol were found to be intoxicated with other drugs.)
Freund KM, Bak SM, Blackhall L: Identifying domestic violence in primary care practice. J Gen Intern Med 1996;11:44.
McCauley J et al: The "battering syndrome": Prevalence and clinical characteristics of domestic violence in primary care internal medicine practices. Ann Intern Med 1995;123:737. (Among 1952 women in four primary care practices, one in every 20 women had experienced domestic violence in the previous year; one in five had experienced violence in her adult life; and one in three had experienced violence either as a child or as an adult.)
Nelson DE et al: Population estimates of household firearm storage practices and firearm carrying in Oregon. JAMA 1996;275:1744. (Ten percent of all households and 6.2% of households with children had firearms that were always or sometimes stored loaded and unlocked. Overall, 4.4% of adults had carried loaded firearms during the previous month.)
Reidelmeier DA et al: Association between cellular telephone calls and motor vehicle collisions. N Engl J Med 1997;336:453. (Use of cellular phones in motor vehicles is associated with a fourfold risk of a collision during the call period.)

SUBSTANCE ABUSE
(See also Chapter 25.)

Substance abuse—including alcohol and illicit drugs—is a major public health problem in the United States and is estimated to be a factor in half of highway fatality accidents. Alcohol abuse affects both adolescents and adults. Approximately two-thirds of high school seniors are regular users of alcohol, and the lifetime prevalence of alcoholism is estimated to be between 12% and 16%. Underdiagnosis of alcoholism is substantial, both because of patient denial and lack of physician alertness to historical and physical clues of the condition. The fact that alcohol-related traffic fatalities declined by 31% from 1982 to 1993 testifies to the success of recent educational and legal efforts to limit drinking and driving. Even so, alcohol-impaired driving remains prevalent, especially among men aged 18–34 years. There appears to be an increase in binge drinking among college students.

As with cigarette use, physician identification and counseling about alcoholism may improve the chances of recovery. Although about 10% of all adults seen in medical practices are problem drinkers, that fact is seldom recognized. An estimated 15–30% of hospitalized patients have problems with alcohol abuse or dependence, but the connection between patients' presenting complaints and their alcohol abuse is often missed. The CAGE test (see Table 1–9) is a simple screening test that is both sensitive and specific. Alternatively, asking the two questions: "Have you ever had a drinking problem?"

Table 1–9. Screening and counseling for alcohol abuse.

1. **CAGE screening test[1]**

   Have you ever felt the
   need to **C**ut down on drinking?

   Have you ever felt **A**nnoyed by criticism of
   your drinking?

   Have you ever felt **G**uilty about your drinking?

   Have you ever taken a
   morning **E**ye opener?

   INTERPRETATION: Two "yes" answers are
   considered a positive screen. One "yes" answer
   should arouse a suspicion of alcohol abuse.

2. **Basic counseling steps[2]**

   Establish a therapeutic relationship

   Make the medical office or clinic off-limits for
   substance abuse

   Present information about negative health
   consequences

   Emphasize personal responsibility and self-efficacy

   Convey a clear message and set goals

   Involve family and other supports

   Establish a working relationship with community treatment resources

   Provide follow-up

[1]Modified from Mayfield D et al: The CAGE questionnaire:
Validation of a new alcoholism screening instrument. Am J
Psychiatry 1974;131:1121.
[2]From the United States Department of Health and Human
Services, U.S. Public Health Service, Office of Disease Prevention and Health Promotion. Clinician's Handbook of Preventive Services: Put Prevention Into Practice. U.S. Government Printing Office, 1994.

and "When did you have your last drink?"—positive
if in the past 24 hours—yields a 91% sensitivity for
alcoholism but is obviously less specific than the
CAGE test. Others recommend asking three questions: (1) How many days per week do you drink?
(To assess frequency.) (2) On a day when you drink
alcohol, how many drinks do you have in one day?
(To assess quantity.) (3) On how many occasions in
the last month did you drink more than five drinks?
(To assess binge drinking.) Treatment of alcoholism
and its complications is discussed in Chapter 25.
Choice of therapy remains controversial. However,
use of screening procedures and brief intervention
methods (see Table 1–9 and Chapter 25) can produce
a 10–30% reduction in long-term alcohol use and alcohol-related problems.

Use of illegal drugs—including cocaine—either
sporadically or episodically remains an important
problem. A disturbing trend is the recent increase in
use of marijuana and inhalants among eighth graders
and high school students. Many drug users are employed, and many use drugs during pregnancy.
Abuse of anabolic-androgenic steroids has been associated with use of other illicit drugs, alcohol, and cigarettes and with violence and criminal behavior. As
with alcohol abuse, the recognition of drug abuse
presents special problems and requires that the physician actively consider the diagnosis. Clinical aspects

of substance abuse and treatment issues are discussed
in Chapter 25.

[National Institute on Alcohol Abuse and Alcoholism Pub-
lications and Databases]
http://www.niaaa.nih.gov/

[National Institute on Drug Abuse information on common
drugs of abuse]
http://www.nida.nih.gov/DrugAbuse.html

Adams WL et al: Screening for problem drinking in older
primary care patients. JAMA 1996;276:1964. (CAGE
questionnaire underestimates prevalence of problem
drinkers in this cohort. Clinicians need to probe about
binge drinking.)

Fuchs CS et al: Alcohol consumption and mortality among
women. N Engl J Med 1995;332:1245. (Light-to-moder-
ate alcohol consumption is associated with reduced mortality rates in women, largely among those at greatest
risk for coronary heart disease.)

Hollander JE et al: Cocaine-associated myocardial infarction. Mortality and complications. Cocaine-Associated
Myocardial Infarction Study Group. Arch Intern Med
1995;155:1081.

Kaban M et al: Effectiveness of physician-based interventions with problem drinkers: A review. Can Med Assoc
J 1995;152:851. (Meta-analysis of 11 studies concluding
that brief interventions by physicians were effective
among men and equivocal among women with drinking
problems in reducing alcohol consumption.)

Kitchens JM: Does this patient have an alcohol problem?
JAMA 1994;272:1782. (Good clinical review of approaches to diagnosis.)

Marzuk PM et al: Fatal injuries after cocaine use as a leading cause of death among young adults in New York
City. N Engl J Med 1995;332:1753.

Mendelson JH, Mello NK: Management of cocaine abuse
and dependence. N Engl J Med 1996;334:965.

Samet JH, Rollnick S, Barnes H: Beyond CAGE: A brief
clinical approach after detection of substance abuse.
Arch Intern Med 1996;156:2287. (Emphasizes motiva-
tional interviewing and a patient-centered counseling
style for enhancing motivation for change, to make brief
interventions more effective by incorporating the patient's readiness to change alcohol or drug use.)

COMMON SYMPTOMS

PAIN

Approach to the Patient

Pain is the most common symptom causing patients to seek medical attention. Information about
the nature, location, timing, severity, and radiation of
pain is crucial for proper treatment; the same is true
for aggravating or alleviating factors.

Many emotional and cultural factors influence the
perception of pain. The primary cause (eg, trauma,
infection), pathogenesis (eg, inflammation, is-

chemia), and contributory factors (eg, recent changes in life situation, symbolic attributes of pain) must all be sought. Fortunately, pain, whether due to trauma, surgery, cancer, or other diseases, can be managed effectively through relatively simple means.

In 1992 and 1994, the Agency for Health Care Policy and Research published two Clinical Practice Guidelines for *Management of Acute Pain* and *Management of Cancer Pain.* Table 1–10 gives the AHCPR's recommended clinical approach to pain management. The AHCPR guidelines emphasize that although pain cannot always be entirely eliminated, appropriate use of drugs and other therapies can effectively relieve pain in the majority of patients. Unfortunately, pain is frequently undertreated, particularly in patients with cancer, AIDS, and previous substance abuse; and in minorities, women, children, and the elderly. Recent studies also document that even patients in hospital intensive care units and nursing homes are too frequently undertreated for pain.

The proper treatment of any patient's pain depends upon a careful diagnosis of its cause, selection of appropriate and cost-effective treatment, and ongoing evaluation of treatment results. Clinicians must be flexible to provide effective pain management, particularly in patients with cancer. Patients differ not only in their diagnosis and stage of disease but also in their responses to pain; their capacity to achieve relief from pain management measures; and in their personal preferences for measures to control pain. A team approach involving patients, their families, and other health professionals is essential for severe chronic pain. The clinician should discuss pain and its management explicitly with patients and their

Table 1–10. Recommended clinical approach to pain management.[1]

A. **A**sk about pain regularly. Assess pain systematically (quality, description, location, intensity or severity, aggravating and ameliorating factors, cognitive responses). Ask about goals for pain control, management preferences.

B. **B**elieve the patient and family in their reports of pain and what relieves it.

C. **C**hoose pain control options appropriate for the patient, family, and setting. Consider drug type, dosage, route, contraindications, side effects. Consider nonpharmacologic adjunctive measures.

D. **D**eliver interventions in a timely, logical, coordinated manner.

E. **E**mpower patients and their families. Enable patients to control their course to the greatest extent possible.

F. **F**ollow up to reassess persistence of pain, changes in pain pattern, development of new pain.

[1]Modified, with permission, from Jacox AK et al: Management of Cancer Pain: Quick Reference Guide No. 9. AHCPR Publication No. 94–0593. Rockville, MD: Agency for Health Care Policy and Research, Public Health Service, U.S. Department of Health and Human Services. March 1994.

families, reassuring them that there are safe and effective methods to relieve the pain and encouraging them to be active partners in its management. Frequent reassessment for changes in pain pattern, development of new pain, or persistence of pain will enable the clinician to order appropriate diagnostic studies, modify the treatment plan, consider other causes (perhaps related to disease progression or treatment), and prescribe alternative, more invasive treatments. Standard pain management scales, based on patient self-report, can be used to assess pain and evaluate the response to interventions (Table 5–4). Finally, effective management of pain includes efforts to improve the patient's quality of life and ability to work productively, to find pleasure in recreational activity, and to engage in normal social relationships. When possible, patients should be encouraged to remain active and to participate in self-care.

Drug Therapy

Drug therapy is effective, relatively low-risk, inexpensive, and rapid in onset. The World Health Organization recommends a three-step hierarchy for use of analgesics. Step 1 agents, used for mild to moderate pain, are nonopioids, such as aspirin, acetaminophen, or NSAIDs, given with or without adjunctive agents. If pain persists or increases, step 2 adds an opioid to the nonopioid, again with or without adjunctive agents (see below). If pain continues or intensifies, step 3 increases the opioid potency or dosage while continuing the nonopioid and adjunctive agents. Medication doses are scheduled regularly "around the clock" to maintain drug levels and prevent recurrence of pain rather than having to subdue it. Additional doses of rapid-onset, short-duration medication are administered on an "as needed" basis for "breakthrough" pain.

A. Drugs for Mild to Moderate Pain: Most people can manage minor aches and pains with OTC analgesics, including aspirin, acetaminophen, and ibuprofen or naproxen in the 200 mg dosage formulation. For moderate pain, salicylates, NSAIDs, or acetaminophen in higher doses often suffice; if not, the clinician can prescribe drugs such as codeine or oxycodone.

1. Aspirin–Aspirin is often the drug of first choice for management of mild to moderate pain and is an effective antipyretic and anti-inflammatory agent. Analgesia is achieved with much lower doses and blood levels than are needed for anti-inflammatory action. Aspirin is available in many forms for oral administration—in a single 325 mg unit dose, as well as smaller (eg, 81 mg) and larger (eg, 500 mg) doses. The usual dose is one or two tablets (325–650 mg) every 4 hours as needed, taken with fluid. Gastrointestinal irritation can be reduced by ingestion with food or with an antacid. Enteric-coated aspirin, which is more expensive (Ecotrin; many others), can be used to avoid gastric irritation, but absorption is delayed.

The main untoward effect of aspirin—especially in large doses or when taken chronically—is gastric irritation and microscopic blood loss from the gut. Rarely, there may be massive gastrointestinal hemorrhage, most commonly in heavy drinkers or patients with a history of peptic ulcer disease.

Aspirin allergy occurs infrequently and may be manifested as rhinorrhea, nasal polyps, asthma, and—very rarely—anaphylaxis. The incidence is less than 0.1%. Aspirin in high doses may produce a vitamin K-responsive prolongation of the prothrombin time.

Because of a possible association with Reye's syndrome, salicylates are best avoided by children and teenagers with febrile viral illnesses such as influenza and chickenpox.

2. Acetaminophen–Acetaminophen in the same dosage as aspirin (650 mg orally every 4 hours) has comparable analgesic and antipyretic effects but lacks the anti-inflammatory property of aspirin. It is useful for people who cannot tolerate aspirin, for those with bleeding disorders, and for those at risk for Reye's syndrome. In very large doses (eg, > 4 g/d chronically, > 7 g/d acutely), acetaminophen can be hepatotoxic, manifested by hepatic necrosis with markedly elevated serum aminotransferase levels. Toxicity may occur at considerably lower doses in the chronic alcoholic.

See Chapter 39 for further details on salicylate and acetaminophen poisoning.

3. Nonsteroidal Anti-inflammatory Drugs (NSAIDs)–Table 1–11 lists the most commonly used NSAIDs along with dosages and pertinent comments. All NSAIDs are analgesic, antipyretic, and anti-inflammatory in a dose-dependent fashion. Their principal uses are in the control of moderate pain of various musculoskeletal disorders, menstrual cramps, and other—mainly self-limited—conditions, including moderate postoperative discomfort.

The activity of NSAIDs is mediated through inhibition of the biosynthesis of prostaglandins. All of these drugs to varying degrees inhibit platelet aggregation and may cause gastric irritation (the risk of associated upper gastrointestinal bleeding is about 1.5 times normal and may be considerably higher than that in elderly patients); kidney damage (including acute renal failure, decreased glomerular filtration, nephrotic syndrome, papillary necrosis, interstitial nephritis, and type IV renal tubular acidosis); and bone marrow suppression, rashes, anorexia, and nausea. Kidney damage is more apt to occur in old men, diuretic users, and patients with heart disease. NSAIDs should generally not be prescribed to patients receiving oral anticoagulant therapy. The principal advantages of the newer NSAIDs over aspirin are the longer duration of action—permitting less frequent dosing and better compliance—and the de-creased frequency of gastrointestinal side effects. (Aspirin is much less expensive, however.) Patients susceptible to gastric or duodenal ulceration who must take NSAIDs regularly can be given misoprostol, a synthetic prostaglandin E_1 analog, in a dose of 200 µg orally three times daily. However, it is an abortifacient and thus contraindicated during pregnancy; side effects consist of diarrhea and crampy abdominal pain; the risk of gastric irritation is minimal. Enteric-coated aspirin is a reasonable alternative, as is high-dose famotidine (40 mg twice daily). NSAIDs may activate quiescent inflammatory bowel disease. Suicide attempts with overdoses of other NSAIDs are less serious and less often successful than attempts with aspirin.

B. Drugs for Moderate to Severe Pain:

1. Opioids–Opioid analgesics are indicated for moderate to severe pain that cannot be relieved with other agents. Examples include the acute pain of severe trauma, burns, myocardial infarction, ureteral stone, and surgery and the chronic pain of progressive diseases such as cancer and AIDS. Opioids are effective, easily titrated, and have a favorable benefit-to-risk ratio. Large doses of opioids may be needed to control pain if it is severe, and extended courses may be necessary if the pain is chronic. Opioid analgesics can also be useful to treat selected patients with intractable pain due to causes other than malignancy, when efforts to remove its cause or to treat it in other ways have been unsuccessful. Selection of such patients for a trial of opioid therapy must be based on a careful evaluation of the pain and of the consequent disability. Continuation of opioid therapy in this circumstance should be based on the clinician's assessment of the results of treatment (degree of pain relief, changes in physical and psychologic functioning, number of prescription refills, telephone calls, clinic or emergency department visits, hospital stays, etc).

Long-term opioid administration may lead to **tolerance** (escalating opioid doses are needed for the same analgesic effect) and **physical dependence** (withdrawal symptoms occur upon sudden opioid discontinuation, though to varying degrees and after varying periods of use). Tolerance and physical dependence are normal physiologic consequences of extended opioid therapy and must not be confused with **addiction.** Addiction is psychologic dependence and is often manifested as drug abuse (variously defined as manipulative drug-seeking behavior or compulsive use of drugs for nonmedicinal purposes despite harmful effects). Patients and family members must be educated regarding the difference between tolerance, physical dependence, and addiction and about the low risk of addiction from long-term use or high doses of opioids for pain relief. Patients with chronic, severe pain must not consider themselves addicts because they are being treated with opioids. *Concerns about addiction should not*

Table 1–11. Useful nonsteroidal anti-inflammatory drugs.[1]

Drug	Usual Dose for Adults ≥ 50 kg Body Weight	Usual Dose for Adults < 50 kg Body Weight[2]	Cost per Unit	Costs for 30 Days' Treatment Based on Maximum Dosage[3]	Comments[4]
ACETAMINOPHEN AND OTC NSAIDs					
Acetaminophen[5] (Tylenol, Datril, etc)	650 mg q4h or 975 mg q6h	10–15 mg/kg q4h (oral); 15–20 mg/kg q4h (rectal)	$0.02/325 mg	$7.00	Not an NSAID because it lacks peripheral anti-inflammatory effects. Equivalent to aspirin as analgesic and antipyretic agent.
Aspirin[6]	650 mg q4h or 975 mg q6h	10–15 mg/kg q4h (oral); 15–20 mg/kg q4h (rectal)	$0.03/325 mg	$11.00	Available also in enteric-coated form that is more expensive and more slowly absorbed but better tolerated.
Ibuprofen (Motrin, Advil, Rufen, others)	400–800 mg q6h	10 mg/kg q6–8h	$0.12/400 mg; $0.14/600 mg	$28.80 $21.00	Relatively well tolerated. Increases serum lithium levels. Less gastrointestinal toxicity.
Naproxen (Naprosyn, Anaprox, Aleve [OTC], others)	200–500 mg q6–8h	5 mg/kg q8h	$1.10/500 mg	$99.00	Generally well tolerated. Lower doses for elderly.
Naprelan Con-trolled-Release	412.5–550 mg q24h		$1.13/412.5 mg $1.03/550 mg	$33.90 $30.90	Once-daily preparation with effi-cacy comparable to that of naproxen 500 mg bid.
PRESCRIPTION NSAIDs					
Choline magnesium salicylate[7] (Trilasate)	1000–1500 mg tid	25 mg/kg tid	$0.34/500 mg	$92.00	Salicylates cause less gastrointestinal distress and renal impairment than NSAIDs but are probably less effective in pain management than NSAIDs.
Choline salicylate[7] (Arthropan)	870 mg q3–4h		$30.00/480 mL; 174 mg/mL	$45.00	Minimal antiplatelet effects.
Diclofenac (Voltaren, Cataflam, others)	50–75 mg bid–tid		$0.74/50 mg, $0.97/75 mg	$88.80 $87.00	May impose higher risk of hepatotoxicity. Low incidence of gastrointestinal side effects. Enteric-coated product, slow onset.
Diclofenac Sus-tained Release (Voltaren-XR)	100 mg q24h		$2.41/100 mg	$144.60	
Diflunisal[8] (Dolobid)	500 mg q12h		$0.60/500 mg	$54.00	Fluorinated acetylsalicylic acid derivative.
Etodolac (Lodine)	200–400 mg q6–8h		$1.39/300 mg	$166.00	Perhaps less gastrointestinal toxicity.
Fenoprofen calcium (Nalfon)	300–600 mg q6h		$0.39/300 mg	$46.80	Perhaps more side effects than others, including tubulointerstitial nephritis.
Flurbiprofen (Ansaid)	50–100 mg tid–qid		$0.87/50 mg, $1.36/100 mg	$156.00 $122.00	Adverse gastrointestinal effects may be more common among elderly.
Indomethacin (Indocin, Indometh, others)	25–50 mg bid–qid		$0.11/25 mg; $0.19/50 mg	$26.40 $22.80	Higher incidence of dose-related toxic effects, especially gastrointestinal and bone marrow effects.

(continued)

Table 1–11. Useful nonsteroidal anti-inflammatory drugs.[1] (continued)

Drug	Usual Dose for Adults ≥ 50 kg Body Weight	Usual Dose for Adults < 50 kg Body Weight[2]	Cost per Unit	Costs for 30 Days' Treatment Based on Maximum Dosage[3]	Comments[4]
Ketoprofen (Orudis, Oruvail, others, OTC)	25–60 mg q6–8h		$0.86/50 mg; $1.00/75 mg	$154.00 $120.00	Lower doses for elderly. Longer use may be associated with acute renal failure.
Ketorolac tromethamine (Toradol)	10 mg q4–6h to a maximum of 40 mg/d		$1.25/10 mg	Not recommended	Short-term use (< 5 days) only; otherwise, increased risk of gastrointestinal side effects.
Magnesium salicylate (Doan's, Magan, Mobidin, others)	650 mg q4h		$0.13/325 mg	$31.00	
Meclofenamate sodium[9] (Meclomen)	50–100 mg q6h		$0.49/100 mg	$59.00	Diarrhea more common.
Mefenamic acid (Ponstel)	250 mg q6h		$0.96/250 mg	$115.00	
Nabumetone (Relafen)	500–1000 mg once daily		$1.11/500 mg $1.31/750 mg	$118.00	May be less ulcerogenic than ibuprofen, but overall side effects may not be less.
Oxaprozin (Daypro)	600–1200 mg once daily		$1.31/600 mg	$79.00	Similar to ibuprofen. May cause rash, pruritus, photosensitivity.
Piroxicam (Feldene)	20 mg daily		$2.20/20 mg	$66.00	Single daily dose convenient. Long half-life. May cause higher rate of gastrointestinal bleeding and dermatologic side effects.
Sodium salicylate	325–650 q3–4h		$0.02/650 mg	$7.50	
Sulindac (Clinoril)	150–200 mg bid		$0.80/150 mg; $0.99/200 mg	$48.00 $58.00	May cause higher rate of gastrointestinal bleeding. May have less nephrotoxic potential.
Tolmetin (Tolectin)	200–600 mg qid		$0.52/200 mg; $1.09/600 mg	$52.00 $104.00	Perhaps more side effects than others, including anaphylactic reactions.
PARENTERAL NSAIDs					
Ketorolac tromethamine[10] (Toradol)	60 mg initially, then 30 mg q6h IM		$8.80/60 mg	Not recommended	Intramuscular NSAID as alternative to opioid. Lower doses for elderly. Short-term use (< 5 days) only. Longer use may be associated with acute renal failure.

[1]Modified from Jacox AK et al: Management of Cancer Pain: Quick Reference Guide for Clinicians No. 9. AHCPR Publication No. 94–0593. Rockville, MD: Agency for Health Care Policy and Research, Public Health Service, U.S. Department of Health and Human Services. March 1994.
[2]Acetaminophen and NSAID dosages for adults weighing less than 50 kg should be adjusted for weight.
[3]Cost to pharmacist (average wholesale price) for 30 days' treatment based on maximum dosage (generic when possible). Source: First Data Bank, Price Alert, April 1997.
[4]The adverse effects of headache, tinnitus, dizziness, confusion, rashes, anorexia, nausea, vomiting, gastrointestinal bleeding, diarrhea, nephrotoxicity, visual disturbances, etc, can occur with any of these drugs. Tolerance and efficacy are subject to great individual variations among patients.
[5]Acetaminophen lacks the antiplatelet activities of NSAIDs.
[6]May inhibit platelet aggregation for 1 week or more and may cause bleeding.
[7]May have minimal antiplatelet activity.
[8]Administration with antacids may decrease absorption.
[9]Coombs-positive autoimmune hemolytic anemia has been associated with prolonged use.
[10]Has the same gastrointestinal toxicities as oral NSAIDs.

prevent the appropriate use of opioids, especially in the management of terminal illness.

Table 1–12 lists opioid analgesics with some of their characteristics. These drugs all have pharmacologic similarities to opium and suppress cough and gastrointestinal motility as well as relieve pain.

Opioids can be classified as full opioid agonists, partial agonists, or mixed agonist-antagonists, based on the specific central nervous system receptors to which they bind and their actions at these receptors. Full agonists include morphine, hydromorphone, codeine, oxycodone, methadone, levorphanol, and fentanyl. Such agents are preferred in management of cancer pain, since their effectiveness is not generally limited by a "ceiling." Meperidine is an agonist also but generally should be avoided in treating severe, chronic pain (see below). Partial agonists like buprenorphine are less effective analgesics because they are less active at the central nervous system opioid receptor and are limited by a dose-related "ceiling" effect. Mixed agonist-antagonists include pentazocine, butorphanol tartrate, and nalbuphine hydrochloride. Mixed agonist-antagonists block or are neutral at one type of opioid receptor while binding to and activating another. These agents also manifest a "ceiling" effect. In addition, mixed agonist-antagonists are contraindicated for use in patients already receiving opioid agonists because they may precipitate an acute withdrawal and cause increased pain.

C. Frequently Used Opioid Agonist Analgesics:

1. Morphine sulfate–Morphine is the most commonly prescribed opioid agent and is readily available in several forms. Morphine, 8–15 mg subcutaneously or intramuscularly, is effective for control of severe pain in many adults. The effects last 4–5 hours. In acute myocardial infarction or in acute pulmonary edema due to left ventricular failure, 2–6 mg may be injected slowly intravenously in 5 mL of saline solution. Patient-controlled administration of intravenous morphine is discussed below. Long-acting, sustained-release oral morphine preparations have an extended duration of action (8–12 hours) and allow less frequent dosing in chronic pain.

2. Morphine congeners–Examples are hydromorphone and oxymorphone, 2–4 mg of either given orally every 4 hours or 1–3 mg of either given subcutaneously every 4 hours. These drugs give effects equivalent to 10 mg of morphine sulfate and have no specific advantages over morphine.

3. Methadone–Methadone, 15–20 mg orally every 6–8 hours, is most often used for treatment of addiction because of its long duration of action. Its side effects are similar to those of morphine (see below), but tolerance and physical dependence are slower to develop.

4. Codeine (sulfate or phosphate)–Codeine in doses of 15–60 mg orally or subcutaneously every 4–6 hours is somewhat less effective than morphine but also less habit-forming. It is often given together with aspirin or acetaminophen for enhanced analgesic effect. Codeine is a powerful cough suppressant in a dosage of 15–30 mg orally every 4 hours, but it is constipating.

5. Oxycodone and hydrocodone–These drugs are given orally and prescribed with another analgesic. The dosage is 5–7.5 mg every 4–6 hours in tablets that contain aspirin 325 mg (Percodan, Roxiprin) or acetaminophen 325 mg (Percocet, Roxicet) or 500 mg (Vicodin, Lortab, Zydone).

6. Meperidine–Meperidine, 50–150 mg orally or intramuscularly every 3–4 hours, provides analgesia similar to morphine in acute pain, but it should be avoided in treating severe chronic pain because of its short duration of action (2.5–3.5 hours) and in renal insufficiency because accumulation of its toxic metabolite (normeperidine) may predispose to seizures.

7. Fentanyl–Fentanyl transdermal patches also are long-acting (2–3 days). Four patch sizes are available (25 μg/h, 50 μg/h, 75 μg/h, and 100 μg/h) to provide flexibility in dosing. Doses above 25 μg/h are not used in opioid-naive patients. The maximum recommended daily dose is 300 μg/h. Each patch contains a 72-hour supply of the drug, but plasma levels rise slowly over 12–18 hours after initial patch placement. Thus, transdermal fentanyl is used mainly in patients with stable, chronic pain who have infrequent episodes of "breakthrough" pain. The latter can be managed with a supplemental oral or parenteral short-acting opioid agent. The most common adverse effects of fentanyl are nausea, mental clouding, and skin irritation.

8. Tramadol–Tramadol is an atypical analgesic with both opioid and nonopioid features, contributing to a dual mode of action. Tramadol and its metabolite both bind moderately to opioid receptors; in addition, tramadol acts like the tricyclic and SSRI antidepressants to block reuptake of norepinephrine and serotonin. Adverse effects (central nervous system, gastrointestinal) are similar to those associated with opioids, but respiratory depression is less. While it does not interact with anticoagulants or oral hypoglycemic agents, tramadol should not be used in patients receiving monoamine oxidase inhibitors. Tramadol produces synergistic effects when used concurrently with NSAIDs and without increasing NSAID side effects. A reduced dose is recommended when administered with other agents that act upon the central nervous system, including opioid analgesic and sedative-hypnotic agents. Recommended doses are 50–100 mg every 4–6 hours up to a total dose of 400 mg/d (maximum 300 mg/d in patients age 75 or older). In patients with renal insufficiency (creatinine clearance < 30 mL/min), the dosage interval should be increased to every 12 hours and the maximum reduced to 200 mg daily. Abrupt cessation

Table 1–12. Useful opioid agonist analgesics.[1]

Drug	Approximate Equianalgesic Dose[2]		Usual Starting Dose				Potential Advantages	Potential Disadvantages
			Adults ≥ 50 kg Body Weight		Adults < 50 kg Body Weight			
	Oral	Parenteral	Oral	Parenteral	Oral	Parenteral		
OPIOID AGONISTS[3]								
Morphine[4]	30 mg q3–4h (repeat around-the-clock dosing); 60 mg q3–4h (single or intermittent dosing)	10 mg q3–4h	30 mg q3–4h $0.24/10 mg $173.00	10 mg q3–4h $0.78/10 mg 6.24/24 h $187.00	0.3 mg/kg q3–4h	0.1 mg/kg q3–4h	Standard of comparison; multiple dosage forms available.	No unique problems when compared with other opioids.
Morphine controlled-release[4] (MS Contin, Roxanol, Oramorph)	90–120 mg q12h	Not available	90–120 mg q12h $1.57/30 mg $283.00	Not available	Not available	Not available		
Hydromorphone[4] (Dilaudid)	7.5 mg q3–4h	1.5 mg q3–4h	6 mg q3–4h $0.31/2 mg $167.00	1.5 mg q3–4h $0.45/2 mg $81.00	0.06 mg/ q3–4h	0.015 mg/kg q3–4h	Similar to morphine. Available in injectable high-potency preparation, rectal suppository.	Short duration.
Levorphanol (Levo-Dromoran)	4 mg q6–8h	2 mg q6–8h	4 mg q6–8h $0.61/2 mg $146.00	2 mg q6–8h $2.26/2 mg $271.00	0.04 mg/kg q6–8h	0.02 mg q6–8h	Longer-acting than morphine sulfate.	
Meperidine[5] (Demerol)	300 mg q2–3h	100 mg q3h	Not recommended $0.28/50 mg	100 mg q3h $1.75/100 mg	Not recommended	0.75 mg/kg q2–3h	May be useful for acute pain if the patient is intolerant to morphine.	Short duration. Metabolite in high concentrations may cause seizures.
Methadone Dolophine, others)	20 mg q6–8h	10 mg q6–8h	20 mg q6–8h $164.40 (40 mg/24h)	10 mg q6–8h $14.27/200 mg $85.62 (40 mg/24h)	0.2 mg/kg q6–8h	0.1 mg/kg q6–8h	Somewhat longer-acting than morphine. Useful in cases of intolerance to morphine.	Analgesic duration shorter than plasma duration. May accumulate, requiring close monitoring during first weeks of treatment.
Oxymorphone[3] (Numorphan)	Not available	1 mg q3–4h	Not available	1 mg q3–4h 20 mL/10 mg/mL $3.72/1 mL (1 mL = 1 mg)				
COMBINATION OPIOID-NSAID OR ANTIDEPRESSANT PREPARATIONS								
Codeine[6,7] (with aspirin or acetaminophen)[8]	180–200 mg q3–4h	130 mg q3–4h	60 mg q3–h4 $0.15/60 mg $36.00		0.5–1 mg/kg q3–4h	Not recommended	Similar to morphine.	Not useful for severe pain.
Codeine				$0.55/30 mg $132.00 $1.00/60 mg $240.00				

(continued)

Table 1–12. Useful opioid agonist analgesics.[1] (continued)

Drug	Approximate Equianalgesic Dose[2]		Usual Starting Dose				Potential Advantages	Potential Disadvantages
			Adults ≥ 50 kg Body Weight		Adults < 50 kg Body Weight			
	Oral	Parenteral	Oral	Parenteral	Oral	Parenteral		
COMBINATION OPIOID-NSAID OR ANTIDEPRESSANT PREPARATIONS								
Hydrocodone[6] (in Lorcet, Lortab, Vicodin, others)[8]	30 mg q3–4h	Not available	10 mg q3–4h $0.16/5 mg $72.00	Not available	0.2 mg/kg q3–4h	Not available		Combination with acetaminophen limits dosage titration.
Oxycodone[6] (Roxicodone, Percocet, Percodan, Tylox, others)[8]	30 mg q3–4h	Not available	10 mg q3–4h $0.20/5 mg $96.00	Not available	0.2 mg/kg q3–4h	Not available	Similar to morphine.	Combination with acetaminophen and aspirin limits dosage titration.
Tramadol (Ultram)		Not available	50–100 mg q4–6h $0.65/50 mg $156.00 Maximum dose 400 mg/d	Not available	50–100 mg q4–6h maximum dose; 300 mg maximum dose for patients over 75 years of age	Not available	Novel agent. Both opioid and non-opioid (inhibits reuptake of norepinephrine and serotonin).	Withdrawal may occur if abruptly discontinued. Must reduce dose in elderly (age > 75); increase dosing interval in renal insufficiency. Potential for abuse. Seizures and anaphylactoid reactions may occur.

[1]Modified from Jacox AK et al: Management of Cancer Pain: Quick Reference Guide for Clinicians No. 9. AHCPR Publication No. 94–0593. Rockville, MD. Agency for Health Care Policy and Research, Public Health Service, U.S. Department of Health and Human Services. March 1994. Reproduced in part from Hosp Formul 1994;29(8 Part 2)586. (Erstad BL: A rational approach to the management of acute pain states.) Copyright by Advanstar Communications, Inc.

[2]Published tables vary in the suggested doses that are equianalgesic to morphine. Clinical response is the criterion that must be applied for each patient; titration to clinical efficacy is necessary. Because there is not complete cross-tolerance among these drugs, it is usually necessary to use a lower than equianalgesic dose initially when changing drugs and to retitrate to response.

[3]*Caution:* Recommended doses do not apply for adult patients with renal or hepatic insufficiency or other conditions affecting drug metabolism.

[4]*Caution:* For morphine, hydromorphone, and oxymorphone, rectal administration is an alternative route for patients unable to take oral medications. Equianalgesic doses may differ from oral and parenteral doses. A short-acting opioid should normally be used for initial therapy.

[5]Not recommended for chronic pain. Doses listed are for brief therapy of acute pain only. Switch to another opioid for long-term therapy.

[6]*Caution:* Doses of aspirin and acetaminophen in combination products must also be adjusted to the patient's body weight (Table 1–11).

[7]*Caution:* Doses of codeine above 65 mg often are not appropriate because of diminishing incremental analgesia with increasing doses but continually increasing nausea, constipation, and other side effects.

[8]*Caution:* Monitor total acetaminophen dose carefully, including any OTC use. Total APAP dose maximum 4 g/d. If liver impairment or heavy alcohol use, maximum is 2 g/d.

Note: Prices listed represent unit costs and costs to pharmacists (average wholesale prices) for 30 days' treatment based on the maximum dose (generic when possible). Source: First Data Bank, Price Alert, April 1997.

of the drug should be avoided to avoid possible withdrawal effects.

Dosing

Table 1–12 summarizes equianalgesic doses of commonly used opioids by patient body weight. Knowledge of equianalgesic dosages enables the clinician to maintain both patient safety and pain relief when changing routes of administration or types of drugs.

The appropriate opioid dose is the amount required to control the pain without intolerable side effects. The need for increasing doses of opioid in patients with cancer often reflects progression of the disease rather than development of tolerance. If tolerance does develop, the same dose of drug can be taken more frequently. If a change in dose is required, a reasonable titration strategy is to increase or decrease the next dose by one-quarter to one-half of the previous dose. If a change from the oral to the rectal route of administration is required, the clinician should begin with the oral dose, then titrate upward carefully. If changing from the oral to the parenteral route, start with lower than oral doses. However, parenteral doses are similar for subcutaneous, intramuscular, and intravenous routes.

A. Schedule: A common error in management of chronic pain from cancer is to prescribe insufficient doses "prn" rather than adequate doses around-the-clock at specified intervals. Scheduling medication doses regularly "around the clock" maintains plasma drug levels and prevents recurrence of pain.

Patients can also achieve more reliable plasma opioid levels through the self-administration of small, repeated intravenous doses. Such **patient-controlled analgesia (PCA)** permits patients to maintain adequate pain control by allowing them to match drug delivery to the need for analgesia. The amount of medication is limited by preestablished dosing intervals and maximum doses within a defined period. Alternatively, continuous or basal delivery is also possible. Treatment starts with a bolus dose followed by a basal continuous rate to achieve desired baseline levels and to permit sleep. Additional doses are available on demand, within the limits established by the physician. A conventional intermittent dosing regimen is preferred, with a continuous infusion to be used only if pain relief is unsatisfactory. Adverse side effects occur less than half as often with PCA as with conventional therapy. Those who have experienced PCA overwhelmingly prefer it to conventional pain control regimens. Originally developed using a pump to deliver the opioid drug parenterally, the technique has been adapted to the oral route of medication delivery. In this use, oral opioids are kept at the bedside for charted patient self-administration.

B. Route: Given its convenience and low cost, oral administration of pain medications is generally preferred. In patients who cannot take oral agents (eg, those with intractable nausea and vomiting), rectal or transdermal routes of administration should be considered. Rectal administration is safe, inexpensive, and effective. However, the rectal route is inappropriate for the patient who has diarrhea, anal or rectal lesions, or mucositis; who is markedly neutropenic or thrombocytopenic; who cannot manage rectal suppositories; or who prefers other routes. The transdermal route (fentanyl) is not suitable for rapid titration of dosage and thus is generally used in situations of relatively stable pain when rapid increases or decreases of pain medication are unlikely to be required. Parenteral administration of pain medications is more invasive, more costly, and more demanding of professional services in the clinic, hospital, or home environment. The intramuscular route should be avoided because of pain, inconvenience, and unreliable drug absorption. The intravenous route provides the most rapid onset of analgesia, but the duration of analgesia following a bolus dose is shorter than with other routes. Continuous intravenous or epidural opioid infusion requires skill and expertise to manage a dedicated portable pump to deliver the drug safely. An alternative is subcutaneous opioid infusion, which has proved practical in the hospital, hospice, or home. Recently, oral transmucosal fentanyl citrate has been used to provide analgesia to patients with acute postoperative pain.

Contraindications to Opioids

The opioid analgesics are relatively contraindicated in some acute illnesses. In patients with acute abdominal pain, for example, the pattern of pain may provide important diagnostic clues. However, some analgesia may be necessary in order to assess the history and perform an adequate physical examination for diagnostic purposes. In acute head injuries, opioid drugs interfere with interpretation of neurologic findings.

Adverse Effects of Opioids

Patients with hypothyroidism, adrenal insufficiency, hypopituitarism, acute intermittent porphyria, reduced blood volume, and severe debility are particularly apt to suffer adverse effects from opioid analgesics. Adverse effects are easily managed if they occur. The side effects of all opioid narcotics are reversed by naloxone, but small doses of naloxone must be employed to avoid reversal of analgesia and precipitation of acute withdrawal.

A. Respiratory Depression: Respiratory depression is commonly feared as a hazard of parenteral morphine administration. Morphine acts to depress the respiratory center in the brainstem. The respiratory rate decreases gradually; abrupt cessation of breathing does not occur. Severe respiratory depression is uncommon, occurring in 0.05–0.9% of treated patients. Although not usually a problem in patients with normal pulmonary function receiving usual doses, a dose-dependent respiratory depression may occur in patients with respiratory insufficiency, cardiac disease, thoracic or upper abdominal surgery, and age over 70 years. It may be more common in those who have not previously taken opioids and following epidural administration. It is less common in patients receiving long-term opioid analgesics for cancer pain, who generally develop tolerance to the respiratory depressant effects of these agents. Treatment of a mild decrease in respiratory rate can be accomplished by simple visual or auditory stimulation. More severe depression (respiratory rates under 10/min) is treated by repeated bolus injections of naloxone (0.1–0.2 mg), by a continuous naloxone infusion, or (rarely) by endotracheal intubation and mechanical ventilation.

B. Central Nervous System Effects: Central nervous system effects include euphoria, mental clouding, and sedation. Antidepressants, antihistamines, phenothiazines, sedative-hypnotics, and alcohol can potentiate these effects. If persistent, these central nervous system effects can be managed by withholding one or two doses, then reducing the dose by 25% and increasing the frequency of administration. Central nervous system stimulants such as caffeine, dextroamphetamine, pemoline, and methylphenidate are also effective.

C. Gastrointestinal Side Effects: Gastrointestinal side effects are chiefly decreased bowel motility and constipation and nausea and vomiting. Because constipation is an inevitable side effect of opioid administration, the physician should attempt to prevent it by prescribing dietary fiber and regularly scheduled doses of a laxative. Severe constipation can be effectively treated with a stimulating cathartic (eg, bisacodyl, senna concentrate, or sorbitol, orally or via suppository). Nausea and vomiting occur in about one-third of patients given oral, parenteral, or epidural morphine. Nausea and vomiting occur because the opioid stimulates the chemoreceptor trigger zone in the central nervous system, decreases gastrointestinal motility and increases pyloric sphincter tone, and sensitizes the vestibular apparatus. Sometimes it can be controlled by changing the opioid regimen (reducing the dose or switching to another agent). Otherwise, trial of an antiemetic agent may be useful. In continuous nausea (often due to stimulation of the chemoreceptor trigger zone), a phenothiazine such as prochlorperazine may be useful. In postprandial nausea and vomiting (due to decreased gastrointestinal motility), metoclopramide or cisapride may be helpful. In nausea and vomiting precipitated by ambulation or changes in head position (due to vestibular dysfunction), meclizine or transdermal scopolamine may be tried.

D. Urinary Retention: Urinary retention sometimes occurs because morphine inhibits parasympathetic outflow from the spinal cord, causing bladder spasm. It is more common following spinal (epidural)

than parenteral or oral administration and more often a problem in older men with benign prostatic hyperplasia. Discontinuation of the narcotic may relieve the problem. If it does not, bethanechol, 2.5 mg (dose titrated to effect) may be given subcutaneously, or naloxone 0.8 mg can be given intravenously.

E. Pruritus: Pruritus occurs commonly when morphine is administered via the epidural or intrathecal routes, less frequently with intravenous or intramuscular administration, and uncommonly following oral dosing. Its pathogenesis is unknown. If the pruritus is severe, naloxone is effective both for treatment (0.1 mg intravenous boluses every 30 minutes as needed) and for prophylaxis (0.4 mg/L by intravenous infusion over 24 hours). Doses of naloxone must be small to avoid reversal of analgesia. Droperidol 2.5 mg may decrease the incidence and severity of pruritus. Diphenhydramine, hydroxyzine, and cimetidine are also sometimes effective.

F. Hypersensitivity: Enhanced sensitivity to the opioid drugs occurs in patients with hepatic impairment; biliary spasm may cause severe biliary colic.

G. Allergic Response: Allergic manifestations also occur, but rarely.

Special Circumstances

A history of substance abuse in the patient or family may complicate pain management. Interventions in such patients require extra care and monitoring, and consultation with experts in substance abuse or pain management is advisable.

Patients using opioids regularly (eg, patients using heroin, patients on methadone maintenance) or frequently (eg, patients with sickle cell disease) often have already developed some degree of pharmacologic tolerance; thus, they usually require higher starting doses and shorter dosing intervals for effective acute pain management.

In the situation of advanced disease or terminal illness, clinicians are sometimes reluctant to give high enough doses of opioids to relieve the pain, fearing serious side effects. However, the clinician's primary ethical responsibility—to benefit patients by relieving their suffering—supports use of escalating doses even at the risk of side effects. Patients with cancer pain may become tolerant to opioids during long-term therapy but usually tolerate increasing opioid doses without unmanageable side effects, without development of addiction, and without shortening of their lives. Patients who are dying sometimes require very large doses of opioids for control of pain (or dyspnea), even with the risk of unintentional respiratory depression. However, most compassionate physicians are willing to accept this "double effect" and find that patients and families are grateful for the relief provided.

Adjuvant Drugs for Pain Control

Corticosteroids are often helpful in management

of cancer pain. Corticosteroids have potent anti-inflammatory activity and reduce cerebral and spinal cord edema. Because they have antiemetic activity and stimulate appetite, they may be beneficial in management of cachexia and anorexia. They also can cause mood elevation.

Anticonvulsants (eg, phenytoin, carbamazepine), antidepressants (eg, amitriptyline, desipramine), and local anesthetics (eg, bupivacaine) are sometimes useful in management of neuropathic pain. Neuroleptics (eg, methotrimeprazine) are useful in chronic pain syndromes since they have antiemetic and anxiolytic effects and do not inhibit gastrointestinal motility or cause constipation. Hydroxyzine is an antihistamine with mild analgesic, anxiolytic, sedative, and antiemetic properties that is useful in treating anxious patients with pain. Placebos should not be used in the management of severe, intractable pain such as that due to cancer or sickle cell crisis.

Physical, Psychologic, & Other Modalities

A variety of nonpharmacologic interventions can assist in pain alleviation. Noninvasive physical and psychosocial modalities can be used concurrently with drugs and other interventions. Physical measures include massage, cutaneous stimulation, heat, cold, exercise, repositioning, immobilization, and counterstimulation (transcutaneous electrical nerve stimulation and acupuncture). Psychologic modalities include patient education and reassurance; biofeedback, relaxation, and imagery techniques; cognitive distraction and framing; psychotherapy, support groups, and structured support; and prayer and pastoral counseling. For severe chronic pain, such as occurs in metastatic cancer or neuropathic conditions, therapies such as nerve block or neurolysis, rhizotomy or ablative surgery, and neurosurgery may be useful in selected patients. These more invasive measures are generally reserved for situations in which other therapies are ineffective or poorly tolerated.

[AHCPR guideline on acute pain management] http://text.nlm.nih.gov/ftrs/pick?dbName=apmc&ftrsK=45830&cp=1&t=858441491&collect=ahcpr

[AHCPR guideline on management of cancer pain] http://text.nlm.nih.gov/ftrs/pick?dbName=capc&ftrsk=50783cp=1&t=866047409&collect=ahcpr

Barkin RL: Focus on tramadol: A centrally acting analgesic for moderate to moderately severe pain. Formulary 1995;30:321. (New analgesic agent.)

Barkin RL et al: Management of chronic pain. Dis Mon Part I: 1996 Jul;42:389; Part II: 1996 Aug;42:457. (Part I describes pharmacotherapeutic interventions and regional nerve blocks. Part II focuses on psychologic assessment and treatment and physical therapy.)

Carr DB et al: Acute Pain Management Guideline Panel: Acute Pain Management in Adults: Operative Procedures. Quick Reference Guide for Clinicians No. 1. AHCPR Publication No. 92–0019. Rockville, MD: Agency for Health Care Policy and Research, Public Health Service, U.S. Department of Health and Human Services. February 1992.

Cherny NI, Arbit E, Jain S: Invasive techniques in the management of cancer pain. Hematol Oncol Clin North Am 1996;10:121. (Reviews useful anesthetic and neurosurgical techniques.)

Cleeland CS et al: Pain and its treatment in outpatients with metastatic cancer. N Engl J Med 1994;330:592. (Among 1308 outpatients with metastatic cancer, 67% reported daily pain or analgesic use and 36% had pain severe enough to interfere with daily activities; 42% of those with pain were given inadequate analgesia.)

Ferrell BA: Pain evaluation and management in the nursing home. Ann Intern Med 1995;123:681. (Between 45% and 80% of nursing home residents have significant pain causing decreased function or quality of life; such pain can be alleviated by careful use of analgesic agents combined with exercise programs and physical therapy.)

Godfrey RG: A guide to the understanding and use of tricyclic antidepressants in the overall management of fibromyalgia and other chronic pain syndromes. Arch Intern Med 1996;156:1047.

Henry D et al: Variability in risk of gastrointestinal complications with individual non-steroidal anti-inflammatory drugs: Results of a collaborative meta-analysis. BMJ 1996;312:1563. (Of the 12 most commonly used NSAIDs, low-dose ibuprofen had by far the lowest risk for serious gastrointestinal complications requiring hospitalization.)

Jacox AK et al: Management of Cancer Pain: Quick Reference Guide for Clinicians No. 9. AHCPR Publication No. 94–0593. Rockville, MD: Agency for Health Care Policy and Research, Public Health Service, U.S. Department of Health and Human Services. March 1994.

Koch M et al: Prevention of nonsteroidal anti-inflammatory drug-induced gastrointestinal mucosal injury. Arch Intern Med 1996;156:2321. (Both misoprostol and H_2 blockers were effective in long-term prevention of duodenal ulcers, but only misoprostol was beneficial in prevention of gastric ulcers.)

Levey MH: Pharmacologic treatment of cancer pain. N Engl J Med 1996;335:1124.

Practice guidelines for acute pain management in the perioperative setting: A report by the American Society of Anesthesiologists Task Force on Pain Management, Acute Pain Section. Anesthesiology 1995;82:1071.

Radbruch L, Grond S, Lehmann KA: A risk-benefit assessment of tramadol in the management of pain. Drug Saf 1996;15:8.

SUPPORT Principal Investigators: A controlled trial to improve care for seriously ill hospitalized patients. JAMA 1995;274:1591. (Fifty percent of severely ill hospitalized patients who died in the hospital were in moderate to severe pain at least half the time during the last 3 days of life.)

FEVER & HYPERTHERMIA

The average normal oral body temperature is 36.7 °C (range 36–37.4 °C). These ranges include 2 SD and thus encompass 95% of a normal population, measured in midmorning. The normal rectal or vaginal temperature is 0.5 °C higher than the oral temperature, and the normal axillary temperature is correspondingly lower. Rectal temperature is more reliable than oral temperature, particularly in the case of patients who are mouth-breathers or who are tachypneic.

The normal diurnal temperature variation may be as much as 1 °C, being lowest in the early morning and highest in the late afternoon. There is a slight sustained temperature rise following ovulation during the menstrual cycle and in the first trimester of pregnancy.

Fever is a regulated rise to a new "set point" of body temperature. When proper stimuli act on appropriate monocyte-macrophages, these cells elaborate one of several pyrogenic cytokines, which causes elevation of the set point through effects in the hypothalamus. These cytokines include interleukin-1 (IL-1), tumor necrosis factor (TNF), interferon-gamma, and interleukin-6 (IL-6). The elevation in temperature may result from either increased heat production (eg, shivering) or decreased heat loss (eg, peripheral vasoconstriction). Body temperature in interleukin-1-induced fever seldom exceeds 41.1 °C unless there is structural damage in the hypothalamus.

Hyperthermia—not mediated by cytokines—occurs when body metabolic heat production or environmental heat load exceeds normal heat loss capacity or when there is impaired heat loss; heat stroke is an example. Body temperature may rise to alarming levels (> 41.1 °C) capable of producing irreversible brain damage; no diurnal variation is observed.

Neuroleptic malignant syndrome is a rare and potentially lethal idiosyncratic reaction to major tranquilizers, particularly haloperidol and fluphenazine. (See Chapters 25 and 39.)

Effect of Elevated Body Temperature

Fever as a symptom should generally be regarded with appropriate concern. The body temperature may provide important information about the presence of illness, particularly infections, and about changes in the clinical status of the patient. The fever pattern, however, is of little or no use for specific diagnosis. Furthermore, the degree of temperature elevation does not necessarily correspond to the severity of the illness. In general, the febrile response tends to be greater in children than in adults; in elderly persons and neonates and those receiving certain medications (eg, NSAIDs, corticosteroids), the febrile response is less marked or absent even in the face of bacteremia.

Markedly elevated body temperature may result in profound metabolic disturbances. High temperature during the first trimester of pregnancy may cause birth defects, such as anencephaly. Fever may increase insulin requirements and also alter the metabolism and disposition of drugs used for the treatment of the diverse diseases associated with fever.

Diagnostic Considerations

The outline below illustrates the wide variety of clinical disorders that may cause fever. Most febrile illnesses are due to common infections, are short-lived, and are relatively easy to diagnose. In certain instances, however, the origin of the fever may remain obscure ("fever of undetermined origin," FUO) after lengthy diagnostic examination. The term FUO has traditionally been reserved for cases of fever of over 38.3 °C for 3 weeks in patients whose diagnosis is not apparent after 1 week or more of studies (see FUO, Chapter 30). In the United States, fever of unknown origin associated with HIV and HIV-related infections is becoming increasingly important, though HIV infection by itself is rarely a cause of fever. In one study, fever occurred in nearly half of a large group of patients with advanced HIV infection followed for 9 months. Thorough evaluation led to a specific diagnosis in a majority (83%) of episodes. AIDS-defining infections and neoplasms accounted for half of the diagnoses. The most frequent diagnoses in febrile patients requiring more than 2 weeks of evaluation were pneumocystis pneumonia, *Mycobacterium avium* complex infection, and lymphoma.

In a prospective case series of 199 consecutive cases of FUO patients from the 1980s, infections—especially tuberculosis, cytomegalovirus, and abscesses—accounted for 23% of cases; multisystem illnesses—such as giant cell arteritis and Still's disease—for 22%; malignant tumors—hematologic and solid—for 7%; drug-related fever for 3%; factitious fever for 4%; habitual hyperthermia for 3%; and miscellaneous causes—such as pulmonary embolism and Crohn's disease—for 15%. No diagnosis could be firmly established in 26% of cases. Diagnostic ultrasound and CT scans led to specific diagnoses in 8% and 15% of cases, respectively.

Important Causes of Fever & Hyperthermia

A. Infections: Bacterial, viral, rickettsial, fungal, parasitic.

B. Autoimmune Diseases: Systemic lupus erythematosus, polyarteritis nodosa, rheumatic fever, polymyalgia rheumatica, giant cell arteritis, Still's disease, Wegener's granulomatosis, vasculitis, relapsing polychondritis; less prominent in dermatomyositis, adult rheumatoid arthritis.

C. Central Nervous System Disease: Cerebral hemorrhage, head injuries, brain and spinal cord tumors, degenerative central nervous system disease (eg, multiple sclerosis), spinal cord injuries. (This category represents interference with the thermal regulatory process rather than true "fever.")

D. Malignant Neoplastic Disease: Primary neoplasms (eg, colon and rectum, liver, kidney, neuroblastoma), tumors metastatic to the liver.

E. Hematologic Disease: Lymphomas, leukemias, hemolytic anemias.

F. Cardiovascular Disease: Myocardial infarction, thrombophlebitis, pulmonary embolism.

G. Gastrointestinal Disease: Inflammatory bowel disease, liver abscess, alcoholic hepatitis, granulomatous hepatitis.

H. Endocrine Disease: Hyperthyroidism, pheochromocytoma may raise temperature because of altered thermoregulation.

I. Diseases Due to Chemical Agents: Drug reactions (including serum sickness), neuroleptic malignant syndrome, malignant hyperthermia of anesthesia, serotonergic syndrome.

J. Miscellaneous Diseases: Sarcoidosis, familial Mediterranean fever, tissue injury, and hematoma.

K. Factitious Fever.

Treatment

Most fever is well tolerated. When the temperature is greater than 40 °C, particularly if prolonged, symptomatic treatment may be required. *Temperature over 41 °C is a medical emergency.* (See Heat Stroke, Chapter 38.)

A. Measures for Removal of Heat: Alcohol sponges, cold sponges, ice bags, ice-water enemas, and ice baths will lower body temperature and provide physical comfort for patients who complain of feeling hot.

B. Antipyretic Drugs: In most instances, antipyretic therapy by itself is not needed except for reasons of comfort or in patients with marginal hemodynamic status. Aspirin or acetaminophen, 325–650 mg every 4 hours, is quite effective in reducing fever. If given, these drugs are best administered continuously rather than as needed, since "prn" dosing results in periodic chills and sweats due to varying levels of drug.

C. Fluid Replacement: Oral or parenteral fluids must be administered to compensate for increased insensible fluid and electrolyte losses as well as those from perspiration.

D. Antibiotic Therapy: Febrile patients in whom a clinically significant infection can be identified should obviously be started on appropriate antibiotic therapy. Prompt, empiric, broad-spectrum antibiotic therapy is also indicated for febrile patients with potential serious infection, even before infection can be documented. This is particularly true for patients with hemodynamic instability in whom sepsis is suspected, for patients who are profoundly neutropenic (neutrophils less than 500/μL), and for asplenic or immunosuppressed patients (including those taking systemic corticosteroids, azathioprine, cyclosporine, or other immunosuppressive medications, and those who are HIV-infected) (see Chapter 31). In many febrile patients, empiric antibiotic therapy can usually be deferred pending further evaluation.

Cunha BA: Fever of unknown origin. Infect Dis Clin North Am 1996;10:111.

deKleijn EM et al: Utility of scintigraphic methods in patients with fever of unknown origin. Arch Intern Med 1995;155:1989. (Indium 111-labeled polyclonal human immunoglobulin G scintigraphy had a sensitivity of 81%, a specificity of 69%, a positive predictive value of 69%, and a negative predictive value of 82% among 29 patients with FUO.)

Knockaert DC, Dujardin KS, Bobbaers HJ: Long-term follow-up of patients with undiagnosed fever of unknown origin. Arch Intern Med 1996;156:618. (In a cohort of 199 patients with FUO, 61 individuals [30%] who were discharged from the hospital without a causal diagnosis were followed for at least 5 years or until death. Ultimately, a definitive diagnosis was established in 20%, usually within 2 months after discharge; 30% had persisting or recurring fever for months or even years; and half became symptom-free during hospitalization or shortly following discharge. Most symptomatic patients could be treated with NSAIDs; corticosteroids were seldom required. The mortality rate was only 3.2%.)

Knockaert DC et al: Recurrent or episodic fever of unknown origin. Review of 45 cases and survey of the literature. Medicine 1993;74:184. (Cyclic fever with fever-free intervals of at least 2 weeks.)

Saper CB, Breder CD: The neurologic basis of fever. N Engl J Med 1994;330:1880.

WEIGHT LOSS

Marked unexplained involuntary weight loss is often an indication of serious physical or psychologic illness. It should be distinguished from voluntary weight loss.

When the patient complains of weight loss but appears to be adequately nourished, inquiry should be made about exact weight changes (with approximate dates) and about changes in clothing size. Family members may provide confirmation of weight loss, as may old documents such as driver's licenses.

Once it has been established that the patient has marked weight loss, the history, physical examination, and conventional laboratory and radiologic investigations such as chest x-ray, upper gastrointestinal series, complete blood count, serum chemistries, and urinalysis usually reveal the cause. Involuntary weight loss is rarely due to "occult disease." Almost all physical causes are clinically evident during the initial evaluation. Cancer, gastrointestinal disorders, and depression are the most common causes. If the initial evaluation is unrevealing, careful follow-up is recommended rather than further diagnostic testing. Psychiatric consultation should be considered when there is evidence of depression, dementia, anorexia nervosa, or other psychologic problems. In approximately 25% of cases, no cause for the weight loss can be found despite extensive evaluation and prolonged follow-up.

A mild, gradual weight loss occurs in some elderly persons. It is due to physiologic changes in body composition, including loss of height and lean body mass and lower basal metabolic rate, which leads to decreased energy requirements. However, rapid unintentional weight loss is highly predictive of morbidity and mortality in the elderly population. In addition to various disease states, causes include loss of teeth and consequent difficulty with chewing, alcoholism, and social isolation.

Involuntary weight loss is a frequent complication of AIDS. Wasting, indicative of severe protein-calorie malnutrition (HIV wasting syndrome), is one element of the CDC's AIDS case definition (Table 31–1).

Iribarren C et al: Association of weight loss and weight fluctuation with mortality among Japanese American men. N Engl J Med 1995;333:686.

Marton KI, Sox HC Jr, Krupp JR: Involuntary weight loss: Diagnostic and prognostic significance. Ann Intern Med 1981;95:568. (Classic article on diagnostic approach to weight loss.)

Palenicek JP et al: Weight loss prior to clinical AIDS as a predictor of survival. Multicenter AIDS Cohort Study Investigators. J Acquir Immune Defic Syndr Hum Retroviral 1995;10:366. (Men with a self-reported unintentional weight loss of > 4.5 kg during the 3–9 months prior to AIDS diagnosis had significantly poorer survival than men without weight loss.)

Reife CM: Involuntary weight loss. Med Clin North Am 1995;79:299. (The underlying mechanisms probably involve the actions of hormones and cytokines, such as TNF [cachectin], adipsin, interleukin-1, and interleukin-6.)

Wallace JI et al: Involuntary weight loss in older outpatients: Incidence and clinical significance. J Am Geriatr Soc 1995;43:329. (In a 4-year prospective cohort study, involuntary weight loss occurred frequently among 247 community-dwelling male veterans 65 years of age or older [13.1% annual incidence]. Weight loss of greater than 4% of body weight was an independent predictor of increased mortality.)

FATIGUE

Fatigue is one of the most common symptoms confronting the office practitioner. In primary care settings, fatigue as an isolated symptom or diagnosis accounts for 1–3% of visits to generalists. The symptoms of fatigue may be less well defined and explained by patients than symptoms associated with specific functions, such as fever or dyspnea. Fatigue or lassitude and the closely related complaints of weakness, tiredness, and lethargy are most often readily explained by common factors such as overexertion, poor physical conditioning, inadequate quantity or quality of sleep, obesity, undernutrition, stress, and emotional problems. Taking a history of the patient's daily living and working habits may obviate the need for extensive and unproductive diagnostic studies.

Important diseases that can cause fatigue include endocrine disorders such as hyperthyroidism and hypothyroidism, cardiac disease (congestive heart failure, neurally mediated hypotension), infections (endocarditis, hepatitis), respiratory disorders (COPD, sleep apnea), anemia, the arthritides and related disorders, cancer, alcoholism, drug side effects such as from sedatives and beta-blockers, and psychologic conditions such as insomnia, depression, and somatization disorder. However, a recent study suggests that psychiatric disorders may be involved in less than 50% of cases.

In a four-community study of nearly 14,000 individuals, the lifetime prevalence of significant fatigue (present for at least 2 weeks) was 24%. Fatigue was reportedly more often due to unknown cause or to psychiatric illness than to physical illness, injury, medications, drugs, or alcohol. Psychiatric disorders associated with fatigue included depression, dysthymia, somatoform disorders, panic attack, and alcohol abuse.

Chronic Fatigue Syndrome

A syndrome of chronic fatigue has received much recent attention. A working case definition of chronic fatigue syndrome was developed in 1988 (Figure 1–1). Chronic fatigue syndrome is not a homogeneous abnormality, and there is no single pathogenic mechanism. No physical finding or laboratory test can be used to confirm the diagnosis of chronic fatigue syndrome.

Early studies suggested an infectious or immune dysregulation mechanism for the pathophysiology of chronic fatigue syndrome. Subsequent studies have documented that neurologic, affective, and cognitive symptoms also occur frequently. Neuropsychologic, neuroendocrine, and brain imaging studies have now confirmed the occurrence of neurobiologic abnormalities in most patients with the syndrome. For example, the chronic fatigue syndrome is associated with previous psychiatric disorders, partly explained by high rates of current psychiatric disorders.

A 1991 NIH panel recommended a standard panel of laboratory tests for initial patient examination, including complete blood count with differential, erythrocyte sedimentation rate, serum chemistries (BUN, serum electrolytes, glucose, creatinine, calcium, liver and thyroid function tests), antinuclear antibody, urinalysis, and tuberculin skin test, and screening questionnaires for psychiatric disorders. Other tests to be performed as clinically indicated are serum cortisol, rheumatoid factor, immunoglobulin levels, Lyme serology in endemic areas, and tests for HIV antibody. This seems a more

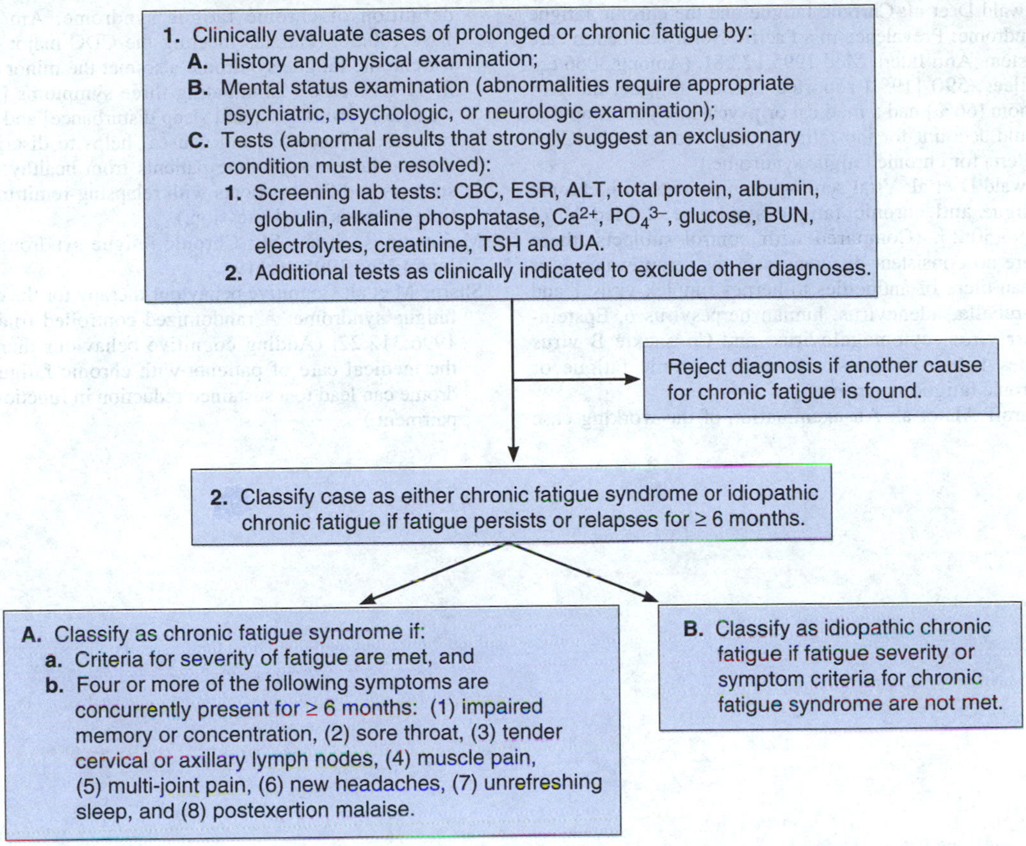

1. Clinically evaluate cases of prolonged or chronic fatigue by:
   A. History and physical examination;
   B. Mental status examination (abnormalities require appropriate psychiatric, psychologic, or neurologic examination);
   C. Tests (abnormal results that strongly suggest an exclusionary condition must be resolved):
      1. Screening lab tests: CBC, ESR, ALT, total protein, albumin, globulin, alkaline phosphatase, Ca^{2+}, PO_4^{3-}, glucose, BUN, electrolytes, creatinine, TSH and UA.
      2. Additional tests as clinically indicated to exclude other diagnoses.

Reject diagnosis if another cause for chronic fatigue is found.

2. Classify case as either chronic fatigue syndrome or idiopathic chronic fatigue if fatigue persists or relapses for ≥ 6 months.

A. Classify as chronic fatigue syndrome if:
   a. Criteria for severity of fatigue are met, and
   b. Four or more of the following symptoms are concurrently present for ≥ 6 months: (1) impaired memory or concentration, (2) sore throat, (3) tender cervical or axillary lymph nodes, (4) muscle pain, (5) multi-joint pain, (6) new headaches, (7) unrefreshing sleep, and (8) postexertion malaise.

B. Classify as idiopathic chronic fatigue if fatigue severity or symptom criteria for chronic fatigue syndrome are not met.

Figure 1–1. Evaluation and classification of unexplained chronic fatigue. (ALT, alanine aminotransferase; BUN, blood urea nitrogen; CBC, complete blood count; ESR, erythrocyte sedimentation rate; PO_4^{3-}, phosphate; TSH, thyroid-stimulating hormone; UA, urinalysis.) (Modified and reproduced, with permission, from Fukuda K et al: The chronic fatigue syndrome: A comprehensive approach to its definition and study. Ann Intern Med 1994;121:953.)

reasonable diagnostic strategy than the more extensive testing others have recommended. Antibody to Epstein-Barr virus is not helpful in evaluation of patients with chronic fatigue. A recent report found an abnormally high rate of postural hypotension with tilt testing. Some of these patients reported dramatic responses to increases in dietary sodium as well as antihypotensive agents such as fludrocortisone, 0.1 mg/d.

A variety of treatments have been tried. Acyclovir does not appear to improve symptoms, nor does oral or vaginal nystatin. There is a greater prevalence of past and current psychiatric diagnoses in patients with this syndrome. Affective disorders are especially common. However, fluoxetine, 20 mg daily, was not found to be beneficial. In all cases, patients should be encouraged to exercise and engage in life's activities to the extent possible and to be reassured that full recovery is eventually possible in most cases.

Bates DW et al: Clinical laboratory test findings in patients with chronic fatigue syndrome. Arch Intern Med 1995;155:97. (Immunologic abnormalities, such as circulating immune complexes, atypical lymphocytosis, and elevated levels of immunoglobulin G, suggest chronic low-level activation of the immune system.)

Bates DW et al: Prevalence of fatigue and chronic fatigue syndrome in a primary care practice. Arch Intern Med 1993;153:2759. (In a prospective cohort of 1000 consecutive patients, 323 [32%] reported fatigue and 271 [27%] complained of at least 6 months of unusual fatigue interfering with normal routines. Of those with fatigue, 186 [57%] had medical or psychiatric conditions causing fatigue and 85 [26%] had no apparent cause. However, only 0.3–1% met various case definitions for chronic fatigue syndrome.)

Bou-Holaigah I et al: The relation between neurally mediated hypotension and the chronic fatigue syndrome. JAMA 1995;274:961. (Twenty-two of 23 patients with the syndrome had abnormal responses to tilt testing compared with four of 14 controls. Nine patients had impressive responses to treatment directed at the postural hypotension.)

Buchwald D et al: Chronic fatigue and the chronic fatigue syndrome: Prevalence in a Pacific Northwest health care system. Ann Intern Med 1995;123:81. (Among 3066 enrollees, 590 [19%] reported chronic fatigue, most of whom [66%] had a medical or psychiatric condition that could account for the fatigue; only three met the CDC criteria for chronic fatigue syndrome.)

Buchwald D et al: Viral serologies in patients with chronic fatigue and chronic fatigue syndrome. J Med Virol 1996;50:25. (Compared with control subjects, there were no consistent differences in the seroprevalence or mean titers of antibodies to herpes simplex virus 1 and 2, rubella, adenovirus, human herpesvirus 6, Epstein-Barr virus, cytomegalovirus, and Coxsackie B virus types 1–6 in patients with either chronic fatigue or chronic fatigue syndrome.)

Komaroff AL et al: An examination of the working case definition of chronic fatigue syndrome. Am J Med 1996;100:56. (Patients meeting the CDC major criteria for chronic fatigue syndrome also met the minor criteria in 91% of cases. Eliminating three symptoms [muscle weakness, arthralgias, and sleep disturbance] and adding two others [anorexia and nausea] helps to discriminate chronic fatigue syndrome patients from healthy control subjects and from patients with relapsing-remitting multiple sclerosis and depression.)

McKenzie R, Straus SE: Chronic fatigue syndrome. Adv Intern Med 1995;40;119.

Sharpe M et al: Cognitive behaviour therapy for the chronic fatigue syndrome: A randomized controlled trial. BMJ 1996;312:22. (Adding cognitive behaviour therapy to the medical care of patients with chronic fatigue syndrome can lead to a sustained reduction in functional impairment.)

Preoperative Evaluation

2

Joshua S. Adler, MD, & Lee Goldman, MD, MPH

Each year, tens of millions of patients in the United States undergo a surgical procedure requiring general or spinal-epidural anesthesia. A disproportionate number of these patients are over age 65. Most patients do not suffer complications as a result of the surgical procedure or the anesthetic. However, about 3–10% of patients do experience significant morbidity, most of which results from cardiac, pulmonary, or infectious complications.

The medical consultant plays a significant role in the evaluation and management of patients before surgery. This role includes clearly defining the patient's medical conditions, evaluating the severity and stability of these conditions, providing a surgical risk assessment, and recommending perioperative measures to reduce surgical risk.

PHYSIOLOGIC EFFECTS OF ANESTHESIA & SURGERY

The complications of anesthesia and surgery are, for the most part, logical results of their known physiologic effects. Both general and spinal or epidural anesthetic agents usually cause peripheral vasodilation, and most of the commonly used general anesthetic regimens also decrease myocardial contractility. These effects often result in transient relative hypotension or, less frequently, prolonged hypotension. The decrease in tidal volume caused by general and spinal-epidural anesthesia can close small airways and lead to atelectasis. Epinephrine and norepinephrine levels increase during surgery and remain elevated for a day or two. The serum cortisol level is generally elevated for 1–3 days, and serum antidiuretic hormone levels may be elevated for up to 1 week postoperatively.

There is no evidence that spinal or epidural anesthesia is preferable to general anesthesia in terms of cardiac outcomes or overall surgical outcomes. In general, the choice of anesthetic technique or agent should be left to the anesthesiologist.

EVALUATION OF THE ASYMPTOMATIC PATIENT

Patients without significant medical problems—especially those under age 50—are at very low risk for perioperative complications. The preoperative evaluation of these patients should include a complete history and physical examination. Special emphasis is placed on the assessment of functional status, exercise tolerance, and cardiopulmonary symptoms and signs in an effort to reveal previously unrecognized disease (especially cardiopulmonary disease) that may require further evaluation prior to surgery. Additionally, a directed bleeding history (Table 2–1) should be taken to uncover disorders of hemostasis that could contribute to excessive surgical blood loss.

Routine testing of patients whose history and physical examination do not disclose significant medical problems should include a 12-lead ECG for men over 40 years of age and women over 50 years of age, specifically to look for evidence of silent myocardial ischemia or infarction. Additional testing of asymptomatic healthy patients has not been found to be helpful and is not recommended. However, the preoperative evaluation may provide an opportunity to perform other tests that are recommended as part of routine health maintenance (see Chapter 1).

Callaghan LC, Edwards ND, Reilly CS: Utilisation of the preoperative ECG. Anesthesia 1995;50:448. (The preoperative ECG is most useful in patients with known heart disease and asymptomatic men over the age of 50 years.)

Velanovich V: Preoperative laboratory evaluation. J Am Coll Surg 1996;183:79. (Overview of the value of routine preoperative testing.)

CARDIAC RISK ASSESSMENT

The cardiac complications of noncardiac surgery are perhaps the major cause of perioperative morbidity and demise. As such, this has been the most ex-

Table 2–1. A directed preoperative bleeding history.[1]

1. Have you ever bled for a long time or developed a swollen tongue or mouth after cutting or biting your tongue, cheek, or lip?
2. Do you develop bruises larger than a silver dollar without being able to remember when or how you injured yourself?
3. Has bleeding ever started up again the day after a tooth extraction?
4. Was bleeding after surgery ever hard to stop? Have you ever developed unusual bruising around an area of surgery or injury?
5. Has any blood relative had a problem with unusual bleeding or bleeding after surgery?

[1]Adapted, with permission, from Rapoport SI: Preoperative hemostatic evaluation. Blood 1982;61:229.

tensively studied area of perioperative medicine. The most important perioperative cardiac complications are myocardial infarction, congestive heart failure, and cardiac death. Older age, preexisting coronary artery disease, and congestive heart failure are the principal risk factors for development of these complications.

Coronary Artery Disease

Approximately one million patients undergoing surgery each year suffer a cardiac complication; 50,000 of these patients have a myocardial infarction. Patients without coronary artery disease are at extremely low risk (< 0.5%) for perioperative ischemic cardiac complications. Patients with known or suspected coronary artery disease, as defined in Table 2–2, have a five- to 50-fold increased risk of perioperative cardiac complications.

The estimated risk of cardiac complications in patients with coronary artery disease can be further refined through an assessment of the severity of anginal symptoms, the use of multifactorial indices, and the judicious use of noninvasive tests for ischemia. The severity of anginal symptoms is most accurately assessed using a standardized scale such as that shown in Table 2–3. Multifactorial indices combine several clinical parameters to estimate an overall risk of cardiac complications. Three of the best-known indices are shown in Table 2–4. Note that these indices are quite similar with respect to the relative

Table 2–2. Characteristics defining patients with known or suspected coronary artery disease.[1]

1. History of myocardial infarction
2. Angiographic evidence of coronary artery disease
3. Evidence of ischemia on prior noninvasive testing
4. Typical angina pectoris
5. Peripheral vascular disease

[1]Adapted, with permission, from Ashton CM et al: The incidence of perioperative myocardial infarction in men undergoing noncardiac surgery. Ann Intern Med 1993;118:504.

Table 2–3. Canadian Cardiovascular Society angina class.[1]

I. Ordinary physical activity, such as walking and climbing stairs, does not cause angina. Angina occurs with strenuous or rapid or prolonged exertion at work or recreation.
II. Slight limitation of ordinary activity. Angina occurs with walking or climbing stairs rapidly, walking uphill, walking or stair climbing after meals, or only during the few hours after awakening. Angina occurs when walking more than two blocks on the level or climbing more than one flight of stairs at a normal pace and in normal conditions.
III. Marked limitation of ordinary physical activity. Angina occurs with walking one to two blocks on the level and climbing one flight of stairs in normal conditions and at a normal pace.
IV. Inability to carry on any physical activity without discomfort; angina may be present at rest.

[1]Reproduced, with permission, from Campeau L: Grading of angina pectoris. [Letter.] Circulation 1975;54:522.

weights given to the severity of coronary artery disease and congestive heart failure. The index of Goldman et al has been validated in an independent prospective series of patients.

Patients who have mild symptoms, defined as Canadian Cardiovascular Society (CCS) class 1 or 2 angina, and a low or intermediate score on one of the multifactorial indices are at low risk for cardiac complications. Noninvasive ischemia testing in these patients is unlikely to improve the accuracy of the clinical risk assessment. Patients with severe symptoms, CCS class 3 or 4 angina, or a high score on one of the multifactorial indices are likely to be at high risk for cardiac complications. Noninvasive ischemia testing in this group of patients is, again, not likely to improve the accuracy of the clinical risk assessment. However, high-risk patients who are candidates for noninvasive ischemia testing independent of the planned noncardiac surgery should have such testing prior to surgery, especially when the test result may lead to a revascularization procedure.

When the patient's medical history is unreliable or when orthopedic or vascular conditions severely limit physical activity, one may consider the use of noninvasive cardiac testing. In patients who are able to exercise, exercise electrocardiography may be very helpful. Patients without ischemia at or above 85% of their maximal predicted heart rate are at low risk for perioperative cardiac complications.

For patients who cannot exercise, an assessment of clinical criteria can help to identify those most likely to benefit from noninvasive testing. One such set of criteria is shown in Table 2–5. Patients who have none of these criteria and a low multifactorial index score are at low risk for cardiac complications. Patients with three or more criteria or a high index score are at high risk. Noninvasive testing in these two groups does not appear to improve the accuracy of risk assessment. Dipyridamole-thallium scintigra-

Table 2–4. Multifactorial cardiac risk indices.[1]

Risk Factor	Points	Interpretation
Goldman et al		Class I: 0–5 points = low risk
Age > 70 years	5	Class II: 6–12 points = intermediate risk
MI in previous 6 months	10	Class III: 13–25 points
S$_3$ gallop or jugular venous distention	11	Class IV: > 26 points } high risk
Important aortic stenosis	3	
Rhythm other than sinus or PACs on last preoperative ECG	7	
> 5 PVCs/min documented at any time before operation	7	
Po$_2$ < 60 or Pco$_2$ > 50 mm Hg; K$^+$ < 3 or HCO$_3^-$ < 20 mEq/L; BUN > 50 or Cr > 3 mg/dL; abnormal AST, signs of chronic liver disease, or bedridden from noncardiac causes; or intraperitoneal, intrathoracic, or aortic operation	3	
Emergency operation	4	
Detsky et al		< 15 points = low risk
MI in previous 6 months	10	> 15 points = high risk
MI more than 6 months previously	5	
Canadian Cardiovascular Society angina		
Class III	10	
Class IV	20	
Unstable angina in previous 6 months	10	
Alveolar pulmonary edema		
Within 1 week	10	
Ever	5	
Suspected critical aortic stenosis	20	
Rhythm other than sinus or sinus plus PACs on last preoperative ECG	5	
> 5 PVCs/min at any time prior to surgery	5	
Poor general medical status	5	
Age > 70 years	5	
Emergency operation	10	
Larsen et al		< 5 points = low risk
Congestive heart failure		5–8 points = intermediate risk
Persistent pulmonary congestion	12	> 8 points = high risk
No, but previous pulmonary edema	8	
Neither, but previous heart failure	4	
Ischemic heart disease		
MI in previous 3 months	11	
No, but older infarction or angina pectoris	3	
Diabetes mellitus	3	
Serum creatinine > 1.6 mg/dL	2	
Emergency operation	3	
Major surgical procedure		
Aortic operation	5	
Other intraperitoneal or intrapleural operation	3	

Key: AST = aspartate aminotransferase; BUN = blood urea nitrogen; Cr = creatinine; ECG = electrocardiogram; K$^+$ = potassium; MI = myocardial infarction; PAC = premature atrial contraction; PVC = premature ventricular contraction

[1]Reproduced, with permission, from Goldman L et al: Multifactorial index of cardiac risk in noncardiac surgical procedures. N Engl J Med 1977;297:845; from Detsky AS et al: Predicting cardiac complications in patients undergoing noncardiac surgery. J Gen Intern Med 1986;1:211 (by permission of Blackwell Science, Inc.); and from Larsen SF et al: Prediction of cardiac risk in non-cardiac surgery. Eur Heart J 1987;8:179.

Table 2–5. Clinical criteria associated with cardiac complications in patients undergoing vascular surgery.[1]

1. History of myocardial infarction
2. Q waves on the ECG
3. History of angina
4. History of ventricular arrhythmias requiring treatment
5. Diabetes mellitus

[1]Adapted, with permission, from Eagle KA et al: Combining clinical and thallium data optimizes preoperative assessment of cardiac risk before major vascular surgery. Ann Intern Med 1989;110:859.

Table 2–6. General approach to patients with angina.[1] (CCS = Canadian Cardiovascular Society)

1. Assess functional capacity by history
2. If the history is reliable and the patient has CCS class I or class II angina, surgery is low risk
3. If the history is unreliable, do an exercise tolerance test
4. If the history is unreliable or unhelpful and the patient is unable to exercise, do dipyridamole thallium scintigraphy, ambulatory ischemia monitoring, or stress echocardiography

[1]Reproduced, with permission, from Goldman L: Cardiac risk in noncardiac surgery: An update. Anesth Analg 1995; 80:810.

phy is most helpful in patients with one or two clinical criteria or an intermediate index score. A normal dipyridamole-thallium scan predicts a low risk of complications (comparable to patients with a low-risk clinical assessment), whereas evidence of thallium redistribution predicts a much higher risk (comparable to patients with a high-risk clinical assessment).

Several recent studies have evaluated preoperative ambulatory ischemia monitoring as a means of cardiac risk assessment. Patients who have evidence of asymptomatic ischemia on 24-hour or 48-hour ambulatory electrocardiographic monitoring are significantly more likely to suffer a cardiac complication compared with patients without evidence of ischemia. Ambulatory ischemia monitoring is likely to be most useful in patients at intermediate risk by clinical assessment. Stress echocardiography using dobutamine or atropine has recently been reported to predict postoperative cardiac complications in patients undergoing vascular surgery. In the largest series, 38% of the vascular surgery patients who demonstrated a new regional wall motion abnormality (RWMA) with the administration of dobutamine with or without supplemental atropine suffered a perioperative cardiac complication, compared with none of the patients who did not have a new RWMA. Similar to dipyridamole-thallium scintigraphy, dobutamine stress echocardiography is likely to be most useful in patients whose symptom severity cannot be assessed by history or exercise testing and who are at intermediate risk based on clinical assessment or a multifactorial index score. At present, too few patients have been studied to permit definitive recommendations regarding the use of this technique for preoperative risk assessment. A general approach to the assessment and testing of patients with coronary artery disease is shown in Table 2–6.

Preoperative Management of Patients With Coronary Artery Disease

A. Low-Risk Patients With Coronary Artery Disease: Patients in this group have roughly a 4% risk of myocardial infarction and about a 1% mortality rate. Results from the CASS trial registry indicate that patients who have undergone prior coronary artery bypass graft surgery are at lower risk for cardiac complications with subsequent noncardiac surgery compared with similar patients treated medically. However, this should not be interpreted as a prescription for the use of prophylactic revascularization. The use of coronary angiography and revascularization in these patients depends on two factors: the urgency of the surgery and whether the patient has indications for such evaluation regardless of the planned surgery. The mortality rate for coronary artery bypass surgery is roughly 1.5%; thus, the routine prophylactic use of this procedure prior to noncardiac surgery is unlikely to decrease total morbidity or mortality rates. However, in patients who are candidates for coronary angiography and subsequent revascularization independent of the planned surgery, it seems prudent to proceed with these prior to noncardiac surgery when feasible. The data on percutaneous transluminal coronary angioplasty (PTCA) suggest that it is not sufficiently different from coronary artery bypass graft surgery to warrant its routine preoperative use, although PTCA is preferable in situations in which coronary revascularization must precede relatively urgent surgery.

Preoperative antianginal medications, including beta-blockers, calcium channel blockers, and nitrates, should be continued preoperatively and during the postoperative period. The institution of prophylactic beta-blockers in the immediate preoperative period has been shown to reduce intraoperative myocardial ischemia and may reduce the incidence of perioperative myocardial infarction. In a recent placebo-controlled, randomized trial, the use of prophylactic atenolol immediately before and for up to 7 days after noncardiac surgery reduced the cardiovascular mortality rate at 6, 12, and 24 months. It is currently recommended for high-risk patients. Prophylactic intraoperative intravenous nitroglycerin may decrease the frequency of ischemia but has not been shown to reduce the rate of postoperative complications. This may be considered for high-risk patients. Too little is known about the effects of the prophylactic use of calcium channel blockers to make any recommendations.

B. High-Risk Patients With Coronary Artery Disease: In this group surgery should be postponed, except in emergency situations, to allow for stabilization of ischemic symptoms. For patients with a recent myocardial infarction, delaying surgery for 3–6 months postinfarction to allow for appropriate stabilization and therapy may significantly reduce perioperative mortality and morbidity rates. Patients with unstable angina should be evaluated and treated as indicated by their cardiac status prior to surgery and then reevaluated with respect to severity of symptoms and functional status. Patients with severe stable angina or worsening angina may be managed in a variety of ways. Like patients with less severe angina, those who are potential candidates for coronary artery bypass graft surgery independently of the planned noncardiac surgery should certainly proceed with this evaluation prior to noncardiac surgery. For patients who are not obvious candidates for revascularization, one approach is to optimize their antianginal medications and reevaluate their symptoms. This approach assumes that an improvement in symptoms correlates with a reduction in perioperative cardiac complication rates—an assumption that is without clear validation at present. An alternative approach is preoperative PTCA. However, it is not known if such a strategy effectively reduces surgical risk. In one series of 50 high-risk patients who had preoperative PTCA, 10% of the patients suffered a major perioperative cardiac complication.

Congestive Heart Failure & Left Ventricular Dysfunction

Decompensated congestive heart failure, manifested by an elevated jugular venous pressure, an audible third heart sound, or evidence of pulmonary edema on physical examination or chest radiography, significantly increases the risk of perioperative pulmonary edema (roughly 15%) and cardiac death (2–10%). Preoperative control of congestive heart failure, including the use of diuretics and afterload reducing agents, is likely to reduce the perioperative risk. One must be cautious not to give too much diuretic, since the volume-depleted patient will be much more susceptible to intraoperative hypotension.

Patients with compensated left ventricular dysfunction are at increased risk for developing perioperative pulmonary edema but are not at excess risk for other cardiac complications. One large study found that patients with a left-ventricular ejection fraction of less than 50% had an absolute risk of 12% for postoperative congestive heart failure compared with 3% for patients with an ejection fraction greater than 50%. Such patients should be maintained on all heart failure medications up to and including the day of surgery. Patients receiving digoxin and diuretics should routinely have serum electrolyte and digoxin levels measured prior to surgery because abnormalities in these levels may increase the risk of perioperative arrhythmias. Preoperative echocardiography or radionuclide angiography to assess left ventricular function should be considered only for patients in whom the results of such testing can be expected to justify a change in perioperative management. The surgeon and anesthesiologist should be made aware of the presence and severity of left ventricular dysfunction so that appropriate decisions can be made regarding perioperative fluid management and intraoperative monitoring.

Valvular Heart Disease

There are few data available regarding the perioperative risks of valvular heart disease independent of associated coronary artery disease or congestive heart failure. Patients with severe symptomatic aortic stenosis are clearly at increased risk for cardiac complications. Such patients who are candidates for valve replacement surgery or, if only short-term relief is needed, for balloon valvuloplasty independent of the planned noncardiac surgery should have the corrective procedure performed prior to noncardiac surgery. On the other hand, in one recent study, patients with asymptomatic aortic stenosis—even those with aortic valve areas < 1 cm^2—tolerated noncardiac surgery with a relatively low nonfatal complication rate (approximately 10%). This may be due to the recent use of invasive intraoperative monitoring, including pulmonary artery catheterization and transesophageal echocardiography. Nevertheless, noncardiac surgery in patients with severe asymptomatic aortic stenosis must be approached with great caution.

The severity of valvular lesions should be defined prior to surgery to allow for appropriate fluid management and consideration of invasive intraoperative monitoring. Echocardiography should also be considered in patients with a previously unexplained heart murmur for those procedures in which a valvular abnormality would require antibiotic prophylaxis. For specific recommendations regarding antibiotic prophylaxis, see Chapter 10.

Arrhythmias

Several early studies on cardiac risk factors reported that both atrial and ventricular arrhythmias were independent predictors of an increased risk of perioperative complications. Recent data have shown these rhythm disturbances to be frequently associated with underlying structural heart disease, especially coronary artery disease and left ventricular dysfunction. The finding of a rhythm disturbance on preoperative evaluation should prompt consideration of further cardiac evaluation, particularly when the finding of structural heart disease would alter perioperative management. Patients found to have a rhythm disturbance without evidence of underlying heart disease are at very low risk for perioperative cardiac complications.

Management of patients with arrhythmias in the preoperative period should be guided by factors independent of the planned surgery. In patients with atrial fibrillation, adequate rate control should be established. Symptomatic supraventricular and ventricular tachycardia must be controlled prior to surgery. There is no evidence that the use of antiarrhythmic medications to suppress an asymptomatic arrhythmia alters perioperative risk.

It seems prudent for patients who have indications for a permanent pacemaker to have it placed prior to noncardiac surgery. When surgery is urgent, these patients may be managed perioperatively with temporary transvenous pacing. Patients with bundle branch block who do not meet recognized criteria for a permanent pacemaker do not require pacing during surgery.

Hypertension

Severe hypertension, defined as a systolic pressure greater than 180 mm Hg or diastolic pressure greater than 110 mm Hg, appears to be an independent predictor of perioperative cardiac complications, including myocardial infarction and congestive heart failure. Mild to moderate hypertension immediately preoperatively is associated with intraoperative blood pressure lability and asymptomatic myocardial ischemia but does not appear to be an independent risk factor for myocardial infarction, unstable angina, or congestive heart failure. It seems wise to delay surgery in patients with severe hypertension until blood pressure can be controlled, though it is not known whether the risk of cardiac complications is reduced with this approach. It is unlikely that treatment of mild to moderate hypertension in the immediate preoperative period will significantly reduce the risk of cardiac complications. However, chronic medications for hypertension should be continued up to and including the day of surgery.

Type of Surgery

Major abdominal, thoracic, and vascular surgical procedures (especially abdominal aortic aneurysm repair) tend to carry a higher risk of postoperative cardiac complications than other procedures. Emergency operations are generally associated with more cardiac complications than elective operations. These high-risk procedures are more often associated with major fluid shifts, hemorrhage, and hypoxemia, which may predispose to cardiac complications.

Ashton CM et al: The incidence of perioperative myocardial infarction in men undergoing noncardiac surgery. Ann Intern Med 1993;118:504.

Baron JF et al: Dipyridamole-thallium scintigraphy and gated radionuclide angiography to assess cardiac risk before abdominal aortic surgery. N Engl J Med 1994; 330:663.

Eagle KA et al: ACC/AHA Task Force Report: Guidelines for perioperative cardiovascular evaluation for noncardiac surgery. Circulation 1996;93:1278. (American Heart Association guidelines for preoperative cardiac evaluation and perioperative management of the cardiac patient.)

Goldman L: Cardiac risk in noncardiac surgery: An update. Anesth Analg 1995;80:810.

L'Italien GJ et al: Development and validation of a Bayesian model for perioperative cardiac risk assessment in a cohort of 1081 vascular surgical candidates. J Am Coll Cardiol 1996;27:779. (An evaluation of simple clinical markers can obviate the need for preoperative dipyridamole-thallium scintigraphy in many patients prior to vascular surgery.)

Mangano DT, Goldman L: Preoperative assessment of the patient with known or suspected coronary artery disease. N Engl J Med 1995;333:1750.

Shaw LJ et al: Meta-analysis of intravenous dipyridamole-thallium-201 imaging (1985 to 1994) and dobutamine echocardiography (1991 to 1994) for risk stratification before vascular surgery. J Am Coll Cardiol 1996;27:787. (Found that the prognostic value of preoperative dipyridamole-thallium scintigraphy and dobutamine echocardiography before vascular surgery are comparable.)

PULMONARY EVALUATION IN NON-LUNG RESECTION SURGERY

Pneumonia, bronchospasm, hypoxemia requiring oxygen supplementation, prolonged mechanical ventilation, and asymptomatic atelectasis or fever have been included as postoperative pulmonary complications in most series. The latter two diagnoses represent a significant percentage (often > 50%) of postoperative pulmonary complications in most studies, yet their clinical significance is not clear. The absolute risk for developing a postoperative pulmonary complication, excluding asymptomatic atelectasis and fever, ranges from 6% to 19%.

Risk Factors for the Development of Postoperative Pulmonary Complications

Numerous series have investigated the risk factors for the development of postoperative pulmonary complications. The risk of developing a pulmonary complication is highest in patients undergoing cardiac, thoracic, and upper abdominal surgery, with reported complication rates ranging from 9% to 76%. The risk in patients undergoing lower abdominal or pelvic procedures ranges from 2% to 5%, and for extremity procedures the range is less than 1–3%. Limited data are available on the pulmonary complication rates associated with laparoscopic and thoracoscopic procedures. In one series of over 1500 patients who underwent laparoscopic cholecystectomy, the pulmonary complication rate was less than 1%, which is much lower than that expected with open cholecystectomy.

Three patient-specific factors have been repeatedly found to increase the risk of postoperative pulmonary complications: chronic lung disease, morbid obesity, and tobacco use. Patients with chronic obstructive pulmonary disease (COPD) have a two- to fourfold increased risk compared with patients without COPD. Various pulmonary function tests and arterial blood gas measurements have been evaluated for their ability to predict postoperative pulmonary complications. Unfortunately, no single test or combination of tests has been found to be particularly useful. Currently available tests lack both sufficient sensitivity and specificity to permit accurate assessments of risk. It does appear, however, that patients with an FEV_1 under 500 mL or an arterial PCO_2 greater than 45 mm Hg are at high risk.

Patients with asthma are at increased risk for bronchospasm during tracheal intubation and extubation and during the postoperative period. However, if patients are at their optimal pulmonary function (as determined by symptoms, physical examination, or spirometry) at the time of surgery, they do not appear to be at increased risk for other pulmonary complications.

Morbidly obese patients—those weighing over 250 lb—are approximately twice as likely to develop postoperative pneumonia as patients weighing less than 250 lb. Mild obesity does not appear to increase the risk of clinically important pulmonary complications.

Several studies have shown that current cigarette smoking is associated with an increased risk for developing postoperative atelectasis. In a single study, cigarette smoking was also found to double the risk of developing postoperative pneumonia, even when controlling for underlying lung disease. A summary of the known risk factors for pulmonary complications is presented in Table 2–7.

Pulmonary Function Testing & Arterial Blood Gas Analysis

The vast majority of studies have shown that preoperative pulmonary function testing in unselected patients is not helpful in predicting postoperative pulmonary complications. The data are conflicting regarding the utility of preoperative pulmonary function testing in certain selected groups of patients: the morbidly obese, those with COPD, and those undergoing upper abdominal or cardiothoracic surgery. No single pulmonary function test value places a patient at prohibitive risk for non-lung resection surgery. At present, definitive recommendations regarding the indications for preoperative pulmonary function testing cannot be made. In general terms, such testing may be helpful to confirm the diagnosis of COPD or asthma, to assess the severity of known pulmonary disease, and perhaps as part of the risk assessment for patients undergoing upper abdominal surgery, cardiac surgery, or thoracic surgery. The current American College of Physicians recommendations for preoperative pulmonary function testing are set forth in Table 2–8.

Arterial blood gas measurement is not routinely recommended except in patients with known lung disease and suspected hypoxemia or hypercapnia.

Perioperative Management

The goal of perioperative management is to reduce the likelihood of postoperative pulmonary complications. Smoking cessation for at least 8 weeks prior to surgery significantly reduces the incidence of pulmonary complications for patients undergoing coronary artery bypass surgery. The use of incentive spirometry and deep breathing exercises begun preoperatively and continued for 3–5 days into the postoperative period reduces the incidence of postoperative atelectasis, and in one study incentive spirometry reduced the length of the hospital stay for patients undergoing upper abdominal surgery. These measures were effective when used for at least 15 minutes four times daily; however, other studies suggest that more frequent use is necessary. Prophylactic continuous positive airway pressure (CPAP) and intermittent positive pressure breathing (IPPB) offer no advantage over incentive spirometry in reducing postoperative pulmonary complications. Given the higher cost of these latter maneuvers, they are not recommended for routine use.

There is some evidence that the incidence of post-

Table 2–7. Risk factors for postoperative pulmonary complications.

1. Upper abdominal or cardiothoracic surgery
2. Anesthetic time > 4 hours
3. Morbid obesity
4. Chronic obstructive pulmonary disease or asthma
5. Tobacco use > 20 pack-years

Table 2–8. American College of Physicians guidelines for preoperative spirometry.[1]

1. Lung resection
2. Coronary artery bypass graft surgery and smoking history or dyspnea
3. Upper abdominal surgery and smoking history or dyspnea
4. Lower abdominal surgery and uncharacterized pulmonary disease,[2] particularly if the surgery will be prolonged or extensive
5. Other surgery and uncharacterized pulmonary disease,[2] particularly in those who might require strenuous postoperative rehabilitation programs

[1]Reproduced, with permission, from: Preoperative pulmonary function testing; American College of Physicians. Ann Intern Med 1990;112:793.
[2]Uncharacterized pulmonary disease is defined as pulmonary symptoms or history of pulmonary disease and no pulmonary function tests within 60 days.

operative pulmonary complications in patients with COPD or asthma may be reduced by preoperative optimization of pulmonary function. Patients who are wheezing will probably benefit from therapy with bronchodilators and, in certain cases, corticosteroids preoperatively. Antibiotics may be of benefit for patients who cough with purulent sputum if the sputum can be cleared prior to surgery. Patients who take oral theophylline should be maintained on it during the intraoperative and postoperative periods, using intravenous theophylline when necessary.

Celli BR: What is the value of preoperative pulmonary function testing? Med Clin North Am 1993;77:309.

Kroenke K et al: Postoperative complications after thoracic and major abdominal surgery in patients with and without obstructive lung disease. Chest 1993;104:1445.

Lawrence VA et al: Risk of pulmonary complications after elective abdominal surgery. Chest 1996;110:744. (Pulmonary complications are common after abdominal surgery and are associated with longer hospital stays.)

Wait J: Southwestern Internal Medicine Conference: Preoperative pulmonary evaluation. Am J Med Sci 1995; 310:118.

EVALUATION OF THE PATIENT WITH LIVER DISEASE

Patients with serious liver disease are generally thought to be at increased risk for perioperative morbidity and demise. Appropriate preoperative evaluation requires consideration of the effects of anesthesia and surgery on postoperative liver function and of the complications associated with anesthesia and surgery in patients with preexisting liver disease.

The Effects of Anesthesia & Surgery on Liver Function

Postoperative elevation of serum aminotransferase levels is a relatively common finding after major surgery. Most of these elevations are transient and not associated with hepatic dysfunction. Studies in the 1960s and early 1970s showed that patients with liver disease are at increased relative risk for postoperative deterioration in hepatic function, though the absolute risk is not known. General anesthetic agents may cause deterioration of hepatic function via intraoperative reduction in hepatic blood flow leading to ischemic injury. It is important to remember that agents for spinal and epidural anesthesia produce similar reductions in hepatic blood flow and thus may be equally likely to lead to ischemic liver injury. Intraoperative hypotension, hemorrhage, and hypoxemia may also contribute to liver injury.

Risk Factors for Surgical Complications

Surgery in the patient with serious liver disease has been associated in several series with a variety of significant complications, including hemorrhage, infection, renal failure, and encephalopathy, and with a substantial mortality rate. A key limitation in interpreting these data is our inability to determine the contribution of the liver disease to the observed complications independently of the surgical procedure.

In three small series of patients with acute viral hepatitis who underwent abdominal surgery, the mortality rate was roughly 10%. Patients undergoing portosystemic shunt surgery who have evidence of alcoholic hepatitis on the preoperative liver biopsy have a significantly increased surgical mortality rate. Although data are quite limited, it seems reasonable to delay elective surgery in patients with acute viral or alcoholic hepatitis, at least until the acute episode has resolved. These data are not sufficient to warrant substantial delays in urgent or emergent surgery.

There are few data regarding the risks of surgery in patients with chronic hepatitis. In a series of 272 patients with chronic hepatitis undergoing a variety of surgical procedures for variceal hemorrhage, the in-hospital mortality rate was less than 2%. It is of note that patients with Child's class C cirrhosis (see Chapter 15) or with serum aminotransferase levels over 150 units/L were excluded. The perioperative risk in patients with asymptomatic chronic hepatitis and elevated serum aminotransferase levels is not known.

Substantial data exist regarding surgery in patients with cirrhosis. In several series, patients with cirrhosis undergoing abdominal surgery had substantial morbidity and mortality rates (7–39% and 7–67%, respectively). Biliary surgery appears to be especially risky. In patients undergoing portosystemic shunt surgery, the degree of hepatic dysfunction roughly correlates with the surgical mortality rate. In general terms, patients with Child's class A cirrhosis have a relatively low mortality rate (roughly 10%) while patients with class C cirrhosis face a substantial mortality rate (roughly 50%). The risks associated with cirrhosis in nonabdominal surgery are not known. A conservative approach would be to avoid elective surgery in patients with severe hepatic dysfunction.

Abu-Elmagd KM et al: Ten years of experience with patients with chronic active liver disease variceal bleeding: Ablative versus selective decompressive therapy. Surgery 1993;114:868. (Major surgery in patients with chronic hepatitis has a relatively low mortality rate.)

Van Thiel DH et al: Preoperative evaluation of a patient for hepatic surgery. J Surg Oncol Suppl 1993;3:49. (General consideration of liver function needed for hepatic surgery.)

PREOPERATIVE HEMATOLOGIC EVALUATION

Several hematologic disorders may have an impact on the outcomes of surgery. A detailed discussion of the preoperative management of patients with complicated hematologic disorders is beyond the scope of this section. Two of the more common clinical situations faced by the medical consultant are the patient with anemia prior to surgery and the assessment of bleeding risk.

The key issues in the anemic patient are to determine the need for preoperative diagnostic evaluation and the need for transfusion. When feasible, the diagnostic evaluation of the patient with previously unrecognized anemia should be done prior to surgery because certain types of anemia (particularly sickle cell disease and immune hemolytic anemias) may have implications for perioperative management. Most data suggest that morbidity and mortality increase as the preoperative hemoglobin level decreases, though none of these data were corrected for the presence of preexisting diseases. Hemoglobin levels below 8 or 9 g/dL appear to be associated with significantly more perioperative complications than higher levels. Determination of the need for preoperative transfusion in an individual patient, however, must consider factors other than the absolute hemoglobin level, including the presence of cardiopulmonary disease, the type of surgery, and the likelihood of surgical blood loss.

The most important component of the bleeding risk assessment is a directed bleeding history (Table 2–1). Patients who are reliable historians and who reveal no suggestion of abnormal bleeding on directed bleeding history and physical examination are at very low risk for having an occult bleeding disorder. Laboratory tests of hemostatic parameters in these patients are generally not needed. When the directed bleeding history is unreliable or incomplete or when abnormal bleeding is suggested, a formal evaluation of hemostasis should be done prior to surgery and should include measurement of the prothrombin time, the activated partial thromboplastin time, the platelet count, and the bleeding time.

Carson JL: Morbidity risk assessment in the surgically anemic patient. Am J Surg 1995;170(6 Suppl):32S. (Review of the perioperative risks of preoperative anemia.)

Houry S et al: A prospective multicenter evaluation of preoperative hemostatic screening tests. Am J Surg 1995;170:19. (Demonstrates that patients without a history or physical examination suggestive of abnormal bleeding do not require hemostatic screening tests [PT, PTT, platelet count, or bleeding time] prior to surgery.)

Messmore HL Jr, Godwin MJ: Medical assessment of bleeding in the surgical patient. Med Clin North Am 1994;78:625.

NEUROLOGIC EVALUATION

Delirium occurs in approximately 9% of patients over the age of 50 years after major surgery. Postoperative delirium has been associated with higher rates of major postoperative cardiac and pulmonary com-

plications, poor functional recovery, and increased length of hospital stay. Several preoperative factors have been associated with the development of postoperative delirium (Table 2–9). Patients with three or more of these factors are at especially high risk. It may be important in high-risk patients to avoid the use of medications in the postoperative period that may increase the risk of developing delirium, including meperidine and most benzodiazepines.

Postoperative stroke is a relatively infrequent complication (< 1%) after noncardiac nonvascular surgery. Stroke may occur in up to 3% of patients undergoing cardiac surgery, carotid artery surgery, or peripheral vascular surgery. Older age, symptomatic carotid stenoses (especially when > 50% occluded), and the occurrence of postoperative atrial fibrillation appear to be independent predictors of postoperative stroke. Most recent studies suggest that asymptomatic carotid bruits and asymptomatic carotid stenoses are associated with little or no increased risk of postoperative stroke. Prophylactic carotid endarterectomy in patients with asymptomatic carotid artery disease is unlikely to be beneficial. On the other hand, patients with carotid disease who are candidates for carotid endarterectomy anyway (Chapter 12) should probably have carotid surgery prior to the elective noncardiac surgery. Some patients require both cardiac and carotid surgery. The ideal timing of these two procedures is not certain and must be decided individually for each patient. In general, the more symptomatic and threatening condition should be addressed first. Adverse neurologic outcomes are especially common after coronary artery bypass surgery. In a recent large multicenter study, the incidence of serious neurologic complications (neurologic death, nonfatal stroke, stupor or coma at discharge, deterioration in intellectual function, memory

Table 2–9. Risk factors for the development of postoperative delirium.[1]

Preoperative factors
Age > 70 years
Alcohol abuse
Poor cognitive status
Poor physical function status
Markedly abnormal serum sodium, potassium, or glucose level[2]
Aortic aneurysm surgery
Noncardiac thoracic surgery

Postoperative factors
Use of meperidine or benzodiazepines

[1]Adapted, with permission, from Marcantonio ER et al: A clinical prediction rule for delirium after elective noncardiac surgery. JAMA 1994;271:134; and from Marcantonio ER et al: The relationship of postoperative delirium with psychoactive medications. JAMA 1994;272:1518. Both copyright © 1994 by American Medical Association.
[2]Defined as follows: sodium < 130 or > 150 mmol/L, potassium < 3 or > 6 mmol/L, glucose < 60 or > 300 mg/dL.

deficit, or seizures) was 6.1%. An adverse neurologic outcome was associated with a significantly increased mortality rate, a longer hospital stay, and an increased likelihood of discharge to a long-term care facility. The most important predictors of adverse neurologic outcomes after coronary artery bypass surgery were the presence of proximal aortic atherosclerosis, a history of neurologic disease, a history of pulmonary disease, and age over 70 years.

Gerraty RP et al: Carotid stenosis and perioperative stroke risk in symptomatic and asymptomatic patients undergoing vascular or coronary surgery. Stroke 1993;24:1115.

Marcantonio ER et al: A clinical prediction rule for delirium after elective noncardiac surgery. JAMA 1994; 271:134.

Marcantonio ER et al: The relationship of postoperative delirium with psychoactive medications. JAMA 1994; 272:1518.

Roach GW et al: Adverse cerebral outcomes after coronary bypass surgery. N Engl J Med 1996;325:1857. (Prospective evaluation of neurologic outcomes after coronary bypass surgery.)

MANAGEMENT OF ENDOCRINE DISEASES

Diabetes Mellitus

Patients with diabetes are at increased risk for postoperative infections. Furthermore, diabetic patients are more likely to have cardiovascular disease and thus are at increased risk for postoperative cardiac complications. The most challenging issue in diabetics, however, is the maintenance of glucose control during the perioperative period.

The increased secretion of cortisol, epinephrine, glucagon, and growth hormone during surgery is associated with insulin resistance and hyperglycemia in diabetic patients. The goal of management is the prevention of severe hyperglycemia or hypoglycemia in the perioperative period.

Although the ideal blood glucose level during surgery is not known, a level between 100 and 250 mg/dL is usually recommended. In vitro studies have shown that cellular immunity may be impaired when the blood glucose level exceeds 250 mg/dL. However, it is not known whether blood glucose levels above 250 mg/dL are associated with more postoperative infections.

All diabetic patients should have serum electrolyte levels measured and abnormalities in any of these levels corrected prior to surgery. Blood urea nitrogen and serum creatinine levels should also be measured to assess renal function. The specific pharmacologic management of diabetes during the perioperative period depends on several factors, including the type of diabetes (insulin-dependent or not), the adequacy of preoperative glucose control, the preoperative diabetes therapy, and the type and length of surgery (Table 2–10).

Table 2–10. The need for intraoperative insulin.[1]

Insulin Generally Required	Insulin Generally Not Required
IDDM[2] patients undergoing any surgical procedure	Diet-controlled diabetics undergoing any surgical procedure
NIDDM[3] patients on insulin undergoing any surgical procedure	NIDDM patients well controlled on oral agents undergoing minor surgery[4] requiring general or spinal anesthesia
NIDDM patients on oral agents undergoing major surgical procedures[5]	

[1]Reprinted by permission of Blackwell Science, Inc., from Schiff RL, Emanuele MA: The surgical patient with diabetes mellitus: Guidelines for management. J Gen Intern Med 1995;10:154.
[2]IDDM = insulin-dependent diabetes mellitus
[3]NIDDM = non-insulin-dependent diabetes mellitus
[4]Minor surgery = procedures such as laparoscopic surgery and transurethral prostatectomy.
[5]Major surgery = thoracotomy, sternotomy, laparotomy, major vascular surgery.

Patients who generally do not require intraoperative insulin still require careful management, including blood glucose monitoring to prevent hypoglycemia and to ensure prompt treatment of severe hyperglycemia (Table 2–11). For patients who require intraoperative insulin, no single regimen has been found to be superior in comparative trials. Intravenous regular insulin usually is preferred over subcutaneous insulin for most patients because of its rapid onset and short duration of action and ease of dose titration. However, the subcutaneous route is

Table 2–11. Management of patients who do not need insulin during surgery.

Patient	Recommended Management
Diabetes well controlled on diet alone	Avoid glucose-containing solutions during surgery Measure blood glucose level every 4–6 hours during surgery
Diabetes well controlled on an oral sulfonylurea or metformin	Discontinue oral agent the day before surgery Measure glucose every 6 hours in the perioperative period and give subcutaneous regular insulin as needed to maintain blood sugar below 250 mg/dL While the patient is fasting, infuse 5% glucose-containing solution at approximately 100 mL/h and continue until the patient is eating Measure blood glucose level every 4–6 hours (or more frequently as indicated) during surgery Resume oral hypoglycemic therapy when the patient returns to baseline diet

easier to implement and is less expensive. Three commonly used insulin administration methods are shown in Table 2–12. Either of the intravenous infusion methods may be continued in the postoperative period until the patient is eating.

Glucocorticoid Replacement

Perioperative complications (predominantly hypotension) resulting from primary or secondary adrenocortical insufficiency are rare. The administration of high-dose glucocorticoids during the perioperative period in patients at risk for adrenocortical insufficiency may decrease the risk of these complications, though clinical trials in humans have not been done to confirm this assumption. There is no consensus regarding the identification of patients at risk for adrenocortical insufficiency. The most conservative approach would be to consider any patient to be at risk for having adrenocortical insufficiency who has received either the equivalent of 20 mg of prednisone daily for 1 week or the equivalent of 7.5 mg of prednisone daily for 1 month within the past year. A commonly used regimen is 100 mg of hydrocortisone given intravenously every 8 hours beginning on the morning of surgery and continuing for 48–72 hours. Tapering the dose is not necessary. Patients being maintained on chronic corticosteroids should then resume their usual dose.

Hypothyroidism

Severe symptomatic hypothyroidism has been associated with several perioperative complications, including intraoperative hypotension, congestive heart failure, cardiac arrest, and death. Elective surgery should be delayed in patients with severe hypothyroidism until adequate thyroid hormone replacement can be achieved. Conversely, patients with asymptomatic or mild hypothyroidism generally tolerate surgery well, with only a slight increase in the incidence of intraoperative hypotension; surgery need not be delayed for the month or more required to ensure adequate thyroid hormone replacement.

Eldridge AJ, Sear JW: Perioperative management of diabetic patients: Any changes for the better since 1985? Anesthesia 1996;51:45. (Survey of anesthesiologist management of diabetes in the perioperative period and review of the relevant data regarding management strategies.)

Mantzoros CS, Evagelopoulou K, Moses AC: Outcome of percutaneous transluminal coronary angioplasty in patients with subclinical hypothyroidism. Thyroid 1995;5:383. (Patients with subclinical hypothyroidism are not at increased risk during angioplasty.)

Salem M et al: Perioperative glucocorticoid coverage: A reassessment 42 years after emergence of a problem. Ann Surg 1994;219:416.

Schiff RL, Emanuele MD: The surgical patient with diabetes mellitus: Guidelines for management. J Gen Intern Med 1995;10:154.

RENAL DISEASE

Although the mortality rate for elective major surgery is low (1–4%) in patients with dialysis-dependent chronic renal failure, the risk for perioperative complications, including postoperative hyperkalemia, pneumonia, fluid overload, and bleeding, is substantially increased. Postoperative hyperkalemia requiring emergent hemodialysis has been reported to occur in 20–30% of patients, and postoperative pneumonia may occur in up to 20% of patients. Patients should be dialyzed preoperatively within 24 hours before surgery, and their serum electrolyte lev-

Table 2–12. Intraoperative insulin administration methods

Method	Insulin Administration	Intravenous Glucose Administration	Blood Glucose Monitoring
Subcutaneous insulin	One-half to two-thirds of the usual dose of insulin is administered on the morning of surgery	Infuse 5% glucose-containing solution at a rate of at least 100 mL/h beginning on the morning of surgery and continuing until the patient begins eating	Every 2–4 hours beginning the morning of surgery
Continuous intravenous insulin infusion in glucose-containing solution	On the morning of surgery, infuse 5–10% glucose solution containing 5–15 units regular insulin per liter of solution at rate of 100 mL/h. This provides 0.5–1.5 units of insulin per hour. Additional insulin may be added as needed to keep blood sugar < 250 mg/dL		Every 2–4 hours during intravenous insulin infusion
Separate intravenous insulin and glucose infusions	Infuse intravenous regular insulin at a rate of 0.5–1.5 units/h, adjusting as needed to keep blood sugar < 250 mg/dL	Infuse 5–10% glucose-containing solution at a rate of 100 mL/h	Every 2–4 hours during intravenous insulin infusion

Table 2–13. Risk factors for the development of postoperative acute renal failure.[1]

Aortic surgery
Cardiovascular surgery
Preoperative jaundice
Preoperative chronic renal insufficiency
Age > 70 years

[1]Modified and reproduced, with permission, from Kellerman PS: Perioperative care of the renal patient. Arch Int Med 1994;154:1674.

els should be measured just prior to surgery and monitored closely during the postoperative period.

The risk for development of a significant reduction in renal function, including dialysis-requiring acute renal failure, after major surgery has been estimated to be between 2% and 20%. The mortality associated with the development of acute renal failure after general, vascular, or cardiac surgery exceeds 50%. Patients found to be at excess risk for the development of postoperative deterioration in renal function are shown in Table 2–13. It is especially important to maintain adequate intravascular volume during the perioperative period.

Kellerman PS: Perioperative care of the renal patient. Arch Intern Med 1994;154:1674. (Review of the risk factors for the development of postoperative acute renal failure and management of chronic renal failure in patients undergoing surgery.)

Novis BK et al: Association of preoperative risk factors with postoperative acute renal failure. Anesth Analg 1994;78:143.

Geriatric Medicine

3

Neil M. Resnick, MD

Of all the people who have ever lived to age 65, more than two-thirds are currently alive. Although the implications of this startling statistic are usually viewed in demographic and economic terms, the impact of age on medical care is also substantial and requires significant alterations in the approach to the older patient.

GENERAL PRINCIPLES OF GERIATRIC MEDICINE

Human aging is best characterized as the progressive constriction of each organ system's homeostatic reserve. This decline, often referred to as "homeostenosis," begins in the third decade and is gradual, linear, and variable among individuals. Each organ system's decline (Table 3–1) is independent of changes in other organ systems and is influenced by diet, environment, and personal habits.

Several principles follow from these facts: Individuals become more dissimilar as they age, belying any stereotype of aging; an abrupt decline in any system or function is always due to disease and not to "normal aging"; "normal aging" can be attenuated to some extent by modification of risk factors (eg, increased blood pressure, smoking, sedentary lifestyle); and "healthy old age" is not an oxymoron. In the absence of disease, the decline in homeostatic reserve should cause no symptoms and impose no restrictions on activities of daily living regardless of age. In short, "old people are sick because they are sick, not because they are old."

Appreciation of these facts may make it easier to understand the striking increases that have occurred in longevity. Average life expectancy is now 17 years at age 65, 11 years at age 75, 6 years at age 85, 4 years at age 90, and 2 years at age 100. Moreover, the bulk of those years is characterized by a lack of significant impairment—only 30% of people over age 85 are impaired in any activity required for daily living, and only 20% reside in a nursing home. These striking and often unappreciated figures have substantial implications for disease screening, patient counseling, and medical decision making.

On the other hand, as individuals age they are more likely to suffer from disease, disability, and drug side effects. Combined with the decrease in physiologic reserve, these added burdens (if present) make the older person more vulnerable to any additional environmental, pathologic, or pharmacologic insult. Understanding the implications of these facts is crucial if one is to provide optimal care to older patients, especially those over age 75–80.

The following principles underlie the remainder of the chapter:

(1) First, disease presentation is often atypical in the elderly. Homeostatic strain caused by a new disease often leads to symptoms associated with a different organ system, especially one compromised by preexisting disease; symptoms will depend on which organ system is the "weakest link." For example, less than one-fourth of older patients with hyperthyroidism present with the classic triad of goiter, tremor, and exophthalmos; more likely are atrial fibrillation, confusion, depression, syncope, and weakness. Because the "weakest link" is so often the brain, the lower urinary tract, or the cardiovascular or musculoskeletal system, a limited number of presenting symptoms predominate—acute confusion, depression, falling, incontinence, and syncope—no matter what the underlying disease. *Thus, regardless of the presenting symptom in older people, the differential diagnosis is often largely the same. The corollary is equally important: the organ system usually associated with a particular symptom is less likely to be the source of that symptom in older individuals than in younger ones.* Thus, compared with middle-aged individuals, acute confusion in older patients is less often due to a new brain lesion, incontinence to a bladder disorder, fracture to osteoporosis, falling to a neuropathy, or syncope to heart disease.

(2) Second, because of their impaired compensatory mechanisms, disease in older patients often presents at an earlier stage. Heart failure may be precipitated by only mild hyperthyroidism, significant cognitive dysfunction by only mild hyperparathyroidism, urinary retention by only mild prostatic enlargement, and nonketotic hyperosmolar coma by only mild glucose intolerance. Thus, paradoxically, treatment of the underlying disease may be easier in the elderly because it is less advanced at the time of

Table 3–1. Selected age-related changes and their consequences.[1]

Organ or System	Age-Related Physiologic Change[2]	Consequences of Age-Related Physiologic Change	Consequences of Disease, Not Age
General	↑ Body fat ↓ Total body water	↑ Volume of distribution for fat-soluble drugs ↓ Volume of distribution for water-soluble drugs	Obesity Anorexia
Eyes and ears	Presbyopia Lens opacification ↓ High-frequency acuity	↓ Accommodation ↑ Susceptibility to glare Difficulty discriminating words if background noise is present	Blindness Deafness
Endocrine	Impaired glucose homeostasis ↓ Thyroxine clearance (and production) ↑ ADH, ↓ renin, and ↓ aldosterone ↓ Testosterone ↓ Vitamin D absorption and activation	↑ Glucose level in response to acute illness ↓ T_4 dose required in hypothyroidism Osteopenia	Diabetes mellitus Thyroid dysfunction ↓ Na^+, ↑ K^+ Impotence Osteomalacia, fractures
Respiratory	↓ Lung elasticity and ↑ chest wall stiffness	Ventilation-perfusion mismatch and ↓ Pao_2	Dyspnea, hypoxia
Cardiovascular	↓ Arterial compliance and ↑ systolic BP → LVH ↓ β-Adrenergic responsiveness ↓ Baroreceptor sensitivity and ↓ SA node automaticity	Hypotensive response to ↑ HR, volume depletion, or loss of atrial contraction ↓ Cardiac output and HR response to stress Impaired blood pressure response to standing, volume depletion	Syncope Heart failure Heart block
Gastrointestinal	↓ Hepatic function ↓ Gastric acidity ↓ Colonic motility ↓ Anorectal function	Delayed metabolism of some drugs ↓ Ca^{2+} absorption on empty stomach Constipation	Cirrhosis Osteoporosis, B_{12} deficiency Fecal impaction Fecal incontinence
Hematologic and immune systems	↓ Bone marrow reserve (?) ↓ T cell function ↑ Autoantibodies	 False-negative PPD response False-positive rheumatoid factor, antinuclear antibody	Anemia Autoimmune disease
Renal	↓ GFR ↓ Urine concentration-dilution (see also Endocrine, above)	Impaired excretion of some drugs Delayed response to salt or fluid restriction or overload; nocturia	↑ Serum creatinine ↓ or ↑ Na^+
Genitourinary	Vaginal or urethral mucosal atrophy Prostate enlargement ↓ Bladder contractility	Dyspareunia, bacteriuria ↑ Residual urine volume	Symptomatic UTI Urinary incontinence; urinary retention Prostate cancer
Musculoskeletal	↓ Lean body mass, muscle ↓ Bone density	↓ Strength Osteopenia	Functional impairment Hip fracture
Nervous system	Brain atrophy ↓ Brain catechol synthesis ↓ Brain dopaminergic synthesis ↓ Righting reflexes ↓ Stage 4 sleep	Benign senescent forgetfulness Stiffer gait ↑ Body sway Early awakening, insomnia	Dementia, delirium Depression Parkinson's disease Falls Sleep apnea

[1]From Resnick NM: Geriatric medicine. In: *Harrison's Principles of Internal Medicine,* 13th ed. Isselbacher K et al (editors). McGraw-Hill, 1994.
[2]Changes generally observed in healthy elderly subjects free of symptoms and detectable disease in the organ system studied. The changes are usually important only when the system is stressed or other factors are added (eg, drugs, disease, or environmental challenge); they rarely result in symptoms otherwise.

presentation. Another ramification of this principle is that drug side effects can occur even with low doses of drugs that usually produce no side effects in younger people. For instance a mild anticholinergic agent (eg, diphenhydramine) may cause confusion, diuretics may precipitate urinary incontinence, digoxin may induce depression even with normal serum levels, and over-the-counter sympathomimetics may precipitate urinary retention in older men with mild prostatic obstruction.

Unfortunately, the predisposition to develop symptoms at an earlier stage of disease is often offset by the change in illness behavior that occurs with age. Raised at a time when symptoms and debility were accepted as normal consequences of aging, the elderly are less likely to seek attention until symptoms become disabling. Thus, any symptom, particularly those associated with a change in functional status, must be taken seriously and evaluated promptly.

(3) Third, since many homeostatic mechanisms are often compromised concurrently, there are usually multiple abnormalities amenable to treatment, and small improvements in each may yield dramatic benefits overall. For instance, cognitive impairment in patients with Alzheimer's disease may be exacerbated by hearing or visual impairment, depression, heart failure, electrolyte imbalance, and anemia. Similarly, urinary incontinence is often worsened by fecal impaction, medications, excess urinary output, and arthritis. In each case, substantial functional improvement can result from treating the contributing factors even if—as in Alzheimer's disease—the disease itself is not treatable.

(4) Fourth, many findings that are abnormal in younger patients are relatively common in older people and may not be responsible for a particular symptom. Such findings include bacteriuria, premature ventricular contractions, low bone mineral density, impaired glucose tolerance, and involuntary bladder contractions. Instead, they may be only incidental findings that result in missed diagnoses and misdirected therapy. For instance, finding bacteriuria should not end the search for a source of fever in an acutely ill older patient, nor should an elevated random blood sugar—especially in an acutely ill patient—be incriminated as the cause of neuropathy. On the other hand, other abnormalities must not be dismissed as due to old age—eg, there is no anemia, impotence, depression, or confusion of old age (Table 3–1).

(5) Fifth, because symptoms in older people are often due to multiple causes, the diagnostic "law of parsimony" often does not apply. For instance, fever, anemia, retinal embolus, and a heart murmur prompt almost a reflex diagnosis of endocarditis in a younger patient but are more apt to reflect aspirin-induced blood loss, a cholesterol embolus, insignificant aortic sclerosis, or a viral illness in an older patient. "Never think of one diagnosis when three will do" is a useful maxim.

Moreover, even when the diagnosis is correct, treatment of a single disease in an older patient is unlikely to result in cure. For instance, in a younger patient, incontinence due to involuntary bladder contractions is treated effectively with a bladder relaxant medication. However, in an older patient whose incontinence is also associated with fecal impaction, who is taking medications that cloud the sensorium, and who has impaired mobility and manual dexterity due to arthritis, treatment of the bladder abnormality alone is unlikely to restore continence. On the other hand, disimpaction, discontinuation of the offending medications, and treatment of the arthritis are likely to restore continence without the need for a bladder relaxant. Failure to recognize these principles often leads to prescribing "ineffective" therapy and unjustified therapeutic nihilism towards older patients.

(6) Sixth, because the older patient is more likely than a younger one to suffer the adverse consequences of disease, treatment—and even prevention—may be equally or even more effective. For instance, the benefits to survival of exercise, as well as thrombolysis and beta-blocker therapy after a myocardial infarction, appear to be at least as impressive in older patients as in younger ones; and treatment of hypertension and transient ischemic attacks, as well as immunization against influenza and pneumococcal pneumonia, is even more effective in older patients than in younger ones. In addition, prevention in older patients often must be seen in a broader context. For instance, although efforts to increase bone density may be futile in older patients, fracture may still be prevented by interventions that improve balance, strengthen legs, treat contributing medical conditions, replete nutritional deficits, remove adverse medications, and reduce environmental hazards.

In summary, optimal treatment of the older person usually requires treating much more than the organ system usually associated with the disease—and often even permits ignoring that organ system entirely.

These principles guide the remainder of the discussion, which focuses on their specific implications for the evaluation and treatment of geriatric patients.

EVALUATION OF THE ELDERLY

Evaluation of the older patient can be spread over several visits, and its extent can be determined by the patient's clinical status. Time invested initially in diagnosis and prevention can reduce subsequent morbidity and resource utilization and enhance satisfaction for patient and physician alike.

Moreover, much can be gleaned from questionnaires filled out by the patient or caregiver in advance, as well as from observation. For instance, it is useful for the physician to greet the patient in the waiting room and to note the affective and cognitive response, the strength of the grip in shaking hands, the ease of rising from the chair without using the arms, the length and steadiness of the stride, and the ability to navigate the corridor and sit safely in the examining room chair. Writing one's note in the room while the patient dresses or undresses affords an opportunity to assess cognition, fine motor skills, balance, and judgment. Such observations facilitate detection of otherwise overlooked conditions, provide more information than standard physical examinations, and often shorten the clinical evaluation.

History Taking

Most older patients can provide a reliable medical history; however, a multitude of complaints may make obtaining a history more difficult, and adequate time must be allotted. For patients unable to comprehend or communicate adequately, data should be sought from family, friends, and caregivers as well as from medical records.

Older people frequently fail to mention several important conditions—not because they do not find them a burden but because they attribute them to aging rather than to disease. Such conditions include falling, depression, cognitive impairment, alcoholism, polypharmacy, incontinence, and sexual dysfunction. Because all are common but treatable sources of morbidity, each must be specifically sought.

Dietary intake should also be assessed. Many elderly patients have limited nutritional intake not only of calories and protein but also of iron, calcium, folate, and vitamin D. In addition to concurrent medical illness, reasons include inadequate income, problems with shopping or preparing meals, eating habits, impaired senses of taste and smell, difficulties with dentures, cognitive impairment, or depression. On the other hand, some elderly people take excess vitamins, many of which (eg, vitamins A and D) may accumulate and cause toxicity. Thus, especially for the older patient with weight loss, the differential diagnosis must go well beyond the usual list of medical causes.

A careful history is essential in any elderly patient who has recently become confused. To assume that confusion is a manifestation of dementia without having inquired into factors such as other illnesses, new medications, or increased doses of drugs that may produce delirium may overlook an easily correctable and serious condition. To make matters worse, if delirium is overlooked and assumed to be dementia with behavioral abnormalities, tranquilizers or psychotropic agents may be prescribed (especially in the nursing home or hospital) that may then further aggravate the delirium.

Advance Directives

All elderly patients should be asked whether they have drafted advance directives, and, if they have, a copy should be placed in the record. Such directives may consist of (1) a health care proxy or durable power of attorney for health care, in which patients designate a surrogate decision-maker who makes health care decisions if the patient cannot; (2) a living will or medical directive, in which patients specify their desires for treatment in specific situations if they cannot communicate at the critical time; or (3) a combination of the two. Different forms are legally binding in different states, and most can be completed by the patient and proxy with witnesses, without the need for legal counsel.

Whether or not the patient has formally drafted these directives, it is useful to indicate in the record who should make health care decisions if the patient is no longer able to do so. Patients should then be encouraged to discuss with the physician as well as the designated proxy their feelings about resuscitation, intubation, feeding tubes, hospitalization, etc, in their current state of health and possible future declining states of health. Although the list of possibilities is potentially endless, it is often possible to predict the situations that might arise, such as intubation for a patient with COPD or a feeding tube in the event of a major stroke for a patient with atrial fibrillation. In addition, such conversations can and should take place over time. The early elicitation of a patient's preferences and values can often help both physicians and families in subsequent difficult decisions by giving all surrogate decision-makers the sense that they are doing as the patient would have wanted.

[Diagnosis and treatment of depression in late life]
  gopher://gopher.nih.gov:70/00/clin/cdcs/individual/
    86.diag
Emanuel LL: Advance directives: Do they work? J Am Coll Cardiol 1995;25:35. (Philosophic and methodologic issues with practical illustrations.)
Johnston SC, Pfeifer MP, McNutt R: The discussion about advance directives: Patient and physician opinions regarding when and how it should be conducted. End of Life Study Group. Arch Intern Med 1995;155:1025. (Patients felt that the discussion should occur earlier than did physicians—at an earlier age, earlier in the natural history of the disease, and earlier in the patient-physician relationship.)
Morrison RS et al: The inaccessibility of advance directives on transfer from ambulatory to acute care settings. JAMA 1995;274:478.
O'Brien LA et al: Nursing home residents' preferences for life-sustaining treatments. JAMA 1995;274:1775. (More than half of residents able to make decisions opted for use of CPR, but few had discussed preferences with their physicians.)

PHYSICAL EXAMINATION

For patients being seen for routine evaluation, it is useful to screen for conditions that could impair function, since functional disability is common and treatable but often goes undetected. A simple inventory is shown in Table 3–2.

Table 3–2. Procedure for functional assessment screening in the elderly.[1]

Target Area	Assessment Procedure	Abnormal Result	Suggested Intervention
Vision	Test each eye with Jaeger card while patient wears corrective lenses (if applicable).	Inability to read greater than 20/40.	Refer to ophthalmologist or optometrist.
Hearing	Whisper a short, easily answered question such as "What is your name?" in each ear while the examiner's face is out of direct view.	Inability to answer question.	Examine auditory canals for cerumen and clean if necessary. Repeat test; if still abnormal in either ear, refer for audiometry and possible prosthesis.
Arm	Proximal: "Touch the back of your head with both hands." Distal: "Pick up the spoon."	Inability to do task.	Examine the arm fully (muscle, joint, and nerve), paying attention to pain, weakness, limited range of motion. Consider referral for physical therapy.
Leg	Observe the patient after instructing as follows: "Rise from your chair, walk 10 feet, return, and sit down."	Inability to walk or transfer out of chair.	Do full neurologic and musculoskeletal evaluation, paying attention to strength, pain, range of motion, balance, and traditional assessment of gait. Consider referral for physical therapy.
Continence of urine	Ask, "Do you ever lose your urine and get wet?"	"Yes."	Ascertain frequency and amount. Search for remediable causes, including local irritations, polyuric states, and medications. Consider urologic referral.
Nutrition	Ask, "Without trying, have you lost 10 lb or more in the last 6 months?" Weigh the patient. Measure height.	"Yes," or weight is below acceptable range for height.	Do appropriate medical evaluation.
Mental status	Instruct as follows: "I am going to name three objects (pencil, truck, book). I will ask you to repeat their names now and then again a few minutes from now." [See text discussion.]	Inability to recall all three objects after 1 minute.	Administer Folstein Mini-Mental Status Examination. If score is less than 24, search for causes of cognitive impairment. Ascertain onset, duration, and fluctuation of overt symptoms. Review medications. Assess consciousness and affect. Do appropriate laboratory tests.
Depression	Ask, "Do you often feel sad or depressed?" or "How are your spirits?"	"Yes" or "Not very good, I guess."	Administer Geriatric Depression Scale. If positive (score above 5), check for antihypertensive, psychotropic, or other pertinent medications. Consider appropriate pharmacologic or psychiatric treatment.
ADL-IADL[2]	Ask, "Can you get out of bed yourself?" "Can you dress yourself?" "Can you make your own meals?" "Can you do your own shopping?"	"No" to any question.	Corroborate responses with patient's appearance; question family members if accuracy is uncertain. Determine reasons for the inability (motivation compared with physical limitation). Institute appropriate medical, social, or environmental interventions.
Home environment	Ask, "Do you have trouble with stairs inside or outside of your home?" Ask about potential hazards inside the home with bathtubs, rugs, or lighting.	"Yes."	Evaluate home safety and institute appropriate countermeasures.
Social support	Ask, "Who would be able to help you in case of illness or emergency?"	. . .	List identified persons in the medical record. Become familiar with available resources for the elderly in the community.

[1]Modified from Lachs MS et al: A simple procedure for general screening for functional disability in elderly patients. Ann Intern Med 1990;112:669.
[2]Activities of daily living–instrumental activities of daily living.

In the remaining patients, the multiple interacting and contributing causes of dysfunction warrant a complete physical examination, including pelvic examination in women and rectal examination in both sexes; some components can be assessed over succeeding visits. Weight and postural blood pressure should be measured at each visit. Vision and hearing should also be checked; if hearing is impaired, excess cerumen should be removed from the external auditory canals. Denture fit should be assessed. The oral cavity should be inspected with the dentures removed, remembering that malignant lesions of the mouth are more often red than white. Although thyroid disease becomes more common with age, because the sensitivity and specificity of related findings are substantially lower than in younger individuals, the physical examination can rarely corroborate or exclude thyroid dysfunction in older patients. The breast examination should not be overlooked, since older women are more likely to have breast cancer and less likely to do breast self-examination than younger women. The systolic murmur of aortic sclerosis is common and may be difficult to differentiate from aortic stenosis, especially since the presence of a fourth heart sound in an elderly patient does not imply clinically significant cardiac disease, and the carotid upstroke normally increases due to age-related arterial stiffening.

In patients with cognitive impairment, it is important to check for asterixis. If deterioration has occurred precipitously, one must also check for signs of nondominant parietal lobe dysfunction, including right-left confusion, neglect, and apraxia.

In inactive patients and those with fecal or urinary incontinence, one should check for fecal impaction. In patients with urinary incontinence—especially men—a distended bladder must be sought, since it may be the only finding in urinary retention; perineal sensation and the bulbocavernosus reflex also should be tested. Patients who fall should be observed standing up from a chair, bending down, reaching up, walking 10 feet, turning, returning, and sitting again; abnormalities of gait and balance should be evaluated, with the patient's eyes open and closed and in response to a sternal push. Careful examination of the feet and assessment of shoe fit are also important in the patient with gait disturbance. If the patient uses a cane or walker, one should make certain it is the correct length or height (ie, equal to the distance from the wrist crease to the ground) and has a good grip. If the patient is chair-bound or bed-bound, the skin should be examined for reddening or evidence of early ulceration over pressure points. Finally, it should be appreciated that "frontal release signs" (eg, "snout," "glabellar," or palmomental reflexes), as well as absent ankle jerks and vibratory sense in the feet, may be found in elderly patients with no other evidence of neurologic disease.

MENTAL STATUS EXAMINATION

In addition to evaluating mood and affect, some form of cognitive testing is essential in all elderly patients, even if it involves only checking different components of the history for consistency; for instance, patients may say that they eat well and enjoy fish but later describe a shopping list that includes no fish and only a limited quantity of other items. Patients with mild degrees of dementia may mask intellectual impairment by a cheerful and cooperative manner. Thus, the examiner should always *probe for content*. For patients who follow the news, ask what stories they're particularly interested in and why; the same applies to reading, social events—even the "soap operas" on television.

If there is any suspicion of a cognitive deficit after this kind of conversational probing, the physician should explain that a mental status evaluation is part of every complete examination, so that the patient will not feel singled out and insulted. An examination that tests only orientation as to person, place, and time is not sufficient to detect mild or moderate intellectual impairment. As a quick screen, simply assessing orientation and asking the patient to draw a clock with the hands at a set time (eg, 10 minutes before 2:00) can be very informative regarding cognitive status, visuospatial deficits, ability to comprehend and execute instructions in logical sequence, and presence or absence of perseveration. For slightly more detailed examinations, many practical mental status tests are available, but the one most widely used is the Mini-Mental Status Examination of Folstein, which provides a numerical score that can be of great value as a baseline test and can be administered by a nonphysician in 5–10 minutes. However, regardless of the test employed, the total score is much less useful diagnostically than is knowledge of the specific domain of the deficit. As a general rule, disproportionate difficulty with recent memory suggests dementia, while predominant difficulty with immediate recall (eg, a list of three items) suggests depression. For patients with deficits of attention—recognized by inability to spell "world" backwards, repeat five digits, or recite the months of the year backwards—delirium is probably present and the accuracy of the remainder of the test is dubious. However, the test can only be interpreted accurately in the context of a comprehensive evaluation, and no single question or task can establish or rule out cognitive impairment. Moreover, these are only screening tests, which must be interpreted in the context of the patient's baseline intellectual function; a few incorrect responses has different connotations in a previously gifted individual: An engineer concerned about recent intellectual mistakes should not be reassured by a perfect score on a screening test.

Callahan CM, Hendrie HC, Tierney WM: Documentation and evaluation of cognitive impairment in elderly primary care patients. Ann Intern Med 1995;122:422. (Owing to the lack of a standard approach to screening, less than 25% of people over age 60 with moderate to severe impairment were identified—even in this excellent primary care setting.)

Mulligan R et al: A comparison of alternative methods of screening for dementia in clinical settings. Arch Neurol 1996;53:532. (Mini-Mental State Examinations [MMSE] as well as informant reports were efficient methods for screening for cognitive impairment.)

Siu A: Screening for dementia and assessing its causes. Ann Intern Med 1991;115:122. (Critical review of usefulness of mental status screening tests. Although laboratory diagnostic tests are also reviewed, the critique's utility is limited by the absence of available data and by cost-benefit considerations.)

EVALUATION OF FUNCTIONAL CAPACITY IN THE ELDERLY

Simply taking a history, performing a physical examination, and listing medical diagnoses are not sufficient for elderly patients: a problem list that includes past stroke, metastatic prostatic cancer, and osteoporosis could describe a Supreme Court justice as well as a bed-bound nursing home patient.

Thus, a clear description of the patient's functional incapacity is essential. Basic activities of daily living (ADLs) should be assessed, including the ability to get in and out of bed and chairs, toilet, bathe, dress, feed, and walk. More advanced function—known as instrumental activities of daily living (IADLs)—should also be evaluated, including the ability to shop, cook, manage money, do housework and laundry, use a telephone, and travel outside the home. Socioeconomic circumstances and social support systems should also be assessed.

For most patients, a questionnaire dealing with these activities can be completed by the patient or family. For frail patients, assessment of the home by a trained observer may be beneficial, not only for identifying problems inapparent in an office setting but also for providing practical advice. For instance, the risk of accidents may be reduced by eliminating environmental obstacles and by installing assistive bars, better lighting, and smoke alarms.

Referrals for community services can be initiated, and families of cognitively impaired patients who are still cooking or driving can be advised to disconnect the stove or to disable or dispose of the car or take possession of the car keys.

Assessment of function and thoughtful attention to what steps can be taken to improve it are often the most important contributions the health team can make in improving the patient's quality of life and preventing or delaying institutionalization.

Fleming KC et al: Practical functional assessment of elderly persons: A primary care approach. Mayo Clin Proc 1995;70:890. (Covers the details of most available screening tools, allowing practitioners to select those most appropriate for their practice setting.)

Ikegami N: Functional assessment and its place in health care. N Engl J Med 1995;332:598.

Landefeld CS et al: A randomized trial of care in a hospital medical unit especially designed to improve the functional outcomes of acutely ill older patients. N Engl J Med 1995;332:1338. (Improvement was noted in basic and advanced ADLs as well as reduction in number of nursing home admissions. Overall cost was $200 per patient.)

Podsialo D, Richardson S: The timed "up and go": A test of basic functional mobility for frail elderly persons. J Am Geriatr Soc 1991;39:142. (Quick, practical assessment of mobility.)

Stuck AE et al: A trial of annual in-home comprehensive geriatric assessments for elderly people living in the community. N Engl J Med 1995;333:1184. (Three-year randomized trial of people over age 75 years found that annual assessments delayed onset of disability and reduced nursing home admissions at a low cost.)

Wasson JH et al: The prescription of assistive devices for the elderly. J Gen Intern Med 1990;5:46. (Practical suggestions every physician should heed.)

LABORATORY EXAMINATIONS & IMAGING

With few exceptions, laboratory values are the same for the elderly as for younger adults. Arterial PO_2 declines as a result of age-associated small airway collapse, which is most marked in the dependent portions of the lung; since these are also the best-perfused areas, ventilation-perfusion mismatch results. The Pao_2 can be estimated by subtracting from 104 the product of the patient's age $\times$ 0.42 (if supine) or age $\times$ 0.27 (if sitting).

The sedimentation rate rises somewhat with age, but the range of normal values is large and its utility in older patients is poorly established. The fasting blood glucose is not significantly altered by age, but the 2- and 3-hour postprandial blood glucose is higher than for younger adults. Hemoglobin A_{1c} is useful in managing the elderly diabetic; however, one must keep in mind that there may be a slight increase in levels in nondiabetic elderly patients. Although glomerular filtration rate declines by an average of 40% with age, the variability among individuals—like that of other physiologic parameters—is great, and healthy elderly persons without hypertension may experience little decline. However, in the absence of renal disease, even patients with an age-related decrease in GFR do not have an increased serum creatinine because creatinine production decreases owing to the decline in lean body mass.

THE FRAIL ELDERLY & THE FIVE *I*'S

Diseases more common in the elderly are listed in Table 3–3 and covered elsewhere in the text. A number of medical problems, however, do not usually present as clear-cut organ-specific diagnoses. These problems are most common in the frail elderly, especially those over 80 years of age, and are often referred to as the "five *I*'s": (1) intellectual impairment, (2) immobility, (3) instability, (4) incontinence, and (5) iatrogenic drug reactions.

INTELLECTUAL IMPAIRMENT

A mild decline in memory and the rate of information processing occurs normally with age but does not affect daily function and does not generally progress. By contrast, dementia is an acquired persistent and progressive impairment of intellectual function with compromise in at least two of the following spheres of mental activity: language, memory, visuospatial skills, emotional behavior or personality, and

Table 3–3. Diseases more common with aging.

1. Atherosclerotic cardiovascular and cerebrovascular diseases with resultant myocardial infarction, strokes, multi-infarct dementia, and abdominal aortic aneurysms and peripheral vascular disease (see Chapters 10, 12, and 24).
2. Cardiac conduction system disease leading to conduction block (see Chapter 10).
3. Senile dementia of the Alzheimer type (see text).
4. Polymyalgia rheumatica (see Chapter 20).
5. Type II diabetes mellitus and nonketotic hyperglycemic coma (see Chapter 27).
6. Cancer, especially of the colon, prostate, lung, breast, and skin (see Chapter 4).
7. Pressure ulcers (see Chapter 6).
8. Tuberculosis (see Chapter 9).
9. Macular degeneration, cataract, and glaucoma (see Chapter 7).
10. Deafness (see Chapter 8).
11. Multiple myeloma, myelodysplasia, and myelofibrosis (see Chapter 13).
12. Constipation, fecal impaction, and fecal incontinence (see Chapter 14).
13. Osteoarthritis, spinal stenosis, osteoporosis, hip fracture, crystal joint disease (gout, pseudogout), and Paget's disease (see Chapter 20).
14. Parkinson's disease (see Chapter 24).
15. Depression and suicide (the latter most common in elderly white men) (see Chapter 25).
16. Chronic obstructive pulmonary disease (see Chapter 9).
17. Benign prostatic hyperplasia (see Chapter 23).
18. Diverticulitis and angiodysplasia (see Chapter 14).
19. Herpes zoster (see Chapters 6 and 32).
20. Systemic hypothermia (see Chapter 38).

cognition (calculation, abstraction, judgment, etc). Because dementia is probably the most feared disease of aging, it is important to reassure older persons with normal age-related memory decline that senile dementia is not inevitable.

Clinically significant intellectual impairment affects an estimated 5–10% of people over age 65 and 20% of people over age 80, though recent estimates are as high as 47% for people over 85. Approximately 60–70% of cases of senile dementia are of the Alzheimer type, and 10–20% are vascular dementias, usually called multi-infarct dementias. These include (1) multiple cortical infarcts, (2) Binswanger's disease (subcortical arteriosclerotic encephalopathy), and (3) lacunar infarcts. Another 10–20% of patients show evidence of both Alzheimer's disease and vascular dementia.

Clinical Features

The earliest manifestation of dementia is usually forgetfulness in the absence of depression and inattentiveness. Many patients with dementia maintain their social graces even in the face of significant cognitive impairment; thus, a clinical impression of preserved intellectual function without mental status testing may miss the diagnosis. As the disease progresses, there is loss of computational ability, word-finding and concentration problems, difficulty with ordinary activities such as dressing, cooking, and balancing the checkbook, then severe memory loss and, ultimately, complete disorientation and social withdrawal. Senile dementia of the Alzheimer type has an insidious onset and is steadily progressive, with death approximately 8–10 years later. Rapid onset of cognitive impairment suggests delirium, depression, drug toxicity, or stroke as the cause. Vascular dementia is more common in men, associated with hypertension with or without a history of transient ischemic attacks or strokes, and is more likely to progress in a series of recognizably distinct steps. The modified Hachinski Ischemia Score (see Table 3–4) is commonly used in making the clinical diag-

Table 3–4. Factors suggesting multi-infarct dementia: Modified Hachinski Ischemia Score.[1]

Characteristic	Point Score[2]
Abrupt onset	2
Stepwise deterioration	1
Somatic complaints	1
Emotional incontinence	1
History or presence of hypertension	1
History of strokes	2
Focal neurologic symptoms	2
Focal neurologic signs	2

[1]Fischer P et al: Prospective neuropathological validation of Hachinski's Ischaemia Score. J Neurol Neurosurg Psychiatry 1991;54:580.
[2]A total score of 6 or more is considered diagnostic of multi-infarct dementia.

nosis, with a score of six or more suggestive of vascular dementia. Although Alzheimer's disease may coexist with vascular dementia, the latter is important to detect since its progression may be slowed by antihypertensive therapy, aspirin therapy, treatment of atrial fibrillation, and smoking cessation.

Diagnosis

Diagnosis is based on the history and on the physical and mental status examinations—supplemented by careful review of the medication list and alcohol intake—and by laboratory investigations to exclude other causes of cognitive impairment. Useful tests include serum electrolytes, calcium, glucose, TSH, vitamin B_{12}, renal and liver function tests, drug levels, and urinalysis as well as arterial oxygen if hypoxemia is suspected. Measurement of serum VDRL is indicated only in selected older individuals who might have tertiary syphilis. A new test, which measures levels of apolipoprotein E4, does not accurately distinguish elderly patients with Alzheimer's disease from those with other causes of dementia.

MRI or CT scan tests should be done in most cases when there are signs of early dementia of relatively short duration (months to 1–2 years). After that time, they should be ordered only upon specific indications. Both tests are useful in ruling out subdural hematoma, frontal lobe tumor, hydrocephalus, stroke or hemorrhage, and vascular dementia, all of which may mimic dementia of the Alzheimer type. However, an MRI or CT scan "consistent with Alzheimer's" is not diagnostic. Similar findings occur in cognitively normal elderly patients and should not keep the physician from doing other tests to rule out treatable dementias.

In difficult cases, neuropsychologic testing can be helpful in differentiating the causes of cognitive impairment, including depression, Alzheimer's disease, stroke, delirium, and Korsakoff's syndrome. In addition, such testing can identify areas of preserved cognitive function even when the cause of cognitive impairment is known. Such knowledge can be helpful in structuring the patient's environment to optimize function.

The significance of Binswanger's disease (subcortical arteriosclerotic encephalopathy) detected by CT scan or MRI remains to be elucidated, since the finding of periventricular white matter hypodensity may be present in normal as well as in demented patients.

Normal-pressure hydrocephalus should be considered in the mildly demented patient who also has a gait disturbance and urinary incontinence. Surgical procedures for cerebrospinal diversion may be helpful, but it is difficult to predict which patients will show clinical improvement. A short duration of symptoms with early gait disturbance and a specific cause correlate best with surgical benefit. Moderately to severely demented patients are seldom helped by surgery.

A very small percentage of patients prove to have a condition whose treatment reverses the dementia. *However, in a far greater proportion cognitive function can be improved significantly by discontinuation of medications that exacerbate confusion and by detection and treatment of contributing disorders such as heart failure, hypoxia, thyroid disease, anemia, medication use, alcoholism, and depression.*

Differential Diagnosis

One of the most important tasks of the physician dealing with older people is to differentiate dementia from depression and from delirium, though they often coexist (see Table 3–5). Delirium is a confusional state characterized by inattention, rapid onset, and fluctuating course that may persist for months if untreated. Unlike delirium tremens, delirium in older patients is often not associated with signs of increased autonomic activity. Thus, in the hospitalized elderly patient, it is easily missed and may be mistaken for dementia. Delirium occurs most commonly in individuals over age 80 with preexisting cognitive impairment. It has multiple causes, the commonest of which are severe illness, drugs, abnormal (either high or low) serum sodium levels, fever, and dehydration.

Table 3–5. *DSM-IIIR* diagnostic criteria for delirium.

A. Reduced ability to maintain attention to external stimuli (eg, questions must be repeated because attention wanders) and to appropriately shift attention to new external stimuli (eg, perseverates answer to a previous question).

B. Disorganized thinking, as indicated by rambling, irrelevant, or incoherent speech.

C. At least two of the following:
   (1) Reduced level of consciousness, eg, difficulty keeping awake during examination.
   (2) Perceptual disturbances: misinterpretations, illusions, or hallucinations.
   (3) Disturbance of sleep-wake cycle with insomnia or daytime sleepiness.
   (4) Increased or decreased psychomotor activity.
   (5) Disorientation to time, place, or person.
   (6) Memory impairment, eg, inability to learn new material, such as the names of several unrelated objects, after 5 minutes, or to remember past events, such as history of current episode of illness.

D. Clinical features develop over a short period of time (usually hours to days) and tend to fluctuate over the course of a day.

E. Either (1) or (2):
   (1) Evidence from the history, physical examination, or laboratory tests of a specific organic factor (or factors) judged to be etiologically related to the disturbance.
   (2) In the absence of such evidence, an etiologic organic factor can be presumed if the disturbance cannot be accounted for by any nonorganic mental disorder, eg, manic episode accounting for agitation and sleep disturbance.

The following other common causes of confusional states may be missed if not specifically looked for.

A. Drugs: A wide variety of agents, including over-the-counter medications, may cause confusion in the elderly. The most common are alcohol, sedatives, hypnotics, H₂ blockers, digoxin, neuroleptics, antidepressants, anticholinergics, antihypertensives, chronic heavy salicylate use, NSAIDs, meperidine, and propoxyphene. If, as sometimes happens, the patient is receiving the same drug under different brand names, there is an increased likelihood of drug-induced confusion.

B. Depression: (See Psychiatric History, above; and Management of Depression, below. See also Chapter 25.) The prevalence of depression (5–10%) does not change with age, but it is often overlooked in those affected, and the highest incidence of suicide is in white men over age 75. The diagnosis requires the presence of a depressed mood for at least two consecutive weeks plus at least four of eight "vegetative" signs, including *S*leep disturbance, lack of *I*nterest, feelings of *G*uilt, decreased *E*nergy, decreased *C*oncentration, decreased *A*ppetite, *P*sychomotor agitation/retardation, and *S*uicidal ideation. These can be recalled using the mnemonic *SIG E CAPS* (as if prescribing energy capsules). Also helpful diagnostically is a personal or family history of depression, past response to an antidepressant, and the presence of anhedonia (ie, little or nothing gives them pleasure). Depression may be superimposed on mild dementia or may even mimic dementia, since decreased attention span, loss of sense of humor, irritability, and poor performance on mental status testing may occur in both conditions. One helpful diagnostic clue is that the depressed patient is more likely to complain of difficulty in answering mental status questions, whereas the demented patient usually is oblivious to the incorrect answers except in the early stages of the disease. Nonetheless, differentiation may be difficult and may warrant a therapeutic trial of antidepressant drugs or psychiatric consultation.

C. Other Psychiatric Problems: Confusion may result from the anxiety and disorienting effect of being in a hospital or other unfamiliar surroundings. Severe anxiety over normal forgetfulness or psychotic behavior may be misdiagnosed as dementia. Sleep deprivation may result in confusion.

D. Sensory Loss: Hearing loss not only leads to social isolation but results in inappropriate answers that may be misinterpreted as evidence of dementia. Behavior resulting from abnormalities of perception in patients with lesions of the nondominant parietal lobe may be mistaken for dementia.

E. Metabolic and Endocrine Disturbances: Hyponatremia is a common cause of confusional state in elderly people because of the age-related increase in antidiuretic hormone (ADH) responsiveness to physiologic stress and the syndrome of inappropriate antidiuretic hormone (SIADH) secretion. Hypernatremia also causes confusion; older persons are predisposed by age-related decreases in thirst and renal concentrating ability, which are exacerbated by renal disease, diuretics, and conditions that reduce access to free water. Hypo- or hyperglycemia, thyroid disorders, hyperparathyroidism, liver failure, renal failure, and cardiopulmonary failure can also cause metabolic confusional states. Confusion due to hypercalcemia is particularly apt to occur in bone disorders that are more often seen in elderly patients (eg, metastatic carcinoma, Paget's disease, multiple myeloma).

F. Bladder and Bowel Disorders: Acute urinary retention and fecal impaction are easily treated causes of delirium, especially in hospitalized elderly patients. These causes are especially important to identify before initiating neuroleptic therapy, which not only may be unnecessary in such cases but may in fact exacerbate them.

G. Nutritional Deficiencies: Cognitive impairment can be produced by vitamin B₁₂, niacin, riboflavin, and thiamin deficiencies.

H. Trauma: Subdural hematoma must always be considered as a possible cause of confusion, since brain size decreases with age while the venous sinuses are fixed to the dura, predisposing them to rupture with minimal trauma. Falls with head injury may be forgotten or not reported by the patient and unknown to the family, and headache is often absent in chronic subdural hematoma.

I. Tumor: Metastatic lesions and gliomas can cause cognitive impairment, as can tumors outside the nervous system (paraneoplastic syndrome).

J. Infections: Acute infection in the elderly may cause confusion even in the absence of fever. Chronic infections of lung, bone, kidneys, skin (associated with pressure sores), and the central nervous system (including AIDS) may also present as dementia. Central nervous system syphilis is now a rare cause of dementia.

K. Cardiovascular or Cerebrovascular Accidents: Myocardial infarction, congestive heart failure, or pulmonary embolism may present as an acute confusional state. Strokes that involve the nondominant parietal lobe or that result in fluent or receptive aphasias are often mistaken for dementia.

Treatment

A. Management of Dementia: The most important first step in management of a "demented" elderly patient is the search for and correction of all treatable factors contributing to cognitive impairment (see above).

Until recently, specific therapy for Alzheimer's disease did not exist, including ergoloid mesylates. However, several recent short-term randomized trials have established the efficacy of tacrine, although only about one-third of patients respond. Moreover, response is more significant statistically than clinically;

the costs are high; the need for weekly monitoring of liver function is strict; and the long-term efficacy of treatment with tacrine is unknown. Thus, tacrine appears to be useful, if at all, only in the healthy patient with mild to moderate cognitive impairment who is able to comply with close monitoring. Preliminary data suggest that donepezil, a similar agent, is as effective as tacrine but less hepatotoxic; only one controlled trial has been published, however.

Despite the limited efficacy of specific therapy, the physician has a substantial role in treating the patient and family. Important steps, which should be repeated whenever mental function abruptly worsens, are as follows:

1. Discontinue nonessential medications, particularly sedatives and hypnotics.

2. Treat coexisting medical and psychiatric problems such as depression, malnutrition, thyroid dysfunction, and even mild infections (eg, subungual toe abscess). Improvement in these conditions may result in striking amelioration of behavioral and functional disturbances, although the maximum benefit may not be achieved for months.

3. Identify and reduce home hazards, and arrange as necessary for community services. (See Functional Assessment, above, and Summary.)

4. After underlying causes are excluded and environmental manipulation maximized, disruptive behavior should be treated pharmacologically as outlined in Chapter 25, albeit generally with lower doses.

5. An advance directive should be drafted as early in the course of the dementia as possible to allow for patient input in difficult future ethical decisions (see above).

6. Help the patient's family cope with this devastating condition. Legal counsel should be sought regarding plans for ongoing management and ultimate disposition of assets. The family should be told that any abrupt change in the patient's function is due to drugs or disease, not to dementia, and the physician should be alerted. They should be urged to read *The Thirty-Six-Hour Day,* by Mace and Rabins (Johns Hopkins University Press, 1981), or one of the many other useful guides. Support groups such as the Alzheimer's Association often are of great value to the family and help to anticipate problems. Day care centers also involve the patient and provide a family respite. Watch for signs of elder abuse by an overstressed caregiver.

B. Management of Depression: For the hospitalized patient—when correction of medical and pharmacologic contributing factors is ineffective and when there is no prior history of mania or major depression—methylphenidate, 5–10 mg at 8 AM and noon (to avoid insomnia), is often very effective, with benefits discernible in just a few days.

For the remainder of patients with major depression, there is no ideal antidepressant drug. All are about equally effective, but there are significant dif-

ferences in side effects (see Chapter 25). Rather than memorizing a list of medications, however, one should become comfortable using one or two agents for depressed patients with psychomotor retardation (eg, desipramine, sertraline) or agitation (eg, nortriptyline, trazodone); because of its potent anticholinergic and orthostatic side effects, amitriptyline should be avoided whenever possible in older patients. Initial dosage should be low, and dosage increases should be made slowly to avoid serious side effects; low doses of each medication (eg, nortriptyline, 10–50 mg daily; desipramine, 25–75 mg daily) are often effective in the elderly. Careful follow-up supervision is required to anticipate and minimize anticholinergic side effects, orthostatic hypotension, sedating effects, confusion, bizarre mental symptoms, cardiovascular complications, and drug overdose with suicidal intent. Adverse drug reactions should not be assumed to be due to the aging process.

Experience with the tetracyclic agents and selective serotonin reuptake inhibitors (SSRIs) in the elderly has been limited. The monoamine oxidase inhibitors are sometimes of benefit when other antidepressants are ineffective. However, they commonly cause or exacerbate orthostatic hypotension (peak risk at 4–5 weeks) and thus should be used with additional caution in the elderly; they should not be used in combination with the cyclic compounds. Electroconvulsive therapy has been successfully used and is usually well tolerated by elderly patients who remain severely depressed despite drug treatment; however, the addition of maintenance pharmacotherapy is usually required.

[Diagnosis and treatment of depression in late life]
gopher://gopher.nih.gov:70/00/clin/cdcs/individual/86.diag

Carlson DL et al: Management of dementia-related behavioral disturbances: A nonpharmacologic approach. Mayo Clin Proc 1995;70:1108.

Cummings JL: Dementia: The failing brain. Lancet 1995;345:1481. (More emphasis on treatment options than on evaluation.)

Fleming KC, Evans MD: Pharmacologic therapies in dementia. Mayo Clin Proc 1995;70:1116.

Geldmacher DS, Whitehouse PJ: Evaluation of dementia. N Engl J Med 1996;335:330.

Inouye SK: The dilemma of delirium: Clinical and research controversies regarding diagnosis and evaluation of delirium in hospitalized elderly medical patients. Am J Med 1994;97:278.

NIH Consensus Development Panel. Diagnosis and treatment of depression in late life. JAMA 1992;268:1018.

IMMOBILITY
(Chair- or Bed-Bound)

The main causes of immobility in the elderly are weakness, stiffness, pain, imbalance, and psychologic problems. Weakness may result from disuse of muscles, malnutrition, electrolyte disturbances, anemia, neurologic disorders, or myopathies. The commonest cause of stiffness in the elderly is osteoarthritis, but Parkinson's disease, rheumatoid arthritis, gout, and pseudogout also occur in this age group, and drugs such as haloperidol may also contribute. Polymyalgia rheumatica should not be overlooked in the elderly patient with pain and stiffness, particularly of the pelvic and shoulder girdle, and with associated systemic symptoms (see Chapter 20). A normal sedimentation rate does not exclude the diagnosis.

Pain, whether from bone (eg, osteoporosis, osteomalacia, Paget's disease, metastatic bone cancer, trauma), joints (eg, osteoarthritis, rheumatoid arthritis, gout), bursa, or muscle (eg, polymyalgia rheumatica, intermittent claudication or "pseudoclaudication"), may immobilize the patient. Foot problems are common and include plantar warts, ulceration, bunions, corns, and ingrown and overgrown toenails. Poorly fitting shoes are a frequent cause of these disorders.

Imbalance and fear of falling are major causes of immobilization. Imbalance often results from several causes present concurrently, including general debility, neurologic disorders (eg, stroke; cervical myelopathy; peripheral neuropathy due to diabetes, alcohol, or malnutrition; vestibulocerebellar abnormalities), anxiety, orthostatic or postprandial hypotension, or drugs (eg, diuretics, antihypertensives, sedatives, neuroleptics, and antidepressants); or it may occur following prolonged bed rest (see Instability, below).

Psychologic conditions such as severe anxiety or depression may contribute to immobilization.

Treatment

A. Consequences: The hazards of bed rest in the elderly are multiple, serious, quick to develop, and slow to reverse. Deconditioning of the cardiovascular system occurs within days and involves fluid shifts, fluid loss, decreased cardiac output, decreased peak oxygen uptake, and increased resting heart rate. Perhaps more striking changes occur in skeletal muscle with loss of contractile velocity and strength. Pressure sores are a third serious complication; mechanical pressure, moisture, friction, and shearing forces all predispose to their development. Thrombophlebitis and pulmonary embolus are additional risks. As a result, within days after being confined to bed, the risk of postural hypotension, falls, aspiration, skin breakdown, and pulmonary embolus rises rapidly in the older patient. Moreover, recovery from these changes usually takes weeks to months.

B. Management: The most important step is preventive—to avoid bed rest whenever possible. When it cannot be avoided, several measures can be employed to minimize its consequences. Adequate nutrition should be ensured, and the skin over pressure points should be inspected frequently. To minimize cardiovascular deconditioning, patients should be positioned as close to the upright position as possible several times daily. To reduce the risks of contracture and weakness, range of motion exercises should begin immediately and isometric and isotonic exercises should be performed while the patient is in bed. Whenever possible, patients should assist with their own positioning, transferring, and self-care. For individuals confined to a wheelchair, ring-shaped devices ("donuts") should not be used to prevent pressure ulcers, since they cause venous congestion and edema and may actually increase the risk. As long as the patient remains immobilized, pharmacologic (eg, low-dose heparin) or nonpharmacologic means (eg, graduated compression stockings) should be employed to reduce the risk of thrombosis.

As mobility becomes feasible, graduated ambulation should begin. Advice from a physical therapist is often helpful. Installing handrails, lowering the bed, and providing chairs of proper height with arms and rubber skid guards may make the patient safely mobile in the home. A properly fitted cane or walker may also be useful.

In treating arthritis in the elderly, NSAIDs (especially indomethacin) cause more serious gastrointestinal bleeding than in younger individuals, as well as central nervous system side effects with resultant confusion or even hallucinations. Enteric-coated aspirin remains a useful and inexpensive drug, though chronic use can lead to salicylism. For osteoarthritis, acetaminophen may be as effective as an NSAID. Exercise has also proved effective.

Bergstrom N et al: Treatment of pressure ulcers. Clinical Practice Guideline, No. 15. Rockville, MD: U.S. Department of Health and Human Services. Public Health Service, Agency for Health Care Policy and Research. AHCPR Publication No. 95-0652. December 1994.

Bradley JD et al: Comparison of an anti-inflammatory dose of ibuprofen, an analgesic dose of ibuprofen, and acetaminophen in the treatment of patients with osteoarthritis of the knee. N Engl J Med 1991;325:87.

Harper CM, Lyles YM: Physiology and complications of bed rest. J Am Geriatr Soc 1988;36:1047.

Hoenig HM, Rubenstein LZ: Hospital-associated deconditioning and dysfunction. J Am Geriatr Soc 1991;39:220.

INSTABILITY
(Physical Instability, Falls, Unstable Gait)

Falls are a major problem for elderly people, especially women. Thirty percent of community-dwelling elderly persons fall each year, and one out of four of those who fall have serious injuries. About 5% of falls result in fractures. Falls are the sixth leading cause of death for older people and a contributing factor in 40% of admissions to nursing homes. Resultant hip problems and fear of falls are major causes of loss of independence. Nonetheless, they must not be viewed as inevitable or untreatable.

Causes of Falls

Balance and ambulation require a complex interplay of cognitive, neuromuscular, and cardiovascular function, and the ability to adapt rapidly to an environmental challenge. Balance becomes impaired, and sway increases with age. The resulting vulnerability predisposes the older person to a fall when challenged by an additional insult to *any* of these systems. Thus, a seemingly minor fall may be due to a serious problem, such as pneumonia or myocardial infarction. Much more commonly, however, falls are due to the complex interaction between a variably impaired patient and an environmental challenge. While a warped floorboard may pose little problem

for a vigorous, unmedicated, cognitively intact person, it may be sufficient to precipitate a fall and hip fracture in the patient with impaired vision, balance, muscle tone, or cognition. Thus, falls in older people are rarely due to a single cause, and effective intervention entails a comprehensive assessment of the patient's intrinsic deficits (usually diseases and medications), the activity engaged in at the time of the fall, and environmental obstacles.

Intrinsic deficits are those that impair sensory input, judgment, blood pressure regulation, reaction time, and balance and gait (Table 3–6). Although some of these may not be treatable, most are, and since the risk of falling is directly related to the number and severity of abnormalities, correction or amelioration of even a few contributory conditions may decrease the risk significantly. As for most geriatric conditions, medications and alcohol use are among

Table 3–6. Intrinsic risk factors for falling and possible interventions.[1]

Risk Factor	Interventions	
	Medical	**Rehabilitative or Environmental**
Reduced visual acuity, dark adaptation, and depth perception	Refraction; cataract extraction	Home safety assessment
Reduced hearing	Removal of cerumen; audiologic evaluation	Hearing aid if appropriate (with training); reduction in background noise
Vestibular dysfunction	Avoidance of drugs affecting the vestibular system; neurologic or ear, nose, and throat evaluation, if indicated	Habituation exercises
Proprioceptive dysfunction, cervical degenerative disorders, and peripheral neuropathy	Screening for vitamin B_{12} deficiency and cervical spondylosis	Balance exercises; appropriate walking aid; correctly sized footwear with firm soles; home safety assessment
Dementia	Detection of reversible causes; avoidance of sedative or centrally acting drugs	Supervised exercise and ambulation; home safety assessment
Musculoskeletal disorders	Appropriate diagnostic evaluation	Balance-and-gait training; muscle-strengthening exercises; appropriate walking aid; home safety assessment
Foot disorders (calluses, bunions, deformities, edema)	Shaving of calluses; bunionectomy; treatment of edema	Trimming of nails; appropriate footwear
Postural hypotension	Assessment of medications; rehydration; possible alteration in situational factors (eg, meals, change of position)	Dorsiflexion exercises; pressure-graded stockings; elevation of head of bed; use of tilt table if condition is severe
Use of medications (sedatives: benzodiazepines, phenothiazines, antidepressants; antihypertensives; others: antiarrhythmics, anticonvulsants, diuretics, alcohol)	Steps to be taken: 1. Attempted reduction in the total number of medications taken 2. Assessment of risks and benefits of each medication 3. Selection of medication, if needed, that is least centrally acting, least associated with postural hypotension, and has shortest action 4. Prescription of lowest effective dose 5. Frequent reassessment of risks and benefits	

[1]Modified slightly from Tinetti ME, Speechley M: Prevention of falls among the elderly. N Engl J Med 1989;320:1055.

the most common, significant, and reversible causes of falling. Other often overlooked but treatable contributors include postprandial hypotension (which peaks 30–60 minutes after a meal), insomnia, urinary urgency, and peripheral edema (which can burden impaired leg strength and gait with an additional 5–10 lb).

Environmental obstacles are listed in Table 3–7 (this list is also useful to give to patients). Since most falls occur in or around the home, a home visit by a visiting nurse, physical therapist, or physician often reaps substantial dividends and is generally reimbursed by third-party payers, including Medicare. Insufficient lighting is an underappreciated factor in many cases. In addition to the number and location of lamps, noting their wattage is also important since—because of a loss of contrast sensitivity—older people often need twice the wattage to maximize acuity; replacement of 60-watt bulbs with 100-watt bulbs may be quite cost-effective.

Complications of Falls

The most common fractures resulting from falls are of the wrist, hip, and vertebrae. There is a high mortality rate (approximately 20% in 1 year) in elderly women with hip fractures, particularly if they were debilitated prior to the time of the fracture.

Fear of falling again is a common but treatable factor in the elderly person's loss of confidence and independence. Referral to a physical therapist for gait training with special devices is often all that is required. Patients are often reassured by the availability of phones at floor level, a portable phone, or a lightweight radio call system.

Subdural hematoma is a treatable but easily overlooked complication of falls that must be considered in any elderly patient presenting with new neurologic signs, including confusion.

Dehydration, electrolyte imbalance, pressure sores, and hypothermia may all occur and endanger the patient's life following a fall.

Prevention & Management

The risk of falling and consequent injury, disability, and potential institutionalization can be reduced by modifying those factors outlined in Tables 3–6 and 3–7. Emphasis should be placed on treating all contributory medical conditions, reducing environmental hazards and the number of medications—particularly those that induce parkinsonism, orthostasis, peripheral edema, confusion, and delayed response—and strength, balance, and gait training.

Table 3–7. Environmental factors affecting the risks of falling.[1]

Environmental Area or Factor	Objective and Recommendations
All areas Lighting	Absence of glare and shadows; accessible switches at room entrances; night light in bedroom, hall, bathroom
Floors	Nonskid backing for throw rugs; carpet edges tacked down; carpets with shallow pile; nonskid wax on floors; cords out of walking path; small objects (eg, clothes, shoes) off floor
Stairs	Lighting sufficient, with switches at top and bottom of stairs; securely fastened bilateral handrails that stand out from wall; top and bottom steps marked with bright, contrasting tape; stair rises of no more than 6 inches; steps in good repair; no objects stored on steps
Kitchen	Items stored so that reaching up and bending over are not necessary; secure step stool available if climbing is necessary; firm, nonmovable table
Bathroom	Grab bars for tub, shower, and toilet; nonskid decals or rubber mat in tub or shower; shower chair with handheld shower; nonskid rugs; raised toilet seat; door locks removed to ensure access in an emergency
Yard and entrances	Repair of cracks in pavement, holes in lawn; removal of rocks, tools, and other tripping hazards; well-lit walkways, free of ice and wet leaves; stairs and steps as above
Institutions	All the above; bed at proper height (not too high or low); spills on floor cleaned up promptly; appropriate use of walking aids and wheelchairs
Footwear	Shoes with firm, nonskid, nonfriction soles; low heels (unless person is accustomed to high heels); avoidance of walking in stocking feet or loose slippers

[1]From Tinetti ME, Speechley M: Prevention of falls among the elderly. N Engl J Med 1989;320:1055.

Greenspan S et al: Fall severity and bone mineral density as risk factors for hip fracture in ambulatory elderly. JAMA 1994;271:128.

Jansen RWMM, Lipsitz LA: Postprandial hypotension: Epidemiology, pathophysiology, and clinical management. Ann Intern Med 1995;122:286.

Kapoor WN: Syncope in older persons. J Am Geriatr Soc 1994;42:426.

King MB, Tinetti ME: A multifactorial approach to reducing injurious falls. Clin Geriatr Med 1996;12:745.

Lipsitz LA: An 85-year-old woman with a history of falls. JAMA 1996;276:59. (Very useful case conference discussion.)

Province MA et al: The effects of exercise on falls in elderly patients: A pre-planned meta-analysis of the FICSIT trials. JAMA 1995;273:1341.

Rubenstein LZ et al: Falls in the nursing home. Ann Intern Med 1994;121:442.

Studenski S (editor): Gait and balance disorders. Clin Geriatr Med 1996;12:635. (Excellent collection of current review articles on most aspects.)

URINARY INCONTINENCE

Loss of bladder control has a major psychologic and social impact and often contributes to institutionalization. Too often, the patient is simply labeled "incontinent of urine," and no attempt is made to discern the type of urinary incontinence, to determine if it is transient or established, or to provide proper treatment.

Classification
(Table 3–8)

A. Transient Causes: Because continence requires adequate mobility, mentation, motivation, and manual dexterity—in addition to integrated control of the lower urinary tract—problems outside the bladder often result in geriatric incontinence. Although known as causes of transient incontinence, the following common conditions may give rise to prolonged incontinence if not identified and treated. Moreover, since they are associated with morbidity that goes beyond urinary incontinence, each should be carefully sought in the incontinent patient.

1. Delirium–A clouded sensorium impedes recognition of both the need to void and the location of the nearest toilet. Delirium is the most common cause of incontinence in hospitalized patients; once it clears, incontinence resolves.

2. Infection–Symptomatic urinary tract infection commonly causes or contributes to incontinence; asymptomatic infection does not.

3. Atrophic urethritis and vaginitis–Because it usually coexists with atrophic vaginitis, atrophic urethritis can be diagnosed presumptively by the presence of vaginal mucosal telangiectasia, petechiae, erosions, erythema, or friability. Urethral inflammation, which often extends to the trigone, commonly contributes to incontinence in women and responds to a short course of low-dose estrogen (eg, 0.3–0.6 mg conjugated estrogens by mouth; topical administration is more expensive and uncomfortable).

Table 3–8. Classification of geriatric incontinence.

Transient
  Delirium/confusional state
  Infection, urinary (symptomatic)
  Atrophic urethritis/vaginitis
  Pharmaceuticals
  Psychologic, especially severe depression
  Excessive urine output (eg, congestive heart failure, hyperglycemia)
  Restricted mobility
  Stool impaction
Established
  Detrusor overactivity
  Detrusor underactivity
  Urethral obstruction
  Urethral incompetence

Table 3–9. Medications that can potentially affect continence.

Type of Medication	Examples	Potential Effects on Continence
Potent diuretics	Furosemide	Polyuria, frequency, urgency
Anticholinergics	Antihistamines, trihexyphenidyl, benztropine, dicyclomine, disopyramide	Urinary retention, overflow incontinence, delirium, impaction
Psychotropics Antidepressants	Amitriptyline, desipramine	Anticholinergic actions, sedation
Antipsychotics	Thioridazine, haloperidol	Anticholinergic actions, sedation, rigidity, immobility
Sedative-hypnotics	Diazepam, flurazepam	Sedation, delirium, immobility
Opioid analgesics	All	Urinary retention, fecal impaction, sedation, delirium
α-Adrenergic blockers	Prazosin, terazosin	Urethral relaxation (stress incontinence in women)
α-Adrenergic agonists	Decongestants	Urinary retention in men
ACE inhibitors	All	Stress incontinence in women (if drug produces coughing)
Calcium channel blockers	All	Urinary retention
Alcohol		Polyuria, frequency, urgency, sedation, delirium, immobility
Vincristine		Urinary retention

4. Pharmaceuticals–Drugs are one of the most common causes of transient incontinence. The most common agents and their mechanisms are listed in Table 3–9.

5. Psychologic–Especially depression or psychosis.

6. Excess urine output–Excess urine output may overwhelm the ability of the older person to reach a toilet in time. In addition to diuretics, common causes include excess fluid intake (many people believe that 8–12 glasses of fluid per day are necessary for good health); metabolic abnormalities (eg, hyperglycemia, hypercalcemia, diabetes insipidus); and disorders associated with peripheral edema (heart failure, venous insufficiency, drugs [eg, nifedipine, NSAIDs]; and low albumin states [eg, malnutrition, cirrhosis]).

7. Restricted mobility–(See immobility and instability sections, above.) If mobility cannot be improved, access to a urinal or commode may restore continence.

8. Stool impaction–This is a common cause of urinary incontinence in hospitalized or immobile patients. Although the mechanism is still unknown, a clinical clue to its presence is the onset of both urinary and fecal incontinence. Disimpaction restores continence.

B. Established Causes: The established causes should be addressed only after the transient causes have been addressed.

1. Detrusor overactivity–Detrusor overactivity is diagnosed when uninhibitable bladder contractions cause leakage that reproduces the patient's symptoms. It is the most common cause of established geriatric incontinence, accounting for two-thirds of cases, regardless of whether patients are demented. Detrusor overactivity can be diagnosed presumptively in a woman when leakage occurs in the absence of stress maneuvers and urinary retention and is preceded by the precipitant onset of an intense urge to urinate that cannot be forestalled. In men, the symptoms are similar, but since detrusor overactivity may be due to coexisting urethral obstruction, urodynamic testing should be done if prescription of a bladder relaxant is planned. Because detrusor overactivity also may be due to bladder stones or tumor, the abrupt onset of otherwise unexplained urge incontinence—especially if accompanied by perineal/suprapubic discomfort or sterile hematuria—should prompt cystoscopy and cytologic examination.

2. Stress incontinence–The second most common cause of established incontinence in older women (it is rare in men), stress incontinence is characterized by *instantaneous* leakage of urine in response to a stress maneuver. Leakage is worse or occurs only during the day unless another abnormality (eg, detrusor overactivity) is also present. To test for stress incontinence, have the patient relax her perineum and cough vigorously (a single cough) while standing with a full bladder. Instantaneous leakage strongly suggests stress incontinence, especially if it reproduces symptoms and urinary retention has been excluded by a postvoiding residual (PVR) determination or by catheterization or ultrasound. A delay of several seconds suggests that leakage is instead caused by an uninhibited bladder contraction induced by coughing.

3. Urethral obstruction–Rarely present in women, urethral obstruction (due to prostatic enlargement, urethral stricture, bladder neck contracture, or prostatic cancer) is the second most common cause of established incontinence in older men. It can present as dribbling incontinence after voiding; urge incontinence due to detrusor overactivity, which coexists in approximately two-thirds of cases; or overflow incontinence due to urinary retention. Renal ul-

trasound is required to exclude hydronephrosis in men whose PVR exceeds 150 mL; in older men for whom surgery is planned, urodynamic confirmation of obstruction is strongly advised in addition to cystoscopy.

4. Detrusor underactivity–Detrusor underactivity is the least common cause of incontinence. It may be idiopathic or due to sacral lower motor nerve dysfunction. When it causes incontinence, detrusor underactivity is associated with urinary frequency, nocturia, and frequent leakage of small amounts. The elevated postvoiding residual (generally over 450 mL) distinguishes it from detrusor overactivity and stress incontinence, but only urodynamic testing (rather than cystoscopy or intravenous urography) differentiates it from urethral obstruction in men; such testing usually is not required in women, in whom obstruction is rarely present.

Treatment

A. Transient Causes: Each identified transient cause should be treated regardless of whether an established cause coexists. For patients with urinary retention induced by an antidepressant or neuroleptic medication, several options are possible. First, since remission is common in both depression (in 6–12 months) and agitation (within days after an underlying illness resolves), discontinuation of the drug should be considered. If this is not feasible, other approaches should be tried, such as psychotherapy or ECT for depression and environmental modification, reorientation, and treatment of precipitants (eg, arthritis, adhesive capsulitis) for agitation. If medication is still required, substituting a nonanticholinergic agent or one with less anticholinergic effect may be useful (eg, sertraline or an MAO inhibitor for depression; haloperidol, trazodone, or a benzodiazepine for agitation). Finally, bethanechol (10–25 mg three times daily) may be helpful but only if the anticholinergic drug must be continued.

B. Established Causes:

1. Detrusor overactivity–The cornerstone of treatment is behavioral therapy. Instruct cooperative patients to void every 1–2 hours while awake. Once daytime continence is restored, increase the interval by 30 minutes, in an iterative process, until the interval reaches 4–5 hours; most patients who become continent during the day on this regimen become continent at night as well.

For patients who are unable to cooperate, caregivers should ask whether they need to void at intervals designed to preempt incontinence. When drugs are necessary, they should be added to these regimens, selected on the basis of side effects, and monitored to avoid inducing urinary retention. Because each drug except the calcium channel blockers has anticholinergic side effects, each should be used at the lowest effective dose. Oxybutynin (2.5–5 mg three or four times daily) has a rapid onset of action, which also makes it useful for episodic use. Imipramine (25–100 mg at bedtime) and doxepin (25–100 mg at bedtime) have a slower onset of action but require less frequent dosing and are useful if the patient is also depressed; orthostatic hypotension must be watched for. Flavoxate has not proved effective, but dicyclomine (10–30 mg three times daily) has. Although widely used, hyoscyamine has not been subjected to clinical trials. Propantheline, which has the most potent anticholinergic side effects, should be avoided in frail or confused older patients.

In refractory cases, where intermittent catheterization is feasible, the physician may choose intentionally to induce urinary retention with a bladder relaxant and have the patient empty the bladder three or four times daily. Clean but not sterile technique is required.

If all measures fail, an external collection device or protective pad or undergarment may be required. A comprehensive, illustrated catalogue of these aids is available (write HIP, PO Box 544, Union, SC 29379).

2. Stress incontinence–Surgery is the most effective treatment for stress incontinence, resulting in a cure rate of 75–85% even in older women. For women who wish to avoid surgery and who can comply indefinitely, pelvic muscle exercises are effective for mild to moderate stress incontinence; they can be combined, if necessary, with biofeedback or vaginal cones. If not contraindicated, an alpha-adrenergic agonist such as phenylpropanolamine (25–50 mg twice daily) is also useful (but uncommonly curative) for mild to moderate stress incontinence, especially if combined with estrogen (eg, conjugated estrogens, 0.3–0.6 mg daily). Occasionally, a pessary or even a tampon (for women with vaginal stenosis) provides some relief, especially for frail women.

3. Urethral obstruction–Surgical decompression is the most effective treatment for obstruction, especially in the setting of urinary retention; a variety of newer, less invasive techniques make decompression feasible even for frail men. For the nonoperative candidate with urinary retention, intermittent or indwelling catheterization is used; a condom catheter is contraindicated. For a man with prostatic obstruction who is not in retention and who either wishes to defer surgery or is not a surgical candidate, treatment with an alpha-adrenergic antagonist (eg, terazosin, 5–10 mg daily) may relieve symptoms; the 5α-reductase inhibitor finasteride may partially relieve symptoms in one-third of patients, but the onset of effect requires many months to a year.

4. Detrusor underactivity–For the patient with a poorly contractile bladder, augmented voiding techniques (eg, double voiding, or adding suprapubic pressure) often prove effective; pharmacologic agents (eg, bethanechol) rarely work. If further emptying is needed, or for the patient with an acontractile bladder, intermittent or indwelling catheterization is the only option. Antibiotics should be used only for symptomatic upper tract infection or as prophylaxis for recurrent symptomatic infections in a patient using intermittent catheterization; they should not be used as prophylaxis with an indwelling catheter.

[AHCPR guideline on urinary incontinence]
  http://text.nlm.nih.gov/ftrs/pick?dbName=cuic&ftrsK=
    46515&cp=1&t=870279781&collect=ahcpr
[Urinary continence in adults]
  gopher://gopher.nih.gov:70/11/clin/cdcs/individual/71.in
    cont
Fantl JA et al: Urinary incontinence in adults: Acute and chronic management. Clinical Practice Guideline, No. 2, 1996 Update. Rockville, MD: US Dept of Health and Human Services. Public Health Service, AHCPR. Publication No. 96-0682.
Hollander JB, Diokno AC: Prostatism: Benign prostatic hyperplasia. Urol Clin North Am 1996;23:75.
Ouslander JG, Schnelle JF: Incontinence in the nursing home. Ann Intern Med 1995;122:438.
Resnick NM: An 89-year-old woman with urinary incontinence. JAMA 1996;276:1832. (Case conference discussion illustrating an effective multifactorial approach.)
Resnick NM: Urinary incontinence. Lancet 1995;346:94.

"IATROGENIC" DRUG REACTIONS

Older patients are two or three times more likely than younger adults to have adverse drug reactions. Drug clearance is often markedly reduced due to a decrease in glomerular filtration rate as well as reduced hepatic clearance. The latter is due to a decrease in activity of the drug-metabolizing microsomal enzymes as well as an overall decrease in blood flow to the liver with aging. The volume of distribution of drugs also is affected. Since the elderly have a decrease in total body water and a relative increase in body fat, water-soluble drugs become more concentrated, and fat-soluble drugs have longer half-lives. In addition, serum albumin levels decrease, especially in sick patients, so that there is some decrease in protein binding of some drugs (eg, warfarin, phenytoin), leaving more free (active) drug available.

In addition to impaired drug clearance, which results in altered pharmacokinetics, older patients have altered responses to similar serum drug levels, a phenomenon known as altered pharmacodynamics. Thus, they are more sensitive to some drugs (eg, opioids) and less sensitive to others (eg, beta-adrenergic agents).

Finally, the older patient with multiple chronic conditions is likely to be receiving many drugs, including nonprescribed agents. Thus, adverse drug reactions and dosage errors are more likely to occur, especially if the patient has visual, hearing, or memory deficits.

Precautions in Administering Drugs

To avoid drug toxicity in the elderly, the following should be kept in mind:

A. Drug Selection and Administration:

1. Ensure that the symptom requiring treatment is not itself due to another drug.

2. Use drug therapy only after nonpharmacologic means have been considered or tried and only when the benefit clearly outweighs the risk.

3. Start with less than the usual adult dosage, and increase the dosage slowly, consistent with its pharmacokinetics in older patients. However, age-related changes in drug distribution and clearance are variable among individuals, and some patients require full doses. Determine acceptable measures of success and toxicity, and increase the dose until encountering one or the other.

4. Keep the dosage schedule as simple and the number of pills as low as possible.

5. Have the patient or a family member bring in all medications at frequent intervals for reinforcing instructions regarding reasons for drug use, dosage, frequency of administration, and possible adverse effects.

6. Serum drug levels are useful for monitoring certain potentially toxic drugs with narrow therapeutic indices such as phenytoin, theophylline, quinidine, aminoglycosides, lithium, and some other psychotropic drugs (eg, nortriptyline). However, one must realize that toxicity can occur even with "normal" therapeutic levels of some drugs (eg, digoxin, phenytoin).

7. Instruct the pharmacist not to use safety cap containers unless the patient is confused or at high risk for suicide or is living with small grandchildren, since it may be difficult or impossible for the patient to open them.

B. Over-the-Counter Drugs: Adverse drug reactions may result from taking over-the-counter drugs or drugs prescribed for others in the household in addition to those prescribed for the patient. Have the patient or a family member bring in for review all over-the-counter drugs as well as prescription drugs the patient may be taking. All over-the-counter hypnotics and most cold pills contain antihistamines that can produce drowsiness or confusion as well as anticholinergic side effects (eg, dryness of mouth, blurring of vision, confusion, urinary hesitancy or retention). In addition, ibuprofen and naproxen are available without prescription and may cause renal or central nervous system side effects.

C. Sedative-Hypnotics: If nonpharmacologic treatment of insomnia is unsuccessful, short-term use of an intermediate-acting agent whose metabolism is not affected by age (eg, oxazepam, 10–30 mg) may be useful. Avoid both long- and short-acting benzodiazepines because of their increased side effects, including confusion. Do not prescribe an antidepressant as a hypnotic unless the patient is depressed. Exercise has recently been shown to be effective for insomnia.

D. Antibiotics: Serum creatinine is not a good index of renal function in old people. Concentrations of toxic agents excreted by the kidney should be measured directly. (See Laboratory Examinations & Imaging, above.)

E. Cardiac Drugs: Digitalis, procainamide, and quinidine have prolonged half-lives in older patients and have narrow therapeutic windows, so toxicity is common at the usual dosages. In addition, digoxin toxicity—especially anorexia, confusion, or depression—can occur with therapeutic digoxin levels.

F. H_2 Receptor Blockers: Cimetidine and ranitidine interfere with hepatic drug metabolism, resulting in a higher incidence of toxicity of drugs metabolized mainly in the liver (eg, propranolol, lidocaine, warfarin, theophylline, phenytoin). In addition, all of the H_2 blockers can produce confusion in the elderly; none is less likely to do so than another. Since they are renally excreted, however, use of lower doses often suffices and minimizes the risk of toxicity.

G. Antidepressants and Antipsychotics: Antidepressants and antipsychotics often produce anticholinergic side effects in old people (eg, confusion, urinary retention, constipation, dry mouth). This can be minimized by switching to a nonanticholinergic agent or one with less anticholinergic effect (see section on depression, above). Moreover, since both depression and agitation usually remit, consider cautious discontinuation of these agents.

H. Glaucoma Medications: Not only can topical beta-blockers cause systemic side effects, but so too can oral carbonic anhydrase inhibitors. The latter commonly cause malaise, anorexia, and weight loss. Such symptoms may occur independently of the induced metabolic acidosis.

I. Anticoagulants: Age is not a contraindication to anticoagulation, and elderly patients benefit from it as much as younger patients.

J. Analgesics: Meperidine and propoxyphene are associated with a disproportionate risk of delirium. Both should be avoided.

K. Avoid Overtreatment: Drugs are not necessarily indicated in some common clinical situations:

1. Asymptomatic bacteriuria–Antibiotics need not be given unless associated with obstructive uropathy, other anatomic abnormalities, or stones.

2. Ankle edema–Often due to venous insufficiency, drugs (eg, NSAIDs or some calcium antagonists), or even inactivity or malnutrition in chairbound patients; diuretics are usually not indicated unless edema is associated with heart failure. Fitted pressure-gradient stockings are often helpful.

3. Claudication–Regular exercise for 30 minutes three times weekly is useful; pentoxifylline is not.

[Treatment of sleep disorders in older people]
  gopher://gopher.nih.gov:70/00/clin/cdcs/individual/
  78.sleep

Avorn J, Gurwitz JH: Drug use in the nursing home. Ann Intern Med 1995;123:195.

Chutka DS at al: Drug prescribing for elderly patients. Mayo Clin Proc 1995;70:685.

King AC et al: Moderate-intensity exercise and self-rated quality of sleep in older adults: A randomized controlled trial. JAMA 1997;277:32. (Insomnia improved in older sedentary adults who did either low-impact aerobics or brisk walking every other day for 16 weeks.)

Kupfer DJ, Reynolds CF: Management of insomnia. N Engl J Med 1997;336:341.

Mendelson W: A 96-year-old woman with insomnia. JAMA 1997;277:990. (Patient-based case discussion and focused review.)

Rochon PA, Gurwitz JH: Drug therapy. Lancet 1995; 346:32.

OVERVIEW OF SPECIAL CONSIDERATIONS IN TREATING THE ELDERLY

Look for Disease, Not Senescence

Always ascribe dysfunction to disease rather than aging. Remember that 80% of patients over age 80 function well and relatively independently in the community and should not be assumed to be demented, helpless, untreatable, or hopeless. Remember also that the average 75-year-old man can expect to live to age 84 and the average 85-year-old woman to age 92. When deciding on the advisability of various interventions, including surgery, age alone should almost never be a contraindication.

Prevention

Much can be done to prevent the progression and even the onset of disease in older people (Table 3–10). Dietary inadequacies should be repleted; daily calcium intake should approximate 1500 mg, and most elderly people should probably take 400–800 IU of vitamin D daily (the amount contained in one or two tablets of most multivitamins). Tobacco and alcohol use should be minimized, since the benefits of discontinuing these noxious habits accrue even to individuals over age 65. The importance of reviewing all of a patient's medications and discontinuing them whenever feasible cannot be overemphasized.

Recent studies have now conclusively documented the benefits to ambulatory elderly patients of treating combined systolic and diastolic hypertension as well as isolated systolic hypertension. Treatment of either one *substantially* reduces the risk of stroke as well as the risk of death due to cardiovascular causes in this group. Depending on the end point, these reductions ranged between 25% and 45%, more benefit than observed with treatment of younger individuals. It is important to realize that conclusive results were achieved using *low* doses of a thiazide or thiazide-like diuretic (eg, chlorthalidone 12.5–25 mg) as the first step and adding *low-dose* reserpine (0.05–0.1 mg) or atenolol (25–50 mg) daily only as needed. Side effects were minimal, cost was trivial, and concerns about potential toxicity were not borne out. Thus, as opposed to more costly and theoretically preferable agents, the benefits of these inexpensive, time-honored agents have now been established in the elderly, and they should be considered the drugs of choice when initiating therapy.

Glaucoma should be detected, though perhaps best by an ophthalmologist, and visual and auditory impairment corrected. Dentures should be assessed for their fit, and oral lesions beneath them should be detected.

Because thyroid dysfunction is common in the elderly, difficult to detect clinically, and treatable, serum TSH should be measured at least once in asymptomatic older people. Serum cholesterol is worth measuring in those with established heart disease, but in those without apparent disease, screening for hypercholesterolemia is controversial. It seems reasonable to screen those who would be willing to comply with therapy, whose quality of life is perceived as good by the patient, whose life expectancy exceeds several years (long enough to potentially benefit from treatment), and whose other risk factors—for which benefit of treatment has been definitely been established—have already been addressed.

A Papanicolaou test should be done in the 15–25% of women who deny having had one in the past decade; it should be repeated triennially in all older women unless two previous tests have been negative. Immunizations for influenza, pneumococcal pneumonia, and tetanus should be current. PPD testing should be done on residents of chronic care facilities and on others at high risk of tuberculosis; if negative, the test should be repeated at 1 week to identify the remainder of exposed patients, and those who have recently converted (not compared with the previous week) should probably be treated.

Elderly women with breast cancer more often die *of* it than *with* it. Screening mammography is indicated every 1–2 years until at least age 75 and thereafter if a positive finding would result in therapeutic intervention.

The relative risks and benefits of low-dose aspirin and (for women) estrogen replacement therapy have not yet been sufficiently elucidated to warrant their use as routine practice, but these agents should be considered on an individual basis and continued if currently used and well-tolerated.

Exercise should be encouraged not only because of its beneficial effects on blood pressure, cardiovascular conditioning, glucose homeostasis, bone density, and even longevity, but also because it improves

Table 3–10. Suggested screening and interventions for people over 70 years of age.[1]

History	
Physical activity/exercise	Yearly
Mobility decline/history of falls	Yearly
Medication review (including OTCs)	Yearly (five or more medications: quarterly)
Nutrition (↓ appetite, weight)	Yearly
Mood	Yearly
Tobacco/alcohol use (CAGE questions)	Initial, then discretionary
Bowel/bladder dysfunction	Yearly
Driving (accidents, "fender benders")	Yearly
Relationships/sexuality	Yearly
Functional assessment (Table 3–2)	Yearly
Social supports	Yearly
Advance directives	Initial, then yearly updates
Physical examination	
Weight, BP (postural, if on relevant drugs)	Yearly (discretionary at each visit)
Skin assessment	Yearly (immobile patients quarterly)
Hearing (observe, whisper test)	Yearly (check for cerumen if impaired)
Breast examination	Yearly
Rectal examination (prostate cancer, note size)	Yearly
Pelvic examination (women), bladder distention (men)	Discretionary
Gait: "Get up and go" test (feet examination if abnormal)	Discretionary (if ↓ mobility or falls)
Folstein Mini-Mental Status Examination	Initial, then discretionary (yearly over age 80)
Geriatric Depression Scale	Discretionary (↓ accuracy in nonhospitalized sick patient)
Screening laboratory and diagnostics	
Urinalysis	Probably initial, then discretionary
Cholesterol	Conflicting data; discretionary (see text)
Glucose (random)	Initial (fasting blood sugar if ≥ 200 mg/dL, then discretionary)
TSH	Initial, then every 3 years unless clinically stable
CBC	Initial, then every 3 years
Vitamin B_{12}	Probably initial, then discretionary
Electrolytes, liver function tests	Probably initial, then discretionary
TB testing (two-step, Mantoux)	Initial, then discretionary (yearly in nursing home patients)
ECG	Initial, then discretionary
Chest x-ray	Discretionary
Cancer screening	
Mammogram	Every 1–2 years until 75, then discretionary
Pap smear	Every 3 years, stop with two negatives
PSA	Discretionary
Fecal occult blood test, sigmoidoscopy/colonoscopy	Discretionary (see Chapter 1)
Referrals	
Ophthalmologist or optometrist	Yearly, or discretionary
Dental evaluation	Yearly
Home safety evaluation (Visiting Nurse Association)	Discretionary
Immunizations	
Influenza	Yearly
Pneumovax	Initial, repeat every 6 years
Tetanus-diphtheria	Initial immunizations if not received; booster discretionary
Hepatitis B	Not specifically indicated

[1]Many may be accomplished by self-administered questionnaire or trained nonprofessionals using validated instruments, such as the Dartmouth COOP charts, or those listed. See text for details.

mood, benefits insomnia and constipation, and prevents falls; spinal flexion exercises should be avoided in patients with osteopenia, and consultation with a physical therapist may be helpful. Resistance training should be emphasized as much as walking programs.

Measures should be taken to prevent falling, as outlined in Tables 3–6 and 3–7. Counseling about driving, especially for patients with cognitive impair-

ment, remains problematic. All older people should be advised of the availability of a "refresher" driving course offered inexpensively through AARP. In those with a recent history of accidents or cognitive impairment, professional evaluation (eg, through the Department of Motor Vehicles or a local rehabilitation facility) should be recommended until better criteria become available.

But perhaps the most valuable procedure for prevention of disease in old people is to take a careful history, focusing not only on the "chief complaint" but also on common and often hidden conditions such as falls, confusion, sexual dysfunction, depression, alcoholism, and incontinence. In addition, one should always identify the complications the specific patient is at risk for and take steps to avert them. For instance, a patient with cognitive impairment who smokes is at risk not only for lung cancer but also for starting a fire, and a patient who requires narcotics is at risk for fecal impaction, delirium, and confusion.

Provide Prompt Medical Care

Because of impaired homeostatic reserve, older people may present with only nonspecific symptoms or a decline in function, even when a serious acute illness is present (eg, confusion, falls, or incontinence—without fever or cough in a patient with pneumonia). Thus, even mild changes in function in the frail elderly mandate *prompt* medical attention.

Identify the "High-Risk" Elderly

The following patients are at greater risk of rapid deterioration and institutionalization than others and should be monitored more closely:

Those over age 80.
Those who live alone.
Those who are bereaved or depressed.
Those who are intellectually impaired.
Those who have fallen several times.
Those with incontinence.
Those who have not coped well in the past.

Encourage Home Care

Every attempt should be made to allow the patient to stay at home. Some community resources that may be of value include the following: Homemaker (to help with housework), Health Care, Day Health Care, Respite Beds (families who care for elderly relatives at home often require periods of relief from that burden if they are to be able to continue to keep the patient at home), Meals on Wheels, Home Health Aides (to assist with personal hygiene), Transportation Services for the Disabled, and Visiting Nurses. Daily telephone contact, emergency radio systems, and communal and sheltered living arrangements all have obvious advantages in overall management of old people needing care and attention.

Assist the Family

If the patient has dementia or other complex medical and psychosocial problems, the family often needs the physician's support even more than the patient does.

Buchner DM: Physical activity and quality of life in older adults. (Editorial.) JAMA 1997;277:64. (Summarizes results of exercise on insomnia and knee osteoarthritis.)

Corti M-C et al: Serum albumin and physical disability as predictors of mortality in older persons. JAMA 1994;272:1036. (Both functional disability and albumin independently predict mortality, even for albumin levels in the "normal" range.)

Danese MD et al: Screening for mild thyroid failure at the periodic health examination. JAMA 1996;276:285. (Cost-effectiveness analysis suggests that it is worth checking TSH every 5 years, especially in the elderly. Since it also detects mild hyperthyroidism, the test seems clearly indicated.)

Denke MA, Winker MA: Cholesterol and coronary heart disease in older adults: No easy answers. JAMA 1995;274:575.

Evans WJ: Exercise, nutrition, and aging. Clin Geriatr Med 1995;11:725.

Fiatarone MA et al: Exercise training and nutritional supplementation for physical frailty in very old people. N Engl J Med 1994;330:1769. (In a randomized trial, resistance training increased muscle strength, mass, and function substantially, even in this group of nonagenarian nursing home residents.)

Flaherty JH: Driving and older persons. Clin Geriatr 1995;3:44.

Guralnik JM et al: Lower-extremity function in persons over the age of 70 years as a predictor of subsequent disability. N Engl J Med 1995;332:556. (Among functionally intact elderly people, inability to walk quickly, balance with one foot in front of the other, and rise quickly from a chair five times in succession [without using arms] predicts subsequent ADL disability.)

Gurley RJ et al: Persons found in their homes helpless or dead. N Engl J Med 1996;334:1710. (Many elderly individuals become acutely disabled and are discovered too late. Many die and most of the rest require intensive care and often cannot return home. Alcohol and use of multiple medications contribute, as does acute illness. More careful monitoring of such individuals, urging them to move to more protected environments, and providing them with portable electronic alert devices are all potentially useful interventions.)

Kerlikowske K et al: Efficacy of screening mammography: A meta-analysis. JAMA 1995;273:149. (Reduced mortality results from screening women under 75 years of age.)

LaCroix AZ et al: Smoking and mortality among older men and women in three communities. N Engl J Med 1991;324:1619. (Corroborates benefit of smoking cessation for cardiovascular, cancer, and all-cause mortality among people over 65 and probably over 75 as well.)

Marottoli RA et al: Predictors of automobile crashes and moving violations among elderly drivers. Ann Intern Med 1994;121:842.

Martinez R: Older drivers and physicians. JAMA 1995;274:1060.

Mulrow CD et al: Hypertension in the elderly. JAMA 1994;272:1932. (Compared with hypertension in younger individuals, fewer elderly needed to be treated to prevent stroke or cardiac disease.)

NIH Consensus Conference: Optimal calcium intake. JAMA 1994;272:1942. (1500 mg/d for those over age 65, though further research is necessary to be certain.)

Psaty BM et al: Health outcomes associated with antihypertensive therapies used as first-line agents: A systematic review and meta-analysis. JAMA 1997;277:739. (Despite theoretical benefits of newer agents, only thiazides and beta-blockers are proved first-line agents.)

Sarkisian CA, Lachs MS: "Failure to thrive" in older adults. Ann Intern Med 1996;124:1072. (Authors suggest abandoning the term and focusing instead on the evaluation and management of the four interacting components usually present: impaired physical function, malnutrition, depression, and cognitive impairment.)

Yoshikawa TT: Tuberculosis in aging adults. J Am Geriatr Soc 1992;40:178.

Cancer

4

Hope S. Rugo, MD

This chapter covers mainly the clinical aspects of cancer: prevention, diagnosis, primary treatment, management of complications, and paraneoplastic syndromes. Further information may be obtained by calling the NCI Cancer Information Service at 1-800-4CANCER or accessing NCI's comprehensive cancer information database "Physician Data Query" (PDQ) via the Internet. PDQ is also available on CD-ROM. The CANCERLIT feature of Medline is a familiar resource for articles about cancer that can be accessed by author or by subject words.

[Physicians' Data Query: Information on cancer]
gopher://gopher.nih.gov/11/clin/cancernet

INCIDENCE & ETIOLOGY

Cancer is the second most common cause of death in the United States, where over 1.3 million new cases of cancer are diagnosed annually, with 550,000 deaths. One out of every two to three individuals in the United States will develop some type of invasive cancer during their lifetime. Table 4–1 summarizes current United States incidence figures for the ten leading types of cancer. Women have an approximately 1:8 lifetime chance of developing breast cancer, and men have an approximately 1:5 chance of developing prostate cancer. Table 4–2 summarizes the lifetime risk of being diagnosed with or dying from the five leading causes of cancer.

The cause of most cancers remains unknown. Recently, however, mutations in DNA sequences leading to amplification of protooncogenes or deletion of tumor suppressor genes—or both processes—have been linked to abnormal cellular proliferation. Oncogenes encode for cellular growth factor receptors, growth factors, or elements of the proliferative machinery of the cancer cell. Tumor suppressor genes govern regulatory proteins that normally suppress cellular proliferation. The consequence of these and other mutations, which may be due to environmental exposure, genetic susceptibility, infectious agents, and other factors, is cancer. Most tumors exhibit chromosomal abnormalities such as deletions, inversions, translocations, or duplications. Although usually nonspecific, certain genetic alterations are strongly associated with specific malignancies. In Burkitt's lymphoma, the c-*myc* oncogene is activated by translocation of genetic material from chromosome 8 to chromosome 14. In colon cancer, loss of the long arm of chromosome 18 predicts a poor outcome. A gene termed *DCC* ("deleted in colorectal cancer") is thought to be inactivated by this loss. Loss of *DCC* expression is associated with a 30% and 20% reduction in the 5-year survival rate from stage II and III colorectal cancer, respectively, when compared with that from tumors expressing *DCC*. Prognostic markers such as these may aid in therapeutic decisions such as whether to use adjuvant therapy or not; however, altered responses to treatment could offset this potential therapeutic benefit. In the presence of aberrant growth signals, the *p53* gene appears to trigger cellular suicide (apoptosis) as a way of regulating uncontrolled cellular proliferation. The *p53* gene product is a transcription factor that binds to DNA to stimulate the growth-inhibiting genes and a gene whose protein product promotes apoptosis. Mutations in the *p53* gene result in loss of the ability of the gene product to bind to DNA, thereby removing its suppressive effect. *p53* can also be inactivated by overexpression of an oncogene whose protein product binds to normal *p53* and prevents its action. This occurs in many soft tissue sarcomas. Another control against abnormal cellular proliferation has been described that contributes to cellular aging. As a cell divides and ages, there is progressive shortening of the ends of the chromosomes, or telomeres. A striking correlation between cancer and the expression of telomerase (an enzyme capable of preventing the shortening of telomeres) suggests that it might be partially responsible for tumor cell immortality.

It is difficult to link exposures to carcinogens with the development of cancer, since latency is long and

65

Table 4–1. Incidence of the ten most common cancers in the USA in males and females (all races).

Rank	Males	Rate[1]	Females	Rate[1]
1	Prostate	187	Breast	111
2	Lung	81	Lung	43
3	Colorectal	56	Colorectal	39
4	Bladder	29	Uterus[2]	30
5	Lymphoma	22	Ovary	15
6	Oropharyngeal	16	Lymphoma	15
7	Melanoma	15	Melanoma	10
8	Kidney	13	Pancreas	8
9	Leukemia	13	Bladder	8
10	Stomach	11	Kidney	8

[1]Rates are per 100,000 in 1992. Both Hodgkin's disease and non-Hodgkin's lymphoma are included under lymphoma.
[2]Uterus includes the cervix and corpus uteri.

the nature of exposure poorly documented. Environmental carcinogens include chemical carcinogens such as benzene and asbestos, oncogenic viruses such as the human papillomavirus and the Epstein-Barr virus, and physical agents such as ionizing radiation and ultraviolet light.

Hereditary predisposition to some cancers has been linked to events within a gene and is manifested by a strong family history of a relatively rare cancer. Examples include familial retinoblastoma, familial adenomatous polyposis, multiple endocrine neoplasia syndromes, and the hereditary breast and ovarian cancer syndromes. Although familial adenomatous polyposis is a rare syndrome, mutations in the af-

Table 4–2. Lifetime risks for the five most common cancers.[1]

Cancer	Risk of Diagnosis (%)	Risk of Death (%)
Prostate	18.5	3.6
Breast (women)	12.6	3.6
Lung		
(men)	8.6	7.1
(women)	5.4	4.2
Colorectal		
(men)	6.2	2.6
(women)	5.9	2.6
Bladder		
(men)	3.3	0.7
(women)	1.2	0.4

[1]Data obtained from the National Cancer Institute's SEER program.

fected gene (adenomatous polyposis coli; *APC*) also occur in more than 60% of patients with colonic carcinomas and in an equal proportion of patients with adenomas. Genetic mutations associated with an increased risk of developing breast and ovarian cancers appear to be much more common than previously thought and are strongly related to age at diagnosis of cancer. It is estimated that 5–10% of all breast cancers and more than 40% of breast cancers occurring in women under 30 are due to inheritance of an abnormal gene. The risk of ovarian cancer is significantly increased in carriers of these susceptibility genes. A tumor suppressor gene termed *BRCA1* on chromosome 17 has been shown to be mutated in families with early-onset breast and ovarian cancer. More than 100 mutations have been identified in the *BRCA1* gene, making identification of high-risk individuals difficult. Two recent population-based studies found that up to 20% of Jewish women with breast cancer at or before the age of 40 and approximately 10% of all women with breast cancer diagnosed before the age of 35 harbor mutations in the *BRCA1* gene; risk was not limited to women with family histories of breast or ovarian cancer. Inheritance of a mutated *BRCA1* gene confers a lifelong risk of 85% for breast cancer and 50% for ovarian cancer. Compared with sporadic ovarian cancers, those associated with the *BRCA1* mutation appeared to have a better clinical course, with a median survival of 77 months in women carrying the mutation compared with 29 months in controls. Inheritance of the *BRCA1* gene also appears to increase the risk of developing both colon and prostate cancers. Another gene, *BRCA2,* has been associated with an increased risk for male breast cancer. Other less common genes have been identified that increase the risk of breast and other cancers.

With the discovery and cloning of more frequent cancer susceptibility genes such as *BRCA1,* commercial testing has been developed for "screening" using linked genetic markers. Tests for genes linked to familial cancer have raised concerns about the impact of their results on patients. One study has evaluated indications for testing of the *APC* gene. Of the patients tested, 85% were felt to have valid indications for testing. However, only 20% received genetic counseling before the test; only 15% gave informed consent; and in 32% of cases the physicians misinterpreted the results. It is essential that physicians recognize the limitations of these tests and that genetic testing be made available.

Other familial clusterings of cancer have been described that have not yet been associated with inheritance of a particular gene. Evaluation of participants in a study of colonic polyps revealed an increased risk of colorectal cancer in the siblings and parents of patients with adenomatous polyps, particularly when the adenoma was diagnosed before age 60 or (for a sibling) when a parent had colorectal cancer.

Certain viral infections may increase the risk of cancer and clearly have a pathogenetic role, such as the association between Epstein-Barr virus infection and endemic Burkitt's lymphoma. Infection with HIV has been associated with non-Hodgkin's lymphoma, Hodgkin's disease, Kaposi's sarcoma, and cervical and anal cancers. The finding of herpesvirus-like DNA sequences in AIDS-related lymphomas and both AIDS-associated and non-AIDS-associated Kaposi's sarcoma supports a causative role of the herpesviruses in the development of some cancers. The sexually transmitted human papillomavirus has also been implicated in cervical carcinoma.

An additional cause is chemotherapy or radiation therapy for a prior malignancy. More aggressive chemotherapeutic and radiation regimens—and especially those combining the two treatment modalities—have been associated with increased rates of both secondary leukemias and solid tumors. The latency period may be short (2–5 years for leukemia) or very long (10–20 years for solid tumors), but the prognosis is uniformly poor. Chemotherapeutic agents known to cause secondary malignancies include alkylating agents (busulfan, cyclophosphamide, mechlorethamine, etc) and topoisomerase II inhibitors (the epipodophyllotoxins: etoposide, teniposide). Secondary leukemias are usually associated with chromosomal aberrations involving chromosomes 5 and 7 in alkylator-induced leukemias and the long arm of chromosome 11 (11q23) in epipodophyllotoxin-induced leukemias. Abnormalities of 11q23 involve a specific breakpoint region thought to control DNA transcription. In addition, the incidence of secondary leukemias caused by epipodophyllotoxins is related to their schedule of administration rather than the total dose given. Giving the drug several times weekly to treat acute lymphoblastic leukemia results in a much higher incidence of secondary leukemia than does giving larger doses less frequently. Alkylating agents used in conjunction with radiation or in small doses over a long period result in a higher incidence of secondary malignancy than either agent alone or alternative schedules of drug. An increase in the rate of secondary acute leukemia has been reported in breast cancer patients treated with dose intensification of cyclophosphamide in combination with doxorubicin (a topoisomerase II active drug) from 1992 to 1994. The incidence is approximately 0.3% in a multicenter study involving over 2500 women with positive axillary nodes, but the follow-up is still short.

Bhatia S et al: Breast cancer and other second neoplasms after childhood Hodgkin's disease. N Engl J Med 1996;334:745. (The risk of solid tumors, especially breast cancer, is high among women surviving childhood Hodgkin's disease who were treated with radiation therapy.)

Chang F, Syrjanen S, Syrjanen K: Implications of the p53 tumor-suppressor gene in clinical oncology. J Clin Oncol 1995;13:1009. (A summary of data on the alterations of the *p53* gene including implications for pathogenesis, diagnosis, prognosis, and therapy in cancers.)

Fitzgerald MG et al: Germ-line *BRCA1* mutations in Jewish and non-Jewish women with early-onset breast cancer. N Engl J Med 1996;334:143. (Two landmark population-based studies screening for this mutation found a 10–20% incidence in young women with breast cancer.)

Foreman KE et al: Propagation of a human herpesvirus from AIDS-associated Kaposi's sarcoma. N Engl J Med 1997;336:163. (Kaposi's sarcoma-associated herpesvirus can be propagated from skin lesions, suggesting a causal role in this cancer.)

Giardiello FM et al: The use and interpretation of commercial *APC* gene testing for familial adenomatous polyposis. N Engl J Med 1997;336:823. (Genetic counseling was infrequently provided, and physicians may misinterpret the results.)

Hines J, Jenson AB, Barnes W: Human papillomaviruses: Their clinical significance in the management of cervical carcinoma. Oncology 1995;9:297. (A comprehensive review of the pathogenesis of papillomavirus-associated carcinoma and novel treatment prospects.)

Moore PS, Chang Y: Detection of herpesvirus-like DNA sequences in Kaposi's sarcoma in patients with and those without HIV infection. N Engl J Med 1995;332:1181. (Herpes-like virus DNA is present in all forms of Kaposi's sarcoma.)

Olopade OI, Cummings S: Genetic counseling for cancer: Parts I and II. PPO Updates: Principles and Practice of Oncology 1996;10:Nos. 1 and 2.

Rubin SC et al: Clinical and pathological features of ovarian cancer in women with germ-line mutations of *BRCA1*. N Engl J Med 1996;335:1413. (Cancers associated with *BRCA1* mutations appear to have a better prognosis than sporadic cancers.)

Shibata D et al: The DCC protein and prognosis in colorectal cancer. N Engl J Med 1996;335:1727. (Loss of expression of the DCC protein is associated with a poorer prognosis.)

Statement of the American Society of Clinical Oncology: Genetic Testing for Cancer Susceptibility. J Clin Oncol 1996;14:1730. (Recommendations for screening.)

PREVENTION OF CANCER

PRIMARY PREVENTION

1. LIFESTYLE MODIFICATIONS

Population studies suggest that lifestyle—including tobacco use, diet, and alcohol consumption—accounts for a majority of avoidable cancer deaths in the United States. Other factors, including obesity, parity, and length of lactation, have also been associated with increased cancer risk. Although prostate and breast cancers are the most common malignancies in men and women, respectively, the most common cause of cancer death in both sexes is still lung cancer. Since 1973, there has been only a 10% increase in the incidence of lung cancer in men compared with a 124% increase in women, reflecting a marked increase in the number of women who smoke. Since tobacco-related cancers account for more than one-third of all fatal forms of cancer, smoking cessation is an important area for continued education and prevention efforts. Strategies for helping patients stop are described in Chapter 1. Programs directed both at cessation of smoking and at reversing the social acceptability of cigarette smoking have been more successful than programs encouraging cessation alone. In California and Massachusetts, increasing the excise tax on cigarettes combined with an antismoking campaign appears to have resulted in a 2–3% decrease in the prevalence of adult smoking. The molecular targets for carcinogens such as alcohol and tobacco have not yet been identified. However, an evaluation of tumor samples from over 100 patients with squamous cell carcinoma of the head and neck has associated cigarette smoking with genetic mutations in the *p53* gene, thought to result in the initiation or progression of this cancer. This supports the epidemiologic evidence that abstinence from smoking is important in preventing head and neck cancer.

Diet is an important area of intervention for primary cancer prevention. Epidemiologic studies suggest an inverse relationship between fruit and vegetable intake and the risk of common carcinomas, indicating a potential protective role of these dietary components. High-fat diets have been associated with an increased risk of breast, colon, prostate, and lung cancer, though these associations are only suggested, not proved. Evaluation of data from seven prospective cohort studies assessing the relationship of fat intake to the risk of breast cancer provided information about 337,819 women with 4980 cases of breast cancer. No evidence of a positive association between total dietary fat intake and the risk of breast cancer could be identified. In addition, there was no reduction in risk even in women with the lowest intake of fat. Another study compared the dietary intake of saturated fat of 1665 men with prostate cancer to the diet of an equal number of men without the disease. A high intake of saturated fat increased the risk of prostate cancer in all four major ethnic groups evaluated. There was no increase in prostate cancer among men with the lowest intake of saturated fats.

The Women's Health Initiative is a large randomized trial begun in 1993 designed to examine the effects of a low-fat eating pattern, hormone replacement therapy, and calcium supplementation on the prevention of cancer, cardiovascular disease, and osteoporosis in about 57,000 women of all races.

The United States has set two priority dietary goals for the year 2000: (1) to double the consumption of carbohydrate and fiber intake and (2) to decrease fat intake so that fat constitutes no more than 30% of total caloric intake.

Another lifestyle factor with important implications for primary prevention is exposure to ultraviolet light. Chronic cumulative exposure to solar ultraviolet radiation is the major risk factor for nonmelanomatous skin cancer. Regular use of sunscreen prevents the development of precancerous solar keratoses and results in regression of existing keratoses. Protection from sunlight and the regular use of sunscreens should be recommended for the primary prevention of skin cancers.

Bal DG, Lloyd JC, Manley MW: The role of the primary care physician in tobacco use prevention and cessation. CA Cancer J Clin 1995;45:369. (Prevention of cigarette smoking depends not only on cessation but also on lowering the social acceptability of smoking.)

Brennan JA et al: Association between cigarette smoking and mutation of the *p53* gene in squamous cell carcinoma of the head and neck. N Engl J Med 1995; 332:712. (Tobacco use is associated with the molecular progression of this cancer, indicating a molecular target of this carcinogen.)

Feldman EB: Dietary intervention and chemoprevention— 1992 perspective. Preventive Med 1993;22:661. (Strategies utilizing diet and directions for future research.)

Frisch M et al: Risk for subsequent cancer after diagnosis of basal-cell carcinoma: A population-based, epidemiological study. Ann Intern Med 1996;125:815. (An increased risk of cancer has been shown in patients with a prior diagnosis of basal cell cancer of the skin from the Danish Cancer Registry.)

2. CHEMOPREVENTION

Chemoprevention focuses on the prevention of cancer by administering chemical compounds that interfere with the multistaged carcinogenic process. Better understanding of the biochemical and molecular mechanisms of carcinogenesis has made possible the identification of potential chemopreventive agents. Four risk groups have been identified for intervention: (1) previous cancer patients (to prevent second malignancies), (2) patients with preneoplastic lesions, (3) patients at high risk for malignancy (family history, lifestyle, occupation), and (4) the general population.

Chemicals used in chemoprevention must be nontoxic and well tolerated by otherwise asymptomatic individuals. In addition, there must be a method of evaluating the efficacy of chemopreventive agents other than waiting for the development of tumors. Biomarkers such as leukoplakia and colonic polyps are currently in clinical use. Molecular susceptibility markers may become useful; nuclear retinoic acid receptors are under investigation in chemoprevention studies of patients with head and neck cancer.

Anticarcinogens under investigation include factors present within the diet (eg, vitamins, speculated to have antioxidant properties), NSAIDs, and hormone-suppressing agents (eg, tamoxifen). Retinoids, the natural derivatives and synthetic analogs of vitamin A, are the best-studied chemopreventive agents. Data from epidemiologic investigations, from studies in vitro and in animals, and now from clinical trials have evaluated the potential role of these agents as cytostatic agents in the prevention of epithelial carcinogenesis.

Isotretinoin

Retinoids are modulators of epithelial cell differentiation both in vivo and in vitro that are thought to act on nuclear receptors to regulate both cellular growth and differentiation and cell death. Isotretinoin has been shown to suppress leukoplakia, a premalignant lesion of the aerodigestive tract. Effectiveness and tolerability of low doses of isotretinoin have been demonstrated. Only patients with a demonstrated response to high-dose induction (1.5 mg/kg/d) were placed on low-dose maintenance therapy (0.5 mg/kg/d). The disease progression rate was only 8% compared with a rate of 55% in a separate group taking beta-carotene.

In contrast, supplemental beta-carotene and vitamins C and E resulted in no difference in the rate of colorectal adenoma in 864 randomly assigned patients. Colonoscopic evaluation was performed 1 year and 4 years after entry into the study, suggesting that long-term changes in diet are necessary to reduce the incidence of this premalignant condition.

Isotretinoin and beta-carotene have been used in an attempt to decrease the risk of primary epithelial malignancy. Beta-carotene can serve as a precursor for retinoid biosynthesis; however, even pharmacologic doses of beta-carotene do not produce measurable increases in tissue retinoid levels. The properties of beta-carotene as an antioxidant are controversial. Studies have found no role for beta-carotene supplementation in the prevention of malignancy. The Alpha-Tocopherol, Beta Carotene (ATBC) Cancer Prevention Study randomized 29,000 Finnish male smokers to receive beta-carotene, vitamin E, both agents, or neither agent for an average of 6 years. A minimal (2%) and statistically insignificant reduction in the incidence of lung cancer was seen in the men who received vitamin E. In contrast, a statistically significant 18% higher incidence of lung cancer was found in the group taking beta-carotene. Vitamin E supplementation reduced prostate cancer incidence by 34% and colorectal cancer by 16%, though only the reduction in prostate cancer incidence was statistically significant. Men in the control group with higher levels of vitamin E or beta-carotene before the study was initiated developed fewer lung cancers, suggesting that other components of foods high in these vitamins may be responsible for some of the protective effects noted in epidemiologic studies.

The interim results of the Beta-Carotene and Retinal Efficacy Trial (CARET), a lung cancer chemoprevention study targeting high-risk populations, have been reported. This trial involved a total of 18,000 smokers, nonsmokers, and workers with extensive occupational exposure to asbestos. Participants were randomized to receive either a combination of 30 mg/d of beta-carotene (as an antioxidant) and 25,000 units/d of retinol (vitamin A, as a tumor suppressor) or placebo. With an average of 4 years and 73,000 person-years of follow-up, the combination of beta-carotene and vitamin A had no benefit on the incidence of lung cancer. In fact, the active treatment group had a 28% higher incidence of lung cancer than the placebo group, and the mortality from all causes and the rate of death from cardiovascular disease were higher by 17% and 26%, respectively. On the basis of these results, the active intervention phase of this study was stopped in January of 1996, though the participants will be followed for an additional 5 years.

The Physician's Health Study investigated 22,000 United States male physicians randomized to receive beta-carotene (50 mg on alternate days) or placebo. The physicians were treated and followed for an average of 12 years; 11% were current smokers and 39% were former smokers at the beginning of the study. In this trial, no evidence either of benefit or of increased risk for cancer was found, even though follow-up was much longer than in the other two studies. There were no differences in the overall incidence of malignant neoplasms, cardiovascular disease, or overall mortality in the group as a whole or in the smokers. One additional randomized study in which a positive effect of beta-carotene supplementation was found evaluated a poorly nourished population group rather than the well-nourished populations described above. Linxian, China, is an area with one of the world's highest rates of esophageal and stomach cancer and a habitually low intake of several nutrients. In nearly 30,000 participants, the mortality rates from cancer were substantially lower among those who received daily supplementation with a combination of beta-carotene, alpha-tocopherol, and selenium over a 5-year period. A marked reduction in the cancer death rate (13%) was observed in the supplemented group, largely due to a 21% decrease in stomach cancer mortality. Over 85% of cancers arose in the esophagus or stomach, but 31 deaths were caused by lung cancer. The risk of death from lung cancer was reduced by 45% among those receiving supplements, though the numbers were very small (11 versus 20 lung cancer deaths), and only 30% of the group were cigarette smokers.

In summary, there is no evidence to support the use of beta-carotene in the primary prevention of cancer in well-nourished populations. The major criticism of the large studies conducted to date is that increasing one type of vitamin—even one stereoisomer of a vitamin—does not reflect the vitamin content of a diet high in vegetables. In addition, intake of beta-carotene is a marker of increased fruit and vegetable consumption. The balanced mixture of antioxidants found in a diet rich in fruit and vegetables may be more important and more effective in reducing cancer risk than beta-carotene supplementation. Collaborative review of the postpublication results will help to confirm the results described above. Other micronutrients such as vitamin E may prove more promising.

The Women's Health Study, begun in 1992, is a randomized, double-blind, placebo-controlled trial testing the risks and benefits of vitamin E, aspirin, and beta-carotene in the primary prevention of cancer and cardiovascular disease in 41,000 healthy women nurses in the USA.

High doses of isotretinoin have been shown to prevent the development of second primary tumors in patients with early squamous cell carcinoma of the head and neck. This information has led to the development of several trials investigating the role of isotretinoin in the prevention of second tumors following treatment of early-stage head and neck cancer or non-small-cell lung cancer. These trials are nearing completion. Because side effects were observed with high doses, the drug is now being given at a lower dose (30 mg/d) for a longer time after diagnosis (3 years). The major toxicity at higher doses includes skin dryness, cheilitis, hypertriglyceridemia, conjunctivitis, and leukoplakia. These toxicities require dose reduction or temporary discontinuation of the drug. Leukoplakia is reversed when the medication is discontinued.

New retinoids have been synthesized that may also be potent chemopreventive agents. Polyprenoic acid inhibits chemically induced hepatocarcinogenesis in rats and spontaneous hepatomas in mice. In patients with hepatocellular carcinoma, the rate of recurrent and second primary hepatomas is high despite curative therapy with surgical resection and ethanol injection therapy. In one study, 89 patients who were free of disease after either method of treatment were randomized to receive either 600 mg/d of polyprenoic acid or placebo for 12 months. After a median follow-up of 38 months, 27% of patients in the polyprenoic acid group versus 49% of the patients in the placebo group had recurrent or new hepatomas, a result which was highly significant statistically. The difference was even greater in the groups that had secondary hepatomas—seven in the treatment group versus 20 in the placebo group. Toxicity was quite modest (headache, nausea), with none of the side effects usually described with isotretinoin. A newer retinoid, fenretinide (4-HPR), is in clinical trials for the chemoprevention of breast and prostate cancers.

Aspirin & Other NSAIDs

Aspirin and other NSAIDs inhibit tumor growth in experimental systems. Prostaglandin inhibitors can reduce the size and number of colon tumors in rats induced by chemicals or radiation. Regular aspirin administration at low doses (16 or more doses per month for at least 1 year) may reduce the risk of fatal colon cancer. Low-dose aspirin may also protect against cancers of the esophagus, stomach, and rectum.

A study evaluating the use of sulindac versus placebo in patients with familial adenomatous polyposis showed reduction of both the number and the size of colorectal adenomas. The effect was incomplete, without complete regression of all polyps in any patient. After the sulindac was discontinued, both polyp size and polyp number increased. A large prospective cohort study was subsequently published evaluating aspirin use and the risk for both colorectal cancer and adenoma in 48,000 male health professionals over a 4-year period. The subsequent risk of developing colorectal cancer and adenomas was lower in men reporting regular use of aspirin (more than twice a week) on the study entry questionnaire even when multiple other variables were taken into account. In the Nurse's Health Study, 90,000 women were evaluated for the risk of colorectal cancer over a 12-year period according to the number of consecutive years of regular aspirin use (two or more tablets per week) reported on three consecutive questionnaires. There was a statistically significant decrease in the risk of colorectal cancer after 20 years of consistent aspirin use, with the maximal reduction seen in women who took four to six tablets per week. A slight reduction in risk was seen in women who took aspirin for 10–19 years as well. Known risk factors such as diet did not influence this risk reduction. Investigation of the use of sulindac and aspirin in the prevention of polyps in patients with a history of adenomatous polyps is ongoing.

Tamoxifen

Tamoxifen is an antiestrogen with an important role in the treatment of both early and advanced breast cancer. Several trials of women taking tamoxifen as adjuvant therapy for unilateral breast cancer have shown a 30–40% reduction in the risk of developing a second primary in the opposite breast. The Breast Cancer Prevention Trial is a nationwide trial that will randomize 16,000 women over 35 who are at increased risk of breast cancer to receive tamoxifen or placebo daily for 5 years. End points will be the development of breast cancer or death from breast cancer, fractures due to osteoporosis, and myocardial infarction, the latter to evaluate known drug toxicities. The NCI is also investigating the combined effects of tamoxifen and the retinoid fenretinide (4-HPR) in women who are at high risk of developing breast cancer or who have carcinoma in situ.

The use of tamoxifen as a chemopreventive agent is controversial, as the prolonged use of tamoxifen is associated with an increased risk of endometrial cancer; however, more than 50% of women in this study took high doses of the drug (40 mg/d). A current subject of debate is whether the use of a chemopreventive agent can be justified if it prevents breast cancer in some women at the cost of inducing endometrial cancer in others. Additional data are required to fully assess this risk in women taking lower doses of tamoxifen (20 mg/d).

Other Current Trials

Other large ongoing chemoprevention trials include the Prostate Cancer Prevention Trial, which is evaluating the use of finasteride to prevent the development of prostate cancer in men with normal digital rectal examinations but elevated prostate-specific antigen (PSA) concentrations. Finasteride, used to treat benign prostatic hyperplasia, inhibits the enzyme responsible for converting testosterone to 5α-dihydrotestosterone, thereby suppressing prostate cell and organ growth. Eighteen thousand men will be randomized in this 5-year study.

Several additional trials are now under way investigating the effect of dietary intervention on high-risk populations. One such trial is evaluating the role of a high-fiber and low-fat diet in preventing the recurrence of bowel adenomas in patients who have had polypectomy procedures. The polyprenols in green tea are thought to play a role in chemoprevention and are under investigation.

Further information about ongoing chemoprevention trials can be obtained from the Chemoprevention Branch of the National Cancer Institute (301-496-8563).

Greenwald P et al: Chemoprevention. CA Cancer J Clin 1995;45:31. (An excellent review of chemopreventive agents, NCI-sponsored trials, and new agents under investigation.)

Hennekens CH et al: Lack of effect of long-term supplementation with beta carotene on the incidence of malignant neoplasms and cardiovascular disease. N Engl J Med 1996;334:1145. (Results of the Physician's Health Study.)

Khuri FR et al: Molecular epidemiology and retinoid chemoprevention of head and neck cancer. J Natl Cancer Inst 1997;89:199. (Review of the data supporting chemoprevention in head and neck cancer as well as current research.)

Krishnan K, Brenner DE: Chemoprevention of colorectal cancer. Gastroenterol Clin North Am 1996;25:821. (A review of chemoprevention data and research for this disease.)

Muto Y et al: Prevention of second primary tumors by an acyclic retinoid, polyprenoic acid, in patients with hepatocellular carcinoma. N Engl J Med 1996;334:1561. (Oral polyprenoic acid prevents second primary hepatomas.)

Omenn GS et al: Effects of a combination of beta carotene and vitamin A on lung cancer and cardiovascular disease. N Engl J Med 1996;334:1150. (Results of the CARET study.)

SECONDARY PREVENTION (Early Detection)

Given the inadequacy of current knowledge concerning the causes of cancer, effective prevention can be achieved for only a minority of malignancies. Other than primary prevention and perhaps chemoprevention, the most effective physician intervention is early diagnosis. Screening is used for early detection of cancer in otherwise asymptomatic populations. Detection of cancer may be achieved through observation (eg, skin, mouth, external genitalia, cervix), palpation (eg, breast, mouth, thyroid, rectum and anus, prostate, testes, ovaries and uterus, lymph nodes), and laboratory tests and procedures (eg, Papanicolaou smear, sigmoidoscopy, mammography). Effective screening requires not only a test that will detect early cancers—there must also be evidence that treatment at an earlier stage of disease will improve the outcome. Screening for breast and cervical cancer alone is projected to result in a 3% reduction in cancer deaths. For most cancers, stage at presentation is related to curability, with the highest cure rates reported when the tumor is small and there is no evidence of metastasis. However, for some tumors (eg, lung or ovarian cancer), distant metastases occur even from a small primary. More sensitive detection methods such as tumor markers are being developed for many forms of cancer, and some tumor markers, such as prostate-specific antigen (PSA), are already a controversial part of routine cancer screening. Screening is not useful if no method of early detection exists (eg, cancer of the pancreas) or if there is no apparent localized stage (eg, leukemia).

Cancers for which screening or early detection has led to an improvement in outcome include cancers of the breast, cervix, colon, oral cavity, and skin. Techniques for early detection for breast cancer include self-examination, clinical examination, and mammography. There is strong evidence that regular mammography and clinical breast examination in women aged 50–69 or with a family history of breast cancer are effective in reducing the number of deaths from this disease. Currently available data are insufficient to evaluate the effect of screening on breast cancer mortality rates in women aged 40–49 and those over age 70. Some palpable breast cancers (10%) are not visible on mammograms. All clinically suspicious lesions should be biopsied regardless of a negative mammogram. Regular screening for cervical cancer (every 3 years in standard risk groups) with Papanicolaou tests has been found to decrease the mortality rate in women who are sexually active or are 18 years of age or older. Routine screening with vaginal Pap smears in women who have previously undergone a hysterectomy for benign gynecologic disease is not as useful owing to the very low incidence of squamous cell cancers of the vagina. Annual fecal occult blood testing and regular screening with sigmoidoscopy in people over age 50 decrease the mortality rate from colorectal cancer. In addition, removing polyps detected by colonoscopy reduces the risk of colorectal cancers. Even adenomatous polyps 5 mm or less in diameter detected in the rectosigmoid by sigmoidoscopy are markers for more advanced proximal neoplasms. These patients should undergo colonoscopy to evaluate the proximal bowel. Unfortunately, screening for ovarian cancer with serum markers (eg, CA 125), transvaginal ultrasound, or pelvic examinations has not been shown to decrease the mortality rate from this disease. A multicenter trial is under way to test whether a multimodality screening program will be more effective than each of these methods alone. Screening for prostate cancer and hepatocellular cancer is discussed in the section on tumor markers.

Kerlikowske K et al: Positive predictive value of screening mammography by age and family history of breast cancer. JAMA 1993;270:2444. (Predictive value highest in women 50 years or older and those with a positive family history.)

Mackey SE, Creasman WT: Ovarian cancer screening. J Clin Oncol 1995;13:783. (Literature review of the value of serum markers, ultrasound, and ultrasonography as screening tools for ovarian cancer.)

Read TE, Read JD, Butterly LF: Importance of adenomas 5 mm or less in diameter that are detected by sigmoidoscopy. N Engl J Med 1997;336:8. (Even tiny distal polyps can predict advanced proximal tumors; these patients require colonoscopic evaluation.)

Toribara NW, Sleisenger MH: Screening for colorectal cancer. N Engl J Med 1995;332:861. (Excellent review of the mechanisms of carcinogenesis and screening.)

Winawer SJ et al: Prevention of colorectal cancer by colonoscopic polypectomy. The National Polyp Study Workgroup. N Engl J Med 1993;329:1977. (A large retrospective study of the risk of colorectal cancer in patients who had previously undergone polypectomy.)

STAGING OF CANCER

Standardized staging for tumor burden at the time of diagnosis is important both for determining prognosis and for making decisions about treatment. The American Joint Committee on Cancer (AJCC) has developed a simple classification scheme that can be incorporated into a form for staging and universally applied. This scheme is designed to encompass the life history of a tumor and is referred to as the TNM system. The untreated primary tumor (T) will gradually increase in size, leading to regional lymph node involvement (N) and, finally, distant metastases (M). The tumor is usually not clinically evident until local invasion or even spread to regional draining lymph nodes has occurred.

TNM staging is used clinically to indicate the extension of cancer before definitive therapy begins. The manner in which staging is accomplished—eg, by clinical examination or pathologic examination of a surgical specimen—must be carefully documented. Certain types of tumors, such as lymphomas and Hodgkin's disease, are usually staged by a different classification scheme that reflects the natural history of this type of tumor spread and helps to direct treatment decisions.

The TNM system allows a numerical assessment of the extent of primary tumor (T), the absence or presence and extent of regional lymph node metastases (N), and the absence or presence of distant metastases (M).

Traditional staging does not take into account the biology or aggressiveness of a particular tumor and may not allow differentiation of prognostic risk groups. For this reason, specific pathologic characteristics are added into the prognostic evaluation for certain tumors (eg, estrogen and progesterone receptors or proliferative index for breast cancer; histologic grade for sarcoma). As these characteristics become standardized and better understood, they may allow us to identify patients with a poorer prognosis early in the course of disease when the patient might benefit from more aggressive therapy.

Oliver H et al (editors): Manual for Staging of Cancer/ American Joint Committee on Cancer, 4th ed. Lippincott, 1992. (The bible of TNM staging.)

PRIMARY CANCER TREATMENT

SURGERY & RADIATION THERAPY

Most cancers present initially as localized tumor nodules and cause local symptoms. Depending on the type of cancer, initial therapy may be directed locally in the form of surgery or radiation therapy. Surgical excision or local radiation (or both) is the treatment of choice for a variety of potentially curable cancers, including most gastrointestinal and genitourinary cancers, central nervous system tumors, and cancers arising from the breast, thyroid, or skin as well as most sarcomas.

Surgery at presentation has both diagnostic and therapeutic effectiveness, since it permits pathologic staging of the extent of local and regional invasion as well as an opportunity for removal of the primary neoplasm. CT and MRI play an increasing role in noninvasive tumor staging. However, it is often necessary for the surgeon to identify patients intraoperatively whose disease can perhaps be cured by local treatment alone.

For certain tumor sites, complete surgical removal of the tumor can be disfiguring, disabling, or unachievable. Under those circumstances, primary local therapy with ionizing radiation may prove to be the treatment of choice. In other instances, surgery and radiation therapy are used in sequence. For stage I and stage II breast cancer, local incision or "lumpectomy" with axillary node dissection combined with radiation results in equivalent 10-year survivals when compared with the more disfiguring and extensive mastectomy procedure. Preoperative or "neoadjuvant" chemotherapy and radiation therapy allow limb-sparing surgery in osteosarcoma and organ preservation in oropharyngeal cancer, among others.

Radiation therapy is usually delivered as brachytherapy or teletherapy. In brachytherapy, the radiation source is placed close to the tumor. This intracavitary approach is used for many gynecologic or oral neoplasms. In teletherapy, supervoltage radiotherapy is usually delivered with a linear accelerator, as this instrument permits more precise beam localization and avoids the complication of skin radiation toxicity. Various beam-modifying wedges, rotational techniques, and other specific approaches are used to increase the radiation dosage to the tumor bed while minimizing toxicity to adjacent normal tissues.

Well-oxygenated tumors are more radiosensitive than hypoxic tumors. Hypoxic tumors are often bulky, implying a potential synergistic role of surgical debulking prior to radiotherapy. Radiation therapy is normally delivered in a fractionated fashion, this method appearing to have radiobiologic superiority by permitting time for recovery of normal host tissues (but not the tumor) from sublethal damage during treatment. Various normal tissues (particularly the skin, mucosal surfaces, spinal cord, bone marrow, and lymphoid system) can exhibit early or late toxicity from radiation therapy and limit radiation dosage. Fractionated radiation doses are usually administered for 5 days a week until the desired total dose has been delivered, usually over the course of 4–6 weeks.

For most tumor types, there is a sigmoid curve of increasing rate of control of the local tumor with increasing radiation dose. Radiosensitive tumors usually exhibit radiosensitivity over the dose range of 3500–5000 cGy.

Currently, more than half of all patients with can-

cer receive radiation therapy during the course of their illness. Radiation therapy is frequently the sole agent used with curative intent for tumors of the larynx (permitting cure without loss of the voice), oral cavity, pharynx, esophagus, uterine cervix, vagina, prostate, skin, Hodgkin's disease, and some tumors of the brain and spinal cord. For more extensive cancers, radiation is combined with surgery (eg, cancer of the breast, ovary, uterus, urinary bladder, rectum, lung, soft tissue sarcomas, and seminoma of the testis). Radiation is used as an adjuvant to chemotherapy for some patients with bulky lymphoma or lung cancer and for several cancers in children. Occasionally, chemotherapy is used to sensitize tumor cells to the toxic effects of radiation. Radiation therapy for palliation of pain or dysfunction (eg, bone pain associated with advanced breast or other cancers) may improve the quality of life of patients suffering from incurable malignancies.

Radiation therapy has both acute and late toxicity. Acute toxicity may include generalized fatigue and malaise, anorexia, nausea and vomiting, local skin changes, diarrhea, and mucosal ulceration of the irradiated area. Radiation of large areas, especially the pelvis and proximal long bones, may result in bone marrow suppression. Radiation of the lungs, heart, and gastrointestinal tract must be approached with appropriate shielding to avoid toxicity such as radiation pneumonitis, congestive heart failure, or radiation gastroenteritis. Long-term toxicity includes hyperpigmentation of the involved skin, decreased function of the irradiated organ, myelopathy, bone necrosis, and secondary malignancies. Both acute and long-term toxicity are dose-related.

Novel modalities are occasionally used to enhance penetrance into large tumors or to specifically target the site of radiation. Regional hyperthermia (40–42 °C) is an adjunct to ionizing irradiation for some tumor sites. The most useful application of hyperthermia to date has been in superficial or easily implantable tumors as well as in relatively bulky hypovascular tumors with some degree of hypoxia. Electron beam therapy has been used effectively to treat superficial tumors in the skin. Radiolabeled antibodies are currently under investigation as a means of delivering high levels of radiation locally to the tumor bed, thereby avoiding systemic toxicity. Increasingly, the primary local therapy of cancer is integrated with systemic therapy, an approach that has proved to be superior for apparently localized tumor types with a high propensity for early metastatic spread and for which anticancer drugs are available.

Damron TA, Pritchard DJ: Current combined treatment of high-grade osteosarcomas. Oncology 1995;9:327. (Neoadjuvant chemotherapy, limb-sparing wide surgical resection, and aggressive surgical treatment of pulmonary metastases appear to have improved the prognosis in this disease.)

Overgaard J: The current and potential role of hyperthermia in radiotherapy. Int J Radiat Oncol Biol Phys 1989;16:535.

Roach M et al: Radiation pneumonitis following combined modality therapy for lung cancer: Analysis of prognostic factors. J Clin Oncol 1995;13:2606. (Fractionation of radiation doses reduces toxicity.)

SYSTEMIC CANCER THERAPY

Use of cytotoxic drugs, hormones, antihormones, and biologic agents has become a highly specialized and increasingly effective means of treating cancer. Therapy is usually administered by a medical oncologist. Selection of specific drugs or protocols for various types of cancer has traditionally been based on results of prior clinical trials. Many patients are treated on protocols to provide optimal therapy for refractory or poorly responsive malignancies. Treatment may be inadequate or ineffective because of drug resistance of the tumor cells. This has been attributed to spontaneous genetic mutations in subpopulations of cancer cells prior to exposure to chemotherapy. After chemotherapy has eliminated the sensitive cells, the resistant subpopulation grows to become the predominant cell type (Goldie-Coldman hypothesis). This has been the basis of alternating non-cross-resistant chemotherapy regimens.

Molecular mechanisms of drug resistance are now the subject of intense study. In many instances, specific drug resistance results from an amplification in the number of gene copies for an enzyme inhibited by a specific chemotherapeutic agent. A more general form of "multidrug resistance" (MDR) has been described in association with expression of a gene (MDR1) encoding a transmembrane glycoprotein of MW 170 (P-glycoprotein) on tumor cells. This protein is an energy-dependent transport pump that facilitates drug efflux from tumor cells and promotes resistance to a broad spectrum of unrelated cancer drugs. Acquired multidrug resistance in multiple myeloma and lymphoma has been reversed clinically by adding the calcium channel blocker verapamil to chemotherapy regimens. Unfortunately, the doses of verapamil required to overcome drug resistance are associated with cardiovascular side effects. High doses of cyclosporine appear to increase the cytotoxicity of etoposide both in vitro and in vivo, probably by inhibiting the function of P-glycoprotein. The use of cyclosporine to enhance the effect of etoposide in purging resistant tumor cells in vitro from autologous bone marrow is under investigation. Cyclosporine has also been shown to enhance the cytotoxic effect of multiagent chemotherapy against resistant multiple myeloma. Verapamil and cyclosporine increase the accumulation and cytotoxicity of daunorubicin in myeloid leukemia cells, enhancing cell kill. MDR modulators will need to be both less toxic and more potent to be clinically useful. An example is the cyclosporine analog PSC 833, with little of the immunosuppressive effects or renal toxicities of cyclosporine but with five- to tenfold greater MDR-modulating activity.

Chemotherapy is used to cure a small percentage of malignancies, as adjuvant therapy to decrease the rate of relapse or improve the disease-free interval, and to palliate symptoms in some patients with incurable malignancies. In addition, chemotherapy may play a role as preoperative or "neoadjuvant" therapy to reduce the size and extent of the primary tumor, thereby allowing complete excision at the time of surgery. Chemotherapy was first shown to be curative in the treatment of advanced stages of choriocarcinoma in women. It is also curative in Hodgkin's disease, diffuse large-cell and some high-grade lymphomas (including Burkitt's), carcinoma of the testis, some cases of acute leukemia, and embryonal rhabdomyosarcoma. When combined with initial surgery—and in some instances with irradiation—chemotherapy increases the cure rate in Wilms' tumor and increases the rate of long-term control and cure of breast cancer, colon cancer, rectal cancer, and osteogenic sarcomas. Combination chemotherapy provides palliation and prolongation of survival in adults with Hodgkin's disease, non-Hodgkin's lymphoma, mycosis fungoides, multiple myeloma and macroglobulinemia, acute and chronic leukemias, and breast, ovary, and small-cell lung carcinoma as well as carcinoid. Patients with incurable tumors who desire aggressive treatment should be referred for experimental protocol therapy. Tumor cell vaccines combined with immune adjuncts are under investigation as specific immunotherapy for chemotherapy-resistant tumors such as malignant melanoma.

High-dose chemotherapy followed by bone marrow transplantation is curative therapy for various types of leukemia, multiple myeloma, and high-risk lymphoma and testicular cancer. Allogeneic or autologous bone marrow or peripheral blood stem cells with or without ex vivo purging is used depending on the disease. The use of growth factors and blood stem cells has decreased the toxicity and cost of bone marrow transplantation. Autologous transplantation may now be used with low morbidity and mortality on selected patients up to age 70. In addition, dose-intense chemotherapy regimens with autologous bone marrow or peripheral blood progenitor cell rescue are currently being investigated in the high-risk adjuvant or early relapse setting for patients with carcinoma of the breast and ovaries. A small study suggests that intensive doses of chemotherapy followed by bone marrow or peripheral blood stem cell infusion in incurable diseases such as metastatic breast cancer may prolong survival. It is possible that this aggressive approach may be useful even when "cure" is not the objective.

While most anticancer drugs are used systemically, there are selected indications for local or regional administration. Regional administration involves direct infusion of active chemotherapeutic agents into the tumor site (eg, intravesical therapy, intraperitoneal therapy, hepatic artery infusion with or without embolization of the main blood supply of the tumor). These treatments can result in palliation and prolonged survival.

A summary of the types of cancer responsive to chemotherapy and the current treatments of choice is offered in Table 4–3. In some instances (eg, Hodgkin's disease), optimal therapy may require a combination of therapeutic resources, eg, radiation plus chemotherapy rather than either modality alone. Patients with stages I, II, and IIIA Hodgkin's disease are often treated with radiation alone, avoiding the potential toxicity of systemic chemotherapy. A small percentage of these patients may require chemotherapy later for disease recurrence.

Table 4–4 sets forth the currently used dosage schedules and toxicities of the most commonly used cancer chemotherapeutic agents. The dosage schedules given are for single-agent therapy. Combination therapy is used for many diseases, including advanced-stage Hodgkin's disease, non-Hodgkin's lymphoma, and testicular carcinoma. Hematologic or other toxicity may limit the therapeutic effectiveness of chemotherapy. It is possible to avoid the need for dose reductions or delay in therapy by using granulocyte colony-stimulating factor (G-CSF; filgrastim) or granulocyte-macrophage colony-stimulating factor (GM-CSF; sargramostim).

Hormonal therapy also plays an important role in cancer management. Hormonal therapy or ablation is important in treatment and palliation of breast and prostatic carcinoma, while added progestins are useful in suppression of endometrial carcinoma. Women with metastatic breast cancer who show objective improvement with hormonal therapy have tumors that contain cytoplasmic estrogen and progesterone receptors. Antiestrogens (eg, tamoxifen) and aromatase inhibitors (eg, anastrazole or megestrol acetate) that block peripheral conversion of adrenal androgens into estrogens have substantial additive effects to—or may obviate the need for—oophorectomy in premenopausal women whose tumors are estrogen- or progesterone receptor-positive. Hormonal approaches are also available to treat prostate cancer, though androgen receptors remain difficult to measure. These include the use of estrogen therapy, gonadotropin-releasing hormone agonists (eg, leuprolide), aromatase inhibitors (eg, aminoglutethimide), and antiandrogens (eg, flutamide). The use of leuprolide plus flutamide can be considered as an alternative to orchiectomy but also causes impotence. High-dose ketoconazole has been used to rapidly suppress adrenal production of steroids in crises such as cord compression. Use of this agent requires hydrocortisone supplementation.

Several recombinant growth factors have been shown to be effective in the treatment of malignancy. Recombinant alpha interferon has marked antitumor effects in hairy cell leukemia and chronic myelogenous leukemia, moderate effects in lymphomas, in the epidemic (AIDS-associated) form of Kaposi's sarcoma, in multiple myeloma, and as adjuvant therapy for malignant melanoma. Alpha interferon has some utility also in metastatic melanoma, renal cell carcinoma, and carcinoid syndrome. Patients with chronic myelogenous leukemia may benefit from treatment with alpha interferon and achieve both a hematologic and cytogenetic remission. Patients with a cytogenetic response to interferon (about 30% of treated patients) have longer survival than patients treated with standard oral chemotherapy. The addition of alpha interferon to systemic chemotherapy for multiple myeloma appears to enhance the degree of cytoreduction achieved as compared with chemotherapy alone; toxicity is additive. Use of alpha interferon for myeloma following chemotherapy or autologous bone marrow transplant has prolonged remission duration, though overall survival may not be altered. Another cytokine, interleukin-2, when administered alone or in combination with lymphocyte-activated killer cells or tumor-infiltrating lymphocytes, exhibits marked antitumor activity in a minority of patients with melanoma or renal cancer, though its use is associated with marked toxicity.

In addition to cytokines, other agents have recently been shown to be efficacious in the treatment of some tumors. For chronic lymphocytic leukemia and low-grade lymphomas, fludarabine phosphate, cladribine (2-chlorodeoxyadenosine; CdA), and pentostatin (2-deoxycoformycin) are effective. Studies using cladribine to treat hairy cell leukemia have resulted in a high remission rate that is durable with tolerable toxicities after a 1-week course of therapy. Pentostatin has been approved for use in hairy cell leukemia. Paclitaxel is a novel agent isolated from the Pacific yew tree that has been found to be effective in reducing tumor size in 20-35% of patients with refractory metastatic ovarian cancer, though most patients experienced rapid disease progression after an initial response; paclitaxel combined with carboplatin appears to be more effective than cyclophosphamide plus carboplatin in the adjuvant setting. Dose intensification as well as intraperitoneal instillation may also be helpful. The toxicity of paclitaxel is primarily hematologic and neurologic. The hematologic toxicity is dose-dependent and can be ameliorated by the use of myeloid growth factors. Effectiveness has been demonstrated in metastatic carcinoma of the breast as well as in other cancers. Docetaxel, a synthetic analog of paclitaxel, has recently been approved and is effective also in the treatment of advanced malignancies, especially breast cancer. Toxicities are similar to those of paclitaxel. Vinorelbine, a semisynthetic vinca alkaloid, has recently

Table 4–3. Treatment choices for cancers responsive to systemic agents.

Diagnosis	Current Treatment of Choice	Other Valuable Agents and Procedures
Acute lymphocytic leukemia	**Induction:** Combination chemotherapy. *Adults:* Vincristine, prednisone, daunorubicin, and asparaginase. *Children:* Vincristine, prednisone with or without asparaginase. **Consolidation:** Multiagent alternating chemotherapy. Allogeneic bone marrow transplant for young adults or high-risk disease or second remission. CNS prophylaxis with intrathecal methotrexate with or without whole brain radiation. **Remission maintenance:** Methotrexate, thioguanine.	Doxorubicin, cytarabine, cyclophosphamide, etoposide, teniposide (VM-26),[1] allopurinol,[2] autologous bone marrow transplantation
Acute myelocytic and myelomonocytic leukemia	**Induction:** Combination chemotherapy with cytarabine and an anthracycline (daunorubicin, idarubicin). Tretinoin for acute promyelocytic leukemia. **Consolidation:** High-dose cytarabine. Autologous (with or without purging) or allogeneic bone marrow transplantation for high-risk disease or second remission.	Mitoxantrone, idarubicin, etoposide, mercaptopurine, thioguanine, azacitidine,[1] amsacrine,[1] methotrexate, doxorubicin, tretinoin, allopurinol,[2] leukapheresis, prednisone
Chronic myelocytic leukemia	Hydroxyurea, alpha interferon. Allogeneic bone marrow transplantation for young patients.	Busulfan, mercaptopurine, thioguanine, cytarabine, plicamycin, melphalan, autologous bone marrow transplantation, allopurinol[2]
Chronic lymphocytic leukemia	Chlorambucil and prednisone or fludarabine (if treatment is indicated).	Vincristine, cyclophosphamide, doxorubicin, cladribine (2-chlorodeoxyadenosine; CdA), androgens,[2] allopurinol[2]
Hairy cell leukemia	Cladribine (2-chlorodeoxyadenosine; CdA).	Pentostatin (deoxycoformycin), alpha interferon
Hodgkin's disease (stages III and IV)	**Combination chemotherapy:** doxorubicin (Adriamycin), bleomycin, vinblastine, dacarbazine (ABVD) or mechlorethamine, vincristine, prednisone, procarbazine (MOPP) or alternating MOPP/ABVD or MOPP/ABV, autologous bone marrow transplant for high-risk patients or relapsed disease.	Carmustine, lomustine, etoposide, thiotepa, autologous bone marrow transplantation
Non-Hodgkin's lymphoma	**Combination therapy** depending on histologic classification but usually including cyclophosphamide, vincristine, doxorubicin, and prednisone (CHOP) with or without other agents. Autologous bone marrow transplantation in high-risk first remission or first relapse.	Bleomycin, methotrexate, etoposide, chlorambucil, fludarabine, lomustine, carmustine, cytarabine, thiotepa, amsacrine, mitoxantrone, allogeneic bone marrow transplantation
Multiple myeloma	**Combination chemotherapy:** melphalan and prednisone or melphalan, cyclophosphamide, carmustine, vincristine, doxorubicin, and prednisone. Autologous bone marrow transplantation in first complete or partial remission. Allogeneic bone marrow transplantation for young patients with poor prognosis disease.	Etoposide, cytarabine, alpha interferon, dexamethasone, autologous bone marrow transplantation
Waldenström's macroglobulinemia	Chlorambucil versus combination chemotherapy: cyclophosphamide, vincristine, prednisone. Allogeneic bone marrow transplantation for high-risk young patients.	Etoposide, alpha interferon, doxorubicin, dexamethasone, plasmapheresis, autologous bone marrow transplantation
Polycythemia vera	Hydroxyurea, phlebotomy	Busulfan, chlorambucil, cyclophosphamide, alpha interferon, radiophosphorus ^{32}P
Carcinoma of lung Small cell	**Combination chemotherapy:** cisplatin and etoposide. Palliative radiation therapy.	Cyclophosphamide, doxorubicin, vincristine
Non-small cell[3]	**Advanced disease:** cisplatin, vinorelbine **Localized disease:** cisplatin, vinblastine	Doxorubicin, etoposide, mitomycin

(*continued*)

Table 4–3. Treatment choices for cancers responsive to systemic agents. (continued)

Diagnosis	Current Treatment of Choice	Other Valuable Agents and Procedures
Carcinoma of the head and neck[3]	**Combination chemotherapy:** cisplatin and fluorouracil	Methotrexate, bleomycin, hydroxyurea, doxorubicin, vinblastine
Carcinoma of the esophagus[3]	**Combination chemotherapy:** fluorouracil, cisplatin, mitomycin	Methotrexate, bleomycin, doxorubicin, mitomycin
Carconoma of the stomach and pancreas[3]	**Stomach:** etoposide, leucovorin,[2] fluorouracil (ELF) **Pancreas:** fluorouracil or ELF, gemcitabine	Carmustine, mitomycin, lomustine, doxorubicin, gemcytidine. Doxorubicin, methotrexate, cisplatin, combinations for stomach
Carcinoma of the colon and rectum[3]	**Colon:** fluorouracil plus levamisole (adjuvant) or with leucovorin.[2] **Rectum:** fluorouracil with radiation therapy (adjuvant)	Methotrexate, mitomycin, carmustine, cisplatin, floxuridine
Carcinoma of the kidney[3]	Floxuridine, vinblastine, IL-2, alpha interferon	Alpha interferon, progestins, infusional FUDR, fluorouracil
Carcinoma of the bladder[3]	Intravesical BCG or thiotepa. Combination chemotherapy: methotrexate, vinblastine, doxorubicin (Adriamycin), cisplatin (M-VAC) or CMV alone	Cyclophosphamide, fluorouracil
Carcinoma of the testis[3]	**Combination chemotherapy:** etoposide and cisplatin. Autologous bone marrow transplantation for high-risk or relapsed disease.	Bleomycin, vinblastine, ifosfamide, mesna,[2] carmustine, carboplatin
Carcinoma of the prostate[3]	Estrogens or LHRH analog (leuprolide) plus an antiandrogen (flutamide)	Ketoconazole, doxorubicin, aminoglutethimide, progestins, cyclophosphamide, cisplatin, estramustine, vinblastine, etoposide, suramin[1]
Carcinoma of the uterus[3]	Progestins or tamoxifen	Doxorubicin, cisplatin, fluorouracil, ifosfamide
Carcinoma of the ovary[3]	**Combination chemotherapy:** cyclophosphamide and cisplatin (or carboplatin) or paclitaxel and cisplatin/carboplatin	Docetaxel, topotecan
Carcinoma of the cervix[3]	**Combination chemotherapy:** methotrexate, doxorubicin, cisplatin, and vinblastine; or mitomycin, bleomycin, vincristine, and cisplatin	Carboplatin, ifosfamide, lomustine
Carcinoma of the breast[3]	**Combination chemotherapy:** cyclophosphamide, doxorubicin, fluorouracil, or cyclophosphamide, methotrexate, fluorouracil. Tamoxifen for estrogen/progesterone receptor-positive tumors. Adjuvant therapy for high-risk patients and for limited metastatic disease: Dose intensification or autologous bone marrow transplantation.	Mitoxantrone, vinblastine, paclitaxel, docetaxel, topotecan, thiotepa, vincristine, carboplatin, cisplatin/carboplatin, mitomycin, vinorelbine, progestins, androgens, aminoglutethimide
Choriocarcinoma (trophoblastic neoplasms)[3]	Methotrexate or dactinomycin (or both) plus chlorambucil	Vinblastine, cisplatin, mercaptopurine, doxorubicin, bleomycin, etoposide
Carcinoma of the thyroid gland[3]	Radioiodine (^{131}I)	Doxorubicin, cisplatin, bleomycin, melphalan
Carcinoma of the adrenal gland[3]	Mitotane	Doxorubicin, suramin[1]
Carcinoid[3]	Fluorouracil plus streptozocin with or without alpha interferon	Doxorubicin, cyclophosphamide, octreotide, cyproheptadine,[2] methysergide[2]
Osteogenic sarcoma[3]	High-dose methotrexate, doxorubicin, vincristine	Cyclophosphamide, ifosfamide, bleomycin, dacarbazine, cisplatin, dactinomycin
Soft tissue sarcoma[3]	Doxorubicin, dacarbazine	Ifosfamide, cyclosphosphamide, etoposide, cisplatin, high-dose methotrexate, vincristine

(continued)

Table 4–3. Treatment choices for cancers responsive to systemic agents. (continued)

Diagnosis	Current Treatment of Choice	Other Valuable Agents and Procedures
Melanoma[3]	Dacarbazine, alpha interferon, IL-2	Carmustine, lomustine, melphalan, thiotepa, cisplatin, paclitaxel,[1] tamoxifen, vincristine
Kaposi's sarcoma	Vincristine alternating with vinblastine or vincristine alone. Palliative radiation therapy.	Alpha interferon, bleomycin, etoposide, doxorubicin
Wilms' tumor (in children)[3]	**Combination chemotherapy:** vincristine and dactinomycin with or without doxorubicin after surgery and radiation therapy	Cyclophosphamide, methotrexate, etoposide, cisplatin
Neuroblastoma[3]	**Combination chemotherapy:** variations of cyclophosphamide, cisplatin, vincristine, doxorubicin, dacarbazine	Melphalan, ifosfamide, autologous or allogeneic bone marrow transplantation

[1]Investigational agent. Treatment is available through qualified investigators and centers authorized by the National Cancer Institute and Cooperative Oncology Groups.
[2]Supportive agent; not oncolytic.
[3]These tumors are generally managed initially with surgery with or without radiation therapy with or without adjuvant chemotherapy. For metastatic disease, the role of palliative radiation therapy is as important as that of chemotherapy.

been approved for use in treating advanced non-small-cell lung cancer. Response rates of 30% have been observed when vinorelbine is used as a single agent in this poorly responsive tumor. Current studies are evaluating combination chemotherapy, including vinorelbine, in the treatment of metastatic breast cancer and other tumors. Newer experimental cancer therapies are discussed briefly at the end of this chapter.

Berkowitz RS, Goldstein DP: Chorionic tumors. N Engl J Med 1996;335:1740. (Review of the clinical presentation and treatment of this curable tumor.)

Chabner BA: Biological basis for cancer treatment. Ann Intern Med 1993;118:633. (A discussion of cancer biology as the basis of drug discovery research and a review of novel cancer therapies.)

O'Brien S, del Giglio A, Keating M: Advances in the biology and treatment of B-cell chronic lymphocytic leukemia. Blood 1995;85:307. (Fludarabine treatment results in high complete remission rates and may allow more aggressive subsequent therapy.)

Philip T et al: Autologous bone marrow transplantation as compared with salvage chemotherapy in relapses of chemotherapy-sensitive non-Hodgkin's lymphoma. N Engl J Med 1995;333:1540. (Bone marrow transplantation for chemotherapy-sensitive relapsed lymphoma markedly improves event-free survival over standard salvage chemotherapy [46% versus 12% at 5 years].)

Pritchard RS, Anthony SP: Chemotherapy plus radiotherapy alone in the treatment of locally advanced, unresectable, non-small-cell lung cancer: A meta-analysis. Ann Intern Med 1996;125:723. (Fourteen articles with 2589 patients suggested a 2-month mean gain in life expectancy when chemotherapy was added to radiation therapy.)

Rowinsky EK, Donehower RC: Paclitaxel (Taxol). N Engl J Med 1995;332:1004. (A thorough review, including mechanisms of action, toxicity, and antitumor effects.)

Saven A, Piro LD: Treatment of hairy cell leukemia. Blood 1992;79:1111. (Current and investigational treatments of hairy cell leukemia, including interferon, deoxycoformycin, and cladribine.)

Yuen A, Sikic BI: Multidrug resistance in lymphomas. J Clin Oncol 1994;12:2453. (Review of multidrug resistance in lymphomas and status of ongoing trials using modulating agents.)

ADJUVANT CHEMOTHERAPY FOR MICROMETASTASES

One of the most important roles of cancer chemotherapy is as adjuvant therapy to eradicate or suppress minimal residual disease after primary field treatment with surgery or irradiation. Failure of primary field therapy to eradicate tumor is due principally to occult micrometastases of tumor stem cells outside the primary field. These distant micrometastases are more likely to be present in patients with positive lymph nodes at the time of surgery (eg, breast cancer), in patients with tumors known to have a propensity for early hematogenous spread (eg, osteogenic sarcoma, Wilms' tumor), and in patients with certain pathologic or molecular risk factors (eg, high proliferative index, vascular invasion, oncogene amplification). Given specific risk factors, the risk of recurrent or metastatic disease can be extremely high (> 80%). Only systemic therapy can adequately prevent micrometastases. Chemotherapeutic regimens that have been shown to be effective in inducing regression of advanced cancers may be curative when combined with surgery for high-risk "early" cancer.

More data are now available to support the use of adjuvant therapy in several neoplasms. Prolongation of survival times has been shown for women (espe-

Table 4–4. Single-agent dosage and toxicity of anticancer drugs.

Drug	Dosage	Acute Toxicity	Delayed Toxicity
Alkylating agents			
Mechlorethamine	6–10 mg/m² IV every 3 weeks	Severe vesicant; severe nausea and vomiting	Moderate suppression of blood counts. Melphalan effect may be delayed 4–6 weeks. Excessive doses produce severe bone marrow suppression with leukopenia, thrombocytopenia, and bleeding. Alopecia and hemorrhagic cystitis occur with cyclophosphamide, while busulfan can cause hyperpigmentation, pulmonary fibrosis, and weakness (see text). Ifosfamide is always given with mesna to prevent cystitis. Acute leukemia may develop in 5–10% of patients receiving prolonged therapy with melphalan, mechlorethamine, or chlorambucil; all alkylators probably increase the risk of secondary malignancies with prolonged use. Most cause either temporary or permanent aspermia/amenorrhea.
Chlorambucil	0.1–0.2 mg/kg/d orally (6–12 mg/d) or 0.4 mg/kg pulse every 4 weeks	None	
Cyclophosphamide	100 mg/m²/d orally for 14 days; 400 mg/m² orally for 5 days; 1–1.5 g/m² IV every 3–4 weeks	Nausea and vomiting with higher doses	
Melphalan	0.25 mg/kg/d orally for 4 days every 6 weeks	None	
Busulfan	2–8 mg/d orally; 150–250 mg/course	None	
Carmustine (BCNU)	200 mg/m² IV every 6 weeks	Local irritant	Prolonged leukopenia and thrombocytopenia. Rarely hepatitis. Acute leukemia has been observed to occur in some patients receiving nitrosoureas. Nitrosoureas can cause delayed pulmonary fibrosis with prolonged use.
Lomustine (CCNU)	100–130 mg orally every 6–8 weeks	Nausea and vomiting	
Procarbazine	100 mg/m²/d orally for 14 days every 4 weeks	Nausea and vomiting	Bone marrow suppression, mental suppression, MAO inhibition, disulfiram-like effect.
Dacarbazine	250 mg/m²/d IV for 5 days every 3 weeks; 1500 mg/m² IV as single dose	Severe nausea and vomiting; anorexia	Bone marrow suppression; flu-like syndrome.
Cisplatin	50–100 mg/m² IV every 3 weeks; 20 mg/m² IV for 5 days every 4 weeks	Severe nausea and vomiting	Nephrotoxicity, mild otic and bone marrow toxicity, neurotoxicity.
Carboplatin	360 mg/m² IV every 4 weeks	Severe nausea and vomiting	Bone marrow suppression, prolonged anemia; same as cisplatin but milder.
Structural analogs or antimetabolites			
Methotrexate	2.5–5 mg/d orally; 20–25 mg IM twice weekly; high-dose: 500–1000 mg/m² IV every 2–3 weeks; 12–15 mg intrathecally every week for 4–6 doses	None	Bone marrow suppression, oral and gastrointestinal ulceration, acute renal failure; hepatotoxicity, rash, increased toxicity when effusions are present. *Note:* Citrovorum factor (leucovorin) rescue for doses over 100 mg/m².
Mercaptopurine	2.5 mg/kg/d orally; 100 mg/m²/d orally for 5 days for induction	None	Well tolerated. Larger doses cause bone marrow suppression.
Thioguanine	2 mg/kg/d orally; 100 mg/m²/d IV for 7 days for induction	Mild nausea, diarrhea	Well tolerated. Larger doses cause bone marrow suppression.
Fluorouracil	15 mg/kg/d IV or 3–5 days every 3 weeks; 15 mg/kg weekly as tolerated; 500–1000 mg/m² IV every 4 weeks	None	Nausea, diarrhea, oral and gastrointestinal ulceration, bone marrow suppression, dacryocystitis.
Cytarabine	100–200 mg/m²/d for 5–10 days by continuous IV infusion; 2–3 g/m² IV every 12 hours for 3–7 days; 20 mg/m² SC daily in divided doses	High-dose; nausea, vomiting, anorexia	Nausea and vomiting; cystitis; severe bone marrow suppression; megaloblastosis; CNS toxicity with high-dose cytarabine.

(continued)

Table 4–4. Single-agent dosage and toxicity of anticancer drugs. (continued)

Drug	Dosage	Acute Toxicity	Delayed Toxicity
Hormonal agents			
Testosterone propionate	100 mg IM 3 times weekly	None	Fluid retention, masculinization, leg cramps. Cholestatic jaundice in some patients receiving fluoxymesterone.
Fluoxymesterone	20–40 mg/d orally	None	
Flutamide	250 mg 3 times a day orally	None	Gynecomastia, hot flushes, decreased libido, mild gastrointestinal side effects.
Diethylstilbestrol	1–5 mg/d orally in divided doses	Occasional nausea and vomiting	Fluid retention, feminization, uterine bleeding, exacerbation of cardiovascular disease, painful gynecomastia, thromboembolic disease.
Ethinyl estradiol	3 mg/d orally	None	
Tamoxifen	20 mg/d orally in 2 divided doses	Transient flare of bone pain	?Increased risk of venous thrombosis; anovulation.
Megestrol acetate	40 mg 4 times a day orally	None	
Anastrazole	1 mg orally daily	None	
Hydroxyprogesterone caproate	1 g IM twice weekly	None	Occasional fluid retention; rare thrombosis, weight gain.
Medroxyprogesterone	100–200 mg/d orally; 200–600 mg orally twice weekly	None	
Adrenocorticosteroid			
Prednisone	20–100 mg/d orally or 50–100 mg every other day orally with systemic chemotherapy	Alteration in mood	Fluid retention, hypertension, diabetes, increased susceptibility to infection, "moon facies," osteoporosis, electrolyte abnormalities, gastritis.
Aromatase inhibitor			
Aminoglutethimide	500 mg/d orally, along with hydrocortisone, 40 mg/d orally	Initial drowsiness	Transient skin rash, which usually subsides with continued therapy; weight gain, fluid retention, leg cramps; cholestatic jaundice.
GnRH analogs			
Leuprolide	7.5 mg IM (depot) once a month; 1 mg/d SC	Local irritation, transient flare of symptoms	Hot flushes, decreased libido, impotence, gynecomastia, mild gastrointestinal side effects.
Goserelin acetate	3.6 mg SC monthly	Transient flare of symptoms	
Biologic response modifiers			
Interferon alfa-2a Interferon alfa-2b	3–5 million units SC 3 times weekly or daily	Fever, chills, fatigue, anorexia	General malaise, weight loss, confusion.
Aldesleukin (IL-2)	600,000 IU/kg IV over 15 minutes every 8 hours for 14 doses, repeated after 9-day rest period. Some doses may be withheld or interrupted because of toxicity. *Caution:* High doses must be administered in an ICU setting by experienced personnel.	Hypotension, fever, chills, rigors, diarrhea, nausea, vomiting, pruritus, liver, kidney, and CNS toxicity, capillary leak (primarily at high doses), pruritic skin rash, infections (can be severe)	Hypoglycemia, anemia.
Peptide hormone inhibitor			
Octreotide acetate	100–600 µg/d SC in 2 divided doses	Local irritant; nausea and vomiting	Diarrhea, abdominal pain, hypoglycemia.
Natural products and miscellaneous agents			
Vinblastine	0.1–0.2 mg/kg or 6 mg/m^2 IV weekly	Mild nausea and vomiting; severe vesicant	Alopecia, peripheral neuropathy, bone marrow suppression, constipation, SIADH, areflexia.

(*continued*)

Table 4–4 Single-agent dosage and toxicity of anticancer drugs. (continued)

Drug	Dosage	Acute Toxicity	Delayed Toxicity
Vincristine	1.5 mg/m² (maximum: 2 mg weekly)	Severe vesicant	Areflexia, muscle weakness, peripheral neuropathy, paralytic ileus, alopecia (see text), SIADH.
Vinorelbine	30 mg/m² IV weekly	Mild nausea and vomiting, fatigue, severe vesicant	Granulocytopenia, constipation, peripheral neuropathy, alopecia.
Paclitaxel	135 mg/m² by continuous infusion over 24 hours every 3 weeks	Hypersensitivity reaction (premedicate with diphenhydramine and dexamethasone), mild nausea and vomiting	Peripheral neuropathy, bone marrow suppression, fluid retention.
Docetaxel	60–100 mg/m² IV every 3 weeks		
Dactinomycin	0.04 mg/kg IV weekly	Nausea and vomiting; severe vesicant	Alopecia, stomatitis, diarrhea, bone marrow suppression.
Daunorubicin	30–60 mg/m² daily IV for 3 days or 30–60 mg/m² IV weekly	Nausea, fever, red urine (not hematuria); severe vesicant; acute cardiotoxicity	Alopecia, stomatitis, bone marrow suppression, late cardiotoxicity. Risk of cardiotoxicity increases with radiation, cyclophosphamide.
Idarubicin	12 mg/m² daily IV for 3 days		
Doxorubicin	60 mg/m² IV every 3 weeks to a maximum total dose of 550 mg/m²		
Liposomal Doxorubicin	20 mg/m² IV every 3 weeks		
Daunorubicin	40 mg/m² IV every 2 weeks		
Etoposide	100 mg/m²/d IV for 5 days or 50–150 mg/d orally	Nausea and vomiting; occasionally hypotension	Alopecia, bone marrow suppression.
Plicamycin (mithramycin)	25–50 µg/kg IV every other day for up to 8 doses	Nausea and vomiting	Thrombocytopenia, diarrhea, hepatotoxicity, nephrotoxicity, stomatitis.
Mitomycin	10–20 mg/m² every 6–8 weeks	Severe vesicant; nausea	Prolonged bone marrow suppression, rare hemolytic-uremic syndrome.
Mitoxantrone	12–15 mg/m²/d IV for 3 days with cytarabine; 8–12 mg/m² IV every 3 weeks	Mild nausea and vomiting	Alopecia, mild mucositis, bone marrow suppression.
Bleomycin	Up to 15 units/m² IM, IV, or SC twice weekly to a total dose of 200 units/m²	Allergic reactions, fever, hypotension	Fever, dermatitis, pulmonary fibrosis.
Hydroxyurea	500–1500 mg/d orally	Mild nausea and vomiting	Hyperpigmentation, bone marrow suppression.
Mitotane	6–12 g/d orally	Nausea and vomiting	Dermatitis, diarrhea, mental suppression, muscle tremors.
Fludarabine	25 mg/m²/d IV for 5 days every 4 weeks	Nausea and vomiting	Bone marrow suppression, diarrhea, mild hepatotoxicity, immune suppression.
Cladribine (CdA)	0.09 mg/kg/d by continuous IV infusion for 7 days	Mild nausea, rash, fatigue	Bone marrow suppression, fever, immune suppression.
Topotecan	1.5 g/kg IV daily for 5 days every 3 weeks	Nausea, vomiting, diarrhea, headache, dyspnea	Alopecia, bone marrow suppression.
Tretinoin	45 mg/m² by mouth until remission or for 90 days	Retinoic acid syndrome (fever, dyspnea, pleural or pericardial effusion) must be treated emergently with dexamethasone; headache, dry skin rash, flushing.	

(continued)

Table 4–4. Single-agent dosage and toxicity of anticancer drugs. (continued)

Drug	Dosage	Acute Toxicity	Delayed Toxicity
Gemcitabine	1000 mg/m^2 every week up to 7 weeks, then 1 week off, then weekly for 3 out of 4 weeks	Nausea, vomiting, diarrhea, fever, dyspnea	Bone marrow suppression, rash, fluid retention, mouth sores, flu-like symptoms, paresthesias.
Supportive agents Allopurinol	300–900 mg/d orally for prevention or relief of hyperuricemia	None	Rash, Stevens-Johnson syndrome; enhances effects and toxicity of mercaptopurine when used in combination.
Mesna	20% of ifosfamide dosage at the time of ifosfamide administration, then 4 and 8 hours after each dose of chemotherapy to prevent hemorrhagic cystitis	Nausea, vomiting, diarrhea	None
Leucovorin	10 mg/m^2 every 6 hours IV or orally until serum methotrexate levels are below 5×10^{-8} mol/L with hydration and urinary alkalinization (about 72 hours)	None	Enhances toxic effects of fluorouracil.
Amifostine	910 mg/m^2 IV daily, 30 minutes prior to chemotherapy	Hypotension, nausea, vomiting, flushing	Decrease in serum calcium.
Dexrazoxanee	10:1 ratio of anthracycline IV, before (within 30 minutes of) chemotherapy infusion	Pain on injection	Increased bone marrow suppression.
Pilocarpine hydrochloride	5–10 mg orally 3 times daily	Sweating, headache, flushing; nausea, chills, rhinitis, dizziness, and urinary frequency at high dosage	
Pamidronate	90 mg IV every month	Symptomatic hypoglycemia (rare), flare of bone pain, local irritation	None
Epoetin alfa (erythropoietin)	100–300 units/kg IV or SC 3 times a week	Skin irritation or pain at injection site	Hypertension, headache, seizures in patients on dialysis (rare).
Filgrastim (G-CSF)	5 μg/kg/d SC or IV	Mild to moderate bone pain, mild hypotension (rare), irritation at injection sites (rare)	?Unknown risk of tumor cell stimulation.
Sargramostim (GM-CSF)	250 μg/kg/d as a 2-hour IV infusion (can be given SC)	Fluid retention, dyspnea, capillary leak (rare), supraventricular tachycardia (rare), mild to moderate bone pain, irritation at injection sites	

cially premenopausal women) with breast cancer and positive or negative axillary lymph nodes (stages I, II, and III) from combination chemotherapy following surgical resection; there are several useful regimens. Node-negative patients are treated with CMF (cyclophosphamide, methotrexate, and fluorouracil) or variants, whereas high-risk, node-positive patients are generally treated with regimens that include dox-

orubicin. Neoadjuvant (preoperative) and perioperative chemotherapy are also used and may improve surgical resectability or time to disease progression. The antiestrogen tamoxifen is used routinely either with or without antecedent chemotherapy if receptors for estrogen and progesterone are present. The role of amplification of the c-*erb*B-2 or Her-2/*neu* oncogene in tamoxifen-resistant breast cancer is a subject of current research. In postmenopausal women, tamoxifen alone may be used. The main challenge in treating women with node-negative (stage I) breast cancer is to identify prognostic factors to determine which patients are at higher risk and therefore more likely to benefit from adjuvant therapy.

Adjuvant chemotherapy with fluorouracil plus levamisole is now indicated in Dukes C (node-positive) colon cancer and has been shown to reduce the risk of cancer recurrence. Earlier clinical trials employing semustine (methyl-CCNU) appeared to result in an increased risk of both leukemia and renal insufficiency. The omission of semustine from combination regimens still results in enhanced cure rates with decreased local and overall tumor recurrence.

Other tumors that have been shown to respond to adjuvant therapy include osteogenic sarcoma, ovarian cancer, and malignant melanoma. Adjuvant therapy remains investigational and unproved for a number of common tumors, including non-small-cell lung cancer and pancreatic cancer. Patients with Hodgkin's disease or testicular carcinoma do not benefit from adjuvant therapy.

Although adjuvant therapy has been shown to reduce the rate of recurrence for some cancers, there is still a high failure rate (up to 80% in high-risk breast cancer despite adjuvant therapy). In most cases, tumor recurrence signifies incurability. There is clear evidence of a dose-response effect of adjuvant chemotherapy in some cancers; however, doses have been limited by bone marrow toxicity. Current studies are investigating the use of dose-intense chemotherapy regimens with or without autologous bone marrow or peripheral blood progenitor cell rescue in the high-risk adjuvant setting for patients with carcinoma of the breast, testis, and ovaries. Otherwise incurable patients with testicular cancer have been cured by this intensive treatment approach. Nonrandomized studies suggest efficacy with tolerable side effects of high-dose chemotherapy with stem cell support in the setting of high-risk breast cancer (more than ten positive lymph nodes). Multicenter trials are now in progress comparing aggressive adjuvant chemotherapy with autologous bone marrow transplantation for high-risk breast cancer. The use of marrow transplantation for high-risk ovarian cancer remains controversial, though long-lived responses in otherwise incurable patients have been documented. Patients with advanced ovarian cancer at high risk for recurrence may now be considered for treatment in a multicenter randomized study comparing transplantation with standard adjuvant chemotherapy. Young patients with high-risk malignancies should be considered for entry into clinical trials investigating this aggressive, potentially curable therapy.

[Physicians' Data query: Information on cancer treatment]
  gopher://gopher.nih.gov.11/clin/cancernet
Bonadonna G et al: Adjuvant cyclophosphamide, methotrexate, and fluorouracil in node-positive breast cancer: The results of 20 years of follow-up. N Engl J Med 1995;332:901. (Long-term improvement in survival in patients with node-positive breast cancer randomized to receive adjuvant chemotherapy following mastectomy.)
Cannistra SA: Cancer of the ovary. N Engl J Med 1993;329:1550. (A review of risk factors, presentation, staging, surgical treatment and chemotherapy, and prognosis.)
Gradishar WJ, Tallman MF, Abrams JS: High-dose chemotherapy for breast cancer. Ann Intern Med 1996;125:599. (A review of this controversial but widely used therapy.)
Moerttel CG: Chemotherapy for colorectal cancer. N Engl J Med 1994;330:1136.
Trimble EL et al: Neoadjuvant therapy in cancer treatment. Cancer 1993;72:3515. (Increasing indications.)

TOXICITY & DOSE MODIFICATION OF CHEMOTHERAPEUTIC AGENTS

A number of cancer chemotherapeutic agents have cytotoxic effects on rapidly proliferating normal cells in bone marrow, mucosa, and skin. Still other drugs such as the vinca alkaloids produce neuropathy, and hormones often have psychologic effects. Acute and chronic toxicities of the various drugs are summarized in Table 4–4. Appropriate dose modification usually minimizes these side effects, so that therapy can be continued with relative safety.

Bone Marrow Toxicity

Depression of bone marrow is usually the most serious limiting toxicity of cancer chemotherapy. Autologous bone marrow or peripheral blood progenitor cell transplantation or rescue can reduce the myelosuppressive toxicity of high-dose chemotherapy; however, cost and toxicity limit its general use. Growth factors that stimulate myeloid proliferation (eg, granulocyte colony-stimulating factor [G-CSF; filgrastim] and granulocyte-macrophage stimulating factor [GM-CSF; sargramostim) or erythroid proliferation (erythropoietin [epoetin alfa]) are now used to ameliorate bone marrow toxicity. G-CSF and GM-CSF have been shown to shorten the period of neutropenia following both standard and high-dose chemotherapy. Mucosal toxicity is also reduced. The myeloid growth factors are also used to stimulate circulation of progenitor cells in the peripheral blood either at steady state or during white blood cell recovery following myelosuppressive chemotherapy. These cells are then harvested using an apheresis machine and frozen for later use. When stimulated peripheral blood progenitor cells are used instead of or in conjunction with bone marrow for autologous transplantation following high-dose chemotherapy and radiotherapy, recovery of both neutrophils and platelets may be hastened by as much as 7–10 days as opposed to the use of bone marrow alone.

Epoetin alfa (erythropoietin) has been shown to improve anemia associated with malignancy. Patients must have adequate iron stores to respond to this agent, and even patients with marrow infiltration with tumor may benefit. Higher doses are necessary for patients with cancer than for patients with renal failure (100–150 units/kg compared with 50 units/kg). It is useful to check the level of erythropoietin before instituting therapy. Very high levels (> 500 ng/mL) predict a poor response. Erythropoietin is usually given by subcutaneous injection three times a week.

Thrombocytopenia remains a problem with high doses of or prolonged exposure to chemotherapeutic agents and may limit therapy. Several agents may help with this problem. Interleukin-3 stimulates myeloid growth and, to a lesser extent, platelet recovery. The megakaryocyte growth factor thrombopoietin has been cloned and is the subject of intense study. Clinical trials using thrombopoietin in a variety of circumstances are under way.

Commonly used short-acting drugs that affect the bone marrow are the alkylating agents (eg, cyclophosphamide, melphalan, chlorambucil), procarbazine, mercaptopurine, methotrexate, vinblastine, fluorouracil, dactinomycin, and doxorubicin. In general, it is preferable to use alkylating agents in intensive "pulse" courses every 3–4 weeks rather than to administer the drugs in continuous daily schedules. This allows for complete hematologic (and immunologic) recovery between courses rather than continuously suppressing the bone marrow with a cytotoxic agent. Pulse therapy reduces side effects to some degree but does not reduce therapeutic efficacy. The standard dosage schedules required to produce tumor responses with these agents often induce bone marrow depression. Continuing some drugs in the face of falling blood counts may result in severe bone marrow aplasia with pancytopenia, bleeding, or infection. Simple guidelines for treatment and follow-up can usually prevent severe marrow depression.

With long-term chemotherapy, counts should be obtained initially at weekly intervals; the frequency of counts may be reduced only after the patient's sensitivity to the drug can be well predicted (eg, 3–4 months) and cumulative toxicity excluded.

In patients with normal blood counts as well as normal liver and kidney function, drugs should be started in full dosages. Bone marrow toxicity is cumulative over time, and this must be anticipated during follow-up. Patients with bone marrow involvement may tolerate chemotherapy poorly initially, with improved counts on future cycles as the tumor burden is reduced.

Drug dosage can usually be modified as a function of the peripheral white blood count or platelet count (or both). These modifications assume that the blood counts are checked shortly before the next course of chemotherapy is to be administered. Dosage modifications are used primarily for repeated courses of oral alkylator or antimetabolite therapy but should be avoided when possible if treatment is given with curative intent. A scheme for dosage modification is presented in Table 4–5. Alternatively, the interval between drug courses can be lengthened, thereby permitting more complete hematologic recovery and repetition of full-dose chemotherapy. Both dosage modification and delay of chemotherapy limit the efficacy of treatment.

ASCO Ad Hoc Colony-Stimulating Factor Guideline Expert Panel: American Society of Clinical Oncology recommendations for the use of hematopoietic colony-stimulating factors: Evidence-based clinical practice guidelines. J Clin Oncol 1994;12:2471. (Standard practice guidelines.)

Kaushansky K: Thrombopoietin: The primary regulator of megakaryocyte and platelet production. Thromb Haemost 1995;74:521. (A review of current preclinical data.)

Vose JM, Armitage JO: Clinical applications of hematopoietic growth factors. J Clin Oncol 1995;13:1023.

Chemotherapy-Induced Nausea & Vomiting

A number of cytotoxic anticancer drugs induce nausea and vomiting. In general, these symptoms are thought to originate in the central nervous system rather than peripherally. Parenteral administration of agents such as doxorubicin, etoposide, or cyclophosphamide frequently is associated with mild to moderate nausea and vomiting, whereas nitrosoureas, dacarbazine, and particularly cisplatin usually cause severe symptoms. Combination chemotherapy can also cause severe symptoms. Antiemetics clearly reduce and often eliminate nausea and vomiting associated with these drugs and are especially useful in conjunction with cisplatin.

Metoclopramide is a particularly useful agent, especially when administered parenterally at a dosage of 1–2 mg/kg both 30 minutes before and again 30 minutes after the administration of chemotherapy. Extrapyramidal signs may be induced with this drug but frequently can be suppressed with 25–50 mg of oral or parenteral diphenhydramine. Dexamethasone

Table 4–5. A common scheme for dose modification of cancer chemotherapeutic agents.[1]

Granulocyte Count	Platelet Count	Suggested Dosage (% of Full Dose)
>2000/µL	>100,000/µL	100%
1000–2000/µL	75,000–100,000/µL	50%
<1000/µL	<50,000/µL	0%

[1]In general, dose modification should be avoided if full recovery is expected within 1–2 weeks. Chemotherapy can be delayed and given after recovery at full dosage to maintain therapeutic efficacy.

has antiemetic effects when administered at a dosage of 6–10 mg either as a single dose prior to or both prior to and every 6 hours following the administration of chemotherapy for two to four total doses. Both of these drugs are more potent than conventional agents such as prochlorperazine, diphenhydramine, and thiethylperazine. Prochlorperazine is given at a dose of 10 mg orally or intravenously every 6 hours. The total dose given over 24 hours should not exceed 40 mg. A 25 mg rectal suppository is available and may be useful for patients who are too nauseated to swallow pills without experiencing further emesis. Unfortunately, all phenothiazines can induce extrapyramidal side effects. Thiethylperazine is given at a dose of 10 mg every 8 hours by mouth and is also available at the same dose in a rectal suppository. Lorazepam has both antiemetic and sedating effects and is administered at a dose of 0.5–1 mg every 4–6 hours by the sublingual route, making it particularly useful in the outpatient setting. Older patients may have intolerable psychologic side effects. Combinations of antiemetics (eg, metoclopramide with dexamethasone and lorazepam) are often more effective than maximal doses of any one agent for blocking cisplatin-induced vomiting.

5-Hydroxytryptamine-3 receptor antagonists (ondansetron, granisetron) have now replaced high-dose metoclopramide in the treatment and prevention of emesis. A new and very potent class of antiemetics, these drugs are serotonin receptor-blocking agents that have few side effects. They are both more effective and less toxic than metoclopramide in cisplatin-treated patients. They are also effective against radiation-induced and postanesthetic vomiting as well as for patients with refractory nausea and vomiting following administration of other chemotherapeutic agents. Ondansetron is administered by the parenteral route at a dose of 0.15 mg/kg for three doses or orally at a dose of 8 mg every 8 hours. The first dose is given 30 minutes before the start of chemotherapy; subsequent doses are given 4 and 8 hours after the first dose. A typical antiemetic regimen might include ondansetron combined with 0.5–1 mg of lorazepam (sublingual) or 10 mg of prochlorperazine orally or intravenously and dexamethasone (10 mg orally), omitting both metoclopramide and diphenhydramine. For less emetogenic regimens, ondansetron alone may be no more effective than metoclopramide and dexamethasone and is usually used only for failure to control nausea with less expensive combination regimens. Granisetron is a long-acting serotonin receptor antagonist that is given as a single dose of 10 µg/kg intravenously 30 minutes before chemotherapy or orally at a dosage of 1–2 mg/d. The half-life of granisetron is 9 hours, and 24-hour dosing is recommended by the manufacturer. Ondansetron may also be effective in a single daily parenteral dose of 32 mg. Both agents appear to be more effective when given in conjunction with dexamethasone.

Dronabinol (Δ^9-tetrahydrocannabinol) is effective in some patients at a dose of 5 mg/m^2 prior to and then every 2–4 hours following chemotherapy for a total of four to six doses a day. Dronabinol may cause undesirable side effects such as dysphoria, and it is available only for oral administration. A patient receiving antiemetics (eg, lorazepam, prochlorperazine, metoclopramide) along with chemotherapy on an outpatient basis must be escorted to and from the clinic, since the antiemetics often induce marked sedation and transient impairment of balance and reflexes. Antiemetics are more effective when given prophylactically. Therefore, regular dosing of an agent such as lorazepam or prochlorperazine is recommended after chemotherapy until the emetogenic effects have dissipated. This is dependent on the patient as well as on the type of chemotherapy administered. One problem with all combinations of antiemetic agents is the development of tachyphylaxis over 4–5 days with continuing highly emetogenic chemotherapy. This limits the effectiveness of any regimen.

Grunberg SM et al: Control of chemotherapy-induced emesis. N Engl J Med 1993;329:1790. (Mechanisms and treatment.)

Perez EA: Review of the preclinical pharmacology and comparative efficacy of 5-hydroxytryptamine-3 receptor antagonists for chemotherapy-induced emesis. J Clin Oncol 1995;13:1036. (This is a highly effective class of antiemetic agents, and all three studied appear to be relatively equivalent.)

Gastrointestinal & Skin Toxicity

Since antimetabolites such as methotrexate and fluorouracil act only on rapidly proliferating cells, they damage the cells of mucosal surfaces such as the gastrointestinal tract. Methotrexate has similar effects on the skin. These toxicities are at times more serious than bone marrow suppression, and they should be looked for routinely when these agents are used.

Erythema of the buccal mucosa is an early sign of mucosal toxicity. If therapy is continued beyond this point, oral ulceration will develop. In general, it is wise to discontinue therapy at the time of appearance of early oral ulceration. This finding usually heralds the appearance of similar but potentially more serious ulceration at other sites lower in the gastrointestinal tract. Therapy can usually be reinstituted when the oral ulcer heals (7–10 days). The dose of drug used may need to be modified downward at this point, with titration to an acceptable level of mucosal toxicity. Adequate mouth care with antimicrobial mouthwashes and attention to dental hygiene are essential and may prevent severe toxicity. Common mouthwashes include the microbicidal oral rinse chlorhexidine and a mixture of salt and bicarbonate of soda in warm water, which aids in debridement of dead mucosa. A prophylactic antifungal mouthwash such as nystatin oral suspension may also be used. High doses of methotrexate require special consideration as noted in the following section.

Radiation therapy may cause xerostomia, which can lead to difficulty in swallowing, discomfort, and gum disease. Pilocarpine hydrochloride, 5–10 mg orally three times a day, can relieve symptoms of dry mouth but must be used regularly.

Miscellaneous Drug-Specific Toxicities

The toxicities of individual drugs have been summarized in Table 4–4. Several of these warrant additional mention, since they occur with commonly administered agents, and special preventive measures are often indicated.

A. Hemorrhagic Cystitis Induced by Cyclophosphamide or Ifosfamide: Metabolic products of cyclophosphamide that retain cytotoxic activity are excreted into the urine. Some patients appear to metabolize more of the drug to these active excretory products. If their urine is concentrated, the toxic metabolite may cause severe bladder damage. Patients receiving cyclophosphamide must be advised to maintain a high fluid intake. Early symptoms of bladder toxicity include dysuria and frequency despite the absence of bacteriuria. Such symptoms develop in about 20% of patients who receive the drug chronically. If microscopic hematuria develops, it is advisable to stop the drug temporarily or switch to a different alkylating agent, increase fluid intake, and administer a urinary analgesic such as phenazopyridine. With severe cystitis, large segments of bladder mucosa may be shed and the patient may have prolonged gross hematuria. Such patients should be observed for signs of urinary obstruction and may require cystoscopy for removal of obstructing blood clots. The risk of developing hemorrhagic cystitis is dose-related. For high doses of cyclophosphamide, preventive continuous bladder irrigation with 0.9% saline solution is used during the period of drug administration and for the following 24 hours.

The cyclophosphamide analog ifosfamide can cause severe hemorrhagic cystitis when used alone. However, when it is used in conjunction with a series of doses of the neutralizing agent mesna, bladder toxicity can be prevented. Mesna can also be used to prevent cystitis in patients receiving cyclophosphamide in high doses.

B. Vincristine-Induced Neuropathy: Neuropathy is a toxic side effect that is peculiar to the vinca alkaloid drugs, especially vincristine. The peripheral neuropathy can be sensory, motor, autonomic, or a combination of these effects. In its mildest form, it consists of paresthesias of the fingers and toes. Occasional patients develop acute jaw or throat pain after vincristine therapy. This may be a form of trigeminal or glossopharyngeal neuralgia.

With continued vincristine therapy, the paresthesias may extend to the proximal interphalangeal joints, hyporeflexia can appear in the lower extremities, and weakness may develop in the quadriceps muscle group. At this point, it is wise to discontinue vincristine therapy until the neuropathy has subsided. A useful means of judging whether peripheral motor neuropathy is severe enough to warrant stopping treatment is to have the patient attempt to do deep knee bends or rise from a chair without using the arm muscles.

Constipation is the most common symptom of autonomic neuropathy associated with vincristine therapy. Patients receiving vincristine should be started on stool softeners and mild cathartics when therapy is begun; otherwise, severe impaction may result along with an atonic bowel.

More serious autonomic involvement can lead to acute intestinal ileus with signs indistinguishable from those of an acute abdomen. Bladder neuropathies are uncommon but may be severe. These two complications are absolute contraindications to continued vincristine therapy. The majority of symptoms from vincristine are mild and resolve slowly after therapy has been completed. Paclitaxel, cisplatin, carboplatin, and vinorelbine can also cause peripheral neuropathy, though as a rule symptoms improve gradually after treatment is stopped.

C. Methotrexate Toxicity and Citrovorum Rescue: In addition to standard uses of methotrexate for cancer chemotherapy, this drug is also used in very high doses that could lead to fatal bone marrow toxicity if given without an antidote. High-dose methotrexate therapy with leucovorin rescue is routinely used to treat osteogenic sarcoma, acute lymphocytic leukemia, and some cases of non-Hodgkin's lymphoma.

The bone marrow and mucosal toxicity of methotrexate can be prevented by early administration of leucovorin. Serum levels of methotrexate are usually monitored and doses of leucovorin adjusted accordingly. Rescue is required for methotrexate doses over 80 mg/m^2 and is usually begun within 4 hours after completing treatment. Up to 100 mg/m^2 of leucovorin is given initially every 6 hours, with further doses adjusted for the serum methotrexate level. Rescue is usually continued orally for 3 days or longer until the serum methotrexate level is below 0.05 μmol/L. If an overdose of methotrexate is administered accidentally, leucovorin therapy should be initiated as soon as possible, preferably within 1 hour. Intravenous infusion should be employed for larger overdosages to ensure adequate drug delivery. It is generally advisable to give leucovorin repeatedly in this situation.

Vigorous hydration and bicarbonate loading also appear to be important in preventing crystallization of high-dose methotrexate in the renal tubular epithelium. Serum creatinine is determined before beginning therapy and daily thereafter, since methotrexate excretion is slowed by renal insufficiency and toxicity will be enhanced. In high doses, methotrexate can itself cause renal injury. Methotrexate doses are reduced in renal insufficiency. Concomitant use of certain drugs will slow methotrexate excretion, and they are avoided during therapy. These drugs include aspirin, NSAIDs, penicillins, sulfonamides, and probenecid.

D. Busulfan Toxicity: The alkylating agent busulfan, occasionally used for the treatment of chronic myelogenous leukemia, has curious delayed toxicities, including increased skin pigmentation, a wasting syndrome similar to that seen in adrenal insufficiency, and progressive pulmonary fibrosis. Patients who develop either of the latter two problems should be switched to a different drug (eg, melphalan) when further therapy is needed. The pigmentary changes are innocuous and will usually regress slowly after treatment is discontinued. Long-term treatment with busulfan also results in an increased risk of secondary leukemias.

E. Bleomycin Toxicity: This antibiotic has found increasing application in cancer chemotherapy in view of its activity in squamous cell carcinomas, Hodgkin's disease, non-Hodgkin's lymphomas, and testicular tumors. Bleomycin can produce edema of the interphalangeal joints and hardening of the palmar and plantar skin. More serious toxicities include an anaphylactic or serum sickness-like reaction and a potentially fatal pulmonary fibrotic reaction (seen especially in elderly patients receiving a total dose of over 300 units). If a nonproductive cough, dyspnea, and pulmonary infiltrates develop, the drug is discontinued, and high-dose corticosteroids are instituted as well as empiric antibiotics pending cultures. Fever alone or with chills is an occasional complication of bleomycin treatment and is not an absolute contraindication to continued treatment. The fever may be avoided by hydrocortisone administration just prior to the injection. Fever alone is not predictive of pulmonary toxicity. About 1% of patients (especially those with lymphoma) may have a severe or even fatal hypotensive reaction after the initial dose of bleomycin. In order to identify and treat such patients, it is wise to administer a test dose of 5 units of bleomycin first and to have adequate monitoring and emergency facilities available. Patients exhibiting a hypotensive reaction should not receive further bleomycin therapy.

F. Doxorubicin-Induced Cardiomyopathy: The anthracycline antibiotics doxorubicin and daunomycin both have acute and delayed cardiac toxicity. The problem is greater with doxorubicin because it has a major role and is used in repeated doses in the treatment of sarcomas, breast cancer, lymphomas, acute leukemia, and certain other solid tumors. Studies of left ventricular function and endomyocardial biopsies indicate that some changes in cardiac dy-

namics occur in most patients by the time they have received 300 mg/m^2 of doxorubicin. The *multiple-gated* ("MUGA") radionuclide cardiac scan is the most useful noninvasive test for assessing toxicity. Doxorubicin should not be used in elderly patients with intrinsic cardiac disease. In general, patients should not receive a total dose in excess of 550 mg/m^2, and 1–10% of patients who receive this dose develop cardiomyopathy. Patients who have had prior chest or mediastinal radiotherapy may develop doxorubicin heart disease at lower total doses. The appearance of a high resting pulse may herald the appearance of cardiac toxicity. Unfortunately, the toxicity may be irreversible and frequently fatal at dosage levels above 550 mg/m^2. At lower doses (eg, 350 mg/m^2), the symptoms and signs of cardiac failure generally respond well to digitalis, diuretics, and cessation of doxorubicin therapy. Recent evidence suggests that cardiac toxicity can be correlated with high peak plasma levels obtained with intermittent high-dose bolus therapy (eg, every 3–4 weeks). Use of weekly injections or low-dose continuous infusion schedules appears to delay the occurrence of cardiac toxicity. Current laboratory studies suggest that cardiac toxicity may be due to a mechanism involving the formation of intracellular free radicals in cardiac muscle. Pretreatment with dexrazoxane, an iron chelator that decreases free radical formation, appears to protect the myocardium from anthracycline-induced injury but may also reduce the anticancer efficacy of the anthracycline. Dexrazoxane is now approved for the prevention of cardiomyopathy in women with metastatic breast cancer receiving cumulative doxorubicin doses > 300 mg/m^2. Liposomally encapsulated doxorubicin and daunorubicin have been FDA-approved and appear to have minimal cardiac toxicity. Their main use to date has been to treat Kaposi's sarcoma. Newer anthracycline analogs include idarubicin, which has shown efficacy against acute nonlymphocytic leukemia and breast cancer when used in combination with other agents. Idarubicin appears to have a similar potential for causing cardiotoxicity when compared with other anthracyclines, though a maximum lifetime dosage recommendation has not yet been made.

G. Cisplatin Nephrotoxicity and Neurotoxicity: Cisplatin is effective in the treatment of testicular, bladder, and ovarian cancer as well as in several other types of tumor. Nausea and vomiting are common, but nephrotoxicity and neurotoxicity are more serious. Vigorous hydration with or without mannitol diuresis may substantially reduce nephrotoxicity. Renal function must be carefully monitored during cisplatin therapy, as should serum magnesium, which may fall during therapy with this agent. Ototoxicity is a potentially serious neurotoxicity that can result in deafness. The neurotoxicity of this drug is delayed and is more common after a total dose of 300 mg/m^2. Other manifestations include peripheral neuropathy of mixed sensorimotor type that may be associated with painful paresthesias. These supportive measures do not appear to reduce the therapeutic effectiveness of cisplatin. The second-generation platinum analog carboplatin is now available and has been shown to be as effective as cisplatin in ovarian cancer. Carboplatin is less nephrotoxic and causes less severe nausea or vomiting, but it does induce myelosuppression. Amifostine, an organic thiophosphate initially developed as a radioprotective agent, has efficacy in preventing renal toxicity from cisplatin. It has recently been approved to reduce cumulative renal toxicity associated with repeat administration of cisplatin in advanced ovarian cancer. In addition, amifostine may reduce cytotoxic chemotherapy-induced hematologic toxicity and neurotoxicity. Glutathione also appears to be a promising agent in preventing cisplatin neurotoxicity. Glutathione was given at a dose of 1.5 g/m^2 intravenously before cisplatin administration, then at a dose of 600 mg by intramuscular injection on days 2–5.

H. Alpha Interferon Toxicities: While alpha interferon is generally tolerated in the standard doses listed in Table 4–4, it has increasing toxicity with increasing doses and is more toxic in elderly patients. Even standard doses may be intolerable to some patients. Fever and chills are initial side effects but are infrequent after continued treatment. These symptoms may be ameliorated or prevented by premedication with acetaminophen and bedtime dosing. However, anorexia, fatigue, and weight loss can be cumulative and with time may become severe. These symptoms may be dose- or treatment-limiting. Thirty percent or more of patients are intolerant of interferon therapy even at low doses. In some patients, central nervous system symptoms develop, usually manifested as confusion or somnolence. Reduction in peripheral blood counts can develop, but this abnormality is usually not clinically important and may even be a desired effect in the treatment of chronic myelogenous leukemia. These interferon-induced side effects are sometimes confused with the symptoms of progressive cancer. The side effects usually clear within 1 week after cessation of interferon therapy.

Borden EC, Parkinson D: Interferons: Effectiveness, toxicities, costs. Ann Intern Med 1996:125; 614. (Discussion of toxicity and how it affects treatment.)

Dorr RT, Von Hoff DD (editors): *Cancer Chemotherapy Handbook.* Appleton and Lange, 1994.

EVALUATION OF TUMOR RESPONSE

Inasmuch as cancer chemotherapy can induce clinical improvement, serious toxicity, or both, it is important to critically assess the beneficial effects of treatment in patients with advanced cancer to determine that the net effect is favorable. The most valuable signs to follow during therapy include the following.

TUMOR SIZE

Shrinkage in tumor size can be demonstrated by physical examination, chest film or other x-ray, sonography, or a radionuclide scanning procedure such as bone scanning (breast, lung, prostate cancer). CT scanning is important for the evaluation of tumor size and location and the extent of distant spread for a wide variety of tumors and sites. MRI is now the best noninvasive means of evaluating posterior fossa brain tumors, spinal cord tumors, spinal cord compression, and pelvic disease, but CT scanning remains useful and may provide additional information. Sonography is also helpful in the evaluation of pelvic neoplasms. A partial response (PR) is defined as a 50% or greater reduction in the original tumor mass. A complete response (CR) refers to the complete disappearance of detectable tumor. Progression is an increase of more than 25% in the size of the tumor or the appearance of any new lesions.

TUMOR MARKERS

A decrease in the quantity of a tumor product or marker substance reflects a reduced amount of tumor in the body. Examples of such markers include paraproteins (abnormal immunoglobulins) in multiple myeloma and macroglobulinemia, human chorionic gonadotropin (hCG) in choriocarcinoma and testicular tumors, prostatic acid phosphatase and prostate-specific antigen (PSA) in prostatic cancer, urinary steroids in adrenal carcinoma and paraneoplastic Cushing's syndrome, and 5-hydroxyindoleacetic acid (5-HIAA) in carcinoid syndrome.

Tumor-secreted fetal antigens are also used to follow the course and response to treatment of cancers. These include alpha$_1$-fetoprotein (AFP) in hepatoma, in teratoembryonal carcinoma, and in occasional cases of gastric carcinoma; ovarian tumor antigen (CA 125) in ovarian cancer; and carcinoembryonic antigen (CEA) in carcinomas of the colon, lung, and pancreas. CA 15-3 may become important in detecting early recurrence of breast cancer but is mainly used to follow response to therapy in metastatic disease. Monoclonal antibodies are now used for measurement of a number of tumor markers and offer the potential of delineating a number of additional markers for diagnostic purposes.

Tumor markers may play an important role in the early detection of some common tumors when combined with good physical examinations. PSA, an immunogenic glycoprotein produced solely by the prostate, is currently the only tumor marker with widespread use in cancer screening, though this practice remains controversial. PSA was initially used only to indicate tumor bulk and disease progression, but it has recently been proposed as a routine screening tool when paired with the digital rectal examination. The American Cancer Society National Prostate Cancer Detection Project is a multicenter study evaluating the use of PSA, rectal examination, and transrectal ultrasound in a large cohort of healthy men. In this and other studies, the combination of a monoclonal PSA greater than 4 ng/mL and an abnormal digital rectal examination was felt to produce a highly sensitive and specific method for detecting prostate cancer. It has not yet been shown that regular screening for prostate cancer using the combination of PSA and the digital rectal examination results in decreased mortality from prostate cancer or improved quality of life.

Nonetheless, an abnormal PSA or digital examination requires further evaluation by transrectal ultrasound and possible biopsy. The increase in screening for prostate cancer over the last few years has markedly increased the reported incidence of this disease. (See Table 4–1.) The PSA may be elevated in benign prostatic hypertrophy and in prostatitis. Levels in benign disease are usually between 4 and 10 ng/mL; a level greater than 10 ng/mL increases the likelihood of finding cancer. In addition, 25–45% of patients with localized prostate cancer may have a normal PSA value.

Tumor markers may be useful to screen populations at high risk for a specific cancer. A recent study has shown that elevated and altered profiles of AFP can serve as predictive markers for the development of hepatocellular carcinoma in patients with cirrhosis. Most tumor markers are not specific or sensitive enough to be useful as screening tools owing to their frequent elevation in benign disease and their absence in some cases of malignancy.

In general, tumor markers are used to follow response to therapy of a specific cancer. In diseases where early treatment of recurrence can influence survival (eg, testicular cancer), tumor markers may be used to screen for recurrent disease before it becomes radiographically or clinically evident.

Coley CM et al: Early detection of prostate cancer. Part I: Prior probability and effectiveness of tests. Ann Intern Med 1997;126:394; and Part II: Estimating the risks, benefits, and costs. Ann Intern Med 1997;126:468. (The lack of direct evidence showing a net benefit of screening in contrast to earlier detection of cancer mandates clinician-patient discussion about this procedure.)

Morgan TO et al: Age-specific reference ranges for serum prostate-specific antigen in black men. N Engl J Med 1996;335:304. (The traditional ranges used may have different specificity and sensitivity within racial groups.)

Rustin GJS et al: Defining response of ovarian carcinoma to initial chemotherapy according to serum CA 125. J Clin Oncol 1996;14:1545. (A 50–75% decrease of CA 125 levels is a reliable definition of response to chemotherapy for ovarian cancer.)

Sato Y et al: Early recognition of hepatocellular carcinoma based on altered profiles of alpha-fetoprotein. N Engl J Med 1993;328:1802. (Screening patients with cirrhosis using alpha-fetoprotein profiles may aid in early diagnosis.)

GENERAL WELL-BEING, PERFORMANCE STATUS, & SUPPORTIVE CARE

The functional status of the cancer patient at diagnosis (or at the start of treatment) is a major prognostic factor and determinant of outcome with or without tumor-directed therapy. It is therefore important to assess functional status as well as tumor burden and symptoms before deciding on possible anticancer therapy. Functional status or performance status evaluates the patient's ability to perform activities of daily living and is clearly related to tumor burden, tumor site, and the patient's underlying physical condition.

Two scales are commonly used to measure performance status. The Karnofsky scale ranges from 100% (asymptomatic and fully functional) through 0% (dead) in steps of 10%. For example, a Karnofsky performance status of 40% implies a patient who is disabled and requires special care and assistance. This patient would be unable to work but able to live at home with special assistance. The more commonly used Eastern Cooperative Oncology Group (ECOG) scale is a five-point system that is simpler and easier to apply to clinical practice. The ECOG scoring system ranges from 0 to 4 as follows: 0, entirely asymptomatic; 1, symptomatic but fully ambulatory; 2, symptomatic and in bed less than 50% of the day; 3, symptomatic and in bed more than 50% of the day but not bedridden; and 4, bedridden. These two systems are often the basis for clinical decisions despite their obvious lack of precision. They are also useful in assessing the impact of therapy and disease progression.

The measures assessing functional status described above do not adequately assess quality of life, a major goal of cancer chemotherapy. Performance status is only one component of quality of life, which is a combination of subjective and objective factors. Factors included in the assessment of general well-being include improved appetite and weight gain and decreased pain as well as improved performance status. In general, cancer patients perceive that they receive inadequate analgesia and have impairment of function because of pain. The adequate use of pain medications is hampered by their sedating side effects. New guidelines for the management of pain and long-acting opioids delivered by a transdermal system may help (eg, fentanyl patch, changed every 3 days). In addition, sedating effects can sometimes be avoided by adding nonsteroidal anti-inflammatory agents or antidepressants to opioid therapy. Occasionally, opioids may be given epidurally to relieve severe pain. As with the use of antiemetics, pain medications work better when given prophylactically on a regular schedule rather than as needed for chronic or severe pain. It is only by completely evaluating all of the factors described above that the physician is able to judge whether the net effect of chemotherapy is worthwhile palliation.

In addition to narcotics, agents that inhibit bone resorption may decrease bone pain and protect against skeletal complications (thereby improving quality of life) in women with breast cancer metastatic to bone and in patients with multiple myeloma and lytic bone lesions. The bisphosphonate pamidronate is well tolerated and is now considered standard therapy in these two groups of patients. Pamidronate is given at a dose of 90 mg intravenously over 2 hours once a month for about 1 year. The use of agents such as pamidronate, growth factors such as erythropoietin, and appetite stimulants such as megestrol acetate (given in dosages ranging from 40 mg orally four times a day up to 800 mg once a day) can improve the quality of life for cancer patients.

Cleeland CS et al: Pain and its treatment in outpatients with cancer. N Engl J Med 1994;330:592. (Cancer patients do not receive adequate analgesia as outpatients.)

Hortobagyi EN et al: Efficacy of pamidronate in reducing skeletal complications in patients with breast cancer and lytic bone metastases. N Engl J Med 1996;335:1785. (Pamidronate as a supplement to chemotherapy can protect against skeletal complications in women with breast cancer metastatic to bone.)

Levy MH: Pharmacologic treatment of cancer pain. N Engl J Med 1996;335:1124. (Review of the agents and guidelines for their use.)

CANCER COMPLICATIONS: DIAGNOSIS & MANAGEMENT

ONCOLOGIC EMERGENCIES

Cancer is a chronic disease, but acute emergencies may occur as a consequence of local involvement (spinal cord compression, superior vena cava syndrome, malignant effusions, etc) or generalized systemic effects (hypercalcemia, opportunistic infections, hypercoagulability, hyperuricemia, etc). These complications may be the presenting manifestation. Two relatively common complications covered elsewhere will not be discussed here: superior vena cava syndrome (Chapter 12) and hypercoagulability (Chapter 13).

Neilan BA: Oncologic emergencies: Treating acute problems resulting from cancer and chemotherapy. Postgrad Med 1994;95:131.

Pimentel L: Medical complications of oncologic disease. Endocrinol Metab Clin North Am 1993;11:407. (Emergency room management of life-threatening oncologic emergencies.)

1. SPINAL CORD COMPRESSION

Spinal cord compression by tumor mass is manifested by back pain, progressive weakness, and sensory loss (usually in the lower extremities). Less commonly, spinal cord disease may present as chest or abdominal pain or as signs of nerve root compression due to the epidural location of the tumor. Bowel and bladder dysfunction are late findings. Spinal cord compression may occur as a complication of metastatic solid tumor, lymphoma, or myeloma. Back pain at the level of the spinal cord lesion occurs in over 80% of cases and may be aggravated by lying down, weight-bearing, sneezing, or coughing. Because back pain may precede the development of neurologic symptoms or signs, it is important to investigate this complaint thoroughly in any patient with cancer.

If neurologic defects are present at diagnosis, they are usually irreversible, though treatment immediately after symptoms develop may result in partial recovery. Neurologic impairment can progress rapidly. Treatment of early lesions may completely avoid significant compromise. Although patients who present with paralysis may not recover function, they should still be treated for pain relief and to limit the extent of progression. In addition, patients may respond to systemic therapy depending on the specific tumor type.

The diagnosis of spinal cord compression has traditionally been made by CT myelography. MRI now provides a noninvasive and extremely sensitive alternative to myelography. It is possible to obtain detailed views of the area in question as well as sagittal images of the entire spinal cord and vertebral canal. This detailed examination is important for detection and treatment of multiple lesions. Bone radiographs and bone scans are useful for detecting vertebral metastases, but they do not aid in assessing spinal cord compromise.

Emergency Treatment

Radiation therapy to the area of spinal cord compression and two adjacent vertebrae above and below the lesion is the treatment of choice. High doses of glucocorticoids (usually dexamethasone, 10–100 mg intravenously) are administered as soon as the diagnosis is suspected or confirmed. A lower dose (eg, 4–6 mg every 6 hours intravenously or orally) is continued throughout the course of radiation therapy and tapered at or near the end of treatment.

Emergency surgery is indicated (1) for spinal cord compression in the absence of a diagnosis of malignancy, (2) for patients who have already received maximal doses of radiation to the involved area of the spine, and (3) for patients who develop progressive neurologic deficits during radiation whose prognosis warrants aggressive therapy. Chemotherapy is useful in treating lymphomas and multiple myeloma in conjunction with or following completion of radiation therapy.

Hill ME et al: Spinal cord compression in breast cancer: A review of 70 cases. Br J Cancer 1993;68:969. (Presenting symptoms and treatment options.)

2. HYPERCALCEMIA

Hypercalcemia occurs in 10–20% of patients with cancer. Common causes include breast, lung, kidney, and head and neck carcinomas as well as multiple myeloma. Although the majority of cancers associated with hypercalcemia metastasize to the bones, approximately 20% of cases are not associated with bony lesions. The recent identification of a novel protein called parathyroid hormone-related protein (PTHrP) has revised some previously held views about the pathogenesis of hypercalcemia. Radioimmunoassays have identified this peptide in the serum of approximately two-thirds of cancer patients with hypercalcemia. High levels have been found in patients with hypercalcemia that was previously thought to be due solely to local osteolysis. PTHrP may become a useful tumor marker in normocalcemic patients. In addition, antibodies to PTHrP may be useful as treatment.

The symptoms and signs of hypercalcemia include nausea, vomiting, constipation, polyuria, muscular weakness and hyporeflexia, confusion, psychosis, tremor, and lethargy. Some patients may be asymptomatic. Electrocardiography often shows a shortening of the QT interval. The presence of hypercalcemia does not invariably indicate a dismal prognosis, especially in breast or prostate cancer and multiple myeloma. In the absence of signs or symptoms of hypercalcemia, a laboratory finding of elevated serum calcium should be rechecked to exclude the possibility of laboratory error.

Emergency Treatment

A. Hydration: Emergency treatment consists of aggressive intravenous hydration with 3–4 L/d of saline followed by diuresis with furosemide. It is essential that the patient be well hydrated before beginning diuretic therapy and that hydration be maintained after diuresis is initiated. Although hydration alone is effective at slowly reducing the calcium level, it is rarely sufficient treatment and can lead to problems with fluid overload.

B. Drug Therapy: There are now several options for the emergent treatment of hypercalcemia used in conjunction with aggressive hydration.

1. Bisphosphonates–Bisphosphonates are potent inhibitors of osteoclast bone resorption and are currently the most important and least toxic agents for the treatment of cancer-related hypercalcemia. Pamidronate disodium is the most potent bisphosphonate available. A single 24-hour intravenous infusion of 60–90 mg with adequate hydration produces complete normalization of serum calcium by day 7 in 70–100% of patients. The drug is often given as a 2- to 4-hour infusion for outpatient management. The most commonly reported side effects have been transient fever, myalgias, and an infusion site reaction. Pamidronate has also been found to reduce the incidence of new skeletal lesions and decrease pain from bone disease in multiple myeloma and breast cancer.

2. Calcitonin–Synthetic salmon calcitonin works immediately to inhibit bone resorption, whereas pamidronate may take 2–3 days to achieve its maximum effect. The usual dose of 4 units/kg intramuscularly or subcutaneously every 12 hours may be increased to 8 units/kg every 12 hours after 1–2 days. Skin testing is usually performed before the first dose to test for hypersensitivity reactions. Calcitonin alone is usually not effective at lowering serum calcium levels but can be added to pamidronate if necessary to achieve normal calcium levels. Repeated treatment with calcitonin is usually not as effective, and tachyphylaxis usually occurs after 1–3 days of treatment.

3. Gallium nitrate–For treatment of hypercalcemia, gallium nitrate is given by continuous intravenous infusion at a dose of 100–200 mg/m^2/d for 5 days. Gallium nitrate is superior to calcitonin both in reducing calcium levels acutely and in keeping the levels low after treatment is completed. Renal function must be carefully monitored.

4. Other drugs–Prednisone has not been shown to be effective as a single agent to treat hypercalcemia, though it can be used in diseases that are responsive to steroids such as multiple myeloma or lymphoma. Refractory hypercalcemia may be treated with intravenous plicamycin, 25 µg/kg/d for 3 or 4 days. Although often effective, its effect may be short-lived, and its use is often associated with hepatic, renal, and bone marrow toxicity.

C. Chemotherapy: Patients with breast cancer

may develop hypercalcemia as a "flare" associated with bone pain after initiation of estrogen or antiestrogen therapy. These patients often achieve excellent tumor response with continued therapy. Tumors may respond to chemotherapy or radiation therapy, leading to resolution of hypercalcemia. If chronic hypercalcemia persists and is refractory to chemotherapy, oral etidronate, phosphates, low-dose prednisone, and aggressive oral hydration may be tried but are unfortunately rarely effective for long. When the more potent bisphosphonates become available in oral formulations, the management of chronic hypercalcemia may improve.

Hall TG et al: Update on the medical treatment of hypercalcemia of malignancy. Clin Pharm 1993;12:117. (Old and new therapies and their relative merits.)

Theriault RL: Hypercalcemia of malignancy: Pathophysiology and implications for treatment. Oncology 1993; 7:47. (Newer agents used to treat hypercalcemia and their relationship to pathophysiology.)

3. HYPERURICEMIA & ACUTE URATE NEPHROPATHY

Hyperuricemia can occur both as a complication of rapidly proliferating malignancies or with treatment-associated tumor lysis of hematologic malignancies such as leukemia, lymphoma, and multiple myeloma. Neoplasms with a high nucleic acid turnover such as acute leukemia and lymphoma may present with elevated serum uric acid and associated renal insufficiency. This problem may be compounded by use of thiazide diuretics, which decrease urate excretion. If a patient presents with hyperuricemia, care must be taken to reduce the uric acid before institution of cancer therapy. Patients at risk for tumor lysis syndrome should be followed with twice-daily measurements of uric acid, phosphate, calcium, and creatinine for the first 2–3 days following initiation of chemotherapy. Rapid elevation of serum uric acid presents the danger of acute urate nephropathy caused by uric acid crystallization in the distal tubules, collecting ducts, and renal parenchyma. A serum urate concentration above 15 mg/dL is associated with a high risk of uric acid nephropathy. Gouty arthritis is usually a problem only in patients with a history of gout.

Prophylactic therapy consists of decreasing the production and increasing the renal excretion of uric acid. Allopurinol is a competitive inhibitor of xanthine oxidase and prevents conversion of highly soluble hypoxanthine and xanthine to the relatively insoluble uric acid. Twelve to 24 hours before beginning therapy, a dose of 600 mg is given, followed by 300 mg/d during the period of high risk. Higher doses (up to 900–1200 mg/d) are used when severe hyperuricemia is anticipated following chemotherapy. Pa-

tients receiving the purine antagonists mercaptopurine or azathioprine should be given only 25–35% of the calculated dose of chemotherapy if they are also receiving allopurinol, since the latter drug will potentiate both the therapeutic effects and the toxicity of these agents. Renal excretion of uric acid is enhanced by maintaining a high urine flow and by alkalinizing the urine to prevent uric acid crystallization, which occurs at acid pH. Alkaline diuresis to maintain a urine pH near 7.0 is required only for prophylaxis in patients expected to have a rapid tumor response with marked hyperuricemia.

Emergency Treatment

Emergency therapy for established severe hyperuricemia consists of (1) hydration with 2–4 L of fluid per day; (2) alkalinization of the urine with 6–8 g of sodium bicarbonate per day; (3) allopurinol, 900–1200 mg/d; and (4) in severe cases, emergency hemodialysis. When severe hyperuricemia is present, adequate therapy may be impossible because of associated renal insufficiency and inadequate urine output. Intravenous allopurinol has recently been approved for use in patients unable to tolerate the oral form of this drug. Even if renal failure occurs and dialysis is required, renal function may return to normal after the acute tumor lysis has resolved.

4. MALIGNANT CARCINOID SYNDROME

Although tumors of argentaffin cells are uncommon, they are important because they secrete a variety of vasoactive materials. These include serotonin, histamine, catecholamines, prostaglandins, and vasoactive peptides. Carcinoid syndrome is usually associated with carcinoid tumors of the small bowel metastatic to the liver and, less commonly, with primary carcinoid tumors in other sites such as the lung or stomach. These tumors tend to metastasize early but have a relatively indolent course, making control of the syndrome important. Related syndromes occur in patients with pancreatic tumors secreting vasoactive peptides, which can cause severe watery diarrhea (pancreatic cholera).

The manifestations of carcinoid syndrome include facial flushing, edema of the head and neck (especially with bronchial carcinoid), abdominal cramps and diarrhea, bronchospasm, cardiac lesions (tricuspid or pulmonary stenosis or regurgitation), telangiectasias, and increased urinary 5-hydroxyindoleacetic acid (5-HIAA). The most common symptoms are flushing and diarrhea. The diagnosis is made by finding elevated levels of 5-HIAA in a 24-hour urine collection. Patients with symptomatic carcinoid usually excrete more than 25 mg of 5-HIAA per day in the urine. Ideally, all drugs and serotonin-rich foods such as bananas should be withheld for several days before beginning the urine collection.

Emergency Treatment

Emergency therapy for patients with symptomatic bronchial carcinoid includes prednisone, 15–30 mg/d. The associated abdominal cramping and diarrhea of intestinal carcinoids can often be managed by hydration and diphenoxylate with atropine. For severe diarrhea, the H_1 histamine receptor antagonist cyproheptadine (4 mg orally three times daily) or an antiserotonin agent such as methysergide maleate (2 mg orally three times daily until 16 mg has been given) may be effective. Other useful agents include cimetidine and the phenothiazines.

The synthetic peptide somatostatin agonist, octreotide acetate, is the most effective agent for reducing symptoms due to the carcinoid syndrome in association with achieving a reduction in levels of urinary 5-HIAA. The dose of octreotide in carcinoid syndrome is 100–600 µg/d in two to four divided doses by subcutaneous injection. Octreotide is also effective in the treatment of symptoms related to vaso-intestinal peptide-secreting pancreatic tumors (VIPomas), markedly reducing the watery diarrhea syndrome associated with this neoplasm. The dose of octreotide used to treat patients with VIPomas is 200–300 µg/d in two to four divided doses.

Surgery is important in the treatment of localized carcinoid. Chemotherapy is used for patients with progressive advanced-stage disease. Active agents include fluorouracil, streptozocin, dacarbazine, cisplatin, doxorubicin, and alpha interferon.

Bajetta E et al: Treatment of metastatic carcinoids and other neuroendocrine tumors with recombinant interferon-alpha-2a. A study by the Italian Trials in Medical Oncology Group. Cancer 1993;72:3099. (Interferon is a useful agent in controlling carcinoid syndrome but has little effect on tumor growth.)

Kvols LK et al: Metastatic carcinoid tumors and the malignant carcinoid syndrome. Acta Oncol 1993;32:197. (Diagnostic and therapeutic advances in the past decade.)

OTHER COMPLICATIONS

1. MALIGNANT EFFUSIONS

The development of effusions in the pleural, pericardial, and peritoneal spaces may be the presenting sign of some tumors or may cause diagnostic and therapeutic problems in patients with advanced neoplasms. Although the cause of an effusion can be elusive in a newly diagnosed asymptomatic patient, it is rarely difficult in the patient with advanced cancer. Approximately half of undiagnosed effusions in patients not known to have cancer will be malignant. The differential diagnosis includes congestive heart failure, pulmonary embolism, trauma, and infections such as tuberculosis. Direct involvement of the serous surface of the involved space with tumor appears to be the most frequent initiating factor, though many other mechanisms such as lymphatic drainage that control the flow of fluid in the pleural space may play a role.

Most patients with pleural or pericardial effusions are symptomatic at presentation with chest pain, shortness of breath, or cough. The diagnosis is made by tapping the involved space. Pericardial effusions are aspirated under fluoroscopic guidance or direct vision through a subxiphoid incision. The fluid should be heparinized and sent for cell count and differential, protein content, lactate dehydrogenase level, and cytologic study. The gross appearance of the fluid is often helpful as well. Bloody effusions are usually due to cancer but occasionally are due to pulmonary embolism, tuberculosis, or trauma. Chylous effusions may be associated with thoracic duct obstruction or may result from enlarged mediastinal lymph nodes in lymphoma. If the cytologic smear is negative on two occasions but the suspicion of tumor is still high, closed pleural biopsy may be helpful.

The management of effusions should be appropriate to the severity of involvement. Treatment of the underlying neoplasm would be ideal but is often not effective in controlling local effusions. Treatment may result in palliation and improve short-term survival when there is substantial pulmonary or cardiac compromise. Diuretics are used as initial treatment for small to moderate-sized peritoneal effusions and as an adjunct to drainage of large effusions to minimize the possibility of reexpansion pulmonary edema that can occur after thoracentesis. Small or loculated effusions may require ultrasonographic localization, but drainage of a large pleural or peritoneal effusion can be accomplished rapidly using an intravenous catheter and phlebotomy tubing connected to a vacuum bottle. Thoracentesis alone controls fewer than 10% of effusions but may be useful in conjunction with systemic chemotherapy for sensitive tumors (eg, lymphoma, small-cell lung cancer, breast cancer). Pleural effusions may occasionally be managed by closed water-seal drainage with a chest tube for 3–4 days, though this procedure is usually performed in conjunction with chemosclerosis (see below). The aim of this procedure is to allow the pleural surfaces to come into close contact and become adherent.

Recurrent symptomatic effusions can often be controlled by drainage followed by chemosclerosis. In this procedure, a chemotherapeutic or nonchemotherapeutic agent is instilled with lidocaine into the involved space. The intended effect is local inflammation and sclerosis to encourage adherence of the serosal surfaces. Many drugs used for this purpose have been abandoned because of severe pain or systemic toxicity, including myelosuppression. Agents commonly used include bleomycin, tetracycline, talc, and the anthracenedione compound mitoxantrone.

Bleomycin is more effective at controlling pleural effusions than tetracycline; when tetracycline was used, the recurrence rate 90 days after sclerosis was almost double, and the side effects were similar. Tetracycline is no longer manufactured or available for intracavitary instillation. The major side effects of bleomycin are pain, fever, and hypersensitivity reactions.

Mitoxantrone has been reported to be effective in controlling malignant pleural effusions, causing minimal fever and local pain. However, one trial evaluated the effectiveness of mitoxantrone versus chest tube alone and found no differences in response or in duration of response. The instillation of sclerosing agents may best be reserved for patients who fail pleural tube drainage alone.

Talc poudrage has been used successfully to control malignant pleural effusions and appears to be relatively painless. For these reasons as well as cost considerations, the use of talc as a sclerosing agent is gaining in popularity.

Intrapleural chemotherapy has been used both to control the effusion and to treat the underlying malignancy with variable results. Sclerosis is generally less useful for the management of malignant ascites, but success has been reported using bleomycin, doxorubicin, thiotepa, and other agents.

Before instilling the sclerosing agent, it is important that the space be drained as thoroughly as possible. For pleural effusions, a small-bore chest tube or pigtail catheter is usually placed and fluid is removed by negative suction until the drainage is under 100 mL per 24 hours and the lung has expanded. Sclerotherapy is ineffective if there is a large residual effusion. The patient is then premedicated with an opioid, and 60 units of bleomycin or 30 mg of mitoxantrone in 50–100 mL of 0.9% saline is instilled directly into the chest tube. The chest tube is then clamped, and the patient is placed in different positions every 15 minutes for 4 hours to distribute the agent equally within the pleural space. At the end of this period, the clamp is removed and the chest tube is allowed to drain with suction. After 24 hours, the chest tube is removed from suction, and when the drainage is minimal, the tube is removed. The whole process takes 3–5 days. Occasionally, repeated doses of the sclerosing agent may be required to stop persistent reaccumulation of the effusion. Talc has been insufflated into the pleural space via a thoracoscope or instilled in a 5 g slurry with iodide via a chest tube. Talc instillation via a thoracoscope under anesthesia can be done quickly, has minimal complications, and appears highly effective. This may become the initial treatment of choice for malignant pleural effusions.

Surgery is infrequently used for patients with pleural or pericardial effusions who have failed sclerosis and who continue to have an expected survival of at least 1 year. Pleuroperitoneal shunting may have limited value in selected patients with high performance status who can participate actively in pumping the shunt the 100 times on five separate oc-

casions each day required for adequate shunt function and fluid drainage. Pleurectomy has a high complication rate but offers excellent control of effusion in carefully selected patients. A pericardial window or stripping also offers good control with a lower complication rate and may also be performed for constrictive pericarditis following radiation therapy to the chest.

Lynch TJ: Management of malignant pleural effusions. Chest 1993;103(4 Suppl):3855. (Etiology, current therapy, and directions for the future.)

Petrou M, Kaplan D, Goldstraw P: Management of recurrent malignant pleural effusions. The complementary role of talc pleurodesis and pleuroperitoneal shunting. Cancer 1995;75:801. (Effective palliation of malignant effusions with talc pleurodesis with the addition of shunting for patients with limited lung expansion.)

Wall TC et al: Diagnosis and management (by subxiphoid pericardiotomy) of large pericardial effusions causing cardiac tamponade. Am J Cardiol 1992;69:1075. (The procedure was effective.)

2. INFECTIOUS COMPLICATIONS

Many patients with cancer have increased susceptibility to both bacterial and opportunistic infections. This may result from impaired host defense mechanisms (eg, Hodgkin's or non-Hodgkin's lymphoma, chronic lymphocytic leukemia, multiple myeloma, acute leukemia or preleukemia) or from the myelosuppressive and immunosuppressive effects of cancer chemotherapy. Impaired host defense mechanisms include defects in neutrophil function, abnormalities in antibody production, depressed cell-mediated immune function, impairment of mechanical barriers by indwelling intravenous catheters, and impairment of mucosal integrity. At least half of the infections seen in neutropenic patients are felt to be endogenous.

The bacterial organisms accounting for the majority of infections in cancer patients include Enterobacteriaceae *(Klebsiella, Enterobacter, Serratia, Escherichia coli), Pseudomonas, Staphylococcus,* and *Streptococcus.* Other important pathogens include *Corynebacterium, Clostridium, Mycobacterium,* and *Legionella.* Patients with prolonged neutropenia or those who have undergone bone marrow transplantation are at risk for infections with fungi such as *Candida* and *Aspergillus,* viral infections such as herpes zoster and cytomegalovirus, and *Pneumocystis carinii.* The incidence of bacteremia rises dramatically when the white count is less than 600/µL or when there are fewer than 200 granulocytes per microliter. In patients with neutropenia, hematologic malignancies, or following bone marrow transplantation, infection must be treated emergently and empirically. Although fever may be due to multiple causes, including mucositis, drugs, and the malignancy itself, infection must be the first consideration and may be present even in the absence of fever, especially in patients who are receiving glucocorticoids. Negative cultures in febrile neutropenic patients do not rule out infection, and treatment should be instituted immediately without waiting for culture results to become available. If an indwelling line is present, blood cultures should be drawn from the periphery as well as through the line itself.

Treatment

Infection management has been aimed at treatment of gram-negative bacterial sepsis, the most rapidly lethal infection. Current concepts have been broadened to include prophylaxis and prevention of the most common infections, including those caused by gram-negative, gram-positive, and fungal pathogens. Until recently, empiric therapy of fever consisted of two- or three-drug combinations, including an aminoglycoside and an antipseudomonal penicillin, with resolution of fever and bacteremia in about 70% of patients. Current results using initial monotherapy with ceftazidime or combination β-lactam appear to yield similar results. Vancomycin or amphotericin B may be added on the basis of clinical suspicion, culture results, or prolonged fever in the absence of positive cultures. Adding aminoglycosides or substituting for ceftazidime a different antibiotic with broad-spectrum gram-negative activity (eg, imipenem) is also indicated for prolonged fever or clinical deterioration.

Prevention

Prophylaxis of infections in high-risk or neutropenic patients can prevent the complications of sepsis. Oral norfloxacin or parenteral ciprofloxacin has been shown to be effective in suppressing gram-negative infections arising from the gastrointestinal tract in neutropenic patients with leukemia or after autologous bone marrow transplantation. Ciprofloxacin may also prevent infections in neutropenic outpatients but can lead to the selection of resistant bacterial strains. Patients undergoing bone marrow transplantation have long-term indwelling catheters and are at high risk for gram-positive bacterial infections. Vancomycin, when given throughout the period of neutropenia as prophylaxis, has been shown to reduce the incidence of gram-positive infections as well as infection morbidity and the number of days of fever following bone marrow transplantation. Trimethoprim-sulfamethoxazole (TMP-SMZ) has been used as prophylaxis in neutropenic patients with variable results. TMP-SMZ is given routinely to prevent infections by *Pneumocystis* in patients with lymphocytic malignancies, AIDS, and following bone marrow transplantation. Other active agents to prevent *Pneumocystis* infection include pentamidine and dapsone. Low-dose amphotericin B and the less toxic triazole fluconazole have been used to prevent fungal infections in immunocompromised patients, though only high-dose amphotericin B is effective against *Aspergillus*. For patients with renal insufficiency, two less nephrotoxic colloidal suspensions of amphotericin B are now available. Because their relative efficacy is unknown and because they are extremely expensive, judicious use is warranted. Patients at high risk for fungal infections include those with prolonged granulocytopenia, those with indwelling catheters, those taking broad-spectrum antibiotics over long periods, and those receiving parenteral nutrition. Viral prophylaxis with acyclovir is usually given only to patients undergoing bone marrow transplantation or those with mucosal ulcerations.

In patients who are severely immunocompromised, some bacterial infections may be prevented with intravenous immune globulin. This is important in patients with chronic lymphocytic leukemia, multiple myeloma, and following bone marrow transplantation if associated immunoglobulin deficiencies are observed.

The availability of recombinant bone marrow growth factors has helped to reduce the morbidity and mortality of infections in immunocompromised hosts. Granulocyte colony-stimulating factor (G-CSF; filgrastim) and granulocyte-macrophage colony-stimulating factor (GM-CSF; sargramostim) have been shown to be effective at reducing the duration of neutropenia and the frequency and severity of infection after myelosuppressive chemotherapy or autologous bone marrow transplantation for nonmyeloid malignancies. These growth patterns improve bone marrow tolerance of escalating doses of chemotherapy, allowing higher doses to be given at shorter intervals. G-CSF and GM-CSF have been used to stimulate bone marrow stem cell production in both the circulating blood and in bone marrow cell populations collected for autologous transplantation. Administration of growth factors may improve survival after the failure of autologous or allogeneic bone marrow grafts. These growth factors are currently being used experimentally to stimulate the growth of refractory myeloid malignancies and thus perhaps enhance cell killing by cytotoxic agents.

Buchanan GR: Approach to treatment of the febrile cancer patient with low-risk neutropenia. Hematol Oncol Clin North Am 1993;7:919. (A population of low-risk patients may be identified for early discharge and outpatient antibiotics.)

De Pauw BE et al: Ceftazidime compared with piperacillin and tobramycin for the empiric treatment of fever in neutropenic patients with cancer. A multicenter randomized trial. The Intercontinental Antimicrobial Study Group. Ann Intern Med 1994;120:834. (Ceftazidime was as effective as and safer than the combination of piperacillin and tobramycin for empiric therapy of febrile neutropenia, even when the neutropenia was severe and prolonged.)

Kantarjian HM et al: Granulocyte colony-stimulating factor supportive treatment following intensive chemotherapy in acute lymphocytic leukemia in first remission. Cancer 1993;72:2950. (G-CSF reduced morbidity and mortality from induction remission of ALL.)

THE PARANEOPLASTIC SYNDROMES

The clinical manifestations of cancer are usually nonspecific—eg, anorexia, malaise, weight loss, fever—or are due to local effects of tumor growth, either in the primary site or at a distant site. The term "paraneoplasia" has been coined to denote the remote effects of malignancy that cannot be attributed either to direct invasion or metastatic lesions. These syndromes may be the first sign of a malignancy and may affect up to 15% of patients with cancer.

The paraneoplastic syndromes are of considerable clinical importance for the following reasons:

(1) They may accompany relatively limited neoplastic growth and provide an early clue to the presence of certain types of cancer.

(2) The course of the paraneoplastic syndrome usually parallels the course of the tumor. Therefore, effective treatment should be accompanied by resolution of the syndrome, and, conversely, recurrence of the cancer may be heralded by return of systemic symptoms.

(3) The metabolic or toxic effects of the syndrome may constitute a more urgent hazard to life than the underlying cancer (eg, hypercalcemia, hyponatremia).

The paraneoplastic syndromes are often considered to be due to aberrant hormonal or metabolic effects not associated with a cancer's normal tissue equivalent. Clinical findings may resemble those of primary endocrine, metabolic, hematologic, or neuromuscular disorders. The mechanisms for such remote effects can be classified into three groups: (1) effects initiated by a tumor product (eg, carcinoid syndrome), (2) effects due to the destruction of normal tissues by tumor (eg, hypercalcemia due to osteolytic skeletal metastases), and (3) effects due to unknown mechanisms such as unidentified tumor products or circulating immune complexes stimulated by the tumor (eg, osteoarthropathy due to bronchogenic carcinoma). Even such nonspecific symptoms as fever and weight loss are truly paraneoplastic and probably are due to the production of specific factors (eg, tumor necrosis factor) by the tumor itself.

Paraneoplastic syndromes associated with ectopic hormone production are among the most common. Tumor tissue secretes a hormone or prohormone that may be of a higher or lower molecular weight than hormones secreted by the more differentiated normal endocrine cell. This ectopic hormone production by cancer cells is believed to result from activation of genes in malignant cells that are normally suppressed in most somatic cells. Neoplastic cells may secrete growth factors that play an autocrine role for tumor growth and also result in paraneoplastic syndromes. A single syndrome such as hypercalcemia may be due to any one or more than one of a variety of causes. Effective antitumor treatment usually results in return of the serum calcium to normal, though additional therapy is often required (see Hypercalcemia, above). In occasional cases, a rapid response to cytotoxic chemotherapy may briefly increase the severity of the paraneoplastic syndrome in association with tumor lysis (eg, hyponatremia with inappropriate antidiuretic hormone excretion). Several neurologic paraneoplastic syndromes have recently been found to be caused by the production of antineuronal antibodies that circulate in the serum and spinal fluid. It is thought that the underlying tumor expresses a similar antigen, resulting in production of a cross-reactive antibody. Treatment of the underlying tumor usually results in only modest improvement of the neurologic deficit. Examples of antineuronal antibodies include the anti-Hu antibody causing sensory neuropathy or encephalitis, associated with small cell cancer of the lung; the anti-Yo antibody causing cerebellar degeneration, associated most often with breast or gynecologic malignancies; and the stiff man syndrome, associated with breast cancer.

The most common cancer associated with paraneoplastic syndromes is small-cell cancer of the lung. This is thought to be due to its neuroectodermal origin. Common paraneoplastic syndromes and associated malignancies are summarized in Table 4–6.

[Physicians' Data Query: Information on cancer complications]
  gopher://gopher.nih.gov/11/clin/cancernet
Conaghan PG, Brooks PM: Rheumatic manifestations of malignancy. Curr Opin Rheumatol 1994;6:105.
Pierce ST: Paraendocrine syndromes. Curr Opin Oncol 1993;5:639.
Posner JB: Paraneoplastic syndromes. Neurol Clin 1991;9:919. (Neuromuscular complications of cancer.)

POTENTIAL FUTURE APPROACHES TO CANCER THERAPY

Topotecan is the first of a new class of drugs called camptothecans to be FDA-approved for use in advanced ovarian cancer and has shown some efficacy in the treatment of several other tumors, including breast cancer. Other camptothecans are in clinical trials.

Tretinoin is a retinoid that induces cytodifferentiation and decreased proliferation and not cytolysis of acute promyelocytic leukemia cells. Use of tretinoin has been approved for induction remission in this unusual form of leukemia.

Liposomal encapsulation of active chemotherapeutic agents may improve drug delivery and decrease systemic toxicity. A liposomally encapsulated

Table 4–6. Paraneoplastic syndromes and certain endocrine secretions associated with cancer.

Hormone Excess or Syndrome	Bronchogenic Carcinoma	Breast Carcinoma	Renal Carcinoma	Adrenal Carcinoma	Hepatoma	Multiple Myeloma	Lymphoma	Thymoma	Prostatic Carcinoma	Pancreatic Carcinoma	Choriocarcinoma	Sarcoma
Hypercalcemia	++	++++	++	++	+	++++	+	+	++	+	+	+
Cushing's syndrome	+++		+	+++				++	+	++		
Inappropriate ADH secretion	+++						+		+	+		
Hypoglycemia				+	++		+					+++
Gonadotropins	+				+						++++	
Thyrotropin											+++	
Polycythemia			+++	+	++							
Erythroid aplasia								++				
Fever		+++			++		+++	++		+		+
Neuromyopathy	++	+						++	+	+		
Dermatomyositis	++	+								+		
Coagulopathy	+	++			+	+			+++	+++		
Thrombophlebitis			+						+	+++		
Humoral immune deficits						+++	+++	+++				

form of the anthracycline doxorubicin has recently been approved for use in Kaposi's sarcoma.

The use of cytotoxic drugs against cancer is limited by a number of factors, including toxicity and tumor resistance. New strategies are now based on improved knowledge of the molecular events responsible for disordered cellular growth and include antibodies directed against abnormal growth-enhancing factors and receptors as well as gene therapy to turn off signaling pathways or provide a missing tumor suppressor. The Her-2/*neu* oncogene (also called c-*erb*B-2), a gene that encodes a receptor tyrosine kinase, is known to be overexpressed in many human cancers and is associated with tumors with poorer prognoses. Antibodies against the Her-2/*neu* gene product are being evaluated in clinical trials designed to suppress tumor growth in breast and ovarian cancers.

Angiogenesis factors such as vascular endothelial growth factor (VEGF) are thought to play an important role in stimulating the growth of new vascular supply necessary for the growth and metastasis of cancer cells. Inhibitors of angiogenesis also exist, and there is great interest in utilizing the concept of angiogenesis inhibition to control neoplastic growth. Early clinical trials of antiangiogenesis factors are under way.

The goal of gene therapy for cancer is to inhibit the constitutive signals that drive tumor growth. Expanding knowledge about signal transduction has provided multiple possible attack points within this complicated pathway. In order to turn off the signaling pathways that drive proliferation within a tumor, it will be necessary to introduce specific genes or other agents. Selective targeting of cells with mutations in oncogenes or tumor suppressor genes, if successful, would allow return of normal growth patterns without toxicity to nonneoplastic cells. One area of active research is to replace the missing function of the mutated tumor suppressor gene, *p53,* or to inhibit the function of a dominant oncogene such as *ras.* One interesting approach is to create a vaccine directed against cells with mutant *p53* or *ras* in order to generate a cytotoxic T cell response to tumor cells expressing the p53 or ras proteins. This vaccine is currently in an NCI clinical trial, though no efficacy data are available. Multiple other trials, including the introduction of new genes that encode inhibitors of oncogene products or enhance tumor cell immunogenicity, are in progress.

Immunotherapy is another exciting new area of investigation of the treatment of cancer. Both radiolabeled and toxin-linked antibodies have been used to treat lymphomas with very encouraging results. An anti-B cell antibody has shown a 50% complete or partial remission in multiply relapsed low-grade B cell lymphoma. This antibody is likely to be available for general clinical use by the end of 1997. Active specific immunotherapy with melanoma vaccines has been evaluated as adjuvant therapy for melanoma with encouraging preliminary results.

New areas of cancer therapy are rapidly expanding, and the next decade could bring important changes in the treatment of common malignancies. Many alternatives to traditional cancer therapy exist (one well-known example is shark cartilage, which is widely available and purported to have anti-angiogenic properties), but there is little evidence to support their efficacy or assess their potential toxicity, and at present there is no federal regulation of these products.

The American Society of Clinical Oncology: The physician and unorthodox cancer therapies. J Clin Oncol 1997;15:401. (Nine percent of patients are estimated to use alternative cancer therapies. Physicians must be educated about these treatments and be able to discuss such issues with their patients.)

Carbone DP, Minna ID: In vivo gene therapy of human lung cancer using wild-type p53 delivery by retrovirus. J Natl Cancer Inst 1994;86:1437. (Retroviruses are used as gene delivery vehicles.)

Folkman I: Angiogenesis in cancer, vascular, rheumatoid and other disease. Nat Med 1995;1:27. (Clinical implications for angiogenesis inhibition.)

Hanania EG et al: Recent advances in the application of gene therapy to human disease. Am J Med 1995;99:537.

Levitzki A, Gazit A: Tyrosine kinase inhibition: An approach to drug development. Science 1995;267:1782. (A review of this new approach to cancer therapy.)

McDonnell WM, Askari FK: Molecular medicine: DNA vaccines N Engl J Med 1996;334:42.

Wilder RB, DeNardo GL, DeNardo S: Radioimmunotherapy: Recent results and future directions. J Clin Oncol 1996;14:1383. (A review of the literature on radiolabeled antibodies in cancer therapy.)

Care at the End of Life

5

Michael W. Rabow, MD, & Robert V. Brody, MD

THE END OF LIFE

DIAGNOSIS OF THE END OF LIFE

Eventually, everyone dies. In the United States, approximately 2.3 million people die each year. Despite all the successes of medical progress, death inevitably comes, and physicians battling to prolong life must recognize when life is ending in order to continue caring well for their patients. While death itself remains a mystery and while caring for the dying has not been well researched or adequately taught as part of medical training, caring for patients at the end of life is an important responsibility and a rewarding opportunity for physicians.

The terms "palliative care," "care of the dying," and "end-of-life care" imply a focus on care of the whole person who is approaching death rather than on an attempt to cure underlying disease. Since it emphasizes that the dying process is part of life, the expression "end-of-life care" is preferable and will be used here. From the medical perspective, the end of life may be defined as that time when death—whether due to terminal illness, acute or chronic illness, or age itself—is expected within weeks to months and can no longer be reasonably forestalled by medical intervention.

Physicians have an important role in helping patients understand that their lives are ending. While certain diseases such as cancer are amenable to prognostic estimates regarding the time course to death, the other common causes of mortality in the United States—including heart disease, stroke, chronic lung disease, and dementia—have variable and difficult to predict prognoses. For such conditions, clinical experience, epidemiologic data, and guidelines from professional organizations* and formal computer-based

modeling and prediction tools[†] may be employed to help patients identify the end period of their lives. Attention must be paid to how predictions are communicated. Although statistically equivalent in the SUPPORT model, a prognosis of 1% survival at 2 months may sound different to a patient than being told he or she has a median survival time of 1 day.

EXPECTATIONS ABOUT THE END OF LIFE

Patients' experiences of the end of life are influenced by their expectations about how they will die and the meaning of death. Many people fear how they will die more than death itself. Patients report fear of dying in pain or of suffocation, of loss of control, indignity, isolation, and being a burden to their families. All of these anxieties can be alleviated with good supportive care provided by an attentive group of caretakers.

For most of human history, death has been regarded as part of the natural process of life. However, with recent technologic advances that serve to forestall the end of life, death has become "medicalized." No longer seen clearly as a profound personal and spiritual event basic to the human condition, death is often regarded as a failure of medical science. The medicalization of death can create or heighten a sense of guilt about the failure to prevent dying. Both the general public and physicians are complicit in denying death, treating dying persons as patients and death as an enemy to be battled furiously in hospitals rather than as an inevitable outcome to be experienced as a part of life at home. Currently in the United States, approximately 80% of people die in hospitals or long-term care facilities.

---

*For example, the National Hospice Organization.

[†]For example, the Acute Physiology and Chronic Health Evaluation (APACHE) system or the Study to Understand Prognoses and Preferences for Outcomes and Risks of Treatment (SUPPORT) model.

THE ROLE OF THE PHYSICIAN AT THE END OF LIFE

Caring for patients at the end of life requires the same skills physicians employ in other tasks of doctoring: eliciting a complete history, examining for signs of physical disease, making careful diagnoses of treatable conditions, providing patient education, sharing in decision-making, and expressing understanding and caring. Communication skills are vitally important. In particular, physicians must become experts at delivering bad news and then dealing with its consequences (Table 5–1).

Three further physician obligations are central to the physician's role at this time. First, physicians must work to identify, understand, and relieve patient suffering. Suffering is experienced by the person as a whole and may include physical, psychologic, social, or spiritual distress. Some authorities argue that the prospect of dying causes suffering because it threatens a person's sense of integrity or intactness. Personality, a past, a cultural and political identity, a set of relationships, a body, a secret life, a perceived future, and a transcendent dimension are some of the components of an intact person, and any of these components may be threatened by disease, disability, and disintegration at the end of life. In assisting with redirection and growth, providing support, assessing meaning, and fostering transcendence, physicians can help ameliorate their patients' suffering.

Second, physicians caring for patients at the end of life have an obligation to serve as a facilitator or catalyst for hope. While a particular outcome may be extremely unlikely (such as cure of advanced cancer following exhaustive conventional and experimental treatments), hope may be defined as the patient's belief in what is still possible. Although hope for a "miraculous cure" may be simplistic and even harmful, hope for relief of pain, for reconciliation with loved ones, for discovery of meaning in the life remaining, and for spiritual transformation is still quite supportable at the end of life. With questions such as "What is still possible for you?"—"What do you wish for before you die?"—"What good might come of this?" physicians can help patients uncover hope, explore meaningful and realistic goals, and develop strategies to realize them.

Third, patients' feelings of isolation and fear engendered by the prospect of dying demand that physicians communicate directly to patients that care will continue to be provided throughout the final stage of life. Perhaps the essential principle of care at the end of life is this promise of nonabandonment: a physician's pledge to an individual patient to serve as a caring partner, a resource for creative problem-solving and relief of suffering, a guide during uncertain times, and a witness to the patient's experiences—no matter what happens. Dying patients need their physicians to offer their presence—not necessarily the ability to solve all problems but rather a commitment to recognize and receive the patients' difficulties and experiences with respect and empathy. At its best, the patient-physician relationship can be a covenant of compassion and a recognition of common humanity.

CARING FOR THE FAMILY

In caring for patients at the end of life, physicians must appreciate the central role played by family, friends, and romantic partners and often must deal with strong emotions of fear, anger, shame, sadness, and guilt experienced by those individuals. While significant others may support and comfort a patient at the end of life, the threatened loss of a loved one may also create or reveal dysfunctional or painful family dynamics. Furthermore, physicians must be attuned to the potential impact of illness on the patient's family: substantial physical caregiving responsibilities and financial burdens as well as increased rates of anxiety, depression, chronic illness, and even mortality.

Physicians can help families confront the imminent loss of a loved one (Table 5–2) and often must negotiate amid complex and changing family needs.

Table 5–1. Suggestions for the delivery of bad news.

Prepare an appropriate place and time.
Address basic information needs.
Be direct; avoid jargon and euphemisms.
Allow for silence and emotional ventilation.
Assess and validate patient reactions.
Respond to immediate discomforts and risks.
Listen actively and express empathy.
Achieve a common perception of the problem.
Reassure about pain relief.
Ensure basic follow-up and make specific plans for the future.

Table 5–2. Physician behaviors helpful to families of dying patients.[1]

Timely, frequent, and consistent communication
Adapting communication to need
Focusing on patient's wishes
Attending to the comfort of the patient
Being aware of family conflict
Accommodating family's grief
Refocusing hope
Encouraging planning
Remaining available
Following up with family after death

[1]Adapted, with permission, from Bascom PB, Tolle SW: Care of the family when the patient is dying. West J Med 1995;163:292.

Identifying a spokesperson for the family, conducting family meetings, allowing all to be heard, and providing time for consensus may help the physician work effectively with the family. However, it is important to remember that the extent of the family's involvement in the receipt of bad news, in the sharing of information, and in medical decision-making is appropriately determined only by the patient. The physician may say to the patient, "I have important new information to discuss with you. Is there anyone you would like to be present while we talk?"

THE LIMITS OF CARE AT THE END OF LIFE

Many physicians find caring for patients at the end of life to be one of the most rewarding aspects of practice. However, working with the dying requires tolerance of great uncertainty, ambiguity, and existential challenges. Physicians must recognize and respect their own limitations and attend to their own needs in order to avoid being overburdened, overly distressed, or emotionally depleted. Open recognition of their own feelings enables physicians to process their emotions and take steps to care for themselves: conferring and consulting with colleagues, retreating, relaxing and recuperating, obtaining informal or professional support, or even—under extraordinary circumstances—transferring the care of a patient to another physician when it is no longer possible to meet the patient's needs or comply with unreasonable requests. Moreover, care of patients at the end of life is not solely the responsibility of physicians. Ideally, physicians, nurses, therapists, clergy, and volunteers can coordinate their efforts to care for patients and can support one another.

Physicians may be limited in caring for persons at the end of life not only by their emotional responses but by a sense of moral obligation as well. While the ethical, legal, and professional controversies over physician-assisted suicide are beyond the scope of this chapter, physicians should be aware of the growing "right to die" movement as an expression, at least in part, of patient dissatisfaction with how people are cared for at the end of life. While individual physicians must decide for themselves within the evolving legal context what their personal limits may be in caring for patients who request aid in dying (eg, physician-assisted suicide), all physicians can reclaim their long-privileged and universally accepted role of caring for the dying. They can do so by dedicating themselves not to abandon their patients and by providing appropriate attention to symptom management, sensitivity to psychologic and social stresses, and unconditional presence and openness to spiritual challenges at the end of life.

Cassel EJ: The nature of suffering and the goals of medicine. N Engl J Med 1982;306:639.

Council on Scientific Affairs, American Medical Association: Good care of the dying patient. JAMA 1996; 275:474.

Covinsky KE et al: The impact of serious illness on patients' families. JAMA 1994;272:1839.

Eisman M, Quill TE: Death and dying. In: *Behavioral Medicine in Primary Care*. Feldman MD, Christensen JF (editors). Appleton & Lange, 1997.

Lynn J, Teno JM: Accurate prognostications of death: Opportunities and challenges for clinicians. West J Med 1995;163:250.

McCue JD: The naturalness of dying. JAMA 1995; 273:1039.

National Hospice Organization: Medical guidelines for determining prognosis in selected non-cancer diseases. Hospice J 1996;11:47.

Quill TE, Cassel CK: Nonabandonment: A central obligation for physicians. Ann Intern Med 1995;122:368.

THE SETTING & STRUCTURE OF CARE

ETHICAL & LEGAL BACKGROUND

Physician care of patients at the end of life is guided by the same ethical and legal principles that inform other types of medical care. Foremost among these are the principles of nonmaleficence, beneficence, autonomy, proportionality, distributive justice, personal integrity, and truth-telling. These are the basic principles that must guide clinicians in helping patients make difficult decisions about care, including decisions about the withdrawal and withholding of support and the hastening of death.

Three additional ethical considerations are relevant to care at the end of life. First, important ethical principles may be in conflict. For example, while a patient may desire a particular medical intervention, the physician may refuse to undertake the intervention if it is of no therapeutic benefit. Moreover, physicians are not bound to offer therapy the patient demands if doing so violates the physician's own moral code (though referral to another physician may then be appropriate).

Second, although physicians and family members often have very different emotional reactions to withholding versus withdrawing support, there is broad consensus among ethicists, supported by legal precedent, of their ethical equivalence. Patients have the same right to stop unwanted medical treatments once begun as they do to refuse those treatments in the first place.

Third, the ethical principle of "double effect" argues that the potential to hasten imminent death is acceptable if it comes as the unintended consequence of a primary intention to provide comfort and relieve suffering. For example, sufficient doses of morphine should be provided to control pain even if there is the potential unintended secondary effect of depressing respiration. In practice, one can almost always find an effective pain regimen without hastening death.

ADVANCE DIRECTIVES

At the end of life, when patients' choices about medical intervention may have life-or-death implications, the principle of autonomy must be emphasized. Well-informed and otherwise competent adults have a right to refuse medical intervention even if refusal is likely to result in death. Many people believe that there are fates worse than death and are willing to sacrifice some quantity of life in exchange for protecting a certain quality of life.

In order to further patient autonomy, physicians are obligated to inform patients about the risks, benefits, alternatives, and expected outcomes of end-of-life medical interventions such as cardiopulmonary resuscitation, intubation and mechanical ventilation, vasopressor medication, hospitalization and ICU care, and artificial nutrition and hydration. It is especially important during discussions about end-of-life care that physicians reassure patients about the ability to control pain and other symptoms and make an explicit pledge not to abandon the patient.

Studies have shown that neither physicians nor families are better than chance at predicting patient preferences for end-of-life care. In order to know what their patients will want when the time comes, physicians must discuss with patients their hopes, values, expectations, philosophies, and choices for end-of-life care. Research has demonstrated that most patients have already thought about end-of-life issues, want to discuss these issues with their physician, want the physician to bring up the subject, and feel better for having had the discussion. Unfortunately, only about 15% of outpatients have had these kinds of discussions with their physicians.

Patient autonomy may be furthered by use of advance directives (eg, a living will or health care proxy) whereby patients express their wishes for or against medical interventions in case they later become incompetent. Advance directives are legally binding documents in all 50 states. Living wills set forth the signatory's preferences for or against particular medical interventions in the event the patient becomes incompetent. The health care proxy or durable power of attorney for health care is a more flexible document that allows a patient to appoint a surrogate decision-maker (an attorney-in-fact, or proxy) who is legally empowered to make medical decisions for the patient if the patient becomes incompetent.

Surrogacy advances patient autonomy because surrogates must try to decide what the patient would have wanted based on the patient's spoken and written wishes, values, and philosophies. In the absence of specific knowledge about what a patient wanted or if it is not possible to make a "substituted judgment" on the patient's behalf, surrogates are responsible for making decisions in the patient's "best interest"—a much more vague and difficult process.

Physicians should educate all patients—ideally, well before the end of life—about the opportunity to formulate an advance directive. The federal Patient Self-Determination Act of 1991 requires that hospitals and other health care institutions receiving Medicare funds inform patients of their rights to formulate an advance directive. Currently, however, only about 10% of people in the United States (including physicians) actually have executed advance directives, and studies have shown that physicians are often unaware of or actually ignore their patients' advance directives.

DNAR ORDERS

Physicians can encourage patients to express their preferences for the use of CPR. Unfortunately, most patients and many physicians are uninformed or misinformed about the nature and success of CPR. Despite the favorable portrayal of CPR in the popular media, only about 15% of all patients who undergo CPR in the hospital survive to hospital discharge. Moreover, among certain populations of patients—especially those with systemic noncardiac disease—the likelihood of survival to hospital discharge following CPR may be nil or extremely slight (Table 5–3).

Table 5–3. Survival to hospital discharge following cardiopulmonary resuscitation of patients with various underlying diseases.[1]

Conditions with highest survival rates:	
Ventricular fibrillation post-MI	26–46%
Drug reaction or overdose	22–28%
Ventricular arrhythmia	19–50%
Conditions with lowest survival rates:	
Malignancy[2]	0–3.5%
Neurologic disease	0–6.7%
Renal failure	0–10%
Respiratory disease	0–7%
Sepsis	0–7%
Nursing home residence	0–1.7%
Out-of-hospital cardiopulmonary arrest[3]	0.6%

[1]Modified, with permission, from Moss AH: Informing the patient about cardiopulmonary resuscitation: When the risks outweigh the benefits. J Gen Intern Med 1989;4:349.
[2]Survival was 0% in patients with metastatic disease in the first nine studies reported.
[3]If return of spontaneous circulation was not obtained after 25 minutes of standard advanced cardiac life support out-of-hospital.

Patients may ask their physician to write an order that CPR not be attempted for them. Although this order initially was referred to as a DNR ("do not resuscitate") order, many physicians now prefer the term DNAR ("do not attempt resuscitation") to emphasize the low likelihood of successful resuscitation.

In addition to mortality statistics, patients deciding about CPR preferences should also be informed about the possible consequences of surviving a CPR attempt. CPR may result in fractured ribs, lacerated internal organs, and neurologic disability, and there is a high likelihood of requiring other aggressive interventions, such as ICU care, if CPR is successful.

For some patients at the end of life, decisions about CPR may be not about whether they will live or die but about how they will die. Physicians should correct the misconception that withholding CPR in appropriate circumstances is tantamount to "not doing everything" or "just letting someone die." Frequently, CPR will not improve the quality of a dying patient's life or alter the patient's underlying prognosis. While respecting the patient's right ultimately to make the decision—and keeping in mind their own biases and prejudices—physicians should offer explicit recommendations about DNAR orders and in that way protect dying patients and their families from feelings of guilt and from the sorrow associated with vain hopes. Finally, physicians should encourage patients and their families to make proactive decisions about what is wanted in end-of-life care rather than focusing only on what is not to be done.

HOSPICE CARE

While most patients die in hospitals, good care of the dying is not the central goal of most hospitals. Instead, it is the focus of hospice, a facility or program designed to provide a caring environment for meeting the physical and emotional needs of the terminally ill. Hospice care focuses on the patient rather than the disease and on providing comfort and pain relief rather than on treating illness or prolonging life. Hospices provide intensive caring with the goal of helping people live well until they die.

The hospice philosophy emphasizes individualized attention, human contact, and a multi-disciplinary team approach involving physicians, nurses, health aides, social workers, psychologists, therapists (physical, occupational, recreational), dietitians, chaplains, and volunteers. Hospice care can include arranging for respite for family caregivers and providing legal, financial, and other services. While some hospice care is provided in hospitals and institutional residences, about 80% of patients receiving hospice care remain at home where they can be cared for by the family and visiting hospice staff. Primary care physicians are strongly encouraged to continue caring for their patients during the time they are receiving hospice care.

Hospice care has been shown to increase patient satisfaction, to ease family anxiety, and even to reduce costs depending on when patients are referred to hospice care. While hospice care may be the appropriate standard of care for the dying, only about 15% of all patients who die receive hospice care (80% of these people have end-stage cancer). Hospice care tends to be utilized late in the course of the end of life. The average length of stay in hospices in the United States is just 36 days, with 15% of patients dying within 7 days after beginning hospice care.

Most hospice organizations require physicians to estimate the patient's probability of survival to be less than 6 months, since this is criterion for eligibility to receive Medicare coverage (a benefit available since 1982). Unfortunately, as currently structured, the hospice benefit tends to be unavailable to people who are homeless, isolated, or with terminal prognoses that are difficult to quantify.

Many of the goals of hospice care, such as relief of suffering and attention to the patient as a person, are relevant to traditional medical care. However, the emphasis on patient well-being rather than on cure, the direct acknowledgment of death and dying issues, and the effort to care for people in their homes make hospice an important alternative to acute hospital care at the end of life. While the initiation of hospice care is often described as a transition from aggressive care to comfort care, hospice care too provides "aggressive" care, though not directed at achieving a cure. It is more appropriate to consider hospice care as one among many health care resources available to patients at the end of life. For the dying, it may be appropriate to "treat" pneumonia with morphine and antipyretics rather than with antibiotics. Helping patients decide when to avail themselves of the resources of hospice care is an important function even for physicians providing the most aggressive and intensive curative medical interventions.

CULTURAL ISSUES

The individual's experience of dying occurs in the context of a complex interaction of personal, philosophic, and cultural influences. Various religious, ethnic, gender, class, and cultural traditions inform patients' styles of communication, comfort in discussing particular topics, expectations about dying and medical interventions, and attitudes about the appropriate disposition of dead bodies. Studies have shown differences in knowledge and beliefs regarding advance directives, autopsy, organ donation, hospice care, and withdrawal of support among patients of different ethnic groups. While each patient must be considered an individual, understanding cultural assumptions and beliefs and respecting ethnic traditions are important responsibilities of the physician caring for a patient at the end of life, especially when the cultures of origin of the physician and patient differ.

[State-specific information about advance directives] http://www.choices.org

Christakis NA, Escarce JJ: Survival of Medicare patients after enrollment in hospice programs. N Engl J Med 1996;335:172.

Council on Ethical and Judicial Affairs, American Medical Association: Decisions near the end of life. JAMA 1992;267:2229.

Council on Ethical and Judicial Affairs, American Medical Association: Guidelines for the appropriate use of do-not-resuscitate orders. JAMA 1991;265:1868.

Diem SJ et al: Cardiopulmonary resuscitation on television: Miracles and misinformation. N Engl J Med 1996;334:1578.

Koenig BA, Gates-Williams J: Understanding cultural differences in caring for dying patients. West J Med 1995;163:244.

THE SPECIFIC TASKS OF CARING

SYMPTOM MANAGEMENT

For patients at the end of life, maximizing the quality of life—rather than postponing death—is the first priority of care. In this context, symptoms that cause disability and suffering must be considered medical emergencies and managed aggressively by frequent elicitation, continuous reassessment, and individualized treatment.

The relief of distressing symptoms at the end of life should not be withheld out of reluctance to use appropriate doses of opioids or sedatives. While physiologic dependence is expected with opioid use, at the end of life, the use of opioids for relief of pain and dyspnea is not associated with a risk of psychologic addiction and abuse. Furthermore, if properly informed, patients or their surrogates may decide to pursue aggressive symptom relief even if the treatments used inadvertently shorten life (ie, have a "double effect").

Pain

Pain is a common problem for patients at the end of life—up to 75% of patients dying of cancer experience pain—and is what many people say they fear most about dying. Pain is under-treated at the end of life. One study has documented that severely ill hospitalized patients spent half of their time during the last 3 days of life in moderate to severe pain.

The experience of pain also includes the patient's emotional reaction to it. Pain is subjective, and physicians cannot reliably detect or quantify pain without asking. A useful means of assessing pain and evaluating the effectiveness of analgesia is to ask the patient to rate the degree of pain along a numeric or visual pain scale (Table 5–4).

Recommendations for the use of analgesic, adjuvant, and nonpharmacologic pain management are reviewed in Chapter 1. The goal of pain management is most properly decided by the patient. While some patients may wish to be completely free of pain even if this entails significant sedation, most will wish to control pain at a level that still allows maximal functioning. Careful attention to pain relief and perseverance in achieving it is indicated for all patients. Hospice physicians regularly report a success rate higher than 90% in relieving pain in terminally ill patients.

There is no maximal allowable dose for opioid agonists such as morphine sulfate. The dose should be increased to whatever is necessary to relieve pain, remembering that certain types of pain (eg, neuropathic pain) may respond better to agents other than opioids. As dosages of opioids are increased, however, increasing difficulty with the three major side effects of opioids is to be expected. The management of constipation and nausea is outlined below. Sedation can be expected with opioids, though tolerance to the sedative effects of opioids may develop within 24–72 hours. Sedation typically appears well before significant respiratory depression. If treatment for sedation is desired, dextroamphetamine (2.5–7.5 mg orally every 6 hours) may be given.

Dyspnea

Dyspnea is the subjective experience of difficulty in breathing and may be characterized by patients as tightness, shortness of breath, or a feeling of suffocation. Dyspnea is common among dying patients—up to one-half of severely ill patients at the end of life experience severe dyspnea.

Treatment of dyspnea is usually first directed at the underlying cause, which may be related to pneumonia, pulmonary embolism, pleural effusion, bronchospasm, tracheal obstruction, neuromuscular disease, restriction of movement of the chest or abdominal walls, cardiac ischemia, congestive heart failure, superior vena cava syndrome, or severe anemia.

At the end of life, dyspnea is often treated nonspecifically with opioids. Immediate-release morphine, preferably via the oral or buccal route, treats dyspnea effectively and typically at doses lower than would be necessary for the relief of moderate pain. Supplemental oxygen may be useful for the dyspneic patient who is hypoxic and may provide subjective benefit to other dyspneic patients as well. However, a nasal cannula and face mask are sometimes not well tolerated, and fresh air from a window or fan may

Table 5–4. Pain assessment scales.

Numeric Scale

No pain   Worst pain

1   2   3   4   5   6   7   8   9   10

Numeric Scale Translated into Word and Behavior Scales

Pain intensity	Word scale	Nonverbal behaviors
0	No pain	Relaxed, calm expression
1–2	Least pain	Stressed, tense expression
3–4	Mild pain	Guarded movement, grimacing
5–6	Moderate pain	Moaning, restless
7–8	Severe pain	Crying out
9–10	Excruciating pain	Increased intensity of above

Visual Faces Scale[1]

0   1   2   3   4   5

[1]Especially useful for patients who cannot read English and for pediatric patients. Modified and reproduced, with permission, from Whaley L, Wong D: *Nursing Care of Infants and Children*, 3rd ed. Mosby, 1987.

provide relief as well. Use of anxiolytics as well as nonpharmacologic relaxation techniques such as meditation and guided imagery may be beneficial for some patients.

Nausea & Vomiting

Nausea and vomiting are common and distressing symptoms. As with pain, the management of nausea may be maximized by around-the-clock dosing. An understanding of the four major inputs to the vomiting center may help direct treatment. (See also Chapter 14.)

The chemoreceptor trigger zone may be stimulated by certain drugs (eg, morphine, NSAIDs), metabolic derangements, and chemotherapeutic agents. Vomiting associated with a particular opioid may be avoided by substitution with an equianalgesic dose of another opioid or a sustained-release formulation. In addition to the other dopamine antagonist antiemetics listed in Table 15–2 that block the trigger zone, haloperidol (0.5–5 mg orally every 4–6 hours) is commonly used.

Vomiting may be due to stimulation of peripheral afferent nerves. Offering patients small amounts of food only when they are hungry may prevent nausea and vomiting. Nasogastric suction may provide rapid relief for vomiting associated with constipation, gastroparesis, or gastric outlet obstruction, with the addition of laxatives, prokinetic agents (metoclopramide,

10–20 mg orally or intravenously four times a day; or cisapride, 10 mg orally four times a day), and high-dose corticosteroids as more definitive treatment. Treatment with high-dose corticosteroids (eg, dexamethasone, 20 mg orally or intravenously), ondansetron (8 mg orally three times daily), or cyclizine (5 mg orally every 8 hours) may be useful for nausea and vomiting due to disease of intra-abdominal or pelvic organs.

Increased intracranial pressure may cause vomiting and may be relieved with high-dose corticosteroids or palliative cranial radiation. Vomiting due to disturbance of the vestibular apparatus may be treated with anticholinergic and antihistaminic agents (see Table 15–2).

The beneficial effects of benzodiazepines for vomiting may derive mainly from their sedative and amnestic effects in the setting of anticipatory vomiting rather than as a primary antiemetic. Many patients find dronabinol (2.5–20 mg orally every 4–6 hours) helpful in the management of nausea and vomiting as well.

Constipation

Given the frequent use of opioids, poor dietary intake, and physical inactivity, constipation is a common problem among the dying. Physicians must inquire about any difficulty with hard or infrequent stools. Constipation is an easily treatable cause of significant discomfort and distress. (See Chapter 14.)

Constipation may be prevented or relieved if patients can increase their activity and their intake of dietary fiber and fluids. Simple considerations such as privacy, undisturbed toilet time, and a bedside commode rather than a bedpan may be important for some patients.

For patients taking opioids, anticipating and preventing constipation is important. A prophylactic bowel regimen of stool softeners (docusate) and stimulants (bisacodyl or senna) should be started when opioid treatment is begun. Lactulose, sorbitol, magnesium citrate, and enemas can be added as needed (Table 5–5).

Delirium & Agitation

Many terminally ill patients die in a state of delirium—a disturbance of consciousness and a change in cognition that develops over a short time and is manifested by misinterpretations, illusions, hallucinations, disturbances in the sleep-wake cycle (eg, sundowning), psychomotor disturbance (eg, lethargy, restlessness), and mood disturbance (eg, fear, anxiety).

Careful attention to patient safety and nonpharma-

Table 5–5. Pharmacologic management of constipation.

Bulk laxatives[1]	
Bran powder	1–2 tbsp orally at bedtime to twice daily
Psyllium fiber	3 g orally at bedtime to 3 times daily
Osmotic laxatives	
Lactulose	15–60 mL orally 1–3 times daily
Sorbitol	15–60 mL orally 1–3 times daily
Magnesium hydroxide	5–10 mL orally 1–4 times daily
Magnesium citrate	8 fluid oz orally daily
Sodium phosphate	30 mL orally daily, may repeat once
Detergent agents	
Docusate sodium	50–300 mg orally at bedtime to 3 times daily[2]
Stimulants	
Bisacodyl	5–15 mg orally at bedtime to 3 times daily or 10–20 mg rectally at bedtime
Senna	5–15 mg orally at bedtime to 3 times daily
Other interventions	
Glycerin suppositories	
Enemas of saline, tap water, oil retention, soapsuds, or milk and molasses	
Digital disimpaction[3]	

[1]Should be avoided in most ill patients and patients with bowel obstruction or impaction.
[2]Acts primarily as a stool softener.
[3]Should be preceded by oil retention enema, adequate lubrication, and premedication with an anxiolytic.

cologic strategies to help the patient remain oriented (clocks, calendars, a familiar environment, reassurance and redirection from caregivers) may be sufficient to prevent or manage minor delirium. Some delirious patients may be "pleasantly confused," and a decision by the patient's family and physician not to treat the delirium may be justified.

More commonly, however, delirium at the end of life is distressing to patients and family and requires treatment. Delirium may interfere with the family's ability to feel comforting to the patient and may prevent a patient from being able to recognize and report important symptoms.

While there are many reversible causes of delirium (see Chapter 25), identifying and correcting the underlying cause at the end of life is often simply a question of attention to the choice and dosing of psychoactive medications.

When the cause of delirium cannot be identified, treated, or corrected rapidly enough, delirium may be treated symptomatically with neuroleptics and benzodiazepines. Haloperidol (1–10 mg orally, subcutaneously, intramuscularly, or intravenously twice or three times a day) is used commonly, but significant extrapyramidal adverse effects may occur. Thioridazine (starting at a dosage of 25 mg orally three times a day) and risperidone (1–3 mg orally twice a day) may be helpful in delirium, but they are only available orally.

As an adjuvant to the above neuroleptics, especially in the setting of anxiety, benzodiazepines such as lorazepam (0.5–2 mg orally, sublingually, subcutaneously, or intravenously every 4–6 hours) may be useful. When delirium is refractory to treatment and remains intolerable, sedation may be required to provide relief and may be achieved rapidly with midazolam (0.5–5 mg/h subcutaneously or intravenously) or barbiturates.

NUTRITION & HYDRATION

Recently, there has been a growing awareness among hospice physicians of the potential medical benefits—without causing or increasing patient discomfort—of forgoing unwanted or artificial nutrition and hydration (including tube feedings, parenteral nutrition, and intravenous hydration) at the end of life.

Without nutrition, the length of life is determined largely by the patient's stores of fat. A normally nourished adult might be expected to die of caloric depletion in about 70 days. At the end of life, eating without hunger and artificial nutrition are associated with a number of potential complications. Force feeding may cause nausea and vomiting in ill patients, and eating will lead to diarrhea in the setting of malabsorption. Nutrition may increase oral and airway secretions and the risk of choking, aspiration, and dyspnea. Nasogastric and gastrostomy tube feeding and total parenteral nutrition impose risks of infection, epistaxis, pneumothorax, electrolyte imbalance, and aspiration—as well as the need to physically restrain the delirious patient to prevent dislodgment of catheters and tubes.

While starvation may cause weakness, lethargy, and apathy, withholding nutrition at the end of life causes remarkably little hunger or distress. Ill people often have no hunger with total starvation, and studies have shown that the ketonemia from starvation produces a sense of well-being, analgesia, and mild euphoria. However, carbohydrate intake even in small amounts (such as that provided by 5% intravenous dextrose solution) blocks ketone production and may blunt the positive effects of total starvation.

Withholding hydration may lead to death in a few days to a month. The quality of life for those at the end of life may be adversely affected by hydration due to its contribution to oral and airway secretions (leading to aspiration or the "death rattle"), polyuria, and the development or worsening of ascites, pleural or other effusions, and peripheral and pulmonary edema.

Although it is unclear to what extent withholding hydration at the end of life creates an uncomfortable sensation of thirst, any such sensation is usually relieved by simply moistening the dry mouth. Ice chips, hard candy, swabs, or a solution of equal parts nystatin solution, viscous lidocaine, diphenhydramine, and minted mouthwash are very effective.

Individuals at the end of life have a right to refuse nutrition and hydration. However, providing or withholding food and water is not simply a medical decision since doing so may have profound social and cultural significance for patients, families, and physicians. Withholding nutrition and hydration challenges the assumption that offering food is an expression of compassion and love. In fact, individuals at the end of life who choose to forgo nutrition and hydration are unlikely to suffer from hunger or thirst. Family and friends can be encouraged to express their love and caring in ways other than intrusive attempts at forced or artificial nutrition and hydration.

WITHDRAWAL OF SUPPORT

Requests for withdrawal of care from appropriately informed and competent patients or their surrogates must be respected. The physician receiving such requests should recognize and explore the significance of this change in health care goals. Alternatively, physicians may determine unilaterally that further medical intervention is medically inappropriate—for example, continuing renal dialysis in a patient dying of multi-organ failure. In such cases, the physician's intention to withdraw a specific interven-

tion should be communicated clearly to the patient and family. If differences of opinion exist about the professional propriety of what is being done, the assistance of institutional ethics committees should be sought.

The withdrawal of life-sustaining interventions such as mechanical ventilation must be approached carefully to avoid needless patient suffering and distress for those in attendance. Physicians should educate the patient and family about the expected course of events and the difficulty of determining the precise timing of death after withdrawal of support. Sedative and analgesic agents should be administered in sufficient dosages and at proper intervals to ensure patient comfort even at the risk of respiratory depression or hypotension. Scopolamine, 10 μg/h subcutaneously or intravenously, is useful for controlling airway secretions and the resultant "death rattle." A guideline for withdrawal of mechanical ventilation is provided in Table 5–6.

PSYCHOLOGIC, SOCIAL, & SPIRITUAL ISSUES

Dying is not exclusively or even primarily a biomedical event. It is an intimate personal experience with profound psychologic, interpersonal, and existential meanings. For many people at the end of life, the prospect of impending death stimulates a deep and urgent assessment of their identity, the quality of their relationships, and the meaning and purpose of

Table 5–6. Guidelines for withdrawal of mechanical ventilation.[1]

1. Stop neuromuscular blocking agents.
2. Administer opiates or sedatives to eliminate distress.
   If not already sedated, begin with Fentanyl 100 μg (or morphine sulfate 10 mg) by intravenous bolus and infusion of Fentanyl 100 μg per hour intravenously (or morphine sulfate 10 mg per hour intravenously).
   Distress is indicated by RR > 24, nasal flaring, use of accessory muscles of respiration, HR increase > 20%, MAP increase > 20%, grimacing, clutching.
3. Discontinue vasoactive agents and other agents unrelated to patient comfort, such as antibiotics, intravenous fluids, and diagnostic procedures.
4. Decrease FiO_2 to room air and PEEP to 0 cm H_2O.
5. Observe patient for distress.
   If patient is distressed, increase opiates by repeating bolus dose and increasing hourly infusion rate by 50 μg Fentanyl (or 5 mg morphine sulfate),[2] then return to observation.
   If patient is not distressed, place on T piece and observe.
   If patient continues without distress, extubate patient and continue to observe for distress.

[1]Adapted, with permission, from San Francisco General Hospital Guidelines for Withdrawal of Mechanical Ventilation/Life Support.
[2]Ventilatory support may be increased until additional opiates have effect.

their existence. As Ira Byock has observed, while the relief of physical symptoms is the "first priority" in caring for patients at the end of life, the "ultimate goal" remains helping patients to die well.

Psychologic Challenges

In 1969, Elisabeth Kübler-Ross identified five psychologic stages or patterns of emotions that patients at the end of life may experience: denial and isolation, anger, bargaining, depression, and acceptance. Not every patient will experience these emotions and not necessarily in an orderly progression. In addition to these five stages are the perpetual challenges of anxiety and fear of the unknown. Simple information, listening, assurance, and support may help patients with these psychologic challenges. Psychotherapy and group support may be beneficial as well.

Social Challenges

At the end of life, patients should be encouraged to discharge personal, professional, and business obligations. This might include completing important work or personal projects, distributing possessions, writing a will, and making funeral and burial arrangements.

The prospect of death often prompts patients to examine the quality of their interpersonal relationships, including their relationship with their physician. Dying may intensify the need for the patient to feel cared for by the doctor, highlighting the physician's obligation of nonabandonment and the need for physician empathy and compassion.

Concern about estranged relationships or "unfinished business" with significant others and interest in reconciliation may become paramount to people who are dying. At the end of life, even healthy interpersonal relationships must reach completion (Table 5–7).

Spiritual Challenges

Spirituality is the attempt to understand or accept the underlying meaning of life, one's relationships to oneself and other people, one's place in the universe, and the possibility of a "higher power" in the universe. Spirituality is distinguished from any particular religious practices or beliefs and is generally considered a universal human concern.

Table 5–7. Five statements often necessary for the completion of important interpersonal relationships.[1]

(1) "Forgive me."	(An expression of regret)
(2) "I forgive you."	(An expression of acceptance)
(3) "Thank you."	(An expression of gratitude)
(4) "I love you."	(An expression of affection)
(5) "Good-bye."	(Leave-taking)

[1]Courtesy of Ira R. Byock, MD.

Perhaps because of an inappropriately exclusive attention to the biologic challenge of forestalling death or perhaps from feelings of discomfort or incompetence, physicians frequently ignore their patients' spiritual concerns or reflexively refer these important issues to psychiatrists or other caretakers (nurses, social workers, clergy).

However, the existential challenges of dying are central to the well-being of people at the end of life and are the proper concern of physicians. Within a biopsychosociospiritual model of medical care, physicians may work to provide more than simple physical comfort and control of bothersome symptoms. Physicians can help patients to die well by providing care to the whole person—by providing physical comfort and social support and by helping patients discover their own unique meaning in the world and an acceptance of death as a part of life.

Unlike physical ailments such as infections and fractures, which usually require a physician's intervention to be treated, the patient's spiritual concerns often require only a physician's attention, listening, and witness. Physicians should routinely inquire about the patient's spiritual concerns and ask whether the patient wishes to discuss them. For example, asking, "How are you within yourself?" communicates that the physician is interested in the patient's whole experience and provides an opportunity for the patient to share perceptions about his or her inner life. Questions that might constitute an existential "review of systems" are presented in Table 5–8.

Attending to the spiritual concerns of patients calls for listening carefully to their stories. Story-telling gives patients the opportunity to verbalize what is meaningful to them and to leave something of themselves behind—the promise of being remembered. Story-telling may be facilitated by suggesting that the patient share his or her life story with family members, record it on audio or video tape, assemble a photo album, organize a scrap book, or write an autobiography.

While dying may be a period of inevitable loss of physical functioning, the end of life also offers an opportunity for psychologic, interpersonal, and spiritual development. Individuals may grow—even achieve a heightened sense of well-being or transcendence—in the process of dying. Through listening, support, and presence, physicians may help foster this learning and be a catalyst for this transformation. Rather than thinking of dying simply as the termination of life, physicians and patients may be guided by a developmental model of dying that recognizes a series of lifelong developmental tasks and landmarks and allows for growth at the end of life.

Byock IR: *Dying Well: The Prospect for Growth at the End of Life.* Riverhead Press, 1997.
Byock IR: The nature of suffering and the nature of opportunity at the end of life. Clin Geriatr Med 1996;12:237.

Table 5–8. An existential review of systems.

Intrapersonal
How are you within yourself?[1]
What does your illness/dying mean to you?
What do you think caused your illness?
How have you been healed in the past?
What do you think is needed for you to be healed now?
What is right with you now?
What do you hope for?

Interpersonal
Who is important to you?
To whom does your illness/dying matter?
Do you have any unfinished business with significant others?

Transpersonal
What is your source of strength, help, or hope?
Do you have spiritual concerns or a spiritual practice?
If so, how does your spirituality relate to your illness/dying and how can I help integrate your spirituality into your health care?[1]
What do you think happens after we die?
What purpose might your illness/dying serve?
What do you think is trying to happen here?[1]

[1]Courtesy of IR Byock, DB Larson, and AL Suchman.

Doyle D et al (editors): *Oxford Textbook of Palliative Medicine.* Oxford Univ Press, 1993.

Jacox AK et al: Management of Cancer Pain. Clinical practice guideline No.9. Agency for Health Care Policy and Research, 1994. Rockville, MD. AHCPR Publication No. 94-0593.

McCann RM et al: Comfort care for terminally ill patients: The appropriate use of nutrition and hydration. JAMA 1994;272:1263.

Miles SH et al: Advance end-of-life treatment planning: A research review. Arch Intern Med 1996;156:1062.

The SUPPORT Principal Investigators: A controlled trial to improve care for seriously ill hospitalized patients: The study to understand prognoses and preferences for outcomes and risks of treatments. JAMA 1995;274:1591.

Sullivan RJ: Accepting death without artificial nutrition and hydration. J Gen Intern Med 1993;8:220.

TASKS AFTER DEATH

After the death of a patient, the physician is called upon to perform a number of tasks, both required and recommended. The physician must plainly and directly inform the family of the death. Providing words of sympathy and reassurance, time for questions and initial grief, and a quiet private room for the family at this time are appropriate and much appreciated.

THE PRONOUNCEMENT & DEATH CERTIFICATE

Physicians are legally required to confirm the death of a patient in a formal process called "pronouncement." The physician must verify the absence of spontaneous respirations and cardiac activity and the presence of fixed and dilated pupils. A note describing these findings and the time of death is entered in the patient's chart.

While the pronouncement may often seem like an awkward and unnecessary formality, physicians may use this time to reassure the patient's loved ones at the bedside that the patient died peacefully and that all appropriate care had been given. Both physicians and families may use the ritual of the pronouncement as an opportunity to process emotionally the death of the patient.

Accurately reporting the underlying cause of death on the death certificate is also legally required and important both for patients and their families (for insurance purposes and an accurate family medical history) and for the epidemiologic study of disease and public health. Unfortunately, recent research has shown that physicians are untrained in and unskilled at correctly completing death certificates.

AUTOPSY & ORGAN DONATION

Discussing the options and obtaining consent for autopsy and organ donation with patients themselves prior to death is usually the best practice. This advances the principle of patient autonomy and lessens the responsibilities of distressed family members during the period immediately following the death of their loved one.

Physicians must be sensitive to ethnic and cultural differences in attitudes about autopsy and organ donation. Patients or their families should be reminded of their right to limit autopsy or organ donation in any way they choose. Pathologists can perform autopsies without interfering with funeral plans or the appearance of the deceased.

The results of an autopsy may help surviving family members (and physicians) understand the exact cause of a patient's death and foster a sense of closure. A physician-family conference to review the results of the autopsy provides a good opportunity for physicians to assess how well families are grieving and to answer questions. Unfortunately, despite the advantages of conducting postmortem examinations, autopsy rates have fallen drastically to less than 15% today.

Most people in the United States support the donation of organs for transplants. Currently, however, organ transplantation is severely limited by the availability of donor organs. Many potential donors and the families of actual donors experience a sense of reward in contributing, even through death, to the lives of others.

FOLLOW-UP & GRIEVING

Proper care of patients at the end of life includes following up with surviving family members after the patient has died. Following up enables the physician to assess how families are grieving and to reassure them about the nature of normal grieving. Physicians can recommend support groups and counseling as needed. A card or telephone call from the physician to the family days to weeks after the patient's death (and potentially on the anniversary of the death) allows the physician to express concern for the family and the deceased.

After a patient dies, the physician too may need to grieve. Although physicians may be relatively unaffected by the deaths of some patients, other deaths may cause distressing feelings of sadness, loss, and guilt. These emotions should be recognized as the first step toward processing them or preventing them in the future.

For physicians, grieving the loss of a patient is normal. Each physician may find solitary or communal activities that best help him or her grieve. Crying, the support of colleagues, time for reflection, and traditional or personal mourning rituals all may be effective. Attending the funeral of a patient who has died can be a satisfying personal experience that is almost universally appreciated by families and may be the final element in caring well for people at the end of life.

McPhee SJ: Maximizing the benefits of autopsy for clinicians and families: What needs to be done. Arch Pathol Lab Med 1996;120:743.

Messite J, Stellman SD: Accuracy of death certificate completion: The need for formalized physician training. JAMA 1996;275:794.

Spielman B, Verhulst S: Discussing organ donations with patients. Fam Med 1996;28:698.

Skin & Appendages

6

Timothy G. Berger, MD

DIAGNOSIS OF SKIN DISORDERS

Morphology

A dermatologic differential diagnosis is based on one feature: the appearance—or morphology—of the skin lesion. In general, specific diseases cause characteristic lesions. All lesions need not have the characteristic feature, but identifying lesions as pustules, vesicles, or scaly plaques will guide the clinician to the right *group* of diseases that will include the correct diagnosis. This chapter will group and discuss diseases according to the types of lesions they cause and guide the reader through appropriate features of the history, physical findings, and laboratory tests that discriminate among the differential diagnoses.

History

A detailed history is important. For example, a history of a change in a pigmented lesion is important in evaluating moles. However, with regard to skin cancer or moles (nevi), for example, the physical examination takes precedence. Important components of a history include systemic disorders, inquiring about prescription or OTC systemic and topical medications, and questioning about specific, not just "new" exposure to physical and chemical agents in the home and work environments. The history is also very important in assessing therapeutic failure. In dermatology, this part of the history includes detailing exactly how the patient is using topical medications.

Physical Examination

If possible, it is best to examine the entire skin surface, including the nails, scalp, palms, soles, and mucous membranes, in bright (preferably natural) light. For some diseases, such as psoriasis, examination of these areas is vital in establishing the diagnosis. Total skin examination is also the best way to detect malignant melanoma. In examining the faces of older individuals at risk for nonmelanoma skin cancer, pay special attention to the lid margins, nose, ears, and lips.

PRINCIPLES OF DERMATOLOGIC THERAPY

Planning Topical Treatment

In general, it is better to be familiar with a few drugs and treatment methods than to attempt to use a great many. In addition, not all generic topical medications are equivalent to their brand-name counterparts, either in potency or in the incorporation of "inert" components that may cause irritation or allergy. This should be kept in mind when assessing unexpected side effects or lack of efficacy. When in doubt about the proper method of treatment, one should *undertreat* rather than overtreat: Inappropriate chronic use of a potent topical corticosteroid without supervision may cause irreversible side effects.

Frequently Employed Treatment Measures

A. General Measures: Soaps and detergents should be used only in the axillae and groin and on the feet by persons with dry or irritated skin. Unless their occupations expose them to oils or soot, most people do not need soaping over all body surfaces. Baths containing a small amount of bath oil may be used but are less effective than application of oils to the skin after bathing (see below).

B. Local Measures: In general, topical agents used by prescription are supplied in only one strength, and thus, with the exception of Table 6–1, concentrations will not be listed in this chapter. Exceptions include hydrocortisone (1% and 2.5%); triamcinolone acetonide cream and ointment (0.025% and 0.1%) or solution (0.1%); fluocinolone cream, ointment, or solution (0.01%), or cream and ointment (0.025%); and desoximetasone (0.05% and 0.25%). In many cases there is little evidence that one concentration has clinical effects that are significantly different from another. Nondermatologists should become familiar with a few agents and use them properly rather than try to master the universe of topical steroids. Tretinoin (Retin-A) is supplied as 0.025%, 0.05%, and 0.1% creams and 0.01% and 0.025% gels, and 0.05% solution. Benzoyl peroxide gels and

Table 6–1. Useful topical dermatologic therapeutic agents.

	Formulations, Strengths, and Prices[1]	Apply	Potency Class	Common Indications	Comments
Corticosteroids Hydrocortisone acetate	Cream 1%: $2.22/30 g Ointment 1%: $2.26/30 g Lotion 1%: $6.47/120 mL	bid	Low	Seborrheic dermatitis. Mild eczema in children. Pruritus ani. Intertrigo.	Not the same as hydrocortisone butyrate or valerate! Not for poison oak! OTC lotion (Aquinil HC). OTC solution (Scalpicin, T Scalp).
	Cream 2.5%: $5.75/30 g Ointment 2.5%: $4.63/20 g Lotion 2.5%: $20.00/120 mL	bid	Low	As for 1% hydrocortisone.	Perhaps better for pruritus ani. Not clearly better than 1%. More expensive. Not OTC.
Alclometasone dipropionate (Aclovate)	Cream 0.05%: $11.77/15 g Ointment 0.05%: $24.54/45 g	bid	Low	As for hydrocortisone.	More efficacious than hydrocortisone. Perhaps causes less atrophy.
Desonide	Cream 0.05%: $11/15 g Ointment 0.05%: $25/60 g Lotion 0.05%: $11/15 mL	bid	Low	As for hydrocortisone. For lesions on face or body folds resistant to hydrocortisone.	More efficacious than hydrocortisone. Can cause rosacea or atrophy. Not fluorinated.
Prednicarbate (Dermatop)	Emollient cream 0.1%: $11.58/15 g	bid	Medium	As for triamcinolone.	May cause less atrophy. No generic formulations. Preservative-free.
Triamcinolone acetonide	Cream 0.1%: $1.78/15 g Ointment 0.1%: $2.00/15 g Lotion 0.1%: $8.90/60 mL	bid	Medium	Eczema on extensor areas. Used for psoriasis with tar. Seborrheic dermatitis and psoriasis on scalp.	Caution in body folds, face. Economical in 0.5 lb and 1 lb sizes for treatment of large body surfaces. Economical as solution for scalp.
	Cream 0.025%: $1.39/15 g Ointment 0.025%: $3.30/80 g	bid	Medium	As for 0.1% strength.	Possibly less efficacy and few advantages over 0.1% formulation.
Fluocinolone acetonide	Cream 0.025%: $2.57/15 g Ointment 0.025%: $3.25/15 g	bid	Medium	As for triamcinolone.	
	Solution 0.01%: $4.55/20 mL	bid	Medium	As for triamcinolone solution.	
Mometasone furoate (Elocon)	Cream 0.1%: $17.14/15 g Ointment 0.1%: $31.40/45 g Lotion 0.1%: $18.60/30 mL	qd	Medium	As for triamcinolone.	Often used inappropriately on the face or in children. Not fluorinated.
Diflorasone diacetate (Florone, Maxiflor)	Cream 0.05%: $22.30/15 g Ointment 0.05%: $67.40/60 g	bid	High	Nummular dermatitis. Allergic contact dermatitis. Lichen simplex chronicus.	Only ultrapotent steroid that can be occluded (but with caution and not with gloves on the hands).
Amcinonide (Cyclocort)	Cream 0.1%: $16.00/15 g Ointment 0.1%: $24.00/30 g Lotion 0.1%: $36.00/60 mL	bid	High	As for betamethasone.	
Fluocinonide	Cream 0.05%: $6.80/15 g Gel 0.05%: $9.60/15 g Ointment 0.05%: $16.50/15 g Solution 0.05%: $23.00/60 mL	bid	High	As for betamethasone. Gel useful for poison oak.	Economical generics. Lidex cream can cause stinging on eczema. Lidex emollient cream preferred.
Betamethasone dipropionate	Cream 0.05%: $6.15/15 g Ointment 0.05%: $6.00/15 g Lotion 0.05%: $3.50/20 mL	bid	Ultra-high	For lesions resistant to medium-potency steroids. Lichen planus. Insect bites.	Economical generics available.

(continued)

Table 6–1. Useful topical dermatologic therapeutic agents. (continued)

	Formulations, Strengths, and Prices[1]	Apply	Potency Class	Common Indications	Comments
Clobetasol propionate	Cream 0.05%: $19.00/15 g Ointment 0.05%: $40.00/45 g Lotion 0.05%: $40.00/50 mL	bid	Ultra-high	As for diflorasone.	Somewhat more potent than diflorasone. Cannot occlude. Limited to 2 continuous weeks of use. Limited to 50 g or less per week. Cream may cause stinging; use "emollient cream" formulation.
Halobetasol pro-pionate (Ultra-vate)	Cream 0.05%: $23.00/15 g Ointment 0.05%: $56.00/50 g	bid	Ultra-high	As for clobetasol.	Marginally more effective than clobetasol in psoriasis. Same restrictions as clobetasol. Cream does not cause stinging.
Flurandrenolide (Cordran)	Tape: $30.00/large roll	q12h	Ultra-high	Lichen simplex chronicus.	Protects the skin and prevents scratching.
Antibiotics (for acne)					
Clindamycin phosphate	Solution 1%: $15.00/30 mL Gel 1%: $21.00/30 mL Lotion 1%: $30.00/60 mL Pledget 1%: $0.50 each	bid	N/A	Mild papular acne.	Lotion is less drying for patients with sensitive skin. No generic formulations.
Erythromycin	Solution 2%: $3.30/60 mL Gel 2%: $14.00/30 g Pledget 2%: $11.00/60	bid	N/A	As for clindamycin.	Many different manufacturers. Economical.
Erythromycin/ben-zoyl peroxide	Gel 3%: $28.00/23.3 g Gel 5%: $52.00/46.6 g	bid	N/A	As for clindamycin. Can help treat come-donal acne.	No generics. More expensive. More effective than other topical antibiotics. Main jar requires refrigeration.
Antibiotics (for impetigo)					
Mupirocin (Bactroban)	Ointment 2%: $16.50/15 g, $31.15/30 g	tid	N/A	Impetigo, folliculitis.	Stop after 10 days to prevent emergence of resistance. Used in the nose twice daily for 5 days to reduce staphylo-coccal carriage.
Antifungals					
Clotrimazole	Cream 1%: $8.30/15 g Lotion 1%: $22.50/30 mL Solution 1%: $10.35/10 mL	bid	N/A	Dermatophyte and *Candida* infections.	Available OTC. Inexpensive generic cream available.
Miconazole	Cream: $3.00/30 g	bid	N/A	As for clotrimazole.	As for clotrimazole.
Other imidazoles					
Econazole (Spectazole)	Cream 1%: $12.60/15 g	qd	N/A	As for clotrimazole.	No generic. Somewhat more effective than clotrimazole and miconazole.
Ketoconazole	Cream 2%: $14.00/15 g	qd	N/A	As for clotrimazole.	No generic. Somewhat more effective than clotrimazole and miconazole.
Oxiconazole (Oxistat)	Cream 1%: $14.40/15 g Lotion 1%: $24.00/30 mL	bid	N/A		
Sulconazole (Exelderm)	Cream 1%: $10.60/15 g Solution 1%: $19.00/30 mL	bid	N/A	As for clotrimazole.	No generic. Somewhat more effective than clotrimazole and miconazole.
Other antifungals					
Ciclopirox (Loprox)	Cream 1%: $11.60/15 g Lotion 1%: $43.40/60 mL	bid	N/A	As for clotrimazole.	No generic. Somewhat more effective than clotrimazole and miconazole.

(continued)

Table 6–1. Useful topical dermatologic therapeutic agents. (continued)

	Formulations, Strengths, and Prices[1]	Apply	Potency Class	Common Indications	Comments
Naftifine (Naftin)	Cream 1%: $16.80/15 g Gel 1%: $44.20/60 mL	qd	N/A	Dermatophytes. Not FDA-approved for *Candida* but probably effective.	No generic. Somewhat more effective than clotrimazole and miconazole.
Terbinafine (Lamisil)	Cream 1%: $28.40/15 g	bid	N/A	For dermatophytes.	Fastest clinical response but most expensive antifungal.
Antipruritics Camphor/menthol	Lotion (0.5% of each)	bid–tid	N/A	For mild eczema, xerosis, mild contact dermatitis.	
Pramoxine hydrochloride (Tronothane, Trondane)	Cream 1%: $3.20/30 g, $5.20/60 g	qid	N/A	As a cream for patients with dry skin, varicella, mild eczema, pruritus ani.	OTC formulations (Aveeno Anti-Itch Cream or Lotion; Itch-X Gel; Tronolane Cream for hemorrhoids). By prescription mixed with 1% or 2% hydrocortisone.
Doxepin (Zonalon)	Cream 5%: $18.20/30 g, $20.00/45 g	qid	N/A	Topical antipruritic, best used in combination with appropriate topical steroid to enhance efficacy.	Can cause sedation.
Emollients Aveeno	Cream: $2.40/30 g Lotion: $5.40/120 mL	qd–tid	N/A	Xerosis, eczema.	Choice is most often based on personal preference by patient.
Aqua glycolic	Lotion, facial moisturizer, shampoo	qd–tid	N/A	Xerosis. Ichthyosis, keratosis pilaris. Mild facial wrinkles. Mild acne or seborrheic dermatitis.	Contains 8% glycolic acid. Available from other makers, eg, Alpha Hydrox, or generic 8% glycolic acid lotion. May cause stinging on eczematous skin.
Aquaphor	Ointment: $12.80/454 g	qd–tid	N/A	Xerosis. Eczema. For protection of area in pruritus ani.	Not as greasy as petrolatum.
Complex 15	Lotion: $3.85/120 mL Cream: $4.50/75 g	qd–tid	N/A	Xerosis. Lotion or cream recommended for split or dry nails.	Active ingredient is a phospholipid.
DML	Cream, lotion, facial moisturizer	qd–tid	N/A	As for Complex 15.	Face cream has sunscreen.
Dermasil	Lotion: $6.00/240 mL Cream: $9.00/45 g	qd–tid	N/A	Xerosis, eczema.	
Eucerin	Cream: $5.50/120 g Lotion: $5.50/240 mL	qd–tid	N/A	Xerosis, eczema.	Many formulations made. Eucerin Plus contains alpha-hydroxy acid and may cause stinging on eczematous skin. Facial moisturizer has SPF 25 sunscreen.
Lac-Hydrin	Lotion: $25.00/225 g	bid	N/A	Xerosis, ichthyosis, keratosis pilaris.	Expensive, not OTC. May protect against corticosteroid-induced atrophy.
Lubriderm	Lotion: $5.28/300 mL	qd–tid	N/A	Xerosis, eczema.	Unscented usually preferred.
Neutrogena	Cream, lotion, facial moisturizer: $7.00/240 mL	qd–tid	N/A	Xerosis, eczema.	Face cream has titanium-based sunscreen.

[1]Cost to pharmacist (average wholesale price) for quantity listed (generic when possible). Source: First Data Bank, Price Alert, April 1997.

washes are supplied in 2.5–10% formulations; the lower concentrations appear to be as efficacious as the higher ones and cause less irritation. All useful antifungals come in only one strength per generic name. Selenium sulfide lotion 2.5% is used to treat tinea versicolor; selenium 1% is used in OTC anti-dandruff shampoos.

1.   Corticosteroids–Representative topical corticosteroid creams, lotions, ointments, gels, and sprays are presented in the following list and in Table 6–1. Topical steroids are divided into classes based on their potency. There is little (except price) to recommend one over another within the same class. The primary use of these agents is to treat inflammatory pruritic dermatoses. It takes an average of 20–30 g to cover the body surface area of an adult once. One should use the rule of nines (as in burn evaluation; see Figure 39–4) to determine the daily amount of steroid required and prescribe an adequate amount for the proposed treatment course.

a.   Lowest potency–Hydrocortisone, desonide, alclometasone dipropionate. Best for chronic use and for the face, groin, and body folds. However, chronic unsupervised use of desonide may result in side effects in some patients.

b.   Mid potency–Flurandrenolide, fluocinolone, triamcinolone, hydrocortisone valerate, hydrocortisone butyrate, betamethasone valerate, mometasone furoate, prednicarbate, etc.

c.   High potency–Desoximetasone, amcinonide, halcinonide, fluocinonide, betamethasone dipropionate, etc.

d.   Highest potency–Betamethasone dipropionate in optimized vehicle, diflorasone, flurandrenolide-impregnated tape (Cordran Tape), clobetasol, and halobetasol. These should be used for brief periods only, on limited areas, and—with rare exceptions—not on the face, breasts, or genitalia or in body folds.

2.   Potentiation of topical corticosteroid creams–By covering selected lesions of psoriasis, lichen planus, and localized eczemas each night, first with the corticosteroid and then with a thin light plastic pliable film (eg, Saran Wrap), the potency of a topical steroid will be increased. For erythrodermic psoriatics or atopics with generalized involvement, the use of a plastic occlusive suit may be most helpful. Complications include miliaria, striae, pyoderma, local skin atrophy, malodor, fungal infections, and, rarely, adrenocortical suppression when extensive areas of body surface are occluded.

3.   Emollients for dry skin–Many types of emollients are available. Petrolatum, mineral oil, Aquaphor, and Eucerin cream are the heaviest and best for very dry skin. They work best when applied to wet skin immediately after a bath to trap the moisture. Mineral oil should be applied while the skin is still wet. Do not rub up and down against the hair but in one direction with the "grain" of the hair to avoid

folliculitis. If the skin is too greasy after application, pat dry again with the damp towel.

In some cases, lotions such as Lubriderm, Nutraderm, Eucerin, Moisturel, DML, and Dermasil may be useful and are not as greasy as the creams and ointments listed above. The pruritus and appearance of dry skin and ichthyosis may be improved by a 12% lactate lotion (Lac-Hydrin) (by prescription) or by a glycolic acid-containing lotion (OTC) provided no inflammation (erythema) is present.

4.   Drying agents for weepy dermatoses–If the skin is weepy from infection or inflammation, drying agents may afford relief. The best drying agent is water, and repeated compresses, with or without such agents as aluminum salts (Burow's solution, Domeboro tablets; follow package instructions) or colloidal oatmeal (Aveeno; dispense one box) are a good first step. Shake lotions (eg, starch or calamine lotions) and powders (especially if the process is acute) may result in messy crusts and are seldom used by dermatologists.

5.   Topical antipruritics–Lotions that contain 0.5% each of camphor and menthol (Sarna) are effective for mild pruritic dermatoses. Pramoxine hydrochloride, 1% cream or lotion, or pramoxine hydrochloride, 1%, with 0.5% menthol, as a surface anesthetic may be an effective antipruritic agent (Prax, Pramegel, Aveeno Anti-Itch lotion). Hydrocortisone, 1% or 2.5%, may be incorporated for its anti-inflammatory effect (Pramosone cream, lotion, or ointment). Doxepin cream 5% may reduce pruritus due to eczematous dermatoses. It appears most effective when applied together with a topical steroid of the appropriate class for the condition or site being treated. Like pramoxine, it is a steroid enhancer, improving response to a given strength of topical steroid. Drowsiness and dry mouth may occur. Monoamine oxidase inhibitors should be discontinued at least 2 weeks before treatment.

6.   Systemic antipruritic drugs–

a.   Antihistamines–In general, H_1 blockers are the agents of choice for pruritus when due to histamine, such as in urticaria. Otherwise, they appear to relieve pruritus only by their sedating and not their antihistamine effects. Different classes of antihistamines differ in their sedating properties, and the less sedating second-generation antihistamines are thus not effective as "antipruritics."

Traditional H_1 antihistamines are usually grouped into six classes. Alkylamines (chlorpheniramine and dexchlorpheniramine) are the least sedating. Ethanolamines (diphenhydramine) are very sedating, as are phenothiazines (promethazine). Piperidines (cyproheptadine), piperazines (hydroxyzine), and ethylenediamines (tripelennamine) cause less sedation. The three least sedating antihistamines are loratadine, terfenadine, and astemizole. Cetirizine is also relatively nonsedating but is more sedating than these three. Some tricyclic antidepressants, such as doxepin, have potent antihistaminic activity and are useful in urticaria.

b. Systemic corticosteroids–(See Chapter 26.)

Greaves MW, Wall PD: Pathophysiology of itching. Lancet 1996;348:938.

Millikan LE: Treating pruritus: What's new in safe relief of symptoms? Postgrad Med 1996;99:173.

Zuckerman E, Schar M, Korula J: Naloxone for intractable pruritus? (Letter.) Am J Gastroenterol 1997;92:183.

Sunscreens

Protection from ultraviolet light should begin at birth but will reduce the incidence of actinic keratoses and basal cell cancers when initiated at any age. The best protection is shelter, but protective clothing, avoidance of direct sun exposure during the 5 peak hours of the day, and the assiduous use of commercially available chemical sunscreens are important. Estimates are that if fair children were to use such sunscreens regularly, their lifetime incidence of skin cancer might be reduced by 75%.

A number of highly effective sunscreens are available in cream, lotion, and nongreasy gel and liquid formulations. Fair-complexioned persons should use a sunscreen with an SPF (sun protective factor) of at least 15 and preferably 30–40. For those who are sensitive to PABA (*p*-aminobenzoic acid), PABA-free formulations are available. Solbar PF (PABA-free) cream with the highest SPF rating of 50 is available. Sunscreens with high SPF values (> 25) afford some protection against UVA as well as UVB light exposure and may be helpful in managing photosensitivity disorders. Many facial moisturizers contain a SPF 15–25 sunscreen in a nongreasy base suitable for daily use.

Physical blockers (titanium dioxide) are available in new vanishing formulations (Ti-Baby Natural, Ti Screen Natural, Neutrogena Chemical-Free Sun Blocker). Zinc oxide used alone is a surprisingly poor sunscreen.

Diffey BL: Sunscreens, suntans and skin cancer: People do not apply enough sunscreen for protection. (Letter.) BMJ 1996;313:942.

Farmer KC, Naylor MF: Sun exposure, sunscreens, and skin cancer prevention: A year-round concern. Ann Pharmacol 1996;30:662.

Pathak MA: Sunscreens: Progress and perspectives on photoprotection of human skin against UVB and UVA radiation. J Dermatol 1996;23:783.

Complications of Topical Dermatologic Therapy

Complications of topical therapy can be largely avoided. They fall into several categories:

A. Allergy: Of the topical antibiotics, neomycin has the greatest potential for sensitization. Diphenhydramine, benzocaine, and ethylenediamine are potential sensitizers in topical medications.

B. Irritation: Preparations of retinoic acid, benzoyl peroxide, and other acne medications should be applied sparingly to the skin when it is dry. Repeated use of lindane (Kwell, etc) and antiseptic soaps can be irritating. Podophyllum resin can be very irritating. Sunscreens may cause irritation or an acne-like eruption.

C. Absorption: Drugs may be absorbed through the skin, especially near mucous membranes, through broken or inflamed skin, or from under occlusive dressings. On average, the systemic dose absorbed by children is three times that of adults. One should determine that the patient is not pregnant before using podophyllum resin. Lindane should not be used in babies, children, or pregnant women, and it should be replaced by permethrin 5% cream (Elimite) in children or with permethrin or precipitated sulfur in pregnant women. Agents containing phenol are contraindicated on open skin or mucous membranes of neonates. Although it has been argued that absorption of tretinoin (Retin-A) is minimal, its prohibition in pregnancy is wise. Injudicious use of medium- and high-potency topical corticosteroids in large amounts or over prolonged periods, especially with occlusive plastic wrapping, can result in significant systemic absorption of steroids, resulting rarely in hypothalamic-pituitary-adrenal axis suppression and aseptic bone necrosis.

D. Overuse: Fluorinated topical corticosteroids may induce acne-like lesions on the face (steroid rosacea) and atrophic striae in body folds.

Funk JO, Dromgoole SH, Maibach HI: Sunscreen intolerance: Contact sensitization, photocontact sensitization, and irritancy of sunscreen agents. Dermatol Clin 1995;13:473.

I. COMMON DERMATOSES

Dermatologic diseases will be classified and discussed here, when possible, according to the types of lesions they cause. Therefore, in order to make a diagnosis, it is best to (1) focus on the type of individual lesion the patient exhibits; (2) choose the morphologic category the lesions seem to fit; and then (3) identify the specific features of the history, physical examination, and laboratory tests that will establish the working diagnosis.

The major morphologic types of skin lesion—and pruritic lesions—are listed in Table 6–2 along with the disorders with which they are most prominently associated. Miscellaneous skin, hair, and nail disor-

Table 6–2. Morphologic categorization of skin lesions and diseases.

Pigmented	Freckle, lentigo, seborrheic keratosis, nevus, blue nevus, halo nevus, dysplastic nevus, melanoma
Scaly	Psoriasis, dermatitis (atopic, stasis, seborrheic, chronic allergic contact or irritant contact), xerosis (dry skin), lichen simplex chronicus, tinea, tinea versicolor, secondary syphilis, pityriasis rosea, discoid lupus erythematosus, exfoliative dermatitis, actinic keratoses, Bowen's disease, Paget's disease, intertrigo
Vesicular	Herpes simplex, varicella, herpes zoster, dyshidrosis (vesicular dermatitis of palms and soles), vesicular tinea, dermatophytid, dermatitis herpetiformis, miliaria, scabies, photosensitivity
Weepy or encrusted	Impetigo, acute contact allergic dermatitis, any vesicular dermatitis
Pustular	Acne vulgaris, acne rosacea, folliculitis, candidiasis, miliaria, any vesicular dermatitis
Figurate (-shaped) erythema	Urticaria, erythema multiforme, erythema migrans, cellulitis, erysipelas, erysipeloid, arthropod bites
Bullous	Impetigo, blistering dactylitis, pemphigus, pemphigoid, porphyria cutanea tarda, drug eruptions, erythema multiforme, toxic epidermal necrolysis
Papular	Hyperkeratotic: warts, corns, seborrheic keratoses Purple-violet: lichen planus, drug eruptions, Kaposi's sarcoma Flesh-colored, umbilicated: molluscum contagiosum Pearly: basal cell carcinoma, intradermal nevi Small, red, inflammatory: acne, miliaria, candidiasis, scabies, folliculitis
Pruritus[1]	Xerosis, scabies, pediculosis, bites, systemic causes, anogenital pruritus
Nodular, cystic	Erythema nodosum, furuncle, cystic acne, follicular (epidermal) inclusion cyst
Photodermatitis (photodistributed rashes)	Drug, polymorphic light eruption, lupus erythematosus
Morbilliform	Drug, viral infection, secondary syphilis
Erosive	Any vesicular dermatitis, impetigo, aphthae, lichen planus, erythema multiforme
Ulcerated	Decubiti, herpes simplex, skin cancers, parasitic infections, syphilis (chancre), chancroid, vasculitis, stasis, arterial disease

[1]Not a morphologic class but included because it is one of the most common dermatologic presentations.

ders and drug eruptions are discussed at the end of the chapter.

PIGMENTED LESIONS

Malignant melanoma accounts for the greatest number of deaths due to skin disease, and such deaths might be prevented by early diagnosis followed by excision. The nondermatologist physician must be able to evaluate pigmented lesions and appropriately refer for evaluation all potentially malignant melanomas. The most relevant question is, "Is this mole suspicious?" If the physician is to avoid overlooking some malignant melanomas, many benign lesions will be properly referred as well. Therefore, clinicians should examine all patients with an eye to spotting the "funny-looking" mole.

In general, a **benign mole** is a small (< 5 mm), well-circumscribed lesion with a well-defined border and a single shade of pigment from beige or pink to dark brown. Most or all of the individual patient's moles often are similar to each other with respect to size and color, or there may be two or three different types of moles on the same patient. The physical examination takes precedence over the history, though a reliable history that a lesion has been present without change for decades is obviously a comfort.

Suspicious moles have an irregular and asymmetric or fuzzy border where the pigment appears to be leaking into the normal surrounding skin; the topography may be irregular, ie, partly raised and partly flat. Color variegation is disturbing, and colors such as pink, blue, gray, white, and black are indications for referral. The American Cancer Society has proposed the mnemonic "ABCD = Asymmetry, Border irregularity, Color variegation, and Diameter greater than 6 mm." Bleeding and ulceration are ominous signs. A mole that stands out from the patient's other moles deserves special scrutiny. A patient with a large number of moles is statistically at increased risk for melanoma and deserves careful and periodic examination, particularly if the lesions are atypical.

The history of a changing mole is the single most important historical reason for close evaluation and possible referral. Referral of suspicious pigmented lesions is always appropriate.

Moles have their own natural history. In the first decade of life, moles often appear as flat, small, brown lesions. They are called **junctional nevi** because the nevus cells are at the junction of the epidermis and dermis. Over the next 2 decades, these moles grow in size and often become raised, reflecting the appearance of a dermal component, giving rise to **compound nevi.** Moles may darken and grow during pregnancy. As Caucasian patients enter their seventh and eighth decades, most moles have lost their junctional component and dark pigmentation and undergo fibrosis or other degenerative changes. Still, at every stage of life, normal moles should be well-demarcated, symmetric, and uniform in contour and color.

CONGENITAL NEVI

The management of small congenital nevi—less than a few centimeters in diameter—is controversial. The vast majority (perhaps > 97%) will never become malignant, but some experts feel that the risk of melanoma in these lesions may be somewhat increased. Since 1% of Caucasians are born with these lesions, management should be conservative and excision advised only for lesions in cosmetically nonsensitive areas where the patient cannot easily see the lesion and note any suspicious changes. Excision should be considered for congenital nevi whose contour (bumpiness, nodularity) or color (different shades) makes it difficult for examiners to note early signs of malignant change. Giant congenital melanocytic nevi (> 25% BSA) are at greater risk for development of melanoma, and surgical removal in stages is often recommended.

DeDavid M et al: A study of large congenital melanocytic nevi and associated malignant melanomas: Review of cases in the New York University Registry and the world literature. J Am Acad Dermatol 1997;36(3 Part 1):409.

Swerdlow AJ et al: The risk of melanoma in patients with congenital nevi: A cohort study. J Am Acad Dermatol 1995;32:595. (High risk of melanoma in patients with nevi covering more than 5% of the body surface area.)

ATYPICAL (DYSPLASTIC) NEVI

The term "atypical nevus" or "atypical mole" has supplanted "dysplastic nevus." Today, the diagnosis of atypical moles is made clinically and not histologically, and moles should be removed if they are suspected to be melanomas—not to document histologic dysplasia, as had been done in the past. Clinically, these moles are large (> 5 mm in diameter), with an ill-defined, irregular border and irregularly distributed pigmentation with erythema and accentuated skin markings. It is estimated that 5–10% of the United States population have one or more atypical nevi, and a patient with a single atypical mole in the absence of a family history of melanoma is thought to be at little increased risk for melanoma. However, the index lesion should be evaluated for melanoma by an expert or by biopsy if indicated—or followed for change. Recent studies have defined an increased risk of melanoma in the following populations: patients with 100 or more nevi with one or more atypical moles and one mole at least 8 mm or larger; patients with at least one atypical mole referred for regular follow-up in a university pigmented lesion clinic, whether or not there is a family history of melanoma; and patients with a few to many definitely atypical moles (with five or six of the features defined above). These patients deserve education and regular (usually every 6–12 months) follow-up. Kindreds with familial melanoma (numerous atypical nevi and a strong family history) deserve even closer attention, as the risk of developing single or even multiple melanomas in some of these individuals can reach 100%.

Bliss JM et al: Risk of cutaneous melanoma associated with pigmentation characteristics and freckling: Systematic overview of 10 case-control studies. The International Melanoma Analysis Group (IMAGE). Int J Cancer 1995;62:367. (Comparing 3000 cases and almost 4000 controls, the authors estimated the relative risk of melanoma associated with aspects of complexion. Compared with individuals with black or dark brown hair, the relative risks for developing melanoma in those with light brown, blond, and red hair were 1.49 [95% CI 1.31, 1.70], 1.84 [95% CI 1.54, 2.21] and 2.38 [95% CI 1.90, 2.97], respectively. Individuals with blue eyes had a risk 1.55 [95% CI 1.35, 1.78] times that for those with brown eyes.)

Ford D et al: Risk of cutaneous melanoma associated with a family history of the disease. The International Melanoma Analysis Group (IMAGE). Int J Cancer 1995;62:377. (In a combined analysis of 2952 melanoma patients and 3618 controls from eight case-control studies, the risk of cutaneous melanoma was 2.24-fold higher [95% CI, 1.76, 2.86] in subjects who reported at least one affected first-degree relative than in subjects who did not.)

Kang S et al: Melanoma risk in individuals with clinically atypical nevi. Arch Dermatol 1994;130:999. (The relative risk was 3 with a 95% confidence interval of 3–83. Melanomas occurred in patients with no family history of melanoma.)

Marghoob AA et al: Risk of cutaneous malignant melanoma in patients with "classic" atypical mole syndrome. Arch Dermatol 1994;130:993. (Ten-year cumulative risk of melanoma was 10.7% compared with 0.62% in case controls.)

Rigel DS: Identification of those at highest risk for development of malignant melanoma. Adv Dermatol 1995;10:151.

Schneider JS et al: Risk factors for melanoma incidence in prospective follow-up. Arch Dermatol 1994;134:1002. (Relative risk was 47 for employees with atypical nevi versus persons with typical moles.)

Slade J et al: Atypical mole syndrome: Risk factor for cutaneous malignant melanoma and implications for management. J Am Acad Derm 1995;32:479. (The risk for the development of melanoma varies from persons with one or two atypical moles and no family history of melanoma at one end of the spectrum to persons with the familial atypical multiple-mole melanoma syndrome at the other.)

Slade J et al: Risk of developing cutaneous malignant melanoma in atypical-mole syndrome: New York University experience and literature review. Recent Results Cancer Res 1995;139:87.

BLUE NEVI

Blue nevi are small, slightly elevated, and blue-black lesions. They are common in persons of Asian descent, and an individual patient may have several of them. If present without change for many years, they may be considered benign, since malignant blue nevi are rare. However, blue-black papules and nodules that are new or growing must be evaluated to rule out nodular melanoma.

Gonzalez-Campora R et al: Blue nevus: Classical types and new related entities. A differential diagnostic review. Pathol Res Pract 1994;190:627.

FRECKLES & LENTIGINES

Freckles (ephelides) and lentigines are flat brown spots. Freckles first appear in young children, darken with ultraviolet exposure, and fade with cessation of sun exposure (in the winter). In older children and adults, depending on the fairness of the complexion, flat brown spots (lentigines), often with smooth borders, gradually appear in sun-exposed areas, particularly the dorsa of the hands. These lesions have increased numbers of melanocytes. They tend not to fade with cessation of sun exposure. They should be evaluated like all pigmented lesions: If the pigmentation is homogeneous and they are symmetric and flat, they are most likely benign. Solar lentigines, so-called liver spots, fade significantly or clear in over 80% of individuals treated with topical 0.1% tretinoin once nightly for 6–10 months.

SEBORRHEIC KERATOSES

Seborrheic keratoses are benign plaques, beige to brown or even black, 3–20 mm in diameter, with a velvety or warty surface. They appear to be stuck or pasted onto the skin. They are relatively common—especially in the elderly—and may be mistaken for melanomas or other types of cutaneous neoplasms. Although they may be frozen with liquid nitrogen or curetted if they itch or are inflamed, no treatment is needed.

MALIGNANT MELANOMA

Essentials of Diagnosis

- May be flat or raised.
- Should be suspected in any pigmented skin lesion with recent change in appearance.
- Examination with good light shows varying colors, including red, white, black, and bluish.
- Borders typically irregular.

General Considerations

Malignant melanoma is the leading cause of death from skin disease. It is estimated that 40,300 cases of melanoma occurred in the USA in 1997, causing melanoma to be ranked as the ninth most common cancer, with 7300 deaths. Although melanomas are more frequently recognized at earlier and more curable stages, the overall death rate for Caucasian men has risen from 2.2 to 3.3 per 100,000 population during the period 1973–1988, and that of Caucasian women from 1.4 to 1.7 per 100,000. Overall survival for melanomas in Caucasians has risen from 60% in 1960–1963 to 85% in 1983–1990.

Tumor thickness (Breslow's classification) is the single most important prognostic factor. Ten-year survival rates—related to thickness in millimeters—are as follows: < 0.76 mm, 96%; 0.76–1.69 mm, 81%; 1.7–3.6 mm, 57%; > 3.6 mm, 31%. With lymph node involvement, the 5-year survival rate is 30%; and with distant metastases, it is less than 10%. These statistics are only of general interest, however, since more accurate prognoses can be made on the basis of thickness, site, histologic features, and sex of the patient using readily available computer databases.

Deaths from malignant melanoma are increasing at a faster rate than death from any other malignant neoplastic disease except lung cancer. There is a trend toward a younger age incidence each year. However, because of increased awareness, most melanomas are being diagnosed at a much earlier stage.

Clinical Findings

Primary malignant melanomas may be classified into various clinicohistologic types, including lentigo maligna melanoma (arising on sun-exposed skin of older individuals); superficial spreading malignant melanoma (the most common type, occurring in two-thirds of individuals developing melanoma); nodular malignant melanoma; acral-lentiginous melanomas (arising on palms, soles, and nail beds); malignant melanomas on mucous membranes; and miscellaneous forms such as amelanotic (nonpigmented) melanoma and melanomas arising from blue nevi (rare) and congenital and giant nevocytic nevi.

While superficial spreading melanoma is largely a disease of Caucasians, persons of other races are at risk for other types of melanoma, particularly acral lentiginous melanoma. These occur as dark, sometimes irregularly shaped lesions on the palms and soles and as new, often broad and solitary, darkly pigmented longitudinal streaks in the nails. Acral lentiginous melanoma may be a difficult diagnosis because benign pigmented lesions of the hands, feet, and nails occur commonly in more darkly pigmented persons and clinicians may hesitate to biopsy the palms and especially the soles and nail beds. As a result, the diagnosis is often delayed until the tumor has become clinically obvious and histologically thick. Clinicians should give special attention to new or changing lesions in these areas.

Melanomas vary from macules to nodules. Variegation of color from flesh tints to pitch black and a frequent admixture of white, blue, purple, and red may occur. The border tends to be irregular, and growth may be rapid or indolent. Superficial melanomas are often larger than 6 mm, but nodular melanomas may be smaller in diameter. Again, one should refer lesions based on a suspicion of melanoma rather than delay until the diagnosis is certain.

Treatment

Treatment of melanoma consists of excision. After histologic diagnosis, the area is usually reexcised with margins dictated by the thickness of the tumor. Large margins (radius ≥ 5 cm) are no longer indicated. Thin low-risk and intermediate-risk tumors require only conservative margins of 1–3 cm. More specifically, surgical margins of 0.5 cm for melanoma in situ and 1 cm for lesions less than 1 mm in thickness are most often recommended.

Elective lymph node dissection in the absence of clinical involvement is an area of great controversy. Sentinel lymph node biopsy (selective lymphadenectomy) using preoperative lymphoscintigraphy and intraoperative lymphatic mapping may be effective for staging melanoma patients with intermediate risk without clinical adenopathy. Alpha interferon and vaccine therapy may reduce recurrences in patients with high-risk melanomas. Referral of intermediate-risk and high-risk patients to centers with expertise in melanoma is strongly recommended.

[Diagnosis and treatment of early melanoma]
gopher://gopher.nih.gov/70/11/clin/cancernet/pdqinfo/soa/Melanoma_Physician

Balch CM, Buzaid AC: Finally, a successful adjuvant therapy for high-risk melanoma. (Editorial and comment.) J Clin Oncol 1996;14:1.

Glass LF et al: The role of selective lymphadenectomy in the management of patients with malignant melanoma. Dermatol Surg 1995;21:979.

Rigel DS: Malignant melanoma: Perspectives on incidence and its effects on awareness, diagnosis, and treatment. (Editorial.) CA Cancer J Clin 1996;46:195.

Schuchter L et al: A prognostic model for predicting 10-year survival in patients with primary melanoma. The Pigmented Lesion Group. Ann Intern Med 1996; 125:369.

SCALING DISORDERS

ATOPIC DERMATITIS (Eczema)

Essentials of Diagnosis

- Pruritic, exudative, or lichenified eruption on face, neck, upper trunk, wrists, and hands and in the antecubital and popliteal folds.
- Personal or family history of allergic manifestations (eg, asthma, allergic rhinitis, atopic dermatitis).
- Tendency to recur, with remission from adolescence to age 20.

General Considerations

Atopic dermatitis looks different at different ages and in people of different races. Because most patients have scaly dry skin at some point, this disease is being discussed under scaly dermatoses. However, acute flares may present with red patches that are weepy, shiny, or lichenified (ie, thickened, with more prominent skin markings) and plaques and papules. Diagnostic criteria for atopic dermatitis must include pruritus, typical morphology and distribution (flexural lichenification in adults; facial and extensor involvement in infants), and a tendency toward chronic or chronically relapsing dermatitis. Also helpful are (1) a personal or family history of atopic disease (asthma, allergic rhinitis, atopic dermatitis), (2) xerosis-ichthyosis, (3) facial pallor with infraorbital darkening, (4) elevated serum IgE, (5) fissures under the ear lobes, (6) a tendency toward nonspecific hand dermatitis, and (7) a tendency toward repeated skin infections.

Clinical Findings

A. Symptoms and Signs: Itching may be extremely severe and prolonged. Dermatitis represents inflammation of the epidermis and presents with erythema but not with the smooth intact epidermal surface of dermal inflammation that characterizes hives.

The epidermal inflammation of acute dermatitis results in rough, red patches without the thickening and discrete demarcation of a proliferative epidermal disorder such as psoriasis. The distribution of the lesions is characteristic, with involvement of the face, neck, and upper trunk ("monk's cowl"). The bends of the elbows and knees are involved. In infants, the eruption usually begins on the cheeks and is often vesicular and exudative. In children (and later) the skin is dry, leathery, and lichenified. Black children tend to present with a papular eruption and poorly demarcated hypopigmented patches (pityriasis alba) are commonly seen on the cheeks and extremities. Adults generally have dry, leathery, hyperpigmented or hypopigmented lesions in typical distribution. In black patients with severe disease, pigmentation may be lost in lichenified areas around the wrists and ankles.

The role of food allergy in causing flares of atopic dermatitis is debatable but is probably significant in about 30% of cases, especially in children. Other patients may be sensitive to dust mites and other antigens.

B. Laboratory Findings: Laboratory findings, including scratch and intradermal tests, often yield many false-positive results leading to unnecessary dietary restriction. Blinded food challenges are the most reliable. RASTs or skin tests may suggest dust mite allergy. Eosinophilia and increased serum IgE levels may be present but are usually not needed for diagnosis.

Differential Diagnosis

In infants, atopic dermatitis must be distinguished from seborrheic dermatitis (frequent scalp and face involvement, greasy and scaly lesions, and quick response to therapy). Contact dermatitis and impetigo may be in the differential, especially for hyperacute, weepy flares of atopic dermatitis (although typically these diseases do not have a chronic course and characteristic distribution). Patients with active lesions are almost always colonized with *Staphylococcus aureus,* and impetiginization of atopic skin should be considered and treated when the patient presents with weepy areas or small erosions that should not be confused with more linear excoriations.

Treatment

Treatment is most effective if the patient is instructed about many aspects of skin care and specific ways to use medications.

A. General Measures: These patients have hyperirritable skin, so one must first explain to the patient or parents that anything that dries or irritates the skin will be a problem. Atopic individuals are sensitive to low humidity and often get worse in the winter, when the air is dry. A reasonable approach is not to let children or adults bathe more than once daily, not to let children sit in soapy water, and not to permit use of bubble bath unless it is shown not to irritate the skin of that child. Soap should be confined to the armpits, groin, and feet and should be used only just before rinsing and ending the bath. Washcloths and brushes should not be used. Soaps should not be drying, and Dove, Eucerin, Aveeno, Basis, Alpha Keri, Purpose, and other soaps or cleansers, such as Cetaphil or Aquanil, may be recommended. After rinsing, the skin should be patted dry (not rubbed) and then immediately—before it dries completely—covered with a thin film of an emollient, such as Aquaphor, Eucerin, Dermasil, DML Cream, Vaseline, mineral oil, or a corticosteroid as needed. Atopic patients may be irritated by scratchy fabrics, including wools and acrylics. Cottons often are preferable, but synthetic blends also are well tolerated. Since some children begin their cycle of itching and scratching with perspiration, one should do what is possible to avoid overheating. Some patients cannot use ointments because they are more occlusive than creams and cause itching. Very hot baths may exacerbate the itching of some patients. Some patients do not tolerate animal danders.

To determine the potential effect of foods, the parent may eliminate one food at a time that is thought to induce flares. Dairy products and wheat are the most common offenders. Foods that are a problem typically cause itching within minutes to a few hours after eating.

B. Local Treatment: Corticosteroids in lotion, cream, or ointment form have almost completely supplanted other topical medications but should not be the only therapy in severe disease. They should be applied sparingly twice to four times daily and rubbed in well. Their potency should be appropriate to the severity of the dermatitis. In general, one should begin with hydrocortisone or another slightly stronger mild steroid (Aclovate, Desonide) and use triamcinolone 0.1% for short periods of time as needed in young children. It is vital that patients taper corticosteroids and substitute emollients when the dermatitis clears to avoid both tachyphylaxis and the side effects of corticosteroids. Tapering is also important to avoid rebound flares of the dermatitis that may follow their abrupt cessation. Doxepin cream 5% may be used up to four times daily to relieve the pruritus. It is best applied simultaneously with the topical steroid. Stinging, burning, and drowsiness were reported in 25%.

Treatment is dictated by the stage of the dermatitis.

1. Acute weeping lesions–Use saline, bicarbonate, or aluminum subacetate solution (Domeboro tablets, one in a pint of cool water) or colloidal oatmeal (Aveeno; dispense one box, and use as directed on box) as soothing or astringent soaks, baths, or wet dressings for 10–30 minutes two to four times daily. Lesions on extremities particularly may be bandaged for protection at night without letting tape touch the skin. Steroid lotions or creams are preferred to ointments for this stage. Adults may use high-potency corticosteroids and children mid-potency steroids, used after bathing and sparing the face and body folds. Systemic corticosteroids may be required (see below).

2. Subacute or scaly lesions–At this stage, the lesions are dry but still red and pruritic. Mid- to high-potency steroids in ointment form if tolerated—creams if not—should be continued until scaling and elevated skin lesions are cleared and itching is decreased substantially. At that point, patients should begin a 2- to 4-week taper from twice-daily to daily to alternate-day dosing with topical steroids to reliance on emollients, with occasional use of steroids on specific itchy areas. Instead of tapering the frequency of usage of a more potent steroid, it may be preferable in children to switch to a low-potency steroid such as hydrocortisone cream or alclometasone.

3. Chronic, dry, lichenified lesions–Thickened and usually well-demarcated, they are best treated with high-potency to highest-potency steroid ointments, sometimes under occlusion for 2–6 weeks initially. Occasionally, tar preparations such as LCD (liquor carbonis detergens) 5% in Aquaphor, or Fototar cream, may be beneficial if corticosteroids are not sufficient.

C. Systemic and Adjuvant Therapy: Systemic corticosteroids are indicated only in extensive and more severe cases. Oral prednisone dosages should be high enough to suppress the dermatitis quickly, usually starting with 40–60 mg daily for adults. The dosage is then tapered to nil over a period of 2–4 weeks. Triamcinolone acetonide suspension, 40–60 mg intramuscularly for adults, used occasionally—but not more frequently than every 4–6 weeks—may exert control but is not a good form of maintenance therapy. Classic antihistamines may be used to aid in the relief of severe pruritus. Hydroxyzine, brompheniramine, or doxepin may be useful, but the dosage must be increased gradually to avoid drowsiness. Fissures, crusts, erosions, or pustules indicate staphylococcal infection clinically. Therefore, antistaphylococcal antibiotics given systemically—such as dicloxacillin or first-generation cephalosporins—may be helpful in management and are often used during flares. Phototherapy can be an important adjunct for severely affected patients, and the properly selected patient with recalcitrant disease may benefit greatly from therapy with UVB, UVB and UVA with or without coal tar, or PUVA.

Complications of Treatment

Patients are at risk of side effects of improperly used corticosteroids, and the physician should monitor for skin atrophy. **Eczema herpeticum,** a generalized herpes simplex infection manifested by monomorphic vesicles, crusts, or erosions superimposed on atopic dermatitis or other extensive eczematous processes, is usually treated successfully with oral acyclovir, 200 mg five times daily for adults, or intravenous acyclovir in a dose of 10 mg/kg intravenously every 8 hours (500 mg/m^2 every 8 hours).

Prognosis

The disease runs a chronic course, often with a tendency to disappear only to recur. Many children outgrow generalized involvement at puberty but develop hand dermatitis as adults. Poor prognostic factors for persistence into adulthood in atopic dermatitis include onset early in childhood, early generalized disease, and asthma. Only 40–60% of these patients have lasting remissions.

Boguniewicz M, Leung DY: New concepts in atopic dermatitis. Compr Ther 1996;22:144.

Rothe MJ, Grant-Kels JM: Atopic dermatitis: An update. J Am Acad Dermatol 1996;35:1. (Diagnostic criteria, epidemiology and genetics, provocative factors, predictors of disease development and markers of disease severity, therapy, and prognosis.)

Tan BB et al: Double-blind controlled trial of effect of housedust-mite allergen avoidance on atopic dermatitis. Lancet 1996;347:15. (The activity of atopic dermatitis was greatly reduced by effective housedust mite avoidance.)

LICHEN SIMPLEX CHRONICUS (Circumscribed Neurodermatitis)

Essentials of Diagnosis

- Chronic itching associated with hyperpigmented lichenified skin lesions.
- Lichenified lesions with exaggerated skin lines overlying a thickened, well-circumscribed scaly plaque.
- Predilection for nape of neck, wrists, external surfaces of forearms, inner thighs, lower legs, popliteal and antecubital areas.

General Considerations

A traditional explanation for lichen simplex chronicus (circumscribed neurodermatitis) is that it represents a self-perpetuating scratch-itch cycle. Hypertrophic nerve fibers have been found in lichenified, thickened lesions of long standing, but it is not known if these are of pathogenetic significance. Patients with very chronic recalcitrant lesions may be depressed or have other psychologic symptoms.

Clinical Findings

Intermittent itching incites the patient to manipulate the lesions. Itching may be so intense as to interfere with sleep. Dry, leathery, hypertrophic, lichenified plaques appear on the neck, wrists, perineum, thighs, or almost anywhere. The patches are well-localized, rectangular, thickened, and pigmented. The lines of the skin are exaggerated and divide the lesion into rectangular plaques.

Differential Diagnosis

This disorder may be confused with plaque-like lesions such as those of psoriasis, which is commonly manifested by redder lesions having whiter scales on the elbows, knees, and scalp and nail findings; with lichen planus, manifested by violaceous, usually smaller polygonal papules; and with nummular (coin-shaped) dermatitis. Similar lesions are seen in atopic dermatitis. Skin biopsy can distinguish among these presentations when necessary, but all respond to high-potency topical steroids.

Treatment

Topical corticosteroids give relief. Clobetasol, halobetasol, diflorasone, and betamethasone dipropionate in augmented vehicle are effective without occlusion and are used twice daily for several weeks. In some patients, flurandrenolide (Cordran) tape may be more effective, since it prevents scratching and rubbing of the lesion. These superpotent steroids are probably the treatment of choice but must be used with careful follow-up to avoid local and systemic side effects. The injection of triamcinolone acetonide suspension (5–10 mg/mL) into the lesions may occasionally be curative. Use of tars, such as 10% LCD (coal tar, liquor carbonis detergens, Fototar) in triamcinolone 0.1% ointment, or continuous occlusion with DuoDerm (occlusive flexible hydrocolloid dressing) for 7 days at a time for 1–2 months, may also be helpful. The area should be protected and the patient encouraged to become aware of when he or she is scratching.

Prognosis

The disease tends to remit during treatment but may recur, or another site may develop.

PSORIASIS

Essentials of Diagnosis

- Silvery scales on bright red, well-demarcated plaques, usually on the knees, elbows, and scalp.
- Nail findings including pitting and onycholysis (separation of the nail plate from the bed).
- Mild itching unless psoriasis is eruptive or occurs in body folds.
- May be associated with psoriatic arthritis.
- Histopathology is not often useful and can be confusing.

General Considerations

Psoriasis is a common benign, acute or chronic inflammatory skin disease that appears to be based upon a genetic predisposition. Injury or irritation of normal skin tends to induce lesions of psoriasis in the site in some patients (Koebner's phenomenon). Psoriasis has several variants—the most common is the plaque type. Eruptive (guttate) psoriasis consisting of myriad lesions 3–10 mm in diameter occurs occasionally in periods of stress or after streptococcal pharyngitis. Grave, occasionally life-threatening forms (generalized pustular and erythrodermic psoriasis) may rarely occur. Plaque type or extensive erythrodermic psoriasis with abrupt onset may accompany HIV infection.

Clinical Findings

There are often no symptoms. Eruptive psoriasis may itch, and psoriasis in body folds and on the vulva may itch severely ("inverse psoriasis"). Although psoriasis may occur anywhere, one should examine the scalp, elbows, knees, palms and soles, and nails. The lesions are red, sharply defined plaques covered with silvery scales. The elbows, knees, and scalp are the most common sites. The glans penis and vulva may be affected. Occasionally, only the flexures (axillae, inguinal areas) are involved. Fine stippling ("pitting") in the nails is highly suggestive of psoriasis. Psoriatics are said to often have a pink or red intergluteal fold. Not all patients have findings in all locations, but the occurrence of a few may help make the diagnosis when other lesions are not typical. Some patients present mainly with hand dermatitis and only minimal findings elsewhere, posing a difficult diagnostic problem. There may be associated arthritis that can resemble the rheumatoid variety but with a negative rheumatoid factor; distal interphalangeal joints are frequently involved.

Differential Diagnosis

The combination of red plaques with silvery scales on elbows and knees, with scaliness in the scalp or nail findings, is diagnostic. Psoriasis lesions are well demarcated and affect extensor surfaces—in contrast to atopic dermatitis, with poorly demarcated plaques in flexural distribution. In the scalp, psoriasis is distinguished from seborrheic dermatitis by well-demarcated red plaques with thick scales, in contrast to diffuse or patchy redness and scaling of seborrheic dermatitis; in body folds, scraping and culture for *Candida* and examination of scalp and nails will distinguish psoriasis from intertrigo and candidiasis. Dystrophic changes in nails may simulate onychomycosis, but again, the general examination combined with a fungal culture will be valuable in diagnosis. The cutaneous features of Reiter's syndrome may mimic psoriasis.

Treatment

There are many therapeutic options in psoriasis, to be chosen according to the extent and severity of disease and with a clear understanding of the risks and benefits of therapy.

A. Limited Disease: For many patients, the easiest regimen is to use a high-potency to highest-potency topical steroid cream or ointment. It is best to restrict the highest-potency steroids to 2–3 weeks of twice-daily use and then use them in a pulse fashion three or four times on weekends or switch to a midpotency corticosteroid and apply a tar overnight, such as Estar or Psorigel or Fototar cream, LCD (coal tar; liquor carbonis detergens), 10% in Nutraderm lotion, or mixed directly with triamcinolone 0.1% cream; it is messier to use than a steroid alone. Topical corticosteroids rarely induce a lasting remission, and some clinicians feel that steroids may make psoriasis more difficult to treat by other measures. Occlusion alone has been shown to clear some isolated plaques in some patients. Patches of occlusive dressings such as thin Duoderm are placed on the lesions and left undisturbed for as long as possible (a minimum of 5 days, up to 7 days) and then replaced. Responses may be seen within several weeks. Perhaps 30–40% of patients respond to this therapy. Anthralin is another agent available for localized disease, but it must be used properly, is irritating, and may stain the skin. Calcipotriene ointment 0.005%, a vitamin D analog, was approved for twice-daily use for treatment of moderate-plaque psoriasis. In a double-blind study of 277 patients, 70% had more than 75% clearing and only 4% failed to respond. Ten percent had an adverse reaction, most often rash, erythema, pruritus, or burning. Initially, patients are treated with twice-daily steroids to rapidly improve the psoriasis. Calcipotriene is then substituted for one of the steroid applications for several weeks. Eventually the topical steroids are stopped, and once- or twice-daily calcipotriene is continued chronically. Calcipotriene cannot be used in the groin or on the face because of frequent irritation. Treatment of extensive psoriasis may result in hypercalcemia. Calcipotriene ointment is very expensive.

For the scalp, start with a tar shampoo (Neutrogena T/Gel regular or extra strength or Ionil T Plus), used daily if possible. For thick scales, use 6% salicylic acid gel (eg, Keralyt), P & S solution (phenol, mineral oil, and glycerin), or fluocinolone acetonide 0.01% in oil (Derma-Smoothe/FS) under a shower cap at night, and shampoo in the morning. In order of increasing potency, triamcinolone 0.1%, or fluocinolone, betamethasone dipropionate, fluocinonide or amcinonide, and clobetasol are available in solution form for use on the scalp twice daily. For psoriasis in the body folds, treatment is much more difficult, since potent steroids cannot be used. When mild corticosteroids are not effective and involvement or itch is severe, some of the modalities described immediately below may be required.

B. Generalized Disease: If psoriasis involves more than 30% of the body surface, it is difficult to treat with topical agents. The treatment of choice is outpatient UVB light exposure three times weekly. Clearing occurs in an average of 7 weeks, and maintenance may be needed since relapses are frequent. Severe psoriasis unresponsive to outpatient ultraviolet light calls for treatment in the hospital or a day care center with the Goeckerman regimen, which involves use of crude coal tar for many hours and exposure to UVB light. Such treatment may offer the best chance for prolonged remissions.

PUVA (psoralen plus ultraviolet A, ie, ultraviolet light in the 320- to 400-nm wavelength range) tends to be a long-term form of treatment, since maintenance therapy is usually required to avoid relapse. Long-term use of PUVA is associated with an increased risk of skin cancer, particularly in persons with fair complexions or those who have received ionizing radiation. Thus, periodic examination of the skin is imperative. Atypical lentigines are common. There can be rapid aging of the skin in fair individuals. Cataracts are a threat but have not been reported with proper use of sunglasses, and there may be a rare conversion to a positive ANA and the even rarer appearance of localized discoid lupus lesions. PUVA is ideally used in combination with other therapy, such as etretinate or methotrexate.

Parenteral corticosteroids should not be used because of the possibility of induction of pustular lesions. Methotrexate is very effective for severe psoriasis in doses up to 25 mg once weekly or in divided doses every 12 hours for three doses once a week. It should be used according to published protocols. Liver biopsy is performed initially after methotrexate has been used long enough by the patient to demonstrate that it is effective and well tolerated, and then at intervals depending on the cumulative dose, usually 1.5–2 g. Administration of folic acid, 5 mg daily, will eliminate nausea caused by methotrexate without compromising efficacy.

Etretinate, a synthetic retinoid, is most effective for pustular psoriasis in dosages of 0.5–1 mg/kg/d, but it also improves erythrodermic and plaque types and psoriatic arthritis. Liver enzymes and serum lipids must be checked periodically. Because etretinate is a teratogen and persists for long periods in fat, only under extraordinary circumstances should it be given to women of childbearing age. When used as single agents, retinoids will flatten psoriatic plaques, but high doses may be required for complete clearing. Retinoids find their greatest use when combined with phototherapy—either UVB or PUVA, with which they are synergistic.

Cyclosporine has shown much promise in the treatment of severe psoriasis, but rapid relapses are the rule after cessation of therapy, and the long-term safety of the drug and the incidence of lymphoma have not been established. Sulfasalazine in dosages of 1 g three times daily markedly improved about one-third of patients in a double-blinded study. Thus, sulfasalazine may be considered for patients who are not candidates for—or who cannot tolerate—more toxic drugs. Thioguanine is another effective alternative for severe disease and is used at doses of 40–80 mg for 2–7 days per week with frequent monitoring of the complete blood count.

Moderate to severe psoriasis in AIDS patients is best initially treated with etretinate, 25–50 mg/d, with the addition of UVB as needed. PUVA and methotrexate are not usually recommended as initial therapies.

Prognosis

The course tends to be chronic and unpredictable, and the disease may be refractory to treatment.

Bruce S et al: Comparative study of calcipotriene (MC 903) ointment and fluocinonide ointment in the treatment of psoriasis. J Am Acad Dermatol 1994;31(5 Part 1):755.

Grossman RM et al: Long-term safety of cyclosporine in the treatment of psoriasis. Arch Dermatol 1996;132:623. (The risk of cyclosporine-induced toxic effects increases with age of the patient and with preexisting hypertension or high serum creatinine levels. The incidence of side effects increases with time. Cyclosporine is not acceptable as long-term monotherapy for psoriasis.)

Lever LR, Farr PM: Skin cancers or premalignant lesions occur in half of high-dose PUVA patients. Br J Dermatol 1994;131:215. (Nineteen percent of 54 patients treated with more than 2000 J/cm^2 of ultraviolet A had developed squamous cell carcinomas. The 13% without lentigines or freckles associated with PUVA therapy had no skin cancers or precancers.)

Menter MA et al: Proceedings of the Psoriasis Combination and Rotation Therapy Conference. J Am Acad Dermatol 1996;34(2 Part 1):315.

Phillips TJ: Current treatment options in psoriasis. Hosp Pract (Off Ed) Apr 1996;31:155.

PITYRIASIS ROSEA

Essentials of Diagnosis

- Oval, fawn-colored, scaly eruption following cleavage lines of trunk.
- Herald patch precedes eruption by 1–2 weeks.
- Occasional pruritus.

General Considerations

This is a common mild, acute inflammatory disease which is 50% more common in females. Young adults are principally affected, mostly in the spring or fall. Concurrent household cases have been reported. The cause is unknown, but it is speculated that a virus may be causative. The attack rate in married couples is less than 2%, so whatever the cause, it is not highly infectious.

Clinical Findings

Itching is common but is usually mild. The diagnosis is made by finding one or more classic lesions. The lesions consist of oval, fawn-colored macules up to 1 cm in diameter. The centers of the lesions have a crinkled or "cigarette paper" appearance and a collarette scale, ie, a thin bit of scale that is bound at the periphery and free in the center. Only a few lesions in the eruption may have this characteristic appearance, however. Lesions follow cleavage lines on the trunk (so-called Christmas tree pattern), and the proximal portions of the extremities are often involved. Variants that affect the flexures (axillae and groin), so called inverse pityriasis rosea, and papular variants, especially in black patients, also occur. An initial lesion ("herald patch") that is often larger than the later lesions often precedes the general eruption by 1–2 weeks. The eruption usually lasts 4–8 weeks and heals without scarring.

Differential Diagnosis

A serologic test for syphilis should be performed if at least a few perfectly typical lesions are not present, if the rash does not itch, and especially if there are palmar and plantar or mucous membrane lesions that are suggestive of secondary syphilis. For the nonexpert, an RPR test in all cases is not unreasonable. Tinea corporis may present with red, slightly scaly plaques, but rarely are there more than a few lesions of tinea corporis compared to the many lesions of pityriasis rosea. A scraping of scale for a KOH test will rapidly make the diagnosis. Seborrheic dermatitis on occasion presents on the body with poorly demarcated patches over the sternum, in the pubic area, and in the axillae. The classic lesions of pityriasis rosea are not present. Tinea versicolor lesions, viral exanthems, and drug eruptions may simulate pityriasis rosea.

Treatment

Pityriasis rosea often requires no treatment. In Asians, Hispanics, or blacks, in whom lesions may remain hyperpigmented for some time, more aggressive management may be indicated. The most effective management consists of daily UVB treatments for a week, or prednisone as used for contact dermatitis. Topical steroids of medium strength (triamcinolone 0.1%) may also be used if pruritus is bothersome.

Prognosis

Pityriasis rosea is usually an acute self-limiting illness that disappears in about 6 weeks.

Leenutaphong V, Jiamton S: UVB phototherapy for pityriasis rosea: A bilateral comparison study. J Am Acad Dermatol 1995;33:996.

SEBORRHEIC DERMATITIS & DANDRUFF

Essentials of Diagnosis

- Dry scales and underlying erythema.
- Scalp, central face, presternal, interscapular areas, umbilicus, and body folds.

General Considerations

Seborrheic dermatitis is an acute or chronic papulosquamous dermatitis. The response of seborrheic dermatitis to the antifungal ketoconazole has raised the possibility that seborrheic dermatitis represents an inflammatory reaction to *Malassezia furfur* yeasts present on the scalp of all humans. However, the effect of ketoconazole in this disease may not be due to its antifungal properties alone.

Clinical Findings

Pruritus is an inconstant finding. The scalp, face, chest, back, umbilicus, eyelid margins, and body folds may be oily or dry, with dry scales or oily yellowish scurf. Fissuring and secondary infection are occasionally present. Patients with Parkinson's disease frequently develop moderately severe seborrheic dermatitis, as do elderly patients who become acutely ill and are hospitalized for a variety of reasons. Patients with HIV infection often present with widespread or well-demarcated plaques of seborrheic dermatitis.

Differential Diagnosis

There is often a clinical spectrum ranging from simple dandruff to seborrheic dermatitis to scalp psoriasis. On the scalp, the presence of well-demarcated red plaques usually is termed psoriasis, and general erythema without tight, thick, silvery scale is usually called seborrheic dermatitis. The presence of mild scaling without any erythema is often termed simple dandruff. Extensive seborrheic dermatitis may simulate intertrigo in flexural areas, but scalp, face, and sternal involvement suggests seborrheic dermatitis. Scaling of the scalp due to tinea capitis may simulate dandruff or seborrheic dermatitis, and brush cultures for tinea should be performed in children.

Treatment

A. Seborrhea of the Scalp: The clinician should suggest several shampoos and let the patient decide which is most acceptable. Shampoos that contain tar, zinc pyrithione, or selenium are used daily if possible, while ketoconazole shampoo is used twice weekly. Topical corticosteroid solutions or lotions are then added if necessary, and are used twice daily intermittently to avoid tachyphylaxis. Atrophy of the scalp is uncommon except in patients with alopecia.

B. Facial Seborrheic Dermatitis: Mild soaps are usually used as described under atopic dermatitis so as not to further irritate the skin. Treatment of the scalp, if involved, is thought to decrease facial involvement. The mainstay of therapy is a mild corticosteroid (hydrocortisone 1%, alclometasone, desonide) used intermittently and not near the eyes. Potent fluorinated corticosteroids used regularly on the face may produce steroid rosacea or atrophy and telangiectasia. These are rarely indicated for seborrheic dermatitis. If the disorder cannot be controlled with intermittent use of a topical steroid alone, ketoconazole (Nizoral) 2% cream is added twice daily.

C. Seborrheic Dermatitis of Nonhairy Areas: Low-potency steroid creams—ie, 1% or 2.5% hydrocortisone, desonide, or alclometasone dipropionate—are highly effective.

D. Seborrhea of Intertriginous Areas: Avoid greasy ointments. Apply low-potency steroid lotions or creams twice daily for 5–7 days and then once or twice weekly for maintenance as necessary. Ketoconazole shampoo may be a useful adjunct.

E. Involvement of Eyelid Margins: "Marginal blepharitis" usually responds to gentle cleaning of the lid margins nightly as needed, with undiluted Johnson and Johnson Baby Shampoo using a cotton swab.

Prognosis

The tendency is to lifelong recurrences. Individual outbreaks may last weeks, months, or years.

Janniger CK, Schwartz RA: Seborrheic dermatitis. Am Fam Physician 1995;52:149.

Peter RJ, Richarz-Barthauer U: Successful treatment and prophylaxis of scalp seborrheic dermatitis and dandruff with 2% ketoconazole shampoo: Results of a multicentre, double-blind, placebo-controlled trial. Br J Dermatol 1995;132:441.

FUNGAL INFECTIONS OF THE SKIN

Mycotic infections are traditionally divided into two principal groups—superficial and deep. In this chapter, we will discuss only the superficial infections: tinea capitis, tinea corporis, and tinea cruris; dermatophytosis of the feet and dermatophytid of the hands; tinea unguium (onychomycosis); and tinea versicolor. See Chapter 36 for discussion of deep mycoses.

The diagnosis of fungal infections of the skin is usually based on the location and characteristics of the lesions and on the following laboratory examinations: (1) Direct demonstration of fungi in 10% potassium hydroxide (KOH) in water or 20% KOH in DMSO preparations of scrapings from suspected lesions. "If it's scaly, scrape it" is a time-honored maxim. (2) Cultures of organisms on dermatophyte test medium (DTM); or one may use a microculture slide that produces color change and allows for direct microscopic identification. Examination of the skin with Wood's light (an ultraviolet light with a special filter), which causes hairs to fluoresce a brilliant green when they are infected by *Microsporum* organisms, used to be a valuable test. However, because most infections of the scalp are not caused by *Microsporum* organisms, this test is rarely positive, and a negative test is meaningless. Histologic sections of nails stained with periodic acid-Schiff (Hotchkiss-McManus) technique may be diagnostic if cultures and scrapings are negative. Serologic and skin tests are of no value in the diagnosis of superficial fungal infections.

Principles of Treatment

In general, treatment follows a diagnosis confirmed by KOH preparation or culture, especially if systemic antifungal therapy is to be used. Many other diseases cause scaling, and use of an antifungal agent without a firm diagnosis makes subsequent diagnosis by a dermatologist more difficult. In general, fungal infections are treated topically except for those involving the scalp or nails or those deep in hair follicles on the face or body.

Griseofulvin is safe and effective for treating dermatophyte infections of the skin (except for the scalp and nails). It is more economical than the newer agents and may be used initially when systemic treatment is required for tinea cruris, tinea pedis, or tinea corporis.

Itraconazole, an azole antifungal, has been approved for use in the USA for treatment of histoplasmosis and blastomycosis and for dermatophytosis. It rapidly accumulates in the nail plate from the matrix and nail bed and persists for 6–9 months after oral administration is discontinued.

Fluconazole is another azole antifungal that is effective in treating cutaneous and mucous membrane candidiasis and dermatophytosis. Itraconazole and fluconazole have been associated with idiosyncratic hepatotoxicity. The recently released suspension is better-absorbed and its use does not require food ingestion (presence of gastric acid) for optimal absorption from the gastrointestinal tract.

Terbinafine is an allylamine oral antifungal. It has excellent activity against dermatophytes. In vitro activity against yeast forms is variable, but the drug is active against hyphal forms. It is well delivered to the nail plate and persists in the nail for long periods after treatment has ended. Loss of taste is a unique unpleasant but uncommon side effect of terbinafine.

Fluconazole, another triazole antifungal, has excellent activity against yeasts and may be the treatment of choice for many forms of mucocutaneous candidiasis. It is not known whether fluconazole is selectively delivered to the keratin compartment, and there have not been sufficient studies to determine effective doses in treating dermatophytosis. Fluconazole appears to require longer treatment courses and so is more expensive than either itraconazole or terbinafine for the treatment of dermatophytosis.

Itraconazole, fluconazole, and terbinafine can all cause elevation of liver function tests and—though rarely in the dosing regimens used for the treatment of dermatophytosis—clinical hepatitis. Ketoconazole is no longer recommended for the treatment of dermatophytosis (except for tinea versicolor) because of the higher rate of hepatitis when it is used for more than a month.

General Measures & Prevention

The skin should be kept dry, since moist skin favors the growth of fungi. Dry the skin carefully after bathing or after perspiring heavily, and let it dry for 10–15 minutes before dressing, or use a hair dryer on low setting. Loose-fitting underwear is advisable. Socks should be changed frequently when moist from perspiration. Sandals or open-toed shoes should be worn if possible. Talc or other drying powders may be useful. The use of topical corticosteroids for other diseases may be complicated by intercurrent tinea or candidal infection, and topical antifungals are often used in intertriginous areas with steroids to prevent this.

Brennan B, Leyden JJ: Overview of topical therapy for common superficial fungal infections and the role of new topical agents. J Am Acad Dermatol 1997;36(2 Part 1):S3.

Lesher JL Jr: Recent developments in antifungal therapy. Dermatol Clin 1996;14:163.

Pierard GE, Arrese JE, Pierard-Franchimont C: Treatment and prophylaxis of tinea infections. Drugs 1996;52:209.

1.   TINEA CAPITIS

Essentials of Diagnosis

- Seborrheic dermatitis-like scaling.
- Impetigo-like lesions with crusting and redness.
- Areas of hair loss with "black dot" broken-off hairs.
- Kerion or inflammatory nodules.
- Lymphadenitis even with subtle scalp disease.
- Positive fungal culture.
- High rate of asymptomatic carriage in certain populations.

General Considerations

We are in the midst of an epidemic of tinea capitis caused by *Trichophyton tonsurans,* particularly among black children, with a peak between ages 2 and 6 years. Spread of infection is promoted by the high carriage rate among asymptomatic individuals—up to 15% of black school children and 30% of asymptomatic adult family contacts are culture-positive on the scalp. Unfortunately, unlike the tinea species *Microsporum audouini* causing infections in the past, *T tonsurans* does not fluoresce, and thus Wood's light screening is not useful. Unlike tinea infections at other sites, the KOH examination is useful only when alopecia is seen. The brush method of culturing is a simple and sensitive test.

Clinical Findings

A.   Symptoms and Signs: The infection is

most often asymptomatic. Impetigo-like lesions and kerions may be marked by soreness. Physical findings include scaling without inflammation in the majority of cases. Scaling may be inapparent if pomades are used in the hair. Alopecia is detected as widening of the area of scalp that is visible when the hair is parted or as areas of thin or absent hair with small broken-off short stubs of hair ("black dot tinea"). When more inflammation is present, erythema, crusts, and pustules may be present, suggesting impetigo. Mixed presentations include alopecia, crusts, and follicular prominence. Patches of alopecia with broken-off dystrophic hairs, or kerions—single boggy tender masses with crusting, pus, and alopecia—represent the least common presentations today, accounting for 20% of cases. Some patients present with multiple smaller nodules.

Cervical lymphadenitis may be very impressive and does not correlate with the extent of scalp inflammation. Tinea corporis is seen in 15% of patients. Well-defined patches of hypopigmentation may be seen on the face. Permanent alopecia may result from kerions or secondarily infected lesions.

B. Laboratory Findings: Scraping the skin for examination with potassium hydroxide may reveal hyphae in scales or chains of arthrospores within dystrophic hairs. All patients must have tinea identified by KOH or by culture prior to treatment. A negative KOH test does not rule out tinea infection, and scrapings from kerions are rarely positive. Cultures are obtained without patient discomfort by using disposable nonsterilized toothbrushes brushed through four or five areas of the scalp and pressed after each area is brushed onto fungal media (a widemouth jar or a fungal plate is needed). If toothbrushes or widemouth jars are not available, cytobrushes used for Papanicolaou smears may be employed.

Differential Diagnosis

Tinea capitis may resemble seborrheic dermatitis, which is uncommon in children 2–8 years of age. In this age range, seborrheic dermatitis is tinea capitis until proved otherwise. Lesions may suggest impetigo and may be culture-positive for *Staphylococcus aureus*. Patients are not uncommonly inappropriately treated with antibiotics, and most cases clear on antifungal therapy alone.

Atopic dermatitis causing scaling in the scalp invariably occurs with severe generalized atopic dermatitis and rarely as an isolated finding. Pityriasis (formerly called tinea) amiantacea presents with a patch or patches of adherent "asbestos-like" scaling. Pityriasis amiantacea is idiopathic and transient or may precede psoriasis. Thick scaling may suggest psoriasis. Bald areas of black dot tinea may suggest alopecia areata, but patches of tinea are never truly "smooth as a baby's bottom" as is described in alopecia areata. Areas of alopecia and broken hairs may also suggest trichotillomania. Patients have also been referred for lymph node biopsies because of lymphadenitis and subtle cutaneous findings. In each case, clinical suspicion and cultures will establish the diagnosis.

Prevention

Tinea capitis is difficult to prevent because of airborne spread of spores and the high rate of asymptomatic carriage in the community. There is no known method for environmental decontamination of spores, which are found on most objects in the home. Keeping patients out of school during treatment is not justified because there are so many undiagnosed cases in the classroom.

Povidone-iodine shampoo can clear over 90% of asymptomatic carriers when used twice weekly for 4 weeks.

Treatment

A. Local Measures: Selenium 2.5% shampoo is used twice weekly to decrease spore shedding during treatment. The use of ketoconazole (Nizoral) shampoo has not been studied. Topical antifungal creams or lotions are not effective primary therapy.

B. Systemic Therapy: Griseofulvin is the current therapy of choice. Eradication of infection requires doses exceeding those recommended in drug information inserts. One begins with a dosage of 15 mg/kg/d of micronized griseofulvin suspension, but 20–25 mg/kg/d is often needed. Patients failing treatment with the suspension may respond to the same doses of ultramicrosize griseofulvin tablets (Gris-PEG) pulverized and mixed in food. Patients return after 6 weeks of therapy for repeat culture, then monthly for repeat cultures, with another repeat culture 1 month after stopping therapy.

Response is slow and may require 3 or more months of therapy. Compliance is poor in the majority of patients without alopecia, who have only asymptomatic scaling. Papular id reactions on the body are commonly seen on the third day and may be misdiagnosed as drug allergy, which is rare.

Itraconazole in preliminary reports appears to be very effective in the treatment of tinea capitis due to *T tonsurans*. The dose is 5 mg/kg/d for 4–8 weeks, or 100 mg/d for most elementary school children (the tinea capitis age group). The oral itraconazole suspension has enhanced bioavailability, so the dosage may be as low as 3 mg/kg/d, and it need not be given with food and does not require gastric acid to enhance absorption. Pulse therapy regimens should not be used for tinea capitis until verified as effective. Oral terbinafine in a dosage of 125 mg daily for 6 weeks also appears to be effective. Neither of these agents is approved for this indication in children.

Prednisone at a dosage of 1 mg/kg/d may be necessary for treatment of kerions, although oral griseofulvin at adequate doses should be sufficient. One should culture four or five areas of the scalp of parents and siblings to detect carriers in the family.

Prognosis

Tinea capitis should be treated whenever detected. Rarely, permanent alopecia may result from kerions.

Drake LA et al: Guidelines of care for superficial mycotic infections of the skin: Tinea capitis and tinea barbae. Guidelines/Outcomes Committee. American Academy of Dermatology. J Am Acad Dermatol 1996;34(2 Part 1):290.

Gianni C et al: Tinea capitis in adults. Mycoses 1995;38:329.

Greer DL: Treatment of tinea capitis with itraconazole. J Am Acad Dermatol 1996;35:637.

Howard R, Frieden IJ: Tinea capitis: New perspectives on an old disease. Semin Dermatol 1995;14:2.

Nejjam F et al: Pilot study of terbinafine in children suffering from tinea capitis: Evaluation of efficacy, safety and pharmacokinetics. Br J Dermatol 1995;132:98. (Report of success in 12 children with tinea capitis treated for 6 weeks with oral terbinafine 125 mg/d.)

Williams JVD et al: Semiquantitative study of tinea capitis and the asymptomatic carrier state in inner-city school children. Pediatrics 1995;96:265. (In one school 3% of African American elementary school children had tinea capitis, and 14% were asymptomatic carriers. Fifty percent of positive cultures were from children in kindergarten and the first grade.)

2. TINEA CORPORIS OR TINEA CIRCINATA (Body Ringworm)

Essentials of Diagnosis

- Ring-shaped lesions with an advancing scaly border and central clearing or scaly patches with a distinct border.
- On exposed skin surfaces or the trunk.
- Microscopic examination of scrapings or culture confirms the diagnosis.

General Considerations

The lesions are often on exposed areas of the body such as the face and arms. A history of exposure to an infected cat may occasionally be obtained, usually indicating *Microsporum* infection. All species of dermatophytes may cause this disease, but *Trichophyton rubrum* is the most common pathogen, usually representing extension of tinea cruris, pedis, or manuum.

Clinical Findings

A. Symptoms and Signs: Itching may be present. In classic lesions, rings of erythema have an advancing scaly border and central clearing, occasionally with hyperpigmentation. More often, tinea corporis lacks this ring shape and presents with scaly patches of 1 to many centimeters.

B. Laboratory Findings: Hyphae can be demonstrated by removing peripheral scale and ex-

amining it microscopically using KOH. The diagnosis may be confirmed by culture.

Material can be obtained for culture on Sabouraud's medium by thoroughly rubbing a cotton swab over the lesion and then rotating the swab while vigorously rubbing it on the medium; this technique is just as accurate as scraping the lesions with a scalpel or curette.

Differential Diagnosis

Positive fungal studies distinguish tinea corporis from other skin lesions with annular configuration, such as the annular lesions of psoriasis, lupus erythematosus, syphilis, erythema multiforme, and pityriasis rosea. Psoriasis has typical lesions on elbows, knees, scalp, and nails. Secondary syphilis is often manifested by characteristic palmar, plantar, and mucous membrane lesions. Erythema multiforme does not have peripheral scale, is mostly acral in distribution, and is often associated with recent herpes simplex infection. Tinea corporis rarely has the large number of lesions seen in pityriasis rosea. Granuloma annulare lacks scales.

Complications

Complications include extension of the disease down the hair follicles (in which case it becomes much more difficult to cure), pyoderma, and dermatophytid.

Prevention

Avoid contact with infected household pets (*Microsporum* infections).

Treatment

A. Local Measures: The following applied topically are effective against dermatophyte infections other than those of the nails: miconazole, 2% cream; clotrimazole, 1% solution, cream, or lotion; ketoconazole, 2% cream; econazole, 1% cream or lotion; sulconazole, 1% cream; oxiconazole, 1% cream; ciclopirox, 1% cream; naftifine, 1% cream or gel; butenafine creams; and terbinafine, 1% cream. Miconazole and clotrimazole are available OTC. Allylamines (naftifine, terbinafine, and butenafine) lead to the most rapid response but are quite expensive. Treatment should be continued for 1–2 weeks after clinical clearing. Betamethasone dipropionate with clotrimazole is often overused by nondermatologists. In general, short-term use of betamethasone-clotrimazole (Lotrisone) does not justify the expense, and chronic improper use may result in side effects from the high-potency steroid component, especially in body folds. Cases of tinea that are clinically resistant to this combination have been reported.

B. Systemic Measures: Griseofulvin (microcrystalline) may be given to children as described for tinea capitis and griseofulvin (ultramicrosize) at 250–500 mg twice daily is used for adults. Typically, only 2–4 weeks of therapy are required. Itraconazole as a single week-long pulse of 200 mg once daily is also effective in tinea corporis. Terbinafine, 250 mg daily for 1 month, is an alternative.

Prognosis

Body ringworm usually responds promptly to conservative topical therapy within 4 weeks or to griseofulvin by mouth.

Drake LA et al: Guidelines of care for superficial mycotic infections of the skin: Tinea corporis, tinea cruris, tinea faciei, tinea manuum, and tinea pedis. Guidelines/Outcomes Committee. American Academy of Dermatology. J Am Acad Dermatol 1996;34(2 Part 1):282.

Pariser DM et al: Double-blind comparison of itraconazole and placebo in the treatment of tinea corporis and tinea cruris. J Am Acad Dermatol 1994;31(2 Part 1):232. (Two weeks of itraconazole 100 mg daily for 2 weeks cured or markedly improved 96% of patients. Similar benefit results from 1 week of 200 mg daily.)

3. TINEA CRURIS
(Jock Itch)

Essentials of Diagnosis

- Marked itching in intertriginous areas, usually sparing the scrotum.
- Peripherally spreading, sharply demarcated, centrally clearing erythematous lesions.
- May have associated tinea infection of feet or toenails.
- Laboratory examination with microscope or culture confirms diagnosis.

General Considerations

Tinea cruris lesions are confined to the groin and gluteal cleft. Intractable pruritus ani may occasionally be caused by a tinea infection.

Clinical Findings

A. Symptoms and Signs: Itching may be severe, or the rash may be asymptomatic. The lesions have sharp margins, cleared centers, and active, spreading scaly peripheries. There rarely may be vesicle formation at the borders. Follicular pustules are sometimes encountered. The area may be hyperpigmented on resolution.

B. Laboratory Findings: Hyphae can be demonstrated microscopically in potassium hydroxide preparations. The organism may be cultured readily.

Differential Diagnosis

Tinea cruris must be distinguished from other lesions involving the intertriginous areas, such as candidiasis, seborrheic dermatitis, intertrigo, psoriasis of body folds ("inverse psoriasis"), erythrasma, and rarely tinea versicolor. Candidiasis is generally bright red and marked by satellite papules and pustules outside of the main border of the lesion. Tinea versicolor can be diagnosed by the KOH preparation, since its causative organisms are distinct from true fungi. Seborrheic dermatitis of the inguinal area also often involves the face, sternum, and axillae. Intertrigo tends to be more red, less scaly, and present in obese individuals in moist body folds with less extension onto the thigh. Inverse psoriasis is characterized by distinct plaques. Other areas of typical psoriatic involvement should be checked, and the KOH examination will be negative. Erythrasma is best diagnosed with Wood's light—a brilliant coral-red fluorescence is seen.

Treatment

A. General Measures: Drying powder (eg, miconazole nitrate [Zeasorb-AF]) should be dusted into the involved area in patients with excessive perspiration or occlusion of skin due to obesity. Avoid overbathing. Underwear should be loose-fitting.

B. Local Measures: Any of the preparations listed in the section on tinea corporis may be used. There is great variation in expense, with miconazole and clotrimazole available OTC and usually at a lower price. Ketoconazole and sulconazole cream may be used daily instead of twice daily. Terbinafine cream is curative in over 80% of cases after twice-daily use for 7 days.

C. Systemic Measures: Griseofulvin ultramicrosize is reserved for severe cases. Give 250–500 mg orally twice daily for 1–2 weeks. One week of either itraconazole, 200 mg daily, or terbinafine, 250 mg daily, is also effective.

Prognosis

Tinea cruris usually responds promptly to topical or systemic treatment. It may leave behind postinflammatory hyperpigmentation.

Drake LA et al: Guidelines of care for superficial mycotic infections of the skin: Tinea corporis, tinea cruris, tinea faciei, tinea manuum, and tinea pedis. Guidelines/Outcomes Committee. American Academy of Dermatology. J Am Acad Dermatol 1996;34(2 Part 1):282.

4. TINEA MANUUM & TINEA PEDIS
(Dermatophytosis, Tinea of Palms & Soles, "Athlete's Foot")

Essentials of Diagnosis

- Most often presenting with asymptomatic scaling.
- May progress to fissuring or maceration in toe web spaces.
- Itching, burning, and stinging of interdigital webs, palms, and soles seen occasionally; deep vesicles in inflammatory cases.

- The fungus is shown in skin scrapings examined microscopically or by culture of scrapings.

General Considerations

Tinea of the feet is an extremely common acute or chronic dermatosis. Certain individuals appear to be more susceptible than others. Most infections are caused by *Trichophyton* and *Epidermophyton* species.

Clinical Findings

A. Symptoms and Signs: The presenting symptom may be itching. However, there may be burning, stinging, and other sensations. Pain may indicate secondary infection with complicating cellulitis, lymphangitis, and lymphadenitis. Tinea pedis has several presentations that vary with the location. On the sole and heel, tinea may appear as chronic noninflammatory scaling, occasionally with thickening and cracking of the epidermis. This may extend over the sides of the feet in a "moccasin" distribution. The KOH preparation is usually positive. Tinea pedis often appears as a scaling or fissuring of the toe webs, perhaps with denudation and sodden maceration. As the web spaces become more macerated, the KOH preparation and fungal culture are less often positive because bacterial species begin to dominate. Finally, there may also be grouped vesicles distributed anywhere on the soles or palms, generalized exfoliation of the skin of the soles, or destructive nail involvement in the form of discoloration and thickening and crumbling of the nail plate.

B. Laboratory Findings: Hyphae can be demonstrated microscopically in skin scales treated with 10% potassium hydroxide. Culture with Sabouraud's medium is simple and often informative but does not always demonstrate pathogenic fungi from macerated areas.

Differential Diagnosis

Differentiate from other skin conditions involving the same areas, such as interdigital erythrasma (use Wood's light). Psoriasis may be a cause of chronic scaling on the palms or soles and may cause nail changes. Repeated fungal cultures should be negative, and the condition will not respond to antifungal therapy. Contact dermatitis (from shoes, powders, nail polish) will often involve the dorsal surfaces and will respond to topical or systemic corticosteroids. Vesicular lesions should be differentiated from pompholyx (dyshidrosis) and scabies by proper scraping of the roofs of individual vesicles. Rarely, gram-negative organisms may cause toe web infections in the setting of prior tinea or in its absence. Culture is not very specific, because gram-negative organisms can be cultured from normal toe webs. This entity is treated with aluminum salts (see below) and imidazole antifungal agents or ciclopirox.

Prevention

The essential factor in prevention is personal hygiene. Use of rubber or wooden sandals in community showers and bathing places is often recommended, though the effectiveness of this practice has not been studied. Careful drying between the toes after showering is essential. A hair dryer used on low setting may be used before dressing. Socks should be changed frequently. Apply dusting and drying powders as necessary. The use of powders containing antifungal agents (eg, Zeasorb-AF) or chronic use of antifungal creams may prevent recurrences of tinea pedis.

Treatment

A. Local Measures: *Caution:* Do not overtreat.

1. Macerated stage–Treat with aluminum subacetate solution soaks for 20 minutes twice daily. It may respond better to 30% aqueous aluminum chloride or to carbolfuchsin paint (this is messy) than to antifungal agents. Broad-spectrum antifungal creams and solutions (containing imidazoles or ciclopirox instead of tolnaftate and haloprogin) will help combat diphtheroids and other gram-positive organisms present at this stage and alone may be adequate therapy.

2. Dry and scaly stage–Use any of the agents listed in the section on tinea corporis.

B. Systemic Measures: Griseofulvin should be used only for severe cases or those recalcitrant to topical therapy. If the infection is cleared by systemic therapy, the patient should be encouraged to begin maintenance with topical therapy, since recurrence is common.

Itraconazole is effective for relief of recalcitrant palm and sole dermatophyte infections. It is expensive and may not prevent recurrences. The dosage is 200 mg daily for 2 weeks or 400 mg daily for 1 week.

Prognosis

For many individuals, tinea pedis becomes a chronic affliction, temporarily cleared by systemic therapy only to recur.

Drake LA et al: Guidelines of care for superficial mycotic infections of the skin: Tinea corporis, tinea cruris, tinea faciei, tinea manuum, and tinea pedis. Guidelines/Outcomes Committee. American Academy of Dermatology. J Am Acad Dermatol 1996;34(2 Part 1):282.

Elewski B et al: Long-term outcome of patients with interdigital tinea pedis treated with terbinafine or clotrimazole. J Am Acad Dermatol 1995;32(2 Part 1):290.

Evans EG: A comparison of terbinafine (Lamasil) 1% cream given for one week with clotrimazole (Canesten) 1% cream given for four weeks, in the treatment of tinea pedis. Br J Dermatol 1994;130(Suppl 43):12. (Terbinafine resulted in higher mycologic cure at 4 weeks—94% versus 73%—and "effective" therapy—90% versus 73%—at 6 weeks. It is many times more expensive, however.)

Leyden JL: Tinea pedis pathophysiology and treatment. J Am Acad Dermatol 1994;31(3 Part 2):S31. (Reviews fungal and bacterial microbiology and immune response.)

5. TINEA VERSICOLOR
(Pityriasis Versicolor)

Essentials of Diagnosis

- Pale macules that will not tan, or hyperpigmented macules.
- Velvety, tan, pink, whitish, or brown macules that scale with scraping.
- Trunk distribution the most frequent site.
- Yeast observed on microscopic examination of scales.

General Considerations

Tinea versicolor is a mild, superficial *Malassezia furfur (Pityrosporum orbiculare)* infection of the skin (usually of the trunk). This yeast is a colonizer of all humans, which accounts for the high 2-year recurrence rate after treatment and initial cure. It is not understood why some patients manifest the spore and hyphal form of the organism and the clinical disease. The eruption is often called to patients' attention by the fact that the involved areas will not tan, and the resulting pseudoachromia may be mistaken for vitiligo. A hyperpigmented form is not uncommon. The disease is not particularly contagious.

Clinical Findings

A. Symptoms and Signs: Lesions are asymptomatic, but a few patients note itching. The lesions are velvety, tan, pink, whitish, or brown macules that vary from 4–5 mm in diameter to large confluent areas. The lesions initially do not look scaly, but scales may be readily obtained by scraping the area. Lesions may appear on the trunk, upper arms, neck, face, and groin.

B. Laboratory Findings: Large, blunt hyphae and thick-walled budding spores ("spaghetti and meatballs") may be seen under the 10× objective when skin scales have been cleared in 10% KOH. Fungal culture is not useful.

Differential Diagnosis

Hypopigmented lesions can be distinguished from vitiligo on basis of appearance. Vitiligo usually presents with periorificial lesions or lesions on the tips of the fingers. Vitiligo (and not tinea versicolor) is characterized by total depigmentation, not just a lessening of pigmentation. Pink and red-brown lesions on the chest are differentiated from seborrheic dermatitis of the same areas by the KOH preparation.

Treatment & Prognosis

Topical treatments include selenium sulfide lotion, which may be applied from neck to waist daily and left on for 5–15 minutes for 7 days; this treatment is repeated weekly for a month and then monthly for maintenance. Ketoconazole shampoo may also be used weekly chronically for maintenance. One must stress to the patient that the raised and scaly aspects of the rash are being treated; the alterations in pigmentation may take months to fade or fill in. One may also use equal parts of propylene glycol and water topically, diluting with water if there is irritation. Other choices are 3% salicylic acid in rubbing alcohol and Tinver lotion (contains sodium thiosulfate). Irritation and odor from these agents are common complaints from patients. Relapses are common.

Sulfur-salicylic acid soap or shampoo (Sebulex) or zinc pyrithrone-containing shampoos used on a continuing basis may be effective prophylaxis.

Ketoconazole, 200 mg daily orally for 1 week or 400 mg as a single oral dose, apparently results in short-term cure of 90% of cases. Patients should be instructed not to shower for 12–18 hours after taking ketoconazole, because it is delivered in sweat to the skin. The single dose may not work in more hot and humid areas, and more protracted therapy carries a small but finite risk of drug-induced hepatitis for a completely benign disease. Without maintenance therapy, recurrences will occur in over 80% of "cured" cases over the subsequent 2 years.

Newer imidazole creams, solutions, and lotions are quite effective for localized areas but are too expensive for use over large areas such as the chest and back.

Drake LA et al: Guidelines of care for superficial mycotic infections of the skin: Pityriasis (tinea) versicolor. Guidelines/Outcomes Committee. American Academy of Dermatology. J Am Acad Dermatol 1996;34(2 Part 1):287.

Faergemann J: Pityriasis versicolor. Semin Dermatol 1993;12:276. (Treatment and prevention of recurrences.)

Savin R: Diagnosis and treatment of tinea versicolor. J Fam Pract 1996;43:127.

DISCOID LUPUS ERYTHEMATOSUS
(Chronic Cutaneous Lupus Erythematosus)

Essentials of Diagnosis

- Red, asymptomatic, localized plaques, usually on the face.
- Scaling, follicular plugging, atrophy, and telangiectasia of involved areas.
- Histology distinctive.
- May be photosensitive.

General Considerations

This type of lupus erythematosus is a localized discoid inflammation of the skin occurring most frequently in areas exposed to solar or ultraviolet irradiation. Permanent hair loss and loss of pigmentation are the most serious sequelae. Systemic lupus erythematosus is discussed in Chapter 20.

Clinical Findings

A. Symptoms and Signs: There are usually no symptoms. The lesions consist of dusky red, well-localized, single or multiple plaques, 5–20 mm in diameter, usually on the face. The scalp, external ears, and oral mucous membranes may be involved. There is atrophy, telangiectasia, and follicular plugging. The lesion may be covered by dry, horny, adherent scales.

B. Laboratory Findings: If ANA is positive in high titer or when the clinical picture suggests systemic involvement, the findings of antibody to double-stranded DNA and hypocomplementemia suggest the diagnosis of systemic lupus erythematosus. Rare patients with marked photosensitivity and a picture otherwise suggestive of lupus have negative ANA tests but are positive for antibodies against Ro/SSA. A direct immunofluorescence test reveals basement membrane antibody but may be falsely positive in sun-exposed skin.

Differential Diagnosis

The diagnosis is based on the clinical appearance confirmed by skin biopsy in the majority of cases. The scales are dry and "thumbtack-like" and can thus be distinguished from those of seborrheic dermatitis and psoriasis. Older lesions that have left depigmented scarring (classically in the concha of the ear) or areas of hair loss will also differentiate lupus from these diseases. A skin biopsy will be diagnostic. Ten percent of patients with systemic lupus erythematosus have discoid skin lesions, and 5% of patients with discoid lesions have SLE.

Treatment

A. General Measures: Protect from sunlight. *Caution:* Do not use any form of radiation therapy. Avoid using drugs that are potentially photosensitizing (eg, thiazides, piroxicam, doxycycline) where possible.

B. Local Treatment: The following should be tried before systemic therapy: high-potency corticosteroid creams applied each night and covered with airtight, thin, pliable plastic film (eg, Saran Wrap); or Cordran tape; or ultra-high-potency corticosteroid cream or ointment applied twice daily without occlusion.

C. Local Infiltration: Triamcinolone acetonide suspension, 2.5–10 mg/mL, may be injected into the lesions once a month. This should be tried before systemic therapy.

D. Systemic Treatment:

1. Antimalarials–*Caution:* These drugs should be used only when the diagnosis is secure, because they have been associated with flares of psoriasis, which may be in the differential diagnosis. They may also cause ocular changes, and ophthalmologic eval-

uation is required before beginning treatment and repeated every 3 months. The use of antimalarials in children is controversial.

a. Hydroxychloroquine sulfate, 0.2–0.4 g orally daily for several months, may be effective and is often used prior to chloroquine. A 3-month trial is recommended.

b. Chloroquine sulfate, 250 mg daily, may be effective in some cases where hydroxychloroquine is not.

c. Quinacrine (Atabrine), 100 mg daily, may be the safest of the antimalarials, since eye damage has not been reported. It colors the skin yellow and is therefore not acceptable to some patients.

2. Dapsone–Dapsone, 50 mg/d orally, may be helpful. (Baseline G6PD levels must be obtained prior to use.)

3. Isotretinoin–Isotretinoin, 1 mg/kg/d, is effective in chronic or subacute cutaneous lupus erythematosus. Recurrences are prompt and predictable on discontinuation of therapy. Because of teratogenicity, the drug is used with caution in women of childbearing age using effective contraception with negative pregnancy tests before and during therapy.

Prognosis

The disease is persistent but not life-endangering unless systemic lupus intervenes, which is uncommon. Treatment with antimalarials is effective in perhaps 60% of cases. Although the only morbidity may be cosmetic, this can be of overwhelming significance in more darkly pigmented patients with widespread disease. Scarring alopecia can be prevented or lessened with close attention and aggressive therapy.

Callen JP: Treatment of cutaneous lesions in patients with lupus erythematosus. Dermatol Clin 1994;12:206. (An approach for treatment of mild to severe disease, including sunscreens, intralesional steroids, antimalarials, azathioprine, retinoids, and other medications.)

CUTANEOUS T CELL LYMPHOMA (Mycosis Fungoides)

Essentials of Diagnosis

- Localized or generalized erythematous scaling plaques.
- Pruritus.
- Lymphadenopathy.
- Distinctive histology.

General Considerations

Mycosis fungoides is a cutaneous T cell lymphoma that begins on the skin and may involve only the skin for years or decades. Certain medications may produce eruptions clinically and histologically identical to those of mycosis fungoides, so this possibility must always be considered.

Clinical Findings

A. Symptoms and Signs: Patients present with localized or generalized erythematous scaling patches or plaques, usually on the trunk. Plaques are almost always over 5 cm in diameter. Pruritus is a frequent complaint. The lesions often begin as nondescript or nondiagnostic patches, and it is not unusual for the patient to have skin lesions for more than a decade before the diagnosis can be confirmed. In more advanced cases, tumors appear. Lymphadenopathy may occur locally or widely. Lymph node enlargement may be due to benign expansion of the node (dermatopathic lymphadenopathy) or by specific involvement with mycosis fungoides.

B. Laboratory Findings: The skin biopsy remains the basis of diagnosis, though at times numerous biopsies are required before the diagnosis can be confirmed. In addition, circulating atypical cells (Sézary cells) can be detected in the blood by sensitive methods. Eosinophilia may be present.

Differential Diagnosis

Mycosis fungoides may be confused with psoriasis, a drug eruption, an eczematous dermatitis, Hansen's disease (leprosy), or tinea corporis. Histologic examination can usually distinguish these conditions.

Treatment

The treatment of mycosis fungoides is complex. Early and aggressive treatment has not been proved to cure or prevent progression of the disease. Topical mechlorethamine ointment or solution, topical steroids, and PUVA are all used for early patches and plaques. Radiation therapy for local lesions and systemic agents such as retinoids, antitumor chemotherapeutic drugs, and alpha interferon are used alone or in various combinations for more advanced disease or in patients who fail topical therapy.

Prognosis

Mycosis fungoides is usually slowly progressive (over decades). Prognosis is better in patients with patch or plaque stage disease and worse in patients with erythroderma, tumors, and lymphadenopathy. Elderly patients with patch and plaque stage disease commonly die of other causes. Overly aggressive treatment may lead to complications and premature death.

Duvic M et al: Combined modality therapy for cutaneous T-cell lymphoma. J Am Acad Dermatol 1996;34:1022.

EXFOLIATIVE DERMATITIS (Exfoliative Erythroderma)

Essentials of Diagnosis

- Scaling and erythema over most of the body.
- Itching, malaise, fever, chills, weight loss.

General Considerations

A preexisting dermatosis has been found as the cause in 25–63% of cases, including psoriasis, atopic dermatitis, contact dermatitis, pityriasis rubra pilaris, and seborrheic dermatitis. Many adult patients with exfoliative dermatitis have psoriasis. Reactions to topical or systemic drugs account for perhaps 16–42% of cases and cancer (cutaneous T cell lymphoma, Sézary syndrome) for 10–20%. Causation of the remainder is indeterminable. At the time of acute presentation, without a clear-cut prior history of skin disease or drug exposure, it is often impossible to make a specific diagnosis of the underlying condition even with skin biopsy, and diagnosis may require follow-up with time.

Clinical Findings

A. Symptoms and Signs: Symptoms may include itching, weakness, malaise, fever, and weight loss. Chills are prominent. Exfoliation may be generalized and sometimes includes loss of hair and nails. Generalized lymphadenopathy may be due to lymphoma or leukemia or may be part of the clinical picture of the skin disease (dermatopathic lymphadenitis). The mucosa is spared.

B. Laboratory Findings: A skin biopsy may show changes of a specific inflammatory dermatitis or cutaneous T cell lymphoma or leukemia. Peripheral leukocytes may show clonal rearrangements of the T cell receptor in Sézary syndrome.

Differential Diagnosis

It may be impossible to identify the cause of exfoliative dermatitis early in the course of the disease, so careful follow-up is necessary. Psoriasis, severe seborrheic dermatitis, and drug eruptions may themselves have an erythrodermic phase.

Complications

Debility (protein loss) and dehydration may develop in patients with generalized inflammatory erythroderma; or sepsis may also occur.

Treatment

A. Topical Therapy: Home treatment is with cool to tepid baths and application of mid-potency steroids under wet dressings or with the use of an occlusive plastic suit (Simmons Co., Chattanooga, Tennessee; or Sleep Sauna, Springhouse, Pennsylvania). If the erythroderma becomes chronic and is not manageable in an outpatient setting, hospitalize the patient. Keep the room at a constant warm temperature and provide the same topical treatment as for an outpatient.

B. Specific Measures: Stop all drugs, if possible. Systemic corticosteroids may provide spectacular improvement in severe or fulminant exfoliative dermatitis, but long-term therapy should be avoided (see Chapter 26). In addition, systemic corticosteroids must be used with caution because some patients with erythroderma have psoriasis and could develop pustular psoriasis. For cases of psoriatic erythroderma and pityriasis rubra pilaris, either etretinate or methotrexate may be indicated. Erythroderma secondary to lymphoma or leukemia requires specific topical or systemic chemotherapy. Suitable antibiotic drugs with coverage for *Staphylococcus* should be given when there is evidence of bacterial infection.

Prognosis

Most patients recover completely or improve greatly over time but may require chronic therapy. Deaths are rare in the absence of cutaneous T cell lymphoma. A minority of patients will suffer from undiminished erythroderma for indefinite periods.

Botella-Estrada R et al: Erythroderma: A clinicopathological study of 56 cases. Arch Dermatol 1994;130:1503. (Presents new data and reviews five previous studies.)

MISCELLANEOUS SCALING DERMATOSES

Isolated scaly patches may represent actinic (solar) keratoses, nonpigmented seborrheic keratoses, or Bowen's or Paget's disease.

Actinic Keratoses

Actinic keratoses are small patches—flesh-colored, pink, or slightly hyperpigmented—that feel like sandpaper and are tender when the finger is drawn over them. They occur on sun-exposed parts of the body in persons of fair complexion. Actinic keratoses are considered premalignant, but only 1:1000 lesions per year progress to become squamous cell carcinomas.

Application of liquid nitrogen is a rapid and effective method of eradication. The lesions crust and disappear in 10–14 days. An alternative treatment is the use of 1–5% fluorouracil cream. This agent may be rubbed into the lesions morning and night until they become first red and sore and then crusted and eroded (usually 2–3 weeks), and then stopped. Similarly, 5% fluorouracil solution may be used two times a day on one or two consecutive days weekly for 7–10 weeks. Any lesions that persist may then be biopsied for histologic examination.

Masoprocol, available as 10% cream, is available for treatment of actinic keratoses. While it seems to cause less inflammation, it also appears to be less effective than fluorouracil and much more likely to cause contact dermatitis.

Kuflik AS, Schwartz RA: Actinic keratosis and squamous cell carcinoma. Am Fam Physician 1994;49:817. (Evolution of lesions and available treatment.)
Thompson SC et al: Reduction of solar keratoses by regular sunscreen use. N Engl J Med 1993;329:1147. (As has been shown for basal cell carcinoma, the number of new actinic keratoses is significantly reduced by the use of sunscreen with a sun protection factor of 17 in adults.)

Bowen's Disease & Paget's Disease

Bowen's disease (intraepidermal squamous cell carcinoma) is relatively uncommon, occurring either on sun-exposed or sun-protected cutaneous surfaces. The lesion is a small (1–3 cm), well-demarcated, slightly raised, pink to red, scaly plaque and may resemble psoriasis or a large actinic keratosis. The course appears to be relatively benign, but these lesions may progress to invasive squamous cell carcinoma. Excision or other definitive treatment is indicated.

Extramammary Paget's disease, considered by some to be a manifestation of apocrine sweat gland carcinoma, resembles chronic eczema and may involve apocrine areas such as the genitalia. There seems to be less likelihood of an underlying sweat gland carcinoma if the lesions are on the vulva than if they are on the perianal area. Mammary Paget's disease of the nipple, a unilateral or rarely bilateral red scaling plaque that may ooze, is associated with an underlying intraductal mammary carcinoma.

Burrows NP et al: Treatment of extramammary Paget's disease by radiotherapy. Br J Dermatol 1995;132:970.

INTERTRIGO

Intertrigo is caused by the macerating effect of heat, moisture, and friction. It is especially likely to occur in obese persons and in humid climates. The symptoms are itching, stinging, and burning. The body folds develop fissures, erythema, and sodden epidermis, with superficial denudation. Candidiasis may complicate intertrigo. "Inverse psoriasis," tinea cruris, erythrasma, and candidiasis must be ruled out.

Maintain hygiene in the area, and keep it dry. Compresses may be useful acutely. If there is evidence of colonization of yeasts or bacteria, apply a topical imidazole antifungal lotion or powder listed above in the section on tinea corporis. Hydrocortisone 1% and an antifungal agent to suppress fungal overgrowth are effective. Recurrences are common.

VESICULAR DERMATOSES

HERPES SIMPLEX
(Cold or Fever Sore; Genital Herpes)

Essentials of Diagnosis

- Recurrent small grouped vesicles on an erythematous base, especially in the orolabial and genital areas.

- May follow minor infections, trauma, stress, or sun exposure; regional lymph nodes may be swollen and tender.
- Tzanck smear is positive for multinucleated epithelial giant cells; viral cultures and direct fluorescent antibody tests are positive.

General Considerations

Over 85% of adults have serologic evidence of herpes simplex type 1 (HSV-1) infections, most often acquired asymptomatically in childhood. Occasionally, primary infections may be manifested as severe gingivostomatitis. Thereafter, the subject may have recurrent self-limited attacks, provoked by sun exposure, orofacial surgery, fever, or a viral infection.

About 25% of the United States population has serologic evidence of infection with herpes simplex type 2 (HSV-2), appearing after the onset of sexual activity. HSV-2 causes lesions whose morphology and natural history are similar to those caused by HSV-1 on the genitalia of both sexes. The infection is initially acquired by sexual contact, and there are usually no symptoms at first. In monogamous heterosexual couples where one partner has HSV-2 infection, seroconversion of the noninfected partner occurs in 10% over a 1-year period. Up to 70% of such infections appeared to be acquired during periods of asymptomatic shedding. Uninfected female partners were at greater risk than males, especially if they were seronegative for HSV-1 antibodies as well. Transverse myelitis, neuropathic pain in the sacral distribution, and encephalitis are rare complications.

Clinical Findings

A. Symptoms and Signs: The principal symptoms are burning and stinging. Neuralgia may precede or accompany attacks. The lesions consist of small, grouped vesicles that can occur anywhere but which most often occur on the vermilion border of the lips, the penile shaft or glans penis, the labia, the perianal skin, and the buttocks. Regional lymph nodes may be swollen and tender. The lesions usually crust and heal in 1 week. It has been demonstrated that patients can be educated to recognize attacks that they previously did not identify as recurrences of herpes simplex. Herpes simplex is the most common cause of painful perianal ulcerations in patients with AIDS.

B. Laboratory Findings: Lesions clinically diagnosed as chancroid, syphilis, pyoderma, or trauma have been found to be herpes simplex virus infections on culture. Direct immunofluorescent antibody slide tests offer rapid, sensitive diagnosis. Viral culture may also be helpful. The Tzanck smear, which demonstrates multinucleated cells, is the least sensitive test. Herpes simplex and varicella-zoster viruses cannot be distinguished on the Tzanck smear.

Complications

Complications include pyoderma, eczema herpeticum, herpetic whitlow, herpes gladiatorum (epidemic herpes in wrestlers transmitted by contact), esophagitis, neonatal infection, keratitis, and encephalitis.

Prevention

Sunscreens are very useful adjuncts in preventing sun-induced recurrences. Prophylactic use of oral acyclovir may prevent some recurrences. Acyclovir should be started at a dosage of 200 mg five times daily beginning 24 hours prior to ultraviolet light exposure.

Treatment

A. Systemic Therapy: Three systemic agents are available for the treatment of herpes infections: acyclovir, its valine analog valaciclovir, and famciclovir. All three agents are very effective and, when used properly, virtually nontoxic. Only acyclovir is available for intravenous administration. In general, with the exception of severe orolabial herpes, only genital disease is treated. For first clinical episodes (including primary) herpes simplex, the dosage of acyclovir is 200 mg orally five times daily (or 800 mg three times daily); of valaciclovir, 1000 mg twice daily; and of famciclovir, 250 mg three times daily. The duration of treatment is from 5 to 10 days depending on the severity of the outbreak. Most cases of recurrent herpes do not require intermittent treatment, and the benefit from treatment is minimal in most patients, reducing the average outbreak by about 12 hours. Recurrent herpes may be treated with 5 days of acyclovir, 200 mg five times daily; valaciclovir, 500 mg twice daily; or famciclovir, 125 mg twice daily—the latter regimen being the least expensive.

In patients with frequent or severe recurrences, suppressive therapy is most effective in controlling disease. Suppressive treatment will reduce outbreaks by 85% and reduces viral shedding by more than 90%. It empowers patients with severe disease, allowing them to cope with herpes more effectively. The recommended suppressive doses, taken continuously, are acyclovir, 400 mg twice daily; valaciclovir, 500 mg once daily; or famciclovir, 250 mg twice daily—the valaciclovir regimen being the cheapest. Long-term suppression appears very safe, and after 5–7 years a substantial proportion of patients can discontinue treatment.

B. Local Measures: In general, topical therapy is not effective. It is strongly urged that 5% acyclovir ointment, if used at all, be limited to the restricted indications for which it has been approved, ie, initial herpes genitalis and mucocutaneous herpes simplex infections in immunocompromised patients. Penciclovir cream, to be applied at the first symptom every 2 hours while awake for 4 days, has been released for treatment of recurrent orolabial herpes. It reduces the average attack duration from 5 days to 4.5 days.

Prognosis

Aside from the complications described above, recurrent attacks last several days, and patients recover without sequelae.

Conant MA et al: Genital herpes: An integrated approach to management. J Am Acad Dermatol 1996;35:601.

Mertz GJ et al: Risk factors for the sexual transmission of genital herpes. Ann Intern Med 1992;116:197. (Study of monogamous couples.)

Pereira FA: Herpes simplex: Evolving concepts. J Am Acad Dermatol 1996;35:503.

Sacks SL et al: Patient-initiated, twice-daily oral famciclovir for early recurrent genital herpes: A randomized, double-blind multicenter trial. Canadian Famciclovir Study Group. JAMA 1996;276:44.

Wald A et al: Suppression of subclinical shedding of herpes simplex virus type 2 with acyclovir. Ann Intern Med 1996;124(1 Part 1):8.

HERPES ZOSTER
(Shingles)

Essentials of Diagnosis

- Pain along the course of a nerve followed by painful grouped vesicular lesions.
- Involvement is unilateral; some lesions may occur outside the affected dermatome.
- Lesions are usually on face or trunk.
- Tzanck smear positive, especially in early lesions.

General Considerations

Herpes zoster is an acute vesicular eruption due to the varicella-zoster virus. It usually occurs in adults. With rare exceptions, patients suffer only one attack of zoster. In immunocompromised patients, generalized, life-threatening dissemination may occur. In patients with HIV infection, zoster often occurs while the patient is otherwise asymptomatic.

Clinical Findings

Pain usually precedes the eruption by 48 hours or more and may persist and actually increase in intensity after the lesions have disappeared. The lesions consist of grouped, tense, deep-seated vesicles distributed unilaterally along a dermatome. The commonest distributions are on the trunk or face. Up to 20 lesions may be found outside the affected dermatomes. Regional lymph glands may be tender and swollen.

Dermatomal herpes zoster does not imply the presence of a visceral malignancy. Generalized disease, however, raises the suspicion of an associated immunosuppressive disorder such as Hodgkin's disease or HIV infection. HIV-infected patients are 20 times more likely to develop zoster, often before other clin-

ical findings of HIV disease are present. A history of HIV risk factors and HIV testing when appropriate should be considered, especially in patients under 55 years of age.

Differential Diagnosis

Since poison oak and poison ivy dermatitis can occur unilaterally and in a streak by a single brush with the plant, it must be differentiated at times from herpes zoster. Tiny, confluent linear vesicles are more typical of allergic contact dermatitis, whereas grouped vesicles are more suggestive of herpetic infection. One must differentiate herpes zoster from lesions of herpes simplex, which occasionally occurs in a dermatomal distribution. One should use doses of antivirals appropriate for zoster in the absence of a clear diagnosis. The pain of preeruptive herpes zoster may lead the clinician to diagnose migraine, myocardial infarction, acute abdomen, herniated nucleus pulposus, etc, depending on the dermatome involved.

Complications

Sacral zoster may be associated with bladder and bowel dysfunction. Persistent neuralgia, anesthesia or scarring of the affected area following healing, facial or other nerve paralysis, and encephalitis may occur. Postherpetic neuralgia is most common after involvement of the trigeminal region, and in patients over the age of 55. Early (within 72 hours after onset) and aggressive antiviral treatment of herpes zoster reduces the severity and duration of postherpetic neuralgia. Zoster ophthalmicus (V_1) can result in visual impairment.

Treatment
A. General Measures:
1. Immunocompetent host–Since early treatment of zoster reduces postherpetic neuralgia, those with a risk of developing this complication should be treated, ie, those over age 55. In addition, younger patients with acute moderate to severe pain may be benefited by effective antiviral therapy. Effective treatment can be given with oral acyclovir, 800 mg five times daily for 7 days; famciclovir, 50 mg three times daily for 7 days; or valaciclovir, 1 g three times daily. For reasons of increased bioavailability and ease of dosing schedule, the preferred agents are those given three times daily. Patients should maintain good hydration, and elderly patients with reduced renal function should be followed closely. The dose of antiviral should be adjusted for renal function as recommended. Nerve blocks may be important in the management of initial severe pain. Ophthalmologic consultation is vital for involvement of the first branch of the trigeminal nerve. Systemic corticosteroids are effective in reducing acute pain and improving quality of life, returning patients to normal activities much more quickly. They do not increase the risk of dissemination in immunocompetent hosts.

If not contraindicated, a tapering 3-week course of prednisone should be considered for its adjunctive benefit in immunocompetent patients. Oral corticosteroids do not reduce the prevalence, severity, or duration of postherpetic neuralgia beyond that achieved by effective antiviral therapy.

2. Immunocompromised host–Given the safety and efficacy of currently available antivirals, most immunocompromised patients with herpes zoster are candidates for antiviral therapy. The dosage schedule is as listed above, but treatment should be continued until the lesions have completely crusted and are healed or almost healed (up to 2 weeks). Corticosteroids should not be given adjunctively in immunosuppressed hosts since they increase the risk of dissemination. Progression of disease may necessitate intravenous therapy with acyclovir, 10 mg/kg intravenously, three times daily. After 3–4 days, oral therapy may be substituted if there has been a good response to intravenous therapy. Adverse effects include decreased renal function from crystallization, nausea and vomiting, and abdominal pain.

Foscarnet, administered in a dosage of 40 mg/kg three times daily intravenously, is indicated for treatment of acyclovir-resistant varicella-zoster virus infections.

B. Local Measures: Calamine or starch shake lotions may be of some help.

C. Postherpetic Neuralgia: The most effective treatment is prevention with early and aggressive antiviral therapy. Once established, postherpetic neuralgia may be treated with capsaicin ointment, 0.025–0.075%. Chronic postherpetic neuralgia may be relieved by regional blocks (stellate ganglion, epidural, local infiltration, or peripheral nerve), with or without corticosteroids added to the injections. Amitriptyline, 25 mg orally three times daily, perphenazine, 4 mg orally three times daily, and fluphenazine, 1 mg four times daily, have also been suggested. Doxepin, 25–50 mg three times daily, has been reported to be helpful. Appropriate cautions should be taken with all of these drugs.

Prognosis

The eruption persists 2–3 weeks and usually does not recur. Motor involvement in 2–3% may lead to temporary palsy.

Balfour HH Jr et al: Management of acyclovir-resistant herpes simplex and varicella-zoster virus infections. J Aquir Immune Defic Synd 1994;7:254. (Suggests that foscarnet be started within 7–10 days after suspicion of acyclovir resistance and used for 10 or more days until clinical resolution occurs.)

Beutner KR: Clinical management of herpes zoster in the elderly patient. Compr Ther 1996;22:183.

Bruxelle J: Prospective epidemiologic study of painful and neurologic sequelae induced by herpes zoster in patients treated early with oral acyclovir. Neurology 1995;45(12

Suppl 8):S78. (Among 301 patients with acute herpes zoster treated early with oral acyclovir, there was no relationship between initial rash severity and either pain incidence or neurologic deficit.)

Donahue JG et al: The incidence of herpes zoster. Arch Intern Med 1995;155:1605.

Tyring S et al: Famciclovir for the treatment of acute herpes zoster: Effects on acute disease and postherpetic neuralgia. A randomized, double-blind, placebo-controlled trial. Collaborative Famciclovir Herpes Zoster Study Group (see comments). Ann Intern Med 1995;123:89.

Whitley RJ et al: Acyclovir with and without prednisone for the treatment of herpes zoster: A randomized, placebo-controlled trial. The National Institute of Allergy and Infectious Diseases Collaborative Antiviral Study Group. Ann Intern Med 1996;125:376.

Wood MJ et al: A randomized trial of acyclovir for 7 days or 21 days with and without prednisolone for treatment of acute herpes zoster (see comments). N Engl J Med 1994;330:896.

POMPHOLYX
(Dyshidrosis, Dyshidrotic Eczema)

Essentials of Diagnosis

- "Tapioca" vesicles of 1–2 mm on the palms, soles, and sides of fingers, associated with pruritus.
- Vesicles may coalesce to form multiloculated blisters.
- Scaling and fissuring may follow drying of the blisters.
- Appearance in the third decade, with lifelong recurrences.

General Considerations

"Dyshidrotic eczema" is a misnomer, suggesting that the vesicles of this condition are related to eccrine sweat ducts and sweating, which they are not. This is an extremely common form of hand dermatitis, preferably called pompholyx (Gr "bubble") or vesicular dermatitis of the palms and soles. Patients often have an atopic background and report flares with stress. Clues to a possible cause of pompholyx are suggested by the following observations. In Scandinavia, women with contact allergy to nickel and pompholyx appear to flare when given oral challenges with nickel. Nickel-free diets have given variable results. The chelator disulfiram has been reported to cause a 25% improvement in one controlled study in nickel-sensitive patients, and oral cromolyn sodium has also been shown to be of benefit. Patients with widespread dermatitis due to any cause may develop pompholyx-like eruptions as a part of an autoeczematization response.

Clinical Findings

Small clear vesicles stud the skin at the sides of the fingers and on the palms or soles. They look like the grains in tapioca. They may be associated with intense itching. Later, the vesicles dry and the area becomes scaly and fissured.

Differential Diagnosis

Unroofing the vesicles and scraping the underside of the roof will reveal hyphae in cases of vesicular tinea. Rarely, blisters extending onto the dorsum of the hands represent true allergic contact dermatitis, and the culprit must be sought by history or by patch testing. Patients with inflammatory tinea pedis may have a vesicular dermatophytid of the palms. NSAIDs may produce an eruption very similar to that of dyshidrosis.

Prevention

There is no known way to prevent attacks.

Treatment

Pompholyx is often not a very steroid-sensitive dermatitis, though topical and systemic corticosteroids help some patients dramatically. Since this is a chronic problem, systemic steroids are generally not appropriate therapy. A high-potency topical steroid used early in the attack may help abort the flare and ameliorate pruritus. Topical steroids are also important in treating the scaling and fissuring that are seen after the vesicular phase. It is essential that patients avoid anything that irritates the skin; they should wear cotton gloves inside vinyl gloves when doing dishes or other wet chores, use long-handled brushes instead of sponges, and use a hand cream after washing the hands. If a history of nickel allergy (rashes with costume jewelry or from watchbands) is obtained, nickel-free diets may be considered. Patients may also slowly respond to PUVA therapy using topical psoralen and special UVA light sources designed to treat hands and feet.

Prognosis

For most patients, the disease is an inconvenience. Even with moderate to severe disease, flares can be controlled with scrupulous care. For some, pompholyx can be incapacitating.

Crosti C, Lodi A: Pompholyx: A still unresolved kind of eczema. Dermatology 1993;186:241.

DERMATOPHYTID
(Allergy or Sensitivity to Fungi)

Essentials of Diagnosis

- Pruritic, grouped vesicular lesions involving the sides and flexor aspects of the fingers and the palms.
- Fungal infection elsewhere on the body, usually the feet.
- No fungus demonstrable in lesions.

General Considerations

Dermatophytid is a rare disorder that must be considered in the differential diagnosis of vesicles on the hands and feet. It is a hypersensitivity reaction to an active focus of inflammatory dermatophytosis elsewhere on the body, usually the feet. Fungi are present in the primary lesions but are not present in the lesions of dermatophytid. The hands are most often affected, but dermatophytid may occur on other areas also.

Clinical Findings

A. Symptoms and Signs: Itching is the only symptom. The lesions consist of grouped vesicles, often involving the thenar and hypothenar eminences. Lesions occasionally involve the backs of the hands or may even be generalized.

B. Laboratory Findings: This entity is best diagnosed morphologically and by response to treatment. The trichophytin skin test is positive, but it may also be positive with other disorders. Culture from the primary site tends to reveal *Trichophyton mentagrophytes* organisms rather than *Trichophyton rubrum*.

Differential Diagnosis

Dermatophytid must be distinguished from all diseases causing vesicular eruptions of the hands—especially contact dermatitis, pompholyx, and photosensitive drug eruptions and "id" reactions due to inflammatory rashes, such as poison oak or other causes of contact dermatitis elsewhere on the body.

Treatment

The lesions should be treated according to type of dermatitis. The primary focus of tinea should be treated with an oral antifungal or by local measures as described for dermatophytosis (see above).

Prognosis

Dermatophytid may occur in an explosive series of episodes, and recurrences are not uncommon; however, it clears with adequate treatment of the primary infection elsewhere on the body.

PORPHYRIA CUTANEA TARDA

Essentials of Diagnosis

- Noninflammatory blisters on sun-exposed sites, especially the dorsal surfaces of the hands.
- Hypertrichosis, skin fragility.
- Associated liver disease.
- Elevated urine porphyrins.

General Considerations

Porphyria cutanea tarda is the most common type of porphyria. Cases are sporadic or hereditary. The disease is associated with ingestion of certain medications, and liver disease from alcoholism or hepatitis C is often present.

Clinical Findings

A. Symptoms and Signs: The condition is generally asymptomatic. However, patients may complain of painless blistering and fragility of the skin of the dorsal surfaces of the hands. Facial hypertrichosis and hyperpigmentation are common.

B. Laboratory Findings: Urinary uroporphyrins are elevated two- to fivefold above coproporphyrins. Patients may also have abnormal liver function tests, evidence of hepatitis C infection, and increased liver iron stores.

Differential Diagnosis

Skin lesions identical to those of porphyria cutanea tarda may be seen in patients being maintained on dialysis and with the ingestion of certain medications (tetracyclines and NSAIDs, especially naproxen). In this so-called pseudoporphyria, the biopsy results are identical to those associated with porphyria cutanea tarda, but urine porphyrins are normal.

Prevention

Although the lesions are triggered by sun exposure, the wavelength of light triggering the lesions is beyond that absorbed by sunscreens, which for that reason are ineffective. Barrier sun protection with clothing is required.

Treatment

Stopping all triggering medications and substantially reducing or stopping alcohol consumption may alone lead to improvement. Phlebotomy without oral iron supplementation at a rate of one unit every 2–4 weeks will gradually lead to improvement. Very low dose antimalarials (as low as 200 mg of hydroxychloroquine twice weekly) will increase the excretion of porphyrins, improving the skin disease. Treatment is continued until the patient is asymptomatic. Urine porphyrins may be monitored.

Prognosis

Most patients improve with treatment. Sclerodermoid skin lesions may develop on the trunk, scalp, and face.

Conry-Cantilena C et al: Porphyria cutanea tarda in hepatitis C virus-infected blood donors. J Am Acad Dermatol 1995;32:512.

DERMATITIS HERPETIFORMIS

Dermatitis herpetiformis is an uncommon disease manifested by pruritic papules, vesicles, and papulovesicles mainly on the elbows, knees, buttocks, posterior neck, and scalp. It appears to have its highest prevalence in Scandinavia and is associated with transplantation antigens HLA-B8, -DR3, and -DQw2. The diagnosis is made by light microscopy, which demonstrates neutrophils at the dermal papillary tips. Direct immunofluorescence studies show granular deposits of IgA along the dermal papillae. Circulating anti-endomysium antibodies can be detected in all cases. Patients have gluten-sensitive enteropathy, but for the great majority it is subclinical. However, ingestion of gluten plays a role in the exacerbation of skin lesions, and strict long-term avoidance of dietary gluten has been shown to decrease the dose of dapsone (usually 100–200 mg/d) required to control the disease and may even eliminate the need for drug treatment. Although adherence to a gluten-free diet is difficult, the availability of many gluten-free foods now makes this easier to accomplish. Patients with dermatitis herpetiformis are at increased risk for development of gastrointestinal lymphoma, and this risk is reduced by a gluten-free diet.

Fry L: Dermatitis herpetiformis. Baillieres Clin Gastroenterol 1995;9:371.

Garioch JJ et al: 25 years' experience of a gluten-free diet in the treatment of dermatitis herpetiformis. Br J Dermatol 1994;131:541. (133 of 212 patients could adhere to a strict diet, and 78 could control their disease with diet alone. Even partial adherence led to decreased requirement for medication in over half. Spontaneous remissions were seen in 10% of those on a normal diet.)

Lewis HM et al: Protective effect of gluten-free diet against development of lymphoma in dermatitis herpetiformis. Br J Dermatol 1996;135:363.

WEEPING OR ENCRUSTED LESIONS

IMPETIGO

Impetigo is a contagious and autoinoculable infection of the skin caused by staphylococci or streptococci (or both). Classically, two forms have been recognized: (1) a vesiculopustular type, with thick golden-crusted lesions caused by group A β-hemolytic *Streptococcus* or coagulase-positive *Staphylococcus aureus*; and (2) a bullous type, generally associated with phage group II *S aureus*. However, most cases of impetigo of either presentation now appear to be due to staphylococci.

Clinical Findings

A. Symptoms and Signs: Itching is the only symptom. The lesions consist of macules, vesicles, bullae, pustules, and honey-colored gummy crusts that when removed leave denuded red areas. The face and other exposed parts are most often involved. **Ec-**

thyma is a deeper form of impetigo caused by staphylococci or streptococci, with ulceration and scarring. It occurs frequently on the legs and other covered areas, often as a complication of debility and local cutaneous trauma.

B. Laboratory Findings: Gram stain and culture confirm the diagnosis.

Differential Diagnosis

The main differential diagnosis is between impetigo and acute allergic contact dermatitis. Contact dermatitis may be suggested by the history or by linear distribution of the lesions, and culture should be negative for staphylococci and streptococci. Herpes simplex infection usually presents with grouped vesicles or discrete erosions and may be associated with a history of recurrences. Viral culture and Tzanck smears of the lesions are positive.

Treatment

Topical antibiotics are not as effective as systemic antibiotics except (in some settings) for 2% mupirocin ointment (Bactroban), dispensed as 15 g and used three times daily for 10 days. If the affected area is large or if there is fever or toxicity—or if there is any concern over the possibility that a nephritogenic strain of *Streptococcus* may be causative—systemic antibiotics should be given. Dicloxacillin, 250 mg four times daily, is usually effective, or one may use cephalexin, 50 mg/kg/24 h. Erythromycin, 250 mg four times daily, is a reasonable alternative depending on the prevalence of erythromycin-resistant staphylococci in the community and as determined by culture and sensitivity tests.

Crusts and weepy areas may be treated with compresses, and washcloths and towels must be segregated and washed separately.

Dagan R: Impetigo in childhood: Changing epidemiology and new treatments. Pediatr Ann 1993;22:235.

Doebbeling BN et al: Long-term efficacy of intranasal mupirocin ointment: A prospective cohort study of *Staphylococcus aureus* carriage. Arch Intern Med 1994;154:1505. (Administration twice daily for 5 days resulted in negative intranasal cultures in 47% versus 28% in treatment versus the placebo group, respectively, at 1 year; negative hand cultures at 6 months were seen in 85% versus 52% in these groups.)

ALLERGIC CONTACT DERMATITIS

Essentials of Diagnosis

• Erythema and edema, with pruritus, often followed by vesicles and bullae in an area of contact with a suspected agent.
• Later, weeping, crusting, or secondary infection.
• Often a history of previous reaction to suspected contactant.
• Patch test with agent usually positive.

General Considerations

Contact dermatitis is an acute or chronic dermatitis that results from direct skin contact with chemicals or allergens. Four-fifths of such disturbances are due to excessive exposure to or additive effects of primary or universal irritants (eg, soaps, detergents, organic solvents) and are called irritant contact dermatitis. Others are due to actual contact allergy such as poison ivy or poison oak. The most common dermatologic compounds causing allergic rashes include antimicrobials (especially neomycin), topical antihistamines, anesthetics (benzocaine), hair dyes, preservatives (eg, parabens), latex, and adhesive tape. Occupational exposure is an important cause of allergic contact dermatitis. Weeping and crusting are typically due to allergic and not irritant dermatitis, which often appears red and scaly. With widespread precautions being taken against HIV infection, contact dermatitis due to latex rubber in gloves and condoms is being seen more frequently.

Clinical Findings

A. Symptoms and Signs: The acute phase is characterized by tiny vesicles and weepy and crusted lesions, whereas resolving or chronic contact dermatitis will present with scaling, erythema, and possibly thickened skin. Itching, burning, and stinging may be severe. The lesions, distributed on exposed parts or in bizarre asymmetric patterns, consist of erythematous macules, papules, and vesicles. The affected area is often hot and swollen, with exudation and crusting, simulating and at times complicated by infection. The pattern of the eruption may be diagnostic (eg, typical linear streaked vesicles on the extremities in poison oak or ivy dermatitis). The location will often suggest the cause: Scalp involvement suggests hair tints, sprays, or tonics; face involvement, creams, cosmetics, soaps, shaving materials, nail polish; neck involvement, jewelry, hair dyes, etc.

B. Laboratory Findings: Gram stain and culture will rule out impetigo or secondary infection (impetiginization). If itching is generalized and impetiginized scabies is considered, a scraping for mites should be done. During the acute episode, patch testing cannot be used, often because the back is involved or because the primary rash will cause many false-positive reactions. After the episode has cleared, the patch test may be useful, but not all potential allergens are available for testing. In the event of a positive reaction, the clinical relevance of the chemical agent and the dermatitis must be determined. In suspected photocontact dermatitis—involvement of face, "V" of the upper chest, and hands, sparing the skin under the nose, chin, and inner upper eyelid—photopatch tests may be done by exposing the traditional patch test site to ultraviolet light after 24 hours.

Differential Diagnosis

Asymmetric distribution, blotchy erythema around the face, linear lesions, and a history of contact help distinguish contact dermatitis from other skin lesions. The most commonly confused diagnosis is impetigo. Differentiation may be difficult if the area of involvement is consistent with that seen in other types of skin disorders such as scabies, dermatophytid, atopic dermatitis, pompholyx, and other eczemas.

Prevention

Prompt and thorough removal of allergens by prolonged washing with water or by dousing with solvents such as isopropyl alcohol or other chemical agents may be effective if done very shortly after exposure to poison oak or ivy. Recently, several barrier creams (eg, Stokogard) have been introduced that may offer some protection to patients at high risk for poison oak and ivy dermatitis. Iodoquinol may benefit nickel allergic patients in a similar manner. Ingestion of *Rhus* antigen is of limited clinical value for the induction of tolerance.

The mainstay of prevention is identification of agents causing the dermatitis and avoidance of exposure or use of protective clothing and gloves. In industry-related cases, prevention may be accomplished by moving the worker to another part of the workplace with different responsibilities.

Treatment

A. Overview: While local measures are important, severe or widespread involvement is difficult to manage without systemic corticosteroids because even the highest-potency topical steroids seem not to work well on vesicular and weepy lesions. Localized involvement (except on the face) can often be managed solely with topical agents. An age-old remedy for itching disorders is repeated exposure to hot water, as in a shower, without soap; this treatment may have the effect of prolonging and aggravating any underlying disorder (eg, atopic or nummular dermatitis). Irritant contact dermatitis is treated by protection from the irritant and use of topical steroids as for atopic dermatitis (described above). The treatment of allergic contact dermatitis is detailed below.

B. Local Measures:

1. Acute weeping dermatitis—Compresses are most often used. It is unwise to scrub lesions with soap and water. Calamine or starch shake lotions may sometimes be used instead of wet dressings or in intervals between wet dressings, especially for involvement of intertriginous areas or when oozing is not marked. Lesions on the extremities may be bandaged with wet dressings for 30–60 minutes several times a day. Potent topical corticosteroids in gel or cream form may help suppress acute contact dermatitis and relieve itching. In cases where weeping is marked or in intertriginous areas, ointments will make the skin even more macerated and should be

avoided. Suggested preparations are fluocinonide gel, 0.05%, used two or three times daily with compresses, or clobetasol or halobetasol cream, used twice daily for a maximum of 2 weeks—for adults only and not in body folds or on the face. This should be followed by tapering of the number of applications per day or use of a mid-potency steroid such as triamcinolone 0.1% cream to prevent rebound of the dermatitis. A soothing formulation is 0.1% triamcinolone acetonide in Sarna lotion (0.5% camphor, 0.5% menthol, 0.5% phenol). Frequent continued use may induce tachyphylaxis.

2. Subacute dermatitis (subsiding)—Mid-potency (triamcinolone 0.1%) to high-potency steroids (amcinonide, fluocinonide, desoximetasone) are the mainstays of therapy.

3. Chronic dermatitis (dry and lichenified)—High- to highest-potency steroids are used in ointment form if acceptable to the patient; creams if not. In some cases, tars (Fototar, or LCD 10%) are useful, often combined with a moderate-strength corticosteroid (eg, 0.1% triamcinolone).

C. Systemic Therapy: For acute severe cases, one may give prednisone orally for 12–21 days. Clinicians use many regimens, and prednisone, 60 mg for 5–7 days, 40 mg for 5–7 days, and 20 mg for 5–7 days without a further taper is one useful regimen. Another is to dispense seventy-eight 5 mg pills to be taken 12 the first day, 11 the second day, and so on. The key is to use enough corticosteroid (and as early as possible) to achieve a clinical effect and to taper slowly enough to avoid rebound. A Medrol Dosepak (methylprednisolone) with 5 days of medication is inappropriate on both counts. Triamcinolone acetonide, 40–60 mg once intragluteally, with 0.5–1 mL of betamethasone for rapid onset of action, may be used instead. (See Chapter 26.)

Prognosis

Allergic contact dermatitis is self-limited if reexposure is prevented but often takes 2–3 weeks for full resolution. Spontaneous desensitization may occur. Increasing sensitivity to industrial contactants may necessitate a change of occupation.

del Savio B, Sherertz EF: Is allergic contact dermatitis being overlooked? Arch Fam Med 1994;3:537. (Reviews irritant and allergic dermatitis and intervention strategies.)

Lepoittevin J-P et al: Studies in patients with corticosteroid contact allergy: Understanding cross-reactivity among different steroids. Arch Dermatol 1995;131:31. (Hydrocortisone, prednisone, and prednisolone show cross-reactivity with betamethasone valerate and clobetasone butyrate but less commonly with triamcinolone and desonide. Administration of systemic steroids to a patient sensitized topically may result in widespread contact dermatitis.)

PUSTULAR DISORDERS

ACNE VULGARIS

Essentials of Diagnosis

- Occurs often at puberty, though onset may be delayed into the third or fourth decade.
- Open and closed comedones are the hallmark of acne vulgaris.
- The most common of all skin conditions.
- Severity varies from purely comedonal to papular/pustular inflammatory acne to cysts to nodules.
- Face and trunk may be affected.
- Scarring may be a sequela of the disease or picking and manipulating by the patient.

General Considerations

Acne vulgaris is discussed under pustular diseases, but it is polymorphic. Open and closed comedones, papules, pustules, and cysts are found. Acne vulgaris is one of the most common diseases of humans. It is of unknown cause and is apparently activated by androgens in those who are genetically predisposed. Similar involvement may occur in identical twins. Acne can present in the neonatal period and may last for weeks to a few months.

The disease is more common and more severe in males. Contrary to popular belief, it does not always clear spontaneously when maturity is reached. If untreated, it may persist into the fourth, fifth, or even sixth decade of life. The skin lesions follow sebaceous activity, plugging of the infundibulum of the follicles, retention of sebum, overgrowth of the acne bacillus (*Propionibacterium acnes*) in incarcerated sebum with resultant release of and irritation by accumulated fatty acids, and foreign body reaction to extrafollicular sebum. The mechanism of antibiotics in controlling acne is not clearly understood, but they may work because of their antibacterial or anti-inflammatory properties. Relapse or resistance may occur after emergence of tetracycline- or erythromycin-resistant strains of *P acnes*. These strains are usually sensitive to minocycline, however.

When a resistant case of acne is encountered in a woman, hyperandrogenism may be suspected. This may or may not be accompanied by hirsutism, irregular menses, or other signs of virilism.

Clinical Findings

There may be mild soreness, pain, or itching. The lesions occur mainly over the face, neck, upper chest, back, and shoulders. Comedones are common, and these are the hallmark of acne vulgaris. Closed comedones are tiny, flesh-colored, noninflamed bumps that give the skin a rough texture or appearance.

Open comedones typically are a bit larger and have black material in them. Inflammatory papules, pustules, ectatic pores, acne cysts, and scarring are also seen.

Acne may have different presentations at different ages. Preteens often present with comedones as their first lesions. Some patients have primarily comedones, with few inflammatory lesions. Inflammatory lesions in young teenagers are often found in the middle of the face, extending outward as the patient becomes older. Women in their third and fourth decades (often with no prior history of acne) commonly present with papular lesions on the chin and around the mouth—so-called perioral dermatitis.

Differential Diagnosis

Other diseases that cause papules and pustules on the face are relatively uncommon compared to acne vulgaris. In adults, acne rosacea will present with papules and pustules in the middle third of the face, but telangiectasia, flushing, and perhaps rhinophyma distinguish this disease from acne vulgaris. A pustular flare on the face in patients receiving antibiotics or with otitis externa should be investigated with culture to rule out an uncommon gram-negative folliculitis. Patients who use systemic steroids or topical fluorinated steroids on the face may develop acne, but comedones are often absent. Acne may be exacerbated or caused by irritating creams or oils, such as coconut oil. The acneiform lesions caused by bromides, iodides, steroids, and contact with chlorinated naphthalenes and diphenyls occur quite rarely, as does perioral acne caused by fluorinated toothpaste. Pustules on the face can also—not commonly—be caused by tinea infections. Lesions on the back are more problematic. When they occur alone, one should suspect staphylococcal folliculitis, miliaria ("heat rash"), or, uncommonly, *Malassezia* folliculitis. Bacterial culture, trial of an antistaphylococcal antibiotic, and observing the response to therapy, will help in the differential diagnosis. In patients with HIV infection, folliculitis is common and often severe and may be due to staphylococcal folliculitis or to eosinophilic folliculitis.

Complications

Cyst formation, pigmentary changes in darkly pigmented patients, severe scarring, and psychologic problems may result.

Treatment

A. General Measures:

1. Education of the patient–When scarring seems out of proportion to the severity of the lesions, one must suspect that the patient is manipulating the lesions. It is essential that the patient be educated in a supportive way about this complication. Although there are exceptions, it is wise to let the patient know that at least 4–6 weeks will be required to see improvement and that old lesions may take months to fade. Therefore, improvement will be judged according to the number of new lesions forming after 6–8 weeks of therapy. Additional time will be required to see improvement on the back and chest, as these areas are slowest to respond. If hair pomades are used, they should contain glycerin and not oil. Avoid topical exposure to oils, cocoa butter (theobroma oil), and greases.

2. Diet–Specific dietary factors are less important than formerly thought in causing acne. If the patient feels that a particular food is exacerbating acne, the food should be avoided for 4–6 weeks and then reintroduced.

B. Comedonal Acne: Treatment of acne is based on the type and severity of lesions. Comedones require treatment different from that of papules, and papules and pustules are treated differently from severe cystic lesions. In assessing severity, one must also take the sequelae of the lesions into account. Therefore, one must treat a more darkly pigmented individual who gets only two new lesions per month that scar or leave postinflammatory hyperpigmentation much more aggressively than a comparable patient whose lesions clear without sequelae. Soaps play little role in acne treatment today, and unless the patient's skin is exceptionally oily, a mild soap should be used to avoid irritation that will limit the usefulness of other topicals, all of which are themselves somewhat irritating.

1. Tretinoin (retinoic acid, Retin-A)–Tretinoin is very effective for comedonal acne or for treatment of the comedonal component of more severe acne, but its usefulness is limited by irritation. Start with 0.025% cream (not gel or liquid) and have the patient use it at first in a test area twice weekly at night, then build up to treat all areas of the face that develop acne as often as nightly. A few patients cannot use even this low-strength preparation more than three times weekly, but even that may cause improvement. A pea-sized amount is sufficient to cover almost half the entire face. It should be put on the skin when dry; to avoid irritation, have the patient wait 20 minutes after washing to let the skin dry. Patients whose skin has become red and irritated from the product will rarely be willing to try it again, so prevention of irritation is essential. Adapalene gel 0.1% and reformulated 0.05% tretinoin (Renova) are other options for patients irritated by standard tretinoin preparations. Some patients—especially teenagers—do best on 0.01% gel. Although the absorption of tretinoin is minimal, its use during pregnancy is *not* recommended. Some patients report photosensitivity with tretinoin. Patients should be warned that they may flare in the first 2 weeks of treatment.

2. Benzoyl peroxide–Commercial preparations include Fostex cream and cake; Acne-Dome cleanser, cream, and lotion; Benzac W gel and wash;

Desquam-X gel and wash; Brevoxyl, Benzagel, Persa-Gel, Clear By Design; and Xerac BP. All of these gels contain benzoyl peroxide. Benzoyl peroxide products are available in concentrations of 2.5%, 4%, 5%, and 10%, but it appears that 2.5% is as effective as 10% and less irritating. In general, water-based and not alcohol-based gels should be used to decrease irritation. Benzoyl peroxide washes such as Desquam-X wash or Benzac W wash may also be used but should be stopped or limited if they are irritating.

3. Antibiotics–Use of topical antibiotics (see below) has been demonstrated to decrease comedonal lesions in controlled studies.

4. Comedo extraction–Open and closed comedones may be removed with a comedo extractor but will recur if not prevented by tretinoin or perhaps benzoyl peroxide.

C. Papular Inflammatory Acne: Antibiotics are the mainstay for treatment of inflammatory acne. They may be used topically or orally. The oral antibiotics of choice are tetracycline and erythromycin. Minocycline is often effective in acne unresponsive or resistant to treatment with these antibiotics but it is expensive. Doxycycline is effective, economical, and easy to take. Rarely, other antibiotics such as trimethoprim-sulfamethoxazole (one double-strength tablet twice daily) and clindamycin (150 mg twice daily) may be tried. Topical clindamycin phosphate and erythromycin are also used (see below). Topicals are probably the equivalent of about 500 mg/d of tetracycline given orally, which is half the usual starting dose. Topical antibiotics are used in three situations: for mild papular acne that can be controlled by topicals alone, for patients who refuse or cannot tolerate oral antibiotics, or to wean patients under good control from oral to topical preparations. There are no studies that have evaluated the usefulness of topical antibiotics while a patient is taking systemic antibiotics, though this is common practice, and there is no study establishing which topical antibiotic to use with each systemic antibiotic. It has been recommended that switching or rotating antibiotics be avoided to decrease resistance and that courses of benzoyl peroxide be used on occasion, since there is an increasing incidence of *P acnes* resistance.

1. Mild acne–The first choice of topical antibiotics in terms of efficacy and relative lack of induction of resistant *P acnes* is the combination of erythromycin with benzoyl peroxide topical gel (benzamycin). It should be kept refrigerated to prevent loss of activity. For patient compliance, a small amount may be stored in a separate jar for 7–10 days at room temperature in the bathroom without significant loss of activity. If this product is not tolerated, either clindamycin (Cleocin T) lotion (least irritating), gel, or solution, or one of the many brands of topical erythromycin gel, solution, or ointment may be used twice daily. The addition of tretinoin 0.025%

cream or 0.01% gel at night may be effective, since it works via a different mechanism.

2. Moderate acne–Tetracycline, 500 mg twice daily, erythromycin, 500 mg twice daily, and minocycline, 50–100 mg twice daily, are all effective though minocycline is more expensive. When initiating minocycline therapy, start at 100 mg in the evening for 4–7 days, then 100 mg twice daily, to decrease the incidence of vertigo. Plan a return visit in 6 weeks and at 3–4 months after that. If the patient's skin is quite clear, instructions should be given for tapering the dose by 250 mg for tetracycline and erythromycin or by 50 mg for minocycline every 6–8 weeks—while treating with topicals—to arrive at the lowest systemic dose needed to maintain clearing. In general, lowering the dose to zero without other therapy results in prompt recurrence of acne. Tetracycline, minocycline, and doxycycline are contraindicated in pregnancy and in young children.

It is important to discuss the issue of contraceptive failure when prescribing antibiotics for women taking oral contraceptives. Case reports and studies of plasma and urinary hormones in women suggest a possible association between tetracycline or erythromycin therapy and oral contraceptive failure. Women may need to consider using barrier methods as well, and should report breakthrough bleeding.

3. Severe acne–

a. Isotretinoin (Accutane) is a vitamin A analog for treatment of severe cystic acne that has not responded to conventional therapy. Informed consent should be obtained before its use in women of childbearing age. A dosage of 0.5–1 mg/kg/d for 20 weeks for a cumulative dose of at least 120 mg/kg is usually adequate for severe cystic acne. Patients should be referred for isotretinoin therapy before they experience significant scarring if they are not promptly and adequately controlled by antibiotics. The drug is *absolutely contraindicated during pregnancy* because of its teratogenicity; serum pregnancy tests should be obtained before starting the drug in a female and every month thereafter. Sufficient medication for only 1 month should be dispensed at each monthly visit. Effective contraception—some authorities say in two forms—must be used. Therapeutic abortion is an alternative for the patient who becomes pregnant during therapy, and the patient's feelings about this option should be discussed before starting therapy. Side effects occur in most patients, usually related to dry skin and mucous membranes (dry lips, nosebleed, and dry eyes). If headache occurs, pseudotumor cerebri must be considered. Depression has been reported. At higher dosage levels, about 25% of patients will develop hypertriglyceridemia, 15% hypercholesterolemia, and 5% a lowering of high-density lipoproteins. Some patients develop minor elevations of aminotransferase levels. Fasting blood sugar may be elevated. Miscellaneous adverse reactions, usually not seen with doses of 0.5–1 mg/kg/d, include de-

creased night vision, musculoskeletal or bowel symptoms, rash, thinning of hair, exuberant granulation tissue in lesions, and bony hyperostoses (seen only with very high doses or with long duration of therapy). Moderate to severe myalgias necessitate decreasing the dosage or stopping the drug. Laboratory tests to be performed in all patients before treatment and after 2–4 weeks on therapy include cholesterol, triglycerides, and liver function studies.

Elevations of liver enzymes and triglycerides return to normal upon conclusion of therapy. The drug may induce long-term remissions in 30–40%, or acne may recur that is more easily controlled with conventional therapy in 40–50%. Occasionally, acne does not respond or promptly recurs after therapy, but it may clear after a second course.

b. Intralesional injection–In otherwise moderate acne, intralesional injection of dilute suspensions of triamcinolone acetonide (2.5 mg/mL, 0.05 mL per lesion), will often hasten the resolution of deeper papules and occasional cysts.

c. Dermabrasion–Cosmetic improvement may be achieved by excision and punch-grafting of deep scars and by abrasion of inactive acne lesions, particularly flat, superficial scars. The technique is not without untoward effects, since hyperpigmentation, hypopigmentation, grooving, and scarring have been known to occur. Dark-skinned individuals do poorly. Dermabrasion within 18 months after isotretinoin therapy may not be advisable.

Prognosis

Untreated acne vulgaris eventually remits spontaneously, but when this will occur cannot be predicted. The condition may persist throughout adulthood and may lead to severe scarring if left untreated. Patients treated with antibiotics continue to improve for the first 3–6 months of therapy. Relapse during treatment may suggest the emergence of resistant *P acnes*. The disease is chronic and tends to flare intermittently in spite of treatment. Remissions following systemic treatment with isotretinoin may be lasting in up to 60% of cases. Relapses after isotretinoin usually occur within 3 years and require a second course in up to 20% of patients.

Driscoll MS et al: Long-term oral antibiotics for acne: Is laboratory monitoring necessary? J Am Acad Dermatol 1993;28:595. (Meta-analysis does not support routine testing.)

Goulden V et al: Long-term safety of isotretinoin as a treatment for acne vulgaris. Br J Dermatol 1994;131:360. (First evidence that there are possible long-term, albeit mild, side effects such as dry skin, dry eyes, and myalgias in a small percentage of patients.)

Goulden V, Layton AM, Cunliffe WJ: Current indications for isotretinoin as a treatment for acne vulgaris. Dermatology 1995;190:284.

Layton AM et al: Isotretinoin for acne vulgaris—10 years later: A safe and successful treatment. Br J Dermatol

1993;129:292. (Eighty-eight patients followed for a mean of 9 years post treatment. Low initial doses and severe truncal acne correlated with relapses, most often within 3 years.)

Miller DM et al: A practical approach to antibiotic treatment in women taking oral contraceptives. J Am Acad Dermatol 1994;30:1008. (Reviews evidence relating antibiotic use to contraceptive failure and suggests an approach to the problem as outlined above.)

Shalita A et al: A comparison of the efficacy and safety of adapalene gel 0.1% and tretinoin gel 0.025% in the treatment of acne vulgaris: A multicenter trial. J Am Acad Dermatol 1996;34:482.

Stainforth JM et al: Isotretinoin for the treatment of acne vulgaris: Which factors may predict the need for more than one course. Br J Dermatol 1993;129:297. (Five year post-treatment follow-up of 299 patients revealed that 23% of patients required re-treatment—most often males younger than 20 years of age.)

ROSACEA

Essentials of Diagnosis

- A chronic facial disorder of middle-aged and older people.
- A vascular component (erythema and telangiectasis) and a tendency to flush easily.
- An acneiform component (papules, pustules, and oily skin) may also be present.
- A glandular aspect accompanied by hyperplasia of the soft tissue of the nose (rhinophyma).

General Considerations

No single factor adequately explains the pathogenesis of this disorder. A statistically significant incidence of migraine headaches accompanying rosacea has been reported.

Potent topical steroids can change trivial dermatoses of the face into recognizable entities called **perioral dermatitis** and **steroid rosacea.** These occur predominantly in young women and may be confused with acne rosacea.

Clinical Findings

The cheeks, nose, and chin—at times the entire face—may have a rosy hue. One sees few or no comedones. Inflammatory papules are prominent, and there may be pustules. Associated seborrhea may be found. The patient often complains of burning or stinging with episodes of flushing. It is not uncommon for patients to have associated ophthalmic disease, including blepharitis and keratitis. This often requires systemic antibiotic therapy.

Differential Diagnosis

Rosacea is distinguished from acne by age, the presence of the vascular component, and the absence of comedones. Bromoderma and iododerma are similar but uncommon. The rosy hue of rosacea is due to inflammation and telangiectases and generally will pinpoint the diagnosis.

Treatment

Medical management is aimed only at the inflammatory papules and pustules and the erythema that surrounds them. The only satisfactory treatment for the telangiectasias is a yellow light laser, eg, pulsed dye or copper vapor laser. Rhinophyma responds only to surgical therapy.

A. Local Therapy: Metronidazole, 0.75% gel applied twice daily, is probably the topical treatment of choice. If metronidazole is not tolerated, topical clindamycin (solution, gel, or lotion) used twice daily is probably effective. Erythromycin as described above may be helpful (see Acne Vulgaris). Five to 8 weeks of treatment are needed for significant response.

B. Systemic Therapy: Tetracycline or erythromycin, 250 or 500 mg orally twice daily on an empty stomach, should be used when topical therapy is inadequate.

Isotretinoin may succeed where other measures fail. A dosage of 0.5–1 mg/kg/d orally for 12–28 weeks is recommended. See precautions above.

Metronidazole, 250 mg twice daily for 3 weeks, may be worth trying but is seldom required. Side effects are few, though metronidazole may produce a disulfiram-like effect when the patient uses alcohol.

Prognosis

Rosacea tends to be a stubborn and persistent process. With the regimens described above, it can usually be controlled adequately.

Thiboutot DM: Acne rosacea. Am Fam Physician 1994;50:1691. (A review of antibiotics, isotretinoin, laser therapy, and surgical therapy.)

FOLLICULITIS
(Including Sycosis)

Essentials of Diagnosis

- Itching and burning in hairy areas.
- Pustules in the hair follicles.
- In sycosis, inflammation of surrounding skin area.

General Considerations

Folliculitis has multiple causes. It may be caused by staphylococcal infection and may be more common in the diabetic. When the lesion is deep-seated, chronic, and recalcitrant on the head and neck, it is called sycosis. Sycosis is usually propagated by the autoinoculation and trauma of shaving. The upper lip is particularly susceptible to involvement in men with chronic nasal discharge from sinusitis or hay fever.

Gram-negative folliculitis, which may develop

during antibiotic treatment of acne, may present as a flare of acne pustules or nodules. *Klebsiella, Enterobacter,* and *Proteus* have been isolated from these lesions.

"Hot tub folliculitis," caused by *Pseudomonas aeruginosa,* is characterized by pruritic or tender follicular or pustular lesions occurring within 1–4 days after bathing in a hot tub, whirlpool, or public swimming pool. Rarely, systemic infections may result.

Nonbacterial folliculitis may also be caused by oils that are irritating to the follicle, and these may be encountered in the workplace (machinists) or at home (various cosmetics and cocoa butter or coconut oils).

Folliculitis may also be caused by occlusion, perspiration, and rubbing, such as that resulting from tight jeans and other heavy fabrics on the upper legs.

Folliculitis on the back that looks like acne but does not respond to acne therapy may be caused by the yeast *Malassezia furfur.* This infection may require biopsy for diagnosis and is treated with oral ketoconazole, 200 mg daily; or topical 2.5% selenium sulfide, 15 minutes daily for 3 weeks.

Folliculitis—so called "steroid acne"—may be seen in the first weeks of systemic steroid therapy or on tapering of the dose.

A form of sterile folliculitis consisting of urticarial papules with prominent eosinophilic infiltration has been reported in patients with AIDS.

Pseudofolliculitis is caused by ingrowing hairs in the beard area and on the nape. In this entity, the papules and pustules are located at the side of and not in follicles. It may be treated by growing a beard or by using chemical depilatories or various proprietary shaving systems (eg, Moore Technique Shaving System).

Clinical Findings

The symptoms range from slight burning and tenderness to intense itching. The lesions consist of pustules of hair follicles. In sycosis, the surrounding skin becomes involved also and so resembles eczema, with redness and crusting.

Differential Diagnosis

It is important to differentiate bacterial from nonbacterial folliculitis. The history is important for pinpointing the causes of nonbacterial folliculitis, and a Gram stain and culture is indispensable. One must differentiate folliculitis from acne vulgaris or pustular miliaria (heat rash) and from infections of the skin such as impetigo or fungal infections. *Pseudomonas* folliculitis is often suggested by the history of hot tub use. Eosinophilic folliculitis in AIDS often requires biopsy for diagnosis.

Complications

Abscess formation is the major complication of bacterial folliculitis.

Prevention

Correct any predisposing local causes (eg, irritations of a mechanical or chemical nature, discharges). Control of blood glucose in diabetes may reduce the number of these infections. Be sure that the water in hot tubs and spas is treated properly with chlorine. If staphylococcal folliculitis is persistent, diagnosis and treatment of nasal or perineal carriage with rifampin, 600 mg daily for 5 days, or with topical mupirocin ointment 2% twice daily for 5 days, may help. The latter may cause stinging in some patients. Chronic oral clindamycin, 150–300 mg/d, is also effective in preventing recurrent staphylococcal folliculitis and furunculosis.

Treatment

A. Local Measures: Cleanse the area gently with chlorhexidine and apply saline or aluminum subacetate soaks or compresses to the involved area for 15 minutes twice daily if very exudative.

Anhydrous ethyl alcohol containing 6.25% aluminum chloride (Xerac AC), applied to lesions and environs and followed by an antibiotic ointment (see above), may be helpful, especially for chronic folliculitis of the buttocks.

B. Specific Measures: For bacterial folliculitis of a limited area, topical 2% mupirocin is effective. It should be applied three times daily for 10 days and protected if possible by dressings; soaks should be applied during the day.

Systemic antibiotics may be tried if the skin infection is resistant to local treatment, if it is extensive or severe and accompanied by a febrile reaction, if it is complicated, or if it involves the nose or upper lip. Extended periods of treatment (4–8 weeks or more) with antistaphylococcal antibiotics are required in some cases.

Hot tub *Pseudomonas* folliculitis virtually always resolves without treatment but may be treated in adults with ciprofloxacin, 500 mg twice daily for 5 days.

Gram-negative folliculitis in acne patients may be treated with isotretinoin in compliance with all precautions discussed above (see Acne Vulgaris).

Irritant folliculitis is best treated by protection from the offending substance and use of drying agents such benzoyl peroxide or Xerac AC.

Eosinophilic folliculitis may be treated initially by the combination of potent topical steroids and oral antihistamines. In more severe cases, treatment is with one of the following: topical permethrin (application for 12 hours every other night for 6 weeks); itraconazole, 200–400 mg daily (tablets) or 200–300 mg daily (suspension); UVB or PUVA phototherapy; or isotretinoin, 0.5 mg/kg/d for up to 5 months. A remission may be induced by some of these therapies, but chronic treatment may be required.

Prognosis

Bacterial folliculitis is occasionally stubborn and

persistent, requiring prolonged or intermittent courses of antibiotics. Steroid folliculitis is treatable by acne therapy and resolves as steroids are discontinued.

Bottone EJ, Perez AA 2nd: *Pseudomonas aeruginosa* folliculitis acquired through use of a contaminated loofah sponge: An unrecognized potential public health problem. J Clin Microbiol 1993;31:480. (A new twist on hot tub folliculitis, also caused by *Pseudomonas*.)

Otley CC, Avram MR, Johnson RA: Isotretinoin treatment of human immunodeficiency virus-associated eosinophilic folliculitis Arch Dermatol 1995;131:1047. (Reviews treatment modalities effective in HIV-associated eosinophilic folliculitis and discusses the use of isotretinoin in this relapsing disorder.)

Sandin RL et al: *Malassezia furfur* folliculitis in cancer patients: The need for interaction of microbiologist, surgical pathologist, and clinician in facilitating identification by the clinical microbiology laboratory. Ann Clin Lab Sci 1993;23:377. (How to diagnose this folliculitis, which is harmless but morphologically similar to *Candida* infection.)

MILIARIA
(Heat Rash)

Essentials of Diagnosis

- Burning, itching, superficial aggregated small vesicles, papules, or pustules on covered areas of the skin, usually the trunk.
- More common in hot, moist climates.
- Rare forms associated with fever and even heat prostration.

General Considerations

Miliaria is an acute dermatitis that occurs most commonly on the upper extremities, trunk, and intertriginous areas. A hot, moist environment is the most frequent cause. Neonates in incubators and bedridden febrile patients are susceptible. Plugging of the ostia of sweat ducts occurs, with consequent ballooning and ultimate rupture of the sweat duct, producing an irritating, stinging reaction. Increase in numbers of resident aerobes, notably cocci, apparently plays a role.

Clinical Findings

The usual symptoms are burning and itching. In severe cases, fever, heat prostration, and even death may result. The lesions consist of small, superficial, reddened, thin-walled, discrete but closely aggregated vesicles (miliaria crystallina), papules (miliaria rubra), or vesicopustules or pustules (miliaria pustulosa). The reaction occurs most commonly on covered areas of the skin.

Differential Diagnosis

Miliaria is to be distinguished from drug rash and folliculitis.

Prevention

Use of an antibacterial preparation such as chlorhexidine prior to exposure to heat and humidity may help prevent the condition. Susceptible persons should avoid exposure to hot, humid environments.

Treatment

Triamcinolone acetonide, 0.1% in Sarna lotion, or a mid-potency corticosteroid in a lotion or cream—but not ointment—base, should be applied two to four times daily. Alternative measures that have been employed with varying success are drying shake lotions and antipruritic powders or other dusting powders. Secondary infections (superficial pyoderma) are treated with erythromycin or dicloxacillin, 250 mg four times daily by mouth. Anticholinergic drugs given by mouth may be very helpful in severe cases, eg, glycopyrrolate, 1 mg twice daily.

Prognosis

Miliaria is usually a mild disorder, but death may occur with the severe forms (tropical anhidrosis and asthenia) as a result of interference with the heat-regulating mechanism.

Lillywhite LP: Investigation into the environmental factors associated with the incidence of skin disease following an outbreak of miliaria rubra at a coal mine. Occup Med (Oxf) 1992;42:183. (Not unexpectedly, there was a positive correlation with increasing temperature and a negative correlation with air quality [air volume per unit of time].)

MUCOCUTANEOUS CANDIDIASIS

Essentials of Diagnosis

- Severe pruritus of vulva, anus, or body folds.
- Superficial denuded, beefy-red areas with or without satellite vesicopustules.
- Whitish curd-like concretions on the oral and vaginal mucous membranes.
- Yeast on microscopic examination of scales or curd.

General Considerations

Mucocutaneous candidiasis is a superficial fungal infection that may involve almost any cutaneous or mucous surface of the body. It is particularly likely to occur in diabetics, during pregnancy, and in obese persons who perspire freely. Antibiotics and oral contraceptive agents may be contributory. Oral candidiasis may be the first sign of HIV infection. Esophageal candidiasis is a frequent AIDS-defining illness in HIV-infected persons (see Chapter 31).

Clinical Findings

A. Symptoms and Signs: Itching may be intense. Burning is reported, particularly around the vulva and anus. The lesions consist of superficially denuded, beefy-red areas in the depths of the body folds such as in the groin and the intergluteal cleft, beneath the breasts, at the angles of the mouth, and in the umbilicus. The peripheries of these denuded lesions are superficially undermined, and there may be satellite vesicopustules. Whitish, curd-like concretions may be present on the surface of the lesions (particularly in the oral and vaginal mucous membranes). Paronychia and interdigital erosions may occur.

B. Laboratory Findings: Clusters of budding cells and hyphae can be seen under the high-power lens when skin scales or curd-like lesions have been cleared in 10% KOH. The organism may be isolated on Sabouraud's medium.

Differential Diagnosis

Intertrigo, seborrheic dermatitis, tinea cruris, "inverse psoriasis," and erythrasma involving the same areas may mimic mucocutaneous candidiasis.

Complications

Systemic invasive candidiasis with candidemia may be seen with immunosuppression and in patients receiving broad-spectrum antibiotic and hypertonic glucose solutions, as in hyperalimentation. There may or may not be clinically evident mucocutaneous candidiasis.

Treatment

A. General Measures: Affected parts should be kept dry and exposed to air as much as possible. If possible, discontinue systemic antibiotics; otherwise, give nystatin by mouth concomitantly in a dose of 1.5 million units three times daily. Fluconazole at a dosage of 100 mg/d is very effective and may be the treatment of choice for mucocutaneous candidiasis. However, the emergence of resistant strains has been noted. Ketoconazole, 200 mg daily by mouth, will also eradicate lesions with minimal side effects except for rare instances of liver damage. Liver function must be monitored. Recurrences follow discontinuance of therapy. For treatment of systemic invasive candidiasis, see Chapter 36.

B. Local Measures:

1. Nails and skin–Apply ciclopirox cream, nystatin cream, 100,000 units/g, or miconazole, econazole, ketoconazole, or clotrimazole cream or lotion three or four times daily. Gentian violet, 1%, or carbolfuchsin paint (Castellani's paint) may be applied once or twice weekly as an alternative, but these preparations are messy.

2. Vulvar and anal mucous membranes–For vaginal candidiasis, use miconazole cream, one applicatorful vaginally at bedtime for 7 days; clotrimazole 10 mg, one suppository vaginally per day for 7 days; terconazole vaginal cream or suppositories; or nystatin, one tablet (100,000 units) vaginally twice daily for 7 days. Topical agents may not be as effective in women with recurrent vaginal candidiasis, and these "intractable" cases may require chronic suppressive therapy. The availability of fluconazole has added new treatment options. Single-dose fluconazole (150 mg) is as effective as ketoconazole (200 mg twice daily for 5 days) for vaginal disease. Itraconazole suspension may be very useful in refractory oropharyngeal candidiasis since it may act locally (as it is held in the mouth and then swallowed) and then has a second systemic action. Even fluconazole-resistant candidiasis may respond to this treatment.

3. Balanitis–This is most frequent in uncircumcised men, and *Candida* usually plays a role. Topical imidazole cream or nystatin ointment is the initial treatment if the lesions are mildly erythematous or superficially erosive. Soaking with dilute aluminum acetate for 15 minutes twice daily may quickly relieve burning or itching. Chronicity and relapses, especially after sexual contact, suggest reinfection from a sexual partner who should be treated. Severe purulent balanitis is usually due to bacteria. If it is so severe that phimosis occurs, oral antibiotics—some with activity against anaerobes—are required; if rapid improvement does not occur, urologic consultation is indicated.

Prognosis

Cases of cutaneous candidiasis range from the easily cured to the intractable and prolonged. It occurs occasionally in children, in whom the disturbance may take the form of a granuloma.

Goldstein SM: Advances in the treatment of superficial *Candida* infections. Semin Dermatol 1993;12:315. (Reviews oral and topical treatments for mucocutaneous candidiasis, including candidal vulvovaginitis.)

Guidelines of care for superficial mycotic infections of the skin: Mucocutaneous candidiasis. Guidelines/Outcome Committee. American Academy of Dermatology. J Am Acad Dermatol 1996;34:110.

FIGURATE ERYTHEMAS

URTICARIA & ANGIOEDEMA

Essentials of Diagnosis

- Eruptions of evanescent wheals or hives.
- Itching is usually intense but may on rare occasions be absent.
- Special forms of urticaria have special features (dermographism, cholinergic urticaria, solar urticaria, or cold urticaria).

- Most incidents are acute and self-limited over a period of 1–2 weeks.
- Chronic urticaria (episodes lasting > 6 weeks) may defy the best efforts of the clinician to find and eliminate the cause.

General Considerations

Urticaria can result from many different stimuli on an immunologic or nonimmunologic basis. The most common immunologic mechanism is hypersensitivity mediated by IgE, seen for most patients with acute urticaria; another involves activation of the complement cascade. Finally, some patients with chronic urticaria demonstrate autoantibodies directed against mast cell IgE receptors, with histamine-releasing activity. In general, extensive costly workups are not indicated in patients who present with urticaria. A careful history and physical examination are more helpful.

Clinical Findings

A. Symptoms and Signs: Lesions are itchy red swellings of a few millimeters to many centimeters. For most types of urticaria, the erythema and the wheal are the same size. The morphology of the lesions may vary over a period of minutes to hours, resulting in geographic or bizarre patterns. With involvement of deeper vessels, there may be swelling of the lips, tongue, eyelids, larynx, palms, soles, and genitalia in association with more typical lesions. For cholinergic urticaria, associated with hot showers or a rise in core body temperature after exercise, there is often a wheal 2–3 mm in diameter with a large surrounding red flare.

B. Laboratory Findings: Laboratory studies are not likely to be helpful in the evaluation of acute or chronic urticaria unless there are suggestive findings in the history and physical examination. The most common causes of acute urticaria are foods, viral and parasitic infections, and medications. The cause of chronic urticaria is rarely found. In patients with individual slightly purpuric lesions that persist past 24 hours, a skin biopsy may help exclude the uncommon entity urticarial vasculitis. Quantitative immunoglobulins, cryoglobulins, cryofibrinogens, and antinuclear antibodies are often sought in cold urticaria but are rarely found. Liver function tests may be of interest, since a serum sickness-like prodrome, with urticaria, may be associated with hepatitis B.

Differential Diagnosis

Papular urticaria resulting from insect bites may persist for long periods. A central punctum can usually be seen, as with flea or gnat bites. Streaked urticarial lesions may be seen in acute allergic plant dermatitis, eg, poison ivy, oak, or sumac. Contact urticaria may be caused by a host of substances, including chemicals, foods, and medications, and may be one type of reaction to latex gloves. Contact urticaria

is often limited to areas exposed to the contactant. Urticarial response to heat, sun, water, and pressure are quite rare. Urticaria may be seen as part of serum sickness, associated with fever and arthralgia, with or without hepatitis B.

In familial angioedema, there is generally a positive family history of angioedema of the extremities and gastrointestinal or respiratory symptoms, but urticaria is not part of the syndrome. Instead, these patients may demonstrate a rapidly expanding annular lesion with an urticarial border.

Treatment

A. General Measures: A detailed search for a cause of acute urticaria should be undertaken, and treatment may then be tailored to include the provocative condition. The chief nonallergic causes are drugs, eg, atropine, pilocarpine, morphine, and codeine; arthropod bites, eg, insect bites and bee stings (though the latter may cause anaphylaxis as well as angioedema); physical factors such as heat, cold, sunlight, injury, and pressure; and, presumably, neurogenic factors such as in cholinergic urticaria induced by exercise, excitement, hot showers, etc.

Allergic causes may include penicillin, aspirin, and other medications; inhalants such as feathers and animal danders; ingestion of shellfish or strawberries; injections of sera and vaccines; external contactants, including various chemicals and cosmetics; and infections such as hepatitis.

B. Systemic Treatment: The mainstay of treatment initially includes H_1 antihistamines (see above). Hydroxyzine, 10 mg twice daily to 25 mg three times daily to even 100 mg three times daily, may be very useful if tolerated. Giving hydroxyzine as one dose of 50–75 mg at night may reduce sedation and other side effects. Antihistamines from different classes should be systematically tried, and doses should be increased weekly to tolerance. Combinations of different antihistamines are often effective, though they have not been systematically investigated. Cyproheptadine, 4 mg four times daily, may be especially useful for cold urticaria. Four "nonsedating" or less sedating antihistamines are available. Astemizole, in a dose of 10 mg/d, is effective, but it may be associated with cardiac arrhythmias, especially if given with medications—macrolide antibiotics and some azole antifungals—interfering with its metabolism. The long half-life of astemizole is a major disadvantage if skin prick testing is needed or if a patient becomes pregnant while on the drug. Loratadine in a dosage of 10 mg/d has a shorter half-life than astemizole and is similar to the other H_1 antihistamines in effectiveness. It appears not to interact with imidazole antifungals or macrolide antibiotics. Cetirizine, a metabolite of hydroxyzine, is less sedating (13% of patients) and is given in a dosage of 10 mg/d. It has a rapid onset of action and does not impose a risk of cardiac arrhythmias when given with other medications. It has been studied in patients with chronic urticaria in doses of 5–20 mg daily, demonstrating efficacy similar to that of astemizole, loratadine, and hydroxyzine. Fexofenadine is given in a dosage of 60 mg twice a day. It does not have cardiovascular toxicity, and its relative efficacy compared with that of other less sedating antihistamines is unknown.

Doxepin (a tricyclic antidepressant), 25 mg three times daily, or, more commonly, 25–75 mg at bedtime, appears to be effective in chronic urticaria. It has anticholinergic side effects.

H_2 antihistamines may rarely be effective if used in combination with H_1 blockers in patients with chronic urticaria unresponsive to H_1 blockers alone, but these are expensive medications, and cimetidine may interact with doxepin and other medications.

Other agents with some promise as adjuvants include calcium channel blockers (used for at least 4 weeks); terbutaline, 1.25–2.5 mg three times daily; colchicine, 0.6 mg twice daily; and attenuated androgens such as danazol. Plasmapheresis and sulfasalazine were reported to help selected patients with chronic urticaria, but these treatments require further study. A few patients with chronic urticaria may respond to a salicylate- and tartrazine-free diet. Although salicylates are ubiquitous in nature, drugs and foods are the most obvious sources. One group has reported curing over 60% of chronic urticaria patients with an allergen elimination diet over a 3-month period. This diet proscribes milk products; beer, wine, and cider; mushrooms, soy sauce, canned tomatoes, pickled and smoked meats, shellfish, vinegar, soured breads, melon, dried fruit, diet soda, chocolate, nuts, peanut products, and strawberries. Systemic steroids in a dose of about 40 mg daily will usually suppress acute and chronic urticaria. However, the use of corticosteroids is rarely indicated, since properly selected combinations of agents with less toxicity are usually effective. Once steroids are withdrawn, the urticaria virtually always returns if it had been chronic. Rather than using systemic steroids in difficult cases, consultation should be sought from a dermatologist or allergist with experience in managing severe urticaria.

C. Local Treatment: Local treatment is rarely rewarding. Starch baths twice daily or Aveeno baths may be useful, prepared by adding one cupful of finely refined cornstarch or a packet of Aveeno to a comfortably warm bath. Alternatively, one may use a lotion containing 0.5% camphor, 0.5% menthol, and 0.5% phenol (Sarna) topically or in addition to the bathing.

Prognosis

Acute urticaria usually lasts only a few days to 6 weeks. Half of patients whose urticaria persists for more than 6 weeks will have it for years.

Breneman D et al: Cetirizine and astemizole therapy for chronic idiopathic urticaria: A double-blind, placebo-controlled, comparative trial. J Am Acad Dermatol 1995;33(2 Part 1):192. (Both cetirizine and astemizole provided effective relief with similar side-effect profiles. However, clinical response occurred more rapidly with cetirizine.)

Charlesworth EN: Urticaria and angioedema: A clinical spectrum. Ann Allergy Asthma Immunol 1996;76:484.

Fox RW: Update on urticaria and angioedema (hives). Allergy Proc 1995;16:289.

Greaves MW: Chronic urticaria. N Engl J Med 1995;332:1767.

Harvell J et al: Contact urticaria and its mechanisms. Food Chem Toxicol 1994;32:103. (Reviews contact urticaria and common causes.)

Kanwar AJ, Greaves MW: Approach to the patient with chronic urticaria. Hosp Pract (Off Ed) 1996 Mar 15;31:175, 183, 187.

Sveum RJ: Urticaria: The diagnostic challenge of hives. Postgrad Med 1996;100:77.

ERYTHEMA MULTIFORME

Essentials of Diagnosis

- Sudden onset of symmetric erythematous skin lesions with history of recurrence.
- May be macular, papular, urticarial, bullous, or purpuric.
- "Target" lesions with clear centers and concentric erythematous rings or "iris" lesions may be noted in erythema minor. These are rare in drug-associated erythema multiforme major (Stevens-Johnson syndrome).
- Mostly on extensor surfaces, palms, soles, or mucous membranes.
- Herpes simplex, systemic infection or disease, and drug reactions are often associated.

General Considerations

Erythema multiforme is an acute inflammatory, polymorphic skin disease due to multiple causes or of undetermined origin. Erythema multiforme is usually divided clinically into minor and major types based on the clinical findings. Approximately 90% of cases of erythema multiforme minor follow outbreaks of herpes simplex and are marked by cutaneous involvement. A few may follow infections caused by *Mycoplasma pneumoniae*. Erythema multiforme major (Stevens-Johnson syndrome), a disease in the differential diagnosis of blisters, is marked by toxicity and involvement of two or more mucosal surfaces (often oral and conjunctival) and is most often caused by drugs, especially sulfonamides, nonsteroidal anti-inflammatory drugs, and anticonvulsants such as phenytoin. Erythema multiforme may also present as recurring oral ulceration, with skin lesions present in only half of the cases, and is diagnosed by oral biopsy. Since erythema multiforme may have its own prodrome, many medications taken for such symptoms have been implicated in its pathogenesis without definitive proof. As in all drug eruptions, the exposure to drugs associated with erythema multiforme may be systemic or topical; any agent should be considered a potential offender.

Clinical Findings

A. Symptoms and Signs: A classic target lesion, found most commonly in herpes-associated erythema multiforme, consists of three concentric zones of color change, most often found acrally on the hands and feet in erythema multiforme minor. Not all lesions will have this appearance. Drug-associated erythema multiforme is manifested by raised target-like lesions, with only two zones of color change and a central blister, or nondescript reddish macules. In erythema multiforme major, mucous membrane ulcerations are present at two or more sites, causing pain on eating, swallowing, and urination.

B. Laboratory Findings: Blood tests are not useful for diagnosis. Skin biopsy is diagnostic. Direct immunofluorescence studies are negative.

Differential Diagnosis

Urticaria and drug eruptions are the chief entities that must be differentiated from erythema multiforme minor. Individual lesions of true urticaria itch, should come and go within 24 hours, are usually responsive to antihistamines, and do not affect the mucosa. In erythema multiforme major, the main differential diagnosis is toxic epidermal necrolysis, and some investigators regard these entities as variants of the same disease. The presence of blisters is always worrisome and dictates the need for consultation. The differential diagnosis of blisters includes pemphigus, pemphigoid, and bullous drug eruptions. Again, skin biopsy is the mainstay of diagnosis.

Complications

Visceral lesions are rare complications (eg, pneumonitis, myocarditis, nephritis). The tracheobronchial mucosa and conjunctiva may be involved in severe cases with resultant scarring (Stevens-Johnson syndrome).

Treatment

A. General Measures: Erythema multiforme major (Stevens-Johnson syndrome) with extensive denudation of skin is best treated in a burn unit. Otherwise, patients need not be admitted unless mucosal involvement interferes with hydration and nutrition. Patients who begin to blister should be seen daily.

B. Specific Measures: Although there are no good data to support the use of corticosteroids in erythema multiforme major, they are still often prescribed. There are retrospective studies showing that children with erythema multiforme treated with large doses of corticosteroids actually have a poorer outcome because of the complications of therapy. These

studies have been criticized because no data were included on when corticosteroids were used. If corticosteroids are to be tried in more severe cases, they should be used early, before blistering occurs, and in moderate to high doses (prednisone, 60–120 mg) and stopped within days if there is no dramatic response. Oral and topical corticosteroids are useful in the oral variant of erythema multiforme. Oral acyclovir prophylaxis of herpes simplex infections may be effective in preventing recurrent herpes-associated erythema multiforme. Antistaphylococcal antibiotics are used for secondary infection, which is uncommon.

C. Local Measures: Topical therapy is not very effective in this disease. For oral lesions, 1% diphenhydramine elixir mixed with Kaopectate or with 1% dyclonine may be used as a mouth rinse several times daily.

Prognosis

Erythema multiforme minor usually lasts 2–6 weeks and may recur. Stevens-Johnson syndrome, in which visceral involvement may occur, may be serious or even fatal in the most severe cases.

Bastuji-Garin S et al: Clinical classification of cases of toxic epidermal necrolysis, Stevens-Johnson syndrome, and erythema multiforme. Arch Dermatol 1993;129:92. (Best attempt to define lesions. Includes examples of target lesions, atypical flat and raised targets, and macules seen in this disease.)

Fabbri P, Panconesi E: Erythema multiforme (minus and maius) and drug intake. Clin Dermatol 1993;11:479. (Review of drugs that have been associated with erythema multiforme.)

Schofield JK, Tatnall FM, Leigh IM: Recurrent erythema multiforme: Clinical features and treatment in a large series of patients. Br J Dermatol 1993;128:542. (Acyclovir led to benefit in 55%—some treatment failures responded to dapsone or to azathioprine.)

ERYTHEMA MIGRANS
(See also Chapter 34.)

Erythema migrans is a unique cutaneous eruption that characterizes the localized or generalized early stage of Lyme disease. Three to 32 days (median: 7 days) after a tick bite, there is gradual expansion of redness around the papule representing the bite site. The advancing border is usually slightly raised, warm, red to bluish-red, and free of any scale. Centrally, the site of the bite may clear, leaving only a rim of peripheral erythema, or it may become indurated, vesicular, or necrotic. The annular erythema usually grows to a median diameter of 15 cm (range: 3–68 cm). It is accompanied by a burning sensation in half of patients; rarely, it is pruritic or painful. Twenty percent of patients will develop multiple secondary annular lesions similar in appearance to the primary lesion but without indurated centers and generally of smaller size. In the southeastern USA, similar lesions are seen in patients without evidence of Lyme borreliosis. The etiology of these cases is unclear.

Without treatment, erythema migrans and the secondary lesions fade in a median of 28 days, though some may persist for months. Ten percent of untreated patients experience recurrences over the ensuing months. Treatment with systemic antibiotics (see Table 34–4) is necessary to prevent systemic involvement. However, only 60–70% of those with systemic involvement experience erythema migrans.

Luft BJ et al: Azithromycin compared with amoxicillin in the treatment of erythema migrans: A double-blind, randomized, controlled trial. Ann Intern Med 1996;124:785.

Maraspin V et al: Treatment of erythema migrans in pregnancy. Clin Infect Dis 1996;22:788.

Nadelman RB et al: The clinical spectrum of early Lyme borreliosis in patients with culture-confirmed erythema migrans. Am J Med 1996;100:502.

ERYSIPELAS

Essentials of Diagnosis

- Edematous, spreading, circumscribed, hot, erythematous area, with or without vesicle or bulla formation.
- Face frequently involved.
- Pain, chills, fever, and systemic toxicity may be striking.

General Considerations

Erysipelas is a superficial form of cellulitis that occurs classically on the cheek, caused by β-hemolytic streptococci.

Clinical Findings

A. Symptoms and Signs: The symptoms are pain, malaise, chills, and moderate fever. A bright red spot appears first, very often near a fissure at the angle of the nose. This spreads to form a tense, sharply demarcated, glistening, smooth, hot area. The margin characteristically makes noticeable advances from day to day. The patch is somewhat edematous and can be pitted slightly with the finger. Vesicles or bullae occasionally develop on the surface. The patch does not usually become pustular or gangrenous and heals without scar formation. The disease may complicate any break in the skin that provides a portal of entry for the organism.

B. Laboratory Findings: Leukocytosis and an increased sedimentation rate are almost invariably present but are not specific; blood cultures may be positive.

Differential Diagnosis

Cellulitis is characterized by a less definite margin and involvement of deeper tissues; erysipeloid is a benign bacillary infection producing redness of the skin of the fingers or the backs of the hands in fishermen and meat handlers.

Complications

Unless erysipelas is promptly treated, death may result from extension of the process and systemic toxicity, particularly in the very young and in the aged.

Treatment

Place the patient at bed rest with the head of the bed elevated, apply hot packs, and give aspirin for pain and fever. Intravenous antibiotics effective against group A beta-hemolytic streptococci and staphylococci are indicated for the first 48 hours in all but the mildest cases. A 7-day course is completed with penicillin VK, 250 mg, dicloxacillin, 250 mg, or a first-generation cephalosporin, 250 mg, orally four times a day. Either erythromycin, 250 mg four times daily for 7–14 days, or clarithromycin, 250 mg twice daily for 7–14 days, is a good alternative in penicillin-allergic patients. Quinolones have poor activity against streptococci and are not recommended.

Prognosis

Erysipelas formerly was a life-threatening infection. It can now usually be quickly controlled with systemic penicillin or erythromycin therapy.

Cox NH et al: Pre-septal cellulitis and facial erysipelas due to *Moraxella* species. Clin Exp Dermatol 1994;19:321. (The patient responded poorly to penicillin. *Moraxella* was isolated from conjunctival swabs.)

Grosshans EM: The red face: Erysipelas. Clin Dermatol 1993;11:307.

Kahn RM, Goldstein EJ: Common bacterial skin infections: Diagnostic clues and therapeutic options. Postgrad Med 1993;93:175.

CELLULITIS

Cellulitis, a diffuse spreading infection of the skin, involves deeper tissues than erysipelas and may be due to one of several organisms, usually gram-positive cocci, though gram-negative rods such as *Escherichia coli* may also be responsible. The lesion is hot and red but has a more diffuse border than does erysipelas. Cellulitis is said to occur after a break in the skin, but this is often not apparent. Attempts to isolate the responsible organism by injecting and then aspirating saline are successful in 20% of cases. In cases of venous stasis, the only clue to cellulitis may be a new localized area of tenderness. Recurrent attacks may sometimes affect lymphatic vessels, producing a permanent swelling called "solid edema." The differential diagnosis includes lipodermatosclerosis, an acute, exquisitely tender red plaque on the medial lower legs above the malleolus in patients with venous stasis or varicosities, and acute severe contact dermatitis on a limb, which produces erythema, vesiculation, and edema as seen in cellulitis, but with itching instead of pain. The erythema and edema are also more superficial than in cellulitis. In cases of cellulitis with crepitus or local cutaneous anesthesia or in which progression is rapid or associated with necrosis, the diagnosis of necrotizing cellulitis-fasciitis (around the male genitals called Fournier's gangrene) must be considered. These diagnoses are established by surgical exploration and debridement, which are vital for treatment and survival.

Intravenous or parenteral antibiotics may be required for the first 24–48 hours. In mild cases or following the initial parenteral therapy, dicloxacillin or cephalexin, 250–500 mg four times daily for 7–10 days, is usually adequate. In patients in whom intravenous treatment is not instituted, the first dose of oral antibiotic can be increased to 750–1000 mg to achieve rapid high blood levels.

Brook I, Frazier EH: Clinical features and aerobic and anaerobic microbiological characteristics of cellulitis. Arch Surg 1995;130:786. (The data highlight the polymicrobial nature of cellulitis.)

Lindbeck G, Powers R: Cellulitis. Hosp Pract (Off Ed) Jul 1993;28(Suppl 2):10. (Most cases can be managed as outpatients after a first parenteral dose of antibiotics.)

Singh N et al: Cutaneous cryptococcosis mimicking bacterial cellulitis in a liver transplant recipient: Case report and review in solid organ transplant recipients. Clin Transplant 1994;8:365. (Presented on the lower extremity and foot; also had cryptococcal septic arthritis.)

ERYSIPELOID

Erysipelothrix insidiosa infection must be differentiated from erysipelas and cellulitis. It is usually a benign infection, seen in fishermen and meat handlers, and characterized by purplish erythema of the skin, most often of a finger or the back of the hand, which gradually extends over a period of several days. Systemic involvement occurs rarely; endocarditis may occur.

Penicillin V potassium, 250–500 mg orally four times daily for 7–10 days, is usually promptly curative. Some strains are resistant to erythromycin but sensitive to ciprofloxacin. Penicillin G, 2–4 million units intravenously every 4 hours, may be used instead if the patient appears toxic, with arthritis or endocarditis.

BLISTERING DISEASES

PEMPHIGUS

Essentials of Diagnosis

- Relapsing crops of bullae.
- Often preceded by mucous membrane bullae, erosions, and ulcerations.
- Superficial detachment of the skin after pressure or trauma variably present (Nikolsky's sign).
- Acantholysis on biopsy.
- Immunofluorescence studies are confirmatory.

General Considerations

Pemphigus is an uncommon intraepidermal blistering disease occurring on skin and mucous membranes and caused by autoantibodies to adhesion molecules in the cadherin family (in pemphigus vulgaris) and to a complex containing desmosomal proteins, including desmoglein I (in pemphigus foliaceus), expressed in skin and mucous membranes. These autoantibodies cause acantholysis, the separation of epidermal cells from each other. The cause is unknown, and in the preantibiotic, presteroid era the condition, if untreated, was usually fatal within 5 years. The bullae appear spontaneously and are relatively asymptomatic, but the lesions become extensive and the complications of the disease lead to great toxicity and debility. The disease occurs almost exclusively in middle-aged or older adults of all races and ethnic groups. Drug-induced autoimmune pemphigus from drugs including penicillamine and captopril has been reported. The pathogenetic role of IgG antibodies has been proved by passive transfer of antibodies to neonatal mice, reproducing the disease, and acantholysis can develop in a culture of normal human skin tissue when pemphigus serum is added. There is an association with HLA-A10 antigen. In addition, more than 95% of patients with pemphigus vulgaris are positive for HLA-DR4/DQw3 or HLA-DRw6/DQw1, and in one series of 13 patients, all of whom were DQw1-positive, all had a single DQ_β allele designated $PV6_\beta$. Pemphigus may present with atypical features, and repeated reevaluation of clinical findings and changes shown by immunofluorescence and histopathologic studies may be necessary.

There are several forms of pemphigus: **pemphigus vulgaris** and its variant, **pemphigus vegetans;** and the more superficially blistering **pemphigus foliaceus** and its variant, **pemphigus erythematosus.** Both forms may occur at any age but most commonly in middle age. The vulgaris form begins in the mouth in over 50% of cases. The foliaceus form is especially apt to be associated with other autoimmune diseases, or it may be drug-induced, eg, by exposure to penicillamine. Paraneoplastic pemphigus, a unique form of the disorder, is associated with numerous types of benign and malignant neoplasms.

Clinical Findings

A. Symptoms and Signs: Pemphigus is characterized by an insidious onset of flaccid bullae in crops or waves. In pemphigus vulgaris, lesions often appear first on the oral mucous membranes, and these rapidly become erosive. In some cases, erosions and crusts predominate over blisters. The scalp is another site of early involvement. Toxemia and a "mousy" odor may develop rapidly. Rubbing a cotton swab or finger laterally on the surface of uninvolved skin may cause easy separation of the epidermis (**Nikolsky's sign**).

B. Laboratory Findings: The diagnosis is made by light microscopy and by direct and indirect immunofluorescence microscopy. Microscopically, acantholysis is the hallmark of pemphigus, but in some patients there may be eosinophilic spongiosis initially. Immunofluorescence microscopy shows deposits of IgG intercellularly in the epidermis, forming a honeycomb pattern. C3 and other immunoglobulins and complement components may be present on occasion. Indirect immunofluorescence microscopy to detect circulating pemphigus antibodies is not necessary for the diagnosis, but antibody titers in some patients may correspond with disease activity and might help in management.

Differential Diagnosis

Blistering diseases include erythema multiforme, drug eruptions, bullous impetigo, contact dermatitis, dermatitis herpetiformis, and bullous pemphigoid, but flaccid blisters are not typical of these diseases, and acantholysis is not seen. In the early stages, pemphigus tends to be treated as impetigo, but bacterial cultures and clinical suspicion leading to early biopsy will clarify the diagnosis. All of these diseases have gross clinical characteristics and different immunofluorescence test results that distinguish them from pemphigus.

Paraneoplastic pemphigus is clinically, histologically, and immunologically distinct from other forms of the disease. Oral erosions and erythematous plaques resembling erythema multiforme are seen. Survival rates are low because of the underlying malignancy.

Complications

Secondary infection commonly occurs; this is a major cause of morbidity and mortality. Disturbances of fluid and electrolyte balance can occur owing to losses through the involved skin in severe cases.

Treatment

A. General Measures: When the disease is severe, hospitalize the patient at bed rest and provide antibiotics and intravenous feedings as indicated. Anesthetic troches used before eating ease painful oral lesions.

B. Systemic Measures: Pemphigus requires systemic therapy as early in its course as possible. However, the main morbidity in this disease today is generally due to the side effects of such therapy. Although high doses of prednisone have been advocated—180–360 mg/d for 6–10 weeks—most clinicians use doses of 80–120 mg to start and increase the dose for rapid progression of the disease or lack of response within a few weeks. A traditional next step has been to add immunosuppressive drugs, described below as "steroid-sparing" agents. However, tetracycline at a dosage of 1.5–3 g/d in divided doses with 500 mg of nicotinamide (*not nicotinic acid or niacin!*) twice to three times daily has been reported to be effective and is probably the preferred adjunctive measure in patients with stable disease, especially those with pemphigus foliaceus. Of the immunosuppressive agents, azathioprine, 100–150 mg/d, is often given concurrently with prednisone. Some clinicians use methotrexate, 25 mg/wk, instead of azathioprine. When control is achieved, the prednisone is slowly tapered. Dapsone at 25–100 mg/d appears to be a useful agent that may allow the tapering of corticosteroids. Plasmapheresis combined with cyclophosphamide or azathioprine may be of use, as well as dapsone, in resistant cases associated with low circulating antibody titers. Gold sodium thiomalate, given as for rheumatoid arthritis, is said to be effective following initial prednisone, but it has been less well studied. Many investigators feel that by initiating and carefully monitoring corticosteroid treatment with concomitant use of methotrexate or azathioprine or with gold, it is possible to reduce the dosage of steroids gradually with fewer of the hazards of long-term steroid therapy. The combined use of prednisone and cyclosporine can also be attempted in refractory cases.

C. Local Measures: In patients with limited disease, skin and mucous membrane lesions should be treated with topical corticosteroids. Complicating infection requires appropriate systemic and local antibiotic therapy.

Prognosis

The course tends to be chronic in most patients, though some appear to experience remission. Infection is the most frequent cause of death, usually from *Staphylococcus aureus* septicemia.

Bystryn JC, Steinman NM: The adjuvant therapy of pemphigus: An update. Arch Dermatol 1996;32:203.

Herrada J et al: A progressive blistering eruption in a patient with lymphoma: Paraneoplastic pemphigus. Arch Dermatol 1997;133:97.

Huilgol SC, Black MM: Management of the immunobullous disorders. II. Pemphigus. Clin Exper Dermatol 1995;20:283.

Lapidoth M et al: The efficacy of combined treatment with

prednisone and cyclosporine in patients with pemphigus: Preliminary study. J Am Acad Dermatol 1994;30(5 Part 1):752. (Sixteen patients were treated for 12 months with cyclosporine at a dosage of 5 mg/kg/d and prednisone at 60–80 mg/d. There was little clinically significant difference in response except cessation of new blister formation.)

Mutasim DF, Pelc NJ, Anhalt GJ: Drug-induced pemphigus. Dermatol Clin 1993;11:463.

OTHER BLISTERING DISEASES

Many other skin disorders are characterized by formation of bullae, or blisters. These include bullous pemphigoid, cicatricial pemphigoid, dermatitis herpetiformis, herpes gestationis, and other less common bullous disorders, including the mechanobullous diseases grouped under epidermolysis bullosa, which are due to defects in epidermal keratin synthesis.

Bullous Pemphigoid

Bullous pemphigoid is a relatively benign pruritic disease characterized by tense blisters in flexural areas, typically in elderly individuals, usually remitting in 5 or 6 years, with a course characterized by exacerbations and remissions. The appearance of blisters may be preceded by urticarial or edematous lesions for months. Oral lesions are present in about one-third of affected persons. Rarely, young people may be affected. The disease may occur in various forms, including localized, vesicular, vegetating, erythematous, erythrodermic, and nodular. There is no statistical association with internal malignant disease.

The diagnosis is made by biopsy and direct immunofluorescence examination. Light microscopy shows a subepidermal blister. With direct immunofluorescence, IgG and C3 are found at the dermal-epidermal junction. Circulating anti-basement membrane antibodies can be found in the sera of patients in about 70% of cases.

If the patient has only a few blisters, ultrapotent steroids, such as clobetasol or halobetasol, may be adequate. Prednisone at dosages of 60–80 mg/d is often used to achieve rapid control of more widespread disease. Although slower in onset of action, tetracycline or erythromycin, 1–1.5 g/d, alone or combined with nicotinamide—*not nicotinic acid!*—(up to 1.5 g/d), if tolerated, may control the disease in patients who cannot use corticosteroids or may allow decreasing or eliminating steroids after control is achieved. If these drugs are not effective, methotrexate, 5–10 mg weekly, or azathioprine, 50 mg one to three times daily, may be used as steroid-sparing agents.

Bouscarat F et al: Treatment of bullous pemphigoid with dapsone: Retrospective study of thirty-six cases. J Am Acad Dermatol 1996;34:683.

Fivenson DP et al: Nicotinamide and tetracycline therapy of bullous pemphigoid. Arch Dermatol 1994;130:753.

(A randomized, open-labeled trial using nicotinamide, 500 mg three times daily, and tetracycline, 500 mg four times daily, in 12 patients versus prednisone in eight patients. There were five complete responses and five partial responses in the nicotinamide plus tetracycline group versus one complete and five partial responses in the prednisone group.)

Huilgol SC, Black MM: Management of the immunobullous disorders. I. Pemphigoid. Clin Exper Dermatol 1995;20:189.

Paul MA et al: Low-dose methotrexate treatment in elderly patients with bullous pemphigoid. J Am Acad Dermatol 1994;31:620. (A retrospective review of 34 patients suggested that methotrexate, 5–10 mg weekly, may lower the amount of prednisone required for control of disease.)

Pereyo NG, Davis LS: Generalized bullous pemphigoid controlled by tetracycline therapy alone. J Am Acad Dermatol 1995;32:138. (Tetracycline, 500 mg twice daily, cleared lesions in 2 weeks in one patient. Other case reports are cited and reviewed.)

Herpes Gestationis

Herpes gestationis occurs in about one in 50,000–60,000 pregnancies. The bullae often appear first in periumbilical distribution, and there may be erythematous papules and plaques, vesicles, and large bullae. It usually begins in the fifth or sixth month of pregnancy, or the onset may be delayed to the postpartum period. The disease is self-limited, but it may recur in subsequent pregnancies. Use of estrogens or progesterone or the onset of menses may trigger flare-ups. The risks to mother and fetus appear to be less significant than was formerly thought but include an increase in prematurity and small-for-gestational-age infants. Blisters are subepidermal, with eosinophils present. Direct immunofluorescence shows C3 at the basement membrane zone in most cases. IgG is found less often.

Corticosteroids are the treatment of choice and are sometimes effective when used topically only.

Tanzi P et al: Herpes gestationis. Int J Gynaecol Obstet 1994;45:47. (A description of three cases and review.)

PAPULES

WARTS

Essentials of Diagnosis

- Verrucous papules anywhere on the skin or mucous membranes, usually no larger than 0.5 cm in diameter.
- Prolonged incubation period (average 2–18 months). Spontaneous "cures" are frequent (50%).
- "Recurrences" (new lesions) are frequent.

General Considerations

Warts are caused by human papillomaviruses. Over 70 different types of human papillomaviruses (HPV) have been identified. The type of mucocutaneous surface infected and the morphology of the wart are closely related to the HPV type causing the infection. Especially in genital warts, simultaneous infection with numerous wart types is common. Genital HPVs are divided into low-risk and high-risk types depending on the likelihood of their association with cervical cancer.

Cervical warts may be transmitted to the newborn via passage through the infected birth canal, causing laryngeal papillomatosis.

Clinical Findings

There are usually no symptoms. Tenderness on pressure occurs with plantar warts; itching occurs with anogenital warts. Occasionally a wart will produce mechanical obstruction (eg, nostril, ear canal, urethra).

Warts vary widely in shape, size, and appearance. Flat warts are most evident under oblique illumination. Subungual warts may be dry, fissured, and hyperkeratotic and may resemble hangnails or other nonspecific changes. Plantar warts resemble plantar corns or calluses.

Differential Diagnosis

Large chronic warts in older individuals should be biopsied to rule out the emergence of squamous cell carcinoma in the wart. Some warty-looking lesions in sun-damaged skin are actually hypertrophic actinic keratoses or squamous cell carcinomas. Some genital warty lesions may be due to secondary syphilis (condylomata lata). The lesions of molluscum contagiosum may be mistaken for warts, especially when they are very large in immunocompromised persons. Seborrheic keratosis may also be confused with warts. In AIDS, wart-like lesions may be caused by varicella-zoster virus.

Prevention

The use of condoms may reduce transmission of genital warts. A person with flat warts should be educated about the infectivity of warts and advised not to scratch or traumatize the areas. Using an electric shaver will in occasional cases prevent the spread of warts in razor scratches.

Treatment

Treatment is aimed at inducing "wart-free" intervals for as long as possible without scarring, since no treatment can guarantee a remission or prevent recurrences. In immunocompromised patients, the goal is even more modest, ie, to control the size and number of lesions present.

A. Removal: For common warts of the hands, patients are usually offered liquid nitrogen or keratolytic agents. The former may work in fewer treatments but requires office visits and is painful. Keratolytic agents are irritating but effective and usually painless if used correctly. They can be used at home but must be applied almost daily for 8–12 weeks for maximum effect.

1. Liquid nitrogen is applied to achieve a thaw time of 20–45 seconds. Two freeze-thaw cycles are given every 2–4 weeks for several visits. Scarring will occur if it is used incorrectly or too aggressively. For example, the face, dorsal hands, and legs are more sensitive than the palms. Improper use along the sides of the fingers has been reported to cause nerve damage and paresthesias. Liquid nitrogen may cause permanent depigmentation in darkly pigmented individuals. It is useful on dry penile warts and on filiform warts involving the face and body. Patients should be warned that its use on the soles and other pressure areas can result in painful and temporarily debilitating blisters. Liquid nitrogen may be used in condylomas, but snipping of perianal lesions followed by light electrodesiccation is more effective.

2. Keratolytic agents–Any of the following salicylic acid products may be used against common warts or plantar warts: Occlusal, Occlusal-HP, Trans-Ver-Sal, Duofilm, and Viranol. Plantar warts may be treated by applying a 40% salicylic acid plaster (Mediplast) after paring. The plaster may be left on for 5–6 days, then removed, the lesion pared down, and another plaster applied. Although it may take weeks or months to eradicate the wart, the method is safe and effective with almost no side effects.

3. Podophyllum resin–Anogenital warts are often initially treated by painting them every 2–3 weeks with 25% podophyllum resin (podophyllin) in compound tincture of benzoin. Apposing normal skin may be protected with petrolatum and by dusting the treated area with cornstarch or talc. Pregnant patients should not be so treated. The purified active component of the resin, podofilox, is available for use at home twice daily three times a week for cycles of 4–6 weeks. After a single 4-week cycle, 45% of patients were wart-free; but of these, 60% relapsed at 6 weeks. Thus, multiple cycles of treatment are often necessary.

4. Operative removal–Plantar warts may be removed by blunt dissection. Local anesthetic is injected into the base, and the wart is then removed with a curette or scissors or by shaving off at the base of the wart with a scalpel. Trichloroacetic acid or Monsel's solution on a tightly wound cotton-tipped applicator may be painted on the wound, or light electrocautery may be used. Excision of warts, however, may result in a permanent painful scar on the foot and is not recommended. For genital warts, snip biopsy (scissors) removal followed by electrocautery is more effective than cryotherapy and does scar. It is often preferred by patients with pedunculated or large lesions that require multiple cryotherapy or podophyllin treatments for removal.

5. Laser therapy—The CO_2 laser is effective for treating recurrent warts, periungual warts, plantar warts, and condylomata acuminata. It leaves open wounds which must fill in with granulation tissue over 4–6 weeks and is best reserved for warts resistant to other modalities. Pulse dye laser treatment may also be used every 3–4 weeks to gradually ablate the wart. For genital warts, it has not been shown that laser therapy is more effective than electrosurgical removal.

6. Other agents—**Bleomycin** diluted to 0.1% with 0.9% saline may be injected under warts, not exceeding 0.1 mL per puncture; with multiple punctures, it has been shown to have a high cure rate for plantar and common warts. It may cause loss of nails and symptoms similar to those of Raynaud's syndrome in individual digits treated.

Intralesional recombinant **interferon alfa-2a** is more effective than placebo in clearing a single condyloma when used three times a week for 3 weeks. Plantar warts do not respond. This treatment is of research interest and is not routinely recommended because of its high cost, its inconvenience, and its low efficacy. It is largely ineffective in immunosuppressed patients.

B. Immunotherapy: Dinitrochlorobenzene (DNCB) may be effective for resistant warts but is not FDA-approved.

C. Retinoids: Tretinoin (Retin-A) cream or gel applied topically twice daily may be effective (anecdotally) for facial or beard flat warts. Extensive warts have been reported to disappear when etretinate was given by mouth for a month. Oral isotretinoin may cure some warts (see Acne Vulgaris).

D. Physical Modalities: Soaking warts in hot (42.2 °C) water for 10–30 minutes daily for 6 weeks has results in dramatic involution in some cases in immunocompromised patients.

E. Cimetidine: Cimetidine, 30–40 mg/kg daily for 3–7 weeks, produces a 50–80% cure rate in flat warts and in common warts in children. It is no more effective than placebo, however, when studied in double-blind trials.

F. Imiquimod: This topical, patient-applied local interferon inducer is effective in the treatment of genital warts, especially in women and on moist nonmucosal surfaces. Initial reports suggest low recurrence rates in the short term. The drug might also find use as a posttreatment adjunct to prevent recurrences.

Prognosis

There is a striking tendency to the development of new lesions. Warts may disappear spontaneously or may be unresponsive to treatment.

Bonnez W et al: Efficacy and safety of 0.5% podofilox solution in the treatment and suppression of anogenital warts. Am J Med 1994;96:420. (After 4 weeks, 68% of warts were gone and 29% of patients had a complete response. Nineteen percent of subjects who used podofilox for the next 8 weeks on healed areas had recurrences versus 50% in the placebo group.)

Glass AT, Solomon BA: Cimetidine therapy for recalcitrant warts in adults. Arch Dermatol 1996;32:680.

Handley J et al: Anogenital warts in prepubertal children: Sexual abuse or not? Int J STD AIDS 1993;4:271. (Forty-two children of mean age 16 months prospectively followed. Sexual abuse suspected in 60%.)

Kaiser JF, Proctor-Shipman LP: Squamous cell carcinoma in situ (Bowen's disease) mimicking subungual verruca vulgaris. J Fam Pract 1994;39:384. (This case report reminds us that wart-like lesions, particularly around the nails and on the feet, that are somewhat atypical and resistant to therapy should be evaluated by biopsy to detect carcinoma.)

Landow K: Nongenital warts: When is treatment warranted? Postgrad Med 1996;99:245.

Miller DM, Brodell RT: Human papillomavirus infection: Treatment options for warts. Am Fam Physician 1996;53:135, 148.

Sterling J: Treating the troublesome wart. Practitioner 1995;239:44.

Yazar S, Basaran E: Efficacy of silver nitrate pencils in the treatment of common warts. J Dermatol 1994;21:329. (Use of silver nitrate sticks every 3 days for three applications resulted in clearing in 43% versus 11% in treatment versus placebo groups, respectively.)

Yilmaz E, Alpsoy E, Basaran E: Cimetidine therapy for warts: A placebo-controlled, double-blind study. J Am Acad Dermatol 1996;34:1005.

CALLOSITIES & CORNS OF FEET OR TOES

Callosities and corns are caused by pressure and friction due to faulty weight-bearing, orthopedic deformities, improperly fitting shoes, or neuropathies.

Tenderness on pressure and "after-pain" are the only symptoms. The hyperkeratotic well-localized overgrowths always occur at pressure points. Dermatoglyphics are preserved over the surface. On paring, a glassy core is found (which differentiates these disorders from plantar warts, which have multiple capillary bleeding points or black dots when pared). A soft corn often occurs laterally on the proximal portion of the fourth toe as a result of pressure against the bony structure of the interphalangeal joint of the fifth toe.

Treatment consists of correcting mechanical abnormalities that cause friction and pressure. Shoes must be properly fitted and orthopedic deformities corrected. Callosities may be removed by careful paring of the callus after a warm water soak or with keratolytic agents as found in various brands of corn pads.

Plantar hyperkeratosis of the heels can be treated successfully by using 20% urea (Ureacin 20) nightly and a pumice stone after soaking in water or by applying equal parts of propylene glycol and water nightly and covering with thin polyethylene plastic film (Baggies).

Women who tend to form calluses and corns should not wear confining footgear and high-heeled shoes.

Singh D, Bentley G, Trevino SG: Callosities, corns, and calluses. BMJ 1996;312:1403.

MOLLUSCUM CONTAGIOSUM

Molluscum contagiosum, caused by a poxvirus, presents as single or multiple rounded, dome-shaped, waxy papules 2–5 mm in diameter that are umbilicated. Lesions at first are firm, solid, and flesh-colored but upon reaching maturity become softened, whitish, or pearly gray and may suppurate. The principal sites of involvement are the face, hands, and lower abdomen and genitals, but the papules are commonly found on other parts of the skin and at times are widely distributed.

The lesions are autoinoculable and spread by wet skin-to-skin contact. In sexually active individuals, they may be confined to the penis, pubis, and inner thighs and are considered a sexually transmitted disease.

Molluscum contagiosum is one of the common viral infections seen in patients with AIDS, and in adults sensitive inquiries should be made about risk factors for HIV infection. AIDS patients tend to develop extensive lesions over the face and neck as well as in the genital area.

The diagnosis is easily established in most instances because of the distinctive central umbilication of the dome-shaped lesion. The best treatment is by curettage or applications of liquid nitrogen as for warts—but more briefly, since molluscum contagiosum is more responsive to therapy than warts. When lesions are frozen, the central umbilication often becomes more apparent. Light electrosurgery with a fine needle is also effective. Cantharidin (no longer available in the USA) may be used on nongenital lesions, applied for 4–6 hours. Lesions in children tend to resolve spontaneously and may be left untreated. It has been estimated that individual lesions persist for about 2 months. They are difficult to eradicate in patients with HIV infection.

Gottlieb SL, Myskowski PL: Molluscum contagiosum. Int J Dermatol 1994;33:453.

BASAL CELL CARCINOMA

Basal cell carcinomas are the most common form of cancer. They occur mostly on sun-exposed skin in otherwise normal fair-skinned individuals beginning in their 20s and 30s but are not frequent after age 50.

The most common presentation is a papule or nodule that may have a central scab or erosion. Occasionally the nodules have a brown-gray color or have stippled pigment (pigmented basal cell carcinoma). Intradermal nevi without pigment on the face of older white individuals may resemble basal cell carcinomas. Basal cell carcinomas grow slowly, attaining a size of 1–2 cm or more in diameter, often after years of growth. There is a waxy, "pearly" appearance, with telangiectatic vessels easily visible. It is the pearly or translucent quality of these lesions that is most diagnostic, and that feature may be best appreciated if the skin is stretched. Less common types include morpheaform or scar-like lesions. These are hypopigmented, somewhat thickened plaques. On the back and chest, basal cell carcinomas appear as reddish, somewhat shiny plaques.

Clinicians should examine the skin routinely, looking for bumps, patches, and scabbed lesions. When examining the face, look at the eyelid margins and medial canthi, the nose and alar folds, the lips, and then around and behind the ears. While metastases almost never occur, therapy of basal cell carcinomas may cause significant cosmetic deformity in these areas, particularly for inadequately treated or recurrent lesions. Neglected lesions may ulcerate and produce great destruction, ultimately invading vital structures and rarely invading the brain, causing death. Basal cell carcinomas of the medial canthi are particularly dangerous. Recurrent lesions around the nose and ears may track along cartilage underneath the skin, requiring treatment of much more extensive areas than are apparent from inspection.

Lesions suspected to be basal cell carcinomas should be biopsied, by shave or punch biopsy. Therapy is then aimed at eradication with minimal cosmetic deformity, often by excision and suturing with recurrence rates of 5% or less. The technique of three cycles of curettage and electrodesiccation depends on the skill of the operator and is not recommended for head and neck lesions. After 4–6 weeks of healing, it leaves a broad, hypopigmented, at times hypertrophic scar. Radiotherapy is effective and often appropriate for older individuals, but recurrent tumors after radiation therapy are more difficult to treat and may be more aggressive. Mohs surgery, ie, removal of the tumor followed by marking of margins, immediate frozen section histopathologic examination of margins with subsequent reexcision of tumor-positive areas, and final closure of the defect, gives the highest cure rates (98%) and results in least tissue loss. It is appropriate therapy for tumors of the eyelids and nose or for recurrent lesions, or where tissue sparing is needed for cosmesis, but it is expensive. Sun avoidance, particularly in children, is essential to lower the incidence of new basal cell cancers. Patients with basal cell carcinomas must be followed for 5 years to detect new or recurrent lesions.

Chorun L et al: Basal cell carcinoma in blacks: A report of 15 cases. Ann Plastic Surg 1994;33:90. (Although unusual, this tumor can occur in blacks.)

Fleming ID et al: Principles of management of basal and squamous cell carcinoma of the skin. Cancer 1995;75(2 Suppl):699.

Frisch M et al: Risk for subsequent cancer after diagnosis of basal-cell carcinoma: A population-based, epidemiologic study (see comments). Ann Intern Med 1996; 125:815.

Goldberg LH: Basal cell carcinoma. Lancet 1996;347:663.

Randle HW: Basal cell carcinoma: Identification and treatment of the high-risk patient. Dermatol Surg 1996;22: 255.

Schottenfeld D: Basal-cell carcinoma of the skin: A harbinger of cutaneous and noncutaneous multiple primary cancer. (Editorial and comment.) Ann Intern Med 1996;125:852.

SQUAMOUS CELL CARCINOMA

Squamous cell carcinoma usually occurs on exposed parts in fair-skinned individuals who sunburn easily and tan poorly. It may arise out of actinic keratoses and tends to develop in the course of a few months. The lesions appear as small red, conical, hard nodules that occasionally ulcerate. They are not as distinctive as basal cell carcinomas and are more easily misdiagnosed clinically. The frequency of metastasis is not precisely known, though metastatic spread is said to be less likely with squamous cell carcinoma arising out of actinic keratoses than with those that arise de novo. In actinically induced squamous cell cancers, rates of metastasis are estimated from retrospective studies to be 3–7%. Squamous cell carcinomas of the lip, oral cavity, tongue, and genitalia have much higher rates of metastasis and require special management.

Keratoacanthomas most often act in benign fashion but resemble squamous cell carcinoma histologically and for all practical purposes should be treated as though they were skin cancers.

Examination of the skin and therapy are essentially the same as for basal cell carcinoma. The preferred treatment of squamous cell carcinoma is excision. Electrodesiccation and curettage and x-ray radiation may be used for some lesions, and fresh tissue microscopically controlled excision (Mohs) is excellent treatment also. Some keratoacanthomas respond to intralesional injection of fluorouracil or methotrexate, but they must be excised if they do not. Follow-up for squamous cell carcinoma must be more frequent and thorough than for basal cell carcinoma, starting at every 3 months, with careful examination of lymph nodes. In addition, palpation of the lips is essential to detect hard or indurated areas that represent early squamous cell carcinoma. All such cases must be biopsied. Multiple squamous cell carcinomas are very common on the sun-exposed skin

of organ transplant patients because of the host's immunosuppressed state. The tumors begin to appear after 5 years of immunosuppression. Biologic behavior may be aggressive, and careful management is required.

Bernstein SC et al: The many faces of squamous cell carcinoma. Dermatol Surg 1996;22:243.

Czarnecki D et al: Metastases from squamous cell carcinoma of the skin in southern Australia. Dermatology 1994;189:52. (A prospective study of 68 immunocompetent patients followed for at least 3 years. Metastases were seen in two patients who had small lesions in sun-damaged skin. The study confirms recent observations that these tumors have metastatic potential, and close follow-up is warranted.)

Marks R: Squamous cell carcinoma. Lancet 1996;347:735.

Schwartz RA: Keratoacanthoma. J Am Acad Dermatol 1994;30:1. (A review of variants and therapy.)

VIOLACEOUS TO PURPLE PAPULES & NODULES

LICHEN PLANUS

Essentials of Diagnosis

- Pruritic, violaceous, flat-topped papules with fine white streaks and symmetric distribution.
- Lacy lesions of the buccal mucosa.
- Commonly seen along linear scratch marks (Koebner phenomenon) on anterior wrists, sacral region, penis, legs.
- Histopathologic examination is diagnostic.

General Considerations

Lichen planus is an inflammatory pruritic disease of the skin and mucous membranes characterized by distinctive papules with a predilection for the flexor surfaces and trunk. It is most often idiopathic. The three cardinal findings are typical skin lesions, mucosal lesions, and histopathologic features of band-like infiltration of lymphocytes, histiocytes, and melanophages in the dermis. Drugs causing lichen planus-like reactions include gold, streptomycin, tetracycline, iodides, chloroquine, quinacrine, quinidine, NSAIDs, phenothiazines, and hydrochlorothiazide. Hepatitis C infection is found with greater frequency in lichen planus patients than in controls in Europe and the USA. Erosive lesions are more common in hepatitis C-associated lichen planus. Lichen planus has been seen after exposure to color film developing solutions.

Clinical Findings

Itching is mild to severe. The lesions are violaceous, flat-topped, angulated papules, 1–4 mm in diameter, discrete or in clusters, with very fine white streaks on the surface (Wickham's striae) on the flexor surfaces of the wrists and on the penis, lips, tongue, and buccal and vaginal mucous membranes. Mucosal lichen planus has been reported in the genital and anorectal areas, the gastrointestinal tract, the bladder, the larynx, and the conjunctiva. The papules may become bullous or ulcerated. The disease may be generalized. Mucous membrane lesions have a lacy white network overlying them that may be confused with leukoplakia. The Koebner phenomenon (appearance of lesions in areas of trauma) may be seen.

A special form of lichen planus is the erosive or ulcerative variety. On palms and soles, it can be disabling. It is a major problem in the mouth, and squamous cell carcinoma may develop.

Differential Diagnosis

Lichen planus must be distinguished from similar lesions produced by sensitivity to medications (see above) and other papular lesions such as psoriasis, lichen simplex chronicus, and syphilis. Lichen planus on the mucous membranes must be differentiated from leukoplakia. Erosive oral lesions require biopsy and often direct immunofluorescence for diagnosis since lichen planus may simulate other bullous diseases. Histologic examination may make the distinction from graft-versus-host disease and in some cases from lichen planus-like drug eruptions.

Treatment

A. Topical Therapy: Superpotent topical corticosteroids such as betamethasone dipropionate in optimized vehicle, diflorasone diacetate, clobetasol propionate, and halobetasol propionate ointments applied twice daily are most helpful for localized disease in nonflexural areas. Alternatively, high-potency corticosteroid cream or ointment may be used nightly under thin pliable plastic film.

Application of tretinoin cream 0.05% to mucosal lichen planus, followed by a corticosteroid ointment, may be helpful. For disabling hypertrophic lichen planus of the soles, tretinoin cream applied and covered with thin, pliable polyethylene film nightly is said to be effective.

B. Systemic Therapy: Corticosteroids (see Chapter 26) may be required in severe cases, or where the most rapid response to treatment is desired. Unfortunately, relapse almost always occurs as the steroids are tapered, making systemic corticosteroid therapy an impractical option for the management of chronic lichen planus.

Isotretinoin and etretinate by mouth appear to be effective for oral and cutaneous lichen planus, though this is not a labeled indication for these drugs. Some clinicians, however, believe that retinoids may be the treatment of choice for widespread disease.

Psoralens plus long-wave ultraviolet light (PUVA) may be effective treatment for lichen planus.

After testing for the presence of glucose-6-phosphate dehydrogenase, erosive lichen planus may be treated with dapsone, 50 mg/d; this may be given over a period of many weeks, if necessary, with appropriate clinical and laboratory monitoring.

Prognosis

Lichen planus is a benign disease, but it may persist for months or years and may be recurrent. Hypertrophic lichen planus and oral lesions tend to be especially persistent, and neoplastic degeneration has been described in chronically eroded lesions. The oral retinoids appear to induce remissions and facilitate healing of erosive lesions in some patients.

Duffey DC, Eversole LR, Abemayor E: Oral lichen planus and its association with squamous cell carcinoma: An update on pathogenesis and treatment implications. Laryngoscope 1996;106(3 Part 1):357.

Eisen D: The therapy of oral lichen planus. Crit Rev Oral Biol Med 1993;4:141. (Corticosteroids, retinoids, griseofulvin, cyclosporine, surgery.)

Lewis FM, Shah M, Harrington CI: Vulval involvement in lichen planus: A study of 37 women. Br J Dermatol 1996;135:89.

Sanchez-Perez J et al: Lichen planus and hepatitis C virus: Prevalence and clinical presentation of patients with lichen planus and hepatitis C virus infection. Br J Dermatol 1996;134:715.

KAPOSI'S SARCOMA

Until recently in the USA, this rare malignant skin lesion was seen mostly in elderly white men, had a chronic clinical course, and was rarely fatal. Kaposi's sarcoma occurs endemically in an often aggressive form in young black men of equatorial Africa, but it is rare in American blacks. Epidemic clusters of Kaposi's sarcoma, predominantly in homosexual men who were infected early in the AIDS epidemic, have been found in large cities of the USA. A novel herpesvirus, human herpesvirus 8, has been found in all forms of Kaposi's sarcoma. Red, purple, or dark plaques or nodules on cutaneous or mucosal surfaces should alert the clinician to the possibility of the disease. Kaposi's sarcoma commonly involves the gastrointestinal tract, but in asymptomatic patients these lesions are not sought or treated. Pulmonary Kaposi's sarcoma may be life-threatening and is managed aggressively. The incidence of AIDS-associated Kaposi's sarcoma appears to be diminishing.

For Kaposi's sarcoma in the elderly, palliative local therapy with intralesional chemotherapy or radiation is usually all that is required. In the setting of iatrogenic immunosuppression, the treatment of Kaposi's sarcoma is primarily reduction of doses of immunosuppressive medications. In AIDS-associated

Kaposi's sarcoma, the patient should first be given effective anti-HIV antiretrovirals (including a protease inhibitor), because in some mild to moderate cases this treatment alone is associated with improvement. Other therapeutic options include cryotherapy or intralesional vinblastine (0.1–0.5 mg/mL) for cosmetically objectionable lesions; radiation therapy for accessible and space-occupying lesions; laser surgery for certain intraoral and pharyngeal lesions; and, for progressive disease, intravenous chemotherapy.

Gao SJ et al: Seroconversion to antibodies against Kaposi's sarcoma-associated herpesvirus-related latent nuclear antigens before the development of Kaposi's sarcoma. N Engl J Med 1996;335:233.

Miles SA: Pathogenesis of AIDS-related Kaposi's sarcoma. Evidence of a viral etiology. Hematol Oncol Clin North Am 1996;10:1011.

Morris AK, Valley AW: Overview of the management of AIDS-related Kaposi's sarcoma. Ann Pharmacother 1996;30:1150.

Northfelt DW et al: Efficacy of pegylated-liposomal doxorubicin in the treatment of AIDS-related Kaposi's sarcoma after failure of standard chemotherapy. J Clin Oncol 1997;15:653.

Tur E, Brenner S: Treatment of Kaposi's sarcoma. (Editorial and comment.) Arch Dermatol 1996;132:327.

PRURITUS
(Itching)

Pruritus is a disagreeable sensation that provokes a desire to scratch. It is a primary sensory impulse carried on unmyelinated C fibers in the spinothalamic tract. It is modulated by central factors, including cortical ones. Not all cases of pruritus are mediated by histamine, though several mediators—bradykinin, neurotensin, secretin, and substance P—release histamine.

Although many cases of generalized pruritus can be attributed to dry skin—whether naturally occurring and precipitated or aggravated by climatic conditions or arising from disease states—there are many other causes: scabies, dermatitis herpetiformis, atopic dermatitis, pruritus vulvae et ani, miliaria, insect bites, pediculosis, contact dermatitis, drug reactions, urticaria, urticarial eruptions of pregnancy, psoriasis, lichen planus, lichen simplex chronicus, exfoliative dermatitis, folliculitis, sunburn, bullous pemphigoid, and fiberglass dermatitis.

Persistent pruritus not explained by cutaneous disease should prompt a staged workup for systemic causes. Perhaps the commonest cause of pruritus associated with systemic disease is uremia in conjunction with hemodialysis. Topical capsaicin may be of benefit. Both this condition and the pruritus of obstructive biliary disease may be helped by phototherapy with ultraviolet B or PUVA. Recently, naloxone has been shown to relieve the pruritus of biliary cholestasis. Endocrine disorders such as hypo- or hyperthyroidism, psychiatric disturbances, lymphoma, leukemia, and other internal malignant disorders, iron deficiency anemia, and certain neurologic disorders may also cause pruritus. Danazol, 400–800 mg daily, may be tried for pruritus associated with myeloproliferative disorders and other systemic illnesses.

Burning or itching involving the face, scalp, and genitalia may be manifestations of primary depression and treatable with antidepressant drugs such as amitriptyline, imipramine, or doxepin.

Prognosis

Elimination of external factors and irritating agents may give complete relief from pruritus. Pruritus accompanying specific skin disease will subside when the disease is controlled. Idiopathic pruritus and that accompanying serious internal disease may not respond to any type of therapy.

Heathcote J: The pruritus of cholestasis is relieved by an opiate antagonist: Is this pruritus a centrally mediated phenomenon? Hepatology 1996;23:1280.

Kolodny L et al: Danazol relieves refractory pruritus associated with myeloproliferative disorders and other diseases. Am J Hematol 1996;51:112.

Lowitt MH, Bernhard JD: Pruritus. Semin Neurol 1992; 12(4):374.

Millikan LE: Treating pruritus. What's new in safe relief of symptoms? Postgrad Med 1996;99:173.

Roger D et al: Specific pruritic diseases of pregnancy: A prospective study of 3192 pregnant women. Arch Dermatol 1994;130:734. (Reviews pruritus gravidarum, herpes gestationis, polymorphic eruption of pregnancy or pruritic urticarial plaques and papules of pregnancy [PUPPP], prurigo gestationis, and pruritic folliculitis.)

ANOGENITAL PRURITUS

Essentials of Diagnosis

- Itching, chiefly nocturnal, of the anogenital area.
- Examination is highly variable, ranging from no skin reactions to excoriations and inflammation of any degree, including lichenification.

General Considerations

Most cases have no obvious cause, but multiple specific causes have been identified. Anogenital pruritus may have the same causes as intertrigo, lichen simplex chronicus, or seborrheic or contact dermatitis (from soaps, colognes, douches, contraceptives, and perhaps scented toilet tissue), or it may be due to irritating secretions, as in diarrhea, leukorrhea, or trichomoniasis, or to local disease (candidiasis, dermatophytosis, erythrasma). Psoriasis or seborrheic dermatitis may be present. Uncleanliness may be at fault. In pruritus ani, hemorrhoids are often found, and leakage of mucus and bacteria from the distal rectum onto the perianal skin may be important in cases in which no other skin abnormality is found.

Many women experience pruritus vulvae. In women, pruritus ani by itself is rare, and pruritus vulvae does not usually involve the anal area, though anal itching will usually spread to the vulva. In men, pruritus of the scrotum is most commonly seen in the absence of pruritus ani. When all possible known causes have been ruled out, the condition is diagnosed as idiopathic or essential pruritus—by no means rare.

Oxyuriasis (pinworm) is a rare cause in adults. Psychologic abnormalities are usually not evident. Lichen sclerosus et atrophicus may at times be the cause. The disease is probably more common than currently thought, especially in young girls. Erythrasma is easily diagnosed by demonstration of coral-red fluorescence with Wood's light; it is easily cured with erythromycin orally and topically.

Clinical Findings

A. Symptoms and Signs: The only symptom is itching, which is chiefly nocturnal. Physical findings are usually not present, but there may be erythema, fissuring, maceration, lichenification, excoriations, or changes suggestive of candidiasis or tinea.

B. Laboratory Findings: Urinalysis and blood glucose testing may lead to a diagnosis of diabetes mellitus. Microscopic examination or culture of tissue scrapings may reveal yeasts, fungi, or parasites. Stool examination may show pinworms.

Differential Diagnosis

The etiologic differential diagnosis consists of *Candida* infection, parasitosis, local irritation from contact with drugs and irritants, and other primary skin disorders of the genital area such as psoriasis, seborrhea, intertrigo, or lichen sclerosus et atrophicus.

Prevention

Instruct the patient in proper anogenital hygiene after treating systemic or local conditions.

Treatment

A. General Measures: Treating constipation, preferably with high-fiber management (psyllium [Metamucil; many others]), may help. Instruct the patient to use very soft or moistened tissue or cotton after bowel movements and to clean the perianal area thoroughly with cool water if possible. Women should use similar precautions after urinating. Instruct the patient regarding the harmful and pruritus-inducing effects of scratching.

B. Local Measures: Pramoxine cream or lotion or hydrocortisone-pramoxine (Pramosone), 1% or 2.5% cream, lotion, or ointment, is helpful in managing pruritus in the anogenital area. The ointment or cream should be applied before and after a bowel movement. Iodochlorhydroxyquin-hydrocortisone creams are useful also but may stain underwear. Potent fluorinated topical corticosteroids may lead to atrophy and striae if used for more than a few days and should in general be avoided. This includes combinations with antifungals. The use of strong steroids on the scrotum may lead to persistent severe burning upon withdrawal of the drug. Soaks with aluminum subacetate solution, 1:20, are of value if the area is acutely inflamed and oozing. Underclothing should be changed daily. Affected areas may be painted with Castellani's solution. Balneol Perianal Cleansing Lotion or Tucks premoistened pads, ointment, or cream (all Tucks preparations contain witch hazel) may be very useful for pruritus ani.

Prognosis

Although benign, anogenital pruritus may be persistent and recurrent.

Daniel GL et al: Pruritus ani: Causes and concerns. Dis Colon Rectum 1994;37:670. (Prospective evaluation of 100 patients. Twenty-three percent had neoplasia—either rectal cancer, anal cancer, adenomatous polyps, or colon cancer in 11%, 6%, 4%, and 2%, respectively. Hemorrhoids or anal fissures were seen in 20% and 12%, respectively. Only 25% had primary pruritus.)

Mazier WP: Hemorrhoids, fissures and pruritus ani. Surg Clin North Am 1994;74:1277. (A review of management.)

SCABIES

Essentials of Diagnosis

- Generalized itching.
- Pruritic vesicles and pustules in "runs" or "galleries," especially on finger webs and the heels of the palms and in wrist creases.
- Mites, ova, and brown dots of feces visible microscopically.
- Red papules or nodules on the penile glans and shaft are pathognomonic.

General Considerations

Scabies is caused by infestation with *Sarcoptes scabiei*. The infestation usually spares the head and neck (though even these areas may be involved in infants, in the elderly, and in patients with AIDS). Scabies is usually acquired by sleeping with or in the bedding of an infested individual or by other close contact. The entire family may be affected.

Clinical Findings

A. Symptoms and Signs: Itching is almost always present and can be quite severe. The lesions consist of more or less generalized excoriations with small pruritic vesicles, pustules, and "runs" or "burrows" on the sides of the fingers and the heels of the palms, wrists, elbows, and around the axillae. Often, burrows are found only on the feet, as they have been scratched off in other locations. The run or gallery appears as a short irregular mark, perhaps 2–3 mm long and the width of a hair. Characteristic lesions may occur on the nipples in females and as pruritic papules on the scrotum or penis in males. Pruritic papules may be seen over the buttocks.

B. Laboratory Findings: The diagnosis should be confirmed by microscopic demonstration of the organism, ova, or feces in a mounted specimen. The success of this procedure depends on choosing the best unexcoriated lesions from interdigital webs, wrists, elbows, or feet. A bit of immersion oil is placed on the lesion and a No. 15 blade is used to scrape the lesion until it is flat. Pinpoint bleeding may result from the scraping. The diagnosis can also be confirmed in most cases with the burrow ink test. Apply ink to the burrow and then do a very superficial shave biopsy by sawing off the burrow with a No. 15 blade, painlessly and bloodlessly. The mite, ova, and feces can be seen under the light microscope.

Differential Diagnosis

Scabies must be distinguished from the various forms of pediculosis and from other causes of pruritus.

Treatment & Prognosis

Treatment is aimed at killing scabies mites and controlling the dermatitis, which can persist for months after effective eradication of the mites, with midpotency topical steroids. Bedding and clothing should be laundered or cleaned or set aside for 14 days in plastic bags. Unless the lesions are complicated by severe secondary pyoderma, treatment consists primarily of disinfestation. If secondary pyoderma is present, it should be treated with systemic antibiotics. Unless treatment is aimed at all infected persons in a family or institutionalized group, reinfestations will probably occur. Resistance to 5% permethrin cream is uncommon.

Disinfestation with lindane (gamma benzene hexachloride), 1% in cream or lotion base, applied from the neck down overnight, may be used in adults. A warning has been issued by the FDA regarding potential neurotoxicity, and any use of lindane in infants and pregnant women or in any patient with widespread excoriations and open skin—as well as overuse in adults—is discouraged. This preparation can be used before secondary infection is controlled.

Permethrin 5% cream is highly effective and safe in the management of scabies. Treatment consists of a single application for 8–12 hours. It may be repeated in 1 week. The drug has been used safely in infants aged 2 months to 5 years and is the treatment of choice in children. An alternative drug is crotamiton cream or lotion, which may be applied in the same way as lindane but is used nightly for 4 nights. It is far less effective if used for only 48 hours.

Pregnant patients should be treated only if they have documented scabies themselves. Permethrin 5% cream once for 12 hours—or 5% or 6% sulfur in petrolatum applied nightly for 3 nights from the collarbones down—may be used for infants and pregnant patients.

Benzyl benzoate may be compounded as a lotion or emulsion in strengths from 20% to 35% and used as generalized applications (from collarbones down) overnight for two treatments 1 week apart. The NF XIV formula is 275 mL benzyl benzoate (containing 5 g of triethanolamine and 20 g of oleic acid) in water to make 1000 mL. It is cosmetically acceptable, clean, and not overly irritating. Patients will continue to itch for several weeks after treatment. Use of triamcinolone 0.1% cream will help resolve the dermatitis. Scabies in nursing home patients, institutionalized or mentally impaired (especially Down's syndrome) patients, and AIDS patients may be much more difficult to treat. Failures with a single application of permethrin may be treated with repeated weekly applications or by the use of ivermectin, 200 µg/kg as a single oral dose.

Persistent pruritic postscabietic papules may be treated with mid- to high-potency steroids or with intralesional triamcinolone acetonide (2.5–5 mg/mL).

Estes SA, Estes J: Therapy of scabies: Nursing homes, hospitals, and the homeless. Semin Dermatol 1993;12:26. (Model treatment plan.)

Meinking TL et al: The treatment of scabies with ivermectin. N Engl J Med 1995;333:26. (The anthelmintic agent ivermectin, given in a single oral dose of 150–200 µg/kg of body weight, was an effective treatment for scabies in both healthy and HIV-infected patients.)

Meinking TL, Taplin D: Safety of permethrin vs lindane for the treatment of scabies. (Editorial and comment.) Arch Dermatol 1996;132:959.

Moore P: Diagnosing and treating scabies. Practitioner 1994;238:632.

Orkin M: Scabies in AIDS: Semin Dermatol 1993;12:9.

Pasternak J et al: Scabies epidemic: Price and prejudice. Infect Control Hosp Epidemiol 1994;15:540. (Stresses that everyone in a facility must be treated simultaneously, and that everyone must be educated.)

Portu JJ et al: Atypical scabies in HIV-positive patients. J Am Acad Dermatol 1996;34(5 Part 2):915.

PEDICULOSIS

Essentials of Diagnosis

- Pruritus with excoriation.
- Nits on hair shafts; lice on skin or clothes.
- Occasionally, sky-blue macules (maculae ceru-

leae) on the inner thighs or lower abdomen in pubic louse infestation.

General Considerations

Pediculosis is a parasitic infestation of the skin of the scalp, trunk, or pubic areas. Body lice usually occur among people who live in overcrowded dwellings with inadequate hygiene facilities. Pubic lice may be acquired by sexual transmission. Head lice may be transmitted by shared use of hats or combs and are epidemic among children of all socioeconomic classes in elementary schools. Head lice are very uncommon among black children.

There are three different varieties: (1) pediculosis pubis, caused by *Pthirus pubis* (pubic louse, "crabs"); (2) pediculosis corporis, by *Pediculus humanus* var *corporis* (body louse); and (3) pediculosis capitis, by *Pediculus humanus* var *capitis* (head louse).

Head and body lice are similar in appearance and are 3–4 mm long. The body louse can seldom be found on the body, because the insect comes onto the skin only to feed and must be looked for in the seams of the clothing. Trench fever, relapsing fever, and typhus are transmitted by the body louse in countries where those diseases are endemic.

Clinical Findings

Itching may be very intense in body louse infestations, and scratching may result in deep excoriations, especially over the upper shoulders, posterior flanks, and neck. In some cases, only itching is present, with few excoriations seen. Pyoderma may be the presenting sign in any of these infestations. Head lice can be found on the scalp or may be manifested as small nits resembling pussy willow buds on the scalp hairs close to the skin. They are easiest to see above the ears and at the nape of the neck. Pubic louse infestations are occasionally generalized, particularly in hairy individuals; the lice may even be found on the eyelashes and in the scalp.

Differential Diagnosis

Head louse infestation must be distinguished from seborrheic dermatitis, body louse infestation from scabies, and pubic louse infestation from anogenital pruritus and eczema.

Treatment

Body lice are treated by disposing of the infested clothing. For pubic lice, lindane lotion (Kwell, Scabene) is used extensively. A thin layer is applied to the infested and adjacent hairy areas. It is removed after 12 hours by thorough washing. Remaining nits may be removed with a fine-toothed comb or forceps. Sexual contacts should be treated. Clothes and bedclothes should be washed and dried at high temperature if possible.

Permethrin 1% cream rinse (Nix) is a topical OTC pediculicide and ovicide and is the treatment of choice for head lice. It is applied to the scalp and hair and left on for 10–30 minutes before being rinsed off with water. Treatment should be repeated in 1 week. Permethrin 1% cream (Nix) is more effective than synergized pyrethrins (RID), OTC products that are applied undiluted until the infested areas are entirely wet. After 10 minutes, the areas are washed thoroughly with warm water and soap and then dried. Nits may be treated as indicated above. For involvement of eyelashes, petrolatum is applied thickly twice daily for 8 days, and remaining nits are then plucked off. Head lice are extremely difficult to eradicate in the epidemic setting, probably because the currently available pediculicides are not uniformly ovicidal when applied as directed.

Forsman KE: Pediculosis and scabies: What to look for in patients who are crawling with clues. Postgrad Med 1995;98:89.

Opaneye AA et al: Pediculosis pubis: A surrogate marker for sexually transmitted diseases. J R Soc Health 1993;113:6. (Thirty-seven percent of patients presenting with pubic lice had another STD.)

Vander Stichele RH, Dezeure EM, Bogaert MG: Systematic review of clinical efficacy of topical treatments for head lice. BMJ 1995;311:604.

SKIN LESIONS DUE TO OTHER ARTHROPODS

Essentials of Diagnosis

- Localized rash with pruritus.
- Furuncle-like lesions containing live arthropods.
- Tender erythematous patches that migrate ("larva migrans").
- Generalized urticaria or erythema multiforme in some patients.

General Considerations

Some arthropods (eg, most pest mosquitoes and biting flies) are readily detected as they bite. Many others are not, eg, because they are too small, because there is no immediate reaction, or because they bite during sleep. Reactions may be delayed for many hours; many are allergic. Patients are most apt to consult a physician when the lesions are multiple and pruritus is intense.

Many persons will react severely only to their earliest contacts with an arthropod, thus presenting pruritic lesions when traveling, moving into new quarters, etc. Body lice, fleas, bedbugs, and local mosquitoes should be considered. Spiders are often incorrectly believed to be the source of bites; they rarely attack humans, though the brown spider (*Loxosceles laeta, Loxosceles reclusa*) may cause severe necrotic reactions and death due to intravascular hemolysis, and the black widow spider (*Latrodectus mactans)* may cause severe systemic symptoms and death. (See also Chapter 39.)

In addition to arthropod bites, the most common lesions are venomous stings (wasps, hornets, bees, ants, scorpions) or bites (centipedes), furuncle-like lesions due to fly maggots or sand fleas in the skin, and a linear creeping eruption due to a migrating larva.

Clinical Findings

The diagnosis may be difficult when the patient has not noticed the initial attack but suffers a delayed reaction. Individual bites are often in clusters and tend to occur either on exposed parts (eg, midges and gnats) or under clothing, especially around the waist or at flexures (eg, small mites or insects in bedding or clothing). The reaction is often delayed for 1–24 hours or more. Pruritus is almost always present and may be all but intolerable once the patient starts to scratch. Secondary infection may follow scratching. Urticarial wheals are common. Papules may become vesicular. The diagnosis is aided by searching for exposure to arthropods and by considering the patient's occupation and recent activities.

The principal arthropods are as follows:

(1) Fleas: Fleas are bloodsucking ectoparasites that feed on dogs, cats, humans, and other species. Flea saliva produces papular urticaria in sensitized individuals. *Ctenocephalides felis* and *Ctenocephalides canis* are the most common species found on cats and dogs, and both species attack humans. The human flea is *Pulex irritans.*

To break the life cycle of the flea, one must treat the home, pets, and outside environment, using quick-kill insecticides, residual insecticides, and a growth regulator. Obviously, this is a repetitive job. Birds and fish are especially sensitive and must be protected during disinfestation.

(2) Bedbugs: In crevices of beds or furniture; bites tend to occur in lines or clusters. Papular urticaria is a characteristic lesion of bedbug *(Cimex lectularius)* bites. The closely related kissing bug (conenose) has been reported with increasing frequency as attacking humans. Its bite is painful.

(3) Ticks: Usually picked up by brushing against low vegetation. Ticks may transmit Rocky Mountain spotted fever, Lyme disease, relapsing fever, and ehrlichiosis.

(4) Chiggers or red bugs: These are larvae of trombiculid mites. A few species confined to particular countries and usually to restricted and locally recognized habitats (eg, berry patches, woodland edges, lawns, brush turkey mounds in Australia, poultry farms) attack humans, often around the waist, on the ankles, or in flexures, raising intensely itching erythematous papules after a delay of many hours. The red chiggers may sometimes be seen in the center of papules that have not yet been scratched.

(5) Bird mites: Larger than chiggers, bird mites infest pigeon lofts or nests of birds in eaves. Bites are multiple anywhere on the body, although poultry handlers are most often attacked on the hands and forearms. Room air conditioning units may suck in bird mites and infest the inhabitants of the room. Rodent mites from mice or rats may cause similar effects. The diagnosis of bird mites, rodent mites, or carpet mites may easily be overlooked and the patient treated for other dermatoses.

(6) Mites in stored products: These are white and almost invisible and infest products such as copra, vanilla pods, sugar, straw, cottonseeds, and cereals. Persons who handle these products may be attacked, especially on the hands and forearms and sometimes on the feet. Infested bedding may occasionally lead to generalized dermatitis.

(7) Caterpillars of moths with urticating hairs: The hairs are blown from cocoons or carried by emergent moths, causing severe and often seasonally recurrent outbreaks after mass emergence. The gypsy moth is a cause in the eastern USA.

(8) Tungiasis: Tungiasis is due to the burrowing flea known as *Tunga penetrans* and is found in Africa, the West Indies, and South and Central America. The female burrows under the skin, sucks blood, swells to 0.5 cm, and then ejects her eggs onto the ground. Ulceration, lymphangitis, gangrene, and septicemia may result, in some cases with lethal effect. Ethyl chloride spray will kill the insect when applied to the lesion, and disinfestation may be accomplished with insecticide applied to the terrain. Simple surgical excision is usually performed.

Differential Diagnosis

Arthropods should be considered in the differential diagnosis of skin lesions showing any of the above symptoms.

Prevention

Arthropod infestations are best prevented by avoidance of contaminated areas, personal cleanliness, and disinfection of clothing, bedclothes, and furniture as indicated. Chiggers, bedbugs, and mites can be killed by lindane (Kwell, Scabene) applied to the head and clothing. (It is not necessary to remove clothing.) Benzyl benzoate and dimethylphthalate are excellent acaricides; clothing should be impregnated by spray or by dipping in a soapy emulsion.

Treatment

Living arthropods should be removed carefully with tweezers after application of alcohol and preserved in alcohol for identification. In endemic Rocky Mountain spotted fever areas, ticks should not be removed with the bare fingers, because infection may occur.

Corticosteroid lotions or creams are helpful. Calamine lotion or a cool wet dressing is always appropriate. Antibiotic creams, lotions, or powders may be applied if secondary infection is suspected.

Localized persistent lesions may be treated with intralesional corticosteroids. Creams containing local anesthetics are not very effective and may be sensitizing.

Stings produced by many arthropods may be alleviated by applying papain powder (Adolph's Meat Tenderizer) mixed with water, or aluminum chloride hexahydrate (Xerac AC).

Extracts from venom sacs of bees, wasps, yellow jackets, and hornets are now available for immunotherapy of patients at risk for anaphylaxis, but they are expensive. Treatment is advisable, however, as there are 50–100 deaths yearly in the USA resulting from this problem.

Reisman RE: Insect stings. N Engl J Med 1994;331:523.

INFLAMMATORY NODULES

ERYTHEMA NODOSUM

Essentials of Diagnosis

- Painful red nodules without ulceration on anterior aspects of legs.
- Slow regression over several weeks to resemble contusions.
- Women are predominantly affected.
- Some cases associated with infection or drug sensitivity.

General Considerations

Erythema nodosum is a symptom complex characterized by tender, erythematous nodules that appear most commonly on the extensor surfaces of the legs. It usually lasts about 6 weeks and may recur. The disease may be associated with various infections—streptococcosis, primary coccidioidomycosis, other deep fungal infections, tuberculosis, *Yersinia pseudotuberculosis* and *Yersinia enterocolitica* infection, or syphilis—or may be due to drug sensitivity. It may accompany leukemia, sarcoidosis, rheumatic fever, and inflammatory bowel disease. Erythema nodosum may be associated with pregnancy or with use of oral contraceptives.

Clinical Findings

A. Symptoms and Signs: The swellings are exquisitely tender and are usually preceded by fever, malaise, and arthralgia. They are most often located on the anterior surfaces of the legs below the knees but may occur (rarely) on the arms, trunk, and face. The lesions, 1–10 cm in diameter, are at first pink to red; with regression, all the various hues seen in a contusion can be observed.

B. Laboratory Findings: The histologic finding of septal panniculitis is characteristic of erythema nodosum. Otherwise, the findings are those of the associated illness.

Differential Diagnosis

Erythema induratum is seen on the posterior surfaces of the legs and may show ulceration. Nodular vasculitis is usually on the calves. Erythema multiforme occurs in generalized distribution. Lupus panniculitis presents as tender nodules on the buttocks and trunk that heal with depressed scars. In the late stages, erythema nodosum must be distinguished from simple bruises and contusions.

Treatment

A. General Measures: One must first identify and treat the underlying cause, eg, systemic infection or exogenous toxin. Primary therapy is with nonsteroidal anti-inflammatory agents in usual doses. Saturated solution of potassium iodide, 5–15 drops three times daily, may result in prompt involution in many cases. Side effects of potassium iodide include salivation, swelling of salivary glands, and headache. Complete bed rest may be advisable if the lesions are very painful. Systemic therapy directed against the lesions themselves may include corticosteroid therapy (see Chapter 26) unless contraindicated by associated infection; salicylates are helpful for several days during the acute painful stage.

B. Local Treatment: This is usually not necessary. Hot or cold compresses may help.

Prognosis

The lesions usually disappear after about 6 weeks, but they may recur.

Fox MD, Schwartz RA: Erythema nodosum. Am Fam Physician 1992;46:818.

FURUNCULOSIS (BOILS) & CARBUNCLES

Essentials of Diagnosis

- Extremely painful inflammatory swelling of a hair follicle that forms an abscess.
- Predisposing condition (diabetes mellitus, HIV disease, injection drug use) sometimes present.
- Coagulase-positive *Staphylococcus aureus* is the causative organism.

General Considerations

A furuncle (boil) is a deep-seated infection (abscess) involving the entire hair follicle and adjacent subcutaneous tissue. The most common sites of occurrence are the hairy parts exposed to irritation and friction, pressure, or moisture or to the plugging action of petroleum products. Because the lesions are autoinoculable, they are often multiple. Thorough investigation usually fails to uncover a predisposing cause; however, diabetes mellitus (especially if using insulin injections), injection drug use, allergy injections, and HIV disease all increase the risk of staphylococcal infections by increasing the rate of nasal carriage.

A carbuncle consists of several furuncles developing in adjoining hair follicles and coalescing to form a conglomerate, deeply situated mass with multiple drainage points.

Clinical Findings

A. Symptoms and Signs: Pain and tenderness may be prominent. The follicular abscess is either rounded or conical. It gradually enlarges, becomes fluctuant, and then softens and opens spontaneously after a few days to 1–2 weeks to discharge a core of necrotic tissue and pus. The inflammation occasionally subsides before necrosis occurs. Infection of the soft tissue around the nails (paronychia) may be due to staphylococci when it is acute. This is a variant of furuncle. Other organisms may be involved, including *Candida* and herpes simplex (herpetic whitlow).

B. Laboratory Findings: There may be slight leukocytosis, but a white blood cell count is rarely required. Although *S aureus* is almost always the cause, pus should be cultured, especially in immunocompromised patients, to rule out methicillin-resistant *S aureus* or other bacteria. Culture of the anterior nares may identify chronic staphylococcal carriage in cases of recurrent cutaneous infection.

Differential Diagnosis

The most common entity in the differential is an inflamed epidermal inclusion cyst that suddenly becomes red, tender, and expands greatly in size over one to a few days. The history of a prior small cyst in the same location, the presence of a clearly visible cyst orifice, and the extrusion of cheesy rather than purulent material helps in the diagnosis. Tinea profunda (deep dermatophyte infection of the hair follicle) may simulate recurrent furunculosis. Furuncle is also to be distinguished from deep mycotic infections such as sporotrichosis (often in gardeners) and blastomycosis, from other bacterial infections such as anthrax and tularemia (rare), and from acne cysts. Hidradenitis suppurativa presents with recurrent tender sterile abscesses in the axillae, groin, on the buttocks, or below the breasts. The presence of old scars or sinus tracts plus negative cultures suggests this diagnosis.

Complications

Serious and sometimes fatal cavernous sinus thrombosis may occur as a complication of a manipulated furuncle on the central portion of the upper lip or near the nasolabial folds. Perinephric abscess, osteomyelitis, and even endocarditis may rarely occur from manipulation of a furuncle.

Treatment

A. Specific Measures: Incision and drainage is recommended for all loculated suppurations and is the mainstay of therapy. Systemic antibiotics are indicated (chosen on the basis of cultures and sensitivity tests if possible). Sodium dicloxacillin, 1 g daily in divided doses by mouth for 10 days, is usually effective. Cephalexin is an effective alternative drug. Erythromycin may be used in penicillin-allergic individuals in communities with low populations of erythromycin-resistant staphylococci or if the particular isolate is sensitive. Ciprofloxacin is effective against strains of staphylococci resistant to other antibiotics.

Recurrent furunculosis may be effectively treated with a combination of dicloxacillin, 250–500 mg four times daily for 2–4 weeks, and rifampin, 300 mg twice daily for 5 days during this period. Family members and intimate contacts may need evaluation for staphylococcal carrier state and perhaps concomitant treatment. Applications of topical 2% mupirocin to the nares, axillae, and anogenital areas three times daily for 5–7 days eliminates the staphylococcal carrier state. Mupirocin may be irritating inside the nose.

B. Local Measures: Immobilize the part and avoid overmanipulation of inflamed areas. Use moist heat to help larger lesions "localize." Use surgical incision and debridement *after* the lesions are "mature." It is not necessary to incise and drain an acute staphylococcal paronychia. Inserting a flat metal spatula or sharpened hardwood stick into the nail fold where it adjoins the nail will release pus from a mature lesion. Inflamed epidermal cysts may be treated in the initial stages with intralesional injections of triamcinolone acetonide into the borders of the lesions, attempting not to puncture the cyst itself. Drainage of fluctuant lesions results in rapid resolution and reduction of pain.

Prognosis

Recurrent crops may harass the patient for months or years.

Feingold DS: Staphylococcal and streptococcal pyodermas. Semin Dermatol 1993;12:331.

Hoss DM, Feder HM Jr: Addition of rifampin to conventional therapy for recurrent furunculosis. Arch Dermatol 1995;131:647.

Levy R et al: Vitamin C for the treatment of recurrent furunculosis in patients with impaired neutrophil functions. J Infect Dis 1996;173:1502.

PHOTODERMATITIS

Essentials of Diagnosis

- Painful or pruritic erythema, edema, or vesiculation on sun-exposed surfaces: the face, neck, hands, and "V" of the chest.
- Inner upper eyelids spared, as is the area under the chin.

General Considerations

Photodermatitis is an acute or chronic inflammatory skin reaction due to hypersensitivity to sunlight or other sources of actinic rays, photosensitization of the skin by certain drugs, or idiosyncrasy to actinic light as seen in some constitutional disorders including the porphyrias and many hereditary disorders (phenylketonuria, xeroderma pigmentosum, and others). Contact photosensitivity may occur with perfumes, antiseptics, and other chemicals.

Photodermatitis is manifested most commonly as photosensitivity—a tendency for the individual to sunburn more easily than usual—or, more rarely, as photoallergy, a true immunologic reaction that often presents with papular or vesicular lesions.

Clinical Findings

A. Symptoms and Signs: The acute inflammatory skin reaction, if severe enough, is accompanied by pain, fever, gastrointestinal symptoms, malaise, and even prostration, but this is very rare. Signs include erythema, edema, and possibly vesiculation and oozing on exposed surfaces. Peeling of the epidermis and pigmentary changes often result. The key to diagnosis is localization of the rash to photo-exposed areas, though these eruptions may become generalized with time to involve even photoprotected areas. The lips are commonly involved in hereditary polymorphous light eruption, a disorder seen in persons of Native American descent.

B. Laboratory Findings: Blood and urine tests are not helpful in diagnosis unless porphyria cutanea tarda is suggested by the presence of blistering, scarring, milia (white cysts 1–2 mm in diameter) and skin fragility of the dorsal hands, and hirsutism. Testing for photosensitivity may be necessary to define the wavelengths of light (long and medium wavelength ultraviolet light or visible light) responsible.

Differential Diagnosis

The differential diagnosis is long. If a clear history of use of a topical or systemic photosensitizer is not available and if the eruption is persistent, then a workup including biopsy and light testing may be required. Photodermatitis must be differentiated from contact dermatitis that may develop from one of the many substances in suntan lotions and oils, as these may often have a similar distribution. This may sometimes be accomplished without photopatch testing by cautiously reapplying the agent to the forearm or back daily for 1–2 weeks and avoiding sun exposure. Sensitivity to actinic rays may also be part of a more serious condition such as porphyria cutanea tarda, variegate porphyria, or lupus erythematosus. These disorders are diagnosed by appropriate blood or urine tests. Erythropoietic protoporphyria is a rare childhood disorder, and pellagra is not commonly seen in the United States. Phenothiazines, sulfones, chlorothiazides, griseofulvin, sulfonylureas, nonsteroidal anti-inflammatory agents, and antibiotics (eg, some tetracyclines) may photosensitize the skin. Polymorphous light eruption is a very common idiopathic photodermatitis that affects both sexes equally and often has its onset in the third to fourth decades except in Native Americans, in whom it commonly presents in childhood. Polymorphous light eruption is chronic in nature. Transitory periods of spontaneous remission do occur, and the risk of developing systemic lupus erythematosus and perhaps other autoimmune disorders is negligible. The action spectrum usually lies in the short (below 320 nm) ultraviolet wavelengths but may also extend into the long ultraviolet wavelengths (320–400 nm).

Complications

Some individuals continue to be chronic light reactors even when they apparently are no longer exposed to photosensitizing or phototoxic drugs.

Prevention

While sunscreeens are useful agents in general and should be used by persons with photosensitivity, patients may react to such low amounts of energy that sunscreens alone may not be sufficient. Protective sunscreening agents (eg, those containing PABA and oxybenzone or dioxybenzone) may be applied before exposure, though PABA and benzophenones themselves may uncommonly cause photosensitivity or allergic contact dermatitis. There are several PABA-free sunscreens of great efficacy, but sunscreens in general provide the best protection against middle-wavelength "burning" UVB rays and not against long-wavelength "tanning" UVA rays that cause most cases of drug-associated phototoxicity. Sunscreens with an SPF of at least 30–50 should be used.

Treatment

A. Specific Measures: Drugs should be suspected in cases of photoallergy even if the particular medication (such as hydrochlorothiazide) has been used for months.

B. Local Measures: When the eruption is vesicular or weepy, treatment is similar to that of any acute dermatitis, using cooling and soothing wet dressing. Ointments should be avoided at this stage.

Sunscreens should be used as described above under prevention. Mid-potency to high-potency topical steroids are of limited benefit in phototoxic reactions but may help in polymorphous light eruption and photoallergic reactions. Since the face is often involved, close monitoring every 2 weeks is necessary to avoid side effects of potent steroids.

C. Systemic Measures: Aspirin may have some value for fever and pain of acute sunburn, as prostaglandins appear to play a pathogenetic role in the early erythema. Systemic corticosteroids in doses as described for acute contact dermatitis may be required for severe photosensitivity reactions. Otherwise, different photodermatoses may be treated in specific ways.

PUVA (psoralen plus UVA light) therapy can actually be a very important therapy for polymorphous light eruption and other idiopathic photosensitive conditions, perhaps by altering immune function in the skin. This is usually administered under strict supervision, using a photosensitizer (psoralen) and artificial light sources or sunlight, and systemic steroids are not uncommonly required to control initial flares. The eyes must be examined prior to treatment, and protective eyewear must be worn while outdoors for 24 hours after psoralen ingestion.

Patients with severe photosensitivity may require immunosuppressives, such as azathioprine, in the range of 50–150 mg/d.

Prognosis

The most common phototoxic sunburn reactions are usually benign and self-limiting except when the burn is severe or when it occurs as an associated finding in a more serious disorder. Polymorphous light eruption and some cases of photoallergy can persist for years.

[Sunlight, ultraviolet light, and the skin]
gopher://gopher.nih.gov/70/11/clin/cdcs/individual/74.skin

Gonzalez E, Gonzalez S: Drug photosensitivity, idiopathic photodermatoses, and sunscreens. J Am Acad Dermatol 1996;35:871.

ULCERS

DECUBITUS ULCERS
(Bedsores, Pressure Sores)

Bedsores (pressure sores) are a special type of ulcer caused by impaired blood supply and tissue nutrition resulting from prolonged pressure over bony or cartilaginous prominences. The skin overlying the sacrum and hips is most commonly involved, but bedsores may also be seen over the occiput, ears, elbows, heels, and ankles. They occur most readily in aged, paralyzed, debilitated, and unconscious patients. Low-grade infection may occur as a complication.

Differential Diagnosis

Herpes simplex virus should be suspected in ulcers in immunocompromised patients, particularly if there is a scalloped border, representing the erosions of herpetic vesicles. Rarely, ulcerated lesions in the perianal area represent actual skin cancers. Rapidly expanding ulcers may also represent pyoderma gangrenosum associated with inflammatory bowel disease in some patients. Ecthyma gangrenosum is an ulcerating lesion associated with sepsis, commonly due to *Pseudomonas,* and observed in neutropenic patients. All ulcerative lesions should be biopsied and cultured if suspicious or if they do not heal properly.

Prevention

Good nursing care, good nutrition, and maintenance of skin hygiene are important preventive measures. The skin and the bed linens should be kept clean and dry. Bedfast, paralyzed, moribund, listless, or incontinent patients who are candidates for the development of decubiti must be turned *frequently* (at least every hour) and must be examined at pressure points for the appearance of small areas of redness and tenderness. Written schedules can be very helpful. Water-filled mattresses, rubber pillows, alternating-pressure mattresses, and thick papillated foam pads are useful in prevention and in the treatment of lesions. "Donut" devices should not be used.

Treatment

A large number of treatments and protocols exist for management of decubiti. Early lesions should be treated with topical antibiotic powders and adhesive absorbent bandage (Gelfoam). Once clean, they may be treated with hydrocolloid dressings such as Duo-Derm. Established lesions require surgical consultation for debridement, cleansing, and dressing. A spongy foam pad placed under the patient may work best in some cases. It must be laundered often. In general, topical antiseptics are not recommended. A continuous dressing of 1% iodochlorhydroxyquin in Lassar's paste may be effective.

Deep infections are commonly present in pressure sores, often requiring systemic antibiotics.

[AHCPR guideline on pressure ulcers in adults]
http://text.nlm.nih.gov/ftrs/gateway

Bennis S, Davis S: An effective approach to treating decubitus ulcers in home healthcare patients. Home Healthcare Nurse 1994;12:47.

Bergstrom N et al: *Pressure Ulcer Treatment.* Clinical Practice Guideline, Quick Reference Guide for Clinicians, No. 15. United States Department of Health and Human Services, Public Health Service, Agency for Health Care Policy and Research. AHCPR Publication No. 95–0653, December 1994.

Granick MS et al: Surgical management of decubitus ulcers. Clin Dermatol 1994;12:71.

LEG ULCERS SECONDARY TO VENOUS INSUFFICIENCY

Essentials of Diagnosis

- Past history of varicosities, thrombophlebitis, or postphlebitic syndrome.
- Irregular ulceration, often on the medial aspect of the lower legs above the malleolus.
- Edema of the legs, varicosities, hyperpigmentation, and red and scaly areas (stasis dermatitis) and scars from old ulcers support the diagnosis.

General Considerations

Patients at risk may have a history of venous insufficiency, either with obvious varicosities or with a past history of thrombophlebitis, or with immobility of the calf muscle group (paraplegics, etc). Red, pruritic patches of stasis dermatitis often precede ulceration. Because venous insufficiency is the most common cause of lower leg ulceration, testing of venous competence is still a required part of the evaluation even when no changes of venous insufficiency are present.

Clinical Findings

A. Symptoms and Signs: Classically, chronic edema is followed by a dermatitis, which is often pruritic. These changes are followed by hyperpigmentation, skin breakdown, and eventually sclerosis of the skin of the lower leg. The ulcer base may be clean, but it often has a yellow fibrin eschar that would appear easy to debride by using compresses but often requires surgical treatment. Ulcers that appear on the feet, toes, or above the knees should be approached with other diagnoses in mind.

B. Laboratory Findings: Thorough evaluation of the patient's vascular system (including measurement of the ankle/brachial index) is essential. Doppler and light rheography examinations as office procedures are usually sufficient (except in the diabetic) to elucidate the cause of most vascular cases of lower leg ulceration.

Differential Diagnosis

The differential includes vasculitis, pyoderma gangrenosum, arterial ulcerations, infection, trauma, insect bites (spiders) and sickle cell anemia. When the diagnosis is in doubt, a punch biopsy from the border (not base) of the lesion may be helpful.

Prevention

Compression stockings to reduce edema are the most important means of prevention. Compression should achieve a pressure of 30 mm Hg below the knee and 40 mm Hg at the ankle. The stockings should not be used in patients with arterial insufficiency with an ankle-brachial pressure index less than 0.7. Pneumatic sequential compression devices may be of great benefit.

Treatment

A. Local Measures: Institution of compression therapy is begun with cleaning of the ulcer. The patient is instructed to clean the base with saline or cleansers such as Saf-clens or Cara-klenz daily. A curette or small scissors can be used to remove the yellow fibrin eschar, under local anesthesia if the areas are very tender.

Once the base is clean, the ulcer is treated with metronidazole gel to reduce gram-negative bacterial growth and odor. Any red dermatitic skin is treated with a medium- to high-potency steroid ointment. The ulcer is then covered with an occlusive hydroactive dressing (Duoderm or Cutinova) or a polyurethan foam (Allevyn) followed by an Unna zinc paste boot. This is changed weekly. The ulcer should begin to heal within weeks, and healing should be complete within 2–3 months. Some ulcerations require grafting. Full- or split-thickness grafts often do not take, and pinch grafts (small shaves of skin laid onto the bed) may be more effective. Cultured epidermal cell grafts, while expensive, are sometimes effective in patients who have failed other therapy.

B. Systemic Therapy: If cellulitis accompanies the ulcer, systemic antibiotics are recommended: both dicloxacillin, 250 mg orally four times a day, and ciprofloxacin, 500 mg orally twice a day, are effective.

Prognosis

The combination of compression stockings and newer dressings enables venous stasis ulcers to heal within weeks or months. Newer modalities appear to be effective in recalcitrant cases. Ongoing control of edema is essential to prevent recurrent ulceration.

Douglas WS, Simpson NB: Guidelines for the management of chronic venous leg ulceration: Report of a multidisciplinary workshop. British Association of Dermatologists and the Research Unit of the Royal College of Physicians. Br J Dermatol 1995;132:446.

Elder DM, Greer KE: Venous disease: how to heal and prevent chronic leg ulcers. Geriatrics 1995;50:30.

Hansson C et al: Repeated treatment with lidocaine/prilocaine cream (EMLA) as a topical anesthetic for the cleansing of venous leg ulcers: A controlled study. Acta Derm Venereol (Stockh) 1993;73:231. (Decreased pain without adverse effects.)

Kirsner RS et al: Split-thickness skin grafting of leg ulcers. The University of Miami Department of Dermatology's experience (1990–1993). Dermatol Surg 1995;21:701.

(Meshed split-thickness skin grafting was a safe and effective therapy for recalcitrant lower extremity ulcers.)

Margolis DJ, Cohen JH: Management of chronic venous leg ulcers: A literature-guided approach. Clin Dermatol 1994;12:19.

Thomson B, Warin A: How to cure non-healing leg ulcers. Practitioner 1995;239:301.

Warburg FE et al: Vein surgery with or without skin grafting versus conservative treatment for leg ulcers: A randomized prospective study. Acta Derm Venereol 1994;74:307. (A study of 47 patients failed to demonstrate an advantage of surgery for incompetent perforating veins with or without excision and grafting of the ulcer versus conservative treatment consisting of compression, treatment of cellulitis with antibiotics, and treatment of stasis dermatitis with topical steroids.)

Zaki I et al: Bacitracin: A significant sensitizer in leg ulcer patients. Contact Dermatitis 1994;31:92. (Sixteen of 85 patients treated with topical antibiotics for venous ulcers had moderate or severe reactions when patch tested to bacitracin. The findings are consistent with long-held views that such patients are easily sensitized and that the minimum number of topical agents should be used.)

II. MISCELLANEOUS DERMATOLOGIC DISORDERS*

PIGMENTARY DISORDERS

Although the color of skin may be altered by many diseases and agents, the vast majority of patients have either an increase or decrease in pigment secondary to some inflammatory disease such as acne or atopic dermatitis.

Other pigmentary disorders include those resulting from exposure to exogenous pigments such as carotenemia, argyria, deposition of other metals (such as gold when given chronically for rheumatoid arthritis), and tattooing. Other endogenous pigmentary disorders are attributable to metabolic substances—including hemosiderin (iron)—in purpuric processes; or to homogentisic acid in ochronosis; bile pigments; and carotenes.

Classification

One should first determine whether the disorder is hyper- or hypopigmentation, ie, an increase or decrease in normal skin colors. Each may be considered to be primary or to be secondary to other disorders.

A. Primary Pigmentary Disorders:

1. Hyperpigmentation—The disorders in this category are nevoid, congenital or acquired, and in-

---

*Hirsutism is discussed in Chapter 26.

clude pigmented nevi, mongolian spots, incontinentia pigmenti, ephelides (juvenile freckles), and lentigines (senile freckles). Hyperpigmentation occurs also in arsenical melanosis or in association with Addison's disease (due to lack of the inhibitory influence of cortisol on the production of MSH by the pituitary gland). Axillary freckling and café au lait spots may be seen in neurofibromatosis. **Melasma (chloasma)** occurs as patterned hyperpigmentation of the face, usually as a direct effect of certain steroid hormones, estrogens, and progesterones in predisposed clones of melanocytes. It occurs not only during pregnancy but also in 30–50% of women taking oral contraceptives.

2. Hypopigmentation and depigmentation—The disorders in this category are vitiligo, albinism, and piebaldism. In vitiligo, pigment cells (melanocytes) are destroyed. The greater the pigment loss, the fewer the number of melanocytes. Vitiligo, present in approximately 1% of the population, may be associated with hyperthyroidism and hypothyroidism, pernicious anemia, diabetes mellitus, and Addison's disease. Albinism represents a number of different genetically determined traits, with different phenotypes. These may be autosomal dominant or recessive and often affect the eye and vision. Piebaldism, a localized hypomelanosis manifested by a white forelock, is an autosomal dominant trait that in some cases may be associated with neurologic abnormalities. Hypopigmented ash leaf spots may be seen in tuberous sclerosis. Hypopigmented halos are common around nevi and may occur around melanomas.

B. Secondary Pigmentary Disorders: Any damage to the skin (irritation, allergy, infection, excoriation, burns, or dermatologic therapy such as curettage, dermabrasion, chemical peels, freezing with liquid nitrogen) may result in hyper- or hypopigmentation. Several disorders of clinical importance are as described below:

1. Hyperpigmentation—The most common type of secondary hyperpigmentation occurs after another dermatologic condition, such as acne, and is most commonly seen in dark-skinned persons. It is called postinflammatory hyperpigmentation.

Berloque hyperpigmentation is the pigmentation left behind by phototoxicity from essential oils in perfumes. Similar hyperpigmentation has been seen in phototoxic reactions to chemicals in the rinds of limes and other citrus fruits and to celery. Pigmentation may be produced by certain drugs, eg, chloroquine, chlorpromazine, minocycline, and amiodarone. Irritation from benzoyl peroxide and tretinoin can result in hyperpigmentation, as may topical fluorouracil. Fixed drug eruptions to phenolphthalein in laxatives, to barbiturates, and to tetracyclines, for example, are further causes.

2. Hypopigmentation—Leukoderma may complicate atopic dermatitis, lichen planus, psoriasis, alopecia areata, discoid lupus erythematosus, lichen simplex chronicus, and such systemic conditions as myxedema, thyrotoxicosis, and syphilis. It may follow local skin trauma of various sorts or may complicate dermatitis due to exposure to gold or arsenic. Physicians must exercise special care in using liquid nitrogen on any patient with olive or darker complexions, since doing so may result in hypopigmentation or depigmentation, at times permanent. Intralesional or intra-articular injections of high concentrations of corticosteroids may also cause localized temporary hypopigmentation.

Differential Diagnosis

One must distinguish true lack of pigment from pseudoachromia, such as occurs in tinea versicolor, pityriasis simplex, and seborrheic dermatitis. The evaluation of pigmentary disorders in Caucasians is helped by Wood's light, which accentuates epidermal pigmentation and highlights hypopigmentation.

Complications

Actinic keratoses and skin cancers are more likely to develop in persons with vitiligo and albinism. There may be severe emotional trauma in extensive vitiligo and other types of hypo- and hyperpigmentation, particularly when they occur in naturally dark-skinned persons.

Treatment & Prognosis

A. Hyperpigmentation: Therapeutic bleaching preparations generally contain hydroquinone. Hydroquinone has occasionally caused unexpected hypopigmentation, hyperpigmentation, or even secondary ochronosis and pigmented milia, particularly with prolonged use.

The role of exposure to ultraviolet light cannot be overstressed as a factor promoting or contributing to most disorders of hyperpigmentation, and such exposure should be minimized. Melasma, ephelides, and postinflammatory hyperpigmentation may be treated with varying success with 3–4% hydroquinone cream, gel, or solution and a sunscreen with an SPF of 15. Solaquin Forte contains both hydroquinone and a sunscreen. Tretinoin cream, 0.025–0.05%, may be added. The superficial melasma responds well, but if there is predominantly dermal deposition of pigment (does *not* enhance with Wood's light), the prognosis is poor. Response to therapy takes months and requires avoidance of sunlight. Hyperpigmentation often recurs after treatment if the skin is exposed to ultraviolet light without potent sunscreens. Solar lentigines are resistant to topicals but respond to liquid nitrogen application or to newer green light lasers. Controlled studies have recently demonstrated that tretinoin, 0.1% cream used over 10 months, will fade solar lentigines (liver spots), hyperpigmented facial macules in Asians, and postinflammatory hyperpigmentation in blacks. New laser systems for the removal of epidermal and dermal pigments are available, and referral should be considered for patients whose responses to medical treatment are inadequate.

B. Hypopigmentation: The pigment dilution is stable in various forms of albinism; spontaneous return of pigment is rare in vitiligo; in secondary hypopigmentation, repigmentation may occur spontaneously. Cosmetics such as Covermark and Dermablend are highly effective for concealing disfiguring patches. Therapy of vitiligo is long and tedious, and the patient must be strongly motivated. If less than 20% of the skin is involved (most cases), topical methoxsalen, 0.1% in ethanol and propylene glycol or in Acid Mantle cream or Unibase, is used, with cautious exposure to long-wavelength ultraviolet light (UVA), followed by thorough washing and application of an SPF 15 sunscreen. With 20–25% involvement, oral methoxsalen, 0.6 mg/kg 2 hours before UVA exposure, is best. Severe phototoxic response (sunburn) may occur with topical or oral psoralens plus UVA. The face and upper chest respond best, and the fingertips and the genital areas do not respond to this treatment. Years of treatment are often required. New techniques of using epidermal autografts and cultured epidermis combined with PUVA therapy give hope for surgical correction of vitiligo with a very low risk of scarring. Potent topical corticosteroids have been advocated for treatment of vitiligo, with daily use for 10 days followed by 10 days of rest, then repetition. However, this strategy is often not successful, and on the face it may result in thinning of the skin and other changes.

Drake LA et al: Guidelines of care for vitiligo. American Academy of Dermatology. J Am Acad Dermatol 1996;35:620.

Grimes PE: Melasma: Etiologic and therapeutic considerations. Arch Dermatol 1995;131:1453.

Grimes PE: Vitiligo: An overview of therapeutic approaches. Dermatol Clin 1993;11:325.

BALDNESS (Alopecia)

Baldness Due to Scarring

Cicatricial baldness may occur following chemical or physical trauma, lichen planopilaris, severe bacterial or fungal infections, severe herpes zoster, chronic discoid lupus erythematosus, scleroderma, and excessive ionizing radiation. The specific cause is often suggested by the history, the distribution of hair loss, and the appearance of the skin, as in lupus erythematosus. Biopsy is useful in the diagnosis of scarring alopecia, but specimens must be taken from the active border and not from the scarred central zone.

Scarring alopecias are irreversible and permanent. There is no treatment except for surgical hair transplants. It is important to diagnose and treat the scarring process as early in its course as possible.

Baldness Not Due to Scarring

Nonscarring alopecia may occur in association with various systemic diseases such as systemic lupus erythematosus, secondary syphilis, hyper- or hypothyroidism, iron deficiency anemia, and pituitary insufficiency. The only treatment necessary is prompt and adequate control of the underlying disorder, in which case hair loss may be reversible.

Male pattern baldness, the most common form of alopecia, is of genetic predetermination. The earliest changes occur at the anterior portions of the calvarium on either side of the "widow's peak." The extent of hair loss is variable and unpredictable. The only available medical treatment at present is Rogaine, a solution containing 20 mg/mL of minoxidil. The best results are achieved in patients under 50 years of age and in those with recent onset (< 5 years) and smaller diameters of alopecia. Approximately 40% of patients treated twice daily for a year will have moderate to dense regrowth of the vertex.

Hair loss or thinning of the hair in women results from the same cause as common baldness in men (androgenetic alopecia) and may be treated with minoxidil (Rogaine). Spironolactone, a synthetic steroidal aldosterone antagonist, has been used successfully for the treatment of diffuse hair loss in women (androgenetic alopecia) in a dose of 25 mg daily by mouth. A workup consisting of determination of serum testosterone, DHEAS, iron, total iron binding capacity, and thyroid function tests and a complete blood count will identify most other causes of hair thinning in premenopausal women. Women who complain of thin hair but show little evidence of alopecia need follow-up, because more than 50% of the scalp hair can be lost before the clinician can perceive it.

Telogen effluvium is transitory increase in the number of hairs in the telogen (resting) phase of the hair growth cycle. This may occur spontaneously, may appear at the termination of pregnancy, may be precipitated by "crash dieting," high fever, stress from surgery or shock, or malnutrition, or may be provoked by hormonal contraceptives. Whatever the cause, telogen effluvium usually has a latent period of 2–4 months. The prognosis is generally good. The condition is diagnosed by the presence of large numbers of hairs with white bulbs coming out upon gentle tugging of the hair. Counts of hairs lost by the patient on combing or shampooing often exceed 150 per day, compared to an average of 70–100. In one study, a major cause of telogen effluvium was found to be iron deficiency, and the hair counts bore a clear relationship to serum iron levels.

Alopecia areata is of unknown cause but is believed to be an immunologic process. Typically, there are patches that are perfectly smooth and without scarring. Tiny hairs 2–3 mm in length, called "exclamation hairs," may be seen. Telogen hairs are easily dislodged from the periphery of active lesions.

The beard, brows, and lashes may be involved. Involvement may extend to all of the scalp hair (alopecia totalis) or to all scalp and body hair (alopecia universalis). Severe forms may be treated by systemic corticosteroid therapy, although recurrences follow discontinuation of therapy. Alopecia areata is occasionally associated with Hashimoto's thyroiditis, pernicious anemia, Addison's disease, and vitiligo.

Intralesional corticosteroids are frequently effective for alopecia areata. Triamcinolone acetonide in a concentration of 2.5–10 mg/mL is injected in aliquots of 0.1 mL at approximately 1- to 2-cm intervals, not exceeding a total dose of 30 mg per month for adults. Alternatively, anthralin 0.5% ointment used daily, may help some patients. Alopecia areata is usually self-limiting, with complete regrowth of hair in 80% of patients, but some mild cases are resistant, as are the extensive totalis and universalis types. Both topical dinitrochlorobenzene (DNCB) and an experimental topical allergen, squaric acid dibutyl ester, have been used to treat persistent alopecia areata. The principle is to sensitize the skin, then intermittently apply weaker concentrations to produce and maintain a slight dermatitis. Hair regrowth in 3–6 months in some patients has been reported to be remarkable. Long-term safety and efficacy have not been established. Support groups for patients with extensive alopecia areata are very beneficial. In **trichotillomania** (the pulling out of one's own hair), the patches of hair loss are irregular and growing hairs are always present, since they cannot be pulled out until they are long enough. The patches are often unilateral, occurring on the same side as the patient's dominant hand. The patient may be unaware of the habit.

Drug-induced alopecia is becoming increasingly important. Incriminated drugs include thallium, excessive and prolonged use of vitamin A, retinoids, antimitotic agents, anticoagulants, clofibrate (rarely), antithyroid drugs, oral contraceptives, trimethadione, allopurinol, propranolol, indomethacin, amphetamines, salicylates, gentamicin, and levodopa. While chemotherapy-induced alopecia is very distressing, it must be emphasized to the patient before treatment that it is invariably reversible.

Drake LA et al: Guidelines of care for androgenetic alopecia. American Academy of Dermatology. J Am Acad Dermatol 1996;35(3 Part 1):465.

Duvic M et al: A randomized trial of minoxidil in chemotherapy-induced alopecia. J Am Acad Dermatol 1996;35:74.

Shupack JI, Stiller MJ: Status of medical treatment for androgenetic alopecia. Int J Dermatol 1993;32:701. (Development and use of minoxidil.)

Whiting DA: Chronic telogen effluvium: Increased scalp hair shedding in middle-aged women. J Am Acad Dermatol 1996;35:899.

NAIL DISORDERS

1. MORPHOLOGIC ABNORMALITIES OF THE NAILS

Classification

Nail disorders may be classified as (1) local, (2) congenital or genetic, and (3) those associated with systemic or generalized skin diseases.

A. Local Nail Disorders:

1. Onycholysis (distal separation of the nail plate from the nail bed, usually of the fingers) is caused by excessive exposure to water, soaps, detergents, alkalies, and industrial keratolytic agents. Candidal infection of the nail folds and subungual area, nail hardeners, and demeclocycline-induced photosensitivity may cause onycholysis, as may hyper- and hypothyroidism and psoriasis.

2. Distortion of the nail occurs as a result of chronic inflammation of the nail matrix underlying the eponychial fold. Such changes may also be caused by warts, tumors, nevi, synovial and mucous cysts, etc, impinging on the nail matrix.

3. Discoloration and crumbly thickened nails are noted in dermatophyte infection and psoriasis.

4. Allergic reactions (to formaldehyde and resins in undercoats and polishes or to nail glues) are characterized by onycholysis or by grossly distorted, hypertrophic, and misshapen nails.

B. Congenital and Genetic Nail Disorders:

1. A longitudinal single nail groove may occur as a result of a genetic or traumatic defect in the nail matrix.

2. Nail atrophy may be congenital.

3. Clubbed fingers may be congenital.

C. Nail Changes Associated With Systemic or Generalized Skin Diseases:

1. Beau's lines (transverse furrows) may follow any serious systemic illness.

2. Atrophy of the nails may be related to trauma or to vascular or neurologic disease.

3. Clubbed fingers may be due to the prolonged hypoxemia associated with cardiopulmonary disorders.

4. Spoon nails may be seen in anemic patients.

5. Stippling or pitting of the nails is seen in psoriasis, alopecia areata, and hand eczema.

6. Nail hyperpigmentation may be caused by zidovudine, doxorubicin, cyclophosphamide, methotrexate, bleomycin, dacarbazine, daunorubicin, fluorouracil, hydroxyurea, melphalan, mechlorethamine, and nitrosoureas.

Differential Diagnosis

It is important to distinguish congenital and genetic disorders from those caused by trauma and environmental disorders. Nail changes due to dermatophyte fungi (see below) may be difficult to differentiate from those due to *Candida* infections. Direct microscopic examination of a specimen cleared with 10% potassium hydroxide—or culture on Sabouraud's medium—may be diagnostic. Onychomycosis may cause nail changes identical to those seen in psoriasis. Careful examination for more characteristic lesions elsewhere on the body is essential to the diagnosis of the nail disorders. Cancer should be suspected (eg, Bowen's disease or squamous cell carcinoma) as the cause of any persistent solitary subungual or periungual lesion.

Complications

Secondary bacterial infection occasionally occurs in onychodystrophies and leads to considerable pain and disability and more serious consequences if circulation or innervation is impaired. Toenail changes may lead to an ingrown nail—in turn often complicated by bacterial infection and occasionally by exuberant granulation tissue. Poor manicuring and poorly fitting shoes may contribute to this complication. Cellulitis may result.

Treatment & Prognosis

Treatment consists usually of careful debridement and manicuring and, above all, reduction of exposure to irritants (soaps, detergents, alkali, bleaches, solvents, etc). Antifungal measures may be used in the case of onychomycosis and candidal onychia. Congenital or genetic nail disorders are usually uncorrectable. Longitudinal grooving due to temporary lesions of the matrix, such as warts, synovial cysts, and other impingements, may be cured by removal of the offending lesion. Intradermal triamcinolone acetonide suspension, 2.5 mg/mL, may be injected in the area of the nail matrix at intervals of 2–4 weeks for the successful management of various types of inflammatory nail dystrophies (psoriasis, lichen planus) but is painful.

If it is necessary to remove dystrophic nails for any reason (eg, fungal nails or severe psoriasis), a nonsurgical method is to apply urea 40%, anhydrous lanolin 20%, white wax 5%, white petrolatum 25%, and silica gel type H. The nail folds are painted with compound tincture of benzoin and covered with cloth adhesive tape. The urea ointment is applied generously to the nail surface and covered with plastic film, and then adhesive tape. The ointment is left on for 5–10 days; then the nail plate may be curetted off. Medication can then be applied that is appropriate for the condition being treated.

2. TINEA UNGUIUM (Onychomycosis)

Tinea unguium is a destructive *Trichophyton* infection of one or more (but rarely all) fingernails or toenails. The species most commonly found is *Trichophyton rubrum.* "Saprophytic" fungi may rarely (< 5%) cause onychomycosis.

There are usually no symptoms. The nails are lusterless, brittle, and hypertrophic, and the substance of the nail is friable and even pithy. Irregular segments of the diseased nail may be broken. Laboratory diagnosis is mandatory. Portions of the nail should be cleared with 10% potassium hydroxide and examined under the microscope for hyphae. Fungi may also be cultured, using Sabouraud's medium. Periodic acid-Schiff stain of a histologic section of the nail plate will also demonstrate the fungus readily.

Onychomycosis is difficult to treat because of the long duration of therapy required and the frequency of recurrences. Fingernails respond more readily than toenails. For toenails, it is in some situations best to discourage therapy and to control discomfort by paring the thickened nail plate.

Topical treatment has relatively low efficacy, but in well-motivated patients with minimally thickened nails it can be useful. Naftifine gel 1% or ciclopirox lotion 1% applied twice daily may clear fingernails in 4–6 months and toenails in 12–18 months.

In general, systemic therapy is required for the treatment of nail onychomycosis. Fingernails can virtually always be cleared, whereas toenails respond in about 60%. For fingernails, ultramicrosize griseofulvin, 750 mg or more daily for 6 months, is often effective. Treatment alternatives are itraconazole, 200 mg daily for 3 months; itraconazole, 400 mg the first 7 days of each month for 2 months; fluconazole, 150 mg 1 day per week for 6 months; and terbinafine, 250 mg daily for 6 weeks. Once clear, fingernails often remain free of disease for years. The efficacy of griseofulvin for toenails is too low to be considered a therapeutic option in most cases. Ketoconazole, with its risk of hepatotoxicity with long-term use, is also not recommended. Itraconazole may be given as 200 mg daily for 3 months or 400 mg for the first 7 days of each month for 3 months for toenail onychomycosis. About 80% of patients will have substantial improvement, and over 50% will be mycologically and clinically cured at 1 year. It interacts with numerous other medications and requires gastric acid to be absorbed. Terbinafine, 250 mg daily for 3 months, has similar efficacy. It is associated with fewer drug interactions and is absorbed in patients with low gastric acid (those receiving H_2 blockers). The rate of long-term recurrences following these forms of treatment is unknown. Fluconazole is currently the least preferred option for the treatment of toenail onychomycosis since it is much more expensive, the long-term results are unclear, and the correct dosage has not been determined. No matter which therapy is used, constant topical treatment for any coexistent tinea pedis is mandatory and should probably be continued for life to attempt to prevent recurrence.

De Doncker P et al: Antifungal pulse therapy for onychomycosis: A pharmacokinetic and pharmacodynamic investigation of monthly cycles of 1-week pulse therapy with itraconazole. Arch Dermatol 1996;132:34.

Degreef HJ, De Doncker PRG: Current therapy of dermatophytosis. J Am Acad Dermatol 1994;31(3 Part 2):S25.

Guidelines of care for nail disorders: American Academy of Dermatology. J Am Acad Dermatol 1996;34:529.

Guidelines of care for superficial mycotic infections of the skin: Onychomycosis. Guidelines/Outcomes Committee. American Academy of Dermatology. J Am Acad Dermatol 1996;34:116.

Itraconazole for onychomycosis: Med Lett Drugs Ther 1996;38:5.

Scher RK: Onychomycosis: A significant medical disorder. J Am Acad Dermatol 1996;35(3 Part 2):S2.

Terbinafine for onychomycosis: Med Lett Drugs Ther 1996;38:72.

DERMATITIS MEDICAMENTOSA (Drug Eruption)

Essentials of Diagnosis

- Usually, abrupt onset of widespread, symmetric erythematous eruption.
- May mimic any inflammatory skin condition.
- Constitutional symptoms (malaise, arthralgia, headache, and fever) may be present.

General Considerations

As is well recognized, only a minority of cutaneous drug reactions result from allergy. True allergic drug reactions involve prior exposure, an "incubation" period, reactions to doses far below the therapeutic range, manifestations different from the usual pharmacologic effects of the drug, involvement of only a small portion of the population at risk, restriction to a limited number of syndromes (anaphylactic and anaphylactoid, urticarial, vasculitic, etc), and reproducibility.

Rashes are among the most common adverse reactions to drugs and occur in 2–3% of hospitalized patients. Amoxicillin, trimethoprim-sulfamethoxazole, and ampicillin or penicillin are the commonest causes of urticarial and maculopapular reactions. Toxic epidermal necrolysis and Stevens-Johnson syndrome are most commonly produced by sulfonamides and anticonvulsants. Phenolphthalein, pyrazolone derivatives, tetracyclines, NSAIDs, trimethoprim-sulfamethoxazole, and barbiturates are the major causes of fixed drug eruptions.

Clinical Findings

A. Symptoms and Signs: The onset is usually abrupt, with bright erythema and often severe itching, but may be delayed. Fever and other constitutional symptoms may be present. The skin reaction usually occurs in symmetric distribution.

Table 6–3 summarizes the types of skin reactions,

Table 6–3. Skin reactions due to systemic drugs.

Reaction	Appearance	Distribution and Comments	Common Offenders
Toxic erythema	Morbilliform, maculo-papular, exanthematous reactions.	The commonest skin reaction to drugs. Often more pronounced on the trunk than on the extremities. In previously exposed patients, the rash may start in 2–3 days. In the first course of treatment, the eruption often appears about the seventh to ninth days. Fever may be present.	Antibiotics (especially ampicillin and trimethoprim-sulfamethoxazole), sulfonamides and related compounds (including thiazide diuretics, furosemide, and sulfonylurea hypoglycemic agents), and barbiturates.
Erythema multiforme major	Target-like lesions. Bullae may occur. Mucosal involvement.	Mainly on the extensor aspects of the limbs.	Sulfonamides, penicillamine, barbiturates, and NSAIDs.
Erythema nodosum	Inflammatory cutaneous nodules.	Usually limited to the extensor aspects of the legs. May be accompanied by fever, arthralgias, and pain.	Oral contraceptives.
Allergic vasculitis	Inflammatory changes may present as urticaria that lasts over 24 hours, hemorrhagic papules ("palpable purpura"), vesicles, bullae, or necrotic ulcers.	Most severe on the legs.	Sulfonamides, indomethacin, phenytoin, allopurinol, and ibuprofen.
Purpura	Itchy, petechial macular rash.	Dependent areas. Results most typically from thrombocytopenia.	Thiazides, sulfonamides, sulfonylureas, barbiturates, quinine, and sulindac.
Eczema	Similar to contact dermatitis.	A rare epidermal reaction in patients previously sensitized by external exposure who are given the same or a related substance systemically.	Penicillin, neomycin, phenothiazines, and local anesthetics.
Exfoliative dermatitis and erythroderma	Red and scaly.	Entire skin surface.	Allopurinol, sulfonamides, isoniazid, gold, or carbamazepine.
Photosensitivity: Increased sensitivity to light, often of ultraviolet A wavelengths, but may be due to UVB or visible light as well	Sunburn, vesicles, papules in photodistributed pattern.	Exposed skin of the face, the neck, and the backs of the hands and, in women, the lower legs. Exaggerated response to ultraviolet light. On occasion, ultraviolet emission from fluorescent lighting may be sufficient.	Sulfonamides and sulfonamide-related compounds (thiazide diuretics, furosemide, sulfonylureas), tetracyclines (especially demeclocycline), phenothiazines, sulindac, amiodarone, NSAIDs, and indomethacin.
Drug-related lupus erythematosus	May present with a photosensitive rash accompanied by fever, polyarthritis, myalgia, and serositis.	Less severe than systemic lupus erythematosus, sparing the kidneys and central nervous system. Recovery often follows drug withdrawal.	Most commonly hydralazine and procainamide; less often, isoniazid and phenytoin.
Lichenoid and lichen planus-like eruptions	Pruritic, erythematous to violaceous polygonal papules that coalesce or expand to form plaques.	May be in photo- or nonphoto-distributed pattern.	Bismuth, carbamazepine, chlordiazepoxide, chloroquine, chlorpropamide, dapsone, ethambutol, furosemide, gold salts, hydroxychloroquine, levamisole, meprobamate, methyldopa, paraphenylenediamine salts, penicillamine, phenothiazines, pindolol, propranolol, quinidine, quinine, quinacrine, streptomycin, sulfonylureas, tetracyclines, thiazides, and triprolidine.
Fixed drug eruptions	Single or multiple demarcated, round, erythematous plaques that often become hyperpigmented.	Recur at the same site when the drug is repeated. Hyperpigmentation, if present, remains after healing.	Numerous drugs, including antimicrobials, analgesics, barbiturates, cardiovascular drugs, heavy metals, antiparasitic agents, antihistamines, phenolphthalein, ibuprofen, and naproxen.

(continued)

Table 6–3. Skin reactions due to systemic drugs. (continued)

Reaction	Appearance	Distribution and Comments	Common Offenders
Toxic epidermal necrolysis	Large sheets of erythema, followed by separation, which looks like scalded skin.	Rare.	In adults, the eruption has occurred after administration of many classes of drugs, particularly barbiturates, phenytoin, sulfonamides, and NSAIDs.
Urticaria	Red, itchy wheals that vary in size from < 1 cm to many centimeters. May be accompanied by angioedema.	Chronic urticaria is rarely caused by drugs.	Acute urticaria: penicillins, NSAIDs, sulfonamides, opiates, and salicylates. Angioedema is common in patients receiving ACE inhibitors.
Pruritus	Itchy skin without rash.		Pruritus ani may be due to overgrowth of *Candida* after systemic antibiotic treatment. NSAIDs may cause pruritus without a rash.
Hair loss		Hair loss most often involves the scalp, but other sites may be affected.	A predictable side effect of cytotoxic agents and oral contraceptives. Diffuse hair loss also occurs unpredictably with a wide variety of other drugs, including anticoagulants, antithyroid drugs, newer antimicrobials, cholesterol-lowering agents, heavy metals, corticosteroids, androgens, NSAIDs, retinoids (isotretinoin, etretinate), and beta-blockers.
Pigmentary changes	Flat hyperpigmented areas.	Forehead and cheeks (chloasma, melasma). The most common pigmentary disorder associated with drug ingestion. Improvement is slow despite stopping the drug.	Oral contraceptives are the usual cause.
	Blue-gray discoloration.	Light-exposed areas.	Chlorpromazine and related phenothiazines.
	Brown or blue-gray pigmentation.	Generalized.	Heavy metals (silver, gold, bismuth, and arsenic). Arsenic, silver, and bismuth are not used therapeutically, but patients who receive gold for rheumatoid arthritis may show this reaction.
	Yellow color.	Generalized.	Usually quinacrine.
	Blue-black patches on the shins.		Minocycline, chloroquine.
	Blue-black pigmentation of the nails and palate and depigmentation of the hair.		Chloroquine.
	Slate-gray color.	Primarily in photoexposed areas.	Amiodarone.
	Brown discoloration of the nails.	Especially in more darkly pigmented patients.	Zidovudine (azidothymidine; AZT).
Psoriasiform eruptions	Scaly red plaques.	May be located on trunk and extremities. Palms and soles may be hyperkeratotic. May cause psoriasiform eruption or worsen psoriasis.	Amodiaquine, chloroquine, debrisoquin, lithium, oxprenolol, pindolol, propranolol, quinacrine, and sulfonamides.
Pityriasis rosea-like eruptions	Oval, red, slightly raised patches with central scale.	Mainly on the trunk.	Barbiturates, bismuth, captopril, clonidine, gold salts, methopromazine, metoprolol, metronidazole, and tripelennamine.
Seborrheic dermatitis-like eruptions	Diffuse redness and loose scale.	On scalp, face, mid chest, axillae, groin.	Cimetidine, gold salts, and methyldopa.
Bullous eruptions	Tense blisters > 1 cm.	Hands, feet, genital areas common; other sites possible.	Aspirin, barbiturates, bromides, chlorpromazine, warfarin, phenytoin, sulfonamides and related compounds, and promethazine.

their appearance and distribution, and the common offenders in each case.

B. Laboratory Findings: Routinely ordered blood work is of no value in the diagnosis of drug eruptions. However, skin biopsies may be helpful in making the diagnosis.

Differential Diagnosis

Observation after discontinuation, which may be a slow process, helps establish the diagnosis. Rechallenge, though of theoretical value, may pose a danger to the patient and is best avoided.

Complications

Some cutaneous drug reactions may be associated with a clinical complex involving other organs (complex drug reactions). The organ systems involved depend on the individual medication or drug class. Most common is an infectious mononucleosis-like illness and hepatitis associated with administration of anticonvulsants.

Treatment

A. General Measures: Systemic manifestations are treated as they arise (eg, anemia, icterus, purpura). Antihistamines may be of value in urticarial and angioneurotic reactions. Epinephrine 1:1000, 0.5–1 mL intravenously or subcutaneously, should be used as an emergency measure. In severe cases, corticosteroids may be used at doses similar to those used for acute contact dermatitis.

B. Local Measures: The varieties and stages of dermatitis are treated according to the major dermatitis present. Extensive blistering eruptions resulting in erosions and superficial ulcerations demand hospitalization and nursing care as for burn patients.

Prognosis

Drug rash usually disappears upon withdrawal of the drug and proper treatment.

Adcock BB, Rodman DP: Ampicillin-specific rashes. Arch Fam Med 1996;5:301.

7

Eye

Paul Riordan-Eva, FRCOphth, & Daniel G. Vaughan, MD

SYMPTOMS OF OCULAR DISEASE

Redness

Redness is the most frequently encountered symptom of ocular disorders. It is due to hyperemia of the conjunctival, episcleral, or ciliary vessels; erythema of the eyelids; or subconjunctival hemorrhage. The major differential diagnoses are conjunctivitis, corneal disorders, acute glaucoma, and acute uveitis (Table 7–1).

Ocular Discomfort

Ocular pain may be caused by trauma (chemical, mechanical, or physical), infection, inflammation, or sudden increase in intraocular pressure.

Foreign body sensation is most commonly due to corneal or conjunctival foreign bodies. Other causes are disturbances of the corneal epithelium and rubbing of eyelashes against the cornea (trichiasis).

Photophobia is commonly due to corneal inflammation, aphakia, iritis, or albinism. A less common cause is fever associated with viral infections.

Itching is characteristically associated with allergic eye disease.

Scratching and burning due to dryness of the eyes are common complaints of older people but may occur at any age. Deficiency of tear film components may be due to dry environment, local ocular disease, systemic disorders (eg, Sjögren's disease), or drugs (eg, atropine-like agents).

Watering (epiphora) is usually due to inadequate tear drainage through obstruction of the lacrimal drainage system or malposition of the lower lid. Reflex tearing occurs with any disturbance of the corneal epithelium.

"Eyestrain" & Headache

Eyestrain is a common complaint that usually means discomfort associated with prolonged reading or close work. Significant refractive error, presbyopia, inadequate illumination, and phoria (usually exophoria with poor convergence) should be ruled out. (A phoria is a latent ocular deviation—discussed further below in the section on extraocular movements.)

Headache is only occasionally due to ocular disorders, but these same conditions should be considered, as well as corneal inflammation, iritis, and acute glaucoma. Headache with scalp tenderness is a major feature of giant cell arteritis, which should always be considered in older patients.

Conjunctival Discharge

Purulent discharge usually indicates bacterial infection of the conjunctiva, cornea, or lacrimal sac. Viral conjunctivitis or keratitis produces watery discharge. Allergic conjunctivitis usually causes tearing and ropy discharge associated with itching.

Visual Loss

The most important causes of blurred vision are refractive error, cataract, macular degeneration, diabetic retinopathy, vitreous hemorrhage, retinal detachment involving the macula, central retinal vein occlusion, central retinal artery occlusion, corneal opacities, and optic nerve disorders.

Monocular field loss indicates disease of the retina or optic nerve. Important causes are retinal detachment, chronic glaucoma, branch retinal artery or vein occlusion, optic neuritis, and anterior ischemic optic neuropathy. (All these conditions may of course produce bilateral visual field loss.) Lesions of the optic chiasm due to pituitary tumors characteristically produce bitemporal field loss. Retrochiasmal lesions cause contralateral homonymous field defects. The more posterior the lesion in the visual pathway, the more congruous (similar in size, shape, and location) are the defects in the two eyes. Cerebrovascular disease and tumors are responsible for most lesions of the retrochiasmal visual pathways.

Lueck CJ: Investigation of visual loss: Neuro-ophthalmology from a neurologist's perspective. J Neurol Neurosurg Psychiatry 1996;60:275. (A review of the management of visual loss for nonophthalmologists.)

Visual Impairment & Blindness

An individual is visually impaired if the best corrected distant visual acuity in the better eye is 20/80

ABBREVIATIONS & SYMBOLS USED IN OPHTHALMOLOGY

A or Acc	Accommodation
Ax or x	Axis of cylindric lens
BI or BO	Base-in or base-out (prism)
CF	Counting fingers
Cyl	Cylindric lens or cylinder
D	Diopter (lens strength)
E	Esophoria
EOG	Electro-oculography
EOM	Extraocular muscles or movements
ERG	Electroretinography
H	Hyperphoria
HM	Hand movements
HT	Hypertropia
IOP	Intraocular pressure
J1, J2, J3, etc	Test types (Jaeger) for testing reading vision
KP	Keratic precipitates
LP	Light perception
L proj	Light projection
NLP	No light perception
NPC	Near point of convergence
OD (R, or RE)	Oculus dexter (right eye)
OS (L, or LE)	Oculus sinister (left eye)
OU	Oculi unitas (both eyes)
PD	Interpupillary distance
PH	Pinhole
PRRE	Pupils round, regular, and equal
S or Sph	Spherical lens
ET	Esotropia (with L or R)
VA	Visual acuity
VER	Visual evoked response
X	Exophoria
XT	Exotropia
+	Plus or convex lens
−	Minus or concave lens
ċ	Combined with
∞	Infinity (6 meters [20 feet] or more distance)
°	Degree (measurement of strabismus angle)
Δ	Prism diopter

blindness worldwide are cataract, trachoma, leprosy, onchocerciasis, and xerophthalmia.

Diplopia

Double vision usually results from extraocular muscle imbalance. This may be caused by disturbance of third, fourth, or sixth cranial nerve function by head injury, vascular disturbance, intracranial tumors, or intraorbital lesions; disease of the neuromuscular junction due to myasthenia; direct involvement of muscle as in dysthyroid eye disease; or entrapment as a result of orbital blowout fracture. Decompensation of a phoria (latent deviation) to a manifest deviation may also be responsible. Monocular diplopia, which persists when the fellow eye is covered, is usually due to lens opacities.

"Spots Before the Eyes" & "Flashing Lights"

Spots before the eyes (floaters) are usually caused by vitreous opacities that have no significance. However, they may also be caused by posterior vitreous detachment, vitreous hemorrhage, or posterior uveitis. Sudden onset of floaters, particularly when associated with flashing lights (photopsia), necessitates dilated fundal examination to exclude a retinal tear or detachment.

OCULAR EXAMINATION

Abbreviations and symbols commonly used in ophthalmology are listed in the accompanying box.

Visual Acuity (VA)

Corrected distant visual acuity should be tested for each eye in turn, using a standardized chart such as the Snellen chart. If appropriate refractive correction is not available, a pinhole will overcome most refractive errors. The Snellen chart is annotated according to the distance at which each line can be read by a normal individual. Visual acuity is expressed as a fraction—the test distance over the figure assigned to the lowest line the patient can read. If the patient is unable to read the top line of the chart, acuity is recorded as counting fingers (CF), hand movements (HM), perception of light (PL), or no light perception (NLP). Distant acuity is usually measured at 20 feet. A corrected acuity of less than 20/30 is abnormal.

If assessment of distant visual acuity is not possible, near acuity should be tested with a reduced Snellen chart or standardized reading test types. The patient must be wearing an appropriate reading correction.

Visual Fields

Confrontation field testing is extremely valuable for rapid assessment of field defects. Use of a red target enhances the detection of neurologic field de-

or less or if visual fields are significantly restricted. Legal blindness (partial) in the USA is defined as visual acuity for distant vision of 20/200 or less in the better eye with best correction or widest diameter of the visual field subtending an angle of less than 20 degrees. There are approximately 500,000 legally blind people in the USA; about half are over the age of 65. The leading causes of blindness are glaucoma, diabetic retinopathy, and macular degeneration.

Most states in the USA require best corrected visual acuity with both eyes of 20/40 for a driving license with no restrictions. Licenses with specific restrictions may be available for those with poorer acuity. Some states also stipulate minimum visual field requirements.

WHO estimates that at least 28 million of the world's population have vision of 10/200 or less, and millions more have loss of sight sufficient to interfere with normal living. The most frequent causes of

Table 7–1. The inflamed eye: Differential diagnosis of common causes.

	Acute Conjunctivitis	Acute Uveitis	Acute Glaucoma[1]	Corneal Trauma or Infection
Incidence	Extremely common	Common	Uncommon	Common
Discharge	Moderate to copious	None	None	Watery or purulent
Vision	No effect on vision	Often blurred	Markedly blurred	Usually blurred
Pain	Mild	Moderate	Severe	Moderate to severe
Conjunctival injection	Diffuse; more toward fornices	Mainly circumcorneal	Mainly circumcorneal	Mainly circumcorneal
Cornea	Clear	Usually clear	Steamy	Clarify change related to cause
Pupil size	Normal	Small	Moderately dilated and fixed	Normal
Pupillary light response	Normal	Poor	None	Normal
Intraocular pressure	Normal	Commonly low but may be elevated	Elevated	Normal
Smear	Causative organisms	No organisms	No organisms	Organisms found only in corneal ulcers due to infection

[1] Angle-closure glaucoma.

fects. Amsler charts are the easiest method of detecting central field abnormalities due to macular disease.

Pupils

The pupils should be examined for absolute and relative size and reactions to both light and accommodation. A large, poorly reacting pupil may be due to third nerve palsy, iris damage caused by acute glaucoma, or pharmacologic mydriasis. A small, poorly reacting pupil is observed in Horner's syndrome (oculosympathetic paralysis), inflammatory adhesions between iris and lens (posterior synechiae), or neurosyphilis (Argyll Robertson pupils). Physiologic anisocoria is a common cause of unequal pupils that react normally.

A relative afferent pupillary defect, in which the pupillary light reaction is of reduced intensity when light is shined into the affected eye compared with the normal eye, is an important objective sign that usually indicates optic nerve disease. It is most easily detected with the "swinging light test," in which the pupillary light reactions are compared as a bright light is moved from one eye to the other. It is only necessary to observe the pupillary reactions of one eye to detect the presence of a relative afferent pupillary defect.

Extraocular Movements

Examination of extraocular movements begins with an assessment of whether the two eyes are cor-

rectly aligned. A misalignment of the visual axes under binocular viewing conditions is known as a manifest deviation, or **tropia.** A deviation that becomes apparent only when binocular function is disrupted is known as a latent deviation, or **phoria.** A manifest deviation may be apparent by comparing the relative positions of the corneal light reflexes. A more reliable test is the **cover test,** in which the deviated eye moves to take up fixation when the other eye is occluded. The correctional movement is in the opposite direction to that of the original manifest deviation. If no manifest deviation is present, occlusion of one eye will elicit any latent deviation because binocular function will have been disrupted. As the occluder is removed **(uncover test),** the presence of a latent deviation is then detected by any correctional movement that occurs to reestablish the normal alignment of the eyes. The presence of a latent deviation is common among normal individuals, but occasionally the effort to control it produces eyestrain.

Horizontal diplopia indicates dysfunction of horizontally acting muscles (medial and lateral recti), and vertical diplopia indicates dysfunction of vertically acting muscles (superior and inferior recti and the obliques). The false outer image arises from the affected eye. If a muscle is underacting, the image separation will be greatest in its normal direction of action. If a muscle is prevented from relaxing, image separation will be greatest in the direction opposite to its normal action. For example, a paretic lateral rectus or a tethered medial rectus of the right eye will cause maximal image separation on looking to the right.

Minor degrees of nystagmus at the extremes of gaze are normal. Other forms of physiologic nystagmus include optokinetic nystagmus and those induced by rotation or caloric stimulation. Exaggerated gaze-evoked nystagmus may be due to drugs or posterior fossa disease. Nystagmus in the primary position is always abnormal. Certain acquired forms specifically localize lesions within the nervous system. Congenital nystagmus may be a benign isolated anomaly or associated with poor vision.

Proptosis (Exophthalmos)

Proptosis may be suspected by observing widening of the palpebral aperture, with exposure of sclera both superiorly and inferiorly. (Eyelid retraction generally causes more exposure superiorly than inferiorly.) By viewing the patient from above, while the patient is asked to look down and the upper lids are lifted by the examiner, a further estimate of the degree of proptosis can be made. Exophthalmometry should be performed for objective assessment. In nonaxial proptosis, there is also horizontal or vertical displacement of the globe, indicating the presence of a mass lesion outside the extraocular muscle cone.

The most frequent cause of proptosis in adults is dysthyroid eye disease. Other causes of (usually unilateral) proptosis include cellulitis, tumors, and pseudotumor of the orbit.

Ptosis

Neurologic causes of ptosis include Horner's syndrome, in which the pupil is constricted, and third nerve palsy, in which there are abnormalities of eye movements and the pupil may be dilated. Local causes include congenital and acquired disorders of the levator muscle complex and tumors and infections of the eyelid. Myasthenia should always be considered.

Anterior Segment Examination

Although slitlamp examination is recommended for accurate documentation of anterior segment abnormalities, examination with a flashlight and loupe usually provides sufficient information for initial diagnosis. Patterns of redness indicate the site of the underlying problem. Conjunctivitis produces redness that extends diffusely across the globe and the inner surface of the lids. Keratitis, intraocular inflammation, and acute glaucoma produce predominantly circumcorneal injection. Episcleritis and scleritis cause localized or diffuse deep injection, which in the case of scleritis is associated with blue discoloration.

Focal lesions of the cornea due to infection or trauma can be differentiated from the diffuse corneal haze of acute glaucoma and from the cloudiness of the anterior chamber and perhaps hypopyon (accumulation of white cells within the anterior chamber) of iritis. Instillation of fluorescein and examination with a blue light aids in detection of corneal epithelial defects. Palpation of the globe will reveal the stony hardness of acute glaucoma.

Direct Ophthalmoscopy

Direct ophthalmoscopy is principally used for examining the retina, but much other useful information can also be gained. Assessment of the red reflex and clarity of fundal details indicates the degree of media opacity. Abnormalities may then be localized to the cornea, lens, or vitreous by variations of focus of the ophthalmoscope and use of parallax.

The optic disk should be examined for swelling, pallor, and glaucomatous cupping. Macular lesions causing poor central vision are usually apparent. The retinal vessels are examined for caliber and wall changes. Retinal hemorrhages, exudates, and cotton-wool spots are noted.

Dilation of the pupil aids direct ophthalmoscopy but should be done with caution in patients with shallow anterior chambers.

Patel KH et al: Incidence of acute angle-closure glaucoma after pharmacologic mydriasis. Am J Ophthalmol 1995;120:709. (If penlight examination did not suggest a shallow anterior chamber and there was no history of glaucoma, the risk of inducing angle closure by pupillary dilation was less than one in 333.)

OPHTHALMOLOGIC REFERRALS

Sudden loss of vision requires urgent or emergency ophthalmologic consultation. The most important causes of sudden visual loss in an uninflamed eye are vitreous hemorrhage, retinal detachment, exudative age-related macular degeneration, retinal artery or vein occlusions, anterior ischemic optic neuropathy, and optic neuritis. Sudden visual loss in an inflamed eye may be due to acute anterior uveitis, acute glaucoma, or corneal ulcer. Other ophthalmologic emergencies include orbital cellulitis, gonococcal keratoconjunctivitis, and major ocular trauma.

Any patient developing gradual loss of vision should be referred for ophthalmologic assessment. Important causes include cataract, atrophic age-related macular degeneration, chronic glaucoma, chronic uveitis, and intraorbital and intracranial tumors.

Patients with diabetes mellitus must undergo regular fundus examination through dilated pupils. Myopic patients should be warned of the increased risk of retinal detachment and made aware of the importance of reporting relevant symptoms. First-degree relatives of patients with glaucoma should be encouraged to undergo annual glaucoma screening once they have reached adulthood.

Reichel E: Vitreoretinal emergencies. Am Fam Physician 1995;52:1415. (Review of the appropriate management of ophthalmic emergencies, particularly those involving the retina and vitreous.)

REFRACTIVE ERRORS

Refractive errors are the most common cause of blurred vision. In **emmetropia** (the normal state), objects at infinity are seen clearly with the unaccommodated eye. Objects nearer than infinity are seen with the aid of accommodation, which increases the refractive power of the lens. In **hyperopia,** objects at infinity are not seen clearly unless accommodation is used, and near objects may not be seen because accommodative capacity is finite. Hyperopia is corrected with plus (convex) lenses. In **myopia,** the unaccommodated eye brings to a focus images of objects closer than infinity, the distance of such objects from the patient becoming shorter and shorter with increasing myopia. (Thus, the high myope is able to focus on very near objects without glasses.) However, objects beyond this distance cannot be seen without the aid of corrective (minus, concave) lenses. In **astigmatism,** the refractive errors in the horizontal and vertical axes differ.

Various surgical techniques are available for the correction of refractive errors, particularly myopia. Photorefractive keratectomy, in which the excimer laser is used to reshape the anterior cornea, is becoming the most widely used, but patient satisfaction is still not optimal.

Presbyopia is the natural loss of accommodative capacity with age. Emmetropes usually notice inability to focus on objects at a normal reading distance at about age 45. Hyperopes experience symptoms at an earlier age. Presbyopia is corrected with plus lenses for near work.

Use of a pinhole will overcome most refractive errors and thus allows their exclusion as a cause of visual loss. Transient refractive errors occur in diabetes—often when diabetic control is erratic—and may be the presenting feature. Autoinoculation of scopolamine from seasickness patches or atropine from vials for parenteral use leads to pupillary dilation and loss of accommodation.

Halliday BL: Refractive and visual results and patient satisfaction after excimer laser photorefractive keratectomy for myopia. Br J Ophthalmol 1995;79:881. (At 1 year following treatment, 47% of patients had lost at least one Snellen line of best-corrected visual acuity and 60% reported problems with glare.)

Seiler T, McDonnell PJ: Excimer laser photorefractive keratectomy. Surv Ophthalmol 1995;40:89. (Review of the applications and efficacy of excimer laser peripheral photorefractive keratectomy.)

Snibson GR et al: One-year evaluation of excimer laser photorefractive keratectomy for myopia and myopic astigmatism. Arch Ophthalmol 1995;113:994. (Outcome of excimer laser peripheral photorefractive keratectomy for low or moderate degrees of myopia, with or without associated astigmatism.)

Contact Lenses

Contact lenses are increasingly being used for correction of refractive errors in addition to their less frequent use in the management of diseases of the cornea, conjunctiva, or lids. It has been estimated that there are at least 24 million contact lens wearers in the USA.

The various types of contact lenses are hard lenses made of polymethylmethacrylate (PMMA), rigid gas-permeable lenses made of cellulose acetate butyrate (CAB) or silicone acrylates, and soft or hydrogel lenses based on hydroxyethylmethacrylate (HEMA). Hard lenses are much more durable and easy to care for than soft lenses but are more difficult to tolerate. Rigid gas-permeable lenses are an effective compromise.

Contact lens care includes cleaning and sterilization whenever the lenses are removed and removal of protein deposits as required. Sterilization may involve thermal or chemical methods. For individuals developing reactions to preservatives in contact lens solutions, various preservative-free systems are available. All contact lenses can be used on a daily-wear basis, ie, they are inserted in the morning and removed at night. Soft lenses are also available for extended wear. Disposable soft lenses to avoid the necessity for lens cleaning and sterilization are available for daily wear or extended wear.

The major risk from contact lens wear is corneal ulceration, which is potentially a blinding condition. Among the contact lens wearers in the USA, there are an estimated 12,000 corneal ulcers per year. Soft lenses present the major hazard, particularly with extended wear, for which there is an approximately eightfold greater risk of corneal ulceration compared with daily wear. The increased risk from extended wear begins with the first night of overnight wear and increases progressively thereafter. Disposable lenses do not overcome the risk of corneal ulceration.

Cosmetic contact lens wearers should be made aware of the risks they face and ways to minimize them, such as avoiding extended-wear soft lenses and maintaining meticulous lens hygiene. Whenever there is ocular discomfort or redness, contact lenses should be removed. If symptoms do not resolve, immediate ophthalmologic care should be sought.

Dart JKG: Diseases and risks associated with contact lenses. Br J Ophthalmol 1993;77:49. (A comprehensive review of the risks associated with contact lens wear.)

Gray TB et al: Acanthamoeba, bacterial, and fungal contamination of contact lens storage cases. Br J Ophthalmol 1995;79:601. (Microbial contamination detected in 81% of contact lens cases and recommendations provided for contact lens care.)

Schein OD et al: The impact of overnight wear on the risk of contact lens-associated ulcerative keratitis. Arch Ophthalmol 1994;112:186. (Eightfold excess risk of ulcerative keratitis with overnight contact lens wear and threefold excess risk with disposable lenses.)

DISORDERS OF THE LIDS & LACRIMAL APPARATUS

Hordeolum

Hordeolum is a common staphylococcal abscess that is characterized by a localized red, swollen, acutely tender area on the upper or lower lid. Internal hordeolum is a meibomian gland abscess that points onto the conjunctival surface of the lid; external hordeolum or sty is smaller and on the margin. The chief symptom is pain of an intensity directly related to the amount of swelling.

Warm compresses are helpful. Incision is indicated if resolution does not begin within 48 hours. An antibiotic ointment (bacitracin or erythromycin) instilled into the conjunctival sac every 3 hours may be beneficial during the acute stage. Internal hordeolum may lead to generalized cellulitis of the lid.

Chalazion

Chalazion is a common granulomatous inflammation of a meibomian gland that may follow an internal hordeolum. It is characterized by a hard, nontender swelling on the upper or lower lid. The conjunctiva in the region of the chalazion is red and elevated. If the chalazion is large enough to impress the cornea, vision will be distorted.

Incision and curettage is done by an ophthalmologist.

Tumors

Verrucae and papillomas of the skin of the lids can often be excised by the general physician if they do not involve the lid margin; otherwise, surgery should be performed by an ophthalmologist so as to avoid permanent notching of the lid. Cancer—including basal cell carcinoma, squamous cell carcinoma, meibomian gland carcinoma, and malignant melanoma—should be ruled out by microscopic examination of the excised material.

Blepharitis

Blepharitis is a common chronic bilateral inflammation of the lid margins. Anterior blepharitis involves the eyelid skin, eyelashes, and associated glands. It may be ulcerative, because of infection by staphylococci; or seborrheic, and associated with seborrhea of the scalp, brows, and ears. Both types are commonly present. Posterior blepharitis is inflammation of the eyelids secondary to dysfunction of the meibomian glands. There may be bacterial infection, particularly with staphylococci, or a primary glandular dysfunction, in which there is a strong association with acne rosacea.

Symptoms are irritation, burning, and itching. In anterior blepharitis, the eyes are "red-rimmed," and scales or "granulations" can be seen clinging to the lashes. In posterior blepharitis, the lid margins are hyperemic with telangiectasias; the meibomian glands and their orifices are inflamed, with dilation of the glands, plugging of the orifices, and abnormal secretions. The lid margin is frequently rolled inward to produce a mild entropion, and the tears may be frothy or abnormally greasy.

Both anterior and, more particularly, posterior blepharitis may be complicated by hordeola or chalazions; abnormal lid or lash positions, producing trichiasis; recurrent conjunctivitis, epithelial keratitis of the lower third of the cornea, marginal corneal infiltrates, and inferior corneal vascularization and thinning.

In anterior blepharitis, cleanliness of the scalp, eyebrows, and lid margins is essential to effective local therapy. Scales must be removed from the lids daily with a damp cotton applicator and baby shampoo. An antistaphylococcal antibiotic eye ointment such as bacitracin or erythromycin is applied daily to the lid margins with a cotton-tipped applicator. Antibiotic sensitivity studies may be required in severe staphylococcal blepharitis.

In mild posterior blepharitis, regular meibomian gland expression may be sufficient to control symptoms. Inflammation of the conjunctiva and cornea indicates a need for more active treatment, including long-term low-dose systemic antibiotic therapy, usually with tetracycline (250 mg twice daily) or erythromycin (250 mg three times daily), and short-term topical steroids, eg, prednisolone, 0.125% twice daily. Topical therapy with antibiotics such as fusidic acid 1% viscous eye drops twice daily (not yet available in USA) may be helpful but should be restricted to short courses because of possible drug toxicity.

Everett SL et al: An in vitro comparison of the susceptibilities of bacterial isolates from patients with conjunctivitis and blepharitis to newer and established topical antibiotics. Cornea 1995;14:382. (No single antibiotic provided 100% broad-spectrum coverage, and newer antibiotics did not appear to provide any advantage over established antibiotics.)

Seal DV et al: Placebo controlled trial of fusidic acid gel and oxytetracycline for recurrent blepharitis and rosacea. Br J Ophthalmol 1995;79:42. (Seventy-five percent success rate.)

Entropion & Ectropion

Entropion (inward turning of usually the lower lid) occurs occasionally in older people as a result of degeneration of the lid fascia, or may follow extensive scarring of the conjunctiva and tarsus. Surgery is indicated if the lashes rub on the cornea.

Ectropion (outward turning of the lower lid) is

fairly common in elderly people. Surgery is indicated if ectropion causes excessive tearing, exposure keratitis, or a cosmetic problem.

Dacryocystitis

Dacryocystitis is infection of the lacrimal sac due to obstruction of the nasolacrimal system. It may be acute or chronic and occurs most often in infants and in persons over 40. It is usually unilateral.

In acute dacryocystitis, the usual infectious organisms are *S aureus* and β-hemolytic streptococci; in chronic dacryocystitis, *Streptococcus pneumoniae* (rarely, *Candida albicans*).

Acute dacryocystitis is characterized by pain, swelling, tenderness, and redness in the tear sac area; purulent material may be expressed. In chronic dacryocystitis, tearing and discharge are the principal signs, and mucus or pus may also be expressed.

Acute dacryocystitis responds well to systemic antibiotic therapy, but recurrences are common if the obstruction is not removed. The chronic form may be kept latent by using antibiotic drugs, but relief of the obstruction is the only cure. The standard procedure for obstruction of the lacrimal drainage system is dacryocystorhinostomy, which involves surgical exploration of the lacrimal sac and formation of a fistula into the nasal cavity. Studies are currently going forward on a less invasive method involving balloon dilation of the site of obstruction under local anesthesia.

Ilgit ET et al: Transluminal balloon dilatation of the lacrimal drainage system for the treatment of epiphora. AJR Am J Roentgenol 1995;165:1517. (Sixty-six percent of patients were free of symptoms after the newly developed balloon dilation technique for obstruction of the lacrimal drainage system.)

Tarbet KJ, Custer PL: External dacryocystorhinostomy: Surgical success, patient satisfaction and economic cost. Ophthalmology 1995;102:1065. (Eighty-seven percent of patients were free of symptoms after the standard surgical treatment for dacryocystitis.)

CONJUNCTIVITIS

Conjunctivitis is the most common eye disease. It may be acute or chronic. Most cases are due to bacterial (including gonococcal and chlamydial) or viral infection. Other causes include keratoconjunctivitis sicca, allergy, and chemical irritants. The mode of transmission of infectious conjunctivitis is usually direct contact via fingers, towels, handkerchiefs, etc, to the fellow eye or to other persons.

Conjunctivitis must be differentiated from acute uveitis, acute glaucoma, and corneal disorders (Table 7–1).

Friedlaender MH: A review of the causes and treatment of bacterial and allergic conjunctivitis. Clin Ther 1995;17:800.

Bacterial Conjunctivitis

The organisms found most commonly in bacterial conjunctivitis are staphylococci, streptococci (particularly *S pneumoniae*), *Haemophilus* spp, *Pseudomonas* spp, and *Moraxella* spp. All may produce a copious purulent discharge. There is no blurring of vision and only mild discomfort. In severe cases, examination of stained conjunctival scrapings and culture studies are recommended.

The disease is usually self-limited, lasting about 10–14 days if untreated. A sulfonamide (eg, sulfacetamide, 10% ophthalmic solution or ointment) instilled locally three times daily will usually clear the infection in 2–3 days.

A. Gonococcal Conjunctivitis: Gonococcal conjunctivitis, usually acquired through contact with infected genital secretions, is manifested by a copious purulent discharge. It is an ophthalmologic emergency because corneal involvement may rapidly lead to perforation. The diagnosis should be confirmed by stained smear and culture of the discharge. If the cornea is not involved, a single intramuscular dose of ceftriaxone, 1 g, is effective. When the cornea is involved, a 5-day course of parenteral ceftriaxone, 1–2 g daily, is required. Topical antibiotics, such as erythromycin and bacitracin, may also be used. In such patients, other sexually transmitted diseases, including chlamydiosis, syphilis, and HIV infection, should be considered.

B. Chlamydial Keratoconjunctivitis:

1. Trachoma–(*Chlamydia trachomatis* serotypes A–C.) Trachoma is a major cause of blindness worldwide. Recurrent episodes of infection in childhood are manifest as bilateral follicular conjunctivitis, epithelial keratitis, and corneal vascularization (pannus). Cicatrization of the tarsal conjunctiva leads to entropion and trichiasis in adulthood, with secondary central corneal scarring.

The specific diagnosis can be made in Giemsa-stained conjunctival scrapings. Treatment should be started on the basis of clinical findings without waiting for laboratory confirmation. Oral tetracycline or erythromycin, 250 mg six times a day, or doxycycline, 100 mg twice a day, is given for 3–5 weeks. Single-dose therapy with azithromycin, 20 mg/kg, may also be effective. Local treatment is not necessary. *Caution:* Tetracyclines are contraindicated during pregnancy and in young children. Surgical treatment includes correction of eyelid deformities and corneal transplantation.

2. Inclusion conjunctivitis–(*C trachomatis* serotypes D–K.) The agent of inclusion conjunctivitis is a common cause of genital tract disease in adults. The eye is usually involved following accidental contact with genital secretions. Adult inclusion conjunctivitis thus occurs most frequently in sexually active young adults. The disease starts with acute redness, discharge, and irritation. The eye findings consist of follicular conjunctivitis with mild keratitis. A nontender preauricular lymph node can often be palpated. Healing usually leaves no sequelae. Cytologic examination of conjunctival scrapings shows a picture similar to that of trachoma. Treatment is with oral tetracycline or erythromycin, 250–500 mg four times a day, or doxycycline, 300 mg initially followed by 100 mg once a day, for 2 weeks. Before treatment, all cases should be appropriately assessed for genital tract infection so that management can be adjusted accordingly.

Tabbara KF et al: Single-dose azithromycin in the treatment of trachoma. Ophthalmology 1996;103:842. (A single oral dose [20 mg/kg] of azithromycin was as effective as tetracycline ointment for 6 weeks in the treatment of active trachoma.)

Viral Conjunctivitis

One of the most common causes of viral conjunctivitis is adenovirus type 3. Conjunctivitis due to this agent is usually associated with pharyngitis, fever, malaise, and preauricular adenopathy (pharyngoconjunctival fever). Locally, the palpebral conjunctiva is red, and there is a copious watery discharge and scanty exudate. Children are more often affected than adults, and contaminated swimming pools are sometimes the source of infection. Epidemic keratoconjunctivitis is caused by adenovirus types 8 and 19. It is more likely to be complicated by visual loss due to corneal subepithelial infiltrates. Local sulfonamide therapy may prevent secondary bacterial infection, hot compresses reduce the discomfort of the associated lid edema, and weak topical steroids (eg, prednisolone, 0.125% four times daily) may be necessary to treat the corneal infiltrates. The disease usually lasts at least 2 weeks.

Tabery HM: Two outbreaks of adenovirus type 8 keratoconjunctivitis with different outcome. Acta Ophthalmol Scand 1995;73:358. (Outbreak of epidemic keratoconjunctivitis successfully controlled by simple measures to interrupt transmission of adenovirus type 8.)

Keratoconjunctivitis Sicca (Dry Eyes)

This is a common disorder, particularly in elderly women. A wide range of conditions predispose to or are characterized by dry eyes. Hypofunction of the lacrimal glands, causing loss of the aqueous component of tears, may be due to aging, hereditary disorders, systemic disease (eg, Sjögren's syndrome, rheumatoid arthritis and other autoimmune disorders), or systemic and topical drugs. Excessive evaporation of tears may be due to environmental factors (eg, a hot, dry, or windy climate) or abnormalities of the lipid component of the tear film, as in blepharitis. Mucin deficiency may be due to malnutrition, infection, burns, or drugs.

The patient complains of dryness, redness, or a scratchy feeling of the eyes. In severe cases there is persistent marked discomfort, with photophobia, difficulty in moving the eyelids, and often excessive mucus secretion. In many cases, gross examination reveals no abnormality, but on slitlamp examination there are subtle abnormalities of tear film stability and reduced volume of the tear film meniscus along the lower lid. In more severe cases, damaged corneal and conjunctival cells stain with 1% rose bengal. (Rose bengal staining should be avoided in severe cases because of the intense pain it may cause.) In the most severe cases there is marked conjunctival injection, loss of the normal conjunctival and corneal luster, epithelial keratitis that may progress to frank ulceration, and mucous strands. Schirmer's test, which measures the rate of production of the aqueous component of tears by the amount of wetting of filter paper strips during a 5-minute period, may be helpful when the diagnosis is in doubt, but false-positive and false-negative results are frequent.

Treatment depends upon the cause. In most early cases, the corneal and conjunctival epithelial changes are reversible. Aqueous deficiency can be treated by replacement of the aqueous component of tears with various types of artificial tears. The simplest preparations are physiologic (0.9%) or hypo-osmotic (0.45%) solutions of sodium chloride. Balanced salt solution is a more physiologic but also more expensive preparation. All these drop preparations can be used as frequently as every half-hour but in most cases are needed only three or four times a day. More prolonged duration of action can be achieved with drop preparations containing methylcellulose (eg, Isopto Plain) or polyvinyl alcohol (eg, Liquifilm Tears or Hypo Tears) or by using petrolatum ointment (Lacri-Lube). Such mucomimetics are particularly indicated when there is mucin deficiency. Artificial tear preparations are generally very safe and without side effects. However, the preservatives necessary to maintain their sterility are potentially toxic and allergenic and may cause keratitis and cicatrizing conjunctivitis in frequent users. Furthermore, the development of such reactions may be misinterpreted by both the patient and the doctor as a worsening of the dry eye state requiring more frequent use of the artificial tears and leading in turn to further deterioration, rather than being recognized as a need to change to a preservative-free preparation. If the mucus is tenacious, mucolytic agents (eg, acetylcysteine, 20% six times a day) may provide some relief. Blepharitis should be treated appropriately (see above).

Allergic Eye Disease

Allergic eye disease takes a number of different forms, but all are expressions of an atopic diathesis, which may also be manifested as atopic asthma, atopic dermatitis, or allergic rhinitis. Symptoms include itching, tearing, redness, stringy discharge, and, in the more severe forms, photophobia and visual loss.

Allergic conjunctivitis is a benign disease, occurring usually in late childhood and early adulthood. It may be seasonal (hay fever conjunctivitis), developing usually during the spring or summer, or perennial. Clinical signs are limited to conjunctival hyperemia and edema (chemosis), the latter occasionally being so marked and sudden in onset as to cause alarm. Vernal keratoconjunctivitis also tends to occur in late childhood and early adulthood. It is usually seasonal, with a predilection for the spring. The conjunctivitis is characterized by large "cobblestone" papillae on the upper tarsal conjunctiva. There may be lymphoid follicles at the limbus. Atopic keratoconjunctivitis is a more chronic disorder of adulthood. Both the upper and the lower tarsal conjunctiva exhibit a fine papillary conjunctivitis with fibrosis, resulting in forniceal shortening and entropion with trichiasis. Staphylococcal blepharitis is a frequent complicating factor. Corneal involvement, including refractory ulceration, is frequent during acute exacerbations of both vernal and atopic keratoconjunctivitis. They are also commonly complicated by herpes simplex keratitis.

Topical lodoxamide four times daily is the recommended treatment for mild and moderately severe allergic eye disease. It is a mast cell stabilizer and is thus better used as prophylaxis than for the treatment of acute episodes. Topical vasoconstrictors and antihistamines are advocated in hay fever conjunctivitis but are of limited efficacy and may produce rebound hyperemia. Systemic antihistamines may be useful in prolonged, severe atopic keratoconjunctivitis. Topical corticosteroids are essential to the control of acute exacerbations of both vernal and atopic keratoconjunctivitis. Steroid-induced side effects, including cataracts, glaucoma, and exacerbation of herpes simplex keratitis, are major problems. Whether topical corticosteroid therapy is justifiable in allergic conjunctivitis is debatable. Systemic steroid therapy and even plasmapharesis may be required in severe atopic keratoconjunctivitis. In allergic conjunctivitis specific allergens may be identifiable and thus avoidable. In vernal keratoconjunctivitis, a cooler climate often provides significant benefit.

Friedlaender MH: Management of ocular allergy. Ann Allergy Asthma Immunol 1995;75:212. (Review of the identification and management of ocular allergic disease, stressing the infrequent need for topical steroid therapy.)

Ghoraishi M et al: Penetrating keratoplasty in atopic keratoconjunctivitis. Cornea 1995;14:610. (Encouragingly good results with corneal grafting in 11 eyes with severe corneal disease due to atopic keratoconjunctivitis.)

PINGUECULA & PTERYGIUM

Pinguecula is a yellow, elevated nodule on either side of the cornea (more commonly on the nasal side) in the area of the palpebral fissure. It is common in persons over age 35.

Pterygium is a fleshy, triangular encroachment of the conjunctiva onto the nasal side of the cornea and is usually associated with constant exposure to wind, sun, sand, and dust. Pterygium may be either unilateral or bilateral. There may be a genetic predisposition, but no hereditary pattern has been described. Pterygium is fairly common in the southwestern USA.

Histologically, pinguecula and pterygium show similar features of which the most important is elastoid degeneration of the conjunctival substantia propria.

Pingueculae rarely grow, but inflammation (pingueculitis) may occur. No treatment is indicated.

Excision of a pterygium is indicated if the growth threatens to interfere with vision by approaching the visual axis. Recurrences are frequent and often more aggressive than the primary lesion. Various forms of treatment are available to reduce the frequency of recurrence.

Chen PP et al: A randomized trial comparing mitomycin C and conjunctival autograft after excision of primary pterygium. Am J Ophthalmol 1995;120:151. (Postoperative topical 0.02% mitomycin C and the surgical procedure of conjunctival autografting were equally effective in reducing the rate of recurrence after pterygium excision.)

Paryani SB et al: Management of pterygium with surgery and radiation therapy. Int J Radiat Oncol Biol Phys 1994;28:101. (Postoperative beta-irradiation [up to 6000 , cGy total dose] with strontium-90 applicator shown to prevent recurrence after pterygium excision.)

CORNEAL ULCER

Corneal ulcers are most commonly due to infection, which may involve bacteria, viruses, fungi, or amebas. Noninfectious causes—all of which may be complicated by infection—include neurotrophic keratitis (resulting from loss of corneal sensation), exposure keratitis (due to inadequate eyelid closure), severe dry eyes, severe allergic eye disease, and various inflammatory disorders that may be purely ocular or part of a systemic vasculitis. These noninfectious conditions will not be discussed further.

Delayed or ineffective treatment of corneal infection may lead to devastating consequences through intraocular infection or corneal scarring. Prompt effective treatment is essential, and for that reason patients must be referred immediately to an ophthalmologist.

Patients present with pain, photophobia, tearing, and reduced vision. The eye is red, with predominantly circumcorneal injection, and there may be purulent or watery discharge. The corneal appearance varies according to the organisms involved.

Kirwan JF et al: Microbial keratitis in intensive care. BMJ 1997;314:433. (Three patients suffering severe bacterial keratitis while unconscious in intensive care.)

Bacterial Keratitis

Bacterial keratitis tends to pursue an aggressive course. Precipitating factors include contact lens wear, especially soft contact lenses worn overnight, and corneal trauma. The pathogens most commonly isolated are *Pseudomonas aeruginosa,* pneumococcus, *Moraxella* sp, and staphylococci. The cornea is hazy, with a central ulcer and adjacent stromal abscess. Sterile hypopyon is often present. The ulcer should be scraped to recover material for Gram's stain and culture prior to starting treatment with high-concentration (fortified) topical antibiotics, given at least every hour night and day for the first 24 hours. The initial choice of antibiotics is based on the Gram stain result. For example, gram-positive cocci are treated with a cephalosporin, such as cefazolin, 100 mg/mL; and gram-negative bacilli are treated with an aminoglycoside, such as tobramycin, 15 mg/mL. If no organisms are seen, these two agents are used in parallel. A fluoroquinolone such as ciprofloxacin, 3 mg/mL, or oxfloxacin, 3 mg/mL, may be used instead of an aminoglycoside.

Bower KS, Kowalski RP, Gordon YJ: Fluoroquinolones in the treatment of bacterial keratitis. Am J Ophthalmol 1996;121:712. (Isolates from 153 cases of bacterial keratitis were more susceptible to combination therapy with cefazolin and a fluoroquinolone than to a fluoroquinolone alone.)

Herpes Simplex Keratitis

Herpes simplex keratitis is an important cause of ocular morbidity in adults. The ability of the virus to colonize the trigeminal ganglion leads to recurrences that may be precipitated by fever, excessive exposure to sunlight, or immunodeficiency (eg, HIV infection).

The dendritic (branching) ulcer is the most characteristic manifestation of epithelial keratitis due to the herpes simplex virus. More extensive ("geographic") ulcers may also occur, particularly if topical corticosteroids have been used. These ulcers are most easily seen after instillation of sterile fluorescein and examination with a blue light. Epithelial disease in itself does not lead to corneal scarring. It responds well to simple debridement and patching. More rapid healing can be achieved by the addition of topical antivirals. Trifluridine drops or idoxuridine drops or ointment are used every 2 hours during the day. Acyclovir ophthalmic ointment may reduce the rates of recurrence and complications but is still not commercially available in the USA. Topical corticosteroids must not be used.

Stromal herpes simplex keratitis produces increasingly severe corneal opacity and irregularity with each recurrence. Topical antivirals alone are usually insufficient to control stromal disease. Thus, topical corticosteroids are frequently used in combination, but steroid dependence is a common consequence.

Corticosteroids may also enhance viral replication, leading to severe epithelial disease. Oral acyclovir, 200–400 mg five times a day, may be helpful in the treatment of severe herpetic keratitis and for prophylaxis against recurrences, particularly in atopic or HIV-infected individuals who are prone to severe herpetic keratitis. Corneal grafting is sometimes necessitated by severe stromal scarring, but the overall outcome is relatively poor. *Caution:* For patients with known or possible herpetic disease, topical corticosteroids should be prescribed only under strict ophthalmologic supervision.

Barron BA et al: Herpetic Eye Disease Study. A controlled trial of oral acyclovir for herpes simplex stromal keratitis. Ophthalmology 1994;101:1871. (Mild improvement in clinical course in immunocompetent patients with herpetic stromal keratitis when treatment with topical trifluridine and steroid drops was supplemented with oral acyclovir.)

Lamholt JA et al: Recurrence and rejection rates following corneal transplantation for herpes simplex keratitis. Acta Ophthalmol Scand 1995;73:29. (Graft survival of 84% at 1 year and only 67% at 2 years after full-thickness corneal grafting for herpes simplex keratitis.)

Uchio E et al: A retrospective study of herpes simplex keratitis over the last 30 years. Jpn J Ophthalmol 1994;38:196. (Lower rates of recurrence and complications with topical acyclovir than with topical idoxuridine in the treatment of herpes simplex keratitis.)

Wilhelmus KR et al: Herpetic Eye Disease Study. A controlled trial of topical corticosteroids for herpes simplex stromal keratitis. Ophthalmology 1994;101:1883. (Addition of topical corticosteroids to topical trifluridine in the treatment of herpes simplex stromal keratitis resulted in shorter and less severe disease but had no effect on rates of recurrence or visual outcome at 6 months.)

Fungal Keratitis

Fungal keratitis tends to occur after corneal injury involving plant material or in an agricultural setting and in immunocompromised patients. There is often an indolent course. The cornea characteristically has multiple stromal abscesses with relatively little epithelial loss. Intraocular infection is common. Corneal scrapings must be cultured on media suitable for fungi whenever the history or corneal appearance is suggestive of fungal disease.

Acanthamoeba Keratitis

Acanthamoeba has recently become a more commonly recognized cause of suppurative keratitis in contact lens wearers. Although severe pain and perineural and ring infiltrates in the corneal stroma are characteristic features, earlier forms of the disease with changes confined to the corneal epithelium are identifiable. Culture requires specialized media. Treatment is severely hampered by the organism's ability to encyst within the corneal stroma. Various agents have been used, including neomycin-polymyxin-gramicidin, the investigational agent propamidine isethionate, and various oral and topical imidazoles such as ketoconazole, miconazole, and itraconazole. Epithelial debridement may be useful in early infections. Corneal grafting may be required in the acute stage to arrest the progression of infection or after resolution of the infection to restore vision.

D'Aversa G, Stern GA, Driebe WT: Diagnosis and successful medical treatment of *Acanthamoeba* keratitis. Arch Ophthalmol 1995;113:1120. (20/50 or better visual acuity in 12 out of 14 eyes treated for *Acanthamoeba* keratitis.)

Radford CF et al: Risk factors for *Acanthamoeba* keratitis in contact lens users: A case-control study. BMJ 1995;310:1567. (Use of disposable lenses and chlorine release disinfection systems for disinfecting conventional soft contact lenses significantly increased the risk of *Acanthamoeba* keratitis.)

Herpes Zoster Ophthalmicus

Herpes zoster frequently involves the ophthalmic division of the trigeminal nerve. It presents with malaise, fever, headache, and burning and itching in the periorbital region. The rash is initially vesicular, quickly becoming pustular and then crusting. Involvement of the tip of the nose or the lid margins indicates a high likelihood of intraocular involvement. Ocular signs include conjunctivitis, keratitis, episcleritis, and anterior uveitis, often with elevated intraocular pressure. Recurrent anterior segment inflammation, neurotrophic keratitis, and posterior subcapsular cataract are possible long-term effects. Optic neuropathy, cranial nerve palsies, acute retinal necrosis, and cerebral angiitis are infrequent complications of the acute stage. HIV infection and AIDS are important risk factors for herpes zoster ophthalmicus and increase the chance of development of complications.

Treatment with high-dose oral acyclovir (800 mg five times a day for 10 days, started within 72 hours after eruption of the rash) reduces the incidence of ocular complications but not of postherpetic neuralgia. Anterior uveitis requires topical steroids and cycloplegics.

Sellitti TP et al: Association of herpes zoster ophthalmicus with acquired immunodeficiency syndrome and acute retinal necrosis. Am J Ophthalmol 1993;116:297. (Fifty-six percent of patients with herpes zoster ophthalmicus aged 45 years or less had HIV infection or AIDS, and 20% of these patients subsequently developed acute retinal necrosis.)

ACUTE (ANGLE-CLOSURE) GLAUCOMA

Essentials of Diagnosis

- Rapid onset in older age groups, particularly hyperopes and Asians.
- Severe pain and profound visual loss.
- Red eye, steamy cornea, dilated pupil.
- Hard eye.

General Considerations

Primary acute angle-closure glaucoma can occur only with closure of a preexisting narrow anterior chamber angle, as is found in elderly persons (owing to physiologic enlargement of the lens), hyperopes, and Asians. About 1% of people over age 35 have narrow anterior chamber angles, but many of these never develop acute glaucoma; thus, the condition is uncommon. Angle closure is associated with pupillary dilation and thus might occur from sitting in a darkened movie theater, at times of stress (owing to increased circulating epinephrine), from pharmacologic mydriasis for ophthalmoscopic examination, or from systemic anticholinergic medications such as atropine (eg, preoperative medication), imipramine, or inhaled ipratropium bromide. Dilation of the pupil should be undertaken with caution if the anterior chamber is shallow (readily determined by oblique illumination of the anterior segment of the eye).

Acute angle-closure glaucoma may also occur secondary to long-standing anterior uveitis or dislocation of the lens. Symptoms are the same as in primary acute angle-closure glaucoma, but differentiation is important because of differences in management.

Clinical Findings

Patients with acute glaucoma usually seek treatment immediately because of extreme pain and blurred vision, though there are subacute cases in which presentation is delayed. The blurred vision is characteristically associated with halos around lights. Nausea and even abdominal pain may occur, and for this reason acute glaucoma must be remembered in the differential diagnosis of abdominal discomfort and vomiting in elderly patients. The eye is red, the cornea steamy, and the pupil moderately dilated and nonreactive to light. Tonometry (or palpation of the globe) reveals elevated intraocular pressure.

Differential Diagnosis

Acute glaucoma must be differentiated from conjunctivitis, acute uveitis, and corneal disorders (Table 7–1).

Treatment

A. Primary: In primary acute angle-closure glaucoma, laser peripheral iridotomy will usually result in permanent cure. Intraocular pressure must be lowered beforehand. A single 500 mg intravenous dose of acetazolamide, followed by 250 mg orally four times a day, is usually sufficient. Osmotic diuretics, such as oral glycerol and intravenous urea or mannitol—the dosage of all three being 1–2 g/kg—can be used if necessary. Once the intraocular pressure has started to fall, topical 4% pilocarpine, 1 drop every 15 minutes for 1 hour and then four times a day, is used to treat the underlying angle closure. The fellow eye should undergo prophylactic iridectomy.

B. Secondary: In secondary acute angle-closure glaucoma, systemic acetazolamide is also used, with or without osmotic agents, to control intraocular pressure. Further treatment is determined by the underlying pathogenesis.

Prognosis

Untreated acute glaucoma results in severe and permanent visual loss within 2–5 days after onset of symptoms.

Dayan M, Turner B, McGhee C: Acute angle closure glaucoma masquerading as systemic illness. BMJ 1996; 313:413. (Three patients with acute angle-closure glaucoma initially were misdiagnosed as having acute abdominal or psychiatric disease.)

Hall SK: Acute angle-closure glaucoma as a complication of combined beta-agonist and ipratropium bromide therapy in the emergency department. Ann Emerg Med 1994;23:884. (A case report illustrating the risk of angle-closure glaucoma with nebulized ipratropium bromide therapy for asthma, presumed to be related to topical absorption rather than a systemic effect.)

Patel KH et al: Incidence of acute angle-closure glaucoma after pharmacologic mydriasis. Am J Ophthalmol 1995;120:709. (If penlight examination did not suggest a shallow anterior chamber and there was no history of glaucoma, the risk of inducing angle closure by pupillary dilation was less than one in 333.)

Ritch R et al: Oral imipramine and acute angle closure glaucoma. Arch Ophthalmol 1994;112:67. (Acute angle-closure glaucoma triggered by oral imipramine in four patients with narrow anterior chamber angles.)

OPEN-ANGLE GLAUCOMA

Essentials of Diagnosis

- Insidious onset in older age groups.
- No symptoms in early stages.
- Gradual loss of peripheral vision over a period of years, resulting in tunnel vision.
- Persistent elevation of intraocular pressure associated with pathologic cupping of the optic disks.
- "Halos around lights" are not present unless the intraocular tension is markedly elevated.

General Considerations

In open-angle glaucoma, the intraocular pressure is consistently elevated. Over a period of months or years, this results in optic atrophy with loss of vision varying from slight constriction of the upper nasal peripheral fields to complete blindness.

The cause of the decreased rate of aqueous outflow in open-angle glaucoma has not been clearly established. The disease is bilateral, and there is an increased prevalence in first-degree relatives of affected individuals. Glaucoma occurs at an earlier age and more frequently in blacks and may result in more severe optic nerve damage. There is increasing evidence that factors other than the level of intraocu-

lar pressure—particularly vascular abnormalities—may play a role in certain individuals in the pathogenesis of glaucomatous optic nerve damage. Elevation of intraocular pressure is also a complication of steroid therapy, whether it be topical (to the eye or periocular skin), oral, inhaled, or administered by nasal spray.

In the USA, it is estimated that 1–2% of people over 40 have glaucoma; about 25% of these cases are undetected. About 90% of all cases of glaucoma are of the open-angle type.

Clinical Findings

Patients with open-angle glaucoma have no symptoms initially. On examination, there may be slight cupping of the optic disk observed as an absolute increase—or an asymmetry between the two eyes—of the ratio of the diameter of the optic cup to the diameter of the whole optic disk (cup-to-disk ratio). Changes in the retinal nerve fiber layer may be observed as an earlier finding in some patients. The visual fields gradually constrict, but central vision remains good until late in the disease.

Tonometry, ophthalmoscopic visualization of the optic nerve, and central visual field testing are the three prime tests for the diagnosis and continued evaluation of glaucoma. The normal intraocular pressure is about 10–21 mm Hg. Except in acute glaucoma, however, the diagnosis is never made on the basis of one tonometric measurement, since various factors can influence the pressure (eg, diurnal variation). Transient elevations of intraocular pressure do not constitute glaucoma (for the same reason that periodic or intermittent elevations of blood pressure do not constitute hypertensive disease). Field testing may prove unreliable in some patients.

Prevention

All persons over age 40, particularly blacks, should have tonometric and ophthalmoscopic examinations every 3–5 years. If there is a family history of glaucoma, annual examination is indicated.

Treatment

Timolol, a β-adrenergic blocking agent, is an effective antiglaucoma agent in a dosage of 1 drop of 0.25% or 0.5% solution every 12 hours, reducing to once daily after 3–6 weeks. Alternative agents are levobunolol, 0.5%, and metipranolol, 0.1–0.6%, each used twice daily. They should not be used in patients with reactive airway disease or heart failure. Betaxolol, 0.25% or 0.5%, a β_1-receptor selective blocking agent, may be safer in patients with reactive airway disease. Epinephrine eye drops, 0.5–1%, or the prodrug dipivefrin, 0.1%, may be used twice a day either alone or in combination with betaxolol (to overcome the reduction in effect of betaxolol compared to the nonselective beta-blocking agents). Apraclonidine,

0.5–1%, an α_2 agonist administered three times a day, is helpful in controlling acute rises in intraocular pressure (such as after laser therapy) and for postponing the need for surgery in patients receiving maximal medical therapy. However its long-term use is limited by the high incidence of allergic reactions. Pilocarpine, which has been the standard drug for a century, is still used in 1–4% concentrations three or four times a day. Because of the induced myopia in younger patients and the pupillary constriction that compromises vision in patients with cataract, it is most often employed when additional therapy to either a beta-blocking agent, epinephrine, or dipivefrin is required. Latanoprost 0.005%, a prostaglandin analogue, used once daily, appears to be as effective as timolol, but permanent changes in iris color have been noted. The topical carbonic anhydrase inhibitor dorzolamide 2% is useful in patients resistant to beta-blockers, as adjunctive therapy twice a day, or when beta-blockers are contraindicated, when it can be used alone three times a day. Oral carbonic anhydrase inhibitors (eg, acetazolamide) may still be used temporarily or long-term if topical therapy is inadequate, but they are likely to be less frequently needed with the availability of dorzolamide. Laser trabeculoplasty is used as an adjunct to topical therapy to postpone the need for surgery. It has also been advocated as primary treatment. Surgical trabeculectomy is necessary for patients whose intraocular pressure remains elevated despite medical and laser therapy and may be used as primary treatment in some individuals. Adjunctive treatment with subconjunctival fluorouracil or mitomycin is used peri- or postoperatively in difficult cases to increase the chances of success of trabeculectomy.

Prognosis

Untreated chronic glaucoma that begins at age 40–45 will probably cause complete blindness by age 60–65. Early diagnosis and treatment will preserve useful vision throughout life in most cases.

Butler P et al: Clinical experience with the long-term use of 1% apraclonidine: Incidence of allergic reactions. Arch Ophthalmol 1995;113:293. (Allergic reactions—periocular contact dermatitis or follicular conjunctivitis—necessitating discontinuation of treatment in 48% of patients treated with apraclonidine.)

Diggory P et al: Avoiding unsuspected respiratory side-effects of topical timolol with cardioselective or sympathomimetic agents. Lancet 1995;345:1604. (Among 80 patients over 60 on timolol and without respiratory complaints, 21 [26%] showed evidence of significant reversible airway obstruction, with improvement in seven after change to betaxolol or dipivefrin.)

Glaucoma Laser Trial Research Group: The glaucoma laser trial (GLT) and glaucoma laser trial follow-up study: 7. Results. Am J Ophthalmol 1995;120:718. (Laser trabeculoplasty produced better reduction in intraocular pressure and better preservation of visual field than medical therapy in the initial treatment of chronic open-angle glaucoma.)

Katz GJ et al: Mitomycin C versus 5-fluorouracil in high-risk glaucoma filtering surgery. Ophthalmology 1995;102:1263. (Single intraoperative application of mitomycin C superior to postoperative subconjunctival injections of 5-fluorouracil in improving the outcome of glaucoma surgery.)

Leske MC et al: Risk factors for open-angle glaucoma. The Barbados Eye Study. Arch Ophthalmol 1995;113:918. (Major risk factors for open-angle glaucoma among black Barbadian-born citizens were age, male gender, high intraocular pressure, and family history of open-angle glaucoma.)

Strahlman E, Tipping R, Vogel R: A double-masked, randomized 1-year study comparing dorzolamide (Trusopt), timolol, and betaxolol. Arch Ophthalmol 1995;113:1009. (Dorzolamide was effective either as a substitute for beta-blockers or as additional therapy.)

Strahlman ER et al: The use of dorzolamide and pilocarpine as adjunctive therapy to timolol in patients with elevated intraocular pressure. Ophthalmology 1996;103:1283. (Dorzolamide 2% produced an effect on intraocular pressure similar to that of pilocarpine 2% when either was used in combination with timolol.)

Watson P, Stjernschantz J, the Latanoprost Study Group: A six-month, randomized, double-masked study comparing latanoprost with timolol in open-angle glaucoma and ocular hypertension. Ophthalmology 1996;103:126. (Once-daily latanoprost was as effective as twice-daily timolol in reducing intraocular pressure, with less systemic side effects but increased iris pigmentation occurring in 10% of patients.)

UVEITIS

Uveitis means inflammation of the uveal tract, which is formed by the iris (iritis), ciliary body (cyclitis), and choroid (choroiditis). Inflammatory eye disease may, however, also originate primarily in the retina (retinitis) or retinal blood vessels (retinal vasculitis).

Intraocular inflammation is classified as anterior uveitis, posterior uveitis, or panuveitis according to whether inflammatory signs are predominantly present in the anterior or posterior segment of the eye or equally distributed between the two. Uveitis may also be categorized as acute or chronic and granulomatous or nongranulomatous. In most cases the pathogenesis of uveitis is primarily immunologic, but in a significant number of patients, particularly those with AIDS or other immunodeficiency states, infection is the primary cause.

Clinical Findings

Anterior uveitis is characterized by inflammatory cells and flare within the aqueous. Cells may also be seen on the corneal endothelium as keratic precipitates (KPs). In granulomatous uveitis, these are large "mutton-fat" KPs, and iris nodules may be seen. In nongranulomatous uveitis, the KPs are smaller and iris nodules are not seen. Occasionally, granulomatous uveitis may initially masquerade as nongranulomatous disease. In severe anterior uveitis, there may be hypopyon (layered collection of white cells) and fibrin within the anterior chamber. In virtually all forms of anterior uveitis, the pupil is small, and with the development of posterior synechiae (adhesions between the iris and anterior lens capsule), it also becomes irregular.

Nongranulomatous anterior uveitis tends to present acutely with unilateral pain, redness, photophobia, and visual loss. Granulomatous anterior uveitis is more likely to present less acutely with blurred vision in a mildly inflamed eye.

In posterior uveitis, there are cells in the vitreous. Inflammatory lesions may be present in the retina or choroid. Fresh lesions are yellow, with indistinct margins, whereas older lesions have more definite margins and are commonly pigmented. Retinal vessel sheathing may occur adjacent to such lesions or more diffusely. In severe cases, vitreous opacity precludes visualization of retinal details.

Posterior uveitis tends to present with gradual visual loss in a relatively quiet eye. Bilateral involvement is common. Visual loss may be due to vitreous haze and opacities, inflammatory lesions involving the macula, macular edema, retinal vein occlusion, or, rarely, associated optic neuropathy.

Etiology

The systemic disorders associated with acute nongranulomatous anterior uveitis are the HLA-B27-related conditions sacroiliitis, ankylosing spondylitis, Reiter's syndrome, psoriasis, ulcerative colitis, and Crohn's disease. Behçet's syndrome produces both anterior uveitis with recurrent hypopyon and posterior uveitis with marked retinal vascular changes. Both herpes simplex and herpes zoster infections may cause nongranulomatous anterior uveitis.

Diseases producing granulomatous anterior uveitis also tend to be causes of posterior uveitis. These include sarcoidosis, which is commonly bilateral; tuberculosis; syphilis; toxoplasmosis; Vogt-Koyanagi-Harada syndrome (bilateral uveitis associated with alopecia, poliosis [depigmented eyelashes, eyebrows, or hair], vitiligo, and hearing loss); and sympathetic ophthalmia. Syphilis produces a characteristic "salt and pepper" fundus, often with surprisingly little visual loss unless there is also primary syphilitic optic atrophy. In congenital toxoplasmosis, there is usually evidence of previous episodes of retinochoroiditis. The principal agents responsible for ocular inflammation in AIDS and other immunodeficiency states are cytomegalovirus, herpes simplex and herpes zoster viruses, mycobacteria, *Cryptococcus, Toxoplasma,* and *Candida.*

Autoimmune retinal vasculitis and pars planitis (intermediate uveitis) are idiopathic conditions that produce posterior uveitis.

Retinal detachment, intraocular tumors, and central nervous system lymphoma may all masquerade as uveitis.

Treatment

Anterior uveitis will usually respond to topical corticosteroids. Occasionally, periocular steroid injections or even systemic steroids may be required. Dilation of the pupil is important to relieve discomfort and prevent posterior synechiae.

Posterior uveitis more commonly requires systemic corticosteroid therapy and occasionally systemic immunosuppression with azathioprine or cyclosporine. Pupillary dilation is not usually necessary.

In all cases if an infective cause is identified, specific chemotherapy may be indicated. In general, the prognosis for anterior uveitis, particularly the nongranulomatous type, is better than that for posterior uveitis.

Management of patients with uveitis must remain primarily in the hands of an ophthalmologist, but the cooperation of other physicians is essential for determining causes and in assisting in the administration of antimicrobials, high-dose systemic corticosteroids, and systemic immunosuppressants.

Rodriguez A et al: Referral patterns of uveitis in a tertiary eye care center. Arch Ophthalmol 1996;114:593. (Retrospective review of 1237 patients at a tertiary referral center reiterates the relatively greater frequency of idiopathic anterior uveitis but also points out the variety of causes of posterior uveitis.)

Rothover A et al: Causes and frequency of blindness in patients with intraocular inflammatory disease. Br J Ophthalmol 1996;80:332. (Thirty-five percent of 582 patients with uveitis had blindness or visual impairment in one or both eyes, with visual loss being particularly associated with panuveitis and disease due to either sarcoidosis or juvenile chronic arthritis.)

Tay-Kearney ML et al: Clinical features and associated systemic diseases of HLA-B27 uveitis. Am J Ophthalmol 1996;121:47. (HLA-B27 uveitis usually presents as an acute recurrent unilateral anterior uveitis in young white men. Nonocular disease was present in 58% of cases.)

CATARACT

Essentials of Diagnosis

- Blurred vision, progressive over months or years.
- No pain or redness.
- Lens opacities (may be grossly visible).

General Considerations

A cataract is a lens opacity. Cataracts are usually bilateral. They may be congenital (owing to intrauterine infections such as rubella and cytomegalovirus, inborn errors of metabolism such as galactosemia, or as yet unidentified hereditary factors); traumatic; or secondary to systemic disease (diabetes, myotonic dystrophy, atopic dermatitis), systemic corticosteroid treatment, or uveitis. Senile cataract is by far the most common type; most persons over age 60 have some degree of lens opacity. Cigarette smoking and heavy alcohol consumption increase the risk of cataract formation.

Clinical Findings

Even in its early stages, a cataract can be seen through a dilated pupil with an ophthalmoscope, a slitlamp, or an ordinary hand illuminator. As the cataract matures, the retina will become increasingly more difficult to visualize, until finally the fundus reflection is absent and the pupil is white.

The degree of visual loss corresponds to the density of the cataract.

Treatment

Functional visual impairment is the prime criterion for surgery. The cataract is usually removed by one of the techniques in which the delicate posterior lens capsule remains (extracapsular). With the development of ultrasonic fragmentation (phacoemulsification) of the lens nucleus, it is now possible to perform cataract surgery through a small incision and without suturing the wound, thus reducing the postoperative complication rate and accelerating the patient's visual rehabilitation.

It is routine practice to implant an intraocular lens at the time of surgery. This dispenses with the need for heavy cataract glasses or contact lenses. With modern techniques and improved intraocular lenses, the success rate is high. Multifocal intraocular lenses have been used with some success to reduce the need for both distance and reading glasses.

Prognosis

If surgery is indicated, lens extraction improves visual acuity in 95% of cases. The remainder either have preexisting retinal damage or develop postoperative complications such as glaucoma, hemorrhage, retinal detachment, or infection.

[AHCPR guideline on cataract in adults]
http://text.nlm.nih.gov/ftrs/pick?dbName=catc&ftrsK=6
4636&cp=1&t=858614505&collect=ahcpr

Javitt JC et al: Cataract surgery in one eye or both—a billion dollar per year issue. Ophthalmology 1995; 102:1583. (Data are presented to demonstrate the greatly increased benefit of bilateral over unilateral cataract surgery.)

Javitt JC et al: National outcomes of cataract extraction: Retinal detachment and endophthalmitis after outpatient cataract surgery. Ophthalmology 1994;101:100. (Cumulative probabilities of 0.8% for retinal detachment within 3 years and 0.08% for endophthalmitis within 1 year after outpatient cataract surgery.)

Klein BE, Klein R, Moss SE: Incidence of cataract surgery in the Wisconsin Epidemiologic Study of Diabetic Retinopathy. Am J Ophthalmol 1995;119:295. (Cataract surgery is shown to be a relatively frequent occurrence in diabetics, occurring in 25% of older diabetics during a 10-year period.)

Koch PS: The evolving technique of cataract surgery. Curr Opin Ophthalmol 1996;7:26.

Schein OD et al: Predictors of outcome in patients who underwent cataract surgery. Ophthalmology 1995;102:817. (The authors identify preoperative factors predictive of poor outcome after cataract surgery.)

RETINAL DETACHMENT

Essentials of Diagnosis

- Blurred vision in one eye becoming progressively worse. ("A curtain came down over my eye.")
- No pain or redness.
- Detachment seen by ophthalmoscopy.

General Considerations

Detachment of the retina is usually spontaneous but may be secondary to trauma. Spontaneous detachment occurs most frequently in persons over 50 years of age. Cataract extraction and myopia are the two most common predisposing causes.

Clinical Findings

As soon as the retina is torn, fluid vitreous is able to pass through the tear and lodge behind the sensory retina. This, combined with vitreous traction and the pull of gravity, results in progressive detachment. The superior temporal area is the most common site of detachment. The area of detachment rapidly increases, causing corresponding progressive visual loss. Central vision remains intact until the macula becomes detached.

On ophthalmoscopic examination, the retina is seen hanging in the vitreous like a gray cloud. One or more retinal tears, usually crescent-shaped and red or orange, are usually present and can be seen by an experienced examiner.

Treatment

All cases of retinal detachment should be referred immediately to an ophthalmologist. During transportation, the patient's head should be positioned so that the detached portion of the retina will fall back with the aid of gravity.

Treatment is directed primarily at closing the retinal tears. A permanent adhesion between the neurosensory retina, the retinal pigment epithelium, and the choroid is produced in the region of the tears by applying cryotherapy to the sclera or laser photocoagulation to the retina. In order to achieve apposition of the neurosensory retina to the retinal pigment epithelium while this adhesion is developing, an indentation may be made in the sclera with a silicone sponge or buckle, the fluid between the neurosensory retina and the retinal pigment epithelium (subretinal fluid) may be drained via an incision in the sclera, and an expansile gas may be injected into the vitreous cavity. Certain types of uncomplicated retinal detachment may be treated by the technique of pneumatic retinopexy, in which an expansile gas is initially injected into the vitreous cavity followed by careful positioning of the patient's head to facilitate reattachment of the retina. Once the retina is repositioned, the retinal tear is sealed by laser photocoagulation or cryotherapy. All the stages of pneumatic retinopexy can be performed under local anesthesia as an office procedure. The last stage is the same as is used to seal retinal tears without associated detachment as prophylaxis against detachment.

In complicated retinal detachments—particularly those in which fibroproliferative tissue has developed on the surface of the retina or within the vitreous cavity—retinal reattachment can be accomplished only by removal of the vitreous, direct manipulation of the retina, and internal tamponade of the retina with air, expansile gases, or even silicone oil. (The presence of an expansile gas within the eye is a contraindication to air travel. Such gases may persist in the globe for weeks after surgery.) (See Chapter 38.)

Prognosis

About 80% of uncomplicated cases can be cured with one operation; an additional 15% will need repeated operations; and the remainder never reattach. The prognosis is worse if the macula is detached or if the detachment is of long duration. Without treatment, retinal detachment often becomes total within 6 months. Spontaneous detachments are ultimately bilateral in 2–25% of cases.

D'Amico DJ: Diseases of the retina. N Engl J Med 1994;331:95. (Includes management of retinal detachment.)

Tielsch JM et al: Risk factors for retinal detachment after cataract surgery: A population-based case-control study. Ophthalmology 1996;103:1537. (Laser posterior capsulotomy significantly elevated the risk of retinal detachment after cataract surgery.)

VITREOUS HEMORRHAGE

Patients with vitreous hemorrhage complain of sudden visual loss, sudden onset of floaters that may progressively increase in severity, or, occasionally, "bleeding within the eye." Visual acuity ranges from 20/20 to light perception only. The eye is not inflamed, and the clue to diagnosis is the inability to see fundal details clearly despite the presence of a clear lens. Causes of vitreous hemorrhage include diabetic retinopathy, retinal tears (with or without retinal detachment), retinal vein occlusions, exudative age-related macular degeneration, blood dyscrasias,

and trauma. In all cases, examination by an ophthalmologist is essential. Retinal tears and detachments necessitate urgent treatment (see above).

Lindgren G et al: A prospective study of dense spontaneous vitreous hemorrhage. Am J Ophthalmol 1995;119:458. (Dense vitreous hemorrhage was found to be most commonly due to vitreous detachment with traction on a retinal blood vessel, proliferative diabetic retinopathy, retinal vein occlusion, or retinal macroaneurysm.)

O'Malley C: Vitreous. In: *General Ophthalmology,* 14th ed. Vaughan D, Asbury T, Riordan-Eva P (editors). Appleton & Lange, 1995. (Many helpful illustrations.)

AGE-RELATED MACULAR DEGENERATION

Age-related macular degeneration is the leading cause of permanent visual loss in the elderly. The exact cause is unknown, but the incidence increases with each decade over age 50 (to almost 30% by age 75). Other associations besides age include race (usually white), sex (slight female predominance), family history, and a history of cigarette smoking.

Age-related macular degeneration includes a broad spectrum of clinical and pathologic findings that can be classified into two groups: atrophic ("dry") and exudative ("wet"). Although both types are progressive and usually bilateral, they differ in manifestations, prognosis, and management.

Atrophic degeneration is characterized by gradually progressive bilateral visual loss of moderate severity due to atrophy and degeneration of the outer retina, retinal pigment epithelium, Bruch's membrane, and choriocapillaris. In exudative degeneration, visual loss is of more rapid onset and greater severity, and the two eyes are usually affected sequentially over a period of a few years. The exudative form accounts for about 90% of all cases of legal blindness due to this disorder. Impairment of the barrier function of Bruch's membrane (between the retinal pigment epithelium and the choriocapillaris) allows serous fluid or blood to leak into the retina to produce elevation of the retinal pigment epithelium from Bruch's membrane (retinal pigment epithelial detachment) or separation of the neurosensory retina from the retinal pigment epithelium (serous retinal detachment). These changes may resolve spontaneously, with variable visual outcome, but are often associated with neovascularization arising from the choroidal vessels and extending between the retinal pigment epithelium and Bruch's membrane (subretinal neovascular membrane). This membrane produces permanent visual loss.

Sudden visual loss in patients with exudative age-related macular degeneration occurs at the time of pigment epithelial or sensory retinal detachment or hemorrhage from a subretinal neovascular membrane. All these changes may occur in previously undiagnosed patients, in patients known to have atrophic changes, and in the other eye of patients with exudative disease. Laser photocoagulation of subretinal neovascular membranes may delay the onset of permanent visual loss but only when the membrane is far enough away from the fovea to permit such treatment. Although laser photocoagulation in patients with disease involving the fovea improves the long-term prognosis for vision, the inevitable immediate reduction in vision from the laser treatment is often not acceptable to the patient. Initial studies have suggested that low-dose radiotherapy may produce regression of subretinal neovascular membranes. Elderly patients developing sudden visual loss due to macular disease—particularly paracentral distortion or scotoma with preservation of central acuity—should be referred urgently to an ophthalmologist for assessment.

There is no specific treatment for atrophic age-related macular degeneration, but—as with the exudative form—patients often benefit from carefully prescribed low vision aids. It is important to reassure all patients that the disorder results in loss of central vision only. Peripheral fields and hence navigational vision are always maintained, though these may become impaired by cataract formation for which surgery may well be helpful. Oral vitamins and minerals, particularly zinc, have been advocated for the prevention and treatment of age-related macular degeneration, but their efficacy has not been substantiated.

Bressler NM, Bressler SB: Preventative ophthalmology: age-related macular degeneration. Ophthalmology 1995;102:1206. (Review of the current knowledge of the pathogenesis of age-related macular degeneration and ways to prevent and treat it.)

Evans J, Wormald R: Is the incidence of registrable age-related macular degeneration increasing? Br J Ophthalmol 1996;80:9. (Reports of blindness due to age-related macular degeneration increased by 30–40% between 1950 and 1990 compared with reports of blindness due to cataract, glaucoma, and optic atrophy.)

Moisseiev J et al: The impact of the macular photocoagulation study results on the treatment of exudative age-related macular degeneration. Arch Ophthalmol 1995; 113:185. (Of 100 consecutive patients with exudative age-related macular degeneration, only 26 were eligible for laser treatment and only four or five were likely to achieve long-term preservation of central vision.)

Seddon JM et al: A prospective study of cigarette smoking and age-related macular degeneration in women. JAMA 1996;276:1141. (Smoking increased the risk of age-related macular degeneration by a factor of 2.4 in women. The next article in the same journal shows the same effect among men.)

CENTRAL & BRANCH RETINAL VEIN OCCLUSIONS

The severity of visual loss in central retinal vein occlusion is variable. Younger patients may present

with near-normal acuity. Older patients present with acuities ranging from 20/40 to hand movements only. The visual impairment is commonly first noticed upon waking in the morning. Ophthalmoscopic signs include disk swelling, venous dilation and tortuosity, retinal hemorrhages, and cotton-wool spots.

In those with initially good acuity (20/60 or better), the visual prognosis is good. In those with poor initial acuity (20/200 or worse), extensive hemorrhages and multiple cotton-wool spots indicate widespread retinal ischemia, which can be confirmed by demonstrating extensive areas of capillary closure on fluorescein angiography. These eyes are at high risk of developing neovascular (rubeotic) glaucoma, typically within 3 months after venous occlusion, and should be monitored carefully by an ophthalmologist so that laser panretinal photocoagulation can be accomplished if neovascularization occurs. The visual prognosis in these cases is poor.

Branch retinal vein occlusions may present in a variety of ways. Sudden loss of vision may occur at the time of occlusion if the fovea is involved or some time afterward from vitreous hemorrhage due to retinal new vessels. More gradual visual loss may occur with development of macular edema or exudate. In a significant proportion, the occlusion is noted incidentally in patients with glaucoma, systemic hypertension, diabetes mellitus, or uveitis.

In acute branch retinal vein occlusion there are signs similar to those of central retinal vein occlusion but affecting only the retina drained by the obstructed vein. There is no specific treatment, but if retinal neovascularization develops, the area of retina affected by the initial occlusion should be laser-photocoagulated. Macular edema may also respond to laser treatment.

All patients with retinal vein occlusion should be referred urgently to an ophthalmologist for confirmation of the diagnosis and further management. It is important to look for glaucoma, systemic hypertension, diabetes mellitus, and hyperlipidemia. In younger patients, levels of protein C, activated protein C resistance, protein S, and antithrombin III should be measured. Hyperviscosity syndromes and other hematologic abnormalities are only rarely associated with retinal vein occlusions but may worsen their prognosis. Branch retinal vein occlusion is an important feature of Behçet's syndrome.

Clarkson JG et al: A randomized clinical trial of early panretinal photocoagulation for ischemic central vein occlusion—the Central Vein Occlusion Study Group report. Ophthalmology 1995;102:1434. (Panretinal photocoagulation for iris or anterior chamber angle neovascularization in ischemic central retinal vein occlusion demonstrated to be more effective when administered as soon as neovascularization has occurred than prophylactically, but this necessitates careful observation with frequent follow-up.)

The Eye Disease Case-Control Study Group: Risk factors

for central retinal vein occlusion. Arch Ophthalmol 1996;114:545. (Risk factors for central retinal vein occlusion included systemic hypertension, diabetes mellitus, open-angle glaucoma, little physical activity, low alcohol consumption, and lack of estrogen replacement therapy in postmenopausal women.)

Larsson J, Olafsdottir E, Bauer B: Activated protein C resistance in young adults with central retinal vein occlusion. Br J Ophthalmol 1996;80:200. (Thirty-six percent of patients younger than 45 years with central retinal vein occlusion had elevated resistance to activated protein C.)

CENTRAL & BRANCH RETINAL ARTERY OCCLUSIONS

Central retinal artery occlusion presents as sudden profound visual loss. Visual acuity is reduced to counting fingers or worse, and visual field is commonly restricted to an island of vision in the temporal field. Ophthalmoscopy reveals pallid swelling of the retina, most obvious in the posterior segment, with a cherry-red spot at the fovea. The retinal arteries are attenuated, and "box-car" segmentation of blood in the veins may be seen. Occasionally, emboli are seen in the central retinal artery or its branches. The retinal swelling subsides over a period of 4–6 weeks, leaving a relatively normal retinal appearance but a pale optic disk and attenuated arterioles.

The patient should be referred as an emergency to an ophthalmologist. If seen within a few hours after onset, emergency treatment—including laying the patient flat, ocular massage, high concentrations of inhaled oxygen, intravenous acetazolamide, and anterior chamber paracentesis—may influence the visual outcome. Thrombolytic therapy by direct infusion into the central retinal artery or by peripheral intravenous infusion may be more effective but is still being evaluated.

The main management problem is identifying any treatable underlying disorder. Giant cell arteritis must be excluded in all older patients, especially because of the risk—highest in the first few days—of involvement of the other eye. If giant cell arteritis is diagnosed, either on the basis of associated symptoms (especially headache or polymyalgia), clinical signs, or a high erythrocyte sedimentation rate, one should give a single dose of methylprednisolone, 250–500 mg intravenously, within 24 hours after onset, followed by high-dose systemic corticosteroids (60–80 mg prednisolone per day). Temporal artery biopsy should be obtained within 5–7 days after starting steroid therapy. Carotid and cardiac sources of emboli must be identified and appropriate treatment given to reduce the risk of stroke.

Branch retinal artery occlusion may also present with sudden loss of vision if the fovea is involved, but more commonly sudden loss of visual field is the presenting complaint. Fundal signs of retinal swelling and adjacent cotton-wool spots are limited to the area of retina supplied by the occluded vessel. Embolic causes are proportionately more common than in central retinal artery occlusion. Migraine, oral contraceptives, and vasculitis must also be considered. Antiphospholipid antibodies have been associated with branch and central retinal artery occlusions in younger patients. Patients with branch retinal artery occlusions should be referred urgently to an ophthalmologist.

Mames RN et al: Peripheral thrombolytic therapy for central retinal artery occlusion. [Letter.] Arch Ophthalmol 1995;113:1094. (Marked improvement in visual acuity in three patients treated within 6 hours after onset of central retinal artery occlusion with intravenous infusion of a thrombolytic agent.)

Schumacher M, Schmidt D, Wakhloo AK: Intra-arterial fibrinolytic therapy in central retinal artery occlusion. Neuroradiology 1993;35:600. (Improvement of visual acuity or field in 52% of patients.)

Vine AK, Samama MM: The role of abnormalities in the anticoagulant and fibrinolytic systems in retinal vascular occlusions. Surv Ophthalmol 1993;37:283. (A comprehensive review including a discussion of the role of protein C, protein S, and antithrombin-III deficiencies and antiphospholipid antibodies in retinal arterial occlusions.)

AMAUROSIS FUGAX

Amaurosis fugax ("fleeting blindness") is characteristically caused by retinal emboli from ipsilateral carotid disease. The visual loss is usually described as a curtain passing vertically across the visual field with complete monocular visual loss lasting a few minutes and a similar curtain effect as the episode passes. In order to reduce the risk of stroke, patients with high-grade stenosis (70–99%) of the ipsilateral internal carotid artery should be considered for carotid endarterectomy. Patients with low-grade stenosis (0–29%) are better treated medically with aspirin or other antiplatelet drugs. The optimal treatment for patients with medium-grade stenosis has not been determined. The assessment of carotid stenosis can be undertaken with carotid Doppler studies, but angiography may be necessary for determining the suitability for surgery of higher grade stenosis. Emboli from cardiac sources may also be responsible for amaurosis fugax. Echocardiography should be undertaken in young patients, in any patient with clinical evidence of a potential cardiac source of emboli, and in all patients being considered for carotid endarterectomy. In patients without carotid or cardiac disease, particularly younger patients, amaurosis fugax is thought to be due to retinal vascular spasm, in which case calcium channel blockers such as nifedipine, 60 mg/d, appear to be effective.

Similar obscurations of vision may occur with

poor ocular perfusion due to severe occlusive carotid disease or to aortic dissection. More transient obscurations (lasting only a few seconds to 1 minute) affecting both eyes occur in patients with raised intracranial pressure. In all cases of episodic visual loss, early ophthalmologic consultation is advisable.

Bruno A et al: Vascular outcome in men with asymptomatic retinal cholesterol emboli. Ann Intern Med 1995;122:249. (Incidentally noted retinal cholesterol emboli found to be associated with a tenfold increased risk of stroke but not with carotid artery disease suitable for endarterectomy.)

Easton JD, Wilterdink JL: Carotid endarterectomy: Trials and tribulations. Ann Neurol 1994;35:5. (A comprehensive and well explained review of the trials of carotid endarterectomy.)

Smit RL, Baarsma GS, Koudstaal PJ: The source of embolism in amaurosis fugax and retinal artery occlusion. Int Ophthalmol 1994;18:83. (In patients suspected of suffering from retinal embolism, no source of emboli was identified in 66%, ipsilateral carotid artery disease was thought to be responsible in 27%, and in only 2% was a cardiac source of emboli thought to be likely.)

Winterkorn MS et al: Brief report: treatment of vasospastic amaurosis fugax with calcium-channel blockers. N Engl J Med 1993;329:396.

RETINAL DISORDERS ASSOCIATED WITH SYSTEMIC DISEASES

Many systemic diseases are associated with retinal manifestations. These include diabetes mellitus, essential hypertension, preeclampsia-eclampsia of pregnancy, blood dyscrasias, and AIDS. The retinal changes caused by these disorders can be easily observed with the aid of the ophthalmoscope.

Diabetic Retinopathy

Diabetic retinopathy is the leading cause of new blindness among US adults aged 20–65. It is broadly classified as nonproliferative and proliferative.

Nonproliferative retinopathy is characterized by dilation of veins, microaneurysms, retinal hemorrhages, retinal edema, and hard exudates. A major subgroup are those patients in which visual loss develops owing to edema, ischemia, or exudates at the macula (diabetic maculopathy). This is the most common cause of legal blindness in maturity-onset diabetes.

Proliferative retinopathy is characterized by neovascularization, arising either from the optic disk or the major vascular arcades. Vitreous hemorrhage is a common sequela. Proliferation into the vitreous of blood vessels, with their associated fibrous component, leads to tractional retinal detachment. Without treatment, the visual prognosis with proliferative retinopathy is generally much worse than that with nonproliferative retinopathy. Severe proliferative retinopathy is often complicated by maculopathy.

Nonproliferative retinopathy is occasionally present at the time of diagnosis in maturity-onset diabetes and may be the presenting feature. Treatment includes optimizing control of blood glucose and any associated systemic hypertension or hyperlipidemia. Laser photocoagulation is particularly helpful in the treatment of focal macular edema but may also be used when there is diffuse macular edema. The presence of macular edema can be detected only by stereoscopic examination of the retina or by fluorescein angiography. The level of visual acuity is a poor guide to the presence of treatable maculopathy—hence the need for regular ophthalmologic follow-up.

Proliferative retinopathy must be recognized early and treated by panretinal laser photocoagulation to prevent blindness. Neovascularization is all too often diagnosed only at the time of vitreous hemorrhage. In some patients, a "preproliferative" retinopathy—characterized by nonproliferative retinopathy plus multiple cotton-wool spots and gross venous abnormalities—may be identified. Whether panretinal laser photocoagulation should be undertaken at this time is determined by the degree of retinal ischemia as assessed by fluorescein angiography.

Surgical treatment (vitrectomy) is being used increasingly either to remove vitreous hemorrhage and thus allow perioperative panretinal laser photocoagulation for the underlying retinal neovascularization, to deal with retinal detachments involving the macula, to manage rapidly progressive proliferative disease, or to treat persistent macular edema. Patients with diabetes mellitus should have at least yearly ophthalmoscopic examination through dilated pupils. Examination by an ophthalmologist is usually advisable in juvenile-onset diabetes of more than 5 years' duration; at the time of diagnosis in maturity-onset diabetes; in early pregnancy or prior to conception in women contemplating pregnancy; if ocular symptoms develop; or if there are suspicious findings of retinopathy, especially neovascularization or macular exudates. Failure to diagnose diabetic retinopathy by ophthalmoscopic examination is common, particularly if the pupils are not dilated. The severity of diabetic retinopathy can be lessened by careful control of blood glucose levels, but good diabetic control is more important in preventing the development of retinopathy than in influencing its subsequent course. Proliferative diabetic retinopathy, especially after successful laser treatment, is not a contraindication to treatment with thrombolytic agents, aspirin, or warfarin unless there has been recent vitreous or preretinal hemorrhage.

Chaudhry NA et al: Early vitrectomy and endolaser photocoagulation in patients with type 1 diabetes with severe vitreous hemorrhage. Ophthalmology 1995;102:1164. (Successful outcome after vitrectomy and perioperative panretinal laser photocoagulation performed within 6 months after severe vitreous hemorrhage in ten diabetics.)

Chew EY et al: Association of elevated serum lipids with retinal hard exudates in diabetic retinopathy. Early Treatment Diabetic Retinopathy (ETDRS) Report 22. Arch Ophthalmol 1996;114:1079. (A further report from the ETDRS showing an association between elevated serum lipid levels and increased risk of retinal exudates in diabetics, suggesting an additional benefit from control of hyperlipidemia apart from reducing the risk of cardiovascular morbidity.)

The Diabetes Control and Complications Trial: The effect of intensive diabetes treatment on the progression of diabetic retinopathy in insulin-dependent diabetes mellitus. Arch Ophthalmol 1995;113:36. (Intensive treatment with at least three times a day injection or pump administration of insulin led to substantially less risk [12% versus 54%] of development of diabetic retinopathy in diabetics started on treatment within 5 years after onset of disease.)

Favard C et al: Full panretinal photocoagulation and early vitrectomy improve prognosis of florid diabetic retinopathy. Ophthalmology 1996;103:561. (Retrospective review of outcome in 20 diabetics with rapidly progressive proliferative retinopathy supporting aggressive treatment with extensive panretinal laser photocoagulation and, when necessary, early vitrectomy.)

Fonseca V et al: Diabetic retinopathy: A review for the primary care physician. South Med J 1996;89:839. (A review of optimal management of diabetic retinopathy and its risk factors in the context of pregnancy.)

Javitt JC, Aiello LP: Cost-effectiveness of detecting and treating diabetic retinopathy. Ann Intern Med 1996; 124:164. (Screening and treatment of diabetic eye disease calculated at $3190 per quality-adjusted life-year.)

Klein R et al: The Wisconsin epidemiologic study of diabetic retinopathy. XV. The long-term incidence of macular edema. Ophthalmology 1995;102:7. (Follow-up over a 10-year period identified the incidence of macular edema to be 20% in patients with diabetes of onset before 30 years of age, 25% in older-onset diabetics on insulin, and 14% in older-onset diabetics not on insulin.)

Murphy RP: Management of diabetic retinopathy. Am Fam Physician 1995;51:785. (A general review of diabetic retinopathy.)

Tachi N, Ogino N: Vitrectomy for diffuse macular edema in cases of diabetic retinopathy. Am J Ophthalmol 1996;122:258. (Resolution of diffuse macular edema after vitrectomy in 57 of 58 diabetic eyes without posterior vitreous detachment.)

Hypertensive Retinochoroidopathy

Systemic hypertension affects both the retinal and choroidal circulations. The clinical manifestations vary according to the degree and rapidity of rise in blood pressure and the underlying state of the ocular circulation. The most florid disease occurs in young patients with abrupt elevations of blood pressure, such as may occur in pheochromocytoma, malignant essential hypertension, acute renal failure, or preeclampsia-eclampsia.

Chronic hypertension accelerates the development of atherosclerosis. The retinal arterioles become more tortuous and narrow and develop abnormal light reflexes ("silver-wiring" and "copper-wiring"). There is increased venous compression at the retinal arteriovenous crossings ("arteriovenous nicking"), which is an important factor predisposing to branch retinal vein occlusions. Flame-shaped hemorrhages occur in the nerve fiber layer of the retina.

Acute elevations of blood pressure result in loss of autoregulation in the retinal circulation, leading to the breakdown of endothelial integrity and occlusion of precapillary arterioles and capillaries. These pathologic changes are manifested as cotton-wool spots, retinal hemorrhages, retinal edema, and retinal exudates, often in a stellate appearance at the macula. In the choroid, vasoconstriction and ischemia result in serous retinal detachments and retinal pigment epithelial infarcts. These infarcts later develop into pigmented lesions that may be focal, linear, or wedge-shaped. The abnormalities in the choroidal circulation may also affect the optic nerve head, producing ischemic optic neuropathy with optic disk swelling. Malignant hypertensive retinopathy was the term previously used to describe the constellation of clinical signs resulting from the combination of abnormalities in the retinal, choroidal, and optic disk circulation. When there is such severe disease, there is likely to be permanent retinal, choroidal, or optic nerve damage. Precipitous reduction of blood pressure may exacerbate such damage.

Blood Dyscrasias

In blood dyscrasias characterized by thrombocytopenia and severe anemia, various types of hemorrhages are present in both the retina and choroid and may lead to visual loss. If the dyscrasia is successfully treated and macular hemorrhages have not occurred, it is possible to regain normal vision.

Proliferative retinopathy (sickle cell retinopathy) is particularly common in hemoglobin SC disease but may also occur with other hemoglobin S variants. Severe visual loss is rare. Retinal photocoagulation reduces the frequency of vitreous hemorrhage. Surgery is occasionally needed for unresolving vitreous hemorrhage or tractional retinal detachment.

AIDS

Cotton-wool spots, retinal hemorrhages, and microaneurysms are the most common ophthalmic abnormalities in AIDS patients. These microvascular changes may be the result of direct retinal infection by HIV. Cotton-wool spots are more commonly seen in patients with advanced HIV disease.

Cytomegalovirus retinitis occurs in many AIDS patients, generally when CD4 counts are below 50/μL. It is characterized by progressively enlarging yellowish-white patches of retinal opacification, which are accompanied by retinal hemorrhages; they usually begin adjacent to the major retinal vascular arcades. Patients are often asymptomatic until there is involvement of the fovea or optic nerve or until retinal detachment develops.

Ganciclovir is useful in cytomegalovirus retinitis. Therapy begins with 5 mg/kg twice a day intravenously for 14–21 days, followed by maintenance therapy of 5 mg/kg/d intravenously or 3 g daily orally. Progression of the disease is common even with treatment. Systemic ganciclovir commonly causes bone marrow suppression, which is particularly a problem if the patient is also receiving zidovudine. Systemic foscarnet, 180 mg/kg/d for 14 days followed by 90–120 mg/kg/d as maintenance therapy, is as effective as systemic ganciclovir and although less well tolerated, foscarnet may be associated with increased life expectancy. Ganciclovir and foscarnet may be used in combination. The new agent cidofovir (formerly HPMPC) has the advantage of needing only twice-weekly infusion for induction treatment and once weekly infusion for maintenance, but there is a high incidence of nephrotoxicity. Ganciclovir, foscarnet, and cidofovir are also effective when given intravitreally, either as repeated injections or, in the case of ganciclovir, as an intraocular implant, but the benefits of systemic treatment, including to the fellow eye, are then lost. Retinal detachments generally require vitrectomy and intravitreal silicone oil. The value of oral ganciclovir for prevention of cytomegalovirus retinitis is being assessed.

Other opportunistic ophthalmic infections occurring in AIDS patients include herpes simplex retinitis, toxoplasmic and candidal chorioretinitis, and herpes zoster ophthalmicus. Kaposi's sarcoma of the conjunctiva and orbital lymphoma may also be seen.

Beiser C: HIV infection—II. BMJ 1997;314:579. (Brief review of opportunistic infections in AIDS, including discussion of options in the treatment of CMV retinitis.)

Masur H et al: Advances in the management of AIDS-related cytomegalovirus retinitis. Ann Intern Med 1996;125:126.

Studies of Ocular Complications of AIDS Research Group, in collaboration with the AIDS Clinical Trials Group: Combination foscarnet and ganciclovir therapy vs monotherapy for the treatment of relapsed cytomegalovirus retinitis in patients with AIDS. The Cytomegalovirus Retreatment Trial. Arch Ophthalmol 1996;114:23. (Combination therapy with foscarnet and ganciclovir appears to be the most effective therapy in patients with relapsed CMV retinitis who can tolerate both drugs.)

Whitcup SM: Ocular manifestations of AIDS. JAMA 1996;275:142. (Case report followed by discussion of the management of various ocular complications of AIDS, particularly CMV retinitis.)

ANTERIOR ISCHEMIC OPTIC NEUROPATHY

Anterior ischemic optic neuropathy—due to inadequate perfusion of the posterior ciliary arteries that supply the anterior portion of the optic nerve—produces sudden visual loss, usually with an altitudinal field defect, and optic disk swelling. In older patients, it is often caused by giant cell arteritis, which necessitates emergency high-dose systemic steroid treatment to prevent visual loss in the fellow eye. (See Central and Branch Retinal Artery Occlusion, above.) In nonarteritic anterior ischemic optic neuropathy, causative factors include systemic hypertension, diabetes mellitus, systemic vasculitis, and inherited deficiencies of protein C, protein S, or antithrombin III. There is a significant risk of subsequent similar involvement of the fellow eye. Optic nerve sheath fenestration (also known as optic nerve sheath decompression) does not appear to provide any benefit and may be harmful. In patients with antiphospholipid antibodies or inherited deficiencies of anticoagulant proteins, warfarin anticoagulation should be considered.

Boone MI et al: Visual outcome in bilateral nonarteritic anterior ischemic optic neuropathy. Ophthalmology 1996;103:1223. (Statistically significant correlation in final outcome between eyes in patients with bilateral nonarteritic anterior ischemic optic neuropathy [NAION].)

The Ischemic Optic Neuropathy Decompression Trial Research Group: Optic nerve decompression surgery for nonarteritic anterior ischemic optic neuropathy (NAION) is not effective and may be harmful. JAMA 1995;273:625. (Results of a multicenter, randomized, single-masked trial of optic nerve fenestration for nonarteritic anterior ischemic optic neuropathy which was terminated early because of lack of benefit and possible adverse effects from surgery.)

Landau K et al: 24-hour blood pressure monitoring in patients with anterior ischemic optic neuropathy. Arch Ophthalmol 1996;114:570. (Consistently lower mean blood pressure and a delay in the usual rise in blood pressure after awakening in the morning compared with controls in patients with nonarteritic anterior ischemic optic neuropathy.)

OPTIC NEURITIS

Optic neuritis is characterized by unilateral loss of vision which usually develops suddenly and may increase during the following few days. At its worst, the level of vision may vary from 20/30 to no perception of light. Visual acuity often then improves within 2–3 weeks and frequently returns to normal. Commonly there is pain in the region of the eye, particularly on eye movements. Field loss is usually a central scotoma, but a wide range of monocular field defects are possible. There is marked loss of color vision and a relative afferent pupillary defect. The optic disk may be swollen, with occasional flame-shaped peripapillary hemorrhages. (In retrobulbar optic neuritis, the optic disk is normal.) In all forms of optic neuritis, optic atrophy subsequently develops if there has been destruction of sufficient optic nerve fibers.

Optic neuritis is particularly associated with demyelinative disease, occurring in patients known to have multiple sclerosis and as a first manifestation of the disease in others. In patients with clinically isolated optic neuritis, as many as 75% will have developed multiple sclerosis within 15 years. MRI of the brain, cerebrospinal fluid analysis, and brain stem and somatosensory evoked potentials may provide more information on the possibility of multiple sclerosis.

Optic neuritis may also occur in association with viral infections (including measles, mumps, influenza, and those caused by the varicella-zoster virus), with various autoimmune disorders, particularly systemic lupus erythematosus, and by spread of inflammation from meninges, orbital tissues, or paranasal sinuses.

Prednisolone alone has no beneficial effect on the visual outcome in acute demyelinative optic neuritis and may increase the risk of recurrent disease. Intravenous methylprednisolone (250 mg every 6 hours for 3 days) followed by oral prednisolone (1 mg/kg for 11 days, then tapered off over 4 days) accelerates visual recovery, but with a small risk of systemic side effects. This regimen reduces the risk of development of multiple sclerosis during the first 3 years after the episode of optic neuritis, particularly in patients with multiple white matter lesions on brain MRI. Whether such therapy is to be used in an individual patient should be determined by the degree of visual loss, the state of the fellow eye, the patient's visual requirements, the results of brain MRI, and the patient's susceptibility to systemic side effects from steroid therapy. Optic neuritis due to herpes zoster or systemic lupus erythematosus generally has a poorer prognosis than other forms of optic neuritis and also requires high-dose intravenous steroid therapy. All patients with optic neuritis should be referred urgently for neuro-ophthalmologic assessment. Any patient with a clinical diagnosis of isolated optic neuritis in which visual recovery does not occur requires further investigation, particularly to exclude a compressive lesion or an intrinsic optic nerve tumor.

Beck RW et al: What we have learned from the Optic Neuritis Treatment Trial. Ophthalmology 1995;102:1504.

Beck RW: The Optic Neuritis Treatment Trial: Three-year follow-up results. Arch Ophthalmol 1995;113:136. (Temporary reduction in the development of clinically definite multiple sclerosis by treatment of isolated optic neuritis with intravenous followed by oral corticosteroids.)

Rodriguez M et al: Optic neuritis: A population-based study in Olmstead County, Minnesota. Neurology 1995;45:244. (Thirty-nine percent of patients presenting with isolated optic neuritis developed clinically definite multiple sclerosis by 10 years of follow-up.)

OPTIC DISK SWELLING

Optic disk swelling may result from intraocular disease, orbital and optic nerve lesions, severe hypertensive retinochoroidopathy, or raised intracranial pressure. Intraocular causes include central retinal vein occlusion, posterior uveitis, and posterior scleritis. Optic nerve lesions causing disk swelling include optic neuritis, anterior ischemic optic neuropathy; optic disk drusen (pseudopapilledema); optic nerve sheath meningioma; and optic nerve infiltration by sarcoidosis, leukemia, or lymphoma. Any orbital lesion causing optic nerve compression may produce disk swelling.

Papilledema (optic disk swelling due to raised intracranial pressure) is usually bilateral and most commonly produces enlargement of the blind spot without loss of acuity. Chronic papilledema, as occurs in idiopathic intracranial hypertension (previously known as benign intracranial hypertension) and dural venous sinus occlusion, may be associated with progressive visual field loss and occasionally profound loss of acuity. All patients with chronic papilledema must be monitored carefully, especially their visual fields, and optic nerve sheath fenestration (also known as optic nerve sheath decompression) or lumboperitoneal shunt should be considered in those with progressive visual failure not controlled by medical therapy (weight loss where appropriate and acetazolamide).

Optic disk drusen should be considered when disk swelling is not associated with any visual disturbance or symptoms of raised intracranial pressure. Exposed optic disk drusen may be obvious clinically or can be demonstrated by their autofluorescence. Buried drusen are best detected by orbital ultrasound or CT scanning. Other family members may be similarly affected.

Kheterpal S et al: Imaging of optic disc drusen: A comparative study. Eye 1995;9:67. (B-mode ultrasonography was more reliable than CT scanning or fluorescein angiography in demonstrating optic disk drusen in four patients.)

Mauriello JA et al: Management of visual loss after optic nerve sheath decompression in patients with pseudotumor cerebri. Ophthalmology 1995;102:441. (Lumboperitoneal shunting resulted in stabilization or recovery of vision in four of five patients suffering visual loss within 1 month after optic nerve sheath fenestration for idiopathic intracranial hypertension.)

Sugerman HJ et al: Effects of surgically induced weight loss on idiopathic intracranial hypertension in morbid obesity. Neurology 1995;45:1655. (Return to normal or almost normal cerebrospinal fluid pressure levels following gastric surgery in eight patients with intracranial hypertension and morbid obesity.)

OCULAR MOTOR PALSIES

In complete **third nerve paralysis,** there is complete ptosis and the eye is divergent and slightly depressed. Extraocular movements are restricted in all directions except laterally (preserved lateral rectus function). Intact fourth nerve (superior oblique) function is detected by the presence of inward rotation on attempted depression of the eye.

Pupillary involvement (dilated pupil that does not react to accommodation or to light shined in either eye) is an important sign differentiating "surgical" from "medical" causes of isolated third nerve palsy. (Compressive lesions of the third nerve, such as aneurysm of the posterior communicating artery and uncal herniation due to a supratentorial mass lesion, characteristically have pupillary involvement.) It is crucial that patients presenting with isolated third nerve palsy with pupillary involvement be assumed to have a posterior communicating artery aneurysm until this has been excluded by cerebral arteriography—and thus they should be referred immediately for neuro-ophthalmologic assessment. Medical causes of isolated third nerve palsy include diabetes, systemic hypertension, syphilis, and giant cell arteritis.

Fourth nerve paralysis causes upward deviation of the eye with failure of depression on adduction. There is vertical diplopia that becomes most apparent on attempted reading and descending stairs. Many cases of isolated fourth nerve palsy are due to decompensation of a congenital lesion. Trauma is a major cause of acquired—particularly bilateral—fourth nerve palsy, but cerebral neoplasms and medical causes such as in third nerve palsies should also be considered.

Sixth nerve paralysis causes convergent squint in the primary position with failure of abduction of the affected eye, producing horizontal diplopia that increases on gaze to the affected side and on looking into the distance. It is an important sign of raised intracranial pressure, particularly in children. Sixth nerve palsy may also be due to trauma, neoplasms, brain stem lesions, or medical causes (see above).

An intracranial or intraorbital mass lesion should be considered in any patient presenting with an isolated ocular motor palsy. In patients with isolated ocular motor nerve palsies presumed to be due to medical causes, CT or MRI must be performed if recovery has not begun within 3 months.

Ocular motor nerve palsies occurring in association with other neurologic signs may be due to lesions in the brain stem, around the cavernous sinus, or in the orbit. Lesions around the cavernous sinus involve the upper divisions of the trigeminal nerve, the ocular motor nerves, and occasionally the optic chiasm. Orbital apex lesions involve the optic nerve and the ocular motor nerves.

Myasthenia and dysthyroid eye disease must always be considered in the differential diagnosis of disordered extraocular movements.

Keane JR: Fourth nerve palsy: Historical review and study of 215 patients. Neurology 1993;43:2439. (Etiology in hospitalized patients.)

Renowden SA, Harris KM, Hourihan MD: Isolated atraumatic third nerve palsy: Clinical features and imaging techniques. Br J Radiol 1993;66:1111. (Clinical findings failed to reliably indicate the etiology, but pupillary involvement was generally indicative of a compressive lesion.)

DYSTHYROID EYE DISEASE

Dysthyroid eye disease is a clinical syndrome caused by deposition of mucopolysaccharides and infiltration with chronic inflammatory cells of the orbital tissues, particularly the extraocular muscles. Patients may have clinical or laboratory evidence of thyroid dysfunction, elevated thyroid autoantibodies, or no detectable abnormality outside the orbit.

The primary clinical features are proptosis, lid retraction and lid lag, conjunctival chemosis and episcleral inflammation, and extraocular muscle abnormalities due to restriction of their actions. Resulting symptoms are cosmetic abnormalities, surface irritation, which usually responds to artificial tears, and diplopia, which should be treated conservatively (eg, with prisms) in the active stages of the disease and only by surgery when the disease has been static for at least 6 months.

The important complications are corneal exposure and optic nerve compression, both of which may lead to profound visual loss. Treatment is by urgent orbital decompression, either medically, with high-dose systemic steroids (prednisolone 80–100 mg/d)—although this is often of only short-term benefit—by radiotherapy, or, most effectively, by surgery, usually consisting of extensive removal of bone from the medial, inferior, and lateral walls of the orbit.

The optimal management of moderately severe dysthyroid eye disease without visual loss is controversial. Oral steroids, radiotherapy, and surgical decompression have all been advocated, but there is a risk of serious local or systemic side-effects from all three. Lateral tarsorrhaphy may be used for moderately severe corneal exposure. Other lid procedures are particularly useful for correcting lid retraction but should not be undertaken until the orbital disease is quiescent and orbital decompression or extraocular muscle surgery has been undertaken if necessary.

Hutchison BM, Kyle PM: Long-term visual outcome following orbital decompression for dysthyroid eye disease. Eye 1995;9:578. (Results of bilateral inferior and medial orbital wall decompression for compressive optic neuropathy in 33 patients with dysthyroid eye disease, 14 requiring further treatment.)

Lyons CJ, Rootman J: Orbital decompression for disfiguring exophthalmos in thyroid orbitopathy. Ophthalmology 1994;101:223. (Results in 34 patients.)

Prummel MF et al: Randomised double-blind trial of prednisone versus radiotherapy in Graves' ophthalmopathy. Lancet 1993;342:949.

Yeatts RP: Graves' ophthalmopathy. Med Clin North Am 1995;79:195. (A review of the various manifestations of dysthyroid eye disease and their management.)

ORBITAL CELLULITIS

Orbital cellulitis is manifested by an abrupt onset of fever, proptosis, restriction of extraocular movements, and swelling and redness of the lids, usually in a child. Infection of the paranasal sinuses is the usual underlying cause. Immediate treatment with intravenous antibiotics is necessary to prevent optic nerve damage and spread of infection to the cavernous sinuses—manifested as increased restriction of extraocular movements, impaired visual acuity, diminished pupillary reflexes, and papilledema, all of which may be bilateral—meninges, and brain. The response to antibiotics is usually excellent, but abscess formation may necessitate surgical drainage.

OCULAR TRAUMA

Conjunctival & Corneal Foreign Bodies

If a patient complains of "something in my eye" and gives a consistent history, a foreign body is usually present on the cornea or under the upper lid even though it may not be readily visible. Visual acuity should be tested before treatment is instituted, as a basis for comparison in the event of complications.

After a local anesthetic (eg, proparacaine, 0.5%) is instilled, the eye is examined with the aid of a hand flashlight, using oblique illumination, and loupe. Corneal foreign bodies may be made more apparent by the instillation of sterile fluorescein. They are then removed with a sterile wet cotton-tipped applicator. Polymyxin-bacitracin ophthalmic ointment should be instilled. It is not necessary to patch the eye, but the patient must be examined 24 hours later for secondary infection of the crater. If a corneal foreign body cannot be removed in this manner, the patient should be referred to an ophthalmologist.

Steel foreign bodies usually leave a diffuse rust ring. This requires excision of the affected tissue and is best done under local anesthesia using a slitlamp. *Caution:* Anesthetic drops should not be given to the patient for self-administration.

If there is no infection, a layer of corneal epithelial cells will line the crater within 24 hours. It should be emphasized that the intact corneal epithelium forms an effective barrier to infection, but once it is disturbed the cornea becomes extremely susceptible to infection. Early infection is manifested by a white necrotic area around the crater and a small amount of gray exudate. These patients should be referred immediately to an ophthalmologist, since untreated corneal infection may lead to severe corneal ulceration, panophthalmitis, and loss of the eye.

In the case of a foreign body under the upper lid, a local anesthetic is instilled and the lid is everted by grasping the lashes gently and exerting pressure on the mid portion of the outer surface of the upper lid with an applicator. If a foreign body is present, it can easily be removed by passing a wet sterile cotton-tipped applicator across the conjunctival surface.

Intraocular Foreign Body

Intraocular foreign body requires emergency treatment by an ophthalmologist. Patients giving a history of "something hitting the eye"—particularly if it happens while hammering on metal or using grinding equipment—must be carefully assessed for the possibility of an intraocular foreign body, especially when no corneal foreign body is seen, a corneal or scleral wound is apparent, or there is marked visual loss or media opacity. Such patients must be treated as for corneal laceration (see below) and referred without delay to an ophthalmologist. Intraocular foreign bodies significantly increase the risk of intraocular infection.

Corneal Abrasions

A patient with a corneal abrasion complains of severe pain and photophobia. There is often a history of trauma to the eye, commonly involving a fingernail, piece of paper, or contact lens. Visual acuity is recorded, and the cornea and conjunctiva are examined with a light and loupe to rule out a foreign body. If an abrasion is suspected but cannot be seen, sterile fluorescein is instilled into the conjunctival sac: the area of corneal abrasion will stain a deeper green than the surrounding cornea.

Treatment includes polymyxin-bacitracin ophthalmic ointment and application of a bandage with firm pressure to prevent movement of the lid. The patient should rest at home, keeping the fellow eye closed, and should be observed the following day to be certain the cornea has healed. Recurrent corneal erosion may follow corneal abrasions.

Contusions

Contusion injuries of the eye and surrounding structures may cause ecchymosis ("black eye"), subconjunctival hemorrhage, edema or rupture of the cornea, hemorrhage into the anterior chamber (hyphema), rupture of the root of the iris (iridodialysis), paralysis of the pupillary sphincter, paralysis of the muscles of accommodation, cataract, dislocation of the lens, vitreous hemorrhage, retinal hemorrhage and edema (most common in the macular area), detachment of the retina, rupture of the choroid, fracture of the orbital floor ("blowout fracture"), or optic nerve injury. Many of these injuries are immediately obvious; others may not become apparent for days or weeks. Patients with moderate to severe contusions should be seen by an ophthalmologist.

Any injury severe enough to cause hyphema involves the danger of secondary hemorrhage, which may cause intractable glaucoma with permanent visual loss. Any patient with traumatic hyphema should be advised to rest quietly until complete resolution has occurred. Daily ophthalmologic assessment is essential. Aspirin and related drugs increase the risk of secondary hemorrhage and must be avoided.

Steinsapir KD, Goldberg RA: Traumatic optic neuropathy. Surv Ophthalmol 1994;38:487. (A comprehensive review of the pathogenesis and treatment of optic nerve trauma.)

Lacerations

A. Lids: If the lid margin is lacerated, the patient should be referred for specialized care, since permanent notching may result. Lacerations of the lower eyelid near the inner canthus often sever the lower canaliculus. Lid lacerations not involving the margin may be sutured just like any other skin laceration.

B. Conjunctiva: In superficial lacerations of the conjunctiva, sutures are not necessary. In order to prevent infection, sulfonamides or other antibiotics are instilled into the eye until the laceration is healed.

C. Cornea or Sclera: Patients with suspected corneal or scleral lacerations must be seen by an ophthalmologist as soon as possible. Manipulation is kept to a minimum, since pressure may result in extrusion of the intraocular contents. The eye is bandaged lightly and covered with a metal shield that rests on the orbital bones above and below. The patient should be instructed not to squeeze the eye shut and to remain as quiet as possible. The eye is routinely studied radiographically to exclude the presence of metallic foreign bodies.

Ultraviolet Keratitis (Actinic Keratitis)

Ultraviolet burns of the cornea are usually caused by use of a sunlamp without eye protection, exposure to a welding arc, or exposure to the sun when skiing ("snow blindness"). There are no immediate symptoms, but about 6–12 hours later the patient complains of agonizing pain and severe photophobia. Slitlamp examination after instillation of sterile fluorescein shows diffuse punctate staining of both corneas.

Treatment consists of binocular patching and instillation of 1–2 drops of 1% cyclopentolate (to relieve the discomfort of ciliary spasm). All patients recover within 24–48 hours without complications. Local anesthetics should not be prescribed.

Chemical Conjunctivitis & Keratitis

Chemical burns are treated by irrigation of the eyes with saline solution or plain water as soon as possible after exposure. Neutralization of an acid with an alkali or vice versa generates heat and may cause further damage. Alkali injuries are more serious and require prolonged irrigation, since alkalies are not precipitated by the proteins of the eye as are acids. It is important to remove any retained particulate matter such as is typically present in injuries involving cement and building plaster. This may require double eversion of the upper lid. The pupil should be dilated with 0.2% scopolamine or 2% atropine, 1 drop twice a day, to relieve discomfort and prophylactic topical antibiotics should be started. In moderate to severe injuries, intensive topical corticosteroids and topical and systemic vitamin C are also necessary. Complications include mucus deficiency, scarring of the cornea and conjunctiva, symblepharon (adhesions between the tarsal and bulbar conjunctiva), tear duct obstruction, and secondary infection.

Desai P et al: Incidence of cases of ocular trauma admitted to hospital and incidence of blinding complications. Br J Ophthalmol 1996;80:592. (A study from Scotland demonstrating that over half of blinding injuries occur in the home.)

PRINCIPLES OF TREATMENT OF OCULAR INFECTIONS

Before one can determine the drug of choice, the causative organisms must be identified, but in most instances empirical treatment, based on clinical experience, is used in the first instance. In the treatment of conjunctivitis and for prophylaxis against ocular infection, it is preferable to use a drug that is not given systemically. Of the available local antibacterial agents, the sulfonamides are effective and inexpensive. Two reliable sulfonamides for ophthalmic use are sulfisoxazole and sodium sulfacetamide. The sulfonamides have the added advantages of low allergenicity and effectiveness against the chlamydial group of organisms. They are available in ointment or solution form. Combined bacitracin-polymyxin ointment is often used prophylactically after corneal foreign body removal for the protection it affords against both gram-positive and gram-negative organisms.

Among the most effective broad-spectrum antibiotics for ophthalmic use are gentamicin, tobramycin, neomycin, and ciprofloxacin. These drugs have some effect against gram-negative as well as gram-positive organisms but are generally not effective against the pneumococcus, for which penicillin G or nafcillin (if beta-lactamase resistance is present) is required. Allergic reactions to neomycin are common. Other antibiotics frequently used are erythromycin, the tetracyclines, and the cephalosporins.

Method of Administration

Most ocular anti-infective drugs are administered locally. Ointments have greater therapeutic effectiveness than solutions, since contact can be maintained longer. However, they do cause blurring of vision; if this must be avoided, solutions should be used.

Systemic administration is required for all intraocular infections, orbital cellulitis, dacryocystitis, gonococcal keratoconjunctivitis, inclusion conjunctivitis, and severe external infection that does not respond to local treatment.

TECHNIQUES USED IN THE TREATMENT OF OCULAR DISORDERS

Table 7–2 lists commonly used ophthalmic drugs and their indications and costs.

Instilling Medications

The patient is placed in a chair with head tilted back, both eyes open, and looking up. The lower lid is retracted slightly, and 2 drops of liquid are instilled into the lower cul-de-sac. The patient looks down while finger contact is maintained, so that the eyes are not squeezed shut. Ointments are instilled in the same general manner.

For self-medication, the same techniques are used except that medications are usually better instilled with the patient lying down.

Eye Bandage

Most eye bandages should be applied firmly enough to hold the lid securely against the cornea. An ordinary patch consisting of gauze-covered cotton is usually sufficient. Tape is applied from the cheek to the forehead.

PRECAUTIONS IN MANAGEMENT OF OCULAR DISORDERS

Use of Local Anesthetics

Unsupervised self-administration of local anesthetics is dangerous because the patient may further injure an anesthetized eye without knowing it. The drug may also interfere with the normal healing process.

Pupillary Dilation

Dilating the pupil can very occasionally precipitate acute glaucoma if the patient has a narrow anterior chamber angle and should be undertaken with caution if the anterior chamber is obviously shallow

(readily determined by oblique illumination of the anterior segment of the eye). A short-acting mydriatic such as tropicamide should be used and the patient warned to report immediately if ocular discomfort or redness develops. Angle closure is probably more likely to occur if pilocarpine is used to overcome pupillary dilation than if the pupil is allowed to constrict naturally.

Talks SJ et al: Angle closure glaucoma and diagnostic mydriasis. Lancet 1993;342:1493. (Only three out of 117 cases of acute angle-closure glaucoma were caused by diagnostic pupillary dilation.)

Local Corticosteroid Therapy

Repeated use of local corticosteroids presents several hazards: herpes simplex (dendritic) keratitis, fungal infection, open-angle glaucoma, and cataract formation. Furthermore, perforation of the cornea may occur when the corticosteroids are used for herpes simplex keratitis.

Contaminated Eye Medications

Ophthalmic solutions are prepared with the same degree of care as fluids intended for intravenous administration, but once bottles are opened there is always a risk of contamination, particularly with solutions of tetracaine, proparacaine, fluorescein, and any preservative-free preparations. The most dangerous is fluorescein, as this solution is frequently contaminated with *P aeruginosa,* an organism that can rapidly destroy the eye. Sterile fluorescein filter paper strips are now available and are recommended for use in place of fluorescein solutions.

Whether in plastic or glass containers, eye solutions should not remain in use for long periods after the bottle is opened. Four weeks after opening is an absolute maximal time to use a solution containing preservatives before discarding. Preservative-free preparations should be kept refrigerated and discarded within 1 week after opening. Any solution should of course be checked for signs of bacterial contamination prior to use.

If the eye has been injured accidentally or by surgical trauma, it is of the greatest importance to use freshly opened bottles of sterile medications or single-use eyedropper units.

Toxic & Hypersensitivity Reactions to Topical Therapy

Patients receiving long-term topical therapy may develop local toxic or hypersensitivity reactions to the active agent or preservatives, especially if there is inadequate tear secretion. Preservatives in contact lens cleaning solutions may produce similar problems. Burning and soreness are exacerbated by drop instillation or contact lens insertion; occasionally, fibrosis and scarring of the conjunctiva and cornea may occur.

Table 7–2. Ophthalmic agents.

Agent	Cost/Size[1]	Sig	Indications
AGENTS FOR GLAUCOMA AND INTRAOCULAR HYPERTENSION			
Sympathomimetics			
Apraclonidine HCl 0.5% solution (Iopidine)	$37.19/5 mL $71.88/10 mL	1 or 2 drops three times daily	To control or prevent elevations of intraocular pressure after laser trabeculoplasty or iridotomy.
Apraclonidine HCl 1% solution (Iopidine)	$12.50/0.2 mL	1 drop 1 hour before and immediately after anterior segment laser surgery	Reduction of intraocular pressure. Expensive. Reserve for treatment of resistant cases.
Dipivefrin HCl 0.1% solution (various)[2]	$13.47/5 mL $24.03/10 mL $35.32/15 mL	1 drop every 12 hours	Open-angle glaucoma
Epinephrine HCl 0.1% solution (Epinephrine Dropperettes)		1 or 2 drops once or twice daily	
Epinephrine HCl 0.25%, 0.5% (Epifrin), 1%, and 2% solution (various)[3]	0.5%: $32.15/15 mL 1%: $34.47/15 mL 2%: $37.72/15 mL	1 or 2 drops once or twice daily	
Epinephryl borate 0.5%, 1% solution (various)	1%: $16.88/7.5 mL	1 or 2 drops once or twice daily	
Beta-adrenergic blocking agents			
Betaxolol HCl 0.5% solution (Betoptic) and 0.25% suspension (Betoptic S)[4]	0.5%: $10.63/2.5 mL, $38.44/10 mL, $57.50/15 mL 0.25%: $10.63/2.5 mL, $20.63/5 mL, $38.44/10 mL, $57.50/15 mL	1 drop twice daily	Reduction of intraocular pressure
Carteolol HCl 1% solution (Ocupress)[5]	$18.17/5 mL $34.28/10 mL	1 drop twice daily	
Levobunolol HCl 0.25% and 8.5% solution (Betagen)	0.25%: $16.72/5 mL or $33.14/10 mL 0.5%: $9.04/2 mL, $19.99/5 mL, $41.56/10 mL, $58.35/15 mL	1 drop once or twice daily	
Metipranolol HCl 0.3% solution (OptiPranolol)	$12.95/5 mL $20.95/10 mL	1 drop twice daily	
Timolol 0.25% and 0.5% solution (Betimol)	0.25%: $10.79/5 mL, $20.85/10 mL, $31.20/15 mL 0.5%: $12.76/5 mL, $24.75/10 mL, $37.06/15 mL	1 drop twice daily	
Timolol maleate 0.25% and 0.5% solution (Timoptic) and 0.25% and 0.5% gel (Timoptic-XE)	0.25% solution: $12.45/5 mL 0.5% solution: $14.73/ 5 mL 0.25% gel: $18.09/ 5 mL 0.5% gel: $21.49/5 mL	1 drop twice daily	
Miotics, direct-acting			
Carbachol, 0.75%, 1.5%, 2.25% (Isopto Carbachol), and 3% solution (various)[6]	0.75%: $18.75/15 mL 1.5%: $19.69/15 mL 2.25%: $20.63/15 mL 3%: $21.87/15 mL	1 or 2 drops up to three times daily	Reduction of intraocular pressure
Pilocarpine HCl 0.25% solution (Isopto Carpine)[7]	$13.75/15 mL	1 or 2 drops up to six times daily	Reduction of intraocular pressure, treatment of acute or chronic angle-closure glaucoma, and pupillary constriction.

(continued)

Table 7–2. Ophthalmic agents. (continued)

Agent	Cost/Size[1]	Sig	Indications
Pilocarpine HCl (various)	0.5%: $4.57/15 mL 1%: $6.13/15 mL 2%: $7.55/15 mL 3%: $7.49/15 mL 4%: $8.16/15 mL 6%: $12.08/15 mL 8%: $18.75/15 mL 10%: $21.25/15 mL	1 or 2 drops up to six times daily[8]	Reduction of intraocular pressure, treatment of acute or chronic angle-closure glaucoma, and pupillary constriction.
Pilocarpine HCl 4% gel (Pilopine HS)	$25.00/4 g	Apply 0.5-inch ribbon in lower conjunctival sac at bedtime.	
Pilocarpine nitrate 1%, 2%, and 4% solution (Pilagan)	1%: $11.59/15 mL 2%: $12.04/15 mL 4%: $12.49/15 mL	1 or 2 drops up to six times daily	
Pilocarpine 20 μg/h for 7 days, and 40 μg/h for 7 days ocular therapeutic system (Ocusert Pilo-20 and Ocusert Pilo-40)[9]	20 μg/h: $39.34/8 each 40 μg/h: $39.34/8 each	Replace each unit every 7 days.	
Miotics, cholinesterase inhibitors Demecarium bromide 0.125% and 0.25% solution (Humorsol)	0.125%: $15.21/5 mL 0.25%: $16.31/5 mL	1 or 2 drops twice weekly to twice daily[10]	Reduction of intraocular pressure
Echothiophate iodide powder for reconstitution to make 0.03%, 0.06%, 0.125%, and 0.25% solution (Phospholine Iodide)	0.03%: $23.58/5 mL 0.06%: $24.70/5 mL 0.125%: $27.71/5 mL 0.25%: $31.23/5 mL	1 or 2 drops twice daily (with one of the two doses at bedtime)[11]	
Isoflurophate 0.025% ointment (Floropryl)	$8.13/3.5 g	0.25-inch strip of ointment into the eye every 8–72 hours[12]	
Physostigmine sulfate 0.25% ointment (various)	$4.53/8 oz.	Apply small quantity to lower fornix up to three times daily.	
Physostigmine salicylate 0.25% and 0.5% solution (Isopto Eserine and Eserine Salicylate)		2 drops once to four times daily	
Carbonic anhydrase inhibitor Dorzolamide HCl 2% solution (Trusopt)[13]	$21.78/5 mL $43.55/10 mL		Reduction of intraocular pressure
Combination product Pilocarpine HCl 1%, 2%, 3%, 4%, and 6% with epinephrine bitartrate 1% solution (various)	1%: $19.07/15 mL 2%: $19.07/15 mL 3%: $20.00/15 mL 4%: $21.25/15 mL 6%: $22.50/15 mL	1 or 2 drops once to four times daily	Additive effects in lowering intraocular pressure. Prevents marked miosis or mydriasis due to their opposing actions on pupilloconstrictors.
ANTI-INFLAMMATORY AGENTS **Nonsteroidal anti-inflammatory agents[14]** Diclofenac sodium 0.1% solution (Voltaren)	$20.31/2.5 mL $31.56/5 mL	1 drop to affected eye four times daily beginning 24 hours after cataract surgery and continuing through first 2 postoperative weeks	Treatment of postoperative inflammation following cataract extraction.
Flurbiprofen sodium 0.03% solution (various)	$8.73–$15.34/2.5 mL	1 drop every half hour beginning 2 hours before surgery	Inhibition of intraoperative miosis. Treatment of cystoid macular edema and inflammation after cataract surgery.

(continued)

Table 7–2. Ophthalmic agents. (continued)

Agent	Cost/Size[1]	Sig	Indications
Ketorolac tromethamine 0.5% solution (Acular)	$20.41/3 mL $34.30/5 mL $61.99/10 mL	1 drop four times daily	Relief of ocular itching due to seasonal allergic conjunctivitis
Suprofen 1% solution (Profenal)	$9.44/2.5 mL	2 drops at 3, 2, and 1 hour prior to surgery	Inhibition of intraoperative miosis
Corticosteroids[15] Dexamethasone sodium phosphate 0.1% solution (various)	$20.00/5 mL $34.37/15 mL	1 or 2 drops as often as indicated by severity. Use every hour during the day and every 2 hours during the night in severe inflammation. Taper off as inflammation decreases.	Treatment of steroid-responsive inflammatory conditions of anterior segment
Dexamethasone 0.1% suspension (various)	$20.00/5 mL $34.38/15 mL		
Dexamethasone sodium phosphate 0.05% ointment (various)	$4.37/3.5 g	Apply thin coating on lower conjunctival sac three or four times daily.	
Fluorometholone 0.1% suspension (various)[16]	$11.65/5 mL $18.25/10 mL $22.70/15 mL	1 or 2 drops as often as indicated by severity. Use every hour during the day and every 2 hours during the night in severe inflammation. Taper off as inflammation decreases.	
Fluorometholone acetate 0.1% suspension (Flarex)[16]	$16.25/5 mL $24.69/10 mL		
Fluorometholone 0.25% suspension (FML Forte)[16]	$14.84/5 mL $26.08/10 mL $36.60/15 mL		
Fluorometholone 0.1% ointment (FML S.O.P.)		Apply thin coating on lower conjunctival sac three or four times daily.	
Medrysone 1% suspension (HMS)	$15.00/5 mL $23.05/10 mL	1 or 2 drops as often as indicated by severity of inflammation. Use every hour during the day and every 2 hours during the night in severe inflammation. Taper off as inflammation decreases.	
Prednisolone acetate 0.12% suspension (Pred Mild)	$16.21/5 mL $23.65/10 mL		
Prednisolone acetate 0.125% suspension (various)	$15.00/5 mL $22.50/10 mL		
Prednisolone sodium phosphate 0.125% solution (various)	$14.41/5 mL $21.19/10 mL		
Prednisolone acetate 1% suspension (various)	$16.40/5 mL $26.10/10 mL		
Prednisolone sodium phosphate 1% solution (various)	$14.41/5 mL $21.19/10 mL $29.30/15 mL		
Rimexolone 1% suspension (Vexol)	$16.13/5 mL $27.00/10 mL		
Mast cell stabilizers Cromolyn sodium 4% solution (Crolom)	$36.25/10 mL	1 drop four to six times daily	Allergic conjunctivitis
Lodoxamide tromethamine 0.1% solution (Alomide)	$37.19/10 mL	1 or 2 drops four times daily (up to 3 months)	Vernal keratoconjunctivitis

(*continued*)

Table 7–2. Ophthalmic agents. (continued)

Agent	Cost/Size[1]	Sig	Indications
ANTIBIOTIC OINTMENTS AND SOLUTIONS			
Bacitracin 500 units/g ointment (various)[17]	$3.62/3.5 g	Refer to package insert (instructions vary)	Infections involving lid, conjunctiva, or cornea
Chloramphenicol 0.5% (5 mg/mL) solution (various)[18]	$3.71/7.5 mL $5.51/15 mL		As above, with both gram-positive and gram-negative coverage
Chloramphenicol 1% (10 mg/g) ointment (various)[18]	$7.67/3.5 g		
Chlortetracycline HCl 1% ointment (Aureomycin)[19]			
Ciprofloxacin HCl 0.3% solution (Cilaxan)	$11.88/2.5 mL $23.13/5 mL		
Erythromycin 0.5% ointment (various)[20]	$4.35/3.5 g		
Gentamicin sulfate 0.3% solution (various)	$6.44/15 mL $8.04/15 mL		
Gentamicin sulfate 0.3% ointment (various)	$10.50/3.5 g		
Norflaxacin 0.3% solution (Chibroxin)	$18.70/5 mL		
Ofloxacin 0.3% solution (Ocuflox)	$22.78/5 mL $45.56/10 mL		
Polymyxin B sulfate 500,000 units, powder for solution (Polymyxin B Sulfate Sterile)[21]	$5.80/500,000 units		
Tetracycline 1% solution (Achromycin)[22]			
Tetracycline 1% ointment (Achromycin)[22]			
Tobramycin 0.3% solution (various)	$14.89/5 mL		
Tobramycin 0.3% ointment (Tobrex)	$21.25/3.5 g		
COMBINATION ANTIBIOTIC PRODUCTS **Ointments and solutions**			
Polymyxin B sulfate 10,000 units/g, neomycin sulfate 3.5 mg/g, and bacitracin zinc 400 units/g ointment (various)[23]	$2.33/1 oz	Refer to package insert (instructions vary)	Infections involving the lids, conjunctiva, or cornea
Polymyxin B sulfate 10,000 units/g, neomycin sulfate 1.75 mg/g, and gramicidin 0.025 mg/mL (various)	$11.52/10 mL		
Polymyxin B sulfate 10,000 units/g and bacitracin zinc 500 units/g ointment (various)	$10.41/3.5 g		
Polymyxin B sulfate 10,000 units/g and oxytetracycline HCl 5 mg/g ointment (various)[24]			

(*continued*)

Table 7–2. Ophthalmic agents. (continued)

Agent	Cost/Size[1]	Sig	Indications
Polymyxin B sulfate 10,000 units/g and trimethoprim 1 mg/mL solution (Polytrim)[25]	$19.80/10 mL		
Steroid and antibiotic solutions and suspensions			
Chloramphenicol 0.25% and hydrocortisone acetate 0.5% suspension (Chloromycetin-Hydrocortisone)		1 or 2 drops every 3–4 hours or more frequently as required	For steroid-responsive inflammatory ocular conditions where bacterial infection or risk of infection exists
Gentamicin base 0.3% and prednisolone acetate 1% suspension (Pred-G Suspension)	$7.09/2 mL $20.53/5 mL $37.17/10 mL		
Neomycin sulfate 0.5% and dexamethasone sodium phosphate 0.1% solution (various)	$9.40/5 mL		
Neomycin sulfate 0.5% and polymyxin B sulfate 10,000 units solution (Statrol)	$36.15/20 mL		
Neomycin sulfate 0.5%, polymyxin B sulfate 10,000 units, and dexamethasone 0.1% suspension (various)	$9.88/5 mL		
Neomycin sulfate 0.5%, polymyxin B sulfate 10,000 units, and hydrocortisone 1% suspension (various)	$10.55/10 mL		
Neomycin sulfate 0.5%, polymyxin B sulfate 10,000 units, and prednisolone acetate 0.5% suspension (Poly-Pred Suspension)	$19.79/5 mL		
Oxytetracycline HCl 0.5% and hydrocortisone acetate 1.5% suspension (Terra-Cortril Suspension)	$18.43/5 mL		
Tobramycin 0.3% and dexamethasone 0.1% suspension (TobraDex)	$12.50/2.5 mL $24.38/5 mL		
Steroid and antibiotic ointments			
Chloramphenicol 1%, polymyxin B sulfate 10,000 units, and hydrocortisone acetate 0.5% ointment (Ophthocor)		Apply ointment to the affected area every 3–4 hours.	For steroid-response inflammatory ocular conditions where bacterial infection or risk of infection exists
Gentamicin base 0.3% and prednisolone acetate 0.6% ointment (Pred-G S.O.P.)	$19.95/3.5 g		
Neomycin sulfate 0.5%, bacitracin zinc 400 units, polymyxin B sulfate, and hydrocortisone 1% ointment (various)	$3.76/3.5 g		
Neomycin sulfate 0.5%, bacitracin zinc 400 units, polymyxin B sulfate, and hydrocortisone 1% acetate ointment (Neotricin HC)	$2.69/3.5 g		
Neomycin sulfate 0.5% and dexa-methasone sodium phosphate 0.05% ointment (Neo-Decadron)	$6.57/3.5 g		

(continued)

Table 7–2. Ophthalmic agents. (continued)

Agent	Cost/Size[1]	Sig	Indications
Neomycin sulfate 0.5% and polymyxin B sulfate 10,000 units ointment (Statrol)		Apply ointment to the affected area every 3–4 hours.	For steroid-response inflammatory ocular conditions where bacterial infection or risk of infection exists
Neomycin sulfate 0.5%, polymyxin B sulfate 10,000 units, and dexamethasone 0.1% ointment (various)	$11.83/3.5 g		
Tobramycin 0.3% and dexamethasone 0.1% ointment (TobraDex)	$24.37/3.5 g		
SULFONAMIDES			
Sulfacetamide sodium 10%, 15%, and 30% solution (various)	10%: $8.50/15 mL 15%: $18.13/15 mL 30%: $21.41/15 mL	1 or 2 drops every 1–3 hours	Conjunctivitis, corneal ulcer, and other superficial ocular infections due to susceptible microorganisms. Used as adjunct to systemic sulfonamide therapy in treatment of trachoma.
Sulfacetamide sodium 10% ointment (various)	$7.28/3.5 g	Apply small amount (0.5 inch) into lower conjunctival sac once to four times daily and at bedtime.	
Sulfisoxazole diolamine 4% solution (Gantrisin)		1 or 2 drops every 1–3 hours	
Sulfonamide and steroid combinations: Suspensions and solutions			
Sodium sulfacetamide 10% and fluorometholone 0.1% suspension (FML-S)	$16.76/5 mL $23.00/10 mL	1–3 drops into conjunctival sac every 1–2 hours during day and at bedtime until responsive	For steroid-responsive inflammatory ocular conditions for which steroids are indicated and where bacterial infection exists
Sodium sulfacetamide 10% and prednisolone acetate 0.2% suspension (various)			
Sodium sulfacetamide 10% and prednisolone acetate 0.25% suspension (various)	$11.50/5 mL $15.18/10 mL		
Sodium sulfacetamide 10% and prednisolone sodium phosphate 0.25% solution (various)			
Sulfonamide and steroid combinations: Ointments			
Sodium sulfacetamide 10% and prednisolone acetate 0.2% ointment (Blephamide)		Apply small amount into conjunctival sac three or four times daily and at bedtime. (Do not prescribe > 8 g initially.)	For steroid-responsive inflammatory ocular conditions for which steroids are indicated and where bacterial infection exists
Sodium sulfacetamide 10% and prednisolone acetate 0.25% ointment (various)			
Sodium sulfacetamide 10% and prednisolone acetate 0.5% ointment (Metimyd)	$24.74/3.5 g		
TOPICAL ANTIFUNGAL AGENTS Natamycin 5% suspension (Natacyn)		1 drop every 1–2 hours	Fungal blepharitis, conjunctivitis, and keratitis caused by susceptible organisms. Drug of choice for *Fusarium solani* keratitis
TOPICAL ANTIVIRAL AGENTS Idoxuridine 0.1% solution (Herplex)		Initially, 1 drop every hour during the day and every 2 hours during the night, reducing the frequency as improvement occurs. (Maximum of 21 days' therapy.)	Treatment for HSV keratitis[26]

(continued)

Table 7–2. Ophthalmic agents. (continued)

Agent	Cost/Size[1]	Sig	Indications
Trifluridine 1% solution (Viroptic)	$53.14/7.5 mL	1 drop onto cornea every 2 hours while awake for a maximum daily dose of 9 drops until resolution occurs. Then an additional 7 days of 1 drop every 4 hours while awake (minimum five times daily).	Primary keratoconjunctivitis and recurrent epithelial keratitis due to HSV types 1 or 2[26]
Vidarabine monohydrate 3% ointment (Vira-A)	$20.77/3.5 g	0.5 inch of ointment into the lower conjunctival sac five times daily at 3-hour intervals	Acute keratoconjunctivitis and recurrent epithelial keratitis due to HSV types 1 or 2[26]
TOPICAL ANTIHISTAMINICS[27] Levocabastine HCl 0.05% ophthalmic solution (Livostin)	$27.50/5 mL $41.88/10 mL	1 drop four times daily (up to 2 weeks)	Allergic conjunctivitis; temporary relief of seasonal allergic conjunctivitis
Combination products[28] Naphazoline HCl 0.025% and pheniramine maleate 0.3% (various)	$7.88/15 mL	Refer to package insert.	"Possibly" effective for relief of ocular irritation or congestion or for treatment of allergic or inflammatory ocular conditions
Naphazoline HCl 0.027% and pheniramine maleate 0.315% (Opcon-A solution)	$8.73/15 mL		
Naphazoline HCl 0.05%, and antazoline phosphate 0.5% (various)	$7.81/15 mL		

[1]Cost to pharmacist (average wholesale price) for maximum dose and regimen listed. Source: First Data Bank Price Alert, April 1997.
[2]Macular edema occurs in 30% of patients.
[3]May (rarely) increase blood pressure. *Caution:* Avoid in patients with sulfite hypersensitivity (some brands contain sulfite).
[4]Cardioselective (β_1) beta-blocker.
[5]Nonselective (β_1 and β_2) beta-blocker. Monitor all patients for systemic side effects, particularly exacerbation of asthma.
[6]Transient stinging, burning, corneal clouding may occur.
[7]Decreased night vision, headaches possible.
[8]Stinging on administration.
[9]Sustained-release preparation. Refrigerate.
[10]Individualize dose to obtain maximal effect. Contraindicated in pregnancy.
[11]Tolerance may develop with prolonged use.
[12]Tolerance may develop.
[13]The only topical carbonic anhydrase inhibitor.
[14]Cross-sensitivity to aspirin and other NSAIDs.
[15]Long-term use may increase intraocular pressure or cause cataracts.
[16]May be less likely to elevate intraocular pressure.

[17]Little efficacy against gram-negative organisms (except *Neisseria*).
[18]Aplastic anemia has been reported with prolonged ophthalmic use. Use only in serious infections for which less toxic drugs are ineffective or contraindicated.
[19]Can use against *Chlamydia trachomatis* in conjunction with oral therapy.
[20]Also indicated for prophylaxis of ophthalmia neonatorum due to *N gonorrhoeae* or *C trachomatis*. Increasing resistance of *S pneumoniae* and *P aeruginosa* has been noted.
[21]No gram-positive coverage.
[22]Indicated for prophylaxis of ophthalmia neonatorum due to *N gonorrhoeae* or *C trachomatis*.
[23]Both gram-positive and gram-negative coverage.
[24]No gram-positive coverage. Good gram-negative coverage.
[25]Both gram-positive and gram-negative coverage.
[26]Recurrences are common and call for additional 7-day treatment.
[27]Antihistamines (topical) are potential sensitizers and may produce local reactions.
[28]Use with caution in persons with narrow angles or a history of glaucoma, since these drugs may produce angle closure.

An antibiotic instilled into the eye can sensitize the patient to that drug and cause a hypersensitivity reaction upon subsequent systemic administration.

Systemic Effects of Ocular Drugs

The systemic absorption of certain topical drugs (through the conjunctival vessels and lacrimal drainage system) must be considered when there is a systemic medical contraindication to the use of the drug. Ophthalmic solutions of the nonselective beta-blockers timolol, levobunolol, and metipranolol may worsen patients with congestive heart failure or asthma. Atropine ointment should be prescribed for children rather than the drops, since absorption of the 1% topical solution may be toxic. Phenylephrine eye drops can precipitate hypertensive crises and angina.

Table 7–3. Adverse ocular effects of systemic drugs.

Drug	Possible Side Effects
Respiratory drugs	
Oxygen	Retinopathy of prematurity.
Cardiovascular system drugs	
Digitalis	Disturbances of color vision, scotomas, photopsia
Quinidine	Optic neuritis (rare).
Thiazides (Diuril, etc)	Xanthopsia (yellow vision), myopia.
Carbonic anhydrase inhibitors (acetazolamide)	Ocular hypotony, transient myopia.
Amiodarone	Corneal deposits.
Gastrointestinal drugs	
Anticholinergic agents	Risk of angle-closure glaucoma due to mydriasis. Blurring of vision due to cycloplegia (occasional).
Central nervous system drugs	
Barbiturates	Extraocular muscle palsies with diplopia, ptosis, cortical blindness.
Chloral hydrate	Diplopia, ptosis, miosis.
Phenothiazines	Deposits of pigment in conjunctiva, cornea, lens and retina. Oculogyric crises.
Amphetamines	Widening of palpebral fissure. Dilation of pupil, paralysis of ciliary muscle with loss of accommodation.
Monoamine oxidase inhibitors	Nystagmus, extraocular muscle palsies, optic atrophy.
Tricyclic agents	Dilation of pupil (risk of angle-closure glaucoma), cycloplegia.
Phenytoin	Nystagmus, diplopia, ptosis, slight blurring of vision (rare).
Neostigmine	Nystagmus, miosis.
Morphine	Miosis.
Haloperidol	Capsular cataract.
Lithium carbonate	Exophthalmos, oculogyric crisis.
Diazepam	Nystagmus.
Hormones	
Corticosteroids	Cataract (posterior subcapsular), local immunologic suppression, causing susceptibility to viral (herpes simplex), bacterial, and fungal infections; steroid-induced glaucoma.
Female sex hormones	Retinal artery occlusion, retinal vein occlusion, papilledema, ocular palsies with diplopia, nystagmus, optic neuropathy, retinal vasculitis, scotomas, migraine, mydriasis and cycloplegia, and macular edema.
Antibiotics	
Chloramphenicol	Optic neuritis and atrophy.
Rifabutin	Uveitis.
Streptomycin	Optic neuritis.
Tetracycline	Pseudotumor cerebri, transient myopia.
Antimalarial agents	
Chloroquine, etc	Macular changes, central scotomas, pigmentary degeneration of the retina, chloroquine keratopathy, ocular palsies, ptosis, ERG depression.
Amebicides	
Iodochlorhydroxyquin	Optic atrophy.
Chemotherapeutic agents	
Sulfonamides	Stevens-Johnson syndrome.
Ethambutol	Optic neuritis and atrophy.
Isoniazid	Optic neuritis and atrophy.
Heavy metals	
Gold salts	Deposits in the cornea and conjunctiva.
Lead compounds	Optic atrophy, papilledema, ocular palsies.
Chelating agents	
Penicillamine	Ocular pemphigold, optic neuritis, ocular myasthenia.
Oral hypoglycemic agents	
Chlorpropamide	Transient change in refractive error, diplopia, Stevens-Johnson syndrome.
Vitamins	
Vitamin A	Papilledema, retinal hemorrhages, loss of eyebrows and eyelashes, nystagmus, diplopia, blurring of vision.
Vitamin D	Band-shaped keratopathy.
Antirheumatic agents	
Salicylates	Nystagmus, retinal hemorrhages, cortical blindness (rare).
Indomethacin	Corneal deposits.
Phenylbutazone	Retinal hemorrhages.

Also to be considered are adverse interactions between systemically administered and ocular drugs. Using only 1 or 2 drops at a time and a few minutes of nasolacrimal occlusion or eyelid closure ensure maximum efficacy and decrease systemic side effects of topical agents.

Edeki TI et al: Pharmacogenetic explanation for excessive beta-blockade following timolol eye drops. JAMA 1995;274:1611. (Poor metabolizers of debrisoquin develop more marked side effects from timolol eyedrop therapy, and this is further exacerbated by oral administration of quinidine.)

ADVERSE OCULAR EFFECTS OF SYSTEMIC DRUGS

Systemically administered drugs produce a wide variety of adverse effects on the visual system. Table 7–3 lists the major examples.

Fraunfelder FT, Mayer SM: Ocular and systemic side effects of drugs. In: *General Ophthalmology,* 14th ed. Vaughan D, Asbury T, Riordan-Eva P (editors). Appleton & Lange, 1995.

Ear, Nose, & Throat

8

Robert K. Jackler, MD, & Michael J. Kaplan, MD

DISEASES OF THE EAR

HEARING LOSS

Classification

A. Conductive Hearing Loss: Conductive hearing loss results from dysfunction of the external or middle ear. There are four mechanisms, each resulting in impairment of the passage of sound vibrations to the inner ear: (1) obstruction (eg, cerumen impaction), (2) mass loading (eg, middle ear effusion), (3) stiffness effect (eg, otosclerosis), and (4) discontinuity (eg, ossicular disruption). Conductive hearing loss is generally correctable with medical or surgical therapy—or in some cases both.

B. Sensory Hearing Loss: Sensory hearing loss results from deterioration of the cochlea, usually due to loss of hair cells from the organ of Corti. Among the many common causes are noise trauma, ototoxicity, and aging (presbyacusis). Sensory hearing loss is not correctable with medical or surgical therapy but often may be prevented or stabilized.

C. Neural Hearing Loss: Neural hearing loss occurs with lesions involving the eighth nerve, auditory nuclei, ascending tracts, or auditory cortex. It is the least common clinically recognized cause of hearing loss. Examples include acoustic neuroma, multiple sclerosis, and cerebrovascular disease.

Nadol JB: Hearing loss. N Engl J Med 1993;329:1092. (Review of anatomy, common causes, diagnosis, and treatment of both conductive and sensorineural hearing loss.)

Epidemiology of Hearing Loss

Conductive losses in adults are most commonly due to cerumen impaction or transient auditory tube dysfunction associated with upper respiratory tract infection. Persistent conductive losses usually result from chronic ear infection, trauma, or otosclerosis.

Sensorineural losses in adults are common. A gradually progressive, predominantly high-frequency loss with advancing age is typical though not invariable. Other than aging effects, common causes of sensorineural loss include excessive noise exposure, head trauma, and systemic diseases such as diabetes mellitus.

Evaluation of Hearing (Audiology)

In a quiet room, the hearing level may be estimated by having the patient repeat aloud words presented in a soft whisper, a normal spoken voice, or a shout. Tuning forks are useful in differentiating conductive from sensorineural losses. A 512-Hz tuning fork is employed, since frequencies below this level elicit a tactile response. In the **Weber test,** the tuning fork is placed on the forehead or front teeth. In conductive losses, the sound appears louder in the poorer-hearing ear, whereas in sensorineural losses it radiates to the better side. In the **Rinne test,** the tuning fork is placed alternately on the mastoid bone and in front of the ear canal. In conductive losses, bone conduction exceeds air conduction; in sensorineural losses, the opposite is true.

Formal audiometric studies are performed in a soundproofed room. Pure-tone thresholds in decibels (dB) are obtained over the range of 250–8000 Hz (the main speech frequencies are between 500 and 3000 Hz) for both air and bone conduction. Conductive losses create a gap between the air and bone thresholds, whereas in sensorineural losses both air and bone conduction are equally diminished. The threshold of normal hearing is from 0 to 20 dB, which corresponds to the loudness of a soft whisper. Mild hearing loss is indicated by a threshold of 20–40 dB (soft spoken voice), moderate loss by a threshold of 40–60 dB (normal spoken voice), severe loss by a threshold of 60–80 dB (loud spoken voice), and profound loss by a threshold of 80 dB (shout). The clarity of hearing is often impaired in sensorineural hearing loss. This is evaluated by speech discrimination testing, which is reported as percentage correct (90–100% is normal). The site of the lesion responsible for sensorineural loss—whether it lies in the cochlea or in the central auditory system—

may be determined with auditory brain stem-evoked responses.

Every patient who complains of a hearing loss should be referred for audiologic evaluation unless the cause is easily remediable (eg, cerumen impaction, otitis media). Audiologic screening is not recommended for adults with apparently normal hearing unless they are exposed to potentially injurious levels of noise or have reached the age of 65, after which screening evaluations should be done every few years.

Lonsbury-Martin BL et al: New approaches to the evaluation of the auditory system and a current analysis of otoacoustic emissions. Otolaryngol Head Neck Surg 1995;112:50. (Useful tools in detection and follow-up.)

Hearing Rehabilitation

Patients with hearing loss not correctable by medical therapy may benefit from hearing amplification. Contemporary hearing aids are comparatively free of distortion and have been miniaturized to the point where they often may be contained entirely within the ear canal. To optimize the benefit, a hearing aid must be carefully selected to conform to the nature of the hearing loss. Digitally programmable hearing aids are now becoming available that promise substantial improvements in speech intelligibility, especially under difficult listening circumstances.

Aside from hearing aids, many assistive devices are available to improve comprehension in individual and group settings, to help with hearing television and radio programs, and for telephone communication. In individuals with profound sensory deafness, the cochlear implant—an electronic device that is surgically implanted to stimulate the auditory nerve—offers socially beneficial auditory rehabilitation to most adults with acquired deafness.

[Noise and hearing loss]
gopher://gopher.nih.gov:70/11/clin/cdcs/individual/76.
noise
Balkany T et al: Update on cochlear implants. Otolaryngol Clin North Am 1996;29:277. (Including outcomes, cost-effectiveness, and ethical issues.)
Byrne D: Key issues in hearing aid selection and evaluation. J Am Acad Audiol 1992;3:67.
Jerger J et al: Hearing impairment in older adults: New concepts. J Am Geriatr Soc 1995;43:928. (Key role of the physician in making appropriate referrals and in helping to overcome negative attitudes toward a hearing handicap.)
Mitchell GW: Otologic devices. Emerg Med Clin North Am 1994;12:787. (Review of common and uncommon complications of hearing aids, ossicular replacements, and implants.)

DISEASES OF THE AURICLE

Disorders of the external ear are for the most part dermatologic. Skin cancers due to actinic exposure are common and may be treated with standard techniques.

Traumatic auricular hematoma must be recognized and drained to prevent significant cosmetic deformity (cauliflower ear) resulting from dissolution of supporting cartilage. Similarly, cellulitis of the auricle must be treated promptly to prevent development of perichondritis and its resultant deformity. Relapsing polychondritis is a systemic disorder often associated with recurrent, frequently bilateral, painful episodes of auricular erythema and edema. Treatment with corticosteroids may help forestall cartilage dissolution. Respiratory compromise may occur as a result of progressive involvement of the tracheobronchial tree. Chondritis and perichondritis may be differentiated from auricular cellulitis by sparing of involvement of the lobule, which does not contain cartilage.

Starck WJ, Kaltman SI: Current concepts in the surgical management of traumatic auricular hematoma. J Oral Maxillofac Surg 1992;50:800. (Early drainage and compression are essential if cosmetic deformity is to be avoided.)
Templer J, Renner GJ: Injuries of the external ear. Otolaryngol Clin North Am 1990;23:1003. (Review of injuries and treatment of injury and complications.)

DISEASES OF THE EAR CANAL

1. CERUMEN IMPACTION

Cerumen is a protective secretion produced by the outer portion of the ear canal. In most individuals, the ear canal is self-cleansing. Recommended hygiene consists of cleaning the external opening with a washcloth over the index finger without entering the canal itself. In most cases, cerumen impaction is self-induced through ill-advised attempts at cleaning the ear. It may be relieved with detergent ear drops (eg, 3% hydrogen peroxide; 6.5% carbamide peroxide), mechanical removal, suction, or irrigation. Irrigation is performed with water at body temperature to avoid a vestibular caloric response. The stream should be directed at the ear canal wall adjacent to the cerumen plug. Irrigation should be performed only when the tympanic membrane is known to be intact.

Use of jet irrigators designed for cleaning teeth (eg, WaterPik) for wax removal should be avoided since they may result in tympanic membrane perforations. Following irrigation, the ear canal should be thoroughly dried (eg, by instilling isopropyl alcohol or using a hair blow drier on low-power setting) to reduce the likelihood of inducing external otitis. Specialty referral for cleaning under microscopic guidance is indicated when the impaction has not responded to routine measures or if the patient has a history of chronic otitis media or tympanic membrane perforation.

Freeman RB: Impacted cerumen: How to safely remove earwax in an office visit. Geriatrics 1995;50:52. (Therapeutic options for the nonspecialist practitioner.)

2. FOREIGN BODIES

Foreign bodies in the ear canal are more frequent in children than in adults. Firm materials may be removed with a loop or a hook, taking care not to displace the object medially toward the tympanic membrane; microscopic guidance is helpful. Aqueous irrigation should not be performed for organic foreign bodies (eg, beans, insects), because water may cause them to swell. Living insects are best immobilized before removal by filling the ear canal with lidocaine.

Bressler K, Shelton C: Ear foreign-body removal: A review of 98 consecutive cases. Laryngoscope 1993;103:367. (Ear canal laceration when removal was performed without microscopic guidance.)

3. EXTERNAL OTITIS

External otitis presents with otalgia, frequently accompanied by pruritus and purulent discharge. There is often a history of recent water exposure or mechanical trauma (eg, scratching, cotton applicators). External otitis is usually caused by gram-negative rods (eg, *Pseudomonas, Proteus*) or fungi (eg, *Aspergillus*), which grow in the presence of excessive moisture.

Examination reveals erythema and edema of the ear canal skin, often with a purulent exudate. Manipulation of the auricle often elicits pain. Because the lateral surface of the tympanic membrane is ear canal skin, it is often erythematous. However, in contrast to acute otitis media, it moves normally with pneumatic otoscopy. When the canal skin is very edematous, it may be impossible to visualize the tympanic membrane. Fundamental to the treatment of external otitis is protection of the ear from additional moisture and avoidance of further mechanical injury by scratching. Otic drops containing a mixture of aminoglycoside antibiotic and anti-inflammatory corticosteroid in an acid vehicle are generally very effective (eg, neomycin sulfate, polymyxin B sulfate, and hydrocortisone). Purulent debris filling the ear canal should be gently removed to permit entry of the topical medication. Drops should be used abundantly (5 or more drops three or four times a day) to penetrate the depths of the canal. When substantial edema of the canal wall prevents entry of drops into the ear canal, a wick is placed to facilitate entry of the medication.

Brook I, Frazier EH, Thompson DH: Aerobic and anaerobic microbiology of external otitis. Clin Infect Dis 1992;15:955. (Although most cases of external otitis are caused by aerobic organisms and are monomicrobial, one-third of patients had polymicrobial infection and one-fourth of cases involved anaerobes.)

Russell JD et al: What causes acute otitis externa? J Laryngol Otol 1993;107:898. (A study of 100 patients confirmed that regular swimming, showering, and hair washing were significantly more common in otitis externa patients.)

4. PRURITUS

Pruritus of the external auditory canal, particularly at the meatus, is a common problem. While it may be associated with external otitis or with dermatologic conditions such as seborrheic dermatitis and psoriasis, most cases are self-induced either from excoriation or by overly zealous ear cleaning. To permit regeneration of the protective cerumen blanket, patients should be instructed to avoid use of soap and water or cotton swabs in the ear canal. Patients with excessively dry canal skin may benefit from application of mineral oil, which helps to counteract dryness and repel moisture. When an inflammatory component is present, topical application of a corticosteroid (eg, 0.1% triamcinolone) may be beneficial. It is axiomatic in persistent pruritus that the patient must cease scratching the ear. In stubborn cases, the fingernails must be kept short and the patient may need to wear cotton gloves at night to avoid manipulation during sleep. Symptomatic reduction of pruritus may be obtained by use of oral antihistamines (eg, diphenhydramine, 25 mg orally at bedtime). Topical application of isopropyl alcohol promptly relieves ear canal pruritus in many patients.

5. MALIGNANT EXTERNAL OTITIS

Persistent external otitis in the diabetic or immunocompromised patient may evolve into osteomyelitis of the skull base, often called malignant external otitis. Usually caused by *Pseudomonas aeruginosa,* osteomyelitis begins in the floor of the ear canal and may extend into the middle fossa floor, the clivus, and even the contralateral skull base. The patient usually presents with persistent foul aural discharge, granulations in the ear canal, deep otalgia, and progressive cranial nerve palsies involving nerves VI, VII, IX, X, XI, or XII. Diagnosis is confirmed by the demonstration of osseous erosion on CT and radionuclide scanning.

Treatment is chiefly medical, requiring prolonged antipseudomonal antibiotic administration, often for several months. Although intravenous therapy is often required, selected patients may be managed with the oral agent ciprofloxacin (500–1000 mg orally twice daily), which has proved effective against many of the causative *Pseudomonas* strains. To avoid relapse, antibiotic therapy should be continued, even in the asymptomatic patient, until gallium scanning indicates a marked reduction in the inflammatory process. Surgical debridement of infected bone is reserved for cases of deterioration despite medical therapy.

Evans P, Hofmann L: Malignant external otitis: A case report and review. Am Fam Physician 1994;49:427. (Most common in elderly diabetic patients and involves *Pseudomonas.*)

Giamarellou H: Malignant otitis externa: The therapeutic evolution of a lethal infection. J Antimicrob Chemother 1992;30:745. (Increasing role of fluroquinolones.)

6. EXOSTOSES & OSTEOMAS

Bony overgrowths of the ear canal are a frequent incidental finding and occasionally have clinical significance. Clinically, they present as skin-covered mounds in the medial ear canal obscuring the tympanic membrane to a variable degree. Solitary osteomas are of no significance as long as they do not cause obstruction or infection. Multiple exostoses, which are generally acquired from repeated exposure to cold water, often progress and require surgical removal.

7. NEOPLASIA

The most common neoplasm of the ear canal is squamous cell carcinoma. When an apparent otitis externa does not resolve on therapy, this should be suspected and biopsy performed. This disease carries a very high 5-year mortality rate and must be treated with wide surgical resection and radiation therapy. Adenomatous tumors, originating from the ceruminous glands, generally follow a more indolent course.

Estrem SA, Renner GJ: Special problems associated with cutaneous carcinoma of the ear. Otolaryngol Clin North Am 1993;26:231. (Points out the poorer prognosis and need for aggressive therapy when skin cancers grow in proximity to the external auditory meatus.)

DISEASES OF THE AUDITORY TUBE

1. AUDITORY TUBE DYSFUNCTION

The tube that connects the middle ear to the nasopharynx—the auditory tube, or eustachian tube—provides ventilation and drainage for the middle ear cleft. It is normally closed, opening only during the act of swallowing or yawning. When auditory tube function is compromised, air trapped within the middle ear becomes absorbed and negative pressure results. The most common causes of auditory tube dysfunction are diseases associated with edema of the tubal lining, such as viral upper respiratory tract infections and allergy. The patient usually reports a sense of fullness in the ear and mild to moderate im-

pairment of hearing. When the tube is only partially blocked, swallowing or yawning may elicit a popping or crackling sound. Examination reveals retraction of the tympanic membrane and decreased mobility on pneumatic otoscopy. Following a viral illness, this disorder is usually transient, lasting days to weeks. Treatment with systemic and intranasal decongestants (eg, pseudoephedrine, 60 mg orally every 4 hours; oxymetazoline, 0.05% spray every 8–12 hours) combined with autoinflation by forced exhalation against closed nostrils may hasten relief. Air travel, rapid altitudinal change, and underwater diving should be avoided. Autoinflation should not be recommended to patients with active intranasal infection, since this maneuver may precipitate middle ear infection. Allergic patients may also benefit from desensitization or intranasal corticosteroids (eg, beclomethasone dipropionate, two sprays in each nostril twice daily for 2–6 weeks).

An overly patent auditory tube is a relatively uncommon problem that may be quite distressing. Typical complaints include fullness in the ear and autophony, an exaggerated ability to hear oneself breath and speak. A patulous auditory tube may develop during rapid weight loss, or it may commence without a discernible cause. In contrast to a hypofunctioning auditory tube, the aural pressure is often made worse by exertion and may diminish during an upper respiratory tract infection. Although physical examination is usually normal, respiratory excursions of the tympanic membrane may occasionally be detected during vigorous breathing. Treatment includes avoidance of decongestant products, insertion of a ventilating tube to reduce the outward stretch of the ear drum during phonation, and surgical narrowing of the auditory tube (rarely).

Kumazawa T et al: Eustachian tube function tests and their diagnostic potential in normal and diseased ears. Acta Otolaryngol 1993;500(Suppl):10. (Use of combinations of tests.)

Monsell EM, Harley RE: Eustachian tube dysfunction. Otolaryngol Clin North Am 1996;29:437. (Management of both hypo- and hyperfunction.)

2. SEROUS OTITIS MEDIA

When the auditory tube remains blocked for a prolonged period, the resultant negative pressure will result in transudation of fluid. This condition, known as serous otitis media, is especially common in children because their auditory tubes are narrower and more horizontal in orientation than adults. It is less common in adults, in whom it usually follows an upper respiratory tract infection or barotrauma. In an adult with persistent unilateral serous otitis media, nasopharyngeal carcinoma must be excluded. The tympanic membrane in serous otitis media is dull and hypomobile, occasionally accompanied by air bubbles in the middle ear and conductive hearing loss. The treatment of serous otitis media is similar to that for auditory tube dysfunction. A short course of oral corticosteroids (eg, prednisone, 40 mg/d for 7 days) has been advocated by some in the management of serous otitis media, as have oral antibiotics (eg, amoxicillin, 250 mg orally three times daily for 7 days)—or even a combination of the two. The role of these regimens remains controversial, but they are probably of little lasting benefit.

When medication fails to bring relief after several months, a ventilating tube placed through the tympanic membrane may restore hearing and alleviate the sense of aural fullness.

Bernstein JM: The role of IgE-mediated hypersensitivity in the development of otitis media with effusion: A review. Otolaryngol Head Neck Surg 1993;109:611. (Suggests that nasal allergy contributes to 35–40% of cases of middle ear effusion.)

Pulec JL: Serous otitis media. Ear Nose Throat J 1993; 72:193.

Sham JST: Serous otitis media: An opportunity for early recognition of nasopharyngeal carcinoma. Arch Otolaryngol 1992;118:794. (More than 40% initially presented with serous otitis.)

3. BAROTRAUMA

Individuals with auditory tube dysfunction due either to congenital narrowness or to acquired mucosal edema may be unable to equalize the barometric stress exerted on the middle ear by air travel, rapid altitudinal change, or underwater diving. The problem is generally most acute during airplane descent, since the negative middle ear pressure tends to collapse and lock the auditory tube. Several measures are useful to enhance auditory tube function and avoid otic barotrauma. The patient should be advised to swallow, yawn, and autoinflate frequently during descent, which may be painful if the auditory tube collapses. Systemic decongestants (eg, pseudoephedrine, 30–60 mg) should be taken several hours before anticipated arrival time so that they will be maximally effective during descent. Topical decongestants such as 1% phenylephrine nasal spray should be administered 1 hour before arrival.

The treatment of acute negative middle ear pressure that persists on the ground is with decongestants and attempts at autoinflation. Myringotomy provides immediate relief and is appropriate in the setting of severe otalgia and hearing loss. Repeated episodes of barotrauma in persons who must fly frequently may be alleviated by insertion of ventilating tubes.

Underwater diving represents even a greater barometric stress to the ear than flying. The problem occurs most commonly during the descent phase, when pain develops within the first 15 feet if inflation of the middle ear via the auditory tube has not occurred. Divers must descend slowly and equilibrate in stages to avoid the development of severely negative pressures in the tympanum that may result in hemorrhage (hemotympanum) or perilymphatic fistulization. In the latter, the oval or round window ruptures, resulting in sensory hearing loss and acute vertigo. Emesis due to acute labyrinthine dysfunction can be very dangerous during an underwater dive. Sensory hearing loss or vertigo, which develops during the ascent phase of a saturation dive, may be the first (or only) symptom of decompression sickness. Immediate recompression will return intravascular gas bubbles to solution and restore the inner ear microcirculation. Patients should be warned to avoid diving when they have upper respiratory infections or episodes of nasal allergy. Tympanic membrane perforation is an absolute contraindication to diving, as the patient will experience an unbalanced thermal stimulus to the semicircular canals and may experience vertigo, disorientation, and even emesis. Finally, individuals with only one hearing ear should be discouraged from diving because of the significant risk of otologic injury.

Brown TP: Middle ear symptoms while flying: Ways to prevent severe outcome. Postgrad Med 1994;96:135. (Avoid flying if symptoms of upper respiratory tract infection are present. Medications may be helpful.)

Clenney TL, Lassen LF: Recreational scuba diving injuries. Am Fam Physician 1996;53:1761. (Distinguishes between the otologic effects of barotrauma and decompression sickness.)

DISEASES OF THE MIDDLE EAR

1. ACUTE OTITIS MEDIA

Acute otitis media is a bacterial infection of the mucosally lined air-containing spaces of the temporal bone. Purulent material forms not only within the middle ear cleft but also within the mastoid air cells and petrous apex when they are pneumatized. Acute otitis media is usually precipitated by a viral upper respiratory tract infection that causes auditory tube edema. This results in accumulation of fluid and mucus, which becomes secondarily infected by bacteria. The most common pathogens both in adults and in children are *Streptococcus pneumoniae*, *Haemophilus influenzae*, and *Streptococcus pyogenes*.

Acute otitis media is most common in infants and children, though it may occur at any age. The patient presents with otalgia, aural pressure, decreased hearing, and often fever. The typical physical findings are erythema and decreased mobility of the tympanic membrane. Occasionally, bullae will be seen on the tympanic membrane. Although it is taught that this represents infection with *Mycoplasma pneumoniae,* most cases involve more common pathogens.

Rarely, when middle ear empyema is severe, the tympanic membrane can be seen to bulge outward. In such cases, tympanic membrane rupture is imminent. Rupture is accompanied by a sudden decrease in pain, followed by the onset of otorrhea. With appropriate therapy, spontaneous healing of the tympanic membrane occurs in most cases. When perforation persists, chronic otitis media frequently evolves. Mastoid tenderness often accompanies acute otitis media and is due to the presence of pus within the mastoid air cells. At this stage, this does not indicate suppurative (surgical) mastoiditis.

The treatment of acute otitis media is specific antibiotic therapy, often combined with nasal decongestants. The first-choice antibiotic treatment is either amoxicillin (20–40 mg/kg/d) or erythromycin (50 mg/kg/d) plus sulfonamide (150 mg/kg/d) for 10 days. Alternatives useful in resistant cases are cefaclor (20–40 mg/kg/d) or amoxicillin-clavulanate (20–40 mg/kg/d) combinations.

Tympanocentesis for bacterial (aerobic and anaerobic) and fungal culture may be performed by any experienced physician. A 20-gauge spinal needle bent 90 degrees to the hub of a 3 mL syringe is inserted through the inferior portion of the tympanic membrane. Interposition of a pliable connecting tube between the needle and syringe permits an assistant to aspirate without inducing movement of the needle. Tympanocentesis is useful for otitis media in immunocompromised patients and when infection recurs despite multiple courses of antibiotics, and in cases of persistent infection despite multiple courses of antibiotics.

Surgical drainage of the middle ear (myringotomy) is reserved for patients with severe otalgia or when complications of otitis (eg, mastoiditis, meningitis) have occurred.

Recurrent acute otitis media may be managed with long-term antibiotic prophylaxis. Single daily doses of sulfamethoxazole (500 mg) or amoxicillin (250 or 500 mg) are given over a period of 1–3 months. Failure of this regimen to control infection is an indication for insertion of ventilating tubes.

Bartelos AI et al: Acute otitis media in adults: A report from the International Primary Care Network. J Am Board Fam Pract 1993;6:333. (Adults complain sooner, have history of tonsillectomy, and have poorer outcome. Tympanic membrane signs are similar.)

Haddad J Jr: Treatment of acute otitis media and its complications. Otolaryngol Clin North Am 1994;27:431.

Weiss JC, Yates GR, Quinn LD: Acute otitis media: Making an accurate diagnosis. Am Family Physician 1996;53:1200. (Erythema of the tympanic membrane alone is not wholly reliable. Pneumatic otoscopy often helpful.)

2. CHRONIC OTITIS MEDIA & CHOLESTEATOMA

Chronic infection of the middle ear and mastoid generally develops as a consequence of recurrent acute otitis media, although it may follow other diseases and trauma. Perforation of the tympanic membrane is usually present. This may be accompanied by mucosal changes such as polypoid degeneration and granulation tissue and osseous changes such as osteitis and sclerosis. The bacteriology of chronic otitis media differs from that of acute otitis media. Common organisms include *P aeruginosa, Proteus* sp, *Staphylococcus aureus,* and mixed anaerobic infections. The clinical hallmark of chronic otitis media is purulent aural discharge. Drainage may be continuous or intermittent, with increased severity during upper respiratory tract infection or following water exposure. Pain is uncommon except during acute exacerbations. Conductive hearing loss results from destruction of the tympanic membrane and ossicular chain. The medical treatment of chronic otitis media includes regular removal of infected debris, use of earplugs to protect against water exposure, and topical antibiotic drops for exacerbations. The activity of ciprofloxacin against *Pseudomonas* may help to dry a chronically discharging ear when given in a dosage of 500 mg orally twice a day for 1–6 weeks.

Definitive management is surgical in most cases. Tympanic membrane repair may be accomplished with temporalis muscle fascia or with homograft middle ear structures. Successful reconstruction of the tympanic membrane may be achieved in about 90% of cases, often with elimination of infection and significant improvement in hearing. When the mastoid air cells are involved by irreversible infection, they should be exenterated through mastoidectomy.

Cholesteatoma is a special variety of chronic otitis media. The most common cause is prolonged auditory tube dysfunction, with resultant chronic negative middle ear pressure that draws inward the upper flaccid portion of the tympanic membrane. This creates a squamous epithelium-lined sac, which—when its neck becomes obstructed—fills with desquamated keratin and becomes chronically infected. Cholesteatomas typically erode bone, with early penetration of the mastoid and destruction of the ossicular chain. Over time, they may erode the inner ear or facial nerve and on rare occasions may spread intracranially. Physical examination reveals an epitympanic retraction pocket or marginal tympanic membrane perforation that exudes keratin debris. The treatment of cholesteatoma is surgical marsupialization of the sac or its complete removal. This often requires creation of a "mastoid bowl" in which the ear canal and mastoid are joined into a large common cavity that must be periodically cleaned.

Campos MA et al: Etiology and therapy of chronic suppurative otitis. J Chemother 1995;7:427. (Ciprofloxacin is usually the initial drug of choice.)

Daly K: Risk factors for otitis media sequelae and chronicity. Ann Otol Rhinol Laryngol 1994;163(Suppl)39. (Male gender, white race, young age, early onset of otitis media, day care attendance, parental smoking.)

Ferlito A: A review of the definition, terminology and pathology of aural cholesteatoma. J Laryngol Otol 1993;107:483.

3. COMPLICATIONS OF OTITIS MEDIA

Mastoiditis

Acute suppurative mastoiditis usually evolves following several weeks of inadequately treated acute otitis media. It is characterized by postauricular pain and erythema accompanied by a spiking fever. Radiography reveals coalescence of the mastoid air cells due to destruction of their bony septa. Initial treatment consists of intravenous antibiotics and myringotomy for culture and drainage. Failure of medical therapy indicates the need for surgical drainage (mastoidectomy).

Gliklich RE et al: A contemporary analysis of acute mastoiditis. Arch Otolaryngol Head Neck Surg 1996;122:135.

Petrous Apicitis

The medial portion of the petrous bone between the inner ear and clivus may become a site of persistent infection when the drainage of its pneumatic cell tracts becomes blocked. This may cause foul discharge, deep ear and retro-orbital pain, and sixth nerve palsy (Gradenigo's syndrome); meningitis may be a complication. Treatment is with prolonged antibiotic therapy (based on culture results) and surgical drainage via petrous apicectomy.

Otogenic Skull Base Osteomyelitis

Infections originating in the external or middle ear may result in osteomyelitis of the skull base, usually due to *P aeruginosa*. The diagnosis and management of this disease are discussed in the section on external otitis.

Facial Paralysis

Facial palsy may be associated with either acute or chronic otitis media. In the acute setting, it results from inflammation of the nerve in its middle ear segment, perhaps mediated through bacterially secreted neurotoxins. Treatment consists of myringotomy for drainage and culture, followed by intravenous antibiotics (based on culture results). The use of corticosteroids is controversial. The prognosis is excellent, with complete recovery in the vast majority of cases.

Facial palsy associated with chronic otitis media usually evolves slowly due to chronic pressure on the nerve in the middle ear or mastoid by cholesteatoma. Treatment requires surgical correction of the underlying disease. The prognosis is less favorable than for facial palsy associated with acute otitis media.

Kangsanarak J et al: Extracranial and intracranial complications of suppurative otitis media: Report of 102 cases. J Laryngol Otol 1993;107:999.

Sigmoid Sinus Thrombosis

Trapped infection within the mastoid air cells adjacent to the sigmoid sinus may cause septic thrombophlebitis. This is heralded by signs of systemic sepsis (spiking fevers, chills), at times accompanied by signs of increased intracranial pressure (headache, lethargy, nausea and vomiting, papilledema). Treatment is with intravenous antibiotics (based on culture results), surgical drainage, and—when emboli are suspected—ligation of the internal jugular vein in the neck.

Grafstein E et al: Lateral sinus thrombosis complicating mastoiditis. Ann Emerg Med 1995;25:420. (Nonotologists need to be aware of the signs of an impending complication of otitis. Late diagnosis is common when the index of suspicion is low.)

Central Nervous System Infection

Otogenic meningitis is by far the most common intracranial complication of ear infection. In the setting of acute suppurative otitis media, it arises from hematogenous spread of bacteria, most commonly *H influenzae* and *S pneumoniae*. In chronic otitis media, it results either from passage of infections along preformed pathways such as the petrosquamous suture line or from direct extension of disease through the dural plates of the petrous pyramid.

Epidural abscesses arise from direct extension of disease in the setting of chronic infection. They are usually asymptomatic but may present with deep local pain, headache, and low-grade fever. They are often discovered as an incidental finding at surgery. Brain abscess may arise in the temporal lobe or cerebellum as a result of septic thrombophlebitis adjacent to an epidural abscess. The predominant causative organisms are *S aureus, S pyogenes,* and *S pneumoniae*. Rupture into the subarachnoid space results in meningitis and often death.

Kangsanarak J et al: Intracranial complications of suppurative otitis media: 13 years' experience. Am J Otol 1995;16:104. (The combination of otorrhea with fever and headache demands investigation.)

4. OTOSCLEROSIS

Otosclerosis is a progressive disease with a marked familial tendency that affects bone surrounding the inner ear. Lesions involving the footplate of the stapes result in increased impedance to the passage of sound through the ossicular chain, producing conductive hearing loss. This may be corrected through surgical replacement of the stapes with a prosthesis (stapedectomy). When otosclerotic lesions impinge on the cochlea, permanent sensory hearing loss occurs. Some evidence suggests that this level of hearing loss may be stabilized by treatment with oral sodium fluoride over prolonged periods of time (Florical—8.3 mg sodium fluoride and 364 mg calcium carbonate—two tablets orally each morning). Fluorides have minimal adverse effects other than occasional mild gastric irritation, which may be eliminated by ingesting the drug with meals.

Lundy L: Otosclerosis update. Otolaryngol Clin North Am 1996;29:257. (Emphasizes the importance of the laser as a tool in stapes surgery.)

Vartiainen E: Surgery in elderly patients with otosclerosis. Am J Otol 1995;16:536. (Results in patients over age 60 equal to those in younger patients.)

5. TRAUMA TO THE MIDDLE EAR

Tympanic membrane perforation may result from impact injury or explosive acoustic trauma. Spontaneous healing occurs in the great majority of cases. Persistent perforation may result from secondary infection brought on by exposure to water. Patients should be advised to wear earplugs while swimming or bathing during the healing period. Hemorrhage behind an intact tympanic membrane (hemotympanum) may follow blunt trauma or extreme barotrauma. Spontaneous resolution over several weeks is the usual course. When a conductive hearing loss greater than 30 dB persists for more than 3 months following trauma, disruption of the ossicular chain should be suspected. Middle ear exploration with reconstruction of the ossicular chain, combined with repair of the tympanic membrane when required, will usually restore hearing.

Berger G et al: Non-explosive blast injury of the ear. J Laryngol Otol 1994;108:395. (Spontaneous closure in 95%. Prognosis good for conductive loss, but 20% have sensorineural loss with poorer prognosis.)

6. MIDDLE EAR NEOPLASIA

Primary middle ear tumors are rare. Glomus tumors arise either in the middle ear (glomus tympanicum) or in the jugular bulb with upward erosion into the hypotympanum (glomus jugulare). They present clinically with pulsatile tinnitus and hearing loss. A vascular mass may be visible behind an intact tympanic membrane. Large glomus jugulare tumors are often associated with multiple cranial neuropathies, especially involving nerves VII, IX, X, XI, and XII. Treatment may require surgery, radiotherapy, or both.

Amble FR et al: Middle ear adenoma and adenocarcinoma. Otolaryngol Head Neck Surg 1993;109:871. (Postulating origin of tumor from paraganglionic tissue.)

EARACHE

External otitis and acute otitis media are both painful conditions. In external otitis, there is often a recent history of swimming, Q-tip use, or physical trauma, while in acute otitis media there is usually an antecedent or concurrent upper respiratory infection. The physical findings also differ. In external otitis, the ear canal skin is erythematous, while in acute otitis media this generally occurs only if the tympanic membrane has ruptured, spilling purulent material into the ear canal. Also, in external otitis the tympanic membrane may be erythematous, but it retains its mobility owing to the normal aeration of the middle ear cavity. Pain out of proportion to the physical findings may be due to herpes zoster oticus, especially when vesicles appear in the ear canal or concha. Chronic otitis media is usually not painful except during acute exacerbations. Persistent pain and discharge from the ear suggest osteomyelitis of the skull base or cancer.

The sensory innervation of the ear is derived from the trigeminal, facial, glossopharyngeal, vagal, and upper cervical nerves. Because of this rich innervation, referred otalgia is quite frequent. Temporomandibular joint dysfunction is a common cause of ear pain. It is often made worse by chewing or psychogenic grinding of the teeth (bruxism) and may be associated with dental malocclusion. Management includes soft diet, local heat to the masticatory muscles, massage, analgesics, and dental referral. Repeated episodes of severe lancinating otalgia may occur in glossopharyngeal neuralgia. Treatment with carbamazepine (100–300 mg orally every 8 hours) often confers substantial symptomatic relief. Severe glossopharyngeal neuralgia, which is refractory to medical management, may respond to microvascular decompression of the ninth nerve. Infections and neoplasia that involve the oropharynx, hypopharynx, and larynx frequently cause otalgia. Persistent earache demands specialty referral to exclude cancer of the upper aerodigestive tract.

Cooper BC, Cooper DL: Recognizing otolaryngologic symptoms in patients with temporomandibular disorders. Cranio 1993;11:260. (Eighty-five percent present with ear symptoms.)

Yanagisawa K, Kveton JF: Referred otalgia. Am J Otolaryngol 1992;13:323. (Nonotologic causes, especially neck cancer, in patients without primary otologic disease.)

DISEASES OF THE INNER EAR

1. SENSORY HEARING LOSS

Diseases of the cochlea result in sensory hearing loss, a condition that is usually irreversible. Most cochlear diseases result in bilateral symmetric hearing loss. The presence of unilateral or asymmetric sensorineural hearing loss suggests a lesion proximal to the cochlea. Lesions affecting the eighth nerve and central auditory system are discussed in the section on neural hearing loss. The primary goals in the management of sensory hearing loss are prevention of further losses and functional improvement with amplification and auditory rehabilitation.

Presbyacusis

Presbyacusis is the progressive, predominantly high-frequency symmetric hearing loss of advancing age. It is difficult to separate the various etiologic factors (eg, noise trauma) that may contribute to presbyacusis, but genetic predisposition appears to play a role. Most patients notice a loss of speech discrimination that is especially pronounced in noisy environments. About 25% of people between the ages of 65 and 75 years and almost 50% of those over 75 experience hearing difficulties.

Nadol JB Jr: Hearing loss. N Engl J Med 1993;329:1092. (Review of anatomy, common causes, diagnosis, and treatment of both conductive and sensorineural hearing loss.)

Noise Trauma

Noise trauma is the second most common cause (after presbyacusis) of sensory hearing loss. Sounds exceeding 85 dB are potentially injurious to the cochlea, especially with prolonged exposures. The loss typically begins in the high frequencies (especially 4000 Hz) and progresses to involve the speech frequencies with continuing exposure. Among the more common sources of injurious noise are industrial machinery, weapons, and excessively loud music. In recent years, monitoring of noise levels in the workplace by regulatory agencies has led to preventive programs that have reduced the frequency of occupational losses. Individuals of all ages, especially those with existing hearing losses, should wear earplugs when exposed to moderately loud noises and specially designed earmuffs when exposed to explosive noises.

Henderson D, Hamernik RP: Biologic bases of noise-induced hearing loss. Occup Med 1995;10:513. (Acoustic trauma shears hair cells. Research indicates that it may be possible for hair cells to regenerate.)
Hetu R, Getty L, Quoc HT: Impact of occupational hearing loss on the lives of workers. Occup Med 1995;10:495.

Physical Trauma

Head trauma has effects on the inner ear similar to those of severe acoustic trauma. Some degree of sensory hearing loss may occur following simple concussion and is frequent after skull fracture.

Fitzgerald DC: Head trauma: Hearing loss and dizziness. J Trauma 1996;40:488. (Evaluation and management of blunt trauma and whiplash injuries from an otologic perspective.)

Ototoxicity

Ototoxic substances may affect both the auditory and vestibular systems. The most common ototoxic medications are salicylates, aminoglycosides, loop diuretics, and several antineoplastic agents, notably cisplatin. The latter three categories may cause irreversible hearing loss even when administered in therapeutic doses. When using these medications, it is important to identify high-risk patients such as those with preexisting hearing losses or renal insufficiency. Patients simultaneously receiving multiple ototoxic agents are at particular risk owing to ototoxic synergy. Useful measures to reduce the risk of ototoxic injury include serial audiometry and monitoring of serum peak and trough levels and substitution of equivalent nonototoxic drugs whenever possible.

Black FO, Pesznecker SC: Vestibular ototoxicity: Clinical considerations. Otolaryngol Clin North Am 1993;26: 713. (Risk minimized by attention to drug selection and dose, monitoring, and antecedent risk factors.)
Campbell KC, Durrant J: Audiologic monitoring for ototoxicity. Otolaryngol Clinics North Am 1993;26(5):903. (Advocates routine audiologic monitoring when potentially ototoxic medications are used.)

Sudden Sensory Hearing Loss

Sudden loss of hearing in one ear may occur at any age but is more common in the elderly. It most probably is the result of sudden vascular occlusion of the internal auditory artery or of a viral inner ear infection. Prognosis is mixed, with many patients suffering permanent deafness in the involved ear while others have complete recovery. Although the subject is controversial, oral corticosteroids are felt by many to improve the odds of recovery. A common regimen is prednisone, 80 mg/d, followed by a tapering dose over a 10-day period.

Fetterman BL et al: Prognosis and treatment of sudden sensorineural hearing loss. Am J Otol 1996;17:5296. (In a study of 837 patients, oral corticosteroid use is correlated with a better prognosis.)
Hughes G et al: Sudden sensorineural hearing loss. Otolaryngol Clin North Am 1996;29:393. (Causation, diagnostic evaluation, and management options.)

Other Causes of Sensory Hearing Loss

There are numerous less common causes of sensory hearing loss. Metabolic derangements (eg, diabetes, hypothyroidism, hyperlipidemia, and renal failure), infections (eg, measles, mumps, syphilis), autoimmune disorders (eg, polyarteritis, lupus erythematosus), physical factors (eg, radiation therapy) and hereditary syndromes are some of the chief examples. Identification of metabolic, infectious, or autoimmune sensory hearing losses is especially important, as these may occasionally be reversible with medical therapy. Meniere's syndrome and labyrinthitis are discussed in the section on vestibular disorders.

Minor LB: Neuro-otology: hearing. Curr Op Neurol 1995;8:89. (Recent advances in the diagnosis and management of hearing disorders.)

2. TINNITUS

Tinnitus is the perception of abnormal ear or head noises. Persistent tinnitus usually indicates the presence of sensory hearing loss. Intermittent periods of mild, high-pitched tinnitus lasting for several minutes are common in normal-hearing persons. When severe and persistent, tinnitus may interfere with sleep and the ability to concentrate, resulting in considerable psychologic distress.

The most important treatment of tinnitus is avoidance of exposure to excessive noise, ototoxic agents, and other factors that may cause cochlear damage. Masking the tinnitus with music or through amplification of normal sounds with a hearing aid may also bring some relief. Although intravenous treatment with antiarrhythmic drugs (eg, lidocaine) suppresses tinnitus in some individuals, evidence suggests no benefit with oral agents that are potentially suitable for long-term symptom relief. Among the numerous drugs that have been tried, oral antidepressants (eg, nortriptyline at an initial dosage of 50 mg orally at bedtime) have proved to be the most efficacious.

Pulsatile tinnitus should be distinguished from tonal tinnitus. Pulsations most often result from conductive hearing loss, which renders transmitted carotid pulsations more apparent. However, it may also indicate a vascular abnormality such as glomus tumor, carotid vaso-occlusive disease, arteriovenous malformation, or aneurysm. CT scan and vascular studies are often necessary to establish a definitive diagnosis.

Ito J, Sakakihara J: Tinnitus suppression by electrical stimulation of the cochlear wall and by cochlear implantation. Laryngoscope 1994;104:752. (Improvement in 69% of patients.)

Murai K et al: Review of pharmacologic treatment of tinnitus. Am J Otol 1992;13:454. (Discouraging experience with lidocaine and other drugs.)

Ogata Y et al: Biofeedback therapy in the treatment of tinnitus. Auris Nasus Larynx 1993;20:95. (Demonstrates some benefit in reducing muscular tension and mental distress in chronic tinnitus sufferers.)

Seidman MD, Jacobson GP: Update on tinnitus. Otolaryngol Clin North Am 1996;29:455. (Causes and management.)

3. VERTIGO
(Table 8–1)

Vertigo is the cardinal symptom of vestibular disease. It is either a sensation of motion when there is no motion or an exaggerated sense of motion in response to a given bodily movement. Thus, vertigo is not just "spinning" but may present, for example, as a sense of tumbling, of falling forward or backward, or of the ground rolling beneath one's feet ("earthquake-like"). It should be distinguished from imbalance, light-headedness, and syncope, all of which are usually nonvestibular in origin. The vertigo that results from peripheral vestibulopathy is usually of sudden onset, may be so severe that the patient is unable to walk or stand, and is frequently accompanied by nausea and vomiting. Tinnitus and hearing loss may be associated and provide strong support for a peripheral origin.

A minimal physical examination of the patient with vertigo includes the Romberg test, an evaluation of gait, and observation for the presence of nystagmus. In peripheral lesions, nystagmus is usually horizontal with a rotatory component; the fast phase usually beats away from the diseased side. Visual fixation tends to inhibit nystagmus except in very acute peripheral lesions or with central nervous system disease. The Nylen-Bárány maneuvers are intended to induce positioning nystagmus but are of limited use when the patient is able to visually fixate. This objection may be overcome either by placing +2-diopter lenses (Fresnel glasses) over the eyes or

Table 8–1. Common vestibular disorders: Differential diagnosis based on classic presentations.

Duration of Typical Vertiginous Episodes	Auditory Symptoms Present	Auditory Symptoms Absent
Seconds	Perilymphatic fistula	Positioning vertigo (cupulolithiasis), vertebrobasilar insufficiency, cervical vertigo
Hours	Endolymphatic hydrops (Meniere's syndrome), syphilis	Recurrent vestibulopathy, vestibular migraine
Days	Labyrinthitis, labyrinthine concussion	Vestibular neuronitis
Months	Acoustic neuroma, ototoxicity	Multiple sclerosis, cerebellar degeneration

by making observations in the dark by means of electronystagmographic recording. The Fukuda test, in which the patient walks in place with eyes closed, is useful for detecting subtle defects. A positive response is observed when the patient rotates, usually toward the side of the diseased labyrinth. Vertigo arising from central lesions tends to develop gradually and then become progressively more severe and debilitating. Nystagmus is not always present but can occur in any direction and may be dissociated in the two eyes. The associated nystagmus is often nonfatigable, vertical rather than horizontal in orientation, without latency, and unsuppressed by visual fixation. Electronystagmography is useful in documenting these characteristics. The evaluation of central audiovestibular dysfunction usually requires imaging of the brain with CT scans or, particularly, MRI.

Episodic vertigo can occur in patients with diplopia from external ophthalmoplegia and is maximal when the patient looks in the direction where the separation of images is greatest. Cerebral lesions involving the temporal cortex may also produce vertigo, which is sometimes the initial symptom of a seizure. Finally, vertigo may be a feature of a number of systemic disorders and can occur as a side effect of certain anticonvulsant, antibiotic, hypnotic, analgesic, and tranquilizing drugs or of alcohol.

Laboratory investigations such as audiologic evaluation, caloric stimulation, electronystagmography, CT scan, and brain stem auditory evoked potential studies are indicated in patients with persistent vertigo or when central nervous system disease is suspected. These studies will help to distinguish between central and peripheral lesions and to identify causes requiring specific therapy. Electronystagmography consists of objective recording of the nystagmus induced by head and body movements, gaze, and caloric stimulation. It is helpful in quantifying the degree of vestibular hypofunction and may help with the differentiation between peripheral and central lesions. Computer-driven rotatory chairs and posturography platforms offer improved diagnostic abilities but are not widely available.

Ruckenstein MJ: A practical approach to dizziness. Postgrad Med 1995;97:70.

Vertigo Syndromes Due to Peripheral Lesions

A. Endolymphatic Hydrops (Meniere's Syndrome): Meniere's syndrome results from distention of the endolymphatic compartment of the inner ear. The primary lesion appears to be in the endolymphatic sac, which is thought to be responsible for endolymph filtration and excretion. Although a precise cause of hydrops cannot be established in most cases, two known causes are syphilis and head trauma. The classic syndrome consists of episodic vertigo, usually lasting 1–8 hours; low-frequency sensorineural hear-

ing loss, often fluctuating; tinnitus, usually low-tone and "blowing" in quality; and a sensation of aural pressure. Symptoms wax and wane as the endolymphatic pressure rises and falls. Caloric testing commonly reveals loss or impairment of thermally induced nystagmus on the involved side.

Specific treatment is intended to lower endolymphatic pressure. A low-salt diet (< 2 g sodium daily), at times supplemented by diuretics, adequately controls symptoms in the great majority of patients. A typical diuretic regimen is hydrochlorothiazide, 50–100 mg daily. In those who have failed medical therapy and remain disabled by their vertigo, surgical decompression of the endolymphatic sac may bring relief.

Episodic vertigo resembling that of Meniere's syndrome but without accompanying auditory symptoms is known as recurrent vestibulopathy. The pathogenic mechanism of this symptom complex is unknown in most cases, though a few patients suffer from a variant of migraine whereas others go on to develop the classic syndrome of endolymphatic hydrops.

B. Labyrinthitis: Patients with labyrinthitis suffer from acute onset of continuous, usually severe vertigo lasting several days to a week, accompanied by hearing loss and tinnitus. During a recovery period that lasts for several weeks, rapid head movements may bring on transient vertigo. Hearing may return to normal or remain permanently impaired in the involved ear. The cause of labyrinthitis is unknown, although it frequently follows an upper respiratory tract infection.

C. Vestibular Neuronitis: In vestibular neuronitis, a paroxysmal, usually single attack of vertigo occurs without accompanying impairment of auditory function and may persist for several days to weeks before clearing. Examination reveals nystagmus and absent responses to caloric stimulation on one or both sides. The cause of the disorder is unclear. Treatment is symptomatic.

D. Traumatic Vertigo: The most common cause of vertigo following head injury is labyrinthine concussion. Symptoms generally diminish within several days but may linger for a month or more. Basilar skull fractures that traverse the inner ear usually result in severe vertigo lasting several days to a week and deafness in the involved ear. Chronic posttraumatic vertigo may result from cupulolithiasis. This occurs when traumatically detached statoconia (otoconia) settle on the ampulla of the posterior semicircular canal and cause an excessive degree of cupular deflection in response to head motion. Clinically, this presents as episodic positioning vertigo. A less common source of posttraumatic vertigo is disruption of the oval or round window with leakage of perilymph into the middle ear. Perilymphatic fistulization may follow physical or barometric trauma or may result from erosion of the inner ear by cholesteatoma or neoplasm. Symptomatic fistulas are usually associated with both vertigo and hearing loss. Surgical repair may be necessary.

E. Positioning Vertigo: This form of vertigo is usually peripheral in origin, though it occasionally occurs with central lesions. Transient vertigo following changes in head position is a frequent complaint. The term "positioning vertigo" is more accurate than "positional vertigo" because it is provoked by changes in head position rather than by the maintenance of a particular posture. Use of the term "*benign positional vertigo*" is discouraged except for cases known to be unassociated with central nervous system disorders. True positional vertigo suggests either vertebrobasilar insufficiency or dysfunction of the cervical spine.

The typical symptoms of positioning vertigo occur in clusters that persist for several days. Typically with peripheral lesions, there is a latency period of several seconds following a head movement before symptoms develop, and they subside within 10–60 seconds. Constant repetition of the positional change leads to habituation. Recent single-session physical therapy protocols, based on the theory that positioning vertigo results from free-floating otoconia within a semicircular canal, have recently been developed. These strive to reposition the offending crystals through a series of head manipulations. New surgical procedures are also being explored which, by interrupting the posterior semicircular canal, attempt to prevent the exaggerated response to angular head motion. In central lesions, there is no latent period, fatigability, or habituation of the sign and symptoms.

Vertigo Syndromes Due to Central Lesions

Central nervous system causes of vertigo include brain stem vascular disease, arteriovenous malformations, tumor of the brain stem and cerebellum, multiple sclerosis, and vertebrobasilar migraine. Vertigo of central origin often becomes unremitting and disabling. There are commonly other signs of brain stem dysfunction (eg, cranial nerve palsies; motor, sensory, or cerebellar deficits in the limbs) or of increased intracranial pressure. Auditory function is generally spared. The underlying cause should be treated.

Management of the Patient With Vertigo

Few specific treatments for labyrinthine disorders have been designed to reverse a known pathogenic mechanism. Examples include low-salt diet and diuretics in Meniere's disease, antibiotic treatment of infectious diseases, and surgical repair of perilymphatic fistulas.

Symptomatic treatment is useful in the vertiginous patient to lessen the abnormal sensation and to alleviate vegetative symptoms such as nausea and vomiting. The most common drug classes employed are the antihistamines, anticholinergics, and sedative-hypnotics. Ample evidence exists that vestibular suppressant medications adversely affect the process of central compensation following acute vestibular disease. For this reason, these drugs should be used only for brief periods. Generally, they are best administered to patients with prominent vegetative symptoms and are best tapered and halted when symptoms are resolved, usually within 1–2 weeks.

In acute severe vertigo, diazepam, 2.5–5 mg intravenously, may abate an attack. Relief from nausea and vomiting usually requires an antiemetic delivered intramuscularly or by rectal suppository (eg, prochlorperazine, 10 mg intramuscularly, or 25 mg rectally every 6 hours). Less severe vertigo may often be successfully alleviated with antihistamines such as meclizine, 25 mg, or cyclizine or dimenhydrinate, 25–50 mg, orally every 6 hours. Scopolamine, administered in low dosage transdermally (0.5 mg/d), has proved beneficial to many patients with recurrent vertigo, although side effects (dry mouth, blurred vision, urinary obstruction) often limit its utility. Sometimes employing one-half or even one-fourth of a patch may allow therapeutic effect without the usual adverse consequences. A combination of drugs sometimes helps when the response to one drug is disappointing.

Bed rest may reduce the severity of acute vertigo. In chronic or recurrent vertigo, one of the most important therapies is exercise. Physical activity substantially enhances the central nervous system's ability to compensate for labyrinthine dysfunction and should be encouraged once nausea and vomiting have resolved. In general, the patient should be instructed to repeatedly perform maneuvers that provoke vertigo—up to the point of nausea or fatigue—in an effort to habituate them. Patients with vertigo and imbalance refractory to conventional therapy may benefit from a formal rehabilitation program under the guidance of a physical therapist. Substantial success has been reported in such patients through use of customized habituation protocols and specialized equipment, including tilt tables. Recently, use of a series of head maneuvers (theoretically intended to reposition free-floating otolithic particles) has gained popularity in the management of positioning vertigo. Such protocols have been shown to be at least as effective as vestibular habituation exercises, and they are less time-consuming.

Surgical remedies are reserved for those who remain substantially disabled despite a prolonged and varied trial of medical therapy and exercises. Selective section of the vestibular portion of the eighth nerve brings relief of vertigo in over 90% of such patients. Surgical removal of the semicircular canals (labyrinthectomy) is also highly effective but is appropriate only for patients with little or no hearing in the involved ear.

Cohen H et al: Disability in Meniere's disease. Arch Oto-laryngol Head Neck Surg 1995;121:29. (Significant disturbance in job performance and activities of daily living.)

Epley JM: Particle positioning maneuver for benign paroxysmal positioning vertigo. Otolaryngol Clin North Am 1996;29:323. (Includes a pictorial description of the procedures employed.)

Gacek RR, Gacek MR: Comparison of labyrinthectomy and vestibular neurectomy in the control of vertigo. Laryngoscope 1996;106:225. (Both are effective in relieving severe vertigo, but vestibular neurectomy is more suitable when useful residual hearing is present.)

LaRouere M: Surgical treatment of Meniere's disease. Otolaryngol Clin North Am 1996;29:311. (Indications for surgical intervention and the technical options.)

Nadol JB Jr: Vestibular neuritis. Otolaryngol Head Neck Surg 1995;112:162. (Natural history is variable. In some patients, complete recovery of acute signs and symptoms, including loss of vestibular response, is seen, whereas in others permanent changes have been reported.)

Steenerson RL, Cronin GW: Comparison of the canalith repositioning procedure and vestibular habituation training in forty patients with benign paroxysmal positional vertigo. Otolaryngol Head Neck Surg 1996;114:61. (Repositioning maneuvers are as effective as habituation protocols but less time-consuming.)

Telian SA, Shepard NT: Update on vestibular rehabilitation therapy. Otolaryngol Clin North Am 1996;29:359. (Reviews central nervous system plasticity and the compensation process as well as the indications and results with rehabilitation protocols.)

DISEASES OF THE CENTRAL AUDITORY & VESTIBULAR SYSTEMS (Table 8–1)

Lesions of the eighth cranial nerve and central audiovestibular pathways produce neural hearing loss and vertigo. One characteristic of neural hearing loss is deterioration of speech discrimination out of proportion to the decrease in pure tone thresholds. Another is auditory adaptation, wherein a steady tone appears to the listener to decay and eventually disappear. Auditory evoked responses are useful in distinguishing cochlear from neural losses and may give insight into the site of lesion within the central pathways.

Vertigo arising from central lesions tends to be more chronic and debilitating than that seen in labyrinthine disease. The associated nystagmus is often nonfatigable, vertical rather than horizontal in orientation, without latency, and unsuppressed by visual fixation. Electronystagmography is useful in documenting these characteristics. The evaluation of central audiovestibular dysfunction usually requires imaging of the brain with CT scans or MRI. The paramagnetic contrast agent gadolinium-DTPA, when used with MRI scanning, substantially improves diagnostic sensitivity in the detection of central audiovestibular lesions.

Gates G et al: Central auditory dysfunction, cognitive dysfunction, and dementia in older people. Arch Otolaryngol Head Neck Surg 1996;122:16. (Central auditory dysfunction often precedes dementia.)

Hirsch BE et al: Localizing retrocochlear hearing loss. Am J Otol 1996;17:537. (Evaluation of patients with suspected eighth nerve and brainstem dysfunction.)

1. VESTIBULAR SCHWANNOMA (Acoustic Neuroma)

Tumors of the cerebellopontine angle, most notably acoustic neuroma, cause central audiovestibular symptoms. Acoustic neuromas are among the most common intracranial neoplasms. These schwannomas generally arise from the vestibular division of the eighth nerve. When small, they may occasionally be excised, with preservation of hearing. Large tumors can also be safely removed in most cases, but cranial nerve palsies—especially facial paralysis and deafness—are common sequelae.

Jackler RK, Pitts LP: Selection of surgical approach to acoustic neuroma. Otolaryngol Clin North Am 1992; 25:361.

Kartush JM, Brackmann DE: Acoustic neuroma update. Otolaryngol Clin North Am 1996;29:377. (Current trends in management.)

NIH Consensus Development Conference Statement on Acoustic Neuroma. Arch Neurol 1994;51:201.

Selesnick SH et al: The changing clinical presentation of acoustic tumors in the MRI era. Laryngoscope 1993;103:431. (Atypical presentations are common; "classic" symptom patterns are the exception, not the rule.)

2. VASCULAR COMPROMISE

Vertebrobasilar insufficiency is a common cause of vertigo in the elderly. It is often triggered by changes in posture or extension of the neck. Reduced flow in the vertebrobasilar system may be demonstrated noninvasively through magnetic resonance angiography. Empirical treatment is with vasodilators, aspirin, and exercise.

Migraine may cause vertiginous attacks. The diagnosis is obvious when vertigo accompanies a typical headache pattern, but this is not always the case. In patients with a history of both migraine headaches and recurrent vertigo, a therapeutic trial of β-adrenergic blocking drugs (propranolol, 80–240 mg orally every 12–24 hours) and ergots (ergotamine, 1 mg orally every 4–6 hours) is reasonable.

Vascular loops that impinge upon the brain stem root entry zone of cranial nerves have been shown to cause dysfunction. Widely recognized examples are hemifacial spasm and tic douloureux. It has been suggested that hearing loss, tinnitus, and disabling positioning vertigo may result from such a loop abutting the eighth nerve.

Aragones JM et al: Migraine: An alternative diagnosis in the diagnosis of unclassified vertigo. Headache 1993;33: 125. (One-third of patients with unclassified vertigo fulfilled the criteria for migraine.)

Kikuchi S et al: Slow flow of the vertebrobasilar system in patients with dizziness and vertigo. Acta Otolaryngol 1993;113:257. (MRI detected slow flow in the posterior circulation in 35% of 102 patients over 50 years of age evaluated for vestibular complaints.)

Odkvist LM et al: Macrovascular causes underlying otoneurological disturbances. Acta Otolaryngol (Stockh) 1995;115:145. (MRI findings in vertebrobasilar ectasia and vascular loops occurring in relation to the eighth nerve.)

3. MULTIPLE SCLEROSIS

Most patients with multiple sclerosis suffer from episodic vertigo and chronic imbalance. Hearing loss in this disease is most commonly unilateral and of rapid onset. Spontaneous recovery may occur.

Drulovic B et al: Sudden hearing loss as the initial monosymptom of multiple sclerosis. Neurology 1993;43: 2703.

OTOLOGIC MANIFESTATIONS OF AIDS

The otologic manifestations of AIDS are protean. The pinna and external auditory canal may be affected by Kaposi's sarcoma as well as persistent and potentially invasive fungal infections, particularly due to *Aspergillus fumigatus*. The most common middle ear manifestation of AIDS is serous otitis media due to auditory tube dysfunction arising from adenoidal hypertrophy (HIV lymphadenopathy), recurrent mucosal viral infections, or an obstructing nasopharyngeal tumor (eg, lymphoma). Experience with middle ear effusion in AIDS patients suggests that ventilating tubes are seldom helpful and may trigger profuse watery otorrhea. Acute otitis media in the AIDS patient is usually caused by the typical bacterial organisms that occur in nonimmunocompromised patients, though *Pneumocystis carinii* otitis has been reported. Complaints referable to the inner ear are common in AIDS patients. Sensorineural hearing loss is common and in some cases appears to result from viral central nervous system infection. In cases of progressive hearing loss, it is important to evaluate for cryptococcal meningitis and syphilitic infection. Acute facial paralysis due to herpes zoster infection (Ramsay Hunt's syndrome) is quite common and follows a clinical course similar to that in nonimmunocompromised patients. Treatment is primarily with high-dose acyclovir. Use of corticosteroids under such circumstances is controversial.

Linstrom OJ et al: Otologic neurotologic manifestations of HIV-related disease. Otolaryngol Head Neck Surg 1993;108:680. (Examples include chronic otitis media, facial paralysis, otosyphilis, and Kaposi's sarcoma of the mastoid.)

DISEASES OF THE NOSE & PARANASAL SINUSES

INFECTIONS OF THE NOSE & PARANASAL SINUSES

1. VIRAL RHINITIS (Common Cold)

The nonspecific symptoms of the ubiquitous common cold are present in the early phases of many diseases that affect the upper aerodigestive tract. Because there are numerous serologic types of rhinoviruses, adenoviruses, and other viruses, patients remain susceptible throughout life. Headache, nasal congestion, watery rhinorrhea, sneezing, and a scratchy throat accompanied by general malaise are typical in viral infections. Nasal examination usually shows reddened, edematous mucosa and a watery discharge. The presence of purulent nasal discharge suggests bacterial infection.

There is no proved specific treatment for a cold, but supportive measures such as decongestants (pseudoephedrine, 30 mg every 4 hours, or 120 mg twice daily) may provide some relief of rhinorrhea and nasal obstruction. Nasal sprays such as oxymetazolone or phenylephrine are rapidly effective. They should not be used for more than a few days at a time, since chronic use leads to a rebound congestion that is often worse than the original symptoms. This chronic nasal stuffiness is known as rhinitis medicamentosa. Treatment requires complete cessation of the sprays. This triggers a period of severe nasal congestion that usually lasts 1–2 weeks. Topical intranasal corticosteroids (flunisolide, two sprays in each nostril twice daily) or a short tapering course of oral prednisone may help during the process of withdrawal.

Other than transient middle ear effusion, complications of viral rhinitis are unusual. Secondary bacterial infection may occur and is suggested by a change in color of the rhinorrhea from clear and watery to mucoid and yellow or green. In such cases, nasal cultures may help treatment. The most common pathogens are the same as those responsible for acute otitis media, ie, *Streptococcus pneumoniae,* other streptococci, *Haemophilus influenzae, Staphylococcus aureus,* and *Moraxella catarrhalis.*

Kirkpatrick GL: The common cold. Prim Care 1996; 23:657.

Luks D, Anderson MR: Antihistamines and the common cold. A review and critique of the literature. J Gen Intern Med 1996;11:240. (Little support for their use.)

2. ACUTE SINUSITIS

Acute sinus infections are uncommon compared to viral rhinitis. Because sinusitis usually has followed an acute respiratory infection and because media advertisements often use the term "sinusitis" when "rhinitis" would be more accurate, it is understandable that patients and physicians alike sometimes confuse these entities. In addition to the symptoms of rhinitis, the diagnosis of sinusitis requires clinical signs and symptoms that indicate involvement of the affected sinus or sinuses such as pain and tenderness over the involved sinus.

Sinusitis occurs when an undrained collection of pus accumulates in a sinus. Diseases that swell the nasal mucous membrane, such as viral or allergic rhinitis, are usually the underlying cause. Edematous mucosa causes obstruction of a sinus drainage tract, resulting in the accumulation of mucous secretion in the sinus cavity that becomes secondarily infected by bacteria. The typical pathogens of bacterial sinusitis are the same as those that cause acute otitis media: *S pneumoniae,* other streptococci, *H influenzae,* and, less commonly, *S aureus* and *Moraxella catarrhalis.*

Clinical Findings

A. Symptoms and Signs: Because the maxillary sinus is the largest of the paranasal sinuses and its ostia into the nose is superiorly placed, thereby failing to take advantage of gravity, it is the most commonly affected sinus. Pain and pressure over the cheek are the usual symptoms. Pain may refer to the upper incisor and canine teeth via branches of the trigeminal nerve, which traverse the floor of the sinus. It is not uncommon for maxillary sinusitis to result from dental infection, and teeth that are tender should be carefully examined for signs of abscess. Discolored nasal discharge and poor response to decongestants may also suggest sinusitis. Other possible causes for facial pain, such as trigeminal neuralgia and optic neuritis, should be kept in mind as well.

Acute ethmoiditis in adults is usually accompanied by maxillary sinusitis. In such cases, the symptoms of maxillary sinusitis generally predominate. Ethmoidal infection presents with pain and pressure over the high lateral wall of the nose that may radiate to the orbit. Periorbital cellulitis may be present.

Sphenoid sinusitis is usually seen in the setting of pansinusitis. The patient may complain of a headache "in the middle of the head" and often points to the vertex. Sixth nerve palsy may occur as the abducens nerve courses just lateral to the sinus.

Acute frontal sinusitis usually causes pain and tenderness of the forehead. This is most easily elicited by palpation of the orbital roof just below the medial end of the eyebrow. Palpation here is more accurate than percussion of the supraorbital area or forehead.

B. Imaging: Although it is often possible to make the diagnosis of sinusitis on clinical grounds alone, radiologic confirmation allows a more definitive diagnosis and is an objective monitor of the course of infection. Transillumination may aid in diagnosis, but variations in soft tissue thickness and technique often make interpretation difficult. The authors have not found it particularly helpful in practice.

The standard set of conventional sinus films and the sinus best seen in each view are Caldwell (frontal), Waters (maxillary), lateral (sphenoid), and submentovertical (ethmoid). Opacification without bone destruction is a typical feature of sinusitis. An air-fluid level may be seen if the films are taken with the patient upright rather than supine. The frontal sinus may occasionally appear normal even in the face of clinically compelling evidence of sinusitis. Limited coronal CT scans have increasingly replaced sinus films for screening sinusitis. They are no more expensive than conventional films and are more sensitive to both inflammatory changes and bone destruction (which would lead one to suspect a tumor). In recurrent sinusitis, CT scanning may help delineate anatomic blockage of the osteomeatal complex and thus suggest a role for functional endoscopic sinus surgery. If, however, malignancy is suspected (eg, because of unilateral cranial neuropathy or a nasoantral mass), then MRI with gadolinium should be ordered. MRI will distinguish tumor from inflammation and inspissated mucus far better than CT.

Treatment

In uncomplicated sinusitis with mild symptoms, outpatient management is usually successful. Oral decongestants (eg, pseudoephedrine, 60–120 mg orally three or four times daily), nasal decongestant sprays (eg, oxymetazoline, 0.05%, one or two sprays each nostril every 6–8 hours for up to 3 days; xylometazoline, 0.05–0.1%, one or two sprays each nostril every 6–8 hours for up to 3 days), and appropriate oral antibiotics are recommended. If purulent discharge is seen in the nose, it should be cultured. Maxillary sinus puncture and aspiration frequently provides a sample for culture; endoscopic sinus lavage may accomplish the same purpose. This is especially important when there is reason to suspect that the pathogen may not be typical, such as in nosocomial sinusitis in an intensive care unit. Although radiologic sinus findings are common, sinusitis in an

ICU is rarely the sole source of fever in this setting. Interestingly, the bacterial spectrum seen in sinusitis in AIDS is similar to that in more common settings; but aspiration for cytology may lead to a diagnosis of lymphoma, a not uncommon finding in apparent "sinusitis" in AIDS patients.

Because amoxicillin (250 mg orally three times a day) achieves better sinus penetration than ampicillin, it is an appropriate first choice. Alternatives include trimethoprim-sulfamethoxazole (4 mg/kg TMP and 20 mg/kg SMZ twice daily; available as tablets containing 80 or 160 TMP and 160 or 800 SMZ); cephalexin (250–500 mg orally daily); cefuroxime (250 mg orally twice daily); and cefaclor (250 mg orally three times a day). Cefixime (400 mg orally daily) is recommended by some on a cost basis, though it fails to cover common β-lactamase-producing organisms. Antibiotic treatment for sinusitis should be continued for 2 weeks, with longer courses sometimes required to prevent relapses.

Failure of sinusitis to resolve after an adequate course of oral antibiotics may necessitate hospital admission for intravenous antibiotics and possible surgical drainage. Frontal sinusitis that does not promptly respond to outpatient care should be managed aggressively, because the posterior sinus wall is adjacent to the dura and because undertreated infection may lead to intracranial extension. If intravenous antibiotics fail to ameliorate symptoms, a frontal sinus trephine may be necessary to drain and irrigate the sinus. Persistent maxillary empyema may be cultured and relieved with a needle inserted through the lateral wall of the nose or anterior wall of the antrum through the gingivobuccal sulcus.

Complications

Local complications of sinusitis include osteomyelitis and mucocele. Mucoceles, a consequence of long-standing ductal obstruction, are more common in the supraorbital ethmoids and frontal sinuses and may become secondarily infected. They appear radiologically as a smoothly expanded sinus filled with homogeneous soft tissue density. Treatment is surgical, requiring either drainage of the mucocele intranasally or its complete excision with fat ablation of the sinus cavity.

Osteomyelitis requires prolonged antibiotics as well as removal of necrotic bone. The frontal sinus is most commonly affected, with bone involvement suggested by a tender puffy swelling of the forehead. Following treatment, secondary cosmetic reconstructive procedures may be necessary.

Intracranial complications of sinusitis occur either through hematogenous spread, as in cavernous sinus thrombosis and meningitis, or by direct extension, as in epidural and intraparenchymal brain abscesses. Fortunately, they are rare today. Cavernous sinus thrombosis is heralded by ophthalmoplegia, chemosis, and visual loss. Frontal epidural abscess is usu-

ally quiescent. It may be detected on CT scan, a study recommended in all cases of atypical or complicated sinusitis.

It should always be kept in mind that paranasal sinus cancer is in the differential diagnosis of sinusitis. The presence of bone destruction radiologically, cranial neuropathies (especially V_2), persistent pain, epistaxis, or a prolonged clinical course should raise the suspicion of possible cancer.

Brook I: Microbiology and management of sinusitis. J Otolaryngol 1996;25:249. (*Streptococcus pneumoniae, Haemophilus influenzae,* and *Moraxella catarrhalis* are predominant in acute sinusitis, anaerobic bacteria and *Staphylococcus aureus* in chronic sinusitis.)

Diaz I, Bamberger DM: Acute sinusitis. Semin Respir Infect 1995;10:14.

Ferguson BJ: Acute and chronic sinusitis: How to ease symptoms and locate the cause. Postgrad Med 1995;97:45, 51, 55.

Knutson JW, Slavin RG: Sinusitis in the aged. Optimal management strategies. Drugs Aging 1995;7:310.

Mafee MF: Modern imaging of paranasal sinuses and the role of limited sinus computerized tomography: Considerations of time, cost and radiation. Ear Nose Throat J 1994;73:532, 536, 540 passim. (Indications for different imaging methods are reviewed, along with a discussion of the role of imaging for endoscopic sinus surgery.)

Reuler JB, Lucas LM, Kumar KL: Sinusitis: A review for generalists. West J Med 1995;163:40.

3. NASAL VESTIBULITIS

Inflammation at the nasal vestibule commonly results from folliculitis of the hairs that line this orifice. Systemic antibiotics effective against *S aureus* (such as dicloxacillin, 250 mg orally four times daily for 7–10 days) are indicated. Topical mupirocin (applied two or three times daily) may be a helpful addition. If recurrent, it is possible that the addition of rifampin (10 mg/kg orally twice daily for the last 4 days of treatment) may eliminate the *S aureus* carrier state. If a furuncle exists, it should be incised and drained, preferably intranasally. Adequate treatment of these infections is important to prevent retrograde spread of infection through valveless veins into the cavernous sinus and intracranial contents.

4. RHINOCEREBRAL MUCORMYCOSIS

Although mucormycosis is rare, any physician seeing patients in a primary care setting must be aware of its presenting signs and symptoms. The fungus *(Mucor, Absidia, Rhizopus)* spreads rapidly through vascular channels and may be lethal if not detected early. Patients with mucormycosis almost invariably have an underlying disease, often diabetes mellitus or uremia. It also occurs following bone marrow transplantation, in patients with lymphoma, in patients who are immunosuppressed for other reasons, and in patients receiving deferoxamine (a metal chelator). Occasional cases have been reported recently in patients with AIDS, though *Aspergillus* is more common in this setting. The initial symptoms may be similar to those of bacterial sinusitis, although facial pain is often more severe. Examination of the nasal mucosa is likely to show black, necrotic eschar adherent to the inferior turbinate, though this may not be present in early stages. Cranial neuropathies and black necrotic skin overlying the ethmoid sinuses are advanced signs. Early diagnosis requires suspicion of the disease and nasal or sinus biopsy, which reveals broad nonseptate hyphae within tissues. Because CT or MRI may initially show only soft tissue changes, intervention should be based on the clinical setting and not on radiologic demonstration of bony destruction—and certainly not intracranial changes.

Mucormycosis represents a medical and surgical emergency. Once recognized, prompt wide surgical debridement and amphotericin B by intravenous infusion are indicated. The use of liposomal amphotericin B may play a role as well. Close management of the underlying disease is also of great importance. Even with early diagnosis and immediate appropriate intervention, the prognosis is guarded. In diabetics, the mortality rate is about 20%; in patients with renal failure, the mortality rate is over 50%; in AIDS, close to 100%.

Harril WC et al: Chronic rhinocerebral mucormycosis. Laryngoscope 1996;106:1292. (A more indolent presentation, usually among diabetics, with an 80% cure rate.)

Nussbaum ES, Hall WA: Rhinocerebral mucormycosis: Changing patterns of disease. Surg Neurol 1994;41:152. (Patients with intracranial infection die. Early diagnosis and aggressive therapy are essential.)

Roithmann R et al: Diagnostic imaging of fungal sinusitis: Eleven new cases and literature review. Rhinology 1995;33:104. (MRI findings of hypo-intense signals on T1-weighted sequences that progress to signal-void area on T2-weighted sequences are characteristic.)

Strasser MD, Kennedy RJ, Adam RD: Rhinocerebral mucormycosis: Therapy with amphotericin B lipid complex. Arch Intern Med 1996;156:337. (Survival of 60-year-old diabetic woman with cavernous sinus involvement.)

Tierney MR, Baker AS: Infections of the head and neck in diabetes mellitus. Infect Dis Clin North Am 1995;9:195.

Yohai RA et al: Survival factors in rhino-orbital-cerebral mucormycosis. Surv Ophthalmol 1994;39:3. (A literature review and analysis of benefits of therapeutic options including aggressive surgery, intravenous amphotericin B, hyperbaric oxygen, and amphotericin B irrigation.)

ALLERGIC RHINITIS

The symptoms of "hay fever" are similar to those of viral rhinitis but are usually more persistent and show seasonal variation. Nasal symptoms are often accompanied by eye irritation, which causes pruritus, erythema, and excessive tearing. Numerous allergens may cause these symptoms: pollens are most common in the spring, grasses in the summer, and ragweed in the fall. Dust and household mites may produce year-round symptoms.

On physical examination, the mucosa of the turbinates is usually pale or violaceous because of venous engorgement—in contrast to the erythema of viral rhinitis. Nasal polyps, which are yellowish boggy masses of hypertrophic mucosa, may be seen.

Treatment is symptomatic in most cases. Oral decongestants alone (eg, pseudoephedrine, 60–120 mg orally three or four times daily) are usually helpful, although antihistamines more specifically counteract allergic mechanisms. Numerous over-the-counter preparations are available. Common antihistamines include brompheniramine or chlorpheniramine (4 mg orally every 6–8 hours, or 8–12 mg orally every 8–12 hours as a sustained-release tablet) and clemastine (1.34–2.68 mg orally twice daily). Nonsedating long-acting antihistamines such as loratidine (10 mg orally daily) or fexofenadine (60 mg orally twice daily), though expensive and by prescription, are especially helpful in patients intolerant of the drowsiness associated with many other classes of antihistamines. Astemizole and terfenadine have been associated with sudden death from presumed QT prolongation, especially in patients receiving erythromycin or ketoconazole concomitantly, and thus should be avoided.

Nasal corticosteroid sprays such as beclomethasone (42 μg/spray) and flunisolide (25 μg/spray) are often remarkably effective if used appropriately. These sprays should be administered as two activations into each nostril twice daily for 1 month. Compliance is poor unless patients know that improvement usually does not begin until 1–2 weeks after starting therapy. Intranasal steroids have a role in seasonal allergies in shrinking nasal polyps, often eliminating the need for surgery. Intranasal cromolyn may be useful, especially when administered before expected contact with an offending allergen.

Maintaining an allergen-free environment by covering pillows and mattresses with plastic covers, substituting synthetic materials (foam mattress, acrylics) for animal products (wool, horsehair), and removing dust-collecting household fixtures (carpets, drapes, bedspreads, wicker) is worth the attempt to help more troubled patients. Air purifiers and dust filters (such as Bionair models) may also aid in maintaining an allergen-free environment. When symptoms are extremely bothersome, a search for offending allergens may prove helpful. This can either be done by skin testing or by serum RAST testing. Desensitization by gradually increasing subdermal exposure to identified allergens may be tried in selected patients, with variable results.

Graft DF: Allergic and nonallergic rhinitis: Directing medical therapy at specific symptoms. Postgrad Med 1996;100:64.

Kobayashi RH et al: Topical nasal sprays: Treatment of allergic rhinitis. Am Fam Physician 1994;50:151, 161. (Reviews the available and newer steroid nasal sprays as well as other topical drugs, such as cromolyn and ipratropium.)

Mabry RL: Allergic and infective rhinosinusitis: Differential diagnosis and interrelationship. Otolaryngol Head Neck Surg 1994;111(3 Part 2):335. (Both infection and allergy may contribute to a patient's symptoms.)

Meltzer EO et al: A pharmacologic continuum in the treatment of rhinorrhea: The clinician as economist. J Allergy Clin Immunol 1995;95(5 Part 2):1147. (Reviews the usage, quality, and cost of major therapies: nasal steroids, antihistamines, and anticholinergics.)

Noble SL, Forbes RC, Woodbridge HB: Allergic rhinitis. Am Fam Physician 1995;51:837. (A practical approach, beginning with clinical recognition and recommended avoidance procedures, decongestant and antihistamine options, and immunotherapy for those unresponsive to simpler methods; cromolyn is the first drug choice in pregnant women.)

Pedinoff AJ: Approaches to the treatment of seasonal allergic rhinitis. Med J 1996;89:1130.

Tan R, Corren J: Optimum treatment of rhinitis in the elderly. Drugs Aging 1995;7:168. (Emphasis on medication side effects in older patients.)

OLFACTORY DYSFUNCTION

The physiology of olfaction is less well understood than that of the other special senses. In the past few years, however, discovery of the family of odor-receptor genes as well as inositol phosphate and cyclic nucleotide signaling pathways have led to a molecular basis of olfactory reception. Clinically, odorant molecules must traverse the nasal vault to reach the cribriform area and become soluble in the mucus overlying the exposed dendrites of receptor cells. Anatomic lack of access to the receptor cells of the first cranial nerve is the most common cause of olfactory dysfunction (hyposmia or anosmia). Polyps, septal deformities, and nasal tumors may all contribute to this inability of air to reach the area of the cribriform plate high in the nose where these receptors are located. Transient olfactory dysfunction often accompanies the common cold, nasal allergies, and perennial rhinitis. About 20% of impaired olfactory function is idiopathic, although it often follows a viral illness. Some have suggested administering large doses of vitamin A and zinc to such patients, although little evidence supports their use. Central nervous system neoplasms, especially those that involve the olfactory groove or temporal lobe, may affect olfaction. Head trauma accounts for less than 5% of cases of hyposmia. Absent, diminished, or distorted smell or taste has been reported in a wide variety of endocrine, nutritional, and nervous disorders. A great many medications have also been implicated.

Evaluation of olfactory dysfunction should include a thorough history of systemic illnesses and medication use as well as a physical examination focusing on the nose and nervous system. Most clinical offices are not set up to test olfaction, but such feats may at times be worthwhile if only to assess whether a patient possesses any sense of smell at all. Odor threshold should be tested in increasing concentrations. For example, use n-butyl alcohol (1-butanolol) in concentrations up to 4% in deionized water. Serial 3:1 dilutions in 12 steps produce an initial test of 46 ppm (v/v) and the maximum of 3055 ppm (at 4%). Odor identification can be tested using standardized choices (see references). In permanent hyposmia, counseling should be offered about seasoning foods with spices (eg, pepper) that stimulate the trigeminal as well as olfactory chemoreceptors and about safety issues such as the use of smoke alarms and electric rather than gas home appliances.

Axel R: The molecular logic of smell. Sci Am 1995;273:154.

Henkin RI: Drug-induced taste and smell disorders: Incidence, mechanisms and management related primarily to treatment of sensory receptor dysfunction. Drug Saf 1994;11:318. (Many drugs impair taste and smell. Loss of acuity occurs primarily by drug inactivation of receptor function through inhibition of tastant-odorant receptor; distortions occur primarily by a drug inducing abnormal persistence of receptor activity.)

Keverne EB: Olfactory learning. Curr Opin Neurobiol 1995;5:482. (Discovery of a huge family of odorant receptor genes is opening new avenues for study of olfaction and may lead to a molecular basis of olfactory perception.)

EPISTAXIS

Bleeding from Kiesselbach's plexus, a vascular plexus on the anterior nasal septum, is by far the most common type of epistaxis encountered. Predisposing factors include nasal trauma (nose picking, foreign bodies, forceful nose blowing), rhinitis, drying of the nasal mucosa from low humidity, deviation of the nasal septum, alcohol use, and antiplatelet medications. Most cases of anterior epistaxis may be successfully treated by direct pressure on the bleeding site. The nasal alae should be firmly compressed for at least 10 minutes. Venous pressure is reduced in the sitting position, and leaning forward lessens the swallowing of blood. Short-acting topical nasal decongestants (eg, phenylephrine, 0.125–1% solution, one or two sprays), which act as vasoconstrictors, may also be helpful. When the bleeding does not readily subside, the nose should be examined, using good illumination and suction, in an attempt to locate the bleeding site. Topical 4% cocaine applied either as a spray or on a cotton strip serves both as an anesthetic and as a vasoconstricting agent. If cocaine is unavailable, a topical decongestant (eg, oxymetazoline) and a topical anesthetic (eg, tetracaine) provide equivalent results. When visible, the bleeding site may be cauterized with silver nitrate, diathermy, or electrocautery. A supplemental patch of Surgicel or Gelfoam may be helpful.

Occasionally, a site of bleeding may be inaccessible to direct control, or attempts at direct control may be unsuccessful. In such cases, nasal packing is necessary. A properly placed anterior pack requires several feet of half-inch iodoform packing lubricated with bacitracin or petroleum ointment. The packing is carefully and systematically placed along the floor and then the vault of the nose. If the equipment necessary to place a pack is not available, various manufactured nasal balloons may serve as either a temporizing or definitive solution.

About 5% of nasal bleeding originates in the posterior nasal cavity. This requires placement of a pack to occlude the choana before placement of a pack anteriorly. Because this is uncomfortable for the patient and because it requires oxygen supplementation to prevent hypoxia, hospitalization for several days is indicated. Narcotic analgesics are needed to reduce the considerable discomfort and elevated blood pressure caused by a posterior pack. Immediate ligation of the nasal arterial supply (internal maxillary artery and ethmoid arteries) is a possible alternative to posterior nasal packing, as is endovascular embolization of the internal maxillary artery. This is certainly necessary when packing fails to control life-threatening hemorrhage. On rare occasions, ligation of the external carotid artery may be necessary.

After control of epistaxis, the patient is advised to avoid vigorous exercise for several days. Avoidance of hot or spicy foods and tobacco is also advisable, as they may cause vasodilation. Avoiding nasal trauma, including digital self-trauma, is an obvious necessity. Lubrication with petroleum jelly or bacitracin ointment and increasing home humidity may be useful ancillary measures.

It is important in all patients with epistaxis to consider underlying causes of the bleeding. Laboratory assessment of bleeding parameters may be indicated, especially in recurrent cases. Other causes of recurrent epistaxis, such as hereditary hemorrhagic telangiectasia (Osler-Weber-Rendu syndrome), should also be considered. Similarly, once the acute episode has passed, careful examination of the nose and paranasal sinuses to rule out neoplasia is wise.

Alvi A, Joyner-Triplett N: Acute epistaxis: How to spot the source and stop the flow. Postgrad Med 1996 May, 99:83. (Cauterization, nasal packing, and intranasal tampon or balloon are often effective, but arterial ligation or angiographic embolization may be necessary.)

Elahi MM et al: Therapeutic embolization in the treatment of intractable epistaxis. Arch Otolaryngol Head Neck Surg 1995;121:65. (Therapeutic embolization using polyvinyl alcohol of the distal branches of the internal maxillary artery is an effective and safe technique.

Anatomic variations occasionally preclude embolization; patients rarely require reembolization.)

McGarry GW, Gatehouse S, Vernham G: Idiopathic epistaxis, haemostasis and alcohol. Clin Otolaryngol 1995;20:174. (Prolonged bleeding time was significantly associated with a history of alcohol use.)

Strong EB et al: Intractable epistaxis: Transantral ligation vs. embolization: Efficacy review and cost analysis. Otolaryngol Head Neck Surg 1995;113:674.

Viducich RA, Blanda MP, Gerson LW: Posterior epistaxis: Clinical features and acute complications. Ann Emerg Med 1995;25:592.

NASAL TRAUMA

The nasal pyramid is the most frequently fractured bone in the body. Fracture is suggested by crepitance or palpably mobile bony segments. Epistaxis and pain are common, as are soft tissue hematomas ("black eye"). It is important to make certain that there is no palpable step-off of the infraorbital rim, which would indicate the presence of a zygomatic complex fracture. Radiologic confirmation may at times be helpful but is not necessary in uncomplicated nasal fractures.

Treatment is aimed at maintaining long-term nasal airway patency and nasal aesthetics. Closed reduction, using topical 4% cocaine and locally injected 1% lidocaine, should be attempted within 1 week of injury. In the presence of marked nasal swelling, it is best to wait several days for the edema to subside before undertaking reduction. Persistent functional or cosmetic defects may be repaired by delayed reconstructive nasal surgery.

Intranasal examination should be performed in all cases to rule out septal hematoma, which appears as a widening of the anterior septum, visible just posterior to the columella. The septal cartilage receives its only nutrition from its closely adherent mucoperichondrium. An untreated subperichondrial hematoma will result in loss of the nasal cartilage with resultant saddlenose deformity. Undrained septal hematomas may become infected, with S aureus the predominant organism. Treatment consists of incision and drainage via an intranasal septal mucosal incision. It is important to be sure that both sides of the septal cartilage are adequately drained. A small Penrose drain sutured in place is helpful. Antibiotics should be given and the drained fluid sent for culture.

Hussain K et al: A comprehensive analysis of craniofacial trauma. J Trauma 1994;36:34.

Owen GO, Parker AJ, Watson DJ: Fractured-nose reduction under local anaesthesia: Is it acceptable to the patient? Rhinology 1992;30:89. (Yes.)

Pollock RA: Nasal trauma: Pathomechanics and surgical management of acute injuries. Clin Plast Surg 1992; 19(1):133. (Biomechanical forces.)

Sharp JF, Denholm S: Routine X-rays in nasal trauma: The influence of audit on clinical practice. J R Soc Med

1994;87:153. (Routine x-rays in simple nasal trauma are of limited value.)

Verwoerd CD: Present day treatment of nasal fractures: Closed versus open reduction. Facial Plast Surg 1992; 8:220.

TUMORS & GRANULOMATOUS DISEASE

1. BENIGN NASAL TUMORS

Nasal Polyps

Nasal polyps are pale, edematous, mucosally covered masses commonly seen in patients with allergic rhinitis. They may result in chronic nasal obstruction and a diminished sense of smell. In patients with nasal polyps and a history of asthma, aspirin should be avoided, as it may precipitate a severe episode of bronchospasm. The presence of polyps in children should alert the physician to the possibility of cystic fibrosis.

Medical treatment with topical nasal steroid sprays (such as beclomethasone, 42 µg/spray) is usually successful for small polyps. A short course of oral corticosteroids (eg, prednisone, 6-day course using twenty-one 5 mg tablets: 30 mg on day 1 and tapering by 5 mg each day) may also be of benefit. When medical management is unsuccessful, polyps should be removed surgically. In healthy persons, this is a minor outpatient procedure. When frequent recurrence is likely or when surgery itself is associated with increased risk (such as in asthmatics), a more complete procedure, such as ethmoidectomy, may be advisable initially. In recurrent polyposis, it may be necessary to remove polyps from the ethmoid, sphenoid, and maxillary sinuses to provide longer-lasting relief. This may be done intranasally, endoscopically, via an anterior transantral route through the gingivolabial sulcus (Caldwell-Luc), or through an external skin incision depending on the extent of disease.

Bernstein JM, Gorfien J, Noble B: Role of allergy in nasal polyposis: A review. Otolaryngol Head Neck Surg 1995;113:724. (A proposed multivariate theory of pathogenesis.)

Cook PR et al: Antrochoanal polyposis: A review of 33 cases. Ear Nose Throat J 1993;72:401, 404. (Choanal polyps account for about 20% of the authors' patients undergoing endoscopic removal, which was successful in all but one instance.)

Hosemann W, Gode U, Wagner W: Epidemiology, pathophysiology of nasal polyposis, and spectrum of endonasal sinus surgery. Am J Otolaryngol 1994;15:85.

Lund VJ, MacKay IS: Outcome assessment of endoscopic sinus surgery. J R Soc Med 1994;87:70.

Inverted Papilloma

Inverted papillomas are benign tumors that usually arise in the common wall between the nose and maxillary sinus. They present with unilateral nasal obstruction and occasionally hemorrhage. Because squamous cell carcinomas are seen in 5–10% of inverted papillomas, complete excision is necessary. All excised tissue (not just a sampling) should be carefully reviewed by the pathologist to be sure no carcinoma is present.

Lawson W et al: Inverted papilloma: A report of 112 cases. Laryngoscope 1995;105(3 Part 1):282. (A summary review of the clinical course and management of inverted papilloma.)

Woodruff WW, Vrabec DP: Inverted papilloma of the nasal vault and paranasal sinuses: Spectrum of CT findings. AJR Am J Roentgenol 1994;162:419. (Reviews the CT findings of this entity.)

Juvenile Angiofibroma

These highly vascular tumors arise in the nasopharynx, typically in adolescent males. Initially, they cause nasal obstruction and hemorrhage. Any adolescent male with recurrent epistaxis should be checked to be sure he is not harboring an angiofibroma. Though benign, these tumors expand locally from the nasopharynx to involve the nasal cavity, the sphenoid and other paranasal sinuses, and the clivus and may extend extradurally or even intradurally at the skull base. Treatment consists of surgical excision, with preoperative embolization to reduce bleeding.

Kaplan MJ: Angiofibroma. In: *Current Therapy in Otolaryngology–Head and Neck Surgery.* Gates GA (editor). Mosby, 1993.

Ungkanont K et al: Juvenile nasopharyngeal angiofibroma: An update of therapeutic management. Head Neck 1996;18:60. (Radiologic assessment with MRI or CT followed by embolization and surgical resection is the most common primary approach.)

Radkowski D et al: Angiofibroma: Changes in staging and treatment. Arch Otolaryngol Head Neck Surg 1996;122: 122. (Surgical excision possible in 95% of cases. Although 20% recur, subsequent surgery may be curative; no craniotomies were required.)

2. MALIGNANT NASOPHARYNGEAL & PARANASAL SINUS TUMORS

Unfortunately, malignant tumors of the nose, nasopharynx, and paranasal sinuses tend to remain asymptomatic until late in their course. In general, the prognosis is poor. Early symptoms are nonspecific, mimicking those of rhinitis or sinusitis. Unilateral nasal obstruction and discharge are common, with pain and recurrent hemorrhage often clues to the diagnosis of cancer. Any patient with unilateral or persistent nasal symptoms should be thoroughly evaluated. A high index of suspicion remains a key to the earlier diagnosis of these tumors. Patients often present with advanced symptoms such as proptosis, expansion of a cheek, or ill-fitting maxillary dentures. Malar hypesthesia, due to involvement of the infraorbital nerve, is common in maxillary sinus tumors. Biopsy is necessary for definitive diagnosis, and MRI or CT scan will usually delineate the extent of disease.

Squamous cell carcinoma is the most common cancer seen in this anatomic region. It is especially common in the nasopharynx, where it obstructs the auditory tube and results in serous otitis media. Nasopharyngeal carcinoma (poorly differentiated squamous cell carcinoma, nonkeratinizing squamous cell carcinoma, or lymphoepithelioma) is usually associated with elevated IgA antibody to the viral capsid antigen of the Epstein-Barr virus. It is particularly common in patients of southern Chinese descent but is seen in all populations. Any adult with persistent serous otitis media, especially when unilateral, requires careful evaluation of the nasopharynx. Adenocarcinomas, mucosal melanomas, sarcomas, and non-Hodgkin's lymphomas are less commonly encountered neoplasms of this area.

Treatment depends on the tumor type and the extent of disease. Nasopharyngeal carcinoma is best treated by radiotherapy and concomitant cisplatin chemotherapy, the latter acting as a radiosensitizer. Other squamous cell carcinomas are best treated—when resectable—with a combination of surgery and irradiation. Numerous protocols investigating the role of chemotherapy are under evaluation. Cranial base surgery appears to be an effective modality in improving the overall prognosis in paranasal sinus malignancies eroding the ethmoid roof.

Alvarez I et al: Prognostic factors in paranasal sinus cancer. Am J Otolaryngol 1995;16:109. (Advanced T-stage and anterior skull base erosion were the most accurate predictors of poor prognosis in this large series.)

Janecka IP et al: Treatment of paranasal sinus cancer with cranial base surgery: Results. Laryngoscope 1994;104(5 Part 1):553.

Osguthorpe JD: Sinus neoplasia: Arch Otolaryngol Head Neck Surg 1994;120:19. (An overview.)

Stelzer KJ et al: Fast neutron radiotherapy. The University of Washington experience. Acta Ontol 1994;33:275. (Neutron radiotherapy results in improved local control compared with conventional irradiation but no improved survival among adenoid cystic carcinomas of the salivary glands.)

3. WEGENER'S GRANULOMATOSIS, NK/T CELL EBV(+) LYMPHOMA, & SARCOIDOSIS

The nose and paranasal sinuses are involved in over 90% of cases of Wegener's granulomatosis. It is often not realized that involvement at these sites is more common than involvement of lungs or kidneys. Examination shows bloodstained crusts and friable

mucosa. Biopsy classically shows necrotizing granulomas and vasculitis, but in practice the differential diagnosis may be more difficult. Sarcoidosis also commonly presents in the paranasal sinuses and is clinically similar to other chronic sinonasal inflammatory processes. Biopsy shows nonnecrotic granulomas.

Polymorphic reticulosis (midline malignant reticulosis, idiopathic midline destructive disease, lethal midline granuloma), as the multitude of apt descriptive terms suggest, is not well understood but appears to be a nasal lymphoma. In contrast to Wegener's granulomatosis, involvement is limited to the mid face, and there may be extensive bone destruction. Its progression in time to a lymphoma is being described with increasing frequency.

Recent studies suggest that these are NK cell/T cell Epstein-Barr-positive lymphomas. Histologically, there is a dense infiltrate of mature lymphocytes, histiocytes, and immunoblasts.

Even with immunohistochemical stains, the differential diagnosis of such lesions may be difficult.

Unlike Wegener's granulomatosis and sarcoidosis, which are treated with drugs such as steroids (and cyclophosphamide, in Wegener's granulomatosis), T cell lymphomas are usually best managed by local irradiation.

Ataman M et al: Wegener's granulomatosis: Case report and review of the literature. Rhinology 1994;32:92.

Burlacoff SG, Wong FS: Wegener's granulomatosis. The great masquerade: A clinical presentation and literature review. J Otolaryngol 1993;22:94.

DeRemee RA: Sarcoidosis and Wegener's granulomatosis: A comparative analysis. Sarcoidosis 1994;11:7.

Finn DG: Lymphoma of the head and neck and acquired immunodeficiency syndrome: Clinical investigation and immunohistological study. Laryngoscope 1995;105(4 Part 2 Suppl 68):1.

Krespi YP, Kuriloff DB, Aner M: Sarcoidosis of the sinonasal tract: A new staging system. Otolaryngol Head Neck Surg 1995;112:221. (A staging system to categorize severity and guide aggressiveness of therapy.)

McDonald TJ, DeRemee RA: Head and neck involvement in Wegener's granulomatosis (WG). Adv Exper Med Biol 1993;336:309. (In a review of 411 patients, head and neck manifestations were common. Six-year survival was 75%.)

Tomita Y et al: Epstein-Barr virus in lymphoproliferative diseases in the sino-nasal region: Close association with CD56+ immunophenotype and polymorphic-reticulosis morphology. Int J Cancer 1997;70:9.

DISEASES OF THE ORAL CAVITY & PHARYNX

LEUKOPLAKIA, ERYTHROPLAKIA, & ORAL CANCER

Leukoplakia is any white lesion that, unlike oral candidiasis, cannot be removed by simply rubbing the mucosal surface. These areas are usually small but may be several centimeters in diameter. Histologically, they may be simple hyperkeratoses occurring in response to chronic irritation (eg, from dentures, tobacco); about 2–6%, however, represent either dysplasia or early invasive squamous cell carcinoma.

Erythroplakia is similar to leukoplakia except that it has a definite erythematous component. The distinction is important, since about 90% of cases of erythroplakia are either dysplasia or carcinoma. Squamous cell carcinoma accounts for 90% of oral cancer. Alcohol and tobacco are the major epidemiologic factors. The differential diagnosis may include oral candidiasis, necrotizing sialometaplasia, pseudoepitheliomatous hyperplasia, median rhomboid glossitis, and vesiculoerosive inflammatory disease such as erosive lichen planus. This should not be confused with the brown-black gingival melanin pigmentation—diffuse or speckled—common in nonwhites, blue-black embedded fragments of dental amalgam, or other systemic disorders associated with general pigmentation (neurofibromatosis, familial polyposis, Addison's disease). Intraoral melanoma is extremely rare.

Any erythroplakic or enlarging leukoplakic area should have an incisional biopsy or an exfoliative cytologic examination done by the clinician who will direct management of a cancer if one is discovered. Specialty referral should be sought early both for diagnosis and treatment. Intraoral staining with 1% toluidine blue may aid in selection of the most suspicious biopsy site. A systematic intraoral examination—including the lateral tongue, floor of the mouth, gingiva, buccal area, palate, and tonsillar fossae—and palpation of the neck for enlarged lymph nodes should be part of any general physical examination, especially in patients over 45 who smoke tobacco or drink immoderately. Indirect or fiberoptic examination of the nasopharynx, oropharynx, hypopharynx, and larynx should also be done by an otolaryngologist–head and neck surgeon or radiation oncologist. Fine-needle aspiration biopsy may be indicated if an enlarged lymph node is found.

Early detection of squamous cell carcinoma is the key to successful management. Lesions less than 4 mm in depth have a low propensity to metastasize. Most patients in whom the tumor is detected before it is 2 cm in diameter are cured. Small lesions are best treated with surgical excision, often with a laser. Radiation is an alternative but is associated with xerostomia, osteonecrosis of the mandible, and inability to use a curative dose again in the treatment field. Large tumors nevertheless are usually treated with a combination of resection and irradiation. Reconstruction, if required, is done at the time of resection and can involve the use of myocutaneous flaps or vascularized free flaps without bone. A number of clinical trials have suggested a role for beta-carotene, vitamin E, and retinoids in producing regression of leukoplakia and reducing the incidence of recurrent squamous cell carcinomas. This area is under intense study.

Benner SE, Lippman SM, Hong WK: Retinoid chemoprevention of second primary tumors. Semin Hematol 1994;31(4 Suppl 5):26. (Reviews the randomized double-blind studies in this field and their implications.)

Garewal HS, Schantz S: Emerging role of beta-carotene and antioxidant nutrients in prevention of oral cancer. Arch Otolaryngol Head Neck Surg 1995;121:141. (Available evidence supports a role for antioxidant nutrients in preventing oral cancer.)

Lippman SM et al: Strategies for chemoprevention study of premalignancy and second primary tumors in the head and neck. Curr Opin Oncol 1995;7:234. (Reviews progress in head and neck cancer chemoprevention: role of retinoids, newer laboratory studies.)

Mashberg A, Samit A: Early diagnosis of asymptomatic oral and oropharyngeal squamous cancers. CA Cancer J Clin 1995;45:328. (Emphasizes the importance of screening asymptomatic individuals at high risk, and categorizes the situations considered "high risk.")

Sciubba JJ: Oral leukoplakia. Crit Rev Oral Biol Med 1995;6:147. (A review of leukoplakia, including possible roles of infectious agents as well as tobacco, as much as chemoprevention.)

Silverman S: Oral cancer. Semin Dermatol 1994;13:132. (An excellent study of methods of early recognition, emphasizing its importance.)

CANDIDIASIS

Oral candidiasis (thrush) is usually painful and looks like creamy-white curd-like patches overlying erythematous mucosa. Because these white areas are easily rubbed off (eg, by a tongue depressor)—unlike leukoplakia or lichen planus—only the underlying irregular erythema may be seen. Oral candidiasis is commonly encountered among denture wearers; in debilitation, diabetes, and anemia; in those undergoing chemotherapy or local irradiation; and in patients receiving corticosteroids or broad-spectrum antibiotics. Candidiasis is often seen prior to other manifestations of HIV infection in high-risk groups. Angular cheilitis is also a manifestation of candidiasis, though it is also seen in nutritional deficiencies.

The diagnosis is usually not difficult—painful intraoral white patches on an erythematous base in a patient at risk for candidiasis. A wet preparation of a smear with potassium hydroxide will confirm spores and may show nonseptate mycelia. Biopsy will show intraepithelial pseudomycelia of *Candida albicans*.

Effective antifungal therapy may be achieved with any of the following: fluconazole (100 mg daily for 7–14 days), ketoconazole (200–400 mg with breakfast [requires acidic gastric environment for absorption] for 7–14 days), clotrimazole troches (10 mg dissolved orally five times daily), or nystatin vaginal troches (100,000 units dissolved orally five times daily) or mouth rinses (500,000 units [5 mL of 100,000 units/mL] held in the mouth before swallowing three times daily). Shorter-duration therapy has also proved effective in many cases, using, for instance, fluconazole. In addition, 0.12% chlorhexidine or half-strength hydrogen peroxide mouth rinses may provide local relief. Nystatin powder (100,000 units/g) applied to dentures three or four times daily for several weeks may help denture wearers.

Challacombe SJ: Immunologic aspects of oral candidiasis. Oral Surg Oral Med Oral Pathol 1994;78:202. (Details current knowledge on the complex humoral and cell-mediated immunologic reaction to different forms of *Candida*.)

Como JA, Dismukes WE: Oral azole drugs as systemic antifungal therapy. N Engl J Med 1994;330:263. (Reviews the relative merits of use of ketoconazole, fluconazole, and itraconazole.)

Garber GE: Treatment of oral *Candida* mucositis infections. Drugs 1994;47:734. (An increasing spectrum of antifungal agents, including imidazoles, are available for treatment and suppression of *Candida*-caused angular cheilitis, leukoplakia, and esophagitis.)

Laskaris G: Oral manifestations of infectious diseases. Dent Clin North Am 1996;40:395. (Presents the clinical features of the most common and important oral infectious diseases.)

Scully C, el-Kabir M, Samaranayake LP: *Candida* and oral candidosis: A review. Crit Rev Oral Biol Med 1994;5:125. (Details current knowledge on *Candida*, oral candidoses, and newer therapeutic regimens.)

GLOSSITIS & GLOSSODYNIA

Inflammation of the tongue with loss of filiform papillae leads to a red, smooth-surfaced tongue (glossitis). Rarely painful, it may be secondary to nutritional deficiencies (eg, niacin, riboflavin, or vitamin E), drug reactions, dehydration, irritants, and possibly autoimmune reactions or psoriasis. Cultures may occasionally be helpful. If the primary cause cannot be identified and corrected, empiric nutritional replacement therapy may be of diagnostic value.

Glossodynia is burning and pain of the tongue; it may occur with or without glossitis. It has been associated with diabetes, drugs (eg, diuretics), tobacco, xerostomia, and candidiasis as well as the sometimes obscure causes of glossitis. Periodontal disease is not

apt to be a factor. Treating possible underlying causes, changing chronic medications to alternative ones, and smoking cessation may resolve symptoms. Reassurance that there is no infection or tumor is likely to be appreciated. Anxiolytic medications and evaluation of possible psychologic status may be considered as well.

Drinka PJ et al: Nutritional correlates of atrophic glossitis: Possible role of vitamin E in papillary atrophy. J Am Coll Nutr 1993;12:14.

Grinspan D et al: Burning mouth syndrome. Int J Dermatol 1995;34:483. (After eliminating patients with local or systemic illnesses, this study reviews the definition of psychosomatic processes causing oral dysesthesia.)

INTRAORAL ULCERATIVE LESIONS

1. NECROTIZING ULCERATIVE GINGIVITIS (Trench Mouth, Vincent's Infection)

Necrotizing ulcerative gingivitis, often caused by an infection of both spirochetes and fusiform bacilli, is common in young adults under stress (classically at examination time). Underlying systemic diseases may also predispose to this disorder. Clinically, there is painful acute gingival inflammation and necrosis, often with bleeding, halitosis, fever, and cervical lymphadenopathy. In addition to altering or removing, if possible, underlying factors and correcting dietary inadequacies, warm half-strength peroxide rinses and oral penicillin (250 mg three times daily for 10 days) may help. Dental gingival curettage may prove necessary.

Necrotizing ulcerative periodontitis is discussed later in this chapter in the section on AIDS.

2. APHTHOUS ULCER (Canker Sore, Ulcerative Stomatitis)

Aphthous ulcers are very common and easy to recognize. Their cause remains uncertain. Found on nonkeratinized mucosa (eg, buccal and labial mucosa and not gingiva or palate), they may be single or multiple, are usually recurrent, and appear as painful small (usually 1–2 mm, but sometimes 1–2 cm) round ulcerations with yellow-gray fibrinoid centers surrounded by red halos. The painful stage lasts 7–10 days; healing is completed in 1–3 weeks.

Treatment is nonspecific. Topical steroids (triamcinolone acetonide, 0.1%, or fluocinonide ointment, 0.05%) in an adhesive base (Orabase Plain) do appear to provide symptomatic relief. A 1-week tapering course of prednisone (40–60 mg/d) has also been used successfully.

Large or persistent areas of ulcerative stomatitis may be secondary to erythema multiforme or drug allergies, acute herpes simplex, pemphigus, pemphigoid, bullous lichen planus, Behçet's disease, or inflammatory bowel disease. Squamous cell carcinoma may occasionally present in this fashion. When the diagnosis is not clear, incisional biopsy is indicated.

Fischman SL: Oral ulcerations. Semin Dermatol 1994; 13:74. (The pathogenesis, clinical appearance, and suggested treatment for the most common ulcerations.)

Korstanje MJ: Drug-induced mouth disorders. Clin Exper Dermatol 1995;20:10.

Main DM, Chamberlain MA: Clinical differentiation of oral ulceration in Behçet's disease. Br J Rheumatol 1992;31:767. (In Behçet's disease, prevalent in the Near East, concurrent ulcers are more common in the oropharynx and soft palate.)

Smith RG, Burtner AP: Oral side-effects of the most frequently prescribed drugs. Special Care Dentistry 1994;14:96. (Oral side effects and their respective prevalence rates for the most commonly prescribed drugs.)

Vincent SD, Lilly GE: Clinical, historic, and therapeutic features of aphthous stomatitis. Oral Surg Oral Med Oral Path 1992;74:79. (Literature review and open clinical trials employing steroids support their use.)

3. HERPETIC STOMATITIS

Herpetic gingivostomatitis is common, mild, and short-lived and requires no intervention in most adults. In immunocompromised individuals, however, reactivation of herpes simplex virus infection is frequent and may be severe. Clinically, there is initial burning, followed by typical small vesicles that rupture and form scabs. Acyclovir (200–800 mg five times daily for 7–14 days) may shorten the course and reduce postherpetic pain. Differential diagnosis includes ulcerative stomatitis (see above) as well as erythema multiforme, syphilitic chancre, and carcinoma. Coxsackievirus-caused lesions (grayish white tonsillar and palatal ulcers of herpangina or buccal and lip ulcers in hand-foot-and-mouth disease) are seen more commonly in children under age 6.

Mattingly G, Rodu B: Differential diagnosis of oral mucosal ulcerations. Compendium 1993;14:136, 138, 140 passim.

Miller CS: Herpes simplex virus and human papillomavirus infections of the oral cavity. Semin Dermatol 1994; 13:108.

Miller CS, Redding SW: Diagnosis and management of orofacial herpes simplex virus infections. Dent Clin North Am 1992;36:879.

Rodu B, Mattingly G: Oral mucosal ulcers: Diagnosis and management. J Am Dent Assoc 1992;123:83.

Spruance SL: The natural history of recurrent oral-facial herpes simplex virus infection. Semin Dermatol 1992;11: 200.

PHARYNGITIS & TONSILLITIS

As common as respiratory tract infections are—and they account for over 10% of all office visits to primary care physicians and 50% of outpatient antibiotics used—one would think the most appropriate management would be a matter of agreement among physicians. However, the issues are deceptively complex. Controversy exists over when to culture an inflamed throat and how long to treat confirmed group A β-hemolytic streptococcal pharyngitis—and with what. Numerous well-conceived and well-controlled studies in the past few years as well as the recent availability of rapid laboratory tests for detection of streptococci (eliminating the delay caused by culturing) appear to make a consensual approach more possible.

The clinical features suggestive of group A β-hemolytic streptococcal pharyngitis include fever, anterior cervical adenopathy, and a pharyngotonsillar exudate. The sore throat may be severe, with odynophagia, tender adenopathy, and a scarlatiniform rash. An elevated white blood count and left shift are consistent with group A β-hemolytic streptococcal pharyngitis. Hoarseness, cough, and coryza are not suggestive of this disease. Marked lymphadenopathy and a shaggy white-purple tonsillar exudate, often extending into the nasopharynx, suggest mononucleosis, especially if present in a young adult. Hepatosplenomegaly and a positive heterophil agglutination test or elevated anti-EBV titer of course are corroborative. It should be kept in mind that about one-third of patients with infectious mononucleosis have secondary streptococcal tonsillitis, requiring treatment. (Ampicillin should be avoided if mononucleosis is suspected because it induces a rash in such patients.) Diphtheria (extremely rare today but described in the alcoholic population) presents with low-grade fever in an ill patient with a gray tonsillar pseudomembrane; it should be distinguished from the more common acute necrotizing ulcerative gingivitis and herpangina.

The most common pathogens other than group A β-hemolytic streptococci in the differential diagnosis of "sore throat" are viruses, *Neisseria gonorrhoeae,* *Mycoplasma,* and *Chlamydia trachomatis.* Rhinorrhea would suggest a virus, as would lack of an exudate, but in practice the most reasonable assumption is that it is not possible to distinguish viral upper respiratory infection from group A β-hemolytic streptococcal infection on clinical grounds alone. Infections with *Corynebacterium diphtheriae,* anaerobic streptococci, and *Corynebacterium haemolyticum* (which responds better to erythromycin than penicillin) may also mimic pharyngitis due to group A β-hemolytic streptococci.

Treatment strategies for a sore throat range from "treat all comers" to "culture all comers, reserving treatment for positive cultures." Issues that affect this decision for an individual include the reliability of cultures and rapid tests for streptococci such as latex agglutination (LA) antigen tests and solid-phase enzyme immunoassays (ELISA), the incidence of pharyngitis not due to group A β-hemolytic streptococci, patient follow-up and medical compliance, and cost. The apparent advantage of the "treat all" approach is the initial short-term cost, savings from elimination of diagnostic tests, and prevention of most streptococcal complications, but such an approach necessarily causes the highest rate of antibiotic use and side effects and therefore overall the highest cost. At the other extreme is the "culture all" approach, which is associated with the fewest penicillin reactions but is more costly than an "antigen test and culture" approach and is also dependent on the excellent follow-up not routinely available in some busy city health clinics. With current sensitivity of rapid group A β-hemolytic streptococcal antigen tests between 80% and 85%, and specificity greater than 90%, the strategy of treating patients with positive antigen test results while culturing (and waiting for results) patients with negative test results appears to be an excellent option. As the sensitivity of newer LA tests, ELISA, or other immunoassays (such as an optical immunoassay for detection of group A streptococcal carbohydrate antigen reported to be 97% sensitive) appears to exceed 90%, the strategy of relying solely on such antigen tests to decide whether to treat is also most attractive. Individual decisions need to be based on the prevalence of streptococcal infection (seasonally and locally); patient allergic history, reliability, and compliance; availability of rapid group A β-hemolytic streptococcal antigen tests; and reliability of available bacteriology laboratories.

Thirty years ago, a single injection of benzathine penicillin or procaine penicillin was standard antibiotic treatment. This remains effective, but the injections are painful. If compliance is an issue, it may be the best choice. Oral treatment, however, is also effective. The controversy over choice of preparation revolves around reducing the already low (10–20%) incidence of treatment failures (positive culture after treatment despite symptomatic resolution) and recurrences. A review of recent controlled studies suggests that penicillin V potassium (250 mg orally three times daily—not once or twice daily—for 10 days) or cefuroxime axetil (250 mg orally twice daily for 5–10 days) are both effective. Erythromycin (active against *Mycoplasma* and *Chlamydia*) is a reasonable alternative to penicillin in allergic patients. Several cephalosporins in their usual dosage schedules are somewhat more effective than penicillin in producing bacteriologic cures; 5-day administration has been successful for selected cephalosporins, such as cefpodoxime or cefuroxime. The macrolide antibiotics have also been reported to be successful in shorter-duration regimens. Azithromycin (500 mg once daily) because of its long half-life, need be taken for only 3 days.

Adequate antibiotic treatment usually avoids the streptococcal complications of scarlet fever, glomerulonephritis, rheumatic myocarditis, and local abscess formation. About 10% of the time, repeat cultures show persistent presence of group A streptococci.

Antibiotic choices for treatment failures are also somewhat controversial. Perhaps surprisingly, penicillin-tolerant strains are not necessarily isolated more frequently in those who fail to improve with treatment than in those treated successfully with penicillin. The reasons for failure appear to be complex, and a second course of treatment with the same drug is therefore not necessarily unreasonable. Alternatives to penicillin include cefuroxime and certain other cephalosporins, dicloxacillin (which is β-lactamase-resistant), and amoxicillin with clavulanate. In penicillin-allergic patients, the usual alternatives should be used, such as erythromycin and cephalosporins. When there is a history of possible penicillin allergy, the usual alternatives should be used, such as erythromycin or cephalosporin. In cases of prior severe penicillin reaction, however, cephalosporins should probably be avoided as the cross-reaction is felt to be higher than the overall 8% rate.

Ancillary treatment of pharyngitis includes appropriate analgesics and anti-inflammatory agents, such as aspirin or acetaminophen. Some patients find that salt water gargling is soothing. In severe cases, anesthetic gargles and lozenges (eg, benzocaine) may provide additional symptomatic relief. Occasionally, odynophagia is so intense that hospitalization for intravenous hydration and antibiotics is warranted.

Blumer JL, Goldfarb J: Meta-analysis in the evaluation of treatment for streptococcal pharyngitis: A review. Clin Ther 1994;16:604; discussion 603. (Oral cephalosporins provide alternatives to penicillin for the treatment of streptococcal pharyngitis, producing bacteriologic cure rates of 92–95% versus 84–87.5%.)

Cohen R et al: Six-day amoxicillin vs. ten-day penicillin V therapy for group A streptococcal tonsillopharyngitis. Pediatr Infect Dis J 1996;15:678. (Compliance was better in the shorter amoxicillin group; efficacy and safety were the same.)

Dagnelie CF, van der Graaf Y, De Melker RA: Do patients with sore throat benefit from penicillin? A randomized double-blind placebo-controlled clinical trial with penicillin V in general practice. Br J Gen Pract 1996;46:589. (Only GABHS-positive patients benefit from penicillin V in their clinical cure [1-2 days more rapid recovery] in the first few days; rapid testing is useful.)

Gehanno P, Chichie D: Tonsillopharyngitis: Evaluation of short-term treatment with cefuroxime axetil versus standard 10-day penicillin V therapy. Br J Clin Pract 1995;49:28. (Short 4- to 5-day courses with oral cephalosporins, such as cefuroxime axetil, have proved to be effective alternatives to 10 days of penicillin.)

Kiselica D: Group A beta-hemolytic streptococcal pharyngitis: Current clinical concepts. Am Fam Physician 1994;49:1147. (Advocates use of rapid antigen tests, early antibiotic use—with penicillin or with erythromycin in penicillin-allergic patients.)

Kline JA, Runge JW: Streptococcal pharyngitis: A review of pathophysiology, diagnosis, and management. J Emerg Med 1994;12:665. (A bibliographic resource for some of the controversies of this topic.)

Pacifico L et al: Comparative efficacy and safety of 3-day azithromycin and 10-day penicillin V treatment of group A beta-hemolytic streptococcal pharyngitis in children. Antimicrob Agents Chemother 1996;40:1005. (Once-daily [10 mg/kg] 3-day oral regimen of azithromycin as safe as 10-day course of penicillin but not an effective alternative to penicillin for group A β-hemolytic streptococcal pharyngitis. Ten days of penicillin, taken at least twice daily, remains the gold standard.)

Pichichero ME: Group A streptococcal tonsillopharyngitis: Cost-effective diagnosis and treatment. Ann Emerg Med 1995;25:390. (Less than 10% of adults and 30% of children presenting with a sore throat have a streptococcal infection; reviews problems with overtreatment, rapid antigen tests, recurrent group A streptococcal tonsillopharyngitis, and treatment strategies.)

Schaad UB, Heynen G: Evaluation of the efficacy, safety and toleration of azithromycin vs. penicillin V in the treatment of acute streptococcal pharyngitis in children: Results of a multicenter, open comparative study. The Swiss Tonsillopharyngitis Study Group. Pediatr Infect Dis J 1996;15:791. (In the present study on GABHS pharyngitis in 343 children, a once-daily (10-mg/kg), 3-day oral regimen of azithromycin was as clinically effective and as safe as traditional penicillin but appeared inferior in eliminating group A β-hemolytic streptococci from the throat.)

Schlager TA et al: Optical immunoassay for rapid detection of group A beta-hemolytic streptococci: Should culture be replaced? Arch Pediatr Adolesc Med 1996;150:245. (Optical immunoassay rapid and performed well but not sensitive enough to replace culture for group A β-hemolytic streptococci.)

PERITONSILLAR ABSCESS & CELLULITIS

When infection penetrates the tonsillar capsule and involves the surrounding tissues, peritonsillar cellulitis results. Peritonsillar abscess and cellulitis present with severe sore throat, odynophagia, trismus, medial deviation of the soft palate and peritonsillar fold, and a "hot potato" voice. Following therapy, peritonsillar cellulitis usually either resolves over several days or evolves into peritonsillar abscess. The existence of an abscess may be confirmed by aspirating pus from the peritonsillar fold just superior and medial to the upper pole of the tonsil. A No. 19 or No. 21 needle should be passed no deeper than 1 cm, because the internal carotid artery passes posterior and deep to the tonsillar fossa. There is controversy about the best way to treat peritonsillar abscesses. Some incise and drain the area and continue with parenteral antibiotics, whereas others aspirate only and follow as an outpatient. At times it is appropriate to consider immediate tonsillectomy (quinsy tonsillectomy) both to drain the abscess and to avoid recurrence. Both approaches are rational and

have support in the literature. Whichever approach is taken, one must be sure the abscess is adequately drained, since complications such as extension to the retropharyngeal, deep neck, and posterior mediastinal spaces are possible. Pus may also be aspirated into the lungs, resulting in pneumonia. While there is controversy about whether a single abscess is sufficient indication for tonsillectomy, most would agree that patients with recurrent abscesses should have their tonsils removed. Overall, about 30% of patients with peritonsillar abscess exhibit relative indications for tonsillectomy.

Herzon FS, Harris P: Mosher Award thesis. Peritonsillar abscess: Incidence, current management practices, and a proposal for treatment guidelines. Laryngoscope 1995; 105(8 Part 3 Suppl 74):1. (An in-depth study, including meta-analysis; needle aspiration recommended for initial surgical drainage procedure unless indications for abscess tonsillectomy are present.)

Savolainen SS et al: Peritonsillar abscess: Clinical and microbiologic aspects and treatment regimens. Arch Otolaryngol Head Neck Surg 1993;119:521. (Ninety-eight patients treated by aspiration had a 19% recurrence rate. These 16 underwent tonsillectomy.)

TONSILLECTOMY

Despite the frequency with which tonsillectomy is performed, the indications for the procedure remain controversial. Most would agree that airway obstruction causing sleep apnea or cor pulmonale is an absolute indication for tonsillectomy. Similarly, persistent marked tonsillar asymmetry should prompt an excisional biopsy to rule out lymphoma. Relative indications include recurrent streptococcal tonsillitis, causing considerable loss of time from school or work, recurrent peritonsillar abscess, and chronic tonsillitis.

Tonsillectomy is not an entirely benign procedure. Postoperative bleeding occurs in 2–8% of cases and on rare occasions can lead to laryngospasm and airway obstruction. Pain may be considerable, especially in the adult. The pros and cons of the procedure need to be discussed with each prospective patient. In addition, there is increasing economic pressure for these procedures to be done as outpatient surgery. Hemorrhage, protracted emesis, or fever appears to occur in about 1% of cases, and such immediate complications usually appear within 6 hours but continue to occur later within the once frequent 24-hour period of hospitalized observation. This topic will continue to receive attention; at present it seems clear that outpatient tonsillectomy is usually safe when followed by a 6-hour period of uneventful observation, but each decision rests on individual circumstances.

Although reports in the 1970s suggested an association of tonsillectomy with Hodgkin's disease, careful review of this literature reveals no causative association whatever.

Bicknell PG: Role of adenotonsillectomy in the management of pediatric ear, nose and throat infections. Pediatr Infect Dis J 1994;13(1 Suppl 1):S75; discussion S78.

Bluestone CD: Current indications for tonsillectomy and adenoidectomy. Ann Otol Rhinol Laryngol 1992;155 (Suppl):58.

Colclasure JB, Graham SS: Complications of outpatient tonsillectomy and adenoidectomy: A review of 3340 cases. Ear Nose Throat J 1990;69:155. (A reminder of the hazards.)

Gerber ME et al: Selected risk factors in pediatric adenotonsillectomy. Arch Otolaryngol Head Neck Surg 1996;122:811. (When snoring is absent, same-day surgery is appropriate since the risk of respiratory compromise is minimal.)

Guida RA, Mattucci KF: Tonsillectomy and adenoidectomy: An inpatient or outpatient procedure? Laryngoscope 1990;100:491. (Discharge home to a reliable environment after uneventful monitoring for several hours is safe.)

Lee WC, Sharp JF: Complications of paediatric tonsillectomy post-discharge. J Laryngol Otol 1996;110:136. (Only one-third of the parents approved of day-case tonsillectomy.)

Myssiorek D, Alvi A: Post-tonsillectomy hemorrhage: An assessment of risk factors. Int J Pediatr Otorhinolaryngol 1996;37:35. (As high as 20% in some series, but this retrospective review found a 3% incidence.)

Pringle MB et al: Day-case tonsillectomy–is it appropriate? Clin Otolaryngol 1996;21:504. (Comprehensive review.)

DEEP NECK INFECTIONS

Deep neck abscesses usually present with marked neck pain and swelling in a toxic febrile patient. They are emergencies because they may rapidly compromise the airway. They may also spread to the mediastinum or cause septicemia. Most commonly, they originate from odontogenic infections. Other causes include suppurative lymphadenitis, direct spread of pharyngeal infection, penetrating trauma, pharyngoesophageal foreign bodies, and intravenous injection of the internal jugular vein, especially in drug abusers. Fundamentals of treatment include securing the airway, intravenous antibiotics, and incision and drainage. The airway may be secured either by intubation or tracheostomy. Tracheostomy is preferable in the patients with substantial pharyngeal edema, since attempts at intubation may precipitate acute airway obstruction. CT scan may be helpful in defining the extent of the abscess. Bleeding in association with a deep neck abscess suggests the possibility of carotid artery or internal jugular vein involvement and requires prompt neck exploration both for drainage of pus and for vascular ligation.

Ludwig's angina is the most commonly encountered neck space infection. It is a cellulitis of the sublingual and submaxillary spaces, often arising from infection of the tooth roots that extend below the mylohyoid line of the mandible. Clinically, there is edema and erythema of the upper neck under the chin and often of the floor of the mouth. The tongue may be displaced upward and backward by the posterior spread of cellulitis. This may lead to occlusion of the airway and necessitate tracheostomy. Microbiologic isolates include streptococci, *Bacteroides,* and *Fusobacterium.* Hospitalization and intravenous antibiotics are necessary. Usual doses of penicillin plus metronidazole, ampicillin-sulbactam, clindamycin, or selective cephalosporins are good initial choices. Culture and sensitivity data will then refine the choice. Dental consultation is advisable. External drainage via bilateral submental incisions is required immediately if the airway is threatened and when medical therapy has not reversed the process.

Har-El G et al: Changing trends in deep neck abscess: A retrospective study of 110 patients. Oral Surg Oral Med Oral Pathol 1994;77:446. (Cause, presentation, diagnostic methods, and bacteriology have changed compared with the earlier literature, but the management principles of airway protection, intravenous antibiotics, and drainage remain the same.).

Johnson JT: Abscesses and deep space infections of the head and neck. Infect Dis Clin North Am 1992;6:705. (Biopsy of tissue for anaerobic bacteriologic culture is critical, as well as drainage of infected neck spaces.)

Peterson LJ: Contemporary management of deep infections of the neck. J Oral Maxillofacial Surg 1993;51:226.

DISEASES OF THE SALIVARY GLANDS

The salivary glands are divided into the two large parotid glands, two submandibular glands, several sublingual glands, and 600–1000 minor salivary glands located throughout the upper aerodigestive tract.

ACUTE INFLAMMATORY SALIVARY GLAND DISORDERS

1. SIALADENITIS

Acute bacterial sialadenitis in the adult most commonly affects either the parotid or submandibular gland. It typically presents with acute swelling of the gland, increased pain and swelling with meals, and tenderness and erythema of the duct opening. Pus often can be massaged from the duct. Sialadenitis often occurs in the setting of dehydration or in association with chronic illness. Underlying Sjögren's syndrome also predisposes. The pathogenesis is ductal obstruction, often by an inspissated mucous plug, followed by salivary stasis and secondary infection. The most common organism recovered from purulent draining saliva is *S aureus*. Treatment consists of intravenous antibiotics such as nafcillin (1 g intravenously every 4–6 hours) and measures to increase salivary flow, including hydration, warm compresses, sialagogues (eg, lemon drops), and massage of the gland. Failure of the process to resolve on this regimen suggests abscess formation, ductal stricture, stone, or tumor causing obstruction. Ultrasound or CT scan may be helpful in establishing the diagnosis. Sialography is best avoided in acute cases.

Brook I: Diagnosis and management of parotitis. Arch Otolaryngol Head Neck Surg 1992;118:469.

Ellies M et al: Surgical management of nonneoplastic diseases of the submandibular gland: A follow-up study. Int J Oral Maxillofac Surg 1996;25:285. (Extirpation of the affected gland proved effective in all. When calculi do not cause inflammation, other options such as lithotripsy might be considered.)

2. SIALOLITHIASIS

Calculus formation is more common in Wharton's duct (draining the submandibular glands) than in Stensen's duct (draining the parotid glands). Clinically, a patient may note postprandial pain and local swelling, often with a history of recurrent acute sialadenitis. Stones in Wharton's duct are usually large and radiopaque, whereas those in Stensen's duct are usually radiolucent and smaller. Those very close to the orifice of Wharton's duct may be palpated manually in the anterior floor of the mouth and removed intraorally by dilating or incising the distal duct. The duct proximal to the stone must be temporarily clamped (using, for instance, a single throw of a suture) to keep manipulation of the stone from pushing it back toward the submandibular gland. Those more than 1.5–2 cm from the duct are too close to the lingual nerve to be removed safely in this manner. Similarly, dilation of Stensen's duct, located on the buccal surface opposite the second maxillary molar, may relieve distal stricture or allow a small stone to pass. The location of the facial nerve makes intraoral retrieval of more proximal parotid stones unsafe.

Repeated episodes of sialadenitis invariably lead to stricture and chronic infection. If the obstruction cannot be safely removed or dilated, excision of the gland may be necessary. In selected cases, piezoelectric shock wave lithotripsy may be successful.

Arzoz E et al: Endoscopic intracorporeal lithotripsy for sialolithiasis. J Oral Maxillofac Surg 1996;54:847. (Another alternative)

Ellies M et al: Surgical management of nonneoplastic diseases of the submandibular gland: A follow-up study. Int J Oral Maxillofac Surg 1996;25:285.

Iro H et al: Shockwave lithotripsy of salivary duct stones. Lancet 1992;339:1333.

McGurk M et al: Laser lithotripsy: A preliminary study on its application for sialolithiasis. Br J Oral Maxillofac Surg 1994;32:218. (The refinement of spectroscopic feedback techniques allows laser lithotripsy to complement ultrasonic lithotripsy.)

CHRONIC INFLAMMATORY & INFILTRATIVE DISORDERS OF THE SALIVARY GLANDS

Numerous infiltrative disorders may cause unilateral or bilateral parotid gland enlargement. Sjögren's disease and sarcoidosis are examples of lymphoepithelial and granulomatous diseases that may affect the salivary glands. Metabolic disorders, including alcoholism, diabetes mellitus, and vitamin deficiencies, may also cause diffuse enlargement. Several drugs have been associated with parotid enlargement, including thioureas, iodine, and drugs with cholinergic effects (eg, phenothiazines), which stimulate flow and cause more viscous saliva.

SALIVARY GLAND TUMORS

Approximately 80% of salivary gland tumors occur in the parotid gland. In adults, about 80% of these are benign. In the submandibular triangle, it is sometimes difficult to distinguish a primary submandibular gland tumor from a metastatic submandibular space node. Only 50–60% of primary submandibular tumors are benign. Tumors of the minor salivary glands are most likely to be malignant, with adenoid cystic carcinoma predominating.

Most parotid tumors present as an asymptomatic mass in the superficial part of the gland. Their presence may have been noted by the patient for months or years. Facial nerve involvement correlates strongly with malignancy. Tumors may extend deep to the plane of the facial nerve or may originate in the parapharyngeal space. In such cases, medial deviation of the soft palate is visible on intraoral examination. MRI and CT scans have largely replaced sialography in defining the extent of tumor.

Although the accuracy of fine-needle aspiration is improving, superficial parotidectomy with facial nerve dissection is required for both diagnosis and treatment of most primary tumors. Similarly, submandibular gland masses generally require excision of the gland. In benign and small low-grade malignant tumors, no additional treatment is needed. Postoperative irradiation is required for larger and high-grade cancers.

Kaplan MJ, Johns ME: Malignant neoplasms (of the salivary glands): In: *Otolaryngology-Head and Neck Surgery,* 2nd ed. Cummings CW, Frederickson J (editors). Mosby, 1992. (Prognostic factors, treatment recommendations, and new developments in imaging and treatment.)

DISEASES OF THE LARYNX

DYSPHONIA, HOARSENESS, & STRIDOR

The primary symptoms of laryngeal disease are hoarseness and stridor. Hoarseness is caused by an abnormal flow of air past the vocal cords. The voice is "breathy" when too much air passes incompletely apposed vocal cords, as in unilateral vocal cord paralysis. The voice is harsh when turbulence is created by irregularity of the vocal cords, as in laryngitis or a mass lesion. Stridor, a high-pitched sound, is produced by lesions that narrow the airway. Airway impairment above the vocal cords produces predominantly inspiratory stridor. Lesions below the vocal cord level produce either expiratory or mixed stridor.

Hagen P, Lyons GD, Nuss DW: Dysphonia in the elderly: Diagnosis and management of age-related voice changes. South Med J 1996;89:204.

COMMON LARYNGEAL DISORDERS

1. EPIGLOTTITIS

Epiglottitis in adults should be suspected when odynophagia seems out of proportion to pharyngeal findings. It may be viral or bacterial in origin. Unlike the case of children, indirect laryngoscopy is generally safe and may demonstrate the swollen, erythematous epiglottis. Initial treatment is hospitalization for intravenous antibiotics—eg, ceftizoxime, 1–2 g intravenously every 8–12 hours; or cefuroxime, 750–1500 mg intravenously every 8 hours; and dexamethasone, usually 4–10 mg as initial bolus, then 4 mg intravenously every 6 hours—and observation of the airway. Steroids may be tapered as signs and symptoms resolve. Similarly, substitution of oral antibiotics may be appropriate to complete a 10-day course. When adult epiglottitis is recognized early, it is usually possible to avoid intubation. In such cases, it would seem prudent to monitor oxyhemoglobin saturation with continuous pulse oximetry.

Barrow HN, Vastola AP, Wang RC: Adult supraglottitis. Otolaryngol Head Neck Surg 1993;109(3 Part 1):474. (Thirty-nine of 46 patients, all older than 8 years, did not require tracheotomy. Rapid development of symptoms correlated with increased likelihood of airway compromise.)

Frantz TD, Rasgon BM, Quesenberry CP Jr: Acute epiglottitis in adults: Analysis of 129 cases. JAMA 1994; 272:1358. (Only 15% required intubation or tracheotomy. Stridor and sitting erect were predictors, and there were no deaths. Sore throat [95%] and odynophagia [94%] were the predominant symptoms, and blood cultures grew *H influenzae* type b in about 10%.)

Kass EG et al: Acute epiglottitis in the adult: Experience with a seasonal presentation. Laryngoscope 1993;103: 841. (Two of 17 patients, both with stridor, required intubation and tracheotomy.)

Wurtele P: Acute epiglottitis in children and adults: A large-scale incidence study. Otolaryngol Head Neck Surg 1990;103:902. (About 25% of cases occur in adults; the incidence in adults is about 1:100,000.)

2. LARYNGEAL PAPILLOMAS

Papillomas are common lesions of the larynx and other sites where ciliated and squamous epithelia meet. Unlike the oral cavity, in the larynx they are likely to be symptomatic, with hoarseness that progresses to stridor over weeks to months. The disease is more common in children but occurs also in adults. Repeated laser excisions via microdirect laryngoscopy are often needed to control the disease. Tracheotomy should be avoided, if possible, since it introduces an iatrogenic additional squamociliary junction where papilloma appear to preferentially grow. A possible role for interferon has been under investigation.

Avidano MA, Singleton GT: Adjuvant drug strategies in the treatment of recurrent respiratory papillomatosis. Otolaryngol Head Neck Surg 1995;112:197. (Adjuvant therapy, including interferon and methotrexate, is of benefit in the treatment of patients with recurrent respiratory papillomatosis, but most otolaryngologists treat these patients successfully with laser surgery alone.)

Kashima H et al: Sites of predilection in recurrent respiratory papillomatosis. Ann Otol Rhinol Laryngol 1993; 102 (8 Part 1):580.

3. ACUTE LARYNGITIS

Acute laryngitis is probably the most common cause of hoarseness, which may persist for a week or so after other symptoms of upper respiratory infection have cleared. The patient should be warned to avoid vigorous use of the voice (singing, shouting) while laryngitis is present, since this may foster the formation of vocal nodules. Although thought to be usually viral in origin, both *Moraxella catarrhalis* and *Haemophilus influenzae* may be isolated from the nasopharynx at higher than expected frequencies, and erythromycin may reduce the severity of hoarseness and cough.

Schalen L et al: Acute laryngitis in adults: Results of erythromycin treatment. Acta Otolaryngol Suppl (Stockh) 1992;492:55.

4. GASTROESOPHAGEAL REFLUX & HOARSENESS

Gastroesophageal reflux into the larynx (laryngopharyngeal reflux) should be considered a possible cause of chronic hoarseness if other causes of abnormal laryngeal airflow (such as tumor) have been excluded by indirect or direct laryngoscopy. As less than half of patients with documented laryngopharyngeal reflux have typical symptoms of heartburn and regurgitation, the lack of such symptoms should not be construed as eliminating this cause. Management should initially exclude more serious laryngeal disease. Twenty-four-hour pH monitoring of the pharynx as well as the esophagus is the diagnostic tool that best documents reflux. A clinical trial of appropriate antireflux measures for a sufficient duration of time has been advocated as an alternative by some. If a clinical trial is to be used, recall that the effect of omeprazole and other proton pump inhibitors is more immediate than cimetidine or ranitidine and that proton pump inhibitors appear to be 90% clinically effective whereas H_2 antagonists are effective in about 70% of cases. Higher doses of omeprazole than are customary in typical gastroesophageal reflux are often needed; 40 mg/d should be the initial dose.

Hanson DG, Kamel PL, Kahrilas PJ: Outcomes of antireflux therapy for the treatment of chronic laryngitis. Ann Otol Rhinol Laryngol 1995;104:550. (Fifty percent responded to nocturnal antireflux precautions alone, while 95% improved if omeprazole or famotidine was added. A few patients required high doses of omeprazole or fundoplication.)
Johnson DA: Medical therapy for gastroesophageal reflux disease. Am J Med 1992;92:88S.
Kamel PL, Hanson D, Kahrilas PJ: Omeprazole for the treatment of posterior laryngitis. Am J Med 1994; 96:321. (The signs and symptoms of posterior laryngitis improve with 40 mg or more of daily omeprazole and recur after discontinuation of therapy.)
Koufman JA: The otolaryngologic manifestations of gastroesophageal reflux disease (GERD): A clinical investigation of 225 patients using ambulatory 24-hour pH monitoring and an experimental investigation of the role of acid and pepsin in the development of laryngeal injury. Laryngoscope 1991;101(4 Part 2 Suppl 53):1.
Massoomi F, Savage J, Destache CJ: Omeprazole: A comprehensive review. Pharmacotherapy 1993;13:46.

TUMORS OF THE LARYNX

1. BENIGN TUMORS OF THE LARYNX

Vocal cord nodules are smooth, paired lesions that form at the junction of the anterior one-third and posterior two-thirds of the vocal cords. They are a common cause of hoarseness resulting from vocal abuse. In adults, they are referred to as "singer's nodules"; in children, "screamer's nodules." Treatment requires modification of voice habits, and referral to a speech therapist is indicated. Recalcitrant nodules may require surgical excision.

Polypoid changes in the vocal cords may result from vocal abuse, smoking, or chemical industrial irritants or may be seen in hypothyroidism. Attention to the underlying problem may resolve the polypoid changes. Inhaled steroid spray (eg, beclomethasone, 42 μg/spray, or dexamethasone, 84 μg/spray, two or three times a day) may hasten resolution. At times, removal of the hyperplastic vocal cord mucosa may be indicated.

A common but often unrecognized cause of hoarseness is contact ulcers on the vocal processes of the arytenoid cartilages secondary to esophageal reflux. Treatment of the underlying reflux with antacids or H_2-receptor blockers (eg, cimetidine, 800 mg orally daily or 300–600 mg orally every 6 hours; or ranitidine, 300 mg orally daily or 150 mg orally twice daily) and elevation of the head of the bed is often curative. Intubation granulomas may also be seen posteriorly between the vocal processes.

2. LARYNGEAL LEUKOPLAKIA

Leukoplakia is a frequent cause of hoarseness, most commonly arising in smokers. Direct laryngoscopy with biopsy is advised. Histologic examination usually demonstrates mild, moderate, or severe dysplasia. Cessation of smoking may reverse dysplastic changes. A certain percentage of patients—estimated to be less than 5% of those with mild dysplasia and about 35–60% of those with severe dysplasia—will subsequently develop squamous cell carcinoma. In some cases, invasive squamous cell carcinoma is present in the initial biopsy.

3. SQUAMOUS CELL CARCINOMA OF THE LARYNX

Squamous cell carcinoma is the most common cancer seen in the larynx. It occurs predominantly in heavy smokers, with alcohol an apparent cocarcinogen. It is most common between ages 50 and 70. Hoarseness is the usual presenting symptom. Any patient with hoarseness that has persisted beyond 2–3 weeks should be evaluated by indirect laryngoscopy. Odynophagia, hemoptysis, weight loss, referred otalgia, vocal cord immobility, and cervical adenopathy suggest more advanced disease.

Early squamous cell carcinoma is best treated with radiation, with cure rates in excess of 85–95%. Conservation surgery or total laryngectomy is necessary for radiation failures and for more advanced disease. Today, the use of tracheoesophageal valves following total laryngectomy restores useful speech for most laryngectomy patients.

VOCAL CORD PARALYSIS

Most cases of vocal cord paralysis result from lesions of the recurrent laryngeal nerve. In the adult, unilateral vocal cord paralysis generally presents as hoarseness with a breathy character. The most common cause is thyroid surgery. In left vocal cord paralysis, it is important to eliminate a mediastinal or pulmonary apical lesion (Pancoast's tumor) as the causative factor. Involvement of the vagus nerve by tumors involving the jugular foramen may cause vocal cord paralysis that is usually accompanied by additional cranial neuropathies (IX, XI). When no cause can be found, function may return spontaneously within 1 year. Hoarseness secondary to unilateral vocal cord paralysis may be improved by injecting Teflon or other substances into the paralyzed cord in order to medialize it, or by laryngoplastic phonosurgery (medialization laryngoplasty or thyroplasty).

Bilateral vocal cord paralysis usually causes stridor. If sudden in onset, the stridor will be inspiratory and expiratory, causing sufficient airway compromise to warrant emergency cricothyrotomy. If insidious in onset, it may (curiously) be asymptomatic at rest. The voice may be quite good, as the cords are apposed in the midline. Thyroid surgery, neck trauma, and tumor invasion from anaplastic thyroid or esophageal carcinoma are among the more common causes. Immobility of the vocal cords may also result from cricoarytenoid arthritis, as seen in advanced rheumatoid arthritis. When airway obstruction is severe, tracheostomy is indicated. Various procedures, which open the glottis by lateralizing a vocal cord, have been used in order to remove the tracheostomy. A less powerful, breathy voice often accompanies these procedures.

Benninger MS et al: Evaluation and treatment of the unilateral paralyzed vocal fold. Otolaryngol Head Neck Surg 1994;111:497. (Multiple modalities are described which allow for restoration of nearly normal phonation.)

Cotter CS et al: Laryngeal complications after type 1 thyroplasty. Otolaryngol Head Neck Surg 199;113:671. (Usually safe, with an extrusion rate of 9% associated with suboptimal prosthesis placement in the smaller female larynx.)

Dedo HH: Injection and removal of Teflon for unilateral vocal cord paralysis. Ann Otol Rhinol Laryngol 1992;101:81. (The standard with which the long-term results of newer techniques must be compared.)

Harries ML: Unilateral vocal fold paralysis: A review of the current methods of surgical rehabilitation. J Laryngol Otol 1996;110:111. (Assesses injection medialisation, laryngeal framework surgery. and reinnervation procedures.)

Kasperbauer JL: Injectable Teflon for vocal cord paralysis. Otolaryngol Clin North Am 1995;28:317. (Injection of Teflon is a reliable technique for rehabilitation of the dysphonia and aspiration related to recurrent laryngeal nerve paralysis.)

Righi PD, Wilson KM, Gluckman JL: Thyroplasty using a silicone elastomer implant. Otolaryngol Clin North Am 1995;28:309. (Silicone elastomer implants remain a viable and safe option in rehabilitating the dysphonia associated with recurrent laryngeal nerve paralysis.)

TRACHEOSTOMY & CRICOTHYROTOMY

There are two primary indications for tracheostomy: airway obstruction at or above the level of the larynx and respiratory failure requiring prolonged mechanical ventilation. In an acute emergency, cricothyrotomy secures an airway more rapidly than tracheostomy, with fewer potential immediate complications such as pneumothorax and hemorrhage. A percutaneous dilation tracheotomy approach is also being evaluated as an alternative to either. In order to reduce the chance of subglottic stenosis, cricothyrotomy should be converted to tracheostomy as soon as the patient is stable.

The most common indication for elective tracheostomy is the need for prolonged mechanical ventilation. There is no firm rule about how many days a patient must be intubated before conversion to tracheostomy should be advised. The incidence of serious complications such as subglottic stenosis increases with extended endotracheal intubation. As soon as it is apparent that the patient will require protracted ventilatory support, tracheostomy should replace the endotracheal tube. Less frequent indications for tracheostomy are life-threatening aspiration pneumonia, the need to improve pulmonary toilet to correct problems related to insufficient clearing of tracheobronchial secretions, and sleep apnea.

Posttracheostomy care requires humidified air to prevent secretions from crusting and occluding the inner cannula of the tracheostomy tube. The tracheostomy tube should be cleaned several times daily. The most frequent early complication of tracheostomy is dislodgment of the tracheostomy tube. Surgical creation of an inferiorly based tracheal flap sutured to the inferior neck skin may make reinsertion of a dislodged tube easier. It should be recalled that the act of swallowing requires elevation of the larynx, which is prevented by tracheostomy. Therefore, frequent tracheal and bronchial suctioning is often required to clear the aspirated saliva as well as the increased tracheobronchial secretions. Care of the skin around the stoma is important to prevent maceration and secondary infection.

Futran ND, Dutcher PO, Roberts JK: The safety and efficacy of bedside tracheotomy. Otolaryngol Head Neck Surg 1993;109:707. (Nine hundred and ninety-six bedside tracheotomies were done between 1983 and 1992 without a higher incidence of complications compared with 92 done in the operating room or, similarly, 346 done in conjunction with other major head and neck procedures.)

Tayal VS: Tracheostomies. Emerg Med Clin North Am 1994;12:707. (A review of tracheostomy tube complications, including obstruction, hemorrhage, and pneumothorax; proper suctioning, cannula removal, cannula insertion, balloon hyperinflation, and endoscopy reduce the incidence of complications.)

Toursarkissian B et al: Percutaneous dilational tracheostomy: Report of 141 cases. Ann Thorac Surg 1994;57:862. (Complication rate was 11%, with one death from bronchospasm and three cases of tracheal stenosis; concludes that percutaneous dilational tracheostomy can be done safely at the bedside, with complication rates comparable to those associated with open tracheotomy.)

FOREIGN BODIES IN THE UPPER AERODIGESTIVE TRACT

FOREIGN BODIES OF THE TRACHEA & BRONCHI

Aspiration of foreign bodies occurs less frequently in adults than in children. The elderly and denture wearers appear to be at greatest risk. Wider familiarity with the Heimlich maneuver has reduced deaths. If the maneuver is unsuccessful, cricothyrotomy may be necessary. Plain chest radiographs may reveal a radiopaque foreign body. Detection of radiolucent foreign bodies may be aided by inspiration-expiration films that demonstrate air trapping distal to the obstructed segment. Atelectasis and pneumonia may occur later.

Tracheal and bronchial foreign bodies should be removed under general anesthesia by a skilled endoscopist working with an experienced anesthesiologist.

Healy GB: Management of tracheobronchial foreign bodies in children: An update. Ann Otol Rhinol Laryngol 1990; 99:889.

Helmers RA, Sanderson DR: Rigid bronchoscopy: The forgotten art. Clin Chest Med 1995;16:393-9. (Describes current indications in adults and children.)

Linegar AG et al: Tracheobronchial foreign bodies: Experience at Red Cross Children's Hospital, 1985–1990. S Afr Med J 1992;82:164.

Limper AH, Prakash UB: Tracheobronchial foreign bodies in adults. Ann Intern Med 1990;112:604. (The setting for adults frequently includes underlying impaired protection of the airway by, for example, sedatives, alcohol, trauma with loss of consciousness, or primary neurologic disorders.)

(The Healy and Linegar references pertain to children but are included for comparison with the clinical setting for adults.)

ESOPHAGEAL FOREIGN BODIES

Foreign bodies in the esophagus create urgent but not life-threatening situations as long as the airway is not compromised. It is a useful diagnostic sign of complete obstruction if the patient is drooling or cannot handle secretions. There is probably time to consult an experienced clinician for management. Patients are likely to have difficulty handling secretions and may be spitting out their saliva. They may often point to the exact level of the obstruction. Indirect laryngoscopy often shows pooling of saliva at the esophageal inlet. Plain films may detect radiopaque foreign bodies such as chicken bones. Coins tend to align in the coronal plane in the esophagus and sagittally in the trachea. If a foreign body is suspected but not certainly known to be present, barium swallow may help make the diagnosis or establish that a foreign body is not (or is no longer) present.

Some have suggested that a Foley catheter may be used to remove an esophageal foreign body. This method risks displacing it into the larynx with resultant airway obstruction. It should be used cautiously, with the patient prone, and only by experienced physicians, and only for proximally located blunt objects. Endoscopic removal with conscious sedation or under general anesthesia is safest. Flexible esophagoscopy is usually successful; right laryngoscopy or esophagoscopy is almost always successful. Highly selected patients with a prior history of food impaction may be treated with a likelihood of success by spasmolytic drugs, such as intravenous glucagon.

Berggreen PJ et al: Techniques and complications of esophageal foreign body extraction in children and adults. Gastrointest Endosc 1993;39:626. (The Foley catheter method is suitable only for proximally located blunt objects.)

O'Flynn P, Simo R: Fish bones and other foreign bodies. Clin Otolaryngol 1993;18:231.

Robbins MI, Shortsleeve MJ: Treatment of acute esophageal food impaction with glucagon, an effervescent agent, and water. AJR Am J Roentgenol 1994;162: 325.

Tibbling L, Stenquist M: Foreign bodies in the esophagus: A study of causative factors. Dysphagia 1991;6:224. (Selected patients may be treated with spasmolytic agents.)

Webb WA: Management of foreign bodies of the upper

gastrointestinal tract: Update. Gastrointest Endosc 1995;41:39. (Experience presented in the successful treatment of 242 foreign bodies of mainly the esophagus and pharynx; the forward-viewing flexible panendoscope has become the instrument of choice in most community and tertiary centers.)

DISEASES PRESENTING AS NECK MASSES

The differential diagnosis of neck masses is heavily dependent on the location in the neck, the age of the patient, and the presence of associated disease processes. Rapid growth and tenderness suggest an inflammatory process, while firm, painless, and slowly enlarging masses are often neoplastic. In young adults, most neck masses are benign (branchial cleft cyst, thyroglossal duct cyst, reactive lymphadenitis), though malignancy should always be considered (lymphoma, metastatic thyroid carcinoma, others). Lymphadenopathy is common in HIV-positive individuals, but a growing mass or a dominant mass may be lymphoma or squamous cell carcinoma metastasis. In adults over 40, cancer is the most common cause of persistent neck mass. A metastasis from squamous cell carcinoma arising within the mouth, pharynx, larynx, or upper esophagus should be suspected, especially if there is a history of tobacco or significant alcohol use. Among patients younger than 30 or older than 70, more consideration of a lymphoma should be given. Most important is a comprehensive otolaryngologic examination. Cytologic evaluation of the neck mass via fine-needle aspiration biopsy is likely to be the next step if an obvious primary tumor is not visible or palpable on physical examination.

CONGENITAL LESIONS PRESENTING AS NECK MASSES IN ADULTS

1. BRANCHIAL CLEFT CYSTS

Branchial cleft cysts usually present as a soft cystic mass along the anterior border of the sternocleidomastoid muscle. These lesions are usually recognized in the second or third decades of life, often when they suddenly swell or become infected. To prevent recurrent infection and possible carcinoma, they should be completely excised, along with their fistulous tracts.

First branchial cleft cysts present high in the neck, sometimes just below the ear. A fistulous connection with the floor of the external auditory canal may be

present. Second cleft cysts, which are far more common, may communicate with the tonsillar fossa. Third cleft cysts, which may communicate with the piriform sinus, are rare.

2. THYROGLOSSAL DUCT CYST

Thyroglossal duct cysts are remnants occurring along the embryologic course of the thyroid's descent from the tuberculum impar of the tongue base to its usual position in the low neck. Although they may occur at any age, they are commonest before age 20. They present as a midline neck mass, often just below the hyoid bone, that moves with swallowing. Surgical excision is recommended to prevent recurrent infection. This requires removal of the entire fistulous tract along with the middle portion of the hyoid bone.

Roback SA, Telander RL: Thyroglossal duct cysts and branchial cleft anomalies. Semin Pediatr Surg 1994;3:142. (Once these congenital cysts become infected, surgical removal is very difficult, and the recurrence rate increases.)

Todd NW: Common congenital anomalies of the neck: Embryology and surgical anatomy. Surg Clin North Am 1993;73:599.

INFECTIOUS & INFLAMMATORY NECK MASSES

1. REACTIVE CERVICAL LYMPHADENOPATHY

The normal cervical lymphatic chain is not palpable. Infections involving the pharynx, salivary glands, and scalp often cause tender enlargement of neck nodes. Enlarged nodes are common in HIV-infected persons. Except for the occasional node that suppurates and requires incision and drainage, treatment is directed against the underlying infection. An enlarged lymph node that persists may warrant fine-needle aspiration biopsy in order to confirm that it is reactive and allay concern about malignancy. An enlarging node unassociated with infection must be further evaluated.

2. NECK INFECTIONS WITH ATYPICAL MYCOBACTERIA (Scrofula)

Granulomatous neck masses are not uncommon. The differential diagnosis includes cat-scratch disease (probably more common than realized), sarcoidosis, and mycobacterial adenitis. Atypical mycobacterial adenitis (scrofula) usually presents as persistent adenopathy and can become fixed to the skin and drain externally. Although fine-needle aspiration may suggest a granulomatous origin, demonstration of mycobacteria by acid-fast staining (of material taken by fine-needle aspiration or open excisional biopsy) or culture is necessary to confirm this diagnosis and address antibiotic sensitivity. Treatment of scrofula is most successful with total excision of the involved nodes and appropriate antituberculous antibiotics for at least 6 months. The antibiotics used will depend on sensitivity studies but are likely to include isoniazid, rifampin, and, for at least the first 2 months, ethambutol in standard doses (see Table 9–11). When total excision might pose formidable surgical risks (eg, facial nerve proximity), a trial of needle aspiration or incision and drainage (along with antituberculosis medication) is worthwhile.

Mycobacterial lymphadenitis among HIV-positive patients is on the rise.

Campbell IA et al: Six months versus nine months chemotherapy for tuberculosis of lymph nodes: Final results. Resp Med 1993;87:621. (Six months is adequate.)

Cleary KR, Batsakis M: Mycobacterial disease of the head and neck: current perspective. Ann Otol Rhinol Laryngol 1995;104(10 Part 1):830. (Early identification of the *Mycobacterium* has been facilitated by molecular diagnostics.)

Gupta SK et al: Cytodiagnosis of tuberculous lymphadenitis: A correlative study with microbiologic examination. Acta Cytol 1993;37:329. (One hundred and two cases of cytodiagnosis were examined. Acid-fast bacilli were seen in 20–32% of smears and cultured in 40–57%. In 8% of cases, the smears were positive when the cultures were negative.)

Lee KC, Schecter G: Tuberculous infections of the head and neck. Ear Nose Throat J 1995;74:395.

Shriner KA, Mathisen GE, Goetz MB: Comparison of mycobacterial lymphadenitis among persons infected with human immunodeficiency virus and seronegative controls. Clin Infect Dis 1992;15:601.

Subrahmanyam M: Role of surgery and chemotherapy for peripheral lymph node tuberculosis. Br J Surg 1993;80:1547. (Many patients respond to chemotherapy alone.)

Williams RG, Douglas-Jones T: *Mycobacterium* marches back. J Laryngol Otol 1995;109:5. (Reviews the features of increasingly prevalent primary and secondary tuberculosis in various head and neck sites.)

3. LYME DISEASE

Lyme disease, caused by the spirochete *Borrelia burgdorferi* and transmitted by an *Ixodes ricinus* tick, may have protean manifestation, but over 75% of patients have symptoms involving the head and neck. Facial paralysis, dysesthesias, dysgeusia, dysesthesias, or other cranial neuropathies are most common. Headache, pain, and cervical lymphadenopathy may occur. See Chapter 34 for a more thorough discussion.

Goldfarb D, Sataloff RT: Lyme disease: A review for the otolaryngologist. Ear Nose Throat J 1994;73:824. (Important in the differential diagnosis of facial paralysis in particular, but also temporal mandibular joint pain, cervical lymphadenopathy, headache, tinnitus, vertigo, decreased hearing, otalgia, and sore throat.)

Moscatello AL et al: Otolaryngologic aspects of Lyme disease. Laryngoscope 1991;101(6 Part 1):592.

Nocton JJ, Steere AC: Lyme disease. Adv Intern Med 1995;40:69. (A detailed review.)

Steere AC: Lyme disease: A growing threat to urban populations. Proc Natl Acad Sci USA 1994;91:2378. (Reviews the epidemiology of Lyme disease, its mimicry of other diseases, and treatment options.)

TUMOR METASTASES

In older adults, 80% of firm, persistent, and enlarging neck masses are metastatic in origin. The great majority of these arise from squamous cell carcinoma of the upper aerodigestive tract. A complete head and neck examination may reveal the tumor of origin, but examination under anesthesia with direct laryngoscopy, esophagoscopy, and bronchoscopy is usually required to fully evaluate the tumor and exclude second primaries.

It is often helpful to obtain a cytologic diagnosis if initial head and neck examination fails to reveal the primary tumor. An open biopsy should be done only if physical examination fails to detect the primary tumor and fine-needle aspiration biopsy has also failed to yield a diagnosis.

Other than thyroid carcinoma, non-squamous cell metastases to the neck are infrequent. While tumors not involving the head and neck seldom metastasize to the middle or upper neck, the supraclavicular region is quite often involved by lung and breast tumors. Infradiaphragmatic tumors, with the exception of renal carcinoma, rarely metastasize to the neck.

LYMPHOMA

About 10% of lymphomas present in the head and neck. Multiple rubbery nodes, especially in the young adult, are suggestive of this disease. A thorough physical examination may demonstrate other sites of nodal or organ involvement. Needle aspiration may be diagnostic, but open biopsy is often required. Lymphoma arising in AIDS patients is an increasing concern.

OTOLARYNGOLOGIC MANIFESTATIONS OF HIV INFECTION
(See also Chapter 31.)

ORAL CAVITY & PHARYNX

Gingivitis (linear gingival erythema, necrotizing ulcerative periodontitis) and stomatitis are frequent presenting symptoms in HIV-infected patients. When CD4 cell counts drop below 200/μL, the incidence of intraoral lesions rises dramatically. In the past few years, the severity of these lesions has slackened, but their incidence or reporting has increased. Candidiasis is common and may require treatment for longer than the usual 1-week course with fluconazole (100 mg daily) or ketoconazole (200–400 mg daily) for control, with clotrimazole or topical nystatin less effective. Giant intraoral ulcers have been seen in some patients. Hairy leukoplakia occurring on the lateral border of the tongue is often an early finding. It may develop quickly and appears as slightly raised leukoplakic areas with a corrugated or "hairy" surface. Histologically, parakeratosis and koilocytes are seen with little or no underlying inflammation. Among HIV-positive patients with oral lesions, hairy leukoplakia was seen in 19% in one study. Although clinical response following administration of zidovudine or acyclovir has been reported, the success of treatment or even the need for treatment is under active investigation. The greater significance of the appearance of hairy leukoplakia among seropositive patients is that it may correlate positively with subsequent more ominous manifestations of AIDS.

Kaposi's sarcoma is most common on the hard palate but may be seen anywhere in the oral cavity and pharynx. It usually appears as a raised violaceous lesion beneath an intact mucosa, although it may be ulcerated, erythematous, and bleeding. Radiation therapy may control the tumor. A brisk mucositis can be expected following radiation therapy.

In addition to Kaposi's sarcoma, an increased incidence of non-Hodgkin's lymphoma is seen in AIDS. An increase in squamous cell carcinoma is also seen in the homosexual population, perhaps related to HIV infection.

Cruz GD et al: The accurate diagnosis of oral lesions in human immunodeficiency virus infection: Impact on medical staging. Arch Otolaryngol Head Neck Surg 1996;122:68. (Forty percent of the HIV-positive homosexual men and 79% of the HIV-positive parenteral drug users with stage-defining oral lesions were not properly identified by the medical examiners. The authors conclude that specific training and a comprehensive oral examination have a significant impact on the diagnoses of oral candidiasis and oral hair leukoplakia and on the medical staging of individuals with HIV infection.)

Dattani I, Ganatra S: Oral manifestations of HIV infections. Oral Health 1993;83:15.

Glick M et al: Necrotizing ulcerative periodontitis: A marker for immune deterioration and a predictor for the diagnosis of AIDS. J Peri 1994;65:393. (HIV-infected patients with necrotizing ulcerative periodontitis very likely to have a CD4 cell count below 200/μL.)

Glick M et al: Oral manifestations associated with HIV-related disease as markers for immune suppression and AIDS. Oral Surg Oral Med Oral Pathol 1994;77:344. (Oral examinations are an essential component for early recognition of disease progression and comprehensive evaluation of HIV-infected patients.)

Greenspan D: Treatment of oral candidiasis in HIV infection. Oral Surg Oral Med Oral Pathol 1994;78:211. (Both topical and systemic drugs are effective, and new slow-release oral topical drug delivery systems may prove to be useful; good clinical descriptions also.)

Greenspan IS: Periodontal complications of HIV infection. Compendium 1994(Suppl 18):S694. (Reviews HIV-related periodontal complications, emphasizing treatment with local and systemic antibiotics.)

Ramirez-Amador VA et al: Prognostic value of oral candidosis and hairy leukoplakia in 111 Mexican HIV-infected patients. J Oral Pathol Med 1996;25:206. (The presence of oral candidiasis, hairy leukoplakia, or both is an indicator of AIDS and calls for initiation of pharmacotherapy.)

Robinson PG et al: The diagnosis of periodontal conditions associated with HIV infection. J Peri 1994;65:236. (Proposes rigid criteria for the accurate diagnosis of periodontal conditions associated with HIV infection.)

Shiboski CH et al: Human immunodeficiency virus-related oral manifestations and gender: A longitudinal analysis. The University of California, San Francisco Oral AIDS Center Epidemiology Collaborative Group. Arch Intern Med 1996;156:2249. (The occurrence of hairy leukoplakia and candidiasis was higher in men [22% and 24%, respectively] than in women [9% and 13%, respectively].)

THE NECK

Persistent generalized lymphadenopathy is extremely common in HIV infection. In this setting, a tender or growing node may represent secondary infection, lymphoma, or other tumor. Fine-needle aspiration for culture and cytology is the best initial diagnostic step. Open biopsy will often be needed if granulomatous disease or lymphoma is suspected, though fine-needle aspiration biopsy may be diagnostic of *M tuberculosis* infection in seropositive patients.

Parotid cysts and benign lymphoepithelial lesions in HIV-positive patients may be seen, often in association with cervical adenopathy.

Burton F, Patete ML, Goodwin WJ Jr: Indications for open cervical node biopsy in HIV-positive patients. Otolaryngol Head Neck Surg 1992;107:367. (Fine-needle aspiration is often sufficient to diagnose tuberculosis. Non-tender or nonenlarging nodes do not require open biopsy.)

Marinoli C et al: Benign lymphoepithelial parotid lesions in HIV-positive patients: Spectrum of findings at gray-scale and Doppler sonography. AJR Am J Roentgenol 1995;165:975.

Som PM, Brandwein MS, Silvers A: Nodal inclusion cysts of the parotid gland and parapharyngeal space: A discussion of lymphoepithelial, AIDS-related parotid, and branchial cysts, cystic Warthin's tumors, and cysts in Sjögren's syndrome. Laryngoscope 1995;105:1122. (Examines CT, MRI, and pathology in 42 patients with inclusion-type cysts of the parotid and parapharyngeal space.)

PARANASAL SINUSES

Sinusitis is common in HIV infection and the causative organisms are diverse, but the same pathogens encountered in nonimmunocompromised patients remain the most common. Early sinus irrigation, with aspirates sent for cytologic examination as well as fungal, viral, *Legionella,* and aerobic and anaerobic culture may be helpful in severe cases, as antibiotic coverage can be based on the aspirate smear, and sensitivity results can help tailor treatment in recurrent or refractory cases. Functional endoscopic surgery to provide sinus drainage is often helpful. Guaifenesin (600 mg orally four times daily), a mucolytic agent, may offer some adjunctive symptomatic relief.

Invasive *Aspergillus* sinusitis is an increasingly reported complication in AIDS. Though this infection is more indolent than mucormycosis, most patients with AIDS and *Aspergillus* sinusitis die as a result of intracranial extension.

Small CB et al: Sinusitis and atopy in human immunodeficiency virus infection. J Infect Dis 1993;167:283.

Tami TA: The management of sinusitis in patients infected with the human immunodeficiency virus (HIV). Ear Nose Throat J 1995;74:360. (Empiric antibiotic therapy in chronic HIV-related sinusitis should cover *Pseudomonas aeruginosa, Staphylococcus aureus,* and anaerobic bacteria; surgical drainage, usually endoscopically, can be a safe and effective management option when medical therapy fails.)

Teh W et al: *Aspergillus* sinusitis in patients with AIDS: Report of three cases and review. Clin Infect Dis 1995;21:529. (Invasive aspergillosis is an uncommon but highly lethal complication of AIDS.)

Upadhyay S et al: Bacteriology of sinusitis in human immunodeficiency virus-positive patients: Implications for management. Laryngoscope 1995;105:1058. (Refractory chronic sinusitis in this setting may be associated with less common pathogens, emphasizing the need for tissue culture when medical therapy fails.)

General References for Otolaryngologic Manifestations of HIV Infection

Barzan L et al: Head and neck manifestations during HIV infection. J Laryngol Otol 1993;107:133. (Eighty-four percent of patients had head and neck manifestations. Otolaryngologic evaluation is frequently helpful.)

Hwang PH et al: Attitudes, knowledge, and practices of otolaryngologists treating patients infected with HIV. Otolaryngol Head Neck Surg 1995;113:733. (Compares attitudes, knowledge, and practices between a lower and a higher geographic prevalence area.)

Murr AH, Lee KC: Universal precautions for the otolaryngologist: Techniques and equipment for minimizing exposure risk. Ear Nose Throat J 1995;74: 338, 341. (A review of various measures to implement universal precautions, and other precautions that can reduce exposure to HIV.)

Roland JT Jr et al: Squamous cell carcinoma in HIV-positive patients under age 45. Laryngoscope 1993;103:509.

Lung

John L. Stauffer, MD

DIAGNOSTIC METHODS

SYMPTOMS OF PULMONARY DISEASES

Dyspnea is the sensation of breathlessness that is excessive for any given level of physical activity. Recording the level of activity that induces dyspnea provides a basis for assessing the results of therapy. Dyspnea of pulmonary origin may be due to disorders of the airway, lung parenchyma, pleura, respiratory muscles, or chest wall. Extrapulmonary disorders causing dyspnea include heart disease (eg, heart failure, angina pectoris), shock, anemia, hypermetabolic states, abdominal distention, physical deconditioning, and anxiety. **Paroxysmal nocturnal dyspnea** (inappropriate breathlessness at night) and **orthopnea** (dyspnea on recumbency) usually are caused by left ventricular dysfunction but may also be observed in asthma, aspiration, and chronic obstructive pulmonary disease. **Platypnea,** the opposite of orthopnea, is dyspnea in the upright position relieved by recumbency. This rare symptom is usually caused by right-to-left intracardiac or pulmonary vascular shunting of venous blood.

Persistent cough should always be considered abnormal. The cough reflex may be triggered by stimulation of receptors located in the tracheobronchial tree, the upper airway, and in other sites such as the sinuses, auditory canal, pleura, pericardium, esophagus, stomach, and diaphragm. Chronic, persistent cough is often caused by cigarette smoking, asthma, bronchiectasis, or chronic obstructive pulmonary disease. Cough may also be caused by drugs (angiotensin-converting enzyme inhibitors), cardiac disease, occupational agents, and psychogenic factors. An upper respiratory tract infection occasionally induces a cough that may persist for as long as 6–8 weeks. However, the physician may encounter patients with this complaint in whom the history, physical examination, chest x-ray, and pulmonary function

tests do not suggest a specific cause. In such cases, the cough is usually found to be caused by postnasal drip from sinusitis, occult asthma, or gastroesophageal reflux. Complications of severe cough include worsening of bronchospasm, vomiting, rib fractures, urinary incontinence, and, occasionally, syncope.

Stridor is a crowing sound during breathing caused by turbulent airflow through a narrowed upper airway. Inspiratory stridor suggests extrathoracic variable airway obstruction, while expiratory stridor indicates intrathoracic variable airway obstruction. Inspiratory and expiratory stridor occurring together suggest fixed obstruction anywhere in the upper airway. Snoring is an inspiratory sound due to vibration in the pharynx during sleep.

Wheezes are continuous musical or whistling noises caused by turbulent airflow through narrowed intrathoracic airways. Most, but not all, complaints of wheezing are due to asthma. Wheezing may be accompanied by a sensation of chest tightness, a nonspecific feeling of labored breathing that implies bronchoconstriction.

Hemoptysis—the expectoration of blood or blood-tinged sputum—is often the first indication of serious bronchopulmonary disease; the history usually distinguishes it from hematemesis and from nasopharyngeal bleeding. Bright red, frothy blood implies a bronchopulmonary origin of bleeding. Though bronchitis and bronchiectasis are more common causes of hemoptysis, carcinoma must always be excluded. Massive hemoptysis, defined arbitrarily as the coughing up of more than 200–600 mL of blood in 24 hours, is often caused by bronchiectasis, tuberculosis (particularly from a Rasmussen aneurysm in cavitary disease), mycetomas, and other chronic suppurative parenchymal diseases. Self-limited minimal hemoptysis occasionally occurs with vigorous coughing accompanying upper or lower respiratory tract infection.

Cahill BC, Ingbar DH: Massive hemoptysis: Assessment and management. Clin Chest Med 1994;15:147. (Review of the broad differential diagnosis of hemoptysis, methods to localize the site of bleeding, and techniques to stop the bleeding.)

Chung KF, Lalloo UG: Diagnosis and management of chronic persistent dry cough. Postgrad Med J 1996; 72:594. (Common causes and diagnostic work-up of chronic cough.)

Colice GL: Hemoptysis. Three questions that can direct management. Postgrad Med 1996;100:227. (Identify the site of bleeding, identify high-risk patients, and distinguish systemic from pulmonary sources of bleeding.)

Mahler DA, Horowitz MB: Clinical evaluation of exertional dyspnea. Clin Chest Med 1994;15:259. (Differential diagnosis, clinical management, and tools to measure dyspnea.)

Manning HL, Schwartzstein RM: Pathophysiology of dyspnea. N Engl J Med 1995;333:1547. (Review of mechanisms of dyspnea, including the role of chemoreceptors and mechanoreceptors.)

Seamens CM, Wrenn K: Breathlessness: Strategies aimed at identifying and treating the cause of dyspnea. Postgrad Med 1995;98:215. (Review of dyspnea and diagnostic approach.)

SIGNS OF PULMONARY DISEASES

Tachypnea, or rapid, shallow breathing, may be defined arbitrarily as a respiratory rate in excess of 18/min, though some would set the limit of normal at 16, 20, or 25 breaths per minute. A sudden onset or persistence of tachypnea is particularly alarming. **Hyperpnea** is rapid, deep breathing. **Hyperventilation** is an increase in the amount of air entering the alveoli, causing hypocapnia (defined as arterial P_{CO_2} < 40 mm Hg).

The thorax is normally symmetric, and both sides expand equally on inspiration. Asymmetry at rest is observed in scoliosis, chest wall deformity, severe fibrothorax, and conditions with unilateral loss of lung volume. Symmetrically reduced chest expansion during deep inspiration is seen in such conditions as neuromuscular disease, emphysema, and ankylosis of the spine. Asymmetric chest expansion during inspiration suggests unilateral airway obstruction, pleural or pulmonary fibrosis, or splinting due to chest pain. Expansion of the chest but collapse of the abdomen on inspiration indicates weakness or paralysis of the diaphragm. If the chest collapses and the abdomen rises on inspiration, airway obstruction, intercostal muscle paralysis, or a flail deformity of the chest wall may be present.

The arterial blood pressure normally falls about 5 mm Hg on inspiration. **Paradoxic pulse,** an exaggeration of the normal response, is defined as a fall in systolic arterial blood pressure of 10 mm Hg or more on inspiration. This occurs in severe asthma or emphysema, upper airway obstruction, pulmonary embolism, pericardial constriction or tamponade, and restrictive cardiomyopathy.

Cyanosis is a bluish discoloration of skin or mucous membranes caused by increased amounts (> 5 g/dL) of unsaturated hemoglobin in the blood. Anemia may preclude detection of cyanosis in a hypoxemic patient. **Central cyanosis,** which is usually caused by hypoxemia from respiratory failure or a right-to-left intracardiac or intrapulmonary shunt, is apparent on inspection of the oral mucous membranes; **peripheral cyanosis** is more likely due to nonrespiratory causes such as reduced cardiac output and vasoconstriction.

Digital clubbing is present when the anteroposterior thickness of the index finger at the base of the fingernail exceeds the thickness of the distal interphalangeal joint. Nail bed sponginess, rounding of the nail plate, and flattening of the angle between the nail plate and proximal nail skin fold are helpful clues to clubbing. Symmetric clubbing occurs in lung cancer, bronchiectasis, lung abscess, pulmonary arteriovenous malformation, idiopathic pulmonary fibrosis, and cystic fibrosis. It is rarely seen in chronic obstructive pulmonary disease and chronic asthma. Nonpulmonary causes of symmetric clubbing include cyanotic congenital heart disease, infective endocarditis, cirrhosis, and inflammatory bowel disease. Clubbing may be congenital.

Hyperresonance to percussion occurs in diseases accompanied by hyperinflation (asthma, emphysema) and in pneumothorax. **Dullness** to percussion is observed in thickening of the chest wall or pleura, pleural effusion, atelectasis, parenchymal infiltration or consolidation, elevation of the diaphragm, or displacement of abdominal contents into the thorax.

Vesicular breath sounds are normal soft, low-pitched sounds heard at the periphery of the lung. The finding of harsh **bronchial (tracheal) breath sounds** in areas where vesicular sounds are normally heard implies consolidation, compression, or infiltration of the lung with a patent bronchus. **Bronchovesicular breath sounds** are intermediate in tone quality between vesicular and bronchial sounds. **Diminished breath sounds** imply inspiratory obstruction to airflow in large airways, pleural disease (especially effusion), pneumothorax, marked obesity, or low tidal volumes.

Adventitious sounds are abnormal sounds on auscultation and may be classified as continuous (**wheezes, rhonchi**) or discontinuous (**crackles, crepitations, or rales**). High-pitched wheezes result from bronchospasm, bronchial or bronchiolar mucosal edema, or airway obstruction by mucus, tumors, or foreign bodies. Low-pitched rhonchi are often caused by sputum in large airways and frequently clear after cough. Crackles are probably generated by the snapping open of small airways during inspiration. Fine crackles are heard in interstitial diseases, early pneumonia or pulmonary edema, patchy atelectasis, and in some patients with asthma or bronchitis. Coarse crackles are heard late in the course of pulmonary edema or pneumonia.

Tactile (vocal) fremitus denotes palpable voice vibrations on the chest wall. This is a normal finding. Localized **reduction in fremitus** occurs in pleural effusion, pneumothorax, or thickening of the chest wall. **Increased fremitus** suggests lung consolidation. **Rhonchal fremitus** means palpable coarse vibrations on the chest wall in patients with loud rhonchi.

Bronchophony refers to increased intensity and clarity of the spoken word during auscultation; it is heard over areas of consolidation or lung compression. **Whispered pectoriloquy** is an extreme form of bronchophony in which softly spoken words are readily heard by auscultation. **Egophony** refers to auscultation of an "a" sound when the patient speaks an "e" sound. It is demonstrated over compressed lung above a pleural effusion, and in consolidation.

Sharma OP: Symptoms and signs in pulmonary medicine: Old observations and new interpretations. Dis Mon 1995 Sep;41:577. (Reemphasizes the importance of the physician's observations from a skillful medical history and physical examination.)

DIAGNOSTIC TESTS: PULMONARY FUNCTION TESTS, PULMONARY EXERCISE STRESS TESTING, & BRONCHOSCOPY

Pulmonary Function Tests

Pulmonary function tests objectively measure the ability of the respiratory system to perform gas exchange by assessing its ventilation, diffusion, and mechanical properties. Indications for pulmonary function testing include the following:

(1) Evaluation of the type and degree of pulmonary dysfunction.

(2) Evaluation of dyspnea, cough, and other symptoms.

(3) Early detection of lung dysfunction.

(4) Surveillance in occupational settings.

(5) Follow-up of response to therapy.

(6) Preoperative evaluation.

(7) Disability assessment.

Relative contraindications to pulmonary function testing include severe acute asthma or respiratory distress, chest pain aggravated by testing, pneumothorax, brisk hemoptysis, and active tuberculosis. Most of the tests depend on the efforts of the patient; some patients may be too impaired to make an optimal effort. Suboptimal effort or test performance by the patient during spirometry limits the validity of spirometry and lung volume calculations derived from spirometry. This is a common cause of misinterpretation of pulmonary function test results. Pulmonary function tests derived from **spirometry** (the measurement of airflow rates and forced vital capacity) and measurement of lung volumes are defined in Table 9–1.

Spirometry and measurement of lung volumes al-

Table 9–1. Definitions of selected pulmonary function tests.

Tests	Definition
Tests derived from spirometry	
Forced vital capacity (FVC)	The volume of gas that can be forcefully expelled from the lungs after maximal inspiration.
Forced expiratory volume in 1 second (FEV$_1$)	The volume of gas expelled in the first second of the FVC maneuver.
Forced expiratory flow from 25% to 75% of the forced vital capacity (FEF$_{25-75}$)	The maximal midexpiratory airflow rate.
Peak expiratory flow rate (PEFR)	The maximal airflow rate achieved in the FVC maneuver.
Maximum voluntary ventilation (MVV)	The maximum volume of gas that can be breathed in 1 minute (usually measured for 15 seconds and multiplied by 4).
Lung volumes	
Slow vital capacity (SVC)	The volume of gas that can be slowly exhaled after maximal inspiration
Total lung capacity (TLC)	The volume of gas in the lungs after a maximal inspiration.
Functional residual capacity (FRC)	The volume of gas in the lungs at the end of a normal tidal expiration.
Residual volume (RV)	The volume of gas remaining in the lungs after maximal expiration.
Expiratory reserve volume (ERV)	The volume of gas representing the difference between functional residual capacity and residual volume.

low determination of the presence and severity of *obstructive* and *restrictive* pulmonary dysfunction. The hallmark of obstructive pulmonary dysfunction is reduction in airflow rates. Causes include asthma, chronic bronchitis, emphysema, small airway dysfunction, bronchiolitis, bronchiectasis, cystic fibrosis, and upper airway obstruction. Some advanced chronic interstitial lung diseases such as sarcoidosis may also cause obstructive dysfunction. Restrictive pulmonary dysfunction is characterized by reduction in lung volumes. Pulmonary infiltrates, lung resection, pleural diseases, chest wall disorders, reduced diaphragm movement, and neuromuscular disease may be responsible. Pulmonary function alterations in obstructive and restrictive disorders are summarized in Table 9–2. The changes in airflow rates and lung volumes in the restrictive category vary according to the specific cause of the disorder.

Obstructive dysfunction is graded according to the reduction in the ratio of **forced expiratory volume in 1 second (FEV$_1$)** to **forced vital capacity (FVC).** Restrictive dysfunction is graded by reduction in the FVC or total lung capacity, comparing observed with predicted values. Predicted values are derived from studies of normals and in general vary with gender, age, and height. Spirometry provides a **spirogram** that displays time (*x*-axis) versus expired volume (*y*-axis) and an expiratory **flow-volume curve** (first derivative of the spirogram) that plots expiratory volume (*x*-axis) versus expiratory airflow rate (*y*-axis) (Figure 9–1). The **flow-volume loop** combines the maximal expiratory and inspiratory flow-volume curves and is especially helpful for determining intrathoracic and extrathoracic airway dynamics and the site of airway obstruction.

Spirometry is adequate for evaluation of most patients with suspected respiratory disease. If airflow

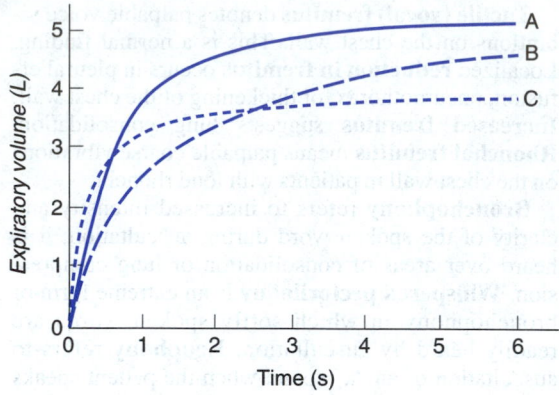
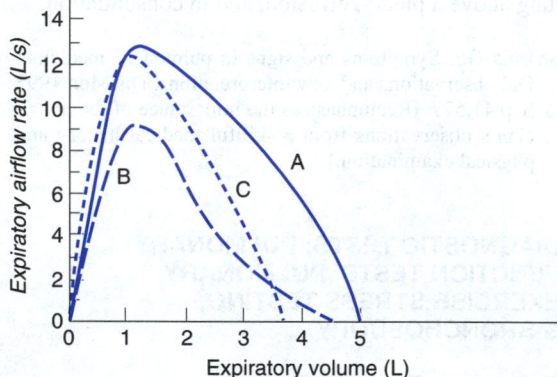

Figure 9–1. Representative spirograms (upper panel) and expiratory flow-volume curves (lower panel) for normal *(A)*, obstructive *(B)*, and restrictive *(C)* patterns.

obstruction is evident, spirometry is repeated 10–20 minutes after an inhaled bronchodilator is administered. This doubles the cost of the study. The absence of improvement in spirometry after inhaled bronchodilator in the pulmonary function laboratory does *not* preclude a successful clinical response to bronchodilator therapy. Measurements of lung volumes and diffusing capacity are useful in selected patients, but these tests are expensive and should not be ordered routinely with spirometry. Total (laboratory and professional) charges are approximately $100–$120 for lung volume measurements and an equal amount for diffusing capacity measurement.

Measurement of the single-breath **diffusing capacity** for carbon monoxide (D$_L$CO), which reflects the ability of the lung to transfer gas across the alveolar/capillary interface, is particularly helpful in evaluation of patients with diffuse infiltrative lung disease or emphysema. The total pulmonary diffusing capacity (D$_L$) depends upon the diffusion properties of the alveolar-capillary membrane and the amount of hemoglobin occupying the pulmonary capillaries. Elevated D$_L$CO is observed in congestive heart fail-

Table 9–2. Results of pulmonary function tests in obstructive and restrictive pulmonary dysfunction.[1]

Tests	Obstructive[2]	Restrictive[2]
Spirometry		
FVC (liters)	N or ↓	↓
FEV$_1$ (liters)	↓	N or ↓
FEV$_1$/FVC (%)	↓	N or ↑
FEF$_{25-75}$ (L/s)	↓	N or ↓
PEFR (L/s)	↓	N or ↑
MVV (L/min)	↓	N or ↓
Lung volumes		
SVC (liters)	N or ↓	↓
TLC (liters)	N or ↑	↓
FRC (liters)	↑	N or ↓
ERV (liters)	N or ↓	N or ↓
RV (liters)	↑	N, ↓, or ↑
RV/TLC ratio	↑	N or ↑

[1]See Table 9–1 for definitions of tests.
[2]N = normal; ↓ = less than predicted; ↑ = greater than predicted.

ure and pulmonary hemorrhage. A diffusing capacity greater than 6 mL CO/mm Hg below the predicted value in women or 8.1 mL CO/mm Hg in men is considered abnormally low (Intermountain Thoracic Society guidelines). The diffusing capacity should be corrected for the blood hemoglobin level.* Reporting the ratio of measured diffusing capacity to alveolar volume ($D_L CO/V_A$) is helpful, because a diminished diffusing capacity may only reflect a reduction in lung volume. In patients with emphysema, the diffusing capacity is characteristically low, the alveolar volume normal or increased, and the $D_L CO/V_A$ ratio is low. In patients with diffuse infiltrative lung disease, both the diffusing capacity and the alveolar volume are characteristically reduced, and the $D_L CO/V_A$ ratio is normal or low.

In patients with AIDS, $D_L CO$ is a highly sensitive screening test for the presence of pulmonary disease, especially *Pneumocystis carinii* pneumonia, but it lacks specificity. A normal $D_L CO$ in an AIDS patient is strong evidence against pneumocystis pneumonia. An abnormal result indicates the need for further diagnostic evaluation. Routine measurement of $D_L CO$ and other pulmonary function tests in AIDS patients with pulmonary disease is not advised, because of expense and lack of specificity.

Arterial blood gas analysis is indicated whenever a clinically important acid-base disturbance, hypoxemia, or hypercapnia is suspected. **Oximetry** provides an inexpensive, noninvasive alternative means of monitoring oxyhemoglobin saturation with oxygen. Oximeters monitor oxygen saturation and not oxygen tension. Table 9–3 displays the normal relationship between oxyhemoglobin saturation and partial pressure of oxygen in blood. This relationship is not linear. The clinical accuracy of pulse oximeters is reduced in such conditions as severe anemia (< 5 g/dL hemoglobin), the presence of abnormal hemoglobin moieties (carboxyhemoglobin, methemoglobin, fetal hemoglobin), the presence of intravascular dyes, motion artifact, and lack of pulsatile arterial blood flow (hypotension, hypothermia, cardiac arrest, simultaneous use of a blood pressure cuff, and cardiopulmonary bypass). The normal arterial P_{O_2} falls with increasing altitude (Table 9–4).

American Thoracic Society: Standardization of spirometry: 1994 update. Am J Respir Crit Care Med 1995;152: 1107. (Current standards for spirometry and peak expiratory flow rate recording.)

Crapo RO: Pulmonary-function testing. N Engl J Med 1994;331:25. (Indications and interpretation.)

Petty TL: The predictive value of spirometry: Identifying patients at risk for lung cancer in the primary care set-

---

*Corrected $D_L CO$ = Measured $D_L CO$ × $\dfrac{[Hb] + 10.22}{1.7\,[Hb]}$

where [Hb] is the measured hemoglobin concentration (g/dL)

Table 9–3. Relationship of oxyhemoglobin saturation and partial pressure of oxygen in blood.[1,2]

Saturation (%)	Partial Pressure (mm Hg)[3]
50	27
60	31
70	37
80	45
85	50
90	58
92	63
94	69
96	81
98	111
99	159

[1]Modified and reproduced, with permission, from Severinghaus JW: Values for a standard blood oxygen dissociation curve: Man. In: *Respiration and Circulation*. Altman PC, Dittmer DS (editors): Federation of American Societies for Experimental Biology, 1971.
[2]This relationship assumes a normal position of the oxyhemoglobin dissociation curve.
[3]Rounded to the nearest whole number.

ting. Postgrad Med 1997;101:128. (Office spirometry can help identify patients at risk for lung cancer.)

Wahr JA, Tremper KK: Noninvasive oxygen monitoring techniques. Crit Care Clin 1995;11:199. (Devices to monitor oxygenation in the critical care setting.)

Pulmonary Exercise Stress Testing

Pulmonary exercise testing is usually performed to evaluate patients with unexplained exertional dyspnea. A bicycle ergometer or treadmill is used. Minute ventilation, expired oxygen and carbon dioxide tension, heart rate, blood pressure, and respiratory rate are monitored. The exercise protocol is determined by the indications for the test and the ability of the patient to exercise. Complications are rare. Total charges for a full exercise study (without arterial catheterization) approximate $400 to $500.

Table 9–4. The effect of altitude on P_{O_2} in normals.

Altitude (feet)	Barometric Pressure (mm Hg)	Atmospheric[1] P_{O_2} (mm Hg)	Tracheal[2] P_{O_2} (mm Hg)	Arterial[3] P_{O_2} (mm Hg)
Sea level	760	159	149	99
2,000	707	148	138	88
4,000	656	137	127	77
6,000	609	127	118	68
8,000	564	118	108	58
10,000	523	109	100	50
15,000	428	90	80	30

[1]Dry gas.
[2]Saturated with water vapor.
[3]Actual values at altitude will be higher, depending on the degree of adaptation (ventilatory response to hypoxia).

Weisman IM, Zeballos RJ: Clinical exercise testing. Clin Chest Med 1994;15:173. [Entire issue.] (Current concepts in cardiopulmonary exercise testing.)

Bronchoscopy

Flexible **fiberoptic bronchoscopy** is an essential tool in the diagnosis and management of many pulmonary diseases. Bronchoscopy is indicated for evaluation of the airway, diagnosis and staging of bronchogenic carcinoma, evaluation of hemoptysis, biopsy of lung infiltrates, diagnosis of pulmonary infections, facilitation of bronchoalveolar lavage, and removal of retained secretions and foreign bodies from the airway. The procedure is contraindicated in patients with severe bronchospasm. A bleeding diathesis is a contraindication to biopsy and brushing. Complications include hemoptysis, fever, and a transient reduction in PO_2 (< 10 mm Hg). The rate of major complications is less than 1% overall, and deaths are rare. The rate of major complications jumps to about 7% when transbronchial lung biopsy is performed. Hospitalization for fiberoptic bronchoscopy is not necessary. The total charges for the procedure range from $600 to over $1500, depending on the need for fluoroscopy, processing of specimens in the laboratory, hospital outpatient stay charges, and other variables.

Rigid bronchoscopy is performed for massive bleeding, extraction of large obstructing objects (foreign bodies, blood clots, tumor masses, broncholiths), biopsy of tracheal or main stem bronchus tumors and bronchial carcinoids, and facilitation of laser therapy. Unlike fiberoptic bronchoscopy, rigid bronchoscopy usually requires general anesthesia.

Borchers SD, Beamis JF Jr: Flexible bronchoscopy. Chest Surg Clin North Am 1996;6:169.

Prakash UBS, Stubbs SE: Optimal bronchoscopy. J Bronchol 1994;1:44. (Overview of current bronchoscopy practice, including indications, methods, and guidelines.)

Silver MR, Balk RA: Bronchoscopic procedures in the intensive care unit. Crit Care Clin 1995;11:97. (The role of fiberoptic bronchoscopy in airway management, hemoptysis, and other critical care problems.)

DISORDERS OF THE AIRWAYS

Diseases of the airways have diverse causes but share certain pathophysiologic and clinical features. Limitation of airflow is characteristic and results from bronchial smooth muscle contraction, intraluminal airway obstruction, thickening of airway walls, or the loss of distending support by interstitial tissues necessary to maintain patency of the airways. Hyper-secretion of mucus, airway irritability, and gas exchange abnormalities result in cough, sputum production, wheezing, and dyspnea.

ASTHMA

Essentials of Diagnosis

- Episodic or chronic wheezing, dyspnea, cough, and feeling of tightness in the chest.
- Prolonged expiration and diffuse wheezing on physical examination.
- Limitation of airflow on pulmonary function testing, or positive bronchoprovocation challenge test.
- Complete or partial reversibility of obstructive dysfunction after bronchodilator therapy.

General Considerations

Asthma is defined as a "disease characterized by an increased responsiveness of the trachea and bronchi to various stimuli, and manifested by widespread narrowing of the airways that changes in severity either spontaneously or as a result of treatment" (American Thoracic Society). Asthma is common in adults and even more common in children. Men and women are equally affected. About 5% of the population, or about 15 million Americans, suffer from asthma. A genetic susceptibility to asthma is recognized.

Asthma is characterized by such pathologic changes as hypertrophy of bronchial smooth muscle, mucosal edema and hyperemia, thickening of epithelial basement membrane, hypertrophy of mucous glands, acute inflammation, and plugging of airways by thick, viscid mucus. These changes result in obstruction of airways of all calibers.

The pathogenesis of asthma is poorly understood. Asthma is now regarded primarily as a subacute inflammatory disease of airways. Multiple complex mechanisms probably are involved in reversible airflow obstruction. Numerous cytokines derived from tissue mast cells, eosinophils, T lymphocytes, macrophages, and other lung cells are critical in initiating and perpetuating the asthmatic response. The sensitized tissue mast cell plays a pivotal role in asthma by degranulating and releasing mediators such as histamine, bradykinin, chemotactic factors, platelet-activating factor, and metabolites of arachidonic acid such as prostaglandins and leukotrienes. Neural factors may augment this response. These mediators act locally to effect bronchoconstriction, cellular infiltration, platelet activation, increased vascular permeability, edema, and increased secretion of mucus. Besides mast cells, other lung cells, including eosinophils, neutrophils, and lymphocytes, play important roles in the immunopathogenesis of airway inflammation in asthma. Airway narrowing in asthma results from a combination of smooth muscle spasm, airway edema and inflammation, and mucus plugging. Successful therapy depends upon reversing each of these factors.

Exercise-induced asthma occurs 5–10 minutes after the patient starts to exercise and may be related to heat loss or water loss from the bronchial surface. **Triad asthma,** a combination of asthma, aspirin sensitivity, and nasal polyposis, occurs in fewer than 10% of asthma patients. Bronchoconstriction in this condition is due to the effects on arachidonic acid metabolism of aspirin and other nonsteroidal anti-inflammatory agents, tartrazine dyes, and other compounds. **Occupational asthma** may be triggered by various agents found in the workplace and occurs a few weeks to many years after initial exposure to an offending agent. Nocturnal cough may be the only symptom. **Cardiac asthma** represents bronchospasm precipitated by congestive heart failure, probably as a result of vasodilation of blood vessels in small airways. **Asthmatic bronchitis** denotes chronic bronchitis with features of bronchospasm that quickly responds to bronchodilator therapy. **Drug-induced asthma** is caused by many commonly used agents (Table 9–23).

Clinical Findings

A. Symptoms and Signs: Asthma is characterized by episodic wheezing, feelings of tightness in the chest, dyspnea, and cough. The frequency of asthma attacks is highly variable. Some patients may have very infrequent, brief attacks of asthma; others may suffer nearly continuous symptoms. Asthma is often worse at night. Nocturnal asthma is usually most severe around 3–4 AM, when circadian variations in bronchomotor tone and bronchial reactivity result in bronchoconstriction.

Asthma attacks occur spontaneously or result from various "trigger factors," including nonspecific irritants (dusts, odors, cold air, sulfur dioxide fumes), emotional stress, upper respiratory infections, sinusitis and postnasal drip, exertion, exposure to aeroallergens, aspiration, and abrupt changes in weather. The antigens of the ubiquitous house dust mite represent an important aeroallergen for many patients with asthma. Inhalation of aeroallergens often initiates wheezing, chest tightness, dyspnea, and cough both immediately (immediate asthmatic response) and 4–6 hours later (late asthmatic response). Aspirin, other nonsteroidal anti-inflammatory drugs, sulfites added to foods and certain medications, beta-blockers, and other drugs (Table 9–23) can trigger attacks of asthma. Patients may present with chronic dry or nonproductive cough rather than with dyspnea and wheezing; baseline pulmonary function tests are normal but bronchial hyperreactivity can be demonstrated with bronchial provocation testing. Inhaled bronchodilators are often effective in controlling cough symptoms in these patients.

Physical findings vary with the severity of the attack. A mild attack may produce only slight tachycardia and tachypnea, with prolonged expiration and mild diffuse wheezing. More severe attacks are associated with use of accessory muscles of respiration, distant breath sounds, loud wheezing, hyperresonance, and intercostal retraction. Ominous signs in severe asthma include fatigue, pulsus paradoxus (> 20 mm Hg), diaphoresis, inaudible breath sounds with diminished wheezing, inability to maintain recumbency, and cyanosis.

B. Laboratory Findings: The total white blood cell count may be slightly increased during an acute attack, and eosinophilia is common. Expectorated sputum is viscid on gross examination; microscopic findings include mucus casts of small airways (Curschmann's spirals), eosinophils, and elongated rhomboid crystals derived from eosinophil cytoplasm (Charcot-Leyden crystals). Pulmonary function tests (Table 9–2) reveal abnormalities typical of obstructive dysfunction, and partial reversibility (improvement in FVC or FEV_1 of at least 15% or improvement in FEF_{25-75} of at least 25%) is often demonstrated after an inhaled bronchodilator is administered. It is important to emphasize that the absence of improvement in the pulmonary function test after bronchodilator does not constitute proof of irreversible airflow obstruction. Measuring the peak expiratory flow rate (PEFR) with a simple, inexpensive hand-held device can also indicate the severity of airflow limitation. Predicted values for PEFR vary with sex, age, and height, and are typically 450–650 L/min in men and 350–500 L/min in women. Values under 100–200 L/min indicate severe ventilatory dysfunction.

Arterial blood gas measurements in asthma may be normal during a mild attack, but respiratory alkalosis and mild hypoxemia are usually observed. In more severe cases, hypoxemia worsens and respiratory alkalosis disappears when respiratory muscle fatigue prevents hyperventilation. Normalization of the PCO_2 or development of respiratory acidosis in this circumstance may indicate the need for mechanical ventilation.

C. Imaging: Routine chest radiographs in adults and children with uncomplicated attacks reveal only hyperinflation; they are unnecessary in acute asthma unless pneumothorax, pneumonia, or another disorder mimicking asthma (see below) is suspected. Bronchial wall thickening and absence of vascular shadows in the periphery of the lung are sometimes observed.

D. Special Examinations: Nonspecific **bronchial provocation testing** with methacholine or histamine is helpful in the evaluation of suspected asthma, particularly when baseline spirometry is normal, and in evaluation of unexplained cough. A positive test is defined as a decrease in FEV_1 of 20% or more after inhalation of the test substance. The test has a sensitivity of about 95% and a specificity of about 70% in the diagnosis of bronchial asthma. Positive results may occur in nonasthmatics with COPD, allergic rhinitis, sarcoidosis, cystic fibrosis, viral respiratory tract infections, and other conditions. A negative result makes the diagnosis of asthma very unlikely. The total charges for bronchial provocation testing are approximately $300–$340. Skin testing for allergens that trigger attacks is most useful in young patients with extrinsic asthma.

Differential Diagnosis

Wheezing occurs not only in bronchial asthma but also in chronic obstructive pulmonary disease (COPD), left ventricular failure, pulmonary embolism, bronchiectasis, anaphylaxis, inhalation lung injury, and partial airway obstruction due to any cause, such as lung cancer and foreign body aspiration. Stridor in upper airway obstruction or in vocal cord dysfunction may simulate wheezing. Asthma must be distinguished from functional disorders of the larynx. Reversible bronchial obstruction with eosinophilia occurs in infections with parasitic infection (particularly *Strongyloides*), bronchopulmonary aspergillosis, and Churg-Strauss syndrome.

Complications

Complications of asthma include exhaustion, dehydration, airway infection, cor pulmonale, and tussive syncope. Pneumothorax is a rare complication. Acute respiratory failure with hypoxemia and hypercapnia occurs in severe disease. In most Western countries, there has been over the last 15 years a gradual increase in the asthma prevalence and mortality rates despite advances in understanding the pathogenesis of this disorder and the availability of new pharmacologic agents. Over 5000 people die from asthma each year in the USA, and the death rate is increasing worldwide. This rise in asthma mortality rates can be explained in large part by socioeconomic conditions affecting urban minorities that result in poor access to health care, excessive environmental risks, psychologic stress, and other factors. Blacks are three times more likely than whites to die from asthma. Overreliance upon inhaled beta-agonist bronchodilators and their excessive use during asthma attacks have also been implicated in the rising asthma mortality rate.

Prevention

Comprehensive patient education, aimed especially at pharmacologic intervention and environmental control, is vital to success in the treatment of asthma. Asthma is often preventable if environmental and occupational agents and other "trigger factors" known to provoke asthma attacks can be identified and eliminated. The importance of environmental control measures in both the home and the workplace cannot be overemphasized. For example, measures to control house dust mite antigen (pillow and mattress covers, removal of carpets, air filtering and condi-

tioning, etc) and animal danders (washing or grooming the pet cat or dog weekly) should be employed. Early treatment of chest infections, recognition and effective management of nasal and paranasal disorders, discontinuance of cigarette smoking, avoidance of exposure to environmental tobacco smoke, and a sympathetic attitude on the part of the physician are essential aspects of preventive care. Pneumococcal and yearly influenza immunization are desirable for patients with moderate to severe asthma. Patient compliance with prescribed medication is essential to prevent flare-ups of asthma. Many patients with asthma will benefit from recording PEFR at home and at work while correlating their symptoms with PEFR values. PEFR values of 60–80% of predicted typically occur with asthma exacerbations of moderate severity, while values of less than 60% predicted indicate severe asthma.

Treatment

A. Ambulatory Patients With Asthma: Management of ambulatory adults with asthma depends upon the severity of the disease. An expert panel of the National Heart, Lung, and Blood Institute has provided some useful guidelines that were updated and revised in 1997. Emphasis must be given to patient education, environmental control, smoking cessation, proper use of metered-dose inhalers, and use of anti-inflammatory therapy. The new NHLBI guidelines call for early control of the disease process with anti-inflammatory therapy, stepping down the therapy thereafter if possible. Table 9–5 summarizes drugs used in the treatment of asthma and COPD.

1. Mild asthma–Adult patients with mild asthma are defined as those with one or more of the following: (1) intermittent, brief symptoms (< 1 hour's duration) up to two times weekly, (2) absence of symptoms between exacerbations, (3) brief (< ½ hour) symptoms with activity, and (4) nocturnal symptoms less than twice per month. These patients typically display baseline PEFR or FEV_1 values greater than 80% (of predicted value or personal best), with less than 20% variability during exacerbations. Such patients may use a short-acting, inhaled β_2 agonist drug, such as albuterol, metaproterenol, bitolterol, terbutaline, or pirbuterol, for symptom relief or before exercise or exposure to other trigger factors. One or two inhalations, delivered by a metered-dose inhaler (MDI) are usually adequate. These drugs have largely replaced older compounds such as isoetharine, isoproterenol, ephedrine, and epinephrine in the management of mild asthma. Oral theophylline is no longer considered useful in the treatment of mild asthma.

2. Moderate asthma–Adult patients with moderate asthma are those with one or more of the following: (1) symptoms more than one or two times weekly, (2) exacerbations affecting sleep and level of

Table 9–5. Selected drugs for obstructive airway diseases.[1]

Drug	Important Formulations	Usual Adult Dosage (Stable Patient)	Cost[2]	Comments
BRONCHODILATORS **Sympathomimetics** Albuterol (Proventil, Ventolin)[3]	Metered-dose inhaler (90 µg/puff; 200 puffs/inhaler)	1–4 puffs every 4–6 hours prn	$25.00/17 g	Preferred formulation in most cases. Clinically similar to metaproterenol but slightly longer duration of action. Proventil HFA brand (albuterol sulfate inhalation aerosol) has a hydrofluoroalkane propellant that replaces the chlorofluorocarbon propellant found in other metered-dose inhalers. Each inhalation delivers 108 µg albuterol sulfate from the mouthpiece (equivalent to 90 µg of albuterol base).
	Nebulized solution (0.5%)	0.5 mL plus 2.5 mL normal saline every 4–6 hours[4]	$15.00/20 mL	Administer with powered nebulizer or, rarely, by IPPB.
	Unit dose solution (0.083%)	One 3 mL dose every 4–6 hours[4]	$7.43/unit	Administer with powered nebulizer.
	Powder (Ventolin Rotocaps) (200 µg)	One 200 µg capsule every 4–6 hours	$26.00/100	Requires Rotohaler to inhale.
	Tablets (2 mg, 4 mg) Syrup (2 mg/5 mL)	2–4 mg orally every 6–8 hours	$25.00/100 2-mg tablets	An extended-release 4-mg tablet is available for use every 12 hours (Proventil Repetab). Volmax extended-release tablets are available in 4 mg and 8 mg strengths.
Salmeterol (Serevent)	Metered-dose inhaler (21 µg/puff; 120 puffs/inhaler)	2 puffs every 12 hours	$55.48/13 g	Long-acting agent for maintenance therapy of asthma. Should not be used for acute relief of symptoms. The most expensive β_2 agonist.
Metaproterenol (Alupent, Metaprel, others)	Metered-dose inhaler (650 µg/puff; 200 puffs/inhaler)	1–4 puffs every 3–4 hours (or more frequently)[4] prn	$21.65/14 g	Preferred formulation in most cases.
	Nebulized solution (5%)	0.3 mL plus 2.5 mL normal saline every 3–4 hours[4]	$15.70/10 mL	Administer with powered nebulizer or, rarely, by IPPB. Also available as single-dose vial.
	Unit dose solution (0.4% and 0.6%)	One 2.5 mL dose every 4–6 hours[4]	$1.78/unit	Administer with powered nebulizer.
	Syrup (10 mg/5 mL)	2 tsp orally every 6–8 hours	$19.00/480 mL	Tremor, nervousness, palpitations common. Oral formulation therefore not recommended.
	Tablets (10 mg, 20 mg)	20 mg orally every 6–8 hours	$21.00/100 20 mg	
Bitolterol (Tornalate)[3]	Metered-dose inhaler (370 µg/puff; 300 puffs/inhaler)	2–3 puffs every 6–8 hours prn	$37.44/15 mL	
	Inhalation solution (0.2%)	1.25 mL every 6–8 hours[3]	$14.60/30 mL	
Pirbuterol (Maxair and Maxaire Autoinhaler)[3]	Metered-dose inhaler (200 µg/puff; 300 puffs/inhaler)	2 puffs every 4–6 hours prn	$29.34/25.6 g	
	Breath-activated metered-dose inhaler (200 µg/puff; 400 puffs/inhaler)	2 puffs every 4–6 hours[4]	$38.74/14 g	

(continued)

Drug	Important Formulations	Usual Adult Dosage (Stable Patient)	Cost[2]	Comments
Terbutaline[3] (Brethaire)	Metered-dose inhaler (200 µg/puff; 300 puffs/inhaler)	2–3 puffs every 4–6 hours[4]	$19.84/7.5 mL	
(Brethine, Bricanyl)	Tablets (2.5 mg, 5 mg)	2.5–5 mg orally 3 times daily	$39.54/100 5-mg tablets	Tremor, nervousness, palpitations common. Oral formulation therefore not recommended.
	Subcutaneous injection (1 mg/mL)	0.25 mg subcutaneously; may be repeated once in 30 minutes	$2.80/1 mg per mL	Slow onset of action (30 minutes). Not limited to β_2-adrenergic stimulation.
Isoetharine (Bronkometer, Bronkosol)	Metered-dose inhaler (340 µg/puff; 200 puffs/10 mL inhaler)	1–4 puffs every 3–4 hours[4]	$32.72/15 mL	
	Nebulized solution (1%)	0.5 mL of 1% solution plus 1.5 mL normal saline every 2–4 hours	$18.56/10 mL	Administer with powered nebulizer or, rarely, by IPPB.
Isoproterenol (Isuprel, others)	Metered-dose inhaler (131 µg/puff; 200 puffs/10 mL)	1–3 puffs every 2–4 hours	$32.46/15 mL	
	Nebulized solution (0.5%; 1% also available)	0.5 mL of 0.5% solution plus 1.5 mL normal saline every 2–4 hours	$24.08/10 mL	Administer with powered nebulizer or, rarely, by IPPB.
Epinephrine (Primatene, Bronitin, many others)	Metered-dose inhaler (200 µg/puff)	1 or 2 puffs every 2–4 hours	$10.63/15 mL	Available without prescription. β_1 and α stimulation limit usefulness.
	Subcutaneous injection (0.1%; 1:1000)	0.3–0.5 mL subcutaneously; may be repeated once in 30 minutes	$0.50/1 mL	Use with caution in older patients or those with tachycardia, hypertension, or arrhythmia. No more effective than inhaled β_2 agonist.
Anticholinergics Ipratropium bromide (Atrovent)	Metered-dose inhaler (18 µg/puff; 200 puffs/inhaler)	2–4 puffs every 6 hours	$31.48/14 g	More potent than sympathomimetics in COPD. Minimal side effects.
	Unit dose inhalation solution (0.02%)	One 2.5 mL dose every 6–8 hours	$2.06/unit	
Theophyllines Theophylline, oral (many brands)	Sustained-release tablets and bead-filled capsules	200 mg orally every 12 hours initially; thereafter, 200–600 mg orally every 8–12 hours	$0.20/200 mg	Maintenance dose is guided by serum theophylline level. Therapeutic level is 10–20 µg/mL. Absorption varies with brand. Formulations are also available for administration every 24 hours.
Aminophylline	Intravenous	Loading dose is 5.6 mg/kg over 30 minutes for a person not using oral theophylline; maintenance dose is 0.7 mg/kg/h by constant infusion pump—lower if patient has liver disease or heart failure or is receiving erythromycin or cimetidine.	$1.00/10 mL of 25 mg/mL	Seldom indicated. Calculate dose from lean body mass. Monitor serum theophylline level.

(continued)

Table 9–5. Selected drugs for obstructive airway diseases.[1] (continued)

Drug	Important Formulations	Usual Adult Dosage (Stable Patient)	Cost[2]	Comments
CORTICOSTEROIDS				
Beclomethasone dipropionate (Beclovent, Vanceril)	Metered-dose inhaler (42 µg/puff; 200 puffs/inhaler)	2 puffs 4 times daily, or 4 puffs twice daily	$34.00/17 g	Rinse mouth with water after use to prevent oral candidiasis; use 30 seconds after inhaled sympathomimetic to control cough and airway irritation. Spacer devices also helpful to prevent oral candidiasis.
Triamcinolone acetonide (Azmacort)	Metered-dose inhaler with spacer (100 µg/puff; 240 puffs/inhaler)	2 puffs 4 times daily, or 4 puffs twice daily	$47.35/20 g	Cough and wheezing after inhalation are reported to be less than after inhalation of beclomethasone.
Flunisolide (AeroBid)	Metered-dose inhaler (250 µg/puff; 100 puffs/inhaler)	2–4 puffs twice daily	$56.80/7 g	Dosing frequency of twice daily offers an advantage.
Fluticasone propionate (Flovent)	Metered-dose inhaler 44 µg/puff; 60 or 120 puffs/inhaler 110 µg/puff; 120 puffs/inhaler 220 µg/puff; 120 puffs/inhaler	2 puffs (88 µg) twice daily up to 880 µg twice daily maximum	44 µg: $43.40/13 g 110 µg: $50.20/13 g 220 µg: $72.00/13 g	No effect on hypothalamic-pituitary-adrenal axis in lower dosage range.
Prednisone (several brands)	Tablets (2.5, 5, 10, 20, and 50 mg)	Acute bronchospasm: 40–60 mg (1 mg/kg) every 24 hours Chronic bronchospasm: 5–40 mg daily to every other day	0.04/5 mg	Discontinue after 14 days if possible.
Methylprednisolone sodium succinate (several brands)	Intravenous injection (vials of 40, 125, 500, 1000, and 2000 mg)	0.5–1 mg/kg every 6 hours	$17.00 for 80 mg/5 mL	Clinical response may be delayed for several hours.
Hydrocortisone sodium succinate (several brands)	Intravenous injection (100, 250, 500, and 1000 mg)	4 mg/kg every 6 hours	$9.50/250 mg	Clinical response may be delayed for several hours.
Fluticasone (Flovent)	Metered-dose inhaler, 55 µg and 220 µg/puff; 120 inhalations/unit	2 puffs twice daily	$43.40/44 µg $50.20/110 µg $75.70/220 µg	High potency, low bioavailability. Adrenal axis suppression possible with > 880 µg/d. May be useful in discontinuing oral maintenance corticosteroids.
ANTIMEDIATORS				
Cromolyn sodium (Intal)	Metered-dose inhaler (800 µg/puff; 200 puffs/14.2 g canister)	2–4 puffs 4 times daily	$66.00/14 g	Clinical response may require 2–4 weeks of treatment. Useful only for prophylaxis; younger patients with asthma are more likely to benefit. To prevent bronchospasm, cromolyn may be used 15–30 minutes before exercise or exposure to cold air or allergens.
	Nebulized solution (20 mg/2 mL ampule)	20 mg 4 times daily by powered nebulizer	$0.80/2 mL	
Nedocromil sodium (Tilade)	Metered-dose inhaler (1.75 mg/puff; 112 puffs/inhaler)	2 puffs 4 times daily	$29.00/16 g	Maintenance therapy for asthma.

(continued)

Table 9–5. Selected drugs for obstructive airway diseases.[1] (continued)

Drug	Important Formulations	Usual Adult Dosage (Stable Patient)	Cost[2]	Comments
ANTILEUKOTRIENES				
Zafirlukast (Accolate)	Tablet (20 mg)	One tablet twice daily	$52.50/30 days	Leukotriene receptor antagonist. For use in adults and children over age 12 as maintenance therapy for chronic asthma. Not advised for acute asthma.
Zileuton (Zyflo)	Tablet (600 mg)	One tablet 4 times daily	$75.00/30 days	A 5-lipoxygenase inhibitor. For use in adults and children over age 12 as maintenance therapy for chronic asthma. Not advised for acute asthma.

[1]Only drugs available in the United States are listed.
[2]Cost to pharmacist (average wholesale price) for unit dose indicated. Source: First Data Bank, Price Alert, April 1997.
[3]Preferential effect is on β_2-adrenergic receptors.
[4]More frequent dosing for acute or severe episodes of bronchoconstriction is acceptable.

activity, (3) exacerbations lasting several days, and (4) requirement for occasional emergency care. These patients typically display baseline PEFR or FEV_1 values 60–80% (of predicted value or personal best), with variability of 20–30% when symptomatic and greater than 30% during the worst exacerbations. Management of these patients consists of daily maintenance therapy with inhaled corticosteroids (200–500 μg daily in two to four divided doses), cromolyn, or nedocromil. A short-acting, inhaled β_2 agonist drug may be used if needed up to three to four times daily for breakthrough symptoms. If symptoms persist, inhaled corticosteroids should be given at a higher dose (800–1000 μg daily), or another agent should be added to the regimen. These additional agents are the oral sustained-release theophylline, an oral β_2 agonist, and the long-acting inhaled β_2 agonist, salmeterol. Any of these three long-acting agents may be tried to control symptoms of nocturnal asthma. An inhaled anticholinergic agent such as ipratropium bromide may be added to the regimen if necessary. Zafirlukast (a leukotriene receptor antagonist) and zileuton (a 5-lipoxygenase inhibitor) are now available for the treatment of moderate asthma induced by allergens, exercise, and aspirin in adults and children over the age of 12 years. These agents are indicated for oral maintenance therapy of chronic asthma, not for treatment of acute asthma. Because these drugs are new, their place in clinical practice guidelines for asthma therapy has not yet been defined. Inhaled corticosteroids are still the drugs of choice for maintenance therapy.

3. Severe asthma–Adult patients with severe asthma are those with one or more of the following: (1) continuous symptoms, (2) frequent exacerbations, (3) limitation of physical activities, (4) frequent nocturnal symptoms, and (5) requirement for occasional emergency care. These patients typically display baseline PEFR or FEV_1 less than 60% (of predicted value or personal best), with variability of 20–30% with routine medication and over 50% during severe exacerbations. Management of severe asthma consists of (1) daily maintenance therapy with inhaled corticosteroids (800–1000 μg daily in two to four divided doses) and (2) daily oral sustained-release theophylline or oral β_2 agonist, or a long-acting inhaled β_2 agonist such as salmeterol. The long-acting agents are especially useful if symptoms of nocturnal asthma are bothersome. An inhaled anticholinergic such as ipratropium bromide may be added to the regimen if necessary. A short-acting, inhaled β_2 agonist drug may be used in severe asthma for breakthrough symptoms as needed up to three to four times daily, but this approach should not be considered as maintenance therapy. If symptoms persist, oral corticosteroids are added with a daily or alternate-day regimen. Management by a specialist is advised for patients with moderately severe or severe asthma.

a. Inhaled sympathomimetics–β_2-Selective agonists are the sympathomimetic agents of choice for relief of bronchospasm. Short-acting β_2 agonists (albuterol, metaproterenol, bitolterol, terbutaline, pirbuterol) are used for control of asthma symptoms, not for maintenance therapy. One or two inhalations are usually sufficient. For severe asthma, up to four inhalations of any of these agents, administered as often as every 3 hours, may be required temporarily. Some patients may benefit from even more than four puffs. Sequential inhalations, separated by at least 1 minute, may enhance the bronchodilator effect. Excessive patient use of inhaled beta-sympathomimetic agents—arbitrarily defined as the use of more than three metered-dose inhalers monthly—should alert both the patient and the physician to the need for more careful evaluation and institution of alternative therapy, particularly anti-inflammatory agents. There is concern that regular excessive use of inhaled sympathomimetics increases the mortality rate in asthma.

Salmeterol, the newest β_2-adrenergic agonist, has the longest duration of action of the inhaled bronchodilators. This agent, administered as two inhalations every 12 hours, is indicated for maintenance therapy of asthma to prevent bronchospasm, *not for relief of acute symptoms of asthma*. Physicians must be certain that their patients understand this important point. Salmeterol has a slower onset of action than short-acting inhaled β_2 agonists. Salmeterol may be particularly useful to control symptoms of nocturnal asthma and asthma triggered by prolonged exercise.

The metered-dose inhaler (MDI) is the preferred means of delivery of sympathomimetic and corticosteroid aerosol drugs. Unfortunately, a metered-dose inhaler may cost the patient as much as $30–$50. Various extension devices ("spacers") may be attached to the inhaler to facilitate use and enhance aerosol deposition in the lung. Unfortunately, MDIs are used incorrectly by at least half of patients, and many physicians are uncertain about the proper technique. Optimal use of these devices requires one actuation (puff) just after beginning a slow, deep breath from functional residual capacity, followed by a 10-second breath-hold to allow deposition of the aerosol in the periphery of the lung. Inspiration should take about 5 seconds. Maximal inspiration to total lung capacity is not required. Careful patient instruction in MDI use and reinforcement of training on follow-up office visits are essential. Physically or mentally handicapped patients may be unable to use MDIs. A breath-activated metered-dose inhaler that overcomes some of these limitations of conventional inhalers is available for delivery of pirbuterol.

Compressed air or oxygen may be used to nebulize certain sympathomimetic drug solutions and cromolyn solution. Jet nebulizers are expensive and inconvenient and have not been demonstrated to be more effective than metered-dose inhalers. Their use should be reserved for patients who are unable to use the metered dose inhaler effectively. Liquid solutions of different medications (eg, a sympathomimetic drug and cromolyn) may be mixed together in the nebulizer unit.

Beta$_2$-agonist drugs should be given orally only in cases of moderate to severe asthma when delivery by inhaler is not feasible or when control of nocturnal asthma symptoms with sustained-release preparations is the therapeutic goal.

b. Corticosteroids–Corticosteroids are effective in asthma because they suppress both acute and chronic airway inflammation. Their complex actions include attenuation of the release of and response to mediators of inflammation. These drugs may also potentiate the action of β_2-adrenergic agents.

Inhaled corticosteroids are now considered first-line maintenance therapy for the majority of patients with moderate asthma and all patients with severe asthma, except those who require high daily doses of oral corticosteroids. They are best started when patients are stable or adequately controlled with other antiasthma medications. Choices include beclomethasone, beginning with two inhalations (84 µg) two to four times daily and progressing, if necessary, to six inhalations four times daily; flunisolide, beginning with two inhalations (500 µg) every 12 hours and progressing to four inhalations every 12 hours; fluticasone, beginning with two inhalations (88 µg) twice daily and progressing to four inhalations (44, 110, or 220 µg per inhalation) twice daily; or triamcinolone, beginning with two inhalations (200 µg) four times daily and progressing to six inhalations four times daily. Corticosteroid aerosols may irritate the airway and stimulate transient cough and wheezing. If this occurs, prescribe these drugs 20 minutes after inhalation of a β_2 agonist. Use of spacer devices for inhalation and mouth rinsing after dosing help prevent oral candidiasis. Too rapid transfer from chronic systemic to inhaled corticosteroids may precipitate adrenal insufficiency.

Oral corticosteroid therapy is effective adjunctive therapy for ambulatory adult patients with moderately severe or severe asthma. Failure to employ oral corticosteroids when indicated may result in substantial morbidity and even death. Prednisone, 40–60 mg/d as a single dose or in divided dose, is given orally for 7 days, followed by a tapering dose over the next 1–2 weeks. Studies have cast doubt on the need to taper the prednisone dose after a burst of 7 days of therapy, but tapering is still considered the standard of care. Early treatment of severe asthma attacks with adequate doses of oral corticosteroids usually relieves symptoms and prevents hospitalization. Chronic maintenance therapy with systemic corticosteroids is unfortunately sometimes necessary and is associated with many adverse effects. Repeated efforts should be made to eliminate daily oral corticosteroids or reduce the dose to the minimal amount necessary to control symptoms. Alternate-day treatment is preferred to daily treatment for corticosteroid-dependent patients to reduce adverse effects, but control of asthma may be difficult. Some patients will experience repeated severe exacerbations of asthma if corticosteroids are tapered too quickly. Inhaled corticosteroids are helpful for many such patients and may eliminate the need for oral corticosteroids or permit a substantial reduction in their dosage.

c. Cromolyn sodium and nedocromil sodium–Inhaled cromolyn sodium and nedocromil sodium are important anti-inflammatory drugs used in preventive maintenance of mild to moderate asthma. Both agents inhibit inflammatory cells in the airway and block both the early and the late asthmatic responses to inhaled antigens. These agents have no direct bronchodilating activity, so they are not effective in relieving acute symptoms of asthma. Both cromolyn and nedocromil are capable of preventing bronchoconstriction induced by exercise or cold air. In management of chronic asthma, neither of these agents has been shown to be superior to inhaled corticosteroids. Either agent is administered by metered-dose inhaler, two inhalations four times daily or 10–15 minutes before exercise. Twice-daily dosing may eventually be adequate. Toxicity is minimal. A nebulizer solution of cromolyn sodium (20 mg/2 mL) is available (Table 9–5).

d. Anticholinergics–Ipratropium bromide antagonizes acetylcholine and prevents increases in intracellular levels of cyclic guanosine monophosphate, a substance that promotes contraction of bronchial smooth muscle. Ipratropium is the bronchodilator drug of choice in patients with COPD, but it is inferior to β_2-adrenergic agonists in the management of asthma. There is no evidence that it adds anything to traditional therapy with inhaled corticosteroids and beta-agonists. A limited clinical trial of ipratropium may be appropriate in patients whose asthma symptoms are poorly controlled despite maximal conventional therapy. The dose of ipratropium is two to four inhalations by metered-dose inhaler every 6 hours. Systemic toxicity is minimal.

e. Oral theophylline–Oral theophyllines are now considered third- or fourth-line agents for this purpose in both children and adults. The mechanism of action of theophylline in producing bronchodilation is unknown. Airway smooth muscle cell adenosine receptor antagonism is the most popular of several proposed mechanisms. Most experts would save theophylline therapy for patients with moderate or severe asthma whose symptoms, especially nocturnal symptoms, persist despite use of an inhaled corticosteroid and a β_2 agonist. Long-acting oral theophylline preparations allow infrequent dosing. The usual starting dose for adults is 400–1000 mg/d in two divided doses given 12 hours apart. Sustained-release preparations intended for dosing once daily are available, the starting dose being 400 mg. Serum theophylline levels should be measured 3–5 days after therapy is started and 4–5 hours after administration of a sustained-release formulation. Therapeutic levels of theophylline are 10–15 µg/mL; concentrations above 20 µg/mL are often associated with gastrointestinal, cardiac, and central nervous system side effects. Theophylline toxicity is common and may be fatal (see Chapter 39). Therapeutic benefits may be seen with levels between 5 and 10 µg/mL. Drug interactions with theophylline are common. Decreases in theophylline clearance accompany the use of cimetidine, erythromycin, and other macrolide antibiotics, quinolone antibiotics, and oral contraceptives. Increases in theophylline clearance are caused by rifampin, phenytoin, barbiturates, and also by cigarette smoking.

f. Antimicrobial drugs–The routine use of antibiotic therapy for acute or chronic asthma is not warranted. In a few cases, bacterial tracheobronchitis may occur simultaneously with an attack of asthma or may follow an attack. Amoxicillin or amoxicillin-potassium clavulanate (500 mg orally every 8 hours for 7–10 days), tetracycline (250–500 mg four times daily by mouth for 7–10 days), and trimethoprim-sulfamethoxazole (160/800 mg orally every 12 hours for 7–10 days) are reasonable choices for empirical therapy.

g. Hyposensitization–Immunotherapy is indicated for selected patients with asthma who fail to respond to environmental control measures and other forms of conventional therapy and who have documented specific reactivity to allergens that have consistently induced asthma attacks. Single-allergen immunotherapy improves symptoms, reduces medication requirements, and alleviates bronchial hyperreactivity but has no beneficial effect on lung function. Overall, only a few adult patients with bronchial asthma are likely to benefit from hyposensitization.

h. Avoiding drugs that worsen symptoms–Beta-blocking drugs may worsen bronchospasm and should be avoided in patients with asthma. Even ophthalmic beta-blocker preparations can cause severe bronchospasm. Angiotensin converting enzyme inhibitors may aggravate cough in patients with bronchial hyperresponsiveness.

B. Emergency Room and Hospitalized Patients With Acute, Severe Asthma: Patients with acute, severe asthma presenting to the emergency room are often exhausted, irritable, and apprehensive. Dehydration and toxic effects resulting from overuse of medications are common. Objective measurement of airflow is important in patients with acute asthma because the intensity of wheezing on auscultation is an unreliable indicator of the extent of airflow limitation; however, in severe cases, patients may be unable to cooperate. The PEFR, the preferred index of airflow in an emergency setting, is measured initially to provide a baseline and at successive intervals during treatment. A PEFR under 100 L/min indicates very severe airway obstruction.

All patients with acute, severe asthma should receive supplemental oxygen, 1–3 L/min by nasal cannula. Monitoring with oximetry is desirable. An inhaled β_2-agonist drug such as metaproterenol (0.3 mL of 5% solution) or albuterol (0.5 mL of 0.5% solution) diluted in 2.5 mL of sterile 0.9% saline, should be given at once, using a powered nebulizer. A metered-dose inhaler is satisfactory if the patient is able to inspire deeply. Up to three nebulizer treatments may be given over 60–90 minutes, using PEFR as a guide. Intravenous aminophylline is not recommended for emergency room management of asthma. Subcutaneous terbutaline (up to three doses of 0.25 mg each over 60–90 minutes) is an alternative form of sympathomimetic therapy, indicated only in young or middle-aged patients unable to use aerosolized drugs.

Corticosteroids are administered intravenously if the patient has very severe acute asthma or fails to respond to sympathomimetic therapy. Hydrocortisone (4 mg/kg) or methylprednisolone (1–2 mg/kg) is given initially and every 6 hours thereafter. A lag period of 4–6 hours before improvement occurs is common. Larger doses have no proved benefit. Although early emergency room treatment with intravenous corticosteroids has not demonstrated benefit in all asthma outcome studies, most physicians readily administer intravenous steroids to emergency room patients with acute, severe asthma. It is not yet clear whether oral therapy is an acceptable alternative to intravenous therapy. Inhaled corticosteroids have no proved role in acute, severe asthma and may worsen bronchospasm. Inhaled cromolyn is also not useful in severe acute asthma. The role of inhalation of nebulized ipratropium bromide aerosol in acute severe asthma is controversial.

The patient should be admitted to the hospital if any of the following are noted: failure to demonstrate objective signs of improvement such as a persistently low PEFR or FEV_1 (< 40% of predicted value) despite vigorous therapy in the emergency room, respiratory acidosis, electrocardiographic abnormalities (supraventricular arrhythmias, including multifocal atrial tachycardia, conduction disturbances, ventricular ectopy), pneumothorax or pneumomediastinum, respiratory fatigue, suspected airway infection, and a history of status asthmaticus or previous intubation for acute respiratory failure.

Status asthmaticus is severe, prolonged asthma refractory to conventional modes of therapy. All patients with status asthmaticus should be managed in the hospital, preferably in an intermediate or intensive care unit. Management consists of close monitoring and specific treatment strategies. Symptoms, vital signs, physical findings, expiratory flow (PEFR or FEV_1), and gas exchange (arterial blood gas or oximetry) should be assessed closely. Treatment consists of supplemental oxygen (to keep oxygen saturation above 90%), systemic corticosteroids (eg, intravenous methylprednisolone, 60 mg every 6 hours), inhaled β_2 agonists as often as every 2 hours until improvement occurs, and intravenous aminophylline (or oral theophylline) to achieve a therapeutic serum concentration of theophylline. Antibiotics are given only if there is purulent sputum or other evidence of infection. Ipratropium bromide nebulizer solution (0.5 mg in 2.5 mL of 0.9% saline, one unit dose three or four times daily) may be added empirically to the above regimen. Chest physical therapy, overhydration, and mucolytic therapy are not indicated in status asthmaticus. Sedation should be avoided unless the patient requires intubation.

Most patients with status asthmaticus improve with this regimen; however, some develop progressive respiratory acidemia and require tracheal intubation and mechanical ventilation. The decision to intubate is based on the general appearance of the patient (fatigue, respiratory distress, apprehension), not on any single laboratory finding. Status asthmaticus not controlled after intubation and mechanical ventilation requires highly aggressive therapy, eg, sedation with a benzodiazepine, general anesthesia with a bronchodilating anesthetic agent, such as halothane, or segmental bronchial lavage to remove plugs of mucus. Fortunately, these extreme measures are rarely necessary.

Prognosis

The outlook for patients with bronchial asthma is excellent despite the small recent increase in the death rate. Attention to general health measures and use of pharmacologic agents permit control of symptoms in nearly all cases. The outlook is better for patients with extrinsic asthma who develop asthma early in life. A rigorous medical regimen may reduce hospitalization rates for patients with frequent exacerbations of asthma.

Abramson MJ, Puy RM, Weiner JM: Is allergen immunotherapy effective in asthma? A meta-analysis of randomized controlled trials. Am J Respir Crit Care Med 1995;151:969. (Selected patients with extrinsic asthma are most likely to benefit.)

Barnes PJ: Inhaled glucocorticoids for asthma. N Engl J Med 1995;332:868. (Mechanisms, pharmacokinetics, efficacy, and side effects.)

Bone RC: Goals in asthma management: A step-care approach. Chest 1996;109:1056. (Treatment based on severity of illness.)

Chan-Yeung M: Assessment of asthma in the workplace. ACCP consensus statement. American College of Chest Physicians. Chest 1995;108:1084. (State-of-the-art report on the evaluation and management of patients with occupational asthma.)

Corbridge TC, Hall JB: The assessment and management of adults with status asthmaticus. Am J Respir Crit Care Med 1995;151:1296. (Diagnostic studies, drug therapy, and mechanical ventilation.)

Drugs for asthma. Med Lett Drugs Ther 1995;37:1.

Goldstein RA et al: Asthma. Ann Intern Med 1994;121:698. (Immunopathogenesis and rationale for therapy.)

Holgate ST, Bradding P, Sampson AP: Leukotriene antagonists and synthesis inhibitors: New directions in asthma therapy. J Allergy Clin Immunol 1996;98:1. (The role of zafirlukast and zileuton in asthma management.)

National Asthma Education and Prevention Program: Expert Panel Report II (EPR-II): Guidelines for the diagnosis and management of asthma. National Heart, Lung, and Blood Institute, National Institutes of Health, Bethesda, MD, February, 1997. Draft. (Update of the 1991 clinical practice guidelines.)

National Asthma Education and Prevention Program, National Heart, Blood, and Lung Institute: National asthma education and prevention program task force on the cost effectiveness, quality of care, and financing of asthma care. Am J Respir Crit Care Med 1996;154:S81. (Economics and quality issues inherent in the management of asthma.)

Nelson HS: β-Adrenergic bronchodilators. N Engl J Med 1995;333:499. (Review of the pharmacology, adverse effects, and role of the six β_2-adrenergic drugs available in the United States.)

Weinberger M, Hendeles L: Theophylline in asthma. N Engl J Med 1996;334:1380. (Pharmacology, use, safety, and role.)

CHRONIC OBSTRUCTIVE PULMONARY DISEASE (COPD)

Essentials of Diagnosis

- History of cigarette smoking (most cases).
- Chronic cough and sputum production (in chronic bronchitis) and dyspnea (in emphysema).
- Rhonchi, decreased intensity of breath sounds, and prolonged expiration on physical examination.
- Airflow limitation on pulmonary function testing (most cases).

General Considerations

Chronic obstructive pulmonary disease (COPD) is defined as a disease state characterized by the presence of airflow obstruction due to chronic bronchitis or emphysema; the airflow obstruction is generally progressive, may be accompanied by airway hyperreactivity, and may be partially reversible (American Thoracic Society). Although emphysema and chronic bronchitis must be diagnosed and treated as specific diseases, most patients with COPD have features of both conditions. About 14 million Americans are affected. Grouped together, COPD and asthma now represent the fourth leading cause of death in the United States, with over 90,000 deaths reported annually. The death rate from COPD is increasing rapidly, especially among elderly men.

Chronic bronchitis is characterized by excessive secretion of bronchial mucus and is manifested by productive cough for 3 months or more in at least 2 consecutive years in the absence of any other disease that might account for this symptom. **Emphysema** denotes abnormal, permanent enlargement of air spaces distal to the terminal bronchiole, with destruction of their walls and without obvious fibrosis (American Thoracic Society). It is worthwhile to note that chronic bronchitis is defined in clinical terms, whereas emphysema is defined in morphologic terms. Cigarette smoking is clearly the most important cause of COPD, even though only 10–15% of smokers develop COPD. Air pollution, airway infection, familial factors, and allergy have also been implicated in chronic bronchitis, and hereditary factors (deficiency of α_1-antiprotease) have been implicated in emphysema. The pathogenesis of emphy-sema may be excessive lysis of elastin and other structural proteins in the lung matrix by elastase and other proteases derived from lung neutrophils, macrophages, and mononuclear cells. Atopy and the tendency for bronchoconstriction to develop in response to nonspecific airway stimuli may be important risks for COPD.

Clinical Findings

A. Symptoms and Signs: The clinical, roentgenographic, and laboratory findings in chronic bronchitis and emphysema are summarized in Table 9–6.

Patients with COPD characteristically present in the fifth or sixth decade of life complaining of excessive cough, sputum production, and shortness of breath that have often been present for 10 years or more. Productive cough usually occurs in the morning. Dyspnea is noted initially only on extreme exertion, but as the condition progresses, it becomes more severe and occurs with mild activity. In severe disease, dyspnea occurs at rest. Frequent exacerbations of illness are common and result in absence from work and eventual disability. Pneumonia, pulmonary hypertension, cor pulmonale, and chronic respiratory failure characterize the late stage of COPD. Death usually occurs during an exacerbation of illness in association with acute respiratory failure. Hemoptysis occurs occasionally.

Clinical findings may be completely absent early in the course of COPD. Diminished breath sounds and prolonged expiration may be detectable during exacerbations of the disease. The physical findings presented in Table 9–6 become apparent as the disease progresses.

B. Laboratory Findings: Secondary polycythemia may be found in advanced COPD as a result of hypoxemia. During exacerbations of illness, examination of the sputum may reveal *Streptococcus pneumoniae, Haemophilus influenzae,* or *Moraxella catarrhalis,* though these may be present in the carrier state between episodes of deterioration. The ECG may show sinus tachycardia, and in advanced disease, chronic pulmonary hypertension may produce electrocardiographic abnormalities typical of cor pulmonale. Supraventricular arrhythmias (multifocal atrial tachycardia, atrial flutter, and atrial fibrillation) and ventricular irritability also occur.

Arterial blood gas measurements characteristically show no abnormalities early in COPD; indeed, they are unnecessary unless hypoxia or hypercapnia is suspected. Hypoxemia occurs in advanced disease, particularly when chronic bronchitis predominates. Compensated respiratory acidosis occurs in patients with chronic respiratory failure, particularly in chronic bronchitis, with worsening of acidemia during acute exacerbations. (See Chapter 21.)

Spirometry provides objective information about pulmonary function and assesses the results of ther-

Table 9–6. Emphysema versus chronic bronchitis: Clinical, roentgenographic, and laboratory findings.[1]

	Emphysema	Chronic Bronchitis
History		
Onset of symptoms	After age 50.	After age 35.
Dyspnea	Progressive, constant, severe.	Intermittent, mild to moderate.
Cough	Absent or mild.	Persistent, severe.
Sputum production	Absent or mild.	Copious.
Sputum appearance	Clear, mucoid.	Mucopurulent or purulent.
Other features	Weight loss.[2]	Airway infections, right heart failure, obesity.
Physical examination		
Body habitus	Thin, wasted.[2]	Stocky, obese.
Central cyanosis	Absent.	Present.[2]
Plethora	Absent.	Present.
Accessory respiratory muscles	Hypertrophied.	Unremarkable.
Anteroposterior chest diameter	Increased.	Normal.
Percussion note	Hyperresonant.	Normal.
Auscultation	Diminished breath sounds.	Wheezes, rhonchi.
Chest x-ray		
Bullae, blebs	Present.	Absent.
Overall appearance	Decreased markings in periphery.	Increased markings ("dirty lungs").
Hyperinflation	Present.	Absent.
Heart size	Normal or small, vertical.	Large, horizontal.
Hemidiaphragms	Low, flat.	Normal, rounded.
Laboratory studies		
Hemotocrit	Normal.	Increased.
ECG	Normal.	Right axis deviation, right ventricular hypertrophy, "P" pulmonale.[2]
Hypoxemia	Absent, mild.	Moderate, severe.
Hypercapnia	Absent.	Moderate, severe.
Respiratory acidosis	Absent.	Present.
Total lung capacity	Increased.	Normal.
Static lung compliance	Increased.	Normal.
Diffusing capacity	Decreased.	Normal.

[1]As noted in the text, most patients with COPD have features of both emphysema and chronic bronchitis.
[2]In advanced disease.

apy. Pulmonary function tests early in the course of COPD reveal only evidence of dysfunction in small airways (abnormal closing volume, reduced midexpiratory flow rate). Reductions in FEV_1 and in the ratio of forced expiratory volume to forced vital capacity (FEV_1:FVC) occur later. In severe disease, the forced vital capacity is markedly reduced. Lung volume measurements reveal an increase in the total lung capacity (TLC), a marked increase in the residual volume (RV), and an elevation of the RV:TLC ratio, indicative of air trapping, particularly in emphysema.

C. Imaging: When emphysema is the main clinical feature, hyperinflation is apparent. Parenchymal bullae or subpleural blebs are pathognomonic of emphysema. Radiographs of patients with chronic bronchitis may show only nonspecific peribronchial and perivascular markings. Pulmonary hypertension becomes evident as enlargement of central pulmonary arteries in advanced disease. Doppler echocardiography is an effective way to estimate pulmonary artery pressure if pulmonary hypertension is suspected.

Differential Diagnosis

It is important to distinguish COPD from a variety of other pulmonary conditions. COPD cannot be diagnosed simply because of a history of heavy cigarette smoking and that the sole finding of obstructive pulmonary dysfunction on spirometry does not establish a diagnosis of COPD.

Clinical, roentgenographic, and laboratory findings should enable the clinician to distinguish COPD from other obstructive pulmonary disorders such as bronchial asthma, bronchiectasis, cystic fibrosis, bronchopulmonary aspergillosis, and central airway obstruction. Bronchiectasis is distinguished from COPD by features such as recurrent pneumonia and hemoptysis, digital clubbing, and radiographic abnormalities. Patients with severe α_1-antiprotease deficiency are recognized by the appearance of panacinar emphysema early in life, usually in the third or fourth decade, and hepatic cirrhosis and hepatocellular carcinoma may occur. Cystic fibrosis occurs in children and younger adults. Rarely, mechanical obstruction of the central airways simulates COPD. Flow-volume loops may help separate patients with central airway obstruction from those with diffuse intrathoracic airway obstruction characteristic of COPD.

Complications

Acute bronchitis, pneumonia, pulmonary embolization, and concomitant left ventricular failure may worsen otherwise stable COPD. Pulmonary hypertension, cor pulmonale, and chronic respiratory failure are common in advanced COPD. Spontaneous pneumothorax occurs in a small fraction of patients with emphysema. Hemoptysis may result from chronic bronchitis or may signal bronchogenic carcinoma.

Prevention

COPD is largely preventable. Many believe that early recognition of small airways dysfunction in patients who smoke, combined with appropriate treatment and cessation of smoking, may prevent relentless progression of the disease. A large multicenter randomized study has demonstrated that smoking cessation slows the decline in FEV_1 in middle-aged smokers with mild airways obstruction. Early treatment of airway infections and vaccination against influenza and pneumococcal disease may also be of benefit but have no effect on the progression of the disease.

Treatment

Management strategies in COPD include discontinuance of cigarette smoking, education of the patient about his or her disease, relief of bronchospasm, aerosol therapy, chest physiotherapy, treatment of complications such as airway infections and heart failure, use of supplemental oxygen, and other measures designed to promote rehabilitation. Standards for the management of patients with COPD have recently been published by the American Thoracic Society. See Chapter 38 for a discussion of air travel in patients with lung disease.

A. Ambulatory Patients: A trial of bronchodilator drugs is warranted in all patients with symptomatic COPD. Inhaled ipratropium bromide or sympathomimetic drugs are the mainstay of this therapy. The response to bronchodilator therapy is assessed with spirometry. Patients with asthmatic bronchitis and those with partially reversible airflow obstruction, frequent acute exacerbations of disease, or wheezing may benefit the most from bronchodilator therapy. The routine use of maintenance bronchodilator drugs in all patients with COPD is controversial. These drugs probably have little value in patients with pure emphysema. If a clinical trial of bronchodilators over several months demonstrates no objective (spirometric) or symptomatic improvement, they may be discontinued; however, this is not often the case.

Ipratropium bromide is superior to sympathomimetic aerosols in achieving bronchodilation in patients with moderate to severe COPD. Ipratropium has a slower onset but a longer duration of action than sympathomimetic agents in stable COPD. In combination with other bronchodilators, it enhances and prolongs bronchodilation. Side effects are minimal, and effects on sputum production and viscosity are negligible. Ipratropium bromide has been shown to confer only a small improvement in FEV_1 in middle-aged smokers with mild airways obstruction, and this benefit is lost when the drug is discontinued. Two to four inhalations (18 μg each) every 6 hours is recommended. Ipratropium bromide may also be administered as an inhalation solution (0.02%) by nebulizer. One unit dose vial (500 μg in 2.5 mL of 0.9% saline) is given every 6–8 hours.

Maintenance therapy with oral theophylline in ambulatory patients with COPD is controversial. Although theophylline has value as a bronchodilator in COPD patients with partial reversibility of airflow limitation, its principal value in COPD may relate to improving respiratory muscle performance. Improvements in dyspnea, exercise performance, and pulmonary function have been reported in some studies but not in others. Sustained-release theophylline improves oxyhemoglobin saturation during sleep in patients with COPD. Oral theophylline is a third-line agent in COPD—behind ipratropium and sympathomimetic agents—and is used in those patients who fail to respond to inhaled bronchodilators or those with sleep-related respiratory disturbances. Once-daily theophylline dosing, preferably at 8 PM, is advocated by some authorities. Patients with moderate or severe COPD often are treated with combinations of ipratropium, β_2 agonists, and theophylline. One study of ambulatory patients with COPD reported that the combination of ipratropium bromide and albuterol given by metered-dose inhaler to ambulatory patients with COPD is slightly more effective in improving FEV_1 than either agent alone, but it is not superior in improving symptoms.

Oral corticosteroids are prescribed in the same fashion as in asthma. Candidates for a trial of oral corticosteroid therapy include patients with asthmatic bronchitis and those with frequent exacerbations or disabling symptoms who fail to respond to conventional therapy with ipratropium bromide, sympathomimetics and theophylline. Corticosteroids should be discontinued after 2–4 weeks if there is no objective (spirometric) improvement. Inhaled corticosteroids may be of value for corticosteroid-responsive patients with chronic bronchitis or chronic asthmatic bronchitis, particularly those requiring less than 20 mg of prednisone (or equivalent) daily. Inhaled corticosteroids may permit discontinuance of systemic therapy. Cromolyn has no role in treatment of chronic bronchitis or emphysema; a trial in those with chronic asthmatic bronchitis may be warranted.

Other measures. Smoking cessation, avoiding airway irritants and allergens, controlling airway infection with broad-spectrum oral antimicrobials and preventing pulmonary aspiration may reduce the production of mucus. Nicotine transdermal patches are effective aids to smoking cessation for patients highly motivated to stop smoking (see Chapter 1). If airway infection is suspected, amoxicillin or amoxicillin-clavulanate (500 mg every 8 hours), ampicillin or tetracycline (250–500 mg four times daily), or trimethoprim-sulfamethoxazole (160/800 mg every 12 hours) may be given orally for 7–10 days. Although routine antibiotic therapy for exacerbations of COPD is controversial, COPD patients with increasing dyspnea and purulent sputum are particularly likely to benefit from antibiotics.

In patients with chronic bronchitis, increased mobilization of secretions may be accomplished through the use of adequate systemic hydration, effective cough training methods, and postural drainage, sometimes with chest percussion or vibration. One effective method of coughing up retained secretions is to have the patient lean forward and "huff" repeatedly, interspersed with relaxed breaths. Forceful paroxysms of cough should be discouraged. Inhalation of bland water aerosols is sometimes helpful. Postural drainage and chest percussion should be used only in selected patients with excessive amounts of retained secretions that cannot be cleared by coughing and other methods; these measures are of no benefit in pure emphysema. Expectorant-mucolytic therapy has generally been regarded as unhelpful in patients with chronic bronchitis. Cough suppressants and sedatives should be avoided as routine measures.

Graded aerobic physical exercise programs (eg, walking 20 minutes three times weekly, or bicycling) are helpful to prevent deterioration of physical condition and to improve the patient's ability to carry out daily activities. Pursed-lip breathing to slow the rate of breathing and abdominal breathing exercises to relieve fatigue of accessory muscles of respiration may reduce dyspnea in some patients. Training of inspiratory muscles by inspiring against progressively larger resistive loads improves exercise tolerance in some but not all patients.

Severe dyspnea in spite of optimal medical management may warrant a clinical trial of an opiate drug. Sedative-hypnotic drugs (eg, diazepam, 5 mg three times daily) are controversial in intractable dyspnea but may benefit very anxious patients. Intermittent negative-pressure (cuirass) ventilation and transnasal positive-pressure ventilation at home to rest the respiratory muscles are promising approaches to improve respiratory muscle function and reduce dyspnea in patients with severe COPD. A bilevel transnasal ventilation system has been reported to reduce dyspnea in ambulatory patients with severe COPD, but the long-term benefits of this approach and compliance with it have not been defined.

Home oxygen therapy is prescribed for selected patients with COPD or other severe lung diseases who have significant hypoxemia. Requirements for Medicare coverage for a patient's home use of oxygen and oxygen equipment are listed in Table 9–7. Arterial blood gas analysis is preferable to ear or pulse oximetry to guide initial oxygen therapy. Oxygen may be prescribed for continuous use, only at night, or with exercise. Hypoxemic patients with pulmonary hypertension, chronic cor pulmonale, erythrocytosis, impaired cognitive function, exercise intolerance, nocturnal restlessness, or morning headache are particularly likely to benefit from home oxygen therapy. Proved benefits of home oxygen therapy in advanced COPD include longer survival, reduced hospitalization needs, and better quality of

Table 9–7. Home oxygen therapy: Requirements for Medicare coverage.[1]

Group I (any of the following):

1. $Pao_2 \leq 55$ mm Hg or $Sao_2 \leq 88\%$ taken at rest breathing room air, while awake.

2. During sleep (prescription for nocturnal oxygen use only):

   a. $Pao_2 \leq 55$ mm Hg or $Sao_2 \leq 88\%$ for a patient whose awake, resting, room air Pao_2 is ≥ 56 mm Hg or $SaO_2 \geq 89\%$,

or

   b. Decrease in $Pao_2 > 10$ mm Hg or decrease in $Sao_2 > 5\%$ associated with symptoms or signs reasonably attributed to hypoxemia (eg, impaired cognitive processes, nocturnal restlessness, insomnia).

3. During exercise (prescription for oxygen use only during exercise):

   a. $Pao_2 \leq 55$ mm Hg or $Sao_2 \leq 88\%$ taken during exercise for a patient whose awake, resting, room air Pao_2 is ≥ 56 mm Hg or $Sao_2 \geq 89\%$.

and

   b. There is evidence that the use of supplemental oxygen during exercise improves the hypoxemia that was demonstrated during exercise while breathing room air.

Group II:[2]

$Pao_2 = 56–59$ mm Hg or $Sao_2 = 89\%$ if there is evidence of any of the following:

1. Dependent edema suggesting congestive heart failure.
2. P pulmonale on ECG (P wave > 3 mm in standard leads II, III, or aVF).
3. Hematocrit > 56%.

[1]Health Care Financing Administration, 1989.
[2]Patients in this group must have a second oxygen test 3 months after the initial oxygen set-up.

life. Survival in hypoxemic patients with COPD treated with supplemental oxygen therapy is directly proportionate to the number of hours per day oxygen is administered. In such patients who are treated with continuous oxygen, the survival after 36 months is about 65%—significantly better than the survival rate of about 45% in those who are treated with only nocturnal oxygen.

Home oxygen may be supplied by liquid oxygen systems (LOX), compressed gas cylinders, or oxygen concentrators. Most patients benefit from having both stationary and portable systems. Oxygen by nasal prongs must be given at least 15 hours a day unless therapy is intended only for exercise or sleep. For most patients, a flow rate of 1–3 L/min achieves a Pao_2 greater than 55 mm Hg. The monthly cost of home oxygen therapy ranges from $300.00 to $500.00 or more, being higher for liquid oxygen systems. Medicare covers approximately 80% of home oxygen expenses. **Transtracheal oxygen** is an alternative method of delivery. Reservoir nasal cannulas or "pendants" and demand (pulse) oxygen delivery systems are also available to conserve oxygen.

The term **"COPD rehabilitation"** has been applied to multidisciplinary, individually tailored outpatient treatment programs designed to restore optimal physiologic and psychologic function in debilitated patients with advanced COPD. Benefits include improved quality of life, greater ability to perform activities of daily living, less need for hospitalization, and reduced affective distress.

Human α_1-proteinase inhibitor is available for replacement therapy of emphysema due to congenital deficiency of α_1-antiproteinase. Patients over 18 years of age with obstructive lung dysfunction and α_1-antiproteinase levels less than 11 μmol/L are potential candidates for replacement therapy. Human α_1-proteinase inhibitor is administered intravenously in a dose of 60 mg/kg body weight once weekly; long-term efficacy of this new agent is unknown.

B. Hospitalized Patients: Hospitalization is indicated for acute worsening of COPD that fails to respond to measures for ambulatory patients. Patients with acute respiratory failure or complications such as cor pulmonale and pneumothorax should also be hospitalized.

Management of the hospitalized patient with an **acute exacerbation of COPD** includes supplemental oxygen, ipratropium bromide, and inhaled sympathomimetics as well as broad-spectrum antibiotics, corticosteroids, and, in selected cases, chest physiotherapy. Oxygen therapy should not be withheld for fear of worsening respiratory acidemia; hypoxemia is more detrimental than hypercapnia. Cor pulmonale usually responds to measures that reduce pulmonary artery pressure, such as supplemental oxygen and correction of acidemia; bed rest, salt restriction, and diuretics may add some benefit. Cardiac arrhythmias, particularly multifocal atrial tachycardia, usually respond to aggressive treatment of COPD itself. atrial flutter may require DC cardioversion after initiation of the above therapy. If progressive respiratory failure ensues, tracheal intubation and mechanical ventilation are necessary. Inspiratory positive-pressure assistance with a face mask is reported as a noninvasive alternative to conventional mechanical ventilation in COPD patients hospitalized for acute respiratory failure.

C. Surgery for COPD:

1. Lung transplantation—Experience with both single and bilateral sequential lung transplantation for severe COPD is accumulating rapidly. Requirements for lung transplantation are severe lung disease, limited activities of daily living, exhaustion of medical therapy, ambulatory status, potential for pulmonary rehabilitation, limited life expectancy without transplantation, adequate function of other organ systems, and a good social support system. Average total charges for lung transplantation through the end of the first postoperative year approximate $300,000. Substantial improvements in pulmonary function and exercise performance have been noted after transplantation. The two-year survival rate after lung transplantation for COPD is 75%. Complications include rejection, opportunistic infection, and obliterative bronchiolitis.

2. Volume reduction surgery (reduction pneumoplasty)—This is a new experimental surgical approach to relief of dyspnea and improvement in exercise tolerance in patients with advanced diffuse emphysema and lung hyperinflation. Bilateral resection of 20–30% of lung volume in these patients may yield modest improvements in pulmonary function, exercise performance, and dyspnea. The optimal technique for volume reduction surgery has not been determined. Both laser and stapling methods are being investigated. Prolonged air leaks occur in up to one-half of patients postoperatively. Mortality rates in centers with the largest experience with volume reduction surgery range from 4% to 10%. The National Heart, Lung and Blood Institute and the Health Care Financing Administration have designated 18 centers in the country as study sites for a clinical trial of lung volume reduction surgery. Candidates for this procedure should be referred to these institutions.

3. Bullectomy—is an older surgical procedure for palliation of severe dyspnea in patients with severe bullous emphysema. In this procedure, the surgeon removes a very large emphysematous bulla that demonstrates no ventilation or perfusion on lung scanning and compresses adjacent lung that has preserved function. Bullectomy can now be performed with a CO_2 laser (**"laser bullectomy"**) via thoracoscopy.

Prognosis

The outlook for patients with clinically significant COPD is poor. The median survival time of patients with severe COPD ($FEV_1 \leq 1$ L) is about 4 years. The degree of pulmonary dysfunction (as measured by FEV_1) at the time the patient is first seen is probably the most important predictor of survival. Comprehensive care programs and cessation of smoking apparently reduce the rate of decline of pulmonary function, but therapy with bronchodilators and other approaches probably has little, if any, impact on the natural course of COPD. Survival time varies widely and cannot be easily predicted. The prognosis is better in the chronic asthmatic form of COPD (chronic asthmatic bronchitis) than in the emphysematous form.

American Thoracic Society: Standards for the diagnosis and care of patients with chronic obstructive pulmonary disease. Am J Respir Crit Care Med 1995;152(Suppl): S77. (A comprehensive consensus statement including definitions, epidemiology, pathophysiology, diagnosis, staging, outpatient and inpatient management, and other considerations.)

Anthonisen NR et al: Effects of smoking intervention and the use of an inhaled anticholinergic bronchodilator on the rate of decline of FEV_1. The Lung Health Study. JAMA 1994;272:1497. (Smoking cessation slows the decline in lung function over time in middle-aged smokers with mild airway obstruction; ipratropium bromide inhaler does not provide any additional long-term benefit.)

Combivent Inhalation Aerosol Study Group: In chronic obstructive pulmonary disease, a combination of ipratropium and albuterol is more effective than either agent alone. An 85-day multicenter trial. Chest 1994;105: 1411. (Slight superiority in FEV_1 with the combination but no improvement in symptoms.)

Weinmann GG, Hyatt R: Evaluation and research in lung volume reduction surgery. Am J Respir Crit Care Med 1996;154:1913. (Concise summary of current thinking in volume reduction surgery.)

CYSTIC FIBROSIS

Essentials of Diagnosis

- Chronic obstructive pulmonary disease in childhood and early adulthood.
- Positive family history of cystic fibrosis.
- Sweat chloride concentration above 80 meq/L in adults (> 60 meq/L under age 20) on two occasions.
- Pancreatic insufficiency, especially in children.
- Chronic *Pseudomonas aeruginosa* or *Staphylococcus aureus* bronchitis and bronchiectasis with recurrent exacerbations.

General Considerations

Cystic fibrosis is a generalized autosomal recessive disorder of the exocrine glands. About one in 2500 Caucasians is affected, and one in 25 is a carrier of the cystic fibrosis gene (transmembrane conductance regulator). Deletion of a single phenylalanine residue from a 1480-amino-acid protein coded by the cystic fibrosis transmembrane conductance regulator *(CFTR)* gene, resulting from a mutation of the long arm of chromosome 7 (band q31), accounts for the large majority (about 70%) of cases of cystic fibrosis. Mutations in the *CFTR* gene result in alterations in chloride transport and water flux across the apical surface of epithelial cells. Almost all exocrine glands are affected by secretion of an abnormal mucus that obstructs glands and ducts in various organs. Obstruction results in dilation of the secretory glands and eventual damage to exocrine tissue. In the respiratory tract, inadequate hydration of the tracheobronchial epithelium impairs mucociliary function. High concentrations of DNA in airway secretions also render the sputum thick and viscous. Pulmonary manifestations, which occur in all patients who survive infancy, include acute and chronic bronchitis, bronchiectasis, pneumonia, atelectasis, and peribronchial and parenchymal scarring. Pneumothorax and mild hemoptysis are common. Cor pulmonale

occurs in advanced cases and signifies a poor prognosis.

Cystic fibrosis is the most common fatal hereditary disorder of Caucasians in the USA and is the most common cause of chronic lung disease in children and young adults. About half of children with cystic fibrosis live beyond age 20. About one-third of the nearly 30,000 cystic fibrosis patients in the USA are adults. Cystic fibrosis may be occult and may present with a variety of pulmonary and nonpulmonary manifestations in the adult.

Patients with cystic fibrosis-like lung disease who do not have diagnostic sweat chloride levels are occasionally seen. A mutation in the cystic fibrosis transmembrane conductance regulator gene has been identified in these patients.

Clinical Findings

A. Symptoms and Signs: The diagnosis should be suspected in a young adult presenting with a history of chronic lung disease (especially bronchiectasis), pancreatitis, or infertility. Cough, exercise intolerance, and recurrent pneumonia are typical. Steatorrhea is common. Digital clubbing, increased anteroposterior chest diameter, hyperresonance to percussion, and basilar crackles are noted on physical examination. Nasal polyps occur in as many as 15% of patients with cystic fibrosis. Biliary cirrhosis and gallstones may occur. Nearly all men with cystic fibrosis have congenital bilateral absence of the vas deferens with azoospermia. Patients with cystic fibrosis have an increased risk of malignancies of the gastrointestinal tract.

B. Laboratory Findings: Arterial blood gas studies reveal hypoxemia. Pulmonary function studies show reduction in forced vital capacity, airflow rates, and total lung capacity. Air trapping (high ratio of residual volume to total lung capacity) and reduction in pulmonary diffusing capacity are common. A mixed obstructive and restrictive pattern of dysfunction characterizes advanced disease.

C. Imaging: Hyperinflation is seen early in the disease process. Peribronchial cuffing, mucus plugging, bronchiectasis (ring shadows and cysts), increased interstitial markings, small rounded peripheral opacities, and focal atelectasis may be seen separately or in various combinations. Thin-section CT scanning may confirm the presence of bronchiectasis.

D. Special Examinations: The pilocarpine iontophoresis "sweat test" reveals elevated sodium and chloride levels (> 60 meq/L) in the sweat of patients with cystic fibrosis. Values higher than 80 meq/L are diagnostic in adults. Two separate tests on consecutive days are required for accurate diagnosis. A normal sweat chloride test does not exclude the diagnosis. Genotyping or other alternative diagnostic studies should be pursued if the test is repeatedly negative but there is a high clinical suspicion of cystic fibrosis.

Treatment

Early recognition and comprehensive, multidisciplinary therapy lengthen survival time and ameliorate symptoms. Referral to one of the regional ambulatory care Cystic Fibrosis Centers with diagnostic and therapeutic expertise in cystic fibrosis is strongly recommended. Treatment of the psychosocial aspects is of paramount importance in young people; genetic and occupational counseling is also critical. Antibiotics are used to treat active airway infections based on results of culture and susceptibility testing of sputum. *S aureus* (including methicillin-resistant strains) and a mucoid variant of *P aeruginosa* are commonly present. *Haemophilus influenzae* and *Burkholderia cepacia*—the latter a highly drug-resistant organism—are occasionally isolated. *Stenotrophomonas maltophilia* is occasionally identified as a cause of chronic airway infection in patients with cystic fibrosis. The use of aerosolized antibiotics (gentamicin and others) for prophylaxis or treatment of lower respiratory tract infections in patients with cystic fibrosis is sometimes helpful. Although some studies demonstrate reduced exacerbations in patients chronically infected with *P aeruginosa,* there is concern about the emergence of drug-resistant organisms, equipment contamination with *B cepacia,* and side effects such as bronchospasm.

Inhaled bland aerosols, chest physiotherapy, and inhaled bronchodilators are used to promote clearance of inspissated airway secretions. Useful chest physiotherapy methods include daily postural drainage and percussion by a caregiver, self-performed postural drainage, positive expiratory pressure (PEP) mask therapy, and other breathing techniques. Cough suppressants should be avoided. Chronic use of mucolytic agents such as acetylcysteine is of no proved benefit and is potentially harmful. Vaccination against pneumococcal infection and annual influenza vaccination are advised. Children with cystic fibrosis who were treated with alternate-day prednisone (2 mg/kg for 4 years) demonstrated improved height, weight, and pulmonary function and reduced hospitalization needs compared to controls in one study.

Care of the adult patient with cystic fibrosis requires a comprehensive approach, including providing adequate nutrition and vitamin supplementation, treatment of glucose intolerance and diabetes mellitus, and management of pancreatic and hepatobiliary disease. Screening of members of the family of a cystic fibrosis patient by DNA analysis may detect the cystic fibrosis gene in 70–75% of carriers.

Lung transplantation is currently the only definitive treatment for cystic fibrosis. Experience with double-lung and heart-lung transplantation is accumulating rapidly, and early results suggest a greatly improved quality of life in survivors. The 3-year survival rate following transplantation is about 57%. The high initial cost of lung transplantation ($150,000–$225,000) and the high frequency of obliterative bronchiolitis in survivors (30–50% within 3–5 years after transplantation) make transplantation for cystic fibrosis debatable.

Recombinant human deoxyribonuclease (rhDNase, or dornase alfa) cleaves the extracellular DNA from neutrophils in sputum, rendering it less viscous and easier to clear. This drug is given by aerosol in a dose of 2.5 mg once or twice daily. The annual cost to the pharmacist exceeds $12,000. Dornase alfa is indicated only for daily maintenance treatment of patients with cystic fibrosis as a supplement to standard therapy. The drug is limited to patients over the age of 5 years and those with FVC values greater than 40% of predicted. Treatment with dornase alfa results in reduced frequency of respiratory tract infections, reduced need for parenteral antibiotics, and shorter hospitalizations. Pharyngitis, laryngitis, and voice alterations are common adverse effects. Gene therapy to transfer the cystic fibrosis transmembrane conductance regulator gene to the airway epithelium with both viral and nonviral vectors is under investigation.

Prognosis

The longevity of patients with cystic fibrosis is increasing, and the median survival age is now 29 years. Few patients survive beyond 35 years. Death occurs from pulmonary complications, eg, pneumonia, pneumothorax, or hemoptysis, or as a result of terminal chronic respiratory failure and cor pulmonale.

Aerosolized deoxyribonuclease for cystic fibrosis. Med Lett Drugs Ther 1994;36:34. (Update on this new therapy for cystic fibrosis.)

Crystal RG (editor): Cystic fibrosis: From the gene to the cure. Am J Respir Crit Care Med 1995;151(3 Part 2):S45.

Davis PB, Drumm M, Konstan MW: Cystic fibrosis. Am J Respir Crit Care Med 1996;154:1229. (Comprehensive review.)

Ramsey BW: Management of pulmonary disease in patients with cystic fibrosis. N Engl J Med 1996;335:179. (Current treatment of children and adults with cystic fibrosis.)

Stern RC: The diagnosis of cystic fibrosis. N Engl J Med 1997;336:487. (Review of sweat testing, genotyping, and other tests.)

UPPER AIRWAY OBSTRUCTION

Acute upper airway obstruction may cause life-threatening asphyxia and must be relieved promptly. Acute upper airway obstruction due to foreign body aspiration is discussed below. Other causes of acute upper airway obstruction include laryngospasm, trauma to the larynx and pharynx, laryngeal edema from airway burns, acute angioedema, and various inflammatory conditions (Ludwig's angina, peritonsillar and retropharyngeal abscess, acute epiglottitis, and acute allergic laryngitis).

Chronic obstruction of the upper airway may be caused by carcinoma of the pharynx or larynx, laryngeal or subglottic stenosis, laryngeal granulomas or webs, or bilateral vocal cord paralysis. Laryngeal or subglottic stenosis may become evident weeks or months following a period of translaryngeal endotracheal intubation. Inspiratory stridor, intercostal retractions on inspiration, and a palpable inspiratory thrill over the throat are characteristic findings. Flow-volume curves may reveal evidence of fixed airway obstruction or variable extrathoracic obstruction. Plain films (soft tissue views of the neck) may demonstrate supra- and infraglottic narrowing, and CT scanning and MRI may be useful to image lesions in the pharynx and larynx. Fiberoptic endoscopy is helpful in diagnosis of upper airway obstruction, but caution is necessary because this procedure may exacerbate upper airway edema, leading to critical airway narrowing.

Occasionally, a functional disorder of the larynx may mimic bronchial asthma. This condition may be distinguished from true asthma by the finding of variable extrathoracic airway obstruction on the flow-volume loop, a normal alveolar-arterial oxygen tension gradient, laryngoscopic evidence of adduction of the vocal cords on both inspiration and expiration, and lack of response to bronchodilator therapy. Pulmonary function testing is normal immediately after the attack resolves. Treatment consists of speech therapy and psychotherapy. Bronchodilator drugs are of no benefit.

Aboussouan LS, Stoller JK: Diagnosis and management of upper airway obstruction. Clin Chest Med 1994;15:35. (Thorough review of the pathophysiology, differential diagnosis, and management of upper airway obstruction.)

LOWER AIRWAY OBSTRUCTION

Tracheal obstruction may be intrathoracic (below the suprasternal notch) or extrathoracic. Fixed tracheal obstruction may be caused by acquired or congenital tracheal stenosis, primary and secondary tracheal neoplasms, compression by extrinsic diseases (tumors of the lung, thymus, or thyroid; lymphadenopathy; congenital vascular rings; aneurysms, etc), foreign body aspiration, tracheal granulomas and papillomas, and tracheal trauma.

Acquired **tracheal stenosis** is usually secondary to tracheostomy or endotracheal intubation. Dyspnea, cough, and inability to clear pulmonary secretions

occur weeks to months after tracheal decannulation or extubation. Physical findings may be absent until tracheal diameter is reduced 50% or more, when wheezing, a palpable tracheal thrill, and harsh breath sounds may be detected. Stridor implies severe stenosis. The diagnosis is usually confirmed by plain films, CT of the trachea when plain films are not adequate, and characteristic findings of the fixed airway obstruction on the flow-volume loop. Complications include recurring pulmonary infection and life-threatening respiratory failure. Management is directed toward ensuring adequate ventilation and oxygenation and avoiding manipulative procedures that may increase edema of the tracheal mucosa. Surgical reconstruction or laser photoresection is required in severe cases.

Bronchial obstruction is caused by retained pulmonary secretions, aspiration, primary lung cancer, compression by extrinsic masses, and (rarely) tumors metastatic to the airway. Clinical and radiographic findings vary depending on the location of the obstruction and the degree of airway narrowing. Symptoms include dyspnea, cough, wheezing, and if infection is present, fever and chills. A history of recurrent pneumonia in the same lobe or segment or slow resolution (> 3 months) of pneumonia on successive x-rays suggests the possibility of bronchial obstruction and the need for bronchoscopy. Complete obstruction of a main stem bronchus may be obvious on physical examination (asymmetric chest expansion, mediastinal shift, absence of breath sounds on the affected side, and dullness to percussion), but partial obstruction is often difficult or impossible to detect. Prolonged expiration and localized wheezing may be the only clues. Alterations of the flow-volume loop may be helpful in diagnosis. Segmental or subsegmental bronchial obstruction may produce no abnormalities on physical examination.

Roentgenographic findings range from **atelectasis** (lung collapse) to air trapping. The latter may be caused by unidirectional expiratory obstruction. Expiratory films may be particularly useful to show air trapping. CT scanning may demonstrate the nature and the exact location of obstruction of the central bronchi. MRI may be superior to CT for delineating the extent of the underlying disease in the hilum, but it is usually reserved for cases in which CT findings are equivocal. Bronchoscopy is the definitive diagnostic study, particularly if tumor or foreign body aspiration is suspected. The finding of tubular breath sounds on physical examination or an air bronchogram on chest x-ray in an area of atelectasis rules out complete airway obstruction. Bronchoscopy is unlikely to be of therapeutic benefit in this situation.

Right middle lobe syndrome is recurrent or persistent atelectasis of the right middle lobe, probably related to inadequate collateral ventilation. Fiberoptic bronchoscopy or CT scan is often necessary to rule out obstructing tumor or foreign body.

ALLERGIC BRONCHOPULMONARY ASPERGILLOSIS

Allergic bronchopulmonary aspergillosis is a pulmonary hypersensitivity disorder that is being recognized with increasing frequency in the USA. It is caused by allergy to antigens of *Aspergillus* species that colonize the tracheobronchial tree and usually occurs in atopic asthmatic individuals who are 20–40 years of age. Primary criteria for the diagnosis of allergic bronchopulmonary aspergillosis include a clinical history of asthma, peripheral eosinophilia, immediate skin reactivity to *Aspergillus* antigen, precipitating antibodies to *Aspergillus* antigen, elevated serum IgE levels, pulmonary infiltrates (transient or fixed), and central bronchiectasis. If the first six of these seven primary criteria are present, the diagnosis is almost certain. Secondary diagnostic criteria include identification of *Aspergillus* in sputum, a history of brown-flecked sputum, and late skin reactivity to *Aspergillus* antigen. Corticosteroids are the treatment of choice, and the response is usually excellent. Bronchodilators (Table 9–5) are also helpful. Complications include hemoptysis, severe bronchiectasis, and pulmonary fibrosis.

Burnie JP: Allergic and invasive aspergillosis. J R Soc Med 1995;25(Suppl):41.

BRONCHIECTASIS

Bronchiectasis is a congenital or acquired disorder of the large bronchi characterized by permanent, abnormal dilation and destruction of bronchial walls. It may be caused by recurrent inflammation or infection of the airways. Cystic fibrosis causes about half of all cases of bronchiectasis. Other causes include lung infection (tuberculosis, fungal infections, lung abscess, pneumonia), abnormal lung defense mechanisms (humoral immunodeficiency, α_1-antiprotease deficiency with cigarette smoking, mucociliary clearance disorders, rheumatic diseases), and localized airway obstruction (foreign body, tumor, mucoid impaction). Immunodeficiency states that may lead to bronchiectasis include congenital or acquired panhypogammaglobulinemia; common variable immunodeficiency; selective IgA, IgM, and IgG subclass deficiencies; and acquired immunodeficiency from cytotoxic therapy, AIDS, lymphoma, multiple myeloma, leukemia, and chronic renal and hepatic diseases. However, most patients with bronchiectasis have panhypergammaglobulinemia, presumably reflecting an immune system response to chronic airway infection. Acquired primary bronchiectasis is now uncommon in the USA because of improved control of bronchopulmonary infections.

Symptoms of bronchiectasis include chronic cough, production of copious amounts of purulent sputum, hemoptysis, and recurrent pneumonia. Weight loss, anemia, and other systemic manifestations are common. Physical findings are nonspecific, but persistent crackles at the lung bases are common. Clubbing is infrequent. Copious, foul-smelling, purulent sputum that separates into three layers in a cup is characteristic. Obstructive pulmonary dysfunction with hypoxemia is seen in moderate or severe disease. Roentgenographic abnormalities include crowded bronchial markings related to peribronchial fibrosis and small cystic spaces at the base of the lungs. Thin-section (1.5 mm) CT scanning may detect moderate to severe cases.

Treatment consists of antibiotics (selected on the basis of sputum smears and cultures), daily chest physiotherapy with postural drainage and chest percussion, and inhaled bronchodilators. Empiric oral antibiotic therapy for 10–14 days with amoxicillin or amoxicillin-clavulanate (500 mg every 8 hours), ampicillin or tetracycline (250–500 mg four times daily), or trimethoprim-sulfamethoxazole (160/800 mg every 12 hours) is reasonable therapy in an acute exacerbation if a specific bacterial pathogen cannot be isolated. Alternating cycles of two or three of these antibiotics, given orally for 2–4 weeks, is sometimes employed in stable bronchiectasis patients with copious, purulent sputum. The role of aerosolized antibiotics has not been established, except in cystic fibrosis. Bronchoscopy is sometimes necessary to evaluate hemoptysis, remove retained secretions and rule out obstructing airway lesions. Surgical resection is reserved for a few patients with localized bronchiectasis and adequate pulmonary function who fail to respond to conservative management. Surgery is also indicated for massive hemoptysis. Complications of bronchiectasis include cor pulmonale, amyloidosis, and secondary visceral abscesses at distant sites, eg, brain.

Marwah OS, Sharma OP: Bronchiectasis: How to identify, treat, and prevent. Postgrad Med 1995;97:149. (Review of diagnostic methods, management, and the role of surgery.)

Nicotra MB: Bronchiectasis. Semin Respir Infect 1994;9:31. (A thorough review with 55 references.)

Smith IE, Flower CD: Review article: Imaging in bronchiectasis. Br J Radiol 1996;69:589. (Value of high-resolution computed tomography in diagnosis.)

BRONCHIOLITIS OBLITERANS

Bronchiolitis is an acute, common, often severe respiratory illness of children under 2 years of age caused by respiratory syncytial virus, other viruses (occasionally), and *Mycoplasma pneumoniae*. An acute infectious bronchiolitis has not been recognized as a distinct entity in adults. However, bronchiolitis obliterans does occur. Once classified as a type of chronic interstitial pneumonia, bronchiolitis obliterans has been reclassified. Five clinical types have been described: (1) toxic fume bronchiolitis obliterans, (2) postinfectious bronchiolitis obliterans, (3) bronchiolitis obliterans associated with connective tissue disease and organ transplantation, (4) bronchiolitis obliterans associated with localized lung lesions, and (5) idiopathic bronchiolitis obliterans with organizing pneumonia.

Bronchiolitis obliterans in adults is probably underrecognized. Cough, dyspnea, crackles on chest auscultation, and obstructive pulmonary dysfunction are characteristic.

Toxic fume bronchiolitis obliterans follows 1–3 weeks after exposure to oxides of nitrogen, phosgene, and other noxious gases. The chest x-ray shows diffuse nonspecific alveolar or "ground-glass" densities.

Postinfectious bronchiolitis obliterans is a late response to mycoplasmal or viral lung infection in adults and has a highly variable radiographic appearance.

Bronchiolitis obliterans may occur in association with rheumatoid arthritis, polymyositis, and dermatomyositis. Penicillamine therapy has been implicated as a possible cause of bronchiolitis obliterans in patients with rheumatoid arthritis. Bronchiolitis obliterans is a common complication of heart-lung transplantation and a rare complication of allogeneic bone marrow transplantation, the latter occurring in the setting of chronic graft-versus-host disease.

Idiopathic bronchiolitis obliterans with organizing pneumonia (BOOP) affects men and women equally. Most patients are between the ages of 50 and 70. Dry cough, dyspnea, and a flu-like illness, ranging in duration from a few days to several months, are typical. Fever and weight loss are common. Physical examination demonstrates crackles in most patients, and wheezing is present in about a third. Clubbing is uncommon. Pulmonary function studies demonstrate restrictive dysfunction and hypoxemia. The chest x-ray typically shows patchy, bilateral, ground glass or alveolar infiltrates. Solitary pneumonia-like infiltrates and a diffuse interstitial pattern have also recently been described.

BOOP is usually a difficult diagnosis to make on clinical grounds alone. The presence of fever and weight loss, abrupt onset of symptoms (often with an upper respiratory tract infection), a relatively short duration of symptoms, the absence of clubbing, and the presence of alveolar infiltrates help the clinician distinguish this entity from idiopathic pulmonary fibrosis. However, open lung biopsy may be necessary. Buds of loose connective tissue and inflammatory cells fill alveoli and distal bronchioles. Corticosteroid therapy is effective in two-thirds of cases, often abruptly. Relapses are common if corticosteroids are stopped prematurely, and most patients require at least 9–12 months of therapy. Prednisone is usually given initially in doses of 1 mg/kg/d for 2–3 months. The dose is then tapered slowly to 20–40 mg/d, depending on response, and eventually to an alternate-day regimen.

Respiratory bronchiolitis is a disorder of small airways in young cigarette smokers. Clinically and radiographically, this disorder resembles idiopathic pulmonary fibrosis. Cough, dyspnea, and crackles on chest auscultation are typical. However, the reduction in lung compliance seen in idiopathic pulmonary fibrosis is not found in this disorder. The condition may be recognized only on open lung biopsy, which demonstrates characteristic metaplasia of terminal and respiratory bronchioles and filling of respiratory and terminal bronchioles, alveolar ducts, and alveoli by pigmented alveolar macrophages.

Diffuse panbronchiolitis is an idiopathic disorder of respiratory bronchioles frequently diagnosed in Japan. The condition appears to be extremely rare in the United States. Men are affected about twice as often as women and are most often between ages 20 and 80. About two-thirds of patients are nonsmokers. The large majority have a history of chronic pansinusitis. Marked dyspnea, cough, and sputum production are cardinal features. Crackles and rhonchi are noted on physical examination. Pulmonary function tests reveal obstructive abnormalities. The chest x-ray shows a distinct pattern of diffuse small nodular shadows and hyperinflation. Open lung biopsy is necessary for diagnosis.

Costabel U, Guzman J, Teschler H: Bronchiolitis obliterans with organising pneumonia: Outcome. Thorax 1995;50:S59. (Review with 57 references.)

Epler GR: Bronchiolitis obliterans organizing pneumonia. Semin Respir Infect 1995;10:65. (Consider BOOP in a febrile patient with clinical features of pneumonia of several weeks' duration and negative cultures.)

Ezri T et al: Bronchiolitis obliterans: Current concepts. Q J Med 1994;87:1. (General review of bronchiolitis obliterans, including BOOP.)

King TE Jr: Bronchiolitis. Clin Chest Med 1993;14:607. (A compendium of articles reviewing different types of bronchiolitis.)

PLEUROPULMONARY INFECTIONS

PNEUMONIA

Pneumonia continues to be a major health problem despite the availability of potent antimicrobial drugs. Microorganisms gain access to the lower respiratory tract by aspiration of oropharyngeal secretions and associated bacterial flora, inhalation of infected aerosols, and hematogenous dissemination. Characteristics of pneumonia caused by specific agents and appropriate antimicrobial therapy are presented in Table 9–8.

Table 9–8. Characteristics and treatment of selected pneumonias.

Organism	Clinical Setting	Gram-Stained Smears of Sputum	Chest Radiograph[1]	Laboratory Studies	Complications	Antimicrobial Therapy[2]
Streptococcus pneumoniae (pneumococcus)	Chronic cardio-pulmonary disease; follows upper respiratory tract infection.	Gram-positive diplococci.	Lobar consolidation.	Gram-stained smear of sputum; culture of blood, pleural fluid	Bacteremia, meningitis, endocarditis, pericarditis, empyema.	Preferred: Penicillin G (or V, oral). Alternative: An erythromycin, cephalosporin.
Haemophilus influenzae	Chronic cardio-pulmonary disease; follows upper respiratory tract infection.	Pleomorphic gram-negative coccobacilli.	Lobar consolidation.	Culture of sputum, blood, pleural fluid.	Empyema, endocarditis.	Preferred: Cefotaxime or ceftriaxone. Alternative: Cefuroxime.
Staphylococcus aureus	Influenza epidemics; nosocomial.	Plump gram-positive cocci in clumps.	Patchy infiltrates.	Culture of sputum, blood, pleural fluid.	Empyema, cavitation.	For non-penicillinase-producing strains: Preferred: Penicillin G (or V, oral). Alternative: A cephalosporin; vancomycin. For penicillinase-producing strains: Preferred: A penicillinase-resistant penicillin. Alternative: A cephalosporin; vancomycin. For methicillin-resistant strains: Preferred: Vancomycin.
Klebsiella pneumoniae	Alcohol abuse, diabetes mellitus; nosocomial.	Plump gram-negative encapsulated rods.	Lobar consolidation.	Culture of sputum, blood, pleural fluid.	Cavitation, empyema.	Preferred: Cefotaxime, ceftriaxone, ceftizoxime, or ceftazidime. For severe infections, a cephalosporin plus an aminoglycoside. Alternative: Ampicillin-sulbactam; imipenem-cilastatin; ticarcillin-clavulanic acid; amoxicillin-clavulanic acid; others.
Escherichia coli	Nosocomial; rarely, community-acquired.	Gram-negative rods.	Patchy infiltrates, pleural effusion.	Culture of sputum, blood, pleural fluid.	Empyema.	Same as for *Klebsiella pneumoniae*.
Pseudomonas aeruginosa	Nosocomial; cystic fibrosis.	Gram-negative rods.	Patchy infiltrates, cavitation.	Culture of sputum, blood.	Cavitation.	Preferred: An antipseudomonal penicillin plus an aminoglycoside. Alternative: Ceftazidime; ciprofloxacin; imipenem-cilastatin or aztreonam plus an aminoglycoside.

(*continued*)

Table 9–8. Characteristics and treatment of selected pneumonias. (continued)

Organism	Clinical Setting	Gram-Stained Smears of Sputum	Chest Radiograph[1]	Laboratory Studies	Complications	Antimicrobial Therapy[2]
Anaerobes	Aspiration, periodontitis.	Mixed flora.	Patchy infiltrates in dependent lung zones.	Culture of pleural fluid or of material obtained by transtracheal or transthoracic aspiration.	Necrotizing pneumonia, abscess, empyema.	Preferred: Penicillin G (for anaerobic streptococci); penicillin G or clindamycin (for oropharyngeral strains of *Bacteroides*), metronidazole (for gastrointestinal strains of *Bacteroides*). Alternative: Clindamycin or a cephalosporin (for anaerobic streptococci); metronidazole, cefoxitin, or ampicillin-sulbactam (for oropharyngeal strains of *Bacteroides*); clindamycin, imipenem-cilastatin, cefoxitin, ticarcillin-clavulanic acid, or others (for gastrointestinal strains of *Bacteroides*).
Mycoplasma pneumoniae	Young adults; summer and fall.	PMNs and monocytes; no bacterial pathogens.	Extensive patchy infiltrates.	Complement fixation titer.[3] Cold agglutinin serum titers are not helpful as they lack sensitivity and specificity.	Skin rashes, bullous myringitis; hemolytic anemia.	Preferred: An erythromycin. Alternative: Tetracycline or doxycycline; clarithromycin; azithromycin.
Legionella species	Summer and fall; exposure to contaminated construction site, water source, air conditioner; community-acquired or nosocomial.	Few PMNs; no bacteria.	Patchy or lobar consolidation.	Direct immunofluorescent examination of sputum or tissue; immunofluorescent antibody titer,[3] culture of sputum or tissue.[4]	Empyema, cavitation, endocarditis, pericarditis.	Preferred: Erythromycin, with or without rifampin. Alternative: Trimethoprim-sulfamethoxazole; azithromycin; clarithromycin; ciprofloxacin.
Chlamydia pneumoniae	Clinically similar to *M pneumoniae*, but prodromal symptoms last longer (up to 2 weeks). Sore throat with hoarseness common. Mild pneumonia in teenagers and young adults.	Nonspecific.	Subsegmental infiltrate, less prominent than in *M pneumoniae* pneumonia. Consolidation rare.	Isolation of the organism is very difficult. Serologic studies include microimmunofluorescence with TWAR antigen and a nonspecific complement fixation antibody test.	Reinfection in older adults with underlying COPD or heart failure may be severe or even fatal.	Preferred: A tetracycline. Alternative: Erythromycin, clarithromycin, or azithromycin.

(continued)

Table 9–8. Characteristics and treatment of selected pneumonias. (continued)

Organism	Clinical Setting	Gram-Stained Smears of Sputum	Chest Radiograph[1]	Laboratory Studies	Complications	Antimicrobial Therapy[2]
Moraxella catarrhalis	Preexisting lung disease; elderly; corticosteroid or immunosup-pressive therapy.	Gram-negative diplococci.	Patchy infil-trates; occa-sional lobar consolidation.	Gram stain and culture of sputum or bronchial aspirate.	Rarely, pleural effusions and bacteremia.	Preferred: Trimetho-prim-sulfamethoxa-zole. Alternative: Amoxicillin-clavulanic acid; an erythromycin; a tetracycline; cefurox-ime; cefotaxime.
Pneumocystis carinii	AIDS, immuno-suppressive or cytotoxic drug therapy, cancer.	Not helpful in diagnosis.	Diffuse inter-stitial and alveolar infil-trates; apical or upper lobe infiltrates in patients on aerosolized pentamidine.	Cysts contain-ing sporo-zoites of *P carinii* on methenamine silver or Giemsa stains of sputum or broncho-alveolar la-vage fluid.	Pneumo-thorax, respi-ratory failure, ARDS, death.	Preferred: Trimetho-prim-sulfamethoxa-zole or pentamidine isethionate plus prednisone. Alternative: Dapsone plus trimethoprim; clindamycin plus primaquine; tri-metrexate plus folinic acid.

[1]X-ray findings lack specificity. See text.
[2]Antimicrobial sensitivities should guide therapy when available. (Modified and reprinted, with permission, from The Medical Letter, Inc.: The choice of antibacterial drugs. Med Lett Drugs Ther 1996;38:25.)
[3]Fourfold rise in titer is diagnostic.
[4]Selective media are required.

Pneumonias are classified as being either community-acquired or hospital-acquired (nosocomial).

Approach to the Immunocompetent Patient With Possible Pneumonia

A chest radiograph is included in the initial evaluation of a patient with symptoms and signs suggestive of pneumonia. The pattern of the infiltrate is not pathognomonic of a specific cause of pneumonia.

Establishing a specific etiologic diagnosis of pneumonia is often difficult. In most cases of both community-acquired and hospital-acquired pneumonia, treatment is empiric. Gram stain of the sputum may be valuable in diagnosis if interpreted cautiously. It is of little value when numerous upper airway epithelial cells are present. The main value of sputum examination is to exclude the presence of certain microorganisms such as mycobacteria, fungi, *Legionella*, and *P carinii* with special smears and cultures. Sputum culture and sensitivity may be helpful in demonstrating the presence of bacteria resistant to particular antibiotics. Routine culturing of sputum for viral pathogens is not advised. A white blood count may help determine which patients should be admitted to the hospital, and the differential count is useful in assessing seriousness of infection and prognosis.

Sputum induction should be performed if sputum examination is considered important to exclude certain organisms as potential pathogens and if the patient cannot produce an adequate sputum specimen by spontaneous cough.

In examining expectorated sputum, one must discriminate between lower respiratory tract pathogens and organisms that colonize the pharynx. For example, the presence of gram-negative bacteria and fungi such as *Candida albicans* and *Aspergillus* species on a smear of expectorated sputum may represent pharyngeal colonization and not lower respiratory tract infection. The absence of a definitive bacterial organism on sputum Gram stain in a patient with pneumonia raises the possibility of lung infection by viruses, *Mycoplasma pneumoniae*, *Chlamydia*, *Legionella*, anaerobic organisms, and fungal or mycobacterial organisms. It is important to emphasize that *the diagnosis of pneumonia cannot be based solely on the results of culture of expectorated sputum.*

In patients appearing especially ill, blood cultures should also be obtained before antimicrobial therapy is started; when positive, the causative organism has been definitively identified.

Thoracentesis should be performed in suspected bacterial pneumonia if pleural effusion is present. Gram-stained smears and cultures of pleural fluid may reveal the causative organism. Pleural fluid with characteristics diagnostic of empyema (see Table 9–27) represents an indication for tube thoracostomy in most cases, depending upon the causative organism.

Antimicrobial therapy should be started after initial diagnostic studies have been performed. Empiric antibiotic therapy is initiated in most cases, because the clinical presentation and initial sputum Gram stain do not commonly indicate infection caused by a specific infectious agent.

1. COMMUNITY-ACQUIRED PNEUMONIA

Guidelines for Management

The American Thoracic Society (1993) has proposed guidelines for the initial treatment of adults with community-acquired pneumonia, based upon limited use of diagnostic tests, categorizing the patient based on four variables (severity of illness, age, comorbid conditions, and need for hospitalization), and the use of empiric broad-spectrum antibiotic therapy.

A. Outpatients Without Comorbidity and Age < 60 Years: The most common pathogens are *Streptococcus pneumoniae, Mycoplasma pneumoniae,* respiratory viruses, *Chlamydia pneumoniae, Haemophilus influenzae,* and miscellaneous organisms (*Legionella, Staphylococcus aureus, Mycobacterium tuberculosis,* endemic fungi, and aerobic gram-negative bacilli). Antibiotic treatment with a macrolide or a tetracycline is advised. Erythromycin (250–500 mg orally four times daily) is the treatment of choice in most cases. This drug is inexpensive, but gastrointestinal intolerance is common. The duration of treatment should probably be about 10–14 days, but firm data supporting this practice are lacking. The recommended duration of treatment for Legionnaires' disease is 14 days (21 days if the patient is immunocompromised).

If the patient is intolerant of erythromycin or if *H influenzae* infection is suspected (eg, in patients with risk factors such as COPD), one of the newer (and more expensive) macrolides, clarithromycin (250 mg orally every 12 hours for 7–14 days) or azithromycin (500 mg orally on the first day and 250 mg orally each day for the next 4 days), should be prescribed. Tetracycline (same dose as erythromycin) is an acceptable alternative for patients intolerant of or allergic to macrolides. Tetracycline and clarithromycin should not be prescribed for pregnant women.

B. Outpatients With Comorbidity or Age > 60 Years: The most common pathogens are *S pneumoniae,* respiratory viruses, *H influenzae,* aerobic gram-negative bacilli, *S aureus,* and miscellaneous organisms (*Legionella, Moraxella catarrhalis, M tuberculosis,* and endemic fungi). The recommended therapy is a second-generation cephalosporin (eg, cefuroxime axetil, 250 or 500 mg orally twice daily for 10 days), or trimethoprim-sulfamethoxazole (160/800 mg orally every 12 hours for 14 days), or a beta-lactam combined with a beta-lactamase inhibitor such as amoxicillin-potassium clavulanate (500 mg

orally every 8 hours for 10 days). A macrolide is advised if Legionnaires' disease is suspected.

C. Hospitalized Patients With Community-acquired Pneumonia: The most common pathogens are *S pneumoniae, H influenzae,* aerobic gram-negative bacilli, *Legionella, S aureus, C pneumoniae,* respiratory viruses, and miscellaneous organisms (*M pneumoniae, M catarrhalis, M tuberculosis,* and endemic fungi). The recommended therapy is a second-generation cephalosporin (such as cefuroxime sodium, 0.75–1.5 g intravenously every 8 hours for 5–10 days); or third-generation cephalosporin (such as ceftriaxone sodium 1–2 g intravenously every 12–24 hours, up to 4 g/d for 5–10 days), or a beta-lactam combined with beta-lactamase inhibitor such as amoxicillin-potassium clavulanate. A macrolide is advised if Legionnaires' disease is suspected.

D. Severely Ill Hospitalized Patients With Community-acquired Pneumonia: The most common pathogens are *S pneumoniae, Legionella,* aerobic gram-negative bacilli, *M pneumoniae,* respiratory viruses, and miscellaneous organisms (*H influenzae, M tuberculosis,* and endemic fungi). Combination therapy is advised with a macrolide plus either a third-generation cephalosporin (eg, ceftazidime sodium, 1–2 g intravenously every 8–12 hours, up to 6 g/d for 7–10 days) with activity against *Pseudomonas* or another antipseudomonal agent.

Criteria for Hospitalization

Many patients can be treated successfully as outpatients. General indications for hospitalization include age over 65, coexisting illnesses (such as alcoholism, diabetes mellitus, COPD), alteration in vital signs, leukopenia or marked leukocytosis, any evidence of respiratory failure, septic appearance, and absence of supportive care at home.

Clearing of lung infiltrates in patients with community-acquired pneumonia may take 6 weeks or longer. Clearance is faster in young patients, nonsmokers, and those with involvement of only one lobe. Radiographic progression of infiltrates in spite of antibiotic therapy is a very poor prognostic sign.

Prevention

Polyvalent pneumococcal vaccine (containing capsular polysaccharide antigens of 23 strains of *S pneumoniae*) has the potential to prevent or lessen the severity of 85–90% of pneumococcal infections in immunocompetent patients. Indications for pneumococcal vaccination include any chronic cardiopulmonary disease (see Chapter 30).

Bartlett JG, Mundy LM: Community-acquired pneumonia. N Engl J Med 1995;333:1618. (Diagnostic tests and treatment recommendations.)
The choice of antibacterial drugs. Med Lett Drugs Ther

1996;38:25. (First-choice and alternative drugs for most important human pathogens.)

Friedland IR, McCracken GH Jr: Management of infections caused by antibiotic-resistant *Streptococcus pneumoniae.* N Engl J Med 1994:331:377. (Increasing resistance of *Streptococcus pneumoniae* to various antibiotics requires the physician to know local patterns of susceptibility of individual strains.)

Mandell LA: Community-acquired pneumonia: Etiology, epidemiology, and treatment. Chest 1995;108(Suppl): 35S. (Reinforces and amplifies the 1993 American Thoracic Society statement.)

Meeker DP, Longworth DL: Community-acquired pneumonia: An update. Cleve Clin J Med 1996;63:16. (Current review of the common pathogens and selection of antibiotics.)

2. HOSPITAL-ACQUIRED PNEUMONIA

Essentials of Diagnosis

- Occurs more than 48 hours after admission to the hospital.
- One or more clinical findings (fever, cough, leukocytosis, purulent sputum) in most patients.
- Especially frequent in patients requiring intensive care and mechanical ventilation.
- Pulmonary infiltrate on chest x-ray.

General Considerations

Hospital-acquired (nosocomial) pneumonia, defined as pneumonia occurring more than 48 hours after admission to the hospital, is a major cause of morbidity and mortality in hospitalized patients, especially those requiring mechanical ventilation. Nosocomial pneumonia is the second most common cause of hospital-acquired infection and has a mortality rate of about 30%. ICU-acquired pneumonia and pneumonia in patients being mechanically ventilated (**"ventilator-associated pneumonia"**) have even higher mortality rates of about 48%. In patients with acute respiratory distress syndrome (ARDS), the mortality rate is 67%.

The most common organisms responsible for nosocomial pneumonia are *Pseudomonas aeruginosa, Staphylococcus aureus, Enterobacter, Klebsiella pneumoniae,* and *Escherichia coli. Proteus, Serratia,* coagulase-negative *S aureus, Streptococcus,* and *Citrobacter* account for most of the remaining cases. Infection by *P aeruginosa* and *Acinetobacter* tend to cause pneumonia in the most debilitated patients, those with previous antibiotic therapy, and those requiring mechanical ventilation. Anaerobic organisms *(Bacteroides,* anaerobic streptococci, *Fusobacterium)* may cause pneumonia in the hospitalized patient; when isolated, they are commonly part of a polymicrobial flora. Mycobacteria, fungi, chlamydiae, viruses, rickettsiae, and protozoal organisms are uncommon causes of nosocomial pneumonia.

Colonization of the pharynx and possibly the stomach with bacteria is the most important step in the pathogenesis of nosocomial pneumonia. Pharyngeal colonization is promoted by exogenous factors (instrumentation of the upper airway with nasogastric and tracheal tubes, contamination by dirty hands and equipment, and treatment with broad-spectrum antibiotic therapy that promotes the emergence of drug-resistant organisms) and patient factors (malnutrition, advanced age, altered consciousness, swallowing disorders, and underlying pulmonary and systemic diseases). Aspiration of infected pharyngeal or gastric secretions delivers bacteria directly to the lower airway, followed by the development of pneumonia in the affected segment or lobe. Impaired cellular and mechanical defense mechanisms in the lung raise the risk of lower respiratory infection after aspiration has occurred. Tracheal intubation increases the risk of lower respiratory infection by mechanical obstruction of the trachea, impairment of mucociliary clearance, trauma to the mucociliary escalator system, and interference with coughing. Tight binding of bacteria such as *Pseudomonas* to the tracheal epithelium makes clearance of these organisms from the lower airway difficult.

Less important pathogenetic mechanisms of nosocomial pneumonia include inhalation of contaminated aerosols and hematogenous dissemination of microorganisms.

Clinical Findings

A. Symptoms and Signs: Precise clinical diagnosis of nosocomial pneumonia is very difficult because of the absence of a standard diagnostic test. However, one or more clinical findings (fever, leukocytosis, purulent sputum, and a new pulmonary infiltrate on chest x-ray) are present in most patients.

B. Laboratory Findings: The minimum evaluation for suspected nosocomial pneumonia includes blood culture and chest x-ray. Blood counts and clinical chemistry tests are not helpful in establishing a specific diagnosis of nosocomial pneumonia. Thoracentesis for pleural fluid examination, including Gram stain and culture, should be performed in patients with pleural effusions.

Examination of expectorated sputum suffers the same disadvantages as in community-acquired pneumonia. Gram stains and cultures of sputum are neither sensitive nor specific in the diagnosis of bacterial nosocomial pneumonia. The identification of a bacterial organism by culture of expectorated or suctioned sputum does not prove that the organism is a lower respiratory tract pathogen. If nosocomial pneumonia from *Legionella pneumophila* is suspected, direct fluorescent antibody staining is performed. Sputum stains and cultures for mycobacteria and certain fungi may be diagnostic, but, as noted above, these are not common causes of nosocomial pneumonia.

Obtaining lower respiratory tract secretions to determine the cause of nosocomial pneumonia is difficult because of contamination of the upper airway by potential pathogens. At best, the cause of nosocomial pneumonia can be determined in only about half of cases.

C. Imaging: Pulmonary infiltrates are nonspecific and are seen in atelectasis, pulmonary edema, aspiration, pulmonary hemorrhage, pleural effusion, and pulmonary thromboembolism in addition to nosocomial pneumonia.

D. Special Examinations: Fiberoptic bronchoscopy has provided a number of techniques that may be helpful in evaluating patients with nosocomial pneumonia, particularly ventilator-associated pneumonia. These techniques use of the **protected specimen brush** and **bronchoalveolar lavage** with quantitative cultures using cutoff levels of 10^4 bacteria colony-forming units per milliliter, respectively. The sensitivity and specificity of these techniques range between 65% and 95% in the hands of experienced investigators. Prior antibiotic treatment reduces sensitivity and specificity to only 36–50%. Clearly, the best results are obtained in patients who have been off antibiotics for 48 hours, limiting the number of suitable candidates for these procedures. Further limitations of these approaches include the time and expense required for bronchoscopy and delays in obtaining the final culture and sensitivity reports. All studies of the diagnosis of hospital-acquired pneumonia suffer from the lack of a "gold standard" for its diagnosis; even those using postmortem tissue cultures and histopathology have some shortcomings.

Treatment

Treatment of nosocomial pneumonia, like treatment of community-acquired pneumonia, is usually empiric. Because of the high mortality rate of nosocomial pneumonia, therapy must be started as soon as pneumonia is suspected. Initial regimens must be broad in spectrum and tailored to the specific clinical setting. There is no uniform consensus on the best empiric antibiotic regimens for nosocomial pneumonia. Empiric therapy for mild to moderate nosocomial pneumonia outside the ICU may consist of one beta-lactam antibiotic such as a second-generation cephalosporin (such as cefuroxime sodium, 0.75–1.5 g intravenously every 8 hours), a nonantipseudomonal third-generation cephalosporin (such as ceftriaxone sodium, 1–2 g intravenously every 12–24 hours, up to 4 g/d), imipenem combined with cilastatin (250–500 mg intravenously every 6–8 hours), or ampicillin combined with sulbactam (1.5–3 g intravenously every 6 hours). Antibiotic choices are listed in Table 9–8.

Empiric therapy for patients with ICU- or ventilator-associated pneumonia should be a combination of antibiotics directed against the most virulent organisms, particularly *P aeruginosa, Acinetobacter,* and *Enterobacter.* The most common regimen is a broad-spectrum beta-lactam (an antipseudomonal penicillin, a third-generation antipseudomonal cephalosporin, or imipenem-cilastatin) plus an aminoglycoside. After results of sputum, blood, and pleural fluid cultures have been obtained, it may be possible to switch to a regimen with a narrower spectrum. Therapy for gram-negative bacillary pneumonia should continue for at least 14 days. In some cases, a fluoroquinolone to which the responsible organism is susceptible (such as ciprofloxacin, 500 or 750 mg orally every 12 hours) may be used to consolidate therapy.

Recommendations for the treatment of hospital-acquired pneumonia have recently been proposed by the American Thoracic Society (1995). Initial empiric therapy with antibiotics is determined by the severity of illness, risk factors, and the length of hospitalization.

American Thoracic Society: Hospital-acquired pneumonia in adults: Diagnosis, assessment of severity, initial antimicrobial therapy, and preventive strategies. Am J Respir Crit Care Med 1995;153:1711. (Consensus statement of experts, using an algorithmic approach to antibiotic therapy.)
The choice of antibacterial drugs. Med Lett Drugs Ther 1996;38:25. (First-choice and alternative drugs for most important human pathogens.)
Meduri GU: Diagnosis and differential diagnosis of ventilator-associated pneumonia. Clin Chest Med 1995;16:61. (Includes review of invasive diagnostic techniques.)
Wunderink RG, editor: Pneumonia in the intensive care unit. Clin Chest Med 1995;16:1. (A compendium of 14 articles.)

3. ANAEROBIC PNEUMONIA & LUNG ABSCESS

Essentials of Diagnosis

- Predisposition to aspiration.
- Fever, weight loss, malaise.
- Poor dental hygiene.
- Foul-smelling sputum (in many patients).
- Infiltrate in dependent lung zone, with single or multiple areas of cavitation or pleural effusion.

General Considerations

Aspiration of small amounts of oropharyngeal secretions occurs during sleep in normal individuals and rarely causes disease. Sequelae of aspiration of larger amounts of material include nocturnal asthma, bronchiectasis, chemical pneumonitis, mechanical obstruction of airways by particulate matter, and pleuropulmonary infection. Individuals predisposed to disease induced by aspiration include those with depressed levels of consciousness due to drug or alcohol use, seizures, general anesthesia, or central nervous system disease; those with impaired deglutition due to esophageal disease or neurologic disorders; and those with tracheal or nasogastric tubes, which disrupt the mechanical defenses of the airways.

Periodontal disease, which increases the number of anaerobic bacteria in aspirated material, is associated with a greater likelihood of anaerobic pleuropulmonary infection. Aspiration of infected oropharyngeal contents initially leads to pneumonia in dependent lung zones, such as the posterior segments of the upper lobes and superior and basilar segments of the lower lobes. Body position at the time of aspiration determines which lung zones are dependent. The onset of symptoms is insidious. By the time the patient seeks medical attention, necrotizing pneumonia, lung abscess, or empyema may be apparent.

About two-thirds of patients with necrotizing pneumonia, lung abscess, and empyema are found to be infected with multiple species of anaerobic bacteria only. Most of the remainder are infected with both anaerobic and aerobic bacteria. *Prevotella melaninogenica* (formerly *Bacteroides melaninogenicus*), anaerobic streptococci, and *Fusobacterium nucleatum* are commonly isolated anaerobic bacteria.

Clinical Findings

A. Symptoms and Signs: Patients with anaerobic pleuropulmonary infection usually present with constitutional symptoms such as fever, weight loss, and malaise. Cough with expectoration of foul-smelling purulent sputum suggests anaerobic infection, though the absence of productive cough does not rule out such an infection. Dental hygiene is poor, but patients are rarely edentulous; if so, an obstructing bronchial lesion is nearly always present.

B. Laboratory Findings: Expectorated sputum is inappropriate for culture of anaerobic organisms because of contaminating mouth flora. Representative material for culture can be obtained only by transtracheal or transthoracic aspiration, thoracentesis, or bronchoscopy with a protected brush. Transthoracic or transtracheal aspiration is rarely indicated, because anaerobic pleuropulmonary infections respond well to penicillin or clindamycin.

C. Imaging: The different types of anaerobic pleuropulmonary infection are distinguished on the basis of their radiographic appearance. **Lung abscess** appears as a thick-walled solitary cavity surrounded by consolidation. An air-fluid level is usually present. Other causes of cavitary lung disease (tuberculosis, mycosis, cancer, infarction, Wegener's granulomatosis) should be excluded. **Necrotizing pneumonia** is distinguished by multiple areas of cavitation within an area of consolidation. **Empyema** is characterized by the presence of pleural fluid (purulent on thoracentesis) and may accompany either of the other two radiographic findings. Ultrasonography is of value in locating fluid and may also reveal pleural loculations.

Treatment

Penicillin G (1–2 million units intravenously every 4 hours) is the usual treatment for anaerobic pleuropulmonary infections caused by anaerobic streptococci or oropharyngeal strains of *Bacteroides* in adults. Penicillin V (0.5–1 g orally every 6 hours) may be used after improvement with intravenous penicillin G has occurred. Clindamycin (600 mg intravenously every 8 hours until improvement, then 300 mg orally every 6 hours) is regarded by most authorities as an acceptable alternative to penicillin for treatment of anaerobic pleuropulmonary infections. Antibiotic therapy should be continued until the chest x-ray stabilizes, a process that may take a month or more. The treatment of anaerobic pleuropulmonary disease requires adequate drainage. Tube thoracostomy is required for the treatment of empyema, but open pleural drainage is sometimes necessary because of the propensity of these infections to produce loculations in the pleural space.

Hammond JM et al: The etiology and antimicrobial susceptibility patterns of microorganisms in acute community-acquired lung abscess. Chest 1995;108:937. (Prospective study based on aspiration of lung abscesses. All nonmycobacterial isolates were susceptible to amoxicillin-clavulanate.)

Vincent MT, Goldman BS: Anaerobic lung infections. Am Fam Physician 1994;49:1815. (Clinical features, diagnosis, and treatment.)

PULMONARY INFILTRATES IN THE COMPROMISED HOST

Pneumonia in immunocompromised patients may be caused by bacterial, mycobacterial, fungal, protozoal, helminthic, or viral pathogens, but not all pulmonary infiltrates in compromised hosts are due to infection. Noninfectious processes such as pulmonary edema, drug reaction, pulmonary infarction, underlying malignant disease, and radiation pneumonitis may mimic infection. Although almost any pathogen can cause pneumonia in a compromised host, two clinical tools help the clinician narrow the differential diagnosis. The first of these is knowledge of the underlying immunologic defect: specific types of immunologic defects predispose to particular infections; eg, defects in humoral immunity predispose mainly to bacterial infections against which antibodies play an important role, whereas defects in cellular immunity predispose to infections with viruses, fungi, mycobacteria, and protozoa. Neutropenia and impaired granulocyte function in conditions such as acute leukemia, chemotherapy administration, and myeloid metaplasia predispose to infections from *S aureus, Aspergillus,* gram-negative bacilli, and *Candida.* Chest radiography is also helpful in clarifying the differential diagnosis. Diffuse infiltrates are usually seen with pneumocystis or viral pneumonias. Bacterial and fungal infections are typically associated with more localized infiltrates.

The time course of infection also provides clues to the etiology of pneumonia in immunocompromised patients. A fulminant pneumonia is probably caused by bacterial infection, whereas an insidious pneumonia is more apt to be caused by viral, fungal, protozoal, or mycobacterial infection. Pneumonia occurring within 2–4 weeks after organ transplantation is most likely to be bacterial, whereas several months or more after transplantation, infection caused by *P carinii,* viruses (CMV, others), and fungi (*Aspergillus,* others) is more likely.

Examination of expectorated sputum for bacteria, fungi, mycobacteria, *Legionella,* and *P carinii* is important and may preclude the need for an expensive, invasive diagnostic procedure. Sputum induction is often necessary for diagnosis.

Frequently, routine evaluation fails to identify the causative organism. The clinician must then either begin empirical antimicrobial therapy or proceed to invasive procedures such as bronchoscopy, transthoracic aspiration, or open lung biopsy. Bronchoalveolar lavage using the flexible fiberoptic bronchoscope is a safe and effective method for obtaining representative pulmonary secretions for microbiologic studies. It involves less risk of bleeding than transbronchial brushing and transbronchial biopsy. Lavage is especially suitable for the diagnosis of *P carinii* pneumonia in patients with AIDS, the yield being 90–97%. Examination of expectorated sputum for *P carinii* is a less expensive and noninvasive alternative to bronchoalveolar lavage. The sensitivity of induced sputum for detection of *P carinii* depends upon institutional expertise, number of specimens analyzed, and detection methods. Selection of the approach to management must be based on the severity of the pulmonary infection, the underlying disease, the risks of empiric therapy, and local expertise and experience with the diagnostic procedures. Open lung biopsy, now performed by video-assisted thoracoscopy, is considered the best procedure for diagnosis of pulmonary infiltrates in the compromised host. Information obtained, however, uncommonly affects the ultimate outcome. Because a specific diagnosis is obtained in only about two-thirds of cases, empiric treatment is generally preferred, especially when the risk-benefit ratio of lung biopsy is high.

Shelhammer JH et al: The laboratory evaluation of opportunistic pulmonary infections. Ann Intern Med 1996;124:585. (Discussion of the appropriate specimens and tests for the diagnosis of lung infection in the immunosuppressed patient population.)

PULMONARY TUBERCULOSIS

Essentials of Diagnosis

- Fatigue, weight loss, fever, night sweats.
- Productive cough. Pulmonary infiltrates on chest radiograph.
- Positive tuberculin skin test reaction (most cases).
- Acid-fast bacilli on smear of sputum.
- Sputum culture positive for *Mycobacterium tuberculosis.*

General Considerations

Infection with *M tuberculosis* begins when aerosolized droplets containing viable organisms are inhaled by a person susceptible to the disease. When they reach the lungs, the organisms are ingested by macrophages and either die or persist and multiply. Widespread lymphatic and hematogenous dissemination of organisms occurs before development of an effective immune response when mycobacteria throughout the body are walled off by granulomatous inflammation. This type of infection, called **primary tuberculosis,** is usually asymptomatic. Uncommonly, the immune response is inadequate, and progressive primary tuberculosis develops, accompanied by both pulmonary and constitutional symptoms. Hematogenous dissemination from the primary focus throughout the lungs ("miliary" tuberculosis), to the pleural space (tuberculous pleural effusion), or to extrapulmonary sites (meninges, bone) is a rare complication of primary tuberculosis. Dormant but viable organisms persist for years, and reactivation of disease in any of these sites may occur if the host's defense mechanisms become impaired. In the past it has been customary to attribute about 90% of cases of tuberculosis in adults to reactivation of disease. However, recent reports of studies using DNA fingerprinting suggest that person-to-person transmission may account for as many as one-third of new cases of tuberculosis in large urban populations. The percentage of patients with atypical presentations— particularly elderly patients, patients with HIV infection, and those in nursing homes—has increased. Extrapulmonary tuberculosis is especially common in patients with HIV infection, who often display lymphadenitis or miliary disease.

Persons infected with the human immunodeficiency virus (HIV), with or without AIDS, are at increased risk of developing tuberculosis. HIV infection has emerged as the most important risk factor for the development of tuberculosis. The increase in the incidence of tuberculosis in the United States, beginning in 1986 but leveling off in the mid nineties, can be attributed to the HIV epidemic and to immigrants from Asia and Central America.

Strains of *M tuberculosis* resistant to one or more first-line antituberculous drugs are being encountered with increasing frequency. Risk factors for drug resistance include immigration from parts of the world with a high prevalence of drug-resistant tuberculosis, close and prolonged contact with individuals with drug-resistant tuberculosis, unsuccessful previous therapy, and patient noncompliance. Resistance to one or more antituberculosis drugs has been found in 15% of tuberculosis patients in the United States, and

New York City accounts for 61.4% of these cases. Outbreaks of multidrug-resistant tuberculosis in hospitals and correctional facilities in Florida and New York have been associated with mortality rates of 70–90% and median survival rates of 4–16 weeks.

Clinical Findings

A. Symptoms and Signs: The patient with reactivated tuberculosis typically presents with constitutional symptoms of fatigue, weight loss, anorexia, low-grade fever, and night sweats. Pulmonary symptoms include cough, which is initially dry but later productive of purulent sputum and (sometimes) blood. Occasionally, there may be no symptoms. On physical examination, patients often appear chronically ill and exhibit evidence of weight loss. Examination of the chest may reveal findings such as posttussive apical rales or may be normal.

B. Laboratory Findings: Definitive diagnosis depends on recovery of *M tuberculosis* from cultures or identification of the organism by DNA probe. Diagnosis therefore starts with collection of an adequate sputum specimen for stain and culture. Three specimens are advised. Induction of sputum may be helpful in patients who cannot voluntarily produce good specimens. Multiple sputum specimens are often required to identify acid-fast bacilli. The fluorochrome rhodamine-auramine stain of concentrated, digested sputum specimens is performed initially as a screening method, with confirmation by the Kinyoun or Ziehl-Neelsen stains. Demonstration of acid-fast bacilli on sputum smear does not confirm a diagnosis of tuberculosis, since saprophytic nontuberculous mycobacteria may colonize the airways or cause pulmonary disease. False-positive sputum cultures of *M tuberculosis* are, however, very rare.

In patients thought to have tuberculosis despite negative sputum smears, fiberoptic bronchoscopy is usually the next diagnostic step. Bronchial washings are particularly helpful. Postbronchoscopy expectorated sputum specimens may also be useful. Early morning aspiration of gastric contents after an overnight fast is an alternative to bronchoscopy. Gastric aspirates are suitable only for culture and not for stained smear, because nontuberculous mycobacteria may be present in the stomach in the absence of tuberculous infection. *M tuberculosis* may also be cultured from blood. *M tuberculosis* bacteremia has been reported in 14% of patients with tuberculosis.

Cultures on solid media to identify *M tuberculosis* require 6–8 weeks. The polymerase chain reaction permits rapid detection of *M tuberculosis* and differentiation of *M tuberculosis* from other mycobacteria. A radiometric culture system (Bactec) may allow detection of mycobacterial growth in as little as several days. Susceptibility testing is now considered routine for the first isolate of *M tuberculosis*, when a treatment regimen is failing, and when sputum cultures remain positive after 3 months of therapy.

Serologic diagnosis of tuberculosis using ELISA methodology to measure IgG antibody against mycobacterial antigens is a new and promising alternative to standard culture techniques. DNA fingerprinting using the polymerase chain reaction technique is available to identify individual strains of *M tuberculosis*, thereby revealing how infection is transmitted from person to person. This methodology demonstrated that exogenous reinfection with multidrug-resistant tuberculosis occurs during treatment for drug-susceptible tuberculosis in patients with AIDS.

In patients with pleural effusions caused by *M tuberculosis*, needle biopsy of the pleura reveals granulomas in up to 80% of patients. Pleural fluid cultures for *M tuberculosis* are positive in less than 25% of cases, but culture of the biopsy specimen affords a much higher yield.

C. Imaging: Because primary tuberculosis is usually asymptomatic, a chest x-ray is infrequently obtained. Radiographic abnormalities in primary tuberculosis are particularly likely to occur in children and include small homogeneous infiltrates (usually in the upper lobe), hilar and paratracheal lymph node enlargement, and segmental atelectasis. Pleural effusion may be present, especially in adults, sometimes as the sole radiographic abnormality. Ghon (calcified primary focus) and Ranke (calcified primary focus and calcified hilar lymph node) complexes are detected as residual evidence of healed primary tuberculosis in a minority of patients.

Postprimary or reactivation tuberculosis is associated with various radiographic manifestations, including fibrocavitary apical disease, nodules, and pneumonic infiltrates. The usual location is in the apical or posterior segments of the upper lobes or in the superior segments of the lower lobes; as many as 30% of patients may present with radiographic evidence of disease in other locations, however. This is especially true in elderly patients, in whom lower lobe infiltrates with or without pleural effusion are encountered with increasing frequency. Lower lung zone tuberculosis, which may occur with endobronchial tuberculosis, may masquerade as pneumonia or lung cancer. In HIV-infected patients who develop pulmonary tuberculosis, the radiographic features of tuberculosis may vary with the stage of HIV disease. In patients with "early" HIV infection, the radiographic features of tuberculosis resemble those in patients without HIV infection. In contrast, atypical radiographic features predominate in patients with "late" stage HIV infection (AIDS). These patients often display lower lung zone, diffuse, or miliary infiltrates, pleural effusions, and enlargement of hilar and mediastinal lymph nodes.

D. Special Examinations: The **tuberculin skin test** identifies individuals who have been infected at some time with *M tuberculosis* but does not distinguish between current disease and past infection. The standard Mantoux test establishes exposure to tuberculosis in individuals, while the multiple puncture test is used for population screening. In the Mantoux test, 0.1 mL of standard purified protein derivative (PPD-S), containing 5 TU, is injected intradermally on the volar surface of the forearm using a 27-gauge needle on a tuberculin syringe. The transverse width (in millimeters) of the induration at the skin test site should be recorded after 48–72 hours. A negative reaction does not rule out the diagnosis of tuberculosis; and the larger the reaction, the greater the likelihood of infection due to *M tuberculosis*. Table 9–9 summarizes American Thoracic Society criteria for interpretation of the Mantoux tuberculin skin test.

A positive skin test reaction in patients with HIV infection or those with defects in cellular immunity is 5 mm or more of induration. In the early (asymptomatic) stage of HIV infection, cutaneous reactivity to tuberculin is intact. Patients with AIDS are commonly anergic.

Both false-positive and false-negative tuberculin reactions occur. False-positive reactions are due to infection with nontuberculous mycobacteria. False-negative reactions occur because of concurrent infection, malnutrition, old age, immunologic disorders,

lymphoreticular malignancies, corticosteroid therapy, chronic renal failure, virus vaccinations or infections, fulminant tuberculosis, and improper testing technique.

"Boosting" of the skin test reaction by serial testing may cause a false impression of conversion, as dormant mycobacterial sensitivity is restored by the antigenic challenge of the initial skin test. This boosting phenomenon may increase the reaction size on a subsequent tuberculin test and is most commonly seen in those over age 55. A two-step testing procedure may identify a boosted tuberculin reaction. If the initial test is negative, it may be repeated a week later. If the second test result is negative, the person is uninfected or anergic. If it is positive, a boosted reaction is most likely. This effect may persist for at least 1 year. BCG (extract of *Mycobacterium bovis*) vaccination renders the PPD positive for 1 year. Thereafter, interpretation is standard. An anergy skin test panel should be placed at the time of tuberculin testing if the patient is judged likely to be anergic for any reason.

Treatment

All possible or proved cases of tuberculosis should be reported to local and state public health departments. Treatment of patients with tuberculosis should be conducted by physicians who are skilled and highly experienced in the management of this condition. This is especially important in cases of drug-resistant tuberculosis.

A. Hospitalization: Hospitalization for initial therapy of tuberculosis is not necessary in most patients, though it should be considered if a patient is incapable of self-care or is likely to expose susceptible individuals to the risk of tuberculosis. Monthly follow-up of compliant outpatients is recommended, including sputum smear and culture until conversion occurs. A private room with appropriate ventilation and instruction in the importance of covering the mouth while coughing are sufficient infection control measures for hospitalized patients receiving effective chemotherapy.

B. Drug Therapy: (Tables 9–10 and 9–11.) (See also Chapter 33.) Standard therapy for pulmonary infection due to *M tuberculosis* has been revised because of the increase in prevalence of drug-resistant tuberculosis in the United States. The treatment recommendations of the Centers for Disease Control and Prevention (CDC) for the initial empiric treatment of tuberculosis are summarized in Table 9–10, and recommended drug dosages are listed in Table 9–11. For patients without HIV infection, three options are suggested by the CDC:

1. The first option is a four-drug regimen consisting of isoniazid, rifampin, pyrazinamide, and either ethambutol or streptomycin. Therapy may be given daily or two or three times weekly if directly observed. Ethambutol or streptomycin may be dis-

Table 9–9. Classification of positive tuberculin skin test reactions.[1,2]

Reaction Size	Group
≥ 5 mm	1. Persons with HIV infection or those at risk for HIV infection. 2. Close contacts of individuals with tuberculosis. 3. Persons with chest x-rays consistent with old healed tuberculosis.
≥ 10 mm	1. Persons from countries with a high incidence of tuberculosis in Asia, Africa, and Latin America. 2. Intravenous drug users. 3. Medically underserved, low-income populations, including blacks, Hispanics, and Native Americans. 4. Long-term residents of correctional institutions, nursing homes, and mental institutions. 5. Persons with the following medical conditions that increase the risk of tuberculosis: gastrectomy, being ≥ 10% below ideal body weight, jejunoileal bypass, diabetes mellitus, silicosis, chronic renal failure, corticosteroid or other immunosuppressive therapy, leukemia, lymphoma, and other malignancies.
≥ 15 mm	6. Other high-risk populations. All other persons.

[1] Recommendations of American Thoracic Society: Am Rev Respir Dis 1990;142:725.
[2] A Mantoux skin test reaction is considered positive if the transverse diameter of the indurated area reaches the size required for the specific group. All other reactions are considered negative.

Table 9–10. Recommended options for the initial treatment of tuberculosis.[1]

	Tuberculosis Without HIV Infection		Tuberculosis With HIV Infection
Option 1	**Option 2**	**Option 3**	
Administer daily isoniazid, rifampin, and pyrazinamide for 8 weeks, followed by 16 weeks of isoniazid and rifampin daily or twice or three times weekly.[2] In areas where the isoniazid resistance rate is not documented to be <4%, ethambutol or streptomycin should be added to the initial regimen until susceptibility to isoniazid and rifampin is demonstrated. Continue treatment for at least 6 months and 3 months beyond culture conversion. Consult a tuberculosis medical expert if the patient is symptomatic or if smear or culture is positive after 3 months.	Administer daily isoniazid, rifampin, pyrazinamide, and streptomycin or ethambutol for 2 weeks followed by twice-weekly[2] directly observed administration of the same drugs for 6 weeks, and subsequently with twice-weekly directly observed administration of isoniazid and rifampin for 16 weeks. Consult a tuberculosis medical expert if the patient is symptomatic or if smear or culture is positive after 3 months.	Treat by directly observed therapy three times a week[2] with isoniazid, rifampin, pyrazinamide, and ethambutol or streptomycin for 6 months.[3] Consult a tuberculosis medical expert if the patient is symptomatic or if the smear or culture is positive after 3 months.	Options 1, 2, or 3 can be used, but treatment regimens should continue for a total of 9 months and at least 6 months beyond culture conversion

[1]Modified from: Initial therapy for tuberculosis in the era of multidrug resistance. Recommendations of the Advisory Council for the Elimination of Tuberculosis. MMWR Morbid Mortal Wkly Rep 1993;42(RR-7):1.
[2]All regimens administered twice or three times a week should be monitored by direct observation for the duration of therapy.
[3]The strongest evidence from clinical trials is for the effectiveness of all four drugs administered for the full 6 months. There is weaker evidence that streptomycin can be discontinued after 4 months if the isolate is susceptible to all drugs. The evidence for stopping pyrazinamide before the end of 6 months is equivocal for the thrice-weekly regimen, and there is no evidence for effectiveness of this regimen with ethambutol for less than the full 6 months.

continued if susceptibility to isoniazid and rifampin is documented. Pyrazinamide should be discontinued after 8 weeks. The total duration of therapy should be at least 6 months and at least 3 months after sputum cultures convert to negative. Fixed-dose combinations of rifampin and isoniazid (Rifamate) and rifampin, isoniazid, and pyrazinamide (Rifater) are available to simplify treatment; they improve compliance but are more expensive than the component drugs purchased individually.

2. The second option calls for daily isoniazid, rifampin, pyrazinamide, and streptomycin or ethambutol for 2 weeks, followed by directly observed twice-weekly administration of the same drugs for 6 weeks,

Table 9–11. Recommended dosages for the initial treatment of tuberculosis.[1]

Drugs	Daily	Cost[2]	Twice a Week	Cost[2]	Three Times a Week	Cost[2]
Isoniazid	5 mg/kg Max: 300 mg/dose	$0.09/300 mg	15 mg/kg Max: 900 mg/dose	$0.54	15 mg/kg Max: 900 mg/dose	$0.81
Rifampin	10 mg/kg Max: 600 mg/dose	$3.25/600 mg	10 mg/kg Max: 600 mg/dose	$6.50	10 mg/kg Max: 600 mg/dose	$9.75
Pyrazinamide	15–30 mg/kg Max: 2 g/dose	$4.48/2 g	50–70 mg/kg Max: 4 g/dose	$17.90	50–70 mg/kg Max: 3 g/dose	$20.15
Ethambutol[3]	5–25 mg/kg Max: 2.5 g/dose	$10.81/2.5 g	50 mg/kg Max: 2.5 g/dose	$21.60	25–30 mg/kg Max: 2.5 g/dose	$32.40
Streptomycin	15 mg/kg Max: 1 g/dose	No charge[4]	25–30 mg/kg Max: 1.5 g/dose	No charge[4]	25–30 mg/kg Max: 1.5 g/dose	No charge[4]

[1]Modified from: Initial therapy for tuberculosis in the era of multidrug resistance. Recommendations of the Advisory Council for the Elimination of Tuberculosis. MMWR Morbid Mortal Wkly Rep 1993;42(RR-7):1.
[2]Cost to pharmacist (average wholesale price) for maximum dose and regimen listed. Source: First Data Bank, Price Alert, April 1997.
[3]Ethambutol is generally not recommended for patients whose visual acuity cannot be monitored. However, ethambutol should be considered for patients with organisms resistant to other drugs when susceptibility to ethambutol has been demonstrated or when susceptibility is likely.
[4]Available from Pfizer Prescription Assistance: 800-254-4445. No charge for specific patient use.

followed by directly observed twice-weekly administration of isoniazid and rifampin for 16 weeks.

3. The third option is directly observed thrice-weekly administration of isoniazid, rifampin, pyrazinamide, and ethambutol or streptomycin for 6 months.

For patients with HIV infection, any of the three options above can be used, but therapy should continue for 9 months and at least 6 months after culture conversion.

The four-drug regimen may be unnecessary if community rates of isoniazid resistance are documented to be less than 4%. The CDC advises consultation with a tuberculosis expert if, after 3 months, the patient is symptomatic or smear or culture positive.

If results of drug susceptibility testing are not available, the decision to continue ethambutol or streptomycin for the total duration of therapy should be based on knowledge of local drug resistance patterns and the patient's HIV status. If the prevalence of isoniazid resistance in a community exceeds 4% or the patient is infected with HIV, ethambutol or streptomycin should be continued for the entire period of therapy.

The CDC recommends that five-drug or six-drug initial regimens be used for outbreaks of tuberculosis resistant to isoniazid and rifampin. In this circumstance, and when resuming therapy in patients previously treated for tuberculosis, the initial regimen should include at least three drugs thought to be active against the organism. Drug susceptibility tests should be used to guide subsequent therapy. If resistance to isoniazid and rifampin is confirmed, a regimen that includes three or more drugs proved to be active against the organism should be continued for 12–24 months after the sputum culture becomes negative.

Directly observed therapy, which requires that a health care worker observe while the patient ingests antituberculous medications in the home, clinic, hospital, or elsewhere, ensures compliance with therapy. Noncompliance is a major cause of treatment failure and drug resistance, which increase the risk of transmission of tuberculosis. The importance of direct observation of drug therapy cannot be overemphasized. Directly observed therapy is advised by the CDC for all patients with drug-resistant tuberculosis and all patients receiving intermittent (twice- or thrice-weekly) therapy.

Treatment of extrapulmonary tuberculosis is the same as for pulmonary tuberculosis. However, 9 months of therapy is advised by many experts. Treatment of skeletal tuberculosis is enhanced by early surgical drainage and debridement of necrotic bone. Corticosteroid therapy is indicated in tuberculous pericarditis and tuberculous meningitis.

Tuberculosis in pregnancy is treated with an initial regimen of isoniazid, rifampin, and ethambutol. Pyrazinamide should be used only if resistance to other drugs is documented or likely and susceptibility to pyrazinamide is likely, because the risk of teratogenicity with pyrazinamide has not been determined. Streptomycin is contraindicated in pregnancy because it may cause congenital deafness. Isoniazid, rifampin, and ethambutol are considered safe in pregnancy.

The physician will occasionally encounter patients with clinical and radiographic abnormalities consistent with tuberculosis, positive tuberculin reactions, and negative bacteriologic findings, even after vigorous attempts have been employed to make a diagnosis of tuberculosis, including sputum induction with hypertonic saline and fiberoptic bronchoscopy. In these patients, the bacillary population is presumed to be lower than in cases where sputum smears or cultures are positive. Evidence suggests the value of treatment of smear- and culture-negative pulmonary tuberculosis. A 4-month regimen of isoniazid and rifampin has been found to be effective. Patients treated in this fashion should have close follow-up. A failure of radiographic improvement within 3 months suggests a diagnosis other than tuberculosis.

Adults should have measurements of serum bilirubin, hepatic enzymes, urea nitrogen, and creatinine and a complete blood count, including platelets, before starting chemotherapy for tuberculosis. Visual acuity and red-green color perception tests are recommended before initiation of ethambutol, and serum uric acid should be measured before starting pyrazinamide. The patient beginning therapy should be cautioned to watch for symptoms of drug toxicity (Table 9–12). Routine monitoring of laboratory tests for evidence of toxicity is not recommended, but monthly questioning for symptoms of drug toxicity is advised.

C. Preventive Therapy (Chemoprophylaxis): Patients infected with *M tuberculosis* but without active disease harbor small numbers of organisms. Isoniazid prophylaxis (300 mg/d for adults and 10–14 mg/kg/d—up to 300 mg/d—for children) for 12 months in such patients may reduce the expected incidence of reactivated tuberculosis by 93%. Six months of isoniazid therapy may offer equal protection and improved patient compliance. Chemoprophylaxis of close contacts of patients with isoniazid-resistant tuberculosis could consist of (1) standard chemoprophylaxis with isoniazid, particularly if there is doubt about isoniazid resistance, (2) treatment with standard doses of rifampin for 6 months (9 months for children), or (3) close observation only. The second approach is advised for those at greatest risk (children, immunocompromised hosts).

The following groups of individuals, regardless of age, should receive preventive therapy *if they have positive tuberculin skin test results as defined in Table 9–9:*

(1) Persons known or suspected to have HIV infection. HIV-infected persons who are at high risk of

Table 9–12. Characteristics of antituberculous drugs.[1]

Drug	Most Common Side Effects	Tests for Side Effects	Drug Interactions	Remarks
Isoniazid	Peripheral neuritis, hepatitis, hypersensitivity.	AST and ALT; neurologic examination	Phenytoin (synergistic); disulfiram (toxicity); warfarin (potentiation).	Bactericidal to both extracellular and intracellular organisms. Pyridoxine, 10 mg orally daily as prophylaxis for neuritis; 50–100 mg orally daily as treatment.
Rifampin	Hepatitis, febrile reaction, purpura (rare).	AST and ALT	Rifampin inhibits the effect of oral contraceptives, quinidine, corticosteroids, warfarin, methadone, digoxin, oral hypoglycemics; aminosalicyclic acid may interfere with absorption of rifampin.	Bactericidal to all populations of organisms. Colors urine and other body secretions orange. Discoloring of contact lenses.
Pyrazinamide	Hyperuricemia, hepatotoxicity.	Uric acid, AST, ALT	. . .	Bactericidal to intracellular organisms. Combination with an aminoglycoside is bactericidal.
Ethambutol	Optic neuritis (reversible with discontinuance of drug; rare at 15 mg/kg); rash.	Red-green color discrimination and visual acuity (difficult to test in children under 3 years of age).	. . .	Bacteriostatic to both intracellular and extracellular organisms. Mainly used to inhibit development of resistant mutants. Use with caution in renal disease or when ophthalmologic testing is not feasible.
Streptomycin	Eighth nerve damage, nephrotoxicity.	Vestibular function (audiograms); BUN and creatinine.	Neuromuscular blocking agents may be potentiated and cause prolonged paralysis.	Bactericidal to extracellular organisms. Use with caution in older patients or those with renal disease.

[1]Modified and reproduced, with permission, from Bailey WC et al: Treatment of tuberculosis and other mycobacterial diseases. Am Rev Respir Dis 1983;127:790.

tuberculosis but have negative skin tests should also be considered for preventive therapy.

(2) Close contacts of persons with newly diagnosed infectious tuberculosis. Household members and other close contacts have a 2–4% risk of developing tuberculosis within the first year of exposure to the index case. Children should be treated even if their initial skin test results are negative, and such tests should be repeated after 3 months of isoniazid therapy. If the skin test reaction becomes positive (> 5 mm), isoniazid preventive therapy should be continued for a total of 9 months.

(3) Recent tuberculin skin test converters. A skin test conversion is defined as an increase in induration of 10 mm or more within 2 years for those under 35 years of age and 15 mm or more for those 35 years of age or older.

(4) Persons with medical conditions that increase the risk of tuberculosis. These conditions include diabetes mellitus, prolonged therapy with corticosteroids (> 15 mg prednisone or equivalent per day), immunosuppressive therapy, hematologic and reticuloendothelial malignancies, intravenous drug users even if known to be HIV-negative, end-stage renal disease, and any medical condition inducing substantial rapid weight loss or chronic undernutrition.

Preventive therapy should also be given to the following groups if the person is under 35 years of age and has a positive tuberculin skin test (> 10 mm):

(1) Foreign-born persons from countries with a high prevalence of tuberculosis, including those in Asia, Africa, and Latin America.

(2) Medically underserved, low-income groups (including racial or ethnic minorities, such as blacks, Hispanics, and Native Americans).

(3) Residents of long-term care facilities (including nursing homes, mental institutions, and prisons). The staffs of such facilities should also be considered candidates for preventive therapy.

Isoniazid preventive therapy is typically given for 12 months, though 6 months of therapy appears to be effective as well. A full 12 months of preventive therapy is required for patients with HIV infection. Children receive 9 months of therapy.

Persons under the age of 35 with no risk factors for tuberculosis who have tuberculin skin test reactions of 15 mm or more should be considered for preventive therapy.

The major risk of isoniazid prophylaxis is drug-induced hepatitis, the incidence of which increases with age. Persons on preventive therapy should be questioned monthly for symptoms of hepatitis and discontinued if clinical evidence of hepatitis develops during therapy. Failure to discontinue the drug may result in progressive hepatic necrosis. The routine monitoring of biochemical tests of liver function periodically during isoniazid prophylaxis is recommended only for persons 35 and older. The risk of fatal isoniazid-induced hepatitis is negligible when such monitoring is performed. Elevations of transaminase up to three times normal without symptoms do not constitute an indication to stop therapy.

D. Vaccine: A number of live tuberculosis vaccines are available and are known collectively as BCG after the original strain of bacterium used in the vaccine (bacillus Calmette-Guérin). BCG vaccination should be considered only if isoniazid chemoprophylaxis cannot be used. Current recommendations are that BCG vaccination be considered for tuberculin-negative persons, especially children, who are repeatedly exposed to individuals with untreated or ineffectively treated tuberculosis and who cannot receive standard preventive therapy. Vaccination should be considered for communities or groups in which a high rate of new infections occurs despite aggressive treatment and surveillance programs. BCG vaccination appears to be effective in reducing the risk of tuberculosis in selected populations.

Prognosis

Almost all properly treated patients with tuberculosis are cured. Relapse rates are less than 5% with current regimens. The main cause of treatment failure is noncompliance.

American Thoracic Society: Diagnostic standards and classification of tuberculosis. Am Rev Respir Dis 1990; 142:725. (Official statement of the American Thoracic Society.)

American Thoracic Society: Treatment of tuberculosis and tuberculosis infection in adults and children. Am J Respir Crit Care Med 1994;149:1359. (Current standards for treatment and for preventive therapy.)

Blumberg HM et al: Preventing the nosocomial transmission of tuberculosis. Ann Intern Med 1995;122:658. (Administrative policies reduced nosocomial transmission of tuberculosis to hospital health care workers.)

Drugs for tuberculosis. Med Lett Drugs Ther 1995;37:67. (This statement summarizes modern treatment of tuberculosis.)

Goodman PC: Tuberculosis and AIDS. Radiol Clin North Am 1995;33:707. (Radiographic presentations of tuberculosis in patients with AIDS are often atypical.)

Hopewell PC: A clinical view of tuberculosis. Radiol Clin North Am 1995;33:641. (Review of the clinical features of tuberculosis in the current era.)

Moffitt MP, Wisinger DB: Tuberculosis. Recommendations for screening, prevention, and treatment. Postgrad Med 1996;100:201. (Emphasis on the tuberculin skin test.)

Sbarbaro JA: Tuberculosis in the 1990s: Epidemiology and therapeutic challenge. Chest 1995;108(Suppl):58S. (Analysis of the causes of the rising incidence of tuberculosis.)

Schluger NW, Rom WN: Current approaches to the diagnosis of active pulmonary tuberculosis. Am J Respir Crit Care Med 1994;149:264. (Techniques to diagnose tuberculosis and recommended management when the sputum smears are negative.)

Schluger NW, Rom WN: The polymerase chain reaction in the diagnosis and evaluation of pulmonary infections. Am J Respir Crit Care Med 1995;152:11. (Review of this DNA amplification technique in the rapid diagnosis of tuberculosis and other lung infections.)

Telzak EE: Tuberculosis and human immunodeficiency virus infection. Med Clin North Am 1997;81:345. (Review with 109 references.)

DISEASE CAUSED BY NONTUBERCULOUS MYCOBACTERIA

Mycobacteria other than *M tuberculosis* ("atypical" mycobacteria) are ubiquitous in nature. Only *Mycobacterium kansasii* and *Mycobacterium avium-intracellulare*—also called *Mycobacterium avium* complex (MAC)—are important causes of pulmonary disease in humans, which is clinically indistinguishable from *M tuberculosis*. The diagnosis rests on recovery of the pathogen from cultures. Infections with MAC are being seen with increasing frequency in patients with AIDS, in whom the disease is likely to be disseminated. In HIV-negative patients, the incidence of pulmonary infections caused by nontuberculous mycobacteria appears to be increasing.

Sputum cultures positive for atypical mycobacteria do not in themselves prove the presence of atypical tuberculosis, because atypical bacteria may exist as saprophytes in the airways or as environmental contaminants. Positive sputum cultures are meaningful if the following criteria are met: (1) The patient has clinical and radiographic evidence of disease compatible with a diagnosis of pulmonary tuberculosis and other causes of the lung disease have been excluded; and (2) four or more sputum specimens or bronchial washings are positive for acid-fast bacilli by smear or culture, the latter with at least ten colonies each. A positive result on culture of material obtained from tissue biopsies or pleural fluid is also diagnostic. Drug susceptibility testing on cultures of nontuberculous mycobacteria is in general unhelpful clinically and not routinely indicated.

Disease caused by *M kansasii* responds well to drug therapy. A daily regimen of rifampin, isoniazid, and ethambutol for 18–24 months is usually sufficient.

In contrast, MAC is resistant in vitro to most antituberculosis drugs. Most nonimmunocompromised patients with lung infection caused by MAC are middle-aged or older men with underlying chronic lung disease. The treatment of MAC infection is controversial. Whether to use a standard or an individualized regimen, whether to use isoniazid, and whether to perform in vitro drug susceptibility testing are debated.

Traditional chemotherapeutic regimens have taken an aggressive approach using five or six drugs, but these have been associated with drug-induced side effects and patient noncompliance.

A three- or four-drug combination of clarithromycin with two or three of five additional drugs (rifampin, ethambutol, clofazimine, amikacin, and ciprofloxacin) is now the treatment of choice for MAC disease. An alternative combination includes rifampin, ethambutol, ciprofloxacin, and clofazimine, with or without amikacin. Other drugs active against MAC include azithromycin, rifabutin (ansamycin), ethionamide, cycloserine, and imipenem. The optimal duration of treatment is unknown, but therapy should be continued for 12 months after sputum conversion to negative. Medical treatment is initially successful in about two-thirds of cases, but relapses after treatment are common. Long-term benefit is demonstrated in about half of all patients treated medically. Those who do not respond favorably generally have active but stable disease. Surgical resection is an alternative for the patient with progressive disease that responds poorly to chemotherapy. The overall success with surgical therapy is favorable.

Dissemination of MAC infection is rare in immunocompetent patients. In contrast, in patients with AIDS, infections with MAC are systemic and tend to occur late in the course. Treatment is difficult. Multiple combinations of drugs such as clarithromycin, isoniazid, ethambutol, rifampin, clofazimine, cycloserine, amikacin, ciprofloxacin, pyrazinamide, and ansamycin have been tried. Combination therapy may provide improvement in symptoms. The current recommendation for treatment of disseminated MAC disease is to use clarithromycin or azithromycin plus one or more of the following: ethambutol, clofazimine, ciprofloxacin, and amikacin; a survival benefit has been reported. Therapy must be continued for at least 18–24 months. Cycloserine and ethionamide should be avoided because of troublesome side effects.

Rifabutin is now available for prevention of disseminated MAC infection in patients with advanced HIV infection and should be given to all patients with CD4 lymphocyte counts of 100 cells/μL or less. Rifabutin (300 mg orally once daily) has been well tolerated, but patients should be watched closely for drug interactions because this drug induces hepatic cytochrome P450 enzymes.

A National Registry for Nontuberculous Mycobacterial Diseases has been established at the National Jewish Center for Immunology and Respiratory Medicine in Denver (800-551-1686).

Drugs for AIDS and associated infections. Med Lett Drugs Ther 1995;37:87. (Current recommendations for treatment of the major infections associated with AIDS.)

Patz EF Jr, Swensen SJ, Erasmus J: Pulmonary manifestations of nontuberculous *Mycobacterium*. Radiol Clin North Am 1995;33:719. (Clinical and radiographic features of atypical mycobacterial infection in immunocompetent patients.)

Wallace RJ Jr et al: Clarithromycin regimens for pulmonary *Mycobacterium avium* complex. The first 50 patients. Am J Respir Crit Care Med 1996;153:1766. (In HIV-negative patients with MAC lung disease, a regimen of clarithromycin, ethambutol, and rifabutin is the treatment of choice.)

NEOPLASTIC & RELATED DISEASES

BRONCHOGENIC CARCINOMA

Essentials of Diagnosis

- Cough, dyspnea, hemoptysis, anorexia, or weight loss in most patients.
- Variable findings on physical examination depending on stage of disease.
- Enlarging mass, infiltrate, atelectasis, cavitation, or pleural effusion on chest x-ray or CT scan in most patients.
- Cytologic or histologic findings diagnostic of (primary) lung cancer in sputum, pleural fluid, or tissue.

General Considerations

About 178,000 new cases of lung cancer are expected in the USA in 1998. Lung cancer accounts for 32% of cancer deaths in men and 25% of cancer deaths in women, and its incidence in women is rising rapidly. Most cases present between the ages of 50 and 70. Fewer than 5% of lung cancer patients are under 40 years of age. Cigarette smoking is the most important cause of lung cancer in both men and women in the USA. Ionizing radiation (indoor radon gas, therapeutic radiation, atomic bomb blasts), asbestos, heavy metals (nickel, chromium), and industrial carcinogens (chloromethyl ether) are established but less potent pulmonary carcinogens. Lung scars, air pollution, and genetic factors are also implicated, but the data supporting these associations are not conclusive. Chronic obstructive pulmonary disease may represent a risk factor for lung cancer even after controlling for cigarette smoking. Primary lung cancer in nonsmokers is uncommon.

More than 20 benign and malignant primary neoplasms of the lung have been identified and classified histologically. Ninety percent of malignant cancers belong to one of the four major cell types of bronchogenic carcinoma, a term denoting primary malignant tumors of the airway epithelium. **Squamous cell carcinoma** and **adenocarcinoma** are the most common types of bronchogenic carcinoma and account for about 30–35% of primary tumors each. **Small cell carcinoma** and **large cell carcinoma** account for about 20–25% and 15%, respectively. Other malignant epithelial tumors of the lung include adenosquamous carcinoma, carcinoid tumor, bronchial gland carcinomas, and a few rare tumors.

Squamous cell carcinoma of the lung tends to originate in the central bronchi as an intraluminal growth and is thus more amenable to early detection through cytologic examination of sputum than are the other types of carcinoma. Squamous cell carcinoma tends to metastasize to regional lymph nodes. About 10% of squamous cell carcinomas cavitate. Small cell carcinoma also occurs centrally and tends to narrow bronchi by extrinsic compression; widespread metastases are common. Adenocarcinoma and large-cell carcinoma resemble each other in their clinical behavior. These tumors usually appear in the periphery of the lung and therefore are not amenable to early detection through examination of sputum. They typically metastasize to distant organs. **Bronchioloalveolar cell carcinoma,** a subtype of adenocarcinoma, is a low-grade carcinoma that represents about 2% of cases of bronchogenic carcinoma and presents as single or multiple pulmonary nodules or an alveolar infiltrate.

Clinical Findings

The clinical features of lung cancer depend on the primary cancer itself, its metastases, systemic effects of the cancer, and any coexisting paraneoplastic syndromes.

A. Symptoms and Signs: Only 10–25% of patients are asymptomatic at the time of diagnosis of lung cancer. Symptomatic lung cancer is generally advanced and often not resectable. Initial symptoms include nonspecific complaints such as cough, weight loss, dyspnea, chest pain, and hemoptysis that are associated with other disorders. Any change in the pattern of cough, blood-streaked sputum, anorexia with weight loss, and hoarseness are symptoms that point to a diagnosis of bronchogenic carcinoma in the appropriate clinical setting.

Physical findings vary and may be totally absent. Central tumors that obstruct segmental, lobar, or main stem bronchi may cause atelectasis and postobstructive pneumonitis with typical physical findings. Peripheral tumors may cause no abnormalities on physical examination. Extension of the tumor to the pleural surface may cause pleural effusion. In one large series, lymphadenopathy, hepatomegaly, and clubbing were noted in about 20% of patients with lung cancer. Superior vena cava syndrome, **Horner's syndrome** (miosis, ptosis, enophthalmos, and loss of sweating on the affected side), **Pancoast's syndrome** (neurovascular complications of superior pulmonary sulcus tumor), recurrent laryngeal nerve palsy with hoarseness, phrenic nerve palsy with hemidiaphragm

paralysis, and skin metastases are each seen in fewer than 5% of cases.

Paraneoplastic syndromes (extrapulmonary organ dysfunction not related to effects of the primary or metastases) occur in 15–20% of lung cancer patients (see Chapter 4). A number of tumor secretory products have been associated with lung cancer. The manifestations of paraneoplastic syndromes may precede, coincide with, or follow the diagnosis of lung cancer. Recognition of paraneoplastic syndromes in lung cancer is important, because treatment of the associated symptoms may improve the patient's well-being even though the primary tumor itself is not curable; occasionally, resection of the tumor is followed by immediate resolution of the paraneoplastic syndrome. Table 9–13 lists important paraneoplastic syndromes associated with lung cancer.

B. Laboratory Findings: Definitive diagnosis requires histologic evidence of cancer. Cytologic examination of expectorated sputum permits definitive diagnosis of lung cancer in 40–60% of cases, especially in centrally located tumors. This test is inexpensive and highly specific. A diagnosis of lung cancer by sputum cytologic examination may spare the

Table 9–13. Paraneoplastic syndromes in lung cancer.

Classification	Syndrome	Common Histologic Type of Cancer
Endocrine and metabolic	Cushing's syndrome	Small cell
	Inappropriate secretion of antidiuretic hormone (SIADH)	Small cell
	Hypercalcemia	Squamous cell
	Gynecomastia	Large cell
Connective tissue and osseous	Clubbing and hypertrophic pulmonary osteoarthropathy	Squamous cell, adenocarcinoma, large cell
Neuromuscular	Peripheral neuropathy (sensory, sensorimotor)	Small cell
	Subacute cerebellar degeneration	Small cell
	Myasthenia (Eaton-Lambert syndrome)	Small cell
	Dermatomyositis	All
Cardiovascular	Thrombophlebitis	Adenocarcinoma
	Nonbacterial verrucous (marantic) endocarditis	
Hematologic	Anemia	All
	Disseminated intravascular coagulation	
	Eosinophilia	
	Thrombocytosis	
Cutaneous	Acanthosis nigricans	All
	Erythema gyratum repens	

patient from having to submit to bronchoscopy or another invasive procedure. Examination of pleural fluid reveals cytologic findings positive for cancer in 40–50% of patients with malignant pleural effusion from lung cancer. Closed pleural biopsy (Cope or Abrams needle) yields a histologic diagnosis of cancer in about 55% of patients. Biopsy and cytologic study of pleural fluid combined establish a diagnosis of cancer in about 80% of patients with malignant pleural effusion.

Tissue for histologic confirmation of lung cancer may be obtained by various techniques, including bronchoscopy, percutaneous needle aspirate, mediastinoscopy, lymph node biopsy, or biopsy of other metastatic sites (eg, skin), and thoracotomy. Biopsy of mediastinal lymph nodes reveals cancer in about a third of lung cancer patients. Fine-needle aspiration of supraclavicular or cervical lymph nodes is useful if these nodes are enlarged on palpation. Thoracotomy is occasionally necessary to diagnose lung cancer when simpler cytologic and histologic evaluations are negative.

C. Imaging: Chest radiography demonstrates abnormal findings in nearly all patients with lung cancer. Comparison of old and current chest radiographs is especially important.

Radiographic abnormalities in primary lung cancer are not specific. Common abnormalities are hilar masses or enlargement, peripheral masses, atelectasis, infiltrates, cavitation, and pleural effusions. Multiple masses, consolidation, and chest wall involvement are unusual. Squamous cell and small cell carcinomas commonly produce a hilar mass and mediastinal widening. Cavitation suggests squamous cell carcinoma and is exceedingly rare in small cell carcinoma. Small peripheral masses usually are adenocarcinomas.

CT scanning, MRI, and ultrasound are useful imaging methods in selected patients with suspected or proved lung cancer. All depend upon initial detection of a suspicious lesion on the plain chest x-ray. CT scanning is particularly useful for evaluation of the lung parenchyma and pleura. MRI may be used for staging the mediastinum when use of an iodinated contrast agent is contraindicated.

D. Special Examinations: Early detection of lung cancer in an asymptomatic stage is feasible with cytologic examination of sputum and chest radiography. However, the mortality rate from lung cancer is not appreciably reduced by early detection except for peripheral coin lesions.

These recommendations, however, do not discount the use of sputum cytology in the evaluation of individual patients whom the physician considers at high risk for lung cancer. Patients with roentgenographically occult non–small cell lung cancer diagnosed by sputum cytology and evaluated by fiberoptic bronchoscopy have a 5-year survival rate of over 50% following surgery or radiation therapy. Small cell carcinoma is nearly always metastatic when first detected.

Staging of lung cancer utilizes the TNM international staging system for lung carcinoma, which was revised in 1996. In this system, T describes the primary tumor, N the nodal involvement, and M any distant metastases (Table 9–14). Small cell carcinoma is staged as "limited" (tumor confined to one hemithorax and hilar, mediastinal, and supraclavicular nodes) or "extensive" (spread to more distant sites). CT scan of the lungs, mediastinum, and upper abdomen (liver, adrenal glands, and periaortic lymph nodes) is usually helpful in staging lung cancer. In a patient with known lung cancer, the finding of mediastinal lymph nodes larger than 2 cm in diameter on CT scan is strong evidence of mediastinal spread of the tumor; however, occasional false-positive results occur with this technique. Nodes smaller than 1 cm have a low probability of tumor involvement. At least 85% of lung cancer patients with negative results on mediastinal CT scans have no evidence of mediastinal lymphadenopathy at the time of surgery.

History, physical examination, and simple laboratory studies are usually sufficient to detect metastases to distant sites such as liver, brain, bone, heart, abdomen, and skin. Routine radionuclide scans are not recommended. Radionuclide bone scanning for asymptomatic skeletal metastases is sensitive but lacks specificity. Patients with skeletal complaints should have bone x-rays. If these are negative, a radionuclide bone scan should be ordered. Those with abnormal central nervous system findings should have a CT scan or MRI of the brain. The latter is preferred for infratentorial lesions. Patients with proved lung cancer who have no clinical features of brain metastases should in general not undergo routine CT scanning of the brain to search for occult metastases. In patients with adenocarcinoma of the lung, however, some authorities still advocate this procedure if the patient is a candidate for pulmonary resection.

Surgical exploration of the mediastinum from the suprasternal or parasternal approach should be strongly considered before thoracotomy if radiographic studies suggest significant mediastinal lymphadenopathy or direct extension of the lung cancer into the mediastinum. This approach reduces the number of thoracotomies that do not permit curative lung resection.

Complications

A. Superior Vena Cava Syndrome: See Chapter 12.

B. Phrenic Nerve Palsy: Tumor destruction of the phrenic nerve, which courses through the mediastinum to innervate the hemidiaphragm, occurs in about 1% of patients with lung cancer and results in hemidiaphragmatic paralysis.

C. Recurrent Laryngeal Nerve Palsy: Recurrent laryngeal nerve palsy due to destruction of the

Table 9–14. TNM staging for lung cancer.[1]

Stage	T	N	M
0	Tis		
IA	T1	N0	M0
IB	T2	N0	M0
IIA	T1	N1	M0
IIB	T2	N1	M0
	T3	N0	M0
IIIA	T3	N1	M0
	T1	N2	M0
	T2	N2	M0
	T3	N2	M0
IIIB	T4	N0	M0
	T4	N1	M0
	T4	N2	M0
	T1	N3	M0
	T2	N3	M0
	T3	N3	M0
	T4	N3	M0
IV	Any	Any	M1

Primary Tumor (T)

TX	Primary tumor cannot be assessed; or tumor proved by the presence of malignant cells in sputum or bronchial washings but not visualized by imaging or bronchoscopy.
T0	No evidence of primary tumor.
Tis	Carcinoma in situ.
T1	A tumor ≤ 3 cm in greatest dimension, surrounded by lung or visceral pleura, and without evidence of invasion proximal to a lobar bronchus at bronchoscopy.
T2	A tumor > 3.0 cm in greatest dimension, or a tumor of any size that either involves a main bronchus (but is ≥ 2 cm distal to the carina), invades the visceral pleura, or has associated atelectasis or obstructive pneumonitis extending to the hilar region. Any associated atelectasis or obstructive pneumonitis must involve less than an entire lung.
T3	A tumor of any size with direct extension into the chest wall (including superior sulcus tumors), the diaphragm, the mediastinal pleura, or the parietal pericardium; or a tumor in the main bronchus < 2 cm distal to the carina without involving the carina; or associated atelectasis or obstructive pneumonitis of the entire lung.
T4	A tumor of any size with invasion of the mediastinum, heart, great vessels, trachea, esophagus, vertebral body, or carina; or with a malignant pleural or pericardial effusion; or with satellite tumor nodules within the ipsilateral lobe of the lung containing the primary tumor.

Regional Lymph Nodes (N)

NX	Regional lymph nodes cannot be assessed.
N0	No demonstrable metastasis to regional lymph nodes.
N1	Metastasis to lymph nodes in the peribronchial or the ipsilateral hilar region, or both, including direct extension.
N2	Metastasis to ipsilateral mediastinal lymph nodes and/or subcarinal lymph nodes.
N3	Metastasis to contralateral mediastinal lymph nodes, contralateral hilar lymph nodes, ipsilateral or contralateral scalene or supraclavicular lymph nodes.

Distant Metastases (M)

MX	Presence of distant metastasis cannot be assessed.
M0	No (known) distant metastasis.
M1	Distant metastasis present.

[1]Adapted from Mountain CF: Revisions in the international system for staging lung cancer. Chest 1997;111:1710.

recurrent laryngeal nerve by tumor causes paralysis of the muscles of the larynx, resulting in hoarseness. This palsy almost always occurs on the left side and is seen in fewer than 3% of patients with lung cancer.

Treatment

The main treatment options in lung cancer include surgery, chemotherapy, and radiation therapy. Photoresection with the Nd:YAG laser is sometimes performed on obstructing central tumors to relieve dyspnea and control hemoptysis.

Surgery remains the treatment of choice for patients with non-small cell carcinoma. Unfortunately, only about 25% of patients with lung cancer are appropriate candidates for surgery, and many of these are found to have unresectable disease at the time of thoracotomy. Contraindications to surgery include extrathoracic metastases; tumor involving the trachea, carina, or proximal main stem bronchi (< 2 cm from the carina); malignant pleural effusion; recurrent laryngeal nerve or phrenic nerve palsy; superior vena cava syndrome; tumor involving the esophagus or pericardium; spread to contralateral mediastinal lymph nodes; poor general health; and extensive involvement of the chest wall. Brain metastases of bronchogenic carcinoma have traditionally been considered unresectable and managed with radiation therapy and corticosteroids. However, one study indicates improved survival and quality of life when selected patients with *solitary* brain metastases are treated with surgical resection followed by radiation therapy compared to those given radiation therapy alone.

Patients with lung cancer often have severe obstructive pulmonary dysfunction. Therefore, pulmonary function testing and measurement of arterial blood gases should be performed before lung resection. Patients whose FEV_1 is less than 2 L, those whose FVC is less than 70% of predicted, and those whose maximum voluntary ventilation is less than 50% of predicted will tolerate pneumonectomy poorly. The preferred approach is to estimate the postresection FEV_1, using preoperative spirometry and a quantitative ventilation/perfusion lung scan. The percentage of total ventilation or perfusion that will remain after resection is estimated and multiplied by the optimal preoperative FEV_1. Values greater than 800 mL or 40% of predicted FEV_1 suggest that the patient will have adequate postoperative ventilatory function. However, the accuracy of such predictions has been questioned, and the cost of ventilation/perfusion lung scanning must be taken into consideration. Patients with hypercapnia ($PaCO_2$ > 45 mm Hg) and those with significant pulmonary hypertension are in general not good candidates for lung resection. Older patients with severe COPD are especially likely to be functionally inoperable.

In patients with non-small cell carcinoma, adjuvant therapy (chemotherapy, radiation therapy, or both given in the postoperative period) has yielded disappointing results. Single agent chemotherapy given postoperatively is of no value. In patients with stage II and stage III adenocarcinoma and large cell carcinoma, chemotherapy with a combination of three drugs for completely resected tumors apparently increases disease-free survival. In patients with incompletely resected non-small cell carcinoma, postoperative radiation therapy is frequently administered, and data suggest that the disease-free survival is further extended when postoperative radiation therapy is used with multidrug chemotherapy. One study suggests that neoadjuvant therapy (combination chemotherapy given prior to surgical resection) improves resectability and survival in patients with non-small cell carcinoma.

In unresectable non-small-cell carcinoma, radiation therapy combined with cisplatin-based chemotherapy appears to be superior to radiation therapy alone in regional control of tumor. Cisplatin is thought to increase sensitization to radiation.

Combination chemotherapy (see Chapter 4) is the treatment of choice for small cell carcinoma and results in considerable improvement in median survival. Single-agent chemotherapy has no proved value. Occasionally, posttreatment surgical debulking of primary lesions is carried out. Prophylactic cranial radiation is performed in patients with small cell carcinoma who have responded to chemotherapy. Although tumor regression in non-small cell carcinoma is possible with combination chemotherapy, median survival is improved only modestly, often at the expense of considerable drug toxicity.

Radiation therapy is often used to palliate symptoms of lung cancer such as cough, hemoptysis, pain due to bone metastases, and dyspnea from bronchial or tracheal obstruction. It is also employed to treat bronchial obstruction (atelectasis, pneumonia). Laser therapy is superior when the obstructing lesion is in a main stem bronchus. Radiation is also useful to treat superior vena cava syndrome resulting from non-small cell carcinoma; small cell carcinoma may be treated with chemotherapy or radiation. Symptomatic brain metastases are treated with radiation therapy and corticosteroids. Selected patients with unresectable lung cancer also receive external beam radiation to the primary tumor site. In patients with limited-stage small cell carcinoma, this improves complete response rates and survival when compared to chemotherapy alone. However, in non-small cell lung cancer, survival is not improved. Intraluminal radiation ("brachytherapy") is an alternative approach to relief of symptoms of recurrent endobronchial lung cancer.

Prognosis

The overall 5-year survival rate for lung cancer is 10–15%. Determinants of survival include the stage of disease at the time of presentation (Table 9–15),

Table 9–15. Approximate 5-year survival rate of treated patients with lung cancer by TNM stage.

TNM Stage	Survival
Occult carcinoma	70–80%
0	No data available
I	50%
II	30%
IIIA	10–15%
IIIB	<5%
IV	<2%

the patient's general health, age, histologic type of tumor, tumor growth rate, and type of therapy. Overall, the 5-year survival rate after "curative" resection of squamous cell carcinoma is 35–40%, compared with 25% for adenocarcinoma and large cell carcinoma. Patients with small cell carcinoma rarely live for 5 years after the diagnosis is made.

Bechtel JJ et al: Outcome of 51 patients with roentgenographically occult lung cancer detected by sputum cytologic testing: A community hospital program. Arch Intern Med 1994;154:975. (Sputum cytology by an expert cytopathologist is valuable in the early detection of lung cancer.)

Cook RM, Miller YE (editors): Lung cancer: Future directions. Sem Respir Crit Care Med 1996;17:283. (Tobacco control, smoking cessation, early detection, staging, treatment, and other topics)

McVie JG (editor): NSCLC: Planning for the future. Chest 1996;109(Suppl):S79. (A compendium of 14 articles on non-small-cell lung cancer.)

Mountain CF: Revisions in the international system for staging lung cancer. Chest 1997;111:1710.

Pugatch RD: Radiologic evaluation in chest malignancies: A review of imaging modalities. Chest 1995;107 (Suppl):294S. (Current practice standards for computed tomography and magnetic resonance imaging in non-small-cell lung cancer.)

Ruckdeschel JC: The Lung Cancer Study Group: Final analysis. Chest 1994;106(Suppl):279S. (Compendium of 32 articles on lung cancer management by Lung Cancer Study Group investigators.)

Wang K-P: Staging of bronchogenic carcinoma by bronchoscopy. Chest 1994;106:588. (Incorporates transbronchial needle aspiration into staging.)

Wang K-P: Transbronchial needle aspiration and percutaneous needle aspiration for staging and diagnosis of lung cancer. Clin Chest Med 1995;16:535. (Transbronchial needle aspiration of mediastinal and hilar lymph nodes is an effective and safe procedure.)

Zeiher BG et al: Predicting postoperative pulmonary function in patients undergoing lung resection. Chest 1995;108:68. (A mathematical formula underestimated postoperative FEV_1 and FVC.)

SOLITARY PULMONARY NODULE

A solitary pulmonary nodule is a round or oval, sharply circumscribed pulmonary lesion (up to 5 cm in diameter; larger lesions are termed "masses") surrounded by normal lung tissue. Central cavitation, calcification, or surrounding ("satellite") lesions may occur. Although mass population screening for lung cancer by chest x-ray is not advised, the finding of a solitary pulmonary nodule on chest x-ray in an individual patient is important. About 25% of cases of bronchogenic carcinoma present as solitary pulmonary nodules, and the 5-year survival rate for bronchogenic carcinoma that is detected in this form approaches 50%, which is considerably higher than the 10–15% 5-year survival rate of lung cancer overall.

In large surgical series, about 60% of solitary pulmonary nodules are benign lesions and 40% are malignant. Infectious granulomas account for most benign lesions, whereas primary lung cancer accounts for more than three-quarters of all malignant solitary pulmonary nodules. Solitary pulmonary nodules occasionally represent metastases from another primary tumor (see below). Determining whether the lesion is likely to be benign or malignant preoperatively is more important than establishing its precise cause.

A lesion is almost certainly benign if the volume doubling time is less than 30 days or more than 500 days or if the lesion is calcified (central, "clustered," or laminated calcium pattern). Factors favoring a benign diagnosis are young age, absence of symptoms, small size (< 2 cm in diameter), smooth margins on CT, and presence of satellite lesions, but none of these criteria are foolproof. Malignant solitary pulmonary nodules are occasionally symptomatic, tend to occur in patients over 45 years of age, are usually larger than 2 cm, often have indistinct margins, and are rarely calcified. Typical features of solitary pulmonary metastases include smooth or lobulated margins, peripheral location, location in the lower lobe, and absence of satellite lesions.

Skin tests and serologic studies for fungal infection are generally not helpful. Cytologic examination of sputum should be considered for evaluation of a large centrally located pulmonary nodule; a positive result might preclude the need for bronchoscopy or needle biopsy. However, sputum cytology is rarely diagnostic of malignancy in small or peripheral pulmonary nodules. Radiographic studies and *comparisons with old chest radiographs* are of utmost importance. CT scanning is particularly useful. Thin section (1.5–5 mm) CT scanning is the preferred method for detection of calcification within the nodule. Investigations for primary cancer elsewhere in the body are not indicated unless abnormal symptoms, signs, and results of simple laboratory studies (complete blood count and differential, urinalysis, stool sample for occult blood) suggest an extrapulmonary cancer. Routine percutaneous needle aspiration of all solitary pulmonary nodules is not advised; it seldom changes subsequent therapy, and false negatives are common. A specific benign diagnosis from a percutaneous needle biopsy is obtained infrequently except in a few centers with great expertise in this procedure. Therefore, in most cases this procedure cannot be justified with the expectation that a specific benign diagnosis will be obtained. Furthermore, if the history, physical examination, and radiographic and laboratory studies indicate that the patient is a candidate for surgical resection, a separate preoperative fiberoptic bronchoscopic procedure for staging purposes is not necessary.

Treatment

The best approaches to this problem are "watchful waiting," fiberoptic bronchoscopy, percutaneous needle aspiration, and resection. All solitary nodules in patients over age 35 should be considered potentially malignant and should be resected unless calcification typical of benign lesions or stability on radiography for 2 years is documented. Prospective evaluation is not appropriate if calcification is not present or if stability cannot be documented.

Strong indications of a benign diagnosis or contraindications to surgery justify a conservative approach. Otherwise, exploratory thoracotomy is advised. **Video-assisted thoracoscopy** is becoming increasingly popular as a safe and accurate way to perform a number of thoracic surgical procedures that previously required thoracotomy, including resection of solitary pulmonary nodules. The morbidity and mortality rates of this procedure are much less than those reported with standard thoracotomy. Decision analysis suggests that the average life expectancy of patients with solitary pulmonary nodules is similar, whether immediate surgery, biopsy, or observation is chosen as the initial approach.

Dholakia S, Rappaport DC: The solitary pulmonary nodule. Is it malignant or benign? Postgrad Med 1996;99:246. (A brief review of diagnostic strategies.)

Lillington GA: Management of solitary pulmonary nodules: How to decide when resection is required. Postgrad Med 1997;101:145. (Practical approach to management.)

Mitruka S et al: Diagnosing the indeterminate pulmonary nodule: Percutaneous biopsy versus thoracoscopy. Surgery 1995;118:676. (Biopsy with thoracoscopy is usually necessary because of the low rate (6%) of specific benign diagnoses with percutaneous biopsy.)

Schwarz CD et al: VATS (video-assisted thoracic surgery) of undefined pulmonary nodules. Preoperative evaluation of videoendoscopic resectability. Chest 1994;106: 1570. (The role of VATS and its limitations in resection of resection of pulmonary nodules.)

SECONDARY LUNG CANCER

Secondary lung cancers represent metastases from extrapulmonary malignant neoplasms that spread to the lungs through vascular or lymphatic channels or by direct extension. Almost any cancer can metastasize to the lung. Metastases to the lung usually occur via the pulmonary artery and typically present as multiple masses on chest radiography. Metastases to the lungs are found in 20–54% of patients dying of various malignancies.

Lymphangitic carcinoma denotes diffuse involvement of the pulmonary lymphatic network by secondary lung cancer, probably a result of extension of tumor from lung capillaries to the lymphatics. **Tumor embolization** from extrapulmonary cancer (renal cell carcinoma, hepatocellular carcinoma, choriocarcinoma) is an uncommon route tumor spread to the lungs. Endobronchial metastases occur in fewer than 5% of patients dying of nonpulmonary cancer; most metastases are intraparenchymal. Carcinoma of the kidney, breast, colon, and cervix and malignant melanoma are the tumors most likely to cause endobronchial metastases. Secondary lung cancer may also present as malignant pleural effusion (see below).

Clinical Findings

A. Symptoms and Signs: Symptoms are uncommon but include cough, hemoptysis, and, in advanced cases, dyspnea. Symptoms are more often referable to the site of the primary tumor.

B. Laboratory Findings: The diagnosis of secondary lung cancer is usually established by identifying the primary tumor. Appropriate studies should be ordered if there is a suspicion of any primary cancer, such as breast, thyroid, testis, or prostate, for which specific treatment is available. Mammography should be considered unless results of a recent mammogram are available. If the history and physical examination fail to reveal the site of the primary tumor, attention is better focused on the lung, where tissue samples obtained by bronchoscopy, needle biopsy, or thoracotomy establish the histologic diagnosis and suggest the most likely primary. Occasionally, cytologic studies of pleural fluid or pleural biopsy reveal the diagnosis. Sputum cytology is rarely helpful.

C. Imaging: Chest radiographs usually show multiple spherical densities with sharp margins. The size of metastatic lesions varies from a few millimeters (miliary densities) to large masses. Nearly all are less than 5 cm in diameter. The lesions are usually bilateral, pleural or subpleural in location, and more common in lower lung zones. Cavitation suggests primary squamous cell tumor; calcification suggests osteosarcoma. Conventional chest radiography is less sensitive than CT scan in detecting pulmonary metastases. The radiographic differential diagnosis of multiple pulmonary nodules includes pulmonary arteriovenous malformation, pulmonary abscesses, granulomatous infection, sarcoidosis, rheumatoid nodules, and Wegener's granulomatosis.

Diffuse lymphangitic spread and the solitary pulmonary nodule are less common radiographic presentations of secondary lung cancer.

Treatment

Once the diagnosis of secondary lung cancer has been established (usually by percutaneous needle biopsy or transbronchial biopsy), management consists of treatment of the primary neoplasm and any pulmonary complications. Surgical resection of a *solitary* pulmonary nodule is often prudent in the patient with known current or previous extrapulmonary cancer. Local resection of one or more pulmonary metastases is feasible in a few carefully selected patients with various sarcomas and carcinomas (breast, testis, colon, kidney, and head and neck). Surgical resection should be considered only if the primary tumor is under control, if the patient is a good surgical risk, if all of the metastatic tumor can be resected, if nonsurgical approaches are not available, and if there are no metastases elsewhere in the body. Relative contraindications to resection of pulmonary metastases include (1) malignant melanoma, (2) requirement for pneumonectomy, (3) pleural involvement, and (4) simultaneous appearance of two or more metastases. The overall 5-year survival rate in secondary lung cancer treated surgically is 20–35%.

Rusch VW: Pulmonary metastasectomy: Current indications. Chest 1995;107(Suppl):322S. (Patient selection and surgical approach.)

MESOTHELIOMA

Mesotheliomas are primary tumors arising from the surface lining of the pleura (80% of cases) or peritoneum (20% of cases). About three-fourths of pleural mesotheliomas are diffuse (usually malignant) tumors, and the remaining one-fourth are localized (usually benign). Men outnumber women by a 3:1 ratio. Numerous studies have confirmed the association of **malignant pleural mesothelioma** with exposure to asbestos (particularly the crocidolite form). The lifetime risk to asbestos workers of developing malignant pleural mesothelioma is about 8%. The physician should inquire about asbestos exposure through mining, milling, manufacturing, shipyard work, insulation, brake linings, building construction and demolition, roofing materials, and a variety of asbestos products (pipe, textiles, paint, tile, gaskets, panels). About 70–80% of patients with malignant pleural mesothelioma report a history of asbestos exposure. Although cigarette smoking increases the risk of bronchogenic carcinoma in asbestos workers and aggravates asbestosis, there is no association between smoking and mesothelioma.

The mean age at onset of symptoms of malignant pleural mesothelioma is about 60 years. The latent period between exposure and onset of symptoms ranges from 20 to 40 years. Symptoms include the insidious onset of shortness of breath, nonpleuritic chest pain, and weight loss. Physical findings include dullness to percussion, diminished breath sounds, and, in some cases, finger clubbing. Radiographic abnormalities consist of nodular, irregular, unilateral pleural thickening and varying degrees of unilateral pleural effusion. CT scan helps demonstrate the extent of pleural involvement.

Pleural fluid is exudative and often hemorrhagic. Open pleural biopsy is usually necessary to obtain an adequate specimen for histologic diagnosis; even then, distinction from benign inflammatory conditions and from metastatic adenocarcinoma may be difficult. The histologic variants of malignant pleural mesothelioma are epithelial and fibrous (sarcomatous). Special stains and electron microscopy may be needed to confirm the diagnosis.

Malignant pleural mesothelioma progresses rapidly as the tumor spreads quickly along the pleural surface to involve the pericardium, mediastinum, and contralateral pleura. The tumor may eventually extend beyond the thorax to involve abdominal lymph nodes and organs. Progressive pain and dyspnea are characteristic. Median survival time from onset of symptoms ranges from 5 months in extensive disease to 16 months in localized disease, and about 75% of patients are dead within 1 year after diagnosis. Treatment with surgery, radiotherapy, chemotherapy, and a combination of methods has been attempted but is generally unsuccessful. Some surgeons claim that extrapleural pneumonectomy is the preferred surgical approach for patients with early stage disease. Drainage of pleural effusions, pleurodesis, radiation therapy, and even resectional surgery may offer palliative benefit in some patients.

Aisner J: Current approach to malignant mesothelioma of the pleura. Chest 1995;107(Suppl):332S. (The role of chemotherapy, surgery, radiation therapy, and intrapleural therapy.)

Antman KH: Natural history and epidemiology of malignant mesothelioma. Chest 1993;103(Suppl):S373. (Overview of asbestos, asbestos-related cancer risk, and diagnosis and management of mesiothelioma.)

Jett JR: Malignant pleural mesothelioma: A proposed new staging system. Chest 1995;108:895. (A basis for future studies of a cancer with a very poor prognosis.)

BENIGN TUMORS OF THE LUNG

Benign neoplasms of the lung typically present as asymptomatic solitary pulmonary nodules detected on routine chest radiography. They account for about 2% of all solitary pulmonary nodules.

Hamartoma is the most common benign lung tumor. Fibromas, lipomas, leiomyomas, hemangiomas, and papillomas account for most of the remainder. The clustered ("popcorn") pattern of calcification on chest x-ray or CT scans is a helpful diagnostic clue to hamartoma.

The medical history, physical examination, and radiographic studies do not permit reliable differentiation of malignant and benign lung tumors. Percutaneous needle biopsy, guided by fluoroscopy or CT scanning and using a needle large enough (18- to 20-gauge) to obtain a core of tissue, is infrequently successful in establishing a *specific* benign diagnosis. However, because of the suspicion of bronchogenic carcinoma, most patients will require thoracotomy for definitive diagnosis. Patients who are poor operative risks may be followed with serial chest films for progression. Even if cancer is present, short periods of observation do not appreciably affect the prognosis.

BRONCHIAL CARCINOID TUMORS

Carcinoid and bronchial gland tumors are sometimes termed bronchial adenomas, but this classification is a misnomer, because it implies that the lesions are benign, when in fact carcinoid tumors and bronchial gland carcinomas are low-grade malignant neoplasms.

Carcinoid tumors are about six times more common than bronchial gland carcinomas, and most of them occur as pedunculated or sessile growths in central bronchi. Men and women are equally affected. Most patients are under 60 years of age. Common symptoms of bronchial carcinoid tumors are hemoptysis, cough, wheezing, and recurrent pneumonia. Peripherally located bronchial carcinoid tumors are rare and present as asymptomatic solitary pulmonary nodules. Carcinoid syndrome (flushing, diarrhea, wheezing, hypotension, etc) is rare. Fiberoptic bronchoscopy reveals a pink or purple tumor in a central airway, and biopsy may be complicated by significant bleeding, because these lesions have a well-vascularized stroma. CT scanning is helpful to localize the lesion and to follow its growth over time. Octreotide scintigraphy is also available for localization of these tumors.

Bronchial carcinoid tumors grow slowly and rarely metastasize. Complications involve bleeding and airway obstruction rather than invasion by tumor and metastases. Surgical excision is necessary in some cases, and the prognosis is generally favorable. Most bronchial carcinoid tumors are resistant to radiation and chemotherapy.

Christin-Maitre S et al: Use of somatostatin analog for localization and treatment of ACTH secreting bronchial carcinoid tumor. Chest 1996;109:845. (Octreotide scintigraphy.)

Davila DG et al: Bronchial carcinoid tumors. Mayo Clin Proc 1993;68:795. (General review of clinical and pathologic features.)

MEDIASTINAL MASSES

Various developmental, neoplastic, infectious, traumatic, and cardiovascular disorders may cause masses that appear in the mediastinum on chest x-ray. A useful convention arbitrarily divides the mediastinum into three compartments—anterior, middle, and posterior—in order to classify mediastinal masses and assist in differential diagnosis. Specific mediastinal masses have a predilection for one or more of these compartments; most are located in the anterior or middle compartment. The differential diagnosis of an anterior mediastinal mass includes thymoma, teratoma, thyroid lesions, lymphoma, and mesenchymal tumors (lipoma, fibroma). The differential diagnosis of a middle mediastinal mass includes lymphadenopathy, pulmonary artery enlargement, aneurysm of the aorta or innominate artery, developmental cyst (bronchogenic, enteric, pleuropericardial), dilated azygous or hemiazygous vein, and foramen of Morgagni hernia. The differential diagnosis of a posterior mediastinal mass includes hiatus hernia, neurogenic tumor, meningocele, esophageal tumor, foramen of Bochdalek hernia, thoracic spine disease, and extramedullary hematopoiesis. The neurogenic tumor group includes neurilemmoma, neurofibroma, neurosarcoma, ganglioneuroma, pheochromocytoma, and others.

Symptoms and signs of mediastinal masses are nonspecific and are usually caused by the effects of the mass on surrounding structures. Insidious onset of retrosternal chest pain, dysphagia, or dyspnea is often an important clue to the presence of a mediastinal mass. In about half of cases, symptoms are absent, and the mass is detected on routine chest x-ray. Physical findings vary depending upon the nature and location of the mass.

CT scanning is helpful in management; additional radiographic studies of benefit include barium swallow if esophageal disease is suspected, Doppler sonography or venography of brachiocephalic veins and the superior vena cava, and arteriography. MRI is also useful; its advantages include distinction between vessels and masses, no need for contrast media, and better delineation of hilar structures. MRI also allows imaging in multiple planes, whereas CT permits only axial imaging. Tissue diagnosis is necessary if a neoplastic disorder is suspected. Treatment and prognosis depend on the underlying cause of the mediastinal mass.

Goldberg M, Burkes RL: Current management of mediastinal tumors. Oncology 1994;8:99. (Current management of benign and malignant mediastinal tumors.)

INTERSTITIAL LUNG DISEASES

Interstitial lung diseases comprise a heterogeneous group of disorders that have in common the features of inflammation and fibrosis of the interalveolar septum, which represent a nonspecific reaction of the lung to injury of diverse cause. About 180 disease entities share the manifestations of interstitial lung disease (Table 9–16). In the majority of patients, no specific cause can be identified. In the remainder, drugs and a variety of inorganic and organic dusts are the predominant causes.

The pathogenesis of interstitial lung disease of un-

Table 9–16. Selected interstitial lung diseases.[1]

Known Cause	Unknown Cause
Inorganic dusts	Cryptogenic fibrosing alveo-
Silica	litis
Silicates (including asbes-	Sarcoidosis
tos)	Langerhans cell
Aluminum	granulomatosis
Antimony	Rheumatic disease-
Carbon	associated
Beryllium	Goodpasture's syndrome
Hard metal dusts	Idiopathic pulmonary
Organic dusts (hypersensi-	hemosiderosis
tivity pneumonitis)	Wegener's granulomatosis
Gases, fumes, vapors	Lymphomatoid
Chlorine	granulomatosis
Sulfur dioxide	Churg-Strauss syndrome
Mercury	Angioimmunoblastic
Drugs	lymphadenopathy
Antineoplastic agents	Inherited diseases
Antibiotics	Tuberous sclerosis
Sulfonamides	Neurofibromatosis
Penicillins	Pulmonary veno-occlusive
Nitrofurantoin	disease
Drugs inducing lupus	Ankylosing spondylitis
erythematosus	Amyloidosis
Sulfonylureas	Chronic eosinophilic
Gold	pneumonia
Phenytoin	Pulmonary
Penicillamine	lymphangiomyomatosis
Amiodarone	Whipple's disease
Poisons	Alveolar proteinosis
Paraquat	Inflammatory bowel disease-
Radiation	associated
Infections	
Disseminated mycobacte-	
rial or fungal infections	
Viral pneumonia	
Pneumocystis carinii	
pneumonia	
Residue of active infection of	
any type	
Pulmonary edema	
Lymphangitic carcinoma	

[1]Modified and reproduced, with permission, from Crystal RG et al: Interstitial lung disease: Current concepts of pathogenesis, staging, and therapy. Am J Med 1981;70:542.

known etiology is believed to be lung injury that leads to inflammation of the interalveolar septum (alveolitis). Persistent alveolitis may lead to eventual irreversible interstitial fibrosis.

Interstitial lung diseases share common clinical, physiologic, and radiographic features. Exertional dyspnea and dry cough of insidious onset are the usual presenting symptoms. Chest examination is often notable for fine inspiratory crackles at the bases of the lung. Digital clubbing is common. Pulmonary function testing reveals a restrictive ventilatory defect and a decreased diffusing capacity for carbon monoxide. Hypoxemia, especially with exercise, is common. Diffuse ground-glass, nodular, reticular, or reticulonodular infiltrates that may progress to "honeycomb lung" are noted on chest x-ray. Infrequently, the chest x-ray is normal when lung biopsy demonstrates interstitial lung disease. Conventional and high-resolution CT scanning of the chest has proved to be valuable in the assessment of patients with chronic diffuse infiltrative lung disease, although a normal high-resolution CT scan does not rule out the presence of interstitial lung disease.

The history, physical examination, chest x-ray, and laboratory studies may provide evidence of a specific cause of interstitial lung disease. Sputum is usually minimal or nonexistent. Induced sputum is likely to yield useful diagnostic information only if pulmonary infection or malignancy is suspected. Lung biopsy via fiberoptic bronchoscopy, thoracotomy, or thoracoscopy and bronchoalveolar lavage are the procedures most commonly used to make a pathologic diagnosis.

Transbronchial biopsy using a fiberoptic bronchoscope is easily performed and is associated with a low morbidity rate, but the tissue specimens obtained are small, and sampling errors are common. Transbronchial biopsies and washings may be adequate to permit the diagnosis of diseases such as sarcoidosis, histiocytosis X, pneumocystis pneumonia, miliary tuberculosis, pulmonary alveolar proteinosis, and lymphangitic carcinomatosis. More acutely ill patients are best served by thoracoscopic biopsy rather than potentially nondiagnostic transbronchial biopsy. It is reasonable to begin with transbronchial biopsy in most patients because of the low rate of complications associated with this procedure. The risks of transbronchial biopsy include all the risks of routine bronchoscopy as well as of pneumothorax (about 5%) and bleeding (1–9%). If the results of bronchoalveolar lavage or transbronchial biopsy are nondiagnostic, surgical lung biopsy by video-assisted thoracoscopy is necessary.

Bronchoalveolar lavage is useful in the diagnosis of *P carinii* pneumonia and in selected patients with lung infection from other organisms (mycobacteria, fungi, cytomegalovirus, and *Legionella* species). It is occasionally employed for specific diagnosis of lung cancer, pulmonary alveolar proteinosis, histiocytosis

X, beryllium-induced lung disease, amiodarone-induced pneumonitis, or pulmonary hemorrhage in thrombocytopenic patients. A very high percentage of T lymphocytes in bronchoalveolar lavage fluid suggests sarcoidosis or hypersensitivity pneumonitis; a predominance of neutrophils, eosinophils, and macrophages suggests idiopathic pulmonary fibrosis. Lung scanning with Ga 67 is nonspecific and has no proved value in diagnosis or management of patients with interstitial lung disease, though it may have some role in the management of outpatients with pneumocystis pneumonia.

Known causes of interstitial lung disease are dealt with in their specific sections. The important idiopathic forms are discussed below.

Orens JB et al: The sensitivity of high-resolution CT in detecting idiopathic pulmonary fibrosis proved by open lung biopsy: A prospective study. Chest 1995;108:109. (High-resolution CT scanning was less sensitive than physiologic testing in detecting interstitial lung disease in symptomatic patients with biopsy-proved idiopathic pulmonary fibrosis.)

Raghu G (editor): Interstitial lung diseases. Part II. Semin Respir Crit Care Med 1994;15:1. (Five articles on diagnostic methods [pulmonary function and exercise tests, imaging, bronchoalveolar lavage], pathology, and management.)

Raghu G: Interstitial lung disease: A diagnostic approach. Are CT scan and lung biopsy indicated in every patient? Am J Respir Crit Care Med 1995;151:909. (The pros and cons of bronchoscopy techniques, CT scan, and surgical lung biopsy in diagnosis of interstitial lung disease.)

Schwarz MI: The acute (noninfectious) interstitial lung diseases. Compr Ther 1996;22:622. (Classification and clinical evaluation.)

CRYPTOGENIC FIBROSING ALVEOLITIS (Idiopathic Pulmonary Fibrosis)

Cryptogenic fibrosing alveolitis is the most common diagnosis among patients presenting with interstitial lung disease. Patients usually present in the sixth or seventh decade with the insidious onset of cough and dyspnea of months' to years' duration. Hamman-Rich syndrome is an uncommon rapidly progressive form of the illness. The disease is more common in men than in women. A familial form of the disease (autosomal dominant trait with variable penetrance) has been described. Some evidence suggests that cryptogenic fibrosing alveolitis is a smoking-related disease. Symptoms, physical findings, and results on pulmonary function tests are typical of those of interstitial lung disease and are described above. Chest x-ray abnormalities are highly variable and correlate poorly with functional and clinical status. Lower lung zone interstitial infiltrates of a reticular pattern are typical when the patient is first seen. High-resolution CT scan best demonstrates the extent of lung parenchymal fibrosis. Patchy subpleural reticular infiltrates and cystic air spaces, most apparent in the lower lung zones, are typical.

Serologic tests for antinuclear antibody and rheumatoid factor are frequently positive (20–40% of cases). The diagnosis of cryptogenic fibrosing alveolitis is usually based on the clinical presentation and exclusion of other specific diagnoses, usually by means of bronchoalveolar lavage or lung biopsy. Histologic examination of lung tissue reveals a combination of cellular infiltration and fibrosis of the alveolar septum. Desquamated mononuclear cells, mainly macrophages, may be observed within alveoli. Open or thoracoscopic lung biopsy for the diagnosis of cryptogenic fibrosing alveolitis is helpful to exclude other specific causes of interstitial lung disease. Its routine use for this purpose is controversial.

Treatment consists of supportive measures, supplemental oxygen, and corticosteroids. A clinical trial of corticosteroids is generally indicated in patients with progressive symptoms or deterioration in lung function. Daily prednisone—beginning at 1–1.5 mg/kg/d (up to 100 mg/d) for 6 weeks and tapering slowly over 3–6 months to a minimum maintenance dose of 0.25 mg/kg/d—is the mainstay of therapy. Cytotoxic drugs such as cyclophosphamide (100–120 mg orally once daily) and azathioprine (3 mg/kg up to 200 mg orally once daily) have also been used.

It is important to distinguish cryptogenic fibrosing alveolitis from bronchiolitis obliterans organizing pneumonia (BOOP) by clinical and radiographic features and lung biopsy if necessary because of the excellent response of the latter disorder to corticosteroid therapy. The PaO_2 at rest and during pulmonary exercise stress testing is superior to traditional pulmonary function tests to monitor the physiologic response to therapy. Almost half of patients experience subjective improvement with corticosteroid therapy, but only about 20–25% demonstrate objective improvement. Younger patients, those with a shorter duration of illness, and those with a histopathologic pattern that is more cellular than fibrotic are more likely to have a favorable response. The finding of a ground-glass pattern in the lung parenchyma on thin-section CT scanning predicts a more favorable response to therapy. Relentless progression of the disease with eventual respiratory insufficiency is inevitable, and the median survival time is about 4 years after the onset of symptoms. The 5-year survival rate is about 50%. Patients with idiopathic pulmonary fibrosis have an increased risk of developing lung cancer. Heart-lung and single-lung transplantation for highly selected patients with end-stage pulmonary fibrosis is available.

Meier-Sydow J et al: Idiopathic pulmonary fibrosis: Current clinical concepts and challenges in management. Semin Respir Crit Care Med 1994;15:77.

Newman LS, Rose CS, Maier LA: Sarcoidosis. N Engl J

Med 1997;336:1224. (Thorough review of epidemiology, pathogenesis, pathology, clinical features, and treatment with 159 references.)

SARCOIDOSIS

Sarcoidosis is a systemic disease of unknown cause characterized by granulomatous inflammation of the lung in about 90% of patients. The incidence is highest in North American blacks and northern European whites; among blacks, women are more frequently affected than men. Onset of disease is usually in the third or fourth decade.

Patients may present with malaise, fever, and dyspnea of insidious onset. Alternatively, sarcoidosis may present with symptoms referable to the skin, eyes, peripheral nerves, liver, kidney, or heart. Some patients are asymptomatic and come to medical attention after abnormal findings (typically bilateral hilar and paratracheal lymphadenopathy) on routine chest radiographs. Physical findings in the chest are typical of those associated with interstitial lung involvement, if the parenchyma is involved. Other findings may include skin rashes, erythema nodosum, parotid gland enlargement, hepatosplenomegaly, and lymphadenopathy.

Laboratory tests may show leukopenia, eosinophilia, an elevated erythrocyte sedimentation rate, and hypercalcemia (about 10% of patients) or hypercalciuria (20%). Angiotensin-converting enzyme (ACE) levels are elevated in 40–80% of patients with active sarcoidosis. This finding is neither sensitive nor specific enough to have diagnostic significance. ACE is derived from the cell membrane of epithelioid cells of the sarcoid granuloma. Its synthesis is controlled by T lymphocytes. Physiologic testing may reveal evidence of airflow obstruction, but restrictive changes of decreased lung volumes and diffusing capacity are more common signs. Skin test anergy is present in 70%.

Radiographic findings are variable and include bilateral hilar adenopathy alone (stage I), hilar adenopathy and parenchymal involvement (stage II), or parenchymal involvement alone (stage III). Parenchymal involvement is usually manifested radiographically by diffuse reticular infiltrates, but focal infiltrates, acinar shadows, nodules, and, rarely, cavitation may be seen. Pleural effusion is noted in fewer than 10% of patients.

The diagnosis of sarcoidosis generally requires histologic demonstration of noncaseating granulomas in biopsies from a patient with other typical associated manifestations. Other granulomatous diseases (eg, berylliosis, tuberculosis) must be ruled out. If indicated, biopsy of easily accessible sites, eg, palpable lymph nodes, skin lesions, or salivary glands, is likely to provide positive findings. Transbronchial lung biopsy has a high yield of positive findings, especially in patients with radiographic evidence of parenchymal involvement. Some clinicians believe that tissue biopsy is not necessary when stage I radiographic findings are detected in a clinical situation that strongly favors the diagnosis of sarcoidosis (eg, a young black woman with erythema nodosum). Biopsy is essential whenever clinical and radiographic findings suggest the possibility of an alternative diagnosis such as lymphoma. Bronchoalveolar lavage is useful in following the activity of sarcoidosis in selected patients but does not provide a specific diagnosis. Bronchoalveolar lavage fluid in sarcoidosis is usually characterized by an increase in lymphocytes and a high CD4/CD8 cell ratio.

Indications for treatment with oral corticosteroids include constitutional symptoms, hypercalcemia, iritis, arthritis, central nervous system involvement, granulomatous hepatitis, cutaneous lesions, and symptomatic pulmonary lesions. Long-term therapy is usually required over months to years. ACE serum levels usually fall with clinical improvement. Immunosuppressive drugs and cyclosporine have been tried, primarily when corticosteroid therapy has been exhausted, but experience with these drugs is limited.

About 20% of patients with lung involvement suffer irreversible lung impairment, characterized by progressive fibrosis, bronchiectasis, and cavitation. Pneumothorax, hemoptysis, mycetoma formation in lung cavities, and respiratory failure often complicate this advanced stage of sarcoidosis. Myocardial sarcoidosis occurs in about 5% of patients, sometimes leading to cardiomyopathy and troublesome cardiac arrhythmias and conduction disturbances. The outlook is best for patients with hilar adenopathy alone; radiographic involvement of the lung parenchyma is associated with a worse prognosis. Death due to pulmonary insufficiency occurs in about 5% of patients.

Newman LS, Rose CS, Maier LA: Sarcoidosis. N Engl J Med 1997;336:1224. (Thorough review of epidemiology, pathogenesis, pathology, clinical features, and treatment, with 159 references.)

INTERSTITIAL LUNG INVOLVEMENT IN OTHER DISEASES

Interstitial lung disease that clinically resembles cryptogenic fibrosing alveolitis has been described in a variety of rheumatic diseases. It also occurs with chronic active hepatitis, inflammatory bowel disease, biliary cirrhosis, autoimmune thrombocytopenia, and hemolytic anemia. Although other manifestations of these diseases usually dominate the clinical picture, interstitial lung disease may be symptomatic and progress to respiratory insufficiency, in which case treatment with anti-inflammatory drugs similar to those used in cryptogenic fibrosing alveolitis should be started. Nonspecific interstitial pneumonitis characterized by diffuse alveolar damage but lacking evidence of infection has been reported to account for one-third of all episodes of clinical pneumonitis in patients with AIDS.

MISCELLANEOUS INFILTRATIVE LUNG DISEASES

PULMONARY ANGIITIS & GRANULOMATOSIS

Wegener's granulomatosis is an idiopathic disease manifested by a combination of glomerulonephritis, necrotizing granulomatous vasculitis of the upper and lower respiratory tracts, and varying degrees of small vessel vasculitis (see Chapter 20). Complaints of chronic sinusitis are a common presentation; pulmonary symptoms occur less often. Arthralgias, fever, skin rash, and weight loss are frequent symptoms. Multiple nodular infiltrates, often with cavitation, are present on chest radiography. Tracheal stenosis and endobronchial disease are sometimes seen. Normochromic, normocytic anemia, mild leukocytosis, and thrombocytosis are common, and virtually all patients have an elevated erythrocyte sedimentation rate. Serum anti-neutrophil cytoplasmic antibodies (ANCAs) are helpful in the diagnosis and differential diagnosis of Wegener's granulomatosis. ANCAs that display a cytoplasmic immunofluorescent staining pattern (C-ANCAs) are elevated in about 90% of patients with active Wegener's granulomatosis and in about 40% of patients in remission. ANCAs that display a perinuclear immunofluorescent staining pattern (P-ANCAs) are not helpful in diagnosing Wegener's granulomatosis. The specificity of C-ANCA is about 90% in the diagnosis of Wegener's granulomatosis. Elevated levels are found in other types of vasculitis, rheumatoid arthritis, liver disease, and inflammatory bowel disease.

Establishing a diagnosis has required biopsy of lung, sinus tissue, or kidney with demonstration of necrotizing granulomatous vasculitis.

Lymphomatoid granulomatosis is a systemic disease manifested by granulomatous angiitis and a polymorphic cellular infiltrate consisting of atypical lymphocytoid and plasmacytoid cells. Any organs may be involved, but lung, brain, and skin are the most frequently affected. In contrast to Wegener's granulomatosis, the upper airway and kidneys are rarely involved clinically, though histologic evidence of cellular infiltration of the kidneys is frequently seen. The glomeruli are spared. Radiographic manifestations may include multiple nodular infiltrates or diffuse reticular infiltrates. The diagnosis is suggested by the characteristic pattern of lung, brain, and skin involvement and is confirmed by histologic findings. Lymphomatoid granulomatosis has a poor prognosis, since it evolves into malignant lymphoma in nearly half of patients.

Allergic angiitis and granulomatosis (Churg-Strauss syndrome) is an idiopathic multisystem vasculitis of small and medium-sized arteries that occurs in patients with asthma. Histologic features include fibrinoid necrotizing epithelioid and eosinophilic granulomas. The skin and lungs are most often involved, but other organs, including the heart, gastrointestinal tract, liver, and peripheral nerves, may also be affected. Marked peripheral eosinophilia is the rule. Abnormalities on chest radiographs range from transient infiltrates to multiple nodules. This illness may be part of a spectrum that includes polyarteritis nodosa.

Treatment of these disorders consists of combination therapy with corticosteroids and cyclophosphamide. Oral prednisone (1 mg/kg ideal body weight per day initially, tapering slowly to alternate-day therapy over 3–6 months) is the corticosteroid of choice; in Wegener's granulomatosis, some clinicians may omit the use of steroids. For fulminant vasculitis, therapy may be initiated with intravenous methylprednisolone for several days. Cyclophosphamide (2 mg/kg ideal body weight per day initially, with dosage adjustments to avoid neutropenia) is given daily by mouth for at least 1 year after complete remission is obtained. Five-year survival rates in patients with these vasculitis syndromes have been improved to about 90% by the combination therapy.

Complete remissions can be achieved in over 90% of patients with Wegener's granulomatosis. Several reports have suggested that the addition of trimethoprim-sulfamethoxazole to standard therapy may bring about remission of Wegener's granulomatosis, but controlled prospective studies of this antibiotic agent have not been reported. The role of trimethoprim-sulfamethoxazole remains controversial. It should be considered only for patients with minimal disease and no renal involvement.

Duna GF, Galperin C, Hoffman GS: Wegener's granulomatosis. Rheum Dis Clin North Am 1995;21:949. (Extensive review of diagnosis and treatment.)

Grotz W et al: Radiographic course of pulmonary manifestations in Wegener's granulomatosis under immunosuppressive therapy. Chest 1994;105:509. (The radiographic abnormalities should improve within 1 week if immunosuppressive therapy is adequate.)

Stegeman CA et al: Trimethoprim-sulfamethoxazole (cotrimoxazole) for the prevention of relapses of Wegener's granulomatosis. N Engl J Med 1996;335:16. (Prospective study suggesting that trimethoprim-sulfamethoxazole reduces the rate of relapses in patients with Wegener's granulomatosis who are in remission.)

ALVEOLAR HEMORRHAGE SYNDROMES

Diffuse alveolar hemorrhage may occur in a variety of immune and nonimmune disorders. Causes of **immune alveolar hemorrhage** have been classified as anti-basement membrane antibody disease (Goodpasture's syndrome), vasculitis and collagen vascular disease (systemic lupus erythematosus, Wegener's granulomatosis, systemic necrotizing vasculitis, and others), and hemorrhage associated with idiopathic rapidly progressive glomerulonephritis. Hemoptysis, alveolar infiltrates on chest x-ray, anemia, dyspnea, and occasionally fever are characteristic. All pulmonary hemorrhage is associated with increased $D_L CO$. **Nonimmune causes** of diffuse hemorrhage include coagulopathy, mitral stenosis, necrotizing pulmonary infection, drugs (penicillamine), toxins (trimellitic anhydride), and idiopathic pulmonary hemosiderosis. Bronchoalveolar lavage is helpful to determine whether diffuse alveolar hemorrhage has an immune or an infectious basis. Rapid clearing of marked diffuse lung infiltrates within 2 days is a clue to the possible diagnosis of diffuse alveolar hemorrhage. Diffuse alveolar hemorrhage is sometimes caused by pulmonary capillaritis, vasculitis of pulmonary capillaries and arterioles marked by infiltration of the alveolar interstitium by neutrophils.

Goodpasture's syndrome is idiopathic recurrent alveolar hemorrhage and rapidly progressive glomerulonephritis. The disease is mediated by antiglomerular basement membrane antibodies detected as a linear fluorescent pattern on immunofluorescence studies of the lung and kidneys. Goodpasture's syndrome occurs mainly in men who are in their 30s and 40s. Hemoptysis is the usual presenting symptom, but pulmonary hemorrhage may be occult. Dyspnea, cough, hypoxemia, and diffuse bilateral alveolar infiltrates are typical features. Iron deficiency anemia and microscopic hematuria are usually present. The diagnosis is based on characteristic linear IgG deposits in glomeruli by immunofluorescence and on the presence of anti-glomerular basement membrane antibody in serum. Goodpasture's syndrome resembles other pulmonary-renal syndromes, which include systemic lupus erythematosus, idiopathic rapidly progressive glomerulonephritis, Wegener's granulomatosis, systemic necrotizing vasculitis, and drug-induced disease (penicillamine, trimellitic anhydride). Combinations of immunosuppressive drugs (methylprednisolone with cyclophosphamide) and plasmapheresis have yielded excellent results in recent years. Long-term remissions are occasionally observed.

Idiopathic pulmonary hemosiderosis is a disease of children or young adults characterized by recurrent pulmonary hemorrhage; in contrast to Goodpasture's syndrome, renal involvement and anti-glomerular basement membrane antibodies are absent. Treatment of acute episodes of hemorrhage with corticosteroids may be useful. Recurrent episodes of pulmonary hemorrhage may result in interstitial fibrosis.

Crausman RS et al: Pulmonary capillaritis and alveolar hemorrhage associated with the antiphospholipid antibody syndrome. J Rheumatol 1995;22:554. (Case report and discussion.)

Green RJ et al: Pulmonary capillaritis and alveolar hemorrhage: Update on diagnosis and management. Chest 1996;110:1305. (Patients with pulmonary capillaritis usually present with diffuse alveolar hemorrhage associated with a variety of underlying disorders for which immunosuppressive therapy is usually required.)

PULMONARY ALVEOLAR PROTEINOSIS

Pulmonary alveolar proteinosis is a disease in which a phospholipid material similar to surfactant accumulates within alveolar spaces. The condition may be primary (idiopathic) or secondary (occurring in immune deficiency, hematologic malignancies, inhalation of mineral dusts, or following lung infections, including tuberculosis and viral infections). Progressive dyspnea is the usual presenting symptom, and chest x-ray shows bilateral alveolar infiltrates suggestive of pulmonary edema. The diagnosis is based on demonstration of characteristic findings on bronchoalveolar lavage (milky appearance and PAS-positive lipoproteinaceous material) in association with typical clinical and radiographic features. In some cases, transbronchial or open lung biopsy (revealing amorphous intra-alveolar phospholipid) is necessary.

The course of the disease varies; some patients experience spontaneous remission, whereas in others, progressive respiratory insufficiency develops. Pulmonary infection with *Nocardia* or fungi may occur. Therapy for alveolar proteinosis consists of periodic whole lung lavage, which is effective in reducing exertional dyspnea.

Wang BM et al: Diagnosing pulmonary alveolar proteinosis: A review and an update. Chest 1997;111:460. (Bronchoalveolar lavage is adequate for diagnosis in most cases.)

EOSINOPHILIC PULMONARY SYNDROMES

The term "chronic eosinophilic pneumonia" denotes a syndrome characterized by peripheral lung infiltrates shown to be eosinophilic by bronchoalveolar lavage or lung biopsy. Blood eosinophilia is present in most cases. Chronic eosinophilic pneumonia is predominantly a disorder of women characterized by fever, night sweats, weight loss, and dyspnea. Therapy with oral prednisone (1 mg/kg daily) usually results in dramatic improvement. An acute form has been described as well.

Löffler's syndrome consists of transient pulmonary infiltrates with cough, fever, and peripheral blood eosinophilia. This condition is associated with exposure to various drugs or infection with roundworm parasites such as filariae, *Ascaris*, or *Strongyloides*. No precipitating cause may be apparent in as many as one-third of cases. If an extrinsic cause is identified, therapy consists of removal of the offending drug or treatment of the underlying parasitic infection. Corticosteroid treatment should be instituted if no treatable extrinsic cause is discovered. The response to corticosteroids is usually dramatic. Recurrences are common.

Allen J, Davis WB: Eosinophilic lung diseases. Am J Respir Crit Care Med 1994;150:1423. (Extensive review of this diverse group of diseases.)

Pope-Harman AL et al: Acute eosinophilic pneumonia: A summary of 15 cases and review of the literature. Medicine 1996;75:334. (Sixty references.)

DISORDERS OF THE PULMONARY CIRCULATION

PULMONARY THROMBOEMBOLISM

Essentials of Diagnosis

- Predisposition to venous thrombosis, usually of the lower extremities.
- Abrupt onset of dyspnea, chest pain, apprehension, hemoptysis, or syncope.
- Acute respiratory alkalosis and hypoxemia in most patients.
- Characteristic defects on ventilation/perfusion lung scan.
- Diagnostic findings on pulmonary angiogram.

General Considerations

Pulmonary emboli arise from thrombi in the venous circulation or right side of the heart (thromboembolism), from tumors that have invaded the venous circulation (tumor emboli), or from other sources (amniotic fluid, air, fat, bone marrow, and foreign intravenous material).

Pulmonary thromboembolism is associated with as many as 250,000 hospitalizations and 50,000 deaths each year in the United States; about 10% of victims die within the first hour. Fewer than 10% of patients who die of pulmonary embolism have received treatment for the condition, a fact underscoring the difficulty encountered in diagnosis.

More than 90% of pulmonary emboli originate as clots in the deep veins of the lower extremities. Most deep venous thrombi originate in the calves, and some 80% of these spontaneously resolve without embolizing. The remainder may propagate into the iliofemoral veins. Fracture of the propagating thrombus in these proximal veins allows a clot to migrate into the inferior vena cava and ultimately to the lungs. One-third to one-half of patients with deep venous thrombosis of the iliofemoral system have clinically significant pulmonary embolism.

Physiologic risk factors for venous thrombosis include venous stasis, venous endothelial injury, and hypercoagulability (eg, oral contraceptives, cancer, protein C or S deficiency, antithrombin III deficiency, and deficiency of factor V Leyden). The latter has been recognized with increasing frequency and may be the most common specifically identified cause of venous hypercoagulability. Clinical risk factors include prolonged bed rest or inactivity, surgery, childbirth, advanced age, stroke, myocardial infarction, congestive heart failure, obesity, and fractures of the hip or femur. Occasionally, in situ thrombosis in the pulmonary arteries occurs without embolization; predisposing factors include sickle cell anemia, chest trauma, and certain congenital cardiac anomalies.

Discharge of thrombus into the pulmonary artery has both hemodynamic and pulmonary consequences. The hemodynamic consequences of pulmonary thromboembolism are related to mechanical obstruction of the pulmonary vascular bed and neurohumoral reflexes causing vasoconstriction. Both factors result in increased pulmonary vascular resistance and, in severe cases, pulmonary hypertension and right ventricular failure. The pulmonary consequences of thromboembolism result from reflex bronchoconstriction in the embolized lung zone, wasted ventilation (increased physiologic dead space), and loss of alveolar surfactant. Frank pulmonary infarction is uncommon.

Clinical Findings

A. Symptoms and Signs: The clinical findings in acute pulmonary thromboembolism (Table 9–17) depend on the size of the embolus and the patient's preexisting cardiopulmonary status. In pulmonary embolism that is less than massive, clot obstructs less than two-thirds of the pulmonary arterial tree. In *massive* pulmonary embolism, acute right ventricular failure and systemic hypotension result. Recognizing pulmonary thromboembolism is more difficult in patients with underlying cardiopulmonary disease. No single symptom or sign or combination of clinical findings is pathognomonic of pulmonary thromboembolism.

Symptoms of pulmonary thromboembolism in-

Table 9–17. Incidence of symptoms and signs of angiographically proved pulmonary thromboembolism in 327 patients.[1]

	(%)
Symptoms	
Chest pain	88
Pleuritic	74
Nonpleuritic	14
Dyspnea	84
Apprehension	59
Cough	53
Hemoptysis	30
Sweats	27
Syncope	13
Signs	
Respiratory rate	92
>16/min	
Crackles	58
Accentuated S_2P	53
Pulse > 100/min	44
Temperature > 37.8 °C	43
Phlebitis	32
Gallop	34
Diaphoresis	36
Edema	24
Murmur	23
Cyanosis	19

[1]Data from Bell WR, Simon TL, DeMets DL: The clinical features of submassive and massive pulmonary emboli. Am J Med 1977;62:355.

clude chest pain, which is often pleuritic, dyspnea, apprehension, cough, hemoptysis, and diaphoresis. Pulmonary embolism occasionally presents as syncope, especially in patients with massive pulmonary embolism.

The signs of pulmonary thromboembolism include tachycardia, tachypnea, crackles, and accentuation of the pulmonary component of the second heart sound. Low-grade fever occurs in about 40% of cases. Thrombophlebitis, diaphoresis, and right-sided cardiac gallop each are noted in about a third of cases. Cyanosis, wheezing, and cardiac arrhythmias are noted in fewer than one-fourth of cases. Shock is unusual. Symptoms and signs do not generally differ between massive and less severe thromboembolism. Pulmonary embolism may mimic pneumonia, myocardial infarction, pneumothorax, and even rib fractures. The clinician should be alert to other conditions that mimic thrombophlebitis of the calf, including cellulitis, muscle strain or rupture, lymphangitis, and rupture of a Baker's cyst.

B. Laboratory Findings: The results of routine laboratory tests are not helpful in diagnosing pulmonary thromboembolism. Arterial blood gas measurements usually reveal acute respiratory alkalosis due to hyperventilation. About 90% of patients with proved pulmonary embolism have an arterial PO_2 under 80 mm Hg. Electrocardiographic findings are likewise not diagnostic. Nearly all patients with pul-

monary thromboembolism have an abnormal ECG. Tachycardia and nonspecific ST–T wave changes are the most common abnormalities, being noted in about 44% and 35–49% of cases, respectively. A pattern of acute right heart strain (S_1Q_3, T wave inversion in leads V_{1-3}) is more characteristic but uncommon. Right axis deviation, right bundle branch block, clockwise rotation, and P pulmonale each are seen in less than 10% of cases of documented pulmonary thromboembolism. Standard pulmonary function tests are helpful only in consideration of alternative diagnoses. Specialized pulmonary function tests may reveal a nonspecific increase in wasted ventilation (increased physiologic dead space) and a failure of the ratio of tidal volume to dead space to fall with exercise, but such tests are not useful clinically. The efficacy and role of testing of blood for D-dimer fragments in evaluation of patients with suspected venous thromboembolism have not been established.

C. Imaging and Special Examinations:

1. Chest radiography–The chest radiograph is usually abnormal in patients with pulmonary embolism, but the abnormalities are often related to chronic pulmonary or cardiac disease. No pathognomonic findings are present. Elevation of a hemidiaphragm and pulmonary infiltration are the most common abnormalities. Plate-like atelectasis, oligemia in the embolized lung zone (Westermark sign), and prominence of the pulmonary artery are sometimes seen. A small unilateral pleural effusion is occasionally present. A homogeneous, wedge-shaped density based on the pleura and pointing toward the hilum (Hampton's hump) is highly suggestive of pulmonary infarction but is uncommon.

2. Lung scanning–Most if not all patients with suspected pulmonary embolism should undergo a ventilation/perfusion scan. Though ventilation/perfusion lung scans may be abnormal in other diseases, including COPD, asthma, pneumonia, and heart failure, their results may be used to direct subsequent pulmonary arteriography and reduce the load of contrast media in these patients.

Ventilation/perfusion lung scans are typically interpreted as being normal, low probability, intermediate (indeterminate) probability, or high probability for the presence of a pulmonary thromboembolism. Criteria for these interpretations are complex.

Some important principles underlie lung scan interpretation. First, a normal perfusion scan rules out clinically significant pulmonary thromboembolism, and no further diagnostic studies are necessary. A perfusion scan is normal if no perfusion defects are present or if the perfusion pattern matches exactly the shape of the lungs as shown on the chest x-ray. A high-probability ventilation/perfusion lung scan is one in which two or more large (or four or more moderate) segmental perfusion defects are present without corresponding ventilation defects or abnormalities on the chest x-ray or are substantially larger than those abnormalities. Interpretation of low and intermediate probabilities requires more expertise. Consultation with a specialist in nuclear medicine is essential when interpreting lung scans.

A "low-probability" ventilation/perfusion scan *does not exclude pulmonary thromboembolism.* Depending on the criteria used for scan interpretation, as many as 31% of patients with "low-probability" scan interpretations demonstrate pulmonary thromboemboli when pulmonary angiograms are performed. However, a high probability (85–90%) of pulmonary embolism exists when there is a lobar perfusion defect with ventilation mismatch. One-third of patients with an "intermediate probability" lung scan have positive pulmonary angiograms. Because of the high frequency of pulmonary embolism in patients with "low" or "intermediate" probability lung scan interpretations, some experts have advocated abandoning the current lung scan classification system and reporting scans as either normal, nondiagnostic, or of high probability. The diagnostic value of lung scanning is enhanced greatly when combined with the clinical estimate of the likelihood of pulmonary embolism or with the results of noninvasive studies for proximal deep vein thrombosis. For example, in patients with low-probability lung scans, pulmonary embolism is present in 40% of those with a high clinical suspicion of pulmonary thromboembolism but only 4% of those with a low clinical suspicion. The role of ventilation/perfusion lung scanning and pulmonary angiography in management of venous thromboembolism is summarized in Figure 9–2.

3. Venous thrombosis studies–Pulmonary thromboembolism can, in general, be thought of as a consequence of deep venous thrombosis of the lower extremities. The term "acute venous thromboembolism" combines the two diagnoses into one entity. This is a reasonable choice of words in view of the finding that about 40% of patients with deep venous thrombosis and no symptoms of pulmonary embolism have radiographic evidence of pulmonary embolism.

Accurate diagnosis of pulmonary thromboembolism often depends on detection of venous thrombi in the lower extremities. One invasive (venography) and four noninvasive (ultrasonography, impedance plethysmography, fibrinogen scanning, radionuclide venography) tests are available for this purpose (Chapter 12). One of these objective tests is often required, because the history and physical examination are neither sensitive nor specific in diagnosis. Documentation of deep venous thrombosis in a patient with suspected pulmonary thromboembolism may preclude the need for pulmonary angiography.

The diagnostic accuracy of these tests depends upon the expertise of the team performing the studies. Practitioners should be aware of which studies are most likely to be accurate in the setting of their own practices.

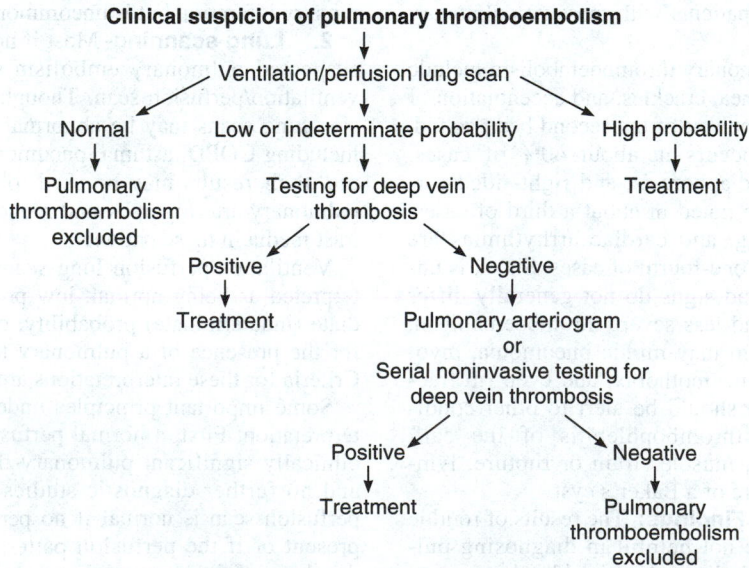

Clinical suspicion of pulmonary thromboembolism

Figure 9–2. A simple algorithm for the management of venous thromboembolism based on the results of ventilation/perfusion lung scanning. The algorithm starts with a clinical suspicion of pulmonary thromboembolism. Management of patients with ventilation/perfusion lung scans of low or indeterminate probability must always be guided by clinical judgment based upon cumulative clinical information and the degree of suspicion of pulmonary thromboembolism.

In most centers, ultrasonography techniques have become the procedure of choice to detect deep venous thrombosis in the femoral and popliteal veins. Properly performed, ultrasonography's sensitivity and specificity both exceed 95%. Duplex ultrasonography is particularly useful in patients without symptoms or signs of deep venous thrombosis in whom there is a high clinical suspicion of acute pulmonary thromboembolism. This test is not sensitive in the detection of thrombi in the iliac or calf veins. It is a highly operator-dependent test that requires considerable technical skill.

Impedance plethysmography is equivalent to ultrasonography for detection of thrombi in the femoral and popliteal veins and is the procedure of choice for suspected iliac vein thrombosis. However, it may miss early, nonocclusive thrombi. Impedance plethysmography is less operator-dependent than ultrasonography. Serial impedance plethysmography over 10–14 days may detect propagation of calf vein thrombi into the popliteal vein.

Because of its high sensitivity and specificity, contrast venography has been considered the standard in testing for venous thrombosis. An intraluminal filling defect is pathognomonic of venous thrombosis. However, about 30% of patients with angiographically proved pulmonary embolism have negative contrast venograms. Disadvantages of contrast venography include discomfort, difficulty in interpretation, expense, difficult technical requirements, and complications such as phlebitis in 3–4% of patients. It is less accurate below the knee. For these reasons, it has been replaced by noninvasive tests (ultrasonography or impedance plethysmography) as the procedure of choice for diagnosis.

If the physician suspects deep venous thrombosis, intravenous heparin should be started if there are no contraindications. Either ultrasonography or impedance plethysmography should be ordered, the choice depending primarily on local expertise. If one of these tests is positive, continued treatment is advised. If the noninvasive study is negative, it should be repeated serially (every 2 days for 7–10 days) until a positive result is obtained; if the results are repeatedly negative, therapy may be terminated. Contrast venography is advised if the noninvasive study yields equivocal results.

4. Pulmonary angiography–Pulmonary angiography—which can detect emboli as small as 3 mm in diameter—remains the definitive test for diagnosis of pulmonary embolism because of its high sensitivity and specificity. Emboli smaller than 3 mm in diameter are unlikely to be of clinical significance. The finding of an intraluminal defect or an arterial cutoff on the pulmonary angiogram is diagnostic. Oligemia and asymmetry of blood flow are suggestive but not specific. After 5 days, negative results on angiography do not rule out the possibility that an embolism has occurred.

Pulmonary angiography is expensive and invasive, occasionally difficult to interpret, and may be associated with complications. For these reasons, it is less than a perfect diagnostic test. In experienced hands, however, the procedure is associated with a morbidity and mortality rate of less than 1%. Used in a diagnostic algorithm with ventilation/perfusion lung scanning, pulmonary angiography is a cost-effective tool in the often difficult diagnosis of pulmonary thromboembolism. The procedure is advised when the diagnosis of pulmonary embolism must be established with certainty, as in situations where anticoagulation is considered especially risky. Ventilation/perfusion lung scans of "intermediate" probability for pulmonary thromboembolism are frequently encountered. Moreover, lung scans of suboptimal quality because of patient performance and technical limitations are commonplace. In these situations, pulmonary angiography is often valuable.

Pulmonary angiography is required if any type of surgical procedure for prevention of recurrent thromboemboli is planned, eg, interruption of the inferior vena cava. It is indicated in patients with suspected embolism whenever the diagnosis remains in doubt after preliminary studies (clinical evaluation, lung scans, tests for deep venous thrombosis) have been performed. Relative contraindications include severe pulmonary hypertension, ventricular arrhythmias, left bundle branch block, and renal failure. As in the use of radiocontrast materials for any purpose, precautions must be taken to prevent radiocontrast-induced acute renal failure and allergic reactions. Spiral CT scanning and MRI are occasionally diagnostic of large thromboemboli in the central pulmonary arteries, but the precise role of these imaging modalities in pulmonary thromboembolism has not yet been defined.

Prevention

Prevention of deep venous thrombosis and pulmonary thromboembolism is critically important. Physicians should institute the appropriate antithrombotic preventive measures whenever a patient is at risk. The current American College of Chest Physicians guidelines for prevention of venous thromboembolism are summarized in Table 9–18.

If low-dose heparin (unfractionated) is indicated, 5000 units subcutaneously is given every 8–12 hours, beginning 2 hours before surgery or upon admission to the hospital and continuing until the risk for deep vein thrombosis has lessened. Continuous monitoring of clotting studies is not necessary, though the partial thromboplastin time and platelet count should be checked occasionally, since some patients show increased sensitivity to heparin. The *adjusted-dose* heparin regimen is to administer just enough heparin subcutaneously every 8 hours to maintain the activated partial thromboplastin time, measured 6 hours after injection, at 31.5–36 seconds.

Table 9–18. Methods for the prevention of venous thromboembolism.[1]

Risk Group	Recommendations for Prophylaxis
Surgical patients	
General surgery	
Low risk (minor operations, age <40, and no clinical risk factors)	Early ambulation.
Moderate risk (major operations, age >40, and no other clinical risk factors)	Elastic stockings, or low-dose heparin (2 hours before surgery and every 12 hours after surgery), or intermittent pneumatic compression; plus intermittent pneumatic compression and elastic stockings (during and after surgery) if possible.
High risk (major operations, age >40, and additional risk factors or myocardial infarction)	Low-dose heparin every 8 hours, or LMW heparin.
Higher risk (major operations, age >40, and additional risk factors) and prone to wound hematoma or infection	Intermittent pneumatic compression.
Very high risk (multiple risk factors)	Low-dose heparin or LMW heparin (started before surgery); plus intermittent pneumatic compression (started during surgery) if possible.
Selected very high risk (major operations, age >40, and additional risk factors)	Perioperative warfarin (INR 2.0–3.0).
Orthopedic surgery	
Total hip replacement surgery	Subcutaneous fixed-dose LMW heparin twice daily, unmonitored (started after surgery); or low-intensity oral anticoagulation (INR 2.0–3.0; started before or immediately after surgery); or adjusted dose heparin (started before surgery); possibly adjuvant elastic stockings or intermittent pneumatic compression.
Total knee replacement surgery	Subcutaneous fixed-dose LMW heparin twice daily, unmonitored (started after surgery); or intermittent pneumatic compression.
Hip fracture surgery	Subcutaneous fixed-dose LMW heparin, unmonitored (started before surgery), or oral anticoagulation (INR 2.0–3.0); possibly adjuvant use of intermittent pneumatic compression.
Selected high-risk orthopedic or trauma patients in whom other preventive measures are not feasible	Consider prophylactic inferior vena cava filter.
Neurosurgery	
Intracranial neurosurgery	Intermittent pneumatic compression with or without elastic stockings; low-dose heparin may be an acceptable alternative; low-dose heparin with intermittent pneumatic compression should be considered in high-risk patients.
Acute spinal cord injury with paralysis	Adjusted-dose heparin, or LMW heparin, or warfarin; intermittent pneumatic compression, elastic stockings, and low-dose heparin may be effective only when used together.
Trauma	
Multiple trauma patients	Intermittent pneumatic compression, warfarin, or LMW heparin; consider serial surveillance with duplex ultrasonography; consider prophylactic inferior vena cava filter in selected very high risk patients.
Medical patients	
Acute myocardial infarction	Low-dose heparin or full-dose anticoagulation; if heparin is contraindicated, intermittent pneumatic compression and perhaps elastic stockings may be useful.
Ischemic stroke with paralysis of lower extremities	Low-dose heparin or LMW heparin; intermittent pneumatic compression and elastic stockings may also be effective.
General medical patients with clinical risk factors, particularly patients with congestive heart failure or chest infections	Low-dose heparin or LMW heparin.
Long-term central venous catheters	Warfarin (1 mg/d).

[1]Modified and reproduced, with permission, from Clagett GP et al: Prevention of venous thromboembolism. Chest 1995; 108(Suppl):312S. Copyright © 1995 by the American College of Chest Physicians.

Low-molecular-weight (LMW) heparin slightly reduces the rate of deep venous thrombosis in patients undergoing elective hip surgery and may be superior to standard heparin in preventing thromboembolism after spinal cord injury. LMW heparin may be preferable to standard heparin in reducing the risks of deep venous thrombosis and pulmonary thromboembolism in patients undergoing orthopedic surgery, as it is less hemorrhagic than standard heparin. Antiplatelet drugs such as aspirin are not recommended for the prevention (or treatment) of venous thrombosis or pulmonary thromboembolism.

Treatment

A. Anticoagulation: Anticoagulation for established pulmonary embolism is really preventive rather than definitive therapy. For acute pulmonary thromboembolism or proximal (thigh) deep venous thrombosis, heparin is the anticoagulant of choice.

Heparin inhibits thrombin and other clotting factors by potentiating antithrombin III; it does not dissolve established thrombi but does prevent their distal propagation. Heparin reduces the rate of recurrence of pulmonary embolism and the incidence of death due to recurrence.

If a diagnosis of venous thromboembolism is suspected and there are no contraindications to heparin, a baseline activated partial thromboplastin time (APTT), complete blood count, and prothrombin time are obtained, followed by administration of a bolus of 5000 units of heparin (American College of Chest Physicians guidelines). After the appropriate imaging study to establish the diagnosis of venous thromboembolism is obtained (Figure 9–2), the patient is given another bolus injection with 5000–10,000 units of heparin. A continuous heparin infusion at 1300 units/h is then started. The activated partial thromboplastin time (APTT) is checked 6 hours later and the infusion adjusted to maintain the APTT at 1.5–2.5 times control. The platelet count is monitored every day, because heparin may induce thrombocytopenia.

Oral anticoagulant therapy with warfarin may be started concurrently with heparin. Institution of warfarin on the first day of anticoagulation with heparin is as effective as the old practice of instituting it several days later. Earlier hospital discharge and cost savings should occur from this change in practice. Warfarin alters the synthesis of vitamin K-dependent procoagulants (factors II, VII, IX, and X) and proteins C and S and usually requires 6–7 days to achieve full effectiveness; treatment is begun with 5–10 mg of warfarin on the first day of heparin therapy and maintained with a daily dose of warfarin thereafter until the INR is 2.0–3.0 without heparin. Heparin is usually stopped after 4–7 days of overlap with warfarin. Maintenance therapy with warfarin may require 2–15 mg daily, the required dose varying widely among patients. Warfarin is contraindicated in pregnancy. Alterations in the prothrombin time in patients receiving warfarin may be caused by a number of drugs (Table 9–19). These effects require the physician to change the dose of warfarin and monitor the prothrombin time closely. If warfarin is contraindicated or inconvenient, subcutaneous heparin may be substituted for warfarin, the dose being adjusted to maintain an APTT of 1.5 times the control value at the mid-dosing interval.

The duration of warfarin therapy after thromboembolic disease has been diagnosed depends on the individual patient's clinical situation, and insufficient data have accrued to define the optimal duration of

Table 9–19. Some important drugs that alter the prothrombin time in patients taking warfarin.

Prothrombin Time Increased By		Prothrombin Time Decreased By
Acetaminophen	Metronidazole	Barbiturates
Amiodarone	Miconazole	Carbamazepine
Anabolic steroids	Omeprazole	Chlordiazepoxide
Aspirin	Phenylbutazone	Cholestyramine
Chloral hydrate	Phenytoin	Contraceptives,
Cimetidine	Piroxicam	oral
Ciprofloxacin	Propafenone	Dicloxacillin
Clofibrate	Propranolol	Griseofulvin
Dextropropoxyphene	Quinidine	Nafcillin
Disulfiram	Simvastatin	Rifampin
Erythromycin	Sulfinpyrazone	Sucralfate
Fluconazole	Tamoxifen	Vitamin K (in
Influenza vaccine	Tetracyclines	polyvitamin
Isoniazid	Trimethoprim-sul-	preparations)
Itraconazole	famethoxazole	

therapy for each circumstance. Three months of therapy at an INR of 2.0–3.0 is routine. Longer treatment is advised if risk factors cannot be quickly eliminated, as in patients with congestive heart failure, prolonged immobility, or venous stasis. If the patient has continuing, unresolvable risk factors, such as cancer, antithrombin III deficiency, or protein C or S deficiency, antiphospholipid antibodies, or recurrent pulmonary embolism after discontinuance of warfarin, permanent anticoagulant therapy is recommended.

Patients with symptomatic deep calf vein thrombosis are anticoagulated for a period of 3 months. If anticoagulation is not feasible, they may be followed for 10–14 days with serial noninvasive studies to look for proximal extension of the thrombus.

The major risk of anticoagulant therapy is bleeding. Independent risk factors for in-hospital bleeding in patients started on long-term anticoagulant therapy include comorbid disorders such as heart, liver, and kidney disease; the use of heparin in patients over age 60; unusually prolonged prothrombin or partial thromboplastin times; and worsening liver function. Major hemorrhage occurs in about 5% of patients receiving intravenous heparin, and the death rate is 0.6%. The risk of hemorrhage is increased in women over 60 years of age and in patients taking aspirin. The rate of major hemorrhage is similar for warfarin (2–10%), but serious hemorrhage is unusual in patients with adequately controlled prothrombin times (INR 2.0–3.0). Longer prothrombin times invite more bleeding complications without enhancing efficacy. Subcutaneous heparin, administered in adjusted doses, may be as effective as warfarin in long-term treatment of deep venous thrombosis and is less likely to cause bleeding.

B. Thrombolytic Therapy: Lysis of pulmonary thromboemboli in situ represents the only available *definitive* medical treatment and is achieved by use of streptokinase, urokinase, and recombinant tissue plasminogen activator, which enhance endogenous fibrinolysis by activating plasminogen, thereby generating plasmin. Plasmin directly lyses thrombi both in the pulmonary artery and in the venous circulation and also has a secondary anticoagulant effect. Thrombolytic therapy, when compared to heparin alone, accelerates the resolution of pulmonary emboli, reduces pulmonary artery and right heart pressures, and improves right and left ventricular function in patients with established pulmonary embolism. Thrombolytic therapy may also preserve the anatomy and function of the valves in deep veins of the lower extremities. It has not been proved to affect the mortality rate from pulmonary thromboembolism, however. Critics of thrombolytic therapy point to its high cost compared to heparin therapy, lack of evidence of improved survival, and risks of bleeding.

While a few experts advocate thrombolysis for all patients with acute venous thromboembolism in the absence of contraindications, most physicians reserve its use for patients with acute massive pulmonary embolism confirmed by pulmonary angiography and for selected patients with established deep venous thrombosis. Suitable candidates include patients with hemodynamic compromise, those with underlying severe cardiopulmonary disease, those with hemodynamic instability when surgical embolectomy is not available, and those who fail to show hemodynamic improvement after heparin therapy.

The duration of symptoms prior to starting thrombolytic therapy should be less than 14 days. Puncture of noncompressible arteries or veins, or intramuscular injections are not permitted during thrombolytic therapy. Anticoagulants and antiplatelet drugs should not be given concurrently. Absolute contraindications to thrombolytic therapy include active internal bleeding and recent (within 2 months) cerebrovascular accident. Other major contraindications include severe hypertension, recent trauma, gastrointestinal bleeding, and major surgical or obstetric procedures. Hemorrhage is the major complication of thrombolytic therapy; the rate of severe bleeding is about 4%. Strict adherence to treatment guidelines reduces the risk. Intracranial bleeding has occurred in 0.3–0.7% of patients given thrombolytic therapy for myocardial infarction.

Pulmonary angiography to confirm the presence of pulmonary thromboembolism is required prior to thrombolytic therapy. An exception is the patient with a high clinical suspicion of pulmonary thromboembolism and a high-probability ventilation/perfusion lung scan. Pulmonary angiography is best performed via the compressible portion (below the inguinal ligament) of the right femoral vein.

Three agents are approved for thrombolytic therapy of pulmonary thromboembolism or deep venous thrombosis: streptokinase, urokinase, and recombinant tissue plasminogen activator. Any of these agents may be administered by continuous infusion into a peripheral vein. Streptokinase is usually preferred because it is less expensive, but development of antibodies may prevent future use of the drug. Streptokinase, 250,000 units intravenously over 30 minutes as a loading dose, is followed by a maintenance dose of 100,000 units/h for 24–72 hours. Urokinase is given as a 2000 units/lb loading dose over 10 minutes, followed by continuous infusion of 2000 units/lb/h for 12–24 hours. Recombinant tissue plasminogen activator is administered in a dose of 100 mg over 2 hours. No tests of coagulation are needed during infusion of any of the thrombolytic agents, because the dosages are fixed. After the thrombolytic agent has been given, standard anticoagulant therapy is resumed. A partial thromboplastin time is obtained at the completion of thrombolytic therapy to guide the infusion of intravenous heparin.

C. Additional Measures: Surgical interruption of the inferior vena cava is indicated when recurrent pulmonary embolism would be life-threatening in a patient with major contraindications to anticoagulation or failure or complications of anticoagulant or thrombolytic therapy. Life-threatening paradoxic thromboembolism or septic thromboembolism may also justify surgical interruption, which may be achieved by ligation, plication, clipping, and insertion of intraluminal filters in the inferior vena cava just below the renal veins. Percutaneous transjugular placement of a filter has become the preferred mode of inferior vena cava interruption when the patient is at continued risk for recurrent pulmonary thromboembolism from pelvic or lower extremity thrombi. The risks of recurrent pulmonary thromboembolism and inferior vena cava occlusion after filter placement are low (2–3%). Infrequent complications have included inferior vena cava thrombosis or trapping of thrombi, hematoma at the insertion site, and, if improper technique has been used, filter migration and perforation of the vena cava wall.

Surgical removal of acute pulmonary thromboemboli (pulmonary embolectomy) is an emergency procedure for patients with life-threatening hemodynamic compromise or cardiac arrest subsequent to massive pulmonary thromboembolism. This procedure is rarely performed, and the outcome is generally dismal.

Prognosis

Pulmonary embolism may cause sudden death, though the prognosis for survivors is generally favorable. The prognosis depends on the underlying disease and on proper diagnosis and treatment. The mortality rate in patients with undiagnosed pulmonary thromboembolism is about 30%. After diagnosis and treatment of pulmonary thromboembolism, death from a recurrence is unusual, occurring in less than 3% of cases. Perfusion defects resolve in most survivors. Pulmonary hypertension may be a complication of chronic recurrent pulmonary thromboembolism.

Becker DM et al: D-dimer testing and acute venous thromboembolism: A shortcut to accurate diagnosis? Arch Intern Med 1996;156:939. (Literature review questions the accuracy of this test.)

Becker RC, Ansell J: Antithrombotic therapy: An abbreviated reference for clinicians. Arch Intern Med 1995; 155:149. (A synopsis of the recommendations of the American College of Chest Physicians Consensus Conference.)

Clagett GP et al: Prevention of venous thromboembolism. Chest 1995;108(Suppl):312S. (A summary of current recommendations on prevention of deep venous thrombosis and pulmonary thromboembolism in a variety of clinical settings, presented by a consensus panel.)

Gefter WB et al: Pulmonary thromboembolism: Recent developments in diagnosis with CT and MR imaging. Radiology 1995;197:561. These studies are not routinely indicated for the diagnosis of pulmonary thromboembolism.)

Ginsberg JS: Management of venous thromboembolism. N Engl J Med 1996;335:1816. (Review of treatment, including during pregnancy; 106 references.)

Goldhaber SZ: Contemporary pulmonary embolism thrombolysis. Chest 1995;107(1 Suppl):45S. (Current guidelines for use of the three thrombolytic agents.)

Goldhaber SZ: Pulmonary embolism: Epidemiology, pathophysiology, diagnosis, and management. Chest 1995; 107(Suppl):1S. [Entire issue.] (A compendium of ten articles that summarize current thinking on different aspects of this disease.)

Hyers TM, Hull RD, Weg JG: Antithrombotic therapy for venous thromboembolic disease. Chest 1995;108 (Suppl):335S. (Current use of anticoagulants, thrombolytic therapy, inferior vena cava interruption, and embolectomy.)

Moser KM et al: Frequent asymptomatic pulmonary embolism in patients with deep venous thrombosis. JAMA 1994;271:223. (Deep venous thrombosis and pulmonary thromboembolism may be thought of as one disorder.)

Tapson VF. Pulmonary embolism: New diagnostic approaches. N Engl J Med 1997;336:1449. (Spiral CT scanning and MRI.)

Wells PS et al: Interactions of warfarin with drugs and food. Ann Intern Med 1994;121:676. (Important drugs with a probable or highly probable interaction with warfarin are summarized in Table 9–19.)

Wheeler HB et al: Diagnostic tests for deep vein thrombosis. Clinical usefulness depends on probability of disease. Arch Intern Med 1994;154:1921. (Ultrasonography is the method of choice.)

PULMONARY HYPERTENSION

Essentials of Diagnosis

- Dyspnea, fatigue, chest pain, and occasionally syncope on exertion.
- Narrow splitting of second heart sound with loud pulmonary component; findings of right ventricular hypertrophy and cardiac failure in advanced disease.
- Hypoxemia: wasted ventilation on pulmonary function tests in most cases.
- Electrocardiographic evidence of right ventricular strain or hypertrophy and right atrial enlargement.
- Enlarged central pulmonary arteries on chest x-ray.

General Considerations

The pulmonary circulation is unique because of its high blood flow, low pressure (normally 25/8 mm Hg, mean 12), and low resistance (normally 200–250 dynes/sec/cm^{-5}). It can accommodate large increases in blood flow during exercise with only modest increases in pressure because of its ability to recruit and distend blood vessels. The normal pulmonary circulation is also largely passive, since its pressures are determined mainly by the function of the right and left ventricles. Contraction of smooth muscle in the walls of pulmonary arteriolar resistance vessels becomes an important factor in numerous pathologic states.

Pulmonary hypertension is present when pulmonary artery pressure rises to a high level inappropriate for a given level of cardiac output. **Primary (idiopathic) pulmonary hypertension** (see Chapter 10) is a rare disorder of the pulmonary circulation occurring mostly in young and middle-aged women; it is characterized by progressive dyspnea, a rapid downhill course, and an invariably fatal outcome. This condition is also called plexogenic pulmonary arteriopathy, in reference to the characteristic histopathologic plexiform lesion found in muscular pulmonary arteries. It has been observed in occasional patients with HIV infection. Secondary pulmonary hypertension is more common.

Selected mechanisms responsible for **secondary pulmonary hypertension** and examples of corresponding clinical conditions are set forth in Table 9–20. Pulmonary hypertension is usually caused by reduction of the cross-sectional area of the pulmonary vasculature at the arterial, capillary, or venous level. Hypoxia of any cause is the most important and potent stimulus of pulmonary arterial vasoconstriction. The mechanisms by which hypoxia causes pulmonary hypertension are poorly understood. Factors operating at the alveolar level and direct stimulation of arteriolar smooth muscle have been implicated. Interest has focused on the release of vasoactive substances from the endothelial cells of pulmonary arteries, such as endothelium-derived relaxing factor and endothelin-1, a potent vasoconstrictor peptide. Hypoxia is partially or fully responsible for the pulmonary hypertension observed in chronic bronchitis, infiltrative lung disease due to various causes, kyphoscoliosis, obesity-hypoventilation syn-

Table 9–20. Mechanisms of pulmonary hypertension and examples of corresponding clinical conditions.

Reduction in cross-sectional area of pulmonary arterial bed
  Vasoconstriction
    Hypoxia from any cause
    Acidosis
  Loss of vessels
    Lung resection
    Emphysema
    Vasculitis
    Pulmonary fibrosis
    Connective tissue disease
  Obstruction of vessels
    Pulmonary embolism (thromboemboli, tumor emboli, foreign body emboli, etc)
    In situ thrombosis
    Schistosomiasis
  Narrowing of vessels
    Secondary structural changes due to pulmonary hypertension
Increased pulmonary venous pressure
  Constrictive pericarditis
  Left ventricular failure or reduced compliance
  Mitral stenosis
  Left atrial myxoma
  Pulmonary veno-occlusive disease
  Mediastinal diseases compressing pulmonary veins
Increased pulmonary blood flow
  Congenital left-to-right intracardiac shunts
Increased blood viscosity
  Polycythmia
Miscellaneous
  Pulmonary hypertension occurring in association with hepatic cirrhosis and portal hypertension

drome, chronic mountain sickness, obstructive sleep apnea, and neuromuscular disease. Acidosis is also a potent stimulus of pulmonary arterial vasoconstriction and exerts a synergistic vasoconstrictive effect with hypoxia.

Extensive obliteration and obstruction of the pulmonary arterial tree may cause pulmonary hypertension. Once present, pulmonary hypertension is self-perpetuating. It introduces secondary structural abnormalities in pulmonary vessels, including smooth muscle hypertrophy and intimal proliferation, and these may eventually stimulate atheromatous changes and in situ thrombosis, leading to further narrowing of the arterial bed.

Increased pulmonary venous pressure, when sustained, may cause "postcapillary" pulmonary hypertension; left ventricular failure (systolic, diastolic, or both) is the most common cause.

Pulmonary veno-occlusive disease is a rare cause of postcapillary pulmonary hypertension occurring in children and young adults. The cause is unknown, but associations with various conditions such as viral infection, bone marrow transplantation, chemotherapy, and malignancy have been described. The disease is characterized by progressive fibrotic occlusion of pulmonary veins and venules, along with

secondary hypertensive changes in the pulmonary arterioles and muscular pulmonary arteries. Nodular areas of pulmonary congestion, edema, hemorrhage, and hemosiderosis are found. Chest radiography reveals prominent, symmetric interstitial markings, Kerley B lines, pulmonary artery dilation, and normally sized left atrium and left ventricle. Premortem diagnosis is often difficult but is occasionally established by open lung biopsy. There is no effective therapy, and most patients die within 2 years as a result of progressive pulmonary hypertension.

Pulmonary hypertension is readily recognized when an obvious cause, such as severe COPD, is present. In adults, pulmonary hypertension in the absence of COPD is often caused by chronic pulmonary thromboembolism, interstitial fibrosis, sleep apnea, or obesity-hypoventilation syndrome. Other disorders listed in Table 9–20 should be excluded before the diagnosis of primary pulmonary hypertension is entertained.

Clinical Findings

A. Symptoms and Signs: Secondary pulmonary hypertension is difficult to recognize clinically in the early stages, when symptoms and signs are primarily those of the underlying disease. Pulmonary hypertension may cause or contribute to dyspnea, which is present initially on exertion and later at rest. Dull, retrosternal chest pain resembling angina pectoris may be present. Fatigue and syncope on exertion also occur, presumably a result of reduced cardiac output related to elevated pulmonary artery pressures or bradycardia.

The signs of pulmonary hypertension include narrow splitting of the second heart sound, accentuation of the pulmonary component of the second heart sound, and a systolic ejection click. In advanced cases, tricuspid and pulmonary valve insufficiency and signs of right ventricular failure and cor pulmonale are found.

B. Laboratory Findings: Polycythemia is found in many cases of pulmonary hypertension that are associated with chronic hypoxemia. Electrocardiographic changes are those of right axis deviation, right ventricular hypertrophy, right ventricular strain, or right atrial enlargement.

C. Imaging and Special Examinations: Radiographic findings depend on the cause of pulmonary hypertension. In chronic disease, dilation of the right and left main and lobar pulmonary arteries and enlargement of the pulmonary outflow tract are seen; in advanced disease, right ventricular and right atrial enlargement are seen. Peripheral "pruning" of large pulmonary arteries is characteristic of pulmonary hypertension in severe emphysema.

Echocardiography is helpful in evaluating patients thought to have mitral stenosis, left atrial myxoma, and pulmonary valvular disease. Echocardiography may also reveal right ventricular enlargement and paradoxic motion of the interventricular septum. Doppler ultrasonography is a reliable noninvasive means of estimating pulmonary artery systolic pressure. However, other precise hemodynamic measurements can only be obtained with right heart catheterization, which is often helpful when postcapillary pulmonary hypertension, intracardiac shunting, or thromboembolic disease is considered as part of the differential diagnosis.

Routine pulmonary function tests reveal no findings diagnostic of pulmonary hypertension. Diminution of the pulmonary capillary bed may cause reduction in the single breath diffusing capacity.

Depending upon the suspected cause of pulmonary hypertension, ventilation/perfusion lung scanning, pulmonary angiography, and surgical lung biopsy are occasionally helpful. Ventilation/perfusion lung scanning is very helpful in identifying patients with pulmonary hypertension caused by recurrent pulmonary thromboemboli, a condition that is often very difficult to recognize clinically. Transbronchial biopsy carries an increased risk of bleeding.

Treatment

Treatment of primary pulmonary hypertension is discussed in Chapter 10. Treatment of secondary pulmonary hypertension consists mainly of treating the underlying disorder, such as COPD, sleep apnea, obesity-hypoventilation syndrome, and mitral stenosis. Early recognition of pulmonary hypertension is crucial to interrupt the self-perpetuating cycle responsible for the rapid progression of this disorder. By the time most patients present with signs and symptoms of pulmonary hypertension, however, the condition is far advanced. If hypoxemia or acidosis is detected, corrective measures should be started immediately. Inhaled nitric oxide has recently been found to be effective in lowering the pulmonary artery pressure in critically ill patients with pulmonary hypertension, asthma, and acute respiratory distress syndrome. This benefit is only temporary, however. Supplemental oxygen administered for at least 15 hours per day has been demonstrated to be of benefit in patients with hypoxemic COPD.

Some clinicians employ permanent anticoagulation therapy in pulmonary hypertension of unknown cause, since multiple, very small pulmonary emboli may produce this picture and be difficult to recognize clinically and because in situ thrombosis may occur. Postcapillary pulmonary hypertension usually responds to treatment of the underlying cardiac disease.

Vasodilator therapy using various pharmacologic agents (eg, calcium antagonists, hydralazine, isoproterenol, diazoxide, nitroglycerin) has been tried in primary pulmonary hypertension and a few patients with secondary pulmonary hypertension with disappointing results. Complications of pulmonary vasodilator therapy have occurred, including systemic hypotension, hypoxemia, and even death. Continuous long-term infusion of prostacyclin (PGI_2; epoprostenol), a potent pulmonary vasodilator, has been shown to confer hemodynamic and symptomatic benefits in selected patients. Epoprostenol is now available for treatment of primary pulmonary hypertension by continuous intravenous infusion using a portable pump.

Primary pulmonary hypertension with pulmonary vasoconstriction, a potentially reversible condition, must be distinguished from fixed obstruction of the pulmonary vascular bed. Patients most likely to benefit from long-term pulmonary vasodilator therapy are those who respond favorably to a vasodilator challenge at right heart catheterization. It is clear that long-term vasodilator therapy should be employed only if hemodynamic benefit is documented. Some experts advise a baseline hemodynamic assessment by right heart catheterization and a repeat study after oral therapy with a vasodilator agent such as a calcium channel blocker. Routine use of vasodilator therapy is not advised.

Patients with marked polycythemia (hematocrit > 60%) should undergo repeated phlebotomy in an attempt to reduce blood viscosity. Cor pulmonale complicating pulmonary hypertension is treated by managing the underlying pulmonary disease and by using diuretics, salt restriction, and, in appropriate patients, supplemental oxygen. The use of digitalis in cor pulmonale remains controversial. Pulmonary thromboendarterectomy may benefit selected patients with pulmonary hypertension secondary to chronic thrombotic obstructions of major pulmonary arteries.

Single or double lung transplantation may be performed on patients with end-stage primary pulmonary hypertension. The two-year survival rate is 49%. Bronchiolitis obliterans is common in those who survive the operation.

Prognosis

The prognosis in secondary pulmonary hypertension depends on the course of the underlying disease. Patients with pulmonary hypertension due to fixed obliteration of the pulmonary vascular bed generally respond poorly to therapy; development of cor pulmonale in these cases implies a poor prognosis. The prognosis is favorable when pulmonary hypertension is detected early and the conditions leading to it are readily reversed.

Barst RJ et al: Survival in primary pulmonary hypertension with long-term continuous intravenous prostacyclin. Ann Intern Med 1994;121:409. (Improved survival compared to historical controls, perhaps serving as a bridge to transplantation.)

Epoprostenol for primary pulmonary hypertension. Med Lett Drugs Ther 1996;38:14. (This drug has been approved by the FDA.)

Fedullo PF et al: Chronic thromboembolic pulmonary hypertension. Clin Chest Med 1995;16:353. (Review of this disease and experience with thromboendarterectomy.)

Lunn RJ: Inhaled nitric oxide therapy. Mayo Clin Proc 1995;70:247. (Review of current use of this vasodilator drug.)

Rubin LJ: Primary pulmonary hypertension. N Engl J Med 1997;336:111. (Review with 53 references.)

DISORDERS DUE TO CHEMICAL & PHYSICAL AGENTS

SMOKE INHALATION

The inhalation of products of combustion may cause serious respiratory complications. As many as one-third of patients admitted to burn treatment units have pulmonary injury from smoke inhalation. Morbidity and deaths due to smoke inhalation exceed those attributed to the burns themselves. The death rate of patients with both severe body burns and smoke inhalation exceeds 50%. All patients suspected to have had significant smoke inhalation should be admitted to the hospital for observation and treatment.

It is important to look for and recognize three consequences of smoke inhalation: impaired tissue oxygenation, thermal upper airway injury, and chemical injury to the lung. Impaired tissue oxygenation results from inhalation of carbon monoxide or cyanide and is an immediate threat to life. The management of patients with carbon monoxide poisoning and cyanide poisoning is discussed in Chapter 39. The clinician must recognize that patients with carbon monoxide poisoning display a normal partial pressure of oxygen in arterial blood (PaO_2) but have a low *measured* (ie, not oximetric) oxyhemoglobin saturation (SaO_2). Immediate treatment with 100% oxygen is essential and should be continued until the measured carboxyhemoglobin level falls to less than 10% and concomitant metabolic acidosis has resolved.

Thermal injury to the mucosal surfaces of the upper airway occurs from inhalation of hot gases. Complications become evident by 18–24 hours. These include impaired ability to clear oral secretions and airway obstruction, producing inspiratory stridor. Respiratory failure with hypercapnia and hypoxemia occurs in severe cases. Early management (see also Chapter 38) includes the use of a high-humidity face mask with supplemental oxygen, gentle suctioning to evacuate oral secretions, elevation of the head 30 degrees to promote clearing of secretions, and topical epinephrine to reduce edema of the oropharyngeal mucous membrane. Helium-oxygen gas mixtures

may reduce labored breathing. Close monitoring with arterial blood gases and later with oximetry is important. Examination of the upper airway with a fiberoptic laryngoscope or bronchoscope is superior to routine physical examination. Endotracheal intubation is often necessary to establish airway patency and is likely to be necessary in patients with deep facial burns, oropharyngeal or laryngeal edema, or respiratory failure. Tracheostomy should be avoided if possible because of an increased risk of pneumonia and death from sepsis.

Chemical injury to the lung results from inhalation of toxic gases and products of combustion, including aldehydes and organic acids. The site of lung injury depends upon the solubility of the gases inhaled, the duration of exposure, and the size of inhaled particles that transport noxious gases to distal lung units. Bronchorrhea and bronchospasm are seen early after exposure along with dyspnea, tachypnea, and tachycardia. Labored breathing and cyanosis may follow. Physical examination at this stage reveals diffuse wheezing and rhonchi. Bronchiolar edema and high-permeability pulmonary edema (ARDS) may develop within 1–2 days after exposure. Sloughing of the bronchiolar mucosa may occur within 2–3 days, leading to airway obstruction, atelectasis and worsening hypoxemia. Bacterial colonization and pneumonia are common by 5–7 days after the exposure.

Treatment of the pulmonary component of smoke inhalation consists of supplemental oxygen, bronchodilators, suctioning of mucosal debris and mucopurulent secretions via an indwelling endotracheal tube, chest physical therapy to aid clearance of secretions, and adequate humidification of inspired gases. Positive end-expiratory pressure (PEEP) has been advocated to treat bronchiolar edema. Judicious fluid management and close monitoring for secondary bacterial infection with daily sputum Gram stains round out the management protocol.

The routine use of corticosteroids for chemical lung injury from smoke inhalation has been shown to be ineffective and may even be harmful. Routine or prophylactic use of antibiotics is not recommended.

Those patients who survive should be watched for the development of late bronchiolitis obliterans.

Demling RH: Smoke inhalation injury. New Horiz 1993;1:422. (Review of therapy.)

Weiss SM, Lakshminarayan S: Acute inhalation injury. Clin Chest Med 1994;15:103. (Pathophysiology and clinical syndromes resulting from inhalation of various toxic chemicals.)

PULMONARY ASPIRATION SYNDROMES

Aspiration of foreign material, such as liquids with pH > 2.5, into the tracheobronchial tree results from various disorders that impair normal deglutition, especially disturbances of consciousness and esophageal dysfunction.

Aspiration of Inert Material

Aspiration of inert material may cause asphyxia if the amount aspirated is massive and if cough is impaired, in which case immediate tracheobronchial suctioning is necessary. Most patients suffer no serious sequelae from aspiration of inert material.

Aspiration of Toxic Material

Aspiration of toxic material into the lung usually results in clinically evident pneumonia. **Hydrocarbon pneumonitis** is caused by ingestion of petroleum distillates, eg, gasoline, kerosene, furniture polish, and other household petroleum products. Lung injury results mainly from vomiting and secondary aspiration. Therapy is supportive. The lung should be protected from repeated aspiration with a cuffed endotracheal tube if necessary. **Lipid pneumonia** is a chronic syndrome related to the repeated aspiration of oily materials, eg, mineral oil, cod liver oil, and oily nose drops; it often occurs in elderly patients with impaired swallowing. Patchy infiltrates in dependent lung zones and lipid-laden macrophages in expectorated sputum are characteristic findings.

"Café Coronary"

Acute obstruction of the upper airway by food is associated with difficulty in swallowing, old age, poor dentition, dental problems that impair chewing, and use of alcohol and sedative drugs. The Heimlich procedure is lifesaving in many cases.

Retention of an Aspirated Foreign Body

Retention of an aspirated foreign body in the tracheobronchial tree may produce various acute and chronic conditions, including recurrent pneumonia, bronchiectasis, lung abscess, atelectasis, and postobstructive hyperinflation. Children are at greater risk than adults for foreign body aspiration. Occasionally, a misdiagnosis of asthma, COPD, or lung cancer is made in adult patients who have aspirated a foreign body. The plain chest x-ray usually suggests the site of the foreign body. In some cases, an expiratory film, demonstrating regional hyperinflation due to a check-valve effect, is helpful. Bronchoscopy is usually necessary to establish the diagnosis and attempt removal of the foreign body.

Chronic Aspiration of Gastric Contents

Chronic aspiration of gastric contents may result from primary disorders of the esophagus, eg, achalasia, esophageal stricture, scleroderma, esophageal carcinoma, esophagitis, and gastroesophageal reflux. In the last condition, relaxation of the tone of the lower esophageal sphincter allows reflux of gastric contents into the esophagus and predisposes to chronic pulmonary aspiration, especially at night. Cigarette smoking, consumption of alcohol, and use of theophylline are known to relax the lower esophageal sphincter. Pulmonary disorders linked to gastroesophageal reflux and chronic aspiration include bronchial asthma, idiopathic pulmonary fibrosis, and bronchiectasis. Even in the absence of aspiration, acid in the esophagus may trigger bronchospasm through reflex mechanisms.

The diagnosis of chronic aspiration is difficult. Ambulatory monitoring of esophageal pH for 24 hours detects gastric aspiration. Esophagogastroscopy and barium swallow are sometimes necessary to rule out esophageal disease. Management consists of elevation of the head of the bed, cessation of smoking, weight reduction, and antacids or H_2 receptor antagonists (eg, cimetidine, 300–400 mg) at night. Metoclopramide (10–15 mg orally four times daily or 20 mg at bedtime), cisapride (10 mg orally before each meal and at bedtime), or bethanechol (10–25 mg at bedtime) may be helpful in some patients with gastroesophageal reflux, as they elevate pressure in the lower esophageal sphincter.

Acute Aspiration of Gastric Contents (Mendelson's Syndrome)

Acute aspiration of gastric contents is often catastrophic. The pulmonary response depends on the characteristics and amount of the gastric contents aspirated. The more acidic the material, the greater the degree of chemical pneumonitis. Aspiration of pure gastric acid (pH < 2.5) causes extensive desquamation of the bronchial epithelium, bronchiolitis, hemorrhage, and pulmonary edema. Acute gastric aspiration is one of the commonest causes of adult respiratory distress syndrome. The clinical picture is one of abrupt onset of respiratory distress, with cough, wheezing, fever, and tachypnea. Crackles are audible at the bases of the lungs. Hypoxemia may be noted immediately after aspiration occurs. Radiographic abnormalities, consisting of patchy alveolar infiltrates in dependent lung zones, appear within a few hours. If particulate food matter has been aspirated along with gastric acid, radiographic features of bronchial obstruction may be observed. Even without superinfection, fever and leukocytosis occur.

Treatment of acute aspiration of gastric contents consists of supplemental oxygen, measures to maintain the airway, and the usual measures for treatment of acute respiratory failure. There is no evidence to support the routine use of corticosteroids or prophylactic antibiotics after gastric aspiration has occurred. Secondary pulmonary infection, which occurs in about one-fourth of patients, typically appears 2–3 days after aspiration. Management of this complication depends upon the observed flora of the tracheobronchial tree (Table 9–8). Hypotension secondary to alveolocapillary membrane injury and intravascular volume depletion is common and is managed with the judicious administration of intravenous fluids.

Tietjen PA, Kaner RJ, Quinn CE: Aspiration emergencies. Clin Chest Med 1994;15:117. (Review of the prevention and management of aspiration of liquid and solid materials.)

OCCUPATIONAL PULMONARY DISEASES

Many acute and chronic pulmonary diseases are directly related to inhalation of noxious substances encountered in the workplace; those disorders that are due to chemical agents may be classified as follows: (1) pneumoconioses, (2) hypersensitivity pneumonitis, (3) obstructive airway disorders, (4) toxic lung injury, (5) lung cancer, (6) pleural diseases, and (7) miscellaneous disorders.

Pneumoconioses

Pneumoconioses are chronic fibrotic lung diseases caused by the inhalation of coal dust and various in-

Table 9–21. Selected pneumoconioses.

Disease	Agent	Occupations
Metal dusts		
Siderosis	Metallic iron or iron oxide	Mining, welding, foundry work
Stannosis	Tin, tin oxide	Mining, tinwork, smelting
Baritosis	Barium salts	Glass and insecticide manufacturing
Coal dust		
Coalworker's pneumoconiosis	Coal dust	Coal mining
Inorganic dusts		
Silicosis	Free silica (silicon dioxide)	Rock mining, quarrying, stone cutting, tunneling, sandblasting, pottery, diatomaceous earth
Silicate dusts		
Asbestosis	Asbestos	Mining, insulation, construction, shipbuilding
Talcosis	Magnesium silicate	Mining, insulation, construction, shipbuilding
Kaolin pneumoconiosis	Sand, mica, aluminum silicate	Mining of china clay; pottery and cement work
Shaver's disease	Aluminum powder	Manufacture of corundum

ert, inorganic, or silicate dusts (Table 9–21). Pneumoconioses due to inhalation of inert dusts are usually asymptomatic disorders with diffuse nodular infiltrates on chest x-ray. Clinically important pneumoconioses include coal workers' pneumoconiosis, silicosis, and asbestosis. Treatment for each is supportive.

A. Coal Worker's Pneumoconiosis: In coal worker's pneumoconiosis, ingestion of inhaled coal dust by alveolar macrophages leads to the formation of coal macules, usually 2–5 mm in diameter, which appear on chest x-ray as diffuse small opacities but are especially prominent in the upper lung. Simple coal worker's pneumoconiosis is usually asymptomatic; pulmonary function abnormalities are unimpressive. Cigarette smoking does not increase the prevalence of coal worker's pneumoconiosis but may have an additive detrimental effect on ventilatory function. In complicated coal worker's pneumoconiosis ("progressive massive fibrosis"), conglomeration and contraction in the upper lung zones occur, with radiographic and clinical features resembling complicated silicosis. **Caplan's syndrome** is a rare condition characterized by the presence of necrobiotic rheumatoid nodules (1–5 cm in diameter) in the periphery of the lung in coal workers with rheumatoid arthritis.

B. Silicosis: In silicosis, extensive or prolonged inhalation of free silica (silicon dioxide) particles in the respirable range (0.3–5 μm) causes the formation of small rounded opacities (silicotic nodules) throughout the lung. Calcification of the periphery of hilar lymph nodes ("eggshell" calcification) is an unusual finding that strongly suggests silicosis. Simple silicosis is usually asymptomatic and has no effect on routine pulmonary function tests; in complicated silicosis, large conglomerate densities appear in the upper lung and are accompanied by dyspnea and obstructive and restrictive pulmonary dysfunction. A chronic lymphocytic alveolitis has been identified in silicosis, and one report suggests that this alveolitis may be responsive to corticosteroids. The incidence of tuberculosis is increased in patients with chronic silicosis. All patients with silicosis should have a tuberculin skin test and a current chest x-ray. If old, healed tuberculosis is suspected, multidrug treatment for tuberculosis (not single-agent preventive therapy) should be instituted.

C. Asbestosis: Asbestosis, a nodular interstitial fibrosis occurring in asbestos workers and miners, is characterized by dyspnea, inspiratory crackles, and in some cases, clubbing and cyanosis. The radiographic features include interstitial fibrosis, thickened pleura, and calcified plaques (pleural) on the diaphragms or lateral chest wall. The lower lungs are more often involved than the upper. High-resolution CT scanning is the best imaging method in asbestosis because of its ability to detect parenchymal fibrosis and define the presence of coexisting pleural plaques.

Cigarette smoking in asbestos workers increases the prevalence of radiographic pleural and parenchymal changes and markedly increases the incidence of lung carcinoma. It may also interfere with the clearance of short asbestos fibers from the lung. Pulmonary function studies show restrictive dysfunction and reduced diffusing capacity.

Hypersensitivity Pneumonitis

The term "hypersensitivity pneumonitis" (or "extrinsic allergic alveolitis") denotes nonatopic, nonasthmatic, allergic pulmonary disease. Hypersensitivity pneumonitis is manifested mainly as occupational disease (Table 9–22), in which exposure to inhaled organic agents leads to acute and eventually chronic pulmonary disease. Antibodies directed against the inhaled agent can be identified in serum. Acute illness is characterized by sudden onset of malaise, chills, fever, cough, dyspnea, and nausea 4–8 hours after exposure to the offending agent. This may occur after the patient has left work or even at night and thus may mimic paroxysmal nocturnal dyspnea. Bibasilar crackles, tachypnea, tachycardia, and (occasionally) cyanosis are noted. Small nodular densities sparing the apices and bases of the lungs are noted on chest x-ray. Pulmonary function studies reveal restrictive dysfunction and reduced diffusing capacity. Laboratory studies reveal an increase in the white blood cell count with a shift to the left, hypoxemia, and the presence of precipitating antibodies to the offending agent in serum. Hypersensitivity pneumonitis antibody panels against common fungal antigens (cost approximately $100) are available.

A subacute hypersensitivity pneumonitis syndrome (15% of cases) has been described that is characterized by the insidious onset of chronic cough and slowly progressive dyspnea, anorexia, and weight loss. Chronic respiratory insufficiency and the appearance of pulmonary fibrosis on radiographs may or may not occur after repeated exposure to the offending agent. Lung biopsy by thoracotomy or thoracoscopy is occasionally necessary for diagnosis. Acute hypersensitivity pneumonitis is characterized by interstitial infiltrates of lymphocytes and plasma cells, with noncaseating granulomas in the interstitium and air spaces. Diffuse fibrosis is the hallmark of the subacute and chronic phases.

Treatment of hypersensitivity pneumonitis consists of identification of the offending agent, avoidance of further exposure, and, in severe acute or protracted cases, oral corticosteroids (prednisone, 0.5 mg/kg daily as a single morning dose, tapered to nil over 4–6 weeks). Change in occupation is advisable in some cases.

Obstructive Airway Disorders

Occupational pulmonary diseases manifested as obstructive airway disorders include occupational asthma, industrial bronchitis, and byssinosis.

A. Occupational Asthma: It has been estimated that from 2% to 5% of all cases of asthma are related to occupation. Offending agents in the workplace are numerous; they include grain dust, wood dust, tobacco, pollens, enzymes, gum arabic, synthetic dyes, isocyanates (particularly toluene diisocyanate), rosin (soldering flux), inorganic chemicals (salts of nickel, platinum, and chromium), trimellitic anhydride, phthalic anhydride, formaldehyde, and various pharmaceutical agents. Diagnosis of occupational asthma depends on a high index of suspicion, an appropriate history, spirometric studies before and after exposure to the offending substance, and peak flow rate measurements in the workplace. Bronchial provocation testing may be helpful in some cases. Treatment consists of avoidance of further exposure to the offending agent and bronchodilators (Table 9–5), but symptoms may persist for years after workplace exposure has been terminated.

B. Industrial Bronchitis: Industrial bronchitis is chronic bronchitis found in coal miners and others exposed to cotton, flax, or hemp dust. Chronic disability does not often occur from industrial bronchitis.

C. Byssinosis: Byssinosis is an asthma-like disorder in textile workers caused by inhalation of

Table 9–22. Selected causes of hypersensitivity pneumonitis.

Disease	Antigen	Source
Farmer's lung	Micropolyspora faeni, Thermoactinomyces vulgaris	Moldy hay
"Humidifier lung"	Thermophilic actinomycetes	Contaminated humidifiers, heating systems, or air conditioners
Bird-fancier's lung ("pigeon-breeder's disease")	Avian proteins	Bird serum and excreta
Bagassosis	Thermoactinomyces sacchari and T vulgaris	Moldy sugar cane fiber (bagasse)
Sequoiosis	Graphium, Aureobasidium, and other fungi	Moldy redwood sawdust
Maple bark stripper's disease	Cryptostroma (Coniosporium) corticale	Rotting maple tree logs or bark
Mushroom picker's disease	Same as farmer's lung	Moldy compost
Suberosis	Penicillium frequentans	Moldy cork dust
Detergent worker's lung	Bacillus subtilis enzyme	Enzyme additives

cotton dust. The pathogenesis is obscure. Chest tightness, cough, and dyspnea are characteristically worse on Mondays or the first day back at work, with symptoms subsiding later in the week. Repeated exposure leads to chronic bronchitis.

Toxic Lung Injury

Toxic lung injury from inhalation of irritant gases is discussed in the section on smoke inhalation. **Silofiller's disease** is acute toxic noncardiogenic pulmonary edema caused by inhalation of nitrogen dioxide encountered in recently filled silos. Bronchiolitis obliterans is a common late complication, which perhaps can be prevented by early treatment of the acute reaction with corticosteroids. Extensive exposure to silage gas may cause sudden death.

Lung Cancer

Many industrial pulmonary carcinogens have been identified, including asbestos, radon gas, arsenic, iron, chromium, nickel, coal tar fumes, petroleum oil mists, isopropyl oil, mustard gas, and printing ink. Cigarette smoking acts as a cocarcinogen with asbestos and radon gas to cause bronchogenic carcinoma. Asbestos alone causes malignant mesothelioma. Almost all histologic types of lung cancer have been associated with these carcinogens. Chloromethylmethyl ether specifically causes small cell carcinoma of the lung.

Pleural Diseases

Occupational diseases of the pleura may result from exposure to asbestos (see above) or talc. Inhalation of talc causes pleural plaques that are similar to those caused by asbestos. Benign asbestos pleural effusion occurs in some asbestos workers and may cause chronic blunting of the costophrenic angle on chest x-ray.

Other Occupational Pulmonary Diseases

Occupational agents are also responsible for other pulmonary disorders. These include **berylliosis,** an acute or chronic pulmonary disorder related to exposure to beryllium, which is absorbed through the lungs or skin and widely disseminated throughout the body. Acute berylliosis is a toxic, ulcerative tracheobronchitis and chemical pneumonitis following intense and severe exposure to beryllium. Chronic berylliosis, a systemic disease closely resembling sarcoidosis, is more common. Chronic pulmonary beryllium disease is thought to be an alveolitis mediated by the proliferation of beryllium-specific helper-inducer T cells in the lung. Exposure to beryllium now occurs in machining and handling of beryllium products and alloys. Beryllium miners are not at risk for berylliosis. Beryllium is no longer used in fluorescent lamp production, which was a source of exposure before 1950.

Cartier A: Definition and diagnosis of occupational asthma. Eur Respir J 1994;7:153. (Clinical evaluation of the most prevalent type of occupational lung disease.)

Kaltreider HB: Hypersensitivity pneumonitis. West J Med 1993;159:570. (Overview with emphasis on immune pathogenesis.)

Madan I: ABC of work related disorders: Occupational asthma and other respiratory diseases. BMJ 1996;313: 291. (Occupational asthma, hypersensitivity pneumonitis, asbestosis, and other disorders.)

Newman LS: Occupational illness. N Engl J Med 1995;333:1128. (Clinical assessment and management of occupational disease.)

Schwartz DA, Peterson MW: Occupational lung disease. Adv Intern Med 1997;42:269. (Review with 161 references.)

DRUG-INDUCED LUNG DISEASE

Typical patterns of pulmonary response to various drugs implicated in drug-induced respiratory disease are summarized in Table 9–23. Pulmonary injury due to drugs occurs as a result of allergic reactions, idiosyncratic reactions, overdose, or undesirable side effects. In most patients, the mechanism of pulmonary injury is unknown.

Precise diagnosis of drug-induced pulmonary disease is often difficult, because results of routine laboratory studies are not helpful and radiographic findings are not specific. A high index of suspicion and a thorough medical history of drug usage are critical to establishing the diagnosis of drug-induced lung disease. The clinical response to cessation of the suspected offending agent is also helpful. Acute episodes of drug-induced pulmonary disease usually disappear 24–48 hours after the drug has been discontinued, but chronic syndromes may take longer to resolve. Challenge tests to confirm the diagnosis are risky and rarely performed.

Treatment of drug-induced lung disease consists of discontinuing the offending agent immediately and managing the pulmonary symptoms appropriately.

Inhalation of freebase (crack) cocaine may cause a spectrum of acute pulmonary syndromes, including pulmonary infiltration with eosinophilia, pneumothorax and pneumomediastinum, bronchiolitis obliterans, and acute respiratory failure associated with diffuse alveolar damage and alveolar hemorrhage. Corticosteroids have been used to treat the latter.

Cooper JA Jr: Drug-induced lung disease. Adv Intern Med 1997;42:231. (Review with 149 references.)

Rosenow EC 3rd: Drug-induced pulmonary disease. Dis Mon 1994 May;40:253. (Thorough review; over 100 drugs have pulmonary toxicity.)

RADIATION LUNG INJURY

The lung is a radiosensitive organ that can be affected by external beam radiation therapy. The pul-

Table 9–23. Pulmonary manifestations of selected drug toxicities.

Asthma	**Pulmonary edema**
Propranolol and other beta-blockers	Noncardiogenic
Aspirin	Aspirin
Nonsteroidal anti-inflammatory drugs	Chlordiazepoxide
	Cocaine
Histamine	Ethchlorvynol
Methacholine	Heroin
Acetylcysteine	Cardiogenic
Aerosolized pentamidine	Propranolol
Any nebulized medication	**Pleural effusion**
Cough	Bromocriptine
Angiotensin-converting enzyme inhibitors	Nitrofurantoin
	Any drug inducing systemic
Inhaled beclomethasone	lupus erythematosus
Inhaled cromolyn	Methysergide
Pulmonary infiltration	Chemotherapeutic agents
Without eosinophilia	**Mediastinal widening**
Amitriptyline	Phenytoin
Azathioprine	Corticosteroids
Amiodarone	Methotrexate
With eosinophilia	**Respiratory failure**
Sulfonamides	Neuromuscular blockade
L-Tryptophan	Aminoglycosides
Nitrofurantoin	Succinylcholine
Penicillin	Gallamine
Methotrexate	Dimethyltubocurarine
Crack cocaine	(metocurine)
Drug-induced systemic	Central nervous system
lupus erythematosus	depression
Hydralazine	Sedatives
Procainamide	Hypnotics
Isoniazid	Narcotics
Chlorpromazine	Alcohol
Phenytoin	Tricyclic antidepressants
Interstitial pneumonitis/	Oxygen
fibrosis	
Nitrofurantoin	
Bleomycin	
Busulfan	
Cyclophosphamide	
Methysergide	
Phenytoin	

monary response is determined by the volume of lung radiated, the dose and rate of therapy, and potentiating factors, eg, concurrent chemotherapy, previous radiation therapy in the same area, and simultaneous withdrawal of corticosteroid therapy. Symptomatic radiation lung injury occurs in about 10% of patients treated with megavoltage therapy for carcinoma of the breast, 5–15% of patients treated for carcinoma of the lung, and 5–35% of patients treated for lymphoma. Two phases of the pulmonary response to radiation are apparent: an acute phase (radiation pneumonitis) and a chronic phase (radiation fibrosis).

Radiation Pneumonitis

Radiation pneumonitis usually occurs 2–3 months (range 1–6 months) after completion of radiotherapy and is characterized by insidious onset of dyspnea,

intractable dry cough, chest fullness or pain, weakness, and fever. The pathogenesis of acute radiation pneumonitis is unknown, but there is speculation that hypersensitivity mechanisms are involved. The dominant histopathologic finding is that of a lymphocytic interstitial pneumonitis. Inspiratory crackles may be heard in the involved area. In severe disease, respiratory distress and cyanosis occur that are characteristic of acute respiratory distress syndrome (ARDS). An increased white blood cell count and elevated sedimentation rate are common. Pulmonary function studies reveal reduced lung volumes, reduced lung compliance, hypoxemia, reduced diffusing capacity, and reduced maximum voluntary ventilation. Chest x-ray, which correlates poorly with the presence of symptoms, usually demonstrates an alveolar or nodular infiltrate with a ground-glass opacification limited to the irradiated area. Air bronchograms are often observed. The sharp borders of the infiltrate help distinguish radiation pneumonitis from other conditions, eg, infectious pneumonia, lymphangitic spread of carcinoma, and recurrent tumor. Treatment consists of aspirin, cough suppressants, and bed rest. Acute respiratory failure, if present, is treated appropriately. Although there is no proof that corticosteroids are effective in radiation pneumonitis, prednisone (1 mg/kg/d orally) is usually given immediately for about 1 week. Thereafter, the dose is reduced and maintained at 20–40 mg/d for several weeks, then slowly tapered. Radiation pneumonitis usually resolves in 2–3 weeks. Death from ARDS is unusual.

Pulmonary Radiation Fibrosis

Pulmonary radiation fibrosis occurs in nearly all patients who receive a full course of radiation therapy for cancer of the lung and breast. Patients who experience radiation pneumonitis develop pulmonary fibrosis after an intervening period (6–12 months) of well-being. Most patients are asymptomatic, though slowly progressive dyspnea occurs in some. Radiation fibrosis may occur with or without antecedent radiation pneumonitis. Cor pulmonale and chronic respiratory failure are rare. Radiographic findings include obliteration of normal lung markings, dense interstitial and pleural fibrosis, reduced lung volumes, tenting of the diaphragm, and sharp delineation of the irradiated area. No specific therapy is necessary, and corticosteroids have no value.

Other Complications of Radiation Therapy

Other complications of radiation therapy directed to the thorax include pericardial effusion, constrictive pericarditis, tracheoesophageal fistula, esophageal candidiasis, radiation dermatitis, and rib fractures. Small pleural effusions, radiation pneumonitis outside the irradiated area, spontaneous pneumothorax, and complete obstruction of central airways are unusual occurrences.

Movsas B et al: Pulmonary radiation injury. Chest 1997;111:1061. (Thorough review of radiation pneumonitis and radiation fibrosis, stressing the role of cytokines; 98 references.)

Salinas FV, Winterbauer RH: Radiation pneumonitis: a mimic of infectious pneumonitis. Semin Respir Infect 1995;10:143. (Pathogenesis, histopathology, and clinical and radiographic features.)

DISORDERS OF VENTILATION

The principal influences on ventilatory control are arterial PCO_2, pH, and PO_2 and cerebrospinal fluid pH. These variables are monitored by **peripheral and central chemoreceptors.** Under normal conditions, the ventilatory control system maintains arterial pH and PCO_2 within narrow limits; arterial PO_2 is more loosely controlled.

PRIMARY ALVEOLAR HYPOVENTILATION

Primary alveolar hypoventilation ("Ondine's curse") is a rare syndrome of unknown cause characterized by inadequate alveolar ventilation despite normal neurologic function and normal airways, lungs, chest wall, and ventilatory muscles. Hypoventilation is even more marked during sleep. Individuals with this disorder are usually nonobese males in their third or fourth decades who present with lethargy, headache, and somnolence. Dyspnea is absent. Physical examination may reveal cyanosis and evidence of pulmonary hypertension and cor pulmonale. Hypoxemia and hypercapnia are present and improve with voluntary hyperventilation. Erythrocytosis is common. Treatment with ventilatory stimulants is usually unrewarding. Augmentation of ventilation by mechanical methods (phrenic nerve stimulation, rocking bed, mechanical ventilators) has been helpful to some patients. Adequate oxygenation should be maintained with supplemental oxygen, but nocturnal oxygen therapy should be prescribed only if diagnostic nocturnal polysomnography has demonstrated its efficacy and safety. Primary alveolar hypoventilation resembles—but should be distinguished from—**central alveolar hypoventilation,** in which impaired ventilatory drive with chronic respiratory acidemia and hypoxemia follows an insult to the brain stem (eg, bulbar poliomyelitis, infarction, meningitis, encephalitis, trauma).

Martin TJ, Sanders MH: Chronic alveolar hypoventilation: A review for the clinician. Sleep 1995;18:617. (Etiology and diagnosis.)

OBESITY-HYPOVENTILATION SYNDROME (Pickwickian Syndrome)

A few obese individuals demonstrate hypoventilation during wakefulness indicative of the obesity-hypoventilation syndrome. This is distinguished from primary alveolar hypoventilation by the presence of extreme obesity. Symptoms, physical findings, and laboratory data are otherwise similar in the two syndromes. Hypercapnia, hypoxemia, and elevated hematocrit are characteristic features. Having the patient voluntarily hyperventilate for about 1 minute causes the PCO_2 and the PO_2 to return toward normal values, in contrast to lung diseases causing chronic respiratory failure such as COPD. In obesity-hypoventilation syndrome, hypoventilation appears to result from a synergistic combination of blunted ventilatory drives and the mechanical load imposed upon the ventilatory apparatus by obesity. Most patients with obesity-hypoventilation syndrome also suffer from obstructive sleep apnea (see below), which must be treated aggressively if identified as a comorbid disorder. Therapy of obesity-hypoventilation syndrome consists mainly of weight loss, which improves hypercapnia and hypoxemia as well as the ventilatory responses to hypoxia and hypercapnia; and medroxyprogesterone acetate, 10–20 mg every 8 hours orally. Marked improvement in hypoxemia, hypercapnia, erythrocytosis, and cor pulmonale may result. The obesity-hypoventilation syndrome should not be confused with **narcolepsy,** a disorder of excessive daytime sleepiness and irresistible sleep attacks (see Chapter 25).

SLEEP-RELATED BREATHING DISORDERS

Abnormal ventilation during sleep is manifested by apnea (breath cessation for at least 10 seconds) or hypopnea (decrement in airflow with drop in oxyhemoglobin saturation of at least 4%). Episodes of apnea are **central** if ventilatory effort is absent for the duration of the apneic episode, **obstructive** if ventilatory effort persists throughout the apneic episode but no airflow occurs because of transient obstruction of the upper airway, and **mixed** if absent ventilatory effort precedes upper airway obstruction during the apneic episode. Pure central sleep apnea is uncommon; it may occur in normals, in patients with primary alveolar hypoventilation, or in patients with lesions of the brain stem. Cheyne-Stokes respiration, an accentuated form of periodic breathing with apnea, is a type of central sleep apnea found in patients with congestive heart failure. Obstructive and mixed sleep apneas are more common and may be associated with life-threatening cardiac arrhythmias, severe hypoxemia during sleep, and daytime consequences of nocturnal hypoxemia, including congestive heart failure, pulmonary hypertension, cor pulmonale, and secondary erythrocytosis. Sleep apnea syndrome (sleep-disordered breathing with daytime hypersomnolence) affects about 4% of men and 2% of women in middle age.

Definitive diagnostic evaluation for a suspected sleep apnea syndrome should include otolaryngologic examination and polysomnography, the monitoring of multiple physiologic factors during sleep. Electroencephalography, electro-oculography, electromyography, electrocardiography, oximetry, and measurement of respiratory effort and airflow are performed in a complete evaluation. Screening may be performed using home nocturnal oximetry, which has a high negative predictive value in ruling out significant sleep apnea.

Obstructive Sleep Apnea

Upper airway obstruction during sleep occurs when loss of normal pharyngeal muscle tone allows the pharynx to collapse passively during inspiration. Patients with anatomically narrowed upper airways (eg, micrognathia, macroglossia, obesity, tonsillar hypertrophy) are also predisposed to the development of obstructive sleep apnea. Alcohol or sedatives before sleeping or nasal obstruction of any type, including the common cold, may precipitate or worsen the condition. Hypothyroidism and cigarette smoking are additional risk factors for obstructive sleep apnea. Before making the diagnosis of obstructive sleep apnea, a drug history should be obtained and a seizure disorder, narcolepsy, or psychiatric depression excluded.

Most patients with obstructive or mixed sleep apnea are obese middle-aged men. Systemic hypertension is common. Patients complain of excessive daytime somnolence, morning sluggishness and headaches, daytime fatigue, cognitive impairment, recent weight gain, and impotence. Bed partners usually report loud cyclical snoring, breath cessation, restlessness, and often thrashing movements of the extremities during sleep. Personality changes, poor judgment, work-related problems, and intellectual deterioration (memory impairment, inability to concentrate) may also be observed.

Physical examination may be normal or may reveal systemic and pulmonary hypertension with cor pulmonale. The patient may appear sleepy or fall asleep during the evaluation. The oropharynx is frequently found to be narrowed by excessive soft tissue folds, large tonsils, pendulous uvula, or prominent tongue. Nasal obstruction by a deviated nasal septum, poor nasal air flow, and a nasal twang to the speech may be observed. A "bull neck" appearance is common. Facial deformities, retrognathia, and pharyngeal tumors are less frequently seen.

Erythrocytosis is common. A hemoglobin level, and thyroid function tests should be obtained. Observation of the sleeping patient reveals loud snoring interrupted by episodes of increasingly strong ventilatory effort that fail to produce airflow. A loud snort accompanies the first breath following an apneic episode. Polysomnography reveals apneic episodes lasting as long as 1–2 minutes. Oxygen saturation falls, often to very low levels. Bradyarrhythmias such as sinus bradycardia, sinus arrest, or atrioventricular block may occur. Tachyarrhythmias, including paroxysmal supraventricular tachycardia, atrial fibrillation, and ventricular tachycardia, are common once airflow is reestablished.

Weight loss and strict avoidance of alcohol and hypnotic medications are the first steps in management and may be curative, but few patients lose weight successfully. Nasal continuous positive airway pressure (nasal CPAP) is very helpful in such circumstances. Polysomnography is necessary to determine what level of CPAP (usually 5–15 cm H_2O) is necessary to abolish obstructive apneas. Patients must use the nasal CPAP system nightly. Unfortunately, only about 75% of patients continue to use nasal CPAP after 1 year. Pharmacologic therapy for obstructive sleep apnea is disappointing. Protriptyline (10–20 mg orally at bedtime) is helpful in a small number of patients. Supplemental oxygen may lessen the severity of nocturnal desaturation but may also lengthen apneas. Polysomnography is necessary to assess the effects of oxygen therapy; it should not be routinely prescribed. Mechanical devices inserted into the mouth at bedtime to hold the jaw forward and prevent pharyngeal occlusion have modest effectiveness in relieving apnea, but patient compliance is not optimal.

Uvulopalatopharyngoplasty, a procedure consisting of resection of pharyngeal soft tissue and amputation of approximately 15 mm of the free edge of the soft palate and uvula, may be helpful in selected patients with retropalatal airway occlusion during sleep. Identifying patients who will benefit is difficult. Only about half of these operations are successful. Uvulopalatopharyngoplasty may now be performed on an outpatient basis with a laser. **Nasal septoplasty** is performed if gross anatomic nasal septal deformity is present. **Tracheostomy** relieves upper airway obstruction and its physiologic consequences and represents the definitive treatment for obstructive sleep apnea. However, it has numerous adverse effects, including granuloma formation, difficulty with speech, and stoma and airway infection. Furthermore, the long-term care of the tracheostomy, especially in obese patients, can be difficult. Tracheostomy and other maxillofacial surgery approaches are reserved for patients with life-threatening arrhythmias or severe disability who have failed to respond to conservative therapy. In severe cases, it is prudent to combine tracheostomy with uvulopalatopharyngoplasty and attempt decannulation at a later time. This avoids the risk of acute airway obstruction due to postoperative edema.

American Thoracic Society: Indications and standards for use of nasal continuous positive airway pressure (CPAP) in sleep apnea syndrome. Am J Respir Crit Care Med 1994;150:1738. (Indications, technology, complications, and compliance in adults and children.)

DeBacker WA: Central sleep apnoea, pathogenesis and treatment: An overview and perspective. Eur Respir J 1995;8:1372. (Review of mechanisms and the limited options for treatment.)

Hla KM et al: Sleep apnea and hypertension: A population-based study. Ann Intern Med 1994;120:382. (The association of hypertension with sleep-disordered breathing is independent of obesity, age, and sex.)

Hudgel DW: Treatment of obstructive sleep apnea: A review. Chest 1996;109:1346. (Thorough discussion of CPAP.)

Johic R, Fitzpatrick MF: Obstructive lung disease and sleep. Med Clin North Am 1996;80:821. (Interrelationship between sleep and the obstructive lung diseases.)

Strohl KP, Redline S: Recognition of obstructive sleep apnea. Am J Respir Crit Care Med 1996;154:279. (State of the art review with 182 references.)

Strollo PJ Jr, Rogers RM: Obstructive sleep apnea. N Engl J Med 1996;334:99.

HYPERVENTILATION SYNDROMES

Hyperventilation is an increase in alveolar ventilation that leads to hypocapnia. It may be caused by a variety of conditions, such as hypoxemia, obstructive and infiltrative lung diseases, sepsis, hepatic dysfunction, fever, and pain. The term "central neurogenic hyperventilation" denotes a monotonous, sustained pattern of rapid and deep breathing seen in comatose patients with brain stem injury of multiple causes. Functional hyperventilation may be acute or chronic. Acute hyperventilation presents with hyperpnea, paresthesias, carpopedal spasm, tetany, and anxiety. Chronic hyperventilation may present with various nonspecific symptoms, including fatigue, dyspnea, anxiety, palpitations, and dizziness. The diagnosis of chronic hyperventilation syndrome is established if symptoms are reproduced during voluntary hyperventilation. Once organic causes of hyperventilation have been excluded, treatment of acute hyperventilation consists of rebreathing expired gas from a paper bag held over the face in order to decrease respiratory alkalemia and its associated symptoms. Anxiolytic drugs are also useful.

Block M, Szidon P: Hyperventilation syndromes. Compr Ther 1994;20:306. (Definition, clinical and physiologic consequences, and disorders associated with hyperventilation.)

ACUTE RESPIRATORY FAILURE

Respiratory failure is defined as respiratory dysfunction resulting in abnormalities of oxygenation or CO_2 elimination severe enough to impair or threaten the function of vital organs. Arterial blood gas criteria for respiratory failure are not absolute but may be arbitrarily established as a P_{O_2} under 60 mm Hg and a P_{CO_2} over 50 mm Hg. Acute respiratory failure may occur in both pulmonary and nonpulmonary disorders (Table 9–24). Respiratory failure may be considered a failure of oxygenation, failure of ventilation, or both. A complete discussion of treatment of acute respiratory failure is beyond the scope of this chapter. Only a few selected general principles of management will be reviewed here.

Clinical Findings

Symptoms and signs of acute respiratory failure are those of the underlying disease combined with those of hypoxemia and hypercapnia. The chief symptom of hypoxemia is dyspnea, though profound hypoxemia may exist in the absence of complaints. Signs of hypoxemia include cyanosis, restlessness, confusion, anxiety, delirium, tachypnea, tachycardia, hypertension, cardiac arrhythmias, and tremor. Dyspnea and headache are the cardinal symptoms of hypercapnia. Signs of hypercapnia include peripheral and conjunctival hyperemia, hypertension, tachycardia, tachypnea, impaired consciousness, papilledema, and asterixis. The symptoms and signs of acute respiratory failure are both insensitive and nonspecific; therefore, the physician must maintain a high index of suspicion and request an arterial blood gas analysis if respiratory failure is suspected.

Treatment

Treatment of the patient with acute respiratory

Table 9–24. Selected causes of acute respiratory failure in adults.

Airway disorders
Asthma
Chronic bronchitis or emphysema in acute exacerbation
Partial obstruction of pharynx, larynx, trachea, or lobar bronchi
Parenchymal lung disorders
Acute respiratory distress syndrome
Congestive heart failure
Pneumonia
Hypersensitivity pneumonitis
Aspiration
Pulmonary vascular disorders
Pulmonary thromboembolism
Chest wall and pleural disorders
Flail chest
Pneumothorax
Neuromuscular disorders
Narcotic or sedative-hypnotic overdose
Guillain-Barré syndrome
Botulism
Spinal cord injury
Myasthenia gravis
Poliomyelitis
Stroke

failure consists of (1) specific therapy directed toward the underlying disease; (2) respiratory supportive care directed toward the maintenance of adequate gas exchange; and (3) general supportive care. Only the last two aspects are discussed below.

A. Respiratory Support: Respiratory support has both nonventilatory and ventilatory aspects.

1. Nonventilatory aspects–*The main therapeutic goal in acute hypoxemic respiratory failure is to ensure adequate oxygenation of vital organs.* Inspired oxygen concentration should be the lowest value that results in an oxygen saturation of $\geq 90\%$ (PaO_2 about 60 mm Hg). Higher arterial oxygen tensions are of no benefit and may cause hypoventilation in patients with chronic hypercapnia; however, *oxygen therapy should not be withheld for fear of causing progressive respiratory acidemia.* Hypoxemia in patients with obstructive airway disease is usually easily corrected by administering low-flow oxygen by nasal cannula (1–3 L/min) or Venturi mask (24–28%). Higher concentrations of oxygen are necessary to correct hypoxemia in patients with acute respiratory distress syndrome (ARDS), pneumonia, and other parenchymal lung diseases.

2. Ventilatory aspects–Ventilatory support consists of maintaining patency of the airway and ensuring adequate alveolar ventilation. Tracheal intubation and mechanical ventilation are often required.

a. Tracheal intubation–Indications for tracheal intubation are (1) hypoxemia which is not quickly reversed by supplemental oxygen, (2) upper airway obstruction, (3) impaired airway protection, (4) poor handling of secretions, and (5) facilitation of mechanical ventilation. In general, orotracheal intubation is preferred to nasotracheal intubation in urgent or emergency situations because it is easier, faster, and less traumatic. Nasotracheal tubes are more comfortable and may be preferable if prolonged intubation is anticipated. The position of the tip of the endotracheal tube at the level of the aortic arch should be verified by chest x-ray immediately following intubation, and auscultation should be performed to verify that both lungs are being inflated. Only tracheal tubes with "floppy" (high-volume, low-pressure) air-filled or foam cuffs should be used. Cuff inflation pressure should be kept below 20 mm Hg if possible to minimize tracheal mucosal injury.

b. Mechanical ventilation–Indications for mechanical ventilation include (1) apnea, (2) acute hypercapnia that is not quickly reversed by appropriate specific therapy, (3) severe hypoxemia, and (4) progressive patient fatigue despite appropriate treatment. In general, positive-pressure, volume-cycled ventilators should be used to provide mechanical ventilatory support. Noninvasive ventilation (mechanical ventilation without tracheal intubation), using such approaches as nasal mask ventilation, is an alternative in highly selected patients.

Several modes of ventilation are available. Assisted mechanical ventilation (AMV), or assist/control (A/C), is a ventilatory mode in which the ventilatory frequency set on the ventilator serves as a backup rate, but the patient may trigger the ventilator to deliver additional positive-pressure breaths, each at the prescribed tidal volume. Continuous mechanical ventilation (CMV) provides ventilation at a specified rate for patients who are apneic. Synchronized intermittent mandatory ventilation (SIMV) is a ventilatory technique in which the rate set on the ventilator serves as a backup rate, but the patient is able to augment the machine ventilation by taking spontaneous breaths through a one-way valve from a reservoir. Intermittent mandatory ventilation may be of value for patients whose breathing cannot be synchronized with the ventilator; for tachypneic or agitated patients who develop respiratory alkalemia on assist/control ventilation; and for patients in whom strictly positive-pressure ventilation results in a reduction of cardiac output and in whom the negative-pressure breaths of intermittent mandatory ventilation produce an improvement in cardiac output. Numerous alternative modes of mechanical ventilation now exist, the most popular being pressure support ventilation (PSV), pressure-controlled ventilation (PCV), inverse ratio ventilation (IRV), and continuous positive airway pressure (CPAP).

Positive end-expiratory pressure (PEEP) is useful in improving oxygenation in patients with diffuse parenchymal lung disease such as ARDS. It should be used cautiously in patients with localized parenchymal disease, hyperinflation, or very high airway pressure requirements during mechanical ventilation.

c. Complications of mechanical ventilation–Potential complications of mechanical ventilation are numerous. Migration of the tip of the endotracheal tube into the right main bronchus can cause atelectasis of the left lung and overdistention of the right lung. **Barotrauma,** manifested by subcutaneous emphysema, pneumomediastinum, subpleural air cysts, pneumothorax, or systemic gas embolism, may occur in patients whose lungs are overdistended by excessive tidal volumes, especially those with hyperinflation caused by airflow obstruction or PEEP. Subtle parenchymal lung injury due to overdistention of alveoli is another potential hazard. Strategies to avoid barotrauma (also recently called "volutrauma") include the use of low mechanical tidal volumes, prolonging the inspiratory time (inverse ratio ventilation); "permissive hypercapnia," or deliberate hypoventilation; PEEP reduction; and improving chest wall compliance (sedation, neuromuscular blockade).

Acute respiratory alkalosis caused by overventilation is common. Hypotension induced by elevated intrathoracic pressure that results in decreased return of systemic venous blood to the heart may occur in patients treated with PEEP, those with severe airflow obstruction, and those with intravascular volume depletion.

Ventilator-associated pneumonia is another serious complication of mechanical ventilation. The mortality rate of this disorder is about 50–60%. Iatrogenic overdistention ("auto-PEEP"), reduced cardiac output, increased intracranial pressure, and psychologic problems are additional complications attributed to mechanical ventilation.

B. General Supportive Care: Maintenance of adequate nutrition is vital; parenteral nutrition should be used only when conventional feeding methods are not possible. Overfeeding, especially with carbohydrate-rich formulas, should be avoided, because it increases CO_2 production and may potentially worsen or induce hypercapnia in patients with limited ventilatory reserve; however, failure to provide adequate nutrition is more common. Hypokalemia and hypophosphatemia may worsen hypoventilation due to muscle weakness. The hematocrit should be determined regularly and transfusions given if necessary. Sedative-hypnotics and narcotic analgesics are avoided if possible. If sedation is necessary, short-acting drugs such as triazolam, lorazepam, or oxazepam are preferred. Temporary paralysis with a nondepolarizing neuromuscular blocking agent is occasionally used to facilitate mechanical ventilation and to lower oxygen consumption. Prolonged muscular weakness is an uncommon but dread complication of these agents.

Psychologic and emotional support, skin care to avoid decubitus ulcers, and meticulous avoidance of nosocomial infection and complications of tracheal tubes are vital aspects of comprehensive care for patients with acute respiratory failure.

Attention must also be paid to preventing complications associated with serious illness. Stress gastritis and ulcers may be avoided by administering sucralfate, antacids, or histamine H_2 receptor antagonists. There is some concern that the latter two agents, which raise the gastric pH, may permit increased growth of gram-negative bacteria in the stomach, predisposing to pharyngeal colonization and ultimately nosocomial pneumonia; many clinicians prefer sucralfate. The risk of deep venous thrombosis and pulmonary embolism may be reduced by subcutaneous administration of heparin (5000 units every 12 hours).

Course & Prognosis

The course and prognosis of acute respiratory failure vary and depend on the underlying disease. The prognosis of acute respiratory failure caused by uncomplicated sedative or narcotic drug overdose is excellent. Acute respiratory failure in patients with COPD who do not require intubation and mechanical ventilation has a good immediate prognosis. On the other hand, ARDS associated with sepsis has an extremely poor prognosis, with mortality rates of about 90%. Overall, adults requiring mechanical ventilation for all causes of acute respiratory failure have sur-

vival rates of 62% to weaning, 43% to hospital discharge, and 30% to 1 year after hospital discharge.

Curtis JR, Hudson LD: Emergent assessment and management of acute respiratory failure in COPD. Clin Chest Med 1994;15:481. (Extensive review of etiology, management, prognosis, ethical and societal issues.)

Meyer TJ, Hill NS: Noninvasive positive pressure ventilation to treat respiratory failure. Ann Intern Med 1994;120:760.

Slutsky AS: Mechanical ventilation. Chest 1993;104:1833. (A thorough review from a consensus conference.)

Tobin MJ, Luce JM: Update in critical care medicine. Ann Intern Med 1996;125:909. (Brief review with 5 references.)

Tobin MJ: Mechanical ventilation. N Engl J Med 1994; 330:1056. (Concise overview of objectives, methods, and complications.)

ACUTE RESPIRATORY DISTRESS SYNDROME (ARDS)

Essentials of Diagnosis

- History of systemic or pulmonary risk factor.
- Acute onset of respiratory distress.
- Bilateral pulmonary infiltrates.
- Normal pulmonary capillary wedge pressure (≤ 18 mm Hg) or clinical absence of evidence of left heart failure.
- Ratio of partial pressure of oxygen in arterial blood (Pa_{O_2}) to fractional concentration of inspired oxygen (F_{IO_2}) < 200 mm Hg.

General Considerations

Acute respiratory distress syndrome (also called adult respiratory distress syndrome) denotes acute respiratory failure following a systemic or pulmonary insult; it is characterized by respiratory distress, bilateral infiltrates, hypoxemia, noncompliant lungs, and normal pulmonary capillary wedge pressure (≤ 18 mm Hg). ARDS may follow a wide variety of catastrophic clinical events (Table 9–25). Common risk factors for ARDS include sepsis, aspiration of gastric contents, shock, infection, lung contusion, nonthoracic trauma, toxic inhalation, near-drowning, and multiple blood transfusions. About one-third of ARDS patients initially have sepsis syndrome. Pro-inflammatory cytokines (eg, tumor necrosis factor, interleukin-1) released from stimulated lymphocytes and macrophages appear to be pivotal in lung injury. Although the mechanism of lung injury varies with the cause, damage to capillary endothelial cells and alveolar epithelial cells (type I pneumocytes) is common to ARDS regardless of cause. Damage to these cells causes increased vascular permeability and inactivation of surfactant; both

Table 9–25. Selected disorders associated with ARDS.

Systemic Insults	Pulmonary Insults
Trauma	Aspiration of gastric contents
Sepsis	Embolism of thrombus, fat,
Pancreatitis	or amniotic fluid
Shock	Miliary tuberculosis
Multiple transfusions	Diffuse pneumonia
Disseminated intravascular	Viral
coagulation	*Mycoplasma*
Burns	Legionnaire's disease
Drugs	(*Legionella pneu-*
Narcotics	*mophila*)
Aspirin	*Pneumocystis*
Chlordiazepoxide	Near-drowning
Phenylbutazone	Toxic gas inhalation
Colchicine	Nitrogen dioxide
Ethchlorvynol	Chlorine
Hydrochlorothiazide	Sulfur dioxide
Paraldehyde	Ammonia
Lidocaine	Smoke inhalation
Thrombotic thrombocytopenic	Oxygen toxicity
purpura	Lung contusions
Cardiopulmonary bypass	Radiation
Venous air embolism	High altitude
Head injury	Hanging
Paraquat	Reexpansion

of these lead to interstitial and alveolar pulmonary edema and alveolar collapse.

Clinical Findings

ARDS is marked by the rapid onset of profound dyspnea that usually occurs 12–48 hours after the initiating event. Labored breathing, tachypnea, intercostal retractions, and crackles are noted on physical examination. Chest radiograph shows diffuse or patchy bilateral infiltrates that are initially interstitial but rapidly become alveolar; these characteristically spare the costophrenic angles. Air bronchograms occur in about 80% of cases. Upper lung zone venous engorgement (flow inversion) is distinctly uncommon. Heart size is normal, and pleural effusions are small or nonexistent. Marked hypoxemia occurs that is refractory to treatment with supplemental oxygen, indicating shunting. Most patients with ARDS demonstrate multiple organ failure, particularly involving the kidneys, liver, gut, central nervous system, and cardiovascular system.

Differential Diagnosis

Since ARDS is a physiologic and radiographic syndrome rather than a specific disease, the concept of differential diagnosis does not strictly apply. Normal-permeability ("cardiogenic") pulmonary edema must be ruled out, however, because specific therapy is available for that disorder. Measurement of pulmonary capillary wedge pressure by means of a flow-directed pulmonary artery catheter may be required, though routine use of the Swan-Ganz catheter in ARDS is discouraged.

Prevention

No measures that effectively prevent ARDS have been identified; specifically, prophylactic use of PEEP in patients at risk for ARDS has not been shown to be effective. Intravenous methylprednisolone does not prevent ARDS when given early to patients with sepsis syndrome or septic shock.

Treatment

Treatment of ARDS must include identification and specific treatment of the underlying condition (eg, sepsis). Aggressive supportive care must then be provided to compensate for the severe dysfunction of the respiratory system associated with ARDS. Supportive therapy almost always includes tracheal intubation and mechanical ventilation. The use of positive end expiratory pressure (PEEP) usually improves oxygenation in patients with ARDS but does not affect the natural history of this condition. PEEP should not be used routinely. The lowest level of PEEP that produces adequate oxygenation combined with an acceptable FIO_2 should be used. The lowest possible FIO_2 to keep the PaO_2 above 60 mm Hg or the SaO_2 above 90% should be used. High levels of PEEP may improve arterial PO_2 but may depress cardiac output and reduce oxygen delivery. Cardiac output must be monitored with a thermodilution pulmonary artery catheter whenever there is concern about adequacy of systemic oxygen transport (a product of cardiac output and arterial oxygen content) or the fluid balance of the patient. Cardiac output that falls when PEEP is used may be improved by reducing the level of PEEP or by administering inotropic drugs (eg, dopamine); administering fluids to increase intravascular volume should be done only with great caution, because doing so may worsen alveolar edema.

Elevated pulmonary capillary pressure worsens pulmonary edema in the presence of increased capillary permeability; therefore, the goal of fluid management is to maintain pulmonary capillary wedge pressure at the lowest possible level compatible with adequate cardiac output. Crystalloid solutions should be used when intravascular volume expansion is necessary. Diuretics should be used to reduce intravascular volume if pulmonary capillary wedge pressure is elevated. Packed red blood cell transfusions (see Chapter 13) are given to keep the hematocrit above 25%, a practice that maintains a reasonable arterial oxygen content.

Oxygenation in patients with ARDS may sometimes be improved by turning them from the supine to the prone position. Inhaled nitric oxide may be administered to lower pulmonary artery pressure in patients with ARDS, resulting in reduced shunting and improved oxygenation, but this therapy is still considered experimental.

Extracorporeal membrane oxygenation, PEEP,

corticosteroids, and prostaglandin E_1 have been shown not to improve survival. Corticosteroid therapy may benefit patients with ARDS due to radiation pneumonitis and possibly fat embolism syndrome. However, in patients with sepsis syndrome and ARDS, intravenous methylprednisolone has been shown to impede reversal of ARDS and increase its mortality rate.

Broad-spectrum antimicrobial treatment should be started promptly when infection is known or suspected (see above).

New treatment approaches under investigation include human recombinant interleukin-1 receptor antagonist, neutrophil inhibitors such as pentoxifylline derivatives, ketoconazole, corticosteroids late in the course of ARDS, small tidal volume mechanical ventilation, and inhaled nitric oxide.

Course & Prognosis

The mortality rate associated with ARDS exceeds 50%. Recent observations suggest that survival is improving. If ARDS is accompanied by sepsis, the mortality rate may reach 90%. The major cause of death in ARDS is nonpulmonary multiple organ system failure, often with sepsis. Median survival is about 2 weeks. Most survivors are asymptomatic within a few months, though abnormalities of oxygenation, diffusing capacity, and lung mechanics may persist in some.

Bernard GR et al: The American-European Consensus Conference on ARDS. Definitions, Mechanisms, Relevant Outcomes, and Clinical Trial Coordination. Am J Respir Crit Care Med 1994;149:818. (A summary of recommendations for future investigation in ARDS.)

Fulkerson WJ et al: Pathogenesis and treatment of the adult respiratory distress syndrome. Arch Intern Med 1996; 156:29. (Pathogenesis, mediators of lung injury, treatment, and experimental therapy.)

Hudson LD: New therapies for ARDS. Chest 1995;108 (Suppl):79S. (Recent developments in ventilator, pharmacologic, and other interventions.)

Schuster DP, Kollef MH: Acute respiratory distress syndrome. Dis Mon 1996 May;42:270. (Thorough review of current concepts; 180 references.)

Temmesfeld-Wollbruck B et al: Prevention and therapy of the adult respiratory distress syndrome. Lung 1995; 173:139. (Current review of therapy, including mechanical ventilation strategies.)

PLEURAL DISEASES

PLEURITIS

Pain due to acute pleural inflammation is caused by irritation of the parietal pleura. Such pain is localized, sharp, and fleeting and is made worse by cough, sneezing, deep breathing, or movement. When the central portion of the diaphragmatic parietal pleura is irritated, pain may be referred to the shoulder. There are numerous causes of pleuritis. The setting in which pleuritic pain develops helps to narrow the differential diagnosis; eg, in young, otherwise healthy individuals, pleuritis is usually caused by viral respiratory infections or pneumonia. The presence of pleural effusion, pleural thickening, or air in the pleural space requires further diagnostic and therapeutic measures. It should also be recalled that simple rib fracture may cause severe pleurisy.

Treatment of pleuritis consists of treating the underlying disease. Simple analgesics and anti-inflammatory drugs (eg, indomethacin, 25 mg orally two or three times daily) are often helpful for pain relief. Codeine (30–60 mg orally every 8 hours) may be used to control cough associated with pleuritic chest pain if retention of airway secretions is not a likely complication. Intercostal nerve blocks are sometimes helpful.

PLEURAL EFFUSION

Essentials of Diagnosis

- Asymptomatic in many cases; pleuritic chest pain if pleuritis is present; dyspnea if effusion is large.
- Decreased tactile fremitus; dullness to percussion; distant breath sounds; egophony if effusion is large.
- Radiographic evidence of pleural effusion.
- Diagnostic findings on thoracentesis.

General Considerations

Pleural fluid is formed in the normal individual mostly on the parietal pleural surface at the rate of about 0.1 mL/kg body weight/h. Absorption of this fluid on the visceral pleural surface is thought to occur, keeping the pleural space nearly dry. However, the parietal pleura may also contribute to absorption. Up to 25 mL of pleural fluid is normally present in the pleural space, an amount not detectable on conventional chest radiographs. Movement of fluid into and out of the pleural space is dependent mostly on hydrostatic and osmotic forces in parietal and visceral pleural capillaries. **Pleural effusion** is an abnormal accumulation of fluid in the pleural space. The five major types of pleural effusion are transudates, exudates, empyema, hemorrhagic pleural effusion or hemothorax, and chylous or chyliform effusion.

Pleural effusions are classified as **transudates** or **exudates** to help in differential diagnosis. An exudate is a pleural fluid having *one or more* of the following features: (1) pleural fluid protein to serum protein ratio > 0.5; (2) pleural fluid LDH to serum

LDH ratio > 0.6; and (3) pleural fluid LDH greater than two-thirds the upper limit of normal serum LDH. Transudates have none of these features.

Causes of transudates and exudates are listed in Table 9–26. Congestive heart failure accounts for most transudates and is the most common cause of pleural effusion. Mechanisms (and examples) leading to formation of transudates include increase in hydrostatic pressure (congestive heart failure), decreased oncotic pressure (hypoalbuminemia), and greater negative intrapleural pressure (acute atelectasis). Bacterial pneumonia and cancer are the commonest causes of exudative effusion. Exudates form as a result of disease of the pleura itself in association with increased capillary permeability (eg, pneumonia) or reduced lymphatic drainage (eg, carcinoma obstructing lymphatic drainage).

The gross appearance of pleural fluid helps to identify the other major types of pleural effusion. **Empyema** is an exudative pleural effusion caused by direct infection of the pleural space, causing the pleural fluid to appear purulent or turbid. **Hemothorax** is the presence of gross blood in the pleural space, usually a result of chest trauma. **Hemorrhagic pleural effusion** is a mixture of blood and pleural fluid. About 10,000 red blood cells per microliter are necessary to create blood-tinged pleural fluid; 100,000 red blood cells per microliter make pleural fluid appear grossly bloody. If the hematocrit of pleural fluid is more than 50% of the hematocrit of peripheral blood, hemothorax is present. In the absence of trauma, grossly bloody pleural fluid suggests cancer or, less commonly, pulmonary embolism.

Table 9–26. Causes of pleural fluid transudates and exudates.

Transudates	Exudates
Congestive heart failure	Pneumonia (parapneumonic effusion)
Cirrhosis with ascites	Cancer
Nephrotic syndrome	Pulmonary embolism
Peritoneal dialysis	Empyema
Myxedema	Tuberculosis
Acute atelectasis	Connective tissue disease
Constrictive pericarditis	Viral infection
Superior vena cava obstruction	Fungal infection
Pulmonary embolism	Rickettsial infection
	Parasitic infection
	Asbestos pleural effusion
	Meigs' syndrome
	Pancreatic disease
	Uremia
	Chronic atelectasis
	Trapped lung
	Chylothorax
	Sarcoidosis
	Drug reaction
	Post-myocardial infarction syndrome

Pleural fluid that is milky in appearance should be centrifuged. Clearing of the milky appearance from the supernatant suggests empyema, whereas persistent cloudy or turbid supernatant signifies **chylous** or **chyliform pleural effusion.** Chylous pleural effusion occurs acutely in chylothorax as a result of disruption of the thoracic duct. Chyliform pleural effusion occurs in pseudochylothorax as a result of accumulation of cholesterol complexes in a chronically thickened pleural space, a phenomenon sometimes seen in cases of trapped lung (entrapment of lung by a fibrous "peel" on the visceral pleura), tuberculous pleuritis (especially with previous therapeutic pneumothorax), or rheumatoid pleural effusion. A chylous pleural effusion has an acute or subacute onset. There is no associated pleural thickening on chest x-ray, and fluid analysis reveals chylomicrons and a high triglyceride level, usually above 100 mg/dL.

Clinical Findings

A. Symptoms and Signs: Small pleural effusions are usually asymptomatic, whereas large pleural effusions may cause dyspnea, particularly in the presence of underlying cardiopulmonary disease. Pleuritic chest pain and dry cough may occur; any pleural fluid found in association with pleuritic chest pain is invariably an exudate. Physical findings are absent if less than 200–300 mL of pleural fluid is present. Findings consistent with the presence of a larger pleural effusion include decrease in tactile fremitus, dullness to percussion, and diminution of breath sounds over the effusion. In large effusions that compress the lung, accentuation of breath sounds and egophony may be noted just above the effusion. A pleural friction rub indicates pleuritis. A massive pleural effusion with high intrapleural pressure may cause contralateral shift of the trachea and bulging of the intercostal spaces.

B. Laboratory Findings: Diagnostic thoracentesis should be performed whenever a pleural effusion is detected and no cause for the effusion is clinically apparent. Not all pleural effusions require diagnostic thoracentesis. More than 1 cm of free pleural fluid should be evident on a lateral decubitus x-ray before diagnostic thoracentesis is attempted. Decubitus films are the preferred method to demonstrate free pleural fluid. Ultrasound examination is useful to find the site for thoracentesis of a loculated pleural effusion.

Transudates lack the distinguishing protein and LDH findings described above and often have other typical characteristics (white blood cell count < 1000/μL, predominance of mononuclear cells in the differential, glucose level in pleural fluid equal to that of serum, and normal pH). Laboratory findings in exudative pleural effusions are more variable and are summarized in Table 9–27. If an exudate is suspected, thoracentesis should be performed quickly.

Table 9–27. Characteristics of important exudative pleural effusions.

Etiology or Type of Effusion	Gross Appearance	White Blood Cell Count (cells/μL)	Differential[1]	Red Blood Cell Count (cells/μL)	Glucose	Comments
Malignant effusion	Turbid to bloody; occasionally serous.	1000 to <100,000	M	100 to several hundred thousand.	Equal to serum levels; <60 mg/dL in 15% of cases.	Eosinophilia uncommon; positive results on cytologic examination.
Uncomplicated parapneumonic effusion	Clear to turbid.	5000–25,000	P	<5000	Equal to serum levels.	Tube thoracostomy unnecessary.
Empyema	Turbid to purulent.	25,000–100,000	P	<5000	Less than serum levels; often very low.	Drainage necessary; putrid odor suggests anaerobic infection.
Tuberculosis	Serous to serosanguineous.	5000–10,000	M	<10,000	Equal to serum levels; occasionally <60 mg/dL.	Protein may exceed 5 g/dL; eosinophils (>10%) or mesothelial cells (>5%) make diagnosis unlikely.
Rheumatoid effusion	Turbid; greenish-yellow.	1000–20,000	M or P	<1000	<40 mg/dL.	Secondary empyema common; high LDH, low complement, high rheumatoid factor, cholesterol crystals are characteristic.
Pulmonary infarction	Serous to grossly bloody.	1000–50,000	M or P	100 to >100,000	Equal to serum levels.	Variable findings; no pathognomonic features.
Esophageal rupture	Turbid to purulent; red-brown	<5000 to >50,000	P	1000–10,000	Usually low.	High amylase level (salivary origin); pneumothorax in 25% of cases; effusion usually on left side; pH <6.0 strongly suggests diagnosis.
Pancreatitis	Turbid to serosanguineous.	1000–50,000	P	1000–10,000	Equal to serum levels.	Usually left-sided; high amylase level.

[1]M = mononuclear cell predominance; P = polymorphonuclear leukocyte predominance.

One should have a low threshold for performing pleural biopsy at this time. The presence of malignant cells or positive results on smear or culture are pathognomonic findings in pleural fluid; determination of other causes depends on a constellation of findings on gross examination and laboratory studies or on biopsy results. Laboratory tests of pleural fluid should include total and differential white blood cell count, protein, glucose, and LDH. Additional tests may be ordered as required after thoracentesis. Pleural fluid pH is helpful in narrowing the differential diagnosis of exudative effusions. A pH less than 7.30 indicates cancer, complicated parapneumonic effusion, lupus or rheumatoid effusion, tuberculosis, or esophageal rupture. A high percentage of lymphocytes in pleural fluid suggests tuberculosis or cancer. Low levels of glucose in pleural fluid point toward cancer, empyema, tuberculosis, esophageal rupture, or connective tissue disease (rheumatoid pleuritis or systemic lupus erythematosus pleuritis). Elevated levels of amylase in pleural fluid suggest one of four diagnoses: pancreatitis, pancreatic pseudocyst, pancreatic cancer, or esophageal rupture.

Closed pleural biopsy with a Cope or Abrams needle should be considered whenever malignancy or tuberculosis is considered in the differential diagnosis of a pleural effusion that is unexplained after routine studies and thoracentesis. Contraindications include bleeding diathesis, poor respiratory reserve, empyema, and absence of pleural fluid. The expected yield of the procedure approximates 55% in pleural malignancy, somewhat less than with cytologic examination of pleural fluid, and over 75% in pleural tuberculosis if the tissue fragments are submitted for culture as well as histology. Open pleural biopsy is sometimes required to establish the diagnosis of pleural malignancy and is especially indicated for the diagnosis of malignant pleural mesothelioma. Thoracoscopy with a flexible or rigid instrument is an alternative procedure with excellent diagnostic accuracy in experienced hands.

C. Imaging: About 250 mL of pleural fluid must be present before effusion can be detected on conventional erect posteroanterior chest x-ray. Lateral decubitus views can detect much smaller amounts of free (nonloculated) pleural fluid. Free pleural fluid collects in the subpulmonary area. Larger amounts of fluid spill over into the costophrenic sulcus to form a meniscus. Thickening of major and minor fissures is common. Atypical collections of pleural fluid are frequently seen. Lateral displacement of the apex of the diaphragm and abrupt obliteration of lung markings at the level of the diaphragm are features of subpulmonary effusion. Pleural fluid may become trapped ("loculated") by pleural adhesions, forming unusual collections along the chest wall or in the lung fissures. Shadows with a broad base on the chest wall that point inward toward the hilum are characteristic of loculated effusions. Round or oval collections of loculated fluid in fissures resemble tumors ("pseudotumors"). Ultrasound is useful to locate loculated or small effusions.

Massive pleural effusion (opacification of an entire hemithorax) is usually caused by cancer but has been observed in tuberculosis and other diseases. CT scanning is sensitive in the detection of small amounts of free or loculated pleural fluid.

Treatment

Treatment should address both the disease causing the pleural effusion and the effusion itself. Because a specific diagnosis can be established in most cases of pleural effusion, a diagnosis of "idiopathic" effusion may delay or even prevent successful therapy.

A. Transudative Pleural Effusion: Transudative pleural effusions generally respond to treatment of the underlying condition; therapeutic thoracentesis is indicated only if massive effusion causes dyspnea. Pleurodesis and tube thoracostomy are rarely if ever indicated. When bilateral pleural effusions are detected in a patient with congestive heart failure, neither diagnostic nor therapeutic thoracentesis is routinely indicated. Such effusions are likely to be transudates and will resolve with treatment of the underlying cardiac disease.

B. Malignant or Paramalignant Pleural Effusion: Pleural effusion in a patient with known cancer may be either malignant or paramalignant. In cancer patients with **malignant pleural effusion,** the pleural surface is directly invaded by malignant cells (pleural fluid cytology or pleural tissue biopsy reveals evidence of malignancy). In such cases the tumor causing the effusion is unresectable, and treatment with chemotherapy or radiotherapy is directed at the underlying cancer. Chemical **pleurodesis** (obliteration of the pleural space by producing fibrous adhesion between the visceral and the parietal pleura) is advised for selected patients with symptomatic malignant pleural effusion who fail to respond to chemotherapy or mediastinal radiation or who are not candidates for these forms of therapy. Chemical pleurodesis is usually performed by instilling bleomycin, mitoxantrone, or talc slurry into the pleural space (see Chapter 4). Repeated therapeutic thoracentesis, pleuroperitoneal shunting, and surgical pleurectomy are alternative approaches for certain patients with rapidly recurring malignant pleural effusion. The term **"paramalignant pleural effusion"** denotes a pleural effusion in a patient with cancer when the pleural space is not directly invaded by tumor and repeated thoracentesis and needle biopsy of the pleura give negative results. In this situation, the underlying tumor may or may not be resectable.

C. Parapneumonic Pleural Effusion: Pleural effusion in the setting of pneumonia ("parapneumonic effusion") usually responds to systemic antibiotic therapy. Management steps include sputum Gram stain and culture, blood cultures, diagnostic thoracentesis, antibiotic therapy, and a decision regarding closed chest drainage (tube thoracostomy). *Effective therapy requires early intervention* to avoid progression of the effusion from the exudative to subsequent (fibrinopurulent and organized) stages. Loculation of pleural fluid collections is likely once organization has occurred. Laboratory findings—especially the pH, glucose concentration, and the white cell count of pleural fluid—are important in guiding additional therapy. In "uncomplicated" parapneumonic effusion, no pleural infection is present, and the pleural fluid glucose and pH are normal. Such effusion is likely to resolve spontaneously, and chest tube drainage is not required. In "complicated" parapneumonic effusion, pleural fluid is either frank empyema or has the potential to organize into a fibrous "peel." A low pH (< 7.2), low glucose (< 50 mg/dL), and high LDH (> 1000 units/L)—but not a high pleural fluid white blood cell count or protein concentration—help to separate complicated from uncomplicated parapneumonic effusions.

Tube thoracostomy is required for parapneumonic effusion if any of the following is present: (1) the fluid resembles frank pus, (2) pleural fluid glucose is < 40 mg/dL, or (3) pleural fluid pH is < 7.0. If the pleural fluid pH is between 7.0 and 7.2 or the LDH is > 1000 units/L, the physician should strongly consider chest tube placement or should monitor the effusion carefully with serial thoracenteses. Serial thoracentesis is not an effective strategy for *treatment* of complicated parapneumonic effusions. The treatment of nonpurulent complicated parapneumonic effusions (Gram stain- or culture-positive and pH < 7.20) requires appropriate antibiotic therapy. However, the routine use of tube thoracostomy in such cases is controversial.

A parapneumonic effusion that does not respond to drainage within 24 hours may have become loculated. The clinician should be aware that localized pockets of empyema may be present in this circumstance, even though thoracentesis from another localized fluid collection did not reveal empyema. In such cases, ultrasound examination is required to guide placement of an additional chest tube in the proper location. Intrapleural injection of streptokinase via the chest tube (250,000 units in 100 mL 0.9% saline daily for up to 10 days) may accelerate drainage. Open surgical drainage may be necessary if these measures are ineffective. A thick pleural "peel" developing after treatment of complicated parapneumonic effusion may resolve slowly over several months. Surgical decortication should be reserved for selected patients with established fibrothorax.

D. Hemothorax: Hemothorax is generally managed by the immediate insertion of one or more large chest tubes in order to control bleeding by causing apposition of pleural surfaces; chest tubes help the physician determine the amount of bleeding and decrease the risk of complications such as empyema and eventual fibrothorax. As much blood as possible should be drained before the chest tube is removed. Thoracotomy is occasionally required to control bleeding, remove large volumes of blood clots, and treat coexisting complications of trauma such as bronchopleural fistula. A very small hemothorax that is stable or improving on chest x-ray can be managed without tube drainage.

E. Other Types of Pleural Effusion: Management of patients with exudative pleural effusion due to other causes consists mainly of treating the underlying disease. A low pleural fluid pH outside the setting of pneumonia is not an automatic indication for chest tube drainage. Patients with rheumatoid pleural effusions should be watched closely for the development of secondary empyema.

Prognosis

The prognosis of patients with pleural effusion depends on the prognosis of the underlying disease. The prognosis of patients with documented malignant pleural effusion is poor, particularly if pleural fluid pH or glucose levels are low.

Daniel TM: Diagnostic thoracoscopy for pleural disease. Ann Thorac Surg 1993;56:639. (Use in malignant pleural effusion.)

LeMense GP, Strange C, Sahn SA: Empyema thoracis: Therapeutic management and outcome. Chest 1995; 107:1532. (Review of experience with 43 cases.)

Light RW: A new classification of parapneumonic effusions and empyema. Chest 1995;108:299. (A proposal for a new classification scheme to guide initial therapy.)

Sahn SA: Management of complicated parapneumonic ef-
fusions. Am Rev Respir Dis 1993;148:813. (Pathophysiology and management.)

Walker-Renard PB, Vaughan LM, Sahn SA: Chemical pleurodesis for malignant pleural effusions. Ann Intern Med 1994;120:56. (Emphasizing the use of doxycycline and minocycline as replacements for tetracycline.)

SPONTANEOUS PNEUMOTHORAX

Essentials of Diagnosis

- Acute onset of ipsilateral chest pain and dyspnea, often of several days' duration.
- Minimal physical findings in mild cases; unilateral chest expansion, decreased tactile fremitus, hyper-resonance, diminished breath sounds, mediastinal shift, cyanosis in tension pneumothorax.
- Presence of pleural air on chest x-ray.

General Considerations

Pneumothorax, or accumulation of air in the pleural space, is classified as spontaneous (primary or secondary) or traumatic. Primary pneumothorax occurs in the absence of an underlying cause, whereas secondary pneumothorax is a complication of preexisting pulmonary disease. Traumatic pneumothorax results from penetrating or nonpenetrating trauma and is often iatrogenic. Iatrogenic pneumothorax may follow procedures such as thoracentesis, pleural biopsy, subclavian line placement, percutaneous lung biopsy, bronchoscopy with transbronchial biopsy, and positive-pressure mechanical ventilation. In tension pneumothorax, the pressure of air in the pleural space exceeds ambient pressure throughout the respiratory cycle. A check-valve mechanism allows air to enter the pleural space on inspiration and prevents egress of air on expiration.

Pneumothorax affects mainly tall, thin men between the ages of 20 and 40 years. It is thought to occur from rupture of subpleural apical blebs in response to high negative intrapleural pressures. Familial factors and cigarette smoking may also be important.

Secondary pneumothorax occurs as a complication of COPD, asthma, cystic fibrosis, tuberculosis, and a wide variety of infiltrative lung diseases, including pneumocystis pneumonia. Aerosolized pentamidine and prior history of pneumocystis pneumonia are considered potential risk factors for the development of pneumothorax. One-half of patients with pneumothorax in the setting of recurrent pneumocystis pneumonia develop contralateral pneumothorax. The mortality rate of pneumothorax in pneumocystis pneumonia is high. Pneumothorax in association with menstruation (catamenial pneumothorax) is another well-established form of secondary pneumothorax. The pathogenesis of catamenial pneumothorax is not well established. Because of underlying disease, secondary pneumothorax is usually a more serious condition than primary spontaneous pneumothorax.

Clinical Findings

A. Symptoms and Signs: Chest pain on the affected side and dyspnea occur in nearly all patients. Symptoms usually begin during rest or sleep. Many patients wait for several days before seeking medical attention. Alternatively, this may be present with life-threatening respiratory failure if underlying COPD or asthma is present; this is true irrespective of the size of the pneumothorax.

If pneumothorax is small, physical findings, other than mild tachycardia, are unimpressive. If pneumothorax is large, diminished breath sounds, decreased tactile fremitus, and hyperresonance are noted. Tension pneumothorax should be suspected in the presence of severe tachycardia, hypotension, and mediastinal or tracheal shift.

B. Laboratory Findings: Arterial blood gas analysis reveals hypoxemia in most patients but is often unnecessary. Left-sided primary pneumothorax may produce QRS axis and precordial T wave changes on the ECG that may be misinterpreted as acute myocardial infarction.

C. Imaging: Demonstration of a visceral pleural line on chest x-ray is diagnostic and is best revealed on an expiratory film. A few patients have secondary pleural effusion that demonstrates a characteristic air-fluid level on chest radiography. In supine patients, pneumothorax on a conventional chest x-ray may appear as an abnormally radiolucent costophrenic sulcus (the "deep sulcus" sign). In patients with tension pneumothorax, chest x-rays show a large amount of air in the affected hemithorax and contralateral shift of mediastinal structures. Tension pneumothorax usually occurs in the setting of penetrating trauma, lung infection, cardiopulmonary resuscitation, or positive-pressure mechanical ventilation.

Differential Diagnosis

If the patient is a young, tall, thin, cigarette-smoking man, the diagnosis of primary spontaneous pneumothorax is usually obvious and can be confirmed by chest x-ray. In secondary pneumothorax, it is sometimes difficult to distinguish loculated pneumothorax from an emphysematous bleb. Occasionally, pneumothorax may mimic myocardial infarction, pulmonary embolization, or pneumonia.

Complications

Tension pneumothorax may result in acute respiratory failure treated with mechanical ventilation. Cardiopulmonary arrest and death are extremely rare. Pneumomediastinum and subcutaneous emphysema may occur as complications of spontaneous pneumothorax. If pneumomediastinum is detected, rupture of the esophagus or a bronchus should be considered.

Treatment

Treatment depends upon the severity of pneumothorax and the nature of the underlying disease. The patient with a new small (< 15%) pneumothorax should be hospitalized and placed at bed rest, treated symptomatically for cough and chest pain, and followed with serial chest x-rays every 12–24 hours. Observation in the hospital for 2 days is adequate in most cases. A patient with a small pneumothorax that has been observed to be stable in size for several days to a week can be followed closely with serial chest x-rays without hospitalization. Many small pneumothoraces resolve spontaneously as air is absorbed from the pleural space; however, pneumothorax may unpredictably progress to tension pneumothorax. Progression to tension pneumothorax is accelerated during positive-pressure mechanical ventilation. In this situation, or in patients who are severely symptomatic or who have a larger pneumothorax (> 15%), chest tube placement (tube thoracostomy) is performed. Small tubes (about 16 gauge) may be effective in cases of small, uncomplicated pneumothorax. The chest tube is placed under water-seal drainage, and suction is applied until the lung expands. Intravenous catheters and emergency pneumothorax treatment tubes should not be used in the hospital setting because of a high rate of technical failures. Air leaks persisting after 3 days are unusual. Tube thoracostomy alone does not cause enough pleural scarification to prevent recurrence of spontaneous pneumothorax. Pulmonary edema on the affected side may follow abrupt evacuation of pneumothorax. If tension pneumothorax is suspected, a large-bore needle should be inserted immediately in the affected side; tube thoracostomy may be performed thereafter.

All patients should be advised to discontinue smoking and warned that the risk of recurrence is 50%. Exposure to high altitudes, flying in unpressurized aircraft, and scuba diving should be avoided. If spontaneous pneumothorax recurs, the second episode should be managed in a manner similar to that of the first episode. Some experts advocate surgery for any recurrence.

Indications for thoracoscopy or open thoracotomy include recurrences of spontaneous pneumothorax (the minimum number of episodes being controversial), any occurrence of bilateral pneumothorax, and failure of tube thoracostomy for the first episode (failure of lung to reexpand or persistent air leak). Surgery permits stapling or laser pleurodesis of the ruptured blebs responsible for the pneumothorax and greatly reduces the risk of recurrence. Pleural symphysis may be obtained by scarification from abrasion of the pleural surface. Pleurectomy is of no particular value. Management of pneumothorax in patients with pneumocystis pneumonia is challenging because of a tendency toward recurrence, and there is no consensus on the best approach. Use of a small chest tube attached to a Heimlich flutter valve has been proposed to allow the patient to leave the hospital. Some clinicians favor its insertion early in the course.

Prognosis

About half of patients with spontaneous pneumothorax experience recurrence of the disorder after either observation or tube thoracostomy for the first episode. Recurrence after surgery is rare. Following successful therapy, there are no long-term complications.

Despars JA, Sassoon CSH, Light RW: Significance of iatrogenic pneumothoraces. Chest 1994;105:1147. (Incidence exceeds that of spontaneous pneumothorax, and the associated morbidity and mortality rates are considerable.)

Jantz MA, Pierson DJ: Pneumothorax and barotrauma. Clin Chest Med 1994;15:75. (Review of mechanisms and management of spontaneous pneumothorax, pneumothorax associated with mechanical ventilation, traumatic and tension pneumothorax, and features of barotrauma.)

Kennedy L, Sahn SA: Talc pleurodesis for the treatment of pneumothorax and pleural effusion. Chest 1994;106: 1215. (The overall success rate is 91%.)

Slabbynck H et al: Thoracoscopic findings in spontaneous pneumothorax in AIDS. Chest 1994;106:1582. (Review of experience with pneumothorax in AIDS.)

Heart

10

Barry M. Massie, MD, & Thomas M. Amidon, MD

SYMPTOMS & SIGNS

COMMON SYMPTOMS

The most common symptoms of heart disease are dyspnea, chest pain, palpitations, presyncope or syncope, and fatigue. None are specific, and interpretation depends on the entire clinical picture and, in many cases, diagnostic testing.

For more complete discussions of the symptoms and signs of heart disease, see references below.

Dyspnea

Dyspnea due to heart disease is precipitated or exacerbated by exertion and results from elevated left atrial and pulmonary venous pressures or hypoxia. The former are most commonly caused by left ventricular systolic dysfunction, left ventricular diastolic dysfunction (due to hypertrophy, fibrosis, or pericardial disease), or valvular obstruction. The acute onset or worsening of left atrial hypertension may result in **pulmonary edema. Hypoxia** may be due to pulmonary edema or intracardiac shunting. Dyspnea should be quantified by the amount of activity that precipitates it. Dyspnea is also a common symptom of pulmonary disease, and the etiologic distinction may be very difficult. Shortness of breath is also found in sedentary or obese individuals, anxiety states, anemia, and many other illnesses.

Orthopnea is dyspnea that occurs in recumbency and results from an increase in central blood volume. Orthopnea may also result from pulmonary disease and obesity. Both are more specific for cardiac diseases than exertional dyspnea, but neither is diagnostic of heart failure. **Paroxysmal nocturnal dyspnea** is shortness of breath that occurs abruptly 30 minutes to 2 hours after going to bed and is relieved by sitting up or standing up; this symptom is more specific for cardiac disease.

Gillespie DJ, Staats BA: Unexplained dyspnea. Mayo Clin Proc 1994;69:657.

Manning HL, Schwartzstein RM: Pathophysiology of dyspnea. N Engl J Med 1995;333:1547.

Chest Pain

Chest pain is a common symptom that can occur as a result of pulmonary or musculoskeletal disease, esophageal or other gastrointestinal disorders, cervicothoracic nerve root irritation, or anxiety states, as well as many cardiovascular diseases. The commonest cause of cardiac chest pain is myocardial ischemia. This is usually described as dull, aching, or as a sensation of "pressure," "tightness," "squeezing," or "gas," rather than as sharp or spasmodic; and it is often perceived as an uncomfortable sensation rather than "pain." **Ischemic pain** usually subsides within 30 minutes but may last longer. Protracted episodes often represent **myocardial infarction.** The pain is commonly accompanied by a sense of anxiety or uneasiness. The location is usually retrosternal or left precordial. Though the pain may radiate to or be localized in the throat, lower jaw, shoulders, inner arms, upper abdomen, or back, it nearly always also involves the sternal region. Ischemic pain is often precipitated by exertion, cold temperature, meals, stress, or combinations of these factors and is usually relieved by rest, but many episodes do not conform to these patterns. It is not related to position or respiration and is usually not elicited by chest palpation. In myocardial infarction, a precipitating factor is frequently not apparent.

Hypertrophy of either ventricle and aortic valvular disease may also give rise to ischemic pain or pain with less typical features. Myocarditis, cardiomyopathy, and mitral valve prolapse are associated with chest pain of a more atypical nature. Pericarditis may produce pain that changes with position or respiration. Aortic dissection produces an instantaneous tearing pain of great intensity that often radiates to the back.

Douglas PS, Ginsburg GS: The evaluation of chest pain in women. N Engl J Med 1996;334:1311. (Interpretation and workup.)

Maseri A et al: Mechanisms and significance of cardiac ischemic pain. Prog Cardiovasc Dis 1992;35:1. (Clinical characteristics of ischemic pain and mechanisms causing it.)

Mayou R et al: Non-cardiac chest pain and benign palpitations in the cardiac clinic. Br Heart J 1994;72:548. (Most patients in a consecutive series were thought to have noncardiac pain, but many nonetheless continued to be disabled by the symptoms.)

Richter JE et al (editors): Unexplained chest pain. Med Clin North Am 1991;75:No. 5. (Differential diagnosis and management.)

Palpitations, Dizziness, Syncope

Awareness of the heartbeat may be a normal phenomenon or may reflect increased cardiac or stroke output in patients with many noncardiac conditions (eg, exercise, thyrotoxicosis, anemia, anxiety). It may also be due to cardiac abnormalities that increase stroke volume (regurgitant valvular disease, bradycardia) or may be a manifestation of cardiac arrhythmias. Ventricular premature beats may be sensed as extra or "skipped" beats. Supraventricular or ventricular tachycardia may be felt as rapid, regular or irregular palpitations or "fluttering"; many patients are asymptomatic, however.

If the abnormal rhythm is associated with a sufficient decline in arterial pressure or cardiac output, it may—especially in the upright position—impair cerebral blood flow, causing dizziness, blurring of vision, loss of consciousness (syncope), or other symptoms.

Cardiogenic syncope most commonly results from sinus node arrest or exit block, atrioventricular conduction block, or ventricular tachycardia or fibrillation. It is associated with few prodromal symptoms and may thus be an occasion for injuries. The absence of premonitory symptoms helps distinguish cardiogenic syncope (often called Stokes-Adams attacks) from vasovagal faint, postural hypotension, or seizure. Although recovery is often immediate, some patients may exhibit seizure-like movements. Aortic valve disease and hypertrophic obstructive cardiomyopathy may also cause syncope, which is usually exertional or postexertional. Another form of syncope that has been the subject of considerable recent attention is termed **neurocardiogenic syncope.** In this syndrome, there is an inappropriate increase in vagal efferent activity, often resulting from a precedent increase in sympathetic cardiac stimulation. Syncope may follow a brief period of diaphoresis and presyncopal symptoms, or it may be abrupt in onset, mimicking arrhythmia-induced syncope.

Brugada P et al: Investigation of palpitations. Lancet 1993;341:1254. (Causes and evaluation.)

Kapoor WN: Workup and management of patients with syncope. Med Clin North Am 1995;79:1153.

Weber BE, Kapoor WN: Evaluation and outcome of patients with palpitations. Am J Med 1996;100:138. (In a series of 190 consecutive patients, the identified cause was cardiac in 43%, psychiatric in 31%, and unclear in 16%. Overall outcome was excellent.)

Edema

Subcutaneous fluid collections appear first in the lower extremities in ambulatory patients or in the sacral region of bedridden individuals. In heart disease, edema results from elevated right atrial pressures. Right heart failure most commonly results from left heart failure, although the right-sided signs may predominate. Other cardiogenic causes of edema include pericardial disease, right-sided valve lesions, and cor pulmonale. Edema may also be due to peripheral venous insufficiency, venous obstruction, nephrotic syndrome, cirrhosis, or premenstrual fluid retention, or it may be idiopathic. Advanced right heart failure can produce ascites, almost always in conjunction with edema.

Ciocon JO, Fernandez BB, Ciocon DG: Leg edema: Clinical clues to the differential diagnosis. Geriatrics 1993;48:34. (Review of the many causes of edema, with focus on the older population.)

FUNCTIONAL CLASSIFICATION OF HEART DISEASE

As a means of quantifying the limitation on activity of cardiac patients imposed by their symptoms, the classification system of the New York Heart Association is commonly employed. In following individual patients, it is important to document specific activities that produce symptoms.

Class I: No limitation of physical activity. Ordinary physical activity does not cause undue fatigue, dyspnea, or anginal pain.

Class II: Slight limitation of physical activity. Ordinary physical activity results in symptoms.

Class III: Marked limitation of physical activity. Comfortable at rest, but less than ordinary activity causes symptoms.

Class IV: Unable to engage in any physical activity without discomfort. Symptoms may be present even at rest.

SIGNS OF HEART DISEASE

Although the cardiovascular examination centers on the heart, peripheral signs are often invaluable.

Appearance

While cardiac patients may appear healthy and comfortable at rest, many with acute myocardial infarction appear anxious and restless. **Diaphoresis** suggests hypotension or a hyperadrenergic state, such as during pericardial tamponade, tachyarrhythmias, or myocardial infarction. Patients with severe congestive heart failure or other chronic low cardiac output states may appear **cachectic.**

Cyanosis may be central, due to arterial desaturation, or peripheral, reflecting impaired tissue delivery of adequately saturated blood in low-output states, polycythemia, or peripheral vasoconstriction. Central cyanosis may be caused by pulmonary disease, left heart failure, or right-to-left shunting; the latter will not be improved by increasing the inspired oxygen concentration. **Pallor** usually indicates anemia but may be a sign of low cardiac output.

Vital Signs

Although the normal **heart rate** ranges from 50 to 100 beats/min, both slower and more rapid rates may occur in normal individuals or may reflect noncardiac conditions such as anxiety or pain, medication effect, thyroid disease, pulmonary disease, anemia, or hypovolemia. If symptoms or clinical suspicion warrants, an electrocardiogram (ECG) should be performed to diagnose arrhythmia, conduction disturbance, or other abnormality. The range of normal **blood pressure** is wide, but even in asymptomatic individuals systolic pressures below 90 mm Hg or above 140 mm Hg and diastolic pressures above 90 mm Hg warrant further clinical evaluation and follow-up. Initially elevated pressures may decline if the patient is allowed to relax and rest comfortably. **Tachypnea** is also nonspecific, but pulmonary disease and heart failure should be considered when respiratory rates exceed 16/min under basal conditions. **Periodic breathing** (Cheyne-Stokes respiration) is not uncommon in severe heart failure.

Peripheral Pulses & Venous Pulsations

Diminished peripheral pulses most commonly result from arteriosclerotic peripheral vascular disease and may be accompanied by localized **bruits.** Asymmetry of pulses should also arouse suspicion of coarctation of the aorta or aortic dissection; previous cardiac catheterization may also be responsible. **Exaggerated pulses** may indicate aortic regurgitation, coarctation, patent ductus arteriosus, or other conditions that increase stroke volume. The carotid pulse is a valuable aid to assessment of left ventricular ejection. It has a **delayed upstroke** in aortic stenosis and a **bisferiens** quality (two palpable peaks) in mixed aortic stenosis and regurgitation or hypertrophic obstructive cardiomyopathy. **Pulsus paradoxus** (a decrease in systolic blood pressure during inspiration greater than the normal 10 mm Hg) is a valuable sign of pericardial tamponade, though it also occurs in asthma and chronic obstructive pulmonary disease.

Jugular venous pulsations provide insight into right atrial pressure. They indicate (1) **elevated central venous pressure** if they are more than 3 vertical centimeters above the angle of Louis, (2) increased central blood volume if they rise more than 1 cm with sustained (30 seconds) right upper quadrant abdominal pressure **(hepatojugular reflux),** (3) tricuspid obstruction or pulmonary hypertension if the *a* wave is exaggerated, and (4) tricuspid regurgitation if **large** *cv* waves are seen. The latter may be associated with hepatic pulsations. Atrioventricular dissociation due to conduction block or ventricular arrhythmia can be recognized by intermittent **cannon** *a* **waves.**

Buttman SM et al: Bedside cardiovascular examination of patients with severe chronic heart failure: Importance of inducible jugular venous distension. J Am Coll Cardiol 1993;22:968.

Cook DJ, Simel DL: Does this patient have abnormal central venous pressure? JAMA 1996;275:630. (Guide to examination of jugular venous pulses.)

Pulmonary Examination

Rales heard at the lung bases are a sign of congestive heart failure but may be caused by similarly localized pulmonary disease. **Wheezing** and **rhonchi** suggest obstructive pulmonary disease but may occur in left heart failure. **Pleural effusions** with bibasilar percussion dullness and reduced breath sounds are common in congestive heart failure.

Precordial Pulsations

A **parasternal lift** usually indicates right ventricular hypertrophy, pulmonary hypertension (pulmonary artery systolic pressure > 50 mm Hg), or left atrial enlargement; pulmonary artery pulsations may also be visible. The left ventricular **apical impulse,** if sustained and enlarged, suggests myocardial hypertrophy or dysfunction. If it is very prominent but not sustained, the apical impulse may indicate volume overload or high-output states. Additional precordial pulsations may reflect regional abnormalities of left ventricular contraction.

Heart Sounds & Murmurs

Auscultation is diagnostic of—or helpful in diagnosis of—many heart diseases, including cardiac failure. Specific findings are discussed under diagnostic headings.

The **first heart sound (S_1)** may be diminished with severe left ventricular dysfunction or accentuated with mitral stenosis or short PR intervals. S_2 is usually split, with the two components (aortic preceding pulmonary) being separated more during inspiration; **splitting** is *fixed* in atrial septal defect, *wide* with right bundle branch block, and *absent* or *reversed* (**paradoxic splitting**) with aortic stenosis, left ventricular failure, or left bundle branch block. With normal splitting, an accentuated P_2 is an important sign of pulmonary hypertension. **Third and fourth heart sounds** (ventricular and atrial gallops, respectively) indicate ventricular volume overload or impaired compliance and may be heard over either ventricle. An apical S_3 is a normal finding in younger individuals and in pregnancy. Additional auscultatory findings include sharp, high-pitched sounds classified as **"clicks."** These may be early systolic and represent **ejection sounds** (as with a bicuspid aortic valve or pulmonary stenosis) or may occur in mid or late systole, indicating myxomatous changes in the mitral valve.

While many **murmurs** indicate valvular disease, a soft, short systolic murmur, usually localized along the left sternal border or toward the apex, may be innocent, reflecting pulmonary flow. **Innocent murmurs** often vary with inspiration, diminish in the upright position, and are most frequently heard in thin individuals. **Systolic murmurs** are **pansystolic (holosystolic)** when they merge with the first sound and persist through all of systole or **"ejection" murmurs** when they begin after the first sound and end before the second sound, with a peak in early or mid systole. The former represent mitral regurgitation if maximal at the apex or in the axilla and tricuspid regurgitation or ventricular septal defect if best heard at the sternal border. Short aortic ejection murmurs with a preserved A_2 are common in older individuals, especially when hypertension has been present, and even if they are moderately loud they usually reflect thickening (sclerosis) of the valve rather than stenosis. Association of murmurs with palpable vibrations **("thrills")** is always clinically significant, as are **diastolic murmurs.**

Edema

Peripheral edema, especially if it is bilateral and associated with other symptoms and signs, may indicate heart failure. Other causes of edema include peripheral venous abnormalities; hepatic, renal, and thyroid disease; and fluid retention due to medications (especially calcium blockers or nonsteroidal agents) or estrogen effect.

Constant J: *Bedside Cardiology,* 4th ed. Little, Brown, 1993. (The disappearing art of clinical assessment.)

Marriott HJ: *Bedside Cardiac Diagnosis.* Lippincott, 1993. (Clinical wisdom from an accomplished teacher.)

Shaver JA: Cardiac auscultation: A cost-effective diagnostic skill. Curr Probl Cardiol 1995;20:441. (Entire issue on approach to and interpretation of the auscultatory examination.)

DIAGNOSTIC TESTING

The **chest x-ray** will provide information about heart size, the pulmonary circulation (with character-

istic signs suggesting both pulmonary artery or pulmonary venous hypertension), primary pulmonary disease, and aortic abnormalities. The **echocardiogram** provides much more reliable information about chamber size, hypertrophy, pericardial effusions, valvular abnormalities, and congenital abnormalities, and where readily available this procedure has replaced the x-ray for evaluation of cardiac disease. The **electrocardiogram (ECG)** indicates cardiac rhythm, reveals conduction abnormalities, and provides evidence of ventricular hypertrophy, myocardial infarction, or ischemia. Nonspecific ST segment and T wave changes may reflect these processes but are also noted with electrolyte imbalance, drug effects, and many other conditions. Routine x-rays and ECGs are not recommended to screen for heart disease and have a limited role in the follow-up of patients with known heart disease. However, a baseline ECG is helpful in older patients.

Goldberger AL: *Clinical Electrocardiography: A Simplified Approach,* 5th ed. Mosby, 1994.

Sox HC: The baseline electrocardiogram. Am J Med 1991;91:573. (When and when not to get it.)

Wagner GS: *Mariott's Practical Electrocardiography,* 9th ed. Williams & Wilkins, 1994.

SPECIAL DIAGNOSTIC PROCEDURES

Noninvasive diagnostic procedures are growing in number and application. However, they are frequently overutilized. The clinician should carefully consider what question is being asked and how the results will alter patient management before ordering these tests. They have limited applicability in screening for asymptomatic disease and should not be substituted for a careful clinical evaluation.

Exercise Electrocardiography

The resting ECG is often insensitive to ischemia, but horizontal or downsloping exercise-induced ST segment depression, particularly when it exceeds 0.15 mV (1.5 mm with usual standardization), is strongly suggestive. Exercise-induced chest pain and hypotension also suggest coronary disease. Exercise testing has a sensitivity of 60–80% and a specificity of 70–80%, and these figures may increase with concomitant imaging procedures. This test helps to diagnose or exclude disease, to estimate its severity, and to provide guidelines for activity in patients with known ischemic heart disease. However, it has not proved very useful in screening asymptomatic individuals, since false-positive results are common (especially in women) and the sensitivity for predicting future events is low.

Fletcher GF et al: Exercise standards: A statement for health professionals from the American Heart Association. Circulation 1995;91:580. (Consensus on procedures, interpretation, and indications for exercise testing. Also discusses risks and procedures for exercise training.)

Jain A, Murray DR: Detection of myocardial ischemia. Curr Probl Cardiol 1995;20:773. (Comprehensive review of exercise testing and other diagnostic procedures.)

Myers J, Froelicher VF: Exercise testing: Procedures and limitations. Cardiol Clin 1993;11:199.

Ambulatory Electrocardiographic Monitoring & Signal-Averaged ECG

Ambulatory electrocardiographic (Holter) monitoring is most useful for determining the need for therapy in patients with symptoms consistent with arrhythmia. Since these symptoms are often nonspecific, their temporal association with a conduction or rhythm disturbance provides a definitive indication for treatment. Documentation of asymptomatic "premonitory" abnormalities such as second-degree atrioventricular block, transient sinus node arrest, or nonsustained ventricular tachycardia may by association suggest the basis for previous symptomatic episodes. Although ambulatory electrocardiographic monitoring is frequently performed in patients with heart disease without symptoms consistent with arrhythmia—and although the detection of frequent or repetitive ventricular ectopy is sometimes associated with a poor prognosis—there are no studies which indicate that interventions alter prognosis. Thus, ambulatory monitoring is rarely indicated except for symptom evaluation.

A number of studies have employed ambulatory monitoring to detect and quantify silent ischemia, which is diagnosed by ST segment shifts. However, the routine clinical use of this approach is not justified by current data, since most patients with silent ischemic episodes also have symptomatic episodes, and the value of treating silent ischemia has not been proved.

Although it has long been appreciated that there are periodical fluctuations in heart rate even under basal conditions, considerable recent interest has been focused on measurements of **heart rate variability.** These measurements can be made under controlled conditions in the electrocardiography laboratory or from recordings obtained during ambulatory monitoring. Greater fluctuations in heart rate correspond to greater parasympathetic activity, and several studies have indicated that greater heart rate variability is associated with a better prognosis and fewer life-threatening arrhythmias in a variety of cardiac conditions. More recently, analyses have employed frequency transformation of RR cycle length variability to provide indices of the relative balance between parasympathetic and sympathetic activity, with the greater contribution of the parasympathetic system being considered to confer a better prognosis.

In studies of postinfarction patients and patients with symptomatic arrhythmias, these indices have had some prognostic value. However, adequate data are not yet available to support routine use of this technique in clinical practice.

Another new technique is the **signal-averaged ECG.** Most commonly, an orthogonal three-lead system is employed to record 300 consecutive beats during basal conditions. Using appropriate electrical filtering and computer averaging of the signal, very low frequency signals called "late potentials" can be identified in the period following the QRS complex. Abnormal late potentials are considered markers for potential ventricular arrhythmias. Adequate data are not yet available to define the role of this technique with confidence, but it may be useful in detecting groups of patients at increased risk for arrhythmic events after myocardial infarction. Approximately one-third of these patients will have abnormal late potentials, and these individuals are at higher risk for arrhythmic events, though the positive predictive value of this finding is relatively low (10–15%). More importantly, the absence of late potentials identifies a group of patients at low risk for arrhythmic events, so post-myocardial infarction patients found to have frequent ventricular ectopy or nonsustained ventricular tachycardia in the absence of late potentials may not require further investigation or treatment. The prognostic value of late potentials in patients with chronic ischemic heart disease who are more than 6–12 months removed from myocardial infarction and in patients with other forms of heart disease is not yet known.

Cain ME et al: Signal-averaged electrocardiography. J Am Coll Cardiol 1996;27:238. (Consensus statement on the methodology and application of this technique.)

Heart rate variability: Standards of measurement, physiologic interpretation, and clinical use. Circulation 1996; 93:1043. (Comprehensive consensus document.)

Kautzner J, Camm AJ: Clinical relevance of heart rate variability. Clin Cardiol 1997;20:162. (So far, a technique in search of an application.)

Mulcahy D et al: Ischemia during ambulatory monitoring as a prognostic indicator in patients with unstable coronary artery disease. JAMA 1997;277:318. (Ambulatory electrocardiographic monitoring did not predict cardiac events in low-risk patients with unstable angina.)

Echocardiography

M-mode and **two-dimensional echocardiograms** yield semiquantitative measurements of left ventricular size, function, and thickness and qualitative information about aortic and mitral stenosis. Left ventricular segmental wall motion can be assessed, and the size of all four cardiac chambers can be determined. Hypertrophic cardiomyopathy, pericardial effusion, mitral valve prolapse, valvular vegetations, and cardiac tumors may all be diagnosed. **Two-dimensional echocardiograms** visualize most of the heart.

Doppler ultrasound provides a quantitative estimation of transvalvular gradients and pulmonary artery pressure and qualitative evaluation of valvular regurgitation and intraventricular shunts. **Color Doppler** visually demonstrates patterns and directionality of flow; it has been particularly useful in evaluating congenital heart disease. Doppler studies frequently detect *clinically insignificant* valvular regurgitation; care should be taken not to overinterpret those findings.

Transesophageal echocardiography is used in an increasing number of centers to improve the quality of echocardiograms, to derive information about posterior structures and prosthetic valves, and to monitor patients during surgery. It is superior to surface echocardiography in diagnosing left atrial thrombi, valvular vegetations, and eccentric mitral regurgitant jets (especially with prosthetic valves). The absence of mural thrombi identifies patients in atrial fibrillation at low risk for embolization, thus facilitating early cardioversion. It is also quite sensitive in detecting aortic dissection and severe atherosclerosis of the ascending aorta, which may be the source for transient ischemic attacks or embolic strokes.

Stress echocardiography is being used increasingly to enhance the information available from ECGs and as an alternative to nuclear medicine procedures. Echocardiograms may be performed during or immediately following exercise. Transient depression of segmental wall motion during or following stress suggests ischemia. Improvement in wall motion during low-dose dobutamine infusions is an indicator of myocardial viability. Dobutamine infusions can also be utilized as a form of stress testing in patients unable to exercise.

ACC/AHA Guidelines for Clinical Applications of Echocardiography. J Am Coll Cardiol 1997;29:862. (Extensive discussion and recommendations.)

Daniel WG, Mügge A: Transesophageal echocardiography. N Engl J Med 1995;332:1268. (Review article for non-cardiologists.)

Pellikka PA et al: Stress echocardiography. Part II. Dobutamine stress echocardiography. Mayo Clinic Proc 1995; 70:16.

Roger VL et al: Stress echocardiography. Part I. Exercise echocardiography. Mayo Clinic Proc 1995;70:5.

Radionuclide Techniques

Several nuclear medicine studies are useful in the assessment of heart disease.

Scintigraphy with **thallium-201** or newer technetium-complexed agents such as technetium-99m sestamibi demonstrates relative myocardial perfusion. It is most commonly employed in conjunction with exercise testing to detect ischemia, which appears as a perfusion defect. After 3–24 hours, a thallium defect will usually fill in or "redistribute" with reversible ischemia but will remain fixed in regions of infarction. A second injection after 3 hours or on another occasion at rest is often required to differentiate viable ischemic myocardium from scar with certainty. (With sestamibi, redistribution does not occur, so a second injection is required.) Scintigraphy following **dipyridamole-** or **adenosine-induced vasodilation** provides similar information in patients unable to exercise. The sensitivity of perfusion scintigraphy is in the 80–90% range, which is somewhat superior to the exercise ECG. However, the specificity of this test can be as low as 50–70% when tomographic imaging procedures (SPECT) are employed, because of artifacts involving the inferoapical region (due to attenuation by the diaphragm), the septum (due to breast attenuation in women), and the outflow track. Because this test carries a large additional cost, its use should be limited to situations in which ordinary exercise testing needs corroboration or is not accurate (eg, bundle branch block, digitalis effect, left ventricular hypertrophy with "strain" pattern, or other baseline repolarization changes) or when regional localization is required. Both exercise and dipyridamole scintigraphy also provide useful prognostic information in patients with prior myocardial infarction and angina pectoris.

The newer technetium-based perfusion agents may provide better image resolution, but no superiority has been demonstrated by clinical criteria. Indeed, data suggest that thallium-201 may be superior in distinguishing viable from infarcted myocardium. They differ from thallium-201 physiologically (with Tc-99m sestamibi remaining "fixed" in the myocardium and Tc-99m teboroxime washing out very rapidly). Dual isotopic imaging protocols using thallium-201 for resting images and Tc-99m sestamibi for stress images allow for rapid, accurate assessment of ischemic heart disease.

Radionuclide angiography provides accurate measurements of left and, in some laboratories, right ventricular ejection fractions. Segmental wall motion may be examined, and semiquantitative estimates of valvular regurgitation are possible. Radionuclide angiography may be performed during exercise, so that changes in global or segmental left ventricular function can be employed to diagnose ischemia or impaired functional reserve. Thallium scintigraphy is a more accurate test for evaluating ischemic heart disease, but the exercise ejection fraction response provides useful prognostic information, especially post-myocardial infarction. Radionuclide angiography can also be used to quantify the pulmonary-to-systemic flow ratio in **left-to-right shunts.** Ratios above 1.3–1.5 can be accurately detected.

Technetium-99m pyrophosphate scintigraphy detects radiotracer uptake in areas of recent infarction. Its usefulness is limited by an 18- to 24-hour lag time after acute infarction before the test becomes positive and a limited sensitivity for small, especially nontransmural infarctions. Radiolabeled antimyosin antibodies have become available to detect myocardial necrosis following myocardial infarction. However, imaging must be performed 24–48 hours after injection. With the availability of assays of troponin T and troponin I, which are more specific for myocardial necrosis than creatine kinase and remain elevated for 5 days or longer, these imaging techniques do not have an important role.

Birnbaum Y, Kloner A: Myocardial viability. West J Med 1996;165:364. (Why assessing viability is important and how to do it—scintigraphy, dobutamine echocardiography, and PET techniques compared.)

Ritchie JL et al: AHA/ACC guidelines for clinical use of cardiac radionuclide imaging. Circulation 1995;91:1278.

Verani MS (editor): Nuclear cardiology. Cardiol Clin 1994;12:169. (Current techniques, applications, and results.)

Zaret BL, Wackers FJ: Nuclear cardiology. (Two parts.) N Engl J Med 1993;329:775, 885.

Newer Imaging Modalities

Many new imaging techniques have been developed, but their application in cardiovascular disease remains to be determined. **Computed tomography (CT scan)** can image the heart and, with contrast medium, the vascular system, but the relatively slow speed of most instruments limits its utility. The main application of CT is the evaluation of pericardial disease. **Ultrafast** or **cine CT** involves a specially designed instrument with high temporal resolution. Its availability is limited, but it provides excellent assessments of cardiac structure and function. Cine CT is increasingly being used to detect and quantify coronary artery calcification, but proper application of this highly sensitive test is uncertain. False-negative studies may occur in patients under 50 years of age, and positive studies in older patients do not necessarily provide a quantitative assessment of the severity of coronary arteriosclerosis. Thus, although this test can stratify patients into lower and higher risk groups, the appropriate management of individual patients with asymptomatic coronary artery calcification—beyond aggressive risk factor modification—is unclear.

Cardiac magnetic resonance imaging (MRI) is an evolving modality that provides high-resolution images of the heart and great vessels without radiation exposure or use of iodinated contrast media. It provides excellent anatomic definition, permitting assessment of pericardial disease, neoplastic disease of the heart, myocardial thickness, chamber size, and many congenital heart defects. It is the best noninvasive test for evaluating dissection of the aorta. Rapid acquisition sequences can produce excellent cine-mode images demonstrating left ventricular function and wall motion, and it is thus a useful alternative when the echocardiogram is suboptimal. Recent advances have been made in imaging the proximal coronary arteries and assessing myocardial perfusion with paramagnetic contrast agents, but these applications remain investigational.

Positron emission tomography (PET) can provide both qualitative and quantitative information concerning myocardial metabolism and blood flow, but its availability is limited, and a nearby cyclotron is required for many applications. PET can accurately distinguish between myocardium which is transiently dysfunctional ("stunned") due to ischemia and infarcted myocardium—a distinction that is important in considering revascularization. However, it is unclear whether this technique provides adequate incremental information over stress and rest perfusion scintigraphy to justify its use.

AHA Scientific Statement: Coronary artery calcification: Pathophysiology, epidemiology, imaging methods, and clinical applications. Circulation 1996;94:1175. (Consensus statement concerning the evolving experience with this controversial approach to screening.)

Blackwell GG, Pohost GM: The usefulness of cardiovascular magnetic resonance imaging. Curr Probl Cardiol 1994;19(3):117. (Imaging, spectroscopy, and new applications.)

Skorton DJ et al (editors): *Cardiac Imaging,* 2nd ed. Saunders, 1996. (All aspects of invasive and noninvasive cardiac imaging.)

Cardiac Catheterization

Right heart catheterization is convenient to perform and allows measurement of right atrial, right ventricular, pulmonary artery and pulmonary capillary wedge pressures (the latter an indicator of left atrial pressure), oxygen saturation, and cardiac output. These data may diagnose intracardiac shunts, physiologically significant pericardial disease, and right-sided valve lesions and can distinguish between cardiac and pulmonary disease. Balloon flotation catheters permit hemodynamic measurements and continuous monitoring at the bedside. These data can be critical in the evaluation and treatment of shock, heart failure, myocardial infarction, respiratory failure, postoperative hemodynamic instability, and many other situations. Bedside echocardiography can also be used in the evaluation and treatment of these entities when continuous monitoring is not required, and it is less invasive. Complications of right heart catheterization include bleeding, pneumothorax, arrhythmias, pulmonary emboli, pulmonary artery rupture, and sepsis. A recent study has suggested that the risk of right heart catheterization and resulting interventions may outweigh the benefits in many individuals.

Left heart catheterization permits quantitative assessment of mitral and aortic stenosis. With contrast angiography, valvular regurgitation and global and regional left ventricular function can be examined. Its main application is to produce selective coronary arteriograms. Since much of this information is available noninvasively, its main role is to confirm assessments of valvular abnormalities preoperatively and to obtain selective coronary arteriograms. Increasingly, the catheterization laboratory is being used for interventional procedures.

Conners AF et al: The effectiveness of right heart catheterization in the initial care of critically ill patients. JAMA 1996;276:889. (In this retrospective analysis, hemodynamic monitoring was associated with increased mortality and resource utilization. A prospective randomized study is needed.)

Grossman W, Baim DS (editors): *Cardiac Catheterization, Angiography, and Intervention,* 5th ed. Lea & Febiger, 1996.

Electrophysiologic Testing

Intracardiac electrocardiographic recording and stimulation studies have revolutionized the diagnosis and treatment of important arrhythmias. Electrophysiologic testing is useful for evaluating recurrent unexplained syncope. The location and severity of atrioventricular conduction disturbances and sinus node dysfunction can be assessed in symptomatic patients in whom diagnostic information cannot be obtained by ambulatory monitoring. The mechanism and optimal therapy of complex supraventricular arrhythmias—particularly those associated with accessory conduction pathways—can be elucidated and the approach to ventricular arrhythmias similarly refined. Catheter ablation procedures can definitively treat many supraventricular arrhythmias and some cases of ventricular tachycardia.

See Arrhythmia section for references.

CONGENITAL HEART DISEASE

Congenital lesions account for only about 2% of heart disease in adults. Only the most common acyanotic lesions are discussed here.

Foster E: Congenital heart disease in adults. West J Med 1995;163:492. (Concise review for primary care physician.)

Perloff JK: *The Clinical Recognition of Congenital Heart Disease,* 4th ed. Saunders, 1994.

Skorton DJ, Garson A Jr (editors): Congenital heart disease in adolescents and adults. Cardiol Clin 1993;11(4). (Entire issue.)

PULMONARY STENOSIS

Essentials of Diagnosis

- No symptoms in patients with mild or moderately severe lesions.

- Severe cases may present with right-sided heart failure and cause sudden death.
- High-pitched systolic ejection murmur maximal in the second left interspace. S_2 delayed and soft or absent. Ejection click often present. Increased right ventricular impulse.
- Right ventricular hypertrophy on ECG; pulmonary artery dilation on x-ray. Echo-Doppler diagnostic.

General Considerations

Stenosis of the pulmonary valve or infundibulum increases the resistance to outflow, raises the right ventricular pressure, and limits pulmonary blood flow. In the absence of associated shunts, arterial saturation is normal, but severe stenosis causes peripheral cyanosis by reducing cardiac output. Clubbing and polycythemia do not develop unless a patent foramen ovale or atrial septal defect is present, permitting right-to-left shunting.

Clinical Findings

A. Symptoms and Signs: Mild cases (right ventricular-pulmonary artery gradient < 30 mm Hg) are asymptomatic. Moderate to severe stenosis (gradients 50 to > 80 mm Hg) may cause dyspnea on exertion, syncope, chest pain, and eventually right ventricular failure.

There is a palpable parasternal lift. A loud, harsh systolic murmur and a prominent thrill are present in the left second and third interspaces parasternally; the murmur is in the third and fourth interspaces in infundibular stenosis. The second sound is obscured by the murmur in severe cases; the pulmonary component is diminished, delayed, or absent. Both components are audible in mild cases. A right-sided S_4 and a prominent *a* wave in the venous pulse are present in severe cases.

B. Electrocardiography and Chest X-Ray: Right axis deviation or right ventricular hypertrophy is noted; peaked P waves provide evidence of right atrial overload. Heart size may be normal on radiographs, or there may be a prominent right ventricle and atrium or gross cardiac enlargement, depending upon the severity. There is often poststenotic dilation of the main and left pulmonary arteries. Pulmonary vascularity is normal or diminished.

C. Other Diagnostic Studies: Echocardiography usually demonstrates the anatomic abnormality and assesses right ventricular size and function. Doppler ultrasound can estimate the gradient accurately; its findings are usually confirmed by cardiac catheterization.

Prognosis & Treatment

Patients with mild pulmonary stenosis may have a normal life expectancy. Severe stenosis is associated with sudden death and can cause heart failure in the 20s and 30s. Moderate stenosis may be asymptomatic in childhood and adolescence, but symptoms increase as patients grow older.

Symptomatic patients or those with evidence of right ventricular hypertrophy and resting gradients over 75–80 mm Hg require correction in most cases. Percutaneous balloon valvuloplasty has proved successful and is usually the treatment of choice. Surgery can be performed with an operative mortality rate of 2–4% and an excellent long-term result in most cases.

Chen C-R et al: Percutaneous balloon valvuloplasty for pulmonic stenosis in adolescents and adults. N Engl J Med 1996;335:21. (Excellent results in a consecutive series of 53 patients.)

COARCTATION OF THE AORTA

Essentials of Diagnosis

- Infants may have severe heart failure; children and adults are usually asymptomatic, presenting with hypertension.
- Absent or weak femoral pulses.
- Systolic pressure higher in upper extremities than in lower extremities; diastolic pressures are similar.
- Harsh systolic murmur heard in the back.
- ECG shows left ventricular hypertrophy; chest x-ray shows rib notching. Echo-Doppler is diagnostic.

General Considerations

Coarctation of the aorta consists of localized narrowing of the aortic arch just distal to the origin of the left subclavian artery. A bicuspid aortic valve is present in 25% of cases. Blood pressure is elevated in the aorta and its branches proximal to the coarctation and decreased distally. Collateral circulation develops through the intercostal arteries and branches of the subclavian arteries.

Clinical Findings

A. Symptoms and Signs: If cardiac failure does not occur in infancy, there are usually no symptoms until the hypertension produces left ventricular failure or cerebral hemorrhage; the latter may also occur from associated cerebral aneurysms. Strong arterial pulsations are seen in the neck and suprasternal notch. Hypertension is present in the arms, but the pressure is normal or low in the legs. This difference is exaggerated by exercise. Femoral pulsations are weak and are delayed in comparison with the brachial pulse. Patients with large collaterals may have relatively small gradients but still have severe coarctation. Late systolic ejection murmurs at the base are often heard better posteriorly, especially over the spinous processes. There may be an associated aortic insufficiency murmur due to a bicuspid aortic valve.

B. Electrocardiography and Chest X-Ray: The ECG usually shows left ventricular hypertrophy. Radiography shows scalloping of the ribs due to enlarged collateral intercostal arteries, dilation of the left subclavian artery and poststenotic aortic dilation, and left ventricular enlargement.

C. Diagnostic Studies: Measurement of the gradient across the lesion by catheterization and aortography remain the primary methods of diagnosis. MRI is a useful imaging adjunct, and Doppler ultrasound can also estimate the severity of obstruction.

Prognosis & Treatment

Cardiac failure is common in infancy and in older untreated patients; it is uncommon in late childhood and young adulthood. Most untreated patients with the adult form of coarctation die before age 50 from the complications of hypertension, rupture of the aorta, infective endarteritis, or cerebral hemorrhage (associated in some cases with congenital cerebral aneurysms). Aortic dissection also occurs with increased frequency in coarctation.

Resection of the coarcted site has a surgical mortality rate of 1–4%. The risks of the disease are such, however, that all coarctations in patients up to age 20 years should be resected. In patients under 40 years of age, surgery is advisable if the patient has refractory hypertension or significant left ventricular hypertrophy. The surgical mortality rate rises considerably in patients over age 50 and is of doubtful value. Balloon angioplasty of the stenosis has been accomplished successfully and may become the procedure of choice, but aortic tears have been described. About one-fourth of corrected patients continue to be hypertensive years after surgery and they have all the complications associated with hypertension.

Phadke K et al: Balloon angioplasty of adult aortic coarctation. Br Heart J 1993;69:36. (Excellent results suggest this may be appropriate first-line therapy.)

Shaddy RE et al: Comparison of angioplasty and surgery for unoperated coarctation of the aorta. Circulation 1993;87:793. (Randomized study in 36 children, raising possibility that restenosis and aneurysm may be complications of angioplasty.)

ATRIAL SEPTAL DEFECT

Essentials of Diagnosis

- Usually asymptomatic until middle age.
- Right ventricular lift; S_2 widely split and fixed.
- Grade I–III/VI systolic ejection murmur at pulmonary area.
- ECG shows right ventricular conduction delay; x-ray shows dilated pulmonary arteries and in-

creased vascularity. Echo-Doppler usually diagnostic.

General Considerations

The most common form of atrial septal defect (80% of cases) is persistence of the ostium secundum in the mid septum; less commonly, the ostium primum (which is low in the septum) persists, in which case mitral or tricuspid abnormalities may also be present. A third form is the sinus venosus defect of the upper part of the septum. This is often associated with partial anomalous drainage of the pulmonary veins into the superior vena cava. In all cases, normally oxygenated blood from the left atrium passes into the right atrium, increasing right ventricular output and pulmonary blood flow.

Clinical Findings

A. Symptoms and Signs: Most patients with small or moderate defects are asymptomatic. With large shunts, exertional dyspnea or cardiac failure may develop, most commonly in the fourth decade or later. Prominent right ventricular and pulmonary artery pulsations are readily visible and palpable. A moderately loud systolic ejection murmur can be heard in the second and third interspaces parasternally as a result of increased pulmonary artery flow. S_2 is widely split and does not vary with breathing.

B. Electrocardiography and Chest X-Ray: Right axis deviation or right ventricular hypertrophy may be present in ostium secundum defects. Incomplete or complete right bundle branch block is present in nearly all cases of atrial septal defect, and superior axis deviation is noted in ostium primum defect. With sinus venosus defects, the P axis is leftward of +15 degrees. The chest radiograph shows large pulmonary arteries, increased pulmonary vascularity, an enlarged right atrium and ventricle, and a small aortic knob.

C. Diagnostic Studies: Echocardiography can demonstrate right ventricular volume overload with a large right ventricle and atrium, and sometimes the defect itself. Echocardiography with saline bubble contrast and Doppler flow studies can demonstrate shunting. A transesophageal echo is helpful when transthoracic echo quality is not optimal, and it improves the sensitivity for small shunts and patent foramen ovale. Radionuclide flow studies quantify left-to-right shunting, and MRI can also elucidate the anatomy. Cardiac catheterization remains the definitive diagnostic procedure, since it can demonstrate an increase in oxygen saturation between the venae cavae and right ventricle due to the admixture of oxygenated blood from the left atrium, quantify the shunt, and measure pulmonary vascular resistance. Right and left ventricular contrast angiography may demonstrate associated valvular abnormalities or anomalous pulmonary venous drainage.

Prognosis & Treatment

Patients with small shunts may live a normal life span. Large shunts cause disability by age 40. Raised pulmonary vascular resistance secondary to pulmonary hypertension rarely occurs in childhood or young adult life in secundum defects but is more common in primum defects; after age 40, pulmonary hypertension, cardiac arrhythmias (especially atrial fibrillation), and heart failure may occur in secundum defects. Paradoxic systemic arterial embolization is a concern, especially in patients with pulmonary hypertension or venous thrombosis. A patent foramen ovale is present in 20-30% of adults and is the lesion responsible for most paradoxic emboli. Infective endocarditis does not occur with increased frequency.

Small atrial septal defects do not require surgery. The risks are now sufficiently low so that patients with left-to-right shunts and pulmonary-to-systemic flow ratios between 1.5 and 2.0 may be operated on if the total clinical picture warrants. Ratios exceeding 2.0 are an indication for surgical closure of the defect.

Surgery should be withheld from patients with pulmonary hypertension with reversed (right-to-left) shunting (Eisenmenger's syndrome) because of the risk of acute right heart failure. Relocation of pulmonary veins is required in patients with partial anomalous venous drainage. In ostium primum defects, in addition to closure of the defect, suture of the valve clefts—especially those of the mitral valve—is advisable if mitral regurgitation of any significant degree is present. The surgical mortality rate is low (< 1%) in patients under age 45 who are not in cardiac failure and those who have systolic pulmonary artery pressures less than 60 mm Hg. It increases to 5–10% in patients over age 40 with cardiac failure or with systolic pulmonary artery pressures greater than 60 mm Hg.

Konstantinides S et al: A comparison of surgical and medical therapy for the atrial septal defect in adults. N Engl J Med 1995;333:469. (Retrospective study of 179 patients with atrial septal defect showing improved survival with surgical repair.)

Ward C: Secundum atrial septal defect: Routine surgical treatment is not of proven benefit. Br Heart J 1994;71:219. (Concluding that the common practice of closing defects with shunt ratios > 1.5 in asymptomatic adults may not be justified.)

PATENT DUCTUS ARTERIOSUS

Essentials of Diagnosis

- Adults with small or moderately large patent ductus are usually asymptomatic at least until middle age.
- Widened pulse pressure; loud S_2.
- Continuous murmur over pulmonary area; thrill common.

- Echo-Doppler is helpful, but the lesion is best visualized by aortography.

General Considerations

The embryonic ductus arteriosus fails to close normally and persists as a shunt connecting the left pulmonary artery and aorta, usually near the origin of the left subclavian artery. Prior to birth, the ductus is kept patent by the effect of circulating prostaglandins; in early infancy, a patent ductus can often be closed by administration of intravenous indomethacin (0.2 mg/kg intravenously). If the defect is not closed, blood flows continuously from the aorta through the ductus into the pulmonary artery in both systole and diastole; the defect is a form of arteriovenous fistula, increasing the work of the left ventricle. If it remains open, obliterative changes in the pulmonary arterioles can cause pulmonary hypertension. Then the shunt is bidirectional or right-to-left (Eisenmenger's syndrome). This complication does not correlate with shunt size.

Clinical Findings

A. Symptoms and Signs: There are no symptoms unless left ventricular failure or pulmonary hypertension develops. The heart is of normal size or slightly enlarged, with a hyperdynamic apical impulse. The pulse pressure is wide, and diastolic pressure is low. A continuous rough "machinery" murmur, accentuated in late systole at the time of S_2, is heard best in the left first and second interspaces at the left sternal border. Thrills are common.

B. Electrocardiography and Chest X-Ray: A normal tracing or left ventricular hypertrophy is found, depending upon the magnitude of shunting. On chest radiographs, the heart is normal in size and contour, or there may be left ventricular and left atrial enlargement. The pulmonary artery, aorta, and left atrium are prominent.

C. Other Diagnostic Studies: Echocardiography quantifies left ventricular and atrial size. MRI can demonstrate the abnormality, and the magnitude of the shunt can also be determined by radionuclide flow studies. Cardiac catheterization establishes the presence and severity of a left-to-right shunt and whether pulmonary hypertension is present; angiography can define its anatomy.

Prognosis & Treatment

Large shunts cause a high mortality rate from cardiac failure early in life. Smaller shunts are compatible with long survival, congestive heart failure being the most common complication. Infective endocarditis or endarteritis may also occur, and antibiotic prophylaxis is required. A small percentage of patients develop pulmonary hypertension and reversal of shunt (right-to-left shunting), such that the lower legs, especially the toes, appear cyanotic and clubbed in contrast to normally pink fingers. At this stage, the patient is inoperable.

Surgical ligation of the patent ductus can be accomplished with excellent results in uncomplicated patients. Recent experience with transcatheter closure has also been favorable, indicating that where available, this newer option is the procedure of choice for most patients. Closure is recommended for children or adults with symptoms or large shunts. Asymptomatic adults with no left ventricular hypertrophy and small left-to-right shunts are at low risk of developing pulmonary hypertension or congestive heart failure. The indications for closure of a patent ductus arteriosus in the presence of pulmonary hypertension are controversial. Opinion favors closure whenever the pulmonary vascular resistance is low and the flow through the ductus is from left to right.

Ing FF et al: Trans-catheter closure of the patent ductus arteriosus in adults using the Gianturco coil. Clin Cardiol 1996;19:875. (Very high success rate.)

VENTRICULAR SEPTAL DEFECT

Essentials of Diagnosis

- Adults asymptomatic if defect is small to moderate.
- Grade II–VI/VI pansystolic murmur maximal at the left sternal border; associated thrill common.
- ECG may show left or right ventricular hypertrophy if shunt is reversed; x-ray shows increased pulmonary vascularity. Echo-Doppler is diagnostic.

General Considerations

In this lesion, a persistent opening in the upper interventricular septum resulting from failure of fusion with the aortic septum permits blood to pass from the high-pressure left ventricle into the low-pressure right ventricle. The subsequent natural history and pathophysiology depend on the size of the defect and the magnitude of left-to-right shunting. Large defects are associated with early left ventricular failure. Chronic but more moderate left-to-right shunts may lead to pulmonary vascular disease and right-sided failure. Many ventricular defects close spontaneously in early childhood.

Clinical Findings

A. Symptoms and Signs: The clinical features are dependent upon the size of the defect and the presence or absence of a raised pulmonary vascular resistance. Large shunts are associated with loud, harsh holosystolic murmurs in the left third and fourth interspaces along the sternum and, in some cases, middiastolic flow murmurs and an S_3 at the apex. Smaller shunts may produce only an early systolic murmur or a diamond-shaped murmur. A systolic thrill is common. Clinical evidence of pulmonary hypertension is often more informative than the murmur itself. High defects may be associated with aortic regurgitation owing to prolapse of a valve leaflet.

B. Electrocardiography and Chest X-Ray: The ECG may be normal or may show right, left, or biventricular hypertrophy, depending on the size of the defect and the pulmonary vascular resistance. With large shunts, the right or left ventricle (or both), the left atrium, and the pulmonary arteries are enlarged, and pulmonary vascularity is increased on chest radiographs. If pulmonary vascular disease evolves, an enlarged pulmonary artery with diminished distal vascularity is seen.

C. Diagnostic Studies: Echocardiography can demonstrate chamber size and may demonstrate the defect. Doppler ultrasound can qualitatively assess the magnitude of shunting and the pulmonary artery pressure. Magnetic resonance imaging can often visualize the defect, while radionuclide flow studies quantify pulmonary-to-systemic flow ratios. Cardiac catheterization permits definitive diagnosis in all but the most trivial defects; it is the only technique that can measure pulmonary vascular resistance.

Prognosis & Treatment

Patients with the typical murmur as the only abnormality have a normal life expectancy except for the threat of infective endocarditis. The latter is more typical of smaller shunts. Antibiotic prophylaxis is mandatory. With large shunts, congestive heart failure may develop early in life, and survival beyond age 40 is unusual. Shunt reversal occurs in an estimated 25%, producing Eisenmenger's syndrome.

Small shunts (pulmonary-to-systemic flow ratio < 1.5) in asymptomatic patients do not require surgery. Defects causing large shunts should be repaired to prevent irreversible pulmonary vascular disease or late heart failure. When severe pulmonary hypertension is present (systolic pulmonary arterial pressures > 85 mm Hg) and the left-to-right shunt is small, the surgical mortality risk is at least 50%. If the shunt is reversed, surgery is contraindicated. If surgery is required because of unrelenting cardiac failure in infancy due to a large left-to-right shunt, early closure of the defect is now the preferred procedure. The surgical mortality rate is 2–3% for primary repair. Some defects (perhaps as many as 40%) close spontaneously. Therefore, surgery should be deferred until late childhood unless the disability is severe or unless pulmonary hypertension is observed to develop or progress. It is now possible to close ventricular septal defects percutaneously in some cases.

Frontera-Izquierdo P, Cabezudo-Huerta G: Natural and modified history of isolated ventricular septal defect: A 17-year study. Pediatr Cardiol 1992;13:193.

VALVULAR HEART DISEASE

While most cases of valvular disease were at one time due to rheumatic heart disease (still true in developing countries), other causes are now more common. The typical findings of each lesion are described in Table 10–1. Table 10–2 shows how to use bedside maneuvers to distinguish murmurs. The references below deal with valve disease in general. Specific lesions are discussed and referenced subsequently.

Carabello BA (editor): Valvular heart disease. Cardiol Clin 1991;9(2):1. (All lesions, diagnostic techniques, and treatment.)
Karalis DG et al: Transesophageal echocardiography in valvular heart disease. Cardiovasc Clin 1993;23:105. (A valuable assessment technique.)
Kotler MN et al: Echo-Doppler in valvular heart disease. Cardiovasc Clin 1993;23:77.
Levine HJ et al: Anti-thrombotic therapy in valvular heart disease. Chest 1995;108:360S. (Rheumatic mitral stenosis, mitral valve prolapse, mitral annular calcification, aortic stenosis, and endocarditis are discussed, with recommendations for use of aspirin and anticoagulation.)

MITRAL STENOSIS

Essentials of Diagnosis

- Dyspnea, orthopnea, and paroxysmal nocturnal dyspnea.
- Symptoms often precipitated by onset of atrial fibrillation or pregnancy.
- Prominent mitral first sound, opening snap (usually), and apical crescendo rumble.
- ECG shows left atrial abnormality and, commonly, atrial fibrillation. Echo-Doppler confirms diagnosis and quantitates severity.

General Considerations

Nearly all patients with mitral stenosis have underlying rheumatic heart disease, though a history of rheumatic fever is often absent.

Clinical Findings

A. Symptoms and Signs: A characteristic finding of mitral stenosis is a localized middiastolic murmur low in pitch whose duration varies with the severity of the stenosis and the heart rate (Table 10–1). Because it is thickened, the valve opens in early diastole with an opening snap. The sound is sharp, is widely distributed over the chest, and occurs early after A_2 in severe and later in milder varieties of mitral stenosis. In severe mitral stenosis with low flow across the mitral valve, the murmur may be soft

Table 10–1. Differential diagnosis of valvular heart disease.

	Mitral Stenosis	Mitral Regurgitation	Aortic Stenosis	Aortic Regurgitation	Tricuspid Stenosis	Tricuspid Regurgitation
Inspection	Malar flush, precordial bulge, and diffuse pulsation in young patients.	Usually prominent and hyperdynamic apical impulse to left of MCL.	Sustained PMI, prominent atrial filling wave.	Hyperdynamic PMI to left of MCL and down. Visible carotid pulsations.	Giant a wave in jugular pulse with sinus rhythm. Often olive-colored skin (mixed jaundice and local cyanosis).	Large v wave in jugular pulse.
Palpation	"Tapping" sensation over area of expected PMI. Middiastolic or presystolic thrill at apex. Small pulse. Right ventricular pulsation left third to fifth ICS parasternally when pulmonary hypertension is present.	Forceful, brisk PMI; systolic thrill over PMI. Pulse normal, small, or slightly collapsing.	Powerful, heaving PMI to left and slightly below MCL. Systolic thrill over aortic area, sternal notch, or carotids. Small and slowly rising carotid pulse.	Apical impulse forceful and displaced significantly to left and down. Prominent carotid pulses. Rapidly rising and collapsing pulses.	Middiastolic thrill between lower left sternal border and PMI. Presystolic pulsation of liver (sinus rhythm only).	Right ventricular pulsation. Occasionally systolic thrill at lower left sternal edge. Systolic pulsation of liver.
Heart sounds, rhythm, and blood pressure	Loud snapping M_1. Opening snap following S_2 along left sternal border or at apex. Atrial fibrillation common. Blood pressure normal.	M_1 normal or buried in murmur. Prominent third heart sound. Atrial fibrillation common. Blood pressure normal. Midsystolic clicks may be present.	A_2 normal, soft, or absent. Paradoxic splitting of S_2 if A_2 is audible. Prominent S_4. Blood pressure normal or systolic pressure normal with high diastolic level.	S_1 normal or reduced, A_2 loud. Wide pulse pressure with diastolic pressure <60 mm Hg.	S_1 often loud.	Atrial fibrillation usually present.
Murmurs Location and transmission	Localized at or near apex. Rarely, short diastolic (Graham Steell) murmur along lower left sternal border in severe pulmonary hypertension.	Loudest over PMI; transmitted to left axilla, left infrascapular area. With posterior papillary muscle dysfunction, may transmit to base.	Right second ICS parasternally or at apex; heard in carotids and occasionally in upper interscapular area.	Loudest along left sternal border in third to fourth interspace. Heard over aortic area and apex. May be associated with low-pitched middiastolic murmur at apex (Austin Flint) in non-rheumatic disease.	Third to fifth ICS along left sternal border out to apex.	As for tricuspid stenosis.
Timing	Onset at opening snap ("middiastolic") with presystolic accentuation if in sinus rhythm. Graham Steell begins with P_2 (early diastole).	Pansystolic: begins with M_1 and ends at or after A_2. May be late systolic in papillary muscle dysfunction.	Midsystolic: begins after M_1, ends before A_2; reaches maximum intensity in mid systole.	Begins immediately after aortic second sound and ends before first sound.	As for mitral stenosis.	As for mitral regurgitation.
Character	Low-pitched, rumbling; presystolic murmur merges with loud M_1 in a "crescendo." Graham Steell high-pitched, blowing.	Blowing, high-pitched; occasionally harsh or musical.	Harsh, rough.	Blowing, often faint.	As for mitral stenosis.	Blowing, coarse, or musical.

(continued)

Table 10-1. Differential diagnosis of valvular heart disease. (continued)

	Mitral Stenosis	Mitral Regurgitation	Aortic Stenosis	Aortic Regurgitation	Tricuspid Stenosis	Tricuspid Regurgitation
Murmurs (cont'd) Optimum auscultatory conditions	After exercise, left lateral recumbency. Bell chest piece lightly applied.	After exercise; diaphragm chest pain. In prolapse, findings most prominent while standing.	Patient resting, leaning forward, breath held in full expiration.	Patient leaning forward, breath held in expiration.	Murmur usually louder during and at peak of inspiration. Patient recumbent.	Murmur usually becomes louder during inspiration.
X-ray	Straight left heart border. Large left atrium sharply indenting esophagus. Elevation of left main stem bronchus. Large right ventricle and pulmonary artery if pulmonary hypertension is present. Calcification occasionally seen in mitral valve.	Enlarged left ventricle and left atrium.	Concentric left ventricular hypertrophy. Prominent ascending aorta, small knob. Calcified valve common.	Moderate to severe left ventricular enlargement. Prominent aortic knob.	Enlarged right atrium only.	Enlarged right atrium and ventricle.
ECG	Broad P waves in standard leads; broad negative phase of diphasic P in V_1. If pulmonary hypertension is present, tall peaked P waves, right axis deviation, or right ventricular hypertrophy appears.	Left axis deviation or frank left ventricular hypertrophy. P waves broad, tall, or notched in standard leads; broad negative phase of diphasic P in V_1.	Left ventricular hypertrophy.	Left ventricular hypertrophy.	Tall, peaked P waves. Normal axis.	Right axis usual.
Echocardiography M mode	Thickened, immobile mitral valve with anterior and posterior leaflets moving together. Slow early diastolic filling slope, left atrial enlargement, normal to small left ventricle.	Thickened mitral valve in rheumatic disease; mitral valve prolapse; flail leaflet or vegetations may be seen. Enlarged left ventricle with above-normal, normal, or decreased function.	Dense persistent echoes from the aortic valve with poor leaflet excursion, left ventricular hypertrophy with preserved contractile function.	Diastolic vibrations of the anterior leaflet of the mitral valve and septum, early closure of the mitral valve when severe, dilated left ventricle with normal or decreased contractility.	Tricuspid valve thickening, decreased early diastolic filling slope of the tricuspid valve. Mitral valve also usually abnormal.	Enlarged right ventricle, prolapsing valve, mitral valve often abnormal.
Two-dimensional	Maximum diastolic orifice size reduced, subvalvular apparatus foreshortened, variable thickening of other valves.	Same as M-mode but more reliable.	Above plus poststenotic dilation of the aorta, restricted opening of the aortic leaflets, bicuspid aortic valve in about 30%.	Above plus may show vegetations in endocarditis, bicuspid valve, root dilation.	Above plus enlargement of the right atrium.	Same as above.
Doppler	Prolonged pressure half-time across mitral valve; indirect evidence of pulmonary hypertension.	Regurgitant flow mapped into left atrium; indirect evidence of pulmonary hypertension.	Increased transvalvular flow velocity, yielding calculated gradient. Valve area estimate using continuity equation.	Demonstrates regurgitation and qualitatively estimates severity.	Prolonged pressure half-time across tricuspid valve.	Regurgitant flow mapped into right atrium and venae cavae; right ventricular systolic pressure estimated.

A_2 = Aortic second sound   MCL = Midclavicular line
ICS = Intercostal space P_2 = Pulmonary second sound
M_1 = Mitral first sound   PMI = Point of maximal impulse

Table 10–2. Effect of various interventions on systolic murmurs.[1]

Intervention	Hypertrophic Obstructive Cardiomyopathy	Aortic Stenosis	Mitral Regurgitation	Mitral Prolapse
Valsalva	↑	↓	↓ or ↔	↑ or ↓
Standing	↑	↑ or ↔	↓ or ↔	↑
Handgrip or squatting	↓	↓ or ↔	↑	↓
Supine position with legs elevated	↓	↑ or ↔	↔	↓
Exercise	↑	↑ or ↔	↓	↑
Amyl nitrite	↑↑	↑	↓	↑

Key: ↑ = increased; ↑↑ = markedly increased; ↓ = decreased; ↔ = unchanged

[1]Modified from Paraskos JA: Combined valvular disease. In: *Valvular Heart Disease.* Dalen JE, Alpert JS (editors). Little, Brown, 1987.

and difficult to find, but the opening snap can usually be heard. If the patient has both mitral stenosis and mitral regurgitation, the dominant features may be the systolic murmur of mitral regurgitation with or without a short diastolic murmur and a delayed opening snap.

When the valve has narrowed to less than 1.5 cm^2 (normal, 4–6 cm^2), the left atrial pressure must rise to maintain normal flow across the valve and a normal cardiac output. This results in a pressure difference between the left atrium and left ventricle during diastole. The pressure gradient and the length of the diastolic murmur reflect the severity of mitral stenosis; they persist throughout the diastole when the lesion is severe or when the ventricular rate is rapid.

In mild cases, left atrial pressure and cardiac output may be essentially normal and the patient asymptomatic, but in moderate stenosis (valve area < 1.5 cm^2)—especially with tachycardia, which shortens diastole and increases mitral flow rate—dyspnea and fatigue appear as the left atrial pressure rises. With severe stenosis, the left atrial pressure is high enough to produce pulmonary venous congestion at rest and reduce cardiac output, with resulting dyspnea, fatigue, and right heart failure. Recumbency at night further increases the pulmonary blood volume, causing orthopnea and paroxysmal nocturnal dyspnea. Severe pulmonary congestion may also be initiated by any acute respiratory infection, excessive salt and fluid intake, endocarditis, or recurrence of rheumatic carditis. As a result of long-standing pulmonary venous hypertension, anastomoses develop between the pulmonary and bronchial veins in the form of bronchial submucosal varices. These often rupture, producing mild or severe hemoptysis. In a few patients, the pulmonary arterioles become narrowed; this greatly increases the pulmonary artery pressure and accelerates the development of right ventricular hypertrophy and failure. These patients have rela-

tively little dyspnea but experience fatigue on exertion.

Fifty to 80 percent of patients develop paroxysmal or chronic atrial fibrillation that, until the ventricular rate is controlled, may precipitate dyspnea or pulmonary edema.

B. Diagnostic Studies: Echocardiography is the most valuable technique for assessing mitral stenosis. The valve is thickened, opens poorly, and closes slowly. The anterior and posterior leaflets are fixed and move together, rather than in opposite directions. Left atrial size can be determined by echocardiography: increased size denotes an increased likelihood of atrial fibrillation or systemic emboli. The mitral valve area can be measured, and the gradient and pulmonary artery pressure can be estimated by Doppler techniques. Echocardiography also detects atrial myxoma, which sometimes presents clinically in a fashion resembling mitral stenosis.

Because echocardiography and careful symptom evaluation provide most of the needed information, cardiac catheterization is employed primarily to detect associated valve, coronary, or myocardial disease—usually after the decision to intervene has been made.

Treatment & Prognosis

Mitral stenosis may be present for a lifetime with few or no symptoms, or it may become severe in a few years. In most cases, there is a long asymptomatic phase, followed by subtle limitation of activity. Pregnancy and its associated increase in cardiac output and the transmitral pressure gradient often precipitates symptoms. The onset of atrial fibrillation often precipitates more severe symptoms, although with return to sinus rhythm (using digoxin and, often, class I or III antiarrhythmic agents) or ventricular rate control, the patient may improve. Conversion to and subsequent maintenance of sinus rhythm is most commonly successful when the duration of atrial fibrillation is brief (< 6–12 months) and the left atrium is not severely dilated (diameter < 4.5 cm). Once atrial fibrillation occurs, the patient should receive warfarin anticoagulation therapy even if sinus rhythm is restored, since 20–30% of these patients will have systemic embolization if untreated. Systemic embolization in the presence of only mild to moderate disease is not an indication for surgery but should be treated with warfarin anticoagulation.

Indications for relieving the stenosis include the following: (1) uncontrollable pulmonary edema; (2) limiting dyspnea and intermittent pulmonary edema; (3) evidence of pulmonary hypertension with right ventricular hypertrophy or hemoptysis; (4) limitation of activity despite ventricular rate control and medical therapy; and (5) recurrent systemic emboli despite anticoagulation with moderate or severe stenosis.

Open mitral commissurotomy may be effective in patients without substantial mitral regurgitation. Replacement of the valve is indicated when combined stenosis and insufficiency are present or when the mitral valve is so distorted and calcified that a satisfactory valvulotomy is not possible. Operative mortality rates are low: 1–3% in most institutions. Balloon valvuloplasty is becoming increasingly popular in patients without accompanying regurgitation. Initial success rates are high, especially if valve calcification is not excessive. The rate of restenosis is lower than that with aortic stenosis. As a result, this option appears to be a suitable alternative to surgery for many patients in experienced centers.

Problems associated with prosthetic valves are thrombosis (especially at the mitral position), paravalvular leak, endocarditis, and degenerative changes in tissue valves. Warfarin anticoagulant therapy is mandatory with mechanical prostheses and is usually employed for at least the initial 3 months with bioprostheses, especially if the patient has significant left atrial enlargement. If atrial fibrillation persists postoperatively, ongoing anticoagulation is required.

MITRAL REGURGITATION
(Mitral Insufficiency)

Essentials of Diagnosis

- Variable causes determine clinical presentation.
- May be asymptomatic for many years (or for life) or may cause left-sided heart failure.
- Pansystolic murmur at the apex, radiating into the axilla; associated with S_3.
- ECG shows left atrial abnormality or atrial fibrillation and left ventricular hypertrophy; x-ray shows left atrial and ventricular enlargement. Echo-Doppler confirms diagnosis and estimates severity.

General Considerations

Mitral regurgitation may result from many processes. Rheumatic disease is associated with a thickened valve with reduced mobility and often a mixed picture of stenosis and regurgitation. Rheumatic disease has been replaced as the commonest cause of mitral regurgitation in most developed countries by other processes, which include myxomatous degeneration (eg, **mitral valve prolapse** with or without connective tissue diseases such as Marfan's syndrome), infective endocarditis, and subvalvular dysfunction (due to papillary muscle dysfunction or ruptured chordae tendineae). Cardiac tumors, chiefly left atrial myxoma, are a rare cause of mitral regurgitation.

Clinical Findings

A. Symptoms and Signs: During left ventricular systole, the mitral leaflets do not close normally, and blood is ejected into the left atrium as well as through the aortic valve. The net effect is an increased volume load on the left ventricle, and the presentation depends on the rapidity with which the lesion develops. In acute regurgitation, left atrial pressure rises abruptly, leading to pulmonary edema if severe. When it is chronic, the left atrium enlarges progressively, but the pressure in pulmonary veins and capillaries rises only transiently during exertion. Exertional dyspnea and fatigue progress gradually over many years.

Mitral regurgitation, like mitral stenosis, predisposes to atrial fibrillation; but this arrhythmia is less likely to provoke acute pulmonary congestion, and fewer than 5% of patients have peripheral arterial emboli. Mitral regurgitation more often predisposes to infective endocarditis.

Clinically, mitral regurgitation is characterized by a pansystolic murmur maximal at the apex, radiating to the axilla and occasionally to the base; a hyperdynamic left ventricular impulse and a brisk carotid upstroke; and a prominent third heart sound. Left atrial enlargement is usually considerable in chronic mitral regurgitation; the degree of left ventricular enlargement usually reflects the severity of regurgitation. Calcification of the mitral valve is less common than in pure mitral stenosis. The same is true of enlargement of the main pulmonary artery on radiographs. Hemodynamically, left ventricular volume overload may ultimately lead to left ventricular failure and reduced cardiac output, but for many years the left ventricular end-diastolic pressure and the cardiac output may be normal at rest, even with considerable increase in left ventricular volume.

Nonrheumatic mitral regurgitation may develop abruptly, such as with papillary muscle dysfunction following myocardial infarction, valve perforation in infective endocarditis, or ruptured chordae tendineae in mitral valve prolapse. In acute mitral regurgitation, patients are in sinus rhythm rather than atrial fibrillation, have little or no enlargement of the left atrium, no calcification of the mitral valve, no associated mitral stenosis, and in many cases little left ventricular dilation.

Myxomatous mitral valve ("floppy" or "billowing" mitral valve, or mitral valve prolapse) is usually asymptomatic but may be associated with nonspecific chest pain, dyspnea, fatigue, or palpitations. Most patients are female, many are thin, and some have minor chest wall deformities. There are characteristic midsystolic clicks, which may be multiple, often but not always followed by a late systolic murmur. These findings are accentuated in the standing position. The diagnosis is primarily clinical but can be confirmed echocardiographically. Its significance is in dispute because of the frequency with which it is diagnosed in healthy young women (up to 10%) and men, but in occasional patients this lesion is not benign. Patients who have only a midsystolic click usually have no sequelae, but patients with a late or pansystolic murmur may develop significant mitral regurgitation, often due to rupture of chordae tendineae. The need for valve replacement is commonest in men and increases with aging, so that approximately 2% of patients with clinically significant regurgitation over age 60 will require surgery. Infective endocarditis may occur, chiefly in patients with murmurs; such patients should have antibiotic prophylaxis prior to dental work and surgical procedures. Sudden death is rare and is probably related to ventricular tachycardias; β-adrenergic blocking agents are often effective for supraventricular arrhythmias. If symptomatic ventricular tachycardia is present, antiarrhythmic therapy and, in many cases, electrophysiologic studies are indicated. An association between mitral prolapse and embolic cerebrovascular events has also been reported. Echocardiographic evidence of marked thickening or redundancy of the valve is associated with a higher incidence of most complications.

Papillary muscle dysfunction or infarction following acute myocardial infarction is less common. When mitral regurgitation is due to papillary dysfunction, it may subside as the infarction heals or left ventricular dilation diminishes. If severe regurgitation persists, these patients have a poor prognosis with or without surgery and a natural history that reflects their underlying heart disease. Transient—but sometimes severe—mitral regurgitation may occur during episodes of myocardial ischemia. Patients with dilated cardiomyopathies of any origin may have **secondary mitral regurgitation** due to papillary muscle dysfunction or dilation of the mitral annulus. In these, mitral valve replacement has been considered contraindicated because of the poor risk:benefit ratio and deterioration of left ventricular function postoperatively. However, several groups have reported good results with mitral valve repair in patients with left ventricular ejection fractions greater than 30% and secondary mitral insufficiency.

B. Diagnostic Studies: Echocardiography is useful in demonstrating the underlying pathologic process (rheumatic, prolapse, flail leaflet), and Doppler techniques provide qualitative and semiquantitative estimates of the severity of mitral regurgitation. It should be noted that Doppler also detects clinically insignificant regurgitation in many normal individuals, and this finding must be interpreted in the context of the clinical presentation. The accompanying information concerning left ventricular size and function, left atrial size, pulmonary artery pressure, and right ventricular function can be invaluable in planning treatment as well as in recognizing associated lesions. Transesophageal echocardiography may reveal the cause of regurgitation and identify candidates for valvular repair. Nuclear medicine techniques as well as MRI permit measurement of left ventricular function and estimation of the severity of regurgitation.

Cardiac catheterization provides accurate assessment of regurgitation and, additionally, of left ventricular function and pulmonary artery pressure. Coronary angiography is often indicated to determine the presence of coronary artery disease prior to valve surgery.

Treatment & Prognosis

Acute mitral regurgitation due to endocarditis, myocardial infarction, and ruptured chordae tendineae often requires emergency surgery. Some patients can be stabilized with vasodilators or intra-aortic balloon counterpulsation, which reduce the amount of regurgitant flow by lowering systemic vascular resistance. Patients with chronic lesions may remain asymptomatic for many years. Operation is necessary when activity becomes limited or if left ventricular function deteriorates progressively. There has been growing success with valve repair in nonrheumatic lesions, which avoids the complications of prosthetic valves described earlier. In addition, left ventricular function is better preserved when the subvalvular structures can be maintained intact by valve repair. Selected patients with poor left ventricular function and severe mitral regurgitation may benefit from this intervention.

Carabello BA: Mitral valve disease. Curr Probl Cardiol 1993;18:423. (Diagnosis, natural history, treatment.)

Lee EM et al: The importance of subvalvular preservation and early operation in mitral valve surgery. Circulation 1996;94:2117. (Repair is superior to replacement, and the subvalvular apparatus should be left in place even if replacement is required.)

Marcus RH et al: The spectrum of severe rheumatic mitral valve disease in a developing country. Ann Intern Med 1994;120:177. (Greater severity is typical.)

Palacios IF et al: Clinical follow-up of patients undergoing percutaneous mitral balloon valvotomy. Circulation 1995;91:671. (In patients free of severe calcification, outcome is excellent.)

Ross J JR: The timing of surgery for severe mitral regurgitation. N Engl J Med 1996;335:1456. (Editorial discussing the strategies of early operation with an emphasis on mitral valve repair.)

Zuppiroli A et al: Natural history of mitral valve prolapse. Am J Cardiol 1995;75:1028. (Follow-up of 316 patients, with low risk of important complications [1% per year] occurring more frequently in men than in women.)

AORTIC STENOSIS

Essentials of Diagnosis

- In adults, usually asymptomatic until middle or old age.
- Delayed and diminished carotid pulses.
- Soft, absent, or paradoxically split S_2.
- Harsh systolic murmur, sometimes with thrill along left sternal border, often radiating to the neck; may be louder at apex in older patients.
- ECG usually shows left ventricular hypertrophy; calcified valve on x-ray or fluoroscopy. Echo-Doppler is diagnostic in most cases.

General Considerations

Aortic valvular stenosis may follow rheumatic fever but is more commonly caused by progressive valvular calcification superimposed upon a congenitally bicuspid valve, or in the elderly, a previously normal valve. In the latter group, the aortic valve becomes sclerotic and, with further calcification, stenotic. Approximately 25% of patients over age 65 and 35% of those over age 70 have echocardiographic evidence of sclerosis, with 2–3% of these exhibiting hemodynamic evidence of stenosis. Thus, aortic stenosis has become the common surgical valve lesion in developed countries. Degenerative valve disease is three to four times more frequent in men than in women and is more common in smokers and hypertensives. Valvular stenosis must be distinguished from supravalvular obstruction and from outflow obstruction of the left ventricular infundibulum, both relatively rare.

Clinical Findings

A. Symptoms and Signs: Slightly narrowed, thickened, or roughened valves (aortic sclerosis) or aortic dilation may produce the typical murmur and thrill without causing significant hemodynamic effects. In mild or moderate cases, the characteristic signs are a systolic ejection murmur at the aortic area transmitted to the neck and apex; in severe cases, a palpable left ventricular heave or thrill, a weak to absent aortic second sound, or reversed splitting of the second sound are present (see Table 10–1). When the valve area is less than 0.8–1 cm² (normal, 3–4 cm²), ventricular systole becomes prolonged and the typical carotid pulse pattern of delayed upstroke and low amplitude is present, but this may be an unreliable finding in older patients with extensive arteriosclerotic vascular disease. Left ventricular hypertrophy increases progressively, with resulting elevations in diastolic pressure. Cardiac output is maintained until the stenosis is severe (with a valve area < 0.8 cm²). Patients may present with left ventricular failure, angina pectoris, or syncope.

Symptoms of failure may be sudden in onset or may progress gradually. Angina pectoris frequently occurs in aortic stenosis. One-half of patients with calcific aortic stenosis and angina have significant associated coronary artery disease, whereas coronary disease is noted at only half this rate in the absence of angina. Syncope is typically exertional and may be due to arrhythmias (usually ventricular tachycardia but sometimes sinus bradycardia), hypotension, or decreased cerebral perfusion resulting from increased blood flow to exercising muscle without compensatory increase in cardiac output. Sudden death may occur but is rarely the initial manifestation of aortic stenosis in previously asymptomatic patients.

B. Diagnostic Studies: The clinical assessment of aortic stenosis may be difficult, especially in older patients. The ECG reveals left ventricular hypertrophy or suggestive repolarization changes in most patients but may be normal in up to 10%. The chest radiograph may show a normal or enlarged cardiac silhouette, calcification of the aortic valve, and dilation and calcification of the ascending aorta. The echocardiogram provides useful data about aortic valve calcification and opening and left ventricular thickness and function, while Doppler can estimate the aortic valve gradient. These data can reliably exclude or diagnose severe stenosis. In patients with moderate obstruction, especially with low cardiac output or concomitant regurgitation, these evaluations may be inaccurate.

Cardiac catheterization is the definitive diagnostic procedure. The valve gradient is measured and the valve area calculated; a valve area below 0.8 cm² indicates severe stenosis. Aortic regurgitation can be quantified by aortic root angiography. Coronary arteriography should be performed in most adults with aortic stenosis.

Prognosis & Treatment

Following the onset of heart failure, angina, or syncope, the prognosis without surgery is poor (50% 3-year mortality rate). Medical treatment may stabilize patients in heart failure, but surgery is indicated for all symptomatic patients, including those with left ventricular dysfunction, which often improves postoperatively. Valve replacement is usually not indicated in asymptomatic individuals. Exceptions are those with declining left ventricular function, very severe left ventricular hypertrophy, and very high gradients (> 80 mm Hg) or severely reduced valve areas (≤ 0.7 cm²).

The surgical mortality rate for valve replacement

is 2–5%, but it rises to 10% above the age of 75. Severe coronary lesions are usually bypassed at the same time. Anticoagulation with warfarin is required for mechanical prostheses but is not essential with bioprostheses. The latter undergo degenerative changes and often require reoperation in 7–10 years. Some centers have begun performing the Ross procedure, which entails switching the patient's pulmonary valve to the aortic position and placing a bioprosthesis in the pulmonary position. Because bioprostheses do not deteriorate as fast on the right side of the heart, this procedure has produced excellent long-term results without anticoagulation.

Although percutaneous balloon valvuloplasty can produce short-term reductions in the severity of aortic stenosis, restenosis occurs rapidly in most adults who have calcified valves. Except in adolescents, balloon valvuloplasty should be reserved for individuals who are poor candidates for surgery or as an intermediate procedure to stabilize high-risk patients prior to surgery.

Faggiano P et al: Progression of valvular aortic stenosis in adults: Literature review and clinical implications. Am Heart J 1996;132:408.

Otto CM et al: Three year outcome after balloon aortic valvuloplasty. Circulation 1995;89:642. (Three-year survival only 23%, in part because of severity of illness in patients undergoing this procedure and in part because of its lack of efficacy.)

Pellikka PA et al: Natural history of adults with asymptomatic hemodynamically significant aortic stenosis. J Am Coll Cardiol 1990;15:1012. (While many become symptomatic, sudden death is rare.)

Stewart BF et al: Clinical factors associated with calcific aortic valve disease. J Am Coll Cardiol 1997;29:630. (Cross-sectional study of bypass in 5201 older patients, describing risk factors for calcific aortic valve disease.)

AORTIC REGURGITATION
(Aortic Insufficiency)

Essentials of Diagnosis
(Chronic Regurgitation)

- Usually asymptomatic until middle age; presents with left-sided failure or chest pain.
- Wide pulse pressure with associated peripheral signs.
- Hyperactive, enlarged left ventricle.
- Diastolic murmur along left sternal border.
- ECG shows left ventricular hypertrophy; x-ray shows left ventricular dilation. Echo-Doppler confirms diagnosis and estimates severity.

General Considerations

Rheumatic aortic regurgitation has become less common than in the preantibiotic era, but nonrheumatic causes are frequent and are the major cause of isolated aortic regurgitation. These include congenitally bicuspid valves, infective endocarditis, and hypertension. Many patients have aortic regurgitation secondary to aortic root diseases such as cystic medial necrosis (especially Marfan's syndrome), aortic dissection, ankylosing spondylitis, Reiter's syndrome, and syphilis.

Clinical Findings

A. Symptoms and Signs: The clinical presentation is determined by the rapidity with which regurgitation develops. In chronic regurgitation, the only sign for many years may be a soft aortic diastolic murmur. As the valve deformity increases, larger amounts regurgitate, diastolic blood pressure falls, and the left ventricle progressively enlarges. Most patients remain asymptomatic even at this point, and an often prolonged plateau phase, characterized by stable left ventricular dilation, occurs. Left ventricular failure is a late event and may be sudden in onset. Exertional dyspnea and fatigue are the most frequent symptoms, but paroxysmal nocturnal dyspnea and pulmonary edema may also occur. Angina pectoris or atypical chest pain may be present. Associated coronary artery disease and syncope are less common than in aortic stenosis.

Hemodynamically, because of compensatory left ventricular dilation, patients eject a large stroke volume which is adequate to maintain forward cardiac output until late in the course of the disease. Left ventricular diastolic pressure remains normal also but may abruptly rise when heart failure occurs. Abnormal left ventricular systolic function, as manifested by reduced ejection fraction and increasing end-systolic left ventricular volume, is a late sign.

The major physical findings relate to the wide arterial pulse pressure. The pulse has a rapid rise and fall (Corrigan's pulse), with an elevated systolic and low diastolic pressure, owing to the large stroke volume and rapid diastolic runoff back into the left ventricle, respectively. The large stroke volume is also responsible for characteristic findings such as Quincke's pulses (subungual capillary pulsations) and Duroziez's sign (diastolic murmur over a partially compressed peripheral artery, commonly the femoral). The apical impulse is prominent, laterally displaced, and usually hyperdynamic and may be sustained. The murmur itself may be quite soft and localized; the aortic diastolic murmur is high-pitched and decrescendo. A mid or late diastolic low-pitched mitral murmur (Austin Flint murmur) may be heard in advanced aortic insufficiency, owing to obstruction of mitral flow produced by partial closure of the mitral valve by the regurgitant jet.

When aortic insufficiency develops acutely (as in aortic dissection or infective endocarditis), left ventricular failure, manifested primarily as pulmonary edema, may develop rapidly, and surgery is urgently required. Patients with acute aortic insufficiency do not have the dilated left ventricle of chronic aortic insufficiency. In the same way, the diastolic murmur is shorter and may be minimal in intensity, and the pulse pressure may not be widened, making clinical diagnosis difficult.

B. Diagnostic Studies: The ECG usually shows moderate to severe left ventricular hypertrophy. Radiographs show cardiomegaly with left ventricular prominence.

Echocardiography can demonstrate whether the lesion involves the aortic root or if valvular disease is present. Serial assessments of left ventricular size and function are critical in determining the timing for valve replacement. Doppler techniques can qualitatively estimate the severity of regurgitation, though it should be noted that "mild" regurgitation is not uncommon and should not be overinterpreted. Scintigraphic studies can quantify left ventricular function and functional reserve during exercise—a useful predictor of prognosis.

Cardiac catheterization can help quantify severity and is used to evaluate the coronary and aortic root anatomy preoperatively.

Treatment & Prognosis

Aortic regurgitation that appears or worsens during or after an episode of infective endocarditis or aortic dissection may lead to acute severe left ventricular failure or subacute progression over weeks or months. The former usually presents as pulmonary edema; surgical replacement of the valve is indicated even during active infection. These patients may be transiently improved or stabilized by vasodilators.

Chronic regurgitation has a long natural history, but the prognosis without surgery becomes poor when symptoms occur. Vasodilators, such as hydralazine, nifedipine, and angiotensin-converting enzyme inhibitors, can reduce the severity of regurgitation, and prophylactic treatment may postpone or avoid surgery in asymptomatic patients with severe regurgitation and dilated left ventricles. Beta-blocker therapy may slow the rate of aortic dilation in Marfan's syndrome. Surgery is usually indicated once aortic regurgitation causes symptoms. Surgery is also indicated for those with few or no symptoms who present with significant left ventricular dysfunction (ejection fraction < 45–50%) or who exhibit progressive deterioration of left ventricular function, irrespective of symptoms. Although the operative mortality rate is higher when left ventricular function is severely impaired, valve replacement or repair is still indicated, since left ventricular function often improves somewhat and the long-term prognosis is thereby enhanced.

The operative mortality rate is usually in the 3–5% range. Surgeons are attempting valve repair more frequently in patients with leaflet prolapse (most frequently in individuals with bicuspid valves). Aortic regurgitation due to aortic root disease requires repair or replacement of the root, a more difficult operation.

Following surgery, left ventricular size usually decreases and left ventricular function improves, except where dysfunction has been present chronically.

Klodas E et al: Aortic regurgitation complicated by extreme left ventricular dilation: Long-term outcome after surgical correction. J Am Coll Cardiol 1996;27:670. (Even in patients with extreme ventricular dilation and impaired ejection fraction, postoperative outcome is acceptable and left ventricular ejection improves.)

Levine RJ, Gaasch WH: Vasoactive drugs in chronic regurgitant lesion of the mitral and aortic valve. J Am Coll Cardiol 1996;28:1083. (Vasodilators are beneficial in aortic regurgitation; their role is less clear in chronic mitral regurgitation.)

Michel PL et al: Degenerative aortic regurgitation. Eur Heart J 1991;12:875. (In one-third of patients undergoing valve replacement for isolated chronic aortic insufficiency, aortic root disease is the cause.)

Tornos NP et al: Clinical outcome of severe asymptomatic chronic aortic regurgitation: A long-term perspective follow-up study. Am Heart J 1995;130:333. (Follow-up of 101 patients indicates that even in severe aortic regurgitation, surgery can be postponed until the appearance of cardiac symptoms or left ventricular dysfunction at rest.)

TRICUSPID STENOSIS

Tricuspid stenosis is usually rheumatic in origin. It should be suspected when "right heart failure" appears in the course of mitral valve disease, marked by hepatomegaly, ascites, and dependent edema. The typical diastolic rumble along the lower left sternal border mimics mitral stenosis. In sinus rhythm, a presystolic liver pulsation may be found.

Hemodynamically, a diastolic pressure gradient of 5–15 mm Hg is found across the tricuspid valve in conjunction with raised pressure in the right atrium and jugular veins, with prominent a waves and with a slow y descent because of slow right ventricular filling.

Echocardiography usually demonstrates the lesion, and Doppler flow studies can measure the gradient; accompanying valve lesions can also be detected. Right heart catheterization is diagnostic.

Acquired tricuspid stenosis may be amenable to valvotomy under direct vision, but it usually requires a prosthetic valve replacement. Although experience is limited, balloon valvuloplasty may be the initial procedure of choice in many patients.

TRICUSPID REGURGITATION

Tricuspid regurgitation may occur in a variety of situations other than disease of the tricuspid valve itself. The most common is right ventricular overload resulting from left ventricular failure due to any cause. Tricuspid insufficiency occurs in association with right ventricular and inferior myocardial infarction. Tricuspid valve endocarditis and resulting regurgitation are common in intravenous drug users. Other causes include the carcinoid syndrome, lupus erythematosus, and myxomatous degeneration of the valve (associated with mitral valve prolapse). Ebstein's anomaly, a congenital defect of the tricuspid valve, often presents in adults as massive right-sided cardiomegaly due to tricuspid regurgitation.

The symptoms and signs of tricuspid insufficiency are identical to those resulting from right ventricular failure due to any cause. In the presence of mitral valve disease, the tricuspid valvular lesion can be suspected on the basis of early onset of right heart failure and a harsh systolic murmur along the lower left sternal border which is separate from the mitral murmur and which often increases in intensity during and just after inspiration.

Hemodynamically, tricuspid insufficiency is characterized by a prominent regurgitant systolic (v) wave in the right atrium and jugular venous pulse, with a rapid y descent and a small or absent x descent. The regurgitant wave, like the systolic murmur, is increased with inspiration, and its size depends upon the size of the right atrium. In tricuspid regurgitation, especially with right ventricular failure, an inspiratory S_3 may be present.

Tricuspid insufficiency secondary to severe mitral valve disease or other left-sided lesions may regress when the underlying disease is corrected. When surgery is required, valve repair or valvuloplasty of the tricuspid ring is often preferable to valve replacement. Replacement of the tricuspid valve is infrequently done now.

Cobanoglu A, Ott GY: Tricuspid valve surgery: Indications, methods, and results. Cardiovasc Clin 1993; 23:265.

Hong YM, Moller JH: Ebstein's anomaly: A long-term study of survival. Am Heart J 1993;125:1419. (Natural history in adults is relatively benign.)

CHOICE & MANAGEMENT OF PROSTHETIC VALVES

Valve repair may be useful for tricuspid, mitral, and occasionally aortic regurgitation. Likewise, percutaneous or open valvulotomy may be indicated in mitral, pulmonary, and tricuspid stenosis. Nonetheless, the number of valve replacement procedures continues to increase as a result of the aging of the population. The choice of a mechanical device versus a bioprosthesis is often a difficult one, balancing the risk of chronic anticoagulation and thromboembolism (mechanical) versus the need for eventual reoperation (bioprosthesis). In general, otherwise healthy patients below age 65 should receive mechanical valves unless anticoagulation is contraindicated because their life expectancy is greater than the durability of tissue prostheses. Furthermore, deterioration of bioprostheses is accelerated in younger patients. In patients with a small left ventricular cavity or aortic annulus, mechanical disk valves have significant hemodynamic advantages. Finally, patients who will require anticoagulation in any case, such as those in atrial fibrillation, should receive mechanical valves. Bioprostheses are preferable in older patients with life expectancies less than 10 years and when anticoagulation is contraindicated. However, hemodialysis patients should not receive tissue valves because they have a high failure rate. As noted previously, the Ross procedure offers another option in younger patients with aortic stenosis.

The identification of valve dysfunction may be difficult, but Doppler echocardiography, especially via the transesophageal approach, can identify regurgitation and stenosis in most cases. In patients with mechanical valves, careful anticoagulation is required with a target INR of 3.0–4.0. Anticoagulation should rarely be discontinued. For elective surgery, oral warfarin can be stopped 2–3 days preoperatively with heparin coverage until effective anticoagulation is resumed. In pregnant women, warfarin should be continued until 2 weeks before expected delivery, when heparin can be substituted, though the risk of fetal hemorrhage is increased somewhat. In one controlled study, aspirin, 100 mg daily, in addition to warfarin, reduced emboli and the mortality rate.

Hammermeister KE et al: A comparison of outcomes in men eleven years after heart-valve replacement with a mechanical valve or bioprosthesis. N Engl J Med 1993;328:1289. (In 575 men followed in a randomized prospective study, survival and complication rates were similar with two types of prostheses, but structural failure occurred only in bioprosthetic valves, whereas bleeding complications were more frequent with mechanical valves.)

Stein PD et al: Anti-thrombotic therapy in patients with mechanical and biological prosthetic heart valves. Chest 1995;108:371S. (Indications and approaches.)

Vongpatanasin W et al: Prosthetic heart valves. N Engl J Med 1996;335:47. (Concise review of the characteristics and the assessment of various prosthetic heart valves. Good discussion of complications and antithrombotic therapy.)

INFECTIVE ENDOCARDITIS

By Henry F. Chambers, MD

Essentials of Diagnosis

- Preexisting organic heart lesion.
- Fever.
- New or changing heart murmur.

- Evidence of systemic emboli.
- Positive blood culture.

General Considerations

Important factors that determine the clinical presentation are (1) the nature of the infecting organism; (2) which valve or valves are infected; and (3) the route of infection, since endocarditis in intravenous drug abusers and infections acquired during open heart surgery have special features.

More virulent organisms—*Staphylococcus aureus* in particular—tend to produce a more rapidly progressive and destructive infection. Patients are more likely to present with acute febrile illnesses, early embolization, and acute valvular regurgitation and myocardial abscess formation. Still, these organisms can produce a more gradual illness, and more indolent organisms can occasionally cause the acute presentation. *Streptococcus viridans,* enterococci, and a variety of other gram-positive and gram-negative bacilli, yeasts, and fungi tend to cause a more subacute picture. Systemic and peripheral manifestations may predominate. Acute deterioration due to valve perforations or large emboli may supervene at any time.

Most patients who develop infective endocarditis have underlying cardiac disease, though this is not the case with intravenous drug users and hospital-acquired infections. Abnormal valves or endocardial changes due to jet flow effects in congenital lesions (most commonly ventricular septal defect, tetralogy of Fallot, coarctation of the aorta, or patent ductus arteriosus) provide a nidus for infection during bacteremic episodes. Predisposing valvular abnormalities include rheumatic involvement of any valve, bicuspid aortic valves, calcific or sclerotic aortic valves (which are very common in elderly hypertensives), hypertrophic subaortic stenosis, and mitral valve prolapse. In the past, rheumatic disease was the commonest predisposing condition; this is no longer the case in developed countries.

The initiating event in infective endocarditis is intravascular contamination by pathogenic organisms. Contamination may occur directly or may result from transient or persistent bacteremia. Transient bacteremia is common during dental, upper respiratory, urologic, and lower gastrointestinal diagnostic and surgical procedures. It is less common during upper gastrointestinal and gynecologic procedures, though a high incidence has been reported during suction abortion.

Approximately 90% of cases of native valve endocarditis are due to viridans streptococci (60%), *S aureus* (20%), and enterococci (5–10%). Gram-negative organisms and fungi account for a small percentage.

The microbiology of native valve endocarditis in intravenous drug users differs from that of other patients. *S aureus* accounts for 60% or more of all cases

and for 80–90% of cases in which the tricuspid valve is infected. Enterococci and streptococci comprise the balance in about equal proportions. Gram-negative aerobic bacilli, fungi, and unusual organisms that rarely infect others may cause endocarditis in intravenous drug users.

The microbiology of prosthetic valve endocarditis also is distinctive. Early infections (ie, those occurring within 2 months after valve implantation) are commonly caused by staphylococci—both coagulase-positive and coagulase-negative—gram-negative organisms, and fungi. Late prosthetic valve endocarditis resembles native valve endocarditis, with the majority of infections caused by streptococci, though coagulase-negative staphylococci still cause a significant proportion of cases.

Clinical Findings

A. Symptoms and Signs: Most patients present with a febrile illness that has lasted several days to 2 weeks. Nonspecific symptoms are common. Cough, dyspnea, arthralgias or arthritis, diarrhea, and abdominal or flank pain may occur as a result of embolization or immunologically mediated phenomena. The initial symptoms or signs of endocarditis may be caused by arterial emboli or cardiac damage.

Most patients have readily documented fever, though fever may be absent in older individuals. Ninety percent have heart murmurs, but murmurs may be absent in patients with right-sided infections. The characteristic peripheral lesions—petechiae (on the palate or conjunctiva or beneath the fingernails); subungual ("splinter") hemorrhages; Osler nodes (painful, violaceous raised lesions of the fingers, toes, or feet); Janeway lesions (painless erythematous lesions of the palms or soles); and Roth spots (exudative lesions in the retina)—occur in 20–25% of patients. Pallor and splenomegaly are other helpful signs.

In acute endocarditis, leukocytosis is common; in subacute cases, anemia of chronic disease and a normal white count are the rule. Hematuria and proteinuria as well as renal dysfunction may result from emboli or immunologically mediated glomerulonephritis.

B. Diagnostic Studies: Blood culture is the single most important procedure for diagnosis of endocarditis. The current recommendation for maximizing the yield of blood cultures is to obtain three sets of blood cultures over a 24-hour period before starting antibiotics unless the patient is acutely ill. Even when this is done, a small but significant number of infected patients (up to 5% of cases) will be culture-negative, which is usually attributable to administration of antimicrobials prior to obtaining cultures. These cases may also be due to a fungus (50% of patients with fungal endocarditis have negative blood cultures), organisms that require special media for growth (eg, *Legionella* species, *Bartonella* species, nutritionally deficient streptococci), organisms that do not grow on artificial media (agents of Q fever, psittacosis), or organisms that are slow-growing and may require several weeks to grow (eg, *Brucella,* anaerobes, certain *Haemophilus* species, *Actinobacillus actinomycetemcomitans, Cardiobacterium hominis, Eikenella corrodens,* and *Kingella* species).

The chest x-ray may show evidence for the underlying cardiac abnormality and, in right-sided endocarditis, pulmonary infiltrates. The ECG is nondiagnostic. Changing conduction abnormalities suggest myocardial abscess formation.

Echocardiography may provide adjunctive information useful for identifying the specific valve or valves that are infected. The sensitivity of transthoracic echocardiography is between 55% and 65%; therefore, it cannot reliably rule out endocarditis but may confirm a clinical suspicion. Transesophageal echocardiography is 90% sensitive in detecting vegetations and is particularly useful for identifying valve ring abscesses as well as pulmonary and prosthetic valve endocarditis.

Clinical criteria (commonly referred to as the Duke criteria) for the diagnosis of endocarditis have been proposed with a weighting scheme of major and minor criteria similar to the Jones criteria used for the diagnosis of rheumatic fever. Major criteria include (1) a positive blood culture for a microorganism that typically causes infective endocarditis from two separate blood cultures; and (2) evidence of endocardial involvement documented by echocardiography (definite vegetation, myocardial abscess, or new partial dehiscence of a prosthetic valve) or development of a new regurgitant murmur. Minor criteria include (1) the presence of a predisposing condition; (2) fever ≥ 38 °C; (3) embolic disease; (4) immunologic phenomena (glomerulonephritis, Osler nodes, Roth spots, rheumatoid factor); (5) positive blood cultures but not meeting the major criteria; and (6) a positive echocardiogram but not meeting the major criteria. A definite diagnosis can be made with 80% accuracy if two major criteria, one major criterion and three minor criteria, or five minor criteria are fulfilled.

Complications

The clinical course of infective endocarditis is determined by the degree of damage to the heart, by the site of infection (right- versus left-sided, aortic versus mitral valve), by whether embolization from the site of infection occurs, and by immunologically mediated processes. Destruction of infected heart valves is especially common and precipitous with *S aureus* and often enterococci but can occur with any organism. The resulting regurgitation can be mild or severe and can progress even after bacteriologic cure. The infection can also extend into the myocardium, resulting in abscesses leading to conduction disturbances, and can also involve the wall of the aorta, creating sinus of Valsalva aneurysms.

Peripheral embolization can occur with any organism. The most catastrophic are cerebral and myocardial embolizations, with resulting infarctions. The spleen and kidneys are also common sites. Peripheral emboli may initiate metastatic infections or may become established in vessel walls, leading to mycotic aneurysms. Right-sided endocarditis, which usually involves the tricuspid valve, often leads to septic pulmonary emboli, causing infarction and lung abscesses.

Prevention

Some cases of endocarditis occur after dental procedures or operations involving the upper respiratory, genitourinary, or intestinal tract. Prophylactic antibiotics should be given to patients with predisposing congenital or valvular anomalies who are to have any of these procedures (Tables 10–3 and 10–4). Current recommendations are given in Table 10–5.

Treatment

Empiric regimens for endocarditis while culture results are pending should include agents active against staphylococci, streptococci, and enterococci. Nafcillin or oxacillin, 1.5 g every 4 hours, plus penicillin, 2–3 million units every 4 hours (or ampicillin, 1.5 g every 4 hours), plus gentamicin, 1 mg/kg every 8 hours, is such a regimen. Vancomycin, 15 mg/kg every 12 hours, may be used instead of the penicillins in the penicillin-allergic patient.

A. Viridans Streptococci: For penicillin-susceptible viridans streptococcal endocarditis (ie, MIC ≤ 0.1 μg/mL), penicillin G, 2–3 million units intravenously every 4 hours for 4 weeks, is recommended. The duration of therapy can be shortened to 2 weeks if gentamicin, 1 mg/kg every 8 hours, is used with penicillin. Ceftriaxone, 2 g once daily intravenously or intramuscularly for 4 weeks, is also effective therapy for penicillin-susceptible strains and is a convenient regimen for home therapy. For the penicillin-allergic patient, either cefazolin, 1 g intravenously every 8 hours for 4 weeks (if the patient does not have an immediate hypersensitivity reaction to penicillin), or vancomycin, 15 mg/kg every 12 hours (in patients with immediate type hypersensitivity) for 4 weeks should be used. Two-week regimens with aminoglycosides have not been studied with any agent other than penicillin. Thus, if cefazolin or vancomycin is used to treat susceptible strains, a 4-week course is needed. The 2-week regimen is not recommended for patients with symptoms of more than 3 months' duration or patients with complications such as myocardial abscess or extracardiac infection. Prosthetic valve endocarditis should be treated with a 6-week course of penicillin with at least 2 weeks of gentamicin.

Viridans streptococci that are relatively resistant to penicillin (ie, MIC > 0.1 μg/mL but ≤ 0.5 μg/mL) should be treated for 4 weeks. Penicillin G, 3 million

Table 10–3. Cardiac lesions for which bacterial endocarditis prophylaxis is or is not recommended.[1,2]

Endocarditis prophylaxis recommended
1. High-risk category
   Prosthetic cardiac valves, including bioprosthetic and homograft valves
   Previous bacterial endocarditis, even in the absence of heart disease
   Complex cyanotic congenital heart disease (eg, single ventricle states, transposition of the great arteries, tetralogy of Fallot)
   Surgically constructed systemic pulmonary shunts or conduits
2. Moderate-risk category
   Most congenital cardiac malformations (other than those listed above and below)
   Rheumatic and other acquired valvular dysfunctions, even after valvular surgery
   Hypertrophic cardiomyopathy
   Mitral valve prolapse with valvular regurgitation[3,4]

Endocarditis prophylaxis not recommended[5]
Isolated secundum septal defect
Surgical repair of atrial septal defect, ventricular septal defect, or patent ductus arteriosus (without residua beyond 6 months)
Previous coronary artery bypass graft surgery
Mitral valve prolapse without valvular regurgitation[6]
Physiologic, functional, or innocent heart murmurs
Previous Kawasaki disease without valvular dysfunction
Previous rheumatic fever without valvular dysfunction
Cardiac pacemakers (intravascular and epicardial) and implanted defibrillators

[1]Modified and reproduced, with permission, from Dajani AS et al: Prevention of bacterial endocarditis. Recommendations by the American Heart Association. JAMA 1997;277:1794. Copyright © 1997 by American Medical Association.
[2]This table lists selected conditions and is not meant to be all-inclusive.
[3]Mitral regurgitation determined by the presence of a murmur or by echo-Doppler.
[4]Men older than 45 without a consistent systolic murmur may warrant prophylaxis even in the absence of resting regurgitation.
[5]Negligible risk category—no greater than in the general population.
[6]Individuals who have a mitral valve prolapse associated with thickening or redundancy of the valve leaflets may be at increased risk for bacterial endocarditis.

Table 10–4. Procedures for which bacterial endocarditis prophylaxis is or is not recommended.[1,2]

Endocarditis prophylaxis recommended[3]
1. Dental
   Dental extractions
   Periodontal procedures
   Dental implant placement or reimplantation
   Endodontic (root canal) instrumentation or surgery only beyond the apex
   Subgingival placement of antibiotic fibers or strips
   Initial placement of orthodontic bands but not brackets
   Intraligamentary local anesthetic injections
   Prophylactic cleaning of teeth or implants where bleeding is anticipated
2. Respiratory tract
   Tonsillectomy, adenoidectomy
   Surgical operations that involve intestinal mucosa
   Bronchoscopy with a rigid bronchoscope
3. Gastrointestinal tract[4]
   Sclerotherapy for esophageal varices
   Esophageal stricture dilation
   Endoscopic retrograde cholangiography with biliary obstruction
   Biliary tract surgery
   Surgical operations that involve intestinal mucosa
4. Genitourinary tract
   Prostatic surgery
   Cystoscopy
   Urethral dilation

Endocarditis prophylaxis not recommended
1. Dental
   Restorative dentistry (filling cavities, operative and prosthodontic) with or without retraction cord[5]
   Local anesthetic injections (nonintraligamentary)

Intracanal endodontic treatment; post placement and buildup
Placement of rubber dams, removable prosthodontic, or orthodontic appliances
Postoperative suture removal
Taking of oral impression
Fluoride treatments
Orthodontic appliance adjustment
2. Respiratory
   Endotracheal intubation
   Bronchoscopy with a flexible bronchoscope, with or without biopsy[6]
   Tympanostomy (insertion)
3. Gastrointestinal
   Transesophageal echocardiography[6]
   Endoscopy with or without gastrointestinal biopsy[6]
4. Genitourinary tract
   Vaginal hysterectomy[6]
   Vaginal delivery[6]
   Cesarean section
   In the absence of infection:
   Urethral catheterization
   Uterine dilation and curettage
   Therapeutic abortion
   Sterilization procedures
   Insertion or removal of intrauterine devices
5. Other
   Cardiac catheterization, including balloon angioplasty
   Implanting cardiac pacemakers or defibrillators and coronary stents
   Incision or biopsy of surgically scrubbed skin
   Circumcision

[1]Modified and reproduced, with permission, from Dajani AS et al: Prevention of bacterial endocarditis. Recommendations by the American Heart Association. JAMA 1997;277:1794. Copyright © 1997 by American Medical Association.
[2]This table lists selected procedures but is not meant to be all-inclusive.
[3]Recommended for individuals with high- and moderate-risk cardiac conditions (Table 10–3).
[4]Prophylaxis is recommended for high-risk patients, optional for moderate-risk patients.
[5]Clinical judgment may indicate antibiotic use in selected circumstances that may create significant bleeding.
[6]Prophylaxis is optional for high-risk patients.

Table 10–5. Endocarditis prophylaxis.[1,2]

DENTAL, RESPIRATORY, OR ESOPHAGEAL PROCEDURES		
Oral	Amoxicillin	2 g 1 hour before procedure
Penicillin allergy	Clindamycin	600 mg 1 hour before procedure
	or	
	Cephalexin or cefadroxil[3]	2 g 1 hour before procedure
	or	
	Azithromycin or clarithromycin	500 mg 1 hour before procedure
Parenteral	Ampicillin	2 g IM or IV 30 minutes before procedure
Penicillin allergy	Clindamycin	600 mg IV 1 hour before procedure
	or	
	Cefazolin[3]	1 g IM or IV 30 minutes before procedure
GASTROINTESTINAL (EXCEPT ESOPHAGEAL) OR GENITOURINARY PROCEDURES		
High-risk patient (Table 10–3)	Ampicillin plus gentamicin	Ampicillin, 2 g IM or IV, plus gentamicin, 1.5 mg/kg (not to exceed 120 mg) 30 minutes before procedure; 6 hours later, ampicillin, 1 g IM or IV, or amoxicillin, 1 g orally
Penicillin allergy	Vancomycin plus gentamicin	Vancomycin, 1 g IV over 1–2 hours, plus gentamicin, 1.5 mg/kg (not to exceed 120 mg) IV or IM; complete infusion or injection 30 minutes before procedure
Moderate-risk patient	Amoxicillin or ampicillin	Amoxicillin, 2 g orally 1 hour before procedure, or ampicillin, 2 g IM or IV 30 minutes before
Penicillin allergy	Vancomycin	Vancomycin, 1 g IV over 1–2 hours; complete infusion 30 minutes before procedure

[1]Modified and reproduced, with permission, from Dajani AS et al: Prevention of bacterial endocarditis. Recommendations by the American Heart Association. JAMA 1997;277:1794. Copyright © 1997 by American Medical Association.
[2]Viridans streptococci are the most common cause of endocarditis occurring after dental or upper respiratory procedures; enterococci are the most common cause after gastrointestinal or genitourinary procedures.
[3]Cephalosporins should not be used in individuals with immediate type hypersensitivity reactions to penicillin.

units intravenously every 4 hours (or cefazolin, 1 g every 8 hours in the penicillin-allergic patient without immediate hypersensitivity), is combined with gentamicin, 1 mL/kg every 8 hours for the first 2 weeks. In the patient with IgE-mediated allergy to penicillin, vancomycin alone, 15 mg/kg every 12 hours for 4 weeks, should be administered.

Viridans streptococci with an MIC > 0.5 μg/mL and nutritionally deficient streptococci should be treated like enterococci (see below).

B. Other Streptococci: Endocarditis caused by *Streptococcus pneumoniae*, *Streptococcus pyogenes* (group A streptococcus), and groups B, C, and G streptococci are unusual causes of endocarditis, and large studies to determine efficacy of antibiotic regimens have not been published. *S pneumoniae* sensitive to penicillin (MIC < 0.1 μg/mL) can be treated with penicillin alone, 2–3 million units every 4 hours for 4–6 weeks. Strains resistant to penicillin (MIC > 0.1 μg/mL) are being reported with increasing frequency, and optimal therapy is not known, though vancomycin should be effective based on in vitro data. Group A streptococcal infection can be treated with penicillin or cefazolin for 4–6 weeks. Groups B, C, and G streptococci tend to be more resistant to penicillin than group A streptococci, and some have recommended adding gentamicin, 1 mg/kg every 8 hours, to penicillin (or cefazolin) for the first 2 weeks of a 4- to 6-week course.

C. Enterococci: For enterococcal endocarditis, the relapse rate is unacceptably high when penicillin is used alone; either streptomycin or gentamicin must be included in the regimen. Because aminoglycoside resistance occurs in enterococci, susceptibility to it should be documented. Gentamicin is the aminoglycoside of choice, because streptomycin resistance is more common than gentamicin resistance and the nephrotoxicity of gentamicin is generally more easily managed than the vestibular toxicity of streptomycin. Ampicillin, 2 g intravenously every 4 hours, or penicillin G, 3–5 million units every 4 hours (or, in the penicillin-allergic patient, vancomycin, 15 mg/kg every 12 hours), plus gentamicin, 1 mg/kg every 8 hours, is recommended. Standard practice is to continue this regimen for at least 4 weeks, and patients at high risk for relapse (those with symptoms of more than 3 months' duration or those with prosthetic valve endocarditis) should be treated for 6 weeks. Experience is more extensive with penicillin and ampicillin than with vancomycin for therapy of enterococcal endocarditis, and penicillin and ampicillin are superior to vancomycin in in vitro studies. Thus, whenever possible, either ampicillin or penicillin should be used. If endocarditis is caused by an organism that demonstrates high-level resistance to aminoglycosides (ie, not inhibited by 500 μg/mL of gentamicin), then the addition of an aminoglycoside will not be beneficial. Therapy with high doses of penicillin or ampicillin is recommended for 8–12 weeks, but the relapse rate may be as high as 50%. Surgery may be the only option in such situations.

D. Staphylococci: For methicillin-susceptible *S aureus,* nafcillin or oxacillin, 2 g every 4 hours for 4–6 weeks, is the preferred therapy. For penicillin-allergic patients, cefazolin, 2 g intravenously every 8 hours, or vancomycin, 15 mg/kg every 12 hours, may be used. For methicillin-resistant strains, vancomycin is the only agent of proved effectiveness.

The role of aminoglycoside combination regimens for *S aureus* endocarditis remains unclear, but they may be useful in shortening the duration of bacteremia. Their maximum benefit is achieved at low doses (1 mg/kg every 8 hours) and in the first 3–5 days of therapy, and they should not be continued beyond the early phase of therapy. An exception is the intravenous drug user with tricuspid valve endocarditis (with or without pulmonary involvement) who does not have serious extrapulmonary sites of infection. In that situation, the total duration of therapy can be shortened from 4 weeks to 2 weeks if an aminoglycoside is added to an antistaphylococcal drug for the entire 2 weeks of therapy. The effect of rifampin with antistaphylococcal drugs is variable, and its routine use is not recommended.

Because coagulase-negative staphylococci—a common cause of prosthetic valve endocarditis—are routinely resistant to methicillin, β-lactam antibiotics should not be used for this infection until the isolate is known to be susceptible. A combination of vancomycin for 6 weeks, rifampin, 300 mg every 8 hours for 6 weeks, and gentamicin, 1 mg/kg every 8 hours for the first 2 weeks, is the regimen of choice. If the organism is sensitive to methicillin, either nafcillin or oxacillin or cefazolin can be used in combination with rifampin and gentamicin. Although clinical data are limited because the mortality rate associated with *S aureus* prosthetic valve endocarditis is so high, most authorities recommend combination therapy with nafcillin or oxacillin (vancomycin for methicillin-resistant strains or patients allergic to β-lactams), rifampin, and gentamicin in this setting.

E. HACEK Organisms: HACEK organisms (*Haemophilus aphrophilus, Haemophilus parainfluenzae, Actinobacillus actinomycetemcomitans, Cardiobacterium hominis, Eikenella corrodens,* and *Kingella kingae*) are slow-growing, fastidious gram-negative bacilli that are normal oral flora and cause about 5–10% of all cases of endocarditis. These organisms can produce β-lactamase, and thus the treatment of choice is ceftriaxone (or some other third-generation cephalosporin), 2 g once daily for 4 weeks. Prosthetic valve endocarditis should be treated for 6 weeks. In the penicillin-allergic patient, experience is limited, but trimethoprim-sulfamethoxazole, quinolones, and aztreonam have in vitro activity and should be considered.

F. Role of Surgery: While most cases can be successfully treated medically, operative management is sometimes required. Valvular regurgitation resulting in acute heart failure that does not resolve promptly after institution of medical therapy is an indication for valve replacement even if active infection is present, especially if the aortic valve is involved. Infections that do not respond to appropriate antimicrobial therapy after 7–10 days are more likely to be eradicated if the valve is replaced. Surgery is nearly always required for fungal endocarditis and is more often necessary with gram-negative bacilli. Surgery is also indicated when the infection involves the sinus of Valsalva or produces septal abscesses. Recurrent infection with the same organism often indicates that surgery is necessary, especially with infected prosthetic valves. Continuing embolization presents a difficult problem when the infection is otherwise responding but may be an indication for surgery. Embolization after bacteriologic cure, however, does not necessarily imply recurrence of endocarditis. Anticoagulation increases the risk of catastrophic intracerebral hemorrhage.

Response to Therapy

Most patients respond rapidly to institution of appropriate antibiotics, with 50% becoming afebrile in 3 days, 72% in 1 week, and 84% by 2 weeks, but this is organism-dependent. If infection is caused by viridans streptococci, enterococci, or coagulase-negative staphylococci, defervescence occurs in 3–4 days on average, whereas if infection is caused by *Staphylococcus aureus* or *Pseudomonas aeruginosa,* patients may remain febrile for 9–12 days. If fevers persist, blood cultures should be obtained to ensure adequacy of therapy. Other causes of persistent fever are myocardial or metastatic abscess, sterile embolization, superimposed nosocomial infection, and drug reaction. Careful posttreatment monitoring is critical. Most relapses occur within 1–2 months after completion of therapy. Obtaining one or two blood cultures during this period allows for early detection of recurrent infection.

Ali AS et al: Culture-negative endocarditis: A historical review and 1990s update. Prog Cardiovasc Dis 1994; 37:149. (Although infrequent, it remains a major diagnostic dilemma.)

Dajani AS et al: Prevention of bacterial endocarditis: Recommendations by the American Heart Association. JAMA 1997;277:1794.

Di Nubile MJ: Short-course antibiotic therapy for right-sided endocarditis caused by *Staphylococcus aureus* in injection drug users. Ann Intern Med 1994;121:873. (Review of published studies showing efficacy.)

Durack DT, Lukes AS, Bright DK: New criteria for diagnosis of infective endocarditis: Utilization of specific echocardiographic findings. Am J Med 1994;96:200.

Durack DT: Prevention of infective endocarditis. N Engl J Med 1995;332:38. (Extensive review of rationale, indications, and results of antibiotic prophylaxis.)

Lindner JR et al: Diagnostic value of echocardiography in suspected endocarditis. Circulation 1996;93:730. (Bayesian approach to the use of transthoracic and transesophageal echocardiography. Echoes should not be used to make the diagnosis in low-probability patients; transthoracic echo should be the initial procedure, except in patients with prosthetic valves.)

Trial JS (editor): Diagnosis and management of infective endocarditis. Cardiol Clin 1996;14. (Entire volume discussing the cardiologic aspects of diagnosing and managing patients with endocarditis.)

Vuille C et al: Natural history of vegetations during successful medical treatment of endocarditis. Am Heart J 1994;128:1200. (Persistent vegetations are common and, in the absence of severe valvular regurgitation, do not predict complications.)

Wilson WR et al: Antibiotic treatment of adults with infective endocarditis due to streptococci, enterococci, staphylococci, and HACEK microorganisms. JAMA 1995;274:1706.

CORONARY HEART DISEASE
(Arteriosclerotic Coronary Artery Disease; Ischemic Heart Disease)

Coronary atherosclerotic heart disease is the commonest cause of cardiovascular disability and death in the USA. Men are more often affected than women by an overall ratio of 4:1, but before age 40 the ratio is 8:1, and beyond age 70 it is 1:1. In men, the peak incidence of clinical manifestations is at age 50–60; in women, at age 60–70.

Risk Factors for Coronary Heart Disease

Epidemiologic studies have identified a number of important risk factors for premature coronary heart disease. These include a positive family history (particularly when onset is before age 50), age, male gender, blood lipid abnormalities, hypertension, physical inactivity, cigarette smoking, diabetes mellitus, and hypoestrogenemia in women. Recent research has focused on abnormalities of lipid metabolism, which play a direct role in the pathophysiology of this condition. Risk increases progressively with higher levels of LDL cholesterol and declines with higher levels of HDL cholesterol. Therefore, the ratio of LDL to HDL cholesterol provides a composite marker of risk, with ratios below 3 indicating a lower risk and ratios above 5 indicating a higher risk. Patients with clinical manifestations of coronary disease before age 50 often have predisposing risk factors, though many do not. These risk factors are less closely linked to the onset of coronary disease in later years.

It is now apparent that other abnormalities of lipid metabolism may also play a role in the pathogenesis of coronary artery disease, and these should be sought in individuals with otherwise unexplained premature coronary atherosclerosis. Among the patterns associated with increased atherosclerosis are elevated levels of apolipoprotein(a) ("little a") and of small, dense LDL lipoprotein particles. These lipoproteins and their accompanying lipids appear more likely to pass into the vessel wall and may be more difficult to clear.

Although the matter is still controversial, accumulating evidence suggests that hypertriglyceridemia is an independent risk factor for coronary artery disease as well. Elevated triglyceride levels often occur in association with other lipid abnormalities, including low levels of HDL cholesterol and elevated concentrations of lipoprotein(a) and small, dense LDL particles.

Pathophysiology

Knowledge concerning the pathophysiology of atherosclerosis and the clinical presentations of coronary artery disease is accumulating rapidly. Abnormal lipid metabolism or excessive intake of cholesterol and saturated fats—especially when superimposed on a genetic predisposition—initiates the atherosclerotic process. The initial step is the "fatty streak," or subendothelial accumulation of lipids and lipid-laden monocytes (macrophages). Low-density lipoproteins (LDLs) are the major atherogenic lipid. High-density lipoproteins (HDLs), in contrast, are protective and probably assist in the mobilization of LDLs. The pathogenetic role of other lipids, including triglycerides, is less clear. LDLs undergo in situ oxidation, which makes them more difficult to mobilize as well as locally cytotoxic.

Macrophages migrate into the subendothelial space and take up lipids, giving them the appearance of "foam" cells. As the plaque progresses, smooth muscle cells also migrate into the lesion. At this stage, the lesion may be hemodynamically insignificant, but endothelial function is abnormal and its ability to limit the entry of lipoproteins into the vessel wall is impaired. If the plaque remains stable, a fibrous cap forms, the lesion becomes calcified, and the vessel lumen may be slowly narrowed.

Although many atherosclerotic plaques remain stable or progress only gradually, others may rupture, with a resulting extrusion of lipids and tissue factors that result in a cascade of events culminating in intravascular thrombosis. The result may be partial or complete vessel occlusion (causing the symptoms of unstable angina or myocardial infarction), or the plaque may become restabilized, often with more severe stenosis.

Several features are associated with enhanced plaque vulnerability, including a higher lipid content, a higher concentration of macrophages, and a very thin fibrous cap. Lesions with these characteristics are often the culprit lesions in young individuals, in whom acute myocardial infarction or sudden death is the first manifestation of coronary disease; and this abrupt progression explains why most infarctions do not occur at the site of preexisting critical stenosis. Conversely, the relatively greater reduction in clinical events than in lesion severity in lipid-lowering treatment trials is probably explained by the regression or prevention of these early nonfibrotic lesions.

Recent observations have resurrected an old theory that atherosclerosis progresses as the result of an inflammatory response in the vessel wall, perhaps initiated or worsened by an infectious agent. A high circulating level of C-reactive protein, a nonspecific inflammatory marker, is associated with a higher rate of ischemic events. Agents as diverse as *Chlamydia pneumoniae,* cytomegalovirus, and *Helicobacter pylori* have been indirectly implicated.

Abrams J, Pasternak RC (editors): Changing the natural history of coronary artery disease. Cardiol Clin 1996; 14:1, 17. (Two chapters of this monograph focus on the endothelial function, vasomotion, and plaque instability.)

Primary & Secondary Prevention of Ischemic Heart Disease

Although many risk factors for coronary artery disease are not modifiable, it is now clear that interventions such as smoking cessation, treatment of hyperlipidemia, lowering of blood pressure, and estrogen replacement therapy can both prevent coronary disease and delay its progression and complications after it is manifest. Treatment of lipid abnormalities delays the progression of atherosclerosis and in some cases produces regression. Even in the absence of regression, fewer new lesions develop, endothelial function may be restored, and the coronary event rate is markedly reduced in patients with clinical evidence of atherosclerosis.

The 4S (Scandinavian Simvastatin Survival Study) and the CARE trials have demonstrated improved outcomes in patients with atherosclerotic disease treated with HMG-CoA reductase inhibitors, even when they have cholesterol levels previously considered satisfactory (LDL cholesterol levels as low as 125 mg/dL). These studies found reductions in cardiac events, cardiovascular deaths, and all cause mortality. This occurred regardless of age, race, or the presence of hypertension. Aggressive lipid-lowering therapy should be implemented in all patients with dyslipidemia and coronary artery or peripheral vascular disease. The West of Scotland Study extended these findings to high-risk individuals without manifest coronary disease, though the cost:benefit ratio of therapy is uncertain when LDL cholesterol is ≤ 160 mg/dL in the absence of multiple risk factors. Treatment of abnormally low HDL levels or elevations of lipoprotein(a) and small, dense LDL particles is more difficult, but oral niacin in high dosages (3 g/d or more) may be effective. The value of reducing elevated triglyceride levels is less clear, but since elevated triglycerides are often associated with other lipid abnormalities, treatment with niacin or gemfibrozil for levels above 400 mg/dL is appropriate. Since LDL oxidation appears to play a role in the atherogenicity of lipid molecules that have passed into the vessel wall, antioxidant therapy has been advocated as a preventive measure. Suggestive but inconclusive data are available to support the use of vitamin E, but more information is required before this approach can be recommended to the general public.

There is also growing evidence that elevated plasma homocysteine is a risk factor for arteriosclerosis and other thrombotic diseases. The prevalence of this risk factor and its pathophysiologic importance remain to be clarified, but when plasma homocysteine levels are elevated or rise following a methionine challenge in patients with premature atherosclerosis who have no other risk factors, treatment is indicated. Homocysteine levels can be reduced with dietary supplements of folic acid (1 mg/d) in combination with vitamin B_6 and vitamin B_{12}.

Another preventive measure is aspirin prophylaxis. Aspirin (325 mg every other day) in males over the age of 50 reduces the incidence of myocardial infarction. Whether this approach should be employed in the general population or only in those at higher risk is unclear, and the optimal dosage is not known. A prudent approach would be to administer 75–325 mg daily to men with at least one risk factor if no contraindication is present. The same approach is probably warranted for women, commencing 5–10 years later. The value of other platelet-inhibiting agents and dietary supplements, such as fish oil or omega-3 fats, is not certain.

Control of blood pressure has now been shown to prevent infarctions in older patients. Although unproved, it seems likely that control of blood pressure in younger individuals also prevents subsequent coronary events. The role of exercise remains controversial. Although individuals who exercise for at least 30 minutes a week are at lower risk for subsequent coronary events, it is difficult to be certain that this outcome relates specifically to exercise rather than a generally healthy lifestyle.

The decrease in number of coronary deaths over the last 2 decades may be due to a decrease in the prevalence of risk factors but probably also reflects improvements in medical therapy, the role of coronary care units, better treatment of angina, arrhythmias, and heart failure, and improved survival after coronary revascularization in some patient subsets.

American College of Physicians: Guidelines for using serum cholesterol, high-density, lipoprotein cholesterol, and triglyceride levels as screening test for preventing coronary heart disease in adults. Ann Intern Med 1996;124:515. (Controversial guidelines discouraging the aggressive approach to cholesterol screening advocated by the National Cholesterol Education Program. An accompanying article by Garber provides the evidence supporting this position, and an accompanying editorial argues the opposite position.)

Andrews TC et al: Effective cholesterol reduction and myocardial ischemia in patients with coronary disease. Circulation 1997;95:324. (Aggressive lowering of cholesterol with HMG Co-A reductase inhibitors not only prevents progression or induces regression of atherosclerotic plaques—it also restores endothelial function. This may be the mechanism of the rapid reduction in ischemic electrocardiographic changes and events following the initiation of lipid-lowering therapy.)

Bostom AG et al: Elevated plasma lipoprotein(a) and coronary heart disease in men aged 55 years and younger. JAMA 1996;276:544. (This atherogenic particle may explain premature coronary artery disease in individuals without other identifiable risk factors.)

Després J-P et al: Hyperinsulinemia as an independent risk factor for ischemic heart disease. N Engl J Med 1996;334:952. (Case-control study indicating that hyperinsulinemia may be an independent risk factor for coronary heart disease, even after correction for obesity and lipid levels.)

Fletcher GF et al: Statement on exercise: Benefits and recommendations for physical activity programs for all Americans. Circulation 1996;94:857. (Consensus recommendation on healthy lifestyle.)

Fuster V et al: Aspirin as a therapeutic agent in cardiovascular disease. Circulation 1993;87:659. (Special report reviewing mechanisms and results of aspirin therapy in ischemic and nonischemic cardiovascular disease.)

Fuster V: Mechanisms leading to myocardial infarction. Insights from studies of vascular biology. Circulation 1994;90:206. (Excellent review of how atherosclerotic plaques form and progress.)

Gardner CD et al: Association of small-low density lipoprotein particles with the incidence of coronary artery disease in men and women. JAMA 1996;276:875. (Case-control study indicating that these particles are atherogenic.)

Gillum RF: Trends in acute myocardial infarction and coronary heart disease depth in the United States. J Am Coll Cardiol 1994;23:1273. (Comments on the remarkable decline in coronary heart disease, morbidity, and mortality. However, it should be remembered that coronary heart disease remains the leading cause of death in the United States.)

Glantz SA, Parmley WW: Passive smoking and heart disease. JAMA 1995;273:1047. (Overview of data supporting the harmful effect of passive smoking.)

Havel RJ, Rapoport E: Management of primary hyperlipidemia. N Engl J Med 1995;332:1491. (Summary of when and how to treat.)

Hlatky M et al: Job strain in the prevalence and outcome of coronary heart disease. Circulation 1995;92:327. (Despite conventional wisdom, severe job strains are not significant predictors of findings on coronary angiography.)

Lee IM et al: Exercise intensity and longevity in men. JAMA 1995;273:1179. (Latest data from Harvard Alumni Study indicating that men engaged in vigorous activities survive longer.)

Levine GN et al: Cholesterol reduction in cardiovascular disease. N Engl J Med 1995;332:512. (Review of primary and secondary prevention trials, including angiographic regression studies and discussion of the pathophysiology.)

Mann JM, Davies MJ: Vulnerable plaque: Relation of characteristics to degree of stenosis in human coronary arteries. Circulation 1996;94:928. (Careful pathologic study delineating the factors within the plaque that seem to predispose to rupture and subsequent thrombotic events.)

Mayer EL et al: Homocysteine and coronary arteriosclerosis. J Am Coll Cardiol 1996;27:517. (Summary of evidence according to elevated homocysteine levels as a risk factor for coronary heart disease.)

O'Keefe JH et al: Insights into the pathogenesis and prevention of coronary artery disease. Mayo Clinic Proc 1995;70:69. (Clinically oriented review with focus on preventive strategies.)

Rich-Edwards JW et al: Primary prevention of coronary heart disease in women. N Engl J Med 1995;332:1758. (In addition to discussing the importance of the usual risk factors, the role of estrogen replacement therapy is discussed.)

Ridker PM et al: Inflammation, aspirin, and the risk of cardiovascular disease in apparently healthy men. N Engl J Med 1997;336:973. (Provocative observation from the Physicians Health Study that elevated C-reactive protein is associated with an increased incidence of ischemic events and that these are prevented by aspirin.)

Scandinavian Simvastatin Survival Study Group: Randomized trial of cholesterol lowering in 4444 patients with coronary heart disease. Lancet 1994;344:1383. (Lowering of moderate cholesterol elevations in patients with angina or prior myocardial infarction reduces mortality, prevents infarction and the need for revascularization, and decreases the rate of stroke and heart failure. Each of these end points is reduced by 30–40%.)

Shepherd J et al: Prevention of coronary heart disease with pravastatin in men with hypercholesterolemia. N Engl J Med 1995;333:1301. (Large-scale primary prevention trial showing that lipid lowering prevents coronary events and deaths. However, the cost:benefit ratio is substantial in patients with only moderate elevations of cholesterol and without multiple risk factors.)

Stampfer MJ et al: A prospective study of triglyceride level, low density lipoprotein particle diameter and risk of myocardial infarction. JAMA 1996;276:882. (Elevated triglycerides and the company they keep appear to be independent risk factors.)

Stephens NG et al: Randomized controlled trial of vitamin E in patients with coronary disease: Cambridge Heart Antioxidant Study (CHAOS). Lancet 1996;347:781. (First study showing that vitamin E therapy can prevent coronary events. In light of multiple negative trials with an antioxidant, this result will require confirmation.)

Superko HR: Lipid disorders contributing to coronary heart disease: An update. Curr Probl Cardiol 1996;21:736.

Twenty-Seventh Bethesda Conference: Matching the intensity of risk factor management and the hazards of coronary disease events. J Am Coll Cardiol 1996;27:957. (Consensus conference report reviewing the pathophysiologic factors associated with risk of coronary heart disease and interventions to prevent its evolution. Emphasis is on matching interventions to level of risk.)

Willard JE et al: The use of aspirin in ischemic heart disease. N Engl J Med 1992;327:175.

Pathophysiology of Symptomatic & Silent Ischemia & Coronary Syndromes

Advanced coronary atherosclerosis and even complete occlusion may remain clinically silent. There is only a modest correlation between the clinical symptoms and the anatomic extent of disease. At present, the only means of determining the location and extent of narrowing is coronary arteriography, although ischemia can be recognized by other less invasive studies. Myocardial ischemia may be provoked by either increased myocardial oxygen requirements (exercise, mental stress, or spontaneous fluctuations in heart rate and blood pressure) or by decreased oxygen supply (caused by coronary vasospasm, platelet plugging, or partial thrombosis). Abnormal endothelial function appears to play a role in the fluctuating threshold for ischemia; impaired release of endothelium-derived relaxing factor (nitrous oxide) may permit unopposed vasoconstriction and facilitate platelet adhesion.

Most studies indicate that in angina pectoris, increased oxygen demand is the most frequent mechanism. In contrast, the acute coronary syndromes of unstable angina and myocardial infarction are caused by plaque disruption, platelet plugging, and coronary thrombosis. Of interest is the predilection for these episodes to occur in the early morning or shortly after arising. The outcome of this series of events is determined by whether the vessel becomes occluded or whether thrombolysis occurs, either spontaneously or as a result of treatment, and whether the plaque subsequently becomes stabilized. Thus, therapy is primarily directed toward inhibition of platelet activity (aspirin) and thrombolysis in acute syndromes and toward minimizing myocardial oxygen requirements—as well as preventive measures—in chronic angina.

Some episodes of myocardial ischemia are painful, causing angina pectoris; others are completely silent. Many silent episodes are brought on by emotional and mental stress. In patients with diagnosed coronary disease, as evidenced by prior myocardial infarction or angina, silent ischemic episodes have the same prognostic import as painful ones. The prognosis for patients with only silent ischemia is not well established, nor is the potential benefit of preventing silent ischemia.

Gabbay FH et al: Triggers of myocardial ischemia during daily life in patients with coronary artery disease: Physical and mental activities, anger, and smoking. J Am Coll Cardiol 1996;27:585. (Mental stress and anger may be more important than physical activity.)

Mulcahy D et al: Ischemia during ambulatory monitoring is not a prognostic indicator in patients with stable coronary artery disease. JAMA 1997;277:318. (Long-term follow-up for 221 patient cohorts, indicating that ambulatory ischemia was a poor predictor of subsequent events, which tended to be caused by new lesions rather than those responsible for ischemia at baseline.)

Selwyn AP et al: Pathophysiology of ischemia in patients with coronary artery disease. Prog Cardiovasc Dis 1992;35:27.

SUDDEN DEATH

Sudden death may be the first clinical manifestation of coronary disease in as many as one-fourth of patients but is more likely to occur in patients with prior infarction and moderate to severe left ventricular dysfunction. In addition, 20% of patients with acute myocardial infarction will die before reaching a hospital. Most of these deaths are caused by ventricular fibrillation. It is noteworthy that transient ischemia (as opposed to infarction or coronary occlusion) is rarely the cause of sudden death.

Note: See section on ventricular arrhythmias and evaluation of survivors of sudden death for management of patients at risk for sudden death and of survivors.

Current perspectives on the problem of sudden cardiac death. Dallas, Texas, September 24–25, 1990. Circulation 1992;85(1 Suppl):I1. (Cupples articles show that underlying coronary artery disease is the main risk factor. Davies article shows that 73% of victims have recent coronary thrombotic lesions.)

Demirovic J, Myerburg RJ: Epidemiology of sudden coronary death: An overview. Prog Cardiovasc Dis 1994; 37:39.

ANGINA PECTORIS

Essentials of Diagnosis

• Precordial chest pain, usually precipitated by stress or exertion, relieved rapidly by rest or nitrates.
• Electrocardiographic or scintigraphic evidence of ischemia during pain or stress testing.
• Angiographic demonstration of significant obstruction of major coronary vessels.

General Considerations

Angina pectoris is usually due to atherosclerotic heart disease. Coronary vasospasm may occur at the site of a lesion or, less frequently, in apparently normal vessels. Other unusual causes of coronary artery obstruction such as congenital anomalies, emboli, arteritis, or dissection may cause ischemia or infarction. Angina may also occur in the absence of coronary artery obstruction as a result of severe myocardial hypertrophy, severe aortic stenosis or insufficiency, or in response to increased metabolic demands, as in hyperthyroidism, marked anemia, or paroxysmal tachycardias with rapid ventricular rates. Rarely, angina occurs with angiographically normal coronary arteries and without other identifiable causes. This presentation has been labeled syndrome X and is felt to be caused by microvascular abnormalities. Although treatment is often not very successful in relieving symptoms, the prognosis of syndrome X is good.

Clinical Findings

A. History: The diagnosis of angina pectoris depends principally upon the history, which should specifically include the following information.

1. Circumstances that precipitate and relieve angina—Angina occurs most commonly during activity and is relieved by resting. Exertion that involves straining the thoracic or upper extremity muscles (eg, lifting) or walking rapidly uphill precipitates attacks most consistently. Patients prefer to remain upright rather than lie down. The amount of activity required to produce angina may be relatively consistent under comparable physical and emotional circumstances or may vary from day to day. It is usually less after meals, during excitement, or on exposure to cold. The threshold for angina is often lower in the morning or after strong emotion; the latter can provoke attacks in the absence of exertion. In addition, discomfort may occur during sexual activity, at rest, or at night as a result of coronary spasm.

2. Characteristics of the discomfort—Patients often do not refer to angina as "pain" but as a sensation of tightness, squeezing, burning, pressing, choking, aching, bursting, "gas," indigestion, or an ill-characterized discomfort. It is often characterized by clenching a fist over the mid chest. The distress of angina is never sharply localized and is not spasmodic.

3. Location and radiation—The distribution of the distress may vary widely in different patients but is usually the same for each patient unless unstable angina or myocardial infarction supervenes. In 80–90% of cases, the discomfort is felt behind or slightly to the left of the mid sternum. When it begins farther to the left or, uncommonly, on the right, it characteristically moves centrally to include the sternum. Although angina may radiate to any dermatome from C8 to T4, it radiates most often to the left shoulder and upper arm, frequently moving down the inner volar aspect of the arm to the elbow, forearm, wrist, or fourth and fifth fingers. Radiation to the right shoulder and distally is less common, but the characteristics are the same. Occasionally, angina may be felt initially in the lower jaw, the back of the neck, the interscapular area, high in the left back, or in the volar aspect of the wrist. If the patient identifies the site of pain by pointing to the area of the apical impulse with one finger, angina is unlikely.

4. Duration of attacks—Angina is of short duration and subsides completely without residual discomfort. If the attack is precipitated by exertion and the patient promptly stops to rest, it usually lasts less than 3 minutes. Attacks following a heavy meal or brought on by anger often last 15–20 minutes. Attacks lasting more than 30 minutes are unusual and suggest the development of unstable angina, myocardial infarction, or an alternative diagnosis.

5. Effect of nitroglycerin—The diagnosis of angina pectoris is strongly supported if sublingual nitroglycerin invariably shortens an attack and if prophylactic nitrates permit greater exertion or prevent angina entirely.

6. Risk factors—The presence of risk factors described previously makes the diagnosis of angina more likely, but their absence does not exclude angina since most patients do not have a risk profile markedly different from that of the general population.

B. Signs: Examination during a spontaneous or induced attack frequently reveals a significant elevation in systolic and diastolic blood pressure, although hypotension may also occur; occasionally, a gallop rhythm and an apical systolic murmur due to transient mitral regurgitation from papillary muscle dysfunction are present during pain only. Supraventricular or ventricular arrhythmias may be present, either as the precipitating factor or as a result of ischemia.

It is important to detect signs of diseases that may contribute to or accompany atherosclerotic heart disease, eg, diabetes mellitus (retinopathy or neuropathy), xanthelasma, tendinous xanthomas, hypertension, thyrotoxicosis, myxedema, or peripheral vascular disease. Aortic stenosis or regurgitation, hypertrophic cardiomyopathy, and mitral valve prolapse should be sought, since they may produce angina or other forms of chest pain.

Differential Diagnosis

With an appropriate history, the diagnosis of angina pectoris is more than 90% certain. When atypical features are present—such as prolonged duration (hours or days); or darting, knifelike pains at the apex or over the precordium—ischemia is less likely.

"Anterior chest wall syndrome" is characterized by sharply localized tenderness of intercostal muscles. Inflammation of the chondrocostal junctions, which may be warm, swollen, and red, may result in diffuse chest pain that is also reproduced by local pressure (Tietze's syndrome). Intercostal neuritis (herpes zoster, diabetes mellitus, etc) also mimics angina.

Cervical or thoracic spine disease involving the dorsal roots produces sudden sharp, severe chest pain suggesting angina in location and "radiation" but related to specific movements of the neck or spine, recumbency, and straining or lifting. Pain due to cervical or thoracic disk disease involves the outer or dorsal aspect of the arm and the thumb and index fingers rather than the ring and little fingers.

Peptic ulcer, chronic cholecystitis, esophageal spasm, and functional gastrointestinal disease may produce pain suggestive of angina pectoris. Reflux esophagitis is characterized by lower chest and upper abdominal pain after heavy meals, occurring in recumbency or upon bending over. The pain is relieved by antacids, sucralfate, or H_2 receptor antagonists. The picture may be especially confusing because ischemic pain may also be associated with upper gastrointestinal symptoms, and esophageal motility disorders may be improved by nitrates and calcium channel blockers. Assessment of esophageal motility may be necessary.

Degenerative and inflammatory lesions of the left shoulder and thoracic outlet syndromes may cause chest pain due to nerve irritation or muscular compression; the symptoms are usually precipitated by movement of the arm and shoulder and are associated with paresthesias.

Spontaneous pneumothorax may cause chest pain as well as dyspnea and may create confusion with angina as well as myocardial infarction. Even the ECG may resemble infarction because of changes in voltage from the pneumothorax. The same is true of pneumonia and pulmonary embolization. Dissection of the thoracic aorta can cause severe chest pain that is commonly felt in the back; it is sudden in onset, reaches maximum intensity immediately, and may be associated with changes in pulses. Other cardiac disorders such as mitral valve prolapse, hypertrophic cardiomyopathy, myocarditis, pericarditis, aortic valve disease, or right ventricular hypertrophy may cause atypical chest pain or even myocardial ischemia. Noninvasive testing and, in many cases, cardiac catheterization may be required to establish the diagnosis.

Castell PO: Chest pain of undetermined origin: Proceedings of a symposium. Am J Med 1992;92(5A):1S.
Sullivan AR et al: Chest pain in women: Clinical investigative and prognostic features. Br Med J 1994;308:883.

Evaluation of Patients With Angina Pectoris

A. Laboratory Findings: Serum lipid levels should be determined in all patients with suspected angina. Anemia and diabetes may also be investigated if clinically appropriate.

B. Electrocardiography: The resting ECG is normal in about a quarter of patients with angina. In the remainder, abnormalities include old myocardial infarction, nonspecific ST–T changes, atrioventricular or intraventricular conduction defects, and changes of left ventricular hypertrophy. During anginal episodes, the characteristic electrocardiographic change is horizontal or downsloping ST segment de-

pression that reverses after the ischemia disappears. T wave flattening or inversion may also occur. Less frequently, ST segment elevation is observed; this finding suggests severe (transmural) ischemia and often occurs with coronary spasm.

C. Exercise Electrocardiography: Exercise testing is the most useful noninvasive procedure for evaluating the patient with angina. Ischemia that is not present at rest is detected by precipitation of typical chest pain or ST segment depression (or, rarely, elevation). Exercise testing is often combined with scintigraphic studies or echocardiography (see below), but in patients without baseline ST segment abnormalities or in whom anatomic localization is not necessary, the exercise ECG should be the initial procedure because of considerations of cost and convenience.

Exercise testing can be done on a motorized treadmill or with a bicycle ergometer. A variety of exercise protocols are utilized, the most common being the Bruce protocol, which increases the treadmill speed and elevation every 3 minutes until limited by symptoms. At least two electrocardiographic leads should be monitored continuously.

1. Precautions and risks–The usually quoted risk of exercise testing is one infarction or death per 1000 tests, but individuals who continue to have pain at rest or minimal activity are at higher risk and should not be tested. Many of the traditional exclusions, such as recent myocardial infarction or congestive heart failure, are no longer employed *if the patient is stable and ambulatory,* but aortic stenosis remains a contraindication. While most tests are carried to a symptom-limited end point (except submaximal testing early postinfarction), the test should be terminated when hypotension, significant ventricular or supraventricular arrhythmias, more than mild to moderate angina, or more than 3- to 4-mm ST segment depression occurs.

2. Indications–Exercise testing is employed (1) to confirm the diagnosis of angina; (2) to determine the severity of limitation of activity due to angina; (3) to assess prognosis in patients with known coronary disease, including those recovering from myocardial infarction, by detecting groups at high or low risk; (4) to evaluate responses to therapy; and (5) less successfully, to screen asymptomatic populations for silent coronary disease. The latter application is controversial. Because false-positive tests often exceed true positives, leading to much patient anxiety and self-imposed or mandated disability, exercise testing of asymptomatic individuals should be done only for those at high risk (usually a strong family history of premature coronary disease or hyperlipidemia), those whose occupations place them or others at special risk (eg, airline pilots), and older individuals commencing strenuous activity.

3. Interpretation–The usual electrocardiographic criterion for a positive test is 1 mm (0.1 mV) horizontal or downsloping ST segment depression (beyond baseline) measured 80 ms after the J point. By this criterion, 60–80% of patients with anatomically significant coronary disease will have a positive test, but 10–20% of those without significant disease will also be positive. False-positives are uncommon when a 2-mm depression is present. Additional information is inferred from the time of onset and duration of the electrocardiographic changes, their magnitude and configuration, blood pressure and heart rate changes, the duration of exercise, and the presence of associated symptoms. In general, patients exhibiting more severe ST segment depression (> 2 mm) at low workloads (< 6 minutes on the Bruce protocol) or heart rates (< 70% of age-predicted maximum)—especially when the duration of exercise and rise in blood pressure are limited or when hypotension occurs during the test—have more severe disease and a poorer prognosis. Depending on symptom status, age, and other factors, such patients should be referred for coronary arteriography and possible revascularization. On the other hand, less impressive positive tests in asymptomatic patients are often "false-positives." Therefore, exercise testing results that do not conform to the clinical picture should be confirmed by stress scintigraphy or echocardiography.

D. Scintigraphic Assessment of Ischemia: Two nuclear medicine studies provide additional information about the presence, location, and extent of coronary disease.

1. Myocardial perfusion scintigraphy–This test provides images in which radionuclide uptake is proportionate to blood flow at the time of injection. Thallium-201 or one of the newer technetium-based imaging agents is used. Areas of diminished uptake reflect relative hypoperfusion (compared to other myocardial regions). If the radiotracer is injected during exercise or dipyridamole- or adenosine-induced coronary vasodilation, scintigraphic defects indicate a zone of ischemia or hypoperfusion. Over time, as relative blood flow equalizes, these defects tend to "fill in" if the abnormality is transient, indicating reversible ischemia. Defects observed when the radiotracer is injected at rest or still present 3–4 hours after an injection during exercise or dipyridamole vasodilation usually indicate myocardial infarction (old or recent) but may be present with severe ischemia. Occasionally, other conditions, including infiltrative diseases (sarcoidosis, amyloidosis), left bundle branch block, and dilated cardiomyopathy, may produce resting or persistent perfusion defects.

In experienced laboratories, stress perfusion scintigraphy is positive in 75–90% of patients with anatomically significant coronary disease and in 20–30% of those without it. False-positive tests in women may be due to attenuation through breast tissue.

Myocardial scintigraphy is indicated (1) when the resting ECG makes an exercise ECG difficult to interpret (LBBB, baseline ST–T changes, low voltage, etc); (2) for confirmation of the results of the exercise ECG when they are contrary to the clinical impression (eg, a positive test in an asymptomatic patient); (3) to localize the region of ischemia; (4) to distinguish ischemic from infarcted myocardium; (5) to assess the completeness of vascularization following bypass surgery or coronary angioplasty; or (6) as a prognostic indicator in patients with known coronary disease.

2. Radionuclide angiography–This procedure images the left ventricle and measures its ejection fraction and wall motion. In coronary disease, resting abnormalities usually represent infarction, and those that occur with exercise usually indicate stress-induced ischemia. Normal subjects usually exhibit an increase in ejection fraction with exercise or no change; patients with coronary disease may exhibit a decrease. Exercise radionuclide angiography has approximately the same sensitivity as thallium-201 scintigraphy, but it is less specific in older individuals and those with other forms of heart disease. The indications are similar to those for thallium-201 scintigraphy.

E. Echocardiography: Echocardiography can image the left ventricle and reveal segmental wall motion abnormalities, which may indicate ischemia or prior infarction. It is a convenient technique for assessing left ventricular function, which is an important indicator of prognosis and determinant of therapy. An increasing number of laboratories are performing echocardiograms during supine exercise or immediately following upright exercise; exercise-induced segmental wall motion abnormalities are used as an additional indicator of ischemia. This technique requires considerable expertise; however, in experienced laboratories, the increment in test accuracy is comparable to that obtained with scintigraphy—though a higher proportion of tests are technically inadequate. Pharmacologic stress with high-dose (20–40 µg/kg/min) dobutamine can be used as an alternative to exercise.

F. Ambulatory Electrocardiographic Monitoring: With current ambulatory electrocardiographic recorders and with trained technicians, episodes of ischemic ST segment depression can be monitored. In patients with coronary artery disease, these episodes usually signify ischemia, even when asymptomatic ("silent"). In many, silent episodes are more frequent than symptomatic ones. In most cases, they occur in patients with other evidence of ischemia, and they respond to the same treatments, so that the role of ambulatory monitoring is unclear, as is the benefit of abolishing all such episodes in patients who are otherwise being managed properly.

G. Coronary Angiography: Selective coronary arteriography is the definitive diagnostic procedure for coronary artery disease. It can be performed with low mortality (about 0.1%) and morbidity (1–5%), but the cost is high, and with currently available noninvasive techniques it is usually not indicated solely for diagnosis.

Coronary arteriography should be performed in the following groups:

(1) Patients being considered for coronary artery revascularization because of limiting stable angina who have failed to improve on an adequate medical regimen.

(2) Patients in whom coronary revascularization is being considered because the clinical presentation (unstable angina, postinfarction angina, etc) or noninvasive testing suggests high-risk disease (see Indications for Revascularization).

(3) Patients with aortic valve disease who also have angina pectoris, in order to determine whether the angina is due to accompanying coronary disease. Coronary angiography is also performed in asymptomatic older patients undergoing valve surgery so that concomitant bypass may be done if the anatomy is propitious.

(4) Patients who have had coronary revascularization with subsequent recurrence of symptoms, to determine whether bypass grafts or native vessels are occluded.

(5) Patients with cardiac failure in whom a surgically correctable lesion, such as left ventricular aneurysm, mitral regurgitation, or reversible ischemic dysfunction, is suspected.

(6) Patients surviving sudden death or with symptomatic or life-threatening arrhythmias in whom coronary artery disease may be a correctable cause.

(7) Patients with chest pain of uncertain cause or cardiomyopathy of unknown cause.

Coronary arteriography visualizes the location and severity of stenoses. Narrowing greater than 50% of the luminal diameter is considered clinically significant, although most lesions producing ischemia are associated with narrowing in excess of 70%. This information has important prognostic value, since mortality rates are progressively higher in patients with one-, two-, and three-vessel disease and those with left main coronary artery obstruction (ranging from 1% per year to 25% per year). Among stable patients, 20%, 30%, and 50% have one-, two-, and three-vessel involvement, respectively, while left main disease is present in 10%. In those with strongly positive exercise ECGs or scintigraphic studies, three-vessel or left main disease may be present in 75–95% depending upon the criteria employed. Coronary arteriography also shows whether the obstructions are amenable to bypass surgery or percutaneous transluminal coronary angioplasty (PTCA).

H. Left Ventricular Angiography: Left ventricular angiography is usually performed at the same time as coronary arteriography. Global and regional left ventricular function are visualized, as well as mitral regurgitation if present. Left ventricular function is the major determinant of prognosis in stable coronary disease and of the risk of bypass surgery.

Abrams J (editor): Angina pectoris: Mechanisms, diagnosis, and therapy. Cardiol Clin 1991;9(1):1.

Chang JA, Froelicher VF: Clinical and exercise test markers of prognosis in patients with stable coronary artery disease. Curr Probl Cardiol 1994;19:533.

Chou TM, Amidon TA: Evaluating coronary artery disease non-invasively: Which test for whom? West J Med 1994;161:173. (Review for primary care physicians.)

Douglas PS, Ginsburg GS: The evaluation of chest pain in women. N Engl J Med 1996;334:1311.

Coronary Vasospasm & Angina With Normal Coronary Arteriograms

Although most symptoms of myocardial ischemia result from fixed stenosis of the coronary arteries or intraplaque hemorrhage or thrombosis at the site of lesions, some ischemic events may be precipitated or exacerbated by coronary vasoconstriction.

Spasm of the large coronary arteries with resulting decreased coronary blood flow may occur spontaneously or may be induced by exposure to cold, emotional stress, or vasoconstricting medications, such as ergot derivative drugs. Spasm may occur both in normal and in stenosed coronary arteries and may be silent or result in angina pectoris. Even myocardial infarction may occur as a result of spasm in the absence of visible obstructive coronary heart disease, although most instances of coronary spasm occur in the presence of coronary stenosis.

Cocaine can induce myocardial ischemia by causing coronary artery vasoconstriction or by increasing myocardial energy requirements.

Prinzmetal's (variant) angina is a clinical syndrome in which chest pain occurs without the usual precipitating factors and is associated with ST segment elevation rather than depression. It often affects women under 50 years of age. It characteristically occurs in the early morning, awakening patients from sleep, tends to involve the right coronary artery, and is apt to be associated with arrhythmias or conduction defects. There may be no fixed stenoses.

Patients with this pattern of pain or any chest pain syndrome associated with ST segment elevation should undergo coronary arteriography to determine whether fixed stenotic lesions are present. If they are, aggressive medical therapy or revascularization is indicated, since this may represent an unstable phase of the disease. If significant lesions are not seen and spasm is suspected, ergonovine may be administered intravenously to precipitate vasospasm. This must be done cautiously and with nitroglycerin prepared for intracoronary administration, since irreversible spasm may lead to infarction. Episodes respond well to nitrates or calcium channel blockers, and both drugs are effective prophylactically. Beta-blockers have exacerbated coronary vasospasm, but they may have a role in management of patients in whom spasm is associated with fixed stenoses.

There is a growing consensus that myocardial ischemia may also occur in patients with normal coronary arteries as a result of disease of the coronary microcirculation. This has been termed syndrome X.

Cannon RO et al: Imipramine in patients with chest pain despite normal coronary angiograms. N Engl J Med 1994;330:1411. (Symptomatic improvement but mechanism unclear.)

Hollander JE: Management of cocaine-associated myocardial ischemia. N Engl J Med 1995;333:1267.

Keavney B et al: Normal coronary angiograms: Financial victory from the brink of clinical defeat? Heart 1996;75:623. (Patients with recurrent, albeit atypical, chest pain consume a large proportion of clinical resources. Obtaining a normal coronary angiogram can profoundly affect subsequent medical management.)

Lichtlen PR et al: Long-term prognosis of patients with angina-like chest pain and normal coronary angiographic findings. J Am Coll Cardiol 1995;25:103. (No matter how characteristic of ischemia the chest pain may be, morbidity and mortality are similar to those of the overall population.)

Treatment

A. Treatment of Acute Attack: Sublingual nitroglycerin is the drug of choice; it acts in about 1–2 minutes. Nitrates decrease arteriolar and venous tone, reduce preload and afterload, and lower the oxygen demand of the heart. Nitrates may also improve myocardial blood flow by dilating collateral channels and, in the presence of increased vasomotor tone, coronary stenoses. As soon as the attack begins, one fresh tablet is placed under the tongue. This may be repeated at 3- to 5-minute intervals. The dosage (0.3, 0.4, or 0.6 mg) and the number of tablets to be used before seeking further medical attention must be individualized. Nitroglycerin buccal spray is also available as a metered (0.4 mg) delivery system. It has the advantage of being more convenient for patients who have difficulty handling the pills and of being more stable. Nitroglycerin should also be used prophylactically before activities likely to precipitate angina. Pain not responding to three tablets or lasting more than 20 minutes may represent evolving infarction, and the patient should be instructed to seek immediate medical attention.

B. Prevention of Further Attacks:

1. Aggravating factors–Angina may be aggravated by hypertension, left ventricular failure, arrhythmia (usually tachycardias), strenuous activity, cold temperatures, and emotional states. These factors should be identified and treated or avoided where possible.

2. Nitroglycerin–Nitroglycerin, 0.3–0.6 mg sublingually or by spray, should be taken 5 minutes before any activity likely to precipitate angina. Sublingual isosorbide dinitrate (2.5–10 mg) is only slightly longer-acting than sublingual nitroglycerin.

3. Long-acting nitrates–A number of longer-acting nitrate preparations are available. These include isosorbide dinitrate, 10–40 mg orally three times daily; isosorbide mononitrate, 10–40 mg orally twice daily or 60–120 mg once daily in a sustained-release preparation; oral sustained-release nitroglycerin preparations, 6.25–12.5 mg two to four times daily; nitroglycerin ointment, 6.25–25 mg applied two to four times daily; and transdermal nitroglycerin patches that deliver nitroglycerin at a predetermined rate (usually 5–20 mg/24 h). The main limitation to chronic nitrate therapy is tolerance, which occurs to some degree in most patients. The degree of tolerance can be limited by utilizing a regimen which includes a minimum 8- to 10-hour period without nitrates. Isosorbide dinitrate given three times daily, with the last dose after dinner, is the most commonly used approach, but longer-acting isosorbide mononitrate is becoming more popular. Because it is the active metabolite of the dinitrate, isosorbide mononitrate has more consistent bioavailability. Transdermal preparations should be removed overnight in most patients.

Nitrate therapy is often limited by headache. Other side effects include nausea, dizziness, and hypotension.

4. Beta-blockers–Beta-blockers prevent angina by reducing myocardial oxygen requirements during exertion and stress. This is accomplished by reducing the heart rate, myocardial contractility, and, to a lesser extent, blood pressure. The beta-blockers are the only antianginal agents that have been demonstrated to prolong life in patients with coronary disease (post-myocardial infarction). They are at least as effective as alternative agents in studies employing exercise testing, ambulatory monitoring, and symptom assessment. As a result, they should be considered for first-line therapy in most patients with chronic angina.

In the United States, only propranolol, metoprolol, nadolol, and atenolol are approved for angina. Nonetheless, all available beta-blockers appear to be effective for angina, though those with intrinsic sympathomimetic activity, such as pindolol, are less desirable because they may exacerbate angina in some individuals and have not been effective in secondary prevention trials. The pharmacology and side effects of the beta-blockers are discussed in Chapter 11 (Table 11–3). The dosages of all these drugs when given for angina are similar. The major contraindications are bronchospastic disease, bradyarrhythmias, and overt heart failure.

5. Calcium entry blocking agents–Verapamil, diltiazem, and the dihydropyridine group of calcium blockers (of which nifedipine is the prototype) are chemically and pharmacologically heterogeneous agents that prevent angina by reducing myocardial oxygen requirements and by inducing coronary artery vasodilation. Myocardial oxygen demand is lessened by reducing blood pressure, left ventricular wall stress, and, in the case of verapamil and diltiazem, resting or exercise heart rate. Though these agents are all potent coronary vasodilators, it is unclear whether they improve myocardial blood flow in most patients with stable exertional angina. In those with coronary vasospasm, the calcium entry blockers may be the agent of choice.

Most calcium channel blockers have negative inotropic, chronotropic, and dromotropic properties in vitro, but the reflex sympathetic response may obscure these effects in vivo (except in the presence of beta blockade or severely depressed left ventricular function). Unlike the beta-blockers, calcium channel blockers have not reduced mortality postinfarction and in some cases have increased ischemia and mortality rates. This appears to be the case with some dihydropyridines and with diltiazem and verapamil in patients with clinical heart failure or moderate to severe left ventricular dysfunction. A recent meta-analysis suggested that short-acting nifedipine in moderate to high doses causes an increase in mortality in patients early after myocardial infarction or with unstable angina. It is uncertain whether these findings are relevant to longer-acting dihydropyridines, and data with verapamil and diltiazem suggest that these latter agents are safe in postinfarction patients with preserved left ventricular function. Nevertheless, considering the uncertainties and the lack of demonstrated favorable effect on outcomes, calcium blockers should be considered third-line anti-ischemic drugs in the postinfarction patient. Similarly, with the exception of amlodipine, which in the PRAISE trial proved safe in patients with heart failure, these agents should be avoided in patients with congestive heart failure or low ejection fractions.

The pharmacologic effects and side effects of the calcium channel blockers are discussed in Chapter 11 and summarized in Table 11–6. Although all have been shown to be efficacious for angina, not all preparations and agents are approved for this indication. By and large, diltiazem and verapamil are preferable as first-line agents because they produce less reflex tachycardia and because the former, at least, may cause fewer side effects. Nifedipine, nicardipine, and amlodipine are also approved agents for angina. Isradipine, felodipine, and nisoldipine are not approved for angina but probably are as effective as the other dihydropyridines. Bepridil is a unique calcium channel blocker similar to verapamil in its effects on automatic tissues but with additional properties similar to those of quinidine (prolonging ventricular refractoriness and the QT interval). It is not approved for hypertension and should be used only for refractory angina because of its potential to induce ventricular arrhythmias.

6. Alternative and combination therapies– Patients who do not respond to one class of antianginal medication often respond to another. It may, therefore, be worthwhile to use an alternative agent before progressing to combinations. If the patient remains symptomatic, a beta-blocker and a long-acting nitrate or a beta-blocker and a calcium channel blocker (other than verapamil, where the risk of atrioventricular block or heart failure is higher) are the most appropriate combinations. A few patients will have a further response to a regimen including all three agents.

7. Anti-platelet drugs–Coronary thrombosis is responsible for most episodes of myocardial infarction and many unstable ischemic syndromes. Several studies have demonstrated the benefit of anti-platelet drugs following unstable angina and infarction. Therefore, unless contraindicated, small doses of aspirin (162–325 mg daily or 325 mg every other day) should be prescribed for patients with angina.

8. Risk reduction–As discussed previously, patients with coronary disease should undergo aggressive risk factor. This approach, with a particular focus on lowering LDL cholesterol to ≤ 100 mg/dL, not only prevents future events but may markedly improve symptomatic angina.

9. Revascularization–The indications for coronary artery revascularization and the choice of procedure are discussed below.

Prognosis

The prognosis of angina pectoris has improved with advances in the understanding of its pathophysiology and in pharmacologic therapy. Mortality rates vary depending on the number of vessels diseased, the severity of obstruction, the status of left ventricular function, and the presence of complex arrhythmias. In patients with stable symptoms and normal ejection fractions (> 55%, depending on the laboratory), the mortality rate is 1–2% per year. However, the outlook in individual patients is unpredictable, and nearly half of the deaths are sudden. Therefore, risk stratification is often attempted. Patients with accelerating symptoms have a poorer outlook. Among stable patients, those whose exercise tolerance is severely limited by ischemia (less than 6 minutes on the Bruce treadmill protocol) and those with extensive ischemia by exercise electrocardiography or scintigraphy have more severe anatomic disease and a poorer prognosis.

Abrams J: The role of nitrates in coronary heart disease. Arch Intern Med 1995;155:357.

Bergelson BA, Tommaso CL: Left main coronary disease: Assessment, diagnosis, and therapy. Am Heart J 1995;129:350. (Because revascularization improves prognosis in patients with symptomatic left main coronary disease, much effort is spent in detecting these individuals. This article reviews by subject and shows how the available data have been extrapolated to situations that have never been studied.)

Drugs for stable angina pectoris. Med Lett Drugs Ther 1994;36:111.

Furberg CD et al: Nifedipine: Dose-related increase in mortality in patients with coronary heart disease. Circulation 1995;92:1326. (Meta-analysis of 16 randomized secondary prevention trials using short-acting nifedipine suggests an increase in mortality from high doses.)

Goldstein S: Beta-blockers in hypertensive and coronary heart disease. Arch Intern Med 1996;156:1267. (Review of the use of beta-blockers for angina, myocardial infarction, and hypertension.)

Gould KL et al: Changes in myocardial perfusion abnormalities by positron emission tomography after long-term, intense risk factor modification. JAMA 1995; 274:894. (Objective evidence that very aggressive risk factor modification can result in improved myocardial perfusion over and above that obtained by antianginal therapy.)

Rodgers WJ et al: Asymptomatic Cardiac Ischemia Pilot (ACIP) Study: Outcome in 1 year for patients with asymptomatic cardiac ischemia randomized to medical therapy or revascularization. J Am Coll Cardiol 1995; 26:594. (Symptoms and events responded significantly more favorably to coronary revascularization.)

Sabonitto S et al: Combination therapy with metoprolol and nifedipine versus monotherapy in patients with stable angina pectoris. J Am Coll Cardiol 1996;27:311. (Findings suggest that nonresponders to a single agent should be tried on medication of another class before combination therapy is instituted.)

REVASCULARIZATION PROCEDURES FOR PATIENTS WITH ANGINA PECTORIS

Indications

The indications for coronary artery revascularization in patients with angina pectoris are often debated. There is general agreement that otherwise healthy patients in the following groups should undergo revascularization. (1) Patients with unacceptable symptoms despite medical therapy to its tolerable limits. (2) Patients with left main coronary artery stenosis greater than 50% with or without symptoms. (3) Patients with three-vessel disease with left ventricular dysfunction (ejection fraction < 50% or previous transmural infarction). (4) Patients with unstable angina who after symptom control by medical therapy continue to exhibit ischemia on exercise testing or monitoring. (5) Post-myocardial infarction patients with continuing angina or severe ischemia on noninvasive testing. (See sections on Unstable Angina and Myocardial Infarction.)

In addition, many cardiologists feel that patients with less severe symptoms should be revascularized if they have two-vessel disease associated with underlying left ventricular dysfunction, anatomically critical lesions (> 90% proximal stenoses, especially of the proximal left anterior descending artery) or physiologic evidence of severe ischemia (early positive exercise tests, large exercise-induced thallium scintigraphic defects, or frequent episodes of ischemia on ambulatory monitoring). This trend toward aggressive intervention has accelerated as a result of the growing use of coronary angioplasty and stenting. While such patients are at increased risk, it has not been proved that their prognosis is better after coronary revascularization by either surgery or angioplasty.

Type of Procedure

A. Coronary Artery Bypass Grafting (CABG): CABG can be accomplished with a very low mortality rate (1–3%) in otherwise healthy patients with preserved cardiac function. However, the mortality rate of this procedure rises to 4–8% in older individuals and in patients who have had a prior CABG. Increasingly, younger individuals with focal lesions of one or several vessels are undergoing coronary angioplasty as the initial revascularization procedure.

Grafts employing one or both internal mammary arteries (usually to the left anterior descending artery or its branches) provide the best long-term results in terms of patency and flow. Segments of the saphenous vein (or, less optimally, other veins) interposed between the aorta and the coronary arteries distal to the obstructions are also utilized. One to five distal anastomoses are commonly performed. After successful surgery, symptoms generally abate. The need for antianginal medications diminishes, and left ventricular function may improve.

The operative mortality rate is increased in patients with poor left ventricular function (left ventricular ejection fraction < 35%) or those requiring additional procedures (valve replacement or ventricular aneurysmectomy). Patients over 70 years of age, patients undergoing repeat procedures, or those with important noncardiac disease (especially renal insufficiency, diabetes, or poor general health) also have higher operative mortality and morbidity rates, and full recovery is slow. Thus, CABG should be reserved for more severely symptomatic patients in this group. Early (1–6 months) graft patency rates average 85–90% (higher for internal mammary grafts), and subsequent graft closure rates are about 4% annually. Early graft failure is common in vessels with poor distal flow, while late closure is more frequent in patients who continue smoking and those with untreated hyperlipidemia. Antiplatelet therapy with aspirin improves graft patency rates. Long-term dipyridamole therapy is expensive, inconvenient, and of limited value. Smoking cessation and vigorous treatment of blood lipid abnormalities is necessary, with a goal for LDL cholesterol of ≤ 100 mg/dL and of HDL cholesterol ≥ 45 mg/dL. Repeat revascularization (see below) is often necessitated by progressive native vessel disease and graft occlusions. Reoperation is technically demanding and less often fully successful than the initial operation.

B. Percutaneous Transluminal Coronary Angioplasty (PTCA): Coronary artery stenoses can be effectively dilated by inflation of a balloon under high pressure. This procedure is performed in the cardiac catheterization laboratory under local anesthesia either at the same time as diagnostic coronary arteriography or at a later time. The mechanism of dilation is rupture of the atheromatous plaque, with subsequent resorption of intraluminal debris.

This procedure was at one time reserved for proximal single-vessel disease, but now it is widely employed in multivessel disease with multiple lesions, though only rarely in left main disease. PTCA is possible but often less successful in CABG stenoses. Optimal lesions for PTCA are relatively proximal, noneccentric, free of significant calcification or plaque dissection, and removed from the origin of large branches. With improved catheter systems, experienced operators are able to successfully dilate 90% of lesions attempted. The major early complication is intimal dissection with vessel occlusion. This can usually be treated by repeat PTCA or by deployment of an intracoronary stent, but urgent CABG is required in 1–2% of cases. Therefore, these procedures must be done in a laboratory where surgery is available on short notice. The major limitation with PTCA has been restenosis, which occurs in the first 6 months in 30–40% of vessels dilated, though it can often be treated successfully by repeat PTCA.

The incidence of restenosis appears to be reduced with intracoronary stent placement. Initially, placement of these devices carried a small risk of acute thrombosis and therefore required aggressive anticoagulation. However, use of high-pressure balloons and intravascular ultrasound for deployment, followed by aggressive antiplatelet therapy with a combination of aspirin and ticlopidine, has eliminated the need for anticoagulation after the immediate periprocedural period, and the acute thrombosis rate has fallen below 1%. Stents are now used in more than 30% of percutaneous revascularization procedures in the United States, and this proportion is increasing. However, ongoing trials will clarify whether this growing use of stents is justified in terms of outcomes.

In the United States, the number of PTCA procedures now exceeds that of CABG operations, but the justification for many of these is unclear. One controlled study showed PTCA to be superior to medical therapy for symptom relief but not in preventing infarction or death.

Several randomized studies of PTCA versus CABG in patients with multivessel disease have been reported. The consistent finding has been comparable mortality and infarction rates over follow-up periods of 1–3 years but a high rate (approximately 40%) of repeat procedures following PTCA. As a result, the choice of revascularization procedure is often a matter of patient preference. However, it should be noted that less than 20% of patients with multivessel disease met the entry criteria, so these results cannot be generalized to all multivessel disease patients.

C. New Devices for Percutaneous Coronary Interventions: A number of atherectomy devices have been developed to remove plaque from coronary arteries and vein grafts. Directional coronary atherectomy shaves plaque, which is collected in a nose cone and removed. This may be useful in large vessels with eccentric, noncalcified lesions. Rotational atherectomy utilizes a high-speed rotational burr that is effective in calcified stenoses. The transluminal extraction catheter is designed to remove large burdens of plaque, particularly from vein grafts. Excimer laser catheters used laser energy in conjunction with angioplasty to open long stenoses or chronic occlusions. Although none of these newer devices have been shown to be uniformly more successful than PTCA, each has a particular niche where it is effective.

Summary of Results of Treatment

Several randomized trials have shown that over follow-up periods of several years, the mortality and infarction rates with PTCA and CABG are generally comparable. An exception may be diabetic patients, who have had better outcomes with CABG. Recovery after PTCA is obviously faster, but the intermediate-term success rate of CABG is higher, because of the high restenosis with PTCA. The increasing popularity of PTCA primarily reflects its lower cost, shorter hospitalization, the perception that CABG is best done only once and can be reserved for later, and the preference of patients for less invasive treatment. These arguments make PTCA the procedure of choice for revascularization of single-vessel disease, though this is not usually indicated except when symptoms are refractory. The situation is less clear with multivessel disease. It should also be noted that the excellent outcome of patients treated medically has made it difficult to show an advantage with either revascularization approach except in patients who remain symptom-limited or have left main lesions or three-vessel disease and left ventricular dysfunction.

Ached E et al: Stents for intracoronary placement: Current status and future directions. J Am Coll Cardiol 1996;27:757. (Review of the history, types, and indications. Results show lower restenosis rates with this procedure compared with PTCA as well as the low thrombotic rate with newer techniques. Authors argue that stenting should become the standard percutaneous coronary intervention.)

Bittl JA: Advances in coronary angioplasty. N Engl J Med 1996;335:1290. (Review of all the new approaches and current results.)

Bypass Angioplasty Revascularization Investigation

(BARI) Investigators: Comparison of coronary bypass surgery with angioplasty in patients with multivessel disease. N Engl J Med 1996;335:217. (Results of the largest comparative trial, showing no difference in 5-year survival between these procedures except in diabetics, who have improved survival with CABG. As in all such studies, subsequent revascularization was required more often after PTCA. Another article from the same trial [JAMA 1997;277:715] showed that the initial advantage in symptom relief with CABG disappears over time.)

Cameron A et al: Coronary bypass surgery with internal thoracic-artery grafts: Effects on survival after a 15-year period. N Engl J Med 1996;334:219. (Analysis of the 15-year follow-up of patients in the CASS study. Patients who had an internal thoracic artery graft have 27% fewer deaths than those who received only vein grafts.)

Gottsauner-Wolf M et al: Restenosis: An open file. Clin Cardiol 1996;19:347. (Review of mechanisms and ongoing attempts to prevent this problem.)

Hasdai D et al: The effect of smoking status on long-term outcome after successful percutaneous coronary revascularization. N Engl J Med 1997;336:755. (Follow-up of more than 5400 patients showed that persistent smokers had an approximately twofold higher incidence of Q-wave myocardial infarction and death.)

Hillis LD: Coronary bypass surgery: Risks and benefits, realistic and unrealistic expectations. J Invest Med 1995; 43:17.

Nwasokwa ON: Coronary artery bypass graft disease. Ann Intern Med 1995;123:528. (Review of this important problem.)

Pocock SJ et al: Meta-analysis of randomized trials comparing coronary angioplasty with bypass surgery. Lancet 1995;346:1184. (Meta-analysis of 3371 patients participating in eight randomized trials, showing similar event rates with CABG and PTCA. However, PTCA patients had a higher rate of residual angina and required considerably more repeat revascularization procedures. The largest trial, BARI, which has not yet been published and is not included in this meta-analysis, found similar results with the exception that diabetics faired significantly better with CABG.)

The Post Coronary Artery Bypass Graft Trial Investigators: The effect of aggressive lowering of low-density lipoprotein cholesterol levels and low-dose anticoagulation on obstructive changes in saphenous-vein coronary artery bypass grafts. N Engl J Med 1997;336:153. (Aggressive lowering of LDL cholesterol with lovastatin reduced the progression of atherosclerosis in grafts, whereas low-dose warfarin did not.)

Yusuf S et al: Effect of coronary artery bypass graft surgery on survival: Overview of 10 year results from randomized trials by the Coronary Artery Bypass Graft Surgery Trialists Collaboration. Lancet 1994;344:563. (Survival is better with CABG in high- and medium-risk patients; there is a trend toward higher mortality in low-risk patients.)

UNSTABLE ANGINA

Most clinicians use the term "unstable angina" to denote an accelerating or "crescendo" pattern of pain in cases where previously stable angina occurs with less exertion or at rest, lasts longer, and is less responsive to medication. Coronary angioscopy has shown that a high proportion of patients with this pattern of symptoms have "complex" coronary stenoses characterized by plaque rupture, ulceration, or hemorrhage with subsequent thrombus formation. This inherently unstable situation may progress to complete occlusion and infarction or may heal, with reendothelialization and a return to a stable though possibly more severe pattern of ischemia. New-onset angina is sometimes considered unstable, but if it is exertional and responsive to rest and medication, it does not carry the same poor prognosis.

Diagnosis

Most patients with unstable angina will exhibit electrocardiographic changes during pain—commonly ST segment depression or T wave flattening or inversion but sometimes, and more ominously, ST segment elevation. They may exhibit signs of left ventricular dysfunction during pain and for a time thereafter.

Treatment

A. General Measures: Treatment of unstable angina should be multifaceted and vigorous. Patients should be hospitalized, maintained at bed rest or at very limited activity, monitored, and given supplemental oxygen. Sedation with a benzodiazepine agent may help. The systolic blood pressure is usually maintained at 100–120 mm Hg, except in previously severe hypertensives, and the heart rate should be lowered to 60/min.

B. Anticoagulation, Antiplatelet, and Thrombolytic Therapy: Because intravascular thrombosis plays a prominent role in the pathophysiology of unstable angina and its progression to myocardial infarction, antithrombotic therapy is an important part of treatment for unstable angina. Heparin may be more effective than aspirin, but it is likely that the two are additive. Aspirin, 325 mg daily (lower doses may be adequate), should be commenced on admission, and intravenous heparin should be started if symptoms have been recent (past 24 hours) or if they recur. Heparin therapy, when necessary, should be continued for at least 2 days. The administration of monoclonal antibodies to the platelet glycoprotein IIB/IIIA receptor appears to be a useful adjunct in patients with unstable angina, particularly when they are undergoing PTCA or stenting. Low-molecular-weight heparin administered subcutaneously and without monitoring of the PTT appears to be at least as effective as, and more convenient than, intravenous heparin. New thrombin inhibitors such as hirulog and hirudin also appear to be promising but remain investigational at present. Probably because the vessel remains patent and the thrombi are undergoing continuous spontaneous formation and thrombolysis, thrombolytic therapy has had little effect on the outcome of unstable angina.

C. Nitroglycerin: The nitrates are first-line anti-ischemic therapy for unstable angina. Nonparenteral therapy with sublingual or oral agents or nitroglycerin ointment is usually sufficient. If pain persists or recurs, intravenous nitroglycerin should be started. The usual initial dosage is 10 µg/min. The dosage should be titrated to 1 µg/kg/min over 30–60 minutes and further increased as tolerated if pain recurs. Dosages up to 10 µg/kg/min or higher may be used. Tolerance to continuous nitrate infusion is common. Careful—usually continuous—blood pressure monitoring is required when intravenous nitroglycerin is used.

D. Beta-Blockers: These agents are also a part of the initial treatment of unstable angina unless otherwise contraindicated. If the patient has no history or physical findings of heart failure, these agents can usually be started without measurements of left ventricular function. Patients with evidence of large or multiple old infarctions are an exception. The pharmacology of these agents is discussed in Chapter 11 and summarized in Table 11–3. Use of agents with intrinsic sympathomimetic activity should be avoided in this setting. The goal of acute treatment is to reduce the heart rate below 60–70/min. Oral medication is adequate in most patients, but intravenous treatment with metoprolol, given as three 5 mg doses, or with esmolol (500 µg/kg followed by 50–200 µg/kg/min), is needed in patients with hemodynamic instability. Oral therapy should be aggressively titrated as blood pressure permits.

E. Calcium Entry Blockers: Calcium blockers have not been shown to favorably affect outcome in unstable angina, and they should be used primarily as third-line therapy in patients with continuing symptoms on nitrates and beta-blockers or those who are not candidates for these drugs. In the presence of nitrates and without accompanying beta-blockers, diltiazem or verapamil is preferred, since nifedipine and the other dihydropyridines are more likely to cause reflex tachycardia or hypotension. The initial dosage should be low, but upward titration should proceed rapidly.

F. Intra-aortic Balloon Counterpulsation (IABC): IABC can both reduce myocardial energy requirements (systolic unloading) and improve diastolic coronary blood flow. This approach is sometimes employed to stabilize patients prior to angiography or revascularization, but with modern techniques it is rarely necessary.

Prognosis & Indications for Revascularization

Over 90% of patients can be rendered pain-free with these measures. Patients who do not become ischemia-free on medical therapy should have early coronary arteriography and revascularization. Controlled trials have not shown any advantage in increased survival or lower infarction rates with CABG or PTCA compared to medical therapy, although many patients treated medically will need revascularization later for recurrent symptoms. Depending on the stringency of the definition of unstable angina, 10–30% of patients will have an early infarction, and the 1-year mortality rate is 10–20%. Elevated troponin T concentrations and "silent" ST segment shifts have both identified patients at higher risk for subsequent myocardial infarction or recurrence of severe ischemia.

Because recurrent episodes, infarction, and sudden death may occur following relief of unstable angina, additional evaluations should be performed in patients who have been stabilized, consisting of either (1) early exercise or pharmacologic stress testing to identify high-risk subsets for further invasive evaluation, or (2) coronary arteriography. The choice of approach should be individualized based on the patient's age and general health as well as the severity of symptoms and signs of ischemia. The artery responsible for the ischemia can usually be determined from electrocardiographic or scintigraphic changes during pain, and the lesion is often amenable to PTCA. If revascularization is not performed, long-term management is the same as that outlined for stable angina pectoris.

[AHCPR guideline on unstable angina]
  http://text.nlm.nih.gov/ftrs/gateway

Anderson HB et al: One-year results of the thrombolysis in myocardial infarction (TIMI) IIIB. J Am Coll Cardiol 1995;26:1643. (Large trial [1473 patients] evaluating the efficacy of t-PA versus placebo and early catheterization versus catheterization only for symptoms. t-PA was ineffective in this trial, as it has been in previous studies of unstable angina and non-Q wave myocardial infarction. The aggressive and conservative strategies produced similar outcomes.)

Braunwald E et al: Diagnosing and managing unstable angina. Circulation 1994;90:613. (Abbreviated version of AHCPR guidelines.)

Califf RM: Acute ischemic syndromes. Med Clin North Am 1995;79:999. (Reviews pathophysiology and treatment.)

Lefkovits J et al: Platelet glycoprotein IIb/IIIa receptors in cardiovascular medicine. N Engl J Med 1995;332:1553. (Reviews the role of this receptor in thrombosis and the growing evidence showing that inhibitors of this receptor are powerful adjuncts in managing unstable ischemic syndromes. Two large trials, EPILOG and CAPTURE, with monoclonal antibodies to this receptor were recently discontinued early because of the significant benefits.)

Lindahall B et al: Relation between troponin T and the risk of subsequent cardiac events in unstable coronary artery disease. Circulation 1996;93:1651. (Elevated troponin T provides a significant and independent marker of risk for subsequent infarction or cardiac death. "Mild" elevations of other cardiac enzymes also identify patients at higher risk.)

Low-molecular-weight heparin during instability in coronary artery disease. Lancet 1996;347:561. (Subcutaneously administered low-molecular-weight heparin significantly reduced the composite end point of death and myocardial infarction compared with placebo. Other studies suggest that low-molecular-weight heparin is at least as effective as intravenous heparin.)

Oler A et al: Adding heparin to aspirin reduces the incidence of myocardial infarction and death in patients with unstable angina: A meta-analysis. JAMA 1996; 276:811. (A meta-analysis of six randomized trials demonstrates a 33% lower risk of myocardial infarction or death in patients with unstable angina treated with heparin in conjunction with aspirin compared with aspirin alone.)

Riberio PA, Shah PM: Unstable angina: New insights into pathophysiological characteristics, prognosis, and management strategies. Curr Probl Cardiol 1996;21:669.

ACUTE MYOCARDIAL INFARCTION

Essentials of Diagnosis

- Sudden but not instantaneous development of prolonged (> 30 minutes) anterior chest discomfort (sometimes felt as "gas") that may produce arrhythmias, hypotension, shock, or cardiac failure.
- Rarely painless, masquerading as acute congestive heart failure, syncope, cerebral vascular accident, or "unexplained" shock.
- Electrocardiography: ST segment elevation or depression, evolving Q waves, symmetric inversion of T waves.
- Elevation of cardiac enzymes (CK-MB, troponin T, or troponin I).
- Appearance of segmental wall motion abnormality by imaging techniques.

General Considerations

Myocardial infarction results from prolonged myocardial ischemia, precipitated in most cases by an occlusive coronary thrombus at the site of a preexisting (though not necessarily severe) atherosclerotic plaque. More rarely, infarction may result from prolonged vasospasm, inadequate myocardial blood flow (eg, hypotension), or excessive metabolic demand. Very rarely, myocardial infarction may be caused by embolic occlusion, vasculitis, aortic root or coronary artery dissection, or aortitis. Cocaine is a cause of infarction, which should be considered in young individuals without risk factors.

The location and extent of infarction depend upon the anatomic distribution of the occluded vessel, the presence of additional stenotic lesions, and the adequacy of collateral circulation. Thrombosis in the anterior descending branch of the left coronary artery results in infarction of the anterior left ventricle and interventricular septum. Occlusion of the left circumflex artery produces anterolateral or posterolateral infarction. Right coronary thrombosis leads to infarction of the posteroinferior portion of the left ventricle and may involve the right ventricular myocardium and interventricular septum. The arteries supplying the atrioventricular node and the sinus node more commonly arise from the right coronary; thus, atrioventricular block at the nodal level and sinus node dysfunction occur more frequently during inferior infarctions. However, because there are great individual variations in coronary anatomy and because associated lesions and collaterals may confuse the picture, prediction of coronary anatomy from the infarct location may be inaccurate.

Infarctions are often classified as transmural, if the classic electrocardiographic evolution of ST segment elevation to Q waves was observed; or nontransmural or subendocardial, if pain, enzyme elevations, and ST–T wave changes occurred in the absence of new Q waves. However, on pathologic examination, most infarctions involve the subendocardium predominantly, and some transmural extension is common even in the absence of Q waves. Thus, the better classification is Q wave versus non-Q wave infarction. The latter generally results from incomplete occlusion or spontaneous lysis of the thrombus and often signifies the presence of additional jeopardized myocardium; it is associated with a higher incidence of reinfarction and recurrent ischemia.

The size and anatomic location of the infarction determine the acute clinical picture, the early complications, and the long-term prognosis. The hemodynamic findings are related directly to the extent of necrosis (together with the amount of damage from previous infarctions). In small infarctions, cardiac function is normal, whereas with more extensive damage, early heart failure and hypotension (cardiogenic shock) may appear. Additional myocardium beyond that initially infarcted is often threatened, being maintained by collateral circulation or by blood flow through a partially recanalized vessel. Thus, preventing extension of the infarct is one of the major goals of early management. The complications of acute infarction are discussed below.

Alpert JS: Myocardial infarction with angiographically normal coronary arteries. Arch Intern Med 1994;154:265. (A continuing mystery in a few percent of patients. Prognosis generally better.)

Giroud D et al: Relation of the site of myocardial infarction to the most severe coronary arterial stenosis at prior angiography. Am J Cardiol 1992;69:729. (Another in a series of articles showing that acute myocardial infarctions are often caused by thrombosis at the site of a noncritical coronary stenosis.)

Hollander KE et al: Cocaine-associated myocardial infarction: Mortality and complications. Arch Intern Med 1995;155:1081. (Retrospective review of 130 patients in 29 hospitals. Most were non-Q wave, and all patients survived.)

Mittleman MA: Triggering of acute myocardial infarction by heavy physical exertion. N Engl J Med 1993; 329:1677. (Heavy exertion actually does precipitate acute myocardial infarctions, though chronic exertion may be protective.)

Muller JE et al: Triggering myocardial infarction by sexual activity: Low absolute risk and prevention by regular physical exertion. JAMA 1996;275:1405.

Reeder GS, Gersh BJ: Modern management of acute myocardial infarction. Curr Probl Cardiol 1996;21:585.

Ryan TJ et al: ACC/AHA guidelines for the management of patients with acute myocardial infarction. A report of the American College of Cardiology/American Heart Association Task Force on Practice Guidelines (Committee on Management of Acute Myocardial Infarction). J Am Coll Cardiol 1996;28:1328. (All aspects of diagnosis, acute management, and postinfarction care.)

Sigurdsson E et al: Unrecognized myocardial infarction: Epidemiology, clinical characteristics, and the prognostic role of angina pectoris. Ann Intern Med 1995;122:96. (One-third of myocardial infarctions not recognized.)

Clinical Findings

A. Symptoms:

1. Premonitory pain–One-third of patients give a history of alteration in the pattern of angina, recent onset of typical or atypical angina, or unusual "indigestion" felt in the chest.

2. Pain of infarction–Most infarctions occur at rest unlike anginal episodes, and more commonly in the early morning. The pain is similar to angina in location and radiation but is more severe, and it builds up rapidly or in waves to maximum intensity over a few minutes or longer. Nitroglycerin has little effect; even narcotics may not relieve the pain.

3. Associated symptoms–Patients may break out in a cold sweat, feel weak and apprehensive, and move about, seeking a position of comfort. They prefer not to lie quietly. Light-headedness, syncope, dyspnea, orthopnea, cough, wheezing, nausea and vomiting, or abdominal bloating may be present singly or in any combination.

4. Painless infarction–In a minority of cases, pain is absent or minor and is overshadowed by the immediate complications. As many as 25% of infarctions are detected on routine ECG without there having been any recallable acute episode.

5. Sudden death and early arrhythmias–Approximately 20% of patients with acute infarction will die before reaching the hospital; these deaths are usually in the first hour and are chiefly due to ventricular fibrillation.

B. Signs:

1. General–Patients usually appear anxious and are often sweating profusely. The heart rate may range from marked bradycardia (most commonly in inferior infarction) to tachycardia resulting from increased sympathetic nervous system activity, low cardiac output, or arrhythmia. The blood pressure may be high, especially in former hypertensives, or low in patients with shock. Respiratory distress usually indicates heart failure. Fever, usually low-grade, may appear after 12 hours and persist for several days.

2. Chest–Clear lung fields are a good prognostic sign, but basilar rales are common and do not necessarily indicate heart failure. More extensive rales or diffuse wheezing suggests pulmonary edema.

3. Heart–The cardiac examination may be unimpressive or very abnormal. An abnormally located ventricular impulse often represents the dyskinetic infarcted region. Jugular venous distention reflects right atrial hypertension, which may indicate right ventricular infarction or elevated left ventricular filling pressures. The absence of elevated central venous pressure, however, does not indicate normal left atrial or left ventricular diastolic pressures. Soft heart sounds may indicate left ventricular dysfunction. Atrial gallops (S_4) are the rule, whereas ventricular gallops (S_3) are less common and indicate significant left ventricular dysfunction. Mitral regurgitation murmurs are not uncommon and usually indicate papillary muscle dysfunction or, rarely, rupture. Pericardial friction rubs are uncommon in the first 24 hours but may appear later.

4. Extremities–Edema is usually not present. Cyanosis and cold temperature indicate low output. The peripheral pulses should be noted, since later shock or emboli may alter the examination.

C. Laboratory Findings:
Leukocytosis of 10,000–20,000/μL often develops on the second day and disappears within a week. The most valuable diagnostic test is serial measurement of cardiac enzymes. A number of new assays have been developed, including quantitative determinations of CK-MB, troponin T, and troponin I. These are all quite specific for cardiac necrosis, though they may be elevated following severe ischemic episodes and with skeletal muscle damage. CK-MB isoforms may be positive within 6 hours after symptom onset, permitting better triage of patients with uncertain diagnoses. Circulating levels of troponin T and troponin I are more specific and remain elevated for 5–7 days or longer postinfarction. These should obviate the use of less specific LDH isoenzyme assays.

D. Electrocardiography:
Most patients with acute infarction have ECG changes, and a normal tracing is rare. The extent of the electrocardiographic abnormalities provides only a crude estimate of the magnitude of infarction. The classic evolution of changes is from peaked ("hyperacute") T waves, to ST segment elevation, to Q wave development, to T wave inversion. This may occur over a few hours to several days. The evolution of new Q waves (> 30 ms in duration and 25% of the R wave amplitude) is diagnostic, but Q waves do not occur in 30–50% of acute infarctions (subendocardial or non-Q wave infarctions). If these patients have an appropriate clinical presentation, characteristic cardiac enzymes, and

ST segment changes (usually depression) or T wave inversion lasting at least 48 hours, they are classified as having non-Q wave infarctions.

E. Chest X-Ray: The chest x-ray may demonstrate signs of congestive heart failure, but these changes often lag behind the clinical findings. Signs of aortic dissection should be sought as a possible alternative diagnosis.

F. Echocardiography: Echocardiography provides convenient bedside assessment of left ventricular global and regional function. This can help with the diagnosis and management of infarction; echocardiography has been used successfully to make judgments about admission and management of patients with suspected infarction, since normal wall motion makes an infarction unlikely. Doppler echocardiography is probably the most convenient procedure for diagnosing postinfarction mitral regurgitation or ventricular septal defect.

G. Scintigraphic Studies: Technetium-99m pyrophosphate scintigraphy can be used to diagnose acute myocardial infarction. When injected at least 18 hours postinfarction, the radiotracer complexes with calcium in necrotic myocardium to provide a "hot spot" image of the infarction. This test is insensitive to small infarctions, and false-positive studies occur, so its use is limited to patients in whom the diagnosis by electrocardiography and enzymes is not possible—principally those who present several days after the event or have intraoperative infarctions. Radiolabeled antimyosin antibody fragments are more sensitive and specific imaging agents, but scintigraphy must be performed 24 and 48 hours postinjection, so this test has limited clinical utility in the diagnosis of acute myocardial infarction.

Scintigraphy with thallium-201 or the newer technetium-based perfusion tracers will demonstrate "cold spots" in regions of diminished perfusion, which usually represent infarction when the radio-tracer is administered at rest, but abnormalities do not distinguish recent from old damage.

Radionuclide angiography demonstrates akinesis or dyskinesis in areas of infarction and also measures ejection fraction, which can be valuable. Right ventricular dysfunction may indicate infarction of this chamber.

H. Hemodynamic Measurements: These can be invaluable in managing the complicated patient. Their use is described below and in Table 10–6.

Goldman L et al: Prediction of the need for intensive care in patients who come to the emergency departments with acute chest pain. N Engl J Med 1996;334:1498. (Electrocardiographic changes, low systolic blood pressure, rales, and prior known ischemic heart disease predicted subsequent complications.)

Ohman EM et al: Cardiac troponin T levels for risk stratification in acute myocardial infarction. N Engl J Med 1996;335:1333. (This measurement provides an additional risk stratification when combined with standard measures such as the ECG and creatine kinase levels.)

Schweitzer P: The electrocardiographic diagnosis of acute myocardial infarction in the thrombolytic era. Am Heart J 1990;119:642. (Review emphasizing limitations.)

Treatment

A. Thrombolytic Therapy: Thrombolytic therapy reduces mortality and limits infarct size. The greatest benefit occurs if treatment is initiated within the first 1–3 hours, when a 50% or greater reduction in mortality rate can be achieved. The magnitude of benefit declines rapidly thereafter, but a 10% mortality reduction can be achieved up to 12 hours after the onset of pain. The benefit is greatest in patients with potentially large infarcts, ie, those with anterior or multifocal electrocardiographic changes, but also occurs with inferior infarctions, which have a relatively good prognosis in any case. Patients with non-Q wave infarctions generally have incomplete or par-

Table 10–6. Hemodynamic subsets in acute myocardial infarction.

Category	CO or SWI	PCWP	Treatment	Comment
Normal	>2.2, >30	<15	None	Mortality rate <5%.
Hyperdynamic	>3.0, >40	<15	Beta-blockers	Characterized by tachycardia; mortality rate <5%.
Hypovolemic	<2.5, <30	<10	Volume expansion	Hypotension, tachycardia, but preserved left ventricular function by echocardiography; mortality rate 4–8%.
Left ventricular failure	<2.2, <30	>15	Diuretics	Mild dyspnea, rales, normal blood pressure; mortality rate 10–20%.
Severe failure	<2.0, <20	>20	Diuretics, vasodilators	Pulmonary edema, mild hypotension; inotropic agents, IABC may be required; mortality rate 20–40%.
Shock	<1.8, <30	>18	Inotropic agents, IABC	IABC early unless rapid reversal; mortality rate >60%.

CI = cardiac index (L/min/m^2); SWI = stroke work index (g-m/m^2, calculated as [mean arterial pressure – PCWP] × stroke volume index × 0.0136); PCWP = pulmonary capillary wedge pressure (in mm Hg; pulmonary artery diastolic pressure may be used instead); IABC = intra-aortic balloon counterpulsation.

tially recanalized occlusions and have not benefited as consistently from thrombolysis; thrombolytic therapy has not improved the prognosis of patients with prior CABG. Serious bleeding complications occur in 0.5–5% of patients. Contraindications include known bleeding diatheses, a history of any cerebrovascular disease, uncontrolled hypertension (> 190/110 mm Hg), pregnancy, and recent trauma or surgery of the head or spine. Relative contraindications include recent major thoracoabdominal surgery or biopsies, gastrointestinal or genitourinary bleeding, diabetic retinopathy, current oral anticoagulant therapy, prolonged cardiopulmonary resuscitation, and noncompressible puncture sites. Older patients have a higher complication rate but also a potentially greater benefit, since they have a much higher hospital mortality rate.

Therefore, the current recommendation is to administer thrombolytic therapy to patients up to age 80—or even older if the benefit-to-risk ratio seems favorable—with ST elevation or Q waves who present within 6–12 hours after onset of pain unless otherwise contraindicated. Adjunctive aspirin causes a further reduction in mortality rate and should there-

fore be administered concomitantly. Therapy can be initiated in the emergency room or ambulance if personnel are appropriately trained and equipped.

Prior to initiating thrombolytic therapy, a large-bore peripheral intravenous line should be established and not removed until 6 hours after the thrombolytic agent is discontinued. Arterial punctures and other invasive procedures should be avoided if possible. Samples should be drawn for baseline coagulation tests (prothrombin time, partial thromboplastin time, fibrinogen level, and platelet count), blood typing, and other blood tests. Automated blood pressure monitoring (preferably noninvasive) should be instituted.

Four thrombolytic agents have been evaluated extensively in acute infarction and are characterized in Table 10–7.

Recombinant tissue plasminogen activator (t-PA) is a naturally occurring thrombolytic factor that is theoretically thrombus-specific. However, bleeding complications have not been less frequent with t-PA, even though fibrinogen levels are better maintained, and hemorrhagic strokes appear to be more frequent. In patients over age 70 or with ele-

Table 10–7. Thrombolytic therapy for acute myocardial infarction.

	Streptokinase	Tissue Plasminogen Activator (t-PA)	Reteplase	Anistreplase (APSAC)
Source	Group C *Streptococcus*	Recombinant DNA	Recombinant DNA	Group C *Streptococcus*
$T_{1/2}$	20 minutes	5 minutes	15 minutes	90 minutes
Usual dose	1.5 million units	100 mg	20 units	30 units
Administration	750,000 units over 20 minutes followed by 750,000 units over 40 minutes	Initial bolus of 15 mg, followed by 50 mg infused over next 30 minutes and 35 mg over the following 60 minutes[1]	10 units as a bolus over 2 minutes, repeated after 30 minutes	Infuse over 2–5 minutes
Anticoagulation after infusion	Aspirin, 325 mg daily. There is no evidence that adjunctive heparin improves outcome following streptokinase.	Aspirin, 325 mg daily. Heparin, 5000 units as bolus, followed by 1000 units per hour infusion, subsequently adjusted to maintain PTT 1½–2 times control.	Aspirin, 325 mg; heparin as with t-PA	Aspirin, 325 mg daily
Clot selectivity	Low	High	High	Moderate
Fibrinogenolysis	+++	+	+	+
Bleeding	+	+[2]	+	+
Hypotension	+++	+	+	+
Allergic reactions	++	0	0	+
Reocclusion	5–20%	10–30%	—	5–20%
Approximate cost[1]	$412.00	$2750.00	$2750.00	$2368.00

[1]Recent studies employing "front-loaded" t-PA (such as the administration of an initial bolus of 15 mg, 50 mg over the next 30 minutes, and 35 mg over the next 60 minutes) have shown higher early patency rates and a modest improvement in 30-day survival compared with streptokinase, especially in younger patients with large anterior infarctions who present within 4 hours after onset of chest pain.
[2]t-PA causes a higher incidence of cerebral hemorrhage than streptokinase when the latter is given with subcutaneous heparin.
[3]Cost for usual doses listed above.

vated blood pressure, the rate of intracranial hemorrhage rises substantially, and t-PA should be avoided in these patients. t-PA produces faster reperfusion, especially when given in the first 4 hours. A regimen consisting of an initial bolus of 15 mg, 50 mg over the next 30 minutes, and 35 mg over the following 60 minutes, achieves higher early patency rates than previous dosing schedules. Reocclusion rates are higher with t-PA because of its shorter half-life, so intravenous heparin is recommended for at least 24 hours. **Reteplase** is a closely related thrombolytic agent made by recombinant technology that has been very effective in restoring patency of the infarct-related artery. Administration of reteplase is convenient—two 10-unit boluses are given 30 minutes apart, with adjunctive aspirin and heparin therapy. A large trial comparing outcomes with t-PA has shown that these agents are comparable.

Streptokinase is more likely to produce allergic reactions, including fever, chills, rashes, and anaphylaxis. This agent should be avoided if the patient has received it previously. Streptokinase also has a tendency to produce severe hypotension and therefore must be administered slowly. Hypotension should be treated by slowing or interrupting the infusion, placing the patient in the Trendelenburg position, and administering fluids. Unlike the experience with t-PA, there is no clear evidence that adjunctive heparin is beneficial in patients given streptokinase.

Anisoylated plasminogen streptokinase activator complex (anistreplase; APSAC) is a conjugate of streptokinase that is inactive until the anisoyl group is hydrolyzed, which occurs gradually after injection (half-time, 90 minutes). The drug is concentrated at the site of the thrombus and is activated locally. Thus, it can be injected as a bolus but will provide continuing thrombolytic activity. This makes APSAC a convenient agent to administer out of the hospital or in a busy emergency room. Otherwise, it has many of the same features of streptokinase, including the potential to produce allergic reactions and hypotension, but it is far more expensive.

Urokinase has not been specifically approved for acute myocardial infarction, but small studies have demonstrated that it induces coronary thrombolysis.

Selection of a thrombolytic agent: Although there is much debate over which agent to utilize, the overriding consideration is the early administration of any one of them. Three large international studies have compared the results with different thrombolytic therapies. The ISIS-3 trial compared three agents (t-PA, streptokinase, and anistreplase) in over 40,000 patients. No difference in mortality rates was observed between treatments, though cerebral hemorrhage was more common with t-PA. GISSI-2 compared the first two of these agents and also failed to show a difference. The GUSTO trial was the only one to use adjunctive intravenous heparin and also employed the accelerated regimen noted above for t-PA. Compared with streptokinase, t-PA produced a small improvement (one case per 100 patients treated) in 30-day and 6-month survival. Reteplase appears to have a similar modest advantage over streptokinase. Since t-PA and reteplase are significantly more expensive than streptokinase, and since intracranial hemorrhage is more frequent with these agents (especially in patients over age 70 and those with hypertension), and since the additional reduction in mortality is relatively small, many physicians limit the use of t-PA—and, by extension, reteplase—to patients in whom the greatest absolute benefits have been noted. These include patients under 70 years of age with anterior myocardial infarctions treated within 4 hours after onset and patients who show evidence of pump failure. Patients who have had streptokinase or APSAC within the past year or recent streptococcal infections and those with borderline blood pressure (systolic pressure < 100 mm Hg) are also better candidates for t-PA, while older patients, especially those with concomitant hypertension (systolic pressure $\geq$ 160 mm Hg) may be better candidates for streptokinase. The only apparent advantage of APSAC is convenience.

Postthrombolytic management: After completion of the thrombolytic infusion, aspirin should be continued. Anticoagulation with intravenous heparin is continued for at least 24 hours after t-PA and reteplase but is optional in patients receiving streptokinase. Prophylactic treatment with antacids and an H_2 blocker is indicated.

Reperfusion rates of 50–80% can be expected, determined primarily by the interval between onset of the infarction and treatment. Reperfusion is recognized clinically by the abrupt cessation of pain, ventricular arrhythmias (most characteristically accelerated idioventricular rhythm), rapid evolution of the ECG to Q waves, and an early peak of CK (by 12 hours); however, all of these signs may be misleading. Even with anticoagulation, 10–20% of reperfused vessels will reocclude during hospitalization. This is usually recognized by the recurrence of pain and ST segment elevation and is treated by readministration of a thrombolytic agent or immediate angiography and PTCA.

The optimal management of myocardial infarction after thrombolysis is controversial but has been clarified considerably by the TIMI 2 trial. Patients with recurrent ischemic pain prior to discharge should undergo catheterization and, if indicated, revascularization. Asymptomatic, clinically stable patients should undergo predischarge evaluation to determine whether residual jeopardized myocardium is present. This can be accomplished by exercise or pharmacologic stress scintigraphy. Those with significantly positive tests or a low threshold for symptomatic ischemia should undergo angiography and revascularization where feasible. Patients with negative tests have an excellent prognosis without intervention, though they may require revascularization for symptoms at a later time.

B. Acute PTCA: A number of centers now manage acute myocardial infarction with primary PTCA (immediate angiography and PTCA of the "infarct-related" vessel), rather than thrombolysis. The results of this approach in specialized centers are excellent, exceeding those obtainable by thrombolytic therapy, but the experience may not be generalizable to centers with less experience or expertise. The use of stents in treating acute myocardial infarction is also under investigation. In the subgroup of patients with cardiogenic shock, early catheterization and PTCA or CABG is the preferred management, because thrombolysis has not improved the dismal prognosis of these individuals.

C. General Measures: CCU monitoring should be instituted as soon as possible. Uncomplicated patients can be transferred to less intensively monitored settings after 24–48 hours. Activity should initially be limited to bed rest, with the availability of a nearby toilet or commode in more stable patients. Progressive ambulation should be started after 24–72 hours if tolerated. Low-flow oxygen therapy (2–4 L/min) is usually given. A liquid diet is recommended during the initial 24 hours.

D. Analgesia: An initial attempt should be made to relieve pain with sublingual nitroglycerin. However, if no response occurs after two or three tablets, intravenous opiates provide the most rapid and effective analgesia. Morphine sulfate, 4–8 mg, or meperidine, 50–75 mg, should be given. Subsequent small doses can be given every 15 minutes until pain abates.

E. Beta-Adrenergic Blocking Agents: Several studies have shown modestly improved short-term survival when intravenous beta-blockers are given immediately after acute myocardial infarction. These agents reduce the duration of ischemic pain and the incidence of ventricular fibrillation. A favorable effect appears to persist even after thrombolytic therapy. However, the survival benefit is small, so beta-blockers should not be given to patients with relative contraindications. Long-term beta-blocker therapy is discussed below.

F. Nitrates: Nitroglycerin is the agent of choice for recurrent ischemic pain and is useful in lowering blood pressure or relieving pulmonary congestion. However, routine nitrate administration is not recommended, since no improvement in outcome has been observed in the ISIS-4 or GISSI-3 trials, in which a total of over 70,000 patients were randomized to nitrate treatment or placebo.

G. Angiotensin-Converting Enzyme (ACE) Inhibitors: A series of trials (SAVE, AIRE, SMILE, TRACE, GISSI-III, and ISIS-IV) have shown both short- and long-term improvement in survival with ACE inhibitor therapy. The benefits are greatest in patients with low ejection fractions, large infarctions, or clinical evidence of heart failure, and only these patients should receive chronic ACE inhibitor therapy for postinfarction indications. Acute short-term treatment may improve survival in a broader group of patients, but this is uncertain. Treatment should be commenced carefully in the first postinfarction day if the patient is not hypotensive. When there is no evidence of heart failure or when a very large infarction is not present, ACE inhibitors should be considered only after the administration of thrombolytic therapy, aspirin, beta-blockers, and, if the patient has evidence of continuing ischemia, nitrates.

H. Antiarrhythmic Prophylaxis: The incidence of ventricular fibrillation in hospitalized patients is approximately 5%, with 80% of episodes occurring in the first 12–24 hours. Prophylactic lidocaine infusions (1–2 mg/min) prevent most episodes, but this therapy has not reduced the mortality rate and it increases the risk of asystole, so this approach is no longer recommended except in patients with very frequent ectopic beats or nonsustained ventricular tachycardia. Intravenous magnesium sulfate has been effective in one study, but ISIS-4 did not report a benefit with routine magnesium administration.

I. Calcium Channel Blockers: There are no studies to support the use of calcium channel blockers in most acute myocardial infarction patients—and indeed, they have the potential to exacerbate ischemia and cause death from reflex tachycardia or myocardial depression. One exception is that diltiazem and verapamil appear to prevent reinfarction and ischemia in the subset of patients with non-Q wave infarction. The former agent is preferable because it causes less myocardial depression. The dosage is 240–360 mg daily. Otherwise, calcium channel blockers should be reserved for management of hypertension or ischemia as second- or third-line drugs after nitrates and beta-blockers.

J. Anticoagulation: With the exception of patients undergoing thrombolysis and subsequent heparin therapy, the use of full anticoagulation in the acute setting remains controversial. Patients who will be at bed rest or on limited activity status for some time should be given 5000 units of heparin subcutaneously every 8–12 hours unless contraindicated. Aspirin, 325 mg daily, should be given also unless contraindicated.

Aylward PE et al: Relation of increased arterial blood pressure to mortality and stroke in the context of contemporary thrombolytic therapy for acute myocardial infarction: A randomized trial. Ann Intern Med 1996;125:891. (Patients with systolic blood pressures greater than 175 mm Hg have a high rate [3.4%] of stroke. Thrombolysis in such individuals may not be a useful option among those with a low risk of cardiac death, no infarction, and no evidence of hemodynamic instability.)

Cairns JS et al: Coronary thrombolysis. Chest 1995; 108:401S. (History, review of major trials, analysis of subgroups and adjunct therapy, complications, and recommendations.)

Collins R et al: Aspirin, heparin, and fibrinolytic therapy in suspected acute myocardial infarction. N Engl J Med 1997;336:847. (Review arguing for wider use of these therapies.)

Every NR et al: A comparison of thrombolytic therapy with primary coronary angioplasty for acute myocardial infarction. N Engl J Med 1996;335:1253. (In a community setting, there was no difference in mortality when PTCA was compared with thrombolysis.)

Hennekens CH et al: Adjunctive drug therapy of acute myocardial infarction—evidence from clinical trials. N Engl J Med 1996;335:1660. (Extensive review of data supporting the use of a variety of pharmacologic agents after myocardial infarction.)

Kim CB, Braunwald E: Potential benefits of late reperfusion of infarcted myocardium: The open artery hypothesis. Circulation 1993;88:2426. (Provocative perspective suggesting long-term benefit from the maintenance of patent coronary artery.)

Sweeney JP, Schwartz GG: Impact of the result of large clinical trials in the management of acute myocardial infarction. West J Med 1996;164:238. (Excellent review encompassing acute and postdischarge management.)

Complications

Most patients have one or more complications of myocardial infarction, though the response to treatment is usually prompt.

A. Infarct Extension and Postinfarction Ischemia: Recurrent infarction in the region of infarction (infarct extension) in the first 10–14 days occurs in approximately 10% of patients. It may be associated with prolonged or intermittent episodes of chest pain. In many cases, the process is relatively silent, being detected on routine ECG, by laboratory testing, or by onset or worsening of heart failure. Infarct extension is at least twice as common in non-Q wave infarcts and is more likely to occur after successful thrombolytic therapy owing to residual jeopardized myocardium. Diltiazem, 60–90 mg four times daily, has been shown to reduce the rate of extension following non-Q wave infarction.

Approximately 30% of patients will have anginal episodes postinfarction. These are more common in patients with angina prior to infarction and in non-Q wave infarction. Postinfarction angina is associated with increased short- and long-term mortality rates. The underlying mechanism is usually inadequate blood flow through a recanalized vessel or reocclusion. Vigorous medical therapy should be instituted, including nitrates, beta-blockers, and calcium blockers (as a third anti-ischemic agent), as well as aspirin and heparin. Most patients with postinfarction angina—and all who are refractory to medical therapy—should undergo early catheterization and revascularization by PTCA or CABG.

B. Arrhythmias: Abnormalities of rhythm and conduction are common.

1. Sinus bradycardia—This is most common in inferior infarctions or may be precipitated by medications. Observation or withdrawal of the offending agent is usually sufficient. If accompanied by signs of low cardiac output, atropine, 0.5–1 mg intravenously, is usually effective. Temporary pacing is rarely required.

2. Supraventricular tachyarrhythmias—Sinus tachycardia is common and may reflect either increased adrenergic stimulation or hemodynamic compromise due to hypovolemia or pump failure. In the latter, beta blockade is contraindicated. Supraventricular premature beats are common and may be premonitory for atrial fibrillation. Electrolyte abnormalities and hypoxia should be corrected and causative agents (especially aminophylline) stopped. Atrial fibrillation should be rapidly controlled or converted to sinus rhythm. Intravenous diltiazem (0.25 mg/kg over 2 minutes, followed by an infusion of 5–15 mg/h), verapamil (given cautiously in 2- to 5-mg increments up to 20 mg), or the short-acting beta-blocker esmolol (500 µg/kg, followed by 50–200 µg/kg/min) are the agents of choice if cardiac function is adequate. Digoxin (0.5 mg as initial dose, then 0.25 mg every 90–120 minutes [up to 1–1.25 mg] for a loading dose, followed by 0.25 mg daily if renal function is normal) is preferable if heart failure is present with atrial fibrillation, but the onset of action is delayed. Electrical cardioversion (commencing with 100 J) may be necessary if atrial fibrillation is complicated by hypotension, heart failure, or ischemia, but the arrhythmia often recurs. A short course of a class Ia agent such as procainamide or quinidine may be required in addition to digoxin, a beta-blocker, or a calcium channel blocker to maintain sinus rhythm.

3. Ventricular arrhythmias—Ventricular arrhythmias are most common in the first few hours after infarction. Ventricular premature beats (VPBs) may be premonitory for ventricular tachycardia or fibrillation. Prophylactic lidocaine may be started (1 mg/kg bolus followed by an infusion of 2 mg/min) if more than 6 VPB/min, early (R on T wave) VPBs, couplets or nonsustained ventricular tachycardia are observed. Additional boluses of 0.5 mg/kg followed by an increased infusion rate (up to 4 mg/min) may be necessary, but toxicity (tremor, anxiety, confusion, seizures) is common, especially in older patients and those with hypotension, heart failure, or liver disease. The infusion rate should be reduced after 3–4 hours, since blood levels tend to rise, but generally, once initiated, lidocaine should be continued for at least 24 hours.

Ventricular tachycardia should be treated with a 1 mg/kg bolus of lidocaine if the patient is stable or by electrical cardioversion (100–200 J) if not. If the arrhythmia cannot be suppressed with lidocaine, procainamide should be initiated (100 mg boluses over 1–2 minutes every 5 minutes to a cumulative dose of 750–1000 mg, followed by an infusion of 20–80 µg/kg/min). Hypotension may occur acutely, and depression of myocardial function or conduction may complicate maintenance therapy. Refractory ventricular arrhythmias are most effectively treated with intravenous amiodarone (150 mg over 10 minutes, which may be repeated as needed, followed by 360 mg over 6 hours and then 540 mg over 18 hours). Bretylium tosylate (5 mg/kg intravenously over 3–5 minutes, repeated after 20 minutes if necessary, followed by an infusion of 1–2 mg/min) is an alternative. Intravenous amiodarone can be very effective, but in the USA it is available only in a few centers. Ventricular fibrillation is treated electrically (300–400 J). Unresponsive ventricular fibrillation should be treated by bretylium and repeat cardioversion while CPR is administered. Accelerated idioventricular rhythm is a regular, wide complex rhythm at a rate of 70–100/min. It often follows reperfusion after thrombolytic therapy. The need for treating it in the absence of other ventricular arrhythmias is controversial.

4. Conduction disturbances–All degrees of atrioventricular block may occur in the course of acute myocardial infarction. Block at the level of the atrioventricular node is more common than infranodal block and occurs in approximately 20% of inferior myocardial infarctions. First-degree block is the most common and requires no treatment. Second-degree block is usually of the Mobitz type I form (Wenckebach), is often transient, and requires treatment only if associated with a heart rate slow enough to cause symptoms. Complete atrioventricular block occurs in up to 5% of acute inferior infarctions, usually is preceded by second-degree block, and generally resolves spontaneously, though it may persist for hours to several weeks. The escape rhythm originates in the distal atrioventricular node or atrioventricular junction and hence has a narrow QRS complex and is reliable, albeit often slow (30–50 beats/min). Treatment is often necessary because of resulting hypotension and low cardiac output. Intravenous atropine (1 mg) usually restores atrioventricular conduction temporarily, but if the escape complex is wide or if repeated atropine treatments are needed, temporary ventricular pacing is indicated. The prognosis for these patients is only slightly worse than that of patients who do not develop atrioventricular block.

In anterior infarctions, the site of block is distal, below the atrioventricular node, and usually a result of extensive damage of the His-Purkinje system and bundle branches. New first-degree block (prolongation of the PR interval) is unusual in anterior infarction; Mobitz type II atrioventricular block or complete heart block may be preceded by intraventricular conduction defects or may occur abruptly. The escape rhythm, if present at all, is an unreliable wide-complex idioventricular rhythm. Urgent ventricular pacing is mandatory, but even with successful pacing, mortality rates following the onset of complete heart block approach 80% because of the associated extensive myocardial change. New conduction abnormalities such as right or left bundle branch block or fascicular blocks may presage progression, often sudden, to second- or third-degree atrioventricular block. Prophylactic temporary ventricular pacing is recommended for new-onset alternating bilateral bundle branch block, bifascicular block, or bundle branch block with worsening first-degree atrioventricular block. Patients with anterior infarction who progress to second- or third-degree block even transiently should be considered for insertion of a prophylactic permanent ventricular pacemaker before discharge.

C. Myocardial Dysfunction: The severity of cardiac dysfunction is proportionate to the extent of myocardial necrosis but is exacerbated by preexisting dysfunction and ongoing ischemia. Patients who have no signs of heart failure, normal blood pressure, and normal urine output have a good prognosis. Those with hypotension or evidence of more than mild heart failure should have bedside right heart catheterization and continuous measurements of arterial pressure. These measurements permit the accurate assessment of cardiac function, facilitate the correct choice of therapy, and provide important prognostic information. Table 10–3 categorizes patients based upon these hemodynamic findings.

1. Acute left ventricular failure–Basilar rales are common in acute myocardial infarction, but dyspnea, more diffuse rales, and arterial hypoxemia usually indicate left ventricular failure. Since both the physical examination and chest x-ray correlate poorly with hemodynamic measurements and since the central venous pressure does not correlate with the pulmonary capillary wedge pressure (PCWP), right heart catheterization may be essential in monitoring therapy. General measures include supplemental oxygen to increase arterial saturation to above 95% and elevation of the trunk. Diuretics are usually the initial therapy unless right ventricular infarction is present. Intravenous furosemide (10–40 mg) or bumetanide (0.5–1 mg) is preferred because of the reliably rapid onset and short duration of action of these drugs. Higher dosages can be given if an inadequate response occurs. Morphine sulfate (4 mg intravenously followed by increments of 2 mg) is valuable in acute pulmonary edema.

Diuretics are usually effective; however, since most patients with acute infarction are not volume overloaded, the hemodynamic response may be limited and may be associated with hypotension. Vasodilators will reduce PCWP and improve cardiac output by a combination of venodilation (increasing venous capacitance) and arteriolar dilation (reducing afterload and left ventricular wall stress). In mild heart failure, sublingual isosorbide dinitrate (2.5–10 mg every 2 hours) or nitroglycerin ointment (6.25–25 mg every 4 hours) may be adequate to lower PCWP. In more severe failure, especially if cardiac output is reduced, sodium nitroprusside is the preferred agent.

It should be initiated only with hemodynamic monitoring; the initial dosage should be low (0.25 µg/kg/min) to avoid excessive hypotension, but the dosage can be increased by increments of 0.5 µg/kg/min every 5–10 minutes up to 5–10 µg/kg/min until the desired hemodynamic response (PCWP < 18 mm Hg, CI > 2.5) is obtained. Excessive hypotension (mean blood pressure < 65–75 mm Hg) or tachycardia (> 10/min increase) should be avoided. Combination of nitroprusside with inotropic agents may be necessary to preserve blood pressure or maximize benefit.

Intravenous nitroglycerin (starting at 10 µg/min) is usually less effective but may lower PCWP with less hypotension. Oral or transdermal vasodilator therapy with nitrates or angiotensin-converting enzyme inhibitors is often necessary after the initial 24–48 hours (see below).

Inotropic agents should be avoided if possible, because they often increase heart rate and myocardial oxygen requirements. Dobutamine has the best hemodynamic profile, increasing cardiac output and modestly lowering PCWP, usually without excessive tachycardia, hypotension, or arrhythmias. The initial dosage is 2.5 µg/kg/min, and it may be increased by similar increments up to 15–20 µg/kg/min at intervals of 5–10 minutes. Dopamine is more useful in the presence of hypotension (see below), since it produces peripheral vasoconstriction, but it has a less beneficial effect on PCWP. Amrinone is a positive inotrope and vasodilator that produces hemodynamic effects similar to those of dobutamine but with a greater decrease in PCWP. However, its longer duration of action makes it less useful in unstable situations. Milrinone is a more potent and newer congener of amrinone with fewer side effects. It should be commenced in a loading dose of 50 µg/kg over 10 minutes, followed by an infusion of 0.375–0.75 µg/kg/min. Digoxin has not been helpful in acute infarction except to control the ventricular response in atrial fibrillation, but it may be beneficial if chronic heart failure persists.

2. Hypotension and shock–Patients with hypotension (systolic blood pressure < 100 mm Hg, individualized depending on prior blood pressure) and signs of diminished perfusion (low urine output, confusion, cold extremities) should be hemodynamically monitored. Up to 20% will have findings indicative of intravascular hypovolemia (due to diaphoresis, vomiting, decreased venous tone, medications—such as diuretics, nitrates, morphine, beta-blockers, calcium channel blockers, and thrombolytic agents—and lack of oral intake). These should be treated with successive boluses of 100 mL of normal saline until PCWP reaches 15–18 mm Hg to determine whether cardiac output and blood pressure respond. Pericardial tamponade due to hemorrhagic pericarditis (especially after thrombolytic therapy or cardiopulmonary resuscitation) or ventricular rupture should

be considered and excluded by echocardiography if clinically indicated. Right ventricular infarction, characterized by a normal PCWP but elevated right atrial pressure, can produce hypotension. This is discussed below.

Most hypotensive patients will have moderate to severe left ventricular dysfunction; pathologic studies indicate that more than 20% of the left ventricle is infarcted (> 40% in cardiogenic shock). If hypotension is only modest (systolic pressure > 90 mm Hg) and the PCWP is elevated, diuretics and an initial trial of nitroprusside (see above for dosing) are indicated. If the blood pressure falls, inotropic support will need to be added or substituted. Such patients may also be treated with intra-aortic balloon counter-pulsation. This device unloads the left ventricle during systole and increases diastolic coronary artery filling pressure. It often facilitates the use of vasodilators in patients who previously did not tolerate them.

Dopamine is the most appropriate pressor for cardiogenic hypotension. It should be initiated at a rate of 2 µg/kg/min and increased at 5-minute intervals to the appropriate hemodynamic end point. At low dosages (< 5 µg/kg/min), it improves renal blood flow; at intermediate dosages (2.5–10 µg/kg/min), it stimulates myocardial contractility; at higher dosages (> 8 µg/kg/min), it is a potent α_1-adrenergic agonist. In general, blood pressure and cardiac index rise, but PCWP does not fall. Dopamine may be combined with nitroprusside or dobutamine (see above for dosing), or the latter may be used in its place if hypotension is not severe. Amrinone has hemodynamic effects similar to those of dobutamine, but its longer duration of action precludes rapid dosage adjustment. Norepinephrine (0.1–0.5 µg/kg/min) is the usual pressor of last resort, since isoproterenol and epinephrine produce less vasoconstriction, do not increase coronary perfusion pressure (aortic diastolic pressure), and tend to worsen the balance between myocardial oxygen delivery and utilization.

Patients with cardiogenic shock have a poor prognosis. If they do not respond rapidly, the previously described measure—intra-aortic balloon counterpulsation—should be instituted. Early PTCA may preserve enough viable myocardium to reverse the hypotension and should be attempted whenever feasible. Operation to repair mechanical defects (see below), revascularize ischemic myocardium, and resect aneurysms should be considered. Left ventricular assist devices as a bridge to early transplantation can be used in refractory patients under age 60 without other systemic illnesses.

D. Right Ventricular Infarction: Right ventricular infarction is present in one-third of patients with inferior wall infarction but is clinically significant in less than 50% of these. It presents as hypotension with relatively preserved left ventricular function and should be considered whenever patients with inferior infarction exhibit signs of low cardiac output and raised venous pressure. Hypotension is often exacerbated by medications that decrease intravascular volume or produce venodilation, such as diuretics, nitrates, and narcotics. Right atrial pressure and jugular venous pulsations are high, while PCWP is normal or low and the lungs are clear. The diagnosis is suggested by right precordial ST segment elevation using V_1 and leads to the right of the sternum corresponding to the location of V_3 and V_4. The diagnosis can be confirmed by echocardiography or hemodynamic measurements. When hypotension is present, hemodynamic measurements are necessary to monitor therapy. Treatment consists of fluid loading to improve left ventricular filling; inotropic agents may also be useful.

E. Mechanical Defects: Partial or complete rupture of a papillary muscle or of the interventricular septum occurs in less than 1% of acute myocardial infarctions and carries a poor prognosis. These complications occur in both anterior and inferior infarctions, usually 3–7 days after the acute event. They are detected by the appearance of a new systolic murmur and clinical deterioration, often with pulmonary edema. The two lesions are distinguished by the location of the murmur (apical versus parasternal) and by Doppler echocardiography. Hemodynamic monitoring is essential for appropriate management and demonstrates an increase in oxygen saturation between the right atrium and pulmonary artery in ventricular septal defect and, often, a large v wave with mitral regurgitation. Treatment by nitroprusside and, preferably, intra-aortic balloon counterpulsation reduces the regurgitation or shunt, but surgical correction is mandatory. In patients remaining hemodynamically unstable or requiring continuous parenteral pharmacologic treatment or counterpulsation, early surgery is recommended, though mortality rates are high (15% to nearly 100%, depending on residual ventricular function and clinical status). Patients who are stabilized medically can have delayed surgery with lower risks (10–25%).

F. Myocardial Rupture: Complete rupture of the left ventricular free wall occurs in less than 1% of patients and usually results in immediate death. It occurs 2–7 days postinfarction, usually involves the anterior wall, and is more frequent in older women. Incomplete or gradual rupture may be sealed off by the pericardium, creating a **pseudoaneurysm.** This may be recognized by echocardiography, radionuclide angiography, or left ventricular angiography, often as an incidental finding. It demonstrates a narrow-neck connection to the left ventricle. Early surgical repair is indicated, since delayed rupture is common.

G. Left Ventricular Aneurysm: Ten to 20 percent of patients surviving an acute infarction develop a left ventricular aneurysm, a sharply delineated area of scar that bulges paradoxically during systole. This usually follows anterior Q wave infarctions. Aneurysms are recognized by persistent ST segment elevation (beyond 4–8 weeks), and a wide neck from the left ventricle can be demonstrated by echocardiography, scintigraphy, or contrast angiography. They rarely rupture but may be associated with arterial emboli, ventricular arrhythmias, and congestive heart failure. Surgical resection may be performed for these indications if other measures fail. The best results (mortality rates of 10–20%) are obtained when the residual myocardium contracts well and when significant coronary lesions supplying adjacent regions are bypassed.

H. Pericarditis: The pericardium is involved in approximately 50% of infarctions, but pericarditis is often not clinically significant. Twenty percent of patients with Q wave infarctions will have an audible friction rub if examined repetitively. Pericardial pain occurs in approximately the same proportion after 2–7 days and is recognized by its variation with respiration and position (improved by sitting). Often, no treatment is required, but aspirin (650 mg every 4–6 hours) or indomethacin (25 mg three or four times daily) will usually relieve the pain. Anticoagulation should be avoided, since hemorrhagic pericarditis may result.

From 1 to 12 weeks after infarction, Dressler's syndrome (post-myocardial infarction syndrome) occurs in less than 5% of patients. This is an autoimmune phenomenon and presents as pericarditis with associated fever, leukocytosis, and, occasionally, pericardial or pleural effusion. It may recur over months. Treatment is the same as for other forms of pericarditis. A short course of corticosteroids may help if nonsteroidal agents do not relieve symptoms.

I. Mural Thrombus: Mural thrombi are common in large anterior infarctions but not in infarctions at other locations. Arterial emboli occur in approximately 2% of patients with known infarction, usually within 6 weeks. Anticoagulation with heparin followed by short-term (3-month) warfarin therapy prevents most emboli and should be considered in all patients with large anterior infarctions. Mural thrombi can be detected by echocardiography or CT scan (MRI has yielded frequent false-positive results) but with only moderate reliability, and only a small percentage (0–25%) embolize, so these procedures should not be relied upon for determining the need for anticoagulation.

Aronson D et al: Mechanisms determining the course and outcome of diabetic patients who have had acute myocardial infarction. Ann Intern Med 1997;126:296. (Mortality rates of diabetic patients remain 1.5–2 times higher than those of nondiabetics. The mechanism and management of this increased risk are discussed.)

Becker RC et al: A composite view of cardiac rupture in the United States National Registry of Myocardial Infarction. J Am Coll Cardiol 1996;27:1321. (Although the incidence of cardiac rupture was less than 1%, it accounted for 3% of hospital deaths. Cardiac rupture was less common in patients receiving thrombolytic therapy.)

Califf RM, Bengtson JR: Cardiogenic shock. N Engl J Med 1994;330:1724.

Chou TM et al: Cardiogenic shock: Thrombolysis or angioplasty? J Intens Care Med 1996;11:37. (Review of clinical trials dealing with patients with cardiogenic shock.)

Hochman JS et al: Current spectrum of cardiogenic shock and effect of revascularization on mortality. Results of an international registry. Circulation 1995;91:873. (Mortality remains high but appears to be improved by early revascularization.)

Kingh JW, Ryan TJ: Right ventricular infarction. N Engl J Med 1994;330:1211.

Reader GS: Identification and treatment of complications of myocardial infarction. Mayo Clin Proc 1995;70:880. (Concise review for primary care physicians.)

Postinfarction Management

Twenty percent of patients with acute myocardial infarction die before they reach the hospital. Mortality rates in hospitalized patients range from 5% to 15% and are determined chiefly by the size of the infarction and the age and general condition of the patient. Patients developing heart failure or hypotension have high early mortality rates. Several classification criteria have been developed to estimate early prognosis for survival. The most accurate is hemodynamic subsetting (Table 10–3). The prognosis after discharge is determined by three major factors: the degree of left ventricular dysfunction, the extent of residual ischemic myocardium, and the presence of ventricular arrhythmias. The mortality rate in the first year after discharge is approximately 6–8%, with over half of deaths occurring in the first 3 months, chiefly in patients with postinfarction heart failure. Subsequently, the mortality rate averages 4% per year.

A. Risk Stratification: A number of findings indicate increased risk after infarction. These include: (1) postinfarction angina; (2) non-Q wave infarction; (3) heart failure; (4) left ventricular ejection fraction less than 40%; (5) exercise-induced ischemia, diagnosed by electrocardiography or scintigraphy; and (6) ventricular ectopy (> 10 VPB/h). It is less certain whether this information should be collected and how it should be acted upon.

Patients with postinfarction angina should undergo coronary arteriography. Authorities differ about which tests should be performed routinely in other patients, but in most a noninvasive assessment of left ventricular function and residual ischemia is appropriate. Significant left ventricular dysfunction is most likely with anterior infarction or multiple infarctions. In these, noninvasive assessment of left ventricular function by echocardiography or scintigraphy will help assess prognosis and facilitate medical management. If the ejection fraction is less than 40%, coronary angiography may be indicated, as this is a high-risk subset in which revascularization may improve prognosis. ACE inhibitor therapy is also indicated. Submaximal exercise testing before discharge or a maximal test after 3–6 weeks (the latter being more sensitive for ischemia) helps patients and physicians plan the return to normal activity. Imaging in conjunction with stress testing adds additional sensitivity for ischemia and provides localizing information. Both exercise and pharmacologic stress imaging have successfully predicted subsequent outcome. One of these tests should usually be employed prior to discharge in patients who have received thrombolytic therapy as a means of selecting appropriate candidates for coronary angiography.

Ambulatory electrocardiographic monitoring for arrhythmias is of less clear value; though it has some prognostic value beyond measurements of left ventricular function, no benefit from antiarrhythmic therapy for asymptomatic patients has been demonstrated. Ischemia detected during ambulatory monitoring is an indicator of poor prognosis, but it is unclear how much additional information is obtained in patients who have also undergone exercise testing or scintigraphic studies. The role of other procedures such as assessment of heart rate variability or baroreceptor testing is uncertain.

A conservative approach to postinfarction evaluation would include measurement of left ventricular function in patients with signs of heart failure or large infarctions and a test for ischemia in patients without recurrent chest pain. The latter should occur before discharge if the patient has undergone thrombolytic therapy but may be delayed for 3–6 weeks in most other patients.

B. Prophylactic Therapy: Postinfarction management should begin with identification and modification of risk factors. Treatment of hyperlipidemia and smoking cessation both prevent recurrent infarction, and data now exist which confirm that aggressive lipid lowering improves survival in patients with clinical coronary artery disease. Recent guidelines suggest a target LDL cholesterol level below 100 mg/dL for patients with manifest coronary artery disease. Blood pressure control, weight loss, and exercise are recommended, though definite benefit on postinfarction prognosis has not been demonstrated.

Beta-blockers improve survival rates, primarily by reducing the incidence of sudden death in high-risk subsets of patients. Beta-blockers should be given to such individuals, except those with overt heart failure, but are of limited value in uncomplicated patients with small infarctions and normal exercise tests. No advantage of one preparation over another has been demonstrated except that those with intrinsic sympathomimetic activity have not proved beneficial in postinfarction patients.

Antiplatelet agents are beneficial; low-dose aspirin (325 mg daily) is recommended. Warfarin anticoagulation for 3 months reduces the incidence of arterial emboli after large anterior infarctions, and according to the results of at least one study it improves long-term prognosis, but after 6 months any benefit additive to aspirin has not been confirmed.

Calcium channel blockers have not been shown to improve prognoses overall and should not be prescribed purely for secondary prevention. However, these agents may be useful for managing hypertension or subsequent angina pectoris. Based on published studies, verapamil and diltiazem may be preferable to nifedipine (the only dihydropyridine studied) in the postinfarction patient.

Antiarrhythmic therapy other than with betablockers has not been shown to be effective except in patients with symptomatic arrhythmias and, in fact, class Ic agents increase the mortality rate in postinfarction patients. Although several small studies with amiodarone suggested some benefits, this has not been confirmed in two large trials conducted in postinfarct patients with either left ventricular dysfunction or frequent ventricular ectopy. However, amiodarone was not harmful, and it is therefore probably the agent of choice for individuals with symptomatic postinfarction arrhythmias, although emerging data suggest that implantable defibrillators may be a more effective option.

Cardiac rehabilitation programs and exercise training can be of considerable psychologic benefit, but it is not known whether they alter prognosis.

C. ACE Inhibitors in Patients With Left Ventricular Dysfunction: Patients who sustain substantial myocardial damage often experience subsequent progressive left ventricular dilation and dysfunction, leading to clinical heart failure and reduced long-term survival. In patients with ejection fractions less than 40%, captopril (25–50 mg three times daily commencing 3–16 days postinfarction) prevents left ventricular dilation and the onset of heart failure and also reduces the mortality rate. Similar data have been collected with ramipril as well. Although two large trials found a benefit from treating unselected patients beginning on admission, it is unclear if this accrues to patients without left ventricular dysfunction and whether there is any advantage to starting treatment while the patient may be hemodynamically unstable.

D. Revascularization: Because of the increasing use of thrombolytic therapy and accumulating experience with PTCA, the indications for revascularization are rapidly evolving. Postinfarction patients who appear likely to benefit from early revascularization if the anatomy is appropriate are (1) those who have undergone thrombolytic therapy and have residual symptoms or laboratory evidence of ischemia; (2) patients with left ventricular dysfunction (ejection fraction < 30–40%) and evidence of ischemia; (3) patients with non-Q wave infarction and evidence of more than mild ischemia; and (4) patients with markedly positive exercise tests and multivessel disease. The value of revascularization in the following groups is less clear: (1) patients treated with thrombolytic agents, with little evidence of reperfusion or residual ischemia; (2) patients with left ventricular dysfunction but no detectable ischemia; and (3) patients with preserved left ventricular function who have mild ischemia and are not symptom-limited. Patients who survive infarctions without complications, have preserved left ventricular function (ejection fraction > 50%), and have no exercise-induced ischemia have an excellent prognosis and do not require invasive evaluation.

[AHCPR guideline on cardiac rehabilitation]
  http://text.nlm.nih.gov/ftrs/gateway

Aguirre FV et al: Early and 1-year clinical outcome of patients' evolving non-Q-wave versus Q-wave myocardial infarction after thrombolysis. Circulation 1995;91:2541. (There was no difference in outcome with aggressive catheterization strategies compared with a more conservative strategy in either group. The lack of advantage of a more aggressive strategy has been confirmed in the VANQUISH Trial, a recently presented multicenter study.)

Almony GT et al: Anti-platelet and anticoagulant use after myocardial infarction. Clin Cardiol 1996;19:357. (Review of the use of aspirin, heparin, warfarin, and newer agents.)

Balady GL et al: Cardiac rehabilitation programs: An AHA position statement. Circulation 1994;90:1602. (Summary for primary care physicians.)

Camm AJ, Fei L: Risk stratification after myocardial infarction. PACE 1994;17:41. (Review with emphasis on role of arrhythmia monitoring, electrophysiologic testing, and autonomic assessment.)

Deedwania PC et al: Evidence-based, cost-effective risk stratification in management after myocardial infarction. Arch Intern Med 1997;157:273. (Consensus panel review of relevant trials, providing recommendations for testing and treatment of infarct survivors.)

Kuntz KM et al: Cost-effectiveness of routine angiography after acute myocardial infarction. Circulation 1996; 94:957. (In appropriately selected patients, such as those with postinfarction angina and strongly positive stress tests, early coronary angiography and subsequent management guided by its results appears to be a cost-effective strategy.)

O'Rourke RB: Management of patients after myocardial infarction and thrombolytic therapy. Curr Probl Cardiol 1994;19(4):177. (Updated review of strategies in the thrombolytic era.)

Pfeffer M et al: Effect of captopril on mortality and morbidity in patients with left ventricular dysfunction after myocardial infarction: Results of the Survival and Ventricular Enlargement Trial. N Engl J Med 1992;327:669. (Seminal trial supporting use of ACE in patients with ejection fractions < 40%.)

Pitt B: Evaluation of the post-infarct patient. Circulation 1995;91:1855. (Well-supported personal perspective.)

Reeder GS, Gibbons RJ: Acute myocardial infarction: Risk stratification in the thrombolytic era. Mayo Clin Proc 1995;70:87. (Concise review and recommendations.)

Soumerai SB et al: Adverse outcomes of underuse of betablockers in elderly survivors of acute myocardial infarction. JAMA 1997;277:115. (Review of Medicare data base, showing that only 21% of eligible patients were receiving beta-blocker therapy and that these had a 43% lower mortality rate and 22% lower rehospitalization rate. In contrast, an increasing number of elderly patients were receiving calcium channel blockers. These findings suggest a substantial frequency of inappropriate practices.)

Vaitkus PT, Barnathan ES: Embolic potential, prevention

and management of mural thrombus complicating anterior myocardial infarction: A metaanalysis. J Am Coll Cardiol 1993;22:1004. (Meta-analysis suggesting patients with anterior myocardial infarction should receive anticoagulation for at least 3 months to reduce incidence of systemic embolization.)

Viscoli CM et al: Beta-blockers after myocardial infarction: Influence of first year clinical course on long-term effectiveness. Ann Intern Med 1993;118:99. (After 1 year of propranolol therapy, the major additional benefit comes from the treatment of high-risk patients. Low-risk patients do not obtain any further reduction in mortality rate.)

DISTURBANCES OF RATE & RHYTHM

Abnormalities of cardiac rhythm and conduction can be lethal (sudden cardiac death), symptomatic (syncope, near syncope, dizziness, or palpitations), or asymptomatic. They are dangerous to the extent that they reduce cardiac output, so that perfusion of the brain or myocardium is impaired, or tend to deteriorate into more serious arrhythmias with the same consequences. Stable supraventricular tachycardia is generally well tolerated in patients without underlying heart disease but may lead to myocardial ischemia or congestive heart failure in patients with coronary disease, valvular abnormalities, and systolic or diastolic myocardial dysfunction. Ventricular tachycardia, if prolonged (lasting more than 10–30 seconds), often results in hemodynamic compromise and is more likely to deteriorate into ventricular fibrillation.

Whether slow heart rates produce symptoms at rest or on exertion depends upon whether cerebral perfusion can be maintained, which is generally a function of whether the patient is upright or supine and whether left ventricular function is adequate to maintain stroke volume. If the heart rate abruptly slows, as with the onset of complete heart block or transient standstill, syncope or convulsions may result.

Arrhythmias are detected either because they present with symptoms or because they are detected during the course of monitoring. Arrhythmias causing sudden death, syncope, or near syncope require further evaluation and treatment unless they are related to conditions that are unlikely to recur (eg, electrolyte abnormalities or acute myocardial infarction). In contrast, there is controversy over when and how to evaluate and treat rhythm disturbances that are not symptomatic but are possible markers for more serious abnormalities (eg, nonsustained ventricular tachycardia). This uncertainty reflects two issues: (1) the difficulty of reliably stratifying patients into high-risk and low-risk groups; and (2) the lack of treatments which are both effective and safe. Thus, screening patients for these so-called "premonitory" abnormalities is often not productive.

A number of procedures are employed to evaluate patients with symptoms who are felt to be at risk for life-threatening arrhythmias, including in-hospital and ambulatory electrocardiographic monitoring, event recorders (instruments that can be worn for prolonged periods in order to record or transmit rhythm tracings when infrequent episodes occur), exercise testing, intracardiac electrophysiologic studies (to assess sinus node function, atrioventricular conduction, and inducibility of arrhythmias), signal-averaged ECGs, and tests of autonomic nervous system function (especially tilt-table testing). These are discussed below and in the subsequent sections on individual rhythm disturbance and symptomatic presentation. In general, these techniques are more successful in diagnosing symptomatic arrhythmias than in predicting the outcome of asymptomatic ones.

Kastor JA: *Arrhythmias.* Saunders, 1993. (Very practical text, appropriate for physicians without background in electrophysiology.)

Zipes DP, Jalife J (editors): *Cardiac Electrophysiology: From Cell to Bedside.* Saunders, 1995.

MECHANISMS OF ARRHYTHMIAS

Electrophysiologic studies have greatly increased our understanding of the mechanisms underlying most arrhythmias. These include (1) disorders of impulse formation or automaticity, (2) abnormalities of impulse conduction, (3) reentry, and (4) triggered activity.

Altered automaticity is the mechanism for sinus node arrest, many premature beats, and automatic rhythms as well as an initiating factor in reentry arrhythmias.

Abnormalities of impulse conduction can occur at the sinus or atrioventricular node, in the intraventricular conduction system, and within the atria or ventricles. These are responsible for sinoatrial exit block, for atrioventricular block at the node or below, and for establishing reentry circuits.

Reentry is the underlying mechanism for many arrhythmias, including premature beats, most paroxysmal supraventricular tachycardias, and atrial flutter. For reentry to occur, there must be an area of unidirectional block with an appropriate delay to allow repeat depolarization at the site of origin. Reentry is confirmed if the arrhythmia can be terminated by interruption of the circuit by a spontaneous or induced premature beat.

Triggered activity occurs when afterdepolarizations (abnormal electrical activity persisting after repolarization) reach the threshold level required to trigger a new depolarization. This may be the mechanism of ventricular tachycardia in the prolonged QT syndrome and in some cases of digitalis toxicity.

Waldo AL, Witt AL: Mechanisms of cardiac arrhythmias. Lancet 1993;341:1189.

TECHNIQUES FOR EVALUATING RHYTHM DISTURBANCES

Electrocardiographic Monitoring

The ideal way of establishing a causal relationship between a symptom and a rhythm disturbance is to demonstrate the presence of the rhythm during the symptom. Unfortunately, this is not always easy because symptoms are usually sporadic.

Patients with aborted sudden death and recent or recurrent syncope are often monitored in the hospital. Those with less potentially life-threatening symptoms may be monitored as outpatients. When episodes are infrequent, use of an event recorder is preferable. Exercise testing may be helpful when the symptoms are associated with exertion or stress. If symptomatic bradyarrhythmias or supraventricular tachyarrhythmias are detected, therapy can usually be initiated without additional diagnostic studies. Further electrophysiologic studies may be useful in evaluating ventricular tachyarrhythmias.

Extreme caution is required before attributing a patient's symptom to rhythm or conduction abnormalities observed during monitoring without concomitant symptoms. In many cases, the symptoms are due to a different arrhythmia or to noncardiac causes. For instance, in evaluating dizziness or syncope in older patients, bradycardia, sinus node abnormalities, and ventricular ectopy are all commonly found but may have nothing to do with the symptoms. Ambulatory monitoring is frequently used to quantify ventricular ectopy and detect asymptomatic ventricular tachycardia in post-myocardial infarction or heart failure patients. Unfortunately, while asymptomatic ventricular arrhythmias have negative prognostic implications, there are few data to support specific therapeutic intervention. Thus, monitoring in asymptomatic individuals is usually not indicated.

Electrophysiologic Testing

Electrophysiologic testing employing intracardiac electrocardiographic recordings and programmed atrial or ventricular (or both) stimulation is useful in the diagnosis and management of complex arrhythmias. The primary indications for electrophysiologic testing are (1) evaluation of recurrent syncope of possible cardiac origin, when the ambulatory ECG has not provided the diagnosis; (2) differentiation of supraventricular from ventricular arrhythmias; (3) evaluation of therapy in patients with accessory atrioventricular pathways; (4) evaluation of the efficacy of pharmacotherapy in survivors of aborted sudden death or other patients with symptomatic or life-threatening ventricular tachycardia; and (5) evaluation of patients for catheter ablation procedures or antitachycardia devices.

Signal-Averaged ECG

A newer approach to arrhythmia evaluation and prediction is the signal-averaged ECG (SAECG). This procedure sums several hundred cardiac cycles to provide a highly resolved electrocardiographic tracing which is then filtered to maximize detection of high-frequency potentials. The finding of late potentials following the QRS complex indicates a possible substrate for ventricular arrhythmias. They are most common and of greater prognostic value in patients who have myocardial scarring from prior infarctions. In this latter group, absence of late potentials indicates a low risk for serious ventricular arrhythmias and sudden death. While the predictive accuracy of a positive SAECG is relatively low, it has been advocated as a screening test for patients who should undergo electrophysiologic testing. At present, however, data are not adequate to support this approach in asymptomatic postinfarction patients even when they exhibit nonsustained ventricular arrhythmias. Conversely, those with symptoms consistent with arrhythmia require further evaluation and treatment regardless of the SAECG results. The value of the SAECG in patients without ischemic heart disease is unclear.

Autonomic Testing

In many patients with recurrent syncope or near syncope, arrhythmias are not the cause. This is particularly true when the patient has no evidence of associated heart disease by history, examination, standard ECG, or noninvasive testing. Syncope may be neurocardiogenic in origin, mediated by excessive vagal stimulation or an imbalance between sympathetic and parasympathetic autonomic activity. With assumption of upright posture, there is venous pooling in the lower limbs. However, instead of the normal response, which consists of an increase in heart rate and vasoconstriction, a sympathetically mediated increase in myocardial contractility activates mechanoreceptors that trigger reflex bradycardia and vasodilation. Autonomic testing is an important component of the evaluation in these individuals and should usually precede invasive electrophysiologic procedures. Carotid sinus massage in patients who do not have carotid bruits or a history of cerebral vascular disease can precipitate sinus node arrest or atrioventricular block in patients with carotid sinus hypersensitivity. Head-up tilt-table testing can identify patients whose syncope may be on a vasovagal basis. Although different testing protocols are employed, passive tilting to at least 70 degrees for 10–40 minutes—in conjunction with isoproterenol infusion, if necessary—is typical. Syncope due to bradycardia, hypotension, or both will occur in approximately one-third of patients with recurrent syncope. Some recent studies have suggested that, at least with some of the more extreme protocols, false-positive responses may occur.

ACC/AHA Task Force Report: Guidelines for intracardiac electrophysiologic and catheter ablation procedures. J Am Coll Cardiol 1995;26:555.

Benditt DG et al: Tilt-table testing for assessing syncope. J Am Coll Cardiol 1996;28:263. (Consensus document covering the rationale, indications, procedures, and interpretations of tilt-table testing.)

Gomes JA et al: Identification of patients at high risk of arrhythmic mortality: Role of ambulatory monitoring, signal-averaged ECG, and heart rate variability. Cardiol Clin 1993;11:55. (Predictive value of each test is low, but combinations of these tests can identify relatively high-risk groups, albeit at high cost and with still relatively low specificity.)

Stein PK et al: Heart rate variability: A measure of cardiac autonomic tone. Am Heart J 1994;127:1376. (Excellent review of principals and practices.)

Antiarrhythmic Drugs
(Table 10–8)

Antiarrhythmic drugs have limited efficacy and produce frequent side effects. They are often divided into four classes based upon their electropharmacologic actions.

Class I agents block membrane sodium channels. Three subclasses are further defined by the effect of agents on the Purkinje fiber action potential. Class Ia drugs slow the rate of rise of the action potential (V_{max}) and prolong its duration, thus slowing conduction and increasing refractoriness. Class Ib agents shorten action potential duration; they do not affect conduction or refractoriness. Class Ic agents prolong V_{max} and slow repolarization, thus slowing conduction and prolonging refractoriness, but more so than class Ia drugs.

Class II agents are the beta-blockers, which decrease automaticity, prolong atrioventricular conduction, and prolong refractoriness.

Class III agents block potassium channels and prolong repolarization, widening the QRS and prolonging the QT interval. They decrease automaticity and conduction and prolong refractoriness.

Class IV agents are the slow calcium channel blockers, which decrease automaticity and atrioventricular conduction.

Although the in vitro electrophysiologic effects of most of these agents have been defined, their use remains largely empirical. All can exacerbate arrhythmias (proarrhythmic effect), and most depress left ventricular function.

The risk of antiarrhythmic agents has been highlighted by the Coronary Arrhythmia Suppression Trial (CAST), in which two class Ic agents (flecainide, encainide) and a class Ia agent (moricizine) increased mortality rates in patients with asymptomatic ventricular ectopy after myocardial infarction.

A similar result has been reported with D-sotalol, a class III agent with the beta-blocking activity of D,L-sotalol, the currently marketed formulation. Therefore, these agents, and perhaps any antiarrhythmic drug, should not be used except for life-threatening ventricular arrhythmias and symptomatic supraventricular tachyarrhythmias.

The use of antiarrhythmic agents for specific arrhythmias is discussed below.

Drugs for cardiac arrhythmias. Med Lett Drugs Ther 1996;38:75. (Currently available antiarrhythmic agents.)

Podrid PJ: Amiodarone: Re-evaluation of an old drug. Ann Intern Med 1995;122:689.

Roden DM: Risks and benefits of antiarrhythmic therapy. N Engl J Med 1994;331:785. (Appropriately careful review.)

Radiofrequency Ablation for Cardiac Arrhythmias

Catheter ablation techniques have become the primary modality for treatment of many arrhythmias. This growing trend reflects the increasing ability to localize the origin or conduction pathways of many arrhythmias, the improved technology for delivering radiofrequency energy, and growing dissatisfaction with the efficacy and safety of pharmacologic therapy. Ablation has become the primary modality of therapy for many symptomatic supraventricular arrhythmias, including atrioventricular nodal reentry tachycardia, reentry tachycardias involving accessory pathways, paroxysmal atrial tachycardia, inappropriate sinus tachycardia, and automatic junctional tachycardia. Many laboratories have achieved reasonable success rates in preventing atrial flutter with radiofrequency techniques, and experience with atrial fibrillation is accumulating as well.

Catheter ablation of ventricular arrhythmias has proved more difficult. Three specific forms of ventricular tachycardia, however, have proved to be amenable to radiofrequency ablation. These include bundle-branch reentry, tachycardia originating in the right ventricular outflow tract, and some tachycardias originating in the left side of the interventricular septum. Other forms of ventricular tachycardia, particularly in patients with coronary artery disease, may be amenable to ablation, but experience thus far is limited.

These procedures are generally safe, though there is a low incidence of perforation of the atria or right ventricle that results in pericardial tamponade and sufficient damage to the atrioventricular node to require permanent cardiac pacing in up 20% of patients. In addition, some procedures involve transseptal or retrograde left ventricular catheterization, with the attendant potential complications of aortic perforation, damage to the heart valves, or left-sided emboli.

Table 10–8. Antiarrhythmic drugs.

Agent	Intravenous Dosage	Oral Dosage	Therapeutic Plasma Level	Route of Elimination	Side Effects
Class Ia: Action: Sodium channel blockers: Depress phase 0 depolarization; slow conduction; prolong repolarization. **Indications:** Supraventricular tachycardia, ventricular tachycardia, prevention of ventricular fibrillation, symptomatic ventricular premature beats.					
Quinidine	6–10 mg/kg (IM or IV) over 20 min (rarely used parenterally)	200–400 mg every 4–6 h or every 8 h (long-acting)	2–5 µg/mL	Hepatic	GI, ↓LVF, ↑Dig
Procainamide	100 mg/1–3 min to 500–1000 mg; maintain at 2–6 mg/min	50 mg/kg/d in divided doses every 3–4 h or every 6 h (long-acting)	4–10 µg/mL; NAPA (active metabolite), 10–20 µg/mL	Renal	SLE, hypersensitivity, ↓LVF
Disopyramide		100–200 mg every 6–8 h	2–8 µg/mL	Renal	Urinary retention, dry mouth, markedly ↓LVF
Moricizine		200–300 mg every 8 h	*Note:* Active metabolites	Hepatic	Dizziness, nausea, headache, ↓theophylline level, ↓LVF
Class Ib: Action: Shorten repolarization. **Indications:** Ventricular tachycardia, prevention of ventricular fibrillation, symptomatic ventricular beats.					
Lidocaine	1–2 mg/kg at 50 mg/min; maintain at 1–4 mg/min		1–5 µg/mL	Hepatic	CNS, GI
Mexiletine		100–300 mg every 6–12 h. Maximum: 1200 mg/d	0.5–2 µg/mL	Hepatic	CNS, GI, leukopenia
Phenytoin	50 mg/5 min to 1000 mg (12 mg/kg); maintain at 200–400 mg/d	200–400 mg every 12–24 h	5–20 µg/mL	Hepatic	CNS, GI
Class Ic: Action: Depress phase 0 repolarization; slow conduction. *Propafenone* is a weak calcium channel- and beta-blocker and prolongs action potential and refractoriness. **Indications:** Life-threatening ventricular tachycardia or fibrillation; refractory supraventricular tachycardia.					
Flecainide		100–200 mg twice daily	0.2–1 µg/mL	Hepatic	CNS, GI, ↓↓LVF, incessant VT, sudden death
Propafenone		150–300 mg every 8–12 h	*Note:* Active metabolites	Hepatic	CNS, GI, ↓↓LVF, ↑Dig
Class II: Action: Beta-blocker, slows AV conduction. *Note:* Other beta-blockers may also have antiarrhythmic effects but are not yet approved for this indication in the USA. **Indications:** Supraventricular tachycardia; may prevent ventricular fibrillation.					
Esmolol	500 µg/kg over 1–2 min; maintain at 25–200 µg/kg/min	Other beta-blockers may be used	0.15–2 µg/mL	Hepatic	↓LVF, bronchospasm
Propranolol	1–5 mg at 1 mg/min	40–320 mg in 1–4 doses (depending on preparation)	Not established	Hepatic	↓LVF, bradycardia, AV block, bronchospasm
Acebutolol		200–600 mg twice daily	Not established	Hepatic	↓LVF, bradycardia, positive ANA, lupus-like syndrome

(continued)

Table 10–8. Antiarrhythmic drugs. (continued)

Agent	Intravenous Dosage	Oral Dosage	Therapeutic Plasma Level	Route of Elimination	Side Effects
Class III: Action: Prolong action potential. **Indications:** *Amiodarone:* refractory ventricular tachycardia, supraventricular tachycardia, prevention of ventricular tachycardia, ventricular fibrillation; *sotalol:* ventricular tachycardia; *bretylium:* ventricular fibrillation, ventricular tachycardia.					
Amiodarone	150 mg infused rapidly, followed by 1 mg/min infusion for 6 hours (360 mg) and then 0.5 mg/min. Additional 150 mg as needed	800–1600 mg/d for 7–21 days; maintain at 100–400 mg/d (higher doses may be needed)	1–5 µg/mL	Hepatic	Pulmonary fibrosis, hypothyroidism, hyperthyroidism, corneal and skin deposits, hepatitis, ↑Dig, neurotoxicity, GI
Sotalol		80–160 mg every 12 h (higher doses may be used for life-threatening arrhythmias)		Renal (dosing interval should be extended if creatinine clearance is <60 mL/min)	↓LVF, bradycardia, fatigue (and other side effects associated with beta-blockers)
Bretylium	5–10 mg/kg over 5–10 min; maintain at 0.5–2 mg/min. Maximum: 30 mg/kg		0.5–1.5 µg/mL	Renal	Hypotension, nausea
Ibutilide	1 mg over 10 minutes, followed by a second infusion of 0.5–1 mg			Hepatic and renal	Torsade de pointes in up to 5% of patients within 3 hours after administration. Patients must be monitored with defibrillator nearby.
Class IV: Action: Slow calcium channel blockers. **Indications:** Supraventricular tachycardia.					
Verapamil	10–20 mg over 2–20 min; maintain at 5 µg/kg/min	80–120 mg every 6–8 h; 240–360 mg once daily with sustained-release preparation (not approved for arrhythmia)	0.1–0.15 µg/mL	Hepatic	↓LVF, constipation, ↑Dig
Diltiazem	0.25 mg/kg over 2 min; second 0.35 mg/kg bolus after 15 min if response is inadequate; infusion rate, 5–15 mg/h	180–360 mg daily in 1–3 doses depending on preparation (oral forms not approved for arrhythmias)		Hepatic metabolism, renal excretion	Hypotension, ↓LVF
Class V: Indications: Supraventricular tachycardia.					
Adenosine	6 mg rapidly followed by 12 mg after 1–2 min if needed			Adenosine receptor stimulation, metabolized in blood	Transient flushing, dyspnea, chest pain, AV block, sinus bradycardia; effect ↓ by theophylline, ↑ by dipyridamole
Digoxin	0.5 mg over 20 min followed by increment of 0.25 or 0.125 mg to 1–1.5 mg over 24 hours	1–1.5 mg over 24–36 hours in 3 or 4 doses; maintenance, 0.125–0.5 mg/d	0.7–2 mg/mL	Renal	AV block, arrhythmias, GI, visual changes

Key: AV = atrioventricular; CNS = central nervous system; ↑Dig = elevation of serum digoxin level; GI = gastrointestinal (nausea, vomiting, diarrhea); ↓LVF = reduced left ventricular function; SLE = systemic lupus erythematosus; VT = ventricular tachycardia

SUPRAVENTRICULAR ARRHYTHMIAS

1. SINUS ARRHYTHMIA, BRADYCARDIA, & TACHYCARDIA

Sinus arrhythmia is a cyclic increase in normal heart rate with inspiration and decrease with expiration. It results from reflex changes in vagal influence on the normal pacemaker and disappears with breath holding or increase of heart rate due to any cause. It has no clinical significance. It is common in both the young and the elderly.

Sinus bradycardia is a heart rate slower than 50/min due to increased vagal influence on the normal pacemaker or organic disease of the sinus node. The rate usually increases during exercise or administration of atropine. In healthy individuals, and especially in patients who are in excellent physical condition, sinus bradycardia to a rate of 50 or even lower is a normal finding. However, severe sinus bradycardia may be an indication of sinus node pathology (see below), especially in elderly patients and individuals with heart disease. It may cause weakness, confusion, or syncope if cerebral perfusion is impaired. Atrial and ventricular ectopic rhythms are more apt to occur with slow sinus rates. Pacing may be required if symptoms correlate with the bradycardia.

Sinus tachycardia is defined as a heart rate faster than 100 beats/min that is caused by rapid impulse formation from the normal pacemaker; it occurs with fever, exercise, emotion, pain, anemia, heart failure, shock, thyrotoxicosis, or in response to many drugs. Alcohol and alcohol withdrawal are common causes of sinus tachycardia and other supraventricular arrhythmias. The onset and termination are usually gradual, in contrast to paroxysmal supraventricular tachycardia due to reentry. The rate infrequently exceeds 160/min but may reach 180/min in young persons. The rhythm is basically regular, but serial 1-minute counts of the heart rate indicate that it varies five or more beats per minute with changes in position, with breath holding or sedation. Rare individuals have persistent or episodic "inappropriate" sinus tachycardia that may be very symptomatic or may lead to left ventricular contractile dysfunction. Radiofrequency modification of the sinus node has mitigated this problem.

Lee RJ et al: Radiofrequency catheter modification of the sinus node for "inappropriate" sinus tachycardia. Circulation 1995;92:2919.

2. ATRIAL PREMATURE BEATS (Atrial Extrasystoles)

Atrial premature beats occur when an ectopic focus in the atria fires before the next sinus node impulse or a reentry circuit is established. The contour of the P wave usually differs from the patient's normal complex. The subsequent R–R cycle length is usually unchanged or only slightly prolonged. Such premature beats occur frequently in normal hearts and are never a sufficient basis for a diagnosis of heart disease. Speeding of the heart rate by any means usually abolishes most premature beats. Early atrial premature beats may cause aberrant QRS complexes (wide and bizarre) or may be nonconducted to the ventricles because the latter are still refractory.

3. DIFFERENTIATION OF ABERRANTLY CONDUCTED SUPRAVENTRICULAR BEATS FROM VENTRICULAR BEATS

This distinction can be very difficult in patients with a wide QRS complex; it is important because of the differing prognostic and therapeutic implications of each type. Findings favoring a ventricular origin include (1) atrioventricular dissociation; (2) a QRS duration exceeding 0.14 s; (3) capture or fusion beats (infrequent); (4) left axis deviation with right bundle branch block morphology; (5) monophasic (R) or biphasic (qR, QR, or RS) complexes in V_1; and (6) a qR or QS complex in V_6. Supraventricular origin is favored by (1) a triphasic QRS complex, especially if there was initial negativity in leads I and V_6; (2) ventricular rates exceeding 170/min; (3) QRS duration longer than 0.12 s but not longer than 0.14 s; and (4) the presence of preexcitation syndrome.

The relationship of the P waves to the tachycardia complex is helpful. A 1:1 relationship usually means a supraventricular origin, except in the case of ventricular tachycardia with retrograde P waves. If the P waves are not clearly seen, Lewis leads (in which the right arm electrode is placed in the V_1 position two interspaces higher than usual and the left arm electrode is placed in the usual V_1 position) may be employed. This accentuates the size of the P waves. Esophageal leads, in which the electrode is placed directly posterior to the left atrium, achieve the same effect even more clearly. Right atrial electrograms may also help to clarify the diagnosis by accentuating the P waves.

Brugada P et al: A new approach to the differential diagnosis of irregular tachycardia with a wide QRS complex. Circulation 1991;83:1649. (A stepwise approach to making this difficult distinction.)

4. PAROXYSMAL SUPRAVENTRICULAR TACHYCARDIA

This is the commonest paroxysmal tachycardia and often occurs in patients without structural heart disease. Attacks begin and end abruptly and may last a few seconds to several hours or longer. The heart rate may be 140–240/min (usually 160–220/min) and is perfectly regular (despite exercise or change in position). The P wave usually differs in contour from sinus beats. Patients may be asymptomatic except for awareness of rapid heart action, but some experience mild chest pain or shortness of breath, especially when episodes are prolonged, even in the absence of associated cardiac abnormalities. Paroxysmal supraventricular tachycardia may result from digitalis toxicity and then is commonly associated with atrioventricular block.

The most common mechanism for paroxysmal supraventricular tachycardia is reentry, which may be initiated or terminated by a fortuitously timed atrial or ventricular premature beat. The reentry circuit may involve the sinus node, the atrioventricular node, or an accessory pathway. About one-third of patients have aberrant pathways to the ventricles. The pathophysiology and management of arrhythmias due to accessory pathways differs in important ways and is discussed separately below.

Treatment of the Acute Attack

In the absence of heart disease, serious effects are rare, and most attacks break spontaneously. Particular effort should be made to terminate the attack quickly if cardiac failure, syncope, or anginal pain develops or if there is underlying cardiac or (particularly) coronary disease. Because reentry is the most common mechanism for paroxysmal atrial tachycardia, effective therapy requires that conduction be interrupted at some point in the reentry circuit.

A. Mechanical Measures: A variety of methods have been used to interrupt attacks, and patients may learn to perform these themselves. These include Valsalva's maneuver, stretching the arms and body, lowering the head between the knees, coughing, and breath holding. These maneuvers, as is true also of carotid sinus pressure (see below), stimulate the vagus, delay atrioventricular conduction, and block the reentry mechanism, terminating the arrhythmias.

B. Vagal Stimulation With Carotid Sinus Pressure: *Caution: This procedure should not be performed if the patient has carotid bruits or a history of transient cerebral ischemic attacks.* With the patient relaxed in the semirecumbent position, firm but gentle pressure and massage are applied first over the right carotid sinus for 10–20 seconds and then over the other. *Pressure should not be exerted on both carotid sinuses at the same time.* Continuous electrocardiographic or auscultatory monitoring of the heart rate is required so that carotid sinus pressure can be relieved as soon as the attack ceases or if excessive slowing occurs. Carotid sinus pressure will interrupt up to half the attacks, especially if the patient has been digitalized or sedated.

C. Drug Therapy: If mechanical measures fail, two rapidly acting intravenous agents will terminate more than 90% of episodes. Intravenous adenosine has a very brief duration of action and minimal nega-

tive inotropic activity. A 6-mg bolus is administered. If no response is observed after 1–2 minutes, a second and third 12-mg bolus should be given. Since the half-life of adenosine is less than 10 seconds, the drug must be given rapidly (in 1–2 seconds from a peripheral intravenous line). Adenosine is very well tolerated, but nearly 20% of patients will experience transient flushing, and some patients experience severe chest discomfort.

Calcium channel blockers also rapidly induce atrioventricular block and break most reentry supraventricular tachycardia. Intravenous verapamil may be given as a 2.5 mg-bolus, followed by additional doses of 2.5 mg to 5 mg every 1–3 minutes up to a total of 20 mg if blood pressure and rhythm are stable. If the rhythm recurs, further doses can be given. Oral verapamil, 80–120 mg every 4–6 hours, can be used as well in stable patients who are tolerating the rhythm without difficulty. Intravenous diltiazem (0.25 mg/kg over 2 minutes, followed by a second bolus of 0.35 mg/kg if necessary and then an infusion of 5/15 mg/h) may cause less hypotension and myocardial depression.

Esmolol, a short-acting beta-blocker, may also be effective; the initial dose is 500 μg/kg intravenously over 1 minute followed by an infusion of 25–200 μg/min. Parasympathetic stimulating drugs such as edrophonium, 5–10 mg intravenously, which delay atrioventricular conduction, may break the reentry mechanism. Because it frequently causes nausea and vomiting, it should be used only if the previously discussed agents fail. Metaraminol or phenylephrine, alpha-adrenergic stimulants that activate the baroreceptors by raising the blood pressure and causing vagal stimulation, can break attacks but should be used cautiously because they may provoke excessive hypertension. Digoxin is effective, but it often requires several hours to safely administer an adequate dose. An initial dose of 0.5–0.75 mg intravenously, followed by 0.25-mg or 0.125-mg increments every 2–4 hours up to a total of 1–1.25 mg, is used. Intravenous procainamide may terminate supraventricular tachycardia; however, since it facilitates atrioventricular conduction and an initial increase in rate may occur, it is usually not given until after digoxin, verapamil, or a beta-blocker has been administered. In patients with Wolff-Parkinson-White syndrome, in which an accessory pathway is involved, these agents may be contraindicated (see below).

D. Cardioversion: If the patient is hemodynamically stable or if adenosine and verapamil are contraindicated or ineffective, synchronized electrical cardioversion (beginning at 100 J) is almost universally successful. If digitalis toxicity is present or strongly suspected, as in the case of paroxysmal tachycardia with block, electrical cardioversion should be avoided.

Prevention of Attacks

A. Drugs: Digoxin orally is the usual drug of

first choice because of its convenience and efficacy. Verapamil, alone or in combination with digitalis, is a second choice. (*Note:* Verapamil increases digoxin serum levels.) Beta-blockers are also effective. Patients who do not respond to agents that increase refractoriness of the atrioventricular node may be treated with class Ia (disopyramide, quinidine, procainamide), class Ic (propafenone), or class III (sotalol, amiodarone) drugs. In patients with evidence of structural heart disease, either sotalol or amiodarone is probably a better choice because of the lower incidence of ventricular proarrhythmia during chronic therapy.

B. Radiofrequency Ablation: Because of concerns about the safety and the intolerability of antiarrhythmic medications, radiofrequency ablation is the preferred approach to patients with recurrent symptomatic reentry supraventricular tachycardia, whether it is due to dual pathways within the atrial ventricular node or to accessory pathways.

Feld GK: Catheter ablation for treatment of atrial tachycardia. Prog Cardiovasc Dis 1995;37:205. (General review with focus on new applications, such as automatic atrial tachycardia and atrial flutter.)

Ganz LI, Friedman PL: Supraventricular tachycardia. N Engl J Med 1995;332:162.

Kadish A, Goldberger J: Ablative therapy for atrioventricular nodal reentry arrhythmias. Prog Cardiovasc Dis 1995;37:273.

Piper SJ, Stanton MS: Narrow QRS complex tachycardias. Mayo Clin Proc 1995;70:371. (Simplified review for primary care physicians of the recognition and treatment of supraventricular tachycardias.)

5. SUPRAVENTRICULAR TACHYCARDIAS DUE TO ACCESSORY ATRIOVENTRICULAR PATHWAYS (Preexcitation Syndromes)

Pathophysiology & Clinical Findings

Accessory pathways between the atria and the ventricle which avoid the conduction delay of the atrioventricular node predispose to reentry tachycardias, such as paroxysmal supraventricular tachycardia and atrial flutter, and to atrial fibrillation. These may be wholly or partly within the node (Mahaim fibers), yielding a short PR interval and normal QRS morphology (**Lown-Ganong-Levine syndrome**). More commonly, they make direct connections between the atria and ventricle through Kent bundles (**Wolff-Parkinson-White syndrome**). This produces a short PR interval but an early delta wave at the onset of the wide, slurred QRS complex owing to early ventricular depolarization of the region adjacent to the pathway. While the morphology and polarity of the delta wave can suggest the location of the bypass tract, mapping by intracardiac recordings is required for precise anatomic localization.

Accessory pathways occur in 0.1–0.3% of the population and facilitate reentry arrhythmias owing to the disparity in refractory periods of the atrioventricular node and accessory pathway. Whether the tachycardia is associated with a narrow or wide QRS complex is determined by whether antegrade conduction is through the node (narrow) or the bypass tract (wide). Many patients with Wolff-Parkinson-White syndrome never conduct antegrade through the bypass tract which is therefore "concealed." Although reentry supraventricular tachycardias involving the atrioventricular node are commonest, 20–30% of patients with tachyarrhythmias have atrial fibrillation or flutter. Many have no arrhythmia. A minority of patients conduct antegrade through the accessory pathway, but these individuals may develop very fast rates, especially during atrial fibrillation. Patients with RR intervals less than 220 ms are at highest risk. Digoxin and, to a lesser extent, verapamil and beta-blockers may decrease accessory pathway refractoriness and increase ventricular response and should be avoided in atrial fibrillation with accessory pathways.

Treatment

A. Pharmacologic Therapy: Narrow complex reentry rhythms can be managed as discussed for paroxysmal supraventricular tachycardias other than atrial fibrillation or flutter. Adenosine has proved to be very effective; digoxin is best avoided in patients with known Wolff-Parkinson-White syndrome. The class Ia antiarrhythmics, as well as the newer class Ic and class III agents, will increase the refractoriness of the bypass tract and are the drugs of choice for wide-complex tachycardias. If hemodynamic compromise is present, electrical cardioversion is warranted.

Long-term therapy often involves a combination of agents that increase refractoriness in the bypass tract (class Ia or Ic agents) and in the atrioventricular node (verapamil, digoxin, and beta-blockers), provided that atrial fibrillation or flutter with short RR cycle lengths is not present (see above). Sotalol and amiodarone are effective in refractory cases. Patients who are difficult to manage should undergo electrophysiologic evaluation.

B. Radiofrequency Ablation: As with the supraventricular tachycardia with the reentry within the atrioventricular node, radiofrequency ablation has become the procedure of choice in patients with accessory pathways and recurrent symptomatic episodes. Patients with preexcitation syndromes who have episodes of atrial fibrillation or flutter should be tested by induction of atrial fibrillation in the electrophysiologic laboratory, noting duration of the RR cycle; if it is less than 220 ms, a short refractory period is present, and these individuals are at highest risk for sudden death, and prophylactic ablation is indicated. Success rates for ablation of accessory pathways with radiofrequency catheters exceed 90% in appropriate patients.

Cain ME et al: Diagnosis and localization of accessory pathways. PACE Pacing Clin Electrophysiol 1992; 15:801.

Munger TM et al: A population study of the natural history of Wolff-Parkinson-White syndrome in Olmstead County, Minnesota, 1953–1989. Circulation 1993;87: 866. (Sudden death is extremely rare in a population-based patient sample, arguing against overly aggressive intervention.)

Plumb VJ: Catheter ablation of the accessory pathways of the Wolff-Parkinson-White syndrome and its variants. Prog Cardiovasc Dis 1995;37:295.

6. ATRIAL FIBRILLATION

Atrial fibrillation is the commonest chronic arrhythmia. It occurs in rheumatic heart disease, dilated cardiomyopathy, atrial septal defect, hypertension, mitral valve prolapse, and hypertrophic cardiomyopathy as well as in patients with no apparent cardiac disease; it may be the initial presenting sign in thyrotoxicosis. Atrial fibrillation often appears paroxysmally before becoming the established rhythm. Pericarditis, chest trauma or surgery, or pulmonary disease (as well as medications such as theophylline and beta-adrenergic agonists) may cause attacks in patients with normal hearts. Acute alcohol excess and alcohol withdrawal—and, in predisposed individuals, even consumption of small amounts of alcohol—may precipitate atrial fibrillation. This syndrome, which is often termed "holiday heart," is usually transient and self-limited. Short-term rate control with digoxin usually suffices as treatment.

Atrial fibrillation is the only common arrhythmia in which the ventricular rate is rapid and the rhythm very irregular. The atrial rate is 400–600/min, but most impulses are blocked at the atrioventricular node. The ventricular response is completely irregular, ranging from 80 to 180/min in the untreated state. Because of the varying stroke volumes resulting from varying periods of diastolic filling, not all ventricular beats produce a palpable peripheral pulse. The difference between the apical rate and the pulse rate is the "pulse deficit"; this deficit is greater when the ventricular rate is high.

Acute Management

Depending upon the ventricular rate and the status of left ventricular function, the initial presentation of atrial fibrillation may precipitate cardiac decompensation or may be an incidental asymptomatic finding. The short-term complications in atrial fibrillation are primarily hemodynamic. In patients with valvular heart disease or left ventricular diastole or systolic dysfunction, rapid atrial fibrillation may lead to acute heart failure or pulmonary edema. Rapid ventricular rates may themselves cause progressive deterioration of left ventricular function, which is often reversible when the rate is controlled. These patients present with palpitations and a general feeling of discomfort.

Acute management includes determination of whether there is underlying cardiac disease, achieving rate control, and restoring sinus rhythm. Atrial fibrillation may be present in patients with valvular heart disease (particularly mitral stenosis or insufficiency), thyrotoxicosis, pulmonary embolism, and a variety of other cardiac diseases. It may be precipitated by alcohol ("holiday heart"). Atrial fibrillation without chest pain is an infrequent presentation of acute myocardial infarction, though it is not an uncommon finding in patients with coronary artery disease. Except with holiday heart or a transient precipitating cause, most patients with new onset of atrial fibrillation do not revert to sinus rhythm spontaneously. Unless the patient is unstable (either from ischemia or hypotension), the initial approach is usually rate control.

Acute rate control can be obtained with intravenous beta-blockers (metoprolol series in 5 mg boluses, or esmolol if there is concern for hemodynamic decompensation), intravenous verapamil or diltiazem, or intravenous digoxin (0.5–0.75 mg over 30–60 minutes, followed by 0.125–0.25 mg every 2–4 hours until rate is controlled). Electrical or pharmacologic cardioversion may be necessary if rate control cannot be achieved and the patient is experiencing ongoing ischemia or hemodynamic instability. However, if atrial fibrillation has been present for more than 48 hours, the risk of embolization during conversion to normal sinus rhythm increases. Transesophageal echocardiography can exclude atrial thrombi and identify patients at low risk or early cardioversion.

After rate control has been achieved and specific causes excluded, a decision must be made about whether to attempt conversion to sinus rhythm or to allow the patient to remain in atrial fibrillation. In most patients with new onset of atrial fibrillation—particularly if a reversible cause can be identified—at least one attempt at restoring sinus rhythm is warranted.

If the arrhythmia has been present for more than 48 hours, anticoagulation should be initiated and maintained for 3–4 weeks prior to cardioversion. An alternative strategy involves transesophageal echocardiography and early cardioversion in individuals without evidence of left atrial thrombi.

There are now several options for elective cardioversion. In patients who have been anticoagulated for a sufficient time or when thrombi have been excluded, pharmacologic conversion can be attempted. The most immediately effective option is the intravenous administration of the short-acting class III agent ibutilide. This medication is infused rapidly (1 mg followed by an additional 0.5–1 mg if sinus rhythm has not been restored in 10 minutes) and converts approximately 40% of patients in atrial fibrillation to sinus rhythm within a period of 3 hours. Other medical options for cardioversion include class Ic or Ia agents, sotalol, and amiodarone. With the exception of amiodarone, all these drugs should be initiated in the hospital with electrocardiographic monitoring in patients with known cardiac disease. Amiodarone can usually be initiated on an outpatient basis, but it is the agent of choice only when chronic therapy is planned.

Electrical cardioversion is another alternative. It is employed in patients who failed to respond to pharmacologic treatment. An initial shock with 100–200 J is administered in synchrony with the R wave. If sinus rhythm is not restored, an additional attempt with 360 J is indicated. If these attempts are unsuccessful, acute loading with a class I antiarrhythmic, such as procainamide, may be tried.

There is now available another option, ie, the intravenous administration of the short-acting class III agent ibutilide. This medication is infused rapidly (1 mg followed by an additional 0.5–1 mg) and converts approximately 50% of patients to sinus rhythm in a period of 3 hours. Patients who remain in atrial fibrillation are candidates for electrical cardioversion.

Since atrial function returns only gradually following cardioversion, there continues to be an increased incidence of thromboembolic events. Therefore, warfarin anticoagulation is required for 4–6 weeks following cardioversion. Only about 25% of patients who are converted from atrial fibrillation will remain in sinus rhythm after 1 year, and this number can be increased to 40–50% with chronic antiarrhythmic therapy. However, the risks of chronic antiarrhythmic therapy may more than outweigh this small advantage. In patients in whom there is a precipitating factor for the episode of atrial fibrillation or in whom there is no apparent cardiac disease, it may be worthwhile to withhold antiarrhythmic therapy or to utilize a beta-blocker or digoxin. Although these latter agents have not been proved to maintain sinus rhythm, they would at least limit the ventricular response of atrial fibrillation if it recurs. If atrial fibrillation does return, then the choice between chronic atrial fibrillation with anticoagulation and rate control and the use of antiarrhythmic therapy to remain in sinus rhythm must be made. In patients with structural heart disease, the recurrence of atrial fibrillation is likely to warrant prophylactic antiarrhythmic therapy if maintenance of sinus rhythm is the objective. However, in these patients, the risk of class I agents is highest, and for that reason amiodarone may be the agent of choice.

Treatment of Chronic Atrial Fibrillation

The disadvantages of chronic atrial fibrillation are primarily two: symptoms related to the arrhythmias and the increased risk of thromboembolic phenomena. With adequate rate control, most patients are not particularly symptomatic, though exercise tolerance may be limited to some degree in active individuals. Rate control is usually obtained with either digoxin, a beta-blocker, or a calcium channel blocker. Digoxin reduces the ventricular response quite nicely at rest but is less effective in controlling the ventricular rate with exercise or activity. Thus, in active individuals, a beta-blocker or calcium blocker is probably the initial agent of choice, though realistically most patients

with normally functioning atrioventricular nodes will require two agents for optimal rate control. In occasional individuals, rate control cannot be achieved. In these, one may add amiodarone, which at low doses effectively further reduces the ventricular response; or radiofrequency modification of the atrioventricular node may be performed. This latter procedure is sometimes complicated by complete heart block and the requirement for a pacemaker, but in any case ventricular rate control can be achieved.

Atrial fibrillation is a major risk factor for stroke as a result of a multifold increase in thromboembolic phenomena. The risk of stroke and other thrombotic events ranges from as low as 2–3% to as high as 20% per year. The factors that increase the risk of stroke include mitral valve disease, increasing age, reduced left ventricular function and heart failure, hypertension, and diabetes. Patients with "lone" atrial fibrillation (atrial fibrillation in the absence of cardiac disease, hypertension, or diabetes) below the age of 60 are at low risk for embolization and do not require anticoagulation, though many physicians would utilize aspirin 325 mg/d in such individuals. Antithrombotic therapy has been shown to reduce the risk of stroke in virtually all other subgroups of patients with chronic atrial fibrillation. In trials where warfarin and aspirin have been compared, warfarin has been consistently more effective in reducing thromboembolic events. However, the risk of bleeding, including hemorrhagic strokes, is higher with warfarin. Based on the experience of several large trials, it is recommended that patients at higher risk for strokes (patients with hypertension, heart failure and left ventricular dysfunction, prior emboli, and diabetes) should be treated with warfarin. While even in the absence of these risk factors men above the age of 70 have an increased risk for stroke, the bleeding rate with warfarin makes aspirin a suitable alternative. As yet, the evidence is inadequate to show whether aspirin and warfarin are equivalent in women over age 75 without other risk factors for stroke.

Albers GW: Atrial fibrillation and stroke. Arch Intern Med 1994;154:1443. (Review of recent studies, with recommendations for anticoagulation. See analysis of pooled data from five trials on p 1449 of same issue.)

Blackshear JL et al: Management of atrial fibrillation in adults: Prevention of thromboembolism and systematic treatment. Mayo Clin Proc 1996;71:150. (Review of current data and recommendations.)

Gilligan DM et al: The management of atrial fibrillation. Am J Med 1996;101:413. (Concise, practical "how-to" article.)

Hylek EM et al: Analysis of the lowest effective intensity of prophylactic anticoagulation for patients with non-rheumatic atrial fibrillation. N Engl J Med 1996; 335:540. (Optimal INR is between 2.0 and 3.0. Lower levels are associated with increased thromboembolic complications and higher levels with increased rates of hemorrhagic complications.)

Klein AL et al: Cardioversion guided by transesophageal echocardiography: The Acute Pilot Study. Ann Intern

Med 1997;126:200. (Multicenter study involving 126 patients with atrial fibrillation demonstrating that cardioversion can be accomplished more rapidly and without prior anticoagulation in patients without evidence of atrial thrombi on transesophageal echocardiography. However, anticoagulation for at least 1 month postconversion is essential.)

Prystowsky EN et al: Management of patients with atrial fibrillation. Circulation 1996;93:1262. (American Heart Association consensus statement covering epidemiology, pathophysiology, acute therapy, and long-term management of this common disorder.)

Stambler BS et al: Efficacy and safety of repeated intravenous doses of ibutilide for rapid conversion of atrial flutter or fibrillation. Circulation 1996;94:1613. (Multicenter study showing that ibutilide successfully converted 40–50% of patients in atrial fibrillation and a higher percentage of those in atrial flutter.)

Zarembski DG et al: Treatment of resistant atrial fibrillation. Arch Intern Med 1995;155:1885. (This overview of seven prospective studies indicates that 60% of patients treated with amiodarone remain in sinus rhythm at 12 months. This seems superior to class I agents.)

7. ATRIAL FLUTTER

Atrial flutter is less common than fibrillation and usually occurs in patients with COPD, rheumatic or coronary heart disease, congestive heart failure, or atrial septal defect. Ectopic impulse formation occurs at atrial rates of 250–350/min, with transmission of every second, third, or fourth impulse through the atrioventricular node to the ventricles. Ventricular rate control is accomplished using the same agents utilized in atrial fibrillation, but it is much more difficult with atrial flutter than with atrial fibrillation. Conversion of atrial flutter to sinus rhythm with class I antiarrhythmic agents is also difficult to achieve, and administration of these drugs has been associated with slowing of the atrial flutter rate to the point where 1:1 atrioventricular conduction can occur at rates in excess of 200/min, with subsequent hemodynamic collapse. The intravenous class III antiarrhythmic agent ibutilide has been significantly more successful in converting atrial flutter. About 50–70% of patients return to sinus rhythm within 60–90 minutes following the infusion of 1–2 mg of this agent. Electrical cardioversion is also very effective for atrial flutter, with approximately 90% of patients converting following shocks of as little as 25–50 J.

The persistence of atrial contractile function in this arrhythmia provides some protection against thrombus formation, though the risk of systemic embolization remains slightly increased. Precardioversion anticoagulation is usually not necessary for atrial flutter of short duration except in the setting of mitral valve disease. However, anticoagulation is prudent in chronic atrial flutter, particularly since transient periods of atrial fibrillation are common in these patients.

Chronic atrial flutter is often a difficult management problem, since rate control is difficult. Amio-

darone is probably the pharmacologic agent of choice, since it has the potential of both maintaining sinus rhythm and helping with rate control when flutter recurs. Experience with the use of radiofrequency ablation to interrupt the atrial flutter circuit is growing, and it is likely that this will become the procedure of choice for patients with chronic or recurring atrial flutter.

Olshansky B et al: Atrial flutter: Update on the mechanism and treatment. PACE Pacing Clin Electrophysiol 1992;15:2308.

Saxon LA et al: Results of radiofrequency catheter ablation for atrial flutter. Am J Cardiol 1996;77:1014. (Results in 51 patients, showing an 86% initial success rate but a 22% recurrence rate and a 34% requirement for continued antiarrhythmic therapy following ablation.)

8. MULTIFOCAL (CHAOTIC) ATRIAL TACHYCARDIA

This is a rhythm characterized by varying P-wave morphology (by definition, three or more foci) and markedly irregular PP intervals. The rate is usually between 100 and 140/min, and atrioventricular block is unusual. Most patients have severe associated illnesses, especially COPD. Treatment of the underlying condition is the most effective approach; verapamil, 240–480 mg daily in divided doses, is also of value in some patients.

Kastor JA: Multifocal atrial tachycardia. N Engl J Med 1990;322:1713.

9. ATRIOVENTRICULAR JUNCTIONAL RHYTHM

The atrial-nodal junction or the nodal-His bundle junctions may assume pacemaker activity for the heart, usually at a rate of 40–60/min. This may occur in patients with myocarditis, coronary artery disease, and digitalis toxicity as well as in individuals with normal hearts. The rate responds normally to exercise, and the diagnosis is often an incidental finding on electrocardiographic monitoring, but it can be suspected if the jugular venous pulse shows cannon *a* waves. Junctional rhythm is often an escape rhythm because of depressed sinus node function with sinoatrial block or delayed conduction in the atrioventricular node. **Nonparoxysmal junctional tachycardia** results from increased automaticity of the junctional tissues in digitalis toxicity or ischemia and is associated with a narrow QRS complex and a rate usually less than 120–130/min. It is usually considered benign when it occurs in acute myocardial infarction, but the ischemia that induces it may also cause ventricular tachycardia and ventricular fibrillation.

VENTRICULAR ARRHYTHMIAS

1. VENTRICULAR PREMATURE BEATS (Ventricular Extrasystoles)

Ventricular premature beats are similar to atrial premature beats in mechanism and manifestations but are more common. They are characterized by wide QRS complexes that differ in morphology from the patient's normal beats. They are usually not preceded by a P wave, although retrograde ventriculoatrial conduction may occur. Unless the latter is present, there is a fully compensatory pause. Bigeminy and trigeminy are arrhythmias in which every second or third beat is premature. Exercise generally abolishes premature beats in normal hearts, and the rhythm becomes regular. The patient may or may not sense the irregular beat, usually as a skipped beat. Ambulatory electrocardiographic monitoring or monitoring during graded exercise may reveal more frequent and complex ventricular premature beats than occur in a single routine ECG.

Sudden death occurs more frequently (presumably as a result of ventricular fibrillation) when ventricular premature beats occur in the presence of organic heart disease but not in individuals with no known cardiac disease. If no associated cardiac disease is present and if the ectopic beats are asymptomatic, no therapy is indicated. If they are frequent, electrolyte abnormalities (especially hypo- or hyperkalemia and hypomagnesemia), hyperthyroidism, and occult heart disease should be excluded. Pharmacologic treatment is then indicated only for patients who are symptomatic. Because of concerns about worsening arrhythmia and sudden death with most antiarrhythmic agents, beta-blockers are the agents of first choice. If symptoms such as palpations or skipped beats occur, beta-blockers may be helpful in asymptomatic patients with very frequent ventricular ectopy or repetitive forms. If the underlying condition is mitral prolapse, hypertrophic cardiomyopathy, left ventricular hypertrophy, or coronary disease—or if the QT interval is prolonged—a trial of a beta-blocker may be worthwhile even though these agents are often unsuccessful. The class I and III agents (see Table 10–8) are all effective in reducing ventricular premature beats but often cause side effects and may exacerbate arrhythmias in 5–20% of patients. Therefore, every attempt should be made to avoid using class I or III antiarrhythmic agents in patients without symptoms.

Campbell RW: Ventricular ectopic beats and non-sustained ventricular tachycardia. Lancet 1993;341:1454.

Sung RJ et al: Ventricular arrhythmias in the absence of organic heart disease. Cardiovasc Clin 1992;22(1):149. (Prognosis is excellent; treatment indicated only for symptoms.)

2. VENTRICULAR TACHYCARDIA

Ventricular tachycardia is defined as three or more consecutive ventricular premature beats. The usual rate is 160–240/min and is moderately regular but less so than atrial tachycardia. Carotid sinus pressure has no effect. The distinction from aberrant conduction of supraventricular tachycardia may be difficult and is discussed above. The usual mechanism is reentry, but abnormally triggered rhythms occur. Ventricular tachycardia is either *nonsustained* (lasting less than 30 seconds) or *sustained*. It may be asymptomatic or associated with syncope or milder symptoms of impaired cerebral perfusion.

Ventricular tachycardia is a frequent complication of acute myocardial infarction and dilated cardiomyopathy but may occur in hypertrophic cardiomyopathy, mitral valve prolapse, myocarditis, and in most other forms of myocardial disease. **Torsade de pointes,** a form of ventricular tachycardia in which QRS morphology varies, may occur spontaneously or after quinidine or any drug that prolongs the QT interval; it has a particularly poor prognosis. In nonacute settings, most patients with ventricular tachycardia have known or easily detected cardiac disease, and the finding of ventricular tachycardia is an unfavorable prognostic sign.

Treatment

A. Acute Ventricular Tachycardia: The treatment of acute ventricular tachycardia is determined by the degree of hemodynamic compromise and the duration of the arrhythmia. The management of ventricular tachycardia in acute infarction has been discussed. In other patients, if hypotension, heart failure, or angina is present, synchronized DC cardioversion with 100–360 J should be performed immediately. If the patient is tolerating the rhythm, lidocaine, 1 mg/kg as an intravenous bolus injection, may terminate it. If the patient is stable and lidocaine is not effective, a trial of intravenous procainamide, 100 mg intravenously slowly every 5 minutes (up to 1000 mg), followed by an infusion of 20–80 μg/kg/min, or bretylium, 5 mg/kg intravenously over 3–5 minutes, repeated after 20 minutes if necessary, followed by an infusion of 1–2 mg/min, may be successful. Ventricular tachycardia can be terminated by ventricular overdrive pacing, and this approach is useful when the rhythm is recurrent.

Intravenous amiodarone is often effective when these approaches are not. This formulation is much more bioavailable than the oral form, so more rapid loading can be achieved. It is usually initiated with a rapid loading infusion of 150 mg over 10 minutes, followed by a slow infusion of 1 mg/min for 6 hours and then a maintenance infusion of 0.5 mg/min for an additional 18–42 hours. Supplemental infusions of 150 mg over 10 minutes can be given for recurrent ventricular tachycardia. However, because the cost of a full loading dose approaches $1000 a day, rapid oral loading (200 mg every 2 hours for a total of 2400 mg/d) may be sufficient except in unstable patients.

B. Chronic Recurrent Ventricular Tachycardia: The treatment of recurrent, **nonsustained ventricular tachycardia** (runs of three or more beats lasting less than 30 seconds) not associated with symptoms is controversial. In subjects without heart disease, this rhythm is not clearly associated with a poor prognosis, whereas in patients with organic heart disease, it is a marker for increased mortality rates from the underlying disease and, in some studies, from arrhythmias. Whether antiarrhythmic therapy is beneficial in these patients with nonsustained ventricular tachycardia is unclear, but it is often initiated. In the patient with coronary artery disease post myocardial infarction, the risk for developing symptomatic ventricular tachycardia or sudden death can be stratified with moderate success. A major factor is the degree of left ventricular dysfunction, since patients with left ventricular ejection fractions of 35–40% have a low rate of sudden death. In the recently terminated MADIT trial, patients with coronary disease, nonsustained ventricular tachycardia, and reduced left ventricular ejection fraction who were found to have inducible monomorphic ventricular tachycardia that was not suppressed by acute loading with intravenous procainamide were randomized to pharmacologic therapy (predominantly amiodarone) or an implantable cardiac defibrillator. Survival free of life-threatening arrhythmia was significantly better with an implantable defibrillator than with antiarrhythmic drug therapy. However, additional data will be required before devices are routinely used in this potentially large asymptomatic population. The lack of occurrence of late potentials on the noninvasively recorded signal-averaged ECG usually implies a good prognosis; however, many patients with late potentials and left ventricular dysfunction also will not become symptomatic, and late potentials are of little prognostic value in patients without coronary artery disease. One strategy is to perform ventricular stimulation in the high-risk patients. Patients with inducible sustained ventricular tachycardia should be treated. Given current data, treatment of patients with nonsustained ventricular arrhythmias should be limited to patients who are either symptomatic or have inducible sustained arrhythmias. In these, class Ia agents have traditionally been the initial approach; class Ib agents are less successful, and class Ic agents have a greater risk of inducing proarrhythmias (Table 10–8). Beta-blockers are occasionally effective. More recent data favor the class III agents, sotalol or amiodarone, because proarrhythmia may be less frequent and because the latter agent has improved outcomes in some studies. The efficacy of treatment is assessed by ambulatory electrocardiographic monitoring or repeat stimulation studies. The signal-averaged ECG has not proved useful for monitoring therapy.

Patients with symptomatic or asymptomatic **sustained ventricular tachycardia** require effective suppressive therapy. To develop a therapeutic regimen, the rhythm either must be present spontaneously or be induced by programmed stimulation in the electrophysiology laboratory. The recent ESVEM (Electrophysiology Study Versus Electrocardiography Monitoring) study suggests that either approach is appropriate, but neither is optimal. Various antiarrhythmic drugs can then be given in sequence to determine which agents prevent ventricular tachycardia. Drugs that prevent the electrical induction of ventricular tachycardia in the laboratory or suppress its occurrence during monitoring are more likely to be effective in vivo for long-term therapy; some agents, such as sotalol and amiodarone, may still be effective even if the arrhythmia is not fully prevented in the laboratory. This is the case especially with amiodarone, which has emerged as the most effective agent for this select group of patients. The potential of all antiarrhythmia drugs to exacerbate ventricular arrhythmias in some patients should be kept in mind in initiating and monitoring therapy.

Patients with sustained ventricular tachycardia who do not respond to or tolerate antiarrhythmic medications are candidates for an implantable cardioverter defibrillator, which can be programmed to sense tachycardia above a predetermined rate. It then attempts to terminate the arrhythmia by antitachycardia pacing or to deliver a shock if pacing has not been successful or if ventricular fibrillation supervenes. Transvenous lead systems are now satisfactory for most patients. The availability of these more versatile and convenient devices, coupled with growing recognition of the limitations of antiarrhythmic drugs, has increased enthusiasm for implantable cardioverter defibrillator therapy. While data are accumulating suggesting an advantage for this procedure, amiodarone, the most effective antiarrhythmic agent, failed to prolong survival in two recent studies in high-risk post-myocardial infarction patients and in one of two studies in congestive heart failure patients. Thus, these devices are the therapy of choice for patients who survive sudden death episodes not precipitated by acute myocardial infarction. However, controversy persists about whether implantable cardioverter defibrillators or antiarrhythmic medications should be the initial therapy for symptomatic or asymptomatic sustained ventricular tachycardia, particularly in light of the high cost of the devices and their implantation (approximately $30,000).

The Multicenter Automatic Defibrillator Implantation Trial (MADIT) has broadened this controversy to include patients who have never had symptomatic arrhythmia or sustained ventricular arrhythmias. This trial studied post-myocardial infarction patients with an ejection fraction of ≤ 35% and nonsustained ventricular tachycardia. They also had inducible sustained tachycardia that could not be suppressed by acute drug therapy in the electrophysiology laboratory, survival was improved with an implantable cardioverter defibrillator as opposed to a nonspecified regimen of "conventional" therapy. Neither the number nor the outcomes of the patients who were noninducible or who were suppressible are known. Furthermore, only a minority of patients were treated with beta-blocker therapy, and the higher number of nondevice patients receiving potentially deleterious antiarrhythmic drugs for an unconventional indication must be considered. Thus, without collaboration from ongoing trials, implantable cardioverter defibrillator therapy for asymptomatic patients without sustained arrhythmias cannot be recommended.

It is now possible to ablate some forms of ventricular tachycardia, particularly those that originate in the right ventricular outflow tract (appearing as a left bundle branch block with inferior axis morphology), posterior fascicle (RBBB, superior axis morphology), or sustained by bundle branch reentry. As experience grows, it is likely that other forms of ventricular tachycardia, including those that are associated with coronary disease, will be successfully treated by ablation. Surgical resection or isolation of the focus of ventricular tachycardia is performed in a few centers but is associated with substantial risk and mixed results.

3. VENTRICULAR FIBRILLATION

The acute treatment of ventricular fibrillation is discussed under complications of myocardial infarction, and the chronic management of survivors is discussed under survivors of sudden death.

Griffith MJ et al: Ventricular tachycardia as a default diagnosis in broad complex tachycardia. Lancet 1994; 343:386. (LBBB morphology indicates ventricular tachycardia; RBBB with rSR' in V_1 and RS in V_6 suggests supraventricular origin.)

Hamdan M, Scheinman M: Current approaches in patients with ventricular tachyarrhythmias. Med Clin North Am 1995;79:1097. (Practical approach to ventricular ectopy and nonsustained and sustained ventricular tachycardia in patients with and without structural heart disease.)

Klein LS, Miles WM: Ablative therapy for ventricular arrhythmias. Prog Cardiovasc Dis 1995;37:225. (Current review in an evolving area.)

Moss AJ et al: Improved survival with an implanted defibrillator in patients with coronary disease at high risk for ventricular arrhythmia. N Engl J Med 1996;335:1933. (The MADIT trial publication—see text.)

Owens DK et al: Cost-effectiveness of implantable cardioverter defibrillators relative to amiodarone for prevention of sudden cardiac death. Ann Intern Med 1997;126:1. (Economic analysis suggesting that use of an implantable cardioverter defibrillator will cost more than $50,000 per quality-adjusted life year gained unless it reduces all-cause mortality by 30% or more in comparison with amiodarone.)

Saksena F et al: Implantable cardioverter-defibrillators are preferable to drugs as primary therapy in sustained tachyarrhythmias. Prog Cardiovasc Dis 1996;38:445. (Review of current data in support of this argument).

See also references following the section below on evaluation of syncope and survivors of sudden death.

4. ACCELERATED IDIOVENTRICULAR RHYTHM

Accelerated idioventricular rhythm is a relatively regular wide complex rhythm with a rate of 60–120/min, usually with a gradual onset. Because the rate is often similar to the sinus rate, fusion beats and alternating rhythms are common. Two mechanisms have been invoked: (1) an escape rhythm due to suppression of higher pacemakers resulting from sinoatrial and atrioventricular block or from depressed sinus node function; and (2) slow ventricular tachycardia due to increased automaticity or, less frequently, reentry. It occurs commonly in acute infarction and following reperfusion after thrombolytic drugs. The incidence of associated ventricular fibrillation is much less than that of ventricular tachycardia with a rapid rate, and treatment is not indicated unless there is hemodynamic compromise or more serious arrhythmias. This rhythm also is common in digitalis toxicity.

Accelerated idioventricular rhythm must be distinguished from the idioventricular or junctional rhythm with rates less than 40–45/min that occurs in the presence of complete atrioventricular block. Atrioventricular dissociation—where ventricular rate exceeds sinus—but not atrioventricular block occurs in most cases of accelerated idioventricular rhythm.

5. LONG QT SYNDROME

Idiopathic long QT syndrome is an uncommon disease that was first described in deaf siblings. It is characterized by recurrent syncope, a long QT interval (usually 0.5–0.7 s), documented ventricular arrhythmias, and sudden death. The sympathetic nervous system (especially the left stellate ganglion) may be important in pathogenesis.

Beta-blockers are the most effective therapy for "congenital" long QT syndrome, though phenytoin and the class Ib agents have also been beneficial. Agents that prolong the QT (classes Ia, Ic, and III) are contraindicated. Refractory acute arrhythmic episodes may be treated by local anesthetic block of the left stellate ganglion, and recurrent episodes can be treated by resection of this ganglion as well as of the first three to five thoracic ganglia.

Acquired long QT interval secondary to use of antiarrhythmic agents or antidepressant drugs, electrolyte abnormalities, myocardial ischemia, or significant bradycardia may result in ventricular tachycardia (torsade de pointes, ie, twisting about the baseline into varying QRS morphology). The role of a prolonged QT interval is difficult to evaluate because classes Ia, Ic, and III antiarrhythmic agents increase the QT interval and yet are effective in treating the ventricular tachyarrhythmias; it may be the reason that these drugs paradoxically cause ventricular tachycardia in some patients. Acquired QT interval prolongation requires further study, but prudence speaks against continuing therapy that prolongs the QT interval beyond 500 ms.

The management of **torsade de pointes** differs from that of other forms of ventricular tachycardia. Class I, Ic, or III antiarrhythmics, which prolong the QT interval, should be avoided—or withdrawn immediately if being used. Intravenous beta-blockers may be effective, especially in the congenital form; intravenous magnesium has also worked. An effective approach is temporary ventricular or atrial pacing, which can both break and prevent the rhythm.

Ben-David J, Zipes DP: Torsades de pointes and proarrhythmia. Lancet 1993;341:1578.
Schwartz PJ et al: Diagnostic criteria for long QT syndrome: An update. Circulation 1993:88:782.

CONDUCTION DISTURBANCES

Abnormalities of conduction can occur between the sinus node and atrium, within the atrioventricular node, and in the intraventricular conduction pathways.

SICK SINUS SYNDROME

This imprecise diagnosis is applied to patients with sinus arrest, sinoatrial exit block (recognized by a pause equal to a multiple of the underlying PP interval or progressive shortening of the PP interval prior to a pause), or persistent sinus bradycardia. These rhythms are often caused or exacerbated by drug therapy (digitalis, calcium channel blockers, beta-blockers, sympatholytic agents, antiarrhythmics), and agents that may be responsible should be withdrawn prior to making the diagnosis. Another presentation is of recurrent supraventricular tachycardias (paroxysmal reentry tachycardias, atrial flutter, and atrial fibrillation), associated with bradyarrhythmias ("tachy-brady syndrome"). The long pauses that often follow the termination of tachycardia cause the associated symptoms.

The electrocardiographic features of sick sinus syndrome are noted mostly in elderly patients. The pathologic changes are usually nonspecific, characterized by patchy fibrosis of the sinus node and cardiac conduction system. Cardiac amyloidosis also preferentially affects these structures. Sick sinus syndrome may also be caused by other conditions, including sarcoidosis, amyloidosis, Chagas' disease, and various cardiomyopathies. Coronary disease is an uncommon cause.

Most patients with electrocardiographic evidence of sick sinus syndrome are asymptomatic, but rare individuals may experience syncope, dizziness, confusion, palpitations, heart failure, or angina. Because these symptoms are either nonspecific or are due to other causes, it is essential that they be demonstrated to coincide temporally with arrhythmias. This may require prolonged ambulatory monitoring or the use of an event recorder. Pharmacologic therapy for sick sinus syndrome has been difficult, but recent studies have indicated that oral theophylline may be effective, especially when sinus bradycardia is the major manifestation. Most symptomatic patients will require permanent pacing. Dual-chamber pacing is preferred because ventricular pacing is associated with a higher incidence of subsequent atrial fibrillation, and subsequent atrioventricular block occurs at a rate of 2% per year. Treatment of associated tachyarrhythmias is often difficult without first instituting pacing, since digoxin and other antiarrhythmic agents may exacerbate the bradycardia. Unfortunately, symptomatic relief following pacing has not been consistent, largely because of inadequate documentation of the etiologic role of bradyarrhythmias in producing the symptom. Furthermore, many of these patients may have associated ventricular arrhythmias that may require treatment; however, carefully selected patients may become asymptomatic with permanent pacing alone.

Brandt J et al: Natural history of sinus node diseases treated with atrial pacing in 213 patients: Implications for selection of stimulation mode. Am J Cardiol 1992;20:633. (Atrial fibrillation and atrioventricular block both occur fairly frequently, suggesting that dual-chamber pacing is the optimal mode.)
Sneddon JF, Camm AJ: Sinus node disease: Current concepts in diagnosis and therapy. Drugs 1992;44:728.

ATRIOVENTRICULAR BLOCK

Atrioventricular block is categorized as first-degree (PR interval > 0.21 s with all atrial impulses conducted), second-degree (intermittent blocked beats), or third-degree (complete heart block, in which no supraventricular impulses are conducted to the ventricles).

Second-degree block is subclassified. In **Mobitz type I (Wenckebach)** atrioventricular block, the atrioventricular conduction time (PR interval) progressively lengthens, with the RR interval shortening, before the blocked beat; this phenomenon is almost always due to abnormal conduction within the atrioventricular node. **Mobitz type II** atrioventricular block is abrupt and is not preceded by a lengthening atrioventricular conduction time; it is usually due to block within the His bundle system. The classification as Mobitz type I or Mobitz type II is only partially reliable, because patients may appear to have both types on the surface ECG, and one cannot predict the site of origin of the 2:1 atrioventricular block from the ECG. The width of the QRS complexes assists in determining whether the block is nodal or infranodal. When they are narrow, the block is usually nodal; when they are wide, the block is usually infranodal. Electrophysiologic studies may be necessary for accurate localization. Management of atrioventricular block in acute myocardial infarction has already been discussed. This section deals with patients in the nonacute setting.

First-degree and **Mobitz type I block** may occur in normal individuals with heightened vagal tone. They may also occur as a drug effect (especially digitalis, calcium channel blockers, beta-blockers, or other sympatholytic agents), often superimposed on organic disease. These disturbances also occur transiently or chronically due to ischemia, infarction, inflammatory processes, fibrosis, calcification, or infiltration. The prognosis is usually good, since reliable alternative pacemakers arise from the atrioventricular junction below the level of block if higher degrees of block occur.

Mobitz type II block is almost always due to organic disease involving the infranodal conduction system. In the event of progression to complete heart block, alternative pacemakers are not reliable. Thus, prophylactic ventricular pacing is required.

Complete (third-degree) heart block is a more advanced form of block often due to a lesion distal to the His bundle and associated with bilateral bundle branch block. The QRS is wide and the ventricular rate is slower, usually less than 50/min. Transmission of atrial impulses through the atrioventricular node is completely blocked, and a ventricular pacemaker maintains a slow, regular ventricular rate, usually less than 45/min. Exercise does not increase the rate. The first heart sound varies in intensity; wide pulse pressure, a changing systolic blood pressure level, and cannon venous pulsations in the neck are also present. Patients may be asymptomatic or may complain of weakness or dyspnea if the rate is less than 35/min; symptoms may occur at higher rates if the left ventricle cannot increase its stroke output. During periods of transition from partial to complete heart block, some patients have ventricular asystole that lasts several seconds to minutes. Syncope occurs abruptly.

Patients with episodic or chronic infranodal complete heart block require permanent pacing, and temporary pacing is indicated if implantation is delayed.

ATRIOVENTRICULAR DISSOCIATION

When a ventricular pacemaker is firing at a rate faster than or close to the sinus rate (accelerated id-ioventricular rhythm, ventricular premature beats, or ventricular tachycardia), atrial impulses arriving at the atrioventricular node when it is refractory may not be conducted. This phenomenon is atrioventricular dissociation but does not necessarily indicate atrioventricular block. No treatment is required aside from management of the causative arrhythmia.

INTRAVENTRICULAR CONDUCTION DEFECTS

Intraventricular conduction defects, including bundle branch block, are common in individuals with otherwise normal hearts and in many disease processes, including ischemic heart disease, inflammatory disease, infiltrative disease, cardiomyopathy, and postcardiotomy. Below the atrioventricular node and bundle of His, the conduction system trifurcates into a right bundle and anterior and posterior fascicles of the left bundle. Conduction block in each of these fascicles can be recognized on the surface ECG. Although such conduction abnormalities are often seen in normal hearts, they are more commonly due to organic heart disease—either an isolated process of fibrosis and calcification or more generalized myocardial disease. Bifascicular block is present when two of these—right bundle, left anterior and posterior hemibundle—are involved. Trifascicular block is defined as right bundle branch block with alternating left hemiblock, alternating right and left bundle branch block, or bifascicular block with documented prolonged infranodal conduction (long HV interval).

The prognosis of intraventricular block is generally that of the underlying myocardial process. Patients with no apparent heart disease have an overall survival rate similar to that of matched controls. However, left bundle branch block—but not right—is associated with a higher risk of development of overt cardiac disease and cardiac mortality. Even in bifascicular block, the incidence of occult complete heart block or progression to it is low, and pacing is not usually warranted. In patients with symptoms (eg, syncope) consistent with heart block and intraventricular block, pacing should be reserved for those with documented concomitant complete heart block on monitoring or those with a very prolonged HV interval (> 90 ms) with no other cause for symptoms. Even in the latter group, prophylactic pacing has not improved the prognosis significantly, probably because of the high incidence of ventricular arrhythmias in the same population.

PERMANENT PACING

The indications for permanent pacing have been discussed: symptomatic bradyarrhythmias, asymptomatic Mobitz II atrioventricular block, or complete heart block. The versatility of pacemaker generator units has increased markedly, and dual-chamber multiple programmable units being implanted with increasing frequency. A standardized nomenclature for pacemaker generators is employed, usually consisting of four letters. The first letter refers to the chamber which is simulated (A = atrium, V = ventricle, D = dual, for both). The second letter refers to the chamber where sensing occurs (also A, V, or D). The third position refers to the sensory mode (I = inhibition by a sensed impulse, T = triggering by a sensed impulse, D = dual modes of response). The fourth letter refers to the programmability or rate modulation capacity (usually P for programming for two functions, M for programming more than two, and R for rate modulation).

Conceptually, a pacemaker that senses and paces in both chambers is the most physiologic approach to pacing patients who remain in sinus rhythm. However, because of the substantially greater cost and complexity of dual-chamber pacing and the shorter projected battery life, they should be used chiefly in patients in whom atrial contraction produces a substantial increment in stroke volume and to those in whom sensing the atrial rate to provide rate-responsive ventricular pacing is useful. Dual-chamber pacing is most useful for individuals with left ventricular systolic or—perhaps more importantly—diastolic dysfunction and for physically active individuals. In patients with single-chamber pacemakers, the lack of an atrial kick may lead to the so-called pacemaker syndrome, in which the patient experiences signs of low cardiac output while upright. Uncontrolled data suggest that chronic dual-chamber pacing is associated with a lower incidence of chronic atrial fibrillation than single-chamber ventricular pacing. However, patients in whom pacing is primarily prophylactic should undergo ventricular pacing.

Pulse generators are also available that can increase their rate in response to motion or respiratory rate when the atrial rate is not an indication of the optimal heart rate. These are most useful in active individuals. Pacers are also available that can increase their rate in response to motion or respiratory rate when the atrial rate is not an indication of optimal heart rate. However, patients with intermittent or potential bradyarrhythmias or conduction disturbances in whom pacing is primarily prophylactic should undergo ventricular pacing. Follow-up after pacemaker implantation, usually by telephonic monitoring, is essential. All pulse generators and lead systems have an early failure rate that is now below 5% as well as a finite life expectancy varying from 4 to 10 years.

Ellenbogan K et al (editors): *Clinical Cardiac Pacing.* Saunders, 1995. (Monograph covering all aspects of pacing, from technology to clinical applications.)

Fahy GJ et al: Natural history of isolated bundle branch block. Am J Cardiol 1996;77:1185.

Glikson M et al: Expanding indications for permanent pacemakers. Ann Intern Med 1995;123:443. (Literature review on emerging and experimental uses of permanent pacemakers, such as dilated cardiomyopathy, prevention of atrial fibrillation, long QT syndrome, and vasovagal syncope.)

Kusumoto FM, Goldschlager N: Cardiac pacing. N Engl J Med 1996;334:89. (Review of indications and approaches.)

Vukmir RB: Emergency cardiac pacing. Am J Emerg Med 1993;11:166. (What to do with patient who presents with bradyarrhythmia.)

EVALUATION OF SYNCOPE & SURVIVORS OF SUDDEN DEATH

SYNCOPE

Syncope, defined as a transient loss of consciousness and postural tone due to inadequate cerebral blood flow with prompt recovery without resuscitative measures, is a common clinical problem, especially in the elderly. Thirty percent of the adult population will experience at least one episode, and syncope accounts for approximately 3% of emergency room visits. Causes include cardiac abnormalities (either disturbances of rhythm or hemodynamics), vascular disorders, or neurologic processes. A specific cause is identified in about 50% of cases during the initial evaluation. The prognosis is relatively benign except when accompanying cardiac disease is present. Syncope is more likely to occur in patients with known heart disease, older men, and young women (who are prone to vasovagal episodes). Syncope is characteristically abrupt in onset, often resulting in injury, transient (lasting for seconds to a few minutes), and followed by prompt recovery or full consciousness.

Vasomotor syncope may be due to excessive vagal tone or impaired reflex control of the peripheral circulation. The most frequent type of vasodepressor syncope is vasovagal hypotension or the "common faint," which is often initiated by stressful, painful, or claustrophobic experience, especially in young women. Premonitory symptoms, such as nausea, diaphoresis, tachycardia, and loss of color, are usual. Episodes can be aborted by lying down or removing the inciting stimulus. Enhanced vagal tone with resulting hypotension is the cause of syncope in carotid sinus hypersensitivity and postmicturition syncope; vagal-induced sinus bradycardia, sinus arrest, and atrioventricular block are common accompaniments and may themselves be the cause of syncope. Carotid sinus massage under carefully monitored conditions or tilt-table testing may be diagnostic (see above under Autonomic Testing). Treatment consists largely of counseling patients to avoid predisposing situations. Paradoxically, beta-blockers may be helpful in patients with altered autonomic function uncovered by head-up tilt testing. Permanent pacing may benefit patients with documented bradycardiac responses.

Orthostatic (postural) hypotension is another common cause of vasomotor syncope, especially in the elderly, in diabetics or other patients with autonomic neuropathy, in patients with blood loss or hypovolemia, and in patients taking vasodilators, diuretics, and adrenergic blocking drugs. In addition, a syndrome of chronic idiopathic orthostatic hypotension exists primarily in older men. In most of these conditions, the normal vasoconstrictive response to assuming upright posture, which compensates for the abrupt decrease in venous return, is impaired. A greater than normal decline (20 mm Hg) in blood pressure immediately upon arising from the supine to the standing position is observed, with or without tachycardia depending on the status of autonomic (baroreceptor) function. Studying patients with a tilt table can establish the diagnosis with more certainty. Autonomic function can be assessed by observing blood pressure and heart rate responses to Valsalva's maneuver and by tilt testing. In older patients, vasoconstrictor abnormalities and autonomic insufficiency are perhaps the most common causes of syncope. Thus, tilt testing should be employed before proceeding to invasive studies unless clinical and ambulatory electrocardiographic evaluation suggests a cardiac abnormality.

Cardiogenic syncope can occur on a mechanical or arrhythmic basis. Mechanical problems that can cause syncope include aortic stenosis (where syncope may occur from autonomic reflex abnormalities or ventricular tachycardia), pulmonary stenosis, hypertrophic obstructive cardiomyopathy, congenital lesions associated with pulmonary hypertension or right-to-left shunting, and left atrial myxoma obstructing the mitral valve. Episodes are commonly exertional or postexertional. More commonly, cardiac syncope is due to disorders of automaticity (sick sinus syndrome), conduction disorders (atrioventricular block), or tachyarrhythmias (especially ventricular tachycardia and supraventricular tachycardia with rapid ventricular rate).

The evaluation for syncope depends on findings from the history and physical examination (especially orthostatic blood pressure evaluation, examination of carotid and other arteries, cardiac examination, and, if appropriate, carotid sinus massage). The resting ECG may reveal arrhythmias, evidence of accessory pathways, prolonged QT interval, and other signs of heart disease (such as infarction or hypertrophy). If the history is consistent with syncope, ambulatory electrocardiographic monitoring is essential. This may need to be repeated several times, since yields increase with longer periods of monitoring, at least up to 3 days. Event recorder and transtelephone electrocardiographic monitoring may be helpful in patients with intermittent presyncopal episodes. Electrophysiologic studies to assess sinus node function and atrioventricular conduction and to induce supraventricular or ventricular tachycardia are indicated in patients with recurrent episodes and nondiagnostic ambulatory ECGs. They reveal an arrhythmic cause in 20–50% of patients, depending on the study criteria, and are most often diagnostic when the patient has had multiple episodes and has identifiable cardiac abnormalities.

Abboud FM: Neurocardiogenic syncope. N Engl J Med 1993;338:1117.

Calkins H et al: The value of the clinical history and the differentiation of syncope due to ventricular tachycardia, atrioventricular block, and neurocardiogenic syncope. Am J Med 1995;98:365. (Syncope due to ventricular tachycardia and atrioventricular block was clearly distinguished from other causes.)

Kapoor WN et al: Psychiatric illnesses in patients with syncope. Am J Med 1995;99:505. (Frequent and often unrecognized factor in patients presenting with syncope.)

Kapoor WN: Work-up and management of patients with syncope. Med Clin North Am 1995;79:1153. (General approach to diagnosis and management.)

Mader SL: Orthostatic hypotension. Med Clin North Am 1989;73:1337. (A common cause of syncope in the elderly, often exacerbated by medications.)

See also references following the section above on techniques for evaluating rhythm disturbances.

SURVIVORS OF SUDDEN DEATH

Sudden cardiac death is defined as unexpected nontraumatic death in clinically well or stable patients who die within 1 hour after onset of symptoms. The causative rhythm in most cases is ventricular fibrillation, which is usually preceded by ventricular tachycardia except in the setting of acute ischemia or infarction. Complete heart block and sinus node arrest may also cause sudden death. A disproportionate number of sudden deaths occur in the early morning hours. Over 75% of victims of sudden cardiac death have had severe coronary artery disease. Many have old infarctions. Sudden death may be the initial manifestation of coronary disease in up to 20% of patients and accounts for approximately 50% of deaths from coronary disease. When ventricular fibrillation occurs in the initial 24 hours after infarction, longterm management is no different from that of other patients with acute infarction. Other conditions that predispose to sudden death include severe left ventricular hypertrophy, hypertrophic cardiomyopathy, congestive cardiomyopathy, aortic stenosis, pulmonary stenosis, primary pulmonary hypertension, cyanotic congenital heart disease, atrial myxoma, mitral valve prolapse, hypoxia, electrolyte abnormalities, prolonged QT interval syndrome, and conduction system disease. Late potentials (after the QRS complex) on a signal-averaged surface ECG in patients with prior myocardial infarction may identify a group of patients at risk of ventricular arrhythmias and sudden death.

Unless ventricular fibrillation occurred early post-myocardial infarction or an unusual correctable process was present (such as an electrolyte abnormality, drug toxicity, or aortic stenosis), these patients require evaluation and intervention since recurrences are frequent. Exercise testing or coronary arteriography should be performed to exclude coronary disease as the underlying cause. Conduction disturbances should be managed as described above. If prodromal supraventricular arrhythmias or ventricular arrhythmias, such as sustained or nonsustained ventricular tachycardia, are found by ambulatory electrocardiographic monitoring, their elimination by therapy may prevent further episodes. Ventricular stimulation studies are also indicated, especially if monitoring does not reveal significant arrhythmias. If inducibility cannot be prevented by the usual agents or if monitored arrhythmias are not obliterated, amiodarone and beta-blockers may still be effective. Implantable cardioverter defibrillator therapy is thought by most experts to be the treatment of choice in all survivors of aborted sudden death unless a specific correctable cause is identified or unless the event occurred in the acute myocardial infarction setting.

Barron HB, Lesh MD: Autonomic nervous system and sudden cardiac death. J Am Coll Cardiol 1996;27:1053. (Importance of the autonomic nervous system in precipitating sudden death, and the utility of techniques of assessment.)

Gilman JK et al: Predicting and preventing sudden death from cardiac causes. Circulation 1994;90:1083.

Pinski SL, Trohman RY: Implantable cardioverter-defibrillators: Implications to the nonelectrophysiologist. Ann Intern Med 1995;122:770. (How to handle the patient with these increasingly common devices in situations such as surgery, diagnostic procedures, and when devices discharge away from the medical center.)

Weaver FD et al: Cost-effectiveness of implantable defibrillator as first-choice therapy versus electrophysiologically guided, tiered strategy in post-infarct sudden death survivors: A randomized study. Circulation 1996;93:489. (Strong trend toward improved survival with device therapy at a reasonable cost, despite the high cost of the devices themselves.)

Wight JN, Salem D: Sudden death and the "athletic heart." Arch Intern Med 1995;155:1473. (In subjects younger than 35, specific causes such as hypertrophic cardiomyopathy, right ventricular dysplasia, and coronary anomalies are the most frequent underlying cause. Above age 35, atherosclerosis becomes a major factor.)

See also the references following the section above on ventricular tachycardia.

RECOMMENDATIONS FOR RESUMPTION OF DRIVING

An important management problem in patients who have experienced syncope, symptomatic ventricular tachycardia, or aborted sudden death is to provide recommendations concerning automobile driving. According to a survey published in 1991, only eight states had specific laws dealing with this issue, whereas 42 had laws restricting driving in patients with seizure disorders. There are not adequate data to support driving restrictions in patients who have not experienced symptomatic arrhythmias, though patients with frequent nonsustained ventricular tachycardia, associated heart disease, and significant left ventricular dysfunction are at high enough risk to warrant cautioning. Patients with syncope or aborted sudden death thought to have been due to temporary factors (acute myocardial infarction, bradyarrhythmias subsequently treated with permanent pacing, drug effect, electrolyte imbalance) should be permitted to resume driving after recovery and an appropriate period of observation (usually 1 month). Other patients with symptomatic ventricular tachycardia or aborted sudden death, whether treated pharmacologically, with antitachycardia devices, or with ablation therapy, should not drive for a least 6 months. Longer restrictions are warranted in many such patients if spontaneous arrhythmias persist. The physician should comply with local regulations and consult local authorities concerning individual cases.

Epstein AE et al: Personal and public safety issues related to arrhythmias that may affect consciousness: Implications for regulation and physician recommendations. Circulation 1996;94:1147. (Consensus statement with detailed discussion and recommendations concerning this difficult but vitally important subject.)

CARDIAC FAILURE

Essentials of Diagnosis

- Left ventricular failure: Exertional dyspnea, cough, fatigue, orthopnea, paroxysmal nocturnal dyspnea, cardiac enlargement, rales, gallop rhythm, and pulmonary venous congestion.
- Right ventricular failure: Elevated venous pressure, hepatomegaly, dependent edema.
- Both: Combination of above.
- Diagnosis should be confirmed by noninvasive or hemodynamic measurements.

General Considerations

Systolic function of the heart is governed by four major determinants: the contractile state of the myocardium, the preload of the ventricle (the end-diastolic volume and the resultant fiber length of the ventricles prior to onset of the contraction), the afterload applied to the ventricles (the impedance to left ventricular ejection), and the heart rate.

Cardiac function may be inadequate as a result of alterations in any of these determinants. In most instances, the primary derangement is depression of myocardial contractility caused either by loss of functional muscle (due to myocardial infarction, etc) or by processes diffusely affecting the myocardium. However, the heart may fail as a pump because preload is excessively elevated, such as in valvular regurgitation, or when afterload is excessive, such as in aortic stenosis or in severe hypertension. Pump function may also be inadequate when the heart rate is too slow or too rapid. While the normal heart can tolerate wide variations in preload, afterload, and heart rate, the diseased heart often has limited reserve for such alterations. Finally, cardiac pump function may be supranormal but nonetheless inadequate when metabolic demands or requirements for blood flow are excessive. This situation is termed **high-output heart failure** and, though uncommon, tends to be specifically treatable. Causes of high output include thyrotoxicosis, beriberi, severe anemia, arteriovenous shunting, and Paget's disease of bone.

Manifestations of cardiac failure can also occur as a result of isolated or predominant **diastolic dysfunction** of the heart. In these cases, filling of the left or right ventricle is impaired because the chamber is noncompliant ("stiff") due to excessive hypertrophy or changes in composition of the myocardium. Even though contractility may be preserved, diastolic pressures are elevated and cardiac output may be reduced.

Pathophysiology

When the heart fails, a number of adaptations occur both in the heart and systemically. If the stroke volume of either ventricle is reduced by depressed contractility or excessive afterload, end-diastolic volume and pressure in that chamber will rise. This increases end-diastolic myocardial fiber length, resulting in a greater systolic shortening (Starling's law of the heart). If the condition is chronic, ventricular dilation will occur. While this may restore resting cardiac output, the resulting chronic elevation of diastolic pressures will be transmitted to the atria and to the pulmonary and systemic venous circulation. Ultimately, increased capillary pressure may lead to transudation of fluid with resulting pulmonary or systemic edema. Reduced cardiac output, particularly if associated with reduced arterial pressure or perfusion of the kidneys, will also activate several neural and humoral systems. Increased activity of the sympathetic nervous system will stimulate myocardial contractility, heart rate, and venous tone; the latter change results in a rise in the effective central blood volume, which serves to further elevate preload. Though these adaptations are designed to increase cardiac output, they may themselves be deleterious. Thus, tachycardia and increased contractility may precipitate ischemia in patients with underlying coronary artery disease, and the rise in preload may worsen pulmonary congestion. Sympathetic nervous system activation also increases peripheral vascular resistance; this adaptation is designed to maintain perfusion to vital organs, but when it is excessive it may itself reduce renal and other tissue blood flow. Peripheral vascular resistance is also a major determinant of left ventricular afterload, so that excessive sympathetic activity may further depress cardiac function.

One of the more important effects of lower cardiac output is reduction of renal blood flow and glomerular filtration rate, which leads to sodium and fluid retention. The renin-angiotensin-aldosterone system is also activated, leading to further increases in peripheral vascular resistance and left ventricular afterload as well as sodium and fluid retention. Heart failure is associated with increased circulating levels of arginine vasopressin, which also serves as a vasoconstrictor and inhibitor of water excretion. While release of atrial natriuretic peptide is increased in heart failure owing to the elevated atrial pressures, there is evidence of resistance to its natriuretic and vasodilating effects.

Hemodynamic Alterations

Myocardial failure is characterized by two hemodynamic derangements, and the clinical presentation is determined by their severity. The first is reduction in cardiac output, ie, the ability to increase cardiac output in response to increased demands imposed by exercise or even ordinary activity (cardiac reserve). The second abnormality, elevation of ventricular diastolic pressures, is primarily a result of the compensatory processes.

Heart failure may be right-sided or left-sided. Patients with the picture of **left heart failure** have symptoms of low cardiac output and elevated pulmonary venous pressure; dyspnea is the predominant feature. Signs of fluid retention predominate in **right heart failure,** with the patient exhibiting edema, hepatic congestion, and, on occasion, ascites. Most patients exhibit signs or symptoms of both right- and left-sided failure, and left ventricular dysfunction is the primary cause of right ventricular failure. Surprisingly, some individuals with severe left ventricular dysfunction will display few signs of left heart failure and appear to have isolated right heart failure. Indeed, they may be clinically indistinguishable from patients with cor pulmonale, who have right heart failure secondary to pulmonary disease.

Although this section concerns cardiac failure due to systolic left ventricular dysfunction, patients with diastolic dysfunction experience many of the same symptoms and may be difficult to distinguish clinically. Diastolic pressures are elevated even though diastolic volumes are normal or small. These pressures are transmitted to the pulmonary and systemic venous systems, resulting in dyspnea and edema. The most frequent cause of diastolic cardiac dysfunction is left ventricular hypertrophy, commonly resulting from hypertension, but conditions such as hypertrophic or restrictive cardiomyopathy, diabetes, and pericardial disease can produce the same clinical picture. While diuretics are often useful in these patients, the other therapies discussed in this section (digitalis, vasodilators, inotropic agents) may be inappropriate.

Causes & Prevention of Cardiac Failure

The syndrome of cardiac failure can be produced by many diseases. In developed countries, coronary artery disease with resulting myocardial infarction and loss of functioning myocardium (ischemic cardiomyopathy) is the commonest cause. In the 4S study, aggressive lipid-lowering therapy in patients with known coronary disease reduced the incidence of heart failure by 30%. A number of processes may present with dilated or congestive cardiomyopathy, which is characterized by left ventricular or biventricular dilation and generalized systolic dysfunction. These are discussed elsewhere in this chapter, but the most common are alcoholic cardiomyopathy, viral myocarditis (including infections by HIV), and dilated cardiomyopathies with no obvious underlying cause (idiopathic cardiomyopathy). Rare causes of dilated cardiomyopathy include infiltrative diseases (hemochromatosis, sarcoidosis, amyloidosis, etc), other infectious agents, metabolic disorders, cardiotoxins, and drug toxicity.

Systemic hypertension remains an important cause of congestive heart failure and, even more commonly in the USA, an exacerbating factor in patients with cardiac dysfunction due to other causes. In several trials, antihypertensive therapy—particularly when directed to the systolic blood pressure—has been effective in reducing the incidence of new-onset heart failure by 40–60%. Valvular heart disease has become a less frequent cause of heart failure with the declining incidence and severity of rheumatic fever. However, aortic stenosis remains a common and reversible cause. Patients with chronic volume overload of the left ventricle, such as mitral or aortic regurgitation, may develop progressive myocardial dysfunction and have a picture of cardiomyopathy even after the underlying condition is corrected. This form of congestive heart failure is preventable by early diagnosis and treatment of the valvular lesion.

Gaasch WH: Diagnosis and treatment based on left ventricular systolic and diastolic dysfunction. JAMA 1994;271:1276.

Poole-Wilson PA et al (editors): *Heart Failure.* Churchill Livingstone, 1997. (Comprehensive coverage from bench to bedside.)

Vasan RS et al: Congestive heart failure with normal ventricular systolic function. Arch Intern Med 1996; 156:146. (Epidemiology, diagnosis, and treatment.)

Wei JY: Age and the cardiovascular system. N Engl J Med 1992;327:1735. (Pathophysiologic changes with aging cause or exacerbate heart failure in many older patients.)

Clinical Findings

A. Symptoms: The symptoms of cardiac failure have been discussed in part in earlier sections. The most common complaint is shortness of breath, chiefly exertional dyspnea at first and then progressing to orthopnea, paroxysmal nocturnal dyspnea, and rest dyspnea. A more subtle and often overlooked symptom of heart failure is a chronic nonproductive cough, which is often worse in the recumbent position. Nocturia due to excretion of fluid retained during the day and increased renal perfusion in the recumbent position is a common nonspecific symptom of heart failure. Patients with heart failure also complain of fatigue and exercise intolerance. These symptoms correlate poorly with the degree of cardiac dysfunction and result in part from changes in peripheral blood flow and blood flow to skeletal muscle which are part of the syndrome of heart failure. Patients with right heart failure may experience right upper quadrant pain due to passive congestion of the liver, loss of appetite and nausea due to edema of the gut or impaired gastrointestinal perfusion, and peripheral edema.

Cardiac failure may present acutely in a previously asymptomatic patient. Causes include myocardial infarction, myocarditis, and acute valvular regurgitation due to endocarditis or other conditions. These patients usually present with pulmonary edema. The management of acute heart failure has been discussed under myocardial infarction and centers around initial stabilization with diuretics and parenteral vasodilators or inotropic agents.

Patients with episodic symptoms may be having left ventricular dysfunction due to intermittent ischemia. This potentially reversible form of heart failure should be considered, especially in patients with angina pectoris and with diabetes mellitus. Patients may also present with acute exacerbations of chronic, stable heart failure. Exacerbations are usually caused by alterations in therapy (or patient noncompliance), excessive salt and fluid intake, arrhythmias, excessive activity, pulmonary emboli, intercurrent infection, or progression of the underlying disease.

B. Signs: Many patients with heart failure, including some with severe symptoms, appear comfortable at rest. Others will be dyspneic during conversation or minor activity, and those with long-standing severe heart failure may appear cachectic or cyanotic. The vital signs may be normal, but tachycardia, hypotension, and reduced pulse pressure may be present. Patients often show signs of increased sympathetic nervous system activity, including cold extremities and diaphoresis. Important peripheral signs of heart failure can be detected by examination of the neck, the lungs, the abdomen, and the extremities. Right atrial pressure may be estimated through the height of the pulsations in the jugular venous system. In addition to the height of the venous pressure, abnormal pulsations such as regurgitant *v* waves should be sought. Examination of the carotid pulse allows estimation of pulse pressure as well as detection of aortic stenosis. The thyroid examination is important, since occult hyperthyroidism and hypothyroidism are readily treatable causes of heart failure. In the lungs, crackles at the bases reflect transudation of fluid into the alveoli. Pleural effusions may cause bibasilar dullness to percussion. Expiratory wheezing and rhonchi may be signs of heart failure. Patients with severe right heart failure may have hepatic enlargement—tender or nontender—due to passive congestion. Systolic pulsations may be felt in tricuspid regurgitation. Sustained moderate pressure on the liver may increase jugular venous pressure (a positive hepatojugular reflux is an increase of > 1 cm). Ascites may also be present. Peripheral pitting edema is a common sign in patients with right heart failure and may extend into the thighs and abdominal wall.

The cardiac examination has been discussed. Cardinal signs in heart failure are a parasternal lift, indicating pulmonary hypertension; an enlarged and sustained left ventricular impulse, indicating left ventricular dilation and hypertrophy; a diminished first heart sound, suggesting impaired contractility; and S_3 gallops originating in the left and sometimes the right ventricle. Murmurs should be sought to exclude primary valvular disease; secondary mitral regurgitation and tricuspid regurgitation murmurs are common in patients with dilated ventricles. In chronic heart failure, many of the expected signs of heart failure may be absent despite markedly abnormal cardiac function and hemodynamic measurements.

C. Laboratory Findings: A blood count may reveal anemia, a cause of high-output failure and an exacerbating factor in other forms of cardiac dysfunction. Biochemical studies may show renal insufficiency as a possible compounding factor. Renal function tests also determine whether cardiac failure is associated with prerenal azotemia. Electrolytes may disclose heightened neuroendocrine activity with resultant hyponatremia. Thyroid function in older patients should be assessed to detect occult thyrotoxicosis or myxedema. Appropriate biopsies may lead to a diagnosis of amyloidosis. Additional assessment in dilated cardiomyopathy should include iron studies to exclude hemochromatosis. Myocardial biopsy may exclude specific causes of dilated cardiomyopathy but rarely reveals specific reversible diagnoses.

D. Electrocardiography and Chest X-Ray: Electrocardiography may indicate an underlying or secondary arrhythmia, myocardial infarction, or nonspecific changes that often include low voltage, intraventricular conduction defects, left ventricular hypertrophy, and nonspecific repolarization changes. Chest radiographs provide information about the size and shape of the cardiac silhouette. Cardiomegaly is an important finding. Evidence of pulmonary venous hypertension includes relative dilation of the upper lobe veins, perivascular edema (haziness of vessel outlines), interstitial edema, and alveolar fluid. In acute heart failure, these findings correlate moder-

ately well with pulmonary venous pressure, and when present in chronic failure they indicate elevated pressures. However, patients with chronic heart failure may show relatively normal pulmonary vasculature despite markedly elevated pressures. Pleural effusions are common and tend to be bilateral or right-sided.

E. Additional Studies: Many studies have indicated that the clinical diagnosis of systolic myocardial dysfunction is often inaccurate. The primary confounding conditions are diastolic dysfunction of the heart with decreased relaxation and filling of the left ventricle (particularly in hypertension and in hypertrophic states) and pulmonary disease. When myocardial ischemia is suspected as a cause of left of ventricular dysfunction, stress testing should be performed.

The most useful test is the echocardiogram. This will reveal the size and function of both ventricles and of the atria. It will also allow detection of pericardial effusion, valvular abnormalities, intracardiac shunts, and segmental wall motion abnormalities suggestive of old myocardial infarction as opposed to more generalized forms of dilated cardiomyopathy.

Radionuclide angiography measures left ventricular ejection fraction and permits analysis of regional wall motion. This test is especially useful when echocardiography is technically suboptimal, such as in patients with severe pulmonary disease.

F. Cardiac Catheterization: In most patients with heart failure, clinical examination and noninvasive tests can determine left ventricular size and function well enough to confirm the diagnosis. Left heart catheterization is necessary when valvular disease must be excluded and when the presence and extent of coronary artery disease must be determined. The latter is particularly important when surgery to excise a left ventricular aneurysm is contemplated or when it is believed that left ventricular dysfunction may be partially reversible by revascularization. The combination of angina or noninvasive evidence of significant myocardial ischemia with symptomatic heart failure is often an indication for coronary angiography if the patient is a potential candidate for revascularization. Right heart catheterization may be useful to select and monitor therapy in patients refractory to standard therapy.

Butman SM et al: Bedside cardiovascular examination of patients with severe chronic heart failure: Importance of rest or inducible jugular venous distention. J Am Coll Cardiol 1993;22:968.

Stevenson LW, Perloff JK: The limited reliability of physical signs for estimating hemodynamics in chronic heart failure. JAMA 1989;261:884. (Left ventricular filling pressure cannot be estimated by examination.)

Treatment

A. Correction of Reversible Causes: The major reversible causes include ischemic left ventricular dysfunction, thyrotoxicosis, myxedema, valvular lesions, intracardiac shunts, high-output states, arrhythmias, and alcohol- or drug-induced myocardial depression. Calcium channel blockers and antiarrhythmic agents are important causes of worsening heart failure. Some metabolic and infiltrative cardiomyopathies may be partially reversible, or their progression may be slowed; these include hemochromatosis, sarcoidosis, and amyloidosis. Acute myocarditis may respond to immunosuppressive therapy and corticosteroids. Reversible causes of diastolic dysfunction include pericardial disease and left ventricular hypertrophy due to hypertension. Once it is established that there is no reversible component, the measures outlined below are appropriate.

B. Diet and Activity: Patients should routinely be under moderate salt restriction (2 g sodium or 5 g salt). More severe sodium restriction is usually difficult to achieve and unnecessary because of the availability of potent diuretic agents. Alterations in lifestyle reduce symptoms and the need for additional medications. In severe heart failure, restriction of activity often facilitates temporary recompensation. With such limitations, these patients may exhibit profound diuresis even though fluid retention was previously refractory. There is no convincing evidence that prolonged bed rest alters the natural history of congestive heart failure. Indeed, a gradual exercise program is associated with diminished symptoms and substantial increases in exercise capacity.

C. Diuretic Therapy: Diuretics are the most effective means of providing symptomatic relief to patients with moderate to severe congestive heart failure. Few patients with signs or symptoms of fluid retention can be optimally managed without a diuretic. However, excessive diuresis can lead to electrolyte imbalance and neurohormonal activation. A combination of a diuretic and an ACE inhibitor should be the initial treatment in most symptomatic patients. When fluid retention is mild, thiazide diuretics or a similar type of agent (hydrochlorothiazide, 25–50 mg; metolazone, 2.5–15 mg; chlorthalidone, 25–50 mg; etc) may be sufficient. These agents block sodium reabsorption in the cortical diluting segment at the terminal portion of the loop of Henle and in the proximal portion of the distal convoluted tubule. The result is natriuresis and kaliuresis. These agents also have weak carbonic anhydrase inhibitor activity, which results in proximal tubule inhibition of sodium reabsorption.

The thiazides are generally ineffective when the glomerular filtration rate falls below 30 mL/min, a not infrequent occurrence in patients with severe heart failure. Metolazone maintains its efficacy down to a glomerular filtration rate of approximately 10 mL/min. Adverse reactions include hypokalemia and intravascular volume depletion with resulting prerenal azotemia, skin rashes, neutropenia and thrombocytopenia, hyperglycemia, hyperuricemia, and hepatic dysfunction.

Patients with more severe heart failure should be treated with one of the loop diuretics. These include furosemide (20–320 mg daily in single or divided doses), bumetanide (1–8 mg daily in single or divided doses), and torsemide (20–200 mg daily). These agents have a rapid onset and short duration of action. In acute situations or when gastrointestinal absorption is in doubt, they should be given intravenously. The loop diuretics inhibit chloride reabsorption in the ascending limb of the loop of Henle, which results in natriuresis, kaliuresis, and metabolic alkalosis. They are active even in severe renal insufficiency, larger doses (up to 500 mg of furosemide or equivalent) may be required. The major adverse reactions include intravascular volume depletion, prerenal azotemia, and hypotension. Hypokalemia, particularly with accompanying digitalis therapy, is a major problem. Less common side effects include skin rashes, gastrointestinal distress, and ototoxicity (the latter more common with ethacrynic acid and possibly less common with bumetanide).

The potassium-sparing agents spironolactone, triamterene, and amiloride are often useful in combination with the loop diuretics and thiazides. Triamterene and amiloride act on the distal tubule to reduce potassium secretion. Their diuretic potency is only mild and not adequate for most patients with heart failure, but they may minimize the hypokalemia induced by more potent agents. Side effects include hyperkalemia, gastrointestinal symptoms, and renal dysfunction. Spironolactone is a specific inhibitor of aldosterone, which is often increased in congestive heart failure. Its onset of action is slower than the other potassium-sparing agents, and its side effects include gynecomastia. Combinations of potassium supplements or angiotensin converting enzyme inhibitors and potassium-sparing drugs can produce hyperkalemia but have been used with success in patients with persistent hypokalemia.

Patients with refractory edema may respond to combinations of a loop diuretic and thiazide-like agents. Metolazone, because of its maintained activity with renal insufficiency, is the most useful agent for such a combination. Extreme caution must be observed with this approach, since massive diuresis and electrolyte imbalances often occur; 2.5 mg of metolazone should be added to the previous dosage of loop diuretic. In many cases this is necessary only once or twice a week, but dosages up to 10 mg daily have been used in some patients.

D. Angiotensin-Converting Enzyme (ACE) Inhibitors: The ACE inhibitors have become standard therapy for heart failure. Their beneficial effects include both vasodilation and inhibition of increased neurohormonal activity. These agents block the renin-angiotensin-aldosterone system, producing vasodilation by blocking angiotensin II-induced vasoconstriction and decreasing sodium retention by reducing aldosterone secretion. They also inhibit the degradation of bradykinin, increase the production of vasodilating prostaglandins, and indirectly inhibit the adrenergic nervous system. Although the other vasodilators tend to stimulate the renin-angiotensin system and often lose part of their effect due to the resulting fluid retention, tolerance to the ACE inhibitors is uncommon.

A growing number of ACE inhibitors are becoming available (Table 11–5). Captopril and enalapril have been approved in the United States for the treatment of heart failure, both to prolong survival and alleviate symptoms. Several other ACE inhibitors have been approved based only on their ability to reduce symptoms, and it is likely that all agents of this class are effective.

Acute hemodynamic studies show that the ACE inhibitors reduce left ventricular filling pressure and right atrial pressure and moderately increase cardiac output. During long-term follow-up, these hemodynamic benefits are maintained or increased. ACE inhibitors lessen symptoms and increase exercise tolerance. They also correct the electrolyte abnormalities that characterize severe heart failure, such as hyponatremia and diuretic-induced hypokalemia, which may reduce the propensity to arrhythmias. Survival rates are improved by ACE inhibitor therapy in patients with mild, moderate, and severe heart failure. In addition, ACE inhibitors can delay the onset and progression of heart failure in patients with asymptomatic left ventricular dysfunction.

Because the ACE inhibitors may produce significant hypotension, particularly after the initial doses, they must be started with caution. Hypotension is most prominent in patients with hypovolemia, prerenal azotemia (especially if it is diuretic-induced), and hyponatremia (an indicator of activation of the renin-angiotensin system). Before therapy with the ACE inhibitors is started, other vasodilators should be discontinued and the dosages of diuretics should be reduced or the drugs withheld for 24 hours. Captopril is the preferred agent for beginning ACE inhibitor therapy, especially in patients at risk for hypotension, because of its predictable onset and short duration of action (peak effect in 30–90 minutes). Treatment should be started with a low dose: either 12.5 mg or, in patients with hyponatremia or preexisting low blood pressure, 6.25 mg. The blood pressure should be monitored for the first 2 hours after dosing; if symptomatic or clinically significant hypotension does not occur, the patient may be sent home on a dosage of 12.5 mg three times daily. Patients should be questioned about symptoms of hypotension, and renal function should be checked during the first week. The chronically effective dose of captopril appears to be 25–100 mg three times daily, although some patients will not tolerate this high a dose because of hypotension.

Enalapril has been utilized in many of the major trials of ACE inhibitors in heart failure. Like captopril, it should be initiated at 2.5 mg twice daily and titrated upward to 10 mg twice daily. It may be less well tolerated in patients with borderline blood pressure or underlying renal dysfunction. Most of the trials which have led to the widespread use of ACE inhibitors have employed much higher doses (typically 15–20 mg daily of enalapril and 150 mg of captopril) than are used by many practitioners. Treatment should be titrated to these dosages unless limited by side effects, hypotension, or renal dysfunction. The dosages of the other ACE inhibitors used in heart failure have been comparable to the antihypertensive dose.

The major limitation to ACE inhibitor therapy in heart failure is hypotension and renal insufficiency due to inadequate renal perfusion pressures. Other side effects such as dysgeusia, rash, cough, neutropenia, and proteinuria are less serious or very uncommon. Similarly uncommon but perhaps most serious, angioedema may develop at any time during the use of these agents. The ACE inhibitors tend to increase serum potassium concentrations. Potassium-sparing agents should be withdrawn before ACE inhibitor therapy is started; and although potassium supplements may be required in individuals receiving diuretics and digitalis, their dosage should be decreased and subsequently adjusted as needed. Angiotensin II blockers (losartan, valsartan, and others) appear to be effective alternatives to ACE inhibitors in patients who develop intolerable cough and skin rashes, but since these agents do not share the potentially important effects of ACE inhibitors on prostaglandin synthesis, it is not certain that they will prove to be of equivalent efficacy. The recently published ELITE trial, which compared captopril and losartan, found no difference between these agents with regard to symptoms, hospitalization rate, or changes in renal function. Although there were fewer deaths in the losartan group, the number of events was small, and this finding requires further corroboration.

E. Digitalis Glycosides: Although digitalis glycosides were once the mainstay of treatment in congestive heart failure, their use in patients who are in normal sinus rhythm has declined somewhat because of safety concerns. However, at least four multicenter trials have demonstrated that digoxin withdrawal is associated with worsening symptoms and signs of heart failure, more frequent hospitalization, and worse exercise tolerance. The 6800-patient Digitalis Investigators Group (DIG) trial has finally settled the issue of safety. Digoxin neither increased nor decreased total or cardiovascular mortality, but this neutral effect was the result of a significant reduction in heart failure death and an apparent increase in the deaths attributed to arrhythmias. The DIG study also showed a significant reduction in hospitalization in heart failure patients. Based on these results, digoxin should be reserved for patients who remain symptomatic on diuretics and ACE-inhibitors.

1. Mechanism of action–Digitalis has a number of effects on the heart. Its positive inotropic effect is accomplished by increasing intracellular calcium and enhancing actin-myosin cross-bridge formation. Digitalis binds to the sodium-potassium ATPase on the cell membrane and inhibits the sodium pump. The resulting increase in intracellular sodium facilitates sodium-calcium exchange, resulting in increasing intracellular calcium concentrations.

The digitalis glycosides have electrophysiologic effects that may be beneficial or deleterious in individual patients. These effects are primarily the result of enhancement of the cardiac effects of the parasympathetic nervous system. Its primary therapeutic effect is inhibition of atrioventricular conduction. This decreases the ventricular response to supraventricular arrhythmias, such as atrial fibrillation or flutter. In addition, digitalis decreases sinus node automaticity. The increase in intracellular calcium and sodium may enhance automaticity of latent pacemakers. This increased excitability of ventricular myocardium underlies many of the arrhythmias associated with digitalis toxicity. Digitalis effect and toxicity are increased by reduced intracellular potassium concentrations and increased extracellular calcium concentrations.

2. Pharmacokinetics–Digitalis glycosides are available in a variety of preparations, but of these only digoxin (intravenously and orally) and digitoxin (primarily orally) are usually employed. The intravenous route is preferable if a rapid effect is desired; this is necessary chiefly when early control of rapid supraventricular arrhythmias is sought. Intravenous digoxin begins to have an effect after 15–30 minutes, and the peak effect is seen after 1½–3 hours. The usual initial dose is 0.5 mg given slowly over 10–20 minutes. Additional 0.25 or 0.125 mg doses may be administered after 3 hours. A total dosage of 1–1.25 mg is usually required to achieve full digitalis effect, but smaller dosages are sometimes adequate in older patients and in individuals with small lean body masses.

Therapeutic concentrations may also be achieved by the oral route. If a full effect is desired fairly rapidly, 1–1.25 mg are administered in divided dosages over the initial 24 hours. An additional 0.5 mg is added during the second 24 hours. In most instances, maximum effect is accomplished more gradually by administering 0.5 mg daily for 3 days, followed by the usual maintenance dosage. Digoxin is excreted principally by the kidneys and has a half-life ranging from 36 to 48 hours. The oral maintenance dose may range from 0.125 to 0.5 mg daily, depending on renal function, body size, age, thyroid function, and gastrointestinal absorption (ordinarily, approximately 60–70% of the oral dose is absorbed). Smaller doses are necessary in the presence of renal insufficiency. Unless the end point of therapy is control of the ventricular response in atrial fibrillation, it is worthwhile to measure serum digoxin levels after approximately 1 week of maintenance therapy; individual absorption rates and excretion rates may vary considerably. Digitoxin is less frequently used because of its long half-life (4–6 days), which will prolong the duration of toxicity if it occurs. Digitoxin is excreted by the liver, so blood levels may fluctuate less in patients with varying degrees of renal insufficiency.

A number of drugs have been found to affect digoxin pharmacology. Bile acid sequestrants (cholestyramine or colestipol), some broad-spectrum oral antibiotics, antacids, and kaolin-pectin mixtures (eg, Kaopectate) may decrease absorption of digoxin. Quinidine, verapamil, amiodarone, and propafenone increase plasma levels of digoxin by reducing both the volume of distribution and the renal excretion of the agent. As noted previously, hypokalemia, hypercalcemia, and hypomagnesemia enhance the digitalis effect and potentiate its toxicity.

3. Digitalis toxicity–The therapeutic-to-toxic ratio of digitalis is quite narrow, and digitalis toxicity remains a potential problem. Its frequency has diminished as a result of improved understanding of its pharmacology, a trend toward employing lower dosages, and the availability of measurements of digoxin levels. Digoxin toxicity is uncommon with serum levels below 1.4 ng/mL and is present in approximately 50% of patients with levels above 3 ng/mL. Symptoms of digitalis toxicity include anorexia, nausea and vomiting, headache, xanthopsia and verdopsia, and disorientation. These symptoms may precede cardiotoxic effects.

Cardiac toxicity may take many forms, the most common being atrioventricular conduction disturbances, arrhythmias reflecting increased automaticity, and reentry arrhythmias. However, atrial flutter is rarely, if ever, secondary to digitalis toxicity. Arrhythmias due to digitalis toxicity include sinus node arrest, Mobitz type I second-degree atrioventricular block, ventricular premature beats or bigeminy, atrioventricular junctional tachycardia, paroxysmal supraventricular tachycardia with associated atrioventricular block, and ventricular tachycardia or fibrillation. When these arrhythmias are seen, digitalis toxicity should be suspected and the medication withheld. This, together with electrocardiographic monitoring, is adequate for many arrhythmias. Hypokalemia should be corrected, and any associated tachyarrhythmias may resolve after blood potassium levels increase to the high-normal range. Potassium administration may exacerbate atrioventricular block, however. Ventricular tachycardia and very frequent ventricular premature beats should be treated with lidocaine or phenytoin. Class Ia and Ib agents are often less effective, and quinidine may exacerbate toxicity. Second-degree atrioventricular block usually does not require treatment, but complete heart block should be managed with atropine followed by temporary transvenous pacing. Electrical cardioversion for tachyarrhythmias should be avoided if possible, since digitalis toxicity may predispose to intractable ventricular fibrillation or cardiac standstill. If it cannot be avoided, patients should be pretreated with lidocaine (1 mg/kg) and low energy levels (10 J) should be employed initially.

Life-threatening episodes of digitalis toxicity or massive overdosages are characterized by severe hyperkalemia due to Na^+-K^+ ATPase blockade. They can be treated with digoxin-specific Fab antibody fragments. Though expensive, they rapidly reverse all manifestations of digitalis toxicity.

F. Vasodilators: Agents that dilate arteriolar smooth muscle and lower peripheral vascular resistance reduce left ventricular afterload. Medications that diminish venous tone and increase venous capacitance reduce the preload of both ventricles as their principal effect. Since most patients with moderate to severe heart failure have both elevated preload and reduced cardiac output, the maximum benefit of vasodilator therapy can be achieved by an agent or combination of agents with both actions. Many patients with heart failure have mitral or tricuspid regurgitation; agents that reduce resistance to ventricular outflow tend to redirect regurgitant flow in a forward direction.

Vasodilator therapy with ACE inhibitors prolongs life in patients with moderate to severe heart failure. Even in patients who have mild symptoms or asymptomatic left ventricular dysfunction, they delay or prevent the progression to more severe heart failure. This has led to a wider use of these drugs. The combination of hydralazine and isosorbide dinitrate has also improved survival, but to a lesser extent than ACE inhibitors.

The intravenous vasodilating drugs and their dosages have been discussed elsewhere in this chapter (in the section on complications in acute myocardial infarction).

1. Nitrates–Sodium nitroprusside is a potent dilator of both the arteriolar resistance and venous capacitance vessels, and it consistently increases cardiac output and reduces ventricular filling pressures. It is only occasionally employed in the management of chronic heart failure, usually during episodes of acute decompensation. In such cases it may produce excessive hypotension, and it has been combined with dopamine or dobutamine to produce optimal hemodynamic improvement. Intravenous nitroglycerin is less useful in chronic heart failure, since it produces only a limited increase in cardiac output.

Isosorbide dinitrate, 20–80 mg orally three times daily, has proved effective in several small studies. Nitroglycerin ointment, 12.5–50 mg (1–4 in) every 8 hours, appears to be equally effective although somewhat inconvenient for long-term therapy. The nitrates are moderately effective in relieving shortness of breath, especially in patients with mild to moderate symptoms, but less successful—probably because they have little effect on cardiac output—in advanced heart failure. Nitrate therapy is generally well tolerated, but headaches and hypotension may limit the dose of all agents. The development of tolerance to chronic nitrate therapy is now generally acknowledged. This is minimized by intermittent ther-

apy, especially if a daily 8- to 12-hour nitrate-free interval is employed, but probably develops to some extent in most patients receiving these agents. Transdermal nitroglycerin patches have no sustained effect in patients with heart failure and should not be employed for this indication.

2. Hydralazine–Oral hydralazine is a potent arteriolar dilator and markedly increases cardiac output in patients with congestive heart failure. However, as a single agent, it has not been shown to improve symptoms or exercise tolerance during chronic treatment. The combination of nitrates and oral hydralazine produces greater hemodynamic and clinical effects.

Hydralazine therapy is frequently limited by side effects. Approximately 30% of patients are unable to tolerate the relatively high doses required to produce hemodynamic improvement in heart failure (200–400 mg daily in divided doses). The major side effect is gastrointestinal distress, but headaches, tachycardia, hypotension, and the drug-induced lupus syndrome are also relatively common.

3. Alpha-adrenergic blockers–These agents produce vasodilation by blocking postsynaptic alpha receptors. Although they cause short-term hemodynamic improvement, their efficacy is limited by the rapid development of tolerance. There may be some long-term benefit from doxazosin, however.

G. Beta-Blocker Therapy: There is increasing evidence that beta-blockers produce important beneficial effects in patients with chronic congestive heart failure. This approach runs counter to the usual practice of avoiding beta-blockers in heart failure but has been justified by the potentially harmful effects of circulating catecholamines. Studies with metoprolol, bisoprolol, and two additional beta-blockers with vasodilator properties (carvedilol and bucindolol) have all suggested benefit during chronic therapy. The most consistent findings have been an increase in ejection fraction and a decrease in hospitalizations and other evidence of worsening heart failure, suggesting that this approach alters the natural history of this syndrome. There is also a favorable trend toward improved survival with beta-blockers, but the number of events and follow-up times are both limited. Carvedilol is the first beta-blocker to be approved for the treatment of heart failure in the United States. It has been evaluated primarily in stable outpatients with mild to moderate symptoms (New York Heart Association class I, II, or III) who have been receiving usual doses of diuretics and ACE inhibitors. Until further studies have been completed, carvedilol and other beta-blockers should not be initiated in unstable patients. The starting dose is 3.125 mg twice daily and is increased to 6.25, 12.5, and 25 mg twice daily at intervals of approximately 2 weeks as tolerated. Patients must be monitored closely, since heart failure may deteriorate in up to 10% of patients during initiation and up-titration. This can usually be managed by upward adjustment of diuretic doses. A great deal remains to be learned about the selection of optimal candidates for beta-blocker therapy, and these agents should be used only by physicians experienced in managing heart failure.

H. Newer Positive Inotropic Agents: The digitalis derivatives are the only available oral inotropic agents at this time in the USA. However, a number of drugs that increase myocardial contractility in experimental preparations have been or are being investigated. These include beta-adrenergic agonists, dopaminergic agents, and a group of nondigitalis, noncatecholamine agents that increase myocardial contractility by inhibiting myocardial phosphodiesterase. Two of the latter class, milrinone and amrinone, have been approved for intravenous use. However, several trials with newer oral inotropic agents, including milrinone, xamoterol (a beta-adrenergic agonist), ibopamine (a dopaminergic agonist), and vesnarinone (an agent with multiple mechanisms of action) have demonstrated substantial increases in mortality. Further development of potent positive inotropic agents for chronic oral therapy is unlikely.

I. Calcium Channel Blockers: First-generation Ca^{2+} blockers may accelerate the progression of congestive heart failure. However, a recent trial with amlodipine in patients with severe heart failure showed that this agent was safe, though not superior to placebo in most patients. In general, these agents should be avoided unless they are being utilized to treat associated angina or hypertension.

J. Anticoagulation: Patients with severe left ventricular failure are prone to development of systemic arterial emboli, particularly when they are in atrial fibrillation, although in prospective studies, the approximately two per 100 patient-years of follow-up is less than many expected. While these may be catastrophic, the routine use of anticoagulants is controversial, since these patients have short life expectancies and are taking multiple medications that may interfere with optimal regulation of anticoagulation. Most experts prescribe anticoagulants only to appropriate patients who have had embolic episodes or those with atrial fibrillation. Some also anticoagulate patients with severe dilated cardiomyopathy (ejection fraction < 20%) in normal sinus rhythm.

K. Antiarrhythmic Therapy: Patients with moderate to severe heart failure have a high incidence of both symptomatic and asymptomatic arrhythmias. Although fewer than 10% of patients have syncope or presyncope resulting from ventricular tachycardia, ambulatory monitoring reveals that up to 70% of patients have asymptomatic episodes of nonsustained ventricular tachycardia. These arrhythmias indicate a poor prognosis independent of the severity of left ventricular dysfunction, but many of the deaths are probably not arrhythmia-related. Several trials are addressing the question of whether amiodarone, the medication that appears to be both the most effective and least likely to be proarrhythmic, improves the prognosis in patients with frequent ventricular ectopia. Two large randomized control trials had produced contradictory results, with one showing improved survival and the other no effect.

Patients with symptomatic ventricular arrhythmias should be treated vigorously as outlined elsewhere in this chapter. Whether patients with asymptomatic nonsustained ventricular tachycardia warrant therapy remains controversial, largely because of the toxicity of such treatment. Many antiarrhythmic agents depress left ventricular function or themselves worsen the arrhythmia. While most experts do not initiate treatment for frequent ventricular premature beats, they may attempt to suppress frequent episodes of nonsustained ventricular tachycardia. As more evidence accrues that all type I antiarrhythmic drugs can worsen the arrhythmia and exacerbate heart failure, amiodarone has become the agent of choice.

L. Coronary Revascularization: Since underlying coronary artery disease is the cause of heart failure in the majority of patients, coronary revascularization may both improve symptoms and prevent progression. However, trials have not been performed in patients whose major symptom is heart failure. Nonetheless, patients with angina who are candidates for surgery should be evaluated for revascularization, usually by coronary angiography. Noninvasive testing for ischemic but viable myocardium may be a more appropriate first step in patients with known coronary disease but no current clinical evidence of ischemia. The benefit of evaluating patients with heart failure of new onset without angina or prior myocardial infarction is limited. In general, bypass surgery is preferable to PTCA in the setting of heart failure because it provides more complete revascularization.

Prognosis

Despite advances in treatment of patients with congestive heart failure, their prognosis remains poor, with annual mortality rates ranging from 10% in stable patients with mild symptoms to over 50% in patients with advanced, progressive symptoms. Poorer prognosis is associated with severe left ventricular dysfunction (ejection fractions < 20%), prominent symptoms and limitation of exercise capacity (maximal oxygen consumption < 10 mL/kg/min), secondary renal insufficiency, hyponatremia, and elevated plasma catecholamine levels. About 40–50% of patients with heart failure die suddenly, presumably due to ventricular arrhythmias. Nonsustained ventricular tachycardia is a poor prognostic sign, but its prevalence is so high that it cannot be used to predict which individuals are at risk of sudden death.

Cardiac Transplantation

Because of the outlook in patients with advanced heart failure, cardiac transplantation has become widely used. Since the advent of cyclosporine immunosuppressive therapy and more careful screening of donor hearts, the survival of patients after cardiac transplantation has increased considerably. Many centers now have 1-year survival rates exceeding

80–90%, and 5-year survival rates above 70%. Infections, hypertension and renal dysfunction caused by cyclosporine, rapidly progressive coronary atherosclerosis, and immunosuppressant-related cancers have been the major complications. The high cost and limited number of donor organs require careful patient selection early in the course.

[AHCPR guideline on heart failure]
http://text.nlm.nih.gov/ftrs/gateway

Baker DW et al: Management of heart failure: III. The role of revascularization in the treatment of patients with moderate or severe left ventricular systolic dysfunction. JAMA 1994;272:1528.

Baker DW, Wright RF: Management of heart failure: IV. Anticoagulation for patients with heart failure due to left ventricular systolic dysfunction. JAMA 1994;272:1614. (Critical review of very limited data.)

Constanzo MR et al: Selection and treatment of candidates for heart transplantation. Circulation 1995;92:3593. (Consensus statement from the American Heart Association.)

Digitalis Investigators Group: The effect of digoxin on mortality and morbidity in patients with heart failure. N Engl J Med 1997;336:525. (Digoxin had a neutral effect on mortality but reduced the rate of hospitalization for worsening heart failure.)

Elefteriades JA et al (editors): Advanced treatment options for the failing left ventricle. Cardiol Clin 1995;13:1. (Surgical approaches to the failing left ventricle, including revascularization, aneurysmectomy, left ventricular assist devices, and valve replacement.)

Garg R, Yusuf S: Overview of randomized trials of angiotensin-converting enzyme inhibitors on mortality and morbidity in patients with heart failure. JAMA 1995;273:1450.

Massie BM, Shah ND: Future approaches to pharmacologic therapy in congestive heart failure. Curr Opin Cardiol 1995;10:229. (New approaches to managing heart failure, including beta-blockers, calcium blockers, and new inotropic agents.)

Massie BM: Treatment of heart failure 1994: A personal perspective. Curr Opin Cardiol 1994;9:255. (Review of current and investigational medicines emphasizing when and how to employ them.)

McKelvie RS et al: Effects of exercise training in patients with congestive heart failure: A critical review. J Am Coll Cardiol 1995;25:789. (Encouraging activity, if not formal rehabilitation programs, is appropriate.)

Sackner-Bernstein JD, Mancini DM: Rationale for treatment of patients with chronic heart failure with adrenergic blockade. JAMA 1995;274:1462. (Review of the rationale and results of published trials prior to the recent carvedilol experience.)

Stevenson WG et al: Sudden death prevention in patients with advanced ventricular dysfunction. Circulation 1993;88:2953. (Reviews mechanisms and prevention.)

ACUTE PULMONARY EDEMA

Essentials of Diagnosis

- Acute onset or worsening of dyspnea at rest.
- Tachycardia, diaphoresis, cyanosis.
- Pulmonary rales, rhonchi; expiratory wheezing.
- X-ray shows interstitial and alveolar edema with or without cardiomegaly.
- Arterial hypoxemia.

General Considerations

Typical causes of cardiogenic pulmonary edema include acute myocardial infarction or severe ischemia, exacerbation of chronic heart failure, acute volume overload of the left ventricle (valvular regurgitation or ventricular septal defect), and mitral stenosis.

Clinical Findings

Acute pulmonary edema presents with a characteristic clinical picture of severe dyspnea, the production of pink, frothy sputum, and diaphoresis and cyanosis. Rales are present in all lung fields, as are generalized wheezing and rhonchi. Pulmonary edema may appear suddenly in the setting of chronic heart failure or may be the first manifestation of cardiac disease, usually acute myocardial infarction, which may be painful or silent.

A number of noncardiac conditions can also produce pulmonary edema. This occurs either because of imbalance in the Starling forces (either a decrease in plasma proteins or an increase in pulmonary venous pressure) or a functional or anatomic abnormality of the alveolar-capillary membrane. Causes include intravenous narcotics, increased intracerebral pressure, high altitude, sepsis, several medications, inhaled toxins, transfusion reactions, shock, and disseminated intravascular coagulation. These are distinguished from cardiogenic pulmonary edema by the clinical setting, the history, and the physical examination. Conversely, in most patients with cardiogenic pulmonary edema, an underlying cardiac abnormality can usually be detected clinically or by the ECG, chest x-ray, or echocardiogram.

The chest radiograph reveals signs of pulmonary vascular redistribution, blurriness of vascular outlines, increased interstitial markings, and, characteristically, the butterfly pattern of distribution of alveolar edema. The heart may be enlarged or normal in size depending on whether heart failure was previously present. Assessment of cardiac function by echocardiography or right heart catheterization is helpful in determining the cause. In cardiogenic pulmonary edema, the pulmonary capillary wedge pressure is universally elevated, usually over 25 mm Hg. Cardiac output may be normal or depressed. In noncardiogenic pulmonary edema. The wedge pressure may be normal or even low.

Treatment

The patient should be placed in a sitting position with legs dangling over the side of the bed; this facilitates respiration and reduces venous return. Oxygen is delivered by mask to obtain an arterial PO_2 greater than 60 mm Hg. If respiratory distress is severe, endotracheal intubation and mechanical ventilation may be necessary.

Morphine is highly effective in pulmonary edema. The initial dosage is 4–8 mg intravenously (subcutaneous administration is effective in milder cases) and may be repeated after 2–4 hours. Morphine increases venous capacitance, lowering left atrial pressure, and relieves anxiety, which can reduce the efficiency of ventilation. However, morphine may lead to CO_2 retention by reducing the ventilatory drive. It should be avoided in patients with narcotic-induced pulmonary edema, who may improve with narcotic antagonists, and in those with neurogenic pulmonary edema.

Intravenous diuretic therapy (furosemide, 40 mg, or bumetanide, 1 mg—or higher doses if the patient has been receiving chronic diuretic therapy) is usually indicated even if the patient has not exhibited prior fluid retention. These agents produce venodilation prior to the onset of diuresis. Other measures to help reduce left ventricular preload consist of the administration of sublingual or intravenous nitrates and phlebotomy of approximately 500 mL of blood or plasmapheresis. Bronchospasm may occur in response to pulmonary edema and may itself exacerbate hypoxemia and dyspnea. Treatment with inhaled beta-adrenergic agonists or intravenous aminophylline may be helpful, but both may also provoke tachycardia and supraventricular arrhythmias. Particularly in patients with elevated arterial pressures, vasodilators such as intravenous nitroprusside may be worthwhile. In patients with low-output states, particularly when hypotension is present, positive inotropic agents are indicated. These approaches to treatment have been discussed previously.

Gropper MB et al: Acute cardiogenic pulmonary edema. Clin Chest Med 1994;15:501.

Kollef MH, Schuster DP: The acute respiratory distress syndrome. N Engl J Med 1995;352:27. (Review of syndrome often confused with pulmonary edema.)

MYOCARDITIS & THE CARDIOMYOPATHIES

ACUTE MYOCARDITIS

Acute myocarditis causes focal or diffuse inflammation of the myocardium. Most cases are infectious, caused by viral, bacterial, rickettsial, spirochetal, fungal, or parasitic agents; but toxins, drugs, and immunologic reaction can also cause myocarditis.

1. INFECTIOUS MYOCARDITIS

Essentials of Diagnosis

- Often follows an upper respiratory infection.
- May present with chest pain (pleuritic or nonspecific) or signs of heart failure.
- ECG may show sinus tachycardia, other arrhythmias, nonspecific repolarization changes, intraventricular conduction abnormalities.
- Echocardiogram documents cardiomegaly and contractile dysfunction.
- Myocardial biopsy, though not sensitive, may reveal a characteristic inflammatory pattern.

General Considerations

Viral myocarditis is the most common form and is usually caused by coxsackieviruses, but a host of other agents have also been responsible. Rickettsial myocarditis occurs with scrub typhus, Rocky Mountain spotted fever, and Q fever. Diphtheritic myocarditis is caused by the toxin and often is manifested by conduction abnormalities as well as heart failure.

Chagas' disease, caused by the insect-borne protozoan *Trypanosoma cruzi,* is a common form of myocarditis in Central and South America; the major clinical manifestations appear after a latent period of more than a decade. At this stage, patients present with cardiomyopathy, conduction disturbances, and sudden death. Associated gastrointestinal involvement (megaesophagus and megacolon) is the rule. Toxoplasmosis causes myocarditis that is usually asymptomatic but can lead to heart failure. Among parasitic infections, trichinosis is the most common cause of cardiac involvement. The potential for the HIV virus to cause myocarditis is now well recognized, though the prevalence of this complication is not known. In addition, other infectious myocarditides are more common in patients with AIDS.

Clinical Findings

A. Symptoms and Signs: Patients may present several days to a few weeks after the onset of an acute febrile illness or a respiratory infection or with heart failure without antecedent symptoms. Pleural-pericardial chest pain is common. Examination reveals tachycardia, gallop rhythm, and other evidence of heart failure or conduction defect.

B. Electrocardiography and Chest X-Ray: Nonspecific ST–T changes and conduction disturbances are common. Ventricular ectopy may be the initial and only clinical finding. Chest x-ray is nonspecific, but cardiomegaly is frequent.

C. Diagnostic Studies: Echocardiography provides the most convenient way of evaluating cardiac function and can exclude many other processes. Gallium-67 scintigraphy has been reported to yield cardiac uptake in acute or subacute myocarditis. Paired serum viral titers and serologic tests for other agents may indicate the cause.

D. Endomyocardial Biopsy: Pathologic examinations may reveal a round cell inflammatory response with necrosis, but the patchy distribution of abnormalities makes the test relatively insensitive. This picture defines an "active" inflammatory stage and may persist for many months.

Treatment & Prognosis

Specific antimicrobial therapy is indicated when an infecting agent is identified. Immunosuppressive therapy with corticosteroids and other agents have been felt by some to improve the outcome when the process is acute (< 6 months) and if the biopsy suggests ongoing inflammation. However, controlled trials have not been positive, so the value of routine myocardial biopsies in patients presenting with an acute myocarditic picture is uncertain; immunosuppressive therapy without histologic confirmation is unwise. Otherwise, treatment is directed toward the manifestations of heart failure and arrhythmias.

Many cases resolve spontaneously, but in others cardiac function deteriorates progressively and may lead to dilated cardiomyopathy. Many cases of dilated cardiomyopathy may represent the end stage of viral myocarditis.

Brown CA, O'Connoll JB: Myocarditis and idiopathic cardiomyopathy. Am J Med 1995;99:309. (Pathogenesis, clinical presentation, diagnosis, and treatment of myocarditis.)

DeCastro S et al: Frequency of development of acute global left ventricular dysfunction in human immunodeficiency virus infection. J Am Coll Cardiol 1994;24:1018. (Not common, but often a lethal complication.)

Hager JM, Rahimtoola SH: Chagas' heart disease. Curr Probl Cardiol 1995;20:825.

Michaels AD et al: Cardiovascular involvement in AIDS. Curr Probl Cardiol 1997;22:112.

2. DRUG-INDUCED & TOXIC MYOCARDITIS

A variety of medications, illicit drugs, and toxic substances can produce acute or chronic myocardial injury; the clinical presentation varies widely. Doxorubicin and other cytotoxic agents, emetine, and catecholamines (especially with pheochromocytoma) can produce a pathologic picture of inflammation and necrosis together with clinical heart failure and arrhythmias; toxicity of the first two is dose-related. The phenothiazines, lithium, chloroquine, disopyramide, antimony-containing compounds, and arsenicals can also cause electrocardiographic changes, arrhythmias, or heart failure. Hypersensitivity reactions to sulfonamides, penicillins, and aminosalicylic acid as well as other drugs can result in cardiac dysfunction. Radiation can cause an acute inflammatory reaction as well as a chronic fibrosis, usually in conjunction with pericarditis.

The incidence of cocaine cardiotoxicity has increased markedly. Cocaine can cause coronary artery spasm, myocardial infarction, arrhythmias, and myocarditis. Because many of these processes are believed to be mediated by cocaine's inhibitory effect on norepinephrine reuptake by sympathetic nerves, beta-blockers have been used therapeutically. In coronary spasm, calcium channel blockers are more appropriate.

Chakko S, Myerburg RJ: Cardiac complications of cocaine abuse. Clin Cardiol 1995;18:67.

Frishman WH et al: Cardiovascular toxicity with cancer chemotherapy. Curr Probl Cardiol 1996;21:227.

Shan K et al: Anthracyclin-induced cardiotoxicity. Ann Intern Med 1996;125:47.

THE CARDIOMYOPATHIES

The cardiomyopathies are a heterogeneous group of entities affecting the myocardium primarily and not associated with the major causes of cardiac disease, ie, ischemic heart disease, hypertension, valvular disease, or congenital defects. While some have specific causes, many cases are idiopathic. There is now general agreement on a classification based upon general features of presentation and pathophysiology (Table 10–9).

McKenna WJ et al (editors): The cardiomyopathies. Br Heart J 1994;72(6 Suppl):1. (Series of articles covering various forms of cardiomyopathies.)

Richardson P et al: Report of the 1995 World Health Organization/International Society and Federation of Cardiology Task Force on the Definition and Classification of Cardiomyopathies. Circulation 1996;93:841.

Role of Myocardial Biopsy

The indications for this procedure remain controversial, but it is essential for the early detection of transplant rejection. Biopsies have also been helpful in distinguishing restrictive cardiomyopathy from pericardial constriction, an often difficult problem. Occasionally, a specific diagnosis of amyloidosis, sarcoidosis, hemochromatosis, or an unusual infection can be made, but in most cases these conditions are suggested by other cardiac or systemic findings. Biopsies can reveal evidence of acute myocarditis and, if immunosuppressive therapy is contemplated, should be performed in appropriate patients.

1. PRIMARY DILATED CARDIOMYOPATHY

Essentials of Diagnosis

- Symptoms and signs of heart failure.
- ECG may show low QRS voltage, nonspecific repolarization abnormalities, intraventricular conduction abnormalities.
- X-ray shows cardiomegaly.
- Echocardiogram confirms left ventricular dilation, thinning, and global dysfunction.

General Considerations

Dilated cardiomyopathies usually present with symptoms and signs of congestive heart failure (most commonly dyspnea). Occasionally, symptomatic ventricular arrhythmias are the presenting event. Left ventricular dilation and systolic dysfunction are essential for diagnosis. Often no cause can be identified, but chronic alcohol abuse and myocarditis are probably frequent causes. Histologically, the picture is one of extensive fibrosis.

Clinical Findings

A. Symptoms and Signs: In most patients, symptoms of heart failure develop gradually. They may be recognized because of asymptomatic cardiomegaly or electrocardiographic abnormalities, including arrhythmias. The initial presentation may be severe biventricular failure. The physical examination reveals cardiomegaly, S_3 gallop rhythm, and often a murmur of functional mitral regurgitation. Signs of left- and right-sided failure may be present on initial examination, a clue to a process involving the heart diffusely.

B. Electrocardiography and Chest X-Ray: The major findings are listed in Table 10–9.

C. Diagnostic Studies: An echocardiogram is indicated to exclude unsuspected valvular or other lesions and confirm the presence of dilated cardiomyopathy. Exercise thallium-201 scintigraphy may suggest the possibility of underlying coronary disease if a large reversible defect is found, but false-positives occur in cardiomyopathy. Cardiac catheterization is seldom of specific value unless myocardial ischemia or left ventricular aneurysm is suspected. The serum ferritin is an adequate screening study for hemochromatosis.

Treatment

Few cases of cardiomyopathy are amenable to spe-cific therapy. Alcohol use should be discontinued. There is often marked recovery of cardiac function following a period of abstinence in alcoholic cardiomyopathy. Endocrine causes (thyroid dysfunction, acromegaly, pheochromocytoma) should be treated. Immunosuppressive therapy is not indicated in chronic dilated cardiomyopathy. The management of congestive heart failure is outlined in the section on heart failure.

Prognosis

The prognosis of dilated cardiomyopathy without clinical heart failure is variable, with some patients remaining stable, some deteriorating gradually, and others declining rapidly. Once heart failure is manifest, the natural history is similar to that of other causes of heart failure. Arterial and pulmonary emboli are more common in dilated cardiomyopathy than in ischemic cardiomyopathy; suitable candidates may benefit from chronic anticoagulation.

Dec GW, Fuster V: Idiopathic dilated cardiomyopathy. N Engl J Med 1994;331:1564.

Fein FS, Sonnenblick EH: Diabetic cardiomyopathy. Cardiovasc Drugs Ther 1994;8:865.

Kasper EK et al: The causes of dilated cardiomyopathy: A clinicopathologic review of 673 patients. J Am Coll Cardiol 1994;23:586. (Most cases are idiopathic, with specific causes present only in the minority.)

Preedy VR, Richardson PJ: Ethanol-induced cardiovascular disease. Br Med Bull 1994;50:152.

Table 10–9. Classification of the cardiomyopathies.

	Dilated	Hypertrophic	Restrictive
Frequent causes	Idiopathic, alcoholic, myocarditis, postpartum, doxorubicin, endocrinopathies, genetic diseases	Hereditary syndrome, possibly chronic hypertension	Amyloidosis, postradiation, post open heart surgery, diabetes, endomyocardial fibrosis
Symptoms	Left or biventricular CHF	Dyspnea, chest pain, syncope	Dyspnea, fatigue, right-sided CHF
Physical examination	Cardiomegaly, S_3, elevated JVP, rales	Sustained PMI, S_4, variable systolic murmur, bisferiens carotid pulse	Elevated JVP, Kussmaul's sign
ECG	ST–T changes, conduction abnormalities, ventricular ectopy	LVH, exaggerated septal Q waves	ST–T changes, conduction abnormalities, low voltage
Chest x-ray	Enlarged heart, pulmonary congestion	Mild cardiomegaly	Mild to moderate cardiomegaly
Echocardiogram, nuclear studies	LV dilation and dysfunction	LVH, asymmetric septal hypertrophy, small LV size, normal or supranormal function, systolic anterior mitral motion, diastolic dysfunction	Small or normal LV size, normal or mildly reduced LV function
Cardiac catheterization	LV dilation and dysfunction, high diastolic pressures, low cardiac output	Small, hypercontractile LV, dynamic outflow gradient, diastolic dysfunction	High diastolic pressures, "square root" sign, normal or mildly reduced LV function

2. HYPERTROPHIC CARDIOMYOPATHY

Essentials of Diagnosis

- May present with dyspnea, chest pain, syncope.
- Examination shows sustained apical impulse, S_4, systolic ejection murmur.
- ECG shows left ventricular hypertrophy, occasionally septal Q waves in the absence of infarction.
- Echocardiogram shows hypertrophy, which may be asymmetric; usually shows normal or enhanced contractility and signs of dynamic obstruction.

General Considerations

Myocardial hypertrophy unrelated to any pressure or volume overload tends to impinge upon the left ventricular cavity. The interventricular septum may be disproportionately involved (asymmetric septal hypertrophy), but in some cases the hypertrophy is localized to the apex. The left ventricular outflow tract is often narrowed during systole between the bulging septum and an anteriorly displaced anterior mitral valve leaflet, causing a dynamic obstruction (hence the name idiopathic hypertrophic subaortic stenosis; IHSS). The obstruction is worsened by factors that increase myocardial contractility (sympathetic stimulation, digoxin, postextrasystolic beat) or that decrease left ventricular filling (Valsalva's maneuver, peripheral vasodilators).

Hypertrophic cardiomyopathy is in some cases inherited as an autosomal dominant trait with variable penetrance caused by mutations of a number of genes, most of which code for myosin heavy chains or proteins regulating calcium handling. It is becoming clear that the prognosis is related to the specific gene mutation. These patients usually present in early adulthood. Others are elderly, and many of those patients have a long history of hypertension. Some cases occur sporadically.

Except in late stages, hypertrophic cardiomyopathy is characterized by a small, hypercontractile left ventricle. Although dyspnea is a common symptom, it results primarily from markedly impaired diastolic compliance rather than systolic dysfunction or outflow obstruction.

Clinical Findings

A. Symptoms and Signs: The most frequent symptoms are dyspnea and chest pain. Syncope is also common and is typically postexertional, when diastolic filling diminishes and outflow obstruction increases. Arrhythmias are an important problem. Atrial fibrillation is a long-term consequence of chronically elevated left atrial pressures and is a poor prognostic sign. Ventricular arrhythmias are also common, and sudden death may occur, often in athletes after extraordinary exertion.

Features on physical examination are a bisferiens carotid pulse, triple apical impulse (due to the prominent atrial filling wave and early and late systolic im-

pulses), and a loud S_4. In cases with outflow obstruction, a loud systolic murmur is present that increases with upright posture or Valsalva's maneuver and decreases with squatting.

B. Electrocardiography and Chest X-Ray: Left ventricular hypertrophy is nearly universal. Exaggerated septal Q waves inferolaterally may suggest myocardial infarction. The chest x-ray is often unimpressive.

C. Diagnostic Studies: The echocardiogram is diagnostic, revealing asymmetric left ventricular hypertrophy, systolic anterior motion of the mitral valve, early closing followed by reopening of the aortic valve, a small and hypercontractile left ventricle, and delayed relaxation and filling of the left ventricle during diastole. Doppler ultrasound reveals turbulent flow and a dynamic gradient across the aortic valve and, commonly, mitral regurgitation. Cardiac catheterization may confirm the gradient but adds little to echocardiographic studies.

Treatment

Beta-blockers should be the initial drug in symptomatic individuals, especially when dynamic outflow obstruction is noted on the echocardiogram. Dyspnea, angina, and arrhythmias respond in about 50% of patients. Calcium channel blockers, especially verapamil, have also been effective in symptomatic patients. Their effect may be due primarily to improved diastolic function, but their vasodilating actions may also increase outflow obstruction. Excision of part of the myocardial septum has been successful in patients with severe symptoms when performed by surgeons experienced with the procedure. Dual-chamber pacing may prevent the progression of hypertrophy and obstruction. Patients with malignant ventricular arrhythmias and unexplained syncope in the presence of a positive family history for sudden death are probably best managed with an implantable defibrillator.

Prognosis

The natural history of hypertrophic cardiomyopathy is highly variable. Several specific mutations are associated with a higher incidence of early malignant arrhythmias and sudden death, and definition of the genetic abnormality provides the best estimate of prognosis. Some patients remain asymptomatic for many years or for life. Sudden death, especially during exercise, may be the initial event. Indeed, hypertrophic cardiomyopathy is the pathologic feature most frequently associated with sudden death in athletes. Other patients have a history of gradually progressive symptoms. A final stage may be a transition into dilated cardiomyopathy.

Nishimura RA et al: Dual-chamber pacing for cardiomyopathies: A 1996 clinical perspective. Mayo Clin Proc 1996;71:1077. (Cautious review of pacing in hypertrophic cardiomyopathy, with additional information about the still more experimental approach of pacing with short atrioventricular intervals in dilated cardiomyopathy.)

Nishimura RA et al: Dual-chamber pacing for hypertrophic cardiomyopathy: A randomized, double-blind, crossover trial. J Am Coll Cardiol 1997;29:435. (Well-designed trial indicating that pacing reduces outflow gradient, but symptomatic responses are quite variable.)

Spirigo P et al: The management of hypertrophic cardiomyopathy. N Engl J Med 1997;336:775. (Review covering medical management and surgical intervention but with a particular focus on genetic mechanisms.)

3. RESTRICTIVE CARDIOMYOPATHY

Restrictive cardiomyopathy is characterized by impaired diastolic filling with preserved contractile function. This condition is relatively uncommon, with the most frequent causes being amyloidosis, radiation, and myocardial fibrosis after open heart surgery. In Africa, endomyocardial fibrosis, a specific entity in which there is severe fibrosis of the endocardium, often with eosinophilia (Löffler's syndrome) is common. Other causes of a restrictive picture are infiltrative cardiomyopathies (eg, sarcoidosis, hemochromatosis, carcinoid syndrome) and connective tissue diseases (eg, scleroderma).

Amyloidosis can affect the heart in several ways. Although it is a frequent cause of restrictive cardiomyopathy, it more often produces dilated cardiomyopathy with congestive heart failure. Almost invariably, conduction disturbances are present. Low voltages on the ECG combined with ventricular hypertrophy by echo are suggestive. Rectal, abdominal fat, or gingival biopsies—as well as myocardial biopsy—can be diagnostic.

The primary diagnostic problem with restrictive cardiomyopathy is differentiation from constrictive pericarditis. The clinical picture often strongly suggests the diagnosis, but the status of left ventricular function (usually normal with pericarditis, slightly depressed with restrictive cardiomyopathy) can be helpful, as can be evidence of a thickened pericardium. Myocardial biopsies are usually negative with pericarditis but not in restrictive cardiomyopathy. In some cases, only surgical exploration can make the diagnosis.

Unfortunately, little useful therapy is available for either the causative conditions or restrictive cardiomyopathy itself. Diuretics can help, but excessive diuresis can produce worsening symptoms. Steroids may be helpful in sarcoidosis but relieve conduction abnormalities more often than heart failure.

Kushiwaha SS et al: Restrictive cardiomyopathy. N Engl J Med 1997;336:267. (Pathogenesis, diagnosis, and treatment of the diverse causes of restrictive cardiomyopathy.)

ACUTE RHEUMATIC FEVER & RHEUMATIC HEART DISEASE

Essentials of Diagnosis

- Uncommon in USA but may be overlooked.
- Peak incidence ages 5–15 years.
- Diagnosis based on Jones criteria and confirmation of streptococcal infection.
- May involve mitral and other valves acutely, rarely leading to heart failure.

General Considerations

Rheumatic fever is a systemic immune process which is a sequela to hemolytic streptococcal infection of the pharynx. Pyodermic infections are not associated with rheumatic fever. Signs of rheumatic fever usually commence 2–3 weeks after infection but may appear as early as 1 week or as late as 5 weeks. It had become uncommon in the USA, except in recent immigrants. However, there have been recent reports of new outbreaks in several regions of the USA. The peak incidence is between ages 5 and 15; rheumatic fever is rare before age 4 and after age 40. Rheumatic carditis and valvulitis may be self-limited or may lead to slowly progressive valvular deformity. The characteristic lesion is a perivascular granulomatous reaction with vasculitis. The mitral valve is attacked in 75–80% of cases, the aortic valve in 30% (but rarely as the sole valve), and the tricuspid and pulmonary valves in under 5%.

Clinical Findings

Diagnostic criteria first described by Jones are still employed. The presence of two major criteria—or one major and one minor criterion—establishes the diagnosis.

A. Major Criteria:

1. Carditis–Carditis is most likely to be evident in children and adolescents. Any of the following suggests the presence of carditis. (1) Pericarditis. (2) Cardiomegaly, detected by physical signs, radiography, or echocardiography. (3) Congestive failure, right- or left-sided—the former perhaps more prominent in children, with painful liver engorgement due to tricuspid regurgitation. (4) Mitral or aortic regurgitation murmurs, indicative of dilation of a valve ring with or without associated valvulitis. The Carey-Coombs short middiastolic mitral murmur may be present.

In the absence of any of the above definitive signs, the diagnosis of carditis depends upon the following less specific abnormalities. (1) Electrocardiographic changes: The most significant abnormality is PR prolongation greater than 0.04 s above the patient's normal. Changing contour of P waves or inversion of T waves is less useful. (2) Changing quality of heart sounds. (3) Sinus tachycardia persisting during sleep and markedly increased by slight activity. (4) Arrhythmias, shifting pacemaker, or ectopic beats.

2. Erythema marginatum and subcutaneous nodules–The former begin as rapidly enlarging macules that assume the shape of rings or crescents with clear centers. They may be raised, confluent, and either transient or persistent.

Subcutaneous nodules are uncommon except in children. They are small (≤ 2 cm in diameter), firm, and nontender and are attached to fascia or tendon sheaths over bony prominences. They persist for days or weeks, are recurrent, and are indistinguishable from rheumatoid nodules.

3. Sydenham's chorea–Sydenham's chorea—involuntary choreoathetoid movements primarily of the face, tongue, and upper extremities—may be the sole manifestation; only half of cases have other overt signs of rheumatic fever. Girls are more frequently affected, and occurrence in adults is rare. This is the least common (3% of cases) but most diagnostic of the manifestations of rheumatic fever.

4. Arthritis–This is a migratory polyarthritis that involves the large joints sequentially. In adults, only a single joint may be affected. The arthritis lasts 1–5 weeks and subsides without residual deformity. Prompt response of arthritis to therapeutic doses of salicylates or nonsteroidal agents is characteristic.

B. Minor Criteria: These include fever, polyarthralgias, reversible prolongation of the PR interval, rapid erythrocyte sedimentation rate, evidence of an antecedent β-hemolytic streptococcal infection, or a history of rheumatic fever.

C. Laboratory Findings: There is nonspecific evidence of inflammatory disease, as shown by a rapid sedimentation rate. High or increasing titers of antistreptococcal antibodies (antistreptolysin O and anti-DNAse B) are used to confirm recent infection; 10% of cases lack this serologic evidence.

Differential Diagnosis

Rheumatic fever may be confused with the following: rheumatoid arthritis, osteomyelitis, endocarditis, chronic meningococcemia, systemic lupus erythematosus, Lyme disease, sickle cell anemia, "surgical abdomen," and many other diseases.

Complications

Congestive heart failure occurs in severe cases. In the longer term, the development of rheumatic heart disease is the major problem. Other complications include arrhythmias, pericarditis with effusion, and rheumatic pneumonitis.

Treatment

A. General Measures: Bed rest should be enforced until: return of temperature to normal without medications; normal sedimentation rate; normal resting pulse rate (< 100/min in adults); and return of ECG to baseline.

B. Medical Measures:

1. Salicylates–The salicylates markedly reduce fever and relieve joint pain and swelling. They have no effect on the natural course of the disease. Adults may require aspirin, 0.6–0.9 g every 4 hours; children are treated with lower doses. Toxicity includes tinnitus, vomiting, and gastrointestinal bleeding.

2. Penicillin–Penicillin (benzathine penicillin, 1.2 million units intramuscularly once, or procaine penicillin, 600,000 units intramuscularly daily for 10 days) is employed to eradicate streptococcal infection if present. Erythromycin (dosage as above) may be substituted.

3. Corticosteroids–There is no proof that cardiac damage is prevented or minimized by corticosteroids. A short course of corticosteroids (prednisone, 40–60 mg orally daily, with tapering over 2 weeks) usually causes rapid improvement and is indicated when response to salicylates has been inadequate.

Prevention of Recurrent Rheumatic Fever

The initial episode of rheumatic fever can usually be prevented by early treatment of streptococcal pharyngitis. (See Chapter 33.) Prevention of recurrent episodes is critical. Recurrences of rheumatic fever are most common in patients who have had carditis during their initial episode and in children, 20% of whom will have a second episode within 5 years. Recurrences are uncommon after 5 years and infrequent in patients over 25 years of age. Prophylaxis is usually discontinued after these times except in groups with a high risk of streptococcal infection—parents of young children, nurses, military recruits, etc.

A. Penicillin: The preferred method of prophylaxis is with benzathine penicillin G, 1.2 million units intramuscularly every 4 weeks. Oral penicillin (200,000–250,000 units twice daily) is less reliable.

B. Sulfonamides or Erythromycin: If the patient is allergic to penicillin, sulfadiazine (or sulfisoxazole), 1 g daily, or erythromycin, 250 mg orally twice daily, may be substituted.

Prognosis

Initial episodes of rheumatic fever may last months in children and weeks in adults. The immediate mortality rate is 1–2%. Persistent rheumatic carditis with cardiomegaly, heart failure, and pericarditis imply a poor prognosis; 30% of children thus affected die within 10 years after the initial attack. Eighty percent of affected children attain adult life, and half of these have little if any limitation of activity. After 10 years, two-thirds of patients will have detectable valvular disease. In adults, residual heart damage occurs in less than 20%, with mitral regurgitation the commonest; aortic insufficiency is more common than in children. In developing countries, acute rheumatic fever appears earlier in life, and the evolution to chronic valvular disease is accelerated.

Burge DJ, DeHoratus RJ: Acute rheumatic fever. Cardiovasc Clin 1993;23:3.

Dajani A et al: Treatment of acute streptococcal pharyngitis and prevention of rheumatic fever: A statement for health professionals. Pediatrics 1995;96:1158. (Guidelines for prevention.)

RHEUMATIC HEART DISEASE

Chronic rheumatic heart disease results from single or repeated attacks of rheumatic fever that produce rigidity and deformity of valve cusps, fusion of the commissures, or shortening and fusion of the chordae tendineae. Stenosis or insufficiency results, and the two often coexist. The mitral valve alone is affected in 50–60% of cases; combined lesions of the aortic and mitral valves occur in 20%; pure aortic lesions are seen in less. Tricuspid involvement occurs only in association with mitral or aortic disease in about 10% of cases. The pulmonary valve is rarely affected. A history of rheumatic fever is obtainable in only 60% of patients with rheumatic heart disease.

The first clue to organic valvular disease is a murmur. Physical examination permits accurate diagnosis of most valve lesions. Echocardiography will reveal valve cusp thickening with decreased opening in stenosis, estimate the magnitude of regurgitation, and demonstrate the earliest stages of specific chamber enlargement.

Recurrences of acute rheumatic fever can be prevented (see above). The patient should also receive prophylactic antibiotics preceding dental extraction, urologic and surgical procedures, etc, to prevent endocarditis (Table 37–9). With mitral valve disease, it is important to identify the onset of atrial fibrillation in order to institute anticoagulation. The important findings in each of the major valve lesions are summarized in Table 10–1. The hemodynamic changes, symptoms, associated findings, and course have been discussed previously.

DISEASES OF THE PERICARDIUM

ACUTE PERICARDITIS

The pericardium consists of two layers: the inner visceral layer, which is attached to the epicardium; and an outer parietal layer. The pericardium stabilizes the heart in anatomic position and reduces contact between the heart and surrounding structures. It is composed of fibrous tissue, and while it will permit moderate changes in cardiac size, it cannot stretch rapidly enough to accommodate rapid dilation of the heart or accumulation of fluid without increasing intrapericardial (and, therefore, intracardiac) pressure.

The pericardium is often involved by processes that affect the heart, but it may also be affected by diseases of adjacent tissues and may itself be a primary site of disease.

INFLAMMATORY PERICARDITIS

Acute inflammation of the pericardium may be infectious in origin or may be due to systemic diseases (autoimmune syndromes, uremia), neoplasm, radiation, drug toxicity, hemopericardium, or contiguous inflammatory processes in the myocardium or lung. In many of these conditions, the pathologic process involves both the pericardium and the myocardium.

The presentation and course of inflammatory pericarditis depend on its cause, but all syndromes are often (not always) associated with chest pain, which is usually pleuritic and postural (relieved by sitting). The pain is substernal but may radiate to the neck, shoulders, back, or epigastrium. Dyspnea may also be present. A pericardial friction rub is characteristic, with or without evidence of fluid accumulation or constriction (see below). Fever and leukocytosis are often present. The ECG usually shows generalized ST and T wave changes and may manifest a characteristic progression beginning with diffuse ST elevation, followed by a return to baseline and then to T wave inversion. The chest x-ray may show cardiac enlargement if fluid has collected, as well as signs of related pulmonary disease. The echocardiogram may disclose pericardial effusions and indicate their hemodynamic significance, but it is often normal in inflammatory pericarditis.

Several of the specific pericarditis syndromes are discussed below.

Viral Pericarditis

Viral infections (especially infections with coxsackieviruses and echoviruses but also influenza, Epstein-Barr, varicella, hepatitis, mumps, and HIV viruses) are the commonest cause of acute pericarditis and probably are responsible for many cases classified as idiopathic. Males—usually under age 50—are most commonly affected. Pericardial involvement often follows upper respiratory infection. The diagnosis is usually clinical, but rising viral titers in paired sera may be obtained for confirmation. Cardiac enzymes may be slightly elevated, reflecting a myocarditic component. The differential diagnosis is primarily with myocardial infarction.

Treatment is generally symptomatic. Aspirin (650 mg every 3–4 hours) or other nonsteroidal agents (eg, indomethacin, 100–150 mg daily in divided doses) are usually effective. Corticosteroids may be beneficial in unresponsive cases. In general, symptoms subside in several days to weeks. The major early complication is tamponade, which occurs in fewer than 5% of patients. There may be recurrences in the first few weeks or months. Rare patients will continue to experience recurrences chronically, sometimes leading to constrictive pericarditis, when pericardial resection may be required.

Tuberculous Pericarditis

Tuberculous pericarditis has become rare in developed countries but remains common in other areas. It results from direct lymphatic or hematogenous spread; clinical pulmonary involvement may be absent or minor, although associated pleural effusions are common. The presentation tends to be subacute, but nonspecific symptoms (fever, night sweats, fatigue) may be present for days to months. Pericardial effusions are usually small or moderate but may be large. The diagnosis can be inferred if evidence of acid-fast bacilli are found elsewhere. The yield of organisms by pericardiocentesis is low; pericardial biopsy has a higher yield but may also be negative, and pericardiectomy may be required. Standard antituberculous drug therapy is usually successful (see Chapter 9), but constrictive pericarditis can occur.

Other Infectious Pericarditides

Bacterial pericarditis has become rare and usually results from direct extension from pulmonary infections. Signs and symptoms are similar to those of other types of inflammatory pericarditides, but patients appear toxic—often critically ill. *Borrelia burgdorferi,* the organism responsible for Lyme disease, can also cause myopericarditis.

Uremic Pericarditis

This syndrome is a common complication of renal failure whose pathogenesis is uncertain; it occurs both with untreated uremia and in otherwise stable dialysis patients. The pericardium is characteristically "shaggy," and the effusion is hemorrhagic and exudative. Uremic pericarditis can present with or without symptoms; fever is absent. The pericarditis usually resolves with the institution of—or with more aggressive—dialysis. Tamponade is fairly common, and partial pericardiectomy (pericardial window) may be necessary. While anti-inflammatory agents may relieve the pain and fever associated with uremic pericarditis, indomethacin and systemic glucocorticoids do not affect the natural history of uremic pericarditis.

Neoplastic Pericarditis

Spread of adjacent lung cancer as well as invasion by breast cancer, renal cell carcinoma, Hodgkin's disease, and lymphomas are the commonest neoplastic processes involving the pericardium and have become the most frequent cause of pericardial tamponade in many countries. Often the process is painless, and the presenting symptoms relate to hemodynamic compromise or the primary disease. The diagnosis can usually be made by cytologic examination of the effusion or by biopsy, but it may be difficult to establish clinically if the patient has received mediastinal radiation within the previous year. MRI and CT scan can visualize neighboring tumor when present. The prognosis with neoplastic effusion is dismal, with only a small minority surviving 1 year. If it is compromising the patient, the effusion is initially drained. Instillation of chemotherapeutic agents or tetracycline may also prevent recurrence. Pericardial windows are rarely effective, but partial pericardiectomy from a subxiphoid incision may be successful; patients may be too ill to tolerate this.

Postmyocardial Infarction or Postcardiotomy Pericarditis (Dressler's Syndrome)

Pericarditis may occur 2–5 days after infarction due to an inflammatory reaction to transmural myocardial necrosis. It usually presents as a recurrence of pain with pleural-pericardial features. A rub is often audible, and repolarization changes may be confused with ischemia. Large effusions are uncommon, and spontaneous resolution usually occurs in a few days. Aspirin or nonsteroidal agents in the dosages given in the section on viral pericarditis provide symptomatic relief.

Dressler's syndrome occurs weeks to several months after myocardial infarction or open heart surgery, may be recurrent, and probably represents an autoimmune syndrome. Patients present with typical pain, fever, malaise, and leukocytosis. The sedimentation rate is usually high. Large pericardial effusions and accompanying pleural effusions are frequent. Tamponade is rare with Dressler's syndrome after infarction but not when it occurs postoperatively. Nonsteroidal agents are given, but recurrences are common; corticosteroids are effective but may be difficult to withdraw without relapse.

Radiation Pericarditis

Radiation can initiate a fibrinous and fibrotic process in the pericardium, presenting as subacute pericarditis or constriction. The clinical onset is usually within the first year but may be delayed for many years. Radiation pericarditis usually follows treatments of more than 4000 cGy delivered to ports including more than 30% of the heart. Symptomatic therapy is the initial approach, but recurrent effusions and constriction often require surgery.

Other Causes of Pericarditis

These include connective tissue diseases, such as lupus erythematosus, rheumatoid arthritis, and drug-induced pericarditis (minoxidil, penicillins), and myxedema.

Benoff LJ, Schweitzer P: Radiation therapy-induced cardiac injury. Am Heart J 1995;129:1193. (Pericarditis is the most frequent cardiac sequela of radiation therapy, particularly following treatment of Hodgkin's disease).

Sagrista-Sauleda J et al: Purulent pericarditis: Review of a 20-year experience in a general hospital. J Am Coll Cardiol 1993;22:1661. (The diagnosis is often missed, and the most common correlate is empyema.)

PERICARDIAL EFFUSION

Pericardial effusion can develop during any of the processes discussed in the preceding paragraphs. The speed of accumulation determines the physiologic importance of the effusion. Because the pericardium stretches, large effusions (> 1000 mL) that develop slowly may produce no hemodynamic effects. Smaller effusions that appear rapidly can cause tamponade. Tamponade is characterized by elevated intrapericardial pressure (> 15 mm Hg), which restricts venous return and ventricular filling. As a result, the stroke volume and pulse pressure fall, and the heart rate and venous pressure rise. Shock and death may result.

Clinical Findings

A. Symptoms and Signs: Pericardial effusions may be associated with pain if they occur as part of an acute inflammatory process or may be painless, as is often the case with neoplastic or uremic effusion. Dyspnea and cough are common, especially with tamponade. Other symptoms may result from the primary disease.

A pericardial friction rub may be present even with large effusions. In cardiac tamponade, tachycardia, tachypnea, a narrow pulse pressure, and a relatively preserved systolic pressure are characteristic. Pulsus paradoxus—a greater than 10 mm Hg decline in systolic pressure during inspiration due to further impairment of left ventricular filling—is the classic finding, but it may also occur with obstructive lung disease. Central venous pressure is elevated, and edema or ascites may be present; these signs favor a more chronic process.

B. Laboratory Findings: Laboratory tests tend to reflect the underlying processes.

C. Diagnostic Studies: Chest x-ray can suggest effusion by an enlarged cardiac silhouette with a globular configuration. The ECG often reveals nonspecific T wave changes and low QRS voltage. Electrical alternans is present uncommonly but is pathognomonic. Echocardiography is the primary method for demonstrating pericardial effusion. Tamponade presents a characteristic picture of inadequate ventricular filling (diastolic collapse of the right ventricle or right atrium). The echocardiogram readily discriminates pericardial effusion from congestive heart failure. MRI also demonstrates pericardial fluid and lesions. Diagnostic pericardiocentesis or biopsy is often indicated for microbiologic and cytologic studies; a pericardial biopsy may be performed relatively simply through a small subxiphoid incision.

Treatment

Small effusions can be followed clinically and with the aid of echocardiograms. When tamponade is present, urgent pericardiocentesis is required. Removal of a small amount of fluid often produces immediate hemodynamic benefit, but complete drainage with a catheter is preferable. Continued drainage may be indicated.

Additional therapy is determined by the nature of the primary process. Recurrent effusion in neoplastic disease and uremia, in particular, may require partial pericardiectomy.

Ameli S, Shah PK: Cardiac tamponade: Pathophysiology, diagnosis, and management. Cardiol Clin 1991;9:665.

Fowler NO: Cardiac tamponade: A clinical or echocardiographic diagnosis? Circulation 1993;87:1738. (Technology may have obscured one of the most important bedside diagnoses.)

Hancock EW: Neoplastic pericardial disease. Cardiol Clin 1990;8:673.

CONSTRICTIVE PERICARDITIS

Inflammation can lead to a thickened, fibrotic, adherent pericardium that restricts diastolic filling and produces chronically elevated venous pressures. In the past, tuberculosis was the most common cause of constrictive pericarditis, but the process now more often occurs after radiation therapy, cardiac surgery, or viral pericarditis; histoplasmosis is another uncommon cause.

The principal symptoms are slowly progressive dyspnea, fatigue, and weakness. Chronic edema, hepatic congestion, and ascites are usually present. The examination reveals these signs and a characteristically elevated jugular venous pressure with a rapid y descent. Kussmaul's sign—an increase in jugular venous pressure during inspiration—occurs in constrictive pericarditis and restrictive cardiomyopathy. Pulsus paradoxus is unusual. Atrial fibrillation is common.

The chest x-ray may show normal heart size or cardiomegaly. Pericardial calcification is best seen on the lateral view and is common. Echocardiography can demonstrate a thick pericardium and small chambers. CT scans and MRI are helpful in revealing pericardial thickening and may be more sensitive than echocardiography.

The primary differential diagnoses are restrictive cardiomyopathy and tamponade. The former distinction can be difficult and is best made by evaluating left ventricular function (more consistently depressed in cardiomyopathy), measuring hemodynamics (which show more complete equalization of diastolic pressures in all four chambers in constrictive pericarditis), and demonstrating pericardial thickening and calcification.

Initial treatment consists of gentle diuresis. Surgical removal of the pericardium, which should be complete, is usually required in symptomatic patients but is associated with a relatively high mortality rate.

Brockington GM et al: Constrictive pericarditis. Cardiol Clin 1990;8:645.

Vaitkus PT, Kussmaul WG: Constrictive pericarditis versus restrictive cardiomyopathy: A reappraisal and update of diagnostic criteria. Am Heart J 1991;122:1431. (A very difficult problem.)

PULMONARY HYPERTENSION & HEART DISEASE

PRIMARY PULMONARY HYPERTENSION

Primary pulmonary hypertension is defined as pulmonary hypertension and elevated pulmonary vascular resistance in the absence of other disease of the lungs or heart. Pathologically, it is characterized by diffuse narrowing of the pulmonary arterioles. Circumstantial evidence suggests that unrecognized recurrent pulmonary emboli or in situ thrombosis may play a role in some cases. The latter may well be an exacerbating factor (precipitated by local endothelial injury) rather than a cause of the syndrome. Primary pulmonary hypertension must be distinguished from chronic pulmonary heart disease (cor pulmonale), recurrent pulmonary emboli, mitral stenosis, congenital heart disease, and occult mitral stenosis; cirrhosis of the liver is another cause. Exclusion of secondary causes by echocardiography and lung scanning—and, if necessary, pulmonary angiography—is essential.

The clinical picture is similar to that of pulmonary hypertension from other causes. Patients—characteristically young women—present with evidence of right heart failure that is usually progressive, leading to death in 2–8 years. Patients have manifestations of low cardiac output, with weakness and fatigue, as well as edema and ascites as right heart failure advances. Peripheral cyanosis is present, and syncope on effort may occur.

The chest x-ray shows enlarged main pulmonary arteries with reduced peripheral branches. The right ventricle is enlarged. The ECG shows right ventricular and atrial hypertrophy.

Some authorities advocate chronic oral anticoagu-

lation. The efficacy of vasodilator drugs is controversial, in part because the responses are variable. For example, a response in the systemic circulation may worsen the problem by reducing venous return. The calcium channel blockers nifedipine and diltiazem appear to be the preferred agents. The best response may be in patients in the earlier stages of the disease, when a more reversible vasoconstrictive component is present.

The prognosis for patients with primary pulmonary hypertension is generally poor. Once symptoms develop, most patients pursue a downhill course. This outcome may be improved by chronic infusion of prostacyclin, a potent pulmonary vasodilator. This therapy often improves symptoms, sometimes dramatically, in patients who have not responded to other vasodilators. It is initiated only in individuals who have failed to respond to calcium channel blockers. The main application of this therapy may be as a bridge to heart-lung or single-lung transplantation.

Barst RJ et al: Comparison of continuous intravenous epoprostenol (prostacyclin) with conventional therapy for primary pulmonary hypertension. N Engl J Med 1996;334:296. (Multicenter trial in 81 patients demonstrating symptomatic and hemodynamic improvement and prolonged survival with prostacyclin.)

Rubin LJ: Primary pulmonary hypertension. N Engl J Med 1997;336:111. (Incidence, pathogenesis, diagnosis, and treatment.)

PULMONARY HEART DISEASE (Cor Pulmonale)

Essentials of Diagnosis

- Symptoms and signs of chronic bronchitis and pulmonary emphysema.
- Elevated jugular venous pressure, parasternal lift, edema, hepatomegaly, ascites.
- ECG shows tall, peaked P waves (P pulmonale), right axis deviation, and right ventricular hypertrophy.
- Chest x-ray: Enlarged right ventricle and pulmonary artery.
- Echocardiogram or radionuclide angiography excludes primary left ventricular dysfunction.

General Considerations

The term "cor pulmonale" denotes right ventricular hypertrophy and eventual failure resulting from pulmonary disease and attendant hypoxia. Its clinical features depend upon both the primary disease and its effects on the heart.

Cor pulmonale is most commonly caused by chronic obstructive pulmonary disease. Rare causes include pneumoconiosis, pulmonary fibrosis, kyphoscoliosis, primary pulmonary hypertension, repeated episodes of subclinical or clinical pulmonary embolization, Pickwickian syndrome, schistosomiasis, and obliterative pulmonary capillary or lymphangitic infiltration from metastatic carcinoma.

Clinical Findings

A. Symptoms and Signs: The predominant symptoms of compensated cor pulmonale are related to the pulmonary disorder and include chronic productive cough, exertional dyspnea, wheezing respirations, easy fatigability, and weakness. When the pulmonary disease causes right ventricular failure, these symptoms may be intensified. Dependent edema and right upper quadrant pain may also appear. The signs of cor pulmonale include cyanosis, clubbing, distended neck veins, right ventricular heave or gallop (or both), prominent lower sternal or epigastric pulsations, an enlarged and tender liver, and dependent edema.

B. Laboratory Findings: Polycythemia is often present in cor pulmonale secondary to COPD. The arterial oxygen saturation is below 85%; PCO_2 may or may not be elevated.

C. Electrocardiography and Chest X-Ray: The ECG may show right axis deviation and peaked P waves. Deep S waves are present in lead V_6. Right axis deviation and low voltage may be noted in patients with pulmonary emphysema. Frank right ventricular hypertrophy is uncommon except in "primary pulmonary hypertension." The ECG often mimics myocardial infarction; Q waves may be present in leads II, III, and aVF because of the vertically placed heart, but they are rarely deep or wide, as in inferior myocardial infarction. Supraventricular arrhythmias are frequent and nonspecific.

The chest radiograph discloses the presence or absence of parenchymal disease and a prominent or enlarged right ventricle and pulmonary artery.

D. Diagnostic Studies: Pulmonary function tests usually confirm the underlying lung disease. The echocardiogram should show normal left ventricular size and function but right ventricular dilation. Perfusion lung scans are rarely of value, but, if negative, they help to exclude pulmonary emboli, an occasional cause of cor pulmonale. Pulmonary angiography is the most specific method of diagnosis for the pulmonary emboli, but it carries increased risk when performed in patients with pulmonary hypertension.

Differential Diagnosis

In its early stages, cor pulmonale can be diagnosed on the basis of radiologic, echocardiographic, or electrocardiographic evidence. Catheterization of the right heart will establish a definitive diagnosis but is usually performed to exclude left-sided heart failure, which may in some patients be an inapparent cause of right-sided failure. Differential diagnostic considerations relate chiefly to the specific pulmonary disease that has produced right ventricular failure (see above).

Treatment

The details of the treatment of chronic pulmonary disease (chronic respiratory failure) are discussed in Chapter 9. Otherwise, therapy is directed at the pulmonary process responsible for right heart failure. Oxygen, salt and fluid restriction, and diuretics are mainstays; digitalis has no place in right heart failure unless atrial fibrillation is present.

Prognosis

Compensated cor pulmonale has the same outlook as the underlying pulmonary disease. Once congestive signs appear, the average life expectancy is 2–5 years, but survival is significantly longer when uncomplicated emphysema is the cause.

Klinger JR, Hill NS: Right ventricular dysfunction in chronic obstructive pulmonary disease. Evaluation and management. Chest 1991;99:715.

MacNee W: Pathophysiology of cor pulmonale in chronic obstructive pulmonary disease. (Two parts.) Am J Resp Crit Care Med 1994;150:833, 1158.

NEOPLASTIC DISEASES OF THE HEART

Primary cardiac tumors are rare and constitute only a small fraction of all tumors that involve the heart or pericardium. Metastases from malignant tumors elsewhere are more frequent. Tumors involving the heart are bronchogenic carcinoma, carcinoma of the breast, malignant melanoma, the lymphomas, renal cell carcinoma, and, in patients with AIDS, Kaposi's sarcoma. These are often clinically silent but may lead to pericardial tamponade, arrhythmias and conduction disturbances, heart failure, and peripheral emboli. The diagnosis is often made by echocardiography, but MRI and CT scanning are also helpful. Electrocardiography may reveal regional Q waves. The prognosis is dismal; effective treatment is not available.

The commonest primary tumors of the heart are atrial myxomas. These tend to occur in middle age, more often in women than in men. They usually originate in the intraventricular septum, with over 80% growing into the left atrium. Myxomas are benign tumors but can embolize systemically.

Patients with myxoma can present with a picture of a systemic illness, obstruction of blood flow through the heart, or signs of peripheral embolization. The characteristic picture includes fever, malaise, weight loss, leukocytosis, elevated sedimentation rate, and emboli (peripheral or pulmonary, depending on the location of the tumor). This picture is often confused with infective endocarditis, lymphoma, other cancers, or autoimmune diseases. In other cases, the tumor may grow to considerable size and produce symptoms by obstructing mitral flow. Episodic pulmonary edema (classically occurring when an upright posture is assumed) and signs of low output may result. Physical examination may reveal a diastolic sound related to motion of the tumor ("tumor plop") or a diastolic murmur similar to that of mitral stenosis. Right-sided myxomas may cause symptoms of right-sided failure. The diagnosis is established by echocardiography or by pathologic study of embolic material. MRI is also useful. Contrast angiography is usually not necessary. Surgical excision is usually curative.

Other primary cardiac tumors include rhabdomyomas, fibrous histiocytomas, hemangiomas, and a variety of unusual sarcomas. The diagnosis may be supported by an abnormal cardiac contour on x-ray. Echocardiography is usually helpful but may miss tumors infiltrating the ventricular wall. It is likely that MRI will be useful as well.

Reynen K: Cardiac myxomas. N Engl J Med 1995; 333:1610.

Salcedo EE et al: Cardiac tumors: Diagnosis and management. Curr Probl Cardiol 1992;17:75.

CARDIAC INVOLVEMENT IN MISCELLANEOUS SYSTEMIC DISEASES

The heart may be involved in a number of systemic syndromes. Many of these have been mentioned briefly in prior subsections of this chapter. The pericardium, myocardium, heart valves, and coronary arteries may be involved either singly or in various combinations. In most cases the cardiac manifestations are not the dominant feature, but in some it is the primary cause of symptoms and may be fatal.

The most common type of myocardial involvement is an infiltrative cardiomyopathy, such as systemic amyloidosis, sarcoidosis, hemochromatosis, or glycogen storage disease. Cardiac calcinosis can occur in hyperparathyroidism (usually the secondary form) and in primary oxalosis. A number of muscular dystrophies can cause a cardiomyopathic picture (particularly Duchenne's, less frequently myotonic dystrophy, and several rarer forms). In addition to left ventricular dysfunction and heart failure, all of these conditions frequently cause conduction abnormalities, which may be the presenting or only feature. The myocardium may also be involved in inflammatory and autoimmune diseases. It is commonly affected in polymyositis and dermatomyositis, but usually this is subclinical. Systemic lupus erythematosus, scleroderma, and mixed connective tissue disease may cause myocarditis, but these commonly also involve the pericardium, coronary arteries, or valves. Several endocrinopathies, including acromegaly, thyrotoxicosis, myxedema, and pheochromocytoma, can produce cardiomyopathies, though again they are usually not isolated features.

Pericardial involvement is quite common in many of the connective tissue diseases. Systemic lupus erythematosus may present with pericarditis, and pericardial involvement is not uncommon (but is less frequently symptomatic) in active rheumatoid arthritis, systemic sclerosis, and mixed connective tissue disease. Endocardial involvement takes the form of patchy fibrous—predominantly on the right side—or inflammatory or sclerotic changes of the heart valves. Carcinoid heart disease typically is manifested as tricuspid regurgitation, and the same may be the case in systemic lupus erythematosus. The hypereosinophilic syndromes involve the endocardium, leading to restrictive cardiomyopathy. A variety of arthritic syndromes are associated with aortic valvulitis or aortitis, including ankylosing spondylitis, rheumatoid arthritis, and Reiter's syndrome, as is tertiary syphilis also. Disorders of elastic tissue (Marfan's syndrome is the most frequent) often affect the ascending aorta, with resulting aneurysmal dilation and aortic regurgitation.

Virtually any vasculitic syndrome can involve the coronary arteries, leading to myocardial infarction. This is most common with polyarteritis nodosa and systemic lupus erythematosus. Two vasculitic syndromes have a particular predilection for the coronary arteries—Kawasaki's disease and Takayasu's disease. In these, myocardial infarction may be the presenting symptom.

Pellikka PA et al: Carcinoid heart disease: Clinical and echocardiographic spectrum in 74 patients. Circulation 1993;87:1188.

TRAUMATIC HEART DISEASE

Penetrating wounds to the heart are, of course, usually lethal unless surgically repaired. Stab wounds to the right ventricle occasionally lead to hemopericardium without progressing to tamponade. The clinical result may be constrictive pericarditis, so surgery is recommended even if the patient presents in an unstable condition.

Blunt trauma is a more frequent cause of cardiac

injuries, particularly outside of the emergency room setting. This type of injury is quite frequent in motor vehicle accidents and may occur with any form of chest trauma. The most common injuries are myocardial contusions or hematomas. These may be asymptomatic (particularly in the setting of more severe injuries) or may present with chest pains of a nonspecific nature or, not uncommonly, with a pericardial component. A minority of patients will develop left or, less commonly, right ventricle aneurysm. Elevations of cardiac enzymes are frequent, and echocardiography may reveal an akinetic segment. Heart failure is uncommon if there are no associated cardiac or pericardial injuries, and conservative management is usually sufficient.

Severe trauma may also cause cardiac or valvular rupture. Cardiac rupture may involve any chamber, but survival is most likely if injury is to one of the atria or the right ventricle. Hemopericardium or pericardial tamponade is the usual clinical presentation, and surgery is almost always necessary. Mitral and aortic valve rupture may occur during severe blunt trauma—the former presumably if the impact occurs during systole and the latter if during diastole. Patients reach the hospital in shock or severe heart failure. Immediate surgical repair is essential. The same types of injuries may result in transection of the aorta, either at the level of the arch or distal to the takeoff of the left subclavian artery. Transthoracic and transesophageal echocardiography are the most helpful and immediately available diagnostic techniques.

Blunt trauma may also result in damage to the coronary arteries. Acute or subacute coronary thrombosis is the most common presentation. The clinical syndrome is one of acute myocardial infarction with attendant electrocardiographic, enzymatic, and contractile abnormalities. Emergent revascularization is sometimes feasible, either by the percutaneous route or by coronary artery bypass surgery. Left ventricular aneurysms are common outcomes of traumatic coronary occlusions. Coronary artery dissection or rupture may also occur in the setting of blunt cardiac trauma.

Pretre R and Chilcott M: Blunt trauma to the heart and great vessels. N Engl J Med 1997;336:626.

THE CARDIAC PATIENT & SURGERY

Patients with known or suspected cardiac disease undergoing general surgery present a common management problem. Anesthesia and surgery are often associated with marked fluctuations of heart rate and blood pressure, changes in intravascular volume, myocardial ischemia or depression, arrhythmias, decreased oxygenation, increased sympathetic nervous system activity, and alterations in medical regimens and pharmacokinetics. Even with careful monitoring and management, the perioperative period can be very stressful to cardiac patients.

The risk of surgery in patients with heart disease depends primarily on three factors: the type of operation, the nature of the heart disease, and the degree of preoperative stability. The type of anesthesia is less important, though halothane, enflurane, and barbiturates are more severe myocardial depressants, while narcotics have little depressive effect. Spinal and epidural anesthesia were previously thought to be preferable in patients with heart disease, but this has not proved to be the case.

The highest-risk procedures are surgery of the aorta and vascular procedures, in part because these patients often have associated severe coronary disease but also because marked blood pressure and volume changes are common. Major abdominal and thoracic surgery are also associated with substantial cardiovascular risk, especially in older patients with associated cardiovascular disease.

Numerous studies have evaluated the excess risk of surgery in patients with various cardiac diseases. Recent (within 3 months) myocardial infarction, unstable angina, congestive heart failure, and significant aortic stenosis are associated with substantial increases in operative morbidity and mortality rates. Any degree of instability in these conditions magnifies the potential risk. Stable angina, especially in an inactive individual, is also associated with a higher operative risk. Although less common, cyanotic congenital heart disease and severe primary or secondary pulmonary hypertension pose great risks during major surgery. In patients with any of these problems, the risk-to-benefit ratio of the planned surgery should be carefully examined. If the procedure is necessary but elective, consideration should be given to delaying it until full recovery postinfarction and correction or optimal stabilization of the other conditions are achieved. Hypertension should be at least moderately controlled. Patients with severe angina should have increased medical therapy or be considered for revascularization before noncardiac surgery. Symptomatic arrhythmias, nonsustained ventricular tachycardia, or high-grade atrioventricular block and cardiac failure should be treated optimally.

Clinical assessment provides the most useful guidance in determining the risk of noncardiac surgery. Important indicators of high risk have been discussed above. Patients with known but clinically stable heart disease, such as angina pectoris or prior myocardial infarction, are at intermediate risk, particularly for major operations such as vascular surgery. If a history or symptoms of heart failure are present, assessment of left ventricular function can be very helpful in perioperative management. Although frequently advocated, further noninvasive testing for myocardial ischemia for the purpose of risk stratification is probably overutilized. Tests such as stress myocardial perfusion scintigraphy or dobutamine echocardiography should be reserved for situations in which the results may alter patient management. There is no evidence that prophylactic revascularization by either PTCA or coronary artery bypass surgery alters long-term outcome in patients (ie, the combined morbidity and mortality of the two surgical procedures) without the usual indications for these procedures. Only in the case of major vascular operations is perioperative mortality and morbidity high enough that this may be the case in selected individuals.

However, it should be noted that many patients undergoing surgery have not had recent medical follow-up, and this may be an appropriate opportunity to perform a more complete evaluation. Thus, stress testing may be indicated for selected patients with symptomatic angina or prior myocardial infarction with a view to instituting more comprehensive medical management or performing coronary revascularization to reduce long-term (rather than perioperative) mortality and morbidity. At the least, such patients should not be discharged without a plan for an appropriate follow-up and institution of antihyperlipidemic, aspirin, and beta-blocker therapy as indicated.

Once the decision to operate is made, careful management is essential. Most cardiac medications should be continued preoperatively and postoperatively. Institution of beta-blockers in patients who are known to have or be at high risk for developing coronary artery disease is a rational approach supported by some evidence. Monitoring is an important prophylactic measure in high-risk individuals; hemodynamic monitoring can facilitate early intervention in patients with heart failure, severe valve disease, or easily induced myocardial ischemia. Excessive hypertension, hypotension, and myocardial ischemia should be identified and appropriately treated using rapidly acting agents. Transesophageal echocardiography can also be used for intraoperative monitoring of ischemia, but its value has never been established in well-designed studies. Ischemic events, whether symptomatic or silent, should be vigorously treated.

ACC/AHA Task Force Report: Guidelines for peri-operative cardiovascular evaluation for non cardiac surgery. J Am Coll Cardiol 1996;27:910. (Extensive review of existing data and recommendations for management.)

Baron JF et al: Dipyridamole-thallium scintigraphy and gated radionuclide angiography to assess cardiac risk before abdominal aortic surgery. N Engl J Med 1994; 3330:663. (Very large prospective study indicating that the results are not as predictive of outcome as previous smaller studies had suggested.)

Bode RH et al: Cardiac outcome after peripheral vascular surgery: comparison of general and regional anesthesia. Anesthesiology 1996;84:3. (Randomized study in 423 patients indicating that the type of anesthesia does not affect postoperative cardiac morbidity after peripheral vascular surgery.)

Mangano DT et al: Effect of atenolol on mortality and cardiovascular morbidity after noncardiac surgery. N Engl J Med 1996;335:1713. (Randomized trial showing an early reduction in ischemic episodes and—more difficult to explain—long-term improvement in survival in 200 patients treated with atenolol for the perioperative period.)

Mangano DT, Goldman L: Perioperative assessment of patients with no suspected coronary artery disease. N Engl J Med 1995;333:1750. (Data-based review and recommendations.)

Mason JJ et al: The role of coronary angiography and coronary revascularization before vascular surgery. JAMA 1995;273:1919. (Decision analysis indicating that coronary angiography and revascularization are rarely indicated as a preoperative risk reduction strategy.)

Massie BM, Mangano DT: Assessment of perioperative risk: Have we put the cart before the horse? J Am Coll Cardiol 1993;21:1356. (Editorial suggesting that risk stratification with expensive diagnostic tests is often not justified.)

THE CARDIAC PATIENT & PREGNANCY

The management of cardiac disease in pregnancy is discussed in detail in the references listed below. Only a few major points can be covered in this brief section.

CARDIOVASCULAR CHANGES DURING PREGNANCY

Normal physiologic changes during pregnancy can exacerbate symptoms of underlying cardiac disease even in previously asymptomatic individuals. Maternal blood volume rises progressively until the end of the sixth or seventh month. Stroke volume increases over the same time course as a result of the volume change and an increase in ejection fraction. The latter reflects predominantly a decline in peripheral resistance due to vasodilation and the low-resistance shunting through the placenta. The heart rate tends to rise in the third trimester. Overall, cardiac output increases by 30–50%; systolic blood pressure tends to rise slightly or remain unchanged, but diastolic pressure falls significantly.

High cardiac output causes alterations in the cardiac examination. A third heart sound is prominent and normal, and a pulmonary flow murmur is common. Electrocardiographic changes include rate-related decreases in PR and QT intervals, a leftward axis shift, inferior Q waves due to the more horizontal position of the heart, and nonspecific ST–T wave changes.

MANAGEMENT OF PREEXISTING CONDITIONS

The physiologic changes imposed by pregnancy can cause cardiac decompensation in patients with any significant cardiac abnormality, but the most severe problems are encountered in patients with valvular stenosis (especially mitral and aortic stenosis), congenital or acquired abnormalities associated with pulmonary hypertension or right-to-left shunting, congestive heart failure due to any cause, coronary heart disease, and hypertension. Valvular insufficiency or left-to-right shunting often diminishes because of the fall in peripheral resistance and is better tolerated.

Mitral stenosis becomes more hemodynamically severe owing to the increase in diastolic flow and the rate-related shortening of diastole. Left atrial pressures rise, and dyspnea or pulmonary edema can occur in previously asymptomatic individuals. The onset of atrial fibrillation often leads to acute decompensation. Patients with moderate to severe stenosis should have the condition corrected prior to becoming pregnant if possible. Patients who become symptomatic can undergo successful surgery, preferably in the third trimester. Balloon valvuloplasty is an attractive alternative, though radiation exposure to the fetus is unavoidable. Coarctation is usually well tolerated, but patients with symptoms should have corrective surgery before pregnancy. Patients with severe pulmonary hypertension and cyanotic congenital heart disease and those with severe aortic stenosis are at extremely high risk and should attempt to avoid pregnancy.

Asymptomatic arrhythmias should be closely observed unless underlying heart disease is present, in which case they should be treated with drugs. Paroxysmal supraventricular arrhythmias are quite common. Patients with Wolff-Parkinson-White syndrome may have more problems during pregnancy. Therapy is similar to that required for nonpregnant women.

Preexisting systemic hypertension is usually well tolerated and controllable, though the fetal morbidity rate is slightly increased. The incidence of preeclampsia and eclampsia (see Chapter 18) is increased.

Treatment with diuretics is best avoided because hypovolemia may reduce uterine blood flow. Hydralazine and methyldopa are the antihypertensive agents for which there has been the greatest experience during pregnancy. Diuretics have also been used frequently, but concern has been raised that intravascular hypovolemia might impair uterine blood flow. Nonetheless, these agents are relatively safe. More recently, there has been considerable use of the combined alpha-beta-blocker labetalol and of calcium channel blockers, which have been proved effective and safe to both the mother and fetus. On the other hand, atenolol has been associated with lower fetal weights. ACE inhibitors and angiotensin II blockers are contraindicated in pregnancy. Beta-blockers may retard fetal growth, but experience with them has been generally favorable. A recent advisory has noted injury to the fetus with ACE inhibitors. Little is known about the safety of most other antihypertensive agents.

CARDIOVASCULAR COMPLICATIONS OF PREGNANCY

Pregnancy-related hypertension (eclampsia and preeclampsia) is discussed in Chapter 18.

Cardiomyopathy of Pregnancy (Peripartum Cardiomyopathy)

In approximately one out of 4000–15,000 patients, dilated cardiomyopathy develops in the final month of pregnancy or within 6 months after delivery. The cause is unclear, but immune and viral causes have been postulated. The course of the disease is variable; many cases improve or resolve completely over several months, but others progress to refractory heart failure. Immunosuppressive therapy has been advocated, but few supportive data are available. Recently, beta-blockers have been administered judiciously to these patients, with at least anecdotal success. Recurrence in subsequent pregnancies has been reported.

Coronary Artery & Other Vascular Abnormalities

There have been a number of reports of myocardial infarction during pregnancy. It is known that pregnancy predisposes to dissection of the aorta and other arteries, perhaps because of the accompanying connective tissue changes. However, coronary artery dissection is responsible for only a minority of the infarctions, with the majority being caused by atherosclerotic coronary artery disease or coronary emboli. Most of the events occur near term or shortly following delivery. Clinical management is essentially similar to that of other patients with acute infarction.

SPECIAL PROBLEMS

Prophylaxis for Infective Endocarditis

Although there is not universal agreement, many authorities recommend antibiotic prophylaxis during labor for patients at risk for endocarditis, especially if forceps or an episiotomy is employed. Ampicillin (2 g intravenously or intramuscularly) plus gentamicin (1.5 mg/kg intravenously or intramuscularly [up to 80 mg]) followed by amoxicillin, 1.5 g orally every 6 hours, is the recommended regimen.

Management of Labor

While vaginal delivery is usually well tolerated, unstable patients (including patients with severe hypertension and worsening heart failure) should have cesarean section. An increased risk of aortic rupture has been noted during delivery in patients with coarctation of the aorta and severe aortic root dilation with Marfan's syndrome, and vaginal delivery should be avoided in these conditions.

Cardiovascular Drugs During Pregnancy

Experience during pregnancy with many drugs is limited, and the effect on the fetus is often not well defined. Drugs with known potential for teratogenicity or fetal injury include phenytoin and the ACE inhibitors. Warfarin also presents a risk, but—at least in patients with prosthetic heart valves—many recommend that it be continued until the final 2 weeks. Self-injected heparin offers an alternative. Other than antihypertensive agents, which have been discussed above, cardiac drugs that appear safe during pregnancy include the digitalis glycosides, quinidine, procainamide, lidocaine, and short-term verapamil.

Bhagwat AR, Engle TJ: Heart disease in pregnancy. Cardiol Clin 1995;13:163.

Lambert MB, Lange RM: Peri-partum cardiomyopathy. Am Heart J 1995;130:860. (Review covering definition, epidemiology, clinical presentation, treatment, and prognosis.)

Page RL: Treatment of arrhythmias during pregnancy. Am Heart J 1995;130:871.

Roth A, Elkayam U: Acute myocardial infarction associated with pregnancy. Ann Intern Med 1996;125:751. (Review of 125 cases documented in the medical literature.)

Cardiovascular Screening of Competitive Athletes

The sudden death of a competitive athlete inevitably becomes an occasion for local if not national publicity. On each such occasion, the public and the medical community ask whether such events could be prevented by more careful or complete screening. Although each such event is tragic, it must be appreciated that there are approximately 5 million competitive athletes at the high school level or above in any given year. The number of cardiac deaths occurring during athletic participation is unknown, but estimates at the high school level range from one in 300,000 to one in 100,000 participants. Death rates among more mature athletics increase as the prevalence of coronary artery disease rises. These numbers highlight the problem of how to screen individual participants. Even an inexpensive test such as an ECG would generate an enormous cost if required of all athletes, and it is likely that few at-risk individuals would be detected. Echocardiography, either as a routine test or as a follow-up examination for abnormal ECGs, would be prohibitively expensive.

Thus, the most feasible approach is that of a careful medical history and cardiac examination performed by personnel aware of the conditions responsible for most sudden deaths in competitive athletes. In a series of 158 athletic deaths in the United States between 1985 and 1995, hypertrophic cardiomyopathy (36%) and coronary anomalies (19%) were by far the most frequent underlying conditions. Left ventricular hypertrophy was present in another 10%, ruptured aorta (presumably due to Marfan's syndrome or cystic medial necrosis) in 6%, myocarditis or dilated cardiomyopathy in 6%, aortic stenosis in 4%, and arrhythmogenic right ventricular dysplasia in 3%.

It is likely that a careful family and medical history and cardiovascular examination will identify some individuals at risk. A family history of premature sudden death or cardiovascular disease or of any of these predisposing conditions should mandate further workup, including an echocardiogram and ECG. Symptoms of chest pain, syncope, or near-syncope also warrant further evaluation. A Marfan-like appearance, significant elevation of blood pressure or abnormalities of heart rate or rhythm, and pathologic heart murmurs or heart sounds should also be investigated before clearance for athletic participation is given. Such an evaluation is recommended before participation at the high school and college levels and every 2 years during athletic competition. Selective use of routine electrocardiography and stress testing is recommended in men above age 40 and women above age 50 who continue to participate in vigorous exercise and at earlier ages when there is a positive family history for premature coronary artery disease or multiple risk factors.

Maron BJ et al: Cardiovascular pre-participation screening of competitive athletes. Circulation 1996;94:850. (A consensus document developed by the American Heart Association.)

Maron BJ et al: Twenty-sixth Bethesda Conference: Recommendations for determining eligibility for competition in athletics with cardiovascular abnormalities. J Am Coll Cardiol 1994;24:845. (Conference Proceedings, with Task Force reports and recommendations for individuals with various forms of heart disease, as well as presumably healthy patients.)

Systemic Hypertension

11

Barry M. Massie, MD

Approximately 45 million Americans have elevated blood pressure (systolic blood pressure ≥ 140 mm Hg or diastolic blood pressure ≥ 90 mm Hg) or are receiving treatment for high blood pressure. The proportion of individuals who are hypertensive increases with age and is greater in blacks than in whites. Although the majority of hypertensives are aware of their condition, only 25% are controlled to a goal of normotension. The mortality rates for stroke and coronary heart disease, the major complications of hypertension, have declined 40–60% over the past 2–3 decades, in part reflecting the increasing proportion of successfully treated patients.

Until recently, hypertension was diagnosed and categorized primarily based upon diastolic blood pressure readings. However, it has long been recognized that morbidity and mortality increase as both systolic and diastolic blood pressures rise, and that in individuals over age 50 the systolic blood pressure is a better predictor of complications. In a prospective follow-up of 18,700 physicians, even borderline elevations of systolic blood pressure (140–159 mm Hg) were associated with a 42% increase in strokes and a 56% increase in cardiovascular deaths. As shown in Table 11–1, hypertension is now diagnosed based upon elevations of *either* the systolic or diastolic blood pressure, and the objective of management is to achieve normalization of both.

Blood pressure should be measured with a well-calibrated sphygmomanometer with a correctly sized cuff (bladder width approximately 20% greater than arm diameter), after the patient has been resting comfortably in the sitting or supine position. Because blood pressure readings in many individuals are highly variable—especially in the office setting—the diagnosis of hypertension should be made only after elevation is noted on three readings on different occasions, usually over a period of several months unless the elevations are severe or associated with symptoms (see Table 11–1). Transient elevation of blood pressure caused by excitement or apprehension does not constitute hypertensive disease but may indicate a propensity toward its evolution. Ambulatory 24-hour blood pressure monitoring may be helpful in evaluating patients with borderline or variable office blood pressure, approximately 20% of whom will have no evidence of hypertension elsewhere, as well as in assessing resistant hypertension and possible treatment-related hypotensive symptoms. This technique has become convenient and increasingly available, but it should be employed only to address specific management problems because of its cost ($200.00–$300.00).

Continued hypertension does not necessarily indicate the need for pharmacologic treatment. Nonpharmacologic approaches and individualized assessment of the benefit-to-risk ratio of drug therapy should precede pharmacologic management in patients with mild hypertension (diastolic pressure < 100 mm Hg; systolic < 160 mm Hg).

Appel LJ, Stason WB: Ambulatory blood pressure monitoring and blood pressure self-measurement in the diagnosis and management of hypertension. Ann Intern Med 1993;118(11):867. (Review of published data indicates that these modalities have limited clinical application.)

The Fifth Report of the Joint National Committee on Detection, Education, and Treatment of High Blood Pressure (JNC V). Arch Intern Med 1993;153:154. O'Donnell CJ et al: Hypertension and borderline isolated systolic hypertension increase risks of cardiovascular disease and mortality in male physicians. Circulation 1997; 95:1132.

Perloff D et al: Human blood pressure determination by sphygmomanometry (AHA Scientific Statement). Circulation 1993;88:2461.

MANAGEMENT OF HYPERTENSION

Etiology & Classification

A. Primary (Essential) Hypertension: In about 95% of cases, no cause can be established. The condition occurs in 10–15% of white adults and 20–30% of black adults in the USA. The onset of essential hypertension is usually between ages 25 and 55; it is uncommon before age 20. In young people, secondary hypertension resulting from renal insufficiency, renal artery stenosis, or coarctation of the aorta makes up a greater—but still relatively small—proportion of cases.

Table 11–1. Classification and follow-up of blood pressure measurements.[1]

Category[2]	Systolic Blood Pressure (mm Hg)	Diastolic Blood Pressure (mm Hg)	Follow-Up Recommended
Normal	<130	<85	Recheck in 2 years.
High Normal	130–139	85–89	Recheck in 1 year.[3]
Hypertension[4]			
Stage 1 (mild)	140–159	90–99	Confirm within 2 months.
Stage 2 (moderate)	160–179	100–109	Evaluate or refer within 1 month.
Stage 3 (severe)	180–209	110–119	Evaluate or refer within 1 week.
Stage 4 (very severe)	≥210	≥120	Evaluate or refer immediately.

[1]The Fifth Report of the Joint National Committee on Detection, Education, and Treatment of High Blood Pressure (JNC-V). Arch Intern Med 1993;153:154.
[2]When systolic and diastolic pressures fall into different categories, the higher category should be selected to classify the individual's blood pressure. Isolated systolic hypertension is defined as a systolic blood pressure of 140 mm Hg or more and a diastolic blood pressure of less than 90 mm Hg.
[3]Consider offering counseling about life-style modifications.
[4]In individuals aged 18 years or older not taking antihypertensive drugs and not acutely ill. Based on the average of two or more readings on two or more occasions after initial screening.

Elevations in pressure are often transient early in the course of the disease. Even in established cases, the blood pressure fluctuates widely in response to emotional stress and physical activity. Blood pressures taken by the patient at home or during daily activities using a portable apparatus are often lower than those recorded in the office, clinic, or hospital and may be more reliable in estimating prognosis.

The pathogenesis of essential hypertension is multifactorial. Genetic factors play an important role. Children with one—and even more so with two—hypertensive parents tend to have higher blood pressures. Environmental factors also appear to play an important role. Increased salt intake has long been incriminated as a pathogenic factor in essential hypertension. It alone is probably not sufficient to elevate blood pressure to abnormal levels; a combination of too much salt plus a genetic predisposition is required. Other factors that may be involved in the pathogenesis of essential hypertension are the following:

1. Sympathetic nervous system hyperactivity–Sympathetic nervous system hyperactivity is most apparent in younger hypertensives, who may exhibit tachycardia and an elevated cardiac output. However, correlations between plasma catecholamines and blood pressure have generally been poor. Insensitivity of the baroreflexes may play a role in the genesis of adrenergic hyperactivity. Sympathetic activation may also play a role in "labile" hypertension, characterized by marked blood pressure fluctuations under differing, or even similar, circumstances.

2. Renin-angiotensin system–Renin, a proteolytic enzyme, is secreted by the juxtaglomerular cells surrounding afferent arterioles in response to a number of stimuli, including reduced renal perfusion pressure, diminished intravascular volume, circulating catecholamines, increased sympathetic nervous system activity, increased arteriolar stretch, and hypokalemia. Renin acts on angiotensinogen to cleave off the ten-amino-acid peptide angiotensin I. This peptide is then acted upon by angiotensin-converting enzyme to create the eight-amino-acid peptide angiotensin II, a potent vasoconstrictor and a major stimulant of aldosterone release from the adrenal glands. A number of population genetic studies have suggested that the incidence of hypertension and its complications may be increased in individuals with the DD genotype of the allele coding for angiotensin-converting enzyme. Nonetheless, despite the important role of this system in the regulation of blood pressure, it probably does not play a primary role in the pathogenesis of essential hypertension in most individuals. Black hypertensives and older patients tend to have lower plasma renin activity. Patients with low plasma renin activity may have higher intravascular volumes. Plasma renin activity levels can be best classified in relation to dietary sodium intake or urinary sodium excretion. Approximately 10% of essential hypertension patients have relatively high levels, 60% have essentially normal levels, and 30% have relatively low levels. Although such measurements have contributed to our understanding of the pathophysiology of hypertension, there is little clinical utility to measuring plasma renin activity.

3. Defect in natriuresis–Normal individuals increase their renal sodium excretion in response to elevations in arterial pressure and to a sodium or volume load. Hypertensive patients, particularly when their blood pressure is normal, exhibit a diminished ability to excrete a sodium load. This defect may result in increased plasma volume and hypertension. However, during chronic hypertension, a sodium load is usually handled normally.

4. Intracellular sodium and calcium–There is growing evidence that intracellular Na^+ is elevated in blood cells and other tissues in essential hypertension. This may result from abnormalities in Na^+-K^+ exchange and other Na^+ transport mechanisms. Circulating "digitalis-like" substances may be responsible. An increase in intracellular Na^+ may lead to increased intracellular Ca^{2+} concentrations as a result of facilitated exchange. This could explain the increase in vascular smooth muscle tone that is characteristic of established hypertension.

5.   Exacerbating factors–A number of conditions exacerbate or precipitate hypertension in predisposed individuals. The best-documented of these is **obesity,** which is associated with an increase in intravascular volume and an appropriately high output. Weight reduction in the obese lowers blood pressure modestly. Excessive use of **alcohol** also raises blood pressure, perhaps by increasing plasma catecholamines. Hypertension can be difficult to control in patients who consume more than 40 g of ethanol (two drinks) daily or drink in "binges." **Cigarette smoking** acutely raises blood pressure, again by increasing plasma norepinephrine. Although the long-term effect of smoking on blood pressure is less clear, the synergistic effects of smoking and high blood pressure on cardiovascular risk are well documented. Blood pressure should not be measured within 1 hour after smoking or 12 hours after alcohol consumption. The relationship of exercise to hypertension is somewhat controversial. Aerobic exercise lowers blood pressure in previously sedentary individuals, but increasingly strenuous exercise in already active subjects may have a lesser effect. Despite popular preconceptions, the relationship between stress and hypertension is not clearly established. **Polycythemia,** whether primary or due to diminished plasma volume, increases blood viscosity and may raise blood pressure. **Nonsteroidal antiinflammatory agents** produce significant increases in blood pressure, averaging 5 mm Hg, and should be avoided in patients with borderline or elevated blood pressures whenever possible.

B.   Secondary Hypertension: Approximately 5% of patients with hypertension can be found to have specific causes. These secondary causes include the following.

1.   Estrogen use–A small increase in blood pressure occurs in most women taking oral contraceptives, but considerable rises are noted occasionally. This is caused by volume expansion due to increased activity of the renin-angiotensin-aldosterone system. The primary abnormality is an increase in the hepatic synthesis of renin substrate. Approximately 5% of women taking oral contraceptives chronically will exhibit a rise in blood pressure above 140/90 mm Hg; this represents twice the expected prevalence. Contraceptive-related hypertension is more common in women over 35 years of age, in those who have taken contraceptives for more than 5 years, and in obese individuals. It is less common in those taking low-dose estrogen tablets. In most cases, hypertension is reversible by discontinuing the contraceptive, but it may take several weeks. There is no evidence that postmenopausal estrogen use causes hypertension, perhaps because hormone replacement maintains endothelium-mediated vasodilation.

2.   Renal disease–Virtually any disease of the renal parenchyma can cause hypertension, and these conditions are the most common causes of secondary hypertension. The mechanism of renal hypertension is multifaceted, but most instances are related to increased intravascular volume or increased activity of the renin-angiotensin-aldosterone system. Hypertension exaggerates progression of renal insufficiency, so its early recognition and vigorous treatment are important. Hypertension may be reversed if plasma volume is controlled by drugs or dialysis or after bilateral nephrectomy (rarely necessary) and is often improved by renal transplantation. However, post-transplantation hypertension is also a problem; this is now recognized to be in part precipitated by immunosuppressive therapy with cyclosporine. Diabetic nephropathy represents a distinct and better characterized cause of chronic hypertension. The progression of this process is exacerbated by intraglomerular hypertension, which itself is worsened by systemic hypertension. Dilation of the efferent arterioles by angiotensin-converting enzyme inhibition reduces the rate of progression.

3.   Renal vascular hypertension–Renal artery stenosis is a common cause of secondary hypertension and is present in 1–2% of hypertensive patients. The cause in younger individuals is most commonly fibromuscular hyperplasia. This accounts for approximately 30% of renal vascular disease, though it is more common in women under 50. The remainder of renal vascular disease is due to atherosclerotic stenoses of the proximal renal arteries. The mechanism of renal vascular hypertension is excessive renin release due to reduction in renal blood flow and perfusion pressure. Renal vascular hypertension may occur when a single branch of the renal artery is stenotic, but in as many as 25% of patients both arteries are obstructed.

Renal vascular hypertension may present in the same manner as essential hypertension but should be suspected in the following circumstances: (1) if the onset is below age 20 or after age 50; (2) if there are epigastric or renal artery bruits; (3) if there is atherosclerotic disease of the aorta or peripheral arteries (15–26% of patients with symptomatic lower limb atherosclerotic vascular disease have renal artery stenosis); or (4) if there is abrupt deterioration in renal function after administration of angiotensin-converting enzyme inhibitors. Additional evaluation is indicated in patients who present in this manner, especially if hypertension is difficult to control medically.

There is no ideal "screening" test for renal vascular hypertension. All tests are sufficiently nonspecific so that in populations with a low incidence of the disease, false-positive results will exceed true-positives; sensitivity rarely exceeds 80%. If the suspicion of renal vascular hypertension is sufficiently high, renal arteriography, the definitive diagnostic test, is the best approach. Where suspicion is moderate to low, radioisotope renography performed in experienced laboratories before and after administration of an angiotensin-converting enzyme inhibitor is probably the best noninvasive diagnostic test. The baseline study may show a smaller kidney with diminished function on the side of the stenosis. Postdrug (captopril, 50 mg orally, or enalaprilat, 2.5 mg intravenously) uptake and clearance of the radiotracer are delayed. However, bilateral disease may be difficult to detect if both kidneys are equally affected. Other diagnostic approaches, including the measurement of peripheral renin activity following provocation with an angiotensin-converting enzyme inhibitor, Doppler ultrasound, and MRI, and intravenous pyelograms, are favored by some experts. Except when stenosis is critical (> 80–90%) and unifocal, the significance of the stenosis should be assessed by measuring differences in renin activity between the renal veins. If the lesion is not associated with a "step-up" in renin activity, hypertension often persists despite correction.

The treatment of patients with recognized renal vascular hypertension is not always clear-cut. Young individuals and good-risk patients of any age who have not responded to medical therapy should have the lesion corrected. Although the surgical results from renal artery reconstruction are generally good, percutaneous transluminal angioplasty is now the preferred approach for fibromuscular hyperplasia and for discrete stenotic arteriosclerotic lesions that do not involve the renal artery ostium. However, among older individuals with arteriosclerosis, only a minority experience normalization without continued drug therapy. Thus, it is reasonable to manage these patients medically if renal function does not deteriorate. Although converting enzyme inhibitors have improved the success rate of medical therapy of hypertension due to renal artery stenosis, these agents have been associated with marked hypotension and deterioration of renal function in individuals with bilateral renal artery stenosis. Thus, renal function and blood pressure should be closely monitored during the first weeks of therapy in patients in whom this is a consideration.

4. Primary hyperaldosteronism and Cushing's syndrome–Patients with excess aldosterone secretion make up less than 0.5% of all cases of hypertension. The usual lesion is an adrenal adenoma, although a minority of patients have bilateral adrenal hyperplasia. The diagnosis should be suspected when patients present with hypokalemia prior to diuretic therapy and when this is associated with excessive urinary potassium excretion (usually > 40 meq/L on a spot specimen) and suppressed levels of plasma renin activity. Aldosterone concentrations in urine and blood are elevated. The lesion can be demonstrated by CT scanning as well as by MRI and abdominal ultrasound. Less commonly, patients with Cushing's syndrome (glucocorticoid excess) may manifest hypertension as a first sign (see Chapter 26).

5. Pheochromocytoma–Although hypertension due to pheochromocytoma is often thought to be episodic, most patients have sustained blood pressure elevations. The majority of patients have exaggerated orthostatic blood pressure changes, and many develop glucose intolerance. The diagnosis and treatment of this entity are discussed in Chapter 26.

6. Coarctation of the aorta–This uncommon cause of hypertension is discussed in Chapter 10.

7. Hypertension associated with pregnancy–Hypertension occurring de novo or worsening during pregnancy is one of the commonest causes of maternal and fetal morbidity and mortality (see Chapter 18).

8. Other causes of secondary hypertension–Hypertension has also been associated with hypercalcemia due to any cause, acromegaly, hyperthyroidism, hypothyroidism, and a variety of neurologic disorders causing increased intracranial pressure.

Bonelli FF et al: Renal artery angioplasty: Technical results and clinical outcome in 320 patients. Mayo Clin Proc 1995;70:1041. (Large experience showing that "cure" of hypertension is unusual when arteriosclerosis is the underlying cause.)

Canzanello VJ, Textor SC: Noninvasive diagnosis of renovascular disease. Mayo Clin Proc 1994;69:1172.

Cunningham FG, Lindheimer MD: Hypertension in pregnancy. N Engl J Med 1992;326:927.

Gordon RD: Mineralocorticoid hypertension. Lancet 1994;344:240.

Johnson AG, et al: Do non-steroidal anti-inflammatory drugs affect blood pressure? A meta-analysis. Ann Intern Med 1994;121:289. (Clear evidence that they do.)

Kaplan NM: Ethnic aspects of hypertension. Lancet 1994;344:450. (Brief review discusses different mechanisms, prognosis, and treatment approaches for different groups.)

National High Blood Pressure Education Program Working Group Report on Primary Prevention of Hypertension. Arch Intern Med 1993;153:186. (Extensively documented report which discusses population and individual approaches to the prevention and non-drug treatment of hypertension.)

Preston Y et al: Renal parenchymal hypertension: Current concepts of pathogenesis and management. Arch Intern Med 1996;156:602. (Most frequent cause of secondary hypertension.)

Complications of Untreated Hypertension

Complications of hypertension are related either to sustained elevations of blood pressure, with consequent changes in the vasculature and heart, or to atherosclerosis that accompanies and is accelerated by long-standing hypertension. The excess morbidity and mortality related to hypertension are progressive over the whole range of systolic and diastolic blood pressures; the risk approximately doubles for each 6 mm Hg increase in diastolic blood pressure. However, target-organ damage varies markedly between individuals with similar levels of office hypertension.

Ambulatory pressures are more closely related to end-organ damage. Specific complications include the following:

A. Hypertensive Cardiovascular Disease: Cardiac complications are the major causes of morbidity and mortality in essential hypertension, and preventing them is a major goal of therapy. Electrocardiographic evidence of left ventricular hypertrophy is found in 2–10% of chronic hypertensives; echocardiographic criteria are met more commonly, in up to 50% of patients. Once established, left ventricular hypertrophy is an indication of increased risk for morbidity and mortality; for any level of blood pressure, its presence is associated with a several-fold increase in risk. Epidemiologic studies have shown that echocardiographic left ventricular hypertrophy is a powerful predictor of prognosis. Left ventricular hypertrophy may cause or facilitate many cardiac complications of hypertension, including congestive heart failure, ventricular arrhythmias, myocardial ischemia, and sudden death.

Left ventricular diastolic dysfunction, which may present with many of the signs and symptoms of congestive heart failure, is common in patients with long-standing hypertension. Hypertensive left ventricular hypertrophy regresses with therapy. Regression is most closely related to the degree of systolic blood pressure reduction and does not seem to reflect the specific medication employed. In two recent large studies, diuretics produced equal or greater reductions of left ventricular mass when compared with other drug classes.

While hypertension alone can lead to many of these cardiac complications, the combination of hypertension with coronary artery disease or alcohol abuse is synergistic in producing these complications. In patients with additional coronary risk factors, the prevalence of asymptomatic coronary artery disease is increased and is at least as powerful a predictor of subsequent complications as left ventricular hypertrophy.

B. Hypertensive Cerebrovascular Disease and Dementia: Hypertension is the major predisposing cause of stroke, especially intracerebral hemorrhage but also cerebral infarction. Cerebrovascular complications are more closely correlated with the systolic than the diastolic blood pressure. The incidence of these complications is markedly reduced by antihypertensive therapy. There is also epidemiologic evidence that preceding hypertension is associated with a higher incidence of subsequent dementia, both the vascular and the Alzheimer types.

C. Hypertensive Renal Disease: Chronic hypertension leads to nephrosclerosis, a common cause of renal insufficiency. Hypertensive renal damage is limited by successful therapy. Secondary renal disease is more common in blacks than whites. Hypertension also plays an important role in accelerating the progression of other forms of renal disease, of which diabetic nephropathy is the most common. Angiotensin-converting enzyme inhibitors have been shown to be particularly effective in preventing the latter complication.

D. Aortic Dissection: Hypertension is a major cause and exacerbating factor in many patients with dissection of the aorta. The diagnosis and treatment of aortic dissection are discussed in Chapter 12.

E. Atherosclerotic Complications: Most patients in the USA with hypertension die of complications of atherosclerosis, but the linkage between hypertension and atherosclerotic cardiovascular disease is much less close than that with the previously discussed complications. This reflects the multifactorial origin of atherosclerosis. Effective antihypertensive therapy is thus less successful in preventing complications of coronary heart disease, but recent trials have convincingly demonstrated that even coronary events can be reduced in high-risk patients.

F. Malignant and Accelerated Hypertension: Any form of sustained hypertension, primary or secondary, may abruptly become accelerated, with resulting encephalopathy, nephropathy, retinopathy, heart failure, or myocardial ischemia. These complications are discussed below in the section on Hypertensive Urgencies and Emergencies.

Chobanian AV, Alexander W: Exacerbation of atherosclerosis by hypertension: Potential mechanisms and clinical implications. Arch Intern Med 1996;156:1952. (Most of the complications of hypertension involve accelerated atherosclerosis. This paper discusses the mechanism for this interaction and the importance of treating both risk factors.)

Levy D et al: Progression from hypertension to congestive heart failure. JAMA 1996;275:1557. (Using longitudinal collected data, the investigators demonstrated that hypertension precedes the onset of heart failure in a large portion of patients, raising the possibility that many of these cases are preventable.)

Maschio G et al: The effect of the angiotensin-converting-enzyme inhibitor benazepril on the progression of chronic renal insufficiency. N Engl J Med 1996;334:939. (ACE inhibitor therapy may prevent progressive renal insufficiency in a broad group of conditions.)

Massie BM et al: Scintigraphic and electrocardiographic evidence of silent coronary artery disease in asymptomatic hypertension: A case-controlled study. J Am Coll Cardiol 1993;22:1598. (Noninvasive evidence of significant coronary disease is more common in hypertensive men with coronary risk factors than in matched normotensive controls. Subsequent data show that markers of ischemia are powerful predictors of coronary and noncoronary complications.)

National High Blood Pressure Education Program Working Group: 1995 update of the Working Group report on chronic renal failure and renovascular hypertension. Arch Intern Med 1996;156:1938. (More aggressive approach to blood pressure lowering in patients with intrinsic renal disease, particularly in the setting of diabetes and in blacks.)

Skoog I et al: Fifteen year longitudinal study of blood pressure and dementia. Lancet 1996;347:1141. (Hypertension may be a major factor in the development of dementia.)

Clinical Findings

The clinical and laboratory findings are mainly referable to involvement of the "target organs": heart, brain, kidneys, eyes, and peripheral arteries.

A. Symptoms: Mild to moderate essential hypertension is usually associated with normal health and well-being for many years. Vague symptoms often appear after patients learn they have "high blood pressure." Suboccipital pulsating headaches, characteristically occurring early in the morning and subsiding during the day, are characteristic, but any type of headache may occur. Accelerated hypertension may be associated with somnolence, confusion, visual disturbances, and nausea and vomiting (hypertensive encephalopathy).

Patients with pheochromocytomas that secrete predominantly norepinephrine usually have sustained hypertension but may have intermittent hypertension. Attacks (lasting minutes to hours) of anxiety, palpitation, profuse perspiration, pallor, tremor, and nausea and vomiting occur; blood pressure is markedly elevated, and angina or acute pulmonary edema may occur. In primary aldosteronism, patients may have recurrent episodes of generalized muscular weakness or paralysis as well as paresthesias, polyuria, and nocturia due to associated hypokalemia; malignant hypertension, however, is rare.

Chronic hypertension often leads to left ventricular hypertrophy, which may be associated with diastolic or, in late stages, systolic dysfunction. Exertional and paroxysmal nocturnal dyspnea may result. Severe left ventricular hypertrophy predisposes to myocardial ischemia (especially when concomitant coronary artery disease is present), ventricular arrhythmias, and sudden death.

Renal involvement may not produce symptoms, but hematuria is frequent in the malignant phase.

Cerebral involvement causes (1) stroke due to thrombosis or (2) small or large hemorrhage from microaneurysms of small penetrating intracranial arteries. Hypertensive encephalopathy is probably caused by acute capillary congestion and exudation with cerebral edema. The findings are usually reversible if adequate treatment is given promptly. Although there is no strict correlation of diastolic blood pressure with hypertensive encephalopathy, it usually exceeds 130 mm Hg.

B. Signs: Physical findings depend upon the cause of hypertension, its duration and severity, and the degree of effect on target organs.

1. Blood pressure–Blood pressure should be measured after the patient has rested 5 or more minutes in quiet, warm surroundings. On the initial observation, pressure should be examined in both arms and, if lower extremity pulses are diminished, in the legs to exclude coarctation of the aorta. Supine and standing measurements should be made to detect a postural drop, usually present in pheochromocytoma. Elderly patients may have falsely elevated readings by sphygmomanometry because of noncompressible vessels. This may be suspected in the presence of Osler's sign—a palpable brachial or radial artery when the cuff is inflated above systolic pressure. Occasionally, it may be necessary to make direct measurements of intra-arterial pressure, especially in patients with apparent severe hypertension who do not tolerate therapy.

2. Retinas–The Keith-Wagener (KW) classification of retinal changes in hypertension, in spite of deficiencies, presages a worse prognosis when stage II or higher changes are present.

3. Heart and arteries–A loud aortic second sound and an early systolic ejection click may occur. Left ventricular enlargement with a left ventricular heave indicates well-established disease. Older patients frequently have systolic ejection murmurs resulting from aortic sclerosis, and these may evolve to significant aortic stenosis in some individuals. Aortic insufficiency may be auscultated in up to 5% of patients, and hemodynamically insignificant aortic insufficiency can be detected by Doppler echocardiography in 10–20%. A presystolic (S_4) gallop due to decreased compliance of the left ventricle is quite common.

4. Pulses–The timing of upper and lower extremity pulses should be compared to exclude coarctation of the aorta. All major peripheral pulses should be evaluated to exclude aortic dissection and peripheral atherosclerosis, which may be associated with renal artery involvement.

C. Laboratory Findings: Most laboratory examinations are normal in uncomplicated essential hypertension. Testing is recommended to detect secondary hypertension and important associated conditions. Thus, standard testing should include the following: hemoglobin determination, to detect anemia or polycythemia; urinalysis and renal function studies, to detect hematuria, proteinuria, and casts, which may signify primary renal disease or nephrosclerosis; serum K^+, to detect hyperaldosteronism; fasting blood sugar level, to detect diabetes and as evidence for pheochromocytoma; plasma lipids, as an indicator of atherosclerosis risk; and serum uric acid, as an additional guide to risk and, if elevated, a relative contraindication to diuretic therapy.

D. Electrocardiography and Chest X-Ray: Electrocardiographic criteria are highly specific but not very sensitive for left ventricular hypertrophy. The "strain" pattern of ST–T wave changes is a sign of more advanced disease and is associated with a poor prognosis. A chest x-ray is not recommended in the routine evaluation of uncomplicated hypertension, since it usually does not yield additional information.

E. Echocardiography: The echocardiogram is much more sensitive than the ECG in detecting left ventricular hypertrophy, and measurements of left ventricular mass predict prognosis in populations. However, until it is found that these measurements are useful in determining the need for therapy or in selecting therapy, this test should not be employed in uncomplicated patients.

F. Diagnostic Studies: Only if the clinical presentation or routine tests suggest secondary or complicated hypertension are additional diagnostic studies indicated. These may include blood and urinary tests for endocrine causes of hypertension, intravenous urograms, or renal ultrasound to diagnose primary renal disease (polycystic kidneys, obstructive uropathy) or renovascular abnormalities, and isotope renograms for the latter diagnosis. Further evaluation may include abdominal imaging studies (CT scan, or MRI) or renal arteriography.

G. Summary: Since most hypertension is "primary," an extensive diagnostic evaluation is not indicated before starting therapy. Most clinicians obtain only a blood count, renal function test, electrolyte panel and urinalysis, and ECG after establishing the diagnosis. If conventional therapy is unsuccessful or if symptoms suggest a secondary cause, further studies are indicated.

Gifford RW et al: Office evaluation of hypertension. Circulation 1989;79:721. (How to approach the initial evaluation.)

Nonpharmacologic Therapy

All patients with high normal or elevated blood pressures (as defined in Table 11–1), those who have a family history of cardiovascular complications of hypertension, and those who have multiple coronary risk factors should be counseled about nonpharmacologic approaches to lowering blood pressure. Approaches of proved but modest value include weight reduction, reduced alcohol consumption, and in some patients reduced salt intake. Increased activity levels should be encouraged in previously sedentary patients, but strenuous exercise training programs in already active individuals may have less benefit. Stress reduction is of unclear value. Calcium and potassium supplements have been advocated, but their ability to lower blood pressure is limited and probably not applicable to most patients.

Alderman MH: Non-pharmacological approaches of hypertension. Lancet 1994;344:307.
Marmot MG et al: Alcohol and blood pressure: The INTERSALT study. Br Med J 1994;308:1263. (Large prospective evaluation indicates that consumption of three or four drinks a day or more causes significant rises in blood pressure.)

Who Should Be Treated With Medications?

Recommendations concerning which patients should be treated with medications after implementation of nonpharmacologic treatment remain controversial. The decision to initiate drug therapy should be based upon the assessment of overall cardiovascular risk rather than the level of blood pressure alone. Factors that unfavorably influence the prognosis in chronic arterial hypertension and so determine the threshold for drug therapy include the following: (1) the level of diastolic and, especially, systolic blood pressures; (2) a family history of hypertension-related complications; (3) male gender; (4) early age at onset; (5) black race; (6) the presence of additional risk factors for coronary artery disease; (7) accompanying cardiac disease, cerebral vascular disease, or diabetes; (8) left ventricular hypertrophy on ECG or echocardiogram; and (9) renal dysfunction.

Drug treatment of severe (systolic blood pressure ≥ 180 mm Hg or diastolic blood pressure ≥ 110 mm Hg) and moderate (systolic blood pressure 160–179 mm Hg or diastolic blood pressure 100–109 mm Hg) chronic hypertension results in lower morbidity and mortality rates from cardiovascular disease (stroke and heart failure) than occur in untreated patients. Recent trials have also demonstrated that coronary events, including nonfatal myocardial infarctions, can be prevented in severely hypertensive patients, including those with isolated systolic hypertension. In patients with diastolic pressures less than 100 mm Hg without accompanying moderate or severe systolic hypertension, the data are less clear, largely because complications are less frequent. Since insurance data have shown that even slight increases in blood pressure reduce longevity, most patients with diastolic blood pressures over 95 mm Hg should be treated, as should individuals with diastolic pressures of 90 mm Hg or more if there is evidence of target organ damage or associated systolic hypertension or if any of the risk factors listed above are present.

Mulrow CD et al: Hypertension in the elderly: Implications and generalizability of randomized trials. JAMA 1994;272:1932. (Treatment of older persons is highly efficacious and cost-effective.)
See also Joint National Committee and WHO Guidelines referenced above.

Goals of Treatment

The goal of treatment should be to reduce blood pressure to normal levels (ie, < 140/90 mm Hg) with minimal side effects. Since there may be additional benefits from further lowering of blood pressure, most authorities also seek to achieve a minimum of 10 mm Hg reduction in diastolic pressure in patients with mild hypertension (90–99 mm Hg). In older patients with predominantly systolic hypertension, a systolic pressure of less than 160 mm Hg may be an acceptable end point if further reduction cannot be obtained without unacceptable side effects. However, a significant decrease in hypertension-related morbidity from blood pressure reduction is possible even if these therapeutic goals are not achieved. Thus, a compromise between goal blood pressure and an adequately tolerated therapeutic regimen may be necessary in some individuals. Some data indicate that the risk of myocardial infarction and sudden death may rise when the diastolic blood pressure is lowered below 80–85 mm Hg (a phenomenon referred to as the "J" curve of morbidity versus blood pressure reduction), but this concept has not been supported by recent trials.

Fletcher AE, Bulpitt CS: How far should blood pressure be lowered? N Engl J Med 1992;326:251. (Discussion of the controversial questions: Is too low dangerous? How much is enough?)

Antihypertensive Drug Therapy

An ideal antihypertensive drug would be effective as a single agent or in combination with other agents in all classes of patients; would lower blood pressure by a physiologic mechanism; would reduce morbidity and mortality rates; would have no long-term toxicity or unpleasant side effects that affect lifestyles; could be taken once a day; would not require multiple-dose titration steps; and would be of moderate cost. No such agent currently exists, but the growing number of available drugs has allowed the physician to tailor treatment to the needs of individual patients. These agents are listed in Tables 11–2 to 11–6.

A. The Stepped Care Approach: In the 1970s and for most of the 1980s, the "stepped care" approach to treatment of hypertension was advocated. Patients were initially started on a diuretic or beta-blocker, and other drugs were added later if required. This approach was highly effective, with approximately 80% of compliant patients exhibiting adequate blood pressure control. Several trials using this

Table 11–2. Factors that may influence the choice of antihypertensive medications.

	More Effective or Appropriate	Less Effective or Contraindicated
Coexisting conditions		
Prior myocardial infarction	Beta-blocker, ACE inhibitor (if ejection fraction is reduced)	Calcium blocker (if ejection fraction is reduced)
Angina pectoris	Beta-blocker, calcium blocker	Vasodilator (without concomitant beta-blocker)
Congestive heart failure	Diuretic, ACE inhibitor	Calcium blocker, beta-blocker[1]
Diabetes mellitus	ACE inhibitor (with nephropathy)	Beta-blocker (if hypoglycemia occurs), diuretic (if glucose is high in type II diabetes)
Peripheral vascular disease		Beta-blocker (if there is rest pain or severe claudication)
Bronchospasm		Beta-blocker
Prostatism	Alpha-blocker	
Migraine	Beta-blocker	
Arthritis		ACE inhibitor (if on chronic NSAID regimen)
Gout		Diuretic
Osteoporosis	Diuretic	
Pregnancy (current or potential)	Beta-blocker (considerable experience with labetalol; atenolol associated with low birth weight), calcium blocker, methyldopa	ACE inhibitor
Demographic factors		
Older patients	Diuretic (especially for those with increased systolic blood pressure)	ACE inhibitor (especially as single agent for increased systolic blood pressure)
Blacks	Calcium blocker, diuretic	ACE inhibitor, beta-blocker (especially in older patients)
Young whites	Beta-blocker, ACE inhibitor	
Smokers	Diuretic	Beta-blocker

[1]Accumulating evidence supports a role for beta-blockers in some patients with congestive heart failure, but these drugs may cause acute deterioration, particularly in the usual antihypertensive doses, and require careful monitoring by experienced physicians.

Table 11–3. Antihypertensive drugs: Diuretics.

Drug	Proprietary Name	Initial Dosage	Dosage Range	Cost per Unit	Cost for 30 Days' Treatment[1] (Average Dosage)	Adverse Effects	Comments
THIAZIDES AND RELATED DIURETICS							
Hydrochlorothiazide	Esidrix,* HydroDiuril*	12.5 or 25 mg once daily	12.5–50 mg once daily	B: $0.20 G: $0.04	B: $6.00 G: $1.20	$\downarrow K^+$, $\downarrow Mg^{2+}$, $\uparrow Ca^{2+}$, $\downarrow Na^+$, $\uparrow$uric acid, $\uparrow$glucose, $\uparrow$LDL cholesterol, $\uparrow$triglycerides, rash, impotence.	Low dosages effective in many patients without associated metabolic abnormalities; metolazone more effective with concurrent renal insufficiency; indapamide does not alter serum lipid levels.
Chlorthalidone	Hygroton* Thaliton	12.5 or 25 mg once daily	12.5–50 mg once daily	B: $0.82 G: $0.08	B: $24.60 G: $2.40		
Metolazone	Diulo, Zaroxolyn Mykrox	1.25 or 2.5 mg once daily 0.5 mg once daily	1.25–5 mg once daily 0.5–1 mg once daily	B: $0.50	B: $22.00		
Indapamide	Lozol*	2.5 mg once daily	2.5–5 mg once daily	B: $0.90 G: $0.70	B: $27.00 G: $21.00		
LOOP DIURETICS							
Furosemide	Lasix*	20 mg bid	40–320 mg in 2 or 3 doses	B: $0.16 G: $0.04	B: $9.60 G: $2.40	Same as thiazides, but higher risk of excessive diuresis and electrolyte imbalance. Increases calcium excretion.	**Furosemide:** Short duration of action a disadvantage; should be reserved for patients with renal insufficiency or fluid retention. Poor antihypertensive. **Torsemide:** Effective blood pressure medication at low dosage.
Bumetanide	Bumex*	0.25 mg bid	0.5–10 mg in 2 or 3 doses	B: $0.31 G: $0.27	B: $19.00 G: $16.00		
Torsemide	Demadex, Torsemide, Presaril	2.5 mg once daily	5–10 mg once daily	B: $0.48	B: $14.40		
COMBINATION PRODUCTS							
Hydrochlorothiazide and triamterene	Dyazide* (25/50 mg) Maxzide (37.5/25 mg)	1 tab once daily	1 or 2 tabs once daily	B: $0.44 G: $0.27	B: $13.20 G: $8.10	Same as thiazides plus GI disturbances, hyperkalemia rather than hypokalemia, headache; triamterene can cause kidney stones and renal dysfunction; spironolactone causes gynecomastia. Hyperkalemia can occur if this combination is used in patients with renal failure or those taking ACE inhibitors.	Use should be limited to patients with demonstrable need for potassium-sparing agent.
Hydrochlorothiazide and amiloride	Moduretic* (50/5 mg)	½ tab once daily	1 or 2 tabs once daily	B: $0.54 G: $0.35	B: $16.20 G: $10.50		
Hydrochlorothiazide and spironolactone	Aldactazide (25/25 mg)	1 tab once daily	1 or 2 tabs once daily	B: $0.43 G: $0.08	B: $12.90 G: $2.40		

*Generic product available (G). (B) = brand name.
[1]Cost to pharmacist (average wholesale price) for 30 days' treatment based on average dosage (generic when possible). Source: First Data Bank, Price Alert, April 1997.

Table 11–4. Antihypertensive drugs: Beta-adrenergic blocking agents.

Drug	Proprietary Name	Initial Dosage	Dosage Range	Cost per Unit	Cost for 30 Days' Treatment (Based on Average Dosage)[1]	Special Properties					Comments[5]
						β1 Selectivity[2]	ISA[3]	MSA[4]	Lipid Solubility	Renal vs Hepatic Elimination	
Acebutolol	Sectral	200 mg once daily	200–1200 mg in 1 or 2 doses	B: $1.31/400 mg	B: $39.00	+	+	+	+	H > R	Positive ANA; rare LE syndrome; also indicated for arrhythmias. Doses > 800 mg have β1 and β2 effects.
Atenolol	Tenormin*	25 mg once daily	25–200 mg once daily	B: $0.94/50 mg G: $0.72/50 mg	B: $28.00 G: $22.00	+	0	0	0	R	Also indicated for angina pectoris and post-MI. Doses > 100 mg have β1 and β2 effects.
Betaxolol	Kerlone	10 mg once daily	10–40 mg once daily	B: $1.13/20 mg	B: $34.00	+	0	0	+	H > R	
Carteolol	Cartrol	2.5 mg once daily	2.5–10 mg once daily	B: $1.02/5 mg	B: $31.00	0	+	0	+	R > H	
Labetalol	Normodyne, Trandate	100 mg bid	200–1200 mg in 2 doses	B: $0.63	B: $38.00	0	0/+	0	++	H	α;β blocking activity 1:3; more orthostatic hypotension, fever, hepatotoxicity.
Metoprolol	Lopressor*	50 mg in 1 or 2 doses	50–200 mg in 1 or 2 doses	B: $0.55 G: $0.46	B: $33.00 G: $28.00	+	0	+	+++	H	Also indicated for angina pectoris and post-MI. Doses > 100 mg have β1 and β2 effects.
	Toprol XL (SR preparation)	50 mg once daily	50–200 mg once daily	B: $0.70/100 mg	B: $21.00						
Nadolol	Corgard*	20 mg once daily	20–160 mg once daily	B: $1.10/40 mg G: $0.95/40 mg	B: $33.00 G: $29.00	0	0	0	0	R	
Penbutolol	Levatol	20 mg once daily	20–80 mg once daily	B: $1.07/20 mg	B: $32.00	0	+	0	++	R > H	
Pindolol	Visken*	5 mg bid	10–60 mg in 2 doses	B: $0.50/5 mg	B: $48.00	0	++	+	+	H > R	In adults, 35% renal clearance.
Propranolol	Inderal*	20 mg bid	40–320 mg in 2 doses	B: $0.60/40 mg G: $0.10/40 mg	B: $36.00 G: $ 6.00	0	0	++	+++	H	Once-daily SR preparation also available. Also indicated for angina pectoris and post-MI.
Timolol	Blocadren*	5 mg bid	10–40 mg in 2 doses	B: $0.53/10 mg G: $0.34/10 mg	B: $32.00 G: $20.00	0	0	0	++	H > R	Also indicated post-MI. 80% hepatic clearance.

*Generic preparation available.

B = brand name; G = generic; ISA = intrinsic sympathomimetic activity; MSA = membrane-stabilizing activity; 0 = no effect; +, ++, +++ = some, moderate, most effect.

[1] Cost to pharmacist (average wholesale price) for 30 days' treatment based on average dosage (generic when possible). Source: First Data Bank, Price Alert, April 1997.

[2] Agents with β1 selectivity are less likely to precipitate bronchospasm and decreased peripheral blood flow *in low doses*, but selectivity is only relative.

[3] Agents with ISA cause less resting bradycardia and lipid changes.

[4] MSA generally occurs at concentrations greater than those necessary for beta-adrenergic blockade. The clinical importance of MSA by beta-blockers has not been defined.

[5] Adverse effects of all beta-blockers: bronchospasm, fatigue, sleep disturbance and nightmares, bradycardia and atrioventricular block, worsening of congestive heart failure, cold extremities, gastrointestinal disturbances, impotence, ↑triglycerides, ↓HDL cholesterol, rare blood dyscrasias.

Table 11–5. Antihypertensive drugs: ACE inhibitors and angiotensin II blockers.

Drug	Proprietary Name	Initial Dosage	Dosage Range	Cost per Unit	Cost of 30 Days' Treatment (Average Dosage)[1]	Adverse Effects	Comments
ACE inhibitors							
Benazepril	Lotensin	10 mg once daily	5–40 mg in 1 or 2 doses	$0.69/20 mg	$20.70	Cough, hypotension, dizziness, renal dysfunction, hyperkalemia, angioedema; taste alteration and rash (may be more frequent with captopril); rarely, proteinuria, blood dyscrasia. **Contraindicated in pregnancy.**	More **fosinopril** is excreted by the liver in patients with renal dysfunction (dose reduction may or may not be necessary). **Captopril** and **lisinopril** are active without metabolism. **Captopril, enalapril, lisinopril,** and **quinapril** are approved for congestive heart failure.
Captopril	Capoten	25 mg bid	50–300 mg in 2 or 3 doses	$0.64/25 mg	$38.00		
Enalapril	Vasotec	5 mg once daily	5–40 mg in 1 or 2 doses	$1.46/20 mg	$43.80		
Fosinopril	Monopril	10 mg once daily	10–80 mg in 1 or 2 doses	$0.79/20 mg	$23.70		
Lisinopril	Prinivil, Zestril	5–10 mg once daily	5–40 mg once daily	$0.87/20 mg	$26.10		
Moexipril	Univasc	7.5 mg once daily	7.5–30 mg in 1 or 2 doses	$0.50/15 mg	$15.00		
Quinapril	Accupril	10 mg once daily	10–80 mg in 1 or 2 doses	$0.91/20 mg	$27.00		
Ramipril	Altace	2.5 mg once daily	2.5–20 mg in 1 or 2 doses	$0.75/5 mg	$22.00		
Trandolapril	Mavik	1 mg once daily	1–8 mg once daily	$0.60/4 mg	$18.00		
Angiotensin II blockers							
Losartan	Cozaar	50 mg once daily	25–100 mg in 1 or 2 doses	$1.17/50 mg	$35.00 (50 mg once daily)	Incidence of side effects is similar to placebo. Combinations have additional side effects. **Contraindicated in pregnancy.**	Losartan has a very flat dose-response curve. Valsartan has a wider dose-response range and longer duration of action. Addition of low-dose diuretic (separately or as the combination pill) increases the response.
Losartan	Hyzaar	50 mg plus hydrochlorothiazide 12.5 mg once daily	One or 2 tablets once daily	$1.14/ tablet	$34.20 (1 tablet daily)		
Valsartan	Diovan	80 mg once daily	80–320 mg once daily	$1.14/160 mg	$34.20		

[1]Cost to pharmacist (average wholesale price) for 30 days' treatment based on average dosage (generic when possible). Source: First Data Bank, Price Alert, April 1997.

approach demonstrated significant reductions in stroke and, in some cases, myocardial infarction and death.

A number of considerations have led some experts to question stepped care as a universal treatment plan. These include the availability of other effective and well-tolerated agents with different mechanisms of action, the recognition that patients not controlled by one agent may respond to another without moving directly to two-drug therapy, and concerns over the long-term implications of metabolic changes observed with diuretics and beta-blockers (especially unfavorable changes in plasma lipids and insulin sensitivity). However, unlike diuretics and beta-block-

ers, these newer agents have not been proved to prevent the complications of hypertension. Indeed, some of them, such as calcium blockers and alpha-blockers, have not been shown to improve outcomes for any indication. Therefore, the pendulum of opinion has begun to swing back in favor of the drugs with proved benefits.

B. Choice of Initial Medication: Diuretics and beta-blockers should be considered for first-line therapy in most patients, but the choice of medications should be individualized. Additional choices include ACE inhibitors, calcium channel blockers, alpha-blockers, combined alpha- and beta-blockers, and angiotensin II-blocking agents. These medications are

Table 11–6. Antihypertensive drugs: Calcium channel-blocking agents.

Drug	Proprietary Name	Initial Dosage	Dosage Range	Cost for 30 Days' Treatment (Average Dosage)[1]	Special Properties			Adverse Effects	Comments
					Cardiac Peripheral Vasodilation	Automaticity and Conduction	Contractility		
Nondihydropyridine agents									
Diltiazem	Cardizem SR	90 mg bid	180–360 mg in 2 doses	$75.00 (240 mg qd)	++	↓↓	↓↓	Edema, headache, bradycardia, GI disturbances, dizziness, AV block, congestive heart failure, urinary frequency.	Also approved for angina.
	Cardizem CD	180 mg qd	180–360 mg qd	$55.00 (240 mg qd)					
	Dilacor XR	180 or 240 mg qd	180–480 mg daily	$39.60 (240 mg qd)					
	Tiazac SA	240 mg qd	180–540 mg qd	$40.67 (240 mg qd)					
Verapamil	Calan SR Isoptin SR* Verelan	180 mg qd	180–480 mg in 1 or 2 doses	$34.50 $42.60 (Verelan) (240 mg qd)	++	↓↓↓	↓↓↓	Same as diltiazem but more likely to cause constipation and congestive heart failure.	Also approved for angina and arrhythmias.
Dihydropyridines									
Amlodipine	Norvasc	5 mg qd	5–20 mg qd	$65.00 (10 mg qd)	+++	↓/0	↓/0	Edema, dizziness, palpitations, flushing, headache, hypotension, tachycardia, GI disturbances, urinary frequency, worsening of congestive heart failure (may be less common with felodipine, amlodipine).	Amlodipine, nicardipine, and nifedipine also approved for angina.
Felodipine	Plendil	5 mg qd	5–20 mg qd	$46.00 (10 mg qd)	+++	↓/0	↓/0		
Isradipine	DynaCirc	2.5 mg bid	5–10 mg in 2 doses	$55.00 (5 mg bid)	+++	↓/0	→		
Nicardipine	Cardene	20 mg tid	60–120 mg in 3 doses	$40.00 (20 mg tid)	+++	↓/0	→		
Nifedipine	Adalat CC	30 mg qd	30–120 mg qd	$48.00 (60 mg qd)	+++	→	↓↑		
	Procardia XL	30 mg qd	30–120 mg qd	$68.00 (60 mg qd)	+++	→	↑↑		

*Generic preparation available.
[1]Cost to pharmacist (average wholesale price) for 30 days' treatment based on average dosage (generic when possible). Source: First Data Bank, Price Alert, April 1997.

all effective and generally well tolerated (the alpha-blockers less so), but responses vary among demographic groups. Selection is based upon individual factors, which include age, race, lifestyle, cost, the experience of the physician, and the side effects of the agent. Accompanying illnesses are often the major factor in selection of medications, since these may exclude some medications or favor the use of others.

Two large studies have compared different classes of agents in placebo-controlled trials. In a Veterans Administration Cooperative study of 1292 patients, the calcium channel blocker diltiazem was the most broadly effective and well-tolerated agent, but responses varied among demographic subgroups. In older whites, the beta-blocker and calcium channel blocker produced the best responses, but the diuretic was the best agent in lowering systolic pressure. In younger whites, the beta-blocker, ACE inhibitor, and calcium blocker were more effective, and diuretic was quite ineffective for lowering diastolic pressure. The calcium channel blocker was the most potent agent in blacks, although diuretic was also effective in older blacks. The ACE inhibitor had little effect as a single agent in blacks. In a somewhat younger patient group of mixed gender, the Treatment of Mild Hypertension Study (TOMHS) found that representatives of these four classes and an alpha-blocker were similarly effective. As in the Veterans Administration study, the diuretic tended to have greater benefit on systolic blood pressure. Importantly, in both trials, adverse effects on blood lipids were not observed during long-term therapy with any agent, and left ventricular hypertrophy regression tended to be greater with the diuretic. Many patients requiring therapy for hypertension have conditions that favor or contraindicate the use of one or more drugs. Some of these factors are listed in Table 11–2.

C. Current Antihypertensive Agents: (See Tables 11–3 to 11–7 for dosages.)

1. Diuretics–(Table 11–3.) Diuretics are the antihypertensive class that has been most extensively studied in clinical trials, which have revealed a consistent reduction in the rate of strokes and a somewhat less consistent effect on coronary events and total mortality. Diuretics lower blood pressure initially by decreasing plasma volume (by suppressing tubular reabsorption of sodium, thus increasing the excretion of sodium and water) and cardiac output, but during chronic therapy their major hemodynamic effect is reduction of peripheral vascular resistance by an as yet unknown mechanism. Most of the antihypertensive effect of these agents is achieved at lower dosages than used previously (typically, 25 mg of hydrochlorothiazide or equivalent), but their biochemical effects are dose-related. The thiazide diuretics are the most widely used. The loop diuretics (such as furosemide) may lead to electrolyte and volume depletion more readily than the thiazides and have short durations of action; therefore, they are not ordinarily used in hypertension except in the presence of renal dysfunction (serum creatinine above 2.5 mg/dL). Relative to the beta-blockers and the ACE inhibitors, diuretics are more potent in blacks, older individuals, the obese, and other subgroups with increased plasma volume or low plasma renin activity. Interestingly, they are relatively more effective in smokers than in nonsmokers. Chronic diuretic administration also mitigates the loss of bone mineral content in older women at risk for osteoporosis. Overall, diuretics administered alone control blood pressure in 50% of patients and can be used effectively with all other agents. They are perhaps the most effective agents for lowering predominantly systolic hypertension.

The adverse effects of diuretics relate chiefly to the metabolic changes listed in Table 11–3. Impotence, skin rashes, and photosensitivity are also less frequent side effects. Hypokalemia, with the resulting potential for arrhythmias or renal dysfunction, has been a concern but is uncommon at the usual current dosages (12.5–25 mg hydrochlorothiazide). The risk can be minimized by limiting salt intake or eating a high-potassium diet, and potassium replacement is usually not required to maintain serum K^+ at ≥ 3.5 mmol/L. Higher serum levels may be prudent in patients at special risk from intracellular potassium depletion (patients taking digoxin or having ventricular arrhythmias and diabetics in whom insulin release and insulin sensitivity are reduced by hypokalemia). It is noteworthy that several of the trials in which diuretic therapy proved most beneficial employed combinations of thiazide and potassium-sparing agents, such as triamterene or amiloride. These medications are more expensive, have additional side effects (primarily gastrointestinal), and may be dangerous in the presence of oliguria. However, it is reasonable to use these agents in appropriate patients receiving higher doses of diuretics and in place of potassium supplements. Diuretics also increase serum uric acid and may precipitate acute gout. Increases in blood glucose, triglycerides, low-density lipoprotein cholesterol, and plasma insulin may occur but are relatively minor during long-term low-dose therapy. Some experts feel that these lipid changes may limit the beneficial effect of blood pressure reduction on the progression of atherosclerosis.

2. Beta-adrenergic blocking agents–(Table 11–4.) These drugs are effective in hypertension because they decrease the heart rate and cardiac output. Even after continued use of beta-blockers for a number of years, cardiac output remains decreased and systemic vascular resistance increased with agents that do not have intrinsic sympathomimetic or alpha-blocking activity. The beta-blockers also decrease renin release and are in general more efficacious in populations likely to have elevated plasma renin activity, such as younger white patients. They neutralize the reflex tachycardia caused by vasodilators such as hydralazine and alpha-adrenergic blockers in the treatment of hypertension. The beta-blockers are especially useful in patients with associated conditions that benefit from this mode of therapy. These include patients with angina pectoris, patients with previous myocardial infarction, and individuals with migraine headaches and somatic manifestations of anxiety.

Although all beta-blockers appear to be approximately equivalent in antihypertensive potency, controlling 50–60% of patients, they differ in a number of pharmacologic properties (these differences are summarized in Table 11–4), including relatively specific to the cardiac β_1 receptors (cardioselectivity) and whether they also block the β_2 receptors in the bronchi and vasculature; at higher dosages, however, all agents are nonselective. The beta-blockers also differ in their pharmacokinetics and lipid solubility—which determines whether they enter the brain and cause cerebral symptoms—and mechanisms of elimination. The effect on the pulse rate varies; agents with intrinsic sympathetic activity may be preferable in patients who develop more pronounced bradycardia (< 45/min) when given other beta-blockers. Labetalol is a combined alpha- and beta-blocker and, unlike most beta-blockers, decreases peripheral resistance.

The side effects of all beta-blockers include development of bronchial asthma in predisposed patients; bradycardia; atrioventricular conduction defects; left ventricular failure; nasal congestion; Raynaud's phenomenon, especially in women; and central nervous system symptoms with nightmares, excitement, and confusion. Fatigue, lethargy, and impotence may occur. All beta-blockers tend to increase plasma triglycerides. The nonselective and, to a lesser extent, the cardioselective beta-blockers tend to depress the protective HDL fraction of plasma cholesterol. This is not seen in agents with intrinsic sympathomimetic activity, and as with diuretics, the changes are blunted with time and dietary changes. Some experts believe that these lipid changes may have an adverse effect on coronary artery disease.

These agents are contraindicated in patients with congestive heart failure or symptomatic bronchospasm. Beta-blockers are relatively contraindicated in insulin-dependent diabetes, since they inhibit gluconeogenesis and may prolong hypoglycemic episodes. However, recent studies have not confirmed earlier suggestions that they may worsen symptoms of peripheral vascular disease.

3. Angiotensin-converting enzyme (ACE) inhibitors and angiotensin II blockers–(Table 11–5.) These drugs are being increasingly used as the initial medication in mild to moderate hypertension. Their primary mode of action is inhibition of the renin-angiotensin-aldosterone system, but they also inhibit bradykinin degradation, stimulate vasodilating prostaglandin synthesis, and, sometimes, reduce sympathetic nervous system activity. These latter actions may explain why they exhibit some effect even in patients with low plasma renin activity. The ACE inhibitors appear to be most effective in younger whites. They are relatively less effective in blacks and in the elderly and in predominantly systolic hypertension. While as single therapy they achieve adequate antihypertensive control in only about 40–50% of patients, the combination of an ACE inhibitor and a diuretic or calcium channel blocker is potent.

The ACE inhibitors are the agents of choice in type I diabetics with frank proteinuria or evidence of renal dysfunction, because they delay the progression to end-stage renal disease. Many authorities have extrapolated this indication to include type II diabetics and type I diabetics with microalbuminuria, even when they do not meet the usual criteria for antihypertensive therapy, although data confirming the benefits of these interventions are not yet available.

An advantage of the ACE inhibitors and angiotensin II blockers is their relative freedom from troublesome side effects. Severe hypotension can occur in patients with bilateral renal artery stenosis; acute renal failure may ensue. Hyperkalemia may develop in patients with intrinsic renal disease and type IV renal tubular acidosis (commonly seen in diabetics) and in the elderly. A chronic dry cough due to bronchial or laryngeal irritation is seen in 5–15% of patients and may require stopping the drug. Skin rashes and taste alterations are seen more often with captopril than with the non-sulfhydryl-containing agents (enalapril and lisinopril) but often disappear with continued therapy. Angioneurotic edema is an uncommon but potentially dangerous side effect of all agents of this class. Proteinuria and neutropenia are very uncommon at the lower dosages now employed except in individuals with preexisting renal insufficiency or autoimmune disease.

Specific inhibitors of the AT_1 angiotensin II receptor offer an alternative approach to inhibiting the renin-angiotensin system. Two agents, losartan and valsartan, are now available in the United States, and several others will soon be approved. These agents are free of the side effects of cough and skin rash. However, they are somewhat less potent in antihypertensive action and usually must be combined with a low dose of diuretic. Because of their higher cost, limited long-term experience, and lesser efficacy, angiotensin II blockers should be reserved primarily for patients who develop side effects when taking ACE inhibitors.

4. Calcium channel blockers–(Table 11–6.) All the agents of this class reduce blood pressure, and a number of new agents with a longer duration of action and perhaps less negative inotropic activity are available. They act by causing peripheral vasodilation, which is associated with less reflex tachycardia and fluid retention than other vasodilators. These agents are effective as single-drug therapy in approximately 60% of patients and appear to be effective in all demographic groups and all grades of hypertension. As a result, they may be preferable to beta-blockers and ACE inhibitors in blacks and older subjects. Calcium channel blockers and diuretics are less additive when given together than when either is combined with beta-blockers or ACE inhibitors. However, verapamil and diltiazem should be combined cautiously with beta-blockers because of their potential for depressing atrioventricular conduction and sinus node automaticity.

Milbefradil is a new calcium channel blocker that acts both on the L- and T-type channels, the latter primarily located on vascular smooth muscle and the sinus node. As a result, it may have less negative inotropic effects.

There are as yet substantial concerns that therapy with calcium blockers may be associated with an increased incidence of myocardial infarction and other cardiac events as well as being associated with a higher rate of gastrointestinal bleeding and cancer, the latter with short-acting formulations. Nonetheless, these safety questions justify concern over the lack of long-term studies with calcium channel blockers and the absence of clearly improved cardiovascular outcomes with their use. Until such data are available, it is prudent not to use short-acting formulations and to choose calcium blockers as first-line agents only in carefully selected individuals.

The most common side effects of calcium channel blockers are headache, peripheral edema, bradycardia, and constipation (especially with verapamil in the elderly). The dihydropyridine agents—nifedipine, nicardipine, isradipine, felodipine, and amlodipine—are more likely to produce symptoms of vasodilation, such as headache, flushing, palpitations, and peripheral edema. Calcium channel blockers have negative inotropic effects and may cause or exacerbate heart failure in patients with cardiac dysfunction. This tendency may be less with amlodipine. Most of these agents are now available in preparations that can be administered once daily.

5. Alpha-adrenoceptor antagonists–(Table 11–7.) Prazosin, terazosin, and doxazosin block postsynaptic alpha receptors, relax smooth muscle, and reduce blood pressure by lowering peripheral vascular resistance. These agents are effective as single-drug therapy in some individuals, but tachyphylaxis may appear during long-term therapy and side effects are relatively common. The major side effects are marked hypotension and syncope after the first dose, which, therefore, should be small and be given at bedtime. Postdosing palpitations, headache, and nervousness may continue to occur during chronic therapy. These side effects may be less frequent or severe with doxazosin because of its more gradual onset of action. Unlike the beta-blockers and diuretics, the alpha-blockers have no adverse effect on serum lipid levels—in fact, they increase high-density lipoprotein cholesterol

while reducing total cholesterol. Whether this is beneficial in the long term has not been established. These drugs are most useful in combination with other agents in less responsive patients. One interesting attribute is a reduction in symptoms of prostatism in some men, which makes these drugs appropriate first-line agents for symptomatic patients.

6. Drugs with central sympatholytic action–(Table 11–7.) Methyldopa, clonidine, guanabenz, and guanfacine lower blood pressure by stimulating alpha-adrenergic receptors in the central nervous system, thus reducing efferent peripheral sympathetic outflow. These agents are effective as single therapy in some patients, but they are usually employed as second- or third-line agents because of the high frequency of drug intolerance, including sedation, fatigue, dry mouth, postural hypotension, and impotence. An important concern is rebound hypertension following withdrawal. Methyldopa also causes hepatitis and hemolytic anemia and should be avoided except in individuals who have already tolerated chronic therapy. Clonidine is available in patches and may have particular value in patients in whom compliance is a troublesome issue.

7. Arteriolar dilators–(Table 11–7.) Hydralazine and minoxidil relax vascular smooth muscle and produce peripheral vasodilation. When given alone, they stimulate reflex tachycardia, increase myocardial contractility, and cause headache, palpitations, and fluid retention. They are usually given in combination with diuretics and beta-blockers in resistant patients. Hydralazine produces frequent gastrointestinal disturbances and may induce a lupus-like syndrome. Minoxidil causes hirsutism and marked fluid retention; this agent is reserved for the most refractory of patients.

8. Peripheral sympathetic inhibitors–(Table 11–7.) These agents are now used infrequently. Reserpine remains a cost-effective antihypertensive agent. Its reputation for inducing mental depression and its other side effects—sedation, nasal stuffiness, sleep disturbances, and peptic ulcers—have made it unpopular, though these problems are uncommon at low dosages. Guanethidine and guanadrel inhibit catecholamine release from peripheral neurons but frequently cause orthostatic hypotension (especially in the morning or after exercise), diarrhea, and fluid retention. These agents are used chiefly in refractory hypertension.

D. Initiating Therapy: When an initial agent is selected, the patient should be informed of common side effects and the need for diligent compliance. Unless the initial blood pressure is very high (> 180/110), follow-up visits should be at 4- to 6-week intervals to allow for full medication effect to be manifest (especially with diuretics).

E. Combination Therapy: Most patients with hypertension can be controlled with one agent or with two-drug regimens, which combine comple-

Table 11–7. Alpha-adrenoceptor blocking agents, sympatholytics, and vasodilators.

Drug	Proprietary Name	Initial Dosage	Dosage Range	Cost per Unit	Cost for 30 Days' Treatment (Average Dosage)[1]	Adverse Effects	Comments
ALPHA-ADRENOCEPTOR BLOCKERS							
Prazosin	Minipress*	1 mg hs	2–20 mg in 2 or 3 doses	G: $0.57/5 mg B: $1.16/5 mg	G: $34.00 B: $70.00 (5 mg bid)	Syncope with first dose; postural hypotension, dizziness, palpitations, headache, weakness, drowsiness, sexual dysfunction, anticholinergic effects, urinary incontinence; first-dose effects may be less with doxazosin.	May ↑HDL and ↓LDL cholesterol. May provide short-term relief of obstructive prostatic symptoms. Tachyphylaxis may occur when used to treat congestive heart failure.
Terazosin	Hytrin	1 mg hs	1–20 mg in 1 or 2 doses	$1.31/1, 2, 5, 10 mg	$39.00 (5 mg qd)		
Doxazosin	Cardura	1 mg hs	1–16 mg qd	$0.96/4 mg	$29.00 (4 mg qd)		
CENTRAL SYMPATHOLYTICS							
Clonidine	Catapres*	0.1 mg bid	0.2–0.6 mg in 2 doses	G: $0.13/0.1 mg B: $0.57/1 mg	G: $8.00 B: $34.00 (0.1 mg bid)	Sedation, dry mouth, sexual dysfunction, headache, bradyarrhythmias; side effects may be less with guanfacine. Contact dermatitis with clonidine patch. Methyldopa also causes hepatitis, hemolytic anemia, fever.	"Rebound" hypertension may occur even after gradual withdrawal. Methyldopa should be avoided in favor of safer agents.
	Catapres TTS	0.1 mg/d patch weekly	0.1–0.3 mg/d patch weekly	$12.84/0.2 mg	$51.00 (0.2 mg weekly)		
Guanabenz	Wytensin	4 mg bid	8–64 mg in 2 doses	G: $0.53/4 mg B: $0.74	G: $32.00 B: $44.00 (4 mg bid)		
Guanfacine	Tenex	1 mg once daily	1–3 mg qd	G: $0.73/1 mg B: $0.87/1 mg	G: $22.00 B: $26.00 (1 mg qd)		
Methyldopa	Aldomet*	250 mg bid	500–2000 mg in 2 doses	G: $0.32/500 mg B: $0.63/500 mg	G: $19.00 B: $37.80 (500 mg bid)		
PERIPHERAL NEURONAL ANTAGONISTS							
Guanethidine	Ismelin	10 mg once daily	10–100 mg qd	$0.84/25 mg	$25.00 (25 mg qd)	Orthostatic hypotension, diarrhea, exercise hypotension, sexual dysfunction, salt and water retention.	
Guanadrel	Hylorel	5 mg bid	10–70 mg in 2 doses	$0.75/10 mg	$45.00 (10 mg bid)		
Reserpine		0.05 mg once daily	0.05–0.25 mg qd	G: $0.04/0.1 mg	$1.20 (0.1 mg qd)	Depression (less likely at low dosages, ie, <0.25 mg); night terrors, nasal stuffiness, drowsiness, peptic disease, gastrointestinal disturbances, bradycardia.	
DIRECT VASODILATORS							
Hydralazine	Apresoline*	25 mg bid	50–300 mg in 2–4 doses	G: $0.04/25 mg B: $0.31/25 mg	G: $2.40 B: $19.00 (25 mg bid)	GI disturbances, tachycardia, headache, nasal congestion, rash, LE-like syndrome.	May worsen or precipitate angina.
Minoxidil	Loniten	5 mg once daily	5–40 mg qd	G: $0.51/10 mg B: $1.03/10 mg	G: $15.30 B: $31.00 (10 mg qd)	Tachycardia, fluid retention, headache, hirsutism, pericardial effusion, thrombocytopenia.	Should be used in combination with beta-blocker and diuretic.

*Generic preparation available. B = brand name; G = generic.

[1]Cost to pharmacist (average wholesale price) for 30 days' treatment based on average dose as shown in parentheses (generic when possible). Source: First Data Bank. Price Alert, April 1997.

mentary agents, such as (1) a diuretic plus a beta-blocker, (2) a diuretic plus an ACE inhibitor, (3) a diuretic plus a calcium channel blocker, or (4) a calcium channel blocker plus an ACE inhibitor. A minority may require triple-drug therapy. Particularly useful multidrug regimens are (1) a diuretic plus a beta-blocker plus a vasodilator or a calcium channel blocker; (2) a diuretic plus an ACE inhibitor plus either a calcium channel blocker or a sympatholytic (or both); and (3) a calcium channel blocker plus an ACE inhibitor plus either a sympatholytic or a beta-blocker (or both). Patients who are compliant with their medications and who do not respond to these combinations should usually be evaluated for secondary hypertension before proceeding to more complex regimens.

F. Treatment of Hyperlipidemia: A critical element in preventing hypertension-related morbidity is concomitant control of hyperlipidemia.

G. Follow-Up of the Treated Hypertensive: Once blood pressure is controlled on a well-tolerated regimen, follow-up visits can be infrequent and laboratory testing should be limited to tests appropriate for the patient and the medications utilized. Yearly monitoring of blood lipids is recommended in patients with hypertension, and an ECG should be repeated at 2- to 4-year intervals depending on whether initial abnormalities are present, the presence of coronary risk factors, and age.

Patients who have had excellent blood pressure control for several years, especially if they have lost weight and initiated favorable lifestyle modifications, should be considered for "step-down" of therapy to determine if lower doses or discontinuing of medications is feasible.

Drugs for hypertension: Med Lett Drugs Ther 1995;37:45.

The Fifth Report of the Joint National Committee on Detection, Education, and Treatment of High Blood Pressure (JNC V). Arch Intern Med 1993;153:154. (Extensive discussion and tabular presentation of antihypertensive drugs and their use in different patient groups.)

Goodfriend TL et al: Angiotensin receptors and their antagonists. N Engl J Med 1996;334:1649.

Materson BJ et al: Single drug therapy for hypertension in men: A comparison of six antihypertensive agents with placebo. N Engl J Med 1993;328:914. (Landmark study of over 1200 patients.)

Neaton JD et al: Treatment of Mild Hypertension Study: Final results. JAMA 1993;270:718. (Additive benefit of five classes of antihypertensive medications in patients undergoing vigorous nonpharmacologic intervention.)

Swales JD: Pharmacological treatment of hypertension. Lancet 1994;344:380. (Concise discussion of why to treat, whom to treat, and how to treat.)

HYPERTENSIVE URGENCIES & EMERGENCIES

Hypertensive emergencies have become less frequent in recent years but still require prompt recognition and aggressive but careful management. A spectrum of acute presentations exists, and the appropriate therapeutic approach varies accordingly.

Hypertensive urgencies are situations in which blood pressure must be reduced within a few hours. Examples are asymptomatic severe hypertension (systolic pressure > 240 mm Hg, diastolic pressure > 130 mm Hg) and symptomatic moderately severe hypertension (systolic pressure > 200 mg Hg, diastolic pressure > 120 mm Hg, or even lower levels) associated with headache, heart failure, or angina or occurring in the perioperative period. Parenteral therapy is rarely required, and partial reduction of blood pressure with relief of symptoms is the goal.

Hypertensive emergencies require substantial reduction of blood pressure within 1 hour to avoid the risk of serious morbidity or death. Although blood pressure is usually strikingly elevated (diastolic pressure > 130 mm Hg), the correlation between pressure and end-organ damage is often poor. It is the latter that determines the seriousness of the emergency and the approach to treatment. Emergencies include hypertensive encephalopathy (headache, irritability, confusion, and altered mental status due to cerebrovascular spasm), hypertensive nephropathy (hematuria, proteinuria, and progressive renal dysfunction due to arteriolar necrosis and intimal hyperplasia of the interlobular arteries), intracranial hemorrhage, aortic dissection, preeclampsia-eclampsia, pulmonary edema, unstable angina, or myocardial infarction. **Malignant hypertension** is by historical definition characterized by encephalopathy or nephropathy with accompanying papilledema. Progressive renal failure usually ensues if treatment is not provided. The therapeutic approach is identical to that employed with other antihypertensive emergencies.

Parenteral therapy is indicated in most hypertensive emergencies, especially if encephalopathy is present. The initial goal of treatment should be rapid reduction of systolic and diastolic pressure by at least 20–40 mm Hg and 10–20 mm Hg, respectively, to levels below 180–200/110–120 mm Hg. A subsequent more gradual reduction to near-normal levels is appropriate.

Pharmacologic Management

A. Parenteral Agents: A growing number of agents are available for management of acute hypertensive problems. (Table 11–8 lists drugs, dosages, and adverse effects.) Sodium nitroprusside is the agent of choice for the most serious emergencies because of its rapid and easily controllable action, but continuous monitoring is essential when this agent is

Table 11–8. Drugs for hypertensive crises and urgencies.

Agent	Action	Dosage	Onset	Duration	Adverse Effects	Comments
PARENTERAL AGENTS (INTRAVENOUSLY UNLESS NOTED)						
Nitroprusside (Nipride)	Vasodilator	0.25–10 µg/kg/min	Seconds	3–5 minutes	GI, CNS; thiocyanate and cyanide toxicity, especially with renal and hepatic insufficiency; hypotension.	Most effective and easily titratable treatment. Use with beta-blocker in aortic dissection.
Nitroglycerin	Vasodilator	0.25–5 µg/kg/min	2–5 minutes	3–5 minutes	Headache, nausea, hypotension, bradycardia.	Tolerance may develop.
Labetalol (Normodyne, Trandate)	Beta- and alpha-blocker	20–40 mg every 10 minutes to 300 mg; 2 mg/min infusion	5–10 minutes	3–6 hours	GI, hypotension, bronchospasm, bradycardia, heart block.	Avoid in congestive heart failure, asthma. May be continued orally.
Esmolol (Brevibloc)	Beta-blocker	Loading dose 500 µg/kg over 1 minute; maintenance, 25–200 µg/kg/min	1–2 minutes	10–30 minutes	Bradycardia, nausea.	Avoid in congestive heart failure, asthma.
Nicardipine (Cardene)	Calcium channel blocker	5 mg/h; may increase by 1–2.5 mg/h every 15 minutes to 15 mg/h	1–5 minutes	3–6 hours	Hypotension, tachycardia, headache.	May precipitate myocardial ischemia.
Enalaprilat (Vasotec)	ACE inhibitor	1.25 mg every 6 hours	15 minutes	6 hours or more	Excessive hypotension.	Additive with diuretics; may be continued orally.
Furosemide (Lasix)	Diuretic	10–80 mg	15 minutes	4 hours	Hypokalemia, hypotension.	Adjunct to vasodilator.
Hydralazine (Apresoline)	Vasodilator	5–20 mg IV or IM (less desirable); may repeat after 20 minutes	10–30 minutes	2–6 hours	Tachycardia, headache, GI.	Avoid in coronary artery disease, dissection. Rarely used except in pregnancy.
Diazoxide (Hyperstat)	Vasodilator	50–150 mg repeated at intervals of 5–15 minutes, or 15–30 mg/min by IV infusion to a maximum of 600 mg	1–2 minutes	4–24 hours	Excessive hypotension, tachycardia, myocardial ischemia, headache, nausea, vomiting, hyperglycemia. Necrosis with extravasation.	Avoid in coronary artery disease and dissection. Use with beta-blocker and diuretic. Mostly obsolete.
Trimethaphan (Arfonad)	Ganglionic blocker	0.5–5 mg/min	1–3 minutes	10 minutes	Hypotension, ileus, urinary retention, respiratory arrest. Liberates histamine; use caution in allergic individuals.	Useful in aortic dissection. Otherwise rarely used.
ORAL AGENTS						
Nifedipine (Adalat, Procardia)	Calcium channel blocker	10 mg initially; may be repeated after 30 minutes	15 minutes	2–6 hours	Excessive hypotension, tachycardia, headache, angina, myocardial infarction, stroke.	Response unpredictable.
Clonidine (Catapres)	Central sympatholytic	0.1–0.2 mg initially; then 0.1 mg every hour to 0.8 mg	30–60 minutes	6–8 hours	Sedation.	Rebound may occur.
Captopril (Capoten)	ACE inhibitor	25 mg	15–30 minutes	4–6 hours	Excessive hypotension.	

used. In the presence of myocardial ischemia, intravenous nitroglycerin or an intravenous beta-blocker, such as labetalol or esmolol, is preferable.

1. Nitroprusside sodium–This agent is given by controlled intravenous infusion gradually titrated to the desired effect. It lowers the blood pressure within seconds by direct arteriolar and venous dilatation. Monitoring with an intra-arterial line is essential to avoid excessive blood pressure reductions. Nitroprusside—in combination with a beta-blocker—is especially useful in patients with aortic dissection.

2. Nitroglycerin, intravenous–This agent is a less potent antihypertensive than nitroprusside and should be reserved for patients with accompanying acute ischemic syndromes.

3. Labetalol–This combined beta- and alpha-adrenergic blocking agent is the most potent adrenergic blocker for rapid blood pressure reduction. Excessive blood pressure responses are unusual. Experience with this agent in hypertensive syndromes associated with pregnancy has been favorable.

4. Nicardipine–Intravenous nicardipine is the most potent and long-acting of the parenteral calcium channel blockers. As a primarily arterial vasodilator, it has the potential to precipitate reflex tachycardia, and for that reason it should not be used without a beta-blocker in patients with coronary artery disease.

5. Esmolol–This rapidly acting beta-blocker is approved by the FDA only for treatment of supraventricular tachycardia. It is less potent than labetalol, but it is useful in acutely lowering blood pressure, especially when combined with a vasodilator such as nitroprusside, nitroglycerin, or hydralazine. Esmolol is especially useful during myocardial ischemia.

6. Enalaprilat–This is the active form of the oral ACE inhibitor enalapril. The onset of action is usually within 15 minutes, but the peak effect may be delayed for up to 6 hours. Therefore, enalaprilat is useful primarily as an adjunctive agent.

7. Diazoxide–Diazoxide acts promptly as a vasodilator without decreasing renal blood flow. Because the magnitude of response is difficult to control and may be excessive, it is only infrequently used. To avoid hypotension, it should be given in small boluses or as an infusion rather than as the previously recommended large bolus. One use of diazoxide has been in preeclampsia-eclampsia. Hyperglycemia and sodium and water retention may occur. The drug should be used only for short periods and is best combined with a powerful diuretic such as furosemide.

8. Hydralazine–Hydralazine can be given intravenously or intramuscularly, but its effect is less predictable than that of other drugs in this group. It produces reflex tachycardia and should not be given without beta-blockers in patients with possible coronary disease or aortic dissection. Based on historical experience, hydralazine is now used primarily in pregnancy and in children, but even in these situations, newer agents are supplanting it.

9. Trimethaphan–The ganglionic blocking agent trimethaphan is titrated with the patient sitting; its activity depends upon this. The patient can be placed supine if the hypotensive effect is excessive. The effect occurs within a few minutes and persists for the duration of the infusion. This agent has largely been supplanted by nitroprusside and newer medications.

10. Diuretics–Intravenous loop diuretics can be very helpful when the patient has signs of heart failure or fluid retention, but the onset of their hypotensive response is slow, making them an adjunct rather than a primary agent for hypertensive emergencies. Low dosages should be used initially (furosemide, 20 mg; or bumetanide, 0.5 mg). They facilitate the response to vasodilators, which often stimulate fluid retention.

B. Oral Agents: Patients with less severe acute hypertensive syndromes can often be treated with oral therapy. They should be closely monitored until a therapeutic end point is achieved. Abrupt blood pressure lowering is not usually necessary in asymptomatic individuals, and the frequent use of potent agents such as rapid-acting nifedipine probably causes more adverse effects than benefits.

1. Clonidine–Clonidine, 0.2 mg orally initially, followed by 0.1 mg every hour to a total of 0.8 mg, will usually lower blood pressure over a period of several hours. Sedation is frequent, and rebound hypertension may occur if the drug is stopped.

2. Captopril–Captopril, 12.5–25 mg orally, will also lower blood pressure in 15–30 minutes. The response is variable and may be excessive.

3. Nifedipine–Nifedipine, 10 mg orally, will reduce blood pressure within 5–20 minutes in most patients. An additional 10 mg dose may be needed. Excessive hypotensive responses may occur, especially if the drug is given sublingually, and reflex tachycardia may induce angina. This approach is commonly applied because of its simplicity, but more often the physician is "treating himself" rather than the patient.

C. Subsequent Therapy: When the blood pressure has been brought under control, combinations of oral antihypertensive agents can be added as parenteral drugs are tapered off over a period of 2–3 days. Most subsequent regimens should include a diuretic.

Gifford RW Jr: Management of hypertensive crises. JAMA 1991;266:829.

Kaplan NM: Management of hypertensive emergencies. Lancet 1994;344:1335.

12

Blood Vessels & Lymphatics

Lawrence M. Tierney, Jr., MD, & Louis M. Messina, MD

Atherosclerosis is the cause of most degenerative arterial disease. It is a disease of the intima of the arterial wall characterized by extracellular lipid deposition and smooth muscle migration and proliferation. Features of complex lesions include a fibrous cap containing smooth muscle and inflammatory cells that overlie a central core of necrotic debris. These lesions can be complicated by calcification, intraplaque hemorrhage, and luminal thrombosis after cap rupture.

The incidence of atherosclerosis increases with age—people over age 40 (particularly men) are most commonly affected. Risk factors include hypercholesterolemia, diabetes mellitus, smoking, a positive family history, and hypertension. Atherosclerosis is a systemic disease, with some degree of involvement of all major arteries, but it produces its clinical manifestations by critical involvement of a limited number of arteries. Narrowing and occlusion of the artery are the most common manifestations. Weakening of the arterial wall from loss of elastin and collagen may result in aneurysmal dilation. Both processes may be present in the same individual. Less common arterial diseases include vasculitis (of both large and small arteries), thromboangiitis obliterans (Buerger's disease), fibrodysplasia of visceral arteries, syphilitic aortitis, and radiation arteritis.

DISEASES OF THE AORTA

ANEURYSMS OF THE ABDOMINAL AORTA

Essentials of Diagnosis

- Most aneurysms are asymptomatic, detected at incidental physical examination or sonography.
- Severe back or abdominal pain indicates rupture.
- Concomitant atherosclerotic occlusive disease not necessarily associated.

General Considerations

Over 90% of abdominal atherosclerotic aneurysms originate below the renal arteries, and many involve the bifurcation of the aorta. Aneurysms of the upper aorta are much less common. The infrarenal aorta is normally 2 cm in diameter; an aneurysm is considered present when the diameter exceeds 4 cm.

Clinical Findings

A. Symptoms and Signs:

1. Asymptomatic—A pulsating upper abdominal mass may be discovered on a routine physical examination, most frequently in men over 50. More often, sonography done for other purposes detects asymptomatic aneurysms. Sonography is also the most cost-effective test for confirming a suspicion of aneurysm raised by physical examination. Peripheral pulses are often readily palpable as a result of generalized arteriomegaly in these patients. Aneurysms of the popliteal artery often coexist; indeed, detection of the latter should raise the suspicion of abdominal aneurysm, since one is present in more than one-third of patients with popliteal aneurysm.

2. Symptomatic—Pain varies from mild to severe midabdominal or lower back pain (or both) and often is secondary to an inflammatory aortic aneurysm. Inflammatory aneurysms account for less than 5% of aortic aneurysms and are characterized by extensive periaortic and retroperitoneal inflammation. Peripheral emboli may occur, even from small aneurysms, and symptomatic arterial insufficiency in the legs may result.

3. Rupture—Aortic aneurysm rupture results in death before hospitalization in many patients, and others die before they reach the operating room. Those with bleeding confined to the retroperitoneal area may have severe pain in the abdomen, flank, or back and a pulsating abdominal mass; retroperitoneal bleeding can produce local tamponade and permit the patient to come to operation. Free peritoneal (anterior) rupture, though much less common, results in death within minutes if untreated.

B. Laboratory Findings: Electrocardiography

and renal function studies should be obtained to assess concomitant dysfunction in those systems.

C. Imaging: Abdominal ultrasonography is the diagnostic study of choice and is also valuable for following aneurysm size in patients not immediately treated surgically. Curvilinear calcifications outlining portions of the aneurysm wall may be visible on plain films of the aortic area in approximately three-fourths of those with an aneurysm, but this study is less sensitive than ultrasonography. Contrast-enhanced CT scanning precisely defines the extent of the aneurysm. Aortography is helpful in planning repair when arterial occlusive disease of the visceral or lower extremity arteries is suspected but may underemphasize the aneurysm's size if thrombus is present. MRI is as sensitive and specific as CT and does not require administration of contrast.

Treatment

A. Standard Therapy: Surgical excision and grafting is the treatment of choice for most aneurysms of the distal abdominal aorta. Aneurysms usually enlarge and ultimately rupture if left untreated. The size of the aneurysm correlates best with the risk of rupture: In asymptomatic patients, surgery is advised when the aneurysm is 5 or 6 cm in diameter; in symptomatic patients, repair is indicated irrespective of size. Improving surgical techniques and postoperative care have led some to recommend surgical resection even for smaller aneurysms. The risk of rupture cannot be safely predicted for individuals, but it increases as a function of its radius. Opinion differs about whether asymptomatic aneurysms in poor-risk patients should be removed or followed closely by means of ultrasound measurements to detect signs of expansion. Long-term beta-blockade appears to be associated with a decreased rate of growth of aneurysms that are being followed. Patients with significant symptomatic coronary or carotid disease may be more likely to suffer myocardial infarction or stroke during and following aneurysm resection; coronary artery bypass grafting or coronary angioplasty to lessen this risk prior to elective aneurysm repair is advocated by some. However, overall mortality increases with each procedure. Some vascular surgeons believe the aneurysms should be treated first, since there may be a higher rate of rupture in patients postoperative for major surgery such as coronary artery bypass grafting. Likewise, prophylactic carotid endarterectomy has not been established as providing overall benefit given the considerations noted.

In general, individuals over age 80 with minimal preoperative risk factors can undergo elective surgery with an acceptable mortality rate; those with significant associated disease generally should not undergo operation without compelling indications.

B. Endovascular Repair: In the last few years, endovascular prostheses are now employed with increasing frequency. Consisting of Dacron grafts with endoluminal stents, these may be employed in any vessel, including aneurysmal thoracic and abdominal aortas, iliac arteries, and more distal vessels. Operative time is reduced, as is the complication rate and the mortality rate. Complications include migration of portions of the prosthesis. Preoperative measurement of the diseased target vessels is essential to plan device insertion accurately. Clinical trials have confirmed the safety and efficacy of endovascular repair of aortic aneurysms. Long-term durability of endovascular repair needs to be established before widespread application of this technique can be recommended.

Complications

The rate of complications after aortic aneurysm repair is usually between 5% and 10%. They include myocardial infarction, bleeding, respiratory insufficiency, ischemic colitis, limb ischemia, renal insufficiency, and stroke. Late complications include graft infection and graft-enteric fistula and are seen more frequently in cases where the initial surgery was performed on an emergent basis.

Prognosis

The mortality rate following elective surgical resection is 3–8%, though in certain centers it has recently approached 1%; clinicians must be aware of surgical success rates in their own institutions before making the often difficult decision to operate, especially in high-risk patients. Data are not available for endovascular repair, but it is almost certain to improve the statistics cited. Of those who survive surgery, approximately 60% are alive 5 years later, and in those who die, myocardial infarction is the leading cause of death. Among unoperated patients, old studies indicate that less than 20% survive 5 years, and aneurysm rupture is the cause of 60% of the deaths; more recently, a less rapid rate of expansion has been reported, but some surgeons dispute this. In general, a patient with an aortic aneurysm has a three-fold greater chance of dying as a consequence of rupture of the aneurysm than of dying from surgical resection. If coronary or carotid artery surgery is done preoperatively, the added morbidity and mortality of these procedures must be considered in the overall approach to the patient.

Blum U et al: Endoluminal stent-graft for infrarenal abdominal aortic aneurysms. N Engl J Med 1997;336:13. (Early results showing safety and efficacy of endoluminal stent-grafts.)

Ernst CB: Abdominal aortic aneurysm. N Engl J Med 1993;328:1167.

Kahn CE, Quiroz FA: Positive predictive clinical suspicion for abdominal aortic aneurysm. J Gen Intern Med 1996;11:756.

Katz DA, Cronenwett JI: The cost-effectiveness of early surgery versus watchful waiting in the management of small abdominal aortic aneurysms. J Vasc Surg 1994; 19:980.

ANEURYSMS OF THE THORACIC AORTA

Thoracic aortic aneurysms are most commonly due to atherosclerosis; syphilis is now a rare cause. Vasculitis and cystic medial necrosis, as occur in Marfan's syndrome, may also result in thoracic aneurysm. Traumatic aneurysms may occur at the ligamentum arteriosus just beyond the left subclavian artery when the wall of the aorta is incompletely torn as a result of a rapid-deceleration accident. Less than 10% of aortic aneurysms are thoracic.

Clinical Findings

Manifestations depend largely on the size and position of the aneurysm and its rate of growth.

A. Symptoms and Signs: There may be no symptoms or signs if the aneurysm has been diagnosed by chest x-ray done for other reasons. Substernal, back, or neck pain may occur, as well as symptoms and signs due to pressure on (1) the trachea (dyspnea, stridor, a brassy cough), (2) the esophagus (dysphagia), (3) the left recurrent laryngeal nerve (hoarseness), or (4) the superior vena cava (edema in the neck and arms, distended neck veins). Aortic regurgitation may be present.

B. Imaging: Aortography may be necessary to confirm the diagnosis and to delineate the precise location and extent of the aneurysm and its relation to the vessels arising from the arch. CT scan and MRI are more sensitive than ultrasound for thoracic aneurysms. The coronary vessels and the aortic valve should also be studied if the ascending aorta is involved.

Differential Diagnosis

It may be difficult to determine whether a mass in the mediastinum is an aneurysm, a neoplasm, or a cyst. Radioactive isotope studies (^{125}I) may be helpful in diagnosing a substernal goiter.

Treatment

Indications for treatment of thoracic aneurysms include symptomatic or rapidly enlarging aneurysms and those whose greatest diameter exceeds 6 cm. Asymptomatic aneurysms in poor-risk patients are better treated only if progressive enlargement occurs. Control of hypertension may slow progression, and the use of beta-blockers makes empiric good sense. The overall mortality rate of thoracic aneurysmectomy, however, is considerably higher than the 3–5% rate for abdominal aneurysms given the complicated surgery; morbidity is appreciable as well.

If the aortic valve is involved, an aortic valve replacement may be necessary, and reattachment of the coronary arteries or aortocoronary bypass grafts may also be indicated. Paraplegia due to anterior spinal artery compromise is a complication of excision and graft replacement in 5–30% of patients depending on the extent of aortic involvement.

Prognosis

The risk of rupture of thoracic aneurysms is related to their size. Elective repair is usually not considered until the maximum diameter exceeds 6 cm. Prognosis without repair is relatively poor, only 20–25% surviving for 5 years. Most deaths are due to rupture or to the complications of generalized atherosclerosis. Saccular aneurysms, those distal to the left subclavian artery, and those limited to the ascending aorta may be approached surgically in good-risk candidates, with the caveats cited above. Resection of aneurysms of the transverse aortic arch involves major technical problems that can be dealt with only by skilled surgical teams using hypothermia to protect the nervous system.

Acher CW, Wynn MM: Technique of thoracoabdominal aneurysm repair. Ann Vasc Surg 1995;9:585.
Coselli JS et al: Results of contemporary surgical treatment of descending thoracic aortic aneurysms: Experience in 198 patients. Ann Vasc Surg 1996;10:131.

PERIPHERAL ARTERY ANEURYSMS (Popliteal & Femoral)

Popliteal Aneurysms

Popliteal aneurysms account for approximately 85% of all peripheral artery aneurysms. Patients with peripheral artery aneurysms are thought to have a generalized disorder of the arterial wall. For example, in half of cases of popliteal and femoral aneurysms, the contralateral artery is involved as well. One-third of patients with popliteal aneurysms and two-thirds of those with femoral aneurysms harbor aortoiliac artery aneurysms also. Peripheral aneurysms occur almost exclusively in men. More than half are symptomatic at the time of diagnosis. Symptoms are rarely due to rupture but rather result from thrombosis, peripheral embolization, or compression of adjacent structures with resultant venous thrombosis or neuropathy.

Ultrasound is the diagnostic study of choice to measure the diameter of the aneurysm as well as to search for other arterial aneurysms. Arteriography is required to define the anatomy of the outflow arteries in preparation for operative repair.

Repair of popliteal aneurysms is recommended for all asymptomatic aneurysms whose diameter exceeds 2 cm and for aneurysms less than 2 cm in diameter which become symptomatic.

A reversed saphenous vein bypass graft with proximal and distal ligation of the aneurysm is generally employed. In large aneurysms with manifestations of vein or nerve compression, resection of the aneurysm with grafting of the arterial defect may be necessary.

Femoral Aneurysms

Femoral aneurysms, as manifested by a pulsatile mass on one or both sides, have the potential for the same complications as popliteal aneurysms. Because the incidence of these complications in asymptomatic patients is less than for popliteal aneurysms, there is more reason to follow rather than operate on smaller, asymptomatic femoral aneurysms and to deal first with aortoiliac and then popliteal aneurysms in preference to femoral aneurysms when aneurysmal disease exists in all of these areas. Pseudoaneurysms often develop at distal anastomotic sites from previous aortic surgery and should be repaired when their diameter exceeds 2 cm.

Raggo A et al: The continuing challenge of aneurysms of the popliteal artery. Surg Gynecol Obstet 1993;177:565. (One center's experience over a 25-year period.)

Seddon AM: Popliteal artery aneurysm: Prompt intervention prevents tragic consequences. Postgrad Med 1993;94:125. (Uncommon, yet important, cause of lower extremity ischemia.)

AORTIC DISSECTION

Essentials of Diagnosis

- A history of hypertension or Marfan's syndrome is often present.
- Sudden severe chest pain with radiation to the back, occasionally migrating to the abdomen and hips.
- Patient appears to be in shock, but blood pressure is normal or elevated; pulse discrepancy in many patients.
- Acute aortic regurgitation may develop.

General Considerations

Aortic dissection is the most common aortic catastrophe requiring admission to a hospital. It originates at the site of an intimal tear and then propagates distally. Over 95% of intimal tears occur either in the ascending aorta just distal to the aortic valve (type A) or just distal to the left subclavian artery (type B). The initial intimal tear probably results from the constant torque applied to the ascending and proximal descending aorta occurring at these two points associated with the pulsatile blood flow from the heart. Dissection occurs on rare occasions in an aorta without an apparent intimal tear; these aortas invariably show histologic abnormalities of the media. Proximal dissections are encountered more often in aortas involved with abnormalities of the smooth muscle, elastic tissue, or collagen; distal dissections occur in patients with long-standing hypertension.

Pregnancy, bicuspid aortic valve, and coarctation are associated with an increased risk of type A and type B dissections; Marfan's syndrome makes a type A dissection more likely. Both hypertension and the rate of acceleration of pulsatile flow (dp/dt) are important in propagation of dissection, which may extend from the ascending aorta to the abdominal aorta or beyond. Alternatively, dissection may remain limited to the ascending aorta and the aortic valve area, especially if hypertension is not present or controlled early; furthermore, dissection may progress not only distally but also proximally.

When not appropriately diagnosed and treated, aortic dissection is a lethal disease. Of patients with type A dissections, 50% are dead within 48 hours and 90% at 1 month. Death is usually due to rupture of the aorta into the pericardial sac or pleural space or to acute aortic regurgitation with left ventricular failure. Deaths due to type B dissection are less common and usually secondary to free rupture in the pleural space, or they may occur as a consequence of acute mesenteric and renal ischemia.

Clinical Findings

A. Symptoms and Signs: Severe, persistent chest pain of sudden onset, nearly always anterior but often also posterior, later progressing to the abdominal and hip areas, is characteristic. Radiation down the arms or into the neck may or may not occur. Usually there is only a mild decrease in the prerupture level of blood pressure. Partial or complete occlusion of the arteries arising from the aortic arch or of the intercostal and lumbar arteries may lead to such nervous system findings as syncope, hemiplegia, or paralysis of the lower extremities. Peripheral pulses and blood pressures may be diminished or unequal. An aortic diastolic murmur may develop as a result of dissection close to the aortic valve, resulting in valvular regurgitation, heart failure, and cardiac tamponade.

B. Laboratory Findings: Electrocardiographic changes indicating left ventricular hypertrophy from long-standing hypertension are often present; acute changes may not develop unless the dissection involves the coronary ostium. In that case, inferior wall abnormalities predominate, since dissection leads to compromise of the right rather than the left coronary artery. In some, the ECG may be normal.

C. Imaging: Chest radiographs often reveal an abnormal aortic contour or a wide superior mediastinum, with changes in the configuration and thickness of the aortic wall in successive films. There may be findings of pleural or pericardial effusion. Diagnosis of dissection can be made by a variety of modalities, including dynamic CT scanning, angiography, MRI, and transesophageal echocardiography (TEE). The latter has been used with increasing frequency because of its high sensitivity (98%) and specificity (99%) and because it can be performed rapidly and relatively noninvasively. The best initial study is the one most readily available that can be interpreted accurately in a given hospital setting. MRI has not played a major role in the initial diagnosis but is ideal for serial follow-up.

Differential Diagnosis

Aortic dissection is most commonly confused with myocardial infarction (see Chapter 10) as well as other causes of chest pain, such as pulmonary embolization. However, it may simulate numerous neurologic lesions and even various abdominal conditions related to renal-visceral ischemia.

Treatment

A. Medical Measures: If hypertension is present, aggressive measures to lower the pressure should probably be initiated even before diagnostic studies have been completed, and while the need for surgery is being contemplated. Treatment generally includes the simultaneous reduction of the systolic blood pressure to 100 mm Hg and reduction of the pulsatile aortic flow (dp/dt) by means of the following:

(1) A rapid-acting antihypertensive agent as an intravenous infusion at a flow rate regulated by very frequent blood pressure determinations. Nitroprusside or trimethaphan may be given as follows: (a) Nitroprusside (50 mg in 1000 mL of 5% dextrose in water) is started at a rate of 0.5 mL/min and the infusion rate increased by 0.5 mL every 5 minutes until adequate control of the pressure has been achieved. Thiocyanate levels should be obtained if treatment is continued for 48 hours, and the infusion should be stopped if the drug level reaches 10 mg/dL; (b) Trimethaphan (1 or 2 mg/mL) may be infused with the patient in the semi-Fowler position.

(2) Intravenous propranolol, 0.15 mg/kg given over a 5-minute period and repeated as necessary to maintain the pulse rate at 60/min. The rapid-acting beta-blocker esmolol may be tried first in patients in whom adverse effects are considered more likely to occur, although propranolol is believed by many to be more effective in this disorder. Intravenous reserpine (0.1–0.2 mg) may be used if beta-blockers are contraindicated.

All patients with type A dissection should undergo emergent surgical repair. Most patients with type B dissection can be managed successfully with aggressive drug therapy. Indications for surgical treatment of type B dissections are severe intractable pain, aortic rupture, mesenteric or renal ischemia, and progression of the dissection.

B. Surgical Measures: For type A dissection, the ascending aorta and, if necessary, the aortic valve and arch may be replaced with reattachment of the coronaries and brachiocephalic vessels. The mortality rate for such operations approaches 20% or more, but this is still less than the rate for untreated type A dissection.

Surgical treatment is increasingly popular for dissections arising in the descending thoracic aorta (type B); it may be delayed until the hypertension and dissection have been stabilized by medical means and oral antihypertensives instituted. The origin of the dissection is then removed; the false lumen is closed; and a graft is inserted to deliver all blood flow through the normal lumen, thus relieving the occlusive pressure on the aortic branches.

Since patients with type B dissections tend to be poor surgical risks, permanent medical therapy may be offered. Indeed, the surgical mortality rate is higher for this operation than for operation on the more technically challenging type A patient. Regimens should include beta-blockers and antihypertensive drugs; vasodilators are contraindicated unless used with beta-blockers.

Prognosis

Without treatment, the mortality rate of aortic dissection at 3 months exceeds 90%; of these, 20% die within a day and 60% die in less than 2 weeks. These figures may be somewhat worse for type A dissections. Although the surgical mortality rate is high in both groups, it is appreciably more so in type B patients because of co-morbid illnesses. Medical therapy of type A dissection is associated with a prohibitively high mortality rate (at least 30% in 24 hours, and up to 75% in 1 week). Survival without treatment, usually due to recanalization, does occasionally occur. Intensive pharmacologic methods to lower the pulse wave and blood pressure have led to healing of the dissected aorta in patients with acute dissection and will convert others to a subacute or chronic form, which may then be treated by surgery.

Cigarroa JE et al: Diagnostic imaging in the evaluation of suspected aortic dissection: Old standards and new directions. N Engl J Med 1993;328:35.

Cohn LH: Aortic dissection: New aspects of diagnosis and treatment. Hosp Pract (Off Ed) 1994 March 15;29:47.

Sommer T et al: Aortic dissection: A comparative study of diagnosis with spiral CT, multiplanar transesophageal echocardiography, and MR imaging. Radiology 1996; 199:347.

Spittell PC et al: Clinical features and differential diagnosis of aortic dissection: Experience with 236 cases (1980 through 1990). Mayo Clin Proc 1993;68:642.

ATHEROSCLEROTIC OCCLUSIVE DISEASE

Occlusive disease of the aorta and its branches is a common cause of disability. It is also a predictor of morbidity for patients with cardiac disease and those undergoing general surgery. It is essential for the primary physician to emphasize its prevention, particularly in light of what is known about etiologic factors. Smoking must be interdicted in all individuals, and serum cholesterol should be determined in all adults under the care of physicians. Discontinuance of smoking and dietary or pharmacologic management when the serum cholesterol exceeds 200 mg/dL are prudent measures likely to reduce morbidity from atherosclerosis (see Chapters 1 and 28). Although peripheral occlusive disease is classified anatomically in the following sections, advances in therapy have made the approach to all such lesions similar irrespective of location.

OCCLUSIVE DISEASE OF THE AORTA & ILIAC ARTERIES

Occlusive disease of the aorta and the iliac arteries begins most frequently just proximal to the bifurcation of the common iliac arteries and at or just distal to the bifurcation of the aorta. Atherosclerotic changes occur in the intima and media, often with associated perivascular inflammation and calcified plaques in the media. Progression involves the complete occlusion of one or both common iliac arteries and then the abdominal aorta up to the segment just below the renal vessels. Although atherosclerosis is a generalized disease, occlusion tends to be segmental in distribution, and when the involvement is in the aortoiliac vessels there may be minimal atherosclerosis in the more distal external iliac and femoral arteries. Patients with localized occlusions less than 10 cm in length at or just beyond the aortic bifurcation with relatively normal vessels proximally and distally are good candidates for angioplasty, atherectomy, and perhaps stenting. Conversely, patients with multisegmented arterial disease usually have more symptoms, are more apt to require surgical treatment, and are at greater risk of losing a limb. Abrupt worsening of limb ischemia symptoms may be associated with plaque rupture (crescendo claudication), as with myocardial ischemia.

Clinical Findings

Intermittent claudication is almost always present in the calf muscles and is usually present in the thighs and buttocks. It is most often bilateral and progressive. Some complain only of weakness in the legs when walking or a feeling of "tiredness" in the buttocks. Impotence is a common complaint in men. Rest pain, by which is meant ischemia even with the absence of exertion, is an infrequent but serious symptom. Rest pain is usually experienced as a nocturnal pain located in the region of the heads of the metatarsal bones of the feet. It is relieved by placing the legs in the dependent position, usually by hanging them over the side of the bed.

Femoral pulses are absent or very weak, and distal pulses are often not palpable. A bruit may be heard over the aorta or over the iliac or femoral arteries. Systolic blood pressure, normally higher in the leg, is greater in the brachial artery than at the ankle; the difference is exaggerated by exercise. Atrophic changes of the skin, subcutaneous tissues, and muscles of the distal leg are usually minimal, as are dependent rubor and coolness of the skin, unless distal arterial disease is also present. Aortography, including oblique views of the thigh and leg arteries, demonstrates the level and extent of the occlusion and the condition of the vessels distal to the block, but it is not indicated unless invasive restoration of flow is contemplated. It may be replaced by magnetic resonance angiography, which does not require contrast. Doppler ultrasonography and transcutaneous oximetry offer noninvasive evaluation of pressure and oxygenation; though not necessary for screening, they can be useful in following progression of disease.

Treatment

Surgical or angioplastic treatment is indicated if claudication interferes appreciably with the patient's essential activities or work. Discontinuation of smoking is essential; some surgeons insist on it as a prerequisite for operation.

Because many of these patients have coexisting ischemic heart disease, their medical management should be maximized preoperatively. The roles of exercise testing and coronary angiography are discussed in Chapter 10 (in the section on the Cardiac Patient and Surgery). Some clinicians obtain these studies with an eye toward prophylactic bypass grafting or coronary angioplasty; this has not been conclusively shown to be of benefit in this situation if patients are minimally symptomatic.

A. Conservative Care: A program of daily walking for fixed periods, stopping for claudication, may improve collateralization and function. Although its use is debated, pentoxifylline, 400 mg three times daily, may help some patients with symptomatic claudication of long duration. It appears to reduce the incidence of invasive therapeutic procedures such as surgery, though the overall cost of care is not affected. Many patients with claudication are receiving beta-blockers for angina or hypertension. Though in theory this may worsen symptoms by allowing unopposed alpha agonism, consensus holds that this is not a clinical problem.

The following therapies are best advanced for disabling symptoms, such as extremity pain at rest and skin ulceration.

B. Arterial Graft (Prosthesis): An arterial prosthesis bypassing the occluded segment or segments is effective treatment for complex aortoiliac occlusive disease. In general, the bifurcation graft extends from the infrarenal abdominal aorta, usually by means of an end-to-end anastomosis, to one or both common femoral arteries as end-to-side anastomoses. A patient may also be treated surgically with less risk but also less favorable results by means of a graft from the axillary artery to one or both femoral arteries or, in the case of unilateral iliac disease, from the femoral artery with normal blood flow to the contralateral femoral artery distal to the stenotic iliac vessel.

C. Thromboendarterectomy: This procedure, which avoids the use of a prosthesis, is generally used when the occlusion is limited to the common iliac arteries and when the external iliac and common femoral arteries are free of significant occlusive disease.

D. Endovascular Surgical Techniques: Occlusive lesions formerly treated as described in paragraphs B and C can under certain circumstances be repaired by percutaneous transluminal angioplasty and endoluminal stent. Atherectomy devices and laser probes have met with little success.

Prognosis

The operative mortality rate is 2–6%—a great deal less for the angioplastic procedure. The immediate and long-term benefits are often impressive. In patients with no distal occlusive disease, improvement is both subjective and objective, with relief of all or most of the claudication and, usually, return of all the pulses in the extremities. Late occlusions in this group of patients are infrequent, and if proper judgment is used in patient selection, results are comparable for angioplasty, endarterectomy, and arterial grafting techniques.

Ahn SS, Eton D: Endovascular surgery for peripheral arterial occlusive disease. Am Fam Physician 1993;47:423.

Clagett GP, Krupski WC: Antithrombotic therapy in peripheral arterial occlusive disease. Chest 1995;108:431S.

Ernst E, Fialka V: A review of the clinical effectiveness of exercise therapy for intermittent claudication. Arch Intern Med 1993;153:2357. (A review of controlled trials, emphasizing that exercise can increase the pain-free walking distance.)

Isner JM, Rosenfield K: Redefining the treatment of peripheral arterial disease: Role of percutaneous revascularization. Circulation 1993;88:1534.

Wolf GL et al: Surgery or balloon angioplasty for peripheral vascular disease: A randomized clinical trial. J Vasc Intervent Radiol 1993;4:639.

OCCLUSIVE DISEASE OF THE FEMORAL & POPLITEAL ARTERIES

In the region of the thigh and knee, the vessels most frequently blocked by occlusive disease are the superficial femoral artery and the popliteal artery. Atherosclerotic changes usually appear first at the most distal point of the superficial femoral artery,

where it passes through the adductor magnus tendon into the popliteal space. In time, the whole superficial femoral artery may become occluded; the disease progresses into the popliteal artery less frequently. The common femoral and deep femoral arteries are usually patent and relatively free of disease, although the origin of the profunda femoris is sometimes narrowed. The distal popliteal and its three terminal branches may also be relatively free of occlusive disease.

Clinical Findings

A. Symptoms and Signs: Intermittent claudication of the calf is typical and is reported occasionally in the foot as well. Atrophic changes in the lower leg and foot are distinct, with loss of hair, thinning of the skin and subcutaneous tissues, and diminution in the size of the muscles. Dependent rubor and blanching on elevation of the foot are usually present. When the leg is lowered after elevation, venous filling on the dorsal aspect of the foot may be slowed to 15–20 seconds or more. The foot is usually cool. The common femoral pulsations are usually of fair or good quality, although a bruit may be heard. No popliteal or pedal pulses can be felt. Pressure measurements in the distal leg, using doppler ultrasound, will supply an objective functional assessment of the circulation. Angiography is indicated only when intervention is being considered.

B. Imaging: If revascularization is being considered, an arteriogram will show the location and extent of the blockages as well as the status of the distal vessels. Lateral or oblique views reveal whether the origin of the profunda femoris is narrow. It is important to know the condition of the aortoiliac vessels also, since a relatively normal inflow as well as an adequate distal "run-off" is important in determining the likelihood of success of an arterial procedure. Magnetic resonance angiography holds promise for a less invasive way to acquire the same information.

Treatment

Walking is the most effective way to develop collateral circulation—ie, walking up to the point of claudication, then continuing after the pain subsides. Smoking must be discontinued.

Surgery is indicated (1) if intermittent claudication is progressive or incapacitating, interfering significantly with the patient's essential physical activities such as ability to work; or (2) if there is rest pain or pregangrenous or gangrenous lesions on the foot.

A. Arterial Graft: An autogenous vein graft using a reversed segment of the saphenous vein is the conduit of choice in the lower extremity to bypass the occluded segment. These bypass procedures are now performed routinely—with patency rates of 75–80% at 5 years—to the level of the dorsalis pedis or posterior tibial artery. Synthetic arterial prostheses provide substantially poorer long-term results except when used to bypass to the above-knee popliteal artery.

B. Thromboendarterectomy: Thromboendarterectomy with removal of the central occluding core may be successful if the occluded and stenotic segment is short.

When significant aortoiliac or common femoral occlusive disease exists as well as superficial femoral and popliteal occlusions, it is usually better to relieve the obstructions in the larger, proximal arteries and deliver more blood flow to the profunda femoris than to operate on the smaller distal vessels. If the origin of the profunda femoris is narrowed, a limited procedure at that site—a profundoplasty—may be successful in improving blood flow to the leg and foot and may be used, especially in poor-risk patients with rest pain.

C. Endovascular Surgery: As for aortoiliac disease, more distal lesions may be treated using one or more nonsurgical approaches, which include balloon angioplasty, mechanical atherectomy, and laser or thermal angioplasty. The results of these procedures remain inferior to open surgical revascularization.

Anticoagulants, antiplatelet drugs, and agents to counteract arterial spasm are also frequently employed acutely. Recurrent stenosis can often be retreated by these techniques, or bypass surgery may be elected.

The most favorable lesions again include single, short discrete stenoses. Less favorable lesions are multiple stenoses in series, those longer than 5 cm, complete occlusions less than 5 cm long, lesions in the smaller arteries, and stenotic arterial anastomoses or grafts, particularly if the patient has diabetes or is a smoker.

After any of these procedures, the patient is generally maintained on permanent antiplatelet medication. A dose of 80–325 mg of aspirin is usually employed, though the optimal amount is debated.

Prognosis

The risk of limb loss for patients with claudication is not as great as might be anticipated: only 7–10% of patients will require amputation. But this low amputation rate is due in part to a 5-year survival rate significantly lower than that of the normal population. Up to 50% die secondary to coronary artery disease. For this reason, operation is usually not recommended for mild or moderate claudication, and approximately 80% of these patients will have relatively stable symptoms and will go for years without much progression. Some may improve as collateral circulation develops. The 5-year overall patency rate for the saphenous vein bypass grafts is in the range of 60–80%. The 2-year patency rate after transluminal angioplasty is less, and this procedure is now reserved for high-risk patients.

Hoch JR et al: Use of magnetic resonance angiography for the preoperative evaluation of patients with infrainguinal arterial occlusive disease. J Vasc Surg 1996;23:792.

OCCLUSIVE DISEASE OF THE ARTERIES IN THE LOWER LEG & FOOT

Occlusive processes in the lower leg and foot may involve, in order of incidence, the tibial and peroneal arteries, the pedal vessels, and occasionally the small digital vessels. Symptoms depend upon the vessels that are narrowed or thrombosed, the suddenness and extent of the occlusion, and the status of the proximal and collateral vessels. The clinical picture may be a rather stable or a slowly progressive form of vascular insufficiency that over months or years may ultimately result in atrophy, ischemic pain, and, occasionally, gangrene.

Clinical Findings

Although all of the possible manifestations of vascular disease in the lower leg and foot cannot be described here, there are certain significant clinical aspects that enter into the evaluation of these patients.

A. Symptoms and Signs: Intermittent claudication is the commonest presenting symptom. Aching fatigue during exertion usually appears first in the calf muscles; in more severe cases, a constant or cramping pain may be brought on by walking only a short distance. Less commonly, the feet are the site of most of the pain. The distance the patient can walk before onset of pain is indicative of the degree of circulatory inadequacy: two blocks (360–460 meters) or more is mild, one block is moderate, and one-half block or less is severe. Rest pain may occur at night and is a dull, persistent ache. It is felt in the area of the heads of the metatarsals. As in the case of femoral and popliteal disease, rest pain implies severe involvement, and indeed suggests impending limb loss. A degree of relief can often be obtained by uncovering the foot and letting it hang over the side of the bed.

On examination, although the popliteal pulses may be present, pedal pulses are usually absent; exercise may make the latter disappear in some patients. Dependent rubor is prominent. The skin is cool, atrophic, and hairless. These findings may be indistinguishable from those of occlusive disease higher in the leg. The presence of a popliteal pulse points to more distal occlusion when these symptoms and signs are present.

B. Imaging: Films of the lower leg and foot may show calcification of the vessels. If there is a draining sinus or an ulcer close to a bone or joint, osteomyelitis may be apparent on the film. If fairly strong popliteal pulses can be felt, arteriography is of little value. Doppler ultrasonography provides an accurate blood pressure assessment in the pedal pulses.

Treatment

A. Medical Measures: Low-dose aspirin (80–325 mg daily) has theoretical value and is given to all patients with severe peripheral vascular disease. Pentoxifylline (400 mg three times daily) may have some usefulness in patients with chronic symptomatology.

B. Circulatory Insufficiency in the Foot and Toes: Historically, lumbar sympathectomy was indicated when ischemic or pregangrenous changes were present in the distal foot or when small ulcers were present in a foot with diminished circulation. Current techniques of arterial bypass allow a direct surgical approach.

ARTERIAL DISEASE IN DIABETIC PATIENTS

Atherosclerosis develops more often and earlier in patients with diabetes mellitus, especially if the patient smokes. Either the large or small vessels may be involved, but occlusion of the smaller vessels is more frequent than in the nondiabetic, and diabetics thus more often have the form of the disease that may not be suitable for arterial surgery. Cigarette smoking must be strongly interdicted. Ulcers, when present, are more likely to be moist and infected; healing, if it occurs at all, may be very slow, and healed areas may break down easily.

Diabetic neuropathy with diminished or absent sensation of the toes or feet may occur, predisposing to injury or pressure ulcerations that may be neglected because of the absence of pain. These patients may not necessarily have diminished circulation to the feet.

Poor vision due to diabetic retinopathy makes the care of the feet more difficult and injury more likely. The best approach to diabetic lower limb loss is prevention, and the incidence can be reduced by up to 50% in communities with diabetic foot clinics.

Lehto S et al: Risk factors predicting lower extremity amputations in patients with NIDDM. Diabetes Care 1996;19:607.

Levin ME: Foot lesions in patients with diabetes mellitus. Emerg Med Clin North Am 1996;25:447.

OCCLUSIVE CEREBROVASCULAR DISEASE

Although episodes of transient cerebral ischemia or stroke may be due to a variety of causes, atherosclerotic occlusive or ulcerative disease accounts for many of these problems. Single or multiple segmental lesions are often located in the extracranial arteries and account for ischemic stroke syndromes in over half of cases. The extracranial areas most often involved are (1) the common carotid bifurcation, including the origins of the internal and external carotid arteries (approximately 90%); (2) the origin of the vertebral artery; (3) the intrathoracic segments of the aortic arch branches; and (4) the aortic arch itself.

Clinical Findings

A. Symptoms: Transient ischemic attacks (TIAs) may be the earliest manifestation of carotid arterial stenosis or ulceration. Episodes usually last for only a few minutes but may continue for up to 24 hours. Significant carotid artery stenosis with temporary diminished blood flow to the brain or ulcerations releasing microemboli to the brain or the ipsilateral retinal artery are responsible for many TIAs and precede a complete stroke in many of these patients. Typical manifestations include contralateral weakness or sensory changes, speech alterations, and visual disturbance (usually temporary partial or complete loss of vision in the ipsilateral eye). Vertebrobasilar TIAs are characterized by brain stem and cerebellar symptoms, including dysarthria, diplopia, vertigo, ataxia, and alternating hemiparesis or quadriparesis.

Dizziness and unsteadiness, particularly when associated with a quick change in position, are nonspecific symptoms and more often the result of postural hypotension than of vertebrobasilar problems. Atypical neurologic symptoms or personality changes are not symptoms of cerebral ischemia.

B. Signs: Bruits in the neck, diminished or absent pulses in the neck or arms, and a blood pressure difference in the two arms of more than 10 mm Hg may be indications of occlusive disease in the brachiocephalic arteries. More significant than a brachiocephalic bruit is one sharply localized high in the lateral neck close to the angle of the jaw (overlying the common carotid bifurcation), but a major stenosis of 70% or more and thus sufficient to reduce the blood flow through the vessel is present in a minority of patients with these bruits. The murmur of aortic stenosis may be heard as a bruit over the subclavian and carotid arteries; when there is no such heart murmur, the bruit generally denotes disease in these arteries. Bruits are often present without symptoms, and the absence of a bruit does not exclude the possibility of carotid artery stenosis. Thus, bruits heard over the carotid arteries are neither sensitive nor specific enough to alter the diagnostic approach in this patient group. Microemboli can arise from ulcerations of arteries to the brain without stenosis or bruit, particularly if the ulcer is large. These emboli may be seen in the optic fundi at arteriolar branch points, appearing as shiny refractile objects referred to as Hollenhorst plaques. Regarding palpation, only the common carotid and superficial temporal pulses can be felt with accuracy; the internal carotid pulses cannot usually be appreciated.

Additional Studies

Studies of the cerebral circulation are both noninvasive and invasive. Of the former, duplex ultrasonography is now the investigation of choice. In duplex ultrasound, the clinician is provided with both physiologic and anatomic information; indeed, ulcerating plaques, hemorrhage into an atherosclerotic lesion, and other abnormalities may be observed in images comparable to those obtained by angiography. Results in combined studies show high specificity and sensitivity for this test—in excess of any other current noninvasive technique. In addition, the hemodynamic degree of stenosis may be accurately determined. When duplex ultrasonography is unavailable, Doppler ultrasound provides an excellent alternative, though the information gleaned concerns mainly changes in blood flow caused by stenosis. Doppler ultrasound is not as sensitive as duplex ultrasonography; it has comparable specificity. When combined with the indirect information obtained by periorbital Doppler ultrasound—which detects collaterals in the periorbital circulation—its sensitivity may be increased. Doppler ultrasound does not identify anatomic abnormalities, however, as reliably as duplex ultrasound. Recently, plaques observed in the aortic arch by transesophageal echocardiography have been shown to be an independent risk for ischemic stroke.

Arteriographic visualization of the cerebral vessels confirms the location and degree of stenoses and plaques, the presence of arterial occlusions, and the nature of collateral flow.

Treatment

A. Medical Measures: Acute strokes, most progressive or evolving strokes, and those with major neurologic deficits are treated by medical means as discussed in the section on cerebrovascular accidents in Chapter 24. Patients with transient ischemic attacks may be treated with antiplatelet drugs (aspirin, 100–325 mg/d) or with oral anticoagulants, though there is now some evidence that the former is safer and more effective than the latter, particularly in men.

B. Surgical Measures:

1. Transient ischemic attacks and stroke– Carotid endarterectomy plus optimal medical therapy is highly effective in preventing stroke and death in symptomatic patients with carotid stenosis greater than 70%. Carotid endarterectomy is most effective when symptoms are specific for cerebral ischemia of recent origin involving the anterior circulation, and it is essential that the vascular surgeon be one who performs carotid endarterectomies regularly with a mortality-complication rate of less than 5%. Primary care physicians are obliged to know this information prior to referral, since an increased risk of neurologic complications after carotid endarterectomy may outweigh the anticipated benefit.

2. Asymptomatic carotid stenosis–Asymptomatic carotid bruits are stronger predictors of death from coronary artery disease than from stroke. Nonetheless, in some patients they may signal the presence of a hemodynamically significant carotid stenosis. Many surgeons believe that with increasing accuracy of the noninvasive evaluation of carotid stenosis, it is possible to identify patients who might be helped by prophylactic endarterectomy. About 2% of patients per year with asymptomatic carotid stenosis suffer a stroke; this approximates 3% if the stenosis exceeds 75%. Thus, the risk of causing stroke from angiography and surgery should be less than 3% if surgery is offered. The American Heart Association has recommended upper limits of acceptable combined morbidity and mortality for carotid endarterectomy. These are 3% for asymptomatic patients and 5% for those with TIAs or stroke. These figures are 7% in patients with previous stroke and 10% in individuals with recurrent carotid stenosis. In 1995, a trial was reported comparing carotid endarterectomy with aspirin in patients with asymptomatic carotid stenosis exceeding 60%. Patients enrolled were under 80 years of age and were considered good surgical risks, and the procedures were performed at centers with excellent staff. Despite an early mortality and morbidity disadvantage in the surgical group, projected 5-year data in these patients were considerably more favorable than the results achieved with aspirin alone. Thus, it now appears that this procedure may be offered to selected asymptomatic patients.

Endarterectomy may be indicated as an emergency procedure in patients with very early and fluctuating neurologic deficits with significant carotid stenosis. It is not useful in acute stroke, progressing stroke, or when there is also severe intracranial vascular disease.

Prognosis

The prognosis and results of therapy are related to the number of vessels involved, the degree of stenosis in each, and the collateral flow in the circle of Willis. Expertly performed surgery may have a mortality rate of 1–2% and with 1–4% permanent major or minor neurologic complications; there is wide institutional variation in these figures. Transient ischemic attacks known to be secondary to significant carotid artery stenosis or ulceration can often be eliminated by surgery, and although future strokes can occur in such patients, other arterial lesions, such as a contralateral carotid stenosis or intracranial arterial lesions, are often responsible. Concomitant coronary artery disease results in an overall mortality rate that is similar in operated and unoperated groups. In the best hands, the operative procedure in patients with transient ischemic attacks or stroke may reduce the chance of developing a permanent neurologic deficit within 5 years from 30% to 5%. The incidence of later stroke after uncomplicated endarterectomy is around 5–15%, and although restenosis may occur in the operated artery, it is usually not symptomatic. Significant carotid artery stenosis without symptoms entails no more than a 10–15% stroke risk over 3–5 years.

Amarenco P et al: Atherosclerotic disease of the aortic arch and the risk of ischemic stroke. N Engl J Med 1994;331:1474. (Plaques detected by transesophageal echo are an important risk factor.)

Executive Committee for the Asymptomatic Carotid Atherosclerosis Study: Endarterectomy for asymptomatic carotid artery stenosis. JAMA 1995;273:1421. (Advantages for surgery in selected patients with stenoses greater than 60%.)

Hirsh J et al: Aspirin and other platelet-active drugs: The relationship among dose, effectiveness, and side effects. Chest 1995;108(4 Suppl):247S.

Mayberg MR et al: Carotid endarterectomy and prevention of cerebral ischemia in symptomatic carotid stenosis. JAMA 1991;266:3289. (Indicates benefit when stenosis is between 70% and 99%.)

Moore WS: Carotid endarterectomy for prevention of stroke. West J Med 1993;159:37. (Areas of investigation and current indications.)

VISCERAL ARTERY INSUFFICIENCY

Chronic intestinal ischemia generally results from atherosclerotic occlusive lesions at or close to the origins of the superior mesenteric, celiac, and inferior mesenteric arteries, leading to a significant reduction of blood flow to the intestines. Symptoms consist of epigastric or periumbilical postprandial pains that last for 1–3 hours. To avoid pain, the patient limits oral intake, and weight loss results; pain at this stage of the process may be less prominent. Such a history in a person over 45 years of age who appears chronically ill and who has peripheral arterial disease is probably an indication for arteriography if the patient is felt to be a candidate for surgery. Angiography usually shows two of the three mesenteric arteries to have significant occlusive disease. Surgical management is directed toward restoration of antegrade visceral arterial flow by bypass or transaortic endarterectomy.

Acute intestinal ischemia results from (1) embolic occlusions of the visceral branches of the abdominal aorta, generally in patients with mitral valvular heart disease or especially with atrial fibrillation, or left ventricular mural thrombus; (2) thrombosis of one or more of the visceral vessels involved with atherosclerotic occlusive changes, sometimes in patients with a history of chronic intestinal ischemia as described above; or (3) nonocclusive mesenteric vascular insufficiency, generally in patients with congestive heart failure receiving recently instituted digitalis with diuretics or in

those who are in shock. The acute onset of crampy or steady epigastric and periumbilical abdominal pain combined with minimal or no findings on abdominal examination and a high leukocyte count should suggest one of these three events in the superior mesenteric system. Pain may be more impressive than physical signs. The combination of lactic acidosis, hypotension, and abdominal distention suggests bowel infarction rather than ischemia. Angiography of the superior mesenteric artery is helpful for early diagnosis. Patients suspected of having acute mesenteric ischemia require emergent laparotomy. Mesenteric duplex scanning is a noninvasive technique for the anatomic and physiologic assessment of the visceral vessels and may be helpful in selecting patients with symptoms of chronic or acute mesenteric ischemia for arteriography. If occlusion is present, antibiotics specific for intestinal flora should be instituted (eg, ampicillin and aminoglycoside plus clindamycin or metronidazole), and laparotomy should be performed to reestablish blood flow to the intestine and remove necrotic bowel. The clinical picture of **acute mesenteric vein occlusion** is similar to that of arterial syndromes but may present in a more subacute manner. Surgical management is usually confined to bowel resection and anticoagulation. In selected patients, venous thrombectomy may be considered. Patients at risk include those with systemic hypercoagulability, such as is observed with paroxysmal nocturnal hemoglobinuria or protein C, protein S, or antithrombin III deficiency.

Through early diagnosis and aggressive treatment, the very poor prognosis of the past should yield somewhat lower morbidity and mortality rates.

Patients who present with chronic mesenteric ischemia often appear ill; weight loss is a common feature.

Ischemic colitis develops when the diminished circulation is most prominent in the distribution of the inferior mesenteric artery. Because of the nature of the collaterals, infarction is uncommon in this instance. However, the patient may have episodic bouts of crampy lower abdominal pain associated with mild diarrhea, often bloody. This picture may be indistinguishable from inflammatory bowel disease. Colonoscopy may reveal segmental inflammatory changes, most often in the rectosigmoid and the splenic flexure where the collateral circulation is most active. Because adequate collateral circulation usually develops, the prognosis is better than when the vascular insufficiency involves the superior mesenteric circulation, and maintenance of hydration may be all that is necessary.

Boley JJ, Brandt LJ (editors): Intestinal ischemia. Surg Clin North Am 1992;72:1. (Topics include diagnostic evaluation, acute mesenteric ischemia, colonic ischemia, and chronic visceral ischemia.)

Scholz FJ: Ischemic bowel disease. Radiol Clin North Am 1993;31:1197.

ACUTE ARTERIAL OCCLUSION

Essentials of Diagnosis

- Symptoms and signs depend on the artery occluded, the organ or region supplied by the artery, and the adequacy of the collateral circulation to the area primarily involved.
- Occlusion in an extremity usually results in pain, paresthesias, and coldness.
- There is pallor or mottling; motor, reflex, and sensory alteration; and collapsed superficial veins.
- Pulsations are absent in arteries distal to the occlusion. Occlusions in other areas result in such conditions as cerebrovascular accidents, intestinal ischemia and gangrene, and renal or splenic infarcts.

Differential Diagnosis

The primary differentiation is between arterial embolism and thrombosis. In an older individual with both arteriosclerotic vascular disease and cardiac disease, the differentiation may be very difficult, and in 10–20% a definite diagnosis either cannot be made or turns out to be incorrect. Many patients with thrombosis have a history of claudication or rest pain. Arterial trauma may result in either occlusion or spasm.

1. ARTERIAL EMBOLISM

Arterial embolism is generally a complication of heart disease; a minority of those with embolism have rheumatic heart disease, but most have ischemic heart disease, with or without myocardial infarction. Atrial fibrillation is often present. Other forms of heart disease and miscellaneous causes account for the rest. In 10%, there is more than one embolism, and recurrent emboli after initial successful treatment may occur.

Emboli tend to lodge at the bifurcation of major arteries, with over half going to the aortic bifurcation or the vessels in the lower extremities; the carotid system is involved in 20%, and the upper extremity and the mesenteric arteries in the remainder. Emboli from arterial ulcerations are usually small, giving rise to transient symptoms in the toes or brain but occasionally to a systemic illness resembling vasculitis (see below).

Clinical Findings

In an extremity, the initial symptoms are usually pain (sudden or gradual in onset), numbness, coldness, and tingling. Signs include absence of pulsations in the arteries distal to the block, coldness, pallor or mottling, hypesthesia or anesthesia, and weakness, muscle spasm, or paralysis. The superficial veins are collapsed. Later, blebs and skin necrosis may appear, and gangrene can result.

Treatment

Immediate embolectomy is the treatment of choice in almost all early cases of emboli in extremities. It is best done within 4–6 hours after the embolic episode; it is occasionally successful after longer delays if the supplied tissue remains viable.

A. Emergency Preoperative Care:

1. Heparin–Heparin sodium, 5000 units intravenously, should be given as soon as the diagnosis is made or suspected in an effort to prevent distal thrombosis and continued until the time of surgery, maintaining the partial thromboplastin time (PTT) at twice the normal level. It may also help relieve associated spasm.

2. Protect the part–The extremity is kept at or below the horizontal plane, and neither heat nor cold is applied. The limb must be protected from hard surfaces and overlying bedclothes.

3. Imaging–Arteriography is often of value either before or during surgery if the distinction between embolism and thrombosis cannot be made on clinical grounds; contrast studies, though still the standard of care and preferred in some centers, may be supplanted by magnetic resonance angiography. There may be more than one embolus in an extremity. Echocardiography may confirm the source; the transesophageal approach increases the test's sensitivity.

B. Surgical Measures: Local anesthesia is generally used if the occlusion is in an artery to an extremity. After the embolus is removed through the arteriotomy, the proximal and distal artery should be explored for additional emboli or secondary thrombi by means of a specially designed catheter with a small inflatable balloon at the tip (Fogarty catheter). An embolus at the aortic bifurcation or in the iliac artery can often be removed under local anesthesia through common femoral arteriotomies with the use of these same catheters. Laparotomy is necessary for emboli to the mesenteric circulation. Heparinization for a week or more postoperatively is indicated, and prolonged anticoagulation with warfarin is essentially desirable after that to prevent recurrence.

Delayed embolectomy carried out more than 12 hours following the embolism or when there is ischemia or necrosis—as evidenced by mottled cyanosis, muscle rigidity, anesthesia, or markedly elevated serum CK—involves a high risk of acute respiratory distress syndrome or acute renal failure (or both). Anticoagulation rather than surgery or catheter embolectomy is the proper initial therapy under such circumstances, accepting urgent or elective amputation as the necessary lifesaving procedure in most instances.

Prognosis

Arterial embolism is a threat not only to the limb (5–25% amputation rate) but also to the life of the patient (25–30% hospital mortality rate, with the underlying heart disease responsible for over half of these deaths).

Emboli in the aortoiliac area are more dangerous than more peripheral emboli, and the mortality rate rises if there are multiple peripheral emboli or carotid or visceral emboli, approaching 100% if all three areas are involved. Emboli associated with hypertensive or arteriosclerotic heart disease have a poorer prognosis than those arising from rheumatic valvular disease.

In patients with atrial fibrillation, an attempt may be made to restore normal rhythm pharmacologically or by cardioversion after the patient has been anticoagulated; restoration of normal rhythm tends to be permanent only in patients with recent onset or transitory fibrillation. Long-term anticoagulant therapy diminishes the danger of further emboli and in the majority of patients is the only long-term prophylactic measure that can be instituted.

If no heart disease exists, arteriography may reveal an atherosclerotic ulcer or small aneurysm to be the origin of the embolus; depending upon location, these may be treated surgically. Three-fourths of the patients surviving the embolic episode and the associated hospital stay may then have a good quality of life.

2. ACUTE ARTERIAL THROMBOSIS

Acute arterial thrombosis generally occurs in an artery in which the lumen has become narrow as a result of arteriosclerotic changes in the wall of the artery. Blood flowing through such a narrow, irregular, or ulcerated lumen may clot, leading to a sudden, complete occlusion of the narrow segment. The thrombosis may then propagate either up or down the artery to a point where the blood is flowing rapidly through a somewhat less diseased artery (usually to a significant arterial branch proximally or one or more functioning collateral vessels distally). Occasionally, the thrombosis is precipitated by the rupture of an arteriosclerotic plaque, blocking the lumen; trauma to the artery may precipitate a similar event. Inflammatory involvement of the arterial wall will also lead to thrombosis. Chronic mechanical irritation of the subclavian artery compressed by a cervical rib leads to complete occlusion. Thrombosis in a diseased artery may be secondary to an episode of hypotension or cardiac failure. Polycythemia and dehydration also increase the chance of thrombosis, as do repeated arterial punctures.

Chronic, incomplete arterial obstruction usually results in the establishment of some collateral flow, and further flow will develop relatively rapidly through the collaterals once complete occlusion has developed. The extremity may be threatened for hours or days, however, while the additional collateral circulation develops around the block.

Clinical Findings

The local findings in the extremity are usually very similar to those described in the section on arterial embolism. The following differential points should be considered: (1) Are there manifestations of advanced occlusive arterial disease in other areas, especially the opposite extremity (bruit, absent pulses, secondary changes)? Is there a history of intermittent claudication? These clinical manifestations are suggestive but not diagnostic of thrombosis. (2) Is there a history or are there findings of rheumatic heart disease or of a recent episode of atrial fibrillation or myocardial infarction? If so, an embolism is more likely than a thrombosis. (3) Electrocardiography, echocardiography, and serum enzyme studies may give added information regarding the presence of a silent myocardial infarction and its likelihood as a source of an embolus. Ultimately, arteriography is necessary for accurate differential diagnosis and for planning therapy.

Treatment

Whereas emergency embolectomy is the usual approach in the case of an early occlusion from an embolus, a nonoperative approach is generally used in the case of thrombosis for two reasons: (1) The segment of thrombosed artery may be quite long, requiring extensive surgery (thromboendarterectomy or artery graft). The removal of a single embolus in a normal artery is, by comparison, relatively easy. (2) The extremity is more likely to survive without development of gangrene because some collateral circulation has usually formed during the slowly progressive stenosing phase before acute thrombosis. With an embolism, this is not usually the case; the block is most often at a major arterial bifurcation, occluding both branches, and the associated arterial spasm is usually more acute. Treatment—particularly if tissue necrosis is present—is as described for emergency preoperative care for arterial embolism. Thrombolytic therapy using streptokinase or the more expensive urokinase or tissue plasminogen activator (t-PA) may be tried in acute thrombosis if no tissue necrosis exists; lysis may be achieved in 50–80% of cases, and direct arterial infusion into the thrombus has fewer bleeding complications than systemic therapy with these drugs since the dose given locally is much smaller. Owing to the relatively slow rate of thrombolysis and the inherent risks of the therapy itself, the rates of complications and amputation (20% and 5%, respectively) remain relatively high. If successful thrombolysis occurs, rethrombosis may be prevented by angioplasty. Otherwise, treatment is as outlined under emergency preoperative care for arterial embolism.

Prognosis

Limb survival usually occurs with acute thrombosis of the iliac or superficial femoral arteries; gangrene is more likely if the popliteal is suddenly occluded, especially if the period between occlusion and treatment is long or if there is considerable arterial spasm or proximal arterial occlusive disease. If the limb does survive the acute occlusion, significant functional recovery may occur gradually over a number of weeks. The later treatment and prognosis are outlined above in the section on occlusive disease of the iliac, femoral, and popliteal arteries.

Vogt MT, Wolfson SK, Kuller LH: Segmental arterial disease in the lower extremities: Correlates of disease and relationship to mortality. J Clin Epidemiol 1993;46: 1267.

Weaver FA et al: Surgical revascularization versus thrombolysis for nonembolic lower extremity native artery occlusions: Results of a prospective randomized trial. The STILE Investigators. Surgery versus thrombolysis for ischemia of the lower extremity. J Vasc Surg 1996;24: 513.

THROMBOANGIITIS OBLITERANS (Buerger's Disease)

Essentials of Diagnosis

- Almost always in young men who smoke.
- Extremities involved with inflammatory occlusions of the more distal arteries, resulting in circulatory insufficiency of the toes or fingers.
- Thromboses of superficial veins may also occur.
- Course is intermittent and amputation may be necessary, especially if smoking is not stopped.

General Considerations

Buerger's disease is an episodic and segmental inflammatory and thrombotic process of the arteries and veins, principally in the limbs. The cause is not known. It is seen most commonly in men under 40 who smoke and is especially common in Ashkenazi Jews of Eastern European background. The effects of the disease are almost solely due to occlusion of the arteries. The symptoms are primarily due to ischemia, complicated in the later stages by infection and tissue necrosis. The inflammatory process is intermittent, with quiescent periods lasting weeks, months, or years.

The arteries most commonly affected are the plantar and digital vessels in the foot and those in the lower leg. The arteries in the hands and wrists may also become involved. Different arterial segments may become occluded in successive episodes; a certain amount of recanalization occurs during quiescent periods. Superficial migratory thrombophlebitis is a common early indication of the disease.

Clinical Findings

The signs and symptoms are primarily those of arterial insufficiency, and the differentiation from arteriosclerotic peripheral vascular disease may be difficult; however, the following findings suggest Buerger's disease:

(1) The patient is a man under 40 who smokes.

(2) There is a history or finding of small, red, tender cords resulting from migratory superficial segmental thrombophlebitis, usually in the saphenous tributaries rather than the main vessel. A biopsy of such a vein provides suggestive evidence of Buerger's disease, though no finding is unambiguously pathognomonic.

(3) Intermittent claudication is common. Rest pain can be frequent and persistent. It tends to be more pronounced than in the patient with atherosclerosis. Numbness, diminished sensation, and pricking and burning pains may be present as a result of ischemic neuropathy.

(4) The digit or the entire distal portion of the foot may be pale and cold, or there may be rubor that may remain relatively unchanged by posture; the skin may not blanch on elevation, and on dependency the intensity of the rubor is often more pronounced than that seen in the atherosclerotic group. The distal vascular changes are often asymmetric, so that not all of the toes are affected to the same degree. Absence or impairment of pulsations in the dorsalis pedis, posterior tibial, ulnar, or radial artery is frequent.

(5) Trophic changes may be present, often with painful indolent ulcerations along the nail margins.

(6) There is usually evidence of disease in both legs and possibly also in the hands and lower arms. There may be a history or findings of Raynaud's phenomenon in the finger or distal foot.

(7) The course is usually intermittent, with acute and often dramatic episodes followed by rather definite remissions. When the collateral vessels as well as the main channels have become occluded, an exacerbation is more likely to lead to gangrene and amputation. The course in the patient with atherosclerosis tends to be less dramatic and more persistent.

Differential Diagnosis

Differences between thromboangiitis obliterans and atherosclerosis obliterans are discussed above.

Raynaud's disease causes symmetric bilateral color changes, primarily in young women. There is no impairment of arterial pulsations. Antiphospholipid antibody syndrome may include vasospasm and livedo reticularis, but arterial pulses are preserved, and the early blanching of the digits seen in Raynaud's disease does not occur. Likewise, cholesterol atheroembolic disease may mimic Buerger's disease, but it is most often observed in older patients with established atherosclerosis.

Treatment

The principles of therapy are the same as those outlined for atherosclerotic peripheral vascular disease, but the long-range outlook is better in patients with Buerger's disease, so that when possible the approach should be more conservative and tissue loss kept to a minimum.

A. General Measures: Smoking must be stopped; the physician must insist on it. The disease will progress if this advice is not followed.

B. Surgical Measures:

1. Sympathectomy–Sympathectomy may be useful in eliminating the vasospastic manifestations of the disease and aiding in the establishment of collateral circulation to the skin. It may also relieve the mild or moderate forms of rest pain. If amputation of a digit is necessary, sympathectomy may aid in healing of the surgical wound.

2. Amputation–The indications for amputation are similar in many respects to those outlined for the atherosclerotic group, although the approach should be more conservative from the point of view of preservation of tissue. Most patients with Buerger's disease who are managed carefully and who stop smoking do not require amputation of the fingers or toes. It is almost never necessary to amputate the entire hand, but amputation below the knee is occasionally necessary because of gangrene or severe pain in the foot.

Prognosis

Except in the case of the rapidly progressive form of the disease—and provided the patient stops smoking and takes good care of the feet—the prognosis for survival of the extremities is good.

Cutler DA, Runge MS: 86 years of Buerger's disease—what have we learned? Am J Med Sci 1995;309:74.
Olin JW: Thromboangiitis obliterans. Curr Opin Rheumatol 1994;6:44.

IDIOPATHIC ARTERITIS OF TAKAYASU ("Pulseless Disease")

Pulseless disease, most frequent in young women, is an occlusive polyarteritis of unknown cause with a special predilection for the branches of the aortic arch. It occurs most commonly in Asians. Manifestations, depending upon the vessel or vessels involved, may include evidence of cerebrovascular insufficiency, with transient ischemic attacks and visual disturbances; and absent pulses in the arms, with a rich collateral flow in the shoulder, chest, and neck areas. The most common clinical finding, however,

is a bruit. The extent of the vascular involvement may be defined by angiography.

Pulseless disease must be differentiated from vascular lesions of the aortic arch due to atherosclerosis, though in the latter instance concomitant lower extremity disease is invariably present. Histologically, the arterial lesions are indistinguishable from those of giant cell arteritis. In the early stage of the disease, the progression of the vascular stenosis may be reversed by steroids; in the more advanced forms, bypass arterial grafts are necessary.

Kerr GS et al: Takayasu arteritis. Ann Intern Med 1994;120:919. (A balanced clinical review.)

GIANT CELL ARTERITIS

This disorder is discussed in Chapter 20.

CHOLESTEROL ATHEROEMBOLIC DISEASE

In some patients with severe atherosclerosis involving the aorta and its branches, a distinct syndrome resulting from repeated microembolization from atherosclerotic plaques has been observed. This syndrome occurs spontaneously or following transfemoral aortographic procedures. Virtually any organ or extremity may be affected. Patients may complain of pain in the abdomen and legs and of mottled lower extremities. Physical examination may reveal cholesterol plaques in the optic fundi, livedo reticularis, and reduced arterial pulses (with or without bruits). Laboratory investigations disclose microhematuria, renal insufficiency, eosinophilia, and an accelerated sedimentation rate, with hypocomplementemia during the first days of the clinical course. Biopsies of the kidney and other tissues show cholesterol clefts in the small vessels.

Misdiagnosis of systemic vasculitis may result in inappropriate use of immunomodulating drugs. The only treatment is identification of the responsible lesion by arteriography and its removal by endarterectomy or exclusion of the arterial segment by a bypass procedure. When atheroemboli are confined to the calf or foot, surgical treatment is a good option.

O'Keeffe ST et al: Blue toe syndrome: Causes and management. Arch Intern Med 1992;152:2197.
Rosman HS et al: Cholesterol embolization: Clinical findings and implications. J Am Coll Cardiol 1990;15:1296. (The presentation of cholesterol embolization may be subtle but should be considered in elderly patients with hypertension and atherosclerosis, especially following invasive vascular procedures.)

VASOMOTOR DISORDERS

RAYNAUD'S DISEASE & RAYNAUD'S PHENOMENON

Essentials of Diagnosis

- Paroxysmal bilateral symmetric pallor and cyanosis followed by rubor of the skin of the digits.
- Precipitated by cold or emotional upset; relieved by warmth.
- Primarily a disorder of young women.

General Considerations

Raynaud's disease is the primary, or idiopathic, form of paroxysmal digital cyanosis. Raynaud's phenomenon, which is more common than Raynaud's disease, may be due to a number of regional or systemic disorders. In Raynaud's disease the digital arteries respond excessively to vasospastic stimuli. The cause is not known, but some abnormality of the sympathetic nervous system seems to be active in this entity.

Clinical Findings

Raynaud's disease and Raynaud's phenomenon are characterized by intermittent attacks of pallor or cyanosis—or pallor followed by cyanosis—in the fingers (and rarely the toes), precipitated by cold or occasionally by emotional upsets. In early attacks of Raynaud's phenomenon, only 1–2 fingertips may be affected; as it progresses, all the fingers down to the distal palm may be involved. The thumbs are rarely affected. During recovery there may be intense rubor, throbbing, paresthesia, and slight swelling. Attacks usually terminate spontaneously or upon returning to a warm room or putting the extremity in warm water. Between attacks there are no abnormal findings. Sensory changes that often accompany vasomotor manifestations include numbness, stiffness, diminished sensation, and aching pain. The condition may progress to atrophy of the terminal fat pads and the digital skin, and gangrenous ulcers may appear near the fingertips; they may heal during warm weather.

Raynaud's disease appears first between ages 15 and 45, almost always in women. It tends to be progressive, and, unlike Raynaud's phenomenon (which may be unilateral and may involve only one or two fingers), symmetric involvement of the fingers of both hands is the rule. Spasm becomes more frequent and prolonged.

Raynaud's disease may be diagnosed if the phenomenon persists for greater than 3 years without evidence of an associated disease (see below). There are no specific laboratory abnormalities; the diagnosis is a clinical one, though studies to exclude the conditions associated with Raynaud's disease are warranted.

Differential Diagnosis

Raynaud's disease must be differentiated from the numerous disorders that may be associated with Raynaud's phenomenon. The history and examination lead to the diagnosis of rheumatoid arthritis, systemic sclerosis (including its more localized CREST variant), systemic lupus erythematosus, and mixed connective tissue disease, with which Raynaud's phenomenon is commonly associated. Raynaud's phenomenon is occasionally the first manifestation of these disorders.

The differentiation from thromboangiitis obliterans is usually not difficult, since thromboangiitis obliterans is generally a disease of men; peripheral pulses are often diminished or absent; and, when Raynaud's phenomenon occurs in association with thromboangiitis obliterans, it is usually in only one or two digits.

Raynaud's phenomenon may occur in patients with the thoracic outlet syndromes. In these disorders, involvement is generally unilateral, and symptoms referable to brachial plexus compression tend to dominate the clinical picture. Carpal tunnel syndrome should also be considered, and nerve conduction tests are appropriate in selected cases.

In acrocyanosis, cyanosis of the hands is permanent and diffuse. Frostbite may lead to chronic Raynaud's phenomenon. Ergot poisoning, particularly due to prolonged or excessive use of ergotamine, must also be considered.

A particularly severe form of Raynaud's phenomenon occurs in up to one-third of patients receiving bleomycin and vincristine in combination, often for testicular cancer. Treatment is unsuccessful, and the problem persists even with discontinuance of the drugs.

Finally, Raynaud's phenomenon may be mimicked by cryoglobulinemia, in which serum proteins aggregate in the cooler distal circulation. Cryoglobulinemia may be idiopathic or associated with multiple myeloma and other hyperglobulinemic states.

Treatment

A. General Measures: The body should be kept warm, and the hands especially should be protected from exposure to cold; gloves should be worn when out in the cold. The hands should be protected from injury at all times; wounds heal slowly, and infections are consequently hard to control. Softening and lubricating lotion to control the fissured dry skin should be applied to the hands frequently. Smoking should be stopped.

B. Vasodilators: Vasodilator drugs are of limited value but may be of some benefit in those patients who are not adequately controlled by general measures and when there is peripheral vasoconstriction without significant organic vascular disease. Shortening of temperature recovery time may occur with the use of transdermal nitroglycerin or a longer-acting oral nitrate. Low doses of nifedipine (sustained-release, 30 mg/d) have been employed with good effect in the treatment of Raynaud's phenomenon and disease.

C. Surgical Measures: Sympathectomy may be indicated when attacks have become frequent and severe, interfering with work and well-being—and particularly if trophic changes have developed and medical measures have failed. In the lower extremities, complete and permanent relief may result, whereas dorsal sympathectomies generally result in only temporary improvement in most patients treated with operation. Although vascular tone of the vessels in the hands usually ultimately reappears, the symptoms in the fingers that may thus recur in 1–5 years are usually milder and less frequent. Sympathectomies are of very limited value in far-advanced cases, particularly if significant digital artery obstructive disease with scleroderma is present.

Prognosis

Raynaud's disease is usually benign, causing mild discomfort on exposure to cold and progressing very slightly over the years. In a few cases rapid progression does occur, so that the slightest change in temperature may precipitate color changes. It is in this situation that sclerodactyly and small areas of gangrene may be noted, and such patients may become quite disabled by severe pain, limitation of motion, and secondary fixation of distal joints. The prognosis of Raynaud's phenomenon is that of the associated disease.

Wigley FM, Flavahan NA: Raynaud's phenomenon. Rheum Dis Clin North Am 1996;22:765.

LIVEDO RETICULARIS

Livedo reticularis is an uncommon vasospastic disorder of unknown cause that results in mottled discoloration on large areas of the extremities, generally in a fishnet pattern with reticulated cyanotic areas surrounding a paler central core. It occurs primarily in young women. It may be associated with an occult malignant neoplasm, polyarteritis nodosa, atherosclerotic microemboli to the skin, or antiphospholipid antibody syndrome (Sneddon's syndrome).

Livedo reticularis is most apparent on the thighs and forearms and occasionally on the lower abdomen and is most pronounced in cold weather. The color may change to a reddish hue in warm weather but does not entirely disappear. A few patients complain of paresthesias, coldness, or numbness in the involved areas. Recurrent ulcers in the lower extremities may occur in severe cases.

Bluish mottling of the extremities is diagnostic. The peripheral pulses are normal. The extremity may be cold, with increased perspiration.

Treatment consists of protection from exposure to cold; use of vasodilators is seldom indicated. In most instances, livedo reticularis is entirely benign. In the rare patient who develops ulcerations or gangrene, underlying systemic disease should be considered.

See reference below.

ACROCYANOSIS

Acrocyanosis is an uncommon symmetric condition involving the skin of the hands and feet and, to a lesser degree, the forearms and legs. It is associated with arteriolar vasoconstriction combined with dilation of the subpapillary venous plexus of the skin, through which deoxygenated blood slowly circulates. It is worse in cold weather but does not completely disappear during the warm season. It occurs in either gender, is most common in the teens and 20s, and usually improves with advancing age or during pregnancy. It is characterized by coldness, sweating, slight edema, and cyanotic discoloration of the involved areas. Pain, trophic lesions, and disability do not occur, and the peripheral pulses are present. The individual may thus be reassured and encouraged to dress warmly in cold weather.

Naldi L et al: Cutaneous manifestations associated with antiphospholipid antibodies in patients with suspected primary antiphospholipid syndrome. Ann Rheum Dis 1993;52:219. (Livedo reticularis and acrocyanosis were significantly associated with antiphospholipid antibodies.)

ERYTHROMELALGIA

Erythromelalgia is a paroxysmal bilateral vasodilatory disorder of unknown cause. Idiopathic (primary) erythromelalgia occurs in otherwise healthy persons, rarely in children, and affects men and women equally. A secondary type is occasionally seen in patients with polycythemia vera, hypertension, gout, and organic neurologic diseases.

The chief symptom is bilateral burning distress that lasts minutes to hours, involving circumscribed areas on the soles or palms first and, as the disease progresses, the entire extremity. The attack occurs in response to stimuli producing vasodilation (eg, exercise, warm environment), especially at night when the extremities are warmed under bedclothes. Reddening or cyanosis as well as heat may be noted. Relief may be obtained by cooling the affected part and by elevation.

No findings are generally present between attacks.

With onset of an attack, heat and redness are noted in association with the typical pain. Skin temperature and arterial pulsations are increased, and the involved areas may sweat profusely.

In primary erythromelalgia, aspirin, 650 mg every 4–6 hours, may give excellent relief. The patient should avoid warm environments. In severe cases, if medical measures fail, section of peripheral nerves may be necessary to relieve pain.

Primary idiopathic erythromelalgia is uniformly benign.

Drenth JP et al: Cutaneous pathology in primary erythermalgia. Am J Dermatopathol 1996;18:30.

REFLEX SYMPATHETIC DYSTROPHY

Essentials of Diagnosis

- Burning or aching pain of a severity greater than expected following trauma to an extremity.
- Manifestations of vasomotor instability are generally present and include temperature, color, and texture alterations of the skin of the involved extremity.

General Considerations

Pain—usually burning or aching—in an injured extremity is the single most common finding, and the disparity between the severity of the inciting injury and the degree of pain experienced is the most characteristic feature. Crushing injuries with lacerations and soft tissue destruction are the most common causes, but closed fractures, simple lacerations, burns (especially electric), and elective operative procedures are also responsible for this syndrome. It may also involve the left upper extremity after intrathoracic diseases such as myocardial infarction. The manifestations of pain and the associated objective changes may be relatively mild or quite severe, and the initial manifestations often change if the condition proceeds to a chronic stage.

Clinical Findings

In the early stages, the pain, tenderness, and hyperesthesia may be strictly localized to the injured area, and the extremity may be warm, dry, swollen, and red or slightly cyanotic. The involved extremity is held in a splinted position by the muscles, and the nails may become ridged. In advanced stages, the pain is more diffuse and worse at night; the extremity becomes cool and clammy and intolerant of temperature changes (particularly cold); and the skin becomes glossy and atrophic. The joints become stiff, generally in a position that makes the extremity useless. Radiographs of the involved extremity reveal severe osteopenia in excess of that anticipated due to disuse. The dominant concern of the patient may be

to avoid the slightest stimuli to the extremity and especially to the trigger points that may develop.

Prevention

During operations on an extremity, peripheral nerves should be handled only when absolutely necessary and then with utmost gentleness. Splinting of an injured extremity for an adequate period during the early, painful phase of recovery, together with adequate analgesics, may help prevent this condition.

Treatment & Prognosis

A. Conservative Measures: It is most important that the condition be recognized and treated in the early stages, when the manifestations are most easily reversed and major secondary changes have not yet developed. In mild, early cases with minimal skin and joint changes, physical therapy involving active and passive exercises combined with diazepam, 2 mg twice daily, or alprazolam, 0.125–0.25 mg every 12 hours, may relieve symptoms. Protecting the extremity from irritating stimuli is important, and the use of nonaddicting analgesics may be necessary.

B. Surgical Measures: If the condition fails to respond to conservative treatment or if there are more severe or advanced objective findings, sympathetic blocks (stellate ganglion or lumbar) may be helpful. Intensive physical therapy may be used during the pain-free periods following effective blocks. Patients who achieve significant temporary relief of symptoms after sympathetic blocks but fail to obtain permanent relief by the blocks may be cured by sympathectomy. In the advanced forms—particularly in association with major local changes and emotional reactions—the prognosis for a useful life is poor. The newer neurosurgical approaches using implantable electronic biostimulator devices to block pain impulses in the cervical spinal cord have met with some success.

Veldman PH et al: Signs and symptoms of reflex sympathetic dystrophy: Prospective study of 829 patients. Lancet 1993;342:1012. (In the early phase, pain, hypesthesia, and hyperpathy were the most common findings. In advanced disease, pain, tissue atrophy, tremor, and incoordination were most common.)

VENOUS DISEASES

VARICOSE VEINS

Essentials of Diagnosis

- Dilated, tortuous superficial veins in the lower extremities.

- May be asymptomatic or may be associated with fatigue, aching discomfort, or pain.
- Edema, pigmentation, and ulceration of the skin of the distal leg may develop.
- Increased frequency after pregnancy.

General Considerations

Varicose veins develop predominantly in the lower extremities. They consist of abnormally dilated, elongated, and tortuous alterations in the saphenous veins and their tributaries. These vessels lie immediately beneath the skin and superficial to the deep fascia; they therefore do not have as adequate support as the veins deep in the leg, which are surrounded by muscles. An inherited defect seems to play a major role in the development of varicosities in many instances, but it is not known whether the basic valvular incompetence that exists is secondary to defective valves in the saphenofemoral veins or to a fundamental weakness of the walls of the vein, resulting in dilation of the vessel. Periods of high venous pressure related to prolonged standing or heavy lifting are contributing factors, and the highest incidence is in women who have been pregnant. Fifteen percent of adults develop varicosities.

Secondary varicosities can develop as a result of obstructive changes and valve damage in the deep venous system following thrombophlebitis, or occasionally as a result of proximal venous occlusion due to neoplasm. Congenital or acquired arteriovenous fistulas are also associated with varicosities.

The long saphenous vein and its tributaries are most commonly involved, but the short saphenous vein may also be affected. There may be one or many incompetent perforating veins in the thigh and lower leg, so that blood can reflux into the varicosities not only from above, by way of the saphenofemoral junction, but also from the deep system of veins through the incompetent perforators in the mid thigh or lower leg. Largely because of these valvular defects in the most proximal valve of the long saphenous vein or in the distal communicating veins, high venous pressures from within the deep system (> 300 mm Hg) that occur during calf compression of walking are transmitted to these superficial veins. Over the years, the veins progressively enlarge, and the surrounding tissue and skin may develop secondary changes such as fibrosis, chronic edema, and skin pigmentation and atrophy.

Clinical Findings

A. Symptoms: The severity of the symptoms caused by varicose veins is not necessarily correlated with the number and size of the varicosities; extensive varicose veins may produce no subjective symptoms, whereas minimal varicosities may produce many symptoms. Dull, aching heaviness or a feeling of fatigue brought on by periods of standing is the most common complaint. One must be careful to dis-

tinguish between the symptoms of arteriosclerotic peripheral vascular disease, such as intermittent claudication and coldness of the feet, and symptoms of venous disease, since occlusive arterial disease usually contraindicates the operative treatment of varicosities distal to the knee. Indeed, reduced blood flow due to atherosclerosis may improve varicosities by reducing blood flow through the veins. Itching from an associated eczematoid dermatitis may occur above the ankle.

B. Signs: Dilated, tortuous, elongated veins beneath the skin in the thigh and leg are generally readily visible in the standing individual, although in very obese patients palpation may be necessary to detect their presence and location. Secondary tissue changes may be absent even in extensive varicosities; but if the varicosities are of long duration, brownish pigmentation and thinning of the skin above the ankle are often present. Swelling may occur, but signs of severe chronic venous stasis such as extensive swelling, fibrosis, pigmentation, and ulceration of the distal lower leg usually denote the postphlebitic state. Doppler ultrasonography or the duplex scanner is useful diagnostically in detecting the precise location of incompetent valves. These incompetent valves allow reflux of blood from the femoral, popliteal, or more peripheral deep veins into the superficial veins; such knowledge allows more precise corrective surgery with better results.

Differential Diagnosis

Primary varicose veins should be differentiated from those secondary to (1) chronic venous insufficiency of the deep system of veins (the postphlebitic syndrome); (2) retroperitoneal vein obstruction from extrinsic pressure or fibrosis; (3) arteriovenous fistula (congenital or acquired)—a bruit is present and a thrill is often palpable; and (4) congenital venous malformation. Pain or discomfort secondary to arthritis, radiculopathy, or arterial insufficiency should be distinguished from symptoms associated with coexistent varicose veins.

Complications

If thin, atrophic, pigmented skin has developed at or above the ankle, secondary ulcerations may occur—often as a result of little or no trauma. An ulcer will occasionally extend into the varix, and the resulting fistula will be associated with profuse hemorrhage unless the leg is elevated and local pressure is applied to the bleeding point.

Chronic stasis dermatitis with fungal and bacterial infection may be a problem.

Thrombophlebitis may develop in the varicosities, particularly in postoperative patients, pregnant or postpartum women, or those taking oral contraceptives. Local trauma or prolonged periods of sitting may also lead to superficial venous thrombosis. Extension of the thrombosis into the deep venous system by way of the perforating veins or through the saphenofemoral junction may occur, resulting in deep thrombophlebitis and the risk of pulmonary embolism.

Treatment

A. Nonsurgical Measures: The use of elastic stockings (medium or heavy weight) to give external support to the veins of the proximal foot and leg up to but not including the knee is the best nonoperative approach to the management of varicose veins. These may be useful in early varicosities as well, in preventing progression of disease. When elastic stockings are worn during the hours that involve much standing and when this is combined with the habit of elevation of the legs when possible, reasonably good control can be maintained and progression of the condition and the development of complications can often be avoided. This approach may be used in elderly patients, in those who refuse or wish to defer surgery, sometimes in women with mild or moderate varicosities who plan to have more children, and in those with mild asymptomatic varicosities.

B. Surgical Measures: The surgical treatment of varicose veins consists of interruption or removal of the varicosities and the incompetent perforating veins. Accurate delineation and division of the latter are required to prevent formation of recurrent varicosities in previously uninvolved veins. Venous segments that are not demonstrated to be incompetent and varicosed should not be ligated or removed; they may be needed as artery grafts later in the patient's life.

Varicose ulcers that are small generally heal with local care, frequent periods of elevation of the extremity, and compression bandages or some form of compression boot dressing for the ambulatory patient. It is best to defer a stripping procedure until healing has been achieved and stasis dermatitis has been controlled. Some ulcers require skin grafting.

C. Compression Sclerotherapy: Sclerotherapy to obliterate and produce permanent fibrosis of the involved veins is generally reserved for the treatment of residual small varicosities following definitive varicose vein surgery. The injection of the sclerosing solution into the varicosed vein is followed by a period of compression of the segment, resulting in obliteration of the vein. Complications such as phlebitis, tissue necrosis, or infection may occur, and vary in incidence with the skill of the operator.

Prognosis

Patients should be informed that even extensive and carefully performed surgery may not prevent the development of additional varicosities and that further (though usually more limited) surgery or sclerotherapy may become necessary. Good results with relief of symptoms are usually obtained in most patients. If extensive varicosities reappear after surgery, the completeness of the high ligation should be questioned, and reexploration of the saphenofemoral area may be necessary. Even after adequate treatment, secondary tissue changes may not regress.

Bergan JJ: Saphenous vein stripping and quality of outcome. Br J Surg 1996;83:1027.

Goldman MP, Weiss RA, Bergan JJ: Diagnosis and treatment of varicose veins: A review. J Am Acad Dermatol 1994;31(3 Part 1):393.

THROMBOPHLEBITIS

Thrombophlebitis is partial or complete occlusion of a vein by a thrombus with inflammatory changes in the wall of the vein. Trauma to the endothelium of the vein wall resulting in exposure of subendothelial tissues to platelets in the venous blood may initiate thrombosis, especially if a degree of venous stasis also exists. Platelet aggregates form on the vein wall followed by the deposition of fibrin, leukocytes, and finally erythrocytes; a thrombus results that can then propagate along the veins as a free-floating clot. Within 7–10 days, this thrombus becomes adherent to the vein wall, and secondary inflammatory changes develop, although a free-floating tail may persist. The thrombus is ultimately invaded by fibroblasts, resulting in scarring of the vein wall and destruction of the valves. Central recanalization may occur later, with restoration of flow through the vein; however, because the valves do not recover function, directional flow is not reestablished, leading in turn to secondary functional and anatomic problems.

1. THROMBOPHLEBITIS OF THE DEEP VEINS

Essentials of Diagnosis

- Pain in the calf or thigh, occasionally associated with swelling; alternatively, there may be no symptoms.
- History of congestive heart failure, recent surgery, neoplasia, oral contraceptive use, or varicose veins; prolonged inactivity also predisposes.
- Physical signs unreliable.
- Duplex ultrasound or venography is diagnostic.

General Considerations

Acute deep venous thrombosis is a common vascular disorder that is diagnosed in up to 800,000 new patients per year. The deep veins of the lower extremities and pelvis are most frequently involved. The process begins approximately 80% of the time in the deep veins of the calf, although it can arise in the femoral or iliac veins. When the process begins in the calf, propagation into the popliteal and femoral veins takes place in approximately 25% of these cases. About 3% of patients undergoing major general surgical procedures will develop clinical manifestations of thrombophlebitis, which may develop up to 2 weeks postoperatively; many others (up to 30%) with the process will have no detectable findings. Certain operations, such as total hip replacement, are associated with appreciably higher incidences of thromboembolic complications. Illnesses that involve periods of bed rest, such as cardiac failure or stroke, are associated with a high incidence of thrombophlebitis. Use of oral contraceptive drugs, especially by women over 30 and by those who smoke, may be associated with hypercoagulability, resulting in thrombophlebitis in some women. These drugs should not be prescribed for women with a history of phlebitis. Hypercoagulability is also observed in cancer, particularly adenocarcinoma and especially in tumors of the pancreas, prostate, breast, and ovary. Finally, rare conditions such as protein C and S deficiencies and antithrombin III deficiency should be considered in young patients with positive family histories and recurrent venous thrombosis. Homocystinuria and paroxysmal nocturnal hemoglobinuria are also associated with venous hypercoagulability.

Clinical Findings

Approximately half of patients with thrombophlebitis have no symptoms or signs in the extremity in the early stages. The patient may suffer a pulmonary embolism, presumably from the leg veins, without symptoms or demonstrable abnormalities in the extremities.

A. Symptoms: The patient may complain of a dull ache, a tight feeling, or frank pain in the calf or, in more extensive cases, the whole leg, especially when walking.

B. Signs: Typical findings, though variable and unreliable and in about half of cases absent, are as follows: slight swelling in the involved calf, distention of the superficial venous collaterals; and slight fever and tachycardia. Any of these signs may occur without deep vein thrombosis. When the femoral and iliac veins are also involved, there may be tenderness over these veins, and the swelling in the extremity may be marked. The skin may be cyanotic if venous obstruction is severe, or pale and cool if a reflex arterial spasm is superimposed.

C. Diagnostic Techniques: Because of the difficulty in making a precise diagnosis by history and examination and because of the morbidity associated with treatment, diagnostic studies are essential. Duplex ultrasonography, because of its high sensitivity, specificity, and repeatability, is rapidly supplanting venography as the most widely used diagnostic test in the initial evaluation of patients suspected of having this disorder. (See Disorders of the Pulmonary Circulation in Chapter 9.)

1. The Doppler ultrasound blood flow detector and impedance plethysmography make it possible to examine noninvasively the major veins in an extremity for thrombosis. Doppler ultrasound may be particularly helpful in detecting an extension of small thrombi in the calf veins into the popliteal and femoral veins on follow-up examinations. It is inexpensive but operator-dependent. Each venous segment is assessed for incompressibility of the vein during light probe pressure and the presence of abnormal doppler flow signals, including absence of spontaneous flow, loss of flow variation with respiration, and failure to increase flow velocity with distal augmentation. An acute clot is usually anechoic (cannot be visualized directly), but its presence is inferred from a lack of compressibility. Incompetence of venous valves in the legs may also be inferred from this investigation. Impedance plethysmography may be used to detect the alteration of venous flow by obstruction of thrombi; in symptomatic patients, Doppler ultrasound is of superior sensitivity and may be used rather than phlebography to confirm positive or equivocal findings of plethysmography. These examinations may miss small thrombi in the calf veins when collateral channels are present; likewise, occasional false-positives are encountered.

2. Ascending contrast venography, the most accurate method of diagnosis, will define the location, extent, and degree of attachment of the thrombosis (thrombi in the profunda femoris and internal iliac veins will not be demonstrated). Because of the risk, expense, and discomfort involved, this test is not used as a screening study and is unsuitable for repeated monitoring. It is particularly useful when the clinical picture strongly suggests calf vein thromboses but noninvasive tests are equivocal. It may on occasion produce or exacerbate a thrombotic process, but this occurs in less than 5% of patients. It is the most accurate study for detection of calf vein or intra-abdominal venous thrombosis.

Differential Diagnosis

Calf muscle strain or contusion may be difficult to differentiate from thrombophlebitis; phlebography may be required to determine the correct diagnosis.

Cellulitis may be confused with thrombophlebitis; with infection, there is usually an associated wound, and inflammation of the skin is more marked.

Obstruction of the lymphatics or the iliac vein in the retroperitoneal area from tumor or irradiation may lead to unilateral swelling, but it is usually more chronic and painless. An acute arterial occlusion is more painful, the distal pulses are absent, there is usually no swelling, and the superficial veins in the foot fill slowly when emptied.

Bilateral leg edema is more likely to be due to heart, kidney, or liver disease.

Occasionally, a ruptured Baker cyst may produce unilateral pain and swelling in the calf. A history of arthritis in the knee of the same leg is a clue to diagnosis, and the patient may report disappearance of the popliteal cyst at the time symptoms develop.

Complications

A. Pulmonary Thromboembolism: See Chapter 9.

B. Chronic Venous Insufficiency: Chronic venous insufficiency with or without secondary varicosities is a late complication of deep thrombophlebitis. (See Chronic Venous Insufficiency.)

Prevention

Prophylactic measures may diminish the incidence of venous thrombosis in hospitalized patients.

A. Nonpharmacologic Means: Venous stasis may be avoided by the following measures:

1. Elevation of the foot of the bed 15–20 degrees will encourage venous flow from the legs, particularly if the head of the bed is kept low or horizontal. Slight flexion of the knees is desirable. This position is also maintained on the operating table and in the recovery room. Sitting in a chair for long periods in the early postoperative period should be avoided.

2. Leg exercises, carried out by the surgical team immediately following major surgery and during the early postoperative period and practiced by the patient when in bed, are important. Intermittent pneumatic compression of the legs may be used prophylactically and may be the preventive measure of choice in patients in whom all anticoagulants are contraindicated, such as in patients undergoing neurosurgery. In addition, it is the most effective of all nonpharmacologic methods of prophylaxis.

3. Elastic antiphlebitic stockings may be employed, particularly in patients with varicose veins or a history of phlebitis who will require bed rest for a number of days. Walking for brief but regular periods postoperatively and during long airplane and automobile trips should be encouraged.

B. Anticoagulation: Anticoagulants may be used in patients considered at high risk for venous thrombosis.

1. Low-dose heparin, 5000 units every 8–12 hours subcutaneously 2 hours preoperatively and during the postoperative period of bed rest and limited ambulation, appears to be effective in reducing the incidence of thromboembolic complications in moderate-risk patients, although its effectiveness in major pelvic and hip procedures has been disappointing for these high-risk patients. Adjusted-dose heparin to a PTT in the upper half of the normal range—or warfarin to an INR of 1.5–2.0—is recommended. LMW heparin is being used increasingly in this setting and appears to be as effective as the standard formulation of heparin or warfarin. It is not necessary to follow clotting parameters in patients receiving low-molecular-weight heparin, and this may offset the greater cost of the drug in overall cost-benefit analysis. Likewise, there does not appear to be any increase in bleeding complications using this agent when compared with standard heparin and warfarin

therapy. External pneumatic compression is significantly less effective than anticoagulation in this setting.

2. Aspirin, 80–325 mg daily, may have a prophylactic value when used both pre- and postoperatively in surgical patients.

Treatment

A. Local Measures: As for prophylaxis, the legs should be elevated 15–20 degrees, the trunk should be kept horizontal, and the head and shoulders may be supported with pillows. The legs should be slightly flexed at the knees. The duration of bed rest now recommended is considerably less than the 7–14 days suggested in previous years and is tailored to individual patients depending on the overall clinical picture.

B. Medical Measures (Anticoagulants): Therapy with anticoagulants is considered to be the preferred treatment in most cases of deep thrombophlebitis with or without pulmonary embolism. There is evidence that the incidence of fatal pulmonary embolism secondary to venous thrombosis is reduced by adequate anticoagulant therapy, and the incidence of death from additional emboli following an initial embolism is reduced. Progressive thrombosis with its associated morbidity is also reduced considerably, and the chronic secondary changes in the involved leg are probably also less severe. Heparin acts rapidly and must be considered the anticoagulant of choice for short-term therapy; it inhibits thrombin formation and the release of granules from platelets. There may be a marginal preference for low-molecular-weight heparin over the standard drug. LMW heparin is given subcutaneously and does not require PTT monitoring. Studies continue to show equal efficacy with standard heparin, and overall cost may be no different. LMW heparin may be administered safely and effectively for proximal leg vein thromboses on an outpatient basis. After the initial phase of therapy with heparin—and if a prolonged period of anticoagulation is advisable—warfarin can be used. Because warfarin also inhibits synthesis of protein C and protein S and because protein C has a short half-life, a hypercoagulable state can occur during the first few days of warfarin administration. Warfarin should be given after the patient is fully anticoagulated with heparin, and heparin is discontinued only after the prothrombin time has been prolonged by warfarin.

Treatment with heparin does not dissolve thrombi per se but stops propagation and allows natural fibrinolysis to occur. The usual duration of therapy for uncomplicated deep vein thrombosis is 3 months. Most clinicians administer heparin for 7–10 days and oral anticoagulants for at least 11 weeks. Permanent anticoagulation may be considered if the stimulus to thrombosis is chronic—eg, congestive heart failure, postphlebitic syndrome—or if previous episodes have occurred. As experience with thrombolysis develops, it may replace heparin as the treatment of first choice; there is evidence that it reduces the incidence of postphlebitic syndrome.

Details on the use of heparin, oral anticoagulants, and thrombolytics may be found in Chapter 9.

Prognosis

With adequate treatment the patient usually returns to normal health and activity within 3–6 weeks. The prognosis in most cases is good once the period of danger of pulmonary embolism has passed. Occasionally, recurrent episodes of phlebitis will occur in spite of good local and anticoagulant management. Such cases may even have recurrent pulmonary emboli as well. Chronic venous insufficiency may result, with its associated complications; this is less likely when thrombolytics are used to treat acute phlebitis.

Koopman MMW et al: Treatment of venous thrombosis with intravenous unfractionated heparin administered in the hospital as compared with subcutaneous low-molecular-weight heparin administered at home. N Engl J Med 1996;334:682. (LMW heparin is efficacious and safe in the outpatient setting.)

Nachman RL, Silverstein R: Hypercoagulable states. Ann Intern Med 1993;119:819. (Overview of both pathophysiology and clinical material.)

Richlie DL: Noninvasive imaging of the lower extremity for deep venous thrombosis. J Gen Intern Med 1993; 8:271. (Practical information.)

Verstraete M: The diagnosis and treatment of deep-vein thrombosis. (Editorial.) N Engl J Med 1993;329:1418.

2. THROMBOPHLEBITIS OF THE SUPERFICIAL VEINS

Essentials of Diagnosis

- Induration, redness, and tenderness along a superficial vein.
- Often a history of recent intravenous line or trauma. No significant swelling of the extremity.

General Considerations

Superficial thrombophlebitis may occur spontaneously, as in pregnant or postpartum women or in individuals with varicose veins or thromboangiitis obliterans; or it may be associated with trauma, as in the case of a blow to the leg or following intravenous therapy with irritating solutions. It may also be a manifestation of abdominal cancer such as carcinoma of the pancreas and may be the earliest sign. The long saphenous vein is most often involved. Superficial thrombophlebitis may be associated with occult deep vein thrombosis in about 20% of cases. Pulmonary emboli are rare.

Short-term plastic venous catheterization of superficial arm veins is now in routine use. The catheter should be observed daily for signs of local inflammation. It should be removed if a local reaction develops in the veins. Serious thrombotic or septic complications can occur if this policy is not followed. The steel intravenous needle with the anchoring flange (butterfly needle) is less likely to be associated with phlebitis and infection than the plastic catheter, but this may be due to its remaining in place for shorter periods.

Clinical Findings

The patient usually experiences a dull pain in the region of the involved vein. Local findings consist of induration, redness, and tenderness along the course of a vein. The process may be localized, or it may involve most of the long saphenous vein and its tributaries. The inflammatory reaction generally subsides in 1–2 weeks; a firm cord may remain for a much longer period. Edema of the extremity and deep calf tenderness are absent unless deep thrombophlebitis has also developed. Chills and high fever suggest septic phlebitis and are often encountered when the phlebitis is secondary to an indwelling intravenous catheter.

Differential Diagnosis

The linear rather than circular nature of the lesion and the distribution along the course of a superficial vein serve to differentiate superficial phlebitis from cellulitis, erythema nodosum, erythema induratum, panniculitis, and fibrositis. Lymphangitis and deep thrombophlebitis must also be considered.

Treatment

If the process is well localized and not near the saphenofemoral junction, local heat and bed rest with the leg elevated are usually effective in limiting the thrombosis. Nonsteroidal anti-inflammatory drugs relieve symptoms.

If the process is very extensive or is progressing upward toward the saphenofemoral junction, or if it is in the proximity of the saphenofemoral junction initially, ligation and division of the saphenous vein at the saphenofemoral junction are indicated. The inflammatory process usually regresses following this procedure, though removal of the involved segment of vein (stripping) may result in a more rapid recovery.

Anticoagulation therapy is usually not indicated unless the disease is rapidly progressing. It is indicated if there is extension into the deep system.

Septic thrombophlebitis requires excision of the involved vein up to its junction with an uninvolved vein in order to control the infection. *Staphylococcus* is the commonest pathogen, and antibiotics with antistaphylococcal activity should be instituted pending results of blood cultures. If cultures are positive, therapy should be continued for 7–10 days—or for 4–6 weeks if complicating endocarditis cannot be excluded. Other organisms, including fungi, may also be responsible.

Prognosis

The course is generally benign and brief, and the prognosis depends on the underlying pathologic process. Phlebitis of a saphenous vein occasionally extends to the deep veins, in which case pulmonary embolism may occur.

CHRONIC VENOUS INSUFFICIENCY

Essentials of Diagnosis

- History of phlebitis or leg injury.
- Ankle edema is the earliest sign.
- Stasis pigmentation, dermatitis, subcutaneous induration, and often varicosities occur later.
- Ulceration at or above the ankle is common (stasis ulcer).

General Considerations

Chronic venous insufficiency generally results from changes secondary to deep thrombophlebitis, although a definite history of phlebitis is not obtainable in about 25% of these patients. There is often a history of leg trauma. It can also occur in association with varicose veins and as a result of neoplastic obstruction of the pelvic veins or congenital or acquired arteriovenous fistula.

When insufficiency is secondary to deep thrombophlebitis (the postphlebitic syndrome), the valves in the deep venous channels of the lower leg have been damaged or destroyed by the thrombotic process. The recanalized, nonelastic deep veins are functionally inadequate because of the damaged valves in the deep and perforating veins. The antegrade venous flow ensured by the valves and the calf muscle pump is lost, resulting in bidirectional flow and abnormally high ambulatory venous pressures in the calf veins in particular. The high ambulatory venous pressure transmitted through the communicating veins to the subcutaneous veins and tissues of the calf and ankle areas results in a series of deleterious secondary changes, including edema, fibrosis of subcutaneous tissue and skin, pigmentation of skin, and later, dermatitis, cellulitis, and ulceration. Dilation of the superficial veins may occur, leading to varicosities. Whereas primary varicose veins with no abnormality of the deep venous system may be associated with some similar changes, the edema is more pronounced in the postphlebitic extremities, and the secondary changes are more extensive and encircling.

Clinical Findings

Chronic venous insufficiency is characterized first by progressive edema of the leg (particularly the lower leg) and later also by secondary changes in the skin and subcutaneous tissues. The usual symptoms are itching, a dull discomfort made worse by periods of standing, and pain if an ulceration is present. The skin is usually thin, shiny, atrophic, and cyanotic; and a brownish pigmentation often develops. Eczema may be present, with superficial weeping dermatitis. The subcutaneous tissues become thick and fibrous. Recurrent ulcerations may occur, usually just above the ankle, on the medial or anterior aspect of the leg; healing results in a thin scar on a fibrotic base that often breaks down with minor trauma. Varicosities frequently appear that are associated with incompetent perforating veins.

Differential Diagnosis

Congestive heart failure and chronic renal disease may result in bilateral edema of the lower extremities, but generally there are other clinical or laboratory findings of heart or kidney disease.

Lymphedema is associated with a brawny thickening in the subcutaneous tissue that does not respond readily to elevation; varicosities are absent, and there is often a history of recurrent cellulitis.

Primary varicose veins may be difficult to differentiate from the secondary varicosities that often develop in this condition, as discussed above. It may be impossible to exclude superimposed acute phlebitis from chronic venous insufficiency without diagnostic tests.

Other conditions associated with chronic ulcers of the leg include autoimmune diseases (eg, Felty's syndrome), arterial insufficiency (often very painful), sickle cell anemia, erythema induratum (bilateral and usually on the posterior aspect of the lower part of the leg), and fungal infections (cultures specific; no chronic swelling or varicosities).

Prevention

Irreversible tissue changes and associated complications in the lower legs can be minimized through early and energetic treatment of acute thrombophlebitis with anticoagulants that may minimize the occlusive and valve damage, particularly in the calf, and specific measures to avoid chronic edema in subsequent years, as described in A, below. Thrombolytic therapies of acute phlebitis may be of greater value than other anticoagulants in prevention of chronic venous insufficiency.

Treatment

A. General Measures: Bed rest, with the legs elevated to diminish chronic edema, is fundamental in the treatment of the acute complications of chronic venous insufficiency. Measures to control the tendency toward edema include (1) intermittent elevation of the legs during the day and elevation of the legs at night (kept above the level of the heart with pillows under the mattress); (2) avoidance of long periods of sitting or standing; and (3) the use of well-fitting, heavy-duty elastic supports worn from the mid foot to just below the knee during the day and evening if there is any tendency for swelling to develop.

B. Stasis Dermatitis: Eczematous eruption may be acute or chronic; treatment varies accordingly.

1. Acute weeping dermatitis–

a. Wet compresses for 1 hour four times daily of solutions containing boric acid, buffered aluminum acetate (Burow's solution), or isotonic saline.

b. Compresses are followed with a local corticosteroid such as 0.5% hydrocortisone cream in a water-soluble base. (Neomycin and nystatin may be incorporated into this cream.)

c. Systemic antibiotics are indicated only if active infection is present.

2. Subsiding or chronic dermatitis–

a. Continue hydrocortisone cream for 1–2 weeks or until no further improvement is noted. Cordran tape, a plastic tape impregnated with flurandrenolide, is a convenient way to apply both medication and dressing.

b. Zinc oxide ointment with ichthammol, 3%, once or twice daily, cleaned off as desired with mineral oil.

c. Broad-spectrum antifungal such as clotrimazole cream (1%) or miconazole cream (2%) may be used.

3. Energetic treatment of chronic edema, as outlined in sections A and C, with almost complete bed rest is important during the acute phase of stasis dermatitis.

C. Ulceration: Ulcerations are preferably treated with compresses of isotonic saline solution, which aid the healing of the ulcer or may help prepare the base for a skin graft. A lesion can often be treated on an ambulatory basis by means of a semirigid boot applied to the leg after much of the swelling has been reduced by a period of elevation. The pumping action of the calf muscles on the blood flow out of the lower extremity is enhanced by a circumferential nonelastic bandage on the ankle and lower leg. The boot must be changed every 1–2 weeks, depending to some extent on the amount of drainage from the ulcer. The ulcer, tendons, and bony prominences must be adequately padded. Special ointments on the ulcer are not necessary. The semirigid boot may be made with Unna's paste (Gelocast, Medicopaste) or Gauztex bandage (impregnated with a nonallergenic self-adhering compound). After the ulcer has healed, heavy below-the-knee elastic stockings are used in an effort to prevent recurrent edema and ulceration. Occasionally, the ulcer is so large and chronic that total excision of the ulcer, with skin graft of the defect, is the best approach. This is often combined with ligation of all incompetent perforating veins.

D. Secondary Varicosities: Varicosities secondary to damage to the deep system of veins may in turn contribute to undesirable changes in the tissues of the lower leg. Varicosities should occasionally be removed and the incompetent veins connecting the superficial and deep system ligated, but the tendency toward edema will persist, because the chronic high venous pressure is usually not effectively lowered during walking by the procedure, and thus the measures outlined above (¶A) will be required for life. Varicosities can often be treated along with edema by elastic stockings and other nonoperative measures, and only about 15–20% require surgery. If the obstructive element in the deep system appears to be severe, B-mode ultrasonography, bidirectional Doppler velocity studies, or phlebography may be of value in mapping out the areas of venous obstruction or incompetence in the deep system as well as the number and location of the damaged perforating veins. A decision about whether to treat with surgery may be influenced by such a study; if the varicosities furnish the chief route of venous return, they should not be removed. Venous valvular reconstructive surgery is now in an investigative stage.

Prognosis

Individuals with chronic venous insufficiency often have recurrent problems, particularly if measures to counteract persistent venous hypertension, edema, and secondary tissue changes are not conscientiously adhered to throughout life. Additional episodes of acute thrombophlebitis may occur, and in reliable patients permanent anticoagulation is a reasonable therapeutic objective.

Ciacon JO et al: Leg edema: Clinical clues to the differential diagnosis. Geriatrics 1993;48:34.

Hansson C: Optimal treatment of venous (stasis) ulcers in elderly patients. Drugs Aging 1994;5:323.

Miller WL: Chronic venous insufficiency. Curr Opin Cardiol 1995;10:543.

SUPERIOR VENA CAVAL OBSTRUCTION

Partial or complete obstruction of the thin-walled superior vena cava is a relatively rare condition that is usually secondary to the neoplastic or inflammatory process in the superior mediastinum. The most frequent causes are (1) neoplasms, such as lymphomas, primary malignant mediastinal tumors, or carcinoma of the lung with direct extension (over 80%); (2) chronic fibrotic mediastinitis, either of unknown origin or secondary to tuberculosis, histoplasmosis, pyogenic infections, or drugs, especially methysergide; (3) thrombophlebitis, often by extension of the process from the axillary or subclavian vein into the innominate vein and vena cava and often associated with catheterization of these veins for central venous pressure measurements or for hyperalimentation; (4) aneurysm of the aortic arch; and (5) constrictive pericarditis.

Clinical Findings

A. Symptoms and Signs: The onset of symptoms is acute or subacute. Symptoms include swelling of the neck and face, headache, dizziness, visual disturbances, stupor, and syncope. There is progressive obstruction of the venous drainage of the head, neck, and upper extremities. The cutaneous veins of the upper chest and lower neck become dilated, and flushing of the face and neck develops. Brawny edema of the face, neck, and arms occurs later, and cyanosis of these areas then appears. Cerebral and laryngeal edema ultimately results in impaired function of the brain as well as respiratory insufficiency. Bending over or lying down accentuates the symptoms; sitting quietly is generally preferred. The manifestations are more severe if the obstruction develops rapidly and if the azygos junction or the vena cava between that vein and the heart is obstructed.

B. Laboratory Findings: The venous pressure is elevated in the arm and is normal in the leg. Since lung cancer is a common cause, bronchoscopy is often performed; transbronchial biopsy, however, is relatively contraindicated because of venous hypertension and the risk of bleeding.

C. Imaging: Chest radiographs and a CT scan will define the location and often the nature of the obstructive process, and phlebography will map out the extent and degree of the venous obstruction and the collateral circulation. Doppler ultrasound can demonstrate the presence of collaterals, and MRI may delineate the site of thrombosis as well as the nature of the cause. Brachial venography or radionuclide scanning following intravenous injection of technetium Tc 99m pertechnetate demonstrates a block to the flow of contrast material into the right heart and enlarged collateral veins. These techniques also allow estimation of blood flow around the occlusion as well as serial evaluation of the response to therapy.

Treatment

Though empiric therapy for neoplasm is occasionally warranted, the clinician should be aware of benign causes, especially histoplasmosis.

Urgent treatment for neoplasm consists of (1) cautious use of intravenous diuretics and (2) mediastinal irradiation, starting within 24 hours, with a treatment plan designed to give a high daily dose but a short total course of therapy to rapidly shrink the local tumor even further. Intensive combined therapy will palliate the process in up to 90% of patients. In patients with a subacute presentation, radiation therapy alone usually suffices. Chemotherapy is added if lymphoma or small-cell carcinoma is diagnosed.

Surgical procedures to bypass the obstruction are complicated by bleeding relating to high venous pressure. In cases secondary to mediastinal fibrosis or pericardial constriction, excision of the fibrous tissue around the great vessels may reestablish flow.

Prognosis

The prognosis depends upon the nature and degree of obstruction and its speed of onset. Slowly developing forms secondary to fibrosis may be tolerated for years. A high degree of obstruction of rapid onset secondary to cancer is often fatal in a few days or weeks because of increased intracranial pressure and cerebral hemorrhage, but treatment of the tumor with radiation and chemotherapeutic drugs may result in significant palliation.

Abner A: Approach to the patient who presents with superior vena cava obstruction. Chest 1993;103(4 Suppl): 394S.

Urban T et al: Superior vena cava syndrome in small cell cancer. Arch Intern Med 1993;153:384. (Intensive chemotherapy was the first line of therapy.)

DISEASES OF THE LYMPHATIC CHANNELS

LYMPHANGITIS & LYMPHADENITIS

Essentials of Diagnosis

- Red streak from wound or area of cellulitis toward regional lymph nodes, which are usually enlarged and tender.
- Chills, fever, and malaise may be present.

General Considerations

Lymphangitis and lymphadenitis are common manifestations of a bacterial infection that is usually caused by hemolytic streptococci or staphylococci (or by both organisms) and usually arises from an area of cellulitis, generally at the site of an infected wound. The wound may be very small or superficial, or an established abscess may be present, feeding bacteria into the lymphatics. The involvement of the lymphatics is often manifested by a red streak in the skin extending in the direction of the regional lymph nodes, which are, in turn, generally tender and enlarged. Systemic manifestations include fever, chills, and malaise. The infection may progress rapidly, often in a matter of hours, and may lead to septicemia and even death.

Clinical Findings

A. Symptoms and Signs: Throbbing pain is usually present in the area of cellulitis at the site of bacterial invasion. Malaise, anorexia, sweating, chills, and fever of 37.8–40°C develop rapidly. The red streak, when present, may be definite or may be very faint and easily missed, especially in dark-skinned patients. It is not usually tender or indurated, as is the area of cellulitis. The involved regional lymph nodes may be significantly enlarged and are usually quite tender. The pulse is often rapid.

B. Laboratory Findings: Leukocytosis with a left shift is usually present. Later, a blood culture may be positive, most often for staphylococcal or streptococcal species. Culture and sensitivity studies on the wound exudate or pus may be helpful in treatment of the more severe or refractory infections but are often difficult to interpret because of skin contaminants.

Differential Diagnosis

Lymphangitis may be confused with superficial thrombophlebitis, but the erythematous reaction associated with thrombosis overlies the induration of the inflammatory reaction in and around the thrombosed vein. Venous thrombosis is not associated with lymphadenitis, and a wound of entrance with the secondary cellulitis is generally absent. Superficial thrombophlebitis frequently arises as a result of intravenous therapy, particularly when the needle or catheter is left in place for more than 2 days; if bacteria have also been introduced, suppurative thrombophlebitis may develop.

Cat-scratch fever should be considered when lymphadenitis is present in which the nodes, though often very large, are relatively nontender. Exposure to cats is common, but the scratch may be forgotten by the patient.

It is extremely important to differentiate cellulitis from soft tissue infections that require early and aggressive incision and often resection of necrotic infected tissue, eg, acute streptococcal hemolytic gangrene, necrotizing fasciitis, gram-negative anaerobic cutaneous gangrene, and progressive bacterial synergistic gangrene. These are deeper infections that are more anatomically extensive; patients appear more seriously ill, and subcutaneous crepitus may be palpated or auscultated using the diaphragm with light pressure over the involved area.

Treatment

A. General Measures: Prompt treatment should include heat (hot, moist compresses or heating pad), elevation when feasible, and immobilization of the infected area. Analgesics may be prescribed for pain.

B. Specific Measures: Antibiotic therapy should always be instituted when local infection becomes invasive, as manifested by cellulitis and lymphangitis. Because the causative organism is so frequently the streptococcus, penicillin G is usually the drug of choice, although antistaphylococcal peni-

cillins (eg, nafcillin) or cephalosporins are favored by some. If the patient is allergic to penicillin, erythromycin may be substituted. (See Chapter 37.)

C. Wound Care: Drainage of pus from an infected wound should be carried out, generally after the above measures have been instituted and only when it is clear that there is an abscess associated with the site of initial infection. An area of cellulitis should not be incised, because the infection may be spread by attempted drainage when pus is not present.

Prognosis

With proper therapy and particularly with the use of an antibiotic effective against the invading bacteria, control of the infection can usually be achieved in a few days. Delayed or inadequate therapy can still lead to overwhelming infection with septicemia.

LYMPHEDEMA

Essentials of Diagnosis

- Painless edema of one or both lower extremities, primarily in young women.
- Initially, pitting edema, which becomes brawny and often nonpitting with time.
- Ulceration, varicosities, and stasis pigmentation do not occur. There may be episodes of lymphangitis and cellulitis.

General Considerations

The underlying mechanism in lymphedema is impairment of the flow of lymph from an extremity. When due to congenital developmental abnormalities consisting of hypo- or hyperplastic involvement of the proximal or distal lymphatics, it is referred to as the primary form. The obstruction may be in the pelvic or lumbar lymph channels and nodes when the disease is extensive and progressive. The secondary form results when an inflammatory or mechanical obstruction of the lymphatics occurs from trauma, regional lymph node resection or irradiation, or extensive involvement of regional nodes by malignant disease or filariasis. Secondary dilation of the lymphatics that occurs in both forms leads to incompetence of the valve system, disrupting the orderly flow along the lymph vessels, and results in progressive stasis of a protein-rich fluid with secondary fibrosis. Episodes of acute and chronic inflammation may be superimposed, with further stasis and fibrosis. Hypertrophy of the limb results, with markedly thickened and fibrotic skin and subcutaneous tissue and diminution in the fatty tissue.

Lymphangiography and radioactive isotope studies are often useful in defining the specific lymphatic defect.

Treatment

The treatment of lymphedema is often not very

satisfactory. The majority of patients can be treated conservatively with some of the following measures: (1) The flow of lymph out of the extremity, with a consequent decrease in the degree of stasis, can be aided through intermittent elevation of the extremity, especially during the sleeping hours (foot of bed elevated 15–20 degrees, achieved by placing pillows beneath the mattress); the constant use of elastic bandages or carefully fitted heavy-duty elastic stockings; and massage toward the trunk—either by hand or by means of pneumatic pressure devices designed to milk edema out of an extremity. (The Wright linear pump delivers sequential pressure cycles that effectively milk fluid out of the foot and leg and then out of the thigh.) (2) Secondary cellulitis in the extremity should be avoided by means of good hygiene and treatment of any trichophytosis of the toes. Once an infection starts, it should be treated by adequate periods of rest, elevation, and antibiotics, with coverage of *Staphylococcus* and *Streptococcus*. Infection can be a serious and recurring problem and is often difficult to control. Intermittent prophylactic antibiotics may occasionally be necessary; dicloxacillin is a good choice. (3) Intermittent courses of diuretic therapy, especially in those with premenstrual or seasonal exacerbations. (4) In carefully selected cases, there are operative procedures that may give satisfactory functional results. Lymphaticovenous anastomosis using microsurgery has yielded some satisfactory cosmetic and functional results, particularly if lymph channels can be localized by lymphoscintigraphy and several lymphovenous anastomoses are made. This technique may replace the more deforming procedures and those aimed at introducing lymphatic bridges or lymphatic venous connections. Amputation is used as a last resort in very severe forms or when lymphangiosarcoma develops in the extremity.

HYPOTENSION & SHOCK

Essentials of Diagnosis

- Low systemic blood pressure and tachycardia.
- Peripheral hypoperfusion and, in most, vasoconstriction.
- Altered mental status.
- Oliguria or anuria.
- Metabolic acidosis in many.

General Considerations

Shock occurs when the circulation of arterial blood is inadequate to meet tissue metabolic needs. Treatment must be directed both at the manifestations of shock and at its cause.

Classification
(Table 12–1)

A. Hypovolemic Shock: Decreased intravascular volume resulting from loss of blood, plasma, or fluids and electrolytes may be obvious (eg, external hemorrhage) or subtle (eg, sequestration in a "third space," as in pancreatitis). Compensatory vasoconstriction temporarily reduces the size of the vascular bed and may temporarily maintain the blood pressure, but if fluid is not replaced, hypotension occurs, peripheral resistance increases, capillary and venous beds collapse, and the tissues become progressively more hypoxic. Even a moderate sudden loss of circulating fluids can result in severe damage to vital centers.

B. Cardiogenic Shock: See discussion in Chapter 10.

Table 12–1. Classification of shock by mechanism and common causes.[1]

Hypovolemic shock
  Loss of blood (hemorrhagic shock)
    External hemorrhage
      Trauma
      Gastrointestinal tract bleeding
    Internal hemorrhage
      Hematoma
      Hemothorax or hemoperitoneum
  Loss of plasma
    Burns
    Exfoliative dermatitis
  Loss of fluid and electrolytes
    External
      Vomiting
      Diarrhea
      Excessive sweating
      Hyperosmolar states (diabetic ketoacidosis, hyperosmolar nonketotic coma)
    Internal ("third spacing")
      Pancreatitis
      Ascites
      Bowel obstruction
Cardiogenic shock
  Dysrhythmia
    Tachyarrhythmia
    Bradyarrhythmia
  "Pump failure" (secondary to myocardial infarction or other cardiomyopathy)
  Acute valvular dysfunction (especially regurgitant lesions)
  Rupture of ventricular septum or free ventricular wall
Obstructive shock
  Tension pneumothorax
  Pericardial disease (tamponade, constriction)
  Disease of pulmonary vasculature (massive pulmonary emboli, pulmonary hypertension)
  Cardiac tumor (atrial myxoma)
  Left atrial mural thrombus
  Obstructive valvular disease (aortic or mitral stenosis)
Distributive shock
  Septic shock
  Anaphylactic shock
  Neurogenic shock
  Vasodilator drugs
  Acute adrenal insufficiency

[1]Reproduced, with permission, from Saunders CE, Ho MT (editors): *Current Emergency Diagnosis & Treatment,* 4th ed. Appleton & Lange, 1992.

C. Obstructive Shock: Obstruction of the systemic or pulmonary circulation, the aortic and mitral valves, or venous inflow, as in pericardial disease, may reduce cardiac output sufficiently to cause shock. Cardiac tamponade, tension pneumothorax, and massive pulmonary embolism are medical emergencies requiring prompt diagnosis and treatment. Tamponade calls for immediate echocardiography and pericardiocentesis. The prognosis for patients with massive pulmonary embolism is guarded despite therapy with anticoagulants or thrombolytics; surgical embolectomy adds little. A less common cause of obstructive shock is myxoma with pulmonary hypertension.

D. Distributive Shock: Reduction in systemic vascular resistance from such diverse causes as sepsis, anaphylaxis, or acute adrenal insufficiency may result in inadequate cardiac output despite normal circulatory volume.

1. Septic shock–Most commonly, vascular shock is due to gram-negative bacteremia (so-called septic shock). In overwhelming infection, there is an initial short period of vasoconstriction followed by vasodilation, with venous pooling of blood in the microcirculation. The vasodilation of septic shock may be mediated by nitrous oxide. The mortality rate is high (40–80%). Responsible organisms are most commonly gram-negative rods (*Escherichia coli, Klebsiella, Proteus,* and *Pseudomonas*) as well as gram-positive cocci *(Staphylococcus, Streptococcus)* and gram-negative anaerobes (eg, *Bacteroides*). Septic shock occurs more often in the very young and the very old; in diabetes, hematologic cancers, and diseases of the genitourinary, hepatobiliary, and intestinal tracts; and in association with immunosuppressive therapy. Immediate precipitating factors may be urinary, biliary, or gynecologic manipulations.

Septic shock is suspected when a febrile patient has chills associated with hypotension. Early, the skin may be warm and the pulse full ("warm shock"). Hyperventilation results in respiratory alkalosis. The sensorium and urinary output are often initially normal, with classic signs of shock becoming manifest later. The symptoms and signs of the inciting infection are not invariably present.

The development of monoclonal antibodies to endotoxin has opened a potential new avenue of therapy. To date, however, data on its efficacy are conflicting.

2. Neurogenic shock–Neurogenic or psychogenic factors, eg, spinal cord injury, pain, trauma, fright, gastric dilation, or vasodilator drugs, may also cause distributive shock due to reflex vagal stimulation with decreased cardiac output, hypotension, and decreased cerebral blood flow.

Diagnosis of Shock & Impending Shock

Shock may be impending if the following signs are present.

A. Hypotension: Hypotension in adults is tra-ditionally defined as a systolic blood pressure of 90 mm Hg or less. However, some normal adults may have levels that low without ill effects, and some hypertensive persons develop shock with what would ordinarily be considered normal blood pressures.

B. Orthostatic Changes in Vital Signs: Patients who are not clearly hypotensive when tested supine should have readings while sitting up with the legs dangling. If no change occurs, repeat the measurements with the patient standing. A drop in systolic pressure of more than 10–20 mm Hg with an increase in pulse of more than 15 suggests depleted intravascular volume. Some normovolemic patients with peripheral neuropathies or those taking certain medications (eg, some antihypertensive drugs) may demonstrate an orthostatic fall in blood pressure, but without associated increase in pulse rate.

C. Peripheral Hypoperfusion: Patients in shock often have cool or mottled extremities and weak or absent peripheral pulses.

D. Altered Mental Status: Patients may demonstrate normal mental status or may be restless, agitated, confused, lethargic, or comatose as a result of inadequate perfusion of the brain.

Treatment

Treatment depends upon prompt assessment of the cause, type, severity, and duration of shock as well as an accurate appraisal of underlying conditions that may influence the onset or maintenance of shock.

A. Position: The patient is placed in the Trendelenburg or supine position with legs elevated to maximize cerebral blood flow.

B. Oxygenation: Oxygen should be given because shock—especially septic shock—may result in hypoxia caused by pulmonary ventilation-perfusion mismatch or, in severe cases, by acute respiratory distress syndrome (see Chapter 9).

C. Analgesics: Severe pain is treated promptly with analgesic drugs. Morphine sulfate, 8–15 mg subcutaneously, is appropriate for severe pain; since subcutaneous absorption is poor in patients in shock, 4–8 mg slowly intravenously may be used as an alternative. Morphine should not be given to unconscious patients, to those who have head injuries, to those with severe hypotension or unstable blood pressure, or to those with respiratory depression.

D. Laboratory Studies: A complete blood count is obtained immediately, and a blood specimen is sent for typing and cross-matching. Electrolytes, blood glucose, serum creatinine, and urinalysis are also important diagnostically. Arterial blood gases (or finger oximeter oxygen saturation) are obtained routinely.

E. Urine Flow: Both oliguric and nonoliguric renal failure may occur in shock. In the patient without preexisting renal disease, urine output is a reliable indication of organ perfusion. An indwelling catheter to monitor urine flow (which should be kept above 0.5

mL/kg/h) may be indicated. Urine flow of less than 25 mL/h indicates inadequate renal perfusion, which, if not corrected, can result in renal tubular necrosis.

F. Monitor Cardiac Rhythm: Periodic electrocardiography or continuous automated monitoring will permit early detection and prompt treatment of myocardial ischemia from hypoperfusion, and arrhythmias from similar causes or from electrolyte and acid-base disturbances.

G. Central Venous Pressure (CVP) or Pulmonary Capillary Wedge Pressure (PCWP): Monitoring of central venous pressure or pulmonary capillary wedge pressure is helpful in treating shock. Central venous pressure determination is relatively simple but is not as reliable as the pulmonary capillary wedge pressure (PCWP) measured by the Swan-Ganz catheter technique, which theoretically provides a better index of left ventricular function. Determination of PCWP has been used traditionally in patients in whom there is uncertainty about the role of cardiac function in the genesis of shock or in myocardial infarction with shock. It is also useful in guiding volume resuscitation in shock patients with a history of heart disease or in such patients in whom pulmonary disease has produced high central venous pressure. Finally, it has a role in the therapy of right ventricular infarction. However, recent prospective studies have not shown benefit and provide some evidence of increased morbidity and mortality in patients receiving pulmonary artery catheters.

In central venous pressure determination, a catheter is inserted percutaneously (or by cutdown) through a major vein. Normal values range from 5 to 8 cm of water. A low central venous pressure suggests the need for fluid replacement. A high central venous pressure (above 15 cm of water) suggests volume overload, cardiac failure, pericardial tamponade, or pulmonary hypertension. The PCWP catheter is inserted in a similar fashion, with localization of its tip determined by monitoring the morphology of the pressure tracing as it is advanced. A PCWP over 14 mm Hg may serve as a warning of impending pulmonary edema. Catheter insertion requires a skilled and experienced physician and is expensive. Surveillance for complications of hemorrhage, sepsis, pneumothorax, arrhythmias, and pulmonary infarction is obligatory.

H. Volume Replacement: Initial or emergency needs may be determined by the history, general appearance, vital signs, and hematocrit. There is no simple technique by which to accurately judge the fluid requirements. An estimate of total fluid losses is an essential first step. Response to therapy—particularly the effect of carefully administered, gradually increasing amounts of intravenous fluids on the central venous pressure or PCWP—is a valuable index.

Selection of the proper fluid for restoration and maintenance of hemodynamic stability is often difficult and controversial. It will depend upon the type of fluid that has been lost (whole blood, plasma, water, electrolytes), associated medical problems, availability of the various replacement solutions, clinical and laboratory monitoring facilities, and, in some circumstances, expense. The most effective replacement fluid in case of hemorrhage is packed red cells with saline, but other available fluids should be given immediately pending return of laboratory studies.

Rapid volume replacement in blood loss will often prevent shock. If central venous pressure or PCWP is low and the hematocrit greater than 35%—and if there is no clinical evidence to suggest occult blood loss—blood volume should be supported with crystalloid solutions or colloids.

1. Crystalloid solutions–Isotonic (0.9%) sodium chloride solution 500–2000 mL, is given rapidly intravenously—ideally under central venous pressure or pulmonary capillary wedge pressure monitoring. The crystalloids are readily available for emergencies and mass casualties. They may obviate the need for blood or colloids. They are often effective, at least temporarily, when given in adequate doses.

2. Colloids–Colloids are high-molecular-weight substances that do not diffuse readily across normal capillary membranes. Colloidal solutions increase the plasma oncotic pressure and thus in theory can draw fluid from the interstitial space into the intravascular space to cause additional fluid volume expansion. However, capillary membranes in the lungs are often damaged in the patient in shock, so that larger molecules may leak from the intravascular space into the interstitium and have an adverse effect on pulmonary function (adult respiratory distress syndrome).

a. Blood–Packed or frozen red cells are preferred to whole blood, since remaining blood products may be used for other purposes. The amount of blood given depends on the clinical course, the hematocrit, and hemodynamic findings. Each unit raises the hematocrit by roughly 3%.

Screening of blood donors for hepatitis B and C infection and for HIV has reduced the frequency of those infections following transfusion. The risk of HIV infection from transfused blood is now estimated to be approximately 1:100,000 in industrialized countries that screen appropriately. The risk for contracting hepatitis B is 1:200,000 transfusions. Hepatitis C remains the commonest infectious complication of transfusion; with the advent of diagnostic tests for hepatitis C, the risk is diminishing but still of concern (1:3300 transfusions).

b. Plasma fractions–Group-specific frozen plasma is a satisfactory colloidal volume expander and occasionally can correct specific coagulation defects. Because of its expense, risk (same as blood transfusion), and relative ineffectiveness, however, its use should be limited. Unit-bagged plasma is preferable to pooled plasma. Albumin 5% in saline, albumin 25% in concentrate, or plasma protein fraction (containing 80–85% albumin) may be rapidly set up for emergencies, and blood typing is not required. These substances have been heat-treated to minimize the risk of infectious hepatitis, which in any case is trivial.

c. Dextrans–Dextrans are high-molecular-weight polysaccharide colloids that are fairly effective plasma expanders. Because they can impair blood coagulation and interfere with blood typing and because they may cause anaphylactoid reactions, dextrans are used very infrequently now.

I. Vasoactive Drugs: Some adrenergic drugs can be useful in the adjunctive therapy of shock. *The adrenergic drugs should not be considered a primary form of therapy in shock.* Simple blood pressure elevation produced by the vasopressor drugs has little beneficial effect on the underlying disturbance, and in many instances the effect may be detrimental. Pressors are given only when hypotension persists after volume deficits are corrected and obstructive causes excluded or remedied.

1. Dopamine hydrochloride has an advantage over other adrenergic drugs because it has a beneficial effect on renal blood flow (at low dose) and because it increases cardiac output and blood pressure. Dopamine hydrochloride, 200 mg in 500 mL of sodium chloride injection USP (400 µg/mL), is given initially at a rate of 1–2 µg/kg/min. This dosage stimulates both the dopaminergic receptors, which increase the renal blood flow and urinary output, and the β-adrenergic cardiac receptors, which increase the cardiac output. If shock persists, gradually increasing doses of dopamine may be required. If dopamine alone fails to maintain adequate perfusion pressure, it may sometimes be necessary to use it in combination with another appropriate adrenergic drug.

Adverse reactions include ventricular arrhythmias, anginal pain, nausea and vomiting, headache, hypotension, azotemia, and rare cases of peripheral gangrene. Special care should be exercised when dopamine is used in the treatment of shock following myocardial infarction, because the drug's inotropic effect may increase myocardial oxygen demand. Dopamine should not be used in patients with pheochromocytoma or uncorrected tachyarrhythmias or in those who are receiving monoamine oxidase inhibitors.

2. Dobutamine, a synthetic catecholamine similar to dopamine but with greater inotropic effect, may be useful when filling pressures are high because of fluid overload or heart failure. Though dopamine at higher doses is a vasoconstrictor, dobutamine has no net effect on peripheral vascular resistance.

J. Corticosteroids: Corticosteroids are life-saving in the treatment of shock associated with acute adrenal insufficiency (see Chapter 26). In other types of shock, however, corticosteroids are of no benefit.

K. Diuretics: Diuretics are not employed until volume deficits are corrected or obstructive causes remedied. There is no evidence that diuretics reduce the overall incidence of renal failure, though some believe they may convert oliguric renal insufficiency to a nonoliguric type.

Atkinson TB, Kahiner MA: Anaphylaxis. Med Clin North Am 1992;76:841.

Mercier JC: New treatment for sepsis. Crit Care Med 1993;21(9 Suppl):S310.

Parrillo JE: Pathogenetic mechanisms for septic shock. N Engl J Med 1993;328:1471.

Zaloga GP et al: Pharmacologic cardiovascular support. Crit Care Clin 1993;9:335. (Entire issue on circulatory shock.)

Blood

13

Charles A. Linker, MD

ANEMIAS

General Approach to Anemias

Anemia is present in adults if the hematocrit is less than 41% (hemoglobin < 13.5 g/dL) in males or 37% (hemoglobin < 12 g/dL) in females. In taking the history, congenital anemia may be suggested by the patient's personal and family history. Poor diet results in folic acid deficiency and may contribute to iron deficiency. Bleeding should always be considered in iron deficiency. Physical examination includes careful attention to signs of primary hematologic diseases (lymphadenopathy, hepatosplenomegaly, or bone tenderness). Mucosal changes such as a smooth tongue raise the possibility of megaloblastic anemia.

Anemias are classified according to their pathophysiologic basis, ie, whether related to diminished production or accelerated loss of red blood cells (Table 13–1); or according to cell size (Table 13–2). The diagnostic possibilities in microcytic anemia are iron deficiency, thalassemia, and anemia of chronic disease. A severely microcytic anemia (MCV < 70 fL) is always due either to iron deficiency or to thalassemia. Macrocytic anemia may be due to megaloblastic (folate or vitamin B_{12} deficiency) or nonmegaloblastic causes. A severely macrocytic anemia (MCV > 125 fL) is almost always due to megaloblastic causes; rare exceptions are the myelodysplastic syndromes, either before or after chemotherapy.

Williams WJ (editor): *Hematology*, 5th ed. McGraw-Hill, 1995.

IRON DEFICIENCY ANEMIA

Essentials of Diagnosis

- Both pathognomonic: absent bone marrow iron stores or serum ferritin < 12 µg/L.
- Nearly always caused by bleeding in adults.
- Response to iron therapy.

General Considerations

Iron deficiency is the most common cause of anemia worldwide. The anemia is usually mild, but it may become moderate or even severe. It is important to make the diagnosis so that the underlying cause (usually gastrointestinal blood loss) can be identified and treated (Table 13–3).

Iron is necessary for the formation of heme and other enzymes. Total body iron ranges between 2 g and 4 g: approximately 50 mg/kg in men and 35 mg/kg in women. The majority (70–95%) of total body iron is present in hemoglobin in circulating red blood cells. One milliliter of packed red blood cells (not whole blood) contains approximately 1 mg of iron. In men, red blood cell volume is approximately 30 mL/kg. A 70-kg man will therefore have approximately 2100 mL of packed red blood cells and consequently 2100 mg of iron in his circulating blood. In women, the red cell volume is about 27 mL/kg; a 50-kg woman will thus have 1350 mg of iron circulating in her red blood cells. Only 200–400 mg of iron is present in myoglobin and nonheme enzymes. The amount of iron present in plasma is negligible. Aside from circulating red blood cells, the major location of iron in the body is the storage pool. Iron is deposited either as ferritin or as hemosiderin and is located largely in macrophages. The range for storage iron is wide (0.5–2 g); approximately 25% of women in the USA have none.

The average American diet contains 10–15 mg of iron per day. About 10% of this amount is absorbed. Absorption occurs in the stomach, duodenum, and upper jejunum. Dietary iron present as heme is efficiently absorbed (10–20%) but nonheme iron less so (1–5%), largely because of interference by phosphates, tannins, and other food constituents. Small amounts of iron—approximately 1 mg/d—are normally lost though exfoliation of skin and mucosal cells. There is no mechanism for increasing normal body iron losses.

Menstrual blood loss in women plays a major role in iron metabolism. The average monthly menstrual blood loss is approximately 50 mL, or about 0.7 mg/d. However, menstrual blood loss may be five

Table 13–1. Classification of anemias by pathophysiology.

Decreased production
Hemoglobin synthesis: Iron deficiency, thalassemia, anemia of chronic disease
DNA synthesis: Megaloblastic anemia
Stem cell: Aplastic anemia, myeloproliferative leukemia
Bone marrow infiltration: Carcinoma, lymphoma
Pure red cell aplasia
Increased destruction
Blood loss
Hemolysis (intrinsic)
Membrane: Hereditary spherocytosis, elliptocytosis
Hemoglobin: Sickle cell, unstable hemoglobin
Glycolysis: Pyruvate kinase deficiency, etc
Oxidation: G6PD deficiency
Hemolysis (extrinsic)
Immune: Warm antibody, cold antibody
Microangiopathic: Thrombotic thrombocytopenic purpura, hemolytic-uremic syndrome, mechanical cardiac valve, paravalvular leak
Infection: Clostridial
Hypersplenism

Table 13–3. Causes of iron deficiency.

Deficient diet
Decreased absorption
Increased requirements
Pregnancy
Lactation
Blood loss
Gastrointestinal
Menstrual
Blood donation
Hemoglobinuria
Iron sequestration
Pulmonary hemosiderosis

times the average. In order to maintain adequate iron stores, women with heavy menstrual losses must absorb 3–4 mg of iron from the diet each day. This strains the upper limit of what may reasonably be absorbed, and women with menorrhagia of this degree will almost always become iron-deficient.

In general, iron metabolism is balanced between absorption of 1 mg/d and loss of 1 mg/d. Pregnancy may also upset the iron balance, since requirements increase to 2–5 mg of iron per day during pregnancy and lactation. Normal dietary iron cannot supply these requirements, and medicinal iron is needed during pregnancy and lactation. Repeated pregnancy (especially with breast feeding) is a common cause of iron deficiency if increased requirements are not met with supplemental medicinal iron.

It is possible to become iron-deficient because of dietary deficiency, though this is rare in adults. Decreased iron absorption can cause iron deficiency and is usually due to gastric surgery.

By far the most important cause of iron deficiency anemia is blood loss, especially gastrointestinal

Table 13–2. Classification of anemias by MCV.

Microcytic
Iron deficiency
Thalassemia
Anemia of chronic disease
Macrocytic
Megaloblastic
Vitamin B_{12} deficiency
Folate deficiency
Nonmegaloblastic
Myelodysplasia, chemotherapy
Liver disease
Increased reticulocytosis
Myxedema
Normocytic
Many causes

blood loss. Chronic aspirin use may cause chronic iron loss even without a documented structural lesion. Iron deficiency should prompt a search for a potential source of gastrointestinal bleeding unless another cause is identified. Other sources of blood loss include menorrhagia or other uterine bleeding and repeated blood donation.

Chronic hemoglobinuria may lead to iron deficiency, since more than 1 mg/d of iron can be lost by this route. The most common cause is traumatic hemolysis due to an abnormally functioning cardiac valve. Other causes of intravascular hemolysis (eg, paroxysmal nocturnal hemoglobinuria) should also be considered if hemoglobinuria is documented.

Rare causes of iron deficiency include sequestration of iron in pulmonary macrophages in the syndrome of idiopathic pulmonary hemosiderosis.

Clinical Findings

A. Symptoms and Signs: As a rule, the only symptoms of iron deficiency anemia are those of the anemia itself (easy fatigability, tachycardia, palpitations and tachypnea on exertion). Severe iron deficiency (uncommon in the USA) causes progressive skin and mucosal changes. These include a smooth tongue, brittle nails, and cheilosis. Advanced iron deficiency may cause dysphagia because of the formation of esophageal webs (Plummer-Vinson syndrome). Many iron-deficient patients develop pica, an unusual craving for specific foods (ice cubes, etc) that may or may not contain iron.

B. Laboratory Findings: Iron deficiency develops slowly and in stages. The first stage is depletion of iron stores. At this point, there is anemia and no changes in red blood cell size. The serum ferritin will become abnormally low. A ferritin value less than 30 µg/L nearly always indicates absent iron stores and is a highly reliable indicator of iron deficiency. The serum total iron-binding capacity (TIBC) rises.

After iron stores have been depleted, red blood cell formation will continue with deficient supplies of iron. Serum iron values will begin to fall to less than 30 µg/dL, and transferrin saturation will fall to less than 15%.

In the early stages, the MCV remains normal. Subsequently, the MCV falls and the blood smear shows hypochromic microcytic cells. With further progression, anisocytosis (variations in red blood cell size) followed by poikilocytosis (variation in shape of red cells) will develop. Severe iron deficiency will produce a bizarre peripheral blood smear, with severely hypochromic cells, target cells, hypochromic pencil-shaped cells, and occasionally small numbers of nucleated red blood cells. The platelet count is usually normal in mild iron deficiency anemia but is typically elevated in more severe cases.

Differential Diagnosis

Other causes of microcytic anemia include anemia of chronic disease, thalassemia, and (less commonly) sideroblastic anemia. Anemia of chronic disease is characterized by normal or increased iron stores in the bone marrow and a normal or elevated ferritin level. The TIBC is either normal or low. Thalassemia characteristically produces a greater degree of microcytosis for any given level of anemia than does iron deficiency. Red blood cell morphology on the peripheral smear becomes abnormal earlier in the evolution of anemia, and iron parameters should be normal.

Treatment

To make the diagnosis of iron deficiency anemia, one can either demonstrate an iron-deficient state or evaluate the response to a therapeutic trial of iron replacement.

Since the anemia itself is rarely life-threatening, the most important part of treatment is identification of the cause—especially a source of occult blood loss. Iron deficiency cannot be overcome by increasing dietary iron; medicinal iron is always required.

A. Oral Iron: There is no better treatment than ferrous sulfate, 325 mg three times daily, which provides 180 mg of iron daily of which 10–20 mg is usually absorbed (though absorption may exceed this amount in cases of severe deficiency). Although ferrous sulfate is optimally taken three times a day on an empty stomach, compliance is often improved by introducing the medicine more slowly in a gradually escalating dose. Patients who cannot tolerate iron on an empty stomach should take it with food. An appropriate response is a return of the hematocrit level halfway toward normal within 3 weeks. It is advisable to see the patient after 3 weeks both to monitor the hematologic response and to answer questions about the medication that may improve compliance. In general, hematologic values return to normal after 2 months of treatment. Iron therapy should continue for 3–6 months after restoration of normal hematologic values in order to replenish iron stores. Failure of response to iron therapy is usually due to noncompliance, although occasional patients may absorb iron poorly. Other reasons for failure to respond include

incorrect diagnosis (anemia of chronic disease, thalassemia) and ongoing gastrointestinal blood loss that exceeds the rate of new erythropoiesis.

B. Parenteral Iron: The indications are intolerance to oral iron, refractoriness to oral iron (poor absorption), gastrointestinal disease (usually inflammatory bowel disease) precluding the use of oral iron, and continued blood loss that cannot be corrected. Because of the possibility of severe and even fatal hypersensitivity reactions, parenteral iron therapy should be used only in cases of clinically significant documented iron deficiency after every reasonable attempt has been made to use oral therapy.

The dose may be calculated by estimating the decrease in volume of red blood cell mass and then supplying 1 mg of iron for each milliliter of volume of red blood cells below normal. One should then add approximately 1 g for storage iron. The total dose is typically 1.5–2 g. The entire dose may be given as an intravenous infusion over 4–6 hours. A test dose of a dilute solution is given first, and the patient should be observed closely during the entire infusion in a setting in which anaphylaxis can be treated.

Finch C: Regulators of iron balance in humans. Blood 1994;84:1697.
Gordon S, Bensen S, Smith R: Long-term follow-up of older patients with iron deficiency anemia after a negative GI evaluation. Am J Gastroenterol 1996;91:885. (Favorable prognosis of iron deficiency anemia in older patients after a negative gastrointestinal evaluation.)
Newton W: Laboratory diagnosis of iron deficiency anemia. J Fam Pract 1995;41:404.

ANEMIA OF CHRONIC DISEASE

Many chronic systemic diseases are associated with mild or moderate anemia. Common causes include chronic infection or inflammation, cancer, and liver disease. The anemia of chronic renal failure is somewhat different in pathophysiology and is usually more severe.

Red blood cell survival is modestly reduced, and the bone marrow fails to compensate adequately by increasing red blood cell production. Failure to increase red cell production is largely due to sequestration of iron within the reticuloendothelial system. Decrease in erythropoietin is rarely an important cause of underproduction of red cells except in renal failure, when decreased erythropoietin is the rule.

Clinical Findings

A. Symptoms and Signs: The clinical features are those of the anemia, which is usually modest. The diagnosis should be suspected in patients with known chronic diseases; it is confirmed by the findings of low serum iron, low TIBC, and normal or increased serum ferritin (or normal or increased bone marrow iron stores). In cases of significant anemia, coexistent iron deficiency or folic acid deficiency should be suspected. Decreased dietary intake of folate or iron is common in these ill patients, and many will also have ongoing gastrointestinal blood losses. Patients undergoing hemodialysis regularly lose both iron and folate during dialysis.

B. Laboratory Findings: The hematocrit rarely falls below 25% (except in renal failure). The MCV is usually normal but may be slightly reduced. Red blood cell morphology is nondiagnostic, and the reticulocyte count is neither strikingly reduced nor increased. Characteristically, both the serum iron values and the TIBC are reduced. Serum iron values may be unmeasurable, and transferrin saturation may be extremely low. A mistaken diagnosis of iron deficiency anemia may be made if overemphasis is placed on the reduced serum iron. A low serum iron and percentage saturation are diagnostic of iron deficiency only when the TIBC is also increased. In contrast to iron deficiency, serum ferritin values should be normal or increased. A serum ferritin value of less than 25 µg/L should suggest coexistent iron deficiency.

Treatment

In most cases no treatment is necessary. In some, however, red blood cell transfusions are required for symptomatic anemia. Purified recombinant erythropoietin has been shown to be safe and effective for treatment of the anemia of renal failure and other secondary anemias such as anemia related to cancer or inflammatory disorders (eg, rheumatoid arthritis). In renal failure, optimal response to erythropoietin requires adequate intensity of dialysis. Erythropoietin is commercially available as epoetin alfa; however, it must be injected subcutaneously three or more times weekly (usual dose 10,000 units) and is very expensive. This agent should be used to alleviate anemia only when the patient is transfusion-dependent or when the quality of life is clearly improved by the hematologic response.

Ifudu O, Feldman J, Friedman EA: The intensity of hemodialysis and the response to erythropoietin in patients with end-stage renal disease. N Engl J Med 1996;334:420.

Krantz SB: Pathogenesis and treatment of the anemia of chronic disease. Am J Med Sci 1994;307:353. (Review of evidence that cytokines directly inhibit erythroid precursor maturation in the bone marrow, erythropoietin action, and erythropoietin production and that, in some cases, anemia can be overcome with administration of recombinant erythropoietin [epoetin alfa].)

Schreiber S et al: Recombinant erythropoietin for the treatment of anemia in inflammatory bowel disease. N Engl J Med 1996;334:619.

THE THALASSEMIAS

Essentials of Diagnosis

- Microcytosis out of proportion to the degree of anemia.

- Positive family history or lifelong personal history of microcytic anemia.
- Abnormal red blood cell morphology with microcytes, acanthocytes, and target cells.
- In beta thalassemia, elevated levels of hemoglobin A_2 or F.

General Considerations

The thalassemias are hereditary disorders characterized by reduction in the synthesis of globin chains (alpha or beta). Reduced globin chain synthesis causes reduced hemoglobin synthesis and eventually produces a hypochromic microcytic anemia because of defective hemoglobinization of red blood cells. Thalassemias can be considered among the hypoproliferative anemias, the hemolytic anemias, and the anemias related to abnormal hemoglobin, since all of these factors may play a role.

Normal adult hemoglobin is primarily hemoglobin A, which represents approximately 98% of circulating hemoglobin. Hemoglobin A is formed from a tetramer—two alpha chains and two beta chains—and can be designated $\alpha_2\beta_2$. Two copies of the α-globin gene are located on chromosome 16, and there is no substitute for α-globin in the formation of hemoglobin. The β-globin gene resides on chromosome 11 adjacent to genes encoding the beta-like globin chains, delta and gamma. The tetramer of $\alpha_2\delta_2$ forms a hemoglobin A_2, which normally comprises 1–2% of adult hemoglobin. The tetramer $\alpha_2\gamma_2$ forms hemoglobin F, which is the major hemoglobin of fetal life but which comprises less than 1% of normal adult hemoglobin.

Alpha thalassemia is due primarily to gene deletion directly causing reduced α-globin chain synthesis (Table 13–4). Since all adult hemoglobins are alpha-containing, alpha thalassemia produces no change in the percentage distribution of hemoglobins A, A_2, and F. In severe forms of alpha thalassemia, excess beta chains may form a β_4 tetramer called hemoglobin H. Hemoglobin H has high oxygen affinity and delivers oxygen to tissues poorly. It is also unstable and subject to oxidative denaturation under conditions of infection or exposure to oxidative drugs (sulfonamides, etc).

Beta thalassemias are usually caused by point mutations rather than large deletions (Table 13–5).

Table 13–4. Alpha thalassemia syndromes.

Alpha Globin Genes	Syndrome	Hematocrit	MCV
4	Normal	Normal	
3	Silent carrier	Normal	
2	Thalassemia minor	32–40%	60–75 fL
1	Hemoglobin H disease	22–32%	60–70 fL
0	Hydrops fetalis		

Table 13–5. Beta thalassemia syndromes.

	Beta Globin Genes	Hgb A	Hgb A$_2$	Hgb F
Normal	Homozygous β	97–99%	1–3%	< 1%
Thalassemia major	Homozygous β^0	0	4–10%	90–96%
	Homozygous β$^+$	0–10%	4–10%	90–96%
Thalassemia intermedia	Homozygous β$^+$ (mild)	0–30%	0–10%	6–100%
Thalassemia minor	Heterozygous β^0	80–95%	4–8%	1–5%
	Heterozygous β$^+$	80–95%	4–8%	1–5%

These mutations result in premature chain termination or in problems with transcription of RNA and ultimately result in reduced or absent β-globin chain synthesis. The molecular defects leading to beta thalassemia are numerous and heterogeneous. Defects that result in absent globin chain expression are termed β^0, whereas defects causing reduced synthesis are termed β$^+$. The reduced β-globin chain synthesis in beta thalassemia results in a relative increase in the percentages of hemoglobins A$_2$ and F compared to hemoglobin A, as the beta-like globins (gamma and delta) substitute for the missing beta chains. In the presence of reduced beta chains, the excess alpha chains are unstable and precipitate, leading to damage to red blood cell membranes. This damage causes marked intramedullary hemolysis (destruction of developing erythroid cells within the bone marrow) as well as hemolysis in the peripheral blood. The bone marrow becomes markedly hyperplastic under the drive of severe anemia and the ineffective erythropoiesis that results from destruction of the developing erythroid cells. This marked expansion of the erythroid element in the bone marrow causes severe bony deformities, osteopenia, and pathologic fractures.

Clinical Findings

A. Symptoms and Signs: The alpha thalassemia syndromes are seen primarily in persons from southeast Asia and China, and, less commonly, in blacks. Normally, adults have four copies of the α-globin chain. When three α-globin genes are present, the patient is hematologically normal and is called a silent carrier. When two α-globin genes are present, the patient is said to have alpha thalassemia trait, one form of thalassemia minor. These patients are clinically normal and have normal life expectancy and performance status. They have a very mild microcytic anemia. When only one α-globin chain is present, the patient has hemoglobin H disease. This is a chronic hemolytic anemia of variable severity (thalassemia minor or intermedia). Physical examination will reveal pallor and splenomegaly. Although affected individuals do not usually require transfusions, they may do so during periods of hemolytic exacerbation caused by infection or other

stresses. When all four α-globin genes are deleted, the affected fetus is stillborn as a result of hydrops fetalis.

Beta thalassemia affects persons of Mediterranean origin (Italian, Greek) and to a lesser extent Chinese, other Asians, and blacks. Patients homozygous for beta thalassemia have the syndrome of thalassemia major. Affected children are normal at birth but during the first year of life develop severe anemia requiring transfusion. Signs of thalassemia typically develop after 6 months of age, because this is the time when hemoglobin synthesis switches from hemoglobin F to hemoglobin A. Numerous clinical problems ensue, including growth failure, bone deformities (abnormal facial structure, pathologic fractures), hepatosplenomegaly, and jaundice. The clinical course has been modified significantly by transfusion therapy. Children with severe thalassemia may grow normally until puberty, when they experience hypogonadism, growth failure, and clinical consequences of iron overload from years of transfusion. The transfusional iron overload (hemosiderosis) results in cardiomyopathy, progressive hepatomegaly, and numerous endocrine dysfunctions. Death from cardiac failure usually occurs between ages 20 and 30.

Patients homozygous for a milder form of beta thalassemia (allowing a higher rate of globin gene synthesis) may have the syndrome of thalassemia intermedia. These patients have chronic hemolytic anemia but usually do not require transfusions except under periods of stress. These patients develop iron overload because of increased gut absorption of iron and periodic transfusion. They survive into adult life but with hepatosplenomegaly and bony deformities.

Patients heterozygous for beta thalassemia have thalassemia minor. These patients have a mild microcytic anemia that is not clinically significant.

Prenatal diagnosis is available for couples at risk of producing a child with one of the severe thalassemia syndromes. Asian couples whose parents on both sides have alpha thalassemia trait are at risk of producing an infant with hydrops fetalis. Mediterranean people (and, less commonly, Chinese or blacks) with two parents heterozygous for beta thalassemia are at risk of producing a homozygous child. Genetic counseling should be offered, and the opportunity for prenatal diagnosis should be discussed.

B. Laboratory Findings:

1. Alpha thalassemia trait–Patients with two α-globin genes have mild anemia, with hematocrits between 28% and 40%. The MCV is strikingly low (60–75 fL) despite the modest degree of anemia, and the red blood count is normal or increased. The peripheral blood smear shows mild abnormalities, including microcytes, hypochromia, occasional target cells, and acanthocytes (cells with irregularly spaced bulbous projections). The reticulocyte count and iron parameters are normal. Hemoglobin electrophoresis will show no increase in the percentage of hemoglobins A_2 or F and no hemoglobin H. Alpha thalassemia trait is usually diagnosed by exclusion in a patient with modest anemia, significant microcytosis, and no elevation of hemoglobins A_2 or F. Definitive diagnosis depends upon hemoglobin gene mapping demonstrating a reduced number of α-globin genes, but this procedure is unnecessary for clinical diagnosis.

2. Hemoglobin H disease–These patients have a variably severe hemolytic anemia, with hematocrits between 22% and 32%. The MCV is strikingly low (69–70 fL). The peripheral blood smear is markedly abnormal, with hypochromia, microcytosis, target cells, and poikilocytosis. The reticulocyte count is elevated. Hemoglobin electrophoresis will show the presence of a fast migrating hemoglobin (hemoglobin H), which comprises 10–40% of the hemoglobin. A peripheral blood smear can be stained with supravital dyes to demonstrate the presence of hemoglobin H.

3. Beta thalassemia minor–Like patients with alpha thalassemia trait, these patients have a modest anemia with hematocrit between 28% and 40%. The MCV ranges from 55 to 75 fL, and the red blood cell count is normal or increased. The peripheral blood smear is mildly abnormal, with hypochromia, microcytosis, and target cells. In contrast to alpha thalassemia, basophilic stippling may be present. The reticulocyte count may be normal or slightly elevated. Hemoglobin electrophoresis (using quantitative techniques) may show an elevation of hemoglobin A_2 to 4–8% and occasional elevations of hemoglobin F to 1–5%.

4. Beta thalassemia major–Beta thalassemia major produces a severe life-threatening anemia, and without transfusion the hematocrit may fall to less than 10%. The peripheral blood smear is bizarre, showing severe poikilocytosis, hypochromia, microcytosis, target cells, basophilic stippling, and nucleated red blood cells. Little or no hemoglobin A is present. Variable amounts of hemoglobin A_2 are seen, and the major hemoglobin present is hemoglobin F.

Differential Diagnosis

Mild forms of thalassemia must be differentiated from iron deficiency. Compared to iron deficiency anemia, patients with thalassemia have a lower MCV, a more normal red blood count, and a more abnormal peripheral blood smear at modest levels of anemia. Iron parameters are normal. The diagnosis of beta thalassemia can be shown by demonstrating increased levels of hemoglobin A_2 (or, less commonly, hemoglobin F), while the diagnosis of alpha thalassemia is made by exclusion. Severe forms of thalassemia may be confused with other hemoglobinopathies. The diagnosis will be made by hemoglobin electrophoresis.

Treatment

Patients with mild thalassemia (alpha thalassemia trait or beta thalassemia minor) are clinically normal and require no treatment. Most importantly, patients with microcytosis should be identified so that they will not be subjected to repeated evaluations for iron deficiency and inappropriately given supplemental iron. Patients with hemoglobin H disease should take folate supplementation and avoid medicinal iron and oxidative drugs such as sulfonamide drugs. They may occasionally need transfusion during pregnancy or under periods of stress. Patients with severe thalassemia should be maintained on a regular transfusion schedule and should receive folate supplementation. Splenectomy is occasionally performed when hypersplenism causes a marked increase in the transfusion requirement. Deferoxamine is routinely given as an iron-chelating agent to avoid or postpone hemosiderosis. Oral iron chelators are now undergoing testing in an investigational setting and may have a major impact. They appear to be effective, but toxicity (agranulocytosis) will limit their general use.

Allogeneic bone marrow transplantation has been introduced as treatment for beta thalassemia major. Children who have not yet experienced iron overload and chronic organ toxicity do well, with long-term survival in more than 80% of cases.

Cao A et al: Clinical experience of management of thalassemia: The Sardinian experience. Semin Hematol 1996;33:66.

Lucarelli G et al: Marrow transplantation for patients with thalassemia: Results in class 3 patients. Blood 1996; 87:2082.

Oliver NF, Brittenham GM: Iron-chelating therapy and the treatment of thalassemia (comprehensive review). Blood 1997;89:739.

Weatherall DJ, Clegg JB: Thalassemia—a global public health problem. Nat Med 1996;2:847.

SIDEROBLASTIC ANEMIA

The sideroblastic anemias are a heterogeneous group of disorders in which hemoglobin synthesis is reduced because of failure to incorporate heme into protoporphyrin to form hemoglobin. Iron accumulates, particularly in the mitochondria. A Prussian blue stain of the bone marrow will reveal ringed sideroblasts, cells with iron deposits (in the mitochondria) encircling the red cell nucleus. The disorder is usually acquired. Sometimes it represents a stage in evolution of a generalized bone marrow disorder (myelodysplasia) that may ultimately terminate in acute leukemia. Other important causes include chronic alcoholism, drug toxicity (antituberculous agents, chloramphenicol), and lead poisoning.

Patients have no specific clinical features other than those related to anemia. The anemia is usually moderate, with hematocrits of 20–30%, but transfusions may occasionally be required. Although the MCV is usually normal or slightly increased, it may occasionally be low, leading to confusion with iron deficiency. The peripheral blood smear characteristically shows a dimorphic population of red blood cells, one normal and one hypochromic. It is the presence of hypochromic cells on peripheral smear combined with a low MCV that may raise the consideration of iron deficiency. In cases of lead poisoning, coarse basophilic stippling of the red cells is seen.

The diagnosis is made by examination of the bone marrow. Characteristically, there is marked erythroid hyperplasia, a sign of ineffective erythropoiesis (expansion of the erythroid compartment of the bone marrow that does not result in the production of reticulocytes in the peripheral blood). The iron stain of the bone marrow shows a generalized increase in iron stores and the presence of ringed sideroblasts. Other characteristic laboratory features include a high serum iron and a high transferrin saturation. In the presence of lead poisoning, serum lead levels will be elevated.

When lead toxicity is causative, it may be treated with chelation therapy. Occasional patients will respond to pharmacologic doses of pyridoxine (200 mg/d), but most patients do not respond to therapy. Anecdotal responses to chloroquine have been reported but require confirmation. Occasionally, the anemia is so severe that support with red cell transfusion is required. These patients usually do not respond to erythropoietin therapy.

Drenou B et al: Treatment of sideroblastic anemia with chloroquine. N Engl J Med 1995;332:614.

VITAMIN B₁₂ DEFICIENCY

Essentials of Diagnosis
- Macrocytic anemia.
- Macro-ovalocytes and hypersegmented neutrophils on peripheral blood smear.
- Serum vitamin B_{12} level less than 100 pg/mL.

General Considerations
Vitamin B_{12} belongs to the family of cobalamins

and serves as a cofactor for two important reactions in humans. As methylcobalamin, it serves as a cofactor for methionine synthetase in the conversion of homocysteine to methionine. As adenosylcobalamin, it serves as a cofactor for the conversion of methylmalonyl-CoA to succinyl-CoA. All vitamin B_{12} comes from the diet, and vitamin B_{12} is present in all foods of animal origin. The daily absorption of vitamin B_{12} is 5 μg.

After being ingested, vitamin B_{12} becomes bound to intrinsic factor, a protein secreted by gastric parietal cells. Other cobalamin-binding proteins (called R factors) compete with intrinsic factor for vitamin B_{12}. Vitamin B_{12} bound to R factors cannot be absorbed. The vitamin B_{12}-intrinsic factor complex travels through the intestine and is absorbed in the terminal ileum by cells with specific receptors for the complex. It is then transported through plasma and stored in the liver. Three plasma transport proteins have been identified. Transcobalamins I and III (differing only in carbohydrate structure) are secreted by white blood cells. Although approximately 90% of plasma vitamin B_{12} circulates bound to these proteins, only transcobalamin II is capable of transporting vitamin B_{12} into cells. The liver contains 2000–5000 μg of stored vitamin B_{12}. Since daily losses are 3–5 μg/d, the body usually has sufficient stores of vitamin B_{12} so that vitamin B_{12} deficiency develops more than 3 years after vitamin B_{12} absorption ceases.

Since vitamin B_{12} is present in all foods of animal origin, dietary vitamin B_{12} deficiency is extremely rare and seen only in vegans—strict vegetarians who avoid all dairy products as well as meat and fish (Table 13–6). Abdominal surgery may lead to vitamin B_{12} deficiency in several ways. Gastrectomy will eliminate that site of intrinsic factor production; blind loop syndrome will cause competition for vitamin B_{12} by bacterial overgrowth in the lumen of the intestine; and surgical resection of the ileum will eliminate the site of vitamin B_{12} absorption. Rare causes of vitamin B_{12} deficiency include fish tapeworm (*Diphyllobothrium latum*) infection, in which the parasite uses luminal vitamin B_{12}, pancreatic in-

Table 13–6. Causes of vitamin B_{12} deficiency.

Dietary deficiency (rare)
Decreased production of intrinsic factor
Pernicious anemia
Gastrectomy
Competition for vitamin B_{12} in gut
Blind loop syndrome
Fish tapeworm (rare)
Pancreatic insufficiency
Decreased ileal absorption of vitamin B_{12}
Surgical resection
Crohn's disease
Transcobalamin II deficiency (rare)

sufficiency (with failure to inactivate competing cobalamin-binding proteins), and severe Crohn's disease, causing sufficient destruction of the ileum to retard vitamin B_{12} absorption.

The most common cause of vitamin B_{12} deficiency is that associated with **pernicious anemia.** This is a hereditary autoimmune disorder historically seen in patients of Scandinavian or northern European ancestry but now increasingly recognized in young black and Hispanic women. Although the disease is hereditary, it is rarely manifested before age 35. Pernicious anemia produces a number of clinical findings in addition to vitamin B_{12} deficiency. Atrophic gastritis is invariably present and results in histamine-fast achlorhydria. These patients may also have a number of other autoimmune diseases, including IgA deficiency, as well as polyglandular endocrine insufficiency. Over time, the atrophic gastritis is associated with an increased risk of gastric carcinoma.

Clinical Findings

A. Symptoms and Signs: The hallmark of vitamin B_{12} deficiency is megaloblastic anemia. The anemia may be severe, with hematocrits as low as 10–15%. The megaloblastic state also produces changes in mucosal cells, leading to glossitis, as well as other vague gastrointestinal disturbances such as anorexia and diarrhea. Vitamin B_{12} deficiency also leads to a complex neurologic syndrome. Peripheral nerves are usually affected first, and patients complain initially of paresthesias. The posterior columns next become impaired, and patients complain of difficulty with balance. In more advanced cases, cerebral function may be altered as well, and on occasion dementia and other neuropsychiatric changes may precede hematologic changes.

On examination, patients are usually pale and may be mildly icteric. Neurologic examination will reveal decreased vibration and position sense.

B. Laboratory Findings: The megaloblastic state produces an anemia of variable severity that on occasion may be very severe. The MCV is usually strikingly elevated, between 110 and 140 fL. However, it is possible to have vitamin B_{12} deficiency with a normal MCV. Occasionally, the normal MCV may be explained by coexistent thalassemia or iron deficiency, but in other cases the reason for the normal MCV is obscure. Patients with neurologic symptoms and signs that suggest possible vitamin B_{12} deficiency should be thoroughly evaluated for the possibility of that deficiency despite a normal MCV and the absence of anemia. The peripheral blood smear is usually strikingly abnormal, with anisocytosis and poikilocytosis. A characteristic finding is the macro-ovalocyte, but numerous other abnormal shapes are usually seen. Because of the strikingly abnormal red blood cell morphology, it is often mistakenly assumed that the anemia is hemolytic. The neu-

trophils are hypersegmented. Typical features include a mean lobe count greater than four or the finding of six-lobed neutrophils. The reticulocyte count is reduced. Because vitamin B_{12} deficiency affects all hematopoietic cell lines, in severe cases the white blood cell count and platelet count are reduced, and pancytopenia is present.

Bone marrow morphology is characteristically abnormal. Marked erythroid hyperplasia is present as a response to defective red blood cell production (ineffective erythropoiesis). Characteristic megaloblastic changes in the erythroid series include abnormally large cell size and asynchronous maturation of the nucleus and cytoplasm—ie, cytoplasmic maturation continues while impaired DNA synthesis causes retarded nuclear development. In the myeloid series, giant metamyelocytes are characteristically seen.

Other laboratory abnormalities include elevated serum LDH and a modest increase in indirect bilirubin. These two findings are a reflection of intramedullary destruction of developing abnormal erythroid cells.

The diagnosis of vitamin B_{12} deficiency is made by finding an abnormally low vitamin B_{12} serum level. Whereas the normal vitamin B_{12} level is 150–350 pg/mL, most patients with overt vitamin B_{12} deficiency will have serum levels less than 100 pg/mL. The Schilling test is used to document the decreased absorption of oral vitamin B_{12} characteristic of pernicious anemia. Initially, a large intramuscular dose of vitamin B_{12} is given to saturate plasma transport proteins. Radiolabeled vitamin B_{12} is given orally, and a 24-hour urine collection is performed to determine how much vitamin B_{12} is absorbed and subsequently excreted. Normally, more than 7% of an administered dose is present in the urine; most patients with impaired absorption will have less than 3% of the dose present in the urine. The second stage of the Schilling test is to administer radiolabeled vitamin B_{12} together with intrinsic factor. If pernicious anemia (a lack of intrinsic factor) is the cause of vitamin B_{12} deficiency, the combined use of vitamin B_{12} and intrinsic factor should correct the abnormally low absorption. However, the full-blown megaloblastic state causes abnormalities in intestinal epithelium that may lead to generalized malabsorption. In these cases, the second stage of the Schilling test will remain abnormal until the intestinal mucosal defect is first corrected by vitamin B_{12} replacement (in approximately 2 months). The repeat evaluation should thus be deferred until there has been time for correction. If the deficiency is caused by bacterial overgrowth in a blind loop, a course of antibiotics will reverse the abnormal second stage of the Schilling test. If the cause of the deficiency is pancreatic insufficiency, a course of pancreatic enzymes will reverse the abnormality. If a tapeworm is the cause, an anthelmintic agent is indicated.

Differential Diagnosis

Vitamin B_{12} deficiency should be differentiated from folic acid deficiency, the other common cause of megaloblastic anemia, in which red blood cell folate is low while vitamin B_{12} levels are normal. The distinction between vitamin B_{12} deficiency and myelodysplasia (the other common cause of macrocytic anemia with abnormal morphology) is based on the characteristic morphology and the low vitamin B_{12} level.

It should be emphasized that any neurologic symptoms or signs suggestive of vitamin B_{12} deficiency should be evaluated for that disorder even in the absence of anemia or macrocytosis.

Treatment

Patients with pernicious anemia are generally treated with parenteral therapy. Intramuscular injections of 100 µg of vitamin B_{12} are adequate for each dose. Replacement is usually given daily for the first week, weekly for the first month, and then monthly for life. It should be stressed that pernicious anemia is a lifelong disorder and that if patients discontinue their monthly therapy, the vitamin deficiency will recur. In some cases, oral cobalamin in high doses (1000 µg/d) can replace parenteral therapy but must be daily and continuous.

Patients respond to therapy with an immediate improvement in their sense of well-being. Hypokalemia may complicate the first several days of therapy, particularly if the anemia is severe. A brisk reticulocytosis occurs in 5–7 days, and the hematologic picture normalizes in 2 months. Central nervous system symptoms and signs are reversible if they are of relatively short duration (less than 6 months), but they may be permanent if treatment is not initiated promptly.

Green R: Screening for vitamin B_{12} deficiency: Caveat emptor. (Editorial and comment.) Ann Intern Med 1996;124:509.

Schilling RE, Williams WJ: Vitamin B_{12} deficiency: Underdiagnosed, overtreated? Hosp Pract (Off Ed) 1995 Jul;30:47.

Sumner AE et al: Elevated methylmalonic acid and total homocysteine levels show high prevalence of vitamin B_{12} deficiency after gastric surgery. Ann Intern Med 1996;124:467.

Swain R: An update of vitamin B_{12} metabolism and deficiency states. J Fam Pract 1995;41:595.

FOLIC ACID DEFICIENCY

Essentials of Diagnosis

- Macrocytic anemia.
- Macro-ovalocytes and hypersegmented neutrophils on peripheral blood smear.
- Normal serum vitamin B_{12} levels.
- Reduced folate levels in red blood cells or serum.

General Considerations

Folic acid is the term commonly used for pteroylmonoglutamic acid. In its reduced form of tetrahydrofolate, it serves as an important mediator of many reactions involving one-carbon transfers. Important reactions include the conversion of homocysteine to methionine and of deoxyuridylate to thymidylate, an important step in DNA synthesis.

Folic acid is present in most fruits and vegetables (especially citrus fruits and green leafy vegetables) and daily requirements of 50–100 µg/d are usually met in the diet. Total body stores of folate are approximately 5000 µg, enough to supply requirements for 2–3 months.

By far the most common cause of folate deficiency is inadequate dietary intake (Table 13–7). Alcoholics, anorectic patients, elderly persons who do not eat fresh fruits and vegetables, and persons who overcook their food are candidates for folate deficiency. Reduced folate absorption is rarely seen, since absorption occurs from the entire gastrointestinal tract. However, drugs such as phenytoin, trimethoprim-sulfamethoxazole, or sulfasalazine may interfere with folate absorption. Folic acid requirements are increased in pregnancy, hemolytic anemia, and exfoliative skin disease, and in these cases the increased requirements (five to ten times normal) may not be met by a normal diet. Patients with increased folate requirements should receive supplementation with 1 mg/d of folic acid.

Clinical Findings

A. Symptoms and Signs: The clinical features are similar to those of vitamin B_{12} deficiency, with megaloblastic anemia and megaloblastic changes in mucosa. However, there are none of the neurologic abnormalities associated with vitamin B_{12} deficiency.

B. Laboratory Findings: The megaloblastic anemia is identical to that resulting from vitamin B_{12} deficiency (see above). However, the serum vitamin B_{12} level is normal. In contrast, the serum folic acid level is low, usually less than 3 ng/mL. The red blood cell folate level is more reliable and has replaced serum folate as the appropriate test. A red

Table 13–7. Causes of folate deficiency.

Dietary deficiency
Decreased absorption
  Tropical sprue
  Drugs: Phenytoin, sulfasalazine, trimethoprim-sulfamethoxazole
Increased requirement
  Chronic hemolytic anemia
  Pregnancy
  Exfoliative skin disease
Loss: Dialysis
Inhibition of reduction to active form
  Methotrexate

blood cell folate level of less than 150 ng/mL is diagnostic of folate deficiency.

Differential Diagnosis

The megaloblastic anemia of folate deficiency should be differentiated from vitamin B_{12} deficiency by the finding of a normal vitamin B_{12} level and a reduced red blood cell folate or serum folate level. Alcoholics, who often have folate deficiency, may also have anemia of liver disease. This latter macrocytic anemia does not cause megaloblastic morphologic changes but rather produces target cells in the peripheral blood. Patients with HIV-related illnesses being treated with zidovudine frequently develop macrocytosis but do not manifest typical megaloblastic morphology. Hypothyroidism is also associated with mild macrocytosis.

Treatment

Folic acid deficiency is treated with folic acid, 1 mg/d orally. The response is similar to that seen in the treatment of vitamin B_{12} deficiency, with rapid improvement and a sense of well-being, reticulocytosis in 5–7 days, and total correction of hematologic abnormalities within 2 months. Large doses of folic acid may produce hematologic responses in cases of vitamin B_{12} deficiency but will allow neurologic damage to progress.

Hercberg S, Galan P: Nutritional anaemias. Baillieres Clin Haematol 1992;5:143. (Discusses iron and folate requirements, intake and assessment of deficiency in different populations.)

PURE RED CELL APLASIA

Adult acquired pure red cell aplasia is extremely rare. It appears to be an autoimmune disease in which an IgG antibody specifically attacks erythroid precursors. A congenital form (Diamond-Blackfan syndrome) has been identified. In adults, the disease is usually idiopathic. However, cases have been seen in association with systemic lupus erythematosus, chronic lymphocytic leukemia, lymphomas, or thymoma. Some drugs (phenytoin, chloramphenicol) may cause red cell aplasia. Transient episodes of red cell aplasia are probably common in response to viral infections, especially parvovirus infections, but also in viral hepatitis. However, these acute episodes will go unrecognized unless the patient has a chronic hemolytic disorder, in which case the hematocrit may fall precipitously.

Clinically, the only signs are those of anemia, unless the patient has an associated autoimmune or lymphoproliferative disorder. The anemia is often severe and is normochromic. Reticulocytes are very low or absent. Red blood cell morphology is normal, and the myeloid and platelet lines are unaffected. The bone marrow is normocellular. All elements present are normal, but erythroid precursors are markedly reduced or absent. In some cases, chest imaging studies will reveal a thymoma.

The disorder should be distinguished from aplastic anemia (in which the marrow is generally hypocellular and other cell lines are affected) and from myelodysplasia. This latter disorder is recognized by the presence of morphologic abnormalities that should not be present in pure red cell aplasia.

Possible offending drugs should be stopped. If a thymoma is present, resection results in amelioration of anemia in some instances. In cases associated with autoimmune disorders, immunosuppressive treatment with cyclophosphamide or prednisone (or both) is indicated. High-dose intravenous immune globulin has produced excellent responses in a small number of cases, especially in parvovirus-related cases. The duration of response remains to be determined, and more experience is needed before this treatment can be generally recommended. For most cases, the treatment of choice is immunosuppressive therapy with a combination of antithymocyte globulin and cyclosporine—similar to therapy of aplastic anemia.

Casadevall N et al: Autoantibodies against erythropoietin in a patient with pure red-cell aplasia. N Engl J Med 1996;334:630.
Charles RJ et al: The pathophysiology of pure red cell aplasia: Implications for therapy. Blood 1996;87:4831.
Lacy MQ, Kurtin PJ, Tefferi A: Pure red cell aplasia: Association with large granular lymphocyte leukemia and the prognostic value of cytogenetic abnormalities. Blood 1996;87:3000.

HEMOLYTIC ANEMIAS

The hemolytic anemias are a group of disorders in which red blood cell survival is reduced, either episodically or continuously. The bone marrow has the ability to increase erythroid production up to eightfold in response to reduced red cell survival, so anemia will be present only when the ability of the bone marrow to compensate is outstripped. This will occur when red cell survival is extremely short or when the ability of the bone marrow to compensate is impaired for some second reason.

Since red blood cell survival is normally 120 days, in the absence of red cell production the hematocrit will fall at the rate of approximately 1/100 of the hematocrit per day, which translates to a decrease in the hematocrit reading of approximately 3% per week. For example, a fall of hematocrit from 45% to 36% over 3 weeks' time need not indicate hemolysis, since this rate of fall would result simply from cessation of red blood cell production. If the hematocrit is falling at a faster rate than that due to decreased production, blood loss or hemolysis is the cause.

Reticulocytosis is an important clue to the presence of hemolysis, since in most hemolytic disorders the bone marrow will respond with increased red blood cell production. However, hemolysis can be present without reticulocytosis when a second disorder (infection, folate deficiency) is superimposed on hemolysis; in these circumstances, the hematocrit will fall rapidly. However, reticulocytosis also occurs during recovery from hypoproliferative anemia or bleeding. Hemolysis is correctly diagnosed (when bleeding is excluded) when the hematocrit is either falling or stable despite reticulocytosis.

Hemolytic disorders are generally classified according to whether the defect is intrinsic to the red cell or due to some external factor (Table 13–8). Intrinsic defects have been described in all components of the red blood cell, including the membrane, glycolytic and other enzymes, and hemoglobin. Most of these disorders are hereditary. The vast majority of hemolytic anemias due to external factors arc the immune hemolytic anemias.

Certain laboratory features are common to all the hemolytic anemias. Haptoglobin, a normal plasma protein that binds and clears hemoglobin released into plasma, may be depressed in hemolytic disorders. However, haptoglobin levels are influenced by many factors and, by themselves, are not a reliable indicator of hemolysis. When intravascular hemolysis occurs, transient hemoglobinemia occurs. Hemoglobin is filtered through the glomerulus and usually reabsorbed by tubular cells. Hemoglobinuria will be present only when the capacity for reabsorption of hemoglobin by these cells is exceeded. In the absence of hemoglobinuria, evidence for prior intravascular hemolysis is the presence of hemosiderin in shed renal tubular cells (positive urine hemosiderin). With severe intravascular hemolysis, hemoglobinemia and methemalbuminemia may be present. Hemolysis increases the indirect bilirubin, and the total bilirubin may rise to as high as 4 mg/dL. Bilirubin

levels higher than this indicate some degree of hepatic dysfunction. Serum LDH levels are strikingly elevated in cases of microangiopathic hemolysis (thrombotic thrombocytopenic purpura, hemolytic-uremic syndrome) and may be elevated in other hemolytic anemias. Iron levels are usually not affected by hemolysis, since the iron from sequestered red cells is recycled through the reticuloendothelial system. Only causes of intravascular hemolysis will lead to iron deficiency due to hemoglobinemia.

Diehl LF, Bolan CD, Weiss RB: Hemolytic anemia and cancer. Cancer Treat Rev 1996;22:33.

HEREDITARY SPHEROCYTOSIS

Essentials of Diagnosis
- Positive family history.
- Splenomegaly.
- Spherocytes and increased reticulocytes on peripheral blood smear.
- Negative Coombs test.

General Considerations
Hereditary spherocytosis is a disorder of the red blood cell membrane, leading to chronic hemolytic anemia. Normally, the red blood cell is a biconcave disk with a diameter of 7–8 μm. The red blood cells must be both strong and deformable—strong to withstand the stress of circulating for 120 days and deformable so as to pass through capillaries 3 μm in diameter and splenic fenestrations in the cords of the red pulp of approximately 2 μm. The red blood cell skeleton, made up primarily of the proteins spectrin and actin, gives the red cells these characteristics of strength and deformability.

The membrane defect in hereditary spherocytosis has not been defined but is most likely an abnormality in spectrin, the protein providing most of the scaffolding for the red blood cell membranes. The result is a decrease in surface-to-volume ratio that results in a spherical shape of the cell. These spherical cells are less deformable and unable to pass through 2-μm fenestrations in the splenic red pulp. Hemolysis takes place because of trapping of red blood cells within the spleen.

Clinical Findings
A. Symptoms and Signs: Hereditary spherocytosis is an autosomal dominant disease of variable severity. It is often diagnosed during childhood, but milder cases may be discovered incidentally late in adult life. Anemia may or may not be present, since the bone marrow may be able to compensate for shortened red cell survival. Severe anemia (aplastic crisis) may occur when bone marrow compensation is impaired by infection or folate deficiency. Chronic hemolysis may cause jaundice and pigment (calcium

---

Table 13–8. Classification of hemolytic anemias.

Intrinsic
  Membrane defects: Hereditary spherocytosis, hereditary elliptocytosis, paroxysmal nocturnal hemoglobinuria
  Glycolytic defects: Pyruvate kinase deficiency, severe hypophosphatemia
  Oxidation vulnerability: G6PD deficiency, methemoglobinemia
  Hemoglobinopathies: Sickle syndromes, unstable hemoglobins, methemoglobinemia

Extrinsic
  Immune: Autoimmune, lymphoproliferative disease, drug toxicity
  Microangiopathic: Thrombotic thrombocytopenic purpura, hemolytic-uremic syndrome, disseminated intravascular coagulation, valve hemolysis, metastatic adenocarcinoma, vasculitis
  Infection: *Plasmodium, Clostridium, Borrelia*
  Hypersplenism
  Burns

binate) gallstones, leading to attacks of chole-cystitis. Examination may reveal icterus and a palpable spleen.

B. Laboratory Findings: The anemia is of variable severity, and the hematocrit may be normal. Reticulocytosis is always present. The peripheral blood smear shows the presence of spherocytes, small cells that have lost their central pallor. Spherocytes usually make up only a small percentage of red blood cells on the peripheral smear. Hereditary spherocytosis is the only important disorder associated with increased MCHC, often greater than 36 g/dL. As with other hemolytic disorders, there may be an increase in indirect bilirubin. The Coombs test is negative.

The presence of spherocytes may be confirmed by the osmotic fragility test. Spherocytes are red cells that have lost some membrane surface and are abnormally vulnerable to swelling induced by hypotonic media. Increased osmotic fragility merely reflects the presence of spherocytes and does not distinguish hereditary spherocytosis from other spherocytic hemolytic disorders such as autoimmune hemolytic anemia.

Treatment

These patients should receive uninterrupted supplementation with folic acid, 1 mg/d. The treatment of choice is splenectomy, which will not correct the membrane defect or correct the spherocytosis but will eliminate the site of hemolysis. In very mild cases discovered late in adult life, splenectomy may not be necessary.

Cynober T, Mohandas N, Tchernia G: Red cell abnormalities in hereditary spherocytosis: Relevance to diagnosis and understanding of the variable expression of clinical severity. J Lab Clin Med 1996;128:259.

Hassoun H et al: Hereditary spherocytosis with spectrin deficiency due to an unstable truncated beta spectrin. Blood 1996;87:2538.

Shilling RF: Estimating the risk for sepsis after splenectomy in hereditary spherocytosis. Ann Intern Med 1995;122:187.

HEREDITARY ELLIPTOCYTOSIS

Hereditary elliptocytosis is a congenital disorder of the red blood cell membrane and probably is due to abnormalities in spectrin tetramer formation. The disorder is autosomal dominant and of variable severity. In the most common form of hereditary elliptocytosis, the mild hemolytic disorder is well compensated, and there is little or no anemia. However, more severe varieties do produce anemia, splenomegaly, and pigment (calcium bilirubinate) gallstones.

In the common mild variety, the hallmark of the disorder is the elliptical shape of the majority of red blood cells on peripheral blood smear. Reticulocytosis may be present. In the rare severe varieties of the disorder (hereditary pyropoikilocytosis), the periph-

eral blood smear is extremely bizarre; and in addition to elliptocytes, microspherocytes and a variety of unusually shaped red cells are present.

No treatment is usually indicated. Severe variants are treated with splenectomy and folate supplementation.

Gallagher PG et al: Molecular basis and haplotyping of the alpha II domain polymorphisms of spectrin: Application to the study of hereditary elliptocytosis and pyropoikilocytosis. Am J Hum Genet 1996;59:351.

PAROXYSMAL NOCTURNAL HEMOGLOBINURIA

Paroxysmal nocturnal hemoglobinuria is an acquired clonal stem cell disorder that results in abnormal sensitivity of the red blood cell membrane to lysis by complement. The defect involves both increased binding of C3b and increased vulnerability to lysis by complement, and is expressed as a deficiency in proteins normally linked to the cell by phosphoinositol. Paroxysmal nocturnal hemoglobinuria is a very rare disorder and should be suspected in confusing cases of hemolytic anemia.

The best screening test for paroxysmal nocturnal hemoglobinuria is the sucrose hemolysis test. The diagnosis can be confirmed by Ham's (acidified serum) test. Flow cytometric assays for CD59 (deficient in paroxysmal nocturnal hemoglobinuria cells) may come to replace these tests.

Clinical Findings

A. Symptoms and Signs: The anemia is of variable severity and may be severe. Classically, patients report episodic hemoglobinuria resulting in reddish brown urine. Hemoglobinuria may be present in the first morning urine, since the mild respiratory acidosis of sleep leads to enhanced complement activity. In addition to anemia, these patients are prone to thrombosis, especially mesenteric and hepatic vein thromboses. The reason for thrombus formation is unclear but may be related to platelet activation by complement. As this is a stem cell disorder, paroxysmal nocturnal hemoglobinuria may progress either to aplastic anemia or to acute myelogenous leukemia.

B. Laboratory Findings: Anemia is of variable severity, and reticulocytosis may or may not be present. Abnormalities on the blood smear are nondiagnostic and may include macro-ovalocytes. As with other hemolytic disorders, haptoglobin may be decreased or absent. Since the episodic hemolysis in paroxysmal nocturnal hemoglobinuria is intravascular, the finding of urine hemosiderin is a useful test. Serum LDH is characteristically elevated. Iron deficiency is commonly present and is related to chronic iron loss from hemoglobinuria, since hemolysis is primarily intravascular.

The white blood cell count and platelet count may

be decreased. A decreased leukocyte alkaline phosphatase—evidence for qualitative abnormality in the myeloid series—is good evidence for paroxysmal nocturnal hemoglobinuria. Bone marrow morphology is variable and may show either hypoplasia or erythroid hyperplasia.

Research laboratories may be helpful in confirming the disorder by functional and antigenic assays.

Treatment

Iron replacement is often indicated for treatment of iron deficiency. This may improve the anemia but may also cause a transient increase in hemolysis. For unclear reasons, prednisone is effective in decreasing hemolysis, and some patients can be managed effectively with alternate-day steroids. In severe cases, allogeneic bone marrow transplantation has been used to correct the disorder.

Hall SE, Rosse WF: The use of monoclonal antibodies and flow cytometry in the diagnosis of paroxysmal nocturnal hemoglobinuria. Blood 1996;87:5332.

Hillmen P et al: Natural history of paroxysmal nocturnal hemoglobinuria. N Engl J Med 1995;333:1253.

Kinoshita T, Inoue N, Takeda J: Role of phosphatidylinositol-linked proteins in paroxysmal nocturnal hemoglobinuria pathogenesis. Annu Rev Med 1996;47:1.

Posse WF, Waire RE: The molecular basis of paroxysmal nocturnal hemoglobinuria. Blood 1995;86:3277.

PYRUVATE KINASE DEFICIENCY

The red blood cell obtains 90% of its energy from anaerobic glycolysis. Defects in glycolytic enzymes produce a chronic hemolytic anemia because of depletion of ATP. Severe hypophosphatemia may result in hemolysis for the same reason.

Pyruvate kinase deficiency is a very rare autosomal recessive disorder that causes chronic hemolytic anemia, usually with onset in childhood. In addition to the anemia, splenomegaly and pigment gallstones may be present. The red blood cell smear is normal, and the diagnosis is made by specific enzyme assays available only in specialized laboratories. Splenectomy is the treatment of choice.

Miwa S et al: Pyruvate kinase deficiency: Historical perspective and recent progress of molecular genetics. Am J Hematol 1993;42:31. (Detailed report of genetic variations in pyruvate kinase genes and their enzymatic characteristics.)

GLUCOSE-6-PHOSPHATE DEHYDROGENASE DEFICIENCY

Essentials of Diagnosis

- X-linked recessive disorder seen commonly in American black men.
- Episodic hemolysis in response to oxidant drugs or infection.
- Minimally abnormal peripheral blood smear.
- Reduced levels of G6PD between hemolytic episodes.

General Considerations

Glucose-6-phosphate dehydrogenase (G6PD) deficiency is a hereditary enzyme defect that causes episodic hemolytic anemia because of decreased ability of red blood cells to deal with oxidative stresses. The hexose monophosphate shunt is not an important source of energy generation in red cells but is important in generating reduced glutathione, which protects hemoglobin from oxidative denaturation. The first step in this pathway is the generation of NADPH by the action of G6PD on glucose 6-phosphate. NADPH serves as a cofactor for glutathione reductase in generating reduced glutathione, which detoxifies hydrogen peroxide. In the absence of reduced glutathione, hemoglobin may become oxidized. Oxidized hemoglobin denatures and forms precipitants called Heinz bodies. These Heinz bodies cause membrane damage, which leads to removal of these cells by the spleen.

Numerous types of G6PD enzymes have been described. The normal type found in Caucasians is designated G6PD-B. Most American blacks have G6PD-A, which is normal in function. Ten to 15 percent of American blacks have the variant G6PD designated A⁻, in which there is only 15% of normal enzyme activity, and enzyme activity declines rapidly as the red blood cell ages past 40 days, a fact that explains many of the clinical findings in this disorder. Many other G6PD variants have been described, including some Mediterranean variants with extremely low enzyme activity.

Clinical Findings

G6PD deficiency is an X-linked recessive disorder affecting 10–15% of American black males. Female carriers are rarely affected—only when an unusually high percentage of cells producing the normal enzyme are inactivated.

A. Symptoms and Signs: Patients are usually healthy, without chronic hemolytic anemia or splenomegaly. Hemolysis occurs as a result of oxidative stress on the red blood cells, generated either by infection or exposure to certain drugs. Common drugs initiating hemolysis include dapsone, primaquine, quinidine, quinine, sulfonamides, and nitrofurantoin. When hemolysis occurs, the patient may become jaundiced and have dark urine. Even with continuous use of the offending drug, the hemolytic episode is self-limited because older red blood cells (with low enzyme activity) are removed and replaced with a population of young red blood cells with adequate functional levels of G6PD.

Severe G6PD deficiency (as in Mediterranean

variants) may produce a chronic hemolytic anemia, and hemolytic crises may be severe or even fatal.

B. Laboratory Findings: Between hemolytic episodes, the blood is normal. During episodes of hemolysis, there is reticulocytosis and increased serum indirect bilirubin. The red blood cell smear is not diagnostic but may reveal a small number of "bite" cells—cells that appear to have had a bite taken out of their periphery. This in fact indicates pitting of hemoglobin aggregates by the spleen. Heinz bodies may be demonstrated by staining a peripheral blood smear with crystal violet. (They are not visible on the usual Wright-stained blood smear.) Specific enzyme assays for G6PD may reveal a low level. Results for G6PD assays may be misleading if they are performed shortly after a hemolytic episode when the enzyme-deficient cohort of cells has been removed and replaced with a young cohort with nearly normal enzyme activity. In these cases, the enzyme assays should be repeated weeks after hemolysis has resolved. In severe cases of G6PD deficiency, enzyme levels are always low.

Treatment

No treatment is necessary except to avoid known oxidant drugs.

Beutler E: G6PD deficiency. Blood. 1994;84:3613. (Clinical manifestations, genetics, and treatment.)

Chang JG, Liu TC: Glucose-6-phosphate dehydrogenase deficiency. Crit Rev Oncol Hematol 1995;20:1.

SICKLE CELL ANEMIA & RELATED SYNDROMES

Essentials of Diagnosis

- Irreversibly sickled cells on peripheral blood smear.
- Positive family history and lifelong history of hemolytic anemia.
- Recurrent painful episodes.
- Hemoglobin S is the major hemoglobin seen on electrophoresis.

General Considerations

Sickle cell anemia is an autosomal recessive disorder in which an abnormal hemoglobin (hemoglobinopathy) leads to chronic hemolytic anemia with a variety of severe clinical consequences. The disorder is a classic example of disease caused by a point mutation in DNA. A single DNA base change leads to an amino acid substitution of valine for glutamine in the sixth position on the β-globin chain. The abnormal beta chain is designated β^s and the tetramer of $\alpha_2\beta^s_2$ is designated hemoglobin S.

When in the deoxy form, hemoglobin S forms polymers that damage the red blood cell membrane. Both polymer formation and early membrane damage are reversible. However, red blood cells that have undergone repeated sickling are damaged beyond repair and become irreversibly sickled cells.

The rate of sickling is influenced by a number of factors, most importantly by the concentration of hemoglobin S in the individual red blood cell. Red cell dehydration makes the cell quite vulnerable to sickling. Sickling is also strongly influenced by the presence of other hemoglobins within the cell. Hemoglobin F cannot participate in polymer formation, and its presence markedly retards sickling. Other factors that increase sickling are those which lead to formation of deoxyhemoglobin S, eg, acidosis and hypoxemia, either systemic or locally in tissues.

Prenatal diagnosis is now available for couples at risk of producing a child with sickle cell anemia. DNA from fetal cells can be directly examined, and the presence of the sickle cell mutation can be accurately and definitively diagnosed. Genetic counseling should be made available to such couples.

Clinical Findings

A. Symptoms and Signs: The hemoglobin S gene is carried in 8% of American blacks, and one birth out of 400 in American blacks will produce a child with sickle cell anemia. The disorder has its onset during the first year of life, when hemoglobin F levels fall as a signal (of unknown nature) is sent to the bone marrow to switch from γ-globin to β-globin production.

Chronic hemolytic anemia produces jaundice, pigment (calcium bilirubinate) gallstones, splenomegaly, and poorly healing ulcers over the lower tibia. The chronic anemia may become life-threatening when severe anemia is produced by hemolytic or aplastic crises. Aplastic crises occur when the ability of the bone marrow to compensate is reduced by viral or other infection or by folate deficiency. Hemolytic crises may be related to splenic sequestration of sickled cells (primarily in childhood, before the spleen has been infarcted) or with coexistent disorders such as G6PD deficiency.

Acute painful episodes due to acute vaso-occlusion may occur spontaneously or be provoked by infection, dehydration, or hypoxia. Clusters of sickled red cells occlude the microvasculature of the organs involved. These episodes last hours to days and produce acute pain and low-grade fever. Common sites of acute painful episodes include the bones (especially the back and long bones) and the chest. Acute vaso-occlusion may also cause strokes and priapism. Vaso-occlusive episodes are not associated with increased hemolysis.

Repeated episodes of vascular occlusion affect a large number of organs, especially the heart and liver. Ischemic necrosis of bone occurs, rendering the bone susceptible to osteomyelitis due to staphylococci or (less commonly) salmonellae. In adult life, the spleen is infarcted. Infarction of the papillae of the renal medulla causes renal tubular concentrating defects and gross hematuria. Retinopathy is often present and may lead to blindness.

These patients are prone to delayed puberty and may rarely have an increased incidence of infection. Infections are related to hyposplenism as well as to defects in the alternative pathway of complement.

On examination, patients are often chronically ill and jaundiced. There is hepatomegaly, but the spleen is not palpable in adult life. The heart is enlarged, with a hyperdynamic precordium and systolic murmurs. Nonhealing ulcers of the lower leg and retinopathy may be present.

Sickle cell anemia becomes a chronic multisystem disease, with death from organ failure. With improved supportive care, average life expectancy is now between ages 40 and 50.

B. Laboratory Findings: Chronic hemolytic anemia is present. The hematocrit is usually 20–30%. The peripheral blood smear is characteristically abnormal, with irreversibly sickled cells comprising 5–50% of red cells. Other findings include reticulocytosis (10–25%), nucleated red blood cells, and hallmarks of hyposplenism such as Howell-Jolly bodies and target cells. The white blood cell count is characteristically elevated to 12,000–15,000/µL, and thrombocytosis may occur. Indirect bilirubin levels are high and haptoglobin is absent.

Most clinical laboratories offer a screening test for sickle cell hemoglobin, and the diagnosis of sickle cell anemia is then confirmed by hemoglobin electrophoresis (Table 13–9). Hemoglobin S has an abnormal migration pattern on electrophoresis and will usually comprise 85–98% of hemoglobin. In homozygous S disease, no hemoglobin A will be present. Hemoglobin F levels are variably increased, and high hemoglobin F levels are associated with a more benign clinical course.

Treatment

No specific treatment is available for the primary disease. However, both longevity and quality of life may be improved by comprehensive medical management by a concerned physician. Patients are maintained chronically on folic acid supplementation and should not routinely be given transfusions. Transfusions are indicated for aplastic or hemolytic crises and during the third trimester of pregnancy.

When acute painful episodes occur, precipitating factors should be identified and infections treated if present. The patient should be kept well hydrated, and oxygen should be given if the patient is hypoxic. Otherwise, treatment is supportive (hydration and analgesics).

Acute vaso-occlusive crises can be treated with exchange transfusion. Exchange transfusions are primarily indicated for the treatment of intractable crises, priapism, and stroke and as a preventive measure for patients undergoing general anesthesia. Hypertransfusion should be avoided because of the potential for further sickling by oxygen steal by the transfused red cells from those that are sickled.

Cytotoxic agents such as hydroxyurea have been shown to increase hemoglobin F levels (by stimulating erythropoiesis in more primitive erythroid precursors). Clinical trials have established the effectiveness of hydroxyurea (500–750 mg/d) in reducing the frequency of painful crises. This therapy is now indicated in patients whose quality of life is disrupted by frequent pain crises, but long-term safety is uncertain and there remains concern about the potential of causing secondary malignancies. Allogeneic bone marrow transplantation is being studied as a possible curative option for severely affected young patients.

[AHCPR guideline on sickle cell disease]
  http://text.nlm.nih.gov/ftrs/dbaccess/scdc
Bellet PS, Kalinyak KA, Shukla R: Incentive spirometry to prevent acute pulmonary complications in sickle cell diseases. N Engl J Med 1995;333;699.
Charache E et al: Effect of hydroxyurea on the frequency of painful crises in sickle cell anemia. Investigators of the Multicenter Study of Hydroxyurea in Sickle Cell Anemia. N Engl J Med 1995;332:1317.
Claster S, Vichinsky E: First report of reversal of organ dysfunction in sickle cell anemia by the use of hydroxyurea: Splenic regeneration. Blood 1996;88:1951.
Embury SH: New treatments of sickle cell disease. West J Med 1996;164:444.
Haberkorn CM et al: Cholecystectomy in sickle cell anemia patients: Perioperative outcome of 364 cases from the National Preoperative Transfusion Study. Blood 1997; 89:1533.
Lane PA: Sickle cell disease. Pediatr Clin North Am 1996;43:639.
Vichinsky EP et al: Acute chest syndrome in sickle cell disease: Clinical presentation and course. Blood 1997; 89:1787.

Table 13–9. Hemoglobin distribution in sickle cell syndromes.

Genotype	Clinical Diagnosis	Hgb A	Hgb S	Hgb A$_2$	Hgb F
AA	Normal	97–99%	0	1–2%	< 1%
AS	Sickle trait	60%	40%	1–2%	< 1%
SS	Sickle cell anemia	0	85–98%	1–3%	5–15%
Sβ^0 thalassemia	Sickle β thalassemia	0	70–80%	3–5%	10–20%
Sβ$^+$ thalassemia	Sickle β thalassemia	10–20%	60–75%	3–5%	10–20%
AS, α thalassemia	Sickle trait	70–75%	25–30%	1–2%	< 1%

Walters MC et al: Bone marrow transplantation for sickle cell disease. N Engl J Med 1996;335:369.

SICKLE CELL TRAIT

Patients with the heterozygous genotype (AS) have sickle cell trait. These persons are clinically normal and have acute painful episodes only under extreme conditions such as vigorous exertion at high altitudes (or in unpressurized aircraft). The patients are hematologically normal, with no anemia and normal red blood cells on peripheral blood smear. They may, however, have a defect in renal tubular function, causing an inability to concentrate the urine, and experience episodes of gross hematuria. A screening test for sickle hemoglobin will be positive, and hemoglobin electrophoresis will reveal that approximately 40% of hemoglobin is hemoglobin S (Table 13–9).

No treatment is necessary. These patients should be considered normal in all respects.

Brewer GJ: Risks in sickle cell trait. J Lab Clin Med 1993;122:354.

SICKLE THALASSEMIA

Patients with homozygous sickle cell anemia and alpha thalassemia have a somewhat milder form of hemolysis because of a slower rate of sickling related to reduced hemoglobin concentration (MCHC) within the red blood cell.

Patients who are double heterozygotes for sickle cell anemia and beta thalassemia are clinically affected with sickle cell syndromes. Sickle β^0 thalassemia is clinically very similar to homozygous SS disease. Vaso-occlusive crises may be somewhat less severe, and the spleen is usually not infarcted. Hematologically, the MCV is usually low—in contrast to the normal MCV of sickle cell anemia—and the smear usually reveals fewer irreversibly sickled cells. Hemoglobin electrophoresis (Table 13–9) reveals no hemoglobin A but will show an increase in hemoglobin A_2 which is not present in sickle cell anemia.

Sickle β^+ thalassemia is a milder disorder than homozygous SS disease, with fewer crises. The spleen is usually palpable. The hemolytic anemia is less severe, and the hematocrit is usually 30–38%, with reticulocytes of 5–10%. Hemoglobin electrophoresis shows the presence of some hemoglobin A.

HEMOGLOBIN C DISORDERS

Hemoglobin C is formed by a single amino acid substitution at the same site of substitution as in sickle hemoglobin but with lysine instead of valine substituted for glutamine at the β_6 position. Hemoglobin C is nonsickling but may participate in polymer formation in association with hemoglobin S. Homozygous hemoglobin C disease produces a mild hemolytic anemia with splenomegaly, mild jaundice, and pigment (calcium bilirubinate) gallstones. The peripheral blood smear shows numerous target cells as well as occasional cells with rectangular crystals of hemoglobin C. Persons heterozygous for hemoglobin C are clinically normal.

Patients with hemoglobin SC disease are double heterozygotes for beta S and beta C. These patients, like those with sickle β^+ thalassemia, have a milder hemolytic anemia and milder clinical course than those with homozygous SS disease. There are fewer vaso-occlusive events, and the spleen remains palpable in adult life. However, persons with hemoglobin SC disease have more retinopathy and more ischemic necrosis of bone than those with SS disease. The hematocrit is usually 30–38%, with 5–10% reticulocytes and few irreversibly sickled cells on the blood smear. Target cells are more numerous than in SS disease. Hemoglobin electrophoresis will show approximately 50% hemoglobin C, 50% hemoglobin S, and no increase in hemoglobin F levels.

Olson JF et al: Hemoglobin C disease in infancy and childhood. J Pediatr 1994;125(5 Part 1):745.

UNSTABLE HEMOGLOBINS

Unstable hemoglobins are prone to oxidative denaturation even in the presence of a normal G6PD system. The disorder is autosomal dominant and of variable severity. Most patients have a mild chronic hemolytic anemia with splenomegaly, mild jaundice, and pigment (calcium bilirubinate) gallstones. Less severely affected patients are not anemic except under conditions of oxidative stress.

The diagnosis is made by the finding of Heinz bodies and a normal G6PD level. Hemoglobin electrophoresis is usually normal, since these hemoglobins characteristically do not have a change in their migration pattern. These hemoglobins can be shown to precipitate in isopropanol. Usually no treatment is necessary. Patients with chronic hemolytic anemia should receive folate supplementation and avoid known oxidative drugs. In rare severe cases, splenectomy may be required.

AUTOIMMUNE HEMOLYTIC ANEMIA

Essentials of Diagnosis

- Acquired anemia caused by IgG autoantibody.
- Spherocytes and reticulocytosis on peripheral blood smear.
- Positive Coombs test.

General Considerations

Autoimmune hemolytic anemia is an acquired disorder in which an IgG autoantibody is formed that binds to the red blood cell membrane. The antibody is most commonly directed against a basic component of the Rh system and is present on virtually all human red blood cells. When IgG antibodies coat the red blood cell, the Fc portion of the antibody is recognized by macrophages (with Fc receptor) present in the spleen and other portions of the reticuloendothelial system. The interaction between splenic macrophage and the antibody-coated red blood cell results in removal of red blood cell membrane and the formation of a spherocyte because of the decrease in surface-to-volume ratio of the red blood cell. These spherocytic cells have decreased deformability and become trapped in the red pulp of the spleen because of their inability to squeeze through the 2-μm fenestrations. When large amounts of IgG are present on red blood cells, complement may be fixed. Direct lysis of cells is rare, but the presence of C3b on the surface of red blood cells allows Kupffer cells in the liver to participate in the hemolytic process because of the presence of C3b receptors on Kupffer cells.

Approximately half of all cases of autoimmune hemolytic anemia are idiopathic. The disorder may also be seen in association with systemic lupus erythematosus, chronic lymphocytic leukemia, or diffuse lymphomas. It must be distinguished from drug-induced hemolytic anemia. Methyldopa commonly stimulates the production of an autoantibody with the same specificity as that in idiopathic autoimmune hemolytic anemia. Other drugs (penicillin, quinidine) become associated with the red blood cell membrane, and the antibody is directed against the membrane-drug complex.

The Coombs antiglobulin test forms the basis for diagnosis of these immune hemolytic disorders. The Coombs reagent is a rabbit IgM antibody raised against human IgG or human complement. The direct Coombs test is performed by mixing the patient's red blood cells with the Coombs reagent and looking for agglutination, which indicates the presence of antibody on the red blood cell surface. The indirect Coombs test is performed by mixing the patient's serum with a panel of type O red blood cells. After incubation of the test serum and panel red blood cells, the Coombs reagent is added. Agglutination in this system indicates the presence of free antibody in the patient's serum. Because the traditional Coombs test relies on visible agglutination as an end point, the test is not very sensitive and will not detect immune hemolytic anemias in which only a small amount of IgG is present on red blood cells. More sensitive tests (micro-Coombs) are now available.

Clinical Findings

A. Symptoms and Signs: Autoimmune hemolytic anemia typically produces an anemia of rapid onset that may be life-threatening in severity. Patients complain of fatigue and may present with angina or congestive heart failure. On examination, jaundice and splenomegaly are usually present. If the patient has an underlying disorder such as systemic lupus erythematosus or chronic lymphocytic leukemia, features of these diseases may be present.

B. Laboratory Findings: The anemia is of variable severity but may be severe, with hematocrit of less than 10%. Reticulocytosis is usually present, and spherocytes are seen on the peripheral blood smear. In cases of severe hemolysis, the stressed bone marrow may also release nucleated red blood cells. As with other hemolytic disorders, indirect bilirubin is increased. Approximately 10% of patients with autoimmune hemolytic anemia have coincident immune thrombocytopenia (Evans's syndrome).

The direct Coombs test is positive, and the indirect Coombs test may or may not be positive. A positive indirect Coombs test indicates the presence of a large amount of autoantibody that has saturated binding sites in the red blood cell and consequently appears in the serum. A patient with acquired spherocytic hemolytic anemia that may be of the autoimmune variety who has a negative Coombs test should be tested with a micro-Coombs test (which is necessary to make the diagnosis in approximately 10% of cases). Because the patient's serum usually contains the autoantibody, it may be difficult to obtain a compatible cross-match with donor's cells. Suitable donors may be selected by special laboratory methods.

Treatment

Initial treatment is with prednisone, 1–2 mg/kg/d in divided doses. If anemia is life-threatening, transfusions should be given cautiously. Most transfused blood will survive no more poorly than the patient's own red blood cells. However, because of difficulty in performing the cross-match, it is possible that incompatible blood will be given, and patients must be monitored carefully during transfusion. Decisions regarding transfusions should be made in consultation with a hematologist (or blood bank physician). If prednisone is ineffective or if the disease recurs on tapering the dose of prednisone to an acceptable chronic dose, splenectomy should be performed. Patients with autoimmune hemolytic anemia refractory to prednisone and splenectomy may be treated with a variety of immunosuppressive agents.

High-dose intravenous immune globulin (500 mg/kg daily for 1–4 days) may be highly effective in controlling hemolysis. However, the benefit is short-lived (1–3 weeks), and the drug is very expensive. Treatment with IGIV should be given only in emergency situations or when prednisone is contraindicated.

The long-term prognosis for patients with this disorder is good. Splenectomy is often successful in controlling or at least ameliorating the disorder.

Flores G et al: Efficacy of intravenous immunoglobulin in the treatment of autoimmune hemolytic anemia. Am J Hematol 1993;44:237. (Only 40% response rate found; lower pretreatment hemoglobin and hepatomegaly correlated with response. IGIV is recommended only for severe cases as adjunctive therapy in situations when prednisone is contraindicated, in emergent situations, and in refractory cases.)

Jefferies LC: Transfusion therapy in autoimmune hemolytic anemia. Hematol Oncol Clin North Am 1994;8:1087.

COLD AGGLUTININ DISEASE

Essentials of Diagnosis

- Increased reticulocytes and spherocytes on peripheral blood smear.
- Coombs test positive only for complement.
- Positive cold agglutinin test.

General Considerations

Cold agglutinin disease is an acquired hemolytic anemia due to an IgM autoantibody usually directed against the I antigen on red blood cells. These IgM autoantibodies characteristically will not react with cells at 37 °C but only at lower temperatures. Since the blood temperature (even in the most peripheral parts of the body) rarely goes lower than 20 °C, only antibodies active at higher temperatures than this will produce clinical effects. In the cooler parts of the body (fingers, nose, ears), agglutination of red blood cells by the IgM antibodies will transiently occur. Hemolysis results indirectly from attachment of IgM, which in the cooler parts of the circulation binds and fixes complement. When the red blood cell returns to a warmer temperature, the IgM antibody dissociates, leaving complement on the cell. Lysis of cells rarely occurs. Rather, C3b present on the red cells is recognized by Kupffer cells (which have receptors for C3b), and red blood cell sequestration ensues.

Most cases of chronic cold agglutinin disease are idiopathic. Others occur in association with Waldenström's macroglobulinemia, in which a monoclonal IgM paraprotein is produced. Acute postinfectious cold agglutinin disease occurs following mycoplasmal pneumonia or infectious mononucleosis (with antibody directed against antigen i rather than I).

Clinical Findings

A. Symptoms and Signs: In chronic cold agglutinin disease, symptoms related to red blood cell agglutination occur on exposure to cold, and patients may complain of mottled or numb fingers or toes. Hemolytic anemia is rarely severe, but episodic hemoglobinuria may occur on exposure to cold. The hemolytic anemia in acute postinfectious syndromes is rarely severe.

B. Laboratory Findings: Mild anemia is present with reticulocytosis and spherocytes. The direct Coombs test will be positive for complement only. Occasionally, a micro-Coombs test is necessary to reveal bound complement (low-titer cold agglutinin disease). Bedside cold agglutinin studies are often falsely positive or falsely negative and should be confirmed by the clinical laboratory.

Treatment

Treatment is largely symptomatic, based on avoiding exposure to cold. Patients with severe involvement may be treated with alkylating agents such as chlorambucil. Splenectomy is ineffective, since hemolysis takes place in the liver. Prednisone is ineffective in reducing Kupffer cell function.

High-dose intravenous immunoglobulin (2 g/kg) may be effective temporarily. Interferon may be of benefit for some patients.

MICROANGIOPATHIC HEMOLYTIC ANEMIAS

The microangiopathic hemolytic anemias are a group of disorders in which red blood cell fragmentation takes place. The anemia is intravascular, producing hemoglobinemia, hemoglobinuria, and, in severe cases, methemalbuminemia. The hallmark of the disorder is the finding of fragmented red blood cells (schistocytes, helmet cells) on the peripheral blood smear.

These fragmentation syndromes can be caused by a variety of disorders (Table 13–8). Thrombotic thrombocytopenic purpura (see below) is the most important of these and is discussed below. Clinical features of the fragmentation syndromes are variable and depend on the underlying disorder. Coagulopathy and thrombocytopenia are variably present.

Chronic microangiopathic hemolytic anemia (such as is present with a malfunctioning cardiac valve prosthesis) may cause iron deficiency anemia because of continuous low-grade hemoglobinuria.

Mach-Pascual S, Samii K, Beris P: Microangiopathic hemolytic anemia complicating FK506 (tacrolimus) therapy. Am J Hematol 1996;52:310.

HEMOLYSIS RELATED TO INFECTION

Clostridial infections may cause severe intravascular hemolysis, presumably because of the action of a clostridial toxin on the red blood cell membrane. Malaria may cause intravascular hemolysis because of parasitism of red blood cells; falciparum malaria causes the severest form (blackwater fever). Other infections associated with hemolysis are bartonellosis and babesiosis.

APLASTIC ANEMIA

Essentials of Diagnosis

- Pancytopenia.
- No abnormal cells seen.
- Hypocellular bone marrow.

General Considerations

All hematopoietic cells are derived from a pluripotent stem cell that gives rise to precursors of erythroid, myeloid, and platelet forms. Injury to or suppression of this hematopoietic stem cell will result in pancytopenia—reduction in all three hematopoietic cell lines (red blood cells, neutrophils, and platelets). Aplastic anemia is a condition of bone marrow failure that arises from injury to or abnormal expression of the stem cell. The bone marrow becomes hypoplastic, and pancytopenia develops.

There are a number of causes of aplastic anemia (Table 13–10). Direct stem cell injury may be caused by radiation, chemotherapy, toxins, or pharmacologic agents. Systemic lupus erythematosus may rarely cause suppression of the hematopoietic stem cell by an IgG autoantibody directed against the stem cell. However, the most common pathogenesis of aplastic anemia appears to be autoimmune suppression of hematopoiesis by a T cell–mediated cellular mechanism.

Clinical Findings

A. Symptoms and Signs: Patients come to medical attention because of the consequences of bone marrow failure. Anemia leads to symptoms of weakness and fatigue; neutropenia causes vulnerability to bacterial infections; and thrombocytopenia results in mucosal and skin bleeding. Physical examination may reveal signs of pallor, purpura, and petechiae. Other abnormalities such as hepatosplenomegaly, lymphadenopathy, or bone tenderness should *not* be present, and their presence should lead one to question the diagnosis of aplastic anemia.

B. Laboratory Findings: The hallmark of aplastic anemia is pancytopenia. However, early in the evolution of aplastic anemia, only one or two cell lines may be reduced.

Anemia may be severe and is always associated with decreased reticulocytes. Red blood cell morphology is unremarkable. The MCV is usually normal but occasionally may be increased. Neutrophils and platelets are reduced in number, and no immature or abnormal forms are seen. The bone marrow aspirate and the bone marrow biopsy appear hypocellular, with only scant amounts of normal hematopoietic progenitors. No abnormal cells are seen.

Differential Diagnosis

The diagnosis of aplastic anemia is made in cases of pancytopenia with a hypocellular marrow biopsy containing no abnormal cells. Aplastic anemia must be differentiated from other causes of pancytopenia (Table 13–11). Myelodysplastic disorders or acute leukemia may occasionally be confused with aplastic anemia. These are differentiated by the presence of morphologic abnormalities or increased blasts. Hairy cell leukemia has been misdiagnosed as aplastic anemia and should be recognized by a high incidence of splenomegaly and by the presence of abnormal lymphoid cells on the bone marrow biopsy. Pancytopenia in the presence of a normocellular bone marrow is usually due to systemic lupus erythematosus, disseminated infection, or hypersplenism. Isolated thrombocytopenia may occur early as aplastic anemia develops and be confused with immune thrombocytopenia.

Treatment

Mild cases of aplastic anemia may be treated with supportive care. Red blood cell transfusions and platelet transfusions are given as necessary, and antibiotics are used to treat infections.

Severe aplastic anemia is defined by the presence of neutrophils less than 500/μL, platelets less than 20,000/μL, reticulocytes less than 1%, and bone marrow cellularity less than 20%. When this constellation of features is present (or three of the four), the median survival without treatment is approximately 3 months, and only 20% of patients survive for 1 year. The treatment of choice for young adults (under age 50) who have HLA-matched siblings is allogeneic bone marrow transplantation. The best results are achieved in younger patients who have not had

---

Table 13–10. Causes of aplastic anemia.

Congenital (rare)
"Idiopathic" (probably autoimmune)
Systemic lupus erythematosus
Chemotherapy, radiotherapy
Toxins: Benzene, toluene, insecticides
Drugs: Chloramphenicol, phenylbutazone, gold salts,
  sulfonamides, phenytoin, carbamazepine, quinacrine,
  tolbutamide
Posthepatitis
Pregnancy
Paroxysmal nocturnal hemoglobinuria

Table 13–11. Causes of pancytopenia.

Bone marrow disorders
  Aplastic anemia
  Myelodysplasia
  Acute leukemia
  Myelofibrosis
  Infiltrative disease: Lymphoma, myeloma, carcinoma,
    hairy cell leukemia
  Megaloblastic anemia
Nonmarrow disorders
  Hypersplenism
  Systemic lupus erythematosus
  Infection: Tuberculosis, AIDS, leishmaniasis, brucellosis

blood transfusions. Prior transfusion increases the risk of graft rejection, apparently because of sensitization to antigens present on hematopoietic progenitors.

For adults over age 50 or those without HLA-matched siblings, the treatment of choice for severe aplastic anemia is immunosuppression with antithymocyte globulin (ATG). ATG is given in the hospital in conjunction with transfusion and antibiotic support. A useful regimen is 40 mg/kg/d for 4 days in combination with cyclosporine, 6 mg/kg orally twice daily. ATG must be used in combination with corticosteroids (prednisone 1–2 mg/kg/d initially, followed by a rapid taper) to avoid complications of serum sickness. Responses usually occur in 4–12 weeks. Responses to ATG are usually only partial, but the blood counts rise high enough to give patients a safe and transfusion-free life.

For patients in whom neutropenia is the dominant abnormality, the myeloid growth factors G-CSF (filgrastim), 5 μg/kg daily, or GM-CSF (sargramostim), 250 μg/m^2/d, may be effective in raising the neutrophil count and decreasing infections. However, they will not benefit other cell lines or provide definitive treatment.

Androgens have been widely used in the past, with a low response rate. However, a few patients can be maintained successfully with this form of treatment. One regimen is oxymetholone, 2–3 mg/kg orally daily. In the rare syndrome of systemic lupus erythematosus causing humorally mediated aplastic anemia, the combination of plasmapheresis and high-dose prednisone may be successful.

Course & Prognosis

Patients with severe aplastic anemia have a rapidly fatal illness if left untreated. Allogeneic bone marrow transplantation is highly successful in previously untransfused children and young adults with HLA-matched siblings. For this group of patients, the durable complete response rate exceeds 80%. For older adults or those who have previously been exposed to blood products, long-term survival rates are between 50% and 80% with new preparative regimens for transplantation giving the improved results due to a lower risk of graft rejection. ATG treatment leads to partial response in approximately 60% of adults, and the long-term prognosis of responders appears to be good. There is increasing evidence that some fraction (as many at 25%) of these nontransplanted patients may develop clonal hematologic disorders such as paroxysmal nocturnal hemoglobinuria or myelodysplasia after many years of follow-up.

Brodsky RA, Sensenbrenner LL, Jones RJ: Complete remission in severe aplastic anemia after high-dose cyclophosphamide without bone marrow transplantation. Blood 1996;87:491.

Kojima S, Matsuyama T: Stimulation of granulopoiesis by high-dose recombinant human granulocyte colony stimulating factor in children with aplastic anemia and very severe neutropenia. Blood 1994;83:1474.

Maciejewski JP et al: A severe and consistent deficit in marrow and circulating primitive hematopoietic cells (long-term culture-initiating cells) in acquired aplastic anemia. Blood 1996;88:1983.

Paquette RL et al: Long-term outcome of aplastic anemia in adults treated with antithymocyte globulin: Comparison with bone marrow transplantation. Blood 1995;85:283.

Rosenfeld SJ et al: Intensive immunosuppression with antithymocyte globulin and cyclosporine as treatment for severe acquired aplastic anemia. Blood 1995;85:3058.

Wagner JL et al: Bone marrow transplantation for severe aplastic anemia from genotypically HLA-nonidentical relatives: An update of the Seattle experience. Transplantation 1996;61:54.

Young NS, Barrett AJ: The treatment of severe acquired aplastic anemia. Blood 1995;85:3367.

NEUTROPENIA

Neutropenia exists when the neutrophil count falls below 1500/μL. However, blacks and other specific population groups may normally have neutrophil counts as low as 1200/μL. The neutropenic patient is increasingly vulnerable to infection by gram-positive and gram-negative bacteria and by fungi. The risk of infection is related to the severity of neutropenia. Patients with "chronic benign neutropenia" are free of infection for years despite very low neutrophil levels.

A variety of bone marrow disorders and nonmarrow conditions may cause neutropenia (Table 13–12). All the causes of aplastic anemia (Table 13–10) and pancytopenia (Table 13–11) may cause neutropenia. Isolated neutropenia is often due to an idiosyncratic reaction to a drug, and agranulocytosis (complete absence of neutrophils in the peripheral

Table 13–12. Causes of neutropenia.

Bone marrow disorders
  Aplastic anemia
  Pure white cell aplasia
  Congenital (rare)
  Cyclic neutropenia
  Drugs: Sulfonamides, chlorpromazine, procainamide, penicillin, cephalosporins, cimetidine, methimazole, phenytoin, chlorpropamide, antiretrovirals
  Benign chronic
Peripheral disorders
  Hypersplenism
  Sepsis
  Immune
  Felty's syndrome
  HIV infection

blood) is almost always due to a drug reaction or to exposure to a variety of chemicals (eg, pesticides). In these cases, examination of the bone marrow shows virtual absence of myeloid precursors, with other cell lines undisturbed. Pure white cell aplasia is a rare condition in which an autoantibody is formed against myeloid progenitors. **Felty's syndrome**—neutropenia associated with seropositive nodular rheumatoid arthritis and splenomegaly—is another cause. Neutropenia in the presence of a normal bone marrow may be due to immunologic peripheral destruction, sepsis, or hypersplenism.

Clinical Findings

Neutropenia results in stomatitis and in infections. Infections are usually due to gram-positive or gram-negative aerobic bacteria or to fungi such as *Candida* or *Aspergillus*. The most common infections are septicemia, cellulitis, and pneumonia. In the presence of severe neutropenia, the usual signs of inflammatory response to infection may be absent. Nevertheless, fever in the neutropenic patient should always be assumed to be of infectious origin.

Treatment

Potential causative drugs are discontinued. Infections are treated with many combinations of broad-spectrum antibiotics, but particular attention should be paid to enteric gram-negative bacteria. Third-generation cephalosporins such as ceftazidime, 2 g intravenously every 8 hours, are effective as single-agent therapy, obviating the need for an aminoglycoside.

When Felty's syndrome leads to repeated bacterial infections, splenectomy is the treatment of choice. Splenectomy usually leads to healing of leg ulcers and to reduction in the rate of infection whether or not the neutrophil count rises.

The prognosis of patients with neutropenia depends on the underlying cause. Most patients with drug-induced agranulocytosis can be supported with broad-spectrum antibiotics and will recover completely. With improved antibacterial antibiotics, the prognosis of these patients has improved considerably. For selected low-risk patients, outpatient management with oral antibiotics or daily intravenous antibiotics may be feasible. The myeloid growth factors G-CSF (filgrastim) and GM-CSF (sargramostim) may be useful in shortening the duration of neutropenia associated with chemotherapy. However, once infection has occurred, they do not increase the survival rate.

Freifeld AG, Pizzo PA: The outpatient management of febrile neutropenia in cancer patients. Oncology 1996; 10:599, 611; discussion, 615.

Krishnaswamy G et al: Resolution of the neutropenia of Felty's syndrome by longterm administration of recombinant granulocyte colony stimulating factor. J Rheumatol 1996;23:763.

Malik IA et al: Feasibility of outpatient management of fever in cancer patients with low-risk neutropenia: Results of a prospective randomized trial. Am J Med 1995;98:224.

Vellenga E et al: Randomized placebo-controlled trial of granulocyte-macrophage colony-stimulating factor in patients with chemotherapy-related febrile neutropenia. J Clin Oncol 1996;14:619.

Welte K, Dale D: Pathophysiology and treatment of severe chronic neutropenia. Ann Hematol 1996;72:158.

LEUKEMIAS & OTHER MYELOPROLIFERATIVE DISORDERS

Myeloproliferative disorders are due to acquired clonal abnormalities of the hematopoietic stem cell. Since the stem cell gives rise to myeloid, erythroid, and platelet cells, one sees qualitative and quantitative changes in all these cell lines. In some disorders (chronic myelogenous leukemia), specific characteristic chromosomal changes are seen. In others, although the disorder is presumed to be related to a defect in DNA, no characteristic cytogenetic abnormalities are seen.

Classically, the myeloproliferative disorders produce characteristic syndromes with well-defined clinical and laboratory features (Tables 13–13 and 13–14). However, these disorders are grouped together because the disease may evolve from one form into another and because hybrid disorders are commonly seen. All of the myeloproliferative disorders may progress to acute myelogenous leukemia.

POLYCYTHEMIA VERA

Essentials of Diagnosis

- Increased red blood cell mass.
- Splenomegaly.
- Normal arterial oxygen saturation.
- Usually elevated white blood count and platelet count.

Table 13–13. Classification of myeloproliferative disorders.

Myeloproliferative syndromes
Polycythemia vera
Myelofibrosis
Essential thrombocytosis
Chronic myeloid leukemia
Myelodysplastic syndromes
Acute myeloid leukemia

Table 13–14. Laboratory features of myeloproliferative disorders.

	White Count	Hematocrit	Platelet Count	Red Cell Morphology
Chronic myeloid leukemia	↑↑	N	N or ↑	N
Myelofibrosis	N or ↓ or ↑	N or ↓	↓ or N or ↑	Abn
Polycythemia vera	N or ↑	↑	N or ↑	N
Essential thrombocytosis	N or ↑	N	↑↑	N

General Considerations

Polycythemia vera is an acquired myeloproliferative disorder that causes overproduction of all three hematopoietic cell lines, most prominently the red blood cells. The hematocrit is elevated (at sea level) when values exceed 54% in males or 51% in females (Table 13–15).

When the hematocrit is elevated, the red blood cell mass should be measured to determine whether true polycythemia or relative polycythemia exists. Normal values for red blood cell mass are 26–34 mL/kg in men and 21–29 mL/kg in women. Relative ("spurious") polycythemia characteristically presents in middle-aged men who are overweight and hypertensive (often on diuretic therapy); the hematocrit is almost always less than 60%.

If the red blood cell mass is increased, one must determine whether the increase is primary or secondary. Primary polycythemia (polycythemia vera) is a bone marrow disorder characterized by autonomous overproduction of erythroid cells. Erythroid production is independent of erythropoietin, and the serum erythropoietin level is low. In vitro, erythroid progenitor cells grow without added erythropoietin, a finding not seen in normal individuals.

Polycythemia vera is a relatively common disorder. Sixty percent of patients are male, and the median age at presentation is 60. Polycythemia vera rarely occurs in adults under age 40.

Clinical Findings

A. Symptoms and Signs: Most patients present with symptoms related to expanded blood volume and increased blood viscosity. Common complaints include headache, dizziness, tinnitus, blurred vision, and fatigue. Generalized pruritus, especially

Table 13–15. Causes of polycythemia.

Spurious polycythemia
Secondary polycythemia
  Hypoxia: Cardiac disease, pulmonary disease, high
    altitude
  Carboxyhemoglobin: Smoking
  Renal lesions
  Erythropoietin-secreting tumors (rare)
  Abnormal hemoglobins (rare)
Polycythemia vera

that occurring following a warm shower or bath, may be a striking symptom and is related to histamine release from the increased number of basophils present. Patients may also initially complain of epistaxis. This is probably related to engorgement of mucosal blood vessels in combination with abnormal hemostasis due to qualitative abnormalities in platelet function.

Physical examination reveals plethora and engorged retinal veins. The spleen is palpably enlarged in 75% of cases, but splenomegaly is nearly always present when imaged. Less commonly, the liver is mildly enlarged.

Thrombosis is the most common complication of polycythemia vera and the major cause of morbidity and death in this disorder. Thrombosis appears to be related to increased blood viscosity and abnormal platelet function. Uncontrolled polycythemia leads to a very high incidence of thrombotic complications of surgery, and elective surgery should be deferred until the condition has been treated. Paradoxically, in addition to thrombosis, increased bleeding also occurs. There is a high incidence of peptic ulcer disease as well as gastrointestinal bleeding. Overproduction of uric acid may lead to gout.

B. Laboratory Findings: The hallmark of polycythemia vera is a hematocrit above normal, at times greater than 60%. Red blood cell morphology is normal. The white blood count is characteristically elevated to 10,000–20,000/μL and the platelet count is variably elevated, sometimes with counts exceeding 1,000,000/μL. Platelet morphology is usually normal, but large hypogranular forms may be seen. White blood cells are usually normal, but basophilia is frequently present. By definition, the red blood cell mass is elevated.

The bone marrow is hypercellular, with panhyperplasia of all hematopoietic elements. A characteristic finding is increased numbers of megakaryocytes. Iron stores are usually absent from the bone marrow, having been transferred to the increased circulating red blood cell mass. Iron deficiency may result from chronic gastrointestinal blood loss. Bleeding may lower the hematocrit to the normal range (or lower), creating diagnostic confusion.

Vitamin B_{12} levels are strikingly elevated because of increased levels of transcobalamin III (secreted by white blood cells). The leukocyte alkaline phosphatase is characteristically elevated as a marker of qualitative abnormalities in the myeloid line. Uric acid levels may be increased. There is no characteristic chromosomal abnormality in this disorder.

Although red blood cell morphology is usually normal at presentation, microcytosis, hypochromia, and poikilocytosis may result from iron deficiency following treatment by phlebotomy (see below). Progressive hypersplenism may also lead to elliptocytosis.

Differential Diagnosis

Spurious polycythemia, in which an elevated hematocrit is due to contracted plasma volume rather than increased red cell mass, may be related to diuretic use or may occur without obvious cause.

A secondary cause of polycythemia should be suspected if splenomegaly is absent and the high hematocrit is not accompanied by increases in other cell lines. Arterial oxygen saturation should be measured to determine if hypoxia is the cause. A smoking history should be taken and carboxyhemoglobin levels measured when indicated. A renal sonogram may be indicated to look for an erythropoietin-secreting cyst or tumor. A positive family history should lead to investigation for congenital high-oxygen-affinity hemoglobin.

Polycythemia vera should be differentiated from other myeloproliferative disorders (Table 13–14). Marked elevation of the white blood count (above 30,000/μL) should lead to consideration of chronic myelogenous leukemia. This disorder is confirmed by the finding of a low leukocyte alkaline phosphatase and by the presence of the Philadelphia chromosome. Abnormal red blood cell morphology and nucleated red blood cells in the peripheral blood should lead to the consideration of myelofibrosis. This condition is diagnosed by bone marrow biopsy showing fibrosis of the marrow. Essential thrombocytosis is diagnosed when the platelet count is strikingly elevated and the red blood cell count is normal.

Treatment

The treatment of choice is phlebotomy. One unit of blood (approximately 500 mL) is removed weekly until the hematocrit is less than 45%; the hematocrit is maintained at less than 45% by repeated phlebotomy as necessary. Because repeated phlebotomy produces iron deficiency, the requirement for phlebotomy should gradually decrease. It is important to avoid medicinal iron supplementation, as this can thwart the goals of a phlebotomy program. It is not necessary to manipulate the diet to decrease iron intake. Patients will usually feel much better as soon as the hematocrit is lowered. Maintaining the hematocrit at normal levels has been shown to decrease the incidence of thrombotic complications.

Occasionally, myelosuppressive therapy is indicated. Indications include a high phlebotomy require-

ment, thrombocytosis, and intractable pruritus. There is evidence that reduction of the platelet count to less than 700,000/μL will reduce the risk of thrombotic complications that are the major cause of morbidity and mortality in this disorder. Alkylating agents and radiophosphorus (^{32}P) have been shown to increase the risk of conversion of this disease to acute leukemia and should be avoided. Hydroxyurea is now being widely used when myelosuppressive therapy is indicated because of the presumption that it will not be leukemogenic. The usual dose is 500–1500 mg/d orally, adjusted to keep platelets < 500,000/μL without reducing the neutrophil count to < 2000/μL. Busulfan may also be used in a dose of 4–6 mg/d for 4–8 weeks. Care must be taken to avoid prolonged severe myelosuppression. Alpha interferon has recently been shown to have some ability to control the disease. The usual dose is 2–5 million units subcutaneously three times weekly. Anagrelide has recently been approved for use in treatment of thrombocytosis and should be another useful agent.

The role of antiplatelet agents such as aspirin in preventing thrombotic complications is controversial. High doses of aspirin (325 mg three times daily) plus dipyridamole (25 mg three times daily) cause a marked increase in gastrointestinal bleeding and should not be given routinely. However, antiplatelet treatment may be warranted in selected patients who have recurrent thromboses despite control of their platelet counts with myelosuppressive therapy. One aspirin tablet daily (325 mg) may be effective therapy.

Allopurinol may be indicated for hyperuricemia. Antihistamine therapy with diphenhydramine or other H_1 blockers may be helpful for control of pruritus.

Prognosis

Polycythemia is an indolent disease with median survival of 11–15 years. The major cause of morbidity and mortality is arterial thrombosis. Over time, polycythemia vera may convert to myelofibrosis or to chronic myelogenous leukemia. In approximately 5% of cases, the disorder progresses to acute myelogenous leukemia, which is usually refractory to therapy.

Anagrelide Study Group: Anagrelide, a therapy for thrombocythemic states: Experience in 577 patients. Am J Med 1992;92:69. (Anagrelide is an investigational agent that satisfactorily controls the platelet count in more than 90% of patients. Side effects are moderate and dose-related.)

Foa P et al: Role of interferon alpha-2a in the treatment of polycythemia vera. Am J Hematol 1995;48:55.

Najean Y et al: The very-long-term course of polycythemia: A complement to the previously published data of the Polycythemia Vera Study Group. Br J Haematol 1994;86:233. (The risks of leukemia after ^{32}P or chemotherapy are high for 10 years after treatment but low thereafter. Phlebotomy is unacceptable as long-term treatment because of poor tolerance and because up to 50% progress toward myelofibrosis after 15 years.)

Nand S et al: Leukemogenic risk of hydroxyurea therapy in polycythemia vera, essential thrombocythemia, and myeloid metaplasia with myelofibrosis. Am J Hematol 1996;52:42.

Polycythemia vera: the natural history of 1213 patients followed for 20 years. Gruppo Italiano Studio Policitemia. Ann Intern Med 1995;123:656.

MYELOFIBROSIS

Essentials of Diagnosis

- Teardrop poikilocytosis on peripheral smear.
- Leukoerythroblastic blood picture; giant abnormal platelets.
- Hypercellular bone marrow with reticulin or collagen fibrosis.

General Considerations

Myelofibrosis (myelofibrosis with myeloid metaplasia, agnogenic myeloid metaplasia) is a myeloproliferative disorder characterized by fibrosis of the bone marrow, splenomegaly, and a leukoerythroblastic peripheral blood picture with teardrop poikilocytosis. It is widely believed that fibrosis occurs in response to increased secretion of platelet-derived growth factor (PDGF). In response to bone marrow fibrosis, extramedullary hematopoiesis (hematopoietic cell development outside the bone marrow) takes place in the liver, spleen, and lymph nodes. In these sites, mesenchymal cells responsible for fetal hematopoiesis can be reactivated.

Clinical Findings

A. Symptoms and Signs: Myelofibrosis develops in adults over age 50 and is usually insidious in onset. Patients most commonly present with fatigue related to their anemia or abdominal fullness related to splenomegaly. Uncommon presentations include bleeding and bone pain. On examination, splenomegaly is almost invariably present and is sometimes massive. The liver is enlarged in more than half of cases.

Later in the course of the disease, progressive bone marrow failure takes place as the marrow becomes progressively more fibrotic. Anemia becomes severe, and red cell transfusion becomes necessary. Progressive thrombocytopenia leads to bleeding. The spleen continues to enlarge, which leads to early satiety. Painful episodes of splenic infarction may occur. Late in the course, the patient becomes cachectic and may experience severe bone pain, especially in the lower legs. Hematopoiesis in the liver leads to portal hypertension with ascites, esophageal varices, and eventually liver failure.

B. Laboratory Findings: Patients are almost invariably anemic at presentation. The white blood count is variable—either low, normal, or elevated—and may be increased to 50,000/μL. The platelet count is variable. The peripheral blood smear is characteristic, consisting of significant poikilocytosis with numerous teardrop forms. Immature myeloid and erythroid forms are present (leukoerythroblastic blood picture). Nucleated red blood cells are present and the myeloid series is less strikingly shifted, with immature forms including a small percentage of promyelocytes or myeloblasts. Platelet morphology may be bizarre, and giant degranulated platelet forms (megakaryocyte fragments) may be seen. The triad of teardrop poikilocytosis, leukoerythroblastic blood, and giant abnormal platelets is almost diagnostic of myelofibrosis.

The bone marrow usually cannot be aspirated (dry tap), though early in the course of the disease it is hypercellular, with a marked increase in megakaryocytes. Fibrosis at this stage is detected only by a silver stain demonstrating increased reticulin fibers. Later, biopsy reveals more severe fibrosis, with eventual replacement of hematopoietic precursors by collagen. There is no characteristic chromosomal abnormality.

Differential Diagnosis

A leukoerythroblastic blood picture from other causes may be seen in response to severe infection or inflammation. However, teardrop poikilocytosis and giant abnormal platelet forms will not be present. Bone marrow fibrosis may be seen in metastatic carcinoma, Hodgkin's disease, and hairy cell leukemia. These disorders are diagnosed by characteristic tissue morphology.

Myelofibrosis is distinguished from other myeloproliferative disorders by the characteristic constellation of findings (Table 13–14). Chronic myelogenous leukemia is diagnosed when there is marked elevation of the white blood count, a low leukocyte alkaline phosphatase, normal red blood cell morphology, and the presence of the Philadelphia chromosome. Polycythemia vera is characterized by an elevated hematocrit, and patients with essential thrombocytosis should have normal red blood cells.

Treatment

There is no specific treatment for this disorder. Anemic patients are supported with red blood cells in transfusion. Androgens such as oxymetholone, 200 mg orally daily, or testosterone help reduce the transfusion requirement in one-third of cases but are poorly tolerated by women. Splenectomy is not routinely performed but is indicated for splenic enlargement that causes recurrent painful episodes, severe thrombocytopenia, or an unacceptably high red blood cell transfusion requirement. Alpha interferon (2–5 million units subcutaneously three times weekly) leads to subjective and objective improvement in some cases.

Course & Prognosis

It is often hard to date the onset of myelofibrosis, but the median survival from time of diagnosis is approximately 5 years. End-stage myelofibrosis is a wasting illness characterized by generalized debility, liver failure, and bleeding from thrombocytopenia. Some cases may terminate in acute myelogenous leukemia.

Bourantas KL et al: Combination therapy with recombinant human erythropoietin, interferon-alpha-2b and granulocyte-macrophage colony-stimulating factor in idiopathic myelofibrosis. Acta Haematol 1996;96:79.

Nand S et al: Leukemogenic risk of hydroxyurea therapy in polycythemia vera, essential thrombocythemia, and myeloid metaplasia with myelofibrosis. Am J Hematol 1996;52:42.

CHRONIC MYELOGENOUS LEUKEMIA

Essentials of Diagnosis

- Markedly elevated white blood count.
- Markedly left-shifted myeloid series with a low percentage of promyelocytes and blasts.
- Presence of Philadelphia chromosome or *bcr-abl* gene.

General Considerations

Chronic myelogenous leukemia is a myeloproliferative disorder characterized by overproduction of myeloid cells. These myeloid cells retain the capacity for differentiation, and normal bone marrow function is retained during the early phases. The disease usually remains stable for years and then transforms to a more overtly malignant disease.

Chronic myelogenous leukemia is associated with a characteristic chromosomal abnormality, the Philadelphia chromosome, and was the first disease associated with a specific karyotypic abnormality. The Philadelphia chromosome is now recognized to be a reciprocal translocation between the long arms of chromosomes 9 and 22. A large portion of 22q is translocated to 9q, and a smaller piece of 9q is moved to 22q. This translocation is thought to be pathogenically significant, based on recent evidence that oncogene activation occurs. The portion of 9q that is translocated contains *abl,* a proto-oncogene that is the cellular homologue of the Ableson murine leukemia virus. The *abl* gene is received at a specific site on 22q, the break point cluster (bcr). The fusion gene *bcr-abl* produces a novel protein that differs from the normal transcript of the *abl* gene in that it possesses tyrosine kinase activity (a characteristic activity of transforming genes).

Usually at the time of diagnosis, the Philadelphia chromosome-positive clone dominates and may be the only one detected. However, a normal clone is present and may express itself either in vivo, after certain forms of therapy, or in vitro, in long-term bone marrow cultures. Approximately 5% of cases of chronic myelogenous leukemia are Philadelphia chromosome-negative. In almost all cases, although the characteristic karyotype is not seen at the light microscopic level, molecular studies demonstrate translocation of *abl* to 22q. In other cases of Philadelphia-negative chronic myelogenous leukemia, the disease is atypical and is better described as chronic myelomonocytic leukemia. Philadelphia chromosome-negative disease has a poor prognosis.

Early chronic myelogenous leukemia ("chronic phase") does not behave like a malignant disease. Normal bone marrow function is retained, white blood cells differentiate, and, despite some qualitative abnormalities (low leukocyte alkaline phosphatase), the neutrophils combat infection normally. However, chronic myelogenous leukemia is inherently unstable, and the disease progresses to accelerated phase and finally after several years, to blast crisis. This progression of the disease is often associated with added chromosomal defects superimposed on the Philadelphia chromosome. Blast crisis chronic myelogenous leukemia is an overtly malignant process that becomes indistinguishable from acute leukemia.

Clinical Findings

A. Symptoms and Signs: Chronic myelogenous leukemia is a disorder of middle age (median age at presentation is 42 years). Patients usually present with fatigue, night sweats, and low-grade fever related to the hypermetabolic state caused by overproduction of white blood cells. At other times, the patient complains of abdominal fullness related to splenomegaly, or an elevated white blood count is discovered incidentally. Rarely, the patient will present with a clinical syndrome related to leukostasis with blurred vision, respiratory distress, or priapism. The white blood count in these cases is usually greater than 500,000/μL.

On examination, the spleen is enlarged (often markedly so), and sternal tenderness may be present as a sign of marrow overexpansion.

Acceleration of the disease is often associated with fever in the absence of infection, bone pain, and splenomegaly. In blast crisis, patients may experience bleeding and infection related to bone marrow failure.

B. Laboratory Findings: The hallmark of chronic myelogenous leukemia is an elevated white blood count; the median white blood count at diagnosis is 150,000/μL. The peripheral blood is characteristic. The myeloid series is left-shifted, with mature forms dominating and with cells usually present in proportion to their degree of maturation. Blasts are usually less than 5%. Basophilia of granulocytes may be present. The peripheral blood smear gives the impression that the bone marrow has spilled over into the blood. At presentation, the patient is usually not anemic. Red blood cell morphology is normal, and nucleated red blood cells are rarely seen. The platelet count may be normal or elevated (sometimes to strikingly high levels). Platelet morphology is usually normal, but abnormally large forms may be seen.

The bone marrow is hypercellular, with markedly left-shifted myelopoiesis. Myeloblasts comprise less than 5% of marrow cells.

The leukocyte alkaline phosphatase score is invariably low and is a sign of qualitative abnormalities in neutrophils. The vitamin B_{12} level is usually markedly elevated because of increased secretion of transcobalamin III. Uric acid levels may be high.

The Philadelphia chromosome is almost invariably present and may be detected in either the peripheral blood or the bone marrow. The *bcr-abl* gene may be reliably detected in peripheral blood by molecular techniques (Southern blot) and is well enough established to substitute for cytogenetics if the only question is whether the Philadelphia chromosome is present.

With progression to the accelerated and blast phases, progressive anemia and thrombocytopenia occur, and the percentage of blasts in the blood and bone marrow increases. Blast phase chronic myelogenous leukemia is diagnosed when blasts comprise more than 30% of bone marrow cells.

Differential Diagnosis

Early chronic myelogenous leukemia must be differentiated from the reactive leukocytosis associated with infection, inflammation, or cancer. In these reactive disorders, the white blood count is usually less than 50,000/μL, splenomegaly is absent, the leukocyte alkaline phosphatase is normal or increased, and the Philadelphia chromosome is not present. If one is in doubt whether leukocytosis is due to chronic myelogenous leukemia or a reactive condition, the patient should be observed, since there is no advantage to early therapy for asymptomatic patients.

Chronic myelogenous leukemia must be distinguished from other myeloproliferative disease (Table 13–14). The hematocrit should not be elevated, the red blood cell morphology should be normal, and nucleated red blood cells should be rare or absent. Definitive diagnosis is made by finding the Philadelphia chromosome or *bcr-abl*.

Treatment

Treatment is usually not emergent even with white blood counts over 200,000/μL, since the majority of circulating cells are mature myeloid cells that are smaller and more deformable than primitive leukemic blasts. In the rare instances in which symptoms result from extreme hyperleukocytosis (pri-

apism, respiratory distress, visual blurring, altered mental status), leukapheresis should be performed on an emergency basis in conjunction with myelosuppressive therapy.

Standard therapy consists of administration of hydroxyurea. The initial dose is usually 2–4 g/d orally, and the maintenance dose varies between 0.5 and 2 g/d as necessary to maintain the white blood count at 5000–10,000/μL. Hydroxyurea must be given without interruption, since the white blood count will rise within days after discontinuing this medication. The response to hydroxyurea is usually gratifying. The white blood count decreases, the spleen decreases in size, and the patient becomes asymptomatic. Most patients in the chronic phase of chronic myelogenous leukemia will have no symptoms either from the disease or their chemotherapy.

Recombinant alpha interferon has largely replaced hydroxyurea as the initial treatment of choice and can prolong both the duration of the chronic phase and overall survival. Up to 80% of patients have a good hematologic response. Interferon, unlike other palliative agents, has the ability to suppress the Philadelphia chromosome and to allow cytogenetically normal cells to appear. This biologic effect may be complete (5–10% of cases) or partial (15–30% of cases). It usually occurs after 1 year (6–18 months) of treatment. Motivated patients should be offered a trial of interferon therapy. Because of the constitutional symptoms associated with full-dose therapy, only some patients will tolerate prolonged use of 5×10^6 units/d. Those patients with good cytogenetic responses will benefit from continued interferon with marked prolongation of survival, whereas others can do equally well with hydroxyurea.

Although the response to myelosuppressive therapy of the chronic phase is gratifying, the treatment is only palliative, and the disease is invariably fatal. The only available curative therapy is allogeneic bone marrow transplantation. This treatment is available for adults under age 60 who have HLA-matched siblings. Approximately 60% of adults have long-term disease-free survival following bone marrow transplantation and appear to be cured of their disease. The best results (70–80% success rate) are obtained in patients who are transplanted within 1 year after initial diagnosis. All young patients should be given the opportunity for allogeneic bone marrow transplantation in the chronic phase if they have suitable bone marrow donors. For young patients without sibling donors, HLA-matched unrelated donors may be located through computer-based registries of volunteer bone marrow donors (National Marrow Donors Program). Results are inferior to those achieved with matched sibling transplants but offer a cure rate of 40–60% for patients with an otherwise invariably fatal disease. For chronic myelogenous leukemia patients who relapse after transplantation, immunologic therapy with infusion of T lymphocytes from the bone marrow donor may produce long-lasting remissions.

Blast crisis of chronic myelogenous leukemia is a notoriously difficult form of acute leukemia to treat. Lymphoid blast crisis (present in one-third of cases) should be identified because chemotherapy for this disorder is less toxic and more effective. Therapy with daunorubicin, vincristine, and prednisone (used in treatment of acute lymphoblastic leukemia) will lead to remission—usually short-lived—in 70% of these cases.

Course & Prognosis

Median survival is 3–4 years. Once the disease has progressed to the accelerated or blast phase, survival is measured in months. Approximately 60% of young adults who have successful allogeneic bone marrow transplantation appear to be cured.

Appelbaum FB et al: Bone marrow transplantation for chronic myelogenous leukemia. Semin Oncol 1995;22: 405.

Collins RH Jr et al: Donor leukocyte infusions in 140 patients with relapsed malignancy after allogeneic bone marrow transplantation. J Clin Oncol 1997;15:433.

Italian Cooperative Study Group on Chronic Myeloid Leukemia: Interferon alfa-2a as compared with conventional chemotherapy for the treatment of chronic myeloid leukemia. N Engl J Med 1994;330:820. (Interferon improves survival and delays progression to blast crisis when compared with conventional therapy with hydroxyurea or busulfan.)

Kantarjian HM et al: Prolonged survival in chronic myelogenous leukemia after cytogenetic response to interferon-alpha. The Leukemia Service. Ann Intern Med 1995;122:254. (Those patients who achieve a complete cytogenetic response to interferon with disappearance of the Philadelphia chromosome have unexpectedly good [90%] 5-year survival. However, only a limited fraction of patients achieve this good response to interferon.)

MYELODYSPLASTIC SYNDROMES

Essentials of Diagnosis

- Cytopenias with a hypercellular bone marrow.
- Morphologic abnormalities in two or more hematopoietic cell lines.

General Considerations

The myelodysplastic syndromes are a group of acquired clonal disorders of the hematopoietic stem cell. They are characterized by the constellation of cytopenias, a hypercellular marrow, and a number of morphologic and cytogenetic abnormalities. The disorders are usually idiopathic but may be seen after cytotoxic chemotherapy—especially procarbazine for Hodgkin's disease and melphalan for multiple myeloma or ovarian carcinoma.

Despite the presence of adequate numbers of hematopoietic progenitor cells, "ineffective hemato-poiesis" occurs, resulting in various cytopenias. Ultimately, the disorder may evolve into frank acute myelogenous leukemia, and the term "preleukemia" has been used to describe these disorders. Although no specific chromosomal abnormality is seen in myelodysplasia, there are frequently abnormalities involving the long arm of chromosome 5 (which contains a number of genes encoding both growth factors and receptors involved in myelopoiesis) as well as deletions of chromosomes 5 and 7.

Myelodysplasia encompasses several heterogeneous syndromes. Those without excess bone marrow blasts are termed "refractory anemia," with or without ringed sideroblasts. Those with excess blasts are diagnosed as "refractory anemia with excess blasts" (RAEB 5–19% blasts) and "refractory anemia with excess blasts in transition" (RAEB-T 20–29% blasts). Those with a proliferative syndrome including peripheral blood monocytosis greater than 1000/μL are termed chronic myelomonocytic leukemia (CMML).

Clinical Findings

A. Symptoms and Signs: Patients are usually over age 60. Many are diagnosed while asymptomatic because of the finding of abnormal blood counts. Patients usually present with fatigue, infection, or bleeding related to bone marrow failure. The course may be indolent, and the disease may present as a wasting illness with fever, weight loss, and general debility. On examination, splenomegaly may be present in combination with pallor, bleeding, and various signs of infection.

B. Laboratory Findings: Anemia may be severe and may require transfusion support. The MCV is normal or increased, and macro-ovalocytes may be seen on the peripheral blood smear. The reticulocyte count is usually reduced. The white blood cell count is usually normal or reduced, and neutropenia is common. The neutrophils may exhibit morphologic abnormalities, including deficient numbers of granules or a bilobed nucleus (Pelger-Huet). The myeloid series may be left-shifted, and small numbers of promyelocytes or blasts may be seen. The platelet count is normal or reduced, and hypogranular platelets may be present.

The bone marrow is characteristically hypercellular. Erythroid hyperplasia is common, and signs of abnormal erythropoiesis include megaloblastic features, nuclear budding, or multinucleated erythroid precursors. The Prussian blue stain may demonstrate ringed sideroblasts. The myeloid series is often left-shifted, with variable increases in blasts. Deficient or abnormal granules may be seen. A characteristic abnormality is the presence of dwarf megakaryoctyes with a unilobed nucleus.

Differential Diagnosis

In subtle cases, cytogenetic evaluation of the bone

marrow may help distinguish this clonal disorder from other causes of cytopenias. As the number of blasts increases in the bone marrow, myelodysplasia is arbitrarily separated from acute myelogenous leukemia by the presence of less than 30% blasts.

Treatment

Patients affected primarily by anemia are best supported with red blood cell transfusions. Patients with severe neutropenia or thrombocytopenia or those with marked constitutional symptoms may be treated with low-dose chemotherapy, although the results of therapy are often inadequate. Erythropoietin (epoetin alfa), 10,000 units subcutaneously three times weekly, reduces the red cell transfusion requirement in some patients. The response rate is 20% or less, but a 4-week trial of erythropoietin is reasonable since it will be of benefit and cost-effective for the subgroup of responders. The combination of myeloid growth factors and high doses of erythropoietin produces a higher response rate, but the cost is prohibitive. The myeloid growth factors C-CSF (filgrastim) and GM-CSF (sargramostim), 5 mg/kg/d, reliably raise the neutrophil count and reduce the incidence of infections. However, they do not usually benefit other cell types and appear not to change the course of the disease.

Investigational drugs such as azacitidine are being evaluated as potential therapeutic agents.

Young patients (under age 60) with matched sibling donors can be successfully treated with ablative chemotherapy and allogeneic bone marrow transplantation. Cure rates are approximately 30–50%.

Course & Prognosis

Myelodysplasia is an ultimately fatal disease. Patients most commonly succumb to infections or bleeding. The risk of transformation to acute myelogenous leukemia depends on the percentage of blasts in the bone marrow. Patients with refractory anemia may survive many years, and the risk of leukemia is low (< 10%). Those with excess blasts or CMML have short survivals (usually < 2 years) and have a higher (20–50%) risk of developing acute leukemia. The finding of deletions of chromosomes 5 and 7 is associated with a poor prognosis. Allogeneic bone marrow transplantation is the only definitive therapy, though its optimal timing given the wide spectrum of prognostic possibilities may be difficult to determine.

Anderson JE et al: Allogeneic marrow transplantation for myelodysplastic syndrome with advanced disease morphology: A phase II study of busulfan, cyclophosphamide, and total-body irradiation and analysis of prognostic factors. J Clin Oncol 1996;14:220.

Anderson JE et al: Allogeneic bone marrow transplantation for 93 patients with myelodysplastic syndromes. Blood 1993;82:677. (Offers curative potential, with 40% disease-free long-term survival. Patients under age 40 without excess marrow blasts do particularly well with 60% long-term survival.)

Rose EH et al: The use of r-HuEpo in the treatment of anaemia related to myelodysplasia (MDS). Br J Haematol 1995;89:831.

Taylor KM et al: Myelodysplasia. Curr Opin Oncol 1994; 6:32. (Current biology, diagnosis, classification, and treatment options.)

ACUTE LEUKEMIA

Essentials of Diagnosis

- Cytopenias or pancytopenia.
- Bone marrow failure causing infection, bleeding, or fatigue.
- More than 30% blasts in the bone marrow.
- Blasts in peripheral blood in 90%.

General Considerations

Acute leukemia is a malignancy of the hematopoietic progenitor cell. The malignant cell loses its ability to mature and differentiate. These cells proliferate in an uncontrolled fashion and ultimately replace normal bone marrow elements. Most cases arise with no clear cause. However, radiation and some toxins (benzene) are clearly leukemogenic. In addition, a number of chemotherapeutic agents (especially procarbazine, melphalan, other alkylating agents, and etoposide) may cause leukemia. The leukemias seen after toxin or chemotherapy exposure often develop from a myelodysplastic prodrome and are associated with abnormalities in chromosomes 5 and 7. Although a number of other cytogenetic abnormalities are seen in certain types of acute leukemia, their exact role in pathogenesis remains unclear.

Most of the clinical findings in acute leukemia are due to bone marrow failure, which results from replacement of normal bone marrow elements by the malignant cell. Less common manifestations include direct organ infiltration (skin, gastrointestinal tract, meninges). Acute leukemia is one of the outstanding examples of a once invariably fatal disease that is now treatable and potentially curable with combination chemotherapy.

Acute lymphoblastic leukemia (ALL) comprises 80% of the acute leukemias of childhood. The peak incidence is between 3 and 7 years of age. However, ALL is also seen in adults and comprises approximately 20% of adult acute leukemias. Acute myelogenous leukemia (AML; acute nonlymphocytic leukemia [ANLL]) is chiefly an adult disease with a median age at presentation of 50 years and an increasing incidence with advanced age. However, it is also seen in young adults and children.

Clinical Findings

A. Symptoms and Signs: Most patients with acute leukemia present with an acute illness and have been ill only for days or weeks. Bleeding (usually due to thrombocytopenia) is usually in the skin and mucosal surfaces, manifested as gingival bleeding, epistaxis, or menorrhagia. Less commonly, widespread severe bleeding is seen in patients with disseminated intravascular coagulation (seen in acute promyelocytic leukemia and monocytic leukemia). Infection is due to neutropenia, with the risk of infection becoming high as the neutrophil count falls below 500/μL. Patients with neutrophil counts less than 100/μL almost invariably become infected within several days. The most common pathogens are gram-negative bacteria (E coli, Klebsiella, Pseudomonas) or fungi (Candida, Aspergillus). Common presentations include cellulitis, pneumonia, and perirectal infections. Septicemia in severely neutropenic patients can cause death within a few hours if treatment with appropriate antibiotics is delayed.

Patients may also seek medical attention because of gum hypertrophy and bone and joint pain. The most dramatic presentation is hyperleukocytosis, in which a markedly elevated circulating blast count (usually > 200,000/μL) leads to impaired circulation, presenting as headache, confusion, and dyspnea. Such patients require emergent leukapheresis and chemotherapy.

On examination, patients are usually pale and have purpura, petechiae, and various signs of infection. Stomatitis and gum hypertrophy may be seen in patients with monocytic leukemia. There is variable enlargement of the liver, spleen, and lymph nodes. Bone tenderness, particularly in the sternum and tibia, may be present.

B. Laboratory Findings: The hallmark of acute leukemia is the combination of pancytopenia with circulating blasts. However, blasts may be absent from the peripheral smear in as many as 10% of cases ("aleukemic leukemia").

The bone marrow is usually hypercellular and dominated by blasts. More than 30% blasts are required to make a diagnosis of acute leukemia.

A number of other laboratory abnormalities may be present. Hyperuricemia may be seen. If disseminated intravascular coagulation is present, the fibrinogen level will be reduced, the prothrombin time prolonged, and fibrin degradation products or fibrin D-dimers present. Patients with acute lymphoblastic leukemia (especially T cell) may have a mediastinal mass visible on chest radiograph. Patients with meningeal leukemia will have blasts present in the spinal fluid. This is seen in approximately 5% of cases at diagnosis and is more common in monocytic types of acute myelogenous leukemia.

Acute leukemia should be classified as either acute lymphoblastic or acute myelogenous leukemia, also called acute nonlymphocytic leukemia. Patients with acute myelogenous leukemia may have granules visible in the blast cells. The Auer rod, an eosinophilic needle-like inclusion in the cytoplasm, is pathognomonic of acute myelogenous leukemia. To confirm the myeloid nature of the cells, histochemical stains demonstrating myeloid enzymes such as peroxidase or chloroacetate esterase may be useful. Monocytic lineage can be demonstrated by the finding of butyrate esterase. Acute lymphoblastic leukemia should be considered when there is no morphologic or histochemical evidence of myeloid or monocytic lineage. The diagnosis is confirmed by demonstrating surface markers characteristic of primitive lymphoid cells. Terminal deoxynucleotidal transferase (TdT) is present in 95% of cases of acute lymphoblastic leukemia. A variety of monoclonal antibodies have been used to define other phenotypes of acute lymphoblastic leukemia. Primitive B lymphocyte antigens include CD10 and CD19. T cell acute lymphoblastic leukemia is diagnosed by the finding of CD2, CD5, and CD7.

Acute myelogenous leukemia is usually categorized on the basis of morphology and histochemistry as follows: Acute undifferentiated leukemia (M0), acute myeloblastic leukemia (M1), acute myeloblastic leukemia with differentiation (M2), acute promyelocytic leukemia (M3), acute myelomonocytic leukemia (M4), acute monoblastic leukemia (M5), erythroleukemia (M6), and megakaryoblastic leukemia (M7).

Acute lymphoblastic leukemia is most usefully classified by immunologic phenotype as follows: common, early B lineage, and T cell.

Cytogenetic studies have emerged as the most powerful prognostic factor in the acute leukemias. Favorable cytogenetics in acute myeloid leukemia include t(8;21), t(15;17), and inv(16)(p13;q22). These patients have a higher chance of achieving both short- and long-term disease control. Favorable cytogenetics in acute lymphoblastic leukemia are the hyperdiploid states. Unfavorable cytogenetics are monosomy 5 and 7, Philadelphia chromosome, and abnormalities of 11q23.

Differential Diagnosis

Acute myelogenous leukemia must be distinguished from other myeloproliferative disorders, chronic myelogenous leukemia, and myelodysplastic syndromes. It is important to distinguish acute leukemia from a left-shifted bone marrow that is recovering from a previous toxic insult. If the question is in doubt, a bone marrow study should be repeated in several days to see if maturation has taken place. Acute lymphoblastic leukemia must be distinguished from other lymphoproliferative disease such as chronic lymphocytic leukemia, lymphomas, and hairy cell leukemia. It may also be confused with the atypical lymphocytosis of mononucleosis. An experienced observer can distinguish these entities based on morphology.

Treatment

Most young patients with acute leukemia are

treated with the objective of effecting a cure. The first step in treatment is to obtain complete remission, defined as normal peripheral blood with resolution of cytopenias, normal bone marrow with no excess in blasts, and normal clinical status. However, complete remission is not synonymous with cure, and leukemia will invariably recur if no further treatment is given.

Acute myelogenous leukemia is treated initially with intensive combination chemotherapy, including daunorubicin and cytarabine. Effective treatment produces aplasia of the bone marrow, which takes 2–3 weeks to recover. During this period, intensive supportive care, including transfusion and antibiotic therapy, is required. Once complete remission has been achieved, several different types of postremission therapy are potentially curative. Options include repeated intensive chemotherapy, high-dose chemoradiotherapy with allogeneic bone marrow transplantation, and high-dose chemotherapy with autologous bone marrow transplantation. Recently, progress has been made in the treatment of acute promyelocytic leukemia (M3). The addition of all-*trans* retinoic acid to initial chemotherapy has improved the results of both initial treatment and long-term survival. Retinoic acid appears to induce terminal differentiation in the malignant cell and hence to induce remission without cytotoxic effect.

Acute lymphoblastic leukemia is treated initially with combination chemotherapy, including daunorubicin, vincristine, prednisone, and asparaginase. Remission induction therapy for acute lymphoblastic leukemia is less myelosuppressive than treatment for acute myelogenous leukemia and does not necessarily produce marrow aplasia. After achieving complete remission, patients receive central nervous system prophylaxis so that meningeal sequestration of leukemic cells does not develop. As with acute myelogenous leukemia, patients may be treated with either chemotherapy or high-dose chemotherapy plus bone marrow transplantation.

Prognosis

Approximately 70–80% of adults with acute myelogenous leukemia under age 60 achieve complete remission. High-dose postremission chemotherapy leads to cure in 30–40% of these patients, and high-dose cytarabine has been shown to be superior to therapy with lower doses. Allogeneic bone marrow transplantation (for younger adults with HLA-matched siblings) is curative in approximately 60% of cases. Autologous bone marrow transplantation is a promising new form of therapy that may cure 50–70% of patients in first remission. One recent study demonstrated the superiority of this approach to nonablative chemotherapy. Older adults with acute myelogenous leukemia reportedly achieve complete remission approximately 50% of the time. In selected cases, older patients may be treated with intensive chemotherapy with curative intent.

Ninety percent of adults with acute lymphoblastic leukemia achieve complete remission. Subsequent postremission chemotherapy is curative in 30–50% of adults. Acute lymphoblastic leukemia in children is much more responsive to therapy, with 95% achieving complete remission and 60–70% of these being cured with postremission treatment that is far less toxic than that necessary for adults.

Once leukemia has recurred ("relapsed") after initial chemotherapy, bone marrow transplantation (BMT) is the only curative option. Allogenic BMT can be used for those under age 55 with histocompatible sibling donors and is successful in 30–40% of cases. Autologous BMT may be curative in 30–50% of cases after a second remission is achieved.

Bishop JF et al: A randomized study of high-dose cytarabine in induction in acute myeloid leukemia. Blood 1996;87:1710.

Cortes JE, Kantarjian H, Freireich EJ: Acute lymphocytic leukemia: A comprehensive review with emphasis on biology and therapy. Cancer Treat Res 1996;84:291.

Degos L et al: *All-trans*-retinoic acid as a differentiating agent in the treatment of acute promyelocytic leukemia. Blood 1995;85:2643.

Keating S et al: Prognostic factors of patients with acute myeloid leukemia (AML) allografted in first complete remission: An analysis of the EORTC-GIMEMA AML 8A trial. The European Organization for Research and Treatment of Cancer (EORTC) and the Gruppo Italiano Malattie Ematologiche Maligne dell' Adulto (GIMEMA) Leukemia Cooperative Groups. Bone Marrow Transplant 1996;17:993.

Linker CA et al: Autologous bone marrow transplantation for acute myeloid leukemia using busulfan plus etoposide as a preparative regimen. Blood 1993;81:311. (Using an intensified preparative regimen and in vitro bone marrow purging, 5-year disease-free survival is greater than 70% in first remission patients and greater than 50% in second remission patients. Updated results in 50 patients confirm these findings, with 70% long-term disease-free survival and a 4% mortality rate for first remission patients.)

Mayer RJ et al: Intensive postremission chemotherapy in adults with acute myeloid leukemia. N Engl J Med 1994;331:896. (A cooperative group study confirming previous reports that in adults under age 60, postremission therapy with high-dose cytarabine is superior to treatment with standard-dose cytarabine. Standard doses are no longer recommended.)

Stein AS et al: In vivo purging with high-dose cytarabine followed by high-dose chemoradiotherapy and reinfusion of unpurged bone marrow for adult acute myelogenous leukemia in first complete remission. J Clin Oncol 1996;14:2206.

Zittoun RA et al: Autologous or allogeneic bone marrow transplantation compared with intensive chemotherapy in acute myelogenous leukemia. N Engl J Med 1995; 32:217. (Autologous bone marrow transplantation produces a superior disease-free survival in first remission patients: 48% at 4 years.)

CHRONIC LYMPHOCYTIC LEUKEMIA

Essentials of Diagnosis

- Lymphocytosis > 5000/μL.
- "Mature" appearance of lymphocytes.
- Co-expression of CD19, CD5.

General Considerations

Chronic lymphocytic leukemia (CLL) is a clonal malignancy of B lymphocytes (rarely T lymphocytes). The disease is usually indolent, with slowly progressive accumulation of long-lived small lymphocytes. These cells are immunoincompetent and respond poorly to antigenic stimulation.

Chronic lymphocytic leukemia is manifested clinically by immunosuppression, bone marrow failure, and organ infiltration with lymphocytes. Immunosuppression, bone marrow failure, and infiltration of organs account for most clinical manifestations. Immunodeficiency is also related to inadequate antibody production by the abnormal B cells. With advanced disease, chronic lymphocytic leukemia may cause damage by direct tissue infiltration.

Clinical Findings

A. Symptoms and Signs: Chronic lymphocytic leukemia is a disease of the elderly, with 90% of cases occurring after age 50 and a median age at presentation of 65. Many patients will be incidentally discovered to have lymphocytosis. Others present with fatigue or lymphadenopathy. On examination, 80% of patients will have lymphadenopathy and half will have enlargement of the liver or spleen.

A prognostically useful staging system has been developed as follows: stage 0, lymphocytosis only; stage I, lymphocytosis plus lymphadenopathy; stage II, organomegaly; stage III, anemia; stage IV, thrombocytopenia.

Chronic lymphocytic leukemia usually pursues an indolent course but occasionally will present as a rapidly progressive disease. These patients usually have larger, less mature-appearing lymphocytes and are said to have "prolymphocytic" leukemia. In 5–10% of cases, chronic lymphocytic leukemia may be complicated by autoimmune hemolytic anemia or autoimmune thrombocytopenia. In approximately 5% of cases, while the systemic disease remains stable, an isolated lymph node will be transformed into an aggressive large cell lymphoma (**Richter's syndrome**).

B. Laboratory Findings: The hallmark of chronic lymphocytic leukemia is isolated lymphocytosis. The white blood count is usually greater than 20,000/μL and may be markedly elevated. Usually 75–98% of the circulating cells are lymphocytes. Lymphocytes appear small and "mature," with condensed nuclear chromatin, and are morphologically indistinguishable from normal small lymphocytes. The hematocrit and platelet count are usually normal at presentation. The bone marrow is variably infiltrated with small lymphocytes. The malignant cells weakly express surface immunoglobulin, and the monoclonal nature of the cells can be demonstrated by the finding of a single light chain type on the surface. The immunophenotype of CLL is unique in that it co-expresses B lymphocyte lineage markers such as CD19 with the T lymphocyte marker CD5. Other B cell malignancies do not express CD5.

Hypogammaglobulinemia is present in half of cases and becomes more common with advanced disease. In some instances, a small amount of IgM paraprotein is present in the serum. Pathologic changes in lymph nodes are the same as in diffuse small cell lymphocytic lymphoma.

Differential Diagnosis

Few syndromes can be confused with chronic lymphocytic leukemia. Viral infections producing lymphocytosis should be obvious from the presence of fever and other clinical findings. Other lymphoproliferative diseases such as Waldenström's macroglobulinemia, hairy cell leukemia, or lymphoma in the leukemic phase are distinguished on the basis of the morphology of circulating lymphocytes and bone marrow.

Treatment

Most cases of early indolent chronic lymphocytic leukemia require no specific therapy. Indications for treatment include progressive fatigue, troublesome lymphadenopathy, or the development of anemia or thrombocytopenia. These patients have either symptomatic and progressive stage II disease or stage III/IV disease. Initial therapy is with chlorambucil, 0.6–1 mg orally every 3 weeks. Complications such as autoimmune hemolytic anemia or immune thrombocytopenia may be treated with high-dose prednisone but often require splenectomy for control. Fludarabine is a new agent which is useful in treating disease refractory to other agents. As initial therapy, fludarabine produces faster and more complete responses than chlorambucil, and the duration of remissions is considerably longer. However, fludarabine causes long-term immunosuppression, and it remains to be determined if it should be used as primary therapy or reserved for use later in the disease. The rare young patient (age under 50) with aggressive disease may be a candidate for allogeneic bone marrow transplantation.

Prognosis

Median survival is approximately 6 years, and 25% of patients live more than 10 years. Patients with stage 0 or I disease have a median survival of 10 years. It is important to reassure these patients that despite the frightening diagnosis of "leukemia" they can live a normal life for many years. Patients with stage III or IV disease have a median survival of less than 2 years. Chronic lymphocytic leukemia is managed in palliative fashion. Patients with advanced disease benefit only briefly from intensive therapy.

Cheson BD et al: National Cancer Institute-sponsored Working Group guidelines for chronic lymphocytic leukemia: Revised guidelines for diagnosis and treatment. Blood 1996;87:4990.

Michallet M et al: HLA-identical sibling bone marrow transplantation in younger patients with chronic lymphocytic leukemia. European Group for Blood and Marrow Transplantation and the International Bone Marrow Transplant Registry. Ann Intern Med 1996;124:311.

O'Brien S, del Giglio A, Keating M: Advances in the biology and treatment of B-cell chronic lymphocytic leukemia. Blood 1995;85:307.

Tallman MS et al: Cladribine in the treatment of relapsed or refractory chronic lymphocytic leukemia. J Clin Oncol 1995;13:983.

HAIRY CELL LEUKEMIA

Essentials of Diagnosis
- Pancytopenia.
- Splenomegaly, often massive.
- Hairy cells present on blood smear and bone marrow biopsy.

General Considerations
Hairy cell leukemia, an uncommon form of leukemia, is an indolent cancer of B lymphocytes.

Clinical Findings
A. Symptoms and Signs: The disease characteristically presents in middle-aged men. The median age at presentation is 55 years, and there is a striking 5:1 male predominance. Most patients present with gradual onset of fatigue, but others complain of symptoms related to markedly enlarged spleen and still others come to attention because of infection.

On physical examination, splenomegaly is almost invariably present and may be massive. The liver is enlarged in half of cases, but lymphadenopathy is uncommon.

B. Laboratory Findings: The hallmark of hairy cell leukemia is pancytopenia. Anemia is nearly universal, and 75% of patients have thrombocytopenia and neutropenia as well. Nearly all patients have striking monocytopenia, which is encountered in almost no other condition. The "hairy cells" are usually present in small numbers on the peripheral blood smear and have a characteristic appearance with numerous cytoplasmic projections. Less commonly, a "leukemic form" of the disorder exists in which large numbers of hairy cells dominate the peripheral blood smear. The bone marrow is usually inaspirable (dry tap), and the diagnosis is made by characteristic morphology on bone marrow biopsy. The hairy cells have a characteristic histochemical staining pattern, with tartrate-resistant acid phosphatase (TRAP). On immunophenotyping, the cells co-express the antigens CD11c and CD22. Pathologic examination of the spleen shows marked infiltration of the red pulp with hairy cells. This is in marked contrast to the usual predilection of lymphomas to involve the white pulp of the spleen.

Hairy cell leukemia is usually an indolent disorder whose course is dominated by pancytopenia and recurrent infections, including mycobacterial infections.

Differential Diagnosis
Hairy cell leukemia should be distinguished from other lymphoproliferative diseases such as Waldenström's macroglobulinemia and non-Hodgkin's lymphomas. It also may be confused with other causes of pancytopenia, including hypersplenism due to any cause or paroxysmal nocturnal hemoglobinuria.

Treatment
The treatment of hairy cell leukemia has been dramatically changed by the development of new effective agents. The treatment of choice is with cladribine (2-chlorodeoxyadenosine; CdA), 0.14 mg/kg daily for 7 days. This is a relatively nontoxic drug that produces benefit in 95% of cases and complete remission in more than 80%. Responses are long-lasting, with few patients relapsing in the first few years. Interferon and splenectomy are rarely used now.

Course & Prognosis
The development of new effective therapies appears to have changed the prognosis of this disease. Formerly, median survival was 6 years, and only one-third of patients survived longer than 10 years. Although longer follow-up will be required, it now appears that most patients with hairy cell leukemia will live longer than 10 years. With current trends in treatment, the prognosis appears open-ended at this time.

Frassoldati A et al: Hairy cell leukemia: A clinical review based on 725 cases of the Italian Cooperative Group. Leukemia Lymphoma 1994;13:307. (Five-year survival rates were 58.9% before 1985 and 87.5% after 1985.)

Saven A, Piro LD: Drug therapy: Newer purine analogue for the treatment of hairy-cell leukemia. N Engl J Med 1994;330:691. (Pentostatin and cladribine inhibit action of adenosine deaminase and produce long-term remission; more rapid recovery from immunosuppression with cladribine.)

Tallman MS et al: Relapse of hairy cell leukemia after 2-chlorodeoxyadenosine: Long-term follow-up of the Northwestern University experience. Blood 1996;88:1954.

Wheaton S et al: Minimal residual disease may predict bone marrow relapse in patients with hairy cell leukemia treated with 2-chlorodeoxyadenosine. Blood 1996;87: 1556.

LYMPHOMAS

NON-HODGKIN'S LYMPHOMAS

The non-Hodgkin's lymphomas are a heterogeneous group of cancers of lymphocytes. The disorders are variable in clinical presentation and course, varying from indolent disease to rapidly progressive devastating illnesses.

Results of studies using techniques of molecular biology have provided clues to the pathogenesis of these disorders. The best-studied example is Burkitt's lymphoma, in which a characteristic cytogenetic abnormality of translocation between the long arms of chromosomes 8 and 14 has been identified. The proto-oncogene c-*myc* is translocated from its normal position on chromosome 8 to the heavy chain locus on chromosome 14. Cells committed to B cell differentiation are likely to have enhanced expression of this heavy chain locus, and it is likely that overexpression of c-*myc* (in its new anomalous position) is related to malignant transformation. In the follicular lymphomas, translocations of a possible oncogene *bcl*-2 from chromosome 8 to the heavy chain locus on chromosome 14 may play a similar role.

Classification of the lymphomas is a controversial area still undergoing evolution. Recently, the National Cancer Institute has sponsored a "working formulation" that characterizes these lymphomas according to their biologic behavior, whether indolent or aggressive (Table 13–16).

Clinical Findings

A. Symptoms and Signs: Patients with indolent lymphomas usually present with painless lymphadenopathy, which may be isolated or widespread. Involved lymph nodes may be present in the retroperitoneum, mesentery, and pelvis. However, the indolent lymphomas are often disseminated at the time of diagnosis, and bone marrow involvement is frequent.

Patients with intermediate and high-grade lymphomas may present with adenopathy or with constitutional symptoms such as fever, drenching night sweats, or weight loss. On examination, lymphadenopathy may be isolated, or extranodal sites of disease (skin, gastrointestinal tract) may be found. Patients with Burkitt's lymphoma frequently present with abdominal pain or abdominal fullness because of the predilection of the disease for the abdomen. Patients with HIV disease also have an increased in-

Table 13–16. Classification of lymphomas: "working formulation."

Low-grade
Small lymphocytic
Small lymphocytic, plasmacytoid
Follicular small cleaved cell
Follicular mixed cell
Intermediate-grade
Follicular large cell
Diffuse small cleaved cell
Diffuse mixed cell
Diffuse large cell
High-grade
Immunoblastic
Small noncleaved (Burkitt's)
Small noncleaved (non-Burkitt's)
Lymphoblastic
True histiocytic
Other
Cutaneous T cell (mycosis fungoides)
Adult T cell leukemia/lymphoma
T γ lymphocytosis

cidence of non-Hodgkin's lymphoma; it may be isolated to the central nervous system in such individuals.

Once a pathologic diagnosis is established, the patient should be staged. Physical examination is supplemented by chest x-ray and CT scan of the abdomen and pelvis. The bone marrow should be biopsied, and—in selected cases such as high-risk morphology—a lumbar puncture should be performed.

B. Laboratory Findings: The peripheral blood is usually normal, but a number of lymphomas may present in a "leukemic" phase. In these situations, the distinction between leukemia and lymphoma is arbitrary, as the malignant cell has the same characteristics. Examples of the diseases that may present as lymphoma or leukemia are small cell lymphoma (chronic lymphocytic leukemia), small cell plasmacytic lymphoma (Waldenström's macroglobulinemia), follicular small cleaved cell lymphoma (lymphosarcoma cell leukemia), cutaneous T cell lymphoma (Sézary syndrome), lymphoblastic lymphoma (T cell acute lymphoblastic leukemia), and Burkitt's lymphoma (B cell acute lymphoblastic leukemia).

Bone marrow involvement is usually manifested as paratrabecular lymphoid aggregates. In some high-grade lymphomas, the meninges may be involved and the spinal fluid may contain malignant cells. The chest radiograph may show a mediastinal mass in lymphoblastic lymphoma.

The serum LDH level is useful in evaluating the extent of disease and the aggressiveness of tumor behavior, with higher levels indicating more widespread disease.

The diagnosis of lymphoma is made by tissue

biopsy. Needle aspiration may yield suspicious results, but usually a lymph node biopsy (or biopsy of involved extranodal tissue) is required.

Treatment

The indolent lymphomas are usually not curable and are approached with palliative therapy. If patients are asymptomatic, no initial treatment may be necessary. However, in 1–3 years, the disease will usually progress and require treatment. Treatment decisions are individualized depending on the patient's age and performance status and the extent of disease. Initial therapy is based on the alkylating agents. Appropriate regimens include chlorambucil, 0.6–1 mg/kg every 3 weeks, or combination therapy with cyclophosphamide, vincristine, and prednisone (CVP). Patients with more aggressive or resistant disease may require more intensive therapy, and allogeneic bone marrow transplantation may be appropriate for selected younger patients. The role of autologous transplantation for indolent lymphomas is controversial at this time. Those with apparently localized disease may be treated initially with local radiation. Low-grade MALT (mucosa-associated lymphoid tissue) lymphomas may be related to *Helicobacter pylori* infection, and disease confined to the stomach has responded completely to antibiotic therapy.

Patients with intermediate and high-grade lymphomas should be treated with curative intent. Irradiation is occasionally used for localized disease (supplemented by brief intensive chemotherapy), but the mainstay of therapy is combination chemotherapy. The traditional treatment regimen has been cyclophosphamide, doxorubicin, vincristine, and prednisone (CHOP) (see Tables 5–2 and 5–3). It remains to be proved that newer and more intensive regimens produce superior results. For patients who relapse following initial treatment with chemotherapy, the treatment of choice is autologous stem cell (or bone marrow) transplantation. The role of autologous transplantation or initial therapy for high-risk patients is promising.

Prognosis

The median survival of patients with indolent lymphomas is 6–8 years. These diseases ultimately become refractory to chemotherapy. This often occurs at the time of histologic progression of the disease to a more aggressive form of lymphoma. The prognosis of patients with high-grade lymphomas depends on their response to chemotherapy. Depending on the initial pathologic subtype and initial bulk of disease, these patients are variably curable.

With appropriate therapy, approximately 50% of patients with disseminated large-cell lymphomas may be cured. Results are better in those who are young, are in good clinical condition, and have less advanced stages of disease. Salvage therapy with au-

tologous bone marrow transplantation may be effective in 50% of cases if the disease is still responsive to chemotherapy and the patient comes to transplant in good condition and with minimal tumor bulk.

The International Non-Hodgkin's Lymphoma Prognostic Factors Project: A predictive model for aggressive non-Hodgkin's lymphoma. N Engl J Med 1993;329:987. (International index and age-adjusted international index based on tumor stage, serum LDH, and performance status among others useful in predicting survival.)

Philip T et al: Autologous bone marrow transplantation as compared with salvage chemotherapy in relapses of chemotherapy-sensitive non-Hodgkin's lymphoma. N Engl J Med 1995;333:1540.

Roggero E et al: Eradication of *Helicobacter pylori* infection in primary low-grade gastric lymphoma of mucosa-associated lymphoid tissue. Ann Intern Med 1995; 122:767.

HODGKIN'S DISEASE

Essentials of Diagnosis

- Painless lymphadenopathy.
- Constitutional symptoms may be present.
- Pathologic diagnosis by lymph node biopsy.

General Considerations

Hodgkin's disease is a group of cancers characterized by Reed-Sternberg cells in an appropriate reactive cellular background. The nature of the malignant cell is a subject of controversy, but recent evidence suggests that it is of macrophage origin.

Clinical Findings

There is a bimodal age distribution, with one peak in the 20s and a second peak over age 50. Most patients present because of a painless mass, commonly in the neck. Others may seek medical attention because of constitutional symptoms such as fever, weight loss, or drenching night sweats, or because of generalized pruritus. An unusual symptom of Hodgkin's disease is pain in an involved lymph node following alcohol ingestion.

An important clinical feature of Hodgkin's disease is its tendency to arise within lymph node areas and to spread in an orderly fashion to contiguous areas of lymph nodes. Only late in the course of the disease will vascular invasion lead to widespread hematogenous dissemination.

The diagnosis is made by examination of lymph node tissue by an experienced hematopathologist. Hodgkin's disease is divided into several subtypes: lymphocyte predominance, nodular sclerosis, mixed cellularity, and lymphocyte depletion. Hodgkin's disease should be distinguished pathologically from other malignant lymphomas. It may also occasionally be confused with reactive lymph nodes seen in infectious mononucleosis, cat-scratch disease, or drug reactions (eg, phenytoin).

Patients should initially undergo a "staging" evaluation to determine the extent of disease. The purpose of this evaluation is to determine whether localized treatment (radiotherapy) is indicated or if systemic chemotherapy must be given. The staging nomenclature is as follows: stage I, one lymph node region involved; stage II, involvement of two lymph node areas on one side of the diaphragm; stage III, lymph node regions involved on both sides of the diaphragm; stage IV, disseminated disease with bone marrow or liver involvement. In addition, patients are designated stage A if they lack constitutional symptoms and stage B if significant weight loss, fever, or night sweats are present.

Treatment

Patients with localized disease (stages IA, IIA) are treated with radiation therapy. Patients with disseminated disease (IIIB, IV) are treated with aggressive combination chemotherapy. The treatment of choice appears to be Adriamycin (doxorubicin), bleomycin, vincristine, dacarbazine (ABVD) (see Tables 5–2 and 5–3). The optimal management of patients with stages IIB or IIIA is controversial, but current evidence suggests an advantage to combination chemotherapy.

Prognosis

Virtually all patients with both localized and disseminated disease should be treated with curative intent. The prognosis of patients with stage IA or IIA disease treated by radiotherapy is excellent, with 10-year survival rates in excess of 80%. Patients with disseminated disease (IIIB, IV) have 5-year survival rates of 50–60%. Poorer results are seen in patients who are elderly, those who have bulky disease, and those with lymphocyte depletion or mixed cellularity on histologic examination. Patients whose disease recurs after initial radiotherapy treatment may still be curable with chemotherapy. Patients who relapse after initial chemotherapy may be cured with intensive therapy involving autologous bone marrow transplantation. Cure rates of 40–60% are seen in those who are still responsive to chemotherapy.

Horning SJ et al: High-dose therapy and autologous hematopoietic progenitor cell transplantation for recurrent or refractory Hodgkin's disease: Analysis of the Stanford University results and prognostic indices. Blood 1997;89:801.

Mauch PM et al: Second malignancies after treatment for laparotomy staged IA-IIIB Hodgkin's disease: Long-term analysis of risk factors and outcome. Blood 1996;87:3625.

Viviani S et al: Alternating versus hybrid MOPP and ABVD combinations in advanced Hodgkin's disease: Ten-year results. J Clin Oncol 1996;14:1421.

Yuen AR et al: Comparison between conventional salvage

therapy and high-dose therapy with autografting for recurrent or refractory Hodgkin's disease. Blood 1997; 89:814.

MULTIPLE MYELOMA

Essentials of Diagnosis

- Bone pain, often in the lower back.
- Monoclonal paraprotein by serum or urine protein electrophoresis or immunoelectrophoresis.
- Replacement of bone marrow by malignant plasma cells.

General Considerations

Multiple myeloma is a malignancy of plasma cells characterized by replacement of the bone marrow, bone destruction, and paraprotein formation. Myeloma is a complex disease that causes clinical symptoms and signs through a variety of mechanisms.

Replacement of the bone marrow (and perhaps humoral suppression of myelopoiesis) leads initially to anemia and later to general bone marrow failure. Bone destruction causes bone pain, osteoporosis, lytic lesions, and pathologic fractures. Hypercalcemia is common and appears to be mediated by osteoclast activating factor (OAF) or similar lymphokines. The malignant plasma cells can form tumors (plasmacytomas) that have a predilection for causing spinal cord compression.

The paraproteins secreted by the malignant plasma cells may cause problems in their own right. Very high paraprotein levels (either IgG or IgA) may cause the hyperviscosity syndrome, though this is more often caused by IgM in Waldenström's macroglobulinemia. The light chain component of the immunoglobulin may cause renal failure (often aggravated by hypercalcemia). Light chain components may be deposited in tissues as amyloid, worsening renal failure and causing a vast array of systemic symptoms.

Myeloma patients are prone to recurrent infections for a number of reasons, including neutropenia and the immunosuppressive effects of chemotherapy. Additionally, there is a failure of antibody production in response to antigen challenge, and myeloma patients are especially prone to infections with encapsulated organisms such as *Streptococcus pneumoniae* and *Haemophilus influenzae*.

Clinical Findings

A. Symptoms and Signs: Myeloma is a disease of older adults (median age at presentation, 60 years). The most common presenting complaints are those related to anemia, bone pain, and infection. Bone pain is most common in the back or ribs or may present as a pathologic fracture, especially of the femoral neck. Patients may also come to medical attention because of renal failure; spinal cord compression, or the hyperviscosity syndrome (mucosal bleeding, vertigo, nausea, visual disturbances, alterations in mental status). Occasionally, patients are diagnosed as having myeloma because of initial laboratory findings of hypercalcemia, proteinuria, elevated sedimentation rate, or abnormalities on serum protein electrophoresis.

Examination may reveal pallor, bone tenderness, and soft tissue masses. Patients may have neurologic signs related to neuropathy or spinal cord compression. Patients with amyloidosis may have an enlarged tongue, neuropathy, or congestive heart failure.

B. Laboratory Findings: Anemia is nearly universal. Red blood cell morphology is normal, but rouleau formation is common and may be marked. The neutrophil and platelet counts are usually normal at presentation. Only rarely will plasma cells be visible on peripheral smear (plasma cell leukemia).

The hallmark of myeloma is the finding of a paraprotein on serum protein electrophoresis (SPEP). The majority of patients will have a monoclonal spike visible in the beta or gamma globulin region. Immunoelectrophoresis (IEP) will reveal this to be a monoclonal protein. Approximately 15% of patients will have no demonstrable paraprotein in the serum. In these, IEP of the urine will reveal either complete immunoglobulin or light chains. Overall, approximately 60% of myeloma patients will have an IgG paraprotein, 25% an IgA, and 15% light chains only.

The bone marrow will be infiltrated by variable numbers of plasma cells ranging from 5% to 100%. Occasionally, the plasma cells may be morphologically indistinguishable from normal cells but more commonly will appear abnormal. Bone radiographs are important in establishing the diagnosis of myeloma. Lytic lesions are most commonly seen in the axial skeleton: skull, spine, proximal long bones, and ribs. At other times, only generalized osteoporosis is seen. The radionuclide bone scan is not useful in detecting bone lesions in myeloma, as there is usually no osteoblastic component.

Other laboratory features include hypercalcemia, renal failure, and an elevated erythrocyte sedimentation rate. Some patients have proximal renal tubular acidosis, with phosphaturia, glycosuria, and uricosuria. The urinalysis may reveal proteinuria, but the dipstick test (which detects primarily albumin) is unreliable for light chains. Often there is a narrow anion gap when the paraprotein is cationic. On occasion, the abnormal protein is cryoprecipitatable, resulting in positive studies for cryoglobulins.

Differential Diagnosis

When a patient is discovered to have a monoclonal paraprotein, the distinction between myeloma and monoclonal gammopathy of unknown significance (MGUS) must be made. MGUS is present in 1% of all adults and 3% of adults over age 70. Thus, if one considers all patients with paraproteins, MGUS is far more common than myeloma. Most commonly, patients with MGUS will have a monoclonal IgG spike less than 2.5 g/dL, and the height of the spike remains stable. In approximately 25% of cases, MGUS progresses to overt malignant disease, but this may take years or even decades.

Myeloma is distinguished from MGUS by findings of replacement of the bone marrow, bone destruction, and progression over time. Although the height of the paraprotein spike should not be used by itself to distinguish benign from malignant disease, in practice all patients with IgG spikes greater than 3.5 g/dL prove to have myeloma. An IgA spike of greater than 2 g/dL is almost always due to myeloma. If there is doubt about whether paraproteinemia is benign or malignant, the patient should be observed without therapy, since there is no advantage to early treatment of asymptomatic multiple myeloma.

Myeloma should be distinguished from polyclonal hypergammaglobulinemia seen in reactive conditions. The distinction is made by finding the polyclonal as opposed to the monoclonal spike. Myeloma may also need to be distinguished from other malignant lymphoproliferative diseases such as Waldenström's macroglobulinemia, lymphomas, and primary amyloidosis.

Treatment

The goal of treatment of myeloma is usually palliation. Patients with minimal disease or in whom the diagnosis of malignancy is in doubt should be observed without treatment. Most commonly, patients require treatment at diagnosis because of bone pain or other symptoms related to the disease. In the past, standard therapy has been melphalan plus prednisone; more recently, combination chemotherapy with alkylating agents has been used. The optimal chemotherapy regimen has not been determined. The height of the paraprotein spike on SPEP is a useful marker for monitoring response to therapy. Patients who fail to respond to standard therapy may be effectively salvaged with low-dose continuous infusion therapy, the VAD (vincristine, Adriamycin [doxorubicin], dexamethasone) regimen (see Tables 5–2 and 5–3).

A number of other ancillary measures are important in the treatment of myeloma. Localized radiotherapy may be useful for palliation of bone pain or for eradicating tumor at the site of pathologic fracture. Hypercalcemia should be treated aggressively and prolonged immobilization and dehydration avoided. The bisphosphonate pamidronate, 90 mg intravenously monthly, has been shown to reduce pathologic fractures and other skeletal events in patients with significant bony disease.

Autologous bone marrow transplantation is useful in the management of advanced disease. It should be strongly considered as initial management of aggressive disease in patients under age 65 since it has been shown to prolong both initial remission and overall survival. Allogeneic transplantation plays a limited role but may be considered for young patients (under age 50) with matched sibling donors.

Prognosis

The median survival of patients with myelomas is 3 years. The prognosis is markedly affected by a number of prognostic features, with shorter survivals in those with high paraprotein spikes, renal failure, hypercalcemia, or extensive bony disease. Patients are said to have a "low tumor burden" if the IgG spike is less than 5 g/dL and there is no more than one lytic bone lesion and no evidence of severe anemia, hypercalcemia, or renal failure. These patients have a median survival of 5–6 years. Conversely, patients with a "high tumor burden" have an IgG spike greater than 7 g/dL, hematocrit less than 25%, calcium greater than 12 mg/dL, or more than three lytic bone lesions. Median survival for this group is approximately 1 year. Early intervention with autologous stem cell transplantation appears to prolong survival in these high-risk patients.

Alexanian R, Dimopoulos M: The treatment of multiple myeloma. N Engl J Med 1994;330:484. (Current chemotherapy results in response in 80% of patients but not cure; use of BMT reviewed.)

Attal M et al: A prospective, randomized trial of autologous bone marrow transplantation and chemotherapy in multiple myeloma. Intergroupe Français du Myélome. N Engl J Med 1996;335:91.

Berenson JR et al: Efficiency of pamidronate in reducing skeletal events in patients with advanced multiple myeloma. N Engl J Med 1996;334:488.

Interferon-alpha 2b added to melphalan-prednisone for initial and maintenance therapy in multiple myeloma: A randomized, controlled trial. The Nordic Myeloma Study Group. Ann Intern Med 1996;124:212.

WALDENSTRÖM'S MACROGLOBULINEMIA

Essentials of Diagnosis

- Symptoms nonspecific: splenomegaly common on examination.
- Monoclonal IgM paraprotein.
- Infiltration of bone marrow by plasmacytic lymphocytes.
- Absence of lytic bone disease.

General Considerations

Waldenström's macroglobulinemia is a malignant disease of B cells that appear to be a hybrid of lymphocytes and plasma cells. These cells characteristically secrete an IgM paraprotein, and many clinical manifestations of the disease are related to this macroglobulin.

Clinical Findings

A. Symptoms and Signs: This disease characteristically presents insidiously in patients in their 60s or 70s. Patients usually present with fatigue related to anemia. Hyperviscosity of serum may be manifested in a number of ways. Mucosal and gastrointestinal bleeding is related to engorged blood vessels and platelet dysfunction. Other complaints include nausea, vertigo, and visual disturbances. Alterations in consciousness vary from mild lethargy to stupor and coma. The IgM paraprotein may also cause symptoms of cold agglutinin disease or peripheral neuropathy.

On examination, there may be hepatosplenomegaly or lymphadenopathy. The retinal veins are characteristically engorged. Purpura may be present. There should be no bone tenderness.

B. Laboratory Findings: Anemia is nearly universal, and rouleau formation is common. The anemia is related in part to expansion of the plasma volume by 50–100% due to the presence of the paraprotein. Other blood counts are usually normal. The abnormal plasmacytic lymphocytes usually appear in small numbers on the peripheral blood smear. The bone marrow is characteristically infiltrated by the plasmacytic lymphocytes.

The hallmark of macroglobulinemia is the presence of a monoclonal IgM spike seen on serum protein electrophoresis (SPEP) in the beta or gamma globulin region. The serum viscosity is usually increased above the normal of 1.4–1.8 times that of water. Symptoms of hyperviscosity usually develop when the serum viscosity is over four times that of water, and marked symptoms usually arise when the viscosity is over six times that of water. Because paraproteins vary in their physicochemical properties, there is no strict correlation between the concentration of paraprotein and serum viscosity. However, after a certain threshold, viscosity rises exponentially with small increments in paraprotein amounts.

The IgM paraprotein may cause a positive Coombs test or have cold agglutinin or cryoglobulin properties. If one suspects macroglobulinemia but the SPEP shows only hypogammaglobulinemia, one should repeat the test while taking special measures to maintain the blood at 37 °C, since the paraprotein may precipitate out at room temperature.

Bone radiographs are normal, and there is no evidence of renal failure.

Differential Diagnosis

Waldenström's macroglobulinemia is differentiated from monoclonal gammopathy of unknown significance by the finding of bone marrow infiltration. It is differentiated from chronic lymphocytic leukemia and multiple myeloma by bone marrow morphology and the finding of the characteristic IgM spike, and also on clinical grounds.

Treatment

Patients who present with marked hyperviscosity syndrome (stupor or coma) should be treated on an emergency basis with plasmapheresis. Pheresis will usually rapidly reduce the paraprotein level below the threshold required to produce symptoms. On a chronic basis, some patients can be managed with periodic plasmapheresis alone. Others are treated with intermittent chemotherapy with chlorambucil or cyclophosphamide. New agents such as fludarabine and cladribine have produced encouraging results.

Prognosis

Waldenström's macroglobulinemia is an indolent disease with a median survival rate of 3–5 years. However, patients may survive 10 years or longer.

Dimopoulos MA, Alexanian R: Waldenström's macroglobulinemia. Blood 1994;83:1452.

Dimopoulos MA et al: Treatment of Waldenström macroglobulinemia with 2-chlorodeoxyadenosine. Ann Intern Med 1993;118:195. (Fifty-nine percent of patients responded with few adverse effects and only one relapse at median 7 months follow-up.)

Zinzani PL et al: Fludarabine treatment in resistant Waldenström's macroglobulinemia. Eur J Haematol 1995;54:120.

DISORDERS OF HEMOSTASIS

Disorders of hemostasis may be due to defects in either platelet number or function or to problems in formation of a fibrin clot (coagulation). Bleeding due to platelet disorders is typically mucosal or skin bleeding. Common problems include epistaxis, gum bleeding, menorrhagia, gastrointestinal bleeding, purpura, and petechiae. Petechiae are seen almost exclusively in conditions of thrombocytopenia and not platelet dysfunction. Bleeding due to coagulopathy may occur as deep muscle hematomas as well as skin bleeding. Spontaneous hemarthroses are seen only in severe hemophilia.

IDIOPATHIC (AUTOIMMUNE) THROMBOCYTOPENIC PURPURA

Essentials of Diagnosis

- Isolated thrombocytopenia.
- Other hematopoietic cell lines normal.
- No systemic illness.
- Spleen not palpable.
- Normal bone marrow with normal or increased megakaryocytes.

General Considerations

Idiopathic thrombocytopenic purpura is an autoimmune disorder in which an IgG autoantibody is formed that binds to platelets. It is not clear which antigen on the platelet surface is involved. Although the antiplatelet antibody may bind complement, platelets are not destroyed by direct lysis. Rather, destruction takes place in the spleen, where splenic macrophages with Fc receptors bind to antibody-coated platelets. Since the spleen is the major site both of antibody production and platelet sequestration, splenectomy is highly effective.

Clinical Findings

A. Symptoms and Signs: Idiopathic thrombocytopenic purpura occurs commonly in childhood, frequently precipitated by viral infection and usually self-limited. In contrast, the adult form is usually a chronic disease and only infrequently follows a viral infection. It is a disease of young persons, with peak incidence between ages 20 and 50, and there is a 2:1 female predominance.

Patients are systemically well and not febrile. The presenting complaint is mucosal or skin bleeding. Common types of bleeding are epistaxis, oral bleeding, menorrhagia, purpura, and petechiae.

On examination, the patient appears well, and there are no abnormal findings other than those related to bleeding. An enlarged spleen should lead one to doubt the diagnosis. Common signs of bleeding are purpura, petechiae, and hemorrhagic bullae in the mouth.

B. Laboratory Findings: The hallmark of the disease is thrombocytopenia, which may be less than 10,000/μL. Other counts are usually normal except for occasional mild anemia, which can be explained by bleeding or associated hemolysis. Peripheral blood cell morphology is normal except that platelets are slightly enlarged (megathrombocytes). These larger platelets are young platelets produced in response to enhanced platelet destruction. Approximately 10% of patients will have coexistent autoimmune hemolytic anemia **(Evans' syndrome),** and in these cases one will see anemia, reticulocytosis, and spherocytes on peripheral smear. Red blood cell fragmentation should not be seen.

The bone marrow will appear normal, with a normal or increased number of megakaryocytes. Coagulation studies will be entirely normal. Tests now available to quantitate platelet-associated IgG may help in the diagnosis. At present, although these tests are highly sensitive (95%), they are very nonspecific, and 50% of all patients with thrombocytopenia from any cause may have increased levels of IgG on the platelet.

Differential Diagnosis

Thrombocytopenia may be produced either by abnormal bone marrow function or by peripheral destruction (Table 13–17). Although most bone marrow disorders produce abnormalities in addition to isolated thrombocytopenia, diagnoses such as myelodysplasia can only be excluded by examining the bone marrow. Most causes of thrombocytopenia resulting from peripheral destruction can be ruled out by initial evaluation. Disorders such as disseminated intravascular coagulation, thrombotic thrombocytopenic purpura, hemolytic-uremic syndrome, hypersplenism, and sepsis are easily excluded by the absence of systemic illness. Thus, patients with isolated thrombocytopenia with no other abnormal findings almost certainly have immune thrombocytopenia. Patients should be questioned regarding drug use, especially sulfonamides, quinidine, quinine, thiazides, cimetidine, gold, and heparin. Heparin is now the most common cause of drug-induced thrombocytopenia in hospitalized patients. Systemic lupus erythematosus and chronic lymphocytic leukemia are common causes of secondary idiopathic thrombocytopenic purpura.

Treatment

Few adults with idiopathic thrombocytopenic purpura will have spontaneous remissions, and most will require treatment. Initial treatment is with prednisone, 1–2 mg/kg/d. Prednisone works primarily by decreasing the affinity of splenic macrophages for antibody-coated platelets. High-dose prednisone therapy also reduces the binding of antibody to the platelet surface, and long-term therapy may decrease antibody production. Bleeding will often diminish within 1 day after beginning prednisone—even before the platelet count begins to rise. This effect has been attributed to enhanced vascular stability. The platelet count will usually begin to rise within a week, and responses are almost always seen within 3 weeks. About 80% of patients will respond, and the

Table 13–17. Causes of thrombocytopenia.

Bone marrow disorders
  Aplastic anemia
  Hematologic malignancies
  Myelodysplasia
  Megaloblastic anemia
  Chronic alcoholism
Nonmarrow disorders
  Immune disorders
    Idiopathic thrombocytopenic purpura
    Drug-induced
    Secondary (CLL, SLE)
    Posttransfusion purpura
  Hypersplenism
  Disseminated intravascular coagulation
  Thrombotic thrombocytopenic purpura
  Hemolytic-uremic syndrome
  Sepsis
  Hemangiomas
  Viral infection, AIDS

platelet count will usually return to normal. High-dose therapy should be continued until the platelet count is normal, and the dose should then be gradually tapered. In most patients, thrombocytopenia will recur if prednisone is completely withdrawn, and one aims to find a low prednisone dose that will maintain an adequate platelet count. It is not necessary for the platelet count to be entirely normal; the risk of bleeding is small with platelet counts above 50,000/μL.

Splenectomy is the most definitive treatment for idiopathic thrombocytopenic purpura, and most adult patients will ultimately undergo splenectomy. High-dose prednisone therapy should not be continued indefinitely in an attempt to avoid surgery. Splenectomy is indicated if patients do not respond to prednisone initially or require unacceptably high doses to maintain an adequate platelet count. Other patients may be intolerant of prednisone or may simply prefer the surgical alternative. Splenectomy can be performed safely even with platelet counts less than 10,000/μL. Approximately 80% of patients benefit from splenectomy with either complete or partial remission.

High-dose intravenous immunoglobulin, 400 mg/kg/d for 3–5 days, is highly effective in rapidly raising the platelet count. The response rate is approximately 90%, and the platelet count rises within 1–5 days. However, this treatment is very expensive (approximately $5000), and the beneficial effect lasts only 1–2 weeks. Immunoglobulin treatment should be reserved for emergency situations such as preparing a severely thrombocytopenic patient for surgery.

For patients who fail to respond to prednisone and splenectomy, danazol, 600 mg/d, has been used, with responses obtained in about half of cases. Immunosuppressive agents employed in refractory cases include vincristine, vinblastine infusions, azathioprine, and cyclophosphamide. In using any of these more toxic treatments, one must carefully balance the risks against the anticipated benefits.

Platelet transfusions are rarely used in the treatment of idiopathic thrombocytopenic purpura, since exogenous platelets will survive no better than the patient's own platelets and in many cases will survive less than a few hours. Platelet transfusion should be reserved for cases of life-threatening bleeding in which enhanced hemostasis for even an hour may be of benefit.

Prognosis

The prognosis for remission is good. In most cases, the disease is initially controlled with prednisone, and splenectomy offers definitive therapy for most patients. The major concern during the initial phases is cerebral hemorrhage, which becomes a risk when the platelet count is less than 5000/μL. These patients usually exhibit warning signs of mucosal bleeding. However, even at these very low platelet counts, fatal bleeding is rare. Chronic disease that has failed to respond to prednisone and splenectomy has a waxing and waning course over years and usually requires continued management.

George JN et al: Idiopathic thrombocytopenic purpura: A practice guideline developed by explicit methods for the American Society of Hematology. Blood 1996;88:3.

McMillan R: Therapy for adults with refractory chronic immune thrombocytopenic purpura. Ann Intern Med 1997;126:307.

Reiner A, Gernsheimer T, Slichter SJ: Pulse cyclophosphamide therapy for refractory autoimmune thrombocytopenic purpura. Blood 1995;85:351.

Stasi R et al: Long-term observation of 208 adults with chronic idiopathic thrombocytopenic purpura. Am J Med 1995;98:436.

Warkentin TE, Kelton JG: A 14-year study of heparin-induced thrombocytopenia. Am J Med 1996;101:502. (Documents high risk of thrombosis in this setting.)

THROMBOTIC THROMBOCYTOPENIC PURPURA

Essentials of Diagnosis

- Microangiopathic hemolytic anemia.
- Thrombocytopenia.
- Neurologic abnormalities.
- Renal abnormalities.
- Fever in the absence of infection.
- Normal coagulation tests.
- Elevated serum LDH.

General Considerations

Thrombotic thrombocytopenic purpura is an uncommon syndrome characterized by the pentad of microangiopathic hemolytic anemia, thrombocytopenia, and neurologic abnormalities, as well as fever and renal abnormalities. The cause is unknown. A platelet-agglutinating factor has recently been identified in the plasma of these patients. Its role in pathogenesis remains controversial.

Thrombotic thrombocytopenic purpura is seen primarily in young adults between ages 20 and 50, and there is a slight female predominance. The syndrome is occasionally precipitated by estrogen use or pregnancy, and is increasingly encountered in association with HIV disease.

Clinical Findings

A. Symptoms and Signs: Patients come to medical attention because of anemia, bleeding, or neurologic abnormalities. The neurologic symptoms and signs are unusual in that they may wax and wane over minutes. Neurologic symptoms include headache, confusion, aphasia, and alterations in consciousness from lethargy to coma. With more advanced disease, one may see hemiparesis and seizures.

On examination, the patient appears acutely ill and is usually febrile. One may detect pallor, purpura, petechiae, and signs of neurologic dysfunction. Patients may have abdominal pain and tenderness due to pancreatitis.

B. Laboratory Findings: Anemia is universal and may be extremely severe. There is usually marked reticulocytosis and occasional circulating nucleated red blood cells. The hallmark is a microangiopathic blood picture with fragmented red blood cells (schistocytes, helmet cells, triangle forms) on the smear. One cannot make the diagnosis without significant red blood cell fragmentation. Thrombocytopenia is invariably present and may be severe. White blood cells may show increased band neutrophils.

Hemolysis may be manifested by increasing indirect bilirubin, absent haptoglobin, and occasionally hemoglobinemia and hemoglobinuria. In severe cases, methemalbuminemia may impart a brown color to the plasma. The LDH is usually markedly elevated in proportion to the severity of hemolysis. The Coombs test should be negative.

Coagulation tests (prothrombin time, partial thromboplastin time, fibrinogen) are normal. Elevated fibrin degradation products may be seen, as in other acutely ill patients. Renal insufficiency may be present, and the urinalysis may be abnormal.

Pathologically, one may see thrombi in capillaries and small arteries, with no evidence of inflammation.

Differential Diagnosis

The normal values of coagulation tests differentiate thrombotic thrombocytopenic purpura from disseminated intravascular coagulation (DIC). Other conditions causing microangiopathic hemolysis (Table 13–18) should be excluded. Evans's syndrome is characterized by the combination of autoimmune thrombocytopenia and autoimmune hemolytic anemia, but the peripheral smear will show spherocytes and not red blood cell fragments. Skin or muscle biopsy is usually not necessary for diagnosis but may be helpful when vasculitis is a consideration. Endocarditis may also closely simulate thrombotic thrombocytopenic purpura.

Treatment

Thrombotic thrombocytopenic purpura should be treated on an emergency basis with large-volume

Table 13–18. Causes of microangiopathic hemolytic anemia.

Thrombotic thrombocytopenic purpura
Hemolytic-uremic syndrome
Disseminated intravascular coagulation
Prosthetic valve hemolysis
Metastatic adenocarcinoma
Malignant hypertension
Vasculitis

plasmapheresis. Sixty to 80 mL/kg of plasma should be removed and replaced with fresh-frozen plasma. Treatment should be continued daily until the patient is in complete remission. Prednisone and antiplatelet agents (aspirin [325 mg three times daily] and dipyridamole [75 mg three times daily]) have been used in addition to plasmapheresis, but their role is unclear.

Patients who do not respond to plasmapheresis or who have rapid recurrences require splenectomy. The combination of splenectomy, corticosteroids, and dextran has been used with success. Splenectomy performed in remission may prevent subsequent relapses.

Prognosis

With the advent of plasmapheresis, the formerly dismal prognosis of thrombotic thrombocytopenic purpura has been dramatically changed. Eighty to 90 percent of patients now recover completely. Neurologic abnormalities are almost always completely reversed. Most complete responses are durable, but in 20% of cases the disease will be chronic and relapsing.

Crowther MA et al: Splenectomy done during hematologic remission to prevent relapse in patients with thrombotic thrombocytopenic purpura. Ann Intern Med 1996;125: 294.

Rock G et al: Cryosupernatant as replacement fluid for plasma exchange in thrombotic thrombocytopenic purpura. Members of the Canadian Apheresis Group. Br J Haematol 1996;94:383.

Rose M et al: The changing course of thrombotic thrombocytopenic purpura and modern therapy. Blood Rev 1993;7:94. (Most respond to therapy, but about half relapse with usually milder disease.)

Ruggenenti P, Remuzzi G: The pathophysiology and management of thrombotic thrombocytopenic purpura. Eur J Haematol 1996;56:191.

Shumak KH, Rock GA, Nair RC: Late relapses in patients successfully treated for thrombotic thrombocytopenic purpura. Ann Intern Med 1995;122:569.

HEMOLYTIC-UREMIC SYNDROME

Essentials of Diagnosis

- Microangiopathic hemolytic anemia.
- Thrombocytopenia.
- Renal failure.
- Elevated serum LDH.
- Normal coagulation tests.
- Absence of neurologic abnormalities.

General Considerations

Hemolytic-uremic syndrome is an uncommon disorder consisting of microangiopathic hemolytic anemia, thrombocytopenia, and renal failure due to microangiopathy (with decreased glomerular filtration, proteinuria, and hematuria). The cause is unclear. The disease is similar to thrombotic thrombocytopenic purpura except that different vascular beds are involved. The pathogenesis of the two disorders is probably similar, and a platelet-agglutinating factor found in plasma may be involved. In children, hemolytic-uremic syndrome frequently occurs after a diarrheal illness secondary to infections with *Shigella, Salmonella, E coli* strain O157:H7, or viral agents. The mortality rate of this form is low (< 5%). In adults, this syndrome is frequently precipitated by estrogen use or pregnancy (especially postpartum) or occurs as a complication of malignant hypertension or renal transplantation. A familial (hereditary) type has been identified in which members of a family have recurrent episodes over several years.

Clinical Findings

A. Symptoms and Signs: Patients present with anemia, bleeding, or renal failure. The renal failure may or may not be oliguric. In contrast to thrombotic thrombocytopenic purpura, there are no neurologic manifestations other than those due to the uremic state.

B. Laboratory Findings: As in thrombotic thrombocytopenic purpura, there is microangiopathic hemolytic anemia and thrombocytopenia, but the thrombocytopenia is often less severe. The peripheral blood smear should show striking red blood cell fragmentation, and the diagnosis of hemolytic-uremic syndrome is untenable without this finding. The LDH is usually strikingly elevated in proportion to the severity of hemolysis, and the Coombs test is negative. Coagulation tests are normal with the exception of elevated fibrin degradation products.

Renal insufficiency is invariably present, and anuric renal failure requiring dialysis may be seen. Kidney biopsy will show endothelial hyaline thrombi in the afferent arterioles and glomeruli. Ischemic necrosis in the renal cortex may occur with obstruction from intravascular coagulation.

Differential Diagnosis

Disseminated intravascular coagulation is excluded by normal coagulation results. Other causes of microangiopathic hemolytic anemia (Table 13–18) should be considered. Occasionally, vasculitis or acute glomerulonephritis is considered, and in these cases renal biopsy may be necessary to establish the diagnosis if the platelet count will allow it.

Hemolytic-uremic syndrome is arbitrarily distinguished from thrombotic thrombocytopenic purpura by the consistent presence of renal failure and the lack of neurologic findings.

Treatment

In children, hemolytic-uremic syndrome is almost always self-limited and requires only conservative management of acute renal failure. In adults, however, without treatment, there is a high rate of permanent renal insufficiency and death. The treatment of choice (as in thrombotic thrombocytopenic purpura) is large-volume plasmapheresis with fresh-frozen replacement (exchange of up to 80 mL/kg), repeated daily until remission is achieved.

Prognosis

The prognosis of hemolytic-uremic syndrome in adults remains unclear. Without effective therapy, up to 40% of patients have died, and 80% have had chronic renal insufficiency. Early institution of aggressive therapy with plasmapheresis promises to be beneficial. Survival and correction of hematologic abnormalities are the rule, but restoration of renal function requires that treatment be initiated early.

Cohen MB: *Escherichia coli* O157:H7 infections: A frequent cause of bloody diarrhea and the hemolytic-uremic syndrome. Adv Pediatr 1996;43:171.

Matsumae T, Takebayashi S, Naito S: The clinico-pathological characteristics and outcome in hemolytic-uremic syndrome of adults. Clin Nephrol 1996;45:153.

Melnyk AM, Solez K, Kjellstrand CM: Adult hemolytic-uremic syndrome: A review of 37 cases. Arch Intern Med 1995;155:2077.

Rondeau E, Peraldi MN: *Escherichia coli* and the hemolytic-uremic syndrome. (Editorial and comment.) N Engl J Med 1996;335:660.

CONGENITAL QUALITATIVE PLATELET DISORDERS

Bleeding disorders characterized by prolonged bleeding times despite a normal platelet count are called qualitative platelet disorders. Patients have a positive family history or lifelong personal history of the defect. The disorders may be classified as (1) von Willebrand's disease, a congenital disorder of a plasma protein necessary for platelet adhesion; and (2) congenital disorders intrinsic to the platelet (Table 13–19). When an intrinsic qualitative platelet disorder is suspected, platelet aggregation studies should be evaluated to make a specific diagnosis.

Table 13–19. Qualitative platelet disorders.

Congenital
Glanzmann's thrombasthenia
Bernard-Soulier syndrome
Storage pool disease
Acquired
Myeloproliferative disorders
Uremia
Drugs: Aspirin, anti-inflammatory agents
Autoantibody
Paraproteins
Acquired storage pool disease
Fibrin degradation products
Von Willebrand's disease

1. VON WILLEBRAND'S DISEASE

Essentials of Diagnosis

- Family history with autosomal dominant pattern of inheritance.
- Prolonged bleeding time, either at baseline or after challenge with aspirin.
- Reduced levels of factor VIII antigen or ristocetin cofactor.
- May have reduced levels of factor VIII coagulant activity.

General Considerations

Von Willebrand's disease is the most common congenital disorder of hemostasis. It is transmitted in an autosomal dominant pattern. It is a group of disorders characterized by deficient or defective von Willebrand factor (vWF), a protein that mediates platelet adhesion. Adhesion is a process separate from platelet aggregation. Platelets adhere to the subendothelium via vWF, which is bound to a specific receptor on the platelet composed of glycoprotein Ib (and missing in Bernard-Soulier syndrome). Platelets aggregate via fibrinogen, which binds to a different receptor composed of glycoproteins IIb and IIIa (deficient in Glanzmann's thrombasthenia). The platelet aggregation system is entirely normal in von Willebrand's disease.

Von Willebrand factor is synthesized in megakaryocytes and endothelial cells and circulates in plasma as multimers of varying size. Only the large multimeric forms are functional in mediating platelet adhesion. Von Willebrand factor has a separate function of binding the factor VIII coagulant protein and protecting it from degradation. The factor VIII coagulant protein (factor VIII:C), a protein encoded by a gene on the X chromosome, is the protein deficient in classic hemophilia. Any of the multimeric forms of vWF can bind and protect factor VIII:C. Von Willebrand's disease, which is primarily a disorder of platelet function, may secondarily cause a coagulation disturbance because of deficient levels of factor VIII:C. However, this coagulopathy is rarely severe.

There are several subtypes of von Willebrand's disease. The most common type (type I, 80% of all cases) is caused by a quantitative decrease in vWF. Type IIa is caused by a qualitative abnormality in protein that prevents multimer formation. Only small multimers are present, and both intermediate and large forms that mediate platelet adhesion are missing. Type IIb von Willebrand's disease is caused by a qualitative abnormality in the protein that causes rapid clearance of the large multimeric forms. Type III von Willebrand's disease is a rare autosomal recessive disorder in which vWF is nearly absent. Pseudo-von Willebrand disease is a rare disorder in which an abnormal platelet membrane has excessive avidity for the large multimeric forms of vWF, causing their clearance from plasma.

Clinical Findings

A. Symptoms and Signs: Von Willebrand's disease is a common disorder affecting both men and women. Most cases are mild. Most bleeding is mucosal (epistaxis, gingival bleeding, menorrhagia), but gastrointestinal bleeding may occur. In most cases, incisional bleeding occurs after surgery or dental extractions. Von Willebrand's disease is rarely as severe as hemophilia, and spontaneous hemarthroses do not occur.

The bleeding tendency is exacerbated by aspirin. Characteristically, bleeding decreases during pregnancy or estrogen use.

B. Laboratory Findings: Platelet number and morphology are normal, and the bleeding time is usually (not always) prolonged. The bleeding time should be ascertained whenever this diagnosis is considered and correlates most closely with the clinical bleeding tendency. When the bleeding time is normal, it is prolonged markedly by aspirin. Normal persons will prolong their bleeding time to a minor extent with aspirin but rarely out of the normal range. In the most common form of von Willebrand's disease (type I), vWF levels in plasma are reduced. This may be measured by factor VIII antigen, which measures the immunologic presence of vWF, or by ristocetin cofactor activity, which measures functional properties of vWF in mediating platelet adhesion.

When factor VIII antigen is reduced, one may also see a decrease in factor VIII coagulant (factor VIII:C) levels. When factor VIII:C levels are less than 25%, the partial thromboplastin time (PTT) will be prolonged. Platelet aggregation studies with standard agonists (ADP, collagen, thrombin) are normal, but platelet aggregation in response to ristocetin is usually subnormal.

In difficult cases, it may be helpful to assay directly the multimeric composition of vWF.

Differential Diagnosis

When patients present with a prolonged bleeding time, one must distinguish von Willebrand's disease from other qualitative platelet disorders (Table 13–19). Acquired qualitative platelet disorders can usually be diagnosed by recent onset of the bleeding tendency and other characteristic clinical features. Congenital intrinsic platelet disorders may present with a positive family history and lifelong history of bleeding episodes. Von Willebrand's disease is diagnosed by the finding of abnormal measurements of vWF and by normal results of platelet aggregation.

When patients present with a prolonged PTT, measurements of factor VIII:C will distinguish von Willebrand's disease from all disorders except hemophilia (Table 13–20). Hemophilia is diagnosed when factor VIII:C is reduced but all measurements of vWF (factor VIII antigen, ristocetin cofactor activity) are normal.

Patients with a suspicious bleeding history but with normal bleeding time and PTT pose a diagnostic problem. On occasion, the postaspirin bleeding time can be used to unmask a bleeding disorder. At other times, one must perform further plasma assays of vWF to make the diagnosis. Von Willebrand's disease waxes and wanes in severity and may be difficult to diagnose, especially in a woman taking estrogens (which raise vWF levels).

It is often useful to distinguish between subtypes of von Willebrand's disease (Table 13–21), because only type I usually responds to desmopressin and because type IIb may be aggravated by its use.

Treatment

The bleeding disorder is characteristically mild, and no treatment is routinely given other than avoidance of aspirin. However, patients often need to be prepared for surgical or dental procedures. The bleeding time is probably the best indicator of the likelihood of bleeding, and prophylactic therapy may be reasonably withheld if the procedure is minor and the bleeding time is normal.

Desmopressin acetate is useful for mild type I von Willebrand's disease and should be considered first. The dose is 0.3 µg/kg, after which vWF levels usually rise two- to threefold in 30–90 minutes. Desmopressin acetate appears to cause release of stored vWF from endothelial cells. The treatment can be given only every 24 hours as stores of vWF become depleted. The drug is not effective in type IIa von Willebrand's disease, in which no endothelial stores are present, and may be harmful in type IIb or may lead to thrombocytopenia and increased bleeding.

New factor VIII concentrates are now available that replace cryoprecipitate as the treatment of choice for von Willebrand's disease when factor replacement is required. Some (not all) of these products now contain functional vWF and, unlike cryoprecipitate, do not transmit HIV or hepatitis. One appropri-

Table 13–20. Causes of prolonged partial thromboplastin time.

Congenital factor deficiencies
Contact factors
Factor XII
Factor XI
Factor IX (hemophilia B)
Factor VIII
Hemophilia A
Von Willebrand's disease
Anticoagulants
Anti-VIII
Lupus
Heparin

Table 13–21. Types of von Willebrand's disease.

	Bleeding Time	Factor VIII Antigen	Ristocetin Cofactor Activity	Factor VIII Coagulant Activity	Multimer
Type I	↑ or N[1]	↓ or N	↓ or N	↓ or N	N
Type IIa	↑	↓ or N	0	↓ or N	Abn
Type IIb	↑	↓ or N	↓ or N	↓ or N	Abn
Type III	↑	0	0	0	...
Pseudo-vW disease	↑	↓ or N	↓ or N	↓ or N	Abn
Hemophilia A	N	N	N	↓	N

[1]Increases with aspirin.

ate product is Humate-P (Armour). The dose is 20–50 units/kg depending on disease severity.

The antifibrinolytic agent tranexamic acid is useful as adjunctive therapy during dental procedures. After either cryoprecipitate or desmopressin acetate, the patient is given 25 mg/kg three times daily for 5–7 days to reduce the likelihood of bleeding.

Prognosis

The prognosis is excellent. In most cases, the bleeding disorder is mild, and in the more serious cases replacement therapy is effective.

Castaman G, Rodeghiero F: Current management of von Willebrand's disease. Drugs 1995;50:602.

Hemophilia and von Willebrand's disease: 1. Diagnosis, comprehensive care and assessment. Association of Hemophilia Clinic Directors of Canada. Can Med Assoc J 1995;153:19.

Hemophilia and von Willebrand's disease: 2. Management. Association of Hemophilia Clinic Directors of Canada. Can Med Assoc J 1995;153:147.

Ruggeri ZM: Von Willebrand's disease and the mechanisms of platelet function. Ciba Found Symp 1995; 189:35.

Scott JP, Montgomery RR: Therapy of von Willebrand disease. Semin Thromb Hemost 1993;19:37. (Choice of therapy depends on subtype and severity of disease; desmopressin for type I, Humate P for moderate to severe type I, type IIA, and type IIB.)

2. DISORDERS INTRINSIC TO THE PLATELETS

Glanzmann's Thrombasthenia

This is a rare autosomal recessive intrinsic platelet disorder causing bleeding. Platelets are unable to aggregate because of lack of receptors (containing glycoproteins IIb and IIa) for fibrinogen, which forms the bridges between platelets during aggregation. Clinically, it is manifested chiefly as mucosal bleeding (epistaxis, gingival bleeding, menorrhagia) and postoperative bleeding. The bleeding defect is of variable severity but may be severe.

Platelet numbers and morphology are normal, but the bleeding time is markedly prolonged. Platelets fail to aggregate in response to typical agonists (ADP, collagen, thrombin) but aggregate normally in response to ristocetin, which causes platelet clumping by a separate mechanism.

Patients are treated with platelet transfusions when necessary. Platelet transfusion therapy is limited by the tendency of these patients to develop multiple alloantibodies.

Bernard-Soulier Syndrome

This is a rare autosomal recessive intrinsic platelet disorder causing bleeding. Platelets cannot adhere to subendothelium because they lack receptors (composed of glycoprotein Ib) for von Willebrand factor, which mediates platelet adhesion. This is often a severe bleeding disorder with mucosal and postoperative bleeding.

Thrombocytopenia may be present, and platelets on smear are abnormally large. The bleeding time is markedly prolonged. Platelet aggregation is normal in response to standard agonists (collagen, ADP, thrombin), but platelets fail to aggregate in response to ristocetin. Measurements of von Willebrand factor in the plasma are normal. Patients are treated with platelet transfusion when necessary.

Storage Pool Disease

This is a group of mild bleeding disorders characterized by defective secretion of platelet granule contents (especially ADP) that stimulate platelet aggregation. Most patients are mildly affected and have increased bruising and postoperative bleeding.

Platelets are normal in number and morphology, but the bleeding time is slightly prolonged. In some cases, the baseline bleeding time is normal, but it becomes markedly prolonged after aspirin. There are variable abnormalities in platelet aggregation studies.

Most patients do not require treatment but should avoid aspirin. Platelet transfusions transiently correct the bleeding tendency. Some patients respond to infusions of cryoprecipitate, and some respond transiently to desmopressin acetate, 0.3 µg/kg every 24 hours.

Peretz H et al: Glanzmann's thrombasthenia associated with deletion-insertion and alternative splicing in the glycoprotein IIb gene. Blood 1995;85:414.

ACQUIRED QUALITATIVE PLATELET DISORDERS

A number of acquired disorders lead to abnormal platelet function (Table 13–19).

Uremia

Uremia causes abnormal platelet function by unknown mechanisms. The severity of the bleeding tendency is roughly proportionate to the degree of renal insufficiency. Bleeding is most commonly mucosal and gastrointestinal and may occasionally be severe. Dialysis is effective in reducing the bleeding tendency but may not completely eliminate it. Patients appear to respond to transfusion with cryoprecipitate, ten units every 12 hours. Desmopressin acetate, 0.3 µg/kg every 24 hours, appears to be just as effective as cryoprecipitate.

Myeloproliferative Disorders

All the myeloproliferative disorders can produce abnormalities in platelet function. A number of biochemical abnormalities are present in these platelets, but the cause of the bleeding tendency is unclear. The severity of the bleeding tendency correlates roughly with the height of the platelet count, although conditions causing reactive thrombocytosis of normal platelets are not associated with abnormal function. Bleeding decreases when the platelet count is controlled with myelosuppressive therapy. In cases of life-threatening bleeding with high platelet counts, plateletpheresis may be necessary to control bleeding. Platelet transfusion will also be helpful temporarily.

Other Disorders

Aspirin causes a mild bleeding tendency by irreversibly acetylating cyclooxygenase, an enzyme that participates in platelet aggregation. The effect lasts for the life of the platelet and may be manifest for 7–10 days, although the major effect lasts only 3–5 days. The effect is not dose-dependent, and 65 mg of aspirin is sufficient.

Aspirin by itself does not cause significant bleeding, but it may unmask bleeding disorders such as mild von Willebrand's disease or mild thrombocytopenia. Certain antibiotics (ticarcillin, some cephalosporins) cause a mild bleeding tendency, presumably by coating the surface of platelets. Nonsteroidal anti-inflammatory drugs cause a transient aspirin-like effect.

Patients with autoantibodies against platelets may have prolonged bleeding times even in the absence of thrombocytopenia. Platelet-associated IgG levels should be high, and the bleeding tendency responds quickly to modest doses of prednisone such as 20 mg/d. Acquired storage pool disease refers to the circulation of "exhausted platelets" that have been stimulated to release their granule contents and hence are no longer functional. Such granule release occurs in response to cardiopulmonary bypass and severe vasculitis.

Bick RL: Platelet function defects associated with hemorrhage or thrombosis. Med Clin North Am 1994;78:577. (Review of clinical features and treatment of inherited and acquired platelet defects.)

Eberst ME, Berkowitz CR: Hemostasis in renal disease: Pathophysiology and management. Am J Med 1994; 96:168.

HEMOPHILIA A

Essentials of Diagnosis

- X-linked recessive pattern of inheritance with only males affected.
- Low factor VIII coagulant (VIII:C) activity.
- Normal factor VIII antigen.
- Spontaneous hemarthroses.

General Considerations

Hemophilia A (classic hemophilia, factor VIII deficiency hemophilia) is a hereditary disorder in which bleeding is due to deficiency of the coagulation factor VIII (VIII:C). In most cases, the factor VIII coagulant protein is quantitatively reduced, but in a small number of cases the coagulant protein is present by immunoassay but defective.

Hemophilia is a classic example of an X-linked recessive disease, and as a rule only males are affected. In rare instances, female carriers are clinically affected if their normal X chromosomes are disproportionately inactivated. Females may also become affected if they are the offspring of a hemophiliac father and carrier mother.

Hemophilia is classified as severe if factor VIII:C levels are less than 1%, moderate if levels are 1–5%, and mild if levels are greater than 5%. Families tend to breed true in the severity of hemophilia produced.

Clinical Findings

A. Symptoms and Signs: Hemophilia A is the most common severe bleeding disorder and after von Willebrand's disease is the most common congenital bleeding disorder overall. Approximately one in 10,000 males is affected. The bleeding tendency is related to factor VIII:C levels. Bleeding may occur anywhere. The most common sites of bleeding are into joints (knees, ankles, elbows), into muscles, and from the gastrointestinal tract. Spontaneous hemarthroses are so characteristic of severe hemophilia that they are almost diagnostic of the disorder. Patients with mild hemophilia bleed only in response to major trauma or surgery. Patients with moderately severe hemophilia bleed in response to mild trauma or surgery, and those with severe hemophilia bleed spontaneously.

Unfortunately, many hemophiliacs are now seropositive for HIV infection transmitted via factor VIII concentrate, and many have already developed AIDS. HIV-associated immune thrombocytopenia may aggravate the bleeding tendency.

B. Laboratory Findings: The partial thromboplastin time (PTT) is prolonged, and other measures of coagulation, including prothrombin time, bleeding time, and fibrinogen level, are normal. Levels of factor VIII:C are reduced, but measurements of von Willebrand factor are normal (Table 13–21).

If one mixes plasma from a hemophiliac patient with normal plasma, the PTT will become normal. Failure of the PTT to normalize in such a mixing test is diagnostic of the presence of a factor VIII inhibitor.

A low platelet count should raise a suspicion of HIV-associated immune thrombocytopenia.

Differential Diagnosis

The finding of a reduced factor VIII:C level will distinguish this disorder from other causes of prolonged PTT (Table 13–20). Clinically, factor VIII hemophilia is indistinguishable from factor IX hemophilia, and only specific factor assays can distinguish these disorders. In cases of mild hemophilia, the disorder needs to be distinguished from von Willebrand's disease by VIII:A assay, which shows normal levels of factor VIII antigen in the former.

An important issue for the families of hemophiliac patients is identifying which females are carriers. Female carriers can usually be identified by the presence of low or normal levels of factor VIII:C with normal levels of factor VIII antigen.

Treatment

Patients with hemophilia should try to live as nearly normal lives as possible. Activities associated with a risk of trauma should be avoided, however, and aspirin should never be used.

Standard treatment is based on infusion of factor VIII concentrates, now heat-treated to reduce the likelihood of transmission of HIV. Recombinant factor VIII appears safe and effective, though expensive, and should impose no risk of transmitting HIV or other viruses. The level of factor VIII one aims to achieve in plasma depends on the severity of the bleeding problem. In response to minor bleeding, it may be necessary only to raise factor VIII:C levels to 25% with one infusion. For moderate bleeding (such as deep muscle hematomas), it is adequate to raise

the level initially to 50% and maintain the level at greater than 25% with repeated infusion for 2–3 days. When major surgery is to be performed, one raises the factor VIII:C level to 100% and then maintains the factor level at greater than 50% continuously for 10–14 days. Head injuries (with or without neurologic signs) should be emergently treated as though major bleeding were present.

The dose of factor VIII concentrate is calculated on the basis that one unit of factor VIII is the amount present in 1 mL of plasma. Plasma volume is 40 mL/kg, and the volume of distribution of factor VIII:C is 1.5 times the plasma volume. Thus, to raise the level 100%, the dose should be $40 \times 1.5 = 60$ units/kg, or approximately 4000 units for a 70-kg individual. To raise the levels to 25% would require 1000 units. The half-life of factor VIII:C is approximately 12 hours. Thus, during major surgery, to achieve an initial level of 100% and maintain it continuously at greater than 50%, a dose of 60 units/kg (approximately 4000 units) initially followed by 30 units/kg (approximately 2000 units) every 12 hours should be adequate. During surgery, one should initially verify that these doses give the anticipated factor VIII levels. If factor VIII levels fail to rise as expected, one should suspect an inhibitor. Patients with inhibitors require specialized therapy under direction of an experienced hematologist.

For mild hemophiliacs, desmopressin acetate, 0.3 µg/kg every 24 hours, may be useful in preparing for minor surgical procedures. Desmopressin acetate causes release of factor VIII:C and will raise the factor VIII:C levels two- to threefold for several hours. In the management of persistent bleeding following use of either desmopressin acetate or factor VIII concentrate, patients may be treated with aminocaproic acid (EACA; Amicar), 4 g orally every 4 hours for several days.

The ongoing care of patients with hemophilia should be coordinated with an orthopedic surgeon who can help manage the chronic joint deformities of these patients.

Prognosis

The prognosis of patients with hemophilia has been transformed by the availability of factor VIII replacement. The major limiting factors are disability from recurrent joint bleeding and viral infections (hepatitis B and C, HIV) from recurrent transfusion. Approximately 15% of patients develop inhibitors to factor VIII, and these patents may die of bleeding because they cannot be adequately supported with factor VIII.

Cohen AJ, Kessler CM: Treatment of inherited coagulation disorders. Am J Med 1995;99:675.

Furie B et al: A practical guide to the evaluation and treatment of hemophilia. Blood 1994;84:3. (Guide for treatment of bleeding complications and surgical prophylaxis.)

Hoyer LW: Hemophilia A. N Engl J Med 1994;330:38. (Pathophysiology, genetics, clinical features, diagnosis, and treatment.)

Lozier JN, Brinkhous KM: Gene therapy and the hemophilias. JAMA 1994;271:47. (Genes for both hemophilia A and B have been cloned, and vectors have been developed; ex vivo and in vivo delivery systems are currently being developed.)

ACQUIRED FACTOR VIII ANTIBODIES

Antibodies to factor VIII may develop either postpartum or with no underlying illness. Factor VIII antibodies also develop in 15% of patients with factor VIII hemophilia who have received infusions of plasma concentrates.

Acquired factor VIII antibodies usually produce a severe bleeding disorder. The PTT is prolonged, and the fibrinogen level, prothrombin time, and platelet count are not affected. A plasma mixing test will usually reveal the presence of an inhibitor by the failure of normal plasma to correct the prolonged PTT. However, the mixing test may require incubation for 2–4 hours to reveal the inhibitor. Factor VIII coagulant levels are low.

Factor VIII antibodies should be suspected in any acquired severe bleeding disorder associated with a prolonged PTT. Factor VIII antibodies are distinguished from lupus anticoagulants both by the presence of clinical bleeding and more importantly by the reduced factor VIII:C level. The diagnosis is confirmed by mixing tests and in vivo by the failure of factor VIII concentrates to raise the factor VIII:C levels by the expected amount.

The treatment of choice is cyclophosphamide, usually combined with prednisone. In the interim, aggressive factor VIII replacement may be necessary. Plasmapheresis to reduce inhibitor levels may be useful. Treatment of factor VIII antibodies is complex and should be done in consultation with a hematologist.

The prognosis of these patients is variable, and many die of overwhelming bleeding.

Kessler CM: An introduction to factor VIII inhibitors: The detection and quantitation. Am J Med 1991;91(5A):1S. (Series of articles reviewing pathophysiology, diagnosis, and natural history.)

HEMOPHILIA B

Essentials of Diagnosis

- X-linked recessive inheritance, with only males affected.
- Low levels of factor IX coagulant activity.
- Spontaneous hemarthroses.

General Considerations

Hemophilia B (Christmas disease, factor IX hemophilia) is a hereditary bleeding disorder due to deficiency of coagulation factor IX. Most commonly, factor IX is quantitatively reduced, but in one-third of cases an abnormally functioning molecule is immunologically present. Factor IX deficiency is one-seventh as common as factor VIII deficiency hemophilia but is otherwise clinically and genetically identical.

The PTT is prolonged, and factor IX levels are reduced when measured by specific factor assays. Other laboratory features are the same as for factor VIII hemophilia.

Treatment

Factor IX hemophilia is managed with factor IX concentrates. Factor VIII concentrates are ineffectual in this type of hemophilia; therefore it is imperative to distinguish between the two. The same dosing considerations apply as in factor VIII hemophilia, with the exception that the volume of distribution of factor IX is twice the plasma volume, so that 80 units/kg are necessary to achieve a 100% level. In addition, the half-life of factor IX is 18 hours. Thus, to maintain a patient through major surgery, the dosage should be 80 units/kg (approximately 6000 units) initially followed by 40 units/kg (3000 units) every 18 hours. Factor IX levels should be measured to ensure that expected levels are achieved and that an inhibitor is not present.

Unlike factor VIII concentrates, factor IX concentrates contain a number of other proteins, including activated coagulating factors that appear to contribute to a risk of thrombosis with recurrent usage of factor IX concentrates. Because of the risk of thrombosis, more care is needed in deciding to use these concentrates. Desmopressin acetate is not useful in this disorder.

Prognosis

The prognosis for these patients is the same as for those with factor VIII hemophilia.

Roberts HR, Eberst ME: Current management of hemophilia B. Hematol Oncol Clin North Am 1993;7:1269. (Main goal of replacement therapy is to achieve a hemostatic circulating level of factor IX with the lowest dose of concentrate; duration of therapy varies with the clinical scenario.)

Djulbegovic B et al: Safety and efficacy of purified factor IX concentrate and antifibrinolytic agents for dental extractions in hemophilia B. Am J Hematol 1996;51:168.

Hemophilia and von Willebrand's disease: 1. Diagnosis, comprehensive care and assessment. Association of Hemophilia Clinic Directors of Canada. Can Med Assoc J 1995;153:19.

Hemophilia and von Willebrand's disease: 2. Management. Association of Hemophilia Clinic Directors of Canada. Can Med Assoc J 1995;153:147.

Scharrer I: The need for highly purified products to treat hemophilia B. Acta Haematol 1995;94(Suppl 1):2.

OTHER CONGENITAL COAGULATION DISORDERS

Factor XI Deficiency

This disorder is seen primarily among Ashkenazi Jews and is autosomal recessive. The PTT may be markedly prolonged, and specific assays of factor XI will show reduced levels. This is usually a mild bleeding disorder manifested primarily by postoperative bleeding. Factor replacement is given with fresh-frozen plasma when necessary.

Afibrinogenemia

In this rare disorder, fibrinogen is absent and both prothrombin time and partial thromboplastin time are markedly prolonged. These patients may have a severe bleeding disorder similar to hemophilia. Fibrinogen is replaced with cryoprecipitate.

Other Coagulation Disorders

Bleeding disorders due to isolated deficiency of factors II, V, X, or VII are extremely rare. Deficiencies of factor XII and the contact pathway factors cause a markedly prolonged PTT but are not associated with any increased bleeding.

Factor XIII deficiency results in delayed bleeding after trauma or surgery. All coagulation tests are normal. The disorder is diagnosed by showing instability of the fibrin clot in 8-molar urea. Factor XIII is replaced with cryoprecipitate or plasma. A rare cause of bleeding is deficiency of the normal inhibitors of fibrinolytic activity: α_2-antiplasmin and plasminogen activator inhibitor.

Al-Mondhiry H, Ehmann WC: Congenital afibrinogenemia. Am J Hematol 1994;46:343. (Rare inherited disorder with bleeding of all types—especially splenic rupture—but with lower event rate than other coagulation disorders.)

COAGULOPATHY OF LIVER DISEASE

Essentials of Diagnosis

- Prothrombin time more prolonged than PTT.
- No response to vitamin K.

General Considerations

The liver is the site of synthesis of all the coagulation factors except factor VIII. As hepatic insufficiency develops, the vitamin K-dependent factors (factors II, VII, IX, X) and factor V are the first to be affected. Because of its rapid turnover (half-life 6 hours), factor VII levels are the first to decline. Conversely, fibrinogen levels are remarkably well conserved, and decreased fibrinogen synthesis does not occur unless liver disease is very severe.

Liver disease has a number of other effects on the hemostatic system. Increased fibrinolysis occurs because the liver synthesizes α_2-antiplasmin (the main inhibitor of fibrinolysis), which is responsible for the clearance of plasminogen activator. Biliary tract disease may lead to malabsorption of vitamin K, and congestive splenomegaly may produce mild thrombocytopenia. A variety of chronic liver diseases cause abnormal posttranslation modification of fibrinogen with resultant dysfibrinogenemia.

Clinical Findings

A. Symptoms and Signs: The coagulopathy of liver disease may lead to bleeding at any site. Excessive fibrinolysis may lead to oozing at venipuncture sites.

B. Laboratory Findings: Hepatic coagulopathy produces a more marked abnormality in the prothrombin time (PT) than in the partial thromboplastin time (PTT). Early in the course of liver disease, only the PT will become affected. Fibrinogen levels should be normal, and the thrombin time should be normal unless dysfibrinogenemia is present. The platelet count should be normal unless production is suppressed by acute alcohol ingestion or unless hypersplenism is present. The peripheral blood smear may show target cells.

Differential Diagnosis

Hepatic coagulopathy can be distinguished from vitamin K deficiency only by demonstrating the failure of vitamin K to correct the abnormal values. Liver disease is distinguished from disseminated intravascular coagulation by the normal fibrinogen level and lack of thrombocytopenia. End-stage liver disease almost invariably leads to some element of disseminated intravascular coagulation, and the disorders overlap (Tables 13–22 and 13–23).

Treatment

Long-term treatment of hepatic coagulopathy with factor replacement is usually ineffective. Fresh-frozen plasma is the treatment of choice, and volume overload will limit one's ability to maintain hemostatic factor levels. For example, to maintain factor levels greater than 25%, one must initially raise the level to 50% with 50% of the plasma volume (20 mL/kg) and then replace 10 mL/kg every 6 hours to

Table 13–22. Causes of isolated prolonged prothrombin time.

Liver disease
Vitamin K deficiency
Warfarin therapy
Factor VII deficiency

Table 13–23. Causes of prolonged prothrombin time and partial thromboplastin time.

Liver disease
Vitamin K deficiency
Disseminated intravascular coagulation
Heparin
Warfarin
Isolated factor deficiencies (rare): II, V, X, I

maintain adequate factor VII levels. In average-sized persons, this will require transfusion of 1400 mL of plasma initially followed by 700 mL every 6 hours. Factor IX concentrates are contraindicated in liver disease because of their tendency to cause disseminated intravascular coagulation. If thrombocytopenia is present, platelet transfusion may be of some help, but platelet recovery is usually disappointing because of hypersplenism.

Prognosis

The prognosis is that of the underlying liver disease.

VITAMIN K DEFICIENCY

Essentials of Diagnosis

- Prothrombin time more prolonged than PTT.
- Rapid correction with vitamin K replacement.
- Underlying dietary deficiency or antibiotic use.

General Considerations

Vitamin K plays a role in coagulation by acting as a cofactor for the posttranslational γ-carboxylation of zymogens II, VII, IX, and X. The modified zymogens (with γ-carboxyglutamic acid residues) are able to bind to platelets in a calcium-dependent reaction and consequently better participate in the complex reactions that activate factors X and II. Without γ-carboxylation, these reactions on the platelet surface occur slowly and hemostasis is impaired.

Vitamin K is supplied in the diet primarily in leafy vegetables and endogenously from synthesis by intestinal bacteria. Factors that contribute to vitamin K deficiency include poor diet, malabsorption, and broad-spectrum antibiotics suppressing colonic flora. A characteristic setting for vitamin K deficiency is a postoperative patient who is not eating and who is receiving antibiotics. Body stores of vitamin K are small, and deficiency may develop in as little as 1 week.

Clinical Findings

A. Symptoms and Signs: There are no specific clinical features, and bleeding may occur at any site.

B. Laboratory Findings: The prothrombin

time is prolonged to a greater extent than the PTT, and with mild vitamin K deficiency only the PT is defective (Tables 13–22 and 13–23). Fibrinogen level, thrombin time, and platelet count are not affected.

Differential Diagnosis

Vitamin K deficiency can be distinguished from hepatic coagulopathy only by assessing the response to vitamin K therapy. Surreptitious warfarin use will produce laboratory features indistinguishable from those of vitamin K deficiency.

Vitamin K deficiency is distinguished from disseminated intravascular coagulation by the normal platelet count and normal fibrinogen level in the former.

Treatment

Vitamin K deficiency responds rapidly to subcutaneous vitamin K, and a single dose of 15 mg will completely correct laboratory abnormalities in 12–24 hours.

Prognosis

The prognosis is excellent, as vitamin K deficiency can be completely corrected with replacement.

Lipsky JJ: Nutritional sources of vitamin K. Mayo Clin Proc 1994;65:462. (Antibiotics do not cause hypoprothrombinemia except in those with renal failure, cancer, or poor oral intake; poor diet alone even with normal intestinal flora can produce vitamin K deficiency.)

DISSEMINATED INTRAVASCULAR COAGULATION (DIC)

Essentials of Diagnosis

- Hypofibrinogenemia, thrombocytopenia, fibrin degradation products, and prolonged prothrombin time.
- Underlying serious illness.
- Microangiopathic hemolytic anemia may be present.

General Considerations

Coagulation is usually confined to a localized area by the combination of blood flow and circulating inhibitors of coagulation, especially antithrombin III. If the stimulus to coagulation is too great, these control mechanisms can be overwhelmed, leading to the syndrome of disseminated intravascular coagulation. In pathophysiologic terms, disseminated intravascular coagulation can be thought of as the consequence of the presence of circulating thrombin (normally confined to a localized area). The effects of thrombin are to cleave fibrinogen to fibrin monomer, stimulate platelet aggregation, activate factors V and VIII, and release plasminogen activator, which generates plasmin. Plasmin in turn cleaves fibrin, generating fibrin degradation products, and further inactivates factors V and VIII. Thus, the excess thrombin activity produces hypofibrinogenemia, thrombocytopenia, depletion of coagulation factors, and fibrinolysis.

Disseminated intravascular coagulation can be caused by a number of serious illnesses, including sepsis (especially with gram-negative bacteria but possible with any widespread bacterial or fungal infection), severe tissue injury (especially burns and head injury), obstetric complications (amniotic fluid embolus, septic abortion, retained dead fetus), cancer (acute promyelocytic leukemia, mucinous adenocarcinomas), and major hemolytic transfusion reactions.

Clinical Findings

A. Symptoms and Signs: Disseminated intravascular coagulation leads to both bleeding and thrombosis. Bleeding is far more common than thrombosis, but the latter may dominate if coagulation is activated to a far greater extent than fibrinolysis. Bleeding may occur at any site, but spontaneous bleeding and oozing at venipuncture sites or wounds are important clues to the diagnosis. Thrombosis is most commonly manifested by digital ischemia and gangrene, but catastrophic events such as renal cortical necrosis and hemorrhagic adrenal infarction may occur. Disseminated intravascular coagulation may also secondarily produce microangiopathic hemolytic anemia.

Subacute disseminated intravascular coagulation is seen primarily in cancer patients and is manifested primarily as recurrent superficial and deep venous thromboses (**Trousseau's syndrome**).

B. Laboratory Findings: Disseminated intravascular coagulation produces a complex coagulopathy with the characteristic constellation of hypofibrinogenemia, elevated fibrin degradation products, thrombocytopenia, and a prolonged prothrombin time. Of the fibrin degradation products, the D-dimer is the most sensitive, since its cross-linking implies origin from fibrin in a clot. All fibrin degradation products are cleared by the liver and thus may be elevated in hepatic dysfunction. Hypofibrinogenemia is another important diagnostic laboratory feature, because only a few other disorders (congenital hypofibrinogenemia, severe liver disease) will lower the fibrinogen level. In some cases of disseminated intravascular coagulation, when the patient's baseline fibrinogen level is markedly elevated, the initial fibrinogen level may be normal. However, since the half-life of fibrinogen is approximately 4 days, a noticeably falling fibrinogen level will confirm the diagnosis of disseminated intravascular coagulation.

Other laboratory abnormalities are variably present. The partial thromboplastin time may or may not be prolonged. In approximately one-fourth of cases, a microangiopathic hemolytic anemia is present, and fragmented red blood cells are seen on the peripheral smear. Antithrombin III levels may be markedly depleted. When fibrinolysis is activated, levels of plasminogen and α_2-antiplasmin may be low.

Subacute disseminated intravascular coagulation produces a very different laboratory picture. Thrombocytopenia and elevated D-dimer are usually the only abnormalities. Fibrinogen levels are normal, and the PTT may be normal.

Differential Diagnosis

Liver disease may prolong both the PT and PTT, but fibrinogen levels are usually normal, and the platelet count is usually normal or only slightly reduced. However, severe liver disease may be difficult to distinguish from disseminated intravascular coagulation. Vitamin K deficiency will not affect the fibrinogen level or platelet count and will be completely corrected by vitamin K replacement.

Sepsis may produce thrombocytopenia and digital ischemia, and coagulopathy may be present because of vitamin K deficiency. However, in these cases, the fibrinogen level should be normal.

Thrombotic thrombocytopenic purpura may produce fever and microangiopathic hemolytic anemia. However, fibrinogen levels and other coagulation tests should be normal.

Treatment

The primary focus should be the diagnosis and treatment of the underlying disorder that has given rise to disseminated intravascular coagulation. In many cases, disseminated intravascular coagulation will produce laboratory abnormalities with only mild clinical manifestations, and in these cases no specific therapy is required.

When the underlying cause of disseminated intravascular coagulation is rapidly reversible (such as in obstetric cases), replacement therapy alone may be indicated. The role of heparin in the treatment of disseminated intravascular coagulation is controversial. In some cases, when any increase in bleeding is unacceptable (neurosurgical procedures), heparin therapy is contraindicated. However, when disseminated intravascular coagulation is producing serious clinical consequences and the underlying cause is not rapidly reversible, heparin therapy may be necessary to control the syndrome. Such therapy is routinely used in the treatment of acute promyelocytic leukemia. In cases where disseminated intravascular coagulation causes thrombosis, heparin therapy is mandatory.

In replacement therapy, platelet transfusion should be used to maintain a platelet count greater than 30,000/μL, and 50,000/μL if possible. Fibrinogen is replaced with cryoprecipitate, and one should aim for a plasma fibrinogen level of 150 mg/dL. One unit of cryoprecipitate usually raises the fibrinogen level by

6–8 mg/dL, so that 15 units of cryoprecipitate will raise the level from 50 to 150 mg/dL. Coagulation factor deficiency may require replacement with fresh-frozen plasma.

Heparin therapy must be used in combination with replacement therapy, since administering heparin on its own will lead to an unacceptable increase in bleeding. Heparin therapy usually requires a dose of 500–750 units per hour. Heparin cannot be effective if antithrombin III levels are markedly depleted. Antithrombin III levels should be measured, and fresh-frozen plasma should be used to raise levels to greater than 50%. In using heparin, it is not necessary to prolong the PTT. Successful therapy is indicated by a rising fibrinogen level. Fibrin degradation products will decline over 1–2 days. Improvement in the platelet count may lag as much as 1 week behind control of the coagulopathy.

In some cases, when disseminated intravascular coagulation is complicated by excessive fibrinolysis, even the combination of heparin and replacement therapy may not be adequate to control bleeding. In these cases, aminocaproic acid, 1 g intravenously per hour, or tranexamic acid, 10 mg/kg intravenously every 8 hours, should be added to decrease the rate of fibrinolysis, raise the fibrinogen level, and control bleeding. *Caution:* It must be emphasized that aminocaproic acid can *never* be used without heparin in disseminated intravascular coagulation, since fatal thrombosis may occur.

Prognosis

The prognosis is that of the underlying disease. Severe disseminated intravascular coagulation can be lethal.

Bick RL: Disseminated intravascular coagulation: Objective clinical and laboratory diagnosis, treatment, and assessment of therapeutic response. Semin Thromb Hemost 1996;22:69.

Baglin T: Disseminated intravascular coagulation: Diagnosis and treatment. BMJ 1996;312:683.

HYPERCOAGULABLE STATES

In many cases, thrombosis is related to local factors causing stasis of blood flow or damage to a blood vessel. Common examples are deep venous thrombosis in the legs following prolonged sitting in one position and thrombosis in the femoral and iliac veins following hip surgery. However, in other cases a systemic disorder causes a general increase in the risk of thrombosis (Table 13–24).

Cancer is associated with an increased risk of both venous and arterial thrombosis. In some cases, low-grade disseminated intravascular coagulation appears to be responsible. In unusual cases, a unique cancer procoagulant stimulates the clotting system. Myeloproliferative disorders such as polycythemia vera, essential thrombocytosis, and paroxysmal nocturnal hemoglobinuria are associated with a high incidence of thrombosis, caused by qualitative platelet abnormalities. For the indolent diseases polycythemia vera and essential thrombocytosis, thrombosis is the major cause of morbidity and deaths. Venous thrombosis may occur in unusual locations such as the mesenteric, hepatic, or splenic venous beds. Arterial thrombosis occurs as well and may be manifested as large vessel occlusion (stroke, myocardial infarction) or as microvascular events with painful burning in the hands and feet.

Heparin is an uncommon but important cause of hypercoagulability. Heparin has been associated with thrombocytopenia in about 10% of treatment courses. Often the thrombocytopenia is modest and resolves spontaneously. However, in some cases severe thrombocytopenia occurs. It is most often in this setting that arterial thrombosis occurs as a complication. The arteries involved are often large ones, such as the iliac artery or even the aorta. It is imperative that heparin be discontinued in this setting, since continuing the drug almost always leads to a fatal outcome.

A number of congenital biochemical defects have also been associated with hypercoagulability (Table 13–24). A family history is usually present. The thromboses are almost always venous and may occur in the large veins of the abdomen. Thromboses often occur during early adulthood rather than in childhood and are often precipitated by factors such as trauma or pregnancy. The most common of these disorders is an abnormal factor V (factor V Leiden), which is resistant to degradation by activated protein C. Dysfibrinogenemia is diagnosed by a prolonged reptilase time.

Table 13–24. Causes of hypercoagulability.

Acquired
Cancer
Inflammatory disorders: Ulcerative colitis
Myeloproliferative disorders
Postoperative
Estrogens, pregnancy
Lupus anticoagulant
Heparin-induced thrombocytopenia
Anticardiolipin antibodies
Congenital
Antithrombin III deficiency
Factor V Leiden
Protein C deficiency
Protein S deficiency
Dysfibrinogenemia
Abnormal plasminogen

The syndrome of **warfarin-induced skin necrosis** may occur in patients with undiagnosed protein C deficiency. Protein C is vitamin K-dependent and has a shorter half-life than the coagulation proteins. Warfarin, by creating a vitamin K-dependent state, will transiently deplete protein C before it leads to anticoagulation. During the period of hypercoagulability due to unopposed protein C depletion, thrombosis of skin vessels may lead to infarction and necrosis. The syndrome can be prevented by the use of heparin for 5–7 days until warfarin induces anticoagulation.

Treatment

If a patient is recognized to be at increased risk of thrombosis, effective prophylactic therapy is usually available. Preoperatively, minidose heparin (5000 units every 8–12 hours) may be useful in reducing the risk of thrombosis in the perioperative period. The hypercoagulable state associated with cancer may benefit from treatment with heparin, 10,000 units subcutaneously every 12 hours. Low-molecular-weight heparin is a more convenient agent which is equally effective and requires less laboratory monitoring. Warfarin is usually ineffective in preventing thrombosis in this situation, most likely because low-grade disseminated intravascular coagulation is the cause. In patients with myeloproliferative disease who have had symptoms of thrombosis, antiplatelet therapy may be helpful. However, such therapy should not be used indiscriminately, because these patients are also at increased risk of bleeding. For patients with **erythromelalgia** (painful redness and burning of the hands), aspirin, 325 mg daily, is almost always effective.

For patients with congenital biochemical defects such as deficiency of antithrombin III or the vitamin K-dependent proteins C and S, warfarin is effective and should probably be given for life. Family members should be screened for the presence of the defect so that their increased risk of thrombosis can be noted and acted upon.

De Stefano V, Finazzi G, Mannucci PM: Inherited thrombophilia: Pathogenesis, clinical syndromes, and management. Blood 1996;87:3531. (Excellent comprehensive review.)

Ginsberg JS: Management of venous thromboembolism. N Engl J Med 1996;335:1816.

den Heijer M et al: Hyperhomocysteinemia as a risk factor for deep-vein thrombosis. N Engl J Med 1996;334:759.

Hillarp A, Zoller B, Dahlback B: Activated protein C resistance as a basis for venous thrombosis. Am J Med 1996;101:534.

Le DT et al: The international normalized ratio (INR) for monitoring warfarin therapy: Reliability and relation to other monitoring methods. Ann Intern Med 1994;120: 552.

Macik BG, Ortel TL: Clinical and laboratory evaluation of the hypercoagulable states. Clin Chest Med 1995;16: 375.

Toglia MR, Weg JG: Venous thromboembolism during pregnancy. N Engl J Med 1996;335:108.

Wells PS et al: Interactions of warfarin with drugs and food. Ann Intern Med 1994;121:676. (Reviews drugs and foods that have known potentiating, inhibiting, or no effect.)

LUPUS ANTICOAGULANT

The lupus anticoagulant is an IgM or IgG immunoglobulin that produces a prolonged PTT by binding to the phospholipid used in the in vitro PTT assay. As such, it is a laboratory artifact and does not cause a clinical bleeding disorder. The "lupus anticoagulant" is seen in 5–10% of patients with systemic lupus erythematosus. More commonly, it is seen without an underlying disorder or in patients taking phenothiazines.

There is no bleeding defect unless a second disorder such as thrombocytopenia, hypoprothrombinemia, or a prolonged bleeding time is present. Paradoxically, the lupus anticoagulant has been associated with an increased risk of thrombosis and of recurrent spontaneous abortions.

The PTT is prolonged and fails to correct when the patient's plasma is mixed in a 1:1 dilution with normal plasma. The PT is either normal or slightly prolonged. The fibrinogen level and thrombin time are normal. The Russell viper venom (RVV) time is a more sensitive assay and is specifically designed to demonstrate the presence of a lupus anticoagulant. An antiphospholipid, the lupus anticoagulant will cause a false-positive VDRL test for syphilis. A related autoantibody, anticardiolipin, can be detected by separate assays.

Lupus anticoagulant should be suspected in cases of a markedly prolonged PTT without clinical bleeding (other causes are factor XII or contact factor deficiency). The plasma mixing test will demonstrate the presence of an inhibitor by the failure of normal plasma to correct the PTT. When acquired factor VIII inhibitors are being considered, a factor VIII:C level may be measured; this will be normal in patients with lupus anticoagulant.

No specific treatment is necessary. Prednisone will usually rapidly eliminate the lupus anticoagulant, and it has been suggested that prednisone therapy reduces spontaneous abortions in this syndrome. It is not clear whether prednisone has any effect on the thrombotic tendency associated with lupus anticoagulant. Patients with thromboses should be treated with anticoagulation in standard doses. Because of the artificially prolonged PTT, heparin therapy is difficult to monitor properly. The dose of warfarin administered may also be inadequate if the baseline PT is prolonged.

Ginsberg JS et al: Antiphospholipid antibodies and venous thromboembolism. Blood 1995;86:3685.

Khamashta MA et al: The management of thrombosis in the antiphospholipid-antibody syndrome. N Engl J Med 1995;332:993.

Shapiro SS: The lupus anticoagulant/antiphospholipid syndrome. Annu Rev Med 1996;47:533.

BLOOD TRANSFUSIONS

RED BLOOD CELL TRANSFUSIONS

Red blood cell transfusions are given to raise the hematocrit levels in patients with anemia or to replace losses after acute bleeding episodes. Because of the inherent risks, blood transfusions should never be given to correct anemia when simpler measures such as administration of iron, folate, or vitamin B_{12} can be used instead. Several types of components containing red blood cells are available.

(1) Fresh whole blood: The major advantage of this component is the simultaneous presence of red blood cells, plasma, and fresh platelets. Fresh whole blood is never absolutely necessary, since all the above components are available separately. The major indications for use of whole blood are cardiac surgery or massive hemorrhage when more than ten units of blood are required in a 24-hour period.

(2) Packed red blood cells: Packed red cells are the component most commonly used to raise the hematocrit. Each unit has a volume of about 300 mL, of which approximately 200 mL consists of red blood cells. One unit of packed red cells will usually raise the hematocrit by approximately 4%. The expected rise in hematocrit can be calculated using an estimated red blood cell volume of 200 mL/unit and a total blood volume of about 70 mL/kg. For example, a 70-kg man will have a total blood volume of 4900 mL, and each unit of packed red blood cells will raise the hematocrit by 200 ÷ 4900 equals 4%.

(3) Leukopoor blood: Patients with severe leukoagglutinin reactions to packed red blood cells may require depletion of white blood cells and platelets from transfused units. White blood cells can be removed either by centrifugation or by washing. Preparation of leukopoor blood causes additional expense and leads to some loss of red cells.

(4) Frozen blood: Red blood cells can be frozen and stored for up to 3 years, but the technique is cumbersome and expensive, and frozen blood should be used sparingly. The major application is for the purpose of maintaining a supply of rare blood types. Patients with very rare blood types may donate units for autologous transfusion should the need

arise. Frozen red cells are also occasionally needed for patients with severe leukoagglutinin reactions or anaphylactic reactions to plasma proteins, since frozen blood has essentially all white blood cells and plasma components removed.

(5) Autologous packed red blood cells: Patients scheduled for elective surgery may donate blood for autologous transfusion. These units may be stored for up to 35 days.

Compatibility Testing

Before transfusion, the recipient's and the donor's blood are cross-matched to avoid hemolytic transfusion reactions. Although many antigen systems are present on red blood cells, only the ABO and Rh systems are specifically tested prior to all transfusions. The A and B antigens are the most important, because everyone who lacks one or both red cell antigens has isoantibodies against the missing antigen or antigens in his or her plasma. These antibodies activate complement and can cause rapid intravascular lysis of the incompatible red cells. In emergencies, type O blood can be given to any recipient, but only packed cells should be given to avoid transfusion of donor plasma containing anti-A or anti-B antibodies.

The other important antigen routinely tested for is the D antigen of the Rh system. Approximately 15% of the population lack this antigen. In patients lacking the antigen, anti-D antibodies are not naturally present, but the antigen is highly immunogenic. A recipient whose red cells lack D and who receives D-positive blood may develop anti-D antibodies that can cause severe lysis of subsequent transfusions of D-positive red cells.

Blood typing includes assay of recipient serum for unusual antibodies by mixing the serum with panels of red cells representing commonly occurring weak antigens. The screening is particularly important if the recipient has had previous transfusions.

Hemolytic Transfusion Reactions

Major hemolytic transfusion reactions are the most dread complication of transfusion and can be fatal. The most severe reactions are those involving mismatches in the ABO system. Most of these cases are due to clerical errors and mislabeled specimens. Hemolysis is rapid and intravascular, releasing free hemoglobin into the plasma. The severity of these reactions depends on the dose of red blood cells given. The most severe reactions are those seen in surgical patients under anesthesia. They will be unable to give early warning signs of myalgias and chills.

Hemolytic transfusion reactions caused by minor antigen systems are typically less severe. The hemolysis usually takes place at a slower rate and is extravascular. Sometimes these transfusion reactions may be delayed for 5–10 days after transfusion. In such cases, the recipient has received blood containing an immunogenic action, and in the time since transfusion, a new alloantibody has been formed. The most common antigens involved in such reactions are Duffy, Kidd, Kell, and C and E loci of the Rh system.

A. Symptoms and Signs: Major hemolytic transfusion reactions cause fever and chills and severe backache and headache. In severe cases, there may be apprehension, dyspnea, hypotension, and vascular collapse. Such symptoms will usually lead to recognition of a transfusion reaction. *The transfusion must be stopped immediately!* In severe cases, disseminated intravascular coagulation or acute renal failure from tubular necrosis can occur, or both may occur.

Patients under general anesthesia will not give such signs, and the first indication may be generalized bleeding and oliguria.

B. Laboratory Findings and Management: Identification of the recipient and of the blood should be checked. The donor transfusion bag with its pilot tube must be returned to the blood bank, and a fresh sample of the recipient's blood must accompany the donor bag for retyping of donor and recipient blood samples and for repeat of the cross-match.

The hematocrit will fail to rise by the expected amount. Coagulation studies will reveal evidence of renal failure and disseminated intravascular coagulation in severe cases. Hemoglobinemia will turn the plasma pink and eventually result in hemoglobinuria. In cases of delayed hemolytic reactions, the hematocrit will fall and the indirect bilirubin will rise. In these cases, the new offending alloantibody is easily detected in the patient's serum.

C. Treatment: If a hemolytic transfusion reaction is suspected, the transfusion should be stopped at once. A sample of anticoagulated blood from the recipient should be centrifuged to detect free hemoglobin in the plasma. If hemoglobinemia is present, the patient should be vigorously hydrated to prevent acute tubular necrosis. There is some evidence that forced diuresis with mannitol may help prevent renal damage.

Leukoagglutinin Reactions

Most transfusion reactions are not hemolytic but represent reactions to antigens present on white blood cells in patients who have been sensitized to the antigens through previous transfusions or pregnancy. Most commonly, patients will develop fever and chills within 12 hours after transfusion. In severe cases, cough and dyspnea may occur and the chest x-ray may show transient pulmonary infiltrates. Because no hemolysis is involved, the hematocrit rises by the expected amount despite the reaction.

Leukoagglutinin reactions may respond to acetaminophen and diphenhydramine. In severe cases, corticosteroids are of value. In the future, the removal of leukocytes by filtration before blood storage will reduce the incidence of these reactions.

Anaphylactic Reactions

Rarely, patients will develop hives or bronchospasm during a transfusion. These reactions are almost always due to plasma proteins rather than white blood cells. Patients who are IgA-deficient may develop these reactions because of antibodies to IgA. Patients with such reactions may require transfusion of washed or even frozen red blood cells to avoid future severe reactions.

Contaminated Blood

Rarely, blood is contaminated with gram-negative bacteria. Transfusion can lead to septicemia and shock from endotoxin. If this is suspected, the offending unit should be cultured and the patient treated with antibiotics as indicated.

Diseases Transmitted Through Transfusion

Despite the use of only volunteer blood donors and the routine screening of blood, transfusion-associated viral diseases remain a problem. All blood products (red blood cells, platelets, plasma, cryoprecipitate) can transmit viral diseases. All blood donors are screened with questionnaires designed to detect donors at high risk of transmitting diseases. All blood is now routinely screened with a variety of tests including hepatitis B surface antigen, antibody to hepatitis B core antigen, syphilis, p24 antigen and antibody to HIV, antibody to HCV, and antibody to HTLV.

With improved screening, the risk of posttransfusion hepatitis has steadily decreased. The risk of hepatitis B is 1:200,000 per unit and of HIV 1:250,000 per unit. The risk of seroconversion to HTLV is 1:70,000, but clinical sequelae when this occurs are rare. The major infectious risk of blood products is hepatitis C, with a seroconversion rate of 1:3300 per unit transfused. Most of these cases are clinically silent, but there is a long-term risk of chronic hepatitis.

Platelet Transfusion

Platelet transfusions are indicated in cases of thrombocytopenia due to decreased platelet production. They are not useful in immune thrombocytopenia, since transfused platelets will last no longer than the patient's endogenous platelets. The risk of spontaneous bleeding rises when the platelet count falls to less than 20,000/μL, and the risk of life-threatening bleeding increases when the platelet count is less than 5000/μL. Because of this, prophylactic platelet transfusions are often given at these very low levels. Platelet transfusions are also given prior to invasive procedures or surgery, and the goal should be to raise the platelet count to over 50,000/μL.

Platelets are most commonly derived from donated blood units. One unit of platelets (derived from

1 unit of blood) usually contains $5–7 \times 10^{10}$ platelets suspended in 35 mL of plasma. Ideally, 1 platelet unit will raise the recipient's platelet count by 10,000/μL, and transfused platelets will last for 2 or 3 days. However, responses are often suboptimal, with poor platelet increments and short survival times. This may be due to sepsis, splenomegaly, or alloimmunization. Most alloantibodies causing platelet destruction are directed at HLA antigens. Patients requiring long periods of platelet transfusion support should be monitored to document adequate responses to transfusions so that the most appropriate product can be used. Patients may benefit from HLA-matched platelets derived from either volunteer donors or family members, with platelets obtained by plateletpheresis. Recently, techniques of cross-matching platelets have been developed and appear to identify suitable platelet donors (nonreactive with the patient's serum) without the need for HLA typing. Such single-donor platelets usually contain the equivalent of six units of random platelets, or 30–50 $\times 10^{10}$ platelets suspended in 200 mL of plasma. Ideally, these platelet concentrates will raise the recipient's platelet count by 60,000/μL. Preliminary reports suggest that leukocyte-depleted platelets may be less immunogenic and that their use may delay the onset of alloimmunization.

Granulocyte Transfusions

Granulocyte transfusions are seldom indicated and have largely been replaced by the use of myeloid growth factors (G-CSF and GM-CSF) that speed neutrophil recovery. However, they may be beneficial in patients with profound neutropenia (< 100/μL) who have gram-negative sepsis or progressive soft tissue infection despite optimal antibiotic therapy. In these cases, it is clear that progressive infection is due to failure of host defenses. In such situations, daily granulocyte transfusions should be given and continued until the neutrophil count rises to above 500/μL. Such granulocytes must be derived from ABO-matched donors. Although HLA matching is not necessary, it is preferred, since patients with alloantibodies to donor white blood cells will have severe reactions and no benefit.

The donor cells usually contain some immuno-competent lymphocytes capable of producing graft-versus-host disease in HLA-incompatible hosts whose immunocompetence may be impaired. Irradiation of the units of cells with 1500 cGy will destroy the lymphocytes without harm to the granulocytes or platelets.

Bordin JO et al: Biologic effects of leukocytes present in transfused cellular blood products. Blood 1994;84:1703.

(Associated with febrile reactions, graft versus host disease, alloimmunization, immunomodulation, transmission of infection; may have some beneficial effects in neutropenia and for immunosuppression; clinical benefit of leukodepletion is unclear.)

Heddle NM et al: The role of plasma from platelet concentrates in transfusion reactions. N Engl J Med 1994; 331:625.

Kampe CE: Clinical syndromes associated with lupus anticoagulants. Semin Thromb Hemost 1994;20:16. (Immunologically distinct from anticardiolipin antibodies but similar clinical syndromes with strong association of arterial and venous thrombosis, thrombocytopenia, and neurologic disorders in patients with SLE and lupus-like disorders.)

Tong MJ et al: Clinical outcomes after transfusion-associated hepatitis C. N Engl J Med 1995;332:1463.

Williamson LM et al: Bedside filtration of blood products in the prevention of HLA alloimmunization: A prospective, randomized study. Blood 1994;83:3028. (This study failed to document a decrease in alloimmunization with the use of filtered blood products. There was no decrease in leukoagglutinin reactions. The optimal method of white blood cell depletion from blood products probably involves removal prior to blood or platelet storage.)

TRANSFUSION OF PLASMA COMPONENTS

Fresh-frozen plasma is available in units of approximately 200 mL. Fresh plasma contains normal levels of all coagulation factors (about 1 unit/mL). Fresh-frozen plasma is used to correct coagulation factors deficiency and to treat thrombotic thrombocytopenic purpura. The risk of transmitting viral disease is comparable to that associated with transfusion of red blood cells.

Cryoprecipitate is made from fresh plasma. One unit has a volume of approximately 20 mL and contains approximately 250 mg of fibrinogen and between 80 and 100 units of factor VIII and von Willebrand factor. Cryoprecipitate is used to treat factor VIII deficiency and von Willebrand's disease and to supplement fibrinogen in cases of congenital deficiency of fibrinogen or disseminated intravascular coagulation. One unit of cryoprecipitate will raise the fibrinogen level by about 8 mg/dL.

College of American Pathologists: Practice parameter for the use of fresh frozen plasma, cryoprecipitate, and platelets. JAMA 1994;271:777.

Koretz RL et al: Non-A, non-B post-transfusion hepatitis: Looking back on the second decade. Ann Intern Med 1993;119:110.

Mollison PL: *Blood Transfusions in Clinical Medicine,* 9th ed. Blackwell, 1993.

14

Alimentary Tract

Kenneth R. McQuaid, MD

SYMPTOMS & SIGNS OF GASTROINTESTINAL DISEASE

DYSPEPSIA

Dyspepsia is an imprecise term that refers to a host of upper abdominal or epigastric symptoms such as pain, discomfort, fullness, bloating, early satiety, belching, heartburn, regurgitation, or, simply, "indigestion." It occurs in one-fourth of the adult population, though most never seek medical attention for this complaint. Even so, it is one of the most common medical complaints, accounting for 3% of general medical office visits.

Etiology

A wide variety of disorders may cause dyspepsia.

A. Drug Intolerance: Examples include aspirin, NSAIDs, antibiotics (metronidazole, erythromycin), corticosteroids, digoxin, theophylline, iron, narcotics, alcohol, and caffeine.

B. Luminal Gastrointestinal Tract Dysfunction: Of patients with dyspepsia who undergo endoscopy, gastroesophageal reflux disease is present in 5–15% and peptic ulcer disease in 15–25%. Gastric cancer is identified in 1% but is rare in persons under age 45 years. Other causes include gastroparesis (especially in diabetes mellitus), lactose intolerance and malabsorptive conditions, and parasitic infection *(Giardia, Strongyloides)*. The role of chronic *Helicobacter pylori*-associated gastritis as a cause of dyspepsia remains unproved and controversial.

C. Pancreatic Disease: Pancreatic carcinoma, chronic pancreatitis.

D. Biliary Tract Disease: The abrupt, severe pain of biliary colic due to cholelithiasis or choledocholithiasis should be distinguishable from dyspepsia in most instances.

E. Other Conditions: Diabetes mellitus, thyroid disease, coronary ischemia, collagen vascular disease, intra-abdominal malignancy, and pregnancy, among others.

F. Functional or "Nonulcer" Dyspepsia: This is the most common cause of chronic dyspepsia. Up to two-thirds of dyspeptic patients have no obvious organic or biochemical cause for their symptoms that can be determined by upper endoscopy or abdominal ultrasonography. Symptoms may arise from a complex interaction of increased visceral afferent sensitivity, delayed gastric emptying or impaired accommodation to food, or psychosocial stressors.

Clinical Findings

A. Symptoms and Signs: Because of the nonspecific nature of dyspeptic symptoms, the clinical history has limited diagnostic utility. The history should clarify the chronicity, location, and quality of the discomfort. The presence of "alarming" symptoms should be elicited, such as weight loss, persistent vomiting, dysphagia, hematemesis, melena, or anemia. If present, these symptoms warrant urgent evaluation with endoscopy or abdominal imaging. Potentially offending medications and excessive alcohol use should be identified and discontinued if possible. The patient's reason for seeking professional attention at this time should be determined. Many patients report a fear of having a serious underlying condition, which must be addressed. Recent changes in employment, marital stress, physical and sexual abuse, anxiety, and depression may all contribute to the development and reporting of symptoms.

The symptom profile is unable to differentiate reliably between nonulcer dyspepsia, peptic ulcer disease, and gastroesophageal reflux disease. Even experienced clinicians are wrong as often as right in their initial clinical impression. Nevertheless, patients with peptic ulcer disease are more likely to be older (> 45 years), to smoke, and to have pain relieved by food or antacids. Patients are more likely to have nonulcer dyspepsia if they are younger, if they report a variety of abdominal and extra-gastrointestinal complaints, show signs of anxiety or depression, or have a history of use of psychotropic medications. The complaint of heartburn as the predominant symptom is 90% specific for the diagnosis of gastroesophageal reflux disease. It is increasingly clear, however, that there are many patients with reflux disease who have dyspepsia (ie, epigastric discomfort) as their main complaint without heartburn.

The physical examination is mandatory but rarely helpful. Signs of serious organic disease such as weight loss, organomegaly, abdominal mass, or fecal occult blood warrant further investigation. In patients over age 45, initial laboratory work should include a complete blood count, serum electrolytes, liver enzymes, serum calcium, and thyroid function tests.

B. Special Examinations: In evaluating patients with dyspepsia, the physician attempts to distinguish organic causes from functional dyspepsia. The level of appropriate evaluation depends upon the chronicity of symptoms, the suspicion of organic disease, the response to empirical treatment, and the level of patient anxiety. Urgent upper endoscopy is indicated in all patients with dyspepsia who have "alarming" symptoms to look for evidence of peptic ulcer disease, gastroesophageal reflux disease, or upper gastrointestinal tract malignancy. It is also helpful for those patients who are worried about the presence of serious underlying disease. In others with uncomplicated dyspepsia, the clinician must decide between pursuing an early definitive diagnosis with upper endoscopy and a trial of empirical medical treatment.

In 1985, the American College of Physicians recommended a trial of empirical therapy with H_2-receptor antagonists for 6–8 weeks for patients with uncomplicated dyspepsia, reserving endoscopic evaluation for those whose symptoms failed to improve or relapsed after discontinuation of therapy. Subsequent clinical outcome trials have shown that although initial improvement of dyspepsia with H_2 antagonists is common, almost two-thirds of patients experience a symptomatic relapse within 1 year and require endoscopic evaluation. Evidence indicates that the long-term costs of management with initial endoscopy compared with empirical H_2 antagonists are approximately the same.

The recent recognition of *H pylori* has led to a dramatic shift in the treatment of peptic ulcer disease and is beginning to alter the initial approach to dyspepsia. The role of noninvasive testing for *H pylori* (IgG serology, urea breath test) is undergoing evaluation. A negative test for *H pylori* in a patient not taking an NSAID virtually excludes the possibility of peptic ulcer disease. The majority of these *H pylori*-negative patients have functional dyspepsia (for which no proved treatment exists) and could be given initial empirical treatment with either an H_2 antagonist or a prokinetic agent. In patients testing positive for *H pylori*, empirical antibiotic treatment should result in definitive treatment for patients with underlying peptic ulcer disease and conceivably may improve symptoms in some patients with nonulcer dyspepsia. Recent decision analytic models suggest that a dyspepsia management strategy based upon initial testing for *H pylori* may be the most cost-effective approach. However, these models remain to be validated by clinical trials.

At present, the optimal cost-effective approach to dyspepsia is unclear. The physician should discuss with the patient the risks and benefits of early endoscopy versus empirical H_2 antagonists versus initial noninvasive testing for *H pylori* with antibiotic therapy of infected patients.

Abdominal ultrasonography is only warranted when biliary or pancreatic disease is suspected. Gastric emptying studies are not recommended in the routine evaluation of dyspepsia.

Treatment of Functional Dyspepsia

The treatment of dyspepsia is directed at the underlying cause. In patients with functional dyspepsia, the following should be considered:

A. General Measures: A stable physician-patient interaction is the most important aspect of therapy. Patients require reassurance that the condition is not serious but may be chronic. Alcohol and caffeine should be eliminated. A food diary, in which patients record their food intake, symptoms, and daily events, may reveal dietary or psychosocial precipitants of pain.

B. Pharmacologic Agents: Over half of patients derive relief from placebo, demonstrating the importance of the therapeutic relationship or the natural history of the illness. H_2 antagonists (ranitidine, 150 mg twice daily; famotidine, 20 mg twice daily; or cimetidine, 400–800 mg twice daily) are only marginally better than placebo but offer benefit to those with symptoms suggestive of gastroesophageal reflux. Prokinetic agents (cisapride, 10 mg, or metoclopramide, 10 mg, three to four times daily before meals) improve symptoms in 60–80% and are significantly better than placebo. Symptom improvement does not correlate with the presence or absence of gastric emptying delay. Drug treatment should be discontinued after 4–8 weeks and the patient observed for symptomatic relapse.

C. Anti-*H pylori* Treatment: Eradication of *H pylori* has not been shown convincingly to improve symptoms in patients with functional dyspepsia in trials with long-term follow-up. Nevertheless, based upon anecdotal reports of dramatic improvement in a subset of infected patients, some authorities have recommended a trial of antibiotic therapy.

Camilleri M: Nonulcer dyspepsia: A look into the future. Mayo Clin Proc 1996;71:614.

Ofman JJ et al: Management strategies for *Helicobacter py-*

lori-seropositive patients with dyspepsia: Clinical and economic consequences. Ann Intern Med 1997;126:280.

NAUSEA & VOMITING

Nausea is a vague, intensely disagreeable sensation of sickness or "queasiness" that may or may not be followed by vomiting. It should be distinguished from anorexia. Vomiting is often preceded by nausea and by retching, spasmodic respiratory and abdominal movements ("dry heaves"). Vomiting should be distinguished from regurgitation, which is the effortless reflux of liquid or food stomach contents.

The act of vomiting is controlled by a center in the medulla that coordinates the respiratory and vasomotor centers and the vagus nervous innervation of the gastrointestinal tract. The vomiting center may be stimulated by four different sources of afferent input: (1) Afferent vagal fibers (rich in serotonin 5-HT$_3$ receptors) and splanchnic fibers from the gastrointestinal viscera; these may be stimulated by biliary or gastrointestinal distention, mucosal or peritoneal irritation or infections. (2) The vestibular system, which may be stimulated by motion or infections. These fibers have high concentrations of histamine H$_1$ and muscarinic cholinergic receptors. (3) Higher central nervous system centers. Disorders of the central nervous system or certain sights, smells, or emotional experiences may induce vomiting. For example, patients receiving chemotherapy may develop vomiting in anticipation of chemotherapy. (4) The "chemoreceptor trigger zone," located outside the blood-brain barrier in the area postrema of the medulla. This area has chemoreceptors that may be stimulated by drugs and chemotherapeutic agents, toxins, hypoxia, uremia, acidosis, and radiation therapy. This region is rich in serotonin 5-HT$_3$ and dopamine D$_2$ receptors. Although the causes of vomiting are many, a simplified list is provided in Table 14–1.

Complications of vomiting include dehydration, hypokalemia, metabolic alkalosis, pulmonary aspiration, rupture of the esophagus (Boerhaave's syndrome), and bleeding secondary to a mucosal tear at the gastroesophageal junction (Mallory-Weiss syndrome).

Clinical Findings

A. Symptoms and Signs: The history and physical examination are important in distinguishing among the causes of vomiting. Acute symptoms without abdominal pain are typically caused by food poisoning, infectious gastroenteritis, or drugs. Inquiry should be made into recent changes in medications, food ingestions, other viral symptoms of malaise or diarrhea, or similar illnesses in family members. The acute onset of severe pain and vomiting suggests peritoneal irritation, acute intestinal obstruction, or pancreaticobiliary disease. Examination

Table 14–1. Causes of nausea and vomiting.

Visceral afferent stimulation	**Mechanical obstruction**
	  Gastric outlet obstruction: peptic ulcer disease, malignancy
	  Small intestinal obstruction: adhesions, hernias, volvulus, Crohn's disease, carcinomatosis
	Dysmotility
	  Gastroparesis: diabetic, medications, postviral, postvagotomy
	  Small intestine: scleroderma, amyloidosis, chronic intestinal pseudo-obstruction, familial myoneuropathies
	Peritoneal irritation
	  Peritonitis: perforated viscus, appendicitis, spontaneous bacterial peritonitis
	Infections
	  Viral gastroenteritis: Norwalk agent, rotavirus
	  "Food poisoning": toxins from *B cereus, S aureus, C perfringens*
	  Hepatitis A, B, or C
	  Acute systemic infections
	Hepatobiliary or pancreatic disorders
	  Acute pancreatitis
	  Cholecystitis or choledocholithiasis
	Topical gastrointestinal irritants
	  Alcohol, NSAIDs, oral antibiotics
	Other
	  Cardiac disease: acute myocardial infarction, congestive failure
	  Urologic disease: stones, pyelonephritis

Central nervous system disorders	**Vestibular disorders**
	  Labyrinthitis, Meniere's syndrome, motion sickness
	Increased intracranial pressure
	  CNS tumors, subdural or subarachnoid hemorrhage
	Infections
	  Meningitis, encephalitis
	Psychogenic
	  Anticipatory vomiting, bulimia, psychiatric disorders

Irritation of chemoreceptor trigger zone	**Antitumor chemotherapy**
	Medications
	  Opioids
	Radiation therapy
	Systemic disorders
	  Diabetic ketoacidosis, uremia, adrenocortical crisis

may reveal fever, focal tenderness, guarding, or rebound tenderness. More chronic vomiting suggests pregnancy, gastric outlet obstruction, gastroparesis, intestinal dysmotility, psychogenic disorders, and central nervous system or systemic disorders. Vomiting immediately after meals suggests bulimia or psychogenic causes. Vomiting of undigested food 1 to several hours after meals suggests gastroparesis or a gastric outlet obstruction. Physical examination in these patients may reveal a succussion splash. Patients with either acute or chronic symptoms should be asked about neurologic symptoms such as headaches, stiff neck, vertigo, and focal paresthesias or weakness. Neurologic and funduscopic examinations are required.

B. Special Examinations: In acute vomiting, flat and upright abdominal radiographs are obtained in patients with severe pain or suspicion of mechanical obstruction to look for free intraperitoneal air or dilated loops of small bowel. In patients with suspected mechanical small intestinal or gastric obstruction, a nasogastric tube should be placed for relief of symptoms. Aspiration of more than 200 mL of residual material in a fasting patient suggests obstruction or gastroparesis. This may be confirmed by a saline load test showing more than 400 mL residual on gastric aspiration performed 30 minutes after nasogastric instillation of 750 mL of 0.9% saline. The cause of the gastric outlet obstruction is best demonstrated by upper endoscopy. Gastroparesis is confirmed by nuclear scintigraphic studies, which show delayed gastric emptying and either upper endoscopy or barium upper GI series showing no evidence of mechanical gastric outlet obstruction. Abnormal liver function tests or elevated amylase suggests pancreaticobiliary disease, which may be investigated with an abdominal sonogram or computerized tomography. Central nervous system symptoms should be investigated by brain CT or MRI.

Treatment

A. General Measures: The treatment of vomiting should be directed primarily at finding and correcting the underlying cause. Most causes of acute vomiting are mild, self-limited, and require no specific treatment. Patients should ingest clear liquids (broths, tea, soups, carbonated beverages) and small quantities of dry foods (soda crackers). For more severe acute vomiting, hospitalization is usually required. Owing to inability to eat and loss of gastric fluids, patients may become dehydrated and develop hypokalemia and metabolic alkalosis. Intravenous 0.45% saline solution with 20 meq/L of potassium chloride is given in most cases to maintain hydration. A nasogastric suction tube for gastric decompression improves patient comfort and permits monitoring of fluid loss.

B. Antiemetic Medications: Medications may be given either to prevent or to control vomiting (see above). Given the complexity of the various pathways that control and stimulate vomiting, it is not surprising that no single medication is effective in all patients. Combinations of drugs from different classes may provide better control of symptoms with less toxicity in some patients. All of these medications should be avoided in pregnancy. (For dosages, see Table 14–2.)

1. Serotonin 5-HT$_3$ receptor antagonists– Ondansetron or graniseton, when initiated prior to treatment, is effective in the prevention of chemotherapy-induced emesis.

2. Dopamine antagonists–The phenothiazines, butyrophenones, and substituted benzamides have antiemetic properties which are due, at least in

Table 14–2. Common antiemetic dosing regimens.

	Dosage	Route
Serotonin 5-HT$_3$ antagonists		
Ondansetron	0.15 mg/kg 15 minutes before chemotherapy, then every 4 hours for two doses or 32 mg once	IV
	8 mg three times daily	PO
Granisetron	10 µg/kg	IV
	1 mg twice daily	PO
Dopamine antagonists		
Prochlorperazine	5–10 mg every 4–6 hours	PO, IM
	25 mg suppository every 6 hours	PR
Promethazine	25 mg every 4–6 hours	PO, IM, PR
Droperidol	1–2.5 mg	IV
Metoclopramide	10–20 mg every 6 hours	PO
	0.5–2 mg/kg every 6–8 hours	IV
Antihistamine and anticholinergics		
Diphenhydramine	25–50 mg every 4–6 hours	PO, IM, IV
Scopolamine patch	1.5 mg every 3 days	Patch
Dimenhydrinate	50 mg every 4 hours	PO
Meclizine	25–50 mg every 24 hours	PO
Corticosteroids		
Dexamethasone	20 mg	IV
Sedatives		
Diazepam	2–5 mg every 4–6 hours	PO, IV
Lorazepam	1–2 mg every 4–6 hours	PO, IV

part, to dopaminergic blockade as well as to their sedative effects. High doses of these agents are associated with antidopaminergic side effects, including extrapyramidal reactions and depression. These agents are commonly used antiemetics for a variety of situations.

3. Antihistamines–These drugs (eg, meclizine) have weak antiemetic properties but are useful in the prevention of vomiting due to motion sickness.

4. Sedatives–Benzodiazepines may be helpful in patients with psychogenic and anticipatory vomiting.

5. Corticosteroids–The corticosteroids may be used in combination with other agents in the treatment of chemotherapy-induced vomiting.

Morrow G et al: Progress in reducing nausea and emesis. Comparisons of ondansetron, granisetron, and tropisetron. Cancer 1995;76:343. (The three drugs are equally effective in preventing emesis. Addition of dexamethasone increases efficacy.)

Roila F and the Italian Group for Antiemetic Research: Dexamethasone, granisetron, or both for the prevention of nausea and vomiting during chemotherapy for cancer. N Engl J Med 1995;332:1. (Combination of granisetron 3 mg intravenous and dexamethasone 8 mg intravenous was superior to granisetron alone in prevention of vomiting and nausea after chemotherapy.)

HICCUPS

Though usually a benign and self-limited annoyance, hiccups may be persistent and a sign of serious underlying illness. Chronic hiccups appear to be without major consequences. Reports that hiccups lead to exhaustion, weight loss, or death are unsubstantiated. In patients being maintained on mechanical ventilation, however, hiccups can trigger a full respiratory cycle and may result in respiratory alkalosis.

Causes of benign, self-limited hiccups include gastric distention (carbonated beverages, air swallowing, overeating), sudden temperature changes (hot/cold liquids, cold shower), alcohol ingestion, and emotional states (excitement, stress, laughing). Over 100 causes of recurrent or persistent hiccups have been reported. These may be grouped into the following categories:

(1) Central nervous system: Neoplasms, infections, cerebrovascular accident, trauma.

(2) Metabolic: Uremia, hypocapnia (hyperventilation), electrolyte imbalance.

(3) Irritation of the vagus or phrenic nerve: (a) Head, neck: Foreign body in ear, goiter, neoplasms. (b) Thorax: Pneumonia, empyema, neoplasms, myocardial infarction, pericarditis, aneurysm, esophageal obstruction, reflux esophagitis. (c) Abdomen: Subphrenic abscess, hepatomegaly, hepatitis,

cholecystitis, gastric distention, gastric neoplasm, pancreatitis, or pancreatic malignancy.

(4) Surgical: General anesthesia, postoperative.

(5) Psychogenic and idiopathic.

Clinical Findings

Evaluation of the patient with persistent hiccups should include a history and physical examination (including neurologic examination), complete blood count, electrolytes, creatinine, liver chemistry tests, and a chest radiograph. When the cause remains unclear, further testing may include CT of the head, chest, and abdomen, echocardiography, bronchoscopy, and upper endoscopy.

Treatment

A number of simple remedies may be helpful in patients with acute, benign hiccups. (1) Irritation of the nasopharynx by tongue traction, lifting the uvula with a spoon, catheter stimulation of the nasopharynx, and eating one teaspoon of dry granulated sugar. (2) Interruption of the respiratory cycle by breath holding, Valsalva's maneuver, sneezing, gasping (fright stimulus), or rebreathing into a bag. (3) Irritation of the vagus by supraorbital pressure, carotid massage. (4) Irritation of the diaphragm by holding knees to chest or by continuous positive airway pressure during mechanical ventilation. (5) Relief of gastric distention by belching or insertion of a nasogastric tube.

In patients with persistent hiccups, therapy should be directed at relieving the predisposing cause.

A number of drugs have been promoted as being useful in the treatment of hiccup, but none have been tested in a controlled fashion. Chlorpromazine, 25–50 mg orally or intramuscularly, is most commonly used. Other agents that have been reported to be effective in some cases include anticonvulsants (phenytoin, carbamazepine), metoclopramide, baclofen, and occasionally general anesthesia.

Rousseau P: Hiccups. South Med J 1995;88:175.

CONSTIPATION

Constipation is an extremely common complaint. The term is used variably by patients to refer to stools that are too hard, small, or infrequent or to excessive straining during defecation. Therefore, the first step in evaluating the patient is to determine what is meant by "constipation." In the general population, the "normal" frequency of bowel movements is broad, ranging from 3 to 12 per week. In many patients, the complaint may reflect a mistaken perception of what constitutes a normal bowel pattern. From a medical perspective, constipation is present when a patient has two or fewer bowel movement per week or excessive difficulty and straining at defecation. The many causes of constipation may be classified as discussed below and summarized in Table 14–3.

Common Identifiable Causes of Constipation

A. Poor Dietary and Behavioral Habits: The overwhelming majority of constipated patients have mild symptoms that cannot be attributed to any structural abnormalities, intestinal motility disorders, or systemic disease. A careful dietary review will reveal that most of these patients do not consume adequate fiber and fluids. Ingestion of 10–12 g of fiber per day either by dietary changes or the addition or commercial fiber supplementation is often all that is needed. At least one or two glasses of fluid should be taken with meals. Patients should be encouraged to heed the "call to stool" that typically occurs after meals (gastrocolic reflex). The elderly in particular are predisposed to constipation because of poor eating habits, a variety of medications that cause constipation, decreased colonic motility, and, in some cases, inability to sit on a toilet (bed-bound patients).

Table 14–3. Causes of constipation in adults.

Most common
  Low-fiber diet
  Poor bowel habits
Structural abnormalities
  Perianal disease: fissure, abscess, thrombosed
    hemorrhoid
  Colonic mass lesion with obstruction: adenocarcinoma
  Colonic stricture: diverticulosis, radiation, ischemia
  Hirschsprung's disease
  Idiopathic megarectum
Systemic disease
  Endocrine: hypothyroidism, hyperparathyroidism, diabetes
    mellitus
  Metabolic: hypokalemia, hypercalcemia, uremia
  Neurologic: paraplegia, Parkinson's disease, multiple
    sclerosis, prior pelvic surgery with disruption of pelvic
    nerves
  Other: amyloidosis, scleroderma
Medications
  Narcotics
  Diuretics
  Calcium channel blockers
  Anticholinergics
  Psychotropic agents
  Antacids
  Calcium and iron supplements
  NSAIDs
Slow colonic transit
  Idiopathic: isolated to colon or part of generalized disorder
  Psychogenic
  Chronic intestinal pseudo-obstruction
Outlet delay
  Rectocele
  Rectal intussusception
  Rectal prolapse
  Perineal descent
  Anismus (pelvic floor dysfunction)
  Solitary rectal ulcer syndrome

B. Structural Abnormalities: Colonic lesions that obstruct fecal passage must be excluded in patients with constipation. Particular concern is raised in patients with lifelong constipation (Hirschsprung's disease) and patients over age 50 with new-onset constipation, progressive thinning of stool, or associated weight loss or hematochezia (colon carcinoma).

C. Systemic Diseases: Medical diseases can cause constipation due to neurologic gut dysfunction, myopathies, endocrine disorders, and electrolyte abnormalities.

Causes of Severe or Refractory Constipation

Patients whose constipation cannot be attributed to the above causes and who do not respond to conservative dietary management present difficult management problems. Conceptually, these patients can be divided into two categories:

A. Colonic Inertia (Slow Colonic Transit): Some patients have an idiopathic delayed transit of stool through the large bowel. Normal colonic transit time is approximately 35 hours; more than 72 hours is significantly abnormal. Severe colonic inertia is more common in women, some of whom have a history of psychosocial problems or sexual abuse. Colonic inertia may be part of a more generalized gastrointestinal dysmotility syndrome. It may also be attributable to years of cathartic abuse ("cathartic colon").

B. Outlet Disorders: Patients with disorders of the rectum or pelvic floor may have difficulty in moving stool out of the rectum. They may complain of excessive straining with a sense of incomplete evacuation, the need for digital pressure on the vagina or perineum, or even digital disimpaction. Most of these patients are women. Defecatory difficulties can be due to a variety of anatomic problems that impede or obstruct flow, some of which may benefit from surgery. In other patients, there is a failure of the pelvic floor to relax during straining ("anismus"); this may be treated with relaxation exercises and biofeedback training.

Evaluation

A. First Level of Investigation: All patients should undergo a careful history and physical examination, including stool testing for occult blood. Routine laboratory studies should include a complete blood count, serum electrolytes including calcium, and serum TSH. In otherwise healthy patients with mild symptoms who are under age 50, a conservative trial of treatment with fiber is reasonable. In patients over age 50, those who have failed conservative treatment, or those with anemia or occult blood in the stools, colonoscopy or flexible sigmoidoscopy and barium enema are obtained to look for structural colonic lesions. Patients without evident structural, medical, or neurologic disease can be treated initially with fiber supplementation (and osmotic laxatives, if needed).

B. Second Level of Investigation: Patients with refractory constipation not responding to conservative measures may require further investigation.

1. Colonic transit study–To confirm that the patient truly has constipation and to measure the transit time, 24 radiopaque plastic markers are swallowed on 3 consecutive days. An abdominal radiograph is taken on days 4 and 7, and the total number of markers remaining in the colon is counted.

2. Studies of pelvic floor function–To diagnose outlet disorders of the anorectum, defecography (a video study taken during straining and defecation) and anal manometry are helpful. However, these studies are not widely available.

Standard Treatment of Chronic Constipation

A. Dietary Measures: Proper dietary fluid and fiber intake should be emphasized. Fiber may be given through dietary alterations or through fiber supplements. Increased dietary fiber may cause temporary distention and flatulence. Whereas fiber benefits the majority of patients with constipation, it normally does not benefit patients with severe colonic inertia or outlet disorders. Fiber supplements include the following:

1. Bran powder–One to 2 tbsp of bran powder twice daily, mixed with fluids or sprinkled over foods, is an excellent inexpensive means of providing 10–20 g/d of fiber. It may produce gas.

2. Pharmaceutical supplements–A variety of pharmaceutical fiber supplements are available, however, they are much more expensive than bran powder. They come in a variety of flavored powders, cookies, or tablets that are easy to ingest, making them attractive to some patients. Furthermore, they may be less gas-producing than bran. Preparations include psyllium, 3.4 g, and methylcellulose, 2 g, one to three times daily (both are natural fibers derived from vegetable matter); and polycarbophil, 1 g one to four times daily (a synthetic fiber).

B. Osmotic Laxatives: These agents, used to soften stools, may be given alone or in combination with fiber supplements. They are commonly employed in elderly nonambulatory patients or institutionalized patients to prevent constipation and fecal impaction. They may be safely used long-term and do not induce dependency. The agents are typically titrated to a dose that results in soft to semi-liquid stools.

1. Nonabsorbable sugars–Either sorbitol or lactulose, 15–60 mL daily, is equally efficacious, but sorbitol is less expensive. These malabsorbed sugars may result in increased bloating, cramps, and flatulence.

2. Magnesium hydroxide–Commonly given at a dosage of 15–30 mL daily. It should not be given to patients with renal insufficiency.

C. Stool Surfactant Agents: Surfactant agents (docusate sodium, 50–200 mg/d) may be given orally or rectally to promote softening of the stools.

Treatment of Chronic or Refractory Constipation

Most of the patients in this category will benefit from referral to a center with an interest and expertise in these difficult problems.

A. Colonic Inertia: Many patients require chronic use of enemas and cathartic agents (see below). Patients with psychologic problems or a history of sexual abuse may benefit from psychiatric therapy. In particularly severe cases, subtotal colectomy may be necessary.

B. Outlet Disorders: Some anatomic problems (eg, rectal prolapse, vaginal rectocele) may benefit from surgical correction. Relaxation techniques and biofeedback are being used in patients with pelvic floor dysfunction.

Treatment of Acute Constipation

Normal people and patients with chronic constipation can become acutely constipated in response to acute medical or surgical illness, dietary changes, medications, travel, etc. If several days have passed since the last bowel movement, the therapies described above for chronic constipation will not be sufficient to induce a prompt evacuation and relief of discomfort. In such cases, the following may be given. (*Caution:* these agents should not be given to patients with a possible large bowel obstruction or fecal impaction.)

A. Cathartic Laxatives: These agents stimulate fluid secretion and colonic contraction, resulting in a bowel movement within 6–12 hours after oral ingestion or 15–60 minutes after rectal administration. They may cause severe cramps and diarrhea. Agents used in the medical setting include cascara sagrada, 4–8 mL orally; bisacodyl, 5–15 mg orally or 10 mg as suppository; and castor oil, 15–45 mL orally. Senna and phenolphthalein are common OTC laxatives. *Note:* Chronic use of any of these agents is discouraged and may result in loss of normal colonic neuromuscular function.

B. Osmotic Laxatives: Osmotic laxatives produce a prompt evacuation in 0.5–3 hours, generally with less discomfort than when cathartic laxatives are given. They are used in the medical setting for purgation prior to surgery or colonic examinations. Preparations include magnesium citrate, 18 g/10 oz; magnesium sulfate, 10–30 g ("Epsom salts"); sodium phosphate, 15–30 g (2–45 mL); and balanced polyethylene glycol lavage solution, 1–4 L over 1–4 hours (GoLYTELY, CoLyte).

C. Enemas: Enemas provide a simple and almost immediate means of relieving acute constipation. In some cases of severe constipation, it is best to treat with an enema first in order to promote comfortable fecal movement prior to giving laxatives. Enemas vary in size and content: saline enemas, 120–240 mL (nonirritating); tap water enemas, 500–1000 mL (irritating); and oil retention enemas 120 mL (useful for hard or impacted stool).

Treatment of Fecal Impaction

Severe impaction of stool in the rectal vault may result in obstruction of further fecal flow leading to a partial or complete large bowel obstruction. Predisposing factors include severe psychiatric disease, prolonged bed rest and debility, neurogenic diseases of the colon, and spinal cord disorders. Clinical presentation includes decreased appetite, nausea, vomiting, and abdominal pain and distention. There may be paradoxic "diarrhea" as liquid stool leaks around the impacted feces. Firm feces are palpable on digital examination in the rectal vault. Initial treatment is directed at relieving the impaction with enemas or digital disruption of the impacted fecal material. Care should be taken not to injure the anal sphincter. Rarely, spinal or general anesthesia is required as an aid to manual disimpaction. Long-term care is directed at maintaining soft stools and regular bowel movements (as above).

Camilleri M et al: Clinical management of intractable constipation. Ann Intern Med 1994;121:520.

Romero Y et al: Constipation and fecal incontinence in the elderly population. Mayo Clin Proc 1996;71:81.

GASTROINTESTINAL GAS

Belching

Belching (eructation) is the involuntary or voluntary release of gas from the stomach or esophagus. It occurs most frequently after meals, when gastric distention results in transient lower esophageal sphincter relaxation. Belching is a normal reflex and does not itself denote gastrointestinal dysfunction. Virtually all stomach gas is derived from swallowed air. With each swallow, 2–5 mL of air are ingested. Swallowing of excessive amounts of air may result in distention, flatulence, and abdominal pain. Increased air swallowing may occur with rapid eating, gum chewing, smoking, and the ingestion of carbonated beverages. Some patients may consciously or unconsciously engage in forceful air swallowing (aerophagia). Chronic excessive belching is almost always caused by aerophagia, which is seen most commonly in anxious individuals and institutionalized patients. Evaluation of belching should be restricted to patients who have other complaints such as dysphagia, heartburn, early satiety, or vomiting.

Belching and aerophagia may be reduced by behavioral changes that include chewing and eating food slowly, not drinking through a straw, and not chewing gum or drinking carbonated beverages.

Once patients understand the relationship between aerophagia and belching, most can deal with the problem by behavioral modification. Physical defects that hamper normal swallowing (ill-fitting dentures, nasal obstruction) should be corrected. Antacids and simethicone are of no value.

Flatus

The rate and volume of expulsion of flatus is highly variable. Normal frequency ranges from six to 20 times a day, and normal volumes from 500 to 1500 mL/d. Flatus is derived from two sources: swallowed air and bacterial fermentation of undigested carbohydrate. The majority of swallowed air that is not belched passes through the gut and leaves as flatus. Swallowed air may contribute up to 500 mL of flatus per day (primarily nitrogen). Bacterial fermentation of undigested carbohydrates leads to the additional production of gas, particularly hydrogen and, in one-third of adults, methane. Except for situations in which there is small intestine bacterial overgrowth, the majority of this fermentation takes place in the colon. Under normal circumstances, a small substrate of fermentable substrates reaches the colon. These substances include lactose, fructose, bean starch, and the complex carbohydrates of fiber, wheat, oats, corn, and potatoes. Gas production may be increased dramatically with diseases of malabsorption (eg, celiac sprue) or with the ingestion of poorly absorbed carbohydrates (eg, lactose, lactulose, or sorbitol). Gases derived from plant carbohydrates (hydrogen and methane) have relatively little odor. In contrast, gases derived from meats and eggs tend to be malodorous. Determining abnormal from normal amounts of flatus is difficult. Excessive amounts of flatus may suggest malabsorption, especially if accompanied by diarrhea or weight loss.

An initial trial of a lactose-free diet should be given. Common gas-producing foods should be reviewed and the patient given an elimination trial. These commonly include brown beans, cauliflower, Brussels sprouts, broccoli, cabbage, onions, beer, red wine, and eggs. For patients with persistent complaints, fructose and complex carbohydrates may be eliminated, but such restrictive diets are unacceptable to most patients. The utility of activated charcoal or simethicone is dubious. The nonprescription agent Beano (α-D-galactosidase enzyme) reduces gas production associated with baked beans. Simethicone is of no value.

The complaints of chronic abdominal distention or bloating are common but do not correlate with increased intra-abdominal gas volumes. Most of these patients have an underlying functional gastrointestinal disorder such as irritable bowel syndrome or nonulcer dyspepsia.

Furne J, Levitt MD: Factors influencing frequency of flatus emission by healthy subjects. Dig Dis Sci 1996;41:1631.

DIARRHEA

Diarrhea is a common symptom that can range in severity from an acute, self-limited annoyance to a severe, life-threatening illness. Patients may use the term "diarrhea" to refer to increased frequency of bowel movements, increased stool liquidity, a sense of fecal urgency, or fecal incontinence. To properly evaluate the complaint, the physician must determine the patient's normal bowel pattern and the nature of the current symptoms.

In the normal state, approximately 10 L of fluid enter the duodenum daily, of which all but 1.5 L are absorbed by the small intestine. The colon absorbs most of the remaining fluid, with only 100 mL lost in the stool. From a medical standpoint, diarrhea is defined as a stool weight of more than 250 g/24 h. In reality, quantification of stool weight is necessary only in some patients with chronic diarrhea. In most cases, the physician's working definition of diarrhea is an increased stool frequency (more than two or three bowel movements per day) or liquidity of feces.

The causes of diarrhea are myriad. In clinical practice, it is helpful to distinguish acute from chronic diarrhea, as the evaluation and treatment are entirely different (Tables 14–4 and 14–6).

Table 14–4. Causes of acute infectious diarrhea.

Noninflammatory Diarrhea	Inflammatory Diarrhea
Viral	**Viral**
Norwalk virus	Cytomegalovirus
Norwalk-like virus	
Rotavirus	
Protozoal	**Protozoal**
Giardia lamblia	Entamoeba histolytica
Cryptosporidium	
Bacterial	**Bacterial**
1. Preformed enterotoxin production	1. Cytotoxin production Enterohemorrhagic E coli O157:H5 (EHEC)
Staphylococcus aureus	Vibrio parahaemolyticus
Bacillus cereus	
Clostridium perfringens	Clostridium difficile
2. Enterotoxin production	2. Mucosal invasion
Enterotoxigenic E coli (ETEC)	Shigella
Vibrio cholerae	Campylobacter jejuni
	Salmonella
	Enteroinvasive E coli (EIEC)
	Aeromonas
	Plesiomonas
	Yersinia enterocolitica
	Chlamydia
	Neisseria gonorrhoeae
	Listeria monocytogenes

1. ACUTE DIARRHEA

Etiology & Clinical Findings

Diarrhea that is acute in onset and persists for less than 3 weeks is most commonly caused by infectious agents, bacterial toxins (either ingested preformed in food or produced in the gut), or drugs. Epidemiologic information may provide clues to the etiologic agent (Table 29–3). Similar recent illness in family members suggests an infectious origin. Recent ingestion of improperly stored or prepared food implicates food poisoning, especially if other people were similarly affected. Exposure to unpurified water (camping, swimming) may result in infection with *Giardia* or *Cryptosporidium*. Recent foreign travel suggests "traveler's diarrhea" (see Chapter 30). Antibiotic administration within the preceding several weeks increases the likelihood of *Clostridium difficile* colitis. Finally, risk factors for HIV infection or sexually transmitted diseases should be determined. (AIDS-associated diarrhea is discussed in Chapter 31.) Persons practicing unprotected anal intercourse are at risk for a variety of infections that cause proctitis and rectal discharge, including gonorrhea, syphilis, lymphogranuloma venereum, and herpes simplex. A variety of medications may cause diarrhea through various mechanisms and should not be overlooked; these will not be discussed further here.

The nature of the diarrhea helps distinguish among different infectious causes (Table 14–4).

A. Noninflammatory Diarrhea: Watery, non-bloody diarrhea associated with periumbilical cramps, bloating, nausea, or vomiting (singly or in any combination) suggests small bowel enteritis caused by either a toxin-producing bacterium (enterotoxigenic *E coli* [ETEC], *Staphylococcus aureus, Bacillus cereus, C perfringens*) or other agents (viruses, *Giardia*) that disrupt the normal absorption and secretory process in the small intestine. Prominent vomiting suggests viral enteritis or *S aureus* food poisoning. Though typically mild, the diarrhea (which originates in the small intestine) may be voluminous (ranging from 10 to 200 mL/kg/24 h) and result in dehydration with hypokalemia and metabolic acidosis due to loss of HCO_3^- in the stool (eg, cholera). Because tissue invasion does not occur, fecal leukocytes are not present.

B. Inflammatory Diarrhea: The presence of fever and bloody diarrhea (dysentery) indicates colonic tissue damage caused by invasion (shigellosis, salmonellosis, *Campylobacter* or *Yersinia* infection, amebiasis) or a toxin (*C difficile, E coli* O157:H7). Because these organisms involve predominantly the colon, the diarrhea is small in volume (< 1 L/d) and associated with left lower quadrant cramps, urgency, and tenesmus. Fecal leukocytes are present in infections with invasive organisms. *E coli* O157:H7 is a toxigenic, noninvasive organisms that may be acquired from contaminated meat or unpasteurized juice and has resulted in several outbreaks of an acute, often severe hemorrhagic colitis. In immunocompromised and HIV-infected patients, cytomegalovirus may result in intestinal ulceration with watery or bloody diarrhea.

Infectious dysentery must be distinguished from acute ulcerative colitis, which may also present acutely with fever, abdominal pain, and bloody diarrhea.

C. Enteric Fever: A severe systemic illness manifested initially by prolonged high fevers, prostration, confusion, respiratory symptoms followed by abdominal tenderness, diarrhea, and a rash is due to infection with *Salmonella typhi* or *Salmonella paratyphi,* which causes bacteremia and multiorgan dysfunction.

Evaluation

In over 90% of patients with acute diarrhea, the illness is mild and self-limited and responds within 5 days to simple rehydration therapy or antidiarrheal agents. In such cases, a laboratory investigation to determine the etiologic agent is unnecessary because it is costly, often unrevealing, and does not affect therapy or outcome. Indeed, the isolation rate of bacterial pathogens from stool cultures in patients with acute diarrhea is under 3%. Thus, the goal of initial evaluation is to distinguish these patients from those with more serious illness. Microscopic examination of the stool for fecal leukocytes distinguishes noninflammatory from inflammatory diarrhea. This test is easily performed and inexpensive. The presence of leukocytes suggests an inflammatory diarrhea and warrants a stool bacterial culture.

Patients with signs of inflammatory diarrhea manifested by any of the following require prompt medical attention: high fever (> 38.5 °C), bloody diarrhea, abdominal pain, or diarrhea not subsiding after 4–5 days. Similarly, patients with symptoms of dehydration must be evaluated (excessive thirst, dry mouth, decreased urination, weakness, lethargy). Physical examination should note the patient's general appearance, mental status, volume status, and the presence of abdominal tenderness or peritonitis. Peritoneal findings may be present in *C difficile* and enterohemorrhagic *E coli.* Hospitalization is required in patients with severe dehydration, toxicity, or marked abdominal pain. Stool specimens should be sent in all cases for examination for fecal leukocytes and bacterial cultures (Table 14–5). The rate of positive bacterial cultures in patients with dysentery is 60–75%. A wet mount examination of the stool for amebiasis should also be performed in patients with dysentery who have a history of recent travel to endemic areas or those who are homosexuals. In patients with a history of antibiotic exposure, a stool sample should be sent for *C difficile* toxin. If *E coli* O157:H7 is suspected, the laboratory must be alerted to do specific serotyping. In patients with diarrhea that persists for more than 10 days, three stool examinations for ova and parasites also should be performed. Rectal swabs may be sent for *Chlamydia, Neisseria gonorrhoeae,* and herpes simplex virus in sexually active patients with severe proctitis.

Sigmoidoscopy is warranted acutely in patients with symptoms of severe proctitis (tenesmus, discharge, rectal pain) and in patients with suspected *C difficile* colitis who appear ill. It may also be helpful in distinguishing infectious diarrhea from ulcerative colitis or ischemic colitis.

Treatment

A. Diet: The overwhelming majority of adults have mild diarrhea that will not lead to dehydration provided the patient takes adequate oral fluids containing carbohydrates and electrolytes. Patients will find it more comfortable to rest the bowel by avoiding high-fiber foods, fats, milk products, caffeine, and alcohol. Frequent feedings of fruit drinks, tea, "flat" carbonated beverages, and soft, easily digested foods (eg, soups, crackers) are encouraged.

B. Rehydration: In more severe diarrhea, dehydration can occur quickly, especially in children. Oral rehydration with fluids containing glucose, Na+,

Table 14–5. Fecal leukocytes in intestinal disorders.

Infectious			Noninfectious
Present	**Variable**	**Absent**	**Present**
Shigella	Salmonella	Norwalk virus	Ulcerative colitis
Campylobacter	Yersinia	Rotavirus	Crohn's disease
Enteroinvasive	Vibrio parahaemolytica	Giardia lamblia	Radiation colitis
E coli (EIEC)	Clostridium difficile	Entamoeba histolytica	Ischemic colitis
	Aeromonas	Cryptosporidium	
		"Food poisoning"	
		Staphylococcus aureus	
		Bacillus cereus	
		Clostridium perfringens	
		Escherichia coli	
		Enterotoxigenic (ETEC)	
		Enterohemorrhagic (EHEC)	

K$^+$, Cl$^-$, and bicarbonate or citrate is preferred in most cases to intravenous fluids because it is inexpensive, safe, and highly effective in almost all awake patients. An easy mixture is ½ tsp salt (3.5 g), 1 tsp baking soda (2.5 g NaHCO$_3$), 8 tsp sugar (40 g), and 8 oz orange juice (1.5 g KCl), diluted to 1 L with water. Alternatively, oral electrolyte solutions (eg, Pedialyte) are readily available. Fluids should be given at rates of 50–200 mL/kg/24 h depending on the hydration status. Intravenous fluids (lactated Ringer's solution) are preferred acutely in patients with severe dehydration.

C. Antidiarrheal Agents: Antidiarrheal agents may be used safely in patients with mild to moderate diarrheal illnesses to improve patient comfort. Opioid agents help decrease the stool number and liquidity and control fecal urgency. However, they should not be used in patients with bloody diarrhea, high fever, or systemic toxicity for fear of worsening the disease. Similarly, they should be discontinued in patients whose diarrhea is worsening despite therapy. With these provisos, these agents provide excellent symptomatic relief. Loperamide is the preferred drug in a dosage of 4 mg initially, followed by 2 mg after each loose stool (maximum: 16 mg/24 h).

Bismuth subsalicylate (Pepto-Bismol), two tablets or 30 mL four times daily, reduces symptoms in patients with traveler's diarrhea by virtue of its anti-inflammatory and antibacterial properties; its role in other settings is poorly studied. Scores of other agents touted for their antidiarrheal action have undergone little or no controlled testing but appear to have minimal or no symptomatic benefit (lactobacilli, kaolin, pectin). Anticholinergic agents are contraindicated in acute diarrhea (eg, diphenoxylate with atropine) because of the rare development of megacolon.

D. Antibiotic Therapy:

1. Empiric treatment–Because the overwhelming majority of patients have mild, self-limited disease due to viruses or noninvasive bacteria, empiric antibiotic treatment of all patients with acute diarrhea is not warranted. Even patients with inflammatory diarrhea caused by invasive pathogens usually have mild disease that will resolve within several days without specific treatment. Conversely, in patients who appear to have signs of an invasive pathogen with moderate to severe symptoms of fever, tenesmus, bloody stools, and fecal leukocytes, empiric treatment is recommended while the stool bacterial culture is incubating. The drugs of choice are the fluoroquinolones (eg, ciprofloxacin, 500 mg twice daily) for 5–7 days. These agents provide good antibiotic coverage against most invasive bacterial pathogens, including *Shigella, Salmonella, Campylobacter, Yersinia,* and *Aeromonas.* Alternative agents are trimethoprim-sulfamethoxazole, 160/800 mg twice daily, or erythromycin, 250–500 mg four times daily.

2. Specific antimicrobial treatment–Antibiotics are not generally recommended in patients with nontyphoid *Salmonella, Campylobacter,* or *Yersinia* infection except in severe or prolonged disease because they have not been shown to hasten recovery or reduce the period of fecal bacterial excretion. The infectious diarrheas for which treatment is clearly recommended are shigellosis, cholera, extraintestinal salmonellosis, "traveler's" diarrhea, *C difficile* infection, giardiasis, amebiasis, and the sexually transmitted infections (gonorrhea, syphilis, chlamydiosis, and herpes simplex infection). Specific treatment of these infections and AIDS-related diarrhea are presented in other chapters of this book.

Dalton C et al: An outbreak of gastroenteritis and fever due to *Listeria monocytogenes* in milk. N Engl J Med 1997;336:100. (This organism was identified in a large outbreak of noninvasive gastroenteritis related to contaminated milk. Four cases of sporadic invasive illness were reported, resulting in sepsis, meningitis, and cerebral abscess.)

Park SI, Giannella RA: Approach to the adult patient with acute diarrhea. Gastroenterol Clin North Am 1993;22:483.

Schiller L: Anti-diarrhoeal pharmacology and therapeutics. Aliment Pharmacol Ther 1995;9:87.

Su C, Brandt L: *Escherichia coli* O157:H7 infection in humans. Ann Intern Med 1995;123:698.

Talal A, Murray J: Acute and chronic diarrhea: How to keep laboratory testing to a minimum. Postgrad Med 1994;96:30.

2. CHRONIC DIARRHEA

Etiology

The causes of chronic diarrhea may be grouped into six major pathophysiologic categories (Table 14–6):

A. Osmotic Diarrheas: As stool leaves the colon, fecal osmolality is equal to the serum osmolality, ie, approximately 290 mosm/kg. Under normal circumstances, the major osmoles are Na$^+$, K$^+$, Cl$^-$, and HCO$_3^-$. The stool osmolality may be estimated by multiplying the stool (Na$^+$ + K$^+$) × 2 (multiplied by 2 to account for the anions). The **osmotic gap** is the difference between the *measured* osmolality of the stool (or serum) and the *estimated* stool osmolality and is normally less than 50 mosm/kg. An increased osmotic gap implies that the diarrhea is caused by ingestion or malabsorption of an osmotically active substance. The most common causes of osmotic diarrhea are disaccharidase deficiency (lactase deficiency), laxative abuse, and malabsorption syndromes (see below). Osmotic diarrheas resolve during fasting. Osmotic diarrheas caused by malabsorbed carbohydrates are characterized by abdominal distention, bloating, and flatulence due to increased colonic gas production.

Table 14–6. Causes of chronic diarrhea.

Osmotic diarrhea
CLUES: Stool volume decreases with fasting; increased stool osmotic gap
1. Medications: antacids, lactulose, sorbitol
2. Disaccharidase deficiency: lactose intolerance
3. Factitious diarrhea: magnesium (antacids, laxatives)

Secretory diarrhea
CLUES: Large volume (>1 L/d); little change with fasting; normal stool osmotic gap
1. Hormonally mediated: VIPoma, carcinoid, medullary carcinoma of thyroid (calcitonin), Zollinger-Ellison syndrome (gastrin)
2. Factitious diarrhea (laxative abuse); phenolphthalein, cascara, senna
3. Villous adenoma
4. Bile salt malabsorption (ileal resection; Crohn's ileitis; postcholecystectomy)
5. Medications

Inflammatory conditions
CLUES: Fever, hematochezia, abdominal pain
1. Ulcerative colitis
2. Crohn's disease
3. Microscopic colitis
4. Malignancy: lymphoma, adenocarcinoma (with obstruction and pseudodiarrhea)
5. Radiation enteritis

Malabsorption syndromes
1. Weight loss, abnormal laboratory values; fecal fat > 7–10 g/24 h, tropical sprue, Whipple's disease, eosinophilic gastroenteritis, Crohn's disease, small bowel resection (short bowel syndrome)
2. Lymphatic obstruction: lymphoma, carcinoid, infectious (TB, MAI), Kaposi's sarcoma, sarcoidosis, retroperitoneal fibrosis
3. Pancreatic disease: chronic pancreatitis, pancreatic carcinoma
4. Bacterial overgrowth: motility disorders (diabetes, vagotomy, scleroderma), fistulas, small intestinal diverticula

Motility disorders
CLUES: Systemic disease or prior abdominal surgery
1. Postsurgical: vagotomy, partial gastrectomy, blind loop with bacterial overgrowth
2. Systemic disorders: scleroderma, diabetes mellitus, hyperthyroidism
3. Irritable bowel syndrome

Chronic infections
1. Parasites: *Giardia lamblia, Entamoeba histolytica, Cyclospora*
2. AIDS-related:
   Viral: Cytomegalovirus, HIV infection (?)
   Bacterial: *Clostridium difficile, Mycobacterium avium* complex
   Protozoal: Microsporida (*Enterocytozoon bieneusi*), *Cryptosporidium, Isospora belli*

Disaccharidase deficiencies are extremely common and should always be considered in patients with chronic diarrhea. Lactase deficiency occurs in three-fourths of nonwhite adults and up to 25% of Caucasians. It may also be acquired after an episode of viral gastroenteritis, medical illness, or gastrointestinal surgery. Sorbitol is commonly used as a sweetener in gums, candies, and some medications that may cause diarrhea in some patients. The diagnosis of sorbitol or lactose malabsorption may be established by an elimination trial for 2–3 weeks. The diagnosis may be confirmed by measuring a rise in breath hydrogen of more than 20 ppm after lactose or sorbitol ingestion, but this is seldom necessary.

Ingestion of magnesium- or phosphate-containing compounds (laxatives, antacids) should be considered in enigmatic chronic diarrhea. Surreptitious use should be considered, especially in young women with possible eating disorders and patients with psychiatric problems, a long history of vague or mysterious medical ailments, or employment in the medical field.

B. Malabsorptive Conditions: The major causes of malabsorption are small mucosal intestinal diseases, intestinal resections, lymphatic obstruction, small intestinal bacterial overgrowth, and pancreatic insufficiency. The hallmarks of malabsorption are weight loss, osmotic diarrhea, and nutritional deficiencies. Significant diarrhea in the absence of weight loss is not likely to be due to malabsorption. The physical and laboratory abnormalities related to

deficiencies of vitamins or minerals are discussed in Chapter 29. Briefly, they include anemia (microcytic or macrocytic), hypoalbuminemia, low serum cholesterol, hypocalcemia, and an elevated prothrombin time.

In patients with suspected malabsorption, quantification of fecal fat should be performed.

C. Secretory Conditions: Increased intestinal secretion or decreased absorption results in a watery diarrhea that may be large in volume (1–10 L/d) but with a normal osmotic gap. There is little change in stool output during the fasting state. In serious conditions, significant dehydration and electrolyte imbalance may develop. Major causes include endocrine tumors (stimulating intestinal or pancreatic secretion), bile salt malabsorption (stimulating colonic secretion), and laxative abuse.

D. Inflammatory Conditions: Diarrhea is present in most patients with inflammatory bowel disease (ulcerative colitis, Crohn's disease, microscopic colitis). A variety of other symptoms may be present, including abdominal pain, fever, weight loss, and hematochezia. (See Inflammatory Bowel Disease, below.)

E. Motility Disorders: Abnormal intestinal motility secondary to systemic disorders or surgery may result in diarrhea due to rapid transit or to stasis of intestinal contents with bacterial overgrowth resulting in malabsorption.

Perhaps the most common cause of chronic diarrhea is irritable bowel syndrome (see Irritable Bowel

Syndrome, below). Although many of these patients complain of "diarrhea," the majority in fact have a normal stool weight.

F. Chronic Infections: Chronic parasitic infections may cause diarrhea through a number of mechanisms. Although the list of parasitic organisms is a long one, agents most commonly associated with diarrhea include the protozoans *Giardia, E histolytica, Cyclospora,* and the intestinal nematodes.

Immunocompromised patients, especially those with AIDS, are susceptible to a number of infectious agents that can cause acute or chronic diarrhea (see Chapter 31). Chronic diarrhea in AIDS is commonly caused by Microsporida, *Cryptosporidium,* cytomegalovirus, *Isospora belli, Cyclospora,* and *Mycobacterium avium* complex.

G. Factitial Diarrhea: Approximately 15% of patients with chronic diarrhea have factitial diarrhea caused by surreptitious laxative abuse or factitious dilution of stool.

Evaluation

A great many tests are available for the evaluation of chronic diarrhea. In most cases, however, a careful history and physical examination suggest the underlying pathophysiologic category that guides the subsequent diagnostic workup (Figure 14–1). The following tests are commonly employed in the evaluation of chronic diarrhea. The evaluation of AIDS-associated diarrhea is discussed in Chapter 31.

A. Stool Analysis:

1. Twenty-four-hour stool collection for weight and quantitative fecal fat–A stool weight of more than 300 g/24 h confirms the presence of diarrhea, justifying further workup. A weight greater than 1000–1500 g suggests a secretory process. A fecal fat in excess of 10 g/24 h indicates a malabsorptive process. (See Celiac Sprue and specific tests for malabsorption, below.)

2. Stool osmolality–An osmotic gap confirms osmotic diarrhea. A stool osmolality less than the

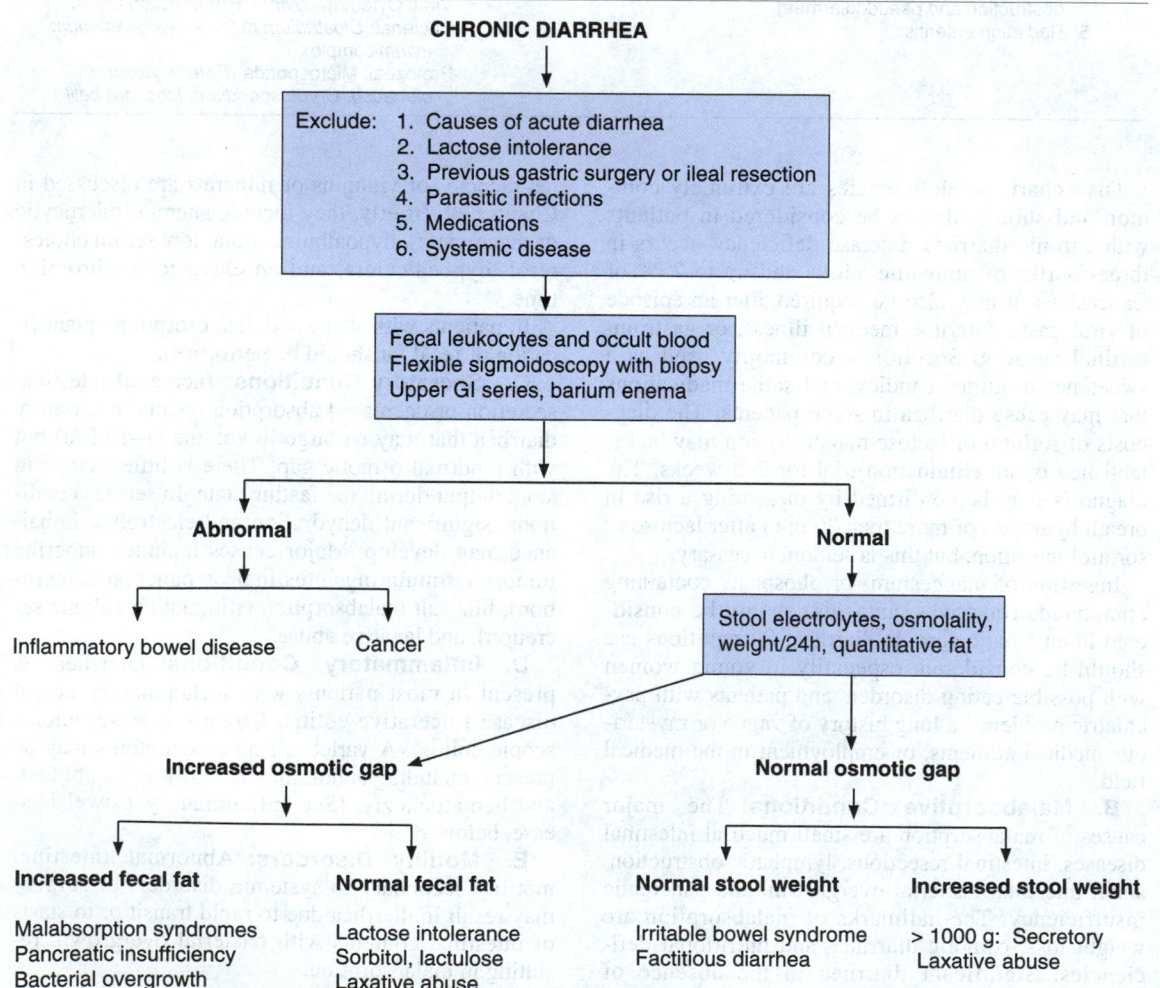

Figure 14–1. Decision diagram for diagnosis of causes of chronic diarrhea.

serum osmolality implies that water or urine has been added to the specimen (factitious diarrhea).

3. Stool laxative screen–In cases of suspected laxative abuse, stool magnesium, phosphate, and sulfate levels may be measured. Phenolphthalein, senna, and cascara are indicated by the presence of a bright-red color after alkalinization of the stool or urine. Bisacodyl can be detected in the urine.

4. Fecal leukocytes–The presence of leukocytes in a stool sample implies an underlying inflammatory diarrhea.

5. Stool for ova and parasites–The presence of *Giardia* and *E histolytica* is detected in routine wet mounts. *Cryptosporidium* and *Cyclospora* are detected with modified acid-fast staining.

B. Blood Tests:

1. Routine laboratory tests–CBC, serum electrolytes, liver function tests, calcium, phosphorus, albumin, TSH, total T_4, beta-carotene, and prothrombin time should be obtained. Anemia occurs in malabsorption syndromes (vitamin B_{12}, folate, iron) and inflammatory conditions. Hypoalbuminemia is present in malabsorption, protein-losing enteropathies, and inflammatory diseases. Hyponatremia and non–anion gap metabolic acidosis may occur in profound secretory diarrheas. Malabsorption of fat-soluble vitamins may result in an abnormal prothrombin time, low serum calcium, low carotene, or abnormal serum alkaline phosphatase.

2. Other laboratory tests–In patients with suspected secretory diarrhea, serum VIP (VIPoma), gastrin (Zollinger-Ellison syndrome), calcitonin (medullary thyroid carcinoma), cortisol (Addison's disease), and urinary 5-HIAA (carcinoid syndrome) levels should be obtained.

C. Proctosigmoidoscopy With Mucosal Biopsy: Examination may be helpful in detecting inflammatory bowel disease (including microscopic colitis) and melanosis coli, indicative of chronic use of anthraquinone laxatives.

D. Imaging: After the above studies have been completed, the cause of the diarrhea will generally be clear and further imaging studies can be ordered as indicated. Calcification on a plain abdominal radiograph confirms the diagnosis of chronic pancreatitis. An upper gastrointestinal series or enteroclysis study is helpful in evaluating Crohn's disease, lymphoma, or carcinoid syndrome. Colonoscopy is helpful in evaluating colonic inflammation due to inflammatory bowel disease. Upper endoscopy with small bowel biopsy is useful in suspected malabsorption due to mucosal diseases. Upper endoscopy with a duodenal aspirate and small bowel biopsy is also useful in patients with AIDS and to document *Cryptosporidium,* Microsporida, and *M avium-intracellulare* infection. Abdominal CT is helpful to detect chronic pancreatitis or pancreatic endocrine tumors.

Treatment

Treatment of chronic diarrhea is directed at the underlying condition. A number of antidiarrheal agents may be used in certain situations in patients with chronic diarrheal conditions and are listed below. Opioids may be used safely in most patients with chronic, stable symptoms.

A. Loperamide: 4 mg initially, then 2 mg after each loose stool (maximum: 16 mg/d).

B. Diphenoxylate With Atropine: One tablet three or four times daily.

C. Codeine, Paregoric: Because of their addictive potential, these drugs are generally avoided except in cases of chronic, intractable diarrhea. Codeine may be given in a dosage of 15–60 mg every 4 hours as needed; the dosage of paregoric is 4–8 mL after each liquid bowel movement.

D. Clonidine: α_2-Adrenergic agonists inhibit intestinal electrolyte secretion. A clonidine patch that delivers 0.1–0.2 mg/d for 7 days may be useful in some patients with secretory diarrheas, cryptosporidiosis, and diabetes.

E. Octreotide: This somatostatin analog stimulates intestinal fluid and electrolyte absorption and inhibits secretion. Furthermore, it inhibits the release of gastrointestinal peptides. It is very useful in treating secretory diarrheas due to VIPomas and carcinoid tumors and in some cases of diarrhea associated with AIDS. Effective doses range from 50 μg to 250 μg subcutaneously three times daily.

F. Cholestyramine: This bile salt binding resin may be useful in patients with bile salt-induced diarrhea secondary to intestinal resection or ileal disease. A dosage of 4 g one to three times daily is recommended.

American Gastroenterological Association Medical Position Statement: Guidelines for the management of malnutrition and cachexia, chronic diarrhea, and hepatobiliary disease in patients with human immunodeficiency virus infection. Gastroenterology 1996;111:1722.

Donowitz M, Kokke ET, Saidi R: Evaluation of patients with chronic diarrhea. (Current Concepts.) N Engl J Med 1995;332:725.

Huang P et al: The first reported outbreak of diarrheal illness associated with *Cyclospora* in the United States. Ann Intern Med 1995;123:409.

Phillips S et al: Stool composition in factitial diarrhea: A 6-years experience with stool analysis. Ann Intern Med 1995;123:97.

GASTROINTESTINAL BLEEDING

1. ACUTE UPPER GASTROINTESTINAL BLEEDING

Essentials of Diagnosis

- Hematemesis (bright red blood or "coffee grounds").
- Melena in most cases; hematochezia in massive upper gastrointestinal bleeds.
- Assess volume status to determine severity of

blood loss; hematocrit is a poor indicator of acute blood loss.
- Endoscopy is diagnostic and may be therapeutic.

General Considerations

There are over 350,000 hospitalizations a year in the USA for acute upper gastrointestinal bleeding, with a mortality rate of 10%. Approximately half of patients are over 60 years of age, and in this age group the mortality rate is even higher. Patients seldom die of exsanguination but rather from complications of an underlying disease.

The most common presentation of upper gastrointestinal bleeding is with hematemesis or melena. Hematemesis may be either bright red blood or brown "coffee grounds" material. Melena develops after as little as 50–100 mL of blood in the upper gastrointestinal tract, whereas hematochezia develops with an acute loss of more than 1000 mL. Although hematochezia generally suggests a lower bleeding source (eg, colonic), massive upper gastrointestinal bleeding may present with hematochezia.

Upper gastrointestinal bleeding is self-limited in 80% of patients, in whom morbidity and mortality rates are low. Conversely, in patients with continued or recurrent bleeding, urgent medical therapy and endoscopic evaluation are warranted.

Etiology

Acute upper gastrointestinal bleeding may originate from a number of sources. These are listed below in order of the frequency with which they cause significant upper gastrointestinal bleeding. Each of these entities is covered in greater detail elsewhere in the chapter.

A. Peptic Ulcer Disease: Peptic ulcers account for half of major upper gastrointestinal bleeding with an overall acute mortality rate of 6–10%.

B. Portal Hypertension: Portal hypertension may result in bleeding from varices (most commonly esophageal; rarely, gastric or duodenal) or portal hypertensive gastropathy. Bleeding esophageal varices account for 10–20% of significant gastrointestinal hemorrhages, with a hospital mortality rate of 15–40%. If untreated, almost half will rebleed during hospitalization. Less than one-third of patients with portal hypertension and varices will develop acute variceal bleeding. A mortality rate of 60–80% is expected at 1–4 years. Bleeding from the gastric mucosa in portal hypertensive gastropathy may account for up to 20% of cases of upper gastrointestinal bleeding in patients with cirrhosis.

C. Mallory-Weiss Tears: Lacerations of the gastroesophageal junction account for 5–10% of cases of upper gastrointestinal bleeding. Over half of patients report a history of heavy alcohol use or retching. Less than 10% have continued or recurrent bleeding.

D. Vascular Anomalies: Vascular anomalies may be found throughout the gastrointestinal tract and may be the source of chronic or acute upper or lower gastrointestinal bleeding. They account for 7% of cases of acute upper tract bleeding. **Vascular ectasias** (angiodysplasias) have a bright red stellate or fern-like appearance. They may be part of systemic conditions (hereditary hemorrhagic telangiectasia, CREST) or may occur sporadically. There is an increased incidence in patients with chronic renal failure.

E. Gastric Neoplasms: Gastric neoplasms account for 1% of significant upper gastrointestinal hemorrhages.

F. Erosive Gastritis: Erosive gastritis is implicated in up to 20% of cases of acute upper tract bleeding, but because the lesions are superficial ones they are a relatively unusual cause of severe gastrointestinal bleeding (< 5% of cases). Gastric mucosal erosions may be due to NSAIDs, alcohol, or severe medical or surgical illness ("stress gastritis").

G. Erosive Esophagitis: Severe erosive esophagitis due to chronic gastroesophageal reflux may rarely cause significant upper gastrointestinal bleeding.

H. Others: An aortoenteric fistula may complicate 2% of abdominal aortic grafts. Usually located between the upper aspects of the aortic graft and the third portion of the duodenum, these fistulas characteristically present with a "herald," nonexsanguinating initial bleed, with melena and hematemesis or with chronic intermittent bleeding. The diagnosis may be confirmed by upper endoscopy or abdominal CT. Surgery is mandatory in patients with suspected or confirmed aortoenteric fistulas to prevent exsanguinating hemorrhage. Rare causes of upper gastrointestinal bleeding include bleeding from a hepatic tumor or vascular lesion (hemobilia), from a pancreatic malignancy or pseudoaneurysm (hemosuccus pancreaticus), and Dieulafoy's lesion (aberrant gastric submucosal artery).

Initial Evaluation & Management

A. Stabilization: Patients who present with gastrointestinal bleeding require rapid evaluation and treatment. The first and most important step is assessment of the hemodynamic status by blood pressure and heart rate. A systolic blood pressure less than 100 mm Hg (irrespective of heart rate) identifies a high-risk patient with severe acute bleeding (20–25% intravascular volume loss) and is an emergency. A heart rate over 100 /min with a systolic blood pressure over 100 mm Hg signifies a moderate acute blood loss. A normal systolic blood pressure and heart rate identifies a patient with a relatively minor hemorrhage. Postural vital signs are poorly reproducible and of undocumented utility. Because the hematocrit may take 24–72 hours to equilibrate with the extravascular fluid, it is not a reliable indicator of the severity of acute bleeding.

In patients with significant bleeding, two 18-gauge or larger intravenous lines should be started prior to further diagnostic tests. Blood is sent immediately for a complete blood count, prothrombin time with INR, serum creatinine, liver enzymes, and cross-matching for two to four units or more of packed red blood cells. In patients without hemodynamic compromise or overt active bleeding, aggressive fluid repletion can be delayed until the extent of the bleeding is further clarified. Patients with evidence of hemodynamic compromise should be given immediate volume replacement with 0.9% saline or lactated Ringer's solution and crossmatched blood as soon as it becomes available. It is rarely necessary to administer type-specific or O-negative blood. Although central venous pressure monitoring is desirable in some cases, it is usually not necessary, and line placement should not interfere with rapid patient resuscitation.

A nasogastric tube should be placed in all patients with suspected upper tract bleeding. The finding of red blood or "coffee grounds" material on nasogastric aspirate confirms an upper gastrointestinal source of bleeding, though 10% of patients with confirmed upper tract sources of bleeding have non-bloody aspirates—especially when bleeding originates in the duodenum. An aspirate of bright red blood indicates active bleeding and is associated with the highest risk of further bleeding, complications, and death, while a clear aspirate identifies patients at lower initial risk. Efforts to stop or slow bleeding by gastric lavage with large volumes of fluid are of no benefit and may expose the patient to an increased risk of aspiration. Periodic reaspiration of the nasogastric tube serves as an indicator of ongoing bleeding or rebleeding.

B. Blood Replacement: The amount of fluid and blood products required is based upon assessment of vital signs, evidence of active bleeding from nasogastric aspirate, and laboratory tests. Sufficient packed red blood cells should be given to maintain a hematocrit of 25–30%. In the absence of continued bleeding, the hematocrit should rise 3% for each unit of transfused packed red cells. Transfusion of blood should not be withheld from patients with brisk active bleeding regardless of the hematocrit. It is desirable to transfuse blood anticipating the nadir hematocrit. When the blood pressure and pulse rate have been restored to normal limits, the rate of transfusion can be slowed. In actively bleeding patients, platelets should be transfused if the platelet count is under 50,000/μL and should be considered if there is impaired platelet function due to aspirin or NSAID use (regardless of the platelet count). Uremic patients (who also have dysfunctional platelets) with active bleeding should be given desmopressin (DDAVP). Fresh frozen plasma should be given for actively bleeding patients with a coagulopathy and an INR > 1.5. In the face of massive bleeding, one unit of fresh frozen plasma should be given for each five units of packed red blood cells transfused.

C. Initial Triage: Risk assessment and resuscitation proceed simultaneously when a patient presents with gastrointestinal hemorrhage. A preliminary assessment of risk based upon several clinical factors aids in the resuscitation as well as the rational triage of the patient. Outcome studies suggest that in patients with gastrointestinal hemorrhage, the presence of advanced age, serious comorbid illness, advanced liver disease, shock or hypotension, hematemesis, low initial hematocrit, or coagulopathy at presentation is predictive of a higher risk of persistent or recurrent bleeding and a poorer outcome.

1. Very low risk–Reliable patients without serious comorbid medical illnesses or advanced liver disease who have normal hemodynamics, no evidence of overt bleeding (hematemesis or melena) within 48 hours, a negative nasogastric lavage, and normal laboratory tests do not require hospital admission and can undergo further evaluation as outpatients as deemed necessary.

2. High risk–Patients with active bleeding manifested by hematemesis or bright red blood on nasogastric aspirate, persistent hemodynamic derangement despite fluid resuscitation, serious comorbid medical illness, or evidence of advanced liver disease require ICU admission.

3. Low to moderate risk–All other patients should be admitted to a regular hospital unit after appropriate stabilization for further evaluation and treatment. In some centers, these patients undergo upper endoscopy either in the emergency room or in the endoscopy unit prior to hospital admission. Based upon the findings at endoscopy, patients deemed to be at low risk of rebleeding may be discharged and followed as outpatients, whereas patients at high risk are admitted to the hospital for further observation (see below).

Subsequent Evaluation & Treatment

Specific treatment of the various causes of upper gastrointestinal bleeding is discussed elsewhere in this chapter. The following general comments apply to most patients with bleeding:

A. History and Physical Examination: The physician's diagnostic impression of the bleeding source is correct in only 40% of cases. Signs of chronic liver disease implicate bleeding due to portal hypertension, but a different source is identified in 25–50% of patients with cirrhosis. A history of dyspepsia, NSAID use, or peptic ulcer disease suggests peptic ulcer. Acute bleeding preceded by heavy alcohol ingestion or retching suggests a Mallory-Weiss tear.

B. Upper Endoscopy: Virtually all patients with upper tract bleeding should undergo upper endoscopy. Endoscopy should be performed after the patient is hemodynamically stable, usually within 12 hours after admission. Patients with continued active bleeding require more urgent endoscopic evaluation. The benefits of endoscopy in this setting are threefold.

1. To identify the source of bleeding–The appropriate acute and long-term medical therapy is determined by the underlying cause of bleeding. For example, patients with portal hypertension will be treated differently from patients with ulcer disease. If surgery is required for uncontrolled bleeding, the source of bleeding as determined at endoscopy will determine the surgical approach.

2. To determine the risk of rebleeding–Patients with a nonbleeding Mallory-Weiss tear, esophagitis, gastritis, and ulcers that have a clean, white base have a very low risk of rebleeding. Preliminary studies suggest that it may be safe and cost-effective to discharge such patients from the emergency room or endoscopy suite without hospital admission. Patients with ulcers that are actively bleeding or have a visible vessel or with variceal bleeding require initial management in an ICU setting.

3. To render endoscopic therapy–Hemostasis can be achieved in actively bleeding lesions with endoscopic modalities such as cautery or injection. About 90% of actively bleeding varices can be effectively treated acutely with injection of a sclerosant or application of a rubber band to the bleeding varix. Similarly, 90% of actively bleeding ulcers, angiomas, or Mallory-Weiss tears can be controlled with either injection of epinephrine or direct cauterization of the vessel by a heater probe or multipolar electrocautery probe. Certain nonbleeding lesions such as esophageal varices, ulcers with visible blood vessels, and angiomas are also treated with these therapies. Specific endoscopic therapy of varices, peptic ulcers, and Mallory-Weiss tears is dealt with elsewhere.

C. Acute Pharmacologic Therapies:

1. Intravenous H_2 receptor antagonists– These agents are administered to most patients with upper tract bleeding, though they have never been proved to lower the risk of recurrent bleeding during the acute hospitalization—even in patients with peptic ulcer disease. The dose should be sufficient to maintain the intragastric pH above 4.0. Continuous infusions are recommended because they are less expensive and provide better control of pH with lower doses. Starting doses are cimetidine, 37.5–50 mg/h; ranitidine, 6.25 mg/h; or famotidine, 1 mg/h. Doses should be doubled after 4–6 hours if the intragastric pH remains low. Proton pump inhibitors are not recommended in the fasting ICU patient because they have unpredictable absorption and because high doses are required in fasting patients in order to control intragastric pH.

2. Octreotide–Continuous intravenous infusion of octreotide, 25–100 µg/h, reduces splanchnic blood flow and portal blood pressures and is effective in the initial control of bleeding related to portal hypertension. It should be administered as soon as possible to all patients with active upper gastrointestinal bleeding and evidence of liver disease or portal hypertension until the source of bleeding can be determined by endoscopy. Octreotide has not been shown to reduce bleeding from sources not related to portal hypertension.

3. Vasopressin–Because of its many side effects, intravenous vasopressin should no longer be used in the treatment of patients with upper gastrointestinal bleeding. Octreotide has equivalent or superior efficacy but is virtually devoid of acute side effects.

D. Other Treatment:

1. Intra-arterial embolization or vasopressin–Angiographic treatment is used rarely in patients with persistent bleeding from ulcers, angiomas, or Mallory-Weiss tears who have failed endoscopic therapy and are poor operative risks.

2. Transvenous intrahepatic portosystemic shunts (TIPS)–Placement by an angiographer of a wire stent from the hepatic vein through the liver to the portal vein provides effective decompression of the portal venous system and control of acute variceal bleeding. It is indicated in patients in whom endoscopic modalities have failed to control acute variceal bleeding.

Jutabha R, Jensen D: Management of upper gastrointestinal bleeding in the patient with chronic liver disease. Med Clin North Am 1996;80:1035.

Liberman D: Gastrointestinal bleeding: initial management. Gastroenterol Clin North Am 1993;22:723.

Rockall T et al: Selection of patients for early discharge or outpatient care after acute upper gastrointestinal haemorrhage. National Audit of Acute Upper Gastrointestinal Haemorrhage. Lancet 1996;347:1138. (Patients with low risk scores are at low risk for rebleeding [4.3%] and death [0.1%] and can be safely discharged or managed as outpatients.)

2. ACUTE LOWER GASTROINTESTINAL BLEEDING

Essentials of Diagnosis

- Hematochezia usually present.
- 10% of cases of hematochezia due to upper gastrointestinal source.
- Evaluation with colonoscopy in stable patients.
- Massive active bleeding calls for evaluation with sigmoidoscopy, upper endoscopy, and angiography or nuclear bleeding scan.

General Considerations

Lower gastrointestinal bleeding is defined as bleeding arising below the ligament of Treitz, ie, the small intestine or colon. However, the vast majority of cases arise from the colon and particularly the anorectal region. Bleeding that arises in the upper small intestine may be manifested as melena. However, most patents with lower gastrointestinal tract bleeding present with hematochezia (bright red blood per rectum). The severity of bleeding may range from streaks of red blood noted on the stool to massive large-volume hematochezia. The report of bright red blood that drips into the toilet after a bowel movement or that streaks or is mixed with solid stools suggests an anorectal source. At least 50% of cases of hematochezia arise from diseases in this region. Conversely, large-volume bloody stools may arise anywhere in the lower gastrointestinal tract. It must be recognized that up to 10% of patients with significant hematochezia have an upper gastrointestinal source of bleeding (eg, peptic ulcer); a "negative" nasogastric lavage does *not* definitively exclude an upper tract source. Upper gastrointestinal endoscopy is required when there is suspicion of a source in that location.

Etiology

A number of entities may cause lower gastrointestinal tract bleeding. The likelihood of these lesions is partially dependent both upon the age of the patient and the nature and severity of the bleeding. In patients under 50 years of age, the most common causes are infectious colitis, anorectal disease, and inflammatory bowel disease. In older patients, significant hematochezia is most often from diverticulosis, vascular ectasias, malignancy, or ischemia. Each of these entities is discussed in greater detail elsewhere in this chapter.

A. Diverticulosis: This is the most common cause of major lower tract bleeding, accounting for 40% of cases. It most commonly presents as acute, painless, large-volume maroon or bright red hematochezia in patients over age 50. Bleeding subsides spontaneously in 80% but may recur in up to 25% of patients.

B. Vascular Ectasias: Vascular ectasias (or angiodysplasias) may cause painless bleeding that ranges from acute hematochezia to chronic occult blood loss. Bleeding from ectasias is most common in patients over 70 years of age or in patients with chronic renal failure. Most commonly seen in the right colon, they occur throughout the upper and lower gastrointestinal tract.

C. Neoplasms: Benign and malignant neoplasms usually present with chronic, occult blood loss but occasionally with intermittent hematochezia and, rarely, massive lower tract bleeding.

D. Inflammatory Bowel Disease: Patients with inflammatory bowel disease (especially ulcerative colitis) often have diarrhea with variable amounts of hematochezia. Bleeding may vary from occult blood loss to recurrent hematochezia which is usually mixed with stool. Symptoms of abdominal pain, tenesmus, and urgency are often present.

E. Anorectal Disease: Anorectal disease commonly results in small amounts of bright red blood noted on the toilet paper, streaking the stool, or dripping into the toilet bowl. The bleeding is usually slight and seldom results in significant blood loss. Painless bleeding is commonly caused by internal hemorrhoids. Bleeding associated with pain during bowel movements suggests an anal fissure.

F. Ischemic Colitis: This entity is seen in elderly patients, most of whom have known atherosclerotic disease. Acute ischemia results in hematochezia or bloody diarrhea, typically associated with mild cramps. In most cases, the bleeding is mild and self-limited.

G. Others: Radiation-induced colitis may result in intestinal bleeding that can occur years later. Acute infectious colitis due to *Shigella, Campylobacter,* and enterohemorrhagic *E coli* (see Acute Diarrhea, above) commonly causes bloody diarrhea. Rare causes of lower tract bleeding include vasculitis, solitary rectal ulcer syndrome, small bowel diverticula, and colonic varices.

Evaluation & Management

The patient's volume status should be assessed and resuscitation with fluids and blood products instituted as necessary (see Acute Upper Gastrointestinal Tract Bleeding, above). A careful history and physical examination should be performed. Painless large-volume bleeding suggests diverticular bleeding, vascular ectasias, or an upper tract source. Frequent bloody diarrhea associated with tenesmus and urgency may suggest inflammatory bowel disease or infectious colitis. Further workup of lower tract bleeding is determined by the severity of the bleeding and whether it is active or has subsided.

A. Exclude an Upper Tract Source: A nasogastric tube and lavage (see above) should be performed in all patients with massive or submassive hematochezia to look for evidence of an upper gastrointestinal tract source. If blood is not seen and bile is aspirated, an upper source is unlikely.

B. Anoscopy and Sigmoidoscopy: In otherwise healthy patients under age 50 with small-volume bleeding, anoscopy and sigmoidoscopy are performed to look for evidence of anorectal disease, inflammatory bowel disease, or infectious colitis. If a likely source of bleeding is found, no further evaluation is needed immediately unless the bleeding persists or is recurrent. In patients over age 50 with small-volume hematochezia, the entire colon must be evaluated with either colonoscopy or a sigmoidoscopy and barium enema to exclude a neoplastic process.

C. Colonoscopy: An urgent colonoscopy should be performed in all patients with significant lower tract bleeding (ie, bleeding associated with a fall in hematocrit) when the bleeding has subsided or slowed (requiring less than two units of packed red blood cells per 24 hours). Colonoscopy is usually performed within 6–24 hours after admission once the colon has been cleansed with a standard oral lavage solution. A possible bleeding source is identified in over 80% of cases; however, active bleeding usually is not seen. When nonbleeding diverticula or vascular ectasias are identified, it is not certain that these are the source of bleeding.

D. Angiography or Nuclear Bleeding Scans: The presence of continued significant bleeding (more than two units of packed red cells transfused per 24 hours) limits the diagnostic utility of colonoscopic examination. In these patients, surgery may become necessary to control bleeding. It is helpful to localize the bleeding site in order to guide the surgical approach. Unfortunately, these studies are frequently nondiagnostic, either because the bleeding is intermittent or because it is too slow. ^{99m}Tc-labeled red cell scans can detect bleeding that requires at least two to four units of packed red cells per 24 hours and can grossly localize the bleeding site to the small intestine or to the right or left colon. Selective mesenteric angiography requires more significant bleeding (> 60 mL/h or bleeding requiring four units per 24 hours), but when positive it can specifically identify the bleeding vessel. Where available, it is preferable in most cases to nuclear studies.

Treatment

Treatment is directed at the underlying lesion. The following general principles apply:

A. Discontinue Aspirin and Other NSAIDs: Over 80% of patients with lower gastrointestinal tract bleeding have evidence of recent aspirin or NSAID ingestion. These agents potentiate bleeding through inhibition of platelet function.

B. Therapeutic Colonoscopy: Endoscopic electrocoagulation techniques are useful in treating vascular ectasias of the colon.

C. Intra-arterial Vasopressin or Embolization: At angiography, the intra-arterial infusion of vasopressin, 0.2 units/min, may arrest bleeding in up to 90% of patients with active bleeding from a diverticulum or vascular ectasia. Embolization may be used in patients with continued bleeding who are poor operative candidates but is associated with intestinal infarction in 15% of cases.

D. Surgery: The nature of surgical therapy depends upon the nature and location of the bleeding source. Surgery is generally indicated in patients with recurrent or persistent diverticular bleeding or transfusion requiring bleeding due to ectasias. In some patients with recurrent but intermittent bleeding, the precise bleeding source cannot be identified. A right hemicolectomy or subtotal colectomy may be necessary in these cases.

Manten HD, Green JA: Acute lower gastrointestinal bleeding: A guide to initial management. Postgrad Med 1995;97:154.

Reinus J, Brandt L: Vascular ectasias and diverticulosis: Common causes of lower intestinal bleeding. Gastroenterol Clin North Am 1994;23:1.

Richter JM et al: Effectiveness of current technology in the diagnosis and management of lower gastrointestinal hemorrhage. Gastrointest Endosc 1995;41:93.

Sharma R, Gorbien MJ: Angiodysplasia and lower gastrointestinal tract bleeding in elderly patients. Arch Intern Med 1995;155:807.

3. OCCULT GASTROINTESTINAL BLEEDING

Essentials of Diagnosis

- No overt gastrointestinal bleeding (hematochezia, melena).
- Detected by fecal occult blood testing or iron deficiency anemia in adult without other source of blood loss.
- Evaluation of colon with colonoscopy or barium enema mandatory.
- Evaluation of upper gastrointestinal tract with endoscopy or barium upper GI series guided by presence of symptoms.

General Considerations

Occult gastrointestinal bleeding is the loss of small amounts of blood into the gastrointestinal tract which is not apparent to the patient because it does not result in gross signs of hematochezia, melena, or hematemesis. Occult gastrointestinal bleeding is typically detected in one of two settings: (1) a positive fecal occult blood test or (2) the presence of iron deficiency anemia in an adult.

A. Fecal Occult Blood Testing (FOBT): Many patients over age 50 undergo annual routine testing of stool specimens for occult blood as a screen for colorectal neoplasms (see Colorectal Cancer Screening, below). From 1% to 2.7% of patients in screening programs will have a positive FOBT warranting investigation of the colon to exclude carcinoma. The positive predictive value of a nonrehydrated positive guaiac test is only 6–17%.

B. Iron Deficiency Anemia: In Western society, men and postmenopausal women with iron deficiency anemia should be presumed to have occult gastrointestinal bleeding unless another cause of anemia is readily apparent. Nutritional causes of iron deficiency are uncommon in Western society. Potential gastrointestinal causes of blood loss can be identified in over 60% of patients with iron deficiency from both the upper and lower gastrointestinal tracts. Gastrointestinal malignancy is present in up to 15%. Celiac sprue may also present with iron deficiency.

Causes of Occult Blood Loss

The most common causes of occult gastrointestinal bleeding are similar to the causes of clinically apparent bleeding cited above. These include (1) neoplasms (colorectal cancers and polyps, gastric cancers, lymphomas), (2) infections (nematodes, especially hookworm; amebiasis, tuberculosis), (3) vascular abnormalities (ectasias, angiodysplasias, portal hypertensive gastropathy), (4) acid-peptic lesions (peptic ulcer, reflux esophagitis, large hiatal hernias with erosions), (5) medications (especially NSAIDs, aspirin, or anticoagulants), and (6) other causes such as inflammatory bowel disease and malabsorption disorders.

Evaluation

A. Upper Endoscopy: Patients should be asked about symptoms such as heartburn, dyspepsia, nausea, vomiting, weight loss, early satiety, diarrhea, constipation, or change in bowel habits. In patients under age 50 years with obvious symptoms referable to the upper gastrointestinal tract, it is reasonable to proceed first with upper endoscopy to look for a source of acute or chronic bleeding. In asymptomatic patients with positive fecal occult blood tests whose colon evaluations are negative, the cost-effectiveness of evaluation of the upper tract is uncertain, and currently this procedure is not recommended. If iron deficiency anemia is present, the patients should undergo upper endoscopy after colonoscopy (see below). If no significant abnormality is found, a small bowel biopsy should be obtained during endoscopy to exclude celiac sprue and other malabsorptive disorders.

B. Colonoscopy Versus Barium Enema: In virtually all other patients with positive occult blood tests or iron deficiency anemia, the colon should be evaluated first with either colonoscopy or a combination of barium enema and sigmoidoscopy. (The latter is required to view the rectum and distal sigmoid adequately, since they are not well visualized by barium enema.) Colonoscopy detects over 95% of colorectal polyps or cancers and permits polypectomy, tumor biopsy, or endoscopic cautery of vascular ectasias. Barium enema examinations have only an 85–90% sensitivity for colorectal polyps, and up to 30–40% of patients with positive occult blood tests will have polyps detected on barium enema or sigmoidoscopy, which then necessitates colonoscopy to remove the polyps. Thus, although colonoscopy is more expensive than barium enema, the overall cost of these two diagnostic strategies is approximately the same. The optimal approach depends upon local expertise and costs (see section on adenomatous polyps).

C. Small Intestine Evaluation: Evaluation of the small intestine is unnecessary in most patients with positive fecal occult blood tests or iron deficiency anemia who have negative evaluation of the colon and upper gastrointestinal tract. With persistent chronic gastrointestinal blood loss that responds poorly to iron supplementation or requires transfusion, further evaluation for a small intestinal source of blood loss is needed. A small intestinal enteroclysis study is useful for detecting mucosal diseases such as Crohn's disease. Small bowel enteroscopy is now available at many centers and permits visualization of the upper one-third to one-half of the small intestine for vascular ectasias. Rarely, angiography or intraoperative endoscopy of the entire small intestine is necessary.

Dachman AH: How effective is enteroclysis in detecting the source of occult bleeding when an upper and lower endoscopy are negative? AJR Am J Roentgenol 1994; 163:1261.

Fine KD: The prevalence of occult gastrointestinal bleeding in celiac sprue. N Engl J Med 1996;334:1163.

Kepczyk T, Kadakia SC: Prospective evaluation of gastrointestinal tract in patients with iron-deficiency anemia. Dig Dis Sci 1995;40:1283.

DISEASES OF THE PERITONEUM

APPROACH TO THE PATIENT WITH ASCITES

Etiology of Ascites

The term "ascites" denotes the pathologic accumulation of fluid in the peritoneal cavity. Healthy men have little or no intraperitoneal fluid, but women normally may have up to 20 mL depending on the phase of the menstrual cycle. The causes of ascites may be classified into two broad pathophysiologic categories: that which is associated with a normal peritoneum and that which occurs due to a diseased peritoneum (Table 14–7). The most common cause of ascites is portal hypertension secondary to chronic liver diseases, which accounts for over 80% of patients with ascites. The management of portal hypertensive ascites is discussed in Chapter 16. The most common causes of non-portal hypertensive ascites include infections (tuberculosis), intra-abdominal malignancy, inflammatory disorders of the peritoneum, and ductal disruptions (chylous, pancreatic, biliary).

Clinical Features

A. Symptoms and Signs: The history usually is one of abdominal pain which is diffuse, constant, and occurs in association with increasing abdominal girth due to accumulation of ascites. Because most ascites is secondary to chronic liver disease with portal hypertension, patients should be asked about risk factors for liver disease, especially ethanol consumption, blood transfusions, tattoos, intravenous drug

Table 14–7. Causes of ascites.

NORMAL PERITONEUM
Portal hypertension (SAAG ≥ 1.1 g/dL)
1. Hepatic congestion[1]
Congestive heart failure
Constrictive pericarditis
Tricuspid insufficiency
Budd-Chiari syndrome
Veno-occlusive disease
2. Liver disease[2]
Cirrhosis
Alcoholic hepatitis
Fulminant hepatic failure
Massive hepatic metastases
Hepatic fibrosis
Acute fatty liver of pregnancy
3. Portal vein occlusion
Hypoalbuminemia (SAAG < 1.1 g/dL)
Nephrotic syndrome
Protein-losing enteropathy
Severe malnutrition with anasarca
Miscellaneous conditions (SAAG < 1.1 g/L)
Chylous ascites
Pancreatic ascites
Bile ascites
Nephrogenic ascites
Urine ascites
Myxedema (SAAG ≥ 1.1 g/dL)
Ovarian disease
DISEASED PERITONEUM (SAAG < 1.1 g/dL[2])
Infections
Bacterial peritonitis
Tuberculous peritonitis
Fungal peritonitis
HIV-associated peritonitis
Malignant conditions
Peritoneal carcinomatosis
Primary mesothelioma
Pseudomyxoma peritonei
Massive hepatic metastases
Hepatocellular carcinoma
Other conditions
Familial Mediterranean fever
Vasculitis
Granulomatous peritonitis
Eosinophilic peritonitis

[1]Hepatic congestion usually associated with SAAG ≥ 1.1 g/dL and ascitic fluid total protein > 2.5 g/dL.
[2]There may be cases of "mixed ascites" in which portal hypertensive ascites is complicated by a secondary process such as infection. In these cases, the SAAG is ≥ 1.1 g/dL.

use, a history of viral hepatitis or jaundice, and birth in an endemic area for hepatitis. A history of cancer or marked weight loss arouses suspicion of malignant ascites. Fevers may suggest infected peritoneal fluid, including bacterial peritonitis (spontaneous or secondary). Patients with chronic liver disease and ascites are at greatest risk of developing spontaneous bacterial peritonitis. In immigrants or immunocompromised hosts with fever, tuberculous peritonitis should be considered.

Physical examination should emphasize signs of portal hypertension and chronic liver disease. Elevated jugular venous distention may suggest right-sided congestive heart failure or constrictive pericarditis. A large tender liver may suggest acute alcoholic hepatitis or Budd-Chiari syndrome. The presence of large abdominal wall veins that flow away from the umbilicus and splenomegaly also suggests portal hypertension. Signs of chronic liver disease include palmar erythema, cutaneous spider angiomas, gynecomastia, and muscle wasting. Asterixis secondary to hepatic encephalopathy may be present. Widespread anasarca may be due to cardiac failure or nephrotic syndrome with hypoalbuminemia. Finally, firm lymph nodes in the left supraclavicular region or umbilicus may suggest intra-abdominal malignancy.

The physical examination is relatively insensitive for detecting ascitic fluid. The most sensitive means of determining whether ascitic fluid is present is to test for "shifting dullness." In general, patients must have at least 1500 mL of fluid to be detected reliably by this method. In many cases, even the experienced clinician may find it difficult to distinguish between obesity and small-volume ascites. In such instances, abdominal ultrasound is useful.

B. Laboratory Testing:

1. Abdominal paracentesis–Abdominal paracentesis should be performed as part of the diagnostic evaluation in all patients with the new onset of ascites. Approximately 30–50 mL of ascitic fluid should be removed for diagnostic studies.

a. Inspection–Cloudy fluid suggests infection. Milky fluid is seen with chylous ascites due to high triglyceride levels. Bloody fluid is most commonly attributable to a traumatic paracentesis, but up to 20% of cases of malignant ascites may be bloody.

b. Routine studies–

(1) Cell count–A white blood cell count is the most important test. Normal ascitic fluid contains less than 250 leukocytes/μL and < 250 PMNs/μL. Any inflammatory condition can cause an elevated ascitic white blood count. A polymorphonuclear neutrophil count of > 250/μL (neutrocytic ascites) is highly suspicious for bacterial peritonitis, either spontaneous primary peritonitis or secondary peritonitis (ie, peritonitis caused by an intra-abdominal source of infection, such as a perforated viscus or appendicitis). An elevated white count with a predominance of lymphocytes is suspicious for tuberculosis or peritoneal carcinomatosis.

(2) Albumin and total protein–The serum-ascites albumin gradient (SAAG) is the best single test for the classification of ascites into portal hypertensive and non–portal hypertensive causes (Table 14–7). Calculated by subtracting the ascitic fluid albumin from the serum albumin, the gradient correlates directly with the portal pressure. A SAAG > 1.1 g/dL strongly suggests underlying portal hypertension, while gradients < 1.1 g/dL implicate non-portal hypertensive causes of ascites.

The accuracy of the SAAG exceeds 95% in classifying ascites. It should be recognized, however, that approximately 4% of patients have "mixed ascites," ie, underlying cirrhosis with portal hypertension complicated by a second cause for ascites formation (such as malignancy or tuberculosis). Thus, a high SAAG is indicative of portal hypertension but does not exclude concomitant malignancy.

The ascitic fluid total protein provides some additional clues to etiology. An elevated SAAG and a high protein level (> 2.5 g/dL) is seen in most cases of hepatic congestion secondary to cardiac disease or Budd-Chiari syndrome. However, an elevated ascitic fluid protein is also found in up to 20% of cases of uncomplicated cirrhosis. Two-thirds of patients with malignant ascites have a total protein level greater than 2.5 g/dL.

(3) Culture and Gram stain–The optimal technique for the culture of ascitic fluid consists of the inoculation of blood culture bottles with 5–10 mL of ascitic fluid at the patient's bedside, which increases the sensitivity for detecting bacterial peritonitis to over 85% in patients with neutrocytic ascites (> 250 polymorphonuclear neutrophils/μL), compared with approximately 50% sensitivity by conventional agar plate or broth cultures.

c. Optional studies–Other laboratory tests are of utility in specific clinical situations but need not be ordered in the routine evaluation of ascites. Glucose and LDH may be helpful in distinguishing spontaneous bacterial peritonitis from secondary bacterial peritonitis (see below). Glucose levels are reduced in patients with tuberculous peritonitis. An elevated amylase may suggest pancreatic ascites or a perforation of the gastrointestinal tract with leakage of pancreatic secretions into the ascitic fluid. Perforation of biliary origin is suspected with an ascitic bilirubin concentration that is greater than the serum bilirubin. An elevated ascitic creatinine suggests leakage of urine from the bladder or ureters. Ascitic fluid cytology should be obtained in patients in whom an intra-abdominal malignancy or peritoneal carcinomatosis are suspected.

C. Imaging: Abdominal ultrasound is useful in confirming the presence of ascites and in the guidance of paracentesis. Both ultrasound and CT imaging are useful in distinguishing between causes of portal hypertensive and non–portal hypertensive ascites. Doppler ultrasound and CT can detect thrombosis of the hepatic veins (Budd-Chiari syndrome) or portal veins. In patients with non–portal hypertensive ascites, these studies are useful in detecting lymphadenopathy, masses of the mesentery and of solid organs such as the liver, ovaries, and pancreas. Furthermore, they permit directed percutaneous needle biopsies of these lesions. Both ultrasound and CT are notoriously poor for the detection of peritoneal carcinomatosis.

D. Laparoscopy: Laparoscopy is an important test in the evaluation of some patients with non–portal hypertensive ascites (low SAAG) or mixed as-cites. It permits direct visualization and biopsy of the peritoneum, liver, and some intra-abdominal lymph nodes. Cases of suspected peritoneal tuberculosis or suspected malignancy with nondiagnostic CT imaging and ascitic fluid cytology are best evaluated by this method. At laparoscopy, up to three-fourths of patients with exudative ascites have peritoneal carcinomatosis.

Jaffe DL, Chung RT, Friedman LS: Management of portal hypertension and its complications. Med Clin North Am 1996;80:1021.

SPONTANEOUS BACTERIAL PERITONITIS

Essentials of Diagnosis

- Occurs in patients with chronic liver disease and ascites.
- Fever and abdominal pain.
- Neutrocytic ascites (> 250 PMNs/μL).
- Must be distinguished from secondary causes of peritonitis.

General Considerations

"Spontaneous" bacterial infection of ascitic fluid occurs in the absence of an apparent intra-abdominal source of infection. It is seen almost exclusively in patients with ascites caused by chronic liver disease. Translocation of enteric bacteria across the gut wall or mesenteric lymphatics leads to seeding of the ascitic fluid. Patients with ascitic total protein levels less than 1 g/dL appear to be at greatest risk of spontaneous infection due to decreased ascitic fluid opsonic activity.

Virtually all cases of spontaneous bacterial peritonitis are caused by a monomicrobial infection. The most common pathogens are enteric gram-negative bacteria (*Escherichia coli, Klebsiella pneumoniae, Enterococcus* species) or gram-positive bacteria (*Streptococcus pneumoniae,* viridans streptococci). Anaerobic bacteria are not associated with spontaneous bacterial peritonitis.

Clinical Findings

A. Symptoms and Signs: Eighty to 90 percent of patients with spontaneous bacterial peritonitis are symptomatic; however, in some cases the presentation may be subtle. Hence, the clinician should have a low index of suspicion for spontaneous bacterial peritonitis in all patients with ascites secondary to liver disease. Clinical deterioration in such patients may be indicative of underlying infection. Spontaneous bacterial peritonitis may be present in 20% of patients hospitalized with chronic liver disease in the absence of any suggestive symptoms or signs.

The most common symptoms are fever and abdominal pain, present in one-half to two-thirds of patients. Spontaneous bacterial peritonitis may also present with a change in mental status due to an exacerbation of underlying hepatic encephalopathy. Physical examination typically demonstrates signs of chronic liver disease with ascites. Significant abdominal tenderness is present in less than half of patients. Peritoneal findings of percussion tenderness or rebound tenderness are present in less than 15%.

B. Laboratory Findings: The most important diagnostic test is abdominal paracentesis. Ascitic fluid should be sent for cell count, and blood culture bottles should be inoculated at the bedside. Gram's stain is insensitive in the detection of spontaneous bacterial peritonitis. An ascitic fluid total protein of more than 1 g/dL is strong evidence against spontaneous bacterial peritonitis.

In the proper clinical setting, an ascitic fluid PMN count of > 250 cells/μL (neutrocytic ascites) is presumptive evidence of bacerial peritonitis. The percentage of PMNs is almost always greater than 50–70% of the ascitic fluid white blood cells. Patients with neutrocytic ascites are presumed to be infected and should be started—regardless of symptoms—on empiric antibiotics in most instances. Although 10–30% of patients with neutrocytic ascites have negative ascitic bacterial cultures ("culture-negative neutrocytic ascites"), it is presumed nonetheless that most of these patients have bacterial peritonitis, and they should all be treated empirically.

Differential Diagnosis

Spontaneous bacterial peritonitis must be distinguished from secondary bacterial peritonitis, in which ascitic fluid has become secondarily infected by an intra-abdominal infection. Even in the presence of perforation, clinical symptoms and signs of peritonitis may be lacking in up to 30% of patients owing to the separation of the visceral and parietal peritoneum by the ascitic fluid. Causes of secondary bacterial peritonitis include appendicitis, diverticulitis, perforated peptic ulcer, perforated bowel, and perforated gallbladder. Secondary bacterial infection may account for up to 15% of infected ascites.

Ascitic fluid total protein, LDH, and glucose are useful in distinguishing spontaneous bacterial peritonitis from secondary infection. Up to two-thirds of patients with secondary bacterial peritonitis have at least two of the following: decreased glucose level (< 50 mg/dL), an elevated LDH level (greater than serum), and total protein greater than 1 g/dL. Ascitic neutrophil counts of over 10,000/μL also are suspicious; however, most cases of secondary peritonitis have neutrophil counts well within the range of spontaneous peritonitis. The presence of multiple organisms on ascitic fluid Gram stain or culture is diagnostic of secondary peritonitis.

If secondary bacterial peritonitis is suspected, plain films, abdominal CT imaging, and water-soluble contrast studies of the upper and lower gastrointestinal tracts should be obtained to look for evidence of an intra-abdominal source of infection. If these studies are negative and secondary peritonitis still is suspected, repeat paracentesis should be performed after 48 hours of antibiotic therapy to confirm that the polymorphonuclear neutrophil count is decreasing. Secondary bacterial peritonitis should be suspected in patients in whom the polymorphonuclear neutrophil count is not below the pretreatment value at 48 hours.

Neutrocytic ascites may also be seen in some patients with peritoneal carcinomatosis, pancreatic ascites, or tuberculous ascites. In these circumstances, however, polymorphonuclear neutrophils account for less than 50% of the ascitic white blood cells.

Treatment

Empirical therapy for spontaneous bacterial peritonitis should be initiated with a third-generation cephalosporin such as cefotaxime, which covers 98% of causative agents in this disorder. If *Enterococcus* infection is suspected, ampicillin may be added. Because of a high risk of nephrotoxicity in patients with chronic liver disease, aminoglycosides should not be used. Although the optimal duration of therapy is unknown, a course of 10 days has been recommended. Recent studies suggest that 5 days of therapy may be sufficient in most patients, or therapy until the ascites fluid PMN count decreases to < 250 cells/μL. Patients with suspected secondary bacterial peritonitis should be started on broad-spectrum coverage for enteric aerobic and anaerobic flora with a third-generation cephalosporin and metronidazole pending identification and definitive (usually surgical) treatment of the underlying cause of infection.

Prognosis

The mortality rate of spontaneous bacterial peritonitis exceeds 50% in many series. However, if the disease is recognized and treated early, the rate is less than 10%. As most patients with spontaneous bacterial peritonitis have severe liver disease, patients may die from liver failure, hepatorenal syndrome, or bleeding complications from portal hypertension.

Two-thirds of patients who survive have a recurrent episode of spontaneous bacterial peritonitis within 1 year. Prophylactic therapy with norfloxacin, 400 mg daily, or trimethoprim-sulfamethoxazole, one double-strength tablet daily, significantly reduces the incidence of recurrent infection in this high-risk group and is now recommended.

Spontaneous bacterial peritonitis develops in over 20% of patients with cirrhosis and ascites. Patients with low-protein ascites (< 1 g/dL) are at greatest risk of developing infection. Recently, trimethoprim-sulfamethoxazole (five double-strength tablets per week) or ciprofloxacin (750 mg once weekly) has been shown to reduce the incidence of spontaneous peritonitis to less than 5% after 6 months in patients without a prior infection. This primary prophylaxis regimen remains investigational, however, and is not yet widely applied in clinical practice.

Gilbert JA, Kamath PS: Spontaneous bacterial peritonitis: An update. Mayo Clinic Proc 1995;70:365.

Rolachon A et al: Ciprofloxacin and long-term prevention of spontaneous bacterial peritonitis: Results of a prospective controlled trial. Hepatology 1995;22(4 Part 1):1171.

Singh N et al: Trimethoprim-sulfamethoxazole for the prevention of spontaneous bacterial peritonitis in cirrhosis: A randomized trial. Ann Intern Med 1995;122:595.

TUBERCULOUS PERITONITIS

Abdominal involvement occurs in 2% of patients with tuberculosis. Patients at increased risk of extrapulmonary infection are those who are HIV-infected, immigrants from underdeveloped countries, the urban poor, prisoners, and nursing home residents. Abdominal tuberculosis can involve the peritoneum, omentum, intestinal tract, liver, spleen, and female genital tract. The onset of peritoneal disease is insidious, with symptoms present over several months. Typical clinical features are low-grade fevers, anorexia, weight loss, and abdominal tenderness. Eighty percent present with abdominal swelling and clinically apparent ascites; over 95% have ascites evident on ultrasound examination. Half of patients in the United States have underlying cirrhosis and portal hypertension, resulting in "mixed" ascites. Chest radiographs are abnormal in half of patients, but active tuberculous pulmonary disease is evident in less than 15%. Skin tests are positive in 70% of patients. Paracentesis usually reveals an elevated ascitic fluid leukocyte count of 250–4000 cells/µL with a lymphocyte predominance. The ascitic fluid protein is over 2.5 g/dL in 85% of patients. Smears of ascitic fluid for acid-fast bacilli are rarely positive, and cultures are positive in only 20%. Laparoscopy is the definitive means for establishing the diagnosis, permitting a presumptive visual diagnosis in the majority of cases. Suggestive findings include scattered white nodules over the parietal surfaces and adhesions between adjacent organs. Biopsies document caseating granulomas in over 85%.

Treatment with two or three drug regimens for 6 months generally is sufficient.

Shakil AO et al: Diagnostic features of tuberculous peritonitis in the absence and presence of chronic liver disease: A case control study. Am J Med 1996;100:179.

PERITONEAL CARCINOMATOSIS

Peritoneal involvement by the spread of primary neoplasms is common. The most common tumors are adenocarcinomas originating from tumors of the ovary, uterus, pancreas, stomach, colon, lung, or breast. Patients present with nonspecific abdominal discomfort and weight loss associated with increased abdominal girth owing to the development of malignant ascites. As the tumor progresses, they may develop partial or complete intestinal obstruction manifested by acute nausea and vomiting. Paracentesis usually demonstrates a low SAAG (< 1.1 mg/dL) and an elevated white count (often both polymorphonuclear neutrophils and mononuclear cells) but with a lymphocyte predominance. Cytology is positive in the vast majority of patients with proved carcinomatosis. Radiologic imaging studies are notoriously poor in the detection of peritoneal carcinomatosis. In difficult cases, laparoscopy may be required to confirm the diagnosis and to exclude tuberculous peritonitis, with which it may be confused. Malignant ascites does not respond to diuretic agents. Patients may be treated with periodic large-volume paracentesis for symptomatic relief from distention. Intraperitoneal chemotherapy is sometimes used to shrink the tumor. The overall prognosis is extremely poor, with only 12% survival at 6 months. Ovarian cancers represent an exception to this rule. With newer treatments consisting of surgical debulking and intraperitoneal chemotherapy, long-term survival from ovarian cancer is reported.

Parsons SL, Watson SA, Steele RJ: Malignant ascites. Br J Surg 1996;83:6.

FAMILIAL MEDITERRANEAN FEVER

This is a rare autosomal recessive disorder of unknown pathogenesis that almost exclusively affects people of Mediterranean ancestry, especially Sephardic Jews, Armenians, Turks, and Arabs. Most patients present with symptoms before the age of 20. It is characterized by episodic bouts of acute peritonitis that may be associated with serositis involving the joints and pleura. Peritoneal attacks are marked by the sudden onset of fever, severe abdominal pain, and abdominal tenderness with guarding or rebound tenderness. If left untreated, attacks resolve within 24–48 hours. Because symptoms resemble those of surgical peritonitis, patients may undergo unnecessary exploratory laparotomy. Colchicine, 0.6 mg two or three times daily, has been shown to decrease the frequency and severity of attacks. Secondary amyloidosis with renal or cardiac involvement may occur in 25% of cases. In the absence of amyloidosis, the prognosis is excellent.

Matzner Y: Biologic and clinical advances in familial Mediterranean fever. Crit Rev Oncol Hematol 1995;18: 472.

MESOTHELIOMA

Primary malignant mesothelioma is a rare tumor. More than 70% of cases have a remote history of asbestos exposure. Patients present with a recent onset of abdominal pain, bowel obstruction, increased abdominal girth, and small to moderate ascites. The chest x-ray reveals evidence of pulmonary asbestosis in over 50%. The ascitic fluid is characteristically hemorrhagic with a low SAAG. Cytology is often negative. Abdominal CT may reveal sheet-like masses involving the mesentery and omentum. Diagnosis is made at laparotomy or laparoscopy. The prognosis is extremely poor; however, long-term survivors have been described with a combination of radiation therapy and systemic or intraperitoneal chemotherapy.

Auerbach A, Sugarbaker P: Peritoneal mesothelioma: Treatment approach based on natural history. Cancer Treat Res 1996;81:193.

MISCELLANEOUS PERITONEAL DISEASES

Chylous ascites is the accumulation of lipid-rich lymph in the peritoneal cavity. The ascitic fluid is characterized by a milky appearance with a triglyceride level greater than 1000 mg/dL. The usual cause in adults is lymphatic obstruction or leakage caused by malignancy, especially lymphoma. Nonmalignant causes include postoperative trauma, cirrhosis, tuberculosis, pancreatitis, and adenitis.

Pancreatic ascites is the intraperitoneal accumulation of massive amounts of pancreatic secretions due to either disruption of the pancreatic duct or a pancreatic pseudocyst. It therefore is most commonly seen in patients with chronic pancreatitis and complicates up to 3% of cases of acute pancreatitis. Because the pancreatic enzymes are not activated, patients present with increased abdominal girth, but pain often is absent. The ascitic fluid is characterized by a high protein level (> 2.5 g/dL) but a low SAAG. Ascitic fluid amylase levels are in excess of 10,000 units/mL. In nonsurgical cases, initial treatment consists of bowel rest, total parenteral nutrition, and octreotide to decrease pancreatic secretion. Persistent leakage requires treatment with either endoscopic placement of stents into the pancreatic duct or surgical drainage.

Bile ascites is caused most commonly by complications of biliary tract surgery, percutaneous liver biopsy, or abdominal trauma. Unless the bile is infected, bile ascites usually does not cause abdominal pain, fever, or leukocytosis. Paracentesis reveals yellow fluid with a ratio of ascites bilirubin to serum bilirubin greater than 1.0. Treatment is dependent upon the location and rate of bile leakage. Postchole-

cystectomy cystic duct leaks may be treated with endoscopic sphincterotomy or biliary stent placement to facilitate bile flow across the sphincter of Oddi. Other leaks may be treated with either percutaneous drainage by interventional radiologists or surgical closure.

Deviere J et al: Complete disruption of the main pancreatic duct: Endoscopic management. Gastrointest Endosc 1995;42:445.

Grauer L, Borkin S: Role of somatostatin and octreotide in the treatment of pancreatic pseudocysts, fistula, and ascites. Digestion 1994;55(Suppl 1):24.

Kozarek RA et al: Endoscopic treatment of biliary injury in the era of laparoscopic cholecystectomy. Gastrointest Endosc 1994;40:10.

DISEASES OF THE ESOPHAGUS

EVALUATION OF ESOPHAGEAL DISORDERS

Symptoms

The clinical history is extremely important in the diagnosis of esophageal disease. Heartburn, dysphagia, and odynophagia virtually always indicate a primary esophageal disorder.

A. Heartburn: Heartburn (pyrosis) is the feeling of substernal burning, often radiating to the neck. Caused by the reflux of acidic (or, rarely, alkaline) material into the esophagus, it is highly specific for gastroesophageal reflux disease.

B. Dysphagia: Difficulties in swallowing may arise from problems in transferring the food bolus from the oropharynx to the upper esophagus (oropharyngeal dysphagia) or from impaired transport of the bolus through the body of the esophagus (esophageal dysphagia). A careful history usually leads to the correct diagnosis.

1. Oropharyngeal dysphagia–The oropharyngeal phase of swallowing is a complex process requiring elevation of the tongue, closure of the nasopharynx, relaxation of the upper esophageal sphincter, closure of the airway, and pharyngeal peristalsis. A brain stem medullary swallowing center integrates cranial nerves V, VII, IX, X, and XII. A variety of mechanical and neuromuscular conditions can disrupt this process (Table 14–8). Oropharyngeal dysphagia is characterized by coughing, choking, and regurgitation that occurs immediately upon initiating swallowing. Liquids are more difficult to swallow than soft foods. There may be associated dysphonia, dysarthria, or other neurologic symptoms.

2. Esophageal dysphagia–Esophageal dysphagia may be caused by **mechanical lesions** ob-

Table 14–8. Causes of oropharyngeal dysphagia.

Neurologic disorders
  Brain stem cerebrovascular accident, mass lesion
  Pseudobulbar palsy
  Amyotrophic lateral sclerosis, multiple sclerosis,
    poliomyelitis
  Myasthenia gravis
Muscular disorders
  Myopathies, polymyositis
  Hypothyroidism
Motility disorders
  Upper esophageal sphincter dysfunction
Structural defects
  Zenker's diverticulum
  Malignancy, surgery, radiation to oropharynx

structing the esophagus or by **motility disorders** (Table 14–9). Patients with mechanical obstruction experience dysphagia, primarily for solids. This is recurrent, predictable, and, if the lesion progresses, will worsen as the lumen narrows. Patients with motility disorders have dysphagia for both solids and liquids. It is episodic, unpredictable, and nonprogressive or progresses at a slow rate.

C. Odynophagia: Odynophagia is sharp substernal pain on swallowing that may limit oral intake. It usually reflects severe erosive disease. It is most commonly associated with infectious esophagitis due to *Candida,* herpesviruses, or cytomegalovirus, especially in immunocompromised patients. It may also be caused by corrosive injury due to caustic ingestions and by pill-induced ulcers.

Diagnostic Studies

A. Upper Endoscopy: Endoscopy is the study of choice for evaluating persistent heartburn, odynophagia, and structural abnormalities detected on barium esophagography. In addition to direct visualization, it allows biopsy of mucosal abnormalities and dilation of strictures.

Table 14–9. Causes of esophageal dysphagia.

Cause	Clues
Mechanical obstruction	**Solid foods worse than liquids**
Schatzki's ring	Intermittent dysphagia; not progressive
Peptic stricture	Chronic heartburn; progressive dysphagia
Esophageal cancer	Progressive dysphagia; age over 50
Motility disorder	**Solid and liquid foods**
Achalasia	Progressive dysphagia
Diffuse esophageal spasm	Intermittent; not progressive; may have chest pain
Scleroderma	Chronic heartburn; Raynaud's phenomenon

B. Videoesophagography: Oropharyngeal dysphagia is best evaluated with rapid sequence videoesophagography conducted by an experienced radiologist or speech pathologist.

C. Barium Esophagography: Patients with esophageal dysphagia often are evaluated first with a radiographic barium study to differentiate between mechanical lesions and esophageal motility disorders. In contrast to endoscopy, it provides limited information about esophageal motility. In patients in whom there is a high suspicion of a mechanical lesion, many clinicians will proceed first to endoscopic evaluation without a barium study. In patients with esophageal dysphagia and a suspected motility disorder, barium esophagoscopy should be obtained first.

D. Esophageal Manometry: Esophageal motility is best studied using manometric techniques. A small pressure-sensing catheter assembly is passed nasally into the esophagus, allowing manometric assessment of the lower and upper esophageal sphincters and esophageal body. It is the optimal study for evaluating dysphagia in patients in whom endoscopy or barium study has excluded a mechanical obstruction.

E. Ambulatory Esophageal pH Monitoring: Esophageal pH may be monitored continuously by means of a small pH probe passed transnasally and attached to a portable pH recording device. The probe and recorder are worn by the patient for up to 24 hours. The recording can be analyzed to determine the amount of gastroesophageal acid reflux and whether a patient's symptoms correlate with documented reflux.

American Gastroenterological Association medical position statement on the clinical use of esophageal manometry. Gastroenterology 1994;107:1865.

American Gastroenterological Association medical position statement: Guidelines on the use of esophageal pH recording. Gastroenterology 1996;110:1981.

INFLAMMATORY ESOPHAGEAL CONDITIONS

1. GASTROESOPHAGEAL REFLUX DISEASE

Essentials of Diagnosis

- Heartburn; may be exacerbated by meals, bending, or recumbency.
- Clinical diagnosis; typical uncomplicated cases do not require diagnostic studies.
- Endoscopy demonstrates abnormalities in < 50% of patients.
- Barium esophagography seldom helpful.

General Considerations

"Gastroesophageal reflux disease" is the term applied to the symptoms or tissue damage caused by the reflux of gastric contents (usually acidic) into the esophagus. It is extremely common, with one-third of adults reporting occasional heartburn and 10% complaining of daily symptoms. It is this more symptomatic group that is likely to seek medical attention. Most patients have mild disease. A few patients develop esophageal mucosal damage (reflux esophagitis) or more severe complications.

Several factors, either alone or in combination, may contribute to gastroesophageal reflux disease.

A. Incompetent Lower Esophageal Sphincter: In most patients, reflux occurs during spontaneous, transient relaxations of the lower esophageal sphincter, even though the baseline lower esophageal sphincteric pressures (10–30 mm Hg) are adequate. Patients with more severe involvement (especially those with strictures or Barrett's esophagus) generally have an incompetent lower esophageal sphincter (< 10 mm Hg), resulting in free reflux or stress reflux during abdominal straining, lifting, or bending.

B. Irritant Effects of Refluxate: Esophageal mucosal damage is related to the potency of the refluxate and the amount of time it is in contact with the mucosa. Acidic gastric fluid (pH < 3.9) is extremely caustic to the esophageal mucosa and is the major injurious agent in the majority of cases. In a few patients, reflux of bile or pancreatic secretions may be contributory.

C. Abnormal Esophageal Clearance: Acid refluxate normally is cleared and neutralized by esophageal peristalsis and salivary bicarbonate. During sleep, swallowing-induced peristalsis is infrequent, prolonging acid exposure. One-third of patients with severe gastroesophageal reflux disease also have diminished peristaltic clearance. Certain medical conditions such as Raynaud's phenomenon, CREST syndrome, and scleroderma, are frequently associated with diminished peristalsis. Conditions associated with impaired salivation such as Sjögren's syndrome, anticholinergic medications, and oral radiation therapy may exacerbate gastroesophageal reflux disease.

Hiatal hernias are common and of no significance in asymptomatic people. They are present in over 90% of patients with severe erosive esophagitis, especially when complicated by the development of strictures or Barrett's esophagus. The hernia sac appears to retard esophageal acid clearance.

D. Delayed Gastric Emptying: Impaired gastric emptying due to gastroparesis or partial gastric outlet obstruction potentiates gastroesophageal reflux disease.

Clinical Findings

A. Symptoms and Signs: The typical symptom of gastroesophageal reflux disease is heartburn. This most often occurs 30–60 minutes after meals and upon reclining. Patients often report relief from taking antacids or baking soda. When this symptom

is dominant, the diagnosis is established with a high degree of reliability. Many patients, however, have less specific dyspeptic symptoms with or without heartburn. Overall, a clinical diagnosis of gastroesophageal reflux has a sensitivity of 78% but a specificity of only 68%. The severity of heartburn is not correlated with the severity of esophageal tissue damage. In fact, some patients with severe esophagitis are almost asymptomatic. Patients may complain of regurgitation—the spontaneous reflux of sour or bitter gastric contents into the mouth. Less common symptoms include dysphagia, which may be due to abnormal peristalsis or the development of complications such as stricture or Barrett's metaplasia.

Gastroesophageal reflux disease may also be manifested by atypical symptoms such as asthma, chronic cough, sore throat, chronic laryngitis, and atypical (noncardiac) chest pain.

Physical examination and laboratory data are normal in uncomplicated disease.

B. Special Examinations: Uncomplicated patients with typical symptoms of heartburn and regurgitation may be treated empirically for 4 weeks for gastroesophageal reflux disease without the need for diagnostic studies. Further investigation is required in patients with complicated disease and those unresponsive to empiric therapy.

1. Upper endoscopy–Upper endoscopy with biopsy is the standard procedure for documenting the type and extent of tissue damage in gastroesophageal reflux disease. Approximately 50% of patients with proved acid reflux will have visible mucosal abnormalities such as erythema and friability of the squamocolumnar junction and erosions, known as reflux esophagitis. However, endoscopy is normal in up to half of symptomatic patients and does not exclude mild disease. Esophageal abnormalities are graded on a scale of I (mild) to IV (severe erosions, stricture, or Barrett's esophagus). Endoscopy is warranted in patients with severe reflux symptoms unresolved by empirical medical therapy and in complicated disease as suggested by dysphagia, hematemesis, guaiac-positive stools, or iron deficiency anemia.

2. Barium esophagography–This study plays a limited role in the evaluation of gastroesophageal reflux disease in most centers because of its limited ability to identify reflux or mucosal abnormalities. In patients with severe dysphagia, it is sometimes obtained prior to endoscopy to identify a stricture.

3. Ambulatory esophageal pH monitoring–Ambulatory pH monitoring is the best study for documenting acid reflux, but it is unnecessary in most patients with gastroesophageal reflux disease. It is useful and indicated in the following situations: (1) to document abnormal esophageal acid exposure in a patient being considered for antireflux surgery who has a normal endoscopy (ie, no evidence of reflux esophagitis); (2) to evaluate patients with a normal endoscopy who have reflux symptoms that are unresponsive to therapy with a proton pump inhibitor; (3) to detect either abnormal amounts of reflux or an association between reflux episodes and atypical symptoms such as noncardiac chest pain, asthma, chronic cough, laryngitis, and sore throat. It is recommended, however, that most patients with atypical symptoms first be given an empirical trial of antireflux therapy with a proton pump inhibitor for 4 weeks.

4. Esophageal manometry–This study is indicated (1) to determine the location of the lower esophageal sphincter before placement of an esophageal pH probe, and (2) for the preoperative assessment of peristaltic function in patients being considered for antireflux surgery. It is not useful in the diagnosis or management of most patients with gastroesophageal reflux disease.

Differential Diagnosis

Symptoms of gastroesophageal reflux disease may be similar to those of other diseases such as esophageal motility disorders, peptic ulcer, cholelithiasis, nonulcer dyspepsia, and angina pectoris. Reflux erosive esophagitis may be confused with pill-induced damage, radiation esophagitis, or infections (CMV, herpes, *Candida*).

Complications

A. Barrett's Esophagus: This is a condition in which the normal squamous epithelium of the esophagus is replaced by a metaplastic columnar epithelium containing goblet and columnar cells. Present in about 10% of patients with gastroesophageal reflux disease, it is believed to arise from chronic reflux-induced injury to the squamous epithelium. Barrett's esophagus invariably involves the most distal esophagus (at the gastroesophageal junction) and extends from one to several centimeters proximally in a circumferential or tongue-like fashion. Biopsies should be obtained to confirm the endoscopic diagnosis. Three types of columnar epithelium may be identified: gastric cardiac, gastric fundic, and specialized columnar (intestinal type). Only the specialized columnar type is of clinical significance.

Barrett's esophagus does not provoke specific symptoms. Rather, symptoms are a consequence of gastroesophageal reflux disease. Most patients have a long history of reflux symptoms, such as heartburn and regurgitation. Dysphagia due to impaired motility is common. Paradoxically, one-third of patients report minimal or no symptoms of gastroesophageal reflux disease, suggesting decreased acid sensitivity of Barrett's epithelium. Indeed, over 90% of individuals with Barrett's esophagus in the general population do not seek medical attention and go unrecognized. Barrett's esophagus may be complicated by stricture formation or deep ulcerations, which can bleed.

Barrett's esophagus is indicative of severe gastroesophageal reflux disease and should be treated aggressively with proton pump inhibitors to heal any active erosive esophagitis. Surgical fundoplication may be desirable in some situations. Medical or surgical therapy may prevent progression of Barrett's esophagus, but there is no convincing evidence that regression occurs. Recently, endoscopic ablation of Barrett's epithelium with cautery probes or the argon laser has resulted in partial or complete regression of columnar epithelium. Further studies are needed before such treatment can be recommended.

The most serious complication of Barrett's esophagus is esophageal adenocarcinoma, which develops at a rate of about one case per 125 patient-years of follow-up, representing a 40-fold risk compared with patients without Barrett's esophagus. Virtually all adenocarcinomas of the esophagus and many such tumors of the gastric cardia arise from Barrett's metaplasia. Although the matter is still being debated, most gastroenterologists recommend that patients with Barrett's esophagus undergo endoscopic surveillance with mucosal biopsies every 2 years. Early adenocarcinoma should be resected. Patients with low-grade dysplasia should be treated with aggressive medical management and endoscopic surveillance every 6 months. The management of high-grade dysplasia is controversial. Because up to 25% may progress to invasive adenocarcinoma within 6 months, surgery is usually recommended for good operative candidates.

B. Peptic Stricture: Stricture formation occurs in about 10% of patients with esophagitis. It is manifested by the gradual development of solid food dysphagia, which progresses over months to years. Often there is a reduction in heartburn because the stricture acts as a barrier to reflux. Most strictures are located at the gastroesophageal junction. Strictures located above this level usually occur in the presence of Barrett's metaplasia. Endoscopy with biopsy is mandatory in all cases to differentiate peptic stricture from other benign or malignant causes of esophageal stricture (Schatzki's ring, esophageal carcinoma). Active erosive esophagitis is often present. Up to 90% of symptomatic patients are effectively treated with dilation. Dilation is continued over one to several sessions. A luminal diameter of 14–15 mm is usually sufficient to relieve dysphagia. Chronic therapy with a proton pump inhibitor (omeprazole or lansoprazole) is required to decrease the likelihood of stricture recurrence. Some patients require intermittent stricture dilation to maintain luminal patency. With the advent of proton pump inhibitors, operative management for strictures that do not respond to dilation is seldom required.

Treatment

A. Medical Treatment: The goal of treatment is to provide symptomatic relief, to heal esophagitis (if present), and to prevent complications. Most patients with mild to moderate symptoms and no evidence of complications are treated in a stepwise fashion as outlined below.

1. Step 1: Lifestyle modifications and antacids–The majority of patients have mild, intermittent symptoms that are effectively treated with lifestyle modifications (to decrease the occurrence of reflux events) and antacids as needed for symptomatic occurrences. Recommended lifestyle modifications include elimination of smoking, moderation in alcohol use, reduction of meal size, weight loss, avoidance of tight-fitting clothes, and refraining from lying down within 3 hours after eating (the period of greatest reflux). Elevation of the head of the bed on 6-inch blocks or by a foam wedge under the mattress is recommended for patients with nocturnal symptoms to reduce reflux and enhance esophageal acid clearance. Patients should avoid foods that lower esophageal sphincteric pressure, especially fried or fatty foods, caffeine, peppermint, chocolate, and alcohol, and foods that cause direct mucosal irritation, such as citrus fruits, tomatoes, coffee, and soft drinks.

Antacids are the mainstay for rapid relief of occasional symptoms. Commonly used formulations are Maalox TC or Mylanta-II, either as liquid (10–15 mL) or tablets (two to four). Gaviscon (two to four tablets) is an alginate-antacid combination that decreases reflux in the upright position and may be superior to antacids alone. Over-the-counter H_2 antagonists (ranitidine or nizatidine 75 mg, famotidine 10 mg, cimetidine 200 mg) may also be used. These agents provide relief of symptoms within 30 minutes that may last for several hours.

2. Step 2: H_2 receptor antagonists or promotility agents–Patients with more frequent, mild to moderate symptoms usually are given a trial of H_2 receptor antagonists or promotility agents. Dosing two times daily is necessary for all of these agents for effective symptom control. "Standard" doses of H_2 receptor antagonists (ranitidine or nizatidine, 150 mg twice daily; cimetidine, 400–800 mg twice daily; famotidine, 20 mg twice daily) afford symptomatic improvement in up to two-thirds of patients but are ineffective in the healing of erosive esophagitis. Therefore, patients with endoscopically documented erosive esophagitis should be treated with proton pump inhibitors. Higher doses of H_2 receptor antagonists (ranitidine or nizatidine, 150–300 mg four times daily; cimetidine, 800 mg twice daily) afford greater symptomatic relief and higher esophagitis healing rates but are more costly (and less effective) than proton pump therapy and for that reason are not recommended.

Promotility agents (cisapride, metoclopramide, bethanechol) increase lower esophageal pressure and enhance esophageal clearance and gastric emptying. These agents are preferred to H_2 receptor antagonists in the treatment of patients with predominant regur-

gitation, other dyspeptic symptoms (bloating, nausea, early satiety), or nocturnal symptoms. They are used also in combination with H_2 receptor antagonists or proton pump inhibitors in patients with reflux due to gastroparesis (eg, diabetic gastropathy or scleroderma). Side effects of bethanechol and metoclopramide limit their long-term use. Cisapride is a serotonin $5-HT_4$ agonist that enhances release of acetylcholine from the gut myenteric plexus. Cisapride (10 mg four times daily or 20 mg twice daily) is equivalent to H_2 receptor antagonists for symptom relief in mild to moderate gastroesophageal reflux. Like H_2 receptor antagonists, it is not effective in the healing of erosive esophagitis.

Successful initial therapy with H_2 receptor antagonists or promotility agents should be discontinued after 8–12 weeks. Patients whose symptoms relapse after discontinuation of therapy may be treated with continuous or intermittent courses of therapy. Persistent mild to moderate symptomatology despite 4–8 weeks of empiric H_2 receptor antagonists or cisapride warrants endoscopy to document the presence and severity of esophagitis.

3. Step 3: Proton pump inhibitors–Proton pump inhibitors are the drugs of choice for patients with (1) severe symptoms, (2) mild to moderate symptoms unresponsive to initial H_2 receptor antagonists or cisapride therapy, (3) endoscopically documented erosive esophagitis, or (4) reflux complications (peptic stricture, Barrett's esophagus). Omeprazole, 20–40 mg daily, or lansoprazole, 30 mg daily, achieves symptomatic relief with complete healing of esophagitis in over 85% of patients with 8 weeks of therapy.

After discontinuation of proton pump inhibitors, symptom relapse within 6 months occurs in the majority of patients with erosive esophagitis. Therefore, chronic maintenance treatment with a proton pump inhibitor (omeprazole, 20–40 mg daily, or lansoprazole, 15–30 mg daily) is needed in most patients to control symptoms and maintain mucosal healing. Cisapride and H_2 receptor antagonists are ineffective for maintenance therapy of erosive disease.

B. Unresponsive Disease: Patients with symptoms of gastroesophageal reflux who do not respond to proton pump inhibitors and who do not have endoscopic evidence of reflux esophagitis should undergo ambulatory esophageal pH monitoring to determine the amount of esophageal acid reflux and whether symptoms are truly acid-related. Approximately 10% of patients with erosive reflux esophagitis do not respond to standard doses of proton pump inhibitors. These patients may benefit from higher proton pump dosages or from combination therapy with a proton pump inhibitor and cisapride. Truly refractory disease may be caused by gastric acid hypersecretion (Zollinger-Ellison syndrome), bile reflux, pill-induced esophagitis, or medical noncompliance.

C. Surgical Treatment: Surgical fundoplication is indicated for patients who fail or are noncompliant with medical therapy, complicated peptic strictures requiring repeated dilations, and patients with respiratory complications of reflux (laryngitis, asthma). In younger patients requiring chronic proton pump inhibitor therapy, it may be the preferred option. Fundoplication is successful in over 85% of patients and may now be performed laparoscopically in most patients.

DeVault K, Castell D, for the Practice Parameters Committee of the American College of Gastroenterology: Guidelines for the diagnosis and treatment of gastroesophageal reflux disease. Arch Intern Med 1995;115: 2165.

Over-the-counter H$_2$-receptor antagonists for heartburn. Med Lett Drugs Ther 1995;37:95.

Provenzale D et al: A guide for surveillance of patients with Barrett's esophagus. Am J Gastroenterol 1994; 89:670. (Decision analysis assessing the cost-effectiveness of various endoscopic screening strategies for patients with Barrett's esophagus. Estimated cost for each year of life saved with yearly surveillance is $300,000. Surveillance may not be cost-effective.)

Richardson W et al: Laparoscopic antireflux surgery. Surg Clin North Am 1996;76:437.

Richter S: Typical and atypical presentations of gastroesophageal reflux disease. Gastroenterol Clin North Am 1996;25:75.

Robinson M et al: Effective maintenance treatment of reflux esophagitis with low-dose lansoprazole. N Engl J Med 1996;124:859. (Among patients with healed esophagitis followed for 1 year, esophagitis and symptoms recurred in 76% of the placebo group, 21% of patients treated with lansoprazole 15 mg daily, and 10% treated with lansoprazole 30 mg daily.)

Spechler S, Goyal R: The columnar-lined esophagus, intestinal metaplasia, and normal Barrett. Gastroenterology 1996;110:614.

Vigneri S et al: A comparison of five maintenance therapies for reflux esophagitis. N Engl J Med 1995; 333:1106. (In patients with erosive esophagitis healed with omeprazole, H$_2$ receptor antagonist or cisapride was ineffective in maintaining mucosal healing. Omeprazole, 20 mg daily, was equivalent to combination therapy with ranitidine, 150 mg twice daily, and cisapride, 10 mg four times daily. Combination therapy with omeprazole and cisapride was superior to combination therapy with H$_2$ receptor antagonists and cisapride but not superior to omeprazole alone.)

INFECTIOUS ESOPHAGITIS

Essentials of Diagnosis

- Immunosuppressed patient.
- Odynophagia, dysphagia, and chest pain.
- Endoscopy with biopsy establishes diagnosis.

General Considerations

Infectious esophagitis occurs most commonly in immunosuppressed patients. Patients with AIDS, solid organ transplants, leukemia, lymphoma, and those receiving immunosuppressive drugs are at particular risk for opportunistic infections. *Candida albicans,* herpes simplex, and cytomegalovirus are the most common pathogens. *Candida* infection may also occur in patients who have uncontrolled diabetes and those being treated with systemic corticosteroids, radiation therapy, or systemic antibiotic therapy. Herpes simplex can affect normal hosts, in which case the infection is generally self-limited.

Clinical Findings

A. Symptoms and Signs: The most common symptoms are odynophagia and dysphagia. Substernal chest pain occurs in some patients. Patients with candidal esophagitis are sometimes asymptomatic. Oral thrush is present in only 75% of patients with candidal esophagitis and 25–50% of patients with viral esophagitis and is therefore an unreliable indicator of the cause of esophageal infection. Patients with esophageal CMV infection may have infection at other sites such as the colon and retina. Oral ulcers (herpes labialis) are often associated with herpes simplex esophagitis.

B. Special Examinations: Treatment may be empiric. For diagnostic certainty, endoscopy with biopsy and cytologic brushings is preferred because of its high diagnostic accuracy. The endoscopic signs of candidal esophagitis are diffuse, linear, yellow-white plaques adherent to the mucosa. Cytomegalovirus esophagitis is characterized by one to several large, shallow, superficial ulcerations. Herpes esophagitis results in multiple, small, deep ulcerations.

Treatment

A. Candidal Esophagitis: Treatment depends on the immune status of the patient and the severity of the illness. Options include topical agents (nystatin, 1–3 million units "swish and swallow" five times daily; clotrimazole troches, 10 mg dissolved in mouth five times daily), oral agents (ketoconazole, fluconazole), and intravenous agents (amphotericin B, fluconazole). Topical therapy is used initially in patients with a normal immune system. Initial therapy for immunocompromised patients (including AIDS) generally is with fluconazole, 100–200 mg/d orally. Ketoconazole should no longer be used because of its lower efficacy, unpredictable absorption, and greater risk of adverse effects. Patients not responding to oral therapy are treated with low-dose amphotericin B, 0.3–0.5 mg/kg/d intravenously for 7 days.

B. Cytomegalovirus Esophagitis: Initial therapy is with ganciclovir, 5 mg/kg intravenously every 12 hours for 3–4 weeks. Neutropenia is a frequent dose-limiting side effect. If resolution of symptoms occurs, the drug may be discontinued. If the condition has improved but not resolved, full-dose therapy may be continued for an additional 2–3 weeks. In some cases (especially in patients with AIDS), continuous ganciclovir, 5 mg/kg intravenously daily, is required for suppressive therapy. The role of oral ganciclovir in the maintenance treatment of CMV gastrointestinal disease is not established. Patients who either do not respond to or cannot tolerate ganciclovir are treated acutely with foscarnet, 90 mg/kg intravenously every 12 hours for 3–4 weeks. The principal toxicity is renal failure.

C. Herpetic Esophagitis: Immune-competent patients may be treated symptomatically and generally do not require specific antiviral therapy. Immunosuppressed patients may be treated with oral acyclovir, 200 mg orally five times daily, or 250 mg/m^2 intravenously every 8–12 hours, usually for 7–10 days. Nonresponders require therapy with foscarnet, 40 mg/kg intravenously every 8 hours for 21 days.

Prognosis

Most patients with infectious esophagitis can be effectively treated with complete symptom resolution. Depending on the patient's underlying immunodeficiency, relapse of symptoms off therapy can raise difficulties. Chronic suppressive therapy is sometimes required.

Dieterich DT, Wilcox CM, the Practice Parameters Committee of the American College of Gastroenterology: Diagnosis and treatment of esophageal diseases associated with HIV infection. Am J Gastroenterol 1996;91:2265.

Wilcox M et al: Esophageal ulceration in human immunodeficiency virus infection. Ann Intern Med 1995;122:143. (In 100 patients with AIDS and esophageal ulcers, 45 were attributed to CMV, 40 were idiopathic, and 5 were due to HSV.)

PILL-INDUCED ESOPHAGITIS

A number of different medications may injure the esophagus, presumably through direct, prolonged mucosal contact. The most commonly implicated are the NSAIDs, potassium chloride pills, quinidine, zalcitabine, zidovudine, alendronate, iron, vitamin C, and antibiotics. Because injury is most likely to occur if pills are swallowed without water or while supine, hospitalized or bed-bound patients are at greater risk. Symptoms include severe retrosternal chest pain, odynophagia, and dysphagia, often beginning several hours after taking a pill. These may occur suddenly and persist for days. Some patients (especially the elderly) have relatively little pain, presenting with dysphagia. Endoscopy may reveal one to several discrete ulcers that may be shallow or deep. Chronic injury may result in severe esophagitis with stricture, hemorrhage, or perforation. Healing occurs rapidly when the offending agent is eliminated. To prevent pill-induced damage, patients should take pills with 4 oz of water and remain upright for 30 minutes after ingestion. Known offenders should not be given to patients with esophageal dysmotility, dysphagia, or strictures.

Boszymski E, Isaacs K: Miscellaneous diseases of the esophagus. In: *Textbook of Gastroenterology*, 2nd ed. Yamada T (editor). Lippincott, 1995. (Review of pill-induced esophagitis and caustic esophageal injury.)

de Groen PC et al: Esophagitis associated with the use of alendronate. N Engl J Med 1996;335:1016. (Alendronate is approved for the treatment of postmenopausal osteoporosis. A significant side effect is severe ulcerative esophagitis. Patients must be educated about the proper means of ingestion.)

CAUSTIC ESOPHAGEAL INJURY

Caustic esophageal injury occurs from accidental (usually children) or deliberate (suicidal) ingestion of liquid or crystalline alkali (drain cleaners, etc) or acid. Ingestion is followed almost immediately by severe burning and varying degrees of chest pain, gagging, dysphagia, and drooling. Aspiration results in stridor and wheezing. Patients require urgent emergency room attention. Initial examination should be directed to circulatory status and to prompt assessment of airway status, including laryngoscopy. Subsequently, there should be a careful examination of the oral cavity, chest, and abdomen. Chest and abdominal radiographs are obtained looking for pneumonitis or free perforation. Initial treatment is supportive, with intravenous fluids and analgesics. Nasogastric lavage and oral antidotes may be dangerous and should generally not be administered. Most patients may be managed medically. Endoscopy is usually performed within the first 24 hours to assess the extent of injury. Many patients are discovered not to have any mucosal injury to the esophagus or stomach, allowing prompt discharge and psychiatric referral. Abnormal endoscopic appearance does not accurately predict the likelihood of transmural injury and perforation. All patients with mucosal damage must therefore be observed carefully in the first 72 hours for signs of deterioration. Circumferential injury to the esophagus portends an increased risk of stricture formation. Previously, antibiotics and corticosteroids were used acutely in an effort to decrease the incidence of stricture formation, but these have not been found to be effective. Surgery is indicated for sepsis, shock, perforation, or progressive deterioration.

Christesen H: Caustic ingestion in adults: Epidemiology and prevention. J Toxicol 1994;32:557.

BENIGN ESOPHAGEAL LESIONS

1. MALLORY-WEISS SYNDROME (Mucosal Laceration of Gastroesophageal Junction)

Essentials of Diagnosis

- Hematemesis; usually self-limited.
- Prior history of vomiting, retching in 50%.
- Endoscopy establishes diagnosis.

General Considerations

Mallory-Weiss syndrome is characterized by a nonpenetrating mucosal tear at the gastroesophageal junction which is hypothesized to arise from events that suddenly raise transabdominal pressure, such as lifting, retching, or vomiting. Alcoholism is a strong predisposing factor. Mallory-Weiss tears are responsible for approximately 5% of cases of upper gastrointestinal bleeding.

Clinical Findings

A. Symptoms and Signs: Patients usually present with hematemesis with or without melena. A history of antecedent retching, vomiting, or straining is obtained in about 50% of cases.

B. Special Examinations: As with other causes of upper gastrointestinal hemorrhage, upper endoscopy should be performed after the patient has been appropriately resuscitated. The diagnosis is established by identification of a 0.5–4 cm linear mucosal tear usually located either at the gastroesophageal junction or, more commonly, just below the junction in the gastric mucosa.

Differential Diagnosis

At endoscopy, other potential causes of upper gastrointestinal hemorrhage are found in over 35% of patients with Mallory-Weiss tears, including peptic ulcer disease, erosive gastritis, arteriovenous malformations, and esophageal varices. Patients with underlying portal hypertension are at higher risk of continued or recurrent bleeding.

Treatment

Patients are initially treated as needed with fluid resuscitation and blood transfusions. Most patients stop bleeding spontaneously and require no therapy. Endoscopic hemostatic therapy is employed in patients who have continued, active bleeding. Injection with epinephrine (1:10,000) or cautery with a bipolar or heater probe coagulation device is effective in 90–95%. Angiographic arterial embolization or operative intervention is required in patients who fail endoscopic therapy.

Bataller R et al: Endoscopic sclerotherapy in upper gastrointestinal bleeding due to the Mallory-Weiss syndrome. Am J Gastroenterol 1994;89:2147.

2. LOWER ESOPHAGEAL RING (Schatzki's Ring)

Schatzki's ring is a circumferential, thin, symmetric mucosal ring (< 4 mm in thickness) that occurs in the distal esophagus at the squamocolumnar junction. It is always associated with a hiatal hernia. Most are over 20 mm in diameter and are asymptomatic. Solid food dysphagia most often occurs with rings less than 13 mm in diameter. Characteristically, the dysphagia is intermittent and not progressive. Large, poorly chewed food boluses such as steak are most likely to cause dysphagia. Obstructing food boluses may pass by drinking extra liquids or are relieved by regurgitation. In some cases, an impacted bolus must be extracted endoscopically. Absence of gastroesophageal reflux symptoms and the nonprogressive nature of the dysphagia helps to distinguish Schatzki's ring from reflux-induced peptic strictures. Lower esophageal rings may be diagnosed by barium swallow or upper endoscopy.

The majority of symptomatic patients can be effectively and permanently treated with the passage of large (17–20 mm) bougie dilators, which disrupt the mucosal ring. A single dilation session usually suffices, but repeat dilations are sometimes necessary.

Rohrmann CA Jr: When is a Schatzki ring clinically significant, and what is the best maneuver to demonstrate it on barium swallow? Does the abnormality progress if it is not treated? AJR Am J Roentgenol 1994;163:215.

3. ESOPHAGEAL WEBS

Webs are thin membranes of squamous mucosa that typically occur in the mid or upper esophagus. They may be asymptomatic or cause intermittent solid food dysphagia. An association with iron deficiency anemia (Plummer-Vinson syndrome) has been noted but is extremely rare. The diagnosis is established by barium esophagography or upper endoscopy. Symptomatic webs are effectively treated with bougienage.

4. ESOPHAGEAL DIVERTICULA

Zenker's Diverticulum

Zenker's diverticulum is a protrusion of pharyngeal mucosa that develops at the pharyngoesophageal junction between the inferior pharyngeal constrictor and the cricopharyngeus. The cause is believed to be loss of elasticity of the upper esophageal sphincter, resulting in restricted opening during swallowing. Symptoms of dysphagia and regurgitation tend to develop insidiously over years in middle-aged to elderly patients. Initial symptoms include vague oropharyngeal dysphagia with coughing or throat discomfort. As the diverticulum enlarges and retains food, patients may note halitosis, spontaneous regurgitation of undigested food, nocturnal choking, gurgling in the throat, or a protrusion in the neck. Complications include aspiration pneumonia, bronchiectasis, and lung abscess. The diagnosis is best established by a barium esophagogram.

Symptomatic patients require surgical diverticulectomy and, in most cases, upper esophageal myotomy. Small asymptomatic diverticula may be observed.

Castell JA, Castell DO: Upper esophageal sphincter and pharyngeal function and oropharyngeal (transfer) dysphagia. Gastroenterol Clin North Am 1996;25:35.

Esophageal Diverticula

Diverticula may occur in the mid or distal esophagus. These may arise secondary to motility disorders (diffuse esophageal spasm, achalasia) or may develop above esophageal strictures. Diverticula are seldom symptomatic, and treatment is directed at the underlying disorder.

Ferraro P, Durancean A: Esophageal diverticula. Chest Surg Clin North Am 1994;4:741.

5. BENIGN ESOPHAGEAL NEOPLASMS

Benign tumors of the esophagus are quite rare. They are submucosal, the most common being leiomyomas. Most are asymptomatic and picked up incidentally on endoscopy or barium esophagography. Larger lesions can cause dysphagia. The major clinical importance of these lesions is to distinguish them from malignant neoplasms. At endoscopy, a smooth, sessile nodule is observed with normal overlying mucosal. Because the lesion is submucosal, endoscopic biopsies are generally nonrevealing. Endoscopic ultrasonography is extremely helpful to confirm the submucosal origin of the tumor.

6. ESOPHAGEAL VARICES

Essentials of Diagnosis

- Develop secondary to portal hypertension.
- Found in 50% of patients with cirrhosis.
- One-third of patients with varices develop upper gastrointestinal bleeding.
- Diagnosis established by upper endoscopy.

General Considerations

Esophageal varices are dilated submucosal veins that develop in patients with underlying portal hypertension and may result in serious upper gastrointestinal bleeding. The causes of portal hypertension are discussed elsewhere (Chapter 15). Under normal circumstances, there is a 2–6 mm Hg pressure gradient between the portal vein and the inferior vena cava. When the gradient exceeds 10 mm Hg, significant portal hypertension exists. Esophageal varices are the most common cause of important gastrointestinal bleeding due to portal hypertension, though gastric varices and, rarely, intestinal varices may also bleed. Bleeding from esophageal varices most commonly occurs in the distal 5 cm of the esophagus.

The most common cause of portal hypertension is cirrhosis. While approximately 50% of patients with cirrhosis have esophageal varices, only one-third of patients with varices develop serious bleeding from the varices. Bleeding esophageal varices have a higher morbidity and mortality rate than any other source of upper gastrointestinal bleeding. The mortality rate associated with acute bleeding episodes ranges from 15% to 40%, and over 60% of patients are dead within 5 years.

A number of factors have been identified that may portend an increased risk of bleeding from esophageal varices. The most important are (1) the size of the varices; (2) the presence at endoscopy of red wale markings on the varix (longitudinal markings that resemble whip marks); (3) the severity of liver disease (as assessed by Child scoring); and (4) active alcohol abuse—alcoholic cirrhotics who continue to drink have an extremely high risk of bleeding. The risk of bleeding correlates poorly with the absolute portosystemic pressure gradient, though bleeding almost never occurs with a gradient under 12 mm Hg.

Clinical Findings

A. Symptoms and Signs: Patients with esophageal varices that develop bleeding present with symptoms and signs of acute gastrointestinal bleeding (see Acute Upper Gastrointestinal Bleeding, above). Most commonly, patients present with spontaneous emesis of either bright red blood or "coffee grounds" material which is typically accompanied by melena or hematochezia. Rarely, varices present with hematochezia or melena alone in the absence of hematemesis. In some cases, there may be preceding retching or dyspepsia attributable to alcoholic gastritis or withdrawal. Varices per se do not cause symptoms of dyspepsia, dysphagia, or retching. Variceal bleeding usually is severe, resulting in hypovolemia manifested by postural vital signs or shock. Although the majority of patients with variceal bleeding have signs of chronic liver disease (eg, palmar erythema, spider angiomas, gynecomastia, asterixis, muscle wasting, splenomegaly, ascites, jaundice), 20–30% of patients with chronic liver disease are bleeding from a source other than esophageal varices.

B. Laboratory Findings: A complete blood count, platelet count, prothrombin time, and partial thromboplastin time, liver function tests, serum electrolytes, and serum albumin should be obtained in all patients. The initial hematocrit is a poor indicator of the severity of acute blood loss. Patients with underlying chronic liver disease often have an abnormal bilirubin, AST, ALT, a prolonged prothrombin time, and a low serum albumin.

Initial Management

A. Acute Resuscitation: The initial management of patients with acute upper gastrointestinal bleeding is discussed in the section on acute upper gastrointestinal bleeding (see above). Variceal hemorrhage may be life-threatening. Rapid patient assessment and resuscitation with fluids or blood products is essential. Many patients with bleeding esophageal varices have coagulopathy due to underlying cirrhosis; fresh frozen plasma or platelets should be administered to patients with an INR > 1.5 or platelets < 50,000/µL in the presence of active bleeding. Patients with advanced liver disease are at high risk of poor outcome regardless of the bleeding source and should be transferred to an ICU where constant monitoring can be provided. A nasogastric tube should be placed to evacuate the stomach (reducing nausea and vomiting) and to monitor for ongoing bleeding. Approximately 60–80% of variceal bleeders will stop spontaneously; however, without therapy, over half of these will rebleed within 1 week.

B. Emergent Endoscopy: Emergent endoscopy should be performed after the patient's hemodynamic status has been appropriately stabilized (usually within 2–12 hours). In patients with active bleeding, endotracheal intubation is commonly performed to protect against aspiration during endoscopy. A vigorous gastric lavage through a large-bore tube is performed prior to endoscopy to facilitate visualization. A careful endoscopic examination is then performed to exclude other causes of upper gastrointestinal bleeding such as a Mallory-Weiss tear, peptic ulcer disease, and portal hypertensive gastropathy. In most patients, variceal bleeding has stopped spontaneously by the time of endoscopy, and the diagnosis of variceal bleeding is made presumptively. Acute endoscopic treatment of the varices is performed with either banding or sclerotherapy. These techniques can arrest active bleeding in 90% of patients. Multiple trials indicate that these techniques can reduce the chance of early recurrent bleeding from 70% to 30–40%, but their impact upon in-hospital mortality is less clear.

To perform banding, a plastic hood encircled by small rubber bands is placed on the end of the endoscope. The varix is drawn into the hood by suction, and a rubber band is released by a trip wire around the varix. Several bands may be applied near the gastroesophageal junction and up to 5 cm proximally. Repeat banding sessions are repeated at intervals of 1–2 weeks until the varices are obliterated or reduced to a small size. Banding has been shown to achieve lower rates of rebleeding, complications, and death than sclerotherapy and should be considered the endoscopic treatment of choice for esophageal variceal bleeding.

Sclerotherapy is performed by advancing through the endoscope a disposable catheter with a retractable 25-gauge needle and injecting the variceal trunks with a sclerosing agent (eg, ethanolamine, tetradecyl sulfate). A repeat session is given at 3–7 days, followed by sessions at 1- to 3-week intervals, until the varices are obliterated. Complications occur in 20–30% and include chest pain, fever, bacteremia, esophageal ulceration, stricture, and perforation. However, sclerotherapy is still preferred by some endoscopists in the actively bleeding patient (in whom visualization for banding may be difficult) and by those with insufficient experience in banding.

C. Pharmacologic Therapy:

1. Antibiotic prophylaxis–Several randomized trials support the administration of prophylactic antibiotics to cirrhotic patients with gastrointestinal hemorrhage to reduce the incidence of infectious complications such as spontaneous bacterial peritonitis, bacteremia, pneumonia, and urinary tract infections. Administration of a quinolone (norfloxacin, ofloxacin, or ciprofloxacin, either intravenously or orally) for 3–10 days with a broad-spectrum antibiotic administered intravenously before endoscopy (amoxicillin-clavulanate or a third-generation cephalosporin) reduces the incidence of infections in this population from over 50% to less than 15%.

2. Octreotide–Somatostatin (not clinically available) and its long-acting synthetic analog, octreotide (25–100 µg/h), reduce splanchnic and hepatic blood flow and portal pressures in cirrhotic patients. These agents provide acute control of variceal bleeding in up to 80% of patients. Meta-analysis of multiple comparative trials has demonstrated that they are superior to vasopressin in the control of variceal bleeding and are without significant side effects. Moreover, two recent studies have demonstrated that a combination of octreotide and endoscopic therapy resulted in a significant reduction in rebleeding and transfusion requirements compared with endoscopic treatment alone. In patients with advanced liver disease and upper gastrointestinal hemorrhage, it is reasonable to initiate therapy with octreotide on admission. If bleeding is determined by subsequent endoscopy not to be secondary to portal hypertension, the infusion can be discontinued.

Vasopressin is a nonselective vasoconstrictor that reduces splanchnic flow and portal pressures but achieves control of variceal hemorrhage in only 50% of cases. Side effects occur in up to one-fourth of patients and include abdominal pain, myocardial or mesenteric ischemia, stroke, bradycardia, hypertension, and hyponatremia. Given the superior efficacy and safety of octreotide, the use of vasopressin can no longer be recommended.

3. Vitamin K–In cirrhotic patients with an abnormal prothrombin time, vitamin K (10 mg) should be administered subcutaneously.

4. Lactulose–Encephalopathy may complicate an episode of gastrointestinal bleeding in patients with severe liver disease. Lactulose, 30 mL twice daily, may be given to prevent encephalopathy, increasing the dose as needed to induce two or three stools per day (see Chapter 15).

D. Balloon Tube Tamponade: Mechanical tamponade with specially designed nasogastric tubes containing large gastric and esophageal balloons (Minnesota or Sengstaken-Blakemore tubes) provides initial control of active variceal hemorrhage in 60–90% of patients; however, rebleeding occurs in 50%. The gastric balloon is inflated first, followed by the esophageal balloon if bleeding continues. After balloon inflation, tension is applied to the tube to directly tamponade the varices. Complications of prolonged balloon inflation include esophageal and oral ulcerations, perforation, aspiration, and airway obstruction (due to a misplaced balloon). Endotracheal intubation is recommended before placement. Given its high rate of complications, mechanical tamponade should be used as a temporizing measure only in patients with bleeding that cannot be controlled with pharmacologic or endoscopic techniques until more definitive decompressive therapy (eg, TIPS) can be provided.

E. Portal Decompressive Procedures: In patients with variceal bleeding that cannot be controlled with pharmacologic or endoscopic therapy, emergency portal decompression is necessary.

1. Transvenous intrahepatic portosystemic shunts (TIPS)–A technique has been devised whereby angiographers pass via a transjugular route a needle-tip catheter into the hepatic vein, through the liver, and into the portal vein. Over a wire that is passed through the catheter, an expandable wire mesh stent (8–12 mm in diameter) is passed through the liver parenchyma, creating a portosystemic shunt from the portal vein to the hepatic vein. The rate of severe complications is only 1–2%. TIPS can control acute hemorrhage in over 90% of patients actively bleeding from gastric or esophageal varices. TIPS is indicated in the 10% of patients with acute variceal bleeding who cannot be controlled with pharmacologic and endoscopic therapy. It is not indicated as initial therapy to control variceal hemorrhage.

2. Emergency portosystemic shunt surgery–In most series, emergency portosystemic shunt surgery is associated with a 40–60% mortality rate. At centers where TIPS is available, that procedure has become the preferred means of providing emergency portal decompression.

Prevention of Rebleeding

Once the initial bleeding episode has been controlled, the risk of rebleeding is 60–80%. The highest incidence of rebleeding is in the first six weeks. Several options are available to decrease the likelihood of rebleeding, though their relative merits are controversial. Use of these approaches varies in different medical centers.

A. Endoscopic Techniques: Multiple trials demonstrate that long-term treatment with sclerotherapy or band ligation reduces the incidence of rebleeding to 30–50%. Meta-analysis of these trials suggests that the mortality rate is also reduced. Band ligation of the varix appears to be equal or superior to sclerotherapy in preventing rebleeding and is associated with a significantly lower complication rate. In most patients, four to six treatment sessions are needed to eradicate the varices. Where expertise is available, endoscopic therapy is generally the preferred approach to long-term therapy of esophageal varices.

B. Beta-Blockers: Multiple trials have demonstrated that nonselective beta-adrenergic blockers (propranolol, nadolol) are effective in reducing the incidence of rebleeding from esophageal varices and portal hypertensive gastropathy compared with placebo. An improvement in mortality statistics has not been shown. In comparative trials and meta-analyses, the efficacy is comparable to that of sclerotherapy. Combination therapy with beta-blockers and sclerotherapy appears to be superior to sclerotherapy alone. Therefore, patients without contraindications to beta-blockers should be started on propranolol, 20 mg twice daily, or nadolol, 40 mg once daily. The dosage is increased gradually until the heart rate falls by 25% or reaches 55 beats/min. An average dose is propranolol or nadolol, 80 mg once daily.

C. TIPS: TIPS is reserved for patients who have recurrent variceal bleeding (more than two episodes) despite the above therapies. The rate of rebleeding at 1 year after placement is less than 20% and is superior to endoscopic therapy. Despite this greater efficacy, a National Digestive Diseases Advisory Board has stated that TIPS is not indicated in the initial therapy to prevent recurrent bleeding until endoscopic or pharmacologic therapies have failed. Stenosis and thrombosis of the stents occurs in over 30% of patients but can be successfully treated. Encephalopathy occurs in 25% of patients. TIPS is also used in patients with recurrent bleeding from gastric varices or portal hypertensive gastropathy (for which sclerotherapy cannot be used). TIPS should also be considered in patients who are noncompliant with other therapies or who live in remote locations (without access to emergency care).

D. Surgical Portosystemic Shunts: Shunt surgery has a significantly lower rate of rebleeding compared with endoscopic therapy but also a higher incidence of encephalopathy. Selective (distal splenorenal) shunts have a lower incidence of encephalopathy than portacaval shunts but are more difficult to perform. In most centers, shunt surgery has been reserved for patients who have failed sclerotherapy or for noncompliant patients. With the advent of TIPS, the role of surgical shunts is unclear.

E. Liver Transplantation: Candidacy for orthotopic liver transplantation should be assessed in all patients with chronic liver disease and bleeding due to portal hypertension. Transplant candidates should be treated with sclerotherapy or TIPS to control bleeding pretransplant.

Prevention of First Episodes of Variceal Bleeding

Because of the high mortality rate associated with variceal hemorrhage, prevention of the initial bleeding episode is desirable. Nonselective beta-adrenergic blockers (nadolol, propranolol) have been shown in multiple trials to decrease the long-term risk of bleeding to 16% (compared with 27% in placebo-treated patients). Up to 15% of patients do not tolerate beta-blocker therapy. Because variceal bleeding occurs in only one-third of cirrhotics, it may be reasonable to use beta-blockers in compliant higher-risk patients, ie, patients with large varices or red wale markings. Prophylactic sclerotherapy in those who have never had a variceal hemorrhage has been shown to result in a higher mortality rate than placebo or treatment with beta-blockers and should not be done.

Besson I et al: Sclerotherapy with or without octreotide for acute variceal bleeding. N Engl J Med 1995;333:55.

Imperiale T et al: A meta-analysis of somatostatin versus vasopressin in the management of acute new esophageal variceal hemorrhage. Gastroenterology 1995;109:1289.

Jutabha R, Jensen DM: Management of upper gastrointestinal bleeding in the patient with chronic liver disease. Med Clin North Am 1996;80:1035.

Kamath PS, McKusick MA: Transvenous intrahepatic portosystemic shunts. Gastroenterology 1996;111:1700.

Laine L, Cook D: Endoscopic ligation compared with sclerotherapy for treatment of esophageal variceal bleeding: A meta-analysis. Ann Intern Med 1995;123:280.

Villanueva C et al: Nadolol plus isosorbide mononitrate compared with sclerotherapy for the prevention of variceal rebleeding. N Engl J Med 1996;334:1624. (As compared with sclerotherapy, nadolol plus isosorbide mononitrate significantly decreased the risk of rebleeding from esophageal varices.)

MALIGNANT ESOPHAGEAL LESIONS (Cancer of the Esophagus)

Essentials of Diagnosis

- Progressive solid food dysphagia.
- Weight loss common.
- Endoscopy with biopsy establishes diagnosis.

General Considerations

Esophageal cancer usually develops in persons be-

tween 50 and 70 years of age. The overall ratio of men to women is 3:1. There are two histologic types: squamous cell carcinoma and adenocarcinoma. In the United States, squamous cell cancer is much more common in blacks than whites. Chronic alcohol and tobacco use are strongly associated with an increased risk of squamous cell carcinoma. The risk of cancer is also increased in patients with tylosis, achalasia, caustic-induced esophageal stricture, and other head and neck cancers. Approximately half of cases occur in the distal third of the esophagus and the other half in the proximal two-thirds. Adenocarcinoma is more common in whites. It is increasing dramatically in incidence and now is as common as squamous carcinoma. The vast majority of adenocarcinomas develop as a complication of Barrett's metaplasia due to chronic gastroesophageal reflux. Thus, most adenocarcinomas arise in the distal third of the esophagus.

Clinical Findings

A. Symptoms and Signs: Most patients with esophageal cancer present with advanced, incurable disease. More than 90% of patients have solid food dysphagia, which progresses over weeks to months. Odynophagia is sometimes present. Significant weight loss is common. Local tumor extension into the tracheobronchial tree may result in a tracheoesophageal fistula, characterized by coughing on swallowing or pneumonia. Chest or back pain suggests mediastinal extension. Recurrent laryngeal involvement may produce hoarseness. Physical examination is often unrevealing. The presence of supraclavicular or cervical lymphadenopathy or of hepatomegaly implies metastatic disease.

B. Laboratory Findings: Laboratory findings are nonspecific. Anemia related to chronic disease or occult blood loss is common. Abnormal aminotransferase or alkaline phosphatase concentrations suggest hepatic or bony metastases. Hypoalbuminemia may result from malnutrition.

C. Imaging: Chest x-rays may show adenopathy, a widened mediastinum, pulmonary or bony metastases, or signs of tracheoesophageal fistula such as pneumonia. A barium esophagogram often is obtained by clinicians as the first study to evaluate dysphagia. The appearance of a polypoid, infiltrative, or ulcerative lesion is suggestive of carcinoma and requires endoscopic evaluation. However, even lesions felt to be benign by radiography warrant endoscopic evaluation.

D. Upper Endoscopy: Endoscopy with biopsy establishes the diagnosis of esophageal carcinoma with a high degree of reliability. In some cases, significant submucosal spread of the tumor may yield nondiagnostic mucosal biopsies. Repeated biopsy may be necessary.

Differential Diagnosis

Esophageal carcinoma must be distinguished from

other causes of progressive dysphagia, including peptic stricture, achalasia, and adenocarcinoma of the gastric cardia with esophageal involvement. Benign-appearing peptic strictures should be biopsied at presentation to exclude occult malignancy.

Staging of Disease

After confirmation of the diagnosis of esophageal carcinoma, the stage of the disease should be determined since doing so influences the choice of therapy. Patients should undergo evaluation with CT of the chest and liver to look for evidence of pulmonary or hepatic metastases, lymphadenopathy, and local tumor extension. If there is no evidence of distant metastases or extensive local spread on CT, endoscopic ultrasonography should be performed, which is superior to CT in demonstrating the level of local mediastinal extension and local lymph node involvement. Bronchoscopy is sometimes required in proximal esophageal cancer to exclude tracheobronchial extension. Apart from distant metastasis, the two most important predictors of poor survival are lymph node involvement and adjacent mediastinal spread.

Stages are determined by the TNM classification as set forth in the accompanying box.

Staging Criteria for Esophageal Cancer

Primary Tumor (T)
  T1: Invasion of lamina propria or submucosa
  T2: Invasion of muscularis propria
  T3: Invasion of adventitia
  T4: Invasion of adjacent structures
Regional Lymph Nodes (N)
  N0: No regional lymph node involvement
  N1: Regional lymph node involvement
Distant Metastasis (M)
  M1: Distant metastasis
  M0: No metastasis
Based upon these parameters, the tumor is classified as:
  Stage I: T1, N0, M0
  Stage IIA: T2 or T3, and N0, M0
  Stage IIB: T1 or T2, and N1, M0
  Stage III: T3, N1, M0 or T4, any N, M0
  Stage IV: Any T or N, M1

Treatment

The approach to esophageal cancer depends upon the tumor stage as well as the local opinions of the attending surgeons, oncologists, and radiotherapists. There is no consensus about the optimal treatment approach. It is helpful, however, to classify patients into two general categories.

A. Palliative Therapy: Patients with extensive local tumor spread (T4) or distant metastases (M1) are incurable, ie, most patients with stage III and all with stage IV tumors. The goal in these patients is to provide relief from dysphagia and pain. The optimal palliative approach depends upon the patient's ex-

pected survival, patient preference, and local institutional experience. None of these modalities prolong survival.

1. Surgical resection–Palliative resection of the esophagus provides the most rapid and durable relief of dysphagia. For reasonably well nourished patients without other serious comorbid medical problems (ie, suitable surgical candidates) who have an expected survival of more than 6–12 months, this may be recommended provided there is no significant involvement of mediastinal structures.

2. Radiation therapy–For patients with unresectable disease and for poor operative candidates, radiation therapy may afford significant short-term palliation of pain and dysphagia. During therapy, esophagitis may lead to worsening of dysphagia and odynophagia.

3. Local tumor therapy–Palliation of dysphagia may be achieved by peroral placement of expandable, permanent wire stents or by application of endoscopic laser therapy. Although dysphagia is improved significantly, patients can seldom eat normally. Complications of stents include perforation, migration, and tumor ingrowth. These are most suitable for patients with a short life expectancy; patients who have failed radiation therapy; or patients in locations where optimal surgical or radiation modalities are not available.

B. "Curable" Disease: The approach to the remainder of patients is controversial and highly dependent upon institutional experience. Currently, there are three broad categories of therapy that may be considered.

1. Surgery alone–There is controversy over the optimal surgical approach. The procedure with the lowest morbidity is transhiatal esophagectomy with anastomosis of the stomach to the cervical esophagus. Critics of this approach note that because it does not involve sampling or removal of mediastinal lymph nodes, it is not suitable as a "curative" approach for node-positive disease. Alternatively, many surgeons recommend transthoracic excision of the esophagus with nodal resection. Critics of this approach note that it has a higher morbidity and no better survival than the transhiatal approach. Regardless of the approach elected, overall 3-year survival after surgery is less than 15% in most series.

2. Chemotherapy plus radiation therapy–Combined therapy with chemotherapy and radiation therapy is superior to radiation therapy alone and has achieved overall survival rates that equal or exceed those of historical surgical cohorts, though there have been no trials specifically comparing these approaches. However, severe side effects occur commonly with combined therapy. The most promising chemotherapeutic agents have been cisplatin and fluorouracil.

3. Surgery with neoadjuvant chemotherapy and radiation therapy–In recent trials, patients have been treated with radiation therapy and chemotherapy (cisplatin and fluorouracil) prior to surgical resection. Trials comparing surgery preceded by neoadjuvant therapy with surgery alone report 3-year survival rates of 32% in the combined treatment group versus 6% in the group receiving surgery alone. Further comparisons of this multimodal treatment versus surgery are needed, and this approach currently should not be used outside of clinical trials.

Prognosis

The overall 5-year survival rate of esophageal carcinoma is less than 15%. Despite improvements in surgical mortality and increased surgical resectability rates, the prognosis of this disease has not changed for years, in part because most patients present with advanced disease. This suggests that surgical approaches alone are inadequate for most patients.

[National Cancer Institute PDQ Internet Information for Esophageal Cancer]
   gopher://gopher.nih.gov:70/00/clin/cancernet/pdqinfo/ soa/Esophageal%20cancer_Physician
Hennessy TP: Cancer of the esophagus. Postgrad Med J 1996;72:458.
Kelsen DP, Ilson DH: Chemotherapy and combined-modality therapy for esophageal cancer. Chest 1995;107(6 Suppl):224S.
Sibille A et al: Long-term survival after photodynamic therapy for esophageal cancer. Gastroenterology 1995;108: 337.
Stahl M et al: Combined preoperative chemotherapy and radiotherapy in patients with locally advanced esophageal cancer: Interim analysis of a Phase II trial. J Clin Oncol 1996;14:829.
Swisher S et al: Changes in the surgical management of esophageal cancer from 1970 to 1993. Am J Surg 1995;169:609.
Walsh TN et al: A comparison of multimodal therapy and surgery for esophageal adenocarcinoma. N Engl J Med 1996;335:462.

ESOPHAGEAL MOTILITY DISORDERS

1. ACHALASIA

Essentials of Diagnosis

- Gradual, progressive dysphagia for solids and liquids.
- Regurgitation of undigested food.
- Barium esophagogram with "bird's beak" distal esophagus.
- Esophageal manometry confirms diagnosis.

General Considerations

Achalasia is an idiopathic motility disorder characterized by loss of peristalsis in the distal two-thirds (smooth muscle) of the esophagus and impaired relaxation of the lower esophageal sphincter. There appears to be denervation of the esophagus resulting from loss of ganglion cells in Auerbach's plexus and degeneration of the vagus nerve and dorsal motor nucleus.

Clinical Findings

A. Symptoms and Signs: Symptoms usually develop in patients between the ages of 25 and 60 years. Patients complain of the gradual onset of dysphagia for solid foods and, in the majority, of liquids also. Symptoms at presentation may have persisted for months to years. Substernal discomfort or fullness may be noted after eating. Many patients eat more slowly and adopt specific maneuvers such as lifting the neck or throwing the shoulders back in order to enhance esophageal emptying. Regurgitation of undigested food is common and may occur during meals or up to several hours later. Nocturnal regurgitation can provoke coughing or aspiration. Weight loss is common. Physical examination is unhelpful.

B. Imaging: Chest x-rays may show an air-fluid level in the enlarged, fluid-filled esophagus. Barium esophagography has characteristic findings, including esophageal dilation, loss of esophageal peristalsis, poor esophageal emptying, and a smooth, symmetric "bird's beak" tapering of the distal esophagus. Without treatment, the esophagus may become markedly dilated ("sigmoid esophagus").

C. Special Examinations: After esophagography, endoscopy is always performed to evaluate the distal esophagus and gastroesophageal junction in order to exclude a distal stricture or a submucosal infiltrating carcinoma. The diagnosis is confirmed by esophageal manometry. The typical manometric features are as follows: (1) Complete absence of peristalsis; swallowing results in simultaneous waves which are usually of low amplitude. (2) Incomplete lower esophageal sphincteric relaxation with swallowing. Whereas the normal sphincter relaxes by over 90%, relaxation with most swallows in patients with achalasia is less than 50%. In many patients, the baseline lower esophageal sphincteric pressure is quite elevated. (3) Intraesophageal pressures are greater than gastric pressures due to a fluid- and food-filled esophagus.

Differential Diagnosis

Chagas' disease is associated with esophageal dysfunction that is indistinguishable from idiopathic achalasia and should be considered in patients from endemic regions (Central and South America). Primary or metastatic tumors can invade the gastroesophageal junction, resulting in a picture resembling that of achalasia, called "pseudoachalasia." Endoscopic ultrasonography and chest CT may be required to examine the distal esophagus in suspicious cases. Achalasia must be distinguished from other motility disorders such as diffuse esophageal spasm and scleroderma esophagus with a peptic stricture.

Treatment

A. Botulinum Toxin Injection: Endoscopically guided injection of botulinum toxin directly into the lower esophageal sphincter results in a marked reduction in lower esophageal sphincter pressure and sustained improvement in symptoms in two-thirds of patients for 6–24 months. Two-thirds of initial responders have improvement after a second injection. The efficacy of further treatments is not established. At present, this therapy may be most appropriate for elderly patients or those with multiple medical problems who are poor candidates for more invasive procedures.

B. Pneumatic Dilation: Over two-thirds of patients derive good to excellent relief of dysphagia after one or two sessions of pneumatic dilation of the lower esophageal sphincter. Under fluoroscopic guidance, 3- to 4-cm diameter balloons are inflated across the gastroesophageal junction in an effort to permanently disrupt the sphincter. Perforations occur in 5% of dilations and may require operative repair.

C. Surgical Myotomy: Surgical therapy is generally reserved for patients who have failed to improve after pneumatic dilation or botulinum toxin injection. A Heller myotomy of the lower esophageal sphincter results in symptomatic relief in over 85% of patients but results in gastroesophageal reflux and esophagitis in 10% of patients. Myotomy is now performed with a laparoscopic or thoracoscopic approach. Patients with a tortuous, markedly dilated "sigmoid" esophagus may require complete esophagectomy.

Prognosis

If treatment is provided before marked esophageal dilation develops, swallowing is near normal in most patients. The incidence of squamous carcinoma of the esophagus is increased 16-fold regardless of therapy.

Oddsdottir M: Laparoscopic management of achalasia. Surg Clin North Am 1996;76:451.

Pasricha PJ et al: Botulinum toxin for achalasia: Long-term outcome and predictors of response. Gastroenterology 1996;110:1410.

Sandler R et al: The risk of esophageal cancer in patients with achalasia. JAMA 1995;274:1359.

2. DIFFUSE ESOPHAGEAL SPASM

Diffuse esophageal spasm is an uncommon motility disorder characterized by intermittent dysphagia for solids and liquids which is generally nonprogressive. Periods of normal swallowing may alternate with periods of dysphagia, which is generally mild. Dysphagia may be provoked by stress, large boluses, or hot or cold liquids. Patients may also note anterior chest pain, which can be confused with angina pectoris but is not usually exertional. The pain is often unrelated to eating. Barium esophagography may detect simultaneous ("tertiary") contractions characterized as a "corkscrew" or "rosary bead" appearance. On esophageal manometry, intermittent simultaneous contractions (> 10% of swallows) are recorded along with periods of normal peristalsis.

Diffuse esophageal spasm is generally a mild condition that is not life-threatening. Therapy is directed at symptom reduction and reassurance. Nitrates (isosorbide dinitrate, 10–30 mg four times daily; nitroglycerin, 0.4 mg sublingually as needed) and calcium channel blockers (nifedipine, 10–30 mg four times daily; diltiazem, 60–90 mg four times daily) are reported to be effective, though no controlled trials have been conducted. Dilation with Maloney bougies provides symptomatic relief in some cases for unclear reasons. Rarely, a long surgical myotomy is required in debilitated patients.

Allen ML, Di Marino AJ Jr: Manometric diagnosis of diffuse esophageal spasm. Dig Dis Sci 1996;41:1346.

3. SCLERODERMA ESOPHAGUS

Esophageal involvement is common in patients with progressive systemic sclerosis or the CREST syndrome, especially those who have Raynaud's phenomenon. Atrophy and fibrosis of the esophageal smooth muscle results in loss of lower esophageal sphincteric competency and markedly diminished esophageal peristaltic amplitude. Acid gastroesophageal reflux results and can cause a severe erosive esophagitis, sometimes resulting in the development of Barrett's esophagus or peptic stricture. Patients report heartburn or dysphagia. The dysphagia may be secondary to impaired peristalsis or may be due to peptic stricture. Barium esophagography demonstrates absent peristalsis in the distal esophagus and a patulous lower esophageal sphincter with free reflux. Esophageal manometry confirms a low or absent lower esophageal sphincteric pressure and markedly diminished peristaltic amplitude in the distal two-thirds of the esophagus. Aggressive therapy for the acid gastroesophageal reflux with antisecretory therapy and cisapride (see above) is given in order to prevent reflux complications. Peptic strictures may require dilation.

4. OTHER MOTILITY DISORDERS

A variety of other motility disorders have been characterized by manometry. These include nutcracker esophagus, hypertensive lower esophageal sphincter, and nonspecific motility abnormalities. These manometric findings are commonly identified in patients complaining of dysphagia or noncardiac chest pain. A cause-and-effect relationship between these manometric disorders and the patients' symptoms, however, is unproved. Symptomatic patients with these manometric abnormalities have a high incidence of psychiatric disorders, including depression, anxiety, panic disorder, and tendencies toward somatization and hypochondriasis. These esophageal manometric findings may represent markers of chronic psychologic stress and a clinical pain syndrome.

Dent J, Holloway RH: Esophageal motility and reflux testing: State-of-the-art and clinical role in the twenty-first century. Gastroenterol Clin North Am 1996;25:51.

Parkman HP et al: Optimal evaluation of patients with nonobstructive esophageal dysphagia: Manometry, scintigraphy, or videoesophagography? Dig Dis Sci 1996;41:1355. (Manometry is the most accurate means of diagnosing esophageal motility disorders; however, videoesophagography has excellent accuracy, lower cost, and better patient acceptance.)

CHEST PAIN OF UNDETERMINED ORIGIN

Approximately 30% of patients with chest pain who undergo cardiac evaluation do not have an apparent cardiac cause of their symptoms. Patients with recurrent noncardiac chest pain can pose a difficult clinical problem. Because coronary artery disease is common and serious and can present in atypical fashion, it is imperative that it be excluded prior to evaluation for other noncardiac causes.

Causes of noncardiac chest pain may include the following.

A. Chest Wall and Thoracic Spine Disease: These are easily diagnosed by history and physical examination.

B. Gastroesophageal Reflux: Up to 25% of patients have increased amounts of gastroesophageal acid reflux. An empirical trial of acid suppressive therapy with omeprazole 40 mg or lansoprazole 30 mg for 4 weeks is recommended, especially in patients with reflux symptoms. In some cases, an ambulatory esophageal pH study is warranted in an effort to document a relationship between acid reflux episodes and chest pain events.

C. Heightened Visceral Sensitivity: Recent studies suggest that most patients with noncardiac chest pain report pain in response to a variety of minor noxious stimuli such as intraesophageal acid infusion, inflation of balloons within the esophageal lumen, injection of intravenous edrophonium (a cholinergic stimulus), or intracardiac catheter manipulation. Controlled treatment trials demonstrate efficacy of low doses of antidepressants such as trazodone or imipramine 50 mg in reducing chest pain symptoms. These agents are hypothesized to reduce visceral afferent awareness.

D. Psychologic: A significant number of patients have underlying depression, anxiety, and panic disorder. Such patients may benefit from appropriate therapy. Patients reporting dyspnea, sweating, tachycardia, a sense of suffocation, dizziness, or fear of dying should be evaluated for panic disorder.

E. Esophageal Dysmotility: Esophageal motility abnormalities such as diffuse esophageal spasm are a rare cause of noncardiac chest pain. Stationary or ambulatory manometry is not recommended in the routine evaluation of this disorder because of the low specificity of these procedures and the unlikelihood of finding a clinically significant disorder. In patients with chest pain and dysphagia, a barium swallow x-ray should be obtained initially to look for evidence of achalasia or diffuse esophageal spasm.

Cannon RO et al: Imipramine in patients with chest pain despite normal coronary angiograms. N Engl J Med 1994;330:1411.

Frobert O et al: Diagnostic value of esophageal studies in patients with angina-like chest pain and normal coronary angiograms. Ann Intern Med 1996;124:959.

Goyal RK: Changing focus of unexplained esophageal chest pain. Ann Intern Med 1996;124:1008.

Rao SS et al: Unexplained chest pain: The hypersensitive, hyperreactive, and poorly compliant esophagus. Ann Intern Med 1996;124:950.

DISEASES OF THE STOMACH & DUODENUM

GASTRITIS & GASTROPATHY

The term "gastritis" is beset by semantic confusion. Endoscopists employ the term to denote a number of gross mucosal features such as erythema, subepithelial hemorrhages, and erosions; to the pathologist, the term denotes histologic inflammation. The term "gastropathy" is used increasingly to denote conditions in which there is epithelial or endothelial damage without inflammation. Gastritis may be divided into three categories: (1) erosive and hemorrhagic gastritis; (2) nonerosive, nonspecific (histologic) gastritis; and (3) specific types of gastritis, characterized by distinctive histologic and endoscopic features that may be diagnostic of a disorder.

1. EROSIVE & HEMORRHAGIC GASTRITIS

Essentials of Diagnosis

- Most commonly seen in alcoholics, critically ill patients, or patients taking NSAIDs.

- Often asymptomatic; may cause epigastric pain, nausea, and vomiting.
- May cause hematemesis; usually not significant bleeding.

General Considerations

The most common causes of erosive gastritis are drugs (especially NSAIDs), alcohol, stress due to severe medical or surgical illness ("stress gastritis"), and portal hypertension ("portal gastropathy"). Uncommon causes include caustic ingestion and radiation. Erosive and hemorrhagic gastritis typically are diagnosed at endoscopy, often being performed because of dyspepsia or upper gastrointestinal bleeding. Endoscopic findings include subepithelial hemorrhages, petechiae, and erosions. These lesions are superficial, vary in size and number, and may be focal or diffuse. There usually is no significant inflammation on histologic examination, though gastropathy may be present.

Clinical Findings

A. Symptoms and Signs: Erosive gastritis is usually asymptomatic. Symptoms, when they occur, include anorexia, epigastric pain, nausea, and vomiting. There is poor correlation between symptoms and the number or severity of endoscopic abnormalities. The most common clinical manifestation of erosive gastritis is upper gastrointestinal bleeding, which presents as hematemesis, "coffee grounds" emesis, or bloody aspirate in a patient receiving nasogastric suction, or as melena. Because erosive gastritis is superficial, hemodynamically significant bleeding is rare.

B. Laboratory Findings: The laboratory findings are nonspecific. The hematocrit is low if significant bleeding has occurred.

C. Special Examination: Upper endoscopy is the most sensitive method of diagnosis. Although bleeding from gastritis is usually insignificant, it cannot be distinguished on clinical grounds from more serious lesions such as peptic ulcers or esophageal varices. Hence, endoscopy is generally performed within 24 hours in patients with upper gastrointestinal bleeding to identify the source. An upper gastrointestinal series is sometimes obtained in lieu of endoscopy in patients with hemodynamically insignificant upper gastrointestinal bleeds to exclude serious lesions but is insensitive for the detection of gastritis.

Differential Diagnosis

Epigastric pain may be due to peptic ulcer, gastroesophageal reflux, gastric cancer, biliary tract disease, food poisoning, viral gastroenteritis, and functional dyspepsia. With severe pain, one should consider a perforated or penetrating ulcer, pancreatic disease, esophageal rupture, ruptured aortic aneurysm, gastric volvulus, and myocardial colic. Causes of upper gastrointestinal bleeding include peptic ulcer disease, esophageal varices, Mallory-Weiss tear, and arteriovenous malformations.

Specific Causes & Treatment
A. Stress Gastritis:

1. Prophylaxis—Stress-related mucosal erosions and subepithelial hemorrhages develop within 18 hours in the majority of critically ill patients. Clinically overt bleeding occurs in 6% but clinically important bleeding in less than 2–3%. Bleeding is associated with a higher mortality rate but is seldom the cause of death. Major risk factors include trauma, burns, hypotension, sepsis, central nervous system injury, coagulopathy, mechanical respiration, hepatic or renal failure, and multiorgan failure.

Pharmacologic prophylaxis with sucralfate or H_2 receptor antagonists in critically ill patients has been shown to reduce the incidence of clinically overt and significant bleeding by 50%. Prophylaxis should be routinely administered upon admission to critically ill patients with risk factors for significant bleeding. In multiple regression analyses, two of the most important risk factors are coagulopathy and respiratory failure with the need for mechanical ventilation. When these two risk factors are absent, the risk of significant bleeding is only 0.1%. Most ICU patients are at low risk of stress-related bleeding and do not require pharmacologic prophylaxis.

There is ongoing debate whether sucralfate or H_2 receptor antagonists are the preferred prophylactic agent. Sucralfate suspension (1 g orally every 4–6 hours) is comparable in efficacy to H_2 receptor antagonists in the prevention of stress-related bleeding and is associated with a 20% lower incidence of nosocomial pneumonia. Given its comparable efficacy, lower cost, and lower incidence of side effects, it is now the preferred prophylactic agent in many ICUs. Alternatively, infusions of H_2 receptor antagonists at a dose sufficient to maintain intragastric pH above 4.0 may be given. Cimetidine (900–1200 mg), ranitidine (150 mg), or famotidine (20 mg) by continuous intravenous infusion over 24 hours is adequate to control pH in most patients. After 4 hours of infusion, the pH should be checked by nasogastric aspirate and the dose doubled if the pH is under 4.0. Proton pump inhibitors should not be used in the ICU for prophylaxis owing to unpredictable oral absorption in such patients.

2. Treatment—Patients in whom stress gastritis results in clinically significant bleeding should receive continuous infusions of an H_2 receptor antagonist as well as sucralfate suspension. Because bleeding is diffuse, endoscopic hemostasis techniques are not helpful. Nevertheless, endoscopy is often performed in such patients to look for other treatable causes of upper gastrointestinal bleeding.

B. NSAID Gastritis: Although half of patients receiving NSAIDs on a chronic basis have gastritis at endoscopy, symptoms of dyspepsia develop in less than one-fourth. Furthermore, of patients with dyspepsia, up to half do not have significant mucosal abnormalities. Given the frequency of dyspeptic symptoms in patients taking NSAIDs, it is neither feasible nor desirable to investigate all such patients. Symptoms may improve with discontinuation of the agent, reduction to the lowest effective dose, or administration with meals. Patients with persistent symptoms despite conservative measures or patients at high risk for NSAID-induced ulcers (see section on peptic ulcer disease) should undergo diagnostic endoscopy. Those without significant NSAID ulceration may be treated symptomatically with sucralfate (1 g four times daily), with H_2 receptor antagonists given twice daily (cimetidine 400 mg, ranitidine 150 mg, or famotidine 20 mg), or with proton pump inhibitors once daily (omeprazole 20 mg or lansoprazole 30 mg). Upper gastrointestinal bleeding due to NSAID gastritis is usually not severe.

C. Alcoholic Gastritis: Erosive and hemorrhagic gastritis account for 20% of episodes of upper gastrointestinal bleeding in chronic alcoholics. These episodes are usually mild and respond to withdrawal of alcohol. Therapy with H_2 receptor antagonists or sucralfate for 2–4 weeks often is prescribed.

D. Portal Hypertensive Gastropathy: Portal hypertension results in gastric mucosal and submucosal congestion of capillaries and venules. Bleeding from congestive gastropathy accounts for 25% of episodes of upper gastrointestinal bleeding in patients with portal hypertension. It may present suddenly with hematemesis or insidiously with iron deficiency anemia. Recurrent acute bleeding is common. Treatment with propranolol reduces the incidence of recurrent acute bleeding by lowering portal pressures. Patients who fail propranolol therapy may be successfully treated with portal decompressive procedures (see section on treatment of esophageal varices).

Carpenter HA, Talley NJ: Gastroscopy is incomplete without biopsy: Clinical relevance of distinguishing gastropathy from gastritis. Gastroenterology 1995;108:917.

Cook DJ et al: Risk factors for gastrointestinal bleeding in critically ill patients. N Engl J Med 1994;330:377.

Cook DJ et al: Stress ulcer prophylaxis in critically ill patients: Resolving discordant meta-analyses. JAMA 1996;275:308.

Miller TA: Stress erosive gastritis: What is optimal therapy and who should undergo it? Gastroenterology 1995; 109:626.

2. NONEROSIVE, NONSPECIFIC GASTRITIS

The diagnosis of nonerosive gastritis is based upon histologic assessment of mucosal biopsies. Endoscopic findings are normal in many cases and do not reliably predict the presence of histologic inflammation. The main types of nonerosive gastritis are those due to *H pylori* infection, those associated with pernicious anemia, and lymphocytic gastritis. (See Specific Types of Gastritis.)

Helicobacter pylori Gastritis

H pylori is a spiral gram-negative rod that resides beneath the gastric mucus layer adjacent to gastric epithelial cells. Although it is not invasive, it causes gastric mucosal inflammation with polymorphonuclear neutrophils and lymphocytes. The mechanisms of injury and inflammation may in part be related to the products of two genes, *vacA* and *cagA*.

In the United States, the prevalence of infection rises from less than 10% in Caucasians under age 30 to over 50% in those over age 60. The prevalence is higher in non-Caucasians and immigrants from developing countries and is correlated inversely with socioeconomic status. Transmission is from person to person, but the mode of spread is not known. The majority of infections are probably acquired in childhood.

Acute infection with *H pylori* may cause a transient clinical illness characterized by nausea and abdominal pain that may last for several days and is associated with acute histologic gastritis with polymorphonuclear neutrophils. After these symptoms resolve, it is believed that the majority progress to chronic infection with chronic, diffuse mucosal inflammation characterized by polymorphonuclear neutrophils and lymphocytes. Inflammation may be confined to the superficial gastric epithelium or may extend deeper into the gastric glands, resulting in varying degrees of gland atrophy (atrophic gastritis) and metaplasia of the gastric epithelium to intestinal type epithelium.

Although chronic *H pylori* infection with gastritis is present in 30–50% of the population, the vast majority are asymptomatic and suffer no sequelae. *H pylori* infection is strongly associated with peptic ulcer disease; however, only 15% of people with chronic infection develop a peptic ulcer (see section on peptic ulcer disease). Chronic *H pylori* gastritis is associated with a four- to sixfold increased risk of gastric adenocarcinoma and low-grade B cell gastric lymphoma (MALToma). There is no convincing evidence that chronic *H pylori*-associated gastritis is a cause of dyspeptic symptoms in patients without ulcer disease.

The only indication for investigating for *H pylori* infection is in patients with peptic ulcer disease. *H pylori* is detected by a variety of invasive and noninvasive means, all of which have greater than 90% sensitivity and specificity. At endoscopy, gastric mucosal biopsies can be assessed for urease activity by placing them in a pH-sensitive medium. Production of ammonia by the urease-secreting organism produces a color change in the medium within 3 hours—presumptive evidence of *H pylori*. This simple, inexpensive test is the preferred method of endoscopic diagnosis. Histologic assessment of gastric biopsies is more definitive but more expensive than the rapid urease test. The absence of chronic antral gastritis on histologic examination definitively excludes *H pylori*. *H pylori* cultures of mucosal biopsies are less sensitive and more expensive tests than other endoscopic tests and are seldom used.

Serum IgG antibodies to *H pylori* are detectable by ELISA, and kits are commercially available. Highly sensitive, these tests do not necessarily denote ongoing, active infection. After successful *H pylori* eradication with antibiotics, antibody levels decline slowly over 6–12 months but may remain positive. Noninvasive ^{14}C- and ^{13}C-urea breath tests have been developed. Because these urease breath tests indicate active infection, they may become the tests of choice for noninvasive screening for *H pylori* infection or for verifying eradication after antibacterial therapy.

Successful eradication of *H pylori* infection may be achieved in over 85% of patients (see section on peptic ulcer disease). After eradication, the chronic gastritis resolves. At present, the only indications for treating *H pylori* gastritis is in patients with peptic ulcer disease and low-grade B cell gastric lymphoma.

Kuipers EG et al: Long-term sequelae of *Helicobacter pylori* gastritis. Lancet 1995;345:1525.
Marshall BJ: *Helicobacter pylori*. Am J Gastroenterol 1994;89:S116. (Outstanding review by the man who discovered *H pylori* and its clinical associations.)
NIH Consensus Development Panel: *Helicobacter pylori* in peptic ulcer disease. JAMA 1994;272:65.
Walsh JH: Unanswered questions about *Helicobacter pylori*. Aliment Pharmacol Ther 1995;9(Suppl 1):31.

Pernicious Anemia Gastritis

Pernicious anemia gastritis is an autoimmune disorder involving the fundic glands with resultant achlorhydria and vitamin B_{12} malabsorption. Fundic histology is characterized by severe gland atrophy. Parietal cell antibodies directed against the H^+-K^+ ATPase pump are present in 90% of patients. Achlorhydria leads to pronounced hypergastrinemia (> 1000 pg/mL) due to loss of acid inhibition of gastrin G cells. Hypergastrinemia may induce hyperplasia of gastric enterochromaffin-like cells that may lead to the development of small, multicentric carcinoid tumors in 5% of patients. Metastatic spread is uncommon in lesions smaller than 2 cm. The risk of adenocarcinoma is also slightly increased but has been overemphasized. Endoscopy with biopsy is indicated in patients with pernicious anemia at the time of diagnosis. Patients with dysplasia or small carcinoids require periodic endoscopic surveillance. Pernicious anemia is discussed in detail in Chapter 13.

Carmel R: Prevalence of undiagnosed pernicious anemia in the elderly. Arch Intern Med 1996;156:1097.

3. SPECIFIC TYPES OF GASTRITIS

A number of disorders are associated with specific mucosal histologic features.

Infections

Acute bacterial infection of the gastric submucosa and muscularis with a variety of aerobic or anaerobic organisms produces a rare, rapidly progressive, life-threatening condition known as phlegmonous or necrotizing gastritis which requires emergency gastric resection and antibiotic therapy. Viral infection with CMV is commonly seen in patients with AIDS and after bone marrow or solid organ transplantation. Endoscopic findings include thickened gastric folds and ulcerations. Fungal infection with *Candida* may occur in immunocompromised patients. Larvae of *Anisakis marina* ingested in raw fish or sushi may become embedded in the gastric mucosa, producing severe abdominal pain. Pain persists for several days until the larvae die. Endoscopic removal of the larvae provides rapid symptomatic relief.

Granulomatous Gastritis

Chronic granulomatous inflammation may be caused by a variety of systemic diseases, including tuberculosis, syphilis, fungi, sarcoidosis, or Crohn's disease. These may be asymptomatic or associated with a variety of gastrointestinal complaints.

Eosinophilic Gastritis

This is a rare disorder in which eosinophils infiltrate the antrum and sometimes the proximal intestine. Infiltration may involve the mucosa, muscularis, or serosa. Peripheral eosinophilia is prominent. Symptoms include anemia from mucosal blood loss, abdominal pain, early satiety, and postprandial vomiting. Treatment with corticosteroids is beneficial in the majority of patients.

Lymphocytic Gastritis

This is an idiopathic condition characterized by fluctuating abdominal pain, nausea, and vomiting. Endoscopic features include mucosal erosions and a varioliform appearance. Biopsies reveal a diffuse lymphocytic gastritis. There is no established effective therapy.

Ménétrier's Disease (Hypertrophic Gastropathy)

This is an idiopathic entity characterized by giant thickened gastric folds predominantly involving the body. Patients complain of nausea, epigastric pain, weight loss, and diarrhea. Because of chronic protein loss, patients may develop severe hypoproteinemia and anasarca. The cause is unknown. Treatment is directed at symptoms. Gastric resection is required in severe cases. There are case reports of resolution of symptoms and improvement in histologic appearance after *H pylori* eradication.

Yardley J, Hendrix T: Gastritis, duodenitis, and associated ulcerative lesions. In: Yamada T (editor): *Textbook of Gastroenterology,* 2nd ed. Lippincott, 1995.

PEPTIC ULCER DISEASE

Essentials of Diagnosis

- History of epigastric pain present in 80–90% of patients but is nonspecific. Relationship to meals is variable.
- Ulcer symptoms characterized by rhythmicity and periodicity.
- 10–20% of patients present with ulcer complications without antecedent symptoms.
- Of NSAID-induced ulcers, 30–50% are asymptomatic.
- Upper endoscopy with antral biopsy for *H pylori* is diagnostic procedure of choice in most patients.
- Gastric ulcer biopsy or documentation of complete healing necessary to exclude gastric malignancy.

General Considerations

Peptic ulcer is a break in the gastric or duodenal mucosa that arises when the normal mucosal defensive factors are impaired or are overwhelmed by aggressive luminal factors such as acid and pepsin. By definition, ulcers extend through the muscularis mucosae and are usually over 5 mm in diameter. In the United States, there are about 500,000 new cases per year of peptic ulcer and 4 million ulcer recurrences; the lifetime prevalence of ulcers in the adult population is approximately 10%. Ulcers occur five times more commonly in the duodenum, where over 95% are in the bulb or pyloric channel. In the stomach, benign ulcers are located most commonly in the antrum (60%) and at the junction of the antrum and body on the lesser curvature (25%).

Ulcers occur slightly more commonly in men than in women (1.3:1). Although ulcers can occur in any age group, duodenal ulcers most commonly occur between the ages of 30 and 55, whereas gastric ulcers are more common between the ages of 55 and 70. Ulcers are more common in smokers and in patients receiving NSAIDs on a chronic basis (see below). Alcohol and dietary factors do not appear to cause ulcer disease. The role of stress is uncertain. The incidence of duodenal ulcer disease has been declining dramatically for the past 30 years, but the incidence of gastric ulcers appears to be increasing, perhaps as a result of the widespread use of NSAIDs.

Etiology

Three major causes of peptic ulcer disease are now recognized: NSAIDs, chronic *H pylori* infection, and acid hypersecretory states such as Zollinger-Ellison syndrome. Evidence of *H pylori* infection or NSAID ingestion should be sought in all patients with peptic ulcer. NSAID- and *H pylori*-associated ulcers will be considered in the present section; Zollinger-Ellison syndrome will be discussed subsequently.

A. *H pylori*-Associated Ulcers: *H pylori* appears to be a necessary cofactor for the overwhelming majority of duodenal and gastric ulcers not associated with NSAIDs. Ninety to 95 percent of duodenal ulcer patients have associated *H pylori* gastritis. It is not known how chronic *H pylori* gastritis potentiates ulcers in the duodenum. The association with gastric ulcers is less clear, but *H pylori* is found in the majority in whom NSAIDs cannot be implicated. Overall, it is estimated that one in six infected patients will develop ulcer disease.

The natural history of peptic ulcer disease is well-defined. After standard therapies, 70–85% of patients will have an endoscopically documented recurrence within 1 year. Half of these will be asymptomatic. In multiple trials, successful eradication of *H pylori* decreases the ulcer recurrence rate to less than 5% per year. At least some of these recurrences are due to NSAID use or failure to eradicate the organism. Although the pathogenetic mechanisms of ulcer formation by *H pylori* are unclear, its importance in ulcer formation is undeniable.

B. NSAID-Induced Ulcers: There is a 10–20% prevalence of gastric ulcers and a 2–5% prevalence of duodenal ulcers in chronic NSAID users. The relative risk of gastric ulcers is increased 40-fold, but the risk of duodenal ulcers is only slightly increased. Users of NSAIDs are at least three times more likely than nonusers to suffer serious gastrointestinal complications from these ulcers such as bleeding, perforation, or death. It is noteworthy that gastric ulcers and duodenal ulcers cause about the same number of complications. Approximately 1–2% of chronic NSAID users will have a major complication within 1 year. Aspirin is the most ulcerogenic NSAID. The risk appears to be dose-related, with some risk even at doses as low as 325 mg every other day. A higher risk of NSAID complications is associated with higher NSAID dosage; with the first 3 months of administration; and with advanced age, a prior history of ulcer disease, concomitant corticosteroid administration, or serious medical illness. At equivalent anti-inflammatory doses, there is no clear evidence that any particular NSAIDs are safer than others. Newer NSAIDs such as nabumetone and etodolac may be associated with a reduced incidence of ulcers because of relative sparing of gastric mucosal prostaglandin synthesis.

H pylori does not increase the likelihood of development of NSAID-associated ulcers. It is increasingly apparent that NSAIDs may cause small intestinal ulcerations and perforations, colitis, and colonic strictures.

Clinical Findings

A. Symptoms and Signs: Epigastric pain (dyspepsia), the hallmark of peptic ulcer disease, is present in 80–90% of patients. However, this complaint is not sensitive or specific enough to serve as a reliable diagnostic criterion for peptic ulcer disease. The clinical history cannot accurately distinguish duodenal from gastric ulcers. Less than one-quarter of patients with dyspepsia have ulcer disease at endoscopy. Up to 20% of patients with ulcer complications such as bleeding have no antecedent symptoms ("silent ulcers"). In patients with NSAID-induced ulcers, up to half are asymptomatic. Up to 60% of patients with complications do not have prior symptoms.

Pain is typically well localized to the epigastrium and not severe. It is described as gnawing, dull, aching, or "hunger-like." Classic features of peptic ulcer pain are rhythmicity and periodicity. Rhythmicity means that the pain fluctuates in intensity throughout the day and night. Approximately half of patients report relief of pain with food or antacids (especially duodenal ulcers) and a recurrence of pain 2–4 hours later. However, many patients deny any relationship to meals or report worsening of pain. Two-thirds of duodenal ulcers and one-third of gastric ulcers cause nocturnal pain that awakens the patient. A change from a patient's typical rhythmic discomfort to constant or radiating pain may reflect ulcer penetration or perforation. Most patients have symptomatic periods lasting up to several weeks with intervals of months to years in which they are pain-free (periodicity).

Nausea and anorexia may occur with gastric ulcers. Significant vomiting and weight loss are unusual with uncomplicated ulcer disease and suggest gastric outlet obstruction or gastric malignancy.

The physical examination is often unremarkable in uncomplicated peptic ulcer disease. Mild, localized epigastric tenderness to deep palpation may be present. Fecal occult blood testing is positive in one-third of patients.

B. Laboratory Findings: Laboratory tests are normal in uncomplicated peptic ulcer disease but are ordered to exclude ulcer complications or confounding disease entities. Anemia may occur with acute blood loss from a bleeding ulcer or less commonly from chronic blood loss. Leukocytosis suggests ulcer penetration or perforation. An elevated serum amylase in a patient with severe epigastric pain suggests ulcer penetration into the pancreas. A fasting serum gastrin level to screen for Zollinger-Ellison syndrome is obtained in some patients (see below). H_2 receptor antagonists should be removed for 24 hours before the gastrin level is measured.

C. Endoscopy: Upper endoscopy is the procedure of choice for the diagnosis of duodenal and gastric ulcers. Endoscopy provides better diagnostic accuracy than barium radiography and the ability to biopsy for the presence of malignancy and H pylori

infection. In most cases of both gastric and duodenal ulcers, gastric mucosal biopsies are required to assess for the presence of H pylori (see above). Duodenal ulcers are virtually never malignant and do not require biopsy. Three to 5 percent of benign-appearing gastric ulcers prove to be malignant. Hence, cytologic brushings and biopsies of the ulcer margin are almost always performed. All patients with gastric ulcers require follow-up endoscopy 12 weeks after the start of therapy to document complete healing even if the first biopsies were negative; nonhealing ulcers are suspicious for malignancy.

D. Imaging: Barium upper gastrointestinal series is an acceptable alternative to screening of uncomplicated patients with dyspepsia. However, because it has limited accuracy in distinguishing benign from malignant gastric ulcers, all gastric ulcers diagnosed by x-ray should be reevaluated with endoscopy after 8–12 weeks of therapy.

E. Testing for H pylori: Given the importance of H pylori in ulcer pathogenesis, testing for this organism should be performed in all patients with peptic ulcers (see section above on Helicobacter pylori gastritis). In patients in whom an ulcer is diagnosed by endoscopy, gastric mucosal biopsies should be obtained for both a rapid urease test and histology. The specimens for histology are discarded if the urease test is positive.

In patients with a history of peptic ulcer or when an ulcer is diagnosed by upper gastrointestinal series, noninvasive assessment for H pylori with urease breath testing or serologic testing is usually done. However, given the high prevalence of H pylori infection in uncomplicated duodenal ulcers (without NSAID use), negative tests have a poor predictive value, ie, they are more likely to be false-negative than true-negative. Although controversial, empiric antibiotic therapy without H pylori testing is a reasonable alternative for duodenal ulcer patients.

Differential Diagnosis

Peptic ulcer disease must be distinguished from other causes of epigastric distress (dyspepsia). Over half of patients with dyspepsia have no obvious organic explanation for their symptoms and are classified as having functional dyspepsia (see section above on functional dyspepsia). Atypical gastroesophageal reflux may be manifested by epigastric symptoms. Biliary tract disease is characterized by discrete, intermittent episodes of pain that should not be confused with other causes of dyspepsia. Severe epigastric pain is atypical for peptic ulcer disease unless complicated by a perforation or penetration. Other causes include acute pancreatitis, acute cholecystitis or choledocholithiasis, esophageal rupture, gastric volvulus, and ruptured aortic aneurysm.

Pharmacologic Agents

The pharmacology of several agents that enhance

the healing of peptic ulcers is briefly discussed here. They may be divided into three categories: (1) acid-antisecretory agents, (2) mucosal protective agents, and (3) agents that promote healing through eradication of *H pylori*. Recommendations for their use are provided in subsequent sections.

A. Acid-Antisecretory Agents:

1. Proton pump inhibitors–Proton pump inhibitors covalently bind the acid-secreting enzyme H^+-K^+ ATPase, or "proton pump," permanently inactivating it. Restoration of acid secretion requires synthesis of new pumps, which have a half-life of 18 hours. Thus, although these agents have a serum half-life of less than 60 minutes, their duration of action exceeds 24 hours. The two available agents, omeprazole 20 mg and lansoprazole 15–30 mg, inhibit over 90% of 24-hour acid secretion, compared with under 65% for H_2 receptor antagonists in standard dosages. Proton pump inhibitors should be administered 30 minutes before meals (usually breakfast).

Omeprazole, 20 mg/d, and lansoprazole, 15 mg/d, are highly effective in the treatment of duodenal ulcers, resulting in over 90% ulcer healing after 4 weeks. Omeprazole, 40 mg/d, and lansoprazole, 30–60 mg/d, heal over 90% of gastric ulcers after 8 weeks. Compared with H_2 receptor antagonists, proton pump inhibitors provide faster pain relief and more rapid ulcer healing. However, nearly equivalent overall healing rates may be achieved with longer courses of H_2 receptor antagonists.

These drugs are remarkably safe in short-term therapy. Serum gastrin levels rise significantly (> 500 pg/mL) in 10% of patients receiving chronic proton pump inhibitor therapy, which is associated with the development of gastric enterochromaffin-like cell hyperplasia in humans and gastric carcinoid tumors in rats. Although the question of safety of long-term therapy with proton pump inhibitors is unresolved, clinical experience in patients taking these agents for up to 5 years has not demonstrated toxicity. Long-term use is unnecessary in peptic ulcer disease but is frequently required in gastroesophageal reflux disease.

2. H_2 receptor antagonists–Four H_2 receptor antagonists are available: cimetidine, ranitidine, famotidine, and nizatidine. These agents competitively inhibit histamine binding to the H_2 receptor on the gastric parietal cell, thereby reducing intracellular cAMP levels and acid secretion. They profoundly inhibit basal and nocturnal acid output but are less effective at inhibiting meal-stimulated acid secretion. Thus, administration of these agents two to four times daily markedly raises nocturnal intragastric pH but has only a modest impact upon the daytime pH profile. For uncomplicated peptic ulcers, H_2 receptor antagonists may be administered twice daily or once daily at bedtime with equivalent efficacy. Recommended doses (once daily at bedtime) for the treat-

ment of acute peptic ulcers are as follows: cimetidine 800 mg; ranitidine and nizatidine 300 mg; and famotidine 40 mg. Complete ulcer symptom relief usually occurs within 2 weeks. Duodenal ulcer healing rates of 85–90% are obtained within 6–8 weeks of therapy. Gastric ulcer healing rates are delayed by 2–4 weeks compared with duodenal ulcers, but 8 weeks of therapy is sufficient in most patients.

The H_2 receptor antagonists are extremely well tolerated, and serious side effects are rare. Central nervous system symptoms of headache, confusion, and lethargy occur with all agents in 1% of patients, especially with intravenous administration. Cimetidine inhibits hepatic P450 drug metabolism, raising the serum concentration of warfarin, theophylline, lidocaine, and phenytoin. Ranitidine binds P450 with only one-tenth the avidity of cimetidine; famotidine and nizatidine have negligible effects. Cimetidine inhibits estradiol metabolism and dihydrotestosterone metabolism and may cause gynecomastia or impotence, especially at higher doses.

B. Agents Enhancing Mucosal Defenses:

1. Sucralfate–Sucralfate is a complex salt of sucrose containing aluminum and sulfate. The negatively charged sulfate groups bind to positively charged proteins in the ulcer base, forming a protective barrier against acid, bile, and pepsin. In addition, sucralfate stimulates mucus and bicarbonate secretion, stimulates prostaglandin production, and binds fibroblast growth factor. Sucralfate is unabsorbed and virtually devoid of side effects except for constipation. Because it binds some medications and inhibits their absorption, it should be administered at least 2 hours apart.

Sucralfate, 1 g four times daily, is equivalent in efficacy to H_2 receptor antagonists in the treatment of duodenal ulcers. Its efficacy in gastric ulcers is less well established.

2. Bismuth–Bismuth compounds in a variety of formulations have been used to treat dyspepsia, peptic ulcer disease, and diarrhea. The only agents currently available in the United States are bismuth subsalicylate and a combination of ranitidine plus bismuth citrate. Bismuth promotes ulcer healing through stimulation of mucosal bicarbonate and prostaglandin production. In addition, bismuth has direct antibacterial action against *H pylori*, eradicating the organism in up to one-third of patients. Less than 1% of bismuth is absorbed and is renally excreted. Salicylate is freely absorbed but does not achieve excessive levels at standard doses. In short-term use, bismuth compounds have excellent safety profiles. Darkening of the feces is expected. Rare cases of encephalopathy are reported in overdoses or after protracted courses of high-dose therapy.

3. Prostaglandin analogs (misoprostol)–Prostaglandin analogs promote ulcer healing by stimulating mucus and bicarbonate secretion and modest inhibition of acid secretion. Misoprostol is the only clinically available agent. It is less effective than other antiulcer agents in the treatment of active ulcers (including NSAID-induced ulcers). It is used solely as a prophylactic agent to prevent NSAID-induced ulcers. Misoprostol causes a dose-related diarrhea in 10–20% of patients. It also may stimulate uterine contractions and induce abortion.

4. Antacids–Low-dose aluminum- and magnesium-containing antacid regimens (120–240 mmol/d) promote ulcer healing through stimulation of gastric mucosal defenses, not by neutralization of gastric acidity. Given the greater compliance and efficacy of other antiulcer regimens, antacids are no longer used as first-line agents in the treatment of acute ulcers. Because of the rapid relief of ulcer symptoms that they provide, they are commonly used as needed to supplement other antiulcer therapies. High-dose regimens are associated with diarrhea, hypophosphatemia, and hypermagnesemia, but at standard low doses these adverse effects are infrequent.

C. *H pylori* Eradication Therapy: Eradication of *H pylori* has proved difficult. The agents that have demonstrated the greatest efficacy against *H pylori* are clarithromycin, metronidazole, amoxicillin, tetracycline, proton pump inhibitors, and bismuth. None of these agents, however, achieves acceptable rates of *H pylori* eradication when used as monotherapy. Furthermore, resistance rapidly develops to metronidazole and clarithromycin but not to amoxicillin or tetracycline. Combination regimens that employ two antibiotics with either bismuth or proton pump inhibitors are required to achieve adequate rates of eradication and to decrease failures due to antibiotic resistance. Although myriad regimens have been tested, none is yet established as the optimal treatment. All currently recommended regimens should achieve greater than 85–90% rates of eradication after 1–2 weeks of treatment. Treatment regimens may be divided into two categories:

1. Regimens using proton pump inhibitors–Combination therapy with a proton pump inhibitor and two antibiotics (clarithromycin plus either amoxicillin or metronidazole) is highly efficacious in *H pylori* eradication. Omeprazole and lansoprazole both have direct antimicrobial action against *H pylori*. Furthermore, by raising intragastric pH, they suppress bacterial growth and optimize antibiotic efficacy. The two treatment regimens that currently are favored are listed in Table 14–10. These regimens achieve eradication rates of over 85%. The amoxicillin-based regimen is preferable in areas in which there is high resistance of *H pylori* to metronidazole. Although a dual eradication therapy regimen of omeprazole and clarithromycin has been approved by the FDA, its efficacy is only 70% and it cannot be recommended.

2. Regimens using bismuth compounds–Combinations of bismuth subsalicylate plus two antibiotics (tetracycline plus either metronidazole or

---

Table 14–10. Treatment options for peptic ulcer disease.

Active *Helicobacter pylori*-associated ulcer:
1. Treat with proton pump inhibitor-based *H pylori* eradication regimen. Administer omeprazole 20 mg twice daily or lansoprazole 30 mg twice daily with one of the following regimens for 10–14 days:
   (1) metronidazole 500 mg twice daily
       clarithromycin 500 mg twice daily

   or–

   (2) amoxicillin 1 g twice daily
       clarithromycin 500 mg twice daily

   or–

   (3) bismuth subsalicylate 2 tablets four times daily
       tetracycline 500 mg four times daily
       metronidazole 250 mg four times daily

(Proton pump inhibitor administered before meals. All antibiotics and bismuth administered with meals. Avoid metronidazole-based regimens in areas of known high metronidazole resistance or in patients who have failed a course of treatment that included metronidazole.)

2. After completion of a 2-week course of *H pylori* eradication therapy, continue treatment with proton pump inhibitor or H_2 receptor antagonist for 4–8 weeks to promote ulcer healing (as below).

Active ulcer not attributable to *H pylori*:
Consider other causes: NSAIDs, Zollinger-Ellison syndrome, gastric malignancy. Treatment options:
1. Proton pump inhibitors:
   a. Uncomplicated duodenal ulcer: omeprazole 20 mg or lansoprazole 15 mg once daily for 4 weeks
   b. Gastric ulcer or complicated ulcer: omeprazole 20 mg twice daily or lansoprazole 30 mg daily for 6–8 weeks
2. H_2 receptor antagonists:
   a. Uncomplicated duodenal ulcer: cimetidine 800 mg, ranitidine or nizatidine 300 mg, or famotidine 40 mg once daily at bedtime for 6 weeks
   b. Gastric ulcer: cimetidine 400 mg twice daily, ranitidine or nizatidine 150 mg twice daiy, or famotidine 20 mg twice daily for 8–12 weeks
   c. Complicated ulcers: H_2 receptor antagonists not recommended
3. Sucralfate 1 g four times daily for uncomplicated duodenal ulcers

Prevention of ulcer relapse
1. NSAID-induced ulcer: prophylactic therapy reserved for high-risk patients (prior ulcer disease or ulcer complications, use of corticosteroids or anticoagulants, age > 70 years):
       Misoprostol 100–200 µg four times daily

       or–

       Proton pump inhibitor twice daily (for high-risk patients intolerant of misoprostol)

2. Chronic "maintenance" therapy: H_2 receptor antagonist at bedtime (cimetidine 400–800 mg, ranitidine or nizatidine 150–300 mg, or famotidine 20–40 mg). (Treatment indicated in patients with recurrent ulcers who are *H pylori*-negative or who have failed attempts at eradication, and in patients with a history of ulcer complications.)

clarithromycin) also achieve eradication rates of over 85% after 2 weeks of therapy. However, these regimens require four times daily dosing and are associated with a higher incidence of side effects than proton pump inhibitor regimens. The addition of a twice-daily proton pump inhibitor to this regimen (ie, "quadruple" therapy) may further enhance eradication rates to over 95%. The regimens that currently can be recommended are listed in Table 14–10. In areas in which there is high metronidazole resistance, clarithromycin, 500 mg three times daily, may be substituted.

Medical Treatment

Patients should be encouraged to eat balanced meals at regular intervals. There is no justification for bland or restrictive diets. Moderate alcohol intake is not harmful. Smoking retards the rate of ulcer healing and increases the frequency of recurrences and should be discouraged.

A. Treatment of H pylori-Associated Ulcers: The goals of treatment of active H pylori-associated ulcers are to relieve dyspeptic symptoms, to promote ulcer healing, and to eradicate H pylori infection. Uncomplicated H pylori-associated ulcers should be treated for the first 10–14 days with one of the proton pump inhibitor-based H pylori eradication regimens described above. In addition to eliminating H pylori, the antisecretory effects of omeprazole provide rapid, effective symptom relief. Although these 2-week treatment regimens heal duodenal ulcers as effectively as 4 weeks of omeprazole therapy, it is still recommended that "conventional" antiulcer therapy be administered for an additional period after completion of antibiotic therapy for both gastric and duodenal ulcers to ensure symptom relief and ulcer healing. For duodenal ulcers, this is most conveniently done by continuing a proton pump inhibitor (omeprazole 20 mg or lansoprazole 15 mg) once daily for an additional 2 weeks (4 weeks total). For gastric ulcers, omeprazole 40 mg or lansoprazole 30 mg should be continued for 6 additional weeks (8 weeks total). Alternatively, after completion of the 2-week course of H pylori eradication therapy, H_2 receptor antagonists or sucralfate can be given for 6–8 weeks (as listed below and in Table 14–10). Confirmation of H pylori eradication in patients with uncomplicated ulcers is not recommended.

In patients with peptic ulcers complicated by gastrointestinal bleeding, significant nausea, or severe pain, initial treatment of H pylori infection should be deferred to avoid potentially confounding issues of drug side effects. Therapy should be initiated with a proton pump inhibitor (omeprazole 20–40 mg, lansoprazole 30 mg) to promote rapid symptom relief. A 1-week course of H pylori eradication therapy can subsequently be administered.

B. Therapy to Prevent Recurrence: Prior to the recognition of the importance of H pylori in ulcer pathogenesis, the recurrence rate of peptic ulcers was over 80% per year. For that reason, patients with frequent ulcer recurrences or ulcer complications were maintained on continuous therapy with half-dose bedtime H_2 receptor antagonists (cimetidine 400 mg, ranitidine 150 mg, famotidine 20 mg). These "maintenance" regimens reduced the symptomatic ulcer recurrence rate to less than 15% per year and the rate of ulcer complications.

Since successful eradication reduces ulcer recurrence rates to less than 10%, all patients with a history of peptic ulcer disease (active or inactive) and H pylori infection should be given a course of eradication therapy. The most common cause of ulcer recurrence after antibiotic therapy is failure to achieve successful eradication, which should be evaluated. Once cure has been achieved, reinfection rates are less than 0.5% per year. Although H pylori eradication has dramatically reduced the need for maintenance H_2 receptor antagonist therapy, there remains a subset of patients who require chronic treatment. These include patients with H pylori-negative recurrent ulcers, patients with H pylori-positive recurrent ulcers who have failed eradication therapy, and patients with a history of H pylori-positive ulcers who have recurrent ulcers despite successful eradication. Surreptitious NSAID ingestion and hypersecretory states (such as gastrinoma) should be excluded in these patients.

C. Treatment of NSAID-Associated Ulcers:
1. Treatment of active ulcers–In patients with NSAID-induced ulcers, the offending agent should be discontinued whenever possible. Both gastric and duodenal ulcers respond rapidly to therapy with H_2 receptor antagonists, proton pump inhibitors, or sucralfate (as outlined above) once NSAIDs are eliminated. In some patients with severe inflammatory diseases, it may not be feasible to discontinue NSAIDs. Although most uncomplicated ulcers will heal with twice-daily H_2 receptor antagonists despite continued NSAID ingestion, ulcer healing is delayed. Therefore, ulcers should be treated with twice-daily proton pump inhibitors (omeprazole 20 mg or lansoprazole 30 mg twice daily), the healing efficacy of which does not appear to be compromised by continued NSAID ingestion. Misoprostol is not effective in the treatment of active NSAID-induced ulcers.

H pylori infection does not appear to increase the risk of NSAID-induced ulcers. Nevertheless, about half of patients who develop ulcers while using NSAIDs are infected with H pylori, and in such cases it is impossible to be certain which is the primary pathogenetic factor. Therefore, antibiotic eradication therapy should be given for NSAID-induced ulcers when H pylori tests are positive.

2. Prevention of NSAID-induced ulcers–The prostaglandin analog misoprostol is effective in the prevention of NSAID-induced gastric and duodenal ulcers and is the only agent approved by the FDA for this purpose. When coadministered with NSAIDs, misoprostol, 200 µg four times daily, reduces the incidence of endoscopically visualized peptic ulcers from 20% to less than 5%. Misoprostol has recently been demonstrated to reduce NSAID-induced ulcer complications by 40% in a clinical setting. Preliminary reports suggest that proton pump inhibitors are equivalent or superior to misoprostol for the prevention of endoscopically visible ulcers, but their impact upon NSAID-induced ulcer complications is untested. Standard doses of H_2 receptor antagonists and sucralfate are ineffective for the prevention of NSAID-induced ulcers. Recently, high-dose famotidine, 40 mg twice daily, has been shown to reduce the incidence of NSAID-induced ulcers. However, this therapy is more costly and not more effective than proton pump inhibitors and is thus not recommended.

Determining the most cost-effective approach to the prevention of NSAID-induced complications is difficult. Although the incidence of NSAID-induced ulcers is high, most of these are clinically silent and of no consequence. The goal of prophylactic therapy is to prevent ulcer complications, which occur in only 1–2% of NSAID-treated patients per year. Therefore, prophylactic therapy should be reserved for patients at high risk of developing complications. Risk factors include a history of ulcer disease or complications, concurrent therapy with corticosteroids or anticoagulants, serious underlying medical illness, and age over 70 years. Whenever possible, NSAIDs should be avoided in this high-risk population. If NSAIDs must be given, prophylactic therapy with misoprostol is recommended, beginning at a dosage of 100 µg four times daily and increasing to 200 µg as tolerated. In patients in whom misoprostol is not tolerated because of cramps or diarrhea, a proton pump inhibitor should be given. Newer NSAIDs such as salsalate, etodolac, or nabumetone may be preferred because they are associated with a lower incidence of endoscopic ulcerations.

D. Refractory Ulcers: Ulcers that are truly refractory to medical therapy are now uncommon. Approximately 10% of ulcers are unhealed after 8–12 weeks of therapy with H_2 receptor antagonists or sucralfate. Noncompliance is the most common cause of ulcer nonhealing. Cigarettes retard ulcer healing and should be proscribed. NSAID and aspirin use, sometimes surreptitious, are commonly implicated in refractory ulcers and must be eliminated. *H pylori* eradication enhances healing and decreases the high recurrence rates of refractory ulcers. Therefore, evidence of *H pylori* infection should be sought and the infection treated, if present, in all refractory ulcer patients. Fasting serum gastrin levels should be obtained to exclude gastrinoma with acid hypersecretion (Zollinger-Ellison syndrome). Nonhealing gastric ulcers raise concerns that an undiagnosed gastric malignancy may be masquerading as a benign gastric ulcer. Repeat ulcer biopsies are mandatory after 2–3 months of therapy in all nonhealed gastric ulcers, and they should be followed with serial endoscopies to verify complete healing. Almost all benign refractory ulcers heal within 8 weeks with a proton pump inhibitor twice daily (omeprazole 20 mg twice daily or lansoprazole 30 mg twice daily). Ulcer relapse rates are high in *H pylori*-negative patients, and most require chronic maintenance therapy with an H_2 antagonist in full doses. Patients with persistent nonhealing ulcers should be referred for surgical therapy after careful exclusion of NSAID use and persistent *H pylori* infection.

[*Helicobacter pylori* in peptic ulcer disease]
  gopher://gopher.nih.gov/11/clin/cdcs/individual/94.hpyl
Marshall BS: *Helicobacter pylori.* Am J Gastroenterol 1994;89:516. (Excellent review by the physician who discovered *H pylori*.)
Scherman J: NSAIDs, gastrointestinal injury, and cytoprotection. Gastroenterol Clin North Am 1996;25:279.
Silverstein FE et al: Misoprostol reduces serious gastrointestinal complications in patients with rheumatoid arthritis receiving nonsteroidal anti-inflammatory drugs. Ann Intern Med 1995;123:241. (Large trial showing that misoprostol reduces NSAID complications by 40%.)
Smalley WE, Griffin M: The risks and costs of upper gastrointestinal disease attributable to NSAIDs. Gastroenterol Clin North Am 1996;25:373.
Soll AH: Medical treatment of peptic ulcer disease. JAMA 1996;275:622. (Practice guidelines issued by a committee of the American College of Gastroenterology.)
Taha AS et al: Famotidine for the prevention of gastric and duodenal ulcers caused by nonsteroidal antiinflammatory drugs. N Engl J Med 1996;334:1435.
Walsh J, Peterson W: The treatment of *Helicobacter pylori* infection in the management of peptic ulcer disease. N Engl J Med 1995;333:984. (Concise review. More specific recommendations, however, are provided in the Soll reference above.)

COMPLICATIONS OF PEPTIC ULCER DISEASE

1. GASTROINTESTINAL HEMORRHAGE

Essentials of Diagnosis

- "Coffee grounds" emesis, hematemesis, melena, or hematochezia.
- Emergent upper endoscopy is diagnostic and therapeutic.

General Considerations

Approximately 50% of all episodes of upper gastrointestinal bleeding are due to peptic ulcers. Clinically significant bleeding occurs in 10–20% of ulcer patients. About 80% of patients stop bleeding spontaneously and generally have an uneventful recovery. Twenty percent of patients have more severe bleeding. The overall mortality rate for ulcer bleeding is

6–10%, but it is higher in the elderly or in patients with other medical problems.

Clinical Findings

A. Symptoms and Signs: Up to 20% of patients have no antecedent symptoms of pain; this is particularly true of patients receiving NSAIDs. Common presenting signs include melena and hematemesis. Massive upper gastrointestinal bleeding or rapid gastrointestinal transit may result in hematochezia rather than melena; this may be misinterpreted as signifying a lower tract bleeding source. Nasogastric lavage that demonstrates "coffee grounds" or bright red blood confirms an upper tract source. Recovered nasogastric lavage fluid that is negative for blood does not exclude active bleeding from a duodenal ulcer.

B. Laboratory Findings: The hematocrit may fall as a result of bleeding or expansion of the intravascular volume with intravenous fluids. The BUN may rise as a result of absorption of blood nitrogen from the small intestine and prerenal azotemia.

Treatment

The assessment and initial management of bleeding from the upper gastrointestinal tract is discussed elsewhere in this chapter. Specific issues pertaining to ulcer bleeding are described below.

A. Medical Therapy: Bleeding stops spontaneously within a few hours after admission in 80% of cases. Intravenous H_2 receptor antagonists are administered by continuous infusions at a dose sufficient to maintain the intragastric pH greater than 4.0. (See treatment of stress gastritis, above.) Vasopressin and intravenous octreotide should not be used for ulcer bleeding.

B. Endoscopy: Endoscopy is the preferred diagnostic procedure in virtually all cases of upper gastrointestinal bleeding because of its high diagnostic accuracy, its ability to predict the likelihood of recurrent bleeding, and its capability for therapeutic intervention in high-risk lesions. In patients with severe bleeding, endoscopy is usually performed within 6–8 hours after admission once resuscitative efforts have been initiated and hemodynamic stability has been restored. Endoscopy is also performed urgently in patients with continued active bleeding.

The appearance of the ulcer base is predictive of the chance of rebleeding. Ulcers with a base that is clean or that appears only as a flat red or black spot impose a less than 5% risk of significant bleeding. Such patients may be transferred quickly from the ICU, resume a normal diet, and begin oral medications. Conversely, ulcers with an adherent clot have a 33% chance and those with a visible vessel a 50% chance of significant rebleeding. Actively bleeding ulcers have a high probability of continuing to bleed.

Endoscopic therapy with a variety of hemostatic injection and coagulation techniques is now considered standard therapy for patients with clinical evidence of a major bleeding episode who have a visible vessel or active ulcer bleeding at endoscopy. Injection is performed into and around the ulcer vessel with epinephrine (1:10,000), ethanol, or saline. Coagulation may also be achieved with contact cautery probes. Using any of these injection or cautery modalities, successful hemostasis is achieved in 90% of actively bleeding lesions. Significant rebleeding occurs in 10–20% of cases. Endoscopic therapy decreases the number of transfusions required and the need for surgery. Less than 10% of patients treated with hemostatic therapy will require surgery.

C. Surgery: All patients with ulcer bleeding severe enough to warrant ICU admission or blood transfusion should be evaluated by a surgeon. Criteria for emergency surgery are reviewed in the section on acute upper gastrointestinal bleeding. The overall surgical mortality rate for emergency ulcer bleeding is less than 6%. The prognosis is much poorer, however, for patients over age 60, those with serious underlying medical illnesses, those with chronic renal failure, and those receiving multiple transfusions.

2. ULCER PERFORATION

Perforations develop in 5% of ulcer patients, usually from ulcers on the anterior wall of the stomach or duodenum. The incidence of perforations may be increasing, perhaps as a consequence of using NSAIDs or crack cocaine. Zollinger-Ellison disease should be considered in patients who present with ulcer perforation. Perforation results in a chemical peritonitis that causes sudden, severe generalized abdominal pain that prompts most patients to seek immediate attention. Elderly or debilitated patients and those receiving chronic steroid therapy may experience minimal initial symptoms, presenting late with bacterial peritonitis, sepsis, and shock. On physical examination, patients appear ill, with a rigid, quiet abdomen and rebound tenderness. Hypotension is not a feature of early ulcer perforation but develops later after bacterial peritonitis has developed. If hypotension is present early with the onset of pain, one should consider other abdominal catastrophes such as a ruptured aortic aneurysm, mesenteric infarction, or acute pancreatitis. Leukocytosis is almost always present. A mildly elevated serum amylase (less than twice normal) is sometimes seen. Upright or decubitus films of the abdomen reveal free intraperitoneal air in 75% of cases, and in most cases this establishes the diagnosis without need for further studies. In the remainder of cases, adjacent omentum seals the perforation before significant leakage occurs. The absence of free air may lead to a misdiagnosis of pancreatitis, cholecystitis, or appendicitis. Upper gastrointestinal radiography with water-soluble contrast may be useful in this setting. Barium studies are contraindicated in patients with possible perforation.

The majority of patients with perforated ulcers should undergo emergency surgery. Closure of the perforation is performed with an omental patch. In most cases, proximal gastric vagotomy is performed to decrease the chance of ulcer recurrence. Although traditionally performed by laparotomy, vagotomy may now be done through a laparoscope.

The overall mortality rate in patients treated surgically is about 5%. Selected patients may be managed nonoperatively. Patients considered to be poor operative candidates and patients who present more than 24 hours after perforation who are stable and who have no evidence of leakage on gastroduodenography may be followed closely on fluids, nasogastric suction, and broad-spectrum antibiotics. If their condition deteriorates in the first 12–24 hours, they should be taken to the operating room. The mortality rate in medically treated patients is less than 5%.

3. ULCER PENETRATION

An ulcer located along the posterior wall of the duodenum or stomach may perforate into contiguous structures such as the pancreas, liver, or biliary tree. Patients complain of a change in the intensity and rhythmicity of their ulcer symptoms. The pain becomes more severe and constant, may radiate to the back, and is unresponsive to antacids or food. Physical examination and laboratory tests are nonspecific. Mild amylase elevations may sometimes occur. Endoscopy and barium x-ray studies confirm the ulceration but are not diagnostic of an actual penetration. Patients should be placed on intravenous H_2 receptor antagonists (as above) or omeprazole, 40 mg/d, and followed closely. Patients who fail to improve should be considered for surgical therapy.

4. GASTRIC OUTLET OBSTRUCTION

Gastric outlet obstruction occurs in 2% of patients with ulcer disease and is due to edema or cicatricial narrowing of the pylorus or duodenal bulb. Most patients have a prior known history of ulcer disease. Obstruction is less commonly caused by gastric neoplasms or extrinsic duodenal obstruction by intra-abdominal neoplasms. The most common symptoms are early satiety, vomiting, and weight loss. Early symptoms are epigastric fullness or heaviness after meals. Later, vomiting may develop that typically occurs one to several hours after eating and consists of partially digested food contents. Chronic obstruction may result in a grossly dilated, atonic stomach, severe weight loss, and malnutrition. Patients may develop dehydration, metabolic alkalosis, and hy-

pokalemia. On physical examination, a succussion splash may be heard in the epigastrium. In most cases, nasogastric aspiration will result in evacuation of a large amount (> 200 mL) of foul-smelling fluid, which establishes the diagnosis. More subtle obstruction is diagnosed by a saline load test or by a nuclear gastric emptying study. Patients are treated initially with intravenous isotonic saline and KCl to correct fluid and electrolyte disorders, intravenous H_2 receptor antagonists (see treatment of stress gastritis, above), and nasogastric decompression of the stomach. Severely malnourished patients should receive total parenteral nutrition. Upper endoscopy is performed after 24–72 hours to define the nature of the obstruction and to exclude a gastric neoplasm. At 72 hours, all patients should be evaluated with a saline load test. A positive test consists of more than 400 mL of residual volume 30 minutes after instillation of 750 mL of 0.9% saline into the stomach by nasogastric tube. Patients with a negative load test may be started on clear liquids and their diet advanced as tolerated. The remainder should remain on nasogastric suction for 5–7 days. Traditionally, patients unimproved after that time have been recommended for surgical treatment with vagotomy and either pyloroplasty or antrectomy. Recently, upper endoscopy with dilation of the gastric obstruction by hydrostatic balloons passed through the instrument has achieved success in two-thirds of patients. It may be reasonable to pursue dilation first in patients with milder symptoms, reserving surgery for those who fail to respond.

Jiranek GC, Kozarek RA: A cost-effective approach to the patient with peptic ulcer bleeding. Surg Clin North Am 1996;76:83.

Laine L, Peterson WL: Bleeding peptic ulcer. N Engl J Med 1994;331:717. (Pathogenesis and treatment.)

Svanes C et al: Adverse effects of delayed treatment for perforated peptic ulcer. Ann Surg 1994;220:168.

Zuccaro G Jr: Bleeding peptic ulcer: Pathogenesis and endoscopic therapy. Gastroenterol Clin North Am 1993; 22:737.

ZOLLINGER-ELLISON SYNDROME (Gastrinoma)

Essentials of Diagnosis

- Peptic ulcer disease; may be severe.
- Gastric acid hypersecretion.
- Diarrhea common.
- Gastrinoma; may be metastatic.
- Most sporadic; 25% with MEN I.

General Considerations

Zollinger-Ellison syndrome is caused by gastrin-secreting tumors (gastrinomas), which result in hypergastrinemia and acid hypersecretion. Less than 1% of peptic ulcer disease is caused by gastrinomas.

Gastrinomas may arise in the pancreas (40%), duodenal wall (40%), or lymph nodes (5–15%). Approximately 90% arise within the "gastrinoma triangle" bounded by the porta hepatis, the neck of the pancreas, and the third portion of the duodenum. Most gastrinomas are solitary or multifocal nodules that are potentially resectable. Over half of gastrinomas are malignant, and up to 40% of patients develop metastatic disease. Approximately 25% of patients have small multicentric gastrinomas associated with MEN that are more difficult to resect.

Clinical Findings

A. Symptoms and Signs: More than 90% of patients with Zollinger-Ellison syndrome develop peptic ulcers. In most cases, the symptoms are indistinguishable from other causes of peptic ulcer disease and therefore may go undetected for years. Ulcers usually are solitary and located in the duodenal bulb, but they may be multiple or occur more distally in the duodenum. Gastroesophageal reflux symptoms occur often. Diarrhea occurs in over half of patients, in some cases in the absence of peptic symptoms. Gastric acid hypersecretion can cause direct intestinal mucosal injury and pancreatic enzyme inactivation resulting in diarrhea, steatorrhea, and weight loss. Screening for Zollinger-Ellison syndrome with fasting gastrin levels should be obtained in patients with ulcers that are refractory to standard therapies, giant ulcers (> 2 cm), ulcers located distal to the duodenal bulb, multiple duodenal ulcers, frequent ulcer recurrences, ulcers associated with diarrhea, ulcers occurring after ulcer surgery, and patients with ulcer complications. Ulcer patients with hypercalcemia or family histories of ulcers (suggesting MEN I) should also be screened. Finally, patients with peptic ulcers who are *H pylori*-negative and who are not taking NSAIDs should be screened.

B. Laboratory Findings: The most sensitive and specific method for identifying Zollinger-Ellison syndrome is demonstration of an increased fasting serum gastrin concentration (> 150 pg/mL). Levels should be obtained with patients not taking H_2 receptor antagonists for 24 hours or omeprazole for 6 days. Hypochlorhydria with increased gastric pH is a much more common cause of hypergastrinemia than is gastrinoma. Therefore, a measurement of gastric pH (and, where available, gastric secretory studies) should be performed in patients with fasting hypergastrinemia. Most patients have a basal acid output of over 15 meq/h. A gastric pH of > 3.0 implies hypochlorhydria and excludes gastrinoma. In a patient with a serum gastrin level of > 1000 pg/mL and acid hypersecretion, the diagnosis of Zollinger-Ellison syndrome is established. With lower gastrin levels (150–1000 pg/mL) and acid secretion, a secretin stimulation test is performed to distinguish Zollinger-Ellison syndrome from other causes of hypergastrinemia. Intravenous secretin (2 units/kg) produces a rise in serum gastrin of over 200 pg/mL within 2–30 minutes in 85% of patients with gastrinoma. An elevated serum calcium suggests hyperparathyroidism and MEN I syndrome. In patients with Zollinger-Ellison syndrome, a serum PTH, prolactin, LH-FSH, and GH level should be obtained to exclude MEN I.

C. Imaging: Imaging studies are obtained in an attempt to localize the tumor and determine whether there is metastatic disease. Preoperative localization can be extremely difficult. Somatostatin receptor scintigraphy (SRS) is the most sensitive test for gastrinoma, detecting over 60% of primary tumors and 90% of hepatic metastases. It should be the first test obtained. If SRS is positive for localization of the tumor, further imaging studies are not indicated. If negative, further studies should be done only if surgery is being considered. MRI of the abdomen is the next most useful procedure, followed by abdominal CT, endoscopic ultrasonography of the pancreas and duodenum, and angiography. These additional studies may increase the overall yield of localization by an additional 10%. There remain approximately 30% of patients whose primary tumors cannot be localized preoperatively.

Differential Diagnosis

Zollinger-Ellison syndrome must be distinguished from other causes of hypergastrinemia. Atrophic gastritis with decreased acid secretion is detected by gastric secretory analysis. Other conditions such as routine peptic ulcer disease, antral G cell hyperfunction, and gastric outlet obstruction are associated with negative secretin stimulation tests.

Treatment

A. Metastatic Disease: In patients with multiple hepatic metastases, gastrinoma resection is not attempted. Patients may have prolonged survival, though many die within 5 years. Initial therapy is directed at controlling the gastric acid hypersecretion. Omeprazole is given at a dose of 40–120 mg/d, which is titrated to achieve a basal acid output of < 10 meq/h. At this dose, there is complete symptomatic relief and ulcer healing. Chemotherapy has been disappointing in this disease but may be considered in patients with symptomatic metastases.

B. Localized Disease: Cure can only be achieved if the gastrinoma is detected and removed before metastatic spread has occurred. Laparotomy should be considered in all patients in whom preoperative studies either fail to localize a tumor or suggest an isolated, resectable lesion. It may also be considered in patients with isolated hepatic metastases. Careful operative palpation combined with intraoperative sonography can identify gastrinomas in the majority of patients. Cure is achieved in over 30% of cases.

Gibril F et al: Somatostatin receptor scintigraphy: Its sensitivity compared with that of other imaging methods in detecting primary and metastatic gastrinomas. A prospective study. Ann Intern Med 1996;125:26.

Modlin IM, Tang LH: Approaches to the diagnosis of gut neuroendocrine tumors: The last word (today). Gastroenterology 1997;112:583.

Termanini B et al: Value of somatostatin receptor scintigraphy: Prospective study in gastrinoma and its effect on clinical management. Gastroenterology 1997;112:335.

BENIGN TUMORS OF THE STOMACH

Gastric epithelial polyps are usually detected incidentally at endoscopy. The majority are hyperplastic polyps, which are small, single or multiple, have no malignant potential, and do not require removal or endoscopic surveillance. Adenomatous polyps account for 10–20% of gastric polyps. They are usually solitary lesions. In rare instances they ulcerate, causing chronic blood loss. Because of their premalignant potential, endoscopic removal is indicated. Annual endoscopic surveillance is recommended to screen for further polyp development. Submucosal gastric polypoid lesions include leiomyoma and pancreatic rests.

MALIGNANT TUMORS OF THE STOMACH

1. GASTRIC ADENOCARCINOMA

Essentials of Diagnosis

- Dyspeptic symptoms with weight loss in patients over age 40.
- Iron deficiency anemia; occult blood in stools.
- Abnormality detected on upper gastrointestinal series or endoscopy.

General Considerations

Although gastric adenocarcinoma is the most common cancer (other than skin cancer) worldwide, its incidence in the United States has declined by two-thirds over the last 30 years to 20,000 cases annually. Gastric cancer is uncommon under age 40; the mean age at diagnosis is 63 years. Men are affected twice as often as women. The incidence is higher in Hispanics, African Americans, and Asian Americans. Certain regions such as Chile, Colombia, Central America, and Japan have rates as high as 80 per 100,000 population. Although most gastric cancers arise in the antrum, the incidence of proximal tumors of the cardia and fundus is increasing.

Chronic *H pylori* gastritis is a strong risk factor for gastric carcinoma of the distal (but not proximal) stomach, increasing the relative risk four- to sixfold. It is estimated that 35–89% of cases of distal gastric carcinoma may be attributable to *H pylori*. It is of note that less than 1% of chronically infected individuals will develop carcinoma. Other risk factors for gastric cancer include chronic atrophic gastritis with intestinal metaplasia (often secondary to chronic *H pylori* infection), pernicious anemia, and a history of partial gastric resection more than 15 years previously.

Gastric cancer may occur in a variety of morphologic types: (1) polypoid or fungating intraluminal masses; (2) ulcerating masses; (3) diffusely spreading (linitis plastica), in which the tumor spreads through the submucosa, resulting in a rigid, atonic stomach with thickened folds (prognosis dismal); and (4) superficially spreading or "early" gastric cancer—confined to the mucosa or submucosa (with or without lymph node metastases) and associated with an excellent prognosis.

Clinical Findings

A. Symptoms and Signs: Gastric carcinoma is generally asymptomatic until the disease is quite advanced. Symptoms are nonspecific and are determined in part by the location of the tumor. Dyspepsia, vague epigastric pain, anorexia, early satiety, and weight loss are the presenting symptoms in most patients. Patients may derive initial symptomatic relief from over-the-counter remedies, further delaying diagnosis. Ulcerating lesions can lead to acute gastrointestinal bleeding with hematemesis or melena. Pyloric obstruction results in postprandial vomiting. Lower esophageal obstruction causes progressive dysphagia. Physical examination is rarely helpful. A gastric mass is palpated in less than one-fifth of patients. Signs of metastatic spread include a left supraclavicular lymph node (Virchow's node), an umbilical nodule (Sister Mary Joseph nodule), a rigid rectal shelf (Blumer's shelf), and ovarian metastases (Krukenberg tumor). Guaiac-positive stools may be detectable.

B. Laboratory Findings: Iron deficiency anemia due to chronic blood loss or anemia of chronic disease is common. Liver function test abnormalities may be present if there is metastatic liver spread. Other tumor markers are of no value.

C. Endoscopy: Upper endoscopy should be obtained in all patients over age 40 with new onset of epigastric symptoms that are persistent or fail to respond to a short trial of antisecretory therapy. Endoscopy with cytologic brushings and biopsies of suspicious lesions is highly sensitive for detecting gastric carcinoma. It can be difficult to obtain adequate biopsy specimens in linitis plastica lesions. Because of the high incidence of gastric carcinoma in Japan, screening upper endoscopy is performed to detect early gastric carcinoma. Approximately 40% of tumors detected by screening are early, with a 5-year survival rate of almost 90%. Screening programs are not recommended in the USA.

D. Imaging: A barium upper gastrointestinal series is an acceptable alternative when endoscopy is not readily available but may not detect small or superficial lesions and cannot reliably distinguish benign from malignant ulcerations. Any abnormalities detected with this procedure require endoscopic confirmation.

Once a gastric cancer is diagnosed, preoperative evaluation with abdominal CT and endoscopic ultrasonography is indicated to delineate the local extent of the primary tumor as well as nodal or distant metastases. Abdominal CT is valuable in identifying distant metastases and direct invasion of adjacent structures. Endoscopic ultrasound imaging is superior to CT in determining the depth of tumor penetration and nodal metastases.

E. Staging: Staging is defined according to the TNM system, in which T1 tumors invade to the submucosa, T2 invade the muscularis propria, T3 penetrate the serosa, and T4 invade adjacent structures. Nodes are graded as N0 if there is no involvement, N1 if there are metastases to perigastric nodes within 3 cm of the tumor, and N2 if nodes more than 3 cm from the tumor are involved. The stages are defined as shown in the accompanying box.

Staging Criteria for Gastric Adenocarcinoma

Stage I: T1N0, T1N1, T2N0, all M0
Stage II: T1N2, T2N1, T3N0, all M0
Stage III: T2N2, T3N1, T4N0, all M0
Stage IV: T4N2M0, any M1

Differential Diagnosis

Ulcerating gastric adenocarcinomas are distinguished from benign gastric ulcers by biopsies. Approximately 3% of gastric ulcers initially felt to be benign later prove to be malignant. To exclude malignancy, all gastric ulcers should be followed with endoscopy to complete healing, and nonhealing gastric ulcers should be resected. Infiltrative carcinoma with thickened gastric folds must be distinguished from lymphoma and other hypertrophic gastropathies such as Ménétrier's disease. Obtaining adequate biopsy specimens can be difficult, and an open, full-thickness biopsy is sometimes required.

Treatment

A. Curative Surgical Resection: Surgical resection is the only therapy with curative potential. However, after preoperative staging, fewer than 30% of patients will be found to have disease that is amenable to this approach. For patients with adenocarcinoma located in the distal two-thirds of the stomach, patients with stage I and stage II disease and selected patients with stage III disease (who have only local nodal involvement) should undergo radical subtotal distal gastrectomy with regional lym-

phadenectomy. Patients with cancer involving the cardia or proximal stomach or linitis plastica require total gastrectomy. Meta-analysis of postoperative chemotherapy or radiation therapy after gastric resection demonstrates no survival benefit.

B. Palliative Modalities: Most patients present with advanced disease (stage IIIB or stage IV) for which "curative" surgical approaches are not indicated. When possible, palliative surgical resection of the tumor should be performed since it removes the risk of bleeding and obstruction and leads to improved quality of life and survival. For patients with unresectable disease, gastrojejunostomy should be performed to prevent obstruction. Tumor bleeding may be treated with endoscopic laser therapy, radiation therapy, or angiographic embolization. Single-agent chemotherapy with fluorouracil, mitomycin, or doxorubicin and combination therapy with fluorouracil, doxorubicin, and cisplatin may provide palliation in 20–30% but do not prolong survival.

Prognosis

The overall 5-year survival rate of gastric carcinoma is only 10–15%. Long-term survival is related to the tumor stage, location, and histologic features. Stage I and stage II tumors resected for cure yield up to 50% long-term survival rates. Tumors of the diffuse type and signet ring carcinomas have a worse prognosis than the intestinal type. Tumors of the proximal stomach (fundus, cardia) have a far worse prognosis than distal lesions. Even with apparently localized disease, proximal tumors have a 5-year survival rate of less than 15%.

[NCI Internet address for gastric cancer]
gopher://gopher.nih.gov:70/00/clin/cancernet/pdqinfo/soa/Gastric%20cancer_Physician

Fuchs CS, Mayer RJ: Gastric carcinoma. N Engl J Med 1995;333:22

Sawyers JL: Gastric carcinoma. Curr Probl Surg 1995; 32:101.

2. LYMPHOMA

Secondary involvement of the gastrointestinal tract is the most common extranodal site of non-Hodgkin's lymphoma, occurring in over 20% of cases, although most patients do not have gastrointestinal symptoms. Primary gastrointestinal lymphomas are the most commonly involved extranodal site of non-Hodgkin's lymphoma, of which two-thirds are gastric. Lymphomas account for less than 3% of gastric malignancies. The majority are high-grade non-Hodgkin's lymphomas of the B cell type.

About 10% of gastric lymphomas derive from mucosa-associated lymphoid tissue (MALT), which tend to be low-grade, indolent tumors that have a low risk of dissemination to lymph nodes or bone marrow and carry an extremely favorable prognosis. Evidence of *H pylori* infection is found in over 85% of patients with primary gastric lymphomas and nearly all with low-grade MALT lymphomas. The risk of primary gastric lymphoma (both high-grade and MALT-related) in *H pylori*-infected individuals is increased sevenfold. *H pylori*-associated chronic gastritis is believed to result in some people in monoclonal, multifocal lymphoproliferation that gives rise to MALT lymphoma. The relation between low-grade MALT lymphoma and high grade B cell gastric lymphomas is unclear.

The clinical presentation and endoscopic appearance of gastric lymphoma is similar to those of adenocarcinoma. Diagnosis is established with endoscopic biopsy. Treatment is controversial. Patients with disease limited to the stomach (stage IE) should undergo surgical resection, but the role of adjuvant chemotherapy is unclear. Patients with disease extending to local lymph nodes (stage IIE), adjacent organs, or with distant spread (stage IV) should undergo chemotherapy as the primary therapeutic modality. Surgical resection may be beneficial in some situations to decrease the risk of perforation and bleeding during chemotherapy and of local recurrence. Overall 5-year survival is 50% but exceeds 80% in patients with stage I or stage II disease. In patients with stage IE low-grade MALT lymphoma, successful eradication of *H pylori* with antibiotics induces regression of lymphoma in at least 60% of cases over a 1-year period. Further follow-up is needed to determine whether these patients are completely cured.

Bayerdorffer E et al: Regression of primary gastric lymphoma of mucosa-associated lymphoid tissue type after cure of *Helicobacter pylori* infection. MALT Lymphoma Study Group. Lancet 1995;345:1591.

Cooper DL, Doria R, Salloum E: Primary gastrointestinal lymphomas. Gastroenterologist 1996;4:54.

Imrie K et al: HIV-associated lymphoma of the gastrointestinal tract: The University of Toronto AIDS-lymphoma study group experience. Leuk Lymphoma 1995;16:343. (The gastrointestinal tract is involved in over one-fourth of HIV-associated lymphomas. Most present with extensive disease. The prognosis, even for apparently limited disease, is poor.)

Roggero E et al: Eradication of *Helicobacter pylori* infection in primary low-grade gastric lymphoma of mucosa-associated lymphoid tissue. Ann Intern Med 1995;122:767. (Disappearance of lymphomatous tissue observed in 15 of 25 patients after *H pylori* eradication.)

CARCINOID TUMORS

Gastric carcinoids are rare tumors that occur sporadically and in 3–5% of patients with Zollinger-Ellison syndrome and pernicious anemia due to chronic hypergastrinemia. They may be solitary or multicentric. Although they may secrete a variety of gut peptides, including serotonin, gastrin, pituitary hormones, and catecholamines, most are clinically silent and are detected incidentally at endoscopy. Symptom development generally reflects hepatic metastases. The majority are small, slow-growing, and benign in their behavior. Tumors larger than 2 cm in diameter have a greater potential for malignant spread and should be surgically excised. Small, solitary lesions may be removed endoscopically. Regression of small carcinoids occurs after antrectomy with resolution of hypergastrinemia.

Thirlby RC: Management of patients with gastric tumors. Gastroenterology 1995;108:296.

DISEASES OF THE SMALL INTESTINE

MALABSORPTION

"Malabsorption" is a broad term that comprises many disease processes. In clinical practice, it generally denotes disorders in which there is a disruption of digestion and nutrient absorption. The clinical and laboratory manifestations of malabsorption are summarized in Table 14–11. Normal digestion and absorption may be divided into three phases:

(1) Intraluminal phase: Dietary fats, proteins, and carbohydrates are hydrolyzed and solubilized by pancreatic and biliary secretions. Fats are broken down by pancreatic lipase to monoglycerides and fatty acids that form micelles with bile salts. Micelles are important for the solubilization and absorption of fat-soluble vitamins (A, D, E, K). Proteins are hydrolyzed by pancreatic proteases to di- and tripeptides and amino acids. Impaired intraluminal digestion may be caused by insufficient intraluminal concentrations of pancreatic enzymes or bile salts. These conditions will not be covered in detail here (see Chapter 15).

Pancreatic insufficiency may be caused by chronic pancreatitis, cystic fibrosis, or pancreatic cancer. Pancreatic enzymes may also be inactivated within the intestinal lumen by acid hypersecretion (Zollinger-Ellison syndrome). Significant pancreatic enzyme insufficiency generally results in significant steatorrhea (triglycerides)—often more than 20–40 g/24 hours—resulting in weight loss, gaseous distention and flatulence, and large, greasy, foul-smelling stools. The digestion of proteins and carbohydrates is affected to a far lesser degree and is generally not clinically significant. Because micellar function and intestinal absorption are normal, signs of other nutrient or vitamin deficiencies are rare.

Table 14–11. Clinical and laboratory manifestations of malabsorption.[1]

Manifestation	Laboratory Findings	Malabsorbed Nutrients
Steatorrhea (bulky, light-colored stools)	Increased fecal fat; decreased serum cholesterol	Fat
Diarrhea (increased fecal water)	Increased fecal fat or positive bile salt breath test	Fatty acids or bile salts
Weight loss; malnutrition (muscle wasting); weakness, fatigue Abdominal distention	Increased fecal fat and nitrogen; decreased glucose and xylose absorption	Calories (fat, protein, carbohydrates)
Iron deficiency anemia	Hypochromic anemia; low serum iron	Iron
Megaloblastic anemia	Macrocytosis; decreased vitamin B_{12} absorption (^{67}Co-labeled B_{12}); decreased serum vitamin B_{12} and red cell folate	Vitamin B_{12} or folic acid
Paresthesia; tetany; positive Trousseau and Chvostek signs	Decreased serum calcium, magnesium, and potassium	Calcium, vitamin D, magnesium, potassium
Bone pain; pathologic fractures; skeletal deformities	Osteoporosis on x-ray; osteomalacia on biopsy	Calcium, protein
Bleeding tendency (ecchymoses, melena, hematuria)	Prolonged prothrombin time	Vitamin K
Edema	Decreased serum albumin; increased fecal loss of α_1-antitrypsin (antiprotease)	Protein (or protein-losing enteropathy)
Nocturia; abdominal distention	Increased small bowel fluid on x-ray	Water
Milk intolerance (cramps, bloating, diarrhea)	Flat lactose tolerance test; decreased mucosal lactase levels	Lactose

[1]Modified from Bayless TM: Malabsorption in the elderly. Hosp Pract (Aug) 1979;14:57.

Decreased bile salt concentrations may be due to biliary obstruction or cholestatic liver diseases. Because bile salts are resorbed in the terminal ileum, resection or disease of this area (eg, Crohn's disease) can lead to insufficient intraluminal bile salts. Finally, destruction or loss of bile salts may be caused by bacterial overgrowth, massive acid hypersecretion, or medications that bind bile salts (eg, cholestyramine). (Bacterial overgrowth is discussed below.) Insufficient concentrations of intraluminal bile salts lead to mild steatorrhea (fatty acids and monoglycerides), though generally less than 20 g/d. Weight loss is minimal. Impaired absorption of fat-soluble vitamins (A, D, E, K) is common, resulting in bleeding tendencies, osteoporosis, and hypocalcemia (Table 14–11). Other nutrient absorption is intact. Intestinal loss of bile salts into the colon may cause a watery secretory diarrhea.

(2) Mucosal phase: The mucosal phase requires a sufficient surface area of intact small intestinal epithelium. Brush border enzymes are important in the hydrolysis of disaccharides and di- and tripeptides. Malabsorption of specific nutrients may occur as a result of deficiency in an isolated brush border enzyme. With the exception of lactase deficiency, these are rare congenital disorders that are evident in childhood. Malabsorption due to primary mucosal diseases, extensive intestinal resections (short bowel syndrome), or lymphoma is discussed below. These disorders result in malabsorption of all nutrients: fats, proteins, and amino acids. Depending upon the severity of malabsorption, patients may manifest a number of symptoms and signs, as outlined in Table 14–11.

(3) Absorptive phase: Obstruction of the lymphatic system results in impaired absorption of chylomicrons and lipoproteins. This may lead to steatorrhea and significant enteric protein losses or "protein-losing enteropathy," discussed below.

1. CELIAC SPRUE

Essentials of Diagnosis

- Weight loss.
- Distention, flatulence, greasy stools.
- Increased fecal fat (> 7 g/24 h).
- Abnormal small bowel biopsy.
- Clinical improvement on gluten-free diet.

General Considerations

Also known as gluten enteropathy or celiac disease, celiac sprue is characterized by diffuse damage to the proximal small intestinal mucosa that results in malabsorption of most nutrients. Although generally manifest in infancy, it may have its first clinical onset in the second to fourth decades, or even later. It occurs largely in whites of Northern European ancestry and is rare in Africans and Asians. It is strongly associated with selected HLA class II antigens: HLA-DR3 and HLA-DQw2. While the precise mechanism of damage is unknown, it is clear that removal of gluten from the diet results in resolution of symptoms and intestinal healing in most patients. Gluten refers to the protein component of grains such as wheat, rye, barley and oats—but not rice or corn. It is hypothesized that in a genetically susceptible host, gluten—perhaps in conjunction with a viral infection—incites a humoral and cell-mediated inflammatory response that results in mucosal inflammation and destruction.

Clinical Findings

A. Symptoms and Signs: The symptoms and signs of malabsorption depend upon the length of small intestine that is involved. Most patients report diarrhea, pronounced flatulence (due to colonic bacterial digestion of malabsorbed nutrients), weight loss, and weakness. The stools are characteristically loose to soft, large, floating, oily or greasy, and foul-smelling. However, they may also be watery and frequent in number (up to 10–12 daily). Patients with minimal involvement of only the duodenum and proximal jejunum may have no diarrhea or even constipation. Patients are often hyperphagic, and the severity of weight loss is highly variable. Physical examination may be entirely normal in mild cases or may reveal signs of malabsorption, such as loss of muscle mass or subcutaneous fat, pallor due to anemia, easy bruising due to vitamin K deficiency, hyperkeratosis due to vitamin A deficiency, or bone pain due to osteomalacia. Abdominal examination may reveal distention with hyperactive bowel sounds.

Dermatitis herpetiformis, a characteristic skin rash, occurs in less than 10% of patients with celiac sprue. Pruritic papulovesicles occur over the extensor surfaces of the extremities and over the trunk, scalp, and neck. Of patients with dermatitis herpetiformis however, over 85% have evidence of celiac disease on intestinal mucosal biopsy, though this may not be clinically evident.

B. Laboratory Findings:

1. Routine laboratory tests—Laboratory abnormalities depend upon the extent of intestinal involvement. A complete blood count, serum iron, red cell folate, vitamin B_{12} level, serum calcium, alkaline phosphatase, albumin, beta-carotene, and prothrombin time should be obtained in all patients with suspected malabsorption. Limited proximal involvement may result only in microcytic anemia due to iron deficiency. More extensive involvement results in a megaloblastic anemia due to folate deficiency. Low serum calcium or elevated alkaline phosphatase may reflect impaired calcium or vitamin D absorption with osteomalacia. Elevations of prothrombin time or a decreased serum beta-carotene reflect impaired fat-soluble vitamin absorption. Severe diarrhea may result in a non–anion gap acidosis and hypokalemia.

2. Specific tests for malabsorption—Steatorrhea is usually present but may be absent in mild disease. It may be detected by a qualitative (Sudan stain) or quantitative stool assessment for fecal fat. A positive Sudan stain is strong evidence of steatorrhea and usually obviates the need for quantitative analysis, but it is falsely negative in 25%. A quantitative 72-hour stool collection taken while patients are consuming a 100 g fat diet is a more sensitive means of detecting fat malabsorption. Excretion of more than 10 g/d of fat is abnormal and warrants further evaluation for malabsorption. Other tests of malabsorption such as the D-xylose test to provide evidence of mucosal malabsorption are no longer required with the availability of serologic screening for celiac disease.

3. Antibodies—A number of serologic tests can be used to screen for celiac disease and to monitor for patient adherence to the gluten-free diet. IgG and IgA anti-gliadin antibodies are present in over 90% of patients with celiac sprue but are elevated also in other mucosal diseases. The IgG antibody is more sensitive, and the IgA antibody is more specific. A combination of the two tests provides a sensitivity and specificity of over 95%. Thus, they are useful for screening for sprue in patients with suspected malabsorption. The IgA endomysial antibody is also less sensitive but more specific than the IgG anti-gliadin test. A combination of all three tests has a greater than 99% positive and negative predictive value. Given this high degree of reliability, it is possible that mucosal biopsy will not be required in the future for confirmation of the diagnosis. All of these antibodies fall rapidly on a gluten-free diet.

C. Mucosal Biopsy: Mucosal biopsy of the distal duodenum or proximal jejunum is the standard method for the diagnosis of celiac sprue. The endoscopic biopsy has supplanted the use of a suction biopsy tube. At endoscopy, atrophy or scalloping of the duodenal folds may be observed. Histology reveals loss of intestinal villi, hypertrophy of the intestinal crypts, and extensive infiltration of the lamina propria with lymphocytes and plasma cells. An adequate normal biopsy excludes the diagnosis. Reversion of these abnormalities on repeat biopsy after a patient is placed upon a gluten-free diet establishes the diagnosis. However, if a patient with a compatible biopsy demonstrates a prompt clinical improvement on a gluten-free diet and a decrease in antigliadin antibodies, a repeat biopsy is unnecessary.

Differential Diagnosis

Celiac sprue must be distinguished from other causes of malabsorption, as outlined above. Severe panmalabsorption of multiple nutrients is almost always caused by mucosal disease. In a patient with steatorrhea, a normal D-xylose test points to pancreatic insufficiency, reduced bile salts, or lymphatic obstruction. If the D-xylose test, however, is also abnormal, it strongly implicates mucosal disorders or bacterial overgrowth. Other mucosal diseases include tropical sprue, Whipple's disease, eosinophilic gastroenteritis, Crohn's disease, and intestinal lymphoma.

Treatment

Removal of all gluten from the diet is essential to therapy. All wheat, rye, barley, and oat products must be eliminated. Rice, soybean, potato, and corn flours are safe. Because of the pervasive use of gluten products in manufactured foods and additives and by restaurants, it is imperative that patients and their families meet with a knowledgeable dietician in order to comply satisfactorily with this lifelong diet. Several excellent dietary guides are available. Most patients with celiac disease also have lactose intolerance either temporarily or permanently and should avoid dairy products until the intestinal symptoms have improved on the gluten-free diet.

Improvement in symptoms should be evident within a few weeks on the gluten-free diet. The most common reason for failure is incomplete removal of gluten.

Prognosis & Complications

If appropriately diagnosed and treated, patients with celiac sprue have an excellent prognosis. Intestinal T cell lymphoma occurs in over 10% of patients with celiac sprue. The disorder should be suspected in patients previously responsive to the gluten-free diet who develop pain or new weight loss and malabsorption. Strict dietary compliance may reduce the risk of lymphoma development. In some patients, the disease may evolve and become refractory to the gluten-free diet. These patients generally have a poor prognosis, though some may respond to corticosteroids or immunosuppression with cyclosporine.

Garst PM, Lawson LM: Living with celiac sprue: The gluten free diet. M. Stevens Agency, PO Box 3004, Frankfurt, KY 40603. (Compiled from newsletters published by the Midwestern Celiac Sprue Association.)

Longstreth G: Successful treatment of refractory sprue with cyclosporine. Ann Intern Med 1993;119:1014. (Review of causes of refractory sprue. First case of response in adults to cyclosporine.)

Misra S, Ament ME: Diagnosis of coeliac sprue in 1994. Gastroenterol Clin North Am 1995;24:133.

O'Mahony S, Howdle PD, Losowsky MS: Management of patients with non-responsive coeliac disease. Aliment Pharmacol Ther 1996;10:671.

2. WHIPPLE'S DISEASE

Essentials of Diagnosis

- Malabsorption.
- Multisystemic disease.
- Fever, lymphadenopathy, arthralgias.
- Duodenal biopsy with PAS-positive macrophages with characteristic bacillus.

General Considerations

Whipple's disease is a rare multisystemic illness caused by infection with the bacillus *Tropheryma whippelii*. It may occur at any age but most commonly affects white men in the fourth to sixth decades. The source of infection is unknown, but no cases of human-to-human spread have been documented.

Clinical Findings

A. Symptoms and Signs: The clinical manifestations are protean. Gastrointestinal symptoms occur in approximately 75% of cases. They include diarrhea and some degree of malabsorption with distention, flatulence, and steatorrhea and weight loss. Loss of protein due to intestinal or lymphatic involvement may result in protein-losing enteropathy with hypoalbuminemia and edema. In the absence of gastrointestinal symptoms, the diagnosis often is delayed for several years. Intermittent low-grade fever occurs in over 50% of cases. Arthralgias or a migratory, nondeforming arthritis occur in 80%. Chronic cough is common. There may be generalized lymphadenopathy that resembles sarcoidosis. Myocardial or valvular involvement may lead to congestive failure or valvular regurgitation. Ocular findings include uveitis, vitreitis, keratitis, retinitis, and retinal hemorrhages. In approximately 10% of cases, central nervous system involvement occurs, manifested by a variety of findings such as dementia, lethargy, coma, seizures, myoclonus, or hypothalamic signs. Cranial nerve findings include ophthalmoplegia or nystagmus.

Physical examination may reveal evidence of malabsorption (see Table 14–11). Lymphadenopathy is present in 50%. Heart murmurs due to valvular involvement may be evident. Peripheral joints may be enlarged or warm. Neurologic findings are cited above.

B. Laboratory Findings: If significant malabsorption is present, patients may have laboratory abnormalities as outlined in Table 14–11. There may be steatorrhea.

C. Histologic Evaluation: The diagnosis of Whipple's disease is established by histologic evaluation of the involved tissues. In most cases, the diagnosis is established by endoscopic biopsy of the duodenum, which demonstrates infiltration of the lamina propria with PAS-positive macrophages that contain gram-positive bacilli (which are not acid-fast) and dilation of the lacteals. The Whipple bacillus has a characteristic electron microscopic appearance. In some patients who present with nongastrointestinal symptoms, the duodenal biopsy rarely may be normal, and biopsy of other involved organs or lymph nodes may be necessary. Because the PAS stain is less sensitive and specific for extraintestinal Whipple's disease, PCR is now used to confirm the diagnosis by demonstrating the presence of 16S ribosomal RNA of *T whippelii*.

Differential Diagnosis

Whipple's disease should be considered in patients who present with signs of malabsorption, fever of unknown origin, lymphadenopathy, seronegative arthritis, or multisystemic disease. Small bowel biopsy readily distinguishes Whipple's disease from other mucosal malabsorptive disorders, such as celiac sprue. Patients with AIDS and infection of the small intestine with *Mycobacterium avium* complex may have a similar clinical and histologic picture; although both conditions are characterized by PAS-positive macrophages, they may be distinguished by the acid-fast stain, which is positive for MAC and negative for the Whipple bacillus. Other conditions that may be confused with Whipple's disease include sarcoidosis, Reiter's syndrome, familial Mediterranean fever, systemic vasculitides, Behçet's disease, intestinal lymphoma, and subacute infective endocarditis.

Treatment

Antibiotic therapy results in a dramatic clinical improvement within several weeks, even in some patients with neurologic involvement. The optimal regimen is unknown. Complete clinical response usually is evident within 1–3 months; however, relapse may occur in up to one-third of patients after discontinuation of treatment. Therefore, prolonged treatment for at least 1 year is required. Drugs that cross the blood-brain barrier are preferred. Trimethoprim-sulfamethoxazole (one double-strength tablet twice daily for 1 year) is recommended as first-line therapy. In patients allergic to sulfonamides, ceftriaxone or chloramphenicol may be reasonable.

Prognosis

If untreated, the disease is fatal. Because some neurologic signs may be permanent, the goal of treatment is to prevent this progression. Patients must be followed closely after treatment for signs of symptom recurrence.

Cerebral Whipple's disease. BMJ 1996;312:371.

Dobbins WO: The diagnosis of Whipple's disease. N Engl J Med 1995;332:390. (PCR is now used to document the presence of *T whippelii* in infected tissues or blood and may be very useful in difficult cases.)

Feurle GE, Marth T: An evaluation of antimicrobial treatment for Whipple's disease: Tetracycline versus trimethoprim-sulfamethoxazole. Dig Dis Sci 1994;39:1642.

3. BACTERIAL OVERGROWTH

The small intestine normally contains a small number of bacteria. Bacterial overgrowth in the small intestine of whatever cause may result in malabsorption via a number of mechanisms. Bacterial deconjugation of bile salts may lead to inadequate micelle formation, resulting in decreased fat absorption with steatorrhea. Microbial uptake of specific nutrients reduces absorption of vitamin B_{12} and carbohydrates. Bacterial proliferation also causes direct damage to intestinal epithelial cells and the brush border, further impairing absorption of proteins and carbohydrates. Passage of the malabsorbed bile acids and carbohydrates into the colon leads to an osmotic and secretory diarrhea.

Causes of bacterial overgrowth include the following: (1) gastric achlorhydria (especially if other predisposing conditions present); (2) anatomic abnormalities of the small intestine with stagnation (afferent limb of Billroth II gastrojejunostomy, small intestine diverticula, obstruction, blind loop, radiation enteritis); (3) small intestine motility disorders (scleroderma, diabetic enteropathy, chronic intestinal pseudo-obstruction); (4) gastrocolic or coloenteric fistula (Crohn's disease, malignancy, surgical resection); and (5) miscellaneous disorders (AIDS, chronic pancreatitis). Bacterial overgrowth is an important cause of malabsorption in the elderly, perhaps because of decreased gastric acidity or impaired intestinal motility.

Clinical Findings

Many patients with bacterial overgrowth are asymptomatic. Patients with severe overgrowth have symptoms and signs of malabsorption, including distention, weight loss, and steatorrhea (Table 14–11). Watery diarrhea is common. Megaloblastic anemia or neurologic signs due to vitamin B_{12} deficiency are a common finding and may be a presenting manifestation. Qualitative or quantitative fecal fat assessment typically is abnormal. D-Xylose absorption is also abnormal owing to bacterial uptake of the carbohydrate. The Schilling test given without and with intrinsic factor may be abnormal, even in patients with normal serum vitamin B_{12} levels.

The diagnosis can be established firmly only by an aspirate and culture of proximal intestinal secretion that demonstrates over 10^5 organisms/mL. However, this is an invasive and laborious test and seldom done in most clinical settings. A number of noninvasive breath tests have been developed but lack sufficient sensitivity and specificity to be of great utility. The ^{14}C-xylose breath test is the most reliable. In this test, bacterial uptake and degradation of the isotope lead to the release of $^{14}CO_2$, which can be measured in exhaled breath. This test is not widely available.

Owing to the lack of an optimal test for bacterial overgrowth, most clinicians employ an empiric antibiotic trial as a diagnostic and therapeutic maneuver in patients with predisposing conditions for bacterial overgrowth who develop unexplained diarrhea or steatorrhea.

Treatment

Where possible, the anatomic defect that has potentiated bacterial overgrowth should be corrected. In many cases, this is not possible. Empiric treatment with broad-spectrum antibiotics usually leads to dramatic clinical improvement. Treatment with 1–2 weeks of an antibiotic (ciprofloxacin, 500 mg twice daily; trimethoprim-sulfamethoxazole, one double-strength tablet twice daily; doxycycline, 100 mg twice daily; or metronidazole, 250 mg three times daily) is recommended.

In patients in whom symptoms recur off antibiotics, cyclic therapy (eg, 1 week out of 4) may be sufficient. Continuous antibiotics should be avoided, if possible, to avoid development of bacterial antibiotic resistance.

In patients with severe intestinal dysmotility, treatment with small doses of octreotide has been shown to be of benefit in preliminary studies.

Kaye SA et al: Small bowel bacterial overgrowth in systemic sclerosis: Detection using direct and indirect methods and treatment outcome. Br J Rheumatol 1995;34:265.
Lewis SJ et al: Altered bowel function and duodenal bacterial overgrowth in patients treated with omeprazole. Aliment Pharmacol Ther 1996;10:557.

4. SHORT BOWEL SYNDROME

Short bowel syndrome is the malabsorptive condition that arises secondary to removal of significant segments of the small intestine. The most common causes in adults are Crohn's disease, mesenteric infarction, radiation enteritis, and trauma. The type and degree of malabsorption depend upon the length and site of the resection and the degree of adaptation of the remaining bowel.

Terminal Ileal Resection

Resection of the terminal ileum results in malabsorption of bile salts and vitamin B_{12}, which are normally absorbed in this region. Patients with low serum vitamin B_{12} levels, an abnormal Schilling test, or resection of over 50 cm of ileum require monthly intramuscular vitamin B_{12} injections. In patients with less than 100 cm of ileal resection, bile salt malabsorption stimulates fluid secretion from the colon, resulting in a watery diarrhea. This may be treated with bile salt binding resins (cholestyramine, 2–4 g three times daily with meals). Resection of over 100 cm of ileum leads to a reduction in the bile salt pool that results in steatorrhea and malabsorption of fat-soluble vitamins. Treatment is with a low-fat diet and vitamins supplemented with medium-chain triglycerides, which do not require micellar solubilization. Unabsorbed fatty acids bind with calcium, reducing its absorption and enhancing the absorption of oxalate. Oxalate kidney stones may develop. Calcium supplements should be administered to bind oxalate and in-

crease serum calcium. Cholesterol gallstones due to decreased bile salts are common also. In patients with resection of the ileocolonic valve, bacterial overgrowth may occur in the small intestine, further complicating malabsorption (as outlined above).

Extensive Small Bowel Resection

Loss of significant small intestine results in loss of absorptive area, resulting in nutrient and water and electrolyte malabsorption in addition to the deficits described above. After resection, the remaining intestine has a remarkable ability to adapt, increasing its absorptive capacity up to fourfold. As little as 100 cm of proximal jejunum may be sufficient to maintain adequate nutrition with oral feedings alone, though fluid and electrolyte losses still may be significant. Adaptation occurs gradually over 1 year. Patients with less than 100 cm of proximal jejunum remaining almost always require supplementation with either enteral supplements (elemental diets or polymeric) or total parenteral nutrition. Lactose should be eliminated. Levels of minerals such as zinc, magnesium, and calcium should be monitored. Parenteral vitamin supplementation may be necessary. Antidiarrheal agents (loperamide, 2–4 mg three times daily) slow transit and reduce diarrheal volume. Octreotide reduces intestinal transit time and fluid and electrolyte secretion. Gastric hypersecretion usually complicates intestinal resection and should be treated with H_2 receptor antagonists. Small intestine transplantation is now being successfully performed in some centers.

Grant D: Current results of intestinal transplantation. The International Intestinal Transplant Registry. Lancet 1996;347:1801. (Small bowel transplantation may be a lifesaving option for patients with short bowel syndrome who cannot tolerate TPN.)
Thompson J. Management of the short bowel syndrome. Gastroenterol Clin North Am 1994;23:403.
Wilmore DW: The short-bowel syndrome: New vistas. Gastroenterology 1996;110:1318. (Using a diet high in complex carbohydrates, low in fat, and supplemented with glutamine and subcutaneous growth hormone injections, 56% of people with short bowel syndrome were able to discontinue TPN.)

5. LACTASE DEFICIENCY

Lactase is a brush border enzyme that hydrolyzes the disaccharide, lactose, into glucose and galactose. Congenital lactase deficiency is common in premature infants of less than 30 weeks' gestation. In full-term infants it is rare, usually inherited as an autosomal recessive trait. The concentration of lactase enzyme levels is high at birth but declines steadily in most people of non-European ancestry during childhood and adolescence and into adulthood. Thus, approximately 50 million people in the USA have partial to complete lactose intolerance. As many as 90% of Asian-Americans, 70% of African-Americans, 95% of Native Americans, 50% of Mexican-Americans, and 60% of Jewish Americans are lactose-intolerant compared with less than 25% of other Caucasian adults. Lactase deficiency may also arise secondary to other gastrointestinal disorders that affect the proximal small intestinal mucosa. These include Crohn's disease, sprue, Whipple's disease, eosinophilic gastroenteritis, viral gastroenteritis, giardiasis, radiation enteritis, AIDS enteropathy (Microsporida infection, *Mycobacterium avium* complex infection, cryptosporidiosis), short bowel syndrome, and malnutrition. Malabsorbed lactose is fermented by intestinal bacteria, producing gas and organic acids. The nonmetabolized lactose and organic acids result in an increased stool osmotic load with an obligatory fluid loss.

Clinical Findings

A. Symptoms and Signs: Patients have great variability in clinical symptoms, depending both on the severity of lactase deficiency and the amount of lactose ingested. Most patients with lactose intolerance can tolerate up to 8 oz of milk without symptoms, though rare patients may have almost complete intolerance. With mild to moderate amounts of lactose malabsorption, patients may experience bloating, abdominal cramps, and flatulence. With higher lactose ingestions, an osmotic diarrhea will result. Isolated lactase deficiency does not result in other signs of malabsorption or weight loss. If these findings are present, other gastrointestinal disorders should be pursued. Diarrheal specimens reveal an increased osmotic gap and a pH of less than 6.0.

B. Laboratory Findings: The most widely available test for the diagnosis of lactase deficiency is the hydrogen breath test. After ingestion of 50 g of lactose, a rise in breath hydrogen of greater than 20 ppm within 90 minutes is a positive test, indicative of bacterial carbohydrate metabolism. In clinical practice, many physicians perform an empirical trial of a lactose-free diet for 2 weeks. Resolution of symptoms (bloating, flatulence, diarrhea) is highly suggestive of lactase deficiency (though a placebo response cannot be excluded) and may be confirmed, if necessary, with a breath hydrogen study.

Differential Diagnosis

The symptoms of late-onset lactose intolerance are nonspecific and may mimic a number of gastrointestinal disorders, such as inflammatory bowel disease, mucosal malabsorptive disorders, irritable bowel syndrome, and pancreatic insufficiency. Furthermore, lactase deficiency frequently develops secondary to other gastrointestinal disorders (as listed above). Concomitant lactase deficiency should always be considered in these gastrointestinal disorders.

Treatment

The goal of treatment in patients with isolated lactase deficiency is achieving patient comfort. Patients usually find their "threshold" of intake at which symptoms will occur. Foods that are high in lactose include milk (12 g/cup), ice cream (9 g/cup), and cottage cheese (8 g/cup). Aged cheeses have a lower lactose content (0.5 g/oz). Unpasteurized yogurt contains bacteria that produce lactase and is generally well tolerated.

Many patients will choose simply to restrict or eliminate milk products. By spreading dairy product intake throughout the day in quantities of less than 12 g of lactose (1 cup of milk), most patients can take dairy products without symptoms and do not require lactase supplements. Calcium supplementation should be considered in susceptible patients to prevent osteoporosis. Most grocery stores provide milk that has been pretreated with lactase, rendering it over 70% lactose-free. Lactase enzyme replacement is commercially available as a nonprescription formulation (Lactaid). Caplets of lactase may be taken with milk products, improving lactose absorption and eliminating symptoms. The number of caplets ingested depends upon the degree of lactose intolerance.

Malagelada J: Lactose intolerance. N Engl J Med 1995; 333:53.

Suarez FL et al: Review article: The treatment of lactose intolerance. Aliment Pharmacol Ther 1995;9:589.

ACUTE SMALL INTESTINAL OBSTRUCTION

Essentials of Diagnosis

- Cramping abdominal pain, vomiting.
- Tender distended abdomen.
- Dilated loops of small bowel; decreased air in colon.

General Considerations

Mechanical obstruction of the small intestine is a common surgical disorder that must be distinguished from adynamic ileus (see below). The most common causes of obstruction are adhesions (almost always in patients with prior abdominal surgery), external hernias, internal hernias, volvulus, Crohn's disease, radiation enteritis, intestinal wall hematomas (after trauma or anticoagulants), and, rarely, neoplasms. Most obstructions result in simple occlusion of the intestinal lumen that results in distention and enormous losses of fluid into the gut. If strangulation occurs, there is necrosis of the intestine with toxicity and the risk of perforation.

Clinical Findings

A. Symptoms and Signs: Cramping periumbilical pain occurs initially in waves lasting a few seconds to minutes but later becomes constant and diffuse as distention develops. Vomiting follows the onset of pain within minutes (proximal obstruction) to hours (distal obstruction). Obstipation soon develops in complete obstruction. With continued vomiting and intraluminal loss of fluids, dehydration develops. There is minimal or no fever. Abdominal distention is minimal in proximal obstruction but pronounced in distal obstruction. Mild tenderness is present, but peritoneal findings are absent. Peristaltic rushes and high-pitched tinkles occur during pain paroxysms. Visible peristalsis may be noted. Careful examination for abdominal wall hernias should be performed.

B. Laboratory Findings: In the initial stages, laboratory findings are normal. Progression is accompanied by hemoconcentration, electrolyte abnormalities, and leukocytosis.

C. Imaging: Plain film radiography reveals a ladder-like pattern of dilated small bowel with air-fluid levels. These findings may be minimal in proximal or closed-loop obstruction. With complete obstruction, the colon and rectum have little or no air. With strangulation, thickening and thumbprinting of the intestinal wall may be seen. In situations in which there is uncertainty about the diagnosis, barium radiography confirms the presence and location of small bowel obstruction.

Differential Diagnosis

Small intestinal obstruction must be distinguished from adynamic ileus and chronic intestinal pseudo-obstruction. It may be confused with other abdominal conditions such as pancreatitis, acute gastroenteritis, appendicitis, and acute mesenteric ischemia.

Complications

Strangulation with necrosis of the bowel wall can occur. This is difficult to detect clinically. Fever, severe tenderness with peritoneal irritation, and leukocytosis should raise suspicion for this possibility. Strangulation may lead to perforation, peritonitis, and sepsis.

Treatment

Initial therapy is directed toward fluid resuscitation and stabilization of the patient. Nasogastric suction is vital to relieve vomiting and abdominal distention. Isotonic fluids are administered as needed to restore intravascular volume and correct electrolyte disorders. If strangulation is suspected, broad-spectrum antibiotics should be given to provide anaerobic and gram-negative coverage.

Surgery is performed in all patients with complete bowel obstruction after appropriate supportive measures have been provided. In patients with incomplete obstruction or self-limited obstruction, the need to perform a surgical procedure is determined by the underlying disorder. For example, in patients with a known history of multiple adhesions, surgeons often prefer to avoid surgery unless symptoms are recurrent. In patients with Crohn's disease and an ileal stricture, an initial trial of medical management may be indicated.

Prognosis

Appropriately treated simple obstruction has a low mortality rate (< 2%). Strangulation is associated with a mortality rate of up to 25% if surgery is delayed.

INTESTINAL MOTILITY DISORDERS

1. ACUTE PARALYTIC ILEUS

Essentials of Diagnosis

- Precipitating factors: surgery, peritonitis, electrolyte abnormalities, severe medical illness.
- Nausea, vomiting, obstipation, distention.
- Minimal abdominal tenderness; decreased bowel sounds.
- Plain abdominal radiography with gas and fluid distention in small and large bowel.

General Considerations

Adynamic ileus is a condition in which there is neurogenic failure or loss of peristalsis in the intestine in the absence of any mechanical obstruction. It is commonly seen in hospitalized patients as a result of (1) intra-abdominal processes such as recent gastrointestinal or abdominal surgery or peritoneal irritation (peritonitis, pancreatitis, ruptured viscus, hemorrhage); (2) severe medical illness such as pneumonia, respiratory failure requiring intubation, sepsis or severe infections, uremia, diabetic ketoacidosis, and electrolyte abnormalities (hypokalemia, hypercalcemia, hypomagnesemia, hypophosphatemia); and (3) medications that affect intestinal motility (opioids, anticholinergics, phenothiazines).

Clinical Findings

A. Symptoms and Signs: Patients who are conscious report mild diffuse, continuous abdominal discomfort with nausea and vomiting. Generalized abdominal distention is present with minimal abdominal tenderness but no signs of peritoneal irritation (unless due to the primary disease). Bowel sounds are diminished to absent.

B. Laboratory Findings: The laboratory abnormalities are attributable to the underlying condition. Serum electrolytes, including potassium, magnesium, phosphorus, and calcium should be obtained to exclude abnormalities as contributing factors.

C. Imaging: Plain film radiography of the abdomen demonstrates distended gas-filled loops of small and large intestine. Air-fluid levels may be seen. Under some circumstances, it may be difficult to distinguish ileus from partial small bowel obstruction. A limited barium small bowel series or a CT scan may be useful in such instances to exclude mechanical obstruction, especially in postoperative patients.

Differential Diagnosis

Adynamic ileus must be distinguished from mechanical obstruction of the small bowel or proximal colon. Pain from small bowel mechanical obstruction is usually intermittent, cramping, and associated initially with profuse vomiting. Acute gastroenteritis, acute appendicitis, and acute pancreatitis all may present with ileus.

Treatment

The primary medical or surgical illness that has precipitated adynamic ileus should be treated. Most cases of ileus respond to restriction of oral intake with gradual liberalization of diet as bowel function returns. Severe or prolonged ileus require nasogastric suction and parenteral administration of fluids and electrolytes.

Frager D: Distinction between postoperative ileus and mechanical small-bowel obstruction: Value of CT compared with clinical and other radiographic findings. AJR Am J Roentgenol 1995;164:891.

2. ACUTE COLONIC PSEUDO-OBSTRUCTION (Ogilvie's Syndrome)

Essentials of Diagnosis

- Severe abdominal distention.
- Arises in postoperative state or with severe medical illness.
- May be precipitated by electrolyte imbalances, medications.
- Absent to mild abdominal pain; minimal tenderness.
- Massive dilation of cecum or right colon.

General Considerations

Spontaneous massive dilation of the cecum and proximal colon may occur in a number of different settings in hospitalized patients. Progressive cecal dilation may lead to spontaneous perforation with dire consequences. The risk of perforation correlates poorly with absolute cecal size. Colonic pseudo-obstruction is most commonly detected in surgical patients after trauma or burns or in the postoperative period and in medical patients with respiratory failure, metabolic imbalance, malignancy, myocardial infarction, congestive heart failure, pancreatitis, or recent neurologic catastrophe (cerebrovascular accident, subarachnoid hemorrhage, trauma). Liberal use of narcotics or anticholinergic agents may precipitate colonic pseudo-obstruction in susceptible patients. It may also occur as a manifestation of colonic ischemia. The etiology of colonic pseudo-obstruction is unknown, but an imbalance between gut sympathetic activity and sacral parasympathetic innervation of the distal colon is hypothesized.

Clinical Findings

A. Symptoms and Signs: Many patients are on ventilatory support or are unable to report symptoms due to altered mental status. Abdominal distention is frequently noted by the clinician as the first sign, often leading to a plain film radiograph that demonstrates colonic dilation. Some patients are asymptomatic, though most report mild, constant abdominal pain. Nausea and vomiting may be present. Bowel movements may be absent, though passage of flatus and diarrhea may continue. Abdominal tenderness with some degree of guarding or rebound tenderness may be detected; however, signs of peritonitis are absent unless perforation has occurred. Bowel sounds may be normal or increased.

B. Laboratory Findings: Laboratory findings reflect the underlying medical or surgical problems. Serum glucose, potassium, magnesium, phosphorus, and calcium should be obtained. Significant fever or leukocytosis raises concern for colonic perforation.

C. Imaging: Plain film radiographs demonstrate colonic dilation, usually confined to the cecum and proximal colon. The upper limits of normal for cecal size is 9 cm. A cecal diameter greater than 10–12 cm is worrisome for the possibility of colonic perforation. Varying amounts of small intestinal dilation and air-fluid levels due to adynamic ileus may be seen.

Differential Diagnosis

The appearance of the colon often raises concern for a colonic mechanical obstruction due to malignancy, volvulus, or fecal impaction. In many centers a Hypaque (diatrizoate meglumine) enema is performed both to exclude colonic obstruction and in an attempt to decompress the colon and evacuate distal fecal material. Colonic pseudo-obstruction should be distinguished from toxic megacolon, which is acute dilation of the colon due to inflammation (inflammatory bowel disease) or infection (pseudomembranous colitis, cytomegalovirus). Patients with toxic megacolon manifest fever, dehydration, significant abdominal pain, leukocytosis, and diarrhea, which is often bloody.

Treatment

The underlying illness should be treated aggressively. A nasogastric tube and a rectal tube should be placed. Patients should not remain in one position but should be periodically rolled from side to side and to the prone position. All electrolyte abnormalities should be corrected, and respiratory function should be optimized. All drugs that reduce intestinal motility, such as narcotics, anticholinergics, and calcium channel blockers, should be discontinued if at all possible. Enemas may be administered judiciously if large amounts of stool are evident on radiography. Oral laxatives are not helpful and may be dangerous. Intravenous cisapride has been reported to be helpful in case reports, but the intravenous formulation is not yet clinically available.

Patients must be watched carefully for signs of worsening distention or abdominal tenderness. Cecal size should be assessed by abdominal radiographs every 12 hours. Intervention to decompress the colon should be considered in patients with progressive dilation despite aggressive medical therapy, with sustained (48–72 hours) dilation without improvement, or with signs of clinical deterioration. Although worrisome, a single radiograph demonstrating an enlarged cecum of greater than 10–12 cm does not in itself warrant emergent decompression. Colonic decompression with aspiration of air or placement of a decompression tube is successful in up to 90% of patients. However, the procedure is technically difficult in an unprepared bowel and has been associated with perforations in the distended colon. Dilation recurs in up to half of patients. In patients in whom colonoscopy is unsuccessful, a tube cecostomy can be performed through a small laparotomy or with percutaneous radiologically guided placement.

Prognosis

In most cases, the prognosis is related to the underlying illness. With aggressive therapy, the development of perforation is unusual.

Rex DK: Acute colonic pseudo-obstruction (Ogilvie's syndrome). Gastroenterologist 1994;2:233.

CHRONIC INTESTINAL PSEUDO-OBSTRUCTION

Chronic intestinal pseudo-obstruction is a syndrome characterized by symptoms and signs of intestinal obstruction in the absence of any mechanical lesions to account for the findings. It is caused by a heterogeneous group of systemic conditions and disorders of the visceral smooth muscle or myenteric plexus. Systemic conditions include hypothyroidism, progressive systemic sclerosis, muscular dystrophy, Chagas' disease, Ehlers-Danlos syndrome, amyloidosis, porphyria, paraneoplastic syndromes, myotonic dystrophy, neurofibromatosis, and Parkinson's disease. In addition, there are a large number of primary visceral myopathies and neuropathies that may be inherited or occur sporadically.

Clinical Findings

The diagnosis is based upon a compatible clinical history and physical examination and the exclusion of mechanical obstruction by radiologic studies.

A. Symptoms and Signs: The type and severity of symptoms vary according to the underlying cause and the extent of gastrointestinal involvement. Symptoms of systemic disease should be sought. A family history should be elicited.

Symptoms of gastrointestinal dysfunction often wax and wane over time. Acute exacerbations may simulate bowel obstruction, and many patients undergo exploratory laparotomy before the diagnosis is recognized. Patients with predominant small bowel involvement have variable amounts of abdominal distention, ranging from unnoticeable to massive. Abdominal pain is common and often parallels the severity of distention. Vomiting—occurring hours after meals—and diarrhea are typical. Patients commonly curtail their oral intake, resulting in malnutrition. Bacterial overgrowth in the stagnant intestine may result in steatorrhea and malabsorption. With colonic involvement, there may be constipation or alternating periods of constipation and diarrhea. Gastric involvement leads to symptoms of gastroparesis with early satiety, nausea, and postprandial vomiting.

Physical abnormalities may include cachexia, signs of dehydration, abdominal distention, and a fluid succussion splash. Bowel sounds range from absent to increased. Laboratory findings reflect the severity of malnutrition and malabsorption. Anemia due to decreased folate, iron, or vitamin B_{12} is common. In cases of unclear origin, thyroid function tests, urinary porphobilinogen, ANA, anti-SCL-70, and serum CK are obtained, as indicated, to exclude underlying systemic disease.

B. Imaging: Plain film radiography demonstrates dilation of small intestine or colon with air-fluid levels. The appearance may resemble that of adynamic ileus or mechanical small or large bowel obstruction. A dilated esophagus, stomach, duodenum, or colon may all be present. Barium radiography of the entire gastrointestinal tract is imperative to exclude mechanical obstruction and to evaluate the extent of gastrointestinal involvement.

C. Manometry: Esophageal manometry demonstrates diminished peristaltic amplitude or aperistalsis in the majority of patients with primary visceral disease. Small intestinal manometry is available at specialized centers and may be able to distinguish patients with visceral myopathy from those with neuropathy.

Treatment

There is no specific therapy for pseudo-obstruction. Difficult cases should be referred to centers with expertise in this area. Treatment is directed at maintaining nutrition. All agents that reduce intestinal motility (opioids, anticholinergics) should be eliminated. Cisapride, 10–20 mg three times daily, may improve symptoms in many patients. Bacterial overgrowth should be treated with intermittent or cyclic antibiotics (see above). The diet should be low in fiber and fat. Vitamin and mineral deficiencies should be corrected. Episodes of acute exacerbation are treated with nasogastric suction and intravenous fluids. Patients with persistent distention may require a venting gastrostomy to relieve distress. Some patients may tolerate enteral nutrition through surgical jejunostomy tubes. Patients unable to maintain adequate nutrition require intermittent or permanent total parenteral nutrition. Small bowel transplantation is an option in some patients.

Prognosis

The prognosis depends upon the underlying cause and the severity of gastrointestinal dysfunction. Many patients survive for many years on parenteral nutrition.

Quigley E: Gastric and small intestinal motility in health and disease. Gastroenterol Clin North Am 1996;25:113.

TUMORS OF THE SMALL INTESTINE

Benign and malignant tumors of the small intestine are rare. They often cause no symptoms or signs. However, they may cause acute gastrointestinal bleeding with hematochezia or melena or chronic gastrointestinal blood loss resulting in fatigue and iron deficiency anemia. Small bowel tumors may cause obstruction due to luminal narrowing or intussusception of a polypoid mass. Small bowel tumors usually are identified by barium radiographic studies, either enteroclysis or a small bowel series. Visualization and biopsy of duodenal and proximal jejunal mass lesions is performed with a long upper endoscope known as an enteroscope.

1. BENIGN TUMORS OF SMALL INTESTINE

Benign polyps may be symptomatic or may be incidental findings detected on endoscopy or radiographic study. With the exception of lipomas, surgical excision usually is recommended. Adenomatous polyps are the most common benign mucosal tumor. The majority are asymptomatic, though acute or chronic bleeding may occur. Malignant transformation does occur. Villus adenomas occur most commonly in the periampullary region of the duodenum and carry a high risk for development of invasive cancer. Lipomas occur commonly in the ileum. Rarely, they may cause obstruction with intussusception. Leiomyomas are found at all levels of the intestine. These submucosal lesions may ulcerate and cause acute or chronic bleeding or may cause obstruction. It is difficult to distinguish these from

leiomyosarcomas except by surgical excision. Benign polyps may also occur as part of familial polyposis syndromes, which are discussed under Diseases of the Colon and Rectum.

2. MALIGNANT TUMORS OF SMALL INTESTINE

Malignant tumors of the small intestine are extremely rare. They may present with anemia, bleeding, obstruction, or evidence of metastatic disease.

Adenocarcinoma

These are aggressive tumors that occur most commonly in the duodenum or proximal jejunum. They account for 30–40% of small bowel cancers. At the time of diagnosis, 80% have already metastasized. Resection is recommended (when possible) for control of symptoms.

Lymphoma

Gastrointestinal lymphomas may arise in the gastrointestinal tract or involve it secondarily with disseminated disease. In Western countries, primary gastrointestinal lymphomas account for 5% of lymphomas and up to one-third of small bowel malignancies. They occur most commonly in the distal small intestine. The majority are non-Hodgkin's B cell lymphomas. However, T cell lymphomas may arise in patients with celiac sprue. In the Middle East, lymphomas also may arise in the setting of IPSID (immunoproliferative small intestinal disease). In this condition, there is diffuse lymphoplasmacytic infiltration of the mucosa and submucosa that results in weight loss, diarrhea, and malabsorption that may lead to lymphomatous transformation. A characteristic feature of the disease is the presence of alpha heavy chains in the serum in 70%.

Presenting symptoms or signs of primary lymphoma include abdominal pain, weight loss, nausea and vomiting, distention, anemia, and occult blood in the stool. Fevers are unusual. Protein-losing enteropathy may result in hypoalbuminemia, but other signs of malabsorption are unusual. Barium radiography helps to localize the site of the lesion. The diagnosis requires endoscopic, percutaneous, or laparoscopic biopsy. In order to determine tumor stage, patients must undergo chest and abdominal CT, bone marrow biopsy, and, in some cases, lymphangiography.

Treatment depends on the stage of disease. Surgical resection of primary intestinal lymphoma (when possible) is usually recommended. Even in cases of stage III or stage IV disease, surgical debulking may improve survival. In patients with limited disease (stage IE) which is resected, the role of adjuvant chemotherapy is unclear. Most patients with more extensive disease are treated with systemic chemotherapy with or without radiation therapy.

Carcinoid

Carcinoids account for up to 30–40% of small intestinal tumors. Over 95% of gastrointestinal carcinoids occur in one of three sites: the rectum, the appendix, or the small intestine. Rectal carcinoids are usually detected incidentally as submucosal nodules during proctoscopic examination. Similarly, appendiceal carcinoids are identified in 0.3% of appendectomies. Almost 80% of these tumors are less than 1 cm in size, and 90% are less than 2 cm. Rectal carcinoids less than 1.5 cm and appendiceal carcinoids less than 2 cm virtually never metastasize and are treated effectively with local excision or simple appendectomy. Tumors larger than 1.5–2 cm are associated with the development of metastasis in over 20% of appendiceal carcinoids and up to 100% of rectal carcinoids. Hence, in younger patients who are good operative risks, a more extensive cancer resection operation is warranted.

Small intestinal carcinoids most commonly arise in the ileum. Up to one-third are multicentric. Although 60% are less than 2 cm in size, even these small carcinoids may metastasize. Almost all tumors over 2 cm are associated with metastasis. Most smaller lesions are asymptomatic, though intussusception with obstruction occurs rarely. Carcinoids may extend locally into the muscularis, serosa, and mesentery, where they engender a fibroblastic reaction with contraction and kinking of the bowel. This may lead to symptoms of partial small bowel obstruction with intermittent abdominal pain. Small bowel barium studies may reveal kinking, but because the lesion is extraluminal the diagnosis may be overlooked for several years. Encasement of the mesenteric vessels can lead to bowel infarction. Further extension occurs to the local lymph nodes and to the liver. Abdominal CT may demonstrate a mesenteric mass with tethering of the bowel, lymphadenopathy, and hepatic metastasis. Carcinoid involvement of the heart (resulting in tricuspid regurgitation) is a late manifestation of metastatic disease. Carcinoid syndrome (see Chapter 4) is seen only in patients with hepatic metastasis. Virtually all patients with carcinoid syndrome have obvious signs of cancer with liver metastasis on abdominal imaging. The optimal initial hepatic imaging study is somatostatin receptor scintigraphy, which is positive in over 90% of patients with metastatic carcinoid. A normal urinary 5-HIAA and serum serotonin excludes carcinoid syndrome with over 99% certainty.

Small intestinal carcinoids are extremely indolent tumors with slow spread; however, true cure is seldom achieved. Patients with disease confined to the small intestine should have local excision, for which the cure rate exceeds 85%. In patients with resectable disease who have lymph node involvement, the 5-year disease-free survival is 80%; however, by 25 years less than 25% remain disease-free. Even in patients with hepatic metastases, the median survival is 3 years. In patients with advanced disease, therapy should be deferred until the patient is symptomatic. Surgery should be directed toward palliation of obstructive symptoms. In patients with carcinoid symptoms, resection of hepatic metastases may provide dramatic symptomatic improvement. Octreotide represents a major advance in the treatment of severe carcinoid syndrome and diarrhea. Hepatic artery occlusion and chemotherapy may provide symptomatic improvement in some patients with hepatic metastases.

Lambert P et al: Treatment and prognosis of primary malignant small bowel tumors. Am Surg 1996;62:709.

Modlin IM, Tang LH: Approaches to the diagnosis of gut neuroendocrine tumors: The last word (today). Gastroenterology 1997;112:583.

Solcia E et al: Endocrine tumors of the small and large intestine. Pathol Res Pract 1995;191:366.

Kaposi's Sarcoma

Kaposi's sarcoma is a common complication in AIDS, though the incidence appears to be declining. Recently, a newly recognized herpesvirus known as human herpesvirus 8 has been implicated as the infectious agent causing this disease. Kaposi's sarcoma is the most common intestinal tumor in HIV-infected patients. Lesions may be present anywhere in the intestinal tract. Visceral involvement usually is associated with cutaneous disease. Most lesions are clinically silent; however, large lesions may be symptomatic. Lesions of the gingiva, palate, and hypopharynx can lead to painful mastication and dysphagia. Lesions of the stomach or small intestine may lead to bleeding, obstruction, or even perforation. Obstruction of peritoneal lymph nodes can lead to protein-losing enteropathy and malabsorption. The diagnosis may be confirmed at endoscopy by the characteristic visual appearance and by biopsy. Oral complications can be treated with the CO_2 laser or radiation. Limited bleeding or obstructing lesions in the stomach or anus can be treated with the YAG laser or radiation therapy. Widespread involvement may be best treated with systemic chemotherapy with combinations of vincristine, bleomycin, or doxorubicin, to which the tumor is very responsive.

Foreman K et al: Propagation of a human herpesvirus from AIDS-associated Kaposi's sarcoma. N Engl J Med 1997;336:163.

Morris A, Valley A: Overview of the management of AIDS-related Kaposi's sarcoma. Ann Pharmacother 1996;30:1950.

APPENDICITIS

Essentials of Diagnosis

- Early: periumbilical pain; later: right lower quadrant pain and tenderness.
- Anorexia, nausea and vomiting, obstipation.
- Low-grade fever and leukocytosis.

General Considerations

Appendicitis is the most common abdominal surgical emergency, affecting approximately 10% of the population. It occurs most commonly between the ages of 10 and 30 years. It is initiated by obstruction of the appendix by a fecalith, inflammation, foreign body, or neoplasm. Obstruction leads to increased intraluminal pressure, venous congestion, infection, and thrombosis of intramural vessels. If untreated, gangrene and perforation develop within 36 hours.

Clinical Findings

A. Symptoms and Signs: Appendicitis usually begins with vague, often colicky periumbilical or epigastric pain. Within 12 hours the pain shifts to the right lower quadrant, manifested as a steady ache that is worsened by walking or coughing. Almost all patients have nausea with one or two episodes of vomiting. Protracted vomiting suggests another diagnosis. A sense of constipation is typical, and some patients administer cathartics in an effort to relieve their symptoms—though some report diarrhea. Low-grade fever (< 38 °C) is typical; high fever or rigors suggest another diagnosis or appendiceal perforation.

On physical examination, localized tenderness with guarding in the right lower quadrant can be elicited with gentle palpation with one finger. When asked to cough, patients may be able to precisely localize the painful area, a sign of peritoneal irritation. Light percussion may also elicit pain. Although rebound tenderness is also present, it is unnecessary to elicit this finding if the above signs are present. Psoas and obturator signs are indicative of adjacent inflammation and strongly suggestive of appendicitis.

B. Laboratory Findings: Moderate leukocytosis (10,000–20,000/µL) with neutrophilia is common. Microscopic hematuria and pyuria is present in one-fourth of patients.

C. Imaging: No imaging studies are necessary in patients with typical appendicitis. Studies may be useful in patients in whom the diagnosis is uncertain. Abdominal or transvaginal ultrasound has a diagnostic accuracy of over 85% and is especially useful in the exclusion of adnexal disease in younger women. Abdominal CT is useful in cases of suspected appendiceal perforation to diagnose a periappendiceal abscess.

Atypical Presentations of Appendicitis

Owing to the variable location of the appendix, there are a number of "atypical" presentations. Because the retrocecal appendix does not touch the anterior abdominal wall, the pain remains less intense and poorly localized; abdominal tenderness is minimal and may be elicited in the right flank. The psoas sign may be positive. With pelvic appendicitis there is pain in the lower abdomen, often on the left, with an urge to urinate or defecate. Abdominal tenderness is absent, but tenderness is evident on pelvic or rectal examination; the obturator sign may be present. In the elderly, the diagnosis of appendicitis is often delayed because patients present with minimal, vague symptoms and mild abdominal tenderness. Appendicitis in pregnancy may present with pain in the right lower quadrant, periumbilical area, or right subcostal area owing to displacement of the appendix by the uterus.

Differential Diagnosis

Given its frequency and myriad presentations, appendicitis should be considered in the differential diagnosis of all patients with an acute abdominal problem. It can be extremely difficult to reliably diagnose appendicitis in some cases. The lack of the classic migration of pain (from the epigastrium to the right lower abdomen), right lower quadrant pain, fever, or guarding makes appendicitis less likely. Approximately 10–20% of patients with suspected appendicitis have either a negative examination at laparotomy or have an alternative surgical diagnosis. The widespread use of ultrasonography and CT has reduced the number of incorrect diagnoses. Still, in some cases diagnostic laparotomy or laparoscopy is required. The most common causes of diagnostic confusion are gastroenteritis and gynecologic disorders. Viral gastroenteritis presents with nausea, vomiting, low-grade fever, and diarrhea and can be difficult to distinguish from appendicitis. The onset of vomiting before pain makes appendicitis less likely. As a rule, the pain of gastroenteritis is more generalized and the tenderness less well localized. Acute salpingitis or tubo-ovarian abscess should be considered in young, sexually active women with fever and bilateral abdominal or pelvic tenderness. A twisted ovarian cyst may also cause sudden severe pain. The sudden onset of lower abdominal pain in the middle of the menstrual cycle suggests mittelschmerz. Sudden severe abdominal pain with diffuse pelvic tenderness and shock suggests a ruptured ectopic pregnancy. A positive pregnancy test and pelvic ultrasonography are diagnostic. Retrocecal or retroileal appendicitis (often associated with pyuria or hematuria) may be confused with ureteral colic or pyelonephritis. Other conditions that may resemble appendicitis include: diverticulitis, perforated colonic cancer, Crohn's ileitis, perforated peptic ulcer, cholecystitis, and mesenteric adenitis. It is virtually impossible to distinguish appendicitis from Meckel's diverticulitis;

the distinction, however, is academic, as both require surgical treatment.

Complications

Perforation occurs in 20% of patients and should be suspected in patients with pain persisting for over 36 hours, high fever, diffuse abdominal tenderness or peritoneal findings, a palpable abdominal mass, or marked leukocytosis. Localized perforation results in a contained abscess, usually in the pelvis. A free perforation leads to suppurative peritonitis with toxicity. Septic thrombophlebitis (pylephlebitis) of the portal venous system is rare. It is suggested by high fever, chills, bacteremia, and jaundice.

Treatment

The treatment of uncomplicated appendicitis is surgical appendectomy. This may be performed through a laparotomy or by laparoscopy. Prior to surgery, patients should be given systemic antibiotics, which reduce the incidence of postoperative wound infections. Emergency appendectomy is also required in patients with perforated appendicitis with generalized peritonitis.

The optimal treatment of stable patients with perforated appendicitis and a contained abscess is controversial. Surgery in this setting can be difficult. Many recommend percutaneous CT-guided drainage of the abscess with intravenous fluids and antibiotics to allow the inflammation to subside. An interval appendectomy may be performed after 6 weeks to prevent recurrent appendicitis.

Prognosis

The mortality rate from uncomplicated appendicitis is extremely low. Even with perforated appendicitis, the mortality rate in most groups is less than 1% but approaches 15% in the elderly.

Panton ON et al: A four-year experience with laparoscopy in the management of appendicitis. Am J Surg 1996; 171:538.

Temple CL et al: The natural history of appendicitis in adults: A prospective study. Ann Surg 1995;221:278.

Wagner JM, McKinney WP, Carpenter JL: Does this patient have appendicitis? JAMA 1996;276:1589.

INTESTINAL TUBERCULOSIS

Intestinal tuberculosis is common in underdeveloped countries. Previously rare in the United States, its incidence has been rising in immigrant groups and patients with AIDS. It is caused by both *M tuberculosis* and *M bovis*. Active pulmonary disease is present in less than 50% of patients. The most frequent site of involvement is the ileocecal region; however, any region of the gastrointestinal tract may be involved. Intestinal tuberculosis may cause mucosal ulcerations or scarring and fibrosis with narrowing of the lumen. Patients may complain of chronic abdominal pain, obstructive symptoms, weight loss, and diarrhea. An abdominal mass may be palpable. Complications include intestinal obstruction, hemorrhage, fistula formation, and bacterial overgrowth with malabsorption. The PPD skin test may be negative, especially in patients with weight loss or AIDS. Barium radiography may demonstrate mucosal ulcerations, thickening, or stricture formation. The differential diagnosis includes Crohn's disease, carcinoma, and intestinal amebiasis. The diagnosis is established by either endoscopic or surgical biopsy revealing acid-fast bacilli within involved tissue.

Treatment with standard regimens is effective.

Leder RA, Low VN: Tuberculosis of the abdomen. Radiol Clin North Am 1995;33:691.

PROTEIN-LOSING ENTEROPATHY

Protein-losing enteropathy comprises a number of conditions that result in excessive loss of serum proteins into the gastrointestinal tract. The essential diagnostic features are hypoalbuminemia and an elevated fecal α_1-antitrypsin level.

The normal intact gut epithelium prevents the loss of serum proteins. Proteins may be lost through one of three mechanisms: (1) mucosal disease with ulceration, resulting in the loss of proteins across the disrupted mucosal surface; (2) lymphatic obstruction, resulting in the loss of protein-rich chylous fluid from mucosal lacteals; and (3) idiopathic change in permeability of mucosal capillaries and conductance of interstitium, resulting in "weeping" of protein-rich fluid from the mucosal surface (Table 14–12).

Hypoalbuminemia is the sine qua non of protein-losing enteropathy. However, a number of other serum proteins such as α_1-antitrypsin also are lost from the gut epithelium. In protein-losing enteropathy caused by lymphatic obstruction, loss of lymphatic fluid commonly results in lymphocytopenia ($< 1000/\mu L$), reduced serum gamma globulins, and reduced cholesterol.

In most cases, protein-losing enteropathy is recognized as a sequela of a known gastrointestinal disorder. In patients in whom the cause is unclear, evaluation is indicated and is guided by the clinical suspicion. Protein-losing enteropathy must be distinguished from other causes of hypoalbuminemia, which include liver disease and nephrotic syndrome; and from congestive heart failure. Protein-losing enteropathy is confirmed by determining the gut α_1-antitrypsin clearance (24-hour volume of feces × stool concentration of α_1-antitrypsin ÷ serum α_1-antitrypsin concentration). A clearance of more than 13 mL/24 h is abnormal.

Table 14–12. Causes of protein-losing enteropathy.

Mucosal disease with ulceration
    Chronic gastric ulcer
    Gastric carcinoma
    Lymphoma
    Inflammatory bowel disease
    Idiopathic ulcerative jejunoileitis
Lymphatic obstruction
    Primary intestinal lymphangiectasia
    Secondary obstruction
        Cardiac disease: constrictive pericarditis, congestive
            heart failure
        Infections: tuberculosis, Whipple's disease
        Neoplasms: lymphoma, Kaposi's sarcoma
        Retroperitoneal fibrosis
        Sarcoidosis
Idiopathic mucosal transudation
    Ménétrier's disease
    Zollinger-Ellison syndrome
    Acute viral gastroenteritis
    Celiac sprue
    Eosinophilic gastroenteritis
    Allergic protein-losing enteropathy
    Parasite infection: giardiasis, hookworm
    Amyloidosis
    Common variable immunodeficiency
    Systemic lupus erythematosus

Laboratory evaluation of protein-losing enteropathy consists of serum protein electrophoresis, lymphocyte count, and serum cholesterol to look for evidence of lymphatic obstruction. Serum ANA and C3 levels are useful to screen for collagen vascular disorders. Stool samples should be examined for ova and parasites. Evidence of malabsorption is evaluated by means of a stool qualitative fecal fat determination. Intestinal imaging is performed with an upper endoscopy with small bowel biopsy and a small bowel barium series. Colonic diseases are excluded with barium enema or colonoscopy. A CT scan of the abdomen is performed to look for evidence of neoplasms or lymphatic obstruction. Rarely, lymphangiography is helpful. In some situations, laparotomy with full-thickness intestinal biopsy is required to establish a diagnosis.

Treatment is directed at the underlying cause.

DISEASES OF THE COLON & RECTUM

IRRITABLE BOWEL SYNDROME

Essentials of Diagnosis

- Chronic functional disorder characterized by abdominal pain, alterations in bowel habits.
- Limited evaluation to exclude organic causes of symptoms.
- Symptoms usually begin in late teens to early 20s.

General Considerations

The functional gastrointestinal disorders are characterized by a variable combination of chronic or recurrent gastrointestinal symptoms *not explained by structural or biochemical abnormalities*. Several clinical entities are included under this broad rubric, including chest pain of unclear origin (noncardiac chest pain), nonulcer dyspepsia, and biliary dyskinesia (sphincter of Oddi dysfunction). There is a large overlap between these entities. For example, over half of patients with noncardiac chest pain and over one-third with nonulcer dyspepsia also have symptoms compatible with irritable bowel syndrome. In none of these cases is there a definitive diagnostic process or test. Rather, the diagnosis is a subjective one based upon the presence of a compatible profile and the exclusion of other "organic" disorders.

Irritable bowel syndrome can be defined, therefore, as an idiopathic clinical entity characterized by some combination of chronic symptoms, including the following: (1) abdominal pain, (2) altered or fluctuating bowel frequency and stool consistency, (3) abdominal distention or bloating, and (4) varying degrees of anxiety or depression. This constellation of symptoms may also be called "spastic colitis" or "mucous colitis." Patients may also have other functional complaints such as dyspepsia, heartburn, chest pain, fatigue, urologic dysfunction, and gynecologic problems.

Irritable bowel syndrome is an idiopathic clinical entity characterized by some combination of chronic (more than 3 months) lower abdominal symptoms and bowel complaints that may be continuous or intermittent. The current working definition of irritable bowel syndrome is based on one or both of the following complaints: (1) **abdominal pain** that is relieved by defecation or is associated with a change in the frequency or consistency of stool, and (2) **disturbed defecation** evidenced by at least two of the following: altered stool frequency (> 3 movements per day or < 3 per week), altered stool form (lumpy-hard, watery), altered stool passage (straining, urgency, incomplete evacuation), bloating or abdominal distention, passage of mucus.

Patients may also have a number of other somatic and psychologic complaints such as dyspepsia, heartburn, chest pain, fatigue, urologic dysfunction, gynecologic symptoms, anxiety, and depression.

This disorder is extremely common. Up to 20% of the adult population has symptoms compatible with the diagnosis, but most never seek medical attention. It is a common problem presenting to both the gastroenterologist and the primary care physician.

Pathogenesis

Irritable bowel syndrome probably represents a common clinical manifestation of a heterogeneous group of disorders. A number of pathophysiologic mechanisms have been identified and may have varying importance among different individuals.

A. Abnormal Motility: A variety of abnormal myoelectrical and motor abnormalities have been identified in the colon and small intestine. In some cases, these are temporally correlated with episodes of abdominal pain or emotional stress. Whether they represent a primary motility disorder or are secondary to psychosocial stress is debated. Differences between patients with constipation-predominant and diarrhea-predominant syndromes are reported.

B. Heightened Visceral Nociception: Patients often have a lower visceral pain threshold, reporting abdominal pain at lower volumes of colonic gas insufflation or colonic balloon inflation than controls. Although many patients complain of bloating and distention, washout studies have shown that their absolute intestinal gas volume is normal. Many patients report rectal urgency despite small rectal volumes of stool.

C. Psychosocial Abnormalities: More than half of patients with irritable bowel who seek medical attention have underlying depression, anxiety, or somatization. By contrast, those who do not seek medical attention are similar psychologically to normal individuals. Psychologic abnormalities may influence how the patient perceives or reacts to illness and minor visceral sensations.

Clinical Findings

A. Symptoms and Signs: Irritable bowel is a chronic, lifelong condition. Symptoms usually begin in the late teens to twenties. Symptoms should have been present for at least 3 months before the diagnosis is considered. The diagnosis is established in the presence of compatible symptoms and after the exclusion of organic disease. Although patients report a variety of symptoms, four in particular are more common in this disorder than in organic disease: (1) abdominal distention, (2) abdominal pain which is relieved by defecation, (3) more frequent stools with the onset of abdominal pain, and (4) looser stools with the onset of pain. Over 90% of patients have two or more of these symptoms, compared with 30% of patients with organic disorders. In patients over age 60, however, in whom organic disease is more common, the predictive value of these criteria is much lower.

Abdominal pain usually is intermittent, crampy, and in the lower abdominal region. It may be relieved by defecation, worsened by stress, and worse for 1–2 hours after meals. It does not usually occur at night or interfere with sleep. Patients may report predominant problems with constipation, diarrhea, or alternating constipation and diarrhea. It is important to clarify what the patient means by these complaints. The patient may use the term constipation to refer to hard or small stools, straining, or reduced stool frequency. Diarrhea may refer to loose stools, frequent stools, urgency, or fecal incontinence. Many patients report that they have a firm stool in the morning followed by progressively looser movements. Mucus is commonly seen. Complaints of visible distention and bloating are common, though these are not clinically evident.

The acute onset of symptoms raises the likelihood of organic disease. Nocturnal diarrhea, hematochezia, weight loss, and fever are incompatible with a diagnosis of irritable bowel syndrome and warrant investigation for underlying disease.

A thorough physical examination should be performed to look for evidence of organic disease and to allay the patient's anxieties. The physical examination usually is unremarkable. Abdominal tenderness, especially in the lower abdomen, is common but not pronounced. A new onset of symptoms in a patient over age 40 warrants further examination.

B. Laboratory Findings and Special Examinations: In a patient 20–50 years of age with a presumptive clinical diagnosis of irritable bowel syndrome, a limited series of examinations is warranted to screen for organic disease. The complete blood count, serologic tests, serum albumin, erythrocyte sedimentation rate, and stool occult blood test all should be normal. In patients with diarrhea, thyroid function tests and stool examination for ova and parasites should be performed. If diarrhea is predominant, a 24-hour stool collection is useful. Stool weight in excess of 300 g/d is atypical of irritable bowel and warrants further evaluation. In patients under age 40, a flexible sigmoidoscopy should be performed. In patients over age 40 who have not had a previous evaluation, barium enema or colonoscopy should be considered.

Differential Diagnosis

These common symptoms may have multiple organic origins that should not be overlooked. Examples are colonic neoplasia, inflammatory bowel disease, causes of chronic constipation, causes of chronic diarrhea, endometriosis, and lactase deficiency. Psychiatric disorders such as depression and anxiety must be considered as well.

Treatment

A. General Measures: As with other functional disorders, the most important interventions the physician can offer are reassurance and a forthright explanation of the functional nature of the symptoms. Indeed, an ongoing therapeutic relationship may be the most important factor in successful management of this disorder. Patients should be told that their symptoms arise from either increased sensitivity to minor stimuli or increased reactivity resulting in spasm or abnormal motility. Although the "mind-gut" interaction should be mentioned, it should be emphasized that the symptoms are real, lest the patient conclude that the physician is implying that "it's all in my head." Physicians will earn the confidence of their patients by being nonjudgmental and attentive. Fears that the symptoms will progress, require surgery, or degenerate into serious illness should be allayed. The patient should understand that irritable bowel syndrome is a chronic disorder characterized by periods of exacerbation and quiescence. The physician can help but cannot "cure" such a disorder. The emphasis should be shifted from finding the cause of the symptoms to finding a way to cope with them. Physicians must resist the temptation to chase chronic complaints with new or repeated diagnostic studies.

B. Dietary Therapy: Patients commonly report dietary intolerances, though the role of dietary triggers in irritable bowel syndrome has never been convincingly proved. Nevertheless, the physician should be open to the idea that dietary changes—for whatever reason—may provide symptomatic benefit. In some patients, a food diary, in which symptoms, food intake, and life events are recorded, may reveal dietary or psychosocial factors that precipitate symptoms. Malabsorption of lactose, fructose, and sorbitol may cause bloating, distention, flatulence, and diarrhea. Lactose intolerance should be excluded in all patients with a trial of a lactose-free diet. Sorbitol is present in a number of artificially sweetened foods and some medications. A variety of foods are flatulogenic, producing pain and distention in some patients. These include brown beans, brussels sprouts, cabbage, cauliflower, raw onions, grapes, plums, raisins, coffee, red wine, and beer. Caffeine is poorly tolerated by most patients with irritable bowel syndrome.

A trial of a high-fiber diet (20–30 g/d) should be recommended for most patients. This may be accomplished by giving 1 tbsp of bran powder two or three times daily with food or in 8 oz of liquid. Some patients report increased gas and distention with fiber supplementation with bran. Fiber supplements with psyllium, methylcellulose, or polycarbophil may be better tolerated (see section on constipation).

C. Pharmacologic Measures: More than two-thirds of patients with irritable bowel syndrome have mild symptoms that respond readily to education, reassurance, and dietary interventions. Drug therapy should be reserved for patients with more severe symptoms that do not respond to these conservative measures. These agents should be viewed as being adjunctive rather than curative. Given the wide spectrum of symptoms, no single agent is expected to provide relief in all or even most patients. Indeed, there is no convincing evidence that any of these agents are superior to placebo therapies, which result in symptomatic improvement in up to 70% of patients. Nevertheless, therapy targeted at the specific dominant symptom (pain, constipation, or diarrhea) may be beneficial.

1. Antispasmodic agents–Anticholinergic agents may ameliorate postprandial abdominal pain when given 30–60 minutes before meals. Side effects include urinary retention, tachycardia, and dry mouth. Available agents include dicyclomine, 10–20 mg orally three or four times daily; hyoscyamine, 0.125 mg orally (or sublingually as needed); or propantheline, 15 mg orally three times daily. Although calcium channel blockers relax gastrointestinal smooth muscle, they have not been well tested in patients with irritable bowel syndrome.

2. Antidiarrheal agents–Opioid and other antidiarrheal agents may be useful in patients with frequent loose stools (see section on chronic diarrhea). They may best be used "prophylactically" in situations where diarrhea is anticipated (such as stressful situations) or would be inconvenient (social engagements). Agents include loperamide, 2 mg orally three or four times daily, and diphenoxylate with atropine, 2.5 mg orally four times daily.

3. Anticonstipation agents–A trial of fiber supplementation with bran, psyllium, methylcellulose, or polycarbophil is beneficial in most cases. Patients who are unresponsive to fiber may be extremely difficult to manage. The prokinetic agent cisapride, 5–10 mg three times daily, may benefit patients with colonic inertia (see section on constipation).

4. Psychotropic agents–Some patients complain of chronic, unremitting abdominal pain. This small subset has a high incidence of underlying psychiatric disturbances and functional impairment and requires frequent office visits. These patients may benefit from tricyclic antidepressants. Amitriptyline may be started at a dosage of 25–50 mg at bedtime and increased gradually to 75–150 mg as tolerated.

5. Other agents–Anxiolytics and narcotics should not be used chronically in irritable bowel syndrome because they have addictive potential. Agents that reduce visceral afferent sensation (serotonin 5-HT_3 receptor antagonists) are currently under investigation.

D. Other Therapies: Behavioral modification with relaxation techniques and hypnotherapy may be beneficial in some patients. Patients with underlying psychologic abnormalities may benefit from evaluation by a psychiatrist or psychologist. Patients with severe disability should be referred to a pain treatment center.

Prognosis

The overwhelming majority of patients with irritable bowel syndrome learn to cope with their symptoms and lead productive lives.

Clouse RE: Antidepressants for functional gastrointestinal syndromes. Dig Dis Sci 1994;38:2352.

Drossman DA: Diagnosing and treating patients with refractory functional gastrointestinal disorders. Ann Intern Med 1995;123:688.

Drossman DA et al: Sexual and physical abuse and gastrointestinal disease. Ann Intern Med 1995;123:782. (Physical or sexual abuse may have occurred in over one-third of patients with irritable bowel syndrome. Physicians should question patients with refractory disease about such abuse.)

Lynn RB, Friedman LS: Irritable bowel syndrome: Managing the patient with abdominal pain and altered bowel habits. Med Clin North Am 1995;79:373.

ANTIBIOTIC-ASSOCIATED COLITIS

Essentials of Diagnosis

- Most cases of antibiotic-associated diarrhea are not attributable to *C difficile* and are usually mild and self-limited.
- Symptoms of antibiotic-associated colitis vary from mild to fulminant; almost all attributable to *C difficile*.
- Diagnosis in mild to moderate cases established by stool toxin assay.
- Flexible sigmoidoscopy provides most rapid diagnosis in severe cases.

General Considerations

Antibiotic-associated diarrhea is a common clinical occurrence. It is particularly common after use of particular antibiotics, such as ampicillin and clindamycin. Characteristically, the diarrhea occurs during the period of antibiotic exposure, is dose-related, and resolves spontaneously after discontinuation of the antibiotic. In most cases, this diarrhea is mild and does not require any specific laboratory evaluation or treatment. Stool examination usually reveals no fecal leukocytes, and stool cultures reveal no pathogens. Although *C difficile* is identified in the stool of 15–25% of cases of antibiotic-associated diarrhea, it is also identified in 5–10% of patients treated with antibiotics who do not have diarrhea. Most cases of antibiotic-associated diarrhea are due to changes in colonic bacterial fermentation of carbohydrates and are not due to *C difficile*.

Antibiotic-associated colitis is a significant clinical problem almost always caused by *C difficile*. Hospitalized patients are the most susceptible. This anaerobic bacterium colonizes the colon of 2–3% of healthy adults. In hospitalized patients, however, it is present in over 20% of patients, most of whom have received antibiotics that disrupt the normal bowel flora and allows the bacterium to flourish. The majority of these patients are asymptomatic. The organism is spread in a fecal-oral fashion. It is found throughout hospitals in patient rooms and bathrooms and is readily transmitted from patient to patient by hospital personnel. Fastidious hand washing and use of disposable gloves are helpful in minimizing transmission.

In some colonized patients, *C difficile*-induced colitis may develop. *C difficile* colitis is the major cause of diarrhea in patients hospitalized for more than 3 days, affecting 7:1000 patients. Although virtually all antibiotics have been implicated, colitis most commonly develops after use of ampicillin, clindamycin, and cephalosporins. Symptoms usually begin during or shortly after antibiotic therapy but may be delayed for several weeks. Thus, it is important to ask all patients with acute diarrhea about recent antibiotic exposure.

Clinical Findings

A. Symptoms and Signs: Most patients report mild to moderate watery diarrhea with lower abdominal cramps. Physical examination is normal or reveals mild left lower quadrant tenderness. With more serious illness, there is abdominal pain and profuse watery diarrhea with up to 30 stools per day. The stools may have mucus but seldom gross blood. There is often a low-grade fever, abdominal tenderness, and leukocytosis. Finally, a small number of patients develop fulminant colitis with lethargy, fever, tachycardia, and abdominal pain and distention.

B. Special Examinations:

1. Stool studies–Pathogenic strains of *C difficile* produce two toxins: toxin A is an enterotoxin and toxin B a cytotoxin. In most patients, the diagnosis of antibiotic-associated colitis is established by the demonstration of *C difficile* toxins in the stool. A stool cytotoxin assay (toxin B) has a specificity of 90% and a sensitivity of 95%. This is the definitive test, but it takes 24 hours. Rapid ELISA assays (2–4 hours) for toxins A and B have been developed that have a 70–85% sensitivity. In a recent study, either the ELISA or the cytotoxin assay was positive in only 81% of patients on the first stool sample and in 91% after two stool samples. Thus, one negative test does not exclude the diagnosis if the patient has typical symptoms and signs. Culture for *C difficile* is not recommended because it is slow, costly, and cannot identify toxicogenic strains. Fecal leukocytes are present in only 50% of patients with colitis.

2. Flexible sigmoidoscopy–Flexible sigmoidoscopy is performed in patients with more severe symptomatology when a rapid diagnosis is desired so that therapy can be initiated. In patients with mild to moderate symptoms, there may be no abnormalities or only patchy or diffuse, nonspecific colitis indistinguishable from other causes. In patients with severe illness, true pseudomembranous colitis is seen. This has a characteristic appearance, with yellow adherent plaques 2–10 mm in diameter scattered over the colonic mucosa interspersed with hyperemic mucosa. Biopsies reveal epithelial ulceration with a classic "volcano" exudate of fibrin and neutrophils. In 10% of cases, pseudomembranous colitis is confined to the proximal colon and may be missed at sigmoidoscopy.

3. Imaging studies–Abdominal radiographs are obtained in patients with fulminant symptoms to look for evidence of toxic dilation or megacolon. Mucosal edema or "thumbprinting" may be evident.

Differential Diagnosis

Other infectious causes of acute diarrhea are unusual in hospitalized patients. Inflammatory bowel disease and ischemic colitis should be considered as well.

Complications

Fulminant disease may result in dehydration, electrolyte imbalance, toxic megacolon, perforation, and death. Chronic, untreated colitis may result in weight loss and protein-losing enteropathy.

Treatment

A. Acute Therapy: If possible, antibiotic therapy should be discontinued. In patients with mild symptoms, doing so may result in prompt resolution of symptoms without specific treatment. If diarrhea is persistent or symptoms severe, specific therapy is warranted. The drug of choice is metronidazole, 250 mg orally four times daily for 10 days. Vancomycin, 125 mg orally four times daily, is equally effective but significantly more expensive.

In patients unable to take oral medications and patients with severe illness, intravenous metronidazole, 500 mg every 6 hours, should be given; intravenous vancomycin does not penetrate the bowel and should not be used. Symptomatic improvement should occur within 72 hours.

B. Treatment of Relapse: Up to 20% of patients have a relapse of diarrhea from *C difficile* within 1 or 2 weeks after stopping initial therapy. This may be due to reinfection or failure to eradicate the organism. Most relapses respond promptly to a second course of metronidazole therapy. Some patients have recurrent relapses that can be difficult to treat. A 4- to 6-week treatment course of vancomycin followed by a slow taper over 1–2 months may be successful.

Kelly C, Pothoulakis C, LaMont JT: *Clostridium difficile* colitis. N Engl J Med 1994;330:257.

Manabe Y et al: *Clostridium difficile* colitis: An efficient clinical approach to diagnosis. Ann Intern Med 1995; 123:835. (Of patients with *C difficile* colitis, the sensitivity of one stool specimen was 81%, of two stool specimens 91%. Cytotoxin assay had a 10% greater yield than ELISA. The negative predictive value of the first stool specimen was 97%.)

INFLAMMATORY BOWEL DISEASE

The term "chronic idiopathic inflammatory bowel disease" includes ulcerative colitis and Crohn's disease. Ulcerative colitis is a chronic, recurrent disease characterized by diffuse mucosal inflammation involving only the colon. Ulcerative colitis invariably involves the rectum and may extend proximally in a continuous fashion to involve part or all of the colon. Crohn's disease is a chronic, recurrent disease characterized by patchy transmural inflammation involving any segment of the gastrointestinal tract from the mouth to the anus.

Drug Therapies for Inflammatory Bowel Disease

Although ulcerative colitis and Crohn's disease appear to be distinct entities, the same pharmacologic agents are used to treat both. Despite intense research, there are still no specific therapies for these diseases. The mainstays of therapy remain 5-aminosalicylic acid derivatives, corticosteroids, and mercaptopurine.

A. 5-Aminosalicylic Acid: 5-Aminosalicylic acid is a topically active agent that has a variety of anti-inflammatory effects. It is used in the active treatment of ulcerative colitis and Crohn's disease and during disease inactivity in order to maintain remission. It is readily absorbed from the small intestine but demonstrates minimal colonic absorption. A number of oral and topical compounds have been designed to deliver 5-aminosalicylic acid to the colon or small intestine while minimizing absorption. Formulations of 5-aminosalicylic acid currently available are sulfasalazine, olsalazine, and mesalamine.

1. Sulfasalazine–Sulfasalazine consists of 5-aminosalicylic acid linked to a sulfapyridine moiety by an azo bond. It is largely unabsorbed in the small intestine. In the colon, bacterial azoreductases cleave 5-aminosalicylic acid from the sulfapyridine group. It is unclear whether the sulfapyridine group has any anti-inflammatory effects. One gram of sulfasalazine contains 400 mg of 5-aminosalicylic acid. The 5-aminosalicylic acid works topically and is largely unabsorbed. The sulfapyridine group, however, is absorbed and may cause side effects in 15–30% of patients. Dose-related side effects include nausea, headaches, leukopenia, oligospermia, and impaired folate metabolism. Allergic and idiosyncratic side effects are fever, rash, hemolytic anemia, neutropenia, worsened colitis, hepatitis, pancreatitis, and pneumonitis. Sulfasalazine is significantly less expensive than other 5-aminosalicylic acid agents.

2. Oral mesalamine agents–These 5-aminosalicylic acid agents are coated in various pH-sensitive resins or packaged in timed-release capsules. Mesalamine tablets dissolve at pH 7.0, releasing 5-aminosalicylic acid in the terminal small bowel and proximal colon. Pentasa releases 5-aminosalicylic acid slowly throughout the small intestine and colon. Side effects of these compounds are uncommon but include nausea, headache, pancreatitis, and nephropathy. Eighty percent of patients intolerant of sulfasalazine can tolerate 5-aminosalicylic acid.

3. Olsalazine–Olsalazine consists of two 5-aminosalicylic acid moieties linked by a diazo bond. Similar to sulfasalazine, it is not absorbed in the small intestine. In the colon, it is cleaved by bacteria, liberating the 5-aminosalicylic acid. Serious side effects are rare. A mild, dose-related secretory diarrhea that occurs in 20% of patients improves if the drug is administered with food.

4. Topical mesalamine–5-Aminosalicylic acid is provided in the form of suppositories (500 mg) and enemas (4 g/60 mL). These formulations can deliver much higher concentrations of 5-aminosalicylic acid to the distal colon than oral compounds. Side effects are extremely uncommon.

B. Corticosteroids: A variety of intravenous, oral, and topical steroid formulations have been used in inflammatory bowel disease. They have utility in the short-term treatment of moderate to severe disease. However, long-term use is associated with serious, potentially irreversible side effects and is to be avoided. The agents, route of administration, duration of use, and tapering regimens employed are based more upon personal bias and experience than upon data from rigorous clinical trials. The most commonly used intravenous formulations have been hydrocortisone or methylprednisolone, which are given by continuous infusion or every 6 hours. Oral formulations are prednisone or methylprednisolone. Topical preparations are provided as hydrocortisone suppositories (100 mg), foam (90 mg), and enemas (100 mg).

C. Mercaptopurine and Azathioprine: Mercaptopurine and azathioprine are used in 10–15% of patients with refractory Crohn's disease. Side effects occur in 10%, including pancreatitis, bone marrow suppression, infections, allergies, and, potentially, a higher risk of neoplasm. After therapy is started, complete blood counts should be obtained weekly for 1 month, then at least monthly.

Social Support for Inflammatory Bowel Disease

Inflammatory bowel disease is a lifelong illness that can have profound emotional and social impacts on the individual. Patients should be encouraged to become involved in the Crohn's and Colitis Foundation of America (CCFA). National headquarters may be contacted at 444 Park Avenue South, 11th Floor, New York, NY 10016–7374; phone 212-685-3440.

1. CROHN'S DISEASE

Essentials of Diagnosis

- Insidious onset.
- Intermittent bouts of low-grade fever, diarrhea, and right lower quadrant pain.
- Right lower quadrant mass and tenderness.
- Perianal disease with abscess, fistulas.

- Radiographic evidence of ulceration, stricturing, or fistulas of the small intestine or colon.

General Considerations

Crohn's disease is an idiopathic inflammatory process that can affect any portion of the alimentary tract from the mouth to the anus. One-third of cases involve only the small bowel, most commonly the terminal ileum (ileitis). About half of cases involve the small bowel and colon, most often the terminal ileum and adjacent proximal ascending colon (ileocolitis). In 15–20% of cases, the colon alone is affected. Unlike ulcerative colitis, Crohn's disease is a transmural process that can result in mucosal inflammation and ulceration, stricturing, fistula development, and abscess formation.

Clinical Findings

A. Symptoms and Signs: Because of the variable location of involvement and severity of inflammation, Crohn's disease may present with a variety of symptoms and signs. In eliciting the history, the clinician should take particular note of fevers, the patient's general sense of well-being, the presence of abdominal pain, the number of liquid bowel movements per day, and prior surgical resections. Physical examination should focus upon the patient's temperature, weight, and nutritional status, the presence of abdominal tenderness or an abdominal mass, rectal examination, and extraintestinal manifestations. Most commonly, there is one or a combination of the following clinical constellations.

1. Chronic inflammatory disease–This is the most common presentation and is often seen in patients with ileitis or ileocolitis. Patients report low-grade fever, malaise, weight loss, and loss of energy. There may be diarrhea, which is nonbloody and often intermittent. Cramping or steady right lower quadrant or periumbilical pain is present. Physical examination reveals focal tenderness, usually in the right lower quadrant. A palpable, tender mass may be present in the lower abdomen which represents thickened or matted loops of inflamed intestine.

2. Intestinal obstruction–Narrowing of the small bowel may occur as a result of inflammation, spasm, or fibrotic stenosis. Patients report postprandial bloating, cramping pains, and loud borborygmi. This sometimes occurs in patients with active inflammatory symptoms (as above). More commonly, however, it occurs later in the disease from chronic fibrosis without other systemic symptoms or signs of inflammation.

3. Fistulization with or without infection–A subset of patients develop sinus tracts that penetrate through the bowel and form fistulas to a number of locations. Fistulas to the mesentery are usually asymptomatic but can result in intra-abdominal or retroperitoneal abscesses manifested by fevers, chills, a tender abdominal mass, and leukocytosis. Fistulas from the colon to the small intestine or stomach can result in bacterial overgrowth with diarrhea, weight loss, and malnutrition. Fistulas to the bladder or vagina produce recurrent infections. Enterocutaneous fistulas usually occur at the site of surgical scars.

4. Perianal disease—One-third of patients with either large or small bowel involvement develop perianal disease manifested by anal fissures, perianal abscesses, and fistulas. This can be a distressing problem.

5. Extraintestinal manifestations—The extracolonic manifestations described above with ulcerative colitis may also be seen with Crohn's disease, particularly Crohn's colitis. Other problems may also arise. Oral aphthous lesions are common. There is an increased prevalence of gallstones due to malabsorption of bile salts from the terminal ileum. Nephrolithiasis with urate or calcium oxalate stones may occur.

B. Laboratory Findings: There is a poor correlation between laboratory studies and the patient's clinical picture. Laboratory values may reflect inflammatory activity or nutritional complications of disease. A complete blood count and serum albumin should be obtained in all patients. Anemia may reflect chronic inflammation, mucosal blood loss, iron deficiency, or vitamin B_{12} malabsorption secondary to terminal ileal inflammation or resection. Leukocytosis may reflect inflammation or abscess formation or may be secondary to corticosteroid therapy. Hypoalbuminemia may be due to intestinal protein loss (protein-losing enteropathy), malabsorption, or chronic inflammation. The sedimentation rate or C-reactive protein level is elevated in many patients during active inflammation. Stool specimens are sent for examination for routine pathogens, ova and parasites, and *C difficile* toxin.

C. Special Diagnostic Studies: In most patients, the initial diagnosis of Crohn's disease is based upon a compatible clinical picture with supporting radiographic findings. An upper gastrointestinal series with small bowel follow-through is obtained in all patients. Suggestive findings include ulcerations, strictures, and fistulas. To evaluate the colon, a barium enema or colonoscopy is obtained. Colonoscopy offers the advantage of obtaining mucosal biopsies of the colon or terminal ileum. Typical endoscopic findings include aphthoid ulcers, linear or stellate ulcers, strictures, and segmental involvement with areas of normal-appearing mucosa adjacent to inflamed mucosa. In 10% of cases, it may be impossible to distinguish ulcerative colitis from Crohn's disease. The presence of granulomas on biopsy are seen in less than 25% of patients but are highly suggestive of Crohn's disease.

Complications

A. Abscess: The presence of a tender abdominal mass with fever and leukocytosis suggests an abscess. Emergent CT of the abdomen is necessary to confirm the diagnosis. Patients should be given broad-spectrum antibiotics and, if malnourished, maintained on TPN. Percutaneous drainage or surgery is usually required.

B. Obstruction: Small bowel obstruction may develop secondary to active inflammation or chronic fibrotic stricturing and is often acutely precipitated by dietary indiscretion. Patients should be given intravenous fluids with nasogastric suction for several days. Systemic steroids are indicated in patients with symptoms or signs of active inflammation but are unhelpful in patients with inactive, fixed disease. Patients unimproved on medical management require surgical resection of the stenotic area or stricturoplasty.

C. Fistulas: The majority of enteromesenteric and enteroenteric fistulas are asymptomatic and require no specific therapy. Most symptomatic fistulas require surgical therapy, particularly when there is evidence of intestinal stricturing below the fistula. Medical therapy is effective in a subset of patients and is usually tried before surgery. Many fistulas close temporarily in response to TPN but recur when oral feedings are resumed. Mercaptopurine heals fistulas in 30–40% of patients but requires 3–6 months.

D. Perianal Disease: Patients with fissures, fistulas, and skin tags have perianal discomfort that is treated conservatively with sitz baths and cotton pads to absorb drainage. Control of diarrhea is important. Metronidazole, 250 mg three or four times daily, and mercaptopurine may help some patients with perianal disease. Surgical treatment of perianal fistulas is unnecessary and to be avoided in most patients. Patients with abscesses require conservative surgical incision and drainage.

E. Carcinoma: Patients with colonic Crohn's disease are at increased risk of developing colon carcinoma. Screening colonoscopy is recommended by some authorities.

F. Hemorrhage: Unlike ulcerative colitis, severe hemorrhage is unusual in Crohn's disease.

G. Malabsorption: Malabsorption may arise from bacterial overgrowth in patients with enterocolonic fistulas, strictures and stasis, extensive jejunal inflammation, and prior surgical resections.

Differential Diagnosis

Chronic cramping abdominal pain and diarrhea are typical of both irritable bowel syndrome and Crohn's disease, but x-ray examinations are normal in the former. Acute fever and right lower quadrant pain may resemble appendicitis or *Yersinia enterocolitica* enteritis. Intestinal lymphoma causes fever, pain, weight loss, and abnormal small bowel radiographs that may mimic Crohn's disease. Patients with undiagnosed AIDS may present with fever and diarrhea. Segmental colitis may be caused by tuberculosis, *Entamoeba histolytica*, *Chlamydia*, or ischemic colitis.

Diverticulitis with abscess formation may be difficult to distinguish acutely from Crohn's disease.

Treatment of Active Disease

Crohn's disease is a chronic lifelong illness characterized by exacerbations and periods of remission. As no specific therapy exists, current treatment is directed toward symptomatic improvement and controlling the disease process. The treatment must address the specific problems of the individual patient.

A. Nutrition:

1. Diet–Patients should eat a well-balanced diet. Because lactose intolerance is common, a trial off dairy products is warranted. Patients with mainly colonic involvement benefit from fiber supplementation. Conversely, patients with obstructive symptoms should be placed on a low-roughage diet, ie, no raw fruits or vegetables, popcorn, nuts, etc. Resection of more than 100 cm of terminal ileum results in fat malabsorption. A low-fat diet with medium-chain triglyceride supplementation is used.

2. Enteral therapy–Enteral therapy with elemental diets (eg, Vivonex) for 4 weeks is as effective as corticosteroids in inducing remission, but the relapse rate after return to a normal diet is high.

3. Total parenteral nutrition–TPN is used short-term in patients with active disease and severe malnutrition; in patients with fistulas while medical therapy is being introduced; and preoperatively to improve nutritional status. It is required long-term in a small subset of patients with extensive intestinal resections resulting in short bowel syndrome with malnutrition.

B. Symptomatic Medications:

1. Antidiarrheals–Chronic diarrhea may respond dramatically to antidiarrheal agents. Loperamide (2–4 mg), diphenoxylate with atropine (one tablet), and tincture of opium (8–15 drops) may be given as needed up to four times daily. Patients with active terminal ileal disease or terminal ileal resection of less than 100 cm may benefit from cholestyramine (2–4 g) or colestipol (5 g) once or twice daily to bind malabsorbed bile salts.

2. Antispasmodics–Propantheline (15 mg), dicyclomine (10–20 mg), or hyoscyamine (0.125 mg) given before meals may reduce abdominal cramps. Patients should discontinue these agents at the first sign of intestinal obstruction.

C. Specific Drug Therapy:

1. 5-aminosalicylic acid agents–Sulfasalazine, 1.5–2 g twice daily, is effective in reducing clinical signs of disease activity in patients with colonic involvement but confers little benefit in small intestine disease. Although mesalamine (Asacol) and its slow-release form (Pentasa) are approved only for the treatment of ulcerative colitis, their release in the small intestine offers usefulness in the treatment of small bowel Crohn's disease. Recent studies have confirmed their efficacy in the treatment of small

bowel and ileocecal disease, particularly when they are used at high dosages (Pentasa 1 g four times daily; Asacol 0.8–1.2 g four times daily).

2. Corticosteroids–Corticosteroids dramatically suppress the acute clinical symptoms or signs in most patients with both small and large bowel disease. However, steroids do not appear to alter the underlying disease diathesis. Prednisone, 40–60 mg/d, is generally administered to patients with an active flare-up of Crohn's disease. After improvement at 2–3 weeks, tapering proceeds at 5 mg/wk until a dosage of 20 mg/d is being given. Thereafter, very slow tapering of 2.5 mg/wk or every other week is recommended. Some patients cannot be completely withdrawn from steroids without experiencing a symptomatic flare-up. Chronic low steroid doses (2.5–10 mg/d) are often required. These may be associated with serious complications such as aseptic necrosis of the hips, osteoporosis, cataracts, diabetes, and hypertension. For these reasons, chronic steroids are to be avoided where possible. Budesonide is a topically active steroid with low systemic activity. A special formulation that releases this agent in the terminal ileum has been shown to reduce disease activity in patients with ileocolitis. Budesonide is not yet available for oral use in the USA.

Patients with more severe disease manifested by severe weight loss or malnutrition should be hospitalized and treated with intravenous steroids (as described for ulcerative colitis). In patients with a tender, palpable inflammatory abdominal mass, a CT scan of the abdomen should be obtained prior to administering steroids in order to rule out an abscess. Even if no abscess is identified, steroids should be administered cautiously along with broad-spectrum antibiotics.

3. Immunomodulatory drugs–Azathioprine (1–2 mg/kg) and mercaptopurine (50–100 mg) are effective in the long-term treatment of Crohn's disease. They are most useful in the management of patients with unresponsive disease, those requiring chronic corticosteroids, and those with symptomatic fistulas. These agents permit elimination or reduction of steroids in over 75% and fistula closure in 30%. Blood counts should be monitored weekly for the first month, then monthly. Drug dosages should be monitored to maintain a white blood cell count > 3000/μL. Side effects requiring withdrawal of the drug occur in about 10%, the most common being pancreatitis. The mean time to symptomatic response is 4 months, so these agents are not useful for acute exacerbations. Once patients achieve remission, these drugs reduce the 3-year relapse rate from over 60% to less than 25%. Other immunosuppressive agents have been investigated in the treatment of Crohn's disease, including cyclosporine and methotrexate; however, efficacy has been modest and toxicity greater than with mercaptopurine. Preliminary reports suggest that cyclosporine may be useful in the treatment of fistulas, but relapse rates have been high.

Maintenance of Remission

Crohn's disease is characterized by recurrent symptomatic flare-ups and remissions. All patients should be counseled firmly to stop smoking, as smokers appear to have a significantly higher recurrence rate. Although earlier trials of sulfasalazine (with or without corticosteroids) did not demonstrate efficacy of this agent in preventing disease recurrence, recent trials have shown that Pentasa 500 mg four times daily or Asacol 800 mg three times daily reduces disease recurrence rates, especially in those with a recent flare and those with ileal disease. Although chronic low doses of corticosteroids are often needed to control activity, they should not be used in patients with inactive disease to maintain remission. The topically active steroid budesonide has not yet demonstrated convincing efficacy as maintenance therapy at 1 year. As discussed above, azathioprine and mercaptopurine have had a definite impact on maintaining remission and should be used in patients with frequent recurrences and patients who require chronic corticosteroids. Recently, an experimental enteric-coated formulation of fish oil containing n-3 fatty acids has also been shown to decrease disease recurrence.

Indications for Surgery

Over half of patients will require at least one surgical procedure. The main indications for surgery are intractability to medical therapy, intra-abdominal abscess, massive bleeding, and obstruction with fibrous stricture. Patients with active inflammation who are unresponsive to medical therapy or who require chronic prednisone in doses exceeding 15 mg/d may achieve dramatic relief from limited surgical excision for 5–15 years before disease recurs.

Prognosis

With proper medical and surgical treatment, the majority of patients are able to cope with this chronic disease and its complications and lead productive lives. Few patients die as a direct consequence of the disease.

Belluzzi A et al: Effect of an enteric-coated fish-oil preparation on relapses in Crohn's disease. N Engl J Med 1996;334:1557.

Glotzar D: Surgical therapy for Crohn's disease. Gastroenterol Clin North Am 1995;24:527.

Griffin M, Mines P: Conventional drug therapy in inflammatory bowel disease. Gastroenterol Clin North Am 1995;24:509.

Kelly D, Fleming R: Nutritional considerations in inflammatory bowel disease. Gastroenterol Clin North Am 1995;24:597.

Pearson DC et al: Azathioprine and 6-mercaptopurine in Crohn's disease: A meta-analysis. Ann Intern Med 1995;123:132.

Thiesen A, Thomson AB: Older systemic and newer topical glucocorticoids and the gastrointestinal tract. Aliment Pharmacol Ther 1996;10:487.

Urrutia RD, Magno E: Maintenance therapy for Crohn's disease. Gastroenterology 1996;110:299.

2. ULCERATIVE COLITIS

Essentials of Diagnosis

- Bloody diarrhea.
- Lower abdominal cramps and urgency.
- Anemia, low serum albumin.
- Negative stool cultures.
- Sigmoidoscopy is the key to diagnosis.

General Considerations

Ulcerative colitis is an idiopathic inflammatory condition that involves the mucosal surface of the colon, resulting in diffuse friability and erosions with bleeding. Approximately 50% of patients have disease confined to the rectosigmoid region (proctosigmoiditis); 30% extend to the splenic flexure (left-sided colitis); and less than 20% extend more proximally (extensive colitis). There is some correlation between disease extent and symptom severity. In the majority of patients, the extent of colonic involvement does not progress over time. In most patients, the disease is characterized by periods of symptomatic flare-ups and remissions.

Clinical Findings

A. Symptoms and Signs: The clinical profile in ulcerative colitis is highly variable. Bloody diarrhea is the hallmark. On the basis of several clinical and laboratory parameters, it is clinically useful to classify patients as having mild, moderate, or severe disease (Table 14–13). Patients should be asked about stool frequency, the presence and amount of rectal bleeding, cramps, abdominal pain, fecal urgency, and tenesmus. Physical examination should focus upon the patient's volume status as determined

Table 14–13. Ulcerative colitis: Assessment of disease activity.

	Mild	Moderate	Severe
Stool frequency (per day)	< 4	4–6	> 6 (mostly bloody)
Pulse (beats/min)	< 90	90–100	> 100
Hematocrit (%)	Normal	30–40	< 30
Weight loss (%)	None	1–10	> 10
Temperature (°F)	Normal	99–100	> 100
ESR (mm/h)	< 20	20–30	> 30
Albumin (g/dL)	Normal	3–3.5	< 3.0

by orthostatic blood pressure and pulse measurements and by nutritional status. On abdominal examination, the clinician should look for tenderness and evidence of peritoneal inflammation. Red blood may be present on digital rectal examination.

1. Mild to moderate disease–Patients with mild disease have a gradual onset of infrequent diarrhea (less than five movements per day) with intermittent rectal bleeding and mucus. Stools may be formed to loose in consistency. Because of rectal inflammation, there is fecal urgency and tenesmus. Left lower quadrant cramps relieved by defecation are common, but there is no significant abdominal tenderness. Patients with moderate disease have more severe diarrhea with frequent bleeding. Abdominal pain and tenderness may be present but are not severe. There may be mild fever, anemia, and hypoalbuminemia.

2. Severe disease–Patients with severe disease have more than six to ten bloody bowel movements per day, resulting in severe anemia, hypovolemia, and impaired nutrition with hypoalbuminemia. Abdominal pain and tenderness are present. "Fulminant colitis" is a subset of severe disease characterized by rapidly worsening symptoms with signs of toxicity.

3. Extracolonic manifestations–Ulcerative colitis is associated with extraintestinal manifestations in 25% of cases. Some extracolonic signs are associated with disease activity. These include erythema nodosum, pyoderma gangrenosum, episcleritis, thromboembolic events, and an oligoarticular, nondeforming arthritis. In patients who are HLA B27-seropositive, there may be anterior uveitis or ankylosing spondylitis which is independent of colitis activity. Sclerosing cholangitis can occur in colitis patients even after total colectomy. Patients with this entity are at higher risk of developing cholangiocarcinoma.

B. Laboratory Findings: The degree of abnormality of the hematocrit, sedimentation rate, and serum albumin reflect disease severity.

C. Endoscopy: In acute colitis, the diagnosis is readily established by sigmoidoscopy. The mucosal appearance is characterized by edema, friability, mucopus, and erosions. Colonoscopy should not be performed in patients with severe disease because of the risk of perforation. After patients have been on therapy and the acute symptoms have improved, colonoscopy is sometimes performed to determine the extent of disease, which will dictate the need for subsequent cancer surveillance.

D. Imaging: Plain abdominal radiographs are obtained in patients with severe colitis to look for significant colonic dilation. Barium enemas are of little utility in the evaluation of acute ulcerative colitis and may precipitate toxic megacolon in patients with severe disease.

Differential Diagnosis

The initial presentation of ulcerative colitis is in-distinguishable from other causes of colitis, clinically as well as endoscopically. Thus, the diagnosis of idiopathic ulcerative colitis is reached after excluding other known causes of colitis. Infectious colitis should be excluded by sending stool specimens for routine bacterial cultures (to exclude *Salmonella, Shigella,* and *Campylobacter*), ova and parasites (to exclude amebiasis), and stool toxin assay for *C difficile.* Mucosal biopsy can distinguish amebic colitis from ulcerative colitis. Enteroinvasive *E coli* and *E coli* O157:H7 will not be detected on routine bacterial cultures. CMV colitis occurs in immunocompromised patients (especially those with AIDS) and is diagnosed on mucosal biopsy. Gonorrhea, chlamydial infection, herpes, and syphilis are considerations in sexually active patients with proctitis. In elderly patients with cardiovascular disease, ischemic colitis may involve the rectosigmoid. A history of radiation to the pelvic region can result in proctitis months to years later. Crohn's disease involving the colon but not the small intestine may be confused with ulcerative colitis. In 10% of patients, a distinction between Crohn's disease and ulcerative colitis is not possible.

Treatment
(Table 14–14)

There are two main treatment objectives: (1) to terminate the acute, symptomatic attack and (2) to prevent recurrence of attacks. The treatment of acute ulcerative colitis is dependent upon the extent of colonic involvement and the severity of illness.

Patients with mild to moderate disease should eat a regular diet, but caffeine and gas-producing vegetables are restricted. Fiber supplements decrease diarrhea and rectal symptoms (psyllium, 3.4 g twice daily; methylcellulose, 2 g twice daily; bran powder, 1 tbsp twice daily). Antidiarrheal agents should not be given in the acute phase of illness but are safe and helpful in patients with mild chronic symptoms. Lo-

Table 14–14. Treatment of ulcerative colitis.

Distal colitis
Proctitis
  Mesalamine suppositories, 500 mg per rectum twice daily, or–
  Hydrocortisone foam, 90 mg per rectum daily, or–
  Hydrocortisone suppositories, 100 mg per rectum daily
Proctosigmoiditis
  Mesalamine enema, 4 g per rectum daily, or–
  Hydrocortisone enema, 100 mg per rectum daily
Extensive colitis
Mild to moderate
  Sulfasalazine, 1.5–3 g orally twice daily, or–
  Mesalamine tablets (delayed release), 2.4–4 g/d
  Olsalazine, 0.75–1.5 g orally twice daily
  If no response after 2–4 weeks, add prednisone, 40–60 mg/d (taper by 5 mg/wk)
Severe
  Methylprednisolone, 48–60 mg IV daily

peramide (2 mg), diphenoxylate with atropine (one tablet), or tincture of opium (8–15 drops) may be given up to four times daily. Such remedies are particularly useful at nighttime and when taken prophylactically for occasions when patients may not have reliable access to toilet facilities.

A. Distal Colitis: Patients with disease confined to the rectum or rectosigmoid region generally have mild but distressing symptoms. Acute therapy is best approached with topical agents. Topical mesalamine is the drug of choice and is superior to topical corticosteroids. Mesalamine is administered as a suppository, 500 mg twice daily for proctitis, and as an enema, 4 g at bedtime for proctosigmoiditis, for 3–12 weeks, with 75% of patients improving. Topical steroids are a less expensive alternative to mesalamine but are also less effective. Hydrocortisone suppository or foam is prescribed for proctitis and hydrocortisone enema (80–100 mg) for proctosigmoiditis. Systemic effects from short-term use are very slight. It is not known whether combination therapy with mesalamine and hydrocortisone is advantageous. Patients with distal disease who fail to improve with topical therapy should be considered for systemic steroids or immunosuppressives as described below.

Patients whose acute symptoms resolve with acute therapy have an 80–90% chance of a symptomatic relapse within 1 year. Maintenance therapy with mesalamine suppositories (500 mg daily) or with oral agents (see below) reduce the relapse rate to less than 20% per year.

B. Mild to Moderate Colitis: Disease extending above the sigmoid colon is best treated with oral agents. The currently available agents—sulfasalazine and mesalamine—result in symptomatic improvement in 50–75% of patients. These drugs appear to be comparable in efficacy. To minimize side effects, sulfasalazine is begun at a dose of 500 mg twice daily and increased gradually over 1–2 weeks to 1.5–2 g twice daily. Most patients improve within 3 weeks, though some require 2–3 months. Total doses of 5–6 g/d may have greater efficacy but are poorly tolerated. Because of their greater cost, olsalazine and mesalamine should be reserved for patients who are intolerant of sulfasalazine. Mesalamine, 800 mg three times daily or 1 g four times daily, is approved for active disease. Higher doses of 1.2–1.6 g three times daily may be required in some patients. Olsalazine, 1 g two or three times daily, is effective but tends to cause a mild secretory diarrhea, making it unsuitable for active disease.

Patients with mild to moderate disease who fail to improve after 2–3 weeks of mesalamine therapy should have the addition of corticosteroid therapy. Topical therapy with hydrocortisone foam or enemas (80–100 mg twice daily) is tried first. Patients who fail to improve after 2 more weeks require systemic steroid therapy. Prednisone and methylprednisolone are most commonly used. Depending on the severity of illness, the initial oral dose of prednisone is 20–30 mg twice daily. Rapid improvement is observed in most cases. One can usually begin to taper prednisone after 2 weeks. Tapering of prednisone should proceed by no more than 5 mg/wk. After tapering to 15 mg/d, slower tapering is sometimes required. Complete tapering without symptomatic flare-ups is possible in the majority of patients.

C. Severe Colitis: About 10–15% of ulcerative colitis patients have a more severe course. Because they may deteriorate rapidly, hospitalization is generally required.

1. General measures–
a. Discontinue all oral intake. Total parenteral nutrition is indicated in patients with poor nutritional status.
b. Avoid all opiate or anticholinergic agents.
c. Restore circulating volume with fluids and blood as needed. Correct electrolyte abnormalities.
d. Perform frequent abdominal examinations to look for evidence of worsening distention or pain.
e. Obtain a plain abdominal radiograph on admission to look for evidence of colonic dilation.
f. Obtain surgical consultation in all patients with severe disease.
g. Send stools for bacterial (including *C difficile*) culture and examination for ova and parasites.

2. Corticosteroid therapy–Methylprednisolone, 48–80 mg, or hydrocortisone, 300 mg, is administered in four divided doses or by continuous infusion over 24 hours. Higher or "pulse" doses are of no benefit. Hydrocortisone enemas should also be administered twice daily as a drip, 100 mg over 30 minutes. In patients who have not previously received corticosteroids, administration of ACTH, 120 units/24 h, may be superior to corticosteroids. Approximately 50–75% of patients achieve remission with systemic steroids within 7–10 days. Once symptomatic improvement has occurred, oral fluids are reinstituted. If well tolerated, the patient is then converted to oral predisone (as described for moderate disease).

3. Cyclosporine–Intravenous cyclosporine benefits over 75% of patients with severe colitis who have not improved after 7–10 days of corticosteroids. This therapy should now be considered in patients with severe steroid-resistant colitis as an alternative to colectomy.

4. Surgical therapy–Patients with severe disease who fail to improve after 7–10 days of corticosteroid therapy are unlikely to respond to continued steroids, and surgery is recommended. Patients with fulminant disease or toxic megacolon who worsen or fail to improve within 48–72 hours should undergo surgery to prevent perforation. If operation is performed before perforation, the mortality rate should be extremely low.

D. Fulminant Colitis and Toxic Megacolon:

A subset of patients with severe disease have a more "fulminant" course with rapid progression of symptoms over 1–2 weeks and signs of severe toxicity. These patients appear quite ill, with prominent hypovolemia, hemorrhage requiring transfusion, and abdominal distention with tenderness. They are at a higher risk of perforation or development of toxic megacolon and must be followed closely. Broad-spectrum antibiotics should be administered to cover anaerobes and gram-negative bacteria.

Toxic megacolon develops in less than 2% of cases of ulcerative colitis. It is characterized by colonic dilation of more than 6 cm on plain films with signs of toxicity. In addition to the therapies outlined above, nasogastric suction should be initiated. Patients should be instructed to roll from side to side and onto the abdomen in an effort to decompress the distended colon. Serial abdominal plain films should be obtained to look for worsening dilation or ischemia.

Maintenance of Remission

Without chronic therapy, 75% of patients who initially go into remission on medical therapy will experience a symptomatic relapse within 1 year. Chronic maintenance therapy with sulfasalazine, 1–1.5 g twice daily; olsalazine, 500 mg twice daily; and mesalamine, 800 mg three times daily or 500 mg four times daily have been shown to reduce relapse rates to less than 33%. Therapy with azathioprine or mercaptopurine may be tried in patients who do not respond to 5-aminosalicylic acid or corticosteroids or who require chronic corticosteroid therapy. The risks of chronic immunosuppressive therapy, however, must be weighed against the certainty of cure with surgical resection.

Risk of Colon Cancer

In ulcerative colitis patients with disease proximal to the sigmoid colon, there is a markedly increased risk of developing colon carcinoma. In patients who have had colitis for more than 10 years, the risk of developing colon cancer increases approximately 0.5–1% per year. Ingestion of folic acid, 1 mg/d, is associated with a decreased risk of cancer development. Colonoscopies are recommended every 1–2 years in patients with extensive colitis, beginning 8–10 years after diagnosis. At colonoscopy, multiple random biopsies are taken as well as biopsies of mass lesions to look for dysplasia or carcinoma. Because of the relatively high incidence of concomitant carcinoma in patients with dysplasia, colectomy is recommended.

Surgery in Ulcerative Colitis

Surgery is required in 25% of patients. Severe hemorrhage, perforation, and documented carcinoma are absolute indications for surgery. Surgery is indicated also in patients with fulminant colitis or toxic megacolon that does not improve within 48–72 hours, (as outlined above); in patients with dysplasia on surveillance colonoscopy; and in patients with refractory disease requiring chronic steroids to control symptoms.

Although total proctocolectomy provides a complete cure of the disease, most patients seek to avoid it out of concern for the impact it may have upon their bowel function, their self-image, and their social interactions. After complete colectomy, patients may have a standard ileostomy with an external appliance, a continent ileostomy, or an internal ileal pouch which is anastomosed to the anal canal (ileoanal anastomosis). The latter maintains intestinal continuity, thereby obviating an ostomy. Under optimal circumstances, patients have five to seven loose bowel movements per day without incontinence.

Prognosis

Ulcerative colitis is a lifelong disease characterized by exacerbations and remissions. For most patients, the disease is readily controlled by medical therapy without need for surgery. The majority never require hospitalization. A subset of patients with more severe disease will require surgery, which results in complete cure of their disease. Properly managed, most ulcerative colitis patients lead close to normal productive lives.

Connell WR et al: Factors affecting the outcome of endoscopic surveillance for cancer in ulcerative colitis. Gastroenterology 1994;107:934. (Several cancers not detected despite colonoscopic surveillance. Both low- and high-grade dysplasia predict high risk of having or developing cancer.)

Hanauer S: New therapeutic approaches. Gastroenterol Clin North Am 1995;24:523.

Lashner BA et al: The effect of folic acid supplementation on the risk of cancer or dysplasia in ulcerative colitis. Gastroenterology 1997;112:29.

Lichtiger S et al: Cyclosporine in severe ulcerative colitis refractory to steroid therapy. N Engl J Med 1994; 330:1841. (Eighty-two percent of patients with severe ulcerative colitis refractory to intravenous steroids responded to cyclosporine.)

Sandborn WJ: A review of immune modifier therapy for inflammatory bowel disease: Azathioprine, 6-mercaptopurine, cyclosporine, and methotrexate. Am J Gastroenterol 1996;91:423.

Weiss E, Wexner S: Surgical therapy for ulcerative colitis. Gastroenterol Clin North Am 1995;24:559.

VASCULAR ECTASIAS

Vascular ectasias, also called angiodysplasias and arteriovenous malformations, occur throughout the upper and lower intestinal tract. However, they most commonly occur in the cecum and ascending colon in elderly individuals (see sections on acute upper and lower gastrointestinal bleeding). They may be a cause of acute or chronic blood loss from the upper or lower gastrointestinal tract. Uncommonly, they are congenital, part of an inherited syndrome such as hereditary hemorrhagic telangiectasia, or related to autoimmune disorders such as scleroderma.

Most colonic ectasias are degenerative lesions that are hypothesized to arise from chronic colonic muscular contraction that obstructs the venous mucosal drainage. Over time, the mucosal capillaries dilate and become incompetent, and an arteriovenous communication forms. The cause of gastric and small intestine ectasias is unknown. Bleeding from vascular ectasias is commonly associated with a number of medical conditions, including valvular heart disease (especially aortic stenosis) and chronic renal failure. Von Willebrand's disorder has been detected in some patients, which may potentiate bleeding.

Clinical Findings

Bleeding from vascular ectasias may present with acute or chronic gastrointestinal blood loss. Most patients are over age 70. Approximately 10% of patients have chronic or intermittent occult blood loss that may result in iron deficiency anemia. More commonly, patients develop recurrent, self-limited gastrointestinal bleeding that is not hemodynamically significant but is manifested by hematochezia, melena, or hematemesis. In a few patients, bleeding may be massive. Bleeding in younger patients is more apt to arise from the small intestine.

The evaluation and treatment of upper and lower gastrointestinal bleeding is discussed elsewhere. In patients with chronic or self-limited lower gastrointestinal bleeding, panendoscopy is the preferred means of identifying colonic, gastric, or duodenal vascular ectasias. However, ectasias can be identified in over 25% of subjects over age 60, which means that their mere presence does not *prove* that the lesion is the source of bleeding because active bleeding is uncommonly seen. Ectasias of the small intestine are extremely difficult to diagnose. Special long-push enteroscopes have been developed recently that permit evaluation of much of the jejunum. Even so, however, a large portion of the small intestine remains inaccessible to inspection. On occasion, the patient is taken to the operating room for laparotomy and intraoperative endoscopy of the small bowel.

Treatment

A. Medical Management: Patients with chronic gastrointestinal blood loss should receive iron supplementation. Some patients require intermittent transfusions. Uncontrolled trials have suggested that hormonal therapy with estrogen-progesterone (norethindrone, 1 mg, plus ethinyl estradiol, 0.05 mg) reduces the incidence of recurrent bleeding and the need for transfusions. A recent controlled trial, however, did not demonstrate any benefit from the conjugated estrogens, 0.625 mg/d, or birth control pills in patients with small intestine ectasias.

B. Endoscopic Therapies: Gastric, duodenal, and colonic ectasias may be treated with endoscopic applications of cautery (bipolar cautery or heater probe) or with laser therapy. The incidence of recurrent bleeding episodes and the need for transfusions is reduced by these therapies. Distal small intestinal ectasias are not accessible to these therapies.

C. Angiography: In patients with severe active lower gastrointestinal bleeding, colonoscopic therapy usually is not feasible. Selective superior mesenteric angiography may be able to identify the bleeding source and control hemorrhage in up to 80% of patients with vasopressin. Transcatheter embolization of the bleeding ectasia may also be used but is complicated by colonic infarction in 15% of patients.

D. Surgery: Right hemicolectomy is performed in patients with recurrent bleeding attributed to colonic ectasias who have failed endoscopic ablation or in patients with severe bleeding that cannot be controlled with angiography. Where possible, it is highly desirable to localize the bleeding source to the right colon with angiography, scintigraphy, or colonoscopy prior to surgery. Because many of these patients are elderly and have concomitant medical problems, surgery has a significant risk. In up to 25% of patients, bleeding recurs after surgery from ectasias in the upper gastrointestinal tract. In patients with recurrent bleeding attributed to small intestinal ectasias, resection may be helpful if preoperative angiography can localize a single bleeding lesion. Alternatively, intraoperative endoscopy with resection or oversewing of identifiable ectasias may be necessary.

Reinus JF, Brandt LJ: Vascular ectasias and diverticulosis: Common causes of lower intestinal bleeding. Gastroenterol Clin North Am 1994;23:1.

Sharma R, Gorbien MJ: Angiodysplasia and lower gastrointestinal tract bleeding in elderly patients. Arch Intern Med 1995;155:807.

DIVERTICULAR DISEASE OF THE COLON

Colonic diverticular disease is prevalent in over one-third of patients over 60 years of age. Most are asymptomatic, discovered incidentally at endoscopy or on barium enema. Complications in one-third include lower gastrointestinal bleeding and diverticulitis.

Colonic diverticula may vary in size from a few millimeters to several centimeters and in number from one to several dozen. These acquired abnormalities are extremely common in Western countries, rising in prevalence from 10% at 40 years to over one-third of patients over age 60. By way of contrast, diverticulosis is very uncommon in developing nations. Almost all patients with diverticulosis have involvement in the sigmoid colon; however, only one-third have proximal colonic disease.

In most patients, diverticulosis is believed to arise after many years of a diet deficient in fiber. The undistended, contracted segments of colon have higher intraluminal pressures. Over time, the contracted colonic musculature, working against greater pressures to move small, hard stools, develops hypertrophy, thickening, rigidity, and fibrosis. Diverticula may develop more commonly in the sigmoid because intraluminal pressures are highest in this region. The extent to which abnormal motility and hereditary factors contribute to diverticular disease is unknown. Patients with diffuse diverticulosis may have an inherent weakness in the colonic wall. Patients with abnormal connective tissue are also disposed to development of diverticulosis, including Ehlers-Danlos syndrome, Marfan's syndrome, and scleroderma.

1. UNCOMPLICATED DIVERTICULOSIS

More than two-thirds of patients with diverticulosis have uncomplicated disease and no specific symptoms. The majority of these will never be aware of the diverticula. In some patients, diverticulosis may be an incidental finding detected during colonoscopic examination or barium enema examination. Some patients have nonspecific complaints of chronic constipation, abdominal pain, or fluctuating bowel habits. It is unclear whether these symptoms are due to alterations in the colonic musculature or underlying irritable bowel syndrome. Physical examination is usually normal but may reveal mild left lower quadrant tenderness with a thickened, palpable sigmoid and descending colon. Screening laboratory studies should be normal in uncomplicated diverticulosis.

There is no reason to perform imaging studies for the purpose of diagnosing uncomplicated disease. Diverticula are best seen on barium enema. Involved segments of colon may also be narrowed and deformed. Colonoscopy is a less sensitive means of detecting diverticula.

Asymptomatic patients in whom diverticulosis is discovered and patients with a history of complicated disease (see below) should be treated with a high-fiber diet or fiber supplements (bran powder, 1–2 tbsp twice daily; psyllium or methylcellulose) (see section on constipation). Retrospective studies suggest that such treatment may decrease the likelihood of subsequent complications.

2. DIVERTICULITIS

Essentials of Diagnosis

• Acute abdominal pain and fever.

• Left lower abdominal tenderness and mass.
• Leukocytosis.

Clinical Findings

A. Symptoms and Signs: Perforation of a colonic diverticulum results in an intra-abdominal infection that may vary from microperforation (most common) with localized paracolic inflammation to macroperforation with either abscess or generalized peritonitis. Thus, there is a range from mild to severe disease. Most patients with localized inflammation or infection report mild to moderate aching abdominal pain usually in the left lower quadrant. Constipation or loose stools may be present. Nausea and vomiting are frequent. In many cases, symptoms are so mild that the patient may not seek medical attention until several days after onset. Physical findings include a low-grade fever, left lower quadrant tenderness, and a palpable mass. Stool occult blood is common, but hematochezia rare. Leukocytosis is mild to moderate. Patients with free perforation present with a more dramatic picture of generalized abdominal pain and peritoneal signs.

B. Imaging: Plain abdominal films are obtained in all patients to look for evidence of free abdominal air (signifying free perforation), ileus, and small or large bowel obstruction. In patients with mild symptoms and a presumptive diagnosis of diverticulitis, empiric medical therapy is started without further imaging in the acute phase. Patients who respond to acute medical management should undergo sigmoidoscopy and barium enema after 7–10 days to corroborate the diagnosis and to exclude other disorders. If barium enema reveals a stricture or mass, colonoscopic evaluation should be performed to exclude malignancy. In patients who do not improve rapidly after 2–4 days of empiric therapy and in patients with severe disease, CT scan of the abdomen is obtained to look for evidence of a free or contained abscess. Flexible sigmoidoscopy and barium enemas are contraindicated during the initial stages of an acute attack because there is a risk of free perforation.

Differential Diagnosis

Localized diverticulitis must be distinguished from perforated colonic carcinoma, Crohn's disease, appendicitis, ischemic colitis, and gynecologic disorders.

Complications

Fistula formation may involve the bladder, ureter, vagina, uterus, bowel, and abdominal wall. Diverticulitis may result in stricturing of the colon with partial or complete obstruction.

Treatment

A. Medical Management: Most patients can be managed with conservative measures. Patients with mild symptoms may be managed initially as outpatients on a low-residue diet and metronidazole, 500 mg orally three times daily, plus either ciprofloxacin, 500 mg twice daily, or trimethoprim-sulfamethoxazole, 160/800 mg twice daily orally for 14 days. Most cases of diverticulitis will require hospitalization acutely. Patients should be given nothing by mouth and should receive intravenous fluids. If ileus is present, a nasogastric tube should be placed. Intravenous antibiotics should be given to cover anaerobic and gram-negative bacteria. A suitable regimen is a second- or third-generation cephalosporin plus metronidazole. Alternatively, an aminoglycoside plus clindamycin provides good coverage. The antibiotics should be continued for 7–10 days, at which time elective evaluation with barium enema should be performed.

B. Surgical Management: Approximately 20–30% of patients with diverticulitis will require surgical management. Surgical consultation should be obtained on all patients with severe disease or those who fail to improve after 72 hours of medical management. Indications for emergent surgical management include free peritonitis and large abscesses. Patients with fistulas or colonic obstruction due to chronic disease will required elective surgery.

Patients with a localized abdominal abscess can be treated acutely with a percutaneous catheter drain placed by an interventional radiologist. This permits control of the infection and resolution of the immediate infectious inflammatory process. In this manner, a subsequent single-stage elective surgical operation can be performed in which the diseased segment of colon is removed and a primary colonic anastomosis performed. In patients in whom catheter drainage is not possible or helpful or in cases requiring emergency surgery, it is necessary to perform surgery in two stages. In the first stage, the diseased colon is resected and the proximal colon brought out to form a temporary colostomy. The distal colonic stump is either closed (forming a Hartmann pouch) or exteriorized as a mucous fistula. Weeks later, after the inflammation and infection have completely subsided, the colon can be reconnected electively.

Prognosis

Diverticulitis recurs in one-third of patients treated with medical management. Recurrent attacks warrant elective surgical resection, which carries a lower morbidity and mortality risk than emergency surgery.

Rothenberg DA, Wiltz O: Surgery for complicated diverticulitis. Surg Clin North Am 1993;73:975.

Schoetz D Jr: Uncomplicated diverticulitis: Indications for surgery and surgical management. Surg Clin North Am 1993;73:965.

3. DIVERTICULAR BLEEDING

Essentials of Diagnosis

- Acute onset of hematochezia without antecedent symptoms.
- Large volume of bright red to maroon blood.
- No distinctive features to distinguish from other causes of lower gastrointestinal bleeding.

Clinical Findings

A. Symptoms and Signs: Lower gastrointestinal bleeding develops in up to 5% of patients with diverticulosis. Although diverticula are much more prevalent on the left side of the colon, bleeding more commonly originates on the right side. Bleeding typically begins without warning in otherwise asymptomatic individuals. Patients experience an acute onset of abdominal cramping followed by the passage of a large volume of bright red or maroon blood mixed with clots. If voluminous, there may be signs of hypovolemia, with postural vital signs or shock. The abdominal examination, however, should be normal. Bleeding may stutter along for hours to days before resolving spontaneously in most cases. Chronic gastrointestinal blood loss or recurrent passage of small amounts of blood per rectum should never be attributed to diverticulosis.

The initial evaluation, resuscitation, and management of patients with lower gastrointestinal bleeding are discussed elsewhere in this chapter (see section on acute lower gastrointestinal bleeding). Briefly, a nasogastric tube should be placed to look for evidence of an upper gastrointestinal source of bleeding. In patients in whom the bleeding has subsided, colonoscopy should be performed within 4–12 hours after purging the colon with a lavage solution. In most cases in which bleeding has stopped, the diagnosis of diverticular hemorrhaging is made presumptively after identifying diverticula at colonoscopy but no other obvious source of acute blood loss. Colonic diverticula rarely are seen to be actively bleeding at colonoscopy.

B. Imaging: In patients with continued active bleeding, emergent evaluation with either a nuclear ^{99m}Tc-labeled red blood cell scan or mesenteric angiography should be performed. Scintigraphy can localize the bleeding site to the right or left colon but cannot identify the cause or pinpoint the exact site. Angiography is frequently nondiagnostic because the bleeding has stopped or is too slow. It may identify the bleeding site in up to half of patients with continued active bleeding.

Differential Diagnosis

Other causes of acute lower gastrointestinal bleeding include vascular ectasias (angiodysplasias), ischemic colitis, and aortoenteric fistulas. Up to 10% of apparent lower gastrointestinal hemorrhages originate in the upper intestinal tract.

Treatment

Bleeding stops spontaneously in up to 90% of cases of diverticular bleeding, requiring no further therapy. In patients with continued bleeding, the therapeutic options are surgery and angiography—the choice depending in part upon the local expertise available. Upper endoscopy should be performed to definitely exclude an upper gastrointestinal source of blood loss. Where available, angiography generally is performed first in the stable patient. At angiography, intra-arterial vasopressin can arrest active diverticular bleeding up to 90% of the time. Surgery is indicated for bleeding that persists despite angiographic maneuvers. However, it is extremely helpful to localize the bleeding site by scintigraphic studies or angiography, as this allows a more limited colonic resection of the involved colon. In situations in which efforts to localize the bleeding site have failed and the bleeding is definitely felt to be arising from the colon, total abdominal colectomy is performed.

Prognosis

Approximately 80% of patients with diverticular bleeding have only one episode. However, patients who experience a second episode have a high likelihood of experiencing further episodes of bleeding. If the bleeding site can be localized, elective surgical resection is warranted.

Bono MJ: Lower gastrointestinal bleeding. Emerg Med Clin North Am 1996;14:547.
McGuire HH Jr: Bleeding colonic diverticula: A reappraisal of natural history and management. Ann Surg 1994;220:653.

POLYPS OF THE COLON & SMALL INTESTINE

Polyps are discrete mass lesions that protrude into the intestinal lumen. Although most commonly sporadic, they may be inherited as part of a familial polyposis syndrome. Polyps may be divided into three major pathologic groups: mucosal neoplastic (adenomatous) polyps, mucosal nonneoplastic polyps (hyperplastic, juvenile polyps, hamartomas, inflammatory polyps), and submucosal lesions (lipomas, lymphoid aggregates, carcinoids, pneumatosis cystoides intestinalis). The nonneoplastic mucosal polyps have no malignant potential and usually are discovered incidentally at colonoscopy or barium enema. Only the adenomatous polyps have significant clinical implications and will be considered further here. Of polyps removed at colonoscopy, over 70% are adenomatous; most of the remainder are hyperplastic. Hyperplastic polyps are generally small (< 5 mm) and of no consequence. Their only importance is that they cannot be reliably distinguished from adenomatous lesions except by biopsy.

NONFAMILIAL ADENOMATOUS POLYPS

Histologically, adenomas are classified as tubular, villous, or tubulovillous. They may be sessile or pedunculated (containing a stalk). They are present in 30% of adults over 50 years of age. Their significance is that most cases of adenocarcinoma of the colon are believed to arise from adenomas. It is proposed that there is an adenoma → carcinoma sequence whereby colorectal cancer develops through a continuous process from normal mucosa to adenoma to carcinoma. Approximately 3% of adenomas contain invasive carcinoma. Malignant potential correlates with the polyp size, villous features, and degree of dysplasia. Most adenomas are less than 1 cm, and fewer than 4% of these enlarge with time. These small adenomas have only a 1% chance of harboring cancer and pose little risk. About 15–35% of adenomas are 1–3 cm in size. These large adenomas have a much higher risk of harboring malignancy (1–2 cm: 10%; > 2 cm: 46%) or of becoming malignant over time. The risk of developing cancer in a 1 cm adenoma is estimated to be 8% after 10 years. It has been estimated from longitudinal studies that it takes an average of 5 years for a medium-sized adenoma to develop from normal-appearing mucosa and 10 years for a gross cancer to arise.

Clinical Findings

A. Symptoms and Signs: Most patients with adenomatous polyps are completely asymptomatic. Chronic occult blood loss may lead to iron deficiency anemia. Large polyps may ulcerate, resulting in intermittent hematochezia.

B. Fecal Occult Blood Testing: Fecal occult blood tests are commonly performed as part of colorectal cancer screening programs. Unfortunately, these tests detect less than 40% of adenomas larger than 1 cm. Of patients with positive tests, approximately one-third have adenomas (only slightly higher than the expected prevalence in the adult population) (see section on colorectal cancer screening, below). Thus, these tests are insensitive and nonspecific for adenomas.

C. Special Tests: Polyps are identified with barium enema examination, flexible sigmoidoscopy, or colonoscopy. Double contrast barium enema can detect up to 90% of polyps, especially those larger than 1 cm. Lesions identified on barium enema require colonoscopic removal or biopsy. Flexible sigmoidoscopy is commonly performed as part of colorectal cancer screening programs. Approximately one-third to one-half of colonic adenomas are within reach of a flexible sigmoidoscope. Polyps are seen in 10–20% of patients undergoing screening sigmoidoscopy and should be biopsied. Hyperplastic polyps require no further evaluation. Patients with adenomatous polyps at sigmoidoscopy should undergo colonoscopy to remove the polyps and to look for other synchronous polyps in the proximal colon (20–40% of patients). Colonoscopy is the best means of detecting polyps, identifying 90% of polyps smaller than 8 mm and over 98% of larger polyps.

Treatment

Because of the adenoma → cancer sequence, all patients with polyps detected at sigmoidoscopy or barium enema should undergo colonoscopy accompanied by polyp removal by electrocautery techniques (polypectomy). The management of patients found to have a solitary small (≤ 5 mm) adenoma on screening sigmoidoscopy is controversial. Some studies suggest that the prevalence of adenomas found in the proximal colon at colonoscopy is not increased. Therefore, the decision to pursue colonoscopy varies among different physicians.

Most adenomatous polyps are amenable to safe colonoscopic removal. Large sessile lesions (> 2–3 cm) may be removed either in a piecemeal fashion or may require primary surgical resection. Once all adenomatous polyps have been removed, repeat "surveillance" colonoscopy is recommended in 3 years to look for missed polyps or new adenomas. If colonoscopy is negative after 3 years, subsequent surveillance may be increased to 5 years.

Malignant polyps may be considered to be adequately treated if (1) the polyp is completely excised and submitted for pathologic examination; (2) it is well differentiated; (3) the margin is not involved; or (4) there is no vascular or lymphatic involvement. The excision site of these "favorable" malignant polyps should be checked at 3 months for residual tissue. In patients with malignant polyps with unfavorable characteristics, surgical cancer resection is advised if the patient is a good operative candidate.

Prolonged regular use of aspirin (325 mg twice a week or oftener) or NSAIDs is associated with a 30–50% decrease in incidence of colorectal cancer and may reduce the number of colorectal adenomas. Pending results of aspirin chemoprevention trials, patients with colorectal adenomas may be advised to take aspirin 325 mg every other day prophylactically (see Chapter 1).

Prognosis

The results of a National Polyp Study involving over 1400 patients with adenomatous polyps treated with colonoscopic removal demonstrated a decline in the expected development of adenocarcinoma of almost 90% over a 13-year period. All but one cancer that did arise were Dukes A lesions.

Bond JH: Polyp guideline: Diagnosis, treatment, and surveillance for patients with nonfamilial colorectal polyps. Ann Intern Med 1993;119:836.

DuBois RN, Giardiello FM, Smalley WE: Non-steroidal antiinflammatory drugs, eicosanoids, and colorectal cancer prevention. Gastroenterol Clin North Am 1996;25: 773.

Marcus AS: Aspirin as prophylaxis against colorectal cancer. N Engl J Med 1995;333:656.

Winawer S et al: Prevention of colorectal cancer by colonoscopic polypectomy. N Engl J Med 1993;329:1977.

FAMILIAL POLYPOSIS SYNDROMES

Gastrointestinal polyposis syndromes refer to a variety of inherited conditions that result in the development of multiple polyps throughout the gastrointestinal tract and an increased risk of carcinoma. These are rare conditions that account for less than 1% of colorectal cancers.

1. FAMILIAL ADENOMATOUS POLYPOSIS

Familial adenomatous polyposis is an autosomal dominant disease characterized by the development of hundreds to thousands of adenomas in the colon and by various extracolonic features. It is due to a defect in the adenomatous polyposis coli gene (APC), which is located on the long arm of chromosome 5. Eighty percent of families have been found to have a genetic mutation in this gene. There is some evidence that the location of the mutation affects the number of polyps and the risk of cancer development.

Polyps occur at a mean age of 16 years, and almost all affected individuals have adenomas by age 35 years. Colon cancer is inevitable by age 50 unless prophylactic colectomy is performed. Gastric fundic gland polyps occur in over 50% but have no malignant potential. In contrast, duodenal adenomatous polyps occur in over 90% and have a 10% lifetime risk of malignancy, most commonly in the periampullary region. Extraintestinal manifestations of familial adenomatous polyposis in some families include osteomas, soft tissue tumors of the skin, dermoid tumors, and congenital hypertrophy of the retina. The combination of familial adenomatous polyposis and extraintestinal lesions used to be called Gardner's syndrome. The distinction between familial adenomatous polyposis and Gardner's syndrome is now questionable, as the same genetic defects have been found in both. When central nervous system tumors are found with familial adenomatous polyposis, the condition has been called Turcot's syndrome. Two-thirds of these families have a defect in the APC gene. An attenuated variant of familial adenomatous polyposis has also been recognized in which families form an average of only 30 polyps and therefore have a lower risk of cancer. These families appear to have a specific defect on the 5' end of the APC gene.

In families known to be affected, screening sigmoidoscopy to detect the development of polyps should begin at age 10–12 and be repeated every 1–2 years. Genetic testing can now be offered, followed by appropriate counseling. Genetic testing is indicated to confirm the diagnosis in patients with a compatible clinical profile and in first-degree family members of affected patients with a proved gene mutation. The cost of genetic screening is $500–$750 per individual. Testing should not be performed in children under the age of 12. Affected family members should undergo total colectomy with either ileoanal or ileorectal anastomosis. Patients with ileorectal anastomosis require frequent sigmoidoscopy for cancer surveillance and obliteration of rectal polyps. The risk of subsequent rectal cancer is over 10%. Sulindac, 150 mg twice daily, has been shown to decrease the number and size of adenomatous polyps in the rectal stump.

Burt R: Familial risk and colorectal cancer. Gastroenterol Clin North Am 1996;25:763.

Giardiello FM et al: Sulindac induced regression of colorectal adenomas in familial adenomatous polyposis: Evaluation of predictive factors. Gut 1996;38:578.

Giardiello FM et al: The use and interpretation of commercial *APC* gene testing for familial adenomatous polyposis. N Engl J Med 1997;336:823.

Vasen HF et al: Molecular genetic tests as a guide to surgical management of familial adenomatous polyposis. Lancet 1996;348:433.

2. OTHER POLYPOSIS SYNDROMES

Peutz-Jeghers syndrome is an autosomal dominant condition characterized by hamartomatous polyps throughout the gastrointestinal tract (most notably in the small intestine) as well as mucocutaneous pigmented macules on the lips, buccal mucosa, and skin. The hamartomas may become quite large, leading to bleeding, intussusception, or obstruction. Although hamartomas are not premalignant, up to 50% of these patients develop malignancies of the gastrointestinal tract (especially the stomach and duodenum) and nonintestinal organs (breasts, gonads, pancreas).

Familial juvenile polyposis is also autosomal dominant and characterized by several—more than ten—juvenile hamartomatous polyps, located most commonly in the colon. There is an increased risk of adenocarcinoma due to synchronous adenomatous polyps or mixed hamartomatous-adenomatous polyps.

COLORECTAL CANCER

Essentials of Diagnosis

- Symptoms or signs dependent upon tumor location.
- Proximal colon: fecal occult blood, anemia.
- Distal colon: change in bowel habits, hematochezia.
- Characteristic findings on barium enema.
- Diagnosis established with colonoscopy.

General Considerations

Colorectal cancer is the second leading cause of death due to malignancy in the United States. Approximately 5% of Americans will develop colorectal cancer. An estimated 134,000 new cases and 55,000 deaths occur annually. Colorectal cancers are almost all adenocarcinomas, which tend to form bulky exophytic masses or annular constricting lesions. Approximately half of cancers are located within the rectosigmoid region; one-fourth are located proximally in the cecum and ascending colon. It is currently believed that the majority of colorectal cancers arise from malignant transformation of an adenomatous polyp.

Risk Factors

A number of factors increase the risk of developing colorectal cancer. Recognition of these has impact upon screening strategies. However, 75% of all new cases occur in people with no known predisposing factors.

A. Age: The incidence of colorectal cancer rises sharply after age 40, and 90% of cases occur in persons over age 50.

B. Personal History of Neoplasia: A history of adenomatous polyps (especially if multiple or larger than 1 cm) increases the risk of subsequent adenomas and carcinoma and therefore requires periodic colonoscopic surveillance (see section on adenomatous polyps, above). Hyperplastic polyps are not deemed to be an important risk factor. Patients with a history of colon cancer have a relative risk of 1.45 of developing a second cancer compared with the general population.

C. Family History: A family history of colorectal cancer is present in 25% of patients with colon cancer. The risk of colon cancer is proportionate to the number of affected first-degree relatives. A person with one family member has a twofold to threefold increased risk; if the affected family member was under 55 years of age at the time of diagnosis, the risk is much greater. People with two first-degree relatives have a 25–35% risk of developing colon cancer. An increased risk is also found in close relatives of people diagnosed with an adenomatous polyp before age 60.

D. Familial Polyposis Syndromes: These autosomal dominant conditions dramatically increase the risk of developing colon cancer. However, they account for less than 1% of cases of colon carcinoma (see section on familial polyposis syndromes, above).

E. Hereditary Nonpolyposis Colorectal Cancer: Two autosomal dominant conditions have been described in which there is a markedly increased risk of developing colon cancer. Unlike the polyposis syndromes, these patients have few or no adenomatous polyps. The genetic defect in 80% of these kindreds has been located to one of four genes that are important in the detection and repair of DNA base pair mismatches. Hereditary nonpolyposis colorectal cancer develops often at an early age and has a predilection for the right colon. In many families there are also a number of extracolonic tumors, especially of the ovary, uterus, urologic tract, and stomach. The risk of colon cancer in affected individuals is over 70% by age 65, and the risk of endometrial cancer is 37–40%. A thorough family history is vital to identify these families and to initiate appropriate screening. At the present time, the "formal" diagnosis is based upon three criteria: (1) three or more first-degree family members with colon cancer, (2) colon cancer involving at least two generations, and (3) at least one colon cancer diagnosed before age 50. These stringent criteria may underestimate the number of affected kindreds. Patients with a family history consistent with hereditary nonpolyposis colorectal cancer must undergo biennial colonoscopic screening beginning at age 25 years, or 5 years younger than the earliest diagnosis of colon cancer in the family. Genetic testing for this disorder is now commercially available but should only be done after genetic counseling, preferably as part of a clinical research program.

F. Inflammatory Bowel Disease: The risk of adenocarcinoma of the colon begins to rise about 7–10 years after disease onset in patients with ulcerative colitis. The cumulative risk may approach 5–10% after 20 years and 20% after 30 years.

G. Other Risk Factors: Patients with a family or personal history of gynecologic cancer and patients with Barrett's esophagus have a moderately increased risk.

Clinical Findings

A. Symptoms and Signs: Adenocarcinomas grow slowly and may be present for several years before symptoms appear. However, asymptomatic tumors may still be detected by the presence of fecal occult blood (see Colorectal Cancer Screening, below). Symptoms depend upon the location of the carcinoma. Chronic blood loss from right-sided colonic cancers may cause iron deficiency anemia, manifested by fatigue and weakness. Obstruction, however, is uncommon because of the large diameter of the right colon and the liquid consistency of the fecal material. Lesions of the left colon often involve the bowel circumferentially. Because the left colon has a smaller diameter and the fecal matter is solid, obstructive symptoms may develop with colicky abdominal pain and a change in bowel habits. Constipation may alternate with periods of increased frequency and loose stools. The stool may be streaked with blood, though marked bleeding is un-

usual. With rectal cancers, patients note tenesmus, urgency, and recurrent hematochezia. Physical examination is usually normal except in advanced disease. A mass may be palpable in the abdomen. The liver should be examined for hepatomegaly, suggesting metastatic spread.

B. Laboratory Findings: A complete blood count is obtained to look for evidence of anemia. Elevated liver function tests are suspicious for metastatic disease. Carcinoembryonic antigen (CEA) should be obtained in all patients with proved colorectal cancer. Levels are elevated in 70% of patients but are poorly correlated with cancer stage. After complete surgical resection, CEA levels should normalize; persistently elevated levels portend a poor prognosis. A rise in CEA levels that had normalized initially after surgery is suggestive of cancer recurrence. However, the cost-effectiveness of CEA screening after colorectal cancer resection has not been proved.

C. Inspection of the Colon: Cancers may be detected with a high degree of reliability with either barium enema or colonoscopy. Colonoscopy is the diagnostic procedure of choice in patients with a clinical history suggestive of colon cancer or in patients with an abnormality suspicious for cancer detected on barium enema. Colonoscopy permits biopsy for pathologic confirmation of malignancy. In patients in whom colonoscopy is unable to reach the cecum (5% of cases) or when a nearly obstructing tumor precludes passage of the colonoscope, barium enema examination should be performed.

D. Imaging: Chest x-ray is obtained to look for evidence of metastatic disease. Most surgeons prefer to obtain an abdominal CT scan to assist in preoperative staging. Endorectal ultrasound provides important information about the depth of invasion of rectal cancers into or through the bowel wall.

Differential Diagnosis

The nonspecific symptoms of colon cancer may be confused with those of irritable bowel syndrome, diverticular disease, ischemic colitis, inflammatory bowel disease, infectious colitis, and hemorrhoids. Neoplasm must be excluded in any patient over age 50 who reports a change in bowel habits or hematochezia or who has an unexplained iron deficiency anemia or occult blood in the stools.

Staging

Determination of the stage of colorectal cancer is important not only because it correlates with the patient's long-term survival but also because it is used to determine which patients should receive adjuvant therapy (Table 14–15). Although the Dukes classification has been widely employed in the past, the TNM system is now commonly used.

Treatment

Surgical resection is the treatment of choice for

Table 14–15. Staging of colorectal cancer.

American Joint Committee Classification	TNM			Dukes Class[1]
Stage 0				
Carcinoma in situ	Tis	N0	M0	
Stage I				
Tumor invades submucosa	T1	N0	M0	Dukes A
Tumor invades muscularis propria	T2	N0	M0	Dukes B_1
Stage II				
Tumor invades into subserosa or into nonperitonealized pericolic or perirectal tissues	T3	N0	M0	Dukes B_1 or B_2
Tumor perforates the visceral peritoneum or directly invades other organs or structures	T4	N0	M0	Dukes B_2
Stage III				
Any degree of bowel wall perforation with lymph node metastasis				
One to three pericolic or perirectal lymph nodes involved	Any T	N1	M0	Dukes C_1
Four or more pericolic or perirectal lymph nodes involved	Any T	N2	M0	Dukes C_2
Metastasis to lymph nodes along a vascular trunk	Any T	N3	M0	
Stage IV				
Presence of distant metastasis	Any T	Any N	M1	Dukes D

[1]Gastrointestinal Tumor Study Group modification of Dukes classification.

virtually all patients who have resectable lesions and can tolerate general anesthesia. Regional lymph node dissection should be performed to determine staging, which guides decisions about adjuvant therapy. Up to 20% of patients with isolated hepatic metastases may be cured with resection or cryosurgical ablation of the hepatic lesion. Even patients with extensive metastatic disease may benefit from resection of the colonic tumor to reduce the likelihood of intestinal obstruction or serious bleeding.

For rectal carcinoma, the operative approach depends upon the level of the tumor above the anal verge, the size and depth of penetration, and the patient's overall condition. In carefully selected patients with small, well-differentiated rectal tumors that appear on endosonography and CT imaging to be localized to the rectal wall, transanal excision may be performed. All other patients will require either a low anterior resection with a colorectal anastomosis or an abdominoperineal resection with a colostomy, depending upon how far above the anal verge the tumor is located and the extent of local tumor spread. With unresectable rectal cancer, the patient may be palliated with a diverting colostomy, laser fulguration, or placement of an expandable wire stent.

A. Adjuvant Therapy for Colon Cancer: Adjuvant chemotherapy and radiotherapy have been demonstrated to improve overall and tumor-free survival in selected patients with colorectal cancer.

1. Stage I–Because of the excellent 5-year survival rate (80–100%), no adjuvant therapy is recommended.

2. Stage II (node-negative disease)–The expected 5-year survival rate is 50–75%. A benefit of adjuvant chemotherapy has not been demonstrated in controlled trials for stage II colon cancer. Patients with advanced local stage II disease (T3–T4) should

be considered for study protocols looking at the role of adjuvant chemotherapy or radiotherapy for control of local recurrence.

3. Stage III (node-positive disease)–The expected 5-year survival rate is 30–50%. Adjuvant chemotherapy with fluorouracil and either levamisole or leucovorin has been shown to reduce mortality by up to 33%. Pending results of comparative trials of levamisole versus leucovorin, the combination of fluorouracil and levamisole is still considered the standard adjuvant regimen. Selected patients with locally advanced colon cancer (T3–T4) may benefit from radiotherapy to reduce the risk of local recurrence.

4. Stage IV (metastatic disease)–Approximately 20% of patients have metastatic disease at the time of initial diagnosis, and another 30% eventually develop distant metastasis. The long-term survival rate of these patients is only 5%. Resection or ablation (cryosurgery, embolization, ultrasound) of isolated (one to three) liver or lung metastases may result in long-term (> 5 years) survival in up to 20% of cases. Systemic chemotherapy with fluorouracil may offer palliation for some patients but does not prolong survival.

B. Adjuvant Therapy for Rectal Cancer: Combined postoperative adjuvant therapy with pelvic radiation and chemotherapy with fluorouracil is recommended for both stage II and stage III rectal cancers. Such therapy has been shown to improve both the overall and the disease-free survival rate and to decrease pelvic recurrences. Where possible, patients should be enrolled in clinical trials that seek to identify the optimal combined modality regimen.

Follow-Up After Surgery

Patients who have undergone resections for cure are followed closely to look for evidence of tumor recurrence. Colonoscopy is performed 6 months to 1 year after surgery to look for evidence of local recurrence. If no tumor or other adenomas are found, it is performed every 3–5 years thereafter to look for metachronous polyps or tumors. Those with multiple polyps or cancers or age under 40 at the time of surgery warrant more frequent examinations. If the patient had an elevated CEA at the time of surgery, repeat levels are drawn at least every 3 months for the first year and every 6 months thereafter for 3 or 4 years. A rising CEA is suggestive of tumor recurrence, which usually requires colonoscopy and abdominal CT scan to look for recurrent or metastatic disease that may be amenable to therapy.

Prognosis

The overall survival rate of colorectal cancer is only 35%. However, patients undergoing "curative" resection have a 55% long-term survival. The stage of the disease at presentation is one of the most important determinants of survival. In addition, the biology of the tumor appears to affect the likelihood of developing metastatic disease. For example, the presence of a mutation of the *p53* gene and the loss of expression of the *DCC* gene in colorectal tumors are independent risk factors for the development of metastatic disease. A variety of other factors such as tumor differentiation and degree of aneuploidy may be important in determining the likelihood of metastatic spread.

Screening for Colorectal Neoplasms

Because virtually all colorectal cancers arise from adenomas, it is theoretically possible to prevent colon cancer by the early detection and removal of adenomas or to improve survival from colon cancer by detecting it at an earlier, presymptomatic stage. Various strategies have been endorsed, including fecal occult blood testing, flexible sigmoidoscopy, and screening colonoscopy. At present, the optimal cost-effective strategy has not been agreed upon.

In 1996, the United States Preventive Services Task Force issued the following recommendation for colorectal cancer screening: "Screening for colorectal cancer is recommended for all persons aged 50 and older with annual fecal occult blood testing (FOBT), or sigmoidoscopy [periodicity unspecified], or both. There is insufficient evidence to determine which of these screening methods is preferable or whether the combination of FOBT and sigmoidoscopy produces greater benefits than does either test alone. There is also insufficient evidence to recommend for or against routine screening with digital rectal examination, barium enema, or colonoscopy, although recommendations against such screening in average-risk persons can be made on other grounds. Persons with a family history of hereditary syndromes associated with a high risk of colon cancer should be referred for diagnosis and management."

A. Fecal Occult Blood Testing (FOBT): The normal gastrointestinal tract loses less than 2 mL/d of blood. Most cancers and some adenomas result in increased chronic blood loss that may be detectable. A variety of tests have been developed that have varying sensitivities for fecal occult blood. The test that has been the subject of most extensive testing and clinical use is a guaiac-based test (Hemoccult II). Red meats, aspirin, NSAIDs, and vegetables with peroxidase activity (turnips, horseradish) should be avoided for 72 hours before the test, since they can cause false-positive test results. Vitamin C may cause a false-negative test. When administered to the general population as part of a colorectal cancer screening program, 1–2.5% of tests are positive; if the slides are rehydrated, the incidence of positive tests rises to 10%.

Patients with positive fecal occult blood tests should undergo colonoscopy with removal of any polyps identified. The sensitivity of nonrehydrated slides for colorectal cancer is 50–80%, and the specificity is 98%. Rehydrating slides increases the sensitivity to 80–90% but decreases the specificity to 90%. The positive predictive value for colorectal cancer of a positive test is 6–17% for unhydrated slides but only 2.2% for rehydrated slides. The cancers that are detected are more likely to be earlier stage lesions (Dukes A or B). Adenomatous polyps are identified in 25–50% of patients with positive tests. The finding of these polyps in most instances is fortuitous, since most are < 1 cm in size and unlikely to cause bleeding.

The impact of fecal occult blood testing on the colorectal cancer mortality rate has been assessed in several large, prospective studies in which fecal occult blood testing was performed either yearly or biennially. Three studies have confirmed a reduction in colorectal cancer mortality of 15–33% after 8–13 years. The estimated cost per year of life saved is less than $20,000. Although in one study one-third of patients ultimately underwent colonoscopy for positive fecal occult blood tests (usually false-positives), less than 5% of patients in the other two studies required colonoscopy over the length of the study.

B. Flexible Sigmoidoscopy: Use of a flexible 60-cm sigmoidoscope permits visualization of the descending and rectosigmoid colon and identifies up to 60% of adenomatous polyps and colorectal cancers. At screening sigmoidoscopy, adenomatous polyps are identified in 10–20% and colorectal cancers in 1% of patients. Polyps less than 5–10 mm in diameter should be biopsied. Patients found to have adenomatous polyps should undergo pancolonoscopy (to look for synchronous polyps in the proximal colon) with polypectomy. As discussed previously, the need for colonoscopy in the patient found to have a solitary small adenoma (< 5–10 mm in diameter) at sigmoidoscopy is controversial. In several studies, such patients have not been found to have a higher prevalence of proximal polyps.

Retrospective studies of populations in which sigmoidoscopy was performed have demonstrated a reduced incidence of subsequent rectosigmoid carcinoma. Prospective screening sigmoidoscopy studies are ongoing. The estimated cost per year of life saved is under $20,000.

C. Recommendations in Average-Risk Patients: In accordance with the United States Preventive Services Task Force guidelines, all average-risk patients over age 50 should be offered screening for colorectal cancer with FOBT, flexible sigmoidoscopy, or both. Annual FOBT testing has resulted in greater reductions in mortality than biennial screening and is thus recommended. The optimal interval for screening sigmoidoscopy is unknown. Five-year intervals currently are recommended, though examinations up to every 10 years may be sufficient. A combination of FOBT and screening sigmoidoscopy corrects some of the limitations of each method used alone; however, it is unclear whether the increased costs and risks will result in corresponding improvements in outcome.

D. Screening in High-Risk Patients: The screening of patients with ulcerative colitis, patients from families with familial adenomatous polyposis and hereditary nonpolyposis colon cancer, and patients with prior histories of adenomatous polyps or cancer is discussed above.

Consensus recommendations for colorectal screening have been issued for patients with a family history of colon cancer. Patients with a single family member who developed colon cancer after age 55 should undergo routine screening with FOBT, sigmoidoscopy, or both but beginning at age 40. Patients with two or more first-degree relatives with colon cancer or one first-degree member who developed colon cancer before age 55 should be considered for screening with colonoscopy. Patients with negative results at colonoscopy may defer further screening for 10 years.

[Adjuvant therapy for colon and rectum cancer] gopher://gopher.nih.gov/11/clin/cdcs/individual/ 79.colon

[National Cancer Institute PDQ Internet Information for Colon and Rectal Cancer] gopher://gopher.nih.gov:70/00/clin/cancernet/pdqinfo/ soa/Colon%20cancer_Physician

Burke W et al: Recommendations for follow-up care of individuals with an inherited predisposition to cancer: I. Hereditary non-polyposis colon cancer. JAMA 1997; 277:915.

Burt R: The familial risk and colorectal cancer. Gastroenterol Clin North Am 1996;25:793.

Eckhauser F, Knol JA: Surgery for primary and metastatic colorectal cancer. Gastroenterol Clin North Am 1997; 26:103.

Levin B, Bond J: Colorectal cancer screening: Recommendations of the U.S. Preventive Services Task Force. Gastroenterology 1996;111:1381.

Sinicrope FA, Sugarman SM: Role of adjuvant therapy in surgically resected colorectal cancer. Gastroenterology 1995;109:984.

Winawer S et al: Colorectal cancer screening: Clinical guidelines and rationale. Gastroenterology 1997;112: 594. (Consensus of an expert multidisciplinary panel convened to make recommendations regarding colorectal cancer screening and surveillance. Reviews evidence and performs cost-effectiveness analysis for multiple screening strategies. A definitive work that summarizes all data through 1996.)

Zauber A, Winawer S: Initial management and follow-up surveillance of patients with colorectal adenomas. Gastroenterol Clin North Am 1997;26:85.

ANORECTAL DISEASES

HEMORRHOIDS

Essentials of Diagnosis

- Bright red blood per rectum
- Protrusion, discomfort
- Characteristic findings on external anal inspection and anoscopic examination

General Considerations

Internal hemorrhoids are a plexus of superior hemorrhoidal veins located above the dentate line which are covered by mucosa. They are a normal anatomic entity, occurring in all adults. Internal hemorrhoids form a vascular cushion in the lower rectum that may contribute to normal continence. They occur in three primary locations—right anterior, right posterior, and left lateral—though smaller hemorrhoids may occur between these primary locations. External hemorrhoids arise from the inferior hemorrhoidal veins located below the dentate line and are covered with squamous epithelium of the anal canal or perianal region.

Hemorrhoids may become symptomatic as a result of activities that increase venous pressure, resulting in distention and engorgement. Straining at stool, constipation, prolonged sitting, pregnancy, obesity, and low-fiber diets all may contribute. With time, redundancy and enlargement of the venous cushions may develop and result in bleeding or protrusion.

Clinical Findings

A. Symptoms and Signs: Patients often attribute a variety of perianal complaints to "hemorrhoids." However, the primary problems attributable to internal hemorrhoids are bleeding and mucoid discharge. Bleeding is manifested by bright red blood that may range from streaks of blood visible on the toilet paper or stool to bright red blood that drips into the toilet bowl after a bowel movement. Rarely is bleeding severe enough to result in anemia. Initially, internal hemorrhoids are confined to the anal canal (stage I). Over time, the internal hemorrhoids may gradually enlarge and protrude from the anal opening. At first, this prolapse occurs during straining and reduces spontaneously (stage II). With progression over time, the prolapsed hemorrhoids may require manual reduction after bowel movements (stage III) or may remain chronically protruding (stage IV). Chronically prolapsed hemorrhoids may result in mucoid perianal discharge, resulting in irritation and soiling of underclothes. Discomfort and pain are unusual with internal hemorrhoids, occurring only when there is extensive inflammation and thrombosis of irreducible tissue or with thrombosis of an external hemorrhoid (see below).

B. Examination: External hemorrhoids are readily visible on perianal inspection. Nonprolapsed internal hemorrhoids are not visible but may protrude through the anus with gentle straining while the physician spreads the buttocks. Prolapsed hemorrhoids are visible as protuberant purple nodules covered by mucosa. The perianal region should also be examined for other signs of disease such as fistulae, fissures, skin tags, or dermatitis. On digital examination, uncomplicated internal hemorrhoids are neither palpable nor painful. Anoscopic evaluation, best performed in the prone jackknife position, provides optimal visualization of internal hemorrhoids.

Differential Diagnosis

Rectal bleeding may be caused by colorectal neoplasms, ulcerative colitis or Crohn's colitis, infectious proctitis, and diverticular disease. Rectal prolapse, in which a full thickness of rectum protrudes concentrically from the anus, is readily distinguished from mucosal hemorrhoidal prolapse. Proctosigmoidoscopy should be performed in all patients with hematochezia to exclude disease in the rectum or sigmoid colon that could be misinterpreted in the presence of hemorrhoidal bleeding. Patients with iron deficiency anemia should undergo colonoscopy or barium enema to exclude disease proximal to the sigmoid colon.

Treatment

A. Conservative Measures: Most patients with early (stage I and stage II) disease can be managed with conservative treatment. To decrease straining with defecation, patients should be given instructions for a high-fiber diet and told to increase fluid intake with meals. Dietary fiber may be supplemented with bran powder (1–2 tbsp twice daily added to food or in 8 oz of liquid) or with commercial psyllium bulk laxatives (eg, Metamucil, Citru-

cel). Suppositories and rectal ointments have no demonstrated utility in the management of mild disease. Mucoid discharge may be treated effectively by the local application of a cotton ball tucked next to the anal opening after bowel movements. For edematous, prolapsed hemorrhoids, gentle manual reduction may be supplemented by suppositories (Anusol) that have anesthetic and astringent properties and by warm sitz baths.

B. Surgical Treatment: Patients with stage I or stage II hemorrhoids and recurrent bleeding despite conservative measures may be treated with injection sclerotherapy or rubber band ligation. However, recurrence is common unless patients alter their dietary habits. Surgical excision (hemorrhoidectomy) is reserved for patients with chronic severe bleeding due to stage III or stage IV hemorrhoids or patients with acute thrombosed stage IV hemorrhoids.

Thrombosed External Hemorrhoid

Thrombosis of the external hemorrhoidal plexus results in a perianal hematoma. It most commonly occurs in otherwise healthy young adults and may be precipitated by coughing, heavy lifting, or straining at stool. The condition is characterized by the relatively acute onset of an exquisitely painful, tense and bluish perianal nodule covered with skin which may be up to several centimeters in size. The pain is greatest within the first few hours but gradually eases over 2–3 days as the edema subsides. Symptoms may be relieved with warm sitz baths, analgesics, and ointments. If the patient is evaluated in the first 24–48 hours, removal of the clot may hasten symptomatic relief. With the patient in the lateral position, the skin around and over the lump is injected subcutaneously with 1% lidocaine. An ellipse of skin is then excised and the clot evacuated. A dry gauze dressing is applied for 12–24 hours, and daily sitz baths are then begun.

Mazier WP: Hemorrhoids, fissures, and pruritus ani. Surg Clin North Am 1995;74:1277.

Metcalf A: Anorectal disorders: Five common causes of pain, itching and bleeding. Postgrad Med 1995;98:81.

ANORECTAL INFECTIONS

A number of organisms can cause inflammation of the anal and rectal mucosa. Proctitis is defined as inflammation of the distal 15 cm of rectum and is characterized by anorectal discomfort, tenesmus, constipation, and discharge. Most cases of proctitis are caused by sexual transmission, especially anal-receptive intercourse. Proctocolitis implies inflammation that extends above the rectum to the sigmoid colon or more proximally and is caused by entirely different organisms such as *Campylobacter, Entamoeba histolytica, Shigella,* and enteroinvasive *E coli.* These organisms are discussed earlier in the section on diarrhea. Symptoms include frequent, small-volume, bloody or watery diarrhea, urgency, cramps, and tenesmus.

Etiology & Management

Several organisms may cause infectious proctitis.

A. *Neisseria gonorrhoeae:* Gonorrhea may cause itching, burning, tenesmus, and a mucopurulent discharge. Blind swabs of the anal canal have a sensitivity of less than 60%. Swabs should be taken for Gram staining and culture during anoscopy, expressing mucopus from the anal crypts. Cultures should also be taken from the urethra and pharynx in men and from the cervix in women. Complications of untreated infections include strictures, fissures, fistulas, and perirectal abscesses.

B. *Treponema pallidum:* Anal syphilis may be asymptomatic or may lead to perianal pain and discharge. With primary syphilis, the chancre may be at the anal margin or within the anal canal and may mimic a fissure, fistula, or ulcer. Proctitis or inguinal lymphadenopathy may be present. With secondary syphilis, condylomata lata (pale-brown, flat verrucous lesions) may be seen, with secretion of foul-smelling mucus. The diagnosis is established with dark-field microscopy of scrapings from the chancre or condylomas. The VDRL test is positive in 75% of primary cases and in 99% of secondary cases.

C. *Chlamydia trachomatis:* Chlamydial infection may cause proctitis similar to gonorrheal proctitis or may cause lymphogranuloma venereum, characterized by proctocolitis with fever and bloody diarrhea, painful perianal ulcerations, anorectal strictures and fistulas, and inguinal adenopathy (buboes). The diagnosis is established by culture of rectal discharge or rectal biopsy, which is over 80% sensitive.

D. Herpes Simplex II: HSV is a common cause of anorectal infection. Symptoms occur 4–21 days after exposure and include severe pain, itching, constipation, tenesmus, urinary retention, and radicular pain from involvement of lumbar or sacral nerve roots. Small vesicles or ulcers may be seen in the perianal area or anal canal. Sigmoidoscopy is not usually necessary but may reveal vesicular or ulcerative lesions in the distal rectum. Diagnosis is established by viral culture or antigen detection assays of vesicular fluid. Symptoms resolve within 2 weeks, but viral shedding may continue for several weeks. Patients may remain asymptomatic with or without viral shedding or may have recurrent mild relapses. Treatment of acute infection with acyclovir, 400 mg orally five times daily for 5–10 days, has been shown to reduce the duration of symptoms and viral shedding. Patients with AIDS and recurrent relapses may benefit from chronic suppressive therapy (see Chapter 32).

E. Venereal Warts: Venereal warts (condylomata acuminata) are a significant cause of anorectal symptoms. Caused by the human papillomavirus, they are seen in up to 50% of homosexual men. The warts are located on the perianal skin and extend within the anal canal up to 2 cm above the dentate line. Patients may have no symptoms or may report itching, bleeding, and pain. The warts may form a confluent mass that may obscure the anal opening. Treatment can be difficult. Topical application of podophyllum resin is effective for small perianal lesions. Anal lesions and large lesions may require CO_2 laser surgery or cryosurgery.

Tobin R, Surawicz C: Infectious proctitis in the immunocompetent. In: Snape W (editor). *Consultations in Gastroenterology.* Saunders, 1996.

RECTAL PROLAPSE & SOLITARY RECTAL ULCER SYNDROME

Rectal prolapse is protrusion through the anus of some or all of the layers of the rectum. It is most commonly seen in the elderly. Although surgical and traumatic injuries are causative in some patients, in most cases rectal prolapse arises from chronic, excessive straining at stool in conjunction with weakening of pelvic support structures. Although prolapse initially reduces spontaneously after defecation, with time the rectal mucosa becomes chronically prolapsed, resulting in mucous discharge, bleeding, incontinence, and sphincteric damage. Patients with complete prolapse require surgical correction.

Solitary rectal ulcer syndrome is characterized by anal pain, excessive straining at stool, and passage of mucus and blood. It is most commonly seen in young adults, especially women. Proctoscopic examination reveals a shallow rectal ulcer, usually located anteriorly about 6–10 cm above the anal verge. It may be caused by rectal intussusception with straining. Treatment is directed at decreasing straining through education of the patient and use of bulking agents.

FECAL INCONTINENCE

Fecal incontinence is present in up to 10% of the elderly. There are five general requirements for bowel continence: (1) solid or semisolid stool (even healthy young adults have difficulty maintaining continence with liquid rectal contents); (2) a distensible rectal reservoir (as sigmoid contents empty into the rectum, the vault must expand to accommodate); (3) a sensation of rectal fullness (if the patient cannot sense this, overflow may occur before the patient can take appropriate action); (4) intact pelvic nerves and muscles; and (5) the ability to reach a toilet in a timely fashion.

Minor Incontinence

Many patients complain of slight soilage of under-garments that tends to occur after bowel movements or with straining or coughing. This may be due to lo-cal anal problems such as hemorrhoids and skin tags that make it difficult to form a tight anal seal, espe-cially if stools are somewhat loose. Patients should be treated with fiber supplements to provide greater stool bulk. Loose application of a cotton ball near the anal opening may absorb small amounts of fecal leakage. Conditions such as ulcerative proctitis that cause tenesmus and urgency, chronic diarrheal condi-tions, and irritable bowel syndrome may result in dif-ficulty in maintaining complete continence, espe-cially if a toilet is not readily available. Similarly, the elderly may require more time or assistance to reach a toilet, which may lead to incontinence. Elderly pa-tients with chronic constipation may develop stool impaction leading to "overflow" incontinence.

Major Incontinence

Complete uncontrolled loss of stool reflects a sig-nificant problem with sphincteric or neurologic dam-age. Causes of sphincteric damage include traumatic childbirth (especially forceps delivery), episiotomy, prolapse, prior anal surgery, and physical trauma. Neurologic disruption may be caused by obstetric trauma (with pudendal nerve damage), aging, dia-betes mellitus, dementia, multiple sclerosis, spinal cord injury, and cauda equina syndrome.

Physical examination should include careful in-spection of the perianal area for hemorrhoids, rectal prolapse, fissures, and fistula. The perianal skin should be stimulated to confirm an intact anocuta-neous reflex. Digital examination during relaxation and squeezing gives valuable information about rest-ing tone (due to the internal sphincter) and external sphincter function and excludes fecal impaction. Proctosigmoidoscopy is useful to exclude rectal car-cinoma or proctitis.

Management is directed at the underlying cause. Patients who are incontinent only of loose or liquid stools are treated with bulking agents and antidiar-rheal drugs (eg, loperamide, 2 mg before meals and prophylactically before shopping trips). Patients with incontinence of solid stool benefit from scheduled toilet use after glycerin suppositories or tap water en-emas. Biofeedback training with anal sphincter exer-cises is helpful in motivated patients to lower the threshold for awareness of rectal filling, or to im-prove anal sphincter squeeze function, or both. Oper-ative management is seldom needed but should be considered in patients with gross incontinence who have failed medical therapy.

Romero Y et al: Constipation and fecal incontinence in the elderly population. Mayo Clin Proc 1996;71:81.

OTHER ANAL CONDITIONS

Anal Fissures

Anal fissures are linear ulcers that extend from the anal verge to the dentate line. They occur most com-monly in the posterior midline, but 10% occur anteri-orly. Fissures are believed to arise from trauma to the anal canal during defecation, perhaps caused by straining, constipation, or high internal sphincter tone. Patients complain of severe, tearing pain during defecation followed by throbbing discomfort that may lead to constipation due to fear of recurrent pain. There may be mild associated hematochezia, with blood on the stool or toilet paper. Anal fissures are confirmed by visual inspection of the anal verge while gently separating the buttocks. Acute fissures look like cracks in the epithelium. Chronic fissures result in fibrosis and the development of a skin tag at the outermost edge (sentinel pile). Digital and anoscopic examinations may cause severe pain and may not be possible. Medical management is di-rected at promoting effortless, painless bowel move-ments. Fiber supplements and sitz baths should be prescribed. Topical anesthetics (eg, mesalamine sup-positories) may provide pain relief. Patients with chronic or recurrent fissures sometimes benefit from partial lateral internal sphincterotomy; however, mi-nor incontinence may complicate this procedure.

Perianal Abscess & Fistula

The anal glands located at the base of the anal crypts at the dentate line may become infected, lead-ing to abscess formation. Other causes of abscess in-clude anal fissure and Crohn's disease. Abscesses may extend upward or downward through the inter-sphincteric plane. Symptoms of perianal abscess are throbbing, continuous perianal pain. Erythema, fluc-tuance, and swelling may be found in the perianal re-gion on external examination or in the ischiorectal fossa on digital rectal examination. Perianal ab-scesses are treated with local incision and drainage, while ischiorectal abscesses require drainage in the operating room. After drainage of an abscess, most patients are found to have a fistula in ano.

Most fistulas in ano arise in an anal crypt and are preceded by an anal abscess. In patients with fistulas that connect to the rectum, other disorders such as Crohn's disease, lymphogranuloma venereum, rectal tuberculosis, and cancer should be considered. Fistu-las are associated with purulent discharge that may lead to itching, tenderness, and pain. Treatment is by surgical incision or excision under anesthesia. Care must be taken to preserve the anal sphincters.

Pruritus Ani

Pruritus ani is characterized by perianal itching and discomfort. It may be caused by poor anal hy-giene associated with fistulas, fissures, prolapsed hemorrhoids, skin tags, and minor incontinence.

Conversely, overzealous cleansing with soaps may contribute to local irritation or contact dermatitis. Pinworms, candidal infection (especially in diabetics), scabies, and condylomata acuminata must be excluded. In patients with idiopathic pruritus ani, examination may reveal erythema, excoriations, or lichenified, eczematous skin. Education is vital to successful therapy. After bowel movements, the perianal area should be cleansed with nonscented wipes premoistened with lanolin followed by gentle drying. A piece of cotton ball should be tucked next to the anal opening to absorb perspiration or fecal seepage. Anal ointments and lotions may exacerbate the condition and should be avoided.

Metcalf A: Anorectal disorders. Five common causes of pain, itching, and bleeding. Postgrad Med 1995;98:81.

SQUAMOUS CELL CARCINOMA OF THE ANUS

These tumors are relatively rare, comprising only 1–2% of all cancers of the anus and large intestine. Bleeding, pain, and local tumor are the commonest symptoms. The lesion is often confused with hemorrhoids or other common anal disorders. These tumors tend to become annular, invade the sphincter, and spread upward into the rectum; they are encountered regularly in AIDS patients.

Except for very small lesions (which can be adequately excised locally), treatment is by combined abdominoperineal resection. Radiation therapy is reserved for palliation and for patients who refuse or cannot withstand operation. Metastases to the inguinal nodes are treated by radical groin dissection when clinically evident. The 5-year survival rate after resection is about 50%.

15

Liver, Biliary Tract, & Pancreas

Lawrence S. Friedman, MD

JAUNDICE
(Icterus)

Jaundice results from the accumulation of bilirubin—a red pigment product of heme metabolism—in the body tissues; it has nonhepatic as well as hepatic causes. Hyperbilirubinemia may be due to abnormalities in the formation, transport, metabolism, and excretion of bilirubin. Total serum bilirubin is normally 0.2–1.2 mg/dL, and jaundice may not be clinically recognizable until levels are about 3 mg/dL.

Pathophysiologically, jaundice may result from predominantly unconjugated or conjugated bilirubin in the serum (Table 15–1). Unconjugated hyperbilirubinemia may result from overproduction of bilirubin because of hemolysis; impaired hepatic uptake of bilirubin due to certain drugs; or impaired conjugation of bilirubin by glucuronide, as in Gilbert's syndrome, which is due to mild decreases in glucuronyl transferase, or Crigler-Najjar syndrome, due to moderate decreases or absence of glucuronyl transferase. Predominantly conjugated hyperbilirubinemia may result from impaired excretion of bilirubin from the liver due to hepatocellular disease, drugs, sepsis, hereditary disorders such as Dubin-Johnson syndrome, or extrahepatic biliary obstruction. Features of some hyperbilirubinemic syndromes are summarized in Table 15–2. The term "cholestasis" denotes retention of bile in the liver, and the term "cholestatic jaundice" is often used when conjugated hyperbilirubinemia results from impaired bile flow.

Manifestations of Diseases
Associated With Jaundice

A. Unconjugated Hyperbilirubinemia: Weakness or abdominal or back pain may occur with acute hemolytic crises. Stool and urine color are normal, and there is mild jaundice, indirect (unconjugated) hyperbilirubinemia with no bilirubin in the urine, and splenomegaly, except in sickle cell anemia. Hepatomegaly is variable.

B. Conjugated Hyperbilirubinemia:

1. Hereditary cholestatic syndromes or in-trahepatic cholestasis–The patient may be asymptomatic; intermittent cholestasis is often accompanied by pruritus, light-colored stools, and, occasionally, malaise.

2. Hepatocellular disease–Malaise, anorexia, low-grade fever, and right upper quadrant discomfort are frequent. Dark urine, jaundice, and amenorrhea occur. An enlarged, tender liver; vascular spiders; palmar erythema; ascites; gynecomastia; sparse body hair; fetor hepaticus; and asterixis may be present, depending on the cause, severity, and chronicity of liver dysfunction.

C. Biliary Obstruction: There may be colicky right upper quadrant pain, weight loss (suggesting carcinoma), jaundice, dark urine, and light-colored stools. Symptoms and signs may be intermittent owing to a stone or to carcinoma of the ampulla or junction of the hepatic ducts. Pain may be absent early in pancreatic cancer. Occult blood in the stools suggests cancer, particularly of the ampulla. Hepatomegaly, visible and palpable gallbladder (Courvoisier's sign), ascites, rectal (Blumer's) shelf, and weight loss also suggest cancer. Fever and chills suggest cholangitis.

Diagnostic Methods for
Evaluation of Liver Disease
& Jaundice
(Table 15–3)

A. Laboratory Studies: Elevated serum aminotransferase levels (AST, ALT) result from hepatocellular necrosis or inflammation; ALT is more specific for the liver than AST, but an AST level at least twice that of the ALT is typical of alcoholic liver injury. Elevated alkaline phosphatase levels suggest cholestasis or infiltrative liver disease (eg, tumor, abscess, granulomas). Alkaline phosphatase elevations of hepatic rather than bone, intestinal, or placental origin are suggested by concomitant elevation of γ-glutamyl transpeptidase or 5′-nucleotidase levels.

B. Liver Biopsy: Percutaneous liver biopsy is the definitive study for determining the cause and extent of hepatocellular dysfunction or infiltrative liver

Table 15–1. Classification of jaundice.

Type of Hyperbilirubinemia	Location and Cause
Unconjugated hyperbilirubinemia (predominant indirect-acting bilirubin)	Increased bilirubin production (eg, hemolytic anemias, hemolytic reactions, hematoma, infarction)
	Impaired bilirubin uptake and storage (eg, posthepatitis hyperbilirubinemia, Gilbert's syndrome, Crigler-Najjar syndrome, drug reactions)
Conjugated hyperbilirubinemia (predominant direct-acting bilirubin)	**HEREDITARY CHOLESTATIC SYNDROMES**
	Faulty excretion of bilirubin conjugates (eg, Dubin-Johnson syndrome, Rotor's syndrome)
	HEPATOCELLULAR DYSFUNCTION
	Biliary epithelial damage (eg, hepatitis, hepatic cirrhosis)
	Intrahepatic cholestasis (eg, certain drugs, biliary cirrhosis, sepsis, postoperative jaundice)
	Hepatocellular damage or intrahepatic cholestasis resulting from miscellaneous causes (eg, spirochetal infections, infectious mononucleosis, cholangitis, sarcoidosis, lymphomas, industrial toxins)
	BILIARY OBSTRUCTION
	Choledocholithiasis, biliary atresia, carcinoma of biliary duct, sclerosing cholangitis, choledochal cyst, external pressure on common duct, pancreatitis, pancreatic neoplasms

Table 15–2. Hyperbilirubinemic disorders.

	Nature of Defect	Type of Hyper-bilirubinemia	Clinical and Pathologic Characteristics
Gilbert's syndrome	Glucuronyl transferase deficiency	Unconjugated (indirect) bilirubin	Benign, asymptomatic hereditary jaundice. Hyperbilirubinemia increased by 24- to 36-hour fast. No treatment required. Prognosis excellent.
Familial chronic idiopathic jaundice (Dubin-Johnson syndrome)	Faulty excretory function of liver cells (hepatocytes)	Conjugated (direct) bilirubin	Benign, asymptomatic hereditary jaundice. Gallbladder does not visualize on oral cholecystography. Liver darkly pigmented on gross examination. Biopsy shows centrilobular brown pigment. Prognosis excellent.
Rotor's syndrome			Similar to Dubin-Johnson syndrome, but liver is not pigmented and the gallbladder is visualized on oral cholecystography. Prognosis excellent.
Benign intermittent cholestasis	Cholestasis of uncertain pathogenesis, often on a familial basis	Unconjugated plus conjugated (total) bilirubin	Benign intermittent idiopathic jaundice, itching, and malaise. Onset in early life and may persist for lifetime. Alkaline phosphatase increased. Cholestasis found on liver biopsy. (Biopsy is normal during remission.) Prognosis excellent.
Recurrent jaundice of pregnancy			Benign cholestatic jaundice of unknown cause, usually occurring in the third trimester of pregnancy. Itching, gastrointestinal symptoms, and abnormal liver excretory function tests. Cholestasis noted on liver biopsy. Prognosis excellent, but recurrence with subsequent pregnancies or use of birth control pills is characteristic.

Table 15–3. Liver function tests: Normal values and changes in two types of jaundice.

Tests	Normal Values	Hepatocellular Jaundice	Uncomplicated Obstructive Jaundice

Bilirubin
  Direct
  Indirect
	0.1–0.3 mg/dL
	0.2–0.7 mg/dL
		Increased
		Increased
			Increased
			Increased

Urine bilirubin	None	Increased	Increased
Serum albumin/total protein	Albumin, 3.5–5.5 g/dL Total protein, 6.5–8.4 g/dL	Albumin decreased	Unchanged
Alkaline phosphatase	30–115 IU/L	Increased (+)	Increased (++++)
Prothrombin time	INR[1] of 1.0–1.4. After vitamin K, 10% increase in 24 hours	Prolonged if damage severe and does not respond to parenteral vitamin K	Prolonged if obstruction marked, but responds to parenteral vitamin K
ALT, AST	ALT, 5–35 units/L; AST, 5–40 units/L	Increased in hepatocellular damage, viral hepatitis	Minimally increased

[1]INR = International Normalized Ratio.

disease. In patients with suspected metastatic disease or a hepatic mass, liver biopsy should be performed under ultrasound or CT guidance.

C. Imaging: Demonstration of dilated bile ducts by ultrasonography or CT scan indicates biliary obstruction (90–95% sensitivity). Ultrasonography, CT scan, and MRI can be used to demonstrate hepatomegaly, intrahepatic tumors, and changes of portal hypertension. Helical arterial-phase CT scanning, in which the liver is imaged during the brief period when intravenously administered contrast material reaches the hepatic artery branches, and CT arterial portography, in which imaging follows intravenous contrast infusion via a catheter placed in the superior mesenteric artery, are the most sensitive techniques available for preoperative detection of small hepatic lesions. Because of its much lower cost, ultrasonography ($350) is preferable to CT ($1200–$1400) or MRI ($2000) as a screening test. Ultrasonography can detect gallstones with a sensitivity of 95%.

Endoscopic retrograde cholangiopancreatography (ERCP) or percutaneous transhepatic cholangiography (PTC) can identify the cause, location, and extent of biliary obstruction. Complications of PTC occur in about 3% of cases and include fever, bacteremia, bile peritonitis, and intraperitoneal hemorrhage. ERCP requires a skilled endoscopist and may be utilized to demonstrate pancreatic or ampullary causes of jaundice, to carry out papillotomy and stone extraction, or to insert a stent through an obstructing lesion. Complications of ERCP include pancreatitis in 4% of cases and, less commonly, cholangitis, bleeding, or duodenal perforation after papillotomy. Endoscopic ultrasonography, where available, appears to be the most sensitive test for detecting small lesions of the ampulla or pancreatic head and for detecting portal vein invasion by pancreatic cancer. Magnetic resonance cholangiography, recently introduced, appears to be a sensitive, nonin-

vasive method of detecting bile duct stones, strictures, and dilation, though without the therapeutic applications of ERCP.

Berk PD, Noyer C (editors): Bilirubin metabolism and the hereditary hyperbilirubinemias. Semin Liver Dis 1994;14:321. (Reviews biochemistry, pathophysiology, genetics, and management.)

Bosma PJ et al: The genetic basis of the reduced expression of bilirubin UDP-glucuronosyltransferase in Gilbert's syndrome. N Engl J Med 1995;333:1171. (Abnormality in the promoter region of the gene is necessary but not sufficient.)

Kamath PS: Clinical approach to the patient with abnormal liver test results. Mayo Clin Proc 1996;71:1089. (Useful algorithms.)

Oliver JH III, Baron RL: Helical biphasic contrast-enhanced CT of the liver: Technique, indications, interpretation, and pitfalls. Radiology 1996;201:1. (Improves detection of hypervascular tumors.)

Soto JA et al: Magnetic resonance cholangiography: Comparison with endoscopic retrograde cholangiopancreatography. Gastroenterology 1996;110:589. (Compared with ERCP, the sensitivity for detecting bile duct stones, strictures, and dilation was 100%, 90%, and 96%, respectively, and the specificity was 94%.)

DISEASES OF THE LIVER

VIRAL HEPATITIS

Essentials of Diagnosis

- Prodrome of anorexia, nausea, vomiting, malaise, symptoms of upper respiratory infection or flu-like syndrome, aversion to smoking.
- Fever, enlarged and tender liver, jaundice.

- Normal to low white cell count; abnormal liver tests, especially markedly elevated aminotransferases early in the course.
- Liver biopsy shows characteristic hepatocellular necrosis and mononuclear infiltrate but is rarely indicated.

General Considerations

Hepatitis can be caused by many drugs and toxic agents as well as by numerous viruses, the clinical manifestations of which may be quite similar. The specific viruses causing viral hepatitis are (1) hepatitis A virus (HAV); (2) hepatitis B virus (HBV); (3) hepatitis C virus (HCV); (4) hepatitis D virus (delta agent); and (5) hepatitis E virus (an enterically transmitted hepatitis seen in epidemic form in Asia, North Africa, and Mexico). The designation hepatitis G virus (HGV) has recently been applied to an agent that rarely, if ever, causes frank hepatitis. In immunocompromised hosts, cytomegalovirus, Epstein-Barr virus, and herpes simplex virus should be considered in the differential diagnosis of hepatitis.

A.   Hepatitis A: (Figure 15–1.) HAV is a 27-nm RNA hepatovirus (in the picornavirus family) that may cause epidemics or sporadic cases of hepatitis. Transmission of the virus is usually by the fecal-oral route, and spread is enhanced by crowding and poor sanitation. Common source outbreaks may result from contaminated water or food. The excretion of hepatitis A virus (HAV) occurs up to 2 weeks prior to clinical illness. HAV is rarely demonstrated in feces after the first week of illness. Blood and stools

are infectious during the incubation period (2–6 weeks) and early illness until aminotransferase levels peak. The mortality rate for hepatitis A is low, and fulminant hepatitis A is uncommon. Chronic hepatitis does not occur and there is no carrier state. Clinical illness is more severe in adults than in children, in whom hepatitis A is often asymptomatic.

Antibody to hepatitis A (anti-HAV) appears early in the course of the illness. Both IgM and IgG anti-HAV are detectable in serum soon after the onset of the illness. Peak titers of IgM anti-HAV occur during the first week of clinical disease and usually disappear within 3–6 months. Detection of IgM anti-HAV is an excellent test for diagnosing acute hepatitis A. Titers of IgG anti-HAV peak after 1 month of the disease and may persist for years. The presence of IgG anti-HAV alone indicates previous exposure to HAV, noninfectivity, and immunity to recurring HAV infection.

B.   Hepatitis B: (Figure 15–2.) Hepatitis B virus (HBV) is a 42-nm hepadnavirus with a partially double-stranded DNA genome, inner core protein (hepatitis B core antigen, HBcAg), and outer surface coat (hepatitis B surface antigen, HBsAg). HBV is usually transmitted by inoculation of infected blood or blood products or by sexual contact and is present in saliva, semen, and vaginal secretions. HBsAg-positive mothers may transmit HBV to their neonates at the time of delivery; the risk of chronic infection in the infant is as high as 90%. Hepatitis B virus (HBV) is highly prevalent in homosexuals and intravenous

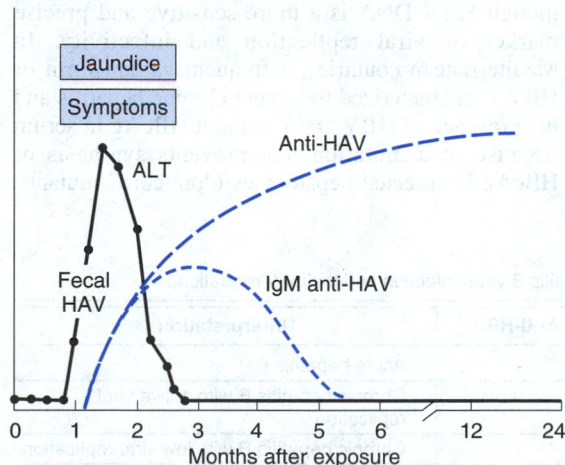

Figure 15–1. The typical course of acute type A hepatitis. (HAV, hepatitis A antigen; anti-HAV, antibody to hepatitis A virus; ALT, alanine aminotransferase.) (Reproduced, with permission, from Schafer DF, Hoofnagle JH: View Dig Dis 1982;14:5.)

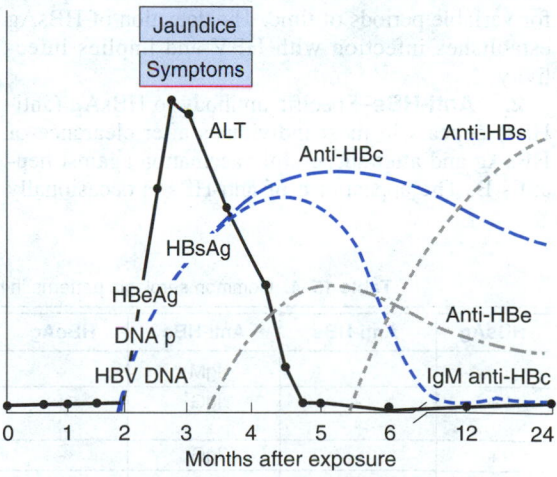

Figure 15–2. The typical course of acute type B hepatitis. (HBsAg, hepatitis B surface antigen; anti-HBs, antibody to HBsAg; HBeAg, hepatitis B e antigen; anti-HBe, antibody to HBeAg; anti-HBc, antibody to hepatitis B core antigen; DNA p, DNA polymerase; ALT, alanine aminotransferase.) (Reproduced, with permission, from Hoofnagle JH, Schafer DF: Serologic markers of hepatitis B virus infection. Semin Liver Dis 1986;6:1.)

drug abusers, but most cases reported in the USA now result from heterosexual transmission. Other groups at high risk include patients and staff at hemodialysis centers, physicians, dentists, nurses, and personnel working in clinical and pathology laboratories and blood banks. The incubation period of hepatitis B is 6 weeks to 6 months (average 12–14 weeks). Administration of hepatitis B immune globulin prolongs the incubation period but attenuates the severity of illness. Clinical features of hepatitis A and B are similar; however, the onset in hepatitis B tends to be more insidious and the aminotransferase levels higher. The risk of fulminant hepatitis is less than 1%, with a mortality rate of up to 60%. Following acute hepatitis B, HBV infection may persist in 1–2% of immunocompetent adults but a higher percentage of immunocompromised adults or children. Persons with chronic hepatitis B, particularly when HBV infection is acquired early in life, are at substantial risk of cirrhosis and hepatocellular carcinoma (up to 25–40%). Infection caused by HBV may be associated with arthritis, glomerulonephritis, and polyarteritis nodosa.

There are three distinct antigen-antibody systems that relate to HBV infection and a variety of circulating markers that are useful in diagnosis. Interpretation of common serologic patterns is shown in Table 15–4.

1. HBsAg–The appearance of HBsAg is the first evidence of HBV infection, appearing before biochemical evidence of liver disease. HBsAg persists throughout the clinical illness. Persistence of HBsAg after the acute illness may be associated with clinical and laboratory evidence of chronic hepatitis for variable periods of time. The detection of HBsAg establishes infection with HBV and implies infectivity.

2. Anti-HBs–Specific antibody to HBsAg (anti-HBs) appears in most individuals after clearance of HBsAg and after successful vaccination against hepatitis B. The appearance of anti-HBs is occasionally delayed until after clearance of HBsAg. During this serologic gap (window period), infectivity has been demonstrated. Disappearance of HBsAg and the appearance of anti-HBs signals recovery from HBV infection, noninfectivity, and protection from recurrent HBV infection.

3. Anti-HBc–IgM anti-HBc appears shortly after HBsAg is detected. (HBcAg itself does not appear free in serum.) Its presence in the setting of acute hepatitis indicates a diagnosis of acute hepatitis B, and it fills the serologic gap in patients who have cleared HBsAg but do not yet have detectable anti-HBs. IgM anti-HBc can persist for 3–6 months or more. IgM anti-HBc may also reappear during flares of previously inactive chronic hepatitis B. IgG anti-HBc also appears during acute hepatitis B but persists indefinitely, whether the patient recovers (with the appearance of anti-HBs in serum) or develops chronic hepatitis B (with persistence of HBsAg). In asymptomatic blood donors, an isolated anti-HBc with no other positive HBV serologic results is often a falsely positive result.

4. HBeAg–HBeAg is a soluble protein found only in HBsAg-positive sera. It represents a secretory form of HBcAg that appears during the incubation period shortly after the detection of HBsAg. HBeAg indicates viral replication and infectivity. Persistence of HBeAg in serum beyond 3 months suggests an increased likelihood of chronic hepatitis B. Disappearance of HBeAg is often followed by the appearance of anti-HBe, signifying diminished viral replication and decreased infectivity.

5. HBV DNA–The presence of HBV DNA in serum generally parallels the presence of HBeAg, though HBV DNA is a more sensitive and precise marker of viral replication and infectivity. In Mediterranean countries, a frequent variant form of HBV is characterized by severe chronic hepatitis and the presence of HBV DNA without HBeAg in serum because of a mutation that prevents synthesis of HBeAg in infected hepatocytes ("pre-core" mutant).

Table 15–4. Common serologic patterns in hepatitis B virus infection and their interpretation.

HBsAg	Anti-HBs	Anti-HBc	HBeAg	Anti-HBe	Interpretation
+	–	IgM	+	–	Acute hepatitis B
+	–	IgG[1]	+	–	Chronic hepatitis B with active viral replication
+	–	IgG	–	+	Chronic hepatitis B with low viral replication
+	+	IgG	+ or –	+ or –	Chronic hepatitis B with heterotypic anti-HBs (≈ 10% of cases)
–	–	IgM	+ or –	–	Acute hepatitis B
–	+	IgG	–	+ or –	Recovery from hepatitis B (immunity)
–	+	–	–	–	Vaccination (immunity)
–	–	IgG	–	–	False-positive; less commonly, infection in remote past

[1]Low levels of IgM anti-HBc may also be detected.

The pre-core mutant may appear during the course of chronic "wild-type" HBV infection, presumably as a result of immune pressure.

C. Hepatitis D (Delta Agent): Hepatitis D virus (HDV) is a defective RNA virus that causes hepatitis only in association with hepatitis B infection and specifically only in the presence of HBsAg; it is cleared when the latter is cleared.

HDV may co-infect with HBV or may superinfect a person with chronic hepatitis B. When acute hepatitis D is coincident with acute HBV infection, the infection is generally similar in severity to acute hepatitis B alone. In chronic hepatitis B, superinfection by HDV appears to carry a more severe prognosis, often resulting in fulminant hepatitis or severe chronic hepatitis that progresses rapidly to cirrhosis. HDV is endemic in some areas, such as Mediterranean countries, where up to 80% of HBV carriers may be superinfected with it. In the USA, infection has occurred primarily among intravenous drug users. Diagnosis is by detection of antibody to hepatitis D antigen (anti-HDV) or, where available, HDV RNA in serum.

At present, hepatitis D is best prevented by prevention of hepatitis B (eg, with HBV vaccine).

D. Hepatitis C (HCV): (Figure 15–3.) The hepatitis C virus is a single-stranded RNA virus with properties similar to those of flavivirus. At least six major genotypes of HCV have been identified. HCV is responsible for over 90% of cases of posttransfusion hepatitis, yet only 4% of cases of hepatitis C are attributable to blood transfusions. Up to 50% of cases are related to intravenous drug use. The risk of sexual and maternal-neonatal transmission is small and may be limited to a subset of patients with high circulating levels of HCV RNA. An outbreak of hepatitis C in patients with immune deficiencies occurred recently in some recipients of intravenous immune globulin. In many patients, the source of infection is uncertain. The incubation period averages 6–7 weeks, and clinical illness is often mild, usually asymptomatic, and characterized by waxing and waning aminotransferase elevations and a high rate (> 50%) of chronic hepatitis. HCV may be a pathogenic factor in cryoglobulinemia, glomerulonephritis, autoimmune thyroiditis, lymphocytic sialadenitis, idiopathic pulmonary fibrosis, and sporadic porphyria cutanea tarda.

Diagnosis of hepatitis C is based on an enzyme immunoassay that detects antibodies to HCV (anti-HCV). Limitations of the enzyme immunoassay include moderate sensitivity for the diagnosis of acute hepatitis C (false-negatives) and low specificity (50%) in healthy blood donors and some persons with elevated gamma globulin levels (false-positives) early in the course. In these situations, a diagnosis of hepatitis C may be confirmed by use of a supplemental recombinant immunoblot assay (RIBA). Most RIBA-positive persons are potentially infectious, as confirmed in research laboratories by use of polymerase chain reaction to detect HCV RNA. Testing of donated blood for HCV has helped reduce the risk of transfusion-associated hepatitis C from 10% a decade ago to less than 0.1% today.

E. Hepatitis E (HEV): Formerly termed enterically transmitted non-A, non-B hepatitis, HEV is a 29- to 32-nm RNA virus similar to calicivirus and responsible for waterborne hepatitis outbreaks in India, Burma, Afghanistan, Algeria, and Mexico. Illness is self-limited (no carrier state) with a high mortality rate (10–20%) in pregnant women.

F. Hepatitis G: The designation hepatitis G virus (HGV) has been applied to a recently identified flavivirus that is percutaneously transmitted and associated with chronic viremia lasting at least 10 years. HGV has been detected in 50% of intravenous drug users, 30% of hemodialysis patients, 20% of hemophiliacs, and 15% of patients with chronic hepatitis B or C, but it does not appear to cause important liver disease.

Clinical Findings

The clinical picture of viral hepatitis is extremely variable, ranging from asymptomatic infection without jaundice to a fulminating disease and death in a few days.

A. Symptoms:

1. Prodromal phase–The onset may be abrupt or insidious, with general malaise, myalgia, arthralgia, easy fatigability, upper respiratory symptoms (nasal discharge, pharyngitis), and anorexia. A distaste for smoking, paralleling anorexia, may occur

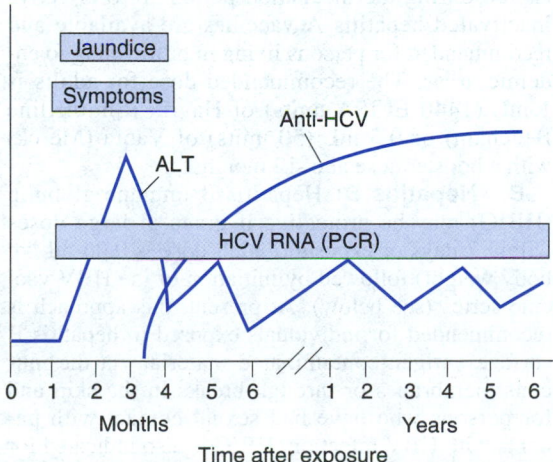

Figure 15–3. The typical course of acute and chronic hepatitis C. (ALT, alanine aminotransferase; Anti-HCV, antibody to hepatitis C virus by enzyme immunoassay; HCV RNA [PCR], hepatitis C viral RNA by polymerase chain reaction.)

early. Nausea and vomiting are frequent, and diarrhea or constipation may occur. Skin rashes, arthritis, or serum sickness may be seen early in acute hepatitis B. Fever is generally present but is rarely over 39.5 °C save in occasional cases of hepatitis A. Defervescence often coincides with the onset of jaundice. Chills or chilliness may mark an acute onset.

Abdominal pain is usually mild and constant in the right upper quadrant or epigastrium and is often aggravated by jarring or exertion. (On rare occasions, upper abdominal pain may be severe enough to simulate cholecystitis or cholelithiasis.)

2. Icteric phase–Clinical jaundice occurs after 5–10 days but may appear at the same time as the initial symptomatology. Most patients never develop clinical icterus. With the onset of jaundice, there is often worsening of the prodromal symptoms, followed by progressive clinical improvement.

3. Convalescent phase–There is an increasing sense of well-being, return of appetite, and disappearance of jaundice, abdominal pain and tenderness, and fatigability.

4. Course and complications–The acute illness usually subsides over 2–3 weeks with complete clinical and laboratory recovery by 9 weeks in hepatitis A and by 16 weeks in hepatitis B. In 5–10% of cases, the course may be more protracted, and less than 1% will have an acute fulminant course. In some cases of acute hepatitis A, clinical, biochemical, and serologic recovery may be followed by one or two relapses, but ultimate recovery is the rule. Hepatitis B, D, and C (and G) may become chronic (see below).

B. Signs: Hepatomegaly—rarely marked—is present in over half of cases. Liver tenderness is usually present. Splenomegaly is reported in 15% of patients, and soft, enlarged lymph nodes—especially in the cervical or epitrochlear areas—may occur. Signs of general toxemia vary from minimal to severe.

C. Laboratory Findings: The white blood cell count is normal to low, especially in the preicteric phase. Large atypical lymphocytes, such as are found in infectious mononucleosis, may occasionally be seen. Mild proteinuria is common, and bilirubinuria often precedes the appearance of jaundice. Acholic stools are often present during the icteric phase. Blood studies reflect hepatocellular damage with often strikingly elevated AST or ALT values. Bilirubin and alkaline phosphatase are elevated and, in a minority of patients, remain so after aminotransferase levels have normalized. Cholestasis is occasionally marked in acute hepatitis A. Marked prolongation of the prothrombin time in severe hepatitis correlates with increased mortality.

Differential Diagnosis

The differential diagnosis of hepatitis includes other viral diseases such as infectious mononucleosis, cytomegalovirus infection, and herpes simplex virus infection; spirochetal diseases such as leptospirosis and secondary syphilis; brucellosis; rickettsial diseases such as Q fever; drug-induced liver disease; and shock liver (ischemic hepatitis). Occasionally, autoimmune hepatitis (see below) may have an acute onset mimicking acute viral hepatitis. Rarely, metastatic cancer of the liver may present with a hepatitis-like picture.

The prodromal phase of viral hepatitis must be distinguished from other infectious disease such as influenza, upper respiratory infections, and the prodromal stages of the exanthematous diseases. Occasionally, cholestasis may be prominent in viral hepatitis and mimic obstructive jaundice.

Prevention

Strict isolation of patients is not necessary, but hand washing after bowel movements is required. Thorough hand washing by medical attendants who come into contact with contaminated utensils, bedding, or clothing is essential. Careful handling of disposable needles—including not recapping used needles—is important for medical personnel. Screening of donated blood for HBsAg, anti-HBc, and anti-HCV has reduced the risk of transfusion-associated hepatitis markedly. All pregnant women should undergo testing for HBsAg. Unnecessary transfusions and commercially obtained blood should be avoided. HBV- and HCV-infected persons should practice "safe sex," but there is little evidence that HCV is spread easily by sexual contact.

A. Hepatitis A: Immune globulin should be given routinely to all *close* (eg, household) personal contacts of patients with hepatitis A. The recommended dose of 0.02 mL/kg intramuscularly has been found to be protective for hepatitis A if administered during the incubation period. Two effective inactivated hepatitis A vaccines are available and recommended for persons living in or traveling to endemic areas. The recommended dose for adults is 1 mL (1440 ELISA units) of Havrix (SmithKline Beecham) or 0.5 mL (50 units) of Vaqta (Merck) with a booster dose at 6–12 months.

B. Hepatitis B: Hepatitis B immune globulin (HBIG) may be protective if given in large doses within 7 days of exposure (adult dose is 0.06 mL/kg body weight) followed by initiation of the HBV vaccine series (see below). At present, this approach is recommended for individuals exposed to hepatitis B surface antigen-contaminated material via the mucous membranes or through breaks in the skin and for persons who have had sexual contact with patients with HBV infection. HBIG is also indicated for newborn infants of HBsAg-positive mothers followed by initiation of the vaccine series (see below).

The currently used vaccine is recombinant-derived. Until recently, the vaccine was targeted to persons at high risk, including renal dialysis patients and attending personnel, patients requiring repeated transfusions, spouses of HBsAg-positive individuals, male homosexuals, intravenous drug abusers, newborns of HBsAg-positive mothers, entering medical and nursing students, as well as all medical technologists. Because this strategy failed to lower the incidence of hepatitis B, the CDC has recommended universal vaccination of infants and children in the USA. Over 90% of recipients of the vaccine mount protective antibody to hepatitis B. The dose for adults is 10–20 µg initially (depending on the formulation) and again at 1 and 6 months; for greatest reliability of absorption, the deltoid muscle is the preferred site of injection. When documentation of seroconversion is considered desirable, postimmunization anti-HBs titers may be checked. Protection appears to be excellent even if the titer wanes—at least for 10 years—and booster reimmunization is not routinely recommended.

Treatment

Bed rest is recommended only on an as-needed basis during the acute initial phase of the disease, when symptoms are most severe. Return to normal activity during the convalescent period should be gradual. If nausea and vomiting are pronounced or if oral intake is substantially decreased, intravenous administration of 10% glucose solution is indicated. If the patient shows signs of encephalopathy or severe coagulopathy, fulminant hepatic failure should be suspected, and hospitalization is mandatory (see below).

In general, dietary management consists of giving palatable meals as tolerated, without overfeeding. Patients should avoid strenuous physical exertion, alcohol, and hepatotoxic agents. While the administration of small doses of oxazepam is safe (metabolism not affected by liver disease), it is recommended that morphine sulfate be avoided.

In controlled studies, corticosteroids have demonstrated no benefit in patients with viral hepatitis, including those with fulminant hepatitis. Treatment of patients with acute hepatitis C with alpha interferon appears to decrease the risk of chronic hepatitis.

Prognosis

In most cases, clinical recovery is complete in 3–16 weeks. Laboratory evidence of liver dysfunction may persist for a longer period, but most patients recover completely. The overall mortality rate is less than 1%, but the rate is reportedly higher in older people.

Hepatitis A does not progress to chronic liver disease, though hepatitis A may persist for up to 1 year, and clinical and biochemical relapses may occur before full recovery. The mortality rate is less than 0.2%. The mortality rate for acute hepatitis B is 0.1–1%, and it is even higher for superimposed hepatitis D. Fulminant hepatitis C is rare in the USA. For unknown reasons, the mortality rate for hepatitis E is especially high in pregnant women (10–20%).

Chronic hepatitis, characterized by elevated aminotransferase levels for more than 6 months, occurs in 1–2% of immunocompetent adult patients with hepatitis B but in as many as 90% of neonates and infants and a substantial proportion of immunocompromised adults with hepatitis B and over 70% of all persons with hepatitis C. Ultimately, cirrhosis may develop in up to 30% of those with chronic hepatitis C and 40% of those with chronic hepatitis B. These patients are also at risk for hepatocellular carcinoma.

Lemon SM, Thomas DL: Vaccines to prevent viral hepatitis. N Engl J Med 1997;336:196. (Emphasizes formulation, efficacy, and indications for hepatitis A and B vaccines.)

Margolis HS et al: Prevention of hepatitis B virus transmission by immunization: An economic analysis of current recommendations. JAMA 1995;274:1201. (Supports routine vaccination of infants.)

Martin P, Friedman LS (editors): Viral hepatitis. Gastroenterol Clin North Am 1994;23:429.

Schreiber GB et al: The risk of transfusion-transmitted viral infections. N Engl J Med 1996;334:1685. (The current risk of transmitting hepatitis B and C by transfusion of screened blood is 1:63,000 and 1:103,000, respectively.)

Sharara AJ et al: Hepatitis C. Ann Intern Med 1996;125:658. (Reviews virology, epidemiology, diagnosis, clinical features, pathogenesis, and treatment.)

FULMINANT HEPATIC FAILURE

Fulminant hepatic failure is characterized by the development of hepatic encephalopathy within 8 weeks after the onset of acute liver disease. Coagulopathy is invariably present. Subfulminant hepatic failure is the term used when encephalopathy occurs between 8 weeks and 6 months after the onset of acute liver disease and carries an equally poor prognosis.

About 70% of all cases of fulminant hepatic failure are caused by acute viral hepatitis. Up to 50% of cases of fulminant viral hepatitis are due to hepatitis B—in some cases detectable only by molecular techniques (polymerase chain reaction). Most of the remainder are due to hepatitis A or unknown viruses. In endemic areas, hepatitis D and hepatitis E may cause fulminant hepatitis. Hepatitis C appears to be a rare cause of fulminant hepatitis in the USA. Nonviral causes of fulminant hepatic failure include drugs, shock, hyper- or hypothermia, Budd-Chiari syndrome, malignancy, Wilson's disease, Reye's syndrome, and fatty liver of pregnancy.

In fulminant hepatic failure due to hepatitis, extensive necrosis of large areas of the liver gives the typical pathologic picture of acute liver atrophy. Toxemia, gastrointestinal symptoms, and hemorrhagic phenomena are common. Jaundice may be absent or minimal, but laboratory tests show severe hepatocellular damage. In fulminant hepatic failure due to microvesicular steatosis (eg, Reye's syndrome), serum aminotransferase elevations may be modest (< 300 units/L).

The treatment of fulminant hepatitis is directed toward correcting metabolic abnormalities associated with severe liver cell dysfunction. They include coagulation defects; disordered fluid, electrolyte, and acid-base balance; renal failure; hypoglycemia; and encephalopathy. Prophylactic antibiotic therapy decreases the risk of infection, which is as high as 90%, but has no effect on survival and is not routinely recommended. For suspected sepsis, broad coverage is indicated pending culture results. The most frequent isolates are *Staphylococcus aureus, Streptococcus* species, coliforms, and, later in the course, *Candida* species. Early administration of acetylcysteine is indicated for acetaminophen toxicity. Early transfer to a liver transplantation center is essential. Extradural sensors may be placed to monitor intracranial pressure for the development of cerebral edema and decreased cerebral perfusion.

Mannitol 100–200 mL of a 20% solution by rapid intravenous infusion, may decrease cerebral edema. Hepatic-assist devices that use living hepatocytes and liver xenografts have shown promise in animal models and are undergoing clinical trials. The mortality rate of fulminant hepatitis with severe encephalopathy is as high as 80%. Emergency liver transplantation has been associated with an 80% survival rate at 1 year. Compared with chronic hepatitis B, liver transplantation for fulminant hepatitis B is less likely to result in reinfection of the graft with HBV.

Caracenci P, Van Thiel DH: Acute liver failure. Lancet 1995;345:163. (Up-to-date overview of management.)

Hoofnagle JH et al: Fulminant hepatic failure: Summary of a workshop. Hepatology 1995;21:240.

Izumi S et al: Coagulation V levels as a prognostic indicator in fulminant hepatic failure. Hepatology 1996; 23:1507. (Low factor V levels proved less predictive of mortality than the "King's College criteria" based on acidosis [pH < 3.1], INR > 6.5, and serum creatinine > 300/μmol/L for acetaminophen-induced fulminant hepatic failure.)

Langnas AN et al: Parvovirus B19 as a possible causative agent of fulminant liver failure and associated aplastic anemia. Hepatology 1995;22:1661. (Evidence in support of role of parvovirus B19 in occasional cases of non-A, B, C, D, E hepatitis associated with aplastic anemia.)

Williams R (ed): Fulminant hepatic failure. Semin Liv Dis 1996;16:341. (Entire issue devoted to the subject.)

CHRONIC HEPATITIS

Chronic hepatitis is defined as a chronic inflammatory reaction of the liver of more than 3–6 months' duration, as demonstrated by persistently abnormal serum aminotransferase levels and characteristic histologic findings. The causes of chronic hepatitis include HBV, HCV, and HDV, autoimmune hepatitis, chronic hepatitis associated with certain medications (including methyldopa and isoniazid), Wilson's disease, α_1-antiprotease (α_1-antitrypsin) deficiency, and hemochromatosis. Traditionally, chronic hepatitis has been categorized histologically as chronic persistent hepatitis and chronic active hepatitis. However, with improved serologic and autoimmune markers, more precise categorization is preferred, based on etiology; the grade of portal, periportal, and lobular inflammation (minimal, mild, moderate, or severe); and the stage of fibrosis (none, mild, moderate, severe, cirrhosis).

Clinical Findings & Diagnosis

A. Autoimmune Hepatitis: This is generally a disease of young women but can occur in either sex at any age. Affected persons are often positive for HLA-B8 and -DR3 or, in older patients, HLA-DR4. The onset is usually insidious, but about 25% of cases present as an acute attack of hepatitis and some cases follow a viral illness such as hepatitis A, Epstein-Barr infection, or measles. The serum bilirubin is usually increased, but 20% of patients are anicteric. Examination often reveals a healthy-appearing young woman with multiple spider nevi, cutaneous striae, acne, hirsutism, and hepatomegaly. Amenorrhea may be a feature of this disease. Extrahepatic features include arthritis, Sjögren's syndrome, thyroiditis, nephritis, and Coombs-positive hemolytic anemia. In classic (type I) autoimmune hepatitis, antinuclear antibody (ANA) or smooth muscle antibody (either or both) is detected in serum. Serum gamma globulin levels are typically elevated (up to 5–6 g/dL). In patients with high gamma globulin levels, the enzyme immunoassay for antibody to HCV may be falsely positive. A second type (II), rarely seen in the United States but more common in Europe, is characterized by circulating antibody to liver-kidney microsomes (anti-LKM1) without anti-smooth muscle antibody or ANA.

B. Chronic Hepatitis B: Chronic hepatitis B chiefly affects males. It may be noted as a continuum of acute hepatitis or may be diagnosed on evaluation of persistently elevated aminotransferase levels.

Early in the course, HBeAg and HBV DNA are present in serum, indicative of active viral replications. Low-level IgM anti-HBc is also present in about 70%. In some patients, clinical and biochemical improvement coincides with disappearance of HBeAg and HBV DNA from serum, appearance of anti-HBe, and integration of the HBV genome into the host genome in infected hepatocytes. Such patients are still at increased risk for the development of cirrhosis and hepatocellular carcinoma. As discussed above, infection by a pre-core mutant of HBV or spontaneous mutation of the pre-core region of the HBV genome during the course of chronic hepatitis caused by wild-type HBV may result in particularly severe chronic hepatitis with rapid progression to cirrhosis, particularly when additional mutations in the core gene of HBV are present.

C. Delta Agent in Hepatitis B: Acute delta infection superimposed on chronic HBV infection may result in severe chronic hepatitis, which may progress rapidly to cirrhosis and may be fatal. The diagnosis is confirmed by detection of anti-HDV in serum.

D. Chronic Hepatitis C: At least 70% of patients with acute hepatitis C develop chronic hepatitis C. It is clinically indistinguishable from chronic hepatitis due to other causes and may be the most common. The diagnosis is confirmed by detection of anti-HCV by enzyme immunoassy (EIA). In rare cases of suspected chronic hepatitis C but a negative EIA, the diagnosis may be confirmed by a positive recombinant immunoblot assay (RIBA) or detection of HCV RNA in serum by polymerase chain reaction.

Treatment

Activity should be modified according to the patient's symptoms, but strict bed rest is not necessary. The diet should be well balanced, without specific limitations other than sodium or protein restriction as dictated by fluid overload or encephalopathy.

Prednisone with or without azathioprine has been shown to improve symptoms, decrease the serum bilirubin, aminotransferase, and gamma globulin levels, and reduce hepatic inflammation in patients with **autoimmune hepatitis.** Symptomatic patients with serum aminotransferase levels elevated tenfold (or fivefold if the serum globulins are elevated at least twofold) are optimal for therapy, and patients with more modest enzyme elevations may be considered for therapy depending on the clinical circumstances. The mortality rate in patients with severe autoimmune hepatitis treated with corticosteroids is significantly reduced.

Prednisone or an equivalent drug is given initially in doses of 30 mg orally daily with azathioprine or mercaptopurine, 50 mg/d orally, which is generally well tolerated and permits the use of lower corticosteroid doses. Nevertheless, complete blood counts should be monitored weekly for the first 8 weeks of therapy and monthly thereafter because of the small risk of bone marrow suppression. The dose of prednisone is lowered from 30 mg/d after 1 week to 20 mg/d and again after 2 or 3 weeks to 15 mg/d. Ultimately, a maintenance dose of 10 mg/d is achieved. While symptomatic improvement is often prompt, biochemical improvement is more gradual, with normalization of serum aminotransferase levels after 6–12 months in many cases. Histologic resolution of inflammation may take up to 18–24 months, the time at which repeat liver biopsy is recommended. Failure of aminotransferase levels to normalize invariably predicts lack of histologic resolution.

The response rate to therapy with prednisone and azathioprine is 80–90%. Cirrhosis, however, does not reverse with therapy and may even develop after apparent biochemical and histologic remission (absence of inflammation). Once remission is achieved, therapy may be withdrawn, but the subsequent relapse rate is 50–90%. Relapses may again be treated in the same manner as the initial episode, with an expected remission rate of again 80–90%. After successful treatment of a relapse, the patient may be kept indefinitely on azathioprine up to 2 mg/kg and the lowest dose of prednisone needed to maintain aminotransferase levels as close to normal as possible. Nonresponders to prednisone and azathioprine may be considered for a trial of cyclosporine.

Patients with **chronic hepatitis B** and active viral replication (HBeAg and HBV DNA in serum; elevated aminotransferase levels) may be treated with recombinant human interferon alfa-2b in a dose of 5 million units a day or 10 million units three times a week intramuscularly for 4 months. About 40% of treated patients will respond with normalization of aminotransferase levels, disappearance of HBeAg and HBV DNA from serum, appearance of anti-HBe, and improved survival. A response is most likely in patients with an HBV DNA level under 200 pg/mL and high aminotransferase levels. Moreover, over 60% of these responders may eventually clear HBsAg from serum and liver, develop anti-HBs in serum, and thus be cured of the infection. Relapses are uncommon in such complete responders. The nucleoside analogs lamivudine and famciclovir, which are taken orally, have shown promise in the treatment of chronic hepatitis B and are well tolerated, even in patients with decompensated cirrhosis, though viral resistance to lamivudine has been reported. Recombinant interferon alfa-2a (9 million units three times a week for 48 weeks) may lead to normalization of serum aminotransferase levels, histologic improvement, and elimination of HDV RNA from serum in about 50% of patients with **chronic hepatitis D,** but relapse is common after therapy is stopped.

Recombinant human interferon alfa-2b in a dose of 3 million units three times a week for 24 weeks has been shown to induce biochemical and histologic improvement in up to 50% of patients with **chronic hepatitis C.** Factors that predict an increased chance of responding to therapy include the absence of cirrhosis on liver biopsy, low serum HCV RNA levels, and possibly infection by genotypes of HCV other than 1a and 1b. After stopping the medication at 24 weeks, only 30–50% of the treated responders will maintain the improvement. More prolonged treatment (eg, for 12–18 months) has been shown to increase the durability of remission and is now generally recommended. The use of higher doses of interferon alfa-2b (eg, 6 million units three times a week) increases toxicity and does not appear to increase the rate of sustained responses. Addition of the experimental nucleoside analog ribavirin may result in higher sustained response rates but should be considered only in the context of a controlled trial. Interferon alfa-2a may be beneficial in the treatment of cryoglobulinemia associated with chronic hepatitis C. Treatment with interferon alfa-2b is costly, and side effects, which include flu-like symptoms, are almost universal; more serious side effects, ie, psychiatric symptoms (irritability, depression), thyroid dysfunction, and bone marrow suppression, are less common. Interferon is contraindicated in patients with decompensated cirrhosis, profound cytopenias, psychiatric disease, and autoimmune diseases.

Prognosis

The course of chronic hepatitis is variable and unpredictable. Untreated autoimmune hepatitis has a 5-year mortality rate of 50%, which decreases markedly with treatment. The sequelae of chronic hepatitis secondary to hepatitis B include cirrhosis, liver failure, and hepatocellular carcinoma. Up to 40–50% of patients with chronic hepatitis B and cirrhosis die within 5 years after the onset of symptoms, though predictive models suggest that therapy with interferon improves the prognosis in responders. Chronic hepatitis C is an indolent, often subclinical disease that may lead to cirrhosis and hepatocellular carcinoma after decades. In one study, the mortality rate from transfusion-associated hepatitis C was no different from that of an age-matched control population. The impact of interferon on the natural history and mortality rate of hepatitis C remains to be seen.

Desmet VJ et al: Classification of chronic hepatitis: Diagnosis, grading and staging. Hepatology 1994;19:1513. (New system based on etiology, degree of inflammation [grade], and extent of fibrosis [stage]; replaces less helpful classification of chronic persistent and chronic active hepatitis.)

Hoofnagel JH, Di Bisceglie AM: The treatment of chronic viral hepatitis. (Drug Therapy.) N Engl J Med 1997; 336:347. (Reviews indications for and results with interferon alfa and discusses promising new agents.)

Niederau C et al: Long-term follow-up of HBeAg-positive patients treated with interferon alfa for chronic hepatitis B. N Engl J Med 1996;334:1422. (Clearance of HBeAg after treatment is associated with fewer complications and improved survival.)

Nishiguchi S et al: Randomized trial of effects of interferon-α on incidence of hepatocellular carcinoma in chronic active hepatitis C. Lancet 1995;346:1051. (Intriguing study suggesting that in this subgroup interferon alpha may prevent or delay the development of hepatocellular carcinoma.)

Poynard T et al: Meta-analysis of interferon randomized trials in the treatment of viral hepatitis C: Effects of dose and duration. Hepatology 1996;24:778. (Based on 37 randomized controlled studies, the authors conclude that for patients with chronic hepatitis C, the efficacy/risk ratio is best for a regimen of 3 million units three times per week for at least 12 months.)

ALCOHOLIC HEPATITIS

Alcoholic hepatitis is characterized by acute or chronic inflammation and parenchymal necrosis of the liver induced by alcohol. While alcoholic hepatitis is often a reversible disease, it is the most common precursor of cirrhosis in the USA, and cirrhosis ranks among the most common causes of death of adults in this country.

The frequency of alcoholic cirrhosis is estimated to be about 8–15% among persons who consume an average of 120 g of alcohol (8 oz of 100-proof whiskey, 30 oz of wine, or eight 12-oz cans of beer) daily for over 10 years. Genetic factors may account in part for differences in susceptibility. Women appear to be more susceptible than men, in part because of lower gastric mucosal alcohol dehydrogenase levels. Although alcoholic hepatitis may not develop in many patients even after several decades of alcohol abuse, it appears in a few individuals within a year after onset of excessive drinking. In general, over 80% of patients with alcoholic hepatitis have been drinking 5 years or more before developing any symptoms that can be attributed to liver disease; the longer the duration of drinking (10–15 or more years) and the larger the alcoholic consumption, the greater the probability of developing alcoholic hepatitis and cirrhosis. While drinking large amounts of alcoholic beverages is essential for the development of alcoholic hepatitis, drunkenness is not. In individuals who drink alcohol excessively, the rate of ethanol metabolism can be sufficiently high to permit the consumption of large quantities of spirits without raising the blood alcohol level over 80 mg/dL, the concentration at which the conventional breath analyzer begins to detect ethanol.

The role of deficiencies in vitamins and calories in the development of alcoholic hepatitis or in the progression of this lesion to cirrhosis remains controversial but is at least contributory. Concurrent HBV or HCV infection also enhances the severity of alcoholic liver disease.

Only liver biopsy can establish the diagnosis with certainty, since any of the clinical and biochemical manifestations of alcoholic hepatitis can be seen in alcoholic fatty liver or cirrhosis, as well as liver disease due to other causes.

Clinical Findings

A. Symptoms and Signs: The clinical presentation of alcoholic hepatitis can vary from an asymptomatic patient with an enlarged liver to a critically ill individual who dies quickly. A recent period of heavy drinking, complaints of anorexia and nausea, and the demonstration of hepatomegaly and jaundice strongly suggest the diagnosis. Abdominal pain and tenderness, splenomegaly, ascites, fever, and encephalopathy may be present.

B. Laboratory Findings: Anemia (usually

macrocytic) may be present. Leukocytosis with shift to the left is common in patients with severe disease. Leukopenia is occasionally seen and disappears after cessation of drinking. About 10% of patients have thrombocytopenia related to a direct toxic effect of alcohol on megakaryocyte production or to hypersplenism.

AST is usually elevated but rarely above 300 units/L. AST is almost invariably greater than ALT, often by a factor of 2 or more. Serum alkaline phosphatase is generally elevated, but rarely more than three times the normal value. Serum bilirubin is increased in 60–90% of patients. Both serum GGTP and mean corpuscular volume are elevated in 90% of alcoholics. Serum bilirubin levels greater than 10 mg/dL and marked prolongation of the prothrombin time ($\geq$ 6 seconds above control) indicate severe disease with a mortality rate as high as 50%. The serum albumin is depressed, and the gamma globulin level is elevated in 50–75% of individuals with alcoholic hepatitis, even in the absence of cirrhosis.

Liver biopsy is usually diagnostic and demonstrates macrovesicular fat, PMN infiltration with hepatic necrosis, and Mallory bodies (alcoholic hyaline). Micronodular cirrhosis may be present as well.

C. Special Procedures: Ultrasound is often helpful in ruling out biliary obstruction or to assess for subclinical ascites. CT scanning with intravenous contrast or MRI may be indicated in selected cases to evaluate patients for collateral vessels, space-occupying lesions of the liver, or concomitant disease of the pancreas.

Differential Diagnosis

Alcoholic hepatitis may be closely mimicked by cholecystitis and cholelithiasis and by injury from certain drugs such as amiodarone. In selected cases, other causes of hepatitis or chronic liver disease may be excluded by serologic or biochemical testing, by imaging studies, or by liver biopsy.

Complications

Ascites may develop during the course of alcoholic hepatitis and should resolve as the hepatitis improves; diuretics are not generally indicated. Bleeding due to coagulopathy is a potential complication. Clinical deterioration and worsening abdominal pain and tenderness may be mistaken for an acute abdominal crisis and result in the unfortunate decision to perform laparotomy. The postoperative mortality rate of acutely ill patients with alcoholic hepatitis is far greater than that for intra- or extrahepatic cholestasis. This is related to the poor nutritional status of these patients and the compromised synthetic function of the liver.

Treatment

A. General Measures: Discontinue all alcoholic beverages. During periods of anorexia, every effort should be made to provide sufficient amounts of carbohydrates and calories to reduce endogenous protein catabolism and to promote gluconeogenesis and prevent hypoglycemia. Nutritional support improves survival in patients with malnutrition. Use of liquid formulas rich in branched-chain amino acids does not improve survival beyond that achieved with less expensive caloric supplementation. The administration of vitamins, particularly folic acid and thiamin, is indicated, especially when deficiencies are noted.

B. Corticosteroids: Several studies have shown that methylprednisolone, 32 mg/d for 1 month, is beneficial in patients with alcoholic hepatitis and either encephalopathy or greatly elevated bilirubin concentrations and prolonged prothrombin times (specifically, when the difference between the patient's prothrombin time minus the control prothrombin time times 4.6 plus the total bilirubin in mg/dL is > 32).

Prognosis

A. Short-Term: When the prothrombin time is short enough to permit performance of liver biopsy without risk (< 3 seconds above control), the 1-year mortality rate is 7.1%, rising to 18% if there is progressive prolongation of the prothrombin time during hospitalization. Individuals in whom the prothrombin time is so prolonged that liver biopsy cannot be attempted have a 42% mortality rate at 1 year. Other unfavorable prognostic factors are a serum bilirubin greater than 10 mg/dL, hepatic encephalopathy, and azotemia.

B. Long-Term: In the USA, the 3-year mortality rate of persons who recover from acute alcoholic hepatitis is ten times greater than that of control individuals of comparable age. Histologically severe disease is associated with continued excessive mortality rates after 3 years, whereas the death rate is not increased after the same period in those whose liver biopsies show only mild alcoholic hepatitis. Complications of portal hypertension (ascites, varices) following recovery from acute alcoholic hepatitis also suggest a poor long-term prognosis.

The most important prognostic consideration is the indisputable fact that continued excessive drinking is associated with reduction of life expectancy in these individuals. The prognosis is indeed poor if the patient is unable to abstain from drinking.

Lieber CS: Alcohol and the liver: 1994 update. Gastroenterology 1994;106:1085. (State-of-the-art review.)

Lumeng L, Crabb DW: Genetic aspects and risk factors in alcoholism and alcoholic liver disease. Gastroenterology 1994;107:572. (Reviews compelling evidence for a genetic predisposition to alcoholism and possibly alcoholic liver disease.)

Mathurin P: Survival and prognostic factors in patients with severe alcoholic hepatitis treated with prednisolone. Gastroenterology 1996;110:1847. (One of several studies showing improved short-term mortality in patients with severe alcoholic hepatitis treated with cortico-steroids; the benefit was especially evident in a subgroup with an elevated blood polymorphonuclear neutrophil count and a neutrophilic infiltrate on liver biopsy.)

Sherlock S: Alcoholic liver disease. Lancet 1995;345:227. (Terse overview.)

DRUG- & TOXIN-INDUCED LIVER DISEASE

The continuing synthesis, testing, and introduction of new drugs into clinical practice has resulted in an increase in toxic reactions of many types. Many widely used therapeutic agents may cause hepatic injury. The diagnosis of drug-induced liver injury is not always easy. Drug-induced liver disease can mimic viral hepatitis or biliary tract obstruction. In any patient with liver disease, the clinician must inquire carefully about the use of potentially hepatotoxic drugs or exposure to hepatotoxins. Drug toxicity may be categorized on the basis of pathogenesis or histologic appearance.

Direct Hepatotoxic Group

The liver lesion caused by this group of drugs is characterized by (1) dose-related severity, (2) a latent period following exposure, and (3) susceptibility in all individuals. Examples include acetaminophen, alcohol, carbon tetrachloride, chloroform, heavy metals, mercaptopurine, phosphorus, tetracyclines, valproic acid, and vitamin A.

Idiosyncratic Reactions

Reactions of this type are sporadic, not related to dose, and occasionally associated with features suggesting an allergic reaction, such as fever and eosinophilia. In some cases, toxicity results directly from a metabolite that is produced only in certain individuals on a genetic basis. Examples include amiodarone, aspirin, carbamazepine, chloramphenicol, diclofenac, halothane, isoniazid, ketoconazole, methyldopa, oxacillin, phenylbutazone, phenytoin, pyrazinamide, quinidine, and streptomycin.

Cholestatic Reactions

There are two general categories that differ in clinical presentation and histopathologic features. These reactions are dose-dependent, but marked differences in individual susceptibility exist:

A. Noninflammatory: Probable direct effect of agent on bile secretory mechanisms: azathioprine, estrogens, or anabolic steroids containing an alkyl or ethinyl group at carbon 17, mercaptopurine, methyltestosterone.

B. Inflammatory: Inflammation of portal areas, with allergic features, eg, eosinophilia: amoxicillin-clavulanic acid, chlorothiazide, chlorpromazine, chlorpropamide, erythromycin, penicillamine, prochlorperazine, sulfadiazine, thiouracils.

Chronic Hepatitis

Histologically and in some cases clinically indistinguishable from autoimmune hepatitis: aspirin, isoniazid, methyldopa, nitrofurantoin, sulfonamides.

Other Reactions

A. Fatty Liver:

1. Large fatty inclusions–Alcohol, amiodarone, corticosteroids, methotrexate.

2. Small cytoplasmic droplets–Tetracyclines, valproic acid.

B. Granulomas: Allopurinol, quinidine, quinine, phenylbutazone, phenytoin.

C. Fibrosis and Cirrhosis: Methotrexate.

D. Peliosis Hepatis (Blood-Filled Cavities): Anabolic steroids, azathioprine, oral contraceptive steroids.

E. Neoplasms: Oral contraceptive steroids, estrogens (hepatic adenoma but not focal nodular hyperplasia); vinyl chloride (angiosarcoma).

De Vriese AS et al: Carbamazepine hypersensitivity syndrome: Report of 4 cases and review of the literature. Medicine 1995;74:144. (Fever and lymphadenopathy are invariable, eosinophilia is common, and fulminant hepatitis can occur.)

García Rodriquez LA et al: Acute liver injury associated with nonsteroidal anti-inflammatory drugs and the role of risk factors. Arch Intern Med 1994;154:311. (This study from England found a low rate of hepatotoxicity from NSAIDs and no fatal cases.)

Kowalski TE et al: Vitamin A hepatotoxicity: A cautionary note regarding 25,000 IU supplements. Am J Med 1994;97:523. (Toxicity may result from massive doses or daily doses as low as 25,000 IU taken for an extended period.)

Lee WM: Drug-induced hepatotoxicity. N Engl J Med 1995;333:1118. (Elegant review.)

Zimmerman HJ, Maddrey WC: Acetaminophen (paracetamol) hepatotoxicity with regular intake of alcohol: Analysis of instances of therapeutic misadventure. Hepatology 1995;22:767. (In some cases, hepatotoxicity occurred in alcoholics taking less than 4 g/d of acetaminophen, the recommended safe upper dose.)

FATTY LIVER & NONALCOHOLIC STEATOHEPATITIS

It was formerly believed that malnutrition rather than ethanol was responsible for hepatic steatosis (fatty liver) in the alcoholic. It is now clear, however, that ethanol is hepatotoxic in the absence of malnutrition. Nevertheless, inadequate diets—specifically, those deficient in choline, methionine, and dietary protein—can contribute to liver damage caused by ethanol.

Other nonalcoholic causes of steatosis are obesity

(the commonest cause), starvation, diabetes mellitus, corticosteroids, poisons (carbon tetrachloride and yellow phosphorus), endocrinopathies such as Cushing's syndrome, hyperlipidemia, and total parenteral nutrition. In addition to macrovesicular steatosis, histologic features may include focal infiltration by polymorphonuclear neutrophils and Mallory's hyalin, a picture indistinguishable from that of alcoholic hepatitis and referred to as nonalcoholic steatohepatitis. In many cases, risk factors such as obesity or diabetes are absent.

Microvesicular steatosis is seen with Reye's syndrome, valproic acid toxicity, high-dose tetracycline, or acute fatty liver of pregnancy and may result in fulminant hepatic failure.

There are apparently at least five factors, acting in varying combinations, that are responsible for the accumulation of fat in the liver: (1) increased mobilization of fatty acids from peripheral adipose depots; (2) decreased utilization or oxidation of fatty acids by the liver; (3) increased hepatic fatty acid synthesis; (4) increased esterification of fatty acids into triglycerides; and (5) decreased secretion or liberation of fat from the liver. Some women in whom fatty liver of pregnancy develops have been found to have a defect in fatty acid oxidation due to reduced long-chain 3-hydroxyacyl-CoA dehydrogenase activity.

Liver function studies may show mildly elevated aminotransferase and alkaline phosphatase levels. Macrovascular steatosis may be readily demonstrated on MRI. Percutaneous liver biopsy is diagnostic but seldom needed.

Treatment consists of removing or modifying the offending factor. The benefit of weight loss in obese patients is inconsistent. Ursodeoxycholic acid, 13–15 mg/kg/d, may improve liver function test results, but the benefit of this agent on liver histology requires further study. Recent experience suggests that hepatic steatosis due to total parenteral nutrition may be ameliorated—and perhaps prevented—with supplemental choline.

Prognosis depends on the underlying condition.

Bacon BR et al: Nonalcoholic steatohepatitis: An expanded clinical entity. Gastroenterology 1994;107:1103. (Of 33 patients, 14 were neither diabetic nor obese.)

Knox TA, Olans LB: Liver disease in pregnancy. N Engl J Med 1996;335:569. (Includes a discussion of acute fatty liver of pregnancy.)

Reyes H et al:Acute fatty liver of pregnancy: A clinical study of 12 episodes in 11 patients. Gut 1994;35:101. (Maternal prognosis is excellent with early recognition and delivery, but fetal mortality remains high.)

Sheth SG et al: Nonalcoholic steatohepatitis. Ann Intern Med 1997;126:137. (Reviews pathogenesis, clinical features, diagnosis, and management.)

Teli MR et al: The natural history of nonalcoholic fatty liver: A follow-up study. Hepatology 1995;22:1714. (The condition is benign in the absence of associated hepatic inflammation or fibrosis.)

CIRRHOSIS

Cirrhosis is the end result of hepatocellular injury that leads to both fibrosis and nodular regeneration throughout the liver. Cirrhosis is a serious and irreversible disease and is the eleventh leading cause of death in the USA, with an age-adjusted death rate of 9.2 per 100,000 per year, over 45% of cases alcohol-related. The clinical features of cirrhosis result from hepatic cell dysfunction, portosystemic shunting, and portal hypertension.

The most common histologic classification divides cirrhosis into micronodular, macronodular, and mixed forms. These are descriptive terms rather than separate diseases, and each form may be seen in the same patient at different stages of the disease.

(1) In micronodular cirrhosis, the regenerating nodules are no larger than the original lobules, ie, approximately 1 mm in diameter or less.

(2) Macronodular cirrhosis is characterized by larger nodules, which can measure several centimeters in diameter and may contain central veins. This form corresponds more or less to postnecrotic (posthepatitic) cirrhosis but does not necessarily follow episodes of massive necrosis and stromal collapse.

(3) Mixed macro- and micronodular cirrhosis signifies that the features of cirrhosis are variable.

There is a limited interrelationship among the histologic form of cirrhosis, the etiology, and the prognosis. Alcoholics who continue to drink tend to have micronodular cirrhosis, and the presence of fatty micronodular cirrhosis is strongly suggestive of chronic alcoholism. Furthermore, there is a higher incidence of hepatocellular carcinoma in macronodular than in micronodular cirrhosis, perhaps because of increased regenerative activity in the liver in macronodular cirrhosis.

Clinical Findings

A. Symptoms and Signs: Micronodular (Laennec's) cirrhosis may cause no symptoms for long periods. The onset of symptoms may be insidious or, less often, abrupt. Weakness, fatigability, muscle cramps, and weight loss are common. In advanced cirrhosis, anorexia is usually present and may be extreme, with associated nausea and occasional vomiting. Abdominal pain may be present and is related either to hepatic enlargement and stretching of Glisson's capsule or to the presence of ascites. Menstrual abnormalities (usually amenorrhea), impotence, loss of libido, sterility, and painfully enlarged breasts in men may occur. Hematemesis is the presenting symptom in 15–25%.

In 70% of cases, the liver is enlarged, palpable, and firm if not hard and has a blunt or nodular edge; the left lobe may predominate. Skin manifestations consist of spider nevi (usually only on the upper half of the body), palmar erythema (mottled redness of the thenar and hypothenar eminences), and evidence of vitamin deficiencies (glossitis and cheilosis). Weight loss, wasting, and the appearance of chronic illness are present. Jaundice—usually not an initial sign—is mild at first, increasing in severity during the later stages of the disease. Ascites, pleural effusions, peripheral edema, and ecchymotic lesions are late findings. Encephalopathy characterized by day-night reversal, asterixis, tremor, dysarthrias, delirium, drowsiness, and ultimately coma also occur late except when precipitated by an acute hepatocellular insult or an episode of gastrointestinal bleeding. Fever may be present in 35% on presentation and usually reflects associated alcoholic hepatitis, spontaneous bacterial peritonitis, cholangitis, or some other intercurrent event. Clinical splenomegaly is present in 35–50% of cases. The superficial veins of the abdomen and thorax may be dilated, reflecting the intrahepatic obstruction to portal blood flow, as do rectal varices.

B. Laboratory Findings: Laboratory abnormalities are either absent or minimal in latent or quiescent cirrhosis. Anemia, a frequent finding, is often macrocytic; causes include suppression of erythropoiesis by alcohol as well as folate deficiency, hemolysis, hypersplenism, and insidious or overt blood loss from the gastrointestinal tract. The white blood cell count may be low, elevated, or normal, reflecting hypersplenism or infection; thrombocytopenia may be secondary to alcoholic marrow suppression, sepsis, folate deficiency, or splenic sequestration. Coagulation abnormalities may result from failure of synthesis of clotting constituents by the liver.

Blood chemical studies reflect hepatocellular injury and dysfunction, manifested by modest elevations of AST and alkaline phosphatase and progressive elevation of the bilirubin. Serum albumin is low; gamma globulin is increased and may be as high as in autoimmune hepatitis.

Liver biopsy may show inactive cirrhosis (fibrosis with regenerative nodules) with no specific features to suggest the underlying cause. Alternatively, there may be additional features of alcoholic liver disease, chronic hepatitis, or other specific causes of cirrhosis.

C. Imaging: Plain films of the abdomen may reveal hepatic or splenic enlargement. Barium studies of the upper gastrointestinal tract may reveal the presence of esophageal or gastric varices, though endoscopy is more sensitive. Ultrasound is helpful for assessing liver size and detecting ascites or hepatic nodules, including small hepatocellular carcinomas. Together with Doppler studies, ultrasound is used to evaluate patency of the splenic, portal, and hepatic veins. Hepatic nodules may be characterized further by CT scan with intravenous bolus contrast injection or MRI along with serum alpha-fetoprotein levels. Nodules suspicious for malignancy may be biopsied under ultrasound or CT guidance.

D. Special Examinations: Esophagogastros-

copy demonstrates or confirms the presence of varices and detects specific causes of bleeding in the esophagus, stomach, and proximal duodenum. In some centers, liver biopsy is performed by laparoscopy, which may be helpful in judging the type of cirrhosis. In selected cases, wedged hepatic vein pressure measurement may be needed to establish the presence and cause of portal hypertension.

Differential Diagnosis

Determining the cause of cirrhosis is important both for prognostic and, potentially, therapeutic reasons. After alcohol, the most common causes of cirrhosis are chronic hepatitis B and C. Hemochromatosis may be associated with "bronzing" of the skin, arthritis, heart failure, and diabetes mellitus; greater than 50% saturation of serum transferrin or serum ferritin level above the upper limit of normal, and special staining for iron and quantitation of the iron on liver biopsy are required to confirm the diagnosis. Other metabolic diseases that may lead to cirrhosis include Wilson's disease and α_1-antiprotease (α_1-antitrypsin) deficiency. Primary biliary cirrhosis occurs more frequently in women and is associated with pruritus, significant elevation of alkaline phosphatase, elevated immunoglobulin (IgM) and cholesterol levels, and antimitochondrial antibodies. Secondary biliary cirrhosis may result from chronic biliary obstruction due to a stone, stricture, or neoplasm and is not associated with antimitochondrial antibody. Congestive heart failure and constrictive pericarditis may lead to hepatic fibrosis ("cardiac cirrhosis") complicated by ascites and may be mistaken for cirrhosis.

Complications

Upper gastrointestinal tract bleeding may occur from varices, portal hypertensive gastropathy, or gastroduodenal ulcer (see Chapter 14). Hemorrhage may be massive, resulting in fatal exsanguination or portosystemic encephalopathy. Varices may also result from portal vein thrombosis. Liver failure may be precipitated by alcoholism, surgery, and infection. Carcinoma of the liver occurs more frequently in patients with cirrhosis but is uncommon in the USA. Hepatic Kupffer cell (reticuloendothelial) dysfunction and decreased opsonic activity lead to an increased risk of systemic infection. Cardiomyopathy may result from alcohol abuse, impairment of cardiac β-adrenergic receptors, and altered hemodynamics due to portal hypertension.

Treatment

A. General Measures: The most important principle of treatment is abstinence from alcohol. The diet should be palatable, with adequate calories and protein (75–100 g/d) and, if there is fluid retention, sodium restriction. In the presence of hepatic encephalopathy, precoma or coma, protein intake should be reduced to 60 g/d. Vitamin supplementation is desirable.

B. Complications:

1. Ascites and edema–Diagnostic paracentesis is usually indicated. Abdominal paracentesis is rarely associated with serious complications such as bleeding, infection, or bowel perforation even in patients with severe coagulopathy. In addition to a cell count and culture, the ascitic albumin level should be determined; a serum-ascites albumin gradient (serum albumin minus ascitic albumin) > 1.1 suggests portal hypertension (Table 15–7). An elevated ascitic adenosine deaminase level is suggestive of tuberculous peritonitis, but the sensitivity of the test is reduced in patients with portal hypertension.

Ascites in patients with cirrhosis is thought to result from portal hypertension (increased hydrostatic pressure); hypoalbuminemia (decreased oncotic pressure); peripheral vasodilation, perhaps mediated by endotoxin-induced release of nitric oxide, with resulting increases in renin and angiotensin levels and sodium retention by the kidneys; impaired liver inactivation of aldosterone; and increased aldosterone secretion secondary to increased renin production. Free water excretion is also impaired in cirrhosis, and hyponatremia may develop.

In all patients with cirrhotic ascites, dietary sodium intake may initially be restricted to 400–800 mg/d; the intake of sodium may be liberalized slightly after diuresis ensues. Restriction of fluid intake (800–1000 mL/d) is required for patients with hyponatremia (serum sodium < 125 meq/L). In some patients, there is a rapid diminution of ascites on bed rest and dietary sodium restriction alone. In individuals with severe fluid retention or those who are considered to have "intractable" ascites, the urinary excretion of sodium is usually less than 10 meq/L.

a. Diuretics–Spironolactone should be used in patients who do not respond to salt restriction alone. After starting with 100 mg daily and monitoring the aldosterone antagonist effect, reflected by an increase in the urinary sodium concentration, the dose may be increased by 100 mg every 3 days (up to a maximal conventional single daily dose of 400 mg/d, though higher doses have been used) until diuresis is achieved, typically preceded by a rise in the urinary sodium concentration. Monitoring for hyperkalemia is important. In patients who cannot tolerate spironolactone because of side effects such as painful gynecomastia, amiloride, another potassium-sparing diuretic, may be used in a dose of 5–10 mg daily. Diuresis may be augmented by the addition of a loop diuretic such as furosemide. This potent diuretic, however, will maintain its effect even with a falling glomerular filtration rate, with resultant prerenal azotemia. The dose of furosemide ranges from 40 to 240 mg/d, and the drug should be administered with careful monitoring of blood pressure, urine output, mental status, and serum electrolytes, especially potassium.

The goal of weight loss in the ascitic patient without associated peripheral edema should be no more than 1–1.5 lb/d (0.5–0.7 kg/d).

b. Large-volume paracentesis–In patients with massive ascites and respiratory compromise, ascites refractory to diuretics, or intolerable diuretic side effects, large-volume paracentesis (4–6 L) is effective; when this is done, it is safest to give intravenous albumin concomitantly at a dosage of 10 g/L of ascites fluid removed to protect the intravascular volume. Large-volume paracentesis can be repeated daily until ascites is largely resolved. The procedure is expensive (albumin is $15.00 per gram), but it may decrease the need for hospitalization. If possible, diuretics should be continued in the hope of preventing recurrent ascites.

c. Transjugular intrahepatic portosystemic shunts (TIPS)–TIPS is a promising alternative to surgical portosystemic shunting in selected cases of variceal bleeding refractory to standard therapy (eg, endoscopic band ligation or sclerotherapy) and has shown benefit in the treatment of severe refractory ascites. The technique involves insertion of an expandable metal stent between a branch of the hepatic vein and portal vein over a catheter inserted via the internal jugular vein. Complications include hepatic encephalopathy in 20% of cases, infection, shunt stenosis in up to 60%, and shunt occlusion in up to 30% of cases; the long-term patency rate is unknown. In most cases, shunt patency can be restored by balloon dilation, local thrombolysis, or placement of an additional stent. Because of the complications associated with TIPS and uncertainty about its long-term efficacy, it is currently preferred in patients who require short-term control of variceal bleeding or ascites until liver transplantation can be performed—as opposed to patients in need of definitive control of bleeding or ascites but in whom liver transplantation is not a consideration.

d. Peritoneovenous shunts–Peritoneovenous shunts have been advocated for use in patients with refractory ascites. These shunts may be effective but carry a considerable complication rate: disseminated intravascular coagulation in 65% of patients (25% symptomatic; 5% severe), bacterial infections in 4–8%, congestive heart failure in 2–4%, and variceal bleeding from sudden expansion of intravascular volume.

2. Hepatic encephalopathy–Hepatic encephalopathy is a state of disordered central nervous system function resulting from failure of the liver to detoxify noxious agents of gut origin because of hepatocellular dysfunction and portosystemic shunting. Ammonia is the most readily identified toxin but is not solely responsible for the disturbed mental status. Pathogenic factors may include enhanced sensitivity of central nervous system neurons to the inhibitory neurotransmitter γ-aminobutyric acid (GABA) or an increase in circulating levels of endogenous benzodiazepines. Bleeding into the intestinal tract may significantly increase the amount of protein in the bowel and may precipitate rapid development of encephalopathy. Other precipitants include alkalosis, potassium deficiency induced by diuretics, narcotics, hypnotics, and sedatives; medications containing ammonium or amino compounds; paracentesis with attendant hypovolemia; and hepatic or systemic infection.

Dietary protein should be withheld during acute episodes. When the patient resumes oral intake, protein is restricted to 60–80 g/d, and vegetable protein is better tolerated than meat protein. Gastrointestinal bleeding should be controlled and blood purged from the gastrointestinal tract. This can be accomplished with 120 mL of magnesium citrate by mouth or nasogastric tube every 3–4 hours until the stool is free of gross blood or with administration of lactulose.

Lactulose, a nonabsorbable synthetic disaccharide, is digested by bacteria in the colon to short-chain fatty acids, resulting in acidification of colon contents. This acidification favors the formation of ammonium ion in the $NH_4^+ \leftrightarrow NH_3 + H^+$ equation; NH_4^+ is not absorbable, whereas NH_3 is absorbable and thought to be neurotoxic. Lactulose also leads to a change in bowel flora so that less ammonia-forming organisms are present. When given orally, the initial dose of lactulose for acute hepatic encephalopathy is 30 mL three or four times daily. The dose should be titrated so that two or three soft stools per day are produced. When rectal use is indicated because of the patient's inability to take medicines orally, the dose is 300 mL of lactulose in 700 mL of saline or sorbitol as a retention enema for 30–60 minutes; it may be repeated every 4–6 hours.

The ammonia-producing intestinal flora may also be controlled with neomycin sulfate, 0.5–1 g orally every 6 or 12 hours for 5–7 days. Side effects of neomycin include diarrhea, malabsorption, superinfection, ototoxicity, and nephrotoxicity, usually only after prolonged use. Alternative antibiotics are vancomycin, 1 g orally twice daily, or metronidazole, 250 mg orally three times daily.

Avoid narcotics, tranquilizers, and sedatives metabolized or excreted by the liver. If agitation is marked, oxazepam, 10–30 mg, which is not metabolized by the liver, may be given cautiously by mouth or by nasogastric tube. The benzodiazepine competitive antagonist flumazenil is effective in a minority of patients with severe hepatic encephalopathy, but the drug is short-acting and intravenous administration is required.

3. Anemia–For iron deficiency anemia, give ferrous sulfate, 0.3 g enteric-coated tablets, one tablet three times daily after meals. Folic acid, 1 mg/d orally, is indicated in the treatment of macrocytic anemia associated with alcoholism.

4. Hemorrhagic tendency–A bleeding tendency due to hypoprothrombinemia may be treated with vitamin K preparations (eg, phytonadione, 5 mg orally or subcutaneously daily). This treatment is ineffective in the presence of severe hepatic disease when synthesis of coagulation factors is impaired. Transfusions with packed red blood cells may be necessary to replace blood loss. Correcting the prolonged prothrombin time in these situations requires large volumes of fresh frozen plasma, and the effect is transient; for that reason, plasma infusions are not indicated unless there is active bleeding or before an invasive procedure.

5. Hemorrhage from esophageal varices–See Chapter 14.

6. Spontaneous bacterial peritonitis–This occurs in cirrhotic patients with ascites. Abdominal pain, increasing ascites, fever, and progressive encephalopathy suggest the possibility, though symptoms may be mild. Paracentesis reveals an ascitic fluid with, most commonly, a total white cell count of more than 500 cells/μL with more than 250 PMNs/μL and a protein concentration of 1 g/dL or less, corresponding to decreased ascitic opsonic activity. Cultures of ascites give the highest yield—80–90% positive—when blood culture bottles are inoculated at the bedside. Common isolates are E coli and pneumococci, but anaerobes are rare. Pending culture results, if there are 250 or more PMNs/μL, intravenous antibiotic therapy should be initiated with cefotaxime, 2 g intravenously every 8–12 hours for at least 5 days. Response to therapy can be documented by a decrease in the PMN count of at least 50% on repeat paracentesis 48 hours after initiation of therapy. The mortality rate is high. In survivors, the risk of recurrent peritonitis may be decreased by long-term norfloxacin, 400 mg orally daily. In high-risk cirrhotics (eg, ascitic protein < 1 g/dL), first episodes of peritonitis may be prevented by prophylactic norfloxacin, trimethoprim-sulfamethoxazole (one double-strength tablet five times a week), or ciprofloxacin (750 mg per week).

7. Hepatorenal syndrome–Hepatorenal syndrome is characterized by azotemia, oliguria, hyponatremia, low urinary sodium, and hypotension in a patient with end-stage liver disease. It is diagnosed only when other causes of renal failure have been excluded. The cause is unknown, but the pathogenesis involves intense renal vasoconstriction, possibly because of impaired synthesis of renal vasodilators such as prostaglandin E_2; histologically, the kidneys are normal. Treatment is ineffective except for liver transplantation in selected cases, and death is commonly due to complicating infection or hemorrhage.

8. Hepatopulmonary syndrome–The hepatopulmonary syndrome is the triad of liver disease, an increased alveolar-arterial gradient while the patient is breathing room air, and intrapulmonary vascular dilations that result in a right-to-left intrapulmonary shunt. The syndrome is presumed to result from failure of the diseased liver to clear circulating pulmonary vasodilators. Patients often have dyspnea and arterial deoxygenation in the upright position and relieved by recumbency. Contrast-enhanced echocardiography is the most sensitive test for detecting the intrapulmonary shunts. Medical therapy has been disappointing, but the shunts may reverse with liver transplantation. TIPS may provide palliation in patients awaiting transplantation.

C. Liver Transplantation: Liver transplantation is indicated in selected cases of irreversible, progressive chronic liver disease, fulminant hepatic failure, and certain metabolic diseases in which the metabolic defect is in the liver. Absolute contraindications include sepsis, malignancy (except small hepatocellular carcinomas in a cirrhotic liver), advanced cardiopulmonary disease (except pulmonary arteriovenous shunting due to portal hypertension and cirrhosis), HIV infection, and lack of patient understanding. Relative contraindications include portal and mesenteric vein thrombosis, chronic hepatitis B with viral replication, and active alcohol or drug abuse. Alcoholics should be abstinent for 6 months. Liver transplantation should be considered in patients with worsening functional status, rising bilirubin, decreasing albumin, worsening coagulopathy, refractory ascites, recurrent variceal bleeding, or worsening encephalopathy. Five-year survival rates as high as 80% are now reported. Hepatocellular carcinoma, hepatitis B and C, and Budd-Chiari syndrome may recur in the transplanted liver, but other chronic liver diseases generally do not. Immunosuppression is achieved with cyclosporine or tacrolimus (FK506), corticosteroids, and azathioprine and may be complicated by infections, renal failure, and neurologic disorders as well as graft rejection, vascular occlusion, or bile leaks.

Prognosis

The prognosis in advanced cirrhosis has shown little change over the years. Factors determining survival include the patient's ability to stop the intake of alcohol as well as the Child class (Table 15–5). In established cases with severe hepatic dysfunction, only 50% survive 2 years and 35% survive 5 years. Hematemesis, jaundice, and ascites are unfavorable signs. Liver transplantation has markedly improved the outlook for patients who are acceptable candidates.

Arroyo V et al: Definition and diagnostic criteria of refractory ascites and hepatorenal syndrome in cirrhosis. Hepatology 1996;23:164. (Refractory ascites may be either unresponsive to diuretics or responsive but at the expense of diuretic-induced complications.)

Gilbert JA, Kamath PS: Spontaneous bacterial peritonitis: An update. Mayo Clin Proc 1995;70:365. (Reviews pathophysiology, diagnosis, variants, and management.)

Jalan R, Seery JP, Taylor-Robinson SD: Review article: Pathogenesis and treatment of chronic hepatic encephalopathy. Aliment Pharmacol Ther 1996;10:681. (Critical review that questions the efficacy of commonly used treatments.)

Kamath PS, McKusick MA: Transvenous intrahepatic portosystemic shunts. Gastroenterology 1996;111:1700. (While TIPS is now generally considered the treatment of choice for recurrent variceal bleeding in patients who have failed endoscopic and pharmacologic therapy, refractory ascites, hepatic hydrothorax, and Budd-Chiari syndrome are also considered possible indications.)

Lange PA, Stoller JK: The hepatopulmonary syndrome. Ann Intern Med 1995;122:521. (Reviews clinical features, pathophysiology, diagnosis, and treatment.)

Ochs A et al: The transjugular intrahepatic portosystemic stent-shunt procedure for refractory ascites. N Engl J Med 1995;332:1192. (May lead to resolution of ascites, increase in creatinine clearance, and improvement in nutritional status.)

Roberts LR, Kamath PS: Ascites and hepatorenal syndrome: pathophysiology and management. Mayo Clin Proc 1996;71:874. (Reviews diuretic management, large-volume paracentesis, and role of transjugular intrahepatic shunt.)

PRIMARY BILIARY CIRRHOSIS

Primary biliary cirrhosis is a chronic disease of the liver characterized by autoimmune destruction of intrahepatic bile ducts and cholestasis. It is insidious in onset, occurs usually in women aged 40–60, and is often detected by the chance finding of elevated alkaline phosphatase levels. The disease is progressive and may be complicated by steatorrhea, xanthomas,

Table 15–5. Child's criteria for hepatic functional reserve.[1]

	A Minimal	B Moderate	C Advanced
Serum bilirubin (mg/dL)	<2.0	2.0–3.0	>3.0
Serum albumin (g/dL)	>3.5	3.0–3.5	<3.0
Ascites	None	Easily controlled	Poorly controlled
Neurologic disorder	None	Minimal	Advanced, "coma"
Nutrition	Excellent	Good	Poor, "wasting"

[1]Modified, with permission, from Child CG III, Turcotte J: In: *The Liver and Portal Hypertension*. Child CG III (editor). Saunders, 1965.

xanthelasma, osteoporosis, osteomalacia, and portal hypertension. It may be associated with scleroderma, Sjögren's syndrome, and hypothyroidism.

Clinical Findings

A. Symptoms and Signs: Many patients are asymptomatic for years. Survival averages 10 years after symptoms appear. The onset of clinical illness is insidious and is heralded by pruritus. As the disease progresses, physical examination reveals hepatosplenomegaly. Xanthomatous lesions may occur in the skin and tendons and around the eyelids. Jaundice and signs of portal hypertension are usually late findings.

B. Laboratory Findings: Hemograms are normal early in the disease. Liver function tests reflect cholestasis with elevation of alkaline phosphatase, cholesterol (especially high-density lipoproteins), and, in later stages, bilirubin. Antimitochondrial antibodies (directed against pyruvate dehydrogenase or other 2-oxo-acid enzymes in mitochondria) are present in 95% of patients, and serum IgM levels are elevated. In advanced disease, adverse prognostic markers are older age, high serum bilirubin, edema, low albumin, prolonged prothrombin time, and variceal hemorrhage.

Differential Diagnosis

The disease must be differentiated from chronic biliary tract obstruction (stone or stricture), carcinoma of the bile ducts, primary sclerosing cholangitis, sarcoidosis, drug toxicity (eg, chlorpromazine), and in some cases chronic hepatitis. Patients with a clinical and histologic picture of primary biliary cirrhosis but no antimitochondrial antibodies are said to have "autoimmune cholangitis," which in some studies has been associated with lower serum IgM levels and a greater frequency of smooth muscle and antinuclear antibodies.

Treatment

Treatment is symptomatic. Cholestyramine (4 g) or colestipol (5 g) in water or juice three times daily may be beneficial for the pruritus. Rifampin, 150–300 mg orally twice daily, has been of benefit in some studies, but not others. Opiate antagonists (eg, naloxone, 0.2 μg/kg/min by intravenous infusion) show promise in the treatment of pruritus, but a long-acting oral opiate antagonist is not commercially available. Deficiencies of vitamins A, K, and D may occur if steatorrhea is present and may be further aggravated when cholestyramine or colestipol is administered. Replacement dosages of these vitamins must be individualized. Calcium supplementation (500 mg three times daily) may be helpful to prevent osteomalacia but is of uncertain benefit in osteoporosis. Penicillamine, corticosteroids, and azathioprine have proved to be of no benefit. Colchicine (0.6 mg twice daily), and methotrexate (15 mg/wk) have had some

reported benefit in reducing elevated serum levels of alkaline phosphatase and bilirubin. Because of its lack of toxicity, ursodeoxycholic acid (10–15 mg/kg/d in one or two doses) is preferred and has been shown to slow the progression of disease. Liver transplantation for advanced primary biliary cirrhosis is associated with a 1-year survival rate of 85–90%.

Combes B et al: A randomized, double-blind, placebo controlled trial of ursodeoxycholic acid in primary biliary cirrhosis. Hepatology 1995;22:759. (Treatment led to improved liver tests and prevented histologic and symptomatic progression in patients with an initial serum bilirubin level < 2 mg/dL.

Kaplan MM: Primary biliary cirrhosis. N Engl J Med 1996;335:1570. (Epidemiology, pathology, clinical features, diagnosis, and treatment.)

Lindor KD et al: Ursodeoxycholic acid in the treatment of primary biliary cirrhosis. Gastroenterology 1994;106: 1284. (In this trial, ursodeoxycholic acid delayed the progression of disease but did not affect symptoms, liver histology, or the need for liver transplantation compared with placebo.)

Metcalf JV et al: Natural history of early primary biliary cirrhosis. Lancet 1996;348:1399. (Most persons who are positive for antimitochondrial antibody eventually develop symptoms of primary biliary cirrhosis.)

Poupon RE et al: Ursodiol for the long-term treatment of primary biliary cirrhosis. N Engl J Med 1994;330:1342. (After 2 years, the risk of hyperbilirubinemia or clinical complications was three times higher with placebo than with ursodeoxycholic acid.)

HEMOCHROMATOSIS

Hemochromatosis is an autosomal recessive disease with linkage in many cases to HLA-A3 and HLA-B14 or HLA-A3 and HLA-B7. Recently, the genetic defect has been identified as a mutation in a newly recognized gene, HLA-H, adjacent to HLA-A on chromosome 6. The alteration leads to substitution of tyrosine for cysteine at position 282 in a region of the gene involved in interaction with β_2-microglobulin. The disorder is characterized by increased accumulation of iron as hemosiderin in the liver, pancreas, heart, adrenals, testes, pituitary, and kidneys. Eventually the patient may develop hepatic, pancreatic, and cardiac insufficiency and hypogonadism. The disease usually occurs in males and is rarely recognized before the fifth decade. The clinical disease appears in affected women 10–20 years postmenopause. Heterozygotes do not develop complications of iron overload in the absence of associated disorders such as viral hepatitis.

Clinical Findings

Clinical manifestations include arthropathy, hepatomegaly and evidence of hepatic insufficiency (late finding), occasional skin pigmentation (combination of slate gray due to iron and brown due to melanin, sometimes resulting in bronze color), cardiac enlargement with or without heart failure or conduction defects, diabetes mellitus with its complications, and impotence in the male. Bleeding from esophageal varices may occur, and in patients who develop cirrhosis, there is a 15–20% incidence of hepatocellular carcinoma. The disease should be considered in patients with a family history or otherwise unexplained mild liver test abnormalities.

Laboratory findings include mildly abnormal liver tests (AST, alkaline phosphatase), an elevated plasma iron with greater than 50% saturation of the transferrin, and an elevated serum ferritin (although a normal ferritin does not exclude the diagnosis). CT and MRI may show changes consistent with iron overload of the liver, but these techniques are not sensitive enough for screening asymptomatic persons. The liver biopsy characteristically shows extensive iron deposition in hepatocytes and usually in bile ducts, vessel walls, and supporting tissues. Diagnosis is confirmed by determination of the hepatic iron index on a liver biopsy specimen (hepatic iron content per gram of liver converted to micromoles and divided by the patient's age). In the absence of secondary iron overload due to severe hemolysis, a hepatic iron index greater than 1.9 suggests hemochromatosis.

Treatment

Early diagnosis and treatment in the precirrhotic phase of hemochromatosis is of great importance. Treatment consists initially of weekly phlebotomies of 500 mL of blood (about 250 mg of iron), continued for up to 2–3 years to achieve depletion of iron stores. This process is monitored by hematocrit and serum iron determinations. When iron store depletion is achieved, maintenance phlebotomies (every 2–4 months) are continued. The chelating agent deferoxamine, administered intravenously or subcutaneously in a dose of 40–50 mg/kg/d infused over 12 hours, can mobilize 30 mg of iron per day. The drug is indicated for patients with hemochromatosis and anemia or with secondary iron overload due to thalassemia who cannot tolerate phlebotomies. However, treatment is painful and not always practical. Complications of hemochromatosis—arthropathy, diabetes mellitus, heart disease, portal hypertension, and hypopituitarism—may require treatment.

The course of the disease is favorably altered by phlebotomy therapy. In precirrhotic patients, cirrhosis may be prevented. Cardiac conduction defects and insulin requirements improve with treatment. In patients with cirrhosis, varices may reverse, and the risk of bleeding declines. However, cirrhotic patients must be monitored for the development of hepatocellular carcinoma. Liver transplantation for advanced cirrhosis due to hemochromatosis is associated with lower survival rates than for other types of liver disease because of cardiac complications. Family members should be screened with serum iron studies and, in siblings, HLA typing; a genetic test will probably be available in the near future. Screening all white men over age 30 by measurement of the transferrin saturation has been recommended.

Baer DM et al: Hemochromatosis screening in asymptomatic ambulatory men 30 years of age and older. Am J Med 1995;98:464. (Among 3977 men screened, 40 had a transferrin saturation > 62% and eight of these had hemochromatosis, supporting the utility of screening.)

Bulaj ZJ et al: Clinical and biochemical abnormalities in people heterozygous for hemochromatosis. N Engl J Med 1996;335:1799. (Complications of iron overload are rare in heterozygotes.)

Feder JN et al: A novel MHC class I-like gene is mutated in patients with hereditary haemochromatosis. Nat Genet 1996;13:399. (Reports the discovery of the gene for this disorder.)

Niederau C et al: Long-term survival in patients with hereditary hemochromatosis. Gastroenterology 1996; 110:1107. (Early diagnosis and therapy largely prevents the adverse consequences of iron overload.)

WILSON'S DISEASE

Wilson's disease (hepatolenticular degeneration) is a rare autosomal recessive disorder that usually occurs between the first and third decades. The condition is characterized by excessive deposition of copper in the liver and brain. The genetic defect, localized to chromosome 13, has been shown to involve a copper-transporting protein in the liver.

Awareness of the entity is important, since it may masquerade as chronic hepatitis, psychiatric disorders, or neurologic disease. It is potentially reversible, and appropriate therapy will prevent neurologic and hepatic damage.

The major physiologic aberration in Wilson's disease is excessive absorption of copper from the small intestine and decreased excretion of copper by the liver, resulting in increased tissue deposition, especially in the liver, brain, cornea, and kidney. Serum ceruloplasmin, the plasma copper-carrying protein, is low. Urinary excretion of copper is high.

Clinical Findings

Wilson's disease tends to present as liver disease in adolescents and neuropsychiatric disease in young adults, but there is great variability. The diagnosis should always be considered in any child or young adult with hepatitis, splenomegaly with hypersplenism, hemolytic anemia, portal hypertension, and neurologic or psychiatric abnormalities. Wilson's disease should also be considered in persons under 40 years of age with chronic or fulminant hepatitis.

Hepatic involvement may range from elevated liver tests to cirrhosis and portal hypertension. The neurologic manifestations are related to basal ganglia dysfunction and are characterized by rigidity or parkinsonian tremor. The pathognomonic sign of the condition is the brownish or gray-green Kayser-Fleischer ring, which represents fine pigmented granular deposits in Descemet's membrane in the cornea close to the endothelial surface. The ring is usually most marked at the superior and inferior poles of the cornea. It can frequently be seen with the naked eye and almost invariably by slit lamp examination. It may be absent in patients with hepatic manifestations only but is almost invariably present in those with neuropsychiatric disease.

The diagnosis is based on demonstration of increased urinary copper excretion (> 100 µg/24 h) or low serum ceruloplasmin levels (< 20 µg/dL), and elevated hepatic copper concentration (> 100 µg/g of dry liver). Liver biopsy may show acute or chronic hepatitis or cirrhosis.

Treatment

Early treatment to remove excess copper is essential before it can produce neurologic or hepatic damage. Early in the treatment phase, restriction of dietary copper (shellfish, organ foods, and legumes are rich in copper) may be of value. Oral penicillamine (0.75–2 g/d in divided doses) is the drug of choice, making possible urinary excretion of chelated copper. Pyridoxine, 50 mg per week, is added, since penicillamine is an antimetabolite of this vitamin. If penicillamine treatment cannot be tolerated because of gastrointestinal, hypersensitivity, or autoimmune reactions, consider the use of trientine, 250–500 mg three times a day. Oral zinc acetate, 50 mg three times a day, promotes fecal copper excretion and may be used as maintenance therapy after decoppering with a chelating agent or as first-line therapy in presymptomatic or pregnant patients.

Treatment should continue indefinitely. The prognosis is good in patients who are effectively treated before liver or brain damage has occurred. Liver transplantation is indicated for fulminant hepatitis, end-stage cirrhosis, and, in selected cases, intractable neurologic disease. Family members, especially siblings, require screening with serum ceruloplasmin, liver function tests, and slit-lamp examination.

Brewer GJ: Practical recommendations and new therapies for Wilson's disease. Drugs 1995;50:240. (Discusses mechanisms and efficacy of drugs used in treatment.)

Cuthbert JA: Wilson's disease: A new gene and an animal model for an old disease. J Invest Med 1995;43:323. (Reviews discovery of gene, animal models, clinical features, diagnosis, and management.)

Ferenci P et al: An international symposium on Wilson's and Menkes' diseases. Hepatology 1996;24:952. (Emphasizes recent developments in the understanding of pathogenesis, genetics, diagnosis, and treatment.)

HEPATIC VEIN OBSTRUCTION (Budd-Chiari Syndrome)

Occlusion of the hepatic veins may occur from a variety of causes. Many cases are associated with polycythemia vera or other myeloproliferative diseases, which may be subclinical. Hepatovenous obstructions may be associated with caval webs, right-sided heart failure or constrictive pericarditis, neoplasms causing hepatic vein occlusions, paroxysmal nocturnal hemoglobinuria, use of birth control pills, and pregnancy. In some cases, an underlying predisposition to thrombosis (eg, protein C or S or antithrombin deficiency or the factor V Leiden mutation) can be identified. Some cytotoxic agents and pyrrolizidine alkaloids ("bush teas") may cause hepatic veno-occlusive disease (occlusion of terminal venules), which mimics Budd-Chiari syndrome clinically. Veno-occlusive disease, often associated with cardiopulmonary and renal failure, is common in patients who have undergone bone marrow transplantation, particularly those with pretransplant aminotransferase elevations or fever during cytoreductive therapy with cyclophosphamide, azathioprine, carmustine, busulfan, or etoposide or those receiving high-dose cytoreductive therapy or high-dose total body irradiation.

Clinical manifestations may include tender, painful hepatic enlargement; jaundice; splenomegaly; and ascites. With advanced disease, bleeding varices and hepatic coma may be evident. Hepatic imaging studies may show a prominent caudate lobe, since its venous drainage may not be occluded. Caval venogram can delineate caval webs and occluded hepatic veins. Percutaneous liver biopsy frequently shows a characteristic centrilobular congestion.

Ascites should be treated with fluid and salt restriction and diuretics. Treatable causes of Budd-Chiari syndrome should be sought. Surgical decompression (mesocaval or mesoatrial shunt) of the congested liver may be required. In some cases, placement of a transjugular intrahepatic portosystemic shunt may be feasible. Balloon angioplasty is preferred in patients with an inferior vena caval web. Liver transplantation is considered in patients with marked hepatocellular dysfunction. Patients often require lifelong anticoagulation and treatment of the underlying myeloproliferative disease.

Dilawari JB et al: Hepatic outflow obstruction (Budd-Chiari syndrome): Experience with 177 patients and review of the literature. Medicine 1994;73:21. (Classifies Budd-Chiari syndrome as acute, characterized by extensive blockage of major hepatic veins, congestive liver cell necrosis, and need for immediate portosystemic shunt; and chronic, characterized by abnormal vascular anatomy, often with a vena caval web, portal hypertension, and the possibility of a therapeutic response to interventional radiology, eg, balloon angioplasty.)

Fried MW et al: Transjugular intrahepatic portosystemic

shunt for the management of severe veno-occlusive disease following bone marrow transplantation. Hepatology 1996;24:588. (A new treatment modality for a complication that occurs in up to 50% of bone marrow transplant recipients.)

Hemming AW et al: Treatment of Budd-Chiari syndrome with portosystemic shunt or liver transplantation. Am J Surg 1996;171:176. (Portosystemic shunt may be effective even in patients with inferior vena caval compression or cirrhosis; liver transplantation is indicated for inferior vena caval occlusion or hepatic decompensation.)

THE LIVER IN HEART FAILURE

Shock liver, or ischemic hepatitis, results from an acute fall in cardiac output due, for example, to acute myocardial infarction or arrhythmia, often in the setting of passive congestion of the liver. The hallmark is a rapid and striking elevation of serum aminotransferase levels (often > 5000 units/L); elevations of serum alkaline phosphatase and bilirubin are usually slight. The mortality rate due to the underlying disease is high, but in patients who recover, the aminotransferase levels return to normal quickly, usually within 1 week.

In patients with passive congestion of the liver due to right-sided heart failure, the serum bilirubin level may be elevated, occasionally as high as 20 mg/dL, due in part to hypoxia of perivenular hepatocytes. Serum alkaline phosphatase levels are normal or slightly elevated. Hepatojugular reflux is present, and with tricuspid regurgitation the liver may be pulsatile. Ascites may be out of proportion to peripheral edema, with a high serum ascites-albumin gradient (> 1.1) and a protein content of more than 2.5 g/dL. In severe cases, signs of encephalopathy, reflecting both hepatic and cerebral anoxia, may develop.

Kamiyama T et al: Ischemic hepatitis in cirrhosis: Clinical features and prognostic implications. J Clin Gastroenterol 1996;22:126. (Suggests that ischemic hepatitis may complicate variceal hemorrhage in patients with cirrhosis more commonly than appreciated.)

Mohacsi P, Meier B: Hypoxic hepatitis in patients with cardiac failure. J Hepatol 1994; 21:693. (Shock liver is the most frequent cause of a serum AST > 1000 units/L in hospitalized patients.)

NONCIRRHOTIC PORTAL HYPERTENSION

Noncirrhotic portal hypertension must be considered in the differential diagnosis of splenomegaly or upper gastrointestinal bleeding due to esophageal or gastric varices and normal liver function. This syndrome may be due to portal vein obstruction, splenic vein obstruction (presenting as gastric varices without esophageal varices), schistosomiasis, noncirrhotic intrahepatic portal sclerosis, or arterial-portal vein fistula. Other than for splenomegaly, the physi-

cal findings are not remarkable. Endoscopy shows esophageal or gastric varices. The liver tests are usually normal, but there may be findings of hypersplenism. Angiography of the portal system is confirmatory, as is needle biopsy of the liver, particularly for schistosomiasis and noncirrhotic intrahepatic portal sclerosis.

If splenic vein thrombosis is the cause, splenectomy is curative. In other cases, sclerotherapy or band ligation is initiated for variceal bleeding, and portosystemic shunting is reserved for failures of endoscopic therapy.

Bernard P-H et al: Progression from idiopathic portal hypertension to incomplete septal cirrhosis with liver failure requiring liver transplantation. J Hepatol 1995; 22:495. (Rare occurrence.)

Orloff M et al: Long-term results of radical esophagogastrectomy for bleeding varices due to unshuntable extrahepatic portal hypertension. Am J Surg 1994;167:96. (May be only option in failures of endoscopic therapy when major veins leading to portal vein are occluded and when devascularization procedure has failed.)

HEPATIC ABSCESS

1. AMEBIC LIVER ABSCESS

Amebic liver abscess is most common in tropical and subtropical regions. In the USA, it is typically seen in young Hispanic adults. The presentation is with right upper quadrant pain, often with associated fever, and right pleuritic chest pain—on average, of 2 weeks' duration. Associated dysentery is uncommon, but 20% of patients will have had a recent diarrheal episode. Usually there is a history of travel to endemic areas.

Clinical Findings

Physical examination discloses fever in most cases, toxic appearance of varying degree, and a tender palpable liver with marked "punch" tenderness. Right lung base abnormalities and localized intercostal tenderness are common.

Laboratory findings usually consist of mild to moderate anemia, moderate leukocytosis with a shift to the left, and slightly abnormal liver tests. Serologic testing, most commonly with indirect hemagglutination tests for *Entamoeba histolytica,* are positive in 95% of patients but may be nondiagnostic on presentation, with a marked rise in titer over the subsequent 3–4 weeks.

An elevated right hemidiaphragm is frequently seen on chest radiograph. Ultrasonography, CT scan, or MRI is helpful in delineating the location and number of abscesses. Most are in the right lobe.

Treatment

Metronidazole, 750 mg three times per day orally

for 5–10 days, is the drug of choice. Occasionally, a second course is necessary. In the acutely toxic patient, percutaneous needle aspiration and decompression of the abscess bring immediate relief and allow for demonstration of the ameba in over 50% of cases; if the patient is not acutely toxic, aspiration is unnecessary. Following completion of treatment for the abscess, the patient needs to take iodoquinol, 650 mg three times a day after meals for 20 days (for adults), to eradicate the intestinal cyst phase of amebiasis.

Fever usually subsides rapidly once treatment is initiated. The hepatic defect may persist on imaging studies for over 6 months.

Complications include rupture of the abscess transcutaneously, into the peritoneal cavity, pleural space, lungs, or pericardium, with a significant associated mortality rate if undiagnosed. Rarely, distal embolization has been reported.

Ravdin JI: Amebiasis. Clin Infect Dis 1995;20:1453. (Comprehensive review.)

2. PYOGENIC ABSCESS

The liver can be invaded by bacteria via (1) the portal vein (pyelephlebitis); (2) the common duct (ascending cholangitis); (3) the hepatic artery, secondary to bacteremia; (4) direct extension from an infectious process; and (5) traumatic implantation of bacteria through the abdominal wall.

Ascending cholangitis resulting from biliary obstruction due to a stone, stricture, or neoplasm is the most common identifiable cause of hepatic abscess in the USA. In 10% of cases, liver abscess is secondary to appendicitis or diverticulitis. Ten to 40 percent of abscesses have no demonstrable cause and are classified as cryptogenic. The most frequently encountered organisms are *Escherichia coli, Proteus vulgaris, Enterobacter aerogenes,* and multiple anaerobic species. Hepatic candidiasis is seen in immunocompromised patients.

Clinical Findings

The presentation is often insidious. Fever is almost always present and may antedate other symptoms or signs. Pain may be a prominent complaint and is localized to the right hypochondrium or epigastric area. Jaundice, tenderness in the right upper abdomen, and either steady or swinging fever are the chief physical findings.

Laboratory examination reveals leukocytosis with a shift to the left. Liver function studies are nonspecifically abnormal. Chest roentgenograms usually reveal elevation of the diaphragm if the abscess is on the right side. Ultrasound, CT, or MRI may reveal the presence of intrahepatic defects. On MRI, characteristic findings include high signal intensity on T2-weighted images and rim enhancement. Hepatic can-

didiasis is seen usually in the setting of systemic candidiasis, and on CT scan the characteristic appearance is that of multiple "bulls-eyes," but imaging studies may be negative in neutropenic patients.

Treatment

Treatment should consist of antimicrobial agents (a third-generation cephalosporin and metronidazole) that are effective against coliform organisms and anaerobes. If the abscess is at least 5 cm in diameter or the response to antibiotic therapy is not rapid, catheter or surgical drainage should be undertaken. The mortality rate is still substantial (10–25%) and is highest in patients with underlying biliary malignancy or severe multiorgan dysfunction. Hepatic candidiasis often responds to intravenous amphotericin B (total dose of 2–9 g).

Chu K-M et al: Pyogenic liver abscess: An audit of experience over the past decade. Arch Surg 1996;131:148. (Mortality rate in a referral center is still as high as 18%.)

Seeto RK, Rockey DC: Pyogenic liver abscess: Changes in etiology, management, and outcome. Medicine 1996; 75:99. (Biliary tract disease is the most common identifiable cause of pyogenic liver abscess, but a substantial number are cryptogenic. Percutaneous catheter drainage and antibiotics are the treatment of choice.)

NEOPLASMS OF THE LIVER

1. HEPATOCELLULAR CARCINOMA

Neoplasms of the liver that arise from parenchymal cells are called hepatocellular carcinomas; those that originate in the ductular cells are called cholangiocarcinomas.

Hepatocellular carcinomas are associated with cirrhosis in general and hepatitis B or C in particular. In Africa and most of Asia, hepatitis B is of major etiologic significance, whereas in western countries and Japan hepatitis C and alcoholic cirrhosis are the most common causes. Other associations include hemochromatosis, aflatoxin exposure (associated with mutation of the *p53* gene), α_1-antiprotease (α_1-antitrypsin) deficiency, and tyrosinemia. The fibrolamellar variant of hepatocellular carcinoma occurs in young women and is characterized by a distinctive histologic picture, absence of risk factors, and an indolent course.

Histologically, hepatocellular carcinoma is made up of cords or sheets of cells that roughly resemble the hepatic parenchyma. Blood vessels such as portal or hepatic veins are commonly involved by tumor.

The presence of a hepatocellular carcinoma may be unsuspected until there is deterioration in the condition of a cirrhotic patient who was formerly stable. Cachexia, weakness, and weight loss are associated symptoms. The sudden appearance of ascites, which may be bloody, suggests portal or hepatic vein thrombosis by tumor or bleeding from the necrotic tumor.

Physical examination may show tender enlargement of the liver, with an occasionally palpable mass. In Africa, young patients typically present with a rapidly expanding abdominal mass. Auscultation may reveal a bruit over the tumor or a friction rub when the process has extended to the surface of the liver.

Laboratory tests may reveal leukocytosis, as opposed to the leukopenia that is frequently encountered in cirrhotic patients. A normal or elevated hematocrit may be found, owing to elaboration of erythropoietin by the tumor. Sudden and sustained elevation of the serum alkaline phosphatase in a patient who was formerly stable is a common finding. Hepatitis B surface antigen is present in a majority of cases in endemic areas, whereas in the United States anti-HCV is found in up to 40% of cases. Alpha-fetoprotein levels are elevated in up to 60% of patients with hepatocellular carcinoma. Cytologic study of ascitic fluid rarely reveals malignant cells.

Arteriographic findings are characteristic, revealing a tumor "blush" that reflects the highly vascular nature of the tumor. Almost as helpful is CT scanning when done with and without intravenous contrast or MRI to characterize the location and vascularity of the tumor. Liver biopsy is diagnostic. Staging in the TNM classification includes the following definitions: T0: no evidence of primary tumor; T1: solitary tumor ≤ 2.0; T2: solitary tumor ≤ 2.0 cm with vascular invasion or > 2.0 cm without vascular invasion or ≤ 2.0 cm and multiple in one lobe; T3: solitary tumor > 2.0 cm with vascular invasion or ≤ 2.0 cm and multiple in one lobe with vascular invasion or multiple in one lobe with any > 2.0 cm with or without vascular invasion; and T4: multiple tumors in more than one lobe or involving a major branch of the portal or hepatic veins.

Attempts at surgical resection are usually fruitless if concomitant cirrhosis is present and if the tumor is multifocal. Surgical resection of solitary hepatocellular carcinomas may result in cure if the unaffected liver is normal. Overall 5-year survival rates are up to 56% for patients with localized resectable disease (T1, T2, T3, selected T4; N0; M0) but virtually nil for those with localized unresectable or advanced disease. Liver transplantation may be appropriate for small unresectable tumors in a patient with advanced cirrhosis, with reported 5-year survival rates of up to 75%. Chemotherapy has not been shown to prolong life, but chemoembolization via the hepatic artery may be palliative. Injection of small tumors (< 3 cm) with absolute ethanol may prolong survival.

In the chronic HBV or HCV carrier, surveillance for the development of hepatocellular carcinoma should be considered and has been practiced in areas endemic for HBV with regular (eg, every 6 months) alpha-fetoprotein testing and ultrasonography. In the USA, experience with surveillance has been sporadic and of uncertain benefit.

2. MISCELLANEOUS LIVER NEOPLASMS

Benign and malignant neoplasms have been encountered in women taking oral contraceptives. Two distinct benign entities with characteristic clinical, radiologic, and histopathologic features have been described. **Focal nodular hyperplasia** occurs at all ages but is questionably related to oral contraceptives. It is often asymptomatic and hypervascular on CT scan or MRI. Microscopically, focal nodular hyperplasia consists of hyperplastic units of hepatocytes with a centrally placed "stellate" scar containing proliferating bile ducts. **Liver cell adenoma** occurs most commonly in the third and fourth decades of life; the clinical presentation is often one of acute abdominal pain due to necrosis of the tumor with hemorrhage. The tumor is hypovascular and reveals a cold defect on liver scan. Grossly, the cut surface appears structureless. As seen microscopically, the liver cell adenoma consists of sheets of hepatocytes without portal tracts or central veins. The only physical finding in focal nodular hyperplasia or liver cell adenoma is a palpable abdominal mass in some cases. Liver function is usually normal.

Treatment of focal nodular hyperplasia is resection only in the symptomatic patient. The prognosis is excellent. Liver cell adenoma often undergoes necrosis and rupture; resection is advised. Regression of benign hepatic tumors may follow cessation of oral contraceptives.

The most common benign neoplasm of the liver is the **cavernous hemangioma,** often an incidental finding on CT scan. This lesion must be differentiated from other space-occupying intrahepatic lesions, usually by MRI. Fine-needle biopsy may be necessary to differentiate these lesions and does not appear to carry an increased risk. Cavernous hemangiomas rarely require treatment.

Cherqui D et al: Management of focal nodular hyperplasia and hepatocellular adenoma in young women: A series of 41 patients with clinical, radiological, and pathological correlations. Hepatology 1995;22:1674. (Focal nodular hyperplasia is more common than adenoma and can be diagnosed by MRI in 70% of cases, obviating the need for surgical biopsy.)

International Working Party: Terminology of nodular hepatocellular lesions. Hepatology 1995;22:983. (Definitions and diagnostic criteria.)

Mazzaferro V et al: Liver transplantation for the treatment of small hepatocellular carcinomas in patients with cirrhosis. N Engl J Med 1996;334:693. (The actuarial 4-year survival rate was 75% for 48 patients with otherwise unresectable tumors.)

Sarasin F et al: Cost-effectiveness of screening for detection of small hepatocellular carcinoma in Western patients with Child-Pugh class A cirrhosis. Am J Med 1996;171:422. (Only for patients with very well compensated cirrhosis and a projected survival rate above 80% at 5 years was screening predicted to be cost-effective.)

DISEASES OF THE BILIARY TRACT

CHOLELITHIASIS
(Gallstones)

Gallstones are more common in women than in men and increase in incidence in both sexes and all races with aging. In the USA, over 10% of men and 20% of women have gallstones by age 65; the total exceeds 20 million people. Although gallstones are less common in black people, cholelithiasis attributable to hemolysis occurs in over a third of individuals with sickle cell anemia. Native Americans of both the Northern and Southern Hemispheres have a high rate of cholesterol cholelithiasis, probably because of a genetic predisposition. As many as 75% of Pima women over the age of 25 years have cholelithiasis. Obesity is a risk factor for gallstones, especially in women, and rapid weight loss, particularly in obese persons, increases the risk of symptomatic gallstone formation. The incidence of gallstones is also high in individuals with Crohn's disease; approximately one-third of individuals with inflammatory involvement of the terminal ileum have gallstones due to disruption of bile salt resorption that results in decreased solubility of the bile. The incidence of cholelithiasis is also increased in patients with diabetes mellitus and in those with cirrhosis. Pregnancy is associated with an increased risk of gallstones and of symptomatic gallbladder disease.

Pathogenesis of Gallstones

Gallstones are classified according to chemical composition: stones containing predominantly cholesterol and those containing predominantly calcium bilirubinate. The latter comprise less than 20% of the stones found in Europe or the USA but 30–40% of stones found in Japan.

Three compounds comprise 80–95% of the total solids dissolved in bile: conjugated bile salts, lecithin, and cholesterol. Cholesterol is a neutral sterol, and lecithin is a phospholipid; both are almost completely insoluble in water. However, bile salts in combination with lecithin are able to form multimolecular aggregates (and micelles) or vesicles that solubilize cholesterol in an aqueous solution. Precipitation of cholesterol microcrystals may come about

because of increased biliary secretion of cholesterol, defective formation of vesicles, an excess of factors promoting the nucleation of cholesterol crystals (or deficiency of antinucleating factors), or delayed emptying of the gallbladder.

Presentation
(Table 15–6)

Cholelithiasis is frequently asymptomatic and is discovered fortuitously in the course of routine radiographic study, operation, or autopsy. There is generally no need for prophylactic cholecystectomy in an asymptomatic person. Ultimately, symptoms (biliary colic) develop in 10–25% of patients by 10 years. "Symptomatic" cholelithiasis usually means characteristic right upper quadrant discomfort or pain (biliary colic). Other sources of the symptoms should be considered. Treatment is usually indicated for symptomatic cholelithiasis.

Treatment

Laparoscopic cholecystectomy has become the treatment of choice for symptomatic gallbladder disease. The minimal trauma to the abdominal wall makes it possible for patients to go home within 2 days after the procedure and to return to work within 7 days (instead of weeks for those undergoing standard open cholecystectomy). This procedure is suitable in most patients, including those with acute cholecystitis. If problems are encountered, the surgery can be converted to a conventional open cholecystectomy. Bile duct injuries occur in 0.1% of cases done by experienced surgeons.

Persistence of symptoms after removal of the gallbladder (postcholecystectomy syndrome) implies either mistaken diagnosis, functional bowel disorder, technical error, retained or recurrent common bile duct stone, or spasm of the sphincter of Oddi (see below).

Cheno- and ursodeoxycholic acids are bile salts that when given orally for up to 2 years dissolve some cholesterol stones and may be considered in selected patients who refuse laparoscopic cholecystectomy. The dose is 7 mg/kg/d of each or 8–13 mg/kg of ursodeoxycholic acid in divided doses daily. They are most effective in patients with a functioning gallbladder, as determined by gallbladder visualization on oral cholecystography (representing not more than 15% of patients with gallstones), and multiple small "floating" gallstones. In half of patients, gallstones recur within 5 years after treatment is stopped.

Lithotripsy in combination with bile salt therapy for single radiolucent stones less than 20 mm in diameter was an option in the past but is no longer generally employed in the USA.

Gebhard RL et al: The role of gallbladder emptying in gallstone formation during diet-induced rapid weight loss. Hepatology 1996;24:544. (Stone formation is more

Table 15–6. Diseases of the biliary tract.

	Clinical Features	Laboratory Features	Diagnosis	Treatment
Gallstones	Asymptomatic	Normal	Ultrasound	None
Gallstones	Biliary colic	Normal	Ultrasound	Laparascopic cholecystectomy
Cholesterolosis of gallbladder	Usually asymptomatic	Normal	Oral cholecystography	None
Adenomyomatosis	May cause biliary colic	Normal	Oral cholecystography	Laparascopic cholecystectomy if symptomatic
Porcelain gallbladder	Usually asymptomatic, high risk of gallbladder cancer	Normal	X-ray or CT	Laparoscopic cholecystectomy
Acute cholecystitis	Epigastric or right upper quadrant pain, nausea, vomiting, fever, Murphy's sign	Leukocytosis	Ultrasound, HIDA scan	Antibiotics, laparoscopic cholecystectomy
Chronic cholecystitis	Biliary colic, constant epigastric or right upper quadrant pain, nausea	Normal	Ultrasound (stones), oral cholecystography (nonfunctioning gallbladder)	Laparoscopic cholecystectomy
Choledocholithiasis	Asymptomatic or biliary colic, jaundice, fever; gallstone pancreatitis	Cholestatic liver function tests; leukocytosis and positive blood cultures in cholangitis; elevated amylase and lipase in pancreatitis	Ultrasound (dilated ducts), ERCP	Endoscopic sphincterotomy and stone extraction; antibiotics for cholangitis

ERCP = endoscopic retrograde cholangiopancreatography; HIDA = iminodiacetic acid.

likely with severe restriction of dietary fat to 2 g/d than with moderate fat restriction of 30 g/d, which stimulates more frequent gallbladder emptying.)

Majeed AW et at: Randomised, prospective, single-blind comparison of laparoscopic versus small-incision cholecystectomy. Lancet 1996;347:989. (No difference in hospital stay or time back to work, but most surgeons still favor the laparoscopic approach.)

Tait N, Little JM: The treatment of gallstones. BMJ 1995;311:99. (Reviews epidemiology, pathogenesis, diagnosis, and treatment; the principles of treatment have not changed with the advent of laparoscopic cystectomy.)

ACUTE CHOLECYSTITIS

Essentials of Diagnosis

- Steady, severe pain and tenderness in the right hypochondrium or epigastrium.
- Nausea and vomiting.
- Fever and leukocytosis.

General Considerations

Cholecystitis is associated with gallstones in over 90% of cases. It occurs when a stone becomes impacted in the cystic duct and inflammation develops behind the obstruction. Acalculous cholecystitis should be considered when unexplained fever or right upper quadrant pain occurs within 2–4 weeks of major surgery or in a critically ill patient who has had no oral intake for a prolonged period. Primarily as a result of ischemic changes secondary to distention, gangrene may develop, resulting in perforation. Although generalized peritonitis is possible, the leak usually remains localized and forms a chronic, well-circumscribed abscess cavity. Acute cholecystitis caused by infectious agents (eg, cytomegalovirus, cryptosporidiosis, or microsporidiosis) may occur in patients with AIDS.

Clinical Findings

A. Symptoms and Signs: The acute attack is often precipitated by a large or fatty meal and is characterized by the relatively sudden appearance of severe, steady pain which is localized to the epigastrium or right hypochondrium and which in the uncomplicated case may gradually subside over a period of 12–18 hours. Vomiting occurs in about 75% of patients and in half of instances affords variable relief. Right upper quadrant abdominal tenderness is almost always present and is usually associated with muscle guarding and rebound pain. A palpable gallbladder is present in about 15% of cases. Jaundice is present in about 25% of cases and, when persistent or severe, suggests the possibility of choledocholithiasis. Fever is usually present.

B. Laboratory Findings: The white blood cell count is usually high (12,000–15,000/μL). Total serum bilirubin values of 1–4 mg/dL may be seen even in the absence of common duct obstruction. Serum aminotransferase and alkaline phosphatase are often elevated—the former as high as 300 units/mL, or even higher when associated with ascending cholangitis. Serum amylase may also be moderately elevated.

C. Imaging: Plain films of the abdomen may show radiopaque gallstones in 15% of cases. ^{99m}Tc hepatobiliary imaging (using iminodiacetic acid compounds), also known as the HIDA scan, is useful in demonstrating an obstructed cystic duct, which is the cause of acute cholecystitis in most patients. This test is reliable if the bilirubin is under 5 mg/dL (98% sensitivity and 81% specificity for acute cholecystitis). Right upper quadrant abdominal ultrasound may show the presence of gallstones but is not specific for acute cholecystitis (67% sensitivity, 82% specificity).

Differential Diagnosis

The disorders most likely to be confused with acute cholecystitis are perforated peptic ulcer, acute pancreatitis, appendicitis in a high-lying appendix, perforated colonic carcinoma or diverticulum of the hepatic flexure, liver abscess, hepatitis, and pneumonia with pleurisy on the right side. Definite localization of pain and tenderness in the right hypochondrium, with radiation around to the infrascapular area, strongly favors the diagnosis of acute cholecystitis. True cholecystitis without stones raises the question of polyarteritis nodosa (rarely).

Complications

A. Gangrene of the Gallbladder: Continuation or progression of right upper quadrant abdominal pain, tenderness, muscle guarding, fever, and leukocytosis after 24–48 hours suggests severe inflammation and possible gangrene of the gallbladder. Necrosis may occasionally develop without definite signs in the obese, diabetic, elderly, or immunosuppressed patient.

B. Cholangitis: Cholangitis classically presents with Charcot's triad, namely, fever and chills, right upper quadrant pain, and jaundice. Although 95% of patients who present with this picture will have common duct stones, only a minority of patients with acute cholecystitis have common duct stones that will present in this manner.

Treatment

Acute cholecystitis will usually subside on a conservative regimen (withholding of oral feedings, intravenous alimentation, analgesics, and antibiotics). Meperidine may be preferable to morphine for pain because of less spasm of the sphincter of Oddi. Because of the high risk of recurrent attacks, cholecystectomy should generally be performed within 2–3 days after hospitalization. If nonsurgical treatment has been elected, the patient (especially if diabetic or elderly) should be watched carefully for recurrent symptoms, evidence of gangrene of the gallbladder, or cholangitis. In high-risk patients, ultrasound-guided aspiration of the gallbladder may postpone or even avoid the need for surgery. Operation is mandatory when there is evidence of gangrene or perforation.

Barie PS, Fischer E: Acute acalculous cholecystitis. J Am Coll Surg 1995;180:232. (Reviews clinical presentation, pathogenesis, diagnosis, treatment, and complications.)

Hobbs KEF: Laparoscopic cholecystectomy. Gut 1995; 36:161. (Reviews indications, technical aspects, complications, and results.)

CYSTIC DUCT SYNDROMES

Precholecystectomy

In a small group of patients (mostly women), right upper quadrant abdominal pain occurs frequently following meals, and conventional radiographic study of the upper gastrointestinal tract and gallbladder—including cholangiography—is unremarkable. However, using cholecystokinin (CCK) as a gallbladder stimulant, contraction and evacuation of the gallbladder does not take place, as usually occurs in the 3- to 5-minute period after injection of the hormone. Instead, the gallbladder assumes a "golf ball" configuration, and biliary-type pain is reproduced. At the time of cholecystectomy, the gallbladder is often enlarged and cannot be emptied by manual compression. Anatomic and histologic examination of the operative specimen reveals obstruction of the cystic duct because of fibrotic stenosis or adhesions and kinking. Additional diagnostic considerations are ampullary spasm and biliary dyskinesia (see below).

Postcholecystectomy

Following cholecystectomy, some patients complain of continuing symptoms, ie, right upper quadrant pain, flatulence, and fatty food intolerance. The persistence of symptoms in this group of patients suggests the possibility of an incorrect diagnosis prior to cholecystectomy, eg, esophagitis, pancreatitis, radiculopathy, or functional bowel disease. It is important to rule out the possibility of choledocholithiasis or common duct stricture as a cause for persistent symptoms in the postoperative period.

Pain has been associated with dilation of the cystic duct remnant, neuroma formation in the ductal wall, foreign body granuloma, or traction on the common duct by a long cystic duct. The clinical presentation of colicky pain, chills, fever, or jaundice should suggest biliary tract disease. Biliary colic associated with elevated liver tests or amylase suggests the possibility of spasm of the ampulla of Vater. Abdominal or endoscopic ultrasonography or retrograde cholangiography may be necessary to demonstrate or exclude biliary tract disease. Biliary manometry during ERCP may be useful in documenting elevated baseline sphincter of Oddi pressures typical of sphincter dysfunction. Endoscopic sphincterotomy or surgical sphincteroplasty with common duct exploration for stones or removal of the cystic duct remnant may be necessary.

Freeman ML et al: Complications of endoscopic biliary sphincterotomy. N Engl J Med 1996;335:909. (Overall rate of complications is 9.8%—but as high as 21.7% in patients with sphincter of Oddi dysfunction.)

Ponchon T et al: Biopsies of the ampullary region in patients suspected to have sphincter of Oddi dysfunction. Gastrointest Endosc 1995;42:296. (Ampullary carcinoma was found in 4%.)

CHRONIC CHOLECYSTITIS

Chronic cholecystitis is characterized pathologically by varying degrees of chronic inflammation of the gallbladder. Calculi are usually present. In about 4–5% of cases, the villi of the gallbladder undergo polypoid enlargement due to deposition of cholesterol that may be visible to the naked eye ("strawberry gallbladder," cholesterolosis). In other instances, adenomatous hyperplasia of all or part of the gallbladder wall may be so marked as to give the appearance of a myoma (pseudotumor). Hydrops of the gallbladder results when acute cholecystitis subsides but cystic duct obstruction persists, producing distention of the gallbladder with a clear mucoid fluid.

Clinical Findings

A. Symptoms and Signs:

1. Pain–Attacks of biliary colic may persist for as long as several hours or be as brief as 15–20 minutes. Pain may be referred to the interscapular area or shoulder. Fatty food intolerance, belching, flatulence, a sense of epigastric heaviness, upper abdominal pain of varying intensity, and heartburn are often erroneously considered to be suggestive of cholelithiasis and cholecystitis but are usually not relieved by cholecystectomy.

2. Physical examination–Physical examination is nonspecific, revealing abdominal tenderness which may be localized to the right hypochondrium and epigastric area but which may also be diffuse. A gallbladder that is palpable in the right upper abdomen suggests hydrops or a Courvoisier gallbladder (see below). The presence of jaundice in a patient with biliary colic suggests choledocholithiasis. Occasionally, a stone in the neck of the gallbladder may compress the bile duct (Mirizzi's syndrome).

B. Laboratory Findings: Routine laboratory studies (white count, liver tests, amylase) are often normal or minimally elevated. Microscopic examination of bile obtained by biliary drainage is occasionally helpful in confirming calculous disease of the gallbladder when no stones are seen on ultrasonography. (The test is valid only in the absence of hepatic disease.)

C. Imaging: Plain films of the abdomen may reveal opacification of the gallbladder caused by high concentrations of calcium carbonate (limy bile) or radiopaque stones. Nonvisualization of the gallbladder on oral cholecystography implies cholecystitis (95% accuracy) provided there is radiologic evidence that the oral contrast material has been absorbed and excreted. Technical reasons for nonvisualization must be excluded: failure to ingest the dye, vomiting or diarrhea, gastric outlet obstruction or esophageal stricture, intestinal malabsorption, abnormal location of the gallbladder, liver disease (including preicteric hepatitis), Dubin-Johnson syndrome, fat-free diet prior to cholecystography, and previous cholecystectomy.

Ultrasound examination of the gallbladder is useful in detecting stones. The sensitivity of diagnosis of cholelithiasis (but not cholecystitis) is high (96%) and the incidence of false-positive results low (2%).

Differential Diagnosis

Upper gastrointestinal distress may be caused by peptic ulcer disease, chronic relapsing pancreatitis, irritable bowel syndrome, and malignant neoplasms of the stomach, pancreas, hepatic flexure, or gallbladder.

Complications

Cholelithiasis with chronic cholecystitis may be associated with acute exacerbations of gallbladder inflammation, common duct stone, fistulization to the bowel, pancreatitis, and, rarely, carcinoma of the gallbladder. Calcified (porcelain) gallbladder has a high association with gallbladder carcinoma and is an indication for cholecystectomy.

Treatment

Surgical treatment is the same as for acute cholecystitis. If indicated, cholangiography can be performed during laparoscopic cholecystectomy. Choledocholithiasis can also be excluded by either pre- or postoperative ERCP.

Prognosis

The overall mortality rate of cholecystectomy is less than 1%, but hepatobiliary tract surgery is a more formidable procedure in the elderly, in whom the mortality rate is 5–10%. A technically successful surgical procedure in an appropriately selected patient is generally followed by complete resolution of symptoms.

Mort EA et al: The influence of age on clinical and patient-reported outcomes after cholecystectomy. J Gen Intern Med 1994;9:61. (Patients over age 60 experience more postoperative complications, less frequent recurrence of preoperative pain, and a decline in postoperative work performance compared with younger patients.)

CHOLEDOCHOLITHIASIS & CHOLANGITIS

Essentials of Diagnosis

- Often a history of biliary colic or jaundice.
- Sudden onset of severe right upper quadrant or

epigastric pain, which may radiate to the right scapula or shoulder.

- Occasional patients present with painless jaundice.
- Nausea and vomiting.
- Fever, which may be followed by hypothermia and gram-negative shock, jaundice, and leukocytosis.
- Abdominal films may reveal gallstones.

General Considerations

About 15% of patients with gallstones have choledocholithiasis. The percentage rises with age, and the frequency in elderly people with gallstones may be as high as 50%. Common duct stones usually originate in the gallbladder but may also form spontaneously in the common duct postcholecystectomy. The stones are frequently "silent" as no symptoms result unless there is obstruction.

Clinical Findings

A. Symptoms and Signs: A history suggestive of biliary colic or prior jaundice may be obtained. Biliary colic results from rapid increases in common bile duct pressure due to obstructed bile flow. The additional features that suggest the presence of a common duct stone are (1) frequently recurring attacks of right upper abdominal pain that is severe and persists for hours: (2) chills and fever associated with severe colic; and (3) a history of jaundice associated with episodes of abdominal pain. The combination of pain, fever (and chills), and jaundice represents **Charcot's triad** and denotes the classic picture of cholangitis. The presence of altered sensorium, lethargy, and septic shock connotes acute suppurative cholangitis accompanied by pus in the obstructed duct and represents an endoscopic or surgical emergency.

Hepatomegaly may be present in calculous biliary obstruction, and tenderness is usually present in the right hypochondrium and epigastrium.

B. Laboratory Findings: Bilirubinuria and elevation of serum bilirubin are present if the common duct is obstructed; levels commonly fluctuate. Serum alkaline phosphatase elevation is especially suggestive of obstructive jaundice. Not uncommonly, serum amylase elevations are present because of secondary pancreatitis. On occasion, acute obstruction of the bile duct produces a transient striking increase in serum aminotransferase levels (> 1000 units/L). Prolongation of the prothrombin time occurs when there is prolonged interruption of the flow of bile to the intestine. When extrahepatic obstruction persists for more than a few weeks, differentiation of obstruction from chronic cholestatic liver disease becomes progressively more difficult.

C. Imaging: Ultrasonography, CT scan, and radionuclide imaging may demonstrate dilated bile ducts and impaired bile flow. Both endoscopic ultra-

sonography and MR cholangiography have been found to be accurate in demonstrating common duct stones. Percutaneous transhepatic cholangiography or endoscopic retrograde cholangiopancreatography (ERCP) provides the most direct and accurate means of determining the cause, location, and extent of obstruction. If the obstruction is thought to be due to a stone, ERCP is the procedure of choice because it permits papillotomy with stone extraction or stent placement.

Differential Diagnosis

The most common cause of obstructive jaundice is common duct stone. Next in frequency is carcinoma of the pancreas, ampulla of Vater, or common duct. Extrinsic compression of the common duct may result from metastatic carcinoma (usually from the gastrointestinal tract) involving porta hepatis lymph nodes or, rarely, from a large duodenal diverticulum. Gallbladder cancer extending into the common duct often presents as obstructive jaundice. Chronic cholestatic liver diseases (primarily biliary cirrhosis, sclerosing cholangitis, drug-induced) must be considered. Hepatocellular jaundice can usually be differentiated by the history, clinical findings, and liver tests, but liver biopsy is necessary on occasion.

Complications

A. Biliary Cirrhosis: Common duct obstruction lasting longer than 30 days results in liver damage leading to cirrhosis. Hepatic failure with portal hypertension occurs in untreated cases.

B. Hypoprothrombinemia: Patients with obstructive jaundice or liver disease may bleed excessively as a result of prolonged prothrombin times. In contrast to hepatocellular dysfunction, hypoprothrombinemia due to obstructive jaundice will respond to 10 mg of parenteral vitamin K or water-soluble oral vitamin K (phytonadione, 5 mg) within 24–36 hours.

Treatment

Common duct stone in a patient with cholelithiasis is usually treated by endoscopic papillotomy followed by laparoscopic cholecystectomy. In some cases, choledocholithiasis discovered at laparoscopic cholecystectomy may be managed via laparoscopic removal or, if necessary, conversion to open surgery (see below). In the postcholecystectomy patient with choledocholithiasis, endoscopic papillotomy with stone extraction is preferable to transabdominal surgery. Lithotripsy, endoscopic or external, or biliary stenting may be a therapeutic consideration for large stones.

A. Preoperative Preparation: Emergency intervention is rarely necessary unless severe ascending cholangitis is present. Liver function should be evaluated thoroughly. Prothrombin time should be restored to normal by parenteral administration of vitamin K (see above). Nutrition should be restored by a high-carbohydrate, high-protein diet and vitamin supplementation. Cholangitis, if present, should be controlled with antimicrobials—eg, mezlocillin, 3 g intravenously every 4 hours, plus either metronidazole, 500 mg intravenously every 6 hours (if no prior manipulation of duct), or gentamicin, 2 mg/kg intravenously as loading dose, plus 1.5 mg/kg every 8 hours adjusted for renal function (if prior manipulation of duct)—but urgent decompression may also be required. Recent experience suggests that ciprofloxacin, 250 mg intravenously every 12 hours, penetrates into bile well and is effective treatment for cholangitis.

B. Indications for Common Duct Exploration: At every operation for cholelithiasis, the advisability of exploring the common duct must be considered. Operative cholangiography via the cystic duct is a useful procedure for demonstrating common duct stones. In patients undergoing laparoscopic cholecystectomy, preoperative ERCP or intraoperative cholangiography may be considered.

1. Preoperative findings suggestive of choledocholithiasis include jaundice, cholangitis, and preoperative ultrasound showing a stone in the common duct. Although biliary pancreatitis results from choledocholithiasis, the stone has usually passed by the time of cholecystectomy.

2. Operative findings of choledocholithiasis are palpable stones in the common duct, dilation or thickening of the wall of the common duct, and gallbladder stones small enough to pass through the cystic duct.

3. For the patient with a T tube and a common duct stone, manipulation with various special instruments via the T tube or T tube sinus tract is often successful in extracting the stone.

4. For the poor-risk patient, endoscopic sphincterotomy has become the treatment of choice even if cholecystectomy for cholelithiasis is considered too risky.

C. Postoperative Care:

1. Antibiotics–Postoperative antibiotics are not administered routinely after biliary tract surgery. Cultures of the bile are always taken at operation. If biliary tract infection was present preoperatively or is apparent at operation, ampicillin (500 mg every 6 hours intravenously) with gentamicin (1.5 mg/kg every 8 hours) and metronidazole (500 mg every 6 hours) or ciprofloxacin (250 mg intravenously every 12 hours) or a third-generation cephalosporin (eg, cefoperazone, 1–2 g intravenous every 12 hours) is administered postoperatively until the results of sensitivity tests on culture specimens are available.

2. Management of the T tube–Following choledochostomy, a simple catheter or T tube is placed in the common duct for decompression. A properly placed tube should drain bile at the operating table and continuously thereafter; otherwise, it should be considered blocked or dislocated. The volume of bile drainage varies from 100 to 1000 mL daily (average, 200–400 mL). Above-average drainage may be due to obstruction at the ampulla (usually by edema).

3. Cholangiography–A T-tube cholangiogram should be done on about the seventh or eighth postoperative day. If the cholangiogram shows no stones in the common duct and the opaque medium flows freely into the duodenum, the tube is clamped overnight and removed by simple traction the following day. A small amount of bile frequently leaks from the tube site for a few days.

Abboud P-AC et al: Predictors of common bile duct stone prior to cholecystectomy: A meta-analysis. Gastrointest Endosc 1996;44:450. (Major predictors are cholangitis, jaundice, and ultrasound evidence of common duct stones.)

Leung JWL et al: Antibiotics, biliary sepsis and bile duct stones. Gastrointest Endosc 1994;40:716. (Of various antibiotics studied, only ciprofloxacin penetrates into bile when duct is obstructed.)

Prat F et al: Prospective controlled study of endoscopic ultrasonography and endoscopic retrograde cholangiography in patients with suspected common-bile duct lithiasis. Lancet 1996;347:75. (Endoscopic ultrasonography is as sensitive as endoscopic cholangiography and could be used to screen patients with suspected choledocholithiasis.)

Targarona EM et al: Randomised trial of endoscopic sphincterotomy with gallbladder left in situ versus open surgery for common bile duct calculi in high-risk patients. (A contrary view showing similar mortality rates but a higher frequency of recurrent biliary symptoms in patients undergoing sphincterotomy.)

BILIARY STRICTURE

Benign biliary strictures are the result of surgical trauma in about 95% of cases. The remainder are caused by blunt external injury to the abdomen, pancreatitis, or erosion of the duct by a gallstone.

Signs of injury to the duct may or may not be recognized in the immediate postoperative period. If complete occlusion has occurred, jaundice will develop rapidly; more often, however, a tear has been accidentally made in the duct, and the earliest manifestation of injury may be excessive or prolonged loss of bile from the surgical drains. Bile leakage may predispose to localized infection, which in turn accentuates scar formation and the ultimate development of a fibrous stricture.

Cholangitis is the most common complication of stricture. Typically, the patient experiences episodes of pain, fever, chills, and jaundice within a few weeks to months after cholecystectomy. Physical findings may include jaundice during an attack of cholangitis and right upper quadrant abdominal tenderness.

Serum alkaline phosphatase is usually elevated. Hyperbilirubinemia is variable, fluctuating during exacerbations and usually remaining in the range of 5–10 mg/dL. Blood cultures may be positive during an episode of cholangitis. Percutaneous transhepatic cholangiography or endoscopic retrograde cholangiopancreatography can be valuable in demonstrating the stricture, permitting biopsy and cytologic specimens, and allowing dilation and stent placement.

Differentiation from cholangiocarcinoma may require surgical exploration. Operative treatment of a stricture frequently necessitates performance of choledochojejunostomy or hepaticojejunostomy to reestablish bile flow into the intestine.

Significant hepatocellular disease due to secondary biliary cirrhosis will inevitably occur if a biliary stricture is not treated. The death rate for untreated stricture ranges from 10% to 15%.

Rossi RL et al: Use of expandable metal stents for benign biliary strictures: Need for balanced multidisciplinary approach. Gastrointest Endosc 1996;43:73. (Currently available metal stents are generally not removable and are avoided in benign [as opposed to malignant] strictures where long-term survival is anticipated; removable stents are being developed.)

PRIMARY SCLEROSING CHOLANGITIS

Primary sclerosing cholangitis is an uncommon disease characterized by a diffuse inflammation of the biliary tract leading to fibrosis and strictures of the biliary system. The disease is most common in men aged 20–40 and is closely associated with ulcerative colitis, which is present in approximately two-thirds of patients with primary sclerosing cholangitis; however, only 1–4% of patients with ulcerative colitis develop clinically significant sclerosing cholangitis. As for ulcerative colitis, smoking is associated with a decreased risk of primary sclerosing cholangitis. Patients with primary sclerosing cholangitis often (60–80%, versus 25% for controls) have the histocompatible antigen HLA-B8, suggesting that genetic factors may play an etiologic role. Antineutrophil cytoplasmic antibodies (ANCA), with fluorescent staining characteristics and target antigens distinct from those found in patients with Wegener's granulomatosis or vasculitis, are found in 70% of patients. In patients with AIDS, sclerosing cholangitis may result from infections caused by CMV, *Cryptosporidium,* or *Microsporum.*

The diagnosis of primary sclerosing cholangitis is made by endoscopic retrograde cholangiography; biliary obstruction by a stone or tumor should be excluded. The disease may be confined to small intrahepatic bile ducts, in which case ERCP is normal, and the diagnosis is suggested by liver biopsy. In general, the diagnosis of primary sclerosing cholangitis is difficult to make after biliary surgery or intrahepatic artery chemotherapy, which may result in bile duct injury. Cholangiocarcinoma may complicate the course of primary sclerosing cholangitis in 10% of cases and may be difficult to diagnose by cytologic examination or biopsy because of false-negative results.

Clinically, the disease presents as progressive obstructive jaundice, frequently associated with malaise, pruritus, anorexia, and indigestion. Some patients are diagnosed in a presymptomatic phase because of an elevated alkaline phosphatase. Survival averages 10 years once symptoms appear. Adverse prognostic markers are older age, higher serum bilirubin, advanced histologic stage, and portal hypertension.

Treatment with corticosteroids and broad-spectrum antimicrobial agents has been employed with inconsistent and unpredictable results. Ursodeoxycholic acid may improve liver function test results but does not appear to alter the natural history. Careful endoscopic evaluation of the biliary tree may permit balloon dilation of localized strictures. If there is a major stricture, stenting is a possibility. For patients with cirrhosis and clinical decompensation, liver transplantation is the procedure of choice. Actuarial survival rates with liver transplantation for this disease are as high as 85% at 3 years, but rates are much lower once cholangiocarcinoma has developed.

The prognosis is poor, with most individuals requiring liver transplantation within a few years after the appearance of symptoms.

Lee JG et al: Endoscopic therapy of sclerosing cholangitis. Hepatology 1995;21:661. (Leads to improvement in symptoms, liver tests, and cholangiograms in nearly 80% of selected patients.)

Lee Y-M, Kaplan MM: Primary sclerosing cholangitis. N Engl J Med 1995;332:924. (Reviews pathology, pathogenesis, diagnosis, clinical features, natural history, and treatment.)

Ramage JK et al: Serum tumor markers for the diagnosis of cholangiocarcinoma in primary sclerosing cholangitis. Gastroenterology 1995;108:865. (Elevated serum CA 19-9 and CEA levels suggest cholangiocarcinoma.)

CARCINOMA OF THE BILIARY TRACT

Carcinoma of the gallbladder occurs in approximately 2% of all people operated on for biliary tract disease. It is notoriously insidious, and the diagnosis is often made unexpectedly at surgery. Cholelithiasis is usually present. Spread of the cancer—by direct extension into the liver or to the peritoneal surface—may be the initial manifestation. The TNM classification includes the following stages: Tis, carcinoma in situ; T1, invasion of mucosa (T1a) or muscle layer (T1b); T2, invasion of perimuscular connective tissue; T3, extension into serosa or into an adjacent organ; T4: invasion > 2 cm into liver or two or more adjacent organs; N1: metastasis in cystic duct, peri-choledochal, or hilar nodes; N2: metastasis in peripancreatic head, periduodenal, periportal, celiac, or superior mesenteric nodes.

Carcinoma of the extrahepatic bile ducts accounts for 3% of all cancer deaths in the USA. It affects both sexes equally but is more prevalent in individuals aged 50–70. Tumors often arise at the confluence of the hepatic ducts (Klatskin tumors). Staging is similar to that for carcinoma of the gallbladder. The frequency of carcinoma in persons with choledochal cysts has been reported to be 2–8%, and surgical excision is recommended. There is an increased incidence in patients with ulcerative colitis. In southeast Asia, infection of the bile ducts with helminths (*Clonorchis sinensis, Fasciola hepatica*) is associated with chronic cholangitis and an increased risk of cholangiocarcinoma.

Clinical Findings

Progressive jaundice is the most common and usually the first sign of obstruction of the extrahepatic biliary system. Pain is usually present in the right upper abdomen and radiates into the back. Anorexia and weight loss are common and frequently associated with fever and chills. Rarely, hematemesis or melena results from erosion of tumor into a blood vessel (hemobilia). Fistula formation between the biliary system and adjacent organs may also occur. The course is usually one of rapid deterioration, with death occurring within a few months.

Physical examination reveals profound jaundice. A palpable gallbladder with obstructive jaundice usually is said to signify malignant disease (Courvoisier's law); however, this clinical generalization has been proved to be accurate only about 50% of the time. Hepatomegaly is usually present and is associated with liver tenderness. Ascites may occur with peritoneal implants. Pruritus and skin excoriations are common.

Laboratory examination reveals predominantly conjugated hyperbilirubinemia, with total serum bilirubin values ranging from 5 to 30 mg/dL. There is usually concomitant elevation of the alkaline phosphatase and serum cholesterol. AST is normal or minimally elevated. An elevated CA 19-9 level may help distinguish cholangiocarcinoma from a benign biliary stricture (in the absence of cholangitis).

The most helpful diagnostic studies before surgery are either percutaneous transhepatic or endoscopic retrograde cholangiography with biopsy and cytologic specimens.

Treatment

In young and fit patients, curative surgery may be attempted if the tumor is well localized. The 5-year survival rate for localized carcinoma of the gallbladder (stage 1, T1a, N0, M0) is as high as 80% but drops to 15% if there is muscular invasion (T1b). If the tumor is unresectable at laparotomy, cholecystoduodenostomy or T-tube drainage of the common duct can be performed. Carcinoma of the bile ducts is curable by surgery in less than 10% of cases. Palliation can be achieved by placement of a self-expandable metal stent via the endoscopic or percutaneous transhepatic route. The prognosis is poor, with few patients surviving for more than 6 months after surgery.

Nakeeb A et al: Cholangiocarcinoma: A spectrum of intrahepatic, perihilar, and distal tumors. Ann Surg 1996;224:463. (Retrospective review suggesting that postoperative adjuvant radiation does not improve survival.)

Nordback IH et al: Unresectable hilar cholangiocarcinoma: Percutaneous versus operative palliation. Surgery 1994;115:597. (In fit patients, surgery was associated with a lower frequency of cholangitis and delayed hepatic failure.)

Sung JJY et al: Endoscopic stenting for palliation of malignant biliary obstruction: A review of progress in the last 15 years. Dig Dis Sci 1995;40:1167. (Self-expandable metal stents are more costly than plastic stents but remain patent longer.)

DISEASES OF THE PANCREAS

ACUTE PANCREATITIS

Essentials of Diagnosis

- Abrupt onset of deep epigastric pain, often with radiation to the back.
- Nausea, vomiting, sweating, weakness.
- Abdominal tenderness and distention, fever.
- Leukocytosis, elevated serum amylase, elevated serum lipase.
- History of previous episodes, often related to alcohol intake.

General Considerations

Acute pancreatitis is thought to result from "escape" of activated pancreatic enzymes from acinar cells into surrounding tissues. Most cases are related to biliary tract disease (a passed gallstone) or heavy alcohol intake. The exact pathogenesis is not known but may include edema or obstruction of the ampulla of Vater, resulting in reflux of bile into pancreatic ducts or direct injury to the acinar cells. Among the numerous other causes or associations are hypercalcemia, hyperlipidemias (chylomicronemia, hypertriglyceridemia, or both), abdominal trauma (including surgery), drugs (including sulfonamides and thiazides), vasculitis, viral infections (eg, mumps), and ERCP. In patients with pancreas divisum, a congenital anomaly in which the dorsal and ventral pancreatic ducts fail to fuse, acute pancreatitis may result from stenosis of the minor papilla with obstruction to flow from the accessory pancreatic duct. Apparently "idiopathic" acute pancreatitis is often caused by occult biliary microlithiasis.

Pathologic changes vary from acute edema and cellular infiltration to necrosis of the acinar cells, hemorrhage from necrotic blood vessels, and intra- and extrapancreatic fat necrosis. All or part of the pancreas may be involved.

Clinical Findings

A. Symptoms and Signs: Epigastric abdominal pain, generally abrupt in onset, is steady and severe and often made worse by walking and lying supine and better by sitting and leaning forward. The pain usually radiates into the back but may radiate to the right or left. Nausea and vomiting are usually present. Weakness, sweating, and anxiety are noted in severe attacks. There may be a history of alcohol intake or a heavy meal immediately preceding the attack, or a history of milder similar episodes or biliary colic in the past.

The abdomen is tender mainly in the upper abdomen, most often without guarding, rigidity, or rebound. The abdomen may be distended, and bowel sounds may be absent with associated paralytic ileus. Fever of 38.4–39 °C, tachycardia, hypotension (even true shock), pallor, and cool clammy skin are often present. Mild jaundice is common. Occasionally, an upper abdominal mass due to the inflamed pancreas or a pseudocyst may be palpated. Acute renal failure (usually prerenal) may occur early in the course of acute pancreatitis.

B. Assessment of Severity: Ranson's criteria are generally used in assessing the severity of acute alcoholic pancreatitis on presentation (pancreatitis due to other causes is assessed by similar criteria). When three or more of the following are present on admission, a severe course complicated by pancreatic necrosis can be predicted:

1. Age over 55 years.
2. White blood cell count over 16,000/μL.
3. Blood glucose over 200 mg/dL.
4. Base deficit over 4 meq/L.
5. Serum LDH over 350 units/L.
6. AST over 250 units/L.

Development of the following in the first 48 hours indicates a worsening prognosis:

1. Hematocrit drop of more than ten percentage points.
2. BUN rise greater than 5 mg/dL.
3. Arterial PO_2 of less than 60 mm Hg.
4. Serum calcium of less than 8 mg/dL.
5. Estimated fluid sequestration of more than 6 L.

Mortality rates correlate with the number of criteria present:

Number of Criteria	Mortality Rate
0–2	1%
3–4	16%
5–6	40%
7–8	100%

The Acute Physiology and Chronic Health (APACHE) II scoring system may also be used to assess severity.

C. Laboratory Findings: Leukocytosis (10,000–30,000/μL), proteinuria, granular casts, glycosuria (10–20% of cases), hyperglycemia, and elevated serum bilirubin may be present. Blood urea nitrogen and serum alkaline phosphatase may be elevated and coagulation tests abnormal. Decrease in serum calcium may reflect saponification and correlates well with severity of disease. Levels lower than 7 mg/dL (when serum albumin is normal) are associated with tetany and an unfavorable prognosis.

Serum amylase and lipase are elevated within 24 hours in 90% of cases; their return to normal is variable depending on the severity of disease. In those who develop ascites or left pleural effusions, fluid amylase content is high. An elevated C-reactive protein level suggests the development of pancreatic necrosis.

D. Imaging: Plain radiographs of the abdomen may show gallstones, a "sentinel loop" (a segment of air-filled small intestine most commonly in the left upper quadrant), the "colon cutoff sign" (a gas-filled segment of transverse colon abruptly ending at the area of pancreatic inflammation), or linear focal atelectasis of the lower lobe of the lungs with or without pleural effusion. CT scan is useful in demonstrating an enlarged pancreas when the diagnosis of pancreatitis is uncertain, in detecting pseudocysts, and in differentiating pancreatitis from other possible intra-abdominal catastrophes. Dynamic bolus CT is of particular value in identifying areas of pancreatic necrosis that may require surgical debridement, although the use of intravenous contrast may increase the risk of renal failure; the presence of a fluid collection in the pancreas correlates with an increased mortality rate. CT-guided needle aspiration of areas of pancreatic necrosis may disclose infection, usually by enteric organisms, which invariably leads to death unless surgical debridement is performed. The presence of gas bubbles on CT scan implies that infection by gas-forming organisms is present. Ultrasonography is less reliable, because the echoes are deflected by the gas-distended small intestine frequently associated with pancreatitis.

E. Electrocardiographic Findings: ST–T wave changes may occur, but they usually differ from those of myocardial infarction. Abnormal Q waves do not occur as a result of pancreatitis.

Differential Diagnosis

Acute pancreatitis must be differentiated from an acutely perforated duodenal ulcer, acute cholecystitis, acute intestinal obstruction, leaking aortic aneurysm, renal colic, and acute mesenteric vascular insufficiency or thrombosis. Serum amylase may also be elevated in high intestinal obstruction, in mumps not involving the pancreas (salivary amylase), in ectopic pregnancy, after administration of narcotics, and after abdominal surgery.

Complications

Intravascular volume depletion secondary to leakage of fluids in the pancreatic bed and ileus with fluid-filled loops of bowel may result in prerenal azotemia and even acute tubular necrosis without overt shock. This usually occurs within 24 hours of the onset of acute pancreatitis and lasts 8–9 days. Some patients require peritoneal dialysis or hemodialysis.

As mentioned above, sterile or infected pancreatic neurosis may complicate the course of 10% of cases and accounts for most of the deaths. The risk of infection correlates with the extent of necrosis. Pancreatic necrosis is often associated with fever, leukocytosis, and, in some cases, shock. Because infected pancreatic necrosis is an absolute indication for operative treatment, necrotic tissue should be aspirated under CT guidance for Gram stain and culture. A serious complication of acute pancreatitis is acute respiratory distress syndrome (ARDS); cardiac dysfunction may be superimposed. It usually occurs 3–7 days after the onset of pancreatitis in patients who have required large volumes of fluid and colloid to maintain blood pressure and urine output. Most patients with ARDS require assisted respiration with positive end-expiratory pressure.

Pancreatic abscess is a suppurative process characterized by rising fever, leukocytosis, and localized tenderness and epigastric mass 2–3 weeks into the course of acute pancreatitis. This may be associated with a left-sided pleural effusion or an enlarging spleen secondary to splenic vein thrombosis.

Pseudocysts, encapsulated fluid collections with high enzyme content, commonly appear in pancreatitis when CT scans are used to monitor the evolution of an acute attack. Although the natural history of pseudocysts is still not well delineated, it appears that those less than 6 cm in diameter often resolve spontaneously. They most commonly are within or adjacent to the pancreas but can present anywhere (eg, mediastinal, retrorectal), by extension along anatomic planes. Pseudocysts are multiple in 14% of cases. Pseudocysts may become secondarily infected, necessitating drainage as for an abscess. Erosion of the inflammatory process into a blood vessel can result in a major hemorrhage into the cyst.

Pancreatic ascites may present after recovery from acute pancreatitis as a gradual increase in abdominal girth and persistent elevation of the serum amylase level. Marked elevations in the ascitic protein (> 3 g/dL) and amylase (> 1000 units/L) concentrations are typical. The condition results from rupture of the pancreatic duct or drainage of a pseudocyst into the peritoneal cavity.

Chronic pancreatitis develops in about 10% of cases. Permanent diabetes mellitus and exocrine pancreatic insufficiency occur uncommonly after a single acute episode.

Treatment

A. Management of Acute Disease: In most patients, acute pancreatitis is a mild disease that subsides spontaneously within several days. The pancreatic rest program includes withholding food and liquids by mouth, bed rest, and, in patients with moderately severe pain or ileus, nasogastric suction. Pain is controlled with meperidine, up to 100–150 mg intramuscularly every 3–4 hours as necessary. In those with severe hepatic or renal dysfunction, the dose may need to be reduced. No fluid or foods should be given orally until the patient is largely free of pain and has bowel sounds. Clear liquids are then given, and gradual advancement to a regular low-fat diet is prescribed, guided by the patient's tolerance and by the absence of pain.

In more severe pancreatitis, there may be considerable leakage of fluids, necessitating large amounts of intravenous fluids to maintain intravascular volume. Infusions of fresh frozen plasma or serum albumin may be necessary. With colloid solutions, there may be an increased risk of developing adult respiratory distress syndrome. If shock persists after adequate volume replacement (including packed red cells), pressors may be required. For the patient requiring a large volume of parenteral fluids, central venous pressure and blood gases should be monitored at regular intervals. The role of intravenous somatostatin in severe acute pancreatitis is uncertain, but octreotide is thought to have no benefit.

Calcium gluconate must be given intravenously if there is evidence of hypocalcemia with tetany (Table 22–10). Antibiotics are generally reserved for documented infections. Cultures of blood, urine, sputum, and pleural effusion (if present) and needle aspirations of areas of pancreatic necrosis (with CT guidance) should be obtained.

The patient with severe pancreatitis requires attention in an intensive care unit. Close follow-up of white blood count, hematocrit, serum electrolytes, serum calcium, serum creatinine, BUN, serum AST and LDH, and arterial blood gases is mandatory.

B. Treatment of Complications and Follow-Up: Pancreatitis complicated by prolonged ileus (24 hours or more), abdominal distention, or vomiting requires nasogastric suction until symptoms subside; in some cases, parenteral nutrition may be required.

A surgeon should be consulted in all cases of severe acute pancreatitis. If the diagnosis is in doubt and investigations indicate a strong possibility of a serious surgically correctable lesion (eg, perforated peptic ulcer), exploration is indicated. When acute pancreatitis is unexpectedly found on exploratory laparotomy, it is usually wise to close without intervention of any kind. If the pancreatitis appears mild and cholelithiasis is present, cholecystostomy or cholecystectomy may be justified. When severe pancreatitis results from choledocholithiasis, endoscopic sphincterotomy and stone extraction is indicated.

Aggressive surgery and enteral or parenteral hyperalimentation may increase survival in patients with severe and unresolving pancreatic necrosis and is always indicated for infected necrosis. Initially, enterostomy tubes and drainage are established. Subsequent surgery is performed to debride necrotic pancreas and surrounding tissue. Peritoneal lavage has not been shown to improve survival in severe acute pancreatitis, in part because late septic complications are unaffected.

The development of a pancreatic abscess is an indication for prompt drainage, usually through the flank. Chronic pseudocysts require drainage when infected or associated with persisting pain, pancreatitis, or common duct obstruction. For pancreatic infections, imipenem, 500 mg every 8 hours intravenously, is a good antibiotic because it achieves bactericidal levels in pancreatic tissue for most causative organisms. Imipenem or cefuroxime (1.5 g intravenously three times daily, then 250 mg orally twice daily) administered to patients with sterile pancreatic necrosis may also reduce the risk of pancreatic infection.

Prognosis

The mortality rate for severe acute pancreatitis (more than three Ranson criteria) is high, especially when hepatic, cardiovascular, or renal impairment is present or when pancreatic necrosis develops. Recurrences are common in alcoholic pancreatitis.

de Beaux AC et al: Factors influencing morbidity and mortality in acute pancreatitis; an analysis of 279 cases. Gut 1995;37:121. (The mortality rate was 7.6% and was influenced by age, cause (greater if unknown), presence of organ failure, and need for transfer to tertiary center.)

Fölsch UR et al: Early ERCP and papillotomy compared with conservative treatment for acute biliary pancreatitis. N Engl J Med 1997;336:237. (In contrast to a previous study, papillotomy did not reduce the frequency of complications in patients without biliary obstruction.)

Lankisch PG et al: Drug induced acute pancreatitis: Incidence and severity. Gut 1995;37:565. (Drugs rarely cause acute pancreatitis, and when they do the course is usually benign.)

Sainio V et al: Early antibiotic treatment in acute necrotising pancreatitis. Lancet 1995;346:663. (Randomized and controlled—but not blinded—trial showing decreased mortality rate with cefuroxime.)

Skaife P, Kingsnorth AN: Acute pancreatitis: Assessment and management. Postgrad Med J 1996;72:277. (Concise review.)

CHRONIC PANCREATITIS

Chronic pancreatitis occurs most often in patients with alcoholism, severe malnutrition, or untreated hyperparathyroidism. It may be hereditary or idiopathic. Recently, a gene for hereditary pancreatitis, transmitted as an autosomal dominant trait with variable penetrance, has been identified on chromosome 7. Progressive fibrosis and destruction of functioning glandular tissue occur. Pancreaticolithiasis and obstruction of the duodenal end of the pancreatic duct are often present.

Differentiation of chronic from recurrent acute pancreatitis is important in that recurrent pancreatitis is initiated by a specific event (eg, alcoholic binge, passage of a stone), whereas chronic pancreatitis is a self-perpetuating disease characterized by pain and ultimately by pancreatic exocrine or endocrine insufficiency.

Clinical Findings

A. Symptoms and Signs: Persistent or recurrent episodes of epigastric and left upper quadrant pain with referral to the upper left lumbar region are typical. Anorexia, nausea, vomiting, constipation, flatulence, and weight loss are common. Abdominal signs during attacks consist chiefly of tenderness over the pancreas, mild muscle guarding, and paralytic ileus. Attacks may last only a few hours or as long as 2 weeks; pain may eventually be almost continuous. Steatorrhea (as indicated by bulky, foul, fatty stools) may occur late in the course.

B. Laboratory Findings: Serum amylase and lipase may be elevated during acute attacks; normal amylase does not exclude the diagnosis, however. Serum alkaline phosphatase and bilirubin may be elevated owing to compression of the common duct. Glycosuria may be present. Excess fecal fat may be demonstrated on chemical analysis of the stool; pancreatic insufficiency may be confirmed by response to therapy with pancreatic enzyme supplements, by a bentiromide (NBT-PABA) test or secretin stimulation test, or, where the tests are available, by decreased fecal chymotrypsin or elastase levels.

C. Imaging: Plain films often show calcifications due to pancreaticolithiasis and mild ileus. CT may show calcifications not seen on plain films. Endoscopic ultrasonography has shown promise in detecting changes of chronic pancreatitis. Endoscopic retrograde cholangiopancreatography may show dilated ducts, intraductal stones, strictures, or pseudocyst, but the results may be normal in patients with so-called minimal change pancreatitis.

Complications

Narcotic addiction is common. Other frequent complications include often brittle diabetes mellitus, pancreatic pseudocyst or abscess, cholestatic liver enzymes with or without jaundice, common bile duct stricture, steatorrhea, malnutrition, and peptic ulcer. Pancreatic cancer develops in 4% of patients after 20 years.

Treatment

Correctable coexistent biliary tract disease should be treated surgically.

A. Medical Measures: A low-fat diet should be prescribed. Alcohol is forbidden because it frequently precipitates attacks. Narcotics should be avoided if possible. Steatorrhea is treated with pancreatic supplements that are selected on the basis of their high lipase activity. The usual dose is 30,000 units of lipase in capsules given before, during, and after meals (Table 15–7). Concurrent administration of sodium bicarbonate, 650 mg before and after meals, H_2 receptor antagonists (eg, ranitidine, 150 mg twice daily), or a proton pump inhibitor (eg, omeprazole, 20–60 mg daily) decreases the inactivation of lipase by acid and may thereby further decrease steatorrhea. In selected cases of alcoholic pancreatitis and in cystic fibrosis, enteric-coated microencapsulated preparations may offer an advantage. In patients with cystic fibrosis, high-dose pancreatic enzyme therapy has been associated with strictures of the ascending colon. Pain secondary to idiopathic chronic pancreatitis may be alleviated by the use of pancreatic enzymes or octreotide, 200 µg subcutaneously three times daily. Associated diabetes should be treated in the usual manner.

B. Surgical and Endoscopic Treatment: Surgery may be indicated in chronic pancreatitis to drain persistent pseudocysts, treat other complications, or, rarely, attempt to relieve pain. The objectives of surgical intervention are to eradicate biliary tract disease, ensure a free flow of bile into the duodenum, and eliminate obstruction of the pancreatic duct. When obstruction of the duodenal end of the duct can be demonstrated by endoscopic retrograde cholangiopancreatography, dilation of the duct or resection of the tail of the pancreas with implantation of the distal end of the duct by pancreaticojejunostomy may be successful. When the pancreatic duct is diffusely dilated, anastomosis between the duct after it is split longitudinally and a defunctionalized limb of jejunum (Puestow procedure), in some cases combined with local resection of the head of the pancreas, is associated with relief of pain in 80% of cases. In advanced cases, subtotal or total pancreatectomy may be considered as a last resort but is associated with variable results and a high rate of pancreatic insufficiency. Endoscopic or surgical drainage is indicated for symptomatic pseudocysts. Recent experience suggests that pancreatic ascites or pancreaticopleural fistulas due to a disrupted pancreatic duct can be managed by endoscopic placement of a stent across the disrupted duct. Fragmentation of stones in the pancreatic duct by lithotripsy and endoscopic removal of stones from the duct at ERCP or placement of a stent across pancreatic duct strictures may relieve pain. For patients with chronic pain and nondilated ducts, a percutaneous celiac plexus nerve block may be considered, but results are often disappointing.

Prognosis

This is a serious disease and often leads to chronic disability. The prognosis is best in patients with recurrent acute pancreatitis caused by a remediable condition such as cholelithiasis, choledocholithiasis, stenosis of the sphincter of Oddi, or hyperparathyroidism. Medical management of the hyperlipidemias frequently associated with the condition may also prevent recurrent attacks of pancreatitis. In alcoholic pancreatitis, pain relief is most likely when a dilated pancreatic duct can be decompressed. In patients with disease not amenable to decompressive surgery, addiction to narcotics is a frequent outcome of treatment.

Table 15–7. Selected pancreatic enzyme preparations.[1]

Product	Enzyme Content Per Unit Dose		
	Lipase	Amylase	Protease
Conventional preparations			
Viokase	8,000	30,000	30,000
Ilozyme	11,000	≥30,000	≥30,000
Cotazym	8,000	30,000	30,000
Enteric-coated microencapsulated preparations			
Creon	8,000	30,000	13,000
Creon 10	10,000	33,200	37,500
Creon 20	20,000	66,400	75,000
Creon 25	25,000	74,700	62,500
Pancrease	4,000	20,000	25,000
Pancrease MT16	16,000	48,000	48,000
Pancrease MT25	25,000	75,000	75,000
Cotazym-S	5,000	20,000	20,000

[1]Modified from *Drug Facts and Comparisons,* 1997.

Bruno MJ et al: Maldigestion associated with exocrine pancreatic insufficiency: Implications of gastrointestinal physiology and properties of enzyme preparations for a cause-related and patient-tailored treatment. Am J Gastroenterol 1995;90:1383. (The ins and outs of pancreatic replacement therapy.)

Dumonceau J-M et al: Endoscopic pancreatic drainage in chronic pancreatitis associated with ductal stones: Long-term results. Gastrointest Endosc 1996;43:547. (Relief of pain is likely when the pancreatic duct can be cleared of stones.)

Steer ML et al: Chronic pancreatitis. N Engl J Med 1995;332:1482. (Balanced review.)

Whitcomb DC et al: A gene for hereditary pancreatitis maps to chromosome 7q35. Gastroenterology 1996; 110:1975. (Genetic basis of one of the more common causes of pancreatitis beginning in childhood.)

CARCINOMA OF THE PANCREAS & THE PERIAMPULLARY AREA

Essentials of Diagnosis

- Obstructive jaundice (may be painless).
- Enlarged gallbladder (may be painful).
- Upper abdominal pain with radiation to back, weight loss, and thrombophlebitis are usually late manifestations.

General Considerations

Carcinoma is the commonest neoplasm of the pancreas. About 75% are in the head and 25% in the body and tail of the organ. Carcinomas involving the head of the pancreas, the ampulla of Vater, the common bile duct, and the duodenum are considered together, because they are usually indistinguishable clinically; of these, carcinomas of the pancreas constitute over 90%. They comprise 2% of all cancers and 5% of cancer deaths.

Clinical Findings

A. Symptoms and Signs: Pain is present in over 70% of cases and is often vague, diffuse, and located in the epigastrium or left upper quadrant when the lesion is in the tail. Radiation of pain into the back is common and sometimes predominates. Sitting up and leaning forward may afford some relief, and this usually indicates that the lesion has spread beyond the pancreas and is inoperable. Diarrhea, as a relatively early symptom, is seen occasionally. Migratory thrombophlebitis is a rare sign. Weight loss is a common but late finding and may be associated with depression. Occasionally a patient presents with acute pancreatitis in the absence of an alternative cause. Jaundice, which may be associated with a palpable gallbladder, is indicative of obstruction by neoplasm (Courvoisier's law), but there are frequent exceptions. In addition, a hard, fixed, occasionally tender mass may be present.

B. Laboratory Findings: There may be mild anemia. Glycosuria, hyperglycemia, and impaired glucose tolerance or true diabetes mellitus are found in 10–20% of cases. The serum amylase or lipase level is occasionally elevated. Liver function tests may suggest obstructive jaundice. Steatorrhea in the absence of jaundice is uncommon. Occult blood in the stool is suggestive of carcinoma of the ampulla of Vater. CA 19-9, with a sensitivity of 70% and a specificity of 87%, has not proved sensitive enough for early detection; increased values are also found in acute and chronic pancreatitis and cholangitis. Point mutations in codon 12 of the *Ki-ras* oncogene are found in 70–100% of patients.

C. Imaging: With carcinoma of the head of the pancreas, the upper gastrointestinal series may show a widening of the duodenal loop, mucosal abnormalities in the duodenum ranging from edema to invasion or ulceration, or spasm or compression. Ultrasound is not reliable because of interference by intestinal gas. Dynamic contrast spiral CT and MRI detect a mass in over 80% of cases and are helpful in delineating the extent of the tumor and allowing for percutaneous fine-needle aspiration for cytologic studies and tumor markers. Selective celiac and superior mesenteric arteriography may demonstrate vessel invasion by tumor, a finding that would interdict attempts at surgical resection, but it is less widely used since the advent of dynamic CT and endoscopic ultrasonography, which is emerging as the most accurate means of demonstrating venous or gastric invasion. ERCP may clarify an ambiguous CT or MRI study by delineating the pancreatic duct system or confirming an ampullary or biliary neoplasm. With obstruction of the splenic vein, splenomegaly or gastric varices are present, the latter delineated by endoscopy, endoscopic ultrasonography, or angiography.

Staging by the TNM classification includes the following definitions: T1: tumor limited to the pancreas (T1a if < 2 cm, T1b if > 2 cm); T2: extension into duodenum, bile duct, or peripancreatic tissues; T3: extension to stomach, spleen, colon, or adjacent large vessels.

Treatment

Abdominal exploration is usually necessary when cytologic diagnosis cannot be made or if resection is to be attempted, which includes about 30% of patients. In a patient with a localized mass in the head of the pancreas and without jaundice, laparoscopy may be used to detect tiny peritoneal or liver metastases and thereby avoid resection. Radical pancreaticoduodenal resection is indicated for lesions strictly limited to the head of the pancreas, periampullary zone, and duodenum (T1, N0, M0). Adjuvant radiation therapy and chemotherapy are of uncertain benefit. When resection is not feasible, cholecystojejunostomy or endoscopic stenting of the bile duct is performed to relieve jaundice. A gastrojejunostomy is also done if duodenal obstruction is expected to develop later. Combined irradiation and chemotherapy may be used for palliation of unresectable cancer confined to the pancreas. However, chemotherapy has been disappointing in metastatic pancreatic cancer. Celiac plexus nerve block may improve pain control.

Prognosis

Carcinoma of the pancreas, especially in the body or tail, has a poor prognosis. Reported 5-year survival rates range from 2% to 5%. Lesions of the ampulla have a better prognosis, with reported 5-year survival rates of 20–40% after resection. The reported operative mortality rate of radical pancreaticoduodenectomy is 10–15%.

Azar C et al: Intraductal papillary mucinous tumours of the pancreas: Clinical and therapeutic issues in 32 patients.

Gut 1996;39:457. (Distinctive features include frequent presentation with acute pancreatitis and very slow growth with a low recurrence rate if resection is performed before invasive carcinoma has developed.)

Hammel P et al: Preoperative cyst fluid analysis is useful for the differential diagnosis of cystic lesions of the pancreas. Gastroenterology 1995;108:1230. (Pseudocysts are characterized by high amylase levels in the cyst fluid; serous cystadenomas, which are benign, by low CEA levels; and mucinous tumors, which are potentially malignant, by high CA 19-9 levels.)

Tan HP et al: Pancreatic carcinoma: An update. J Am Coll Surg 1996;183:164. (Comprehensive review.)

16

Breast

Armando E. Giuliano, MD

BENIGN BREAST DISORDERS

MAMMARY DYSPLASIA
(Fibrocystic Disease)

Essentials of Diagnosis

- Painful, often multiple, usually bilateral masses in the breast.
- Rapid fluctuation in the size of the masses is common.
- Frequently, pain occurs or increases and size increases during premenstrual phase of cycle.
- Most common age is 30–50. Rare in postmenopausal women not receiving hormonal replacement.

General Considerations

This disorder, also known as fibrocystic disease or chronic cystic mastitis, is the most frequent lesion of the breast. It is common in women 30–50 years of age but rare in postmenopausal women who are not taking hormonal replacement medications; this suggests that it is related to ovarian activity. Estrogen hormone is considered a causative factor. The term "mammary dysplasia," or "fibrocystic disease," is imprecise and encompasses a wide variety of pathologic entities. These lesions are always associated with benign changes in the breast epithelium, some of which are found so commonly in normal breasts that they are probably variants of normal breast histology but have unfortunately been termed a "disease."

The microscopic findings of fibrocystic disease include cysts (gross and microscopic), papillomatosis, adenosis, fibrosis, and ductal epithelial hyperplasia. Although mammary dysplasia has generally been considered to increase the risk of subsequent breast cancer, only the variants in which proliferation (especially with atypia) of epithelial components is demonstrated represent true risk factors.

Clinical Findings

A. Symptoms and Signs: Mammary dyspla-

sia may produce an asymptomatic lump in the breast that is discovered by accident, but pain or tenderness often calls attention to the mass. There may be discharge from the nipple. In many cases, discomfort occurs or is increased during the premenstrual phase of the cycle, at which time the cysts tend to enlarge. Fluctuation in size and rapid appearance or disappearance of a breast mass are common in cystic disease. Multiple or bilateral masses are common, and many patients will give a history of a transient lump in the breast or cyclic breast pain.

B. Diagnostic Tests: Because a mass due to mammary dysplasia is frequently indistinguishable from carcinoma on the basis of clinical findings, suspicious lesions should be biopsied. Fine-needle aspiration cytology may be used, but if a suspicious mass that is nonmalignant on cytologic examination does not resolve over several months, it must be excised. Surgery should be conservative, since the primary objective is to exclude cancer. Simple mastectomy or extensive removal of breast tissue is rarely, if ever, indicated for mammary dysplasia.

Differential Diagnosis

Pain, fluctuation in size, and multiplicity of lesions are the features most helpful in differentiation from carcinoma. However, if a dominant mass is present, the diagnosis of cancer should be assumed until disproved by biopsy. Final diagnosis often depends on excisional biopsy. Mammography may be helpful, but the breast tissue in these young women is usually too radiodense to permit a worthwhile study. Sonography is useful in differentiating a cystic from a solid mass.

Treatment

When the diagnosis of mammary dysplasia has been established by previous biopsy or is practically certain because the history is classic, aspiration of a discrete mass suggestive of a cyst is indicated in order to alleviate pain and, more importantly, to confirm the cystic nature of the mass. The patient is reexamined at intervals thereafter. If no fluid is obtained or if fluid is bloody, if a mass persists after aspiration, or if at any time during follow-up a persistent lump is noted, biopsy examination should be performed.

Breast pain associated with generalized mammary dysplasia is best treated by avoiding trauma and by wearing (night and day) a brassiere that gives good support and protection. Hormone therapy is not advisable, because it does not cure the condition and has undesirable side effects. Danazol (100–200 mg twice daily orally), a synthetic androgen, has been used for patients with severe pain. This treatment suppresses pituitary gonadotropins, but androgenic effects (acne, edema, hirsutism) usually make this treatment intolerable; it should therefore be reserved for the unusual severe case, and in practice, it is rarely used.

The role of caffeine consumption in the development and treatment of fibrocystic disease is controversial. Some studies suggest that eliminating caffeine from the diet is associated with improvement. Many patients are aware of these studies and report relief of symptoms after giving up coffee, tea, and chocolate. Similarly, many women find vitamin E (400 IU daily) helpful. However, these observations have been difficult to confirm and are anecdotal.

Prognosis

Exacerbations of pain, tenderness, and cyst formation may occur at any time until the menopause, when symptoms usually subside, except in patients receiving hormonal replacement therapy. The patient should be advised to examine her own breasts each month just after menstruation and to inform her physician if a mass appears. The risk of breast cancer in women with mammary dysplasia showing proliferative or atypical changes in the epithelium is higher than that of women in general. These women should be followed carefully with physical examinations and mammography.

Colditz GA et al: The use of estrogens and progestins and the risk of breast cancer in postmenopausal women. N Engl J Med 1995;332:1589.

Fiorica JV: Fibrocystic changes. Obstet Gynecol Clin North Am 1994;12:445.

Gately CA et al: Drug treatments for mastalgia: 17 years experience in the Cardiff Mastalgia Clinic. J R Soc Med 1992;85:12.

London SJ et al: A prospective study of benign breast disease and the risk of breast cancer. JAMA 1992;267:941.

McDivitt RW et al: Histologic types of benign breast disease and the risk for breast cancer. Cancer 1992; 69:1408.

Meyer JE et al: Image-guided aspiration of solitary occult breast "cysts." Arch Surg 1992;127:433.

FIBROADENOMA OF THE BREAST

This common benign neoplasm occurs most frequently in young women, usually within 20 years after puberty. It is somewhat more frequent and tends to occur at an earlier age in black than in white women. Multiple tumors in one or both breasts are found in 10–15% of patients.

The typical fibroadenoma is a round, rubbery, discrete, relatively movable, nontender mass 1–5 cm in diameter. The tumor is usually discovered accidentally. Clinical diagnosis in young patients is generally not difficult. In women over 30, cystic disease of the breast and carcinoma of the breast must be considered. Cysts can be identified by aspiration or ultrasonography. Fibroadenoma does not normally occur after the menopause, but postmenopausal women may occasionally develop fibroadenoma after administration of hormones.

No treatment is usually necessary if the diagnosis can be made by needle biopsy or cytologic examination. At times, treatment is by excision under local anesthesia as an outpatient procedure, with pathologic examination of the specimen.

Cystosarcoma phyllodes is a fibroadenoma-like tumor with cellular stroma that tends to grow rapidly. This tumor may reach a large size and if inadequately excised will recur locally. The lesion is rarely malignant. Treatment is by local excision of the mass with a margin of surrounding breast tissue. The treatment of malignant cystosarcoma phyllodes is more controversial. In general, complete removal of the tumor and a rim of normal tissue should avoid recurrence. Since these tumors may be large, simple mastectomy is sometimes necessary to achieve complete control. Lymph node dissection is not necessary, since the sarcomatous portion of the tumor may metastasize directly to the lungs and not the lymph nodes.

Cant PJ et al: Non-operative management of breast masses diagnosed as fibroadenoma. Br J Surg 1995;82;792.

Cross MJ et al: Stereotactic breast biopsy as an alternative to open excisional biopsy. Ann Surg Oncol 1995;2:195.

Dupont WD et al: Long-term risk of breast cancer in women with fibroadenoma. N Engl J Med 1994;331:10.

Isaacs JH: Benign tumors of the breast. Obstet Gynecol Clin North Am 1994;21:487. A variety of benign tumors of the breast and their operative and nonoperative management.

McGregor GI, Knowling MA, Este FA: Sarcoma and cystosarcoma phyllodes tumors of the breast: A retrospective review of 58 cases. Am J Surg 1994;167:477. (Sarcoma and phyllodes tumors of the breast. Wide excision remains the only standard therapy for these unusual tumors.)

Reinfuss M et al: The treatment and prognosis of patients with phyllodes tumors of the breast: An analysis of 170 cases. Cancer 1996;77:910.

NIPPLE DISCHARGE

In order of increasing frequency, the following are the commonest causes of nipple discharge in the nonlactating breast: carcinoma, intraductal papilloma, and mammary dysplasia with ectasia of the ducts. The important characteristics of the discharge and some other factors to be evaluated by history and physical examination are as follows:

(1) Nature of discharge (serous, bloody, or other).
(2) Association with a mass or not.
(3) Unilateral or bilateral.
(4) Single duct or multiple duct discharge.
(5) Discharge is spontaneous (persistent or intermittent) or must be expressed.
(6) Discharge produced by pressure at a single site or by general pressure on the breast.
(7) Relation to menses.
(8) Premenopausal or postmenopausal.
(9) Patient taking contraceptive pills or estrogen.

Unilateral, spontaneous serous or serosanguineous discharge from a single duct is usually caused by an intraductal papilloma or, rarely, by an intraductal cancer. In either case, a mass may not be palpable. The involved duct may be identified by pressure at different sites around the nipple at the margin of the areola. Bloody discharge is more suggestive of cancer but is usually caused by a benign papilloma in the duct. Cytologic examination may identify malignant cells, but negative findings do not rule out cancer, which is more likely in women over age 50. In any case, the involved duct—and a mass if present—should be excised. Ductography may identify a filling defect prior to excision of the duct system but is of limited value since excision of the bloody duct system is indicated regardless of ductography findings.

In premenopausal women, spontaneous multiple duct discharge, unilateral or bilateral, most marked just before menstruation, is often due to mammary dysplasia. Discharge may be green or brownish. Papillomatosis and ductal ectasia are usually seen on biopsy. If a mass is present, it should be removed.

Milky discharge from multiple ducts in the nonlactating breast occurs in certain endocrine syndromes, presumably as a result of increased secretion of pituitary prolactin. Serum prolactin and TSH levels should be obtained to search for a pituitary tumor or hypothyroidism. Phenothiazines and contraceptive pills may also cause milky discharge that ceases on discontinuance of the medication.

Oral contraceptive agents or estrogen replacement therapy may cause clear, serous, or milky discharge from a single duct, but multiple duct discharge is more common. The discharge is more evident just before menstruation and disappears on stopping the medication. If it does not and is from a single duct, exploration should be considered.

Purulent discharge may originate in a subareolar abscess and require excision of the abscess and related lactiferous sinus.

When localization is not possible, no mass is palpable, and the discharge is nonbloody, the patient should be reexamined every 2 or 3 months for a year. Mammography should be done. Cytologic examination of nipple discharge for exfoliated cancer cells may rarely be helpful in diagnosis.

Chronic unilateral nipple discharge, especially if bloody, is an indication for resection of the involved ducts.

Gulay H et al: Management of nipple discharge. J Am Coll Surg 1994;178:471.

FAT NECROSIS

Fat necrosis is a rare lesion of the breast but is of clinical importance because it produces a mass, often accompanied by skin or nipple retraction, that is indistinguishable from carcinoma. Trauma is presumed to be the cause, though only about half of patients give a history of injury to the breast. Ecchymosis is occasionally seen near the tumor. Tenderness may or may not be present. If untreated, the mass associated with fat necrosis gradually disappears. As a rule, the safest course is to obtain a biopsy. The entire mass should be excised, primarily to rule out carcinoma. Fat necrosis is common after segmental resection and radiation therapy.

BREAST ABSCESS

During nursing, an area of redness, tenderness, and induration not infrequently develops in the breast. The organism most commonly found in these abscesses is *Staphylococcus aureus*. In the early stages, the infection can often be reversed while nursing is continued from that breast by administering an antibiotic such as dicloxacillin or oxacillin, 250 mg four times daily for 7–10 days (see Puerperal Mastitis, Chapter 18). If the lesion progresses to form a localized mass with local and systemic signs of infection, an abscess is present and should be drained, and nursing should be discontinued.

A subareolar abscess may develop (rarely) in young or middle-aged women who are not lactating. These infections tend to recur after incision and drainage unless the area is explored in a quiescent interval with excision of the involved lactiferous duct or ducts at the base of the nipple. Except for the subareolar type of abscess, infection in the breast is very rare unless the patient is lactating. In the nonlactating breast, inflammatory carcinoma must always be considered. Therefore, findings suggestive of abscess in the nonlactating breast are an indication for incision and biopsy of any indurated tissue. If the abscess can be percutaneously drained and completely resolves, the patient may be followed.

Schein M: Subareolar breast abscesses. Surgery 1996; 120:902. (Highly successful nonoperative ultrasound-guided aspiration and antibiotic therapy of breast abscesses. This should probably be the first choice for treatment of small lesions.)

DISORDERS OF THE AUGMENTED BREAST

Since the development of the silicone breast implant in the early 1960s, estimates are that nearly 4 million American women have had breast implants. Breast augmentation is performed by placing implants usually under the pectoralis muscle or, less desirably, in the subcutaneous tissue of the breast. Most implants are made of an outer silicone shell filled with a silicone gel, saline, or some combination of the two. About 15–25% of the patients develop capsule contraction or scarring around the implant, leading to a firmness and distortion of the breast that can be painful. Some require removal of the implant and capsule.

Implant rupture may occur in as many as 5–10% of women, and bleeding of gel through the capsule may occur even more commonly. While silicone gel may be an adjuvant for autoimmune reactions, there are no clinical data proving an increased incidence of connective tissue disorders in patients with silicone gel breast implants. A retrospective cohort study from the Mayo Clinic showed no increased incidence of autoimmune disorders among women with silicone implants. In April of 1992, the FDA concluded that the safety and effectiveness of silicone gel breast implants had not been established by manufacturers of these devices and called for additional preclinical and clinical studies. They advised symptomatic women with ruptured implants to discuss the need for surgical removal with their physicians. However, they noted that the risk of removal was probably greater than the risk of retention in asymptomatic women. Thus, women who are asymptomatic and have no evidence of rupture of a silicone gel prosthesis should probably not undergo removal of the implant. However, those in whom the implant has ruptured or who have symptoms suggestive of autoimmune disorder should discuss with a physician the risks and benefits of surgical removal.

Two large epidemiologic studies have failed to show any association between implants and an increased incidence of breast cancer. However, breast cancer may develop in any patient with a silicone gel prosthesis. The detection of breast cancer in patients with implants for augmentation mammoplasty is made more difficult since mammography is less able to detect early lesions. However, local recurrence after breast reconstruction for cancer is usually cutaneous or subcutaneous and is easily detectable by palpation. If a cancer develops, it should be treated in the same manner as in women without implants. Such women should be offered the option of mastectomy or breast-conserving therapy, which may require removal or replacement of the implant. Adjuvant treatments should be given for the same indications as for women who have no implants.

Bryant H, Brasher P: Breast implants and breast cancer: Reanalysis of a linkage study. N Engl J Med 1995; 332:1535.

Council on Scientific Affairs, AMA: Silicone gel breast implants. JAMA 1993;270:2602.

Gabriel SE et al: Complications leading to surgery after breast implantation. N Engl J Med 1997;336:677.

Gabriel SE et al: Risk of connective tissue diseases and other disorders after breast implantation. N Engl J Med 1994;330:1697.

Press RI et al: Antinuclear autoantibodies in women with silicone breast implants. Lancet 1992;340:1304.

Sanchez-Guerrero J et al: Silicone breast implants and the risk of connective-tissue diseases and symptoms. N Engl J Med 1995;332:1666.

CARCINOMA OF THE FEMALE BREAST

Essentials of Diagnosis

- Risk factors are delayed childbearing, positive family history of breast cancer, and personal history of breast cancer or some types of mammary dysplasia. Most women with breast cancer do not have identifiable risk factors.
- Early findings: Single, nontender, firm to hard mass with ill-defined margins; mammographic abnormalities and no palpable mass.
- Later findings: Skin or nipple retraction; axillary lymphadenopathy; breast enlargement, redness, edema, pain; fixation of mass to skin or chest wall.

INCIDENCE & RISK FACTORS

Aside from skin cancer, the breast is the most common site of cancer in women, and cancer of the breast is second only to lung cancer as a cause of death from cancer among women. The probability of developing breast cancer increases throughout life. The mean and the median age of women with breast cancer is between 60 and 61 years.

There will be about 182,000 new cases of breast cancer and about 46,000 deaths from this disease in women in the USA in 1998. At the present rate of incidence, the American Cancer Society predicts that one of every eight or nine American women will develop breast cancer during her lifetime. Women whose mothers or sisters had breast cancer are three to four times more likely to develop the disease than others. Risk is increased in patients whose mothers' or sisters' breast cancers occurred before menopause or was bilateral and in those with a family history of breast cancer in two or more first-degree relatives. However, there is no history of breast cancer among female relatives in over 90% of breast cancer patients. Nulliparous women and women whose first full-term pregnancy was after age 35 have a 1.5 times higher incidence of breast cancer than multiparous women. Late menarche and artificial menopause are associated with a lower incidence of breast cancer, whereas early menarche (under age 12) and late natural menopause (after age 50) are associated with a slight increase in risk of developing breast cancer. Mammary dysplasia (fibrocystic disease of the breast), when accompanied by proliferative changes, papillomatosis, or atypical epithelial hyperplasia, is associated with an increased incidence of cancer. A woman who has had cancer in one breast is at increased risk of developing cancer in the other breast. Such women develop a contralateral cancer at the rate of 1% or 2% per year. Women with cancer of the uterine corpus have a breast cancer risk significantly higher than that of the general population, and women with breast cancer have a comparably increased endometrial cancer risk. In the USA, breast cancer is more common in whites than in non-whites. The incidence of the disease among non-whites (mostly blacks), however, is increasing, especially in younger women. In general, rates reported from developing countries are low, whereas rates are high in developed countries, with the notable exception of Japan. Some of the variability may be due to underreporting in the developing countries, but a real difference probably exists. Dietary factors, particularly increased fat content, may account for some differences in incidence. Oral contraceptives do not appear to increase the risk of breast cancer. There is some evidence that administration of estrogens to postmenopausal women may result in a slightly increased risk of breast cancer, but only with higher, long-term doses of estrogens. Other studies suggest that only women with a family history of breast cancer who take postmenopausal estrogens or those who take estradiol or unconjugated estrogens do slightly increase their risk of breast cancer. Alcohol consumption may increase the risk of breast cancer slightly. Some inherited breast cancers have been found to be associated with a gene on chromosome 17. This gene, *BRCA1*, has been shown to be mutated in families with early-onset breast cancer and ovarian cancer. It is estimated that about 85% of women with *BRCA1* gene mutations will develop breast cancer in their lifetime. Other genes have recently been identified that are associated with increased risk of breast and other cancers, such as *BRCA2*, ataxia-telangiec-

tasia mutation, and *TP53*, the tumor suppressor gene. *TP53* mutations have been found in approximately 1% of breast cancers in women under 40 years of age. Genetic testing is now commercially available for women at high risk of breast cancer. Such genetic testing is highly controversial, as problems associated with management of patients with identified mutations, their insurability, and potential social conflicts are anticipated.

Women who are at greater than normal risk of developing breast cancer (Table 16–1) should be identified by their physicians, taught the techniques of breast self-examination, and followed carefully. Those with an exceptional family history should be counseled and given the option of genetic testing. Some of these high-risk women may consider prophylactic mastectomy.

There is no known way to prevent breast cancer. However, the NSABP began actually comparing tamoxifen with placebo for patients who show no evidence of breast cancer but who are at high risk for its occurrence. Perhaps because of recent adverse publicity concerning tamoxifen use and the increased risk of endometrial cancer, this controversial trial has not yet completed patient accrual. However, when completed, it may identify a pharmacologic means of preventing the disease in young women.

Beckhardt S for the American Society of Clinical Oncology. Statement of the American Society of Clinical Oncology: Genetic testing for cancer susceptibility. J Clin Oncol 1996;14:1730. (Summarizes the position of the American Society of Clinical Oncology on genetic testing for cancer susceptibility.)

Collaborative Group on Hormonal Factors in Breast Cancer (Radcliffe Infirmary, Oxford, England): Breast cancer and hormonal contraceptives: Collaborative reanalysis of individual data on 53,297 women with breast cancer and 100,239 women without breast cancer from 54 epidemiological studies. Lancet 1996;347:1713. (Examines the effect of oral contraceptives on the incidence of breast cancer. The relationship appears more complex than previously appreciated.)

Table 16–1. Factors associated with increased risk of breast cancer.[1]

Race	White
Age	Older
Family history	Breast cancer in mother, sister, or daughter (especially bilateral or premenopausal)
Genetics	*BRCA1* or *BRCA2* mutation
Previous medical history	Endometrial cancer Some forms of mammary dysplasia Cancer in other breast
Menstrual history	Early menarche (under age 12) Late menopause (after age 50)
Pregnancy	Nulliparous or late first pregnancy

[1]Normal lifetime risk in white women = 1 in 8 or 9.

Henderson BE, Ross RK, Pike MC: Hormonal chemoprevention of cancer in women. Science 1993;259:633.

Henrich JB: The postmenopausal estrogen/breast cancer controversy. JAMA 1992;268:1900.

Madigan MP et al: Proportion of breast cancer cases in the United States explained by well-established risk factors. J Natl Cancer Inst 1995;87:1681. (Known breast cancer risk factors and the estimated percentage of cases attributed to them.)

Marcus IN et al: Hereditary breast cancer: Pathobiology, prognosis, and BRCA1 and BRCA2 gene linkage. Cancer 1996;77:697.

The National Advisory Council for Human Genome Research: Statement on use of DNA testing for presymptomatic identification of cancer risk. JAMA 1994;271:785.

Page DL, Jensen RA: Evaluation and management of high risk and premalignant lesions of the breast. World J Surg 1994;18:32. (Breast cancer risks associated with benign breast disease, and recommended management based on risk.)

Pritchard KI, Sawka CA: Menopausal estrogen replacement therapy in women with breast cancer. Cancer 1995;75:1.

Thompson WD: Genetic epidemiology of breast cancer. Cancer 1994;74(1 Suppl):279.

EARLY DETECTION OF BREAST CANCER

Screening Programs

A number of mass screening programs consisting of physical and mammographic examination of the breasts of asymptomatic women have been conducted. Such programs frequently identify about ten cancers per 1000 women older than age 50 and about two cancers per 1000 women younger than age 50. About 80% of these women have negative axillary lymph nodes at the time of surgery, whereas only 45% of nonscreened women found in the course of usual medical practice have uninvolved axillary nodes. Detecting breast cancer before it has spread to the axillary nodes greatly increases the chance of survival, and about 85% of such women will survive at least 5 years.

Both physical examination and mammography are necessary for maximum yield in screening programs, since about 35–50% of early breast cancers can be discovered only by mammography and another 40% can be detected only by palpation. About one-third of the abnormalities detected on screening mammograms will be found to be malignant when biopsy is performed. Women 20–40 years of age should have a breast examination as part of routine medical care every 2–3 years. Women over age 40 should have yearly breast examinations. The sensitivity of mammography varies from approximately 60% to 90%. This sensitivity depends on several factors, including patient age (breast density), tumor size, location, and mammographic appearance. In young women with dense breasts, mammography is less sensitive than in older woman with fatty breasts, in whom mammography can detect at least 90% of malignancies.

Smaller tumors, particularly those without calcifications, are more difficult to detect, especially in dense breasts. The lack of sensitivity in young women has led to questions concerning the value of mammography for screening in women 40–50 years of age. The specificity of mammography in women under 50 years of age varies from about 30% to 40% for nonpalpable mammographic abnormalities to 85% to 90% for clinically evident malignancies.

In February 1993, the National Cancer Institute held an international workshop on screening for breast cancer. The purpose of this workshop was to undertake critical review of clinical screening trials. The conference examined only randomized studies and focused on clinical evidence related to the efficacy of breast cancer screening in various age groups. Of the eight randomized trials identified, only the Health Insurance Plan Project (HIP) demonstrated a beneficial effect of screening for women between ages 40 and 49 years. This benefit was seen between 10 and 18 years after entry into the study and resulted in a 25% decrease in deaths from breast cancer. Several Swedish trials showed a 13% decrease in breast cancer mortality for women in this age group after 12 years of follow-up; however, this decrease was not statistically significant. In a meta-analysis of five randomized trials, the breast cancer death rates were virtually identical in women aged 40–49 whether screened or not. The beneficial effect of screening in women aged 50–69 is undisputed and has been confirmed by all clinical trials. The efficacy of screening in older women—those older than 70—is inconclusive and is difficult to determine because of the very few women over 70 screened. Once the HIP study was published, there was general agreement that women older than 50 should have annual physical examination and mammography. This opinion was codified by various groups, including the National Cancer Institute, the American Cancer Society, and the American College of Radiology. However, serious doubt exists about the beneficial effect of screening in women under age 50. Questions such as the potential harmful effects of x-rays in a large population of young women and the general value of early detection were raised and largely ignored as various groups supported screening between ages 40 and 50. While the HIP study did show a beneficial effect of screening in such women, a recent Canadian trial demonstrated an unexplained shortening of survival time from time of random assignment to death in the screening group. The small number of patients in this study experienced no beneficial effect, but the 95% confidence interval included a potential lifesaving effect as well as a potential harmful effect. A very large number of patients is necessary to show a beneficial effect of screening among patients age 40–49, where the incidence of breast cancer is low. In addition, the problems of crossover of patients in the control group with women undergoing physician examination and nonscreening mammograms, problems with mammography quality, and problems in recruitment, randomization, and compliance make the interpretation of such trials extremely difficult.

Until recently, the policy of the NCI was simply that there is no agreement about the role of screening mammography for women aged 40–49. This uncertainty and the recommendation of a recent Swedish consensus panel led the NCI to reconsider its position on screening mammography for women in their 40s. In January 1997, and NCI consensus panel convened to reexamine this issue. Two of the Swedish trials now showed a statistical advantage for screening women in their 40s, and a meta-analysis similarly showed a statistical survival advantage for screened women with longer follow-up. In March 1997, the National Cancer Advisory Board recommended that women with average risk factors should have screening mammography every 1–2 years in their 40s and that women at higher risk should seek expert medical advice on when to begin screening. The American Cancer Society then recommended screening every year for asymptomatic women starting at age 40.

Screening of women older than age 70 should be performed after consideration by the physician of the patient's comorbid conditions and her overall state of health.

Ductography is occasionally useful to evaluate the cause of nipple discharge. In this study, the radiologist injects contrast medium into the discharging duct and obtains a mammogram. The injected duct may contain a filling defect (most commonly an intraductal papilloma) or may have a dilated or cystic appearance in patients with duct ectasia or fibrocystic disease. Malignancy may appear as an abrupt obstruction or filling defect. However, in the patient with a bloody discharge, ductography is not useful since operation is indicated regardless of the ductography findings.

Self-Examination

All women over age 20 should be advised to examine their breasts monthly. Premenopausal women should perform the examination 7–8 days after the menstrual period. The breasts should be inspected initially while standing before a mirror with the hands at the sides, overhead, and pressed firmly on the hips to contract the pectoralis muscles. Masses, asymmetry of breasts, and slight dimpling of the skin may become apparent as a result of these maneuvers. Next, in a supine position, each breast should be carefully palpated with the fingers of the opposite hand. Physicians should instruct women in the technique of self-examination and advise them to report at once for medical evaluation if a mass or other abnormality is noted.

Some women discover small breast lumps more readily when their skin is moist while bathing or showering.

Most women do not practice self-examination, and its value is controversial. Clearly, however, it is not harmful, it is inexpensive, and it may be beneficial.

Mammography

Mammography is the most useful technique for the detection of early breast cancer. The two methods of mammography in common use are ordinary film screen radiography and xeroradiography. From the standpoint of diagnosing breast cancer, the two methods give comparable results. Using film screen techniques, it is now possible to perform a high-quality mammogram while delivering less than 0.4 cGy to the mid breast per view, and for this reason film screen mammography has largely replaced the xeromammographic technique, which delivers more radiation.

Mammography is the only reliable means of detecting breast cancer before a mass can be palpated in the breast. Slowly growing breast cancers can be identified by mammography at least 2 years before reaching a size detectable by palpation.

Calcifications are the most easily recognized mammographic abnormality. The most common mammographic abnormalities associated with carcinoma of the breast are clustered polymorphic microcalcifications. Such calcifications are usually at least five to eight in number, aggregated in one part of the breast and differing from each other in size and shape, often including branched or V- or Y-shaped configurations. There may be an associated mammographic mass density or, at time, only a mass density with no calcifications. Such a density usually has irregular or ill-defined borders and may lead to architectural distortion within the breast. A small mass or architectural distortion, particularly in a dense breast, may be subtle and difficult to detect.

Indications for mammography are as follows: (1) to screen at regular intervals women who are at high risk for developing breast cancer (see above); (2) to evaluate each breast when a diagnosis of potentially curable breast cancer has been made, and at yearly intervals thereafter; (3) to evaluate a questionable or ill-defined breast mass or other suspicious change in the breast; (4) to search for an occult breast cancer in a woman with metastatic disease in axillary nodes or elsewhere from an unknown primary; (5) to screen women prior to cosmetic operations or prior to biopsy of a mass, to examine for an unsuspected cancer; and (6) to follow those women with breast cancer who have been treated with breast-conserving surgery and radiation.

Patients with a dominant or suspicious mass must undergo biopsy despite mammographic findings. The mammogram should be obtained prior to biopsy so that other suspicious areas can be noted and the contralateral breast can be checked. Mammography is never a substitute for biopsy, because it may not reveal clinical cancer in a very dense breast, as may be seen in young women with mammary dysplasia, and may not reveal medullary type cancers.

Communication and documentation between the patient, the referring physician, and the interpreting physician are critical for high-quality screening and diagnostic mammography. The patient should be informed about *how* she will receive timely results of her mammogram; that mammography does not "rule out" cancer, and that she should expect a correlative examination at the mammography facility if referred for a suspicious lesion. She should also be aware of the technique and need for breast compression and that this may be uncomfortable. The mammography facility should be informed *in writing* of abnormal physical examination findings. It is strongly recommended in the AHCPR Clinical Practice Guideline that all mammography reports be communicated with the patient as well as the health care provider in writing. Additional phone communication about any abnormal findings should take place between the interpreting and referring physicians.

Baines CJ: The Canadian National Breast Screening Study: A perspective on criticisms. Ann Intern Med 1994; 120:326.

Brenner RJ: Breast MR imaging: An analysis of its role with respect to other imaging and interventional modalities. MRI Clin North Am 1994;2:705.

Feig SA: Doubtful results in the Canadian national breast screening study. Breast Diseases 1996;6:354.

Feig SA: Estimation of currently obtainable benefit from mammographic screening of women aged 40–49 years. Cancer 1995;75:2412.

Kopans DB: Screening for breast cancer and mortality reductions among women 40–49 years of age. Cancer 1994;74:311.

Leitch MA et al: American Cancer Society guidelines for the early detection of breast cancer: Update 1997. CA Cancer J Clin 1997;47:150. (Includes the most recent recommendations of the American Cancer Society, similar to but not identical with those of the National Cancer Institute.)

Mettler FA et al: Benefits versus risks from mammography: A critical reassessment. Cancer 1996;77:903.

Tabar L et al: Efficacy of breast cancer screening by age: New results from the Swedish two-county trial. Cancer 1995;75:2507.

Clinical Clues to Early Detection of Breast Cancer

A. Symptoms and Signs: The presenting complaint in about 70% of patients with breast cancer is a lump (usually painless) in the breast. About 90% of breast masses are discovered by the patient herself. Less frequent symptoms are breast pain; nipple discharge; erosion, retraction, enlargement, or itching of the nipple; and redness, generalized hardness, enlargement, or shrinking of the breast. Rarely, an axillary mass or swelling of the arm may be the first symptom. Back or bone pain, jaundice, or weight loss may be the result of systemic metastases,

but these symptoms are rarely seen on initial presentation.

The relative frequency of carcinoma in various anatomic sites in the breast is shown in Figure 16–1.

Inspection of the breast is the first step in physical examination and should be carried out with the patient sitting, arms at sides and then overhead. Abnormal variations in breast size and contour, minimal nipple retraction, and slight edema, redness, or retraction of the skin can be identified. Asymmetry of the breasts and retraction or dimpling of the skin can often be accentuated by having the patient raise her arms overhead or press her hands on her hips in order to contract the pectoralis muscles. Axillary and supraclavicular areas should be thoroughly palpated for enlarged nodes with the patient sitting (Figure 16–2). Palpation of the breast for masses or other changes should be performed with the patient both seated and supine with the arm abducted (Figure 16–3). Some authorities recommend palpation with a rotary motion of the examiner's fingers as well as a horizontal stripping motion.

Breast cancer usually consists of a nontender, firm or hard mass with poorly delineated margins (caused by local infiltration). Slight skin or nipple retraction is an important sign. Minimal asymmetry of the breast may be noted. Very small (1–2 mm) erosions of the nipple epithelium may be the only manifestation of Paget's carcinoma. Watery, serous, or bloody discharge from the nipple is an occasional early sign but is more often associated with benign disease.

A lesion smaller than 1 cm in diameter may be dif-

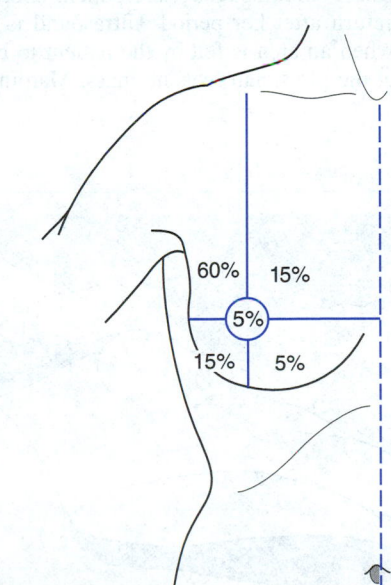

Figure 16–1. Frequency of breast carcinoma at various anatomic sites.

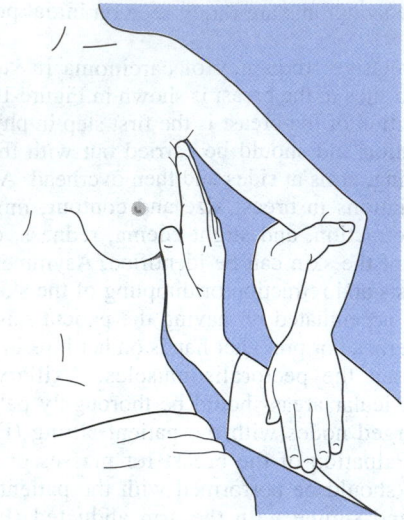

Figure 16–2. Palpation of axillary region for enlarged lymph nodes.

ficult or impossible for the examiner to feel and yet may be discovered by the patient. She should always be asked to demonstrate the location of the mass; if the physician fails to confirm the patient's suspicions, the examination should be repeated in 2–3 months, preferably 1–2 weeks after the onset of menses. During the premenstrual phase of the cycle, increased innocuous nodularity may suggest neoplasm or may obscure an underlying lesion. If there is any question regarding the nature of an abnormality under these circumstances, the patient should be asked to return after her period. Ultrasound is often valuable when an area is felt by the patient to be abnormal but the physician feels no mass. Mammogra-

phy must always be performed if the patient suspects an abnormality.

The following are characteristic of advanced carcinoma: edema, redness, nodularity, or ulceration of the skin; the presence of a large primary tumor; fixation to the chest wall; enlargement, shrinkage, or retraction of the breast; marked axillary lymphadenopathy; supraclavicular lymphadenopathy; edema of the ipsilateral arm; and distant metastases.

Metastases tend to involve regional lymph nodes, which may be clinically palpable. With regard to the axilla, one or two movable, nontender, not particularly firm lymph nodes 5 mm or less in diameter are frequently present and are generally of no significance. Firm or hard nodes larger than 1 cm in diameter usually contain metastases. Axillary nodes that are matted or fixed to skin or deep structures indicate advanced disease (at least stage III). Histologic studies show that microscopic metastases are present in about 30% of patients with clinically negative nodes. On the other hand, if the examiner thinks that the axillary nodes are involved, that impression will be borne out by histologic section in about 85% of cases. The incidence of positive axillary nodes increases with the size of the primary tumor. Noninvasive cancers do not metastasize.

In most cases no nodes are palpable in the supraclavicular fossa. Firm or hard nodes of any size in this location or just beneath the clavicle (infraclavicular nodes) are suggestive of metastatic cancer and should be biopsied. Ipsilateral supraclavicular or infraclavicular nodes containing cancer indicate that the tumor is in an advanced stage (stage IV). Edema of the ipsilateral arm, commonly caused by metastatic infiltration of regional lymphatics, is also a sign of advanced (stage IV) cancer.

B. Laboratory Findings: A consistently elevated sedimentation rate may be the result of disseminated cancer. Liver or bone metastases may be associated with elevation of serum alkaline phosphatase. Hypercalcemia is an occasional important finding in advanced cancer of the breast. Carcinoembryonic antigen (CEA) and CA15-3 may be used as markers for recurrent breast cancer.

C. Imaging for Metastases: Chest radiographs may show pulmonary metastases. CT scanning of the liver and brain is of value only when metastases are suspected in these areas. Bone scans utilizing technetium Tc 99m-labeled phosphates or phosphonates are more sensitive than skeletal x-rays in detecting metastatic breast cancer. Bone scanning has not proved to be of clinical value as a routine preoperative test in the absence of symptoms, physical findings, or abnormal alkaline phosphatase levels. The frequency of abnormal findings on bone scan parallels the status of the axillary lymph nodes on pathologic examination. Bone scan should be performed for patients with symptoms and for those with elevated calcium or alkaline phosphatase levels.

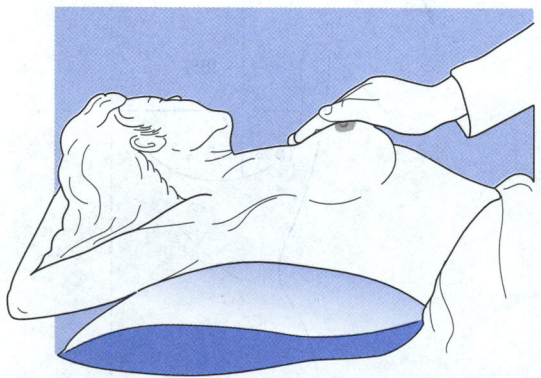

Figure 16–3. Palpation of breasts. Palpation is performed with the patient supine and arm abducted.

Positron emission tomography (PET) is being clinically evaluated and may prove to be an effective single scan for bone and soft tissue or visceral metastases in patients with signs or symptoms of metastatic disease.

D. Diagnostic Tests:

1. Biopsy—The diagnosis of breast cancer depends ultimately upon examination of tissue or cells removed by biopsy. Treatment should never be undertaken without an unequivocal histologic or cytologic diagnosis of cancer. The safest course is biopsy examination of all suspicious masses found on physical examination or, in the absence of a mass, of suspicious lesions demonstrated by mammography. About 60% of lesions thought to be definitely cancer prove on biopsy to be benign, and about 30% of lesions believed to be benign are found to be malignant. These findings demonstrate the fallibility of clinical judgment and the necessity for biopsy. A breast mass should not be followed without histologic diagnosis, except perhaps in the premenopausal woman with a nonsuspicious mass presumed to be fibrocystic disease. A lesion such as this could be observed through one or two menstrual cycles. However, if the mass does not completely resolve during this time, it must be biopsied. Figures 16–4 and 16–5

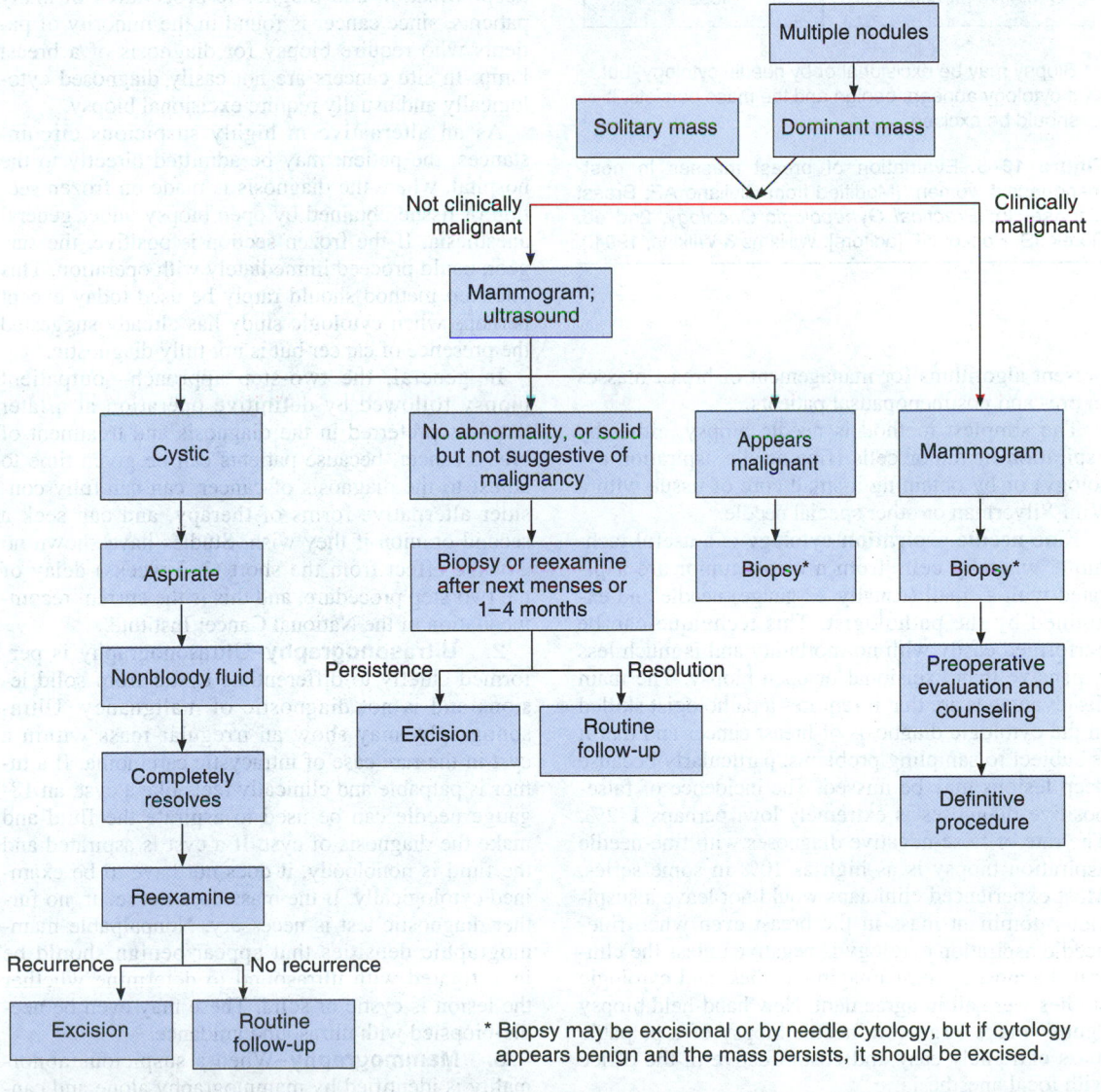

Figure 16–4. Evaluation of breast masses in premenopausal women. (Modified from Giuliano AE: Breast disease. In: *Practical Gynecologic Oncology,* 2nd ed. Berek JS, Hacker NF [editors]. Williams & Wilkins, 1994.)

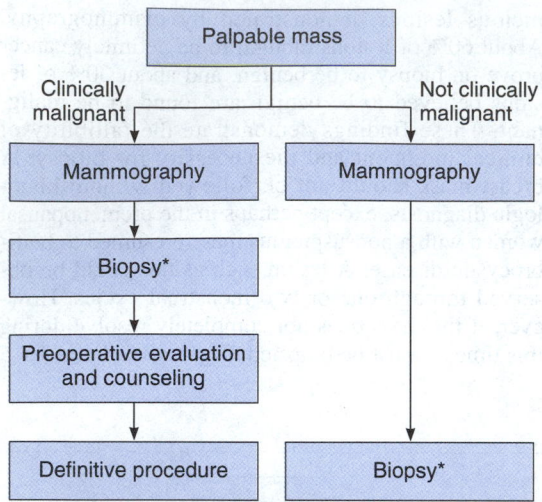

* Biopsy may be excisional or by needle cytology, but
if cytology appears benign and the mass persists, it
should be excised.

Figure 16–5. Evaluation of breast masses in postmenopausal women. (Modified from Giuliano AE: Breast
disease. In: *Practical Gynecologic Oncology*, 2nd ed.
Berek JS, Hacker NF [editors]. Williams & Wilkins, 1994.)

present algorithms for management of breast masses
in pre- and postmenopausal patients.

The simplest method is needle biopsy, either by
aspiration of tumor cells (fine-needle aspiration cytology) or by obtaining a small core of tissue with a
Vim-Silverman or other special needle.

Fine-needle aspiration cytology is a useful technique whereby cells from a breast tumor are aspirated with a small (usually 22-gauge) needle and examined by the pathologist. This technique can be
performed easily with no morbidity and is much less
expensive than excisional or open biopsy. The main
disadvantages are that it requires a pathologist skilled
in the cytologic diagnosis of breast cancer and that it
is subject to sampling problems, particularly because
deep lesions may be missed. The incidence of false-
positive diagnoses is extremely low, perhaps 1–2%.
The rate of false-negative diagnoses with fine-needle
aspiration biopsy is as high as 10% in some series.
Most experienced clinicians would not leave a suspicious dominant mass in the breast even when fine-
needle aspiration cytology is negative unless the clinical diagnosis, breast imaging studies, and cytologic
studies were all in agreement. New hand-held biopsy
"guns" make large-core needle biopsy of a palpable
mass extremely easy and cost-effective in the office
with local anesthesia.

Large-needle (core needle) biopsy is an accepted
diagnostic technique in which a core of tissue is removed with a large cutting needle. As in the case of
any needle biopsy, the main problem is sampling error due to improper positioning of the needle, giving
rise to a false-negative test result.

Open biopsy under local anesthesia as a separate
procedure prior to deciding upon definitive treatment
is the most reliable means of diagnosis. Needle
biopsy or aspiration, when positive for malignancy,
offers a more rapid approach with less morbidity, but
when nondiagnostic it must be followed by excisional biopsy.

Decisions on additional workup for metastatic disease and on definitive therapy can be made and discussed with the patient after the histologic or cytologic diagnosis of cancer has been established. This
approach has the advantage of avoiding unnecessary
hospitalization and diagnostic procedures in many
patients, since cancer is found in the minority of patients who require biopsy for diagnosis of a breast
lump. In situ cancers are not easily diagnosed cytologically and usually require excisional biopsy.

As an alternative in highly suspicious circumstances, the patient may be admitted directly to the
hospital, where the diagnosis is made on frozen section of tissue obtained by open biopsy under general
anesthesia. If the frozen section is positive, the surgeon could proceed immediately with operation. This
one-step method should rarely be used today except
perhaps when cytologic study has already suggested
the presence of cancer but is not fully diagnostic.

In general, the two-step approach—outpatient
biopsy followed by definitive operation at a later
date—is preferred in the diagnosis and treatment of
breast cancer, because patients can be given time to
adjust to the diagnosis of cancer, can carefully consider alternative forms of therapy, and can seek a
second opinion if they wish. Studies have shown no
adverse effect from the short (1–2 weeks) delay of
the two-step procedure, and this is the current recommendation of the National Cancer Institute.

2. Ultrasonography–Ultrasonography is performed chiefly to differentiate cystic from solid lesions and is not diagnostic of malignancy. Ultrasonography may show an irregular mass within a
cyst in the rare case of intracystic carcinoma. If a tumor is palpable and clinically feels like a cyst, an 18-
gauge needle can be used to aspirate the fluid and
make the diagnosis of cyst. If a cyst is aspirated and
the fluid is nonbloody, it does not have to be examined cytologically. If the mass does not recur, no further diagnostic test is necessary. Nonpalpable mammographic densities that appear benign should be
investigated with ultrasound to determine whether
the lesion is cystic or solid. These may even be nee-
dle-biopsied with ultrasound guidance.

3. Mammography–When a suspicious abnormality is identified by mammography alone and cannot be palpated by the clinician, the patient should be
studied by **computerized stereotactic modifica-**

tions, which have been added to mammographic units in order to localize abnormalities and perform needle biopsy without surgery. Under mammographic guidance, a biopsy needle can be inserted into the lesion in the mammographer's suite, and a core of tissue for histologic examination or cells for cytology can be examined.

Mammographic localization biopsy is performed by obtaining a mammogram in two perpendicular views and placing a needle or hook-wire near the abnormality so that the surgeon can use the metal needle or wire as a guide during operation to locate the lesion. After mammography confirms the position of the needle in relation to the lesion, an incision is made and the subcutaneous tissue is dissected until the needle is identified. Using the films as a guide, the abnormality can then be localized and excised. It often happens that the abnormality cannot even be palpated through the incision—this is the case with microcalcifications—and it is thus essential to obtain a mammogram of the specimen to document that the lesion was excised. At that time, a second marker needle can further localize the lesion for the pathologist. Studies of stereotactic core needle biopsies show results equivalent to mammographic localization biopsies. Core biopsy is preferable to mammographic localization for accessible lesions.

4. Other imaging modalities–Other modalities of breast imaging have been investigated. Automated breast ultrasonography is very useful in distinguishing cystic from solid lesions but should be used only as a supplement to physical examination and mammography in screening for breast cancer. Ductography may be useful to define the site of a lesion causing a bloody discharge, but since biopsy is always indicated, ductography may be omitted and the blood-filled nipple system excised. Diaphanography (transillumination of the breasts) and thermography are of no proved screening value.

5. Cytology–Cytologic examination of nipple discharge or cyst fluid may be helpful on rare occasions. As a rule, mammography (or ductography) and breast biopsy are required when nipple discharge or cyst fluid is bloody or cytologically questionable.

Cox CE et al: Analysis of residual cancer after diagnostic breast biopsy: An argument for fine-needle aspiration cytology. Ann Surg Oncol 1995;2:201.

Israel PZ, Fine RE: Stereotactic needle biopsy for occult breast lesions: A minimally invasive alternative. Am Surg 1995;61:87.

Jansson T et al: Positron emission tomography studies in patients with locally advanced and/or metastatic breast cancer: A method for early therapy evaluation? J Clin Oncol 1995;13:1470.

Liberman L et al: Atypical ductal hyperplasia diagnosed at stereotactic core biopsy of breast lesions: An indication for surgical biopsy. AJR Am J Roentgenol 1995; 164:1111.

Parker SH et al: Percutaneous large-core breast biopsy: A multi-institutional study. Radiology 1994;193:359.

Sailors DM et al: Needle localization for nonpalpable breast lesions. Am Surg 1994;60:186.

Stavros AT et al: Solid breast nodules: Use of sonography to distinguish between benign and malignant lesions. Radiology 1995;196:123.

DIFFERENTIAL DIAGNOSIS

The lesions to be considered most often in the differential diagnosis of breast cancer are the following, in descending order of frequency: mammary dysplasia (cystic disease of the breast), fibroadenoma, intraductal papilloma, lipoma, and fat necrosis. The differential diagnosis of a breast lump should be established without delay by biopsy, by aspiration of a cyst, or by observing the patient until disappearance of the lump within a period of a few weeks.

STAGING

The extent of disease evident from physical findings and special preoperative studies is used to determine its clinical stage. Currently, the American Joint Committee on Cancer and the International Union Against Cancer have agreed on a TNM (Tumor, Regional Lymph Nodes, Distant Metastases) staging system for breast cancer. The use of this uniform TNM staging system will enhance communication among investigators and clinicians. Table 16–2 sets forth the TNM classification.

Giuliano AE et al: Lymphatic mapping and sentinel lymphadenectomy for breast cancer. Ann Surg 1994;220: 391.

Giuliano AK et al: Improved axillary staging of breast cancer with sentinel lymphadenectomy. Ann Surg 1995; 222:394.

Loprinzi CL et al: Do American oncologists know how to use prognostic variables for patients with newly diagnosed primary breast cancer? J Clin Oncol 1994;12: 1422.

Piccirillo JF, Feinstein AR: Clinical symptoms and co-morbidity: Significance for the prognostic classification of cancer. Cancer 1996;77:834.

PATHOLOGIC TYPES

Numerous pathologic subtypes of breast cancer can be identified histologically (Table 16–3). These types are distinguished by the histologic appearance and growth pattern of the tumor. In general, breast cancer arises either from the epithelial lining of the large or intermediate-sized ducts (ductal) or from the epithelium of the terminal ducts of the lobules (lobular). The cancer may be invasive or in situ. Most breast cancers arise from the intermediate ducts and

Table 16–2. TNM staging for breast cancer.[1]

Stage	T	N	M
0	Tis	N0	M0
I	T1	N0	M0
IIA	T0	N1	M0
	T1	N1	M0
	T2	N0	M0
IIB	T2	N1	M0
	T3	N0	M0
IIIA	T0	N2	M0
	T1	N2	M0
	T2	N2	M0
	T3	N1, N2	M0
IIIB	T4	Any N	M0
	Any T	N3	M0
IV	Any T	Any N	M1

Tumor Size (T)

TX	Primary tumor cannot be assessed.
T0	No evidence of primary tumor.
Tis	Carcinoma in situ; intraductal carcinoma, lobular carcinoma in situ, or Paget's disease of the nipple with no tumor.
T1	Tumor 2 cm or less in greatest dimension.
	T1a 0.5 cm or less in greatest dimension.
	T1b More than 0.5 cm but not more than 1 cm in greatest dimension.
	T1c More than 1 cm but not more than 2 cm in greatest dimension.
T2	Tumor more than 2 cm but not more than 5 cm in greatest dimension.
T3	Tumor more than 5 cm in greatest dimension.
T4	Tumor of any size with direct extension to chest wall or skin.
	T4a Extension to chest wall.
	T4b Edema, ulceration, or skin satellite nodules (same breast).
	T4c Both (T4a and T4b).

Regional Lymph Nodes (N)

NX	Regional lymph nodes cannot be assessed (eg, previously removed).
N0	No regional lymph node metastases.
N1	Metastasis to movable ipsilateral axillary lymph node(s).
N2	Metastasis to ipsilateral axillary lymph node(s) fixed to one another or to other structures.
N3	Metastasis to ipsilateral internal mammary lymph node(s).

Distant Metastases (M)

MX	Presence of distant metastasis cannot be assessed.
M0	No distant metastasis.
M1	Distant metastasis (includes metastasis to ipsilateral supraclavicular lymph node[s]).

[1]American Joint Committee on Cancer: *Manual for Staging of Cancer,* 4th ed. Lippincott, 1992.

Table 16–3. Histologic types of breast cancer.

Type	Frequency of Occurrence
Infiltrating ductal (not otherwise specified)	80–90%
Medullary	5–8%
Colloid (mucinous)	2–4%
Tubular	1–2%
Papillary	1–2%
Invasive lobular	6–8%
Noninvasive	4–6%
Intraductal	2–3%
Lobular in situ	2–3%
Rare cancers	<1%
Juvenile (secretory)	
Adenoid cystic	
Epidermoid	
Sudoriferous	

are invasive (invasive ductal, infiltrating ductal), and most histologic types are merely subtypes of invasive ductal cancer with unusual growth patterns (colloid, medullary, scirrhous, etc). Ductal carcinoma that has not invaded the extraductal tissue is intraductal or in situ ductal. Lobular carcinoma may be either invasive or in situ.

Except for the in situ cancers, the histologic subtypes have only a slight bearing on prognosis when outcomes are compared after accurate staging. Various histologic parameters, such as invasion of blood vessels, tumor differentiation, invasion of breast lymphatics, and tumor necrosis have been examined, but they too seem to have little prognostic value.

The noninvasive cancers by definition are confined by the basement membrane of the ducts and lack the ability to spread. However, in patients whose biopsies show noninvasive intraductal cancer, associated invasive ductal cancers are present in about 1–3% of cases. Lobular carcinoma in situ (LCIS) is a premalignant lesion that is not a true cancer but is a risk factor associated with subsequent development of invasive cancer in at least 20% of cases.

SPECIAL CLINICAL FORMS OF BREAST CANCER

Paget's Carcinoma

The basic lesion is usually an infiltrating ductal carcinoma, usually well differentiated, or a ductal carcinoma in situ (DCIS). The ducts of the nipple epithelium are infiltrated, but gross nipple changes are often minimal, and a tumor mass may not be palpable. The first symptom is often itching or burning of the nipple, with superficial erosion or ulceration. The diagnosis is established by biopsy of the erosion.

Paget's carcinoma is not common (about 1% of all breast cancers), but it is important because the nipple changes appear innocuous. These are frequently diagnosed and treated as dermatitis or bacterial infection, leading to unfortunate delay in detection. When the lesion consists of nipple changes only, the incidence of axillary metastases is less than 5%, and the prognosis is excellent. When a breast mass is also present, the incidence of axillary metastases rises, with an associated marked decrease in prospects for cure by surgical or other treatment.

Inflammatory Carcinoma

This is the most malignant form of breast cancer and constitutes less than 3% of all cases. The clinical findings consist of a rapidly growing, sometimes painful mass that enlarges the breast. The overlying skin becomes erythematous, edematous, and warm. Often there is no distinct mass, since the tumor infiltrates the involved breast diffusely. The diagnosis should be made when the redness involves more than one-third of the skin over the breast and biopsy shows infiltrating carcinoma with invasion of the subdermal lymphatics. The inflammatory changes, often mistaken for an infection, are caused by carcinomatous invasion of the subdermal lymphatics, with resulting edema and hyperemia. If the physician suspects infection but the lesion does not respond rapidly (1–2 weeks) to antibiotics, biopsy examination must be performed. Metastases tend to occur early and widely, and for this reason inflammatory carcinoma is rarely curable. Mastectomy is seldom indicated unless chemotherapy and radiation have resulted in clinical remission with no evidence of distant metastases. In these cases, residual disease in the breast may be eradicated. Radiation, hormone therapy, and anticancer chemotherapy are the measures most likely to be of value rather than operation.

Breast Cancer Occurring During Pregnancy or Lactation

Only 1–2% of breast cancers occur during pregnancy or lactation. Breast cancer complicates approximately one in 3000 pregnancies. The diagnosis is frequently delayed, because physiologic changes in the breast may obscure the lesion. This results in a tendency of both patients and physicians to misinterpret findings and to procrastinate in deciding on biopsy. When the cancer is confined to the breast, the 5-year survival rate after mastectomy is about 70%. Axillary metastases are already present in 60–70% of patients, and for them the 5-year survival rate after mastectomy is only 30–40%. Pregnancy (or lactation) is not a contraindication to operation, and treatment should be based on the stage of the disease as in the nonpregnant (or nonlactating) woman. Overall survival rates have improved, since cancers are now diagnosed in pregnant women earlier than in the past. Breast-conserving surgery, radiation, and even chemotherapy may be performed usually after delivery of the infant.

Bilateral Breast Cancer

Clinically evident simultaneous bilateral breast cancer occurs in less than 1% of cases, but there is a 5–8% incidence of later occurrence of cancer in the second breast. Bilaterality occurs more often in familial breast cancer, and women under age 50 and is more frequent when the tumor in the primary breast is lobular. The incidence of second breast cancers increases directly with the length of time the patient is alive after her first cancer—about 1% per year.

In patients with breast cancer, mammography should be performed before primary treatment and at regular intervals thereafter, to search for occult cancer in the opposite breast. Routine biopsy of the opposite breast is usually not warranted even for lobular cancer.

Noninvasive Cancer

Noninvasive cancer can occur within the ducts (ductal carcinoma in situ) or lobules (lobular carcinoma in situ). While ductal carcinoma in situ behaves as an early malignancy, lobular carcinoma in situ would perhaps be better called lobular neoplasia. Ductal carcinoma in situ tends to be unilateral and most likely would progress to invasive cancer if untreated. Approximately 40–60% of women who have ductal carcinoma in situ treated with biopsy alone will develop invasive cancer within the same breast. Lobular carcinoma in situ, however, appears to be more of a risk factor calling attention to the probability of developing invasive cancer in either breast. Approximately 20% of women with lobular carcinoma in situ will develop invasive cancer. This invasive cancer may occur in either breast regardless of the side of the original biopsy and is usually ductal.

The treatment of intraductal lesions is controversial. Ductal carcinoma can be treated with total mastectomy or breast conservation with wide excision with or without radiation therapy. Lobular carcinoma in situ is probably best managed with careful observation. However, patients who are unwilling to accept the increased risk of breast cancer may be offered bilateral total mastectomy. Axillary metastases from in situ cancers should not occur unless there is an occult invasive cancer.

Barth A, Brenner RJ, Giuliano EA: Current management of ductal carcinoma in situ. West J Med 1995;163:360. (The biology, diagnosis, and natural history of breast carcinoma in situ, summarizing various approaches to management.)

Fisher ER et al: Pathologic findings from the National Surgical Adjuvant Breast Project (NSABP) Protocol B-17: Intraductal carcinoma (ductal carcinoma in situ). Cancer 1995;75:1310.

Glass JL, Frazee RC: Inflammatory breast cancer. Am Surg 1995;61:121.

Perez CA et al: Management of locally advanced carcinoma of the breast: II. Inflammatory carcinoma. Cancer 1994;74:466.

Silverstein MJ et al: Prognostic classification of breast ductal carcinoma in situ. Lancet 1995;354:1154.

Solin LJ et al: Fifteen-year results of breast conserving surgery and definitive breast irradiation for the treatment of ductal carcinoma in situ of the breast. J Clin Oncol 1996;14:754. (Showing that breast conservation is feasible in this group of patients.)

HORMONE RECEPTOR SITES

The presence or absence of estrogen and progesterone receptors in the cytoplasm of tumor cells is of paramount importance in managing patients with breast cancer. Patients whose primary tumors are receptor-positive have a more favorable course than those whose tumors are receptor-negative. Receptors are of proved value in determining adjuvant therapy and therapy for patients with advanced disease. Up to 60% of patients with metastatic breast cancer will respond to hormonal manipulation if their tumors contain estrogen receptors. However, fewer than 5% of patients with metastatic, estrogen receptor-negative tumors can be successfully treated with hormonal manipulation.

Receptor status is not only valuable for the management of metastatic disease but helps in the selection of patients for adjuvant therapy. Adjuvant hormonal therapy (tamoxifen) for patients with receptor-positive tumors and adjuvant chemotherapy for patients with receptor-negative tumors improve survival rates even in the absence of lymph node metastases (see Adjuvant Therapy, below).

Progesterone receptors may be an even more sensitive indicator than estrogen receptors of patients who may respond to hormonal manipulation. Up to 80% of patients with metastatic progesterone receptor-positive tumors seem to respond to hormonal manipulation. Receptors probably have no relationship to response to chemotherapy.

Estrogen and progesterone receptor assays should be done routinely for every breast cancer at the time of initial diagnosis, either by quantitative assay or by immunohistochemistry. Receptor status may change after hormonal therapy, radiotherapy, or chemotherapy.

Khan SA et al: Estrogen expression of benign breast epithelium and its association with breast cancer. Cancer Res 1994;54:993.

Li BDL et al: Estrogen and progesterone receptor concordance between primary and recurrent breast cancer. J Surg Oncol 1994;57:71.

Roodi N et al: Estrogen receptor gene analysis in estrogen receptor-positive and receptor-negative primary breast cancer. J Natl Cancer Inst 1995;87:446.

CURATIVE TREATMENT

Treatment may be curative or palliative. Curative treatment is advised for clinical stage I and stage II disease (Table 16–2). Patients with locally advanced (stage III) and even inflammatory tumors may be cured with multimodality therapy, but in most cases palliation is all that can be expected. Palliative treatment is appropriate for all patients with stage IV disease and for previously treated patients who develop distant metastases or who have unresectable local cancers.

The growth potential of tumors and host resistance factors vary over a wide range from patient to patient and may be altered during the course of the disease. The doubling time of breast cancer cells ranges from several weeks in a rapidly growing lesion to nearly a year in a slowly growing one. Assuming that the rate of doubling is constant and that the neoplasm originates in one cell, a carcinoma with a doubling time of 100 days may not reach clinically detectable size (1 cm) for about 8 years. On the other hand, rapidly growing cancers have a much shorter preclinical course and a greater tendency to metastasize to regional nodes or more distant sites by the time a breast mass is discovered.

The relatively long preclinical growth phase and the tendency of breast cancers to metastasize have led many clinicians to believe that breast cancer is a systemic disease at the time of diagnosis. Although it may be true that breast cancer cells are released from the tumor prior to diagnosis, variations in the host-tumor relationship may prohibit the growth of disseminated disease in many patients. Clearly, not all breast cancer is systemic at the time of diagnosis. For this reason, a pessimistic attitude concerning the management of localized breast cancer is not warranted, and many patients can be cured with proper treatment.

Controversy surrounds the timing of surgery with respect to the menstrual cycle. Some studies suggest that operation during the time of unopposed estrogen adversely affects survival. Despite the media attention, most studies support no effect of the timing of surgery on prognosis. Scheduling of surgery on the basis of the menstrual cycle is unjustifiable.

Choice of Primary Therapy

The extent of disease and its biologic aggressiveness are the principal determinants of the outcome of primary therapy. Clinical and pathologic staging help in assessing extent of disease (Table 16–2), but each is to some extent imprecise. Other factors such as DNA flow cytometry, tumor grade, hormone receptor assays, and oncogene amplification may be of prognostic value but are not important in determining the type of local therapy. Since about two-thirds of patients eventually manifest distant disease regardless of the form of primary therapy, there is a tendency to think of breast carcinoma as being systemic in most patients at the time they first present for treatment.

There is a great deal of controversy regarding the optimal method of primary therapy of stage I, II, and

III breast carcinoma, and opinions on this subject have changed considerably in the past decade. Legislation initiated in California and Massachusetts and now adopted in numerous states requires physicians to inform patients of alternative treatment methods in the management of breast cancer.

Breast-Conserving Therapy

Many nonrandomized trials and the results of the Milan trial and a large randomized trial conducted by the National Surgical Adjuvant Breast Project (NSABP) in the USA showed that disease-free survival rates were similar for patients treated by partial mastectomy plus axillary dissection followed by radiation therapy and for those treated by modified radical mastectomy (total mastectomy plus axillary dissection). All patients whose axillary nodes contained tumor received adjuvant chemotherapy.

In the NSABP trial, patients were randomized to three treatment types: (1) "lumpectomy" (removal of the tumor with *confirmed* tumor-free margins) plus whole breast irradiation, (2) lumpectomy alone, and (3) total mastectomy. All patients underwent axillary lymph node dissection. Some patients in this study had tumors as large as 4 cm with (or without) palpable axillary lymph nodes. The lowest local recurrence rate was among patients treated with lumpectomy and postoperative irradiation; the highest—nearly 40% at 8 years of follow-up—was among patients treated with lumpectomy alone. However, no statistically significant differences were observed in overall or disease-free survival among the three treatment groups. This study shows that lumpectomy and axillary dissection with postoperative radiation therapy is as effective as modified radical mastectomy for the management of patients with stage I and stage II breast cancer.

The results of these and other trials have demonstrated that much less aggressive surgical treatment of the primary lesion than has previously been thought necessary gives equivalent therapeutic results and may preserve an acceptable cosmetic appearance.

Tumor size is a major consideration in determining the feasibility of breast conservation. The lumpectomy trial of the NSABP randomized patients with tumors as large as 4 cm. To achieve an acceptable cosmetic result, the patient must have a breast of sufficient size to enable excision of a 4 cm tumor without considerable deformity. Therefore, large size is only a relative contraindication. Subareolar tumors are also difficult to excise without considerable deformity, but this location is not a contraindication to breast conservation. Clinically detectable multifocality is a relative contraindication to breast-conserving surgery, as is fixation to the chest wall or skin or involvement of the nipple or overlying skin. However, the patient and not the surgeon should be the judge of what is cosmetically acceptable; some patients would prefer breast deformity rather than complete absence of the breast or even reconstruction.

It is important to recognize that axillary dissection is valuable in preventing axillary recurrences, in staging cancer, and in planning therapy. Recently, intraoperative lymphatic mapping and sentinel node dissection, which identifies the lymph node most likely to harbor metastases if they are present in the axillary nodes, has been reported. This technique identifies one or two lymph nodes in the axilla that indicate with a high degree of accuracy the presence or absence of lymph node metastases. Several studies have confirmed the validity of this technique. Ongoing trials are examining the replacement of formal axillary dissection with sentinel node dissection.

Current Recommendations

A 1990 NIH consensus statement asserts that breast-conserving surgery with radiation is the preferred form of treatment for patients with early-stage breast cancer. However, this technique has still not gained wide acceptance by physicians or patients. Despite the numerous randomized trials showing no survival benefit of mastectomy over breast-conserving partial mastectomy and irradiation, breast-conserving surgery appears underutilized and mastectomy remains the more common treatment. About 25% of patients in the United States with stage I or stage II breast cancer are treated with breast-conserving surgery and radiation therapy, compared with 75% treated with mastectomy. Use of breast-conserving surgery and radiation therapy seems to vary by region of the country, ranging from 15% in the South Central United States to approximately 30% in the Pacific Region.

Modified radical mastectomy (total mastectomy plus axillary lymph node dissection) has been the standard therapy for most patients with breast cancer. This operation removes the entire breast, overlying skin, nipple, and areolar complex as well as the underlying pectoralis fascia with the axillary lymph nodes in continuity. The major advantage of modified radical mastectomy is that radiation therapy is usually not necessary. The disadvantage, of course, is the psychologic trauma associated with breast loss. Radical mastectomy, which removes the underlying pectoralis muscle, should be performed rarely if at all. Axillary node dissection is not indicated for noninfiltrating cancers, because nodal metastases are rarely present. Radiotherapy after partial mastectomy consists of 5–6 weeks of five daily fractions to a total dose of 5000–6000 cGy. Some radiotherapists use a boost dose, but the value of this practice is controversial.

Preoperatively, full discussion with the patient regarding the rationale for operation and various alternative forms of treatment is essential. Breast-conserving surgery and radiation should be offered whenever possible, since most patients would prefer to save the breast. Breast reconstruction should be discussed with patients who choose or require mastectomy, and the option of simultaneous mastectomy with immediate reconstruction should be discussed. Time spent preoperatively in educating the patient and her family about these matters is time well spent.

Adjuvant Systemic Therapy

Following surgery and radiation therapy, chemotherapy or hormonal therapy is advocated for most patients with curable breast cancer. The objective of adjuvant systemic therapy is to eliminate the occult metastases responsible for late recurrences while they are microscopic and theoretically most vulnerable to anticancer agents.

Numerous clinical trials with various adjuvant chemotherapeutic regimens have been completed. The most extensive clinical experience to date is with the CMF (cyclophosphamide, methotrexate, and fluorouracil) regimen. Cyclophosphamide can be given either orally, in a dose of 100 mg/m^2 daily for 14 days; or intravenously, in a dose of 600 mg/m^2 on days 1 and 8. Methotrexate is given intravenously, 40 mg/m^2 on days 1 and 8; and fluorouracil is given intravenously, 600 mg/m^2 on days 1 and 8. This cycle is repeated every 4 weeks. Some clinicians prefer to give the drugs on 1 day only every 3 weeks. There appears to be no obvious advantage except that patient compliance is assured when the cyclophosphamide is give intravenously. The regimen should be continued for 6 months in patients with axillary metastases. Premenopausal women with positive axillary nodes definitely benefit from adjuvant chemotherapy. The recurrence rate in premenopausal patients who received no adjuvant chemotherapy was more than 1½ times that of those who received such therapy. No therapeutic effect with CMF has been shown in postmenopausal women with positive nodes, perhaps because therapy was modified so often in response to side effects that the total amount of drugs administered was less than planned. Other trials with different agents support the value of adjuvant chemotherapy in postmenopausal women. There are many forms of combination chemotherapy that are effective. Most are variations of CMF or AC (Adriamycin [doxorubicin] plus cyclophosphamide).

Selection of patients to receive chemotherapy must take into account other common health problems that older women may have and the effects of chemotherapy on the patient's overall health. Tamoxifen can be given with few side effects even in the elderly. Tamoxifen appears to increase bone density and favorably affect lipid and lipoprotein profiles, which may explain the observed decreased mortality rate from coronary artery disease seen in patients taking tamoxifen.

The addition of hormonal therapy, usually with tamoxifen, may improve the results of adjuvant therapy. For example, tamoxifen has been shown to enhance the beneficial effects of melphalan and fluorouracil in postmenopausal women whose tumors are ER-positive. Tamoxifen alone in a dosage of 10 mg orally twice a day has been the recommended treatment for postmenopausal women with ER-positive tumors. However, an NSABP trial showed that tamoxifen plus chemotherapy (Adriamycin [doxorubicin] plus cyclophosphamide [AC] or prednisone plus Adriamycin plus fluorouracil [PAF]) lowered recurrence rates more than tamoxifen alone in postmenopausal women with ER-positive tumors.

The length of time adjuvant therapy must be administered remains uncertain. Several studies suggest that shorter treatment periods may be as effective as longer ones. For example, one study compared 6 versus 12 cycles of postoperative CMF and found 5-year disease-free survival rates to be comparable. One of the earliest adjuvant trials used a 6-day perioperative regimen of intravenous cyclophosphamide alone; follow-up at 15 years shows a 15% improvement in disease-free survival rates for treated patients, suggesting that short-term therapy may be effective. A recent NSABP study shows that 5 years of treatment with tamoxifen may be superior to 10 years of adjuvant tamoxifen.

Several studies of adjuvant therapy in node-negative women have now been published and show a beneficial effect of adjuvant chemotherapy or tamoxifen in delaying recurrence and improving survival. A number of protocols, including CMF with leucovorin rescue as well as tamoxifen alone, have increased disease-free survival times. The magnitude of this improvement is about one-third, ie, a group of women with an estimated 30% recurrence rate would have a 20% recurrence rate after adjuvant systemic therapy. Quality of life while receiving chemotherapy does not appear to be greatly altered.

The current recommendations for adjuvant chemotherapy are summarized in Tables 16–4 and 16–5).

A 1990 consensus statement from the NIH on early-stage breast cancer recommends (1) that all patients who are candidates for clinical trials be offered the opportunity to participate, and (2) that node-negative patients who are not candidates for clinical trials ". . . should be made aware of the benefits and

Table 16–4. Adjuvant chemotherapy for premenopausal women.[1]

Nodal Involvement	Estrogen Receptors	Adjuvant Systemic Therapy
Yes	Positive	Combination chemotherapy
Yes	Negative	Combination chemotherapy
No	Positive	Tamoxifen
No	Negative	Combination chemotherapy

[1]Summary of NIH Consensus Conference, June 18–21, 1990.

Table 16–5. Adjuvant chemotherapy for postmenopausal women.[1]

Nodal Involvement	Estrogen Receptors	Adjuvant Systemic Therapy
Yes	Positive	Tamoxifen
Yes	Negative	Combination chemotherapy
No	Positive	Tamoxifen
No	Negative	Combination chemotherapy

[1]Summary of NIH Consensus Conference, June 18–21, 1990.

risks of adjuvant systemic therapy. The decision to use adjuvant treatment should follow a thorough discussion with the patient regarding the likely risk of recurrence without adjuvant therapy, the expected reduction in risk with adjuvant therapy, toxicities of therapy, and its impact on quality of life." These recommendations have not changed. In practice, most medical oncologists are currently using systemic adjuvant therapy for patients with early-stage breast cancer. Other prognostic factors being used to determine the patient's risks are tumor size, estrogen and progesterone receptor status, nuclear grade, histologic type, proliferative rate, and oncogene expression. Table 16–6 summarizes these prognostic factors. The assumption is made that patients with node-negative aggressive tumors should receive adjuvant therapy. Only patients who have serious coexistent medical problems are currently not receiving adjuvant systemic therapy. Few patients cannot at least tolerate tamoxifen.

Important questions remaining to be answered are the timing and duration of adjuvant chemotherapy, which chemotherapeutic agents should be applied for which subgroups of patients, how best to coordinate adjuvant chemotherapy with postoperative radiation therapy, the use of combinations of hormonal therapy

Table 16–6. Prognostic factors in node-negative breast cancer.

Prognostic Factor	Increased Recurrence	Decreased Recurrence
Size	T3, T2	T1, T0
Hormone receptors	Negative	Positive
DNA flow cytometry	Aneuploid	Diploid
Histologic grade	High	Low
Tumor labeling index	<3%	>3%
S phase fraction	>5%	<5%
Lymphatic or vascular invasion	Present	Absent
Cathepsin D	High	Low
HER-2/*neu* oncogene	High	Low
Epidermal growth factor receptor	High	Low

and chemotherapy, and the value of prognostic factors other than hormone receptors in predicting response to adjuvant therapy. Adjuvant systemic therapy is not currently indicated for patients with small tumors and those with negative lymph nodes who have favorable tumor markers.

Appelbaum FR: The use of bone morrow and peripheral blood stem cell transplantation in the treatment of cancer. CA Cancer J Clin 1996;46:142.

Ayash LJ et al: Prognostic factors for a prolonged progression-free survival with high-dose chemotherapy with autologous stem-cell support for advanced breast cancer. J Clin Oncol 1995;13:2043.

Cooke AL et al: Tamoxifen with and without radiation after partial mastectomy in patients with involved nodes. Int J Radiat Oncol Biol Phys 1995;31:777.

Dale PS, Giuliano AK: Nipple-areolar preservation during breast-conserving therapy for subareolar breast carcinomas. Ann Surg 1996;131:430.

Decensi A et al: Effect of tamoxifen on endometrial proliferation. J Clin Oncol 1996;14:440.

Early Breast Cancer Trialists' Collaborative Group: Systemic treatment of early breast cancer by hormonal cytotoxic or immune therapy: 133 randomized trials involving 31,000 recurrences and 24,000 deaths among 75,000 women. Lancet 1992;339:1, 71.

Fisher B et al: Reanalysis and results after 12 years of follow-up in a randomized clinical trial comparing total mastectomy with lumpectomy with or without irradiation in the treatment of breast cancer. N Engl J Med 1995;333:1456. (At 12 years there are no differences in survival among the various forms of local regional treatment, confirming the value of lumpectomy and radiation therapy.)

Garne JP et al: Primary prognostic factors in invasive breast cancer with special reference to ductal carcinoma and histologic malignancy grade. Cancer 1994;73:1438.

Guenther JM, Tokita KM, Giuliano AK: Breast-conserving surgery and radiation after augmentation mammoplasty. Cancer 1994;73:2613.

Haftty BG et al: Ipsilateral breast tumor recurrence as a predictor of distant disease: Implications for systemic therapy at the time of local relapse. J Clin Oncol 1996;14:52.

Henderson IC: Adjuvant systemic therapy for early breast cancer. Cancer 1994;74:401.

Hillner BE et al: Trade-offs between survival and breast preservation for three initial treatments of ductal carcinoma-in-situ of the breast. J Clin Oncol 1996;14:70.

Leborgne F et al: Breast conservation treatment of early stage breast cancer: Patterns of failure. Int J Radiat Oncol Biol Phys 1995;31:7655.

Ravdin PM et al: Phase II trial of docetaxel in advanced anthracycline resistant or anthracenedione resistant breast cancer. J Clin Oncol 1995;13:2879.

Scottish Cancer Trials Breast Group and ICRF Breast Unit, Guy's Hospital, London: Adjuvant ovarian ablation versus CMF chemotherapy in premenopausal women with pathological stage II breast carcinoma: The Scottish Trial. Lancet 1993;341:1293.

Tomas E et al: Comparison between the effects of tamoxifen and toremifene on the uterus in postmenopausal breast cancer patients. Gynecol Oncol 1995;59:261. (Effects endometrial proliferation.)

Veronesi U et al: Conservation surgery after primary chemotherapy in large carcinomas of the breast. Ann Surg 1995;222:612. (Preoperative chemotherapy for large tumors enables breast conservation to be performed.)

PALLIATIVE TREATMENT

This section covers palliative therapy of disseminated disease incurable by surgery (stage IV).

Radiotherapy

Palliative radiotherapy may be advised for locally advanced cancers with distant metastases in order to control ulceration, pain, and other manifestations in the breast and regional nodes. Irradiation of the breast and chest wall and the axillary, internal mammary, and supraclavicular nodes should be undertaken in an attempt to cure locally advanced and inoperable lesions when there is no evidence of distant metastases. A small number of patients in this group are cured in spite of extensive breast and regional node involvement. Neoadjuvant chemotherapy should be considered for such patients.

Palliative irradiation is of value also in the treatment of certain bone or soft tissue metastases to control pain or avoid fracture. Radiotherapy is especially useful in the treatment of isolated bony metastasis, chest wall recurrences, brain metastases, and acute spinal cord compression.

Hormone Therapy

Disseminated disease may shrink—or grow less rapidly—after endocrine therapy such as administration of hormones (eg, estrogens, androgens, progestins; see Table 16–7); ablation of the ovaries, adrenals, or pituitary; or administration of drugs that block hormone receptor sites (eg, antiestrogens) or drugs that block the synthesis of hormones (eg, aminoglutethimide). Hormonal manipulation is usually more successful in postmenopausal women even if they have received estrogen replacement therapy.

If treatment is based on the presence of estrogen receptor protein in the primary tumor or metastases, however, the rate of response is nearly equal in premenopausal and postmenopausal women. A favorable response to hormonal manipulation occurs in about one-third of patients with metastatic breast cancer. Of those whose tumors contain estrogen receptors, the response is about 60% and perhaps as high as 80% for patients whose tumors contain progesterone receptors as well. Because only 5–10% of women whose tumors do not contain estrogen receptors respond, they should not receive hormonal therapy except in unusual circumstances such as an elderly patient who could not tolerate chemotherapy.

Since the quality of life during a remission induced by endocrine manipulation is usually superior to a remission following cytotoxic chemotherapy, it is usually best to try endocrine manipulation first in cases where the estrogen receptor status of the tumor is unknown. However, if the estrogen receptor status is unknown but the disease is progressing rapidly or involves visceral organs, endocrine therapy is rarely successful, and introducing it may waste valuable time.

In general, only one type of therapy should be given at a time unless it is necessary to irradiate a destructive lesion of weight-bearing bone while the patient is on another regimen. The regimen should be changed only if the disease is clearly progressing but not if it appears to be stable. This is especially important for patients with destructive bone metastases, since changes in the status of these lesions are difficult to determine radiographically. A plan of therapy that would simultaneously minimize toxicity and maximize benefits is often best achieved by hormonal manipulation.

The choice of endocrine therapy depends on the menopausal status of the patient. Women within 1 year of their last menstrual period are considered to be premenopausal, while women whose menstruation ceased more than a year ago are postmenopausal. If endocrine therapy is the initial choice of therapy, it is referred to as primary hormonal manipulation; subsequent endocrine treatment is called secondary or tertiary hormonal manipulation.

Table 16–7. Agents commonly used for hormonal management of metastatic breast cancer.

Drug	Action	Usual Oral Dose	Major Side Effects
Tamoxifen (Nolvadex)	Antiestrogen	10 mg twice daily	Hot flushes, uterine bleeding, thrombophlebitis, rash
Diethylstilbestrol (DES)	Estrogen	5 mg three times daily	Fluid retention, uterine bleeding, thrombophlebitis, nausea
Megestrol acetate (Megace)	Progestin	40 mg four times daily	Fluid retention
Aminoglutethimide (Cytadren)[1]	Aromatase inhibitor	250 mg four times daily	Adrenal suppression, skin rashes, neurologic reactions

[1]Used with hydrocortisone.

A. The Premenopausal Patient:

1. Primary hormonal therapy–The potent antiestrogen tamoxifen is the endocrine treatment of choice in the premenopausal patient. Tamoxifen is usually given orally in a dose of 10 mg twice a day. At least two randomized clinical trials have now shown no significant difference in survival or response between tamoxifen therapy and bilateral oophorectomy. Most physicians prefer to use tamoxifen rather than perform oophorectomy, since it can be given with little morbidity and few side effects. Controversy continues about whether a response to tamoxifen is predictive of probable success with other forms of endocrine manipulation.

Bilateral oophorectomy is an alternative to primary hormonal manipulation in premenopausal women but is rarely indicated since tamoxifen is so well tolerated. It can be achieved rapidly and safely by surgery or, if the patient is a poor operative risk, by irradiation of the ovaries. Ovarian radiation therapy should be avoided in otherwise healthy patients, however, because of the high rate of complications and the longer time necessary to achieve results. Oophorectomy presumably works by eliminating estrogens, progestins, and androgens, which stimulate growth of the tumor. Tamoxifen is by far the most common and preferred method of hormonal manipulation for both pre- and postmenopausal women. The average remission is about 12 months.

2. Secondary or tertiary hormonal therapy–Although patients who do not respond to tamoxifen or oophorectomy should be treated with cytotoxic drugs, those who respond and then relapse may subsequently respond to another form of endocrine treatment (Table 16–7). The initial choice for secondary endocrine manipulation has not been clearly defined.

Patients who respond initially to oophorectomy but subsequently relapse should receive tamoxifen. If tamoxifen fails, use of aminoglutethimide or megestrol acetate should be considered. Aminoglutethimide is an inhibitor of adrenal hormone synthesis and, when combined with a corticosteroid, provides a therapeutically effective "medical adrenalectomy." Megestrol is a progestational agent. Both drugs cause less morbidity and mortality than surgical adrenalectomy; can be discontinued once the patient improves; and are not associated with the many problems of postsurgical hypoadrenalism, so that patients who require chemotherapy are more easily managed. Adrenalectomy or hypophysectomy induces regression in approximately 30–50% of patients who have previously responded to oophorectomy. However, pharmacologic hormonal manipulation has replaced these invasive procedures.

B. The Postmenopausal Patient:

1. Primary hormonal therapy–Tamoxifen, 10 mg twice daily, is the initial therapy of choice for postmenopausal women with metastatic breast cancer amenable to endocrine manipulation. It has fewer side effects than diethylstilbestrol, the former therapy of choice, and is just as effective. The main side effects of tamoxifen are nausea, vomiting, and skin rash. Rarely, it may induce hypercalcemia in patients with bony metastases.

2. Secondary or tertiary hormonal therapy–Postmenopausal patients who do not respond to tamoxifen should be given cytotoxic drugs such as cyclophosphamide, methotrexate, and fluorouracil (CMF) or Adriamycin (doxorubicin) and cyclophosphamide (AC). Postmenopausal women who respond initially to tamoxifen but later manifest progressive disease could be given diethylstilbestrol or megestrol acetate. Some authorities use aminoglutethimide. Megestrol has fewer side effects than either aminoglutethimide or diethylstilbestrol. Androgens have many side effects and should rarely be used. In general, neither hypophysectomy nor adrenalectomy is still being performed. Anastrazole, 1 mg daily, is being used as secondary hormonal manipulation after tamoxifen in postmenopausal women. Response rates of about 30% have been reported.

Chemotherapy

Cytotoxic drugs should be considered for the treatment of metastatic breast cancer (1) if visceral metastases are present (especially brain or lymphangitic pulmonary); (2) if hormonal treatment is unsuccessful or the disease has progressed after an initial response to hormonal manipulation; or (3) if the tumor is ER-negative. The most useful single chemotherapeutic agent to date is doxorubicin (Adriamycin), with a response rate of 40–50%. Single agents are rarely used but are usually given in combination with other cytotoxic drugs. The remissions tend to be brief, and single-agent chemotherapy has generally been abandoned in patients with disseminated disease.

Combination chemotherapy using multiple agents has proved to be more effective, with objectively observed favorable responses achieved in 60–80% of patients with stage IV disease. Various combinations of drugs have been used, and clinical trials are continuing in an effort to improve results and reduce undesirable side effects. Nausea and vomiting are now well controlled with drugs that directly affect the central nervous system, such as ondansetron and granisetron. These drugs are selective antagonists of serotonin receptors in the central nervous system and are extremely effective at blocking nausea caused by cytotoxic chemotherapy. Doxorubicin (40 mg/m^2 intravenously on day 1) and cyclophosphamide (200 mg/m^2 orally on days 3–6) produce an objective response in about 85% of patients so treated. Other chemotherapeutic regimens have consisted of various combinations of drugs, including cyclophosphamide, vincristine, methotrexate, and fluorouracil, with response rates ranging up to 60–70%. Prior adjuvant chemotherapy does not seem to alter response rates in patients who relapse. Growth factors such as epoetin alfa, which stimulates red blood cell production and mimics the effect of erythropoietin, and filgrastim (granulocyte colony-stimulating factor; G-CSF), which stimulates proliferation and differentiation of hematopoietic cells, are now used to prevent life-threatening anemia and neutropenia seen commonly with high doses of chemotherapy. These agents greatly diminish the incidence of infections that may complicate the use of myelosuppressive chemotherapy.

Paclitaxel, given by intravenous infusion in a dose of 135–175 mg/m^2, has been shown to be very effective for patients with breast cancer. It is usually given after failure of combination chemotherapy for metastatic disease or relapse shortly after completion of adjuvant chemotherapy. Paclitaxel has been shown to have response rates of 30–40% in patients with metastatic disease.

Docetaxel is a new agent that shows promise for treatment of patients with anthracycline-resistant tumors.

Recently, high-dose chemotherapy and autologous bone marrow or stem cell transplantation have aroused widespread interest for the treatment of metastatic breast cancer. With this technique, the patient receives high doses of cytotoxic agents. These cause severe side effects, including bone marrow suppression, for which the patient subsequently undergoes autologous bone marrow or stem cell transplantation. Reported complete response rates are as high as 30–35%—considerably better than what can be achieved with conventional chemotherapy. However, median survival times and overall survival rates do not appear to be significantly different from those reported with conventional chemotherapy. No randomized controlled clinical trial has been published that compares conventional chemotherapy with high-dose chemotherapy followed by stem cell support. A study is under way to evaluate these two options in a controlled prospective manner. Several randomized studies are currently examining high-dose chemotherapy with bone marrow autotransplantation or stem cell support in an adjuvant setting for patients at extremely high risk of recurrence of breast cancer. Some studies have shown a lower recurrence rate than that of historical controls, but the validity of this approach awaits randomized trial results. It is extremely costly, and the treatment itself is associated with a mortality rate of about 3–7%.

Malignant Pleural Effusion

This condition develops at some time in almost half of patients with metastatic breast cancer (see Chapter 9).

Bezwoda WR, Seymour L, Dansey RD: High-dose chemotherapy with hematopoietic rescue as primary treatment for metastatic breast cancer: A randomized trial. J Clin Oncol 1995;13:2483. (The first reported randomized trial comparing high-dose chemotherapy with standard-dose therapy for metastatic breast cancer. The authors show increased response and survival with high-dose chemotherapy, making this a reasonable option especially for young women with metastatic disease.)

Dhodapkar MV et al: Prognostic factors in elderly women with metastatic breast cancer treated with tamoxifen: An analysis of patients entered on four prospective clinical trials. Cancer 1996;77:683.

Falkson G et al: Ten-year follow-up study of premenopausal women with metastatic breast cancer: An Eastern Cooperative Oncology Group Study. J Clin Oncol 1995;13:1453.

Jaiyesimi IA et al: Use of tamoxifen for breast cancer: Twenty-eight years later. J Clin Oncol 1995;13:513.

Seidman AD et al: Paclitaxel as second and subsequent therapy for metastatic breast cancer: Activity independent for prior anthracycline response. J Clin Oncol 1995;13:1152.

Von Schoultz E et al: Influence of prior and subsequent pregnancy on breast cancer prognosis. J Clin Oncol 1995;13:430.

PROGNOSIS

The stage of breast cancer is the single most reliable indicator of prognosis (Table 16–8). Patients with disease localized to the breast and no evidence of regional spread after microscopic examination of the lymph nodes have by far the most favorable prognosis. Axillary lymph node status is the single best prognostic factor studied to date and correlates with survival at all tumor sizes. In addition, the number of axillary nodes involved correlates directly with lower survival rates. Estrogen and progesterone receptors appear to be an important prognostic variable, because patients with hormone receptor-negative tumors and no evidence of metastases to the axillary lymph nodes have a much higher recurrence rate than do patients with hormone receptor-positive tumors and no regional metastases. The histologic subtype of breast cancer (eg, medullary, lobular, colloid) seems

Table 16–8. Approximate survival (%) of patients with breast cancer by TNM stage.

TNM Stage	Five Years	Ten Years
0	95	90
I	85	70
IIA	70	50
IIB	60	40
IIIA	55	30
IIIB	30	20
IV	5–10	2
All	65	30

to have little, if any, significance in prognosis once these tumors are truly invasive. Flow cytometry of tumor cells to analyze DNA index and S-phase frequency aid in prognosis. Tumors with marked aneuploidy have a poor prognosis (Table 16–6). HER-2/*neu* oncogene amplification, epidermal growth factor receptors, and cathepsin D may have some prognostic value, but no markers are as significant as lymph node metastases in predicting outcome.

The mortality rate of breast cancer patients exceeds that of age-matched normal controls for nearly 20 years. Thereafter, the mortality rates are equal, although deaths that occur among breast cancer patients are often directly the result of tumor. Five-year statistics do not accurately reflect the final outcome of therapy.

When cancer is localized to the breast, with no evidence of regional spread after pathologic examination, the clinical cure rate with most accepted methods of therapy is 75–90%. Exceptions to this generalization may be related to the hormonal receptor content of the tumor, tumor size, host resistance, or associated illness. Patients with small mammographically detected estrogen and progesterone receptor-positive tumors and no evidence of axillary spread probably have a 5-year survival rate greater than 90%. When the axillary lymph nodes are involved with tumor, the survival rate drops to 40–50% at 5 years and probably around 25% at 10 years. In general, breast cancer appears to be somewhat more malignant in younger than in older women, and this may be related to the fact that fewer younger women have ER-positive tumors.

Berg JW, Hutter RVP: Breast cancer. Cancer 1995;75:257.

Dorr FA: Prognostic factors observed in current clinical trials. Cancer 1993;71:2163.

Garne JP et al: Primary prognostic factors invasive breast cancer with special reference to ductal carcinoma and histologic malignancy grade. Cancer 1994;73:1438.

Offit K: *BRCA1:* A new marker in the management of patients with breast cancer? Cancer 1996;77:599.

FOLLOW-UP CARE

After primary therapy, patients with breast cancer should be followed for life for at least two reasons: to detect recurrences and to observe the opposite breast for a second primary carcinoma. Local and distant recurrences occur most frequently within the first 3 years. During this period, the patient is examined every 3–4 months. Thereafter, examination is done every 6 months until 5 years postoperatively and then every 6–12 months. Special attention is given to the remaining breast, because 10% of patients will develop a contralateral primary malignancy. The patient should examine her own breast monthly, and a mammogram should be obtained annually. In some cases, metastases are dormant for long periods and may appear up to 10–15 years or longer after removal of the primary tumor. Estrogen and progestational agents are rarely used for a patient free of disease after treatment of primary breast cancer, particularly if the tumor was hormone receptor-positive. However, studies have failed to show an adverse effect of hormonal agents in patients who are free of disease. Indeed, even pregnancy has not been clearly associated with shortened survival of patients rendered disease-free—yet most oncologists are reluctant to advise a young patient with breast cancer that she may become pregnant, and most are reluctant to prescribe hormone replacement therapy for the postmenopausal breast cancer patient. Estrogen replacement therapy may be prescribed for a woman with a history of breast cancer after discussion of the benefits and risks of such therapy for such conditions as severe osteoporosis and hot flushes.

Local Recurrence

The incidence of local recurrence correlates with tumor size, the presence and number of involved axillary nodes, the histologic type of tumor, the presence of skin edema or skin and fascia fixation with the primary, and the type of initial local (breast) therapy. About 8% of patients develop local recurrence on the chest wall after total mastectomy and axillary dissection. When the axillary nodes are not involved, the local recurrence rate is 5%, but the rate is as high as 25% when they are heavily involved. A similar difference in local recurrence rate was noted between small and large tumors. Factors that affect the rate of local recurrence in patients who had partial mastectomies are not yet determined. However, early studies show that such things as multifocal cancer, in situ tumors, positive resection margins, chemotherapy, and radiotherapy are important.

Chest wall recurrences usually appear within the first 2 years but may occur as late as 15 or more years after mastectomy. Suspicious nodules and skin lesions should be biopsied. Local excision or localized radiotherapy may be feasible if an isolated nodule is present. If lesions are multiple or accompanied by evidence of regional involvement in the internal mammary or supraclavicular nodes, the disease is best managed by radiation treatment of the entire chest wall including the parasternal, supraclavicular, and axillary areas.

Local recurrence after mastectomy usually signals the presence of widespread disease and is an indication for bone scans, abdominal CT or liver ultrasound, posteroanterior and lateral chest x-rays, and other examinations as needed to search for evidence of metastases. Most patients with locally recurrent tumor will develop distant metastases within 2 years. When there is no evidence of metastases beyond the chest wall and regional nodes, irradiation for cure or complete local excision should be attempted. Patients with local recurrence may be cured with local resection or radiation. After partial mastectomy, local recurrence may not have as serious a prognostic significance as after mastectomy. However, those patients who do develop a breast recurrence have a worse prognosis than those who do not. It is speculated that the ability of a cancer to recur locally after radiotherapy is a sign of aggressiveness. Completion of the mastectomy should be done for local recurrence after partial mastectomy; some of these patients will survive for prolonged periods, especially if the breast recurrence is DCIS or more than 5 years after initial treatment. Systemic chemotherapy or hormonal treatment should be used for women who develop disseminated disease or those in whom local recurrence occurs following total mastectomy.

Edema of the Arm

Significant edema of the arm occurs in about 10–30% of patients after radical mastectomy. Edema of the arm occurs more commonly if radiotherapy has been given or if there was postoperative infection. Partial mastectomy with radiation to the axillary lymph nodes is followed by chronic edema of the arm in 10–20% of patients. To avoid this complication, many authorities advocate axillary lymph node sampling rather than complete axillary dissection. However, since axillary dissection is a more accurate staging operation than axillary sampling, we recommend axillary dissection, with removal of at least level I and II lymph nodes, in combination with partial mastectomy. Sentinel lymph node dissection may offer accurate staging without the risk of lymphedema for node-negative patients. Judicious use of radiotherapy, with treatment fields carefully planned to spare the axilla as much as possible, can greatly diminish the incidence of edema, which will occur in only 5% of patients if no radiotherapy is given to the axilla after a partial mastectomy and lymph node dissection.

Late or secondary edema of the arm may develop years after treatment, as a result of axillary recurrence or of infection in the hand or arm, with obliteration of lymphatic channels. Infection in the arm or hand on the dissected side should be treated promptly with antibiotics, rest, and elevation. When edema develops, careful examination of the axilla should be done to detect a regional recurrence. If there is no sign of recurrence, the swollen extremity should be treated with rest and elevation. A mild diuretic may be helpful for a few weeks. If there is no improvement, a compressor pump should be used to decrease the swelling, and the patient should then be fitted with an elastic glove or sleeve. Most patients are not bothered enough by mild edema to wear an uncomfortable glove or sleeve and will treat themselves with elevation alone. Benzopyrones have been reported to decrease lymphedema but are not approved for this use in the USA. Rarely, edema may be severe enough to interfere with use of the limb.

Breast Reconstruction

Breast reconstruction, with the implantation of a prosthesis, is usually feasible after standard or modified radical mastectomy. Reconstruction should probably be discussed with patients prior to mastectomy, because it offers an important psychologic focal point for recovery. However, most patients who are initially interested in reconstruction decide later that they no longer wish to undergo the procedure. Reconstruction is not an obstacle to the diagnosis of recurrent cancer. The most common breast reconstruction has been implantation of a silicone gel prosthesis in the subpectoral plane between the pectoralis minor and pectoralis major muscles. Recently, the Food and Drug Administration has placed a moratorium on the use of silicone gel implants because of possible leakage of silicone and associated autoimmune disorders. This remote possibility should not prevent the cancer patient from having a reconstruction, and breast cancer patients are exempt from the moratorium. Most plastic surgeons currently would place a saline-filled prosthesis rather than a silicone gel implant. Alternatively, autologous tissue can be used for reconstruction. Autologous tissue flaps are aesthetically superior to implant reconstruction in most patients. They also have the advantage of not feeling like a foreign body to the patient. The most popular autologous technique currently is the transrectus abdominis muscle flap (TRAM flap), which is done by rotating the rectus abdominis muscle with attached fat and skin cephalad to make a breast mound. A latissimus dorsi flap can be swung from the back but offers less fullness than the TRAM flap and is therefore less acceptable cosmetically. Reconstruction may be performed immediately (at the time of initial mastectomy) or may be delayed until later, usually when the patient has completed adjuvant therapy.

Risks of Pregnancy

Data are insufficient to determine whether interruption of pregnancy improves the prognosis of patients who are discovered during pregnancy to have potentially curable breast cancer and who receive definitive treatment. Theoretically, the increasingly high levels of estrogen produced by the placenta as the pregnancy progresses could be detrimental to the patient with occult metastases of hormone-sensitive breast cancer. Moreover, occult metastases are present in most patients with positive axillary nodes, and treatment by adjuvant chemotherapy could be potentially harmful to the fetus, although chemotherapy has been given to pregnant women. Under these circumstances, interruption of early pregnancy seems reasonable, with progressively less rationale for the procedure as term approaches. Obviously, the decision must be highly individualized and will be affected by many factors, including the patient's desire to have the baby and the generally poor prognosis when axillary nodes are involved.

Equally important is the advice regarding future pregnancy (or abortion in case of pregnancy) to be given to women of child-bearing age who have had definitive treatment for breast cancer. Under these circumstances, one must assume that pregnancy will be harmful if occult metastases are present, though this has not been demonstrated. Patients whose tumors are ER-negative probably would not be affected by pregnancy. A number of studies have shown no adverse effect of pregnancy on survival of pregnant women who have had breast cancer, although most oncologists advise against it.

In patients with inoperable or metastatic cancer (stage IV disease), induced abortion is usually advisable because of the possible adverse effects of hormonal treatment, radiotherapy, or chemotherapy upon the fetus.

Buzdar A: Anastrozole, a potent and selective aromatase inhibitor versus megestrol acetate in postmenopausal women with advanced breast cancer: Results of overview analysis of two phase II trials. J Clin Oncol 1996;14:2000. (Anastrozole is as effective as megestrol in women whose disease progressed after tamoxifen therapy.)

Carlson IS et al: The importance of the lumpectomy surgical margin status in long term results of breast conservation. Cancer 1995;76:259.

Casley-Smith JR, Morgan RG, Piller NB: Treatment of lymphedema of the arms and legs with 5,6-benzo[α]pyrone. N Engl J Med 1993;329:1158.

Johnson JE et al: Recurrent mammary carcinoma after local excision: A segmental problem. Cancer 1995;75:1612.

CARCINOMA OF THE MALE BREAST

Essentials of Diagnosis

- A painless lump beneath the areola in a man usually over 50 years of age.
- Nipple discharge, retraction, or ulceration may be present.

General Considerations

Breast cancer in men is a rare disease; the incidence is only about 1% of that in women. The average age at occurrence is about 60—somewhat older than the commonest presenting age in women. The prognosis, even in stage I cases, is worse in men than in women. Blood-borne metastases are commonly present when the male patient appears for initial treatment. These metastases may be latent and may not become manifest for many years. As in women, hormonal influences are probably related to the development of male breast cancer. There is a high incidence of both breast cancer and gynecomastia in Bantu men, theoretically owing to failure of estrogen inactivation by a damaged liver associated with vitamin B deficiency.

Clinical Findings

A painless lump, occasionally associated with nipple discharge, retraction, erosion, or ulceration, is the chief complaint. Examination usually shows a hard, ill-defined, nontender mass beneath the nipple or areola. Gynecomastia not uncommonly precedes or accompanies breast cancer in men. Nipple discharge is an uncommon presentation for breast cancer in men, as it is in women. However, nipple discharge in a man is an ominous finding associated with carcinoma in nearly 75% of cases.

Breast cancer staging is the same in men as in women. Gynecomastia and metastatic cancer from another site (eg, prostate) must be considered in the differential diagnosis of a breast lesion in a man. Biopsy settles the issue.

Treatment

Treatment consists of modified radical mastectomy in operable patients, who should be chosen by the same criteria as women with the disease. Irradiation is the first step in treating localized metastases in the skin, lymph nodes, or skeleton that are causing symptoms. Examination of the cancer for hormone receptor proteins may prove to be of value in predicting response to endocrine ablation. Adjuvant chemotherapy is used for the same indications as in breast cancer in women.

Since breast cancer in men is frequently a disseminated disease, endocrine therapy is of considerable importance in its management. Castration in advanced breast cancer is the most successful palliative measure and more beneficial than the same procedure in women. Objective evidence of regression may be seen in 60–70% of men who are castrated—approximately twice the proportion in women. The average duration of tumor growth remission is about 30 months, and life is prolonged. Bone is the most frequent site of metastases from breast cancer in men (as in women), and castration relieves bone pain in most patients so treated. The longer the interval between mastectomy and recurrence, the longer the tumor growth remission following castration. As in women, there is no correlation between the histologic type of the tumor and the likelihood of remission following castration.

Tamoxifen (10 mg orally twice daily) is becoming increasingly popular and should replace castration as the initial therapy for metastatic disease. However, little clinical experience is available with tamoxifen in male breast cancers. Aminoglutethimide (250 mg orally four times a day) should replace adrenalectomy in men as it has in women. Corticosteroid therapy alone has been considered to be efficacious but probably has no value when compared with major endocrine ablation.

Estrogen therapy—5 mg of diethylstilbestrol three times daily orally—may be effective as secondary hormonal manipulation after medical adrenalectomy (with aminoglutethimide). Androgen therapy may exacerbate bone pain. Tamoxifen should be the initial treatment for metastatic breast cancer in men. Castration and tamoxifen are the main therapeutic resources for advanced breast cancer in men at present. Chemotherapy should be administered for the same indications and using the same dosage schedules as for women with metastatic disease.

Prognosis

The prognosis of breast cancer is poorer in men than in women. The crude 5- and 10-year survival rates for clinical stage I breast cancer in men are about 58% and 38%, respectively. For clinical stage II disease, the 5- and 10-year survival rates are approximately 38% and 10%. The survival rates for all stages at 5 and 10 years are 36% and 17%.

Friedman LS et al: Mutation analysis of *BRCA1* and *BRCA2* in a male breast cancer population. Am J Hum Genet 1997;60:313. (Reports *BRCA* genetic mutations in male breast cancer.)

Joshi MG et al: Male breast carcinoma: An evaluation of prognostic factors contributing to a poor outcome. Cancer 1996;77:490.

Salvadori B et al: Prognosis of breast cancer in males: An analysis of 170 cases. Eur J Cancer 1994;30:930.

Winchester DJ: Male breast cancer. Semin Surg Oncol 1996;12:364. (Diagnosis, pathogenesis, and clinical course.)

Gynecology

H. Trent MacKay, MD

ABNORMAL PREMENOPAUSAL BLEEDING

Normal menstrual bleeding lasts an average of 4 days (range, 2–7 days), with a mean blood loss of 40 mL. Blood loss of over 80 mL per cycle is abnormal and frequently produces anemia. Excessive bleeding, often with the passage of clots, may occur at regular menstrual intervals (**menorrhagia**) or irregular intervals (**dysfunctional uterine bleeding**). When there are fewer than 21 days between the onset of bleeding episodes, the cycles are likely to be anovular. **Ovulation bleeding**, a single episode of spotting between regular menses, is quite common. Heavier or irregular intermenstrual bleeding warrants investigation.

Dysfunctional uterine bleeding is usually caused by overgrowth of endometrium due to estrogen stimulation without adequate progesterone to stabilize growth; this occurs in anovular cycles. Anovulation associated with high estrogen levels commonly occurs in teenagers, in women aged late 30s to late 40s, and in extremely obese women or those with polycystic ovaries.

Clinical Findings

A. Symptoms and Signs: The diagnosis of the disorders underlying the bleeding usually depends upon the following: (1) A careful description of the duration and amount of flow, related pain, and relationship to the last menstrual period (LMP). Pad counts are an unreliable measure of blood loss, since pads or tampons, even of the same brand, may vary in their absorbency. The presence of blood clots or the degree of inconvenience caused by the bleeding may be more useful indicators. (2) A history of pertinent illnesses. (3) A history of all medications the patient has taken in the past month, so that possible inhibition of ovulation or endometrial stimulation can be assessed. (4) A careful pelvic examination to look for pregnancy, uterine myomas, adnexal masses, infection, or evidence of endometriosis.

B. Laboratory Studies: Cervical smears should be obtained as needed for cytologic and culture studies. Blood studies should include a complete blood count, sedimentation rate, and glucose levels to rule out diabetes. Diabetes may occasionally initially present with abnormal bleeding. A test for pregnancy and studies of thyroid function and blood clotting should be considered in the clinical evaluation. Tests for ovulation in cyclic menorrhagia include basal body temperature records, serum progesterone measured 1 week before the expected onset of menses, and analysis of an endometrial biopsy specimen for secretory activity shortly before the onset of menstruation.

C. Imaging: Pelvic ultrasound may be useful to diagnose intrauterine or ectopic pregnancy, subserous or intrauterine myomas, endometriosis, or adnexal masses that may be related to abnormal bleeding. Hysterosalpingography can outline endometrial polyps, submucous myomas, or uterine synechiae. MRI can definitively diagnose submucous myomas and adenomyosis.

D. Cervical Biopsy and Endometrial Curettage: Biopsy, curettage, or aspiration of the endometrium and curettage of the endocervix are often necessary to diagnose the cause of bleeding. These and other invasive gynecologic diagnostic procedures are described in Table 17–1. Polyps, tumors, and submucous myomas are commonly identified in this way. If cancer of the cervix is a possibility, multiple quadrant biopsies (or colposcopically directed biopsies) and endocervical curettage are indicated as first steps.

E. Hysteroscopy: Hysteroscopy can visualize endometrial polyps, submucous myomas, and exophytic endometrial cancers. It is useful immediately before D&C.

Treatment

Premenopausal patients with abnormal uterine bleeding include those with submucous myomas, infection, early abortion, or pelvic neoplasms. The history, physical examination, and laboratory findings should identify such patients, who require definitive therapy depending upon the cause of the bleeding. A large group of patients remains, most of whom have dysfunctional uterine bleeding on a hormonal basis.

Table 17–1. Common gynecologic diagnostic procedures.

Colposcopy
Visualization of cervical, vaginal, or vulvar epithelium under 5–50× magnification to identify abnormal areas requiring biopsy. Used to identify genital warts on males as well as females. An office procedure.

D&C
Dilation of the cervix and curettage of the entire endometrial cavity, using a metal curette or suction cannula and often using forceps for the removal of endometrial polyps. Performed to diagnose endometrial disease and to stop heavy bleeding. Can usually be done in the office under local anesthesia.

Endometrial biopsy
Removal of one or more areas of the endometrium by means of a curette or small aspiration device without cervical dilation. Less accurate diagnostically than D&C. An office procedure performed under local anesthesia.

Endocervical curettage
Removal of endocervical epithelium with a small curette for diagnosis of cervical dysplasia and cancer. An office procedure performed under local anesthesia.

Hysteroscopy
Visual examination of the uterine cavity with a small fiberoptic endoscope passed through the cervix. Biopsies, excision of myomas, and other procedures can be performed. Can be done in the office under local anesthesia or in the operating room under general anesthesia.

Hysterosalpingography
Injection of radiopaque dye through the cervix to visualize the uterine cavity and oviducts. Mainly used in investigation of infertility.

Laparoscopy
Visualization of the abdominal and pelvic cavity through a small fiberoptic endoscope passed through a subumbilical incision. Permits diagnosis, tubal sterilization, and treatment of many conditions previously requiring laparotomy. General anesthesia is usually used.

Dysfunctional uterine bleeding can usually be treated hormonally; progestins, which limit and stabilize endometrial growth, are generally effective. Office D&C is usually not necessary in women under age 40. Medroxyprogesterone acetate, 10 mg/d, or norethindrone acetate, 5 mg/d, should be given for 10–14 days starting on day 15 of the cycle, following which withdrawal bleeding (so-called medical curettage) will occur. The treatment is repeated for several cycles; it can be reinstituted if amenorrhea or dysfunctional bleeding recurs. In young women who are bleeding actively, any of the combination oral contraceptives can be given four times daily for one or 2 days followed by two pills daily through day 5 and then one pill daily through day 20; after withdrawal bleeding occurs, pills are taken in the usual dosage for three cycles. In cases of intractable heavy bleeding, danazol, 200 mg four times daily, is sometimes used to create an atrophic endometrium. Alternatively, a GnRH agonist such as depot leuprolide, 3.75 mg intramuscularly monthly, or nafarelin, 0.2–0.4 mg intranasally twice daily, can be used for up to 6 months to create a temporary cessation of menstru-

ation by ovarian suppression. Symptoms of hypoestrinism are common and occur early in treatment, while use beyond 6 months is associated with significant osteopenia that is reversible after therapy is terminated.

In cases of heavy bleeding, intravenous conjugated estrogens, 25 mg every 4 hours for three or four doses, can be used, followed by oral conjugated estrogens, 2.5 mg daily, or ethinyl estradiol, 20 µg daily, for 3 weeks, with the addition of medroxyprogesterone acetate, 10 mg daily for the last 10 days of treatment, or a combination oral contraceptive daily for 3 weeks. This will thicken the endometrium and control the bleeding. If the abnormal bleeding is not controlled by hormonal treatment, a D&C is necessary to check for incomplete abortion, polyps, submucous myomas, or endometrial cancer. In women over age 40, a D&C or careful endometrial biopsy is generally indicated to rule out neoplasm before beginning hormonal therapy.

Endometrial ablation through the hysteroscope with laser photocoagulation or electrocautery is an option; this technique is designed to reduce or prevent any future menstrual flow.

Nonsteroidal anti-inflammatory drugs such as ibuprofen, naproxen, or mefenamic acid in the usual anti-inflammatory doses will often reduce blood loss in menorrhagia—even that associated with an IUD.

Prolonged use of a progestin, as in a minipill, in injectable contraceptives, or in the therapy of endometriosis, can also lead to intermittent bleeding, sometimes severe. In this instance, the endometrium is atrophic and fragile. If bleeding occurs, it should be treated with estrogen as follows: ethinyl estradiol, 20 µg, or conjugated estrogens, 1.25 mg/d for 7 days.

It is useful for the patient and the physician to discuss stressful situations or life-styles that may contribute to anovulation and dysfunctional bleeding, such as prolonged emotional turmoil or excessive use of drugs or alcohol.

Brenner PF: Differential diagnosis of abnormal uterine bleeding. Am J Obstet Gynecol 1996;175:766. (Brief but complete summary of causes.)

MacKay HT: Non-pregnancy-related vaginal bleeding. In: *The Clinical Practice of Emergency Medicine,* 3rd ed. Harwood-Nuss AL et al (editors). Lippincott-Raven, 1996. (Diagnosis and treatment recommendations.)

POSTMENOPAUSAL VAGINAL BLEEDING

Vaginal bleeding that occurs 6 months or more following cessation of menstrual function should be investigated. The most common causes are atrophic endometrium, endometrial proliferation, hyperplasia, endometrial or cervical cancer, and administration of estrogens without added progestin. Other causes include atrophic vaginitis, trauma, endometrial polyps, trophic ulcers of the cervix associated with prolapse of the uterus, and blood dyscrasias. Uterine bleeding is usually painless, but pain will be present if the cervix is stenotic, if bleeding is severe and rapid, or if infection or torsion or extrusion of a tumor is present. The patient may report a single episode of spotting or profuse bleeding for days or months.

Diagnosis

The vulva and vagina should be inspected for areas of bleeding, ulcers, or neoplasms. A cytologic smear of the cervix and vaginal pool should be taken. An unstained wet mount of vaginal fluid in saline and potassium hydroxide may reveal white blood cells, infective organisms, or basal epithelial cells indicative of a low estrogen effect. Endocervical curettage and sampling by aspiration of the endometrium, preferably preceded by hysteroscopy, should be performed next, and careful search for endometrial polyps should be made. The tissue obtained in the course of the hysteroscopic examination may reveal atrophy, polyps, endometrial hyperplasia (with or without an atypical glandular pattern), or cancer.

Transvaginal sonography can be used to measure endometrial thickness (< 5 mm indicating atrophy, > 15 mm indicating hypertrophy).

Treatment

Aspiration curettage (with polypectomy if indicated) will frequently be curative. If simple endometrial hyperplasia is found, give cyclic progestin therapy (medroxyprogesterone acetate, 10 mg/d, or norethindrone acetate, 5 mg/d) for 21 days of each month for 3 months. A repeat D&C or endometrial biopsy can then be performed, and if tissues are normal and estrogen replacement therapy is reinstituted, a progestin should be prescribed (as above) for the last 10–14 days of each estrogen cycle, followed by 5 days with no hormone therapy, so that the uterine lining will be shed. If endometrial hyperplasia with atypical cells or carcinoma of the endometrium is found, hysterectomy is necessary.

Bakos O et al: Transvaginal ultrasonography for identifying endometrial pathology in postmenopausal women. Maturitas 1994;20:181.

Gredmark T et al: Histopathological findings in women with postmenopausal bleeding. Br J Obstet Gynecol 1995;102:133. (Among 457 women with postmenopausal bleeding, 8% had cancer and 7% significant hyperplasia.)

PREMENSTRUAL SYNDROME (Premenstrual Tension)

The premenstrual syndrome is a recurrent, variable cluster of troublesome physical and emotional symptoms that develop during the 7–14 days before the onset of menses and subside when menstruation occurs. The syndrome intermittently affects about one-third of all premenopausal women, primarily those 25–40 years of age. In about 10% of affected women, the syndrome may be recurrent and severe. Although not every woman experiences all the symptoms or signs at one time, many describe bloating, breast pain, ankle swelling, a sense of increased weight, skin disorders, irritability, aggressiveness, depression, inability to concentrate, libido change, lethargy, and food cravings.

The pathogenesis of premenstrual syndrome is still uncertain. Psychosocial factors may play a role. Suppression of ovarian function with a GnRH agonist has been shown to diminish all symptoms during therapy. Add-back therapy with estrogen and progestin may allow extended use of a GnRH agonist. Suppression of ovulation with an oral contraceptive is sometimes helpful, but the patient often complains that she still has premenstrual syndrome.

Current treatment methods are mainly empiric. The physician should provide the best support possible for the patient's emotional and physical distress. This includes the following:

(1) Careful evaluation of the patient, with understanding, explanation, and reassurance, is of first importance.

(2) Advise the patient to keep a daily diary of all symptoms for 2–3 months, to help in evaluating the timing and characteristics of the syndrome. If her symptoms occur throughout the month rather than in the 2 weeks before menses, she may be depressed or may have other emotional problems in addition to premenstrual syndrome. Psychotherapy and self-help groups are helpful for many women or couples.

(3) A diet emphasizing complex carbohydrates can be recommended. Foods high in sugar content and alcohol should be avoided to minimize reactive hypoglycemia. Use of caffeine should be minimized whenever tension and irritability predominate.

(4) A variety of vitamins and minerals in relatively high doses have been suggested for this syndrome, but none have proved useful in double-blind studies, and some have undesirable side effects. If a supplement is desired, use a single daily dose of a multivitamin-multimineral containing the RDA for these substances.

(5) A program of regular conditioning exercise, such as jogging, has been found to decrease depression, anxiety, and fluid retention premenstrually in several studies.

(6) Natural progesterone taken daily or by vaginal suppositories in doses of 50–400 mg daily during the luteal phase is widely used for premenstrual syndrome. Double-blind studies have not confirmed its efficacy, nor has the safety of this treatment been evaluated.

(7) Serotonin reuptake inhibitors such as fluoxe-

tine, 20 mg/d, are effective in relieving tension, irritability, and dysphoria with few side effects. Short-acting benzodiazepines have also been used, but the potential for addiction to these drugs makes their use problematic in this recurrent disorder.

Barnhart KT et al: A clinician's guide to the premenstrual syndrome. Med Clin North Am 1995;79:1457. (Serotonin reuptake inhibitors are becoming first-line therapy for severe PMS.)

Steiner M et al: Fluoxetine in the treatment of premenstrual dysphoria. N Engl J Med 1995;322:1529. (Low-dose fluoxetine was effective at reducing PMS symptoms.)

DYSMENORRHEA

1. PRIMARY DYSMENORRHEA

Primary dysmenorrhea is menstrual pain associated with ovular cycles in the absence of pathologic findings. The pain usually begins within 1–2 years after the menarche and may become more severe with time. The frequency of cases increases up to age 20 and then decreases with age and markedly with parity. Fifty to 75 percent of women are affected at some time, and 5–6% have incapacitating pain.

Primary dysmenorrhea is low, midline, wave-like, cramping pelvic pain often radiating to the back or inner thighs. Cramps may last for 1 or more days and may be associated with nausea, diarrhea, headache, and flushing. The pain is produced by uterine vasoconstriction, anoxia, and sustained contractions mediated by prostaglandins.

Clinical Findings

The pelvic examination is normal between menses; examination during menses may produce discomfort, but there are no pathologic findings.

Treatment

Nonsteroidal anti-inflammatory drugs (ibuprofen, ketoprofen, mefenamic acid, naproxen) are generally helpful. Drugs should be started at the onset of bleeding to avoid inadvertent drug use during early pregnancy. Medication should be continued on a regular basis for 2–3 days. Ovulation can be suppressed and dysmenorrhea usually prevented by oral contraceptives.

2. SECONDARY DYSMENORRHEA

Secondary dysmenorrhea is menstrual pain for which an organic cause exists. It usually begins well after menarche, sometimes even as late as the third or fourth decade of life.

Clinical Findings

The history and physical examination commonly suggest endometriosis or pelvic inflammatory disease. Other causes may be submucous myoma, IUD use, cervical stenosis with obstruction, or blind uterine horn (rare).

Diagnosis

Laparoscopy is often needed to differentiate endometriosis from pelvic inflammatory disease. Submucous myomas can be detected most reliably by MRI but also by hysterogram, by hysteroscopy, or by passing a sound or curette over the uterine cavity during D&C. Cervical stenosis may result from induced abortion, creating crampy pain at the time of expected menses with no blood flow; this is easily cured by passing a sound into the uterine cavity after administering a paracervical block.

Treatment

A. Specific Measures: Periodic use of analgesics, including the nonsteroidal anti-inflammatory drugs given for primary dysmenorrhea, may be beneficial, and oral contraceptives may give relief, particularly in endometriosis. Danazol and GnRH agonists are effective in the treatment of endometriosis (see below).

B. Surgical Measures: If disability is marked or prolonged, laparoscopy or exploratory laparotomy is usually warranted. Definitive surgery depends upon the degree of disability and the findings at operation.

MacKay HT, Chang RJ: Dysmenorrhea. In: *Current Therapy, 1993.* Rakel RE (editor). Saunders, 1993.

Smith RP: Cyclic pain and dysmenorrhea. Obstet Gynecol Clin North Am 1993;20;753. (History and physical examination are the most sensitive tests for distinguishing secondary from primary dysmenorrhea.)

VAGINITIS

Inflammation and infection of the vagina are common gynecologic problems, resulting from a variety of pathogens, allergic reactions to vaginal contraceptives or other products, or the friction of coitus. The normal vaginal pH is 4.5 or less, and *Lactobacillus* is the predominant organism. At the time of the midcycle estrogen surge, clear, elastic, mucoid secretions from the cervical os are often profuse. In the luteal phase and during pregnancy, vaginal secretions are thicker, white, and sometimes adherent to the vaginal walls. These normal secretions can be confused with vaginitis by concerned women.

Clinical Findings

When the patient complains of vaginal irritation, pain, or unusual discharge, a careful history should be taken, noting the onset of the last menstrual period; recent sexual activity; use of contraceptives, tampons, or douches; and the presence of vaginal burning, pain, pruritus, or unusually profuse or malodorous discharge. The physical examination should include careful inspection of the vulva and speculum examination of the vagina and cervix. The cervix is cultured for gonococcus or *Chlamydia* if applicable. A specimen of vaginal discharge is examined under the microscope in a drop of 0.9% saline solution to look for trichomonads or clue cells and in a drop of 10% potassium hydroxide to search for *Candida*. The vaginal pH can be tested; it is frequently greater than 4.5 in infections due to trichomonads and bacterial vaginosis. A bimanual examination to look for evidence of pelvic infection should follow.

A. Candida albicans: Pregnancy, diabetes, and use of broad-spectrum antibiotics or corticosteroids predispose to *Candida* infections. Heat, moisture, and occlusive clothing also contribute to the risk. Pruritus, vulvovaginal erythema, and a white curd-like discharge that is not malodorous are found. Microscopic examination with 10% potassium hydroxide reveals filaments and spores. Cultures with Nickerson's medium may be used if *Candida* is suspected but not demonstrated.

B. Trichomonas vaginalis: This protozoal flagellate infects the vagina, Skene's ducts, and lower urinary tract in women and the lower genitourinary tract in men. It is transmitted through coitus. Pruritus and a malodorous frothy, yellow-green discharge occur, along with diffuse vaginal erythema and red macular lesions on the cervix in severe cases. Motile organisms with flagella are seen by microscopic examination of a wet mount with saline solution.

C. Bacterial Vaginosis: This condition is considered to be a polymicrobial disease which is not sexually transmitted. An overgrowth of *Gardnerella* and other anaerobes is often associated with increased malodorous discharge without obvious vulvitis or vaginitis. The discharge is grayish and sometimes frothy, with a pH of 5.0–5.5. An amine-like ("fishy") odor is present if a drop of discharge is alkalinized with 10% potassium hydroxide. On wet mount in saline, epithelial cells are covered with bacteria to such an extent that cell borders are obscured (clue cells). Vaginal cultures are generally not useful in diagnosis.

D. Condylomata Acuminata (Genital Warts): Warty growths on the vulva, perianal area, vaginal walls, or cervix are caused by various types of the human papillomavirus. They are sexually transmitted. Pregnancy and immunosuppression favor growth. Vulvar lesions may be obviously wart-like or may be diagnosed only after application of 4% acetic acid (vinegar) and colposcopy, when they appear whitish, with prominent papillae. Fissures may be present at the fourchette. Vaginal lesions may show diffuse hypertrophy or a cobblestone appearance. Cervical lesions may be visible only by colposcopy after pretreatment with 4% acetic acid. These lesions may be related to dysplasia and cervical cancer. Vul-

var cancer is also currently considered to be associated with the human papillomavirus.

Treatment

A. Candida albicans: Effective treatment includes 3-day regimens of butoconazole (2% cream, 5 g), clotrimazole (200 mg vaginal tablet), terconazole (0.8% cream, 5 g, or 80 mg suppository), or miconazole (200 mg vaginal suppository); 7-day regimens of clotrimazole (1% cream or 100 mg vaginal tablet), or miconazole (2% cream, 5 g, or 100 mg vaginal suppository); or single-dose regimens of clotrimazole (500 mg tablet) or tioconazole ointment (6.5%, 5 g). Fluconazole, 150 mg orally in a single dose, is also effective. Ketoconazole, 100 mg orally once daily, for up to 6 months, is effective for suppression of recurrent vulvovaginitis.

B. Trichomonas vaginalis: Treatment of both partners simultaneously is necessary; metronidazole, 2 g as a single dose or 500 mg twice daily for 7 days, is usually employed. In the case of treatment failure, the patient should be retreated with metronidazole, 500 mg twice a day for 7 days. If repeated failure occurs in the absence of infection, treat with a single dose of 2 g of metronidazole once daily for 3–5 days. If this is not effective in eradicating the organisms, metronidazole susceptibility testing can be arranged with the CDC.

C. Bacterial Vaginosis: The recommended regimen is metronidazole, 500 mg twice daily for 7 days. A 2 g single-dose regimen is slightly less efficacious than the 7-day regimen but is probably equally effective in actual clinical practice because compliance is better. Other regimens include clindamycin vaginal cream (2%, 5 g) once daily for 7 days, metronidazole gel (0.75%, 5 g) twice daily for 5 days, or clindamycin, 300 mg orally twice daily for 7 days.

D. Condylomata Acuminata: A variety of modalities are available for treatment. Treatment for small vulvar warts is with podophyllum resin 25% in tincture of benzoin (do not use during pregnancy or on bleeding lesions) or 50–90% trichloroacetic acid, carefully applied to avoid the surrounding skin. The pain of trichloroacetic acid application can be lessened by a sodium bicarbonate paste applied immediately after treatment. Podophyllum resin must be washed off after 2–4 hours. Podofilox, an active lignan from the crude podophyllum resin, can be safely and comfortably applied by the patient. Freezing with liquid nitrogen or a cryoprobe and electrocautery are also effective. Vaginal warts may be treated with cryotherapy with liquid nitrogen, trichloroacetic acid, or podophyllum resin. Extensive warts may require treatment with CO_2 laser under local or general anesthesia. Interferon is not recommended because it is very expensive and no more effective than other therapies. Therapy with fluorouracil has not been studied in controlled trials, frequently causes local irritation, and is not recommended. Treatment of sex partners is not necessary for management of genital warts, since the role of reinfection appears to be a small one.

Bonnes W et al: Efficacy and safety of podofilox solution in the treatment and suppression of anogenital warts. Am J Med 1994;96:420. (Podofilox solution is effective and well tolerated and can be self-administered for the treatment of vulvar warts.)

1993 Sexually transmitted diseases treatment guidelines. MMWR Morb Mortal Wkly Rep 1993;42(RR-14):1.

CERVICITIS

Infection of the cervix must be distinguished from physiologic ectopy of columnar epithelium, which is common in young women. Cervicitis is characterized by a red edematous cervix with purulent, often blood-streaked discharge and tenderness on cervical motion. The infection may follow tears during delivery or abortion or may result from a sexually transmitted pathogen such as *Neisseria gonorrhoeae, Chlamydia,* or herpesvirus (which presents with vesicles and ulcers on the cervix during a primary herpetic infection). Yellow mucopurulent endocervical secretions and the presence of ten or more polymorphonuclear leukocytes per high dry field are suggestive of chlamydial infection.

Mucopurulent cervicitis is an insensitive predictor of either gonorrheal or chlamydial infection and in addition has a low positive predictive value. Presumptive antibiotic treatment of mucopurulent cervicitis is not indicated unless there is a high prevalence of either *N gonorrhoeae* or *Chlamydia* in the population. (See Chapter 33 for discussion.) Three months after treatment, approximately 20% of women will have persistent or recurrent mucopus in the cervix, not explained by relapse or reinfection. This may be related to cervical ectopy and an inflammatory reaction caused by columnar cell contact with the vaginal environment.

Thorpe EM Jr et al: Chlamydial cervicitis and urethritis: Single dose treatment compared with doxycycline for seven days in community-based practises. Genitourin Med 1996;72:93. (Single-dose azithromycin and doxycycline for 7 days are equally effective.)

CERVICAL POLYPS

Cervical polyps commonly occur after the menarche and are occasionally noted in postmenopausal women. The cause is not known, but inflammation may play an etiologic role. The principal symptoms are discharge and abnormal vaginal bleeding. However, abnormal bleeding should not be ascribed to a cervical polyp without sampling the endocervix and endometrium. The polyps are visible in the cervical os on speculum examination.

Cervical polyps must be differentiated from polypoid neoplastic disease of the endometrium, small submucous pedunculated myomas, and endometrial polyps. Cervical polyps rarely contain malignant foci.

Treatment

Cervical polyps can generally be removed in the office by avulsion with a uterine packing forceps or ring forceps. If the cervix is soft, patulous, or definitely dilated and the polyp is large, surgical D&C is required (especially if the pedicle is not readily visible). Exploration of the cervical and uterine cavities with the polyp forceps and curette may reveal multiple polyps. All tissue removed should be submitted for microscopic examination.

CYST & ABSCESS OF BARTHOLIN'S DUCT

Trauma or infection may involve Bartholin's duct, causing obstruction of the gland. Drainage of secretions is prevented, leading to pain, swelling, and abscess formation. The infection usually resolves and pain disappears, but stenosis of the duct outlet with distention often persists. Reinfection causes recurrent tenderness and further enlargement of the duct.

The principal symptoms are periodic painful swelling on either side of the introitus and dyspareunia. A fluctuant swelling 1–4 cm in diameter in the inferior portion of either labium minus is a sign of occlusion of Bartholin's duct. Tenderness is evidence of active infection.

Pus or secretions from the gland should be cultured for gonorrhea, *Chlamydia,* and other pathogens and treated accordingly (see Chapter 33); frequent warm soaks may be helpful. If an abscess develops, aspiration or incision and drainage are the simplest forms of therapy, but the problem may recur. Marsupialization, incision and drainage with the insertion of an indwelling Word catheter, or laser treatment will establish a new duct opening. An asymptomatic cyst does not require therapy.

EFFECTS OF EXPOSURE TO DIETHYLSTILBESTROL IN UTERO

Between 1947 and 1971, diethylstilbestrol (DES) was widely used in the USA for diabetic women during pregnancy and to treat threatened abortion. It is estimated that 2–3 million fetuses were exposed. A relationship between fetal DES exposure and clear cell carcinoma of the vagina was later discovered, and a number of other related anomalies have since been noted. In one-third of all exposed women, there are changes in the vagina (adenosis, septa), cervix (deformities and hypoplasia of the vaginal portion of the cervix), or uterus (T-shaped cavity).

At present, all exposed women are advised to have an initial colposcopic examination to outline vaginal and cervical areas of abnormal epithelium, followed by cytologic examination of the vagina (all four quadrants of the upper half of the vagina) and cervix at yearly intervals. Lugol's iodine stain of the vagina and cervix will also outline areas of metaplastic squamous epithelium.

Many women are not aware of having been exposed to DES. Therefore, in the age groups at risk (26–50 years), examiners should pay attention to structural changes of the vagina and cervix that may signal the possibility of DES exposure and indicate the need for follow-up.

The incidence of clear cell carcinoma is approximately one in 1000 exposed women, and the incidence of cervical and vaginal intraepithelial neoplasia (dysplasia and carcinoma in situ) is twice as high as in unexposed women. DES daughters have more difficulty conceiving and have an increased incidence of early abortion, ectopic pregnancy, and premature births. In addition, mothers treated with DES in pregnancy appear to have a small increase in the incidence of breast cancer, beginning 20 years after exposure.

Noller KL: Role of colposcopy in the examination of diethylstilbestrol-exposed women. Obstet Gynecol 1993;20:165. (Colposcopy should be part of initial gynecologic examination for DES-exposed women.)

CERVICAL INTRAEPITHELIAL NEOPLASIA (CIN; Dysplasia of the Cervix)

The squamocolumnar junction of the cervix is an area of active squamous cell proliferation. In childhood, this junction is located on the exposed vaginal portion of the cervix. At puberty, because of hormonal influence and possibly because of changes in the vaginal pH, the squamous margin begins to encroach on the single-layered, mucus-secreting epithelium, creating an area of metaplasia (transformation zone). Factors associated with coitus (see Prevention, below) may lead to cellular abnormalities, which over a period of time can result in the development of squamous cell dysplasia or cancer. There are varying degrees of dysplasia (Table 17–2), defined by the degree of cellular atypia; all types must be observed and treated if they persist or become more severe. At present, the malignant potential of a specific lesion cannot be predicted. Some lesions remain stable for long periods of time; some regress; and others advance.

Clinical Findings

There are no specific signs or symptoms of cervi-

Table 17–2. Classification systems for Papanicolaou smears.

Numerical	Dysplasia	CIN	Bethesda System
1	Benign	Benign	Normal
2	Benign with inflammation	Benign with inflammation	Normal
3	Mild dysplasia	CIN I	Low-grade SIL
3	Moderate dysplasia	CIN II	
3	Severe dysplasia	CIN III	High-grade SIL
4	Carcinoma in situ		
5	Invasive cancer	Invasive cancer	Invasive cancer

CIN = cervical intraepithelial neoplasia; SIL = squamous intraepithelial lesion.

cal intraepithelial neoplasia. The presumptive diagnosis is made by cytologic screening of an asymptomatic population with no grossly visible cervical changes. All visibly abnormal cervical lesions should be biopsied.

Diagnosis

A. Cytologic Examination (Papanicolaou Smear): Specimens should be taken from a nonmenstruating patient, spread on a single slide, and fixed. A specimen should be obtained from the squamocolumnar junction with a wooden or plastic spatula and from the endocervix with a cotton swab or nylon brush.

Cytologic reports from the laboratory may describe findings in one of several ways (see Table 17–2). While use of class I–IV is decreasing, the CIN classification continues to be used along with a description of abnormal cells, including evidence of human papillomavirus (HPV). The term "squamous intraepithelial lesions (SIL)," low-grade or high-grade, is increasingly used. Cytopathologists consider a Papanicolaou smear to be a medical consultation and will recommend further diagnostic procedures, treatment for infection, and comments on factors that prevent adequate evaluation of the specimen. The role of HPV testing of cytologic smears remains undefined, and this procedure is not currently recommended for routine use.

B. Colposcopy: Viewing the cervix with 10–20× magnification allows for assessment of the size and margins of an abnormal transformation zone and determination of extension into the endocervical canal. The application of 3–5% acetic acid (vinegar) dissolves mucus, and the acid's desiccating action sharpens the contrast between normal and actively proliferating squamous epithelium. Abnormal changes include white patches and vascular atypia, which indicate areas of greatest cellular activity. Paint the cervix with Lugol's solution (strong iodine solution [Schiller's test]). Normal squamous epithelium will take the stain; nonstaining squamous epithelium should be biopsied. (The single-layered, mucus-secreting endocervical tissue will not stain either but can readily be distinguished by its darker pink, shinier appearance.)

C. Biopsy: Colposcopically directed punch biopsy and endocervical curettage are office procedures. If colposcopic examination is not available, the normal-appearing cervix shedding atypical cells can be evaluated by endocervical curettage and multiple punch biopsies of nonstaining squamous epithelium or biopsies from each quadrant of the cervix.

Data from both cervical biopsy and endocervical curettage are important in deciding on treatment.

Prevention

Current data suggest that cervical infection with the human papillomavirus (HPV) is associated with a high percentage of all cervical dysplasias and cancers. There are over 60 recognized HPV subtypes, of which types 6 and 11 tend to cause mild dysplasias, while types 16, 18, 31, and others cause higher grade cellular changes.

Cervical cancer almost never occurs in virginal women; it is epidemiologically related to the number of sexual partners a woman has had and the number of other female partners a male partner has had. Use of the diaphragm or condom has been associated with a protective effect. Long-term oral contraceptive users develop more dysplasias and cancers of the cervix than users of other forms of birth control, and smokers are also more at risk. Preventive measures include the following:

(1) Regular cytologic screening to detect abnormalities.

(2) Limiting the number of sexual partners.

(3) Using a diaphragm or condom for coitus.

(4) Stopping smoking.

Women with HIV infection appear to be at increased risk of the disease and of recurrent disease after treatment. Women with HIV infection should receive regular cytologic screening and should be followed closely after treatment for cervical intraepithelial neoplasia.

Treatment

Treatment varies depending on the degree and extent of cervical intraepithelial neoplasia. Biopsies should always precede treatment.

A. Cauterization or Cryosurgery: The use of either hot cauterization or freezing (cryosurgery) is effective for noninvasive small lesions visible on the cervix without endocervical extension.

B. CO_2 Laser: This well-controlled method minimizes tissue destruction. It is colposcopically directed and requires special training. It may be used with large visible lesions. In current practice it involves the vaporization of the transformation zone on the cervix and the distal 5–7 mm of endocervical canal.

C. Loop Resection: When the CIN is clearly visible in its entirety, a wire loop can be used for excisional biopsy. Cutting and hemostasis are effected with a low-voltage electrosurgical machine (Bovie). This office procedure with local anesthesia is quick and uncomplicated.

D. Conization of the Cervix: Conization is surgical removal of the entire transformation zone and endocervical canal. It should be reserved for cases of severe dysplasia or cancer in situ (CIN III), particularly those with endocervical extension. The procedure can be performed with the scalpel, the CO_2 laser, or by large-loop excision.

E. Follow-Up: Because recurrence is possible—especially in the first 2 years after treatment—and because the false-negative rate of a single cervical cytologic test is 20%, close follow-up is imperative. Vaginal cytologic examination should be repeated at 3-month intervals. After 2 years, yearly examinations suffice.

Cuzick J et al: Human papillomavirus testing in primary cervical screening. Lancet 1995;345:1533. (HPV testing could augment cytologic screening, but further studies are needed.)

Kurman RJ et al: Interim guidelines for management of abnormal cervical cytology. JAMA 1994;271:1866. (Recommended management of low-grade abnormal lesions by the Bethesda System.)

Maiman M et al: Recurrent cervical intraepithelial neoplasia in human immunodeficiency virus-seropositive women. Obstet Gynecol 1993;82:170. (Recurrence of CIN occurred in 39% of HIV-positive and 9% of HIV-negative women.)

Pearce KF et al: Cytopathological findings on vaginal Papanicolaou smears after hysterectomy for benign gynecologic disease. N Engl J Med 1996;335:1559. (Because of the very low rate of abnormal Papanicolaou smears in women who have had a hysterectomy for benign disease, routine Papanicolaou smear screening is not justified in this population.)

CARCINOMA OF THE CERVIX

Essentials of Diagnosis

- Abnormal uterine bleeding and vaginal discharge.
- Cervical lesion may be visible on inspection as a tumor or ulceration.
- Vaginal cytology usually positive; must be confirmed by biopsy.

General Considerations

Cancer appears first in the intraepithelial layers (the preinvasive stage, or carcinoma in situ). Preinvasive cancer (CIN III) is a common diagnosis in women 25–40 years of age and is etiologically related to infection with the human papillomavirus. Two to 10 years are required for carcinoma to penetrate the basement membrane and invade the tissues. After invasion, death usually occurs within 3–5 years in untreated or unresponsive patients.

Clinical Findings

A. Symptoms and Signs: The most common signs are metrorrhagia, postcoital spotting, and cervical ulceration. Bloody or purulent, odorous, nonpruritic discharge may appear after invasion. Bladder and rectal dysfunction or fistulas and pain are late symptoms.

B. Cervical Biopsy and Endocervical Curettage, or Conization: These procedures are necessary steps after a positive Papanicolaou smear to determine the extent and depth of invasion of the cancer. Even if the smear is positive, treatment is never justified until definitive diagnosis has been established through biopsy.

C. "Staging," or Estimate of Gross Spread of Cancer of the Cervix: The depth of penetration of the malignant cells beyond the basement membrane is a reliable clinical guide to the extent of primary cancer within the cervix and the likelihood of metastases. It is customary to stage cancers of the cervix under anesthesia as shown in Table 17–3. Further assessment may be carried out by abdominal and pelvic CT scanning or MRI.

Complications

Metastases to regional lymph nodes occur with increasing frequency from stage I to stage IV. Paracervical extension occurs in all directions from the cervix. The ureters are often obstructed lateral to the cervix, causing hydroureter and hydronephrosis and consequently impaired kidney function. Almost two-thirds of patients with untreated carcinoma of the cervix die of uremia when ureteral obstruction is bilateral. Pain in the back, in the distribution of the lumbosacral plexus, is often indicative of neurologic involvement. Gross edema of the legs may be indicative of vascular and lymphatic stasis due to tumor.

Vaginal fistulas to the rectum and urinary tract are severe late complications. Hemorrhage is the cause of death in 10–20% of patients with extensive invasive carcinoma.

Treatment

A. Emergency Measures: Vaginal hemorrhage originates from gross ulceration and cavitation in stage II–IV cervical carcinoma. Ligation and suturing of the cervix are usually not feasible, but ligation of the uterine or hypogastric arteries may be lifesaving when other measures fail. Styptics such as negatol, Monsel's solution, or acetone are effective, although delayed sloughing may result in further bleeding. Wet vaginal packing is helpful. Emergency irradiation usually controls bleeding.

Table 17–3. International classification of cancer of the cervix.[1]

Preinvasive carcinoma	
Stage 0	Carcinoma in situ, intraepithelial carcinoma.

Invasive carcinoma	
Stage I	Carcinoma strictly confined to the cervix (extension to the corpus should be disregarded).
IA	Preclinical carcinomas of the cervix, ie, those diagnosed only by microscopy.
IA1	Minimal microscopically evident stromal invasion.
IA2	Lesions detected microscopically that can be measured. The upper limits of the measurement should not show a depth of invasion of > 5 mm taken from the base of the epithelium, either surface or glandular, from which it originates; and a second dimension, the horizontal spread, must not exceed 7 mm. Larger lesions should be classified as stage IB.
Stage II	Carcinoma extends beyond the cervix but has not extended to the pelvic wall. The carcinoma involves the vagina but not as far as the lower third.
IIA	No obvious parametrial involvement.
IIB	Obvious parametrial involvement.
Stage III	Carcinoma has extended either to the lower third of the vagina or to the pelvic sidewall. All cases of hydronephrosis or nonfunctioning kidney, unless known to be due to other causes.
IIIA	Involvement of lower third of vagina. No extension to pelvic sidewall.
IIIB	Extension onto the pelvic wall and/or hydronephrosis or nonfunctioning kidney.
Stage IV	Carcinoma extended beyond the true pelvis or clinically involving the mucosa of the bladder or rectum. Does not include edema of bladder mucosa.
IVA	Spread of growth to adjacent organs (ie, rectum or bladder with positive biopsy from those organs).
IVB	Spread of growth to distant organs.

[1]International Federation of Gynecology and Obstetrics: *Annual Report on the Results of Treatment in Gynecological Cancer*, vol 20. FIGO, 1988.

B. Specific Measures:

1. Carcinoma in situ (stage 0)–In women who have completed childbearing, total hysterectomy is the treatment of choice. In women who wish to retain the uterus, acceptable alternatives include cervical conization or, in experienced hands, ablation of the lesion with cryotherapy or laser. Close follow-up with Papanicolaou smears every 4 months for 1 year and every 6 months for another year is necessary after cryotherapy or laser.

2. Invasive carcinoma–Microinvasive carcinoma (stage IA) is treated with simple, extrafascial hysterectomy. Stage IB and stage IIA cancers may be treated with either radical hysterectomy or radiation therapy. Stage IIB and stage III and IV cancers must be treated with radiation therapy. Because radical surgery results in fewer long-term complications than irradiation and may allow preservation of ovarian function, it may be the preferred mode of therapy in younger women without contraindications to major surgery.

Prognosis

The overall 5-year relative survival rate for carcinoma of the cervix is 68% in white women and 55% in black women in the United States. Survival rates are inversely proportionate to the stage of cancer: stage 0, 99–100%; stage IA, > 95%; stage IB-IIA, 80–90%; stage IIB, 65%; stage III, 40%; stage IV, < 20%.

Cannistra SA, Niloff JM: Cancer of the uterine cervix. (Medical Progress.) N Engl J Med 1996;334:1030.

LEIOMYOMA OF THE UTERUS (Fibroid Tumor)

Essentials of Diagnosis

- Irregular enlargement of the uterus (may be asymptomatic).
- Heavy or irregular vaginal bleeding, dysmenorrhea.
- Acute and recurrent pelvic pain if the tumor becomes twisted on its pedicle or infarcted.
- Symptoms due to pressure on neighboring organs (large tumors).

General Considerations

Uterine leiomyomas are the most common benign neoplasm of the female genital tract. It is a discrete, round, firm, often multiple uterine tumor composed of smooth muscle and connective tissue. The most convenient classification is by anatomic location: (1) intramural, (2) submucous, (3) subserous, (4) intraligamentous, (5) parasitic (ie, deriving its blood supply from an organ to which it becomes attached), and (6) cervical. A submucous myoma may become pedunculated and descend through the cervix into the vagina.

Clinical Findings

A. Symptoms and Signs: In nonpregnant women, myomas are frequently asymptomatic. However, they can cause urinary frequency, dysmenorrhea, heavy bleeding (often with anemia), or other complications due to the presence of an abdominal mass. Occasionally, degeneration occurs, causing intense pain. Infertility may be due to a myoma that significantly distorts the uterine cavity.

In pregnant women, myomas occasionally cause additional hazards: abortion, malpresentation, failure of engagement, premature labor, localized pain (from degeneration or torsion), obstructed labor, and postpartum hemorrhage.

B. Laboratory Findings: Hemoglobin levels

may be decreased as a result of blood loss, but in rare cases polycythemia is present, presumably as a result of the production of erythropoietin by the myomas.

C. Imaging: Ultrasonography will confirm the presence of uterine myomas and can be used sequentially to monitor growth. When multiple subserous or pedunculated myomas are being followed, ultrasonography is important to exclude ovarian masses. MRI can delineate intramural and submucous myomas accurately. Hysterography or hysteroscopy can also confirm cervical or submucous myomas.

Differential Diagnosis

Irregular myomatous enlargement of the uterus must be differentiated from the similar but symmetric enlargement that may occur with pregnancy or adenomyosis (the presence of endometrial glands and stroma in the myometrium). Subserous myomas must be distinguished from ovarian tumors. Leiomyosarcoma is an unusual tumor occurring in 0.5% of women operated on for symptomatic myoma. It is very rare under the age of 40 and increases in incidence thereafter.

Treatment

A. Emergency Measures: If the patient is markedly anemic as a result of long, heavy menstrual periods, preoperative treatment with depot medroxyprogesterone acetate, 150 mg intramuscularly every 28 days, or danazol, 400–800 mg/d, will slow or stop bleeding, and medical treatment of anemia can be given prior to surgery. Emergency surgery is required for acute torsion of a pedunculated myoma. The only emergency indication for myomectomy during pregnancy is torsion; abortion is not an inevitable result.

B. Specific Measures:

1. Nonpregnant women–In women who are not pregnant, small asymptomatic myomas should be observed at 6-month intervals. Elective myomectomy can be done to preserve the uterus. Myomas do not require surgery on an urgent basis unless they cause significant pressure on the ureters, bladder, or bowel or severe bleeding leading to anemia or unless they are undergoing rapid growth. Cervical myomas larger than 3–4 cm in diameter or pedunculated myomas that protrude through the cervix must be removed. Submucous myomas can be removed using a hysteroscope and laser or resection instruments.

GnRH analogues such as depot leuprolide, 3.75 mg intramuscularly monthly, or nafarelin, 0.2–0.4 mg intranasally twice a day, are used preoperatively for 2- to 3-month periods to induce reversible hypogonadism, which reduces the size of myomas, suppresses their further growth, and reduces surrounding vascularity. If the patient does not undergo surgery, regrowth of myomas occurs within several months after termination of GnRH.

2. Pregnant patients–If the uterus is no larger

than a 6-month pregnancy by the fourth month of gestation, an uncomplicated course may be anticipated. If the mass (especially a cervical tumor) is the size of a 5- or 6-month pregnancy by the second month, abortion will probably occur. If possible, defer myomectomy or hysterectomy until 6 months after delivery, at which time involution of the uterus and regression of the tumor will be complete.

C. Surgical Measures: Surgical measures available for the treatment of myoma are myomectomy and total or subtotal abdominal or vaginal hysterectomy. Myomectomy is the treatment of choice during the childbearing years.

Prognosis

Surgical therapy is curative. Future pregnancies are not endangered by myomectomy, although cesarean delivery may be necessary after wide dissection with entry into the uterine cavity.

Christiansen JK: The facts about fibroids. Postgrad Med 1993;94:129. (Medical or surgical management depending on age and symptoms.)
Strobelt N et al: Natural history of uterine leiomyomas in pregnancy. J Ultrasound Med 1994;13:399. (In a series of 134 pregnant women with leiomyomas, only 15% experienced enlargement of the leiomyoma.)

CARCINOMA OF THE ENDOMETRIUM

Adenocarcinoma of the uterine corpus is the second most common cancer of the female genital tract. It occurs most often in women 50–70 years of age. Some patients will have taken unopposed estrogen in the past; their increased risk appears to persist for 10 or more years after stopping the drug. Obesity, nulliparity, diabetes, and polycystic ovaries with prolonged anovulation and the extended use of tamoxifen for the treatment of breast cancer are also risk factors.

Abnormal bleeding is the presenting sign in 80% of cases. Endometrial carcinoma may cause obstruction of the cervix with collection of pus (pyometra) or blood (hematometra) causing lower abdominal pain. However, pain generally occurs late in the disease, with metastases or infection.

Papanicolaou smears of the cervix occasionally show atypical endometrial cells but are an insensitive diagnostic tool. Endocervical and endometrial sampling is the only reliable means of diagnosis. Adequate specimens of each can usually be obtained during an office procedure performed following local anesthesia (paracervical block). Simultaneous hysteroscopy can be a valuable addition in order to localize polyps or other lesions within the uterine cavity. Vaginal ultrasonography may be used to determine the thickness of the endometrium as an indication of hypertrophy and possible neoplastic change.

Pathologic assessment is important in differentiat-

ing hyperplasias, which often can be treated with cyclic oral progestins.

Prevention

Prompt endometrial sampling for patients who report abnormal menstrual bleeding or postmenopausal uterine bleeding will reveal many incipient as well as clinical cases of endometrial cancer. Postmenopausal women taking estrogens or younger women with prolonged anovulation can be given oral progestins for 13 days at the end of each estrogen cycle in order to promote periodic shedding of the uterine lining; this has been associated with a decreased incidence of uterine adenocarcinoma.

Staging

Examination under anesthesia, endometrial and endocervical sampling, chest x-ray, intravenous urography, cystoscopy, sigmoidoscopy, transvaginal sonography, and MRI will help determine the extent of the disease and its appropriate treatment. The staging is based on the surgical and pathologic evaluation.

Treatment

Treatment consists of total hysterectomy and bilateral salpingo-oophorectomy. Peritoneal material for cytologic examination is routinely taken. Preliminary external irradiation or intracavitary radium therapy is indicated if the cancer is poorly differentiated or if the uterus is definitely enlarged in the absence of myomas. If invasion deep into the myometrium has occurred or if sampled preaortic lymph nodes are positive for tumor, postoperative irradiation is indicated.

Palliation of advanced or metastatic endometrial adenocarcinoma may be accomplished with large doses of progestins, eg, medroxyprogesterone, 400 mg intramuscularly weekly, or megestrol acetate, 80–160 mg daily orally.

Prognosis

With early diagnosis and treatment, the 5-year survival is 80–85%.

Photopopulos GJ: Surgicopathologic staging of endometrial adenocarcinoma. Curr Opin Obstet Gynecol 1994;6:92. (Required to fully assess extent of disease and to predict survival.)
Rose PG: Endometrial carcinoma. (Medical Progress.) N Engl J Med 1996;335:640. (Epidemiology, diagnosis, and treatment.)

CARCINOMA OF THE VULVA

Essentials of Diagnosis

- History of genital warts.
- History of prolonged vulvar irritation, with pruritus, local discomfort, or slight bloody discharge.

- Early lesions may suggest or include nonneoplastic epithelial disorders.
- Late lesions appear as a mass, an exophytic growth, or a firm, ulcerated area in the vulva.
- Biopsy is necessary to make the diagnosis.

General Considerations

The vast majority of cancers of the vulva are squamous lesions that classically have occurred in women over 50 years of age. Several subtypes (particularly 16, 18, and 31) of the human papillomavirus have been identified in some but not all vulvar cancers. As with squamous cell lesions of the cervix, a grading system of vulvar intraepithelial neoplasia (VIN) from mild dysplasia to carcinoma in situ has been established.

Differential Diagnosis

Biopsy is essential for the diagnosis of vulvar cancer and should be performed with any localized atypical vulvar lesion, including white patches. Multiple skin-punch specimens can be taken in the office under local anesthesia, with care to include tissue from the edges of each lesion sampled.

Benign vulvar disorders that must be excluded in the diagnosis of carcinoma of the vulva include chronic granulomatous lesions (eg, lymphogranuloma venereum, syphilis), condylomas, hidradenoma, or neurofibroma. Lichen sclerosus and other associated leukoplakic changes in the skin should be biopsied. The likelihood that a superimposed vulvar cancer will develop in a woman with a nonneoplastic epithelial disorder (vulvar dystrophy) ranges from 1% to 5%.

Treatment

A. General Measures: Early diagnosis and treatment of irritative or other predisposing or contributing causes to carcinoma of the vulva should be pursued. A 7:3 combination of betamethasone and crotamiton is particularly effective for itching. After an initial response, fluorinated steroids should be replaced with hydrocortisone because of their skin atrophying effect. Testosterone propionate (1–2% in petrolatum), applied to the vulva twice daily for 6 weeks, offers the best results in lichen sclerosus and can be used chronically in decreasing amounts and frequency.

B. Surgical Measures:

1. In situ squamous cell carcinoma of the vulva and small, invasive basal cell carcinoma of the vulva should be excised with a wide margin. If the squamous carcinoma in situ is extensive or multicentric, laser therapy or superficial surgical removal of vulvar skin may be required. In this way, the clitoris and uninvolved portions of the vulva may be spared. Skin grafting may be necessary, but mutilating vulvectomy is avoided.

2. Invasive carcinoma confined to the vulva

without evidence of spread to adjacent organs or to the regional lymph nodes will necessitate radical vulvectomy and inguinal lymphadenectomy if the patient is able to withstand surgery. Debilitated patients may be candidates for palliative irradiation only.

Prognosis

Basal cell carcinomas very seldom metastasize, and carcinoma in situ by definition has not metastasized. With adequate excision, the prognosis for both lesions is excellent. Patients with invasive vulvar carcinoma 3 cm in diameter or less without inguinal lymph node metastases who can sustain radical surgery have about a 90% chance of a 5-year survival. If the lesion is greater than 3 cm and has metastasized, the likelihood of 5-year survival is less than 25%.

Johnson PR, Carson LF: Contemporary management of vulvar cancer. In: Rock JA et al (editors). *Advances in Obstetrics and Gynecology,* vol 3. Mosby-Year Book, 1996.

ENDOMETRIOSIS

Aberrant growth of endometrium outside the uterus, particularly in the dependent parts of the pelvis and in the ovaries, is a common cause of abnormal bleeding and secondary dysmenorrhea. This condition is known as endometriosis. Its causes, pathogenesis, and natural course are poorly understood. The prevalence in the USA is 2% among fertile women and three- to fourfold greater than that in the infertile. Depending on the location and extent of the endometrial implants, infertility, dyspareunia, or rectal pain with bleeding may result. Aching pain tends to be constant, beginning 2–7 days before the onset of menses, and becomes increasingly severe until flow slackens. Pelvic examination may disclose tender indurated nodules in the cul-de-sac, especially if the examination is done at the onset of menstruation.

Endometriosis must be distinguished from pelvic inflammatory disease, ovarian neoplasms, and uterine myomas. In general, only in salpingitis and endometriosis are the symptoms aggravated by menstruation. Bowel invasion by endometrial tissue may produce clinical findings, including blood in the stool, that must be distinguished from bowel neoplasm. Differentiation in these instances depends upon proctosigmoidoscopy and biopsy.

Ultrasound examination will often reveal complex fluid-filled masses that cannot be distinguished from neoplasms. MRI is more sensitive and specific than ultrasound, particularly in the diagnosis of adnexal masses. Barium enema may delineate colonic involvement of endometriosis. However, the clinical diagnosis of endometriosis is presumptive and must be confirmed by laparoscopy or laparotomy.

Treatment

A. Medical Treatment: The goal of medical treatment is to preserve the fertility of women wanting future pregnancies, ameliorate symptoms, and simplify future surgery or make it unnecessary. Medications are designed to inhibit ovulation over 4–9 months and lower hormone levels, thus preventing cyclic stimulation of endometriotic implants and decreasing their size. The optimum duration of therapy is not clear, and the relative merits in terms of pregnancies, side effects, and long-term risks and benefits show insignificant differences when compared with each other, with surgery (including laser surgery), and, in mild cases, with placebo.

1. The GnRH analogues such as nafarelin nasal spray, 0.2–0.4 mg twice daily, or long-acting injectable leuprolide acetate, 3.75 mg intramuscularly monthly, used for 6 months, suppress ovulation. Side effects consisting of vasomotor symptoms and bone demineralization may be relieved by "add-back" therapy with norethindrone, 5–10 mg daily.

2. Danazol is used for 6–9 months in the lowest dose necessary to suppress menstruation, usually 200–400 mg twice daily. Side effects are androgenic and include decreased breast size, weight gain, acne, and hirsutism.

3. Any of the combination oral contraceptives may be given, one daily continuously for 6–12 months. Breakthrough bleeding can be treated with conjugated estrogens, 1.25 mg daily for 1 week, or estradiol, 2 mg daily for 1 week.

4. Medroxyprogesterone acetate, 100 mg intramuscularly every 2 weeks for four doses; then 100 mg every 4 weeks; add oral estrogen or estradiol valerate, 30 mg intramuscularly, for breakthrough bleeding. Use for 6–9 months.

5. Low-dose oral contraceptives can be given for 21 days out of each 28; prolonged suppression of ovulation will often inhibit further stimulation of residual endometriosis, especially if taken after one of the therapies mentioned above.

6. Analgesics, with or without codeine, may be needed during menses. Nonsteroidal anti-inflammatory drugs may be helpful.

B. Surgical Measures: The surgical treatment of moderately extensive endometriosis depends upon the patient's age and symptoms and her desire to preserve reproductive function. If the patient is under 35, resect the lesions, free adhesions, and suspend the uterus. At least 20% of patients so treated can become pregnant, although some must undergo surgery again if the disease progresses. If the patient is over 35 years old, is disabled by pain, and has involvement of both ovaries, bilateral salpingo-oophorectomy and hysterectomy will probably be necessary.

Foci of endometriosis can be treated at laparoscopy by bipolar coagulation or laser vaporization. Because pelvic endometriosis can take forms other than the classic powder burns and hemorrhagic cysts, a meticulous survey of the peritoneum is required.

Prognosis

The prognosis for reproductive function in early or moderately advanced endometriosis is good with conservative therapy. Bilateral ovariectomy is curative for patients with severe and extensive endometriosis with pain. Following hysterectomy and oophorectomy, estrogen replacement therapy is indicated.

Olive DL, Swartz LB: Endometriosis. N Engl J Med 1993;24:1759. (Review of etiology, diagnosis, and management.)

Witt BR, Barad DH: Management of endometriosis in women older than 40 years of age. Obstet Gynecol Clin North Am 1993;20:349.

GENITAL PROLAPSE
(Cystocele, Rectocele, Enterocele)

Cystocele, rectocele, and enterocele are vaginal hernias commonly seen in multiparous women. Cystocele is a hernia of the bladder wall into the vagina, causing a soft anterior fullness. Cystocele may be accompanied by urethrocele, which is not a hernia but a sagging of the urethra following its detachment from the symphysis during childbirth. Rectocele is a herniation of the terminal rectum into the posterior vagina, causing a collapsible pouch-like fullness. Enterocele is a vaginal vault hernia containing small intestine, usually in the posterior vagina and resulting from a deepening of the pouch of Douglas. Enterocele may also accompany uterine prolapse or follow hysterectomy, when weakened vault supports or a deep unobliterated cul-de-sac containing intestine protrudes into the vagina. One or more of the three types of hernias often occur in combination.

Supportive measures include a high-fiber diet. Weight reduction in obese patients and limitation of straining and lifting are helpful. Pessaries may reduce cystocele, rectocele, or enterocele temporarily and are helpful in women who do not wish surgery or are chronically ill.

The only cure for symptomatic cystocele, rectocele, or enterocele is corrective surgery. The prognosis following an uncomplicated procedure is good.

DeLancey JOL (editor): Pelvic organ prolapse: Clinical management and scientific foundations. Clin Obstet Gynecol 1993;36:895. (A series of ten articles providing comprehensive information on genital prolapse.)

UTERINE PROLAPSE

Uterine prolapse most commonly occurs as a delayed result of childbirth injury to the pelvic floor (particularly the transverse cervical and uterosacral ligaments). Unrepaired obstetric lacerations of the levator musculature and perineal body augment the weakness. Attenuation of the pelvic structures with aging and congenital weakness can accelerate the development of prolapse.

In slight prolapse, the uterus descends only part way down the vagina; in moderate prolapse, the corpus descends to the introitus and the cervix protrudes slightly beyond; and in marked prolapse (procidentia), the entire cervix and uterus protrude beyond the introitus and the vagina is inverted. Inability to walk comfortably because of protrusion or discomfort from the presence of a vaginal mass is an indication that surgical treatment should be considered.

Treatment

The type of surgery depends upon the extent of prolapse and the patient's age and her desire for menstruation, pregnancy, and coitus. The simplest, most effective procedure is vaginal hysterectomy with appropriate repair of the cystocele and rectocele. If the patient desires pregnancy, a partial resection of the cervix with plication of the cardinal ligaments can be attempted. For elderly women who do not desire coitus, partial obliteration of the vagina is surgically simple and effective. Abdominal uterine suspension or ventrofixation will fail in the treatment of prolapse.

A well-fitted vaginal pessary (eg, inflatable doughnut type, Gellhorn pessary) may give relief if surgery is refused or contraindicated.

Zeitlin MP, Lebherz TB: Pessaries in the geriatric patient. J Am Geriatr Soc 1992;40:635. (Practical advice on indications, management, and prevention of complications.)

PELVIC INFLAMMATORY DISEASE (PID; Salpingitis, Endometritis)

Essentials of Diagnosis

- Lower abdominal adnexal and cervical motion tenderness.
- Cervical or vaginal discharge.
- Laboratory evidence of cervical infection with *Neisseria gonorrhoeae* or *Chlamydia trachomatis.*
- Tubo-ovarian abscess on sonography or laparoscopic abnormalities consistent with pelvic inflammatory disease.

General Considerations

Pelvic inflammatory disease is a polymicrobial infection of the upper genital tract associated with the sexually transmitted organisms *N gonorrhoeae* and *C trachomatis* as well as endogenous organisms, including anaerobes, *H influenzae*, enteric gram-negative rods, and streptococci. It is most common in young, nulliparous, sexually active women with multiple partners. Other risk markers include nonwhite race, douching, and smoking. The use of oral contraceptives or barrier methods of contraception may provide significant protection.

Tuberculous salpingitis is rare in the USA but more common in developing countries; it is characterized by pelvic pain and irregular pelvic masses not responsive to antibiotic therapy. It is not sexually transmitted.

Clinical Findings

A. Symptoms and Signs: Patients with pelvic inflammatory disease may have lower abdominal pain, chills and fever, menstrual disturbances, purulent cervical discharge, and cervical and adnexal tenderness. Right upper quadrant pain (Fitz-Hugh and Curtis syndrome) may indicate an associated perihepatitis. However, diagnosis of PID is complicated by the fact that many women may have subtle or mild symptoms, not readily recognized as PID. Women with lower abdominal, adnexal, or cervical motion tenderness should be considered to have PID and be treated with antibiotics unless there is a competing diagnosis such as ectopic pregnancy or appendicitis.

B. Laboratory Findings: The white blood cell count and sedimentation rate are not consistently elevated. Gram stain of endocervical discharge may reveal *N gonorrhoeae*, with gram-negative intracellular diplococci, or suggest the presence of *C trachomatis*, with over 10 WBC/hpf. Endocervical culture should be performed routinely.

C. Imaging Studies: Pelvic ultrasound may help to distinguish pelvic masses associated with PID from those of endometriosis, uterine myomas, ovarian cysts or tumors, and ectopic pregnancy. Endovaginal ultrasound may reveal thickened, fluid-filled uterine tubes.

Differential Diagnosis

Appendicitis, ectopic pregnancy, septic abortion, hemorrhagic or ruptured ovarian cysts or tumors, twisted ovarian cyst, degeneration of a myoma, and acute enteritis must be considered. Pelvic inflammatory disease is more likely to occur when there is a history of pelvic inflammatory disease, recent sexual contact, recent onset of menses, or an IUD in place or if the partner has a sexually transmitted disease. Acute pelvic inflammatory disease is highly unlikely when recent intercourse has not taken place or an IUD is not being used. A sensitive serum pregnancy test should be obtained to rule out ectopic pregnancy. Culdocentesis will differentiate hemoperitoneum (ruptured ectopic pregnancy or hemorrhagic cyst) from pelvic sepsis (salpingitis, ruptured pelvic abscess, or ruptured appendix). Pelvic and vaginal ultrasound is helpful in the differential diagnosis of ectopic pregnancy of over 6 weeks. Laparoscopy is often utilized to diagnose pelvic inflammatory disease, and it is imperative if the diagnosis is not certain or if the patient has not responded to antibiotic therapy after 48 hours. The appendix should be visualized at laparoscopy to rule out appendicitis. Cultures obtained at the time of laparoscopy are often specific and helpful.

Treatment

A. Hospitalization: Patients with acute pelvic inflammatory disease should be admitted for intravenous antibiotic therapy if: (1) the diagnosis is uncertain and surgical emergencies such as appendicitis or ectopic pregnancy cannot be ruled out; (2) a pelvic abscess is suspected; (3) the patient is pregnant; (4) the patient is an adolescent; (5) the patient is unable to follow or tolerate an outpatient regimen; (6) the patient has failed to respond clinically to outpatient therapy; (7) clinical follow-up within 72 hours cannot be arranged; (8) the patient is HIV-positive. Many experts recommend that all patients with acute PID be hospitalized for intravenous antibiotic therapy. Women who are HIV-positive may have a greater likelihood of requiring operative treatment, but they generally respond to the inpatient regimens listed below.

B. Antibiotics: Early treatment with appropriate antibiotics effective against *N gonorrhoeae, C trachomatis,* and the endogenous organisms listed above is essential to prevent long-term sequelae. The sexual partner should be examined and treated appropriately.

Two inpatient regimens have been shown to be effective in the treatment of acute pelvic inflammatory disease: (1) Cefoxitin, 2 g intravenously every 6 hours, or cefotetan, 2 g every 12 hours, plus doxycycline, 100 mg intravenously or orally every 12 hours. This regimen is continued for at least 48 hours after the patient shows significant clinical improvement. Doxycycline, 100 mg twice daily, should be continued to complete a total of 14 days therapy. (2) Clindamycin, 900 mg intravenously every 8 hours, plus gentamicin intravenously in a loading dose of 2 mg/kg followed by 1.5 mg/kg every 8 hours. This regimen is continued for at least 48 hours after the patient shows significant clinical improvement and is followed by either clindamycin, 450 mg four times daily, or doxycycline, 100 mg twice daily, to complete a total of 14 days of therapy.

Two outpatient regimens are recommended: (1) Ofloxacin, 400 mg orally twice daily for 14 days, plus either clindamycin, 450 mg orally four times daily, or metronidazole, 500 mg orally twice daily, for 14 days. (2) Either a single dose of cefoxitin, 2 g intramuscularly, with probenecid, 1 g orally, or ceftriaxone, 250 mg intramuscularly, plus doxycycline, 100 mg orally twice daily, for 14 days.

C. General Measures: Bed rest in a semi-Fowler position and adequate fluid intake are recommended. Pain is controlled with mild analgesics. Sexual intercourse should be avoided until recovery is complete, often for 2–3 months. Subsequent use of a condom or a diaphragm with spermicide and avoidance of coitus during menses may reduce the risk of reinfection.

D. Surgical Measures: Tubo-ovarian abscesses may require surgical excision or transcutaneous or transvaginal aspiration. Unless rupture is suspected, institute high-dose antibiotic therapy in the hospital, and monitor therapy with ultrasound. In 70% of cases, antibiotics are effective; in 30%, there is inadequate response in 48–72 hours, and intervention is required. Unilateral adnexectomy in the presence of unilateral abscess is acceptable. Hysterectomy and bilateral salpingo-oophorectomy may be necessary for overwhelming infection or in cases of chronic disease with intractable pelvic pain.

Prognosis

In spite of treatment, one-fourth of women with acute disease develop long-term sequelae, including repeated episodes of infection, chronic pelvic pain, dyspareunia, ectopic pregnancy, or infertility. The risk of infertility increases with repeated episodes of salpingitis: it is estimated at 10% after the first episode, 25% after a second episode, and 50% after a third episode.

McCormack WM: Pelvic inflammatory disease. N Engl J Med 1994;330:115.

1993 Sexually transmitted diseases treatment guidelines. MMWR Morb Mortal Wkly Rep 1993;42(RR-14):1.

OVARIAN TUMORS

Essentials of Diagnosis

- Vague gastrointestinal discomfort.
- Pelvic pressure and pain.
- Many cases of early-stage cancer are asymptomatic.
- Pelvic examination, CA 125, and ultrasound are mainstays of diagnosis.

General Considerations

Ovarian tumors are common. Most are benign, but malignant ovarian tumors are the leading cause of death from gynecologic cancer. The wide range of types and patterns of ovarian tumors is due to the complexity of ovarian embryology and differences in tissues of origin (Table 17–4).

In women with no family history of ovarian cancer, the lifetime risk is 1.6%, whereas a woman with one affected first-degree relative has a 5% lifetime risk. With two or more affected first-degree relatives, the risk is 7%. Approximately 3% of women with two or more affected first-degree relatives will have a hereditary ovarian cancer syndrome with a lifetime

Table 17–4. Ovarian functional and neoplastic tumors.

Tumor	Incidence	Size	Consistency	Menstrual Irregularities	Endocrine Effects	Potential for Malignancy	Special Remarks
Follicle cysts	Rare in childhood; frequent in menstrual years; never in postmenopausal years.	< 6 cm, often bilateral.	Moderate	Occasional	Occasional anovulation with persistently proliferative endometrium.	0	Often disappear after a 2-month regimen of oral contraceptives.
Corpus luteum cysts	Occasional, in menstrual years.	4–6 cm, unilateral.	Moderate	Occasional delayed period	Prolonged secretory phase.	0	Functional cysts. Intraperitoneal bleeding occasionally.
Theca lutein cysts	Occurs with hydatidiform mole, choriocarcinoma; also with gonadotropin or clomiphene therapy.	To 4–5 cm, multiple, bilateral. (Ovaries may be ≥ 20 cm in diameter.)	Tense	Amenorrhea	hCG elevated as a result of trophoblastic proliferation.	0	Functional cysts. Hematoperitoneum or torsion of ovary may occur. Surgery to be avoided.
Inflammatory (tuboovarian abscess)	Concomitant with acute salpingitis.	To 15–20 cm, often bilateral.	Variable, painful	Menometrorrhagia	Anovulation usual.	0	Unilateral removal indicated if possible.
Endometriotic cysts	Never in preadolescent or postmenopausal years. Most common in women age 20–40 years.	To 10–12 cm, occasionally bilateral.	Moderate to softened	Rare	0	Very rare	Associated pelvic endometriosis. Medical treatment or conservative surgery recommended.
Teratoid tumors: Benign teratomas (dermoid cysts)	Childhood to postmenopause.	< 15 cm; 15% are bilateral.	Moderate to softened	0	0	Rare	Torsion can occur. Partial oophorectomy recommended.
Malignant teratomas	< 1% of ovarian tumors. Usually in infants and young adults.	> 20 cm, unilateral.	Irregularly firm	0	Occasionally, hCG elevated.	All	Unresponsive to any therapy.

Type	Frequency	Size & bilaterality	Consistency	Menstrual abnormalities	Hormone output	Malignant potential	Special features
Cystadenoma, cystadenocarcinoma	Common in reproductive years.	Serous; <25 cm, 33% bilateral. Mucinous; up to 1 meter, 10% bilateral.	Moderate to softened	0	0	> 50% for serous. About 5% for mucinous.	Peritoneal implants often occur with serous tumors, rarely occur with mucinous tumors. If mucinous tumor is ruptured, pseudomyxoma peritonei may occur.
Endometrioid carcinoma	15% of ovarian carcinomas.	Moderate, 13% bilateral.	Firm	0	0	All	Adenocarcinoma of endometrium coexists in 15–30% of cases.
Fibroma	< 5% of ovarian tumors.	Usually < 15 cm.	Very firm	0	0	Rare	Ascites in 20% (rarely, pleural fluid).
Arrhenoblastoma	Rare. Average age 30 years or more.	Often small (< 10 cm), unilateral.	Firm to softened	Amenorrhea	Androgens elevated.	< 20%	Recurrences are moderately sensitive to irradiation.
Theca cell tumor (thecoma)	Uncommon.	< 10 cm, unilateral.	Firm	Occasionally irregular periods	Estrogens or androgens elevated.	< 1%	
Granulosa cell tumor	Uncommon. Usually in prepubertal girls or women older than 50 years.	May be very small.	Firm to softened	Menometrorrhagia	Estrogens elevated.	15–20%	Recurrences are moderately sensitive to irradiation.
Dysgerminoma	About 1–2% of ovarian tumors.	< 30 cm, bilateral in one-third of cases.	Moderate to softened	0	0	All	Very radiosensitive.
Brenner tumor	About 1% of ovarian tumors.	< 30 cm, unilateral.	Firm	0	0	Very rare	> 50% occur in postmenopausal years.
Secondary ovarian tumors	10% of fatal malignant disease in women.	Varies, often bilateral.	Firm to softened	Occasional	Very rare (thyroid, adrenocortical origin).	All	Bowel or breast metastases to ovary common.

risk of 40%. These women should be screened annually with transvaginal ultrasound (TVS) and CA 125, and prophylactic oophorectomy is recommend by age 35 or whenever childbearing is completed because of the high risk of disease. The benefits of such screening for women with one or no affected first-degree relatives are unproved, and the risks associated with unnecessary surgical procedures may outweigh the benefits in low-risk women. In women at increased risk of ovarian cancer, the long-term use of oral contraceptives may decrease the risk.

Clinical Findings

A. Symptoms and Signs: Unfortunately, most women with both benign and malignant ovarian neoplasms are either asymptomatic or experience only mild nonspecific gastrointestinal symptoms or pelvic pressure. Women with early disease are typically detected on routine pelvic examination. Women with advanced malignant disease may experience abdominal pain and bloating, and a palpable abdominal mass with ascites is often present.

B. Laboratory Findings: An elevated serum CA 125 (> 35 units) indicates a greater likelihood that a ovarian tumor is malignant. CA 125 is elevated in 80% of women with epithelial ovarian cancer overall but in only 50% of women with early disease. Furthermore, serum CA 125 may be elevated in premenopausal women with benign disease such as endometriosis.

C. Imaging Studies: TVS is useful for screening high-risk women and but has inadequate sensitivity for screening low-risk women. Ultrasound is helpful in differentiating ovarian masses that are benign and likely to resolve spontaneously from those with malignant potential. Color Doppler imaging may further enhance the specificity of ultrasound diagnosis.

Differential Diagnosis

Once an ovarian mass has been detected, it must be categorized as functional, benign neoplastic, or potentially malignant. Predictive factors include age, size of the mass, ultrasound configuration, CA 125 levels, the presence of symptoms, and whether the mass is unilateral or bilateral. In a premenopausal woman, an asymptomatic, mobile, unilateral, simple cystic mass less than 8–10 cm may be observed for 4–6 weeks. Most will resolve spontaneously. If the mass is larger or unchanged on repeat pelvic examination and TVS, surgical evaluation is required.

Most ovarian masses in postmenopausal women require surgical evaluation. However, a postmenopausal woman with an asymptomatic unilateral simple cyst less than 5 cm in diameter and a normal CA 125 level may be followed closely with TVS. All others require surgical evaluation.

Exploratory laparotomy has been the standard approach. The use of laparoscopy for evaluation of ovarian masses is controversial. While performed commonly, there are no data on the safety and efficacy of this approach. If malignancy is suspected, preoperative workup should include chest x-ray, evaluation of liver and kidney function, and hematologic indices.

Treatment

If a malignant ovarian mass is suspected, surgical evaluation should be performed by a gynecologic oncologist. For benign neoplasms, tumor removal or unilateral oophorectomy is usually performed. For ovarian cancer in an early stage, the standard therapy is complete surgical staging followed by abdominal hysterectomy and bilateral salpingo-oophorectomy with omentectomy and selective lymphadenopathy. With more advanced disease, aggressive removal of all visible tumor improves survival. Except for women with low-grade ovarian cancer in an early stage, postoperative chemotherapy is indicated. Several chemotherapy regimens are effective, such as the combination of cisplatin and cyclophosphamide with or without doxorubicin, with clinical response rates of up to 60–70%.

Prognosis

Unfortunately, approximately 75% of women with ovarian cancer are diagnosed with advance disease after regional or distant metastases have become established. The overall 5-year survival is approximately 17% with distant metastases, 36% with local spread, and 89% with early disease.

[Ovarian cancer: screening, treatment, and follow-up] gopher://gopher.nih.gov/00/clin/cdcs/individual/96.ovca

Cannistra SA: Cancer of the ovary. N Engl J Med 1993;329:1550. (Review article with extensive references.)

Carlson KJ et al: Screening for ovarian cancer. Ann Intern Med 1994;121:124. (For patients without family history or evidence of hereditary cancer syndrome, routine screening is not recommended.)

Nguyen HN et al: Ovarian carcinoma. Cancer 1994;74:545. (For patients with hereditary cancer syndrome, prophylactic oophorectomy may be warranted.)

NIH Consensus Conference: Ovarian cancer: Screening, treatment and followup. JAMA 1995;273:491.

PERSISTENT ANOVULATION (Polycystic Ovary Syndrome, Stein-Leventhal Syndrome)

Essentials of Diagnosis

- Chronic anovulation.
- Infertility.
- Elevated plasma testosterone and LH values and a reversed FSH/LH ratio.
- Hirsutism (in 70% of patients).

General Considerations

Polycystic ovary syndrome is a common endocrine disorder affecting 2–5% of women of reproductive age. The primary lesion is unknown. These patients have a relatively steady state of high estrogen, androgen, and LH levels rather than the fluctuating condition seen in ovulating women. Increased levels of estrone come from obesity (conversion of ovarian and adrenal androgens to estrone in body fat) or from excessive levels of androgens seen in some women of normal weight. The high estrone levels are believed to cause suppression of pituitary FSH and a relative increase in LH. Constant LH stimulation of the ovary results in anovulation, multiple cysts, and theca cell hyperplasia with excess androgen output. The polycystic ovary has a thickened, pearly white capsule and may not be enlarged.

Women with Cushing's syndrome, congenital adrenal hyperplasia, and androgen-secreting adrenal tumors also tend to have high circulating androgen levels and anovulation with polycystic ovaries.

Clinical Findings

Polycystic ovary syndrome is manifested by hirsutism (70% of cases), obesity (40%), and virilization (20%). Fifty percent of patients have amenorrhea, 30% have abnormal uterine bleeding, and 20% have normal menstruation. Additionally, they show insulin resistance and hyperinsulinemia when infused with glucose, and these women are at increased risk of early-onset NIDDM. The patients are generally infertile, although they may ovulate occasionally. They have an increased long-term risk of cancer of the breast and endometrium because of unopposed estrogen secretion.

Differential Diagnosis

Anovulation in the reproductive years may also be due to (1) premature menopause (high FSH and LH levels); (2) rapid weight loss, extreme physical exertion (normal FSH and LH levels for age), or obesity; (3) discontinuation of oral contraceptives (anovulation for 6 months or more occasionally occurs); (4) pituitary adenoma with elevated prolactin (galactorrhea may or may not be present); (5) hyper- or hypothyroidism. Always check FSH, LH, prolactin, TSH, testosterone, and dehydroepiandrosterone sulfate (DHEAS) levels when amenorrhea has persisted for 6 months or more without a diagnosis. A 10-day course of progestin (eg, medroxyprogesterone acetate, 10 mg/d) will cause withdrawal bleeding if estrogen levels are high. This will aid in the diagnosis and prevent endometrial hyperplasia. In long-term anovular patients over age 35, it is wise to search for an estrogen-stimulated cancer with mammography and endometrial aspiration.

Treatment

In obese patients with polycystic ovaries, weight reduction is often effective; a decrease in body fat will lower the conversion of androgens to estrone and thereby help to restore ovulation.

If the patient wishes to become pregnant, clomiphene or other drugs can be employed for ovulatory stimulation. The addition of dexamethasone 0.5 mg at bedtime to a clomiphene regimen may increase the likelihood of ovulation by suppression of ACTH and circulating adrenal androgens. Wedge resection of the ovary is often successful in restoring ovulation and fertility, although this procedure is used less commonly now that medical treatments are available.

If the patient does not desire pregnancy, give medroxyprogesterone acetate, 10 mg/d for the first 10 days of each month. This will ensure regular shedding of the endometrium so that hyperplasia will not occur. If contraception is desired, a low-dose combination oral contraceptive can be used; this is also useful in controlling hirsutism, for which treatment must be continued for 6–12 months before results are seen.

Hirsutism may be managed with epilation and electrolysis. Dexamethasone, 0.5 mg each night, is helpful in women with excess adrenal androgen secretion. If hirsutism is severe, some patients will elect to have a hysterectomy and bilateral oophorectomy followed by estrogen replacement therapy. Spironolactone, an aldosterone antagonist, is also useful for hirsutism in doses of 25 mg three or four times daily.

Haseltine FP et al: An NICHD Conference: Androgens and Women's Health. Am J Med 1995;98(Suppl 1A):1S. (A series of articles providing comprehensive coverage of androgen disorders in women.)

PAINFUL INTERCOURSE (Dyspareunia)

Questions related to sexual functioning should be asked as part of the reproductive history. Two helpful questions are, "Are you sexually active?" and "Are you having any sexual difficulties at this time?" The physician should be able to provide basic sex counseling and should allow adequate time for a discussion of problems related to sexuality, personal relationships, contraception, and fears of pregnancy.

Painful intercourse may be caused by vulvovaginitis; vaginismus; an incompletely stretched hymen; insufficient lubrication of the vagina; vaginal atrophy; endometriosis; or tumors or other pathologic conditions. During the pelvic examination, the patient should be placed in a half-sitting position and given a hand-held mirror and then asked to point out the site of pain and describe the type of pain.

Etiology

A. Vulvovaginitis: Vulvovaginitis is inflammation or infection of the vagina. Areas of marked tenderness in the vulvar vestibule without visible inflammation occasionally show lesions resembling small condylomas on colposcopy (see Vaginitis, above).

B. Vaginismus: Vaginismus is voluntary or involuntary contraction of muscles around the introitus. It results from fear, pain, sexual trauma, or having learned negative attitudes toward sex during childhood.

C. Remnants of the Hymen: The hymen is usually adequately stretched during initial intercourse, so that pain does not occur subsequently. In some women, the pain of initial intercourse may produce vaginismus. In others, a thin or thickened rim or partial rim of hymen remains after several episodes of intercourse, causing pain.

D. Insufficient Lubrication of the Vagina: See Vaginal Atrophy, below.

E. Infection, Endometriosis, Tumors, or Other Pathologic Conditions: Pain occurring with deep thrusting during coitus is usually due to acute or chronic infection of the cervix, uterus, or adnexa; endometriosis; adnexal tumors; or adhesions resulting from prior pelvic disease or operation. Careful history taking and a pelvic examination will generally help in the differential diagnosis.

F. Dyspareunia Due to Unknown Cause: Occasionally, no organic cause of pain can be found. These patients may have psychosexual conflicts or a history of childhood sexual abuse.

Treatment

A. Vulvovaginitis: Lesions resembling warts on colposcopy or biopsy should be treated in the appropriate way (see Vaginitis). The sexual partner should also be treated to prevent recurrence. Irritation from spermicides may be a factor. The couple may be helped by a discussion of noncoital techniques to achieve orgasm until the infection subsides.

B. Vaginismus: Sexual counseling and education on anatomy and sexual functioning may be appropriate. The patient can be instructed in self-dilation, using a lubricated finger or test tubes of graduated sizes. Before coitus (with adequate lubrication) is attempted, the patient—and then her partner—should be able to easily and painlessly introduce two fingers into the vagina. Penetration should never be forced, and the woman should always be the one to control the depth of insertion during dilation or intercourse.

C. Remnants of the Hymen: In rare situations, manual dilation of a remaining hymen under general anesthesia is necessary. Surgery should be avoided.

D. Insufficient Lubrication of the Vagina: If inadequate sexual arousal is the cause, sexual counseling for the woman—and her partner if possible—

is helpful. Lubricants may be used during sexual foreplay. For women with low plasma estrogen levels, use of a lubricant during coitus is sometimes sufficient. If not, use conjugated estrogen cream, one-eighth applicatorful daily for 10 days and then every other day. Using the applicator or a finger, the patient can apply the cream directly to the most tender area, usually the hymenal ring. Testosterone cream 1–2% in a water-soluble base is also helpful.

E. Infection, Endometriosis, Tumors, or Other Pathologic Conditions: Medical treatment of acute cervicitis, endometritis, or salpingitis and temporary abstention from coitus usually relieve pain. Hormonal or surgical treatment of endometriosis may be helpful. Dyspareunia resulting from chronic pelvic inflammatory disease or any condition causing extensive adhesions or fixation of pelvic organs is difficult to treat without extirpative surgery. Couples can be advised to try coital positions that limit deep thrusting and to use manual and oral sexual techniques.

F. Dyspareunia Due to Unknown Cause: Colposcopy in discrete areas of pain without obvious lesions may be useful to rule out papilloma virus infections. Biopsies should be taken if there is an identifiable lesion. Supportive, understanding discussion may be helpful. Small amounts of topical remedies such as 1% testosterone cream, estrogen cream, or topical lidocaine gel may relieve pain. Resolution of psychosexual problems or problems relating to traumatic sexual experiences may be necessary.

Bornstein J et al: Polymerase chain reaction search for viral etiology of vulvar vestibulitis syndrome. Am J Obstet Gynecol 1996:175;139. (Fifty-four percent of 86 women with vulvar vestibulitis had detectable human papillomavirus DNA in excised vulvar tissue compared with 4% of 25 women without that disorder.)

Steege JF, Ling FN: Dyspareunia: A special type of chronic pelvic pain. Obstet Gynecol Clin North Am 1993;20:779.

INFERTILITY

A couple is said to be infertile if pregnancy does not result after 1 year of normal sexual activity without contraceptives. About 25% of couples experience infertility at some point in their reproductive lives; the incidence of infertility increases with age. The male partner contributes to about 40% of cases of infertility, and a combination of factors is common.

Diagnostic Survey

During the initial interview, the physician can present an overview of infertility and discuss a plan of study. Separate private consultations are then conducted, allowing appraisal of psychosexual adjustment without embarrassment or criticism. Pertinent details (eg, sexually transmitted disease or prior pregnancies) must be obtained. The ill effects of excess caffeine, cigarettes, alcohol, and other recreational drugs on fertility in both men and women should be discussed. Prescription drugs that impair male potency should be noted. The gynecologic history should include queries regarding the menstrual pattern. The present history includes use and types of contraceptives, douches, libido, sex techniques, frequency and success of coitus, and correlation of intercourse with time of ovulation. Family history includes repeated abortions and maternal DES use.

General physical and genital examinations are performed on both partners. Basic laboratory studies include complete blood count, urinalysis, cervical culture for *Chlamydia,* serologic test for syphilis, rubella antibody determination, and thyroid function tests. Tay-Sachs screening should be offered if both parents are Jews and sickle cell screening if both parents are black.

The woman is instructed to chart her basal body temperature orally daily on arising and to record on a graph episodes of coitus and days of menstruation. Self-performed urine tests for the midcycle LH surge can be used to enhance temperature observations relating to ovulation. Couples should be advised that coitus resulting in conception occurs during the 6-day period ending with the day of conception.

The man is instructed to bring a complete ejaculate for analysis. Sexual abstinence for at least 3 days before the semen is obtained is emphasized. A clean, dry, wide-mouthed bottle for collection is preferred. Condoms should not be employed, as the protective powder or lubricant may be spermicidal. Semen should be examined within 1–2 hours after collection. Semen is considered normal with the following minimum values: volume, 3 mL; concentration, 20 million sperm per milliliter; motility, 50% after 2 hours; and normal forms, 60%. If the sperm count is abnormal, further evaluation includes a search for exposure to environmental and workplace toxins, alcohol or drug abuse, and hypogonadism.

A. First Testing Cycle: While the contribution of cervical factors to infertility is controversial, most gynecologists include a postcoital test in their workup. The test is scheduled for just before ovulation (eg, day 12 or 13 in an expected 28-day cycle). Preovulation timing can be enhanced by serial urinary LH tests. The patient is examined within 6 hours after coitus. The cervical mucus should be clear, elastic, and copious owing to the influence of the preovular estrogen surge. (The mucus is scantier and more viscid before and after ovulation.) A good spinnbarkeit (stretching to a fine thread 4 cm or more in length) is desirable. A small drop of cervical mucus should be obtained from within the cervical os and examined under the microscope. The presence of five or more active sperm per high-power field constitutes a satisfactory postcoital test. If no spermatozoa are found, the test should be repeated (assuming that active spermatozoa were present in the semen analysis). Sperm agglutination and sperm immobilization tests should be considered if the sperm are immotile or show ineffective tail motility.

The presence of more than three white blood cells per high-power field in the postcoital test suggests cervicitis in the woman or prostatitis in the man. When estrogen levels are normal, the cervical mucus dried on the slide will form a fern-like pattern when viewed with a low-power microscope. This type of mucus is necessary for normal sperm transport.

The serum progesterone level should be measured at the midpoint of the secretory phase (21st day); a level of 10–20 ng/mL confirms adequate luteal function.

B. Second Testing Cycle: Hysterosalpingography using an oil dye is performed within 3 days following the menstrual period. This x-ray study will demonstrate uterine abnormalities (septa, polyps, submucous myomas) and tubal obstruction. A repeat x-ray film 24 hours later will confirm tubal patency if there is wide pelvic dispersion of the dye. This test has been associated with an increased pregnancy rate by some observers. If the woman has had prior pelvic inflammation, give doxycycline, 100 mg twice daily, beginning immediately before and for 7 days after the x-ray study.

C. Further Testing:

1. Gross deficiencies of sperm (number, motility, or appearance) require repeat analysis. Zona-free hamster egg penetration tests are available to evaluate the ability of human sperm to fertilize an egg.

2. Obvious obstruction of the uterine tubes requires assessment for microsurgery or in vitro fertilization.

3. Absent or infrequent ovulation requires additional laboratory evaluation. Elevated FSH and LH levels indicate ovarian failure causing premature menopause. Elevated LH levels in the presence of normal FSH levels confirm the presence of polycystic ovaries. Elevation of blood prolactin (PRL) levels suggests pituitary microadenoma.

4. Major histocompatibility antigen typing of both partners will confirm human leukocyte antigen-B locus homozygosity, which is found in greater than expected numbers among couples with unexplained infertility.

5. Ultrasound monitoring of folliculogenesis may reveal the occurrence of unruptured luteinized follicles.

6. Endometrial biopsy in the luteal phase associated with simultaneous serum progesterone levels will rule out luteal phase deficiency.

D. Laparoscopy: Approximately 25% of women whose basic evaluation is normal will have findings on laparoscopy explaining their infertility (eg, peritubal adhesions, endometriotic implants).

Treatment

A. Medical Measures: Fertility may be restored by appropriate treatment in many patients with endocrine imbalance, particularly those with hypo- or hyperthyroidism. Antibiotic treatment of cervicitis is of value. In women with abnormal postcoital tests and demonstrated antisperm antibodies causing sperm agglutination or immobilization, condom use for up to 6 months may result in lower antibody levels and improved pregnancy rates.

Women who engage in vigorous athletic training often have low sex hormone levels; fertility improves with reduced exercise and some weight gain.

B. Surgical Measures: Excision of ovarian tumors or ovarian foci of endometriosis can improve fertility. Microsurgical relief of tubal obstruction due to salpingitis or tubal ligation will reestablish fertility in a significant number of cases. In special instances of cornual or fimbrial block, the prognosis with newer surgical techniques has become much better. Peritubal adhesions or endometriotic implants often can be treated via laparoscopy or via laparotomy immediately following laparoscopic examination if prior consent has been obtained.

With varicocele in the male, sperm characteristics are often improved following surgical treatment.

C. Induction of Ovulation:

1. Clomiphene citrate–Clomiphene citrate stimulates gonadotropin release, especially LH. Consequently, plasma estrone (E_1) and estradiol (E_2) also rise, reflecting ovarian follicle maturation. If E_2 rises sufficiently, an LH surge occurs to trigger ovulation.

After a normal menstrual period or induction of withdrawal bleeding with progestin, give 50 mg of clomiphene orally daily for 5 days. If ovulation does not occur, increase the dose to 100 mg orally daily for 5 days. If ovulation still does not occur, repeat the course with 150 and then 200 mg daily for 5 days and add chorionic gonadotropin, 10,000 units intramuscularly, 7 days after clomiphene.

The rate of ovulation following this treatment is 90% in the absence of other infertility factors. The pregnancy rate is high. Twinning occurs in 5% of these patients, and three or more fetuses are found in rare instances (< 0.5% of cases). An increased incidence of congenital anomalies has not been reported. Painful ovarian cyst formation occurs in 8% of patients and may warrant discontinuation of therapy. Several recent studies have suggested a two- to threefold increased risk of ovarian cancer with the use of clomiphene for more than 1 year.

In the presence of increased androgen production (DHEA-S > 200 μg/dL), the addition of dexamethasone, 0.5 mg, or prednisone, 5 mg, at bedtime, improves the response to clomiphene. Dexamethasone should be discontinued after pregnancy is confirmed.

2. Bromocriptine–Use only if PRL levels are elevated and there is no withdrawal bleeding following progesterone administration (otherwise use clomiphene). To minimize side effects (nausea, diarrhea, dizziness, headache, fatigue), bromocriptine should be taken with meals. Begin with 2.5 mg once daily and increase to two or three times daily in increments of 1.25 mg. The drug is discontinued once pregnancy has occurred.

3. Human menopausal gonadotropins (hMG)–hMG is indicated in cases of hypogonadotropism and most other types of anovulation (exclusive of ovarian failure). Because of the complexities, laboratory tests, and expense associated with this treatment, patients who require hMG for the induction of ovulation should be referred to a specialist.

4. Gonadotropin-releasing hormone (GnRH)–Hypothalamic amenorrhea unresponsive to clomiphene will be reliably and successfully treated with subcutaneous pulsatile gonadotropin-releasing hormone (GnRH). Use of this substance will avoid the dangerous ovarian complications and the 25% incidence of multiple pregnancy associated with hMG, though the overall rate of ovulation and pregnancy is lower than hMG.

D. Treatment of Endometriosis: See above.

E. Treatment of Inadequate Transport of Sperm:

1. Cervical mucus will provide better transport following administration of 0.3 mg of conjugated equine estrogens from days 5 to 15 of the ovarian cycle (ovulation may be delayed).

2. Intrauterine insemination of concentrated washed sperm has been used to bypass a poor cervical environment associated with scant or hostile cervical mucus. The sperm must be handled by sterile methods, washed in sterile saline or tissue culture solutions, and centrifuged. A small amount of fluid (0.5 mL) containing the sperm is then instilled into the uterus.

F. Artificial Insemination in Azoospermia: If azoospermia is present, artificial insemination by a donor usually results in pregnancy, assuming female function is normal. Both partners must consent to this method. The use of frozen sperm is currently preferable to fresh sperm because the frozen specimen can be held pending cultures and blood test results for sexually transmitted diseases, including AIDS.

G. Assisted Reproductive Technologies: Couples who have failed to respond to traditional infertility treatments, including those with tubal disease, severe endometriosis, oligospermia, and immunologic or unexplained infertility, may benefit from the newer technologies of in vitro fertilization (IVF), gamete intrafallopian transfer (GIFT), and zygote intrafallopian transfer (ZIFT). These techniques are complex and require a highly organized team of specialists. All of the procedures involve ovarian stimulation to produce multiple oocytes, oocyte retrieval by transvaginal ultrasound-guided needle aspiration, and handling of the oocytes outside the body. With IVF, the eggs are fertilized in vitro and the embryos transferred to the uterine fundus. Extra embryos may be cryopreserved for subsequent cycles. The average delivery rate per retrieval for 249 programs in the USA and Canada in 1994 was

20.7%. Age is an important determinant of success; for couples under the age of 40, without additional infertility problems in the male partner, the average delivery rate per retrieval was 24.5%, while the rate for women over 40 was 9%. The use of donor oocytes will increase the likelihood of pregnancy for older women. In 1994, 36.3% of pregnancies were multiple. Ectopic pregnancy may occur in women with tubal disease.

GIFT involves the placement of sperm and eggs in the fallopian tube by laparoscopy or minilaparotomy. While GIFT is a more invasive procedure than IVF, the success rate is higher, 28.4% overall in 1994. For women under 40, the delivery rate per retrieval cycle without a male factor was 33.5%. For women over 40, the rate was 12.3%. GIFT is not appropriate for women with severe tubal disease and is less successful than IVF with male factor infertility, since fertilization cannot be documented. With ZIFT, fertilization occurs in vitro, and the early development of the embryo occurs in the natural site, the fallopian tube, after transfer by laparoscopy or minilaparotomy. The average delivery rate per retrieval in 1994 was 29.1%.

Prognosis

The prognosis for conception and normal pregnancy is good if minor (even multiple) disorders can be identified and treated; it is poor if the causes of infertility are severe, untreatable, or of prolonged duration (over 3 years).

It is important to remember that in the absence of identifiable causes of infertility, 60% of couples will achieve a pregnancy within 3 years. Couples with unexplained infertility who do not achieve pregnancy within 3 years should be offered ovulation induction or assisted reproductive technology. Also, offering appropriately timed information about adoption is considered part of a complete infertility regimen.

Bristow RE, Karlan BY: Ovulation induction, infertility, and ovarian cancer risk. Fertil Steril 1996;66:499. (Critical review of published data suggesting that association between ovulation induction and ovarian cancer is not necessarily causal and that infertility itself is an independent risk factor. There is no consistent dose-effect relationship, and latency is highly variable.)

Jones HW, Toner JP: The infertile couple. N Engl J Med 1993;329:1710. (Review of evaluation and treatment options and success rates of various methods.)

Society for Assisted Reproductive Technology, American Society for Reproductive Medicine: Assisted reproductive technology in the United States and Canada: 1994 results generated from the ASRM/SART Registry. Fertil Steril 1996;66:697.

CONTRACEPTION

Voluntary control of childbearing benefits women, men, and the children born to them. Contraception should be available to all women and men of repro-ductive ages. Education about contraception and access to contraceptive pills or devices are especially important for sexually active teenagers and for women following childbirth or abortion.

Education about sexually transmitted disease, especially AIDS, should be given to all sexually active people, along with information that condoms with spermicide offer a high degree of protection (but not complete protection) to both sexes against sexually transmitted disease as well as pregnancy. The worldwide AIDS epidemic should cause a significant shift toward the use of condoms plus spermicide.

Kaunitz AM et al: Contraception, a clinical review for internists. Med Clin North Am 1995;79:1377.

1. ORAL CONTRACEPTIVES

Combined Oral Contraceptives

A. Efficacy and Methods of Use: Oral contraceptives have a theoretical failure rate of less than 0.5% if taken absolutely on schedule and a typical failure rate of 3%. Their primary mode of action is suppression of ovulation. The pills are initially started on the first or fifth day of the ovarian cycle and taken daily for 21 days, followed by 7 days of placebos or no medication, and this schedule is then continued for each cycle. The pills are often initially started on the first Sunday after the onset of menses, to help patients remember their starting day and to avoid menses on the weekend. If a pill is missed at any time, two pills should be taken the next day, and another method of contraception should be used for the rest of the cycle (eg, condoms or foam). A backup method should also be used during the first cycle if the pills are started later than the fifth day. Low-dose oral contraceptives is no longer contraindicated in women aged 35–50 who are nonsmokers and have no risk factors for cardiovascular disease.

B. Benefits of Oral Contraceptives: There are many noncontraceptive advantages to oral contraceptives. Menstrual flow is lighter, resultant anemia is less common, and dysmenorrhea is relieved for most women. Functional ovarian cysts generally disappear with oral contraceptive use, and new cysts do not occur. Pain with ovulation and postovulatory aching are relieved. The risk of ovarian and endometrial cancer is decreased. The risks of salpingitis and ectopic pregnancy may be diminished. Acne is usually improved. The frequency of developing myomas is lower in long-term users (> 4 years). There is a beneficial effect on bone mass.

C. Selection of an Oral Contraceptive: Any of the combination oral contraceptives containing less than 50 μg of estrogen are suitable for most women. Women taking pills containing 50 μg or more of estrogen should be switched to lower-dosage pills, since many of the adverse side effects are dose-related. There is some variation in potency of the various progestins in the pills, but there are essentially no clinically significant differences for most women among the progestins in the low-dose pills. Women who have acne or hirsutism may benefit from use of one of the pills containing the newer progestins, desogestrel or norgestimate, as they are the least androgenic. The dose of estrogen in oral contraceptives is four or more times higher than that in estrogen preparations used in menopause, and for that reason more side effects can be expected from oral contraceptives. The low-dose oral contraceptives commonly used in the United States are listed in Table 17–5.

D. Drug Interactions: Several drugs interact with oral contraceptives to decrease their efficacy by causing induction of microsomal enzymes in the liver, by increasing sex hormone-binding globulin, and by other mechanisms. Some commonly prescribed drugs in this category are phenytoin, phenobarbital (and other barbiturates), primidone, carbamazepine, and rifampin. Women taking these drugs

should use another means of contraception for maximum safety.

E. Contraindications and Adverse Effects: Oral contraceptives have been associated with many adverse effects; they are contraindicated in some situations and should be used with caution in others (Table 17–6).

1. Myocardial infarction–The risk of heart attack is higher with use of oral contraceptives, particularly with pills containing 50 µg of estrogen or more. Cigarette smoking, obesity, hypertension, diabetes, or hypercholesterolemia increases the risk. Young nonsmoking women have minimal increased risk. Smokers over age 40 and women with other cardiovascular risk factors should use other methods of birth control.

2. Thromboembolic disease–An increased rate of venous thromboembolism is found in oral contraceptive users, especially if the dose of estrogen is 50 µg or more. While the overall risk is very low (15 per 100,000 woman-years), several recent studies have reported a twofold increased risk in women us-

Table 17–5. Commonly used low-dose oral contraceptives.

Name	Type	Progestin	Estrogen (Ethinyl Estradiol)	Cost per Month[1]
Loestrin 1/20	Combination	1 mg norethindrone acetate	20 µg	$27.69
Lo/Ovral	Combination	0.3 mg dl-norgestrel	30 µg	$22.00
Nordette and Levlen	Combination	0.15 mg levonorgestrel	30 µg	$21.25
Norinyl 1/35 and Ortho-Novum 1/35	Combination	1 mg norethindrone	35 µg	$24.30
Loestrin 1.5/30	Combination	1.5 mg norethindrone acetate	30 µg	$27.69
Demulen 1/35	Combination	1 mg ethynodiol diacetate	35 µg	$25.59
Brevicon, Modicon, and Jenest	Combination	0.5 mg norethindrone	35 µg	$25.06
Ovcon 35	Combination	0.4 mg norethindrone	35 µg	$25.33
Ortho-Cept and Desogen	Combination	0.15 mg desogestrel	30 µg	$26.38
Ortho-Cyclen	Combination	0.25 mg norgestimate	35 µg	$25.05
Tricyclen	Triphasic	0.15 mg norgestimate (days 1–7) 0.215 mg norgestimate (days 8–14) 0.25 mg norgestimate (days 15–21)	35 µg	$25.05
Ortho-Novum 7/7/7	Triphasic	0.5 mg norethindrone (days 1–7) 0.75 mg norethindrone (days 8–14) 1 mg norethindrone (days 15–21)	35 µg	$24.98
Tri-Norinyl	Triphasic	0.5 mg norethindrone (days 1–7) 1 mg norethindrone (days 8–16) 0.5 mg norethindrone (days 17–21)	35 µg	$24.16
Triphasil and Tri-Levlen	Triphasic	0.05 mg levonorgestrel (days 1–6) 0.0075 mg levonorgestrel (days 7–11) 0.125 mg levonorgestrel (days 12–21)	30 µg 40 µg 30 µg	$25.75
Micronor and Nor-QD	Progestin-only minipill	0.35 mg norethindrone to be taken continuously		$29.22
Ovrette	Progestin-only minipill	0.075 mg dl-norgestrel to be taken continuously		$28.05

[1]Cost to pharmacist (average wholesale price) for 30 days' treatment. Source: First Data Bank, Price Alert, April 1997.

Table 17–6. Contraindications to use of oral contraceptives.

Absolute contraindications
Pregnancy
Thrombophlebitis or thromboembolic disorders (past or present)
Stroke or coronary artery disease (past or present)
Cancer of the breast (known or suspected)
Undiagnosed abnormal vaginal bleeding
Estrogen-dependent cancer (known or suspected)
Benign or malignant tumor of the liver (past or present)

Relative contraindications
Age over 35 years and heavy cigarette smoking (> 15 cigarettes daily)
Migraine or recurrent persistent, severe headache
Hypertension
Cardiac or renal disease
Diabetes
Gallbladder disease
Cholestasis during pregnancy
Active hepatitis or infectious mononucleosis
Sickle cell disease (S/S or S/C type)
Surgery, fracture, or severe injury
Lactation
Significant psychologic depression

ing oral contraceptives containing the progestins gestodene (not available in the United States) or desogestrel compared with women using oral contraceptives with levonorgestrel and norethindrone. Women with any risk factors for thromboembolism should not use these oral contraceptives. Established users without risk factors may continue using them after receiving counseling about the increased risk. Women who develop thrombophlebitis should stop using this method, as should those at risk of thrombophlebitis because of surgery, fracture, serious injury, or immobilization.

3. Cerebrovascular disease–Overall, a small increased risk of hemorrhagic stroke and subarachnoid hemorrhage and a somewhat greater increased risk of thrombotic stroke has been found; smoking, hypertension, and age over 35 years are associated with increased risk. Women who develop warning symptoms such as severe headache, blurred or lost vision, or other transient neurologic disorders should stop using oral contraceptives.

4. Carcinoma–A relationship between long-term (3–4 years) oral contraceptive use and occurrence of cervical dysplasia and cancer has been found in various studies. No confirmed relationship has been found between use of oral contraceptives and cancer of the breast. Combination oral contraceptives reduce the risk of endometrial carcinoma by 40% after 2 years of use and 60% after 4 or more years of use. The risk of ovarian cancer is reduced by 30% with pill use for less than 4 years, by 60% with use for 5–11 years, and by 80% after 12 or more years. Rarely, oral contraceptives have been associated with the development of benign or malignant hepatic tumors; this may lead to rupture of the liver,

hemorrhage, and death. The risk increases with higher dosage, longer duration of use, and older age.

5. Metabolic disorders–A decrease in glucose tolerance and an increase in triglyceride levels is seen in pill takers, and women with diabetes using this method should be carefully monitored.

6. Hypertension–Oral contraceptives may cause hypertension in some women; the risk is increased with longer duration of use and older age. Women who develop hypertension while using oral contraceptives should use other contraceptive methods. However, with regular blood pressure monitoring, nonsmoking women under the age of 40 with well-controlled mild hypertension may use oral contraceptives.

7. Headache–Migraine or other vascular headaches may occur or worsen with pill use. If severe or frequent headaches develop while using this method, it should be discontinued.

8. Amenorrhea–Postpill amenorrhea lasting a year or longer occurs occasionally, sometimes with galactorrhea. PRL levels should be checked; if elevated, a pituitary prolactinoma may be present.

9. Disorders of lactation–Combined oral contraceptives can impair the quantity and quality of breast milk. While it is preferable to avoid the use of combination oral contraceptives during lactation, the effects on milk quality are small and are not associated with developmental abnormalities in infants. Combination oral contraceptives should be started no earlier than 6 weeks postpartum to allow for establishment of lactation. Progestin-only pills, levonorgestrel implants, and depot medroxyprogesterone acetate are alternatives with no adverse effects on milk quality.

10. Other disorders–Depression may occur or be worsened with oral contraceptive use. Fluid retention may occur. Patients who had cholestatic jaundice during pregnancy may develop it while taking birth control pills.

F. Minor Side Effects: Nausea and dizziness may occur in the first few months of pill use. A weight gain of 2–5 lb commonly occurs. Spotting or breakthrough bleeding between menstrual periods may occur, especially if a pill is skipped or taken late; this may be helped by switching to a pill of slightly greater potency (see ¶C, above). Missed menstrual periods may occur, especially with low-dose pills. A pregnancy test should be performed if pills have been skipped or if two or more menstrual periods are missed. Depression, fatigue, and decreased libido can occur. Chloasma may occur, as in pregnancy, and is increased by exposure to sunlight.

Progestin Minipill

A. Efficacy and Methods of Use: Formulations containing 0.35 mg of norethindrone or 0.075 mg of norgestrel are available in the USA. Their efficacy is slightly lower than that of combined oral contraceptives, with failure rates of 1–4% being reported. The minipill is believed to prevent conception by causing thickening of the cervical mucus to make it hostile to sperm, alteration of ovum transport (which may account for the higher rate of ectopic pregnancy with these pills), and inhibition of implantation. Ovulation is inhibited inconsistently with this method. The minipill is begun on the first day of a menstrual cycle and then taken continuously for as long as contraception is desired.

B. Advantages: The low dose and absence of estrogen make the minipill safe during lactation; it may increase the flow of milk. It is often tried by women who want minimal doses of hormones and by patients who are over age 35. The minipill can be used by women with uterine myomas or sickle cell disease (S/S or S/C). Like the combined pill, the minipill decreases the likelihood of pelvic inflammatory disease by its effect on cervical mucus.

C. Complications and Contraindications: Minipill users often have bleeding irregularities (eg, prolonged flow, spotting, or amenorrhea); such patients may need monthly pregnancy tests. Ectopic pregnancies are more frequent, and complaints of abdominal pain should be investigated with this in mind. The absolute contraindications and many of the relative contraindications listed in Table 17–6 apply to the minipill. Exceptions are mentioned in ¶E, above. Minor side effects of combination oral contraceptives such as weight gain and mild headache may also occur with the minipill.

Colpitz GA: Oral contraceptive use and mortality during 12 years of follow-up: The Nurses' Health Study. Ann Intern Med 1994;120:821. (No increase in mortality rate noted with use of oral contraceptives. Some increase of breast cancer risk in current users and decreased risk of ovarian and endometrial cancer.)

DeCherney A: Bone-sparing properties of oral contraceptives. Am J Obstet Gynecol 1996;174:15. (The most important benefit of oral contraceptives for women over 35 may be prevention of loss of bone mass.)

Faculty of Family Planning and Reproductive Health Care, RCOG. Guidelines for prescribing combined oral contraceptives. BMJ 1996;312:121. (Addresses the risks of thromboembolism in oral contraceptive users.)

WHO Collaborative Study of Cardiovascular Disease and Steroid Hormone Contraception: Ischaemic stroke and combined oral contraceptives: Result of an international, multicentre, case-control study. Lancet 1996;348:498. (The risk of ischemic stroke in reproductive-aged women is low, and the attributable risk due to oral contraceptive use is small.)

2. CONTRACEPTIVE INJECTIONS & IMPLANTS (Long-Acting Progestins)

The injectable progestin medroxyprogesterone acetate is approved for contraceptive use in the USA. There is extensive worldwide experience with this method over the past 2 decades. The medication is given as a deep intramuscular injection of 150 mg every 3 months and has a contraceptive efficacy of 99.7%. Common side effects include irregular bleeding, amenorrhea, weight gain, and headache. Bone mineral loss may occur. Users commonly have irregular bleeding initially and subsequently develop amenorrhea. Ovulation may be delayed after the last injection. Contraindications are similar to those for the minipill.

The other available long-acting progestin is the Norplant system, a contraceptive implant containing levonorgestrel. The system consists of six small Silastic capsules that are inserted subcutaneously in the inner aspect of the upper arm. They release daily and provide highly effective contraception for 5 years. In the first year of use, Norplant is 99.8% effective. Contraceptive effectiveness drops slightly in succeeding years, but even in the fifth year it is more effective than the combination pill. The most common side effects include irregular bleeding and spotting, amenorrhea, headache, acne, and weight gain. Irregular bleeding is the most common reason for discontinuation. Hormone levels drop rapidly after removal of the implants, and there is no delay in the return of fertility. Contraindications are similar to those for the minipill. Insertion of the implants requires a minor surgical procedure under local anesthesia. Removal is also done under local anesthesia and may be more difficult than insertion. Removal may be facilitated by the "U" technique, involving use of a modified vasectomy clamp through a 4 mm incision parallel to the implants between implants three and four.

Kaunitz AM: Long-acting injectable contraception with depot medroxyprogesterone acetate. Am J Obstet Gynecol 1994;170:1543. (Contraceptive efficacy greater than 99%. Long-term use may cause bone loss and lipid alterations.)

Rosenberg MJ et al: A comparison of "U" and standard techniques for Norplant removal. Obstet Gynecol 1997;89:168. (This recently developed technique for Norplant removal is more easily performed than the standard technique, especially for inexperienced clinicians.)

3. INTRAUTERINE DEVICES (IUDs)

The only IUDs currently manufactured in the USA are the Progestasert (which secretes progesterone into the uterus) and the Copper T380A. Some all-plastic IUDs (Lippes Loop) are also still in use. Failure rates of most IUDs are 1–2%; the mechanism of action is thought to be related to impaired fertilization due to effects on sperm motility and to abnormal development in the oviduct of those ova that may have been fertilized.

The all-plastic IUDs do not need to be replaced at a specific time, and some women use them for 10 years or more. The copper-bearing IUDs must be replaced every 8 years for maximum efficacy. The progesterone-secreting IUDs must be replaced yearly but have the advantage of causing decreased cramping and menstrual flow.

The IUD is often an excellent contraceptive method for parous women with one sexual partner. It is less desirable for young nulliparas because of the greater threat of pelvic inflammatory disease in young women and the possible impairment of future fertility.

Insertion

Insertion can be performed during or after the menses, at midcycle to prevent implantation, or later in the cycle if the patient has not become pregnant. Most clinicians wait for 6–8 weeks postpartum before inserting an IUD. When insertion is performed during lactation, there is greater risk of uterine perforation or embedding of the IUD. Insertion immediately following abortion is acceptable if there is no sepsis and if follow-up insertion a month later will not be possible; otherwise, it is wise to wait until 4 weeks postabortion. Because of the risk of pelvic inflammation, a single prophylactic dose of doxycycline (200 mg) 1 hour before insertion is often used.

Contraindications & Complications

Contraindications to use of IUDs are outlined in Table 17–7.

A. Pregnancy: An IUD can be inserted within 5 days following a single episode of unprotected mid-cycle coitus as a postcoital contraceptive. An IUD should not be inserted into a pregnant uterus. If pregnancy occurs as an IUD failure, there is a greater chance of spontaneous abortion if the IUD is left in situ (50%) than if it is removed (25%). Spontaneous

Table 17–7. Contraindications to IUD use.

Absolute contraindications
Pregnancy
Acute or subacute pelvic inflammatory disease or purulent cervicitis
Relative contraindications
History of pelvic inflammatory disease since the last pregnancy
History of ectopic pregnancy (progestin-containing IUD only)
Multiple sexual partners
Nulliparous woman concerned about future fertility
Lack of available follow-up care
Menorrhagia or severe dysmenorrhea
Cervical or uterine neoplasia
Abnormal size or shape of uterus, including myomas distorting cavity
Valvular heart disease

abortion with an IUD in place is associated with a high risk of severe sepsis, and death can occur rapidly. Women using an IUD who become pregnant should have the IUD removed if the string is visible. It can be removed at the time of abortion if this is desired. If the string is not visible and the patient wants to continue the pregnancy, she should be informed of the serious risk of sepsis and, occasionally, death with such pregnancies. She should be informed that any flu-like symptoms such as fever, myalgia, headache, or nausea warrant immediate medical attention for possible septic abortion.

Since the ratio of ectopic to intrauterine pregnancies is increased among IUD wearers, clinicians should search for adnexal masses in early pregnancy and should always check the products of conception for placental tissue following abortion.

B. Pelvic Infection: There is an increased risk of pelvic infection during the first month following insertion. The subsequent risk of pelvic infection appears to be primarily related to the risk of acquiring sexually transmitted infections. The risk of infection at the time of insertion may be reduced by the use of antibiotic prophylaxis such as 200 mg of doxycycline. The threat of sexually transmitted pelvic infection can be essentially eliminated by limiting the use of the IUD to parous women with a single sexual partner. The use of IUDs by young nulliparas is undesirable because of the increased risk of sexually transmitted disease and the threat to future fertility.

C. Menorrhagia or Severe Dysmenorrhea: The IUD can cause heavier menstrual periods, bleeding between periods, and more cramping, so it is generally not suitable for women who already suffer from these problems. However, progesterone-secreting IUDs can be tried in these cases, as they often cause decreased bleeding and cramping with menses. Nonsteroidal anti-inflammatory drugs are also helpful in decreasing bleeding and pain in IUD users.

D. Complete or Partial Expulsion: Spontaneous expulsion of the IUD occurs in 10–20% of cases during the first year of use. Remove any IUD if the body of the device can be seen or felt in the cervical os.

E. Missing IUD Strings: If the transcervical tail cannot be seen, this may signify unnoticed expulsion, perforation of the uterus with abdominal migration of the IUD, or simply retraction of the string into the cervical canal or uterus owing to movement of the IUD or uterine growth with pregnancy. Once pregnancy is ruled out, one should probe for the IUD with a sterile sound or forceps designed for IUD removal, after administering a paracervical block. If the IUD cannot be detected, pelvic ultrasound will demonstrate the IUD if it is in the uterus. Alternatively, obtain anteroposterior and lateral x-rays of the pelvis with another IUD or a sound in the uterus as a marker, to confirm an extrauterine IUD. If the IUD is in the abdominal cavity, it should generally be removed by laparoscopy or laparotomy. Open-looped all-plastic IUDs such as the Lippes Loop can be left in the pelvis without danger, but ring-shaped IUDs may strangulate a loop of bowel and copper-bearing IUDs may cause tissue reaction and adhesions.

Perforations of the uterus are less likely if insertion is performed slowly, with meticulous care taken to follow directions applicable to each type of IUD.

Chi I: What we have learned from recent IUD studies. Contraception 1993;48:81. (Newer IUDs are safe, effective means of contraception in selected patients. No increased risk of pelvic inflammatory disease or infertility.)

4. DIAPHRAGM & CERVICAL CAP

The diaphragm (with contraceptive jelly) is a safe and effective contraceptive method with features that make it acceptable to some women and not others. Failure rates range from 2% to 20%, depending on the motivation of the woman and the care with which the diaphragm is used. The advantages of this method are that it has no systemic side effects and gives significant protection against pelvic infection and cervical dysplasia as well as pregnancy. The disadvantages are that it must be inserted near the time of coitus and that pressure from the rim predisposes some women to cystitis after intercourse.

The cervical cap (with contraceptive jelly) is similar to the diaphragm but fits snugly over the cervix only (the diaphragm stretches from behind the cervix to behind the pubic symphysis). The cervical cap is more difficult to insert and remove than the diaphragm. The main advantages are that it can be used by women who cannot be fitted for a diaphragm because of a relaxed anterior vaginal wall or by women who have discomfort or develop repeated bladder infections with the diaphragm.

Because of the small risk of toxic shock syndrome, a cervical cap or diaphragm should not be left in the vagina for over 12–18 hours, nor should these devices be used during the menstrual period (see above).

5. CONTRACEPTIVE FOAM, CREAM, JELLY, & SUPPOSITORY

These products are available without prescription, are easy to use, and are fairly effective, with reported failure rates of 2–30%. All contain the spermicides nonoxynol 9 or octoxynol 9, which also have some virucidal and bactericidal activity. Spermicides may alter the vaginal bacterial flora and allow overgrowth of E coli with an increased risk of bacteriuria. The products have the advantages of being simple to use

and easily available. Their disadvantage is a slightly higher failure rate than the diaphragm or condom.

McGroarty JA et al: The influence of nonoxynol-9-containing spermicides on urogenital infection. J Urol 1994; 152:831. (Nonoxynol-9 may decrease lactobacilli in vagina and urethra and predispose to bacteriuria.)

6. CONDOM

The male sheath of latex or animal membrane affords good protection against pregnancy—equivalent to that of a diaphragm and spermicidal jelly; latex (but not animal membrane) condoms also offer protection against sexually transmitted disease and cervical dysplasia. Men and women seeking protection against HIV transmission are advised to use a latex condom along with spermicide during vaginal or rectal intercourse. When a spermicide such as vaginal foam is used with the condom, the failure rate approaches that of oral contraceptives. Condoms coated with spermicide are available in the USA. The disadvantages of condoms are dulling of sensation and spillage of semen due to tearing, slipping, or leakage with detumescence of the penis.

A female condom made of polyurethane is now available in the USA. The reported failure rate in preventing pregnancy (26%) is somewhat higher than other barrier methods. However, it is the only female-controlled method that offers significant protection from both pregnancy and sexually transmitted diseases.

Roper WL, Peterson HB, Curran JW: Commentary: Condoms and HIV/STD prevention: Clarifying the message. Am J Public Health 1993;83:501. (When used correctly and consistently, condoms are highly effective in preventing HIV infection and other STDs.)

Trussel J et al: Comparative contraceptive efficacy of the female condom and other barrier methods. Fam Plann Perspect 1994;26:66. (Data are inadequate for making definite conclusions about comparative efficacy, but based on historical controls it is likely that the efficacy is similar to that of the diaphragm or sponge.)

7. CONTRACEPTION BASED ON AWARENESS OF FERTILE PERIODS

There is renewed interest in methods to identify times of ovulation and avoidance of unprotected intercourse at that time as a means of family planning. These methods are most effective when the couple restricts intercourse to the postovular phase of the cycle or uses a barrier method at other times. Women benefit from learning to identify their fertile periods. Well-instructed, motivated couples may achieve low pregnancy rates with fertility awareness, but in many field trials, the pregnancy rates were as high as 20%.

"Symptothermal" Natural Family Planning

The basis for this approach is patient-observed increase in clear elastic cervical mucus, brief abdominal midcycle discomfort ("mittelschmerz"), and a sustained rise of the basal body temperature about 2 weeks after onset of menstruation. Unprotected intercourse is avoided from shortly after the menstrual period, when fertile mucus is first identified, until 48 hours after ovulation, as identified by a sustained rise in temperature and the disappearance of clear elastic mucus.

Calendar Method

After the length of the menstrual cycle has been observed for at least 8 months, the following calculations are made: (1) The first fertile day is determined by subtracting 18 days from the shortest cycle; (2) the last fertile day is determined by subtracting 11 days from the longest cycle. For example, if the observed cycles run from 24 to 28 days, the fertile period would extend from the sixth day of the cycle (24 minus 18) through the 17th day (28 minus 11).

Basal Body Temperature Method

This method indicates the safe time for intercourse after ovulation has passed. The temperature must be taken immediately upon awakening, before any activity. A slight drop in temperature often occurs 1–1½ days before ovulation, and a rise of about 0.4 °C occurs 1–2 days after ovulation. The elevated temperature continues throughout the remainder of the cycle. New data suggest that the risk of pregnancy increases starting 5 days prior to the day of ovulation, peaks on the day of ovulation, and then rapidly decreases to zero by the day after ovulation.

Prospective European Multicenter Study of Natural Family Planning: Interim Results. The European Natural Family Planning Study Groups. Adv Contracept 1993;9:269. (The symptothermal method used with periodic abstinence and fertility awareness with the use of barriers during the fertile phase can be an effective contraceptive method.)

Wilcox AJ et al: Timing of sexual intercourse in relation to ovulation. N Engl J Med 1995;333:1517. (Among 221 women attempting conception, all pregnancies occurred with coitus during the 6-day period ending on the day of ovulation.)

8. POSTCOITAL CONTRACEPTION

If unprotected intercourse occurs in midcycle and the woman is certain she has not inadvertently become pregnant earlier in the cycle, the following regimens are effective in preventing implantation. The failure rate is less than 1.5%. These methods should be started within 72 hours after coitus. (1) Ethinyl estradiol, 2.5 mg twice daily for 5 days. (2) Ovral (50

μg of ethinyl estradiol with 0.5 mg of norgestrel), two tablets at once followed by two tablets 12 hours later, or four pills twice, 12 hours apart, of Lo/Ovral, Nordette, Levlen, or the yellow pills in the Triphasil or Tri-Levlen regimens. Antinausea medication may be necessary with these regimens. Bleeding should occur within 3–4 weeks. If pregnancy occurs, abortion is advisable because of fetal exposure to possibly teratogenic doses of sex steroids. Mifepristone (RU 486), in a single 600 mg dose within 72 hours after unprotected intercourse, appears to be an excellent postcoital contraceptive with minimal side effects. Unfortunately, mifepristone is not currently available in the United States.

IUD insertion within 5 days after one episode of unprotected midcycle coitus will also prevent pregnancy; copper-bearing IUDs have been tested for this purpose. The disadvantage of this method is possible infection, especially in rape cases; the advantage is ongoing contraceptive protection if this is desired in a patient for whom the IUD is a suitable choice.

9. ABORTION

Since the legalization of abortion in the USA in 1973, the related maternal mortality rate has fallen markedly, because illegal and self-induced abortions have been replaced by safer medical procedures. Abortions in the first trimester of pregnancy are performed by vacuum aspiration under local anesthesia. A similar technique, dilation and evacuation, is often used in the second trimester, with general or local anesthesia. Techniques utilizing intra-amniotic instillation of hypertonic saline solution or prostaglandins are also occasionally used after 18 weeks from the LMP but are more difficult for the patient. Abortions are rarely performed after 20 weeks from the LMP. It is currently believed that fetal viability begins at about 24 weeks. Legal abortion has a mortality rate of 1:100,000. Rates of morbidity and mortality rise with length of gestation. Currently in the USA, 90% of abortions are performed before 12 weeks' gestation and only 3–4% after 17 weeks. Every effort should be made to continue the trend toward earlier abortion.

Complications resulting from abortion include retained products of conception (often associated with infection and heavy bleeding) and unrecognized ectopic pregnancy. Immediate analysis of the removed tissue for placenta can exclude or corroborate the diagnosis of ectopic pregnancy. Women presenting with fever, bleeding, or abdominal pain after abortion should be examined; use of broad-spectrum antibiotics and reaspiration of the uterus are frequently necessary. Hospitalization is advisable if acute salpingitis requires intravenous administration of antibiotics. Complications following illegal abortion often need emergency care for hemorrhage, septic shock, or uterine perforation.

Rh immune globulin should be given to all Rh-negative women following abortion. Contraception should be thoroughly discussed and contraceptive supplies or pills provided at the time of abortion. In women with a past history of pelvic inflammatory disease, prophylactic antibiotics are indicated: A one-dose regimen is doxycycline, 200 mg orally 1 hour before the procedure, or aqueous penicillin G, 1 million units intravenously 30 minutes before. In the second trimester, use cefazolin, 1 g intravenously 30 minutes before the procedure. Many clinics prescribe tetracycline, 500 mg four times daily for 5 days after the procedure for all patients.

Long-term sequelae of repeated induced abortions have been studied, but as yet there is no consensus on whether there are increased rates of fetal loss or premature labor. It is felt that such adverse sequelae can be minimized by performing early abortion with minimal cervical dilation or by the use of osmotic dilators to induce gradual cervical dilation. A recent population-based study showed no evidence of an increased risk of breast cancer in women who had undergone an induced abortion.

An oral abortifacient, mifepristone (RU 486), 600 mg as a single dose followed in 36–48 hours by a prostaglandin vaginally or orally, is 95% successful in spontaneously terminating pregnancies of up to 9 weeks' duration with minimum complications. The drug acts as an antihormone to progesterone and glucocorticoids without producing adrenal insufficiency. Currently available in some European countries, it is not approved for use in the USA. Although not approved by the FDA for this indication, a combination of intramuscular methotrexate, 50 mg/m^2 of body surface area, followed 7 days later by vaginal misoprostol, 800 μg, was 98% successful in terminating pregnancy at 8 weeks or less.

Creinin MD et al: A randomized trial comparing misoprostol three and seven days after methotrexate for early abortion. Am J Obstet Gynecol 1995;173:1578. (This combination of readily available drugs may be an alternative to RU-486 regimens for medical termination of pregnancy.)

El-Refaey H et al: Induction of abortion with mifepristone (RU-486) and oral or vaginal misoprostol. N Engl J Med 1995;332:983. (Highly effective at terminating pregnancy at 9 weeks or less.)

Melbye M et al: Induced abortion and the risk of breast cancer. N Engl J Med 1997;336:81. (A large population-based study demonstrating that induced abortion has no overall effect on the subsequent risk of breast cancer.)

10. STERILIZATION

In the USA, sterilization is the most popular method of birth control for couples who want no more children. Although sterilization is reversible in some instances, reversal surgery in both men and woman is costly, complicated, and not always successful. Therefore, patients should be counseled carefully before sterilization and should view the procedure as final.

Vasectomy is a safe, simple procedure in which the vas deferens is severed and sealed through a scrotal incision under local anesthesia. Long-term follow-up studies on vasectomized men show no excess risk of cardiovascular disease. Several studies have shown a possible association with prostate cancer, but the evidence is weak and inconsistent.

Female sterilization is currently performed via laparoscopic bipolar electrocoagulation or plastic ring application on the uterine tubes or via minilaparotomy with Pomeroy tubal resection. The advantages of laparoscopy are minimal postoperative pain, small incisions, and rapid recovery. The advantage of minilaparotomy is that it can be performed with standard surgical instruments under local or general anesthesia. However, there is more postoperative pain and a longer recovery period. Failure rates after tubal sterilization are approximately 0.5%; this fact should be discussed with women preoperatively. Some studies have found an increased risk of menstrual irregularities as a long-term complication of tubal ligation, but findings in different studies have been inconsistent.

Raspa RF: Complications of vasectomy. Am Fam Physician 1993;48:1264. (Compared with tubal ligation, vasectomy has similar efficacy but a lower complication rate.)

Rulin MC et al: Long-term effects of tubal sterilization on menstrual indices and pelvic pain. Obstet Gynecol 1993;82:118. (This study of 500 women followed for up to 1½ years disclosed no significant long-term effects on menstrual function.)

RAPE

Rape, or sexual assault, is legally defined in different ways in various jurisdictions. Physicians and emergency room personnel who deal with rape victims should be familiar with the laws pertaining to sexual assault in their own state. From a medical and psychologic viewpoint, it is essential that persons treating rape victims recognize the nonconsensual and violent nature of the crime. About 95% of reported rape victims are women. Penetration may be vaginal, anal, or oral and may be by the penis, hand, or a foreign object. The absence of genital injury does not imply consent by the victim. The assailant may be unknown to the victim or may be an acquaintance or even the spouse.

"Unlawful sexual intercourse," or statutory rape, is intercourse with a female before the age of majority even with her consent.

Rape represents an expression of anger, power, and sexuality on the part of the rapist. The rapist is usually a hostile man who uses sexual intercourse to terrorize and humiliate a woman. Women neither secretly want to be raped nor do they expect, encourage, or enjoy rape.

Rape involves severe physical injury in 5–10% of cases and is always a terrifying experience in which most victims fear for their lives. Consequently, all victims suffer some psychologic aftermath. Moreover, some rape victims may acquire sexually transmissible disease or become pregnant.

Because rape is a personal crisis, each patient will react differently. The rape trauma syndrome comprises two principal phases:

(1) Immediate or acute: Shaking, sobbing, and restless activity may last from a few days to a few weeks. The patient may experience anger, guilt, or shame or may repress these emotions. Reactions vary depending on the victim's personality and the circumstances of the attack.

(2) Late or chronic: Problems related to the attack may develop weeks or months later. The lifestyle and work patterns of the individual may change. Sleep disorders or phobias often develop. Loss of self-esteem can rarely lead to suicide.

Physicians and emergency room personnel who deal with rape victims should work with community rape crisis centers whenever possible to provide ongoing supportive, skilled counseling.

General Office Procedures

The physician who first sees the alleged rape victim should be empathetic. Begin with a statement such as, "This is a terrible thing that has happened to you. I want to help."

(1) Secure written consent from the patient, guardian, or next of kin for gynecologic examination; for photographs if they are likely to be useful as evidence; and for notification of police. If police are to be notified, do so, and obtain advice on the transfer of evidence.

(2) Obtain and record the history in the patient's own words. The sequence of events, ie, the time, place, and circumstances, must be included. Note the date of the LMP, whether or not the woman is pregnant, and the time of the most recent coitus prior to the sexual assault. Note the details of the assault such as body cavities penetrated, use of foreign objects, and number of assailants.

Note whether the victim is calm, agitated, or confused (drugs or alcohol may be involved). Record whether the patient came directly to the hospital or whether she bathed or changed her clothing. Record findings but do not issue even a tentative diagnosis lest it be erroneous or incomplete.

(3) Have the patient disrobe while standing on a white sheet. Hair, dirt, and leaves; underclothing; and any torn or stained clothing should be kept as evidence. Scrape material from beneath fingernails and comb pubic hair for evidence. Place all evidence in separate clean paper bags or envelopes and label carefully.

(4) Examine the patient, noting any traumatized areas that should be photographed. Examine the body and genitals with a Wood light to identify semen, which fluoresces; positive areas should be swabbed with a premoistened swab and air-dried in order to identify PSA from prostatic secretions. Colposcopy can be used to identify small areas of trauma from forced entry especially at the posterior fourchette.

(5) Perform a pelvic examination, explaining all procedures and obtaining the patient's consent before proceeding gently with the examination. Use a narrow speculum lubricated with water only. Collect material with sterile cotton swabs from the vaginal walls and cervix and make two air-dried smears on clean glass slides. Swab the mouth (around molars and cheeks) and anus in the same way, if appropriate. Label all slides carefully. Collect secretions from the vagina, anus, or mouth with a premoistened cotton swab, place at once on a slide with a drop of saline, and cover with a coverslip. Look for motile or nonmotile sperm under high, dry magnification, and record the percentage of motile forms.

(6) Perform appropriate laboratory tests as follows. Culture the vagina, anus, or mouth (as appropriate) for *N gonorrhoeae* and *Chlamydia.* Perform a Papanicolaou smear of the cervix, a wet mount for *T vaginalis,* a baseline pregnancy test, and VDRL test. A confidential test for HIV antibody can be obtained if desired by the patient and repeated in 2–4 months if initially negative. Repeat the pregnancy test if the next menses is missed, and repeat the VDRL test in 6 weeks. Obtain blood (10 mL without anticoagulant) and urine (100 mL) specimens if there is a history of forced ingestion or injection of drugs or alcohol.

(7) Transfer clearly labeled evidence, eg, laboratory specimens, directly to the clinical pathologist in charge or to the responsible laboratory technician, in the presence of witnesses (never via messenger), so that the rules of evidence will not be breached.

Treatment

(1) Give analgesics or tranquilizers if indicated.

(2) Administer tetanus toxoid if deep lacerations contain soil or dirt particles.

(3) Give ceftriaxone, 125 mg intramuscularly, to prevent gonorrhea. In addition, give metronidazole, 2 g as a single dose, and doxycycline, 100 mg twice daily for 7 days to treat chlamydial infection. Incubating syphilis will probably be prevented by these medications, but the VDRL test should be repeated 6 weeks after the assault.

(4) Prevent pregnancy by using one of the methods discussed under Postcoital Contraception, if necessary (see above).

(5) Vaccinate against hepatitis B.

(6) Make sure the patient and her family and friends have a source of ongoing psychologic support.

Dunn SFM, Gilchrist VJ: Sexual assault. Prim Care 1993;20:359. (Reviews appropriate initial evaluation of sexual assault victim and long-term sequelae.)

Hampton HL: Care of the woman who has been raped. (Current Concepts.) N Engl J Med 1995;332:234.

MENOPAUSAL SYNDROME

Essentials of Diagnosis

- Cessation of menses due to aging or to bilateral oophorectomy.
- Elevation of FSH and LH levels.
- Hot flushes and night sweats (in 80% of women).
- Decreased vaginal lubrication; thinned vaginal mucosa with or without dyspareunia.

General Considerations

The term "menopause" denotes the final cessation of menstruation, either as a normal part of aging or as the result of surgical removal of both ovaries. In a broader sense, as the term is commonly used, it denotes a 1- to 3-year period during which a woman adjusts to a diminishing and then absent menstrual flow and the physiologic changes that may be associated—hot flushes, night sweats, and vaginal dryness or soreness with coitus.

The average age at menopause in Western societies today is 51 years. Premature menopause is defined as ovarian failure and menstrual cessation before age 40; this often has a genetic or autoimmune basis. Surgical menopause due to bilateral oophorectomy is common and can cause more severe symptoms owing to the sudden rapid drop in sex hormone levels.

There is no objective evidence that cessation of ovarian function is associated with severe emotional disturbance or personality changes. However, mood changes toward depression and anxiety can occur at this time. Furthermore, the time of menopause often coincides with other major life changes, such as departure of children from the home, a midlife identity crisis, or divorce. These events, coupled with a sense of the loss of youth, may exacerbate the symptoms of menopause and cause psychologic distress.

Clinical Findings

A. Symptoms and Signs:

1. Cessation of menstruation–Menstrual cycles generally become irregular as menopause approaches. Anovular cycles occur more often, with irregular cycle length and occasional menorrhagia. Menstrual flow usually diminishes in amount owing to decreased estrogen secretion, resulting in less abundant endometrial growth. Finally, cycles become longer, with missed periods or episodes or spotting only. When no bleeding has occurred for one year, the menopausal transition can be said to have occurred. Any bleeding after this time warrants investigation by endometrial curettage or aspiration to rule out endometrial cancer.

2. Hot flushes–Hot flushes (feelings of intense heat over the trunk and face, with flushing of the skin and sweating) occur in 80% of women as a result of the decrease in ovarian hormones. Hot flushes can begin before the cessation of menses. An increase in pulsatile release of gonadotropin-releasing hormone from the hypothalamus is believed to trigger the hot flushes by affecting the adjacent temperature-regulating area of the brain. Hot flushes are more severe in women who undergo surgical menopause. Flushing is more pronounced late in the day, during hot weather, after ingestion of hot foods or drinks, or during periods of tension. Occurring at night, they often cause sweating and insomnia and result in fatigue on the following day.

3. Vaginal atrophy–With decreased estrogen secretion, thinning of the vaginal mucosa and decreased vaginal lubrication occur and may lead to dyspareunia. The introitus decreases in diameter. Pelvic examination reveals pale, smooth vaginal mucosa and a small cervix and uterus. The ovaries are not normally palpable after the menopause. Continued sexual activity will help prevent tissue shrinkage; use of lubricants, estrogen or testosterone cream, or oral estrogen therapy can prevent or relieve pain.

4. Osteoporosis–Osteoporosis may occur as a late sequela of menopause.

B. Laboratory Findings:
Serum FSH and LH levels are elevated. Vaginal cytologic examination will show a low estrogen effect with predominantly parabasal cells, indicating lack of epithelial maturation due to hypoestrinism.

Treatment

A. Natural Menopause:
Education and support from health providers, midlife discussion groups, and reading material will help most women having difficulty adjusting to the menopause. Physiologic symptoms can be treated as follows:

1. Vasomotor symptoms–Give conjugated estrogens, 0.3 mg or 0.625 mg; estradiol, 0.5 or 1 mg; or estrone sulfate, 0.625 mg; or estradiol can be given transdermally (Estraderm) as skin patches that are changed twice weekly and secrete 0.05–0.1 mg of hormone daily. When either form of estrogen is used, add a progestin (medroxyprogesterone acetate) to prevent endometrial hyperplasia or cancer. The hormones can be given in several differing regimens. Give estrogen on days 1–25 of each calendar month, with 5–10 mg of medroxyprogesterone acetate added on days 14–25. Withhold hormones from day 26 until the end of the month, when the endometrium will be shed, producing a light, generally painless monthly period. Alternatively, give the estrogen along with 2.5 mg of medroxyprogesterone acetate daily, without stopping. This regimen causes some initial bleeding or spotting, but within a few months it produces an atrophic endometrium that will not bleed. If the patient has had a hysterectomy, a progestin need not be used. Explain to the patient that hot flushes will probably return if the hormone is discontinued. When women wish to stop hormone therapy, the dose should be tapered.

Clonidine, an α-adrenergic agonist, has been found to be effective in reducing hot flushes when given orally or transdermally in doses of 100–150 μg daily. Side effects include dry mouth, drowsiness, and blood pressure decrease, but the effects are usually mild at these low dosages. Natural methods to decrease the severity of hot flushes include daily exercise, electroacupuncture, relaxation practices, and avoiding caffeine and alcohol.

2. Vaginal atrophy–This problem can be treated with hormone therapy as outlined above. Alternatively, topical use of hormone creams in small doses will often relieve pain with minimal systemic absorption. Use conjugated estrogen vaginal cream, one-eighth applicatorful (0.3 mg of conjugated estrogen) nightly for 7–10 nights. Thereafter, use every other night or twice weekly. Testosterone propionate 1–2%, 0.5–1 g, in a vanishing cream base used in the same manner is also effective if estrogen is contraindicated. A bland lubricant such as unscented cold cream or water-soluble gel can be helpful at the time of coitus.

3. Osteoporosis–Women should ingest at least 800 mg of calcium daily throughout life. Nonfat or low-fat milk products, calcium-fortified orange juice, green leafy vegetables, corn tortillas, and canned sardines or salmon consumed with the bones are good dietary sources. In addition, 1 g of elemental calcium should be taken as a daily supplement at the time of the menopause and thereafter; calcium supplements should be taken with meals to increase their absorption. Vitamin D, 400 units/d from food, sunlight, or supplements, is necessary to enhance calcium absorption. A daily program of energetic walking and exercise to strengthen the arms and upper body helps maintain bone mass.

Women most at risk for osteoporotic fractures should consider hormone replacement therapy. This includes Caucasian and Asian women, especially if they have a family history of osteoporosis; are thin, short, cigarette smokers, and physically inactive; or have had a low calcium intake in adult life.

B. Advantages and Risks of Hormone Therapy: Long-term estrogen therapy has been shown to decrease a woman's risk of fatal heart attack, probably by decreasing LDL cholesterol, increasing HDL cholesterol, and increasing the elasticity of blood vessel walls. Estrogen replacement therapy may prevent or delay the onset of Alzheimer's disease. The dose of estrogen is much lower than that found in oral contraceptives, and side effects such as hypertension and other cardiovascular disorders are not seen. However, there may be a small increase in the risk of thromboembolic disease. Progestins counteract some but not all of these favorable effects. Estrogen helps to prevent osteoporosis, hot flushes, and dyspareunia and may elevate mood. The risks of estrogen include a probable small increase in breast cancer, especially in women with a close family history of the disease. Endometrial cancer can occur unless adequate progestin is used. Estrogen may cause the growth of uterine myomas, which otherwise shrink after the menopause. (See also discussion of hormone replacement therapy in Chapter 26.)

C. Surgical Menopause: The abrupt hormonal decrease resulting from oophorectomy generally results in severe vasomotor symptoms and rapid onset of dyspareunia and osteoporosis unless treated. Estrogen replacement is generally started immediately after surgery. Conjugated estrogen, 1.25 mg, estrone sulfate, 1.25 mg, or estradiol, 2 mg, is given for 25 days of each month. After age 45–50 years, this dose can be tapered to 0.625 mg of conjugated estrogen or equivalent.

Belchetz PE: Hormonal treatment of postmenopausal women. N Engl J Med 1994;330:1062. (Review of data on benefits and risks of hormonal replacement therapy.)

Cauley JA et al: Estrogen replacement therapy and fractures in older women. Ann Intern Med 1995;122:9. (Study of elderly women showing decrease in nonspinal fractures with current use of estrogen, with effect greater if started within 5 years after menopause.)

Grodstein F et al: Postmenopausal estrogen and progestin use and the risk of cardiovascular disease. N Engl J Med 1996;335:453. (Addition of a progestin to estrogen replacement therapy does not appear to reduce the cardioprotective effect of estrogen.)

Grodstein F et al: Prospective study of exogenous hormones and the risk of pulmonary embolism in women. Lancet 1996;348:983. (While primary pulmonary embolism in the study cohort was rare, current though not past use of estrogen replacement therapy was associated with a twofold increased risk.)

Paganini-Hill A, Henderson VW: Estrogen replacement therapy and risk of Alzheimer disease. Arch Intern Med 1996;156:2213. (Postmenopausal estrogen use was associated with a significant decrease in the risk of Alzheimer's disease.)

18

Obstetrics*

William R. Crombleholme, MD

DIAGNOSIS & DIFFERENTIAL DIAGNOSIS OF PREGNANCY

It is advantageous to diagnose pregnancy as promptly as possible when a sexually active woman misses a menstrual period or has symptoms suggestive of pregnancy. In the event of a desired pregnancy, prenatal care can begin early, and potentially harmful medications and activities, such as drug and alcohol use, smoking, and occupational chemical exposure, can be halted. In the event of an unwanted pregnancy, counseling about termination of the pregnancy can be provided at an early stage.

Pregnancy Tests

All urine or blood pregnancy tests rely on the detection of hCG produced by the placenta. hCG levels increase shortly after implantation, double approximately every 48 hours, reach a peak at 50–75 days, and fall to lower levels in the second and third trimesters. Laboratory and home pregnancy tests now use monoclonal antibodies specific for hCG. These tests are performed on urine or serum and are accurate at the time of the missed period or shortly after it.

Compared with intrauterine pregnancies, ectopic pregnancies may show lower levels of hCG, which level off or fall in serial determinations. Quantitative assays of hCG repeated at 48- to 72-hour intervals are used in the diagnosis of ectopic pregnancy, as well as in cases of molar pregnancy, threatened abortion, and missed abortion. Comparison of hCG levels between laboratories may be misleading in a given patient because different international standards may produce results that vary by a factor of two.

Manifestations of Pregnancy

The following symptoms and signs are usually due to pregnancy, but none are diagnostic. A record of the time and frequency of coitus is helpful for diagnosing and dating a pregnancy.

A. Symptoms: Amenorrhea, nausea and vomiting, breast tenderness and tingling, urinary frequency and urgency, "quickening" (noted at about the 18th week), weight gain.

B. Signs (in Weeks From LMP): Breast changes (enlargement, vascular engorgement, colostrum), abdominal enlargement, cyanosis of vagina and cervical portion (about the seventh week), softening of the cervix (seventh week), softening of the cervicouterine junction (eighth week), generalized enlargement and diffuse softening of the corpus (after eighth week).

The uterine fundus is palpable above the pubic symphysis by 12–15 weeks from the LMP and reaches the umbilicus by 20–22 weeks. Fetal heart tones can be heard by Doppler at 10–12 weeks of gestation and by 20 weeks with an ordinary fetoscope.

Differential Diagnosis

The nonpregnant uterus enlarged by myomas can be confused with the gravid uterus, but it is usually very firm and irregular. An ovarian tumor may be found midline, displacing the nonpregnant uterus to the side or posteriorly. Ultrasonography and a pregnancy test will provide accurate diagnosis in these circumstances.

ESSENTIALS OF PRENATAL CARE

The first prenatal visit should occur as early as possible after the diagnosis of pregnancy and should include the following.

History

Age, ethnic background, occupation. Onset of LMP and its normality, possible conception dates, bleeding after LMP, medical history, all prior pregnancies (duration, outcome, and complications), symptoms of present pregnancy. Use of drugs, alcohol, tobacco, caffeine, nutritional habits (Table

---

*Parts of this chapter are reprinted from Brown JS, Crombleholme WR (editors): *Handbook of Gynecology/Obstetrics.* Appleton & Lange, 1993.

Table 18–1. Common drugs that are teratogenic or fetotoxic.[1]

Alcohol	Estrogens
Amantadine	Griseofulvin
Androgens	Hypoglycemics, oral
Anticonvulsants (third trimester):	Isotretinoin
Aminoglutethimide	Lithium
Ethotoin	NSAIDs (third trimester)
Phenytoin	Opioids (prolonged use)
Paramethadione	Progestins
Valproic acid	Radioiodine (antithyroid)
Aspirin and other salicylates (third trimester)	Reserpine
Benzodiazepines	Ribavirin
Carbarsone (amebicide)	Sulfonamides (third trimester)
Chloramphenicol (third trimester)	Tetracycline (third trimester)
Diazoxide	Tobacco smoking
Diethylstilbestrol	Trimethoprim (third trimester)
Disulfiram	Warfarin and other coumarin anticoagulants
Ergotamine	

[1]Many other drugs are also contraindicated during pregnancy. Evaluate any drug for its need versus its potential adverse effects. Further information can be obtained from the manufacturer or from any of several teratogenic registries around the country.

18–1). Family history of congenital anomalies and heritable diseases. History of childhood varicella.

Physical Examination

Height, weight, blood pressure, general physical examination. Abdominal and pelvic examination: (1) estimate uterine size or measure fundal height; (2) evaluate bony pelvis for symmetry and adequacy; (3) evaluate cervix for structural anatomy, infection, effacement, dilation; (4) detect fetal heart sounds by ultrasound after 6 weeks or with Doppler device after 10 weeks.

Laboratory Tests

Urinalysis, culture of a clean-voided midstream urine sample, complete blood count with red cell indices, serologic test for syphilis, rubella antibody titer, blood group, Rh type, atypical antibody screening, and HBsAg evaluation. Human immunodeficiency virus (HIV) screening should be offered to all pregnant women. Cervical cultures are usually obtained for *Neisseria gonorrhoeae* and *Chlamydia,* along with a Papanicolaou smear of the cervix. All black women should have sickle cell screening. Women of African, Asian, or Mediterranean ancestry with anemia or low MCV values should have hemoglobin electrophoresis performed to identify abnormal hemoglobins (Hb S, C, F, α-thalassemia, β-thalassemia). Tuberculosis skin testing is increasingly indicated for immigrant and inner city populations. Genetic counseling with the option of chorionic villus sampling or genetic amniocentesis should be offered to all women who will be 35 years of age or older at delivery and those who have had prior offspring with chromosomal abnormalities. Tay-Sachs blood screening is offered to Jewish women with Jewish partners.

Pregnant women who work in medical-dental health care or the public safety field and those who are household contacts of a hepatitis B virus carrier or a hemodialysis patient and are HBsAg-negative at prenatal screening are at high risk of acquiring hepatitis B. They should be vaccinated during pregnancy.

Advice to Patients

A. Prenatal Visits: Prenatal care should begin early and maintain a schedule of regular prenatal visits: 0–28 weeks: every 4 weeks; 28–36 weeks: every 2 weeks; 36 weeks on: weekly.

B. Diet:

1. Eat a balanced diet containing the major food groups.

2. Take prenatal vitamins with iron and folic acid.

3. Expect to gain 20–40 lb. Do not diet to lose weight during pregnancy.

4. Decrease caffeine intake to 0–1 cup of coffee, tea, or cola daily.

5. Avoid eating raw or rare meat, and wash hands after handling raw meat.

6. Eat fresh fruits and vegetables and wash them before eating.

C. Medications: Do not take medications unless prescribed or authorized by your physician.

D. Alcohol and Other Drugs: Abstain from alcohol, tobacco, and all recreational ("street") drugs. No safe level of alcohol intake has been established for pregnancy. Fetal effects are manifest in the **fetal alcohol syndrome,** which includes growth restriction, facial abnormalities, and serious central nervous system dysfunction. These effects are thought to result from direct toxicity of ethanol itself as well as of its metabolites such as acetaldehyde. Characteristic findings include shortened palpebral fissures, low-set ears, midfacial hypoplasia, a smooth philtrum, a thin upper lip, microcephaly, mental retardation, and attention deficit disorder. Skeletal and cardiac abnormalities may also be seen.

Cigarette smoking results in fetal exposure to carbon monoxide and nicotine, which is thought to eventuate in a number of adverse pregnancy outcomes. An increased risk of abruptio placentae, placenta previa, and premature rupture of the membranes is documented among women who smoke. Premature delivery may occur 20% more frequently among smoking pregnant women, and the birth weights of their infants are on average 200 g lower than infants of nonsmokers. Women who smoke should quit or at least reduce the number of cigarettes smoked per day to as few as possible. Sometimes compounding the above effects on pregnancy outcome are the independent adverse effects of illicit drugs. Cocaine use in pregnancy is associated with an increased risk of premature rupture, preterm delivery, placental abruption, intrauterine growth restriction, neurobehavioral deficits, and sudden infant death syndrome. Similar adverse pregnancy effects are associated with amphetamine use, perhaps reflecting the vasoconstrictive potential of both amphetamines and cocaine. Adverse effects associated with opioid use include intrauterine growth restriction, prematurity, stillbirth, and fetal death.

E. X-Rays and Noxious Exposures: Avoid x-rays unless essential and approved by a physician. Inform your dentist and your other physicians that you are pregnant. Avoid chemical or radiation hazards. Avoid excessive heat in hot tubs or saunas. Avoid handling cat feces or cat litter. Wear gloves when gardening.

F. Rest and Activity: Obtain adequate rest each day. Abstain from strenuous physical work or activities, particularly when heavy lifting or weight bearing is required. Exercise regularly at a mild to moderate level. Avoid exhausting or hazardous exercises or new athletic training programs during pregnancy. Heart rate should be kept below 140 beats/min during exercise.

G. Birth Classes: Enroll with your partner in a childbirth preparation class well before your due date.

Tests & Procedures

A. Each Visit: Weight, blood pressure, fundal height, fetal heart rate, urine specimen for protein and glucose. Review patient's concerns about pregnancy, health, and nutrition.

B. 6–12 Weeks: Confirm uterine size and growth by pelvic examination. Document fetal heart tones (audible at 10–12 weeks of gestation by Doppler). Chorionic villus sampling between 10 and 12 weeks when indicated.

C. 12–18 Weeks: Genetic counseling for women 35 years or older at EDC, or those with a family history of congenital anomalies, a previous child with a chromosomal abnormality, metabolic disease, or neural tube defect. Amniocentesis is performed as indicated and requested by the patient.

D. 12–24 Weeks: Fetal ultrasound examination when indicated to determine pregnancy dating or evaluate fetal anatomy. An earlier examination provides the most accurate dating, while a later examination demonstrates fetal anatomy in greater detail. The best compromise is at 18–20 weeks of gestation.

E. 16–20 Weeks: Maternal serum alpha-fetoprotein testing is offered to all women to screen for neural tube defects. In some states, such testing is mandatory. In some institutions, serum alpha-fetoprotein is combined with measurement of estriol and hCG (triple screen) for the detection of fetal Down's syndrome.

F. 20–24 Weeks: Instruct patient in signs and symptoms of preterm labor and rupture of membranes.

G. 24 Weeks to Delivery: Ultrasound examination is performed as indicated. Typically, fetal size and growth are evaluated when fundal height is 3 cm less than or more than expected for gestational age. In multiple pregnancies, ultrasound should be performed every 4 weeks to evaluate for discordant growth.

H. 26–28 Weeks: Screening for gestational diabetes by a 50-g glucose load (Glucola) and a 1-hour post-Glucola blood glucose determination. A blood glucose concentration less than 140 mg/dL is normal. Abnormal values should be followed up with a 3-hour glucose tolerance test unless the Glucola screen value is greater than 200 mg/dL, in which case the diagnosis is established.

I. 28 Weeks: Repeat antibody testing for Rh-negative, unsensitized patients. If still Rh antibody-negative, Rh_o (D) immune globulin is administered.

J. 28–32 Weeks: Repeat the complete blood count to evaluate for anemia of pregnancy.

K. 28 Weeks to Delivery: Determination of fetal position and presentation. Question the patient at each visit for signs or symptoms of preterm labor or rupture of membranes. Assess maternal perception of fetal movement at each visit. Antepartum fetal testing is performed as medically indicated.

L. 36 Weeks to Delivery: Repeat HIV testing and cervical cultures for *N gonorrhoeae* in at-risk patients. Discuss with the patient the indicators of onset of labor, admission to hospital, management of labor and delivery, and options for analgesia and anesthesia. Weekly cervical examinations are not necessary unless indicated to assess a specific clinical situation. Elective delivery (whether by induction or cesarean section) prior to 39 weeks of gestation requires confirmation of fetal lung maturity.

The CDC has recently approved two approaches—screening-based and risk factor-based—for management of group B streptococcal colonization in pregnancy:

1. In the screening-based approach, a single standard culture of the distal vagina and anorectum is collected at 35–37 weeks. No prophylaxis is needed if the screening culture is negative. Patients whose cultures are positive receive intrapartum penicillin prophylaxis with labor. Patients with risk factors such as a previous infant with invasive group B streptococcal disease, or group B streptococcal bacteriuria during the pregnancy, or delivery at less than 37 weeks of gestation also receive intrapartum prophylaxis. Patients whose cultures at 35–37 weeks were not done or whose results are not known receive prophylaxis only with the risk factors of intrapartum temperature greater than 38 °C or membrane rupture greater than 18 hours.

2. In the risk factor approach, no screening cultures are performed, and all patients with any of the risk factors noted above are treated.

3. The routine recommended regimen for prophylaxis is penicillin G, 5 million units intravenously as loading dose and then 2.5 million units intravenously every 4 hours until delivery. In penicillin-allergic patients, clindamycin, 900 mg intravenously every 8 hours until delivery, is substituted.

M. 41 Weeks and Beyond: Cervical examination to determine probability of successful induction of labor. Based on this, induction of labor is undertaken if the cervix is favorable; if unfavorable, antepartum fetal testing is begun.

American College of Obstetricians and Gynecologists: *Substance Abuse in Pregnancy.* ACOG Technical Bulletin 195, 1994.

Briggs G et al: *Drugs in Pregnancy and Lactation.* Williams & Wilkins, 1994.

D'Alton ME, DeCherney AH: Prenatal diagnosis. N Engl J Med 1993;328:114.

Ewigman BG et al: Effect of prenatal ultrasound screening on perinatal outcome. RADIUS Study Group. N Engl J Med 1993;329:821.

Kuller JA, Laifer SA: Preconceptual counseling and intervention. Arch Intern Med 1994;154:2273.

Macri J et al: Prenatal maternal dried blood screening with alpha-fetoprotein and free beta-human chorionic gonadotropin for open neural tube defect and Down syndrome. Am J Obstet Gynecol 1996;174:566.

Prevention of perinatal group B streptococcal disease: A public health perspective. MMWR Morb Mortal Wkly Rep 1996;45(RR-7).

NUTRITION IN PREGNANCY

Nutrition in pregnancy significantly affects maternal health and infant size and well-being. Pregnant women should have nutrition counseling early in prenatal care and access to supplementary food programs if they lack funds for adequate nutrition. Counseling should stress abstention from alcohol, smoking, and drugs. Caffeine and artificial sweeteners should be used only in small amounts. "Empty calories" should be avoided, and the diet should contain the following foods: protein foods of animal and vegetable origin, milk and milk products, whole-grain cereals and breads, and fruits and vegetables—especially green leafy vegetables.

Weight gain in pregnancy should be 20–40 lb, which includes the added weight of the fetus, placenta, and amniotic fluid and of maternal reproductive tissues, fluid, blood, increased fat stores, and increased lean body mass. Maternal fat stores are a caloric reserve for pregnancy and lactation; weight restriction in pregnancy to avoid developing such fat stores may affect the development of other fetal and maternal tissues and is not advisable. Obese women can have normal infants with less weight gain (15–20 lb) but should be encouraged to eat high-quality foods. Normally, a pregnant woman gains 2–5 lb in the first trimester and slightly less than 1 lb/wk thereafter. She needs approximately an extra 200–300 kcal/d (depending on energy output) and 30 g/d of additional protein for a total protein intake of about 75 g/d. Appropriate caloric intake in pregnancy helps prevent the problems associated with low birth weight.

Rigid salt restriction is not necessary. While the consumption of highly salted snack foods and prepared foods is not desirable, 2–3 g/d of sodium is permissible. The increased calcium needs of pregnancy (1200 mg/d) can be met with milk, milk products, green vegetables, soybean products, corn tortillas, and calcium carbonate supplements.

The increased need for iron and folic acid should be met from foods as well as vitamin and mineral supplements. (See section on anemia in pregnancy.) Megavitamins should not be taken in pregnancy, as they may result in fetal malformation or disturbed metabolism. However, a balanced prenatal supplement containing 30–60 mg of elemental iron, 0.5–0.8 mg of folate, and the recommended daily allowances of various vitamins and minerals is widely used in the USA and is probably beneficial to many women with marginal diets. There is evidence that periconceptional folic acid supplements can decrease the risk of neural tube defects in the fetus. For this reason, the United States Public Health Service recommends the consumption of 0.4 mg of folic acid per day for all women capable of becoming pregnant. Women with a prior neural tube defect-affected pregnancy may require higher supplemental doses as determined by their physician. Lactovegetarians and ovolactovegetarians do well in pregnancy; vegetarian women who eat neither eggs nor milk products should have their diets assessed for adequate calories and protein and should take oral vitamin B_{12} supplements during pregnancy and lactation.

Abrams BF, Berman CA: Nutrition during pregnancy and lactation. Prim Care 1993;20:585.

Institute of Medicine, National Academy of Sciences: *Nutrition During Pregnancy.* Part I, *Weight Gain;* Part II, *Nutrient Supplements.* National Academy Press, 1990.

Recommendations for the use of folic acid to reduce the number of cases of spina bifida and other neural tube defects. MMWR Morb Mortal Wkly Rep 1992;41(RR-14):1.

TRAVEL & IMMUNIZATIONS DURING PREGNANCY

During an otherwise normal low-risk pregnancy, travel can be planned most safely between the 18th and 32nd weeks. Commercial flying in pressurized cabins does not pose a threat to the fetus. An aisle seat in the nonsmoking section will allow frequent walks. Adequate fluids should be taken during the flight.

It is not advisable to travel to endemic areas of yellow fever in Africa or Latin America or to areas of Africa or Asia where chloroquine-resistant falciparum malaria is a hazard, since complications of malaria are more common in pregnancy.

Ideally, all immunizations should precede pregnancy. Live virus products are contraindicated (measles, rubella, yellow fever). Inactivated poliovaccine (Salk) can be used instead of the oral vaccine. Vaccines against pneumococcal pneumonia and meningococcal meningitis can be used, but their safety during pregnancy has not been conclusively proved.

Pooled gamma globulin to prevent hepatitis A is safe and does not carry a risk of HIV transmission. Chloroquine can be used for malaria prophylaxis in pregnancy, and proguanil is also safe.

Water should be purified by boiling, since iodine purification may provide more iodine than is safe during pregnancy.

Do not use prophylactic antibiotics or bismuth subsalicylate during pregnancy to prevent diarrhea. Use oral rehydration fluids, and treat bacterial diarrhea with erythromycin or ampicillin if necessary.

Macleod CL: The pregnant traveler. Med Clin North Am 1992;76:1313.

VOMITING OF PREGNANCY
(Morning Sickness)
& HYPEREMESIS GRAVIDARUM
(Pernicious Vomiting of Pregnancy)

Morning or evening nausea and vomiting usually begin soon after the first missed period and cease after the fourth to fifth months of gestation. At least half of women, most of them primiparas, complain of nausea and vomiting during early pregnancy. This problem exerts no adverse effects on the pregnancy and does not presage other complications, though it

is particularly common with multiple pregnancy and hydatidiform mole. The cause of vomiting during pregnancy is believed to be high estrogen levels.

Persistent, severe vomiting during pregnancy—hyperemesis gravidarum—can be disabling and require hospitalization. Dehydration, acidosis, and nutritional deficiencies may develop with protracted vomiting. Thyroid dysfunction can be associated with hyperemesis gravidarum, so it is advisable to determine TSH and free T_4 values in these patients.

Treatment

A. Mild Nausea and Vomiting of Pregnancy: Reassurance and dietary advice are all that is required in most instances. Because of possible teratogenicity, drugs used during the first half of pregnancy should be restricted to those of major importance to life and health. Antiemetics, antihistamines, and antispasmodics are generally unnecessary to treat nausea of pregnancy. Vitamin B_6 (pyridoxine), 50–100 mg/d orally, is nontoxic and may be helpful in some patients.

B. Hyperemesis Gravidarum: Hospitalize the patient in a private room at bed rest. Give nothing by mouth for 48 hours, and maintain hydration and electrolyte balance by giving appropriate parenteral fluids and vitamin supplements as indicated. Rarely, total parenteral nutrition may become necessary. As soon as possible, place the patient on a dry diet consisting of six small feedings daily with clear liquids 1 hour after eating. Prochlorperazine rectal suppositories may be useful. After in-patient stabilization, the patient can be maintained at home even if she requires intravenous fluids in addition to her oral intake.

Kousen M: Treatment of nausea and vomiting in pregnancy. Am Fam Physician 1993;48:1279.

SPONTANEOUS ABORTION

Abortion is defined as termination of gestation before the 20th week of pregnancy. About three-fourths of spontaneous abortions occur before the 16th week; of these, three-fourths occur before the eighth week. Almost 20% of all clinically recognized pregnancies terminate in spontaneous abortion.

More than 60% of spontaneous abortions result from chromosomal defects due to maternal or paternal factors; about 15% appear to be associated with maternal trauma, infections, dietary deficiencies, diabetes mellitus, hypothyroidism, or anatomic malformations. There is no reliable evidence that abortion may be induced by psychic stimuli such as severe fright, grief, anger, or anxiety. In about one-fourth of cases, the cause of abortion cannot be determined. There is no evidence that video display terminals or associated electromagnetic fields are related to an increased risk of spontaneous abortion.

It is important to differentiate women with a history of incompetent cervix from those with more typical early abortion and those with premature labor or rupture of the membranes. Characteristically, incompetent cervix presents as "silent" cervical dilation (ie, with minimal uterine contractions) between 16 and 28 weeks of gestation. Women with incompetent cervix often present with significant cervical dilation (2 cm or more) and minimal symptoms. When the cervix reaches 4 cm or more, active uterine contractions or rupture of the membranes may occur secondary to the degree of cervical dilation. This does not change the primary diagnosis. Factors that predispose to incompetent cervix are a history of incompetent cervix with a previous pregnancy; cervical conization or surgery; cervical injury; DES exposure; and anatomic abnormalities of the cervix. Prior to pregnancy or during the first trimester, there are no methods for determining whether the cervix will eventually be incompetent. After 14–16 weeks, ultrasound may be used to evaluate the internal anatomy of the lower uterine segment and cervix for the funneling and shortening abnormalities consistent with cervical incompetence.

Clinical Findings

A. Symptoms and Signs:

1. Threatened abortion–Bleeding or cramping occurs, but the pregnancy continues. The cervix is not dilated.

2. Inevitable abortion–The cervix is dilated and the membranes may be ruptured, but passage of the products of conception has not occurred. Bleeding and cramping persist, and passage of the products of conception is considered inevitable.

3. Complete abortion–The fetus and placenta are completely expelled. Pain ceases, but spotting may persist.

4. Incomplete abortion–Some portion of the products of conception (usually placental) remain in the uterus. Only mild cramps are reported, but bleeding is persistent and often excessive.

5. Missed abortion–The pregnancy has ceased to develop, but the conceptus has not been expelled. Symptoms of pregnancy disappear. There is a brownish vaginal discharge but no free bleeding. Pain does not develop. The cervix is semifirm and slightly patulous; the uterus becomes smaller and irregularly softened; the adnexa are normal.

B. Laboratory Findings:
Pregnancy tests show low or falling levels of hCG. A complete blood count should be obtained if bleeding is heavy. Determine Rh type, and give Rh_o (D) immune globulin if the type is Rh-negative. All tissue recovered should be assessed by a pathologist and may be sent for genetic analysis in selected cases.

C. Ultrasonographic Findings:
The gestational sac can be identified at 5–6 weeks from the LMP, a fetal pole at 6 weeks, and fetal cardiac activity at 6–7 weeks. Serial observations are often required to evaluate changes in size of the embryo. A small, irregular sac without a fetal pole with accurate dating is diagnostic of an abnormal pregnancy.

Differential Diagnosis

The bleeding that occurs in abortion of a uterine pregnancy must be differentiated from the abnormal bleeding of an ectopic pregnancy and anovular bleeding in a nonpregnant woman. The passage of hydropic villi in the bloody discharge is diagnostic of hydatidiform mole.

Treatment

A. General Measures:

1. Threatened abortion–Place the patient at bed rest for 24–48 hours followed by gradual resumption of usual activities, with abstinence from coitus and douching. Hormonal treatment is contraindicated. Antibiotics should be used only if there are signs of infection.

2. Missed or inevitable abortion–This calls for counseling regarding the fate of the pregnancy and planning for its elective termination at a time chosen by the patient and physician. Insertion of a laminaria to dilate the cervix followed by aspiration is the method of choice for a missed abortion. Prostaglandin vaginal suppositories are an effective alternative.

B. Surgical Measures:

1. Incomplete abortion–Prompt removal of any products of conception remaining within the uterus is required to stop bleeding and prevent infection. Analgesia and a paracervical block are useful, followed by uterine exploration with ovum forceps or uterine aspiration.

2. Cerclage and restriction of activities–These are the treatment of choice for incompetent cervix. A variety of suture materials including a 5 mm Mersilene band can be used to create a purse-string type of stitch around the cervix, using either the McDonald or Shirodkar method. Cerclage should be undertaken with caution when there is advanced cervical dilation or membranes are prolapsed into the vagina. Rupture of the membranes and infection are specific contraindications to cerclage. Cervical cultures for *N gonorrhoeae*, *Chlamydia*, and group B streptococci should be obtained before or at the time of cerclage.

Apgar BS, Churgay CA: Spontaneous abortion. Prim Care 1993;20:621.

RECURRENT (HABITUAL) ABORTION

Recurrent, or habitual, abortion has been defined for years as the loss of three or more previable (< 500 g) pregnancies in succession. Recurrent or chronic abortion occurs in about 0.4–0.8% of all pregnancies. Abnormalities related to repeated abortion can be identified in approximately half of the couples. If a woman has lost three previous pregnancies without identifiable cause, she still has a 70–80% chance of carrying a fetus to viability. If she has aborted four or five times, the likelihood of a successful pregnancy is 65–70%.

Recurrent abortion is a clinical rather than pathologic diagnosis. The clinical findings are similar to those observed in other types of abortion (see above).

Treatment

A. Preconception Therapy: Preconception therapy is aimed at detection of maternal or paternal defects that may contribute to abortion. A thorough general and gynecologic examination is essential. Polycystic ovaries should be ruled out. A random blood glucose test and thyroid function studies (including thyroid antibodies) should be done. Lupus anticoagulant detection and an antinuclear antibody test may be indicated. Endometrial tissue should be examined in the postovulation stage of the cycle to determine the adequacy of the response of the endometrium to hormones. The competency of the cervix must be determined and hysteroscopy or hysterography used to exclude submucous myomas and congenital anomalies. Chromosomal (karyotype) analysis of both partners rules out balanced translocations (found in 5% of infertile couples).

Recent experiments have focused on the major histocompatibility complex (MHC) of chromosome 6, which carries HLA loci and other genes that may influence reproductive success. Many couples who experience habitual abortion share a significant number of HLA antigens, and some women demonstrate a lack of maternal antibody response to paternal lymphocytes, which is customarily found in normal women after successful childbearing. Centers where HLA typing can be performed will identify couples whose unusual gene sharing may play a role in habitual abortion. The immunologic approach of enhancing maternal antibody response to paternal lymphocytes is still experimental.

B. Postconception Therapy: Provide early prenatal care and schedule frequent office visits. Complete bed rest is justified only for bleeding or pain. Empiric sex steroid hormone therapy is contraindicated.

Prognosis

The prognosis is excellent if the cause of abortion can be corrected.

Daya S: Issues in the etiology of recurrent spontaneous abortion. Curr Opin Obstet Gynecol 1994;6:153.

Rand SE: Recurrent spontaneous abortion: Evaluation and management. Am Fam Physician 1993;48:1451.

ECTOPIC PREGNANCY

Any pregnancy arising from implantation of the ovum outside the cavity of the uterus is ectopic. Ectopic implantation occurs in about one out of 150 live births. About 98% of ectopic pregnancies are tubal. Other sites of ectopic implantation are the peritoneum or abdominal viscera, the ovary, and the cervix. Any condition that prevents or retards migration of the fertilized ovum to the uterus can predispose to an ectopic pregnancy, including a history of infertility, pelvic inflammatory disease, ruptured appendix, and prior tubal surgery. Combined intra- and extrauterine pregnancy (heterotopic) may occur rarely. In the USA, undiagnosed or undetected ectopic pregnancy is currently the most common cause of maternal death in pregnancies with abortive outcomes.

Clinical Findings

A. Symptoms and Signs: The cardinal symptoms and signs of tubal pregnancy are (1) amenorrhea or irregular bleeding and spotting, followed by (2) pelvic pain, and (3) pelvic (adnexal) mass formation. They may be acute or chronic.

1. Acute (40%)–Severe lower quadrant pain occurs in almost every case. It is sudden in onset, lancinating, intermittent, and does not radiate. Backache is present during attacks. Shock occurs in about 10%, often after pelvic examination. At least two-thirds of patients give a history of abnormal menstruation; many have been infertile.

2. Chronic (60%)–Blood leaks from the tubal ampulla over a period of days, and considerable blood may accumulate in the peritoneum. Slight but persistent vaginal spotting is reported, and a pelvic mass can be palpated. Abdominal distention and mild paralytic ileus are often present.

B. Laboratory Findings: Blood studies may show anemia and slight leukocytosis. Quantitative serum pregnancy tests will show levels generally lower than expected for normal pregnancies of the same duration. If pregnancy tests are followed over a few days, there may be a slow rise or a plateau rather than the doubling every 2 days associated with normal early intrauterine pregnancy or the falling levels that occur with spontaneous abortion.

C. Imaging: Ultrasonography can reliably demonstrate a gestational sac 6 weeks from the LMP and a fetal pole at 7 weeks if located in the uterus. An empty uterine cavity raises a strong suspicion of extrauterine pregnancy, which can occasionally be revealed by endovaginal ultrasound. Specified levels of serum hCG have been reliably correlated with ultrasound findings of an intrauterine pregnancy. For example, an hCG level of 6500 mIU/mL (1st I.R.) with an empty uterine cavity by transabdominal ultrasound is virtually diagnostic of an ectopic pregnancy. Similarly, an hCG value of 2000 mIU/mL or more (1st I.R.) can be indicative of an ectopic pregnancy if no products of conception are detected within the uterine cavity by transvaginal ultrasound.

D. Special Examinations: With the advent of high-resolution transvaginal ultrasound, culdocentesis is rarely used in evaluation of possible ectopic pregnancy. Laparoscopy is the surgical procedure of choice to both confirm an ectopic pregnancy and in most cases to permit pelviscopic removal of the ectopic pregnancy without the need for exploratory laparotomy.

Differential Diagnosis

Clinical and laboratory findings suggestive or diagnostic of pregnancy will distinguish ectopic pregnancy from many acute abdominal illnesses such as acute appendicitis, acute pelvic inflammatory disease, ruptured corpus luteum cyst or ovarian follicle, and urinary calculi. Uterine enlargement with clinical findings similar to those found in ectopic pregnancy is also characteristic of an aborting uterine pregnancy or hydatidiform mole. Ectopic pregnancy should be suspected when postabortal tissue examination fails to reveal placenta. Steps must be taken for immediate diagnosis, including prompt microscopic tissue examination, ultrasonography, and serial hCG titers every 48 hours. Patients must be warned of possible ectopic pregnancy problems and followed very closely.

Treatment

The patient is hospitalized if there is a reasonable likelihood of ectopic pregnancy. Blood is typed and cross-matched. Ideally, diagnosis and operative treatment should precede frank rupture of the tube and intra-abdominal hemorrhage.

Surgical treatment is definitive. In a stable patient, diagnostic laparoscopy is the initial surgical procedure performed. Depending on the size of the ectopic pregnancy and whether or not it has ruptured, a salpingostomy with removal of the ectopic or a partial or complete salpingectomy can usually be performed pelviscopically through the laparoscope. Clinical conditions permitting, patency of the contralateral tube can be established by the injection of indigo carmine into the uterine cavity and flow through the contralateral tube confirmed visually by the surgeon.

Methotrexate—given systemically as single or multiple doses—is now acceptable medical therapy of early ectopic pregnancy. Favorable criteria are that the pregnancy should be less than 3.5 cm and unruptured, with no active bleeding.

Iron therapy for anemia may be necessary during convalescence. Give Rh$_o$ (D) immune globulin to Rh-negative patients.

Prognosis

Repeat tubal pregnancy occurs in about 12% of cases. This should not be regarded as a contraindication to future pregnancy, but the patient requires careful observation and early ultrasound confirmation of an intrauterine pregnancy.

Carson SA, Buster TE: Ectopic pregnancy. N Engl J Med 1993;329:1174.

Lawlor HK, Rubin BJ: Early diagnosis of ectopic pregnancy. West J Med 1993;159:195.

Stovall T, Ling F: Single-dose methotrexate: An expanded clinical trial. Am J Obstet Gynecol 1993;168:1759.

PREECLAMPSIA-ECLAMPSIA

Preeclampsia-eclampsia can occur any time after 20 weeks of gestation and up to 6 weeks postpartum. It is a disease unique to pregnancy, with the only cure being delivery of the fetus and placenta. Approximately 7% of pregnant women in the United States develop preeclampsia-eclampsia. Primiparas are most frequently affected; however, the incidence of preeclampsia-eclampsia is increased with multiple pregnancies, chronic hypertension, diabetes, renal disease, collagen-vascular and autoimmune disorders, and gestational trophoblastic disease. Uncontrolled eclampsia is a significant cause of maternal death. Five percent of women with preeclampsia progress to eclampsia.

The basic cause of preeclampsia-eclampsia is not known. Epidemiologic studies suggest an immunologic cause for preeclampsia, since it occurs predominantly in women who have had minimal exposure to sperm (having used barrier methods of contraception) or have new consorts; in primigravidas; and in women both of whose parents have similar HLA antigens. Preeclampsia is an endothelial disorder resulting from poor placental perfusion, which releases a factor that injures the endothelium, causing activation of coagulation and an increased sensitivity to pressors. Before the syndrome becomes clinically manifest in the second half of pregnancy, there has been vasospasm in various small vessel beds, accounting for the pathologic changes in maternal organs and the placenta with consequent adverse effects on the fetus.

The use of diuretics, dietary restriction or enhancement, sodium restriction, and vitamin-mineral supplements has not been shown to be useful in clinical studies. The only cure is termination of the pregnancy at a time as favorable as possible for fetal survival.

Despite encouraging initial findings, large prospective randomized studies have failed to show a benefit of low-dose aspirin in preventing preeclampsia in low- or high-risk women.

Definition

Preeclampsia is defined as the presence of the triad of elevated blood pressure, proteinuria, and edema during pregnancy. Eclampsia occurs with the addition of seizures to this triad. The three abnormalities of preeclampsia-eclampsia are defined as follows:

A. Blood Pressure: An elevation of at least 30 mm Hg systolic or 15 mm Hg diastolic (or both) over baseline values established prior to 20 weeks of gestation. In the absence of baseline values, blood pressures of 140/90 mm Hg or more (in the absence of chronic hypertension) after 20 weeks of gestation are abnormal. An alternative definition is a 20 mm Hg increase in mean arterial pressure (MAP) or an absolute MAP of 105 mm Hg alone. All abnormal blood pressure readings must be confirmed with two separate readings at least 6 hours apart.

B. Proteinuria: At least 0.3 g/24 h as determined by 24-hour urine collection.

C. Edema: Clinically apparent fluid retention, or increase in weight of 5 lb or more in 1 week. The edema may involve the upper extremities and face rather than just the lower extremities.

Classically, the presence of all three elements is required for the diagnosis of preeclampsia-eclampsia. Clinically, however, there is a great deal of variation in presentation. Hypertension occurs most frequently, but proteinuria or edema may be the dominant abnormality at presentation. Subtle elevations in blood pressure that meet the 30/15 mm Hg criteria but with the reading still under 140/90 mm Hg are significant but may be overlooked. The absence of one or two components does not exclude the diagnosis of preeclampsia-eclampsia, and many women with the disorder are asymptomatic early. Diagnosis at an early stage thus requires careful attention to details and a high index of suspicion.

Clinical Findings

Clinically, the severity of preeclampsia-eclampsia can be measured with reference to the six major sites in which it exerts its effects: the central nervous system, the kidneys, the liver, the hematologic and vascular systems, and the fetal-placental unit. By evaluating each of these areas for the presence of mild to moderate versus severe preeclampsia-eclampsia, the degree of involvement can be assessed, and an appropriate management plan can be formulated that is integrated with gestational age assessment (Table 18–2).

A. Preeclampsia:

1. Mild to moderate–Precise differentiation between mild and moderate preeclampsia-eclampsia is difficult because the abnormalities that define the disease are quite variable and fail to accurately predict progression to more severe disease. Symptoms are generally minimal or mild. With mild preeclampsia, patients usually have few complaints, and the diastolic blood pressure is less than 90–100 mm Hg. Edema is usually more pronounced with moderate disease, and diastolic blood pressures are in the range

Table 18–2. Indicators of mild to moderate versus severe preeclampsia-eclampsia.

Site	Indicator	Mild to Moderate	Severe
Central nervous system		Hyperreflexia Headache	Seizures Blurred vision Scotomas Headache Clonus Irritability
Kidney	Proteinuria	0.3–4.0 g/24 h	>5 g/24 h or catheterized urine with 4+ protein
	Urine output	>20–30 mL/h	<20–30 mL/h
Liver	AST, ALT, LDH	Normal	Elevated Epigastric pain Ruptured liver
Hematologic	Platelets Hemoglobin	>100,000/μL Normal range	<100,000/μL Elevated
Vascular	Blood pressure Retina	<160/110 mm Hg Arteriolar spasm	>160/110 mm Hg Retinal hemorrhages
Fetal-placental unit	Growth retardation Oligohydramnios Fetal distress	Absent May be present Absent	Present Present Present

of 90–110 mm Hg. The platelet count is over 100,000/μL, antepartum fetal testing is reassuring, central nervous system irritability is minimal, epigastric pain is not present, and liver enzymes are not excessively elevated.

2. Severe–Symptoms are more dramatic and persistent. The blood pressure is often quite high, with readings over 160/110 mm Hg. Thrombocytopenia (platelet counts < 100,000/μL) may be present and progress to disseminated intravascular coagulation. Severe epigastric pain may be present from hepatic subcapsular hemorrhage with significant stretch or rupture of the liver capsule. The HELLP syndrome (hemolysis, elevated liver enzymes, low platelets) is a form of severe preeclampsia.

B. Eclampsia: The occurrence of seizures defines eclampsia. It is a manifestation of severe central nervous system involvement. The other abnormal findings of severe preeclampsia are also observed with eclampsia.

Differential Diagnosis

Preeclampsia-eclampsia can mimic and be confused with many other diseases, including (among many others) chronic hypertension, chronic renal disease, primary seizure disorders, gallbladder and pancreatic disease, immune or thrombotic thrombocytopenic purpura, and hemolytic uremic syndrome. It must always be considered as a disease of exclusion in any pregnant women beyond 20 weeks of gestation. It is particularly difficult to diagnose when preexisting disease such as hypertension present. Uric acid values can be quite helpful in such situations, since hyperuricemia is uncommon in pregnancy except with gout, renal failure, or preeclampsia-eclampsia.

Treatment

A. Preeclampsia: Early recognition is the key to treatment. This requires careful attention to the details of prenatal care—especially subtle changes in blood pressure and weight. The objectives are to prolong pregnancy if possible to fetal lung maturity while preventing progression to severe disease and eclampsia. The critical factors are the gestational age of the fetus, fetal pulmonary maturity status, and the severity of maternal disease. Preeclampsia-eclampsia at 36 weeks or more of gestation is managed by delivery regardless of how mild the disease is judged to be. Prior to 36 weeks, severe preeclampsia-eclampsia requires delivery except in unusual circumstances associated with extreme fetal prematurity, in which case prolongation of pregnancy may be attempted. Epigastric pain, thrombocytopenia, and visual disturbances are strong indications for delivery of the fetus. For mild to moderate preeclampsia-eclampsia, bed rest is the cornerstone of therapy. This increases central blood flow to the kidneys, heart, brain, liver, and placenta and may stabilize or even improve the degree of preeclampsia-eclampsia for a period of time.

Bed rest may be attempted at home or in the hospital. Prior to making this decision, the physician should evaluate the six sites of involvement listed in Table 18–2 and make an assessment about the severity of disease.

1. Home management–Home management with bed rest may be attempted for patients with mild preeclampsia and a stable home situation. This requires homemaking assistance, rapid access to the hospital, a reliable patient, and the ability to obtain frequent blood pressure readings. A home health nurse can often provide frequent home visits and assessment.

2. Hospital care–Hospitalization is required for women with moderate or severe preeclampsia or those with unreliable home situations. Regular assessment of blood pressure, reflexes, urine protein, and fetal heart tones and activity are required. A complete blood count, platelet count, and electrolyte panel including liver enzymes should be checked every 1 or 2 days. A 24-hour urine collection for creatinine clearance and total protein should be obtained on admission and repeated as indicated. Sedatives and opioids should be avoided because the fetal central nervous system depressant effects interfere with fetal testing. Magnesium sulfate is not used until the diagnosis of severe preeclampsia-eclampsia is made or until labor occurs.

Fetal evaluation should be obtained as an integral part of the workup. If the patient is being admitted to the hospital, fetal testing must be performed on the same day to make certain that the fetus is safe. This may be done by fetal heart rate testing with nonstress or stress testing or by biophysical profile. A regular schedule of fetal surveillance must then be followed. Daily fetal kick counts can be recorded by the patient herself. Consideration should be given to amniocentesis to evaluate fetal lung maturity status if hospitalization occurs at 30–37 weeks of gestation. If immaturity is present, steroids (betamethasone 12 mg or dexamethasone 16 mg, two doses intramuscularly 12–24 hours apart) can be administered. Fetuses between 26 and 30 weeks of gestation can be presumed to be immature and given steroids.

The method of delivery is determined by the maternal and fetal status. Cesarean section is reserved for the usual fetal indications.

B. Eclampsia:

1. Emergency care–If the patient is convulsing, she is turned on her side to prevent aspiration and to improve blood flow to the placenta. Fluid or food is aspirated from the glottis or trachea. The seizure may be stopped by giving an intravenous bolus of either magnesium sulfate, 4 g, or diazepam, 5–10 mg, over 4 minutes or until the seizure stops. A continuous intravenous infusion of magnesium sulfate is then started at a rate of 2–3 g/h unless the patient is known to have significantly reduced renal function. Magnesium blood levels are then checked every 4–6 hours and the infusion rate adjusted to maintain a therapeutic blood level. Deep tendon reflexes, the respiratory rate and depth, and urine output are checked hourly to monitor for magnesium toxicity, which can be reversed with calcium gluconate.

2. General care–The occurrence of eclampsia necessitates delivery once the patient is stabilized. It is important, however, that assessment of the status of the patient and fetus take place first. Continuous fetal monitoring must be performed and blood typed and cross-matched quickly. A urinary catheter is inserted to monitor urine output, and blood is sent for complete blood count, platelets, liver enzymes, uric acid, creatinine or urea nitrogen, and electrolytes. If hypertension is present with diastolic values over 110 mm Hg, antihypertensive medications should be administered to reduce the diastolic blood pressure to 90–100 mm Hg. Lower blood pressures than this may induce placental insufficiency through reduced perfusion. Hydralazine given in 5- to 10-mg increments intravenously every 20 minutes is frequently used to lower blood pressure. Nifedipine, 10 mg sublingually or orally, or labetalol, 10–20 mg intravenously, can also be used.

3. Delivery—Except in unusual circumstances, delivery is mandated once eclampsia has occurred. Vaginal delivery may be attempted if the patient has already been in active labor or the cervix is quite favorable *and* the patient is clinically stable. The rapidity with which delivery must be achieved depends on the fetal and maternal status following the seizure and the availability of laboratory data on the patient. Oxytocin may be used to induce or augment labor. Regional analgesia or anesthesia is acceptable. Cesarean section is used for the usual obstetric indications or when rapid delivery is necessary for maternal or fetal indications.

4. Postpartum—Magnesium sulfate infusion (2–3 g/h) should be continued until preeclampsia-eclampsia has begun to resolve postpartum. This may take 1–7 days. The most reliable indicator of this is the onset of diuresis with urine output of over 100–200 mL/h. When this occurs, magnesium sulfate can be discontinued. Late-onset preeclampsia-eclampsia can occur during the postpartum period. It is usually manifested by either hypertension or seizures. Treatment is the same as prior to delivery—ie, with magnesium sulfate—though other antiseizure medications can be used since the fetus is no longer present.

Collaborative Low-Dose Aspirin Study in Pregnancy Collaborative Group. CLASP: A randomized trial of low-dose aspirin for the prevention and treatment of preeclampsia among 9,364 pregnant women. Lancet 1994;343:619.

Cunningham FG, Lindheimer MD: Hypertension in pregnancy. (Current Concepts.) N Engl J Med 1992;326:927.

Roberts JM, Redman CWG: Pre-eclampsia: More than pregnancy induced hypertension. Lancet 1993;341:1447.

Sibai BH et al: Prevention of preeclampsia with low dose aspirin in healthy, nulliparous pregnant women. N Engl J Med 1993;329:1213.

Smith MA: Pre-eclampsia. Prim Care 1993;20:655.

GESTATIONAL TROPHOBLASTIC NEOPLASIA
(Hydatidiform Mole & Choriocarcinoma)

Gestational trophoblastic neoplasia is a spectrum of disease that includes hydatidiform mole, invasive mole, and choriocarcinoma. Partial moles generally show evidence of an embryo or gestational sac, are polypoid, slower-growing and less symptomatic, and are often present clinically as a missed abortion. Partial moles tend to follow a benign course, while complete moles have a greater tendency to become choriocarcinomas.

The highest rates of gestational trophoblastic neoplasia occur in some developing countries, with rates of 1:125 pregnancies in certain areas of Asia. In the USA, the frequency is 1:1500 pregnancies. Risk factors include low socioeconomic status, a history of

mole, and age below 18 or above 40. Approximately 10% of women require further treatment after evacuation of the mole; 5% develop choriocarcinoma.

Clinical Findings

A. Symptoms and Signs: Excessive nausea and vomiting occur in over one-third of patients with hydatidiform mole. Uterine bleeding, beginning at 6–8 weeks, is observed in virtually all instances and is indicative of threatened or incomplete abortion. In about one-fifth of cases, the uterus is larger than would be expected in a normal pregnancy of the same duration. Intact or collapsed vesicles may be passed through the vagina. These grape-like clusters or enlarged villi are diagnostic. Bilaterally enlarged cystic ovaries are sometimes palpable. They are the result of ovarian hyperstimulation due to excess of hCG.

Preeclampsia-eclampsia, frequently of the fulminating type, may develop during the second trimester of pregnancy, but this is unusual.

Choriocarcinoma may be manifested by continued or recurrent uterine bleeding after evacuation of a mole or following a delivery, abortion, or ectopic pregnancy. The presence of an ulcerative vaginal tumor, pelvic mass, or evidence of distant metastatic tumor may be the presenting observation. The diagnosis is established by pathologic examination of curettings or by biopsy.

B. Laboratory Findings: A serum hCG β-subunit value above 40,000 mIU/mL or a urinary hCG value in excess of 100,000 units/24 h increases the likelihood of hydatidiform mole, though such values are occasionally seen with a normal pregnancy (eg, in multiple gestation).

C. Imaging: Ultrasound has virtually replaced all other means of preoperative diagnosis of hydatidiform mole. The multiple echoes indicating edematous villi within the enlarged uterus and the absence of a fetus and placenta are pathognomonic. A preoperative chest film is indicated to rule out pulmonary metastases of trophoblast.

Treatment

A. Specific (Surgical) Measures: Empty the uterus as soon as the diagnosis of hydatidiform mole is established, preferably by suction. Do not resect ovarian cysts or remove the ovaries; spontaneous regression of theca lutein cysts will occur with elimination of the mole.

If malignant tissue is discovered at surgery or during the follow-up examination, chemotherapy is indicated.

Thyrotoxicosis indistinguishable clinically from that of thyroid origin may occur. While hCG usually has minimal TSH-like activity, the very high hCG levels associated with moles can account for clinically significant TSH activity. Patients thyrotoxic on this basis should be stabilized with beta-blockers prior to induction of anesthesia for their surgical evacuation. Surgical removal of the mole promptly corrects the thyroid overactivity.

B. Follow-Up Measures: Effective contraception (preferably birth control pills) should be prescribed. Weekly quantitative hCG level measurements are initially required. Moles show a progressive decline in hCG. After two negative weekly tests (< 5 mIU/mL), the interval may be increased to monthly for 6 months and then to every 2 months for a year. If levels plateau or begin to rise, the patient should be evaluated by repeat chest film and D&C before the initiation of chemotherapy.

C. Antitumor Chemotherapy: For low-risk patients with a good prognosis, give methotrexate, 0.4 mg/kg intramuscularly over a 5-day period, or dactinomycin, 10–12 μg/kg/d intravenously over a 5-day period (see Chapter 4). Refer patients with a poor prognosis to a tumor center, where multiple-agent chemotherapy probably will be given. The side effects—anorexia, nausea and vomiting, stomatitis, rash, diarrhea, and bone marrow depression—usually are reversible in about 3 weeks and can be ameliorated by the administration of leucovorin (0.1 mg/kg). Repeated courses of methotrexate 2 weeks apart generally are required to destroy the trophoblast and maintain a zero chorionic gonadotropin titer, as indicated by hCG β-subunit determination.

D. Supportive Measures: Prescribe oral contraceptives (if acceptable) or another reliable birth control method to avoid the hazard and confusion of elevated hCG from a new pregnancy. hCG levels should be negative for a year before pregnancy is again attempted. In the pregnancy following a mole, the hCG level should be checked 6 weeks postpartum.

Prognosis

Five years' survival after courses of chemotherapy, even when metastases have been demonstrated, can be expected in at least 85% of cases of choriocarcinoma.

Lewis JL Jr: Diagnosis and management of gestational trophoblastic disease. Cancer 1993;71:1639.

THIRD-TRIMESTER BLEEDING

Five to ten percent of women have vaginal bleeding in late pregnancy. The physician must distinguish between placental causes (placenta previa, placental abruption, vasa previa) and nonplacental causes (infection, disorders of the lower genital tract, systemic disease). The approach to bleeding in late pregnancy should be conservative and expectant unless fetal distress or risk of maternal hemorrhage occurs.

The patient should be hospitalized and placed at bed rest with continuous fetal monitoring. A complete blood count should be obtained and two to four units of blood typed and cross-matched. If an ultrasound examination has been performed earlier in the pregnancy, it may be possible to exclude placenta previa as a cause. If not, one should be performed to determine placental location. A speculum and digital pelvic examination is done only after ultrasound study has ruled out placenta previa. Continuous electronic fetal monitoring is required to exclude fetal distress. Uterine contractions, pain, or tenderness, if present, often indicate associated abruptio placentae. A negative ultrasound, however, does not exclude it. If vaginal bleeding is profuse and the uterus painful or contracting, the patient is prepared for cesarean section, and blood is available when the vaginal examination is performed.

If the patient is less than 36 weeks of gestation, continued hospitalization and bed rest may be necessary, especially with placenta previa during the initial 7–10 days following vaginal bleeding. If the patient has close proximity to the hospital and immediate access, can be on strict bed rest, and has complete resolution of bleeding and uterine contractions, home management may be considered. She must be well instructed and counseled regarding the risks. Patients with vaginal bleeding at less than 36 weeks of gestation should also be considered for amniocentesis to test for fetal lung maturity. Steroid therapy (betamethasone 12 mg intramuscularly, two doses 12–24 hours apart) is indicated at less than 34 weeks if fetal lung immaturity is present.

Patients with placenta previa should be offered phlebotomy for autologous blood banking.

MEDICAL CONDITIONS COMPLICATING PREGNANCY

Anemia

Plasma volume increases 50% during pregnancy, while red cell volume increases 25%, causing lower hemoglobin and hematocrit values, which are maximally changed around the 24th to 28th weeks. Anemia in pregnancy is often defined as a hemoglobin measurement below 10 g/dL or hematocrit below 30%. Anemia is very common in pregnancy, causing fatigue, anorexia, dyspnea, and edema. Prevention through optimal nutrition and iron and folic acid supplementation is desirable.

A. Iron Deficiency Anemia: Many women enter pregnancy with low iron stores resulting from heavy menstrual periods, previous pregnancies, breast feeding, or poor nutrition. It is difficult to meet the increased requirement for iron through diet, and anemia often develops unless iron supplements are given. Red cells may not become hypochromic and microcytic until the hematocrit has fallen significantly. When this occurs, a serum iron level below

40 μg/dL, and a transferrin saturation less than 10% suggest iron deficiency anemia. Treatment consists of a diet containing iron-rich foods and 60 mg of elemental iron (eg, 300 mg of ferrous sulfate) three times a day with meals. Iron is best absorbed if taken with a source of vitamin C (raw fruits and vegetables, lightly cooked greens). All pregnant women should take daily iron supplements.

B. Folic Acid Deficiency Anemia: Folic acid deficiency anemia is the main cause of macrocytic anemia in pregnancy, since vitamin B_{12} deficiency anemia is rare in the childbearing years. The daily requirement doubles from 400 μg to 800 μg in pregnancy. Twin pregnancies, infections, malabsorption, and use of anticonvulsant drugs such as phenytoin can precipitate folic acid deficiency. The anemia may first be seen in the puerperium owing to the increased need for folate during lactation.

The diagnosis is made by finding macrocytic red cells and hypersegmented neutrophils in a blood smear. However, blood smears in pregnancy may be difficult to interpret, since they frequently show iron deficiency changes as well. Because the deficiency is hard to diagnose and folate intake is inadequate in some socioeconomic groups, 0.8–1 mg of folic acid is given as a supplement in pregnancy; the dose in established deficiency is 1–5 mg/d.

Good sources of folate in food are leafy green vegetables, orange juice, peanuts, and beans. Cooking and storage of food destroy folic acid. Strict vegetarians who eat no eggs or milk products should take vitamin B_{12} supplements during pregnancy and lactation.

C. Sickle Cell Anemia: Women with sickle cell anemia are subject to serious complications in pregnancy. The anemia becomes more severe, and crises may occur more frequently. Complications include infections, bone pain, pulmonary infarction, congestive heart failure, and preeclampsia. There is an increased rate of spontaneous abortion and higher maternal and perinatal mortality rates. Intensive medical treatment may improve the outcome for mother and fetus. Frequent indicated transfusions of packed cells or leukocyte-poor washed red cells lower the level of hemoglobin S and elevate the level of hemoglobin A; this minimizes the severity of anemia and the risk of sickle cell crises.

Genetic counseling should be offered to patients with sickle cell disease or sickle trait. They may wish to undergo first-trimester chorionic villus biopsy or second-trimester amniocentesis to determine whether the abnormality has been passed on to the fetus. IUDs and oral contraceptives are contraindicated, but progestin-only contraceptives may be used. Women with sickle cell trait alone usually have an uncomplicated gestation except for an increased risk of urinary tract infection. Sickle cell-hemoglobin C disease in pregnancy is similar to sickle cell anemia and is treated similarly.

Lupus Anticoagulant-Anticardiolipin Antibody Syndrome

The presence of antibodies to phospholipids and a variety of clinical symptoms, including vascular thromboses, thrombocytopenia, and recurrent pregnancy loss, characterize the lupus anticoagulant-anticardiolipin antibody syndrome. Many of these patients have SLE-like symptoms but do not meet specific diagnostic criteria for that disease. The lupus anticoagulant and anticardiolipin antibody may occur in these patients, and both may cause arterial and venous thromboses. Detection of these antiphospholipid antibodies may require a combination of laboratory tests. The lupus anticoagulant will prolong both the partial thromboplastin time (PTT) and the Russell viper venom time. The latter is a more sensitive predictor of disease. Such patients should also be screened for the presence of the recently identified factor V Leiden mutation. Anticardiolipin antibody may be detected with ELISA testing. Either antibody may cause false-positive syphilis serologic tests.

This syndrome may require treatment with immunosuppressive or anticoagulant medications. In a small number of patients with recurrent pregnancy loss and a diagnosis of lupus anticoagulant syndrome, improved outcomes have been reported following treatment with daily high-dose prednisone (40 mg/d) and low-dose aspirin (81 mg) or heparin anticoagulation (see references for dosages) and low-dose aspirin begun before or early in pregnancy and continued until the postpartum period. Although complications have been reported with both regimens, current opinion seems to favor the heparin and low-dose aspirin combination.

Branch DW et al: Outcome of treated pregnancies in women with antiphospholipid syndrome: An update of the Utah experience. Obstet Gynecol 1992;80:614. (The total daily dose of heparin given in two or three doses is 10,000–20,000 units.)

Cowchock FS et al: Repeated fetal losses associated with antiphospholipid antibodies: A collaborative randomized trial comparing prednisone to low dose heparin treatment. Am J Obstet Gynecol 1992;166:1318. (The total daily dose of heparin given in two doses is 17,000 units.)

Kutteh W: Antiphospholipid antibody-associated recurrent pregnancy loss: Treatment with heparin and low-dose aspirin is superior to low-dose aspirin alone. Am J Obstet Gynecol 1996;174:1584. (The total daily dose of heparin given in two doses ranged from 8000 to 20,000 units.)

Lynch A et al: Antiphospholipid antibodies in predicting adverse pregnancy outcome: A prospective study. Ann Intern Med 1994;120:470.

Asthma

The effect of pregnancy on asthma is unpredictable. About 50% of patients have no change, 25% improve, and 25% get worse. Management of acute and chronic asthma during pregnancy does not differ significantly from that of nonpregnant women. The goal is to maintain maternal $P_{O_2} > 80$ mm Hg to sustain normal fetal oxygenation.

Clark SL: Asthma in pregnancy. National Asthma Education Program Working Group on Asthma and Pregnancy. National Institutes of Health, National Heart, Lung and Blood Institute. Obstet Gynecol 1993; 82:1036.

AIDS During Pregnancy

In the USA at present, 83% of women with AIDS are intravenous drug users or partners of HIV-infected men. Recipients of HIV-contaminated blood transfusions (5%) and women with no risk reported or identified (12%) constitute the remainder of cases. Asymptomatic infection is not associated with a decreased pregnancy rate or increased risk of adverse pregnancy outcomes. There is no evidence that pregnancy causes AIDS progression.

The rates of transplacental transmission of AIDS have varied from 10% to 40%, apparently related to the stage of the mother's illness. Most cases of transmission occur close to or at delivery. The use of zidovudine prophylactically during the antepartum period (after 12 weeks of gestation), during the intrapartum period in labor, and to the infant for the first 6 weeks of life reduces the transmission risk of HIV from mother to fetus by approximately two-thirds, from 25% to 8%. HIV-infected women should be advised not to breast-feed their infants.

Appropriate counseling of HIV antibody-positive pregnant women includes the option of pregnancy termination.

Obstetric caregivers should meticulously observe the established protocols for skin and eye protection against blood and internal secretions, particularly at the time of delivery.

Connor E et al: Reduction of maternal-infant transmission of human immunodeficiency virus type 1 with zidovudine treatment. Pediatric AIDS Clinical Trials Group Protocol 076 Study Group. N Engl J Med 1994; 331:1173.

Lindsay M: HIV infection in women. Clin Obstet Gynecol 1996;39:277.

Peckham CS: Human immunodeficiency virus infection and pregnancy. Sex Transm Dis 1994;21:S28.

Diabetes Mellitus

Pregnancy is associated with increased tissue resistance to insulin, resulting in increased levels of blood insulin as well as glucose and triglycerides. These changes are due to placental lactogen and elevated circulating estrogens and progesterone. Although pregnancy does not appear to alter the long-term consequences of diabetes, retinopathy and nephropathy may first appear or become worse during pregnancy. The White classification (Table 18–3)

Table 18–3. Modified White classification of diabetes mellitus.[1]

Class A:	Chemical diabetes diagnosed *before* pregnancy; managed by diet *alone;* any age of onset or duration.
Class B:	Insulin treatment necessary *before* pregnancy; onset after age 20; duration of less than 10 years.
Class C:	Onset at age 10–19; or duration of 10–19 years.
Class D:	Onset before age 10; or duration of 20 or more years; or chronic hypertension; or background retinopathy.
Class F:	Renal disease.
Class H:	Coronary artery disease.
Class R:	Proliferative retinopathy.
Class T:	Renal transplant.

[1]Reproduced, with permission, from DeCherney AH, Pernoll ML (editors): *Current Obstetric & Gynecologic Diagnosis & Treatment,* 8th ed. Appleton & Lange, 1994.

summarizes the pathologic features of diabetes complicating pregnancy. It is also important to recognize the practical overlap between pregestational and gestational diabetes categorized as class A. Debate continues over whether gestational diabetics are women whose glucose intolerance is solely a function of their pregnant compared to their nonpregnant state. Alternatively, pregnancy may merely serve to unmask their underlying propensity for glucose intolerance, which will be evident even in the nonpregnant state at some time in the future if not in the immediate postpartum period. In part as an aid in the long-term management of such women, patients categorized as class A are commonly subdivided into A_1 and A_2 diabetes. A_1 diabetics are those patients whose fasting blood glucose is under 105 mg/dL but have two abnormal values among the remaining three glucose determinations. A_2 diabetics are those patients whose fasting blood glucose is 105 mg/dL or more and in addition have one or more elevations among the remaining three glucose determinations. A_1 diabetics typically can be managed by diet alone, while A_2 diabetics will most often require insulin therapy during their pregnancy.

Prepregnancy counseling and evaluation of diabetic women should include a complete chemistry panel, HbA_{1c} determination, 24-hour urine collection for total protein and creatinine clearance, funduscopic examination, and an ECG. Any medical problems should be addressed, and HbA_{1c} levels of less than 8–9% should be achieved before pregnancy. Euglycemia should be established before conception and maintained during pregnancy with daily home glucose monitoring by the patient. A well-planned dietary program is a key component, with an intake of 1800–2200 kcal/d divided into three meals and three snacks. Insulin is given subcutaneously in a split-dose regimen with frequent dosage adjustments. The use of continuous insulin pump therapy is currently limited to women with difficult (brittle) diabetes.

Congenital anomalies result from hyperglycemia during the first 4–8 weeks of pregnancy. They occur in 4–10% of diabetic pregnancies (two to three times the rate in nondiabetic pregnancies). Euglycemia in the early weeks of pregnancy, when organogenesis is occurring, reduces the rate of anomalies to near-normal levels. Even so, because few women with diabetes begin a rigorous program to achieve euglycemia until well after they have become pregnant, congenital anomalies are the principal cause of perinatal fetal deaths in diabetic pregnancies. All women with diabetes should receive counseling about pregnancy and, when the decision has been made to start a family, should receive prepregnancy management by physicians experienced in diabetic pregnancies.

Fasting and preprandial glucose values are lower during pregnancy in both diabetic and nondiabetic women. Euglycemia is considered to be 60–80 mg/dL while fasting and 30–45 minutes before meals and < 120 mg/dL 1 hour after meals. This is the target for good diabetic control during pregnancy. Glycosylated hemoglobin levels help determine the quality of glucose control both before and during pregnancy.

While perinatal problems for mother and baby are decreased by fastidious diabetic control, the incidence of hydramnios, preeclampsia-eclampsia, infections, and prematurity is increased even in carefully managed diabetic pregnancies. Diabetes is an inherently unstable disease characterized by fluctuations of blood glucose levels, particularly late in pregnancy. The risk of fetal demise in the third trimester

(stillbirth) and neonatal death increases with the level of hyperglycemia. Consequently, pregnant women with type I diabetes must receive regular antepartum fetal testing (nonstress testing, contraction stress testing, biophysical profile) during the third trimester. The timing of delivery is dictated by the quality of diabetic control, the presence or absence of medical complications, and fetal status. The goal is to achieve 39 weeks (38 completed weeks) and then proceed with delivery. Confirmation of lung maturity is necessary only for delivery prior to 39 weeks. Cesarean sections are performed for obstetric indications.

Because 15% of patients with gestational diabetes require insulin during pregnancy and because the infants of gestational diabetics have some risks similar to those of infants of diabetic mothers (particularly macrosomia), screening of all pregnant women for glucose intolerance has been recommended between the 24th and 28th weeks of pregnancy (Table 18–4). Patients with gestational diabetes should be evaluated 6–8 weeks postpartum by a 2-hour oral glucose tolerance test (75 g glucose load).

Kitzmiller JL: Sweet success with diabetes. Diabetes Care 1993;16:107.

Landon M: Diabetes in pregnancy. Clin Perinatol 1993;20:507.

Heart Disease

Most cases of heart disease complicating pregnancy in the USA are congenital, with 5% of maternal deaths due to heart disease. Normal pregnancy causes a faster pulse, an increase of cardiac output of more than 30%, and a rise in plasma volume greater than red cell mass with relative hemodilution. Both vital capacity and oxygen consumption rise only slightly.

For practical purposes, the functional capacity of the heart is the best single measurement of cardiopulmonary status.

Table 18–4. Screening and diagnostic criteria for gestational diabetes mellitus.

Screening for gestational diabetes

1. 50-g oral glucose load, administered between the 24th and 28th weeks, without regard to time of day or time of last meal, to all pregnant women who have not been identified as having glucose intolerance before the 24th week.
2. Venous plasma glucose measured 1 hour later.
3. Value of 140 mg/dL (7.8 mmol/L) or above in venous plasma indicates the need for a full diagnostic glucose tolerance test.

Diagnosis of gestational diabetes mellitus

1. 100-g oral glucose load, administered in the morning after overnight fast lasting at least 8 hours but not more than 14 hours, and following at least 3 days of unrestricted diet (>150 g carbohydrate) and physical activity.
2. Venous plasma glucose is measured fasting and at 1, 2, and 3 hours. Subject should remain seated and not smoke throughout the test.
3. Two or more of the following venous plasma concentrations must be equaled or exceeded for positive diagnosis: fasting, 105 mg/dL (5.8 mmol/L); 1 hour, 190 mg/dL (10.6 mmol/L); 2 hours, 165 mg/dL (9.2 mmol/L); 3 hours, 145 mg/dL (8.1 mmol/L).

Functional Cardiac Assessment

Class I	Ordinary physical activity causes no discomfort (perinatal mortality rate about 5%).
Class II	Ordinary activity causes discomfort and slight disability (perinatal mortaility rate 10–15%).
Class III	Less than ordinary activity causes discomfort or disability; patient is barely compensated (perinatal mortality rate about 35%).
Class IV	Patient decompensated; any physical activity causes acute distress (perinatal mortality rate over 50%).

In general, patients with class I or class II functional disability (80% of pregnant women with heart disease) do well obstetrically, with four-fifths of maternal deaths due to heart disease occurring in women with class III or class IV disability. Congestive failure is the usual cause of death. Most deaths occur in the early puerperium. Pregnancy is contraindicated in Eisenmenger's complex; in primary pulmonary hypertension; in severe mitral stenosis with secondary pulmonary hypertension; and in Marfan's syndrome, in which the aorta is prone to dissection and rupture. In addition, pregnancy is poorly tolerated in patients with aortic stenosis, aortic coarctation, tetralogy of Fallot, and active rheumatic carditis.

Therapeutic abortion and elective sterilization should be offered to patients with significant cardiac disease. Cesarean section should be performed only for obstetric indications. Women with valvular heart disease, mitral valve prolapse associated with mitral insufficiency, or idiopathic hypertrophic subaortic stenosis should receive appropriate antibiotic prophylaxis against infective endocarditis during labor and delivery or termination of pregnancy.

Peripartum Cardiomyopathy

Cardiac failure that develops during pregnancy or during the first 6 months postpartum in a woman without a history of heart disease and with no cause for heart failure other than pregnancy is termed peripartum cardiomyopathy. The incidence varies from 1:4000 to 1:1000. It is higher in Africa. It occurs more often in older women, those with twins, and in patients with pregnancy-induced hypertension. The cause of peripartum cardiomyopathy is unknown. In patients who continue to have signs and symptoms of disease for more than 6 months postpartum, the mortality rate is high, and subsequent pregnancy is especially dangerous.

Symptoms of peripartum cardiomyopathy are those of congestive heart failure. An electrocardiogram may reveal tachycardia and atrial or ventricular arrhythmias. Death may occur as a result of arrhythmia or embolism. Autopsy usually reveals an enlarged, dilated heart, and mural thrombi (the source of pulmonary and systemic emboli) are often found.

The treatment of peripartum cardiomyopathy is that of congestive cardiomyopathy (see Chapter 10). Patients with persistent cardiomegaly or mural thrombi shown by echocardiography require anticoagulant therapy. The long-term prognosis in these patients depends on whether cardiomegaly resolves within 6 months after the onset of symptoms. If it does not resolve, the 5-year mortality rate is 35%. If it does resolve, the mortality rate is still about 15%. If cardiomegaly does not resolve and another pregnancy intervenes, cardiomyopathy recurs in 50% of cases, with an almost 100% mortality rate.

McMullan MR, Moore CK, O'Connell JB: Diagnosis and management of peripartum cardiomyopathy. Hosp Pract (Off Ed) 1993 Nov 15;28:89.

Herpes Genitalis
(See also Chapter 6.)

Infection of the lower genital tract by herpes simplex virus type 2 (HSV-2) is a common sexually transmitted disease of potential seriousness to pregnant women and their newborn infants. Although up to 20% of women in an obstetric practice may have antibodies to HSV-2, a history of the infection is unreliable and the incidence of neonatal infection is low (1:20,000–1:3000 live births). Most infected neonates are born to women with no symptoms, signs, or history of infection.

Women who have had *primary* herpes infection late in pregnancy are at high risk of shedding virus at delivery. Some authors suggest screening by means of weekly cultures during the last month of pregnancy, because the neonatal attack rate is 50%.

Women with a history of *recurrent* genital herpes have a neonatal attack rate of 5% and should be followed by clinical observation and culture of any suspicious lesions. Since asymptomatic viral shedding is not predictable by antepartum cultures, current recommendations do not include routine cultures in individuals with a history of herpes without active disease. However, when labor begins, vulvar and cervical inspection and cultures should be performed, with prompt treatment of a newborn after a positive culture.

For treatment, see Chapter 32. The use of acyclovir in pregnancy is acceptable when there is significant fetal or neonatal risk.

Cesarean section is indicated at the time of labor if there are prodromal symptoms, active genital lesions, or a positive cervical culture obtained within the preceding week.

Cone RW et al: Frequent detection of genital herpes simplex virus DNA by polymerase chain reaction among pregnant women. JAMA 1994;272:792.

Maccato M: Herpes in pregnancy. Clin Obstet Gynecol 1993;36:869.

Prober CG et al: Use of routine viral cultures at delivery to identify neonates exposed to herpes simplex virus. N Engl J Med 1988;318:887.

Hypertensive Disease

Hypertensive disease in women of childbearing age is usually essential, but secondary causes should be considered: coarctation of the aorta, pheochromocytoma, aldosteronism, and renovascular and renal hypertension.

Preeclampsia is superimposed on 20% of pregnancies in hypertensive women and appears earlier, is more severe, and is more often associated with intrauterine growth retardation. It may be difficult to determine whether or not hypertension in a pregnant woman precedes or derives from the pregnancy if she is not examined until after the 20th week. Serum uric acid can help differentiate, since it is elevated with preeclampsia and normal in chronic hypertension. If hypertension persists for 6–8 weeks postpartum, essential hypertension is likely.

Pregnant women with chronic hypertension require medication only if the diastolic pressure is sustained at or above 100 mm Hg. For initiation of treatment, methyldopa is still the drug of choice. Start with 250 mg orally twice daily and increase in divided doses as needed to as much as 3 g daily. The goal is to keep the diastolic pressure between 80 and 100 mm Hg.

If a hypertensive woman is being managed successfully by medical treatment when she registers for antenatal care, one may generally continue the antihypertensive medication. Diuretics may be continued in pregnancy. ACE inhibitors should be replaced with a drug of another class because of reports of fetal and neonatal renal failure with these compounds.

Continued use of antihypertensive medications in preeclampsia remains controversial. This should be attempted only with significant fetal prematurity, absence of fetal compromise, and close supervision of the patient.

Therapeutic abortion may be indicated in cases of severe hypertension during pregnancy. If pregnancy is allowed to continue, the risk to the fetus must be assessed periodically in anticipation of early delivery. An early second-trimester ultrasound examination will confirm the duration of pregnancy, and follow-up examinations after 28 weeks will evaluate intrauterine growth retardation.

Maternal Hepatitis B Carrier State

There are an estimated 200 million chronic carriers of hepatitis B virus worldwide. Among these people there is an increased incidence of chronic active hepatitis, cirrhosis, and hepatocellular carcinoma. The frequency of the hepatitis B carrier state varies from 1% in the USA and Western Europe to 35% in parts of Africa and Asia. All pregnant women should be screened for hepatitis B surface antigen (HBsAg). Transmission of the virus to the baby after delivery is likely if both surface antigen and e antigen are positive. Vertical transmission can be blocked by the immediate postdelivery administration to the newborn of 0.5 mL of hepatitis B immunoglobulin and hepatitis B vaccine intramuscularly. The vaccine dose is repeated at 1 and 6 months of age.

Pastorek J: The ABC's of hepatitis in pregnancy. Clin Obstet Gynecol 1993;36:843.
Simms J, Duff P: Viral hepatitis in pregnancy. Semin Perinatol 1993;17:384.

Acute Fatty Liver of Pregnancy

Acute fatty liver of pregnancy is a disorder limited to the gravid state. It occurs in the third trimester of pregnancy and involves acute hepatic failure. The mortality rate has been reported to be as high as 85%, but with improved recognition and immediate delivery, the mortality range is 20–30%. The disorder is usually seen after the 35th week of gestation and is more common in primigravidas and those with twins. The incidence is about 1:14,000 deliveries.

The cause of acute fatty liver of pregnancy is not known. Pathologic findings are unique to the disorder, with fatty engorgement of hepatocytes. Clinical onset is gradual, with flu-like symptoms that progress to the development of abdominal pain, jaundice, encephalopathy, disseminated intravascular coagulation, and death. On examination, the patient shows signs of hepatic failure.

Laboratory findings show marked elevation of alkaline phosphatase but only moderate elevations of ALT and AST. Prothrombin time and bilirubin are also elevated. The white blood cell count is elevated, and the platelet count is depressed. Hypoglycemia may be profound.

The differential diagnosis is that of fulminant hepatitis. However, liver aminotransferases for fulminant hepatitis are higher (> 1000 units/mL) than those for acute fatty liver of pregnancy (usually < 500 units/mL). It is also important to review the appropriate history and perform the appropriate tests for toxins that cause liver failure. Preeclampsia may involve the liver but typically does not cause jaundice. The elevations in liver function tests in patients with preeclampsia usually do not reach the levels seen in patients with acute fatty liver of pregnancy.

Diagnosis of acute fatty liver of pregnancy mandates immediate delivery. Supportive care during labor includes administration of glucose, platelets, and fresh frozen plasma as needed. Vaginal delivery is preferred. Resolution of encephalopathy occurs over days, and supportive care with a low-protein diet is needed.

Recurrence rates for this liver disorder are unclear. Most authorities advise against subsequent pregnancy, but there have been reported cases of successful outcomes in later pregnancies.

Usta IM et al: Acute fatty liver of pregnancy: An experience in the diagnosis and management of fourteen cases. Am J Obstet Gynecol 1994;171:1342.

Seizure Disorders

Women contemplating pregnancy who have not had a seizure for 5 years should consider a prepregnancy trial of withdrawal from seizure medication. Those with recurrent epilepsy should use a single drug with blood level monitoring. Trimethadione and valproate are contraindicated during pregnancy; phenytoin and carbamazepine may be teratogenic in the first trimester and should not be used unless absolutely necessary. Phenobarbital is considered the drug of choice. Serum levels should be measured in each trimester and dosage adjustments made to keep serum levels in the low normal therapeutic range. Pregnant women taking these drugs should receive vitamin supplements, including folic acid and vitamin D, throughout pregnancy. Vitamin K, 20 mg/d, is administered during the last month to help prevent bleeding problems in the newborn, who are at risk of bleeding tendencies due to decreased levels of clotting factors. Such infants should receive an injection of vitamin K_1, 1 mg given subcutaneously immediately after delivery, and should have clotting studies 2–4 hours later. Breast feeding is not contraindicated.

Yerby MS: Epilepsy and pregnancy: New issues for an old disorder. Neurol Clin 1993;11:777.

Syphilis, Gonorrhea, & *Chlamydia trachomatis* Infection
(See also Chapters 33 and 34.)

These sexually transmitted diseases have significant consequences for mother and child. Untreated syphilis in pregnancy will cause late abortion stillbirth from or transplacental infection with congenital syphilis. Gonorrhea will produce large-joint arthritis by hematogenous spread as well as newborn eye damage. Maternal chlamydial infections are largely asymptomatic but are manifested in the newborn by inclusion conjunctivitis and, at age 2–4 months, by pneumonia. The diagnosis of each can be reliably made by appropriate laboratory tests, which should be included in all prenatal care. The sexual partners of women with sexually transmitted diseases should be identified and treated also if that can be done.

Group B Streptococcal Infection

Group B streptococci frequently colonize the lower female genital tract, with an asymptomatic carriage rate in pregnancy of 5–30%. This rate depends on maternal age, gravidity, and geographic variation. Vaginal carriage is asymptomatic and intermittent, with spontaneous clearing in approximately 30% and recolonization in about 10% of women. Adverse perinatal outcomes associated with group B streptococcal colonization include urinary tract infection, intrauterine infection, premature rupture of membranes, preterm delivery, and postpartum endometritis.

Women with postpartum endometritis due to infection with group B streptococci, especially after cesarean section, develop fever, tachycardia, and abdominal distention, usually within 24 hours after delivery. Approximately 35% of these women are bacteremic.

Group B streptococcal infection is a common cause of neonatal sepsis. Transmission rates are high, yet the rate of neonatal sepsis is surprisingly low at less than 4:1000 live births. Unfortunately, the mortality rate associated with early-onset disease can be as high as 50% in premature infants and approaches 25% even in those at term. Moreover, these infections can contribute markedly to chronic morbidity, including mental retardation and neurologic disabilities. Late-onset disease develops through contact with hospital nursery personnel. Up to 45% of these health care workers can carry the bacteria on their skin and transmit the infection to newborns.

See Tests and Procedures, p 726, ¶L, for CDC recommendations for screening and prophylaxis of group B streptococcal colonization.

Varicella

Commonly known as chickenpox, varicella-zoster virus (VZV) infection has a fairly benign course when incurred during childhood but may result in serious illness in adults, particularly during pregnancy. Infection results in lifelong protective immunity. Approximately 95% of women born in the USA have VZV antibodies by the time they reach reproductive age. The incidence of VZV infection during pregnancy has been reported as up to 7:10,000.

The incubation period for this infection is 10–20 days. A primary infection follows and is characterized typically by a flu-like syndrome with malaise, fever, and development of a pruritic maculopapular rash on the trunk which becomes vesicular and then crusts. Pregnant women are prone to the development of VZV pneumonia, often a fulminant infection sometimes requiring respiratory support. After primary infection, the virus becomes latent, ascending to dorsal root ganglia. Subsequent reactivation can occur as zoster, often under circumstances of immunocompromise, though this is rare during pregnancy.

Two types of fetal infection have been documented. The first is congenital VZV syndrome, which typically occurs in 2–3% of fetuses exposed to primary VZV infection during the first trimester. Anomalies include limb and digit abnormalities, microphthalmos, and microcephaly.

Infection during the latter two trimesters is less threatening. Maternal IgG crosses the placenta, protecting the fetus. The only infants at risk for severe infection are those born after maternal viremia but before development of maternal protective antibody. Maternal infection manifesting 5 days before or after delivery is the time period arbitrarily determined to be most hazardous for transmission to the fetus.

Diagnosis is commonly made on clinical grounds. Laboratory verification of recent infection is made most often by antibody detection techniques, including ELISA, fluorescent antibody, and hemagglutination inhibition. Serum obtained by cordocentesis may be tested for VZV IgM to document fetal infection.

There is no drug known to eradicate VZV. Varicella zoster immune globulin (VZIG) has been shown to prevent or modify the symptoms of infection in some women. Treatment success depends on identification of susceptible women at or just following exposure. Women with a questionable or negative history of chickenpox should be checked for antibody, since the overwhelming majority will have been exposed previously. If the antibody is negative, VZIG (625 units intramuscularly) should be given within 96 hours after exposure. There are no known adverse effects of VZIG administration during pregnancy. Infants born within 5 days of onset of maternal infection should also receive VZIG (125 units).

Infected pregnant women should be closely observed and hospitalized at the earliest signs of pulmonary involvement. Intravenous acyclovir (10–15 mg/kg every 8 hours for 7–10 days) is recommended in the treatment of VZV pneumonia.

Enders G et al: Consequences of varicella and herpes zoster in pregnancy: Prospective study of 1739 cases. Lancet 1994;343:1548.

Pastuszak AL et al: Outcome after maternal varicella infection in the first 20 weeks of pregnancy. N Engl J Med 1994;330:901.

Thyrotoxicosis

Thyrotoxicosis during pregnancy may result in fetal anomalies, late abortion, or preterm labor and fetal hyperthyroidism with goiter. Thyroid storm in late pregnancy or labor is a life-threatening emergency.

Radioactive isotope therapy must never be given during pregnancy. The thyroid inhibitor of choice is propylthiouracil, which acts to prevent further thyroxine formation by blocking iodination of tyrosine. There is a 2 to 3-week delay before the pretreatment hormone level begins to fall. The initial dose of propylthiouracil is 100–150 mg three times a day; the dose is lowered as the euthyroid state is approached. It is desirable to keep free T_4 in the high normal range during pregnancy. A maintenance dose of 100 mg/d minimizes the chance of fetal hypothyroidism and goiter.

Recurrent postpartum thyroiditis is a newly recognized entity occurring 3–6 months after delivery. A hyperthyroid state of 1–3 months' duration is followed by hypothyroidism, sometimes misdiagnosed as depression. Microsomal thyroid antibodies and thyroglobulin antibodies are present. Recovery is spontaneous in over 90% of cases after 3–6 months.

Burrow GN et al: Maternal and fetal thyroid function. N Engl J Med 1994;331:1072.

Tuberculosis

The diagnosis of tuberculosis in pregnancy is made by history taking, physical examination, and skin testing, with special attention to women from ethnic groups with a high prevalence of the disease (such as women from southeast Asia). Chest films should not be obtained as a routine screening measure in pregnancy but should be used only in patients with a skin test conversion or with suggestive findings in the history and physical examination. Abdominal shielding must be used if a chest film is obtained.

If adequately treated, tuberculosis in pregnancy has an excellent prognosis. There is no increase in spontaneous abortion, fetal problems, or congenital anomalies.

Treatment is with isoniazid and ethambutol or isoniazid and rifampin (see Chapter 33). Because isoniazid therapy may result in vitamin B_6 deficiency, a supplement of 50 mg/d of vitamin B_6 should be given simultaneously. Streptomycin, ethionamide, and most other antituberculous drugs should be avoided in pregnancy.

Urinary Tract Infection

The urinary tract is especially vulnerable to infections during pregnancy because the altered secretions of steroid sex hormones and the pressure exerted by the gravid uterus upon the ureters and bladder cause hypotonia and congestion and predispose to urinary stasis. Labor and delivery and urinary retention postpartum also may initiate or aggravate infection. *Escherichia coli* is the offending organism in over two-thirds of cases.

From 2% to 8% of pregnant women have asymptomatic bacteriuria, which some believe to be associated with an increased risk of prematurity. It is estimated that 20–40% of these women will develop pyelonephritis during pregnancy if untreated.

A first-trimester urine culture is indicated in women with a history of recurrent or recent episodes of urinary tract infection. If the culture is positive, treatment should be initiated as a prophylactic measure. Nitrofurantoin, penicillins, and cephalosporins are acceptable medications for 3–7 days. Sulfonamides should not be given in the third trimester because they interfere with bilirubin binding and thus impose a risk of neonatal hyperbilirubinemia and kernicterus. If bacteriuria returns, suppressive medication (one daily dose of an appropriate antibiotic) for the remainder of the pregnancy is indicated. Acute pyelonephritis requires hospitalization for intravenous administration of antibiotics until the patient is afebrile; this is followed by a full course of oral antibiotics.

Abbott J: Medical illness during pregnancy. Emerg Med Clin North Am 1994;12:115.

Jaff MR: Medical aspects of pregnancy. Cleve Clin J Med 1994;61:263.

Rouse DJ et al: Screening and treatment of asymptomatic bacteriuria of pregnancy to prevent pyelonephritis: A cost-effectiveness and cost-benefit analysis. Obstet Gynecol 1995;86:119.

SURGICAL COMPLICATIONS DURING PREGNANCY

Elective major surgery should be avoided during pregnancy. Normal uncomplicated pregnancy does not alter operative risk except as it may interfere with the diagnosis of abdominal disorders and increase the technical problems of intra-abdominal surgery. Abortion is not a serious hazard after operation unless peritoneal sepsis or other significant complications occur. During the first trimester, congenital anomalies may be induced in the developing fetus by hypoxia. Thus, the second trimester is usually the optimal time for operative procedures.

Appendicitis

Appendicitis occurs in about one of 5000 pregnancies. Diagnosis is difficult, since the appendix is carried high and to the right, away from McBurney's point, as the uterus enlarges, and localization of pain does not usually occur. Nausea, vomiting, fever, and leukocytosis occur regularly. Any right-sided abdominal pain associated with these symptoms should arouse the suspicion. In at least 20% of obstetric patients, the diagnosis of appendicitis is not made until rupture occurs and peritonitis has become established. Such a delay may lead to premature labor or abortion. With early diagnosis and appendectomy, the prognosis is good for mother and baby.

Carcinoma of the Breast

Cancer of the breast (see also Chapter 16) is diagnosed approximately once in 3500 pregnancies. Pregnancy may accelerate the growth of cancer of the breast, and delay in diagnosis affects the outcome of treatment. Inflammatory carcinoma is an extremely virulent type of breast cancer that occurs most commonly during lactation. Prepregnancy mammography should be encouraged for women over age 35 who are anticipating a pregnancy.

Breast enlargement during pregnancy obscures parenchymal masses, and breast tissue hyperplasia decreases the accuracy of mammography. Any discrete mass should be evaluated by aspiration to verify its cystic structure, with fine-needle biopsy if it is solid. A definitive diagnosis may require excisional biopsy under local anesthesia. If breast biopsy confirms the diagnosis of cancer, surgery should be done regardless of the stage of the pregnancy. If spread to the regional glands has occurred, irradiation or chemotherapy should be considered. Under these circumstances, the alternatives are termination of an early pregnancy or delay of therapy for fetal maturation.

Choledocholithiasis, Cholecystitis, & Idiopathic Cholestasis of Pregnancy

Severe choledocholithiasis and cholecystitis are not uncommon during pregnancy. When they do occur, it is usually in late pregnancy or in the puerperium. About 90% of patients with cholecystitis have gallstones; 90% of stones will be visualized by ultrasonography. Symptomatic relief may be all that is required.

Gallbladder surgery in pregnant women should be attempted only in extreme cases (eg, obstruction), because it increases the perinatal mortality rate to about 15%. Cholecystostomy and lithotomy may be all that is feasible during advanced pregnancy, cholecystectomy being deferred until after delivery. On the other hand, withholding surgery may result in necrosis and perforation of the gallbladder and peritonitis. Cholangitis due to impacted common duct stone requires surgical removal of gallstones and establishment of biliary drainage. Endoscopic retrograde cholangiopancreatography and endoscopic retrograde sphincterotomy can be performed safely in pregnant women if precautions are taken to minimize exposure to radiation.

Idiopathic cholestasis of pregnancy is due to a hereditary metabolic (hepatic) deficiency aggravated by the high estrogen levels of pregnancy. It causes intrahepatic biliary obstruction of varying degrees. The rise in bile acids is sufficient in the third trimester to cause severe, intractable, generalized itching and sometimes clinical jaundice. There may be mild elevations in blood bilirubin and alkaline phosphatase levels. The fetus is also threatened by this condition. An increased incidence of preterm delivery has been reported as well as unexplained intrauterine fetal demise. For this reason, antenatal surveillance of the fetus is mandatory in patients with this diagnosis. Resins such as cholestyramine (4 g three times a day) absorb bile acids in the large bowel and relieve pruritus but are difficult to take and may cause constipation. Their use requires vitamin K supplementation. The disorder is relieved once the infant has been delivered, but it recurs in subsequent pregnancies and sometimes with the use of oral contraceptives.

Ovarian Tumors

The most common adnexal mass in early pregnancy is the corpus luteum, which may become cystic and enlarge to 6 cm in diameter. Any persistent mass over 6 cm should be evaluated by ultrasound examination; unilocular cysts are likely to be corpus luteum cysts, whereas septated or semisolid tumors are likely to be neoplasms. The incidence of malignancy in ovarian masses over 6 cm in diameter is 2.5%. Ovarian tumors may undergo torsion and cause abdominal pain and nausea and vomiting and must be differentiated from appendicitis, other bowel disease, and ectopic pregnancy. Patients with suspected ovarian cancer should be referred to a tertiary perinatal center to determine whether the pregnancy can progress to fetal viability or whether treatment should be instituted without delay.

Kort B et al: The effect of nonobstetric operation during pregnancy. Surg Gynecol Obstet 1993;177:371.

PREVENTION OF HEMOLYTIC DISEASE OF THE NEWBORN (Erythroblastosis Fetalis)

The antibody anti-Rh_o (D) is responsible for most severe instances of hemolytic disease of the newborn (erythroblastosis fetalis). About 15% of whites and much lower proportions of blacks and Asians are Rh_o (D)-negative. If an Rh_o (D)-negative woman carries an Rh_o (D)-positive fetus, she may develop antibodies against Rh_o (D) when fetal red cells enter her circulation during small fetomaternal bleeding episodes in the early third trimester or during delivery, abortion, ectopic pregnancy, abruptio placentae, or other antepartum bleeding problems. This antibody, once produced, remains in the woman's circulation and poses the threat of hemolytic disease for subsequent Rh-positive fetuses.

Passive immunization against hemolytic disease of the newborn is achieved with Rh_o (D) immune globulin, a purified concentrate of antibodies against Rh_o (D) antigen. The Rh_o (D) immune globulin (one vial of 300 μg intramuscularly) is given to the mother within 72 hours after delivery (or spontaneous or induced abortion or ectopic pregnancy). The antibodies in the immune globulin destroy fetal Rh-positive cells so that the mother will not produce anti-Rh_o (D). During her next Rh-positive gestation, erythroblastosis will be prevented. An additional safety measure is the administration of the immune globulin at the 28th week of pregnancy. The passive antibody titer that results is too low to significantly affect an Rh-positive fetus. The maternal clearance of the globulin is slow enough that protection will continue for 12 weeks.

Hemolytic disease of varying degrees, from mild to serious, continue to occur in association with Rh subgroups (C, c, or E) or Kell, Kidd, and other factors. Therefore, atypical antibodies should be checked in the third trimester of all pregnancies.

Gollin Y, Copel J: Management of the Rh-sensitized mother. Clin Perinatol 1995;22:545.

PREVENTION OF PRETERM (PREMATURE) LABOR

Preterm (premature) labor is labor that begins before the 37th week of pregnancy; it is responsible for 85% of neonatal illnesses and deaths. The onset of labor is a result of a complex sequence of biologic events involving regulatory factors that are still poorly understood. Significant risk factors for the onset of preterm labor are a past history of preterm delivery, premature rupture of the membranes, urinary tract infection, or exposure to diethylstilbestrol. In addition, multiple gestation and abdominal or cervical surgery are especially important.

Low rates of preterm delivery are associated with success in educating patients to identify regular, frequent uterine contractions and in alerting medical and nursing staff to evaluate these patients early and initiate treatment if cervical changes can be identified. Cessation of work or physical activities that seem related to increased uterine activity is mandatory. Resting at home will often suffice to slow contractions. Portable lightweight monitors of uterine contractions permit a woman to record uterine activity at will or on a schedule and to transmit the data by telephone to a central terminal for analysis.

In more acute situations, intravenous magnesium sulfate is effective, as are intravenous beta-adrenergic drugs. Magnesium sulfate is given as a 4- or 6-g bolus, followed by a continuous infusion of 2–3 g/h. The rate may be increased by 1 g/h every 1½–2 hours until contractions cease or a blood magnesium concentration of 6–8 mg/dL is reached. Magnesium levels are determined every 4–6 hours to monitor the therapeutic blood level. After contractions have ceased for 12–24 hours, magnesium can be stopped and the situation reassessed.

Uterine smooth muscle is largely under sympathetic nervous system control, and stimulation of β_2 receptors relaxes the myometrium. Consequently, inhibition of uterine contractility often can be accomplished by the administration of beta-adrenergic drugs such as ritodrine or terbutaline.

Ritodrine can be administered by intravenous infusion in lactated Ringer's solution, beginning at a rate of 50 μg/min and increasing by 50 μg/min every 20 minutes until contractions cease or become less frequent than every 10 minutes, or until an infusion rate of 350 μg/min is reached. After 1 hour of satisfactory tocolysis, the infusion rate can be decreased by 50 μg/min every 30 minutes to the lowest rate that continues inhibition for 12 hours. Oral therapy with terbutaline (5 mg every 4 hours) is started 30 minutes before stopping intravenous ritodrine. Oral terbutaline (5 mg orally every 3–4 hours) is continued for varying periods of time after intravenous therapy depending on physician preference. If labor resumes, the step-up and step-down regimen can be reinstituted.

A dose-related elevation of heart rate of 20–40 beats/min may occur. An increase of systolic blood pressure up to 10 mm Hg is likely, and the diastolic pressure may fall 10–15 mm Hg during the infusion. Nonetheless, cardiac output increases considerably. Transient elevation of blood glucose, insulin, and fatty acids together with slight reduction of serum potassium have been reported. Fetal tachycardia may be slight or absent. No drug-caused perinatal deaths have been reported with beta-agonists. Maternal side effects requiring dose limitation are tachycardia ($\geq$ 120 beats/min), palpitations, and nervousness. Fluids should be limited to 2500 mL/24 h. Serious side effects (pulmonary edema, chest pain with or without electrocardiographic changes) are often idiosyncratic, not dose-related, and warrant termination of therapy.

One must identify cases in which untimely delivery is the sole threat to the life or health of the infant. An effort should be made to eliminate (1) maternal conditions that compromise the intrauterine environment and make premature birth the lesser risk, eg, preeclampsia-eclampsia; (2) fetal conditions that either are helped by early delivery or render attempts to stop premature labor meaningless, eg, severe erythroblastosis fetalis; and (3) clinical situations in which it is likely that an attempt to stop labor will be futile, eg, ruptured membranes with chorioamnionitis, cervix fully effaced and dilated more than 3 cm, strong labor in progress.

In pregnancies of less than 34 weeks' duration, betamethasone (12 mg intramuscularly repeated in 12–24 hours) is administered to hasten fetal lung maturation and permit delivery 48 hours after initial treatment when further prolongation of pregnancy is contraindicated.

Johnson P: Suppression of preterm labour: Current Concepts. Drugs 1993;45:684.

Lefevre ML, Hueston WJ: Preterm birth. Prim Care 1993;20:639.

LACTATION

Breast feeding should be encouraged by educative measures throughout pregnancy and the puerperium. Mothers should be told the benefits of breast feeding—it is emotionally satisfying, promotes mother-infant bonding, is economical, and gives significant immunity to the infant. The period of amenorrhea associated with frequent and consistent breast feeding provides good birth control until menstruation begins at 6–12 months postpartum or the intensity of breast feeding diminishes. If the mother must return to work, even a brief period of nursing is beneficial. Transfer of immunoglobulins in colostrum and breast milk protects the infant against many systemic and enteric infections. Macrophages and lymphocytes transferred to the infant from breast milk play an immunoprotective role. The intestinal flora of breast-fed infants inhibits the growth of pathogens. Breast-fed infants have fewer bacterial and viral infections, less severe diarrhea, fewer allergy problems, and less subsequent obesity than bottle-fed infants.

Frequent breast feeding on an infant demand schedule enhances milk flow and successful breast feeding.

Mothers breast feeding for the first time need help and encouragement from physicians, nurses, and other nursing mothers. Milk supply can be increased by increased suckling and increased rest.

Nursing mothers should have a fluid intake of over 2 L/d. The United States RDA calls for 21 g of extra protein (over the 44 g/d baseline for an adult woman) and 550 extra kcal/d in the first 6 months of nursing. Calcium intake should be 1200 mg/d. Continuation of a prenatal vitamin and mineral supplement is wise. Strict vegetarians who eschew both milk and eggs should always take vitamin B_{12} supplements during pregnancy and lactation.

Effects of Drugs in a Nursing Mother

Drugs taken by a nursing mother may accumulate in milk and be transmitted to the infant. The amount of a drug entering the milk depends on the drug's lipid solubility, mechanism of transport, and degree of ionization (Table 18–5).

Suppression of Lactation

A. Mechanical Suppression: The simplest and safest method of suppressing lactation after it has started is to gradually transfer the baby to a bottle or a cup over a 3-week period. Milk supply will decrease with decreased demand, and minimal discomfort ensues. If nursing must be stopped abruptly, the mother should avoid nipple stimulation, refrain from expressing milk, and use a snug brassiere. Ice packs and analgesics can be helpful. If suppression is desired before nursing has begun, use this same technique. Engorgement will gradually recede over a 2- to 3-day period.

B. Hormonal Suppression: Oral and long-acting injections of hormonal preparations were used at one time to suppress lactation. Because of their questionable efficacy and particularly because of associated side effects such as thromboembolic episodes and hair growth, their use for this purpose has largely been abandoned in recent years. Similarly, lactation suppression with bromocriptine is to be avoided because of reports of severe hypertension, seizures, strokes, and myocardial infarctions associated with its use.

Ito S et al: Prospective follow-up of adverse reactions in breastfed infants exposed to maternal medications Am J Obstet Gynecol 1993;168:1393.

Melnikow J, Bedinghaus JM: Management of common breastfeeding problems. J Fam Pract 1994;39:56.

PUERPERAL MASTITIS
(See also Chapter 16.)

Postpartum mastitis occurs sporadically in nursing mothers shortly after they return home, or it may oc-

Table 18–5. Drugs or substances to be used cautiously or not at all by nursing mothers.[1] (Other drugs are also contraindicated during pregnancy and lactation. Evaluate any drug for its need and its potential adverse effects.)

Drugs or Substances	Effect on Nursing Infant
Alcohol	No harmful effects unless taken in excess, when it can be associated with decreased linear growth and sedation.
Antibiotics	
Aminoglycosides	Not advised; will alter infant's bowel flora.
Nitrofurantoin	May cause hemolytic anemia in infant with glucose-6-phosphate dehydrogenase (G6PD) deficiency.
Tetracycline	Effects are dose-related; amount infant receives from milk is too small to cause discoloration of teeth. Safe.
Chloramphenicol[2]	Neonate may be unable to conjugate the drug; potential harm to bone marrow, leading to anemia, shock, and death.
Sulfonamides[2]	May cause jaundice in the neonatal period; may cause hemolytic anemia in infant with glucose-6-phosphate dehydrogenase (G6PD) deficiency.
Metronidazole	Nursing may be resumed 48 hours after last dose.
Anticoagulants	
Phenindione[2]	Can use heparin or warfarin instead.
Antihistamines	Contraindicated because of increased sensitivity of newborns and infants to antihistamines.
Antineoplastics[2]	Suspend nursing if these drugs are taken.
Antithyroids	
Thiouracil,[2] methimazole[2]	Contraindicated; may cause goiter or agranulocytosis.
Propylthiouracil	Considered safe.
Cardiac drugs	
Quinidine[2]	Contraindicated; may cause arrhythmia in infant.
Cimetidine,[2] ranitidine	Concentrated in breast milk; may suppress gastric acidity and cause central nervous system stimulation.
Ergot alkaloids	
Ergotamine (in doses to treat migraine)[2]	Causes vomiting, diarrhea, convulsions. May suppress lactation.
Bromocriptine[2]	Suppresses lactation.
Gold salts[2]	Contraindicated.
Hormones	
Oral contraceptives (low-dose)	May cause reduction of milk supply. Progestin-only minipill may be used.
Laxatives	
Cascara, senna	Can cause diarrhea in infant.
Lithium carbonate[2]	Contraindicated because of toxicity.
Nicotine	Increased respiratory disease in infants exposed to smoke.
Radioactive materials for testing[2]	
^{67}Ga	Insignificant amount excreted in milk; no nursing for 2 weeks.
^{125}I	Discontinue nursing for 48 hours.
^{131}I	After a test dose, nursing may be resumed after 24–36 hours; after a treatment dose, nursing may be resumed after 2–3 weeks.
^{99m}Tc	Discontinue nursing for 72 hours (half-life, 6 hours).
Sedatives and tranquilizers	Can cause sedation in infant. Benzodiazepines should be avoided.
Other drugs	
Caffeine	Irritability, poor sleep pattern with large amounts.
Cannabis;[2] cocaine;[2] polyhalogenated biphenyls[2] (eg, PCBs, PBBs); D-lysergic acid[2] (LSD)	Contraindicated; may interfere with mother's caretaking abilities and nutrition.

[1]Modified and reproduced, with permission, from Sahu S: Drugs and the nursing mother. Am Fam Physician (Dec) 1981;24:137.
[2]Absolutely contraindicated.

cur in epidemic form in the hospital. *Staphylococcus aureus* is usually the causative agent. Inflammation is generally unilateral, and women nursing for the first time are more often affected. Rarely, inflammatory carcinoma of the breast can be mistaken for puerperal mastitis.

Mastitis frequently begins within 3 months after delivery and may start with a sore or fissured nipple. There is obvious cellulitis in an area of breast tissue, with redness, tenderness, local warmth, and fever. Treatment consists of antibiotics effective against penicillin-resistant staphylococci (dicloxacillin or a cephalosporin, 500 mg orally ever 6 hours for 5–7 days) and regular emptying of the breast by nursing followed by expression of any remaining milk by hand or with a mechanical suction device.

If the mother begins antibiotic therapy before suppuration begins, infection can usually be controlled in 24 hours. If delay is permitted, breast abscess can result. Incision and drainage are required for abscess formation. Despite puerperal mastitis, the baby usually thrives without prophylactic antimicrobial therapy.

19 Allergic & Immunologic Disorders

Daniel C. Adelman, MD, & Abba Terr, MD

A wide variety of diseases are associated with disordered immune responses. Knowledge of immunoglobulin structure and function and of the cellular basis of immunity has resulted in a better understanding of these disorders. Diseases of immunity are usually caused by pathologic imbalances resulting from either excesses or deficiencies of immunocompetent cells or their products that disrupt normal homeostasis.

IMMUNOGLOBULINS & ANTIBODIES

IMMUNOGLOBULIN STRUCTURE & FUNCTION

Disorders of immune function are the basis of many human illnesses. The basic unit of all immunoglobulins consists of four polypeptide chains linked by disulfide bonds. There are two identical heavy chains (MW 55,000–70,000) and two identical light chains (MW about 23,000). Both heavy and light chains have a carboxyl terminal constant (C) region and an amino terminal variable (V) region. A hypervariable portion of the V regions of heavy and light chains folded together in a three-dimensional conformation form the combining site, which is responsible for the specific interaction with antigen.

Antibodies contain one of five classes of heavy chains (γ, α, μ, δ, ϵ) and one of two types of light chains (κ and λ). Either type of light chain can be associated with each of the heavy chain classes. Approximately 60% of human immunoglobulins have κ light chains, and 40% have λ light chains. About 10 million different antibody specificities are thought to exist in a given individual.

Immunoglobulin Classes

A. Immunoglobulin M (IgM): IgM is made up of five identical basic immunoglobulin units. These units are connected to one another by disulfide bonds and a small polypeptide known as the J chain. The molecular weight of IgM is about 900,000. The IgM molecule is found predominantly in the intravascular compartment and on the surface of B lymphocytes and does not normally cross the placenta. IgM antibody predominates early in immune responses; carbohydrate antigens such as blood group substances stimulate IgM.

B. Immunoglobulin A (IgA): IgA is present in blood and in relatively high concentrations in saliva, colostrum, tears, and secretions of the bronchi and gastrointestinal tract. Serum IgA is a single immunoglobulin unit, whereas secretory IgA is made up of two units connected to each other by a J chain. A 70,000-MW molecule called secretory component is attached to the Fc portion. It is necessary to transport IgA into the lumens of exocrine glands, and it confers resistance to enzymatic destruction. Secretory IgA plays an important role in host defense against viral and bacterial infections by blocking transport of microbes across mucosa.

C. Immunoglobulin G (IgG): IgG is a single immunoglobulin unit of MW 150,000 that comprises about 85% of total serum immunoglobulins. IgG is distributed in the extracellular fluid and is the only immunoglobulin that normally crosses the placenta. IgG binds complement via an Fc receptor present in the constant region of the heavy chain. IgG binds to the surface of cells and microbes, which allows them to be phagocytosed or killed by cytotoxic cells.

D. Immunoglobulin E (IgE): IgE is present in serum in very low concentrations as a single immunoglobulin unit with ϵ heavy chains. Approximately 50% of patients with allergic diseases have increased serum IgE levels. IgE is a skin-sensitizing or reaginic antibody by virtue of attachment to mast cells. The specific interaction between antigen and IgE bound to the surface of mast cells results in the release of inflammatory products such as histamine, leukotrienes, proteases, chemotactic factors, and cytokines. These mediators can produce bronchospasm, vasodilation, smooth muscle contraction, and chemoattraction of other inflammatory and immune cells.

E. Immunoglobulin D (IgD): IgD is present in the serum in very low concentrations as a single basic immunoglobulin unit with heavy chains. IgD is found on the surface of most B lymphocytes in association with IgM, where it probably serves as a receptor for antigen.

Clamen HN: The biology of the immune response. JAMA 1992;268:2790.

Janeway CA: How the immune system recognizes invaders. Sci Am 1993;269:73.

Schindler LW: The immune system: How it works. NIH Publication No. 92–3229. (Information for patients.)

Schindler LW: Understanding the immune system. USD-HHS, PHS, NIH Publication No. 92–529. (Information for health care personnel.)

Unanue ER: Overview of the immune system. In: *Samter's Immunologic Diseases,* 5th ed. Frank MM et al (editors). Little, Brown, 1995.

Immunoglobulin Genes

Genes that code for immunoglobulin light and heavy chain molecules undergo rearrangements in the DNA of B cells, which result in the synthesis and expression of the highly diverse group of immunoglobulin molecules. Clonal rearrangements of immunoglobulin genes in B cells are useful for determining the lineage of many leukemias and lymphomas.

Parlsow TG: Immunoglobulin genes, B cells, and the humoral immune response. In: *Basic & Clinical Immunology,* 8th ed. Stites DP, Terr AI, Parslow TG (editors). Appleton & Lange, 1994.

Tests for Immunoglobulins

Immunoglobulin levels can be elevated or reduced in a large number of diseases. In some diseases, particularly the gammopathies (see below), increased serum immunoglobulins, especially monoclonal types, are critical for diagnosis. In other diseases such as chronic liver diseases, chronic infection, or idiopathic inflammatory states, polyclonal increases in immunoglobulins are incidental or of unknown significance. If immunodeficiency is suspected in the presence of recurrent bacterial infections, measurement of serum immunoglobulins provides an essential test of B cell and plasma cell function. In acquired immune deficiencies such as AIDS, with many recurrent infections, paradoxical increases in immunoglobulins may occur.

Antibodies and immunoglobulins can be measured in three ways: (1) by quantitative and qualitative determinations of serum immunoglobulins; (2) by determination of isohemagglutinin and febrile agglutinin titers; and (3) by determination of antibody titers following immunization with tetanus toxoid, diphtheria toxoid, or pneumococcal polysaccharide vaccines. The first method tests for the presence of serum immunoglobulins but not for the functional adequacy of the immunoglobulins. The second method tests for functional antibodies that are present in the serum of almost all individuals as a consequence of exposure to blood group substances or infection. The third method examines functional antibody activity in the serum after intentional immunization. Commonly used clinical tests of antibody immunity, for many diseases, are protein electrophoresis, immunoelectrophoresis, and quantitative immunoglobulin determinations.

Protein Electrophoresis & Immunoelectrophoresis

Protein electrophoresis is a screening test to measure semiquantitatively various proteins in body fluids, usually serum or urine. Proteins are electrically separated on a strip of cellulose acetate on the basis of charge into albumin, α_1, α_2, β, and γ globulins. This test is useful to screen for diseases with excess or deficiency of immunoglobulins, although the method should not be used to diagnose antibody deficiency disorders.

Immunoelectrophoresis is used to identify the specific immunoglobulin class in a body fluid. Serum, for example, is separated electrophoretically and then reacted with appropriate antisera directed against IgG, IgA, or IgM. The resulting patterns produced allow identification of abnormal immunoglobulins such as myeloma (M) proteins. This method is also useful in differentiation of monoclonal from polyclonal increases in immunoglobulins. It is only semiquantitative and thus cannot be used to determine immunoglobulin levels precisely, eg, in Waldenström's macroglobulinemia.

Another similar technique called immunofixation electrophoresis has to a large extent replaced immunoelectrophoresis. With this technique, serum proteins are separated electrophoretically in a gel and then immunoprecipitated in situ with monospecific antisera. This method has the advantages of more rapid results and slightly higher resolution of low levels of monoclonal immunoglobulin chains. If protein electrophoresis is normal despite suspicion of an M protein, immunoelectrophoresis or immunofixation electrophoresis of both serum and concentrated urine should be performed because of the greater sensitivity of these tests.

Quantitative Immunoglobulin Determinations

Quantitative determinations of serum IgG, IgA, and IgM levels can be made rapidly and accurately by nephelometry. The measurement of immunoglobulin levels alone does not distinguish monoclonal immunoglobulins, as does the immunoelectrophoresis or immunofixation electrophoresis procedure.

IgD levels have no recognized clinical use, and IgE levels must be measured with more sensitive techniques such as radioimmunoassay or enzyme-linked immunoassay.

Hamilton RG, Adkinson NF: Serologic assays for antigens and antibodies: Immunol Allergy Clin North Am 1994;14:351. (Describes immunoassays for antigen and antibody measurement.)

DISEASES OF IMMUNOGLOBULIN OVERPRODUCTION (Gammopathies)

The monoclonal gammopathies include those disease entities in which there is a disproportionate proliferation of a single clone of immunoglobulin-forming cells that produce a homogeneous heavy chain, light chain, or complete molecule. The amino acid sequence of the variable (V) regions is fixed, and only one type (κ or λ) of light chain is produced. Polyclonal gammopathies result from proliferation of many B cell clones, resulting in a diffuse increase of immunoglobulins.

Monoclonal Gammopathy of Uncertain Significance (MGUS)

The diagnosis is made upon finding a homogeneous (monoclonal) immunoglobulin (with either κ or λ chains, but not both) in immunoelectrophoresis of the serum. The incidence of homogeneous serum immunoglobulins increases with age and may approach 3% in persons 70 years of age or older. As many as a third of individuals with apparently benign monoclonal gammopathies will eventually develop lymphoid malignancies, amyloidosis, or multiple myelomas. No specific therapy is necessary, but indefinite observation for the development of lymphoproliferation is required. Actuarial risk for the development of a malignant disorder is 33% at 20 years. Parameters that suggest a favorable prognosis in benign monoclonal gammopathy include the following: (1) concentration of homogeneous immunoglobulin less than 2 g/dL, (2) no significant increase in the concentration of the homogeneous immunoglobulin from the time of diagnosis, (3) no decrease in the concentration of normal immunoglobulins, (4) absence of a homogeneous light chain in the urine, and (5) normal hematocrit and serum albumin concentration.

Multiple Myeloma (See also Chapter 13.)

This disease is characterized by the overproduction and spread of neoplastic plasma cells throughout the bone marrow. Myeloma cells sometimes express molecules of early B cell or myelomonocytic lineages. Rarely, extraosseous plasmacytomas may be found. Anemia, hypercalcemia, increased susceptibility to infection, and bone pain are frequent. Diagnosis depends upon the presence of the following: (1) radiographic findings of osteolytic lesions or diffuse osteoporosis, (2) the presence of a homogeneous serum immunoglobulin (myeloma protein) or a single type of light chain in the urine (Bence Jones proteinuria), and (3) finding of an abnormal plasma cell infiltrate in the bone marrow biopsy (see Chapter 13). The presence of over 20% bone marrow plasma cells reliably differentiates early myeloma from MGUS. There is an approximate correlation between the incidence of immunoglobulin type in myeloma and the normal serum concentration of the immunoglobulin involved. That is, IgG > IgA > IgD > IgE. IgM myeloma does not occur for all practical purposes. Multiple myeloma remains difficult to treat and is rarely, if ever, cured.

Waldenström's Macroglobulinemia

Waldenström's macroglobulinemia is characterized by a proliferation of abnormal lymphoid cells that have morphologic features of both B cells and plasma cells. These cells secrete a homogeneous macroglobulin (IgM) detectable by immunoelectrophoresis. Monoclonal light chains are present in 10% of cases. Clinical manifestations depend upon the physicochemical characteristics of the macroglobulin. Raynaud's phenomenon and peripheral vascular occlusions are associated with cold-insoluble proteins (cryoglobulins). Retinal hemorrhages, visual impairment, and transient neurologic deficits are common with high-viscosity serum. Bleeding diatheses or hemolytic anemia can occur when the macroglobulin complexes with coagulation factors or binds to the surface of red blood cells.

Amyloidosis

Amyloidosis is a group of disorders manifested by impaired organ function from infiltration of tissues with insoluble protein fibrils or proteins complexed with polysaccharides. Variations in composition of the fibrils can be largely correlated with the clinical syndromes (Table 19–1). Amyloid occurs in a primary form or in company with plasmacytosis in bone marrow or lymphoid tissues. The protein fibrils in these entities are composed of immunoglobulin light chains or fragments of light chains, particularly the V region. This form of amyloid has been designated AL.

Symptoms and signs of amyloid infiltration are related to malfunction of the organ involved (eg, nephrotic syndrome in 35%, chronic renal failure, cardiomyopathy and cardiac conduction defects in 35%, intestinal malabsorption, intestinal obstruction, carpal tunnel syndrome, macroglossia in 22%, peripheral neuropathy in 17%, end-organ insufficiency of endocrine glands, respiratory failure, obstruction to ventilation, and capillary damage with ecchymosis). Amyloidosis due to deposition of β_2-microglobulin in joints and bones occurs in chronic hemodialysis patients. Table 19–1 lists organs characteristically involved with each type of amyloid.

Table 19–1. Classification of amyloidosis.[1]

	Clinical Type	Common Sites of Deposition
Familial	Amyloid polyneuropathy (Portuguese, dominant inheritance)	Peripheral nerves, viscera
	Familial Mediterranean fever (recessive)	Liver, spleen, kidneys, adrenals
Generalized	Primary	Tongue, heart, gut, skeletal and smooth muscles, nerves, skin, ligaments
	Associated with plasma cell dyscrasia	Liver, spleen, kidneys, adrenals
	Secondary (infection, inflammation, etc)	Any site
Localized	Lichen amyloidosis	Skin
	Endocrine-related (eg, thyroid carcinoma)	Endocrine organ (thyroid)
Senile		Heart, brain

[1]Reproduced, with permission, from Stites DP, Terr AI, Parslow TG (editors): *Basic & Clinical Immunology,* 8th ed. Appleton & Lange, 1994.

The diagnosis of amyloidosis is based on clinical suspicion, family history, and preexisting long-standing infection or debilitating illness. The diagnosis of amyloidosis is confirmed by protein electrophoresis and established by microscopic examination of biopsy specimens. In patients with systemic disease, rectal or gingival biopsies show a sensitivity of about 80%, bone-marrow biopsy about 50%, and abdominal fat aspiration between 70% and 80%. Fine-needle biopsy of subcutaneous abdominal fat is a simple and reliable method for diagnosing secondary systemic amyloidosis.

Treatment of localized amyloid tumors is by surgical excision. There is no effective treatment of systemic amyloidosis, and death usually occurs within 1–3 years. Patients who develop renal failure requiring dialysis have a median survival of less than 1 year, and usually die due to extrarenal progression of their systemic amyloidosis. Treatment of the predisposing disease may cause a temporary remission or slow the progress of the disease, but it is unlikely that the established metabolic process is altered. Patients with amyloid due to plasma cell dyscrasia may occasionally respond to treatment with melphalan and prednisone. Colchicine is of use in familial Mediterranean fever to slow the development of amyloidosis. Early and adequate treatment of pyogenic infections may prevent secondary amyloidosis.

Heavy Chain Disease
(α, γ, μ)

These are rare disorders in which the abnormal serum and urine protein is a part of a homogeneous α, γ, or μ heavy chain. The clinical presentation is more typical of lymphoma than multiple myeloma, and there are no destructive bone lesions. Gamma chain disease presents as a lymphoproliferative disorder commonly with autoimmune features or in the context of a lymphoid malignancy. Alpha chain disease is frequently associated with severe diarrhea and infiltration of the lamina propria of the small intestine with abnormal plasma cells. Mu chain disease is associated with chronic lymphocytic leukemia.

Baklogie B et al: Plasma cell dyscrasias. JAMA 1992;268:2946. (Review of multiple myeloma, Waldenström's macroglobulinemia, light chain and heavy chain disease.)

Gertz MA, Kyle RA, O'Fallon WM: Dialysis support of patients with primary systemic amyloidosis. Arch Intern Med 1992;152:2245. (Eighteen percent of patients undergo dialysis, which is best predicted by 24-hour creatinine clearance and protein at the time of diagnosis; median survival of these patients is 1 year, and most deaths result from cardiac involvement.)

Kyle RA: "Benign" monoclonal gammopathy—after 20 to 35 years of follow-up. Mayo Clin Proc 1993;68:26. (About one-fourth of patients eventually develop multiple myeloma, amyloidosis, macroglobulinemia, or related disorders.)

Kyle RA, Greipp PR: Amyloidosis (AL): Clinical and laboratory features in 229 cases. Mayo Clin Proc 1983;58:665.

Linke RP: Therapy of amyloid diseases. Renal Failure 1993;15:395.

Stone MJ: Amyloidosis: A final common pathway for protein deposition in tissues. Blood 1990;75:531.

Ucci G et al: Presenting features of monoclonal gammopathies: An analysis of 684 newly diagnosed cases. J Intern Med 1993;234:165. (Multiple myeloma may be safely distinguished from MGUS by using criterion of > 20% bone marrow plasma cell for multiple myeloma.)

Vogelgesang SA, Klirple GL: The many guises of amyloidosis: Clinical presentations and disease associations. Postgrad Med 1994;96:126. (General review of primary and secondary amyloidosis.)

CELLULAR IMMUNITY

CELLS INVOLVED IN IMMUNITY

Development of T & B Lymphocytes

Lymphocytes interact with antigens via specific receptors and thereby initiate immune responses. The thymus-derived cells (T lymphocytes) are involved in cellular immune responses; the bone marrow-derived cells (B lymphocytes) are involved in antibody responses.

Both T and B lymphocytes are derived from precursor or stem cells in the marrow. Precursors of T cells migrate to the thymus, where they develop some of the functional and cell surface characteristics of mature T cells. Clones of autoreactive T cells are eliminated, and mature antigen-reactive T cells then migrate to the peripheral lymphoid tissues and enter the pool of long-lived lymphocytes that recirculate from the blood to the lymph.

B cell maturation has antigen-independent and antigen-dependent stages. Antigen-independent maturation includes development from precursor cells in the marrow through the virgin B cell (a cell that has not been exposed to antigen previously) found in the peripheral lymphoid tissues. The production and maturation of virgin B cells are ongoing processes even in adult animals. Antigen-dependent maturation occurs following the interaction of antigen with virgin B cells. The final products of B cell development are circulating long-lived memory B cells and plasma cells that secrete copious amounts of specific antibody. Mature B cells in the periphery are found predominantly in primary follicles and germinal centers of the lymph nodes and spleen.

Subpopulations of T Cells

T lymphocytes are heterogeneous with respect to their cell surface features (Table 19–2) and func-

Table 19–2. Selected surface antigens detected by monoclonal antibodies on T and B cells.

Cluster of Differentiation	Antibody Designation	Distribution
CD2	Leu-5	Pan T cell marker, NK cells
CD3	Leu-4, OKT3	TcR-associated antigen
CD4	Leu-3, T4	Mature helper-inducer T cells
CD8	Leu-2, T8	Cytotoxic-suppressor T cells
CD19	B4	Pan B cell marker
CD25	Tac	One chain in the IL-2 receptor; seen on activated T cells and some B and NK cells
CD45RA	2H4	"Naive" CD4 and CD8 T cells; some B cells and monocytes
CD45RO	UCH-1	"Memory" CD4 and CD8 T cells

tional characteristics. At least four subpopulations of T cells are now recognized.

A. Helper-Inducer T Cells: These cells help to amplify the production of antibody-forming cells from B lymphocytes after interaction with antigen. Helper T cells also amplify the production of effector T cells that mediate cytotoxicity. The several different functions of these T cells may reflect various stages of development rather than unique or separate lineages of these lymphocytes. Two subsets of helper T cells can be identified on the basis of their pattern of cytokine production. The subsets are called type 1 T helper (TH1) cells, which produce interleukin-2 and gamma interferon; and type 2 T helper (TH2) cells, which produce interleukins-4, -5, and -6, among others. TH1 and TH2 subsets of helper T cells are important cellular components of cellular and humoral immune responses, respectively. TH2 helper T cells play a central role in the generation of IgG-mediated responses to allergen.

B. Cytotoxic or Killer T Cells: These cells are generated after mature T cells interact with certain antigens such as those present on the surface of foreign cells. These cells are responsible for organ graft rejection and for killing of virally infected cells and some tumor cells.

C. Suppressor T Cells: These cells suppress the formation of antibody-forming cells from B lymphocytes. Suppressor T cells are regarded as regulatory cells that modulate antibody formation. Cell-mediated immunity (ie, organ graft rejection) is also regulated by suppressor cells.

D. Suppressor-Inducer T Cells: These cells, which have helper cell (not suppressor cell) surface antigens, amplify the development of suppressor T cells.

Identification of T Cell Subpopulations With Monoclonal Antibodies

Monoclonal antibodies to T cell subpopulations are produced by immunizing animals with human T cells and then fusing the spleen cells of the animal with mouse myeloma cells to develop hybridoma cell lines. These hybridoma lines secrete monoclonal antibodies that identify cell surface antigens common to all human T cells (Table 19–2). The term CD (cluster of differentiation) is used to designate various lymphocyte types. About 75% of the peripheral blood lymphocytes of normal individuals are T cells; 50% are helper-inducer T cells, and 25% are suppressor or cytotoxic T cells.

Changes in the number or ratio of various T cell subsets occur in a wide variety of clinical conditions. For example, the ratio of helper to suppressor (H/S) cells in healthy individuals is about 1.6–2.2. In many acute viral infections, this ratio falls temporarily both as a result of decrease in helper/inducer cells and of increase in suppressor/cytotoxic cells. In AIDS and related HIV infections, H:S ratios are nearly always reduced (probably irreversibly) by the destructive effects of this lymphotropic virus. Among other clinical applications of the enumeration of these cells are the diagnosis of some immunodeficiencies, phenotyping of leukemias and lymphomas, and monitoring of immunologic changes following organ transplantation.

Cytokines

Many T cell functions are mediated by cytokines, which are humoral factors secreted by lymphocytes among numerous other cells. Cytokines are secreted when cells are activated by antigens or other cytokines. Table 19–3 lists some examples of cytokines and their functions. The cytokines can be functionally organized into groups according to their major activities: (1) those that promote and mediate natural immunity, such as IL-1, IL-6, interferon (IFN)-γ, and IL-8; (2) those that support allergic inflammation, such as IL-4, which acts to promote IgE production, IL-3, -4, -9, and -10, which act to promote mast cell growth, and IL-3, IL-5, and granulocyte-macrophage colony stimulating factor (GM-CSF), which promote the growth of eosinophils; (3) those that exert lymphocyte regulatory activity, such as IL-10 produced by the TH2 helper T cell, and IFN-γ, which is produced by the TH1 T helper cell; and (4) those that act as hematopoietic growth factors (IL-7 and GM-CSF). This complicated network of interacting cytokines

functions to modulate and regulate cellular function so that the host may survive in an otherwise hostile environment.

Therapeutically, cytokines are being used experimentally both to evaluate immune function and to treat disease. Receptors for IL-2 circulate in blood and are a measure of generalized immune stimulation. IL-2 in combination with autologous lymphocytes has been tested as an anti-cancer treatment in selected patients with limited success. Aldesleukin is now available and approved for treatment of metastatic renal cell carcinoma in adults.

T Cell Antigen Receptors

T cells interact with several different types of cells during the regulation and mediation of immune responses. These interactions include presentation of antigens to T cells by macrophages or other cells, T cell-induced differentiation of B cells into antibody-secreting cells, and T cell killing of a variety of other cells. In all of these cell-cell interactions, T cells recognize foreign antigens on the surface of the target cell in association with other cell surface antigens that are coded for by the major histocompatibility gene complex of the non-T cell. T cells have cell surface receptors that recognize at least two different molecules; one recognition site binds to any single foreign antigen (viral, bacterial, etc.), and the other binds to major histocompatibility antigens. An exam-

Table 19–3. Major sources and activities of selected cytokines.

Cytokine	Primary Cellular Source	Primary Biologic Activity
IL-1	Macrophages	Immunologic and inflammatory mediator; acute phase reactant; augments immune responses.
IL-2	T lymphocytes	Promotes T lymphocyte activation, growth.
IL-3	T lymphocytes	Hematopoietic growth factor, "multicolony stimulating factor."
IL-4	T lymphocytes	T and B lymphocyte, mast cell growth factor; promotes IgE isotype switching.
IL-5	T lymphocytes	B cell growth factor; promotes IgA production; promotes eosinophil growth and differentiation.
IL-6	Macrophages, T lymphocytes	B cell differentiation factors; acute phase reactant.
IL-7	Stromal cells of the spleen and thymus	Growth factor for very early B and T lymphocytes.
IL-8	Macrophages, T cells	Chemotactic factor for neutrophils, lymphocytes; up-regulates integrin expression.
IL-9	T lymphocytes	Hematopoietic enhancing factor with IL-2, IL-3, IL-4.
IL-10	T lymphocytes	Down-regulates cellular activation; inhibits production of proinflammatory cytokines by monocytes and macrophages.
TNF	Macrophages, T cells, mast cells, NK cells	Overlaps activity with IL-1 but has more antitumor activity.
IFN-α IFN-β IFN-γ	B lymphocytes, macrophages Fibroblasts, epithelial cells T lymphocytes	Antiviral and antitumor activities; activates macrophages; enhances cytotoxic lymphocyte and NK activity.
GM-CSF	T lymphocytes, fibroblasts, endothelial cells	Growth factor for granulocytes, macrophage and eosinophil colonies; activates neutrophil phagocytosis; enhances eosinophil-mediated cytotoxicity; promotes basophil histamine release.

Key: IL = interleukin; GM-CSF = granulocyte-macrophage colony-stimulating factor (sargramostin); NK = natural killer cells.

ple of this dual recognition is observed in the killing of virus-infected target cells by cytolytic T cells. Cytolytic T cells taken from humans immunized to a given virus will kill virus-infected target cells if the target cells carry the same histocompatibility antigens as the immunized host.

The structure of T cell antigen receptors and the genes that encode these glycoproteins have been defined. The antigen recognition structure is a complex of two molecules, one containing variable α and β or γ and δ chains and the other the monomorphic T3 (CD3) molecule. Genes encoding the β chain have homology to immunoglobulin genes. Clonal rearrangement of T cell receptor genes proceeds during T cell development to generate diversity for antigen recognition in a fashion similar to that of immunoglobulin genes in B cells. T cell receptor gene rearrangements have been used to identify T cell leukemias, lymphomas, and mycosis fungoides, a rare malignant neoplasm of the skin.

Adelman DC: Functional assessment of mononuclear leukocytes. Immunol Allergy Clin North Am 1994; 14:241.

Griesser H, Mak TW: The T-cell receptor: Structure, function, and clinical application. Hematol Pathol 1994;8:1. (Understanding T cell receptor may hold clues to reactive and malignant disorders of T cells.)

Janeway CA Jr, Bottomly K: Signals and signs for lymphocyte responses. Cell 1994;76:275. (Effector responses of T cells depend on the interplay of the T cell receptor with costimulatory molecules and cytokines, which may have implications in modulating the immune response.)

Shelhamer JH (moderator): Airway inflammation. Ann Intern Med 1995;123:288. (Airway production of cytokines may play an important role in the generation and perpetuation of airway inflammation.)

B Lymphocytes

B cells express different characteristic surface molecules (Table 19–2). The majority of B cells express both IgM and IgD on the surface and are derived from pre-B cells found mainly in the bone marrow. Pre-B cells contain intracytoplasmic IgM but do not express surface immunoglobulin. Patients with X-linked hypogammaglobulinemia frequently show a developmental arrest at the stage of the pre-B cell. The majority of patients with acquired hypogammaglobulinemia have a block of transition from the mature B cell to the plasma cell. Thus, most patients with this disease have normal numbers of circulating mature B cells but reduced numbers of plasma cells.

B cells have been commonly identified by other surface markers in addition to immunoglobulins. These include the receptor for the Fc portion of immunoglobulins, B cell-specific antigens CD19 and CD20, and surface antigens coded for by the HLA-D genetic region in humans (Table 19–2). All mature B cells bear surface immunoglobulin that is the antigen-specific receptor. The major role of B cells is

differentiation to antibody-secreting plasma cells. However, B cells may also release cytokines and function as antigen-presenting cells.

Other Cells Involved in Immune Responses

A. Macrophages: Macrophages are involved in the ingestion, processing, and presentation of particulate antigens for interaction with lymphocytes. They play an important role in T and B lymphocyte cooperation in the induction of antibody responses. In addition, they are effector cells for certain types of tumor immunity.

B. NK (Natural Killer) Cells: These lymphocytic cells, which are indirectly related to the T cell lineage, can kill a wide spectrum of target cells. They are recognized by the presence of specific surface antigens and Fc receptors. Many appear as large granular lymphocytes. Their role in host defense is probably the killing of virally infected cells and tumor cells in the absence of prior sensitization and without MHC restriction.

Murphy WJ et al: Natural killer cells and bone marrow transplantation. J Natl Cancer Inst 1993;85:1475. (Review of basic biology of NK cells and effects on hematopoiesis and on outcome of marrow graft, including graft-versus-host disease and graft-versus-tumor response.)

TESTS FOR CELLULAR IMMUNITY

Identification of Human B & T Cells

A. B Cells: Cell surface structures that characterize B cells include the following: (1) easily detectable surface immunoglobulin, (2) specific antigens (CD19, CD20), (3) a receptor for the Fc portion of immunoglobulins that have been aggregated or complexed with antigen, and (4) MCH class I, or DR antigens (Table 19–2).

B. T Cells: T cell markers include surface antigens identified by specific monoclonal antibodies (Table 19–2). T cells can also be detected in tissue sections or suspensions using enzyme-labeled antibodies. Approximately 75% of human peripheral blood lymphocytes are T cells, and up to 20% are B cells. The remainder are NK cells.

Procedures for Testing Cell-Mediated Immunity, or T Cell Function

A. Skin Testing: Cell-mediated immunity can be assessed qualitatively by evaluating skin reactivity following intradermal injection of a battery of antigens to which humans are frequently sensitized (ie, streptokinase, streptodornase, purified protein derivative, *Trichophyton, Dermatophyton,* or *Candida*). Intradermal injections of 0.1 mL of recommended test strengths are observed for maximal induration and erythema at 24 and 48 hours. A positive reaction varies in size with particular antigens but is generally at least 10 mm in diameter. Anergy or lack of skin reactivity to all of these substances usually indicates a depression of cell-mediated immunity. Delayed hypersensitivity skin tests depend on complex interactions of T cells, macrophages, and other immunoreactants; thus, failure to respond cannot specifically identify a defect in a particular cell type.

B. In Vitro Stimulation of Peripheral Blood Lymphocytes With Mitogens or Antigens: T lymphocytes are transformed to blast cells upon short-term incubation with mitogens such as phytohemagglutinin or recall antigens in vitro. T cell activation can be determined quantitatively by following the cellular uptake of [^{3}H]thymidine introduced into the culture medium. The in vitro uptake of [^{3}H]thymidine by human peripheral blood lymphocytes indicates T cell function and correlates well with other manifestations of cell-mediated immunity as measured by delayed hypersensitivity skin tests. These functional tests can detect abnormalities in T cells despite normal or slightly reduced cell counts, particularly following bone marrow transplantation or in congenital immunodeficiency diseases. Stimulation of transplant recipients' lymphocytes or donor lymphocytes (the mixed lymphocyte reaction) is a critical test for determining histocompatibility, especially in renal and bone marrow transplantation.

APPLICATIONS OF T & B CELL TESTS

Immunodeficiency Diseases

Thymic hypoplasia is associated with a marked decrease in the number of T cells in the peripheral blood. On the other hand, the absence of B cells in the blood is frequently found in X-linked hypogammaglobulinemia. Marked reduction of both T and B cells occurs in severe combined immunodeficiency disease (SCID). Patients with HIV infection and particularly the acquired immunodeficiency syndrome (AIDS) have reduced numbers of T cells and reduced T helper-to-suppressor ratios.

Lymphoproliferative Diseases

A marked increase in the number of peripheral blood lymphocytes that bear immunoglobulin of a single heavy chain class and light chain type represents a monoclonal proliferation of cells. Blood lymphocytes from almost all patients with chronic lymphocytic leukemia and non-Hodgkin's lymphoma with blood involvement show this abnormality. On the other hand, lymphocytosis secondary to viral or bacterial infection is associated with a normal percentage of B cells and the usual distribution of immunoglobulin classes on the cell surface.

Lymphocytic leukemias can be classified by phenotyping T and B cells, with implications for prognosis and, sometimes, treatment. Monitoring various T cell subsets is also useful in following patients with organ transplants.

Adelman DC: Functional assessment of mononuclear leukocytes. Immunol Allergy Clin North Am 1994; 14:241. (Review of delayed hypersensitivity testing, measures of lymphocyte activation and proliferation and antibody production, natural killer cells and monocyte function, and detection of cytokines and other products of immune cells.)

IMMUNOLOGIC DEFICIENCY DISEASES

The primary immunologic deficiency diseases include congenital and acquired disorders of humoral immunity (B cell function) or cell-mediated immunity (T cell function). Most of these diseases are rare and since they are genetically determined, occur primarily in children.

Classification

Some immunodeficiency disorders affect adults, and several are discussed below. The WHO classification of immunodeficiency disorders more often affecting adults includes the following:

A. Primary Immunodeficiency Disorders:

1. Selective IgA deficiency (see below).

2. Common variable immunodeficiency (see below).

3. X-linked immunodeficiency with hyper-IgM.

4. Immunodeficiency with normal serum globulins or hyperimmunoglobulinemia.

5. Immunodeficiency with thymoma.

6. Acquired immunodeficiency syndrome (AIDS) (see below).

B. Secondary Immunodeficiency Disorders:

1. AIDS (see below).

2. Iatrogenic (eg, cancer chemotherapy).

3. Immunodeficiency associated with sarcoidosis.

4. Immunodeficiency associated with Hodgkin's disease.

Rosen FS, Cooper MD, Wedgewood RJP: The primary immunodeficiencies. N Engl J Med 1995;333:431. (Review of primary immunodeficiency disorders with correlations to cellular ontogeny.)

Sheaker WT et al: Laboratory assessment of immune deficiency disorders. Immunol Allergy Clin North Am

1994;14:265. (Discusses molecular basis for primary immunodeficiency, laboratory evaluation of defects in antibody function, lymphocyte function, phagocyte function, and complement function and how these relate to primary and secondary immunodeficiencies.)

COMMON VARIABLE IMMUNODEFICIENCY

The prevalence of common variable immunodeficiency is about 1:80,000 in the United States. Onset is typically late in adolescence or early in adulthood. Increased susceptibility to pyogenic infections is the hallmark of the disease, which if left untreated often leads to recurrent sinusitis and pneumonia progressing to bronchiectasis. Patients may also develop a sprue-like syndrome with diarrhea, steatorrhea, malabsorption, protein-losing enteropathy, and hepatosplenomegaly.

Arthritis of the type associated with congenital hypogammaglobulinemia and autoimmune diseases may occur. Diagnosis is confirmed in patients with recurrent infections (eg, sinopulmonary, gastrointestinal) by demonstration of functional or quantitative defects in antibody production. Serum IgG levels are usually less than 250 mg/dL; serum IgA and IgM levels are subnormal. Decreased to absent function responses to protein antigen immunizations establish the diagnosis of common variable immunodeficiency. Lymph nodes may be enlarged in these patients, yet biopsies show marked reduction in plasma cells. Noncaseating granulomas are frequently found in the spleen, liver, lungs, or skin. There is an increased propensity for the development of B cell neoplasms, gastric carcinomas, and skin cancers.

The cause of the panhypogammaglobulinemia in the overwhelming majority of common variable immunodeficiency patients is an intrinsic B cell defect in antibody production. In a small number of patients, excessive suppressor T cell activity which inhibits B cells—or helper T cell activity inadequate to assist B cells to make antibody—has been identified. The absolute B cell count in the peripheral blood in most patients, despite the underlying cellular defect, is normal. A subset of these patients have concomitant T cell immunodeficiency with increased numbers of activated CD8 cells, splenomegaly, and decreased delayed-type hypersensitivity. Therapy at present is similar to that of congenital hypogammaglobulinemia, with infusions of 300–500 mg/kg of intravenous immune globulin at about monthly intervals. Adjustment of dosage or infusion interval is made on the basis of clinical responses and steady state trough serum IgG levels. Such therapy is effective in decreasing the incidence of (or preventing) potentially life-threatening infections. It is important that the diagnosis be unequivocally established, because the yearly cost of monthly infusions can be in excess of $20,000–$30,000.

Sneller MC et al: New insights into common variable immunodeficiency. Ann Intern Med 1993;118:720. (Characterized by hypogammaglobulinemia, recurrent infection, and an increased incidence of autoimmune disease and malignancy; pathogenesis related to defect in B cell function due to B cell itself, lack of lymphokine signals, or increased number of CD8 cells.)

SELECTIVE IMMUNOGLOBULIN A DEFICIENCY

Selective IgA deficiency is the most common primary immunodeficiency disorder and is characterized by the absence of serum IgA with normal levels of IgG and IgM; its prevalence is about 1:700 to 1:500 individuals. Most patients have minimal or absent symptoms, but some have frequent and recurrent infections typically involving the paranasal sinuses, bronchi, and lungs. Some cases of IgA deficiency may spontaneously remit. When IgG_2 subclass deficiency occurs in combination with IgA deficiency, recurrent sinusitis and bronchopulmonary infections are common. Patients with a combined IgA and IgG subclass deficiency should be assessed for functional antibody responses to glycoprotein antigen immunization. Occasionally, a sprue-like syndrome with steatorrhea has been associated with an isolated IgA deficit. Treatment with commercial immune globulin is ineffective, since IgA and IgM are present only in small quantities in these preparations. Frequent infusions of plasma (containing IgA) or unwashed blood transfusions are hazardous, since anti-IgA antibodies may develop, resulting in systemic anaphylaxis or serum sickness.

Koskinen S et al: Long-term persistence of selective IgA deficiency in healthy adults. J Clin Immunol 1994;14:116. (Follow-up of 204 healthy blood donors with initial IgA deficiency showed 78% with no IgA present and 21% with lower than normal levels of IgA after a median time of 19 years.)

ACQUIRED IMMUNODEFICIENCY SYNDROME (AIDS)
(See also Chapter 31.)

AIDS is a chronic retroviral infection with human immunodeficiency virus (HIV) that produces severe, life-threatening T cell defects. In addition to reduction of CD4 (helper T cells), there is an increase in CD8 (suppressor/cytotoxic T cells), most of which have a cytotoxic phenotype.

B cell function is altered so that many infected individuals have marked hypergammaglobulinemia, and AIDS patients fail to respond normally to antigens when immunized. Autoantibodies and circulating immune complexes are present. Most infected individuals progress from health to AIDS over several years. The immunologic determinants of the clinical fate of persons infected with HIV are unknown.

In AIDS, immunologic tests reveal a severe selective deficiency of T lymphocyte function and number, with little alteration in B lymphocyte numbers. Patients are frequently anergic. In vitro tests of peripheral blood T cell function such as proliferative responses to antigens and mitogens are markedly reduced or absent. The absolute lymphocyte count is severely decreased (frequently < 500 cells/μL), and the ratio of helper to suppressor/cytotoxic T cells is considerably lower than normal. Although T cell depletion in HIV infection is a consequence of destruction of CD4 cells by the virus, other mechanisms to deplete T cells and suppress immune responses are also operative. The immunologic changes that occur in asymptomatic HIV seropositive individuals are usually not as marked as those in AIDS patients.

Chernoff D: Human immunodeficiency virus disease and related opportunistic infections. In: *Manual of Allergy and Immunology,* 3rd ed. Lawlor GJ, Fischer TJ, Adelman DC (editors). Little, Brown, 1994.

Pantaleo G et al: New concepts in the immunopathogenesis of human immunodeficiency virus infection. N Engl J Med 1993;328:327. (Review of immunopathogenic mechanisms of HIV infection; poorly understood mechanisms of depletion of CD4 cells not entirely understood and may be related to virus itself or other mechanisms, including appropriate cell signaling apoptosis and superantigen stimulation.)

SECONDARY IMMUNODEFICIENCY

Deficiencies in T cell immunity, antibody immunity, or both have been associated with many diseases. Two examples of altered immunity secondary to underlying disease are discussed below.

Immunodeficiency Associated With Sarcoidosis

The immunodeficiency associated with sarcoidosis is characterized by a partial deficit in T cell function with intact or increased B cell function. Patients with sarcoidosis often are relatively nonreactive to intradermal injections of common antigens. However, complete lack of skin reactivity is infrequent. A positive reaction to purified protein derivative is usually noted during active infection with *Mycobacterium tuberculosis.* Serum immunoglobulin levels are normal or high, and specific antibody formation is generally normal.

Immunodeficiency Associated With Hodgkin's Disease

A moderate to severe deficit in T cell function with intact B cell function is frequently found in Hodgkin's disease. Only 10–20% of patients with Hodgkin's disease show skin reactivity to common antigens, as compared to 70–90% of controls. Many patients show depressed responses to in vitro stimulation of peripheral blood lymphocytes with phytohemagglutinin. Serum immunoglobulins are normal, and specific antibody formation is intact except in agonal cases.

The clinical significance of depressed cell-mediated immunity in Hodgkin's disease is difficult to evaluate, since most patients are treated with potent immunosuppressive agents. Nevertheless, frequent infections with herpes zoster and *Cryptococcus* are probably related to immunodeficiency associated with the underlying disease.

Buckley RH: Immunodeficiency disease. JAMA 1992;268:2797.(A concise review of the major immunodeficiency diseases, including a practical approach to the patient with recurrent infections).

AUTOIMMUNITY

Autoimmune diseases cannot be explained by a solitary cause or mechanism. Small amounts of autoantibodies are normally produced and may have physiologic roles in cellular interactions. The major theories regarding the development of autoimmune disease are (1) release of normally sequestered antigens, (2) the presence of abnormal autoreactive cellular clones, (3) shared antigens between the host and microorganisms, and (4) defects in helper or suppressor T cell function. A genetic susceptibility is also a likely determinant of autoimmune disease. In nearly all autoimmune diseases, multiple mechanisms of autoimmunity are operative and the exact underlying causes are unknown.

Cell-Mediated Autoimmunity

Certain autoimmune diseases are mediated by T cells that have become specifically immunized to autologous tissues. Cytotoxic or killer T cells generated by this aberrant immune response attack and injure specific organs in the absence of serum autoantibodies.

Diminished suppressor T cell activity results in disordered regulation of immune responses and may promote overactivity of other autoreactive mechanisms. The immune damage in systemic (non-organ-specific) specific diseases such as systemic lupus erythematosus may be in part due to such a mechanism.

Antibody-Mediated Autoimmunity

Several autoimmune diseases have been shown to be caused by autoantibodies in the absence of cell-mediated autoimmunity. The autoimmune hemolytic anemias, idiopathic thrombocytopenia, and Goodpasture's syndrome appear to be mediated solely by autoantibodies directed against autologous cell membrane constituents. In these diseases, antibody attaches to cell membranes, fixes complement, and the ensuing inflammatory reaction severely injures the cells.

The existence of anti-receptor antibodies that compete with or mimic various physiologic agonists for cellular receptors is a specific autoimmune mechanism in several diseases. In Graves' disease, antibodies are present that bind to thyroid cells' TSH receptors and thereby stimulate thyroid hormone production. In rare instances of type I diabetes mellitus, anti-insulin receptor antibodies cause insulin resistance in peripheral target tissues. In contrast, the anti-islet cell antibodies that are usually found in type I diabetes produce insulin deficiency by destroying islet cells in the pancreas. In myasthenia gravis, antibodies to acetylcholine receptors of the myoneural junction block neuromuscular transmission and thereby produce muscle weakness.

Immune Complex Disease

In this group of diseases (systemic lupus erythematosus, rheumatoid arthritis, some drug-induced hemolytic anemias and thrombocytopenias), autologous tissues are injured as innocent bystanders. Autoantibodies are not directed against cellular components of the target organ but rather against autologous or heterologous antigens in the serum. The resultant antigen-antibody complexes bind nonspecifically to autologous membranes (eg, glomerular basement membrane) and fix complement. Fixation and subsequent activation of complement components produce a local inflammatory response that results in tissue injury.

AUTOIMMUNE DISEASES
(See also Chapter 20.)

The diagnosis and treatment of specific autoimmune diseases are described elsewhere in this book. Autoantibodies associated with certain autoimmune diseases may not be implicated in the pathogenesis of tissue injury but are thought instead to be by-products of the injury (eg, autoimmune thyroiditis and antithyroglobulin antibody).

TESTS FOR AUTOANTIBODIES ASSOCIATED WITH AUTOIMMUNE DISEASES

Assays for autoantibodies are similar to those used for detection of antibodies to foreign antigens. Four commonly used methods are discussed below.

Many of the autoantibodies are not specific for a single disease entity (eg, antinuclear antibody, rheumatoid factor). Tests for the latter autoantibodies are best used when the clinical diagnosis is uncertain, in that a negative result makes the diagnosis of certain autoimmune diseases unlikely. For example, a negative antinuclear antibody test makes the diagnosis of systemic lupus erythematosus unlikely, since this antibody is detected in the serum of more than 95% of lupus patients. The disease associations of several autoantibodies are summarized in Table 19–4.

Agglutination of Antigen-Coated Red Blood Cells

Red cells (human, sheep, etc) are incubated with tannic acid or other chemicals so that the cell surface becomes sticky. The red cells are subsequently incubated with purified specific antigen (eg, thyroglobulin), which is adsorbed to the cell surface. The antigen-coated cells are suspended in the patient's serum, and antibody is detected by red cell agglutination. Antigen-coated latex particles are substituted for red cells in the latex fixation tests.

Enzyme-Linked Immunoassays (ELISA)

Antibodies to various tissue antigens can be readily detected by ELISA tests. Extracted and purified antigens are fixed to a plastic microtiter well or beads. Patient's serum is added, and excess proteins are removed by washing and centrifugation. A second antibody coupled to an enzyme (eg, alkaline phosphatase) is added. The enzyme's substrate is then added, and color forms that is measured in a spectrophotometer. This test can also be adapted to antigen detection by placing the antibody on the plastic surface. ELISA assays are very widely applied in clinical laboratory testing.

Immunofluorescence Microscopy

This technique is most frequently used for detection of antinuclear antibody. Frozen sections of mouse liver or other substrates are cut and placed on glass slides. A patient's serum is placed over the sections and washed away. Fluorescein-conjugated rabbit anti-human immunoglobulin is then applied and washed. Antinuclear antibody specifically binds to the nucleus, and the fluorescein conjugate binds to the human antibody. Fluorescence of the cell nucleus observed by fluorescence microscopy indicates a positive test.

Complement Fixation

Specific antigen, unknown serum, and complement are reacted together. Sheep red blood cells coated with anti-sheep cell antibody are subsequently added to the above reaction mixture for 30 minutes at 37 °C. Lysis of sheep cells indicates that complement is present (attaches to sheep cell surface). Lack of lysis indicates that complement has been fixed by the interaction of antibody in the unknown serum with the specific antigen. Lack of lysis is a positive test for the presence of specific antibody.

Table 19–4. Autoantibodies: Associations with connective tissue diseases.[1]

Suspected Disease State	Test	Primary Disease Association (Sensitivity, Specificity)	Other Disease Associations	Comments
CREST[2] syndrome	Anticentromere antibody	CREST (70–90%, high)	Scleroderma (10–15%), Raynaud's disease (10–30%)	Predictive value of a positive test is >95% for scleroderma or related disease (CREST, Raynaud's). Diagnosis of CREST is made clinically.
Systemic lupus erythematosus (SLE)	Antinuclear antibody (ANA)	SLE (>95%, low)	Rheumatoid arthritis (30–50%), discoid lupus, scleroderma (60%), drug-induced lupus (100%), Sjögren's syndrome (80%), miscellaneous inflammatory disorders.	Often used as a screening test; a negative test virtually excludes SLE; a positive test, while nonspecific, increases posttest probability of SLE. Titer does not correlate with disease activity.
	Anti-double-stranded-DNA (anti-ds-DNA)	SLE (60–70%, high)	Lupus nephritis, rarely rheumatoid arthritis, connective tissue disease, usually in low titer.	Predictive value of a positive test is >90% for SLE if present in high titer; a decreasing titer may correlate with worsening renal disease. Titer generally correlates with disease activity.
	Anti-Smith antibody (anti-Sm)	SLE (30–40%, high)		SLE-specific. A positive test substantially increases posttest probability of SLE. Test rarely indicated.
Mixed connective tissue disease (MCTD)	Anti-ribonucleoprotein antibody (RNP)	Scleroderma (20–30%, low), MCTD (95–100%, low)	SLE (30%), Sjögren's syndrome, rheumatoid arthritis (10%), discoid lupus (20–30%).	A negative test essentially excludes MCTD; a positive test in high titer, while nonspecific, increases posttest probability of MCTD.
Rheumatoid arthritis	Rheumatoid factor (RF)	Rheumatoid arthritis (50–90%)	Other rheumatic diseases, chronic infections, some malignancies, some healthy individuals, elderly patients.	Titer does not correlate with disease activity.
Scleroderma	Anti-Scl-70 antibody	Scleroderma (15–20%, low)		Predictive value of a positive test is >95% for scleroderma.
Sjögren's syndrome	Anti-SS-A/Ro antibody	Sjögren's (60–70%, low)	SLE (30–40%), rheumatoid arthritis (10%), subacute cutaneous lupus, vasculitis.	Useful in counseling women of childbearing age with known connective tissue disease, since a positive test is associated with a small but real risk of neonatal SLE and congenital heart block.
Wegener's granulomatosis	Anti-neutrophil cytoplasmic antibody (ANCA)	Wegener's granulomatosis (systemic necrotizing vasculitis) (56–96%, high)	Crescentic glomerulonephritis or other systemic vasculitis (eg, polyarteritis nodosa).	Ability of this assay to reflect disease activity remains unclear.

[1]Modified, with permission, from Harvey AM et al (editors): *The Principles and Practice of Medicine*, 22nd ed. Appleton & Lange, 1988; White RH, Robbins DL: Clinical significance and interpretation of antinuclear antibodies. West J Med 1987;147:210; and Tan EM: Autoantibodies to nuclear antigens (ANA): Their immunobiology and medicine. Adv Immunol 1982,33:167.
[2]CREST = calcinosis, Raynaud's phenomenon, esophageal dysmotility, sclerodactyly, and telangiectasia.

Treatment of Autoimmune Diseases

Therapy of autoimmune diseases involves a variety of approaches. Suppression of production of autoantibodies with corticosteroids and cytotoxic agents is often effective. Anti-inflammatory drugs such as aspirin, NSAIDs, colchicine, and corticosteroids relieve tissue damage from immune complexes. Plasmapheresis to remove offending autoantibodies and circulating immune complexes, when combined with cytotoxic drugs, has been useful in some diseases. All of these modalities are directed at symptoms, since the underlying cause of these disorders remains unknown.

Borland P, Lipstein E: Selection and use of laboratory tests in the rheumatic diseases. Am J Med 1996;100:165.

Ruddy S, Moxley G: Clinical utility of assays for immune complexes and complement. Immunol Allergy Clin North Am 1994;14:387. (Describes assays available for immune complexes and complement; lack of standardization, interassay variation, low sensitivity, and poor correlation with disease activity limit the clinical utility of immune complex assays, but complement assays are well standardized and sensitive to changes in etiology.)

Weigle WO: Immunologic tolerance: Development and disruption. Hosp Pract (Off Ed) Feb 15, 1995;30:81. (Loss of tolerance can lead to autoimmunity. Mechanisms involve changes in antigen presentation, the physical form of the antigen, different T helper subsets, and stimulatory signals involved in B cell differentiation.)

IMMUNOGENETICS & TRANSPLANTATION

GENETIC CONTROL OF THE IMMUNE RESPONSE

The ability to mount a specific immune response is under the direct control of genes closely associated on the same chromosome with the structural genes for the major transplantation antigens. The major transplantation antigens are the cell surface glycoproteins (found on most cells of the body), which elicit the strongest transplantation rejection reaction when tissues are exchanged between two members of a particular species. These molecules function to present antigens to various immunocompetent cells. In humans, this genetic region has been designated the **human leukocyte antigen (HLA)** complex because these antigens were first detected on peripheral blood lymphocytes. The complex includes antigens HLA-A, -B, -C, -DR and others, each with many alleles.

The HLA region has been localized to chromosome 6, and the order of the different HLA loci is shown in Figure 19–1. Most (98%) of the time, the HLA complex is inherited intact as two haplotypes (one from each parent), and within any particular family, therefore, the number of different combinations found will be fairly small (eg, siblings have a 1:4 chance of being HLA-identical). In contrast, the number of antigen combinations among unrelated individuals is huge, resulting in probabilities of fewer than one in several thousand, depending upon the phenotype involved, of finding HLA-compatible individuals in a random donor pool. This is particularly important when compatible donors are needed for allosensitized patients requiring platelet transfusions or organ transplantation. Family members have the highest likelihood of being compatible donors, whereas HLA compatibility between two unrelated individuals has a very low probability. HLA-A and -B typing or cross-matching is utilized for selection of compatible donors for platelet transfusions to allosensitized, thrombocytopenic recipients. Typing for these class I antigens as well as for HLA-DR (class II) antigens is important in determining compatibility for organ transplantation. Typing for HLA markers is of value in studying associations between the HLA system and genetic control of disease susceptibility.

In the genetic region determining the major transplantation antigen complex, there are genes determining the ability to mount a specific immune response. These are called immune response, or Ir, genes. Although the exact mechanism of action of Ir genes is not yet known, it is clear that they affect the

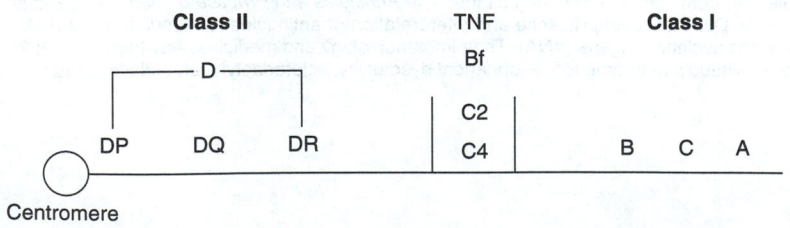

Figure 19–1. Genetic map of the HLA region. The centromere is to the left. (Bf, C2, and C4 are genes for components of the complement system. TNF is the tumor necrosis factor gene.)

ability to recognize foreign antigens and to initiate the development of T and B cell immunity to these antigens. Genes with such a strong effect on specific immune responsiveness might be expected to have major effects on resistance or susceptibility to a wide variety of infectious, neoplastic, and autoimmune diseases.

Polka MS: Histocompatibility antigens: Transplantation and HLA disease associations. Immunol Allergy Clin North Am 1994;14:323. (Reviews genetics, nomenclature, and molecular biology of HLA molecules as well as serologic typing and relevance to transplantation and association with diseases.)

HLA TYPING

The standard method for detecting HLA-A, -B, and -C antigens is that of lymphocyte microcytotoxicity. Lymphocytes isolated from peripheral blood or lymph nodes are added to each well of a typing tray that has been preloaded with sera containing the appropriate cytotoxic alloantibody. When complement is added, cells to which antibody has been specifically bound will have complement activated at the cell surface, resulting in cell death or lysis. It is thus possible to type for all of the known HLA-A, -B, and -C specificities. The vast majority of typing serum samples are obtained from multiparous women since they form antibodies to fetal alloantigens.

Typing for the class II antigens HLA-DR and -DQ is performed similarly. Antigens of the HLA-D, -DR, -DQ, and -DP series are also detected by in vitro cellular reactivity. Lymphocytes of one individual ("responder" cells) will undergo DNA synthesis and proliferation upon encountering lymphocytes from another individual ("stimulator" cells) possessing foreign HLA-DR and -DQ antigens. A responder lacking the stimulator's DR and DQ antigens will respond by brisk DNA synthesis and proliferation that can readily be measured by DNA incorporation of tritiated thymidine. Responders possessing the DR and DQ antigens of the donor will remain nonreactive.

Increasingly, HLA class II typing is being performed by molecular technology. The DNA sequences for the HLA genes and their flanking sequences are known. Selected primers that amplify the gene of interest using the polymerase chain reaction (PCR) technique are known as sequence-specific primers.

Although technically demanding and requiring viable lymphoid cells and experienced laboratories, HLA typing is available at most large medical centers or blood banks.

Colombe BW: Histocompatibility testing. In: *Basic & Clinical Immunology,* 8th ed. Stites DP, Terr AI, Parslow TG (editors). Appleton & Lange, 1994.
Colombe BW: Transplantation immunology: Histocompati-

bility testing and the HLA system in humans. In: *Manual of Allergy and Immunology,* 3rd ed. Lawlor GJ, Fischer TJ, Adelman DC (editors). Little, Brown, 1995.

CLINICAL TRANSPLANTATION

Organ transplants are commonly used in the treatment of many diseases. The main limitations to their more widespread use are the scarcity of donor organs and the expense of these procedures. Failure to achieve completely successful grafts is primarily due to histoincompatibility and lack of totally safe and effective immunosuppressive regimens to halt rejection. Great care in avoiding transmission of infectious agents (eg, HIV, HBV, HCV, CMV) from donor to recipient requires extensive pretransplant serologic testing.

Kidney Transplantation

End-stage renal disease is the indication for kidney transplantation. Kidneys from living related donors who are HLA-identical and also red blood cell ABO-matched have 90% survival at 1 year; less identical grafts and grafts from living unrelated donors have a somewhat lower survival rate. Transplants with matched cadaver kidney donors survive nearly as long, especially if the recipient does not contain antibodies to donor antigens. A positive cross-match by cytotoxicity testing between recipient serum and donor cells is considered a contraindication to that transplant. Donor screening is performed in all cases to avoid transmission of HIV and other infectious agents. Pretreatment of recipients with blood transfusions from the donor appears to extend graft survival even longer. Graft rejection is manifested by diminishing renal function and is treated with immunosuppressive drugs, especially cyclosporine (see below).

Terasaki PI et al: High survival rates of kidney transplants from spousal and living unrelated donors. N Engl J Med 1995;333:333. (Excellent outcomes from use of spousal donors—equal to that of parental donors.)

Heart Transplantation

The indication for heart transplantation is end-stage cardiac disease clearly refractory to medical treatment. Donors and recipients are matched by excluding anti-HLA antibodies in the recipient, since there is rarely time for HLA typing. Rejection is diagnosed by endomyocardial biopsy and treated with immunosuppressants, particularly cyclosporine. Five-year survival is as high as 80% at selected centers.

Sharples LD et al: Risk factors for survival following combined heart-lung transplantation: The first 100 patients. Transplantation 1994;57:218.

Lung Transplantation

Lung transplantation is most often combined with

heart transplantation because of the poorer results achieved with lung grafts alone. Combined heart-lung transplants have a one year survival of approximately 65%, whereas for single lung transplants, survival is approximately 60%.

Jenkinson SG, Levine SM: Lung transplantation. Dis Mon (Jan) 1994;40:1. (Review of history of lung transplants recipient and donor selection, surgical technique, immunosuppression, postoperative care, and complications.)

Liver Transplantation

The major indications for liver transplantation are severe liver dysfunction as manifested by synthetic or regulatory abnormalities which are likely to progress to death within 2 years, and the absence of serious systemic complications of hepatic failure. Children with developmental defects (eg, extrahepatic biliary atresia, inborn errors of metabolism) are typical recipients. The indications for liver transplantation in adults in selected cases include chronic active hepatitis (although the risk of recurrent disease in the graft is substantial), primary biliary cirrhosis, sclerosing cholangitis and inborn errors of metabolism. Recipients are selected on the basis of ABO matching and organ size. HLA typing has not achieved practical results. One-year survival rates range between 70% and 85%.

Keefe EB, Esquivel CO: Controversies in patient selection for liver transplantation. West J Med 1993;159:586. (Discussion of controversies surrounding transplantation for alcoholic liver disease, chronic hepatitis B, and hepatocellular carcinoma. Argues for continued use of transplant in carefully selected patients with these disorders.)

Krom RAF, Kondo M, Moore SB: Liver transplantation and the lymphocytic crossmatch. Transpl Rev 1995;9:207. (Although cross-matching is not routinely performed, a negative result suggests a better prognosis.)

Lidofsky SD: Liver transplantation for fulminant hepatic failure. Gastroenterol Clin North Am 1993;22:257. (Early decision regarding need for transplant and supportive care for complications of liver failure while awaiting transplant are important in improving outcome of patients with fulminant hepatic failure.)

Pancreas & Islet Cell Transplants

Although these procedures currently are largely experimental, the indications are pancreatic insufficiency and, in some cases, diabetes mellitus. These procedures are typically performed at the time of kidney transplantation. Clinical results have improved, with 1-year graft survival at selected centers of up to 80%.

High-Dose Chemotherapy With Hematopoietic Progenitor Cell Transplantation

Transient myelosuppression after cancer chemotherapy is a well-established adverse effect of such treatments. For most regimens commonly utilized, this myelosuppression is rapidly reversible and requires no intervention. Some malignancies (eg, many leukemias, lymphomas, and chemotherapy-sensitive breast and small-cell lung carcinomas) may demonstrate a higher cure rate with higher-dose therapy; however, associated with this approach is an increase in hematologic toxicity. Administering the maximal tolerated chemotherapy dose and thus restoring all hematopoietic functions as rapidly as possible has led to evolution of the concept of hematopoietic progenitor cell (HPC) transplant. HPC transplants have also expanded somewhat into the therapy of certain nonmalignant disorders of hematopoiesis and hematologic function; examples are aplastic anemia, sickle cell anemia, myelodysplasia, and paroxysmal nocturnal hemoglobinuria.

The two sources of HPC are the bone marrow and the peripheral blood. While these pluripotent cells are still incompletely characterized, they comprise less than 0.5–1% of all nucleated bone marrow cells. Until recently, such cells were "harvested" by repeated aspirations of the bone marrow, filtered, cryopreserved, and administered usually within a day after completion of the chemotherapy regimen. Recently, it has become common practice to harvest the HPC from the peripheral blood by apheresis. As the peripheral blood has approximately one-fortieth the number of circulating HPC as the bone marrow, these cells must be "mobilized" by the administration of cytotoxic chemotherapy (with the harvest being performed during the recovery phase), or the administration of hematopoietic growth factors such as granulocyte colony stimulating factor (G-CSF; filgrastim) or granulocyte-monocyte colony stimulating factor (GM-CSF; sargramostim). As before, the cells are frozen and administered at a later date.

Because syngeneic (twin to twin) transplants are rare, the two predominant transplants are autologous, where the HPCs are harvested from and returned to the patient; or allogeneic, where the source is an HLA-matched donor, ideally a sibling. The goals of the two procedures—and their associated adverse effects—are frequently different. Allogeneic transplants are most commonly offered to patients with malignant and nonmalignant disorders involving the bone marrow. Chemotherapy is given to ablate the marrow, resulting in maximal suppression or eradication of the recipient's native immune system and replacement by donor cells that contain not only HPCs but also functional donor T lymphocytes. These T cells can cause subsequent development of graft-versus-host disease, in which the recipient's tissues are recognized as nonself. While this is occasionally desirable, as in the "graft-versus-leukemia" effect, it is the cause of considerable morbidity and can be fatal. There are two separate phases of graft-versus-host disease: acute disease, secondary to cytokine-mediated cytotoxicity against the cells of the liver, the mucosa of the gastrointestinal tract, and skin; and chronic disease, characterized by fibrosis and collagen deposition and resembling autoimmune disease such as scleroderma. The incidence of graft-versus-host disease can be decreased by depleting the donor marrow of T cells, but this is associated with a higher incidence of graft failure and, in the case of leukemia, a higher relapse rate. Though only a few allogeneic peripheral HPC transplants have been reported, graft-versus-host disease in such cases does not appear to be as severe, though experience is still very limited.

Autologous HPC transplants are performed solely for the treatment of malignancies. In these cases the chemotherapy is intensively myelosuppressive though not necessarily myeloablative. One prominent exception is patients with chronic myelogenous leukemia in the accelerated phase or "blast crisis," who receive their autologous HPC in an effort to return their disease to the chronic phase. Since patients usually have some residual immune function and are receiving their own HPC—and thus do not require posttransplant immunosuppression—the risk of opportunistic infections and immunosuppression-related neoplasia is markedly reduced.

The success rates of HPC transplantation depend mostly upon the underlying disease and the associated risk of relapse (in cases of leukemia), the level of matching between donor and recipient, and thus the likelihood of graft-versus-host disease, the age of the recipient (over age 30, the incidence increases), and the complications associated with conditioning (veno-occlusive liver disease and infection). Overall, the success rates are about 60–70% in aplastic anemia, 40–75% survival at 1 year in various forms of leukemia and other neoplasms such as non-Hodgkin's lymphomas and breast carcinomas. Success rates are extremely variable in immunologic deficiency diseases.

Other Organs & Tissues

Transplantation of other organs or tissues (ie, skin, cornea, bone, and heart valves) is now a routine surgical procedure. Much further research remains to be done on transplantation of other organs, particularly neural tissue.

Chandler C, Passaro E Jr: Transplant rejection: Mechanisms and treatment. Arch Surg 1993;128:279. (Review of cellular and molecular events involved in organ transplantation rejection. Covers current and possible future therapies.)

Kerman RH: Relevance of histocompatibility testing in clinical transplantation. Surg Clin North Am 1994; 74:1015. (Effect of HLA matching and cross-matching on graft survival is often center-dependent as well as dependent on immunosuppressive regimen given.)

Stadtmauer EA, Schneider CJ, Silberstein LE: Peripheral blood progenitor cell generation and harvesting. Semin Oncol 1995;22:291. (Review of the current practice of HPC harvest techniques and outcomes.)

Takemoto S et al: Survival of nationally shared, HLA-matched kidney transplants from cadaveric donor. The UNOS Scientific Renal Transplant Registry. N Engl J Med 1992;327:834. (Report of a prospective trial from all US transplantation centers on nationwide shipment of cadaveric organs to HLA-A, -B, and -DR matched recipients.)

MECHANISM OF ACTION OF IMMUNOSUPPRESSIVE DRUGS

Despite advances in tissue type techniques and donor-recipient matching, allograft rejection remains a central issue in the management of organ transplant recipients. Clear understanding of the underlying cellular and molecular events involved in graft rejection will improve the selection of specific immunosuppressive therapies, which in turn will lead to prolongation of graft survival and minimization of adverse side effects. The most frequently used immunosuppressor drugs and their modes of action are briefly summarized below. Many new drugs with potent immunosuppressive actions and reduced toxicities are under development and in clinical trials.

Corticosteroids

This group of drugs has potent anti-inflammatory and direct effects on immunocompetent cells. Corticosteroids inhibit cell-mediated immune responses more severely than antibody responses. T helper cells are preferentially reduced owing to redistribution. Neutrophils are increased owing to demargination and bone marrow release. Monocytes and eosinophils are reduced. These cellular changes result in reduced inflammatory responses. Disruption of the interaction between T cells and macrophages appears to be an important mechanism, and corticosteroids have been shown to block the activation of T cells by interleukin-1 (IL-1) derived from macrophages. In addition, corticosteroids inhibit the expression of class II histocompatibility antigens on the macrophage surface, thereby interfering with presentation of antigen to T cells.

Cytotoxic Drugs

The most frequently used cytotoxic drugs are azathioprine and cyclophosphamide. Azathioprine is a structural analogue of mercaptopurine, an antagonist of purine synthesis. Azathioprine is a phase-specific drug that kills rapidly replicating cells. It inhibits proliferation of both T and B cells as well as macrophages. Cyclophosphamide is an alkylating agent that damages cells by cross-linking DNA. Although this cycle-specific drug is most effective in killing cells going through the mitotic cycle, it can also cause intermitotic cell injury and death. Cyclophosphamide can inhibit both T and B cell immunity as well as inflammation. Azathioprine and cyclophosphamide are effective inhibitors of the production of serum antibodies.

Antimetabolites

The most commonly used antimetabolite is methotrexate, an inhibitor of folic acid synthesis. Methotrexate inhibits rapidly proliferating cells in S phase and suppresses both cell-mediated and humoral immunity as well as inflammation. Without immunosuppression, the incidence of graft-versus-host disease after allogeneic HPC transplant is almost 100%; this can be reduced to 20–30% when these two drugs are given in combination. Cyclosporine prevents T cell activation, while methotrexate inhibits the function of T cells that are already activated.

Cyclosporine

This cyclic polypeptide derived from a fungus has been used recently as an immunosuppressive drug in organ transplant recipients. Cyclosporine interferes with the secretion of interleukin-2 (IL-2) by T lymphocytes. Since IL-2 is necessary for T cell replication, this drug is a potent inhibitor of T cell proliferation and thereby inhibits T cell-mediated immune responses. Little effect has been shown on direct B cell immune responses or on inflammation. Its toxic effects are primarily on renal and hepatic function. In addition to methotrexate, methylprednisolone has also been utilized with cyclosporine to treat graft-versus-host disease, though T cell-directed immunotoxins have not proved to be of any benefit.

Tacrolimus (FK506)

This drug was developed for use in transplantation and is a macrolide with potent anti-T cell properties and a mode of action similar to that of cyclosporine. Like cyclosporine, tacrolimus inhibits IL-2 and interferon-γ production and T cell activation. It has been approved for use in liver transplantation. Both cyclosporine and tacrolimus block the intracellular pathway of calcineurin dephosphorylation of nuclear transcription factors. Clinical trials are under way in kidney, liver, and heart transplantation.

Tacrolimus is approximately ten times more potent than cyclosporine. While rates of graft-versus-host disease are lower for tacrolimus-based regimens when compared with cyclosporine-based regimens, it remains to be determined by ongoing randomized trials if either drug is truly superior to the other.

Mycophenolate Mofetil

Mycophenolate mofetil was approved in 1995 for use in kidney transplantation. By blocking lymphocyte production of guanine nucleotides, it inhibits T and B lymphocyte proliferation. Its use in combination with cyclosporine has led to a lower incidence of acute graft rejection.

Anderlini P, Przepiorka D: Allogeneic marrow transplantation. In: *Medical Oncology: A Comprehensive Review,* 2nd ed. Pazdur R (editor). PRR, 1995. (Experience at one large cancer center and a review of the literature.)

Sollinger HW: Mycophenolate mofetil for the prevention of acute rejection in primary cadaveric renal allograft recipients. Transplantation 1995;60:225. (The incidence of acute rejection was reduced from 47% to 31% during the first 6 months after grafting.)

Thomson AW, Forrester SV: Therapeutic advances in immunosuppression. Clin Exp Immunol 1994;98:351. (Discussion of new agents being investigated for transplantation, autoimmune disease, and asthma.)

U.S. Multicenter FK506 Liver Study Group: A comparison of tacrolimus (FK 506) and cyclosporine for immunosuppression in liver transplantation. N Engl J Med 1994;331:1110. (Open-label randomized trial comparing two drugs at 1-year posttransplant. There were no significant differences in patient or graft survival. Tacrolimus was associated with lower rates of acute, corticosteroid-resistant, or refractory rejection but substantially more adverse events, especially neurotoxicity and nephrotoxicity, requiring discontinuation of the drug.)

Wallemacq PE, Reding R: FK 506 (tacrolimus), a novel immunosuppressant in organ transplantation: Clinical, biomedical, and analytical aspects. Clin Chem 1993;39:2219.

Winkelstein A: Immunosuppressive therapy. In: *Basic & Clinical Immunology,* 8th ed. Stites DP, Terr AI, Parslow TG (editors). Appleton & Lange, 1994.

ASSOCIATIONS BETWEEN HLA ANTIGENS & SPECIFIC DISEASES

In humans, very striking associations are observed between particular HLA antigens and specific diseases. These facts are important in relating HLA to diseases: HLA antigen frequencies vary substantially among different ethnic groups, and therefore control populations must be carefully selected. Appropriate statistical corrections must be made to compensate for the large number of antigens tested. Accurate clinical definition of disease is necessary to avoid diluting an HLA-disease association by mixing together diseases that are pathogenetically different but clinically similar. If the disease studied has a fatal outcome, then the proper disease phase must be selected to demonstrate associations. Some quantitative measure of strength of association is necessary to compare different HLA-disease relationships.

Table 19–5 is a partial list of HLA-disease associations. Studies have revealed that the strongest association is between HLA-B27 and ankylosing spondylitis, which holds in all ethnic groups but is more striking in Japanese people than in Caucasians studied. Other spondyloarthropathies (eg, Reiter's syndrome, arthritis following *Salmonella* or *Yersinia*

Table 19–5. HLA and disease associations.

Disease	Antigen	Frequency		Relative Risk
		Patients (%)	Controls (%)	
Ankylosing spondylitis				
Caucasians	B27	89	4–13	69
Japanese	B27	85	<1	207
Reiter's disease	B27	80	9	37
Salmonella arthritis	B27	60–92	8–14	30
Rheumatoid arthritis	DR4	68	25	3.8
Psoriasis vulgaris	Cw6	27	4	8.5
Graves' disease				
Caucasians	Dw3	56	25	3.7
Japanese	Dw12	48	16	5
Diabetes mellitus		DR3 heterozygotes		3
Diabetes mellitus		DR4 heterozygotes		3.6
Diabetes mellitus		DR3/DR4 heterozygotes		33
Acute lymphocytic leukemia	A2	83	44	6
Systemic lupus erythematosus	DR4	73	33	5
Narcolepsy	DR2	100	34	358

infection) are also strongly associated with B27, suggesting that despite apparently different causes the pathogeneses of these diseases share some common factor related to the B27 marker. B27 is not specific for all arthritis; eg, rheumatoid arthritis associates not with that antigen but with DR4. Furthermore, disease associations are not restricted to B and DR: eg, psoriasis vulgaris is associated with a C locus antigen and acute lymphocytic leukemia with an A locus antigen. In diabetes mellitus, heterozygote individuals possess both the DR3 and the DR4 antigens and have a relative risk of 33, far greater than expected by simple addition of risks for DR3 plus DR4. It also appears that a single mechanism may associate with different antigens in different ethnic groups. Among Caucasians studied in whom the Dw12 antigen is almost absent, Dw3 is associated with Graves' disease. Among Japanese people where Dw3 is almost completely lacking, Dw12 is associated with Graves' disease.

Sometimes combinations of antigens exhibit disease associations. This suggests either interaction among different genes affecting susceptibility or unusual linkage between the known HLA genes and some nearby gene actually responsible for the disease susceptibility.

Felttkamp TE, Khan MA, Lopez de Castro JA: The pathogenetic role of HLA-B27. Immunol Today 1996;17:5.

Paul WE, Fathman CG, Metzger H (editors): *Annual Review of Immunology,* 1984–present. (Annual entire issue.)

ALLERGIC DISEASES

Allergy is defined as an immunologically (IgE antibody) mediated reaction to a foreign antigen (allergen), causing tissue inflammation and organ dysfunction. It may be local or systemic. Because the allergen is foreign (ie, environmental), the skin and respiratory tract are the organs most frequently involved in allergic disease. Allergic reactions may also localize to the vasculature, gastrointestinal tract, or other visceral organs. Anaphylaxis is the most extreme form of systemic allergy.

CLASSIFICATION

Hypersensitivity diseases can be classified according to (1) the immunologic mechanism involved in pathogenesis, (2) the organ system affected, and (3) the nature and source of the allergen. An immunologic classification is preferred, because it serves as a rational basis for diagnosis and treatment.

Immunologic Mechanisms

The two major pathways of immunologically induced inflammation involve the reaction of the antigen with T cells and with B cell products (antibodies). Of the five immunoglobulin classes of antibodies, only three, IgG, IgM, and IgE, are known to be involved in hypersensitivity reactions. Classification of the hypersensitivity disorders helps elucidate the underlying pathogenic mechanism of clinical symptoms. A common classification of the hypersensitivity diseases is as follows: type I, IgE-mediated reactions (eg, allergic rhinitis, asthma, anaphylaxis); type II, antibody-antigen-mediated hypersensitivity reactions (eg, hemolytic anemia or Rh hemolytic disease); type III, antigen-antibody complex-mediated hypersensitivity (eg, serum sickness and Arthus reactions); and type IV, mediated by helper T lymphocytes, not by antibodies (eg, contact dermatitis, tuberculin reactions).

A. Type I, or IgE-Mediated (Immediate) Hypersensitivity: IgE antibodies occupy receptor sites on mast cells. Within minutes after exposure to the allergen, vasoactive and inflammatory mediators are activated and released from the mast cell, causing vasodilation, visceral smooth muscle contraction, and mucus secretory gland stimulation. Other mediators induce a late-phase inflammatory response that appears several hours later. There are two clinical subgroups of IgE-mediated allergy: atopy and anaphylaxis.

1. Atopy–The term atopy denotes a group of diseases (allergic rhinitis, allergic asthma, atopic dermatitis, and allergic gastroenteropathy) that occur in certain persons with an inherited tendency to develop IgE antibodies to multiple common organic environmental allergens. The reaction is localized to a susceptible target organ, but more than one of these diseases may occur in an allergic individual. There is a strong familial tendency.

2. Anaphylaxis–Certain allergens, especially drugs, insect venom, and foods, may induce an IgE antibody response that causes a generalized release of mediators from mast cells, resulting in systemic anaphylaxis. This is characterized by (1) hypotension or shock from widespread vasodilation, (2) bronchospasm, (3) gastrointestinal and uterine muscle contraction, and (4) urticaria or angioedema (see Chapter 6). The condition is potentially fatal. Unlike atopy, anaphylactic sensitivities are rarely multiple. The condition affects both nonatopic and atopic persons. Urticaria and angioedema are cutaneous forms of anaphylaxis and are much more common. Like anaphylaxis, they are usually caused by a drug, food, or insect venom. These disorders are generally benign unless extensive enough to cause hypotension or unless angioedema obstructs the larynx or hypopharynx, causing respiratory obstruction.

B. Type II, Antibody-Mediated (Cytotoxic) Hypersensitivity: Cytotoxic reactions involve the specific reaction of either IgG or IgM antibody to cell-bound antigens. This results in activation of the complement cascade and the destruction of the cell to which the antigen is bound. Examples of tissue injury by this mechanism include immune hemolytic anemia and Rh hemolytic disease in the newborn.

C. Type III, Immune Complex-Mediated Hypersensitivity: Antibodies of the IgG or IgM isotype can form complexes with the allergen and thereby activate complement to generate mediators of inflammation. Under conditions of similar concentrations of both allergen and antibody, the clinical manifestations of disease include the Arthus reaction, a localized cutaneous and subcutaneous inflammatory response to injected allergen, and serum sickness, a systemic disease characterized by fever, arthralgias, and dermatitis.

D. Type IV, T Cell-Mediated Hypersensitivity (Delayed Hypersensitivity, Cell-Mediated Hypersensitivity): The most common expression of T cell-mediated allergy is allergic contact dermatitis (see Chapter 6), in which the allergen causes dermal inflammation on direct contact with the skin. The reaction occurs after a latent period of 1–2 days from the time of contact. Hypersensitivity pneumonitis (extrinsic allergic alveolitis) is a pulmonary T cell-mediated hypersensitivity disease.

Organ System

Patients present to the physician with symptoms and physical findings that may be either localized or generalized. Knowledge of the organs involved may help to determine the type of allergy and the nature of the allergen (see Table 19–6).

Allergens & Antigens

Although any exogenous (environmental) material can theoretically be allergenic, certain antigens are encountered more frequently than are others. It is convenient to classify them by route of exposure.

A. Inhalants: Pollens, mold spores, animal products (danders, saliva, urine), house dust, and insect and arthropod emanations (especially the house dust mite) are the usual allergens that cause atopic disease. The house dust mite (*Dermatophagoides* species) may be the most prevalent allergen for atopic allergy worldwide. Hypersensitivity pneumonitis (see Chapter 9) can be caused by many airborne organic dusts, microorganisms, some organic chemicals, and by some drugs such as minocycline. Occasionally, allergens causing contact dermatitis may reach the skin via atmospheric fumes. Immunologic analysis of bronchoalveolar lymphocytes from patients with drug-induced hypersensitivity pneumonitis suggests a central role for T lymphocytes in the pathogenesis of this disease.

B. Ingestants: Foods cause allergic gastroenteropathy and may cause atopic dermatitis, asthma, anaphylaxis, and urticaria or angioedema. Allergic reactions to drugs are most commonly urticaria and anaphylaxis. Drug-induced nonurticarial dermatitis or fixed drug eruptions are suspected to be allergic in origin, though the immunologic mechanism is uncertain. Serum sickness is classically caused by injected foreign protein (eg, antilymphocyte globulin), but

Table 19–6. Allergic diseases classified according to the involved organ or tissue.

Organ or Tissue	Disease	Mechanism			
		T Cell	IgE	Immune Complex	Uncertain
Skin	Allergic contact dermatitis	•			
	Atopic dermatitis		•		
	Urticaria and angioedema		•		
	Arthus reaction			•	
	Generalized drug eruption				•
	Fixed drug eruption				•
Upper respiratory tract	Allergic rhinitis		•		
Bronchi	Asthma		•		
	Allergic bronchopulmonary aspergillosis		•	•	
Alveoli	Hypersensitivity pneumonitis				
	Acute			•	
	Chronic	•			
Eyes	Allergic conjunctivitis		•		
Gastrointestinal tract	Allergic gastroenteropathy		•		
Liver	Hepatic drug reaction				•
Kidney	Allergic interstitial nephritis				•
Systemic	Anaphylaxis		•		
	Serum sickness			•	

mild reactions may occur after oral administration of drugs such as penicillin.

C. Injectants: Drugs, Hymenoptera venom, and injected atopic allergens account for most cases of anaphylaxis and acute urticaria or angioedema.

D. Contactants: Plant oils, cosmetics and perfumes, nickel in jewelry or on buckles and undergarment fasteners, hair dyes, topical medications including their additives, and occupational chemicals are the most common causes of T cell–mediated (type IV) contact dermatitis.

Occasionally, urticaria or anaphylaxis may be induced by direct skin contact with the allergen. The number of cases of anaphylaxis and urticaria from contact with gloves, catheters, dental dams, and other medical devices has increased dramatically. These disorders are caused by allergy to a protein in the latex and affect both patients and health care workers.

Kaliner MA: How the current understanding of the pathophysiology of asthma influences our approach to therapy. J Allergy Clin Immunol 1993;92(1 Part 2):144. (Critique of role of immunotherapy in allergic asthma.)

Klau MV, Wieselthier JS: Contact dermatitis. Am Fam Physician 1993;48:629. (Types include allergic contact dermatitis, irritant contact dermatitis, contact photodermatitis, and contact urticaria. Diagnosis made by localization of eruption and history of exposure to offending agent.)

Marks DR, Marks LM: Food allergy. Manifestations, evaluation, and management. Postgrad Med 1993;93:191. (More common in children than adults. Workup may include skin testing and double-blind oral food challenge in addition to history and physical. Avoidance of offending agent is most important feature of treatment.)

Reisman RE: Insect stings. N Engl J Med 1994;331:523. (Discusses pathogenesis, diagnosis, and treatment. Venom immunotherapy is effective in decreasing risk of anaphylactic reactions in people at risk to 2% after 3 years of therapy.)

Sussman GL, Beezhold DH: Allergy to latex rubber. Ann Intern Med 1995;122:43. (Prevalence in health care workers about 7–10%. Can be manifested as irritant contact dermatitis, allergic contact dermatitis, and, less commonly, as type I allergic responses. Algorithm for diagnosis and treatment presented.)

DIAGNOSIS

The clinical manifestations of allergy can also occur in the absence of an immunologic mechanism. For example, nonallergic (intrinsic) asthma is triggered by the nonimmunologic effect of inhaled dusts and fumes, weather changes, stress, etc; irritant contact dermatitis is the result of physical or chemical damage to the skin; and anaphylactoid reactions are produced nonimmunologically by iodinated contrast media, by certain drugs, and by physical exercise. Therefore, the diagnosis of allergy requires answers to the following questions: (1) What is the nature of the disease? (2) Is the disease caused by allergy? (3) What specific allergens (one or several) are responsible?

The history must include a survey of allergens associated with home, work, hobbies, and habits as well as medications. Physical examination is most useful if performed during a period of allergen exposure. Imaging studies may be necessary to supplement the physical examination. In some cases, physiologic testing such as pulmonary function tests is required to establish the diagnosis.

Tests of Specific Immune Responses

Allergy tests reveal an immune response to a particular allergen. A positive test result must be correlated with the history before one can conclude that the allergen caused the illness. The type of immune response must be consistent with the nature of the disease, for example, IgE antibody causes allergic rhinitis but not allergic contact dermatitis.

A. IgE Antibody Tests: IgE antibodies are detected by in vivo (skin tests) or in vitro methods.

1. Skin tests–Epicutaneous or cutaneous allergen testing produces a localized pruritic wheal and erythema which is maximal at 15–20 minutes. It is used most commonly in the diagnosis of allergic respiratory disease (rhinitis and asthma). Patients with symptoms of pruritus, congestion, or paroxysms of sneezing as well as chronic cough or chest tightness should be considered reasonable candidates for allergy skin testing. Standard sets of allergen extracts are available commercially for pollens, fungi, animal danders, dust, and dust mites. The pollen and mold allergens must be appropriate to the patient's geographic area.

To avoid a systemic reaction, most allergists perform epicutaneous (prick) testing first, followed by selected intradermal tests to allergens that were negative by prick testing. Special allergenic extracts can be prepared for other allergens where indicated. Skin testing for food allergy is appropriate only if the patient has symptoms consistent with IgE-mediated allergy within 2 hours after eating the suspect food.

Skin testing for allergy to drugs is reliable for protein drugs (eg, heterologous serum, insulin) but not for haptenic drugs (low-molecular-weight organic compounds). An important exception is penicillin skin testing, which is highly predictive of anaphylactic allergy in patients allergic to this drug. The combination of skin testing with the major and minor metabolic determinants of penicillin (the minor determinants are not available commercially, though they may be synthesized and are often available at specialized centers) and assessment of the severity and type of previous penicillin allergic reaction may allow the designation of patients into high and low risk groups for subsequent reactions. The negative predictive value of skin tests for IgE-mediated reactions to subsequently administered penicillin is good. Few data are available for determining the cross-reactivity between the cephalosporin antibiotics and penicillins. There appears to be no allergic cross-reactivity between the monobactam antibiotics (aztreonam) and the penicillins and no adverse reactions have been reported in patients with true IgE-mediated penicillin reactions administered a monobactam

antibiotic. A high degree of cross-reactivity exists between the penicillin and the carbapenem, imipenem, so this drug should be given to the penicillin-allergic patient with the same degree of caution as if the patient were to receive penicillin.

Some drugs, notably opiates, cause nonimmunologic release of mast cell mediators and thereby give universal wheal-and-erythema reactions. A negative diluent control test is essential. A positive control with histamine or a histamine liberator, such as morphine, is desirable.

Skin testing is preferred to in vitro methods (discussed below) because it detects the presence of IgE antibody in tissue and shows biologic activity. It is convenient, inexpensive, and provides an immediate result. Any drug with antihistamine effect must be withdrawn prior to testing. Extensive active dermatitis may limit the availability of skin for testing. There is an exceedingly small risk of inducing a systemic reaction when skin testing is conducted properly. Skin testing for anaphylactic reactions to Hymenoptera venom or a drug is performed by serial titration, starting with appropriately diluted solutions to avoid a systemic reaction. Some physicians use serial titration of inhalant allergens in testing for atopic diseases.

2. In vitro tests of IgE antibody–IgE antibodies can be detected in serum by radioallergosorbent test (RAST) or enzyme-linked immunosorbent assay (ELISA). Protein allergens are covalently linked to the immunosorbent. Haptenic allergens must first be coupled to a nonallergenic protein carrier such as human serum albumin, which is then linked to the immunosorbent. Many of the usual atopic allergens are available commercially for RAST or ELISA testing.

In vitro tests detect allergen-specific antibody in serum. Since IgE-mediated allergy is caused by IgE antibodies bound to mast cells (not by circulating IgE), in vitro tests generally are less sensitive than skin tests for diagnostic use. They are not affected by antihistamine therapy, but they can give false-positive results in patients with high total serum IgE and false-negative results in patients treated with immunotherapy who have significant allergen-specific IgG antibodies. There is no risk of a systemic reaction. The test is significantly more expensive than skin testing, and results are not immediately available. The RAST or ELISA method is particularly useful for detecting IgE antibodies to certain occupational chemicals or potentially toxic allergens.

The total IgE level in serum is higher on average in atopic patients than it is in nonatopic individuals. There is considerable overlap, so that it is not a satisfactory diagnostic test for atopy.

B. Tests for Immune Complex Allergic Diseases: The IgG antibody may be present in sufficient quantity in serum to be detected by the precipitin-in-gel method. ELISA will detect antibodies present in lesser amounts. Reduced serum levels of

C3, C4, or CH50 may be sought as evidence of complement activation.

C. Tests for T Cell-Mediated Hypersensitivity: Cell-mediated immunity or hypersensitivity is detected by intradermal (tuberculin-type) skin tests which elicit 48-hour inflammatory induration or by patch testing in the diagnosis of allergic contact dermatitis. The patch test is performed by topical application of the suspected contactant allergen. A positive test at 48–72 hours consists of erythema, swelling, and papules. Concentrations of allergens for patch testing must be screened in nonallergic subjects to avoid false-positive irritant responses.

Cell-mediated hypersensitivity can be detected in vitro by exposing peripheral blood mononuclear cells to allergen to detect the release of cytokines or inhibition of cell migration, but such tests are rarely useful for diagnosis.

Provocation Tests

Occasionally, direct allergen challenge of the target organ or tissue under controlled conditions is required for definitive diagnosis. Such challenges may be bronchial, nasal, conjunctival, oral, or cutaneous. A positive test confirms that the reaction can be caused by the test substance, but it does not prove that an immunologic mechanism is responsible.

A. Bronchoprovocation Testing: An aerosolized solution of the allergen is delivered by inhalation through a dosimeter in graded increasing dosages. The response in FEV_1 or FEV_1/FVC is measured by spirometry, and the provoking dose (PD_{20}) producing a 20% fall in FEV_1 is determined. This test should be done in a facility where the patient can be monitored for 6–24 hours after allergen inhalation because of the possibility of a late-phase response. Bronchoprovocation is not necessary in the routine diagnosis of allergic asthma, but it may be helpful in some cases of occupational asthma.

Natural provocation field testing can be done by having the patient make serial determinations of peak expiratory flow rate (PEFR) using a portable peak flowmeter during periods of natural exposure to a suspected airborne allergen.

Bronchial provocation with exercise or with inhalation of methacholine, histamine, or cold air documents the nonspecific bronchial hyperirritability of asthma. These procedures do not detect allergic sensitivities.

B. Nasal Provocation Testing: This procedure is similar to bronchial provocation except that the allergen is inhaled through the nose and changes in nasal airway resistance or symptoms are measured. The procedure is complicated by significant excursions of nasal airway resistance that occur normally.

C. Conjunctival Provocation: A drop of allergen extract is instilled into one conjunctival sac. An allergic reaction produces itching, conjunctival injec-

tion, swelling, and tearing within minutes. The control contralateral eye is not affected. The method is unpleasant and therefore rarely used.

D. Oral Provocation: In most cases of suspected allergy to a food or drug, double-blind placebo-controlled oral challenge is the definitive test. For a positive test, the reported clinical findings must be reproduced. Freeze-dried foods in large opaque capsules provide a sufficient dose of allergen for testing. It should not be done in patients with suspected food-induced anaphylaxis.

Kishiyama JL, Adelman DC: The cross reactivity and immunology of beta-lactam antibiotics. Drug Saf 1994;10:318.

Kniker WT: Multi-test skin testing in allergy: A review of published findings. Ann Allergy 1993;71:485. (Reliable, convenient method for skin testing for diagnosis of allergic sensitization with high sensitivity and good reproducibility. Also correlates with in vitro testing.)

Muller BA et al: Comparisons of specific and nonspecific bronchoprovocation in subjects with asthma, rhinitis and healthy subjects. J Allergy Clin Immunol 1993;91:758. (Update on definitive diagnostic procedure in allergic asthma diagnosis.)

Smith TF: Allergy testing in clinical practice. Ann Allergy 1992;68:293. (Discussion of principles of allergy testing and available in vivo and in vitro tests.)

Sogn DD et al: Results of the National Institute of Allergy and Infectious Diseases Collaborative Clinical Trial to test the predictive value of skin testing with major and minor penicillin derivatives in hospitalized adults. Arch Intern Med 1992;152:1025. (Negative skin tests have good negative predictive value for penicillin allergy, while positive skin tests to both major and minor derivatives have high positive predictive value for penicillin reactions.)

MANAGEMENT

Allergic disease management requires both symptomatic therapy and allergen-specific treatment. General measures for treating each of the diseases are presented elsewhere in this book. This section will discuss only the management of the allergic causes.

The three basic principles of allergy management are (1) avoidance of the allergen, (2) symptomatic therapy, and (3) immunotherapy.

Avoidance Therapy

Avoidance is the most effective treatment for any allergic condition, and it should always be considered in addition to pharmacologic and immunologic treatment. Avoidance of allergen exposure cures the specific problem, but it may or may not reduce the underlying immunologic sensitivity to that allergen. Success requires accurate diagnosis of the causative allergens in each case.

A. Pollens: Remaining in air-conditioned environments avoids exposure to pollens but is impractical.

B. Animal Danders: If the allergy is slight, the patient may benefit from merely keeping the animal out of the bedroom; usually, however, it is necessary to remove the animal from the home altogether. Washing or otherwise treating the fur of a live animal has not been proved to reduce allergenicity.

C. House Dust and Dust Mites: The mattress and pillows should be encased in dust-proof material, and the bedroom floor should be uncarpeted. The room should be dusted frequently. Electronic air purifiers are of unproved effectiveness. Acaricides to eliminate dust mites are under investigation.

D. Mold Spores: Out of doors, mold spores are unavoidable. Indoor mold contamination can be controlled by repairing leaks and cleaning mold buildup on sinks, shower curtains, pipes, etc.

E. Insect Stings: Sensitive patients should not walk barefoot outdoors, because yellow jackets nest in the ground. Garbage cans should be well covered, and affected individuals should avoid outdoor eating.

F. Drugs: It is necessary to avoid all cross-reacting drugs. Allergy to penicillin or to sulfonamides often encompasses most if not all penicillin or sulfonamide derivatives, respectively. Rarely, a patient exquisitely sensitive to penicillin may react to penicillin in milk products.

G. Foods: Most persons with well-documented food allergy are allergic to one or a small number of foods. Persons with peanut anaphylaxis can have a fatal reaction to ingestion of a minute amount of the food. The presence of peanut proteins can be unsuspected in some foods, so that the patient must be vigilant in restaurants or at parties. Soy-based formulas are available for infants with milk allergy.

H. Contactants: Patients with poison ivy, poison oak, or other plant oil allergy must learn to identify the plant. In California, poison oak allergen is often transmitted to human skin by pets. Nickel-containing jewelry, buckles, etc., can be coated with clear nail polish. Protective clothing and gloves may be necessary for occupational contact dermatitis.

Drug Therapy

Pharmacotherapy of the immune response to reduce the allergic manifestations is achieved with drugs that inhibit inflammation.

A. IgE-Mediated Allergy: Three classes of drugs are useful for IgE-mediated diseases, based on (1) inhibition of release of mediators from mast cells, (2) inhibition of the action of mediators on their target cells, and (3) reversal of the vascular and inflammatory responses in the target tissues.

1. Cromolyn–Pretreatment with this drug prevents the response to allergen by stabilizing the mast cell, though the specific molecular mechanism of action is unknown. Cromolyn is effective only when applied directly to the involved organ, and its action is short-lived. It is available as a bronchial inhaler or a nasal spray. It is administered four times daily on a continuous maintenance schedule as long as there is exposure to the allergen. Not all patients respond, but the drug has very few side effects and a wide margin of safety. A high-dose oral form of the drug has been released for use in treating systemic mastocytosis, but its effectiveness in preventing food-induced allergic gastroenteropathy is not known. A new cromolyn-like drug, nedocromil, has been released for clinical use in asthma.

2. Antimediator drugs–Of the numerous mediators released from mast cells by reaction of allergen with IgE antibody, histamine is the only one that can be effectively blocked by drugs currently available. Antihistamine drugs are competitive inhibitors for the histamine receptors. Those that inhibit H_1 receptors are used to treat IgE-mediated allergy. There are a number of such drugs on the market (Table 19–7), but their use is limited by side effects, primarily sedation and dryness. Rare complications are convulsions and tachyarrhythmias. Terfenadine and astemizole are nonsedating and have prolonged action. Rare complications of antihistamine overdosage, especially for those two drugs, are ventricular tachyarrhythmias and QT interval prolongation. Concomitant use of ketoconazole or macrolide antibiotics (erythromycin) with terfenadine or astemizole may cause QT prolongation, torsades de pointes, other ventricular arrhythmias, cardiac arrest and death. A new nonsedating histamine H_1 receptor-blocking drug, loratidine, appears not to be associated with arrhythmias.

Antihistamine therapy is helpful in allergic rhinitis and in urticaria but not in all patients. It does not alleviate asthma, though it is not contraindicated when used to treat concomitant rhinitis or pruritus. The antipruritic effect of antihistamines may be a useful adjunct in treatment of eczematous diseases. Intramuscular or intravenous antihistamines are used in systemic anaphylaxis as adjunctive treatment only. They relieve cutaneous and gastrointestinal symptoms but have no effect on vascular collapse or airway obstruction.

3. Sympathomimetic drugs–Adrenergic agonists are used for both α-adrenergic (vasoconstricting) and β-adrenergic (bronchodilating) properties. Injected epinephrine is initial therapy in anaphylaxis, because it has both effects and acts rapidly. Alpha-adrenergic agonists are used orally as nasal decongestants and conjunctivally as vasoconstrictors in allergic rhinitis and conjunctivitis, respectively. Beta-adrenergic drugs are primarily used for reversal of acute asthma, and they can be given by aerosol, by metered-dose inhaler, or orally. Some studies suggest that regular multiple-dose daily β-adrenergic drugs given by inhalation as primary treatment of chronic asthma may worsen disease morbidity, so as-needed

Table 19–7. H_1 antihistamines.

Chemical Class and Representative Drugs	Usual Daily Dosage	Cost per Unit	Cost for 30 Days' Treatment Based on Maximum Dosage[1]
Ethanolamine			
Diphenhydramine	25–50 mg every 4–6 hours	$0.04/25 mg	$10.00
Clemastine	0.34–2.68 mg every 12 hours	$0.33/1.34 mg	$39.60
Ethylenediamine			
Tripelennamine	25–50 mg every 4–6 hours	$0.25/25 mg	$18.00
Alkylamine			
Brompheniramine	4 mg every 4–6 hours 8–12 mg of SR form every 8–12 hours	$0.18/4 mg; $0.34/12 mg	$4.00 $20.40
Chlorpheniramine	4 mg every 4–6 hours 8–12 mg of SR form every 8–12 hours	$0.05/4 mg; $0.35/12 mg	$6.00 $21.00
Triprolidine (1.25 mg/5 mL)	2.5 mg every 4–6 hours	$0.05/5 mL	$12.00
Phenothiazine			
Promethazine	25 mg at bedtime	$0.07/25 mg	$2.10
Piperazine			
Hydroxyzine	25 mg every 6–8 hours	$0.10/25 mg	$12.00
Piperidines			
Astemizole (nonsedating)	10 mg/d	$1.99/10 mg	$59.70
Azatadine	1–2 mg every 12 hours	$0.91/1 mg	$109.00
Cetirizine	10 mg/d	$0.77/10 mg	$23.00
Cyproheptadine	4 mg every 6–8 hours	$0.04/4 mg	$4.80
Fexofenadine (nonsedating)	60 mg every 12 hours	$0.86/60 mg	$51.60
Loratidine (nonsedating)	10 mg every 24 hours	$2.08/10 mg	$62.40

[1]Cost to pharmacist (average wholesale price) for 30 days' treatment based on maximum dosage (generic when possible). Source: First Data Bank, Price Alert, April 1997.

dosing is now recommended by many specialists. The main side effect is muscle tremor, especially when the drug is taken orally, but tolerance usually develops with continued use.

4. Theophylline–This drug is used as a bronchodilator. Its mechanism of action is unknown, but it may involve inhibition of the bronchoconstricting effect of endogenous adenosine, liberated during the allergic reaction. Long-term continuous dosing with slow-release oral preparations to achieve a blood level of 10–20 μg/mL is effective for some asthmatic patients.

5. Glucocorticoids–These drugs have a therapeutic role in virtually all types of allergic diseases because of their anti-inflammatory action, rather than by their immunosuppressive effects. They are extremely effective, but they do not modify the underlying disease. Their use in allergy requires close attention to side effects and toxicity. Corticosteroid drugs are available in oral, intramuscular, intravenous, intranasal, and bronchial inhalational forms, as eye drops, and in topical formulations for dermatologic use. Short-term systemic burst therapy is indicated for treatment of severe asthma, allergic contact dermatitis, and acute exacerbations of hypersensitivity pneumonitis and allergic bronchopulmonary aspergillosis. Steroid eye drops are used for short-term treatment of acute allergic conjunctivitis, but the patient must be monitored for signs of corneal ulceration, keratitis, and glaucoma. Corticosteroid nasal spray is effective and probably safe for long-term use, but epistaxis can occur and nasal septal perforation is a possible complication. Flunisolide, beclomethasone, and triamcinolone are similarly efficacious, often requiring only a single daily dose after an initial period of therapy with four doses daily for 1 week. Long-term high-dose inhaled corticosteroid therapy for asthma is currently considered an important aspect of management of the inflammatory phase of the disease. Systemic absorption may occur. Oral candidiasis is a complication that is usually prevented by immediate mouth washing after each application. Topical steroid therapy is the primary treatment of atopic dermatitis. It may be sufficient for mild cases of contact dermatitis.

6. Treatment of anaphylaxis–At the first suspicion, aqueous epinephrine 1:1000 in a dose of 0.2–0.5 mL (0.2–0.5 mg) is injected subcutaneously or intramuscularly. Repeated injections can be given every 20–30 minutes when necessary.

The definitive therapy of anaphylactic shock is the rapid intravenous infusion of large volumes of fluids (saline, lactated Ringer's, plasma, colloid solutions, or plasma expanders) to replace loss of intravascular plasma into tissues. Other vasopressor drugs (dopamine, dobutamine, norepinephrine, phenylephrine) may be necessary if the patient remains hypotensive despite epinephrine.

Airway obstruction may be caused by edema of the larynx and hypopharynx or by bronchospasm. The former is treated by maintenance of an airway with endotracheal intubation or tracheostomy. Bronchospasm responds to subcutaneous epinephrine or terbutaline. Inhalation of selective β_2-adrenergic agonists such as albuterol or terbutaline and intravenous administration of theophylline are given for bronchospasm.

Antihistamines (H_1 and H_2 receptor antagonists) may be useful as adjuvant therapy for alleviating the cutaneous manifestations of urticaria or angioedema and pruritus and for the gastrointestinal and uterine smooth muscle spasms. Corticosteroids will not reverse respiratory obstruction or shock even when given intramuscularly or intravenously, but these drugs may be helpful in moderating later sequelae of the vascular damage. Long-term combined oral antihistamine-prednisone therapy has been shown to reduce the number and severity of attacks in patients with frequent life-threatening episodes of idiopathic anaphylaxis.

There may be a clinical late-phase IgE response in anaphylaxis, as there is in atopy. Since this begins some hours after exposure to the allergen and after subsidence of the immediate-phase response, all patients with anaphylaxis should be monitored for up to 24 hours.

Anaphylaxis in a patient being treated with β-adrenergic blocker drugs is a special problem because of refractoriness to epinephrine and selective β-adrenergic agonists. Higher than usual doses of these drugs may be required for the desired effect; using glucagon in those patients taking beta-blockers may be additionally beneficial.

B. Immune Complex Allergic Diseases:

1. Serum sickness—This disease is self-limited, so treatment is usually conservative and symptomatic only. Aspirin will relieve the arthralgias. Antihistamines and topical steroids will control the dermatitis. Corticosteroid therapy is rarely necessary. Because the disease is usually free of long-term sequelae, these drugs should be given in dosages sufficient to control symptoms.

2. Allergic bronchopulmonary aspergillosis—Patients with this disease have asthma complicated by periodic episodes of *Aspergillus* bronchitis and pneumonitis. (See Chapter 9.)

3. Hypersensitivity pneumonitis—See Chapter 9.

C. T Cell-Mediated Hypersensitivity: Aller-gic contact dermatitis is treated with systemic steroids and topical emollients.

D. Radiocontrast Media Reactions: Reactions to radiocontrast media do not appear to be mediated by IgE antibodies, yet clinically they are similar to anaphylaxis and are referred to as anaphylactoid reactions. If a patient has had an anaphylactoid reaction to conventional radiocontrast media, then the risk for a second reaction upon reexposure may be as high as 30%. The management of patients experiencing radiocontrast media reactions includes the use of the lower osmolar preparations and prophylactic pretreatment with prednisone (50 mg orally every 6 hours beginning 18 hours before the procedure), diphenhydramine (25–50 mg intramuscularly), and ephedrine (25 mg orally 60 minutes prior to the procedure). The use of the lower-osmolality radiocontrast media in combination with the pretreatment regimen decreases the incidence of reactions to less than 1%.

Immunotherapy

Treatment of atopy, especially allergic rhinitis, by the repeated long-term injection of allergen has been shown in many controlled clinical trials to be an effective method for reducing or eliminating symptoms and signs of the allergic disorder.

A. Indications: This treatment is recommended for patients with severe allergic rhinitis who respond poorly to drug therapy and whose allergens are not avoidable. It is also used for allergic asthma, though there are few definitive clinical trials in that disease. There is no current evidence for an effect on atopic dermatitis. Inhalant allergens only are used. Food allergy is treated by avoidance.

Immunotherapy of systemic anaphylaxis to Hymenoptera venom has been shown to be extremely effective. The duration of treatment required to achieve permanent immunity is currently under investigation. The current recommendations for continued protection are that venom immunotherapy should be continued indefinitely, until conclusive data are available. Risk factors for recurrent allergic reactions to insect stings if immunotherapy is discontinued include a presenting history of a severe systemic reaction and systemic reactions to the therapy.

Short-course desensitization for IgE allergy to certain drugs, especially penicillin and insulin, has been successful in many cases. This is usually accomplished by a course of injections of increasing doses over a period of hours rather than the weeks or months as required for atopic disease treatment. Oral, injected, or topical desensitization for contact dermatitis has been attempted without evidence that it is efficacious.

B. Immunologic Effects: The term allergen immunotherapy is usually used instead of desensitization, because the immunologic basis for this form of treatment is currently unknown. Nevertheless, certain immunologic changes can be induced by these injections. Circulating levels of IgE antibodies specific to the injected allergens increase slightly during the first few months, then decrease, eventually to substantially lower levels than before treatment. Seasonal rises in IgE antibodies to pollens are blunted or eliminated. IgG blocking antibody is produced. Changes in regulatory T cells favoring suppression of IgE antibody production have been reported. All of these effects are allergenically specific.

C. Clinical Effects: Most patients with allergic rhinitis caused by pollen become more tolerant to natural pollen exposure during successive seasons while on immunotherapy; some become completely asymptomatic, while a few patients derive no benefit. A beneficial response may or may not persist after treatment is stopped. Clinical effects, like immunologic responses, are specific for the injected allergens only.

Treatment

A. Procedure: Based on the clinical evaluation, a sterile aqueous solution of the allergen or allergens responsible for the individual patient's disease is administered repeatedly by subcutaneous injection in increasing doses once or twice a week until a maintenance dose is reached. The maintenance dose is determined individually based on improvement in symptoms and signs of the allergic disease and without systemic or excessive local reactions to the injected allergen. Thereafter, the same dose is injected every 2–4 weeks indefinitely.

B. Adverse Effects: Reactions to treatment may be local or systemic. Localized immediate and late-phase skin reactions occur at injection sites. These are not harmful, but the dose must be adjusted to avoid excessively large or prolonged local reactions. Immediate systemic reactions or anaphylaxis are a potential problem with each injection and must be prevented by careful monitoring of dosage. The patient must remain for at least 30 minutes after each injection visit at the treatment facility where drugs and equipment for treating anaphylaxis are available. Exacerbation of the patient's allergic manifestations (rhinitis, asthma, eczema) also calls for reducing the subsequent dosage.

No long-term adverse immunologic or nonimmunologic consequences of aqueous allergen extract immunotherapy are known.

Busse WW: Role of antihistamines in allergic disease. Ann Allergy 1994;72:371. (Better than placebo against sneezing and rhinitis. Second-generation medications have less side effects.)

Frew AJ: Injection immunotherapy. British Society for Allergy and Immunology Working Party. Br Med J 1993;307:919. (Recommended only for summer hay fever uncontrolled by conventional medicines and wasp and venom hypersensitivity but not asthma or allergic rhinitis from other allergies.)

Platts-Mills TA: How environment affects patients with allergic disease: Indoor allergens and asthma. Ann Allergy 1994;72:381. (Sensitization to indoor allergens is strongly associated with development of asthma, and making changes in the indoor environment has been shown to decrease bronchial hypersensitivity in asthmatics.)

20 Arthritis & Musculoskeletal Disorders

David B. Hellmann, MD

DIAGNOSIS & EVALUATION

Examination of the Patient

The diagnosis of a rheumatic disease can often be made in the office or at the bedside by history and physical examination. In general, the two clinical clues most helpful for diagnosis are the joint pattern and the presence or absence of extra-articular manifestations. The joint pattern is defined by answering three questions: (1) Is inflammation present? (2) How many joints are involved? and (3) What specific joint sites are affected? Joint inflammation is manifested by redness, warmth, swelling, and morning stiffness of at least 30 minutes' duration. Both the number of affected joints and the specific sites of involvement help determine the differential diagnosis (Table 20–1). Some diseases—gout, for example— are characteristically monarticular, whereas other diseases, such as rheumatoid arthritis, are chiefly polyarticular (Table 20–1). The location of joint involvement can also be distinctive. Only two diseases cause prominent involvement of the distal interphalangeal joint (DIP): osteoarthritis and psoriatic arthritis. As will be detailed in the discussion of specific diseases, the presence or absence of extra-articular manifestations such as fever, rash, nodules, or neuropathy helps narrow the differential diagnosis (see Table 20–1).

Laboratory procedures complete the evaluation, most commonly including sedimentation rate, tests for rheumatoid factor and antinuclear or other antibodies, synovial fluid analysis, and x-rays of affected joints. These studies are important for diagnosis and as a baseline for judging the results of therapy.

Arthrocentesis & Examination of Joint Fluid

Synovial fluid examination (Table 20–2) may provide specific diagnostic information in joint disease. Contraindications to arthrocentesis include infection of the overlying skin, bleeding disorder, or inability of the patient to cooperate. Most large joints are easily aspirated (Figure 20–1).

A. Types of Studies: When synovial fluid is examined, the following studies should be included:

1. Gross examination–If fluid is green or purulent, a Gram's stain is indicated. If grossly bloody, consider a bleeding disorder, trauma, or traumatic tap.

2. Microscopic examination–Compensated polarized light microscopy identifies and distinguishes monosodium urate (gout) and calcium pyrophosphate (pseudogout) crystals.

3. Culture–Routine bacterial cultures as well as special studies for gonococci, tubercle bacilli, or fungi when indicated.

B. Interpretation: (See Table 20–2.) Although synovial fluid analysis is diagnostic in infectious or microcrystalline arthritis, there is considerable overlap in the cytologic and biochemical values obtained in these and other diseases (Table 20–3). These studies do make possible, however, a differentiation according to severity of inflammation. Inflammatory joint fluids have more than 3000 white blood cells per microliter, of which 50% or more are polymorphonuclear neutrophils (Table 20–2). Noninflammatory disease fluids have fewer than 3000/µL and less than 25% polymorphonuclear neutrophils. Synovial fluid glucose and protein levels (Table 20–2) add little information and, therefore, should not be ordered.

Baker DB, Schumacher HR: Acute monarthritis. N Engl J Med 1993;329:1013. (Clues to differential diagnosis.)

Pinals RS: Polyarthritis and fever. N Engl J Med 1994;330:769. (Clues to differential diagnosis.)

Table 20–1. Diagnostic value of the joint pattern.

Characteristic	Status	Representative Disease
Inflammation	Present	Rheumatoid arthritis, systemic lupus erythematosus, gout
	Absent	Osteoarthritis
Number of involved joints	Monarticular	Gout, trauma, septic arthritis, Lyme disease
	Oligoarticular (2–4 joints)	Reiter's disease, psoriatic arthritis, inflammatory bowel disease
	Polyarticular (≥ 5 joints)	Rheumatoid arthritis, systemic lupus erythematosus
Site of joint involvement	Distal inter-phalangeal	Osteoarthritis, psoriatic arthritis (not rheumatoid arthritis)
	Metacarpopha-langeal, wrists	Rheumatoid arthritis, systemic lupus erythematosus (not osteoarthritis)
	First metatarsal phalangeal	Gout, osteoarthritis

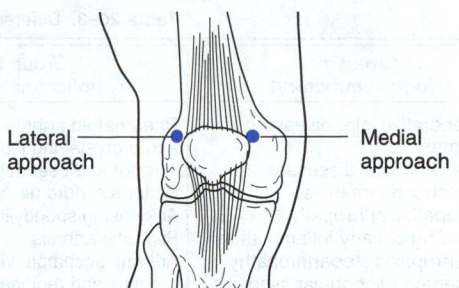

Figure 20–1. Aspiration of the knee joint. The knee joint—the most commonly aspirated joint—can be entered either medially or laterally. The patient should be supine, with the leg fully extended. Apply pressure on the side of the joint opposite to the puncture site to assist in directing the needle toward the bulging synovium. From the lateral approach, the needle (held parallel to the examining table) is directed medially, just beneath the patella, into the suprapatellar space. From the medial approach, the needle (held parallel to the examining table) is introduced between the patella and the medial condyle and advanced upward and laterally, beneath the patella and into the joint space. (Reproduced, with permission, from Detmer W et al: *Pocket Guide to Diagnostic Tests.* Appleton & Lange, 1992.)

DEGENERATIVE & CRYSTAL-INDUCED ARTHRITIS

DEGENERATIVE JOINT DISEASE (Osteoarthritis)

Essentials of Diagnosis

- A degenerative disorder without systemic manifestations.
- Pain relieved by rest; morning stiffness brief; articular inflammation minimal.
- X-ray findings: narrowed joint space, osteophytes,

increased density of subchondral bone, bony cysts.
- Commonly secondary to other articular disease.

General Considerations

Osteoarthritis is the most common form of joint disease, sparing no age, race, or geographic area. At least 20 million adults in the USA suffer from the effects of this condition at any one time, and 90% of all people will have radiographic features of osteoarthritis in weight-bearing joints by age 40. Symptomatic disease also increases with age.

This arthropathy is characterized by degeneration of cartilage and by hypertrophy of bone at the articular margins. Inflammation is usually minimal. Hered-

Table 20–2. Examination of joint fluid.

Measure	Normal	Group I (Noninflammatory)	Group II (Inflammatory)	Group III (Septic)
Volume (mL) (knee)	< 3.5	Often > 3.5	Often > 3.5	Often > 3.5
Clarity	Transparent	Transparent	Translucent to opaque	Opaque
Color	Clear	Yellow	Yellow to opalescent	Yellow to green
WBC (per μL)	< 200	200–300	3000–50,000	> 50,000[1]
Polymorphonuclear leukocytes (%)	< 25%	< 25%	50% or more	75% or more[1]
Culture	Negative	Negative	Negative	Usually positive
Glucose (mg/dL)	Nearly equal to serum	Nearly equal to serum	> 25, lower than serum	< 25, much lower than serum

[1]Counts are lower with infections caused by organisms of low virulence or if antibiotic therapy has been started.

Table 20–3. Differential diagnosis by joint fluid groups.[1]

Group 1 (Noninflammatory)	Group II (Inflammatory)	Group III (Purulent)	Hemorrhagic
Degenerative joint disease Trauma[2] Osteochondritis dissecans Osteochondromatosis Neuropathic arthropathy[2] Subsiding or early inflammation Hypertrophic osteoarthropathy[3] Pigmented villonodular synovitis[2]	Rheumatoid arthritis Acute crystal-induced synovitis (gout and pseudogout) Reiter's syndrome Ankylosing spondylitis Psoriatic arthritis Arthritis accompanying ulcerative colitis and regional enteritis Rheumatic fever[3] Systemic lupus erythematosus[3] Progressive systemic sclerosis (scleroderma)[3] Tuberculosis Mycotic infections	Pyogenic bacterial infections	Hemophilia or other hemorrhagic diathesis Trauma with or without fracture Neuropathic arthropathy Pigmented villonodular synovitis Synovioma Hemangioma and other benign neoplasms

[1]Reproduced from Rodnan GP (editor): Primer on the rheumatic diseases, 7th ed. JAMA 1973;224(Suppl):662.
[2]May be hemorrhagic.
[3]Group I or II.

itary and mechanical factors may be variably involved in the pathogenesis.

Degenerative joint disease is traditionally divided into two types: (1) primary, which most commonly affects some or all of the following: the terminal interphalangeal joints (Heberden's nodes) and less commonly the proximal interphalangeal joints (Bouchard's nodes), the metacarpophalangeal and carpometacarpal joints of the thumb, the hip, the knee, the metatarsophalangeal joint of the big toe, and the cervical and lumbar spine; and (2) secondary, which may occur in any joint as a sequela to articular injury resulting from either intra-articular (including rheumatoid arthritis) or extra-articular causes. The injury may be acute, as in a fracture; chronic, as that due to occupational overuse of a joint, metabolic disease (eg, hyperparathyroidism, hemochromatosis, ochronosis), or neurologic disorders (tabes dorsalis; see below). Obesity is a risk factor for knee osteoarthritis and probably for the hip as well. Recreational running does not increase the incidence of osteoarthritis, but participation in competitive contact sports does.

Pathologically, the articular cartilage is first roughened and finally worn away, and spur formation and lipping occur at the edge of the joint surface. The synovial membrane becomes thickened, with hypertrophy of the villous processes; the joint cavity, however, never becomes totally obliterated, and the synovial membrane does not form adhesions. Inflammation is prominent only in occasional patients with acute interphalangeal joint involvement.

Clinical Findings

A. Symptoms and Signs: The onset is insidious. Initially, there is articular stiffness, seldom lasting more than 15 minutes; this develops later into pain on motion of the affected joint and is made worse by activity or weight bearing and relieved by rest. Deformity may be absent or minimal; however, bony enlargement of the interphalangeal joints is occasionally prominent, and flexion contracture or varus deformity of the knee is not unusual. There is no ankylosis, but limitation of motion of the affected joint or joints is common. Coarse crepitus may often be felt in the joint. Joint effusion and other articular signs of inflammation are mild. There are no systemic manifestations.

B. Laboratory Findings: Elevated sedimentation rate and other laboratory signs of inflammation are not present.

C. Imaging: Radiographs may reveal narrowing of the joint space, sharpened articular margins, osteophyte formation and lipping of marginal bone, and thickened, dense subchondral bone. Bone cysts may also be present.

Differential Diagnosis

Because articular inflammation is minimal and systemic manifestations are absent, degenerative joint disease should seldom be confused with other arthritides. The distribution of joint involvement in the hands also helps distinguish osteoarthritis from rheumatoid arthritis. Osteoarthritis chiefly affects the distal and proximal interphalangeal joints and spares the wrist and metacarpophalangeal joints (except at the thumb); rheumatoid arthritis chiefly involves the wrists and metacarpophalangeal joints and spares the distal interphalangeal joints. Furthermore, the joint enlargement is bony-hard and cool in osteoarthritis but spongy and warm in rheumatoid arthritis. One must be cautious in attributing all skeletal symptoms to degenerative changes in joints, especially in the spine, where metastatic neoplasia, osteoporosis, multiple myeloma, or other bone disease may coexist.

Prevention

Weight reduction has been shown in women to reduce the risk of developing symptomatic knee osteoarthritis.

Treatment

A. General Measures: Education is the cornerstone of treatment and may be all that is needed for osteoarthritis of the hands. For patients with mild to moderate osteoarthritis of weight-bearing joints, a supervised walking program may result in clinical improvement of functional status without aggravating the joint pain. Dietary fads such as taking chondroitin sulfate have never been shown to be effective.

B. Analgesic and Anti-inflammatory Drugs: For many patients, acetaminophen in doses of 2.6–4 g/d is as effective as and less toxic than other NSAIDs. (See discussion of NSAID toxicity in the section on treatment of rheumatoid arthritis.) Patients who fail to improve with acetaminophen and nonpharmacologic therapies described above can be treated with salicylates or other NSAIDs (see Chapter 1). High doses of salicylates, as used in more inflammatory arthritides, are unnecessary. The need to continue any drug treatment for patients with osteoarthritis should be reviewed periodically. For many patients, it is possible eventually to reduce the dosage or limit use of the drug to periods of exacerbation. For patients with knee osteoarthritis and effusion, intra-articular injection of triamcinolone (20–40 mg) may obviate the need for analgesics or NSAIDs. Capsaicin cream 0.25% applied twice daily can also reduce knee pain without NSAIDs.

C. Surgical Measures: Total hip replacement provides excellent symptomatic and functional improvement when that joint is seriously afflicted, as indicated by severely restricted walking and pain at rest, particularly at night. Knee replacement is also usually effective. Although arthroscopic surgery for knee osteoarthritis is commonly performed, its long-term efficacy is unestablished. Experimental techniques to repair focal cartilage loss in the knee by autologous chondrocyte transplantation have achieved promising results.

Prognosis

Marked disability is less common than in rheumatoid arthritis, but symptoms may be quite severe and limit activity considerably (especially with involvement of the hips, knees, and cervical spine). Proper treatment may relieve symptoms and improve function.

Ettinger WH et al: A randomized trial comparing aerobic exercise and resistance exercise with a health education program in older adults with knee osteoarthritis. The fitness arthritis and seniors trial (FAST). JAMA 1997;277:25. (Either walking or resistance exercise moderately reduces pain and disability.)

Felson DT et al: The incidence and natural history of knee osteoarthritis in the elderly. The Framingham osteoarthritis study. Arthritis Rheum 1995;38:1500. (In this elderly cohort [age range 63–91], knee osteoarthritis developed 1.7 times more often in women than men. Among women, 1% per year developed symptomatic knee osteoarthritis.)

Hochberg MC et al: Guidelines for the medical management of osteoarthritis. Part I. Osteoarthritis of the hip. Arthritis Rheum 1995;38:1535. (American College of Rheumatology guidelines: nonpharmacologic modalities and acetaminophen given first; if inadequate, then ibuprofen [up to 400 mg four times daily] or nonacetylated salicylates; if inadequate, then full doses of NSAIDs; if inadequate, consider joint surgery.)

Hochberg MC et al: Guidelines for the medical management of osteoarthritis. Part II. Osteoarthritis of the knee. Arthritis Rheum 1995;38:1541. (Similar to guidelines for hip except consider intra-articular triamcinolone injection before acetaminophen if effusion present, and consider topical capsaicin cream if acetaminophen inadequate.)

CRYSTAL DEPOSITION ARTHRITIS

1. GOUTY ARTHRITIS

Essentials of Diagnosis

- Acute onset, typically nocturnal and usually monarticular, often involving the first metatarsophalangeal joint.
- Postinflammatory desquamation and pruritus.
- Hyperuricemia in most; identification of urate crystals in joint fluid or tophi is diagnostic.
- Asymptomatic periods between acute attacks.
- Dramatic therapeutic response to NSAIDs or colchicine.
- With chronicity, urate deposits in subcutaneous tissue, bone, cartilage, joints, and other tissues.

General Considerations

Gout is a metabolic disease of heterogeneous nature, often familial, associated with abnormal amounts of urates in the body and characterized early by a recurring acute arthritis, usually monarticular, and later by chronic deforming arthritis. The associated hyperuricemia is due to overproduction or underexcretion of uric acid—sometimes both. The disease is especially common in Pacific islanders, eg, Filipinos and Samoans. It is rarely caused by a specifically determined genetic aberration (eg, Lesch-Nyhan syndrome). Secondary gout, which may have a heritable component, is related to acquired causes of hyperuricemia, eg, diuretic use, cyclosporine use, myeloproliferative disorders, multiple myeloma, hemoglobinopathies, chronic renal disease, hypothyroidism, and lead poisoning.

About 90% of patients with primary gout are men, usually over 30 years of age. In women the onset is usually postmenopausal. The characteristic histologic lesion is the tophus, a nodular deposit of monosodium urate monohydrate crystals, with an associated foreign body reaction. These may be found in cartilage, subcutaneous and periarticular tissues, tendon, bone, the kidneys, and elsewhere. Urates have been demonstrated in the synovial tissues (and fluid) during acute arthritis; indeed, the acute inflammation of gout is believed to be activated by the phagocytosis by polymorphonuclear cells of urate crystals with the ensuing release from the neutrophils of chemotactic and other substances capable of mediating inflammation. The precise relationship of hyperuricemia to acute gouty arthritis is still obscure, since chronic hyperuricemia is found in people who never develop gout or uric acid stones (Table 20–4). Rapid fluctuations in serum urate levels, either increasing or decreasing, are important factors in precipitating acute gout. The mechanism of the late, chronic stage of gouty arthritis is better understood. This is characterized pathologically by tophaceous invasion of the articular and periarticular tissues, with structural derangement and secondary degeneration (osteoarthritis).

Uric acid kidney stones are present in 5–10% of patients with gouty arthritis. The term "gouty kidney" denotes kidney disease due to sodium urate deposition in the renal interstitium. Uric acid stones are not related to its pathogenesis, and a relationship to renal insufficiency or to the severity of gout has not been established.

Unless there is a rapid breakdown of cellular nucleic acid following aggressive treatment of leukemia or lymphoma, uric acid-lowering drugs need not be instituted until arthritis, renal calculi, or tophi become apparent. Psoriasis, sarcoidosis, and diuretic drugs are commonly overlooked causes of hyperuricemia and may precipitate attacks in patients with gout. Asymptomatic hyperuricemia should not be treated.

Clinical Findings

A. Symptoms and Signs: The acute arthritis is characterized by its sudden onset, frequently nocturnal, either without apparent precipitating cause or following rapid fluctuations in serum urate levels from food and alcohol excess, surgery, infection, diuretics, chemicals (eg, meglumine diatrizoate, Urografin), or uricosuric drugs. The metatarsophalangeal joint of the great toe is the most susceptible joint ("podagra"), although others, especially those of the feet, ankles, and knees, are commonly affected. Hips and shoulders are rarely involved in gouty arthritis. More than one joint may occasionally be affected during the same attack; in such cases, the distribution of the arthritis is usually asymmetric. As the attack progresses, the pain becomes intense. The involved joints are swollen and exquisitely tender and the overlying skin tense, warm, and dusky red. Fever is common and may reach 39 °C. Local desquamation and pruritus during recovery from the acute arthritis are characteristic of gout but are not always present. Tophi may be found in the external ears, hands, feet, olecranon, and prepatellar bursas. They are usually seen only after several attacks of acute arthritis.

Asymptomatic periods of months or years commonly follow the initial acute attack. Later, gouty arthritis may become chronic, with symptoms of progressive functional loss and disability. Gross deformities, due usually to tophaceous invasion, are seen. Signs of inflammation may be absent or superimposed.

B. Laboratory Findings: The serum uric acid is elevated (> 7.5 mg/dL) in 95% of patients who have serial measurements during the course of an attack. However, a single uric acid determination is normal in up to 25% of cases, so a normal level does not exclude gout, especially in patients taking uricopenic drugs. During an acute attack, the erythrocyte sedimentation rate and white cell count are frequently elevated. Examination of the material aspirated from a tophus shows the typical crystals of sodium urate and confirms the diagnosis. Further confirmation is obtained by identification of sodium urate crystals by compensated polariscopic examination of wet smears prepared from joint fluid aspirates. Such crystals are negatively birefringent and needle-like and may be found free or in neutrophils.

C. Imaging: Early in the disease, radiographs show no changes. Later, punched-out erosions with an overhanging rim of cortical bone ("rat bite") develop. When these are adjacent to a soft tissue tophus, they are diagnostic of gout.

Table 20–4. Origin of hyperuricemia.[1]

Primary hyperuricemia
A. Increased production of purine:
  1. Idiopathic.
  2. Specific enzyme defects (eg, Lesch-Nyhan syndrome, glycogen storage disease).
B. Decreased renal clearance of uric acid (idiopathic).

Secondary hyperuricemia
A. Increased catabolism and turnover of purine:
  1. Myeloproliferative disorders.
  2. Lymphoproliferative disorders.
  3. Carcinoma and sarcoma (disseminated).
  4. Chronic hemolytic anemias.
  5. Cytotoxic drugs.
  6. Psoriasis.
B. Decreased renal clearance of uric acid:
  1. Intrinsic kidney disease.
  2. Functional impairment of tubular transport:
    a. Drug-induced (eg, thiazides, probenecid).
    b. Hyperlactiacidemia acid (eg, lactic acidosis, alcoholism).
    c. Hyperketoacidemia (eg, diabetic ketoacidosis, starvation).
    d. Diabetes insipidus (vasopressin-resistant).
    e. Bartter's syndrome.

[1]Modified from Rodnan GP: Gout and other crystalline forms of arthritis. Postgrad Med (Oct) 1975;58:6.

Differential Diagnosis

Acute gout is often confused with cellulitis. Appropriate bacteriologic studies should exclude acute pyogenic arthritis. Pseudogout is distinguished by the identification of calcium pyrophosphate crystals (strong positive birefringence) in the joint fluid, usually normal serum uric acid, the x-ray appearance of chondrocalcinosis, and the relative therapeutic ineffectiveness of colchicine.

Chronic tophaceous arthritis may rarely mimic chronic rheumatoid arthritis. In such cases, the diagnosis of gout is suggested by an earlier history of monarthritis and is established by the demonstration of urate crystals in a suspected tophus. Likewise, hips and shoulders are generally spared in tophaceous gout. Biopsy may be necessary to distinguish tophi from rheumatoid nodules. An x-ray appearance similar to that of gout may be found in rheumatoid arthritis, sarcoidosis, multiple myeloma, hyperparathyroidism, or Hand-Schüller-Christian disease. Chronic lead intoxication may result in attacks of gouty arthritis (saturnine gout); abdominal pain, peripheral neuropathy, and renal insufficiency are clues to the diagnosis.

Treatment

A. Acute Attack: The most common mistake in managing gout is starting drug treatment for both the acute arthritis and the hyperuricemia simultaneously. Treatment must be separated by treating the acute arthritis first and hyperuricemia later, if at all. Sudden reduction of serum uric acid often precipitates further episodes of gouty arthritis.

1. Nonsteroidal anti-inflammatory drugs– NSAIDs have become the treatment of choice for acute gout. Traditionally, indomethacin has been the most frequently used agent, but all of the other newer NSAIDs are probably equally effective. Indomethacin is initiated at a dosage of 25–50 mg every 8 hours and continued until the symptoms have resolved (usually 5–10 days). Active peptic ulcer disease, impaired renal function, and a history of allergic reaction to NSAIDs are contraindications to the use of these drugs.

2. Colchicine–Colchicine is also effective for acute gout but is less favored, since 80% of treated patients develop significant abdominal cramping, diarrhea, nausea, or vomiting. Colchicine is thought to work by inhibiting chemotaxis and thereby interfering with the inflammatory response to urate crystals; thus, it is most effective when given in the first few hours after onset of symptoms. The dose is 0.5 or 0.6 mg by mouth every hour until pain is relieved or until nausea or diarrhea appears; the drug is then stopped. The usual total dose required is 4–6 mg and should not exceed 8 mg. The incidence of gastrointestinal side effects of colchicine can be reduced by intravenous administration. Use of intravenous colchicine, however, is discouraged because of potential severe toxicity, including local pain, tissue damage from extravasation during injection, bone marrow suppression, disseminated intravascular coagulation, and death. The initial dose is 2 mg in 20–50 mL of saline solution given through an intravenous catheter. Two additional doses of 1 mg each can be administered at 6-hour intervals. The total dose should not exceed 4 mg; and no additional colchicine should be given by mouth for 3 weeks. Dosages must be reduced by at least 50% in the presence of renal or hepatic disease or old age. Combined renal and hepatic disease contraindicates the use of intravenous colchicine. Intravenous administration of colchicine is inadvisable if the oral route can be used. Oral colchicine should not be used in patients with inflammatory bowel disease.

3. Corticosteroids–Corticosteroids often give dramatic symptomatic relief in acute episodes of gout and will control most attacks. They are best reserved for patients unable to take oral NSAIDs. If the patient's gout is monarticular, intra-articular administration (eg, triamcinolone, 10–40 mg depending on the size of the joint) is most effective. For polyarticular gout, corticosteroids may be given intravenously (eg, methylprednisolone, 40 mg/d tapered off over 7 days) or orally (eg, prednisone, 40–60 mg/d tapered off over 7 days). It should be recognized that gouty and septic arthritis can coexist, albeit rarely. Therefore, joint aspiration and Gram stain of synovial fluid should be performed before corticosteroids are given.

4. Analgesics–At times the pain of an acute attack may require opioids. Aspirin should be avoided (see below).

5. Bed rest is important in the management of the acute attack and should be continued for about 24 hours after the acute attack has subsided. Early ambulation may precipitate a recurrence.

Physical therapy is of little value acutely, though hot compresses to or elevation of the affected joints makes some patients more comfortable.

B. Management Between Attacks: Treatment during symptom-free periods is intended to minimize urate deposition in tissues, which causes chronic tophaceous arthritis, and to reduce the frequency and severity of recurrences.

1. Diet–Potentially reversible causes of hyperuricemia are a high-purine diet, obesity, frequent alcohol consumption, and use of certain medications (see below). Although dietary purines usually contribute only 1 mg/dL to the serum uric acid level, moderation in eating foods with high-purine content is advisable (Table 20–5). Moderating alcohol use is particularly important, since alcohol is not only a source of purines but also inhibits the renal excretion of purines. A high liquid intake and, more importantly, a daily urinary output of 2 L or more will aid urate excretion and minimize urate precipitation in the urinary tract.

Table 20–5. The purine content of foods.[1,2]

Low-purine foods
Refined cereals and cereal products, cornflakes, white bread, pasta, flour, arrowroot, sago, tapioca, cakes
Milk, milk products, and eggs
Sugar, sweets, and gelatin
Butter, polyunsaturated margarine, and all other fats
Fruit, nuts, and peanut butter
Lettuce, tomatoes, and green vegetables (except those listed below)
Cream soups made with low-purine vegetables but without meat or meat stock
Water, fruit juice, cordials, and carbonated drinks

High-purine foods
All meats, including organ meats, and seafood
Meat extracts and gravies
Yeast and yeast extracts, beer, and other alcoholic beverages
Beans, peas, lentils, oatmeal, spinach, asparagus, cauliflower, and mushrooms

[1]Reproduced, with permission, from Emmerson BT: The management of gout. N Engl J Med 1996;334:445.
[2]The purine content of a food reflects its nucleoprotein content and turnover. Foods containing many nuclei (eg, liver) have many purines, as do rapidly growing foods such as asparagus. The consumption of large amounts of a food containing a small concentration of purines may provide a greater purine load than consumption of a small amount of a food containing a large concentration of purines.

2. Avoidance of hyperuricemic medications–Thiazide and loop diuretics inhibit renal excretion of uric acid, thereby producing or increasing hyperuricemia. Whenever possible, these diuretics should be avoided in patients with gout. Similarly, low doses of aspirin (< 3 g daily) also inhibit renal excretion of uric acid and aggravate hyperuricemia. Nicotinic acid is yet another medication that produces hyperuricemia.

3. Colchicine–The decision to begin chronic pharmacologic treatment of gout should be based on an estimate of the likelihood of further attacks. Patients with a single episode of gout who are willing to lose weight and stop drinking alcohol are at low risk of another attack and therefore unlikely to benefit from chronic medical therapy. In contrast, older individuals with mild chronic renal failure who require diuretic use and have a history of multiple attacks of gout are more likely to benefit from pharmacologic treatment. In general, the higher the uric acid level and the more frequent the attacks, the more likely that chronic medical therapy will be beneficial.

There are two indications for daily colchicine administration: (1) The drug can be used by itself to prevent future attacks of gout. The drug does not affect the uric acid level but reduces the frequency of attacks. For the person who has mild hyperuricemia and has had several attacks of gouty arthritis, chronic colchicine prophylaxis may be all that is needed. The usual dose is 0.6 mg twice a day. Patients who have coexisting moderate renal insufficiency or heart failure should have the dose reduced to once a day in or-

der to avoid the development of a mixed peripheral neuropathy and myositis that can complicate the use of higher doses. (2) It is also used when uricosuric drugs or allopurinol (see below) are started, to suppress the acute attacks that can be precipitated by abrupt changes in the serum uric acid level.

4. Reduction of serum uric acid–Indications include frequent acute arthritis not controlled by colchicine prophylaxis, tophaceous deposits, or renal damage. Hyperuricemia with infrequent attacks of arthritis may not require treatment; asymptomatic hyperuricemia should not be treated. If instituted, the goal of medical treatment is to maintain the serum uric acid below 6 mg/dL, which should prevent crystallization of urate.

Two classes of agents may be used to lower the serum uric acid—the uricosuric drugs and allopurinol (neither is of value in the treatment of acute gout). The choice of one or the other depends on the result of a 24-hour urine uric acid determination. A value under 800 mg/d indicates undersecretion of uric acid, which is amenable to uricosuric agents. Patients with more than 800 mg of uric acid in a 24-hour urine collection are overproducers of uric acid who require allopurinol.

a. Uricosuric drugs–These drugs, by blocking tubular reabsorption of filtered urate and reducing the metabolic pool of urates, prevent the formation of new tophi and reduce the size of those already present. Furthermore, when administered concomitantly with colchicine, they may lessen the frequency of recurrences of acute gout. The indication for uricosuric treatment is the increasing frequency or severity of acute attacks. Uricosuric agents are ineffective in patients with renal insufficiency, as manifested by a serum creatinine of more than 2 mg/dL.

The following uricosuric drugs may be employed: (1) Probenecid, 0.5 g daily initially, with gradual increase to 1–2 g daily; or (2) sulfinpyrazone, 50–100 mg twice daily initially, with gradual increase to 200–400 mg twice daily. Hypersensitivity to either uricosuric drug in the form of fever and rash occurs in 5% of cases; gastrointestinal complaints occur in 10%. Note that probenecid inhibits the excretion of penicillin, indomethacin, dapsone, and acetazolamide.

Precautions with uricosuric drugs. It is important to maintain a daily urinary output of 2000 mL or more in order to minimize the precipitation of uric acid in the urinary tract. This can be further prevented by giving alkalinizing agents (eg, potassium citrate, 30–80 meq/d) to maintain a urine pH of above 6.0. Uricosuric drugs are best avoided in patients with a history of uric acid lithiasis. Salicylates in low doses antagonize the action of uricosuric agents; doses greater than 3 g daily are themselves uricosuric, but aspirin should be avoided by patients with gout.

b. Allopurinol–The xanthine oxidase inhibitor

allopurinol promptly lowers plasma urate and urinary uric acid concentrations and facilitates tophus mobilization. The drug is of special value in uric acid overproducers; in tophaceous gout; in patients unresponsive to the uricosuric regimen; and in gouty patients with uric acid renal stones. It should be used in low doses in patients with renal insufficiency and is not indicated in asymptomatic hyperuricemia. The most frequent adverse effect is the precipitation of an acute gouty attack. However, the commonest sign of hypersensitivity to allopurinol (occurring in 2% of cases) is a pruritic rash that may progress to toxic epidermal necrolysis, a potentially fatal complication. Vasculitis and hepatitis are other rare but serious complications.

The daily dose is determined by the serum uric acid response. The initial dose of allopurinol is 100 mg/d for 1 week; the dose is increased if the serum uric acid is still high. A normal serum uric acid level is often obtained with a daily dose of 200–300 mg. Occasionally (and in selected cases) it may be helpful to continue the use of allopurinol with a uricosuric drug. Neither of these drugs is useful in acute gout.

Allopurinol can interact with other drugs. The combined use of allopurinol and ampicillin causes a drug rash in 20% of patients. Allopurinol can increase the half-life of probenecid, while probenecid increases the excretion of allopurinol. Thus, a patient taking both drugs may need to use slightly higher than usual doses of allopurinol and lower doses of probenecid. Allopurinol potentiates the effect of azathioprine. If allopurinol cannot be avoided, the dose of azathioprine should be reduced by 75% before allopurinol is started.

C. Chronic Tophaceous Arthritis: Tophaceous deposits can be made to shrink and disappear altogether with allopurinol therapy. Resorption of extensive tophi may require maintaining a serum uric acid below 5 mg/dL, which may be achievable only with concomitant use of allopurinol and a uricosuric agent. Surgical excision of large tophi offers immediate mechanical improvement in selected deformities but is rarely required.

D. Gout in the Transplant Patient: Since many transplant patients have decreased renal function and require drugs that inhibit uric acid excretion (especially cyclosporine and diuretics), these patients commonly develop hyperuricemia and gout. Treating these patients is challenging: NSAIDs are usually contraindicated because of renal impairment; intravenous colchicine should be avoided for the same reason; and corticosteroids are already being used. Often the best approach for monarticular gout—after excluding infection—is injecting corticosteroids into the joint (see above). For polyarticular gout, increasing the dose of systemic corticosteroid may be the only alternative. Since transplant patients often have multiple attacks of gout, long-term relief requires lowering the serum uric acid with allopurinol. Renal impairment seen in many transplant patients would make uricosuric agents ineffective. As noted above, azathioprine must be stopped or reduced by 75% before allopurinol is started.

Prognosis

Without treatment, the acute attack may last from a few days to several weeks, but proper treatment quickly terminates the attack. The intervals between acute attacks vary up to years, but the asymptomatic periods often become shorter if the disease progresses. Chronic tophaceous arthritis occurs after repeated attacks of acute gout, but only after inadequate treatment. Although the deformities may be marked, only a small percentage of patients become bedridden. The younger the patient at the onset of disease, the greater the tendency to a progressive course. Destructive arthropathy is rarely seen in patients whose first attack is after age 50.

Patients with gout have an increased incidence of hypertension, renal disease (eg, nephrosclerosis, tophi, pyelonephritis), diabetes mellitus, hypertriglyceridemia, and atherosclerosis, although these relationships are not well understood.

Emmerson BT: The management of gout. N Engl J Med 1996;334:445. (Annual incidence of gouty arthritis is 0.1–0.5% for serum urate < 7 mg/dL and about 5% for serum urate > 9 mg/dL.)

Erickson AR et al: The prevalence of hypothyroidism in gout. Am J Med 1994;97:231. (Fifteen percent of gout patients had a history of hypothyroidism or serum TSH > 6 μU/mL.)

Vandenberg MK et al: Gout attacks in chronic alcoholics occur at lower serum urate levels than in nonalcoholics. J Rheumatol 1994;21:700. (Uric acid level of less than 8.5 mg/dL during gout attacks found in 66% of alcoholics and 30% of nonalcoholics.)

2. CHONDROCALCINOSIS & PSEUDOGOUT (Calcium Pyrophosphate Dihydrate [CPPD] Deposition Disease)

The term chondrocalcinosis refers to the presence of calcium-containing salts in articular cartilage. It is most often first diagnosed radiologically. It may be familial and is commonly associated with a wide variety of metabolic disorders, eg, hemochromatosis, hyperparathyroidism, ochronosis, diabetes mellitus, hypothyroidism, Wilson's disease, and true gout. Pseudogout, most often seen in persons age 60 or older, is characterized by acute, recurrent and rarely chronic arthritis that usually involves large joints (principally the knees and the wrists) and is almost always accompanied by chondrocalcinosis of the affected joints. Pseudogout, like gout, frequently develops 24–48 hours after major surgery. Identification of calcium pyrophosphate crystals in joint aspirates is diagnostic of pseudogout. With light microscopy, the rhomboid-shaped pseudogout crystals can usually be distinguished from the needle-shaped gout crystals. A red compensator is used for positive identification, since pseudogout crystals are blue when parallel and yellow when perpendicular to the axis of the compensator. Urate crystals give the exact opposite color pattern. X-ray examination shows not only calcification (usually symmetric) of cartilaginous structures but also signs of degenerative joint disease (osteoarthritis). Unlike gout, pseudogout is usually associated with normal serum urate levels and is not dramatically improved by colchicine.

Treatment of chondrocalcinosis is directed at the primary disease, if present. Some of the nonsteroidal anti-inflammatory agents (salicylates, indomethacin, naproxen, and other drugs) are helpful in the treatment of acute episodes. Colchicine, 0.6 mg orally twice daily, appears to be more effective for prophylaxis than for acute attacks. Aspiration of the inflamed joint and intra-articular injection of triamcinolone, 10–40 mg, depending on the size of the joint, are also of value in resistant cases.

Handy JR: Pyrophosphate arthropathy in the knees of elderly persons. Arch Intern Med 1996;156:2426-2432. (Thorough review.)

PAIN SYNDROMES

CERVICOBRACHIAL PAIN SYNDROMES

A large group of articular and extra-articular disorders is characterized by pain that may involve simultaneously the neck, shoulder girdle, and upper extremity. Diagnostic differentiation is often difficult. Some of these entities and clinical syndromes represent primary disorders of the cervicobrachial region; others are local manifestations of systemic disease. The clinical picture is further complicated when two or more of these conditions occur coincidentally.

Clinical Findings

A. Symptoms and Signs: Neck pain may be limited to the posterior neck region or, depending upon the level of the symptomatic joint, may radiate segmentally to the occiput, anterior chest, shoulder girdle, arm, forearm, and hand. It may be intensified by active or passive neck motions. The general distribution of pain and paresthesias corresponds roughly to the involved dermatome in the upper extremity. Radiating pain in the upper extremity is often intensified by hyperextension of the neck and deviation of the head to the involved side. Limitation of cervical

movements is the most common objective finding. Neurologic signs depend upon the extent of compression of nerve roots or the spinal cord. Compression of the spinal cord may cause long-tract involvement resulting in paraparesis or paraplegia.

B. Imaging: The radiographic findings depend on the cause of the pain; many plain x-rays are completely normal in patients who have suffered an acute cervical strain. Loss of the normal anterior convexity of the cervical curve (loss of cervical lordosis) is frequently seen but is a nonspecific result of paraspinal muscle spasm. In osteoarthritis, comparative reduction in height of the involved disk space is a frequent finding. The most common late x-ray finding is osteophyte formation anteriorly, adjacent to the disk; other late changes occur around the apophysial joint clefts, chiefly in the lower cervical spine. Use of advanced imaging techniques is indicated in the patient who has severe pain of unknown cause that fails to respond to conservative therapy or in the patient who has evidence of myelopathy. MRI is more sensitive than CT in detecting disk disease, extradural compression, and intramedullary cord disease.

Differential Diagnosis & Treatment

The causes of neck pain include acute and chronic cervical strain or sprains, herniated nucleus pulposus, osteoarthritis, ankylosing spondylitis, rheumatoid arthritis, osteomyelitis, neoplasms, spinal stenosis, compression fractures, and functional disorders.

A. Acute or Chronic Cervical Musculotendinous Strain: Cervical strain is generally caused by mechanical postural disorders, overexertion, or injury (eg, whiplash). Acute episodes are associated with pain, decreased cervical spine motion, and paraspinal muscle spasm, resulting in stiffness of the neck and loss of motion. Muscle trigger points can often be localized. Management includes neck and head immobilization by traction, a cervical collar, and administration of analgesics. Corticosteroid injection into cervical facet joints is ineffective. Gradual return to full activity is encouraged.

Patients with chronic symptoms often have few objective findings. Mechanical stress due to work or recreational activities is often implicated. Chronic pain, especially that radiating into the upper extremity, may require additional treatment such as bracing.

B. Herniated Nucleus Pulposus: Rupture or prolapse of the nucleus pulposus of the cervical disks into the spinal canal causes pain that radiates to the arms at the level of C6–7. When intra-abdominal pressure is increased by coughing, sneezing, or other movements, symptoms are aggravated, and cervical muscle spasm may often occur. Neurologic abnormalities may include decreased reflexes of the deep tendons of the biceps and triceps and decreased sensation and muscle atrophy or weakness in the forearm or hand. Cervical traction, bed rest, and other conservative measures are usually successful. Radicular symptoms usually respond to conservative therapy, including NSAIDs, activity modification, intermittent cervical traction, and neck immobilization. Cervical epidural steroid injections may help those who fail. Surgery is indicated for unremitting pain and progressive weakness despite a full trial of conservative therapy and if a surgically correctable abnormality is identified by MRI or CT myelography. Surgical decompression achieves excellent results in 70–80% of such patients.

C. Arthritic Disorders: Cervical spondylosis (degenerative arthritis) is a collective term describing degenerative changes that occur in the apophysial joints and intervertebral disk joints, with or without neurologic signs. Osteoarthritis of the articular facets is characterized by progressive thinning of the cartilage, subchondral osteoporosis, and osteophytic proliferation around the joint margins. Degeneration of cervical disks and joints may occur in adolescents but is more common after age 40. Degeneration is progressive and is marked by gradual narrowing of the disk space, as demonstrated by x-ray. Osteocartilaginous proliferation occurs around the margin of the vertebral body and gives rise to osteophytic ridges that may encroach upon the intervertebral foramina and spinal canal, causing compression of the neurovascular contents.

Osteoarthritis of the cervical spine is often asymptomatic but may cause diffuse neck pain, radicular pain, or myelopathy. Myelopathy develops insidiously and is manifested by numb, clumsy hands. Some patients also complain of unsteady walking, urinary frequency and urgency, or electrical shock sensations with neck flexion or extension (Lhermitte's sign). Weakness, sensory loss, and spasticity with exaggerated reflexes develop below the level of spinal cord compression. Motor neuron disease, multiple sclerosis, syringomyelia, spinal cord tumors, and tropical spastic paresis from HTLV-1 infection can mimic myelopathy from cervical arthritis. The mainstay of conservative therapy is immobilizing the cervical spine with a collar. With moderate to severe symptoms, surgical treatment is indicated.

Ankylosing spondylitis is discussed below. Atlantoaxial subluxation may occur in patients with rheumatoid arthritis, regardless of the severity of disease. Inflammation of the synovial structures resulting from erosion and laxity of the transverse ligament can lead to neurologic signs of spinal cord compression. Treatment may vary from use of a cervical collar or more rigid bracing to operative treatment, depending on the degree of subluxation and neurologic progression. Surgical treatment may involve stabilization of the cervical spine.

D. Other Disorders: Osteomyelitis and neoplasms are discussed below. Osteoporosis is discussed in Chapter 26.

Lord SM et al: Percutaneous radio-frequency neurotomy for chronic cervical zygapophyseal-joint pain. N Engl J Med 1996;335:1721. (In such patients, the procedure can provide lasting relief.)

McCormack BM, Weinstein PR: Cervical spondylosis: An update. West J Med 1996;165:43. (Diagnosis and management.)

THORACIC OUTLET SYNDROMES

Thoracic outlet syndromes include those disorders that result in compression of the neurovascular structures supplying the upper extremity. Patients often have a history of trauma to the head and neck areas.

Symptoms and signs arise from intermittent or continuous pressure on elements of the brachial plexus and the subclavian or axillary vessels by a variety of anatomic structures of the shoulder girdle region. The neurovascular bundle can be compressed between the anterior or middle scalene muscles and a normal first thoracic rib or a cervical rib. Descent of the shoulder girdle may continue during adulthood and cause compression. Faulty posture, chronic illness, and occupation may be other predisposing factors. The components of the median nerve that encircle the axillary artery may cause compression and vascular symptoms. Sudden or repetitive strenuous physical activity may initiate "effort thrombosis" of the axillary or subclavian vein.

Pain may radiate from the point of compression to the base of the neck, the axilla, the shoulder girdle region, arm, forearm, and hand. Paresthesias are frequently present and are commonly distributed to the volar aspect of the fourth and fifth digits. Sensory symptoms may be aggravated at night or by prolonged use of the extremities. Weakness and muscle atrophy are the principal motor abnormalities. Vascular symptoms consist of arterial ischemia characterized by pallor of the fingers on elevation of the extremity, sensitivity to cold, and, rarely, gangrene of the digits or venous obstruction marked by edema, cyanosis, and engorgement.

Deep reflexes are usually not altered. When the site of compression is between the upper rib and clavicle, partial obliteration of subclavian artery pulsation may be demonstrated by abduction of the arm to a right angle with the elbow simultaneously flexed and rotated externally at the shoulder so that the entire extremity lies in the coronal plane. Neck or arm position has no effect on the diminished pulse, which remains constant in the subclavian steal syndrome.

Chest x-ray will identify patients with cervical rib. MRI with the arms held in different positions is useful in identifying sites of impaired blood flow. Intraarterial or venous obstruction is confirmed by angiography. Determinations of the conduction velocities of the ulnar and other peripheral nerves of the upper extremity may help to localize the site of their compression.

Thoracic outlet syndrome must be differentiated

from osteoarthritis of the cervical spine, tumors of the cervical spinal cord or nerve roots, and periarthritis of the shoulder.

Treatment is directed toward relief of compression of the neurovascular bundle. Overhead pulley exercises are useful to improve posture. Shoulder bracing, although uncomfortable, provides a constant stimulus to improve posture. When lying down, the shoulder girdle should be bolstered by arranging pillows in an inverted "V" position.

Symptoms may disappear spontaneously or may be relieved by conservative treatment. Operative treatment is more likely to relieve the neurologic rather than the vascular component that causes symptoms.

CALCIFIC TENDINITIS OF THE SHOULDER

Calcific tendinitis of the shoulder joint is an acute or chronic inflammatory disorder of the capsulotendinous cuff (especially the supraspinatus portion) characterized by deposits of calcium salts among tendon fibers. It is a common cause of acute pain near the lateral aspect of the shoulder joint in men over age 30. The calcium deposit may be restricted to the tendon substance or may rupture into the overlying bursa.

Symptoms consist of pain (at times severe), tenderness to pressure, and restriction of shoulder joint motion. Radiographic examination confirms the diagnosis and demonstrates the site of the lesion.

Calcific tendinitis must be differentiated from other cervicobrachial pain syndromes, pyogenic arthritis, osteoarthritis, gout, Pancoast tumors, and tears of the rotator cuff.

The aim of treatment is to relieve pain and restore shoulder joint function. Pain is best treated by injection of the lesion with a local anesthetic with corticosteroid. NSAIDs are also effective. Acute symptoms occasionally subside after spontaneous rupture of the calcium deposit into the subacromial bursa. Chronic symptoms may be treated by analgesics, exercises, and injection of local anesthetics with 20–40 mg of triamcinolone; repeated injections should be avoided. Rarely, calcific deposits may require surgical evacuation.

When x-ray examination shows disappearance of a deposit, recurrence is rare. Symptoms persist if shoulder joint motion is not fully regained.

SCAPULOHUMERAL PERIARTHRITIS (Adhesive Capsulitis, Frozen Shoulder)

Periarthritis of the shoulder joint is an inflammatory disorder primarily involving the soft tissues. The condition may be divided into a primary type, in which no obvious cause can be identified, and a secondary type associated with an organic lesion (eg, rheumatoid arthritis, osteoarthritis, fracture or dislocation). The primary type is most common among women after the fourth decade. It may be manifested as inflammation of the articular synovia, the tendons around the joint, the intrinsic ligamentous capsular bands, the paratendinous bursae (especially the subacromial), or the bicipital tendon sheath. Calcific tendinitis and attritional disease of the rotator cuff, with or without tears, are incidental lesions.

The onset of pain, which is aggravated by extremes of shoulder joint motion, may be acute or insidious. Pain may be most annoying at night and may be intensified by pressure on the involved extremity when the patient sleeps in the lateral decubitus position. Tenderness upon palpation is often noted near the tendinous insertions into the greater tuberosity or over the bicipital groove. Although a sensation of stiffness may be noted only at onset, restriction of shoulder joint motion soon becomes apparent and is likely to progress unless effective treatment is instituted.

Pain can often be controlled with nonsteroidal anti-inflammatory agents. Passive exercise of the shoulder by an overhead pulley mechanism should be repeated slowly for about 2 minutes four times daily. Injection of tender areas with corticosteroids gives transitory relief. Operative treatment should be reserved for the occasional refractory case.

LOW BACK PAIN

Low back pain is exceedingly common, experienced at some time by up to 80% of the population, and ranks second among reason for doctor office visits. The differential diagnosis is broad and includes primary spine disease (eg, disk herniation, degenerative arthritis), systemic diseases (eg, metastatic cancer), and regional diseases (eg, aortic aneurysm). A precise diagnosis cannot be made in the majority of cases. Even when anatomic defects—such as vertebral osteophytes or a narrowed disk space—are present, clinical disease cannot be assumed since such defects are common in asymptomatic patients. The majority of patients will improve in 1–4 weeks and need no evaluation beyond the initial history and physical examination. The diagnostic challenge is to identify those patients who require more extensive or urgent evaluation.

In practice, this means identifying those patients with pain caused by (1) infection, (2) cancer, (3) inflammatory back disease such as ankylosing spondylitis, (4) or nonrheumatologic conditions, especially leaking aortic aneurysm. Significant or progressive neurologic deficits also require identification. If there is no evidence of these problems, conservative therapy is called for.

1. CLINICAL APPROACH TO DIAGNOSIS

General History & Physical Examination

The most common mistake in evaluating patients with low back pain is failing to perform a detailed physical examination. Low back pain is a final common pathway of many processes; the pain of vertebral osteomyelitis, for example, is not very different in quality and intensity from the pain due to back strain of the weekend gardener. Historical factors of importance include smoking, weight loss, age over 50, and cancer, all of which are risk factors for vertebral body metastasis. Osteomyelitis most frequently occurs in adults with a history of recurrent urinary tract infections and is especially common in diabetics.

Previous peptic ulcer disease suggests that a patient's back pain is due to a penetrating ulcer. A history of cardiac murmurs should raise concern about endocarditis, since back pain is a not uncommon manifestation. A history of renal stones might indicate another serious cause of referred back pain.

History of the Back Pain

Certain qualities of a patient's pain can indicate a specific diagnosis. Low back pain radiating down the buttock and below the knee suggests a herniated disk causing nerve root irritation. Other conditions—including sacroiliitis, facet joint degenerative arthritis, spinal stenosis, or irritation of the sciatic nerve from a wallet—can also cause this pattern.

The diagnosis of disk herniation is further suggested by physical examination (see below) and confirmed by imaging techniques. Disk herniation can be asymptomatic, so its presence does not invariably link it to the symptom.

Low back pain at night, unrelieved by rest or the supine position, should suggest the possibility of malignancy, either vertebral body metastasis (chiefly from prostate, breast, lung, multiple myeloma, or lymphoma) or a cauda equina tumor. Similar pain can also be caused by compression fractures (from osteoporosis or myeloma).

Symptoms of large or rapidly evolving neurologic deficits identify patients who need urgent evaluation for possible cauda equina tumor, epidural abscess, or, rarely, massive disk herniation. Even with a herniated disk and nerve root impingement, pain is the most prominent symptom; numbness and weakness are less commonly reported and when present are of the magnitude consistent with compression of a single nerve root. Thus, symptoms of bilateral leg weakness (from multiple lumbar nerve root compressions) or of saddle area anesthesia, bowel or bladder incontinence, or impotence (indicating multiple sacral nerve root compressions) indicate a cauda equina process.

Low back pain that worsens with rest and improves with activity is characteristic of ankylosing spondylitis or other seronegative spondyloarthropathies, especially when the onset is insidious and begins before age 40. Most degenerative back diseases produce precisely the opposite pattern, with rest alleviating and activity aggravating the pain.

Low back pain causing the patient to writhe occurs in renal colic but can also indicate a leaking aneurysm.

Low back pain associated with pseudoclaudication often indicates spinal stenosis. The typical patient is bothered less by back pain than by a discomfort occurring in the buttock, thigh, or leg that (like true claudication) is brought on by walking but (unlike claudication) can also be elicited by prolonged standing. The discomfort is frequently bilateral. Classically, the pain is improved with rest or with flexion of the lumbar spine; patients have less difficulty walking uphill than downhill. Some patients complain less about leg discomfort and more about an exercise-dependent weakness, unsteadiness, or stiffness of the legs.

Physical Examination of the Back

Although examination of the back usually does not suggest a specific cause, several physical findings should be sought because they do help identify those few patients who need more than just conservative management.

Neurologic examination of the lower extremities will detect the small deficits produced by disk disease and the large deficits complicating such problems as cauda equina tumors. A positive straight leg raising test indicates nerve root irritation. The examiner performs the test on the supine patient by passively raising the patient's leg. The test is positive if radicular pain is produced with the leg raised 60 degrees or less. The test is has a specificity of 40% but is 95% sensitive in patients with herniation at the L4–5 or L5–S1 level (the sites of 95% of disk herniations). It can be falsely negative, especially in patients with herniation above the L4–5 level.

The crossed straight leg sign is only 25% sensitive but is 90% specific for disk herniation and is positive when raising the contralateral leg reproduces the sciatica.

Detailed examination of the sacral and lumbar nerve roots, especially L5 and S1, is essential for detecting neurologic deficits associated with back pain. Disk herniation produces deficits predictable for the site involved (Table 20–6). Deficits of multiple nerve roots suggest a cauda equina tumor, an epidural abscess, or some other important process that requires urgent evaluation and treatment.

Measurement of spinal motion in the patient with acute pain is rarely of diagnostic utility and usually simply confirms that pain limits motion. An excep-

Table 20–6. Neurologic testing of lumbosacral nerve disorders.

Nerve Root	Motor	Reflex	Sensory Area
L4	Dorsiflexion of foot	Knee jerk	Medial calf
L5	Dorsiflexion of great toe	None	Medial fore-foot
S1	Eversion of foot	Ankle jerk	Lateral foot

tion to this general rule is that evidence of decreased range of motion in multiple regions of the spine (cervical, thoracic, and lumbar) indicates a diffuse spinal disease such as ankylosing spondylitis. But by the time the patient has such limits, the diagnosis is usually not a mystery.

If the back pain is not severe and does not itself limit motion, Schober's test of lumbar motion is helpful in early diagnosis of ankylosing spondylitis. To perform this test, two marks are made, one 10 cm above S1 and another 5 cm below. The patient then bends forward as far as possible, and the distraction between the points is measured. Normally, the points distract at least 5 cm. Anything less indicates reduced lumbar motion, which in the absence of severe pain is most commonly due to ankylosing spondylitis or other seronegative spondyloarthropathies.

Palpation of the spine usually does not yield diagnostic information. Point tenderness over a vertebral body is reported to suggest osteomyelitis, but this association is uncommon. A step-off noted between the spinous process of adjacent vertebral bodies may indicate spondylolisthesis, but the sensitivity of this finding is extremely low. Tenderness of the soft tissues overlying the greater trochanter of the hip is a manifestation of trochanteric bursitis.

Inspection of the spine is not often of value in identifying serious causes of low back pain. The classic posture of ankylosing spondylitis is a late finding. Scoliosis of mild degree is not associated with an increased risk of clinical back disease. Cutaneous neurofibromas can identify the very rare patient who has nerve root encasement.

Examination of the hips should be part of the complete examination. While hip arthritis usually produces groin pain, some patients have buttock or low back symptoms.

Further Examination

If the history and physical examination do not suggest the presence of infection, cancer, inflammatory back disease, major neurologic deficits, or pain referred from abdominal or pelvic disease, further evaluation can be eliminated or deferred while conservative therapy is tried. The great majority of patients will spontaneously improve with conservative care over 1–4 weeks.

Regular radiographs of the lumbosacral spine give 20 times the radiation dose of a chest x-ray and provide limited, albeit important, information. X-rays can provide evidence of vertebral body osteomyelitis, cancer, fractures, or ankylosing spondylitis. Degenerative changes in the lumbar spine are ubiquitous in patients over 40 and do not prove clinical disease. Plain x-rays have very low sensitivity or specificity for disk disease. Thus, plain x-rays are warranted promptly for patients suspected of having infection, cancer, fractures, or inflammation; selected other patients who fail to improve after 2–4 weeks of conservative therapy are also candidates.

MRI provides exquisite anatomic detail but is reserved for patients in whom the information would change therapy. It is needed urgently in any patient suspected of having an epidural mass or cauda equina tumor but not if a patient is suspected of having a routine disk herniation, since most such patients will improve over 4–6 weeks of conservative therapy. Noncontrast CT does not image cauda equina tumors or other intradural lesions, and if used instead of MRI it must include intrathecal contrast.

Radionuclide bone scanning has limited utility. It is most useful for early detection of vertebral body osteomyelitis or metastases. The bone scan is often normal in multiple myeloma because lytic lesions do not take up isotope.

2. MANAGEMENT

While any management plan must be individualized, key elements of most conservative treatments for back pain include analgesia and education. Analgesia can usually be provided with NSAIDs, but severe pain may require opioids. Rarely does the need for opioids extend beyond 1–2 weeks, and they are contraindicated in the management of chronic low back pain.

Limited evidence supports the use of "muscle relaxants" such as diazepam, cyclobenzaprine, carisoprodol, and methocarbamol. These drugs should be reserved for patients who fail NSAIDs and should also be limited to courses of 1–2 weeks. Their use should be avoided in older patients, who are at risk of falling. All patients should be taught how to protect the back in daily activities—ie, not to lift heavy objects, to use the legs rather than the back when lifting, to use a chair with arm rests, and to rise from bed by first rolling to one side and then using the arms to push to an upright position. Back manipulation for benign, mechanical low back pain appears safe and as effective as therapies provided by physicians.

Rest and back exercises, once thought to be cornerstones of conservative therapy, are now known to be ineffective for acute back pain. Two days of bed rest gives better results than 7 days. Indeed, no bed rest with continuation of ordinary activities as tolerated is superior to either 2 days of bed rest or back mobilizing exercises. The value of corsets or traction is dubious. The efficacy of epidural corticosteroid injections in treating sciatica is still being debated. Corticosteroid injections into facet joints are ineffective for chronic low back pain.

Surgical consultation is needed urgently for any patient with a large or evolving neurologic deficit. Surgery for disk disease is indicated when there is documentation of herniation by some imaging procedure, a consistent pain syndrome, and a consistent neurologic deficit that has failed to respond to 4–6 weeks of conservative therapy. Percutaneous lumbar discectomy, performed under local anesthesia, is a safe and effective (up to 75%) alternative to laminectomy. The percutaneous procedure is contraindicated in the presence of tumor, infection, spondylolisthesis, foraminal stenosis, loose disk fragments, or severe facet joint arthritis.

Complaints without objective findings suggest a psychologic role in symptom formation. Treatment includes reassurance and nonopioid analgesics.

[AHCPR guideline on acute low back problems in adults] http://text.nlm.nih.gov/ftrs/gateway

Carey TS et al: The outcomes and costs of care for acute low back pain among patients seen by primary care practitioners, chiropractors, and orthopedic surgeons. N Engl J Med 1995;333:913. (Outcomes are similar. Primary care physicians provide the least expensive care.)

Deen HG Jr: Diagnosis and management of lumbar disk disease. Mayo Clin Proc 1996;71:283.

Katz JN et al: Degenerative lumbar spinal stenosis: Diagnostic value of the history and physical examination. Arthritis Rheum 1995;38:1236. (Severe lower extremity pain, absence of pain when seated, wide-based gait, and thigh pain following 30 seconds of lumbar extension help identify patients with lumbar spinal stenosis.)

Malmivaara A et al: The treatment of acute low back pain—bed rest, exercises, or ordinary activity? N Engl J Med 1995;332:351. (Continuing ordinary activities as tolerated better than 2 days of bed rest or back-mobilizing exercises.)

FIBROSITIS

Essentials of Diagnosis

- Chronic widespread musculoskeletal pain syndrome with multiple tender points.
- Fatigue, headaches, numbness common.
- Most frequent in women aged 20–50.
- Objective signs of inflammation absent; laboratory studies normal.
- Partially responsive to exercise, amitriptyline.

General Considerations

Fibrositis (also called fibromyalgia) is one of the most common rheumatic syndromes in ambulatory general medicine affecting 3–10% of the general population. It shares many features with the chronic fatigue syndrome, namely, an increased frequency among women aged 20–50, absence of objective findings, and absence of diagnostic laboratory tests. While many of the clinical features of the two conditions overlap, musculoskeletal pain predominates in fibrositis whereas lassitude dominates the chronic fatigue syndrome.

The cause is unknown, but sleep disorders, depression, viral infections, and aberrant perception of normal stimuli have all been proposed. Fibrositis can be a complication of hypothyroidism, rheumatoid arthritis, or, in men, sleep apnea.

Clinical Findings

The patient complains of chronic aching pain and stiffness, frequently involving the entire body but with prominence of pain around the neck, shoulders, low back, and hips. Fatigue, sleep disorders, subjective numbness, chronic headaches, and irritable bowel symptoms are common. The patient feels incapable of performing normal activities, and even minor exertion aggravates pain and increases fatigue. Patients occasionally trace the onset of symptoms to an acute event or viral-like illness. Physical examination is normal except for "trigger points" of pain produced by palpation of various areas such as the trapezius, the medial fat pad of the knee, and the lateral epicondyle of the elbow.

Differential Diagnosis

Fibrositis is a diagnosis of exclusion. A detailed history and repeated physical examination can obviate the need for extensive laboratory testing. Rheumatoid arthritis and systemic lupus erythematosus virtually always present with objective physical findings or abnormalities on routine testing, including the erythrocyte sedimentation rate. Thyroid function tests are useful, since hypothyroidism can produce a secondary fibromyalgia syndrome. Polymyositis produces weakness rather than pain. The diagnosis of fibrositis probably should be made hesitantly in a patient over age 50 and should never be invoked to explain fever, weight loss, or any other objective signs. Polymyalgia rheumatica produces shoulder and girdle pain, is associated with anemia and an elevated sedimentation rate, and occurs after age 50.

Treatment

Patient education is of paramount importance. Patients can be comforted by the knowledge that they have a recognizable diagnosable syndrome that can be managed by means of specific though imperfect therapies and that the course is not progressive. Placebo-controlled trials have demonstrated modest efficacy of amitriptyline, fluoxetine, chlorpromazine, or cyclobenzaprine. Amitriptyline is initiated at a dosage of 10 mg at bedtime and gradually increased to 40–50 mg depending on its efficacy and toxicity. Exercise programs are also beneficial. NSAIDs are generally ineffective. Opioids and corticosteroids are ineffective and should never be used to treat fibrositis.

Prognosis

Most patients have chronic symptoms. With treatment, however, many do eventually resume increased activities. Progressive or objective findings do not develop.

Carette S et al: Comparison of amitriptyline, cyclobenzaprine, and placebo in the treatment of fibromyalgia: A randomized, double-blind clinical trial. Arthritis Rheum 1994;37:32. (Both more effective than placebo, but only one-third significantly improved after 6 months of therapy.)

Goldenberg D et al: A randomized double-blind crossover trial of fluoxetine and amitriptyline in the treatment of fibromyalgia. Arthritis Rheum 1996;39:1852. (Both work; the combination is better.)

CARPAL TUNNEL SYNDROME

Carpal tunnel syndrome is a common painful disorder caused by compression of the median nerve between the carpal ligament and other structures within the carpal tunnel (entrapment neuropathy). The volume of the contents of the tunnel can be increased by organic lesions such as synovitis of the tendon sheaths or carpal joints, recent or malhealed fractures, tumors, and occasionally congenital anomalies. Even though no anatomic lesion is apparent, flattening or even circumferential constriction of the median nerve may be observed during operative section of the ligament. The disorder may occur in pregnancy, is seen in individuals with a history of repetitive use of the hands, and may follow injuries of the wrists. A familial type of carpal tunnel syndrome has been reported in which no etiologic factor can be identified.

Carpal tunnel syndrome can also be a feature of many systemic diseases: rheumatoid arthritis and other rheumatic disorders (inflammatory tenosynovitis); myxedema, amyloidosis, sarcoidosis, and leukemia (tissue infiltration); acromegaly; hyperparathyroidism, hypocalcemia, and diabetes mellitus.

Clinical Findings

Pain in the distribution of the median nerve, which may be burning and tingling (acroparesthesia), is the initial symptom. Aching pain may radiate proximally into the forearm and occasionally proximally to the shoulder, neck, and chest. Pain is exacerbated by manual activity, particularly by extremes of volar flexion or dorsiflexion of the wrist. It may be most bothersome at night. Impairment of sensation in the median nerve distribution may not be apparent. Subtle disparity between the affected and opposite sides can be demonstrated by testing for two-point discrimination or by requiring the patient to identify different textures of cloth by rubbing them between the tips of the thumb and the index finger. Tinel's or Phalen's sign may be positive. (Tinel's sign is tingling or shock-like pain on volar wrist percussion; Phalen's sign, pain or paresthesia in the distribution of the median nerve when the patient flexes both wrists to 90 degrees with the dorsal aspects of the hands held in apposition for 60 seconds.) The carpal compression test, performed by applying direct pressure on the carpal tunnel, may be more sensitive and specific than the Tinel and Phalen tests. Muscle weakness or atrophy, especially of the abductor pollicis brevis, appears later than sensory disturbances. Useful special examinations include electromyography and determinations of segmental sensory and motor conduction delay. Distal median sensory conduction delay may be evident before motor delay.

Differential Diagnosis

This syndrome should be differentiated from other cervicobrachial pain syndromes, from compression syndromes of the median nerve in the forearm or arm, and from mononeuritis multiplex. When left-sided, it may be confused with angina pectoris.

Treatment

Treatment is directed toward relief of pressure on the median nerve. When a primary lesion is discovered, specific treatment should be given. When soft tissue swelling is a cause, elevation of the extremity may relieve symptoms. Splinting of the hand and forearm at night may be beneficial. Injection of corticosteroid into the carpal tunnel can alleviate symptoms in some patients, particularly those with synovitis of the wrist. To reduce the chance of nerve injury, this injection should be performed by a physician thoroughly familiar with the anatomy of the carpal tunnel.

Operative division of the volar carpal ligament gives lasting relief from pain, which usually subsides within a few days. Muscle strength returns gradually, but complete recovery cannot be expected when atrophy is pronounced.

EPICONDYLITIS
(Tennis Elbow, Epicondylalgia)

Epicondylitis is a pain syndrome affecting the mid portion of the upper extremity; no single causative lesion has been identified. It has been postulated that chronic strain of the forearm muscles due to repetitive grasping or rotatory motions of the forearm causes microscopic tears and subsequent chronic inflammation of the common extensor or common flexor tendon at or near their respective osseous origins from the epicondyles.

Epicondylitis occurs most frequently in the dominant extremity during middle life. Pain is predominantly on the medial or lateral aspect of the elbow region, may be aggravated by grasping, and may radiate proximally into the arm or distally into the forearm. The point of maximal tenderness to pressure is 1–2 cm distal to the epicondyle but may also be present in the muscle bellies more distally. Resisted dorsiflexion or volar flexion of the wrist may accentuate the pain. The elbow joint has normal range of motion, is not swollen, and appears normal on x-ray.

Treatment is directed toward relief of pain. Most symptoms can be relieved by rest and NSAIDs. An elastic bandage applied about the proximal forearm may ameliorate discomfort when the patient is grasping forcefully. Infiltration of "trigger points" by local anesthetic solutions with corticosteroids may be helpful. Operative treatment is reserved for severe, refractory cases.

DUPUYTREN'S CONTRACTURE

This relatively common disorder is characterized by hyperplasia of the palmar fascia and related structures, with nodule formation and contracture of the palmar fascia. The cause is unknown, but the condition has a genetic predisposition and occurs primarily in white men over 50 years of age. The incidence of Dupuytren's contracture is higher among alcoholics and patients with chronic systemic disorders (eg, cirrhosis, diabetes, epilepsy, tuberculosis). The onset may be acute, but slowly progressive chronic disease is more common.

Dupuytren's contracture manifests itself by nodular or cord-like thickening of one or both hands, with the fourth and fifth fingers most commonly affected. The patient may complain of tightness of the involved digits, with inability to satisfactorily extend the fingers, and on occasion there is tenderness. The resulting functional and cosmetic problems may be extremely disabling, but in general the contracture is well tolerated since it exaggerates the normal position of function of the hand. Fasciitis involving other areas of the body may lead to plantar fibromatosis (10% of patients) or Peyronie's disease (1–2%).

If the palmar nodule is growing rapidly, injections of triamcinolone into the nodule may be of benefit. Surgical intervention is indicated in patients with significant flexion contractures, depending on the location, but recurrence is not uncommon.

REFLEX SYMPATHETIC DYSTROPHY

Reflex sympathetic dystrophy is a syndrome of pain and swelling of an extremity accompanied by signs of trophic skin changes in the extremity (eg, skin atrophy, hyperhidrosis) and signs and symptoms of vasomotor instability. Any extremity can be involved, but the disorder most commonly occurs in the hand and is associated with ipsilateral restricted shoulder motion (shoulder-hand syndrome). The swelling in reflex sympathetic dystrophy is diffuse ("catcher's mitt hand") and not restricted to joints. Pain is often described as burning in quality. The **shoulder-hand variant** of reflex sympathetic dystrophy is common after neck or shoulder injuries or following myocardial infarction. Direct trauma to the hand or foot can also provoke this syndrome. Reflex sympathetic dystrophy can also develop after a knee injury or after arthroscopic knee surgery. There are no systemic symptoms, and x-rays reveal severe generalized osteopenia. The severe osteoporosis occurring in the posttraumatic variant of reflex sympathetic dystrophy is known as Sudeck's atrophy. Bone scans also show increased uptake. In a significant minority of cases, symptoms and findings are bilateral.

This syndrome should be differentiated from other cervicobrachial pain syndromes, rheumatoid arthritis, polymyositis, scleroderma, and gout.

In addition to specific treatment of the underlying disorder, treatment is directed toward restoration of function. For most patients, physical therapy is the cornerstone of treatment. Patients who have restricted shoulder motion may benefit from the treatment described for scapulohumeral periarthritis. In resistant cases, prednisone, 30–40 mg/d for 2 weeks and then tapered off over 2 weeks, may be effective. Stellate ganglion block can also be effective for reflex sympathetic dystrophy.

The prognosis depends in part upon the stage in which the lesions are encountered and the extent and severity of associated organic disease. Early treatment offers the best prognosis for recovery.

BURSITIS

Inflammation of the synovium-like cellular membrane overlying bony prominences may be secondary to trauma, infection, or arthritic conditions such as gout, rheumatoid arthritis, or osteoarthritis. The most common locations are the subdeltoid, olecranon, ischial, trochanteric, semimembranous-gastrocnemius (Baker's cyst) and prepatellar bursae.

There are several ways to distinguish bursitis from arthritis. Bursitis is more likely than arthritis to begin abruptly and cause focal tenderness and swelling. Olecranon bursitis, for example, causes a "goose egg" swelling at the tip of the elbow, whereas elbow joint inflammation causes more diffuse swelling. Similarly, a patient with prepatellar bursitis has a small focus of swelling over the kneecap and no distention of the knee joint itself. Active and passive range of motion are usually much more limited in arthritis than in bursitis. A patient with trochanteric bursitis will have normal internal rotation of the hip, whereas a patient with hip arthritis will not. Bursitis caused by trauma responds to local heat, rest, immobilization, NSAIDs, and local corticosteroid injections.

Bursitis can result from infection. The two most common sites are the olecranon and prepatellar bursae. Acute bursitis at these two sites calls for aspiration to rule out infection. The absence of fever does not exclude infection, and one-third of those with septic olecranon bursitis have no fever. A bursal fluid white blood cell count of greater than 1000/μL indicates inflammation from infection, rheumatoid arthritis, or gout. In septic bursitis, the white cell count averages over 50,000/μL. Most cases are caused by *Staphylococcus aureus;* Gram stain is positive in only two-thirds. Treatment involves antibiotics and repeated aspiration for tense effusions.

A bursa can also become symptomatic when it ruptures. This is particularly true for Baker's cyst, whose rupture can cause calf pain and swelling that mimic thrombophlebitis. The ruptured cyst can be imaged with sonography, MRI, or arthrography. In most cases, none of these tests are necessary because Baker's cyst or the frequently associated knee effusion is detectable on physical examination. Often it is more important to exclude thrombophlebitis than it is to visualize Baker's cyst. Treatment of a ruptured cyst includes rest, leg elevation, and injection of triamcinolone, 20–40 mg into the knee (which communicates with the cyst). Rarely, Baker's cyst can compress vascular structures and cause leg edema and true thrombophlebitis.

JOGGING INJURIES

The beneficial effects on cardiovascular function and the sense of well-being associated with aerobic activity have led to considerable enthusiasm for jogging and running. This has resulted in a large number of transient musculoskeletal injuries, which are estimated to occur in about 75% of runners. Many of the deleterious effects can be prevented by appropriate precautions, such as stretching exercises, proper footwear, avoidance of overexertion, and prompt attention to injuries. After an injury has healed, a graduated schedule for returning to training is necessary to avoid recurrence. Since injuries occur frequently in long-distance runners, it is most important that these individuals avoid overexertion, and, when early signs of injury appear, reduce the distance run.

Fries JF et al: Relationship of running to musculoskeletal pain with age: A six-year longitudinal study. Arthritis Rheum 1996;39:64. (Running not associated with an increase in musculoskeletal pain with age and is associated with decreased disability and mortality rates.)

AUTOIMMUNE DISEASES

The autoimmune disorders are a protean group of acquired diseases in which genetic factors appear to play a role. They have in common widespread immunologic and inflammatory alterations of connective tissue.

These illnesses share certain clinical features, and differentiation among them is often difficult because of this. Common findings include synovitis, pleuritis, myocarditis, endocarditis, pericarditis, peritonitis, vasculitis, myositis, skin rash, alterations of connective tissues, and nephritis. Laboratory tests may reveal Coombs-positive hemolytic anemia, thrombocytopenia, leukopenia, immunoglobulin excesses or deficiencies, antinuclear antibodies (which include antibodies to many nuclear constituents, including DNA and extractable nuclear antigen), rheumatoid factors, cryoglobulins, false-positive serologic tests for syphilis, elevated muscle enzymes, and alterations in serum complement.

Some of the laboratory alterations that occur in this group of diseases (eg, false-positive serologic tests for syphilis, rheumatoid factor) occur in asymptomatic individuals. These changes may also be demonstrated in certain asymptomatic relatives of patients with connective tissue diseases, in older persons, in patients using certain drugs, and in patients with chronic infectious diseases.

RHEUMATOID ARTHRITIS

Essentials of Diagnosis

- Prodromal systemic symptoms of malaise, fever, weight loss, and morning stiffness.
- Onset usually insidious and in small joints; progression is centripetal and symmetric; deformities common.
- Radiographic findings: juxta-articular osteoporosis, joint erosions, and narrowing of the joint spaces.
- Rheumatoid factor usually present.
- Extra-articular manifestations: subcutaneous nodules, pleural effusion, pericarditis, lymphadenopathy, splenomegaly with leukopenia, and vasculitis.

General Considerations

Rheumatoid arthritis is a chronic systemic inflammatory disease of unknown cause, chiefly affecting synovial membranes of multiple joints. The disease has a wide clinical spectrum with considerable variability in joint and extra-articular manifestations. The prevalence in the general population is 1–2%; female patients outnumber males almost 3:1. The usual age at onset is 20–40 years, although rheumatoid arthritis may begin at any age. Susceptibility to rheumatoid arthritis is genetically determined. Most patients have a class 2 human leukocyte antigen (HLA) with an identical five-amino-acid sequence.

The pathologic findings in the joint include chronic synovitis with pannus formation. The pannus erodes cartilage, bone, ligaments, and tendons. In the acute phase, effusion and other manifestations of inflammation are common. In the late stage, organization may result in fibrous ankylosis; true bony ankylosis is rare. In both acute and chronic phases, inflammation of soft tissues around the joints may be prominent and is a significant factor in joint damage.

The microscopic findings most characteristic of rheumatoid arthritis are those of the subcutaneous nodule. This is a granuloma with a central zone of fibrinoid necrosis, a surrounding palisade of radially arranged elongated connective tissue cells, and a periphery of chronic granulation tissue. Pathologic alterations indistinguishable from those of the subcutaneous nodule are occasionally seen in the myocardium, pericardium, endocardium, heart valves, visceral pleura, lungs, sclera, dura mater, spleen, and larynx as well as in the synovial membrane, periarticular tissues, and tendons. Nonspecific pericarditis and pleuritis are found in 25–40% of patients at autopsy. Additional nonspecific lesions associated with rheumatoid arthritis include inflammation of small arteries, pulmonary fibrosis, mononuclear cell infiltration of skeletal muscle and perineurium, and hyperplasia of lymph nodes. Secondary amyloidosis may also be present.

Clinical Findings

A. Symptoms and Signs: The clinical manifestations of rheumatoid disease are highly variable. The onset of articular signs of inflammation is usually insidious, with prodromal symptoms of malaise, weight loss, and vague periarticular pain or stiffness. Less often, the onset is acute, apparently triggered by a stressful situation such as infection, surgery, trauma, emotional strain, or the postpartum period. There is characteristically symmetric joint swelling with associated stiffness, warmth, tenderness, and pain. Stiffness is prominent in the morning and subsides during the day; its duration is a useful indicator of activity of disease. Stiffness may recur after daytime inactivity and may be much more severe after strenuous activity. Although any joint may be affected in rheumatoid arthritis, the proximal interphalangeal and metacarpophalangeal joints of the fingers as well as the wrists, knees, ankles, and toes are most often involved. Monarticular disease is occasionally seen early. Synovial cysts and rupture of tendons may occur. Entrapment syndromes are not unusual—particularly entrapment of the median nerve at the carpal tunnel of the wrist. Palmar erythema is noted occasionally, as are tiny hemorrhagic infarcts in the nail folds or finger pulps, which are signs of vasculitis. Twenty percent of patients have subcutaneous nodules, most commonly situated over bony prominences but also observed in the bursas and tendon sheaths; these nearly always occur in seropositive patients, as do most other extra-articular manifestations. A small number of patients have splenomegaly and lymph node enlargement. Low-grade fever, anorexia, weight loss, fatigue, and weakness often persist; chills are rare. After months or years, deformities may occur; the most common are ulnar deviation of the fingers, "swan-neck" deformity (hyperextension of the distal interphalangeal joint with flexion of the proximal interphalangeal joint), boutonnière deformity (flexion of the distal interphalangeal with extension of the proximal interphalangeal joint), and valgus deformity of the knee. Atrophy of skin or muscle is common. Dryness of the eyes, mouth, and other mucous membranes is found especially in advanced disease (see Sjögren's Syndrome). Other ocular manifestations include episcleritis and scleromalacia, often due to scleral nodules. Pericarditis and pleural disease, when present, are frequently silent clinically. Aortitis is a rare late complication that can result in aortic regurgitation or rupture and is usually associated with evidence of rheumatoid vasculitis elsewhere in the body.

B. Laboratory Findings: Serum protein abnormalities are often present. Rheumatoid factor, an IgM antibody directed against the Fc fragment of IgG, is present in the sera of more than 75% of patients. High titers of rheumatoid factor are commonly associated with severe rheumatoid disease. Titers may also be significantly elevated in a number of diverse conditions, including syphilis, sarcoidosis, infective endocarditis, tuberculosis, leprosy, and parasitic infections; in advanced age; and in asymptomatic relatives of patients with autoimmune diseases. Antinuclear antibodies are demonstrable in 20% of patients, though their titers are lower in rheumatoid arthritis than in systemic lupus erythematosus.

During both the acute and chronic phases, the erythrocyte sedimentation rate and the gamma globulins (most commonly IgM and IgG) are typically elevated. A moderate hypochromic normocytic anemia is common. The white cell count is normal or slightly elevated, but leukopenia may occur, often in the presence of splenomegaly (eg, Felty's syndrome). The platelet count is often elevated, roughly in proportion to the severity of overall joint inflammation. Joint fluid examination is valuable, reflecting abnormalities that are associated with varying degrees of inflammation. (See Tables 20–1 and 20–2.)

C. Imaging: Of all the laboratory tests, x-ray changes are the most specific for rheumatoid arthritis. X-rays, however, are not sensitive in that most of those taken during the first 6 months are read as normal. The earliest changes occur in the wrists or feet and consist of soft tissue swelling and juxta-articular demineralization. Later, diagnostic changes of uniform joint space narrowing and erosions develop. The erosions are often first evident at the ulnar styloid and at the juxta-articular margin, where the bony surface is not protected by cartilage. Diagnostic changes also occur in the cervical spine, with C1–2 subluxation, but these changes usually take several years to develop.

Differential Diagnosis

The differentiation of rheumatoid arthritis from other diseases of connective tissue can be difficult. However, certain clinical features are helpful. Rheumatic fever is characterized by the migratory nature of the arthritis, an elevated antistreptolysin titer, and a more dramatic and prompt response to aspirin; carditis and erythema marginatum may occur in adults, but chorea and subcutaneous nodules virtually never do. Butterfly rash, discoid lupus erythematosus, photosensitivity, alopecia, high titer to anti-DNA, renal disease, and central nervous system abnormalities point to the diagnosis of systemic lupus erythematosus. Degenerative joint disease (osteoarthritis) is not associated with constitutional manifestations, and the joint pain is characteristically relieved by rest, in contrast to the morning stiffness of rheumatoid arthritis. Signs of articular inflammation, prominent in rheumatoid arthritis, are usually minimal in degenerative joint disease. Osteoarthritis—in contrast to rheumatoid arthritis—spares the wrist and the metacarpophalangeal joints. While in the early years gouty arthritis is almost always intermittent and monarticular, in later years it can become a chronic polyarticular process that mimics rheumatoid arthritis. Gouty tophi can at times resemble rheumatoid nodules. The early history of intermittent monarthritis and the presence of synovial urate crystals are distinctive features of gout. Pyogenic arthritis can be distinguished by chills and fever, demonstration of the causative organism in joint fluid, and the frequent presence of a primary focus elsewhere, eg, gonococcal arthritis. Chronic Lyme disease typically involves only one joint, most commonly the knee, and is associated with positive serologic tests (see Chapter 34). Human parvovirus B19 infection in adults can occasionally mimic rheumatoid arthritis. The mean age at onset is 35–37; arthralgias are much more prominent than arthritis; and rash—on the cheeks, torso, or extremities—is common. The patients are rheumatoid factor-negative, do not have erosions, and have serologic evidence of recent human parvovirus B19 infection (ie, serum positive for anti-parvovirus B19 IgM antibody). Polymyalgia rheumatica occasionally causes polyarthritis in patients over age 50, but these patients remain rheumatoid factor-negative and have chiefly proximal muscle pain and stiffness. A variety of cancers produce paraneoplastic syndromes, including polyarthritis. One form is hypertrophic pulmonary osteoarthropathy most often produced by lung and gastrointestinal carcinomas, characterized by a rheumatoid-like arthritis associated with clubbing, periosteal new bone formation, and a negative rheumatoid factor. Diffuse swelling of the hands with palmar fasciitis has also been reported with a variety of cancers, especially ovarian carcinoma.

Treatment

A. Basic Program (Nonpharmacologic Management): The primary objectives in treating rheumatoid arthritis are reduction of inflammation and pain, preservation of function, and prevention of deformity. To a large extent, patient satisfaction and the success of therapy depend on how effectively the physician utilizes the nonpharmacologic measures outlined in the following paragraphs.

1. Education and emotional factors–Chronic diseases such as rheumatoid arthritis challenge the belief that individuals have control over their lives. This feeling of helplessness may be more disabling than the disease itself. The physician should explain the disease, describe its fluctuations, and involve the patient in how decisions about therapy will be made. Most patients think of "treatment" as a brief course of drug followed by rapid recovery. The concept of chronic disease control and empiric treatment employing different agents in series must be explained if the patient is to have confidence in the physician. Education of the family and loved ones serves as a source of the emotional support so critical to the patient's long-term well-being.

2. Physical and occupational therapies–Physical and occupational therapists understand nonpharmacologic treatments of arthritis (described below) and can effectively teach them. The therapist can develop a program the patient can follow at home, with only periodic monitoring.

3. Systemic rest–The amount of systemic rest required depends upon the presence and severity of inflammation. Complete bed rest may be desirable in patients with profound systemic and articular inflammation, as can occur in rheumatoid arthritis, systemic lupus erythematosus, or psoriatic arthritis. With mild inflammation, 2 hours of rest each day may suffice. In general, rest should be continued until significant improvement is sustained for at least 2 weeks; thereafter, the program may be liberalized. However, the increase of physical activity must proceed gradually and with appropriate support for any involved weight-bearing joints.

4. Articular rest–Decrease of articular inflammation may be expedited by articular rest. Relaxation and stretching of the hip and knee muscles, to prevent flexion contractures, can be accomplished by having the patient lie in the prone position for 15 minutes several times daily. Sitting in a flexed position for prolonged periods is a poor form of joint rest. Appropriate adjustable supports provide rest for inflamed weight-bearing joints, relieve spasm, and may reduce deformities, soft tissue contracture, or instability of the ligaments. The supports must be removable to permit daily range of motion and exercise of the affected extremities (see below). When ambulation is started, care must be taken to avoid weight bearing, which may aggravate flexion deformities. This is accomplished with the aid of crutches or braces until the tendency toward contracture has subsided.

5. Exercise—Exercises are designed to preserve joint motion, muscular strength, and endurance. Initially, for inflammatory disease, passive range of motion and isometric exercises (such as straight leg raising) are best tolerated. The buoyancy of water permits maximum isotonic and isometric exercise with no more stress on joints than active range of motion exercises. Although ideal for arthritic patients, the cost of hydrotherapy often precludes its use. As tolerance for exercise increases and the activity of the disease subsides, progressive resistance exercises may be introduced. Patients should follow the general rule of eliminating any exercise that produces increased pain 1 hour after the exercise has ended.

6. Heat and cold—These are used primarily for their muscle-relaxing and analgesic effects. Radiant or moist heat is generally most satisfactory. The ambulatory patient will find warm tub baths convenient. Exercise may be better performed after exposure to heat. Some patients derive more relief of joint pain from local application of cold.

7. Assistive devices—Patients with significant hip or knee arthritis may benefit from having a raised toilet seat, a gripping bar, or a cane. Patients hold the cane in the hand opposite to the affected knee or hip, thus leaning away from the affected joint. Crutches or walkers may be needed for patients with more extensive disease.

8. Splints—Splints may provide joint rest, reduce pain, and prevent contracture, but certain principles should be adhered to.

a. Night splints of the hands or wrists (or both) should maintain the extremity in the position of optimum function. The elbow and shoulder lose motion so rapidly that other local measures and corticosteroid injections are usually preferable to splints.

b. The best "splint" for the hip is prone-lying for several hours a day on a firm bed. For the knee, prone-lying may suffice, but splints in maximum tolerated extension are frequently needed. Ankle splints are of the simple right-angle type.

c. Splints should be applied for the shortest period needed, should be made of lightweight materials for comfort, and should be easily removable for range-of-motion exercises once or twice daily to prevent loss of motion.

d. Corrective splints, such as those for overcoming knee flexion contractures, should be used under the guidance of a physician familiar with their proper use.

Note: Avoidance of prolonged sitting or knee pillows may decrease the need for splints.

9. Weight loss—For overweight patients, achieving ideal body weight will reduce the wear and tear placed on arthritic joints of the lower extremities.

B. Nonsteroidal Anti-inflammatory Drugs (NSAIDs): The first drug used to treat rheumatoid arthritis is an NSAID. These agents have analgesic and anti-inflammatory effects but are believed not to be capable of preventing erosions or altering progression of the disease.

A number of NSAIDs are available, including ibuprofen, fenoprofen, naproxen, tolmetin, sulindac, meclofenamate sodium, piroxicam, flurbiprofen, diclofenac, oxaprozin, nabumetone, etodolac, and ketoprofen (see Table 1–11). In terms of efficacy for groups of patients, all of the nonsteroidal anti-inflammatory drugs—including aspirin—are equivalent. With a few exceptions noted below, all NSAIDs have similar side effects. Thus, the choice of an NSAID depends mostly upon cost, convenience, and patient preference. Aspirin, for example, has become less popular as the initial choice of NSAID not because it is less effective or substantially more toxic (at least in the enteric-coated preparation) but because the dosing of aspirin (typically two to four 325 mg tablets four times daily) is less convenient than that of other NSAIDs.

In terms of toxicity, gastrointestinal side effects are most frequent. All the NSAIDs inhibit cyclooxygenase and thereby decrease production of gastric prostaglandin E, a local hormone responsible for gastric mucosal cytoprotection. Consequently, these drugs can produce gastric ulceration and bleeding. The overall rate of bleeding with NSAID use in the general population appears to be low (1:6000 users or less). The frequency of bleeding is increased by chronic use, concomitant use of corticosteroids or anticoagulants, the presence of rheumatoid arthritis, a history of peptic ulcer disease or alcoholism, and old age. Approximately 25% of all hospitalizations and deaths from peptic ulcer disease result from NSAID therapy. Some reports suggest that each year 1:1000 patients with rheumatoid arthritis will require hospitalization for gastrointestinal NSAID-related bleeding or perforation. Although all NSAIDs can cause massive gastrointestinal bleeding, the risk may be higher with indomethacin and piroxicam. There are different isomers of cyclooxygenase in inflammatory cells than in the stomach. The increased gastrointestinal toxicity of indomethacin and piroxicam may be traced to their preferential inhibition of stomach cyclooxygenase. Other NSAIDs—eg, ibuprofen and nabumetone—inhibit both stomach and inflammatory cyclooxygenase equally and appear to have less gastrointestinal toxicity. It is hoped that development of NSAIDs that selectively inhibit the cyclooxygenase of inflammatory cells will result in even safer drugs.

To reduce gastrointestinal toxicity, patients should

take NSAIDs with food rather than on an empty stomach. Misoprostol, a synthetic analog of prostaglandin E, and high-dose famotidine (ie, 40 mg twice daily) significantly reduce the risk of gastric ulcer in patients taking NSAIDs. H_2 blockers and carafate lack this effect but ameliorate dyspepsia. The efficacy of concomitant antacids has not been formally tested. Misoprostol should be reserved for patients who must take an NSAID and have risk factors for gastrointestinal complications (ie, age > 75, previous gastrointestinal bleeding, previous peptic ulcer disease, and a history of cardiac disease). Unfortunately, 20% of patients will not tolerate diarrhea and bloating associated with full doses (200 μg four times daily). Smaller amounts (eg, 100 μg four times daily) or less frequent doses (eg, 200 μg twice daily) improves tolerance while reducing efficacy only modestly. Misoprostol is an abortifacient and is contraindicated in patients who are or might become pregnant.

NSAIDs can also affect the lower intestinal tract, causing perforation or aggravating inflammatory bowel disease.

Acute liver injury from NSAIDs is rare, occurring in about one out of every 25,000 patients using these agents. Having rheumatoid arthritis or taking sulindac may increase the risk. Minor transient increases in aminotransferase levels do not predict risk for NSAID-associated hepatotoxicity.

All of the NSAIDs, including aspirin, can produce renal toxicity, resulting in interstitial nephritis, nephrotic syndrome, reversible renal failure, and aggravation of baseline hypertension. Hyperkalemia due to hyporeninemic hypoaldosteronism may also be seen. The risk of renal toxicity is low but is increased by age over 60, a history of renal disease, congestive heart failure, ascites, and diuretic use.

All NSAIDs except the nonacetylated salicylates interfere with platelet function and prolong bleeding time. For all NSAIDs but aspirin, the effect on bleeding time resolves as the drug is cleared. Aspirin irreversibly inhibits platelet function, so the bleeding time effect resolves only as new platelets are made. Indomethacin is probably no more effective than the salicylates in rheumatoid arthritis, and its untoward effects are greater. Phenylbutazone is not advised for chronic therapy because of its toxicity.

C. Additional Drugs: If the patient fails to respond to the basic regimen with a reduction in morning stiffness, fatigue, and joint swelling, additional medications are added. They should be added early and used aggressively to maximize the chance of achieving a good outcome.

1. Methotrexate–Many now believe that methotrexate is the treatment of choice for patients with severe rheumatoid arthritis who fail to respond to NSAIDs. Methotrexate is generally well-tolerated and often produces a beneficial effect in 2–6 weeks—compared with the 2- to 6-month onset of action for drugs such as gold, penicillamine, and antimalarials. The usual initial dose is 7.5 mg of methotrexate orally once weekly. If the patient has tolerated methotrexate but has not responded in 1 month, the dose can be increased to 15 mg orally once per week. The maximal dose is approximately 20 mg/wk. The most frequent side effects are gastric irritation and stomatitis. If needed to minimize gastrointestinal toxicity, methotrexate can be administered by subcutaneous or intramuscular injection. A severe, potentially life-threatening interstitial pneumonitis occurs rarely and usually responds to cessation of the drug and institution of corticosteroids. Hepatotoxicity with fibrosis and cirrhosis is another important toxic effect of methotrexate that fortunately appears to be very rare, with a risk of approximately 1:1000 after 5 years of methotrexate therapy. Still, methotrexate is contraindicated in a patient with any form of chronic hepatitis. Diabetes, obesity, and renal disease appear to increase the risk of hepatotoxicity. Liver function tests should be monitored every 4–8 weeks, along with the CBC, serum creatinine, and serum albumin. Heavy alcohol use increases the hepatotoxicity, so patients should be advised not to drink. In a patient with no risk factors for hepatotoxicity, liver biopsy is not needed initially but is performed if aminotransferase levels are elevated, despite dosage reduction, in 6 out of 12 monthly determinations or if the serum albumin falls below normal. Cytopenia due to bone marrow suppression and infection are other important potential problems. Side effects, including hepatotoxicity, may be reduced by prescribing either daily folate (1 mg) or weekly leucovorin calcium (2.5–5 mg taken 24 hours after the dose of methotrexate). To date, methotrexate has not been proved to increase the risk of malignancy. The combination of methotrexate and other folate antagonists, such as trimethoprim-sulfamethoxazole, should be used cautiously, since pancytopenia can result. Probenecid should also be avoided since it increases methotrexate drug levels and toxicity.

2. Antimalarials–Hydroxychloroquine sulfate is the antimalarial agent most often used against rheumatoid arthritis. It should be reserved for patients with mild disease, since only 25–50% will respond and in some of those cases only after 3–6 months of therapy. The advantage of hydroxychloroquine is its comparatively low toxicity. A dosage of 200–400 mg/d minimizes the likelihood of toxic reactions. The most important reaction, pigmentary retinitis causing visual loss, is fortunately rare when the dosage is kept low. Biannual ophthalmologic examinations are required when this drug is employed for long-term therapy. Other reactions include neuropathies and myopathies of both skeletal and cardiac muscle, which usually improve when the drug is withdrawn.

3. Gold salts (chrysotherapy)–For patients

who fail to improve on or who cannot tolerate methotrexate, treatment with gold salts may be effective. About 60% of patients may be expected to benefit from gold therapy, although complete remissions are uncommon. Their mode of action is not known.

a. **Indications**–Disease responding unfavorably to conservative management; erosive disease.

b. **Contraindications**–Previous gold toxicity; significant renal, hepatic, or hematopoietic dysfunction.

c. **Preparations of choice**–Intramuscular gold sodium thiomalate or aurothioglucose; oral auranofin. Intramuscular gold is used most often because it is more effective than oral gold.

d. **Dosage**–Intramuscular gold is given as a 10 mg test dose the first week and a 25 mg dose the second week before reaching the maintenance dose of 50 mg weekly, which is then continued (for up to 20 weeks) unless toxic reactions appear. If there is no response after 800 mg has been administered, the drug should be discontinued. If the response is good, a total dose of 1 g should be given, followed by a regimen of 50 mg every 2 weeks and, with continued improvement, every 3 and then every 4 weeks for an indefinite period.

The oral dose of auranofin is 3 mg twice daily until benefit or toxicity occurs.

e. **Toxic reactions**–About one-third of patients (range: 4–50%) experience toxic reactions to gold therapy; the mortality rate is less than 0.4%. The manifestations of toxicity are similar to those of poisoning by other heavy metals (notably arsenic) and include dermatitis (mild to exfoliative, and pruritic), stomatitis, neutropenia, proteinuria, and nitritoid reactions (especially to gold thiomalate and presumably due to its vehicle). Auranofin causes side effects less frequently than intramuscular gold, though diarrhea is common. In order to prevent or reduce the severity of toxic reactions, gold should not be given to patients with any of the contraindicating disorders listed above. Periodic urinalyses and complete blood counts should be obtained.

Severe toxicity may require corticosteroids for control, and failure to respond might then be an indication for the cautious use of penicillamine or dimercaprol (BAL) as chelating agents for the gold. Worsening of articular symptoms after the initial dose is often temporary and is not an indication for withdrawal of the drug. Patients so affected may ultimately respond favorably if treatment is continued.

4. **Corticosteroids**–Although corticosteroids usually produce an immediate and dramatic anti-inflammatory effect in rheumatoid arthritis, they do not alter the natural progression of the disease; furthermore, clinical manifestations of active disease commonly reappear when the drug is discontinued. The serious problem of untoward reactions resulting from prolonged corticosteroid therapy greatly limits its long-term use. Another disadvantage that might stem from the use of steroids lies in the tendency of the patient and the physician to neglect the less spectacular but proved benefits derived from general supportive treatment, physical therapy, and orthopedic measures.

Corticosteroids may be used on a short-term basis to tide patients over acute disabling episodes, to facilitate other treatment measures (eg, physical therapy), or to manage serious extra-articular manifestations (eg, pericarditis, perforating eye lesions). Corticosteroids may also be indicated for active and progressive disease that does not respond favorably to conservative management and when there are contraindications to or therapeutic failure of methotrexate, gold salts, or other disease-modifying agents.

The least amount of steroid that will achieve the desired clinical effect should be given, but not more than 10 mg of prednisone or equivalent per day is appropriate for articular disease. Many patients do reasonably well on 5–7.5 mg daily. (The use of 1 mg tablets is to be encouraged.) When the steroids are to be discontinued, they should be phased out gradually on a planned schedule appropriate to the duration of treatment. All patients receiving chronic corticosteroid therapy should take measures to prevent osteoporosis.

Intra-articular corticosteroids may be helpful if one or two joints are the chief source of difficulty. Intra-articular triamcinolone, 10–40 mg depending on the size of the joint to be injected, may be given for symptomatic relief, but no more often than four times a year.

5. **Sulfasalazine**–This drug has become established as a second-line agent for rheumatoid arthritis, with an efficacy similar to that of gold and penicillamine. Sulfasalazine is usually introduced at a dosage of 0.5 g twice daily and then increased each week by 0.5 g until the patient improves or the daily dose reaches 3 g. Side effects, particularly neutropenia and thrombocytopenia, occur in 10–25% and are serious in 2–5%. Sulfasalazine also causes hemolysis in patients with glucose-6-phosphate dehydrogenase (G6PD) deficiency. Patients taking sulfasalazine should have complete blood counts monitored every 2–4 weeks for the first 3 months, then every 3 months.

6. **Azathioprine**–This agent, like methotrexate, is an antimetabolite that is effective for severe rheumatoid arthritis not responsive to gold or antimalarials. The usual initial dose is 1 mg/kg, gradually increased as needed to a maximum of 2.5–3 mg/kg. Its potential for severe toxicity, including immunosuppression complicated by opportunistic infection, restricts its use.

7. **Penicillamine**–Penicillamine may be used in patients with severe rheumatoid arthritis who have continuing rheumatic activity in spite of therapy with the agents discussed above. This agent may prove effective in a number of such patients, although toxicity is substantial. The mechanism of action is not understood. Up to one-half of patients experience some side effects such as oral ulcers, loss of taste, fever, rash, thrombocytopenia, leukopenia, and aplastic anemia. Proteinuria and nephrotic syndrome may occur. Immune complex diseases (eg, myasthenia gravis, systemic lupus erythematosus, polymyositis, Goodpasture's syndrome) appear to be induced by the drug. It should not be used during pregnancy.

If penicillamine is employed, one should start with small doses: 250 mg daily, increasing by 125 mg every 2–3 months up to a maximum of 0.75–1 g/d. Penicillamine is given between meals to enhance absorption. Careful monitoring for toxicity is essential.

8. Minocycline–Minocycline has been shown to be more effective than placebo for rheumatoid arthritis. This agent should be reserved for mild cases, since its efficacy is modest. The mechanism of action is not clear, but tetracyclines do have anti-inflammatory properties, including the ability to inhibit destructive enzymes such as collagenase. The dose of minocycline is 200 mg/d. Adverse effects are uncommon except for dizziness, which occurs in about 10%.

9. Combination therapy–Combination therapy can be considered for patients who have failed to respond to individual agents. The combination of methotrexate, hydroxychloroquine, and sulfasalazine appears more effective than methotrexate alone. The combination of cyclosporine (2.5–5 mg/kg/d) plus methotrexate also appears more effective than methotrexate alone. However, regimens should be considered experimental until the long-term effects have been assessed.

D. Experimental Therapy: Cyclophosphamide, chlorambucil, cyclosporine, total lymph node irradiation, immunization with allogeneic mononuclear white blood cells, and monoclonal antibodies directed against cytokines or T cells have been used with success in experimental studies. Only patients who fail to respond to all other measures should be considered for these treatments, which should be provided by physicians familiar with their toxicities. Dietary modification, especially supplementation with n-3 fatty acids in doses of 2.5–3 g/d, has been helpful to some patients, as has oral administration of collagen from articular cartilage.

E. Surgical Measures: See below.

Course & Prognosis

Determining the best initial treatment is difficult because patients suspected of having rheumatoid arthritis can follow two widely divergent courses. Of all patients who present with polyarthritis that appears to be (but probably is not) rheumatoid arthritis, 50–75% experience remission within 2 years. These patients are often negative for rheumatoid factor, have good functional status even during disease activity, and are commonly seen in community prac-

tices but rarely in academic centers. Clearly, conservative therapy makes good sense for this patient population.

For patients whose joint symptoms persist beyond 2 years the outcome is not so favorable. Patients in this group die, on average, 10–15 years earlier than people without rheumatoid arthritis. In fact, for patients who have persistent symptoms and poor functional status, the mortality curve resembles that for stage IV Hodgkin's disease or triple-vessel coronary artery disease. The most common causes of death are infection, heart disease, respiratory failure, renal failure, and gastrointestinal disease. Factors that identify those at particular risk of early death include positive rheumatoid factor, poor functional status, more than 30 inflamed joints, and extra-articular manifestations (eg, rheumatoid lung disease). These patients, then, need aggressive therapy and probably need it early, since extensive bone damage can occur during the first 2 years. Patients at risk of developing severe disease may possibly be identified by genotypes for HLA-DRB1 alleles. If so, then it will be possible to determine whether earlier institution of potent second-line agents such as methotrexate or use of agents in combination will improve the outcome in this unfortunate population.

American College of Rheumatology Ad Hoc Committee on Clinical Guidelines: Guidelines for monitoring drug therapy in rheumatoid arthritis. Arthritis Rheum 1996;39:723.

American College of Rheumatology Ad Hoc Committee on Clinical Guidelines: Guidelines for the Management of Rheumatoid arthritis. Arthritis Rheum 1996;39:713. (Early treatment with disease-modifying drugs advocated.)

American College of Rheumatology Task Force on Osteoporosis Guidelines: Recommendations for the prevention and treatment of glucocorticoid-induced osteoporosis. Arthritis Rheum 1996;39:1791. (Prevent osteoporosis with education and with daily vitamin D and calcium supplements; estrogen is added for postmenopausal women.)

MacGregor A et al: HLA-DRB1*0401/0404 genotype and rheumatoid arthritis: Increased association in men, young age at onset, and disease severity. J Rheumatol 1995;22:1032. (Certain HLA-DRB1 alleles increase the risk of developing rheumatoid arthritis by four- to 30-fold depending on the allele. Some genotypes, especially 0401/0404, are markers for severe disease.)

O'Dell JR et al: Treatment of rheumatoid arthritis with methotrexate alone, sulfasalazine and hydroxychloroquine, or a combination of all three medications. N Engl J Med 1996;334:1287. (Combination therapy with methotrexate, sulfasalazine, and hydroxychloroquine is more effective than either methotrexate alone or a combination of sulfasalazine and hydroxychloroquine.)

Rodriguez LAG et al: Acute liver injury associated with nonsteroidal anti-inflammatory drugs and the role of risk factors. Arch Intern Med 1994;154:311. (In a retrospective cohort study of 625,307 persons the risk of acute liver injury was estimated to be about one in every 25,000 patients.)

Saag KG et al: Low dose long-term corticosteroid therapy in rheumatoid arthritis: An analysis of serious adverse events. Am J Med 1994;96:115. (More than 5 mg of prednisone daily increases risk of fracture, infection, ulcer or bleeding, and cataracts.)

Silverstein FE et al: Misoprostol reduces serious gastrointestinal complications in patients with rheumatoid arthritis receiving nonsteroidal anti-inflammatory drugs: A randomized, double-blind, placebo-controlled trial. Ann Intern Med 1995;123:241. (Misoprostol reduces by 40% the risk of a serious gastrointestinal complication. Four risk factors for gastrointestinal complications are age > 75, previous gastrointestinal hemorrhage, previous ulcer disease, and history of heart disease. Accompanying editorial [p 309] notes that patients with no risk factors had an 0.4% risk of gastrointestinal complication, whereas patients with all four risk factors had a 9% risk. The cost of preventing one complication was $276,916 in the former and $12,486 in the latter.)

Taha AS et al: Famotidine for the prevention of gastric and duodenal ulcers caused by nonsteroidal antiinflammatory drugs. N Engl J Med 1996;334:1435. (Famotidine 40 mg orally twice daily significantly reduces the risk of ulcers caused by NSAIDs.)

van der Heide A et al: The effectiveness of early treatment with "second-line" antirheumatic drugs: A randomized, controlled trial. Ann Intern Med 1996;124:699. (Compared with delayed use of second-line agents, early and aggressive treatment improves disability, pain, joint score, and ESR—but not x-ray findings—after 1 year.)

JUVENILE CHRONIC ARTHRITIS

Rheumatoid-like disease with onset before age 17 is referred to as juvenile chronic arthritis. Synovitis that persists for at least 6 weeks is the essential criterion of the diagnosis. Four forms are recognized:

The **polyarticular form** resembles adult rheumatoid arthritis in joint distribution, seropositivity, and prognosis.

The **oligoarticular form** affects chiefly young girls during the peak ages of 2–4, is seronegative, has a good chance for complete remission, and may be associated with a positive ANA test, which in turn is associated with uveitis. Since the uveitis is often initially silent, all children with the oligoarticular form and a positive ANA test should be examined by an ophthalmologist.

Systemic-onset disease, or **Still's disease,** is characterized by high spiking fevers that may antedate arthritis by months; a characteristic evanescent, salmon-colored morbilliform rash; and—commonly but not always—hepatosplenomegaly, lymphadenopathy, pleuropericarditis, anemia, and leukocytosis.

The fourth form of juvenile chronic arthritis is a juvenile form of **ankylosing spondylitis** characterized initially by inflammatory arthritis involving a few peripheral joints, particularly in a lower extremity, that later extends to the spine.

Systemic-onset disease (Still's disease) can occur in adults and may present initially as fever of undetermined origin. While there is no diagnostic laboratory test, the constellation of signs and symptoms—especially the very characteristic rash—may suggest the diagnosis. The rash is often missed because it is present chiefly during episodes of fever, which characteristically occur during the night.

In many children with polyarticular chronic arthritis, the apophysial joints of the cervical spine, especially C2–3, are affected. Abnormalities of bony growth and development are related to active disease and may be transient and reversible or, with chronic disease activity, may be irreversible and result in premature closure of epiphyses or ossification centers; micrognathia is one consequence.

The differential diagnosis of juvenile chronic arthritis includes leukemia or lymphoma, inflammatory bowel disease, and chronic infectious disease (eg, Lyme disease; see Chapter 34). Joint fluid examination, culture, serologic tests, and synovial biopsy may be useful in diagnosis.

The treatment of juvenile chronic arthritis must be individualized; in general, the approach to therapy is similar to that for adult rheumatoid arthritis.

Sampalis JS et al: A controlled study of the long-term prognosis of adult Still's disease. Am J Med 1995;98:384. (Fifty percent still required medication 10 years after diagnosis.)

SYSTEMIC LUPUS ERYTHEMATOSUS

Essentials of Diagnosis

- Occurs mainly in young women.
- Rash over areas exposed to sunlight.
- Joint symptoms in 90% of patients. Multiple system involvement.
- Depression of hemoglobin, white blood cells, platelets.
- Serologic findings: antinuclear antibody with high titer to native DNA.

General Considerations

Systemic lupus erythematosus (SLE) is an inflammatory autoimmune disorder that may affect multiple organ systems. Many of its clinical manifestations are secondary to the trapping of antigen-antibody complexes in capillaries of visceral structures or to autoantibody-mediated destruction of host cells (eg, thrombocytopenia). The clinical course is marked by spontaneous remission and relapses. The severity may vary from a mild episodic disorder to a rapidly fulminating fatal illness.

Before making a diagnosis of spontaneous SLE, it is imperative to ascertain that the condition has not been induced by a drug. A host of pharmacologic agents have been implicated as causing a lupus-like syndrome, but only a few cause the disorder with appreciable frequency (Table 20–7). Procainamide, hydralazine, and isoniazid are the best-studied drugs. While antinuclear antibody tests and other serologic findings become positive in many persons receiving these agents, in only a few do clinical manifestations occur.

The prevalence of SLE is influenced by many factors, including gender, race, and genetic inheritance. About 85% of patients are women. Sex hormones appear to play some role, since most cases develop after menarche and before menopause. Among the patients who develop SLE during childhood or after the age of 50, the preponderance of women is less. Race is also a factor, as SLE occurs in 1:1000 white women but in 1:250 black women. Familial occurrence of SLE has been repeatedly documented, and the disorder is concordant in 25–70% of identical twins. If a mother has SLE, her daughters' risk of developing the disease is 1:40 and her sons' risk is 1:250. Aggregation of serologic abnormalities (positive antinuclear antibody) is seen in asymptomatic family members, and the prevalence of other rheumatic diseases is increased among close relatives of patients. The importance of specific genes in SLE is emphasized by the high frequency of certain HLA haplotypes, especially DR2 and DR3, and null complement alleles.

Four features of drug-induced lupus separate it from spontaneously occurring disease: (1) the sex ratio is nearly equal; (2) nephritis and central nervous system features are not ordinarily present; (3) depressed serum complement and antibodies to native DNA are absent; and (4) the clinical features and most laboratory abnormalities often revert toward normal when the offending drug is withdrawn.

The diagnosis of SLE should be suspected in patients having a multisystem disease with serologic positivity (eg, antinuclear antibody, false-positive serologic test for syphilis). Differential diagnosis includes rheumatoid arthritis, vasculitis, scleroderma, chronic active hepatitis, acute drug reactions, polyarteritis, and drug-induced lupus.

The diagnosis of SLE can be made with reasonable probability if 4 of the 11 criteria set forth in Table 20–8 are met. These criteria should be viewed as rough guidelines that do not supplant clinical judgment in the diagnosis of SLE.

Clinical Findings

A. Symptoms and Signs: The systemic features include fever, anorexia, malaise, and weight loss. Most patients have skin lesions at some time; the characteristic "butterfly" rash affects fewer than half of patients. Other cutaneous manifestations are discoid lupus, typical fingertip lesions, periungual erythema, nail fold infarcts, and splinter hemorrhages. Alopecia is common. Mucous membrane lesions tend to occur during periods of exacerbation.

Table 20–7. Drugs associated with lupus erythematosus.[1]

Definite association

Chlorpromazine	Methyldopa
Hydralazine	Procainamide
Isoniazid	Quinidine

Possible association

Acebutolol	Nitrofurantoin
Atenolol	Oxprenolol
Captopril	Penicillamine
Carbamazepine	Phenytoin
Cimetidine	Pindolol
Ethosuximide	Practolol
Hydrazines	Propranolol
Labetalol	Propylthiouracil
Levodopa	Sulfasalazine
Lithium	Sulfonamides
Mephenytoin	Trimethadione
Methimazole	
Metoprolol	

Unlikely association

Allopurinol	Penicillin
Chlorthalidone	Phenylbutazone
Gold salts	Reserpine
Griseofulvin	Streptomycin
Methysergide	Tetracyclines
Oral contraceptives	

[1]Modified and reproduced, with permission, from Hess EV, Mongey AB: Drug-related lupus. Bull Rheum Dis 1991;40:1.

Table 20–8. Criteria for the classification of SLE.[1] (A patient is classified as having SLE if any 4 or more of 11 criteria are met.)

1. Malar rash
2. Discoid rash
3. Photosensitivity
4. Oral ulcers
5. Arthritis
6. Serositis
7. Renal disease
   a. > 0.5 g/d proteinuria, or—
   b. ≥ 3 + dipstick proteinuria, or—
   c. Cellular casts
8. Neurologic disease
   a. Seizures, or—
   b. Psychosis (without other cause)
9. Hematologic disorders
   a. Hemolytic anemia, or—
   b. Leukopenia (< 4000/μL), or—
   c. Lymphopenia (< 1500/μL), or—
   d. Thrombocytopenia (< 100,000/μL)
10. Immunologic abnormalities
   a. Positive LE cell preparation, or—
   b. Antibody to native DNA, or—
   c. Antibody to Sm, or—
   d. False-positive serologic test for syphilis
11. Positive antinuclear antibody (ANA)

[1]Modified and reproduced, with permission, from Tan EM et al: The 1982 revised criteria for the classification of systemic lupus erythematosus. Arthritis Rheum 1982;25:1271.

Raynaud's phenomenon, present in about 20% of patients, often antedates other features of the disease.

Joint symptoms, with or without active synovitis, occur in over 90% of patients and are often the earliest manifestation. The arthritis is seldom deforming; erosive changes are almost never noted on x-ray study. Subcutaneous nodules are rare.

Ocular manifestations include conjunctivitis, photophobia, transient blindness, and blurring of vision. Cotton-wool spots on the retina (cytoid bodies) represent degeneration of nerve fibers due to occlusion of retinal blood vessels.

Pleurisy, pleural effusion, bronchopneumonia, and pneumonitis are frequent. Restrictive lung disease is often demonstrated.

The pericardium is affected in the majority of patients. Cardiac failure may result from myocarditis and hypertension. Cardiac arrhythmias are common. Atypical verrucous endocarditis of Libman-Sacks is usually clinically silent but occasionally can produce acute or chronic valvular incompetence—most commonly mitral regurgitation—and can serve as a source of emboli.

Abdominal pains, ileus, and peritonitis may result from vasculitis; the right colon is especially susceptible. Nonspecific reactive hepatitis or that induced by salicylates may alter liver function.

Neurologic complications of SLE include psychosis, organic brain syndrome, seizures, peripheral and cranial neuropathies, transverse myelitis, and strokes. Severe depression and psychosis are sometimes exacerbated by the administration of large doses of corticosteroids.

Several forms of glomerulonephritis may occur, including mesangial, focal proliferative, diffuse proliferative, and membranous. Some patients may also have interstitial nephritis. With appropriate therapy, the survival rate even for patients with serious renal disease (proliferative glomerulonephritis) is favorable.

Other clinical features include arterial and venous thrombosis, lymphadenopathy, splenomegaly, Hashimoto's thyroiditis, hemolytic anemia, and thrombocytopenic purpura.

B. Laboratory Findings: (Tables 20–9 and 20–10.) SLE is characterized by the production of many different autoantibodies (eg, positive Coombs), some of which produce specific laboratory abnormalities (eg, hemolytic anemia). Antinuclear antibody tests are sensitive but not specific for systemic lupus—ie, they are positive in virtually all patients with lupus but are positive also in many patients with nonlupus conditions such as rheumatoid arthritis, various forms of hepatitis, and interstitial lung disease. Antibodies to double-stranded DNA and to Sm are specific for systemic lupus but not sensitive, since they are present in only 60% and 30% of patients, respectively. Depressed serum complement—a finding suggestive of disease activity—often returns toward normal in remission. Anti-native DNA antibody levels also correlate with disease activity; anti-Sm levels do not.

Three types of antiphospholipid antibodies occur (Table 20–10): The first causes the biologic false-positive tests for syphilis; the second is the lupus anticoagulant, which despite its name is a risk factor for venous and arterial thrombosis and miscarriage. It is most commonly identified by prolongation of the activated partial thromboplastin time, though other phospholipid-dependent coagulation tests, such as Russell's viper venom time, are more sensitive. Anticardiolipin antibodies are the third type of antiphospholipid antibodies and may be a risk factor for fetal death in pregnant patients with lupus. In many cases, the "anticardiolipin antibody" appears to be directed at a serum cofactor (β_2-glycoprotein-I) rather than at

Table 20–9. Frequency (%) of autoantibodies in rheumatic diseases.

	ANA	Anti-Native DNA	Rheumatoid Factor	Anti-Sm	Anti-Ro	Anti-La	Anti-SCL-70	Anti-Centromere	Anti-Jo-1	ANCA
Rheumatoid arthritis	30–60	0–5	72–85	0	0–5	0–2	0	0	0	0
Systemic lupus erythematosus	95–100	60	20	10–25	15–20	5–20	0	0	0	0–1
Sjögren's syndrome	95	0	75	0	60–70	60–70	0	0	0	0
Diffuse scleroderma	80–95	0	25–33	0	0	0	33	1	0	0
Limited scleroderma (CREST syndrome)	80–95	0	25–33	0	0	0	20	50	0	0
Polymyositis/dermatomyositis	80–95	0	33	0	0	0	10	0	20–30	0
Wegener's granulomatosis	0–15	0	50	0	0	0	0	0	0	93–96[1]

ANA = antinuclear antibodies; ANCA = anti-neutrophil cytoplasmic antibody.
[1]Frequency for generalized, active disease.

Table 20–10. Frequency of laboratory abnormalities in systemic lupus erythematosus.[1]

Anemia	60%
Leukopenia	45%
Thrombocytopenia	30%
Biologic false-positive tests for syphilis	25%
Lupus anticoagulant	7%
Anti-cardiolipin antibody	25%
Direct Coombs-positive	30%
Proteinuria	30%
Hematuria	30%
Hypocomplementemia	60%
ANA	95–100%
Anti-native DNA	50%
Anti-Sm	20%

[1]Modified and reproduced, with permission, from Hochberg MC et al: Systemic lupus erythematosus: A review of clinico-laboratory features and immunologic matches in 150 patients with emphasis on demographic subsets. Medicine 1985; 64:285.

phospholipid itself. A primary **antiphospholipid antibody syndrome** is diagnosed in patients who have recurrent venous or arterial occlusions, recurrent fetal loss, or thrombocytopenia in the presence of antiphospholipid antibodies but without specific features of SLE. Other features of the primary antiphospholipid antibody syndrome include livedo reticularis, skin ulcers, mental status changes, and mitral regurgitation.

Abnormality of urinary sediment is almost always found in association with renal lesions. Showers of red blood cells, with or without casts, and mild proteinuria are frequent during exacerbation of the disease; these usually abate with remission.

Treatment

Some patients with SLE have a benign form of the disease requiring only supportive care and need little or no medication. Emotional support, as described for rheumatoid arthritis, is especially important for patients with lupus. Patients with photosensitivity should be cautioned against sun exposure and should apply a protective lotion to the skin while out of doors. Skin lesions often respond to the local administration of corticosteroids. Minor joint symptoms can usually be alleviated by rest and NSAIDs. Every drug that may have precipitated the condition should be withdrawn if possible.

Antimalarials (hydroxychloroquine) may be helpful in treating lupus rashes or joint symptoms that do not respond to NSAIDs. When these are used, the dose should not exceed 400 mg/d, and biannual monitoring for retinal changes is necessary. Drug-induced neuropathy and myopathy may be erroneously ascribed to the underlying disease.

Corticosteroids are required for the control of certain serious complications. These include thrombocy-topenic purpura, hemolytic anemia, myocarditis, pericarditis, convulsions, and nephritis. Forty to 60 mg of prednisone is often needed initially; however, the lowest dose of corticosteroid that controls the condition should be employed. Central nervous system lupus may require higher doses of corticosteroids than are usually given; however, steroid psychosis may mimic lupus cerebritis, in which case reduced doses are appropriate. In lupus nephritis, sequential studies of serum complement and antibodies to DNA often permit early detection of disease exacerbation and thus prompt increase in corticosteroid therapy. Such studies also allow for lowering the dosage of the drugs and withdrawing them when they are no longer needed. Immunosuppressive agents such as cyclophosphamide, chlorambucil, and azathioprine are used in cases resistant to corticosteroids. The exact role of immunosuppressive agents is controversial. Cyclophosphamide improves renal survival. Overall patient survival, however, is no better than in the prednisone-treated group. Very close follow-up is needed to watch for potential side effects when immunosuppressants are employed; these agents should be given by physicians experienced in their use. The androgenic steroid danazol may be effective therapy for thrombocytopenia not responsive to corticosteroids. Dehydroepiandrosterone (DHEA) is also being studied. Anticoagulation, most commonly with warfarin to achieve an INR > 3, is prescribed for patients who have antiphospholipid antibodies and clotting of the arterial or venous systems. Systemic steroids are not usually given for minor arthritis, skin rash, leukopenia, or the anemia associated with chronic disease. Positive serologic findings in asymptomatic patients are not an indication for treatment.

Course & Prognosis

The prognosis for patients with systemic lupus appears to be considerably better than older reports implied. From both community settings and university centers, 10-year survival rates exceeding 85% are routine. In most patients, the illness pursues a relapsing and remitting course. Corticosteroids, often needed in doses of 40 mg/d or more during severe flares, can usually be tapered to low doses (10–15 mg/d) during disease inactivity. However, there are some in whom the disease pursues a virulent course, leading to serious impairment of vital structures such as lung, heart, brain, or kidneys, and the disease may lead to death. With improved control of lupus activity and with increasing use of corticosteroids and immunosuppressive drugs, the mortality and morbidity patterns in lupus have changed. Infections—especially with opportunistic organisms—have become the leading cause of death, followed by active SLE, chiefly due to renal or central nervous system disease. Although such manifestations are more likely to be seen in the early phases of the illness, one must be alert to the possibility of their occurrence at any time. Accelerated atherosclerosis attributed, in part, to corticosteroid use, has been responsible for a rise in late deaths due to myocardial infarction. With more patients living longer, it has become evident that avascular necrosis of bone, affecting most commonly the hips and knees, is responsible for substantial morbidity. Still, it must be emphasized that the outlook for most patients with SLE has become increasingly favorable.

Abu-Shakra M et al: Mortality studies in systemic lupus erythematosus: Results from a single center. I. Causes of death. J Rheumatol 1995;22:1259. (The most common causes of death were infection [32%], active SLE [16%], and acute vascular events [15%]. Death from active SLE was more likely to occur early [in the first 5 years], whereas death from acute vascular events more commonly occurred late [after the first 5 years].)

Boumpas DT et al: Systemic lupus erythematosus: Emerging concepts. Part 1: Renal, neuropsychiatric, cardiovascular, pulmonary, and hematologic disease; and Part 2: Dermatologic and joint disease, the antiphospholipid antibody syndrome, pregnancy and hormonal therapy, morbidity and mortality, and pathogenesis. Ann Intern Med 1995;122:940 and 1995;123:42.

Drenkard C et al: Remission of systemic lupus erythematosus. Medicine 1996;75:88. (One hundred and fifty-six out of 667 patients went into remission at a rate of 3% per year.)

Petri M: Systemic lupus erythematosus and pregnancy. Rheum Dis Clin North Am 1994;20:87. (Thorough review with 243 references. In the author's experience, pregnancy was associated with a twofold increased risk of flare; 45% of babies were preterm.)

Sanchez-Guerrero J et al: Postmenopausal estrogen therapy and the risk for developing systemic lupus erythematosus. Ann Intern Med 1995;122:430. (Prospective cohort study of nearly 70,000 postmenopausal women who did not initially have SLE. Users of postmenopausal hormones were roughly twice as likely to develop SLE as never-users.)

PROGRESSIVE SYSTEMIC SCLEROSIS (Scleroderma)

Essentials of Diagnosis

- Diffuse thickening of skin, with telangiectasia and areas of increased pigmentation and depigmentation.
- Raynaud's phenomenon in 90% of patients.
- Systemic features of dysphagia, hypomotility of gastrointestinal tract, pulmonary fibrosis, and cardiac and renal involvement.

General Considerations

Progressive systemic sclerosis is a chronic disorder characterized by diffuse fibrosis of the skin and internal organs. The causes of scleroderma are not known, but autoimmunity, fibroblast disregulation, and occupational exposure to silica have been impli-

cated. Symptoms usually appear in the third to fifth decades, and women are affected two to three times as frequently as men.

Scleroderma may be localized or systemic. Localized scleroderma—morphea, linear scleroderma—is not associated with visceral organ involvement and is therefore benign. Two forms of systemic scleroderma are generally recognized: diffuse (20% of patients) and limited (80%). Patients with limited systemic scleroderma frequently have calcinosis cutis, Raynaud's phenomenon, esophageal involvement, sclerodactyly, and telangiectasia (CREST syndrome). Patients with CREST syndrome differ from those with diffuse systemic scleroderma in having skin tightening limited to the hands and face (versus the trunk), a lower risk of renal involvement, a higher risk of pulmonary hypertension, and an overall better prognosis.

Rapid progression of visceral organ disease leading to death within a few years is much more common in diffuse systemic scleroderma than in CREST syndrome.

Clinical Findings

A. Symptoms and Signs: Most frequently, the disease makes its appearance in the skin, although visceral involvement may precede cutaneous alteration. Polyarthralgia and Raynaud's phenomenon (present in 90% of patients) are early manifestations. Subcutaneous edema, fever, and malaise are common. With time the skin becomes thickened and hidebound, with loss of normal folds. Telangiectasia, pigmentation, and depigmentation are characteristic. Ulceration about the fingertips and subcutaneous calcification are seen. Dysphagia due to esophageal dysfunction is common and results from abnormalities in motility and later from fibrosis. Fibrosis and atrophy of the gastrointestinal tract cause hypomotility, and malabsorption results from bacterial overgrowth. Large-mouthed diverticula occur in the jejunum, ileum, and colon. Diffuse pulmonary fibrosis and pulmonary vascular disease are reflected in low diffusing capacity and decreased lung compliance. Cardiac abnormalities include pericarditis, heart block, myocardial fibrosis, and right heart failure secondary to pulmonary hypertension. Hypertensive uremic syndrome, resulting from obstruction to smaller renal blood vessels, indicates a grave prognosis.

B. Laboratory Findings: Mild anemia is often present, and it is occasionally hemolytic because of mechanical damage to red cells from diseased small vessels. Elevation of the sedimentation rate and hypergammaglobulinemia are also common. Proteinuria and cylindruria appear in association with renal involvement. Antinuclear antibody tests are frequently positive (Table 20–8). The scleroderma antibody (SCL-70) is found in one-third of patients with diffuse scleroderma and in 20% of those with CREST syndrome; an anticentromere antibody is seen in 50% of those with CREST syndrome and in 1% of individuals with diffuse scleroderma (Table 20–8). Though these tests may be of academic interest, their lack of sensitivity and (usually) specificity precludes cost-effective application in diagnosis.

Differential Diagnosis

Eosinophilic fasciitis is a rare disorder presenting with skin changes that appear to be like those in diffuse systemic scleroderma. The inflammatory abnormalities, however, are limited to the fascia rather than the dermis and epidermis. Patients with eosinophilic fasciitis are further distinguished from those with systemic scleroderma by the presence of peripheral blood eosinophilia, the absence of Raynaud's phenomenon, the good response to prednisone, and an increased risk of developing aplastic anemia.

The eosinophilia-myalgia syndrome was first noted in patients who ingested tryptophan, an essential amino acid that was sold—until banned by the Food and Drug Administration—as an over-the-counter remedy for insomnia and premenstrual symptoms. Weeks to months after beginning ingestion, affected patients developed a syndrome of severe generalized myalgias, and cutaneous abnormalities ranging from hives to generalized swelling and induration of the arms and legs similar to that seen in scleroderma or eosinophilic fasciitis. Peripheral eosinophilia (> 1000/µL) is characteristic. Other common clinical manifestations have included pulmonary symptoms, fever, myopathy, lymphadenopathy, and ascending polyneuropathy. Besides eosinophilia, laboratory features include mild elevations of aldolase with normal creatine kinase levels and, frequently, positive ANA tests. Full-thickness biopsies reveal at times features of scleroderma and at other times evidence of fasciitis or myositis or small vessel vasculitis. While some patients improve after discontinuing tryptophan, others progress and have required corticosteroid therapy, which is not always effective. Deaths have been reported, especially from neurologic involvement. Therefore, anyone with a scleroderma or an eosinophilic fasciitis-like syndrome should be asked about tryptophan use.

Case reports have suggested that silicone breast implants can cause scleroderma or other rheumatic diseases, including SLE and undifferentiated autoimmune diseases. However, controlled population studies have not confirmed these associations.

Treatment

Treatment of progressive systemic sclerosis is symptomatic and supportive. Severe Raynaud's syndrome may respond to calcium channel blockers, eg, nifedipine, 30–60 mg/d. Intravenous iloprost, a prostacyclin analog that causes vasodilation and platelet inhibition, is moderately effective in healing digital ulcers. Patients with esophageal disease should take medications in liquid or crushed form. Esophageal reflux can be reduced and scarring prevented by avoiding late-night meals, elevating the head of the bed, and using antacids and H_2 blockers. Proton pump inhibitors (eg, omeprazole, 20–40 mg/d) are the only drugs that achieve near-complete inhibition of gastric acid production, and they are remarkably effective for refractory esophagitis. Patients with delayed gastric emptying maintain their weight better if they eat small, frequent meals and remain upright for at least 2 hours after eating. Prokinetic drugs (eg, cisapride) infrequently produce a meaningful improvement in gastric emptying and are ineffective in promoting esophageal emptying. Octreotide, a somatostatin analog, has helped a few patients with bacterial overgrowth and pseudo-obstruction. Malabsorption due to bacterial overgrowth also responds to antibiotics, eg, tetracycline, 500 mg four times daily. The hypertensive crises seen chiefly in diffuse systemic scleroderma can often be treated with angiotensin-converting enzyme inhibitors, eg, captopril, 37.5–75 mg/d in three divided doses. The ability of drugs to prevent the development of visceral disease is controversial. The best evidence, however imperfect, suggests that penicillamine in doses as for rheumatoid arthritis (see above) may be helpful for patients at high risk of developing early visceral involvement, ie, those with rapidly progressive diffuse systemic scleroderma. Prednisone has little or no role in the treatment of scleroderma. Cyclophosphamide, a drug with many important side effects, may improve severe interstitial lung disease.

The prognosis tends to be worse in blacks, in males, and in older patients. In most cases, death results from renal, cardiac, or pulmonary failure. Breast and lung cancer may be more common in patients with scleroderma.

Abu-Shakra M, Guillemin F, Lee P: Gastrointestinal manifestations of systemic sclerosis. Semin Arthritis Rheum 1994;24:29. (Esophageal dysmotility [58%] and reflux [15%], bacterial overgrowth [10%], and widemouth colonic diverticula [7%] most frequent.)

Palmieri GMA et al: Treatment of calcinosis with diltiazem. Arthritis Rheum 1995;38:1646. (Diltiazem but not verapamil effectively treats calcinosis.)

Roca RB, Wigley FM, White B: Depressive symptoms associated with scleroderma. Arthritis Rheum 1996; 39:1035. (Nearly two-thirds depressed; 17% with moderate to severe symptoms. Depression linked more to personality than to objective measures of severity of disease.)

Wigley FM et al: Intravenous iloprost infusion in patients with Raynaud phenomenon secondary to systemic sclerosis: A multicenter, placebo-controlled, double-blind study. Ann Intern Med 1994;120:199. (Moderately effective for severe Raynaud's and digital ulcers.)

POLYMYOSITIS-DERMATOMYOSITIS

Essentials of Diagnosis

- Bilateral proximal muscle weakness (all cases).
- Heliotrope suffusion of upper eyelids, characteristic rash, papules over knuckles (many cases).
- Diagnostic tests: elevated CK and other muscle enzymes, muscle biopsy, electromyogram.
- Increased incidence of malignancy, especially when rash is present and with late age of onset.

General Considerations

Polymyositis is a systemic disorder of unknown cause whose principal manifestation is muscle weakness. It is the most frequent primary myopathy in adults. When skin manifestations are associated with it, the entity is designated dermatomyositis. The true incidence is not known, since milder cases are frequently not diagnosed. The disease may affect persons of any age group, but the peak incidence is in the fifth and sixth decades of life. Women are affected twice as commonly as men. There is an increased risk of malignancy, especially in patients with dermatomyositis. The malignancy may be evident initially or may not become evident for months after the muscle disease presents. Ovarian cancer appears to be especially common, found in some series to affect more than 20% of women aged over 40 with dermatomyositis.

Clinical Findings

A. Symptoms and Signs: Polymyositis may begin abruptly, although often it is gradual and progressive. The characteristic rash is dusky red and may be seen over the butterfly area of the face, neck, shoulders, and upper chest and back. Periorbital edema and a purplish (heliotrope) suffusion over the upper eyelids are typical signs. Subungual erythema, cuticular telangiectases, and scaly patches over the dorsum of the proximal interphalangeal and metacarpophalangeal joints (Gottron's sign) are highly suggestive. Muscle weakness chiefly involves proximal groups, especially of the extremities. Leg weakness (eg, difficulty rising from a chair or climbing steps) precedes arm symptoms. Neck flexor weakness occurs in two-thirds of cases. Pain and tenderness of affected muscles occur in one-fourth of cases, and Raynaud's phenomenon and joint symptoms may be associated. Atrophy and contractures occur late. Associated myocarditis is uncommon. Interstitial pulmonary disease, usually mild, is sometimes associated, and calcinosis may be observed, especially in children. Polymyositis may occur in association with Sjögren's syndrome, SLE, or scleroderma.

B. Laboratory Findings: Measurement of serum levels of muscle enzymes, especially creatine phosphokinase and aldolase, is most useful in diagnosis and in assessment of disease activity. Anemia is uncommon. The sedimentation rate is not appreciably elevated in half of the patients. Rheumatoid factor is found in a minority of patients. Antinuclear antibodies are present in many patients, and anti-Jo-1 antibodies are seen in the subset of patients who have associated interstitial lung disease (Table 20–8). Chest x-rays are usually normal, though interstitial fibrosis is occasionally seen. Electromyographic abnormalities consisting of polyphasic potentials, fibrillations, and high-frequency action potentials are helpful in establishing the diagnosis. None of the studies are specific. The search for an occult malignancy should begin with a history and physical examination and include the cancer screening tests that would be routine for that patient (see Chapter 1). If these evaluations are unrevealing, then a more invasive or extensive laboratory evaluation is not cost-effective. No matter how extensive the initial screening, some malignancies will not become evident for months after the initial presentation.

C. Muscle Biopsy: Biopsy of clinically involved muscle, usually proximal, is the only specific diagnostic study. Findings include necrosis of muscle fibers associated with inflammatory cells, sometimes located near blood vessels. The muscle biopsy may, however, reveal little change in spite of significant muscle weakness owing to the patchy distribution of pathologic abnormalities.

Differential Diagnosis

Most endocrine diseases can be associated with proximal muscle weakness. This is particularly true for hyper- and hypothyroidism, and the latter is associated also with elevations of creatinine phosphokinase. Patients with polymyalgia rheumatica are over the age of 50 and—in contrast to patients with polymyositis—have pain but no objective weakness. Disorders of the peripheral and central nervous systems (eg, chronic inflammatory polyneuropathy, multiple sclerosis, myasthenia gravis, Eaton-Lambert disease, and amyotrophic lateral sclerosis) can produce weakness but are distinguished by characteristic symptoms and neurologic signs and often by distinctive electromyographic abnormalities. Many drugs, including corticosteroids, alcohol, clofibrate, penicillamine, tryptophan, and hydroxychloroquine, can produce proximal muscle weakness. Chronic use of colchicine at doses as low as 0.6 mg twice a day in elderly patients with mild to moderate renal insufficiency can produce a mixed neuropathy-myopathy that mimics polymyositis. The weakness and muscle enzyme elevation reverse with cessation of the drug. Lovastatin, a drug increasingly used to treat hypercholesterolemia, also can rarely produce myositis, especially when used in combination with gemfibrozil. Polymyositis can occur as a complication of HIV or HTLV-I infection and with zidovudine therapy as well. Inclusion body myositis is distinguished from polymyositis in that most patients are over 50 years old, have involvement of distal muscles, experience slow progression of disease over years, may not respond to prednisone, and have characteristic inclusion bodies in the muscle identifiable by electron microscopy.

Treatment

Most patients respond to corticosteroids. Often a daily dose of 40–60 mg or more of prednisone is required initially. The dose is then adjusted downward according to the response of sequentially observed serum levels of muscle enzymes. Long-term use of steroids is often needed, and the disease may recur or reemerge when they are withdrawn. Patients with an associated neoplasm have a poor prognosis, although remission may follow treatment of the tumor; steroids may or may not be effective in these patients. In patients resistant or intolerant to corticosteroids, therapy with methotrexate or azathioprine may be helpful, but these agents should be used with caution in view of their adverse effects. Intravenous immune globulin has also been shown to be effective for dermatomyositis resistant to prednisone, but leukapheresis and plasma exchange are not.

Plotz PH et al: Myositis: Immunologic contributions to understanding cause, pathogenesis, and therapy. Ann Intern Med 1995;122:715. (Thorough review. Dermatomyositis differs from polymyositis in inflaming vessels of muscles via complement activation.)

Vazquez-Abad D, Rothfield NF: Sensitivity and specificity of anti-Jo-1 antibodies in autoimmune diseases with myositis. Arthritis Rheum 1996;39:292. (Jo-1 antibody 20% sensitive and 100% specific for polymyositis and dermatomyositis.)

Zantos D, Zhang Y, Felson D: The overall and temporal association of cancer with polymyositis and dermatomyositis. J Rheumatol 1994;21:1855. (Meta-analysis showing association of cancer with both dermatomyositis [odds ratio = 4.4] and polymyositis [odds ratio = 2.1].)

OVERLAP (OR MIXED) CONNECTIVE TISSUE DISEASE

Not infrequently, patients have features of more than one rheumatic disease. Special attention has been drawn to patients who have overlapping features of SLE, scleroderma, and polymyositis. Initially, these patients were thought to have a distinct entity ("mixed connective tissue disease") defined by a specific autoantibody to ribonuclear protein (RNP). With time in many patients, the manifestations evolve to one predominant disease, such as scleroderma, and many patients with antibodies to RNP have clear-cut SLE. Therefore, "overlap connective tissue disease" is the preferred designation for patients having features of different rheumatic diseases.

SJÖGREN'S SYNDROME

Essentials of Diagnosis

- 90% of patients are women; the average age is 50 years.
- Dryness of eyes and dry mouth (sicca components) are the most common features; they occur alone or in association with rheumatoid arthritis or other connective tissue disease.
- Rheumatoid factor and other autoantibodies common.
- Increased incidence of lymphoma.

General Considerations

Sjögren's syndrome, an autoimmune disorder, is the result of chronic dysfunction of exocrine glands in many areas of the body. It is characterized by dryness of the eyes, mouth, and other areas covered by mucous membranes and is frequently associated with a rheumatic disease, most often rheumatoid arthritis. The disorder is predominantly a disease of women, in a ratio of 9:1, with greatest incidence between age 40 and 60 years.

Disorders with which Sjögren's syndrome is frequently associated include rheumatoid arthritis, SLE, primary biliary cirrhosis, scleroderma, polymyositis, Hashimoto's thyroiditis, polyarteritis, and interstitial pulmonary fibrosis. When Sjögren's syndrome occurs without rheumatoid arthritis, HLA-DR2 and -DR3 antigens are present with increased frequency.

Clinical Findings

A. Symptoms and Signs: Keratoconjunctivitis sicca results from inadequate tear production caused by lymphocyte and plasma cell infiltration of the lacrimal glands. Symptoms include burning, itching, ropy secretions, and impaired tear production during crying. Parotid enlargement, which may be chronic or relapsing, develops in one-third of patients. Dryness of the mouth (xerostomia) leads to difficulty in speaking and swallowing and to severe dental caries. There may be loss of taste and smell. Desiccation may involve the nose, throat, larynx, bronchi, vagina, and skin.

Systemic manifestations include dysphagia, pancreatitis, pleuritis, neuropsychiatric dysfunction, and vasculitis; they may be related to the associated diseases noted above. Renal tubular acidosis (type I, distal) occurs in 20% of patients. Chronic interstitial nephritis, which may result in impaired renal function, may be seen. A glomerular lesion is rarely observed but may occur secondary to associated cryoglobulinemia.

A spectrum of lymphoproliferation ranging from benign to malignant may be found. Malignant lymphomas and Waldenström's macroglobulinemia occur nearly 50 times more frequently than can be explained by chance alone in primary Sjögren's syndrome.

B. Laboratory Findings: Laboratory findings include mild anemia, leukopenia, and eosinophilia. Rheumatoid factor is found in 70% of patients. Heightened levels of gamma globulin, antinuclear antibodies, and antibodies against RNA, salivary gland, lacrimal duct, and thyroid may be noted. Antibodies against cytoplasmic antigens SS-A (or Ro) and SS-B (or La) are found predominantly in Sjögren's syndrome alone, whereas antibodies against salivary ducts and the RANA antigen are found in Sjögren's syndrome in association with rheumatoid arthritis (Table 20–8). When SS-A antibodies are present, extraglandular manifestations of Sjögren's syndrome are far more common.

Useful ocular diagnostic tests include the Schirmer test, which measures the quantity of tears secreted. Labial biopsy, a simple procedure, is the only specific diagnostic technique and has minimal risk; if lymphoid foci are seen in accessory salivary glands, the diagnosis is confirmed. Biopsy of the parotid gland should be reserved for patients with atypical presentations such as unilateral gland enlargement.

Treatment & Prognosis

Treatment is symptomatic and supportive. Artificial tears applied frequently will relieve ocular symptoms and avert further desiccation. The mouth should be kept well lubricated. Atropinic drugs and decongestants decrease salivary secretions and should be avoided. A program of oral hygiene is essential in order to preserve dentition. If there is an associated rheumatic disease, its treatment is not altered by the presence of Sjögren's syndrome.

The disease is usually benign and may be consistent with a normal life span; it is influenced mainly by the nature of the associated disease.

Kruize AA et al: Long-term followup of patients with Sjögren's syndrome. Arthritis Rheum 1996;39:297. (Primary Sjögren's syndrome usually follows a stable and mild course over 10 years except that 10% died of lymphoma.)

Tzioufas AG et al: Mixed monoclonal cryoglobulinemia and monoclonal rheumatoid factor cross-reactive idiotypes as predictive factors for the development of lymphoma in primary Sjögren's syndrome. Arthritis Rheum 1996;39:767. (The presence of mixed monoclonal cryoglobulinemia was associated with a high risk of developing lymphoma.)

VASCULITIS SYNDROMES

The vasculitis syndromes are a heterogeneous group of disorders characterized by the pathologic features of inflammation and necrosis of blood vessels. The cause of most forms of vasculitis is not known. Infection is important in the pathogenesis of some forms of vasculitis. In polyarteritis, 30–50% of patients have evidence of hepatitis B or C. Most patients with mixed cryoglobulinemia are infected with hepatitis C. Infective endocarditis and syphilis can be associated with vasculitis, and cases of herpes zoster can rarely be followed by central nervous system vasculitis. Drug reactions—especially to penicillins, sulfonamides, and allopurinol—can produce serum sickness associated with vasculitis. No common pathogenic link has been identified for these disorders, though the deposition of immune complexes in the vascular system occurs in many.

Although vasculitis is seen in multiple disorders, only the major vasculitides will be discussed here.

POLYARTERITIS NODOSA

Essentials of Diagnosis

- Clinical findings depend on arteries involved.
- Affects kidneys, muscles, joints, nerves, heart, gastrointestinal tract in most patients; cutaneous and pulmonary involvement unusual but possible.
- Manifestations include fever, hypertension, abdominal pain, livedo reticularis, mononeuritis multiplex, anemia, hematuria, elevated sedimentation rate.
- Diagnostic confirmation by biopsy or angiogram.

General Considerations

Polyarteritis is characterized by focal or segmental lesions of blood vessels, especially arteries of small to medium size, resulting in a variety of clinical presentations depending upon the specific site of the blood vessel involved. The pathologic hallmark of the disease is acute necrotizing inflammation of the arterial media, with fibrinoid necrosis and extensive inflammatory cell infiltration of all coats of the vessel and surrounding tissue. Aneurysmal dilations occur; hemorrhage, thrombosis, and fibrosis may lead to occlusion of the lumen. Arterial lesions may be seen in all stages—acute, healing, and healed. Such vascular lesions may involve virtually every organ of the body but are especially prominent in the kidney, heart, liver, gastrointestinal tract, muscle, and testes.

The cause of polyarteritis is unknown. Hepatitis B and hepatitis C have been strongly implicated, with 30–50% of patients having serologic evidence of these infections. In addition, immune complexes consisting in part of hepatitis B antigens have been identified in the serum and in the inflamed vessels of some patients. It is not surprising, therefore, that polyarteritis nodosa is more common in intravenous drug abusers and in other groups who have a high prevalence of hepatitis B or C infection. Yet at least half of patients with polyarteritis have no evidence of current or previous hepatitis. Polyarteritis may occur at any age but is more frequent in young adults, and men are affected three times as frequently as women.

Clinical Findings

A. Symptoms and Signs: The clinical onset is usually insidious, with fever, malaise, weight loss, and other symptoms developing over weeks to months. Abrupt onset over a few days of multiorgan inflammation is much more typical of toxic shock syndrome, sepsis, or thrombotic thrombocytopenia purpura than of polyarteritis. Extremity pain is often a prominent early feature of polyarteritis, caused by arthralgia, myalgia (particularly affecting the calves), or neuropathy. In fact, the combination of mononeuritis multiplex (with lesions including foot drop) and any other systemic feature such as fever or weight loss is one of the earliest specific clues that the patient has polyarteritis. A wide variety of cutaneous abnormalities develop. Livedo reticularis, subcutaneous nodules, and palpable purpura are most common; skin ulcers and digital gangrene are less so. Occlusion of retinal vessels results in cotton-wool spots (cytoid bodies). Kidney involvement occurs eventually in more than 80% of cases, with abnormal renal function tests (see below) or hypertension. Indeed, newly acquired hypertension develops in 50% of patients with polyarteritis but is rare in Wegener's granulomatosis. The renal lesion is a segmental necrotizing glomerulonephritis with extracapillary proliferation, often with localized intravascular coagulation. Abdominal pain, especially diffuse pain beginning about 30 minutes after meals (so-called abdominal angina), and nausea and vomiting are common. Infarction due to the arteritis compromises the function of major viscera and may lead to cholecystitis and appendicitis. A few patients present dramatically with an acute abdomen and hypotension caused by rupture of a microaneurysm in the kidney, liver, or other areas of the mesenteric circulation. Cardiac involvement usually occurs late and is manifested by pericarditis, myocarditis, and arrhythmias; myocardial infarction secondary to coronary vasculitis also may be observed. Polyarteritis is an occasional cause of fever of unknown origin.

B. Laboratory Findings: Laboratory findings include proteinuria, hematuria, and red cell casts. Most patients manifest anemia and leukocytosis. Eosinophilia is more frequently encountered if there are pulmonary manifestations, including fleeting infiltrates and bronchospasm; this may represent a different disease process (Churg-Strauss vasculitis), though overlap occurs. The sedimentation rate is almost always elevated. Rheumatoid factor, antinuclear antibody, positive serologic test for syphilis, and increased serum concentration of gamma globulin are neither sensitive nor specific. Serum complement is often normal or elevated. Serologic tests for hepatitis C or for hepatitis B, such as HBsAg and HBeAg, are positive in 30–50%.

The role of anti-neutrophil cytoplasmic antibodies (ANCA) in the diagnosis of polyarteritis is not yet fully defined. A cytoplasmic pattern (cANCA) is produced by antibodies to a proteinase and is seen chiefly in patients with Wegener's granulomatosis. A perinuclear pattern (pANCA) is caused by antibodies specific for myeloperoxidase. pANCA is found in 30% of patients with polyarteritis but can also be found in other conditions, including SLE, inflammatory bowel disease, and vasculitis limited to the kidney (microscopic polyarteritis). Given the limited sensitivity and specificity of pANCA, the diagnosis of polyarteritis requires histopathologic or angiographic confirmation.

C. Biopsy and Angiography: Biopsy of symptomatic sites (such as muscle, nerve, or testicle) is sensitive (70%) and specific (95%), with low morbidity. If these biopsies are negative or if there is no symptomatic site, the patient should undergo visceral angiography to look for characteristic aneurysmal dilation of the renal, mesenteric, or hepatic arteries. Visceral angiography has sensitivity and specificity similar to those of biopsy of symptomatic sites, but angiography can produce complications such as a rise in creatinine and, rarely, death.

Treatment

Corticosteroids in high doses (up to 60 mg of prednisone daily) may control fever and constitutional symptoms and heal vascular lesions. Immunosuppressive agents, especially cyclophosphamide, appear to improve the survival of patients when given with steroids. These drugs may be required chronically, and relapses are not infrequent when they are withdrawn. Some patients who have polyarteritis in association with replicating hepatitis B, as reflected in a positive test for HBeAg, may respond to a short course of prednisone followed by antiviral therapy.

Prognosis

Without treatment, the 5-year survival rate is 20%. Corticosteroids alone improve the 5-year survival to 50%. With corticosteroids and immunosuppressive drugs, the 5-year survival has improved to 60–90%.

Fortin PR et al: Prognostic factors in systemic necrotizing vasculitis of the polyarteritis nodosa group: A review of 45 cases. J Rheumatol 1995;22:78. (Five-year survival 58%; cardiac or renal disease increases risk of death.)

Guillevin L et al: Polyarteritis nodosa related to hepatitis B virus: A prospective study with long-term observation of 41 patients. Medicine 1995;74:238. (When treated with 2 weeks of corticosteroid followed by plasma exchange and antiviral therapy, 80% of patients survived [mean follow-up 69 months] and 56% seroconverted.)

Guillevin L et al: Prognostic factors in polyarteritis nodosa and Churg-Strauss syndrome: A prospective study in 342 patients. Medicine 1996;75:17. (Argues that patients with idiopathic polyarteritis nodosa and a good prognosis should be treated with prednisone alone; those with bad prognosis [ie, those with cardiac, central nervous system, renal, or gastrointestinal involvement] should be treated with prednisone and cyclophosphamide. Those with hepatitis B-associated polyarteritis nodosa should be treated with prednisone briefly, then plasmapheresis and antiviral therapy.)

POLYMYALGIA RHEUMATICA & GIANT CELL ARTERITIS

Polymyalgia rheumatica and giant cell arteritis probably represent a spectrum of one disease: Both affect the same population (patients over the age of 50), show preference for the same HLA haplotypes, and show similar patterns of cytokines in blood and arteries. Polymyalgia rheumatica and giant cell arteritis also frequently coexist. Clinically, the important difference between the two conditions is that polymyalgia rheumatica alone does not cause blindness and responds to low-dose (10–20 mg/d) prednisone therapy, whereas giant cell arteritis can cause blindness and requires high-dose therapy (40–60 mg/d).

Polymyalgia rheumatica is a clinical diagnosis based on pain and stiffness of the shoulder and pelvic girdle area, frequently in association with fever, malaise, and weight loss. Anemia and a markedly elevated sedimentation rate are almost always present. Because of the shoulder and pelvic area stiffness and pain, patients have trouble combing their hair, putting on a coat, or getting up out of a chair. In contrast to polymyositis, polymyalgia rheumatica does not cause muscular weakness. A few patients have joint swelling, particularly of the knees, wrists, and sternoclavicular joints. The differential diagnosis of malaise, anemia, and a markedly elevated sedimentation rate includes multiple myeloma, other malignant disorders, and chronic infections such as bacterial endocarditis. Patients with polymyalgia rheumatica by itself are treated with prednisone, 10–20 mg/d. If the patient fails to experience a dramatic improvement within 72 hours, the diagnosis should be doubted. Within 1–2 months after beginning treatment, the patient's symptoms and laboratory abnormalities will resolve. Slow tapering of the prednisone reduces the likelihood of relapse. The total duration of treatment varies considerably but ranges from 6 months to more than 2 years.

Giant cell arteritis is a systemic panarteritis affecting medium-sized and large vessels in patients over the age of 50. The condition is also called temporal arteritis, since that artery is frequently involved, as are other extracranial branches of the carotid artery. About 50% of patients with giant cell arteritis also have polymyalgia rheumatica. The classic symptoms suggesting that a patient has arteritis are headache, scalp tenderness, visual symptoms, jaw claudication, or throat pain. The temporal artery is usually normal on physical examination but may be nodular, enlarged, tender, or pulseless. Blindness results from occlusive arteritis of the posterior ciliary branch of the ophthalmic artery. The ischemic optic neuropathy of giant cell arteritis may produce no funduscopic findings for the first 24–48 hours after the onset of blindness. The murmur of aortic regurgitation or bruits heard near the clavicle identify the occasional patient in whom giant cell arteritis has affected the aorta or its major branches. Indeed, 40% of patients will have nonclassic presentations chiefly with respiratory tract problems (most frequently dry cough), mononeuritis multiplex (most frequently with painful paralysis of a shoulder), or fever of unknown origin. Giant cell arteritis accounts for 15% of all cases of fever of unknown origin in patients over the age of 65. The fever can be as high as 40 °C and is frequently associated with rigors and sweats. In contrast to patients with infection, patients with giant cell arteritis and fever almost always have a normal white blood count (before prednisone is started). Thus, in an older patient with fever of unknown origin, a very high erythrocyte sedimentation rate, and a normal white blood count, giant cell arteritis must be considered even in the absence of specific features such as headache or jaw claudication.

The main reason to diagnose and treat giant cell arteritis is to prevent blindness. Once blindness develops, it is usually permanent. Therefore, when a patient has symptoms and findings suggestive of temporal arteritis, therapy with prednisone, 60 mg daily, is initiated immediately, and temporal artery biopsy is promptly obtained. How quickly the histologic changes in the temporal artery resolve after initiation of therapy is unclear, but biopsies obtained within 1–2 weeks after initiation of therapy should be reliable. Typically, a positive biopsy shows inflammatory infiltrate in the media and adventitia with lymphocytes, histiocytes, plasma cells, and giant cells. An adequate biopsy specimen (3–5 cm in length) is essential, because the disease tends to be segmental. Unilateral temporal artery biopsy is positive in approximately 80–85% of patients; bilateral biopsies add 10–15% to the yield. Ten to 15 percent of patients have vasculitis of other major arteries. Prednisone should be continued in a dosage of 60 mg/d for 1–2 months before tapering. When only the symptoms of polymyalgia rheumatica are present, temporal artery biopsy is not necessary.

In adjusting the dosage of steroid, the erythrocyte sedimentation rate is a useful but not absolute guide to disease activity. Blindness rarely occurs when the ESR has reached the normal range. The drug may be slowly tapered when disease activity ceases, although the disorder may recur and in some patients remains active for years. Thoracic aortic aneurysm with rupture is a complication of giant cell arteritis that can occur at any time but typically develops 7 years after the diagnosis of giant cell arteritis.

Achkar AA et al: How does previous corticosteroid treatment affect the biopsy findings in giant cell (temporal) arteritis? Ann Intern Med 1994;120:987. (Temporal artery biopsies can remain positive even after 2 weeks of corticosteroid therapy.)

Evans JM et al: Thoracic aortic aneurysm and rupture in giant cell arteritis: A descriptive study of 41 cases. Arthritis Rheum 1994;37:1539. (Thoracic aortic aneurysm occurred a median of 7 years after diagnosis of giant cell arteritis, causing congestive heart failure, dyspnea, and sudden death.)

Gonzalez-Gay MA et al: Polymyalgia rheumatica without significantly increased erythrocyte sedimentation rate: A more benign syndrome. Arch Intern Med 1997;157:317. (Suggests that polymyalgia rheumatica with an ESR < 40 mm/h is more common than previously thought, especially in men.)

Helfgott SM, Kieval RI: Polymyalgia rheumatica in patients with a normal erythrocyte sedimentation rate. Arthritis Rheum 1996;39:304. (Polymyalgia rheumatica with an ESR < 30 mm/h found in 20%, especially men.)

Matteson EL et al: Long-term survival of patients with giant cell arteritis in the American College of Rheumatology giant cell arteritis classification criteria cohort. Am J Med 1996;100:193. (Giant cell arteritis does not decrease life expectancy.)

WEGENER'S GRANULOMATOSIS

Wegener's granulomatosis is a rare disorder (prevalence of three per 100,000) characterized by vasculitis, necrotizing granulomatous lesions of both upper and lower respiratory tract, and glomerulonephritis. Without treatment it is invariably fatal, most patients surviving less than a year after diagnosis. It occurs most commonly in the fourth and fifth decades of life and affects men and women with equal frequency.

Clinical Findings

A. Symptoms and Signs: The disorder usually develops over 4–12 months, with 90% of patients presenting with upper or lower respiratory tract symptoms or both. Upper respiratory tract symptoms can include nasal congestion, sinusitis, otitis media, mastoiditis, gum hypertrophy, or stridor due to subglottic stenosis. Since many of these symptoms are common, the underlying disease is not often suspected until the patient develops systemic symptoms or the original problem is refractory to treatment. The lung is affected initially in 40% and eventually in 80%, with symptoms including cough, dyspnea, and hemoptysis. Other early symptoms can include unilateral proptosis (from pseudotumor), red eye from scleritis, arthritis, purpura, and dysesthesia due to neuropathy. Renal involvement, which develops in three-fourths of the cases, usually does not cause symptoms before the diagnosis is established. Fever, malaise, and weight loss are common.

Physical examination can be remarkable for congestion, crusting, ulceration, bleeding, and even perforation of the nasal mucosa. Destruction of the nasal cartilage with "saddle nose" deformity occurs late. Otitis media, proptosis, and scleritis are other common findings. Newly acquired hypertension, a frequent feature of polyarteritis, is rare in Wegener's granulomatosis.

Although limited forms of Wegener's granulomatosis have been described in which the kidney is spared initially, most untreated patients will develop renal disease. In such cases the urinary sediment invariably contains red cells, with or without white cells, and red cell casts. Renal biopsy discloses a segmental necrotizing glomerulonephritis with multiple crescents; this is characteristic but not diagnostic. Granulomas are observed in 10%.

B. Laboratory Findings: Most patients have slight anemia, mild leukocytosis, and an elevated erythrocyte sedimentation rate. Chest CT is a good deal more sensitive than chest x-ray; lesions include infiltrates, nodules, masses, and cavities. Often the radiographs prompt concern about lung cancer. Hilar adenopathy is very rare in Wegener's granulomatosis; if present, sarcoidosis, tumor, or infection is more likely. Other common laboratory abnormalities include sinus destruction, hematuria, and red cell casts.

Histologic features of Wegener's granulomatosis include vasculitis, granuloma, geographic necrosis, and acute and chronic inflammation. The full range of pathologic changes are usually evident only on thoracoscopic lung biopsy. Nasal biopsies often do not show vasculitis but can show the other changes, which in the appropriate setting and when interpreted by an experienced pathologist can offer convincing evidence of the diagnosis.

Over 90% of patients with active Wegener's granulomatosis are positive for anti-neutrophil cytoplasmic antibody (ANCA). cANCA is more common and specific for this disorder, but some patients have the less specific pANCA. Previously, experts insisted on a tissue diagnosis, usually from open lung biopsy. cANCA has not obviated the need for a tissue diagnosis but has reduced the once frequent requirement for open lung biopsy. That is, the diagnosis of Wegener's syndrome can be confidently established in the patient with typical clinical findings, a biopsy that is suggestive but not necessarily definitive (eg, from skin, nose, or mastoids), and a positive cANCA test.

Treatment

It is essential that the diagnosis be made early, since treatment may be lifesaving. Early treatment is also crucial in preventing renal failure. While Wegener's granulomatosis may involve the sinuses or lung for months, once proteinuria or hematuria develops, progression to renal failure can be rapid (over several weeks). Remissions have been induced in up to 75% of patients treated with cyclophosphamide and prednisone. though half of such patients have a recurrence of the disease. Most patients also have serious morbidity from the disease or its treatment. The risk of cancer—particularly bladder cancer and lymphoma—is increased in patients treated with cyclophosphamide. The cyclophosphamide is best given daily by mouth; intermittent high-dose intravenous cyclophosphamide is less effective. Studies suggest that methotrexate, 20 mg/wk, is as effective as oral cyclophosphamide for patients who do not have immediately life-threatening disease. Thus, for these patients, the combination of methotrexate and prednisone has become the initial treatment of choice. Trimethoprim-sulfamethoxazole (one double-strength tablet twice daily) is ineffective for life-threatening Wegener's disease; however, the drug has been shown to be effective in helping to keep patients in remission. Trimethoprim-sulfamethoxazole and methotrexate are both folate and antagonist; the combination can cause aplastic anemia and should be used with great care. ANCA levels correlate erratically with disease activity, so the titer by itself should not dictate changes in treatment.

Hoffman GS et al: Wegener granulomatosis: An analysis of 158 patients. Ann Intern Med 1992;116:488. (A sobering review of the complications of the disease and its treatment. Eighty-five percent of patients had serious morbidity from irreversible features of the disease, and half had serious adverse effects of therapy. Cyclophosphamide was associated with a 2.4-fold increase in all malignancies, a 30-fold increase in bladder cancers, and an 10-fold increase in lymphomas.)

Rao JK et al: The role of antineutrophil cytoplasmic antibody (c-ANCA) testing in the diagnosis of Wegener granulomatosis: A literature review and meta-analysis. Ann Intern Med 1995;123:925. (c-ANCA sensitivity ranged from 34% to 92%, and specificity ranged from 88% to 100%.)

Sneller MC et al: An analysis of forty-two Wegener's granulomatosis patients treated with methotrexate and prednisone. Arthritis Rheum 1995;38:608. (Suggests that methotrexate is an acceptable alternative to cyclophosphamide in this selected group of patients.)

Stegeman CA et al: Trimethoprim-sulfamethoxazole (cotrimoxazole) for the prevention of relapses of Wegener's granulomatosis. N Engl J Med 1996;335:16. (Co-trimoxazole [800 mg of sulfamethoxazole and 160 mg of trimethoprim] given twice daily to patients in remission helps prevent relapses. However, 20% of patients stopped the drug because of toxicity.)

Talar-Williams C et al: Cyclophosphamide-induced cystitis and bladder cancer in patients with Wegener granulomatosis. Ann Intern Med 1996;124:477. (Incidence of bladder cancer was 5% at 10 years and 16% at 15 years. Nonglomerular hematuria identified group at high risk.)

CRYOGLOBULINEMIA

Vasculitis secondary to cryoglobulinemia is uncommon but should be considered when patients present with palpable purpura on the lower extremities, glomerulonephritis (reflected by hematuria, proteinuria, and red blood cell casts), and peripheral neuropathy. Abnormal liver function tests, abdominal pain, cardiac disease, and pulmonary disease may also occur. The diagnosis is based on a compatible clinical picture and a positive serum test for cryoglobulins. Type II (monoclonal antibody with rheumatoid factor activity) and type III (polyclonal antibody with rheumatoid factor activity) cryoglobulins are most common in patients with vasculitis. Type I cryoglobulin (a monoclonal protein that does not have rheumatoid factor activity) is more commonly seen in lymphoproliferative disease associated with a hyperviscosity syndrome. Although the cause of cryoglobulinemia in vasculitis is unknown, the majority of patients have evidence of hepatitis C infection. Prednisone and immunosuppressive drugs are, at best, moderately effective for visceral complications such as renal insufficiency and neuropathy.

Cacoub P et al: Mixed cryoglobulinemia and hepatitis C virus. Am J Med 1994; 96:124. (Most patients with mixed cryoglobulinemia have hepatitis C antibodies or hepatitis C RNA.)

HENOCH-SCHÖNLEIN PURPURA

This is a form of purpura of unknown cause; the underlying pathologic feature is vasculitis, which principally affects small blood vessels. Although the disease is predominantly seen in children, adults are also affected. Hypersensitivity to aspirin and food and drug additives has been reported. The purpuric skin lesions are typically located on the lower extremities but may also be seen on the hands, arms, and trunk. Localized areas of edema, especially common on the dorsal surfaces of the hands, are frequently observed. Joint symptoms are present in the majority of patients, the knees and ankles being most commonly involved. Abdominal pain secondary to vasculitis of the intestinal tract is often associated with gastrointestinal bleeding. Hematuria signals the presence of a renal lesion that is usually reversible, although it occasionally may progress to renal insufficiency. Biopsy of the kidney reveals segmental glomerulonephritis with crescents and mesangial deposition of IgA and, sometimes, IgG. Aside from an elevated sedimentation rate, most laboratory findings are noncontributory; the platelet count is normal or elevated.

The disease is usually self-limited, lasting 1–6 weeks, and subsides without sequelae if renal involvement is not severe. The efficacy of treatment is not well established. In a small number of patients, high-dose immunoglobulin therapy has been reported to stabilize patients whose nephritis had been progressive.

Rostoker G et al: High-dose immunoglobulin therapy for severe IgA nephropathy and Henoch-Schönlein purpura. Ann Intern Med 1994;120:476–484. (Stabilized 11 patients with severe nephritis.)

Yasui K et al: Successful treatment of Behçet disease with pentoxifylline. Ann Intern Med 1996;124:891. (Worked in three patients.)

RELAPSING POLYCHONDRITIS

This is a rare disease of unknown cause characterized by inflammatory destructive lesions of cartilaginous structures, principally the ears, nose, trachea, and larynx. It may be associated either with other immunologic disorders such as SLE, rheumatoid arthritis, or Hashimoto's thyroiditis or with cancers, especially multiple myeloma. The disease, which is usually episodic, affects males and females equally. The cartilage is painful, swollen, and tender during an attack and subsequently becomes atrophic, resulting in permanent deformity. Biopsy of the involved cartilage shows inflammation and chondrolysis. Noncartilaginous manifestations of the disease include fever, episcleritis, uveitis, deafness, aortic insufficiency, and rarely immune complex-mediated renal disease. In 85% of patients, an arthropathy is seen that tends to be migratory, asymmetric, and seronegative, affecting both large and small joints and the parasternal articulation.

Corticosteroid therapy is often effective. Dapsone may also be effective, sparing the need for chronic high-dose corticosteroid treatment. Involvement of the tracheobronchial tree, leading to its collapse, may cause death if tracheostomy is not done promptly.

BEHÇET'S SYNDROME

Named after the Turkish dermatologist who first described it, this disease of unknown cause is characterized by recurrent oral and genital ulcers, uveitis, seronegative arthritis, and central nervous system abnormalities. Other features include ulcerative skin lesions, erythema nodosum, thrombophlebitis, and vasculitis. Arthritis occurs in about two-thirds of patients, most commonly affecting the knees and ankles. Keratitis, uveitis—often with hypopyon (pus in the anterior chamber)—and optic neuritis are observed. The ocular involvement is often fulminant and may result in blindness. Involvement of the central nervous system often results in serious disability or death. Findings include cranial nerve palsies, convulsions, encephalitis, mental disturbances, and spinal cord lesions. Leukocytosis and a rapid sedimentation rate are common.

The clinical course may be chronic but is often characterized by remissions and exacerbations. Corticosteroids, azathioprine, chlorambucil, pentoxifylline, and cyclosporine have been used with beneficial results. Oral base corticosteroids may be of some help for oral ulcerations.

SERONEGATIVE SPONDYLOARTHROPATHIES

The seronegative spondylarthropathies are ankylosing spondylitis, psoriatic arthritis, Reiter's syndrome (also called reactive arthritis), and colitic arthritis. These disorders are noted for onset usually before age 40, inflammatory arthritis of the spine or the large peripheral joints (or both), uveitis in a significant minority, the absence of autoantibodies in the serum, and a striking association with HLA-B27. Present in only 8% of normal Caucasians and 3% of normal blacks, HLA-B27 is positive in 90% of patients with ankylosing spondylitis and 75% with Reiter's syndrome. HLA-B27 also occurs in 50% of the psoriatic and colitic arthritis patients who have sacroiliitis; patients with only peripheral arthritis in these two syndromes do not show an increase in HLA-B27.

That HLA-B27 itself and not some other nearby gene confers susceptibility to these diseases has been demonstrated by experiments with transgenic rats. When the human HLA-B27 gene is expressed in rats, the animals develop a spinal and peripheral arthritis, psoriasiform nail and skin changes, and bowel inflammation. Thus, having HLA-B27 is crucial to the development of a spondylarthropathy.

Infection also appears to play a key role in some of the spondylarthropathies, especially Reiter's syndrome, which characteristically develops days to weeks after a bacterial dysenteric or nongonococcal venereal infection (see below). The interplay of susceptibility genes and environmental infections is demonstrated by the fact that the risk of developing Reiter's syndrome is 0.2% in the general population, 2% in the HLA-B27 individuals, and 20% in patients with HLA-B27 who become infected with *Salmonella, Shigella,* or enteric organisms. The importance of infection in the pathogenesis of spondylarthropathies is also demonstrated by the transgenic rats that express human HLA-B27; rats raised in germ-free environments do not develop arthritis. Despite these gains in our understanding of the importance of HLA-B27 and infection, the way in which genes and infection cause spondylarthropathy is not yet known.

ANKYLOSING SPONDYLITIS

Essentials of Diagnosis

- Chronic low backache in young adults.
- Progressive limitation of back motion and of chest expansion.
- Transient (50%) or permanent (25%) peripheral arthritis.
- Uveitis in 20–25%.
- Diagnostic x-ray changes in sacroiliac joints.
- Accelerated erythrocyte sedimentation rate and negative serologic tests for rheumatoid factor. HLA-B27 usually positive.

General Considerations

Ankylosing spondylitis is a chronic inflammatory disease of the joints of the axial skeleton, manifested clinically by pain and progressive stiffening of the spine. The age at onset is usually in the late teens or early 20s. The incidence is greater in males than in females, and symptoms are more prominent in men, with ascending involvement of the spine more likely to occur.

Clinical Findings

A. Symptoms and Signs: The onset is usually gradual, with intermittent bouts of back pain that may radiate down the thighs. As the disease advances, symptoms progress in a cephalad direction and back motion becomes limited, with the normal lumbar curve flattened and the thoracic curvature exaggerated. Chest expansion is often limited as a consequence of costovertebral joint involvement. Radicular symptoms due to cauda equina fibrosis may occur years after onset of the disease. In advanced cases, the entire spine becomes fused, allowing no motion in any direction. Transient acute arthritis of the peripheral joints occurs in about 50% of cases, and permanent changes in the peripheral joints—most commonly the hips, shoulders, and knees—are seen in about 25%.

Spondylitic heart disease, characterized chiefly by atrioventricular conduction defects and aortic insufficiency, occurs in 3–5% of patients with long-standing severe disease. Nongranulomatous anterior uveitis is associated in as many as 25% of cases and may be a presenting feature. Pulmonary fibrosis of the upper lobes, with progression to cavitation and bronchiectasis mimicking tuberculosis, may occur, characteristically long after the onset of skeletal symptoms. Constitutional symptoms similar to those of rheumatoid arthritis are absent in most patients.

B. Laboratory Findings: The erythrocyte sedimentation rate is elevated in 85% of cases, but serologic tests for rheumatoid factor are characteristically negative. Anemia may be present but is often mild.

HLA-B27 is found in 90% of patients with ankylosing spondylitis. Because this antigen occurs in 8% of the normal population, it is not a specific diagnos-

tic test. Persons with other rheumatic diseases such as rheumatoid arthritis, degenerative joint disease (osteoarthritis), and gout do not show a higher than normal incidence of HLA-B27.

C. Imaging: The earliest radiographic changes are usually in the sacroiliac joints. In the first few months of the disease process, the sacroiliac changes may be detectable only by CT scanning. Later, erosion and sclerosis of these joints are evident on regular radiographs. Later, involvement of the apophysial joints of the spine, ossification of the annulus fibrosus, calcification of the anterior and lateral spinal ligaments, and squaring and generalized demineralization of the vertebral bodies may occur. The term "bamboo spine" has been used to describe the late radiographic changes.

Additional x-ray findings include periosteal new bone formation on the iliac crest, ischial tuberosities and calcanei, and alterations of the pubic symphysis and sternomanubrial joint similar to those of the sacroiliacs. Radiologic changes in peripheral joints, when present, tend to be asymmetric and lack the demineralization and erosions seen in rheumatoid arthritis.

Differential Diagnosis

In contrast to ankylosing spondylitis, rheumatoid arthritis predominantly affects multiple, small, peripheral joints of the hands and feet, spares the sacroiliac joint, has little effect on the rest of the spine except for C1–C2, causes rheumatoid nodules, is associated with rheumatoid factor, and is not associated with HLA-B27. The history and physical findings of ankylosing spondylitis serve to distinguish this disorder from other causes of low back pain such as disk disease, osteoporosis, soft tissue trauma, and tumors. The single most valuable distinguishing radiologic sign of ankylosing spondylitis is the appearance of the sacroiliac joints, although a similar pattern may be seen in Reiter's syndrome and in the arthritis associated with inflammatory intestinal diseases and psoriasis. A spondyloarthropathy associated with hidradenitis suppurativa has been described in blacks. In ankylosing hyperostosis (diffuse idiopathic skeletal hyperostosis [DISH], Forestier's disease), there is exuberant osteophyte formation. The osteophytes are thicker and more anterior than the syndesmophytes of ankylosing spondylitis, and the sacroiliac joints are not affected. The x-ray appearance of the sacroiliac joints in spondylitis should be distinguished from that in osteitis condensans ilii. In some geographic areas and in persons with appropriate occupations, brucellosis and fluoride poisoning may be important in the differential diagnosis.

Treatment

A. Basic Program: The general principles of managing chronic arthritis (see above) apply equally well to ankylosing spondylitis. The importance of postural and breathing exercises should be stressed.

B. Drug Therapy: The nonsteroidal anti-inflammatory agents are employed in the treatment of this disorder. Of these, indomethacin appears to be the most effective, though it can be quite toxic. The dosage of indomethacin is usually 25–50 mg three times a day, but the least amount should be used that will provide symptomatic improvement. Agents such as naproxen, fenoprofen, tolmetin, sulindac, piroxicam, and other newer NSAIDs are valuable alternatives and may be used as primary therapy. Indomethacin may produce a variety of untoward reactions, including headache, giddiness, nausea and vomiting, peptic ulcer, renal insufficiency, depression, and psychosis. Sulfasalazine (see above) can be effective in patients who do not respond to NSAIDs.

C. Physical Therapy: See above.

Prognosis

Almost all patients have persistent symptoms over decades; rare individuals experience long-term remissions. The severity of disease varies greatly, with about 10% of patients having work disability after 10 years. Developing hip disease within the first 2 years of disease onset presages a worse prognosis.

Amor B et al: Predictive factors for the longterm outcome of spondyloarthropathies. J Rheumatol 1994;21:1883. (Seven entry variables correlated with poor prognosis: hip arthritis, ESR > 30 mm/h, poor response to NSAIDs, limitation of lumbar spine, sausage digit, oligoarthritis, and onset at 16 years of age or younger.)

Creemers MCW et al: Methotrexate in severe ankylosing spondylitis: An open study. J Rheumatol 1995;22:1104. (In an open study of 11 patients, methotrexate appeared effective.)

Clegg DO et al: Comparison of sulfasalazine and placebo in the treatment of ankylosing spondylitis: A Department of Veterans Affairs Cooperative Study. Arthritis Rheum 1996;39:2004. (Sulfasalazine 2000 mg/d is effective for peripheral arthritis but not for long-standing spinal disease.)

PSORIATIC ARTHRITIS

Essentials of Diagnosis

- Psoriasis precedes onset of arthritis in 80% of cases.
- Arthritis usually asymmetric, with "sausage" appearance of fingers and toes; resembles rheumatoid arthritis; rheumatoid factor is absent from serum.
- Sacroiliac joint involvement common; ankylosing spondylitis may be associated.
- X-ray findings: osteolysis; pencil-in-cup deformity; relative lack of osteoporosis; bony ankylosis; asymmetric sacroiliitis and atypical syndesmophytes.

General Considerations

In 15–20% of patients with psoriasis, arthritis coexists. The patterns or subsets of arthritis that may accompany psoriasis include the following:

(1) Joint disease that resembles rheumatoid arthritis in which polyarthritis is symmetric. Usually, fewer joints are involved than in rheumatoid arthritis, and rheumatoid factor is absent from the serum.

(2) An oligoarticular form that may lead to considerable destruction of the affected joints.

(3) A pattern of disease in which the distal interphalangeal joints are primarily affected. Early, this may be monarticular, and often the joint involvement is asymmetric. Pitting of the nails and onycholysis are frequently associated.

(4) A severe deforming arthritis (arthritis mutilans) in which osteolysis is marked.

(5) A spondylitic form with sacroiliitis and spinal involvement predominating; 50% of these patients are HLA-B27 positive.

Clinical Findings

A. Symptoms and Signs: Although psoriasis usually precedes the onset of arthritis, in 20–25% of patients the arthritis precedes the skin disease. Arthritis is at least five times more common in patients with severe skin disease than in those with only mild skin findings. Occasionally, however, patients may have a single patch of psoriasis (typically hidden in the scalp, gluteal cleft, or umbilicus) and are unaware of its connection to the arthritis. Thus, a detailed search for cutaneous lesions is essential in patients with arthritis of new onset. Also, the psoriatic lesions may have cleared when arthritis appears—in such cases, the history is most useful in diagnosing previously unexplained cases of mono- or oligoarthritis. Nail pitting, a residue of previous psoriasis, is sometimes the only clue.

B. Laboratory Findings: Laboratory studies show an elevation of the sedimentation rate, but rheumatoid factor is not present. Uric acid levels may be high, reflecting the active turnover of skin affected by psoriasis. There is a correlation between the extent of psoriatic involvement and the level of uric acid, but gout is no more common than in patients without psoriasis. Desquamation of the skin may also reduce iron stores.

C. Imaging: Radiographic findings are most helpful in distinguishing the disease from other forms of arthritis. There are marginal erosions of bone and irregular destruction of joint and bone, which, in the phalanx, may give the appearance of a sharpened pencil. Fluffy periosteal new bone may be marked, especially at the insertion of muscles and ligaments into bone. Such changes will also be seen along the shafts of metacarpals, metatarsals, and phalanges. Paravertebral ossification occurs, which may be distinguished from ankylosing spondylitis by the absence of ossification in the anterior aspect of the spine.

Treatment

Treatment regimens are symptomatic. Nonsteroidal anti-inflammatory drugs are useful. Antimalarials may exacerbate the psoriasis. Gold therapy is often effective. In resistant cases, methotrexate has been used with some success, but it should be employed only by those fully conversant with its use. Successful treatment of the skin lesions commonly—though not invariably—is accompanied by an improvement in peripheral articular symptoms. Sulfasalazine may also be effective.

Clegg DO et al: Comparison of sulfasalazine and placebo in the treatment of psoriatic arthritis: A Department of Veterans Affairs Cooperative Study. Arthritis Rheum 1996;39:2013. (Sulfasalazine 2000 mg/d moderately more effective than placebo.)

REITER'S SYNDROME (Reactive Arthritis)

Reiter's syndrome, also called "reactive arthritis," is a clinical tetrad of urethritis, conjunctivitis (or, less commonly, uveitis), mucocutaneous lesions, and arthritis. It occurs most commonly in young men, is associated with HLA–B27 in 80% of white patients and 50–60% of blacks, and often follows infection (see above). Most cases of Reiter's syndrome develop within days or weeks of either a dysenteric infection (with *Shigella, Salmonella, Yersinia, Campylobacter*) or a sexually transmitted infection (with *Chlamydia trachomatis* or perhaps *Ureaplasma urealyticum*). Whether the inciting infection is sexually transmitted or dysenteric does not affect the subsequent manifestations but does influence the sex ratio: The ratio is 1.0 after enteric infections but 9:1 with male predominance after sexually transmitted infections.

Although affected joints are culture-negative, fragments of putative organisms have been identified in swollen joints. The exact role of infection remains unclear.

The arthritis is most commonly asymmetric and frequently involves the large weight-bearing joints (chiefly the knee and ankle); sacroiliitis or ankylosing spondylitis is observed in at least 20% of patients, especially after frequent recurrences. Systemic symptoms including fever and weight loss are common at the onset of disease. The mucocutaneous lesions may include balanitis, stomatitis, and keratoderma blennorrhagicum, resembling pustular psoriasis with involvement of the skin and nails. Carditis and aortic regurgitation may occur. While most signs of the disease disappear within days or weeks, the arthritis may persist for several months or

even years. Recurrences involving any combination of the clinical manifestations are common and are sometimes followed by permanent sequelae, especially in the joints.

X-ray signs of permanent or progressive joint disease may be seen in the sacroiliac as well as the peripheral joints.

Gonococcal arthritis can initially mimic Reiter's syndrome, but the marked improvement after 24–48 hours of antibiotic administration and the culture results distinguish the two disorders. Rheumatoid arthritis, idiopathic ankylosing spondylitis, and psoriatic arthritis must also be considered. The association of Reiter's syndrome and HIV has been debated, but evidence now indicates Reiter's syndrome is equally common in sexually active men regardless of HIV status.

NSAIDs have been the mainstay of therapy. Antibiotics may also have some role. Antibiotics given at the time of a nongonococcal venereal infection reduce the chance that the individual will develop Reiter's syndrome and the chance of a relapse in those who have a history of Reiter's syndrome. Tetracycline given for 3 months to patients with Reiter's syndrome associated with *C trachomatis* reduces the duration of symptoms. Tetracyclines have anti-inflammatory properties, so the response need not be attributed solely to an antimicrobial effect. Patients with enteric Reiter's syndrome do not respond to antibiotics. Patients who fail NSAIDs and antibiotics may respond to sulfasalazine.

Clegg DO et al: Comparison of sulfasalazine and placebo in the treatment of reactive arthritis (Reiter's syndrome): A Department of Veterans Affairs Cooperative Study. Arthritis Rheum 1996;39:2021. (Sulfasalazine 2000 mg/d is well tolerated and effective.)

Gaston JSH et al: Identification of 2 *Chlamydia trachomatis* antigens recognized by synovial fluid T cells from patients with *Chlamydia* induced reactive arthritis. J Rheumatol 1996;23:130. (That Reiter's syndrome may be caused by an immune response to chronic joint infections is suggested by finding synovial T cells that respond to chlamydial antigens.)

Nanagara R et al: Alteration of *Chlamydia trachomatis* biologic behavior in synovial membranes: Suppression of surface antigen production in reactive arthritis and Reiter's syndrome. Arthritis Rheum 1995;38:1410. (Presents evidence that chlamydial organisms undergo alteration allowing them to escape immune surveillance and to cause reactive arthritis.)

ARTHRITIS & INFLAMMATORY INTESTINAL DISEASES

One-fifth of patients with inflammatory bowel disease have arthritis, making it second only to anemia as the most common extraintestinal manifestation. Arthritis complicates Crohn's disease somewhat more frequently than it does ulcerative colitis. In both diseases, two distinct forms of arthritis occur. The first is peripheral arthritis—usually a nonde-forming asymmetric oligoarthritis of large joints—in which the activity of the joint disease parallels that of the bowel disease. The arthritis usually begins months to years after the bowel disease, but occasionally the joint symptoms develop earlier and may be prominent enough to cause the patient to overlook intestinal symptoms. The second form of arthritis is a spondylitis that is indistinguishable by symptoms or x-ray from ankylosing spondylitis and follows a course independent of the bowel disease. About 50% of these patients are HLA-B27-positive.

Controlling the intestinal inflammation usually eliminates the peripheral arthritis. The spondylitis often requires NSAIDs, which need to be used cautiously since these agents may activate the bowel disease in a few patients. Range-of-motion exercises as prescribed for ankylosing spondylitis can be helpful.

About two-thirds of patients with Whipple's disease experience arthralgia or arthritis, most often an episodic, large-joint polyarthritis. The arthritis usually precedes the gastrointestinal manifestations by years. In fact, the arthritis resolves as the diarrhea develops. Thus, Whipple's disease should be considered in the differential diagnosis of unexplained episodic arthritis.

About 15% of patients who have jejunoileal bypass surgery for morbid obesity develop an inflammatory symmetric polyarticular disorder. The arthritis is usually acute in onset and nonmigratory and may affect the small as well as the large joints. The sedimentation rate is elevated, and antinuclear antibody and rheumatoid factor tests may be positive. Nonsteroidal anti-inflammatory agents are often effective, although some patients require prednisone.

INFECTIOUS ARTHRITIS*

NONGONOCOCCAL ACUTE BACTERIAL (SEPTIC) ARTHRITIS

Essentials of Diagnosis

- Sudden onset of acute arthritis, usually monarticular, most often in large weight-bearing joints and wrists.
- Previous joint damage or intravenous drug abuse common risk factors.
- Infection with causative organisms commonly found elsewhere in body.

*Lyme disease is discussed in Chapter 34.

- Joint effusions are usually large, with white blood counts commonly > 100,000/μL.

General Considerations

Nongonococcal acute bacterial arthritis is a disease of an abnormal host. The key risk factors are persistent bacteremia (eg, intravenous drug abuse, endocarditis) and damaged joints (eg, rheumatoid arthritis). *Staphylococcus aureus* is the most common cause of nongonococcal septic arthritis, followed by group A and group B streptococci. Gram-negative septic arthritis, once rare, has become more common, especially in intravenous drug abusers and in other immunocompromised hosts. *Escherichia coli* and *Pseudomonas aeruginosa* are the most common gram-negative isolates in adults.

The widespread use of arthroscopy and prosthetic joint surgery has also increased the frequency of septic arthritis. In the latter conditions, *Staphylococcus epidermidis* is the usual offending organism. Pathologic changes include varying degrees of acute inflammation, with synovitis, effusion, abscess formation in synovial or subchondral tissues, and, if treatment is not adequate, articular destruction.

Clinical Findings

A. Symptoms and Signs: The onset is usually sudden, with acute pain, swelling, and heat of one joint—most frequently the knee. Other commonly affected sites are the hip, wrist, shoulder, and ankle. Unusual sites, such as the sternoclavicular or sacroiliac joint, can be involved in intravenous drug abusers. Chills and fever are common but are absent in up to 20% of patients. Infection of the hip usually does not produce apparent swelling but results in groin pain greatly aggravated by walking.

B. Laboratory Findings: Blood cultures are positive in approximately 50% of patients. The leukocyte count of the synovial fluid may be greater than 100,000/μL, with 90% or more polymorphonuclear cells. Synovial fluid glucose is usually low. Gram stain of the synovial fluid is positive in 75% of staphylococcal infections and in 50% of gram-negative infections.

C. Imaging: Radiographs are usually normal early in the disease, but evidence of demineralization may be present within days of onset. Bony erosions and narrowing of the joint space followed by osteomyelitis and periostitis may be seen within 2 weeks.

Differential Diagnosis

The septic course with chills and fever, the acute systemic reaction, the joint fluid findings, evidence of infection elsewhere in the body, and the evidence of response to appropriate antibiotics are diagnostic of bacterial arthritis. Gout and pseudogout are excluded by the failure to find crystals on synovial fluid analysis. Acute rheumatic fever and rheumatoid arthritis commonly involve many joints; Still's disease may mimic septic arthritis, but laboratory evidence of infection is absent. Pyogenic arthritis may be superimposed on other types of joint disease, notably rheumatoid arthritis, and must be excluded (by joint fluid examination) in any apparent acute relapse of the primary disease, particularly when a joint has been needled or when one is more strikingly inflamed than the others.

Treatment

Prompt systemic antibiotic therapy of any septic arthritis should be based on the best clinical judgment of the causative organism and the results of smear and culture of joint fluid, blood, urine, or other specific sites of potential infection. If the organism cannot be determined clinically, treatment should be started with bactericidal antibiotics effective against staphylococci, pneumococci, and gram-negative organisms.

Frequent (even daily) local aspiration is indicated when synovial fluid rapidly reaccumulates and causes symptoms. Immediate surgical drainage is reserved for septic arthritis of the hip, because that site is inaccessible to repeated aspiration. For most other joints, surgical drainage is used only if medical therapy fails over 2–4 days to improve the fever and the synovial fluid volume, white blood count, and culture results. Pain can be relieved with local hot compresses and by immobilizing the joint with a splint or traction. Rest, immobilization, and elevation are used at the onset of treatment. Early active motion exercises within the limits of tolerance will hasten recovery.

Prognosis

With prompt antibiotic therapy and no serious underlying disease, functional recovery is usually good. Five to 10 percent of patients with an infected joint die, chiefly from respiratory complications of sepsis. The mortality rate is 30% for patients with polyarticular sepsis. Bony ankylosis and articular destruction commonly also occur if treatment is delayed or inadequate.

Kaandorp CJE et al: Risk factors for septic arthritis in patients with joint disease. Arthritis Rheum 1995;38:1819. (Risk factors for infection were age > 80, diabetes, rheumatoid arthritis, prosthetic hip or knee, joint surgery, and skin infection.)

GONOCOCCAL ARTHRITIS

Essentials of Diagnosis

- Prodromal migratory polyarthralgias.
- Tenosynovitis most common sign.
- Purulent monarthritis in 50%.
- Characteristic skin rash.

- Most common in young women during menses or pregnancy.
- Symptoms of urethritis frequently absent.
- Dramatic response to antibiotics.

General Considerations

Disseminated gonococcal infection is the most common cause of infectious arthritis in large urban areas. In contrast to nongonococcal bacterial arthritis, gonococcal arthritis chiefly occurs in otherwise healthy individuals. Host factors, however, influence the expression of the disease: gonococcal arthritis is two to three times more common in women than in men, is especially common during menses and pregnancy, and is rare after age 40. Gonococcal arthritis is also common in male homosexuals, whose high incidence of asymptomatic gonococcal pharyngitis and proctitis predisposes them to disseminated gonococcal infection. Some of the signs of disseminated gonococcal infection may result from an immunologic reaction to nonviable fragments of the organism's cell wall; this may explain the frequent inability to culture organisms from skin and joint lesions. Recurrent disseminated gonococcal infection should prompt evaluation for a congenital deficiency of complement components, especially C7 and C8.

Clinical Findings

A. Symptoms and Signs: One to 4 days of migratory polyarthralgias involving the wrist, knee, ankle, or elbow is the most common initial course. Thereafter, two patterns emerge, one (60% of patients) characterized by tenosynovitis and the other (40%) by purulent monarthritis, most frequently involving the knee. Less than half of patients have fever, and less than one-fourth have any genitourinary symptoms. Most patients will have asymptomatic but highly characteristic skin lesions that usually consist of two to ten small necrotic pustules distributed over the extremities, especially the palms and soles.

B. Laboratory Findings: The peripheral blood leukocyte count averages about 10,000 cells/μL and is elevated in less than one-third of patients. The synovial fluid white blood cell count, however, is typically over 50,000 cells/μL. The synovial fluid Gram stain is positive in one-fourth of cases and culture in less than half. Positive blood cultures are seen in 40% of patients with tenosynovitis and virtually never in patients with suppurative arthritis. Urethral, throat, and rectal cultures should be done in all patients, since they are often positive in the absence of local symptoms. Culturing *Neisseria gonorrhoeae* is facilitated by rapid transport to the microbiology laboratory, inoculation on appropriate media, and incubation in carbon dioxide.

C. Imaging: Radiographs are usually normal or show only soft tissue swelling.

Differential Diagnosis

Reiter's syndrome can also produce acute monarthritis in a young person but is distinguished by negative cultures, sacroiliitis, and failure to respond to antibiotics. Lyme disease involving the knee is less acute, does not show positive cultures, and may be preceded by known tick exposure and characteristic rash. The synovial fluid analysis will exclude gout, pseudogout, and nongonococcal bacterial arthritis. Rheumatic fever and sarcoidosis can produce migratory tenosynovitis but have other distinguishing features. Infective endocarditis with septic arthritis can mimic disseminated gonococcal infection.

Treatment

In most cases, patients suspected of having gonococcal arthritis should be admitted to the hospital to confirm the diagnosis, to exclude endocarditis, and to start treatment. While outpatient treatment has been recommended in the past, the rapid rise in gonococci resistant to penicillin makes initial inpatient treatment advisable. Approximately 4–5% of all gonococcal isolates produce a β-lactamase that confers penicillin resistance. An additional 15–20% of gonococcal species have chromosomal mutations that result in relative resistance to penicillin. Therefore, the current recommendations for initial treatment of gonococcal arthritis are to give ceftriaxone, 1 g intravenously daily (or cefotaxime, 1 g intravenously every 8 hours, or ceftizoxime, 1 g intravenously every 8 hours). Once improvement from parenteral antibiotics has been achieved for 24–48 hours, patients can be switched to oral cefixime, 400 mg orally twice daily, or ciprofloxacin, 500 mg orally twice daily, to complete a 7- to 10-day course.

Prognosis

Generally, gonococcal arthritis responds dramatically in 24–48 hours after initiation of antibiotics so that daily joint aspirations are rarely needed. Complete recovery is the rule.

Liebling MR et al: Identification of *Neisseria gonorrhoeae* in synovial fluid using the polymerase chain reaction. Arthritis Rheum 1994;37:702. (Suggests that PCR is 96% specific, 79% sensitive.)

RHEUMATIC MANIFESTATIONS OF HIV INFECTION

Infection with human immunodeficiency virus (HIV) has been associated with various rheumatic disorders, most commonly Reiter's syndrome or reactive arthritis or arthralgias and more rarely myositis, psoriatic arthritis, Sjögren's syndrome, or vasculitis (see Chapter 31). It is possible that these disorders stem directly from HIV infection itself or from the many other infections that occur in immunodeficient patients. The rheumatic syndromes can follow or precede by several months the diagnosis of acquired AIDS. Thus, HIV infection must be considered as a possible cause of Reiter's syndrome, and Reiter's syndrome should be considered a possible early manifestation of HIV infection. The lower extremity joints, especially the knees and ankles, are most commonly affected. Often, as in classic Reiter's syndrome, Achilles tendon inflammation (enthesopathy) or knee periarthritis is a prominent and distinguishing feature. Many patients respond to NSAIDs, though a few are unresponsive and develop progressive deformities. The use of immunosuppressive agents, however, is contraindicated in these immunodeficient patients.

VIRAL ARTHRITIS

Arthritis may be a manifestation of many viral infections. It is generally mild and of short duration, and it terminates spontaneously without lasting ill effects. Mumps arthritis may occur in the absence of parotitis. Rubella arthritis, which occurs more commonly in adults than in children, may appear immediately before, during, or soon after the disappearance of the rash. Its usual polyarticular and symmetric distribution mimics that of rheumatoid arthritis. However, the seronegative tests for rheumatoid factor and the rising rubella titers in convalescent serum help to confirm the diagnosis. Postrubella vaccination arthritis may have its onset as long as 6 weeks following vaccination and occurs in all age groups. In adults, arthritis may follow infection with human parvovirus B19.

Polyarthritis may be associated with type B hepatitis and typically occurs before the onset of jaundice; it may occur in anicteric hepatitis as well. Urticaria or other types of skin rash may be present. Indeed, the clinical picture may be indistinguishable from that of serum sickness. Serum transaminase levels are elevated, and hepatitis B surface antigen is most often present. Serum complement levels are usually low during active arthritis and become normal after remission of arthritis. False-positive tests for rheumatoid factor, when present, disappear within several weeks. The arthritis is mild; it rarely lasts more than a few weeks and is self-limiting and without deformity.

Weibel RE, Benor DE: Chronic arthropathy and musculoskeletal symptoms associated with rubella vaccines: A review of 124 claims submitted to the National Vaccine Injury Compensation Program. Arthritis Rheum 1996; 39:1529. (Eighty-seven percent developed arthritis symptoms within 6 weeks after vaccination.)

INFECTIONS OF BONES

Direct microbial contamination of bones results from open fracture, surgical procedures, gunshot wounds, diagnostic needle aspirations, and therapeutic or self-administered drug injections.

Indirect or secondary infections are first noticed in other areas of the body and extend to bones by hematogenous routes.

ACUTE PYOGENIC OSTEOMYELITIS

Essentials of Diagnosis

- Fever and chills associated with pain and tenderness of involved bone.
- Aspiration of involved bone is usually diagnostic.
- Culture of blood or lesion tissue is essential for precise diagnosis.
- Radiographs early in the course are typically negative.

General Considerations

Initial bone infections are indirectly seeded by a single strain of pyogenic bacteria about 95% of the time. About 75% of hematogenous acute infections of bone are due to staphylococci; group A hemolytic streptococci are the next most common pathogens. Vertebral osteomyelitis, due to more indolent organisms, is being encountered with increasing frequency in elderly patients. Among intravenous drug abusers, gram-positive organisms (eg, *Staphylococcus aureus*) and Enterobacteriaceae (eg, *Escherichia coli*) account for 80% of cases of osteomyelitis. Infections of bone due to trauma are often polymicrobial.

Salmonellae cause many cases of bacteremia associated with sickle cell disease. Among patients with hemoglobinopathies, osteomyelitis is caused by salmonellae almost ten times as often as by other pyogenic bacteria. In otherwise healthy patients with salmonellosis, bone lesions are likely to be solitary. In typhoid fever, however, infections of bones occur as a complication in less than 1% of cases. (See Salmonellosis, Chapter 33.)

Bone infection is an uncommon complication of brucellosis, but the clinical picture when it does occur is characteristic. Bone lesions most commonly occur in the lumbar spine or sacroiliac joints.

Clinical Findings

A. Symptoms and Signs: The onset of acute osteomyelitis in adults is less likely to be striking than the sudden and alarming presentation often seen in children. Generalized toxic symptoms of bacteremia may be absent, and vague or evanescent local pain may be the earliest manifestation. Tenderness may be present or absent, depending upon the extent and duration of bone involvement.

B. Laboratory Findings: Aspiration of bone and periosteum to recover organisms for culture is necessary for accurate diagnosis. Blood cultures are frequently positive, particularly when systemic symptoms are prominent, in which case the white count and sedimentation rate are often elevated.

With infections due to *Salmonella* or *Brucella,* significant rising serologic agglutination titers support a tentative diagnosis during the acute stage. Culture of material from the osteoid focus is specific.

C. Imaging: Early findings may include soft tissue swelling, loss of tissue planes, and periarticular demineralization of bone. About 2 weeks after onset of symptoms, erosion of bone and alteration of cancellous bone appear, followed by periostitis. Radionuclide imaging is 90% sensitive, becoming positive within 1–2 days after onset of acute osteomyelitis, but has low (60–70%) specificity. For example, on the basis of bone scans it is difficult to distinguish overlying cellulitis or septic arthritis from osteomyelitis. CT scans and MRI are also more sensitive than conventional radiographs and are particularly helpful in demonstrating the extent of soft tissue involvement. When osteomyelitis involves the vertebrae, it commonly traverses the disk space—a finding that is not observed in tumor.

Differential Diagnosis

Acute hematogenous osteomyelitis should be distinguished from suppurative arthritis, rheumatic fever, and cellulitis. More subacute forms must be differentiated from tuberculous or mycotic infections of bone and Ewing's sarcoma or, in the case of vertebral osteomyelitis, from metastatic tumor.

Complications

Inadequate treatment of bone infections results in chronicity of infection, and this possibility is increased by delay in diagnosis and treatment. Extension to adjacent bone or joints may complicate acute osteomyelitis. Recurrence of bone infections often results in anemia, weight loss, weakness, and, rarely, amyloidosis or nephrotic syndrome. Pseudoepitheliomatous hyperplasia, squamous cell carcinoma, or fibrosarcoma may occasionally arise in persistently infected tissues.

Treatment

Cultures and antibiotic sensitivity studies should determine the choice of antibiotic agents; the initial selection of drug is based on clinical assessment of the most probable cause. Oral therapy with ciprofloxacin, 750 mg twice daily for 6–8 weeks, has been shown to be as effective as standard parenteral antibiotic therapy for chronic osteomyelitis in adults with susceptible organisms. Open or closed drainage of the local lesion is important when prompt clinical response to initial treatment does not occur. Analgesics, rest, immobilization, and elevation of the part should be used from the beginning of treatment.

Prognosis

If sterility of the lesion is achieved within 2–4 days, a good result can be expected in most cases if there is no compromise of the patient's immune system. However, progression of the disease to a chronic form may occur. It is especially common in the lower extremities and in patients in whom circulation is impaired (eg, diabetics). Surgical saucerization, excision of bone, and debridement of healthy tissues are often necessary.

Aliabadi P, Nikpoor N: Imaging osteomyelitis. Arthritis Rheum 1994;37:617. (Review of techniques.)

MYCOTIC INFECTIONS OF BONES & JOINTS

Fungal infections of the skeletal system are usually secondary to a primary infection in another organ, frequently the lungs (see Chapter 36). Although skeletal lesions have a predilection for the cancellous extremities of long bones and the bodies of vertebrae, the predominant lesion—a granuloma with varying degrees of necrosis and abscess formation—does not produce a characteristic clinical picture.

Differentiation from other chronic focal infections depends upon culture studies of synovial fluid or tissue obtained from the local lesion. Serologic tests provide presumptive support of the diagnosis.

1. COCCIDIOIDOMYCOSIS

Coccidioidomycosis of bones and joints is usually secondary to primary pulmonary infection. Arthralgia with periarticular swelling, especially in the knees and ankles, occurring as a nonspecific manifestation of systemic coccidioidomycosis, should be distinguished from actual bone or joint infection. Osseous lesions commonly occur in cancellous bone of the vertebrae or near the ends of long bones at tendinous insertions. These lesions are initially osteolytic and thus may mimic metastatic tumor or myeloma.

The precise diagnosis depends upon recovery of *Coccidioides immitis* from the lesion or histologic examination of tissue obtained by open biopsy. Rising titers of complement-fixing antibodies also provide evidence of the disseminated nature of the disease.

Itraconazole, 200 mg twice daily for 6–12 months, has become the treatment of choice for bone and joint coccidioidomycosis. Chronic infection may require operative excision of infected bone and soft tis-

sue; amputation may be the only solution for stubbornly progressive infections. Immobilization of joints by plaster casts and avoidance of weight bearing provide benefit. Synovectomy, joint debridement, and arthrodesis are reserved for more advanced joint infections.

Stevens DA: Coccidioidomycosis. N Engl J Med 1995; 332:1077. (Disseminated disease most commonly affects bones of skull, hands, feet, spine, and tibia. Most common joints are ankles and knees.)

2. HISTOPLASMOSIS

Focal skeletal or joint involvement in histoplasmosis is rare and generally represents dissemination from a primary focus in the lungs. Skeletal lesions may be single or multiple and are not characteristic.

TUBERCULOSIS OF BONES & JOINTS

Essentials of Diagnosis

- A disease of children, the elderly, or those with HIV infection.
- In most cases, a single site of bone or joint is infected.
- Spine—especially lower thoracic—or knee most common sites.
- Chest x-ray abnormal in less than half.

General Considerations

Most tuberculous infections in the USA are caused by the human strain of *Mycobacterium tuberculosis* (see Chapter 9). Infection of the musculoskeletal system is caused by hematogenous spread from a primary lesion of the respiratory tract; it may occur shortly after primary infection or may be seen years later as a reactivation disease. Tuberculosis of the thoracic or lumbar spine (Pott's disease) usually occurs in the absence of extraspinal infection. It is a disease of children in developing nations and of the elderly in the United States. Tuberculosis of peripheral joints is almost always monarticular, with the knee the most common site. Extra-articular tuberculosis occurs in only 20%.

Clinical Findings

A. Symptoms and Signs: The onset of symptoms is generally insidious and not accompanied by general manifestations of fever, sweating, toxicity, or prostration. Pain may be mild at onset, is usually worse at night, and may be accompanied by stiffness. As the disease process progresses, limitation of joint motion becomes prominent because of muscle contractures and destruction of the joint. The knee is the most commonly involved peripheral joint. Symptoms of pulmonary tuberculosis may also be present.

Local findings during the early stages may be limited to tenderness, soft tissue swelling, joint effusion, and increase in skin temperature about the involved area. As the disease progresses without treatment, muscle atrophy and deformity become apparent. Abscess formation with spontaneous drainage externally leads to sinus formation. Progressive destruction of bone in the spine may cause a gibbus, especially in the thoracolumbar region.

B. Laboratory Findings: The precise diagnosis rests upon recovery of the acid-fast organism from joint fluid, pus, or tissue specimens. Biopsy of the bony lesion, synovium, or a regional lymph node may demonstrate the characteristic histopathologic picture of caseating necrosis and giant cells.

C. Imaging: There is a latent period between the onset of symptoms and the initial positive radiographic finding. The earliest changes of tuberculous arthritis are those of soft tissue swelling and distention of the capsule by effusion. Subsequently, bone atrophy causes thinning of the trabecular pattern, narrowing of the cortex, and enlargement of the medullary canal. As joint disease progresses, destruction of cartilage, both in the spine and in peripheral joints, is manifested by narrowing of the joint cleft and focal erosion of the articular surface, especially at the margins. Where the lesion is limited to bone, especially in the cancellous portion of the metaphysis, the x-ray picture may be that of single or multilocular cysts surrounded by sclerotic bone. With spinal tuberculosis, CT scanning is helpful in demonstrating any associated paraspinal soft tissue infection (eg, psoas abscess, epidural extension).

Differential Diagnosis

Tuberculosis of the musculoskeletal system must be differentiated from all subacute and chronic infections, rheumatoid arthritis, gout, and, occasionally, osseous dysplasia. In the spine, metastatic tumor may be suggested.

Complications

Destruction of bones or joints may occur in a few weeks or months if adequate treatment is not provided. Deformity due to joint destruction, abscess formation with spread into adjacent soft tissues, and sinus formation are common. Paraplegia is the most serious complication of spinal tuberculosis. As healing of severe joint lesions takes place, spontaneous fibrous or bony ankylosis follows.

Treatment
(See also Chapter 37.)

A. General Measures: General care is especially important when prolonged recumbency is necessary; skillful nursing care must be provided.

B. Chemotherapy: Because of the rise of resis-

tant organisms, the new recommendation for treating bony tuberculosis is to begin with four drugs: isoniazid, 300 mg/d; rifampin, 600 mg/d; pyrazinamide, 25 mg/kg/d; and ethambutol, 15 mg/kg/d. If the isolate is sensitive to isoniazid and rifampin, the ethambutol can be stopped, with the pyrazinamide maintained for 2 months. Isoniazid and rifampin are continued for a total of 6 months. Cure without need for surgical intervention may be effected in most cases, even with extensive disease.

C. Surgical Measures: In acute infections where synovitis is the predominant feature, treatment can be conservative, at least initially. Immobilization by splint or plaster, aspiration, and chemotherapy may suffice to control the infection. This treatment is especially desirable for the management of infections of large joints of the lower extremities in children during the early stage of the infection. Synovectomy may be valuable for less acute hypertrophic lesions that involve tendon sheaths, bursae, or joints.

Puttick MPE et al: Soft tissue tuberculosis. A series of 11 cases. J Rheumatol 1995;22:1321. (Most common site was tenosynovitis of hand or foot. Almost all patients were immigrants, and about 50% were immunosuppressed.)

TUMORS & TUMOR-LIKE LESIONS OF BONE

Essentials of Diagnosis

- Persistent pain, swelling, or tenderness of a skeletal part.
- Pathologic ("spontaneous") fractures.
- Suspicious areas of bony enlargement, deformity, radiodensity, or radiolucency on x-ray.
- Histologic evidence of bone neoplasm on biopsy specimen.

General Considerations

Primary tumors of bone are relatively uncommon in comparison with secondary or metastatic neoplasms. They are, however, of great clinical significance because of the possibility of cancer and because some of them grow rapidly and metastasize widely.

Although tumors of bone have been categorized classically as primary or secondary, there is some disagreement about which tumors are primary to the skeleton. Tumors of mesenchymal origin that reflect skeletal tissues (eg, bone, cartilage, and connective tissue) and tumors developing in bones that are of hematopoietic, nerve, vascular, fat cell, and notochordal origin should be differentiated from secondary malignant tumors that involve bone by direct extension or hematogenous spread. Because of the great variety of bone tumors, it is difficult to establish a satisfactory simple classification of bone neoplasms.

Clinical Findings

Persistent skeletal pain and swelling, with or without limitation of motion of adjacent joints or spontaneous fracture, are indications for prompt clinical, x-ray, laboratory, and possibly biopsy examination. X-rays may reveal the location and extent of the lesion and certain characteristics that may suggest the specific diagnosis. The so-called classic x-ray findings of certain tumors (eg, punched-out areas of the skull in multiple myeloma, "sun ray" appearance of osteogenic sarcoma, and "onion peel" effect of Ewing's sarcoma), although suggestive, are not pathognomonic. Even histologic characteristics of the tumor, when taken alone, cannot provide infallible information about the nature of the process. The age of the patient, the duration of complaints, the site of involvement and the number of bones involved, and the presence or absence of associated systemic disease—as well as the histologic characteristics—must be considered collectively for proper management.

The possibility of benign developmental skeletal abnormalities, metastatic neoplastic disease, infections (eg, osteomyelitis), posttraumatic bone lesions, or metabolic disease of bone must always be kept in mind. If bone tumors occur in or near the joints, they may be confused with the various types of arthritis, especially monarticular arthritis.

Specific Bone Tumors

Tumors arising from osteoblastic connective tissue include osteoid osteoma and osteogenic sarcoma. Osteoid osteomas are benign tumors of children and adolescents that should be surgically removed. Osteogenic sarcomas usually involve the knees or long bones and are treated by resection and chemotherapy, with improving survival in recent years. Fibrosarcomas, which are derived from nonosteoblastic connective tissue, have an outlook similar to that of the osteogenic sarcomas. Tumors derived from cartilage include enchondromas, chondromyxoid fibromas, and chondrosarcomas. Histologic examination is confirmatory in this group, and the outlook with appropriate curettement or surgery is generally good.

Other bone tumors include giant cell tumors (osteoclastomas), chondroblastomas, and Ewing's sarcoma. Of these, chondroblastomas are almost always benign. About 50% of giant cell tumors are benign, while the rest may be frankly malignant or recur after excision. Ewing's sarcoma, which affects children, adolescents, and young adults, has a 50% mortality rate in spite of chemotherapy, irradiation, and surgery.

Treatment

Although prompt action is essential for optimal treatment of certain bone tumors, accurate diagnosis is required because of the great potential for harm that may result either from temporization or from radical or ablative operations or unnecessary irradiation.

NEUROGENIC ARTHROPATHY (Charcot's Joint)

Neurogenic arthropathy is joint destruction resulting from loss or diminution of proprioception, pain, and temperature perception. Although traditionally associated with tabes dorsalis, it is more frequently seen in diabetic neuropathy, syringomyelia, spinal cord injury, pernicious anemia, leprosy, and peripheral nerve injury. Prolonged administration of hydrocortisone by the intra-articular route may also cause Charcot's joint. As normal muscle tone and protective reflexes are lost, a marked secondary degenerative joint disease ensues; this results in an enlarged, boggy, painless joint with extensive erosion of cartilage, osteophyte formation, and multiple loose joint bodies. X-ray changes may be degenerative or hypertrophic in the same patient.

Treatment is directed against the primary disease; mechanical devices are used to assist in weight bearing and prevention of further trauma. In some instances, amputation becomes unavoidable.

ARTHRITIS IN SARCOIDOSIS

The frequency of arthritis among patients with sarcoidosis is variously reported between 10% and 35%. It is usually acute in onset, but articular symptoms may appear insidiously and often antedate other manifestations of the disease. Knees and ankles are most commonly involved, but any joint may be affected. Distribution of joint involvement is usually polyarticular and symmetric. The arthritis is commonly self-limiting after several weeks or months; infrequently, the arthritis is recurrent or chronic. Despite its occasional chronicity, the arthritis is rarely associated with joint destruction or significant deformity. Although sarcoid arthritis is often associated with erythema nodosum, the diagnosis is contingent upon the demonstration of other extra-articular manifestations of sarcoidosis and, notably, biopsy evidence of noncaseating granulomas. In chronic arthritis, x-ray shows rather typical changes in the bones of the extremities with intact cortex and cystic changes.

Treatment of arthritis in sarcoidosis is usually symptomatic and supportive. Colchicine may be of value. A short course of corticosteroids may be effective in patients with severe and progressive joint disease.

Mana J et al: Periarticular ankle sarcoidosis: A variant of Lofgren's syndrome. J Rheumatol 1996;23:874. (Periarticular ankle inflammation with bilateral hilar adenopathy is an acute form of sarcoidosis that follows a benign course.)

OTHER RHEUMATIC DISORDERS

OSTEOGENESIS IMPERFECTA
(Fragilitas Ossium, Brittle Bones)

Osteogenesis imperfecta is a heritable disorder of connective tissue usually transmitted as an autosomal dominant, although some cases may be autosomal recessive. Two recognized clinical types may occur: osteogenesis imperfecta congenita (fetal type), in which fractures occur in utero and skeletal deformities are apparent at birth; and osteogenesis imperfecta tarda, in which fractures and deformities occur after birth. Fragility of bones is the single most obvious diagnostic criterion. Clearness or blue coloration of the scleras, conduction deafness, and spinal deformities (scoliosis and kyphosis) are often present. Milder cases of the late form may simulate idiopathic juvenile or menopausal osteoporosis. Unfortunately, there is no treatment for the inadequate formation of osteoid.

RHEUMATIC MANIFESTATIONS OF CANCER

Rheumatologic syndromes may be the presenting manifestations for a variety of cancers. Dermatomyositis in adults, for example, is not infrequently associated with cancer. Middle-aged or older patients with polyarthritis that mimics rheumatoid arthritis but is associated with new onset of clubbing and periosteal new bone formation should be suspected of having hypertrophic pulmonary osteoarthropathy, a disorder commonly associated with both malignant diseases (eg, lung and intrathoracic cancers) and nonmalignant ones (eg, cyanotic heart disease, cirrhosis, and lung abscess). Palmar fasciitis is characterized by bilateral palmar swelling and finger contraction and may be the first indication of cancer, particularly ovarian carcinoma. Palpable purpura due to leukocytoclastic vasculitis may be the presenting complaint in myeloproliferative disorders. Hairy cell leukemia can be associated with medium-sized vessel vasculitis such as polyarteritis nodosa. Acute leukemia can produce joint pains that are disproportionately severe in comparison to the minimal swelling and heat that are present. Leukemic arthritis complicates approximately 15% of childhood leukemia cases and 5% of adult cases. Rheumatic manifestations of myelodysplastic syndromes include cutaneous vasculitis, lupus-like syndromes, neuropathy, and episodic intense arthritis. Erythromelalgia, a painful warmth and redness of the extremities that (unlike Raynaud's) improves with cold exposure or with elevation of the extremity, is often associated with myeloproliferative diseases.

Jacobson AF: Musculoskeletal pain as an indicator of occult malignancy: Yield of bone scintigraphy. Arch Intern Med 1997;157:105. (Bone scan useful in detecting occult malignancy in patients over 50 with enigmatic diffuse musculoskeletal pain or in patients with focal pain out of proportion to plain x-ray findings.)

PALINDROMIC RHEUMATISM

Palindromic rheumatism is a disease of unknown cause characterized by frequent recurring attacks (at irregular intervals) of acutely inflamed joints. Periarticular pain with swelling and transient subcutaneous nodules may also occur. The attacks cease within several hours to several days. The knee and finger joints are most commonly affected, but any peripheral joint may be involved. Systemic manifestations other than fever do not occur. Although hundreds of attacks may take place over a period of years, there is no permanent articular damage. Laboratory findings are usually normal. Palindromic rheumatism must be distinguished from acute gouty arthritis and an atypical, acute onset of rheumatoid arthritis.

Symptomatic treatment with NSAIDs is usually all that is required during the attacks. Hydroxychloroquine may be of value in preventing recurrences.

AVASCULAR NECROSIS OF BONE

Avascular necrosis of bone is a complication of corticosteroid use, trauma, SLE, pancreatitis, alcoholism, gout, sickle cell disease, infiltrative diseases (eg, Gaucher's disease), and caisson disease. The most commonly affected sites are the proximal and distal femoral heads, leading to hip or knee pain. Many patients with hip disease actually first present with pain referred to the knee. Physical examination will reveal that it is internal rotation of the hip—not movement of the knee—that is painful. Other commonly affected sites include the ankle, shoulder, and elbow. Initially, plain x-rays are often normal; MRI, CT scan, and bone scan are all more sensitive techniques. Treatment involves avoidance of weight bearing on the affected joint for several weeks at least. The merit of surgical core decompression is controversial, but the procedure at least allows the tissue diagnosis of clinically similar problems.

Holman AJ et al: Quantitative magnetic resonance imaging predicts clinical outcome of core decompression for osteonecrosis of the femoral head. J Rheumatol 1995; 22:1929. (If less than 21% of the femoral head is involved, core decompression usually works. If more is involved, the procedure fails.)

SOME ORTHOPEDIC PROCEDURES FOR ARTHRITIC JOINTS

Synovectomy

This procedure has been used for over 50 years to attempt to retard joint destruction by invasive synovial pannus of rheumatoid arthritis. However, its prophylactic effect has not been documented, and inflammation of regenerated synovial membrane occurs. Thus, the only indication for synovectomy is intractable pain in an isolated joint, most commonly the knee.

Joint Replacement (See also Total Joint Arthroplasty, below.)

Total hip replacement has been highly successful. Infection, the major complication, is uncommon. The long-term effects of replacement of the knee—and more recently the ankle, shoulder, and other joints—have not been fully determined.

Arthroplasty

Realignment and reconstruction of the knee, wrist, and small joints of the hand are feasible in a small number of selected patients.

Tendon Rupture

This is a fairly common complication in rheumatoid arthritis and requires immediate orthopedic referral. The most common sites are the finger flexors and extensors, the patellar tendon, and the Achilles tendon.

Arthrodesis

Arthrodesis (fusion) is being used less now than formerly, but a chronically infected, painful joint may be an indication for this surgical procedure.

Total Joint Arthroplasty

In the last 3 decades, remarkable progress has been made in the replacement of severely damaged joints with prosthetic materials. Although many different joints can be replaced, the largest experience and greatest success have been with hip and knee replacement. Indication for total joint arthroplasty is severe pain (usually including pain at rest) accompanied by loss of function and severe destruction of the joint on x-ray. Age is also a consideration, as the durability of artificial joints beyond 10–15 years is limited with older surgical techniques and unproved with newer techniques. Thus, patients over 65 are less likely than younger ones to face the challenge of revision.

Whatever the patient's age, success of the replacement depends upon the amount of physical stress to which the prosthetic components are subjected. Vigorous impact activity, even with the most advanced biomaterials and design, will result in failure of the prosthesis with time. Revision operations are technically more difficult, and the results may not be as good as with the primary procedure. The patient, therefore, must understand the limitations of joint replacement and the consequences of unrestrained joint usage.

A. Total Hip Arthroplasty: Hip replacement was originally designed for use in patients over 65 years of age with severe osteoarthritis. In these patients—usually less active physically—the prosthesis not only functioned well but outlasted the patients. Severe arthritis that fails to respond to conservative measures remains the principal indication for hip arthroplasty. Hip arthroplasty may also be indicated in younger patients severely disabled by painful hip disease (eg, rheumatoid arthritis), since in such cases it can be assumed that stress on the prosthetic joint will not be great. Contraindications to the operation include active infection and neurotrophic joint disease. Obesity is a relative contraindication. Serious complications may occur in about 1% of patients and include thrombophlebitis, pulmonary embolization, infection, and dislocation of the joint. Extensive experience has now been accumulated, and the short-term results are highly successful in properly selected patients. The long-term success has been limited by loosening of the prosthesis, a complication seen in 30–50% of patients 10 years after replacement with "first generation" techniques. Although loosening and periprosthetic osteolysis were blamed on the cement, second-generation cementing techniques for prosthetic hips have proved more durable than cementless hips.

B. Total Knee Arthroplasty: The indications and contraindications for total knee arthroplasty are similar to those for hip arthroplasty, but experience with the artificial knee is not as extensive. Results are slightly better in osteoarthritis patients than in those with rheumatoid arthritis. Knee arthroplasty is probably not advisable in younger individuals. Complications are similar to those with hip arthroplasty.

The failure rate of knee arthroplasty is slightly higher than that of hip arthroplasty.

Harris WH: Total hip replacement: "Cement versus cementless" resolution. Bull Rheum Dis 1994;43:1. ("Second-generation" cementing techniques for the femoral component are superior to cementless replacement. With modern femoral cementing, the risk of femoral loosening is 2% after 14 years.)

Mahomed N, Katz JN: Revision total hip arthroplasty: Indications and outcomes. Arthritis Rheum 1996;39:1939. (Patients with loosening should be considered for revision.)

21

Fluid & Electrolyte Disorders

Toshihiro Okuda, MD, PhD, Kiyoshi Kurokawa, MD, MACP, & Maxine A. Papadakis, MD

DIAGNOSIS OF FLUID & ELECTROLYTE DISORDERS

Approach to the Patient

A. History and Physical Examination:

1. Alterations in body fluid volume—Causes of changes in body fluid volume can usually be determined by the history and physical examination. **Volume overload** is manifested by an increase in weight and peripheral edema or ascites. Edema from local obstruction of venous return must be differentiated from systemic processes (congestive heart failure, cirrhosis, and nephrotic syndrome). A history of increased dietary sodium intake and use of medications that affect the renin-angiotensin system (converting enzyme inhibitors, prostaglandin synthesis inhibitors, mineralocorticoids, calcium channel blockers) should be sought. **Volume depletion** is characterized by weight loss, excessive thirst, and dry mucous membranes. There may be resting tachycardia, orthostatic hypotension, or shock. Causes include vomiting or diarrhea, diuretic use, renal disease, diabetes mellitus or diabetes insipidus, dehydration from inadequate oral intake associated with altered mental status, and excessive insensible losses from sweating or fever.

B. Further Evaluation: Treatment of fluid and electrolyte disorders is based on (1) assessment of total body water and its distribution, (2) electrolyte concentrations, and (3) serum osmolality.

1. Body water—Table 21–1 shows the sex difference in total body water and the decrease in total body water that occurs with aging.

2. Electrolytes—Table 21–2 shows the normal values for serum electrolytes.

3. Serum osmolality—Serum osmolality (normally 285–295 mosm/kg) can be calculated from the following formula:

$$\text{Osmolality} = 2(\text{Na}^+ \text{ meq/L}) + \frac{\text{Glucose mg/dL}}{18} + \frac{\text{BUN mg/dL}}{2.8}$$

(1 mosm of glucose equals 180 mg/L, and 1 mosm of urea nitrogen equals 28 mg/L).

Solute concentration is usually expressed in terms of osmolality. The number of particles in solution (either molecules or ions) determines the number of milliosmoles. Each particle has a unit value of 1, so if a substance ionizes, each ion contributes the same amount as a nonionizable molecule. For example, glucose in solution is nonionizable. Therefore, 1 mmol of glucose has an osmole concentration of 1 mosm/kg H_2O. One mmol of NaCl, however, forms two ions in water (one Na^+ and one Cl^-) and has an osmole concentration of roughly 2 mosm/kg H_2O. Osmole per kilogram of water is termed osmolality; osmole per liter of solution is termed osmolarity. At the solute concentration of body fluids, the two measurements correspond so closely that they are interchangeable.

C. Clinical Implications: In many instances, electrolyte disorders are asymptomatic. However, patients may develop lethargy, weakness, confusion, delirium, and seizures, especially in the presence of an abnormal serum sodium concentration. Often these symptoms are mistaken for primary neurologic or metabolic disorders. Muscle weakness occurs in patients with severe hypokalemia, hyperkalemia, and hypophosphatemia; confusion, seizures, and coma may develop in those with severe hypercalcemia. Measurement of electrolytes (sodium, potassium, chloride, bicarbonate, calcium, magnesium, and phosphorus) is indicated for any patient with even vague neuromuscular symptoms.

Table 21–1. Total body water (as percentage of body weight) in relation to age and sex.

Age	Male	Female
18–40	60%	50%
40–60	60–50%	50–40%
Over 60	50%	40%

TREATMENT OF SPECIFIC FLUID, ELECTROLYTE, & ACID-BASE DISORDERS

DISORDERS OF SODIUM CONCENTRATION

1. HYPONATREMIA

Hyponatremia (defined as a serum sodium concentration less than 130 meq/L) is the most common electrolyte abnormality observed in a general hospitalized population, seen in about 2% of patients. The initial approach to its investigation is the determination of serum osmolality (Figure 21–1).

The Urine Sodium

Measurement of urine sodium helps distinguish renal from nonrenal causes of hyponatremia. Urine sodium exceeding 20 meq/L is consistent with renal salt wasting (diuretics, ACE inhibitors, mineralocorticoid deficiency, salt-losing nephropathy). Hyponatremia in AIDS patients is usually due to the syndrome of inappropriate ADH secretion (SIADH) or gastrointestinal sodium loss but may be due to relative mineralocorticoid or glucocorticoid deficiency. Urine sodium less than 10 meq/L or fractional excretion of sodium less than 1% (unless diuretics have been given) implies avid sodium retention by the kidney to compensate for extrarenal fluid losses from

Table 21–2. Normal values and mass conversion factors.[1]

	Normal Plasma Values	Mass Conversion
Na^+	135–145 meq/L	23 mg = 1 meq
K^+	3.5–5.0 meq/L	39 mg = 1 meq
Cl^-	98–107 meq/L	35 mg = 1 meq
HCO_3^-	22–28 meq/L	61 mg = 1 meq
Ca^{2+}	8.5–10.5 mg/dL	40 mg = 1 mmol
Phosphorus	2.5–4.5 mg/dL	31 mg = 1 mmol
Mg^{2+}	1.8–3.0 mg/dL	24 mg = 1 mmol
Osmolality	280–295 mosm/kg	. . .

[1]Modified and reproduced, with permission, from Cogan MG: *Fluid and Electrolytes: Physiology and Pathophysiology.* Appleton & Lange, 1991.

vomiting, diarrhea, sweating, or third-spacing, as with ascites. Fractional excretion (FE) of sodium or urea is calculated using a random urine (U) sample with simultaneously obtained plasma (P) samples for sodium (or urea) and creatinine (Cr):

$$FE(Na) = \frac{(U/P)Na}{(U/P)Cr} \times 100$$

Isotonic Hyponatremia

In hyperlipidemia and hyperproteinemia, the marked increases in lipids (chylomicrons and triglycerides, but not cholesterol) and proteins (> 10 g/dL) occupy a disproportionately large portion of the plasma volume. Plasma osmolality remains normal because its measurement is unaffected by the lipids or proteins. A decreased volume of water results, so that the sodium concentration in total plasma volume is decreased. Because the sodium concentration in the plasma water is normal, hyperlipidemia and hyperproteinemia cause pseudohyponatremia. Most United States laboratories now measure serum electrolytes using ion-specific electrodes and thus avoid misdiagnosis.

Hypotonic Hyponatremia

The volume status is useful in differentiating the etiology of hypotonic hyponatremia.

A. Hypovolemic Hypotonic Hyponatremia: Hyponatremia with decreased extracellular fluid volume occurs in the setting of renal or extrarenal volume loss (Figure 21–1). Total body sodium is decreased. To increase intravascular volume, antidiuretic hormone (ADH) secretion increases, and free water is retained. The drive to replenish intravascular volume supersedes the need to maintain osmolality; losses of salt and water are replaced by water alone. Since clinicians frequently fail to recognize hypovolemia, the combination of low fractional excretion of sodium (< 0.5%) and low fractional urea clearance (< 55%) is the best biochemical way to predict saline response. Hyponatremia has been shown to develop in patients with intracranial diseases through renal sodium wasting. Unlike those with SIADH, these patients are hypovolemic, though plasma levels of ADH are inappropriately high. The cause of this syndrome is not known.

Treatment consists of replacement of lost volume with isotonic saline or lactated Ringer's infusion. Corticosteroids can be used empirically if hypocortisolism is considered in the differential diagnosis. See Adrenocortical Hypofunction in Chapter 26 for diagnosis (by means of the cosyntropin stimulation test) and treatment of hypocortisolism.

B. Euvolemic Hypotonic Hyponatremia: In this setting, determinations of urine osmolality (Figure 21–1) along with urine sodium are useful for appropriate diagnosis.

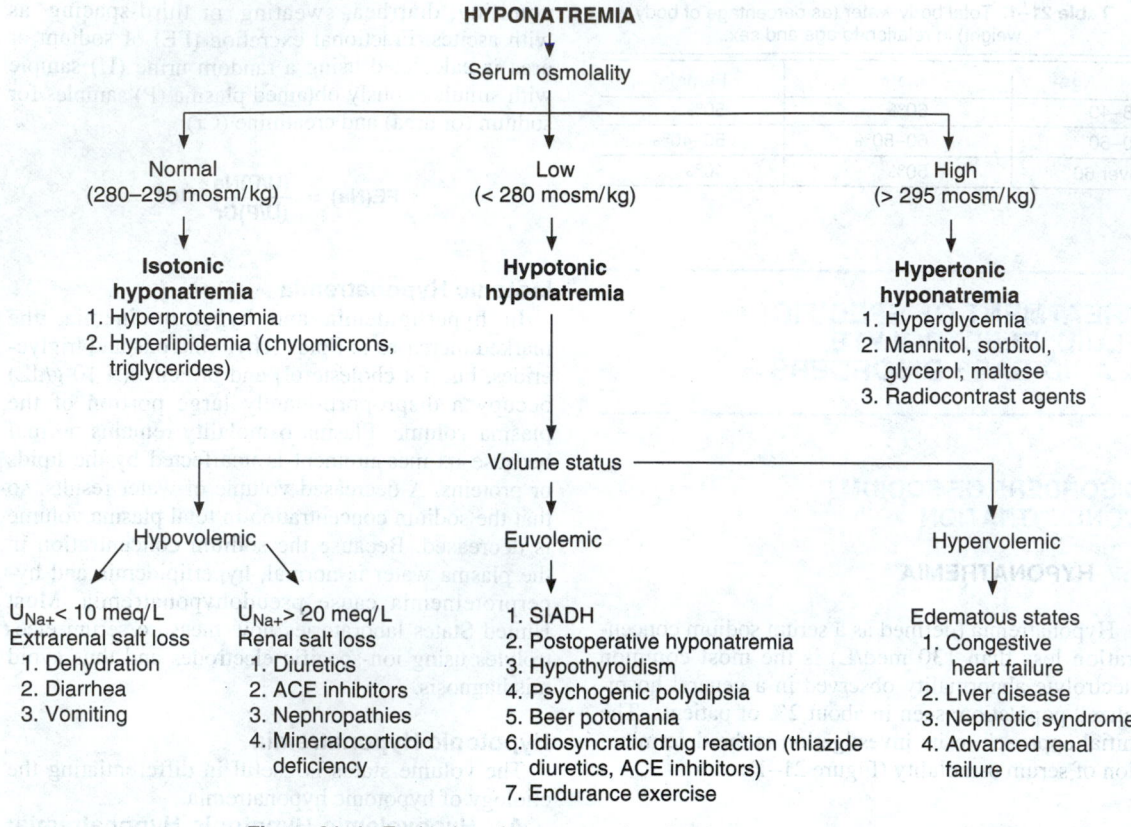

Figure 21–1. Evaluation of hyponatremia using the serum osmolality.

1. Clinical syndromes–

a. Syndrome of inappropriate ADH secretion (SIADH)–Increased ADH secretion is physiologic in hypovolemic states, so the diagnosis of SIADH is made only if the patient is euvolemic. In SIADH, release of ADH occurs without osmolality-dependent or volume-dependent physiologic stimulation. Normal regulation of ADH release occurs from both the central nervous system and the chest via baroreceptors and neural input. It follows that the causes of SIADH are disorders affecting the central nervous system—structural, metabolic, psychiatric, or pharmacologic—or the lungs. Furthermore, some carcinomas, such as small cell lung carcinoma, synthesize ADH. Other states associated with SIADH include AIDS (see below) and administration of drugs that either increase ADH secretion or potentiate its action (Table 21–3). Fluoxetine-induced SIADH may be more common in geriatric patients.

(1) Patterns of abnormal ADH secretion–

(a) Random secretion–ADH release is unrelated to osmoregulation. This pattern is seen in carcinomas and central nervous system diseases.

(b) Reset osmostat–This variant is characterized by ADH secretion appropriately suppressed at very low serum osmolalities but has ADH osmoregulation downset to a lower level of "normal." Therefore, ADH is secreted at a subnormal serum osmolality threshold (< 280 mosm/kg). Appropriate urinary dilution can be attained but at low serum osmolalities. This pattern is seen in the elderly, in patients with pulmonary processes, or in drug-induced SIADH.

(c) Leak of ADH–In conditions such as basilar skull fractures, low levels of ADH are "leaked" despite hypo-osmolality. If serum osmolality rises to normal, ADH secretion increases appropriately and then continues to respond normally if osmolality further increases.

(2) Clinical features–SIADH is characterized by (1) hyponatremia; (2) decreased osmolality (< 280 mosm/kg) with inappropriately increased urine osmolality (> 150 mosm/kg); (3) absence of cardiac, renal, or liver disease; (4) normal thyroid and adrenal function (see Chapter 26 for thyroid function tests and cosyntropin stimulation test); and (5) urine sodium usually over 20 meq/L. Natriuresis compensates for the slight increase in volume from ADH secretion. The mechanisms that regulate sodium excretion in response to increases in extracellular volume,

Table 21–3. Causes of drug-induced SIADH.

Increased ADH production
  Antidepressants
    Amitriptyline
    Clomipramine
    Desipramine
    Imipramine
    Monoamine oxidase inhibitors
    Fluoxetine
  Antineoplastics
    Cyclophosphamide
    Vincristine
    Vinblastine
  Carbamazepine
  Clofibrate
  Neuroleptics
    Thiothixene
    Thioridazine
    Fluphenazine
    Haloperidol
    Trifluoperazine
Potentiated ADH action
  Carbamazepine
  Chlorpropamide, tolbutamide
  Cyclophosphamide
  NSAIDs
  Somatostatin and analogues

such as suppression of the sympathetic nervous and renin-angiotensin systems and increased secretion of atrial natriuretic factor, are preserved and account for the increase in urinary sodium. The expansion of extracellular volume is not large enough to cause clinical hypervolemia, hypertension, or edema since the excess water is distributed throughout the total body water. Other changes frequently seen in SIADH include low blood urea nitrogen (BUN) (< 10 mg/dL) and hypouricemia (< 4 mg/dL), which are not only dilutional but result from increased urea and uric acid clearances in response to the volume-expanded state. A high BUN suggests a volume-contracted state, which precludes a diagnosis of SIADH. With the use of the more physiologic tests listed above, serum ADH levels have little utility.

b. Postoperative hyponatremia–Severe postoperative hyponatremia can develop in 2 days or less after elective surgery in healthy patients, especially premenopausal women. Most have received excessive postoperative hypotonic fluid in the setting of elevated ADH levels related to pain or surgery. Patients awake normally from general anesthesia but within 2 days develop nausea, headache, seizures, and even respiratory arrest. Serum sodium levels may be less than 110 meq/L. Premenopausal women who develop hyponatremic encephalopathy are about 25 times more likely than menopausal women to die or to suffer permanent brain damage, suggesting a role of estrogen in the pathophysiology of this disorder. Hyponatremia from the absorption of hypotonic fluids through uterine veins during endometrial ablation in menstruating women has been recently described. The mechanism of fluid absorption is similar to one that occurs during transurethral prostate resection in men. These patients can be symptomatic intraoperatively, with tremulousness, hypothermia, or hypoxia, or upon awakening from anesthesia, with headache, nausea, and vomiting.

c. Hypothyroidism–Hyponatremia is not commonly caused by hypothyroidism, but it can occur with serum sodium levels as low as 103 meq/L. Water retention is the cause, probably both from inappropriately elevated ADH levels and from nonhormonal alterations in the handling of water by the kidneys.

d. Psychogenic polydipsia–Marked excess free water intake (generally > 10 L/d) may produce hyponatremia. Euvolemia is maintained through the renal excretion of sodium. Urine sodium is therefore generally elevated (> 20 meq/L), but unlike SIADH, levels of ADH are suppressed. Urine osmolality is appropriately low (< 300 mosm/kg) as the increased free water is excreted. Hyponatremia from bursts of ADH occur in manic-depressive patients with excess free water intake.

e. Beer potomania–Excessive chronic intake of beer (generally at least 8 L daily) can cause hyponatremia as low as 100 meq/L. This disorder occurs primarily in patients with cirrhosis, who have elevated levels of ADH and decreased glomerular filtration rates. Beer generally has a very low content of sodium (< 10 meq/L), and hyponatremia develops through retention of free water (beer).

f. Idiosyncratic diuretic reaction–In addition to hyponatremia that develops from volume contraction due to diuretic therapy (see above), a less common, but severe, diuretic-induced (generally thiazide) hyponatremia can occur in euvolemic patients. This syndrome is most often seen in healthy older women (over 70 years of age). Serious symptoms often develop after only a few days of therapy. The mechanism for the hyponatremia appears to be a combination of excessive renal sodium loss and water retention.

g. Idiosyncratic ACE inhibitor reactions–ACE inhibitors can cause central polydipsia and increased antidiuretic hormone secretion, both of which can cause severe, symptomatic hyponatremia. Patients given ACE inhibitors who develop polydipsia should have their serum Na+ levels checked.

h. Endurance exercise hyponatremia–Hyponatremia after endurance exercise may not be merely secondary to loss of sodium and water with replacement by hypotonic fluid. In the setting of continued ADH secretion after the exercise has stopped, reperfusion of the exercise-induced ischemic splanchnic bed occurs. Thus, there is delayed absorption of previously ingested hypotonic fluid. The retention of hypotonic fluid may be exacerbated by NSAIDs frequently used by athletes.

2. Treatment–

a. Symptomatic hyponatremia–Symptomatic

hyponatremia is usually seen in patients with SIADH. Serum sodium levels are generally under 115 meq/L. If there are central nervous system symptoms, hyponatremia should be rapidly treated at any level of serum sodium concentration.

(1) Rate and degree of correction–Brain damage, including central pontine myelinolysis, may occur from osmotically induced demyelination from overly rapid correction of serum sodium (to levels above 135 meq/L within the initial 48 hours or an increase of more than 25 meq/L within the first 24 hours of therapy). Hypoxic-anoxic episodes that occur during the hyponatremia may contribute to the demyelination. A reasonable approach is to increase the serum sodium concentration by 0.5–1 meq/L/h, aiming not to exceed 130 meq/L in the first 48 hours. This approach guards against overcorrection.

(2) Saline plus furosemide–Hypertonic (eg, 3%) saline with furosemide is indicated for symptomatic hyponatremic patients. If one administers 3% saline without a diuretic to a patient with SIADH, the serum sodium concentration increases temporarily but excess sodium is then excreted in the urine, because such patients are euvolemic. If one adds furosemide (0.5–1 mg/kg intravenously), however, the kidney cannot concentrate urine even in the presence of high levels of ADH. Infusion of 3% saline is accompanied by excretion of isotonic urine with a net loss of free water. The sodium concentration of 3% saline is 513 meq/L. In order to determine how much 3% saline to administer, one must measure a spot urinary Na^+ after a furosemide diuresis has begun. The excreted Na^+ is replaced with 3% saline, empirically begun at 50–75 mL/h and then adjusted based on urinary output and urinary sodium. For example, after administration of furosemide, urine volume may be 400 mL/h and sodium excretion is 100 meq/L. The excreted Na^+ is 40 meq/h, which is replaced with 78 mL/h of 3% saline (40 meq/h divided by 513 meq/L). Free water loss is the difference between urine volume excreted and 3% saline infused, or 322 mL (400 mL – 78 mL). A rise in plasma sodium concentration of 1.5 meq/L/h can be expected. Measurements of plasma sodium should be done approximately every 4 hours and the patient observed closely.

b. Asymptomatic hyponatremia–

(1) Water restriction–Water intake should be restricted to 0.5–1 L/d. Gradual increase of serum sodium will occur over days.

(2) 0.9% saline–0.9% saline with furosemide may be used in asymptomatic patients whose serum sodium is less than 120 meq/L. Replace urinary sodium and potassium losses as above.

(3) Demeclocycline–Demeclocycline (300–600 mg twice daily) is useful for patients who cannot adhere to water restriction or need additional therapy. Onset of action may require 1 week. Therapy with demeclocycline in cirrhosis appears to increase the

risk of renal failure, and for that reason the drug should not be used in this condition.

(4) Fludrocortisone–Hyponatremia occurring as part of the cerebral salt-wasting syndrome can be treated with fludrocortisone.

C. Hypervolemic Hypotonic Hyponatremia: Hyponatremia with increased extracellular fluid volume is seen when hyponatremia is accompanied by edema-associated disorders such as congestive heart failure, cirrhosis, nephrotic syndrome, and advanced renal disease (Figure 21–1). Total body sodium is increased, yet effective circulating volume is sensed as inadequate by baroreceptors. ADH secretion occurs, which results in a greater retention of water.

The **urine sodium** concentration is generally less than 10 meq/L unless the patient has been taking diuretics.

Treatment

A. Water Restriction: The treatment of hyponatremia is that of the underlying condition (eg, improving cardiac output in congestive heart failure) and water restriction (to < 1–2 L of water daily).

B. Diuretics: To hasten excretion of water and salt, use of diuretics may be indicated. Since diuretics may cause hyponatremia, the hyponatremic patient must be cautioned not to increase free water intake or the hyponatremia may worsen.

C. Hypertonic (3%) Saline: Hypertonic saline administration is dangerous in volume-overloaded states and is not routinely recommended. In patients with severe hyponatremia (serum sodium < 110 meq/L) and central nervous system symptoms, judicious administration of small amounts (100–200 mL) of 3% saline with diuretics may be necessary. Emergency dialysis should also be considered.

Hypertonic Hyponatremia

Hypertonic hyponatremia is most commonly seen with hyperglycemia. When blood glucose becomes acutely elevated, water is drawn from the cells to the extracellular space, diluting the serum sodium. The plasma sodium levels fall 1.6 meq/L for every 100 mg/dL rise in glucose concentration over 200 mg/dL. This dilutional hyponatremia is not pseudohyponatremia, since the sodium concentration does indeed fall, which it does not in the pseudohyponatremia of hyperlipidemia. Infusion of hypertonic solutions containing osmotically active osmoles (eg, mannitol) may also cause hypertonic hyponatremia by drawing water to the extracellular space.

Fenves AZ, Thomas S, Knochel JP: Beer potomania: Two cases and review of the literature. Clin Nephrol 1996; 45:61.

Harrigan MR: Cerebral salt wasting syndrome: A review. Neurosurgery 1996;38:152.

Karp BI, Laureno R: Pontine and extrapontine myelinolysis: A neurologic disorder following rapid correction of hyponatremia. Medicine 1993;72:359.4.

Lipschutz JH, Arieff AI: Reset osmostat in a healthy patient. Ann Intern Med 1994;120:574.

Mulloy AL, Caruana RJ: Hyponatremic emergencies. Med Clin North Am 1995;79:155.

Musch W et al: Combined fractional excretion of sodium and urea better predicts response to saline in hyponatremia than do usual clinical and biochemical parameters. Am J Med 1995;99:348.

Siegler EL et al: Risk factors for the development of hyponatremia in psychiatric inpatients. Arch Intern Med 1995;155:953. (Use of diuretics, fluoxetine, tricyclic antidepressants, and calcium antagonists.)

Terzian C, Frye EB, Piotrowski ZH: Admission hyponatremia in the elderly: Factors influencing prognosis. J Gen Intern Med 1994;9:89. (The in-hospital mortality rate for patients with admission hyponatremia was 16%—twice that for patients without admission hyponatremia.)

Hyponatremia in AIDS

Hyponatremia is seen in up to 50% of patients hospitalized for AIDS and in 20% of ambulatory AIDS patients, often associated with pneumonia and meningitis. If hyponatremia is present at the time of hospital admission, it is just as likely to be due to hypovolemic gastrointestinal loss as to euvolemic SIADH. However, if hyponatremia develops after hospital admission, most patients have euvolemic SIADH. Infrequently, hypovolemic hyponatremia is due to adrenal insufficiency, isolated mineralocorticoid deficiency with hyporeninemic hypoaldosteronism, or an HIV-specific impairment in renal sodium conservation. Hyponatremia from adrenal insufficiency, generally associated with hyperkalemia, may coexist with hypokalemia if the patient also has diarrhea. Adrenal function can be tested with corticotropin stimulation to determine the adequacy of serum cortisol response (see Chapter 26). Patients with isolated hyporeninemic hypoaldosteronism have normal cortisol responses to corticotropin but have decreased serum aldosterone levels. The mortality rate in hospitalized hyponatremic AIDS patients is nearly twice that of normonatremic patients.

Freda P et al: Primary adrenal insufficiency in patients with the acquired immunodeficiency syndrome: A report of five cases. J Clin Endocrinol Metab 1994;79:1540.

Lortholary O et al: Hypothalamo-pituitary-adrenal function in human immunodeficiency virus-infected men. J Clin Endocrinol Metab 1996;81:791.

Perazella MA, Brown E: Electrolyte and acid-base disorders associated with AIDS: An etiologic review. J Gen Intern Med 1994;9:232.

2. HYPERNATREMIA

Hypernatremia (serum sodium > 145 meq/L) develops from excess water loss, frequently accompanied by an impaired thirst mechanism (eg, dehydration, lactulose or mannitol therapy, or diabetes insipidus). Hypokalemia, hypercalcemia, or sickle cell anemia can cause nephrogenic diabetes insipidus. Rarely, excessive sodium intake may cause hypernatremia (eg, accidental intravascular injection of hypertonic saline used for induction of abortion or use of large doses of sodium bicarbonate therapy during cardiac arrest). Since total body sodium content is the major determinant of extracellular fluid volume, one must determine if the hypernatremia is accompanied by a normal, decreased, or increased extracellular fluid volume.

Clinical Findings

A. Symptoms and Signs: Intact thirst usually prevents hypernatremia, and thus its presence is commonly associated with conditions in which access to water is limited, eg, cerebrovascular disease. Orthostatic hypotension and oliguria are typical. Hyperthermia, delirium, and coma may be seen with severe hyperosmolality.

B. Laboratory Findings:

1. Urine osmolality > 400 mosm/kg–Renal water-conserving ability is functioning.

a. Nonrenal losses–Hypernatremia will develop if water ingestion fails to keep up with hypotonic losses from excessive sweating, exertional losses from the respiratory tract, or through stool water. Lactulose causes an osmotic diarrhea with loss of free water.

b. Renal losses–While diabetic hyperglycemia can cause pseudohyponatremia (see above), progressive volume depletion from the osmotic diuresis of glycosuria can result in true hypernatremia. Osmotic diuresis can occur with the use of mannitol or urea.

2. Urine osmolality < 250 mosm/kg–A dilute urine with osmolality less than 250 mosm/kg with hypernatremia is characteristic of central and nephrogenic diabetes insipidus. Nephrogenic diabetes insipidus, seen with lithium or demeclocycline therapy or after relief of prolonged urinary tract obstruction, or with interstitial nephritis, results from renal insensitivity to ADH.

Treatment

Treatment of hypernatremia is directed toward correcting the cause of the fluid loss and replacing water and, as needed, electrolytes. In response to increases in plasma osmolality, brain cells synthesize solutes—or idiogenic osmoles—which increase osmotic flow of water back into the brain cells to regulate their volume. This begins 4–6 hours after dehydration and takes several days to reach a steady state. If hypernatremia is too rapidly corrected, the osmotic imbalance may cause water to preferentially enter brain cells, causing cerebral edema and potentially severe neurologic impairment. Fluid therapy should be administered over a 48-hour period, aiming for a decrease in serum sodium of 1 meq/L/h (1 mmol/L/h). Potassium and phosphate may be added as indicated by serum levels; other electrolytes are also monitored frequently.

A. Choice of Type of Fluid for Replacement:

1. Hypernatremia with hypovolemia–Severe hypovolemia should be treated with isotonic (0.9%) saline to restore the volume deficit and to treat the hyperosmolality, since the osmolality of isotonic saline (308 mosm/kg) is often lower than that of the plasma. This should be followed by 0.45% saline to replace any remaining free water deficit. Milder volume deficit may be treated with 0.45% saline and 5% dextrose in water.

2. Hypernatremia with euvolemia–Water drinking or 5% dextrose and water intravenously will result in excretion of excess sodium in the urine. If GFR is decreased, diuretics will increase urinary sodium excretion but may impair renal concentrating ability, increasing the quantity of water that needs to be replaced.

3. Hypernatremia with hypervolemia–Treatment consists of providing water as 5% dextrose in water to reduce hyperosmolality, but this will expand vascular volume. Thus, loop diuretics such as furosemide (0.5–1 mg/kg) should be administered intravenously to remove the excess sodium. In severe renal insufficiency, hemodialysis may be necessary.

B. Calculation of Water Deficit: When calculating fluid replacement, both the deficit and the maintenance requirements should be added to each 24-hour replacement regimen.

1. Acute hypernatremia–In acute dehydration without much solute loss, free water loss is similar to the weight loss. Initially, 5% dextrose in water may be employed. As correction of water deficit progresses, therapy should continue with 0.45% saline with dextrose.

2. Chronic hypernatremia–Water deficit is calculated to restore normal osmolality for total body water. Total body water (TBW) (Table 21–1) correlates with muscle mass and therefore decreases with advancing age, cachexia, and dehydration and is lower in women than in men. Current TBW equals 0.4–0.6 of current body weight. [Na$^+$] = measured serum Na$^+$.

$$\text{Volume (in L) to be replaced} = \text{Current TBW} \times \frac{[\text{Na}^+] - 140}{140}$$

Palevsky PM, Bhagrath R, Greenberg A: Hypernatremia in hospitalized patients. Ann Intern Med 1996;124:197. (Development of hypernatremia before hospitalization occurs mainly in geriatric patients, while hospital-acquired hypernatremia is mainly iatrogenic regardless of patient age.)

DISORDERS OF POTASSIUM CONCENTRATION

1. HYPOKALEMIA

A total body deficit of about 350 meq occurs for each 1 meq/L decrement in serum potassium concentration below a level of 4 meq/L. However, changes in blood pH and hormones (insulin, β-adrenergic agonists, and aldosterone) independently affect serum potassium levels (Table 21–4). Elevated serum epinephrine may contribute to the hypokalemia commonly seen in trauma patients; this normalizes within 24 hours after injury without significant potassium replacement.

Clinical Findings

A. Symptoms and Signs: Muscular weakness, fatigue, and muscle cramps are frequent complaints in mild to moderate hypokalemia. Smooth muscle involvement may result in constipation or ileus. Flaccid paralysis, hyporeflexia, hypercapnia, tetany, and rhabdomyolysis may be seen with severe hypokalemia (< 2.5 meq/L).

B. Laboratory Findings: The ECG shows decreased amplitude and broadening of T waves, prominent U waves, depressed ST segments, and, in more severe deficits, atrioventricular block and finally cardiac arrest. Hypokalemia also increases the likelihood of digitalis toxicity.

Pathophysiology & Diagnosis

Hypokalemia can occur as a result of shift of potassium from outside to inside the cell, extrarenal potassium loss (or insufficient potassium intake), or renal potassium loss. Potassium uptake by the cell is stimulated by insulin in the presence of glucose. It is also facilitated by adrenergic beta-stimulation, whereas adrenergic alpha-stimulation blocks it (Table 21–4). All of these effects are transient. Urinary potassium concentration is low (< 20 meq/L) as a result of extrarenal fluid loss (eg, diarrhea, vomiting) and inappropriately high (> 40 meq/L) with renal fluid loss (eg, mineralocorticoid excess, Bartter's syndrome, Liddle's syndrome). Genetic mutation of Na-K-2Cl cotransporter in the thick ascending limb

Table 21–4. Factors affecting the transcellular shift of potassium.

From Inside to Outside	From Outside to Inside
Acidosis[1] (mineral acids, HCl)	Alkalosis
Adrenergic alpha-stimulation	Insulin
Digitalis	Adrenergic beta-stimulation
Solvent drag	

[1]In the case of organic acid accumulation (eg, lactic acidosis), a shift of potassium does not occur since organic acid can easily move across the cell membrane.

in the loop of Henle has been shown in some patients with Bartter's syndrome.

Treatment

The safest way to treat mild to moderate deficiency is with oral potassium, which is rapidly absorbed. Liquid potassium chloride has an unpleasant taste and may be better tolerated if added to fruit juice. Rarely, enteric-coated or slow-release tablets or capsules of potassium chloride can cause peptic ulceration.

Intravenous potassium replacement is indicated for patients with severe hypokalemia and in those who cannot take oral supplementation. If the serum potassium level is greater than 2.5 meq/L and there are no electrocardiographic abnormalities characteristic of hypokalemia, potassium can be given at a rate of 10 meq/L/h by peripheral intravenous line in concentrations that should never exceed 40 meq/L. For severe deficiency, potassium may be given through a peripheral intravenous line at rates up to 40 meq/L/h. Continuous electrocardiographic monitoring is indicated, and the serum potassium level should be checked every 3–6 hours.

Occasionally, hypokalemia may be refractory to potassium replacement. Magnesium deficiency may make potassium correction more difficult. Concomitant magnesium repletion avoids this problem.

Hamill-Ruth RJ, McGory R: Magnesium repletion and its effect on potassium homeostasis in critically ill adults: Results of a double-blind, randomized, controlled trial. Crit Care Med 1996;24:38. (Patients treated with magnesium required less potassium, but the results were not statistically significant.)

Simon DB et al: Bartter's syndrome, hypokalemia, alkalosis with hypercalciuria, is caused by mutations in the Na-K-2Cl cotransporter NKCC2. Nat Genet 1996;13: 183.

Vanek VW et al: Serum potassium concentrations in trauma patients. South Med J 1994;87:41. (Self-limited hypokalemia occurs in one-half of trauma patients.)

2. HYPERKALEMIA

Many cases of hyperkalemia are spurious or associated with acidosis (Table 21–5). The common practice of repeatedly clenching and unclenching a fist during venipuncture may raise the potassium concentration by 1–2 meq/L by causing local release of potassium from forearm muscles.

Intracellular potassium shifts to the extracellular fluid in hyperkalemia associated with acidosis. Serum potassium concentration rises about 0.7 meq/L for every decrease of 0.1 pH unit during acidosis. Potassium movement out of cells occurs primarily in metabolic acidosis due to the accumulation of minerals such as NH_4Cl or HCl. The inability of the chloride anion to permeate the cell membrane re-

Table 21–5. Causes of hyperkalemia.

Spurious
Leakage from erythrocytes if separation of serum from clot is delayed (plasma K^+ not affected)
Thrombocytosis, with release of K^+ from platelets (plasma K^+ not affected)
Marked leukocytosis
Repeated fist clenching during phlebotomy, with release of K^+ from forearm muscles
Specimen drawn from arm with K^+ infusion
Decreased excretion
Renal failure, acute and chronic
Severe oliguria due to severe dehydration or shock
Renal secretory defects (may or may not have frank renal failure): renal transplant, interstitial nephritis, SLE, sickle cell disease, amyloidosis, obstructive uropathy
Adrenocortical insufficiency
Hyporeninemic hypoaldosteronism (often with long-term diabetes mellitus) or selective hypoaldosteronism (some patients with AIDS)
Drugs that inhibit potassium excretion (spironolactone, triamterene, ACE inhibitors, trimethoprim, NSAIDs)
Shift of K^+ from tissues
Massive release of intracellular K^+ in burns, rhabdomyolysis, crush injury, hemolysis, severe infection, internal bleeding, vigorous exercise
Metabolic acidosis
Hyperosmolality
Insulin deficiency (metabolic acidosis may not be apparent)
Hyperkalemic periodic paralysis
Drugs: succinylcholine, arginine, digitalis toxicity, β-adrenergic antagonists
Excessive intake of K^+
Overtreatment with K^+, orally or parenterally

sults in the transcellular exchange of H^+ for K^+. Metabolic acidosis from organic acids (keto acids and lactic acid) does not induce hyperkalemia. Unlike the minerals, these organic acids easily permeate cell membranes and retard Na^+-K^+ ATPase. The hyperkalemia frequently observed in diabetic ketoacidosis is not due to the acidosis but to a combination of the hyperosmolality (the intracellular K^+ concentration of the dehydrated cell increases and K^+ diffuses extracellularly) and deficiencies of insulin, catecholamines, and aldosterone. In the absence of acidosis, serum potassium concentration rises about 1 meq/L when there is a a total body potassium excess of 50–200 meq/L. However, the higher the serum potassium concentration, the smaller the excess necessary to raise the potassium levels further.

Trimethoprim is structurally related to amiloride and triamterene, and all three drugs inhibit renal potassium excretion. Serum potassium levels rise progressively over 4–5 days in patients treated with standard or high-dose trimethoprim (combined with sulfamethoxazole or dapsone), especially if they have concurrent renal insufficiency (creatine ± 1.2 mg/dL). Over one-half of inpatients taking this drug have potassium levels over 5 meq/L and 20% have severe hyperkalemia (> 5.5 meq/L). The potassium concentration returns to baseline after drug discontinuation.

Causes of hyperkalemia in AIDS include adrenal insufficiency, hyporeninemic hypoaldosteronism, renal failure, and drugs such as pentamidine and trimethoprim.

Clinical Findings

The elevated K^+ concentration interferes with normal neuromuscular function to produce weakness and flaccid paralysis; abdominal distention and diarrhea may occur. Electrocardiography is not a sensitive method for detecting hyperkalemia, since nearly half of patients with a serum potassium level greater than 6.5 meq/L will not manifest electrocardiographic changes. When electrocardiographic changes of hyperkalemia occur, the ECG reflects impaired conduction by peaked T waves of increased amplitude, atrial arrest, widening of the QRS, and biphasic QRS–T complexes (Figure 21–2). The heart rate may be slow; ventricular fibrillation and cardiac arrest are terminal events.

Treatment
(Table 21–6)

First confirm that the elevated level of serum K^+ is genuine. Potassium concentration can be measured in plasma rather than in serum to avoid leakage of potassium out of cells into the serum of the blood sample in the course of clotting, which may be matched in thrombocytosis. Treatment consists of withholding potassium and giving cation exchange resins by mouth or enema. Sodium polystyrene sulfonate, 40–80 g/d in divided doses, is usually effective. Emergent treatment of hyperkalemia is indicated if cardiac toxicity or muscular paralysis is present or if the hyperkalemia is severe (serum potassium > 6.5–7 meq/L) even in the absence of electrocardiographic changes. Insulin plus 10–50% glucose (5–10 g of glucose per unit of insulin) may be employed to deposit K^+ with glycogen in the liver, and Ca^{2+} may be given intravenously as an antagonist ion. Transcellular shifts of potassium can also be mediated by β_2-adrenergic stimulation. Albuterol, a nebulized β_2 agonist, is effective in decreasing serum potassium in patients on hemodialysis. For such patients, nebulized albuterol can reduce serum K^+ 0.5–1 meq/L within 30 minutes after administration, and this effect is sustained for at least 2 hours. Albuterol and insulin are probably equally efficacious in lowering potassium in uremic patients, and the hypokalemic effects of coadministration of the two drugs (with glucose) are additive and appear not to be a hazard. Sodium bicarbonate can be given intravenously as an emergency measure in severe hyperkalemia; the increase in blood pH results in a shift of K^+ into cells. Hemodialysis or peritoneal dialysis may be required to remove K^+ in the presence of protracted renal insufficiency. Therapy of the precipitating event proceeds concurrently.

Alappan R, Perazella MA, Buller GK: Hyperkalemia in hospitalized patients treated with trimethoprim-sulfamethoxazole. Ann Intern Med 1996;124:316. (Marked hyperkalemia [> 5.5 meq/L] occurred in 20% of patients.)

Liou HH et al: Hypokalemic effects of intravenous infusion or nebulization of salbutamol in patients with chronic renal failure: Comparative study. Am J Kidney Dis 1994;23:266. (Intravenous and inhaled preparations both work well. Intravenous works faster, but inhaled albuterol causes less tachycardia.)

Metcalfe MJ, Seidelin PH: Images in cardiology. ECG changes of severe hyperkalaemia. Br Heart J 1994;72:260.

Oster JR, Singer I, Fishman LM: Heparin-induced aldosterone suppression and hyperkalemia. Am J Med 1995;98:575. (Heparin, regardless of dose, decreases aldosterone levels. One should monitor potassium frequently in patients at high risk for hyperkalemia—renal insufficiency, diabetes, exposure to certain drugs.)

Yu AS: Atypical electrocardiographic changes in severe hyperkalemia. Am J Cardiol 1996;77:906. (A case of severe hyperkalemia associated only with pseudonormalized T waves and sinoatrial exit block.)

DISORDERS OF CALCIUM CONCENTRATION

Calcium constitutes about 2% of body weight, but only about 1% of the total body calcium is in solution in body fluid. In the plasma, calcium is present as a nondiffusible complex with protein (33%); as a diffusible but undissociated complex with anions such as citrate, bicarbonate, and phosphate (12%); and as ionized calcium (55%). The normal total plasma (or serum) calcium concentration is

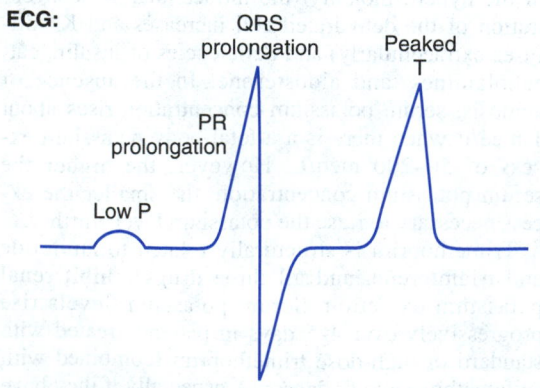

Figure 21–2. Electrocardiographic changes in hyperkalemia. (Reproduced, with permission, from Cogan MG: *Fluid and Electrolytes: Physiology and Pathophysiology.* Appleton & Lange, 1991.)

Table 21–6. Treatment of hyperkalemia.[1]

EMERGENCY

Modality	Mechanism of Action	Onset	Duration	Prescription	K+ Removed From Body
Calcium	Antagonizes cardiac conduction abnormalities	0–5 minutes	1 hour	Calcium gluconate 10%, 5–30 mL IV; or calcium chloride 5%, 5–30 mL IV	0
Bicarbonate	Distributes K+ into cells	15–30 minutes	1–2 hours	NaHCO$_3$, 44–88 meq (1–2 ampules) IV	0
Insulin	Distributes K+ into cells	15–60 minutes	4–6 hours	Regular insulin, 5–10 units IV, plus glucose 50%, 25 g (1 ampule) IV	0
Albuterol	Distributes K+ into cells	15–30 minutes	2–4 hours	Nebulized albuterol, 10–20 mg in 4 mL normal saline, inhaled over 10 minutes	0

NONEMERGENCY

Modality	Mechanism of Action	Duration of Treatment	Prescription	K+ Removed From Body
Loop diuretic	↑Renal K+ excretion	0.5–2 hours	Furosemide, 40–160 mg IV or orally with or without NaHCO$_3$, 0.5–3 meq/kg daily	Variable
Sodium polystyrene sulfonate (Kayexalate)	Ion exchange resin binds K+	1–3 hours	Oral: 15–30 g in 20% sorbitol (50–100 mL). Rectal: 50 g in 20% sorbitol	0.5–1 meq/g
Hemodialysis	Extracorporeal K+ removal	48 hours	Blood flow ≥ 200–300 mL/min. Dialysate [K+] = 0.	200–300 meq
Peritoneal dialysis	Peritoneal K+ removal	48 hours	Fast exchange, 3–4 L/h	200–300 meq

[1]Modified and reproduced, with permission, from Cogan MG: *Fluid and Electrolytes: Physiology and Pathophysiology*. Appleton & Lange, 1991.

9–10.3 mg/dL. It is ionized calcium (normal: 4.7–5.3 mg/dL) which, under physiologic regulation, is necessary for muscle contraction and nerve function. Calcium-sensing protein, a receptor-like protein with the special function of detecting extracellular calcium ion concentrations, has been identified in parathyroid cells and in the kidney. Some diseases (eg, familial hypocalcemia and familial hypocalciuric hypercalcemia) associated with disturbed calcium metabolism are due to functional defects of this protein.

1. HYPOCALCEMIA

Important causes of hypocalcemia are listed in Table 21–7.

The most common cause of hypocalcemia is renal failure, in which decreased production of active vitamin D$_3$ and hyperphosphatemia both play a role. Some cases of primary hypoparathyroidism are due to mutation of calcium-sensing protein in which inappropriate suppression of PTH release leads to

hypocalcemia. Hypocalcemia in pancreatitis is also a marker for severe disease (see Chapter 15).

Clinical Findings

A. Symptoms and Signs: Hypocalcemia increases excitation of nerve and muscle cells, primarily affecting the neuromuscular and cardiovascular systems. Extensive spasm of skeletal muscle causes cramps and tetany. Laryngospasm with stridor can obstruct the airway, causing fatal asphyxia. Convulsions can occur as well as paresthesias of lips and extremities and abdominal pain. Chvostek's sign (contraction of the facial muscle in response to tapping the facial nerve against the bone just anterior to the ear) and Trousseau's sign (carpal spasm occurring after occlusion of the brachial artery with a blood pressure cuff for 3 minutes) are usually readily elicited. Prolongation of the QT interval predisposes to the development of ventricular arrhythmias; heart block and ventricular fibrillation are also encountered. In chronic hypoparathyroidism, cataracts and calcification of basal ganglia of the brain may appear. (See Hypoparathyroidism, Chapter 26.)

Table 21–7. Causes of hypocalcemia.

Decreased intake or absorption
  Malabsorption
  Small bowel bypass, short bowel
  Vitamin D deficit (decreased absorption, decreased
    production of 25-hydroxyvitamin D or 1,25-dihydroxyvita-
    min D)
Increased loss
  Alcoholism
  Chronic renal insufficiency
  Diuretic therapy
Endocrine disease
  Hypoparathyroidism (genetic, acquired; including
    hypo- and hypermagnesemia)
  Sepsis
  Pseudohypoparathyroidism
  Calcitonin secretion with medullary carcinoma of the
    thyroid
Physiologic causes
  Associated with decreased serum albumin[1]
  Decreased end-organ response to vitamin D
  Hyperphosphatemia
  Induced by aminoglycoside antibiotics, plicamycin, loop
    diuretics, foscarnet

[1]Calcium ion concentration is normal.

B. Laboratory Findings: Serum Ca^{2+} is low (< 9 mg/dL). The depressed level of serum Ca^{2+} must be correlated with the simultaneous concentration of serum albumin: When albumin is low, serum Ca^{2+} concentration is also depressed in a ratio of 0.8–1 mg of Ca^{2+} to 1 g of albumin. Serum phosphate is usually elevated. Serum Mg^{2+} is commonly low, and hypomagnesemia reduces both parathyroid hormone release and tissue responsiveness to parathyroid hormone, causing hypocalcemia. In respiratory alkalosis, total serum calcium is normal but ionized calcium is low, which can be measured by use of a Ca^{2+}-sensitive electrode. The ECG shows a prolonged QT interval.

Treatment*
(Table 21–8)
A. Severe, Symptomatic Hypocalcemia: In the presence of tetany, arrhythmias, or seizures, calcium gluconate 10% (10–20 mL) administered intravenously over 10–15 minutes is indicated. Because of the short duration of action, calcium infusion is usually required. Ten to 15 milligrams of calcium per kilogram body weight, or six to eight 10-mL vials of 10% calcium gluconate (558–744 mg of calcium), is added to 1 L of D_5W and infused over 4–6 hours. By monitoring the serum calcium level frequently (every 4–6 hours), the infusion rate is adjusted to maintain the serum calcium level at 7–8.5 mg/dL.
B. Asymptomatic Hypocalcemia: Oral calcium and vitamin D preparations (Table 26–10) are

*See also Chapter 26 for discussion of the treatment of hypoparathyroidism.

used. Calcium carbonate is well tolerated and less expensive than many other calcium tablets. The low serum Ca^{2+} associated with low serum albumin concentration does not require replacement therapy. If serum Mg^{2+} is low, therapy must include replacement of magnesium, which by itself usually will correct hypocalcemia.

Brown EM et al: Calcium-ion-sensing cell-surface receptors. N Engl J Med 1995;333:234.
Guise TA, Numdy GR: Evaluation of hypocalcemia in children and adults. J Clin Endocrinol Metab 1995;80:1473.
Jankowski S, Vincent JL: Calcium administration for cardiovascular support in critically ill patients: When is it indicated? J Intensive Care Med 1995;10:91. (Importance of maintaining ionized calcium and the potential deleterious effects of calcium replacement.)
Reber PM, Heath H 3rd: Hypocalcemic emergencies. Med Clin North Am 1995;79:93.

2. HYPERCALCEMIA

Important causes of hypercalcemia are listed in Table 21–9. The milk-alkali syndrome, which had become rare with the advent of nonabsorbable antacid therapy for ulcer disease, should be considered as a cause of hypercalcemia with the current popularity of calcium ingestion for osteoporosis prevention. In the milk-alkali syndrome, massive calcium and vitamin D ingestion can cause hypercalcemic nephropathy. Because of the decreased GFR, retention of the alkali in the calcium antacid occurs and causes metabolic alkalosis, which can be worsened by the vomiting associated with this disorder.

Clinical Findings
A. Symptoms and Signs: Polyuria and constipation are the most characteristic symptoms, and a variety of neurologic symptoms also are observed. Stupor, coma, and azotemia may develop in severe hypercalcemia. Ventricular extrasystoles and idioventricular rhythm occur and can be accentuated by digitalis.
B. Laboratory Findings: A significant elevation of serum Ca^{2+} is seen; the level must be interpreted in relation to the serum albumin level (see Hypocalcemia). Serum phosphate may or may not be low, depending on the cause. The ECG shows a shortened QT interval.

Treatment
Until the primary disease can be brought under control, renal excretion of calcium with resultant decrease in serum Ca^{2+} concentration is promoted. Excretion of Na^+ is accompanied by excretion of Ca^{2+}; therefore, establishing euvolemia and inducing natriuresis by giving saline with furosemide is the emergency treatment of choice. In dehydrated patients with normal cardiac and renal function, 0.45% saline

Table 21–8. Treatment of hypocalcemia.

Modality	Amount of Ca^{2+}	Onset	Dose
Intravenous calcium Calcium gluconate 10%	93 mg (4.7 meq) per 10 mL	Immediate	93–186 mg over 10–15 minutes; then 10–15 mg/kg over 4–6 hours
Oral calcium Calcium carbonate (generic, Os-Cal, Biocal, Caltrate, Tums)	40% elemental calcium; 250 mg/624 mg tablet or 500 mg/1250 mg tablet or 600 mg/1500 mg tablet	<1 hour	250–500 mg calcium 5 times a day
Vitamin D preparations	See Table 26–10.		

or 0.9% saline can be given rapidly (250–500 mL/h). Intravenous furosemide (20–40 mg every 2 hours) prevents volume overload and enhances Ca^{2+} excretion. Thiazides can actually worsen hypercalcemia (as can furosemide if inadequate saline is given). See Chapter 4 for a discussion of the treatment of hypercalcemia of malignancy; and see Chapter 26 for a a discussion of the treatment of hypercalcemia of hyperparathyroidism.

Beall DP, Scofield RH: Milk-alkali syndrome associated with calcium carbonate consumption. Medicine 1995; 74:89.

Edelson GW, Kleerekoper M: Hypercalcemic crisis. Med Clin North Am 1995;79(1):79.

Kaye TB: Hypercalcemia: How to pinpoint the cause and customize treatment. Postgrad Med 1995;97:153.

Sharma OP: Vitamin D, calcium, and sarcoidosis. Chest 1996;109:535. (Hypercalcemia in sarcoidosis.)

Walls I, Bundred N, Howell A: Hypercalcemia and bone resorption in malignancy. Clin Orthop 1995 Mar (312):51.

Table 21–9. Causes of hypercalcemia.

Increased intake or absorption
 Milk-alkali syndrome
 Vitamin D or vitamin A excess
Endocrine disorders
 Primary hyperparathyroidism (adenoma, hyperplasia, carcinoma)
 Secondary hyperparathyroidism (renal insufficiency, malabsorption)
 Acromegaly
 Adrenal insufficiency
Neoplastic diseases
 Tumors producing PTH-related proteins (ovary, kidney, lung)
 Metastases to bone
 Lymphoproliferative disease, including multiple myeloma
 Secretion of prostaglandins and osteolytic factors
Miscellaneous causes
 Thiazide diuretic-induced
 Sarcoidosis
 Paget's disease of bone
 Hypophosphatasia
 Immobilization
 Familial hypocalciuric hypercalcemia
 Complications of renal transplantation
 Iatrogenic

DISORDERS OF PHOSPHORUS CONCENTRATION

Eighty percent of the phosphorus in the body is combined with calcium in bones and teeth. Only 10% is incorporated into a variety of organic compounds, and 10% is combined with proteins, lipids, carbohydrates, and other compounds in muscle and blood. Organic phosphate is the principal intracellular anion; inorganic phosphate comprises only a small fraction of intracellular phosphorus.

Phosphate is crucial in energy transfer and in the metabolism of carbohydrate, protein, and fat. Phosphate serves as the principal urinary buffer (HPO_4^{2-}, $H_2PO_4^-$), constituting most of titratable acidity.

Renal tubular reabsorption of filtered phosphate is reduced (phosphate excretion increased) by parathyroid hormone, expansion of extracellular fluid volume, increased intake of sodium, hypercalcemia, calcitonin, glucocorticoids, and growth hormone. Likewise, proximal tubular dysfunction such as occurs in myeloma kidney may have a similar effect.

Phosphorus metabolism and homeostasis are intimately related to calcium metabolism. See sections on metabolic bone disease in Chapter 26.

1. HYPOPHOSPHATEMIA

Hypophosphatemia may occur in the presence of normal phosphate stores. Serious depletion of body phosphate stores may exist with low, normal, or high concentrations of phosphorus in serum. Leading causes of hypophosphatemia are listed in Table 21–10.

Hypophosphatemia is a reversible cause of respiratory muscle hypocontractility and impaired tissue oxygenation by causing a decrease in the erythrocyte 2,3-diphosphoglycerate concentration in patients with COPD and asthma. Mechanisms of hypophosphatemia include intracellular shifts of phosphorus related to the correction of respiratory acidosis and the use of drugs that increase renal phosphate excretion such as theophylline, corticosteroids, loop diuretics, and β_2-adrenergic bronchodilators. Transient

Table 21–10. Causes of hypophosphatemia.

Diminished supply or absorption
Starvation
Parenteral alimentation with inadequate phosphate content
Malabsorption syndrome, small bowel bypass
Absorption blocked by oral aluminum hydroxide or bicarbonate
Vitamin D-deficient and vitamin D-resistant osteomalacia
Increased loss
Phosphaturic drugs: theophylline, diuretics, bronchodilators, corticosteroids
Hyperparathyroidism (primary or secondary)
Hyperthyroidism
Renal tubular defects permitting excessive phosphaturia (congenital, induced by monoclonal gammopathy, heavy metal poisoning)
Hypokalemic nephropathy
Inadequately controlled diabetes mellitus
Alcoholism
Intracellular shift of phosphorus
Administration of glucose, fructose (transient)
Anabolic steroids, estrogen, oral contraceptives
Respiratory alkalosis
Salicylate poisoning
Electrolyte abnormalities
Hypercalcemia
Hypomagnesemia
Metabolic alkalosis
Abnormal losses followed by inadequate repletion
Diabetes mellitus with acidosis, particularly during aggressive therapy
Recovery from starvation or prolonged catabolic state
Chronic alcoholism, particularly during restoration of nutrition; associated with hypomagnesemia
Respiratory alkalosis
Recovery from severe burns

---

defects in renal tubular function, such as decreases in the renal threshold of phosphate excretion and increases in the fractional excretion of calcium and magnesium, are common in patients with chronic alcoholism and account in part for the high prevalence of hypophosphatemia, hypomagnesemia, and hypocalcemia in these patients. These renal defects reverse within a month of abstinence.

Clinical Findings

A. Symptoms and Signs: Acute, severe hypophosphatemia (0.1–0.2 mg/dL) can lead to acute hemolytic anemia with increased erythrocyte fragility, impaired oxygen delivery to tissues, increased susceptibility to infection from impaired chemotaxis of leukocytes, and platelet dysfunction with petechial hemorrhages. Rhabdomyolysis, encephalopathy (irritability, confusion, dysarthria, seizures, and coma), and heart failure are uncommon but serious manifestations.

Chronic severe depletion may be manifested by anorexia, pain in muscles and bones, and fractures.

B. Laboratory Findings: In addition to hypophosphatemia, evidence of anemia due to hemolysis may be present (eg, elevated serum lactate dehydrogenase). Rhabdomyolysis results in elevated serum creatine kinase (which contains mostly the MM fraction but also some MB fraction) and, in many cases, myoglobin in the urine. Other values vary according to the cause. Renal glycosuria and hypouricemia together with hypophosphatemia indicate Fanconi's syndrome. In chronic depletion, radiographs and biopsies of bones show changes resembling those of osteomalacia.

Treatment

Treatment is best directed toward prophylaxis by including phosphate in repletion and maintenance fluids. A rapid decline in calcium levels can occur with parenteral administration of phosphate; therefore, when possible, oral replacement of phosphate is preferable. For parenteral alimentation, 620 mg (20 mmol) of phosphorus is required for every 1000 nonprotein kcal to maintain phosphate balance and to ensure anabolic function. A daily ration for prolonged parenteral fluid maintenance is 620–1240 mg (20–40 mmol) of phosphorus. For asymptomatic hypophosphatemia (serum phosphorus 0.7–1 mg/dL), an infusion should provide 279–310 mg (9–10 mmol)/12 h until the serum phosphorus exceeds 1 mg/dL. A magnesium deficit often coexists and should be treated simultaneously. In administering phosphate-containing solutions, serum creatinine and calcium must be monitored to guard against hypocalcemia.

For oral use, phosphate salts are available in skim milk (approximately 1 g [33 mmol]/L). Tablets or capsules of mixtures of sodium and potassium phosphate may be given to provide 0.5–1 g (18–32 mmol) per day.

Contraindications to therapy with phosphate salts include hypoparathyroidism, renal insufficiency, tissue damage and necrosis, and hypercalcemia. When hyperglycemia due to any cause is treated, phosphate accompanies glucose into cells, and hypophosphatemia may ensue.

Bollaert PE et al: Hemodynamic and metabolic effects of rapid correction of hypophosphatemia in patients with septic shock. Chest 1995;107(6):1698. (Severe hypophosphatemia can cause myocardial depression. Rapid correction is well tolerated and has beneficial myocardial and vascular benefits.)

Clark CL et al: Treatment of hypophosphatemia in patients receiving specialized nutrition support using a graduated dosing scheme: Results from a prospective clinical trial. Crit Care Med 1995;23:1504. (A "sliding scale" approach to phosphorus repletion was safe and effective.)

Rosen GH et al: Intravenous phosphate repletion regimen for critically ill patients with moderate hypophosphatemia. Crit Care Med 1995;23:1204. (More aggressive than usual guidelines. If serum phosphorus is < 2 mg/dL, ICU patients received 15 mmol [1425 mg] sodium phosphate in 100 mL 0.9% NaCl intravenously over 2 hours.)

2. HYPERPHOSPHATEMIA

Causes of hyperphosphatemia are given in Table 21–11. Growing children normally have serum phosphate levels higher than those of adults.

Clinical Findings

A. Symptoms and Signs: The clinical manifestations are those of the underlying disorders (eg, chronic renal failure, hypoparathyroidism). Hyperphosphatemia in chronic renal failure leads to secondary hyperparathyroidism and renal osteodystrophy.

B. Laboratory Findings: In addition to elevated phosphate, other blood chemistry values are those characteristic of the underlying disease.

Treatment

Treatment is that of the underlying disease and of associated hypocalcemia if present. In acute and chronic renal failure, dialysis will reduce serum phosphate, but high-flux dialysis is more effective than conventional dialysis. Absorption of phosphate can be reduced by administration of calcium carbonate, 0.5–1.5 g three times daily with meals (500 mg tablets). This approach is preferred to the traditional use of aluminum hydroxide because of concerns about aluminum toxicity.

DISORDERS OF MAGNESIUM CONCENTRATION

About 50% of total body magnesium exists in the insoluble state in bone. Only 5% is present as extracellular cation; the remaining 45% is contained in cells as intracellular cation. The normal plasma concentration is 1.5–2.5 meq/L, with about one-third bound to protein and two-thirds existing as free cation. Excretion of magnesium ion is via the kidney.

Magnesium is an important activator ion, participating in the function of many enzymes involved in phosphate transfer reactions. Magnesium exerts physiologic effects on the nervous system resembling those of calcium. Magnesium acts directly upon the myoneural junction.

Altered concentration of Mg^{2+} in the plasma usually provokes an associated alteration of Ca^{2+}. Hypermagnesemia suppresses secretion of parathyroid hormone with consequent hypocalcemia. Severe and prolonged magnesium depletion impairs secretion of PTH with consequent hypocalcemia. Hypomagnesemia may impair end-organ response to PTH as well.

1. HYPOMAGNESEMIA

Causes of hypomagnesemia are given in Table 21–12. Nearly half of hospitalized patients in whom serum electrolytes are ordered have unrecognized hypomagnesemia; in critically ill patients, arrhythmias and sudden death may be complications. Common causes include use of large volumes of intravenous fluids, diuretics, cisplatin in cancer patients (with concomitant hypokalemia), and administration of nephrotoxic agents such as aminoglycosides and amphotericin B.

Clinical Findings

A. Symptoms and Signs: Common symptoms are weakness, muscle cramps, and tremor. There is marked neuromuscular and central nervous system hyperirritability, with tremors, athetoid movements, jerking, nystagmus, and a positive Babinski response. There may be hypertension, tachycardia, and ventricular arrhythmias. Confusion and disorientation may be prominent features.

Table 21–11. Causes of hyperphosphatemia.

Endocrine disease
  Excessive growth hormone (acromegaly)
  Hypoparathyroidism associated with low calcium
  Pseudohypoparathyroidism associated with low calcium
Decreased excretion
  Chronic renal insufficiency
  Acute renal failure
Catabolic states; tissue destruction
  Stress or injury, rhabdomyolysis (especially if renal insufficiency exists)
  Chemotherapy of malignant disease, particularly lymphoproliferative disease
Excessive intake or absorption
  Laxatives or enemas containing phosphate
  Hypervitaminosis D

Table 21–12. Causes of hypomagnesemia.

Diminished absorption or intake
  Malabsorption, chronic diarrhea, laxative abuse
  Prolonged gastrointestinal suction
  Small bowel bypass
  Malnutrition
  Alcoholism
  Parenteral alimentation with inadequate Mg^{2+} content
Increased loss
  Diabetic ketoacidosis
  Diuretic therapy
  Diarrhea
  Hyperaldosteronism, Bartter's syndrome
  Associated with hypercalciuria
  Renal magnesium wasting
Unexplained
  Hyperparathyroidism
  Postparathyroidectomy
  Vitamin D therapy
  Induced by aminoglycoside antibiotics, cisplatin, amphotericin B

B. Laboratory Findings: In addition to hypomagnesemia, hypocalcemia and hypokalemia are often present. The ECG shows a prolonged QT interval, particularly due to lengthening of the ST segment.

Treatment

Treatment consists of the use of intravenous fluids containing magnesium as chloride or sulfate, 240–1200 mg/d (10–50 mmol/d) during the period of severe deficit, followed by 120 mg/d (5 mmol/d) for maintenance. Magnesium sulfate may also be given intramuscularly in a dosage of 200–800 mg/d (8–33 mmol/d) in four divided doses. Serum levels must be monitored and dosage adjusted to keep the concentration from rising above 2.5 mmol/L. K^+ and Ca^{2+} may be required as well. Magnesium oxide, 250–500 mg by mouth two to four times daily, is useful for repleting stores in those with chronic hypomagnesemia.

al-Ghamdi SM, Cameron EC, Sutton RA: Magnesium deficiency: Pathophysiologic and clinical overview. Am J Kidney Dis 1994;24:737.

Elin RJ. Magnesium: the fifth but forgotten electrolyte. Am J Clin Pathol 1994;102:616.

Tosiello L: Hypomagnesemia and diabetes mellitus: A review of clinical implications. Arch Intern Med 1996; 156:1143. (Hypomagnesemia has been correlated with both poor diabetic control and insulin resistance in elderly patients.)

2. HYPERMAGNESEMIA

Magnesium excess is almost always the result of renal insufficiency and the inability to excrete what has been taken in from food or drugs, especially antacids and laxatives.

Clinical Findings

A. Symptoms and Signs: Muscle weakness, mental obtundation, and confusion are characteristic manifestations. Weakness—even flaccid paralysis—and fall in blood pressure are evident on examination. There may be respiratory muscle paralysis or cardiac arrest.

B. Laboratory Findings: Serum Mg^{2+} is elevated. In the common setting of renal insufficiency, concentrations of BUN and of serum creatinine, phosphate, and uric acid are elevated; serum K^+ may be elevated. Serum Ca^{2+} is often low. The ECG shows increased PR interval, broadened QRS complexes, and elevated T waves, probably related to associated hyperkalemia.

Treatment

Treatment is directed toward alleviating renal insufficiency. Calcium acts as an antagonist to Mg^{2+} and may be given intravenously as calcium chloride, 500 mg or more at a rate of 100 mg (4.5 mmol)/min. Hemodialysis or peritoneal dialysis may be indicated.

Fung MC, Weintraub M, Bowen DL: Hypermagnesemia: Elderly over-the-counter drug users at risk. Arch Fam Med 1995;4:718. (Products that contain significant amounts of magnesium.)

Golzarian J, Scott HW Jr, Richards WO: Hypermagnesemia-induced paralytic ileus. Dig Dis Sci 1994;39: 1138.

Vissers RJ, Purssell R: Iatrogenic magnesium overdose: Two case reports. J Emerg Med 1994;39:1138.

Vissers RJ, Purssell R: Iatrogenic magnesium overdose: Two case reports. J Emerg Med 1996;14:187. (The major life-threatening clinical manifestations are cardiac conduction delays, asystole, apnea, and coma.)

HYPEROSMOLAR DISORDERS & OSMOLAR GAPS

1. HYPEROSMOLALITY WITH ONLY TRANSIENT OR NO SIGNIFICANT SHIFT IN WATER

Urea and alcohol are two substances that readily cross cell membranes and can produce hyperosmolality. Because of its permeant nature, urea has little effect on the shift of water across the cell membrane. Urea may be administered acutely in large doses to "draw" water from cells, but the effect is transient, as is the diuresis, and urea soon equilibrates throughout body water. Alcohol quickly equilibrates between intracellular and extracellular water, adding 22 mosm/L for every 1000 mg/L. This measured hyperosmolality does not produce symptoms by itself because of the equilibrium described, but in any case of stupor or coma in which measured osmolality exceeds that calculated from values of serum Na^+ and glucose and BUN, ethanol intoxication should be considered as a possible explanation of the discrepancy (osmolar gap). Toxic alcohol ingestion, particularly methanol or ethylene glycol, also causes an osmolar gap characterized by anion gap metabolic acidosis (Chapter 39).

The combination of anion gap metabolic acidosis and an osmolar gap exceeding 10 mosm/kg is not specific for toxic alcohol ingestion. Nearly half of patients with alcoholic ketoacidosis or lactic acidosis have similar findings, caused in part by elevations of endogenous glycerol, acetone, and acetone metabolites.

Braden GL et al: Increased osmolal gap in alcoholic acidosis. Arch Intern Med 1993;153:2377.

Glaser S: Utility of the serum osmol gap in the diagnosis of methanol or ethylene glycol ingestion. Ann Emerg Med 1996;27:343. (Limitations of the test.)

Kruse JA, Cadnapaphornchai P: The serum osmole gap. J Crit Care 1994;9:185.

2. HYPEROSMOLALITY ASSOCIATED WITH SIGNIFICANT SHIFTS IN WATER

Increased concentrations of solutes that do not readily enter cells produce a shift of water from the intracellular space to effect a true intracellular dehydration. Sodium and glucose are the solutes commonly involved. In these instances, the hyperosmolality does produce symptoms.

Clinical symptoms are mainly referred to the central nervous system. The severity of symptoms depends on the degree of hyperosmolality and rapidity of development. In acute hyperosmolality, symptoms of somnolence and confusion can appear when the osmolality exceeds 320–330 mosm/L, and coma, respiratory arrest, and death occur when it exceeds 340–350 mosm/L.

ACID-BASE DISORDERS

In order to assess a patient's acid-base status, measurement of arterial pH, partial pressure of carbon dioxide (PCO_2), and plasma bicarbonate (HCO_3^-) is needed. Blood gas analyzers directly measure pH and PCO_2, and the HCO_3^- value is calculated from the Henderson-Hasselbalch equation:

$$pH = 6.1 + \log \frac{[HCO_3^-]}{0.03 \times PCO_2}$$

The total venous CO_2 measurement is a more direct determination of HCO_3^-. Because of the dissociation characteristics of carbonic acid (H_2CO_3) at body pH, dissolved CO_2 is almost exclusively in the form of HCO_3^-, and for clinical purposes the total carbon dioxide content is equivalent (± 3 meq/L) to the HCO_3^- concentration:

$$H^+ + HCO_3^- \leftrightarrow H_2CO_3 \leftrightarrow CO_2 + H_2O$$

The syringe used for taking blood arterial blood gas determinations should be coated with 1 mL of heparin (1000 units/mL) as an anticoagulant, but excessive heparin artificially lowers the PCO_2 and HCO_3^- derived from that sample. If precise measurements of oxygenation are not needed or if oxygen saturation obtained from the pulse oximeter is adequate, venous blood gases generally provide useful information for assessment of acid-base balance and can be used interchangeably with arterial blood gases since the arteriovenous differences in pH and PCO_2 are small and relatively constant. Venous blood pH is usually 0.03–0.04 units lower than that of arterial blood, and venous blood PCO_2 is 7 or 8 mm Hg higher. Calculated HCO_3^- concentration in venous blood is at most 2 meq/L higher than that of arterial blood. An important exception to the rule of inter-changeability between arterial and venous blood gases for determination of acid-base balance is during cardiopulmonary arrest. In this setting, arterial pH may be 7.41 and venous pH 7.15, and arterial blood PCO_2 can be 32 mm Hg with a venous blood PCO_2 of 74 mm Hg.

Types of Acid-Base Disorders

There are two types of acid-base disorders: respiratory and metabolic. Primary respiratory disorders affect blood acidity by causing changes in PCO_2, and primary metabolic disorders are caused by disturbances in the HCO_3^- concentration. The primary disturbances are usually accompanied by compensatory changes, but these changes do not fully compensate for the primary acid-base disorders even if the disorders are chronic. Therefore, if the pH is less than 7.40, the primary process is acidosis (either respiratory or metabolic). If the pH is higher than 7.40, the primary process is either respiratory or metabolic alkalosis. The presence of one disorder with its appropriate compensatory change is a simple disorder.

Mixed Acid-Base Disorders

The presence of more than one simple disorder (not compensatory) is a mixed disorder. Double or triple disorders can coexist but not quadruple ones, since simultaneous respiratory acidosis and alkalosis are not possible.

Clinicians frequently find it difficult to decide if a mixed disorder is present. One useful scheme is to determine if the degree of compensation for the primary disorder is appropriate (Table 21–13). In respiratory disorders, if the magnitude of compensation in HCO_3^- level differs from that which is predicted, the patient has a mixed disorder. Therefore, superimposed metabolic acidosis will decrease HCO_3^- to lower than the predicted level, and a metabolic alkalosis will increase HCO_3^- over the predicted value. For example, a patient with chronic respiratory acidosis and PCO_2 of 60 mm Hg should have a HCO_3^- of 31 meq/L (assuming that normal HCO_3^- is 24 meq/L). If the HCO_3^- is 25 meq/L, a superimposed metabolic acidosis exists, and if the HCO_3^- is 45 meq/L, there is a superimposed metabolic alkalosis. Using data from Table 21–13, similar calculations can be made for primary metabolic disorders.

Laski ME, Kurtzman NA: Acid-base disorders in medicine. Dis Mon 1996;42(2):51.

Williamson JC: Acid-base disorders: Classification and management strategies. Am Fam Physician 1995;52: 584.

1. RESPIRATORY ACIDOSIS

Respiratory acidosis results from decreased alveolar ventilation and subsequent hypercapnia. Pul-

Table 21–13. Primary acid-base disorders and expected compensation.

Disorder	Primary Defect	pH	Compensatory Response	Magnitude of Compensation
Respiratory				
Acidosis				
Acute	$\uparrow P_{CO_2}$	$\downarrow pH$	$\uparrow HCO_3^-$	$\uparrow$1 meq HCO_3^- per 10 mm Hg $\uparrow P_{CO_2}$
Chronic	$\uparrow P_{CO_2}$	$\downarrow pH$	$\uparrow HCO_3^-$	$\uparrow$3.5 meq HCO_3^- per 10 mm Hg $\uparrow P_{CO_2}$
Alkalosis				
Acute	$\downarrow P_{CO_2}$	$\uparrow pH$	$\downarrow HCO_3^-$	$\downarrow HCO_3^-$ 2 meq/L per 10 mm Hg $\downarrow P_{CO_2}$
Chronic	$\downarrow P_{CO_2}$	$\uparrow pH$	$\downarrow HCO_3^-$	$\downarrow HCO_3^-$ 5 meq/L per 10 mm Hg $\downarrow P_{CO_2}$
Metabolic				
Acidosis	$\downarrow HCO_3^-$	$\downarrow pH$	$\downarrow P_{CO_2}$	$\downarrow P_{CO_2}$ 1.3 mm Hg per $\downarrow$1 meq HCO_3^-
Alkalosis	$\uparrow HCO_3^-$	$\uparrow pH$	$\uparrow P_{CO_2}$	$\uparrow P_{CO_2}$ 0.7 mm Hg per 1 meq HCO_3^-

monary as well as nonpulmonary disorders can cause hypoventilation (Table 21–14). The clinician must be mindful of readily reversible causes of respiratory acidosis, especially that due to narcotic-induced central nervous system depression.

Acute respiratory failure is associated with severe acidosis and only a small increase in the plasma bicarbonate. After 6–12 hours, the primary increase in P_{CO_2} evokes a renal compensatory response to generate more HCO_3^-, which tends to ameliorate the respiratory acidosis. This usually takes several days to complete. In acute respiratory acidosis, the serum HCO_3^- level should increase by 1 meq/L for each increment of 10 mm Hg in P_{CO_2} (Table 21–13).

Chronic respiratory acidosis is generally seen in patients with underlying lung disease, such as

Table 21–14. Causes of respiratory acidosis.[1]

Acute	Chronic
Airway obstruction	**Airway obstruction**
Aspiration of foreign body or vomitus	Chronic obstructive lung disease (bronchitis,
Laryngospasm	emphysema)
Generalized bronchospasm	
Obstructive sleep apnea	
Respiratory center depression	**Respiratory center depression**
General anesthesia	Chronic sedative overdosage
Sedative overdosage	Primary alveolar hypoventilation (Ondine's
Cerebral trauma or infarction	curse)
Central sleep apnea	Obesity-hypoventilation syndrome
Circulatory catastrophes	(Pickwickian syndrome)
Cardiac arrest	Brain tumor
Severe pulmonary edema	Bulbar poliomyelitis
Neuromuscular defects	**Neuromuscular defects**
High cervical cordotomy	Polymyositis
Botulism, tetanus	Multiple sclerosis
Guillain-Barré syndrome	Muscular dystrophy
Crisis in myasthenia gravis	Amyotrophic lateral sclerosis
Familial hypokalemic periodic paralysis	Diaphragmatic paralysis
Hypokalemic myopathy	Myxedema
Polymyositis	Myopathic disease
Drugs or toxic agents (eg, curare, succinyl-	
choline, aminoglycosides, organophos-	
phorus)	
Restrictive defects	**Restrictive defects**
Pneumothorax	Kyphoscoliosis
Hemothorax	Fibrothorax
Flail chest	Hydrothorax
Severe pneumonitis	Interstitial fibrosis
Acute respiratory distress syndrome	Decreased diaphragmatic movement (eg,
Mechanical hypoventilation	ascites)
Increased CO$_2$ production with fixed minute	Prolonged pneumonitis
ventilation	Obesity
Parenteral nutrition with high-carbohydrate	
intake	
Sorbent-regenerative hemodialysis	

[1]Modified from Gennari FJ: Respiratory acidosis and alkalosis. In: *Maxwell and Kleeman's Clinical Disorders of Fluid and Electrolyte Metabolism,* 5th ed. Narins RG (editor). McGraw-Hill, 1994.

chronic obstructive disease. In chronic respiratory acidosis, the serum bicarbonate level should increase by 3.5 meq/L for each increment of 10 mm Hg PCO_2. Urinary excretion of acid in the form of NH_4^+ and Cl^- ions results in the characteristic hypochloremia of chronic respiratory acidosis. When chronic respiratory acidosis is corrected suddenly, especially in patients who receive mechanical ventilation, there is a 2- to 3-day lag in renal bicarbonate excretion, resulting in posthypercapnic metabolic alkalosis.

Clinical Findings

A.   Symptoms and Signs: With acute onset, there is somnolence and confusion, and myoclonus with asterixis may be seen. Coma from CO_2 narcosis ensues. Severe hypercapnia increases cerebral blood flow and cerebrospinal fluid pressure. Signs of increased intracranial pressure (papilledema, pseudotumor cerebri) may be seen.

B.   Laboratory Findings: Arterial pH is low, and PCO_2 is increased. Serum HCO_3^- is elevated, but not enough to completely compensate for the hypercapnia. If the disorder is chronic, hypochloremia is seen.

Treatment

Since drug overdose is an important reversible cause of acute respiratory acidosis, administration of naloxone, 0.04–2 mg intravenously (see Chapter 39) should be considered in all such patients if no obvious cause for respiratory depression is present. In all forms of respiratory acidosis, treatment is directed at the underlying disorder to improve ventilation. Mechanical ventilation may be necessary (see Chapter 9 for treatment of respiratory failure).

2.   RESPIRATORY ALKALOSIS

Respiratory alkalosis, or hypocapnia, occurs when hyperventilation reduces the PCO_2, which increases the pH. The most common cause of respiratory alkalosis is hyperventilation syndrome (Table 21–15). Symptoms in acute respiratory alkalosis are related to decreased cerebral blood flow induced by the disorder. The physiologic state of pregnancy is chronic respiratory alkalosis, probably from progesterone stimulation of the respiratory center, with an average PCO_2 of 30 mm Hg.

Determination of appropriate compensatory changes in the HCO_3^- is useful to sort out the presence of an associated metabolic disorder (see above under Mixed Acid-Base Disorders). As in respiratory acidosis, the changes in HCO_3^- values are greater if the respiratory alkalosis is chronic (Table 21–14). In acute respiratory alkalosis, HCO_3^- decreases 2 meq/L for every 10 mm Hg fall in PCO_2. In chronic respiratory alkalosis, there is a compensatory de-

Table 21–15. Causes of respiratory alkalosis.[1]

Hypoxia
   Decreased inspired oxygen tension
   High altitude
   Ventilation/perfusion inequality
   Hypotension
   Severe anemia
CNS-mediated disorders
   Voluntary hyperventilation
      Anxiety-hyperventilation syndrome
   Neurologic disease
   Cerebrovascular accident (infarction, hemorrhage)
   Infection
   Trauma
   Tumor
   Pharmacologic and hormonal stimulation
      Salicylates
      Nicotine
      Xanthines
      Pregnancy (progesterone)
   Hepatic failure
   Gram-negative septicemia
   Recovery from metabolic acidosis
   Heat exposure
Pulmonary disease
   Interstitial lung disease
   Pneumonia
   Pulmonary embolism
   Pulmonary edema
Mechanical overventilation

[1]Adapted from Gennari FJ: Respiratory acidosis and alkalosis. In: *Maxwell and Kleeman's Clinical Disorders of Fluid and Electrolyte Metabolism,* 5th ed. Narins RG (editor). McGraw-Hill, 1994.

crease in renal acid excretion. Serum HCO_3^- decreases by 5 meq/L for every 10 mm Hg drop in PCO_2. While serum HCO_3^- is frequently below 15 meq/L in metabolic acidosis, it is unusual to see such a low level in respiratory alkalosis, and its presence would imply a superimposed (noncompensatory) metabolic acidosis.

Clinical Findings

A.   Symptoms and Signs: In acute cases (hyperventilation), there is light-headedness, anxiety, paresthesias, numbness about the mouth, and a tingling sensation in the hands and feet. Tetany occurs in more severe alkalosis from a fall in ionized calcium. In chronic cases, symptomatic findings are those of the primary disease.

B.   Laboratory Findings: Arterial blood pH is elevated, and PCO_2 is low. Serum bicarbonate is decreased in chronic respiratory alkalosis.

Treatment

Treatment is directed toward the underlying cause. In acute hyperventilation syndrome from anxiety, rebreathing into a paper bag will increase the PCO_2. Sedation may be necessary if the maneuver does not terminate the attack. Rapid correction of chronic respiratory alkalosis may result in metabolic acidosis as P_{CO_2} is increased in the setting of previous compensatory decrease in HCO_3^-.

3. METABOLIC ACIDOSIS

The hallmark of metabolic acidosis is decreased HCO_3^-, seen also in respiratory alkalosis (see above), but the pH distinguishes between the two disorders. Calculation of the anion gap is useful in determining the cause of the metabolic acidosis (Table 21–16). The anion gap represents the difference between readily measured anions and cations.

In plasma,

$$Na + \frac{Unmeasured}{cations} = HCO_3^- + Cl^- + \frac{Unmeasured}{anions}$$

$$Anion\ gap = (Na^+) - (HCO_3^- + Cl^-)$$

The major unmeasured cations are calcium (5 meq/L), magnesium (2 meq/L), gamma globulins, and potassium (4 meq/L). The major unmeasured anions are negatively charged albumin (2 meq/L per g/dL), phosphate (2 meq/L), sulfate (1 meq/L), lactate (1–2 meq/L), and other organic anions (3–4

Table 21–16. Abnormal anion gap.[1]

Decreased (< 6 meq)
Hypoalbuminemia (decreased unmeasured anion)
Plasma cell dyscrasias
   Monoclonal protein (cationic paraprotein) (accompanied by chloride and bicarbonate)
Bromide intoxication
Increased (> 12 meq)
Metabolic anion
   Diabetic ketoacidosis
   Alcoholic ketoacidosis
   Lactic acidosis
   Renal insufficiency (PO_4^{3-}, SO_4^{2-})
   Starvation
   Metabolic alkalosis (increased number of negative charges on protein)
Drug or chemical anion
   Salicylate intoxication
   Sodium carbenicillin therapy
   Methanol (formic acid)
   Ethylene glycol (oxalic acid)
Normal (6–12 meq)
Loss of HCO_3^-
Diarrhea
Recovery from diabetic ketoacidosis
Pancreatic fluid loss
Ileostomy (unadapted)
Carbonic anhydrase inhibitors
Chloride retention
Renal tubular acidosis
Ileal loop bladder
Administration of HCl equivalent or NH_4Cl
Arginine and lysine in parenteral nutrition

[1]Reference ranges for anion gap may vary based on differing laboratory methods.

meq/L). Traditionally, the normal anion gap has been 12 ± 4 meq/L. With the new generation of autoanalyzers (Bechman ASTRA analyzer), the reference range may be lower (6 ± 1 meq/L), primarily from an increase in Cl^- values. Despite its usefulness, the serum anion gap can be misleading. Non-acid-base disorders that may contribute to an error in anion gap interpretation include hypoalbuminemia (see below), antibiotic administration (eg, carbenicillin is an unmeasured anion; polymyxin is an unmeasured cation), hypernatremia, or hyponatremia.

Decreased Anion Gap

A decreased anion gap can occur because of a reduction in unmeasured anions or an increase in unmeasured cations.

A. Decreased Unmeasured Anions: If the sodium concentration remains normal but HCO_3^- and Cl^- increase, the anion gap will decrease. This is seen when there are decreased unmeasured anions, especially in hypoalbuminemia. For every 1 g/dL decline in serum albumin, a 2 meq/L decrease in anion gap will occur. The new reference range for anion gap diminishes the usefulness of a low anion gap categorization except to detect an increased anion gap acidosis mimicking a normal anion gap acidosis.

B. Increased Unmeasured Cations: If the sodium concentration falls because of addition of unmeasured cations but HCO_3^- and Cl^- remain unchanged, the anion gap will decrease (Figure 21–2). This is seen in (1) severe hypercalcemia, hypermagnesemia, or hyperkalemia; (2) IgG myeloma, where the immunoglobulin is cationic in 70% of cases; and (3) lithium toxicity.

Increased Anion Gap Acidosis (Increased Unmeasured Anions)

The hallmark of this disorder is that metabolic acidosis (thus low HCO_3^-) is associated with normal serum Cl^-, so that the anion gap increases. Normochloremic metabolic acidosis generally results from addition to the blood of nonchloride acids such as lactate, acetoacetate, β-hydroxybutyrate, and exogenous toxins. An exception is uremia, with underexcretion of organic acids and anions. Pseudometabolic acidosis is caused by underfilling Vacutainer tubes. If 1 mL of blood is put into a 10-mL red-top Vacutainer tube, a significant decline in HCO_3^- with an increase in anion gap occurs.

A. Lactic Acidosis: Lactic acid is formed from pyruvate in anaerobic glycolysis. Therefore, most of the lactate is produced in tissues with high rates of glycolysis, such as gut (responsible for over 50% of lactate production), skeletal muscle, brain, skin, and erythrocytes. Normally, lactate levels remain low (1 meq/L) because of metabolism of lactate principally by the liver through gluconeogenesis or oxidation via the Krebs cycle. Furthermore, the kidneys metabolize about 30% of lactate.

In lactic acidosis, lactate levels are at least 4–5 meq/L but commonly 10–30 meq/L. The mortality rate exceeds 50%. There are two basic types of lactic acidosis, both associated with increased lactate production and decreased lactate utilization. Type A is characterized by hypoxia or decreased tissue perfusion, whereas in type B there is no clinical evidence of hypoxia. Type A (hypoxic) lactic acidosis is the more common type, resulting from poor tissue perfusion; cardiogenic, septic, or hemorrhagic shock; or carbon monoxide poisoning. These conditions not only cause lactic acid production to increase peripherally but, more importantly, hepatic metabolism of lactate to decrease as liver perfusion declines. In addition, severe acidosis impairs the ability of the liver to extract the perfused lactate.

Type B lactic acidosis may be due to metabolic causes, such as diabetes, ketoacidosis, liver disease, renal failure, infection, leukemia, or lymphoma; or may occur as a result of toxicity from ethanol, methanol, salicylates, isoniazid, or phenformin. AIDS without AIDS-related lymphoma is associated with type B lactic acidosis. It is postulated that tissue oxygen utilization is impaired in these instances.

Idiopathic lactic acidosis, usually in debilitated patients, has an extremely high mortality rate. (For treatment of lactic acidosis, see Chapter 27.)

B. Diabetic Ketoacidosis: This metabolic abnormality is characterized by hyperglycemia and metabolic acidosis (pH < 7.25 or plasma bicarbonate < 16 meq/L). Anion gap metabolic acidosis is the acid-base disturbance generally ascribed to diabetic ketoacidosis:

$$H + B^- + NaHCO_3 \leftrightarrow CO_2 + NaB + H_2O$$

where B^- is β-hydroxybutyrate or acetoacetate.

The anion gap should be calculated from the serum electrolytes as measured, since correction of the serum sodium for the dilutional effect of hyperglycemia will incorrectly exaggerate the anion gap. The increased anion gap is due to hyperketonemia (acetoacetate and β-hydroxybutyrate) and at times to an increase in serum lactate secondary to reduced tissue perfusion and increased anaerobic metabolism. If a rise in anion gap from normal is equal to a fall in HCO_3^-, a diagnosis of simple metabolic acidosis can be made. However, it often happens in the simple anion gap metabolic acidosis of diabetic ketoacidosis or lactic acidosis that the elevation in the anion gap exceeds the fall in the plasma bicarbonate concentration. Since more than half of the excess H^+ is buffered by the cells and not by HCO_3^-, one can see why a change in anion gap/change in HCO_3^- ratio greater than 1.0 is not necessarily diagnostic of a mixed acid-base disorder.

During the recovery phase of diabetic ketoacidosis, anion gap acidosis can be transformed into hyperchloremic non-anion gap acidosis. The mechanism for this is as follows: As GFR increases from NaCl therapy of diabetic ketoacidosis, the retention of Cl^- causes a mild decrease in the anion gap from dilution. More importantly, the increased GFR causes the urinary excretion of ketone salts (NaB), which are formed as bicarbonate is consumed:

$$HB + NaHCO_3^- \rightarrow NaB + H_2CO_3$$

The kidney reabsorbs ketone anions poorly but can compensate for the loss of anions (and therefore Na^+) by increasing the reabsorption of Cl^-. Conversely, even on presentation, patients with diabetic ketoacidosis and normal renal perfusion may have marked ketonuria, severe metabolic acidosis, and only a mildly increased anion gap. Again, the variable relationship between the rise in the anion gap and the fall in the HCO_3^- can occur with the urinary loss of Na^+ or K^+ salts of β-hydroxybutyrate, which will lower the anion gap without altering the H^+ excretion or the severity of the acidosis.

Use of the anion gap during treatment of diabetic ketoacidosis to monitor metabolic improvement can help circumvent some of the diagnostic difficulties encountered with the use of the nitroprusside-containing serum acetone tests (Acetest and Ketostix). Since the nitroprusside reacts to acetoacetate, less to acetone, and not at all to the predominant keto acid, β-hydroxybutyrate, the serum acetone test is most useful in the initial diagnosis of diabetic ketoacidosis (Table 27–11). With therapy, the patient's clinical status and the reduction of the anion gap are better markers of improvement than monitoring the serum acetone test. Clearing of the acetoacetate may lag behind the clearing of β-hydroxybutyrate, leaving the nitroprusside reaction strongly positive despite improvement in the diabetic ketoacidosis. Conversely, in the presence of concomitant lactic acidosis, a shift in the redox state can increase β-hydroxybutyrate and decrease the readily detectable acetoacetate, thus lowering the nitroprusside reaction. As availability of β-hydroxybutyrate measurements becomes more widespread, these difficulties should be ameliorated.

C. Alcoholic Ketoacidosis: This is a common disorder of chronically malnourished patients who consume large quantities of alcohol daily. Most of these patients have mixed acid-base disorders (10% have a triple acid-base disorder). While decreased HCO_3^- is usual, half the patients may have normal or alkalemic pH. The three types of metabolic acidosis seen in alcoholic ketoacidosis are the following: (1) Ketoacidosis due to β-hydroxybutyrate and acetoacetate excess. (2) Lactic acidosis: Alcohol metabolism increases the NADH:NAD ratio, causing increased production and decreased utilization of lactate. Moderate to severe elevations of lactate (> 6 mmol/L) are seen with concomitant disorders such as sepsis, pancreatitis, or hypoglycemia. (3) Hyperchloremic acidosis from bicarbonate loss in the urine associated with ketonuria. Metabolic alkalosis occurs from volume contraction and vomiting. Respiratory alkalosis results from alcohol withdrawal, pain, or associated disorders such as sepsis or liver disease. Half of the patients have either hypoglycemia or hyperglycemia. When serum glucose levels are greater than 250 mg/dL, the distinction from diabetic ketoacidosis is difficult. The diagnosis of alcoholic ketoacidosis is supported by absence of a diabetic history and by no evidence of glucose intolerance after initial therapy.

D. Toxins: (See also Chapter 39.) Multiple toxins and drugs can increase the anion gap by increasing endogenous acid production. Examples include methanol (metabolized to formic acid), ethylene glycol (glycolic and oxalic acid), and salicylates (salicylic acid and lactic acid), which can cause a mixed disorder of metabolic acidosis with respiratory alkalosis.

E. Uremic Acidosis: At glomerular filtration rates below 20 mL/min, the inability to excrete H^+ with retention of acid anions such as PO_4^{3-} and SO_4^{2-} result in an anion gap acidosis, which rarely is severe. The unmeasured anions "replace" HCO_3^- (which is consumed as a buffer). Hyperchloremic normal anion gap acidosis may be seen in milder cases of renal insufficiency.

Normal Anion Gap Acidosis (Table 21–17)

The hallmark of this disorder is that the low HCO_3^- of metabolic acidosis is associated with hyperchloremia, so that the anion gap remains normal. The most common causes are gastrointestinal HCO_3^- loss and defects in renal acidification (renal tubular acidoses). The urinary anion gap can differentiate between these two common causes (see below).

A. Gastrointestinal HCO_3^- Loss: Bicarbonate is secreted in multiple areas in the gastrointestinal tract. Small bowel and pancreatic secretions contain large amounts of HCO_3^-. Therefore, diarrhea or pancreatic drainage can result in HCO_3^- loss because of increased HCO_3^- secretion and decreased absorption. Hyperchloremia occurs because the ileum and colon secrete HCO_3^- in a one-to-one exchange for Cl^- by countertransport. The resultant volume contraction causes increased Cl^- retention by the kidney in the setting of decreased anion, HCO_3^-. Patients with ureterosigmoidostomies can develop hyperchloremic metabolic acidosis because the colon secretes HCO_3^- in the urine in exchange for Cl^-.

B. Renal Tubular Acidosis: In renal tubular acidosis, the defect is either inability to excrete H^+ or inadequate generation of new HCO_3^-. Four discrete types can be differentiated by the clinical setting, urinary pH, urinary anion gap (see below), and serum K^+ level.

1. Classic distal renal tubular acidosis (type I)–This disorder is characterized by hypokalemic hyperchloremic metabolic acidosis and is due to selective deficiency in H^+ secretion in the dis-

tal nephron. Despite acidosis, urinary pH cannot be acidified and is always above 5.5. Urinary excretion of $NH_4^+Cl^-$ is decreased, and the urinary anion gap is positive (see below). Enhanced K^+ excretion occurs probably because there is less competition from H^+ in the distal nephron transport system. Furthermore, as a response to renal salt wasting, hyperaldosteronism occurs. Nephrocalcinosis and nephrolithiasis frequently accompany this disorder.

2. Proximal renal tubular acidosis (type II)–Proximal renal tubular acidosis is a hypokalemic hyperchloremic metabolic acidosis due to a selective defect in the proximal tubule's ability to adequately reabsorb filtered HCO_3^-. Carbonic anhydrase inhibitors (acetazolamide) can cause proximal renal tubular acidosis. About 90% of filtered HCO_3^- is absorbed by the proximal tubule. The distal nephron has a limited ability to absorb HCO_3^- but becomes overwhelmed and does not function adequately when there is increased delivery. Eventually, distal delivery of filtered HCO_3^- declines because the plasma HCO_3^- level has dropped as a result of progressive urinary HCO_3^- wastage. When the plasma HCO_3^- level drops to 15–18 meq/L, delivery of HCO_3^- drops to the point where the distal nephron is no longer overwhelmed and can regain function. At that point, bicarbonaturia disappears, and urinary pH can be acidic. Thiazide-induced volume contraction can be used to decrease distal HCO_3^- delivery and improve bicarbonaturia and renal acidification. The increased delivery of HCO_3^- to the distal nephron also increases K^+ secretion, and hypokalemia results. Proximal renal tubular acidosis often exists with other defects of absorption in the proximal tubule, resulting in glucosuria, aminoaciduria, phosphaturia, and uricaciduria (Fanconi's syndrome).

3. Renal tubular acidosis of glomerular insufficiency (type III)–When GFR decreases to 20–30 mL/min, ability to generate adequate NH_3 is impaired, with subsequent decreased $NH_4^+Cl^-$ excretion. A normokalemic, hyperchloremic metabolic acidosis ensues. Further reduction in GFR results in increased anion gap acidosis of uremia (see above).

4. Hyporeninemic hypoaldosteronemic renal tubular acidosis (type IV)–Type IV is the only type characterized by hyperkalemic, hyperchloremic acidosis. The defect is aldosterone deficiency or antagonism, which impairs distal nephron Na^+ reabsorption and K^+ and H^+ excretion. Renal salt wasting is frequently present. Relative hypoaldosteronism from hyporeninemia is most commonly found in diabetic nephropathy, tubulointerstitial renal diseases, hypertensive nephrosclerosis, and AIDS. In patients with these disorders, caution must be taken when using drugs that can exacerbate the hyperkalemia, such as angiotensin-converting enzyme inhibitors, which will further reduce aldosterone levels, aldosterone receptor blockers such as spironolactone, and NSAIDs.

Table 21-17. Hyperchloremic, normal anion gap metabolic acidoses.[1]

Renal Defect	GFR	Serum [K⁺]	Proximal H⁺ Secretion[2]	Distal H⁺ Secretion		Urinary Anion Gap	Treatment
				Minimal Urine pH	Urinary NH₄⁺ Plus Titratable Acid		
Gastrointestinal HCO₃⁻ loss	None	↓	↓	Normal	<5.5	↑↑	Negative	Na⁺, K⁺, and HCO₃⁻ as required
Renal tubular acidosis								
I. Classic distal	Distal H⁺ secretion	Normal	↓	Normal	>5.5	↓	Zero or positive	NaHCO₃ (1–3 meq/kg/d)
II. Proximal	Proximal H⁺ secretion	Normal	↓	↓³	<5.5	Normal	Zero or positive	NaHCO₃ or KHCO₃ (10–15 meq/kg/d), thiazide
III. Glomerular insufficiency	NH₃ production	↓	Normal	Normal	<5.5	↓	Zero or positive	NaHCO₃ (1–3 meq/kg/d)
IV. Hyporeninemic hypoaldosteronism	Distal Na⁺ reabsorption, K⁺ secretion, and H⁺ secretion	↓	↑	Normal	5.5	↓	Zero or positive	Fludrocortisone (0.1–0.5 mg/d), dietary K⁺ restriction, furosemide (40–160 mg/d), NaHCO₃ (1–3 meq/kg/d)

[1]Reproduced, with permission, from Cogan MG: *Fluid and Electrolytes: Physiology and Pathophysiology.* Appleton & Lange, 1991.
[2]HCO₃⁻ reabsorption during HCO₃⁻ loading.
[3]Fractional excretion of bicarbonate > 15% during bicarbonate loading; usually associated with Fanconi's syndrome.

C. Dilutional Acidosis: Rapid dilution of plasma volume by 0.9% NaCl may cause a mild hyperchloremic acidosis. Greatest retention of NaCl occurs in a volume-contracted state.

D. Recovery From Diabetic Ketoacidosis: See above.

E. Posthypocapnia: In prolonged respiratory alkalosis, HCO_3^- decreases and Cl^- increases from decreased renal $NH_4^+Cl^-$ excretion. If the respiratory alkalosis is corrected quickly, PCO_2 will increase acutely but HCO_3^- will remain low until the kidneys can generate new HCO_3^-, which generally takes several days. In the meantime, the increased PCO_2 with low HCO_3^- causes metabolic acidosis.

F. Hyperalimentation: Hyperalimentation fluids may contain amino acid solutions that acidify when metabolized, such as arginine hydrochloride and lysine hydrochloride.

Urinary Anion Gap to Assess Hyperchloremic Metabolic Acidosis

Increased renal $NH_4^+Cl^-$ excretion to enhance H^+ removal is a normal physiologic response to metabolic acidosis. NH_3 reacts with H^+ to form NH_4^+, which is accompanied by the anion Cl^- for excretion.

$$Cl^- + NH_3 + H^+ \rightarrow NH_4Cl$$

Direct measurement of urine NH_4^+ or, if not available, urinary anion gap from a random urine sample ($[Na^+ + K^+] - Cl^-$) reflects the ability of the kidney to excrete NH_4Cl and aids in the distinction between gastrointestinal and renal causes of hyperchloremic acidosis. If the cause of the metabolic acidosis is gastrointestinal HCO_3^- loss (diarrhea), renal acidification ability remains normal and NH_4Cl excretion increases in response to the acidosis. The urinary anion gap is negative (eg, –30 meq/L). If the cause is distal renal tubular acidosis, the urinary anion gap is positive (eg, +25 meq/L), since the basic lesion in the disorder is inability of the kidney to excrete H^+ and thus inability to increase NH_4Cl excretion. Urinary pH may not as readily differentiate between the two causes. Despite acidosis, if volume depletion from diarrhea causes inadequate Na^+ delivery to the distal nephron and therefore decreased exchange with H^+, urinary pH may not be lower than 5.3. Potassium depletion, which can accompany diarrhea (and surreptitious laxative abuse), may also impair renal acidification. Thus, when volume depletion is present, the urinary anion gap is a better measurement of ability to acidify the urine than urinary pH.

Clinical Findings

A. Symptoms and Signs: Symptoms of metabolic acidosis are mainly those of the underlying disorder. Compensatory hyperventilation is an important clinical sign and may be misinterpreted as a primary respiratory disorder; when severe, Kussmaul respirations (deep, regular, sighing respirations) are seen.

B. Laboratory Findings: Blood pH, serum HCO_3^-, and PCO_2 are decreased. Anion gap may be normal (hyperchloremic) or increased (normochloremic). Hyperkalemia may be seen (see above).

Treatment

A. Increased Anion Gap Acidosis: Treatment is aimed at the underlying disorder, such as insulin and fluid therapy for diabetes and appropriate volume resuscitation to restore tissue perfusion. The metabolism of lactate will produce HCO_3^- and increase pH. The use of supplemental HCO_3^- is indicated for treatment of hyperkalemia (Table 21–6) and some forms of normal anion gap acidosis but has been controversial for treatment of increased anion gap metabolic acidosis. Administration of large amounts of HCO_3^- may have deleterious effects, including hypernatremia and hyperosmolality. Furthermore, intracellular pH may decrease because administered HCO_3^- is converted to CO_2, which easily diffuses into cells. There, it combines with water to create additional hydrogen ions and worsening of intracellular acidosis. Theoretically, this could impair cellular function, but the clinical significance of this phenomenon is uncertain. In any event, bicarbonate is most apt to be helpful in metabolic acidosis caused by gastrointestinal loss or renal tubular acidosis. The amount of HCO_3^- deficit can be calculated as follows:

Amount of HCO_3^- deficit = 0.5 × Body weight × (24 − HCO_3^-)

Half of the calculated deficit should be administered within the first 3–4 hours to avoid overcorrection and volume overload.

B. Normal Anion Gap Acidosis: (Table 21–17.) Each 650 mg tablet of $NaHCO_3$ contains 8 meq of HCO_3^-. Citrate, which is converted to HCO_3^-, is often better tolerated than HCO_3^- but is more expensive. Bicitra (500 mg sodium citrate and 334 mg citric acid per teaspoon) yields the equivalent of 1 meq $NaHCO_3$/mL. The usual adult dose is 10–30 mL dissolved in 1–3 ounces of water after meals and at bedtime.

In distal renal tubular acidosis, supplementation of bicarbonate is necessary since acid accumulates systemically in this disorder. However, in proximal renal tubular acidosis, correction of low serum bicarbonate with bicarbonate is sometimes hazardous and unnecessary except in severe cases. If the blood bicarbonate concentration is elevated in response to bicarbonate administration and bicarbonate concentration in the glomerular filtrate exceeds the capacity of the proximal tubule to reabsorb it, a large quantity of bicarbonate is excreted into the urine accompanied by potassium, exacerbating hypokalemia. Thus, potassium should also be given when bicarbonate therapy is indicated in proximal renal tubular acidosis.

Frassetto L, Sebastian A: Age and systemic acid-base equilibrium: Analysis of published data. J Gerontol A Biol Sci Med Sci 1996;51:B91.

Hanna JD, Scheinman JI, Chan JC: The kidney in acid-base balance. Pediatr Clin North Am 1995;42:1365.

Kitabchi AE, Wall BM: Diabetic ketoacidosis. Med Clin North Am 1995;79:9.

Mikulaschek A et al: Serum lactate is not predicted by anion gap or base excess after trauma resuscitation. J Trauma 1996;40:218.

Okuda Y et al: Counterproductive effects of sodium bicarbonate in diabetic ketoacidosis. J Clin Endocrinol Metab 1996;81:314.

Williamson JC: Acid-base disorders: Clarification and management strategies. Am Fam Physician 1995;52:584.

Stacpoole PW et al: Natural history and course of acquired lactic acidosis in adults. DCA-Lactic Acidosis Study Group. Am J Med 1994;97:47. (Survival is 41% at 3 days and 17% at 30 days.)

4. METABOLIC ALKALOSIS

Classification

Metabolic alkalosis is characterized by high HCO_3^-. The high HCO_3^- is seen also in chronic respiratory acidosis (see above), but pH differentiates the two disorders. It is useful to classify the causes of metabolic alkalosis into two groups based on "saline responsiveness" or urinary Cl^-, which are markers for volume status (Table 21–18). Saline-responsive metabolic alkalosis is a sign of extracellular volume contraction, and saline-unresponsive alkalosis implies a volume-expanded state. It is rare for a compensatory increase in PCO_2 to exceed 55 mm Hg. A higher value implies a superimposed respiratory acidosis.

A. Saline-Responsive Metabolic Alkalosis: Saline-responsive metabolic alkalosis is by far the more common disorder. It is characterized by normotensive extracellular volume contraction and hypokalemia. Less frequently, hypotension or orthostatic hypotension may be seen. In vomiting or nasogastric suction, for example, loss of acid (HCl) initiates the alkalosis, but volume contraction from loss of Cl^- sustains the alkalosis. Volume contraction sustains metabolic alkalosis because the decline in GFR causes avid renal Na^+ and HCO_3^- reabsorption. Since there is Cl^- depletion from loss of HCl, NaCl, and KCl from the stomach, the available anion is HCO_3^-, whose reabsorption is increased proximally. Renal Cl^- reabsorption (as well as Na^+) reabsorption is high, and the urinary Cl^- is therefore low (< 10–20 meq/L). In alkalosis, bicarbonaturia with Na^+ excreted as the accompanying cation may occur even if volume depletion is present. Therefore, urinary Cl^- is preferred to urinary Na^+ as a measure of extracellular volume. An exception to the usefulness of urinary Cl^- is in patients who have recently received diuretics. Their urine may contain high Na^+ and Cl^- despite extracellular volume contraction. If diuretics are discontinued, the urinary Cl^- will decrease.

Metabolic alkalosis is generally associated with hypokalemia, due partly to secondary hyperaldo-

Table 21–18. Metabolic alkalosis.[1]

Saline-Responsive (U_{Cl} < 10 meq/d)	Saline-Unresponsive (U_{Cl} > 10 meq/d)

Excessive body bicarbonate content
Renal alkalosis
  Diuretic therapy
  Poorly reabsorbable anion therapy:
    carbenicillin, penicillin, sulfate, phosphate
  Posthypercapnia
Gastrointestinal alkalosis
  Loss of HCl from vomiting or nasogastric
    suction
  Intestinal alkalosis: chloride diarrhea
Exogenous alkali
  $NaHCO_3$ (baking soda)
  Sodium citrate, lactate, gluconate, acetate
  Transfusions
  Antacids
Normal bicarbonate content
  "Contraction alkalosis"
	Excessive body bicarbonate content
	Renal alkalosis
	A. Normotensive
	  Bartter's syndrome (renal salt wasting
	    and secondary hyperaldosteronism)
	  Severe potassium depletion
	  Refeeding alkalosis
	  Hypercalcemia and hypoparathyroidism
	B. Hypertensive
	  Endogenous mineralocorticoids
	    Primary aldosteronism
	    Hyperreninism
	    Adrenal enzyme deficiency: 11- and
	      17-hydroxylase
	    Liddle's syndrome
	  Exogenous mineralocorticoids
	    Licorice
	    Carbenoxalone
	    Chewing tobacco

[1]Modified and reproduced, with permission, from Narins RG et al: Diagnostic strategies in disorders of fluid, electrolyte and acid-base homeostasis. Am J Med 1982;72:496.

steronism from volume depletion, which further worsens the metabolic alkalosis by increasing bicarbonate reabsorption in the proximal tubule and hydrogen ion secretion in the distal tubule. Administration of KCl will correct the disorder. Repletion of KCl is important to reverse the disorder.

1. Contraction alkalosis–Diuretics can acutely decrease extracellular volume from urinary loss of NaCl and water. There is no associated bicarbonaturia, so that body HCO_3^- content remains normal. However, plasma HCO_3^- increases because of extracellular fluid contraction—the reverse of what occurs in dilutional acidosis.

2. Posthypercapnia alkalosis–In chronic respiratory acidosis, compensatory increases in HCO_3^- occur (Table 21–13). Hypercapnia also directly affects the proximal tubule to decrease NaCl reabsorption, which can cause extracellular volume depletion. If PCO_2 is corrected rapidly, as with mechanical ventilation, metabolic alkalosis will ensue until adequate bicarbonaturia occurs. Hypovolemia will inhibit bicarbonaturia until Cl^- is repleted. Many patients with chronic respiratory acidosis receive diuretics, which further exacerbate the metabolic alkalosis.

B. Saline-Unresponsive Alkalosis:

1. Hyperaldosteronism–Primary hyperaldosteronism causes expansion of extracellular volume with hypertension. Metabolic alkalosis with hypokalemia results from the renal mineralocorticoid effect. In an attempt to decrease extracellular volume, high levels of NaCl are excreted, and for that reason the urinary Cl^- is high (> 20 meq/L). Therapy with NaCl will only increase volume expansion and hypertension and will not treat the underlying problem of mineralocorticoid excess.

2. Alkali administration with decreased GFR–Despite large ingestions of HCO_3^-, enhanced bicarbonaturia almost always prevents a patient with normal renal function from developing metabolic alkalosis. However, with renal insufficiency, urinary excretion of bicarbonate is inadequate. If large

Table 21–19. Daily maintenance rations for average adult (60–100 kg) requiring parenteral fluids.

Glucose	100–200 g
Na^+	80–120 meq
K^+	80–120 meq
Water	2500 mL

amounts of HCO_3^- or metabolizable salts of organic acids such as sodium lactate, sodium citrate, or sodium gluconate are consumed, as with intensive antacid therapy, metabolic alkalosis will occur. In milk-alkali syndrome, large and sustained ingestion of absorbable antacids and milk causes renal insufficiency from hypercalcemia. Decreased GFR prevents appropriate bicarbonaturia from the ingested alkali, and metabolic alkalosis occurs. Volume contraction from renal hypercalcemic effects further exacerbates the alkalosis.

Clinical Findings

A. Symptoms and Signs: There are no characteristic symptoms or signs. Orthostatic hypotension may be encountered. Weakness and hyporeflexia occur if serum K^+ is markedly low. Tetany and neuromuscular irritability occur rarely.

B. Laboratory Findings: The arterial blood pH and bicarbonate are elevated. The arterial PCO_2 is increased. Serum potassium and chloride are decreased. There may be an increased anion gap.

Treatment

Mild alkalosis is generally well tolerated. Severe or symptomatic alkalosis (pH > 7.60) requires urgent treatment.

A. Saline-Responsive Metabolic Alkalosis: Therapy for saline-responsive metabolic alkalosis is aimed at correction of extracellular volume deficit. Depending on the degree of hypovolemia, adequate

Table 21–20. Electrolyte concentrations of commonly used intravenous crystalloid solutions.[1]

	Osmolality (mosm/kg H_2O)	Na^+ (meq/L)	Cl^- (meq/L)	Glucose (g/L)
Isotonic				
0.9% saline	308	154	154	0
$D_5$0.9% saline	560	154	154	50
Ringer's lactate[2]	273	130	109	0
Hypotonic				
D_5W	252	0	0	50
$D_5$0.2% saline	320	34	34	50
0.45% saline	154	77	77	0
$D_5$0.45% saline	405	77	77	50

[1]Modified and reproduced, with permission, from Cogan MG: *Fluid and Electrolytes: Physiology and Pathophysiology.* Appleton & Lange, 1991.
[2]Also contains 28 meq/L lactate (which is converted to HCO_3^-), 4 meq/L K^+, and 2 meq/L Ca^{2+}.

Table 21–21. Replacement guidelines for sweat and gastrointestinal fluid losses.

	Average Electrolyte Composition				Replacement Guidelines per Liter Lost				
	Na^+ (meq/L)	K^+ (meq/L)	Cl^- (meq/L)	HCO_3^- (meq/L)	0.9% saline (mL)	0.45% saline (mL)	D_5W (mL)	KCl (meq/L)	7.5% $NaHCO_3$ (45 meq HCO_3^-/amp)
Sweat	30–50	5	50			500	500	5	
Gastric secretions	20	10	10			300	700	20	
Pancreatic juice	130	5	35	115		400	600	5	2 amps
Bile	145	5	100	25	600		400	5	0.5 amp
Duodenal fluid	60	15	100	10		1000		15	0.25 amp
Ileal fluid	100	10	60	60		600	400	10	1 amp
Colonic diarrhea[1]	140	10	85	60		1000		10	1 amp

[1]In the absence of diarrhea, colonic fluid Na^+ levels are low (40 meq/L).

amounts of 0.9% NaCl and KCl should be administered. Discontinuation of diuretics and administration of H_2-blockers in patients whose alkalosis is due to nasogastric suction can be useful. If impaired pulmonary or cardiovascular status prohibits adequate volume repletion, acetazolamide, 250–500 mg intravenously every 4–6 hours, can be used. Administration of acid can be used as emergency therapy. HCl, 0.1 mol/L, is infused via a central vein (the solution is sclerosing). Dosage is calculated to decrease the HCO_3^- level by one-half over 2–4 hours, assuming a HCO_3^- volume of distribution (L) of 0.5 × body weight (kg). Patients with marked renal insufficiency may require dialysis.

B. Saline-Unresponsive Metabolic Alkalosis: Therapy for saline-unresponsive metabolic alkalosis includes surgical removal of a mineralocorticoid-producing tumor and blockage of aldosterone effect with an angiotensin-converting enzyme inhibitor or with spironolactone.

Cogan MG: *Fluid & Electrolytes. Physiology & Pathophysiology.* Appleton & Lange, 1991.
Laski ME, Kurtzman NA: Acid-base disorders in medicine. Dis Mon 1996;42(2):51.

FLUID MANAGEMENT

Most of those who require water and electrolytes intravenously are relatively normal people who cannot take orally what they require for maintenance. Table 21–19 shows that the range of tolerance for water and electrolytes (homeostatic limits) permits reasonable latitude in therapy provided normal renal function exists to accomplish the final regulation of volume and concentration.

An average adult whose entire intake is parenteral would require for maintenance 2500–3000 mL of 5% dextrose in 0.2% saline solution (34 meq Na^+ plus 34 meq Cl^-/L). To each liter, 30 meq of KCl could be added. In 3 L, the total chloride intake would be 192 meq, which is easily tolerated. Table 21–20 sets forth the composition of commonly used crystalloid solutions. Guidelines for gastrointestinal fluid losses are shown in Table 21–21.

In situations requiring maintenance or maintenance plus replacement of fluid and electrolyte by parenteral infusion, the total daily ration should be administered continuously over the 24-hour period in order to ensure the best utilization by the patient.

If parenteral fluids are the only source of water, electrolyte, and calories for longer than a week, more complex fluids containing amino acids, lipids, trace metals, and vitamins may be indicated. (See Total Parenteral Nutrition, Chapter 29.)

22

Kidney

Gail Morrison, MD

APPROACH TO THE PATIENT WITH SUSPECTED RENAL DISEASE

The history of a patient with suspected renal disease should include a review of recent clinical events and an inventory of all the patient's prescription and nonprescription medications. In both outpatients and hospitalized patients, important information includes blood pressure, pulse rate, alterations in daily weights, daily fluid intake, and urine output. The physical examination will also be helpful in assessing evidence for manifestations of systemic disease. For example, the abdominal and pelvic examinations may disclose a distended bladder suggestive of obstructive uropathy, peripheral vascular disease, inflammatory or neoplastic masses, or an enlarged uterus, all of which can affect renal function. In the skin, palpable purpura or livedo reticularis suggests vasculitis; nonpalpable purpura raises the question of thrombotic thrombocytopenic purpura or hemolytic uremic syndrome, which are associated with vascular compromise of the kidney.

The history and physical examination can help in categorizing the probable type of renal disease. Prerenal azotemia (hypoperfusion of the kidneys) often occurs in patients with a history of cardiac disease or those with conditions associated with extracellular fluid volume depletion. Postrenal (obstructive) nephropathy is observed in patients with a history of cancer of the bladder, pelvic cavity, or prostatic disease. Intrarenal disease is glomerular or tubulointerstitial. The former complicates systemic disease such as diabetes or polyarteritis; the latter is frequently drug-related or seen after a hypotensive episode (acute tubular necrosis).

URINALYSIS

A normal urine sediment occurs in prerenal azotemia. Hematuria, pyuria, or crystals may be seen in obstructive disease. A sediment showing tubular cells, cellular casts, or proteinuria identifies an intrarenal source. Red cell casts and proteinuria are seen in glomerular disease. White cell casts, tubular cells or casts, eosinophiluria, and isosthenuria suggest tubulointerstitial nephritis (Table 22–1). For further discussion, see Dipstick Urinalysis in Chapter 23.

PROTEINURIA

The urine dipstick, performed as a part of the routine urinalysis, is the method that most frequently identifies the presence of proteinuria, specifically albuminuria. However, since the dipstick measurement will vary depending on whether the urine sample is concentrated or dilute, a 24-hour urine collection is the *only* reliable way to quantify proteinuria. The presence of nephrotic syndrome (> 3.5 g/24 h of protein) has significant medical implications. Thus, any individual with persistent proteinuria by dipstick should complete a 24-hour urinary protein determination. A finding of over 150 mg/24 h of protein is the criterion for proteinuria.

Proteinuria is not a disease but a clinical marker signifying that an underlying renal abnormality exists. When caused by a renal or systemic disease, proteinuria is accompanied by other clinical abnormalities—elevated BUN and serum creatinine levels, abnormal urinary sediment, elevated blood pressure measurements, or evidence of systemic illness (eg, fever, rash, vasculitis). Severe proteinuria, generally in the nephrotic range (> 3.5 g/24 h) is usually associated with glomerulonephritis. Lesser amounts of proteinuria, though not excluding glomerulonephritis, usually signify tubulointerstitial nephritis. "Benign" proteinuria includes functional, idiopathic transient, orthostatic, and intermittent proteinuria.

Functional proteinuria occurs in association with conditions such as high fever, strenuous exercise, and congestive heart failure. Up to 10% of patients admitted for acute medical illnesses have transient proteinuria. The proteinuria is glomerular in origin,

Table 22–1. Significance of specific urinary casts.

Type	Significance
Hyaline casts	Concentrated urine, febrile disease, after strenuous exercise, in the course of diuretic therapy (not indicative of renal disease)
Red cell casts	Glomerulonephritis
White cell casts	Pyelonephritis, interstitial nephritis (indicative of infection or inflammation)
Renal tubular cell casts	Acute tubular necrosis, interstitial nephritis
Coarse, granular casts	Nonspecific; represent degeneration of cast with cellular element
Broad, waxy casts	Chronic renal failure (indicative of stasis in collecting tubule)

caused by renal hemodynamic alterations that increase the glomerular filtration of plasma proteins, and clears with resolution of the precipitating event.

Idiopathic transient proteinuria is a benign physiologic phenomenon in children and young adults that comes and goes. Intermittent proteinuria is a condition in which proteinuria is found in half of all urine specimens tested in an individual over a number of years. Most renal biopsies are normal and the condition appears to be benign, especially in young people.

Orthostatic proteinuria is a benign condition that does not require further diagnostic evaluation and usually remits spontaneously. It is confirmed by collecting the 24-hour urine in two 12-hour samples. The first 12-hour specimen is collected during the day, when the patient is active and upright; the second is collected overnight while the patient is resting and supine. Significant proteinuria (150 mg/dL) when the patient is upright (first 12 hours) and under 75 mg/dL during the 12 hours when sleeping and supine establishes the diagnosis.

ASSESSMENT OF GLOMERULAR FILTRATION

The glomerular filtration rate (GFR) is used as a clinical assessment of renal function. The creatinine clearance (C_{cr}) is the clinical measurement that most closely approximates GFR. The BUN and serum creatinine (S_{cr}) often but not always correlate with the GFR.

Blood Urea Nitrogen (BUN)

Amino acids from endogenous (muscle) and exogenous (dietary) protein generate NH_3, which is converted in the liver to urea and measured in the blood as urea nitrogen. Urea is filtered by the glomerulus, and approximately 50% is reabsorbed by the tubules. However, the percentage absorbed varies inversely with urine flow rates, so that in volume-depleted states (prerenal azotemia), the BUN is elevated out of proportion to the fall in GFR. BUN can be affected by other factors as well (Table 22–2), thus making it an unreliable index of GFR.

Serum Creatinine & Its Clearance

Creatinine is produced by the nonenzymatic dehydration of muscle creatine. Because the daily production of creatinine is relatively constant, its clearance is a relatively reliable index of GFR.

If S_{cr} is affected independently of GFR by the conditions listed in Table 22–3, S_{cr} may not accurately reflect GFR.

The measurement of creatinine clearance requires the completion of a 24-hour urine collection. Complete urine collections for males should have total creatinine concentrations of 15–25 mg/kg body weight/24 h and for females 10–20 mg/kg body weight/24 h.

The C_{cr} declines by 1 mL/min/y over the age of 40 as part of the aging process. In individuals with GFRs of 20 mL/min/1.73 m^2 or less, the C_{cr} may overestimate the GFR, since a small portion of the urinary creatinine is due to the secretion of creatinine by the renal tubules.

IMAGING STUDIES

Radionuclide Studies

Radionuclide studies can measure renal function. Technetium diethylenetriamine pentaacetic acid (^{99m}Tc-DTPA) is freely filtered by the glomerulus and not reabsorbed and is used to estimate GFR. Technetium dimercaptosuccinate (^{99m}Tc-DMSA) is bound to the tubules and provides an assessment of functional renal mass. Radioiodinated (^{131}I) orthoiodohippurate is secreted into the renal tubules and assesses renal plasma flow (RPF). The indications for nuclear renography are to measure function and flow; to determine the contribution of each kid-

Table 22–2. Conditions affecting BUN independently of GFR.

Increased BUN
Reduced effective circulating blood volume (prerenal azotemia)
Catabolic states
High-protein diets
Gastrointestinal bleeding
Glucocorticoids
Tetracycline
Decreased BUN
Liver disease
Malnutrition
Sickle cell anemia

Table 22–3. Conditions affecting serum creatinine independently of GFR.

Condition	Mechanism
Conditions causing elevation	
Ketoacidosis	Noncreatinine chromogen
Cephalothin, cefoxitin	Noncreatinine chromogen
Other drugs: aspirin, cimetidine, trimethoprim	Inhibition of tubular creatinine secretion
Conditions causing decrease	
Advanced age	Physiologic decrease in muscle mass
Cachexia	Pathologic decrease in muscle mass
Liver disease	Decreased hepatic creatine synthesis and cachexia

ney to overall renal function; to demonstrate the presence or absence of functioning renal tissue in mass lesions; to detect obstruction; and to evaluate renovascular disease.

Poor flow along with poor function is consistent with acute tubular necrosis or end-stage renal disease. Decreased flow to one kidney suggests arterial occlusion of that kidney. To establish the possibility of renal artery stenosis, the test is done both with and without captopril (see Chapter 11).

Ultrasonography

Ultrasonography noninvasively images the kidney. It can identify the renal cortex, medulla, pyramids, and a distended collection system or ureter. Kidney size can be determined; a kidney less than 9 cm in length indicates significant irreversible renal disease. A difference in size of more than 1.5 cm between the two kidneys is observed in unilateral renal disease. Renal ultrasound is also performed to screen for hydronephrosis, characterize renal mass lesions, screen for autosomal dominant polycystic kidney disease, evaluate the perirenal space, localize the kidney for a percutaneous invasive procedure, and assess postvoiding bladder residual.

Intravenous Urography

The intravenous pyelogram (IVP) has been for many years the standard imaging procedure for evaluating the urinary tract since it provides an assessment of the kidneys, ureters, and bladder. The dye is filtered and secreted by the renal tubules in normal kidneys, resulting in a nephrogram formed by opacification of the renal parenchyma. The density of the nephrogram is dependent on the GFR. Filling of the pelvicaliceal system produces the pyelogram. The IVP can demonstrate differential function between the right and left kidneys by the rate of appearance of the nephrogram phase.

An IVP necessitates the injection of contrast and is relatively contraindicated in patients with an in-

creased risk for developing acute renal failure (eg, diabetes mellitus with serum creatinine > 2 mg/dL, severe volume contraction, or prerenal azotemia); chronic renal failure with serum creatinine greater than 5 mg/dL; and multiple myeloma. IVP is performed to obtain a detailed view of the pelvicaliceal system, assess renal size and shape, detect and localize renal stones, and assess renal function. Ultrasonography has replaced it in many clinical situations.

Computed Tomography

Computed tomography (CT) is required for further investigation of abnormalities detected by ultrasound or IVP. Although the routine study requires radiographic contrast administration, no contrast is necessary if the reason for the study is to demonstrate hemorrhage or calcifications in the kidneys. Since contrast is filtered by the glomeruli and concentrated in the tubules, there is enhancement of parenchymal tissue, making abnormalities such as cysts or neoplasms easily identified and allowing good visualization of renal vessels and ureters. CT is especially useful for evaluation of solid or cystic lesions in the kidney or the retroperitoneal space, particularly if the ultrasound results are suboptimal.

Magnetic Resonance Imaging (MRI)

MRI can easily distinguish renal cortex from medulla. Loss of corticomedullary function, which can be seen in a variety of disorders (glomerulonephritis, hydronephrosis, renal vascular occlusion, and renal failure) will be evident on MRI. Renal cysts seen on a CT scan can also be identified by MRI. For some solid lesions, MRI may be superior to CT scanning. MRI is indicated as an addition or alternative to CT for staging renal cell cancer and as a substitute for CT in the evaluation of a renal mass, especially for patients with tumors in whom contrast is contraindicated; in addition, the adrenals are well imaged.

Arteriography & Venography

Renal arteriography is useful in the evaluation of atherosclerotic or fibrodysplastic stenotic lesions, aneurysms, vasculitis, and renal mass lesions. Venography is useful to diagnose renal vein thrombosis.

Abuelo JG: Diagnosing vascular causes of renal failure. Ann Intern Med 1995;123:601.

RENAL BIOPSY

Percutaneous needle biopsy can be helpful for making a diagnosis, assessing prognosis, monitoring disease progression, and choosing among therapeutic options. Indications include (1) acute renal failure which is unresolving and for which a cause is not evident; (2) nephrotic syndrome if one suspects a primary glomerular disease (see discussion of renal biopsy in the section on nephrotic syndrome); (3) proteinuria of 2 g/24 h/1.73 m^2 along with an abnormal urine sediment with or without functional deterioration; (4) hematuria associated with an abnormal urine sediment or proteinuria; (5) systemic diseases associated with kidney dysfunction, such as systemic lupus erythematosus, Goodpasture's syndrome, and Wegener's syndrome, to confirm the extent of renal involvement and to guide management; and (6) suspected transplant rejection, to differentiate it from other causes of acute renal failure and to guide management. Contraindications include a solitary or ectopic kidney (exception: transplant allografts), horseshoe kidney, uncorrected bleeding disorder, severe uncontrolled hypertension, renal infection, renal neoplasm, hydronephrosis, end-stage kidneys, congenital anomalies, or an uncooperative patient.

When a percutaneous needle biopsy is technically not feasible and renal tissue is necessary for a diagnosis, open renal biopsy under general anesthesia can be done.

Radford MG Jr et al: Renal biopsy in clinical practice. Mayo Clinic Proc 1994;69:983.

ACUTE RENAL FAILURE

Essentials of Diagnosis

- Sudden increase in BUN or serum creatinine.
- Oliguria often associated.
- Symptoms and signs depend on cause.

General Considerations

Acute renal failure is defined as a sudden decrease in renal function resulting in the retention of urea nitrogen and creatinine in the blood. As creatinine is primarily eliminated by glomerular filtration, it is the most convenient laboratory value for assessing renal function. In the absence of kidney function, the serum creatinine concentration will increase by 1–1.5 mg/dL/d. BUN is also used as a marker for acute renal failure. However, since urea nitrogen synthesis in the liver is protein-dependent, both large quantities of exogenous protein (high-protein diet) and endogenous protein (catabolism) can elevate the BUN concentration independently of renal function. Reduced urine flow rates that occur in obstructive uropathy or congestive heart failure result in increased tubular reabsorption of urea, causing a markedly elevated BUN with only a mildly reduced GFR. Therefore, a rise in BUN is a less reliable marker for acute renal failure than a rise in serum creatinine concentration.

Clinical Findings

A. Symptoms and Signs: The symptoms of acute renal failure include those related to azotemia generally and those due to the underlying cause. Azotemic patients often complain of anorexia, nausea, and malaise but may be entirely asymptomatic. Complaints relevant to pre- and postrenal as well as intrarenal disease processes are discussed under the specific entities. Physical examination is similar; patients with acute renal failure may demonstrate pericardial friction rub or asterixis or may have no abnormal signs. Hypertension may or may not be noted. Otherwise, the findings are those of the causative problem.

B. Laboratory Findings: There are no abnormalities in the blood that allow separation of acute from chronic renal failure. Both may exhibit elevated BUN and creatinine, hypocalcemia, and hyperphosphatemia.

Classification & Etiology

Acute renal failure can be divided into three categories (as described below); identifying the cause is the first step in managing the patient.

A. Prerenal Azotemia: Prerenal azotemia is a syndrome associated with a decrease in GFR resulting from renal hypoperfusion (a decrease in renal blood flow). Hypoperfusion can be immediately reversed upon restoration of blood flow. Thus, prerenal azotemia is not associated with structural damage to the kidney. Prerenal azotemia is the most common cause of acute renal failure. In most instances, the history and physical examination will suggest the diagnosis. As the kidney's response to a decrease in blood flow is to avidly reabsorb salt and water, spot urinary indices frequently show a high urine osmolality (> 500 mosm/L), a low sodium concentration (< 20 meq/L), and a fractional excretion of sodium (FE_{Na^+}) $< 1\%$.

The fractional excretion (percent) of sodium is calculated as follows:

$$FE_{Na^+} = \frac{\text{Urine sodium/Plasma sodium}}{\text{Urine creatinine/Plasma creatinine}}$$

Decreased renal perfusion causes a diminished tubular flow rate that results in increased back diffusion of filtered urea from the tubules. The BUN:creatinine ratio will typically exceed 20:1 in prerenal azotemia (Table 22–4).

Since there is no parenchymal damage associated with prerenal azotemia, the urinalysis is typically normal, though hyaline casts may be present. Glomerulonephritis may also have a low FE_{Na^+}, mimicking prerenal azotemia (Table 22–4). The pres-

Table 22–4. Classification and differential diagnosis of renal failure.

	Prerenal Azotemia	Postrenal Azotemia	Intrinsic Renal Disease			
			Acute Tubular Necrosis (Oliguric)	Acute Tubular Necrosis (Polyuric)	Acute Glomerulonephritis	Acute Interstitial Nephritis
Etiology	Hypovolemia, congestive heart failure	Obstruction of the urinary tract	Hypotension, nephrotoxins	Hypotension, nephrotoxins	Poststreptococcal; collagen vascular disease	Allergic reaction; drug reaction
Urinary indices						
Serum BUN: Cr	>20:1	>20:1	<20:1	<20:1	>20:1	<20:1
U_{Na} (meq/L)	<20	Variable	>20	>20	<20	Variable
FE_{Na+} (%)	<1	>1	>1	>1	<1	<1; >1
Urine osmolality (mosm/kg)	>500	<400	250–300	250–300	>500	Variable
Urinary sediment	Hyaline casts	Normal or red cells, white cells, or crystals	Granular casts, renal tubular cells	Granular casts, renal tubular cells	Red cells, red cell casts	White cells, white cell casts ± eosinophiluria

ence of marked glomerular inflammatory changes, as can be seen in poststreptococcal glomerulonephritis or rapidly progressive glomerulonephritis, can significantly reduce the GFR, causing a diminished tubular flow rate, increased back diffusion of filtered urea, and a BUN:creatinine ratio greater than 20:1 and low FE_{Na+}. The urinalysis, unlike the situation in prerenal azotemia, typically shows red cells, red cell casts, and proteinuria (Table 22–4).

A drug history is important because two classes of drugs, NSAIDs and ACE inhibitors, can affect renal hemodynamics and cause prerenal azotemia. Susceptible individuals are those with renal hypoperfusion states due to volume depletion and those with ineffective renal blood flow related to renal artery stenosis, congestive heart failure, or cirrhosis. NSAIDs, by inhibiting prostaglandin-mediated compensatory renal vasodilation, potentiates vasoconstriction, resulting in hypoperfusion and prerenal azotemia.

ACE inhibitors, alternatively, reduce efferent arteriolar tone in the glomerulus, reducing renal perfusion pressure, which results in a lower glomerular capillary filtration pressure. In individuals whose kidneys are dependent on a higher perfusion pressure (ie, those with bilateral renal artery stenosis or unilateral stenosis of a solitary kidney), these drugs can cause acute renal failure. Discontinuation of NSAIDs and ACE inhibitors results in improvement of renal function in individuals susceptible to prerenal azotemia.

B. Postrenal Azotemia: Postrenal azotemia is a syndrome associated with conditions causing obstruction of the urinary tract and, as a consequence, a decrease in GFR. Obstructive uropathy is the least common cause of acute renal failure but the most treatable. Most obstruction is postvesicular; ureteral obstruction must either be bilateral or occur in a patient with only a single functioning kidney to cause acute renal failure. The commonest causes of obstructive uropathy are discussed in Chapter 23.

Urine flow rate may vary from anuria, as with complete obstruction, to polyuria. Urine flow may fluctuate from day to day, suggesting intermittent obstruction.Thus, a normal 24-hour total urine volume does not exclude obstructive renal function. The urinalysis in such cases is frequently normal.

Laboratory findings are variable. Initially, with the onset of obstruction, urinary indices may show a high urine osmolality, a low urine sodium and fractional excretion of sodium, and a high BUN:creatinine ratio similar to what is seen in prerenal azotemia. After several days of obstruction, parenchymal injury occurs and the urinary indices show an isotonic urine with a high fractional excretion of sodium.

Bladder catheterization revealing an increased postvoid residual urine volume documents obstructive uropathy. Renal ultrasound performed prior to catheterization is useful, since the absence of hydronephrosis excludes obstruction and because additional information may be gleaned about the cause of the renal failure.

C. Acute Parenchymal (Intrinsic) Renal Failure: After prerenal and postrenal causes have been excluded, intrinsic or parenchymal causes must be considered. The history, physical examination, and laboratory findings—especially routine urinalysis—should help to diagnose acute glomerulonephritis, vasculitis, and tubulointerstitial nephritis. If these conditions are eliminated, most acute renal failure falls under the category of acute tubular necrosis, which is typically associated with an abrupt decrease in GFR due to tubular cell damage, a consequence of either renal ischemia or nephrotoxic injury. The history often includes evidence for prolonged hypotension, severe trauma with myoglobinuria, intravenous contrast media exposure, major surgery, and aminoglycoside or other nephrotoxin administration. The physical findings will depend upon the history.

Urinalysis shows an active urinary sediment, with renal tubular epithelial cells, cellular debris, pigmented granular casts, renal tubular cell casts, and "muddy brown" coarse granular casts. In the setting of oliguria and azotemia, urinary indices may be very helpful in distinguishing between prerenal azotemia and acute tubular necrosis (Table 22–4). In the latter, the urine osmolality is usually isotonic (< 350 mosm/L), the urine sodium concentration is > 40 meq/L, and the FE_{Na+} and renal failure indices are both > 1% and frequently > 2–3%. The urine/plasma urea nitrogen ratio and the urine/plasma creatinine ratio can also distinguish prerenal azotemia from acute tubular necrosis.

1. Exogenous nephrotoxins–

a. Antibiotics–In hospitalized patients, acute tubular necrosis occurs in up to 25% of patients receiving gentamicin, tobramycin, or amikacin even when the plasma levels of these drugs appear to have been in the therapeutic range. Aminoglycoside-induced acute renal failure is typically nonoliguric and becomes clinically apparent after 5–10 days of drug administration. Advanced age, preexisting renal disease, volume depletion, and recent exposure to other nephrotoxins predispose to aminoglycoside-induced acute tubular necrosis.

Nephrotoxicity occurs in most patients after a cumulative total dose of 2–3 g of amphotericin B. Distal renal tubular acidosis, hypokalemia, and nephrogenic diabetes insipidus may accompany the azotemia.

b. Radiographic contrast media–Acute renal failure due to contrast media is characterized by a low FE_{Na+} and a high urine specific gravity from the contrast media. Advanced age, preexisting renal disease (serum creatinine > 5 mg/dL), volume depletion, diabetes mellitus with renal insufficiency (serum creatinine > 2 mg/dL), large repeated doses of contrast media, and recent exposure to other nephrotoxic agents are associated with an increased risk. New nonionic radiographic contrast agents may be less nephrotoxic. Hydration with 0.45% saline at a rate of 50–100 mL/h 12 hours before and 12 hours after injection of the contrast medium is the most effective means of preventing acute decreases in renal function in patients with chronic renal failure or diabetes mellitus, watching carefully for evidence of congestive heart failure. Neither mannitol nor furosemide offers any benefit over saline hydration. Tests involving contrast media, especially if associated with catheter placement in atherosclerotic vessels, may be associated with cholesterol emboli syndrome (see Chapter 12).

c. Cyclosporine–Cyclosporine nephrotoxicity is usually dose-dependent. High blood levels may help to predict the development of renal failure. In many cases, kidney biopsy may be necessary to distinguish transplant rejection from cyclosporine nephrotoxicity. Renal function generally improves after decreasing or discontinuing the drug.

2. Endogenous nephrotoxins–

a. Pigments–Myoglobinuria as a consequence of rhabdomyolysis is a frequent cause of acute renal failure. The release of large amounts of myoglobin from necrotic muscle tissue in the setting of volume depletion results in acute tubular necrosis. Patients with rhabdomyolysis will frequently complain of muscle pain and have elevated levels of creatine kinase. The urine will appear dark brown. The urine dipstick is positive for blood because of the presence of myoglobin, but there are no red blood cells in the urine on microscopic examination. Hyperkalemia, hyperphosphatemia, hyperuricemia, and hypocalcemia, followed by hypercalcemia are other clinical features associated with rhabdomyolysis, which most often occurs in a setting of alcohol abuse, crush injury, muscle necrosis from prolonged unconsciousness, or seizures. Dehydration, hypokalemia, hypophosphatemia, and acidosis predispose to the development of myoglobinuric acute renal failure.

Massive intravascular hemolysis can be seen in severe transfusion reactions and snake bites and may cause significant hemoglobinuria and acute tubular necrosis.

b. Crystals–Hyperuricemic acute tubular necrosis can occur during chemotherapy for leukemia and lymphomas or for tumors with a rapid cell turnover such as germ cell neoplasia. The plasma uric acid level is frequently above 20 mg/dL. Renal failure occurs as a result of intratubular deposition of uric acid crystals.

c. Bence Jones proteins–Tubular damage resulting in acute tubular necrosis can occur in multiple myeloma from the filtration of Bence Jones proteins and their inspissation. Renal complications also arise from hypercalcemia and hyperviscosity associated with plasma cell dyscrasias.

Course

The clinical course of acute parenchymal renal failure (acute tubular necrosis) depends to a large extent on the underlying cause. Prerenal and postrenal causes, if diagnosed and treated expeditiously, can be corrected, resulting in a return of renal function to normal or to the patient's previous level of function. Depending on the cause of the acute parenchymal (intrinsic) disorder, treatment may be more prolonged (eg, corticosteroids for glomerulonephritis, vasculitides), and renal function may not return to normal. The diagnosis of acute tubular necrosis is made only after all prerenal, postrenal, and other acute parenchymal disorders have been eliminated.

The clinical course of acute renal failure can usually be divided into oliguric, diuretic, and recovery phases. The oliguric phase usually begins within a day after the inciting event but may be delayed up to a week following a nephrotoxic injury. It lasts from a few hours to 3–4 weeks and is followed by the diuretic phase, during which urine volume will increase until it reaches several liters per day. Once the BUN and creatinine stop rising and begin to fall toward normal, the recovery phase has begun. In some individuals with severe oliguric acute tubular necrosis, there may be no diuretic or recovery phase, and dialysis will be required permanently. In others, the initiating event is followed by a nonoliguric phase and then by recovery. Most patients recover renal function within 6 weeks after developing acute tubular necrosis.

Complications

All patients with acute tubular necrosis develop complications resulting from the accumulation of nitrogenous wastes, disordered handling of water and electrolytes, and an inability to excrete acid metabolites. These disturbances develop more rapidly and are more severe in patients who are oliguric and hypercatabolic. Life-threatening complications include hypervolemia, causing hypertension and congestive heart failure; hyperkalemia; metabolic acidosis; hyponatremia, leading to central nervous system dysfunction; uremia, with neurologic dysfunction; gastrointestinal bleeding; platelet dysfunction; pericarditis; and infections, which are the leading cause of death. Less serious but common complications include hyperphosphatemia, hypocalcemia, hypermagnesemia, and anemia.

Treatment

Initial care is focused on reversing the underlying cause and correcting fluid and electrolyte imbalances. Attempts to convert oliguric to nonoliguric acute tubular necrosis with mannitol (12.5–25 g intravenously) are frequently made early to facilitate fluid management. However, mannitol may precipitate congestive heart failure, and high doses of loop diuretics may cause hearing loss. Management consists of restricting fluids to match measurable plus insensitive losses (usually < 1 L/d in oliguric patients), restriction of electrolytes to match measured losses (Na^+ 80–100 meq/d; K^+ 40 meq/d), restriction of protein of high biologic value to 0.6 g/kg/d, and provision of at least 100 g/d of carbohydrates. Even with this regimen, the individual may undergo catabolic weight loss of 0.5 lb/d; if more than this is lost, hyperalimentation may be needed. As part of the plan, hyperkalemia must be treated, magnesium-containing medications avoided, and drug dosages adjusted, particularly for those eliminated via the kidney.

Initial management for myoglobulinuric acute tubular necrosis is directed at reversing factors that can potentiate acute renal failure. Alkalization of the urine with intravenous sodium bicarbonate, 100 meq/L in D_5W, if the urine is acidotic by dipstick, is safe as long as the volume and calcium status of the patient are monitored closely. If attempts at inducing diuresis fail and acute renal failure prevails, peritoneal dialysis or hemodialysis may need to be instituted.

Dialysis—either hemodialysis, continuous arteriovenous hemofiltration, or peritoneal dialysis—may need to be instituted to treat life-threatening complications. These procedures are discussed further below in the section on chronic renal failure.

Prognosis

The mortality rate from acute renal failure is 20–50% in medical illness and as high as 60–70% in a surgical setting. Factors associated with increased mortality rates include advanced age, severe underlying disease, and multiple organ failure. The leading causes of death are infections, fluid and electrolyte disturbances, and progression of underlying disease. Mortality rates have not significantly improved over the past 20 years, making prevention of acute renal failure a high priority.

Albers FJ: Clinical characteristics of atherosclerotic renovascular disease. Am J Kidney Dis 1994;24:636.

Davda RK, Guzman NJ: Acute renal failure: Prompt diagnosis is key to effective management. Postgraduate Med 1994;96:89.

Fischereder M et al: Therapeutic strategies in the prevention of acute renal failure. Semin Nephrol 1994;14:41.

Solomon R et al: Effects of saline, mannitol and furosemide on acute decreases in renal function induced by radiocontrast agents. N Engl J Med 1994;331:1416.

Thadhani R, Pascual M, Bonventre JV: Acute renal failure. N Engl J Med 1996;334:1448. (Diagnosis and management.)

Wardle EN: Acute renal failure and multiorgan failure. Nephron 1994;66:380.

CHRONIC RENAL FAILURE

Essentials of Diagnosis

- Progressive azotemia over weeks or months.
- Isosthenuria is common.
- Hypertension in the majority.
- Bilateral small kidneys on ultrasound are diagnostic.
- Radiologic evidence of renal osteodystrophy confirms the diagnosis.

General Considerations

The symptoms of chronic renal failure depend on the severity and rapidity of the underlying renal disorder. When chronic renal failure develops slowly, most individuals remain asymptomatic until the renal failure is far-advanced (GFR < 10–15 mL/min). The major causes are listed in Table 22–5.

Clinical Findings

A. Symptoms and Signs: The symptoms of chronic renal failure are nonspecific (Table 22–6). Manifestations include fatigue, weakness, malaise, and lassitude. Gastrointestinal complaints such as anorexia, nausea, vomiting, a metallic taste in the

Table 22–5. Major causes of chronic renal failure.

Glomerulopathies
Primary glomerular diseases:
1. Focal and segmental glomerulosclerosis
2. Membranoproliferative glomerulonephritis
3. IgA nephropathy
4. Membranous nephropathy
Secondary glomerular diseases:
1. Diabetic nephropathy
2. Amyloidosis
3. Heroin abuse nephropathy
4. Post infectious glomerulonephritis
5. Collagen vascular diseases
6. Sickle cell nephropathy
Tubulointerstitial nephritis
Drug hypersensitivity
Heavy metals
Analgesic nephropathy
Reflux/chronic pyelonephritis
Idiopathic
Hereditary diseases
Polycystic kidney disease
Medullary cystic disease
Alport's syndrome
Obstructive nephropathies
Prostatic disease
Nephrolithiasis
Retroperitoneal fibrosis/tumor
Congenital
Vascular diseases
Hypertensive nephrosclerosis
Renal artery stenosis

Table 22–6. Symptoms and signs of uremia.

Organ System	Symptoms	Signs
General	Fatigue, weakness	Sallow-appearing, chronically ill
Skin	Pruritus, easy bruisability	Pallor, ecchymoses, excoriations, edema, xerosis
ENT	Metallic taste in mouth, epistaxis	Urinous breath
Eye		Pale conjunctiva
Pulmonary	Shortness of breath	Rales, pleural effusion
Cardiovascular	Dyspnea on exertion, retrosternal pain on inspiration (pericarditis)	Hypertension, cardiomegaly, friction rub
Gastrointestinal	Anorexia, nausea, vomiting, hiccup	
Genitourinary	Nocturia, impotence	Isosthenuria
Neuromuscular	Restless legs, numbness and cramps in legs	
Neurologic	Generalized irritability and inability to concentrate, decreased libido	Stupor, asterixis, myoclonus, peripheral neuropathy

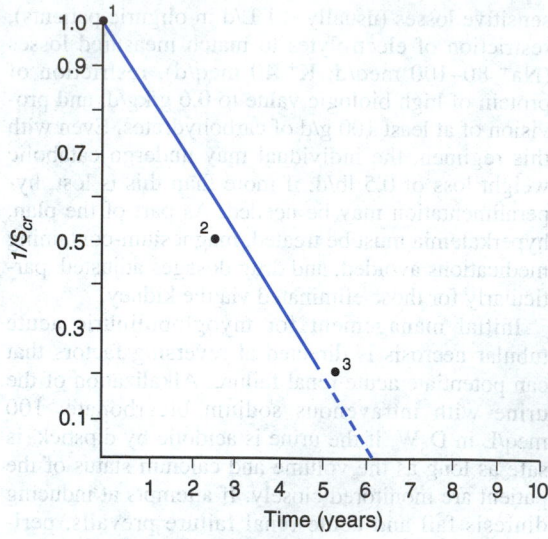

^{1} Value of serum creatinine level = 1.0 mg/dL
^{2} Value of serum creatinine level = 2.0 mg/dL
^{3} Value of serum creatinine level = 5.0 mg/dL

Figure 22–1. Decline in renal function plotted against time to end-stage renal disease. The solid line indicates the linear decline in renal function over time. The dotted line indicates the approximate time to end-stage renal disease.

mouth, and hiccup are common initially. Neuromuscular problems are also common and include decreased ability to concentrate, insomnia, irritability, restless legs, and twitching. As uremia progresses, decreased libido and menstrual irregularities, pruritus, chest pain from pericarditis, easy bruisability, and paresthesias can develop.

On physical examination, the individual may have a sallow complexion and appear chronically ill. The skin may be yellow-brown, with ecchymoses and petechiae. Cardiovascular findings may include hypertension, cardiomegaly, edema, and a pericardial friction rub. Mental status changes may be present and include confusion, stupor, and coma if uremia is severe. Myoclonus and asterixis can be noted as well.

In any patient with renal failure, it is important to eliminate all possible reversible causes, which can result in a more rapid deterioration of renal function than previously observed. It is often helpful to plot the inverse of serum creatinine ($1/S_{cr}$) versus time to determine if the slope of the line representing progressive loss of renal function has declined (Figure 22–1). In all individuals with progressive renal failure, urinary tract infections, obstruction, extracellular fluid volume depletion, nephrotoxins, hypertension, congestive heart failure, and pericarditis should be excluded (Table 22–7). Any one of these factors can worsen the underlying chronic renal failure.

B. Laboratory Findings: The diagnosis of renal failure is made by documenting elevations of the BUN and serum creatinine concentrations. Further

evaluation is then necessary to differentiate between acute and chronic renal failure. Evidence from old records documenting previously elevated BUN and serum creatinine helps to establish a diagnosis of chronic renal failure. Anemia, metabolic acidosis, hyperphosphatemia, and hypocalcemia occur in both acute and chronic renal failure.

Table 22–7. Reversible causes of renal failure.

Reversible Factors	Diagnostic Clues
Infection	Urine culture and sensitivity tests
Obstruction	Bladder catheterization, then renal ultrasound
Extracellular fluid volume depletion	Orthostatic blood pressure and pulse: ↓BP and ↑pulse upon sitting up from a supine position
Hypercalcemia and hyperuricemia (usually > 15 mg/dL)	Serum electrolytes, calcium, phosphate, uric acid
Nephrotoxic agents	Drug history
Pericarditis	Echocardiography, chest x-ray
Hypertension	Blood pressure, chest x-ray
Congestive heart failure	Physical examination, chest x-ray

C. Imaging: The finding of small kidneys bilaterally (< 10 cm) by ultrasonography supports a diagnosis of chronic renal failure, though normal or even large kidneys can be seen with chronic renal failure caused by adult polycystic kidney disease, diabetic nephropathy, multiple myeloma, amyloidosis, and obstructive uropathy. Radiographic evidence of renal osteodystrophy is another helpful finding, since x-ray changes of secondary hyperparathyroidism do not appear unless parathyroid hormone levels have been elevated for at least 1 year. Evidence for subperiosteal reabsorption along the radial sides of the digital bones of the hand confirms hyperparathyroidism.

Complications of Chronic Renal Failure & Their Management

A number of management options are appropriate that may reduce the rate of progression of chronic renal failure as well as the symptoms and long-term complications.

A. Hyperkalemia: Potassium balance is generally intact until the GFR is less than 10 mL/min. However, some individuals may be placed at risk for hyperkalemia before the onset of end-stage renal disease. Low-salt diets with ingestion of salt substitutes (which contain potassium chloride) and administration of drugs that either interfere with renal potassium excretion (triamterene, amiloride, spironolactone, ACE inhibitors, NSAIDs) or block cellular potassium uptake (beta-blockers) can produce hyperkalemia at higher levels of GFR. The presence of hyporeninemic hypoaldosteronism, seen in many patients with chronic renal failure, renders patients more susceptible to hyperkalemia.

Early therapy involves the use of calcium chloride, glucose, insulin, and bicarbonate and is discussed in Chapter 21. Long-standing hyperkalemia is best treated by dietary potassium restriction and, when necessary, sodium polystyrene sulfonate, an orally administered ion exchange resin. The usual dose is 15–30 g once a day in juice or sorbitol.

B. Acid-Base Disorders: Most metabolic acidosis in renal failure is due to inability of damaged kidneys to excrete the 1 meq/kg/d of acid generated by metabolism of dietary proteins. Though patients with chronic renal failure are in positive hydrogen ion balance, the arterial blood pH is maintained at 7.25–7.35 and the serum bicarbonate concentration rarely falls below 15 meq/L. The excess hydrogen ions are buffered by the large calcium carbonate stores in bone that may contribute to uremic osteodystrophy. Generally, maintaining the serum HCO_3^- concentration at 18–20 meq/L is recommended. Sodium bicarbonate can be given as 650 mg tablets three times a day and titrated as needed. Calcium carbonate may also be used, since it addresses both hypocalcemia and the acidosis. Modest dietary restriction of protein is recommended to decrease the daily metabolic acid load.

C. Cardiovascular Complications:

1. Hypertension–As renal failure progresses, hypertension due to salt and water retention usually develops. Since hypertension can accelerate the progression of renal failure, meticulous blood pressure control is necessary. Control of hypertension can be achieved with both salt and water restriction and antihypertensive therapy, such as calcium channel-blocking agents and ACE inhibitors (if serum potassium permits).

The capacity of the kidney to adjust to variations in sodium and water intake becomes limited as renal failure progresses. A sodium chloride intake that is too high leads to sodium retention and congestive heart failure, edema, and hypertension. A salt intake that is too low leads to volume contraction and hypotension. Generally, a 6 g NaCl diet ("no added salt") is a good starting point. If edema or hypertension develops, the NaCl intake should be reduced to 2–4 g.

2. Pericarditis–Pericarditis may develop as a complication of severe uremia when the BUN concentration exceeds 100–150 mg/dL. Symptoms include chest pain and fever, and a friction rub may be auscultated. Lack of a rub may indicate significant pericardial effusion; cardiac tamponade is a possibility in such patients. Pericarditis is an absolute indication for initiation of hemodialysis.

3. Congestive heart failure–If water and salt intakes are not controlled in the patient who is oliguric or anuric, plasma volume expansion and symptoms of congestive heart failure will ultimately ensue. Many patients with renal failure have underlying hypertensive cardiovascular disease that may contribute to the problem. New evidence suggests that elevated levels of PTH can be incriminated in the pathogenesis of the cardiomyopathy of renal failure.

Diuretics may be of value in the patient with chronic renal failure, though thiazides are ineffective when the creatinine clearance is < 10–15 mL/min and should therefore be avoided. Loop diuretics are commonly utilized, but higher doses will be necessary in patients with renal failure. Digoxin should be used with caution given its renal excretion; lower maintenance doses are the rule. Control of hyperphosphatemia, maintenance of normal plasma levels of calcium, and administration of calcitriol should be standard therapy.

D. Hematologic Complications:

1. Anemia–The anemia of renal failure is characteristically normochromic and normocytic; it is due mainly to decreased erythropoietin secretion from damaged kidneys, though low-grade hemolysis may play an additional role.

Erythropoietin (epoetin alfa) is generally used in patients whose hematocrit is less than 30%. The effective dose differs from patient to patient. The medication, in a dosage of 20–50 units/kg (1000–4000 units/dose) three times a week, can be given either intravenously (most commonly by that route in the hemodialysis patient) or subcutaneously (for patients receiving peritoneal dialysis or those who have not yet started dialysis therapy). Iron stores must be adequate to ensure response. Iron supplementation should be given if the serum ferritin is lower than 100 μg/mL, the transferrin saturation is lower than 20%, or more than 10% of red cells are hypochromic. Oral iron, as ferrous sulfate or fumarate, may not be well tolerated, and intravenous iron administration with either iron dextran or ferrous gluconate may be necessary. Aluminum excess from aluminum hydroxide binders prevents response to the drug; deferoxamine can be used to chelate aluminum in such patients. Finally, patients with chronic inflammatory processes may not respond.

Hypertension is a complication of erythropoietin therapy in about 20% of patients. It appears to develop more abruptly in patients with the lowest hematocrit values at the initiation of therapy. Patients receiving erythropoietin may therefore require adjustment of antihypertensive drugs or initiation of medication if they were previously not requiring any.

2. Coagulopathy—Purpura and petechiae are common manifestations of untreated uremia. Platelet counts in most patients are only moderately decreased or within normal limits. Even so, the bleeding time is prolonged, a defect that has been attributed to decreased platelet adhesiveness. This abnormality improves with dialysis, though it does not always completely normalize. Giving platelet transfusions to these patients is of limited value, since the transfused platelets are quickly modified by the uremic environment. Cryoprecipitate (10–15 bags) has occasionally been used but has only a transient effect. Desmopressin (0.03 mg/kg) is quite effective and is often used in preparation for surgery in order to minimize bleeding. Conjugated estrogens, 0.6 mg/kg diluted in 50 mL of 0.9% sodium chloride infused over 30–40 minutes daily for 5 days, have a beneficial effect and a prolonged duration of action (for several days or weeks).

E. Neurologic Complications: Peripheral neuropathy was at one time a major complication of end-stage renal disease. Presumably as a result of the earlier initiation of dialysis, it is now seen less often. The response of peripheral neuropathy to dialysis is variable, however; some cases respond only after transplantation. Other neurologic symptoms such as restless legs, asterixis, myoclonus, generalized irritability, and inability to concentrate dramatically improve with dialysis. PTH may have direct toxic effects on the central nervous system.

F. Disorders of Mineral Metabolism: Renal osteodystrophy is a complex disorder with several pathogenetic features. The most common component is osteitis fibrosa, manifested as subperiosteal resorption of bone. In renal failure, increases in serum phosphorus cause decreases in serum calcium, stimu-

lating the secretion of parathyroid hormone. Because of the phosphaturic effect of parathyroid hormone, the serum phosphorus tends to be normalized but at the expense of a higher circulating PTH level; ultimately, progression of renal disease results in persistent hyperphosphatemia and hypocalcemia, leading to extremely high PTH concentrations. Aluminum hydroxide and calcium carbonate have been used to bind phosphorus in the gut in such patients.

Another important component of renal osteodystrophy is osteomalacia. Diseased kidneys fail to convert 25-hydroxycholecalciferol to 1,25-dihydroxycholecalciferol. This leads to increased losses of calcium in the feces and defective mineralization in bone. Calcitriol or dihydrotachysterol can effectively overcome this problem. Standard vitamin D preparations should be used cautiously in these patients, since hypercalcemia, if it occurs, may be prolonged. In some patients with renal osteodystrophy, phosphate binders and vitamin D preparations are ineffective in reducing the parathyroid hormone level, and subtotal parathyroidectomy is required.

The least common type of renal osteodystrophy is aluminum-induced osteomalacia. In patients who have received aluminum for many years, the element may interfere with mineralization of bone. This diagnosis is confirmed by high serum aluminum levels and demonstration of aluminum in bone biopsy specimens. Chelation with deferoxamine may be effective.

G. Metabolic and Endocrine Disturbances: Glucose intolerance occurs with regularity in the nondiabetic patient once the serum creatinine exceeds 10–12 mg/dL. Its exact cause is controversial, but a dialyzable toxin is suspected since the abnormality seems to disappear after several weeks of adequate dialysis. Conversely, some patients with end-stage renal disease, usually of several years' duration, develop hypoglycemia. Reduced renal gluconeogenesis may play a role in pathogenesis.

Decreased libido and impotence occur in a high percentage of patients with chronic renal failure. Menstrual irregularities or amenorrhea is the rule, and successful pregnancy does not occur. There are many hormonal abnormalities that might play a role in these symptoms: decreased circulating testosterone in men, increased circulating prolactin in women. Sexual function appears to improve in patients whose hematocrits are normalized with erythropoietin.

H. Gastrointestinal Tract Complications: Gastrointestinal bleeding is a relatively common consequence of renal failure. A prolonged bleeding time may play a role. There appears to be increased frequency of angiodysplasia of the upper gastrointestinal tract. There is no increased incidence of peptic disease.

Both hepatitis B and hepatitis C are common in dialysis units. The use of hepatitis B vaccines has decreased the frequency of hepatitis in patients and staff, all of whom should receive this vaccine even though the antibody response to the vaccine in renal failure may be less than ideal. Although ascites may occur in association with chronic liver disease, dialysis patients also manifest on occasion an exudative ascites in the face of normal liver function. Its pathogenesis is unknown.

Treatment

A. Dietary Management: The dietary management of chronic renal failure is complex and must be individualized. For each patient, an evaluation and recommendation should be made for protein, salt and water, potassium intake, and phosphorus intake.

1. Protein restriction–There is some evidence that protein restriction may slow the deterioration of renal function in patients with a variety of renal diseases. Although the practicality as well as the efficacy and nutritional value of such an approach have not been conclusively demonstrated, it is generally recommended that protein intake should be limited to 1 g/kg/d.

2. Salt and water restriction–For patients with hypertension and edema, restriction of salt and water is indicated. In patients who are neither hypertensive nor edematous, salt restriction may not be necessary.

3. Potassium restriction–Potassium restriction is not usually necessary until oliguria develops except for individuals with tubulointerstitial nephritis or with hyporeninemic hypoaldosteronism.

4. Phosphorus restriction–Since the maintenance of normal serum phosphorus levels can prevent renal osteodystrophy and progression of renal failure, the serum phosphorus concentration should be maintained between 3.5 and 4 mg/dL (1.1–1.3 mmol/L). Dietary sources very rich in phosphorus should be restricted (eg, eggs, dairy products, meat). Hyperphosphatemia can be corrected using aluminum hydroxide phosphate binders (15–30 mL three times daily; or in tablet form). However, calcium carbonate (650 mg three times daily) is now the preferred long-term phosphate-binding agent because it prevents aluminum toxicity, which can cause both an irreversible central nervous system neurologic disorder and bone disease. Until the serum phosphorus is controlled, vitamin D should not be given to normalize serum calcium levels; thereafter, therapy with calcitriol may be initiated with a dosage of 0.25 μg/d, which can be increased at intervals once or twice a month until calcium is normalized.

5. Magnesium restriction–Use of all magnesium-containing antacids is contraindicated in chronic renal failure.

B. Dialysis: When conservative management fails to control uremic signs and symptoms, dialysis and kidney transplantation (see below) are alternatives. Indications for dialysis in oliguric patients include the following: (1) volume overload unresponsive to diuretic therapy, (2) severe metabolic acidosis (pH < 7.20), (3) pericarditis, (4) seizures and other neurologic symptoms, and (5) hyperkalemia. At this level of renal function, it is often necessary to modify dosages of some antimicrobial drugs to prevent complications (Table 22–8).

Many patients with chronic renal failure start dialysis when the serum creatinine is approximately 10 mg/dL (or BUN 100 mg/dL); patients with diabetic nephropathy often seem to require dialysis somewhat earlier. When possible, an arteriovenous fistula should be placed several weeks before the anticipated initiation of hemodialysis. This allows maturation of the fistula and a higher blood flow through the dialyzer.

1. Hemodialysis–Most patients will require hemodialysis three times weekly. The procedure takes 3–4 hours depending on the type of membranes used, the size of the patient, and other factors.

Home hemodialysis has the advantage that it can be performed at the patient's convenience. Patients receiving home hemodialysis must become much more knowledgeable about their treatment than patients treated in a center. Many believe that home dialysis patients do better for this reason, but selection bias obviously plays a role. A major disadvantage of home hemodialysis is that a helper must be available, and training is required.

2. Peritoneal dialysis–While the percentage of patients receiving home hemodialysis has declined over the past 10 years, the number of patients receiving continuous ambulatory peritoneal dialysis has greatly increased. Peritoneal dialysis is performed by the patient, and the continual nature of the dialysis leads to better clearance of poorly dialyzable compounds, especially phosphate. This in turn results in less dietary restriction for these patients. Similarly, continuous dialysis is not associated with symptom swings observed in hemodialysis.

When it was first introduced, it was hoped that the cost of continuous ambulatory peritoneal dialysis would be much less than that of hemodialysis. While the equipment costs are indeed less, the total cost of care of these patients is not. Peritonitis remains a major complication of peritoneal dialysis, and its treatment (which sometimes requires hospitalization) is expensive. When vascular access for hemodialysis is technically difficult, such as in small children and in some diabetic patients, continuous ambulatory peritoneal dialysis is a reasonable alternative. Patients who have been treated with both modalities usually prefer peritoneal dialysis.

C. Kidney Transplantation: In most patients who develop chronic renal failure, consideration should be given to kidney transplantation. About two-thirds of kidney transplants performed in the United States come from cadaveric donors and the remainder from living related donors. Posttransplant immunosuppression with corticosteroids, azathio-

Table 22–8. Antimicrobial dosages in renal failure.[1]

	No Change	Moderate Reduction	Marked Reduction	Avoid
Aminoglycosides				
Amikacin			•	
Gentamicin			•	
Netilmicin			•	
Tobramycin			•	
Amphotericin B			•	
Cephalosporins				
First-generation:				
Cefadroxil			•	
Cephradine			•	
Cephalexin	•			
Cephalothin			•	
Cephapirin			•	
Cefazolin			•	
Second-generation:				
Cefaclor		•		
Cefonicid			•	
Cefotetan			•	
Cefoxitin			•	
Cefuroxime			•	
Third-generation:				
Cefoperazone	•			
Cefotaxime			•	
Ceftazidime			•	
Ceftizoxime			•	
Ceftriaxone	•			
Chloramphenicol	•			
Clindamycin	•			
Erythromycin	•			
Monobactams (aztreonam)			•	
Nitrofurantoin				•
Penicillins				
Amoxicillin		•		
Ampicillin		•		
Azlocillin		•		
Carbenicillin	•			
Dicloxacillin		•		
Methicillin		•		
Mezlocillin	•			
Nafcillin	•			
Penicillin G		•		
Piperacillin		•		
Ticarcillin			•	
Quinolones				
Ciprofloxacin		•		
Norfloxacin		•		
Trimethoprim-sulfamethoxazole		•		
Tetracyclines				
Doxycycline	•			
Tetracycline				•
Vancomycin			•	

[1]GFR = < 10 mL/min

prine, and cyclosporine—singly or in combination—are regularly required in cadaveric kidney transplants and generally in living related donor transplants as well, though the number of drugs and the duration of administration depend upon the degree of HLA matching. The 2-year kidney graft survival rate for living related donor transplantations is 85%; the 2-year graft survival rate for cadaveric donor transplantations is 70%.

[Morbidity and mortality of dialysis]
gopher://gopher.nih.gov/11/clin/cdcs/individual/93.dialys

Buckalew VM Jr: Pathophysiology of progressive renal failure. South Med J 1994;87:1028.

Erslev AJ, Besarab A: Erythropoietin in the pathogenesis and treatment of the anemia of chronic renal failure. Kidney Int 1997;51:622. (Production, action, and therapeutic use of erythropoietin for the anemia of chronic renal failure.)

Massry SG, Smogrozewski M: The heart in uremia. Semin Nephrol 1996;16:214.

Michael B, Burke JF Jr: Chronic renal disease: New therapies to delay kidney replacement. Geriatrics 1994;49:33.

Morbidity and mortality of renal dialysis: An NIH Consensus Conference Statement. Consensus Development Conference Panel. Ann Intern Med 1994;121:62.

Remuzzi G, Ruggenenti P, Benigni A: Understanding the nature of renal disease progression. Kidney Int 1997;51:2. (Pathogenesis of renal disease and the rationale for specific treatment modalities.)

Valderrabano F: Erythropoietin in chronic renal failure. Kidney Int 1996;50:1373. (Case presentation and in-depth discussion of erythropoietin use in end-stage renal disease.)

GLOMERULONEPHRITIS

Glomerulonephritis is an inflammatory process primarily involving the glomerulus, though at times the renal vasculature, interstitium, and tubular epithelium may also be affected. Glomerular inflammation can result in damage to any of the three major components of the glomerulus: the basement membrane, the mesangium, or the capillary endothelium. Identification of the specific histopathologic pattern of glomerular injury by renal biopsy is often the most helpful technique available for defining the cause of glomerulonephritis.

Classification

Diseases causing glomerulonephritis can be classified according to whether they present as either a nephritic or a nephrotic syndrome, though some glomerular disease processes can present with components of both.

Glomerular diseases presenting as **nephritic syndromes** are associated with a clinical presentation of hypertension, edema, a urine sample showing red blood cells, red blood cell casts, and a moderate degree of proteinuria. Glomerular diseases presenting as **nephrotic syndromes** are characterized by heavy proteinuria (> 3.5 g/24 h) and frequently hypoalbuminemia, hyperlipidemia, and edema.

Diseases causing glomerulonephritis can also be classified according to whether they cause only renal abnormalities (primary renal diseases) or whether the renal abnormalities result from a systemic disease (secondary renal diseases).

Evaluation of Suspected Glomerulonephritis

In an individual suspected of having glomerulonephritis, the initial evaluation should include the following procedures and determinations:

A. Urinalysis: Dipstick and microscopic evaluation will reveal evidence for hematuria, proteinuria, and cellular elements including red cells, white cells, and casts.

B. Twenty-Four Hour Urine for Protein Excretion and Creatinine Clearance: This quantifies the amount of proteinuria and establishes the presence of nephrotic syndrome and documents the degree of renal dysfunction.

C. Creatinine Clearance: Documents the degree of renal dysfunction.

D. Urine and Serum Protein Electrophoresis: These studies identify monoclonal or Bence Jones proteins suggestive of multiple myeloma or amyloidosis.

E. Further Tests: Depending on the history and the results of the preliminary evaluation, further tests may be warranted, including complement levels (CH50, C3, C4), ASO titer, anti-GBM antibody levels, cryoglobulins, C3 nephritic factor, renal ultrasound, and renal biopsy.

GLOMERULONEPHRITIS PRESENTING WITH NEPHRITIC MANIFESTATIONS

1. POSTSTREPTOCOCCAL GLOMERULONEPHRITIS

Poststreptococcal glomerulonephritis is the result of infection with a nephritogenic strain of group A (β-hemolytic) streptococci, especially type 12. It most commonly presents following infections of the throat (pharyngitis) or skin (impetigo) and occurs both sporadically and in clusters. The latent period between infection and onset of urinary symptoms is 6–21 days. There is a wide spectrum of glomerular disease from subclinical to cases associated with anemia and renal failure.

Clinical Findings

Poststreptococcal glomerulonephritis is characterized by the abrupt onset of tea-colored urine, oliguria, edema, and variable degrees of hypertension. Urinary abnormalities include hematuria and red cell casts and proteinuria, which is usually mild to moderate and not in the nephrotic range (< 3.5 g/24 h). Renal tubular cells, leukocytes, and hyaline and granular casts may be seen. The creatinine clearance is mildly reduced. Urinary sodium is low, with fractional excretion often less than 0.5%. Antistreptolysin O (ASO), antistreptokinase, and antihyaluronidase titers may rise, but this rise may be blunted by previous treatment with antibiotics. There is usually a decrease in serum complement levels, both total hemolytic complement (CH50) and the level of C3.

Poststreptococcal glomerulonephritis is an immune complex-mediated disease presenting on light microscopy as a diffuse proliferative glomerulonephritis. Immunofluorescence shows IgG and C3 in a granular pattern along the capillary basement membrane and in mesangial regions. Electron microscopy shows large, dense subepithelial deposits or "humps" (Table 22–9).

Course & Treatment

The disorder is usually self-limiting, with 95% of individuals recovering normal renal function within 2 months after onset. About 5% develop rapidly progressive glomerulonephritis, with a small number of these individuals progressing to end-stage renal disease.

In some adults, hypertension and proteinuria may persist, and chronic renal failure may develop after

10–20 years. There is no specific treatment except for antihypertensives, salt restriction, and diuretics. Corticosteroids have not been shown to be of any value.

Infections with pathogens other than streptococci can cause a similar postinfectious glomerulonephritis. Glomerulonephritis can occur in association with subacute infective endocarditis, peritoneoventricular shunt infections, and bacterial abscesses of the lung and abdominal cavity. Treatment of the underlying infection may resolve the glomerulonephritis as well.

Buzio C et al: Significance of albuminuria in the follow-up of acute poststreptococcal glomerulonephritis. Clin Nephrol 1994;41:259.

Montseny JJ et al: The current spectrum of infectious glomerulonephritis. Medicine 1995;74:63. (Experience of 76 patients with glomerulonephritis and review of the literature.)

Schlondorff D et al: Limitations of therapeutic approaches to glomerular diseases. Kidney Int 1995;48(Suppl 50):519. (Reviews problems of etiology and diagnosis, limitations of current therapy, and future therapies for specific types of glomerular disease.)

2. IgA NEPHROPATHY & HENOCH-SCHÖNLEIN PURPURA

IgA Nephropathy

IgA nephropathy (Berger's disease) is usually a primary renal disease, but the same renal lesion can be seen in Henoch-Schönlein syndrome. IgA nephropathy is the most common form of acute glomerulonephritis in the USA and is even more common in Asian countries. The cause is unknown.

Table 22–9. Classification and findings in glomerulonephritis: Nephritic syndromes.

Syndrome	Etiology	Histopathology	Pathogenesis
Acute (postinfectious) glomerulonephritis	Streptococci, other bacteria	Light: Diffuse proliferative glomerulonephritis Immunofluorescence: IgG; C3, granular pattern Electron microscopy: Subepithelial deposits or "humps"	Trapped immune complexes
IgA nephropathy (Berger's disease and Henoch-Schönlein purpura)	In association with viral upper respiratory tract infections; gastrointestinal infection or flu-like syndrome	Light: Mesangioproliferative glomerulonephritis Immunofluorescence: IgA (+/– IgG, C3) Electron microscopy: Mesangial deposits	Unknown
Rapidly progressive glomerulonephritis	Lupus erythematosus, mixed cryoglobulinemia, subacute infective endocarditis, shunt infections	Light: Crescentic glomerulonephritis Immunofluorescence: IgG, IgA; C3 granular pattern Electron microscopy: Deposits in subepithelium, subendothelium, or mesangium	Trapped immune complexes
	Goodpasture's syndrome or idiopathic	Light: Crescentic glomerulonephritis Immunofluorescence: IgG; C3, linear pattern Electron microscopy: Widening of basement membrane	Anti-GBM antibodies
	Wegener's granulomatosis, polyarteritis, idiopathic	Light: Crescentic glomerulonephritis Immunofluorescence: No immunoglobulins Electron microscopy: No deposits	Unknown

This disorder tends to present as an episode of macroscopic hematuria, frequently in association with an upper respiratory infection (50%), gastrointestinal symptoms (10%), or a flu-like illness (15%). In contrast to poststreptococcal glomerulonephritis, there is no significant latent period, and hypertension and edema are uncommon. Gross hematuria usually lasts 2–6 days. Proteinuria rarely exceeds 1–2 g/d, though 10% of patients can present with nephrotic syndrome. About half of individuals with gross hematuria will have only a single episode; the remainder will have recurrent episodes over many years. Fifty percent of patients with IgA nephropathy eventually develop progressive loss of renal function, with this course being more common in adults than in children. The presence of hypertension early in the course, male sex, and proteinuria greater than 3 g/d are indicators for progressive disease.

The serum IgA level is increased in 30–50% of patients; in such cases the IgA level is helpful diagnostically, though a normal value does not rule out the diagnosis. Serum complement levels are usually normal. Most individuals will also have granular deposits of IgA in the dermal capillaries of otherwise normal skin.

The typical finding by light microscopy is a focal proliferative glomerulonephritis localized to the mesangium. Small crescents are seen in all individuals biopsied who have macroscopic hematuria and red cell casts. Immunofluorescence reveals diffuse deposition of IgA and often IgG and C3 in the mesangium of all glomeruli. Electron microscopy confirms mesangial deposits (Table 22–9).

A daily dose of 12 g of fish oil (n–3 fatty acids) may retard the rate at which renal function is lost, especially in individuals with mildly impaired renal function.

Henoch-Schönlein Purpura (Anaphylactoid Purpura)

This disease classically presents with palpable purpura caused by a leukocytoclastic vasculitis, arthralgias, and abdominal symptoms, including colic, nausea, and melena. Purpuric skin lesions are often located on the lower extremities, though the platelet count is normal. Males are affected in the greatest numbers, and the disease is commoner in children. Renal insufficiency is common with a nephritic presentation. The renal lesion is identical to that of IgA nephropathy with mesangial deposition of IgA, but the clinical presentations of these disorders are clearly different. Most individuals will recover renal function completely and seldom go on to end-stage renal disease. Further details about Henoch-Schönlein purpura appear in Chapter 20.

Andreoli SP: Chronic glomerulonephritis in childhood. Ped Clin North Am 1995;42:1487. (Membranoproliferative glomerulonephritis, Henoch-Schönlein purpura nephritis, and IgA nephropathy.)

Donadio JV et al: A controlled trial of fish oil in IgA nephropathy. N Engl J Med 1994;331:1194.

Galla JH: IgA nephropathy. Kidney Int 1995;47:377.

Ibels LS, Gyory AZ: IgA nephropathy: Analysis of the natural history, important factors in the progression of renal disease, and a review of the literature. Medicine 1994; 73:79.

3. RAPIDLY PROGRESSIVE GLOMERULONEPHRITIS

Rapidly progressive glomerulonephritis can be defined as any glomerular disease associated with rapid progressive loss of renal function over days or weeks. The manifestations of glomerulonephritis—hypertension, edema, proteinuria, hematuria, and red cell casts—are similar irrespective of the cause. Renal biopsy should be performed in any individual with normal- or large-sized kidneys and no medical contraindications to biopsy (see section on renal biopsy). Rapidly progressive glomerulonephritis should be considered if the renal biopsy reveals the presence of crescents in 50% or more glomeruli. The causes of rapidly progressive glomerulonephritis can be categorized according to the immunofluorescence patterns found on renal biopsy. Granular deposits of immunoglobulin (IgG, IgA) and complement along the glomerular capillary walls and in the mesangium suggest an immune complex disease.

The finding of no or only scanty amounts of detectable immunoglobulin is associated with pauci-immune crescentic glomerulonephritis. Almost 80% of individuals with this form of glomerulonephritis have antineutrophil cytoplasmic autoantibodies (ANCA) and, clinically, Wegener's granulomatosis, polyarteritis nodosa, or "idiopathic" crescentic glomerulonephritis. Electron microscopy confirms the lack of immune complexes and immunoglobulins.

The presence of IgG antibodies with C3 deposition along the glomerular basement membrane in a linear pattern with or without pulmonary involvement defines anti-GBM glomerulonephritis (either Goodpasture's syndrome or idiopathic anti-GBM nephritis). Electron microscopy reveals widening of the basement membrane by amorphous subendothelial material.

Since the prognosis and treatment depend on the cause, early renal biopsy should be done before the start of medical therapy. Immunofluorescence and electron microscopic studies are done on the same tissue sample.

Treatment is directed toward correction of fluid overload, hypertension, and uremia and the inflammatory injury to the kidney. Salt and water restriction, diuretic therapy, and even dialysis may be needed to control and prevent volume overload. Antihypertensive medications are often necessary, and immunosuppressive therapy with corticosteroids and cytotoxic agents reduces the inflammatory injury.

The decision to use immunosuppressive therapy depends on the nature and severity of the disease. Immune complex postinfectious glomerulonephritis is managed by treating the infection with appropriate antibiotics, and immunosuppressive therapy is unwarranted. Immune complex vasculitis without infection, as can occur in systemic lupus and cryoglobulinemia, necessitates immunosuppression for both renal and extrarenal inflammatory injury. Pauci-immune rapidly progressive glomerulonephritis with or without necrotizing arteritis is often treated with cytotoxic drugs, both corticosteroids and cyclophosphamide. Anti-GBM-mediated glomerulonephritis requires aggressive immunosuppression to prevent rapid progression to end-stage renal failure.

Rapidly Progressive Glomerulonephritis Due to Glomerular Immune Complex Formation

About 40% of patients with rapidly progressive glomerulonephritis will have granular deposits of immunoglobulin and complement in the glomeruli suggestive of immune complex glomerulonephritis. On electron microscopy, dense deposits representing immune complexes are found in the subepithelial, subendothelial, or mesangial locations. In such cases, the glomerulonephritis is usually a manifestation of a systemic disease such as systemic lupus erythematosus or cryoglobulinemia, or a primary renal disease such as poststreptococcal (or other postinfectious) glomerulonephritis or membranoproliferative glomerulonephritis.

The prognosis of rapidly progressive glomerulonephritis is dependent on the underlying disease process. Clinical and laboratory features in association with pathologic findings in the kidney can usually distinguish among these conditions and suggest a specific diagnosis. Treatment with high-dose methylprednisolone (for 3 days) is followed by oral prednisone, 2 mg/k/d, which is tapered over several months. In addition, cytotoxic drugs—usually cyclophosphamide, 1–2 mg/kg/d orally, or pulse intravenous cyclophosphamide, 500 mg/m^2 per month—are added. Plasma exchange therapy has also been employed with some favorably reported but uncontrolled results.

Idiopathic (Pauci-immune) Crescentic Glomerulonephritis

This form of rapidly progressive glomerulonephritis may involve only the kidney (idiopathic or pauci-immune crescentic glomerulonephritis) or may be part of a systemic disorder (microscopic polyarteritis nodosa or Wegener's granulomatosis). It is associated with elevated antineutrophil cytoplasmic anti-bodies (ANCA), but there are neither granular nor linear immune deposits in the glomeruli.

In the idiopathic form, males are affected twice as commonly as females. Many patients have had a recent flu-like syndrome with fever, myalgias, and polyarthralgias. Symptoms are nonspecific and include oliguria, dark urine, and occasionally symptoms related to volume overload. Examination may yield hypertension and edema, but no cutaneous or other symptoms are present. These manifestations may also be seen in Wegener's granulomatosis, which is discussed below.

Hematuria and red cell casts are often present, as is proteinuria, though nephrotic syndrome is uncommon. Serum anti-GBM antibodies and circulating immune complexes are absent, and serum complement levels are normal. ANCA levels are generally elevated and parallel disease activity.

On light microscopy, glomerulonephritis is found, with 50% of the glomeruli having crescents. A focal segmental necrotizing glomerular lesion is commonly present. No glomerular immune deposits are identified by immunofluorescence or electron microscopic studies (Table 22–9).

Therapy is the same irrespective of the underlying disease process and the same as that indicated for rapidly progressive glomerulonephritis due to glomerular immune complex formation.

Goodpasture's Syndrome

Goodpasture's syndrome accounts for about 5% of all patients with rapidly progressive glomerulonephritis. It is a rare disease associated with the triad of pulmonary hemorrhage, iron deficiency anemia, and glomerulonephritis due to anti-GBM antibody deposition in the kidneys and lungs. The disease is due to the production and deposition of antibodies to antigens on the alpha-3 chain of type IV collagen. The causative factors for development of anti-GBM antibodies are unknown, though influenza A infection, hydrocarbon solvent exposure, and the presence of HLA-DRw2 and -B7 antigens have been implicated.

The disease frequently occurs in young white male smokers (male:female ratio 6:1). Pulmonary symptoms often appear first and can range from mild hemoptysis with bilateral fluffy alveolar infiltrates to life-threatening pulmonary hemorrhage with hypoxemia and respiratory failure.

Iron deficiency anemia is often present—in contrast to the usual normocytic anemia associated with renal failure—and is thought to be secondary to blood loss and iron sequestration in the lungs. Microscopic hematuria and proteinuria generally develop within 2 weeks after the onset of the pulmonary disease, and progressive loss of renal function ensues. Circulating serum anti-GBM antibodies parallel the activity of the renal disease and are diagnostic of this syndrome.

On light microscopy, the histology is consistent

with a focal proliferative and necrotizing lesion with crescent formation. On immunofluorescence, there is a linear deposition of IgG (or, rarely, IgA) in a continuous uninterrupted pattern along the glomerular basement membrane, often with C3 in a similar pattern. A linear deposit of IgG is also seen along the tubular basement membrane. On electron microscopy, anti-GBM antibody deposits are not seen.

A diagnosis of Goodpasture's is confirmed by finding circulating serum anti-GBM antibodies in an individual with pulmonary hemorrhage or alveolar infiltrates and glomerulonephritis. Early diagnosis is a necessity to reverse the renal lesion, since the response to therapy is poor once there is oliguria or a serum creatinine exceeding 6 mg/dL.

The treatment of choice is a combination of plasma exchange therapy to remove circulating anti-GBM antibody and immunosuppressive drugs—both prednisone, 1 mg/kg/d, and cyclophosphamide, 2–3 mg/kg/d—to inhibit further antibody production.

Over 50% of individuals with rapidly progressive glomerulonephritis caused by anti-GBM antibodies will not have pulmonary hemorrhage or other extrarenal manifestations of disease. Treatment in such cases if circulating serum anti-GBM antibodies are found is the same as for Goodpasture's syndrome.

Kelly PT, Haponik EF: Goodpasture syndrome: Molecular and clinical advances. Medicine 1994;73:171.

Levy JB, Winearls CG: Rapidly progressive glomerulonephritis: What should be first-line therapy? Nephron 1994;67:402.

Mandell BF, Hoffman GS: Differentiating the vasculitides. Rheum Dis Clin North Am 1994;20:409. (Review and algorithms for diagnosing and managing vasculitis.)

Petersson EE, Sundelin B, Heigl ZZ: Incidence and outcome of pauci-immune necrotizing and crescentic glomerulonephritis in adults. Clin Nephrol 1995;43:141. (Seven-year follow-up [1986–1992] of 71 individuals.)

Short AK, Esnault VL, Lockwood CM: Anti-neutrophil cytoplasm antibodies and anti-glomerular basement membrane antibodies: Two co-existing distinct autoreactivities detectable in patients with rapidly progressive glomerulonephritis. Am J Kidney Dis 1995;26:439.

Turner AN, Rees AJ: Goodpasture's disease and Alport's syndrome. Ann Rev Med 1996;47:377. (Pathogenesis of diseases affecting the glomerular basement membrane.)

NEPHROTIC SYNDROME

Essentials of Diagnosis

- Urine protein excretion > 3.5 g/1.73 m^2 per 24 hours.
- Hypoalbuminemia (serum albumin < 3.0 g/dL).
- Peripheral edema (or anasarca with ascites).
- Hypercholesterolemia (fasting level > 200 mg/dL).

General Considerations

In adults, about one-third of patients with nephrotic syndrome will have a systemic disease such as diabetes mellitus, amyloidosis, or systemic lupus erythematosus. The remainder will be categorized as having idiopathic nephrotic syndrome due to one of four forms of glomerular diseases: minimal change, focal glomerular sclerosis, membranous nephropathy, or membranoproliferative glomerulonephritis.

Clinical Findings

A. Symptoms and Signs: Regardless of the cause, peripheral edema is the hallmark of nephrotic syndrome, though it is not evident until the plasma albumin concentration falls below 3 g/dL. Ascites and anasarca generally develop as a consequence of the severity of the hypoalbuminemia. Exertional dyspnea suggests pulmonary edema associated with severe hypoalbuminemia, large pleural effusions, or restriction of the diaphragm by ascitic fluid. Many patients complain of feeling bloated or "tight" as a result of edema or will complain of abdominal fullness if ascites is present. When secondary to a systemic disease, additional manifestations pertinent to those processes are also present.

B. Laboratory Findings:

1. Urine protein–The screening test to determine if abnormal amounts of protein (specifically, albumin) are being excreted in the urine is the urinary protein dipstick analysis. The dipstick can detect as little as 10–15 mg/dL of protein, but the results must be interpreted in light of the urine specific gravity: A 1+ result in a concentrated specimen (eg, specific gravity 1.030) may have no significance, while a 1+ finding in urine with a low specific gravity (eg, 1.002) may indicate significant protein excretion over 24 hours.

2. Microscopic analysis–Glomerular diseases presenting with nephrotic syndrome often have no cellular elements or casts. The finding of hematuria, pyuria, and cellular casts strongly suggests a glomerular disease that also causes the nephritic syndrome, even if heavy proteinuria is also present. Common to all diseases causing nephrotic syndrome is the presence of oval fat bodies in the urine. These degenerating tubular epithelial cells having cholesteryl esters appear under light microscopy as a cell with "grape clusters," and under polarized light these clusters have a "Maltese cross" appearance.

3. Blood chemistries–Characteristic blood chemistries associated with nephrotic syndrome include a decreased serum albumin (< 3 g/dL), a decreased total serum protein (< 6 g/dL), and an elevated serum cholesterol (> 200 mg/dL).

4. Special tests–Other less common tests performed in patients with nephrotic syndrome may include complement levels (C3, C4, CH50), serum and urine electrophoresis, antinuclear antibody (ANA), and hepatitis serology, specifically for hepatitis B antigen. Data obtained from the history and physical examination determine their appropriateness.

5. Renal biopsy–Renal biopsy is the standard procedure for determining in adults the cause of idiopathic nephrotic syndrome in which the presence of a steroid-treatable or steroid-resistant lesion is possible or likely. Empiric therapy with steroids is not usually recommended unless there is a contraindication to renal biopsy. It should be performed in individuals with persistent proteinuria in whom the etiology or the prognosis of the proteinuria is in doubt as long as there are no medical contraindications to the procedure. Nephrotic-range proteinuria, a result of a systemic disease such as diabetes mellitus or amyloidosis, does not necessitate renal biopsy since that degree of proteinuria represents irreversible glomerular damage from the systemic disease process. Each specimen is examined by light microscopy, after immunofluorescence studies, and with the electron microscope. The histologic pattern—ie, the presence or absence of immune complexes and electron-dense deposits—is most helpful in categorizing the renal abnormality and establishing a diagnosis and thus serves as a guide to therapy and prognosis.

Management of Nephrotic Syndrome

Some management problems common to all patients with nephrotic syndrome regardless of the cause are dealt with here.

A. Protein Loss: Since increased protein intake can have an adverse effect on renal function in some disease processes, moderation of intake by patients with nephrotic syndrome seems reasonable. A protein intake of 0.5–0.6 g/kg/d and the optional addition of an angiotensin-converting enzyme inhibitor will often reduce the amount of proteinuria. However, if the urinary protein loss exceeds 10 g/24 h, individuals may develop negative nitrogen balance and protein malnutrition. For these individuals, additional quantities of dietary protein, equivalent to their daily losses, may be needed.

B. Peripheral Edema and Ascites: Dietary salt restriction is the key to success in managing edema. However, most patients will eventually need the addition of diuretics. Although thiazide diuretics are used for mild edema, loop diuretics are often employed for the more refractory fluid retention associated with pleural effusions and ascites. The addition of a diuretic such as metolazone or a thiazide acting distal to the loop of Henle may potentiate the diuretic activity of the loop diuretic if one is needed.

C. Hyperlipidemia: Hypercholesterolemia and hypertriglyceridemia frequently accompany nephrotic syndrome. Increased hepatic production of lipids has been generally considered responsible for the hyperlipidemia. Dietary management appears to be of limited value, but most patients should be maintained on a low-fat diet, with a weight control and exercise program. Since hyperlipidemia may predispose to accelerated atherosclerosis, pharmacologic intervention should be considered and approached somewhat the same way as hyperlipidemia without nephrotic syndrome (Chapter 28).

D. Hypercoagulable State: With nephrotic proteinuria, loss of antithrombin III and other proteins involved in the clotting and fibrinolytic cascades can result in a relative hypercoagulable state. Individuals have an increased incidence of peripheral venous thrombosis and renal vein thrombosis. If thrombosis is detected, heparin therapy followed by warfarin is necessary for at least 6 months.

1. MINIMAL CHANGE DISEASE (Lipoid Nephrosis, Nil Disease)

Minimal change disease, though most common in children, is seen occasionally in adults. Although the pathogenesis is unknown, the disease has occurred following viral upper respiratory tract infections, immunizations, or hypersensitivity to drugs (especially NSAIDs) or bee stings. It is also encountered as a paraneoplastic effect of Hodgkin's disease.

Minimal change disease is so called because the glomeruli appear totally normal under light microscopy. Immunofluorescence tests are usually negative. Under electron microscopy, there is characteristic "fusion" of the epithelial foot processes, which is not a specific finding for this disorder but occurs in all glomerular diseases associated with significant proteinuria (Table 22–10).

Minimal change disease does not progress to renal failure. However, the disorder can result in significant complications, including increased susceptibility to infection with gram-positive organisms; a tendency toward thromboembolic events; severe hyperlipidemia; and protein malnutrition.

A subgroup of patients present with nephrotic syndrome and on light microscopy have varying degrees of mesangial cell proliferation but no sclerotic changes. Immunofluorescence studies may show diffuse mesangial deposits of IgM and C3. These individuals tend to have more hematuria and hypertension, and, in contrast to patients with pure minimal change disease, respond poorly to corticosteroid therapy, though they are treated in somewhat the same way as those with minimal change disease or kidney biopsy.

This disorder tends to respond to prednisone, 1 mg/kg/d, after 4–6 weeks. However, a significant number of individuals will relapse when steroids are discontinued and will require additional doses of steroids; some will become steroid-dependent, relapsing every time steroids are discontinued. For frequent relapses and steroid-dependent individuals, cyclophosphamide and chlorambucil may be needed to induce subsequent remissions.

Table 22–10. Classification and findings in glomerulonephritis: Nephrotic syndromes.

Syndrome	Etiology	Histopathology	Pathogenesis
Minimal change disease (nil disease; lipoid nephrosis)	Associated with allergy, Hodgkin's disease, NSAIDs	Light: Normal (+/– mesangial proliferation) Immunofluorescence: No immunoglobulins Electron microscopy: Fusion foot processes	Unknown
Focal and segmental glomerulosclerosis	Associated with heroin abuse, HIV infection, reflux nephropathy, obesity	Light: Focal segmental sclerosis Immunofluorescence: IgM and C3 in sclerotic segments Electron microscopy: Fusion foot processes	Unknown
Membranous nephropathy	Associated with non-Hodgkin's lymphoma, carcinoma (gastrointestinal, renal, bronchogenic, thyroid), gold therapy, penicillamine, lupus erythematosus	Light: Thickened GBM and spikes Immunofluorescence: Granular IgG and C3 along capillary loops Electron microscopy: Dense deposits in subepithelial area	In situ immune complex formation
Membranoproliferative glomerulonephropathy	Type I associated with upper respiratory infection	Light: Increase mesangial cells and matrix with splitting of basement membrane Immunofluorescence: Granular C3, C1q, C4 with IgG and IgM Electron microscopy: Dense deposits in subendothelium	Unknown
	Type II	Light: Same as type I Immunofluorescence: C3 only Electron microscopy: Dense material in GBM	Unknown

2. FOCAL GLOMERULAR SCLEROSIS

Focal glomerular sclerosis can present as idiopathic nephrotic syndrome; over 80% of patients also have microscopic hematuria at presentation. It is also associated with heroin abuse, AIDS, reflux nephropathy, an idiosyncratic reaction to NSAIDs, and massive obesity. Clinical features that distinguish focal glomerular sclerosis from minimal change disease are the presence of hypertension and decreased renal function in 25–50% of individuals at the time of diagnosis.

On light microscopy, focal segmental glomerular sclerosing lesions are seen, occurring first in the juxtamedullary glomeruli and later in the glomeruli in the superficial cortex. On immunofluorescence, deposits of IgM and C3 are found in the sclerotic segments. Electron microscopy reveals effacement of the foot processes as seen in minimal change disease (Table 22–10).

Prednisone, 60 mg/m^2 for 4 weeks, followed by 40 mg/m^2 every other day for 4 more weeks, is recommended because up to 40% of patients respond. Whether cytotoxic drugs are warranted for steroid-resistant individuals is a matter of controversy at present. Despite therapy, most patients progress to end-stage renal disease within 5–10 years.

3. MEMBRANOUS GLOMERULONEPHRITIS

Membranous glomerulonephritis is the most common cause of primary nephrotic syndrome in adults.

The natural history is variable, with about 50% of individuals developing a slow but progressive loss of renal function over 3–10 years. Membranous glomerulonephritis may be idiopathic or associated with a variety of disorders, including hepatitis B antigenemia; autoimmune diseases, including lupus erythematosus, diabetes, thyroiditis, and mixed connective tissue disease; carcinoma; and use of certain drugs such as gold, penicillamine, and captopril.

This disorder occurs in adults, most commonly in the fifth and sixth decades. Many patients have secondary renal vein thrombosis, and there is a higher than expected incidence of occult neoplasms of the lung, stomach, and colon in individuals over age 50.

By light microscopy, an increase in capillary wall thickness without inflammatory changes or cellular proliferation can be seen. When stained with silver methenamine, a "spike and dome" pattern may be observed due to projections of excess basement membrane between the subepithelial deposits. On immunofluorescence, there are finely granular deposits of IgG and C3 present uniformly along all the capillary loops. Electron microscopy reveals electron-dense deposits in a discontinuous pattern along the subepithelial surface of the basement membrane (Table 22–10).

The natural history of idiopathic membranous glomerulonephritis has been so variable that the influence of treatment is difficult to assess. Poor prognostic indicators include proteinuria in excess of 10 g/d, male gender, hypertension, and decreased renal function. Although treatment remains controversial, a 3-month course of prednisone, 2 mg/kg/d, may induce remission. Cytotoxic agents are often added if there is evidence for renal function deterioration.

4. MEMBRANOPROLIFERATIVE GLOMERULONEPHRITIS

Membranoproliferative glomerulonephritis is a disorder of unknown cause that is responsible for about 10% of all cases of idiopathic nephrotic syndrome. At least two major subgroups are recognized: type I and type II.

In type I, about one-third of patients have a history of a recent upper respiratory tract infection. Characteristically, this disorder is associated with the presence of granular subendothelial and sometimes subepithelial immune complex deposits, low levels of serum complement, and the presence of cryoglobulins and circulating immune complexes. There is an increase in mesangial cells and matrix that interposes itself between the glomerular basement membrane and the endothelial cells, giving a characteristic splitting or double contour to the capillary wall. Immunofluorescence reveals coarsely granular deposits of C3 and often C1q, C4, and properdin in the mesangium and along the capillary wall along with IgG and IgM. Electron microscopy shows electron-dense deposits along the subendothelial surface of the capillary loops and in the mesangium (Table 22–10).

Type II membranoproliferative glomerulonephritis (dense-deposit disease) is a rare disorder characterized by the presence of a circulating IgG antibody termed C3 nephritic factor (C3NeF). Light microscopy is similar to what is seen in type I, but immunofluorescence stains only for C3. Electron microscopy reveals a dense homogeneous osmophilic material replacing the lamina densa of the glomerular basement membrane.

Although steroid therapy and antiplatelet drugs are used, there is no agreement that any form of therapy is of benefit in this disorder. Though some patients may experience a spontaneous remission, the majority will progress to end-stage renal disease within a few years or months.

Cortes L, Tejani A: Dilemma of focal segmental glomerular sclerosis: Kidney Int 1996;49(Suppl):S57. (Difficulty in diagnosing the disorder from clinical parameters.)

Harris RC, Ismail N: Extrarenal complications of the nephrotic syndrome. Am J Kidney Dis 1994;23:477. (Causes of hypoalbuminemia and the associated metabolic abnormalities of the nephrotic syndrome.)

Mallick NP, Brenchley PEC, Webb NJA: Minimal change nephropathy and focal segmental glomerulosclerosis. Kidney Int 1997;51(Suppl):S80. (Differences associated with minimal change nephropathy and focal glomerular sclerosis.)

Pauker SG, Kopelman RI: Hunting for the cause: How far to go? N Engl J Med 1993;328:1621. (An interesting clinical problem-solving case involving a patient with
the nephrotic syndrome with special emphasis on how hard to search for an underlying cause.)

TUBULOINTERSTITIAL NEPHRITIS

Tubulointerstitial nephritis is an inflammatory disorder of the renal interstitium in which the immune system plays a significant role pathogenetically. Although both humoral and cell-mediated reactions have been implicated, the most prevalent forms of interstitial nephritis involve only the cell-mediated immune response. T lymphocytes may damage the interstitium through direct cytotoxicity or by releasing lymphokines that recruit monocytes and inflammatory cells, including eosinophils.

ALLERGIC TUBULOINTERSTITIAL NEPHRITIS

Essentials of Diagnosis

- Fever; occasionally flank pain.
- Transient maculopapular rash.
- Acute renal insufficiency.
- Hematuria and peripheral blood eosinophilia.

General Considerations

Fifteen percent of cases of acute renal failure are caused by acute tubulointerstitial nephritis. If no causative factors are found, the disease is presumed to be autoimmune in origin; most cases are drug-related. (See Table 22–11.)

Clinical Findings

A. Symptoms and Signs: Acute tubulointerstitial nephritis presents as a sudden decrease in renal function in an otherwise asymptomatic patient who has been taking a new medication. Signs and symptoms characteristic of an allergic reaction are common and include fever (85–100%) and transient maculopapular rash (25–50%). Bilateral or unilateral flank pain is often described and occurs as a result of distention of the renal capsule as the kidney swells. Although the classic triad of fever, rash, and eosinophilia is found in less than 30% of patients, when all three features are present the diagnosis of acute tubulointerstitial nephritis is strongly suggested. Renal failure generally evolves over several days to several weeks.

Although a number of drugs are reported to cause acute tubulointerstitial nephritis, those implicated most frequently are the beta-lactam antibiotics (methicillin, ampicillin, cephalosporins) and the

Table 22–11. Causes of acute tubulointerstitial nephritis.

Drug reactions
Antibiotics
  Beta-lactam antibiotics: methicillin, penicillin, ampicillin, cephalosporins
  Ciprofloxacin
  Erythromycin
  Sulfonamides
  Tetracycline
  Vancomycin
  Trimethoprim-sulfamethoxazole
  Ethambutol
  Rifampin
Nonsteroidal anti-inflammatory drugs
Diuretics
  Thiazides
  Furosemide
Miscellaneous
  Allopurinol
  Cimetidine
  Phenytoin
Systemic Infections
  Bacteria
    Streptococcus
    Corynebacterium diphtheriae
    Legionella
  Viruses
    Epstein-Barr virus
  Others
    Mycoplasma
    Rickettsia rickettsii
    Leptospira icterohaemorrhagiae
    Toxoplasma
Idiopathic
  Tubulointerstitial nephritis-uveitis (TIN-U)

NSAIDs. Other responsible drugs are rifampin, sulfonamides, thiazides and furosemide, and cimetidine.

B. Laboratory Findings: Common laboratory findings include gross or microscopic hematuria (95%) and peripheral blood eosinophilia (80%). Pyuria, proteinuria (usually < 1 g/24 h), eosinophiluria, and white blood cell casts occur less frequently. Either Hansel's stain or Wright's stain can be used to examine the urine for eosinophils. An inability to acidify the urine in association with hyperchloremic acidosis (ie, renal tubular acidosis) may indicate tubular damage. A finding of more than 1% eosinophils in the urine yields a sensitivity of 65% and a specificity of 95% for acute tubulointerstitial nephritis. In patients in whom the diagnosis is unclear, renal biopsy may be indicated.

C. Imaging: Ultrasound examination of the kidneys reveals normal-sized or enlarged kidneys with increased cortical echogenicity. Gallium scanning may show bilaterally increased uptake of the isotope by the kidneys, but this is a nonspecific finding.

Differential Diagnosis

A. Infection: Although uncomplicated bacterial pyelonephritis does not cause renal dysfunction, a number of systemic infections are associated with acute tubulointerstitial nephritis. Legionnaires' dis-

ease, Epstein-Barr virus infection, leptospirosis, mycoplasmal pneumonia, and Rocky Mountain spotted fever have been complicated by acute tubulointerstitial nephritis.

B. Other Drugs That Induce Nephropathies: The NSAIDs cause an allergic acute interstitial nephritis associated with the nephrotic syndrome. On biopsy, the glomerular lesion is minimal change disease with epithelial foot process fusion on electron microscopy. Typically absent are the findings of rash, fever, and eosinophilia. Patients with this entity tend to be older and have generally taken these drugs for a prolonged period of time (range: 2 weeks to 18 months). NSAIDs can also cause sodium retention and hyporeninemic hypoaldosteronism with hyperkalemia.

The clinical pattern of rifampin-induced tubulointerstitial nephritis is also somewhat different, with the onset of the renal failure occurring after rechallenge with the drug. Rifampin can also cause a direct proximal tubular injury and minimal change disease with nephrotic syndrome.

C. Idiopathic: There are individuals with acute tubulointerstitial nephritis for which no etiologic factors can be identified. One group composed chiefly of adolescent girls has tubulointerstitial nephritis and uveitis (so-called TIN-U syndrome) but there are no granulomas on renal biopsy or systemic evidence of sarcoidosis or other granulomatous diseases.

Treatment & Prognosis

Treatment consists of discontinuation of the offending drug. Acute dialytic therapy may be necessary in up to one-third of all patients with drug-induced acute interstitial nephritis before resolution of the disorder. Although there are no controlled clinical trials to support a beneficial effect, corticosteroids in high doses (eg, prednisone, 1 mg/kg/d for 4–8 weeks) are often administered if drug discontinuation does not result in return of renal function to baseline levels within a few days. Use of cytotoxic drugs such as cyclophosphamide is controversial and unproved.

Many patients with drug-induced acute tubulointerstitial nephritis will have complete recovery of renal function. However, a prolonged bout of acute renal failure and advanced age at onset are poor prognostic indicators for complete recovery.

CHRONIC TUBULOINTERSTITIAL NEPHRITIS

Essentials of Diagnosis
• Kidney size: small and contracted.
• Decreased urinary concentrating ability.
• Hyperchloremic metabolic acidosis.
• Hyperkalemia.
• Distal renal tubular acidosis (occasionally).

General Considerations

The causes of chronic tubulointerstitial nephritis are numerous (Table 22–11). The most common cause is prolonged obstruction of the urinary tract, followed by reflux nephropathy. Analgesic abuse can be associated with both renal failure and chronic tubulointerstitial nephritis, and its prevalence is often dependent on the region or country of residence. Environmental exposure to heavy metals—particularly lead and cadmium—may also be an important cause.

Clinical Findings

A. Symptoms and Signs: Polyuria and nocturia are the most frequent clinical complaints that occur because of an inability to concentrate the urine. Some individuals may also have a salt-wasting defect, putting them at risk for significant volume depletion following sodium restriction or the use of diuretics.

B. Laboratory Findings: As opposed to acute tubulointerstitial nephritis, urinalysis in chronic tubulointerstitial nephritis is essentially nonspecific, showing mild proteinuria, few cells, and broad granular casts. The most characteristic laboratory finding is evidence for tubular dysfunction (polyuria and sodium wasting) out of proportion to the degree of renal impairment and an inability to acidify the urine in association with hyperchloremic metabolic acidosis (eg, renal tubular acidosis).

Etiology

A. Obstructive Uropathy: In partial obstruction, urine output may alternate between polyuria and oliguria, and there may be evidence of distal tubular dysfunction (eg, a vasopressin-resistant concentrating defect). Azotemia and hypertension are usually present. The major clinical causes are renal stone disease, prostatic disease in older men, locally edematous carcinoma of the cervix in older women, and involvement of the retroperitoneum with other tumors or fibrosis. Although renal ultrasound is the most useful diagnostic screening test for revealing hydronephrosis, antegrade or retrograde pyelography may occasionally have to be done to confirm the diagnosis.

B. Reflux: Reflux nephropathy is primarily a disorder of childhood and occurs when urine passes retrograde from the bladder to the kidneys during voiding. Urine extravasates into the interstitium, an inflammatory response develops against either bacterial antigens or normal urinary components such as Tamm-Horsfall protein, and fibrosis results. Most of the damage occurs before the age of 5, but progressive renal deterioration continues as a result of the early insults. Focal glomerulosclerosis and hypertension are common sequelae.

Most individuals present as adolescents or young adults with hypertension, renal insufficiency, and a history of urinary tract infections as children. Pro-

teinuria (> 1 g/d) and a renal ultrasound or IVP showing renal scarring are frequently seen. Progression to end-stage renal disease is the rule.

C. Heavy Metals: Chronic exposure to lead over a number of years results in progressive azotemia and urinary concentrating defects. This disorder occurs among individuals with an occupational exposure (eg, among battery or smelter workers) or among "moonshine" whiskey drinkers who use automobile radiators to process their liquor. Associated with lead nephropathy is saturnine gout and hypertension. To diagnose lead nephropathy, an edetate (EDTA) test can be performed. Urinary excretion of more than 600 mg of lead in the 24 hours following an intravenous infusion of 1 g of EDTA indicates excessive lead exposure. Occupational exposure to cadmium can also result in chronic tubulointerstitial nephritis. These patients present clinically with proximal tubular dysfunction, hypercalciuria, and nephrolithiasis.

D. Analgesics: Analgesic nephropathy was initially felt to be a result of the ingestion of large quantities of analgesic combinations containing phenacetin. However, it is now believed to occur with prolonged ingestion of acetaminophen, particularly when taken in combination with aspirin and caffeine. This disorder occurs most frequently in women who abuse analgesics for chronic headaches, muscular pain, and arthritis. Many of these individuals deny or underestimate the quantity ingested. A cumulative analgesic intake of 3 kg or more or ingestion of 1 g/d for 3 years strongly supports a diagnosis of analgesic nephropathy.

Both acetaminophen, a phenacetin metabolite, and aspirin are concentrated in the kidney, particularly in the papillae and inner medulla. Acetaminophen is metabolized in the papillae by the prostaglandin hydroperoxidase pathway to reactive intermediates that bind covalently to interstitial cell macromolecules, causing necrosis. Salicylates and other NSAIDs may further the process by decreasing both glutathione levels (which can prevent covalent binding) and medullary blood flow by inhibition of prostaglandin synthesis.

Polyuria, nocturia, hematuria and proteinuria, hypertension, anemia (a consequence of gastrointestinal bleeding), and sterile pyuria are often present. If gross hematuria occurs as a consequence of papillary necrosis, sloughed papillae can frequently be found in the urine.

The IVP may be helpful. If papillary necrosis has occurred, dye will fill the area of the sloughed papillae, leaving a "ring shadow" sign at the papillary tip.

Differential Diagnosis

Because of the nonspecificity of many of the findings of chronic tubulointerstitial nephritis, it is easily mimicked by chronic glomerular diseases such as focal and segmental glomerulosclerosis. Likewise, systemic diseases with renal complications causing end-stage renal disease may simulate this disorder. Most glomerular diseases typically manifest heavy proteinuria on urinalysis even with the development of end-stage renal disease.

Treatment

Treatment depends first upon identifying the underlying disorder responsible for the renal dysfunction. Whether or not recovery of renal function is possible then depends on the degree of interstitial fibrosis that has developed. Once there is evidence for loss of parenchyma (small, shrunken kidneys), nothing will prevent the development of end-stage renal disease, and treatment is then directed toward management of medical complications.

If hydronephrosis is found, temporary or permanent relief of the obstruction should be undertaken since prolonged obstruction leads to tubular damage—particularly in the distal nephron—which may be irreversible even after the obstruction has been relieved. Medical treatment of the specific tubular dysfunction with potassium dietary restriction or sodium and bicarbonate supplements may be necessary if damage is irreversible. Neither surgical correction of reflux nor medical therapy with antibiotics prevents progressive deterioration of renal function once renal scarring has occurred.

For those suspected of having lead nephropathy in whom an EDTA test indicates excessive exposure to lead, treatment consists of ongoing chelation therapy as long as there is no evidence of marked interstitial fibrosis.

Treatment of analgesic nephropathy necessitates withdrawal of all analgesics. This measure may result in stabilization or improvement in renal function if significant interstitial fibrosis has not already resulted.

Dodd S: The pathogenesis of tubulointerstitial disease and mechanism of fibrosis. Curr Top Pathol 1995;88:51.

Fried T: Acute interstitial nephritis: Why do the kidneys suddenly fail? Postgrad Med 1993;93:105, 111, 117.

Hill GS: Tubulointerstitial nephritis and vasculitis. Curr Opin Nephrol Hypertension 1994;3:356.

Kleinknecht D: Interstitial nephritis, the nephrotic syndrome, and chronic renal failure secondary to non-steroidal anti-inflammatory drugs. Semin Nephrol 1995; 15:228.

CYSTIC DISEASES OF THE KIDNEY

Renal cysts are epithelium-lined cavities filled with fluid or semisolid material that develop primarily from renal tubular elements. One or more simple cysts are found in 50% of individuals over the age of 50, but they are rarely symptomatic and have little clinical significance. In contrast, generalized cystic diseases are associated with cysts scattered throughout the cortex and medulla of both kidneys.

The term "polycystic" applies to cysts present throughout the renal cortex and medulla; "medullary cystic" applies to those principally in the medullary and papillary regions of the kidney (Table 22–12).

1. SIMPLE OR SOLITARY CYSTS

Generally seen on the outer portion of the kidney cortex, simple cysts usually contain a clear fluid having a composition similar to that of an ultrafiltrate of plasma. Most simple cysts are found coincidentally on routine urographic examinations. These cysts occasionally become infected but usually remain asymptomatic. The major concern is to differentiate them from a malignant renal mass. Sonography and CT scanning are the recommended procedures for evaluating these cysts.

A simple cyst must meet all the following sonographic criteria to be considered benign: (1) echo-free, (2) smooth wall with good transmission of sound, and (3) an enhanced back wall. Complex cysts demonstrate (1) thick walls, (2) calcifications, (3) solid components, and (4) mixed echogenicity. On CT, renal cell carcinoma appears as a mass of low density (compared with the rest of the parenchyma), which enhances after intravenous contrast but still appears less dense than the rest of the parenchyma. Arteriography can also be used to evaluate the mass preoperatively. A renal cell carcinoma is hypervascular in 80% of cases; 15% are hypovascular and 5% avascular.

If a cyst meets the criteria for being benign, observation and periodic reappraisal is the standard of care. However, if the lesion is considered not consistent with a simple cyst or is a solid mass, surgical exploration is recommended.

2. AUTOSOMAL DOMINANT POLYCYSTIC KIDNEY DISEASE

This disorder exhibits autosomal dominant inheritance with nearly complete penetrance but with some variability of expression, since some individuals develop symptomatic disease by age 20 and others die late in life of unrelated problems. The defective gene is located on the short arm of chromosome 16. The disease causes renal insufficiency in 50% of individuals by age 70 years. It is among the five leading causes of renal failure in adults and accounts for 5–10% of dialysis patients in the USA.

Clinical Findings

Most patients present with episodes of abdominal

Table 22–12. Clinical features of renal cystic disease.

	Simple Renal Cysts	Acquired Renal Cysts	Autosomal Dominant Polycystic Kidney Disease	Medullary Sponge Kidney	Medullary Cystic Kidney
Prevalence	Common	Dialysis patients	1:1000	1:5000	Rare
Inheritance	None	None	Autosomal dominant	None	Autosomal dominant
Age at onset	...	...	20–40	40–60	Adulthood
Kidney size	Normal	Small	Large	Normal	Small
Cyst location	Cortex and medulla	Cortex and medulla	Cortex and medulla	Collecting ducts	Cortico-medullary junction
Hematuria	Occasional	Occasional	Common	Rare	Rare
Hypertension	None	Variable	Common	None	None
Associated complications	None	Adenocarcinoma in cysts	Urinary tract infections, renal stones, cerebral aneurysms 10–15%, hepatic cysts 40–60%	Renal stones, urinary tract infections	Polyuria, salt wasting
Renal failure	Never	Always	Frequently	Never	Always

or flank pain associated with microscopic or gross hematuria. A history of urinary tract infections and kidney stones is frequent. A positive family history can be obtained in 75% of cases. More than 50% will have hypertension (see below), which may antedate the diagnosis of the renal disease. All patients have large palpable kidneys that can often be appreciated by abdominal palpation. Indeed, the combination of hypertension and an abdominal mass should suggest the diagnosis. Forty to 50 percent have concomitant hepatic cysts. The urinalysis may show hematuria and mild proteinuria. The diagnosis is confirmed by ultrasonography, which shows more than five cysts scattered throughout the renal cortex and medulla of each kidney in an individual with a consistent family history. If the sonogram is equivocal, CT is recommended and is highly sensitive.

Complications & Treatment

A. Pain: Abdominal or flank pain is often caused by bleeding into cysts. Bed rest and analgesics are recommended.

B. Hematuria: Gross hematuria is usually due to rupture of a cyst into the renal pelvis, but it may also be caused by a renal stone or urinary tract infection, or in rare circumstances may be secondary to a malignancy. Bed rest, sedation, and hydration are recommended for a ruptured cyst.

C. Renal Infection: Patients presenting with flank pain, fever, and leukocytosis should be suspected of having an infected renal cyst. The urinalysis may be normal, since the cysts may not communicate directly with the urinary tract. A CT scan may be helpful, since an infected cyst may exhibit an increased wall thickness. Bacterial cyst infections are difficult to eradicate and often require at least

2 weeks of a parenteral bactericidal antibiotic followed by long-term oral therapy.

D. Nephrolithiasis: About 10–20% of patients have nephrolithiasis. Renal stones are typically composed of calcium oxalate. High fluid intake (2–3 L/d) is recommended.

E. Hypertension: Most patients will develop hypertension during the course of their disease, and 50% will have hypertension at the time of presentation. Its pathogenesis and treatment are the same as those of the renal disease, though diuretics should be used with caution since it is not known what effect these drugs have on the formation of renal cysts.

F. Cerebral Aneurysms: About 10–15% of patients have arterial aneurysms of the circle of Willis. Arteriography or CT scans are not recommended unless symptoms suggest cerebral hemorrhage. Patients also appear to have an increased incidence of aortic aneurysms and abnormalities of the mitral valve.

Prognosis

No medical therapy has been shown to prevent the development of renal failure, though treatment of hypertension and a low-protein diet may have a beneficial effect on the rate at which the disease progresses.

3. ACQUIRED POLYCYSTIC DISEASE

About 50% of patients treated by either hemodialysis or peritoneal dialysis for longer than 3 years show evidence of acquired polycystic kidney disease. Multiple cysts are found throughout the remnant kidneys, which in 5% of cases contain adenocarcinomas. Diagnosis is made by ultrasonography or CT scanning with contrast. Any suggestion of neoplasm necessitates nephrectomy even though these lesions are usually slow-growing ones. The cysts appear to regress in patients who have undergone successful renal transplantation and become nonazotemic.

4. JUVENILE NEPHRONOPHTHISIS & MEDULLARY CYSTIC DISEASE

These diseases appear to be analogous to inherited polycystic diseases. The childhood type, juvenile nephronophthisis, is probably an autosomal recessive disorder; and the type that appears primarily in adulthood, medullary cystic disease, appears to be an autosomal dominant process. In both cases, there are multiple small cysts at the corticomedullary junction. The kidneys are generally small, the cortex is reduced, and the glomeruli are sclerotic.

Clinical Findings

In juvenile nephronophthisis, there is usually a history of polydipsia, polyuria, pallor, lethargy, and growth retardation. End-stage renal disease occurs before age 20. In adults, medullary cystic disease causes similar symptoms except for growth retardation. Adults generally require large amounts of salt and water to prevent dehydration and volume depletion. Although ultrasonography and CT scan can be useful in making a diagnosis, an open renal biopsy that ensures recovery of tissue from the corticomedullary junction is definitive, though it may not be clinically necessary.

Treatment & Prognosis

There is no medical therapy that will prevent progression to renal failure. Adequate salt and water intake are essential to replenish what is lost through the kidneys. Both diseases progress to end-stage renal disease.

MEDULLARY SPONGE KIDNEY

This disease, though present at birth, is usually not diagnosed until the fourth or fifth decade. It is associated with a marked irregular enlargement of the medullary and interpapillary collecting ducts, giving a "Swiss cheese" appearance to the kidney in these regions.

Clinical Findings

Medullary sponge kidney presents with gross or microscopic hematuria, recurrent urinary tract infections, or nephrolithiasis with renal colic. The most common abnormalities are a decreased urinary con-

centrating ability, nephrocalcinosis, and, rarely, type I distal renal tubular acidosis (inability to acidify the urine maximally). The diagnosis is confirmed by intravenous pyelography, which shows striations in the papillary portions of the kidney produced by the accumulation of contrast in dilated collecting ducts.

Treatment

There is no known therapy. Adequate fluid intake (2 L/d) should be encouraged to prevent calcium stone formation. If hypercalciuria is present, a thiazide diuretic is recommended. Alkali therapy may be needed if renal tubular acidosis is present.

Prognosis

Renal function is well maintained unless there are complications from recurrent urinary tract infections and nephrolithiasis.

Fick GM, Gabow PA: Natural history of autosomal dominant polycystic kidney disease. Ann Rev Med 1994; 45:23. (Genetics, diagnosis, and natural history of the manifestations associated with polycystic kidney disease.)

Fick GM et al: Causes of death in autosomal dominant polycystic kidney disease. J Am Soc Nephrol 1995; 5:2048. (Review of the medical records of 129 patients dying with polycystic kidney disease between 1956 and 1993.)

Gabow PA: Autosomal dominant polycystic kidney disease. N Engl J Med 1993;329:332.

Martinez JR, Grantham JJ: Polycystic kidney disease: Etiology, pathogenesis and treatment. Dis Mon 1995 Nov;41:697. (Up-to-date review of the pathogenesis of cyst formation and etiology, diagnosis, management and prognosis of autosomal dominant and recessive polycystic kidney disease and acquired cystic kidney disease.)

MULTISYSTEM DISEASES WITH VARIABLE KIDNEY INVOLVEMENT

WEGENER'S GRANULOMATOSIS, POLYARTERITIS NODOSA, & ANTINEUTROPHIL CYTOPLASMIC AUTOANTIBODIES

Antineutrophil cytoplasmic autoantibodies have been described in some patients with necrotizing glomerulonephritis, with or without associated pulmonary hemorrhage, and in patients with active Wegener's granulomatosis. Wegener's granulomatosis is discussed in Chapter 20. Two types of antibodies have been described: one in which the staining is largely cytoplasmic and another in which staining is perinuclear. In addition to being potentially useful serologic tests for the diagnosis of these two disorders, the antibodies may be pathogenetically important in the development of some of the necrotizing lesions associated with the diseases.

Cees GM: Antineutrophil cytoplasmic antibody: A still growing class of autoantibodies in inflammatory disorders. Am J Med 1992;93:675.

Geffriaud-Ricouard C et al: Clinical spectrum associated with ANCA of defined antigen specificities in 98 selected patients. Clin Nephrol 1993;39:125. (The presence of ANCA is a good marker of vasculitis. The titer of ANCA is not correlated with the severity of vasculitis, and the disappearance of ANCA is almost always associated with absence of disease activity.)

Jennette JC, Falk RJ: The pathology of vasculitis involving the kidney. Am J Kidney Dis 1994;24:130.

SYSTEMIC LUPUS ERYTHEMATOSUS

Lupus nephritis is a serious complication of systemic lupus erythematosus (Chapter 20). Patients may present with either a nephrotic or a nephritic clinical picture since the urinalysis may correlate poorly with the histologic kidney findings and the severity of the glomerular disease. Renal biopsy is often done to identify the type and severity of disease. One of five possible types of renal biopsy patterns is present: I. normal, II. minimal or mesangial proliferative, III. focal and segmental proliferative, IV. diffuse proliferative, and V. membranous.

Individuals with type I or type II lupus nephritis require no treatment. Transformation of type I or type II to a more active lesion usually results in an increase in lupus serologic activity and evidence of deteriorating renal function (eg, rising serum creatinine, increasing proteinuria). Repeat biopsy in such individuals to confirm the transformation is the standard procedure. Individuals with type III or type IV lupus nephritis should receive aggressive immunosuppressive therapy. Therapy for individuals with type V lupus nephritis is unclear, though a trial of oral steroids is often used.

Serologic evidence of activity includes increased levels of antinuclear antibodies and antibodies to double-stranded DNA and reduced levels of C3, C4, and CH50. The best markers for following the activity of renal disease are the serum creatinine levels, urine protein excretion, and microscopic examination of the urinary sediment.

Oral steroids are of benefit in treating lupus nephritis. The addition of cytotoxic drugs appears to improve the outlook for long-term renal survival in those with type IV lupus nephritis.

Appel GB, Valeri A: The course and treatment of lupus nephritis. Ann Rev Med 1994;45:525. (Course of lupus nephritis and various treatments for it.)

Boumpas DT et al: Systemic lupus erythematosus: Emerging concepts. Part 1: Renal, neuropsychiatric, cardiovascular, pulmonary and hematologic disease. Ann Intern Med 1995;122:940.

Golbus J, McCone WJ: Lupus nephritis: Classification, prognosis, immunopathogenesis and treatment. Rheum Dis Clin North Am 1994;20:213.

DIABETIC NEPHROPATHY

Currently, diabetic nephropathy is the major cause of end-stage renal failure in the United States. Groups at high risk for developing nephropathy include males, blacks, and Native Americans. Approximately 35–45% of patients with type I and 20% of those with type II diabetes will require dialysis or transplantation.

The earliest changes in the kidneys resulting from diabetes mellitus are an increase in kidney size due to cellular hypertrophy and cellular proliferation and an increase (20–50%) in the glomerular filtration rate. Routine biochemical laboratory studies do not detect these abnormalities, and renal function appears normal. Treatment with ACE inhibitors for microalbuminuria, normalization of blood pressure, and strict glycemic control has been shown to prevent or slow the rate of progression to end-stage renal disease. See the detailed discussion of diabetic nephropathy in Chapter 27.

Individuals with diabetic nephropathy are more prone to have papillary necrosis, hyperkalemic urinary retention, and non-anion gap metabolic acidosis (type IV renal tubular acidosis) as a result of hyporeninemic hypoaldosteronism; susceptibility to acute renal failure after exposure to radiographic contrast agents also appears to be increased.

Bauer JH: Diabetic nephropathy: Can it be prevented? Are there real protective antihypertensive drugs of choice? South Med J 1994;87:1043.

Breyer JA: Medical management of nephrology in type I diabetes mellitus: Current recommendations. J Am Soc Nephrol 1995;6:1523. (Discussion of intensive glucose control, lowering of systemic blood pressure, use of ACE inhibitors for microalbuminuria, and new interventions such as aldose reductase inhibitors in slowing the progression of diabetic nephropathy.)

Lewis EJ et al: The effect of angiotensin-converting-enzyme inhibition on diabetic nephropathy. The Collaborative Study Group. N Engl J Med 1993;329:1456.

Materson BJ, Preston RA: Prevention of diabetic nephropathy. Hosp Pract 1997:32:129. (Reviews how normalization of blood pressure and use of ACE inhibitor or AT_1-receptor blockers for abnormal albumin or creatinine level can prevent or slow the rate of progression to end-stage renal disease.)

Perneger TV et al: End-stage renal disease attributable to diabetes mellitus. Ann Intern Med 1994;121:912.

Rossing P et al: Unchanged incidence of diabetic nephropathy in IDDM patients. Diabetes 1995;44:739.

DYSPROTEINEMIAS

Multiple Myeloma

Multiple myeloma is discussed in detail in Chapter 13. Renal involvement may occur as a result of the disease or as a consequence of complications arising during the course of the disease. The most important factor contributing to renal dysfunction is the presence of light chain immunoglobulins (Bence Jones proteinuria) in the urine. Bence Jones proteins may be directly nephrotoxic to the kidney tubules or may cause tubular obstruction by precipitating within the tubules. In about 10% of patients, glomerular amyloidosis complicates multiple myeloma, resulting in nephrotic syndrome, hypertension, and progressive renal insufficiency. The major component of the amyloid fibrils is the light chain immunoglobulin. Both hypercalcemia, which can cause polyuria, nephrocalcinosis, and nephrolithiasis, and hyperuricemia, which can cause uric acid stones, occur frequently with myeloma. Other conditions resulting in renal dysfunction include plasma cell infiltration of the renal parenchyma and a hyperviscosity syndrome associated with myeloma that can compromise renal blood flow.

Choukroun G, Varet B, Grunfeld JP: Multiple myeloma. Part I: Renal involvement. (Clinical Conference.) Nephron 1995;70:11.

Uchida M, Kamata K, Okubo M: Renal dysfunction in multiple myeloma. Internal Medicine 1995;34:364.

23   Urology

Joseph C. Presti, Jr., MD, Marshall L. Stoller, MD, & Peter R. Carroll, MD

UROLOGIC EVALUATION

HISTORY

Systemic Manifestations

Fever when associated with other symptoms of a urinary tract infection (see below) helps to localize the site of infection. In the female, high fevers occur in acute pyelonephritis. Fevers are not typical of uncomplicated cystitis. In the male, a febrile urinary tract infection implies acute pyelonephritis, acute prostatitis, or acute epididymitis. Fever may also be seen associated with malignancy of the kidney, bladder, or testis.

Weight loss and malaise also may be associated with tumor or disease states associated with chronic renal failure.

Pain

Pain in the genitourinary tract is usually associated with distention of a hollow viscus (ureteral obstruction, urinary retention) or the capsule of an organ (acute prostatitis, acute pyelonephritis). Pain may be local or referred. Pain associated with malignancy is usually a late manifestation and indicative of advanced disease.

A. Renal Pain: Pain of renal origin is usually located in the ipsilateral costovertebral angle. It may radiate to the umbilicus and may be referred to the ipsilateral testicle in men or the labium in women. In infection, the pain is typically constant, whereas in obstruction it may come and go. Nausea and vomiting may result from reflex stimulation of the celiac ganglion. Patients with intraperitoneal pathology will typically lie motionless to avoid pain, while patients with renal disease will move about to try to find a more comfortable position.

B. Ureteral Pain: Ureteral pain is usually acute and a result of obstruction. Distention of the ureter and possibly the renal capsule along with hyperperi-

stalsis and spasm of the smooth muscle of the ureter may result in two different pain patterns. The distention may cause a constant dull ache, while the spasms result in colic. The site of obstruction may sometimes be determined by the site of pain. Upper ureteral obstruction may result in pain referred to the scrotum in males or to the labium in females. Midureteral obstruction may cause pain in the lower quadrant and thus may be confused with appendicitis in right-sided ureteral obstruction or diverticulitis in left-sided ureteral obstruction. Lower ureteral obstruction may cause inflammation of the ureteral orifice and thus be associated with symptoms of vesical irritability.

C. Vesical Pain: Acute urinary retention results in severe suprapubic discomfort. Chronic urinary retention is usually painless despite tremendous vesical distention. Suprapubic pain not related to the act of micturition is rarely vesical in origin. Acute cystitis pain is usually referred to the distal urethra and is associated with the act of micturition.

D. Prostatic Pain: Prostatic pain is usually associated with inflammation and is located in the perineum. This pain may radiate to the lumbosacral spine, inguinal canals, or lower extremities. Because of its location near the bladder neck, inflammatory processes of the prostate may result in irritative voiding complaints.

E. Penile Pain: Pain in the flaccid penis is usually secondary to inflammatory processes caused by sexually transmitted diseases or paraphimosis, a condition of the uncircumcised male in which the retracted foreskin is trapped behind the glans penis, resulting in vascular congestion and painful swelling of the glans. Pain in the erect penis may be due to Peyronie's disease (fibrous plaque of the tunica albuginea, resulting in painful curvature of the erect penis) or to priapism (prolonged painful erection necessitating immediate intervention).

F. Testicular Pain: Acute conditions such as trauma, torsion of the testis or one of its appendices, or epididymo-orchitis cause acute pain within the scrotum with radiation to the ipsilateral groin. Chronic pain may persist for months following successful treatment of acute epididymitis. Chronic pain produced by a varicocele or hydrocele usually results in a dull "heaviness" without radiation. Disorders of the kidney, retroperitoneal structures, or inguinal canal may result in pain referred to the testis.

Hematuria

Gross hematuria in adults should be considered a sign of malignancy until proved otherwise.

The character of the hematuria may give a clue to the site of origin. **Initial hematuria,** the presence of blood at the beginning of the urinary stream that clears during the stream, implies an anterior (penile) urethral source. **Terminal hematuria,** the presence of blood at the end of the urinary stream, implies a bladder neck or prostatic urethral source. **Total hematuria,** the presence of blood throughout the urinary stream, implies a bladder or upper tract source.

Associated symptoms may give important clues as to the cause of hematuria. Hematuria associated with renal colic may imply a ureteral stone, yet the passage of blood clots from a bleeding renal tumor may mimic this scenario. Severe irritative voiding symptoms in a young woman may suggest an acute bacterial infection and associated hemorrhagic cystitis, yet the same scenario in an older woman or in any male must raise concerns for neoplasm. In any situation, if urine cultures are negative or symptoms fail to resolve after appropriate therapy, further evaluation is warranted. In the absence of other symptoms, gross hematuria may be more indicative of neoplasm, yet other disorders such as staghorn calculi, glomerulonephropathies, or polycystic kidney disease must be considered.

Irritative Voiding Symptoms

Urgency is the strong, sudden desire to void. It may be observed in inflammatory conditions such as cystitis or in hyperreflexic neuropathic conditions such as neurogenic bladders resulting from upper motor neuron lesions. **Dysuria** (painful urination) is usually associated with inflammation. The pain is typically referred to the tip of the penis in men or to the urethra in women. **Frequency** is the increased number of voids during the daytime, and **nocturia** is nocturnal frequency. Adults normally void five or six times a day and once or not at all during the nighttime hours. Increased numbers of voidings may result from increased urinary output or decreased functional bladder capacity. Diabetes mellitus, diabetes insipidus, excess fluid ingestion, and diuretics (including caffeine and alcohol) are a few of the causes of increased urinary output. Decreased functional bladder capacities may result from bladder outlet obstruction (increased residual urine volume results in a lower functional capacity), neurogenic bladder disorders (spasticity and reduced compliance), extrinsic bladder compression (uterine fibroids, radiation-in-duced fibrosis, pelvic neoplasms), or psychologic factors (anxiety).

Obstructive Voiding Symptoms

Hesitancy is a delay in the initiation of micturition. It results from the increased time required for the bladder to attain the high pressure necessary to exceed that of the urethra in the obstructed setting. **Decreased force of stream** results from the high resistance the bladder faces and is often associated with a decrease in caliber of the stream. **Intermittency** and **postvoid dribbling** are interruption of the urinary stream and the uncontrolled release of the terminal few drops of urine, respectively. Obstructive symptoms are most commonly due to benign prostatic hyperplasia, urethral stricture, or neurogenic bladder disorders. Less commonly, they may result from prostatic or urethral carcinoma or a foreign body.

Incontinence

Urinary incontinence is the involuntary loss of urine. The history permits subclassification into one of four categories of incontinence. Such a distinction is necessary, as the workup and treatment vary with each of the categories. With **total incontinence,** patients lose urine at all times and in all positions. **Stress incontinence** is the loss of urine associated with activities that result in an increase in intra-abdominal pressure (coughing, sneezing, lifting, exercising). The uncontrolled loss of urine that is preceded by a strong urge to void is known as **urge incontinence.** Chronic urinary retention may result in **overflow incontinence.**

Other Symptoms

Hematospermia, the presence of blood in the ejaculate, usually results from inflammation of the prostate or seminal vesicles. Blood in the initial portion of the ejaculate implicates the prostate, whereas terminal hematospermia implies a seminal vesicle origin. Workup should include urinalysis, digital rectal examination with prostate massage, and microscopic evaluation of the expressed prostatic secretions. More invasive procedures such as cystoscopy or transrectal ultrasound with prostate biopsy are reserved for patients with hematuria or abnormal rectal examinations, respectively. Persistent hematospermia warrants similar testing. The risk of malignancy with isolated hematospermia, normal urinalysis, and normal digital rectal examination remains low.

Pneumaturia, the presence of gas in the urine, is almost always secondary to a fistula between the bladder and the gastrointestinal tract. Diverticulitis, carcinoma of the bladder or sigmoid colon, and regional enteritis are some of the more common underlying causes.

Urethral discharge is the most common symptom of sexually transmitted diseases. Dysuria and urethral itching are commonly seen in association with the discharge. A bloody urethral discharge, especially in an elderly patient, suggests urethral carcinoma.

Cloudy urine may be secondary to a urinary tract infection, yet in the absence of infection it is commonly a result of an alkaline urinary pH. Such conditions result in phosphate crystal precipitation. Chyluria, the presence of lymph in the urine, results from a fistula between the urinary tract and the lymphatic system. Filariasis, tuberculosis, and retroperitoneal tumors are some of the possible causes of this rare symptom.

PHYSICAL EXAMINATION

General Examination

Inspection of the skin may reveal pallor associated with anemia. Cachexia may be seen in malignancy. Gynecomastia occurs in testicular carcinomas or may occur as a treatment-related complication of hormonal therapy in prostatic cancer. Hypertension can be a result of renovascular disease or adrenal cancer.

Detailed Examination

A. Kidney: Because of the liver, the right kidney is lower than the left. The lower pole of the right kidney may be palpable in thin patients, yet the left kidney is usually not palpable unless abnormally enlarged. To palpate the kidney, one hand is placed posteriorly in the costovertebral angle to push the kidney anteriorly, while the second hand is placed anteriorly under the costal margin. With inspiration, the kidney may be palpated between the two hands.

Auscultation of the upper abdominal quadrants in hypertensive patients may reveal a systolic bruit associated with renal artery stenosis or an arteriovenous malformation.

Patients presenting with flank pain should be tested for hyperesthesia of the overlying skin by pin testing, as this may be secondary to nerve root irritation and radiculitis rather than being of renal origin.

B. Bladder: The normal adult bladder is not palpable unless it is filled with at least 150 mL of urine. Percussion is better than palpation in diagnosing the distended bladder. Dullness is perceived over the full bladder and changes to tympany over the air-filled bowel.

Bimanual examination under anesthesia is critical in the evaluation of patients with bladder neoplasms. In the male, the bladder is palpated between the abdominal wall and the rectum while in the female it is palpated between the abdominal wall and the vagina. This is the best means of assessing vesical mobility and thus resectability.

C. Penis: The foreskin must be retracted in the uncircumcised male to permit inspection of the urethral meatus and glans. The position of the urethral meatus, the presence of urethral discharge, inflammation, penile tumor, and other skin lesions must be noted. In **phimosis,** the foreskin cannot be retracted over the glans. In **paraphimosis,** the foreskin has been left retracted behind the glans, resulting in painful engorgement and edema of the glans. If not attended to, this may result in glandular ischemia. Congenital anomalies of position of the urethral meatus are called **hypospadias** when the meatus is located on the ventral aspect of the penis, scrotum, or perineum and **epispadias** when it is located on the dorsal aspect of the penis. A thick yellow urethral discharge is seen in gonococcal urethritis, whereas a thin clear or white discharge is noted in nongonococcal urethritis. Palpation of the dorsal penile shaft for plaques of Peyronie's disease and of the ventral surface for urethral tumors should be performed.

D. Scrotum and Its Contents: The most common referral to the urologist involving the scrotum is for evaluation of a scrotal mass. It is thus critical to determine whether the lesion resides within the testicle or whether it is related to the epididymis or cord structures. The testes are palpated between the fingertips of both hands. Normal testes measure 6×4 cm and are rubbery in consistency. The epididymis normally rests posterolateral to the testis and varies in its degree of testicular attachment. Masses arising from within the testes are usually malignant, while those arising from the epididymis and spermatic cord structures are usually benign. Transillumination is critical to the evaluation of any scrotal mass and will distinguish between solid and cystic lesions.

The differential diagnosis of scrotal masses includes both benign and malignant processes. The history and physical examination can make the diagnosis in the majority of cases. Tumors of the testis are usually painless, firm, solid lesions within the substance of the testis. These lesions do not transilluminate.

Acute epididymitis is an acute infectious process of the epididymis and is associated with painful enlargement of the epididymis. Fever and irritative voiding symptoms are common. In advanced states, the infection can spread to the testis, making the distinction between the epididymis and the testicle difficult on physical examination. The entire scrotal contents may be painful on palpation, yet relief may be offered to the supine patient by elevation of the scrotum above the pubic symphysis (Prehn's sign).

A **hydrocele** is a collection of fluid between the two layers of the tunica vaginalis. The diagnosis is readily made by transillumination. Careful evaluation of the testis is necessary, as approximately 10% of testicular tumors may have an associated hydrocele.

A **varicocele** is engorgement of the internal spermatic veins above the testis. These almost always occur on the left side as the left spermatic vein empties into the left renal vein while the right spermatic vein empties into the inferior vena cava. Varicoceles should diminish in size or disappear with the patient in the supine position. The sudden onset of a right varicocele should raise the question of a retroperitoneal malignancy resulting in obstruction of the right spermatic vein.

Torsion of the testis typically occurs in the 10- to 20-year age group and presents with the acute onset of pain and swelling within the testis. Examination may reveal a painful testis that may have a "high lie" in relation to the other testis. The acute onset, lack of voiding symptoms, and the different age distribution may help distinguish it from epididymitis.

Torsion of the appendices of the testis or epididymis may be indistinguishable from torsion of the testis and affects a similar age group as torsion of the testis. On occasion a small palpable lump on the superior pole of the testis or epididymis is discernible that may appear blue when the skin is pulled tautly over it ("blue dot sign").

E. Rectal Examination in the Male: Rectal examinations should be performed with the patient bent over the examining table or in the knee-chest position. Inspection for anal pathology (fissures, warts, carcinoma, hemorrhoids) should be performed. Upon insertion of the finger, anal tone can be estimated and a bulbocavernosus reflex can be elicited. As the anal and urinary sphincter derive from a common innervation, important clues to neurogenic disorders may be obtained. The entire prostate is then examined, with attention being directed toward size and consistency. The normal prostate is approximately 4 × 4 cm and weighs 25 g. Normal consistency is that of the contracted thenar eminence with the thumb opposed to the little finger. Rubbery enlargement of the prostate is noted in benign prostatic hyperplasia. Induration may be perceived with carcinoma but also with chronic inflammation. The remainder of the rectum is then examined to exclude primary rectal disease.

F. Pelvic Examination in the Female: Examination of the introitus should include inspection for atrophic changes, ulcers, discharge, and warts. The urethral meatus can be inspected for caruncles and palpated for tumors or diverticula. Bimanual examination of the bladder, uterus, and adnexa should be performed with two fingers in the vagina and one hand on the abdomen, and attention is directed toward abnormal masses.

URINALYSIS

Collection of Specimens

In the male patient, a clean-catch urine is obtained in separate aliquots. Such a scheme may permit localization of disease. The first 5–10 mL is collected and represents the urethral specimen (VB-1, or voided bladder 1). An aliquot of the midstream specimen (VB-2) represents the bladder and upper urinary tracts. If necessary, the prostate is then massaged and the expressed prostatic secretions are collected. If no fluid is obtained, the next 2–3 mL of urine are collected (VB-3), which reflects the prostate.

Dipstick Urinalysis

A. pH: There is no role for dipstick urinalysis screening for urinary tract disorders in asymptomatic adults except for pregnant women. Urinary pH (range 5.0–9.0) may be helpful in the diagnosis and treatment of some urologic conditions. Alkaline urine in a patient with a urinary tract infection suggests the presence of a urea-splitting organism, most commonly *Proteus mirabilis,* though some strains of *Klebsiella, Pseudomonas, Providencia,* and *Staphylococcus* may also produce urease. Acidic urine in a patient with urolithiasis suggests uric acid or cystine stones. Failure to acidify the urine below a pH of 5.5 despite a metabolic acidosis suggests a distal renal tubular acidosis.

B. Protein: Dipsticks using bromphenol blue can detect protein in concentrations exceeding 10 mg/dL. It measures albumin and is not sensitive for the light chain of immunoglobulins (Bence Jones proteins). False-positive results are seen in urine containing numerous leukocytes or epithelial cells. (See Proteinuria in Chapter 22.)

C. Urobilinogen and Bilirubin: Urobilinogen is formed from the catabolism of conjugated bilirubin in the gut by bacteria, and the majority is cleared by the liver. Normally, only 1–4 mg of urobilinogen is excreted in the urine per day. Hemolytic processes or hepatocellular disease can lead to increased urinary levels, while complete biliary obstruction or broad-spectrum antibiotics that alter the gut bacterial flora may result in absent urinary urobilinogen. Unconjugated bilirubin is not filtered by the glomerulus, while only 1% of conjugated bilirubin is filtered. Normally no bilirubin is detected by urinary dipstick, since only concentrations greater than 0.4 mg/dL are detectable. Conditions manifesting elevated conjugated bilirubin in the serum will result in higher urinary levels. Ascorbic acid may cause false-negative results, while phenazopyridine may cause false-positive results.

D. Glucose and Ketones: Only small amounts of glucose are normally excreted in the urine, and these levels are below the sensitivity of the dipstick. Any positive finding requires medical evaluation to exclude diabetes mellitus. The test is specific for glucose and does not cross-react with any other sugars. Ascorbic acid or elevated ketones may result in false-negative results.

Ketones are not normally found in the urine, but fasting, postexercise states, and pregnancy may result in elevated urinary ketones. Diabetics often demonstrate elevated urinary ketone levels prior to an elevation in serum levels. False-positive results may occur in dehydration or in the presence of levodopa metabolites, mesna (sodium mercaptoethanesulfonate), and other sulfhydryl-containing compounds.

E. Nitrites: Normally, the urine does not contain nitrites. Many gram-negative bacteria can reduce nitrate to nitrite, which is thus an indicator of bacteriuria. However, the low sensitivity of the test requires clarification. Adequate numbers of bacteria must be present (10^5 organisms/mL), nitrates must be available in the urine, and the bacteria must be in contact with the urine for a sufficient time (usually 4 hours). Therefore, the first morning voided sample is preferable. False-negative results may be due to non-nitrate-reducing organisms, frequent urination, dilute or acidic urine (pH < 6.0), and the presence of urobilinogen. False-positive results are usually secondary to contaminated specimens, so that bacteria are indeed present in the sample yet not present in the urinary tract.

F. Leukocyte Esterase: Leukocyte esterase is an enzyme produced by white cells. The dipstick test is thus a means of detecting leukocytes in the urine, which is thus suggestive but not diagnostic for bacteria. False-positive tests result from specimen contamination. False-negative tests result from high specific gravity, glycosuria, the presence of urobilinogen, and medications, including rifampin, phenazopyridine, and ascorbic acid.

G. Blood: The urinary dipstick for blood measures intact erythrocytes, free hemoglobin, and myoglobin. False-positive results in women may occur as a result of contamination at collection with menstrual blood. Concentrated urine may also cause a false-positive result, as patients normally excrete 1000 erythrocytes per milliliter of urine. Vigorous exercise and vitamins or foods associated with high oxidant levels may also give a false-positive result. High ascorbic acid levels may give a false-negative result.

Microscopic Urinalysis

A. Leukocytes: The presence of more than five leukocytes per high-power field is considered significant pyuria. Leukocytes in the urine are indicative of injury to the urinary tract, which may or may not be due to infection. Other causes of pyuria include calculous disease, stricture disease, neoplasm, glomerulonephropathy, or interstitial cystitis. Leukocyte counts will vary by the state of hydration, method of collection, and degree of injury to the urinary tract.

B. Erythrocytes: The presence of more than five erythrocytes per high-power field is considered significant and warrants further investigation. (See Evaluation of Hematuria, below.) The appearance of the red cells sometimes gives a clue to their origin within the urinary tract. Dysmorphic (irregularly shaped) cells have an uneven distribution of hemoglobin and cytoplasm. Such cells tend to favor glomerular origin and have dysmorphic features as a consequence of passage through the nephron. Red cells that are round, with evenly distributed hemoglobin, are epithelial in origin and suggest disease along the epithelial lining of the urinary tract. All patients with hematuria require further diagnostic workup (see below); morphology, though of interest, is not of sufficient accuracy to allow firm diagnostic conclusions.

C. Epithelial Cells: The presence of squamous epithelial cells in the urinary sediment is indicative of contamination and thus requires a repeat collection. Transitional epithelial cells are occasionally noted in normal urinary sediment, but if present in large numbers or clumps they cause concern about possible neoplasm. Experienced cytopathologists are necessary to confirm the finding.

D. Bacteria and Yeasts: The identification of organisms in an uncontaminated specimen implies infection, which must be confirmed by culture. The presence of several organisms per high-power field usually correlates with a culture count of 10^5 organisms per milliliter. Gram staining may further aid in characterizing the organism. *Candida albicans* is the most common yeast seen in the urine, and characteristic budding and clumps are typically observed.

E. Casts: Casts are formed in the distal tubules and collecting ducts as a result of Tamm-Horsfall mucoprotein precipitation. Casts tend to congregate near the edges of the coverslip and are detected best in a fresh specimen viewed under low power. If devoid of cells, hyaline casts are formed. Casts with entrapped red cells are indicative of glomerulonephritis or vasculitis. Leukocyte casts are suggestive of pyelonephritis. Epithelial casts in small numbers are considered normal, but in large numbers they suggest intrinsic renal disease. Granular casts result from degeneration of other cellular casts and also suggest intrinsic renal disease.

F. Crystals: Uric acid, oxalate, and cystine crystals are more often precipitated in acid urine, while phosphate crystals are more commonly seen in alkaline urine. The presence of uric acid, phosphate, and oxalate crystals can be seen in normal patients as well as in stone-formers. Cystine crystals, with a characteristic hexagonal benzene ring shape, are seen only in patients with cystinuria and are thus pathologic.

Pels RJ et al: Dipstick urinalysis screening of asymptomatic adults for urinary tract disorders. II. Bacteriuria. JAMA 1989;262:1221. (Screening recommended only for pregnant women.)

Press SM et al: Incidence of negative hematuria in patients with acute urinary lithiasis presenting to the emergency room with flank pain. Urology 1995;45:753. (Five percent of patients with acute urinary lithiasis had negative dipstick and microscopic urine evaluations.)

Woolhandler S et al: Dipstick urinalysis screening of asymptomatic adults for urinary tract disorders. I. Hematuria and proteinuria. JAMA 1989;262:1215. (A controlled trial of hematuria screening is needed. Proteinuria screening is not recommended in the healthy adult population, since less than 1.5% of dipstick-positive patients have serious treatable disease.)

EVALUATION OF HEMATURIA

Evaluation begins with a history and physical examination. If gross hematuria occurs, a description of the timing (initial, terminal, total) may give a clue to the localization of disease. Associated symptoms (ie, renal colic, irritative voiding symptoms, constitutional symptoms) should be investigated. Drug ingestion and associated medical problems may also provide diagnostic clues. Anticoagulants, analgesic abuse (papillary necrosis), cyclophosphamide (chemical cystitis), antibiotics (interstitial nephritis), diabetes mellitus, sickle cell trait or disease (papillary necrosis), a history of stone disease, or malignancy should all be investigated. The presence of hematuria in patients on anticoagulation therapy warrants a complete evaluation consisting of upper tract imaging, cystoscopy, and urine cytology.

Physical examination should emphasize signs of systemic disease (fever, rash, lymphadenopathy, abdominal or pelvic masses) as well as signs of medical renal disease (hypertension, volume overload). Urologic evaluation may demonstrate an enlarged prostate, flank mass, or urethral disease.

Initial laboratory investigations include a urinalysis and urine culture. Proteinuria and casts suggest renal origin. Irritative voiding symptoms, bacteriuria, and a positive urine culture in the female suggest urinary tract infection, but follow-up urinalysis is important after treatment to ensure resolution of the hematuria.

Further evaluation includes urinary cytology, upper tract imaging, and cystoscopy. Cytology especially assists in the diagnosis of bladder neoplasm, and three voided samples are recommended to maximize sensitivity. Upper tract imaging (usually an intravenous urogram) may identify neoplasms of the kidney or ureter as well as identifying benign conditions such as urolithiasis, obstructive uropathy, papillary necrosis, medullary sponge kidney, or polycystic kidney disease. The role of ultrasonographic evaluation of the urinary tract for hematuria is unclear. While it may provide adequate information for the kidney, its sensitivity in detecting ureteral disease may be lower. In addition, its higher degree of operator dependence may further confound the issue. Cystoscopy can assess for bladder or urethral neoplasm, benign prostatic enlargement, and radiation or chemical cystitis. For gross hematuria, cystoscopy is ideally performed while the patient is actively bleeding to allow better localization (ie, lateralize to one side of the upper tracts, bladder, or urethra).

In patients with gross or microscopic hematuria, an upper tract source (kidneys and ureters) can be identified in 10% of cases. For upper tract sources, stone disease accounts for 42%, medical renal disease (medullary sponge kidney, glomerulonephritis, papillary necrosis) for 19%, renal cell carcinoma for 10%, and transitional cell carcinoma of the ureter or renal pelvis for 7%. In the absence of infection, gross hematuria from a lower tract source is most commonly from transitional cell carcinoma of the bladder. Microscopic hematuria in the male is most commonly from benign prostatic hyperplasia. In patients with negative evaluations, repeat evaluations are warranted to avoid a missed malignancy; however, the ideal frequency of such evaluations is not defined. Urinary cytology can be repeated in 3–6 months, and cystoscopy and upper tract imaging may be repeated in 1 year.

Culclasure TF et al: The significance of hematuria in the anticoagulated patient. Arch Intern Med 1994;154:649. (Anticoagulation at currently recommended levels does not predispose patients to hematuria.)

Hiatt RA, Ordonez JD: Dipstick urinalysis screening, asymptomatic microhematuria, and subsequent urological cancers in a population-based sample. Cancer Epidemiol Biomarkers Prev 1994;3:439. (A retrospective review of over 20,000 asymptomatic adults screened by dipstick urinalysis demonstrated a positive predictive value of 0.5% in the detection of urologic malignancy.)

Messing EM et al: Hematuria home screening: Repeat testing results. J Urol 1995;154:57. (Bladder cancer has a brief preclinical duration, and testing must be repeated annually for screening to provide early detection.)

GENITOURINARY TRACT INFECTIONS

Urinary tract infections are among the most common entities encountered in medical practice. In acute infections, a single pathogen is usually found, whereas two or more pathogens are often seen in chronic infections. Coliform bacteria are responsible for most nonnosocomial, uncomplicated urinary tract infections, with *E coli* being the most common. Such infections typically are sensitive to a wide variety of orally administered antibiotics and respond quickly. Nosocomial infections often are due to more resistant pathogens and may require parenteral antibiotics. Renal infections are of particular concern because if they are inadequately treated, loss of renal function may result. Previously, a colony count $> 10^5$/mL was considered the criterion for urinary tract infection. However, it is now recognized that up to 50% of women with symptomatic infections have lower counts. In addition, the presence of pyuria correlates poorly with the diagnosis of urinary tract infection, and thus urinalysis alone is not adequate for diagnosis. With respect to treatment, soft tissue infections (pyelonephritis, prostatitis) require intensive therapy for 3–4 weeks, while mucosal infections (cystitis) may require 1–3 days of therapy.

Classification & Pathogenesis

First infections—ie, first documented infections—in young women tend to be uncomplicated. **Unresolved bacteriuria** occurs when the urinary tract is never sterilized during therapy. This may result from bacterial resistance to therapy, noncompliance, mixed infections with organisms having different susceptibilities, renal insufficiency, or the rapid emergence of resistance from an initially sensitive organism. **Persistent bacteriuria** occurs when the urinary tract is initially sterilized during therapy but a persistent source of infection in contact with the urinary tract remains. This may result from infected stones, chronic pyelonephritis or prostatitis, vesicoenteric or vesicovaginal fistulas, obstructive uropathy, foreign bodies, or urethral diverticula. **Reinfections** occur when new infections with new pathogens occur following successful treatment.

Ascending infection from the urethra is the most common route. Women are particularly at risk for urinary tract infections because the female urethra is short and the vagina becomes colonized with bacteria. Sexual intercourse is a major precipitating factor in young women and the use of diaphragms and spermicidal creams (alters normal vaginal bacterial flora) further increases the risk for cystitis. Pyelonephritis most commonly results from ascent of infection up the ureter. **Hematogenous spread** to the urinary tract is uncommon, with the exceptions being tuberculosis and cortical renal abscesses. **Lymphogenous spread** is rare. **Direct extension** from other organs may occur, especially from intraperitoneal abscesses in inflammatory bowel disease or pelvic inflammatory disease.

Susceptibility Factors

A. Bacterial Virulence Factors: Over 90% of first infections are caused by *E coli*. While there are over 150 strains of *E coli*, most infections are caused by only five serogroups (O1, O4, O6, O18, and O75). It appears that strains implicated in infection have a higher degree of bacterial adherence, which is mediated by the bacterial fimbriae or pili. A relationship between the type of fimbriae and the type of infection exists. P-fimbriated strains of *E coli* are associated with pyelonephritis in normal urinary tracts, whereas strains without P fimbriae are associated with pyelonephritis only when vesicoureteral reflux is present.

B. Host Susceptibility Factors:

1. Bladder and upper tract factors—Intrinsic defense mechanisms in the bladder include efficient emptying of the bladder with voiding, which decreases colony counts; a protective glycosaminoglycan layer, which interferes with bacterial adherence; and the antimicrobial properties of urine (high osmolality and extremes of pH). The presence of vesi-

coureteral reflux, diminished renal blood flow, or intrinsic renal disease may increase the likelihood of upper tract involvement.

2. Female-specific factors—The anatomically short female urethra facilitates the ascent of organisms from the introitus into the bladder. Women with recurrent urinary tract infections have more adhesin receptors on their genitourinary mucosa and therefore have more binding sites for pathogens. Women whose mucosal secretions lack fucosyltransferase activity ("nonsecretors") are more prone to urinary tract infections. The lack of this enzyme results in lack of expression of the A, B, and H blood group antigens that normally may mask some of the bacterial adhesin receptors, making these receptors more available for pathogen binding.

3. Male-specific factors—A higher incidence of urinary tract infections in the uncircumcised male in comparison to the circumcised male has been observed. The mucosal surface of the foreskin has a propensity for colonization with P-fimbriated bacteria in a fashion analogous to that of the female introitus. The prostate in normal males secretes zinc, which is a potent antibacterial agent and thus prevents ascending infection. Lower zinc levels are seen in prostatic secretions of men with bacterial prostatitis.

Prevention of Reinfections

Prophylactic antibiotic therapy is given to prevent recurrence after treatment of urinary tract infection.

Women who have more than three episodes of cystitis per year are considered candidates for prophylaxis. Prior to institution of therapy, a thorough urologic evaluation is warranted to exclude any anatomic abnormality (stones, reflux, fistula, etc). Only selected antimicrobial agents are effective in prophylaxis. To be successful, the agent must eliminate pathogenic bacteria from the fecal or introital reservoirs and not cause bacterial resistance. Single dosing at bedtime or at the time of intercourse is the recommended schedule. The three most commonly used agents for prophylaxis are trimethoprim-sulfamethoxazole (40 mg/200 mg), nitrofurantoin (100 mg), and cephalexin (250 mg).

Hooton TM: A simplified approach to urinary tract infection. Hosp Pract (Off Ed) 1995 Feb;30:23.

Sanderson PJ: Preventing hospital acquired urinary and respiratory infection. Brit Med J 1995;310:1452.

Stamm WE, Hooton TM: Management of urinary tract infections in adults. N Engl J Med 1993;329:1328.

ACUTE CYSTITIS

Essentials of Diagnosis

- Irritative voiding symptoms.
- Patient usually afebrile.
- Positive urine culture.

General Considerations

Acute cystitis is an infection of the bladder most commonly due to the coliform bacteria (especially *E coli*) and occasionally gram-positive bacteria (enterococci). Viral cystitis due to adenovirus is sometimes seen in children but is rare in adults. The route of infection is typically ascending from the urethra.

Clinical Findings

A. Symptoms and Signs: Irritative voiding symptoms are common (frequency, urgency, dysuria) as well as suprapubic discomfort. Women may demonstrate gross hematuria, and symptoms in women may often appear following sexual intercourse. Physical examination may elicit suprapubic tenderness, but examination is often unremarkable. Systemic toxicity is absent.

B. Laboratory Findings: Urinalysis shows pyuria and bacteriuria and varying degrees of hematuria. The degree of pyuria and bacteriuria does not necessarily correlate with the severity of symptoms. Urine culture is positive for the offending organism, but colony counts exceeding 10^5/mL are not essential for the diagnosis.

C. Imaging: Follow-up imaging is warranted only if pyelonephritis, recurrent infections, or anatomic abnormalities are suspected.

Differential Diagnosis

In women, infectious processes such as vulvovaginitis and pelvic inflammatory disease can usually be distinguished by pelvic examination and urinalysis. In men, urethritis and prostatitis may be distinguished by physical examination (urethral discharge or prostatic tenderness). Cystitis in men is rare and implies a pathologic process such as infected stones, prostatitis, or chronic urinary retention requiring further investigation.

Noninfectious causes of cystitis-like symptoms include pelvic irradiation, chemotherapy (cyclophosphamide), bladder carcinoma, interstitial cystitis, voiding dysfunction disorders, and psychosomatic disorders.

Treatment

Uncomplicated cystitis in women can be treated with short-term antimicrobial therapy, which consists of single-dose therapy or 1–3 days of therapy. Trimethoprim-sulfamethoxazole or cephalexin is often effective (Table 23–1). Because uncomplicated cystitis is rare in men, elucidation of the underlying problem with appropriate investigations is warranted. Hot sitz baths or urinary analgesics (phenazopyridine, 200 mg orally three times daily) may provide symptomatic relief.

Prognosis

Infections typically respond rapidly to therapy, and failure to respond suggests resistance to the se-

lected drug or anatomic abnormalities requiring further investigation.

Farland M: Urinary tract infection: How has its management changed? Postgrad Med 1993;93:71.

Hanno PM: Diagnosis of interstitial cystitis. Urol Clin North Am 1994;21:63. (Volume devoted to various aspects of this controversial entity.)

Hooton TM et al: Randomized comparative trial and cost analysis of 3-day antimicrobial regimens for treatment of acute cystitis in women. JAMA 1995;273:41. (A 3-day regimen of trimethoprim-sulfamethoxazole is more effective and less expensive than 3-day regimens of nitrofurantoin, cefadroxil, or amoxicillin for treatment of uncomplicated cystitis in women.)

ACUTE PYELONEPHRITIS

Essentials of Diagnosis

- Fever.
- Flank pain.
- Irritative voiding symptoms.
- Positive urine culture.

General Considerations

Acute pyelonephritis is an infectious inflammatory disease involving the kidney parenchyma and renal pelvis. Gram-negative bacteria are the most common causative agents including *E coli, Proteus, Klebsiella, Enterobacter,* and *Pseudomonas.* Gram-positive bacteria are less commonly seen, including *Enterococcus faecalis* and *Staphylococcus aureus.* The infection usually ascends from the lower urinary tract—with the exception of *S aureus,* which usually is spread by a hematogenous route.

Clinical Findings

A. Symptoms and Signs: Symptoms include fever, flank pain, shaking chills, and irritative voiding symptoms (urgency, frequency, dysuria). Nausea and vomiting and diarrhea are not uncommon. Signs include fever and tachycardia. Costovertebral angle tenderness is usually pronounced.

B. Laboratory Findings: Complete blood count shows leukocytosis and a left shift. Urinalysis shows pyuria, bacteriuria, and varying degrees of hematuria. White cell casts may be seen. Urine culture demonstrates heavy growth of the offending agent.

C. Imaging: In complicated pyelonephritis, renal ultrasound may show hydronephrosis from a stone or other source of obstruction.

Differential Diagnosis

Acute intra-abdominal disease such as appendicitis, cholecystitis, pancreatitis, or diverticulitis must be distinguished from pyelonephritis. A normal urinalysis is usually seen in gastrointestinal disorders; however, on occasion, inflammation from adjacent

Table 23–1. Empirical therapy for urinary tract infections.

Diagnosis	Antibiotic	Route	Duration	Cost per Duration Noted[1]
Acute pyelonephritis	Ampicillin, 1 g every 6 hours, and gentamicin, 1 mg/kg every 8 hours	IV	21 days	$333.37
	Trimethoprim-sulfamethoxazole, 160/800 mg every 12 hours	Orally	21 days	$8.40
	Ciprofloxacin, 750 mg every 12 hours	Orally	21 days	$242.76
	Ofloxacin, 200–300 mg every 12 hours	Orally	21 days	$164.64
Chronic pyelonephritis	Same as for acute pyelonephritis, but duration of therapy is 3–6 months.			
Acute cystitis	Trimethoprim-sulfamethoxazole, 160/800 mg, two tablets	Orally	Single dose	$0.40
	Cephalexin, 250–500 mg every 6 hours	Orally	1–3 days	$12.00/3 days (500 mg)
	Ciprofloxacin, 250–500 mg every 12 hours	Orally	1–3 days	$20.52/3 days (500 mg)
	Nitrofurantoin (Macrocrystals), 100 mg every 12 hours	Orally	7 days	$15.82
	Norfloxacin, 400 mg every 12 hours	Orally	1–3 days	$16.74/3 days
	Ofloxacin, 200 mg every 12 hours	Orally	1–3 days	$19.80/3 days
Acute bacterial prostatitis	Same as for acute pyelonephritis		21 days	
Chronic bacterial prostatitis	Trimethoprim-sulfamethoxazole, 160/800 mg every 12 hours	Orally	1–3 months	$12.00/1 month
	Ciprofloxacin, 250–500 mg every 12 hours	Orally	1–3 months	$217.00/1 month (400 mg)
	Ofloxacin, 200–400 mg every 12 hours	Orally	1–3 months	$248.40/1 month (100 mg)
Acute epididymitis Sexually transmitted	Ceftriaxone, 250 mg as single dose, plus: Doxycycline, 100 mg every 12 hours	IM Orally	10 days	$11.50/250 mg $8.00
Non-sexually transmitted	Same as for chronic bacterial prostatitis.	Orally	3 weeks	

[1]Cost to pharmacist (average wholesale price) for treatment, duration noted (generic when possible). Source: First Data Bank, Price Alert, April 1997.

bowel (appendicitis or diverticulitis) may result in hematuria or pyuria. Abnormal liver function tests or elevated amylase levels may assist in the differentiation. Lower lobe pneumonia is distinguishable by the abnormal chest radiograph.

In the male patient, the main differential diagnosis for a febrile urinary tract infection includes acute epididymitis, acute prostatitis, and acute pyelonephritis. Physical examination and the location of the pain should permit this distinction.

Complications

Sepsis with shock can occur with acute pyelonephritis. In diabetics, emphysematous pyelonephritis resulting from gas-producing organisms may

be fatal if not adequately treated. Healthy adults usually recover complete renal function, yet if coexistent renal disease is present, scarring or chronic pyelonephritis may result. Inadequate therapy could result in abscess formation.

Treatment

Severe infections or complicating factors require hospital admission. Urine and blood cultures are obtained to identify the causative agent and to determine antimicrobial sensitivity. Intravenous ampicillin and an aminoglycoside are initiated prior to obtaining sensitivity results (Table 23–1). In the outpatient setting, trimethoprim-sulfamethoxazole or quinolones may be initiated (Table 23–1). Antibiotics are adjusted according to sensitivities. Fevers may persist for up to 72 hours; failure to respond warrants radiographic imaging (ultrasound) to exclude complicating factors that may require prompt intervention. Catheter drainage may be necessary in the face of urinary retention, and nephrostomy drainage may be required if there is ureteral obstruction. In inpatients, intravenous antibiotics are maintained for 24 hours after the patient defervesces, and oral antibiotics are then given to complete a 3-week course of therapy. Follow-up urine cultures are mandatory several weeks following the completion of treatment.

Prognosis

With prompt diagnosis and appropriate treatment, acute pyelonephritis carries a good prognosis. Complicating factors, underlying renal disease, and increasing patient age may lead to a less favorable outcome.

Behr MA et al: Fever duration in hospitalized acute pyelonephritis patients. Am J Med 1996;101:277. (Fever in treated pyelonephritis can take 4 days to resolve, and routine urologic investigation after 2–3 days of fever may be unwarranted.)

Bergeron MG: Treatment of pyelonephritis in adults. Med Clin North Am 1995;79:619. (A general review.)

Boam WD, Miser WF: Acute focal bacterial pyelonephritis. Am Fam Physician 1995;52:919. (Sometimes referred to as focal lobar nephronia, this is a focal infection of the kidney that may lead to renal abscess.)

Caceres VM et al: The clinical utility of a day of hospital observation after switching from intravenous to oral antibiotic therapy in the treatment of pyelonephritis. J Fam Pract 1994;39:337. (In a retrospective review of 138 adults hospitalized for acute pyelonephritis, the need for continued hospitalization following the conversion from intravenous to oral antibiotics was assessed. The limited usefulness of such a practice was demonstrated, since less than 5% of patients experienced a relapse.)

ACUTE BACTERIAL PROSTATITIS

Essentials of Diagnosis

- Fever.
- Irritative voiding symptoms.
- Perineal or suprapubic pain; exquisite tenderness common on rectal examination.
- Positive urine culture.

General Considerations

Acute bacterial prostatitis is usually caused by gram-negative rods, especially *E coli* and *Pseudomonas* species and less commonly by gram-positive organisms (eg, *Enterococcus*). The most likely routes of infection include ascent up the urethra and reflux of infected urine into the prostatic ducts. Lymphatic and hematogenous routes are probably rare.

Clinical Findings

A. Symptoms and Signs: Perineal, sacral, or suprapubic pain, fever, and irritative voiding complaints are common. Varying degrees of obstructive symptoms may occur as the acutely inflamed prostate swells, which may lead to urinary retention. High fevers and a warm and tender prostate are detected on examination. Care should be taken in performing a gentle rectal examination, as vigorous manipulations may result in septicemia. Prostatic massage is contraindicated.

B. Laboratory Findings: Complete blood count shows leukocytosis and a left shift. Urinalysis shows pyuria, bacteriuria, and varying degrees of hematuria. Urine cultures will demonstrate the offending pathogen.

Differential Diagnosis

Acute pyelonephritis or acute epididymitis should be distinguishable by the location of pain as well as by physical examination. Acute diverticulitis is occasionally confused with acute prostatitis; however, the history and urinalysis should permit clear distinction. Urinary retention from benign or malignant prostatic enlargement is distinguishable by initial or follow-up rectal examination.

Treatment

Hospitalization is usually required and parenteral antibiotics (ampicillin and aminoglycoside) should be initiated until organism sensitivities are available (Table 23–1). After the patient is afebrile for 24–48 hours, oral antibiotics (trimethoprim-sulfamethoxazole or quinolones) are used to complete 4–6 weeks of therapy. If urinary retention develops, urethral catheterization or instrumentation is contraindicated, and a percutaneous suprapubic tube is required. Follow-up urine culture and examination of prostatic secretions should be performed after the completion of therapy to ensure eradication.

Prognosis

With effective treatment, chronic bacterial prostatitis is rare.

CHRONIC BACTERIAL PROSTATITIS

Essentials of Diagnosis

- Irritative voiding symptoms.
- Perineal or suprapubic discomfort, often dull and poorly localized.
- Positive expressed prostatic secretions and culture.

General Considerations

Although chronic bacterial prostatitis may evolve from acute bacterial prostatitis, many men have no history of acute infection. Gram-negative rods are the most common etiologic agents, but only one gram-positive organism *(Enterococcus)* is associated with chronic infection. Routes of infection are the same as discussed for acute infection.

Clinical Findings

A. Symptoms and Signs: Clinical manifestations are variable. Some patients are asymptomatic, but most have varying degrees of irritative voiding symptoms. Low back and perineal pain is not uncommon. Many patients report a history of urinary tract infections. Physical examination is often unremarkable, though the prostate may feel normal, boggy, or indurated.

B. Laboratory Findings: Urinalysis is normal unless a secondary cystitis is present. Expressed prostatic secretions demonstrate increased numbers of leukocytes (> 10/hpf), especially lipid-laden macrophages. However, this finding is consistent with inflammation and is not diagnostic of bacterial prostatitis. Culture of the secretions or the third midstream bladder specimen is necessary to make the diagnosis.

C. Imaging: Imaging tests are not necessary, though pelvic radiographs or transrectal ultrasound may demonstrate prostatic calculi.

Differential Diagnosis

Chronic urethritis may mimic chronic prostatitis, though cultures of the fractionated urine may localize the source of infection. Cystitis may be secondary to prostatitis, yet again fractionated urine samples should localize the infection. Anal disease may share some of the symptoms of prostatitis, but physical examination should permit a distinction between the two.

Treatment

Few antimicrobial agents attain therapeutic intraprostatic levels in the absence of acute inflammation. Trimethoprim does diffuse into the prostate, and trimethoprim-sulfamethoxazole is associated with the best cure rates (Table 23–1). Other effective agents include carbenicillin, erythromycin, cephalexin, and the quinolones. The optimal duration of therapy remains controversial, ranging from 6 to 12 weeks. Symptomatic relief may be provided by anti-inflammatory agents (indomethacin, ibuprofen) and hot sitz baths.

Prognosis

Chronic bacterial prostatitis is difficult to cure, but its symptoms and tendency to cause recurrent urinary tract infections can be controlled by suppressive antibiotic therapy.

NONBACTERIAL PROSTATITIS

Essentials of Diagnosis

- Irritative voiding symptoms.
- Perineal or suprapubic discomfort, similar to that of chronic bacterial prostatitis.
- Positive expressed prostatic secretions, but culture is negative.

General Considerations

Nonbacterial prostatitis is the most common of the prostatitis syndromes, and its cause is unknown. Speculation implicates chlamydiae, mycoplasmas, *Ureaplasma,* and viruses, but no substantial proof exists. Nonbacterial prostatitis is believed to represent a noninfectious inflammatory disorder. Some investigators believe that it is an autoimmune disease. Nonbacterial prostatitis is thus a diagnosis of exclusion.

Clinical Findings

A. Symptoms and Signs: The clinical presentation is identical to that of chronic bacterial prostatitis; however, no history of urinary tract infections is present.

B. Laboratory Findings: Increased numbers of leukocytes are seen on expressed prostatic secretions, but all cultures are negative.

Differential Diagnosis

The major distinction is from chronic bacterial prostatitis. The absence of a history of urinary tract infection and of positive cultures makes the distinction (Table 23–2). In older men with irritative void-

Table 23–2. Clinical characteristics of prostatitis and prostatodynia syndromes.

Findings	Acute Bacterial Prostatitis	Chronic Bacterial Prostatitis	Nonbacterial Prostatitis	Prostatodynia
Fever	+	–	–	–
Urinalysis	+	–	–	–
Expressed prostatic secretions	Contraindicated	+	+	–
Bacterial culture	+	+	–	–

ing symptoms and negative cultures, the possibility of bladder cancer must be excluded. Urinary cytologic examination and cystoscopy are warranted.

Treatment

Because of the uncertainty regarding the etiology of nonbacterial prostatitis, a trial of antimicrobial therapy directed against *Ureaplasma, Mycoplasma,* or *Chlamydia* is warranted. Erythromycin (250 mg orally four times daily) can be initiated for 14 days yet should only be continued (for 3–6 weeks) if a favorable clinical response ensues. Some symptomatic relief may be obtained with anti-inflammatory agents or sitz baths. Dietary restrictions are not necessary unless the patient relates a history of symptom exacerbation by certain substances such as alcohol, caffeine, and perhaps certain foods.

Prognosis

Annoying, recurrent symptoms are common, but serious sequelae have not been identified.

PROSTATODYNIA

Prostatodynia is a noninflammatory disorder that affects young and middle-aged men and has variable causes, including voiding dysfunction and pelvic floor musculature dysfunction. The term "prostatodynia" is a misnomer, as the prostate is actually normal.

Clinical Findings

A. Symptoms and Signs: Symptoms are the same as those seen with chronic prostatitis, yet there is no history of urinary tract infection. Additional symptoms may include hesitancy and interruption of flow. Patients may relate a lifelong history of voiding difficulty. Physical examination is unremarkable, but increased anal sphincter tone and paraprostatic tenderness may be observed.

B. Laboratory Findings: Urinalysis is normal. Expressed prostatic secretions show normal numbers of leukocytes. Urodynamic testing may show signs of dysfunctional voiding (detrusor contraction without urethral relaxation, high urethral pressures, spasms of the urinary sphincter) and is indicated in patients failing empiric trials of alpha-blockers or anticholinergics.

Differential Diagnosis

Normal urinalysis will distinguish it from acute infectious processes. Examination of expressed prostatic secretions is crucial to distinguish this entity from prostatitis syndromes (Table 23–2).

Treatment

Bladder neck and urethral spasms can be treated by α-blocking agents (terazosin, 1–10 mg orally once a day; or doxazosin, 1–8 mg orally once a day).

Pelvic floor muscle dysfunction may respond to diazepam and biofeedback techniques. Sitz baths may contribute to symptomatic relief.

Prognosis

Prognosis is variable depending upon the specific cause.

Doble A: Chronic prostatitis. Brit J Urol 1994;74:537.

Miller JL et al: Prostatodynia and interstitial cystitis: One and the same? Urology 1995;45:587. (The diagnosis of interstitial cystitis should be considered in patients with nonbacterial prostatitis or prostatodynia.)

Moul JW: Prostatitis: Sorting out the different causes. Postgrad Med 1993;94:191. (Review of the various forms of prostatitis, including acute, chronic, nonbacterial, and prostatodynia.)

Pfau A: Complicated UTI and prostatitis in men. Infection 1994;22(Suppl 1):S58.

ACUTE EPIDIDYMITIS

Essentials of Diagnosis

- Fever.
- Irritative voiding symptoms.
- Painful enlargement of epididymis.

General Considerations

Most cases of acute epididymitis are infectious and can be divided into one of two categories that have different age distributions and etiologic agents. Sexually transmitted forms typically occur in men under age 40, are associated with urethritis, and result from *C trachomatis* or *N gonorrhoeae*. Non-sexually transmitted forms typically occur in older men, are associated with urinary tract infections and prostatitis, and are caused by gram-negative rods. The route of infection is probably via the urethra to the ejaculatory duct and then down the vas deferens to the epididymis.

Clinical Findings

A. Symptoms and Signs: Symptoms may follow acute physical strain (heavy lifting), trauma, or sexual activity. Associated symptoms of urethritis (pain at the tip of the penis and urethral discharge) or cystitis (irritative voiding symptoms) may occur. Pain develops in the scrotum and may radiate along the spermatic cord or to the flank. Fever and scrotal swelling are usually apparent. Early in the course, the epididymis may be distinguishable from the testis; however, later the two may appear as one enlarged, tender mass. The prostate may be tender on rectal examination.

B. Laboratory Findings: Complete blood count shows leukocytosis and a left shift. In the sexually transmitted variety, Gram staining of a smear of urethral discharge may be diagnostic of gram-negative intracellular diplococci *(N gonorrhoeae)*. White cells without visible organisms on urethral smear represent nongonococcal urethritis, and *C trachomatis* is the most likely pathogen. In the non-sexually transmitted variety, urinalysis shows pyuria, bacteriuria, and varying degrees of hematuria. Urine cultures will demonstrate the offending pathogen.

C. Imaging: Scrotal ultrasound may aid in the diagnosis if examination is difficult because of the presence of a large hydrocele or because questions exist regarding the diagnosis.

Differential Diagnosis

Tumors generally cause painless enlargement of the testis. Urinalysis is negative, and examination reveals a normal epididymis. Scrotal ultrasound is helpful to define the pathology. Testicular torsion usually occurs in prepubertal males but is occasionally seen in young adults. Acute onset of symptoms and a negative urinalysis favor testicular torsion or torsion of one of the testicular or epididymal appendages. Prehn's sign (elevation of the scrotum above the pubic symphysis improves pain from epididymitis) may be helpful but is not completely reliable.

Treatment

Bed rest with scrotal elevation is important in the acute phase. Treatment is directed toward the identified pathogen (Table 23–1). The sexually transmitted variety is treated with 10–21 days of antibiotics, and the sexual partner must be treated as well. Non-sexually transmitted forms are treated for 21–28 days with appropriate antibiotics, at which time evaluation of the urinary tract is warranted to identify underlying disease.

Prognosis

Prompt treatment usually results in a favorable outcome. Delayed or inadequate treatment may result in epididymo-orchitis, decreased fertility, or abscess formation.

Barloon TJ et al: Diagnostic imaging of patients with acute scrotal pain. Am Fam Physician 1996;53:1734. (Doppler ultrasound can be useful in distinguishing between epididymitis [increased blood flow] and testicular torsion [decreased blood flow].)

Berger RE: Infection of the male reproductive tract. Curr Ther Endocrinol Metab 1994;5:305. (General review.)

Sadek I et al: Amiodarone-induced epididymitis: Report of a new case and literature review of 12 cases. Can J Cardiol 1993;9:833. (This is a self-limiting reaction with or without amiodarone reduction and does not require antimicrobial drugs.)

URINARY STONE DISEASE

Urinary stone disease is exceeded in frequency as a urinary tract disorder only by infections and prostatic disease and is estimated to afflict 240,000–720,000 Americans per year. Men are more frequently affected by urolithiasis than women, with a ratio of 4:1. Initial presentation predominates in the third and fourth decades. The ratio of men to women approaches parity in the sixth and seventh decades.

Urinary calculi are polycrystalline aggregates composed of varying amounts of crystalloid and a small amount of organic matrix. Stone formation requires saturated urine that is dependent upon pH, ionic strength, solute concentration, and complexation. There are five major types of urinary stones: calcium oxalate, calcium phosphate, struvite, uric acid, and cystine. The most common types are composed of calcium, and for that reason most urinary stones (85%) are radiopaque. Uric acid stones can be radiolucent yet frequently are composed of a combination of uric acid and calcium oxalate and thus are radiopaque. Cystine stones frequently have a smooth-edged ground-glass appearance.

Geographic factors contribute to the development of stones. Areas of high humidity and elevated temperatures appear to be contributing factors, and the incidence of symptomatic ureteral stones is greatest during hot summer months.

Diet and fluid intake may be important factors in the development of urinary stones. Those afflicted with recurrent urinary stone disease should be encouraged to maintain a diet restricted in sodium and protein intake. Sodium should be restricted to 100 meq/d. Increased sodium intake will increase sodium, calcium excretion, monosodium urate saturation (that can act as a nidus for stone growth), the relative saturation of calcium phosphate, and a decrease in urinary citrate excretion. All of these factors encourage stone growth. Protein intake should be limited to 1 g/kg/d. An increased protein load can increase calcium, oxalate, and uric acid excretion and can also decrease urinary citrate excretion—all factors that can exacerbate stone disease. Carbohydrates and fats have not been proved to have any impact on urinary stone disease. Bran can significantly decrease urinary calcium by increasing bowel transit time and mechanically binding to calcium. Excess intake of oxalate and purines can increase the incidence of stones in predisposed individuals. Although a reduction in dietary calcium results in reduced urinary calcium, the concurrent increase in urinary oxalate may promote stone formation. Only type II absorptive hypercalciuric patients (see below) benefit from a low-calcium diet. Additionally, water or other fluid intake is important in preventing urolithiasis. Persons in sedentary occupations have a higher incidence of stones than manual laborers.

Genetic factors may contribute to urinary stone formation. Cystinuria is an autosomal recessive disorder. Homozygous individuals have markedly increased excretion of cystine and frequently have numerous recurrent episodes of urinary stones despite attempts to optimize medical treatment. Distal renal tubular acidosis may be transmitted as a hereditary trait, and urolithiasis occurs in up to 75% of patients affected with this disorder.

Clinical Findings

A. Symptoms and Signs: Obstructing urinary stones usually present with acute colic. Pain usually occurs suddenly and may awaken patients from sleep. It is localized to the flank, is usually severe, and may be associated with nausea and vomiting. Patients are constantly moving—in sharp contrast to those with an acute abdomen. The pain may occur episodically and may radiate anteriorly over the abdomen. As the stone progresses down the ureter, the pain may be referred into the ipsilateral testis or labium. If the stone becomes lodged at the ureterovesical junction, patients will complain of marked urinary urgency and frequency. Stone size does not correlate with the severity of the symptoms.

B. Metabolic Evaluation: Stone analysis should be performed on recovered stones. Much controversy exists in deciding which patients need a thorough metabolic evaluation for stone disease. Uncomplicated first-time stone-formers should probably undergo blood screening for abnormalities of serum calcium, phosphate, electrolytes, and uric acid as a baseline.

More extensive evaluation is required in recurrent stone-formers or patients with a family history of stone disease. A 24-hour urine collection on a random diet should ascertain volume, urinary pH, and calcium, uric acid, oxalate, phosphate, and citrate excretion. A second collection on a restricted calcium (400 mg/d) and sodium (100 meq/d) diet is undertaken to subcategorize patients, if necessary. Serum PTH and calcium load tests can be performed at a third visit. A calcium load test is performed as follows: After a patient has been on a restricted calcium diet for at least 1 week, the patient is told to fast from 9 PM. The patient discards his early morning voided specimen (7 AM). While still fasting, the patient voids at 9 AM, which is the fasting sample. The patient then ingests 1 g of calcium gluconate, and all urine is collected from 9 AM to 1 PM, which is the calcium load sample. Table 23–3 demonstrates the diagnostic criteria for the hypercalciuric states. (See discussion below.)

C. Laboratory Findings: Urinalysis usually reveals microscopic or gross ($\approx 10\%$) hematuria. However, the absence of microhematuria does not exclude urinary stones. Infection must be excluded, because the combination of infection and urinary tract obstruction requires prompt intervention as described below. Urinary pH is a valuable clue as to the cause of the possible stone. Normal urine pH is 5.85. There is a normal postprandial urinary alkaline tide. Numerous dipstick measurements are valuable in the complete workup of a stone patient. Persistent urinary pH below 5.0 is suggestive of uric acid or cystine stones, both relatively radiolucent as seen on plain films of the abdomen. In contrast, a persistent pH above 7.5 is suggestive of a struvite infection stone, radiopaque on plain films.

D. Imaging: A plain film of the abdomen and renal ultrasound examination will diagnose most stones. Stones suspected of being located at the ureterovesical junction can be imaged with abdominal ultrasonography with the aid of the acoustic window of a full bladder. Alternatively, transvaginal or transrectal ultrasonography will help identify calculi near the ureterovesical junction. When the diagnosis remains uncertain, intravenous urography is indicated.

Table 23–3. Diagnostic criteria of different types of hypercalciuria.

	Absorptive Type I	Absorptive Type II	Absorptive Type III	Resorptive	Renal
Serum					
Calcium	N	N	N	↑	N
Phosphorus	N	N	↓	↓	N
PTH	N	N	N	↑	↑
Vitamin D	N	N	↑	↑	↑
Urinary calcium					
Fasting	N	N	↑	↑	↑
Restricted	↑	N	↑	↑	↑
After calcium load	↑	↑	↑	↑	↑

Key: ↑ = elevated
↓ = low
N = normal

Medical Treatment & Prevention

To reduce the recurrence rate of urinary stones, one must attempt to achieve a stone-free status. Small stone fragments may serve as a nidus for future stone development. Selected patients must be thoroughly evaluated to reduce stone recurrence rates. Uric acid stone-formers may have recurrences within months if appropriate therapy is not initiated. If no medical treatment is provided after surgical stone removal, stones will generally recur in 50% of patients within 5 years. Of greatest importance in reducing stone recurrence is an increased fluid intake. Absolute volumes are not targeted, yet doubling previous fluid intake is recommended. Patients are encouraged to ingest fluids during meals, 2 hours after each meal (when the body is most dehydrated), and prior to going to sleep in the evening—enough to awaken the patient to void and to ingest additional fluids during the night. Increasing fluids only during daylight hours may not dilute a supersaturated urine and thus initiate a new stone.

A. Calcium Nephrolithiasis:

1. Hypercalciuric–Hypercalciuric calcium nephrolithiasis (> 200 mg/24 h) can be caused by absorptive, resorptive, and renal disorders.

Absorptive hypercalciuria is secondary to increased absorption of calcium at the level of the small bowel, predominantly in the jejunum, and can be further subdivided into types I, II, and III. Type I absorptive hypercalciuria is independent of calcium intake. There is increased urinary calcium on a regular or even a calcium-restricted diet. Treatment is centered upon decreasing bowel absorption of calcium. Cellulose phosphate, a chelating agent, is an effective form of therapy. An average dose is 10–15 g in three divided doses. It binds to the calcium and impedes small bowel absorption due to its increased bulk. Cellulose phosphate does not change the intestinal transport mechanism. It should be given with meals so it will be available to bind to the calcium. Taking this chelating agent prior to bedtime is ineffective. Postmenopausal women should be treated with caution. It is interesting, however, that there is no enhanced decline in bone density after long-term use. Inappropriate use without an initial metabolic evaluation (see above) may result in a negative calcium balance and a secondary parathyroid stimulation. Long-term use without follow-up metabolic surveillance may result in hypomagnesemia and secondary hyperoxaluria and recurrent calculi. Routine follow-up every 6–8 months will help encourage medical compliance and permit adjustments in medical therapy based upon repeat metabolic studies.

Thiazide therapy is an alternative to cellulose phosphate in the treatment of type I absorptive hypercalciuria. Thiazides decrease renal calcium excretion but have no impact on intestinal absorption. This therapy results in increased bone density of approximately 1% per year. Thiazides have limited long-term utility (< 5 years) as they lose their hypocalciuric effect with continued therapy.

Type II absorptive hypercalciuria is diet-dependent. Decreasing calcium intake by 50% (approximately 400 mg/d) will decrease the hypercalciuria to normal values (150–200 mg/24 h). There is no specific medical therapy.

Type III absorptive hypercalciuria is secondary to a renal phosphate leak. This results in increased vitamin D synthesis and secondarily increased small bowel absorption of calcium. This can be readily reversed by orthophosphates (0.5 g three times per day). Orthophosphates do not change intestinal absorption but rather inhibit vitamin D synthesis.

Resorptive hypercalciuria is secondary to hyperparathyroidism. Hypercalcemia, hypophosphatemia, hypercalciuria, and an elevated parathyroid hormone value are found. Appropriate surgical resection of the adenoma cures the disease and the urinary stones. Medical management is invariably a failure.

Renal hypercalciuria occurs when the renal tubules are unable to efficiently reabsorb filtered calcium, and hypercalciuria results. Spilling calcium in the urine results in secondary hyperparathyroidism. Serum calcium is normal. Hydrochlorothiazides are effective long-term therapy in patients with this disorder.

2. Hyperuricosuric–Hyperuricosuric calcium nephrolithiasis is secondary to dietary excesses or uric acid metabolic defects. Both disorders can be treated with purine dietary restrictions or allopurinol therapy (or both). In contrast to uric acid nephrolithiasis, hyperuricosuric calcium stones will maintain a urinary pH greater than 5.5. Monosodium urates absorb inhibitors and promote heterogeneous nucleation. Hyperuricosuric calcium nephrolithiasis is probably secondary to epitaxy, or heterogeneous nucleation. In such situations, similar crystal structures (ie, uric acid and calcium oxalate) can grow together with the aid of a protein matrix infrastructure.

3. Hyperoxaluric–Hyperoxaluric calcium nephrolithiasis is usually due to primary intestinal disorders. Patients usually present with a history of chronic diarrhea frequently associated with inflammatory bowel disease or steatorrhea. Increased bowel fat combines with intraluminal calcium to form a soap-like product. Calcium is therefore unavailable to bind to oxalate, which is then freely and rapidly absorbed. A small increase in oxalate absorption will significantly increase stone formation. If the diarrhea or steatorrhea cannot be effectively curtailed, oral calcium supplements should be given with meals. It remains controversial whether excess ascorbic acid increases urinary oxalate levels. Emphasis on encouraging increased fluid intake is required for these patients as for all stone-formers.

Any condition that results in metabolic acidosis (including prolonged fasting, hypomagnesemia, and hypokalemia) will decrease urinary citrate excretion, since it will be consumed by the citric acid cycle within the mitochondria of renal cells.

4. Hypocitraturic–Hypocitraturic calcium nephrolithiasis may be secondary to chronic diarrhea, type I (distal tubule) renal tubular acidosis, chronic hydrochlorothiazide treatment, and, in rare cases, is idiopathic. It is frequently associated with other forms of calcium stone formation. Citrate appears to bind to calcium in solution, thereby decreasing available calcium for stone formation. Potassium citrate supplements are usually effective. Urinary citrate is decreased in acidotic situations and is increased during alkalotic conditions. The potassium will supplement the frequent hypokalemic states, and citrate will help to correct the acidosis. A typical dose is 20 meq three times a day (available in solution or in 5 and 10 meq tablets or in crystal formulations).

B. Uric Acid Calculi: The average urinary pH is 5.85. Uric acid stone-formers frequently have urinary pH values less than 5.5. The pK of uric acid is 5.75, at which point half of the uric acid is ionized as a urate salt and is soluble, while the other half is insoluble. Increasing the pH above 6.5 dramatically increases solubility and can effectively dissolve large calculi. Potassium citrate is the most frequently used medication to increase urinary pH. It can be given in liquid preparation, as crystals that need to be taken with fluids, or as tablets (10 meq), two by mouth three or four times daily. Compliant urinary alkalinization may dissolve uric acid calculi at a rate of 1 cm of stone per month as seen on an abdominal radiograph. Patients with uric acid calculi should be given nitrazine pH paper with which to monitor the effectiveness of their urinary alkalinization. Other contributing factors include hyperuricemia, myeloproliferative disorders, malignancy with increased uric acid production, abrupt and dramatic weight loss, and uricosuric medications. If hyperuricemia is present, allopurinol (300 mg.d) should be instituted. Although pure uric acid stones are relatively radiolucent, most have some calcium components and can be visualized on plain abdominal radiographs. Renal ultrasonography is a helpful adjunct for appropriate diagnosis and long-term management.

C. Struvite Calculi: Struvite stones are synonymous with magnesium-ammonium-phosphate stones. They are commonly seen in women with recurrent urinary tract infections recalcitrant to appropriate antibiotics. They rarely form as ureteral stones without prior upper tract endourologic intervention. Frequently they are discovered as a large staghorn calculi forming a cast of the renal collecting system. These stones are radiodense. Urinary pH is high, usually above 7.0–7.5. These stones are formed secondary to urease-producing organisms, including *Proteus, Pseudomonas, Providencia,* and less commonly *Klebsiella,* staphylococci, and *Mycoplasma.* An *E coli* urinary tract infection is not consistent with an infectious reservoir originating from a struvite calculus. These frequently large stones are relatively soft and amenable to percutaneous nephrolithotomy. Appropriate perioperative antibiotics are required. These stones can recur rapidly, and efforts should be taken to render the patient stone-free. Postoperative irrigation through nephrostomy tubes can eliminate small fragments. Acetohydroxamic acid is an effective urease inhibitor. However, because of gastrointestinal side effects, it is poorly tolerated by most patients.

D. Cystine Calculi: Cystine stones are a result of abnormal excretion of cystine, ornithine, lysine, and arginine. Cystine is the only amino acid that becomes insoluble in urine. These stones are particularly difficult to manage medically. Prevention is centered around increased fluid intake, alkalinization of the urine above pH 7.5 (monitored with nitrazine pH paper), and a variety of medications including penicillamine and tiopronin.

Surgical Treatment

Forced intravenous fluids will not push stones down the ureter. Effective peristalsis directing a bolus of urine down the ureter requires opposing ureteral walls to approach each other and touch. Large dilated systems are ineffective, as opposing ureteral walls are unable to approach each other. Massive diuresis is counter-productive and will exacerbate the pain. Appropriate pain medications are required. Associated fever may represent infection, which is a medical emergency. Fever in association with upper tract obstruction requires prompt drainage by a ureteral catheter or a percutaneous nephrostomy tube. Antibiotics alone in the face of impending or florid urosepsis are inadequate.

A. Ureteral Stones: Impediment to urine flow by ureteral stones usually occurs at three sites: (1) at the ureteropelvic junction, (2) at the crossing of the ureter over the iliac vessels, and finally (3) as the ureter enters the bladder at the ureterovesical junction. Prediction of spontaneous stone passage is difficult. Stones less than 6 mm in diameter as seen on a plain abdominal radiograph will usually pass spontaneously. Conservative observation with appropriate pain medications is appropriate for the first 6 weeks. If spontaneous stone passage has failed, therapeutic intervention is required. Distal ureteral stones are best managed either with ureteroscopic stone extraction or in situ extracorporeal shock wave lithotripsy (ESWL). Ureteroscopic stone extraction involves placement of a small endoscope through the urethra and into the ureter. Under direct vision, basket extraction or fragmentation followed by extraction is performed. Complications during endoscopic retrieval increase as the duration of conservative observation increases beyond 6 weeks. Indications for earlier intervention include severe pain unresponsive to medications, fever, persistent nausea and vomiting requiring intravenous hydration, social requirements requiring return to work, or anticipated remote travel. Most upper tract stones that enter the bladder can exit the urethra with minimal discomfort.

In situ ESWL, an alternative, utilizes an external energy source that is focused upon the stone. This focused energy is additive, resulting in minimal tissue insult except at the focus where the stone is positioned with the aid of fluoroscopy or ultrasonography. This can be performed under monitored anesthesia care as an outpatient procedure and usually results in stone fragmentation. It requires time for the stone fragments to pass spontaneously. Most stone fragments will pass uneventfully within 2 weeks. Fragments that have not passed within 3 months are unlikely to pass without intervention. Women of childbearing age are best not treated with ESWL for a stone in the lower ureter, as the impact upon the ovary is unknown.

Proximal and midureteral stones—those above the inferior margin of the sacroiliac joint—can be treated with ESWL or ureteroscopy. ESWL can be delivered directly to the stone (in situ), or the stones can be pushed back into the renal pelvis (via a retrograde ureteral catheter) to allow for a more capacious surrounding space and thus for more efficient fragmentation. To help ensure adequate drainage after ESWL, a double J ureteral stent is frequently placed. Double J stents do not ensure passage of stone fragments after ESWL. Occasionally, stone fragments will obstruct the ureter after ESWL. Conservative management will usually result in spontaneous resolution with eventual passage of the stone fragments. If this is unsuccessful, adequate proximal drainage through a percutaneous nephrostomy tube will facilitate passage. In rare instances, ureteroscopic extraction will be required.

B. Renal Stones: Patients with renal calculi presenting without pain, urinary tract infections, or obstruction need not be treated. They should be followed with serial abdominal radiographs or renal ultrasonographic examinations. If calculi are growing or become symptomatic, intervention should be undertaken. Renal stones less than 3 cm in diameter are best treated with ESWL. Stones located in the inferior calix frequently result in suboptimal stone-free rates as measured at 3 months by x-ray. Such stones and others of larger diameter are best treated via percutaneous nephrolithotomy. Perioperative antibiotic coverage should be given on the basis of preoperative urine cultures.

[Prevention and treatment of kidney stones.]
  gopher://gopher.nih.gov/00/clin/cdcs/individual/
    67.kidney
Brown WW, Wolfson M: Diet as culprit or therapy: Stone disease, chronic renal failure, and nephrotic syndrome. Med Clin North Am 1993;77:783. (Dietary factors that promote urolithiasis and dietary recommendations utilized in the medical management of stone disease.)
Coe FL et al: The pathogenesis and treatment of kidney stones. N Engl J Med 1992;327:1141. (Excellent general review.)
Curhan GC et al: A prospective study of dietary calcium and other nutrients and the risk of symptomatic kidney stones. N Engl J Med 1993;328:833. (In this cohort of men, a high dietary calcium intake was found to decrease the risk of symptomatic kidney stones.)
Gault MH et al: Bacteriology of urinary tract stones. J Urol 1995;153:1164. (Routine stone cultures may be of limited value except for bladder and large renal stones.)
Kupin WL: A practical approach to nephrolithiasis. Hosp Pract (Off Ed) 1995 Mar;30:57. (Stone composition is an important guide for the physician's decision concerning investigation and a rational choice of treatment.)
Parivar F et al: The influence of diet on urinary stone disease. J Urol 1996;155:432. (In an extensive literature review, dietary manipulation was beneficial in the prevention of recurrent urolithiasis in only a selected group of patients.)

URINARY INCONTINENCE

Urinary incontinence is most common in the elderly. Its prevalence varies from 5% to 15% in the community to perhaps more than 50% in long-term care facilities. The normal urinary bladder can store relatively large volumes of urine at low pressures. Continence is dependent upon a compliant reservoir and sphincteric efficiency that has two components: the involuntary smooth muscle of the bladder neck and the voluntary skeletal muscle of the external sphincter. (See also discussion in Chapter 3.)

Classification

Urinary incontinence occurs when urine leaks involuntarily and can be classified into one of four categories as described in the following paragraphs.

A. Total Incontinence: With total incontinence, patients lose urine at all times and in all positions. Total incontinence results when sphincteric efficiency is lost (previous surgery, nerve damage, cancerous infiltration) or when an abnormal connection between the urinary tract and the skin exists that bypasses the urinary sphincter (vesicovaginal or ureterovaginal fistulas).

B. Stress Incontinence: Stress incontinence is the loss of urine associated with activities that result in an increase in intra-abdominal pressure (coughing, sneezing, lifting, exercising). Patients do not leak in the supine position. Laxity of the pelvic floor musculature—most commonly seen in the multiparous woman or in patients who have undergone pelvic surgery—results in urethral sphincteric insufficiency.

C. Urge Incontinence: The uncontrolled loss of urine that is preceded by a strong, unexpected urge to void is known as urge incontinence. It is unrelated to position or activity and is indicative of detrusor hyperreflexia or sphincter dysfunction. Inflammatory conditions or neurogenic disorders of the bladder are commonly associated with urge incontinence.

D. Overflow Incontinence: Chronic urinary retention may result in overflow incontinence. Incontinence results from the chronically distended bladder receiving an additional increment of urine, so that intravesical pressure just exceeds the outlet resistance, allowing a small amount of urine to dribble out.

Clinical Findings

A. Symptoms and Signs: The history is the most important step in the evaluation of urinary incontinence. It may be supplemented with a voiding diary prepared by the patient. Physical examination is important to exclude fistula for cases of total incontinence, neurologic abnormalities in cases of urge incontinence (spasticity, flaccidity, rectal sphincter tone), or the distended bladder in cases of overflow incontinence. Rectal examination will reveal the general function of the pelvic floor. Normal anal tone suggests an intact external sphincter. A tender levator ani suggests an overfacilitated pelvic floor. A lax sphincter suggests a lower motor neuron lesion. The bulbocavernosus reflex further confirms the integrity of the lower motor neurons. This reflex is confirmed by feeling an anal contraction in response to pressure on the glans penis or the clitoris.

B. Laboratory Findings: Urinalysis and urine culture are important to exclude urinary tract infection in cases of urge incontinence. Abnormal renal function may be detected in cases of overflow incontinence. Cystograms may demonstrate fistula sites. Lateral stress cystograms may show descensus of the bladder neck (descent of bladder neck more than 1.5 cm on straining view) in cases of stress incontinence. Those suspected of overflow incontinence can have postvoid residual urine volume assessed by urethral catheterization or ultrasonography.

C. Special Tests: Urinary continence depends upon both bladder and sphincteric mechanisms; dysfunction of either component may result in incontinence. Urodynamic evaluation can assess both bladder and sphincteric function. Such testing is indicated in patients with moderate to severe incontinence, those suspected of having neurologic disease, and those with urge incontinence when infection and neoplasm have been excluded.

Bladder capacity, accommodation, sensation, voluntary control, contractility, and response to pharmacologic intervention can be assessed by cystometry. Cystometry is performed by filling the bladder with water or CO_2 and simultaneously recording intravesical pressure.

During filling, the normal bladder has the ability to maintain a low pressure. As volume increases, compliance increases. Normal sensation is first appreciated with volumes less than 150 mL. There is a strong sensation prior to micturition. Normal capacity in an adult bladder is 350–500 mL. Micturition is consciously initiated starting with pelvic floor relaxation followed by a sustained bladder contraction. Normal bladder function will empty the bladder completely. Uninhibited contractions during the normal filling phase are abnormal and are usually associated with a strong urge to void. Causes of decreased urinary capacity include incontinence, infections, interstitial cystitis, radiation damage, upper motor neuron lesions, and postoperative changes. Increased bladder capacity is seen with chronic urinary tract obstruction, lower motor neuron lesions, and sensory neuropathies.

Responses to routine medications during cystometry will help confirm a diagnosis and facilitate appropriate therapy. Lack of an appropriate detrusor contraction may be secondary to poor bladder muscle function or inadequate filling. Myogenic function can be assessed with bethanechol chloride, a parasympathomimetic drug. Lack of response to intravenous bethanechol suggests intrinsic muscle damage. In contrast, an exaggerated response is suggestive of a lower motor neuron lesion.

Sphincteric function assessment is necessary in the evaluation of urinary incontinence. More formal evaluation of the urinary sphincter may be performed using urethral profilometry, electromyography, or combined video studies.

Treatment

A. Total Incontinence: True incontinence is due to anatomic abnormalities, either congenital or acquired. Congenital defects, including bladder exstrophy, ectopic ureteral orifices, and urethral diverticula, and acquired lesions such as vesicovaginal fistulas require surgical correction. Sphincter injuries following prostatectomy may be managed by surgical reconstruction (bladder neck reconstruction), periurethral collagen injections, or placement of an artificial urinary sphincter.

B. Stress Incontinence: In patients with stress urinary incontinence, the bladder neck will descend below the midportion of the pubic symphysis when viewed on a lateral stress cystogram. Urodynamic investigations usually reveal a shortened functional urethral length, decreased urethral closure pressure, minimal augmentation of closure pressure with stress activities, decreased urethral pressure and length when assuming an upright position, and decreased closure pressure with bladder filling.

If hypoestrogenism of the vagina or urethra is discovered, topical estrogen creams applied locally are indicated. Mild cases can be treated medically with agents directed at increasing urethral resistance (phenylpropanolamine, 50 mg orally daily). Surgical treatment is centered upon placing the bladder neck into an appropriate anatomic location, allowing increased intra-abdominal pressure to be transmitted to both the bladder and the bladder neck. These procedures also lengthen the urethra. Transvaginal or suprapubic (culpocystourethropexy) approaches can pull the bladder neck into proper position. Surgery is usually corrective.

C. Urge Incontinence: The etiology of urge urinary incontinence includes urethral or detrusor instability or a combination of these mechanisms. Treatment is medical rather than surgical. Effective agents include antispasmodic medication (oxybutinin, 5 mg orally three times daily), anticholinergic medication (propantheline 15 mg orally three times daily), or tricyclic antidepressants (imipramine, 25–75 mg orally at bedtime). Alternative experimental treatments include nerve stimulation and acupuncture.

D. Overflow Incontinence: Placement of a urethral catheter is both diagnostic and therapeutic in the acute setting. Further treatment must address the underlying disease. Elderly men with benign prostatic hyperplasia can be treated with medical therapy, prostatectomy, or newer less invasive procedures (see below). Patients with urethral strictures can be treated with a direct internal urethrotomy or open urethroplasty. Neurogenic causes (external sphincteric spasticity) may be managed with intermittent catheterization regimens with or without pharmacotherapy.

[Urinary incontinence in adults.]
  gopher://gopher.nih.gov/00/clin/cdcs/individual/
    71.incont
Fantl JA et al: Estrogen therapy in the management of urinary incontinence in postmenopausal women: A meta analysis. First report of the Hormones and Urogenital Therapy Committee. Obstet Gynecol 1994;83:12. (Estrogen subjectively improves urinary incontinence in postmenopausal women.)
Ouslander JG et al: Does eradicating bacteriuria affect the severity of urinary incontinence in nursing home residents? Ann Intern Med 1995;122:749. (No.)
Resnick NM: Urinary incontinence. Lancet 1995;346:94. (General review.)
Rosenthal AJ et al: Urinary incontinence in the elderly. Often simple to treat when properly evaluated. Postgrad Med 1995;97:109. (Clinicians and patients alike benefit from the realization that urinary incontinence is a treatable problem.)
Swami SK, Abrams P: Urge incontinence. Urol Clin North Am 1996;23:41. (Entire volume dedicated to urinary incontinence.)

MALE ERECTILE DYSFUNCTION & SEXUAL DYSFUNCTION

Impotence is defined as the consistent inability to maintain an erect penis with sufficient rigidity to al-

low sexual intercourse. This condition is thought to affect 10 million American men, and its incidence is age-related. Approximately 25% of all men older than age 65 suffer from this disorder. Most cases of male erectile disorders have an organic rather than a psychogenic cause. Normal male erection is a neurovascular phenomenon relying on an intact autonomic and somatic nerve supply to the penis, smooth and striated musculature of the corpora cavernosa and pelvic floor, and arterial inflow supplied by the paired pudendal arteries. Erection is precipitated and maintained by an increase in arterial flow, active relaxation of the smooth muscle elements of the sinusoids within the corporal bodies of the penis, and an increase in venous resistance. Contraction of the bulbocavernosus and ischiocavernosus muscles results in further rigidity of the penis. The neurotransmitters that initiate the process have not been identified with certainty, though nitric oxide, vasoactive intestinal polypeptide, acetylcholine, and prostaglandins have all been postulated to initiate or contribute to male erection.

Male sexual dysfunction may be manifested in a variety of ways, and the history is critical to the proper classification and subsequent treatment. Androgens have a strong influence on the sexual desire of men. A **loss of libido** may indicate androgen deficiency on the basis of either hypothalamic, pituitary or testicular disease. Serum testosterone and gonadotropin levels may help localize the site of disease. **Loss of erections** may result from arterial, venous, neurogenic, or psychogenic causes. Concurrent medical problems may damage one or more of the mechanisms. In addition, many medications, especially antihypertensives, are associated with erectile dysfunction. Centrally acting sympatholytics (methyldopa, clonidine, reserpine) can result in loss of erection, while vasodilators, alpha-blockers, and diuretics rarely alter erections. Beta-blockers and spironolactone may result in loss of libido. It is important to determine whether the patient ever had any normal erections, such as early morning or during sleep. If normal erections do occur, an organic cause is unlikely. The gradual loss of erections over a period of time is more suggestive of an organic cause. The **loss of emission** (lack of antegrade seminal fluid during ejaculation) may result from several underlying disorders. **Retrograde ejaculation** may occur as a result of mechanical disruption of the bladder neck, especially following transurethral resection of the prostate or sympathetic denervation as a result of medications (alpha-blockers), diabetes mellitus, or radical pelvic or retroperitoneal surgery. Androgen deficiency may also result in lack of emission by decreasing the amount of prostatic and seminal vesicle secretions. If libido and erection are intact, the **loss of orgasm** is usually of psychologic origin. **Premature ejaculation** is usually an anxiety-related disorder and rarely has an organic cause. The history may elucidate the presence of a new partner, unreasonable expectations about performance, or emotional disorders.

Clinical Findings

A. Symptoms and Signs: Impotence should be clearly distinguished from problems of ejaculation, libido, and orgasm. The degree of the dysfunction (whether chronic, occasional, or situational) as well as its timing should be noted. The history should include inquiries about hyperlipidemia, hypertension, neurologic disease, diabetes mellitus, renal failure, and adrenal and thyroid disorders. Trauma to the pelvis or pelvic or peripheral vascular surgery also identifies patients at increased risk of impotence. A complete recording of drug use should be made, since about 25% of all cases of sexual dysfunction may be drug-related. The use of alcohol, tobacco, and recreational drugs should be recorded as well, since each is associated with an increased risk of sexual dysfunction.

During the physical examination, secondary sexual characteristics should be assessed. Neurologic and peripheral vascular examination should be performed. Motor and sensory examination should be performed as well as palpation and quantification of lower extremity vascular pulsations. The genitalia should be examined, noting the presence of penile scarring or plaque formation (Peyronie's disease) and any abnormalities in size or consistency of either testicle. Examination of the prostate is an essential feature of the urologic examination in all adult patients.

B. Laboratory Findings: Laboratory evaluation is limited and should consist of a complete blood count, urinalysis, lipid profile, determination of serum testosterone, glucose, and prolactin. Patients with abnormalities of testosterone or prolactin require further evaluation with measurement of serum FSH and LH, and endocrinologic consultation is advised.

C. Special Tests: Further testing is based on the patient's goals. Patients who will accept only noninvasive forms of therapy may be offered medical therapy or a vacuum constriction device, as described below. Most patients undergo further evaluation with direct injection of vasoactive substances into the penis. Such substances (prostaglandin E_1, papavarine, or a combination of drugs) will induce erections in men with intact vascular systems. Patients who respond with a rigid erection require no further vascular evaluation. However, organic and psychogenic impotence can be differentiated by use of nocturnal penile tumescence testing, where the frequency as well as the rigidity of erections are recorded by a simple device attached to the penis before sleep. Patients with psychogenic impotence will have nocturnal erections of adequate frequency and rigidity.

Additional vascular testing is indicated in patients who fail to achieve an erection with injection of vasoactive substances on serial attempts using increasing doses or combination of drugs and who would consider vascular reconstructive surgery. The diameter and flow in the cavernous arteries can be assessed using duplex ultrasound. Patients with poor arterial inflow in the absence of known peripheral vascular disease (as in patients who have sustained pelvic trauma) are candidates for pelvic arteriography before planned arterial reconstruction. Patients with normal arterial inflow should be suspected of suffering from venous leak. Further testing in this group would include cavernosometry (measurement of flow required to maintain erection) and cavernosography (contrast study of the penis to determine site and extent of venous leak).

Treatment

The vast majority of men suffering from erectile dysfunction can be managed successfully with one of the approaches outlined below. Men who do not suffer from organic dysfunction will probably benefit from behaviorally oriented sex therapy.

A. Medical Treatment: Testosterone injections (200 mg intramuscularly every 3 weeks) are offered to men with documented androgen deficiency who have undergone endocrinologic evaluation as described and in whom prostatic cancer has been excluded by PSA screening and digital rectal examination.

B. Vacuum Constriction Device: The vacuum constriction device is a cylindric device that draws the penis into an erect state by inducing a vacuum within the cylinder. Once adequate tumescence has been achieved, a rubber constriction device or band is placed around the proximal penis to prevent loss of erection, and the cylinder is removed. Such devices are suitable for patients with venous disorders of the penis and those who fail to achieve an adequate erection with injection of vasoactive substances. Complications are rare.

C. Injection Therapy: Direct injection of vasoactive prostaglandins into the penis is an acceptable form of treatment for most men with impotence. These injections are performed using a tuberculin syringe. The base and lateral aspect of the penis is used as the injection site to avoid injury to the superficial blood supply located anteriorly. Complications are rare and include dizziness, local pain, fibrosis, and infection. A prolonged erection requiring aspiration of blood and injection of epinephrine and phenylephrine to achieve detumescence occurs very rarely.

D. Penile Prostheses: Prosthetic devices may be implanted directly into the paired corporal bodies. Such prostheses may be rigid, malleable, hinged, or inflatable. Each is manufactured in a variety of sizes and diameters. Inflatable models may result in a more cosmetic appearance but may be associated with a greater likelihood of mechanical failure.

E. Vascular Reconstruction: Patients with

disorders of the arterial system are candidates for various forms of arterial reconstruction, including endarterectomy and balloon dilation for proximal arterial occlusion and arterial bypass procedures utilizing arterial (epigastric) or venous (deep dorsal vein) segments for distal occlusion. Patients with disorders of venous occlusion may be managed with ligation of certain veins (deep dorsal or emissary veins) or the crura of the corpora cavernosa. Experience with vascular reconstructive procedures is still limited, and many patients so treated still fail to achieve a rigid erection.

[Impotence.]
gopher://gopher.nih.gov/11/clin/cdcs/individual/91.impot
Kirby RS: Impotence: Diagnosis and management of male erectile dysfunction. Br Med J 1994;308:957.
Morley JE, Kaiser FE: Impotence: The internist's approach to diagnosis and treatment. Adv Intern Med 1993; 38:151.
NIH Consensus Conference: Impotence. JAMA 1993;270: 83.
O'Keefe M et al: Assessment and treatment of impotence. Med Clin North Am 1995;79:415.

MALE INFERTILITY

Primary infertility affects 15–20% of married couples. Approximately one-third of cases result from male factors, one-third from female factors, and one-third from combined factors. It is thus critical to have simultaneous evaluation of the female partner. Clinical evaluation is warranted following 6 months of unprotected intercourse. A thorough history and physical examination are critical in the evaluation of the infertile male. Endocrinologic profiles and detailed semen analyses are the cornerstones of laboratory investigations. **Oligospermia** is the presence of less than 20 million sperm/mL of the ejaculate; **azoospermia** is the absence of sperm. As spermatogenesis takes approximately 74 days, it is thus important to review events from the past 3 months.

Clinical Findings

A. Symptoms and Signs: The history should include prior testicular insults (torsion, cryptorchism, trauma), infections (mumps orchitis, epididymitis), environmental factors (excessive heat, radiation, chemotherapy), medications (anabolic steroids, cimetidine, and spironolactone may affect spermatogenesis; phenytoin may lower FSH; sulfasalazine and nitrofurantoin affect sperm motility), and drugs (alcohol, marijuana). Sexual habits, frequency and timing of intercourse, use of lubricants, and each partner's previous fertility experiences are important. Loss of libido and headaches or visual disturbances may indicate a pituitary tumor. The past medical or surgical history may reveal thyroid or liver disease (abnormalities of spermatogenesis), diabetic neuropathy (retrograde

ejaculation), radical pelvic or retroperitoneal surgery (absent seminal emission secondary to sympathetic nerve injury), or hernia repair (damage to the vas deferens or testicular blood supply).

Physical examination should pay particular attention to features of hypogonadism: underdeveloped secondary sexual characteristics, diminished male pattern hair distribution (axillary, body, facial, pubic), eunuchoid skeletal proportions (arm span 2 inches > height; upper to lower body ratio < 1.0), gynecomastia. The scrotal contents should be carefully evaluated. Testicular size should be noted (normal size approximately 4.5 × 2.5 cm, volume 18 mL). Varicoceles should be looked for in the standing position and on occasion may only be appreciated with the Valsalva maneuver. The vas deferens, epididymis, and prostate should be palpated.

B. Laboratory Findings: Semen analysis should be performed after 72 hours of abstinence. The specimen should be analyzed within 1 hour after collection. Abnormal sperm concentrations are less than 20 million/mL. Normal semen volumes range between 1.5 and 5 mL (volumes < 1.5 mL may result in inadequate buffering of the vaginal acidity and may be due to retrograde ejaculation or androgen insufficiency). Normal sperm motility and morphology demonstrate 50–60% motile cells and more than 60% normal morphology. Abnormal motility may result from antisperm antibodies or infection. Abnormal morphology may result from a varicocele, infection, or exposure history.

Endocrinologic evaluation is warranted if sperm counts are low or if there is a clinical basis (from the history and physical examination) for suspecting an endocrinologic origin. Testing should include serum FSH, LH, and testosterone. Elevated FSH and LH and low testosterone (hypergonadotropic hypogonadism) are associated with primary testicular failure, which is usually irreversible. Low FSH and LH associated with low testosterone occur in secondary testicular failure (hypogonadotropic hypogonadism) and may be of hypothalamic or pituitary origin. Such defects may be correctable. Serum prolactin should be checked to exclude pituitary prolactinoma.

C. Imaging: Scrotal ultrasound may detect a subclinical varicocele. Vasography may be required in selected patients with suspected ductal obstruction.

D. Special Tests: Azoospermic patients should have postmasturbation urine samples centrifuged and analyzed for sperm to exclude retrograde ejaculation. Azoospermic patients and patients with ejaculate volumes less than 1 mL should have fructose levels determined on the ejaculate. Fructose is produced in the seminal vesicles and if absent in the ejaculate implies obstruction of the ejaculatory ducts.

Treatment

A. General Measures: Education with respect to the proper timing for intercourse in relation to the female's ovulatory cycle as well as the avoidance of spermicidal lubricants should be discussed. In cases of toxic exposure or medication-related factors, the offending agent should be removed. Patients with active genitourinary tract infections should be treated with appropriate antibiotics.

B. Endocrine Therapy: Hypogonadotropic hypogonadism may be treated with chorionic gonadotropin once primary pituitary disease has been excluded or treated. Dosage is usually 2000 IU intramuscularly three times a week. If sperm counts fail to rise after 12 months, FSH therapy should be initiated. Menotropins (Pergonal) is available as a premixed vial of 75 IU of FSH and 75 IU of LH. The usual dosage ranges from one-half to one vial intramuscularly three times per week.

C. Retrograde Ejaculation Therapy: Oligospermic patients with retrograde ejaculation may benefit from alpha-adrenergic agonists (pseudoephedrine, 60 mg orally three times a day) or imipramine (25 mg orally three times a day). Medical failures may require the collection of postmasturbation urine for intrauterine insemination or electroejaculation in the case of absent emission.

D. Varicocele: Surgical approaches to varicoceles may be accomplished via a scrotal, inguinal, or laparoscopic approach. More recently, percutaneous venographic approaches have been developed, obviating the need for an anesthetic.

E. Ductal Obstruction: The level of obstruction must be delineated via a vasogram prior to operative treatment. Mechanical obstruction of the ejaculatory duct may be corrected by transurethral resection and unroofing of the ducts in the prostatic urethra. Obstruction of the vas deferens is best managed by a microsurgical approach, and a vasovasostomy or vasoepididymostomy may be required.

F. Assisted Reproductive Techniques: Advances in reproductive technology may provide alternatives to patients who have failed other means of treating reduced sperm counts and motility. Such measures include intrauterine insemination, in vitro fertilization, and gamete intrafallopian transfer.

Howard SS: Treatment of male infertility. N Engl J Med 1995;332:312.

Lipshultz LI (editor): Male infertility. Urol Clin North Am 1994;21(3). (Entire volume.)

BENIGN PROSTATIC HYPERPLASIA

Essentials of Diagnosis

- Decreased force and caliber of the urinary stream.
- Nocturia.
- High postvoid residual urine volume.
- Azotemia and urinary retention on occasion.

General Considerations

Benign prostatic hyperplasia is a common disorder, and its incidence is age-related. Its histologic prevalence in autopsy studies rises from approximately 20% in men aged 41–50 years to over 80% in men older than 80 years. Although clinical evidence of disease occurs less commonly, symptoms of prostatic obstruction are also age-related. At age 55, approximately 25% of men report obstructive voiding symptoms. At age 75 years, 50% of men will complain of a decrease in the force and caliber of their urinary stream.

The cause is not completely understood but seems to be multifactorial and under endocrine control. The prostate is composed of both stromal and epithelial elements, and each—alone or in combination—can give rise to hyperplastic nodules and the symptoms associated with hyperplasia of the organ. Indeed, both elements are targets of medical management. Whereas prostatic cancers originate in the peripheral zone of the prostate, benign prostatic hyperplasia originates in the periurethral and transition zones. The natural history is quite variable, and a large number of affected patients may note either improvement or stabilization of their symptoms with time.

Clinical Findings

A. Symptoms and Signs: Benign prostatic hyperplasia may be associated with both obstructive and irritative voiding symptoms. Obstructive symptoms include decreased force and caliber of the urinary stream, an intermittent stream, and urinary hesitancy. Irritative symptoms, which may be a consequence of bladder dysfunction, include urinary frequency, nocturia, and urgency. Symptoms may be quantitated by various scoring classifications, which may aid in selecting patients for various forms of treatment and assessing their response to such treatment. Digital rectal examination may reveal either focal or uniform enlargement of the prostate. Focal areas of induration may represent malignant rather than benign prostatic growth, and further evaluation (transrectal ultrasound and possible biopsy) is indicated in such patients. The volume of the prostate estimated on digital rectal examination should not direct therapy, because the size of the prostate estimated in this manner may not correlate with either the symptoms or signs of the disorder or the need for treatment. Examination of the lower abdomen should be performed to assess for a distended bladder consistent with urinary retention, which may occur in the absence of symptoms. A neurologic examination assessing the sacral nerve roots is also helpful.

B. Laboratory Findings: Serum urea nitrogen and creatinine may be elevated in patients with high postvoid residual volumes and impairment of renal function. Urinalysis should be performed to exclude associated infection or hematuria. Prostate-specific antigen is often measured in order to increase the sensitivity of prostatic cancer detection, although it is elevated in benign prostatic hyperplasia.

C. Imaging: Intravenous urography was at one time performed routinely in the evaluation of men with signs or symptoms of prostatic hypertrophy. Elevation of the bladder base, trabeculation and thickening of the bladder, diverticular formation, elevation of the distal ureters, and poor emptying can often be observed. Evidence of hydronephrosis occurs less commonly. However, intravenous urography is normal in the majority of patients and should be reserved for those with hematuria or when upper urinary tract disease is suspected. A plain film of the abdomen may reveal urinary tract calculi, and ultrasonography can be used to assess bladder or upper tract changes described earlier. In addition, prostate volume can be determined. However, routine imaging is not necessary in patients with mild to moderate symptoms and a normal urinalysis, serum creatinine, and physical examination.

D. Urodynamic Evaluation: Uroflowmetry is perhaps the most useful urodynamic technique for the assessment of benign prostatic hypertrophy. The maximum urinary flow rate is usually recorded, and such a measurement is reliable only if the total volume voided exceeds 150 mL. Most urologists agree that a peak flow rate less than 10 mL per second is indicative of infravesical obstruction. More detailed urodynamic evaluation is indicated in patients with signs or symptoms of hyperplasia and known neurologic disorders; in very young patients; and in those with primarily irritative, rather than obstructive, symptoms.

E. Cystourethroscopy: Cystourethroscopy is an invasive procedure and should be performed when the diagnosis is uncertain and, on occasion, when patients are being evaluated for newer forms of treatment. When prostatectomy is indicated, cystourethrography should be performed immediately before the procedure.

Differential Diagnosis

The symptoms associated with benign prostatic hypertrophy may be produced by other disorders that may also cause bladder outlet obstruction: urethral stricture, bladder neck contracture, bladder calculi, and cancers of the prostate or bladder. Urinary tract infection, which may lead to irritative voiding symptoms, should be excluded. Neurologic disease can lead to voiding disorders and should be considered in patients with a history of such diseases and in those with an abnormal neurologic examination.

Diagnostic Evaluation & Treatment

Clinical practice guidelines have recently been released for the evaluation and treatment of patients with benign prostatic hypertrophy (Figure 23–1). Most patients with benign prostatic hypertrophy may be approached using these guidelines. However, they do not apply to all patients, eg, those who pose a greater surgical risk because of coexistent medical disease.

A detailed history focusing on the urinary tract is obtained, complemented by a physical examination including a digital rectal examination of the prostate and a focused neurologic examination. Urinalysis is then performed and serum creatinine determined. Measurement of PSA is considered optional. Although PSA testing will increase detection of prostate cancer, there is significant overlap in PSA values between patients with benign prostatic hypertrophy and prostate cancer.

Imaging of the upper urinary tract, cystometry, and cystourethroscopy are rarely indicated. Pressure-flow studies, uroflowmetry, and measurement of postvoid residual urine volumes are optional and should be considered in selected cases only.

Patients with refractory urinary retention, recurrent urinary tract infection, recurrent or persistent hematuria, bladder calculi, and renal insufficiency are good candidates for prostatic surgery. Patients without such symptoms or signs are evaluated with a symptom scoring system (American Urological Association Symptom Index; Table 23–4). Patients with mild symptoms (symptom score 0–7) are good candidates for watchful waiting with periodic reevaluation. Patients with moderate (symptom score 8–19) to severe (symptom score 20–35) symptoms are offered treatment options that may be facilitated by giving the patient printed material describing the particular benefits and risks of each treatment option. Table 23–5 reviews outcomes for various treatment options. As one can see, there is considerable uncertainty regarding the likelihood of some outcomes.

A. Medical Treatment: Prostatic enlargement may be a product of stromal or epithelial hyperplasia. Medical management may target either or both elements. It appears that prostatic androgen levels play at least a permissive role in benign hypertrophy, and therapies that reduce their levels will reduce prostatic size and improve obstructive symptoms. Androgen deprivation may be induced at various levels along the hypothalamic-pituitary-testicular axis (Table 23–6). Methods that reduce circulating levels of testosterone will result in loss of libido and sexual function, however. The human prostate and bladder base contains both α_1 and α_2 adrenoceptors, and the prostate will show a contractile response to such agonists. The contractile properties of the prostate are mediated primarily by α_1 receptors. Alpha$_1$ blockade has been shown to result in both objective and subjective improvement in the symptoms and signs of benign prostatic hypertrophy in some patients (Table 23–7). Side effects are related to the antagonism of α adrenoceptors. In placebo-controlled trials, both fi-

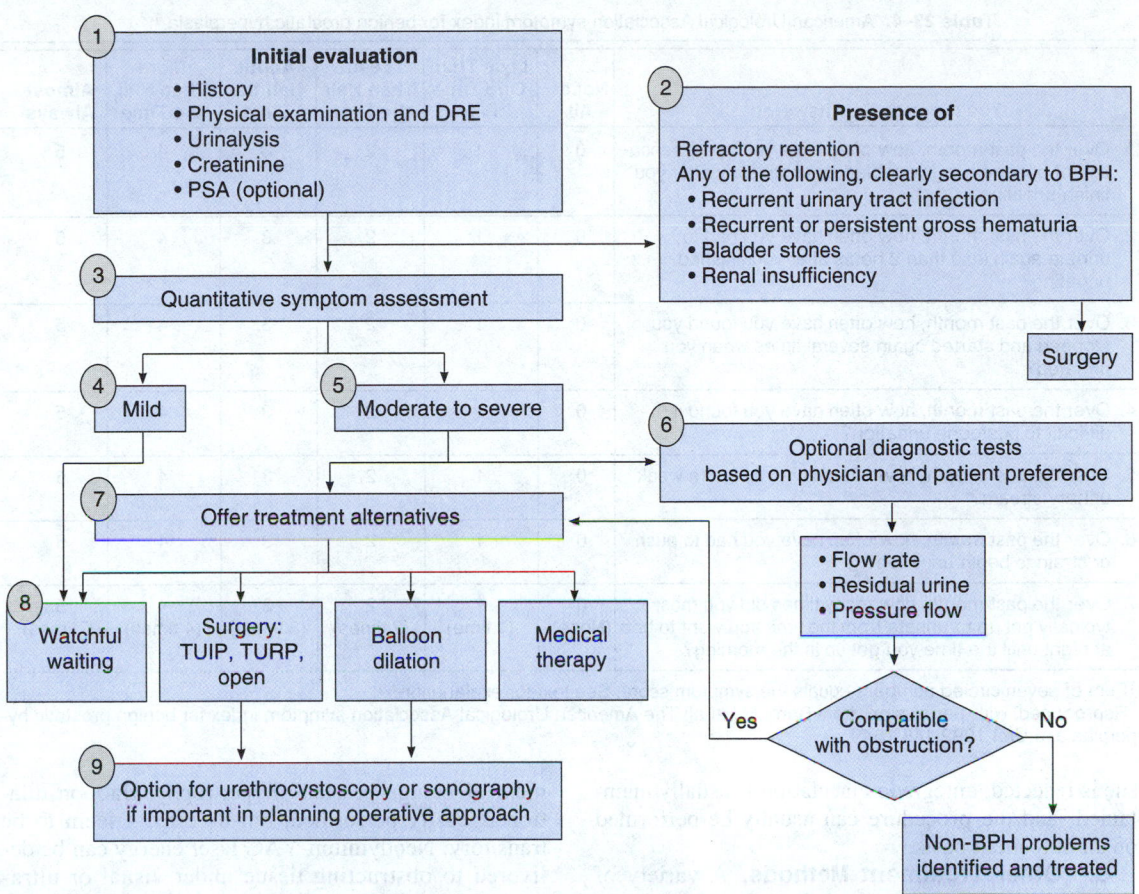

Figure 23–1. Benign prostatic hyperplasia decision diagram. (BPH, benign prostatic hyperplasia; DRE, digital rectal examination; TUIP, transurethral incision of the prostate; TURP, transurethral resection of the prostate.)

nasteride and selective α_1 blockade benefit a small to moderate number of patients with respect to symptom score, urinary flow rates, and residual urine volumes. The long-term benefits of such therapy are unknown at present. In a large multicenter, multi-arm trial investigating the possible benefit of combination medical therapy (alpha-blocker and finasteride), found alpha-blockers were found to be effective therapy for benign prostatic hyperplasia while finasteride had limited efficacy. However, prostatic enlargement was not an entry criterion, which may have favored the alpha-blocker arms of the trial.

B. Surgical Treatment: Removal of obstructing adenomatous prostatic tissue can be accomplished either through an incision or transurethrally. Transurethral resection is associated with a low mortality rate (0.1%), a moderate morbidity rate (18%), and a very high likelihood of both objective and symptomatic improvement in the symptoms and signs of benign prostatic hypertrophy. Retrograde ejaculation occurs in up to 90% of patients after this

procedure. Complications occur uncommonly and include bladder neck contracture (2.7%), urethral stricture disease (2.5%), and incontinence (1.7%). Repeat resection is necessary in less than 10% of men who undergo transurethral prostatectomy. Transurethral resection has come under more intense scrutiny for several reasons. It is the second most common surgical procedure in men over age 60, and its costs have escalated in recent years. The relative risk of death may be higher in patients undergoing transurethral compared to open prostatectomy. Reasons for this discrepancy are not known. In addition, other treatment options are available that may be associated with less morbidity. Whether alternative treatment methods will prove to be equivalent or superior to transurethral prostatectomy for the long-term control of benign prostatic hypertrophy is not known.

Patients with symptoms and signs of benign prostatic hypertrophy associated with smaller glands—especially in younger men—may benefit from transurethral incision of the prostate (TUIP). No tis-

Table 23–4. American Urological Association symptom index for benign prostatic hyperplasia.[1,2]

Questions to Be Answered	Not at All	Less Than One Time in Five	Less Than Half the Time	About Half the Time	More Than Half the Time	Almost Always
1. Over the past month, how often have you had a sensation of not emptying your bladder completely after you finish urinating?	0	1	2	3	4	5
2. Over the past month, how often have you had to urinate again less than 2 hours after you finished urinating?	0	1	2	3	4	5
3. Over the past month, how often have you found you stopped and started again several times when you urinated?	0	1	2	3	4	5
4. Over the past month, how often have you found it difficult to postpone urination?	0	1	2	3	4	5
5. Over the past month, how often have you had a weak urinary stream?	0	1	2	3	4	5
6. Over the past month, how often have you had to push or strain to begin urination?	0	1	2	3	4	5
7. Over the past month, how many times did you most typically get up to urinate from the time you went to bed at night until the time you got up in the morning?	0 (None)	1 (1 time)	2 (2 times)	3 (3 times)	4 (4 times)	5 (5 times)

[1]Sum of seven circled numbers equals the symptom score. See text for explanation.
[2]Reproduced, with permission, from Barry MJ et al: The American Urological Association symptom index for benign prostatic hyperplasia. J Urol 1992;148:1549.

sue is resected, antegrade ejaculation is usually maintained, and the procedure can usually be performed on an outpatient basis.

C. Other Treatment Methods: A variety of minimally invasive procedures have been developed and are currently being evaluated for the management of benign prostatic hypertrophy. Balloon dilation is easily performed, but its effects seem to be transitory. Neodymium-YAG laser energy can be delivered to obstructing tissue under visual or ultrasound guidance. Prostatic tissue may be desiccated using either transurethral or transrectal application of

Table 23–5. Balance sheet for benign prostatic hyperplasia treatment outcomes.[1]

Outcome	TUIP	Open Surgery	TURP	Watchful Waiting	Alpha Blockers	Finasteride[2]
Chance for improvement	78–83%	94–99.8%	75–96%	31–55%	59–86%	54–78%
Degree of symptom improvement (% reduction in symptom score)	73%	79%	85%	Unknown	51%	31%
Morbidity and complications	2.2–33.3%	7–42.7%	5.2–30.7%	1–5%	2.9–43.3%	13.6–18.8%
Death within 30–90 days	0.2–1.5%	1–4.6%	0.5–3.3%	0.8%	0.8%	0.8%
Total incontinence	0.1–1.1%	0.3–0.7%	0.7–1.4%	2%	2%	2%
Need for operative treatment for surgical complications	1.3–2.7%	0.6–14.1%	0.7–10.1%	0	0	0
Impotence	3.9–24.5	4.7–39.2	3.3–34.8	3	3	2.5–5.3
Retrograde ejaculation	6–55%	36–95%	25–99%	0	4–11%	0
Loss of work in days	7–21	21–28	7–21	1	3.5	1.5
Hospital stay in days	1–3	5–10	3–5	0	0	0

TUIP = transurethral incision of the prostate; TURP = transurethral resection of the prostate.
[1]90% confidence interval.
[2]Most of the data reviewed for finasteride is derived from three trials that have required an enlarged prostate for entry. The chance of improvement in men with symptoms yet minimally enlarged prostates may be much less, as noted from the VA Cooperative Trial.

Table 23–6. Androgen ablation and blockade for benign prostatic hyperplasia.

Agent	Action	Effects
Leuprolide, busere-lin, nafarelin (LHRH agonists)	Inhibit pituitary lu-teinizing hormone secretion; de-crease testoste-rone and dihydro-testosterone.	Impotence, loss of libido; hot flashes, gynecomastia.
Megestrol acetate, hydroxyproges-terone caproate (progestational agents)	Inhibit pituitary LH secretion; de-crease testoste-rone and dihydro-testosterone.	Impotence, loss of libido.
Flutamide (anti-an-drogen)	Androgen recep-tor inhibition.	Gynecomastia, diarrhea; libido maintained.
Finasteride (5α-re-ductase inhibitor)	Decreases dihy-drotestosterone.	Libido maintained.

microwave hyperthermia. Self-retaining intraurethral stents have been developed. The use of laser energy, microwave hyperthermia, and stents is still investiga-tional, and their use for the treatment of benign pros-tatic hypertrophy is the subject of several ongoing trials. Early comparative trials between laser and conventional transurethral resections demonstrate more dramatic improvement in symptom score and uroflowmetry with conventional resections at the ex-pense of higher morbidity and longer hospital stays.

Berges RR et al: Randomised, placebo-controlled, double-blind clinical trial of beta-sitosterol in patients with be-nign prostatic hyperplasia. Beta-sitosterol Study Group. Lancet 1995;345:1529. (Beta-sitosterol resulted in sig-nificant improvement in symptom scores and uroflow-metry.)

Cowles RS et al: A prospective randomized comparison of transurethral resection to visual laser ablation of the prostate for the treatment of benign prostatic hyperpla-sia. Urology 1995;46:155. (At 1-year follow-up, patients undergoing TURP had a more significant improvement in symptom score, uroflowmetry, and quality of life than those undergoing a laser procedure; however, the hospi-tal stay was longer and the morbidity rate was higher.)

Kreder KJ: Combination drug therapy for benign prostatic hyperplasia. JAMA 1995;274:359.

Table 23–7. Alpha blockade for benign prostatic hyperplasia.

Agent	Action	Dose
Phenoxybenz-amine	Alpha$_1$ and alpha$_2$ blockade	5–10 mg twice daily
Prazosin	Alpha$_1$ blockade	1–5 mg twice daily
Terazosin	Alpha$_1$ blockade	1–10 mg daily
Doxazosin	Alpha$_1$ blockade	1–8 mg daily

Lepor H: Medical therapy for benign prostatic hyperplasia. Urology 1993;42:483.

McConnell et al: Benign prostatic hyperplasia: Diagnosis and treatment. Clinical Practice Guideline No. 8. AHCPR Publication No. 940582. Agency for Health Care Policy and Research, Public Health Service, U.S. Department of Health and Human Services, February 1994.

Moul JW: Benign prostatic hypertrophy: New concepts for the 1990s. Postgrad Med 1993;94:141. (Medications for mild to moderate disease and transurethral resection of the prostate for severe disease remain the standard of care. Further studies are needed to determine the roles of balloon dilation, laser prostatectomy, prostatic stents, and microwave hyperthermia.)

Oesterling JE: Benign prostatic hyperplasia. Medical and minimally invasive treatment options. N Engl J Med 1995;332:99.

Rittmaster RS: Finasteride. N Engl J Med 1994;330:120.

Wasson JH et al: A comparison of transurethral surgery with watchful waiting for moderate symptoms of benign prostatic hyperplasia. The Veterans Affairs Cooperative Study Group on Transurethral Resection of the Prostate. N Engl J Med 1995;332:75. (Surgery is more effective than watchful waiting in men with moderate symptoms of benign prostatic hyperplasia.)

MALIGNANT GENITOURINARY TRACT DISORDERS

PROSTATE CANCER

Essentials of Diagnosis

- Prostatic induration on digital rectal examination or elevation of PSA.
- Most often asymptomatic.
- Systemic symptoms (weight loss, bone pain) in 20% of patients.

General Considerations

Prostatic cancer is the most common cancer de-tected in American men. In the United States in 1996, over 300,000 new cases of prostate cancer will be diagnosed, and over 41,000 deaths will result. However, the clinical incidence of the disease does not match the prevalence noted at autopsy, where more than 40% of men over 50 years of age are found to have prostatic carcinoma. Most such occult cancers are small and contained within the prostate gland. Few are associated with regional or distant disease. The incidence of prostatic cancer increases with age. Whereas 30% of men age 60–69 will have the disease, autopsy incidence increases to 67% in men aged 80–89 years. Although the prevalence of prostatic cancer in autopsy specimens around the world varies little, the clinical incidence is considerably different (high in North America and European countries, intermediate in South America, and low in the Far East), suggesting that environmental or dietary differences among populations may be important for prostatic cancer growth. A 50-year-old American man has a lifetime risk of 40% for latent cancer, 9.5% for developing clinically apparent cancer, and a 2.9% risk of death due to prostatic cancer. Blacks and others with a family history of prostatic cancer and perhaps men who have undergone vasectomy are at an increased risk of developing it.

Clinical Findings

A. Symptoms and Signs: Most prostatic cancers are detected in asymptomatic men who are found to have focal nodules or areas of induration within the prostate at the time of digital rectal examination.

Rarely, patients present with signs of urinary retention (palpable bladder) or neurologic symptoms as a result of epidural metastases and cord compression. Obstructive voiding symptoms are most often due to benign prostatic hyperplasia, which occurs in the same age group. However, large or locally extensive prostatic cancers can cause obstructive voiding symptoms. Lymph node metastases can lead to lower extremity lymphedema. As the axial skeleton is the most common site of metastases, patients may present with back pain or pathologic fractures.

B. Laboratory Findings:

1. Serum tumor markers—Prostate-specific antigen (PSA) is a glycoprotein produced only in the cytoplasm of benign and malignant prostate cells. The serum level correlates with the volume of both benign and malignant prostatic tissue. Measurement of PSA may be useful in detecting and staging prostatic cancer, monitoring response to treatment, and detecting recurrence before it becomes obvious clinically. As a first-line screening test, PSA will be elevated in approximately 10–15% of men self-referred for screening. Approximately 20–25% of men with intermediate degrees of elevation (4.1–10 ng/mL; normal < 4 ng/mL) will be found to have prostatic cancer. Almost two-thirds of those with elevations greater than 10 ng/mL will have prostatic cancer. (See age-specific PSA reference ranges under Screening for Prostatic Cancer, below.) Patients with intermediate levels of PSA will usually have localized and therefore potentially curable cancers. However, it should be remembered that approximately 20% of patients who undergo radical prostatectomy for localized prostatic cancer will have normal levels of PSA.

In untreated patients with prostatic cancer, the level of PSA correlates with the volume and stage of the disease. Whereas most organ-confined cancers are associated with PSA levels less than 10 ng/mL, more advanced disease (seminal vesicle invasion, lymph node involvement, or occult distant metas-

tases) is more common in patients with PSA levels in excess of 40 ng/mL. Approximately 98% of patients with metastatic prostatic cancer will have elevated PSA. However, there are occasional cancers that are localized despite substantial elevations in PSA. Therefore, treatment decisions in patients with untreated cancers cannot be made on the basis of PSA testing alone. A rising level of PSA after treatment is consistent with progressive disease whether it be locally recurrent or metastatic.

Until the advent of PSA testing, serum acid phosphatase was the standard serum tumor marker used in the evaluation of patients with localized and metastatic prostatic cancer. Because PSA is more sensitive than serum acid phosphatase, it has largely replaced its use. However, an elevated serum acid phosphatase is more predictive of metastatic disease than an elevated PSA, and for this reason it is still used by some. Serum acid phosphatase levels will be normal in approximately 25% of patients with metastatic disease.

2. Miscellaneous laboratory testing—Patients in urinary retention or those with ureteral obstruction due to locally or regionally advanced prostatic cancers may present with elevations in serum urea nitrogen or creatinine. Patients with bony metastases may have elevations in alkaline phosphatase or hypercalcemia. Laboratory and clinical evidence of disseminated intravascular coagulation can occur in patients with advanced prostatic cancers.

3. Prostatic biopsy—Transrectal ultrasound-guided biopsy seems to be a better method for detection of prostatic cancer than finger-guided biopsy. The use of a spring-loaded, 18-gauge biopsy needle has allowed transrectal biopsy to be performed with little patient discomfort and low attendant morbidity. The specimen preserves glandular architecture and allows for accurate grading as described below. Taking biopsy specimens from the apex, midportion, and base of the prostate is recommended by some and should be considered in patients with significant elevations in PSA but a normal digital rectal examination. Patients with abnormalities of the seminal vesicles can have guided biopsies of these structures performed to allow for detection of local tumor invasion. Aspiration biopsies of the prostate, though accurate and associated with low morbidity, have been used rarely since the introduction of the spring-loaded biopsy device but should be considered in patients at an increased risk of bleeding.

C. Imaging: Modern transrectal ultrasound instrumentation provides high-definition images of the prostate. Transrectal ultrasonography has been used largely for the staging of prostatic carcinomas. In addition, transrectal ultrasound-guided—rather than digitally guided—biopsy of the prostate may be a more accurate way to investigate suspicious lesions. Most prostatic cancers are hypoechoic.

MRI of the prostate allows for evaluation of the

prostatic lesion as well as regional lymph nodes. The positive predictive value for detection of both capsular penetration and seminal vesicle invasion is similar for both transrectal ultrasound and MRI. CT scanning plays little role in evaluation because of its inability to accurately identify or stage prostatic cancers.

Radionuclide bone scan is superior to conventional plain skeletal x-rays in detecting bony metastases. Most prostatic cancer metastases are multiple and are most commonly localized to the axial skeleton. Because of the high frequency of abnormal scans in patients in this age group resulting from degenerative joint disease, plain films are often useful in evaluating patients with indeterminate radionuclide findings. Intravenous urography and cystoscopy are not routinely used to evaluate patients with prostatic cancer.

Imaging can be tailored to the likelihood of advanced disease in newly diagnosed patients. Asymptomatic patients with well to moderately well differentiated cancers—thought to be localized to the prostate on digital rectal examination and transurethral ultrasound and associated with normal or only modest elevations of PSA (ie, < 10 ng/mL)—need no further evaluation.

Those with more advanced local lesions, symptoms of metastases (ie, bone pain), and elevations in PSA greater than 10 ng/mL should undergo radionuclide bone scan. Cross-sectional imaging of the prostate is usually indicated only in those patients in the latter group who have negative bone scans in an attempt to detect lymph node metastases. Patients found to have enlarged pelvic lymph nodes are candidates for fine-needle aspiration. Despite application of modern and sophisticated imaging, understaging of prostatic cancer is common.

Screening for Prostatic Cancer

The incidence of prostate cancer is rising in this country, partly due to wider application of detection techniques (transrectal ultrasound and PSA testing). The goal of a screening effort should be to detect and effectively treat only those prostatic carcinomas most likely to cause morbidity or mortality if left untreated. Detection of latent, nonprogressive cancers would expose patients to unnecessary treatment and its attendant complications and costs. Whether screening for prostatic cancer will result in a decrease in yearly mortality rates due to the disease is the subject of much current debate.

The screening tests currently available include digital rectal examination, PSA testing, and transrectal ultrasound. Depending on the patient population being evaluated, detection rates using digital rectal examination alone will vary from 1.5% to 7%. Unfortunately, most cancers detected in this way are advanced (stages T3 or greater). Transrectal ultrasound should not be used as a first-line screening tool because of its expense, its low specificity (and therefore high biopsy rate), and the fact that it increases the detection rate very little when compared with the combined use of digital rectal examination and PSA testing.

PSA testing will increase the detection rate of prostatic cancers compared with digital rectal examination. Approximately 2–2.5% of men older than age 50 will be found to have prostatic cancer using PSA testing compared with a rate of approximately 1.5% using digital rectal examination alone. PSA is not specific for cancer, and there is considerable overlap of values between men with benign prostatic hypertrophy and those with prostatic cancers. The sensitivity, specificity, and positive predictive value of PSA and digital rectal examination are listed in Table 23–8. PSA-detected cancers are more likely to be localized compared with those detected with digital rectal examination alone.

In order to improve the performance of PSA as a screening test, several investigators have developed alternative methods for its use. The measurement of PSA serially (PSA velocity) may increase specificity for cancer detection with little loss in sensitivity. A rate of change in PSA greater than 0.75 ng/mL per year is associated with an increased likelihood of cancer detection. In a patient with a normal digital rectal examination, an elevated PSA, and a normal transrectal ultrasound, the indications for prostate biopsy may be refined by calculating PSA density (serum PSA/volume of the prostate as measured by ultrasound). Patients with high PSA density are more likely to have disease in spite of a normal digital rectal examination and normal transrectal ultrasound. As PSA concentration is directly related to patient age, establishment of age-specific reference ranges would increase specificity (fewer older men with benign prostatic hypertrophy would undergo evaluation) and

Table 23–8. Screening for prostatic cancer: Test performance.[1]

Test	Sensitivity	Specificity	Positive Predictive Value
Abnormal PSA (>4 ng/mL)	0.67	0.97	0.43
Abnormal DRE	0.50	0.94	0.24
Abnormal PSA *or* DRE	0.84	0.92	0.28
Abnormal PSA *and* DRE	0.34	0.995	0.49

Key: DRE = digital rectal examination
PSA = prostate-specific antigen
[1]Modified from Kramer BS et al: Prostate cancer screening: What we know and what we need to know. Ann Intern Med 1993;119:914.

increase sensitivity (more younger men with cancer would undergo evaluation). Age-specific reference ranges have been established: men 40–49, < 2.5 ng/mL; men 50–59, < 3.5 ng/mL; men 60–69, < 4.5 ng/mL; men 70–79, < 6.5 ng/mL (based on a previously normal serum PSA of < 4.0 ng/mL). However, age-specific reference ranges for PSA need to be validated in larger patient populations, including various ethnic groups. The most recent attempt at refining PSA has been the measurement of free serum and protein-bound levels (cancer patients have a lower percentage of free serum PSA). Numerous centers are analyzing this assay to define an optimal cutoff level. Early reports using cutoffs of 18–20% of free PSA resulted in 5–10% lost sensitivity for 15–40% gains in specificity.

Pathology & Staging

The majority of prostatic cancers are adenocarcinomas. Most arise in the periphery of the prostate (peripheral zone), though a small percentage arise in the central (5–10%) and transition zones (20%) of the gland. Most pathologists employ the Gleason grading system whereby a "primary" grade is applied to the architectural pattern of cancerous glands occupying the largest area of the specimen and a "secondary" pattern is assigned to the next largest area of cancerous growth. Grading is based on architectural (rather than histologic) criteria, and five possible "grades" are possible. Adding the score of the primary and secondary patterns gives a Gleason score. Grade correlates well with tumor volume, stage, and prognosis. The TNM classification of the American Joint Cancer Committee for prostatic cancer is shown in Table 23–9.

The patterns of prostatic cancer progression have been well defined. The likelihood of both local invasion and metastases is greater in larger or less well differentiated cancers. Small and well-differentiated cancers (grades 1 and 2) are usually confined within the prostate, whereas large-volume (> 4 mL) or poorly differentiated (grades 4 and 5) cancers are more commonly locally extensive or metastatic to regional lymph nodes or bone. Penetration of the prostatic capsule by cancer is common and often occurs along perineural spaces. Seminal vesicle invasion is associated with a high likelihood of regional or distant disease. Lymphatic metastases are most often identified in the obturator lymph node chain. The axial skeleton, as mentioned previously, is the most common site of distant metastases.

Treatment

A. Localized Disease: What constitutes the optimal form of treatment for patients with clinically localized cancers remains controversial. Treatment decisions are at present made on the basis of tumor grade and stage and the age and health of the patient. Although selected patients may be candidates for sur-

Table 23–9. TNM staging system for prostate cancer.

T: Primary tumor	
Tx	Cannot be assessed
T0	No evidence of primary tumor
Tis	Carcinoma in situ (CIS)
T1a	≤ 3 foci of carcinoma in resection for benign disease; normal digital rectal examination
T1b	≥ 3 foci of carcinoma in resection for benign disease; normal digital rectal examination
T1c	Detected from elevated PSA alone; normal digital rectal examination
T2a	Tumor in less than half of one lobe
T2b	Tumor in more than half of one lobe
T2c	Tumor in both lobes
T3a	Unilateral extracapsular extension
T3b	Bilateral extracapsular extension
T3c	Seminal vesicle involvement
T4	Adjacent organ involvement
N: Regional lymph nodes	
Nx	Cannot be assessed
N0	No regional lymph node metastasis
N1	Metastasis in a single lymph node 2 cm or less
N2	Metastasis in a single lymph node > 2 cm and < 5 cm or multiple nodes none > 5 cm
N3	Metastasis in lymph node > 5 cm
M: Distant metastasis	
Mx	Cannot be assessed
M0	No distant metastasis
M1	Distant metastasis present

veillance based on age or health and the presence of small-volume or well-differentiated cancers, most patients with an anticipated survival in excess of 10 years should be considered for treatment with irradiation or surgery. Both radiation therapy and radical prostatectomy allow for acceptable levels of local control. A randomized trial comparing watchful waiting and radical prostatectomy in men with clinically localized prostate cancer is currently under way in the United States (PIVOT: Prostate Cancer Intervention Versus Observation Trial). This trial will randomize 2000 patients and will run for 15 years. Patients need to be advised of all treatment options (including surveillance) along with their particular benefits, risks, and limitations.

B. Radical Prostatectomy: In radical prostatectomy, the seminal vesicles, prostate, and ampullae of the vas deferens are removed. Refinements in technique have allowed maintenance of urinary continence in almost all patients and erectile function in selected patients. However, the procedure should be used selectively. As capsular penetration is a common finding in patients with presumed localized prostatic cancer, preservation of the neurovascular bundle contiguous with a prostatic cancer may increase the likelihood of local tumor recurrence. Local recurrence is uncommon after radical prostatectomy, and its incidence is related to pathologic stage. Organ-confined cancers rarely recur (2% local, 1% distant). However, cancers found to be locally extensive (capsular penetration, seminal vesicle invasion) are associated with higher local (10–25%) and distant (20–25%) relapse rates.

Ideal candidates for the procedure include healthy patients with stages T1, T2, and selected T3 prostatic cancers. Patients with advanced local tumors (T3 and T4) and those with lymph node metastases are rarely candidates for this procedure.

Patients with positive surgical margins are at an increased risk for local and distant tumor relapse. Such patients are often considered candidates for adjuvant therapy (radiation for positive margins or androgen deprivation for lymph node metastases). Although adjuvant radiation seems to be associated with fewer local recurrences (0–5% with radiation versus 15–30% without), it has little or no impact on distant failure rates (30–35% with radiation versus 30–45% without).

C. Radiation Therapy: Radiation can be delivered by a variety of techniques including use of external beam radiotherapy and transperineal implantation of radioisotopes. Morbidity is limited, and the survival of patients with localized cancers (T1, T2, and selected T3) approaches 65% at 10 years. As with surgery, the likelihood of local failure correlates with technique and tumor stage. The likelihood of a positive, prostatic biopsy more than 18 months after surgery varies between 20% and 60% in selected series. Patients with local recurrence are at an increased risk of cancer progression and cancer death compared with those who have negative biopsies. Ambiguous target definitions, inadequate radiation doses, and understaging of patients may be responsible for the failure noted in some series. Newer techniques of radiation (implantation, conformal therapy using three-dimensional reconstruction of CT-based tumor volumes, heavy particle, charged particle, and heavy charged particle) may improve local control rates.

D. Surveillance: A positive impact of localized prostatic cancer treatment with regard to survival has not been conclusively demonstrated. Surveillance alone may be an appropriate form of management for selected patients with prostatic cancer. However, many patients in such series are older and have very small and well-differentiated cancers. Even in such a selected population, cancer death rates approach 10%. In addition, end points for intervention in patients on surveillance regimens have not been defined.

E. Locally and Regionally Advanced Disease: Prostatic cancers associated with minimal degrees of capsular penetration are candidates for standard irradiation or surgery. Those with locally extensive cancers, including those with seminal vesicle and bladder neck invasion, are at increased risk of both local and distant relapse despite conventional therapy. Currently, a variety of investigational regimens are being tested in an effort to improve local and distant relapse rates in such patients. Combination therapy (androgen deprivation combined with surgery or irradiation), cryosurgery, newer forms of irradiation, and hormonal therapy alone are being tested in such patients. Similarly, patients with lymph node metastases may benefit little from aggressive local therapy and are best treated with androgen deprivation because of the inevitability of distant relapse in the majority of such patients.

F. Metastatic Disease: Since death due to prostatic carcinoma is almost invariably a result of failure to control metastatic disease, research has emphasized efforts to improve control of distant disease. It is well known that most prostatic carcinomas are hormone-dependent, and approximately 70–80% of men with metastatic prostatic carcinoma will respond to various forms of androgen deprivation. Testosterone, the major circulating androgen, is produced by Leydig cells in the testes (95%), with a smaller amount being produced by peripheral conversion of other steroids. Although 98% of serum testosterone is protein-bound, free testosterone enters prostate cells and is converted to dihydrotestosterone, the major intracellular androgen. Dihydrotestosterone binds a cytoplasmic receptor protein, and the complex moves to the cell nucleus, where it modulates transcription. Androgen deprivation may be induced at several levels along the pituitary-gonadal axis using a variety of methods or agents (Table 23–10). Use of LHRH agonists (leuprolide, buserelin, nafarelin)—a new class of drugs delivered monthly by injection—has allowed induction of androgen deprivation without orchiectomy or administration of diethylstilbestrol. Presently, administration of LHRH agonists and orchiectomy are the most common forms of primary androgen blockade used. Because of its rapid onset of action, ketoconazole should be considered in patients with advanced prostatic cancer who present with spinal cord compression, bilateral ureteral obstruction, or disseminated intravascular coagulation. Although testosterone is the major circulating androgen, the adrenal gland secretes the androgens dehydroepiandrosterone, dehydroepiandrosterone sulfate, and androstenedione. Some investigators believe that suppressing both testicular and adrenal androgens will allow for a better initial and longer response than methods that inhibit production of only testicular androgens. Complete androgen blockade can be achieved by combining an antiandrogen with use of an LHRH agonist or orchiectomy. Flutamide is a nonsteroidal antiandrogen that appears to act by com-

Table 23–10. Androgen ablation for prostatic cancer.

Level	Agent	Sequelae	Dose
Pituitary, hypothalamus	Estrogens	Gynecomastia, hot flashes, thromboembolic disease, impotence	1–3 mg daily
	LHRH agonists	Impotence, hot flashes, gynecomastia, rarely anemia	Monthly injection
Adrenal	Ketoconazole	Adrenal insufficiency, nausea, gynecomastia, hepatic toxicity	400 mg 3 times daily
	Aminoglutethimide	Adrenal insufficiency, nausea, rash, ataxia	250 mg 4 times daily
	Glucocorticoids	Gastrointestinal bleeding, fluid retention	Prednisone: 20–40 mg daily
Testis	Orchiectomy	Gynecomastia, hot flashes, impotence	
Prostate cell	Antiandrogens	No impotence when used alone; nausea, diarrhea	Flutamide: 250 mg 3 times daily

petitively binding the receptor for dihydrotestosterone, the intracellular androgen responsible for prostatic cell growth and development. When patients with metastatic prostatic cancer are stratified with regard to extent of disease and performance status, those patients with limited disease and a good performance status treated with combined androgen blockade (LHRH agonist and flutamide) seem to survive longer than those treated with an LHRH agonist alone. However, a recent trial has demonstrated no benefit from the addition of an antiandrogen in patients treated with orchiectomy. Additional trials examining the potential benefits of intermittent androgen deprivation are ongoing, and new antiandrogens are being tested.

Although androgen deprivation is effective, most patients with advanced disease so treated will experience disease relapse, usually within 3 years. In patients on complete androgen blockade, withdrawal of the antiandrogen can result in a secondary response in 20% of patients. The mechanism of this response remains unclear, yet both serologic (PSA) and clinical responses (improvement in bone scan and pain) have been reported. Once relapse has been identified, survival is limited. Palliative care including adequate pain control and focal irradiation of symptomatic or unstable bone disease should be instituted in patients who have failed standard hormonal therapy. Secondary therapy with chemotherapeutic agents has had limited results but should be considered in patients with a reasonable performance status. Preliminary trials of suramin, a growth factor antagonist, suggest that it may have some activity in patients with hormone-refractory prostatic cancer, and dose-escalation studies are currently ongoing. Other agents being investigated in large trials include ketoconazole and mitoxantrone.

Albertsen PC et al: Long-term survival among men with conservatively treated localized prostate cancer. JAMA 1995;274:626. (In this population-based, retrospective cohort study, men aged 65–75 years with conservatively treated low-grade prostate cancer underwent no loss of life expectancy; however, men with higher-grade tumors [Gleason score 5–10] experienced increasing loss of life expectancy. Coexistent disease also impacts upon long-term survival and thus must also be considered when counseling patients about treatment options.)

Catalona WJ et al: Evaluation of percentage of free serum prostate-specific antigen to improve specificity for prostate cancer screening. JAMA 1995;274:1214. (Percentage of free PSA is lower in men with prostate cancer, and its measurement increases the specificity of the test.)

Catalona WJ: Management of cancer of the prostate. N Engl J Med 1994;331:996.

Chodak GW et al: Results of conservative management of clinically localized prostate cancer. N Engl J Med 1994;330:242. (Results from pooled data from six nonrandomized trials since 1985 demonstrate that disease-specific survival for grade 1 or grade 2 tumors, Gleason sum 2–7, is equivalent to that of surgery or radiation therapy, ie, approximately 87%; however, the series are retrospective and may be biased toward older patients.)

Crawford ED, DeAntoni EP: PSA as a screening test for prostate cancer. Urol Clin North Am 1993;20(4):637. (This issue discusses tumor markers.)

Cupp MR, Oesterling JE: Prostate-specific antigen, digital rectal examination, and transrectal ultrasonography: Their roles in diagnosing early prostate cancer. Mayo Clin Proc 1993;68:297. (Algorithm offered.)

Dorr VJ et al: An evaluation of prostate-specific antigen as a screening test for prostate cancer. Arch Intern Med 1993;153:2529. (Studies are needed to demonstrate improved outcomes before universal screening can be recommended.)

Gann PH et al: A prospective evaluation of plasma prostate-specific antigen for detection of prostatic cancer. JAMA 1995;273:289. (This nested case-control study showed that a single PSA measurement above 4.0 ng/mL had a sensitivity of 46% and a specificity of 91% for the detection of prostate cancers that arose within 4 years.)

Garnick MB: Prostate cancer: Screening, diagnosis, and management. Ann Intern Med 1993;118:804.

Kramer BS et al: Prostate cancer screening: What we know and what we need to know. Ann Int Med 1993;119:914.

Perez CA et al: Localized carcinoma of the prostate: Review of management with external beam radiation therapy. Cancer 1993;72:3156.

Pinta KJ, Esper PS: Risk factors for prostate cancer. Ann Intern Med 1993;118:793. (Analysis of literature to date supports age, race, family history, vasectomy, and dietary fat as risk factors.)

Presti JC Jr et al: Local staging of prostatic carcinoma: Comparison of transrectal sonography and endorectal MR imaging. AJR Am J Roentgenol 1996;166:103. (Both imaging modalities had comparable predictive values for the detection of extracapsular extension.)

Woolf SH: Screening for prostate cancer with prostate-specific antigen. N Engl J Med 1995;333:1401. (Until results of screening trials are known, the true benefits and risks of screening remain a matter of opinion rather than fact.)

BLADDER CANCER

Essentials of Diagnosis

- Irritative voiding symptoms.
- Gross or microscopic hematuria.
- Positive urinary cytology in most patients.
- Filling defect within bladder noted on imaging.

General Considerations

Bladder cancer is the second most common urologic cancer, occurs more commonly in men than women (2.7:1), and the mean age at diagnosis is 65 years. Cigarette smoking and exposure to industrial dyes or solvents are risk factors for the disease and account for approximately 60% and 15% of new cases, respectively.

Clinical Findings

A. Symptoms and Signs: Hematuria—gross or microscopic, chronic or intermittent—is the presenting symptom in 85–90% of patients with bladder cancer. Irritative voiding symptoms (urinary frequency and urgency) will occur in a small percentage of patients as a result of the location or size of the cancer. Most patients with bladder cancer will fail to have signs of the disease because of its superficial nature. Masses detected on bimanual examination may be present in patients with large-volume or deeply infiltrating cancers. Hepatomegaly or supraclavicular lymphadenopathy may be present in patients with metastatic disease, and lymphedema of the lower extremities may be present as a result of locally advanced cancers or metastases to pelvic lymph nodes.

B. Laboratory Findings: Urinalysis will reveal hematuria in the majority of cases. On occasion, it may be accompanied by pyuria. Azotemia may be present in a small number of cases associated with ureteral obstruction. Anemia may occasionally be due to chronic blood loss or to bone marrow metastases. Exfoliated cells from normal and abnormal urothelium can be readily detected in voided urine specimens. Cytology may be useful in detecting the disease at the time of initial presentation or to detect recurrence. Cytology is very sensitive in detecting cancers of higher grade and stage (80–90%) but less so in detecting superficial or well-differentiated lesions (50%). Sensitivity of detection using exfoliated cells may be enhanced by flow cytometry.

C. Imaging: Bladder cancers may be detected using intravenous urography, ultrasound, CT, or MRI where filling defects within the bladder are noted. However, the presence of cancer is confirmed by cystoscopy and biopsy, so imaging is useful primarily for evaluating the upper urinary tract and in staging the more advanced lesions.

D. Cystourethroscopy and Biopsy: The diagnosis and staging of bladder cancers is made by cystoscopy and transurethral resection. If cystoscopy—performed usually under local anesthesia—confirms the presence of bladder cancer, the patient is scheduled for transurethral resection under general or regional anesthesia. A careful bimanual examination is performed initially and at the end of the procedure, noting the size, position, and degree of fixation of a mass, if present. Any suspicious lesions are resected using electrocautery. Resection is carried down to the muscular elements of the bladder wall so as to allow complete staging. Random bladder and, on occasion, prostatic urethral biopsies are performed to detect occult disease elsewhere in the bladder and, therefore, identify patients at high risk of recurrence and progression.

Pathology & Selection of Treatment

Ninety-eight percent of primary bladder cancers are epithelial malignancies, with the majority being transitional cell carcinomas (90%). These latter cancers most often appear as papillary growths, but higher-grade lesions are often sessile and ulcerated. Grading is based on histologic architecture: size, pleomorphism, mitotic rate, and hyperchromatism. The frequency of recurrence and progression is strongly correlated with grade. Whereas progression may be noted in few grade I cancers (19–37%), it is common with poorly differentiated lesions (33–67%). Carcinoma in situ is recognizable as a flat, nonpapillary, anaplastic epithelium and may occur focally or diffusely, but it is most often found in association with papillary bladder cancers. Its presence identifies a patient at increased risk of recurrence and progression.

Adenocarcinomas and squamous cell cancers account for approximately 2% and 7% (respectively) of all bladder cancers detected in the USA. The latter is often associated with schistosomiasis, vesical calculi, or chronic catheter use.

Bladder cancer staging is based on the extent of bladder wall penetration and the presence of either regional or distant metastases. The TNM classification of the American Joint Cancer Committee for bladder cancer is shown in Table 23–11.

The natural history of bladder cancer is based on two separate but related processes: tumor recurrence and progression to higher stage disease. Both are related to tumor grade and stage. At initial presentation, approximately 50–80% of bladder cancers will be superficial: Ta, Tis, T1. Lymph node metastases and progression are uncommon in such patients when they are properly treated, and survival is excellent at 81%. Patients with superficial cancers (Ta, T1) are treated with complete transurethral resection and the selective use of intravesical chemotherapy. The latter is used to prevent or delay recurrence. Patients who present with large, high-grade, recurrent Ta lesions, T1 cancers, and those with carcinoma in situ are good candidates for intravesical chemotherapy. Patients with more invasive (T2, T3) but still localized cancers are at risk of both nodal metastases and progression, and they require more aggressive surgery, irradiation, or the combination of chemotherapy and selective surgery or irradiation due to the much higher risk of progression compared to patients with lower-stage lesions. Patients with evidence of lymph node or distant metastases should undergo systemic chemotherapy initially.

Treatment

A. Intravesical Chemotherapy: Immuno- or chemotherapeutic agents can be delivered directly into the bladder by a urethral catheter. They can be used to eradicate existing disease or to reduce the likelihood of recurrence in those who have undergone complete transurethral resection. Such therapy is more effective in the latter situation. Most agents are administered weekly for 6–12 weeks. The use of maintenance therapy after the initial induction regimen may be beneficial. Efficacy may be increased by prolonging contact time to 2 hours. Common agents include thiotepa, mitomycin, doxorubicin, and BCG, the latter being the most effective agent when compared with the others. Side effects of intravesical chemotherapy include irritative voiding symptoms and hemorrhagic cystitis. Systemic effects are rare. Patients who develop symptoms from BCG may require antituberculous therapy.

B. Surgical Treatment: Although transurethral resection is the initial form of treatment for all bladder cancers as it is diagnostic, allows for proper staging, and will control superficial cancers, muscle infiltrating cancers will require more aggressive treatment. Partial cystectomy may be indicated in patients with solitary lesions and those with cancers in a bladder diverticulum. Radical cystectomy entails removal of the bladder, prostate, seminal vesicles, and surrounding fat and peritoneal attachments in men and in women also the uterus, cervix, urethra, anterior vaginal vault, and usually the ovaries. Bilateral pelvic lymph node dissection is performed simultaneously.

Urinary diversion can be performed using a conduit of small or large bowel. However, continent forms of diversion have been developed that avoid the necessity of an external appliance.

C. Radiotherapy: External beam radiotherapy delivered in fractions over a 6- to 8-week period is generally well tolerated, but approximately 10–15% of patients will develop bladder, bowel, or rectal complications. Unfortunately, local recurrence is common after radiotherapy (30–70%). Increasingly, radiotherapy is being combined with systemic chemotherapy in an effort to improve local and distant relapse rates.

D. Chemotherapy: Fifteen percent of patients with newly diagnosed bladder cancer will present with metastatic disease, and 40% of those thought to have localized disease at the time of cystectomy or definitive radiotherapy will develop metastases usually within 2 years after the start of treatment. Cisplatin-based combination chemotherapy will result in partial or complete responses in 15–35% and 15–45% of patients, respectively.

Combination chemotherapy has been integrated into trials of surgery and radiotherapy. It has been used before each in an attempt to preserve the bladder and decrease recurrence rates. Alternatively, it has been employed postoperatively in patients who have undergone cystectomy and have been found to be at high risk of recurrence. In current practice, ad-

Table 23–11. TNM staging system for bladder cancer.

T: Primary tumor	
Tx	Cannot be assessed
T0	No evidence of primary tumor
Tis	Carcinoma in situ (CIS)
Ta	Noninvasive papillary carcinoma
T1	Invasion into lamina propria
T2	Invasion into superficial layer of muscularis propria
T3a	Invasion into deep layer of muscularis propria
T3b	Invasion through serosa into perivesical fat
T4a	Invasion into adjacent organs
T4b	Invasion into pelvic sidewall
N: Regional lymph nodes	
Nx	Cannot be assessed
N0	No regional lymph node metastasis
N1	Metastasis in a single lymph node ≤ 2 cm
N2	Metastasis in a single lymph node >2 cm and <5 cm or multiple nodes none >5 cm
N3	Metastasis in lymph node >5 cm
M: Distant metastasis	
Mx	Cannot be assessed
M0	No distant metastasis
M1	Distant metastasis present

juvant chemotherapy when indicated—ie, when the primary tumor invades perivesical fat or adjacent organs or when lymph nodes are found to have metastatic disease—is being offered mainly to patients being treated with radical cystectomy. It is used less often for patients with unresectable disease (extension to pelvic side wall).

Carroll PR: Urothelial carcinoma: Cancers of the bladder, ureter and renal pelvis. In: *Smith's General Urology,* 14th ed. Tanagho EA, McAninch JW (editors). Appleton & Lange, 1995.

Esrig D et al: Accumulation of nuclear p53 and tumor progression in bladder cancer. N Engl J Med 1994; 331:1259. (In patients undergoing radical cystectomy for invasive transitional cell carcinoma, mutant p53 expression, as detected by immunohistochemistry, predicted risk of relapse or death independently of tumor grade, stage, and lymph node status.)

Hall RR: Superficial bladder cancer. Br Med J 1994; 308:910.

Kaufman DS et al: Selective bladder preservation by combination treatment of invasive bladder cancer. N Engl J Med 1993;329:1377.

Perry JJ et al: Management of disseminated disease in patients with bladder cancer. Urol Clin North Am 1994; 21:661. (The efficacy and toxicity of the most commonly used chemotherapeutic regimens are reviewed.)

Sternberg CN: Neoadjuvant and adjuvant chemotherapy in locally advanced bladder cancer. Semin Oncol 1996; 5:621. (Patients with high-stage or unresectable disease are appropriate candidates for neoadjuvant chemotherapy. Bladder preservation after neoadjuvant chemotherapy is a controversial issue that will require validation in randomized trials. Adjuvant chemotherapy may prolong disease-free survival in patients at high risk for relapse after cystectomy.)

CANCERS OF THE URETER & RENAL PELVIS

Cancers of the renal pelvis and ureter are rare and occur more commonly in smokers, in those with Balkan nephropathy, in those exposed to Thorotrast (a contrast agent with radioactive thorium in use until the 1960s), or those with a long history of analgesic abuse. The majority are transitional cell carcinomas. Gross or microscopic hematuria occurs in most patients, and flank pain secondary to bleeding and obstruction occurs less commonly. Like primary bladder cancers, urinary cytology is often positive. The most common signs identified at the time of intravenous pyelography include an intraluminal filling defect, unilateral nonvisualization of the collecting system, and hydronephrosis. Ureteral and renal pelvic tumors must be differentiated from calculi, blood clots, papillary necrosis, or inflammatory or infectious lesions. On occasion, such lesions are accessible to direct biopsy, fulguration, or resection using a ureteroscope. Treatment is based on the site, size, depth of penetration, and number of tumors present. Most such cancers are excised with nephroureterectomy (renal pelvic and upper ureteral lesions) or segmental excision of the ureter (distal ureteral lesions). Endoscopic resection may be indicated in patients with limited renal function and in the management of focal, low-grade, upper tract cancers.

Melamed MR, Reuter VE: Pathology and staging of urothelial tumors of the kidney and ureter. Urol Clin North Am 1993;20(2):333.

PRIMARY TUMORS OF THE KIDNEY

1. RENAL CELL CARCINOMA

Essentials of Diagnosis

- Gross or microscopic hematuria.
- Flank pain or mass in some patients.
- Systemic symptoms such as fever, weight loss may be prominent.
- Solid renal mass on imaging.

General Considerations

Renal cell carcinoma accounts for 2.3% of all adult cancers. In the United States in 1996, approximately 30,600 cases of renal cell carcinoma will be diagnosed and 12,000 deaths will result. Renal cell carcinoma has a peak incidence in the sixth decade of life and a male-to-female ratio of 2:1.

The cause is unknown. Cigarette smoking is the only significant environmental risk factor that has been identified. Familial settings for renal cell carcinoma have been identified (von Hippel-Lindau syndrome) as well as an association with dialysis-related acquired cystic disease, but sporadic tumors are far more common.

Renal cell carcinoma originates from the proximal tubule cells. Various cell types (clear, granular, spindle) and histologic patterns (acinar, papillary, solid) are observed. However, cell type and histologic pattern do not affect treatment. The TNM classification of the American Joint Cancer Committee for kidney cancer is shown in Table 23–12.

Clinical Findings

A. Symptoms and Signs: Historically, 60% of patients presented with gross or microscopic hematuria. Flank pain or an abdominal mass was detected in approximately 30% of cases. The triad of flank pain, hematuria, and mass was found in only 10–15% of patients and is often a sign of advanced disease. Symptoms of metastatic disease (cough, bone pain) occur in 20–30% of patients at presentation. Because of the more widespread use of ultrasound and CT scanning for diverse indications, renal tumors are being detected incidentally in patients with no urologic symptoms.

Table 23–12. TNM staging system for kidney cancer.

T: Primary tumor

Tx	Cannot be assessed	
T0	No evidence of primary tumor	
T1	Tumor ≤ 2.5 cm limited to kidney	
T2	Tumor > 2.5 cm limited to kidney	
T3a	Tumor invades adrenal gland or perinephric tissue	
T3b	Tumor extends into renal vein or vena cava	
T4	Tumor invades outside of Gerota's fascia	

N: Regional lymph nodes

Nx	Cannot be assessed
N0	No regional lymph node metastasis
N1	Metastasis in a single lymph node ≤ 2 cm
N2	Metastasis in a single lymph node > 2 cm and < 5 cm or multiple nodes none > 5 cm
N3	Metastasis in lymph node > 5 cm

M: Distant metastasis

Mx	Cannot be assessed
M0	No distant metastasis
M1	Distant metastasis present

B. Laboratory Findings: Hematuria is present in 60% of patients. Paraneoplastic syndromes are not uncommon in renal cell carcinoma. Erythrocytosis from increased erythropoietin production occurs in 5%, though anemia is far more common; hypercalcemia may be present in up to 10% of patients. Stauffer's syndrome is a reversible syndrome of hepatic dysfunction in the absence of metastatic disease.

C. Imaging: Renal masses are often first detected by intravenous urography. Further evaluation requires ultrasound to determine whether it is solid or cystic. CT scanning is the most valuable imaging test for renal cell carcinoma. It confirms the character of the mass and further stages the lesion with respect to regional lymph nodes, renal vein, or hepatic involvement. It also gives valuable information on the contralateral kidney (function, bilaterality of neoplasm). Chest radiographs exclude pulmonary metastases, and bone scans should be performed for large tumors and in patients with bone pain or elevated alkaline phosphatase levels. MRI and duplex Doppler ultrasonography are excellent methods of assessing for the presence and extent of tumor thrombus within the renal vein or vena cava in selected patients.

Differential Diagnosis

Solid lesions of the kidney are renal cell carcinoma until proved otherwise. Other solid masses include angiomyolipomas (fat density usually visible by CT); transitional cell cancers of the renal pelvis (more centrally located, involvement of the collecting system, positive urinary cytology reports); adrenal tumors (supero-anterior to the kidney) and oncocytomas (indistinguishable from renal cell carcinoma preoperatively); and renal abscesses.

Treatment & Prognosis

Radical nephrectomy is the primary treatment for localized renal cell carcinoma. Tumors confined to the renal capsule (T1–T2) demonstrate 5-year disease-free survivals of 90–100%. Tumors extending beyond the renal capsule (T3 or T4) and node-positive tumors have 50–60% and 0–15% 5-year disease-free survivals, respectively.

No effective chemotherapy is available for metastatic renal cell carcinoma. Vinblastine is the single most effective agent, with short-term partial response rates of 15%. Biologic response modifiers have received much attention, including alpha interferon and interleukin-2. Partial response rates of 15–20% and 15–35%, respectively, have been reported. Responders tend to have lower tumor burdens, metastatic disease confined to the lung, and a high performance status. Because of these low response rates, new investigations are ongoing with tumor vaccines and gene therapy.

One subgroup of metastatic patients has demonstrated long-term survival, namely, those with solitary resectable metastases. In this setting, radical nephrectomy with resection of the metastasis has resulted in 5-year disease-free survival rates of 15–30%.

Fyfe G et al: Results of treatment of 255 patients with metastatic renal cell carcinoma who received high-dose recombinant interleukin-2 therapy. J Clin Oncol 1995;13:688. (Five percent complete response rate, median duration not reached yet; and a 9% partial response rate, median duration of 19 months.)

Guinan PD et al: Renal cell carcinoma: Tumor size, stage and survival. Members of the Cancer Incidence and End Results Committee. J Urol 1995;153:901. (Tumor size correlated with tumor stage and survival.)

Taneja SS et al: Management of disseminated kidney cancer. Urol Clin North Am 1994;21:625. (Historical review of immunotherapy and logical approach to patients with metastatic renal cell carcinoma.)

Thrasher JB, Paulson DF: Prognostic factors in renal cancer. Urol Clin North Am 1993;20:247. (Volume covering various aspects of kidney tumors.)

2. OTHER PRIMARY TUMORS OF THE KIDNEY

Oncocytomas account for 3–5% of renal tumors and are indistinguishable from renal cell carcinoma by all imaging modalities. The biologic potential of these lesions is not well defined. These tumors are seen in other organs, including the adrenals, the salivary glands, and the thyroid and parathyroid glands.

Angiomyolipomas are rare benign tumors composed of fat, smooth muscle, and blood vessels. They are most commonly seen in patients with tuberous sclerosis (often multiple and bilateral) or in young to middle-aged women. CT scanning may identify the fat component, which is diagnostic for angiomyolipoma. Asymptomatic lesions less than 5 cm in diameter usually do not require intervention.

Lieber MM: Renal oncocytoma. Urol Clin North Am 1993;20(2):355.

Morra MN, Das S: Renal oncocytoma: A review of histogenesis, histopathology, diagnosis, and treatment. J Urol 1993;150(2 Part 1):295.

Weiss LM et al: Adult renal epithelial neoplasms. Am J Clin Pathol 1995;103:624. (Reviews clinicopathologic characteristics of oncocytomas and other histologic variants of renal cell carcinoma.)

SECONDARY TUMORS OF THE KIDNEY

The kidney is not an infrequent site for metastatic disease. Of the solid tumors, the lung is the most common (20%), followed by breast (10%), stomach (10%), and the contralateral kidney (10%). Lymphoma, both Hodgkin's and non-Hodgkin's, may also involve the kidney, though it tends to be a diffusely infiltrative process resulting in renal enlargement rather than a discrete mass.

PRIMARY TUMORS OF THE TESTIS

Essentials of Diagnosis

- Commonest neoplasm in men aged 20–35.
- Typical presentation as a patient-identified painless nodule.
- Orchiectomy necessary for diagnosis.

General Considerations

Malignant tumors of the testis are rare, with approximately two to three new cases per 100,000 males being reported in the United States each year. Ninety to 95 percent of all primary testicular tumors are germ cell tumors (seminoma and nonseminoma), while the remainder are nongerminal neoplasms (Leydig cell, Sertoli cell, gonadoblastoma). The lifetime probability of developing testicular cancer is 0.2% for an American white male. For the purposes of this review, we will only consider germ cell tumors. Survival in testicular cancer has improved dramatically in recent years as a result of the development and application of effective combination chemotherapy.

Testicular cancer is slightly more common on the right than on the left, which parallels the increased incidence of cryptorchism on the right side. One to 2 percent of primary testicular tumors are bilateral, and up to 50% of these men have a history of unilateral or bilateral cryptorchism. Primary bilateral testicular tumors may occur synchronously or asynchronously but tend to be of the same histology. Seminoma is the most common histologic finding in bilateral *primary* testicular tumors, while malignant lymphoma is the most common bilateral testicular tumor.

While the cause of testicular cancer is unknown, both congenital and acquired factors have been associated with tumor development. Approximately 5% of testicular tumors develop in a patient with a history of cryptorchism, with seminoma being the most common. However, 5–10% of these tumors occur in the contralateral, normally descended testis. The relative risk of development of malignancy is highest for the intra-abdominal testis (1:20) and lower for the inguinal testis (1:80). Placement of the cryptorchid testis into the scrotum (orchiopexy) does not alter the malignant potential of the cryptorchid testis; however, it does facilitate examination and tumor detection.

Exogenous estrogen administration during pregnancy has been associated with an increased relative risk for testicular tumors ranging from 2.8 to 5.3. Other acquired factors such as trauma and infection-related testicular atrophy have been associated with testicular tumors; however, a causal relationship has not been established.

Histopathology & Clinical Staging

From a treatment standpoint, testicular carcinoma can be divided into two major categories: (1) nonseminomas, which include embryonal cell carcinomas (20%), teratomas (5%), choriocarcinomas (< 1%), and mixed cell types (40%); and (2) seminomas (35%). In a commonly used staging system for nonseminoma germ cell tumors, a stage A lesion is confined to the testis; stage B demonstrates regional lymph node involvement in the retroperitoneum; and stage C indicates distant metastasis. For seminoma, the M.D. Anderson system is commonly used. In this system, a stage I lesion is confined to the testis, a stage II lesion has spread to the retroperitoneal lymph nodes, and a stage III lesion has supradiaphragmatic nodal or visceral involvement. The TNM classification of the American Joint Cancer Committee for testis cancer is shown in Table 23–13.

Clinical Findings

A. Symptoms and Signs: The most common symptom of testicular cancer is painless enlargement of the testis. Sensations of heaviness are not unusual. Patients are usually the first to recognize an abnormality, yet the typical delay in seeking medical attention ranges from 3 to 6 months. Acute testicular pain resulting from intratesticular hemorrhage occurs in approximately 10% of cases. Ten percent of patients are asymptomatic at presentation, and 10% manifest symptoms relating to metastatic disease such as back pain (retroperitoneal metastases), cough (pulmonary metastases), or lower extremity edema (vena cava obstruction).

Table 23–13. TNM staging system for testicular cancer.

T: Primary tumor

	Tx	Cannot be assessed
	T0	No evidence of primary tumor
	Tis	Intratubular cancer (CIS)
	T1	Limited to testis
	T2	Invades beyond tunica albuginea or into epididymis
	T3	Invades spermatic cord
	T4	Invades scrotum

N: Regional lymph nodes

	Nx	Cannot be assessed
	N0	No regional lymph node metastasis
	N1	Metastasis in a single lymph node 2 cm or less
	N2	Metastasis in a single lymph node >2 cm and <5 cm or multiple nodes none >5 cm
	N3	Metastasis in lymph node >5 cm

M: Distant metastasis

	Mx	Cannot be assessed
	M0	No distant metastasis
	M1	Distant metastasis present

A testicular mass or diffuse enlargement of the testis is found in the majority of cases on physical examination. Secondary hydroceles may be present in 5–10% of cases. In advanced disease, supraclavicular adenopathy may be detected, and abdominal examination may palpate a retroperitoneal mass. Gynecomastia is seen in 5% of germ cell tumors.

B. Laboratory Findings: Several biochemical markers are important in the diagnosis and treatment of testicular carcinoma, including human chorionic gonadotropin (hCG), alpha-fetoprotein, and LDH. Alpha-fetoprotein is never elevated in seminomas, and while hCG is occasionally elevated in seminomas, levels tend to be lower than those seen in nonseminomas. LDH may be elevated in either type of tumor. Liver function tests may be elevated in the presence of hepatic metastases, and anemia may be present in advanced disease. In patients with advanced disease who will receive chemotherapy, renal function is assessed with a 24-hour creatinine clearance urine collection.

C. Imaging: Scrotal ultrasound can readily determine whether the mass is intra- or extratesticular in origin. Once the diagnosis of testicular cancer has been established by inguinal orchiectomy, clinical staging of the disease is accomplished by chest radiograph and abdominal and pelvic CT scanning.

Differential Diagnosis

An incorrect diagnosis is made at the initial examination in up to 25% of patients with testicular tumors. The differential diagnosis of scrotal masses has been discussed previously in this chapter. Scrotal ultrasonography should be performed if any uncertainty exists with respect to the diagnosis. Although most intratesticular masses are malignant, one benign

lesion, an epidermoid cyst, may rarely been seen. Epidermoid cysts are usually very small benign nodules located just underneath the tunica albuginea; on occasion, however, they can be large.

Treatment

Inguinal exploration with early vascular control of the spermatic cord structures is the initial intervention to exclude neoplasm. If cancer cannot be excluded by examination of the testis, radical orchiectomy is warranted. Scrotal approaches and open testicular biopsies should be avoided. Further therapy is dependent upon the histology of the tumor as well as the clinical stage.

The 5-year disease-free survival rates for stage I and IIa (retroperitoneal disease < 10 cm in diameter) seminomas treated by radical orchiectomy and retroperitoneal irradiation are 98% and 92–94%, respectively. High-stage seminomas of stage IIb (> 10 cm retroperitoneal involvement) and stage III receive primary chemotherapy (etoposide and cisplatin or cisplatin, etoposide, and bleomycin). Ninety-five percent of patients with stage III disease will attain a complete response following orchiectomy and chemotherapy. Surgical resection of residual retroperitoneal masses is warranted only if the mass is larger than 3 cm in diameter, under which circumstances 40% will harbor residual carcinoma.

Up to 75% of stage A nonseminomas are cured by orchiectomy alone. Currently, such patients may be treated by modified retroperitoneal lymph node dissections designed to preserve the sympathetic innervation for ejaculation. Selected patients who meet specific criteria may be offered surveillance. These criteria are as follows: (1) tumor is confined within the tunica albuginea (T1); (2) tumor does not demonstrate vascular invasion; (3) tumor markers normalize after orchiectomy; (4) radiographic imaging shows no evidence of disease (chest x-ray and CT); and (5) the patient is reliable. Surveillance should be considered an active process both by the physician and by the patient. Patients are followed monthly for the first 2 years and bimonthly in the third year. Tumor markers are obtained at each visit, and chest x-ray and CT scans are obtained every 3–4 months. Follow-up continues beyond the initial 3 years; however, the majority of relapses will occur within the first 8–10 months. With rare exceptions, patients who relapse can be cured by chemotherapy or surgery. The 5-year disease-free survival rate for patients with stage A disease ranges from 96% to 100%. For low-volume stage B disease, 90% 5-year disease-free survival is attainable.

Patients with bulky retroperitoneal disease (> 3 cm nodes) or metastatic nonseminomas are treated with primary cisplatin-based combination chemotherapy following orchiectomy (etoposide and cisplatin or cisplatin, etoposide, and bleomycin). If tumor markers normalize and a residual mass is apparent on imaging studies, resection of that mass is mandatory because 20% of the time it will harbor residual cancer and 40% of the time it will be teratoma. Even if patients have a complete response to chemotherapy, retroperitoneal lymphadenectomy is advocated by some as 10% of patients may harbor residual carcinoma and 10% may have teratoma in the retroperitoneum. If tumor markers fail to normalize following primary chemotherapy, salvage chemotherapy is required (cisplatin, etoposide, bleomycin, ifosfamide).

Prognosis

Patients with bulky retroperitoneal or disseminated disease treated with primary chemotherapy followed by surgery have a 5-year disease-free survival rate of 55–80%.

Heiken JP et al: Neoplasms of the bladder, prostate and testis. Radiol Clin North Am 1994;32:81. (A review of the imaging tests used to evaluate and stage patients with the above tumors.)

Klein EA, Kay R (editors): Testis cancer in adults and children. Urol Clin North Am 1993;20(1):1. (Entire volume.)

Puc HS et al: Management of residual mass in advanced seminoma: Results and recommendations from the Memorial Sloan-Kettering Cancer Center. J Clin Oncol 1996;14:454. (Patients with advanced seminoma who have normal radiographs or residual masses less than 3 cm after chemotherapy can be observed without further intervention.)

Richie JP: Detection and treatment of testicular cancer. CA Cancer J Clin 1993;43:151. (Testicular cancer is one of the most curable solid tumors, with survival rates increasing from 10% to 90% over the past 20 years.)

SECONDARY TUMORS OF THE TESTIS

Secondary tumors of the testis are rare. Lymphoma is the most common testis tumor in a patient over the age of 50 and is the most common secondary neoplasm of the testis, accounting for 5% of all testicular tumors. It may be seen in three clinical settings: (1) as a late manifestation of widespread lymphoma; (2) as the initial presentation of clinically occult disease; and (3) as primary extranodal disease. Radical orchiectomy is indicated to make the diagnosis. Prognosis is related to the stage of disease.

Metastasis to the testis is rare. The most common primary site is the prostate, followed by the lung, gastrointestinal tract, melanoma, and kidney.

Nervous System

Michael J. Aminoff, MD, FRCP

HEADACHE

Headache is such a common complaint and can occur for so many different reasons that its proper evaluation may be difficult. Although underlying structural lesions are not present in most patients presenting with headache, it is nevertheless important to bear this possibility in mind. About one-third of patients with brain tumors, for example, present with a primary complaint of headache.

The intensity, quality, and site of pain—and especially the duration of the headache and the presence of associated neurologic symptoms—may provide clues to the underlying cause. The onset of severe headache in a previously well patient is more likely than chronic headache to relate to an intracranial disorder such as subarachnoid hemorrhage or meningitis. Headaches that disturb sleep, exertional headaches, and late-onset paroxysmal headaches are also more suggestive of an underlying structural lesion, as are headaches accompanied by neurologic symptoms such as drowsiness, visual or limb problems, seizures, or altered mental status. Chronic headaches are commonly due to migraine, tension, or depression, but they may be related to intracranial lesions, head injury, cervical spondylosis, dental or ocular disease, temporomandibular joint dysfunction, sinusitis, hypertension, and a wide variety of general medical disorders. Depending on the initial clinical impression, the need for such investigations as CT scan or MRI of the head, electroencephalography, and lumbar puncture must be assessed on an individual basis. The diagnosis and treatment of primary neurologic disorders associated with headache are considered separately under these disorders.

Tension Headache

Patients frequently complain of poor concentration and other vague nonspecific symptoms, in addition to constant daily headaches that are often vise-like or tight in quality and may be exacerbated by emotional stress, fatigue, noise, or glare. The headaches are usually generalized, may be most intense about the neck or back of the head, and are not associated with focal neurologic symptoms.

When treatment with simple analgesics is not effective, a trial of antimigrainous agents (see Migraine, below) is worthwhile. Techniques to induce relaxation are also useful and include massage, hot baths, and biofeedback. Exploration of underlying causes of chronic anxiety is often rewarding.

Depression Headache

Depression headaches are frequently worse on arising in the morning and may be accompanied by other symptoms of depression. Headaches are occasionally the focus of a somatic delusional system. Tricyclic antidepressant drugs are often helpful, as may be psychiatric consultation.

Migraine

Classic migrainous headache is a lateralized throbbing headache that occurs episodically following its onset in adolescence or early adult life. In many cases, however, the headaches do not conform to this pattern, although their associated features and response to antimigrainous preparations nevertheless suggest that they have a similar basis. In this broader sense, migrainous headaches may be lateralized or generalized, may be dull or throbbing, and are sometimes associated with anorexia, nausea, vomiting, photophobia, phonophobia, and blurring of vision. They usually build up gradually and may last for several hours or longer. They have been related to dilation and excessive pulsation of branches of the external carotid artery. Focal disturbances of neurologic function may precede or accompany the headaches and have been attributed to constriction of branches of the internal carotid artery. Visual disturbances occur quite commonly and may consist of field defects; of luminous visual hallucinations such as stars, sparks, unformed light flashes (photopsia), geometric patterns, or zigzags of light; or of some combination of field defects and luminous hallucinations (scintillating scotomas). Other focal disturbances such as aphasia or numbness, tingling, clumsiness, or weakness in a circumscribed distribution may also occur.

Patients often give a family history of migraine. Attacks may be triggered by emotional or physical stress, lack or excess of sleep, missed meals, specific foods (eg, chocolate), alcoholic beverages, menstruation, or use of oral contraceptives.

An uncommon variant is **basilar artery migraine,** in which blindness or visual disturbances throughout both visual fields are initially accompanied or followed by dysarthria, disequilibrium, tinnitus, and perioral and distal paresthesias and are sometimes followed by transient loss or impairment of consciousness or by a confusional state. This, in turn, is followed by a throbbing (usually occipital) headache, often with nausea and vomiting.

In **ophthalmoplegic migraine,** lateralized pain—often about the eye—is accompanied by nausea, vomiting, and diplopia due to transient external ophthalmoplegia. The ophthalmoplegia is due to third nerve palsy, sometimes with accompanying sixth nerve involvement, and may outlast the orbital pain by several days or even weeks. The ophthalmic division of the fifth nerve has also been affected in some patients. Ophthalmoplegic migraine is rare; more common causes of a painful ophthalmoplegia are internal carotid artery aneurysms and diabetes.

In rare instances, the neurologic or somatic disturbance accompanying typical migrainous headaches becomes the sole manifestation of an attack ("migraine equivalent"). Very rarely, the patient may be left with a permanent neurologic deficit following a migrainous attack.

The pathophysiology of migraine probably relates to the neurotransmitter serotonin. Headache may result from release of neuropeptides acting as neurotransmitters at trigeminal nerve branches, leading to an inflammatory process; another possible mechanism involves activation of the dorsal raphe nucleus.

Management of migraine consists of avoidance of any precipitating factors, together with prophylactic or symptomatic pharmacologic treatment if necessary.

During acute attacks, many patients find it helpful to rest in a quiet, darkened room until symptoms subside. A simple analgesic (eg, aspirin) taken right away often provides relief, but treatment with extracranial vasoconstrictors or other drugs is sometimes necessary. Cafergot, a combination of ergotamine tartrate (1 mg) and caffeine (100 mg), is often particularly helpful; one or two tablets are taken at the onset of headache or warning symptoms, followed by one tablet every 30 minutes, if necessary, up to six tablets per attack and ten tablets per week. Because of impaired absorption or vomiting during acute attacks, oral medication sometimes fails to help. Cafergot given rectally as suppositories (one-half to one suppository containing 2 mg of ergotamine); ergotamine tartrate given by inhalation (0.36 mg per puff; up to six puffs per attack) or sublingually (2 mg tablets; not more than three tablets per 24 hours); or dihydroergotamine mesylate (0.5–1 mg intravenously or 1–2 mg subcutaneously or intramuscularly) may be useful in such cases. Ergotamine-containing preparations may affect the gravid uterus and thus should be avoided during pregnancy. Sumatriptan is a new, rapidly effective agent for aborting attacks when given subcutaneously by an autoinjection device. It has a high affinity for serotonin$_1$ receptors. It should probably be avoided in pregnancy.

Prophylactic treatment may be necessary if migrainous headaches occur more frequently than two or three times a month. Some of the more common drugs used for this purpose are listed in Table 24–1. Their mode of action is unclear and may involve both an effect on extracerebral vasculature and a cerebral effect, eg, by stabilizing serotonergic neurotransmission. Several drugs may have to be tried in turn before the headaches are brought under control. Once a drug has been found to help, it should be continued for several months. If the patient remains headache-free, the dose can then be tapered and the drug eventually withdrawn.

Calcium channel antagonist drugs may decrease the frequency of attacks after an interval of several weeks, but the severity and duration of attacks are not influenced. They should not be used with beta-blockers.

Cluster Headache
(Migrainous Neuralgia)

Cluster headache affects predominantly middle-aged men. Its cause is unclear but may relate to a vascular headache disorder or a disturbance of serotonergic mechanisms. There is often no family history of headache or migraine. Episodes of severe unilateral periorbital pain occur daily for several weeks and are often accompanied by one or more of the following: ipsilateral nasal congestion, rhinorrhea, lacrimation, redness of the eye, and Horner's syndrome. Episodes usually occur at night, awaken the patient, and last for less than 2 hours. Spontaneous remission then occurs, and the patient remains well for weeks or months before another bout of closely spaced attacks occurs. During a bout, many patients report that alcohol triggers an attack; others report that stress, glare, or ingestion of specific foods occasionally precipitates attacks. In occasional patients, typical attacks of pain and associated symptoms recur at intervals without remission. This variant has been referred to as chronic cluster headache.

Examination reveals no abnormality apart from Horner's syndrome that either occurs transiently during an attack or, in long-standing cases, remains as a residual deficit between attacks.

Treatment of an individual attack with oral drugs is generally unsatisfactory, but subcutaneous sumatriptan (6 mg) or dihydroergotamine (1–2 mg) or use of ergotamine tartrate aerosol or inhalation of 100% oxygen (7 L/min for 15 minutes) may be effective. Butorphanol tartrate, a synthetic opioid agonist-antagonist, may also be helpful when administered by nasal spray. Ergotamine tartrate is an effective pro-

Table 24–1. Prophylactic treatment of migraine.

Drug	Usual Adult Daily Dose	Common Side Effects
Aspirin	650–1950 mg	Dyspepsia, gastrointestinal bleeding.
Propranolol	80–240 mg	Fatigue, lassitude, depression, insomnia, nausea, vomiting, constipation.
Amitriptyline	10–150 mg	Sedation, dry mouth, constipation, weight gain, blurred vision, edema, hypotension, urinary retention.
Imipramine	10–150 mg	Similar to those of amitriptyline (above).
Sertraline	50–200 mg	Anxiety, insomnia, sweating, tremor, gastrointestinal disturbances.
Fluoxetine	20–60 mg	Similar to those of sertraline (above).
Ergonovine maleate	0.6–2 mg	Nausea, vomiting, abdominal pain, diarrhea.
Cyproheptadine	12–20 mg	Sedation, dry mouth, epigastric discomfort, gastrointestinal disturbances.
Clonidine	0.2–0.6 mg	Dry mouth, drowsiness, sedation, headache, constipation.
Methysergide	4–8 mg	Nausea, vomiting, diarrhea, abdominal pain, cramps, weight gain, insomnia, edema, peripheral vasoconstriction. Retroperitoneal and pleuropulmonary fibrosis and fibrous thickening of cardiac valves may occur.
Verapamil[1]	80–160 mg	Headache, hypotension, flushing, edema, constipation. May aggravate atrioventricular nodal heart block and congestive heart failure.

[1]Other calcium channel antagonists (eg, nimodipine, nifedipine, and diltiazem) may also be used.

phylactic and can be given as rectal suppositories (0.5–1 mg at night or twice daily), by mouth (2 mg daily), or by subcutaneous injection (0.25 mg three times daily for 5 days per week). Various prophylactic agents that have been found to be effective in individual patients are propranolol, amitriptyline, cyproheptadine, lithium carbonate (monitored by plasma lithium determination), prednisone (20–40 mg daily or on alternate days for 2 weeks, followed by gradual withdrawal), verapamil (240–480 mg daily), and methysergide (4–6 mg daily).

Giant Cell (Temporal or Cranial) Arteritis

The superficial temporal, vertebral, ophthalmic, and posterior ciliary arteries are often the most severely affected pathologically. Most patients are elderly. The major symptom is headache, often associated with or preceded by myalgia, malaise, anorexia, weight loss, and other nonspecific complaints. Loss of vision is the most feared manifestation and occurs quite commonly. Clinical examination often reveals tenderness of the scalp and over the temporal arteries. Further details, including approaches to treatment, are given in Chapter 20.

Posttraumatic Headache

A variety of nonspecific symptoms may follow closed head injury, regardless of whether consciousness is lost. Headache is often a conspicuous feature. Some authorities believe that psychologic factors may be important because there is no correlation of severity of the injury with neurologic signs.

The headache itself usually appears within a day or so following injury, may worsen over the ensuing weeks, and then gradually subsides. It is usually a constant dull ache, with superimposed throbbing that may be localized, lateralized, or generalized. It is sometimes accompanied by nausea, vomiting, or scintillating scotomas.

Disequilibrium, sometimes with a rotatory component, may also occur and is often enhanced by postural change or head movement. Impaired memory, poor concentration, emotional instability, and increased irritability are other common complaints and occasionally are the sole manifestations of the syndrome. The duration of symptoms relates in part to the severity of the original injury, but even trivial injuries are sometimes followed by symptoms that persist for months.

Special investigations are usually not helpful. The electroencephalogram may show minor nonspecific changes, while the electronystagmogram sometimes suggests either peripheral or central vestibulopathy. CT scans or MRI of the head usually show no abnormal findings.

Treatment is difficult, but optimistic encouragement and graduated rehabilitation, depending upon the occupational circumstances, are advised. Headaches often respond to simple analgesics, but severe headaches may necessitate treatment with amitriptyline, propranolol, or ergot derivatives.

Cough Headache

Severe head pain may be produced by coughing (and by straining, sneezing, and laughing) but, fortunately, usually lasts for only a few minutes or less. The pathophysiologic basis of the complaint is not known, and often there is no underlying structural lesion. However, intracranial lesions, usually in the posterior fossa (eg, Arnold-Chiari malformation, basilar impression), are present in about 10% of cases, and brain tumors or other space-occupying lesions may certainly present in this way. Accordingly, CT scanning or MRI should be undertaken in all patients and repeated annually for several years, since a small structural lesion may not show up initially.

The disorder is usually self-limited, although it may persist for several years. For unknown reasons, symptoms sometimes clear completely after lumbar puncture. Indomethacin (75–150 mg daily) may provide relief.

Headache Due to Other Neurologic Causes

Intracranial mass lesions of all types may cause headache owing to displacement of vascular structures. Posterior fossa tumors often cause occipital pain, and supratentorial lesions lead to bifrontal headache, but such findings are too inconsistent to be of value in attempts at localizing a pathologic process. The headaches are nonspecific in character and may vary in severity from mild to severe. They may be worsened by exertion or postural change and may be associated with nausea and vomiting, but this is true of migraine also. Headaches are also a feature of pseudotumor cerebri (see below). Signs of focal or diffuse cerebral dysfunction or of increased intracranial pressure will indicate the need for further investigation. Similarly, a progressive headache disorder or the new onset of headaches in middle or later life merits investigation if no cause is apparent.

Cerebrovascular disease may be associated with headache, but the mechanism is unclear. Headache may occur with internal carotid artery occlusion or carotid dissection and after carotid endarterectomy. Diagnosis is facilitated by the clinical accompaniments and the circumstances in which the headache developed.

Acute severe headache accompanies subarachnoid hemorrhage and meningeal infections; accompanying signs of meningeal irritation and impairment of consciousness indicate the need for further investigations.

Dull or throbbing headache is a frequent sequela of lumbar puncture and may last for several days. It is aggravated by the erect posture and alleviated by recumbency. The exact mechanism is unclear, but it is commonly attributed to leakage of cerebrospinal fluid through the dural puncture site. Its incidence may be reduced if a small-diameter needle is used for the spinal tap, and perhaps also if the patient lies prone or supine after the procedure.

Moskowitz MA, Macfarlane R: Neurovascular and molecular mechanisms in migraine headaches. Cerebrovasc Brain Metab Rev 1993;5:159. (The pathophysiology of migraine.)

Pearce JMS: Headache. J Neurol Neurosurg Psychiatry 1994;57:134. (Management.)

Silberstein SD: Tension-type and chronic daily headache. Neurology 1993;43:1644.

Welch KMA: Drug therapy of migraine. N Engl J Med 1993;329:1476. (Pharmacotherapy.)

FACIAL PAIN

Trigeminal Neuralgia

Trigeminal neuralgia ("tic douloureux") is most common in middle and later life. It affects women more frequently than men. The disorder is characterized by momentary episodes of sudden lancinating facial pain that commonly arises near one side of the mouth and then shoots toward the ear, eye, or nostril on that side. The pain may be triggered or precipitated by such factors as touch, movement, drafts, and eating. Indeed, in order to lessen the likelihood of triggering further attacks, many patients try to hold the face still while talking. Spontaneous remissions for several months or longer may occur. As the disorder progresses, however, the episodes of pain become more frequent, remissions become shorter and less common, and a dull ache may persist between the episodes of stabbing pain. Symptoms remain confined to the distribution of the trigeminal nerve (usually the second or third division) on one side only.

The characteristic features of the pain in trigeminal neuralgia usually distinguish it from other causes of facial pain. Neurologic examination shows no abnormality except in a few patients in whom trigeminal neuralgia is symptomatic of some underlying lesion, such as multiple sclerosis or a brain stem neoplasm, in which case the finding will depend on the nature and site of the lesion. Similarly, CT scans and radiologic contrast studies are normal in patients with classic trigeminal neuralgia.

In a young patient presenting with trigeminal neuralgia, multiple sclerosis must be suspected even if there are no other neurologic signs. In such circumstances, findings on evoked potential testing and examination of cerebrospinal fluid may be corroborative. When the facial pain is due to a posterior fossa tumor, CT scanning and MRI generally reveal the lesion.

The drug most helpful for treatment of trigeminal neuralgia is carbamazepine, given in a dose of up to 1200 mg/d, with monitoring by serial blood counts and liver function tests. If carbamazepine is ineffective or cannot be tolerated, phenytoin should be tried. (Doses and side effects of these drugs are shown in Table 24–2.) Baclofen (10–20 mg three or four times daily) may also be helpful, either alone or in combination with carbamazepine or phenytoin.

In the past, alcohol injection of the affected nerve, rhizotomy, or tractotomy was recommended if pharmacologic treatment was unsuccessful. More recently, however, posterior fossa exploration has frequently revealed some structural cause for the

Table 24–2. Drug treatment for seizures.

Drug	Usual Adult Daily Dose	Minimum No. of Daily Doses	Time to Steady-State Drug Levels	Optimal Drug Level	Selected Side Effects and Idiosyncratic Reactions
Generalized tonic-clonic (grand mal) or partial (focal) seizures					
Phenytoin	200–400 mg	1	5–10 days	10–20 µg/mL	Nystagmus, ataxia, dysarthria, sedation, confusion, gingival hyperplasia, hirsutism, megaloblastic anemia, blood dyscrasias, skin rashes, fever, systemic lupus erythematosus, lymphadenopathy, peripheral neuropathy, dyskinesias.
Carbamazepine	600–1200 mg	2–3	3–4 days	4–8 µg/mL	Nystagmus, dysarthria, diplopia, ataxia, drowsiness, nausea, blood dyscrasias, hepatotoxicity.
(extended-release formulation)		(2)			
Valproic acid	1500–2000 mg	3	2–4 days	50–100 µg/mL	Nausea, vomiting, diarrhea, drowsiness, alopecia, weight gain, hepatotoxicity, thrombocytopenia, tremor.
Phenobarbital	100–200 mg	1	14–21 days	10–40 µg/mL	Drowsiness, nystagmus, ataxia, skin rashes, learning difficulties, hyperactivity.
Primidone	750–1500 mg	3	4–7 days	5–15 µg/mL	Sedation, nystagmus, ataxia, vertigo, nausea, skin rashes, megaloblastic anemia, irritability.
Felbamate[1,2]	1200–3600 mg	3	4–5 days	?	Anorexia, nausea, vomiting, headache, insomnia, weight loss, dizziness, hepatotoxicity, aplastic anemia.
Gabapentin[2]	900–1800 mg	3	1 day	?	Sedation, fatigue, ataxia, nystagmus.
Lamotrigine[2]	100–500 mg	2	4–5 days	?	Sedation, skin rash, visual disturbances, dyspepsia, ataxia.
Topiramate[2]	200–400 mg	2	4 days	?	Somnolence, nausea, dyspepsia, irritability, dizziness, ataxia, nystagmus, diplopia.
Absence (petit mal) seizures					
Ethosuximide	100–1500 mg	2	5–10 days	40–100 µg/mL	Nausea, vomiting, anorexia, headache, lethargy, unsteadiness, blood dyscrasias, systemic lupus erythematosus, urticaria, pruritus.
Valproic acid	1500–2000 mg	3	2–4 days	50–100 µg/mL	See above.
Clonazepam	0.05–0.2 mg/kg	2	?	20–80 ng/mL	Drowsiness, ataxia, irritability, behavioral changes, exacerbation of tonic-clonic seizures.
Myoclonic seizures					
Valproic acid	1500–2000 mg	3	2–4 days	50–100 µg/mL	See above.
Clonazepam	0.04–0.2 mg/kg	2	?	20–80 ng/mL	See above.

[1]Not to be used as a first-line drug; when used, blood counts should be performed regularly (every 2–4 weeks). Should be used only in selected patients because of risk of aplastic anemia.
[2]Approved as adjunctive therapy for partial and secondarily generalized seizures.

neuralgia (despite normal findings on CT scans, MRI, or arteriograms), such as an anomalous artery or vein impinging on the trigeminal nerve root. In such cases, simple decompression and separation of the anomalous vessel from the nerve root produce lasting relief of symptoms. In elderly patients with a limited life expectancy, radiofrequency rhizotomy is sometimes preferred because it is easy to perform, has few complications, and provides symptomatic relief for a period of time. Surgical exploration generally reveals no abnormality and is inappropriate in patients with trigeminal neuralgia due to multiple sclerosis.

Barker FG et al: The long-term outcome of microvascular decompression for trigeminal neuralgia. N Engl J Med 1996;334:1077.

Atypical Facial Pain

Facial pain without the typical features of trigeminal neuralgia is generally a constant, often burning pain that may have a restricted distribution at its onset but soon spreads to the rest of the face on the affected side and sometimes involves the other side, the neck, or the back of the head as well. The disorder is especially common in middle-aged women, many of them emotionally depressed, but it is not clear whether depression is the cause of or a reaction to the pain. Simple analgesics should be given a trial, as should tricyclic antidepressants, carbamazepine, and phenytoin; the response is often disappointing. Opioid analgesics pose a danger of addiction in patients with this disorder. Attempts at surgical treatment are not indicated.

Glossopharyngeal Neuralgia

Glossopharyngeal neuralgia is an uncommon disorder in which pain similar in quality to that in trigeminal neuralgia occurs in the throat, about the tonsillar fossa, and sometimes deep in the ear and at the back of the tongue. The pain may be precipitated by swallowing, chewing, talking, or yawning and is sometimes accompanied by syncope. In most instances, no underlying structural abnormality is present. Carbamazepine is the treatment of choice and should be tried (in daily doses up to 1200 mg) before any surgical procedures are considered.

Postherpetic Neuralgia

Herpes zoster (shingles) is due to infection of the nervous system by varicella-zoster virus. About 10% of patients who develop shingles suffer from postherpetic neuralgia. This complication seems especially likely to occur in the elderly and when the first division of the trigeminal nerve is affected. A history of shingles and the presence of cutaneous scarring resulting from shingles aid in the diagnosis. Severe pain with shingles correlates with the intensity of postherpetic symptoms.

The incidence of postherpetic neuralgia may be reduced by the treatment of shingles with systemic corticosteroids (prednisone, 60 mg daily for 2 weeks, with rapid taper) but is not influenced by treatment with acyclovir. Management of the established complication is essentially medical. If simple analgesics fail to help, a trial of a tricyclic drug (eg, amitriptyline, up to 100–150 mg/d) in conjunction with a phenothiazine (eg, perphenazine, 2–8 mg/d) is often effective. Other patients respond to carbamazepine (up to 1200 mg/d) or phenytoin (300 mg/d). Topical application of capsaicin cream (eg, Zostrix, 0.025%) may also be helpful, perhaps because of depletion of pain-mediating peptides from peripheral sensory neurons.

Rowbotham MC: Managing post-herpetic neuralgia with opioids and local anesthetics. Ann Neurol 1994;35:S46.

Facial Pain Due to Other Causes

Facial pain may be caused by temporomandibular joint dysfunction in patients with malocclusion, abnormal bite, or faulty dentures. There may be tenderness of the masticatory muscles, and an association between pain onset and jaw movement is sometimes noted. Treatment consists of correction of the underlying problem.

A relationship of facial pain to chewing or temperature changes may suggest a dental disturbance. The cause is sometimes not obvious, and diagnosis requires careful dental examination and x-rays. Pain on mastication may also occur in giant cell arteritis. Sinusitis and ear infections causing facial pain are usually recognized by the history of respiratory tract infection, fever, and, in some instances, aural discharge. There may be localized tenderness. Radiologic evidence of sinus infection or mastoiditis is confirmatory.

Glaucoma is an important ocular cause of facial pain, usually localized to the periorbital region.

On occasion, pain in the jaw may be the principal manifestation of angina pectoris. Precipitation by exertion and radiation to more typical areas establish the cardiac origin.

EPILEPSY

Essentials of Diagnosis

- Recurrent seizures.
- Characteristic electroencephalographic changes accompany seizures.
- Mental status abnormalities or focal neurologic symptoms may persist for hours postictally.

General Considerations

The term epilepsy denotes any disorder characterized by recurrent seizures. A seizure is a transient disturbance of cerebral function due to an abnormal paroxysmal neuronal discharge in the brain. Epilepsy is common, affecting approximately 0.5% of the population in the USA.

Etiology

Epilepsy has several causes. Its most likely cause in individual patients relates to the age at onset.

A. Idiopathic or Constitutional Epilepsy: Seizures usually begin between 5 and 20 years of age but may start later in life. No specific cause can be identified, and there is no other neurologic abnormality.

B. Symptomatic Epilepsy: There are many causes for recurrent seizures.

1. Congenital abnormalities and perinatal injuries may result in seizures presenting in infancy or childhood.

2. Metabolic disorders such as hypocalcemia, hypoglycemia, pyridoxine deficiency, and phenylketonuria are major treatable causes of seizures in newborns or infants. In adults, withdrawal from alcohol or drugs is a common cause of recurrent seizures, and other metabolic disorders such as renal failure and diabetes may also be responsible.

3. Trauma is an important cause of seizures at any age, but especially in young adults. Posttraumatic epilepsy is more likely to develop if the dura mater was penetrated and generally becomes manifest within 2 years following the injury. However, seizures developing in the first week after head injury do not necessarily imply that future attacks will occur. There is suggestive evidence that prophylactic anticonvulsant drug treatment reduces the incidence of posttraumatic epilepsy.

4. Tumors and other space-occupying lesions may lead to seizures at any age, but they are an especially important cause of seizures in middle and later life, when the incidence of neoplastic disease increases. The seizures are commonly the initial symptoms of the tumor and often are partial (focal) in character. They are most likely to occur with structural lesions involving the frontal, parietal, or temporal regions. Tumors must be excluded by appropriate laboratory studies in all patients with onset of seizures after 30 years of age, focal seizures or signs, or a progressive seizure disorder.

5. Vascular diseases become increasingly frequent causes of seizures with advancing age and are the most common cause of seizures with onset at age 60 years or older.

6. Degenerative disorders such as Alzheimer's disease are a cause of seizures in later life.

7. Infectious diseases must be considered in all age groups as potentially reversible causes of seizures. Seizures may occur with an acute infective or inflammatory illness, such as bacterial meningitis or herpes encephalitis, or in patients with more long-standing or chronic disorders such as neurosyphilis or cerebral cysticercosis. In patients with AIDS, they may result from central nervous system toxoplasmosis, cryptococcal meningitis, secondary viral encephalitis, or other infective complications. Seizures are a common sequela of supratentorial brain abscess, developing most frequently in the first year after treatment.

Classification of Seizures

Seizures can be categorized in various ways, but the descriptive classification proposed by the International League Against Epilepsy is clinically the most useful. Seizures are divided into those that are generalized and those affecting only part of the brain (partial seizures).

A. Partial Seizures: The initial clinical and electroencephalographic manifestations of partial seizures indicate that only a restricted part of one cerebral hemisphere has been activated. The ictal manifestations depend upon the area of the brain involved. Partial seizures are subdivided into simple seizures, in which consciousness is preserved, and complex seizures, in which it is impaired. Partial seizures of either type sometimes become secondarily generalized, leading to a tonic, clonic, or tonic-clonic attack.

1. Simple partial seizures–Simple seizures may be manifested by focal motor symptoms (convulsive jerking) or somatosensory symptoms (eg, paresthesias or tingling) that spread (or "march") to different parts of the limb or body depending upon their cortical representation. In other instances, special sensory symptoms (eg, light flashes or buzzing) indicate involvement of visual, auditory, olfactory, or gustatory regions of the brain, or there may be autonomic symptoms or signs (eg, abnormal epigastric sensations, sweating, flushing, pupillary dilation). When psychic symptoms occur, they are usually accompanied by impairment of consciousness, but the sole manifestations of some seizures are phenomena such as dysphasia, dysmnesic symptoms (eg, déjà vu, jamais vu), affective disturbances, illusions, or structured hallucinations.

2. Complex partial seizures–Impaired consciousness may be preceded, accompanied, or followed by the psychic symptoms mentioned above, and automatisms may occur. Such seizures may also begin with some of the other simple symptoms mentioned above.

B. Generalized Seizures: There are several different varieties of generalized seizures, as outlined below. In some circumstances, seizures cannot be classified because of incomplete information or because they do not fit into any category.

1. Absence (petit mal) seizures–These are characterized by impairment of consciousness, sometimes with mild clonic, tonic, or atonic components (ie, reduction or loss of postural tone), autonomic components (eg, enuresis), or accompanying automatisms. Onset and termination of attacks are abrupt. If attacks occur during conversation, the patient may miss a few words or may break off in mid sentence for a few seconds. The impairment of external awareness is so brief that the patient is unaware of it. Absence seizures almost always begin in childhood and frequently cease by the age of 20 years, although occasionally they are then replaced by other forms of generalized seizure. Electroencephalographically, such attacks are associated with bursts of bilaterally synchronous and symmetric 3-Hz spike-and-wave activity. A normal background in the electroencephalogram and normal or above-normal intelligence imply a good prognosis for the ultimate cessation of these seizures.

2. Atypical absences–There may be more marked changes in tone, or attacks may have a more gradual onset and termination than in typical absences.

3. Myoclonic seizures–Myoclonic seizures consist of single or multiple myoclonic jerks.

4. Tonic-clonic (grand mal) seizures–In these seizures, which are characterized by sudden loss of consciousness, the patient becomes rigid and falls to the ground, and respiration is arrested. This tonic phase, which usually lasts for less than a minute, is followed by a clonic phase in which there is jerking of the body musculature that may last for 2 or 3 minutes and is then followed by a stage of flaccid coma. During the seizure, the tongue or lips may be bitten, urinary or fecal incontinence may occur, and the patient may be injured. Immediately after the seizure, the patient may either recover consciousness, drift into sleep, have a further convulsion without recovery of consciousness between the attacks (**status epilepticus**), or after recovering consciousness have a further convulsion (**serial seizures**). In other cases, patients will behave in an abnormal fashion in the immediate postictal period, without subsequent awareness or memory of events (**postepileptic automatism**). Headache, disorientation, confusion, drowsiness, nausea, soreness of the muscles, or some combination of these symptoms commonly occurs postictally.

5. Tonic, clonic, or atonic seizures–Loss of consciousness may occur with either the tonic or clonic accompaniments described above, especially in children. Atonic seizures (**epileptic drop attacks**) have also been described.

Clinical Findings

A. Symptoms and Signs: Nonspecific changes such as headache, mood alterations, lethargy, and myoclonic jerking alert some patients to an impending seizure hours before it occurs. These prodromal symptoms are distinct from the aura which may precede a generalized seizure by a few seconds or minutes and which is itself a part of the attack, arising locally from a restricted region of the brain.

In most patients, seizures occur unpredictably at any time and without any relationship to posture or ongoing activities. Occasionally, however, they occur at a particular time (eg, during sleep) or in relation to external precipitants such as lack of sleep, missed meals, emotional stress, menstruation, alcohol ingestion (or alcohol withdrawal; see below), or use of certain drugs. Fever and nonspecific infections may also precipitate seizures in known epileptics; in infants and young children, it may be hard to distinguish such attacks from febrile seizures. In a few patients, seizures are provoked by specific stimuli such as flashing lights or a flickering television set (**photosensitive epilepsy**), music, or reading.

Clinical examination between seizures shows no abnormality in patients with idiopathic epilepsy, but in the immediate postictal period, extensor plantar responses may be seen. The presence of lateralized or focal signs postictally suggests that seizures may have a focal origin. In patients with symptomatic epilepsy, the findings on examination will reflect the underlying cause.

B. Imaging: CT or MRI scan is indicated for patients with focal neurologic symptoms or signs, focal seizures, or electroencephalographic findings of a focal disturbance; some physicians routinely order imaging studies for all patients with new-onset seizure disorders. Such studies should certainly be performed in patients with clinical evidence of a progressive disorder and in those presenting with seizures after the age of 30 years, because of the possibility of an underlying neoplasm. A chest radiograph should also be obtained in such patients, since the lungs are a common site for primary or secondary neoplasms.

C. Laboratory and Other Studies: In patients older than 10 years, initial investigations should always include a full blood count, blood glucose determination, liver and renal function tests, and serologic tests for syphilis. The hematologic and biochemical screening tests are important both in excluding various causes of seizures and in providing a baseline for subsequent monitoring of long-term effects of treatment.

Electroencephalography may support the clinical diagnosis of epilepsy (by demonstrating paroxysmal abnormalities containing spikes or sharp waves), may provide a guide to prognosis, and may help classify the seizure disorder. Classification of the disorder is important for determining the most appropriate anticonvulsant drug with which to start treatment. For example, absence (petit mal) and complex partial seizures may be difficult to distinguish clinically, but the electroencephalographic findings and treatment of choice differ in these two conditions. Finally, by localizing the epileptogenic source, the electroencephalographic findings are important in evaluating candidates for surgical treatment.

Differential Diagnosis

The distinction between the various disorders likely to be confused with generalized seizures is usually made on the basis of the history. The importance of obtaining an eyewitness account of the attacks cannot be overemphasized.

A. Differential Diagnosis of Partial Seizures:

1. Transient ischemic attacks–These attacks are distinguished from seizures by their longer duration, lack of spread, and symptomatology. There is a loss of motor or sensory function (eg, weakness or numbness) with transient ischemic attacks, whereas positive symptomatology (eg, convulsive jerking or paresthesias) characterizes seizures.

2. Rage attacks–Rage attacks are usually situational and lead to goal-directed aggressive behavior.

3. Panic attacks–These may be hard to distinguish from simple or complex partial seizures unless there is evidence of psychopathologic disturbances between attacks and the attacks have a clear relationship to external circumstances.

B. Differential Diagnosis of Generalized Seizures:

1. Syncope–Syncopal episodes usually occur in relation to postural change, emotional stress, instrumentation, pain, or straining. They are typically preceded by pallor, sweating, nausea, and malaise and lead to loss of consciousness accompanied by flaccidity; recovery occurs rapidly with recumbency, and there is no postictal headache or confusion. Serum creatine kinase measured about 3 hours after the event is generally normal after syncopal episodes but markedly elevated after tonic-clonic seizures.

2. Cardiac dysrhythmias–Cerebral hypoperfusion due to a disturbance of cardiac rhythm should be suspected in patients with known cardiac or vascular disease or in elderly patients who present with episodic loss of consciousness. Prodromal symptoms are typically absent. A relationship of attacks to physical activity and the finding of a systolic murmur is suggestive of aortic stenosis. Repeated Holter monitoring may be necessary to establish the diagnosis; monitoring initiated by the patient ("event monitor") may be valuable if the disturbances of consciousness are rare.

3. Brain stem ischemia–Loss of consciousness is preceded or accompanied by other brain stem signs. Basilar artery migraine and vertebrobasilar vascular disease are discussed elsewhere in this chapter.

4. Pseudoseizures–The term pseudoseizures is used to denote both hysterical conversion reactions and attacks due to malingering when these simulate epileptic seizures. Many patients with pseudoseizures also have true seizures or a family history of epilepsy. Although pseudoseizures tend to occur at times of emotional stress, this may also be the case with true seizures.

Clinically, the attacks superficially resemble tonic-clonic seizures, but there may be obvious preparation before pseudoseizures occur. Moreover, there is usually no tonic phase; instead, there is an asynchronous thrashing of the limbs, which increases if restraints are imposed and which rarely leads to injury. Consciousness may be normal or "lost," but in the latter context the occurrence of goal-directed behavior or of shouting, swearing, etc, indicates that it is feigned. Postictally, there are no changes in behavior or neurologic findings.

Laboratory studies may aid in recognition of pseudoseizures. There are no electrocerebral changes, whereas the electroencephalogram changes during organic seizures accompanied by loss of consciousness. The serum level of prolactin has been found to increase dramatically between 15 and 30 minutes after a tonic-clonic convulsion in most patients, whereas it is unchanged after a pseudoseizure.

Treatment

A. General Measures: For patients with recurrent seizures, drug treatment is prescribed with the goal of preventing further attacks and is usually continued until there have been no seizures for at least 3 years. Epileptic patients should be advised to avoid situations that could be dangerous or life-threatening if further seizures should occur. State legislation may require physicians to report to the state department of public health any patients with seizures or other episodic disturbances of consciousness.

1. Choice of medication–The drug with which treatment is best initiated depends upon the type of seizures to be treated (Table 24–2). The dose of the selected drug is gradually increased until seizures are controlled, blood levels reach the upper limit of the optimal therapeutic range, or side effects prevent further increases. If seizures continue despite treatment at the maximal tolerated dose, a second drug is added and the dose increased until its blood levels are in the therapeutic range; the first drug is then gradually withdrawn. In treatment of partial and secondarily generalized tonic-clonic seizures, the success rate is higher with carbamazepine, phenytoin, or valproic acid than with phenobarbital or primidone. Gabapentin and lamotrigine are newly approved antiepileptic drugs that are effective adjunctive therapy for partial or secondarily generalized seizures. Felbamate is also effective for such seizures but, because it may cause aplastic anemia, should be used only in selected patients unresponsive to other measures. In most patients with seizures of a single type, satisfactory control can be achieved with a single anticonvulsant drug. Treatment with two drugs may further reduce seizure frequency or severity, but usually only at the cost of greater toxicity. Treatment with more than two drugs is almost always unhelpful unless the patient is having seizures of different types.

2. Monitoring–Monitoring plasma drug levels

has led to major advances in the management of seizure disorders. The same daily dose of a particular drug leads to markedly different blood concentrations in different patients, and this will affect the therapeutic response. Steady-state drug levels in the blood should therefore be measured after treatment is initiated, dosage is changed, or another drug is added to the therapeutic regimen and when seizures are poorly controlled. Dose adjustments are then guided by the laboratory findings. The most common cause of a lower concentration of drug than expected for the prescribed dose is poor patient compliance. Compliance can be improved by limiting to a minimum the number of daily doses. Recurrent seizures or status epilepticus may result if drugs are taken erratically, and in some circumstances noncompliant patients may be better off without any medication.

All anticonvulsant drugs have side effects, and some of these are shown in Table 24–2. A complete blood count should be performed at least annually in all patients, because of the risk of anemia or blood dyscrasia. Treatment with certain drugs may require more frequent monitoring or use of additional screening tests. For example, periodic tests of hepatic function are necessary if valproic acid or carbamazepine is used, and serial blood counts are important with carbamazepine, ethosuximide, or felbamate.

3. Discontinuance of medication–Only when patients have been seizure-free for several (at least 3) years should withdrawal of medication be considered. Unfortunately, there is no way of predicting which patients can be managed successfully without treatment, although seizure recurrence is more likely in patients who initially failed to respond to therapy, those with seizures having focal features or of multiple types, and those with continuing electroencephalographic abnormalities. Dose reduction should be gradual over a period of weeks or months, and drugs should be withdrawn one at a time. If seizures recur, treatment is reinstituted with the same drugs used previously. Seizures are no more difficult to control after a recurrence than before.

4. Surgical treatment–Patients with surgically remediable epilepsy or seizures refractory to pharmacologic management may be candidates for operative treatment, which is best undertaken in specialized centers.

B. Special Circumstances:

1. Solitary seizures–In patients who have had only one seizure, investigation should exclude an underlying cause requiring specific treatment. Prophylactic anticonvulsant drug treatment is generally not required unless further attacks occur or investigations reveal some underlying pathology that itself is untreatable. The risk of seizure recurrence varies in different series between about 30% and 70%. Epilepsy should not be diagnosed on the basis of a solitary seizure. If seizures occur in the context of transient, nonrecurrent systemic disorders such as acute cerebral anoxia, the diagnosis of epilepsy is inaccurate, and long-term prophylactic anticonvulsant drug treatment is unnecessary.

2. Alcohol withdrawal seizures–One or more generalized tonic-clonic seizures may occur within 48 hours or so of withdrawal from alcohol after a period of high or chronic intake. If the seizures have consistently focal features, the possibility of an associated structural abnormality, often traumatic in origin, must be considered. Treatment with anticonvulsant drugs is generally not required for alcohol withdrawal seizures, since they are self-limited. Status epilepticus may rarely follow alcohol withdrawal and is managed along conventional lines (see below). Further attacks will not occur if the patient abstains from alcohol.

3. Tonic-clonic status epilepticus–Poor compliance with the anticonvulsant drug regimen is the most common cause; others include alcohol withdrawal, intracranial infection or neoplasms, metabolic disorders, and drug overdose. The mortality rate may be as high as 20%, and among survivors the incidence of neurologic and mental sequelae may be high. The prognosis relates to the length of time between onset of status epilepticus and the start of effective treatment.

Status epilepticus is a medical emergency. Initial management includes maintenance of the airway and 50% dextrose (25–50 mL) intravenously in case hypoglycemia is responsible. If seizures continue, 10 mg of diazepam is given intravenously over the course of 2 minutes, and the dose is repeated after 10 minutes if necessary. (Many authorities prefer a 4 mg intravenous bolus of lorazepam, repeated once after 10 minutes if necessary, rather than diazepam; relative utility is under study.) This is usually effective in halting seizures for a brief period but occasionally causes respiratory depression.

Regardless of the response to diazepam or lorazepam, phenytoin (18–20 mg/kg) is given intravenously at a rate of 50 mg/min; this provides initiation of long-term seizure control. The drug is best injected directly but can also be given in saline; it precipitates, however, if injected into glucose-containing solutions. Because arrhythmias may develop during rapid administration of phenytoin, electrocardiographic monitoring is prudent. Hypotension may complicate phenytoin administration, especially if diazepam has also been given. In the United States, injectable phenytoin has been replaced by fosphenytoin, which is rapidly and completely converted to phenytoin following intravenous administration. No dosing adjustments are necessary because fosphenytoin is in terms of phenytoin equivalents (PE); fosphenytoin is less likely to cause reactions at the infusion site, can be given with all common intravenous solutions, and may be administered at a faster rate (150 mg PE/min). It is also more expensive and has not yet been approved for use in children.

If seizures continue, phenobarbital is then given in a loading dose of 10–20 mg/kg intravenously by slow or intermittent injection. Respiratory depression and hypotension are common complications and should be anticipated; they may occur also with diazepam alone, though less commonly. If these measures fail, general anesthesia with ventilatory assistance and neuromuscular junction blockade may be required. Alternatively, intravenous midazolam may provide control of refractory status epilepticus; the suggested loading dose is 0.2 mg/kg, followed by 0.05–0.2 mg/kg/h.

After status epilepticus is controlled, an oral drug program for the long-term management of seizures is started, and investigations into the cause of the disorder are pursued.

4. Nonconvulsive status epilepticus–Absence (petit mal) and complex partial status epilepticus are characterized by fluctuating abnormal mental status, confusion, impaired responsiveness, and automatism. Electroencephalography is helpful both in establishing the diagnosis and in distinguishing the two varieties. Initial treatment with intravenous diazepam is usually helpful regardless of the type of status epilepticus, but phenytoin, phenobarbital, carbamazepine, and other drugs may also be needed to obtain and maintain control in complex partial status epilepticus.

Benetello P: New antiepileptic drugs. Pharmacol Res 1995;31:155.

McNamara JO: Cellular and molecular basis of epilepsy. J Neurosci 1994;14:3413.

Sabers A, Gram L: Drug treatment of epilepsy in the 1990s. Drugs 1996;52:483.

Shorvon S: Tonic clonic status epilepticus. J Neurol Neurosurg Psychiatry 1993;56:125. (Pathophysiology and treatment.)

NEUROLOGIC CAUSES OF SYNCOPE

The term syncope refers to transient loss of consciousness resulting from pancerebral hypoperfusion. The clinical features and certain general causes of syncope are discussed in detail in Chapter 10, and only the neurologic causes are considered here.

Syncope may occur because of orthostatic (postural) hypotension, which occurs in a variety of neurologic contexts when the baroreceptor reflex arc is interrupted. Spinal cord transection and other myelopathies (eg, due to tumor or syringomyelia) above the T6 level may lead to marked postural hypotension, as also do brain stem lesions such as syringobulbia and posterior fossa tumors. Postural hypotension is occasionally found in neurosyphilis (tabes dorsalis) and is a frequent and conspicuous complication of diabetic neuropathy. Other polyneuropathies associated with orthostatic hypotension include Guillain-Barré syndrome, primary amyloidosis, acute porphyric neuropathy, and that associated with carcinoma. An acute or subacute autonomic neuropathy may also develop on an autoimmune basis.

Primary degenerative disorders of the central nervous system may lead to dysautonomia occurring in isolation (primary autonomic failure) or in association with more widespread neurologic abnormalities (multisystem atrophy) that may include parkinsonian, pyramidal, lower motor neuron, and cerebellar deficits.

McIntosh SJ et al: Clinical characteristics of vasodepressor, cardioinhibitory, and mixed carotid sinus syndrome in the elderly. Am J Med 1993;95:203. (Clinical features.)

SENSORY DISTURBANCES

Patients may complain of either lost or abnormal sensations. The term "numbness" is often used by patients to denote loss of feeling, but the word also has other meanings and the patient's intention must be clarified. Abnormal spontaneous sensations are generally called paresthesias, and unpleasant or painful sensations produced by a stimulus that is usually painless are called dysesthesias.

Sensory symptoms may be due to disease located anywhere along the peripheral or central sensory pathways. The character, site, mode of onset, spread, and temporal profile of sensory symptoms must be established and any precipitating or relieving factors identified. These features—and the presence of any associated symptoms—help identify the origin of sensory disturbances, as do the physical signs as well. Sensory symptoms or signs may conform to the territory of individual peripheral nerves or nerve roots. Involvement of one side of the body—or of one limb in its entirety—suggests a central lesion. Distal involvement of all four extremities suggests polyneuropathy, a cervical cord or brain stem lesion, or—when symptoms are transient—a metabolic disturbance such as hyperventilation syndrome. Short-lived sensory complaints may be indicative of sensory seizures or cerebral ischemic phenomena as well as metabolic disturbances. In patients with cord lesions, there may be a transverse sensory level. "Dissociated sensory loss" is characterized by loss of some sensory modalities with preservation of others. Such findings may be encountered in patients with either peripheral or central disease and must therefore be interpreted in the clinical context in which they are found.

The absence of sensory signs in patients with sensory symptoms does not mean that symptoms have a nonorganic basis. Symptoms are often troublesome before signs of sensory dysfunction have had time to develop.

WEAKNESS & PARALYSIS

Loss of muscle power may result from central disease involving the upper or lower motor neurons; from peripheral disease involving the roots, plexus, or peripheral nerves; from disorders of neuromuscular transmission; or from primary disorders of muscle. The clinical findings help to localize the lesion and thus reduce the number of diagnostic possibilities.

Weakness due to upper motor neuron lesions is characterized by selective involvement of certain muscle groups and is associated with spasticity, increased tendon reflexes, and extensor plantar responses. The site of upper motor neuron (pyramidal) involvement may be indicated by the presence of other clinical signs or by the distribution of the motor deficit. Lower motor neuron lesions lead to muscle wasting as well as weakness, with flaccidity and loss of tendon reflexes, but no change in the plantar responses unless the neurons subserving them are directly involved. Fasciculations may be evident over affected muscles. In distinguishing between a root, plexus, or peripheral nerve lesion, the distribution of the motor deficit and of any sensory changes is of particular importance. In patients with disturbances of neuromuscular transmission, weakness is patchy in distribution, often fluctuates over short periods of time, and is not associated with sensory changes. In myopathic disorders, weakness is usually most marked proximally in the limbs, is not associated with sensory loss or sphincter disturbance, and is not accompanied by muscle wasting or loss of tendon reflexes—at least not until an advanced stage.

TRANSIENT ISCHEMIC ATTACKS

Essentials of Diagnosis

- Risk factors for vascular disease often present.
- Focal neurologic deficit of acute onset.
- Clinical deficit resolves completely within 24 hours.

General Considerations

Transient ischemic attacks are characterized by focal ischemic cerebral neurologic deficits that last for less than 24 hours (usually less than 1–2 hours). About 30% of patients with stroke have a history of transient ischemic attacks, and proper treatment of the attacks is an important means of prevention. The incidence of stroke does not relate to either the number or the duration of individual attacks but is increased in patients with hypertension or diabetes.

Etiology

An important cause of transient cerebral ischemia is embolization. In many patients with these attacks, a source is readily apparent in the heart or a major

extracranial artery to the head, and emboli sometimes are visible in the retinal arteries. Moreover, an embolic phenomenon explains why separate attacks may affect different parts of the territory supplied by the same major vessel. Cardiac causes of embolic ischemic attacks include rheumatic heart disease, mitral valve disease, cardiac arrhythmia, infective endocarditis, atrial myxoma, and mural thrombi complicating myocardial infarction. Atrial septal defects and patent foramen ovale may permit emboli from the veins to reach the brain ("paradoxical emboli"). An ulcerated plaque on a major artery to the brain may serve as a source of emboli. In the anterior circulation, atherosclerotic changes occur most commonly in the region of the carotid bifurcation extracranially, and these changes may cause a bruit. In some patients with transient ischemic attacks or strokes, an acute or recent hemorrhage is found to have occurred into this atherosclerotic plaque, and this finding may have pathologic significance. Patients with AIDS have an increased risk of developing transient ischemic deficits or strokes.

Other (less common) abnormalities of blood vessels that may cause transient ischemic attacks include fibromuscular dysplasia, which affects particularly the cervical internal carotid artery; inflammatory arterial disorders such as giant cell arteritis, systemic lupus erythematosus, polyarteritis, and granulomatous angiitis; and meningovascular syphilis. Hypotension may cause a reduction of cerebral blood flow if a major extracranial artery to the brain is markedly stenosed, but this is a rare cause of transient ischemic attack.

Hematologic causes of ischemic attacks include polycythemia, sickle cell disease, and hyperviscosity syndromes. Severe anemia may also lead to transient focal neurologic deficits in patients with preexisting cerebral arterial disease.

The **subclavian steal syndrome** may lead to transient vertebrobasilar ischemia. Symptoms develop when there is localized stenosis or occlusion of one subclavian artery proximal to the source of the vertebral artery, so that blood is "stolen" from this artery. A bruit in the supraclavicular fossa, unequal radial pulses, and a difference of 20 mm Hg or more between the systolic blood pressures in the arms should suggest the diagnosis in patients with vertebrobasilar transient ischemic attacks.

Clinical Findings

A. Symptoms and Signs: The symptoms of transient ischemic attacks vary markedly among patients; however, the symptoms in a given individual tend to be constant in type. Onset is abrupt and without warning, and recovery usually occurs rapidly, often within a few minutes.

If the ischemia is in the carotid territory, common symptoms are weakness and heaviness of the contralateral arm, leg, or face, singly or in any combination. Numbness or paresthesias may also occur either as the sole manifestation of the attack or in combination with the motor deficit. There may be slowness of movement, dysphasia, or monocular visual loss in the eye contralateral to affected limbs. During an attack, examination may reveal flaccid weakness with pyramidal distribution, sensory changes, hyperreflexia or an extensor plantar response on the affected side, dysphasia, or any combination of these findings. Subsequently, examination reveals no neurologic abnormality, but the presence of a carotid bruit or cardiac abnormality may provide a clue to the cause of symptoms.

Vertebrobasilar ischemic attacks may be characterized by vertigo, ataxia, diplopia, dysarthria, dimness or blurring of vision, perioral numbness and paresthesias, and weakness or sensory complaints on one, both, or alternating sides of the body. These symptoms may occur singly or in any combination. Drop attacks due to bilateral leg weakness, without headache or loss of consciousness, may occur, sometimes in relation to head movements.

The natural history of attacks is variable. Some patients will have a major stroke after only a few attacks, whereas others may have frequent attacks for weeks or months without having a stroke. Attacks may occur intermittently over a long period of time, or they may stop spontaneously. In general, carotid ischemic attacks are more liable than vertebrobasilar ischemic attacks to be followed by stroke.

B. Imaging: CT scan of the head will exclude the possibility of a small cerebral hemorrhage or a cerebral tumor masquerading as a transient ischemic attack. A number of noninvasive techniques, such as ultrasonography, have been developed for studying the cerebral circulation and imaging the major vessels to the head. Carotid duplex ultrasonography is useful for detecting significant stenosis of the internal carotid artery, but arteriography remains important for demonstrating the status of the cerebrovascular system. MR angiography may reveal stenotic lesions of large vessels but is less sensitive than conventional arteriography. Accordingly, if findings on CT scan are normal, if there is no cardiac source of embolization, and if age and general condition indicate that the patient is a good operative risk, bilateral carotid arteriography should be considered in the further evaluation of carotid ischemic attacks, although the ultrasound findings may help in selecting patients for study.

C. Laboratory and Other Studies: Clinical and laboratory evaluation must include assessment for hypertension, heart disease, hematologic disorders, diabetes mellitus, hyperlipidemia, and peripheral vascular disease. It should include complete blood count, fasting blood glucose and serum cholesterol determinations, serologic tests for syphilis, and an ECG and chest x-ray. Echocardiography with bubble contrast is performed if a cardiac source is

likely, and blood cultures are obtained if endocarditis is suspected. Holter monitoring is indicated if a transient, paroxysmal disturbance of cardiac rhythm is suspected.

Differential Diagnosis

Focal seizures usually cause abnormal motor or sensory phenomena such as clonic limb movements, paresthesias, or tingling, rather than weakness or loss of feeling. Symptoms generally spread ("march") up the limb and may lead to a generalized tonic-clonic seizure. The electroencephalogram may help in detecting the epileptogenic source.

Classic migraine is easily recognized by the visual premonitory symptoms, followed by nausea, headache, and photophobia, but less typical cases may be hard to distinguish. The patient's age and medical history (including family history) may be helpful in this regard. Patients with migraine commonly have a history of episodes since adolescence and report that other family members have a similar disorder.

Focal neurologic deficits may occur during periods of hypoglycemia in diabetic patients receiving insulin or oral hypoglycemic agent therapy, and the lack of general hypoglycemic symptoms does not exclude this possibility.

Treatment

When arteriography reveals a surgically accessible high-grade stenosis (70–99% in luminal diameter) on the side appropriate to carotid ischemic attacks and there is relatively little atherosclerosis elsewhere in the cerebrovascular system, operative treatment (carotid thromboendarterectomy) reduces the risk of ipsilateral carotid stroke, especially when transient ischemic attacks are of recent onset (< 2 months). Surgery is not indicated for mild stenosis (< 30%); its benefits are unclear with severe stenosis plus diffuse intracranial atherosclerotic disease. See Chapter 12 for additional discussion.

In patients with carotid ischemic attacks who are poor operative candidates (and thus have not undergone arteriography) or who are found to have extensive vascular disease, medical treatment should be instituted. Similarly, patients with vertebrobasilar ischemic attacks are treated medically and are not subjected to arteriography unless there is clinical evidence of stenosis or occlusion in the carotid or subclavian arteries.

Medical treatment is aimed at preventing further attacks and stroke. Cigarette smoking should be stopped, and cardiac sources of embolization, hypertension, diabetes, hyperlipidemia, arteritis, or hematologic disorders should be treated appropriately. If anticoagulants are indicated for the treatment of embolism from the heart, they should be started immediately, provided there is no contraindication to their use. There is no advantage in delay, and the common fear of causing hemorrhage into a previously infarcted area is misplaced, since there is a far greater risk of further embolism to the cerebral circulation if treatment is withheld. Treatment is initiated with intravenous heparin (in a loading dose of 5000–10,000 units of standard molecular weight heparin, and maintenance infusion of 1000–2000 units per hour depending on the partial thromboplastin time) while warfarin sodium is introduced in a daily dose of 5–15 mg orally, depending on prothrombin time. Alternatively, aspirin (325 mg daily) may be used in patients with nonrheumatic atrial fibrillation to reduce the risk of stroke.

In patients with presumed or angiographically verified atherosclerotic changes in the extracranial or intracranial cerebrovascular circulation, antithrombotic medication is prescribed. The treatment selected will depend upon the patient's age, the likelihood of compliance in taking the drug, and the ready availability of medical and laboratory services. Some physicians use anticoagulant drugs (eg, warfarin, with temporary heparinization until the dose of warfarin is adequate) unless they are medically contraindicated, continuing them for 3–6 months before they are tapered and ultimately replaced with aspirin, which is continued for another year. However, there is no convincing evidence that anticoagulant drugs are of value. Other physicians therefore prefer aspirin from the onset.

The evidence supporting a therapeutic role for aspirin to suppress platelet aggregation is convincing. Platelets adhere to and aggregate around an atherosclerotic plaque and release various substances including thromboxane A_2. One study found that treatment with aspirin significantly reduces the frequency of transient ischemic attacks and the incidence of stroke or myocardial infarcts in high-risk patients. A daily dose of 325 mg is adequate; higher doses may provide added benefit but are associated with a higher incidence of gastrointestinal side effects. Dipyridamole is not as effective, and when added to aspirin does not offer any advantage over aspirin alone for stroke prevention. In patients intolerant of aspirin, ticlopidine (another platelet aggregation inhibitor) may be used in a dose of 250 mg twice daily, but patients must be monitored closely for the development of neutropenia or agranulocytosis.

In recent years, many patients with transient ischemic attacks associated with stenotic lesions of the distal internal carotid or the proximal middle cerebral arteries have undergone surgical extracranial-intracranial arterial anastomosis. However, no benefit of surgical treatment could be demonstrated in a large controlled prospective study.

Besson G, Bogousslavsky J: Current and future options for the prevention and treatment of stroke. CNS Drugs 1995;3:351.

Humphrey P: Stroke and transient ischaemic attacks. J Neurol Neurosurg Psychiatry 1994;47:534. (Management.)

NASCET Investigators: Clinical alert: Benefit of carotid endarterectomy for patients with high-grade stenosis of the internal carotid artery. Stroke 1991;22:816.

STROKE

Essentials of Diagnosis

- Sudden onset of characteristic neurologic deficit.
- Patient often has history of hypertension, diabetes mellitus, valvular heart disease, or atherosclerosis.
- Distinctive neurologic signs reflect the region of the brain involved.

General Considerations

In the USA, stroke remains the third leading cause of death, despite a general decline in the incidence of stroke in the last 30 years. The precise reasons for this decline are uncertain, but increased awareness of risk factors (hypertension, diabetes, hyperlipidemia, cigarette smoking, cardiac disease, AIDS, recreational drug abuse, heavy alcohol consumption, family history of stroke) and improved prophylactic measures and surveillance of those at increased risk have been contributory. A previous stroke makes individual patients more susceptible to further strokes.

For years, strokes have been subdivided pathologically into infarcts (thrombotic or embolic) and hemorrhages, and clinical criteria for distinguishing between these possibilities have been emphasized. However, it is often difficult to determine on clinical grounds the pathologic basis for stroke.

1. LACUNAR INFARCTION

Lacunar infarcts are small lesions (usually < 5 mm in diameter) that occur in the distribution of short penetrating arterioles in the basal ganglia, pons, cerebellum, anterior limb of the internal capsule, and, less commonly, the deep cerebral white matter. Lacunar infarcts are associated with poorly controlled hypertension or diabetes and have been found in several clinical syndromes, including contralateral pure motor or pure sensory deficit, ipsilateral ataxia with crural paresis, and dysarthria with clumsiness of the hand. The neurologic deficit may progress over 24–36 hours before stabilizing.

Lacunar infarcts are sometimes visible on CT scans as small, punched-out, hypodense areas, but in other patients no abnormality is seen. In some instances, patients with a clinical syndrome suggestive of lacunar infarction are found on CT scanning to have a severe hemispheric infarct.

The prognosis for recovery from the deficit produced by a lacunar infarct is usually good, with partial or complete resolution occurring over the following 4–6 weeks in many instances.

2. CEREBRAL INFARCTION

Thrombotic or embolic occlusion of a major vessel leads to cerebral infarction. Causes include the disorders predisposing to transient ischemic attacks (see above) and atherosclerosis of cerebral arteries. The resulting deficit depends upon the particular vessel involved and the extent of any collateral circulation. Cerebral ischemia leads to release of excitatory and other neuropeptides that may augment calcium flux into neurons, thereby leading to cell death and increasing the neurologic deficit.

Clinical Findings

A. Symptoms and Signs: Onset is usually abrupt, and there may then be very little progression except that due to brain swelling. Clinical evaluation always includes examination of the heart and auscultation over the subclavian and carotid vessels to determine whether there are any bruits.

1. Obstruction of carotid circulation—Occlusion of the ophthalmic artery is probably symptomless in most cases because of the rich orbital collaterals, but its transient embolic obstruction leads to amaurosis fugax—sudden and brief loss of vision in one eye.

Occlusion of the anterior cerebral artery distal to its junction with the anterior communicating artery causes weakness and cortical sensory loss in the contralateral leg and sometimes mild weakness of the arm, especially proximally. There may be a contralateral grasp reflex, paratonic rigidity, and abulia (lack of initiative) or frank confusion. Urinary incontinence is not uncommon, particularly if behavioral disturbances are conspicuous. Bilateral anterior cerebral infarction is especially likely to cause marked behavioral changes and memory disturbances. Unilateral anterior cerebral artery occlusion proximal to the junction with the anterior communicating artery is generally well tolerated because of the collateral supply from the other side.

Middle cerebral artery occlusion leads to contralateral hemiplegia, hemisensory loss, and homonymous hemianopia (ie, bilaterally symmetric loss of vision in half of the visual fields), with the eyes deviated to the side of the lesion. If the dominant hemisphere is involved, global aphasia is also present. It may be impossible to distinguish this clinically from occlusion of the internal carotid artery. With occlusion of either of these arteries, there may also be considerable swelling of the hemisphere, leading to drowsiness, stupor, and coma in extreme cases. Occlusions of different branches of the middle cerebral artery cause more limited findings. For example, involvement of the anterior main division leads to a predominantly expressive dysphasia and to contralateral paralysis and loss of sensations in the arm, the face, and, to a lesser extent, the leg. Posterior branch occlusion produces a receptive (Wernicke's) aphasia and a homonymous visual field defect. With involvement of the nondominant hemisphere, speech and comprehension are preserved, but there may be a confusional state, dressing apraxia, and constructional and spatial deficits.

2. Obstruction of vertebrobasilar circulation—Occlusion of the posterior cerebral artery may lead to a thalamic syndrome in which contralateral hemisensory disturbance occurs, followed by the development of spontaneous pain and hyperpathia. There is often a macular-sparing homonymous hemianopia and sometimes a mild, usually temporary, hemiparesis. Depending on the site of the lesion and the collateral circulation, the severity of these deficits varies and other deficits may also occur, including involuntary movements and alexia. Occlusion of the main artery beyond the origin of its penetrating branches may lead solely to a macular-sparing hemianopia.

Vertebral artery occlusion distally, below the origin of the anterior spinal and posterior inferior cerebellar arteries, may be clinically silent because the circulation is maintained by the other vertebral artery. If the remaining vertebral artery is congenitally small or severely atherosclerotic, however, a deficit similar to that of basilar artery occlusion is seen unless there is good collateral circulation from the anterior circulation through the circle of Willis. When the small paramedian arteries arising from the vertebral artery are occluded, contralateral hemiplegia and sensory deficit occur in association with an ipsilateral cranial nerve palsy at the level of the lesion. An obstruction of the posterior inferior cerebellar artery or an obstruction of the vertebral artery just before it branches to this vessel leads ipsilaterally to spinothalamic sensory loss involving the face, ninth and tenth cranial nerve lesions, limb ataxia and numbness, and Horner's syndrome, combined with contralateral spinothalamic sensory loss involving the limbs.

Occlusion of both vertebral arteries or the basilar artery leads to coma with pinpoint pupils, flaccid quadriplegia and sensory loss, and variable cranial nerve abnormalities. With partial basilar artery occlusion, there may be diplopia, visual loss, vertigo, dysarthria, ataxia, weakness or sensory disturbances in some or all of the limbs, and discrete cranial nerve palsies. In patients with hemiplegia of pontine origin, the eyes are often deviated to the paralyzed side, whereas in patients with a hemispheric lesion, the eyes commonly deviate from the hemiplegic side.

Occlusion of any of the major cerebellar arteries produces vertigo, nausea, vomiting, nystagmus, ipsilateral limb ataxia, and contralateral spinothalamic sensory loss in the limbs. If the superior cerebellar artery is involved, the contralateral spinothalamic loss also involves the face; with occlusion of the anterior inferior cerebellar artery, there is ipsilateral spinothalamic sensory loss involving the face, usually in conjunction with ipsilateral facial weakness and deafness. Massive cerebellar infarction may lead to coma, tonsillar herniation, and death.

3. Coma–Infarction in either the carotid or vertebrobasilar territory may lead to loss of consciousness. For example, an infarct involving one cerebral hemisphere may lead to such swelling that the function of the other hemisphere or the rostral brain stem is disturbed and coma results. Similarly, coma occurs with bilateral brain stem infarction when this involves the reticular formation, and it occurs with brain stem compression after cerebellar infarction.

B. Imaging: Radiography of the chest may reveal cardiomegaly or valvular calcification; the presence of a neoplasm would suggest that the neurologic deficit is due to metastasis rather than stroke. A CT scan of the head (without contrast) is important in excluding cerebral hemorrhage, but it may not permit distinction between a cerebral infarct and tumor. CT scanning is preferable to MRI in the acute stage because it is quicker and because intracranial hemorrhage is not easily detected by MRI within the first 48 hours after a bleeding episode.

C. Laboratory and Other Studies: Investigations should include a complete blood count, sedimentation rate, blood glucose determination, and serologic tests for syphilis. Antiphospholipid antibodies (lupus anticoagulants and anticardiolipin antibodies) promote thrombosis and are associated with an increased incidence of stroke. Similarly, elevated serum cholesterol and lipids may indicate an increased risk of thrombotic stroke. Electrocardiography will help exclude a cardiac arrhythmia or recent myocardial infarction that might be serving as a source of embolization. Blood cultures should be performed if endocarditis is suspected, echocardiography if heart disease is suspected, and Holter monitoring if paroxysmal cardiac arrhythmia requires exclusion. Examination of the cerebrospinal fluid is not always necessary but may be helpful if there is diagnostic uncertainty; it should be delayed until after CT scanning.

Treatment

If the neurologic deficit progresses over the following minutes or hours, heparinization may be of value in limiting or arresting further deterioration. Since the signs of progressing stroke may be simulated by an intracerebral hematoma, the latter must be excluded by immediate CT scanning or angiography before the patient is heparinized.

Early management of a completed stroke consists of attention to general supportive measures. During the acute stage, there may be marked brain swelling and edema, with symptoms and signs of increasing intracranial pressure, an increasing neurologic deficit, or herniation syndrome. Corticosteroids have been prescribed in an attempt to reduce vasogenic cerebral edema. Prednisone (up to 100 mg/d) or dexamethasone (16 mg/d) has been used, but the evidence that corticosteroids are of any benefit is conflicting. Dehydrating hyperosmolar agents have also been prescribed in efforts to reduce brain swelling, but there is little evidence of any lasting benefit. Likewise, clinical benefit from treatment with vasodilators such as papaverine is minimal. Neither hypercapnia nor hypocapnia has been shown to have any benefit. Barbiturates are known to decrease neuronal metabolism and energy requirements and have been reported to improve functional recovery in experimental stroke models; their use in humans, however, is experimental. Attempts to lower the blood pressure of hypertensive patients during the acute phase of a stroke should be avoided, since there is loss of cerebral autoregulation and lowering the blood pressure may further compromise ischemic areas.

Anticoagulant drugs have no role in the management of patients with a completed stroke, except when there is a cardiac source of embolization. Treatment is then started with intravenous heparin while warfarin is introduced. The target is an international normalized ratio of 3:4 for the prothrombin time. If the CT scan shows no evidence of hemorrhage and the cerebrospinal fluid is clear, anticoagulant treatment may be started without delay. Some physicians prefer to wait for 2 or 3 days before initiating anticoagulant treatment; the CT scan is then repeated and anticoagulant therapy is initiated if it again shows no evidence of hemorrhagic transformation.

Thrombolytic therapy by administration of tissue plasminogen activator within 3 hours after onset (often difficult to determine) of stroke improves clinical outcome. Preliminary studies suggest that calcium channel blocking drugs such as nimodipine (30 mg orally every 6 hours for 4 weeks) reduce the deficit produced by cerebral ischemia and the morbidity and mortality rates from stroke. Multicenter studies are now in progress to study further the effects of these agents in acute cerebral ischemia.

Blockage of glutamate, an excitatory neurotransmitter, reduces the sensitivity of central neurons to ischemia. The N-methyl-D-aspartate (NMDA) type of glutamate receptors is linked to calcium-permeable channels, and studies in animals have shown that specific NMDA-receptor antagonists reduce stroke size, deficits, and the percentage of severely ischemic neurons. The role of this therapeutic approach in humans is currently under study.

Physical therapy has an important role in the management of patients with impaired motor function. Passive movements at an early stage will help prevent contractures. As cooperation increases and some recovery begins, active movements will improve strength and coordination. In all cases, early mobilization and active rehabilitation are important. Occupational therapy may improve morale and motor skills, while speech therapy may be beneficial in patients with expressive dysphasia or dysarthria. When there is a severe and persisting motor deficit, a device such as a leg brace, toe spring, frame, or cane may help the patient move about, and the provision of other aids to daily living may improve the quality of life.

Prognosis

The prognosis for survival after cerebral infarction is better than after cerebral or subarachnoid hemorrhage. Loss of consciousness after a cerebral infarct implies a poorer prognosis than otherwise. The extent of the infarct governs the potential for rehabilitation. Patients who have had a cerebral infarct are at risk for further strokes and for myocardial infarcts.

American Academy of Neurology, Quality Standards Subcommittee: Thrombolytic therapy for acute ischemic stroke—summary statement. Neurology 1996;47:835. (Practice advisory.)

Brickner ME: Cardioembolic stroke. Am J Med 1996; 100:465. (Review.)

Caplan LR: *Stroke: A Clinical Approach,* 2nd ed. Butterworth-Heinemann, 1993.

Cannegieter SC et al: Optimal oral anticoagulant therapy in patients with mechanical heart valves. N Engl J Med 1995;333:11. (Outcomes at different levels of anticoagulation.)

Fisher M: Potentially effective therapies for acute ischemic stroke. Eur Neurol 1995;35:3. (Emerging therapies.)

National Institutes of Neurological Disorders and Stroke rt-PA Stroke Study Group: Tissue plasminogen activator for acute ischemic stroke. N Engl J Med 1995;333:1581. (Clinical trial.)

Pessin MS et al: Safety of anticoagulation after hemorrhagic infarction. Neurology 1993;43:1298. (Anticoagulants may sometimes be used after hemorrhagic infarcts.)

3. INTRACEREBRAL HEMORRHAGE

Spontaneous intracerebral hemorrhage in patients with no angiographic evidence of an associated vascular anomaly (eg, aneurysm or angioma) is usually due to hypertension. The pathologic basis for hemorrhage is probably the presence of microaneurysms that are now known to develop on perforating vessels of 100–300 μm in diameter in hypertensive patients. Hypertensive intracerebral hemorrhage occurs most frequently in the basal ganglia and less commonly in the pons, thalamus, cerebellum, and cerebral white matter. Hemorrhage may extend into the ventricular system or subarachnoid space, and signs of meningeal irritation are then found. Hemorrhages usually occur suddenly and without warning, often during activity.

In addition to its association with hypertension, nontraumatic intracerebral hemorrhage may occur with hematologic and bleeding disorders (eg, leukemia, thrombocytopenia, hemophilia, or disseminated intravascular coagulation), anticoagulant therapy, liver disease, cerebral amyloid angiopathy, and primary or secondary brain tumors. Bleeding is primarily into the subarachnoid space when it occurs from an intracranial aneurysm or arteriovenous malformation (see below), but it may be partly intraparenchymal as well. In some cases, no specific cause for cerebral hemorrhage can be identified.

Clinical Findings

A. Symptoms and Signs: With hemorrhage into the cerebral hemisphere, consciousness is initially lost or impaired in about one-half of patients. Vomiting occurs very frequently at the onset of bleeding, and headache is sometimes present. Focal symptoms and signs then develop, depending on the site of the hemorrhage. With hypertensive hemorrhage, there is generally a rapidly evolving neurologic deficit with hemiplegia or hemiparesis. A hemisensory disturbance is also present with more deeply placed lesions. With lesions of the putamen, loss of conjugate lateral gaze may be conspicuous. With thalamic hemorrhage, there may be a loss of upward gaze, downward or skew deviation of the eyes, lateral gaze palsies, and pupillary inequalities.

Cerebellar hemorrhage may present with sudden onset of nausea and vomiting, disequilibrium, headache, and loss of consciousness that may terminate fatally within 48 hours. Less commonly, the onset is gradual and the course episodic or slowly progressive—clinical features suggesting an expanding cerebellar lesion. In yet other cases, however, the onset and course are intermediate, and examination shows lateral conjugate gaze palsies to the side of the lesion; small reactive pupils; contralateral hemiplegia; peripheral facial weakness; ataxia of gait, limbs, or trunk; periodic respiration; or some combination of these findings.

B. Imaging: CT scanning (without contrast) is important not only in confirming that hemorrhage has occurred but also in determining the size and site of the hematoma. As indicated earlier, it is superior to MRI for detecting intracranial hemorrhage of less than 48 hours' duration. If the patient's condition permits further intervention, cerebral angiography may be undertaken thereafter to determine if an aneurysm or arteriovenous malformation is present (see below).

C. Laboratory and Other Studies: A complete blood count, platelet count, bleeding time, prothrombin and partial thromboplastin times, and liver and renal function tests may reveal a predisposing cause for the hemorrhage. Lumbar puncture is contraindicated because it may precipitate a herniation syndrome in patients with a large hematoma, and CT scanning is superior in detecting intracerebral hemorrhage.

Treatment

Neurologic management is generally conservative and supportive, regardless of whether the patient has a profound deficit with associated brain stem compression, in which case the prognosis is grim, or a more localized deficit not causing increased intracranial pressure or brain stem involvement. Decompression is helpful, however, when a superficial hematoma in cerebral white matter is exerting a mass effect and causing incipient herniation. In patients with cerebellar hemorrhage, prompt surgical evacuation of the hematoma is appropriate, because spontaneous unpredictable deterioration may otherwise lead to a fatal outcome and because operative treatment may lead to complete resolution of the clinical deficit. The treatment of underlying structural lesions or bleeding disorders depends upon their nature.

4. SUBARACHNOID HEMORRHAGE

Between 5% and 10% of strokes are due to subarachnoid hemorrhage. Although hemorrhage is usually from rupture of an aneurysm or arteriovenous malformation, no specific cause can be found in 20% of cases.

Clinical Findings

A. Symptoms and Signs: Subarachnoid hemorrhage has a characteristic clinical picture. Its onset is with sudden headache of a severity never experienced previously by the patient. This may be followed by nausea and vomiting and by a loss or impairment of consciousness that can either be transient or progress inexorably to deepening coma and death. If consciousness is regained, the patient is often confused and irritable and may show other symptoms of an altered mental status. Neurologic examination generally reveals nuchal rigidity and other signs of meningeal irritation, except in deeply comatose patients. A focal neurologic deficit is occasionally present and may suggest the site of the underlying lesion.

B. Imaging: A CT scan should be performed immediately to confirm that hemorrhage has occurred and to search for clues regarding its source. It is preferable to MRI because it is faster and more sensitive in detecting hemorrhage in the first 24 hours. CT findings sometimes are normal in patients with suspected hemorrhage, and the cerebrospinal fluid must then be examined for the presence of blood or xanthochromia before the possibility of subarachnoid hemorrhage is discounted.

Cerebral arteriography may be undertaken to determine the source of bleeding; it is not performed unless or until the patient's condition has stabilized and is good enough so that operative treatment is feasible. In general, bilateral carotid and vertebral arteriography are necessary because aneurysms are often multiple, while arteriovenous malformations may be supplied from several sources. MR angiography may also permit these vascular anomalies to be visualized but is less sensitive than conventional arteriography.

Treatment

The measures outlined in the section on stupor and coma are applied to comatose patients. Conscious patients are confined to bed, advised against any exertion or straining, treated symptomatically for headache and anxiety, and given laxatives or stool softeners. If there is severe hypertension, the blood pressure can be lowered gradually, but not below a diastolic level of 100 mm Hg. Phenytoin is generally prescribed routinely to prevent seizures. Further comment concerning the specific operative management of arteriovenous malformations and aneurysms follows.

5. INTRACRANIAL ANEURYSM

Saccular aneurysms ("berry" aneurysms) tend to occur at arterial bifurcations, are considerably more common in adults than in children, are frequently multiple (20% of cases), and are usually asymptomatic. They may be associated with polycystic kidney disease and coarctation of the aorta. Most aneurysms are located on the anterior part of the circle of Willis—particularly on the anterior or posterior communicating arteries, at the bifurcation of the middle cerebral artery, and at the bifurcation of the internal carotid artery.

Clinical Findings

A. Symptoms and Signs: Aneurysms may cause a focal neurologic deficit by compressing adjacent structures. However, most are asymptomatic or produce only nonspecific symptoms until they rupture, at which time subarachnoid hemorrhage results. There is often a paucity of focal neurologic signs in patients with subarachnoid hemorrhage, but when present, such signs may relate either to a focal hematoma or to ischemia in the territory of the vessel with the ruptured aneurysm. Hemiplegia or other focal deficit sometimes occurs after a delay of 4–14 days and is due to focal arterial spasm in the vicinity of the ruptured aneurysm. This spasm is of uncertain, probably multifactorial, cause, but it sometimes leads to significant cerebral ischemia or infarction, and it may further aggravate any existing increase in intracranial pressure. Subacute hydrocephalus due to interference with the flow of cerebrospinal fluid may occur after 2 or more weeks, and this leads to a delayed clinical deterioration that is relieved by shunting.

In some patients, "warning leaks" of a small amount of blood from the aneurysm precede the major hemorrhage by a few hours or days. They lead to headaches, sometimes accompanied by nausea and neck stiffness, but the true cause of these symptoms is often not appreciated until massive hemorrhage occurs.

B. Imaging: The CT scan generally confirms that subarachnoid hemorrhage has occurred, but occasionally it is normal. Angiography (bilateral carotid and vertebral studies) generally indicates the size and site of the lesion, sometimes reveals multiple aneurysms, and may show arterial spasm. If subarachnoid hemorrhage is confirmed by lumbar puncture or CT scanning but arteriograms show no abnormality, the examination should be repeated after 2 weeks, because vasospasm may have prevented detection of an aneurysm during the initial study.

C. Laboratory and Other Studies: The cerebrospinal fluid is bloodstained. The electroencephalogram sometimes indicates the side or site of hemorrhage but frequently shows only a diffuse abnormality. Electrocardiographic evidence of arrhythmias or myocardial ischemia has been well described and probably relates to excessive sympathetic activity. Peripheral leukocytosis and transient glycosuria are also common findings.

Treatment

The major aim of treatment is to prevent further hemorrhages. Definitive treatment requires a surgical approach to the aneurysm and ideally consists of clipping of its base. If surgery is not feasible, medical management as outlined above for subarachnoid hemorrhage is continued for about 6 weeks and is followed by gradual mobilization. Endovascular treatment by interventional radiologists is sometimes feasible for inoperable aneurysms.

The risk of further hemorrhage is greatest within a few days of the first hemorrhage; approximately 20% of patients will have further bleeding within 2 weeks and 40% within 6 months. Attempts have been made to reduce this risk pharmacologically. Treatment with an antifibrinolytic agent such as aminocaproic acid during the first 14 days reduces the risk of recurrent hemorrhage but is associated with such an increase in cerebral ischemic complications that the mortality rate and the degree of disability among survivors are unchanged. Thus, early operation (ie, within about 2 days of hemorrhage) is preferred for good operative candidates.

Calcium channel-blocking agents have helped to reduce or reverse experimental vasospasm, and nimodipine has been shown to reduce, in neurologically normal patients, the incidence of ischemic deficits from arterial spasm without producing any side effects. The dose of nimodipine is 60 mg every 4 hours for 21 days. After surgical obliteration of any aneurysms, symptomatic vasospasm may also be treated by intravascular volume expansion, induced hypertension, or transluminal balloon angioplasty of involved intracranial vessels.

With regard to unruptured aneurysms, those that are symptomatic merit prompt surgical treatment, whereas small asymptomatic ones discovered incidentally are often followed arteriographically and corrected surgically only if they increase in size to over 5 mm. The natural history of unruptured aneurysms is not clearly defined.

Kopitnik TA, Sampson DS: Management of subarachnoid haemorrhage. J Neurol Neurosurg Psychiatry 1993; 56:947.
Nichols DA: Endovascular treatment of the acutely ruptured intracranial aneurysm. J Neurosurg 1993;79:1.

6. ARTERIOVENOUS MALFORMATIONS

Arteriovenous malformations are congenital vascular malformations that result from a localized maldevelopment of part of the primitive vascular plexus and consist of abnormal arteriovenous communications without intervening capillaries. They vary in size, ranging from massive lesions that are fed by multiple vessels and involve a large part of the brain to lesions so small that they are hard to identify at arteriography, surgery, or autopsy. In approximately 10% of cases, there is an associated arterial aneurysm, while 1–2% of patients presenting with aneurysms have associated arteriovenous malformations. Clinical presentation may relate to hemorrhage from the malformation or an associated aneurysm or may relate to cerebral ischemia due to diversion of blood by the anomalous arteriovenous shunt or due to venous stagnation. Regional maldevelopment of the brain, compression or distortion of adjacent cerebral tissue by enlarged anomalous vessels, and progressive gliosis due to mechanical and ischemic factors may also be contributory. In addition, communicating or obstructive hydrocephalus may occur and lead to symptoms.

Clinical Findings

A. Symptoms and Signs:

1. Supratentorial lesions–Most cerebral arteriovenous malformations are supratentorial, usually lying in the territory of the middle cerebral artery. Initial symptoms consist of hemorrhage in 30–60% of cases, epilepsy in 20–40%, headache in 5–25%, and miscellaneous complaints (including focal deficits) in 10–15%. Up to 70% of arteriovenous malformations bleed at some point in their natural history, most commonly before the patient reaches the age of 40 years. This tendency to bleed is unrelated to the lesion site or to the patient's sex, but small arteriovenous malformations are more likely to bleed than large ones. Arteriovenous malformations that have bled once are more likely to bleed again. Hemorrhage is commonly intracerebral as well as into the subarachnoid space, and it has a fatal outcome in about 10% of cases. Focal or generalized seizures may accompany or follow hemorrhage, or they may be the initial presentation, especially with frontal or parietal arteriovenous malformations. Headaches are especially likely when the external carotid arteries are involved in the malformation. These sometimes simulate migraine but more commonly are nonspecific in character, with nothing about them to suggest an underlying structural lesion.

In patients presenting with subarachnoid hemorrhage, examination may reveal an abnormal mental status and signs of meningeal irritation. Additional findings may help to localize the lesion and sometimes indicate that intracranial pressure is increased. A cranial bruit always suggests the possibility of a cerebral arteriovenous malformation, but bruits may also be found with aneurysms, meningiomas, acquired arteriovenous fistulas, and arteriovenous malformations involving the scalp, calvarium, or orbit. Bruits are best heard over the ipsilateral eye or mastoid region and are of some help in lateralization but of no help in localization. Absence of a bruit in no way excludes the possibility of arteriovenous malformation.

2. Infratentorial lesions–Brain stem arteriovenous malformations are often clinically silent, but they may hemorrhage, cause obstructive hydrocephalus, or lead to progressive or relapsing brain stem deficits. Cerebellar arteriovenous malformations may also be clinically inconspicuous but sometimes lead to cerebellar hemorrhage.

B. Imaging: In patients presenting with suspected hemorrhage, CT scanning indicates whether subarachnoid or intracerebral bleeding has recently occurred, helps to localize its source, and may reveal the arteriovenous malformation. If the CT scan shows no evidence of bleeding but subarachnoid hemorrhage is diagnosed clinically, the cerebrospinal fluid should be examined.

When intracranial hemorrhage is confirmed but the source of hemorrhage is not evident on the CT scan, arteriography is necessary to exclude aneurysm or arteriovenous malformation. MR angiography is not sensitive enough for this purpose. Even if the findings on CT scan suggest arteriovenous malformation, arteriography is required to establish the nature of the lesion with certainty and to determine its anatomic features so that treatment can be planned. The examination must generally include bilateral opacification of the internal and external carotid arteries and the vertebral arteries. Arteriovenous malformations typically appear as a tangled vascular mass with distended tortuous afferent and efferent vessels, a rapid circulation time, and arteriovenous shunting. Findings on plain radiographs of the skull are often normal unless an intracerebral hematoma is

present, in which case there may be changes suggestive of raised intracranial pressure and displacement of a calcified pineal gland.

In patients presenting without hemorrhage, CT scan or MRI usually reveals the underlying abnormality, and MRI frequently also shows evidence of old or recent hemorrhage that may have been asymptomatic. The nature and detailed anatomy of any focal lesion identified by these means is delineated by angiography, especially if operative treatment is under consideration.

C. Laboratory and Other Studies: Electroencephalography is usually indicated in patients presenting with seizures and may show consistently focal or lateralized abnormalities resulting from the underlying cerebral arteriovenous malformation. This should be followed by CT scanning.

Treatment

Surgical treatment to prevent further hemorrhage is justified in patients with arteriovenous malformations that have bled, provided that the lesion is accessible and the patient has a reasonable life expectancy. Surgical treatment is also appropriate if intracranial pressure is increased or if there is cardiac decompensation, as occurs in children, and to prevent further progression of a focal neurologic deficit. In patients presenting solely with seizures, anticonvulsant drug treatment is usually sufficient, and operative treatment is unnecessary unless there are further developments.

Definitive operative treatment consists of excision of the arteriovenous malformation if it is surgically accessible. Arteriovenous malformations that are inoperable because of their location are sometimes treated solely by embolization; although the risk of hemorrhage is not reduced, neurologic deficits may be stabilized or even reversed by this procedure. Two other new techniques for the treatment of intracerebral arteriovenous malformations are injection of a vascular occlusive polymer through a flow-guided microcatheter and permanent occlusion of feeding vessels by positioning detachable balloon catheters in the desired sites and then inflating them with quickly solidifying contrast material. Proton beam therapy may also be useful in the management of inoperable cerebral arteriovenous malformations.

7. INTRACRANIAL VENOUS THROMBOSIS

Intracranial venous thrombosis may occur in association with intracranial or maxillofacial infections, hypercoagulable states, polycythemia, sickle cell disease, and cyanotic congenital heart disease and in pregnancy or during the puerperium. It is characterized by headache, focal or generalized convulsions, drowsiness, confusion, increased intracranial pressure, and focal neurologic deficits—and sometimes by evidence of meningeal irritation. The diagnosis is confirmed by CT scanning and MRI, MR venography, or angiography.

Treatment includes anticonvulsant drugs if seizures have occurred and antiedema agents (eg, dexamethasone, 4 mg four times daily) to reduce intracranial pressure. Anticoagulation with dose-adjusted intravenous heparin reduces morbidity and mortality of venous sinus thrombosis.

8. SPINAL CORD VASCULAR DISEASES

Infarction of the Spinal Cord

Infarction of the spinal cord is rare. It occurs only in the territory of the anterior spinal artery because this vessel, which supplies the anterior two-thirds of the cord, is itself supplied by only a limited number of feeders. Infarction usually results from interrupted flow in one or more of these feeders, eg, with aortic dissection, aortography, polyarteritis, or severe hypotension, or after surgical resection of the thoracic aorta. The paired posterior spinal arteries, by contrast, are supplied by numerous arteries at different levels of the cord.

Since the anterior spinal artery receives numerous feeders in the cervical region, infarcts almost always occur caudally. Clinical presentation is characterized by acute onset of flaccid, areflexive paraplegia that evolves after a few days or weeks into a spastic paraplegia with extensor plantar responses. There is an accompanying dissociated sensory loss, with impairment of appreciation of pain and temperature but preservation of sensations of vibration and position. Treatment is symptomatic.

Cheshire WP et al: Spinal cord infarction: Etiology and outcome. Neurology 1996;47:321. (Clinical review.)

Epidural or Subdural Hemorrhage

Epidural or subdural hemorrhage may lead to sudden severe back pain followed by an acute compressive myelopathy necessitating urgent myelography and surgical evacuation. It may occur in patients with bleeding disorders or those who are taking anticoagulant drugs, sometimes following trauma or lumbar puncture. Epidural hemorrhage may also be related to a vascular malformation or tumor deposit.

Arteriovenous Malformation of the Spinal Cord

Arteriovenous malformations of the cord are congenital lesions that present with spinal subarachnoid hemorrhage or myeloradiculopathy. Since most of these malformations are located in the thoracolumbar region, they lead to motor and sensory disturbances in the legs and to sphincter disorders. Pain in the legs or back is often severe. Examination reveals an up-per, lower, or mixed motor deficit in the legs; sensory deficits are also present and are usually extensive, although occasionally they are confined to radicular distribution. Cervical arteriovenous malformations lead also to symptoms and signs in the arms. Spinal MRI may not detect the arteriovenous malformation, and negative findings do not exclude the diagnosis. In general, the diagnosis is suggested at myelography (performed with the patient prone and supine) when serpiginous filling defects due to enlarged vessels are found. Selective spinal arteriography confirms the diagnosis. Most lesions are extramedullary, are posterior to the cord (lying either intra- or extradurally), and can easily be treated by ligation of feeding vessels and excision of the fistulous anomaly or by embolization procedures. Delay in treatment may lead to increased and irreversible disability or to death from recurrent subarachnoid hemorrhage.

INTRACRANIAL & SPINAL SPACE-OCCUPYING LESIONS

1. PRIMARY INTRACRANIAL TUMORS

Essentials of Diagnosis

- Generalized or focal disturbance of cerebral function, or both.
- Increased intracranial pressure in some patients.
- Neuroradiologic evidence of space-occupying lesion.

General Considerations

Half of all primary intracranial neoplasms (Table 24–3) are gliomas and the remainder meningiomas, pituitary adenomas, neurofibromas, and other tumors. Certain tumors, especially neurofibromas, hemangioblastomas, and retinoblastomas, may have a familial basis, and congenital factors bear on the development of craniopharyngiomas. Tumors may occur at any age, but certain gliomas show particular age predilections (Table 24–3).

Clinical Findings

A. Symptoms and Signs: Intracranial tumors may lead to a generalized disturbance of cerebral function and to symptoms and signs of increased intracranial pressure. In consequence, there may be personality changes, intellectual decline, emotional lability, seizures, headaches, nausea, and malaise. If the pressure is increased in a particular cranial compartment, brain tissue may herniate into a compartment with lower pressure. The most familiar syndrome is herniation of the temporal lobe uncus through the tentorial hiatus, which causes compression of the third cranial nerve, midbrain, and posterior cerebral artery. The earliest sign of this is ipsilateral pupillary dilation, followed by stupor, coma,

Table 24–3. Primary intracranial tumors.

Tumor	Clinical Features	Treatment and Prognosis
Glioblastoma multiforme	Presents commonly with nonspecific complaints and increased intracranial pressure. As it grows, focal deficits develop.	Course is rapidly progressive, with poor prognosis. Total surgical removal is usually not possible, and response to radiation therapy is poor.
Astrocytoma	Presentation similar to glioblastoma multiforme but course more protracted, often over several years. Cerebellar astrocytoma, especially in children, may have a more benign course.	Prognosis is variable. By the time of diagnosis, total excision is usually impossible; tumor often is not radiosensitive. In cerebellar astrocytoma, total surgical removal is often possible.
Medulloblastoma	Seen most frequently in children. Generally arises from roof of fourth ventricle and leads to increased intracranial pressure accompanied by brain stem and cerebellar signs. May seed subarachnoid space.	Treatment consists of surgery combined with radiation therapy and chemotherapy.
Ependymoma	Glioma arising from the ependyma of a ventricle, especially the fourth ventricle; leads early to signs of increased intracranial pressure. Arises also from central canal of cord.	Tumor is not radiosensitive and is best treated surgically if possible.
Oligodendroglioma	Slow-growing. Usually arises in cerebral hemisphere in adults. Calcification may be visible on skull x-ray.	Treatment is surgical and usually successful.
Brain stem glioma	Presents during childhood with cranial nerve palsies and then with long-tract signs in the limbs. Signs of increased intracranial pressure occur late.	Tumor is inoperable; treatment is by irradiation and shunt for increased intracranial pressure.
Cerebellar hemangioblastoma	Presents with disequilibrium, ataxia of trunk or limbs, and signs of increased intracranial pressure. Sometimes familial. May be associated with retinal and spinal vascular lesions, polycythemia, and hypernephromas.	Treatment is surgical.
Pineal tumor	Presents with increased intracranial pressure, sometimes associated with impaired upward gaze (Parinaud's syndrome) and other deficits indicative of midbrain lesion.	Ventricular decompression by shunting is followed by surgical approach to tumor; irradiation is indicated if tumor is malignant. Prognosis depends on histopathologic findings and extent of tumor.
Craniopharyngioma	Originates from remnants of Rathke's pouch above the sella, depressing the optic chiasm. May present at any age but usually in childhood, with endocrine dysfunction and bitemporal field defects.	Treatment is surgical, but total removal may not be possible.
Acoustic neurinoma	Ipsilateral hearing loss is most common initial symptom. Subsequent symptoms may include tinnitus, headache, vertigo, facial weakness or numbness, and long-tract signs. (May be familial and bilateral when related to neurofibromatosis.) Most sensitive screening tests are MRI and brain stem auditory evoked potential.	Treatment is excision by translabyrinthine surgery, craniectomy, or a combined approach. Outcome is usually good.
Meningioma	Originates from the dura mater or arachnoid; compresses rather than invades adjacent neural structures. Increasingly common with advancing age. Tumor size varies greatly. Symptoms vary with tumor site—eg, unilateral exophthalmos (sphenoidal ridge); anosmia and optic nerve compression (olfactory groove). Tumor is usually benign and readily detected by CT scanning; may lead to calcification and bone erosion visible on plain x-rays of skull.	Treatment is surgical. Tumor may recur if removal is incomplete.
Primary cerebral lymphoma	Associated with AIDS and other immunodeficient states. Presentation may be with focal deficits or with disturbances of cognition and consciousness. May be indistinguishable from cerebral toxoplasmosis.	Treatment is by whole-brain irradiation; chemotherapy may have an adjunctive role. Prognosis depends upon CD4 count at diagnosis.

decerebrate posturing, and respiratory arrest. Another important herniation syndrome consists of displacement of the cerebellar tonsils through the foramen magnum, which causes medullary compression leading to apnea, circulatory collapse, and death. Other herniation syndromes are less common and of less clear clinical importance.

Intracranial tumors also lead to focal deficits depending on their location.

1. Frontal lobe lesions–Tumors of the frontal lobe often lead to progressive intellectual decline, slowing of mental activity, personality changes, and contralateral grasp reflexes. They may lead to expressive aphasia if the posterior part of the left inferior frontal gyrus is involved. Anosmia may also occur as a consequence of pressure on the olfactory nerve. Precentral lesions may cause focal motor seizures or contralateral pyramidal deficits.

2. Temporal lobe lesions–These lesions may produce a variety of disturbances. Tumors of the uncinate region may be manifested by seizures with olfactory or gustatory hallucinations, motor phenomena such as licking or smacking of the lips, and some impairment of external awareness without actual loss of consciousness. Temporal lobe lesions also lead to depersonalization, emotional changes, behavioral disturbances, sensations of déjà vu or jamais vu, micropsia or macropsia, visual field defects (crossed upper quadrantanopia), and auditory illusions or hallucinations. Left-sided lesions may lead to dysnomia and receptive aphasia, while right-sided involvement sometimes disturbs the perception of musical notes and melodies.

3. Parietal lobe lesions–Tumors in this location characteristically cause contralateral disturbances of sensation and may cause sensory seizures, sensory loss or inattention, or some combination of these symptoms. The sensory loss is cortical in type and involves postural sensibility and tactile discrimination, so that the appreciation of shape, size, weight, and texture is impaired. Objects placed in the hand may not be recognized (astereognosis). Extensive parietal lobe lesions may produce contralateral hyperpathia and spontaneous pain (thalamic syndrome). Involvement of the optic radiation leads to a contralateral homonymous field defect that sometimes consists solely of lower quadrantanopia. Lesions of the left angular gyrus cause Gerstmann's syndrome (a combination of alexia, agraphia, acalculia, right-left confusion, and finger agnosia), whereas involvement of the left submarginal gyrus causes ideational apraxia. Anosognosia (the denial, neglect, or rejection of a paralyzed limb) is seen in patients with lesions of the nondominant (right) hemisphere. Constructional apraxia and dressing apraxia may also occur with right-sided lesions.

4. Occipital lobe lesions–Tumors of the occipital lobe characteristically produce crossed homonymous hemianopia or a partial field defect. With left-sided or bilateral lesions, there may be visual agnosia both for objects and for colors, while irritative lesions on either side can cause unformed visual hallucinations. Bilateral occipital lobe involvement causes cortical blindness in which there is preservation of pupillary responses to light and lack of awareness of the defect by the patient. There may also be loss of color perception, prosopagnosia (inability to identify a familiar face), simultagnosia (inability to integrate and interpret a composite scene as opposed to its individual elements), and Balint's syndrome (failure to turn the eyes to a particular point in space, despite preservation of spontaneous and reflex eye movements). The denial of blindness or a field defect constitutes Anton's syndrome.

5. Brain stem and cerebellar lesions–Brain stem lesions lead to cranial nerve palsies, ataxia, incoordination, nystagmus, and pyramidal and sensory deficits in the limbs on one or both sides. Intrinsic brain stem tumors, such as gliomas, tend to produce an increase in intracranial pressure only late in their course. Cerebellar tumors produce marked ataxia of the trunk if the vermis cerebelli is involved and ipsilateral appendicular deficits (ataxia, incoordination and hypotonia of the limbs) if the cerebellar hemispheres are affected.

6. False localizing signs–Tumors may lead to neurologic signs other than by direct compression or infiltration, thereby leading to errors of clinical localization. These false localizing signs include third or sixth nerve palsy and bilateral extensor plantar responses produced by herniation syndromes, and an extensor plantar response occurring ipsilateral to a hemispheric tumor as a result of compression of the opposite cerebral peduncle against the tentorium.

B. Imaging: CT scanning or MRI with gadolinium enhancement may detect the lesion and may also define its location, shape, and size; the extent to which normal anatomy is distorted; and the degree of any associated cerebral edema or mass effect. CT scanning is less helpful with tumors in the posterior fossa, but MRI is of particular value there. The characteristic appearance of meningiomas on CT scanning is virtually diagnostic; ie, a lesion in a typical site (parasagittal and sylvian regions, olfactory groove, sphenoidal ridge, tuberculum sellae) that appears as a homogeneous area of increased density in noncontrast CT scans and enhances uniformly with contrast.

Arteriography may show stretching or displacement of normal cerebral vessels by the tumor and the presence of tumor vascularity. The presence of an avascular mass is a nonspecific finding that could be due to tumor, hematoma, abscess, or any space-occupying lesion. In patients with normal hormone levels and an intrasellar mass, angiography is necessary to distinguish with confidence between a pituitary adenoma and an arterial aneurysm.

C. Laboratory and Other Studies: The electroencephalogram provides supporting information concerning cerebral function and may show either a focal disturbance due to the neoplasm or a more diffuse change reflecting altered mental status. Lumbar puncture is rarely necessary; the findings are seldom diagnostic, and the procedure carries the risk of causing a herniation syndrome.

Treatment

Treatment depends on the type and site of the tumor (Table 24–3) and the condition of the patient. Complete surgical removal may be possible if the tumor is extra-axial (eg, meningioma, acoustic neuroma) or is not in a critical or inaccessible region of the brain (eg, cerebellar hemangioblastoma). Surgery also permits the diagnosis to be verified and may be beneficial in reducing intracranial pressure and relieving symptoms even if the neoplasm cannot be completely removed. Clinical deficits are sometimes due in part to obstructive hydrocephalus, in which case simple surgical shunting procedures often produce dramatic benefit. In patients with malignant gliomas, radiation therapy increases median survival rates regardless of any preceding surgery, and its combination with chemotherapy provides additional benefit. Indications for irradiation in the treatment of patients with other primary intracranial neoplasms depend upon tumor type and accessibility and the feasibility of complete surgical removal. Corticosteroids help reduce cerebral edema and are usually started before surgery. Herniation is treated with intravenous dexamethasone (10–20 mg as a bolus, followed by 4 mg every 6 hours) and intravenous mannitol (20% solution given in a dose of 1.5 g/kg over about 30 minutes). Anticonvulsants are also commonly administered in standard doses (Table 24–2).

Black P McL: Brain tumors. (Two parts.) N Engl J Med 1991;324:1471, 1555. (Epidemiology, pathogenesis, clinical features, and treatment.)

Pollack IF: Brain tumors in children. N Engl J Med 1994;331:1500.

2. METASTATIC INTRACRANIAL TUMORS

Cerebral Metastases

Metastatic brain tumors present in the same way as other cerebral neoplasms, ie, with increased intracranial pressure, with focal or diffuse disturbance of cerebral function, or with both of these manifestations. Indeed, in patients with a single cerebral lesion, the metastatic nature of the lesion may only become evident on histopathologic examination. In other patients, there is evidence of widespread metastatic disease, or an isolated cerebral metastasis develops during treatment of the primary neoplasm.

The most common source of intracranial metastasis is carcinoma of the lung; other primary sites are the breast, kidney, and gastrointestinal tract. Most cerebral metastases are located supratentorially. Laboratory and radiologic studies used to evaluate patients with metastases are those described for primary neoplasms. They include MRI and CT scanning performed both with and without contrast material. Lumbar puncture is necessary only in patients with suspected carcinomatous meningitis (see below). In patients with verified cerebral metastasis from an unknown primary, investigation is guided by symptoms and signs. In women, mammography is indicated; in men under 50, germ cell origin is sought since both have therapeutic implications.

In patients with only a single cerebral metastasis who are otherwise well, it may be possible to remove the lesion and then treat with irradiation; the latter may also be selected as the sole treatment. In patients with multiple metastases or widespread systemic disease, the prognosis is gloomy, and treatment is palliative only.

Leptomeningeal Metastases (Carcinomatous Meningitis)

The neoplasms metastasizing most commonly to the leptomeninges are carcinoma of the breast, lymphomas, and leukemia. Leptomeningeal metastases lead to multifocal neurologic deficits, which may be associated with infiltration of cranial and spinal nerve roots, direct invasion of the brain or spinal cord, obstructive hydrocephalus, or some combination of these factors.

The diagnosis is confirmed by examination of the cerebrospinal fluid. Findings may include elevated cerebrospinal fluid pressure, pleocytosis, increased protein concentration, and decreased glucose concentration. Cytologic studies may indicate that malignant cells are present; if not, spinal tap should be repeated at least twice to obtain further samples for analysis.

CT scans showing contrast enhancement in the basal cisterns or showing hydrocephalus without any evidence of a mass lesion support the diagnosis. Gadolinium-enhanced MRI frequently shows enhancing foci in the leptomeninges. Myelography may show deposits on multiple nerve roots.

Treatment is by irradiation to symptomatic areas, combined with intrathecal methotrexate. The long-term prognosis is poor—only about 10% of patients survive for 1 year.

3. INTRACRANIAL MASS LESIONS IN AIDS PATIENTS

AIDS patients may present with **primary cerebral lymphoma.** This leads to disturbances in cognition or consciousness, focal motor or sensory deficits, aphasia, seizures, and cranial neuropathies. Similar clinical disturbances may result from **cerebral toxoplasmosis,** which is also a common complication in patients with AIDS. Neither CT nor MRI findings distinguish these two disorders, and serologic tests for toxoplasmosis are unreliable in AIDS patients. Accordingly, for neurologically stable patients, a trial of treatment with sulfadiazine (100 mg/kg/d up to 8 g/d in four divided doses) and pyrimethamine (75 mg/d for 3 days, then 25 mg/d) is recommended for 3 weeks; the imaging studies are then repeated, and if any lesion has improved, the antitoxoplasmosis regimen is continued indefinitely. If any lesion does not improve, cerebral biopsy is necessary. Primary cerebral lymphoma is treated with whole-brain irradiation.

Cryptococcal meningitis is also a commonly opportunistic infection in AIDS patients. Clinically, it may resemble cerebral toxoplasmosis or lymphoma, but cranial CT scans are usually normal. The diagnosis is made on the basis of cerebrospinal fluid studies, with positive India ink staining in 75–80% and cryptococcal antigen tests in 95% of cases. Treatment is with amphotericin B, sometimes accompanied by flucytosine, as set forth in Table 36–1.

Berger JR: AIDS and the nervous system. In: *Neurology and General Medicine,* 2nd ed. Aminoff MJ (editor). Churchill Livingstone, 1995. (Clinical review.)

4. PRIMARY & METASTATIC SPINAL TUMORS

Approximately 10% of spinal tumors are intramedullary. Ependymoma is the most common type of intramedullary tumor; the remainder are other types of glioma. Extramedullary tumors may be extradural or intradural in location. Among the primary extramedullary tumors, neurofibromas and meningiomas are relatively common, are benign, and may be intra- or extradural. Carcinomatous metastases, lymphomatous or leukemic deposits, and myeloma are usually extradural; in the case of metastases, the prostate, breast, lung, and kidney are common primary sites.

Tumors may lead to spinal cord dysfunction by direct compression, by ischemia secondary to arterial or venous obstruction, and, in the case of intramedullary lesions, by invasive infiltration.

Clinical Findings

A. Symptoms and Signs: Symptoms usually develop insidiously. Pain is often conspicuous with extradural lesions; is characteristically aggravated by coughing or straining; may be radicular, localized to the back, or felt diffusely in an extremity; and may be accompanied by motor deficits, paresthesias, or numbness, especially in the legs. When sphincter disturbances occur, they are usually particularly disabling. Pain, however, often precedes specific neurologic symptoms from epidural metastases.

Examination may reveal localized spinal tenderness. A segmental lower motor neuron deficit or dermatomal sensory changes (or both) are sometimes found at the level of the lesion, while an upper motor neuron deficit and sensory disturbance are found below it.

B. Imaging: Findings on plain radiography of the spine may be normal but are commonly abnormal when there are metastatic deposits. CT myelography or MRI may be necessary to identify and localize the site of cord compression. The combination of known tumor elsewhere in the body, back pain, and either abnormal plain films of the spine or neurologic signs

of cord compression is an indication to perform these studies on an urgent basis. Some clinicians proceed to myelography based solely on new back pain in a cancer patient. If a complete block is present at lumbar myelography, a cisternal myelogram is performed to determine the upper level of the block and to investigate the possibility of block higher in the cord.

C. Laboratory Findings: The cerebrospinal fluid removed at myelography is often xanthochromic and contains a greatly increased protein concentration with normal cell content and glucose concentration.

Treatment

Intramedullary tumors are treated by decompression and surgical excision (when feasible) and by irradiation. The prognosis depends upon the cause and severity of cord compression before it is relieved.

Treatment of epidural spinal metastases consists of irradiation, irrespective of cell type. Dexamethasone is also given in a high dosage (eg, 25 mg four times daily for 3 days, followed by rapid tapering of the dosage, depending on response) to reduce cord swelling and relieve pain. Surgical decompression is reserved for patients with tumors that are unresponsive to irradiation or have previously been irradiated and for cases in which there is some uncertainty about the diagnosis. The long-term outlook is poor, but radiation treatment may at least delay the onset of major disability.

Sze G: Magnetic resonance imaging in the evaluation of spinal tumors. Cancer 1991;67:1229. (Role of CT scans and MRI.)

5. BRAIN ABSCESS

Cerebral abscess presents as an intracranial space-occupying lesion and arises as a sequela of disease of the ear or nose, may be a complication of infection elsewhere in the body, or may result from infection introduced intracranially by trauma or surgical procedures. The most common infective organisms are streptococci, staphylococci, and anaerobes; mixed infections are not uncommon. Headache, drowsiness, inattention, confusion, and seizures are early symptoms, followed by signs of increasing intracranial pressure and then a focal neurologic deficit. There may be little or no systemic evidence of infection.

A CT scan of the head characteristically shows an area of contrast enhancement surrounding a low-density core. Similar abnormalities may be found in patients with metastatic neoplasms. MRI findings often permit earlier recognition of focal cerebritis or an abscess. Arteriography indicates the presence of a space-occupying lesion, which appears as an avascular mass with displacement of normal cerebral vessels, but this procedure provides no clue to the nature of the lesion.

Treatment consists of intravenous antibiotics, combined with surgical drainage (aspiration or excision) if necessary to reduce the mass effect, or sometimes to establish the diagnosis. Abscesses smaller than 2 cm can often be cured medically. Broad-spectrum antibiotics are used if the infecting organism is unknown. In adults, a common regimen is penicillin G (2 million units every 2 hours intravenously) plus either chloramphenicol (1–2 g intravenously every 6 hours), metronidazole (750 mg intravenously every 6 hours), or both. Nafcillin is added if *Staphylococcus aureus* infection is suspected. Dexamethasone (4–25 mg four times daily, depending on severity, followed by tapering of dose, depending on response) may reduce any associated edema.

Pons V: Acute bacterial infections of the central nervous system. In: *Neurology and General Medicine,* 2nd ed. Aminoff MJ (editor). Churchill Livingstone, 1995.

NONMETASTATIC NEUROLOGIC COMPLICATIONS OF MALIGNANT DISEASE

A variety of nonmetastatic neurologic complications of malignant disease can be recognized:

(1) Metabolic encephalopathy due to electrolyte abnormalities, infections, drug overdose, or the failure of some vital organ may be reflected by drowsiness, lethargy, restlessness, insomnia, agitation, confusion, stupor, or coma. The mental changes are usually associated with tremor, asterixis, and multifocal myoclonus. The electroencephalogram is generally diffusely slowed. Laboratory studies are necessary to detect the cause of the encephalopathy, which must then be treated appropriately.

(2) Immune suppression resulting from either the malignant disease or its treatment (eg, by chemotherapy) predisposes patients to brain abscess, progressive multifocal leukoencephalopathy, meningitis, herpes zoster infection, and other opportunistic infectious diseases. Moreover, an overt or occult cerebrospinal fluid fistula, as occurs with some tumors, may also increase the risk of infection. CT scanning aids in the early recognition of a brain abscess, but metastatic brain tumors may have a similar appearance. Examination of the cerebrospinal fluid is essential in the evaluation of patients with meningitis but is of no help in the diagnosis of brain abscess. Treatment should be specific for the infective organism.

(3) Cerebrovascular disorders that cause neurologic complications in patients with systemic cancer include nonbacterial thrombotic endocarditis and septic embolization. Cerebral, subarachnoid, or subdural hemorrhages may occur in patients with myelogenous leukemia and may be found in association with metastatic tumors, especially malignant melanoma. Spinal subdural hemorrhage sometimes occurs after lumbar puncture in patients with marked thrombocytopenia.

Disseminated intravascular coagulation occurs most commonly in patients with acute promyelocytic leukemia or with some adenocarcinomas and is characterized by a fluctuating encephalopathy, often with associated seizures, that frequently progresses to coma or death. There may be few accompanying neurologic signs.

Venous sinus thrombosis, which usually presents with convulsions and headaches, may also occur in patients with leukemia or lymphoma. Examination commonly reveals papilledema and focal or diffuse neurologic signs. Anticonvulsants, anticoagulants, and drugs to lower the intracranial pressure may be of value.

(4) Paraneoplastic cerebellar degeneration occurs most commonly in association with carcinoma of the lung. Symptoms may precede those due to the neoplasm itself, which may be undetected for several months or even longer. Typically, there is a pancerebellar syndrome causing dysarthria, nystagmus, and ataxia of the trunk and limbs. The disorder probably has an autoimmune basis. Treatment is of the underlying malignant disease.

(5) Encephalopathy, characterized by impaired recent memory, disturbed affect, hallucinations, and seizures, occurs in some patients with carcinomas. The cerebrospinal fluid is often abnormal. EEGs may show diffuse slow-wave activity, especially over the temporal regions. Pathologic changes are most marked in the inferomedian portions of the temporal lobes. There is no specific treatment.

(6) Malignant disease may be associated with sensorimotor polyneuropathy and less commonly with pure sensory neuropathy (ie, dorsal root ganglionitis) or autonomic neuropathy. A subacute motor neuronopathy may be associated with lymphomas.

(7) Dermatomyositis or a myasthenic syndrome may be seen in patients with underlying carcinoma (see Chapter 20). The myasthenic syndrome may have an autoimmune basis and differs clinically from myasthenia gravis.

Posner JB: Paraneoplastic syndromes involving the nervous system. In: *Neurology and General Medicine,* 2nd ed. Aminoff MJ (editor). Churchill Livingstone, 1995.

PSEUDOTUMOR CEREBRI (Benign Intracranial Hypertension)

Symptoms of pseudotumor cerebri consist of headache, diplopia, and other visual disturbances due to papilledema and abducens nerve dysfunction. Examination reveals the papilledema and some enlargement of the blind spots, but patients otherwise look well. Investigations reveal no evidence of a space-occupying lesion, and the CT scan shows small or normal ventricles. Lumbar puncture confirms the presence of intracranial hypertension, but the cerebrospinal fluid is normal.

There are many causes of pseudotumor cerebri. Thrombosis of the transverse venous sinus as a noninfectious complication of otitis media or chronic mastoiditis is one cause, and sagittal sinus thrombosis may lead to a clinically similar picture. MR venography is helpful in screening for these disorders. Other causes include chronic pulmonary disease, endocrine disturbances such as hypoparathyroidism or Addison's disease, vitamin A toxicity, and the use of tetracycline or oral contraceptives. Cases have also followed withdrawal of corticosteroids after long-term use. In many instances, however, no specific cause can be found, and the disorder remits spontaneously after several months.

Untreated pseudotumor cerebri leads to secondary optic atrophy and permanent visual loss. Repeated lumbar puncture to lower the intracranial pressure by removal of cerebrospinal fluid is effective, but pharmacologic approaches to treatment are now more satisfactory. Acetazolamide (250 mg orally three times daily) reduces formation of cerebrospinal fluid and can be used to start treatment. Oral corticosteroids (eg, prednisone, 60–80 mg daily) may also be necessary. Obese patients should be advised to lose weight. Treatment is monitored by checking visual acuity and visual fields, funduscopic appearance, and pressure of the cerebrospinal fluid.

If medical treatment fails to control the intracranial pressure, surgical placement of a lumboperitoneal or other shunt—or optic nerve sheath fenestration—should be undertaken to preserve vision.

In addition to the above measures, any specific cause of pseudotumor cerebri requires appropriate treatment. Thus, hormone therapy should be initiated if there is an underlying endocrine disturbance. Discontinuing the use of tetracycline, oral contraceptives, or vitamin A will allow for resolution of pseudotumor cerebri due to these agents. If corticosteroid withdrawal is responsible, the medication should be reintroduced and then tapered more gradually.

Radhakrishnan K et al: Idiopathic intracranial hypertension. Mayo Clin Proc 1994;69:169. (Epidemiology, clinical features, pathophysiology, and treatment.)

SELECTED NEUROCUTANEOUS DISEASES

Tuberous Sclerosis

Tuberous sclerosis may occur sporadically or on a familial basis with autosomal dominant inheritance. The responsible gene is located on the long arm of chromosome 9 in at least some cases. Its pathogenesis is unknown. Neurologic presentation is with seizures and progressive psychomotor retardation beginning in early childhood. The cutaneous abnormality, adenoma sebaceum, becomes manifest usually between 5 and 10 years of age and typically consists of reddened nodules on the face (cheeks, nasolabial folds, sides of the nose, and chin) and sometimes on the forehead and neck. Other typical cutaneous lesions include subungual fibromas, shagreen patches (leathery plaques of subepidermal fibrosis, situated usually on the trunk), and leaf-shaped hypopigmented spots. Associated abnormalities include retinal lesions and tumors, benign rhabdomyomas of the heart, lung cysts, benign tumors in the viscera, and bone cysts.

The disease is slowly progressive and leads to increasing mental deterioration. There is no specific treatment, but anticonvulsant drugs may help in controlling seizures.

Neurofibromatosis

Neurofibromatosis may occur either sporadically or on a familial basis with autosomal dominant inheritance. Two distinct forms are recognized: Type 1 (**Recklinghausen's disease**) is characterized by multiple hyperpigmented macules and neurofibromas and type 2 by **eighth nerve tumors,** often accompanied by other intracranial or intraspinal tumors. Among familial cases, the gene for type 1 is located on chromosome 17 and that for type 2 on chromosome 22.

Neurologic presentation is usually with symptoms and signs of tumor. Multiple neurofibromas characteristically are present and may involve spinal or cranial nerves, especially the eighth nerve. Examination of the superficial cutaneous nerves usually reveals palpable mobile nodules. In some cases, there is an associated marked overgrowth of subcutaneous tissues (plexiform neuromas), sometimes with an underlying bony abnormality. Associated cutaneous lesions include axillary freckling and patches of cutaneous pigmentation (café au lait spots). Malignant degeneration of neurofibromas occasionally occurs and may lead to peripheral sarcomas. Meningiomas, gliomas (especially optic nerve gliomas), bone cysts, pheochromocytomas, scoliosis, and obstructive hydrocephalus may also occur.

It may be possible to correct disfigurement by plastic surgery. Intraspinal or intracranial tumors and tumors of peripheral nerves should be treated surgically if they are producing symptoms.

Berg BO: Neurocutaneous syndromes. In: *Neurology and General Medicine,* 2nd ed. Aminoff MJ (editor). Churchill Livingstone, 1995. (Clinical review.)

Sturge-Weber Syndrome

Sturge-Weber syndrome consists of a congenital, usually unilateral, cutaneous capillary angioma involving the upper face, leptomeningeal angiomatosis, and, in many patients, choroidal angioma. It has no sex predilection and usually occurs sporadically. The cutaneous angioma sometimes has a more extensive distribution over the head and neck and is often quite disfiguring, especially if there is associated overgrowth of connective tissue. Focal or generalized seizures are the usual neurologic presentation and may commence at any age. There may be contralateral homonymous hemianopia, hemiparesis and hemisensory disturbance, ipsilateral glaucoma, and mental subnormality. Skull x-rays taken after the first 2 years of life usually reveal gyriform ("tramline") intracranial calcification, especially in the parieto-occipital region, due to mineral deposition in the cortex beneath the intracranial angioma.

Treatment is aimed at controlling seizures pharmacologically. Ophthalmologic advice should be sought concerning the management of choroidal angioma and of increased intraocular pressure.

MOVEMENT DISORDERS

1. BENIGN ESSENTIAL (FAMILIAL) TREMOR

The cause of benign essential tremor is uncertain, but it is sometimes inherited in an autosomal dominant manner. Tremor may begin at any age and is enhanced by emotional stress. The tremor usually involves one or both hands, the head, or the hands and head, while the legs tend to be spared. Examination reveals no other abnormalities. Ingestion of a small quantity of alcohol commonly provides remarkable but short-lived relief by an unknown mechanism.

Although the tremor may become more conspicuous with time, it generally leads to little disability, and treatment is often unnecessary. Occasionally, it interferes with manual skills and leads to impairment of handwriting. Speech may also be affected if the laryngeal muscles are involved. In such circumstances, propranolol may be helpful but will need to be continued indefinitely in daily doses of 60–240 mg. However, intermittent therapy is sometimes useful in patients whose tremor becomes exacerbated in specific predictable situations. Primidone may be helpful when propranolol is ineffective, but patients with essential tremor are often very sensitive to it. They are therefore started on 50 mg daily, and the daily dose is increased by 50 mg every 2 weeks depending on the response; a maintenance dose of 125 mg three times daily is commonly effective. Occasional patients fail to respond to these measures but are helped by alprazolam (up to 3 mg daily in divided doses).

2. PARKINSONISM

Essentials of Diagnosis

- Any combination of tremor, rigidity, bradykinesia, progressive postural instability.
- Seborrhea of skin quite common.
- Mild intellectual deterioration is often observed.

General Considerations

Parkinsonism is a relatively common disorder that occurs in all ethnic groups, with an approximately equal sex distribution. The most common variety, idiopathic Parkinson's disease (paralysis agitans), begins most often between 45 and 65 years of age.

Etiology

Postencephalitic parkinsonism is becoming increasingly more rare. Exposure to certain toxins (eg, manganese dust, carbon disulfide) and severe carbon monoxide poisoning may lead to parkinsonism. Typical parkinsonism has occurred in individuals who have taken 1-methyl-4-phenyl-1,2,5,6-tetrahydropyridine (MPTP) for recreational purposes. This compound is converted in the body to a neurotoxin that selectively destroys dopaminergic neurons in the substantia nigra. Reversible parkinsonism may develop in patients receiving neuroleptic drugs (see Chapter 25) and has also been caused by reserpine and metoclopramide. Only rarely is hemiparkinsonism the presenting feature of a brain tumor or some other progressive space-occupying lesion.

In idiopathic parkinsonism, dopamine depletion due to degeneration of the dopaminergic nigrostriatal system leads to an imbalance of dopamine and acetylcholine, which are neurotransmitters normally present in the corpus striatum. Treatment is directed at redressing this imbalance by blocking the effect of acetylcholine with anticholinergic drugs or by the administration of levodopa, the precursor of dopamine.

Clinical Findings

Tremor, rigidity, bradykinesia, and postural instability are the cardinal features of parkinsonism and may be present in any combination. There may also be a mild decline in intellectual function. The tremor of about four to six cycles per second is most conspicuous at rest, is enhanced by emotional stress, and is often less severe during voluntary activity. Although it may ultimately be present in all limbs, the tremor is commonly confined to one limb or to the limbs on one side for months or years before it becomes more generalized. In some patients, tremor is absent.

Rigidity (an increase in resistance to passive movement) is responsible for the characteristically flexed posture seen in many patients, but the most disabling symptoms of parkinsonism are due to bradykinesia, manifested as a slowness of voluntary movement and a reduction in automatic movements such as swinging of the arms while walking. Curiously, however, effective voluntary activity may briefly be regained during an emergency (eg, the patient is able to leap aside to avoid an oncoming motor vehicle).

Clinical diagnosis of the well-developed syndrome is usually simple. The patient has a relatively immobile face with widened palpebral fissures, infrequent blinking, and a certain fixity of facial expression. Seborrhea of the scalp and face is common. There is often mild blepharoclonus, and a tremor may be present about the mouth and lips. Repetitive tapping (about twice per second) over the bridge of the nose produces a sustained blink response (Myerson's sign). Other findings may include saliva drooling from the mouth, perhaps due to impairment of swallowing; soft and poorly modulated voice; a variable rest tremor and rigidity in some or all of the limbs; slowness of voluntary movements; impairment of fine or rapidly alternating movements; and micrographia. There is typically no muscle weakness (provided that sufficient time is allowed for power to be developed) and no alteration in the tendon reflexes or plantar responses. It is difficult for the patient to arise from a sitting position and begin walking. The gait itself is characterized by small shuffling steps and a loss of the normal automatic arm swing; there may be unsteadiness on turning, difficulty in stopping, and a tendency to fall.

Differential Diagnosis

Diagnostic problems may occur in mild cases, especially if tremor is minimal or absent. For example, mild hypokinesia or slight tremor is commonly attributed to old age. Depression, with its associated expressionless face, poorly modulated voice, and reduction in voluntary activity, can be difficult to distinguish from mild parkinsonism, especially since the two disorders may coexist; in some cases, a trial of antidepressant drug therapy may be necessary. The family history, the character of the tremor, and lack of other neurologic signs should distinguish essential tremor from parkinsonism. Wilson's disease can be distinguished by its early age at onset, the presence of other abnormal movements, Kayser-Fleischer rings, and chronic hepatitis, and by increased concentrations of copper in the tissues. Huntington's disease presenting with rigidity and bradykinesia may be mistaken for parkinsonism unless the family history and accompanying dementia are recognized. In Shy-Drager syndrome, the clinical features of parkinsonism are accompanied by autonomic insufficiency (leading to postural hypotension, anhidrosis, disturbances of sphincter control, impotence, etc) and more widespread neurologic deficits (pyramidal, lower motor neuron, or cerebellar signs). In progressive supranuclear palsy, bradykinesia and rigidity are accompanied by a supranuclear disorder of eye movements, pseudobulbar palsy, and axial dystonia. Creutzfeldt-Jakob disease may be accompanied by features of parkinsonism, but dementia is usual, myoclonic jerking is common, ataxia and pyramidal signs may be conspicuous, and the electroencephalographic findings are usually characteristic. In cortical-basal ganglionic degeneration, parkinsonism is accompanied by conspicuous signs of cortical dysfunction (eg, apraxia, sensory inattention, dementia, aphasia).

Treatment

A. Medical Measures: Drug treatment is not required early in the course of parkinsonism, but the nature of the disorder and the availability of medical treatment for use when necessary should be discussed with the patient.

1. Amantadine–Patients with mild symptoms but no disability may be helped by amantadine. This drug improves all of the clinical features of parkinsonism, but its mode of action is unclear. Side effects include restlessness, confusion, depression, skin rashes, edema, nausea, constipation, anorexia, postural hypotension, and disturbances of cardiac rhythm. However, these are relatively uncommon with the usual dose (100 mg twice daily).

2. Anticholinergic drugs–Anticholinergics are more helpful in alleviating tremor and rigidity than bradykinesia. Treatment is started with a small dose (Table 24–4) and gradually increased until benefit occurs or side effects limit further increments. If treatment is ineffective, the drug is gradually withdrawn and another preparation then tried.

Common side effects include dryness of the mouth, nausea, constipation, palpitations, cardiac arrhythmias, urinary retention, confusion, agitation, restlessness, drowsiness, mydriasis, increased intraocular pressure, and defective accommodation.

Anticholinergic drugs are contraindicated in patients with prostatic hypertrophy, narrow-angle glaucoma, or obstructive gastrointestinal disease and are often tolerated poorly by the elderly.

3. Levodopa–Levodopa, which is converted in the body to dopamine, improves all of the major features of parkinsonism, including bradykinesia, but does not stop progression of the disorder. The commonest early side effects of levodopa are nausea, vomiting, and hypotension, but cardiac arrhythmias may also occur. Dyskinesias, restlessness, confusion,

Table 24–4. Some anticholinergic antiparkinsonian drugs.[1]

Drug	Usual Daily Dose (mg)
Benztropine mesylate (Cogentin)	1–6
Biperiden (Akineton)	2–12
Chlorphenoxamine (Phenoxene)	150–400
Cycrimine (Pagitane)	5–20
Orphenadrine (Disipal, Norflex)	150–400
Procyclidine (Kemadrin)	7.5–30
Trihexyphenidyl (Artane)	6–20

[1]Modified, with permission, from Aminoff MJ: Pharmacologic management of parkinsonism and other movement disorders. In: *Basic & Clinical Pharmacology*, 6th ed. Katzung BG (editor). Appleton & Lange, 1994.

and other behavioral changes tend to occur somewhat later and become more common with time. Levodopa-induced dyskinesias may take any conceivable form, including chorea, athetosis, dystonia, tremor, tics, and myoclonus. An even later complication is the "on-off phenomenon," in which abrupt but transient fluctuations in the severity of parkinsonism occur unpredictably but frequently during the day. The "off" period of marked bradykinesia has been shown to relate in some instances to falling plasma levels of levodopa. During the "on" phase, dyskinesias are often conspicuous but mobility is increased.

Carbidopa, which inhibits the enzyme responsible for the breakdown of levodopa to dopamine, does not cross the blood-brain barrier. When levodopa is given in combination with carbidopa, the extracerebral breakdown of levodopa is diminished. This reduces the amount of levodopa required daily for beneficial effects, and it lowers the incidence of nausea, vomiting, hypotension, and cardiac irregularities. Such a combination does not prevent the development of the "on-off phenomenon," and the incidence of other side effects (dyskinesias or psychiatric complications) may actually be increased.

Sinemet, a commercially available preparation that contains carbidopa and levodopa in a fixed ratio (1:10 or 1:4), is generally used. Treatment is started with a small dose—eg, one tablet of Sinemet 25/100 (containing 25 mg of carbidopa and 100 mg of levodopa) three times daily—and gradually increased depending on the response. Sinemet CR is a controlled-release formulation (containing 50 mg of carbidopa and 200 mg of levodopa). It is sometimes helpful in reducing fluctuations in clinical response to treatment and in reducing the frequency with which medication must be taken. Response fluctuations are also reduced by keeping the daily intake of protein at the recommended minimum and taking the main protein meal as the last meal of the day.

The dyskinesias and behavioral side effects of levodopa are dose-related, but reduction in dose may eliminate any therapeutic benefit.

Levodopa therapy is contraindicated in patients with psychotic illness or narrow-angle glaucoma. It should not be given to patients taking monoamine oxidase A inhibitors or within 2 weeks of their withdrawal, because hypertensive crises may result. Levodopa should be used with care in patients with suspected malignant melanomas or with active peptic ulcers.

4. Dopamine agonists–Dopamine agonists act directly on dopamine receptors, and their use in parkinsonism is associated with a lower incidence of the response fluctuations and dyskinesias that occur with long-term levodopa therapy. They were previously reserved for patients who had either become refractory to levodopa or developed the "on-off phenomenon." However, they are now best given with a low dose of Sinemet 25/100 (carbidopa 25 mg and

levodopa 100 mg), one tablet three times daily when dopaminergic therapy is first introduced; the dose of Sinemet is kept constant, while the dose of the agonist is gradually increased. The two most widely used agonists are bromocriptine and pergolide, which are equally effective. The initial dosage of bromocriptine is 1.25 mg twice daily; this is increased by 2.5 mg at 2-week intervals until benefit occurs or side effects limit further increments. The usual daily maintenance dose in patients with parkinsonism is between 10 and 30 mg. Pergolide is similarly started in a low dose (eg, 0.05 mg daily) and built up gradually depending on the response and tolerance.

Side effects include anorexia, nausea, vomiting, constipation, postural hypotension, digital vasospasm, cardiac arrhythmias, various dyskinesias and mental disturbances, headache, nasal congestion, erythromelalgia, and pulmonary infiltrates.

Bromocriptine and pergolide are contraindicated in patients with a history of mental illness or recent myocardial infarction and are probably best avoided in those with peripheral vascular disease or peptic ulcers (as bleeding from the latter has been reported).

Pramipexole and ropinirole are two new dopamine agonists that will become available in the USA in 1997. They are more selective, have fewer side effects, and may produce a longer-lasting therapeutic response than existing agonists.

5. Selegiline–Selegiline is a monoamine oxidase B inhibitor that is sometimes used as adjunctive treatment for parkinsonism in patients receiving levodopa. By inhibiting the metabolic breakdown of dopamine, selegiline has been used to improve fluctuations or declining response to levodopa. In general, however, the response to treatment with it has been disappointing. The drug is taken in a standard dose of 5 mg with breakfast and 5 mg with lunch. It may increase any adverse effects of levodopa.

There are reasons to believe that selegiline may arrest the progression of Parkinson's disease. Studies have failed to establish this conclusively, but this remains an important consideration for patients who are young or have mild disease.

B. General Measures: Physical therapy or speech therapy helps many patients. The quality of life can often be improved by the provision of simple aids to daily living, eg, rails or banisters placed strategically about the home, special table cutlery with large handles, nonslip rubber table mats, and devices to amplify the voice.

C. Surgical Measures: Thalamotomy or pallidotomy may be helpful for patients who become unresponsive to medical treatment or have intolerable side effects from antiparkinsonian agents, especially if they have no evidence of diffuse vascular disease. Surgical implantation of adrenal medullary or fetal substantia nigra tissue into the caudate nucleus has recently been reported to benefit some patients, but other investigators have failed to substantiate such claims or have found only modest benefits, and the procedure is still being evaluated.

Aminoff MJ: Treatment of Parkinson's disease. West J Med 1994;161:303. (Clinical review.)

Jenner P et al: New insights into the cause of Parkinson's disease. Neurology 1992;42:2241.

Koller WC et al: An algorithm for the management of Parkinson's disease. Neurology 1994;44:Supplement 10.

Montrastruc JL et al: New directions in the drug treatment of Parkinson's disease. Drugs Aging 1996;9:169.

Quinn N: Drug treatment of Parkinson's disease. Br Med J 1995;310:575.

3. HUNTINGTON'S DISEASE

Essentials of Diagnosis

- Gradual onset and progression of chorea and dementia.
- Family history of the disorder.
- Responsible gene identified on chromosome 4.

General Considerations

Huntington's disease is characterized by chorea and dementia. It is inherited in an autosomal dominant manner and occurs throughout the world, in all ethnic groups, with a prevalence rate of about 5 per 100,000. The gene responsible for the disease has been located on the short arm of chromosome No. 4. At 4p16.3 there is an expanded and unstable CAG trinucleotide repeat. Symptoms do not usually develop until after 30 years of age, by which time the patient has usually had children, and so the disease continues from one generation to the next. The cause of Huntington's disease is unknown.

Clinical Findings

Clinical onset is usually between 30 and 50 years of age. The disease is progressive and usually leads to a fatal outcome within 15–20 years. The initial symptoms may consist of either abnormal movements or intellectual changes, but ultimately both occur. The earliest mental changes are often behavioral, with irritability, moodiness, antisocial behavior, or a psychiatric disturbance, but a more obvious dementia subsequently develops. The dyskinesia may initially be no more than an apparent fidgetiness or restlessness, but eventually choreiform movements and some dystonic posturing occur. Progressive rigidity and akinesia (rather than chorea) sometimes occur in association with dementia, especially in cases with childhood onset. CT scanning usually demonstrates cerebral atrophy and atrophy of the caudate nucleus in established cases. MRI and positron emission tomography (PET) have shown reduced glucose utilization in an anatomically normal caudate nucleus.

Chorea developing with no family history of choreoathetosis should not be attributed to Huntington's disease, at least not until other causes of chorea have been excluded clinically and by appropriate laboratory studies. In younger patients, self-limiting Sydenham's chorea develops after group A streptococcal infections on rare occasions. If a patient presents solely with progressive intellectual failure, it may not be possible to distinguish Huntington's disease from other causes of dementia unless there is a characteristic family history or a dyskinesia develops.

Treatment

There is no cure for Huntington's disease, progression cannot be halted, and treatment is purely symptomatic. The reported biochemical changes suggest a relative underactivity of neurons containing gamma-aminobutyric acid (GABA) and acetylcholine or a relative overactivity of dopaminergic neurons. Treatment with drugs blocking dopamine receptors, such as phenothiazines or haloperidol, may control the dyskinesia and any behavioral disturbances. Haloperidol treatment is usually begun with a dose of 1 mg once or twice daily, which is then increased every 3 or 4 days depending on the response. Tetrabenazine, a drug that depletes central monoamines, is widely used in Europe to treat dyskinesia but is not available in the USA. Reserpine is similar in its actions to tetrabenazine and may be helpful; the daily dose is built up gradually to between 2 and 5 mg, depending on the response. Behavioral disturbances may respond to clozapine. Attempts to compensate for the relative GABA deficiency by enhancing central GABA activity or to compensate for the relative cholinergic underactivity by giving choline chloride have not been therapeutically helpful. High levels of somatostatin (a neuropeptide) have recently been reported in certain areas of the brain in patients with Huntington's disease, and the therapeutic response to cysteamine (a selective depleter of somatostatin in the brain) is currently under study.

Offspring should be offered genetic counseling. Now that the gene responsible for the disorder has been isolated, an accurate and specific test for the presymptomatic detection and definitive diagnosis of Huntington's disease has become more widely available.

Furtado S, Suchowersky O: Huntington's disease: Recent advances in diagnosis and management. Can J Neurol Sci 1995;22:5.

4. IDIOPATHIC TORSION DYSTONIA

Essentials of Diagnosis

- Dystonic movements and postures.
- Normal birth and developmental history. No other neurologic signs.
- Investigations (including CT scan) reveal no cause of dystonia.

General Considerations

Idiopathic torsion dystonia may occur sporadically or on a hereditary basis, with autosomal dominant, autosomal recessive, and X-linked recessive modes of transmission. The responsible gene has been localized to the long arm of chromosome 9 in the dominantly inherited disorder and to the long arm of the X chromosome in the X-linked recessive form; the responsible gene in the autosomal recessive disorder is unknown. Symptoms may begin in childhood or later and persists throughout life.

Clinical Findings

The disorder is characterized by the onset of abnormal movements and postures in a patient with a normal birth and developmental history, no relevant past medical illness, and no other neurologic signs. Investigations (including CT scan) reveal no cause for the abnormal movements. Dystonic movements of the head and neck may take the form of torticollis, blepharospasm, facial grimacing, or forced opening or closing of the mouth. The limbs may also adopt abnormal but characteristic postures. The age at onset influences both the clinical findings and the prognosis. With onset in childhood, there is usually a family history of the disorder, symptoms commonly commence in the legs, and progression is likely until there is severe disability from generalized dystonia. In contrast, when onset is later, a positive family history is unlikely, initial symptoms are often in the arms or axial structures, and severe disability does not usually occur, although generalized dystonia may ultimately develop in some patients. If all cases are considered together, about one-third of patients eventually become so severely disabled that they are confined to chair or bed, while another one-third are affected only mildly.

Before a diagnosis of idiopathic torsion dystonia is made, it is imperative to exclude other causes of dystonia. For example, perinatal anoxia, birth trauma, and kernicterus are common causes of dystonia, but abnormal movements usually then develop before the age of 5, the early development of the patient is usually abnormal, and a history of seizures is not unusual. Moreover, examination may reveal signs of mental retardation or pyramidal deficit in addition to the movement disorder. Dystonic posturing may also occur in Wilson's disease, Huntington's disease, or parkinsonism; as a sequela of encephalitis lethargica or previous neuroleptic drug therapy; and in certain other disorders. In these cases, diagnosis is based on the history and accompanying clinical manifestations.

Treatment

Idiopathic torsion dystonia usually responds poorly to drugs. Levodopa, diazepam, baclofen, carbamazepine, amantadine, or anticholinergic medication (in high dosage) is occasionally helpful; if not, a trial of treatment with phenothiazines or haloperidol may be worthwhile. In each case, the dose has to be individualized, depending on response and tolerance. However, the doses of these latter drugs that are required for benefit lead usually to mild parkinsonism. Stereotactic thalamotomy is sometimes helpful in patients with predominantly unilateral dystonia, especially when this involves the limbs.

Tsui JKC, Calne DB: *Handbook of Dystonia.* Marcel Dekker, 1995.

5. FOCAL TORSION DYSTONIA

A number of the dystonic manifestations that occur in idiopathic torsion dystonia may also occur as isolated phenomena. They are best regarded as focal dystonias that either occur as formes frustes of idiopathic torsion dystonia in patients with a positive family history or represent a focal manifestation of the adult-onset form of that disorder when there is no family history. Medical treatment is generally unsatisfactory. A trial of the drugs used in idiopathic torsion dystonia is worthwhile, however, since a few patients do show some response. In addition, with restricted dystonias such as blepharospasm or torticollis, local injection of botulinum A toxin into the overactive muscles may produce worthwhile benefit for several weeks or months and can be repeated as needed.

Both blepharospasm and oromandibular dystonia may occur as an isolated focal dystonia. The former is characterized by spontaneous involuntary forced closure of the eyelids for a variable interval. Oromandibular dystonia is manifested by involuntary contraction of the muscles about the mouth causing, for example, involuntary opening or closing of the mouth, roving or protruding tongue movements, and retraction of the platysma.

Spasmodic torticollis, usually with onset between 25 and 50 years of age, is characterized by a tendency for the neck to twist to one side. This initially occurs episodically, but eventually the neck is held to the side. Spontaneous resolution may occur in the first year or so. The disorder is otherwise usually lifelong. Selective section of the spinal accessory nerve and the upper cervical nerve roots is sometimes helpful if medical treatment is unsuccessful. Local injection of botulinum A toxin provides benefit in most cases.

Writer's cramp is characterized by dystonic posturing of the hand and forearm when the hand is used for writing and sometimes when it is used for other tasks, eg, playing the piano, using a screwdriver or eating utensils. Drug treatment is usually unrewarding, and patients are often best advised to learn to use the other hand for activities requiring manual dexterity. Injections of botulinum A toxin are helpful in some instances.

Yoshimura DM et al: Botulinum toxin therapy for limb dystonias. Neurology 1992;42:627.

6. MYOCLONUS

Occasional myoclonic jerks may occur in anyone, especially when drifting into sleep. General or multifocal myoclonus is common in patients with idiopathic epilepsy and is especially prominent in certain hereditary disorders characterized by seizures and progressive intellectual decline, such as the lipid storage diseases. It is also a feature of various rare degenerative disorders, notably Ramsay Hunt syndrome, and is common in subacute sclerosing panencephalitis and Creutzfeldt-Jakob disease. Generalized myoclonic jerking may accompany uremic and other metabolic encephalopathies, result from levodopa therapy, occur in alcohol or drug withdrawal states, or follow anoxic brain damage. It also occurs on a hereditary or sporadic basis as an isolated phenomenon in otherwise healthy subjects.

Segmental myoclonus is a rare manifestation of a focal spinal cord lesion. It may also be the clinical expression of **epilepsia partialis continua,** a disorder in which a repetitive focal epileptic discharge arises in the contralateral sensorimotor cortex, sometimes from an underlying structural lesion. An electroencephalogram is often helpful in clarifying the epileptic nature of the disorder, and CT or MRI scan may reveal the causal lesion.

Myoclonus may respond to certain anticonvulsant drugs, especially valproic acid, or to one of the benzodiazepines, particularly clonazepam (Table 24–2). It may also respond to piracetam (up to 16.8 g daily). Myoclonus following anoxic brain damage is often responsive to oxitriptan (5-hydroxytryptophan), an investigational agent that is the precursor of serotonin, and sometimes to clonazepam. Oxitriptan is given in gradually increasing doses up to 1–1.5 mg daily. In patients with segmental myoclonus, a localized lesion should be searched for and treated appropriately.

Brown P et al: Effectiveness of piracetam in cortical myoclonus. Mov Disord 1993;8:63. (Clinical trial.)

7. WILSON'S DISEASE

In this metabolic disorder, abnormal movement and posture may occur with or without coexisting signs of liver involvement. It is discussed in Chapter 15.

8. DRUG-INDUCED ABNORMAL MOVEMENTS

Phenothiazines and butyrophenones may produce a wide variety of abnormal movements, including parkinsonism, akathisia (ie, motor restlessness), acute dystonia, chorea, and tardive dyskinesia. These complications are discussed in Chapter 25. Chorea may also develop in patients receiving levodopa, bromocriptine, anticholinergic drugs, phenytoin, carbamazepine, lithium, amphetamines, or oral contraceptives, and it resolves with withdrawal of the offending substance. Similarly, dystonia may be produced by levodopa, bromocriptine, lithium, metoclopramide, or carbamazepine; and parkinsonism by reserpine, tetrabenazine, and metoclopramide. Postural tremor may occur with a variety of drugs, including epinephrine, isoproterenol, theophylline, caffeine, lithium, thyroid hormone, tricyclic antidepressants, and valproic acid.

9. GILLES DE LA TOURETTE'S SYNDROME

Essentials of Diagnosis

- Multiple motor and phonic tics.
- Symptoms begin before age 21 years.
- Tics occur frequently for at least 1 year.
- Tics vary in number, frequency, and nature over time.

Clinical Findings

Motor tics are the initial manifestation in 80% of cases and most commonly involve the face whereas in the remaining 20%, the initial symptoms are phonic tics; all patients ultimately develop a combination of different motor and phonic tics. These are noted first in childhood, generally between the ages of 2 and 15. Motor tics occur especially about the face, head, and shoulders (eg, sniffing, blinking, frowning, shoulder shrugging, head thrusting, etc). Phonic tics commonly consist of grunts, barks, hisses, throat-clearing, coughs, etc, but sometimes also of verbal utterances including coprolalia (obscene speech). There may also be echolalia (repetition of the speech of others), echopraxia (imitation of others' movements), and palilalia (repetition of words or phrases). Some tics may be self-mutilating in nature, such as nail-biting, hair-pulling, or biting of the lips or tongue. The disorder is chronic, but the course may be punctuated by relapses and remissions. Obsessive-compulsive behaviors are commonly associated and may be more disabling than the tics themselves.

Examination usually reveals no abnormalities other than the tics. In addition to obsessive-compulsive behavior disorders, psychiatric disturbances may occur because of the associated cosmetic and social embarrassment. Electroencephalography may show minor nonspecific abnormalities of no diagnostic relevance.

The diagnosis of the disorder is often delayed for years, the tics being interpreted as psychiatric illness or some other form of abnormal movement. Patients are thus often subjected to unnecessary treatment before the disorder is recognized. The tic-like character of the abnormal movements and the absence of other neurologic signs should differentiate this disorder from other movement disorders presenting in childhood. Wilson's disease, however, can simulate the condition and should be excluded.

Treatment

Treatment is symptomatic and may need to be continued indefinitely. Haloperidol is generally regarded as the drug of choice. It is started in a low daily dose (0.25 mg) that is gradually increased (by 0.25 mg every 4 or 5 days) until there is maximum benefit with a minimum of side effects or until side effects limit further increments. A total daily dose of between 2 and 8 mg is usually optimal, but higher doses are sometimes necessary. Treatment with clonazepam (in a dose that depends on response and tolerance) or clonidine (2–5 µg/kg/d) may also be helpful, and it seems sensible to begin with one of these drugs in order to avoid some of the long-term extrapyramidal side effects of haloperidol. Phenothiazines, such as fluphenazine (2–15 mg daily), have been used, but patients unresponsive to haloperidol are usually unresponsive to these as well.

Pimozide, an oral dopamine-blocking drug related to haloperidol, may be helpful in patients who cannot tolerate or have not responded to haloperidol. Treatment is started with 1 mg daily and the daily dose increased by 1–2 mg every 10 days; the average dose is between 7 and 16 mg daily.

There are a few anecdotal reports that calcium channel blockers may be helpful, but this requires further study.

Weeks RA et al: Tourette's syndrome: A disorder of cingulate and orbitofrontal function? Q J Med 1996;89:401. (Clinical characteristics and treatment strategies.)

DEMENTIA

Dementia, the symptom complex of progressive global impairment of intellectual function, is a major medical, social, and economic problem that is worsening as the number of elderly people in the general population increases. It is discussed in Chapter 4, and the only point to be reiterated here is the importance of recognizing early any treatable or reversible causes of dementia, such as normal-pressure hydrocephalus, intracranial mass lesions, vascular disease, hypothyroidism, thiamin or vitamin B_{12} deficiency, Wilson's disease, hepatic or renal failure, neurosyphilis, and the chronic meningitides.

MULTIPLE SCLEROSIS

Essentials of Diagnosis

- Episodic symptoms that may include sensory abnormalities, blurred vision, sphincter disturbances, and weakness with or without spasticity.
- Patient usually under 55 years of age at onset.
- Single pathologic lesion cannot explain clinical findings.
- Multiple foci best visualized by MRI.

General Considerations

This common neurologic disorder of unknown cause has its greatest incidence in young adults. Epidemiologic studies indicate that multiple sclerosis is much more common in persons of western European lineage who live in temperate zones. No population with a high risk for multiple sclerosis exists between latitudes 40 °N and 40 °S. Genetic, dietary, and climatic factors cannot account for these differences. There may be a familial incidence of the disease, since affected relatives are sometimes reported. The strong association between multiple sclerosis and specific HLA antigens (HLA-DR2) provides support for a theory of genetic predisposition. Many believe that the disease has an immunologic basis. Pathologically, focal—often perivenular—areas of demyelination with reactive gliosis are found scattered in the white matter of brain and spinal cord and in the optic nerves.

Clinical Findings

A. Symptoms and Signs: The common initial presentation is weakness, numbness, tingling, or unsteadiness in a limb; spastic paraparesis; retrobulbar neuritis; diplopia; disequilibrium; or a sphincter disturbance such as urinary urgency or hesitancy. Symptoms may disappear after a few days or weeks, although examination often reveals a residual deficit.

In most patients, there is an interval of months or years after the initial episode before new symptoms develop or the original ones recur. Eventually, however, relapses and usually incomplete remissions lead to increasing disability, with weakness, spasticity, and ataxia of the limbs, impaired vision, and urinary incontinence. The findings on examination at this stage commonly include optic atrophy, nystagmus, dysarthria, and pyramidal, sensory, or cerebellar deficits in some or all of the limbs.

Less commonly, symptoms are steadily progressive from their onset, and disability develops at a relatively early stage. The diagnosis cannot be made with confidence unless the total clinical picture indicates involvement of different parts of the central nervous system at different times.

A number of factors (eg, infection, trauma) may

precipitate or trigger exacerbations. Relapses are also more likely during the 2 or 3 months following pregnancy, possibly because of the increased demands and stresses that occur in the postpartum period.

B. Imaging: MRI of the brain or cervical cord is often helpful in demonstrating the presence of a multiplicity of lesions. CT scans are less helpful.

In patients presenting with myelopathy alone and in whom there is no clinical or laboratory evidence of more widespread disease, myelography or MRI may be necessary to exclude a congenital or acquired surgically treatable lesion. The foramen magnum region must be visualized to exclude the possibility of Arnold-Chiari malformation, in which part of the cerebellum and the lower brain stem are displaced into the cervical canal and produce mixed pyramidal and cerebellar deficits in the limbs.

C. Laboratory and Other Studies: A definitive diagnosis can never be based solely on the laboratory findings. If there is clinical evidence of only a single lesion in the central nervous system, multiple sclerosis cannot properly be diagnosed unless it can be shown that other regions are affected subclinically. The electrocerebral responses evoked by monocular visual stimulation with a checkerboard pattern stimulus, by monaural click stimulation, and by electrical stimulation of a sensory or mixed peripheral nerve have been used to detect subclinical involvement of the visual, brain stem auditory, and somatosensory pathways, respectively. Other disorders may also be characterized by multifocal electrophysiologic abnormalities.

There may be mild lymphocytosis or a slightly increased protein concentration in the cerebrospinal fluid, especially soon after an acute relapse. Elevated IgG in cerebrospinal fluid and discrete bands of IgG (oligoclonal bands) are present in many patients. The presence of such bands is not specific, however, since they have been found in a variety of inflammatory neurologic disorders and occasionally in patients with vascular or neoplastic disorders of the nervous system.

Treatment

At least partial recovery from acute exacerbations can reasonably be expected, but further relapses may occur without warning, and there is no means of preventing progression of the disorder. Some disability is likely to result eventually, but about half of all patients are without significant disability even 10 years after onset of symptoms.

Recovery from acute relapses may be hastened by treatment with corticosteroids, but the extent of recovery is unchanged. A high dose (eg, prednisone, 60 or 80 mg) is given daily for 1 week, after which medication is tapered over the following 2 or 3 weeks. Such a regimen is often preceded by methylprednisolone, 1 g intravenously for 3 days. Long-term treatment with steroids provides no benefit and does not prevent further relapses.

Several recent studies have suggested that intensive immunosuppressive therapy with cyclophosphamide or azathioprine may help to arrest the course of chronic progressive active multiple sclerosis. The evidence of benefit is incomplete, however, and further clinical trials are in progress. There is little evidence that plasmapheresis enhances any beneficial effects of immunosuppression in multiple sclerosis, and its role in the management of the various clinical forms of the disease is uncertain. In patients with relapsing-remitting multiple sclerosis, treatment with beta interferon has been shown to reduce the annual exacerbation rate, and further studies of this approach are proceeding. Finally, preliminary studies suggest that Cop 1 (a random polymer-simulating myelin basic protein) may be beneficial in patients with the exacerbating-remitting form of multiple sclerosis, and further evaluation of this approach seems warranted.

Treatment for spasticity (see below) and for neurogenic bladder may be needed in advanced cases. Excessive fatigue must be avoided, and patients should rest during periods of acute relapse.

Beck RW et al: A randomized, controlled trial of corticosteroids in the treatment of acute optic neuritis. N Engl J Med 1992;326:581. (Intravenous methylprednisolone followed by oral prednisone speeds recovery after optic neuritis.)

Hughes RAC: Immunotherapy for multiple sclerosis. J Neurol Neurosurg Psychiatry 1994;57:3.

IFNB Multiple Sclerosis Study Group: Interferon beta-1b is effective in relapsing-remitting multiple sclerosis. Neurology 1993;43:655. (Double-blind controlled trial.)

VITAMIN E DEFICIENCY

Vitamin E deficiency may produce a disorder somewhat similar to Friedreich's ataxia (see below). There is spinocerebellar degeneration involving particularly the posterior columns of the spinal cord and leading to limb ataxia, sensory loss, absent tendon reflexes, slurring of speech, and, in some cases, pigmentary retinal degeneration. The disorder may occur as a consequence of malabsorption or on a hereditary basis. Treatment is with alpha-tocopheryl acetate (eg, Aquasol E capsules or drops), as discussed in Chapter 29.

Kayden HJ: The neurologic syndrome of vitamin E deficiency: A significant cause of ataxia. Neurology 1993;43:2167. (Editorial review.)

SPASTICITY

The term "spasticity" is commonly used for an upper motor neuron deficit, but it properly refers to a velocity-dependent increase in resistance to passive movement that affects different muscles to a different extent, is not uniform in degree throughout the range of a particular movement, and is commonly associated with other features of pyramidal deficit. It is often a major complication of stroke, cerebral or spinal injury, static perinatal encephalopathy, and multiple sclerosis.

Physical therapy with appropriate stretching programs is important during rehabilitation after the development of an upper motor neuron lesion and in subsequent management of the patient. The aim is to prevent joint and muscle contractures and perhaps to modulate spasticity.

Drug management is important also, but treatment may increase functional disability when increased extensor tone is providing additional support for patients with weak legs. Dantrolene weakens muscle contraction by interfering with the role of calcium. It may be helpful in the treatment of spasticity but is best avoided in patients with poor respiratory function or severe myocardial disease. Treatment is begun with 25 mg once daily, and the daily dose is built up by 25 mg increments every 3 days, depending on tolerance, to a maximum of 100 mg four times daily. The drug should be withdrawn if no benefit has occurred after treatment with the maximum tolerated dose for about 2 weeks. Side effects include diarrhea, nausea, weakness, hepatic dysfunction (that may rarely be fatal, especially in women older than 35), drowsiness, light-headedness, and hallucinations.

Baclofen seems to be the most effective drug for treating spasticity of spinal origin. It is particularly helpful in relieving painful flexor (or extensor) spasms. The maximum recommended daily dose is 80 mg; treatment is started with a dose of 5 or 10 mg twice daily and then built up gradually. Side effects include gastrointestinal disturbances, lassitude, fatigue, sedation, unsteadiness, confusion, and hallucinations. Diazepam may modify spasticity by its action on spinal interneurons and perhaps also by influencing supraspinal centers, but effective doses often cause intolerable drowsiness and vary with different patients. Tizanidine, a centrally acting α_2-adrenergic agonist, is a short-acting agent that has become available for the acute and intermittent management of spasticity; long-term safety and efficacy are uncertain. The daily dose is built up gradually, usually to 8 mg taken three times daily. Side effects include sedation, lassitude, hypotension, and dryness of the mouth.

Motor-point blocks by intramuscular phenol have been used to reduce spasticity selectively in one or a few important muscles and may permit return of function in patients with incomplete myelopathies. Intramuscular administration of botulinum toxin may also be helpful. Intrathecal injection of phenol or absolute alcohol may be helpful in more severe cases, but greater selectivity can be achieved by nerve root or peripheral nerve neurolysis. These procedures should not be undertaken until the spasticity syndrome is fully evolved, ie, only after about 1 year or so, and only if long-term drug treatment either has been unhelpful or carries a significant risk to the patient.

A number of surgical procedures, eg, adductor or heel cord tenotomy, may help in the management of spasticity. Neurectomy may also facilitate patient management. For example, obturator neurectomy is helpful in patients with marked adductor spasms that interfere with personal hygiene or cause gait disturbances. Posterior rhizotomy reduces spasticity, but its effect may be short-lived, whereas anterior rhizotomy produces permanent wasting and weakness in the muscles that are denervated.

Spasticity may be exacerbated by decubitus ulcers, urinary or other infections, and nociceptive stimuli.

Brown P: Pathophysiology of spasticity. J Neurol Neurosurg Psychiatry 1994;57:773.

Young RR (editor): Role of tizanidine in the treatment of spasticity. Neurology 1994;44(Suppl 9). (Review and clinical trials.)

MYELOPATHIES IN AIDS

Patients with AIDS may develop a subacute or chronic vacuolar myelopathy leading to paraparesis or quadriparesis, sphincter dysfunction, and sensory disturbances. There is no effective treatment. Myelitis or radiculomyelitis may occur also in AIDS patients as a result of opportunistic viral infections. When extradural lymphomatous deposits cause compressive myelopathy, pain and spinal tenderness are conspicuous, and MRI or myelography reveals the underlying lesion. Treatment is with corticosteroids, radiotherapy, and chemotherapy. Lymphomatous meningitis occurring in AIDS patients has the features described above.

MYELOPATHY OF HUMAN T CELL LEUKEMIA VIRUS

Human T cell leukemia virus (HTLV-1), a human retrovirus, is transmitted by breast feeding, sexual contact, blood transfusion, and contaminated needles. Most patients are asymptomatic, but after a variable latent period (may be as long as several years) a myelopathy develops in some instances. The MRI, electrophysiologic, and cerebrospinal fluid findings are similar to those of multiple sclerosis, but HTLV-1 antibodies are present in serum and spinal fluid. There is no specific treatment.

Engstrom JW: HTLV-I infection and the nervous system. In: *Neurology and General Medicine,* 2nd ed. Aminoff MJ (editor). Churchill Livingstone, 1995. (Clinical review.)

SUBACUTE COMBINED DEGENERATION OF THE SPINAL CORD

Subacute combined degeneration of the spinal cord is due to vitamin B_{12} deficiency, such as occurs in pernicious anemia. It is characterized by myelopathy with predominant pyramidal and posterior column deficits, sometimes in association with polyneuropathy, mental changes, or optic neuropathy. Megaloblastic anemia may also occur, but this does not parallel the neurologic disorder, and the former may be obscured if folic acid supplements have been taken. Treatment is with vitamin B_{12}. For pernicious anemia, a convenient therapeutic regimen is 100 mg cyanocobalamin intramuscularly daily for 1 week, then weekly for 1 month, and then monthly for the remainder of the patient's life.

Savage DG, Lindenbaum J: Neurological complications of acquired cobalamin deficiency: Clinical aspects. Baillieres Clin Haematol 1995;8:657.

WERNICKE'S ENCEPHALOPATHY

Wernicke's encephalopathy is characterized by confusion, ataxia, and nystagmus leading to ophthalmoplegia (lateral rectus muscle weakness, conjugate gaze palsies); peripheral neuropathy may also be present. It is due to thiamin deficiency and in the USA occurs most commonly in alcoholics. It may also occur in patients with AIDS. In suspected cases, thiamin (50 mg) is given intravenously immediately and then intramuscularly on a daily basis until a satisfactory diet can be ensured. Intravenous glucose given before thiamin may precipitate the syndrome or worsen the symptoms. The diagnosis is confirmed by the response to treatment, which must not be delayed while laboratory confirmation is obtained.

Messing RO, Greenberg DA: Alcohol and the nervous system. In: *Neurology and General Medicine,* 2nd ed. Aminoff MJ (editor). Churchill Livingstone, 1995. (Clinical review.)

STUPOR & COMA

The patient who is stuporous is unresponsive except when subjected to repeated vigorous stimuli, while the comatose patient is unarousable and unable to respond to external events or inner needs, although reflex movements and posturing may be present.

Coma is a major complication of serious central nervous system disorders. It can result from seizures, hypothermia, metabolic disturbances, or structural lesions causing bilateral cerebral hemispheric dysfunction or a disturbance of the brain stem reticular activating system. A mass lesion involving one cerebral hemisphere may cause coma by compression of the brain stem.

Assessment & Emergency Measures

The diagnostic workup of the comatose patient must proceed concomitantly with management. Supportive therapy for respiration or blood pressure is initiated; in hypothermia, all vital signs may be absent, all such patients should be rewarmed before the prognosis is assessed.

The patient can be positioned on one side with the neck partly extended, dentures removed, and secretions cleared by suction; if necessary, the patency of the airways is maintained with an oropharyngeal airway. Blood is drawn for serum glucose, electrolyte, and calcium levels; arterial blood gases; liver and renal function tests; and toxicologic studies as indicated. Dextrose 50% (25 g), naloxone (0.4–1.2 mg), and thiamine (50 mg) are given intravenously.

Further details are then obtained from attendants of the patient's medical history, the circumstances surrounding the onset of coma, and the time course of subsequent events. Abrupt onset of coma suggests subarachnoid hemorrhage, brain stem stroke, or intracerebral hemorrhage, whereas a slower onset and progression occur with other structural or mass lesions. A metabolic cause is likely with a preceding intoxicated state or agitated delirium. On examination, attention is paid to the behavioral response to painful stimuli, the pupils and their response to light, the position of the eyes and their movement in response to passive movement of the head and ice-water caloric stimulation, and the respiratory pattern.

A. Response to Painful Stimuli: Purposive limb withdrawal from painful stimuli implies that sensory pathways from and motor pathways to the stimulated limb are functionally intact. Unilateral absence of responses despite application of stimuli to both sides of the body in turn implies a corticospinal lesion; bilateral absence of responsiveness suggests brain stem involvement, bilateral pyramidal tract lesions, or psychogenic unresponsiveness. Inappropriate responses may also occur. Decorticate posturing may occur with lesions of the internal capsule and rostral cerebral peduncle, decerebrate posturing with dysfunction or destruction of the midbrain and rostral pons, and decerebrate posturing in the arms accompanied by flaccidity or slight flexor responses in the legs in patients with extensive brain stem damage extending down to the pons at the trigeminal level.

B. Ocular Findings:

1. Pupils—Hypothalamic disease processes may lead to unilateral Horner's syndrome, while bilateral diencephalic involvement or destructive pontine lesions may lead to small but reactive pupils. Ipsilateral pupillary dilation with no direct or consensual response to light occurs with compression of the third cranial nerve, eg, with uncal herniation. The pupils are slightly smaller than normal but responsive to light in many metabolic encephalopathies; however, they may be fixed and dilated following overdosage with atropine, scopolamine, or glutethimide, and pinpoint (but responsive) with opiates. Pupillary dilation for several hours following cardiopulmonary arrest implies a poor prognosis.

2. Eye movements–Conjugate deviation of the eyes to the side suggests the presence of an ipsilateral hemispheric lesion or a contralateral pontine lesion. A mesencephalic lesion leads to downward conjugate deviation. Dysconjugate ocular deviation in coma implies a structural brain stem lesion unless there was preexisting strabismus.

The oculomotor responses to passive head turning and to caloric stimulation relate to each other and provide complementary information. In response to brisk rotation of the head from side to side and to flexion and extension of the head, normally conscious patients with open eyes do not exhibit contraversive conjugate eye deviation (doll's-head eye response) unless there is voluntary visual fixation or bilateral frontal pathology. With cortical depression in lightly comatose patients, a brisk doll's-head eye response is seen. With brain stem lesions, this oculocephalic reflex becomes impaired or lost, depending on the site of the lesion.

The oculovestibular reflex is tested by caloric stimulation using irrigation with ice water. In normal subjects, jerk nystagmus is elicited for about 2 or 3 minutes, with the slow component toward the irrigated ear. In unconscious patients with an intact brain stem, the fast component of the nystagmus disappears, so that the eyes tonically deviate toward the irrigated side for 2–3 minutes before returning to their original position. With impairment of brain stem function, the response becomes perverted and finally disappears. In metabolic coma, oculocephalic and oculovestibular reflex responses are preserved, at least initially.

C. Respiratory Patterns: Diseases causing coma may lead to respiratory abnormalities. Cheyne-Stokes respiration may occur with bihemispheric or diencephalic disease or in metabolic disorders. Central neurogenic hyperventilation occurs with lesions of the brain stem tegmentum; apneustic breathing (in which there are prominent end-inspiratory pauses) suggests damage at the pontine level (eg, due to basilar artery occlusion); and atactic breathing (a completely irregular pattern of breathing with deep and shallow breaths occurring randomly) is associated with lesions of the lower pontine tegmentum and medulla.

1. STUPOR & COMA DUE TO STRUCTURAL LESIONS

Supratentorial mass lesions tend to affect brain function in an orderly way. There may initially be signs of hemispheric dysfunction, such as hemiparesis. As coma develops and deepens, cerebral function becomes progressively disturbed, producing a predictable progression of neurologic signs that suggest rostrocaudal deterioration.

Thus, as a supratentorial mass lesion begins to impair the diencephalon, the patient becomes drowsy, then stuporous, and finally comatose. There may be Cheyne-Stokes respiration; small but reactive pupils; doll's-head eye responses with side-to-side head movements but sometimes an impairment of reflex upward gaze with brisk flexion of the head; tonic ipsilateral deviation of the eyes in response to vestibular stimulation with cold water; and initially a positive response to pain but subsequently only decorticate posturing. With further progression, midbrain failure occurs. Motor dysfunction progresses from decorticate to bilateral decerebrate posturing in response to painful stimuli; Cheyne-Stokes respiration is gradually replaced by sustained central hyperventilation; the pupils become middle-sized and fixed; and the oculocephalic and oculovestibular reflex responses become impaired, perverted, or lost. As the pons and then the medulla fail, the pupils remain unresponsive; oculovestibular responses are unobtainable; respiration is rapid and shallow; and painful stimuli may lead only to flexor responses in the legs. Finally, respiration becomes irregular and stops, the pupils often then dilating widely.

In contrast, a subtentorial (ie, brain stem) lesion may lead to an early, sometimes abrupt disturbance of consciousness without any orderly rostrocaudal progression of neurologic signs. Compressive lesions of the brain stem, especially cerebellar hemorrhage, may be clinically indistinguishable from intraparenchymal processes.

A structural lesion is suspected if the findings suggest focality. In such circumstances, a CT scan should be performed before, or instead of, a lumbar puncture in order to avoid any risk of cerebral herniation. Further management is of the causal lesion and is considered separately under the individual disorders.

2. STUPOR & COMA DUE TO METABOLIC DISTURBANCES

Patients with a metabolic cause of coma generally have signs of patchy, diffuse, and symmetric neurologic involvement that cannot be explained by loss of function at any single level or in a sequential manner, although focal or lateralized deficits may occur in hypoglycemia. Moreover, pupillary reactivity is usually preserved, while other brain stem functions are often grossly impaired. Comatose patients with meningitis, encephalitis, or subarachnoid hemorrhage may also exhibit little in the way of focal neurologic signs, however, and clinical evidence of meningeal irritation is sometimes very subtle in comatose patients. Examination of the cerebrospinal fluid in such patients is essential to establish the correct diagnosis.

In patients with coma due to cerebral ischemia and hypoxia, the absence of pupillary light reflexes at the time of initial examination indicates that there is little chance of regaining independence; by contrast, preserved pupillary light responses, the development of spontaneous eye movements (roving, conjugate, or better), and extensor, flexor, or withdrawal responses to pain at this early stage imply a relatively good prognosis.

Treatment of metabolic encephalopathy is of the underlying disturbance and is considered in other chapters. If the cause of the encephalopathy is obscure, all drugs except essential ones may have to be withdrawn in case they are responsible for the altered mental status.

Bates D: The management of medical coma. J Neurol Neurosurg Psychiatry 1993;56:589. (Causes, prognosis, and management.)

3. BRAIN DEATH

The definition of brain death is controversial, and diagnostic criteria have been published by many different professional organizations. In order to establish brain death, the irreversibly comatose patient must be shown to have lost all brain stem reflex responses, including the pupillary, corneal, oculovestibular, oculocephalic, oropharyngeal, and respiratory reflexes, and should have been in this condition for at least 6 hours. Spinal reflex movements do not exclude the diagnosis, but ongoing seizure activity or decerebrate or decorticate posturing is not consistent with brain death. The apnea test (presence or absence of spontaneous respiratory activity at a $PaCO_2$ of at least 60 mm Hg) serves to determine whether the patient is capable of respiratory activity.

Reversible coma simulating brain death may be seen with hypothermia (temperature < 32 °C) and overdosage with central nervous system depressant drugs, and these conditions must be excluded. Certain ancillary tests may assist the determination of brain death but are not essential. An isoelectric electroencephalogram, when the recording is made according to the recommendations of the American Electroencephalographic Society, is especially helpful in confirming the diagnosis. Alternatively, the demonstration of an absent cerebral circulation by intravenous radioisotope cerebral angiography or by four-vessel contrast cerebral angiography can be confirmatory.

Wijdicks EFM: Determining brain death in adults. Neurology 1995;45:1003. (Diagnostic guidelines.)

4. PERSISTENT VEGETATIVE STATE

Patients with severe bilateral hemispheric disease may show some improvement from an initially comatose state, so that, after a variable interval, they appear to be awake but lie motionless and without evidence of awareness or higher mental activity. This persistent vegetative state has been variously referred to as akinetic mutism, apallic state, or coma vigil. Most patients in this persistent vegetative state will die in months or years, but partial recovery has occasionally occurred and in rare instances has been sufficient to permit communication or even independent living.

American Neurological Association Committee on Ethical Affairs: Persistent vegetative state. Ann Neurol 1993; 33:386. (Diagnostic and management issues.)

5. LOCKED-IN SYNDROME (De-efferented State)

Acute destructive lesions (eg, infarction, hemorrhage, demyelination, encephalitis) involving the ventral pons and sparing the tegmentum may lead to a mute, quadriparetic but conscious state in which the patient is capable of blinking and of voluntary eye movement in the vertical plane, with preserved pupillary responses to light. Such a patient can mistakenly be regarded as comatose. Physicians should recognize that "locked-in" individuals are fully aware of their surroundings. The prognosis is variable, but recovery has occasionally been reported—in some cases including resumption of independent daily life, though this may take up to 2 or 3 years.

HEAD INJURY

Trauma is the most common cause of death in young people, and head injury accounts for almost half of these trauma-related deaths. The prognosis following head injury depends upon the site and severity of brain damage. Some guide to prognosis is provided by the mental status, since loss of consciousness for more than 1 or 2 minutes implies a worse prognosis than otherwise. Similarly, the degree of retrograde and posttraumatic amnesia provides an indication of the severity of injury and thus of the prognosis. Absence of skull fracture does not exclude the possibility of severe head injury. During the physical examination, special attention should be given to the level of consciousness and extent of any brain stem dysfunction.

Note: Patients who have lost consciousness for 2 minutes or more following head injury should be admitted to the hospital for observation, as should patients with focal neurologic deficits, lethargy, or skull fractures. If admission is declined, responsible family members should be given clear instructions about the need for, and manner of, checking on them at regular (hourly) intervals and for obtaining additional medical help if necessary.

Skull radiographs or CT scans may provide evidence of fractures. Because injury to the spine may have accompanied head trauma, cervical spine radiographs (especially in the lateral projection) should always be obtained in comatose patients and in patients with severe neck pain or a deficit possibly related to cord compression. CT scanning has an important role in demonstrating intracranial hemorrhage and may also provide evidence of cerebral edema and displacement of midline structures.

Cerebral Injuries

These are summarized in Table 24–5 along with comments about treatment. Increased intracranial pressure may result from ventilatory obstruction, abnormal neck position, seizures, dilutional hyponatremia, or cerebral edema; an intracranial hematoma requiring surgical evacuation may also be responsible. Other measures that may be necessary to reduce intracranial pressure include induced hyperventilation, intravenous mannitol infusion, and intravenous furosemide; corticosteroids provide no benefit in this context.

Scalp Injuries & Skull Fractures

Scalp lacerations and depressed or compound depressed skull fractures should be treated surgically as appropriate. Simple skull fractures require no specific treatment.

The clinical signs of basilar skull fracture include bruising about the orbit (raccoon sign), blood in the external auditory meatus (Battle's sign), and leakage of cerebrospinal fluid (which can be identified by its glucose content) from the ear or nose. Cranial nerve palsies (involving especially the first, second, third, fourth, fifth, seventh, and eighth nerves in any combination) may also occur. If there is any leakage of cerebrospinal fluid, conservative treatment, with elevation of the head, restriction of fluids, and administration of acetazolamide (250 mg four times daily), is often helpful; but if the leak continues for more than a few days, lumbar subarachnoid drainage may be necessary. Antibiotics are given if infection occurs, based on culture and sensitivity studies. Only very occasional patients require intracranial repair of the dural defect because of persistence of the leak or recurrent meningitis.

Late Complications of Head Injury

The relationship of chronic subdural hemorrhage to head injury is not always clear. In many elderly persons there is no history of trauma, but in other cases a head injury, often trivial, precedes the onset of symptoms by several weeks. The clinical presentation is usually with mental changes such as slowness, drowsiness, headache, confusion, memory disturbances, personality change, or even dementia. Focal neurologic deficits such as hemiparesis or hemisensory disturbance may also occur but are less common. CT scan is an important means of detecting the hematoma, which is sometimes bilateral. Treatment is by surgical evacuation to prevent cerebral compression and tentorial herniation.

Normal-pressure hydrocephalus may follow head injury, subarachnoid hemorrhage, or meningoencephalitis.

Other late complications of head injury include posttraumatic seizure disorder and posttraumatic headache.

Table 24–5. Acute cerebral sequelae of head injury.

Sequelae	Clinical Features	Pathology
Concussion	Transient loss of consciousness with bradycardia, hypotension, and respiratory arrest for a few seconds followed by retrograde and posttraumatic amnesia. Occasionally followed by transient neurologic deficit.	Bruising on side of impact (coup injury) or contralaterally (contrecoup injury).
Cerebral contusion/laceration	Loss of consciousness longer than with concussion. May lead to death or severe residual neurologic deficit.	Cerebral contusion, edema, hemorrhage, and necrosis. May have subarachnoid bleeding.
Acute epidural hemorrhage	Headache, confusion, somnolence, seizures, and focal deficits occur several hours after injury and lead to coma, respiratory depression, and death unless treated by surgical evacuation.	Tear in meningeal artery, vein, or dural sinus, leading to hematoma visible on CT scan.
Acute subdural hemorrhage	Similar to epidural hemorrhage, but interval before onset of symptoms is longer. Treatment is by surgical evacuation.	Hematoma from tear in veins from cortex to superior sagittal sinus or from cerebral laceration, visible on CT scan.
Cerebral hemorrhage	Generally develops immediately after injury. Clinically resembles hypertensive hemorrhage. Surgical evacuation is sometimes helpful.	Hematoma, visible on CT scan.

Alexander MP: Mild traumatic brain injury: Pathophysiology, natural history, and clinical management. Neurology 1995;45:1253.

Miller JD: Head injury. J Neurol Neurosurg Psychiatry 1993;56:440. (Pathophysiology, evaluation, management, and monitoring of head injury.)

SPINAL TRAUMA

While spinal cord damage may result from whiplash injury, severe injury usually relates to fracture-dislocation causing compression or angular deformity of the cord either cervically or in the lower thoracic and upper lumbar regions. Extreme hypotension following injury may also lead to cord infarction.

Total cord transection results in immediate flaccid paralysis and loss of sensation below the level of the lesion. Reflex activity is lost for a variable period, and there is urinary and fecal retention. As reflex function returns over the following days and weeks, spastic paraplegia or quadriplegia develops, with hyperreflexia and extensor plantar responses, but a flaccid atrophic (lower motor neuron) paralysis may be found depending on the segments of the cord that are affected. The bladder and bowels also regain some reflex function, permitting urine and feces to be expelled at intervals. As spasticity increases, flexor or extensor spasms (or both) of the legs become troublesome, especially if the patient develops bed sores or a urinary tract infection. Paraplegia with the legs in flexion or extension may eventually result.

With lesser degrees of injury, patients may be left with mild limb weakness, distal sensory disturbance, or both. Sphincter function may also be impaired, urinary urgency and urgency incontinence being especially common. More particularly, a unilateral cord lesion leads to an ipsilateral motor disturbance with accompanying impairment of proprioception and contralateral loss of pain and temperature appreciation below the lesion (Brown-Séquard's syndrome). A central cord syndrome may lead to a lower motor neuron deficit and loss of pain and temperature appreciation, with sparing of posterior column functions. A radicular deficit may occur at the level of the injury—or, if the cauda equina is involved, there may be evidence of disturbed function in several lumbosacral roots.

Treatment of the injury consists of immobilization and—if there is cord compression—decompressive laminectomy and fusion. Early treatment with high doses of corticosteroids (eg, methylprednisolone, 30 mg/kg by intravenous bolus, followed by 5.4 mg/kg/h for 23 hours) has been shown to improve neurologic recovery if commenced within 8 hours after injury. Treatment with $G_M 1$ ganglioside for 3 or 4 weeks is an experimental approach that has also been helpful. Anatomic realignment of the spinal cord by traction and other orthopedic procedures is also important. Subsequent care of the residual neurologic deficit—paraplegia or quadriplegia—requires treatment of spasticity and care of the skin, bladder, and bowels.

Tator CH: Update on the pathophysiology and pathology of acute spinal cord injury. Brain Pathol 1995;5:407.

Wirtz KM et al: Managing chronic spinal cord injury: Issues in critical care. Crit Care Nurs 1996;16:24.

SYRINGOMYELIA

Destruction or degeneration of gray and white matter adjacent to the central canal of the cervical spinal cord leads to cavitation and accumulation of fluid within the spinal cord. The precise pathogenesis is unclear, but many cases are associated with Arnold-Chiari malformation, in which there is displacement of the cerebellar tonsils, medulla, and fourth ventricle into the spinal canal, sometimes with accompanying meningomyelocele. In such circumstances, the cord cavity connects with and may merely represent a dilated central canal. In other cases, the cause of cavitation is less clear. There is a characteristic clinical picture, with segmental atrophy and areflexia and loss of pain and temperature appreciation in a "cape" distribution owing to the destruction of fibers crossing in front of the central canal. Thoracic kyphoscoliosis is usually present. With progression, involvement of the long motor and sensory tracts occurs as well, so that a pyramidal and sensory deficit develops in the legs. Upward extension of the cavitation (syringobulbia) leads to dysfunction of the lower brain stem and thus to bulbar palsy, nystagmus, and sensory impairment over one or both sides of the face.

Syringomyelia, ie, cord cavitation, may also occur in association with an intramedullary tumor or following severe cord injury, and the cavity then does not communicate with the central canal.

In patients with Arnold-Chiari malformation, there are commonly skeletal abnormalities on plain x-rays of the skull and cervical spine. CT scans show caudal displacement of the fourth ventricle. MRI or positive contrast myelography may demonstrate the malformation itself. Focal cord enlargement is found at myelography or by MRI in patients with cavitation related to past injury or intramedullary neoplasms.

Treatment of Arnold-Chiari malformation with associated syringomyelia is by suboccipital craniectomy and upper cervical laminectomy, with the aim of decompressing the malformation at the foramen magnum. The cord cavity should be drained, and if necessary an outlet for the fourth ventricle can be made. In cavitation associated with intramedullary tumor, treatment is surgical, but radiation therapy may be necessary if complete removal is not possible. Posttraumatic syringomyelia is also treated surgically if it leads to increasing neurologic deficits or to intolerable pain.

MOTOR NEURON DISEASES

This group of disorders is characterized clinically by weakness and variable wasting of affected muscles, without accompanying sensory changes. Certain of these disorders, such as Werdnig-Hoffman disease and Kugelberg-Welander syndrome, occur in infants or children and are not considered further here.

Motor neuron disease in adults generally commences between 30 and 60 years of age. There is degeneration of the anterior horn cells in the spinal cord, the motor nuclei of the lower cranial nerves, and the corticospinal and corticobulbar pathways. The disorder is usually sporadic, but familial cases may occur.

Classification

Five varieties have been distinguished on clinical grounds.

A. Progressive Bulbar Palsy: Bulbar involvement predominates owing to disease processes affecting primarily the motor nuclei of the cranial nerves.

B. Pseudobulbar Palsy: Bulbar involvement predominates in this variety also, but it is due to bilateral corticobulbar disease and thus reflects upper motor neuron dysfunction.

C. Progressive Spinal Muscular Atrophy: This is characterized primarily by a lower motor neuron deficit in the limbs due to degeneration of the anterior horn cells in the spinal cord.

D. Primary Lateral Sclerosis: There is a purely upper motor neuron deficit in the limbs.

E. Amyotrophic Lateral Sclerosis: A mixed upper and lower motor neuron deficit is found in the limbs. This disorder is sometimes associated with dementia or parkinsonism.

Clinical Findings

A. Symptoms and Signs: Difficulty in swallowing, chewing, coughing, breathing, and talking (dysarthria) occur with bulbar involvement. In progressive bulbar palsy, there is drooping of the palate, a depressed gag reflex, pooling of saliva in the pharynx, a weak cough, and a wasted, fasciculating tongue. In pseudobulbar palsy, the tongue is contracted and spastic and cannot be moved rapidly from side to side. Limb involvement is characterized by motor disturbances (weakness, stiffness, wasting, fasciculations) reflecting lower or upper motor neuron dysfunction; there are no objective changes on sensory examination, though there may be vague sensory complaints. The sphincters are generally spared.

The disorder is progressive and usually fatal within 3–5 years; death usually results from pulmonary infections. Patients with bulbar involvement generally have the poorest prognosis.

B. Laboratory and Other Studies: Electromyography may show changes of chronic partial denervation, with abnormal spontaneous activity in the resting muscle and a reduction in the number of motor units under voluntary control. In patients with suspected spinal muscular atrophy or amyotrophic lateral sclerosis, the diagnosis should not be made with confidence unless such changes are found in at least three extremities. Motor conduction velocity is usually normal but may be slightly reduced, and sensory conduction studies are also normal. Biopsy of a wasted muscle shows the histologic changes of denervation. The serum creatine kinase may be slightly elevated but never reaches the extremely high values seen in some of the muscular dystrophies. The cerebrospinal fluid is normal.

A familial form of amyotrophic lateral sclerosis has been described with autosomal dominant inheritance, related to mutations in the copper-zinc superoxide dismutase gene on the long arm of chromosome 21. X-linked bulbospinal neuronopathy is associated with an expanded trinucleotide repeat sequence on the androgen receptor gene and carries a more benign prognosis than other forms of motor neuron disease. There have been recent reports of juvenile spinal muscular atrophy due to hexosaminidase deficiency, with abnormal findings on rectal biopsy and reduced hexosaminidase A in serum and leukocytes. Pure motor syndromes resembling motor neuron disease may also occur in association with monoclonal gammopathy or multifocal motor neuropathies with conduction block. A motor neuronopathy may also develop in Hodgkin's disease and has a relatively benign prognosis.

Treatment

Riluzole, which reduces the presynaptic release of glutamate, may slow progression of amyotrophic lateral sclerosis. There is otherwise no specific treatment except in patients with gammopathy, in whom plasmapheresis and immunosuppression may lead to improvement. Therapeutic trials of various neurotrophic factors to slow disease progression are, however, in progress. Symptomatic and supportive measures may include prescription of anticholinergic drugs (such as trihexyphenidyl, amitriptyline, or atropine) if drooling is troublesome, braces or a walker to improve mobility, and physical therapy to prevent contractures. Spasticity may be helped by baclofen or diazepam. A semiliquid diet or nasogastric tube feeding may be needed if dysphagia is severe. Gastrostomy or cricopharyngomyotomy is sometimes resorted to in extreme cases of predominant bulbar involvement, and tracheostomy may be necessary if respiratory muscles are severely affected; however, in the terminal stages of these disorders, the aim of treatment should be to keep patients as comfortable as possible.

Rose FC (editor): *ALS: From Charcot to the Present and Into the Future.* Smith-Gordon, 1994. (General review.)

PERIPHERAL NEUROPATHIES

Peripheral neuropathies can be categorized on the basis of the structure primarily affected. The predominant pathologic feature may be axonal degeneration (axonal or neuronal neuropathies) or paranodal or segmental demyelination. The distinction may be possible on the basis of neurophysiologic findings. Motor and sensory conduction velocity can be measured in accessible segments of peripheral nerves. In axonal neuropathies, conduction velocity is normal or reduced only mildly and needle electromyography provides evidence of denervation in affected muscles. In demyelinating neuropathies, conduction may be slowed considerably in affected fibers, and in more severe cases, conduction is blocked completely, without accompanying electromyographic signs of denervation.

Peripheral neuropathies may also occur as a result of disorders affecting the connective tissues of the nerves or the blood vessels supplying the nerves, but these are much less common than the preceding varieties.

Nerves may be injured or compressed by neighboring anatomic structures at any point along their course. Common **mononeuropathies** of this sort are considered below. They lead to a sensory, motor, or mixed deficit that is restricted to the territory of the affected nerve. A similar clinical disturbance is produced by peripheral nerve tumors, but these are rare except in patients with Recklinghausen's disease. Multiple mononeuropathies suggest a patchy multifocal disease process such as vasculopathy (eg, diabetes, arteritis), an infiltrative process (eg, leprosy, sarcoidosis), radiation damage, or an immunologic disorder (eg, brachial plexopathy). Diffuse **polyneuropathies** lead to a symmetric sensory, motor, or mixed deficit, often most marked distally. They include the hereditary, metabolic, and toxic disorders; idiopathic inflammatory polyneuropathy (Guillain-Barré syndrome); and the peripheral neuropathies that may occur as a nonmetastatic complication of malignant diseases. Involvement of motor fibers leads to flaccid weakness that is most marked distally; dysfunction of sensory fibers causes impaired sensory perception. Tendon reflexes are depressed or absent. Paresthesias, pain, and muscle tenderness may also occur.

1. POLYNEUROPATHIES & MONONEURITIS MULTIPLEX

The cause of polyneuropathy or mononeuritis multiplex is suggested by the history, mode of onset, and predominant clinical manifestations. Laboratory workup includes a complete blood count and sedimentation rate, serum protein electrophoresis, determination of plasma urea and electrolytes, liver and thyroid function tests, tests for rheumatoid factor and antinuclear antibody, HBsAg determination, a serologic test for syphilis, fasting blood glucose level, urinary heavy metal levels, cerebrospinal fluid examination, and chest radiography. These tests should be ordered selectively, as guided by symptoms and signs. Measurement of nerve conduction velocity is important in confirming the peripheral nerve origin of symptoms and providing a means of following clinical changes, as well as indicating the likely disease process (ie, axonal or demyelinating neuropathy). Cutaneous nerve biopsy may help establish a precise diagnosis (eg, polyarteritis, amyloidosis). In about half of cases, no specific cause can be established; of these, slightly less than half are subsequently found to be heredofamilial.

Treatment is of the underlying cause, when feasible, and is discussed below under the individual disorders. Physical therapy helps prevent contractures, and splints can maintain a weak extremity in a position of useful function. Anesthetic extremities must be protected from injury. To guard against burns, patients should check the temperature of water and hot surfaces with a portion of skin having normal sensation, measure water temperature with a thermometer, and use cold water for washing or lower the temperature setting of their hot-water heaters. Shoes should be examined frequently during the day for grit or foreign objects in order to prevent pressure lesions.

Patients with polyneuropathies or mononeuritis multiplex are subject to additional nerve injury at pressure points and should therefore avoid such behavior as leaning on elbows or sitting with crossed legs for lengthy periods.

Neuropathic pain is sometimes troublesome and may respond to simple analgesics such as aspirin. Narcotics or narcotic substitutes may be necessary for severe hyperpathia or pain induced by minimal stimuli, but their use should be avoided as far as possible. The use of a frame or cradle to reduce contact with bedclothes may be helpful. Many patients experience episodic stabbing pains, which may respond to phenytoin, carbamazepine, or tricyclic antidepressants.

Symptoms of autonomic dysfunction are occasionally troublesome. Postural hypotension is often helped by wearing waist-high elastic stockings and sleeping in a semierect position at night. Fludrocortisone reduces postural hypotension, but doses as high as 1 mg/d are sometimes necessary in diabetics and may lead to recumbent hypertension. Indomethacin (25 or 50 mg three times daily) is sometimes helpful. Impotence and diarrhea are difficult to treat; a flaccid neuropathic bladder may respond to parasympathomimetic drugs such as bethanechol chloride, 10–50 mg three or four times daily.

Inherited Neuropathies

A. Charcot-Marie-Tooth Disease: Several distinct varieties of Charcot-Marie-Tooth disease can be recognized. There is usually an autosomal dominant mode of inheritance, but occasional cases occur on a sporadic, recessive, or X-linked basis. The responsible gene is commonly located on the short arm of chromosome 17 and less often shows linkage to chromosome 1 or the X chromosome. Clinical presentation may be with foot deformities or gait disturbances in childhood or early adult life. Slow progression leads to the typical features of polyneuropathy, with distal weakness and wasting that begin in the legs, a variable amount of distal sensory loss, and depressed or absent tendon reflexes. Tremor is a conspicuous feature in some instances. Pathologic examination reveals segmental demyelination and remyelination of peripheral nerves, an increase in their transverse fascicular area, and hyperplasia of Schwann cells. Electrodiagnostic studies show a marked reduction in motor and sensory conduction velocity (hereditary motor and sensory neuropathy [HMSN] type I).

In other instances (HMSN type II), motor conduction velocity is normal or only slightly reduced, sensory nerve action potentials may be absent, and signs of chronic partial denervation are found in affected muscles electromyographically. The predominant pathologic change is axonal loss rather than segmental demyelination.

A similar disorder may occur in patients with progressive distal spinal muscular atrophy, but there is no sensory loss; electrophysiologic investigation reveals that motor conduction velocity is normal or only slightly reduced, and nerve action potentials are normal.

B. Dejerine-Sottas Disease (HMSN Type III): Most cases are sporadic or autosomal recessive. The recessive form has its onset in infancy or childhood and leads to a progressive motor and sensory polyneuropathy with weakness, ataxia, sensory loss, and depressed or absent tendon reflexes. The peripheral nerves may be palpably enlarged and are characterized pathologically by segmental demyelination, Schwann cell hyperplasia, and thin myelin sheaths. Electrophysiologically, there is slowing of conduction, and sensory action potentials may be unrecordable.

C. Friedreich's Ataxia: Patients generally present in childhood or early adult life with this autosomal recessive disorder, which has been related to a genetic defect on the long arm of chromosome 9. The gait becomes atactic, the hands become clumsy, and other signs of cerebellar dysfunction develop accompanied by weakness of the legs and extensor plantar responses. Involvement of peripheral sensory fibers leads to sensory disturbances in the limbs and depressed tendon reflexes. There is bilateral pes cavus. Pathologically, there is a marked loss of cells in the posterior root ganglia and degeneration of peripheral sensory fibers. In the central nervous system, changes are conspicuous in the posterior and lateral columns of the cord. Electrophysiologically, conduction velocity in motor fibers is normal or only mildly reduced, but sensory action potentials are small or absent.

D. Refsum's Disease (HMSN Type IV): This autosomal recessive disorder is due to a disturbance in phytanic acid metabolism. Clinically, pigmentary retinal degeneration is accompanied by progressive sensorimotor polyneuropathy and cerebellar signs. Auditory dysfunction, cardiomyopathy, and cutaneous manifestations may also occur. Motor and sensory conduction velocity is reduced, often markedly, and there may be electromyographic evidence of denervation in affected muscles. Dietary restriction of phytanic acid and its precursors may be helpful therapeutically.

E. Porphyria: Peripheral nerve involvement may occur during acute attacks in both variegate porphyria and acute intermittent porphyria. Motor symptoms usually occur first, and weakness is often most marked proximally and in the upper limbs rather than the lower. Sensory symptoms and signs may be proximal or distal in distribution. Autonomic involvement is sometimes pronounced. The electrophysiologic findings are in keeping with the results of neuropathologic studies suggesting that the neuropathy is axonal in type. Hematin (4 mg/kg intravenously over 15 minutes once or twice daily) may lead to rapid improvement. A high-carbohydrate diet and, in severe cases, intravenous glucose or levulose may also be helpful. Propranolol (up to 100 mg every 4 hours) may control tachycardia and hypertension in acute attacks. Porphyria is discussed further in Chapter 23.

Neuropathies Associated With Systemic & Metabolic Disorders

A. Diabetes Mellitus: In this disorder, involvement of the peripheral nervous system may lead to symmetric sensory or mixed polyneuropathy, asymmetric motor neuropathy (diabetic amyotrophy), thoracoabdominal radiculopathy, autonomic neuropathy, or isolated lesions of individual nerves. These may occur singly or in any combination.

Sensory polyneuropathy, the most common manifestation, may lead to no more than depressed tendon reflexes and impaired appreciation of vibration in the legs. When symptomatic, there may be pain, paresthesias, or numbness in the legs, but in severe cases distal sensory loss occurs in all limbs. Diabetic amyotrophy is characterized by asymmetric weakness and wasting involving predominantly the proximal muscles of the legs, accompanied by local pain. Thoracoabdominal radiculopathy leads to pain over the trunk. In patients with autonomic neuropathy, postural hypotension, impaired thermoregulatory sweating, postgustatory hyperhidrosis, constipation, flatulence, diarrhea, impotence, urinary retention, and incontinence may occur, and there may be abnormal pupillary responses. Isolated lesions of individual peripheral nerves are common and in the limbs tend to occur at sites of compression or entrapment. Treatment is symptomatic. Entrapment neuropathies may be helped by surgical decompression. Treatment of neuropathic pain is discussed above.

B. Uremia: Uremia may lead to a symmetric sensorimotor polyneuropathy that tends to affect the lower limbs more than the upper limbs and is more marked distally than proximally. The diagnosis can be confirmed electrophysiologically, for motor and sensory conduction velocity is moderately reduced. The neuropathy improves both clinically and electrophysiologically with renal transplantation and to a lesser extent with chronic dialysis.

C. Alcoholism and Nutritional Deficiency: Many alcoholics have an axonal distal sensorimotor polyneuropathy that is frequently accompanied by painful cramps, muscle tenderness, and painful paresthesias and is often more marked in the legs than in the arms. Symptoms of autonomic dysfunction may also be conspicuous. Motor and sensory conduction velocity may be slightly reduced, even in subclinical cases, but gross slowing of conduction is uncommon. A similar distal sensorimotor polyneuropathy is a well-recognized feature of beriberi (thiamin deficiency). In vitamin B_{12} deficiency, distal sensory polyneuropathy may develop but is usually overshadowed by central nervous system manifestations (eg, myelopathy, optic neuropathy, or intellectual changes).

D. Paraproteinemias: A symmetric sensorimotor polyneuropathy that is gradual in onset, progressive in course, and often accompanied by pain and dysesthesias in the limbs may occur in patients (especially men) with multiple myeloma. The neuropathy is of the axonal type in classic lytic myeloma, but segmental demyelination (primary or secondary) and axonal loss may occur in sclerotic myeloma and lead to predominantly motor clinical manifestations. Both demyelinating and axonal neuropathies are also observed in patients with paraproteinemias without myeloma. A small fraction will develop myeloma if serially followed. The demyelinating neuropathy in these patients may be due to the monoclonal protein's reacting to a component of the nerve myelin. The neuropathy of classic multiple myeloma is poorly responsive to therapy. The polyneuropathy of benign monoclonal gammopathy may respond to immunosuppressant drugs and plasmapheresis.

Polyneuropathy may also occur in association with macroglobulinemia and cryoglobulinemia and sometimes responds to plasmapheresis. Entrapment neuropathy, such as carpal tunnel syndrome, is more common than polyneuropathy in patients with (nonhereditary) generalized amyloidosis. With polyneuropathy due to amyloidosis, sensory and autonomic symptoms are especially conspicuous, whereas distal wasting and weakness occur later; there is no specific treatment.

Neuropathies Associated With Infectious & Inflammatory Diseases

A. Leprosy: Leprosy is an important cause of peripheral neuropathy in certain parts of the world. Sensory disturbances are mainly due to involvement of intracutaneous nerves. In tuberculoid leprosy, they develop at the same time and in the same distribution as the skin lesion but may be more extensive if nerve trunks lying beneath the lesion are also involved. In lepromatous leprosy, there is more extensive sensory loss, and this develops earlier and to a greater extent in the coolest regions of the body, such as the dorsal surfaces of the hands and feet, where the bacilli proliferate most actively. Motor deficits result from involvement of superficial nerves where their temperature is lowest, eg, the ulnar nerve in the region proximal to the olecranon groove, the median nerve as it emerges from beneath the forearm flexor muscle to run toward the carpal tunnel, the peroneal nerve at the head of the fibula, and the posterior tibial nerve in the lower part of the leg; patchy facial muscular weakness may also occur owing to involvement of the superficial branches of the seventh cranial nerve.

Motor disturbances in leprosy are suggestive of multiple mononeuropathy, whereas sensory changes resemble those of distal polyneuropathy. Examination, however, relates the distribution of sensory deficits to the temperature of the tissues; in the legs, for example, sparing frequently occurs between the toes and in the popliteal fossae, where the temperature is higher. Treatment is with antileprotic agents (see Chapter 33).

B. AIDS: A variety of neuropathies occur in HIV-infected patients. Patients with AIDS may develop a chronic symmetric sensorimotor axonal **polyneuropathy** associated usually with no abnormal cerebrospinal fluid findings. Treatment is symptomatic. AIDS patients may also develop progressive **polyradiculopathy** or radiculomyelopathy that leads to leg weakness and urinary retention; sensory loss is less conspicuous than in polyneuropathy. The cerebrospinal fluid may show mononuclear pleocytosis and increased protein and low glucose concentrations. Cytomegalovirus is responsible in at least some cases. The prognosis is generally poor, but some patients respond to intravenous ganciclovir (2.5 mg/kg every 8 hours for 10 days, then 7.5 mg/kg daily 5 days per week).

An inflammatory **demyelinating polyradiculoneuropathy** sometimes occurs in HIV-seropositive patients without AIDS and may follow an acute, subacute, or chronic course. Weakness is usually more conspicuous distally than proximally and tends to overshadow sensory symptoms. Tendon reflexes are depressed or absent. The cerebrospinal fluid shows an increased cell count and protein concentration. Treatment with plasmapheresis has helped some patients. Spontaneous improvement may also occur. Seropositive patients without AIDS may also develop a **mononeuropathy multiplex** that sometimes responds to treatment with plasmapheresis.

C. Lyme Borreliosis: The neurologic manifestations of Lyme disease include meningitis, meningoencephalitis, polyradiculoneuropathy, mononeuropathy multiplex, and cranial neuropathy. Serologic tests establish the underlying disorder. Treatment is as described in Chapter 34.

D. Sarcoidosis: Cranial nerve palsies (especially facial palsy), multiple mononeuropathy, and, less commonly, symmetric polyneuropathy may all occur, the latter sometimes preferentially affecting either motor or sensory fibers. Improvement may occur with use of corticosteroids.

E. Polyarteritis: Involvement of the vasa nervorum by the vasculitic process may result in infarction of the nerve. Clinically, one encounters an asymmetric sensorimotor polyneuropathy (mononeuritis multiplex) that pursues a waxing and waning course. Steroids and cytotoxic agents—especially cyclophosphamide—may be of benefit in severe cases.

F. Rheumatoid Arthritis: Compressive or entrapment neuropathies, ischemic neuropathies, mild distal sensory polyneuropathy, and severe progressive sensorimotor polyneuropathy can occur in rheumatoid arthritis.

Neuropathy Associated With Critical Illness

Patients in intensive care units with sepsis and multiorgan failure sometimes develop polyneuropathies. This may be manifested initially by unexpected difficulty in weaning patients from a mechanical ventilator and in more advanced cases by wasting and weakness of the extremities and loss of tendon reflexes. Sensory abnormalities are relatively inconspicuous. The neuropathy is axonal in type. Its pathogenesis is obscure, and treatment is supportive. The prognosis is good provided patients recover from the underlying critical illness.

Toxic Neuropathies

Axonal polyneuropathy may follow exposure to industrial agents or pesticides such as acrylamide, organophosphorus compounds, hexacarbon solvents, methyl bromide, and carbon disulfide; metals such as arsenic, thallium, mercury, and lead; and drugs such as phenytoin, perhexiline, isoniazid, nitrofurantoin, vincristine, and pyridoxine in high doses. Detailed occupational, environmental, and medical histories and recognition of clusters of cases are important in suggesting the diagnosis. Treatment is by preventing further exposure to the causal agent. Isoniazid neuropathy is prevented by pyridoxine supplementation.

Diphtheritic neuropathy results from a neurotoxin released by the causative organism and is common in many areas. Palatal weakness may develop 2–4 weeks after infection of the throat, and infection of the skin may similarly be followed by focal weakness of neighboring muscles. Disturbances of accommodation may occur about 4–5 weeks after infection and distal sensorimotor demyelinating polyneuropathy after 1–3 months.

Neuropathies Associated With Malignant Diseases

Both a sensorimotor and a purely sensory polyneuropathy may occur as a nonmetastatic complication of malignant diseases. The sensorimotor polyneuropathy may be mild and occur in the course of known malignant disease; or it may have an acute or subacute onset, lead to severe disability, and occur before there is any clinical evidence of the cancer, occasionally following a remitting course.

Acute Idiopathic Polyneuropathy (Guillain-Barré Syndrome)

This acute or subacute polyradiculoneuropathy sometimes follows infective illness, inoculations, or surgical procedures. There is an association with preceding *Campylobacter jejuni* enteritis. The disorder probably has an immunologic basis, but the precise mechanism is unclear. The main complaint is of weakness that varies widely in severity in different patients and often has a proximal emphasis and symmetric distribution. It usually begins in the legs, spreading to a variable extent but frequently involving the arms and often one or both sides of the face. The muscles of respiration or deglutition may also be affected. Sensory symptoms are usually less conspicuous than motor ones, but distal paresthesias and dysesthesias are common, and neuropathic or radicular pain is present in many patients. Autonomic disturbances are also common, may be severe, and are sometimes life-threatening; they include tachycardia, cardiac irregularities, hypotension or hypertension, facial flushing, abnormalities of sweating, pulmonary dysfunction, and impaired sphincter control.

The cerebrospinal fluid characteristically contains a high protein concentration with a normal cell content, but these changes may take 2 or 3 weeks to develop. Electrophysiologic studies may reveal marked abnormalities, which do not necessarily parallel the clinical disorder in their temporal course. Pathologic examination has shown that primary demyelination occurs in regions infiltrated with inflammatory cells, and it seems probable that myelin disruption has an autoimmune basis.

When the diagnosis is made, the history and appropriate laboratory studies should exclude the possibility of porphyric, diphtheritic, or toxic (heavy metal, hexacarbon, organophosphate) neuropathies. Poliomyelitis, botulism, and tick paralysis must also be considered. The presence of pyramidal signs, a markedly asymmetric motor deficit, a sharp sensory level, or early sphincter involvement should suggest a focal cord lesion.

Most patients eventually make a good recovery, but this may take many months, and 10–20% of patients are left with persisting disability. Treatment with prednisone is ineffective and may actually affect the outcome adversely by prolonging recovery time. Plasmapheresis is of value; it is best performed within the first few days of illness and is best reserved for clinically severe or rapidly progressive cases or those with ventilatory impairment. Intravenous immunoglobulin (400 mg/kg/d for 5 days) is also helpful and imposes less stress on the cardiovascular system than plasmapheresis. Patients should be admitted to intensive care units if their forced vital capacity is declining, and intubation is considered if the forced vital capacity reaches 15 mL/kg, dyspnea becomes evident, or the oxygen saturation declines. Respiratory toilet and chest physical therapy help prevent atelectasis. Marked hypotension may respond to volume replacement or pressor agents. Low-dose heparin to prevent pulmonary embolism should be considered.

Approximately 3% of patients with acute idiopathic polyneuropathy have one or more clinically similar relapses, sometimes several years after the initial illness. Plasma exchange therapy may produce improvement in chronic and relapsing inflammatory polyneuropathy.

Chronic Inflammatory Polyneuropathy

Chronic inflammatory demyelinating polyneuropathy, an acquired immunologically mediated disorder, is clinically similar to Guillain-Barré syndrome except that it has a relapsing or steadily progressive course over months or years. In the relapsing form, partial recovery may occur after some relapses, but in other instances there is no recovery between exacerbations. Although remission may occur spontaneously with time, the disorder frequently follows a progressive downhill course leading to severe functional disability.

Electrodiagnostic studies show marked slowing of motor and sensory conduction, and focal conduction block. Signs of partial denervation may also be present owing to secondary axonal degeneration. Nerve biopsy may show chronic perivascular inflammatory

infiltrates in the endoneurium and epineurium, without accompanying evidence of vasculitis. However, a normal nerve biopsy result or the presence of nonspecific abnormalities does not exclude the diagnosis.

Corticosteroids may be effective in arresting or reversing the downhill course. Treatment is usually begun with prednisone, 60 mg daily, continued for 2–3 months or until a definite response has occurred. If no response has occurred despite 3 months of treatment, a higher dose may be tried. In responsive cases, the dose is gradually tapered, but most patients become corticosteroid-dependent, often requiring prednisone, 20 mg daily on alternate days, on a long-term basis. Patients unresponsive to corticosteroids may benefit instead from treatment with a cytotoxic drug such as azathioprine. There are increasing anecdotal reports of short-term benefit with plasmapheresis; high-dose intravenous immunoglobulin treatment (eg, 400 mg/kg/d) may produce clinical improvement lasting for weeks to months.

Dyck PJ et al (editors): *Peripheral Neuropathy,* 3rd ed. Saunders, 1993.

Ropper AH: The Guillain-Barré syndrome. N Engl J Med 1992;326:1130.

Said G: Diabetic neuropathy: An update. J Neurol 1996;243:431.

Simpson DM, Olney RK: Peripheral neuropathies associated with human immunodeficiency virus infection. Neurol Clin 1992;10:685.

2. MONONEUROPATHIES

An individual nerve may be injured along its course or may be compressed, angulated, or stretched by neighboring anatomic structures, especially at a point where it passes through a narrow space (entrapment neuropathy). The relative contributions of mechanical factors and ischemia to the local damage are not clear. With involvement of a sensory or mixed nerve, pain is commonly felt distal to the lesion. Symptoms never develop with some entrapment neuropathies, resolve rapidly and spontaneously in others, and become progressively more disabling and distressing in yet other cases. The precise neurologic deficit depends on the nerve involved. Percussion of the nerve at the site of the lesion may lead to paresthesias in its distal distribution.

Entrapment neuropathy may be the sole manifestation of subclinical polyneuropathy, and this must be borne in mind and excluded by nerve conduction studies. Such studies are also indispensable for the accurate localization of the focal lesion.

In patients with acute compression neuropathy such as Saturday night palsy, no treatment is necessary. Complete recovery generally occurs, usually within 2 months, presumably because the underlying pathology is demyelination. However, axonal degeneration can occur in severe cases, and recovery then takes longer and may never be complete.

In chronic compressive or entrapment neuropathies, avoidance of aggravating factors and correction of any underlying systemic conditions are important. Local infiltration of the region about the nerve with corticosteroids may be of value; in addition, surgical decompression may help if there is a progressively increasing neurologic deficit or if electrodiagnostic studies show evidence of partial denervation in weak muscles.

Peripheral nerve tumors are uncommon, except in Recklinghausen's disease, but also give rise to mononeuropathy. This may be distinguishable from entrapment neuropathy only by noting the presence of a mass along the course of the nerve and by demonstrating the precise site of the lesion with appropriate electrophysiologic studies. Treatment of symptomatic lesions is by surgical removal if possible.

Carpal Tunnel Syndrome

See Chapter 20.

Pronator Teres or Anterior Interosseous Syndrome

The median nerve gives off its motor branch, the anterior interosseous nerve, below the elbow as it descends between the two heads of the pronator teres muscle. A lesion of either nerve may occur in this region, sometimes after trauma or owing to compression from, for example, a fibrous band. With anterior interosseous nerve involvement, there is no sensory loss, and weakness is confined to the pronator quadratus, flexor pollicis longus, and the flexor digitorum profundus to the second and third digits. Weakness is more widespread and sensory changes occur in an appropriate distribution when the median nerve itself is affected. The prognosis is variable. If improvement does not occur spontaneously, decompressive surgery may be helpful.

Ulnar Nerve Lesions

Ulnar nerve lesions are likely to occur in the elbow region as the nerve runs behind the medial epicondyle and descends into the cubital tunnel. In the condylar groove, the ulnar nerve is exposed to pressure or trauma. Moreover, any increase in the carrying angle of the elbow, whether congenital, degenerative, or traumatic, may cause excessive stretching of the nerve when the elbow is flexed. Ulnar nerve lesions may also result from thickening or distortion of the anatomic structures forming the cubital tunnel, and the resulting symptoms may also be aggravated by flexion of the elbow, because the tunnel is then narrowed by tightening of its roof or inward bulging of its floor. A severe lesion at either site causes sensory changes in the medial 1½ digits and along the medial border of the hand. There is weakness of the ulnar-innervated muscles in the forearm and hand. With a cubital tunnel lesion, however, there may be relative sparing of the flexor carpi ulnaris muscle. Electrophysiologic evaluation using nerve stimulation techniques allows more precise localization of the lesion.

If conservative measures are unsuccessful in relieving symptoms and preventing further progression, surgical treatment may be necessary. This consists of nerve transposition if the lesion is in the condylar groove, or a release procedure if it is in the cubital tunnel.

Ulnar nerve lesions may also develop at the wrist or in the palm of the hand, usually owing to repetitive trauma or to compression from ganglia or benign tumors. They can be subdivided depending upon their presumed site. Compressive lesions are treated surgically. If repetitive mechanical trauma is responsible, this is avoided by occupational adjustment or job retraining.

Radial Nerve Lesions

The radial nerve is particularly liable to compression or injury in the axilla (eg, by crutches or by pressure when the arm hangs over the back of a chair). This leads to weakness or paralysis of all the muscles supplied by the nerve, including the triceps. Sensory changes may also occur but are often surprisingly inconspicuous, being marked only in a small area on the back of the hand between the thumb and index finger. Injuries to the radial nerve in the spiral groove occur characteristically during deep sleep, as in intoxicated individuals (Saturday night palsy), and there is then sparing of the triceps muscle, which is supplied more proximally. The nerve may also be injured at or above the elbow; its purely motor posterior interosseous branch, supplying the extensors of the wrist and fingers, may be involved immediately below the elbow, but then there is sparing of the extensor carpi radialis longus, so that the wrist can still be extended. The superficial radial nerve may be compressed by handcuffs or a tight watch strap.

Femoral Neuropathy

The clinical features of femoral nerve palsy consist of weakness and wasting of the quadriceps muscle, with sensory impairment over the anteromedian aspect of the thigh and sometimes also of the leg to the medial malleolus, and a depressed or absent knee jerk. Isolated femoral neuropathy may occur in diabetics or from compression by retroperitoneal neoplasms or hematomas (eg, expanding aortic aneurysm). Femoral neuropathy may also result from pressure from the inguinal ligament when the thighs are markedly flexed and abducted, as in the lithotomy position.

Meralgia Paresthetica

The lateral femoral cutaneous nerve, a sensory nerve arising from the L2 and L3 roots, may be compressed or stretched in obese or diabetic patients and during pregnancy. The nerve usually runs under the outer portion of the inguinal ligament to reach the thigh, but the ligament sometimes splits to enclose it. Hyperextension of the hip or increased lumbar lordosis—such as occurs during pregnancy—leads to nerve compression by the posterior fascicle of the ligament. However, entrapment of the nerve at any point along its course may cause similar symptoms, and several other anatomic variations predispose the nerve to damage when it is stretched. Pain, paresthesia, or numbness occurs about the outer aspect of the thigh, usually unilaterally, and is sometimes relieved by sitting. Examination shows no abnormalities except in severe cases when cutaneous sensation is impaired in the affected area. Symptoms are usually mild and commonly settle spontaneously, so patients can be reassured about the benign nature of the disorder. Hydrocortisone injections medial to the anterosuperior iliac spine often relieve symptoms temporarily, while nerve decompression by transposition may provide more lasting relief.

Sciatic & Common Peroneal Nerve Palsies

Misplaced deep intramuscular injections are probably still the most common cause of sciatic nerve palsy. Trauma to the buttock, hip, or thigh may also be responsible. The resulting clinical deficit depends on whether the whole nerve has been affected or only certain fibers. In general, the peroneal fibers of the sciatic nerve are more susceptible to damage than those destined for the tibial nerve. A sciatic nerve lesion may therefore be difficult to distinguish from peroneal neuropathy unless there is electromyographic evidence of involvement of the short head of the biceps femoris muscle. The common peroneal nerve itself may be compressed or injured in the region of the head and neck of the fibula, eg, by sitting with crossed legs or wearing high boots. There is weakness of dorsiflexion and eversion of the foot, accompanied by numbness or blunted sensation of the anterolateral aspect of the calf and dorsum of the foot.

Tarsal Tunnel Syndrome

The tibial nerve, the other branch of the sciatic, supplies several muscles in the lower extremity, gives origin to the sural nerve, and then continues as the posterior tibial nerve to supply the plantar flexors of the foot and toes. It passes through the tarsal tunnel behind and below the medial malleolus, giving off calcaneal branches and the medial and lateral plantar nerves that supply small muscles of the foot and the skin on the plantar aspect of the foot and toes. Compression of the posterior tibial nerve or its branches between the bony floor and ligamentous roof of the tarsal tunnel leads to pain, paresthesias, and numbness over the bottom of the foot, especially at night, with sparing of the heel. Muscle weakness may be hard to recognize clinically. Compressive lesions of the individual plantar nerves may also occur more distally, with similar clinical features to those of the tarsal tunnel syndrome. Treatment is surgical decompression.

Stewart J: *Focal Peripheral Neuropathies,* 2nd ed. Raven Press, 1993.

Facial Neuropathy

An isolated facial palsy may occur in patients with HIV seropositivity, sarcoidosis, or Lyme disease (Chapter 34), but most often it is idiopathic (Bell's palsy).

3. BELL'S PALSY

Bell's palsy is an idiopathic facial paresis of lower motor neuron type that has been attributed to an inflammatory reaction involving the facial nerve near the stylomastoid foramen or in the bony facial canal. A relationship of Bell's palsy to reactivation of herpes simplex virus has recently been suggested, but there is little evidence to support this.

The clinical features of Bell's palsy are characteristic. The facial paresis generally comes on abruptly, but it may worsen over the following day or so. Pain about the ear precedes or accompanies the weakness in many cases but usually lasts for only a few days. The face itself feels stiff and pulled to one side. There may be ipsilateral restriction of eye closure and difficulty with eating and fine facial movements. A disturbance of taste is common, owing to involvement of chorda tympani fibers, and hyperacusis due to involvement of fibers to the stapedius occurs occasionally.

The management of Bell's palsy is controversial. Approximately 60% of cases recover completely without treatment, presumably because the lesion is so mild that it leads merely to conduction block. Considerable improvement occurs in most other cases, and only about 10% of all patients are seriously dissatisfied with the final outcome because of permanent disfigurement or other long-term sequelae. Treatment is unnecessary in most cases but is indicated for patients in whom an unsatisfactory outcome can be predicted. The best clinical guide to progress is the severity of the palsy during the first few days after presentation. Patients with clinically complete palsy when first seen are less likely to make a full recovery than those with an incomplete one. A poor prognosis for recovery is also associated with advanced age, hyperacusis, and severe initial pain. Electromyography and nerve excitability or conduction studies provide a guide to prognosis but not early enough to aid in the selection of patients for treatment.

The only medical treatment that may influence the outcome is administration of corticosteroids, but studies supporting this concept have been criticized. Many physicians nevertheless routinely prescribe corticosteroids for patients with Bell's palsy seen within 5 days of onset. The author prescribes them only when the palsy is clinically complete or there is severe pain. Treatment with prednisone, 60 or 80 mg daily in divided doses for 4 or 5 days, followed by tapering of the dose over the next 7–10 days, is a satisfactory regimen. It is helpful to protect the eye with lubricating drops (or lubricating ointment at night) and a patch if eye closure is not possible. There is no evidence that surgical procedures to decompress the facial nerve are of benefit.

DISCOGENIC NECK & BACK PAIN
(See also Chapter 20.)

1. LOW BACK PAIN

Spinal disease may lead to local pain, root pain, or both. It may also lead to pain that is referred to other parts of the involved dermatomes. Local pain may lead to protective reflex muscle spasm, which in turn causes further pain and may result in abnormal posture and limitation of movement. Radicular pain arises from compression, stretch, or irritation of nerve roots and usually radiates from the back to the territory of the affected root, being exacerbated by coughing, straining, or stretching of the nerve fibers, eg, by straight leg raising. Root disturbances may also lead to paresthesias and numbness in dermatomal (as opposed to peripheral nerve) distribution (Figure 24–1) and to weakness in segmental distribution; reflex changes may accompany involvement of motor or sensory fibers. Only pain due to disk disease is considered here; other causes have been considered in Chapter 20.

Acute Lumbar Intervertebral Disk Prolapse

This cause of low back pain generally involves the L4–5 or the L5–S1 disk and leads to back and radicular (L5 or S1) pain. The L4 root is occasionally affected, but involvement of a higher lumbar root should arouse suspicion of other causes of root compression. There may be accompanying numbness and paresthesias in dermatomal distribution or segmental motor deficit. An L5 radiculopathy causes weakness of dorsiflexion of the foot and toes. With an S1 root lesion, there is weakness of eversion and plantar flex-

ion of the foot and a depressed ankle jerk. A centrally prolapsed disk may lead to bilateral limb disturbances and sphincter involvement. Pelvic and rectal examination and plain x-rays of the spine help to exclude other disorders such as local primary cancers or metastatic deposits. Symptoms are often relieved with simple analgesics, diazepam, and bed rest on a firm mattress. Persisting pain, an increasing neurologic deficit, or any evidence of sphincter dysfunction calls for investigation by CT myelography—or, preferably, by MRI—followed by surgical treatment.

Degenerative Lumbar Osteoarthropathy & Chronic Disk Degeneration

This process leads to local pain, stiffness, and restricted activity. The radiologic findings vary from minor degenerative abnormalities to marked osteophytic spurs, ridges, and other changes. Even minor changes may lead to root or cord dysfunction when there is also a congenitally narrowed spinal canal (spinal stenosis). Pain, sometimes accompanied by weakness or radicular sensory disturbances in the legs, then occurs with activity or with certain postures and is relieved by rest. This has been referred to as neurogenic claudication; surgical decompression may be helpful in selected cases.

Ciricillo SF, Weinstein PR: Lumbar spinal stenosis. West J Med 1993;158:171. (Clinical review.)

Frank A: Low back pain. Br Med J 1993;306:901. (Practical overview.)

2. NECK PAIN

A variety of congenital abnormalities may involve the cervical spine and lead to neck pain; these include hemivertebrae, fused vertebrae, basilar impression, and instability of the atlantoaxial joint. Traumatic, degenerative, infective, and neoplastic disorders may also lead to pain in the neck. When rheumatoid arthritis involves the spine, it tends to affect especially the cervical region, leading to pain, stiffness, and reduced mobility; displacement of vertebrae or atlantoaxial subluxation may lead to cord compression that can be life-threatening if not treated by fixation. Further details are given in Chapter 20, and discussion here is restricted to disk disease.

Acute Cervical Disk Protrusion

Acute cervical disk protrusion leads to pain in the neck and radicular pain in the arm, exacerbated by head movement. With lateral herniation of the disk, motor, sensory, or reflex changes may be found in a radicular (usually C6 or C7) distribution on the affected side; with more centrally directed herniations, the spinal cord may also be involved, leading to spastic paraparesis and sensory disturbances in the legs,

Peripheral nerve

Nerve root

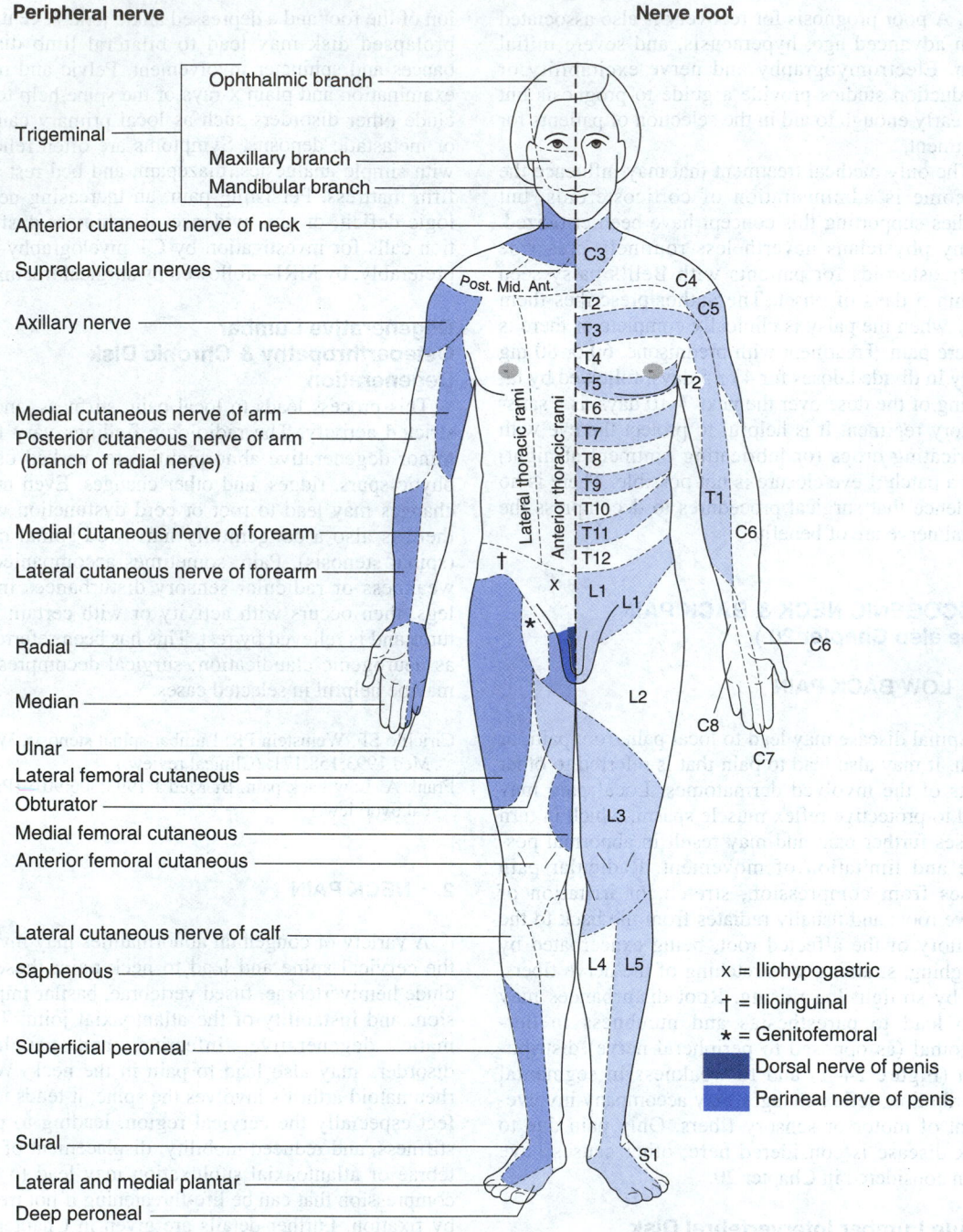

Ophthalmic branch

Trigeminal

Maxillary branch

Mandibular branch

Anterior cutaneous nerve of neck

Supraclavicular nerves

Axillary nerve

Medial cutaneous nerve of arm

Posterior cutaneous nerve of arm
(branch of radial nerve)

Medial cutaneous nerve of forearm

Lateral cutaneous nerve of forearm

Radial

Median

Ulnar

Lateral femoral cutaneous

Obturator

Medial femoral cutaneous

Anterior femoral cutaneous

Lateral cutaneous nerve of calf

Saphenous

Superficial peroneal

Sural

Lateral and medial plantar

Deep peroneal

Post. Mid. Ant.

C3
C4
C5
T2
T3
T4
T5
T6
T7
T8
T9
T10
T11
T12
L1
L2
L3
L4 L5
S1

Lateral thoracic rami

Anterior thoracic rami

T2
T1
C6
C8
C7

†
x
*

x = Iliohypogastric
† = Ilioinguinal
* = Genitofemoral

██ Dorsal nerve of penis
██ Perineal nerve of penis

Figure 24–1. Cutaneous innervation. The segmental or radicular (root) distribution is shown on the left side of the body and the peripheral nerve distribution on the right side. **Above:** anterior view; **facing page:** posterior view. (Reproduced, with permission, from Aminoff MJ, Greenberg DA, Simon RP: *Clinical Neurology,* 3rd ed. Appleton & Lange, 1996.)

Nerve root

Peripheral nerve

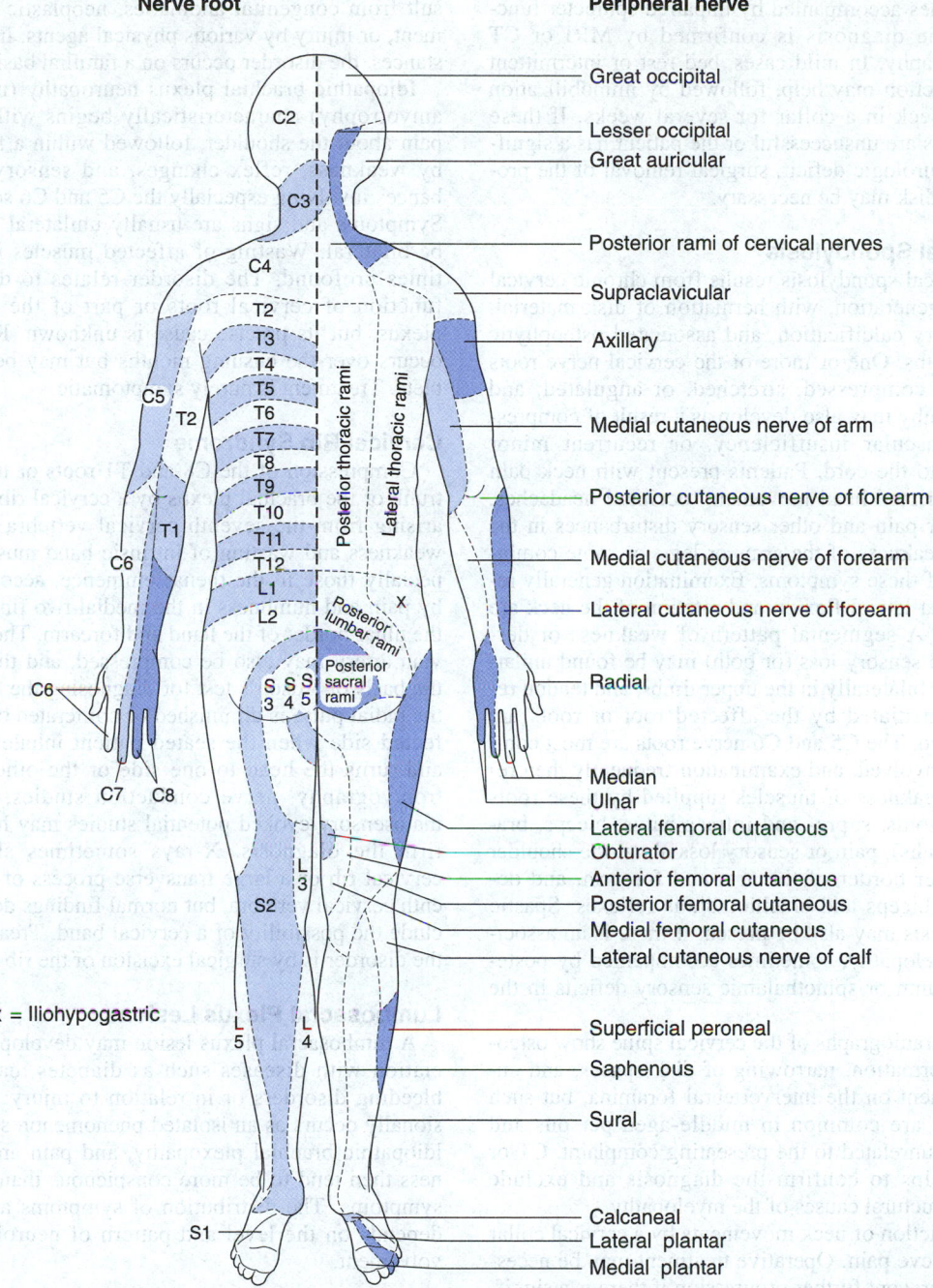

- Great occipital
- Lesser occipital
- Great auricular
- Posterior rami of cervical nerves
- Supraclavicular
- Axillary
- Medial cutaneous nerve of arm
- Posterior cutaneous nerve of forearm
- Medial cutaneous nerve of forearm
- Lateral cutaneous nerve of forearm
- Radial
- Median
- Ulnar
- Lateral femoral cutaneous
- Obturator
- Anterior femoral cutaneous
- Posterior femoral cutaneous
- Medial femoral cutaneous
- Lateral cutaneous nerve of calf
- Superficial peroneal
- Saphenous
- Sural
- Calcaneal
- Lateral plantar
- Medial plantar

C2, C3, C4, T2, T3, T4, T5, T6, T7, T8, T9, T10, T11, T12, L1, L2, C5, T2, C6, T1, C6, C7, C8

Posterior thoracic rami

Lateral thoracic rami

Posterior lumbar rami

Posterior sacral rami

S3 S4 S5

L3, S2, L5, L4, S1

x = Iliohypogastric

Figure 24–1. (Continued)

sometimes accompanied by impaired sphincter function. The diagnosis is confirmed by MRI or CT myelography. In mild cases, bed rest or intermittent neck traction may help, followed by immobilization of the neck in a collar for several weeks. If these measures are unsuccessful or the patient has a significant neurologic deficit, surgical removal of the protruding disk may be necessary.

Cervical Spondylosis

Cervical spondylosis results from chronic cervical disk degeneration, with herniation of disk material, secondary calcification, and associated osteophytic outgrowths. One or more of the cervical nerve roots may be compressed, stretched, or angulated; and myelopathy may also develop as a result of compression, vascular insufficiency, or recurrent minor trauma to the cord. Patients present with neck pain and restricted head movement, occipital headaches, radicular pain and other sensory disturbances in the arms, weakness of the arms or legs, or some combination of these symptoms. Examination generally reveals that lateral flexion and rotation of the neck are limited. A segmental pattern of weakness or dermatomal sensory loss (or both) may be found unilaterally or bilaterally in the upper limbs, and tendon reflexes mediated by the affected root or roots are depressed. The C5 and C6 nerve roots are most commonly involved, and examination frequently then reveals weakness of muscles supplied by these roots (eg, deltoids, supra- and infraspinatus, biceps, brachioradialis), pain or sensory loss about the shoulder and outer border of the arm and forearm, and depressed biceps and brachioradialis reflexes. Spastic paraparesis may also be present if there is an associated myelopathy, sometimes accompanied by posterior column or spinothalamic sensory deficits in the legs.

Plain radiographs of the cervical spine show osteophyte formation, narrowing of disk spaces, and encroachment on the intervertebral foramina, but such changes are common in middle-aged persons and may be unrelated to the presenting complaint. CT or MRI helps to confirm the diagnosis and exclude other structural causes of the myelopathy.

Restriction of neck movements by a cervical collar may relieve pain. Operative treatment may be necessary to prevent further progression if there is a significant neurologic deficit or if root pain is severe, persistent, and unresponsive to conservative measures.

BRACHIAL & LUMBAR PLEXUS LESIONS

Brachial Plexus Neuropathy

Brachial plexus neuropathy may be idiopathic, sometimes occurring in relationship to a number of different nonspecific illnesses or factors. In other instances, brachial plexus lesions follow trauma or result from congenital anomalies, neoplastic involvement, or injury by various physical agents. In rare instances, the disorder occurs on a familial basis.

Idiopathic brachial plexus neuropathy (neuralgic amyotrophy) characteristically begins with severe pain about the shoulder, followed within a few days by weakness, reflex changes, and sensory disturbances involving especially the C5 and C6 segments. Symptoms and signs are usually unilateral but may be bilateral. Wasting of affected muscles is sometimes profound. The disorder relates to disturbed function of cervical roots or part of the brachial plexus, but its precise cause is unknown. Recovery occurs over the ensuing months but may be incomplete. Treatment is purely symptomatic.

Cervical Rib Syndrome

Compression of the C8 and T1 roots or the lower trunk of the brachial plexus by a cervical rib or band arising from the seventh cervical vertebra leads to weakness and wasting of intrinsic hand muscles, especially those in the thenar eminence, accompanied by pain and numbness in the medial two fingers and the ulnar border of the hand and forearm. The subclavian artery may also be compressed, and this forms the basis of Adson's test for diagnosing the disorder; the radial pulse is diminished or obliterated on the affected side when the seated patient inhales deeply and turns the head to one side or the other. Electromyography, nerve conduction studies, and somatosensory evoked potential studies may help confirm the diagnosis. X-rays sometimes show the cervical rib or a large transverse process of the seventh cervical vertebra, but normal findings do not exclude the possibility of a cervical band. Treatment of the disorder is by surgical excision of the rib or band.

Lumbosacral Plexus Lesions

A lumbosacral plexus lesion may develop in association with diseases such as diabetes, cancer, or bleeding disorders or in relation to injury. It occasionally occurs as an isolated phenomenon similar to idiopathic brachial plexopathy, and pain and weakness then tend to be more conspicuous than sensory symptoms. The distribution of symptoms and signs depends on the level and pattern of neurologic involvement.

DISORDERS OF NEUROMUSCULAR TRANSMISSION

1. MYASTHENIA GRAVIS

Essentials of Diagnosis

- Fluctuating weakness of commonly used voluntary muscles, producing symptoms such as diplopia, ptosis, and difficulty in swallowing.
- Activity increases weakness of affected muscles.

- Short-acting anticholinesterases transiently improve the weakness.

General Considerations

Myasthenia gravis occurs at all ages, sometimes in association with a thymic tumor or thyrotoxicosis, as well as in rheumatoid arthritis and lupus erythematosus. It is commonest in young women with HLA-DR3; if thymoma is associated, older men are more commonly affected. Onset is usually insidious, but the disorder is sometimes unmasked by a coincidental infection that leads to exacerbation of symptoms. Exacerbations may also occur before the menstrual period and during or shortly after pregnancy. Symptoms are due to a variable degree of block of neuromuscular transmission caused by autoantibodies binding to acetylcholine receptors; these are found in most patients with the disease and have a primary role in reducing the number of functioning acetylcholine receptors. Additionally, cellular immune activity against the receptor is found. Clinically, this leads to weakness; initially powerful movements fatigue readily. The external ocular muscles and certain other cranial muscles, including the masticatory, facial, and pharyngeal muscles, are especially likely to be affected, and the respiratory and limb muscles may also be involved.

Clinical Findings

A. Symptoms and Signs: Patients present with ptosis, diplopia, difficulty in chewing or swallowing, respiratory difficulties, limb weakness, or some combination of these problems. Weakness may remain localized to a few muscle groups, especially the ocular muscles, or may become generalized. Symptoms often fluctuate in intensity during the day, and this diurnal variation is superimposed on a tendency to longer-term spontaneous relapses and remissions that may last for weeks. Nevertheless, the disorder follows a slowly progressive course and may have a fatal outcome owing to respiratory complications such as aspiration pneumonia.

Clinical examination confirms the weakness and fatigability of affected muscles. In most cases, the extraocular muscles are involved, and this leads to ocular palsies and ptosis, which are commonly asymmetric. Pupillary responses are normal. The bulbar and limb muscles are often weak, but the pattern of involvement is variable. Sustained activity of affected muscles increases the weakness, which improves after a brief rest. Sensation is normal, and there are usually no reflex changes.

The diagnosis can generally be confirmed by the response to a short-acting anticholinesterase. Edrophonium can be given intravenously in a dose of 10 mg (1 mL), 2 mg being given initially and the remaining 8 mg about 30 seconds later if the test dose is well tolerated; in myasthenic patients, there is an obvious improvement in strength of weak muscles lasting for about 5 minutes. Alternatively, 1.5 mg of neostigmine can be given intramuscularly, and the response then lasts for about 2 hours; atropine sulfate (0.6 mg) should be available to reverse muscarinic side effects.

B. Imaging: Lateral and anteroposterior x-rays of the chest and CT scans should be obtained to demonstrate a coexisting thymoma, but normal studies do not exclude this possibility.

C. Laboratory and Other Studies: Electrophysiologic demonstration of a decrementing muscle response to repetitive 2- or 3-Hz stimulation of motor nerves indicates a disturbance of neuromuscular transmission. Such an abnormality may even be detected in clinically strong muscles with certain provocative procedures. Needle electromyography of affected muscles shows a marked variation in configuration and size of individual motor unit potentials, and single-fiber electromyography reveals an increased jitter, or variability, in the time interval between two muscle fiber action potentials from the same motor unit.

Assay of serum for elevated levels of circulating acetylcholine receptor antibodies is another approach—increasingly used—to the laboratory diagnosis of myasthenia gravis and has a sensitivity of 80–90%.

Treatment

Medication such as aminoglycosides that may exacerbate myasthenia gravis should be avoided. Anticholinesterase drugs provide symptomatic benefit without influencing the course of the disease. Neostigmine, pyridostigmine, or both can be used, the dose being determined on an individual basis. The usual dose of neostigmine is 7.5–30 mg (average, 15 mg) taken four times daily; of pyridostigmine, 30–180 mg (average, 60 mg) four times daily. Overmedication may temporarily increase weakness, which is then unaffected or enhanced by intravenous edrophonium.

Thymectomy usually leads to symptomatic benefit or remission and should be considered in all patients younger than age 60, unless weakness is restricted to the extraocular muscles. If the disease is of recent onset and only slowly progressive, operation is sometimes delayed for a year or so, in the hope that spontaneous remission will occur.

Treatment with corticosteroids is indicated for patients who have responded poorly to anticholinesterase drugs and have already undergone thymectomy. It is introduced with the patient in the hospital, since weakness may initially be aggravated. Once weakness has stabilized after 2–3 weeks or any improvement is sustained, further management can be on an outpatient basis. Alternate-day treatment is usually well tolerated, but if weakness is enhanced on the nontreatment day it may be necessary for medication to be taken daily. The dose of corticosteroids is determined on an individual basis, but an initial high daily dose (eg, prednisone, 60–100 mg) can gradually be tapered to a relatively low maintenance level as improvement occurs; total withdrawal is difficult, however. Treatment with azathioprine may also be effective. The usual dose is 2–3 mg/kg orally daily after a lower initial dose.

In patients with major disability in whom conventional treatment is either unhelpful or contraindicated, plasmapheresis or intravenous immunoglobulin therapy may be beneficial. It may also be useful for stabilizing patients before thymectomy and for managing acute crisis.

2. MYASTHENIC SYNDROME
(Lambert-Eaton Syndrome)

Myasthenic syndrome may be associated with small-cell carcinoma, sometimes developing before the tumor is diagnosed, and occasionally occurs with certain autoimmune diseases. There is defective release of acetylcholine in response to a nerve impulse, and this leads to weakness especially of the proximal muscles of the limbs. As is not the case in myasthenia gravis, however, power steadily increases with sustained contraction. The diagnosis can be confirmed electrophysiologically, because the muscle response to stimulation of its motor nerve increases remarkably if the nerve is stimulated repetitively at high rates, even in muscles that are not clinically weak.

Treatment with plasmapheresis and immunosuppressive drug therapy (prednisone and azathioprine) may lead to clinical and electrophysiologic improvement, in addition to therapy aimed at tumor when present. Prednisone is usually initiated in a daily dose of 60–80 mg and azathioprine in a daily dose of 2 mg/kg. Guanidine hydrochloride (25–50 mg/kg/d in divided doses) is occasionally helpful in seriously disabled patients, but adverse effects of the drug include marrow suppression. The response to treatment with anticholinesterase drugs such as pyridostigmine or neostigmine, either alone or in combination with guanidine, is variable.

3. BOTULISM

The toxin of *Clostridium botulinum* prevents the release of acetylcholine at neuromuscular junctions and autonomic synapses. Botulism occurs most commonly following the ingestion of contaminated home-canned food and should be suggested by the development of sudden, fluctuating, severe weakness in a previously healthy person. Symptoms begin within 72 hours following ingestion of the toxin and may progress for several days. Typically, there is diplopia, ptosis, facial weakness, dysphagia, and

nasal speech, followed by respiratory difficulty and finally by weakness that appears last in the limbs. Blurring of vision (with unreactive dilated pupils) is characteristic, and there may be dryness of the mouth, constipation (paralytic ileus), and postural hypotension. Sensation is preserved, and the tendon reflexes are not affected unless the involved muscles are very weak. If the diagnosis is suspected, the local health authority should be notified and a sample of serum and contaminated food (if available) sent to be assayed for toxin. Support for the diagnosis may be obtained by electrophysiologic studies; with repetitive stimulation of motor nerves at fast rates, the muscle response increases in size progressively.

Patients should be hospitalized in case respiratory assistance becomes necessary. Treatment is with trivalent antitoxin, once it is established that the patient is not allergic to horse serum. Guanidine hydrochloride (25–50 mg/kg/d in divided doses) to facilitate release of acetylcholine from nerve endings sometimes helps to increase muscle strength. Anticholinesterase drugs are of no value. Respiratory assistance and other supportive measures should be provided as necessary. Further details are provided in Chapter 33.

4. DISORDERS ASSOCIATED WITH USE OF AMINOGLYCOSIDES

Aminoglycoside antibiotics, eg, gentamicin, may produce a clinical disturbance similar to botulism by preventing the release of acetylcholine from nerve endings, but symptoms subside rapidly as the responsible drug is eliminated from the body. These antibiotics are particularly dangerous in patients with preexisting disturbances of neuromuscular transmission and are therefore best avoided in patients with myasthenia gravis.

MYOPATHIC DISORDERS

Muscular Dystrophies

These inherited myopathic disorders are characterized by progressive muscle weakness and wasting. They are subdivided by mode of inheritance, age at onset, and clinical features, as shown in Table 24–6. In the Duchenne type, pseudohypertrophy of muscles frequently occurs at some stage; intellectual retardation is common; and there may be skeletal deformities, muscle contractures, and cardiac involvement. The serum creatine kinase level is increased, especially in the Duchenne and Becker varieties, and mildly increased also in limb-girdle dystrophy. Electromyography may help to confirm that weakness is myopathic rather than neurogenic. Similarly, histopathologic examination of a muscle biopsy specimen may help to confirm that weakness is due

Table 24–6. The muscular dystrophies.

Disorder	Inheritance	Age at Onset (years)	Distribution	Prognosis
Duchenne type	X-linked recessive	1–5	Pelvic, then shoulder girdle; later, limb and respiratory muscles.	Rapid progression. Death within about 15 years after onset.
Becker's	X-linked recessive	5–25	Pelvic, then shoulder girdle.	Slow progression. May have normal life span.
Limb-girdle (Erb's)	Autosomal recessive (may be sporadic or dominant)	10–30	Pelvic or shoulder girdle initially, with later spread to the other.	Variable severity and rate of progression. Possible severe disability in middle life.
Facioscapulo-humeral	Autosomal dominant	Any age	Face and shoulder girdle initially; later, pelvic girdle and legs.	Slow progression. Minor disability. Usually normal life span.
Distal	Autosomal dominant	40–60	Onset distally in extremities; proximal involvement later.	Slow progression.
Ocular	Autosomal dominant (may be recessive)	Any age (usually 5–30)	External ocular muscles. May also be mild weakness of face, neck, and arms.	
Oculopharyngeal	Autosomal dominant	Any age	As in the ocular form but with dysphagia.	

to a primary disorder of muscle and to distinguish between various muscle diseases.

A genetic defect on the short arm of the X chromosome has been identified in Duchenne dystrophy. The affected gene codes for the protein dystrophin, which is markedly reduced or absent from the muscle of patients with the disease. Dystrophin levels are generally normal in the Becker variety, but the protein is qualitatively altered.

Duchenne muscular dystrophy can now be recognized early in pregnancy in about 95% of women by genetic studies; in late pregnancy, DNA probes can be used on fetal tissue obtained for this purpose by amniocentesis. The gene causing facioscapulo-humeral dystrophy has recently been localized to the long arm of chromosome 4. The genetic defect has been characterized, but the abnormal gene product is not yet known.

There is no specific treatment for the muscular dystrophies, but it is important to encourage patients to lead as normal lives as possible. Prolonged bed rest must be avoided, as inactivity often leads to worsening of the underlying muscle disease. Physical therapy and orthopedic procedures may help to counteract deformities or contractures.

Karpati G, Acsadi G: The potential for gene therapy in Duchenne muscular dystrophy and other genetic muscle diseases. Muscle Nerve 1993;16:1141.

Myotonic Dystrophy

Myotonic dystrophy, a slowly progressive, dominantly inherited disorder, usually manifests itself in the third or fourth decade but occasionally appears early in childhood. The genetic defect has been localized to the long arm of chromosome 19. Myotonia leads to complaints of muscle stiffness and is evidenced by the marked delay that occurs before affected muscles can relax after a contraction. This can often be demonstrated clinically by delayed relaxation of the hand after sustained grip or by percussion of the belly of a muscle. In addition, there is weakness and wasting of the facial, sternocleidomastoid, and distal limb muscles. Associated clinical features include cataracts, frontal baldness, testicular atrophy, diabetes mellitus, cardiac abnormalities, and intellectual changes. Electromyographic sampling of affected muscles reveals myotonic discharges in addition to changes suggestive of myopathy.

Myotonia can be treated with quinine sulfate (300–400 mg three times daily), procainamide (0.5–1 g four times daily), or phenytoin (100 mg three times daily). More recently, tocainide and mexiletine have been used. In myotonic dystrophy, phenytoin is preferred, since the other drugs may have undesirable effects on cardiac conduction. Neither the weakness nor the course of the disorder is influenced by treatment.

Ptacek LJ et al: Genetics and physiology of the myotonic muscle disorders. N Engl J Med 1993;328:482.

Myotonia Congenita

Myotonia congenita is commonly inherited as a dominant trait. The responsible gene may be on the long arm of chromosome 7. Generalized myotonia without weakness is usually present from birth, but symptoms may not appear until early childhood. Patients complain of muscle stiffness that is enhanced by cold and inactivity and relieved by exercise. Muscle hypertrophy, at times pronounced, is also a feature. A recessive form with later onset is associated with slight weakness and atrophy of distal muscles. Treatment with quinine sulfate, procainamide, tocainide, mexiletine, or phenytoin may help the myotonia, as in myotonic dystrophy.

Polymyositis & Dermatomyositis

See Chapter 20.

Inclusion Body Myositis

This disorder, of unknown cause, begins insidiously, usually after middle age, with progressive proximal weakness of first the lower and then the upper extremities. Distal weakness is usually mild. Serum creatine kinase levels may be normal or increased. The diagnosis is confirmed by muscle biopsy. In contrast to polymyositis, corticosteroid therapy is usually ineffective.

Mitochondrial Myopathies

The mitochondrial myopathies are a clinically diverse group of disorders that on pathologic examination of skeletal muscle with the modified Gomori stain show characteristic "ragged red fibers" containing accumulations of abnormal mitochondria. Patients may present with progressive external ophthalmoplegia or with limb weakness that is exacerbated or induced by activity. Other patients present with central neurologic dysfunction, eg, myoclonic epilepsy (myoclonic epilepsy, ragged red fiber syndrome, or MERRF), or the combination of myopathy, encephalopathy, lactic acidosis, and stroke-like episodes (MELAS). These disorders result from separate abnormalities of mitochondrial DNA. (See also Chapter 19.)

Myopathies Associated With Other Disorders

Myopathy may occur in association with chronic hypokalemia, any endocrinopathy, and in patients taking corticosteroids, chloroquine, colchicine, clofibrate, emetine, aminocaproic acid, lovastatin, bretylium tosylate, or drugs causing potassium depletion. Weakness is mainly proximal, and serum creatine kinase is typically normal, except in hypothyroidism and some of the toxic myopathies. Treatment is of the underlying cause. Myopathy also occurs with chronic alcoholism, whereas acute reversible muscle necrosis may occur shortly after acute alcohol intoxication. Inflammatory myopathy may occur in patients taking penicillamine; myotonia may be induced by diazocholesterol or clofibrate; and preexisting myotonia may be exacerbated or unmasked by depolarizing muscle relaxants (eg, suxamethonium), beta-blockers (eg, propranolol), fenoterol, ritodrine, and, possibly, certain diuretics.

PERIODIC PARALYSIS SYNDROME

Periodic paralysis may have a familial (dominant inheritance) basis. Episodes of flaccid weakness or paralysis occur, sometimes in association with abnormalities of the plasma potassium level. Strength is normal between attacks. The **hypokalemic** variety is characterized by attacks that tend to occur on awakening, after exercise, or after a heavy meal and may last for several days. Patients should avoid excessive exertion. A low-carbohydrate and low-salt diet may help prevent attacks, as may acetazolamide, 250–750 mg/d. An ongoing attack may be aborted by potassium chloride given orally or by intravenous drip, provided the ECG can be monitored and renal function is satisfactory. In young Asian men, it is commonly associated with hyperthyroidism; treatment of the endocrine disorder then prevents recurrences. In **hyperkalemic** periodic paralysis, attacks also tend to occur after exercise but usually last for less than an hour. They may be terminated by intravenous calcium gluconate (1–2 g) or by intravenous diuretics (furosemide, 20–40 mg), glucose, or glucose and insulin; daily acetazolamide or chlorothiazide may prevent recurrences. Genetic linkage studies suggest that many families with this disorder have a defect in the sodium channel gene on the long arm of chromosome 17. **Normokalemic** periodic paralysis is similar clinically to the hyperkalemic variety, but the plasma potassium level remains normal during attacks; treatment is with acetazolamide.

Feero WG et al: Hyperkalemic periodic paralysis: Rapid molecular diagnosis and relationship of genotype to phenotype in 12 families. Neurology 1993;43:668. (Genotype-phenotype correlations.)

Psychiatric Disorders

25

Stuart J. Eisendrath, MD

Psychiatric disorders are functional impairments that may result from disturbance of one or more of the following interrelated factors: (1) biologic function, (2) psychodynamic adaptation, (3) learned behavior, and (4) social and environmental conditions. Although the clinical situation at a given time determines which area of dysfunction will be emphasized, proper patient care requires an approach that adequately evaluates all factors.

Biologic Function

Psychiatric disorders of biologic origin may be secondary to identifiable physical illness or caused by biochemical disturbances of the brain. A wide variety of psychiatric disorders (eg, psychosis, depression, delirium, anxiety) as well as nonspecific symptoms are caused by organic brain disease or by derangement of cerebral metabolism resulting from illness, biochemical aberrations (usually neurotransmitter dysfunction), nutritional deficiencies, or toxic agents.

Neurotransmitter functions have been correlated with the major psychiatric disorders. Cholinergic deficiency is present in some dementias, and adrenergic imbalance is important in some psychoses. Serotonergic mechanisms are significantly involved in affective disorders, aggression, autism, and the anxiety disorders, particularly obsessive-compulsive disorders.

Psychodynamic Maladaptation

Psychodynamic maladaptation involves intrapsychic aberrations and is usually treated by a psychotherapeutic approach. There are many forms of psychotherapy: supportive, interpretive, cognitive, persuasive, educative, or some combination of these methods. Depth, duration, intensity, and frequency of sessions may vary.

Learned Behavior

Learned behavior is part of the pathogenetic mechanism in all psychiatric disorders. For example, in somatization disorder, the patient may have learned that being sick is the only way to get attention. Alter-

ing such positive reinforcement may be critical in producing a change in behavior. Personality disorders are examples of failure to learn to incorporate patterns of behavior acceptable in social surroundings.

Social & Environmental Conditions

Social and environmental factors have always been considered of vital importance in the mental balance of the individual. Without encounter with the environment, there can be no socially recognized illness: The exigencies of everyday life contribute both to the development of a stable personality and to the deviations from the norm. There is a constantly changing ethnic influence that determines which types of behavior will be tolerated or considered deviant. Cultural attitudes and fears play key roles in the perception of illness and acceptance of treatment. Changes in the family unit have coincided with changes in work patterns of parents and in schooling and work patterns of young adults. The changes are complex and generally have lengthened the period of dependency and increased stresses in the family unit; this, in turn, affects the underlying social fabric.

Aldrich CK: Psychiatry in 2001. J Fam Pract 1993;36:323. (The authors urge greater commitment by family medicine to psychosocial training and research, especially in areas such as physician-patient and physician-family relationships.)

Gabbard GO: Mind and brain in psychiatric treatment. In: *Synopsis of Treatment of Psychiatric Disorders,* 2nd ed. Gabbard SD, Atkinson SD (editors). American Psychiatric Press, 1996.

PSYCHIATRIC ASSESSMENT

Psychiatric diagnosis rests upon the established principles of a thorough history and examination. All of the forces contributing to the individual's life situation must be identified, and this can be done only if the examination includes the history; mental status; medical conditions (including drugs); and pertinent social, cultural, and environmental factors impinging on the individual.

Interview

Every psychiatric history should cover the following points: (1) complaint, from the patient's viewpoint; (2) the present illness, or the evolution of the complaints; (3) previous disorders and the nature and extent of treatment; (4) the family history—important for genetic aspects and family influences; (5) personal history—childhood development, adolescent adjustment, level of education, and adult coping patterns; (6) sexual history; (7) current life functioning, with attention to vocational, social, educational, and avocational areas; and (8) current medications, alcohol, or other drugs.

It is often essential to obtain additional information from the family. Observing interactions of significant other people with the patient in the context of a family interview may give significant diagnostic information and may even underscore the nature of the problem and suggest a therapeutic approach.

The formal mental status examination should be particularly detailed when there is any evidence or high risk of cognitive dysfunction. The mental status examination includes the following: (1) Appearance: Note unusual modes of dress, use of makeup, etc. (2) Activity and behavior: Gait, gestures, coordination of bodily movements, etc. (3) Affect: Outward manifestation of emotions such as depression, anger, elation, fear, resentment, or lack of emotional response. (4) Mood: The patient's report of feelings and observable emotional manifestations. (5) Speech: Coherence, spontaneity, articulation, hesitancy in answering, and duration of response. (6) Content of thought: Associations, preoccupations, obsessions, depersonalization, delusions, hallucinations, paranoid ideation, anger, fear, or unusual experiences. (7) Cognition: (a) orientation to person, place, time, and circumstances; (b) remote and recent memory and recall; (c) calculations, digit retention (six forward is normal), serial sevens or threes; (d) general fund of knowledge (presidents, states, distances, events); (e) abstracting ability, often tested with common proverbs or with analogies and differences (eg, "How are a lie and a mistake the same, and how are they different?"); (f) ability to identify by naming, reading, and writing specified test names and objects; (g) ideomotor function, which combines understanding and the ability to perform a task (eg, "Show me how to throw a ball"); (h) ability to reproduce geometric constructions (eg, parallelogram, intersecting squares); and (i) right-left differentiation. (8) Judgment regarding commonsense problems such as what to do when one runs out of medicine. (9) Insight into

the nature and extent of the current difficulty and its ramifications in the patient's daily life.

Cognitive tests such as the Mini-Mental Status Examination produce a numerical score with up to 30 points given for correct answers to questions (clearly organic < 20 points). Specific cognitive assessment must be performed, since many patients are able to cover a deficit in routine conversation.

The examination of a psychiatric patient must include a complete medical history and physical examination (with emphasis on the neurologic examination) as well as all necessary laboratory and other special studies. Physical illness may frequently present as psychiatric disease, and vice versa.

Special Diagnostic Aids

Many tests and evaluation procedures are available that can be used to support and clarify initial diagnostic impressions.

A. Psychologic Testing: Testing by a psychologist may measure intelligence and cognitive functioning; provide information about personality, feelings, psychodynamics, and psychopathology; and differentiate psychic problems from organic ones. The place of such tests is similar to that of other tests in medicine—helpful in diagnostic problems but a useless expense when not needed.

1. Objective tests–These tests provide quantitative evaluation compared to standard norms.

a. Intelligence tests–The test most frequently used is the Wechsler Adult Intelligence Scale–Revised (WAIS-R). Intelligence tests often reveal more than IQ. The results, given expert interpretation, can quantify intellectual deterioration that has occurred.

b. Minnesota Multiphasic Personality Inventory (MMPI)–The MMPI is an empirically based test of personality assessment. The patient's scores are interpreted in comparison with data about others with the same response pattern to assess psychopathologic changes.

c. Screening instruments–These tests include the Beck Depression Inventory and the Prime-MD. They quantify dysphoric moods such as anxiety and depression.

d. Neuropsychologic assessment–Such an assessment is made when an organic deficit is present but information on anatomic location and extent of dysfunction is required.

2. Projective tests–These tests are unstructured, so that the patient is forced to respond in ways that reflect fantasies and individual modes of adaptation. They are particularly useful in identifying psychotic disorders and unconscious motivations.

a. Rorschach Psychodiagnostics–This test utilizes ten inkblots to provide important information on psychodynamic themes and aberrations.

b. Thematic Apperception Test (TAT)–This test uses 20 pictures of people in different situations to assess areas of interpersonal conflicts.

B. Neurologic Evaluation: Consultation is often necessary and may include specialized tests. Brain imaging is useful for detecting structural abnormalities in the patient who presents with a nondefinitive history and examination (eg, dissociative episodes, unusual psychotic episodes not explained by drug abuse). MRI is particularly useful in delineating lesions and identifying demyelinating and degenerative diseases (eg, Huntington's disease). Electroencephalography is particularly useful for the diagnosis of seizure disorders and in differentiating delirium from depression or dementia. Typically, delirium is associated with generalized electroencephalographic slowing, while depression and dementia do not have this change. Single photon emission computed tomography (SPECT) is a gamma imaging technology like PET, and both provide tomographic images of brain activity. SPECT is cheaper but has the disadvantages of lower image resolution and lower quantification of regional brain activity.

Formulation of the Diagnosis

A psychiatric diagnosis must be based upon positive evidence accumulated by the above techniques. It must not be based simply on the exclusion of organic findings.

A thorough psychiatric evaluation has therapeutic as well as diagnostic value and should be expressed in ways best understood by the patient, family, and other physicians.

Crum RM et al: Population-based norms for the Mini-Mental State Examination by age and educational level. JAMA 1993;269:2386. (Older or less well educated subjects may score somewhat lower but still may be normal.)

McNiel DE, Binder RL: Correlates of accuracy in the assessment of psychiatric inpatients' risk of violence. Am J Psychiatry 1995;152:901. (Clinicians can accurately classify the potential for violence in the majority of patients at admission.)

Reifler DR et al: Impact of screening for mental health concerns on health service utilization and functional status in primary care patients. Arch Intern Med 1996; 156:2593.

Schuckit MA et al: Difficult differential diagnoses in psychiatry: The clinical use of SPECT. J Clin Psychiatry 1995;56:539.

TREATMENT APPROACHES

The approaches to treatment of psychiatric patients are, in a broad sense, similar to those in other branches of medicine. For example, the internist treating a patient with heart disease uses not only **medical** measures such as digitalis and pacemakers but also **psychologic** techniques to change attitudes and behaviors, **social** and **environmental** manipulation to mitigate deleterious influences, and **behavioral** techniques to change behavior patterns.

Regardless of the methods employed, treatment must be directed toward an objective, ie, it must be **goal-oriented.** This usually involves (1) obtaining active cooperation on the part of the patient; (2) establishing reasonable goals and modifying the goal if failure occurs; (3) emphasizing positive behavior (goals) instead of symptom behavior (problems); (4) delineating the method; and (5) setting a time frame (which can be modified later).

The physician must resist pressures for instantaneous results. In almost all cases, psychiatric treatment involves the active participation of the significant people in the patient's life. Time must be spent with the patient, but the frequency and duration of appointments are highly variable and should be adjusted to meet both the patient's psychologic needs and financial restrictions. Compliance (collaboration) is the end product of many factors, the most important being clear communication, attention to cost, and simple dosage regimens when drugs are prescribed. The physician can unwittingly promote chronic illness by prescribing inappropriate medication. The patient may come to believe that problems respond only to medication, and the more drugs prescribed, the stronger the misconception becomes.

Psychiatric Consultation

All physicians are in an excellent position to meet their patients' emotional needs in an organized and competent way, referring to psychiatrists for consultation or for ongoing treatment of patients whose problems are considered beyond the expertise of the referring physician. The most pressing problems involve evaluation of suicidal or assaultive potential and diagnostic differentiation in mood disorders and psychoses. Psychiatric problems associated with unusual psychopharmacologic therapy and with medications used in other branches of medicine may require pharmacologic consultation. When a psychiatric referral is made, it should be conducted like any other referral: in an open manner, with full explanation of the problem to the patient.

Hospitalization

The need for hospital care may range from admission to a medical bed in a general hospital for an acute situational stress reaction to admission to a psychiatric ward when the patient is in acute psychosis. The trend over recent years has been to admit patients to general hospitals in the community, treat patients aggressively, and discharge them promptly to the next appropriate level of treatment—day hospital, halfway house, outpatient therapy, etc. The decision to propose involuntary hospitalization should be taken only after weighing the potential benefits to the patient and the community against the individual's loss of autonomy. Sixty percent of all psychiatric admissions are readmissions. The total "in residence" population (hospital plus residential) is about the same as the hospital total of 30 years ago. This population does not include the homeless mentally ill, however—a group that would have been institutionalized in past years.

Hospital care may be indicated when patients are too sick to care for themselves or when they present serious threats to themselves or others; when observation and diagnostic procedures are necessary; or when specific kinds of treatment such as complex medication trials or a hospital environment ("milieu therapy") are required. Symptoms calling for hospitalization are self-neglect, violent or bizarre behavior, paranoid ideation or delusions, marked intellectual impairment, and poor judgment.

The disadvantages of psychiatric hospitalization include decreased self-confidence as a result of needing hospitalization; the stigma of being a "psychiatric patient"; possible increased dependency and regression; and the expense. Generally, there is no advantage to prolonged hospital stays for most psychiatric disorders. Partial hospitalization or "day" programs are providing many of the benefits of hospitalization without some of the disadvantages; in these programs, the patient attends daytime treatment but sleeps at home.

Grisso T, Appelbaum PS: Comparison of standards for assessing patients' capacities to make treatment decisions. Am J Psychiatry 1995;52:1033. (Choice of standards for determining competence will affect the identity and proportion of patients classified as impaired.)
Katon W et al: Collaborative management to achieve treatment guidelines. Impact on depression in primary care. JAMA 1995;273:1026. (Collaborative management by the primary care physician and a consulting psychiatrist, intensive patient education, and surveillance of continued refills of antidepressant medication improved adherence to antidepressant regimens in patients with major and with minor depression.)

COMMON PSYCHIATRIC DISORDERS

STRESS & ADJUSTMENT DISORDERS (Situational Disorders)

Essentials of Diagnosis

- Anxiety or depression clearly secondary to an identifiable stress.
- Future symptoms of anxiety or depression commonly elicited by similar stress of lesser magnitude.
- Alcohol and other drugs are commonly used in self-treatment.

General Considerations

Stress exists when the adaptive capacity of the individual is overwhelmed by events. The event may be an insignificant one objectively considered, and even favorable changes (eg, promotion and transfer) requiring adaptive behavior can produce stress. For each individual, stress is subjectively defined, and the response to stress is a function of each person's personality and physiologic endowment.

Classification & Clinical Findings

Opinion differs about what events are most apt to produce stress reactions. The causes of stress are different at different ages—eg, in young adulthood, the sources of stress are found in the marriage or parent-child relationship, the employment relationship, and the struggle to achieve financial stability; in the middle years, the focus shifts to changing spousal relationships, problems with aging parents, and problems associated with having young adult offspring who themselves are encountering stressful situations; in old age, the principal concerns are apt to be retirement, loss of physical capacity, major personal losses, and thoughts of death.

An individual may react to stress by becoming anxious or depressed, by developing a physical symptom, by running away, by having a drink or starting an affair, or in limitless other ways. Common subjective responses are fear (of repetition of the stress-inducing event), rage (at frustration), guilt (over aggressive impulses), and shame (over helplessness). Acute and reactivated stress may be manifested by restlessness, irritability, fatigue, increased startle reaction, and a feeling of tension. Inability to concentrate, sleep disturbances (insomnia, bad dreams), and somatic preoccupations often lead to self-medication, most commonly with alcohol or other central nervous system depressants. Maladaptive behavior to stress is called adjustment disorder, with the major symptom specified (eg, "adjustment disorder with depressed mood").

Posttraumatic stress disorder is a syndrome characterized by "reexperiencing" the traumatic event (eg, rape, severe burns, military combat), along with decreased responsiveness to and avoidance of current events associated with the trauma; and physiologic hyperarousal, which includes startle reactions, intrusive thoughts, illusions, overgeneralized associations, sleep problems, nightmares, dreams about the precipitating event, impulsivity, difficulties in concentration, and hyperalertness. The symptoms may be precipitated or exacerbated by distant events that are a reminder of the original stress (less common with the anxiety disorders). Symptoms frequently arise after a long latency period (eg, child abuse can result in later posttraumatic stress syndrome). The sooner the symptoms arise after the initial trauma and the sooner therapy is initiated, the better the prognosis. The therapeutic approach is to facilitate the normal recovery that was blocked at the time of the trauma. Therapy at that time should be brief, simple (catharsis and working through of the traumatic experience), and expectant (of quick recovery and a rapid return to work).

Treatment initiated later, when symptoms have crystallized, includes programs for cessation of alcohol and other drug abuse, group psychotherapy, and social support systems.

Differential Diagnosis

Adjustment disorders must be distinguished from anxiety disorders, affective disorders, and personality disorders exacerbated by stress and from somatic disorders with psychic overlay.

Treatment

A. Behavioral: Stress reduction techniques include immediate symptom reduction (eg, rebreathing in a bag for hyperventilation) or early recognition and removal from a stress source before full-blown symptoms appear. It is often helpful for the patient to keep a daily log of stress precipitators, responses, and alleviators. Relaxation and exercise techniques are also helpful in reducing the reaction to stressful events.

B. Social: The stress reactions of life crisis problems are—more than any other category—a function of psychosocial upheaval, and patients frequently present with somatic symptoms. While it is not easy for the patient to make necessary changes (or they would have been made long ago), it is important for the therapist to establish the framework of the problem, since the patient's denial system may obscure the issues. Clarifying the problem allows the patient to begin viewing it within the proper context and facilitates the sometimes difficult decisions the patient eventually must make (eg, change of job or relocation of adult dependent offspring).

C. Psychologic: Prolonged in-depth psychotherapy is seldom necessary in cases of isolated stress response or adjustment disorder. Supportive psychotherapy (see above) with an emphasis on the here and now and strengthening of existing defenses is a helpful approach so that time and the patient's own resiliency can restore the previous level of function. Posttraumatic stress syndromes respond to early catharsis and dynamic psychotherapy oriented toward acceptance of the event, with the expectation of quick recovery and return to the previous level of function. Marital problems are a major area of concern, and it is important that the physician have available a dependable referral source when marriage counseling is indicated. In posttraumatic stress disor-

der, group psychotherapy and individual counseling are both helpful.

D. Medical: Judicious use of sedatives (eg, lorazepam, 1–2 mg orally daily) for a limited time and as part of an overall treatment plan can provide relief from acute anxiety symptoms. Problems arise when the situation becomes chronic through inappropriate treatment or when the treatment approach supports the development of chronicity (see Sedative-Hypnotic Drugs, below).

In posttraumatic stress disorder, antidepressant drugs in full dosage are helpful in ameliorating depression, panic attacks, sleep disruption, and startle responses, though there is no way to predict which drug will be most useful. Beta-blockers (eg, propranolol, 80–160 mg daily) are used to lessen the peripheral symptoms of anxiety (eg, tremors, palpitations). Antiseizure medications such as valproic acid (eg, 500–2000 mg daily) will often mitigate symptoms in patients with a history of alcohol and other drug abuse. Benzodiazepines such as clonazepam (1–4 mg daily) will reduce anxiety and panic attacks when used in adequate dosage, but dependency problems are a concern, particularly when the patient has had such problems in the past.

Prognosis

Return to satisfactory function after a short period is part of the clinical picture of this syndrome. Resolution may be delayed if others' responses to the patient's difficulties are thoughtlessly harmful or if the secondary gains outweigh the advantages of recovery. The longer the chronicity, the worse the prognosis.

Bende BC, Philpott RM: Persistent post-traumatic stress disorder. (Clinical conference.) Br Med J 1994;309:526.

Katz L et al: A review of the psychobiology and pharmacotherapy of posttraumatic stress disorder. Can J Psychiatry 1996;41:233.

ANXIETY DISORDERS & DISSOCIATIVE DISORDERS

Essentials of Diagnosis

- Overt anxiety or an overt manifestation of a defense mechanism (such as a phobia), or both.
- Not limited to an adjustment disorder.
- Somatic symptoms referable to the autonomic nervous system or to a specific organ system (eg, dyspnea, palpitations, paresthesias).
- Not a result of physical disorders, psychiatric conditions (eg, schizophrenia), or drug abuse (eg, cocaine).

General Considerations

Stress, fear, and anxiety all tend to be interactive. The principal components of anxiety are **psychologic** (tension, fears, difficulty in concentration, apprehension) and **somatic** (tachycardia, hyperventilation, palpitations, tremor, sweating). Other organ systems (eg, gastrointestinal) may be involved in multiple-system complaints. Fatigue and sleep disturbances are common. Sympathomimetic symptoms of anxiety are both a response to a central nervous system state and a reinforcement of further anxiety. Anxiety can become self-generating, since the symptoms reinforce the reaction, causing it to spiral. This is often the case when the anxiety is an epiphenomenon of other medical or psychiatric disorders.

Anxiety may be free-floating, resulting in acute anxiety attacks, occasionally becoming chronic. When one or several defense mechanisms (see above) are functioning, the consequences are well-known problems such as phobias, conversion reactions, dissociative states, obsessions, and compulsions. Lack of structure is frequently a contributing factor, as noted in those people who have "Sunday neuroses." They do well during the week with a planned work schedule but cannot tolerate the unstructured weekend. Planned-time activities tend to bind anxiety, and many people have increased difficulties when this is lost, as in retirement.

Some believe that various manifestations of anxiety are not a result of unconscious conflicts but are "habits"—persistent patterns of nonadaptive behavior acquired by learning. The "habits," being nonadaptive, are unsatisfactory ways of dealing with life's problems—hence the resultant anxiety. Help is sought only when the anxiety becomes too painful. Exogenous factors such as stimulants (eg, caffeine, cocaine) must be considered as a contributing factor.

Clinical Findings

A. Generalized Anxiety Disorder: This is the most common of the clinically significant anxiety disorders. Initial manifestations appear at age 20–35 years, and there is a slight predominance in women. The disabling anxiety symptoms of apprehension, worry, irritability, hypervigilance (preparation for threat), and somatic complaints are long-lasting and persist for at least 1 month. Manifestations include cardiac (eg, tachycardia, increased blood pressure), gastrointestinal (eg, increased acidity, epigastric pain), and neurologic (eg, headache, near-syncope) systems. Some of the origins or exacerbating causes of the anxiety may be identified in life situations.

B. Panic Disorder: This is characterized by short-lived, recurrent, unpredictable episodes of intense anxiety (with or without agoraphobia) accompanied by marked physiologic manifestations. Distressing symptoms and signs such as dyspnea, tachycardia, palpitations, headaches, dizziness, paresthesias, choking, smothering feelings, nausea, and bloating are associated with feelings of impending doom (alarm response). Recurrent sleep panic attacks (not nightmares) occur in about 30% of panic disorders. Anticipatory anxiety develops in all these patients and further constricts their daily lives. Panic disorder tends to be familial, with onset usually under age 25; it affects 3–5% of the population, and the female-to-male ratio is 2:1. The premenstrual period is one of heightened vulnerability. Patients frequently undergo emergency medical evaluations (eg, for "heart attacks" or "hypoglycemia") before the correct diagnosis is made. Gastrointestinal symptoms are especially common, occurring in about one-third of cases. Myocardial infarction, pheochromocytoma, hyperthyroidism, and various recreational drug reactions can mimic panic disorder. Mitral valve prolapse may be present but is not usually a significant factor. Patients with recurrent panic disorder often become **demoralized, hypochondriacal, agoraphobic,** and **depressed.** These individuals are at increased risk for major depression and the suicide attempts associated with that disorder. Alcohol abuse (about 20%) results from self-treatment and is not infrequently combined with dependence on sedatives. Some patients have atypical panic attacks associated with seizure-like symptoms that often include psychosensory phenomena (a history of stimulant abuse often emerges). About 25% of panic disorder patients also have obsessive-compulsive disorder.

C. Obsessive-Compulsive Disorder (OCD): In the obsessive-compulsive reaction, the irrational idea or the impulse persistently intrudes into awareness. Obsessions (constantly recurring thoughts such as fears of exposure to germs) and compulsions (repetitive actions such as washing the hands many times before peeling a potato) are recognized by the individual as absurd and are resisted, but anxiety is alleviated only by ritualistic performance of the action or by deliberate contemplation of the intruding idea or emotion. The primary underlying concern of the patient is not to lose control. Many patients do not mention the symptoms and must be asked about them. These patients are usually predictable, orderly, conscientious, and intelligent—traits that are seen in many compulsive behaviors such as bulimia and compulsive running. There is an overlapping of obsessive-compulsive disorder and other behaviors ("OCD spectrum"), including tics, trichotillomania (hair pulling), onychophagia (nail biting), hypochondriasis, Tourette's syndrome, and eating disorders (see Chapter 29). The 2–3% incidence of OCD in the general population is much higher than was previously recognized. In addition, there is a high comorbidity of OCD and major depression; two-thirds of OCD patients will develop major depression during their lifetime. Male:female ratios are similar, with the highest rates occurring in the young, divorced, separated, and unemployed (all high stress categories). Neurologic abnormalities of fine motor coordination and involuntary movements are common. Under extreme stress, these patients sometimes exhibit paranoid and delusional behaviors, often associated with depression, and can mimic schizophrenia.

D. Phobic Disorder: Phobic ideation can be considered a mechanism of "displacement" in which patients transfer feelings of anxiety from their true object to one that can be avoided. However, since phobias are ineffective defense mechanisms, there tends to be an increase in their scope, intensity, and number. Social phobias are global or specific; in the former, all social situations are poorly tolerated, while the latter group includes performance anxiety or well-delineated phobias. Agoraphobia (fear of open places and public areas) is frequently associated with severe panic attacks. Patients often develop the agoraphobia in early adult life, making a normal lifestyle difficult.

E. Dissociative Disorder: Fugue (the sudden, unexpected travel away from one's home with inability to recall one's past), amnesia, somnambulism, and multiple personality are the most common dissociative states. The reaction is precipitated by emotional crisis. The symptom produces anxiety reduction and a temporary solution of the crisis. Mechanisms include repression and isolation as well as particularly limited concentration as seen in hypnotic states. This condition is similar in many ways to symptoms seen in patients with temporal lobe dysfunction.

Treatment

In all cases, underlying medical disorders must be ruled out (eg, cardiovascular, endocrine, respiratory, and neurologic disorders and substance-related syndromes, both intoxication and withdrawal states). These and other disorders can coexist with panic disorder.

A. Medical:

1. Anxiety–Benzodiazepines and buspirone are the anxiolytics of choice in most cases of generalized anxiety. The benzodiazepines are most commonly used since they are almost immediately effective. Onset of action is a function of rate of absorption (related to lipophilic property) and varies, with diazepam and clorazepate being the most rapidly absorbed. This characteristic, along with high lipid solubility, may explain the popularity of diazepam. The duration of action of the benzodiazepines varies as a function of the active metabolites they produce. Short-acting benzodiazepines such as lorazepam do not produce active metabolites and have half-lives of 10–20 hours. Ultra-short-acting agents such as triazolam have half-lives of 1–3 hours. Other benzodiazepines such as flurazepam and diazepam produce active metabolites and have half-lives of 20–120 hours.

Buspirone is the only marketed anxiolytic drug that is not a tranquilizer and has the advantage of not causing physiologic dependence problems. There is no evidence that it produces depressant effects or dependence. In fact, it is increasingly being used in the treatment of agitated depression and compulsive be-

haviors. It differs from the other antianxiety agents in that motor skills are not impaired, and it does not potentiate the effects of alcohol or cause a withdrawal syndrome—nor can it be used in benzodiazepine or alcohol withdrawal. There is a 1- to 3-week delay before the drug takes effect, and patients require education regarding this lag.

Beta-blockers such as propranolol may help reduce peripheral somatic symptoms. Ethanol is the most frequently self-administered drug and should be interdicted. Panic disorder does not usually respond to benzodiazepines other than clonazepam and alprazolam. Those high-potency benzodiazepines and the antidepressants are most commonly used for panic disorder.

The highly addicting drugs with a narrow margin of safety such as glutethimide, ethchlorvynol, methyprylon, meprobamate, and the barbiturates (with the exception of phenobarbital) should be avoided. Phenobarbital, in addition to its anticonvulsant properties, is a reasonably safe and very cheap sedative but has the disadvantage of causing hepatic microsomal enzyme stimulation (not the case with benzodiazepines), which markedly reduces its usefulness if any other relevant medications are being used by the patient.

a. Clinical indications–Whether the indications for antianxiety agents are anxiety or insomnia, the drugs should be used judiciously. The longer-acting benzodiazepines are used for the treatment of alcohol withdrawal and anxiety symptoms; the shorter-acting drugs are useful as sedatives for insomnia (eg, lorazepam) and medical procedures such as endoscopy (eg, midazolam).

b. Dosage forms–All of the antianxiety agents may be given orally, and several are available in parenteral form (Table 25–1). Short-acting benzodiazepines like lorazepam are absorbed rapidly when given intramuscularly. In psychiatric disorders, the benzodiazepines are usually given orally; in controlled medical environments (eg, the ICU) where the rapid onset of respiratory depression can be assessed, they are often given intravenously. Antacids significantly alter the absorption of clorazepate and prazepam; this is an important consideration, since many anxious individuals suffer from gastrointestinal disturbances and use both types of drugs concomitantly. Food also modifies the absorption of diazepam (and possibly the other benzodiazepines), initially slowing absorption but resulting in higher levels over many hours. In the average case of anxiety, diazepam, 5–10 mg orally every 6–8 hours as needed, is a reasonable starting regimen. Since people vary widely in their response and since the drugs are long-lasting, one must individualize the dosage. Once this is established, an adequate dose early in the course of symptom development will obviate the need for "pill-popping," which contributes to dependency problems. Flurazepam and temazepam are

Table 25–1. Commonly used antianxiety and hypnotic agents.

	Usual Daily Oral Dose	Usual Daily Maximum Dose	Cost for 30 Days' Treatment Based on Maximum Dosage
Benzodiazepines (used for anxiety)			
Alprazolam (Xanax)[2]	0.5 mg	4 mg	$105.60
Chlordiazepoxide (Librium)[3]	10–20 mg	40 mg	$26.40
Clonazepam (Klonopin)[3]	1–2 mg	10 mg	$166.50
Clorazepate (Tranxene)[3]	15–30 mg	60 mg	$60.00
Diazepam (Valium)[3]	5–15 mg	30 mg	$15.30
Lorazepam (Ativan)[2]	2–4 mg	4 mg	$24.00
Oxazepam (Serax)[2]	10–30 mg	60 mg	$27.00
Benzodiazepines (used for sleep)			
Estazolam (Prosom)[2]	1 mg	2 mg	$31.50
Flurazepam (Dalmane)[3]	15 mg	30 mg	$7.50
Midazolam (Versed IV)[4]	5 mg IV	40 mg	5 mg/mL = $10.00
Quazepam (Doral)[3]	7.5 mg	15 mg	$53.70
Temazepam (Restoril)[2]	15 mg	30 mg	$9.00
Triazolam (Halcion)[1]	0.125 mg	0.25 mg	$19.80
Miscellaneous (used for anxiety)			
Buspirone (Buspar)[2]	10–30 mg	60 mg	$126.00
Phenobarbital[3]	15–30 mg	90 mg	$1.24
Miscellaneous (used for sleep)			
Chloral hydrate (Noctec)[2]	500 mg	1000 mg	$7.80
Hydroxyzine (Vistaril)[2]	50 mg	100 mg	$10.50
Zolpidem (Ambien)[1]	5–10 mg	10 mg	$53.10

[1]Short physical half-life (1–5 hours).
[2]Intermediate physical half-life (10–20 hours).
[3]Long physical half-life (>20 hours).
[4]Intravenously for procedures.

both longer-acting and should be avoided in elderly patients. The latter has a somewhat shorter duration of action but a delayed onset of action in the range of 1–3 hours.

Buspirone is usually given in a dosage of 15–45 mg/d in three divided doses. Higher doses tend to be counterproductive and produce gastrointestinal symptoms and dizziness. Sleep is sometimes negatively affected.

c. Side effects–The side effects of all the antianxiety agents are mainly behavioral and depend on patient reaction and dosage. As the dosage exceeds the levels necessary for sedation, the side effects include disinhibition, ataxia, dysarthria, nystagmus, and errors of commission. (Machinery should not be operated until the patient is well stabilized, and the patient should be so informed.) Agitation, anxiety, psychosis, confusion, mood lability, and anterograde amnesia have been reported, particularly with the shorter-acting benzodiazepines.

The antianxiety agents produce **cumulative** clinical effects with repeated dosage (especially if the patient has not had time to metabolize the previous dose); **additive** effects when given with other classes of sedatives or alcohol (many apparently "accidental" deaths are the result of concomitant use of sedatives and alcohol); and **residual** effects after termina-

tion of treatment (particularly in the case of drugs that undergo slow biotransformation).

Overdosage results in respiratory depression, hypotension, shock syndrome, coma, and death. Fortunately, flumazenil, a benzodiazepine antagonist, is now available. Treatment of overdoses (see Chapter 39) and withdrawal states are medical emergencies.

Serious side effects of chronic excessive dosage are development of tolerance, resulting in increasing dose requirements, and physiologic dependence resulting in withdrawal symptoms similar in morbidity and mortality to alcohol or barbiturate withdrawal (withdrawal effects must be distinguished from reemergent anxiety). Abrupt withdrawal of sedative drugs may cause serious and even fatal convulsive seizures. Psychosis, delirium, and autonomic dysfunction have also been described. Both duration of action and duration of exposure are major factors. Common withdrawal symptoms after low to moderate daily use of benzodiazepines are classified as **somatic** (disturbed sleep, tremor, nausea, muscle aches), **psychologic** (anxiety, poor concentration, irritability, mild depression), or **perceptual** (poor coordination, mild paranoia, mild confusion). The presentation of symptoms will vary depending on the half-life of the drug. There are no significant side effects on organ systems other than the brain, and the drugs are safe in most medical conditions. Benzodiazepine interactions with other drugs are listed in Table 25–2.

2. Panic attacks–Panic attacks may be treated in several ways. A sublingual dose of lorazepam (0.5–2 mg) or alprazolam (0.5–1 mg) is often effective for urgent treatment. For sustained treatment, antidepressants are the initial drugs of choice (adequate blood levels will require dosages similar to those used in the treatment of depression). As in depression, lithium may be used to augment the antidepressant drugs. Serotonin selective reuptake inhibitors (SSRIs) are effective, particularly if obsessive-compulsive disorder is present with the panic disorder (25% of patients). Because of overresponsiveness to the antidepressants, doses should be low initially and very gradually increased. High-potency benzodiazepines may be used for symptomatic treatment as the antidepressant dose is titrated upward. Clonazepam (1–6 mg/d orally) and alprazolam (0.5–6 mg/d orally) are effective alternatives to antidepressants. Both drugs may produce marked withdrawal if stopped abruptly and should always be tapered. Because of chronicity of the disorders and the problem of dependency with benzodiazepine drugs, it is generally desirable to use antidepressant drugs as the principal pharmacologic approach. Antidepressants have been used in conjunction with propranolol (40–160 mg/d orally) in resistant cases. Beta-blockers such as propranolol or atenolol have been used to mute the peripheral symptoms of anxiety without significantly affecting motor performance. They block symptoms mediated by sympathetic stimulation (eg, palpitations, tremulousness) but not nonadrenergic symptoms (eg, diarrhea, muscle tension). Contrary to current belief, they usually do not cause depression as a side effect. Recently valproate has been found to be as effective in panic disorder as the antidepressants and is another useful alternative.

3. Phobic disorder–Phobic disorder may be part of the panic disorder and is treated within that framework. Global social phobias may be treated with fluoxetine or MAO inhibitors in the same dosage as used for depression, while specific phobias such as performance anxiety may respond to moderate doses of beta-blockers. A sustained effect is often not obtained with drugs alone; a combination of drugs, behavioral techniques, and cognitive psychotherapy is most effective. If there is any indication of seizure-like phenomena, carbamazepine or valproic acid should be considered.

4. Obsessive-compulsive disorders–Obsessive-compulsive disorders respond to serotonergic drugs in about 60% of cases. Clomipramine has proved effective in doses equivalent to those used for depression. Fluoxetine (an SSRI drug) has been widely used in this disorder but in doses higher than those used in depression (up to 60–80 mg/d). The other SSRI drugs such as sertraline and paroxetine are being used with early results comparable to those achieved with clomipramine and fluoxetine. The new SSRI, fluvoxamine, is also effective in obsessive-compulsive disorder. Buspirone in doses of 15–60 mg/d appears to be effective primarily as an antiobsessional augmenting agent for the aforementioned drugs. Psychosurgery has a limited place in selected cases of severe unremitting obsessive-compulsive disorder. The stereotactic techniques now being used, including modified cingulotomy, are great improvements over the crude methods of the past.

B. Behavioral: Behavioral approaches are widely used in various anxiety disorders, often in conjunction with medication. Any of the behavioral techniques (see above) can be used beneficially in altering the contingencies (precipitating factors or rewards) supporting any anxiety-provoking behavior. Relaxation techniques can sometimes be helpful in reducing anxiety. Desensitization, by exposing the patient to graded doses of a phobic object or situation, is an effective technique and one that the patient can practice outside the therapy session. Emotive imagery, wherein the patient imagines the anxiety-provoking situation while at the same time learning to relax, helps to decrease the anxiety when the patient faces the real-life situation. Physiologic symptoms in panic attacks respond well to relaxation training.

C. Psychologic: Cognitive approaches have been effective in treatment of panic disorders, phobias, and obsessive-compulsive disorder when erroneous beliefs need correction. The combination of medical and cognitive therapy is more effective than either alone. Group therapy is the treatment of choice when the anxiety is clearly a function of the patient's difficulties in dealing with others, and if these other people are part of the family it is appropriate to include them and initiate family or couples therapy.

D. Social: Peer support groups for panic disorder and agoraphobia have been particularly helpful. Social modification may require measures such as family counseling to aid acceptance of the patient's symptoms and avoid counterproductive behavior in

Table 25–2. Benzodiazepine interactions with other drugs.

Drug	Effects
Antacids	Decreased absorption of benzodiazepines.
Cimetidine	Increased half-life of flurazepam, alprazolam.
Contraceptives	Increased levels of diazepam and triazolam.
Digoxin	Alprazolam and diazepam raise digoxin level.
Disulfiram	Increased duration of action of sedatives.
Isoniazid	Increased plasma diazepam.
Levodopa	Inhibition of antiparkinsonism effect.
Propoxyphene	Impaired clearance of diazepam.
Rifampin	Decreased plasma diazepam.
Warfarin	Decreased prothrombin time.

behavioral training. Any help in maintaining the social structure is anxiety-alleviating, and work, school, and social activities should be maintained. School and vocational counseling may be provided by professionals, who often need help from the physician in defining the patient's limitations.

Prognosis

Anxiety disorders are usually of long standing and may be quite difficult to treat. All can be relieved to varying degrees with medications and behavioral techniques. The prognosis is much better if one can break the commonly observed anxiety-panic-phobia-depression cycle with a combination of the therapeutic interventions discussed above.

Baer L et al: Cingulotomy for intractable obsessive-compulsive disorder. Prospective long-term follow-up of 18 patients. Arch Gen Psychiatry 1995;52:384. (Twenty-five to 30 percent of the patients who previously were unresponsive to medication and behavioral treatments are significantly improved after cingulotomy.)

Greist J et al: Double-blind parallel comparison of three dosages of sertraline and placebo in outpatients with obsessive-compulsive disorder. Arch Gen Psychiatry 1995;52:289. (Results support the safety and efficacy of sertraline in the short-term treatment of patients with obsessive-compulsive disorder.)

Greist JH et al: Efficacy and tolerability of serotonin transport inhibitors in obsessive-compulsive disorder. A meta-analysis. Arch Gen Psychiatry 1995;52:53. (This meta-analysis supports the superiority of clomipramine compared with fluoxetine, fluvoxamine, and sertraline.)

Hornig CD, McNally RJ: Panic disorder and suicide attempt: A reanalysis of data from the Epidemiologic Catchment Area study. Br J Psychiatry 1995;167:76. (Depression increases the likelihood of suicide attempt.)

Papp LA et al: Carbon dioxide hypersensitivity, hyperventilation, and panic disorder. Am J Psychiatry 1993; 150:1149. (Panic disorder may be due to an inherently unstable autonomic nervous system coupled with cognitive distress.)

Woodman CL, Noyes R: Panic disorder: Treatment with valproate. J Clin Psychiatry 1994;55:134.

SOMATOFORM DISORDERS
(Abnormal Illness Behaviors)

Essentials of Diagnosis

- Physical symptoms may involve one or more organ systems and are not intentional.
- Subjective complaints exceed objective findings.
- Correlations of symptom development and psychosocial stresses.
- Matrix of biogenetic and developmental patterns.

General Considerations

A major source of diagnostic confusion in medicine has been to assume cause-and-effect relationships when parallel conditions exist. This problem is particularly vexing in situations where the individual exhibits psychosocial distress that could well be secondary to a chronic illness but has been assumed to be primary and causative. An example is the person with a chronic bowel disease who becomes querulous and demanding. Is this behavior a result of problems of coping with a chronic disease, or is it a personality pattern that causes the gastrointestinal problem?

Vulnerability in one or more organ systems and exposure to family members with somatization problems play a major role in the development of particular symptoms, and the "functional" versus "organic" dichotomy is a hindrance to good treatment. Physicians should suspect psychiatric disorders in a number of conditions. For example, 45% of patients complaining of palpitations had lifetime psychiatric diagnoses including generalized anxiety, depression, panic, and somatization disorders. Similarly, 33–44% of patients who undergo coronary angiography for chest pain but have negative results have been found to have panic disorder.

In any patient presenting with a condition judged to be somatoform, depression must be considered in the diagnosis.

Clinical Findings

A. Conversion Disorder: "Conversion" (formerly "hysterical conversion") of psychic conflict into physical symptoms in parts of the body innervated by the sensorimotor system (eg, paralysis, aphonia) is a disorder that is more common in individuals from lower socioeconomic classes and certain cultures. The defense mechanisms utilized in this condition are repression (a barring from consciousness) and isolation (a splitting of the affect from the idea). The somatic manifestation that takes the place of anxiety is typically paralysis, and in some instances the organ dysfunction may have symbolic meaning (eg, arm paralysis in marked anger). Pseudoepileptic ("hysterical") seizures are often difficult to differentiate from intoxication states or panic attacks. Retention of consciousness, random flailing with asynchronous movements of the right and left sides, and resistance to having the nose and mouth pinched closed during the attack all point toward a pseudoepileptic event. Electroencephalography, particularly in a video-EEG assessment unit, during the attack is the most helpful diagnostic aid in excluding genuine seizure states. Serum prolactin levels rise abruptly in the postictal state only in true epilepsy. La belle indifférence (a lack of affect) is not a significant characteristic, as commonly believed. Important criteria in diagnosis include a history of conversion or somatization disorder, modeling, a serious precipitating emotional event, associated psychopathology (eg, schizophrenia, personality disorders), a temporal correlation between the precipitating event and the symptom, and a temporary "solving of the problem" by the conversion. It is important to identify physical disorders with unusual presentations (eg, multiple sclerosis).

B. Somatization Disorder (Briquet's Syndrome, Hysteria): This is characterized by multiple physical complaints referable to several organ systems. Anxiety, panic disorder, and depression are often present, and **major depression** is an important consideration in the differential diagnosis. There is a significant relationship (20%) to a lifetime history of panic-agoraphobia-depression. It usually occurs before age 30 and is ten times more common in women. Polysurgery is often a feature of the history. Preoccupation with medical and surgical therapy becomes a lifestyle that excludes most other activities. The symptoms are a reflection of maladaptive coping techniques and reactivity of the particular organ system. There is often evidence of long-standing somatic symptoms (particularly dysmenorrhea, a lump in the throat, vomiting, shortness of breath, burning in the sex organs, painful extremities, and amnesia), often with a history of similar organ system involvement in other family members. Multiple symptoms that constantly change and inability of more than three doctors to make a diagnosis are strong clues to the problem.

C. Pain Disorder Associated With Psychologic Factors (Formerly Somatoform Pain Disorder): This involves a long history of complaints of severe pain not consonant with anatomic and clinical signs. This diagnosis must not be one of exclusion and should be made only after extended evaluation has established a clear correlation of psychogenic factors with exacerbations and remissions of complaints.

D. Hypochondriasis: This is a fear of disease and preoccupation with the body, with perceptual amplification and heightened responsiveness. A process of social learning is usually involved, frequently with a role model who was a member of the family and may be a part of the underlying psychodynamic causation. It is common in panic disorders.

E. Factitious Disorders: These disorders, in which symptom production is intentional, are not somatoform conditions. They are characterized by self-induced symptoms or false physical and laboratory findings for the purpose of deceiving physicians or other hospital personnel. The deceptions may involve self-mutilation, fever, hemorrhage, hypoglycemia, seizures, and an almost endless variety of manifestations—often presented in an exaggerated and dramatic fashion (Munchausen syndrome). "Munchausen by proxy" is the term used when a parent creates an illness in a child so the adult (usually the mother) can maintain a relationship with physicians. The duplicity may be either simple or extremely complex and difficult to recognize. The patients are frequently connected in some way with the health professions; they are often migratory; and there is no apparent external motivations other than achieving the patient role.

Complications

A poor doctor-patient relationship, with iatrogenic disorders and "doctor shopping," tends to exacerbate the problem. Sedative and analgesic dependency is the most common iatrogenic complication.

Treatment

A. Medical: Medical support with careful attention to building a therapeutic doctor-patient relationship is the mainstay of treatment. It must be accepted that the patient's distress is real. Every problem not found to have an organic basis is not necessarily a mental disease. Diligent attempts should be made to relate symptoms to adverse developments in the patient's life. It may be useful to have the patient keep a meticulous diary, paying particular attention to various pertinent factors evident in the history. Regular, frequent, short appointments that are not symptom-contingent may be helpful. Drugs (frequently abused) should not be prescribed to replace appointments. One doctor should be the primary physician, and consultants should be used mainly for evaluation. An empathic, realistic, optimistic approach must be maintained in the face of the expected ups and downs. Ongoing reevaluation is necessary, since somatization can coexist with a concurrent physical illness.

B. Psychologic: Psychologic approaches can be used by the primary physician when it is clear that the patient is ready to make some changes in lifestyle in order to achieve symptomatic relief. This is often best approached on a here-and-now basis and oriented toward pragmatic changes rather than an exploration of early experiences that the patient frequently fails to relate to current distress. Group therapy with other individuals who have similar problems is sometimes of value to improve coping, allow ventilation, and focus on interpersonal adjustment. Hypnosis or amobarbital interviews used early are helpful in resolving conversion disorders. If the primary physician has been working with the patient on psychologic problems related to the physical illness, the groundwork is often laid for successful psychiatric referral.

For patients who have been identified as having a factitious disorder, early psychiatric consultation is indicated. There are two main treatment strategies for these patients. One consists of a conjoint confrontation of the patient by both the primary physician and the psychiatrist. The patient's disorder is portrayed as a cry for help, and psychiatric treatment is recommended. The second approach avoids direct confrontation and attempts to provide a face-saving way to relinquish the symptom without overt disclosure of the disorder's origin. Techniques such as biofeedback and self-hypnosis may foster recovery using this strategy. Another face-saving approach is to utilize a double bind with the patient. For example, the patient is told there are two possible diagnoses: (1) an organic disease that should respond to the next medical intervention (usually modest and noninvasive), or (2) factitious disorder for which the patient will need psychiatric treatment. Given these options, many patients will choose to recover and not have to admit the origin of their problem.

C. Behavioral: Behavioral therapy is probably best exemplified by biofeedback techniques. In biofeedback, the particular abnormality (eg, increased peristalsis) must be recognized and monitored by the patient and therapist (eg, by an electronic stethoscope to amplify the sounds). This is immediate feedback, and after learning to recognize it the patient can then learn to identify any change thus produced (eg, a decrease in bowel sounds) and so become a conscious originator of the feedback instead of a passive recipient. Relief of the symptom operantly conditions the patient to utilize the maneuver that relieves symptoms (eg, relaxation causing a decrease in bowel sounds). With emphasis on this type of learning, the patient is able to identify symptoms early and initiate the countermaneuvers, thus decreasing the symptomatic problem. Migrainoid and tension headaches have been particularly responsive to biofeedback methods.

D. Social: Social endeavors include family, work, and other interpersonal activity. Family members should come for some appointments with the patient so they can learn how best to live with the patient. This is particularly important in treatment of somatization and pain disorders. Peer support groups provide a climate for encouraging the patient to accept and live with the problem. Ongoing communication with the employer may be necessary to encourage long-term continued interest in the employee. Employers can become just as discouraged as physicians in dealing with employees who have chronic problems.

Prognosis

The prognosis is much better if the primary physician is able to intervene early before the situation has deteriorated. After the problem has crystallized into chronicity, it is very difficult to effect change.

Barsky AJ et al: Psychiatric disorders in medical outpatients complaining of palpitations. J Gen Intern Med 1994;9:306.

Eisendrath SJ: Factitious physical disorders. West J Med 1994;160:177.

Wilhelmsen I et al: Discriminant analysis of factors distinguishing patients with functional dyspepsia from patients with duodenal ulcer. Significance of somatization. Dig Dis Sci 1995;40:1105. (Compared with patients with duodenal ulcer, patients with functional dyspepsia had higher scores of depression, trait anxiety, general psychopathology, and different somatic complaints.)

CHRONIC PAIN DISORDERS

Essentials of Diagnosis
- Chronic complaints of pain.
- Symptoms frequently exceed signs.
- Minimal relief with standard treatment.
- History of having seen many physicians.
- Frequent use of several nonspecific medications.

General Considerations

A problem in the management of pain is the lack of distinction between acute and chronic pain syndromes. Most physicians are adept at dealing with acute pain problems but have difficulty handling the patient with a chronic pain disorder. This type of patient frequently takes too many medications, stays in bed a great deal, has seen many physicians, has lost skills, and experiences little joy in either work or play. All relationships suffer (including those with physicians), and life becomes a constant search for succor. The search results in complex physician-patient relationships that usually include many drug trials, particularly sedatives, with adverse consequences (eg, irritability, depressed mood) related to long-term use. Treatment failures provoke angry responses and depression from both the patient and the physician, and the pain syndrome is exacerbated. When frustration becomes too great, a new physician is found, and the cycle is repeated. The longer the existence of the pain disorder, the more important become the psychologic factors of anxiety and depression. As with all other conditions, it is counterproductive to speculate about whether the pain is "real." It is real to the patient, and acceptance of the problem must precede a mutual endeavor to alleviate the disturbance.

Clinical Findings

Components of the chronic pain syndrome consist of anatomic changes, chronic anxiety and depression, anger, and changed lifestyle. Usually, the anatomic problem is irreversible, since it has already been subjected to many interventions with increasingly unsatisfactory results. An algorithm for assessing chronic pain and differentiating from other psychiatric conditions is illustrated in Figure 25–1.

Chronic anxiety and depression produce heightened irritability and overreaction to stimuli. A marked decrease in pain threshold is apparent. This pattern develops into a hypochondriacal preoccupation with the body and a constant need for reassurance. The pressure on the doctor becomes wearing and often leads to covert rejection devices, such as not being available or making referrals to other physicians. This is perceived by the patient, who then intensifies the effort to find help, and the typical cycle is repeated. Anxiety and depression are seldom discussed, almost as if there is a tacit agreement not to deal with these issues.

Changes in lifestyle involve some of the so-called

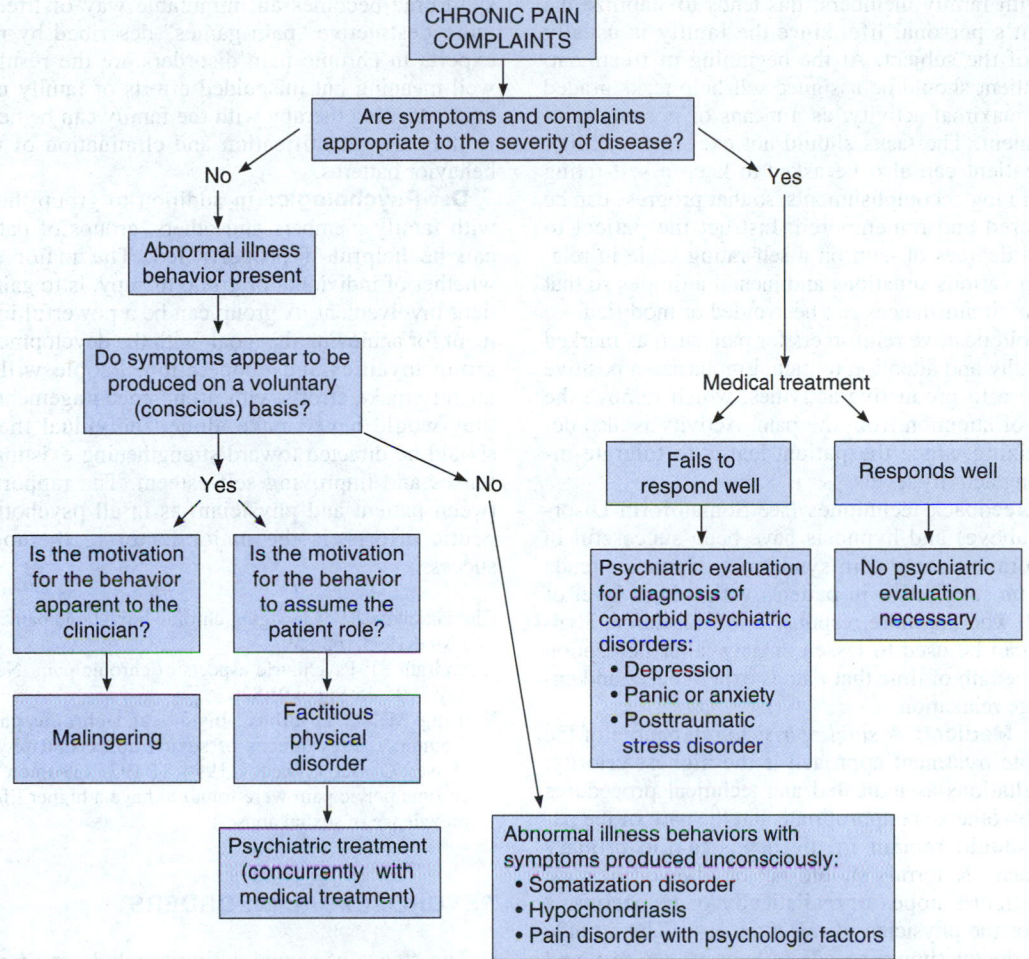

Figure 25–1. Algorithm for assessing psychiatric component of chronic pain. (Modified and reproduced, with permission, from Eisendrath SJ: Psychiatric aspects of chronic pain. Neurology 1995;45[Suppl 9]:S20.)

pain games. These usually take the form of a family script in which the patient accepts the role of being sick, and this role then becomes the focus of most family interactions and may become important in maintaining the family, so that neither the patient nor the family wants the patient's role to change. Demands for attention and efforts to control the behavior of others revolve around the central issue of control of other people (including physicians). Cultural factors frequently play a role in the behavior of the patient and how the significant people around the patient cope with the problem. Some cultures encourage demonstrative behavior, while others value the stoic role.

Another secondary gain that frequently maintains the patient in the sick role is financial compensation or other benefits ("green poultice"). Frequently, such systems are structured so that they reinforce the maintenance of sickness and discourage any attempts

to give up the role. Physicians unwittingly reinforce this role because of the very nature of the practice of medicine, which is to respond to complaints of illness. Helpful suggestions from the physician are often met with responses like, "Yes, but. . . ." Medications then become the principal approach, and drug dependency problems may develop.

Treatment

A. Behavioral: The cornerstone of a unified approach to chronic pain syndromes is a comprehensive behavioral program. This is necessary to identify and eliminate pain reinforcers, to decrease drug use, and to use effectively those positive reinforcers that shift the focus from the pain. It is critical that the patient be made a partner in the effort to alleviate pain. The physician must shift from the idea of biomedical cure to ongoing care of the patient. The patient should agree to discuss the pain only with the physician and not with family members; this tends to stabilize the patient's personal life, since the family is usually tired of the subject. At the beginning of treatment, the patient should be assigned self-help tasks graded up to maximal activity, as a means of positive reinforcement. The tasks should not exceed capability. The patient can also be asked to keep a self-rating chart to log accomplishments, so that progress can be measured and remembered. Instruct the patient to record degrees of pain on a self-rating scale in relation to various situations and mental attitudes so that similar circumstances can be avoided or modified.

Avoid positive reinforcers for pain such as marked sympathy and attention to pain. Emphasize a positive response to productive activities, which remove the focus of attention from the pain. Activity is also desensitizing, since the patient learns to tolerate increasing activity levels.

Biofeedback techniques (see Somatoform Disorders, above) and hypnosis have been successful in ameliorating some pain syndromes. Hypnosis tends to be most effective in patients with a high level of denial, who are more responsive to suggestion. Hypnosis can be used to lessen anxiety, alter perception of the length of time that pain is experienced, and encourage relaxation.

B. Medical: A *single physician* in charge of the multiple treatment approach is the highest priority. Consultations as indicated and technical procedures done by others are appropriate, but the care of the patient should remain in the hands of the primary physician. Referrals should not be allowed to raise the patient's hopes unrealistically or to become a way for the physician to reject the case. The attitude of the doctor should be one of honesty, interest, and hopefulness—not for a cure but for control of pain and improved function. If the patient manifests narcotic addiction, detoxification may be an early treatment goal.

If analgesics or sedatives are prescribed, they should not be given on an "as-needed" schedule (see Chapter 1). A fixed schedule lessens the conditioning effects of these drugs. Tricyclic antidepressants (eg, nortriptyline) in doses up to those used in depression may be helpful, particularly in neuropathic pain syndromes. In other conditions, their effects on pain may be less clear, but ameliorating depression is usually important nonetheless.

In addition to medications, a variety of alternative strategies may be offered, including physical therapy and acupuncture.

C. Social: Involvement of family members and other significant persons in the patient's life should be an early priority. The best efforts of both patient and therapists can be unwittingly sabotaged by other persons who may feel that they are "helping" the patient. They frequently tend to reinforce the negative aspects of the chronic pain disorder. The patient becomes more dependent and less active, and the pain syndrome becomes an immutable way of life. The more destructive "pain games" described by many experts in chronic pain disorders are the results of well-meaning but misguided efforts of family members. Ongoing therapy with the family can be helpful in the early identification and elimination of these behavior patterns.

D. Psychologic: In addition to group therapy with family members and others, groups of patients can be helpful if properly led. The major goal, whether of individual or group therapy, is to gain patient involvement. A group can be a powerful instrument for achieving this goal, with the development of group loyalties and cooperation. People will frequently make efforts with group encouragement that they would never make alone. Individual therapy should be directed toward strengthening existing defenses and improving self-esteem. The rapport between patient and physician, as in all psychotherapeutic efforts, is the major factor in therapeutic success.

Chodakiewitz JW: Managing chronic intractable pain. West J Med 1995;162:259.

Eisendrath SJ: Psychiatric aspects of chronic pain. Neurology 1995;45(Suppl 9):S26.

Walling MK et al: Abuse history and chronic pain in women: I. Prevalences of sexual abuse and physical abuse. Obstet Gynecol 1994;84:193. (Women with chronic pelvic pain were found to have a higher lifetime prevalence of sexual abuse.)

PSYCHOSEXUAL DISORDERS

The stages of sexual activity include **excitement** (arousal), **plateau, orgasm,** and **resolution.** The precipitating excitement or arousal is psychologically determined. Arousal response leading to plateau is a physiologic and psychologic phenomenon of vasocongestion, a parasympathetic reaction causing erection in the male and labial-clitoral congestion in the female. The orgasmic response includes emission in the male and clonic contractions of the analogous striated perineal muscles of both male and female. Resolution is a gradual return to normal physiologic status.

While the arousal stimuli—vasocongestive and orgasmic responses—constitute a single response in a well-adjusted person, they can be considered as separate stages that can produce different syndromes responding to different treatment procedures.

Clinical Findings

There are three major groups of sexual disorders.

A. Paraphilias (Sexual Arousal Disorders): In these conditions, formerly called "deviations" or "variations," the excitement stage of sexual activity is associated with sexual objects or orientations different from those usually associated with adult heterosexual stimulation. The stimulus may be a woman's shoe, a child, animals, instruments of torture, or incidents of aggression. The pattern of sexual stimulation is usually one that has early psychologic roots. Poor experiences with heterosexual activity frequently reinforce this pattern over time.

Exhibitionism is the impulsive behavior of exposing the genitalia in order to achieve sexual excitation. It is a childhood sexual behavior carried into adult life.

Transvestism is the wearing of clothes and the enactment of a role of the opposite sex for the purpose of sexual excitation. Such fetishistic "crossdressing" can be part of masturbation foreplay. Transvestism in homosexuality and transsexualism is not done to cause sexual excitement but is a function of the homosexual preference or gender disorder.

Voyeurism involves the achievement of sexual arousal by secretly watching the activities of the opposite sex, usually in various stages of undress or sexual activity. In both exhibitionism and voyeurism, excitation leads to masturbation as a replacement for heterosexual activity.

Pedophilia is the use of a child of either sex to achieve sexual arousal and, in many cases, gratification. Contact is frequently oral, with either participant being dominant, but pedophilia includes intercourse of any type. Adults of both sexes engage in this behavior, but because of social and cultural factors it is more commonly identified with males. The pedophile has difficulty in adult sexual relationships, and males who perform this act are frequently impotent.

Incest involves a sexual relationship with a person in the immediate family, most frequently a child. In many ways it is similar to pedophilia (intrafamilial pedophilia). Incestuous feelings are fairly common, but cultural mores are usually sufficiently strong to act as a barrier to the expression of sexual feelings.

Bestiality is the attainment of sexual gratification by intercourse with an animal. The intercourse may involve penetration or simply contact with the human genitalia by the tongue of the animal. The practice is more common in rural or isolated areas and is frequently a substitute for human sexual contact rather than an expression of preference.

Sadism is the attainment of sexual arousal by inflicting pain upon the sexual object, and **masochism** is the attainment of sexual excitation by enduring pain. Much sexual activity has aggressive components (eg, biting, scratching). However, forced sexual acquiescence (eg, rape) is considered to be primarily an act of aggression.

Bondage is the achievement of erotic pleasure by being humiliated, enslaved, physically bound, and restrained. It is life-threatening, since neck binding or partial asphyxiation usually forms part of the ritual. It is estimated that bondage is responsible for about 1000 accidental deaths a year in males (the practice is much less common in females).

Necrophilia is sexual intercourse with a dead body or the use of parts of a dead body for sexual excitation, often with masturbation.

B. Gender Identity Variations: Core gender identity reflects a biologic self-image—the conviction that "I am a male" or "I am a female" that is usually well developed by age 3 or 4. Gender dysphoria refers to the development of a sexual identity that is the opposite of the biologic one.

Transsexualism (a gender identity disorder) is an attempt to deny and reverse biologic sex by maintaining sexual identity with the opposite gender. Transsexuals do not alternate between gender roles; rather, they assume a fixed role of attitudes, feelings, fantasies, and choices consonant with those of the opposite sex, all of which clearly date back to early development. For example, male transsexuals in early childhood behave, talk, and fantasize as if they were girls. They do not grow out of feminine patterns; they do not work in professions traditionally considered to be masculine; and they have no interest in their own penises either as evidence of maleness or as organs for erotic behavior. The desire for sex change starts early and may culminate in assumption of a feminine lifestyle, hormonal treatment, and use of surgical procedures, eg, castration and vaginoplasty.

Homosexuality is no longer considered to be a classifiable sexual disorder. Although Kinsey reported higher rates, more recent studies suggest that 6% of men and 3% of women have engaged in homosexual behavior after adolescence. Problems arise when the individual has difficulty accepting his or her sexual orientation or is under stress in a society that is intolerant.

C. Psychosexual Dysfunction: This category includes a large group of vasocongestive and orgasmic disorders. Often, they involve problems of sexual adaptation, education, and technique that are often initially discussed with, diagnosed by, and treated by the family physician.

There are two conditions common in the male: impotence and ejaculation disturbances.

Impotence (erectile dysfunction) is inability to achieve or maintain an erection firm enough for satisfactory intercourse; patients sometimes use the term to mean premature ejaculation. Careful questioning is necessary, since causes of this vasocongestive disorder can be psychologic, physiologic, or both. The majority are pathophysiologic and, to varying degrees, treatable. After onset of the problem, a history of occasional erections—especially nocturnal penile tumescence, which may be evaluated by a simple monitoring device, or a sleep study in the sleep laboratory—is usually evidence that the dysfunction is psychologic in origin, with the caveat that decreased nocturnal penile tumescence occurs in some depressed patients. **Psychologic impotence** is caused by interpersonal or intrapsychic factors (eg, marital disharmony, depression). **Organic factors** (which usually develop gradually) include arteriosclerosis, hypertension, diabetes mellitus, drug abuse (alcohol, nicotine, narcotics, stimulants), pharmacologic agents (anticholinergic drugs, antihypertensive medication, antihistamines, disulfiram, all psychotropic drugs, narcotics, estrogens), organ system failure (circulatory, cardiorespiratory, renal), surgical complications (prostatectomy, vascular and back surgery), trauma (disk and spinal cord injuries), endocrine disturbances (pituitary, thyroid, adrenal, gonadal), zinc deficiency, neurologic disorders (multiple sclerosis, tumors, peripheral neuropathies, injuries, pernicious anemia, syphilis), urologic problems (phimosis), and primary developmental abnormalities (Klinefelter's syndrome).

Ejaculation disturbances include premature ejaculation, inability to ejaculate, and retrograde ejaculation. (One may ejaculate even though impotent.) Ejaculation is usually connected with orgasm, and ejaculatory control is an acquired behavior that is minimal in adolescence and increases with experience. Pathogenic factors are those that interfere with learning control, most frequently sexual ignorance. Intrapsychic factors (anxiety, guilt, depression) and interpersonal maladaptation (marital problems, unresponsiveness of mate, power struggles) are also common. Organic causes include interference with sympathetic nerve distribution (often due to surgery or trauma) and the effects of pharmacologic agents (eg, SSRIs or sympatholytics).

In females, the two most common forms of sexual dysfunction are vaginismus and frigidity.

Vaginismus is a conditioned response in which a spasm of the perineal muscles occurs if there is any stimulation of the area. The desire is to avoid penetration. Sexual responsiveness and vasocongestion may be present, and orgasm can result from clitoral stimulation.

Frigidity is a complex condition in which there is a general lack of sexual responsiveness. The woman has difficulty in experiencing erotic sensation and does not have the vasocongestive response. Sexual activity varies from active avoidance of sex to an occasional orgasm. Orgasmic dysfunction—in which a woman has a vasocongestive response but varying degrees of difficulty in reaching orgasm—is sometimes differentiated from frigidity. Causes for the dysfunctions include poor sexual techniques, early traumatic sexual experiences, interpersonal disharmony (marital struggles, use of sex as a means of control), and intrapsychic problems (anxiety, fear, guilt). Organic causes include any conditions that might cause pain in intercourse, pelvic pathology, mechanical obstruction, and neurologic deficits.

Disorders of sexual desire consist of diminished or absent libido in either sex and may be a function of organic or psychologic difficulties (eg, anxiety, phobic avoidance). Any chronic illness can sap desire. Hormonal disorders, including hypogonadism or use of antiandrogen compounds such as cyproterone acetate, and chronic renal failure contribute to deterioration in sexual activity. Alcohol, sedatives, narcotics, marijuana, and some medications may affect sexual drive and performance.

Treatment

A. Paraphilias and Gender Identity Disorders:

1. Psychologic–Sexual arousal disorders involving variant sexual activity (paraphilia), particularly those of a more superficial nature (eg, voyeurism) and those of recent onset, are responsive to psychotherapy in a moderate percentage of cases. The prognosis is much better if the motivation comes from the individual rather than the legal system; unfortunately, however, judicial intervention is frequently the only stimulus to treatment, because the condition persists and is reinforced until conflict with the law occurs. Therapies frequently focus on barriers to normal arousal response; the expectation is that the variant behavior will decrease as normal behavior increases.

2. Behavioral–Aversive and operant conditioning techniques have been tried frequently in gender role disorders but have only occasionally been successful. In some cases, the sexual arousal disorders improve with modeling, role-playing, and conditioning procedures. Emotive imagery is occasionally helpful in lessening anxiety in fetish problems.

3. Social–Although they do not produce a change in sexual arousal patterns or gender role, self-help groups have facilitated adjustment to an often hostile society. Attention to the family is particularly important in helping persons in such groups to accept their situation and alleviate their guilt about the role they think they had in creating the problem.

4. Medical–Medroxyprogesterone acetate, a suppressor of libidinal drive, is used to mute disruptive sexual behavior in males of all ages. Onset of action is usually within 3 weeks, and the effects are generally reversible. Fluoxetine or other SSRIs may reduce some of the compulsive sexual behaviors including the paraphilias. Although some transsexuals are treated with genital reconstructive surgery, many others are screened out by trial periods of living as females prior to operation.

B. Psychosexual Dysfunction:

1. Medical–Identification of a contributory reversible cause is most important. Even if the condition is not reversible, identification of the specific cause helps the patient to accept the condition. Marital disharmony, with its exacerbating effects, may thus be avoided. Of all the sexual dysfunctions, impotence is the condition most likely to have an organic basis. As part of the evaluation, vascular factors can be assessed in the office by injections of papaverine and alprostadil to produce an erection (apparently by raising nitric oxide levels or relaxing smooth muscle through other pathways). (See Male Erectile Dysfunction in Chapter 23.) Ultrasound examination is helpful in detecting arterial abnormalities. Yohimbine, 18 mg orally daily, has had modest effectiveness in both organic and psychogenic impotence. When the condition is irreversible, penile implants may be considered. Revascularization surgery has been done in patients with impotence due to circulatory problems. Because of their common effect in delaying ejaculation, the SSRIs have been effective in premature ejaculation.

2. Behavioral–Syndromes resulting from conditioned responses have been treated by conditioning techniques, with excellent results. Vaginismus responds well to desensitization with graduated Hegar dilators along with relaxation techniques. Masters and Johnson have used behavioral approaches in all of the sexual dysfunctions, with concomitant supportive psychotherapy and with improvement of the communication patterns of the couple.

3. Psychologic–The use of psychotherapy by itself is best suited for those cases in which interpersonal difficulties or intrapsychic problems predominate. Anxiety and guilt about parental injunctions against sex may contribute to sexual dysfunction. Even in these cases, however, a combined behavioral-psychologic approach usually produces results most quickly.

4. Social–The proximity of other people (eg, a mother-in-law) in a household is frequently an inhibiting factor in sexual relationships. In such cases, some social engineering may alleviate the problem.

[Impotence]
gopher://gopher.nih.gov/00/clin/cdcs/individual/91.impot
Friedman RC, Downey JI: Homosexuality. N Engl J Med 1994;331:923.
Kravitz HM et al: Medroxyprogesterone and paraphiles: Do testosterone levels matter? Bull Am Acad Psychiatry Law 1996;24:73. (Medroxyprogesterone can be effective in preventing relapse in sexual offenders.)
O'Keefe M, Hunt DK: Assessment and treatment of impotence. Med Clin North Am 1995;79:415.
Speckens AE et al: Psychosexual functioning of partners of men with presumed nonorganic erectile dysfunction: Cause or consequence of the disorder? Arch Sex Behav 1995;24:157. (Relationship problems, female psychosexual dysfunction, and the possible effect of relatively high levels of female sexual interest may contribute to the onset, exacerbation, and maintenance of impotence.)

PERSONALITY DISORDERS

Essentials of Diagnosis

- Long history dating back to childhood.
- Recurrent maladaptive behavior.
- Low self-esteem and lack of confidence.
- Minimal introspective ability with a tendency to blame others for all problems.
- Major difficulties with interpersonal relationships or society.
- Depression with anxiety when maladaptive behavior fails.

General Considerations

Personality—a hypothetical construct—is the result of a genetic substrate and the prolonged interaction of an individual with personal drives and with outside influences (parent-child interactions, peer influences, random events). The sum of the effects produces the enduring and unique patterns of behavior that are adopted in order to cope with the environment and that characterize one as an individual. The personality structure, or character, is an integral part of self-image and is important to one's sense of personal identity.

The classification of subtypes depends upon the predominant symptoms and their severity. The most severe disorders—those that bring the patient into greatest conflict with society—tend to be classified as antisocial (psychopathic) or borderline.

Personality disorders can be considered a matrix for some of the more severe psychiatric problems (eg, schizotypal, relating to schizophrenia; avoidance types, relating to some anxiety disorders).

Classification & Clinical Findings

See Table 25–3.

Differential Diagnosis

Patients with personality disorders tend to show anxiety and depression when pathologic techniques fail, and their symptoms can be similar to those occurring with anxiety disorders. Occasionally, the more severe cases may decompensate into psychosis under stress and mimic other psychotic disorders.

Treatment

A. Social: Social and therapeutic environments such as day hospitals, halfway houses, and self-help communities utilize peer pressures to modify the self-destructive behavior. The patient with a personality disorder often has failed to profit from experience, and difficulties with authority impair the learning experience. The use of peer relationships and the repetition possible in a structured setting of a helpful community enhance the behavioral treatment opportunities and increase learning. When problems are detected early, both the school and the home can serve as foci of intensified social pressure to change the behavior, particularly with the use of behavioral techniques.

B. Behavioral: The behavioral techniques used are principally operant conditioning and aversive conditioning. The former simply emphasizes the

Table 25–3. Personality disorders: Classification and clinical findings.

Personality Disorder	Clinical Findings
Paranoid	Defensive, oversensitive, secretive, suspicious, hyperalert, with limited emotional response.
Schizoid	Shy, introverted, withdrawn, avoids close relationships.
Compulsive	Perfectionist, egocentric, indecisive, with rigid thought patterns and need for control.
Histrionic (hysterical)	Dependent, immature, seductive, egocentric, vain, emotionally labile.
Schizotypal	Superstitious, socially isolated, suspicious, with limited interpersonal ability and odd speech.
Narcissistic	Exhibitionist, grandiose, preoccupied with power, lacks interest in others, with excessive demands for attention.
Avoidant	Fears rejection, hyperreacts to rejection and failure, with poor social endeavors and low self-esteem.
Dependent	Passive, overaccepting, unable to make decisions, lacks confidence, with poor self-esteem.
Passive-aggressive	Stubborn, procrastinating, argumentative, sulking, helpless, clinging, negative to authority figures.
Antisocial	Selfish, callous, promiscuous, impulsive, unable to learn from experience, has legal problems.
Borderline	Impulsive; has unstable and intense interpersonal relationships; is suffused with anger, fear, and guilt; lacks self-control and self-fulfillment; has identity problems and affective instability; is suicidal (a serious problem—up to 80% of hospitalized borderline patients make an attempt at some time during treatment, and the incidence of completed suicide is as high as 5%); aggressive behavior, feelings of emptiness, and occasional psychotic decompensation. This group has a high drug abuse rate, which plays a role in symptomatology. There is extensive overlap with other diagnostic categories, particularly mood disorders and posttraumatic stress disorder.

recognition of acceptable behavior and its reinforcement with praise or other tangible rewards. Aversive responses usually mean punishment, though this can range from a mild rebuke to some specific punitive responses such as verbal abuse or deprivation of privileges. Extinction plays a role in that an attempt is made not to respond to inappropriate behavior, and the lack of response eventually causes the person to abandon that type of behavior. Pouting and tantrums, for example, diminish quickly when such behavior elicits no reaction.

C. Psychologic: Psychologic intervention is best conducted in group settings. Group therapy is helpful when specific interpersonal behavior needs to be improved (eg, schizoid and inadequate types, in which involvement with people is markedly impaired). This mode of treatment also has a place with so-called acting-out patients, ie, those who frequently act in an impulsive and inappropriate way. The peer pressure in the group tends to impose restraints on rash behavior. The group also quickly identifies the patient's types of behavior and helps to improve the validity of the patient's self-assessment, so that the antecedents of the unacceptable behavior can be effectively handled, thus decreasing its frequency. Individual therapy should initially be supportive, ie, helping the patient to restabilize and mobilize defenses. If the individual has the ability to observe his or her own behavior, a longer-term and more introspective therapy may be warranted. The therapist must be able to handle countertransference feelings (which are frequently negative), maintain appropriate boundaries in the relationship (no physical contacts, however well-meaning), and refrain from premature confrontations and interpretations.

D. Medical: Hospitalization is rarely indicated except in the case of serious suicidal danger. In most cases, treatment can be accomplished in the day treatment center or self-help community. Antipsychotics may be required for short periods in conditions that have temporarily decompensated into transient psychoses (eg, haloperidol, 2–5 mg orally every 3–4 hours until the patient has quieted down and is regaining contact with reality). In most cases, these drugs are required only for several days and can be discontinued after the patient has regained a previously established level of adjustment. Carbamazepine, 800 mg orally daily in divided doses, decreases the severity of behavioral dyscontrol. Antidepressants have improved anxiety, depression, and sensitivity to rejection in some borderline patients.

Prognosis

Antisocial and borderline categories generally have a guarded prognosis. Those patients with poor outcomes are more likely to have a history of parental abuse and a family history of mood disorder, whereas persons with mild schizoid or passive-aggressive tendencies have a better prognosis with appropriate treatment.

Hubbard JR et al: Recognizing borderline personality disorder in the family practice setting. Am Fam Physician 1995;52:908.

Hueston WJ, Mainous AG 3rd, Schilling R: Patients with personality disorders: Functional status, health care utilization, and satisfaction with care. J Fam Pract 1996;42:54. (Primary care patients with a personality disorder have a greater likelihood of lower functional status, lower satisfaction with health care, and higher risk for depression and alcohol abuse.)

Sansone RA, Sansone LA: Borderline personality disorder. Interpersonal and behavioral problems that sabotage treatment success. Postgrad Med 1995;97:169.

Soloff PH et al: Risk factors for suicidal behavior in borderline personality disorder. Am J Psychiatry 1994; 151(9):1316. (Risk factors for suicidal behavior in patients with borderline personality disorder include older age, prior suicide attempts, antisocial personality, impulsive actions, and depressive moods.)

SCHIZOPHRENIC & OTHER PSYCHOTIC DISORDERS

Essentials of Diagnosis

- Social withdrawal, usually slowly progressive, often with deterioration in personal care.
- Loss of ego boundaries, with inability to perceive oneself as a separate entity.
- Loose thought associations, often with slowed thinking or overinclusive and rapid shifting from topic to topic.
- Autistic absorption in inner thoughts and frequent sexual or religious preoccupations.
- Auditory hallucinations, often of a derogatory nature.
- Delusions, frequently of a grandiose or persecutory nature.
- Symptoms of at least 6 months' duration.

Frequent additional signs:

- Flat affect and rapidly alternating mood shifts irrespective of circumstances.
- Hypersensitivity to environmental stimuli, with a feeling of enhanced sensory awareness.
- Variability or changeable behavior incongruent with the external environment.
- Concrete thinking with inability to abstract; inappropriate symbolism.
- Impaired concentration worsened by hallucinations and delusions.
- Depersonalization, wherein one behaves like a detached observer of one's own actions.

General Considerations

The schizophrenic disorders are a group of syndromes manifested by massive disruption of thinking, mood, and overall behavior as well as poor filtering of stimuli. The characterization and nomenclature of the disorders are quite arbitrary and are influenced by sociocultural factors and schools of psychiatric thought.

It is currently believed that the schizophrenic disorders are of multifactorial cause, with genetic, environmental, and neuroendocrine pathophysiologic components. At present, there is no laboratory method for confirmation of a diagnosis of schizophrenia. There may or may not be a history of a major disruption in the individual's life (failure, loss,

physical illness) before gross psychotic deterioration is evident.

"Other psychotic disorders" are conditions that are similar to schizophrenic disorders in their acute symptoms but have a less pervasive influence over the long term. The individual usually attains higher levels of functioning. The acute psychotic episodes tend to be less disruptive of the person's lifestyle, with a fairly quick return to previous levels of functioning.

Classification

A. Schizophrenic Disorders: Schizophrenic disorders are subdivided on the basis of certain prominent phenomena that are frequently present. **Disorganized (hebephrenic) schizophrenia** is characterized by marked incoherence and an incongruous or silly affect. **Catatonic schizophrenia** is distinguished by a marked psychomotor disturbance of either excitement (purposeless and stereotyped) or rigidity with mutism. Infrequently, there may be rapid alternation between excitement and stupor (see under catatonic syndrome, below). **Paranoid schizophrenia** includes marked persecutory or grandiose delusions often consonant with hallucinations of similar content. **Undifferentiated schizophrenia** denotes a category in which symptoms are not specific enough to warrant inclusion of the illness in the other subtypes. **Residual schizophrenia** is a classification that includes persons who have clearly had an episode warranting a diagnosis of schizophrenia but who at present have no overt psychotic symptoms, though they show milder signs such as social withdrawal, flat affect, and eccentric behaviors.

B. Paranoid (Delusional) Disorders: Paranoid disorders are psychoses in which the predominant symptoms are persistent persecutory delusions, with minimal impairment in daily function (the schizophrenic disorders show significant impairment). Intellectual and occupational activities are little affected, whereas social and marital functioning tend to be markedly involved. Hallucinations are not usually present. Many of these patients are misdiagnosed as paranoid schizophrenics.

C. Schizoaffective Disorders: Schizoaffective disorders are those cases that fail to fit comfortably either in the schizophrenic or in the affective categories. They are usually cases with affective symptoms that precede or develop concurrently with psychotic manifestations.

D. Schizophreniform Disorders: Schizophreniform disorders are similar in their symptoms to schizophrenic disorders except that the duration is less than 6 months but more than 1 week.

E. Brief Reactive Psychotic Disorders: These disorders last less than 1 week. They are the result of psychologic stress. The shorter duration is significant and correlates with a more acute onset and resolution as well as a much better prognosis.

F. Late Life Psychosis: Brain abnormalities occur in 40% of patients who develop psychotic symptoms after age 60. The psychotic symptoms are typical, and there are other findings such as low IQ scores and diminished cognitive function.

G. Atypical Psychoses: This group includes a wide range of conditions with psychotic symptomatology. The cause is often not clear, but later events (eg, new symptoms) may clarify the diagnosis. The most common example is chronic psychosis developing either during periods of heavy abuse of drugs or at some time after the drug use has ceased. Other conditions include temporal lobe dysfunction, HIV infection, and a number of the conditions noted in the differential diagnosis (see below). They often have a good premorbid history, a precipitous onset, and an episodic course with symptom-free intervals.

Clinical Findings

The symptoms and signs vary markedly among individuals as well as in the same person at different times. The patient's **appearance** may be bizarre, though the usual finding is a mild to moderate unkempt blandness. **Motor activity** is generally reduced, though extremes ranging from catatonic stupor to frenzied excitement occur. **Social behavior** is characterized by marked withdrawal coupled with disturbed interpersonal relationships and a reduced ability to experience pleasure. Dependency and a poor self-image are common. **Verbal utterances** are variable, the language being concrete yet symbolic, with unassociated rambling statements (at times interspersed with mutism) during an acute episode. Neologisms (made-up words or phrases), echolalia (repetition of words spoken by others), and verbigeration (repetition of senseless words or phrases) are occasionally present. **Affect** is usually flattened, with occasional inappropriateness. **Depression** is present in almost all cases but may be less apparent during the acute psychotic episode and more obvious during recovery. Depression is sometimes confused with akinetic side effects of antipsychotic drugs. It is also related to **boredom,** which increases symptoms and decreases the response to treatment. Work is generally unavailable and time hangs heavy, providing opportunities for counterproductive activities such as drug abuse, withdrawal, and increased psychotic symptoms.

Thought content may vary from a paucity of ideas to a rich complex of delusional fantasy with archaic thinking. One frequently notes after a period of conversation that little if any information has actually been conveyed. Incoming stimuli produce varied responses. In some cases a simple question may trigger explosive outbursts, whereas at other times there may be no overt response whatsoever (catatonia). When paranoid ideation is present, the patient is often irritable and less cooperative. **Delusions** (false beliefs) are characteristic of paranoid thinking, and they usually take the form of a preoccupation with the supposedly threatening behavior exhibited by other individuals. This ideation may cause the patient to adopt active countermeasures such as locking doors and windows, taking up weapons, covering the ceiling with aluminum foil to counteract radar waves, and other bizarre efforts. Somatic delusions revolve around issues of bodily decay or infestation. **Perceptual distortions** usually include auditory hallucinations—visual hallucinations are more commonly associated with organic mental states—and may include illusions (distortions of reality) such as figures changing in size or lights varying in intensity. Cenesthetic hallucinations (eg, a burning sensation in the brain, feeling blood flowing in blood vessels) occasionally occur. Lack of humor, feelings of dread, depersonalization (a feeling of being apart from the self), and fears of annihilation may be present. Any of the above symptoms generate higher anxiety levels, with heightened arousal and occasional panic and suicidal ideation, as the individual fails to cope.

Schizophrenic symptoms have been classified recently into positive and negative categories. Positive symptoms include hallucinations, delusions, and formal thought disorders. These symptoms appear to be related to increased (D_2) dopaminergic activity in the mesolimbic region. Negative symptoms include diminished sociability, restricted affect, and poverty of speech and appear to be related to decreased dopaminergic activity in the mesocortical system.

Ventricular enlargement and cortical atrophy, as seen on the CT scan, have been correlated with a chronic course, severe cognitive impairment, and nonresponsiveness to neuroleptic medications. Decreased frontal lobe activity on positron emission tomography has been associated with negative symptoms.

The development of the acute episode in schizophrenia frequently is the end product of a gradual decompensation. Frustration and anxiety appear early, followed by depression and alienation, along with decreased effectiveness in day-to-day coping. This often leads to feelings of panic and increasing disorganization, with loss of the ability to test and evaluate the reality of perceptions. The stage of so-called psychotic resolution includes delusions, autistic preoccupations, and psychotic insight, with acceptance of the decompensated state. The process is frequently complicated by the use of caffeine, alcohol, and other recreational drugs. Life expectancy of schizophrenics is as much as 20% shorter than that of cohorts in the general population (usually because of a higher mortality rate in younger people).

Polydipsia may produce water intoxication with hyponatremia—characterized by symptoms of confusion, lethargy, psychosis, seizures, and occasionally death—in any psychiatric disorder, but most commonly in schizophrenia. These problems exacerbate the schizophrenic symptoms. Possible pathogenetic factors include a hypothalamic defect, inappropriate ADH secretion (exclude medical causes of SIADH), neuroleptic medications (anticholinergic effects, stimulation of hypothalamic thirst center, effect on ADH), smoking (nicotine and SIADH), psychotic thought processes (delusions), and other medications (eg, diuretics, antidepressants, lithium, alcohol). Other causes of polydipsia must be ruled out (eg, diabetes mellitus, diabetes insipidus, renal disease).

Differential Diagnosis

One should not hesitate to reconsider the diagnosis of schizophrenia in any person who has received that diagnosis in the past, particularly when the clinical course has been atypical. A number of these patients have been found to actually have atypical episodic affective disorders that have responded well to lithium. Manic episodes often mimic schizophrenia. Furthermore, many individuals have been diagnosed as schizophrenic because of inadequacies in psychiatric nomenclature. Thus, persons with brief reactive psychoses, obsessive-compulsive disorder, paranoid disorders, and schizophreniform disorders were often inappropriately diagnosed as having schizophrenia.

Psychotic depressions, psychotic organic mental states, and any illness with psychotic ideation tend to be confused with schizophrenia, partly because of the regrettable tendency to use the terms interchangeably. Adolescent phases of growth and counterculture behaviors constitute another area of diagnostic confusion. It is particularly important to avoid a misdiagnosis in these groups, because of the long-term implications arising from having such a serious diagnosis made in a formative stage of life.

Medical disorders such as thyroid dysfunction, adrenal and pituitary disorders, reactions to toxic materials (eg, mercury, PCBs), and almost all of the organic mental states in the early stages must be ruled out. Postpartum psychosis is discussed under Mood Disorders. **Complex partial seizures,** especially when psychosensory phenomena are present, are an important differential consideration. Toxic drug states arising from prescription, over-the-counter, and street drugs may mimic all of the psychotic disorders. The chronic use of amphetamines, cocaine, and other stimulants frequently produces a psychosis that is almost identical to the acute paranoid schizophrenic episode. The presence of formication and stereotypy suggests the possibility of stimulant abuse. Phencyclidine (see below) has become a very common street drug, and in many cases a reaction to it is difficult to distinguish from other psychotic disorders. Cerebellar signs, excessive salivation, dilated pupils, and increased deep tendon reflexes should alert the physician to the possibility of a toxic psychosis. Industrial chemical toxicity (both organic and metallic), degenerative disorders, and metabolic deficiencies must be considered in the differential diagnosis.

Catatonic syndrome, frequently assumed to exist solely as a component of schizophrenic disorders, is actually the end product of a number of illnesses, including various organic conditions. Neoplasms, viral and bacterial encephalopathies, central nervous system hemorrhage, metabolic derangements such as diabetic ketoacidosis, sedative withdrawal, and hepatic and renal malfunction have all been implicated. It is particularly important to realize that drug toxicity (eg, overdoses of antipsychotic medications such as fluphenazine or haloperidol) can cause catatonic syndrome, which may be misdiagnosed as a catatonic schizophrenic disorder and inappropriately treated with more antipsychotic medication.

Treatment

A. Medical: Hospitalization is often necessary, particularly when the patient's behavior shows gross disorganization. The presence of competent family members lessens the need for hospitalization, and each case should be judged individually. The major considerations are to prevent self-inflicted harm or harm to others and to provide the patient's basic needs. A full medical evaluation and CT scan or MRI should be considered in first episodes of schizophreniform disorder and other psychotic episodes of unknown cause.

Antipsychotic medications (see below) are the treatment of choice. They block the response to stimulation. The relapse rate can be reduced by 50% with proper maintenance neuroleptic therapy. Long-acting, injectable depot neuroleptics are used in noncompliant patients or nonresponders to oral medication. So-called **positive symptoms** such as hallucinations and delusions respond best, while **negative symptoms** such as withdrawal, psychomotor retardation, and poor interpersonal relationships may show little improvement. Clozapine may reduce these negative symptoms. Antidepressant drugs may be used in conjunction with neuroleptics if significant depression is present. Resistant cases may require concomitant use of lithium, carbamazepine, or valproic acid. The addition of a benzodiazepine drug to the neuroleptic regimen may prove helpful in treating the agitated or catatonic psychotic patient who has not responded to neuroleptics alone—lorazepam, 1–2 mg orally, can produce a rapid resolution of catatonic symptoms; the benzodiazepine may allow maintenance with a lower neuroleptic dose. ECT has also been effective in treating catatonia.

Antipsychotic drugs include **phenothiazines, thioxanthenes** (both similar in structure), **butyrophenones, dihydroindolones, dibenzoxazepines,** and **benzisoxazoles.** Table 25–4 lists the drugs in order of increasing milligram potency and decreasing anticholinergic and adrenergic side effects but increasing extrapyramidal symptoms. For example, chlorpromazine has lower potency and causes more severe anticholinergic and adrenergic side effects.

Table 25–4. Commonly used antipsychotics.

	Chlorproma- zine Ratio	Usual Daily Oral Dose	Usual Daily Maximum Dose[1]	Cost per Unit	Cost for 30 Days' Treat- ment Based on Maximum Dosage[2]
Phenothiazines					
Chlorpromazine (Thor- azine; others)	1:1	100–400 mg	1 g	$0.15/200 mg	$22.50
Thioridazine (Mellaril)	1:1	100–400 mg	600 mg	$0.47/200 mg	$42.30
Mesoridazine (Serentil)	1:2	50–200 mg	400 mg	$1.03/100 mg	$123.60
Perphenazine (Trilafon)[3]	1:10	16–32 mg	64 mg	$1.05/16 mg	$126.00
Trifluoperazine (Stela- zine)	1:20	5–15 mg	60 mg	$1.52/10 mg	$273.60
Fluphenazine (Permitil, Prolixin)[3]	1:50	2–10 mg	60 mg	$1.15/10 mg	$207.00
Thioxanthenes					
Thiothixene (Navane)[3]	1:20	5–10 mg	80 mg	$0.55/10 mg	$132.00
Dihydroindolone					
Molindone (Moban)	1:12	30–100 mg	225 mg	$1.76/50 mg	$237.60
Dibenzoxazepine					
Loxapine (Loxitane)	1:10	20–60 mg	200 mg	$1.65/50 mg	$198.00
Dibenzodiazepine					
Clozapine (Clozaril)	1:1	300–450 mg	900 mg	$3.52/100 mg	$950.40
Butyrophenone					
Haloperidol (Haldol)	1:50	2–5 mg	80 mg	$1.02/20 mg	$122.40
Benzisoxazole					
Risperidone[4] (Risperdal)	1:100	2–6 mg	10 mg	$3.40/2 mg	$510.00
Thienbenzodiazepine					
Olanzapine (Zyprexa)	1:50	5–10 mg	10 mg	$7.73/10 mg	$231.90

[1]Can be higher in some cases.
[2]Cost to pharmacist (average wholesale price) for 30 days' treatment based on maximum dosage (generic when possible). Source: First Data Bank, Price Alert, April 1997.
[3]Indicates piperazine structure.
[4]For risperidone, daily doses above 6 mg increase the risk of extrapyramidal syndrome. Risperidone 6 mg is approximately equivalent to haloperidol 20 mg.

The increased anticholinergic effect of chlorpromazine, however, produces less risk of extrapyramidal symptoms.

The phenothiazines comprise the bulk of the currently used neuroleptic drugs. The only butyrophenone commonly used in psychiatry is haloperidol, which is totally different in structure but very similar in action and side effects to the piperazine phenothiazines such as fluphenazine, perphenazine, and trifluoperazine. These drugs and haloperidol (dopamine [D_2] receptor blockers) have high potency, a paucity of autonomic side effects, and act to markedly lower arousal levels. Molindone and loxapine, while less potent, are similar in action, side effects, and safety to the piperazine phenothiazines.

Clozapine and risperidone are the first agents of a new generation of "atypical" (novel) antipsychotic drugs. Clozapine, a dibenzodiazepine derivative, has dopamine (D_4) receptor-blocking activity as well as central serotonergic, histaminergic, and alpha-noradrenergic receptor-blocking activity. It is effective in the treatment of about 30% of psychoses resistant to other neuroleptic drugs. Risperidone is a new antipsychotic that blocks some serotonin receptors

(5-HT_2) and dopamine receptors (D_2). Risperidone causes fewer extrapyramidal side effects than the typical antipsychotics. It appears to be as effective as haloperidol. It probably is not as effective as clozapine in treatment-resistant patients, though it warrants a trial in this population because of its reduced risk of agranulocytosis and its lower cost. Clozapine, although requiring weekly white blood cell counts, appears uniquely effective in refractory disorders and in patients with tardive dyskinesia.

Olanzapine is a newly released neuroleptic that is a potent blocker of muscarinic, anticholinergic, 5-HT_2, and dopamine D_1, D_2, and D_4 receptors. High doses of olanzapine (12.5–17.5 mg daily) appear to be more effective than lower doses. The drug appears to be more effective than haloperidol in the treatment of negative symptoms. It has, however, been associated with elevated serum alanine aminotransferase than those taking haloperidol. It is associated with a much lower incidence of dystonic reaction than haloperidol and is perhaps less likely to induce tardive dyskinesia. Its most common side effects include agitation, nervousness, headache, insomnia, somnolence, dizziness, weight gain, and dyspepsia.

Its role in treatment-refractory patients remains to be explored.

None of the antipsychotics produce true physical dependency, and they have wide safety margins between therapeutic and toxic effects. All decrease adrenergic responses. Previous patient response, experience with the drug, and its side effects dictate the choice of drug.

Clinical Indications

The antipsychotics are used to treat all forms of the **schizophrenias** as well as **psychotic ideation in organic brain psychoses, drug-induced psychoses, psychotic depression,** and **mania.** They are also effective in Tourette's disorder. They quickly lower the arousal (activity) level and, perhaps indirectly, gradually improve socialization and thinking. The improvement rate is about 80%. Patients whose behavioral symptoms worsen with use of antipsychotic drugs may have an undiagnosed organic condition such as anticholinergic toxicity.

Symptoms that are ameliorated by these drugs include hyperactivity, hostility, aggression, delusions, hallucinations, irritability, and poor sleep. Individuals with acute psychosis and good premorbid function respond quite well. The most common cause of failure in the treatment of acute psychosis is inadequate dosage, and the most common cause of relapse is noncompliance.

Dosage Forms & Patterns

The dosage range is quite broad. For example, haloperidol, 1 mg orally at bedtime, may be sufficient for the elderly person with a mild organic brain syndrome, whereas 60 mg/d may be used in a young schizophrenic patient. A dosage of 10–20 mg/d is adequate initially for most patients. For quick response, one may start with haloperidol, 10 mg intramuscularly, which is absorbed rapidly and achieves an initial tenfold plasma level advantage over equal oral doses. Psychomotor agitation, racing thoughts, and general arousal are quickly reduced. The dose can be repeated every 3–4 hours; when the patient is less symptomatic, oral doses can replace parenteral administration in most cases.

Various factors play a role in the absorption of oral medications. Of particular importance are previous gastrointestinal surgery and concomitant administration of other drugs, eg, antacids (Table 25–5). There are racial differences in metabolizing the neuroleptic drugs—eg, many Asians require only about half the usual dosage. Bioavailability is influenced by other factors such as smoking or hepatic microsomal enzyme stimulation with alcohol or barbiturates and enzyme-altering drugs such as carbamazepine or methylphenidate. Plasma drug level determinations are not currently of major clinical assistance.

Divided daily doses are not necessary after a maintenance dose has been established, and most pa-

Table 25–5. Antipsychotic drug interactions with other drugs.

Drug	Effects
Antacids	Decreased absorption of antipsychotic drugs.
All anticholinergics	Increased anticholinergic effects.
Barbiturates	Central nervous system depression and decreased antipsychotic drug levels.
Carbamazepine	Decreased neuroleptic levels.
Cimetidine	Increased chlorpromazine levels.
Tricyclic antidepressants	Increased antidepressant blood levels.
Guanadrel	Increased hypotensive effect.
Guanethidine	Decreased hypotensive effect.
Indomethacin	Severe drowsiness (with haloperidol).
Levodopa	Decreased antiparkinson effect.
Methyldopa	Decreased hypotensive effect.
Phenytoin	Increased phenytoin levels.
Propranolol	Increased thioridazine levels.
Thiazide diuretics	Increased hypotensive effect.
Trihexyphenidyl	Decreased antipsychotic levels.

tients can then be maintained on a single daily dose, usually taken at bedtime. This is particularly appropriate in a case where the sedative effect of the drug is desired for nighttime sleep, and undesirable sedative effects can be avoided during the day. Risperidone is an exception, being given twice daily. First-episode patients especially should be tapered off medications after about 6 months of stability and carefully monitored; their rate of relapse is lower than that of multiple-episode patients.

Psychiatric patients—particularly paranoid individuals—often neglect to take their medication. In these cases and in nonresponders to oral medication, the enanthate and decanoate (the latter is slightly longer-lasting and has fewer extrapyramidal side effects) forms of fluphenazine or the decanoate form of haloperidol may be given by deep subcutaneous injection or intramuscularly to achieve an effect that will usually last 7–28 days. A patient who cannot be depended on to take oral medication (or who overdoses on minimal provocation) will generally agree to come to the physician's office for a "shot." The usual dose of the fluphenazine long-acting preparations is 25 mg every 2 weeks. Dosage and frequency of administration vary from about 100 mg weekly to 12.5 mg monthly. Use the smallest effective amount as infrequently as possible. A monthly injection of 25 mg of fluphenazine decanoate is equivalent to about 15–20 mg of oral fluphenazine daily. Concomitant use of a benzodiazepine (eg, lorazepam, 2 mg orally twice daily) may permit reduction of the required dosage of oral or parenteral antipsychotic drug.

Intravenous haloperidol, the neuroleptic most commonly used by this route, is often used in critical care units in the management of agitated, delirious patients. Intravenous haloperidol should be given no faster than 1 mg/min to reduce cardiovascular side effects.

Side Effects

The side effects *decrease* as one goes from the sedating, lower milligram potency drugs such as chlorpromazine or thioridazine to those of higher milligram potency such as fluphenazine and haloperidol. However, the extrapyramidal effects *increase* as one goes down the list (consider chlorprothixene as similar to chlorpromazine).

The most common anticholinergic side effects include dry mouth (which can lead to ingestion of caloric liquids and weight gain), blurred near vision, urinary retention (particularly in elderly men with enlarged prostates), delayed gastric emptying, ileus, delirium, and precipitation of acute glaucoma in patients with narrow anterior chamber angles. Other autonomic effects include orthostatic hypotension and sexual dysfunction—problems in achieving erection, ejaculation (including retrograde ejaculation), and orgasm in males (approximately 50% of cases) and females (approximately 30%). Delay in achieving orgasm is often a factor in medication noncompliance. Electrocardiographic changes occur frequently, but clinically significant arrhythmias are much less common. Elderly patients and those with preexisting cardiac disease are at greater risk. The most frequently seen electrocardiographic changes include diminution of the T wave amplitude, appearance of prominent U waves, depression of the ST segment, and prolongation of the QT interval. These electrocardiographic findings usually do not call for any change in treatment. In some critical care patients, however, torsade de pointes has been associated with the use of high-dose intravenous haloperidol (usually > 100 mg/24 h).

Metabolic and endocrine effects include weight gain, hyperglycemia, infrequent temperature irregularities (particularly in hot weather), and water intoxication that may be due to inappropriate antidiuretic hormone secretion. Lactation and menstrual irregularities are common (antipsychotic drugs should be avoided, if possible, in breast cancer patients because of potential trophic effects of elevated prolactin levels on the breast). Both antipsychotic and antidepressant drugs inhibit sperm motility. Bone marrow depression and cholestatic jaundice occur rarely; these are hypersensitivity reactions, and they usually appear in the first 2 months of treatment. They subside on discontinuance of the drug. There is cross-sensitivity among all of the phenothiazines, and a drug from a different group should be used when allergic reactions occur.

Clozapine is associated with a 1.6% risk of **agranulocytosis** (higher in persons of Ashkenazi Jewish ancestry), and its use must be strictly monitored with weekly blood counts. It also lowers the seizure threshold and has many side effects, including sedation, hypotension, increased liver enzyme levels, hypersalivation, respiratory arrest, weight gain, and changes in both ECG and EEG.

Photosensitivity, retinopathy, and hyperpigmentation are associated with use of fairly high dosages of chlorpromazine and thioridazine. The appearance of particulate melanin deposits in the lens of the eye is related to the total dose given, and patients on long-term medication should have periodic eye examinations. Teratogenicity has not been causally related to these drugs, but prudence is indicated particularly in the first trimester of pregnancy. The seizure threshold is lowered, but it is safe to use these medications in epileptics controlled by anticonvulsants.

The **neuroleptic malignant syndrome (NMS)** is a catatonia-like state manifested by extrapyramidal signs, blood pressure changes, altered consciousness, and hyperpyrexia; it is an uncommon but serious complication of neuroleptic treatment. Muscle rigidity, involuntary movements, confusion, dysarthria, and dysphagia are accompanied by pallor, cardiovascular instability, fever, pulmonary congestion, and diaphoresis and may result in stupor, coma, and death. The cause may be related to a number of factors, including poor dosage control of neuroleptic medication, affective illness, decreased serum iron, dehydration, and increased sensitivity of dopamine receptor sites. Lithium in combination with a neuroleptic drug may increase vulnerability, which is already increased in patients with an affective disorder. In most cases, the symptoms develop within the first 2 weeks of antipsychotic drug treatment. The syndrome may occur with small doses of the drugs. Intramuscular administration is a risk factor. Elevated creatine kinase and leukocytosis with a shift to the left are present early in about half of cases. Treatment includes controlling fever and providing fluid support. Dopamine agonists such as bromocriptine, 2.5–10 mg orally three times a day, and amantadine, 100–200 mg orally twice a day, have also been useful. Dantrolene, 50 mg intravenously as needed, is used to alleviate rigidity (do not exceed 10 mg/kg/d). There is ongoing controversy about the efficacy of these three agents as well as the use of calcium channel blockers and benzodiazepines. Electroconvulsive therapy has been used effectively in resistant cases. Clozapine has been used with relative safety and fair success as an antipsychotic drug for patients who have had NMS. The syndrome must be differentiated from acute lethal catatonia, malignant hyperthermia, neurotoxic syndromes (including AIDS), and a variety of other conditions such as viral encephalitis, Wilson's disease, central anticholinergic syndrome, and hypertonic states (eg, tetany, strychnine poisoning).

Akathisia is the most common (about 20%) so-called **extrapyramidal symptom.** It usually occurs early in treatment (but may persist after neuroleptics are discontinued) and is frequently mistaken for anxiety or exacerbation of psychosis. It is characterized by a subjective desire to be in constant motion followed by an inability to sit or stand still and consequent pacing. It may include suicidality or feelings of fright, rage, terror, or sexual torment. Insomnia is often present. In all cases, reevaluate the dosage requirement or the type of neuroleptic drug. One should inquire also about cigarette smoking, which in women has been associated with an increased incidence of akathisia. Antiparkinsonism drugs such as trihexyphenidyl, 2–5 mg orally three times daily, or benztropine mesylate, 1–2 mg twice daily, may be helpful. In resistant cases, symptoms may be alleviated by propranolol, 30–80 mg/d orally; diazepam, 5 mg three times daily; or amantadine, 100 mg orally three times daily.

Acute dystonias usually occur early, though a late (tardive) occurrence is reported in patients (mostly males after several years of therapy) who previously had early severe dystonic reactions and a mood disorder (see below). Younger patients are at higher risk for acute dystonias. The most common signs are bizarre muscle spasms of the head, neck, and tongue. Frequently present are torticollis, oculogyric crises, swallowing or chewing difficulties, and masseter spasms. Laryngospasm is particularly dangerous. Back, arm, or leg muscle spasms are occasionally reported. Diphenhydramine, 50 mg intramuscularly, is effective for the acute crisis; one should then give benztropine mesylate, 2 mg orally twice daily, for several weeks, and then discontinue gradually, since few of the extrapyramidal symptoms require long-term use of the antiparkinsonism drugs (all of which are about equally efficacious—though trihexyphenidyl tends to be mildly stimulating and benztropine mildly sedating).

Drug-induced parkinsonism is indistinguishable from idiopathic parkinsonism, but it is reversible, occurs later in treatment than the preceding extrapyramidal symptoms, and in some cases appears after neuroleptic withdrawal. The condition includes the typical signs of apathy and reduction of facial and arm movements (akinesia, which can mimic depression), festinating gait, rigidity, loss of postural reflexes, and pill-rolling tremor. AIDS patients seem particularly vulnerable to extrapyramidal side effects. High-potency neuroleptics often require antiparkinsonism drugs (Table 24–4). The neuroleptic dosage should be reduced, and immediate relief can be achieved with antiparkinsonism drugs in the same dosages as above. After 4–6 weeks, these antiparkinsonism drugs can often be discontinued with no recurrent symptoms. In any of the extrapyramidal symptoms, amantadine, 100–400 mg daily, may be used instead of the antiparkinsonism drugs. Neuroleptic-induced catatonia is similar to catatonic stupor with rigidity, drooling, urinary incontinence, and cogwheeling. It usually responds slowly to withdrawal of the offending medication and use of antiparkinsonism agents.

Tardive dyskinesia is a syndrome of abnormal involuntary stereotyped movements of the face, mouth, tongue, trunk, and limbs that may occur after months or (usually) years of treatment with neuroleptic agents. The syndrome affects 20–35% of patients who have undergone long-term neuroleptic therapy. Predisposing factors include older age, many years of treatment, cigarette smoking, and diabetes mellitus. Pineal calcification is higher in this condition by a margin of 3:1. There are no known differences among any of the antipsychotic drugs in the development of this syndrome.

Early manifestations include fine worm-like movements of the tongue at rest, difficulty in sticking out the tongue, facial tics, increased blink frequency, or jaw movements of recent onset. Later manifestations may include bucco-linguo-masticatory movements, lip smacking, chewing motions, mouth opening and closing, disturbed gag reflex, puffing of the cheeks, disrupted speech, respiratory distress, or choreoathetoid movements of the extremities (the last being more prevalent in younger patients). The symptoms do not necessarily worsen and in rare cases may lessen even though neuroleptic drugs are continued. The dyskinesias do not occur during sleep and can be voluntarily suppressed for short periods. Stress and movements in other parts of the body will often aggravate the condition.

Early signs of dyskinesia must be differentiated from those reversible signs produced by ill-fitting dentures or nonneuroleptic drugs such as levodopa, tricyclic antidepressants (TCAs), antiparkinsonism agents, anticonvulsants, and antihistamines. Other neurologic conditions such as Huntington's chorea can be differentiated by history and examination.

The emphasis should be on prevention. Use the least amount of neuroleptic drug necessary to mute the psychotic symptoms. Detect early manifestations of dyskinesias. When these occur, stop anticholinergic drugs and gradually discontinue neuroleptic drugs. Weight loss and cachexia sometimes appear on withdrawal of neuroleptics. In an indeterminate number of cases, the dyskinesias will remit. Keep the patient off the drugs until reemergent psychotic symptoms dictate their resumption, at which point they are restarted in low doses and gradually increased until there is clinical improvement. If neuroleptic drugs are restarted, the use of adjunctive agents such as benzodiazepines or lithium may help directly or indirectly by allowing control of psychotic symptoms with a low dosage of neuroleptics. If the dyskinesic syndrome recurs and it is necessary to continue neuroleptic drugs to control psychotic symptoms, informed consent should be obtained. Benzodiazepines, buspirone (in doses of 40–160 mg/d), phosphatidylcholine, clonidine, calcium channel blockers, vitamin E, and propranolol all have had limited usefulness in treating the dyskinetic side effects.

B. Social: Environmental considerations are most important in the individual with a chronic illness, who usually has a history of repeated hospitalizations, a continued low level of functioning, and symptoms that never completely remit. Family rejection and work failure are common. In these cases, board and care homes staffed by personnel experienced in caring for psychiatric patients are most important. There is frequently an inverse relationship between stability of the living situation and the amounts of required antipsychotic drugs, since the most salutary environment is one that reduces stimuli. Nonresidential self-help groups such as Recovery, Inc., should be utilized whenever possible. They provide a setting for sharing, learning, and mutual support and are frequently the only social involvement with which this type of patient is comfortable. Vocational rehabilitation and work agencies (eg, Goodwill Industries, Inc.) provide assessment, training, and job opportunities at a level commensurate with the person's clinical condition.

C. Psychologic: The need for psychotherapy varies markedly depending on the patient's current status and history. In a person with a single psychotic episode and a previously good level of adjustment, supportive psychotherapy may help the patient reintegrate the experience, gain some insight into antecedent problems, and become a more self-observant individual who can recognize early signs of stress. Insight-oriented psychotherapy is often counterproductive in this type of disorder. More importantly, family therapy should be given concomitantly to help alleviate the patient's stress and to assist relatives in coping with the patient.

D. Behavioral: Behavioral techniques (see above) are most frequently used in therapeutic settings such as day treatment centers, but there is no reason why they cannot be incorporated into family situations or any therapeutic setting. Many behavioral techniques are used unwittingly (eg, positive reinforcement—whether it be a word of praise or an approving nod—after some positive behavior), and with some careful thought this approach can be a powerful instrument for helping a person learn behaviors that will facilitate social acceptance. Music from portable cassette players with earphones is one of many ways to divert the patient's attention from auditory hallucinations.

Prognosis

In any psychosis in the large majority of patients, the prognosis is excellent for alleviation of positive symptoms such as hallucinations or delusions treated with medication. Negative symptoms such as diminished affect and sociability are much more difficult to treat and are the principal reason schizophrenic patients do not achieve optimal function. Unavailability of structured work situations and lack of family therapy are two other reasons why the prognosis is so

guarded in such a large percentage of schizophrenic patients. Psychosis connected with a history of serious drug abuse has a guarded prognosis because of the central nervous system damage, usually from the drugs themselves and associated medical illnesses.

Andreasen NC: Symptoms, signs, and diagnosis of schizophrenia. Lancet 1995;346(8973):477. (Discusses positive and negative symptoms.)

Beal M: Clozapine update. West J Med 1994;160:53.

Eisendrath SJ: Psychiatry in the critical care unit. In: *Current Critical Care Diagnosis and Treatment.* Bongard FS, Sue DY (editors). Appleton & Lange, 1994.

Kane JM: Drug therapy: Schizophrenia. N Engl J Med 1996;334:34. (Broad review of current approaches.)

Pickar D: Prospects for pharmacotherapy of schizophrenia. Lancet 1995;345:557.

Wilt JL et al: Torsade de pointes associated with the use of intravenous haloperidol. Ann Intern Med 1993;119:391.

MOOD DISORDERS
(Depression & Mania)

Essentials of Diagnosis

Present in most depressions:

- Lowered mood, varying from mild sadness to intense feelings of guilt, worthlessness, and hopelessness.
- Difficulty in thinking, including inability to concentrate, ruminations, and lack of decisiveness.
- Loss of interest, with diminished involvement in work and recreation.
- Somatic complaints such as headache; disrupted, lessened, or excessive sleep; loss of energy; change in appetite; decreased sexual drive.
- Anxiety.

Present in some severe depressions:

- Psychomotor retardation or agitation.
- Delusions of a hypochondriacal or persecutory nature.
- Withdrawal from activities.
- Physical symptoms of major severity, eg, anorexia, insomnia, reduced sexual drive, weight loss, and various somatic complaints.
- Suicidal ideation.

Present in mania:

- Mood ranging from euphoria to irritability.
- Sleep disruption.
- Hyperactivity.
- Racing thoughts.
- Grandiosity.
- Variable psychotic symptoms.

General Considerations

Depression is extremely common, with up to 30% of primary care patients having depressive symptoms. Depression may be the final expression of (1) genetic factors (neurotransmitter dysfunction), (2) developmental problems (personality defects, childhood events), or (3) psychosocial stresses (divorce, unemployment). It frequently presents in the form of somatic complaints with negative medical workups. Although sadness and grief are normal responses to loss, depression is not. Patients experiencing normal grief tend to produce sympathy and sadness in the physician caregiver; depression often produces frustration and irritation in the physician. Grief is usually accompanied by intact self-esteem, whereas depression is marked by a sense of guilt and worthlessness.

Mania is often combined with depression and may occur alone or in cyclic fashion with depression.

Clinical Findings

In general, there are four major types of depressions, with similar symptoms in each group.

A. Adjustment Disorder With Depressed Mood: Depression may occur in reaction to some identifiable stressor or adverse life situation, usually loss of a person by death (grief reaction), divorce, etc; financial reversal (crisis); or loss of an established role, such as being needed. Anger is frequently associated with the loss, and this in turn often produces a feeling of guilt. The disorder occurs within 3 months of the stressor and causes significant impairment in social or occupational functioning. The symptoms range from mild sadness, anxiety, irritability, worry, lack of concentration, discouragement, and somatic complaints to the more severe symptoms of the next group.

B. Depressive Disorders: The subclassifications include major depressive episodes and dysthymia.

1. A major depressive episode (eg, "endogenous" unipolar disorder, melancholia) is a period of serious mood depression that occurs at any time of life. Many consider a physiologic or metabolic aberration to be causative. Complaints vary widely but most frequently include a loss of interest and pleasure (anhedonia), withdrawal from activities, and feelings of guilt. Also included are inability to concentrate, some cognitive dysfunction, anxiety, chronic fatigue, feelings of worthlessness, somatic complaints (unidentifiable somatic complaints frequently indicate depression), and loss of sexual drive. Diurnal variation with improvement as the day progresses is common. Vegetative signs that frequently occur are insomnia, anorexia with weight loss, and constipation. Occasionally, severe agitation and psychotic ideation (paranoid thinking, somatic delusions) are present. These symptoms are more common in postmenopausal depression (involutional melancholia). Paranoid symptoms may range from general suspiciousness to ideas of reference with delusions. The somatic delusions frequently revolve around feelings of impending annihilation or hypochondriacal beliefs (eg, that the body is rotting away with cancer). Hallucinations are uncommon.

2. Dysthymia is a chronic depressive disturbance. Sadness, loss of interest, and withdrawal from activities over a period of 2 or more years with a relatively persistent course is necessary for this diagnosis. Generally, the symptoms are milder but longer-lasting than those in a major depressive episode.

3. Depressive disorder not otherwise specified—This one includes several subcategories. **Atypical depression** is characterized by hypersomnia, overeating, lethargy, and rejection sensitivity. These patients should be carefully evaluated for bipolar disorder. **Seasonal affective disorder (SAD)** is a dysfunction of circadian rhythms that occurs more commonly in the winter and is believed to be due to decreased exposure to full-spectrum light. Common symptoms include carbohydrate craving, lethargy, hyperphagia, and hypersomnia. **Premenstrual dysphoric disorder** usually has depressive symptoms during the late luteal phase of the menstrual cycles throughout the year.

Prenatal and **postpartum depressive disorders** usually occur 2 weeks to 6 months postpartum. Most women (up to 80%) experience some mild letdown of mood in the postpartum period. For some of these (10–15%), the symptoms are more severe and similar to those usually seen in serious depression, with an increased emphasis on concerns related to the baby (obsessive thoughts about harming it or inability to care for it). When psychotic symptoms occur, there is frequently associated sleep deprivation, volatility of behavior, and manic-like symptoms. Postpartum psychosis is much less common (< 2%) and often occurs within the first 2 weeks. Biologic vulnerability with hormonal changes and psychosocial stressors all play a role. The chances of a second episode are about 25% and may be reduced with prophylactic treatment.

C. Bipolar Disorders: Bipolar disorders (manic and depressive episodes) and individual manic episodes usually occur earlier (late teens or early adult life) than major depressive episodes.

1. A manic episode is a mood change characterized by elation with hyperactivity, overinvolvement in life activities, increased irritability, flight of ideas, easy distractibility, and little need for sleep. The overenthusiastic quality of the mood and the expansive behavior initially attract others, but the irritability, mood lability with swings into depression, aggressive behavior, and grandiosity usually lead to marked interpersonal difficulties. Activities may occur that are later regretted, eg, excessive spending, resignation from a job, a hasty marriage, sexual acting out, and exhibitionistic behavior, with alienation of friends and family. Atypical manic episodes can include gross delusions, paranoid ideation of severe proportions, and auditory hallucinations usually related to some grandiose perception. The episodes begin abruptly (sometimes precipitated by life stresses) and may last from several days to months. Spring and summer tend to be the peak periods. Generally, the manic episodes are of shorter duration than the depressive episodes. In almost all cases, the manic episode is part of a broader bipolar (manic-depressive) disorder. Patients with more than four complete cycles without remission in 1 year are called "rapid cyclers." (Substance abuse, particularly cocaine, can mimic rapid cycling.) These patients have a higher incidence of hypothyroidism. Manic patients differ from schizophrenics in that the former use more effective interpersonal maneuvers, are more sensitive to the social maneuvers of others, and are more able to utilize weakness and vulnerability in others to their own advantage. Creativity has been positively correlated with mood disorders, but the best work done is between episodes of mania and depression.

2. Cyclothymic disorders are chronic mood disturbances with episodes of depression and hypomania. The symptoms must have at least a 2-year duration and are milder than those that occur in depressive or manic episodes. Occasionally, the symptoms will escalate into a full-blown manic or depressive episode, in which case reclassification as bipolar disorder would be warranted.

D. Mood Disorders Secondary to Illness and Drugs: (All are classified as organic mood disorders.) Any illness, severe or mild, can cause significant depression. Conditions such as rheumatoid arthritis, multiple sclerosis, and chronic heart disease are particularly likely to be associated with depression, as are other chronic illnesses. Hormonal variations clearly play a role in some depressions. Varying degrees of depression occur at various times in schizophrenic disorders, central nervous system disease, and organic mental states. **Alcohol dependency** frequently coexists with serious depression.

The classic model of drug-induced depression occurs with the use of reserpine, both in a clinical and a neurochemical sense. Corticosteroids and oral contraceptives are commonly associated with affective changes. Antihypertensive medications such as methyldopa, guanethidine, and clonidine have been associated with the development of depressive syndromes, as have digitalis and antiparkinsonism drugs (eg, levodopa). Infrequently, disulfiram and anticholinesterase drugs may be associated with symptoms of depression. All stimulant use results in a depressive syndrome when the drug is withdrawn. Alcohol, sedatives, opiates, and most of the psychedelic drugs are depressants and, paradoxically, are often used in self-treatment of depression.

Differential Diagnosis

Since depression may be a part of any illness—either reactively or as a secondary symptom—careful attention must be given to personal life adjustment problems, the role of medications (eg, reserpine, corticosteroids, levodopa). Schizophrenia, partial complex seizures, organic brain syndromes, panic disorders, and anxiety disorders must be differentiated. Subtle thyroid dysfunction must be ruled out.

Complications

The longer the depression continues, the more crystallized it becomes—particularly when there is an element of secondary reinforcement. The most important complication is suicide, which often includes some elements of aggression. Suicide rates in the general population vary from 9 per 100,000 in Spain to 20 per 100,000 in the USA to 58 per 100,000 in Hungary. In individuals with depression, the lifetime risk rises to 10–15%. Males tend toward successful suicide, particularly in older age groups, whereas women make more attempts with lower mortality rates. An increased suicide rate is being observed in the younger population, ages 15–35. Patients with cancer, respiratory illnesses, AIDS, and those being maintained on hemodialysis have higher suicide rates. Alcohol is a significant factor in many suicide attempts.

There are four major groups of people who make suicide attempts:

(1) Those who are overwhelmed by problems in living (the despair of ordinary people). By far the greatest number fall into this category. There is often great ambivalence; they don't really want to die, but they don't want to go on as before either. These may be impulsive or aggressive acts not associated with significant depression.

(2) Those who are clearly attempting to control others. This is the blatant attempt in the vicinity of a significant other person in order to hurt or control that person.

(3) Those with severe depressions (high-risk group). This group includes both exogenous conditions (eg, AIDS, whose victims have a suicide rate over 30 times that of the general population) and endogenous conditions (eg, panic disorders). It also includes those who may not be diagnosed as having depression but who are overwhelmed by a serious stressful situation (eg, the man charged with child molestation who hangs himself in his cell). Anxiety, panic, and fear are major findings in suicidal behavior. A patient may seem to make a dramatic improvement, but the lifting of depression may be due to the patient's decision to commit suicide.

(4) Those with psychotic illness (high-risk group). These individuals tend not to verbalize their concerns, are unpredictable, and are often successful but comprise a small percentage of the total. (Suicide is ten times more prevalent in schizophrenics than in the general population, and jumping from bridges is more common. In one study of 100 jumpers, 47% were schizophrenic.)

The immediate goal of psychiatric evaluation is to assess the current suicidal risk and the need for hospitalization versus outpatient management. The intent is less likely to be truly suicidal, for example, if small amounts of poison or drugs were ingested or scratching of wrists was superficial; if the act was performed in the vicinity of others or with early notification of others; or if the attempt was arranged so that early detection would be anticipated. Alcohol, hopelessness, delusional thoughts, and complete or nearly complete loss of interest in life or ability to experience pleasure are all positively correlated with suicide attempts. Other risk factors are previous attempts, a family history of suicide, medical or psychiatric illness (eg, anxiety, depression, psychosis), male sex, older age, contemplation of violent methods, and drug use (including long-term sedative or alcohol use), which contributes to impulsiveness or mood swings. Successful treatment of the patient at risk for suicide cannot be achieved if the patient continues to abuse drugs.

The patient's current mood status is best evaluated by direct evaluation of plans and concerns about the future, personal reactions to the attempt, and thoughts about the reactions of others. The patient's immediate resources should be assessed—people who can be significantly involved (most important), family support, job situation, financial resources, etc.

If hospitalization is not indicated (eg, gestures, impulsive attempts; see above), the physician must formulate and institute a treatment plan or make an adequate referral. Medication should be dispensed in small amounts to at-risk patients. Although tricyclics and SSRIs are associated with an equal incidence of suicide attempts, the risk of successful suicide is higher with tricyclic overdose. Guns and drugs should be removed from the patient's household. Driving should be interdicted until the patient improves. The problem is often worsened by the long-term complications of the suicide attempt, eg, brain damage due to hypoxia; peripheral neuropathies caused by staying for long periods in one position, causing nerve compressions; and medical or surgical problems such as esophageal strictures and tendon dysfunctions.

The reasons for self-mutilation, most commonly wrist cutting (but also autocastration, autoamputation, and autoenucleation, which are associated with psychoses), may be very different from the reasons for a suicide attempt. The initial treatment plan, however, should presume suicidal ideation, and conservative treatment should be initiated as for attempted suicide.

Sleep disturbances in the depressions are discussed below.

Treatment of Depression

A. Medical: Depression associated with reactive disorders usually does not call for drug therapy and can be managed by psychotherapy and the passage of time. In severe cases—particularly when vegetative signs are significant and symptoms have persisted for more than a few weeks—antidepressant drug therapy is often effective. Drug therapy is also suggested by a family history of major depression in first-degree relatives or a past history of prior episodes.

The antidepressant drugs may be conveniently classified into three groups: (1) the tricyclic antidepressants (TCAs) and clinically similar drugs; (2) the newer antidepressants, including the serotonin-selective reuptake inhibitors (SSRIs) and bupropion, venlafaxine, nefazodone, and mirtazapine; and (3) the monoamine oxidase (MAO) inhibitors. These groups are described in greater detail below. Electroconvulsive therapy is effective in all types of depression (particularly involutional melancholia) and will also rapidly resolve a manic episode. It is also very effective for postpartum depression. Megavitamin treatment, acupuncture, and electrosleep are of unproved usefulness for any psychiatric condition.

Hospitalization is necessary if suicide is a major consideration or if complex treatment modalities are required.

Drug selection is influenced by the history of previous responses if that information is available. If a relative has responded to a particular drug, this suggests that the patient may respond similarly. If no background information is available, a drug such as desipramine, starting with 50 mg and gradually increasing to 150 mg daily, or sertraline, 50 mg daily, can be selected and a *full trial* instituted. The medication trial should be monitored every 1–2 weeks until week 6. If successful, the medication should be continued for 6–12 months at the full therapeutic dose before tapering is considered. Current research suggests that antidepressants should be continued indefinitely at full dosage in individuals with more than two episodes after age 40 or one episode after age 50. If the response is inadequate, the serum level is measured and the diagnosis of depression reassessed. If the diagnosis is supported by review and drug levels are adequate, a drug from a different group (eg, fluoxetine) is given a trial. If the second drug fails, augmentation with lithium (eg, 600–900 mg/d) or thyroid medication (eg, liothyronine, 25 μg/d) should be considered. Dysthymia is also treated in this way. The Agency for Health Care Policy and Research has produced clinical practice guidelines that outline one algorithm of treatment decisions (Figure 25–2).

Psychotic depression can be treated with amoxapine, which is metabolized to a neuroleptic; and if that drug is not adequate, a combination of an antipsychotic such as perphenazine (used initially) and an antidepressant such as desipramine is usually effective.

Atypical depression (including SAD) can be treated with an MAO inhibitor or a newer drug such as fluoxetine with good results. Light therapy is preferentially used in SAD.

Stimulants such as dextroamphetamine (5–30 mg/d) and methylphenidate (10–45 mg/d) have enjoyed a resurgence of interest for the short-term treatment of depression in medically ill and geriatric patients. Their 50–60% efficacy rate is slightly below

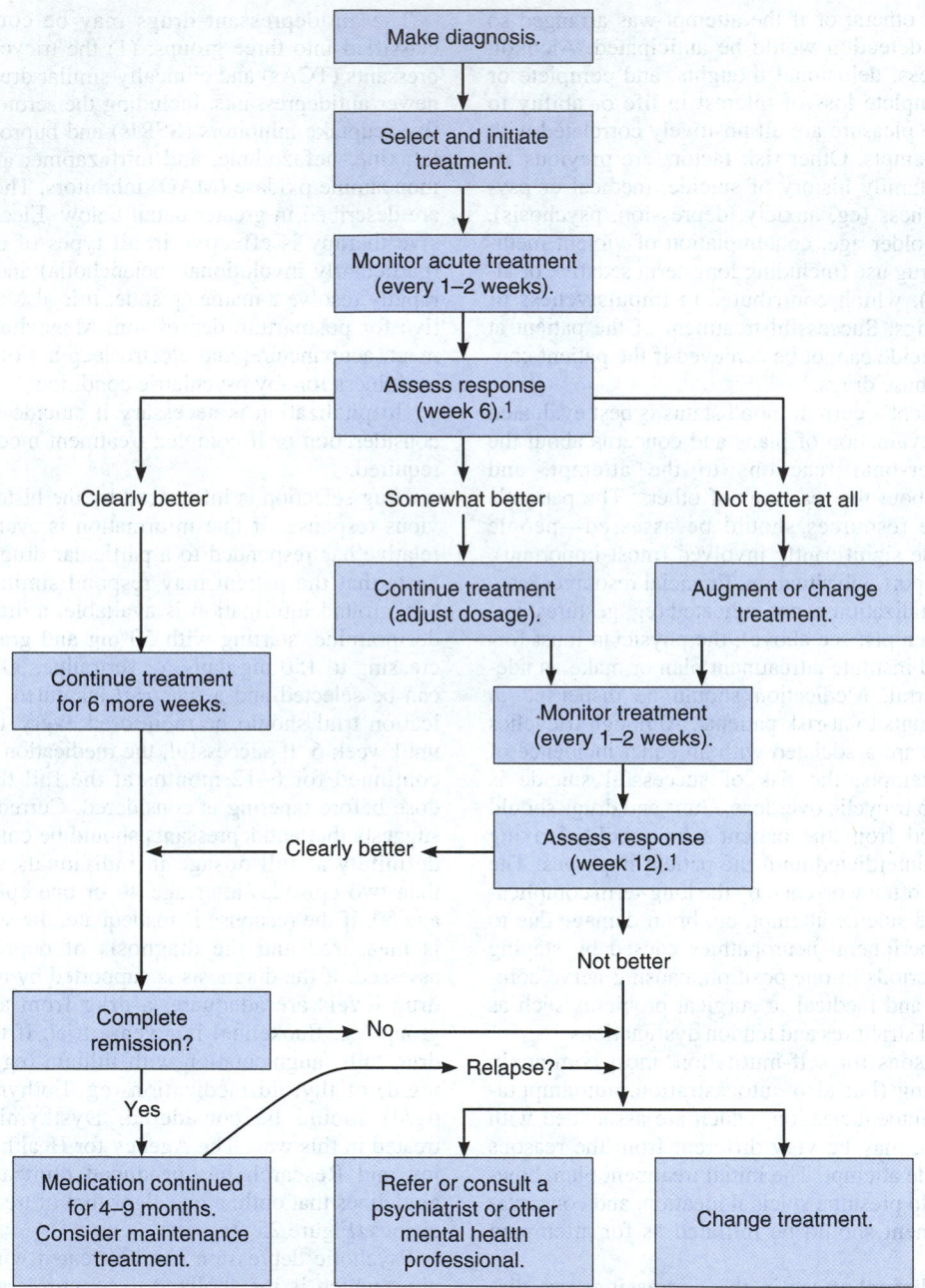

¹Times of assessment (weeks 6 and 12) rest on very modest data. It may be necessary to revise the treatment plan earlier for patients failing to respond at all.

Figure 25–2. Overview of treatment for depression. (Reproduced, with permission, from Agency for Health Care Policy and Research: *Depression in Primary Care*. Vol 2: *Treatment of Major Depression*. United States Department of Health and Human Services, 1993.)

that of other agents. The stimulants are notable for rapid onset of action (hours) and a paucity of side effects (tachycardia, agitation) in most patients. They are usually given in two divided doses early in the day (eg, 7 AM and noon) so as to avoid interfering

with sleep. These agents may also be useful as adjunctive agents in refractory depression.

Caution: Depressed patients may have suicidal thoughts, and the amount of drug dispensed should be appropriately controlled. The older tricyclics have a narrow therapeutic index, and one advantage of the newer drugs is their wider margin of safety. In all cases of pharmacologic management of depressed states, caution is indicated until the risk of suicide is considered minimal.

1. Tricyclic antidepressants and clinically similar drugs–These drugs have been the mainstay of drug therapy for depression for many years. They have also been effective in panic disorders, pain syndromes, and anxiety states. Specific ones have been effective in obsessive-compulsive disorder (clomipramine), enuresis (imipramine), psychotic depression (amoxapine), and reduction of craving in cocaine withdrawal (desipramine).

The tricyclics are characterized more by their similarities than by their differences. There is a lag in clinical response for up to several weeks, partly as a result of side effects that prevent rapid increase in dosage and partly because of their neurotransmitter effects. They tend to affect both serotonin and norepinephrine reuptake; some drugs act mainly on the former and others principally on the latter neurotransmitter system. Individuals receiving the same dosages vary markedly in therapeutic drug levels achieved (elderly patients require smaller doses), and determination of plasma drug levels is helpful when clinical response has been disappointing. Nortriptyline is usually effective when plasma levels are between 50 and 150 ng/mL; imipramine at plasma levels of 200–250 ng/mL; and desipramine at plasma levels of 100–250 ng/mL. High blood levels are not more effective than moderate levels and may be counterproductive (eg, delirium, seizures). Patients with gastrointestinal side effects benefit from plasma level monitoring to assess absorption of the drug. Most of the tricyclics can be given in a single dose at bedtime, starting at fairly low doses (eg, nortriptyline 25 mg orally) and increasing by 25 mg every several days as tolerated until the therapeutic response is achieved (eg, nortriptyline, 100–150 mg) or to maximum dose if necessary (eg, nortriptyline, 300 mg). The most common cause of treatment failure is an inadequate trial. A full trial consists of giving maximum daily dosage for at least 2 weeks. To reach maximum dosage, the trial encompasses a total of about 4 weeks. Because of marked anticholinergic and sedating side effects, clomipramine is started at a low dose (25 mg/d orally) and increased slowly in divided doses up to 100 mg/d, held at that level for several days, and then gradually increased as necessary up to 250 mg/d. Any of the TCA-like drugs should be started at very low doses (eg, 10–25 mg/d) and increased slowly in the treatment of panic disorder.

The tricyclic antidepressants have anticholinergic side effects to varying degrees (amitriptyline 100 mg is equivalent to atropine 5 mg). One must be particularly wary of the effect in elderly men with prostatic hyperplasia. The anticholinergic effects also predispose to other medical problems such as heat stroke or dental problems from xerostomia. Orthostatic hypotension is fairly common, may not remit with time, and is a major problem in elderly women with osteoporosis who may suffer a hip fracture after a fall. Cardiac effects of the TCAs are functions of the anticholinergic effect, direct myocardial depression (quinidine-like effect), and interference with adrenergic neurons. These factors may produce altered rate, rhythm, and contractility, particularly in patients with preexisting cardiac disease, such as bundle-branch or bifascicular block. Electrocardiographic changes range from benign ST segment and T wave changes and sinus tachycardia to a variety of complex and serious arrhythmias, the latter requiring a change in medication. Because TCAs have class I antiarrhythmic effects, they should be used with caution in patients with ischemic heart disease or arrhythmias. SSRIs or bupropion may be better initial choices for this population. TCAs lower the seizure threshold so this is of particular concern in patients with a propensity for seizures (eg, previous head injury, alcohol withdrawal). Loss of libido and erectile, ejaculatory, and orgasmic dysfunction are fairly common and can compromise compliance. Trazodone rarely causes priapism, which requires treatment within 12 hours (epinephrine 1:1000 injected into the corpus cavernosum). Delirium, agitation, and mania are infrequent complications. Sudden discontinuation of some of these drugs can produce "cholinergic rebound," manifested by headaches and nausea with abdominal cramps. Overdoses of the tricyclic compounds are often serious because of the narrow therapeutic index and quinidine-like effects (see Chapter 39).

2. Newer antidepressants–The chief advantages of these agents are that they do not cause significant cardiovascular or anticholinergic side effects or significant weight gain, as do the tricyclic agents. This group includes the serotonin-selective reuptake inhibitors (SSRIs): fluoxetine, sertraline, paroxetine, and fluvoxamine. Also in the group are bupropion, which appears to exert its effect through the dopamine neurotransmitter system; venlafaxine, which inhibits the reuptake of both serotonin and norepinephrine; and nefazodone, which blocks the reuptake of serotonin but also inhibits the 5-HT$_2$ postsynaptic receptors. All of these antidepressants are effective in the treatment of depression, both typical and atypical. The SSRI drugs have shown promise in the treatment of panic attacks, bulimia, and obsessive-compulsive disorders, while bupropion may have some particular effectiveness in the treatment of rapid-cycling bipolar disorder. They do not seem to be as clearly effective in some pain syndromes as the tricyclics.

All of the drugs in this group tend to be activating and are given in the morning so as not to interfere with sleep. Some patients, however, may have sedation, requiring that the SSRI be given at bedtime.

This reaction occurs most commonly with paroxetine. The SSRIs can be given in once-daily dosage. Bupropion and venlafaxine are given in three divided doses daily. Nefazodone is usually given twice daily. There is usually some delay in response; fluoxetine, for example, requires 2–6 weeks to act in depression, 4–8 weeks to be effective in panic disorder, and 6–12 weeks in treatment of obsessive-compulsive disorder. The starting dose (10–20 mg) is the usual daily dose for depression, while obsessive-compulsive disorder may require up to 80 mg daily. Some patients, particularly the elderly, may tolerate and benefit from as little as 10 mg/d or every other day. The other SSRIs (sertraline, paroxetine, and fluvoxamine) have shorter half-lives and a lesser effect on hepatic enzymes, which reduces their impact on the metabolism of other drugs (thus not increasing significantly the serum concentrations of other drugs as much as fluoxetine). The shorter half-lives also allow for more rapid clearing if adverse side effects appear. Venlafaxine appears to be more effective with doses greater than 200 mg/d, although some individuals respond at 75 mg/d.

The side effects common to all of these drugs are headache, nausea, tinnitus, insomnia, and nervousness. Akathisia has been common with the SSRIs; other extrapyramidal symptoms (eg, dystonias) have occurred infrequently but particularly in withdrawal states. Sexual side effects of impotence, retrograde ejaculation, and dysorgasmia are very common. Cyproheptadine, 4 mg orally prior to sexual activity, may be helpful in countering drug-induced anorgasmia. Because of early research with bulimic patients, bupropion has been burdened with an unwarranted reputation for causing seizures. The SSRIs are strong serotonin uptake blockers and may in high dosage or in combination with MAO inhibitors, including the antiparkinsonian drug selegiline, cause a "serotonin syndrome." This syndrome is manifested by rigidity, hyperthermia, autonomic instability, myoclonus, confusion, delirium, and coma. This syndrome can be a particularly troublesome problem in the elderly. Several cases of angina have been reported in association with SSRIs. Although early research raised the possibility that SSRIs might induce vasospasm in the presence of coronary artery disease, there has been little clinical evidence of this. In fact, some recent research has suggested that fluoxetine may have a protective cardiac effect by interfering with coagulation, although the actual clinical significance of this research remains speculative.

Recent research indicates that fluoxetine does not cause an increased risk of major fetal malformation when used in pregnancy. Both TCAs and fluoxetine are associated with a higher risk of miscarriage, but this may be related to the underlying depressive disorder.

Venlafaxine is reported to be well tolerated without significant anticholinergic or cardiovascular side effects. Nausea, nervousness, and profuse sweating appear to be the major side effects. Venlafaxine appears to have few drug-drug interactions. It does require monitoring of blood pressure because some individuals develop a dose-related hypertension. Nefazodone is newly released and appears to lack the anticholinergic effects of the TCAs and the agitation sometimes induced by SSRIs. Nefazodone should not be give with terfenadine, astemizole, or cisapride. Because nefazodone inhibits the liver's cytochrome P450-3A4 isoenzymes, concurrent use of the other medications can lead to serious QT prolongation, ventricular tachycardia, or death.

Mirtazapine is the most recently released antidepressant. It selectively blocks presynaptic α_2-adrenergic receptors and enhances both noradrenergic and serotonergic transmission. Its most common adverse side effects include somnolence, increased appetite, weight gain, and dizziness. There have been reports of agranulocytosis in two of 2796 patients. Although it is metabolized by P450 isoenzymes, it is not an inhibitor of this system. In view of our limited experience at present, mirtazapine should not be a first-line agent. It is given in a single dose at bedtime starting at 15 mg and increasing in 15 mg increments every week or every other week up to 45 mg.

3. Monoamine oxidase inhibitors–The MAO inhibitors are now generally used as third-line drugs for depression (after a failure of tricyclics or the newer agents) because of the dietary and other restrictions required (see below and Table 25–6). They should be considered as drugs of first choice in atypical depression (with rejection sensitivity) or as useful agents for panic disorder or refractory depression.

MAO inhibitors are administered in gradual stepwise dosage and may be given in the morning or evening, depending upon their effect on sleep. They tend to take effect in a fairly low dosage range (Table 25–7). Blood levels are not congruent with therapeutic response.

The MAO inhibitors commonly cause symptoms of orthostatic hypotension (which may persist) and sympathomimetic effects of tachycardia, sweating, and tremor. Nausea, insomnia (often associated with intense afternoon drowsiness), and sexual dysfunction are common. Trazodone, 25–75 mg orally at bedtime, may ameliorate the MAO-induced insomnia. Central nervous system effects include agitation

Table 25–6. Principal dietary restrictions in MAOI use.

1. Cheeses except cream cheese and cottage cheese and fresh yogurt
2. Fermented or aged meats such as bologna, salami
3. Broad bean pods such as Chinese bean pods
4. Liver of all types
5. Meat and yeast extracts
6. Red wine, sherry, vermouth, cognac, beer, ale
7. Soy sauce, shrimp paste, sauerkraut

Table 25–7. Commonly used antidepressants.

	Usual Daily Oral Dose (mg)	Usual Daily Maximum Dose (mg)	Sedative Effects[1]	Anticho-linergic Effects[1]	Cost per Unit	Cost for 30 Days' Treatment Based on Maximum Dosage[2]
TRICYCLIC AND CLINICALLY SIMILAR COMPOUNDS						
Amitriptyline (Elavil)	150–250	300	4	4	G: $0.30/150 mg	$18.00
Amoxapine (Asendin)	150–200	400	2	2	G: $1.43/100 mg	$171.60
Clomipramine (Anafranil)	100	250	3	3	B: $1.09/50 mg	$163.50
Desipramine (Norpramin)	100–250	300	1	1	G: $1.02/100 mg	$91.80
Doxepin (Sinequan)	150–200	300	4	3	G: $0.38/100 mg	$34.20
Imipramine (Tofranil)	150–200	300	3	3	G: $0.05/50 mg	$9.00
Maprotiline (Ludiomil)	100–200	300	4	2	G: $0.62/75 mg	$74.40
Nortriptyline (Aventyl, Pamelor)	100–150	150	2	2	G: $1.48/50 mg	$177.60
Protriptyline (Vivactil)	15–40	60	1	3	B: $0.67/10 mg	$121.00
Trazodone (Desyrel)	100–300	400	4	<1	G: $0.32/100 mg	$38.40
Trimipramine (Surmontil)	75–200	200	4	4	B: $1.57/100 mg	$94.20
Bupropion (Wellbutrin)	300[3]	450[3]		<1	B: $0.75/100 mg	$101.00
Bupropion SR (Wellbutrin SR)					B: $1.18/100 mg B: $1.22/150 mg	$70.80 $73.20
SSRIs AND OTHER NEW COMPOUNDS						
Fluoxetine (Prozac)	5–40	80	<1	<1	B: $2.41/20 mg	$289.00
Fluvoxamine (Luvox)	100–300	300	1	<1	B: $2.73/100 mg	$200.00
Nefazodone (Serzone)	300–600	600	2	<1	B: $0.93/200 mg	$83.70
Paroxetine (Paxil)	20–30	50	1	1	B: $2.00/20 mg	$150.00
Sertraline (Zoloft)	50–150	200	<1	<1	B: $2.15/100 mg	$129.00
Venlafaxine (Effexor)	150–225	375	1	<1	B: $1.15/75 mg	$172.50
Mirtazepine (Remeron)	15–45	45	4	2	B: $2.00/30 mg	$90.00
MONOAMINE OXIDASE INHIBITORS						
Phenelzine (Nardil)	45–60	90	...	...	B: $0.40/15 mg	$72.00
Tranylcypromine (Parnate)	20–30	50	...	...	B: $0.48/10 mg	$72.00

[1]**Key:** 4 = strong effect; 1 = weak effect; B = brand name; G = generic.
[2]Cost to pharmacist (average wholesale price) for 30 days' treatment based on maximum dosage (generic when possible). Source: First Data Bank, Price Alert, April 1997. If there are multiple suppliers, the generic average wholesale price is based on the mean price.
[3]No single dose should exceed 150 mg.

and toxic psychoses. Dietary limitations (Table 25–6) and abstinence from drug products containing phenylpropanolamine, phenylephrine, meperidine, dextromethorphan, and pseudoephedrine are mandatory for MAO-A type inhibitors (those marketed for treatment of depression), since the reduction of available monoamine oxidase leaves the patient vulnerable to exogenous amines (eg, tyramine in foodstuffs).

Treatment for a resultant hypertensive crisis has been the same as for pheochromocytoma (see Chapter 26), but there have been reports of success with nifedipine, 10 mg chewed and placed under the tongue, normalizing blood pressure in 1–5 minutes. The restrictions on the proscribed foodstuffs and sympathomimetic drugs are in effect during treatment and for 1 month after cessation of therapy. Termination of therapy with MAO inhibitors may be associated with anxiety, agitation, cognitive slowing, and headache. Very gradual withdrawal and short-term benzodiazepine therapy will ameliorate symptoms.

4. Switching and combination therapy–If the therapeutic response has been poor after an adequate trial with the chosen drug, one should reassess the diagnosis. Assuming that the trial has been adequate and the diagnosis is correct, a trial with a drug from another group is appropriate. In switching from one group to another, an adequate "washout time" must be allowed. This is critical in certain situations—eg, in switching from an MAO inhibitor to a tricyclic, allow 2–3 weeks between stopping one drug and starting another; in switching from an SSRI to an MAO inhibitor, allow 4–5 weeks. In switching within groups—eg, from one tricyclic to another (amitriptyline to desipramine, etc)—no washout time is needed, and one can rapidly decrease the dosage of one drug while increasing the other. Combining two antidepressants requires caution and is usually reserved for refractory patients after psychiatric consultation.

However, in any of the three groups, one can augment the antidepressant drug if the therapeutic response has been less than satisfactory. Lithium and thyroid hormone (eg, 25 μg daily of liothyronine) are the most commonly used augmenting agents. Lithium is an excellent augmentation agent for the 25–40% of depressed patients who fail to respond to an adequate trial of an antidepressant. One-half of these patients will respond to the addition of lithium (600–900 mg/d) with an enhanced antidepressant effect.

5. Maintenance and tapering–When clinical relief of symptoms is obtained, medication is continued for 12 months in the effective maintenance dosage, which is usually the dosage required in the acute stage. Current research suggests that when an individual is over age 40 with two episodes or over age 50 with one episode, the full dosage should be continued indefinitely. This research suggests that major depression should often be considered as a chronic disease. If the medication is being tapered, it should be done gradually over several months, monitoring closely for relapse.

6. Drug interactions–Interactions with other drugs are listed in Table 25–8.

7. Electroconvulsive therapy (ECT)–ECT causes a generalized central nervous system seizure (peripheral convulsion is not necessary) by means of electric current. The key objective is to exceed the seizure threshold, which can be accomplished by a variety of means. Electrical stimulation is more reliable and simpler than the use of chemical convulsants. The mechanism of action is not known, but it is thought to involve major neurotransmitter responses at the cell membrane. Current insufficient to cause a seizure produces no therapeutic benefit.

Electroconvulsive therapy is the most effective (about 70–85%) treatment of severe depression, particularly the delusions and agitation commonly seen with depression in the involutional period. It is indicated when medical conditions preclude the use of antidepressants or in cases of nonresponsiveness to these medications. Comparative controlled studies of

Table 25–8. Antidepressant drug interactions with other drugs.

Drug	Effects
Tricyclic and other non-MAOI antidepressants	
Antacids	Decreased absorption of antidepressants.
Anticoagulants	Increased hypoprothrombinemic effect.
Cimetidine	Increased antidepressant blood levels and psychosis.
Clonidine	Decreased antihypertensive effect.
Digitalis	Increased incidence of heart block.
Disulfiram	Increased antidepressant blood levels.
Guanadrel	Decreased antihypertensive effect.
Guanethidine	Decreased antihypertensive effect.
Haloperidol	Increased clomipramine levels.
Insulin	Decreased blood sugar.
Lithium	Increased lithium levels with fluoxetine.
Methyldopa	Decreased antihypertensive effect.
Other anticholinergic drugs	Marked anticholinergic responses.
Phenytoin	Increased blood levels.
Procainamide	Decreased ventricular conduction.
Procarbazine	Hypertensive crisis.
Propranolol	Increased hypotension.
Quinidine	Decreased ventricular conduction.
Rauwolfia derivatives	Increased stimulation.
Sedatives	Increased sedation.
Sympathomimetic drugs	Increased pressor effect.
Terfenadine	Torsade
Monoamine oxidase inhibitors	
Antihistamines	Increased sedation.
Belladonna-like drugs	Increased blood pressure.
Dextromethorphan	Same as meperidine.
Guanadrel	Increased blood pressure.
Guanethidine	Decreased blood pressure.
Insulin	Decreased blood sugar.
Levodopa	Increased blood pressure.
Meperidine	Increased agitation, seizures, coma, death.
Methyldopa	Decreased blood pressure.
Pseudoephedrine	Hypertensive crisis (increased blood pressure).
Reserpine	Increased blood pressure and temperature.
Succinylcholine	Increased neuromuscular blockage.
Sulfonylureas	Decreased blood sugar.
Sympathomimetic drugs	Increased blood pressure.

electroconvulsive therapy in severe depression show that it is more effective than chemotherapy. It is also effective in the manic disorders and psychoses during pregnancy (when drugs may be contraindicated). It has not been shown to be helpful in chronic schizophrenic disorders, and it is generally not used in acute schizophrenic episodes unless drugs are not effective and it is urgent that the psychosis be controlled (eg, a catatonic stupor complicating an acute medical condition).

The most common side effects are memory disturbance and headache. Memory loss or confusion is usually related to number and frequency of electroconvulsive therapy treatments and proper oxygenation during treatment. Some memory loss is occasionally permanent, but most memory faculties return to full capacity within several weeks. There have been reports that lithium administration concurrent with electroconvulsive therapy resulted in greater memory loss. Before anesthesia was used, spinal compression fractures and severe anticipatory anxiety were common.

Increased intracranial pressure is a serious contraindication. Other problems such as cardiac disorders, aortic aneurysms, bronchopulmonary disease, and venous thrombosis are relative contraindications and must be evaluated in light of the severity of the medical problem versus the need for electroconvulsive therapy. Serious complications arising from electroconvulsive therapy occur in less than one in 1000 cases. Most of these problems are cardiovascular or respiratory in nature (eg, aspiration of gastric contents). Poor patient understanding and lack of acceptance of the technique by the public are the biggest obstacles to the use of electroconvulsive therapy.

8. Phototherapy is used in seasonal affective disorder (SAD). It consists of exposure (at a 3-foot distance) to a light source of 2500 lux for 2 hours daily. Light visors are an adaptation that provides greater mobility and an adjustable light intensity. The price of these full-spectrum light sources range between $300 and $400. The dosage varies, with some patients requiring morning and night exposure. One effect is alteration of biorhythm through melatonin mechanisms.

B. Psychologic: It is seldom possible to engage an individual in penetrating psychotherapeutic endeavors during the acute stage of a severe depression. While medications may be taking effect, a supportive approach to strengthen existing defenses and appropriate consideration of the patient's continuing need to function at work, to engage in recreational activities, etc, are necessary as the severity of the depression lessens. If the patient is not seriously depressed, it is often quite appropriate to initiate intensive psychotherapeutic efforts, since flux periods are a good time to effect change. A catharsis of repressed anger and guilt may be beneficial. Therapy during or just after the acute stage may focus on coping techniques, with some practice of alternative choices. When lack of self-confidence and identity problems are factors in the depression, individual psychotherapy can be oriented to ways of improving self-esteem, increasing assertiveness, and lessening dependency. As previously noted, numerous studies have shown that the combination of drug therapy plus cognitive psychotherapy is more effective than either modality alone. It is usually helpful to involve the spouse or other significant family members early in treatment.

C. Social: Flexible use of appropriate social services can be of major importance in the treatment of depression. Since alcohol is often associated with depression, early involvement in alcohol treatment programs such as Alcoholics Anonymous can be important to future success (see Alcohol Dependency and Abuse, below). The structuring of daily activities during severe depression is often quite difficult for the patient, and loneliness is often a major factor. The help of family, employer, or friends is often necessary to mobilize the patient who experiences no joy in daily activities and tends to remain uninvolved and to deteriorate. Insistence on sharing activities will help involve the patient in simple but important daily functions. In some severe cases, the use of day treatment centers or support groups of a specific type (eg, mastectomy groups) is indicated. It is not unusual for a patient to have multiple legal, financial, and vocational problems requiring legal and vocational assistance.

D. Behavioral: When depression is a function of self-defeating coping techniques such as passivity, the role-playing approach can be useful. Behavioral techniques, including desensitization, may be used in problems such as phobias where depression is a by-product. When depression is a regularly used interpersonal style, behavioral counseling to family members or others can help in extinguishing the behavior in the patient.

Treatment of Mania

Acute manic or hypomanic symptoms will respond to lithium therapy after several days of treatment, but it is common to use neuroleptic drugs or high-potency benzodiazepines (eg, clonazepam) to immediately treat the excited or psychotic manic stage. Some schizoaffective disorders and some cases of so-called schizophrenia are probably atypical bipolar affective disorder, for which lithium treatment may be effective.

A. Haloperidol: Manic episodes are treated with haloperidol, 5–10 mg orally or intramuscularly every 2–3 hours until symptoms subside. The dosage of haloperidol is gradually reduced after lithium is started (see below).

B. Clonazepam: Clonazepam is an alternative to a neuroleptic such as haloperidol. It is effective in controlling acute behavioral symptoms. Clonazepam has the advantage of causing no extrapyramidal side effects. Although 1–2 mg orally every 4–6 hours may be effective, up to 16 mg/d may be necessary.

C. Lithium: As a prophylactic drug for bipolar affective disorder, lithium significantly decreases the frequency and severity of both manic and depressive attacks in about 70% of patients. A positive response is more predictable if the patient has a low frequency of episodes (no more than two per year with intervals free of psychopathology). A positive response occurs more frequently in individuals who have blood relatives with a diagnosis of manic or hypomanic attacks. Patients who swing rapidly back and forth between manic and depressive attacks (at least four cycles per year) usually respond poorly to lithium prophylaxis initially, but some improve with continued long-term treatment. Carbamazepine (see below) has been used with success in this group.

In addition to its use in manic states, lithium is sometimes useful in the prophylaxis of recurrent unipolar depressions (perhaps undiagnosed bipolar disorder). Lithium may ameliorate nonspecific aggressive behaviors and dyscontrol syndromes. The dosages are the same as used in bipolar disorder. Most patients with bipolar disease can be managed long-term with lithium alone, though some will require continued or intermittent use of a neuroleptic, antidepressant, or carbamazepine. An excellent resource for information pertaining to lithium is the Lithium Information Center, Dean Foundation, 8000 Excelsior Drive, Suite 302, Madison, WI 53717-1914.

Before treatment, the clinical workup should include a medical history and physical examination; complete blood count; T_4, TSH, blood urea nitrogen, serum creatinine, and serum electrolyte determinations; urinalysis; and electrocardiography.

1. Dosage–Lithium carbonate in generally prescribed in the 300 mg unit. In a small minority of patients, a slow release form or units of different dosage may be required. Lithium citrate is available as a syrup. The dosage is that required to maintain blood levels in the therapeutic range. For acute attacks, this ranges from 1 to 1.5 meq/L. Although there is controversy about the optimal chronic maintenance dose, many clinicians reduce the acute level to 0.6–1 meq/L in order to reduce side effects. The dose required to meet this need will vary in different individuals. For acute mania, doses of 1200–1800 mg/d are generally recommended. Augmentation of antidepressants is usually achieved with one-half of these doses. Once-a-day dosage is acceptable, but most patients have less nausea when they take the drug in divided doses with meals.

Lithium is readily absorbed, with peak serum levels occurring within 1–3 hours and complete absorption in 8 hours. Half of the total body lithium is excreted in 18–24 hours (95% in the urine). Blood for lithium levels should be drawn 12 hours after the last dose. Serum levels should be measured 5–7 days after initiation of treatment until stabilization occurs, and then after every change in dosage. For maintenance treatment, lithium levels should be monitored initially every 1–2 months but may be measured every 6–12 months in stable, long-term patients. Levels should be monitored more closely when there is any condition that causes volume depletion (eg, diarrhea; dehydration; use of diuretics).

2. Side effects–Mild gastrointestinal symptoms (take lithium with food), fine tremors (treat with propranolol, 20–60 mg/d orally, only if persistent),

slight muscle weakness, and some degree of somnolence are early side effects that are usually transient. Moderate polyuria (reduced renal responsiveness to antidiuretic hormone) and polydipsia (associated with increased plasma renin concentration) are often present. Potassium administration can blunt this effect. Weight gain (often a result of calories in fluids taken for polydipsia) and leukocytosis not due to infection are fairly common.

Other side effects include goiter (3%; often euthyroid), hypothyroidism (10%; concomitant administration of lithium and iodide or lithium and carbamazepine enhances the hypothyroid and goitrogenic effect of either drug), changes in the glucose tolerance test toward a diabetes-like curve, nephrogenic diabetes insipidus (usually resolving about 8 weeks after cessation of lithium therapy), nephrotic syndrome, edema, folate deficiency, and pseudotumor cerebri (ophthalmoscopy is indicated if there are complaints of headache or blurred vision). A metallic taste, hair loss, and Raynaud's phenomenon have been reported in a few cases. Thyroid and kidney function should be checked at 3- to 4-month intervals. Most of these side effects subside when lithium is discontinued; when residual side effects exist, they are usually not serious. Most clinicians treat lithium-induced hypothyroidism (more common in women) with thyroid hormone while continuing lithium therapy. Hypercalcemia and elevated parathyroid hormone levels occur in some patients. Electrocardiographic abnormalities (principally T wave flattening or inversion) may occur during lithium administration but are not of major clinical significance. Sinoatrial block may occur, particularly in the elderly. It is important that other drugs which prolong intraventricular conduction, such as tricyclics, be used with caution in conjunction with lithium. Lithium impairs ventilatory function in patients with airway obstruction. Lithium alone does not have a significant effect on sexual function, but when combined with benzodiazepines (clonazepam in most symptomatic patients) it causes sexual dysfunction in about 50% of male patients. Lithium may precipitate or exacerbate psoriasis in some patients.

Patients receiving long-term lithium therapy may have cogwheel rigidity and, occasionally, other extrapyramidal signs. Lithium potentiates the parkinsonian effects of haloperidol. Long-term lithium therapy has also been associated with a relative lowering of the level of memory and perceptual processing (affecting compliance in some cases). Some impairment of attention and emotional reactivity has also been noted. Lithium-induced delirium with therapeutic lithium levels is an infrequent complication usually occurring in the elderly and may persist for several days after serum levels have become negligible. Encephalopathy has occurred in patients receiving combined lithium and neuroleptic therapy and in those who have cerebrovascular disease, thus requiring careful evaluation of patients who develop neurotoxic signs at subtoxic blood levels.

The long-term use of lithium may have adverse effects on renal function (with interstitial fibrosis, tubular atrophy, and glomerulosclerosis). A rise in serum creatinine levels is an indication for in-depth evaluation of renal function. Incontinence has been reported in women, apparently related to changes in bladder cholinergic-adrenergic balance.

Lithium exposure in early pregnancy increases the frequency of congenital anomalies, especially Ebstein's and other major cardiovascular anomalies. It is advisable for women using lithium either to avoid pregnancy or not to use lithium at all during a planned pregnancy, particularly during the first trimester. Recent prospective studies suggest that the risk imposed by lithium in pregnancy may be overemphasized. Indeed, the risk of untreated bipolar disorder carries its own risks for pregnancy. Formula feeding should be considered in mothers using lithium, since concentration in breast milk is one-third to one-half that in serum.

Frank toxicity usually occurs at blood lithium levels above 2 meq/L. Because sodium and lithium are reabsorbed at the same loci in the proximal renal tubules, any sodium loss (diarrhea, use of diuretics, or excessive perspiration) results in increased lithium levels. Symptoms and signs include vomiting and diarrhea, the latter exacerbating the problem since more sodium is lost and more lithium is absorbed. Other symptoms and signs, some of which may not be reversible, include tremors, marked muscle weakness, confusion, dysarthria, vertigo, choreoathetosis, ataxia, hyperreflexia, rigidity, lack of coordination, myoclonus, seizures, opisthotonos, and coma. Toxicity is more severe in the elderly, who should be maintained on slightly lower serum levels. Lithium overdosage may be accidental or intentional or may occur as a result of poor monitoring.

Patients with massive ingestions of lithium or blood lithium levels above 2.5 meq/L should be treated with induced emesis and gastric lavage. If renal function is normal, osmotic and saline diuresis increases renal lithium clearance. Urinary alkalinization is also helpful, since sodium bicarbonate decreases lithium reabsorption in the proximal tubule, as does acetazolamide. Aminophylline potentiates the diuretic effect by increasing the glomerular filtration rate of lithium. Drugs affecting the distal loop have no effect on lithium reabsorption. Blood lithium levels above 2.5 meq/L confirmed by cerebrospinal fluid lithium levels should be considered an indication for hemodialysis.

Compliance with lithium therapy is adversely affected by the loss of some hypomanic experiences valued by the patient. These include social extroversion and a sense of heightened enjoyment in many activities such as sex and business dealings, often with increased productivity in the latter.

3. Drug interactions–Patients receiving lithium should use diuretics with caution and only under close medical supervision. The thiazide diuretics cause increased lithium reabsorption from the proximal renal tubules, resulting in increased serum lithium levels (Table 25–9), and adjustment of lithium intake must be made to compensate for this. Reduce lithium dosage by 25–40% when the patient is receiving 50 mg of hydrochlorothiazide daily. Potassium-sparing diuretics (spironolactone, amiloride, triamterene) may also cause increased serum lithium levels and require careful monitoring of lithium levels. Loop diuretics (furosemide, ethacrynic acid, bumetanide) do not appear to alter serum lithium levels. Concurrent use of lithium and ACE inhibitors requires a 50–75% reduction in lithium intake to achieve therapeutic lithium levels.

D. Valproic Acid: Valproic acid (divalproex) is an antiseizure drug whose activity is at least partially related to GABA neurotransmission. It is gaining favor as a first-line treatment for mania because it has a broader index of safety than lithium. This issue is particularly important in AIDS or other medically ill patients prone to dehydration or malabsorption with wide swings in serum lithium levels. Valproic acid has also been utilized effectively in panic disorder and migraine headache. Treatment is often started at a dose of 750 mg/d orally, and dosage is then titrated to achieve therapeutic serum levels. Concomitant use of aspirin, carbamazepine, warfarin, or phenytoin may affect serum levels. Gastrointestinal symptoms are the main side effects. Liver function tests and complete blood counts should be monitored, and teratogenic effects are a concern.

E. Carbamazepine: Carbamazepine, an antiseizure drug that stabilizes the activity of cell membranes, has been used with increasing frequency in the treatment of bipolar patients who cannot be satis-

Table 25–9. Lithium interactions with other drugs.

Drug	Effects
ACE inhibitors	↑Lithium levels
Fluoxetine	↑Lithium levels
Ibuprofen	↑Lithium levels
Indomethacin	↑Lithium levels
Methyldopa	Rigidity, mutism, fascicular twitching
Osmotic diuretics (urea, mannitol)	↑Lithium excretion
Phenylbutazone	↑Lithium levels
Potassium-sparing diuretics (spironolactone, amiloride, triamterene)	↑Lithium levels
Sodium bicarbonate	↑Lithium excretion
Succinylcholine	↑Duration of action of succinylcholine
Theophylline, aminophylline	↑Lithium excretion
Thiazide diuretics	↑Lithium levels
Valproic acid	↓Lithium levels

factorily treated with lithium (nonresponsive, excessive side effects, or rapid cycling). It is often effective at 800–1600 mg/d orally. It has also been used in the treatment of resistant depressions, alcohol withdrawal, and hallucinations (in conjunction with neuroleptics) and in patients with behavioral dyscontrol or panic attacks. It suppresses some phases of kindling (see Stimulants) and has been used to treat residual symptoms in previous stimulant abusers (eg, posttraumatic stress disorder with impulse control problems). Dose-related side effects include sedation and ataxia. Dosages start at 400–600 mg orally daily and are increased slowly to therapeutic levels. Skin rashes and a mild reduction in white count are common. SIADH occurs rarely. Nonsteroidal anti-inflammatory drugs (except aspirin); the antibiotics erythromycin, troleandomycin, and isoniazid; the calcium channel blockers verapamil and diltiazem (but not nifedipine); fluoxetine, propoxyphene, and cimetidine all increase carbamazepine levels. Carbamazepine can be effective in conjunction with lithium, though there have been reports of reversible neurotoxicity with the combination. Carbamazepine stimulates hepatic microsomal enzymes and so tends to decrease levels of haloperidol and oral contraceptives. It also lowers T_4, free T_4, and T_3 levels. Cases of fetal malformation (particularly spina bifida) have been reported along with growth deficiency and developmental delay. Liver tests and complete blood counts should be monitored in patients taking carbamazepine.

F. Calcium Channel Blockers: Calcium channel blockers (eg, verapamil) have been used in bipolar states that have failed to respond to lithium, carbamazepine, or valproic acid. This has come about with the realization that a number of drugs used in psychiatry (eg, lithium, antidepressants, neuroleptics, and carbamazepine) have calcium channel-blocking activity. There is also preliminary evidence that these drugs may be useful in the treatment of tardive dyskinesia and panic attacks. Verapamil may be safer than lithium or carbamazepine during pregnancy, though it decreases uterine contractility and must be discontinued before delivery.

Prognosis

Reactive depressions are usually time-limited, and the prognosis with treatment is good if a pathologic pattern of adjustment does not intervene. Major affective disorders frequently respond well to a full trial of drug treatment.

Mania and bipolar disorder have a good prognosis with adequate treatment.

[AHCPR guideline on depression in primary care]
  http://text.nlm.nih.gov/ftrs/gateway
Agency for Health Care Policy and Research: *Depression in Primary Care.* Vol 2: *Treatment of Major Depres-sion.* United States Department of Health and Human Services, 1993.

Bowden CL et al: Efficacy of divalproex vs. lithium and placebo in the treatment of mania. JAMA 1994;271:918.

Burns MM, Eisendrath SJ: Dextroamphetamine treatment for depression in terminally ill patients. Psychosomatics 1994;35:80.

Cohen LS et al: A reevaluation of risk of in utero exposure to lithium. JAMA 1994;271:146.

Garza-Trevino ES, Overall JE, Hollister MD: Verapamil versus lithium in acute mania. Am J Psychiatry 1992; 149:121.

Glassman AH et al: The safety of tricyclic antidepressants in cardiac patients: Risk-benefit reconsidered. JAMA 1993;269:2673.

Menys VC et al: Platelet 5-hydroxytryptamine is decreased in a preliminary group of depressed patients receiving the 5-hydroxytryptamine re-uptake inhibiting drug fluoxetine. Clin Sci 1996;91:87. (The authors predict a protective effect of fluoxetine against coronary thrombosis.)

Pastuszak A et al: Pregnancy outcome following first-trimester exposure to fluoxetine (Prozac). JAMA 1993; 269:2246.

Price LH, Heninger GR: Lithium in the treatment of mood disorders. N Engl J Med 1994;331:591.

Rickels K et al: Nefazodone and imipramine in major depression: A placebo controlled trial. Br J Psychiatry 1994;164:802.

Rosenthal NE: Diagnosis and treatment of depression: Seasonal affective disorder. JAMA 1993;270:2717.

Song F et al: Selective serotonin reuptake inhibitors: Meta-analysis of efficacy and acceptability. Br Med J 1993; 306:683.

SLEEP DISORDERS

Sleep consists of two distinct states as shown by electroencephalographic studies: REM (rapid eye movement) sleep, also called dream sleep, D state sleep, paradoxic sleep; and NREM (non-REM) sleep, also called S stage sleep, which is divided into stages 1, 2, 3, and 4 recognizable by different electroencephalographic patterns. Stages 3 and 4 are "delta" sleep. Dreaming occurs mostly in REM and to a lesser extent in NREM sleep.

Sleep is a cyclic phenomenon, with four or five REM periods during the night accounting for about one-fourth of the total night's sleep (1½–2 hours). The first REM period occurs about 80–120 minutes after onset of sleep and lasts about 10 minutes. Later REM periods are longer (15–40 minutes) and occur mostly in the last several hours of sleep. Most stage 4 (deepest) sleep occurs in the first several hours.

Age-related changes in normal sleep include an unchanging percentage of REM sleep and a marked decrease in stage 3 and stage 4 sleep, with an increase in wakeful periods during the night. These normal changes, early bedtimes, and daytime naps play a role in the increased complaints of insomnia in older people. Variations in sleep patterns may be due to circumstances (eg, "jet lag") or to idiosyncratic patterns ("night owls") in persons who perhaps because of different "biologic rhythms" habitually go to bed late and sleep late in the morning. Creativity and rapidity of response to unfamiliar situations are impaired by loss of sleep. There are also rare individuals who have chronic difficulty in adapting to a 24-hour sleep-wake cycle (desynchronization sleep disorder), which can be resynchronized by altering exposure to light.

The three major sleep disorders are discussed below.

1. DYSSOMNIAS (Insomnia)

Classification & Clinical Findings

Patients may complain of difficulty getting to sleep or staying asleep, intermittent wakefulness during the night, early morning awakening, or combinations of any of these. Transient episodes are usually of little significance. Stress, caffeine, physical discomfort, daytime napping, and early bedtimes are common factors.

Psychiatric disorders are often associated with persistent insomnia. **Depression** is usually associated with fragmented sleep, decreased total sleep time, earlier onset of REM sleep, a shift of REM activity to the first half of the night, and a loss of slow wave sleep—all of which are nonspecific findings. In **manic disorders,** sleeplessness is a cardinal feature and an important early sign of impending mania in bipolar cases. Total sleep time is decreased, with shortened REM latency and increased REM activity. Sleep-related panic attacks occur in the transition from stage 2 to stage 3 sleep in some patients with a longer REM latency in the sleep pattern preceding the attacks.

Abuse of alcohol may cause or be secondary to the sleep disturbance. There is a tendency to use alcohol as a means of getting to sleep without realizing that it disrupts the normal sleep cycle. Acute alcohol intake produces a decreased sleep latency with reduced REM sleep during the first half of the night. REM sleep is increased in the second half of the night, with an increase in total amount of slow wave sleep (stages 3 and 4). Vivid dreams and frequent awakenings are common. Chronic alcohol abuse increases stage 1 and decreases REM sleep (most drugs delay or block REM sleep), with symptoms persisting for many months after the individual has stopped drinking. Acute alcohol or other sedative withdrawal causes delayed onset of sleep and REM rebound with intermittent awakening during the night.

Heavy smoking (more than a pack a day) causes difficulty falling asleep—apparently independently of the often associated increase in coffee drinking. Excess intake near bedtime of caffeine, cocaine, and other stimulants (eg, OTC cold remedies) causes decreased total sleep time—mostly NREM sleep—with some increased sleep latency.

Sedative-hypnotics—specifically, the benzodiazepines, which are the prescription drugs of choice to promote sleep—tend to increase total sleep time, decrease sleep latency, and decrease nocturnal awakening, with variable effects on NREM sleep. Withdrawal causes just the opposite effects and results in continued use of the drug for the purpose of preventing withdrawal symptoms. Antidepressants decrease REM sleep (with marked rebound on withdrawal in the form of nightmares) and have varying effects on NREM sleep. The effect on REM sleep correlates with reports that REM sleep deprivation produces improvement in some depressions.

Persistent insomnias are also related to a wide variety of medical conditions, particularly delirium, pain, respiratory distress syndromes, uremia, asthma, and hypothyroidism. Adequate analgesia and proper treatment of medical disorders will reduce symptoms and decrease the need for sedatives.

Treatment

In general, there are two broad classes of treatment for insomnia, and the two may be combined: psychologic (cognitive-behavioral) and pharmacologic. In situations of acute distress, such as a grief reaction, pharmacologic measures may be most appropriate. With primary insomnia, however, initial efforts should be psychologically based. This is particularly true in the elderly to avoid the potential adverse reactions of medications. The elderly population is at risk for complaints of insomnia because sleep becomes lighter and more easily disrupted with aging. Medical disorders that become more common with age may also predispose to insomnia.

A. Psychologic: Psychologic strategies should include educating the patient regarding good sleep hygiene: (1) Go to bed only when sleepy. (2) Use the bed and bedroom only for sleeping and sex. (3) If still awake after 20 minutes, leave the bedroom and only return when sleepy. (4) Get up at the same time every morning regardless of the amount of sleep during the night. (5) Discontinue caffeine and nicotine, at least in the evening if not completely. (6) Establish a daily exercise regimen. (7) Avoid alcohol as it may disrupt continuity of sleep. (8) Limit fluids in the evening. (9) Learn and practice relaxation techniques.

The physician should also discuss any myths or misconceptions about sleep that the patient may hold.

B. Medical: When the above measures are insufficient, medications may be useful. Pharmacologic measures currently rely primarily on safe hypnotic medications that are difficult to overdose with. Lorazepam (0.5 mg nightly), temazepam (7.5–15 mg nightly), and zolpidem (2.5–5 mg nightly) are often effective for the elderly population and can be given in larger doses (twice what is prescribed for the elderly) in younger populations. It is important to note that short-acting agents like triazolam or zolpidem may lead to amnestic episodes if used on a daily ongoing basis. Longer-acting agents such as flurazepam (half-life of > 48 hours) may accumulate in the elderly and lead to cognitive slowing, ataxia, falls, and somnolence. In general, it is appropriate to use medications for short courses of 1–2 weeks. The medications described above have largely replaced barbiturates as hypnotic agents because of their greater safety in overdose and their lesser hepatic enzyme induction effects. Antihistamines such as diphenhydramine (25 mg nightly) or hydroxyzine (25 mg nightly) may also be useful for sleep, as they produce no pharmacologic dependency; their anticholinergic effects may, however, produce confusion or urinary symptoms in the elderly.

Triazolam has achieved popularity as a hypnotic drug because of its very short duration of action. Because it has been associated with dependency, transient psychotic reactions, anterograde amnesia, and rebound anxiety, it has been removed from the market in several European countries. If used, it must be prescribed only for short periods of time.

2. HYPERSOMNIAS
(Disorders of Excessive Sleepiness)

The hypersomnias are a more severe problem than insomnia.

Classification & Clinical Findings

A. Sleep Apnea: This disorder is characterized by cessation of breathing for at least 30 episodes (each lasting about 10 seconds) during the night. There are two types: obstructive and central. The obstructive type is discussed in Chapter 9. Central sleep apnea is due to failure during sleep of the respiratory drive mechanism. Obese middle-aged and older men with hypertension and associated congestive heart failure are most often affected. Both types may occur simultaneously. Symptoms include snoring, restless sleep, and excessive daytime sleepiness, which may be associated with headaches, memory impairment, and depression. Cardiac arrhythmias (particularly bradycardia) and blood gas abnormalities occur during episodes. The patients tend to have poor judgment and a history of work-related problems. Definitive diagnostic evaluation may include thyroid evaluation and otolaryngologic examination; polysomnography in the hospital to record sleep, heart rate, and respiratory movement; and oxygen saturation studies. Moderate alcohol intake at bedtime has produced sleep apnea episodes (10–12 nightly) in healthy men.

B. Narcolepsy: Narcolepsy consists of a tetrad of symptoms: (1) Sudden, brief (about 15 minutes) sleep attacks that may occur during any type of activity; (2) cataplexy—sudden loss of muscle tone involving specific small muscle groups or generalized muscle weakness that may cause the person to slump to the floor, unable to move, often associated with emotional reactions and sometimes confused with seizure disorder; (3) sleep paralysis—a generalized flaccidity of muscles with full consciousness in the transition zone between sleep and waking; and (4) hypnagogic hallucinations, visual or auditory, which may precede sleep or occur during the sleep attack. The attacks are characterized by an abrupt transition into REM sleep—a necessary criterion for diagnosis. The disorder begins in early adult life, affects both sexes equally, and usually levels off in severity at about 30 years of age.

REM sleep behavior disorder, characterized by motor dyscontrol and often violent dreams during REM sleep, may be related to narcolepsy.

C. Kleine-Levin Syndrome: This syndrome, which occurs mostly in young males, is characterized by hypersomnic attacks three or four times a year lasting up to 2 days, with hyperphagia, hypersexuality, irritability, and confusion on awakening. It has often been associated with antecedent neurologic insults. It usually remits after age 40.

D. Nocturnal Myoclonus: Periodic lower leg movements occur during sleep with subsequent daytime sleepiness, anxiety, depression, and cognitive impairment.

Treatment

Treatment of sleep apnea may include medical measures such as weight reduction and administration during sleep of air under continuous pressure through the nasopharynx. Surgical treatment is discussed in Chapter 9. Diaphragmatic pacing has also been helpful for central sleep apnea. Trials with protriptyline have improved daytime somnolence and nocturnal oxygenation, with no significant change, however, in the number of apneic episodes. Acetazolamide has shown some promise, probably by creating a metabolic acidosis and the resultant hypercapnic ventilatory response.

Narcolepsy is managed by daily administration of a stimulant such as dextroamphetamine sulfate, 10 mg in the morning, with increased dosage as necessary. Imipramine, 75–100 mg daily, has been effective in treatment of cataplexy but not narcolepsy.

Nocturnal myoclonus and REM sleep behavior disorder can be treated with clonazepam with variable results. There is no treatment for Kleine-Levin syndrome.

3. PARASOMNIAS
(Abnormal Behaviors During Sleep)

These disorders are fairly common in children and less so in adults.

Classification & Clinical Findings

A. Sleep Terror: Sleep terror (pavor nocturnus) is an abrupt, terrifying arousal from sleep, usually in preadolescent boys though it may occur in adults as well. It is distinct from sleep panic attacks. Symptoms are fear, sweating, tachycardia, and confusion for several minutes, with amnesia for the event.

B. Nightmares: Nightmares occur during REM sleep; sleep terrors in stage 3 or stage 4 sleep.

C. Sleepwalking: Sleepwalking (somnambulism) includes ambulation or other intricate behaviors while still asleep, with amnesia for the event. It affects mostly children aged 6–12 years, and episodes occur during stage 3 or stage 4 sleep in the first third of the night and in REM sleep in the later sleep hours. Sleepwalking in elderly people may be a feature of dementia. Idiosyncratic reactions to drugs (eg, marijuana, alcohol) and medical conditions (eg, partial complex seizures) may be causative factors in adults.

D. Enuresis: Enuresis is involuntary micturition during sleep in a person who usually has voluntary control. Like other parasomnias, it is more common in children, usually in the 3–4 hours after bedtime, but is not limited to a specific stage of sleep. Confusion during the episode and amnesia for the event are common.

Treatment

Treatment for sleep terrors is with benzodiazepines (eg, diazepam, 5–20 mg at bedtime), since it will suppress stage 3 and stage 4 sleep. Somnambulism responds to the same treatment for the same reason, but simple safety measures should not be neglected. Enuresis may respond to imipramine, 50–100 mg at bedtime, though desmopressin nasal spray (an antidiuretic hormone preparation) has increasingly become the treatment of choice for nocturnal enuresis. Behavioral approaches (eg, bells that ring when the pad gets wet) have also been successful.

[Treatment of sleep disorders in older people] gopher://gopher.nih.gov/00/clin/cdcs/individual/78.sleep

Becker PM, Jamieson AO: Insomnia: Use of a decision tree to assess and treat. Postgrad Med 1993;93:66.

Farney RJ, Walker JM: Office management of common sleep-wake disorders. Med Clin North Am 1995;79:391.

Gorbien MJ: When your older patient can't sleep: How to put insomnia to rest. Geriatrics 1993;48:65.

Grad RM: Benzodiazepines for insomnia in community-dwelling elderly: A review of benefit and risk. J Fam Pract 1995;41:473. (Clinicians should discontinue long-acting benzodiazepines in the elderly to reduce risk of falls and hip fractures.)

Guilleminault C et al: Nondrug treatment trials in psychophysiologic insomnia. Arch Intern Med 1995; 155:838. (Patients with chronic psychophysiologic insomnia may benefit from a nondrug treatment approach.)

DISORDERS OF AGGRESSION

Acts performed with the deliberate intent of causing physical harm to persons or property have a wide variety of causative features. Aggression and violence are symptoms rather than diseases, and most frequently they are not associated with an underlying medical condition. Clinicians are unable to predict dangerous behavior with greater than chance accuracy. In terms of demographic characteristics, the perpetrator of an act of aggression is often a male under age 25, a member of a socioeconomically deprived group, and a resident of an inner city area. Depression, schizophrenia, personality disorders, mania, paranoia, temporal lobe dysfunction, and organic mental states may be associated. Anabolic steroid usage by athletes has been associated with increased tendencies toward violent behavior.

In the USA, a significant proportion of all violent deaths are alcohol-related. The ingestion of even small amounts of alcohol can result in pathologic intoxication that resembles an acute organic mental condition. Amphetamines, crack cocaine, and other stimulants are frequently associated with aggressive behavior. Phencyclidine is a drug commonly associated with violent behavior that is occasionally of a bizarre nature, partly due to lowering of the pain threshold. Impulse control disorders are characterized by physical abuse, usually of the aggressor's domestic partner or children, pathologic intoxication, impulsive sexual activities, and reckless driving.

Domestic violence and rape are much more widespread than heretofore recognized. Awareness of the problem is to some degree due to increasing recognition of the rights of women and the understanding by women that they do not have to accept abuse. Acceptance of this kind of aggression inevitably leads to more, with the ultimate aggression being murder—20–50% of murders in the USA occur within the family. Police are called in more domestic disputes than all other criminal incidents combined. Children living in such family situations frequently become victims of abuse.

Features of individuals who have been subjected to chronic physical or sexual abuse are as follows: trouble expressing anger, staying angry longer, general passivity in relationships, feeling "marked for life" with an accompanying feeling of deserving to be victimized, lack of trust, and dissociation of affect from experiences. They are prone to express their psychologic distress with somatization symptoms, often pain complaints. They may also have symptoms related to posttraumatic stress, as discussed above. The physician should be suspicious about the origin of any injuries not fully explained, particularly if such incidents recur.

Treatment

A. Psychologic: Management of any violent

individual includes appropriate psychologic maneuvers. Move slowly, talk slowly with clarity and reassurance, and evaluate the situation. Strive to create a setting that is minimally disturbing and eliminate people or things threatening to the violent individual. Do not threaten or abuse and do not touch or crowd the person. Allow no weapons in the area (an increasing problem in hospital emergency rooms). Proximity to a door is comforting to both the patient and the examiner. Use a negotiator the violent person can relate to comfortably. Food and drink are helpful in defusing the situation (as are cigarettes for those who smoke). Honesty is important. Make no false promises, bolster the patient's self-esteem, and continue to engage the subject verbally until the situation is under control. This type of individual does better with strong external controls to replace the lack of inner controls over the long term. Close probationary supervision and judicially mandated restrictions can be most helpful. There should be a major effort to help the individual avoid drug use (eg, Alcoholics Anonymous). Victims of abuse are essentially treated as any victim of trauma and, not infrequently, have evidence of posttraumatic stress disorder.

B. Pharmacologic: Pharmacologic means are often necessary whether or not psychologic approaches have been successful. This is particularly true in the agitated or psychotic patient. The drug of choice in psychotic aggressive states is haloperidol, 10 mg intramuscularly every hour until symptoms are alleviated. Benzodiazepine sedatives (eg, diazepam, 5 mg orally or intravenously every several hours) can be used for mild to moderate agitation, but an antipsychotic drug is preferred for management of the seriously violent and psychotic patient. Chronic aggressive states, particularly in retardation and brain damage (rule out causative organic conditions and medications such as anticholinergic drugs in amounts sufficient to cause confusion), have been ameliorated with propranolol, 40–240 mg/d orally, or pindolol, 5 mg twice daily orally (pindolol causes less bradycardia and hypotension). Carbamazepine and valproic acid are effective in the treatment of aggression and explosive disorders, particularly when associated with known or suspected brain lesions. Lithium and SSRIs are also effective for some intermittent explosive outbursts. Buspirone (10–45 mg/d orally) is helpful for aggression, particularly in mentally retarded patients.

C. Physical: Physical management is necessary if psychologic and pharmacologic means are not sufficient. It requires the active and visible presence of an adequate number of personnel (five or six) to reinforce the idea that the situation is under control despite the patient's lack of inner controls. Such an approach often precludes the need for actual physical restraint. When adequate personnel are not available, however, two people shielded by a mattress (single-bed size) can usually corner and subdue the patient without injury to anyone. Seclusion rooms and restraints should be used only when necessary (ambulatory restraints are an alternative), and the patient must then be observed at frequent intervals. Design of corridors and seclusion rooms is important. Narrow corridors, small spaces, and crowded areas exacerbate the potential for violence in an anxious patient.

D. Other: The treatment of victims (eg, battered women) is challenging and often complicated by their reluctance to leave the situation. Reasons for staying vary, but common themes include the fear of more violence because of leaving; the hope that the situation may ameliorate (in spite of steady worsening); and the financial aspects of the situation, which are seldom to the woman's advantage. Concerns for the children often finally compel the woman to seek help. An early step is to get the woman into a therapeutic situation that provides the support of others in similar straits. Al-Anon is frequently a valuable asset and quite appropriate when alcohol is a factor. The group can support the victim while she gathers strength to consider alternatives without being paralyzed by fear. Many cities now offer temporary emergency centers and counseling. Use the available resources, attend to any medical or psychiatric problems, and maintain a compassionate interest. Some states now require physicians to report injuries caused by abuse to police authorities.

Abbott J et al: Domestic violence against women: Incidence and prevalence in an emergency department population. JAMA 1995;273:1763. (The incidence of acute domestic violence among the 418 women with a current male partner was 11.7%.)

Marwick C: Health and justice professionals set goals to lessen domestic violence. JAMA 1994;271:1147.

Su T-P et al: Neuropsychiatric effects of anabolic steroids in male normal volunteers. JAMA 1993;269:2760.

SUBSTANCE USE DISORDERS
(Drug Dependency, Drug Abuse)

The term "drug dependency" is used in a broad sense here to include both addictions and habituations. It involves the triad of compulsive drug use referred to as drug addiction, which includes (1) a **psychologic dependence** or craving and the behavior included in the procurement of the drug ("hustle"); (2) **physiologic dependence,** with withdrawal symptoms on discontinuance of the drug; and (3) **tolerance,** ie, the need to increase the dose to obtain the desired effects. Drug dependency is a function of the amount of drug used and the duration of usage.

The amount needed to produce dependency varies with the nature of the drug and the idiosyncratic nature of the user. The frequency of use is usually daily, and the duration is inevitably greater than 2–3 weeks. Polydrug abuse is very common. Transgenerational continuity of drug abuse is also common. A large percentage of drug abusers present themselves for something other than treatment (eg, avoiding legal sanctions, obtaining more drugs).

There is accumulating evidence that an impairment syndrome exists in many former (and current) drug users. It is believed that drug use produces damaged neurotransmitter receptor sites and that the consequent imbalance produces symptoms that may mimic other psychiatric illnesses. **"Kindling"**—repeated stimulation of the brain—renders the individual more susceptible to focal brain activity with minimal stimulation. Stimulants and depressants can produce kindling, leading to relatively spontaneous effects no longer dependent on the original stimulus. These effects may be manifested as mood swings, panic, psychosis, and occasionally overt seizure activity. The imbalance also results in personal nonproductivity: frequent job changes, marital problems, and generally erratic behavior. Patients with posttraumatic stress disorder frequently have treated themselves with a variety of drugs. Chronic abusers of a wide variety of drugs exhibit cerebral atrophy on CT scans, a finding that may relate to the above symptoms. Early recognition is important, mainly to establish realistic treatment programs that are chiefly symptom-directed.

The physician faces three problems with substance abuse: (1) the prescribing of substances such as sedatives, stimulants, or narcotics that might produce dependency; (2) the treatment of individuals who have already abused drugs, most commonly alcohol; and (3) the detection of illicit drug use in patients presenting with psychiatric symptoms. The usefulness of urinalysis for detection of drugs varies markedly with different drugs and under different circumstances (pharmacokinetics is a major factor). Water-soluble drugs (eg, alcohol, stimulants, opioids) are eliminated in a day or so. Lipophilic substances (eg, barbiturates, tetrahydrocannabinol) appear in the urine over longer periods of time: several days in most cases, 1–2 months in chronic marijuana users. Sedative drug determinations are quite variable, amount of drug and duration of use being important determinants. False-positives can be a problem related to ingestion of some legitimate drugs (eg, phenytoin for barbiturates, phenylpropanolamine for amphetamines, chlorpromazine for opioids) and some foods (eg, poppy seeds for opioids, coca leaf tea for cocaine). Manipulations can alter the legitimacy of the testing. Dilution, either in vivo or in vitro, can be detected by checking urine specific gravity. Addition of ammonia, vinegar, or salt may invalidate the test, but odor and pH determinations are simple. Hair analysis can determine drug use over longer periods, particularly sequential drug-taking patterns. The sensitivity and reliability of such tests are considered good, and the method may be complementary to urinalysis.

Botvin GJ et al: Long-term follow-up results of a randomized drug abuse prevention trial in a white middle-class population. JAMA 1995;273:1106. (Drug abuse prevention programs conducted during junior high school can produce meaningful and durable reductions in tobacco, alcohol, and marijuana use.)

Finlayson RE, Davis LJ Jr: Prescription drug dependence in the elderly population: Demographic and clinical features of 100 inpatients. Mayo Clin Proc 1994;69:1137. (The most frequent drug dependence involved sedatives or hypnotics.)

Gil-Rivas V et al: Sexual abuse, physical abuse, and posttraumatic stress disorder among women participating in outpatient drug abuse treatment. J Psychoactive Drugs 1996;28:95. (Women are more likely to have suffered abuse but are also more willing to engage in treatment groups that mitigate substance abuse relapses.)

Stewart SH: Alcohol abuse in individuals exposed to trauma: A critical review. Psychol Bull 1996;120:83. (Strong relationship.)

ALCOHOL DEPENDENCY & ABUSE (Alcoholism)

Essentials of Diagnosis

Major criteria:
- Physiologic dependence as manifested by evidence of withdrawal when intake is interrupted.
- Tolerance to the effects of alcohol.
- Evidence of alcohol-associated illnesses, such as alcoholic liver disease, cerebellar degeneration.
- Continued drinking despite strong medical and social contraindications and life disruptions.
- Impairment in social and occupational functioning.
- Depression.
- Blackouts.

Other signs:
- Alcohol stigmas: alcohol odor on breath, alcoholic facies, flushed face, scleral injection, tremor, ecchymoses, peripheral neuropathy.
- Surreptitious drinking.
- Unexplained work absences.
- Frequent accidents, falls, or injuries of vague origin; in smokers, cigarette burns on hands or chest.
- Laboratory tests (elevated values of liver function tests, mean corpuscular volume, serum uric acid and triglycerides).

General Considerations

Alcoholism is a syndrome consisting of two phases: problem drinking and alcohol addiction. Problem drinking is the repetitive use of alcohol, often to alleviate anxiety or solve other emotional problems. Alcohol addiction is a true addiction similar to that which occurs following the repeated use of other sedative-hypnotics. There is a high incidence among homeless individuals. Alcohol and other drug abuse patients have a much higher prevalence of lifetime psychiatric disorders. While male-to-female ratios in alcoholic treatment agencies remain at 4:1, there is evidence that the rates are converging. Women delay seeking help, and when they do they tend to seek it in medical or mental health settings. Adoption and twin studies indicate some genetic influence. Ethnic distinctions are important—eg, 40% of Japanese have aldehyde dehydrogenase deficiency and are more susceptible to the effects of alcohol. Depression is often present and should be evaluated carefully. The majority of suicides and intrafamily homicides involve alcohol, and alcohol is a major factor in rapes and other assaults also.

There are several screening instruments that may help identify alcoholism. One of the most useful is the CAGE questionnaire (Table 1–6).

Clinical Findings

A. Acute Intoxication: The signs of alcoholic intoxication are the same as those of overdosage with any other central nervous system depressant: drowsiness, errors of commission, psychomotor dysfunction, disinhibition, dysarthria, ataxia, and nystagmus. For a 70-kg person, an ounce of whiskey, a glass of wine, or a 12-oz bottle of beer raises the level of alcohol in the blood by 25 mg/dL. For a 50-kg person, the blood alcohol level would rise even higher (35 mg/dL) with the same consumption. Blood alcohol levels below 50 mg/dL rarely cause significant motor dysfunction. Intoxication as manifested by ataxia, dysarthria, and nausea and vomiting indicates a blood level above 150 mg/dL, and lethal blood levels range from 350 to 900 mg/dL. In severe cases, overdosage is marked by respiratory depression, stupor, seizures, shock syndrome, coma, and death. Serious overdoses are frequently due to a combination of alcohol with other sedatives.

B. Withdrawal: There is a wide spectrum of manifestations of alcoholic withdrawal, ranging from anxiety, decreased cognition, and tremulousness through increasing irritability and hyperreactivity to full-blown **delirium tremens.** The latter is an acute organic psychosis that is usually manifest within 25–72 hours after the last drink (but may occur up to 7–10 days later). It is characterized by mental confusion, tremor, sensory hyperacuity, visual hallucinations (often of snakes, bugs, etc), autonomic hyperactivity, diaphoresis, dehydration, electrolyte disturbances (hypokalemia, hypomagnesemia), seizures, and cardiovascular abnormalities. The acute withdrawal syndrome is often completely unexpected and occurs when the patient has been hospitalized for some unrelated problem and presents as a diagnostic problem. Suspect alcohol withdrawal in every unexplained delirium. Seizures occur early (the first 24 hours) and are more prevalent in persons who have a history of withdrawal syndromes. The mortality rate from delirium tremens has steadily decreased with early diagnosis and improved treatment.

In addition to the immediate withdrawal symptoms, there is evidence of persistent longer-term ones, including sleep disturbances, anxiety, depression, excitability, fatigue, and emotional volatility. These symptoms may persist for 3–12 months, and in some cases they become chronic.

C. Alcoholic (Organic) Hallucinosis: This syndrome occurs either during heavy drinking or on withdrawal and is characterized by a paranoid psychosis without the tremulousness, confusion, and clouded sensorium seen in withdrawal syndromes. The patient appears normal except for the auditory hallucinations, which are frequently persecutory and may cause the patient to behave aggressively and in a paranoid fashion.

D. Chronic Alcoholic Brain Syndromes: These encephalopathies are characterized by increasing erratic behavior, memory and recall problems, and emotional instability—the usual signs of organic brain injury due to any cause. Wernicke-Korsakoff syndrome due to thiamin deficiency may develop with a series of episodes. Wernicke's encephalopathy consists of the triad of confusion, ataxia, and ophthalmoplegia (typically sixth nerve). Early recognition and treatment with thiamine can minimize damage. One of the possible sequelae is Korsakoff's psychosis, characterized by both anterograde and retrograde amnesia, with confabulation early in the course. Early recognition and treatment of the alcoholic with intravenous thiamine and B complex vitamins can minimize damage.

Differential Diagnosis

The differential diagnosis of problem drinking is essentially between primary alcoholism (when no other major psychiatric diagnosis exists) and secondary alcoholism, when alcohol is used as self-medication for major underlying psychiatric problems such as schizophrenia or affective disorder. The differentiation is important, since the latter group requires treatment for the specific psychiatric problem.

The differential diagnosis of alcohol withdrawal includes other sedative withdrawals and other causes of delirium. Acute alcoholic hallucinosis must be differentiated from other acute paranoid states such as amphetamine psychosis or paranoid schizophrenia. An accurate history is the most important differentiating factor. The history and laboratory test results (elevated liver function tests, increased mean corpuscular volume, increased serum uric acid and triglycerides, decreased serum potassium and magnesium) are the most important features in differentiating chronic organic brain syndromes due to alcohol from those due to other causes. The form of the brain syndrome is of little help—eg, chronic brain syndromes from lupus erythematosus may be associated with confabulation similar to that resulting from long-standing alcoholism.

Complications

The medical, economic, and psychosocial problems of alcoholism are staggering. The central and peripheral nervous system complications include chronic brain syndromes, cerebellar degeneration, cardiomyopathy, and peripheral neuropathies. Direct effects on the liver include cirrhosis, esophageal varices, and eventual hepatic failure. Indirect effects include protein abnormalities, coagulation defects, hormone deficiencies, and an increased incidence of liver neoplasms.

Fetal alcohol syndrome includes one or more of the following developmental defects in the offspring of alcoholic women: (1) low birth weight and small size with failure to catch up in size or weight; (2) mental retardation, with an average IQ in the 60s; and (3) a variety of birth defects, with a large percentage of facial and cardiac abnormalities. The fetuses are very quiet in utero, and there is an increased frequency of breech presentations. There is a higher incidence of delayed postnatal growth and behavior development. The risk is appreciably higher the more alcohol ingested by the mother each day. Cigarette and marijuana smoking as well as cocaine use can produce similar effects on the fetus.

Treatment of Problem Drinking

A. Psychologic: The most important consideration for the physician is to suspect the problem early and take a nonjudgmental attitude, though this does not mean a passive one. The problem of **denial** must be faced, preferably with significant family members at the first meeting. This means dealing from the beginning with any enabling behavior of the spouse or other significant people. Enabling behavior allows the alcoholic to avoid facing the consequences of his or her behavior.

There must be an emphasis on the things that can be done. This approach emphasizes the fact that the physician cares and strikes a positive and hopeful note early in treatment. Valuable time should not be wasted trying to find out why the patient drinks; come to grips early with the immediate problem of how to stop the drinking. Total abstinence (not "controlled drinking") should be the goal.

B. Social: Get the patient into Alcoholics Anonymous (AA) and the spouse into Al-Anon. Success is usually proportionate to the utilization of AA, religious counseling, and other resources. The patient should be seen frequently for short periods and charged an appropriate fee.

Do not underestimate the importance of religion, particularly since the alcoholic is often a dependent person who needs a great deal of support. Early enlistment of the help of a concerned religious adviser can often provide the turning point for a personal conversion to sobriety.

One of the most important considerations is the patient's job—fear of losing a job is one of the most powerful motivations for giving up drink. The business community has become painfully aware of the problem, with the result that about 70% of the Fortune 500 companies offer programs to their employees to help with the problem of alcoholism. In the latter case, some specific recommendations to employers can be offered: (1) Avoid placement in jobs where the alcoholic must be alone, eg, as a traveling buyer or sales executive. (2) Use supervision but not surveillance. (3) Keep competition with others to a minimum. (4) Avoid positions that require quick decision making on important matters (high stress situations).

C. Medical: Hospitalization is not usually necessary. It is sometimes used to dramatize a situation and force the patient to face the problem of alcoholism, but generally it should be used on medical indications.

Because of the many medical complications of alcoholism, a complete physical examination with appropriate laboratory tests is mandatory, with special attention to the liver and nervous system. Two tests that may provide clues to an alcohol problem are γ-glutamyl transpeptidase measurement (levels above 30 units/L are suggestive of heavy drinking) and mean corpuscular volume (> 95 fL in males and > 100 fL in females). If both are elevated, a serious drinking problem is likely. Use of other recreational drugs with alcohol skews and negates the significance of these tests. HDL cholesterol elevations combined with elevated γ-glutamyl transpeptidase concentrations also can help to identify heavy drinkers.

Use of sedatives as a replacement for alcohol is not desirable. The usual result is concomitant use of sedatives and alcohol and worsening of the problem. Lithium is not helpful in the treatment of alcoholism.

Disulfiram (250–500 mg/d orally) has been used for many years as an aversive drug to discourage alcohol use. Disulfiram inhibits alcohol dehydrogenase, causing toxic reactions when alcohol is consumed. The results have generally been of limited effectiveness and depend on the motivation of the individual to be compliant.

Naltrexone, an opiate antagonist, in a dosage of 50 mg daily, has been helpful in lowering relapse rates over the 3–6 months after cessation of drinking, apparently by lessening the pleasurable effects of alcohol. It has been approved by the FDA for maintenance therapy. Studies indicate that it reduces alcohol craving when used as part of a comprehensive treatment program.

D. Behavioral: Conditioning approaches have been used in some settings in the treatment of alcoholism, most commonly as a type of aversion therapy. For example, the patient is given a drink of whiskey and then a shot of apomorphine, and proceeds to vomit. In this way a strong association is built up between the vomiting and the drinking. Although this kind of treatment has been successful in some cases, many people do not sustain the learned aversive response.

Treatment of Hallucinosis & Withdrawal

A. Medical:

1. Alcoholic hallucinosis—Alcoholic hallucinosis, which can occur either during or on cessation of a prolonged drinking period, is not a typical withdrawal syndrome and is handled differently. Since the symptoms are primarily those of a psychosis in the presence of a clear sensorium, they are handled like any other psychosis: hospitalization (when indicated) and adequate amounts of antipsychotic drugs. Haloperidol, 5 mg orally twice a day for the first day or so, usually ameliorates symptoms quickly, and the drug can be decreased and discontinued over several days as the patient improves. It then becomes necessary to deal with the chronic alcohol abuse, which has been discussed.

2. Withdrawal symptoms—Withdrawal symptoms, ranging from a mild syndrome to the severe state usually called delirium tremens, are a medical problem with a significant morbidity and mortality rate. They usually occur when an intake of at least 7–8 pints of beer or 1 pint of spirits daily for several months has been stopped (onset 12 hours, peak intensity 48–72 hours after cessation of alcohol intake). Providing adequate central nervous system depressants (eg, benzodiazepines) is important to counteract the excitability resulting from sudden cessation of alcohol intake. The choice of a specific sedative is less important than using adequate doses to bring the patient to a level of moderate sedation, and this will vary from person to person. Mild dependency requires "drying out"—a short course of oral benzodiazepines on an outpatient basis with no alcohol intake. In moderate to severe withdrawal, hospitalize the patient and use diazepam orally in a dosage of 5–10 mg hourly depending on the clinical need as judged by withdrawal symptoms, including nausea, tremor, autonomic hyperactivity, agitation; tactile, visual, and auditory hallucinations; and disorientation. This type of symptom-driven medication regimen for withdrawal appears to reduce total benzodiazepine usage over fixed-dose schedules. Antipsychotic drugs such as chlorpromazine should not be used. Monitoring of vital signs and fluid and electrolyte levels is essential for the severely ill patient.

In very severe withdrawal, intravenous administration is necessary. After stabilization, the amount of diazepam required to maintain a sedated state may be given orally every 8–12 hours. If restlessness, tremu-lousness, and other signs of withdrawal persist, the dosage is increased until moderate sedation occurs. The dosage is then gradually reduced by 20% every 24 hours until withdrawal is complete. This usually requires a week or so of treatment. Clonidine, 5 μg/kg orally every 2 hours, or the patch formulation of appropriate dosage strength, suppresses cardiovascular signs of withdrawal and has some anxiolytic effect. Carbamazepine, 400–800 mg daily orally, compares favorably with benzodiazepines for alcohol withdrawal.

Atenolol, as an adjunct to benzodiazepines, can reduce symptoms of alcohol withdrawal. The daily oral atenolol dose is 100 mg when the heart rate is above 80 beats per minute and 50 mg for a heart rate between 50 and 80 beats per minute. Atenolol should not be used when bradycardia is present.

Meticulous examination for other medical problems is necessary. Alcoholic hypoglycemia can occur with low blood alcohol levels (see Chapter 27). Alcoholics commonly have liver disease and associated clotting problems and are also prone to injury—and the combination all too frequently leads to undiagnosed subdural hematoma.

Phenytoin does not appear to be useful in managing alcohol withdrawal seizures per se. Sedating doses of benzodiazepines are effective in treating alcohol withdrawal seizures. Thus, other anticonvulsants are not usually needed unless there is a preexisting seizure disorder.

A general diet should be given, and vitamins in high doses: thiamine, 50 mg intravenously initially, then intramuscularly on a daily basis; pyridoxine, 100 mg/d; folic acid, 1 mg/d; and ascorbic acid, 100 mg twice a day. Intravenous glucose solutions should not be given prior to thiamine for fear of precipitation of Wernicke's syndrome. Thiamine is necessary as a ketolase enzyme cofactor. Concurrent administration is satisfactory, and hydration should be meticulously assessed on an ongoing basis.

Chronic brain syndromes secondary to a long history of alcohol intake are not clearly responsive to thiamine and vitamin replenishment. Attention to the social and environmental care of this type of patient is paramount.

B. Psychologic and Behavioral:
The comments in the section on problem drinking apply here also; these methods of treatment become the primary consideration after successful treatment of withdrawal or alcoholic hallucinosis. Psychologic and social measures should be initiated in the hospital shortly before discharge. This increases the possibility of continued posthospitalization treatment.

Adams WL et al: Screening for problem drinking in older primary care patients. JAMA 1996;276:1964. (The CAGE survey and other questions can identify alcohol abuse in elderly populations.)

Diamond I, Messing RU: Neurologic effects of alcoholism. West J Med 1994;161:279.

Lieber CS: Medical disorders of alcoholism. N Engl J Med 1995;333:1058.

O'Malley SS: Opioid antagonists in the treatment of alcohol dependence: Clinical efficacy and prevention of relapse. Alcohol Alcohol 1996;31:77. (Naltrexone can help reduce craving and prevent relapse in some patients.)

Saitz R et al: Individualized treatment for alcohol withdrawal. JAMA 1994;272:519.

See also Substance Abuse references in Chapter 1.

OTHER DRUG & SUBSTANCE DEPENDENCIES

Opioids

The terms "opioids" and "narcotics" are used interchangeably and include a group of drugs with actions that mimic those of morphine. The group includes natural derivatives of opium (opiates), synthetic surrogates (opioids), and a number of polypeptides, some of which have been discovered to be natural neurotransmitters. The principal narcotic of abuse is heroin (metabolized to morphine), which is not used as a legitimate medication. A large percentage of heroin addicts are infected with HIV because of nonsterile needles. The other common narcotics are prescription drugs and differ in milligram potency, duration of action, and agonist and antagonist capabilities (see Chapter 1). All of the narcotic analgesics can be reversed by the narcotic antagonist naloxone.

The clinical symptoms and signs of mild narcotic intoxication include changes in mood, with feelings of euphoria; drowsiness; nausea with occasional emesis; needle tracks; and miosis. The incidence of snorting and inhaling heroin ("smoking") is increasing, particularly among cocaine users. This coincides with a decrease in the availability of methaqualone (no longer marketed) and other sedatives used to temper the cocaine "high" (see discussion of cocaine under Stimulants, below). Overdosage causes respiratory depression, peripheral vasodilation, pinpoint pupils, pulmonary edema, coma, and death.

Dependency is a major concern when continued use of narcotics occurs, though withdrawal causes only moderate morbidity (similar in severity to a bout of "flu"). Addicts sometimes consider themselves more addicted than they really are and may not require a withdrawal program. Grades of withdrawal are categorized from 0 to 4: grade 0 includes craving and anxiety; grade 1, yawning, lacrimation, rhinorrhea, and perspiration; grade 2, previous symptoms plus mydriasis, piloerection, anorexia, tremors, and hot and cold flashes with generalized aching; grades 3 and 4, increased intensity of previous symptoms and signs, with increased temperature, blood pressure, pulse, and respiratory rate and depth. In withdrawal from the most severe addiction, vomiting, diarrhea, weight loss, hemoconcentration, and spontaneous ejaculation or orgasm commonly occur.

Treatment for overdosage (or suspected overdosage) is naloxone, 2 mg intravenously. If an overdose has been taken, the results are dramatic and occur within 2 minutes. Since the duration of action of naloxone is much shorter than that of the narcotics, the patient must be under close observation. Hospitalization, supportive care, repeated naloxone administration, and observation for withdrawal from other drugs should be maintained for as long as necessary. Complications of heroin administration include infections (eg, pneumonia, septic emboli, hepatitis, and HIV infection), traumatic insults (eg, arterial spasm due to drug injection, gangrene), and pulmonary edema.

Treatment for withdrawal begins if grade 2 signs develop. If a withdrawal program is necessary, use methadone, 10 mg orally (use parenteral administration if the patient is vomiting), and observe. If signs (piloerection, mydriasis, cardiovascular changes) persist for more than 4–6 hours, give another 10 mg; continue to administer methadone at 4- to 6-hour intervals until signs are not present (rarely more than 40 mg of methadone in 24 hours). Divide the total amount of drug required over the first 24-hour period by 2 and give that amount every 12 hours. Each day, reduce the total 24-hour dose by 5–10 mg. Thus, a moderately addicted patient initially requiring 30–40 mg of methadone could be withdrawn over a 4- to 8-day period. Clonidine, 0.1 mg several times daily over a 10- to 14-day period, is an alternative adjunct to methadone detoxification; it is not necessary to taper the dose. Clonidine is helpful in alleviating cardiovascular symptoms but does not significantly relieve anxiety, insomnia, or generalized aching. There is a protracted abstinence syndrome of metabolic, respiratory, and blood pressure changes over a period of 3–6 months.

Methadone maintenance programs are of some value in chronic recidivism. Under carefully controlled supervision, the narcotic addict is maintained on fairly high doses of methadone (40–120 mg/d) that satisfy craving and block the effects of heroin to a great degree.

Narcotic antagonists (eg, naltrexone) can also be used successfully for treatment of the patient who has been free of opioids for 7–10 days. Naltrexone blocks the narcotic "high" of heroin when 50 mg is given orally every 24 hours initially for several days and then 100 mg is given every 48–72 hours. Liver disorders are a major contraindication. Compliance tends to be poor, partly because of the dysphoria that can persist long after opioid discontinuance.

Sedatives (Anxiolytics)

See Antianxiety Drugs, above.

Psychedelics

About 6000 species of plants have psychoactive properties. All of the common psychedelics (LSD, mescaline, psilocybin, dimethyltryptamine, and other derivatives of phenylalanine and tryptophan) can produce similar behavioral and physiologic effects. An initial feeling of tension is followed by emotional release such as crying or laughing (1–2 hours). Later, perceptual distortions occur, with visual illusions and hallucinations, and occasionally there is fear of ego disintegration (2–3 hours). Major changes in time sense and mood lability then occur (3–4 hours). A feeling of detachment and a sense of destiny and control occur (4–6 hours). Of course, reactions vary among individuals, and some of the drugs produce markedly different time frames. Occasionally, the acute episode is terrifying (a "bad trip") which may include panic, depression, confusion, or psychotic symptoms. Preexisting emotional problems, the attitude of the user, and the setting where the drug is used affect the experience.

Treatment of the acute episode primarily involves protection of the individual from erratic behavior that may lead to injury or death. A structured environment is usually sufficient until the drug is metabolized. In severe cases, antipsychotic drugs with minimal side effects (eg, haloperidol, 5 mg intramuscularly) may be given every several hours until the individual has regained control. In cases where "flashbacks" occur (mental imagery from a "bad trip" that is later triggered by mild stimuli such as marijuana, alcohol, or psychic trauma), a short course of an antipsychotic drug (eg, trifluoperazine, 5 mg orally) for several days is usually sufficient. An occasional patient may have "flashbacks" for much longer periods and require small doses of neuroleptic drugs over the longer term.

Phencyclidine

Phencyclidine (PCP, angel dust, peace pill, hog), developed as an anesthetic agent, first appeared as a street drug deceptively sold as tetrahydrocannabinol (THC). Because it is simple to produce and mimics to some degree the traditional psychedelic drugs, PCP has become a common deceptive substitute for LSD, THC, and mescaline. It is available in crystals, capsules, and tablets to be inhaled, injected, swallowed, or smoked (it is commonly sprinkled on marijuana).

Absorption after smoking is rapid, with onset of symptoms in several minutes and peak symptoms in 15–30 minutes. Mild intoxication produces euphoria accompanied by a feeling of numbness. Moderate intoxication (5–10 mg) results in disorientation, detachment from surroundings, distortion of body image, combativeness, unusual feats of strength (partly due to its anesthetic activity), and loss of ability to integrate sensory input, especially touch and proprioception. Physical symptoms include dizziness, ataxia, dysarthria, nystagmus, retracted upper eyelid with blank stare, hyperreflexia, and tachycardia. There are increases in blood pressure, respiration, muscle tone, and urine production. Usage in the first trimester of pregnancy is associated with an increase in spontaneous abortion and congenital defects. Severe intoxication (20 mg or more) produces an increase in degree of moderate symptoms, with the addition of seizures, deepening coma, hypertensive crisis, and severe psychotic ideation. The drug is particularly long-lasting (several days to several weeks) owing to high lipid solubility, gastroenteric recycling, and the production of active metabolites. Overdosage may be fatal, with the major causes of death being hypertensive crisis, respiratory arrest, and convulsions. Acute rhabdomyolysis has been reported and can result in myoglobinuric renal failure.

Differential diagnosis involves the whole spectrum of street drugs, since in some ways phencyclidine mimics sedatives, psychedelics, and marijuana in its effects. Blood and urine testing can detect the acute problem.

Treatment is discussed in Chapter 39.

Marijuana

Cannabis sativa, a hemp plant, is the source of marijuana. The parts of the plant vary in potency. The resinous exudate of the flowering tops of the female plant (hashish, charas) is the most potent, followed by the dried leaves and flowering shoots of the female plant (bhang) and the resinous mass from small leaves of inflorescence (ganja). The least potent parts are the lower branches and the leaves of the female plant and all parts of the male plant. Mercury may be a contaminant in marijuana grown in volcanic soil. The drug is usually inhaled by smoking. Effects occur in 10–20 minutes and last 2–3 hours. "Joints" of good quality contain about 500 mg of marijuana (which contains approximately 5–15 mg of tetrahydrocannabinol with a half-life of 7 days). Marijuana soaked in formaldehyde and dried ("AMP") has produced unusual effects, including autonomic discharge and severe, transient cognitive impairment.

With moderate dosage, marijuana produces two phases: mild euphoria followed by sleepiness. In the acute state, the user has an altered time perception, less inhibited emotions, psychomotor problems, impaired immediate memory, and conjunctival injection. High doses produce transient psychotomimetic effects. No specific treatment is necessary except in the case of the occasional "bad trip," in which case the person is treated in the same way as for psychedelic usage. Marijuana frequently aggravates existing mental illness, adversely affects motor performance, and slows the learning process in children.

Studies of long-term effects have conclusively shown abnormalities in the pulmonary tree. Laryngitis and rhinitis are related to prolonged use, along with chronic obstructive pulmonary disease. Electrocardiographic abnormalities are common, but no long-term cardiac disease has been linked to marijuana use. Chronic usage has resulted in depression of plasma testosterone levels and reduced sperm counts. Abnormal menstruation and failure to ovulate have occurred in some female users. Cognitive impairments are probable, though studies are not conclusive. Health care utilization for a variety of health problems is increased in chronic marijuana smokers. Sudden withdrawal produces insomnia, nausea, myalgia, and irritability. Psychologic effects of chronic marijuana usage are still unclear. Urine testing is reliable if samples are carefully collected and tested. Detection periods span 4–6 days in acute users and 20–50 days in chronic users.

Stimulants: Amphetamines & Cocaine

Stimulant abuse is quite common, either alone or in combination with abuse of other drugs. The **amphetamines,** including Methedrine ("speed")—one variant is a smokable form called "ice," which gives an intense and fairly long-lasting high—methylphenidate, and phenmetrazine, are under prescription control, but street availability remains high. Moderate usage of any of the stimulants produces hyperactivity, a sense of enhanced physical and mental capacity, and sympathomimetic effects. The clinical picture of acute stimulant intoxication includes sweating, tachycardia, elevated blood pressure, mydriasis, hyperactivity, and an acute brain syndrome with confusion and disorientation. Tolerance develops quickly and, as the dosage is increased, hypervigilance, paranoid ideation (with delusions of parasitosis), stereotypy, bruxism, tactile hallucinations of insect infestation, and full-blown psychoses occur, often with persecutory ideation and aggressive responses. Stimulant withdrawal is characterized by depression with symptoms of hyperphagia and hypersomnia.

People who have used stimulants chronically (eg, anorexigenics) occasionally become sensitized (**"kindling"**) to future use of stimulants. In these individuals, even small amounts of mild stimulants such as caffeine can cause symptoms of paranoia and auditory hallucinations.

Cocaine is a stimulant, not a narcotic. It is a product of the coca plant. The derivatives include seeds, leaves, coca paste, cocaine hydrochloride, and the free base of cocaine. Coca paste is a crude extract that contains 40–80% cocaine sulfate and other impurities. Cocaine hydrochloride is the salt and the most commonly used form. Free base, a purer (and stronger) derivative called "crack," is prepared by simple extraction from cocaine hydrochloride.

There are various modes of use. Coca leaf chewing involves toasting the leaves and chewing with alkaline material (eg, the ash of other burned leaves) to enhance buccal absorption. One achieves a mild high, with onset in 5–10 minutes and lasting for about an hour. Intranasal use is simply snorting cocaine through a straw. Absorption is slowed somewhat by vasoconstriction (which may eventually cause tissue necrosis and septal perforation); the onset of action is in 2–3 minutes, with a moderate high (euphoria, excitement, increased energy) lasting about 30 minutes. The purity of the cocaine is a major determinant of the high. Intravenous use of cocaine hydrochloride or free-base cocaine is effective in 30 seconds and produces a short-lasting, fairly intense high of about 15 minutes' duration. The combined use of cocaine and ethanol results in the metabolic production of cocaethylene by the liver. This substance produces more intense and long-lasting cocaine-like effects. Smoking free-base cocaine (volatilized cocaine because of the lower boiling point) acts in seconds and results in an intense high lasting several minutes. The intensity of the reaction is related to the marked lipid solubility of the free-base form and produces by far the most severe medical and psychiatric symptoms.

Cardiovascular collapse, arrhythmias, myocardial infarction, and transient ischemic attacks have been reported. Seizures, strokes, migraine symptoms, hyperthermia, and lung damage may occur, and there are several obstetric complications, including spontaneous abortion, abruptio placentae, teratogenic effects, delayed fetal growth, and prematurity. Cocaine can cause anxiety, mood swings, and delirium, and chronic use can cause the same problems as other stimulants (see above).

Physicians should be alert to cocaine use in patients presenting with unexplained nasal bleeding, headaches, fatigue, insomnia, anxiety, depression, and chronic hoarseness. Sudden withdrawal of the drug is not life-threatening but usually produces craving, sleep disturbances, hyperphagia, lassitude, and severe depression (sometimes with suicidal ideation) lasting days to weeks.

Treatment is imprecise and difficult. Since the high is related to blockage of dopamine reuptake, the dopamine agonist bromocriptine, 1.5 mg orally three times a day, alleviates some of the symptoms of craving associated with acute cocaine withdrawal. Other dopamine agonists such as apomorphine, levodopa, and amantadine are under study for this purpose. There is preliminary evidence that carbamazepine in the usual doses reduces craving in withdrawal (probably owing to its effect on kindling), and desipramine in moderate doses has been useful in helping maintain abstinence in the early stages of treatment. Treatment of psychosis is the same as that of any psychosis: antipsychotic drugs in dosages sufficient to alleviate the symptoms. Any medical symptoms (eg, hyperthermia, seizures, hypertension) are treated specifically. These approaches should be used in conjunction with a structured program, most often based on the AA model. Hospitalization may be required if self-harm or violence toward others is a perceived threat (usually indicated by paranoid delusions).

Caffeine

Caffeine, along with nicotine and alcohol, is one of the most commonly used drugs worldwide. About 10 billion pounds of coffee (the richest source of caffeine) are consumed yearly throughout the world. Tea, cocoa, and cola drinks also contribute to an intake of caffeine that is often astoundingly high in a large number of people. Low to moderate doses (30–200 mg/d) tend to improve some aspects of performance (eg, vigilance). The approximate content of caffeine in a (180 mL) cup of beverage is as follows: brewed coffee, 80–140 mg; instant coffee, 60–100 mg; decaffeinated coffee, 1–6 mg; black leaf tea, 30–80 mg; tea bags, 25–75 mg; instant tea, 30–60 mg; cocoa, 10–50 mg; and 12-oz cola drinks, 30–65 mg. A 2-oz chocolate candy bar has about 20 mg. Some herbal teas (eg, "morning thunder") contain caffeine. Caffeine-containing analgesics usually contain approximately 30 mg per unit. Symptoms of caffeinism (usually associated with ingestion of over 500 mg/d) include anxiety, agitation, restlessness, insomnia, a feeling of being "wired," and somatic symptoms referable to the heart and gastrointestinal tract. It is common for a case of caffeinism to present as an anxiety disorder. It is also common for caffeine and other stimulants to precipitate severe symptoms in compensated schizophrenic and manic-depressive patients. Chronically depressed patients often use caffeine drinks as self-medication. This diagnostic clue may help distinguish some major affective disorders. Withdrawal from caffeine (> 250 mg/d) can produce headaches, irritability, lethargy, and occasional nausea.

Miscellaneous Drugs, Solvents

The principal OTC drugs of concern are phenylpropanolamine and an assortment of antihistaminic agents. Frequently, these drugs are sold in combination with a mild analgesic as cold remedies (eg, Dristan, Triaminic). Most appetite suppressant drugs are combinations of phenylpropanolamine and caffeine (fenfluramine is an exception); these drugs are also heavily marketed as "stay-awake" drugs. Practically all of the so-called sleep aids are now antihistamines. Scopolamine and bromides have generally been removed from OTC products.

The major problem in the use of all these drugs relates to phenylpropanolamine, which has all the side effects of any stimulant, including precipitation of anxiety states, increased pressor effect, auditory and visual hallucinations, paranoid ideation, and, occasionally, delirium. Aggressiveness and some loss of impulse control have been reported. Sleep disturbances are common even with reasonably small doses.

Antihistamines usually produce some central nervous system depression—thus their use as OTC sedatives. Drowsiness may be a problem. The mixture of antihistamines with alcohol usually exacerbates the central nervous system effects.

The abuse of laxatives sometimes can lead to electrolyte disturbances that may contribute to the manifestations of a delirium. The greatest use of laxatives tends to be in the elderly and in those with eating disorders, both of whom are the most vulnerable to physiologic changes.

Anabolic steroids are being abused by people who wish to increase muscle mass for cosmetic reasons or for greater strength. In addition to the medical problems, the practice is associated with significant mood swings, aggressiveness, and paranoid delusions. Alcohol and stimulant use is higher in these individuals. Withdrawal symptoms of steroid dependency include fatigue, depressed mood, restlessness, and insomnia.

Amyl nitrite, a drug useful in angina pectoris, has been used in recent years as an "orgasm expander." The changes in time perception, "rush," and mild euphoria caused by the drug prompted its nonmedical use, and popular lore concerning the effects of inhalation just prior to orgasm has led to increased use. Subjective effects last from 5 seconds to 15 minutes. Tolerance develops readily, but there are no known withdrawal symptoms. Abstinence for several days reestablishes the previous level of responsiveness. Long-term effects may include damage to the immune system and respiratory difficulties.

Sniffing of solvents and inhaling of gases (including aerosols) produce a form of inebriation similar to that of the volatile anesthetics. Agents include gasoline, toluene, petroleum ether, lighter fluids, cleaning fluids, paint thinners, and solvents that are present in many household products (eg, nail polish, typewriter correction fluid). Typical intoxication states include euphoria, slurred speech, hallucinations, and confusion, and with high doses, acute manifestations are unconsciousness and cardiorespiratory depression or failure; chronic exposure produces a variety of symptoms related to the liver, kidney, bone marrow, or heart. Lead encephalopathy can be associated with sniffing leaded gasoline. In addition, studies of workers chronically exposed to jet fuel showed significant increases in neurasthenic symptoms, including fatigue, anxiety, mood changes, memory difficulties, and somatic complaints. These same problems have been noted in long-term solvent abuse.

The so-called designer drugs are synthetic substitutes for commonly used recreational drugs and are produced in small, clandestine laboratories. The most common designer drugs have been methyl analogues of fentanyl and have been used as heroin substitutes. MDMA (methylenedioxymethamphetamine), an amphetamine derivative sometimes called "ecstasy," is also a designer drug with high abuse potential and neurotoxicity. Manufacture and use of these substances are a vexing problem for law enforcement, since the newest drugs have not yet achieved illegal status and there are no tests developed for detection. Furthermore, they present problems for physicians faced with symptoms from a totally unknown cause.

Brookoff D et al: Testing reckless drivers for cocaine and marijuana. N Engl J Med 1994;331:518. (Over half of the reckless drivers who were not intoxicated with alcohol were found to be intoxicated with other drugs.)

Hartel DM et al: Heroin use during methadone maintenance treatment: The importance of methadone dose and cocaine use. Am J Public Health 1995;85:83. (Heroin use during the 3 months prior to interview was shown to be greatest among patients maintained on methadone dosages of less than 70 mg/d and among patients who used cocaine during treatment.)

O'Brien CP: Recent developments in the pharmacotherapy of substance abuse. J Consult Clin Psychol 1996;64:677.

Polen MR et al: Health care use by frequent marijuana smokers who do not smoke tobacco. West J Med 1993;158:596.

Silverman K et al: Withdrawal syndrome after the double-blind cessation of caffeine consumption. N Engl J Med 1992;327:1109. (Lower than previously thought.)

DELIRIUM, DEMENTIA, & OTHER COGNITIVE DISORDERS (Formerly: Organic Brain Syndrome [OBS])

Essentials of Diagnosis

- Transient or permanent brain dysfunction.
- Cognitive impairment to varying degrees: may include impaired recall and recent memory, inability to focus attention, random psychomotor activity such as stereotypy, and problems in perceptual processing, often with psychotic ideation.
- Emotional disorders frequently present: depression, anxiety, irritability.
- Behavioral disturbances may include problems of impulse control, sexual acting-out, attention deficits, aggression, and exhibitionism.

General Considerations

The organic problem may be a primary brain disease or a secondary manifestation of some general disorder. All of the cognitive disorders show some degree of impaired thinking depending on the site of involvement, the rate of onset and progression, and the duration of the underlying brain lesion. Emotional disturbances (eg, depression) are often present as significant comorbidities. The behavioral distur-

bances tend to be more common with chronicity, more directly related to the underlying personality or central nervous system vulnerability to drug side effects, and not necessarily correlated with cognitive dysfunction.

Etiology

A. Intoxication: Alcohol, sedatives, bromides, analgesics (eg, pentazocine), psychedelic drugs, stimulants, and household solvents.

B. Drug Withdrawal: Withdrawal from alcohol, sedative-hypnotics, corticosteroids.

C. Long-Term Effects of Alcohol: Wernicke-Korsakoff syndrome.

D. Infections: Septicemia; meningitis and encephalitis due to bacterial, viral, fungal, parasitic, or tuberculous organisms or to central nervous system syphilis; acute and chronic infections due to the entire range of microbiologic pathogens.

E. Endocrine Disorders: Thyrotoxicosis, hypothyroidism, adrenocortical dysfunction (including Addison's disease and Cushing's syndrome), pheochromocytoma, insulinoma, hypoglycemia, hyperparathyroidism, hypoparathyroidism, panhypopituitarism, diabetic ketoacidosis.

F. Respiratory Disorders: Hypoxia, hypercapnia.

G. Metabolic Disturbances: Fluid and electrolyte disturbances (especially hyponatremia, hypomagnesemia, and hypercalcemia), acid-base disorders, hepatic disease (hepatic encephalopathy), renal failure, porphyria.

H. Nutritional Deficiencies: Deficiency of vitamin B_1 (beriberi), vitamin B_{12} (pernicious anemia), folic acid, nicotinic acid (pellagra); protein-calorie malnutrition.

I. Trauma: Subdural hematoma, subarachnoid hemorrhage, intracerebral bleeding, concussion syndrome.

J. Cardiovascular Disorders: Myocardial infarctions, cardiac arrhythmias, cerebrovascular spasms, hypertensive encephalopathy, hemorrhages, embolisms, and occlusions indirectly cause decreased cognitive function.

K. Neoplasms: Primary or metastatic lesions of the central nervous system, cancer-induced hypercalcemia.

L. Seizure Disorders: Ictal, interictal, and postictal dysfunction.

M. Collagen and Immunologic Disorders: Autoimmune disorders, including systemic lupus erythematosus, Sjögren's syndrome, and AIDS.

N. Degenerative Diseases: Alzheimer's disease, Pick's disease, multiple sclerosis, parkinsonism, Huntington's chorea, normal pressure hydrocephalus.

O. Medications: Anticholinergic drugs, antidepressants, H_2-blocking agents, digoxin, salicylates (chronic use), and a wide variety of other OTC and prescribed drugs.

Clinical Findings

The manifestations are many and varied and include problems with orientation, short or fluctuating attention span, loss of recent memory and recall, impaired judgment, emotional lability, lack of initiative, impaired impulse control, inability to reason through problems, depression (worse in mild to moderate types), confabulation (not limited to alcohol organic brain syndrome), constriction of intellectual functions, visual and auditory hallucinations, and delusions. Physical findings will naturally vary according to the cause. The EEG usually shows generalized slowing in delirium.

A. Delirium: Delirium (acute confusional state) is a transient global disorder of attention, with clouding of consciousness, usually a result of systemic problems (eg, drugs, hypoxemia). Onset is usually rapid. The mental status fluctuates (impairment is usually least in the morning), with varying inability to concentrate, maintain attention, and sustain purposeful behavior. ("Sundowning"—mild to moderate delirium at night—is more common in patients with preexisting dementia and may be precipitated by hospitalization, drugs, and sensory deprivation.) There is a marked deficit of short-term memory and recall. Anxiety and irritability are common. Amnesia is retrograde (impaired recall of past memories) and anterograde (inability to recall events after the onset of the delirium). Orientation problems follow the inability to retain information. Perceptual disturbances (often visual hallucinations) and psychomotor restlessness with insomnia are common. Autonomic changes include tachycardia, dilated pupils, and sweating. The average duration is about 1 week, with full recovery in most cases. Delirium can coexist with dementia.

B. Dementia: (See also Chapter 4.) Dementia is characterized by chronicity and deterioration of selective mental functions. Onset is insidious over months to years in most cases. Dementia is usually progressive, more common in the elderly, and rarely reversible even if underlying disease can be corrected. Dementia can be classified as cortical or subcortical.

There are three types of cortical dementia: (1) primary degenerative dementia (eg, Alzheimer's), accounting for about 50–60% of cases; (2) atherosclerotic (multi-infarct) dementia, 15–20% of cases (this figure is probably low because of the tendency to overuse the diagnosis of Alzheimer's dementia); and (3) mixtures of the first two types or dementia due to miscellaneous causes, 15–20% of cases (see also Chapter 4). Examples of primary degenerative dementia are Alzheimer's dementia (most common) and Pick, Creutzfeldt-Jakob, and Huntington dementias (less common).

In all types, loss of impulse control (sexual and language) is common. The tenuous level of functioning makes the individual most susceptible to minor physical and psychologic stresses. The course depends on the underlying cause, and the general trend is steady deterioration.

HIV infection can produce a primary neurogenic disorder (partially due to neuronal loss) and secondary effects due to opportunistic infections, neoplasias, or the effects of drug therapy. At present there has been a reduction in dementia symptoms in both early and late stages, perhaps due to earlier use of zidovudine. The general trend is variable, and patients require ongoing monitoring of neuropsychiatric status.

Pseudodementia is a term applied to depressed patients who appear to be demented. These patients are often identifiable by their tendency to complain about memory problems vociferously rather than try to cover them up. They usually say they can't complete cognitive tasks but with encouragement can often do so.

C. Amnestic Syndrome: This is a memory disturbance without delirium or dementia. It is usually associated with thiamin deficiency and chronic alcohol use (eg, Korsakoff's syndrome). There is an impairment in the ability to learn new information or recall previously learned information.

D. Substance-Induced Hallucinosis: This condition is characterized by persistent or recurrent hallucinations (usually auditory) without the other symptoms usually found in delirium or dementia. Alcohol or hallucinogens are often the cause. There does not have to be any other mental disorder, and there may be complete spontaneous resolution.

E. Personality Changes Due to a General Medical Condition (Formerly Organic Personality Syndrome): This syndrome is characterized by emotional lability and loss of impulse control along with a general change in personality. Cognitive functions are preserved. Social inappropriateness is common. Loss of interest and lack of concern with the consequences of one's actions are often present. The course depends on the underlying cause (eg, frontal lobe contusion may resolve completely).

Differential Diagnosis

The differential diagnosis consists mainly of schizophrenia and the other psychoses, which are sometimes confused with organic brain syndrome, which itself is often accompanied by psychotic symptoms.

Complications

Chronicity may result from delayed correction of the defect, eg, subdural hematoma, low-pressure hydrocephalus. Accidents secondary to impulsive behavior and poor judgment are a major consideration. Secondary depression and impulsive behavior not infrequently lead to suicide attempts. Drugs—particularly sedatives—may worsen thinking abilities and contribute to the overall problems.

Treatment
(See also Chapter 4.)

A. Medical: Delirium should be considered a syndrome of acute brain dysfunction analogous to acute renal failure. The first aim of treatment is to identify and correct the etiologic medical problem. Evaluation should consist of a comprehensive physical examination including a search for neurologic abnormalities, infection, or hypoxia. Routine laboratory tests may include serum electrolytes, serum glucose, BUN, serum creatinine, liver function tests, thyroid function tests, arterial blood gases, complete blood count, serum calcium, phosphorus, magnesium, vitamin B_{12}, folate, blood cultures, urinalysis, and cerebrospinal fluid analysis. Discontinue drugs that may be contributing to the problem (eg, analgesics, corticosteroids, cimetidine, lidocaine, anticholinergic drugs, central nervous system depressants, mefloquine). Do not overlook any possibility of reversible organic disease. Electroencephalography, CT, MRI, PET, and SPECT evaluations may be helpful in diagnosis. Ideally, the patient should be monitored without further medications while the evaluation is carried out. There are, however, two indications for medication in delirious states: behavioral control (eg, pulling out lines) and subjective distress (eg, pronounced fear due to hallucinations). If these indications are present, medications may be employed. If there is any hint of alcohol or substance withdrawal (the most common cause of delirium in the general hospital), a benzodiazepine such as lorazepam (1–2 mg every hour) can be given parenterally. If there is little likelihood of withdrawal syndrome, haloperidol is often used in doses of 1–10 mg every hour. Given intravenously, it appears to impose slight risk of extrapyramidal side effects. In addition to the medication, a pleasant, comfortable, nonthreatening, and physically safe environment with adequate nursing or attendant services should be provided. Once the underlying condition has been identified and treated, adjunctive medications can be tapered.

Treatment of dementia syndrome usually involves symptomatic management with one exception. Since there is a cholinergic deficiency in Alzheimer's disease, recent research has focused on drugs to increase cholinergic activity (eg, tacrine, phosphatidylcholine). Tacrine (tetrahydroaminoacridine, THA) is a reversible cholinesterase inhibitor that has been released for treatment of cognitive deficits associated with Alzheimer's disease. Studies suggest that tacrine (80–160 mg/d in four divided doses) may improve cognition in 25–42% of patients, with higher doses producing better effects. There was, however, no functional improvement in the subjects. Serum ALT levels increase in 50% of patients, with most returning to normal when the drug is discontinued. Many patients who discontinue tacrine due to elevated liver enzymes may be retried on it successfully with careful monitoring.

Aggressiveness and rage states in central nervous system disease can be reduced with lipophilic beta-blockers (eg, propranolol, metoprolol) in moderate doses. Since the serotonergic system has been implicated in arousal conditions, drugs that affect serotonin have been found to be of some benefit in aggression and agitation. Included in this group are lithium, trazodone, buspirone, and clonazepam. Dopamine blockers (eg, the neuroleptic drugs such as haloperidol) have been used for many years to attenuate aggression. There are recent reports of reduced agitation in Alzheimer's disease from carbamazepine, 100–400 mg/d orally (with slow increase as needed). Emotional lability in some cases responds to small doses of imipramine (25 mg orally one to three times per day) or fluoxetine (5–20 mg/d orally); and depression, which often occurs early in the course of Alzheimer's dementia, responds to the usual doses of antidepressant drugs, preferably those with the least anticholinergic side effects (eg, SSRIs and MAO inhibitors).

Cerebral vasodilators were originally used on the assumption that cerebral arteriosclerosis and ischemia were the principal causes of the dementias. Although there is a slight reduction of blood flow in primary degenerative dementia (probably as a result of the basic disorder), there is no evidence that this is a major factor in this group of disorders or that vasodilators are of value. Ergotoxine alkaloids (ergoloid mesylates: Hydergine, others) have been studied with mixed results; improvement in ambulatory self-care and depressed mood has been noted, but there has been no improvement of cognitive functioning on any standardized tests. Hyperbaric oxygen treatment has not produced significant improvement. Stimulant drugs (eg, methylphenidate) do not change cognitive function but can improve affect and mood, which helps the caretakers cope with the problem.

Failing sensory functions should be supported as necessary, with hearing aids, cataract surgery, etc.

B. Social: Substitute home care, board and care, or convalescent home care may be most useful when the family is unable to care for the patient. The setting should include familiar people and objects, lights at night, and a simple schedule. Counseling may help the family to cope with problems and may help keep the patient at home as long as possible. Information about local groups can be obtained from the Alzheimer's Disease and Related Disorders Association, 70 East Lake Street, Suite 600, Chicago, IL 60601. Volunteer services, including homemakers, visiting nurses, and adult protective services, may be helpful in maintaining the patient at home.

C. Behavioral: Behavioral techniques include operant responses that can be used to induce positive behaviors, eg, paying attention to the patient who is trying to communicate appropriately, and extinction by ignoring inappropriate responses. Alzheimer's patients can learn skills and retain them but do not recall the circumstances in which they were learned.

D. Psychologic: Formal psychologic therapies are not usually helpful and may make things worse by taxing the patient's limited cognitive resources.

Prognosis

The prognosis is good for recovery of mental functioning in delirium when the underlying condition is reversible. For most dementia syndromes, the prognosis is for gradual deterioration, though new drug treatments may prove helpful.

Corey-Bloom J et al: Diagnosis and evaluation of dementia. Neurology 1995;45:211.

Jarrett PG et al: Behavioral problems in nursing home residents. Safe ways to manage dementia. Postgrad Med 1995;97:189. (Environmental changes and monitoring of pharmacologic agents can be highly effective.)

Skoog I et al: A population-based study of dementia in 85-year-olds. N Engl J Med 1993;328:153. (A surprising percentage of vascular dementias with treatment implications.)

Sumner AD, Simons RJ: Delirium in the hospitalized elderly. Cleve Clin J Med 1994;61:258.

Watkins PB et al: Hepatotoxic effects of tacrine administration in patients with Alzheimer's disease. JAMA 1994;271:992.

GERIATRIC PSYCHIATRIC DISORDERS
(See also Chapter 4.)

There are three basic factors in the process of aging: biologic, sociologic, and psychologic.

The complex **biologic** changes depend on inherited characteristics (the best chance of long life is to have long-lived parents), nutrition, declining sensory functions such as hearing or vision, disease, trauma, and lifestyle. A definite correlation between hearing loss and paranoid ideation exists in the elderly. (See Organic Brain Syndrome, above.) As a person ages, relatively minor disorders or combinations of disorders may cause deficits in cognition and affective response. Hypochondriasis is frequently a mechanism of compensating for decreased function (eg, preoccupation with bowel function).

The **sociologic** factors derive from stresses connected with occupation, family, and community. Any or all of these areas may be disrupted in a general phenomenon of "disengagement" and lack of intimacy that older people experience as friends die, the children move away, and the surroundings become less familiar. Retirement commonly precipitates a major disruption in a well-established life structure. This is particularly stressful in the person whose compulsive devotion to a job has inhibited the development of other interests, so that sudden loss of this outlet leaves a void that is not easily filled. New duties, such as caring for a spouse with dementia, may also lead to depression.

The **psychologic** withdrawal of the elderly person is frequently related to a loss of self-esteem, which is based on the economic insecurity of older age with its congruent loss of independence, the recognition of decreasing physical and mental ability, loneliness, and the fear of approaching death. The process of aging is often poorly accepted, and the real or imagined loss of physical attractiveness may have a traumatic impact that the plastic surgeon can only soften for a time. In a culture that stresses physical and sexual attractiveness, it is difficult for some people to accept the change.

Clinical Findings & Complications

The most common psychiatric syndrome in the elderly is dementia (organic brain syndrome) of varying degree. Psychotic ideation (usually paranoid) may coexist with dementia. Frequently, in milder cases, the individual is aware of the deficiency in cognition and becomes depressed about actual or threatened loss of function. Depression may then amplify the apparent cognitive decline.

Overt depression, often presenting as a somatic complaint, is often related to life changes (80% of people over age 65 have some kind of medical problem). Alcoholism is present in approximately 15% of older patients presenting with psychiatric symptoms. The incidence of suicide is higher in elderly people—loneliness, age, and medical problems being directly related. Deprivation of full-spectrum light may be a factor in some patients (eg, nursing home residents). Anxiety, often associated with organic illness, heightens preexisting confusion in the patient with organic brain syndrome.

Abuse of the elderly—both physical neglect (passive) and physical injury (active)—demands early recognition. Bruises, welts, fractures, and debilitation should alert the physician. The battered elderly are probably just as numerous as battered children, but less reported, and require the same diligence in physician recognition.

Polypharmacy (with both prescription and OTC drugs) is a major cause of accidents (often with resultant hip fracture) and illness in the elderly. Cognitive impairment increases as the number of drugs used increases; sedatives and anticholinergic drugs are the major culprits (eg, overuse in sleep problems). The increased and varied complaints are often an attempt to compensate and divert attention from decreased mental function.

Treatment

A. Social: Socialization, a structured schedule of activities, familiar surroundings, continued achievement, and avoidance of loneliness (probably the most important factor) are some of the major considerations in prevention and amelioration of the psychiatric problems of old age. The patient can be supported in the primary environment by various agencies that can help avoid a premature change of habits. For patients with disabilities that make it difficult to cope with the problems of living alone, homemaker services can assist in continuing the day-to-day activities of the household; visiting nurses can administer medications and monitor the physical condition of the patient; and geriatric social groups can help maintain socialization and human contacts. In the hospital or nursing home, attention to the kinds of people placed in the same room is most important (mix active and inactive patients).

B. Medical: Treatment of any reversible components of a dementia syndrome is obviously the major medical consideration. One commonly overlooked factor is self-medication, frequently with nonprescription drugs that further impair the patient's already precarious functioning. Common culprits are antihistamines and anticholinergic drugs, sometimes mixed with ethanol abuse.

Any signs of psychosis, such as paranoid ideation, agitation, and delusions, respond very well to *small doses* of antipsychotics. Trifluoperazine, 2–5 mg orally once a day, or fluphenazine, 1–2 mg orally daily, will usually decrease psychotic ideation markedly.

Do not use drugs that cause significant orthostatic hypotension (resulting in dizziness, falls, fractures).

Antidepressants (in one-third to one-half the doses given to young adults) are used when indicated for depression. Occasionally, a stimulant in small doses (eg, methylphenidate, 5–30 mg orally usually given in two doses at 7 AM and noon) can be used to treat apathy. The stimulant may help increase the patient's energy for social involvement and help the patient to maintain life activities.

The appropriate use of wine and beer for mild sedative effects is quite rewarding in the hospital and other care facilities as well as at home.

C. Behavioral: The impaired cognitive abilities of the geriatric patient necessitate simple behavioral techniques. Positive responses to appropriate behavior encourage the patient to repeat desirable kinds of behavior, and frequent repetition offsets to some degree the defects in recent memory and recall. It also results in participation—a most important element, since there is a tendency in the older population to withdraw, thus increasing isolation and functional decline.

One must be careful not to reinforce and encourage obstreperous behavior by responding to it; in this way, extinction or at least gradual reduction of inappropriate behavior will occur. At the same time, the obstreperous behavior often represents a nondirective response to frustration and inability to function, and a structured program of activity is necessary.

D. Psychologic: Patients may require help in adjusting to changing roles and commitments and in finding new goals and viewpoints. The older person steadily loses an important commodity—the future—and may attempt to compensate by preoccupation with the past. Involvement with the present and psychotherapy on a here-and-now basis can help make the adjustment easier.

Baumgarten M et al: Health of family members caring for elderly persons with dementia. Ann Intern Med 1994;120:126.

Preskorn SH: Recent pharmacologic advances in antidepressant therapy for the elderly. Am J Med 1993; 94(Suppl 5A):2S.

Shorr RI et al: Changes in antipsychotic drug use in nursing homes during implementation of the OBRA-87 regulations. JAMA 1994;271:358. (A substantial decrease in antipsychotic drug use coincided with the implementation of the 1987 United States government regulations.)

PSYCHIATRIC PROBLEMS ASSOCIATED WITH HOSPITALIZATION & MEDICAL & SURGICAL DISORDERS

Diagnostic Categories

A. Acute Problems:

1. Delirium with psychotic features secondary to the medical or surgical problem, or compounded by effect of treatment.

2. Acute anxiety, often related to ignorance and fear of the immediate problem as well as uncertainty about the future.

3. Anxiety as an intrinsic aspect of the medical problem (eg, hyperthyroidism).

4. Denial of illness, which may present during acute or intermediate phases of illness.

B. Intermediate Problems:

1. Depression as a function of the illness or acceptance of the illness, often associated with realistic or fantasied hopelessness about the future.

2. Behavioral problems, often related to denial of illness and, in extreme cases, causing the patient to leave the hospital against medical advice.

C. Recuperative Problems:

1. Decreasing cooperation as the patient sees improvement and compliance is not compelled.

2. Readjustment problems with family, job, and society.

General Considerations

A. Acute Problems:

1. **"Intensive care unit psychosis"** is a delirium. The stressful environment may contribute to the problem. Critical care unit factors include sleep deprivation, increased arousal, mechanical ventilation, and social isolation. Other causes include those common to delirium and require vigorous investigation (see Delirium, above).

2. Pre- and postsurgical anxiety states are common—and commonly ignored. Presurgical anxiety is very common and is principally a fear of death (many surgical patients make out their wills). Patients may be fearful of anesthesia (improved by the preoperative anesthesia interview), the mysterious operating room, and the disease processes that might be uncovered by the surgeon. Such fears frequently cause people to delay examinations that might result in earlier surgery and a greater chance of cure.

The opposite of this is **surgery proneness,** the quest for surgery to escape from overwhelming life stresses. Polysurgery patients are not easily categorized. Dynamic motivations include narcissism, societal pressures (eg, breast implants), unconscious guilt, a masochistic need to suffer, an attempt to deal with another family member's illness, and somatoform disorders and body dysmorphic disorder (an obsession that a body part is disfigured). More apparent reasons may include an attempt to get relief from pain and a lifestyle that has become almost exclusively medically oriented, with all of the risks entailed in such an endeavor.

Postsurgical anxiety states are usually related to pain, procedures, and loss of body image. Acute pain problems are quite different from chronic pain disorders (see Chronic Pain Disorders, above); the former are readily handled with adequate analgesic medication (see Chapter 1). Alterations in body image, as with amputations, ostomies, and mastectomies, often raise concerns about relationships with others.

3. Iatrogenic problems usually pertain to medications, complications of diagnostic and treatment procedures, and impersonal and unsympathetic staff behavior. Polypharmacy is often a factor. Patients with unsolved diagnostic problems are at higher risk. They are desirous of relief, and the quest engenders more diagnostic procedures with a higher incidence of complications. The upset patient and family may be very demanding. Excessive demands usually result from anxiety. Such behavior is best handled with calm and measured responses.

B. Intermediate Problems:

1. Prolonged hospitalization presents unique problems in certain hospital services, eg, burn units, orthopedic services, and tuberculosis wards. The acute problems of the severely burned patient are discussed in Chapter 38. The problems often are behavioral difficulties related to length of hospitalization and necessary procedures. For example, in burn units, pain is a major problem in addition to anxiety about procedures. Disputes with staff are common and often concern pain medication or ward privi-

leges. Some patients regress to infantile behavior and dependency. Staff members must agree about their approach to the patient in order to ensure the smooth functioning of the unit.

Denial of illness may present in the patient with acute myocardial infarction. Intervention by an authority figure (eg, immediate work supervisor) may help the patient accept treatment and eventually abandon the defense of denial.

2. Depression frequently occurs during this period. Therapeutic drugs (eg, corticosteroids) may be a factor. Depression can contribute to irritability and overt anger. Severe depression can lead to anorexia, which further complicates healing and metabolic balance. It is during this period that the issue of disfigurement arises—relief at survival gives way to concern about future function and appearance.

C. Recuperative Problems:

1. Anxiety about return to the posthospital environment can cause regression to a dependent position. Complications increase, and staff forbearance again is tested. Anxiety occurring at this stage usually is handled more easily than previous behavior problems.

2. Posthospital adjustment is related to the severity of the deficits and the use of outpatient facilities (eg, physical therapy, rehabilitation programs, psychiatric outpatient treatment). Some patients may experience posttraumatic stress symptoms (eg, from traumatic injuries or even from necessary medical treatments). Lack of appropriate follow-up can contribute to depression in the patient, who may feel that he or she is making poor progress and may have thoughts of "giving up." Reintegration into work, educational, and social endeavors may be slow. Life is simply much more difficult when one is disfigured, disabled, or disfranchised.

Clinical Findings

The symptoms that occur in these patients are similar to those discussed in previous sections of this chapter, eg, organic brain syndrome, stress and adjustment disorders, anxiety, and depression. Behavior problems may include lack of cooperation, increased complaints, demands for medication, sexual approaches to nurses, threats to leave the hospital, and actual signing out against medical recommendations. The underlying personality structure of the individual is a major factor in coping styles (eg, the compulsive individual increases indecision, the hysterical individual increases dramatic behavior).

Differential Diagnosis

Delirium and dementia (including cases associated with HIV infection and drug abuse) must always be ruled out, since they often present with symptoms resembling anxiety, depression, or psychosis. Personality disorders existing prior to hospitalization often underlie the various behavior problems, but particularly the management problems.

Complications

Prolongation of hospitalization causes increased expense, deterioration of patient-staff relationships, and increased probabilities of iatrogenic and legal problems. The possibility of increasing posthospital treatment problems is enhanced.

Treatment

A. Medical: The most important consideration by far is to have one physician in charge, a physician whom the patient trusts and who is able to oversee multiple treatment approaches (see Somatoform Disorders, above). In acute problems, attention must be paid to metabolic imbalance, alcohol withdrawal, and previous drug use—prescribed, recreational, or OTC. Adequate sleep and analgesia are important in the prevention of delirium.

Most physicians are attuned to the early detection of the surgery-prone patient. Plastic and orthopedic surgeons are at particular risk. Appropriate consultations may help detect some problems and mitigate future ones.

Postsurgical anxiety states can be alleviated by personal attention from the surgeon. Anxiety is not so effectively lessened by ancillary medical personnel, whom the patient perceives as lesser authorities, until after the physician has reassured the patient. Inappropriate use of "as needed" analgesia places an unfair burden on the nurse. "Patient-controlled analgesia" can improve pain control, decrease anxiety, and minimize side effects (see Chapter 1).

Depression should be recognized early. If severe, it may be treated by antidepressant medications (see Antidepressant Drugs, above). High levels of anxiety can be lowered with judicious use of anxiolytic agents. Unnecessary medications tend to reinforce the patient's impression that there must be a serious illness or medication would not be required.

B. Psychologic: Prepare the patient and family for what is to come. This includes the types of units where the patient will be quartered, the procedures that will be performed, and any disfigurements that will result from surgery. Repetition improves understanding. The nursing staff can be helpful, since patients frequently confide a lack of understanding to a nurse but are reluctant to do so to the physician.

Denial of illness is frequently a block to acceptance of treatment. This too should be handled with family members present (to help the patient face the reality of the situation) in a series of short interviews (for reinforcement). Dependency problems resulting from long hospitalization are best handled by focusing on the changes to come as the patient makes the transition to the outside world. Key figures are teachers, vocational counselors, and physical therapists.

Challenges should be realistic and practical and handled in small steps.

Depression is usually related to the loss of familiar hospital supports, and the outpatient therapists and counselors help to lessen the impact of the loss. Some of the impact can be alleviated by anticipating, with the patient and family, the signal features of the common depression to help prevent the patient from assuming a permanent sick role (invalidism).

Suicide is always a concern when a patient is faced with despair. An honest, compassionate, and supportive approach will help sustain the patient during this trying period.

C. Behavioral: Prior desensitization can significantly allay anxiety about medical procedures. A "dry run" can be done to reinforce the oral description. Cooperation during acute problem periods can be enhanced by the use of appropriate reinforcers such as a favorite nurse or helpful family member. People who are positive reinforcers are even more helpful during the intermediate phases when the patient becomes resistant to the seemingly endless procedures (eg, debridement of burned areas).

Specific situations (eg, psychologic dependency on the respirator) can be corrected by weaning with appropriate reinforcers (eg, watching a favorite movie on a videorecorder when disconnected from the ventilator). Behavioral approaches should be employed in a positive and optimistic way for maximal reinforcement.

Relaxation techniques and attentional distraction can be used to block side effects of a necessary treatment (eg, nausea in cancer chemotherapy).

D. Social: A change in environment requires adaptation. Because of the illness, admission and hospitalization may be more easily handled than discharge. Reintegration into society can be difficult. In some cases, the family is a negative influence. A predischarge evaluation must be made to determine whether the family will be able to cope with the physical or mental changes in the patient. Working with the family while the patient is in the acute stage may presage a successful transition later on.

Development of a new social life can be facilitated by various self-help organizations (eg, the stoma club). Sharing problems with others in similar circumstances eases the return to a social life which may be quite different from that prior to the illness.

Prognosis

The prognosis is good in all patients who have reversible medical and surgical conditions. It is guarded when there is serious functional loss that impairs vocational, educational, or societal possibilities—especially in the case of progressive and ultimately life-threatening illness.

Bone RC et al: Recognition, assessment, and treatment of anxiety in the critical care patient. Disease-A-Month

1995 May;41:293. (Anxiety is ubiquitous in critical care units and can interfere with recovery if left untreated.)

Frasure-Smith N et al: Depression following myocardial infarction: Impact on 6-month survival. JAMA 1993; 270:1819. (Major depression represents a mortality risk equal to that of left ventricular dysfunction.)

Travella JI et al: Depression following myocardial infarc-

tion: A one year longitudinal study. Int J Psychiatry Med 1994;24:357. (There may be two types of depression following myocardial infarction: an acute depression associated with greater functional impairment and a prolonged depression that may be associated with inadequate social support.)

Endocrinology

26

Paul A. Fitzgerald, MD

Hormones exert their effects by interacting with receptors on the cell surface (catecholamines and peptide hormones) or inside the cell (thyroid and steroid hormones). Endocrine disorders result from an excess or deficiency of hormonal effects.

COMMON PRESENTATIONS IN ENDOCRINOLOGY

Obesity

Obesity is a common problem, but rarely is there an identifiable endocrine cause. Instead, obesity can usually be attributed to other factors. Physical inactivity can cause some weight gain. Aging also plays a role in obesity, since adults gain an average of 0.1 kg/m^2 per year between ages 20 and 63 years. Genetics is the most important determinant for obesity. Studies of twins indicate that about 70% of obesity is due to genetic factors.

A gene regulating obesity (the *ob* gene) produces leptin, a protein secreted by fat cells in response to fat storage. With fatty weight gain, leptin acts upon the brain to decrease appetite and increase the body's metabolic rate. With weight loss, reduced leptin secretion causes an increased appetite and a reduced metabolic rate. In human obesity, fat cells secrete more leptin, causing serum levels of leptin to be an average of four times higher in obese individuals compared with their nonobese counterparts. This indicates that a major cause for obesity is a relative insensitivity of the brain to leptin.

Several endocrine disorders do cause obesity. Cushing's syndrome causes central obesity (due to intraperitoneal fat) with relatively thin extremities; such patients usually have plethoric, rounded (moon) facies along with prominent supraclavicular and dorsocervical fat pads (buffalo humps), thin skin, and striae that are wider and more purple than those usually seen with simple obesity. Alcoholism causes hypercortisolism and a similar syndrome. Hypothy-

roidism occasionally causes mild weight gain due to edema and fat accumulation. Hyperthyroidism may cause mild weight gain due to hyperphagia. Pancreatic insulinomas secrete excessive amounts of insulin, causing hypoglycemia and compensatory overeating. Growth hormone deficiency usually causes mild obesity in both children and adults.

Estrogen replacement therapy and oral estrogen-containing contraceptives may cause weight gain. Insulin therapy for type II diabetes usually worsens obesity.

Obesity may be associated with other disorders as part of several recognized syndromes. Syndrome X (the cluster of obesity, diabetes, and hypertension) has a 50% hereditary component. Polycystic ovary syndrome refers to the combination of obesity with anovulation, amenorrhea, cystic ovaries, and hirsutism. Hypothalamic lesions can cause massive obesity and are often associated with headache, lethargy, depression, diabetes insipidus, and hypopituitarism. Congenital obesity may be due to various uncommon syndromes of hypothalamic obesity and hypogonadotropic hypogonadism: Prader-Willi syndrome (hyperphagia, hypotonia, mental retardation); Biemond syndrome (polydactyly, diabetes mellitus, iritis); Laurence-Moon-Bardet-Biedel syndrome (polydactyly, renal anomalies, retinitis pigmentosa, mental retardation).

Caro JF et al: Leptin: The tale of an obesity gene. Diabetes 1996;45:1455.

Considine RV et al: Serum immunoreactive-leptin concentrations in normal-weight and obese humans. N Engl J Med 1996;334:292.

Fabitz RR et al: Genetic influences in adult weight gain and maximum body mass index in male twins. Am J Epidemiol 1994;140:711.

Leibel RL et al: Changes in energy expenditure resulting from altered body weight. N Engl J Med 1995;332:621. (Basal metabolic rates fall with weight loss, making dieting difficult.)

Unintended Weight Loss

Uncontrolled diabetes mellitus may be associated with weight loss, polyphagia, polydipsia, and polyuria. Anorexia and nausea may be seen with diabetic ketoacidosis and with adrenal insufficiency (due either to pituitary ACTH deficiency or to Addison's disease). Patients with severe diabetes insipidus may also lose weight. Patients with hyperthyroidism typically lose weight despite increased appetite; some patients with hypothyroidism lose weight because of diminished appetite. Some patients with Cushing's syndrome lose weight as a result of muscle wasting.

A great variety of nonendocrine conditions enter into the differential diagnosis of unintended weight loss (see Chapter 1). Anorexia is frequently a side effect of medications or radiation therapy and is also seen with azotemia, AIDS, and many gastrointestinal conditions. Malignancies typically produce diminished appetite and cachexia. Tuberculosis may cause weight loss even when occult. Chronic respiratory insufficiency is often associated with weight loss. Psychiatric illnesses producing diminished appetite include depressed or agitated affective disorder, catatonia, and anorexia nervosa.

Abnormal Skin Pigmentation or Color

Increased skin pigmentation is often present in conditions associated with ACTH excess such as Addison's disease. It may be very marked after bilateral adrenalectomy for Cushing's disease (Nelson's syndrome). Pregnancy and oral contraceptives may cause symmetric pigmentation of the upper lip, forehead, or malar eminences, known as **chloasma.** Nonendocrine conditions such as sprue, chronic iron deposition, chronic ingestion of chlorpromazine, arsenic poisoning, and severe malnutrition may also be associated with increased skin pigmentation.

Acanthosis nigricans presents as velvety brown thickened skin of the neck and body folds. It may be associated with syndromes of severe insulin resistance type A (young women with ovarian dysfunction and hirsutism) or type B (autoimmune). It may also be familial or associated with obesity, acromegaly, thyroid disease, or polycystic ovaries. Acanthosis presenting after age 40 is often a sign of an underlying malignancy.

Patients with neurofibromatosis may have freckles and café au lait pigmentation with smooth borders associated with a 5% incidence of pheochromocytoma.

Patients with McCune-Albright syndrome have café au lait skin pigmentation with irregular borders associated with multiple bone and endocrine abnormalities.

Hemochromatosis may cause a gray-brown ("bronze") hyperpigmentation associated with endocrine deficiencies such as diabetes mellitus.

Gynecomastia

Gynecomastia is a glandular enlargement of the male breast that may be tender and is often asymmetric or unilateral. It must be distinguished from tumors and from the fatty breast enlargement of obesity.

Pubertal gynecomastia is common and is characterized by tender discoid enlargement of breast tissue 2–3 cm in diameter beneath the areola; the swelling usually subsides spontaneously within a year. Gynecomastia is also common among elderly men, particularly when there is associated weight gain. Gynecomastia can be the first sign of a serious disorder such as a testicular tumor.

The causes of gynecomastia are multiple and diverse (Table 26–1).

The history and physical examination will often clarify the cause of gynecomastia. A careful drug history is important. An adolescent with slight gynecomastia or a man with prostatic carcinoma taking diethylstilbestrol needs no further study. Careful examination of the testes is mandatory to look for a testicular tumor. Small, firm testes are characteristic of Klinefelter's syndrome. Eunuchoid features, signs of liver disease, or the enlarged thyroid of Graves' disease are also helpful.

Laboratory investigation of unclear cases should include the following:

Table 26–1. Causes of gynecomastia.

Idiopathic	Drugs
	Alcohol
Physiologic causes	Alkylating agents
Neonatal period	Amiodarone
Puberty	Amphetamines
Aging	Androgens
Obesity	Busulfan
	Butyrophenones
Endocrine diseases	Chorionic gonadotropin
Androgen resistance	Cimetidine
syndromes	Clomiphene
Hyperprolactinemia	Cyclophosphamide
Hyperthyroidism	Diazepam
Klinefelter's syndrome	Diethylstilbestrol
Male hypogonadism	Digitalis preparations
	Domperidone
Systemic diseases	Estrogens
Chronic liver disease	Ethionamide
Chronic renal disease	Finasteride
Refeeding after starvation	Flutamide
	Hydroxyzine
Neoplasms	Isoniazid
Adrenal tumors	Ketoconazole
Bronchogenic carcinoma	Marijuana
Carcinoma of the breast	Meprobamate
Testicular tumors	Methadone
Hepatocellular carcinoma	Methyldopa
(rare)	Metoclopramide
	Narcotics
	Omeprazole
	Penicillamine
	Phenothiazines
	Progestins
	Reserpine
	Spironolactone
	Testosterone
	Tricyclic antidepressants

(1) A chest x-ray to search for metastatic or bronchogenic carcinoma.

(2) Measurements of plasma levels of the beta subunit of human chorionic gonadotropin (β-hCG). Detectable levels implicate a testicular tumor (germ cell or Sertoli cell) or other malignancy (usually lung or liver). Detectable low levels of serum β-hCG (< 5 mU/mL) may be reported in men with primary hypogonadism and high serum LH levels if the assay for β-hCG cross-reacts with LH.

(3) Measurements of plasma testosterone and luteinizing hormone (LH) are valuable in the diagnosis of primary or secondary hypogonadism. A low testosterone and high LH are seen in primary hypogonadism. High testosterone levels *plus* high LH levels characterize partial androgen resistance.

(4) Serum estradiol is usually normal. Elevated levels may be caused by testicular tumors, increased β-hCG, adrenal tumors (rare), liver disease, obesity, or true hermaphroditism (rare). Many estrogens and substances with estrogen activity are *not* detected by estradiol radioimmunoassay. Other laboratory tests such as serum prolactin, serum thyroxine and TSH, and chromosomal analysis (for Klinefelter's syndrome) can be helpful also.

(5) Needle biopsy with cytologic examination may be performed on suspicious areas of male breast enlargement (especially when unilateral or asymmetric) to distinguish gynecomastia from tumor.

The treatment of gynecomastia is that of the underlying condition. Idiopathic and pubertal gynecomastia usually resolve spontaneously within 1–2 years. Drug-induced gynecomastia resolves after the offending drug is removed. Painful gynecomastia may be treated with tamoxifen (an antiestrogen), 10 mg orally twice daily; discomfort improves, but breast size reduction occurs in only 50% and is usually minor. Surgical correction is reserved for persistent or severe gynecomastia, since results are often disappointing. Subcutaneous liposuction mastectomy by a surgeon experienced in the technique may produce acceptable results.

Braunstein GD: Gynecomastia. N Engl J Med 1993; 328:490.
Green L, Wysowski DK, Fourcroy JL: Gynecomastia and breast cancer during finasteride therapy. N Engl J Med 1996;335:823.
Thompson DF, Carter JR: Drug-induced gynecomastia. Pharmacotherapy 1993;13:37.

Galactorrhea

Lactation that occurs in the absence of nursing is termed galactorrhea. A small amount of breast milk can be expressed from the nipple in many parous women and is not cause for concern. Normal breast milk may be various colors besides white. Galactorrhea requires evaluation when it occurs in significant amounts or in nulliparous women or when it is associated with amenorrhea, headache, visual field abnormalities, or other symptoms implying systemic illness.

Evaluation begins with serum prolactin measurement; a persistently elevated level should prompt further investigation to determine its cause (Table 26–5). MRI of the pituitary and hypothalamus is done for nonpregnant patients with serum prolactin levels over 200 mg/dL, those with headaches or visual field defects, and women with persistently elevated prolactin levels with no discernible cause. Treatment is directed at correcting the cause of the elevated prolactin. Galactorrhea may occur in the absence of elevated serum prolactin levels (idiopathic). Whatever the cause, galactorrhea can be reduced with bromocriptine administration.

Impotence & Lack of Libido in Males

Erectile dysfunction is a frequent problem. Psychogenic factors as well as endocrine, vascular, or neurologic abnormalities may be important. Hypogonadism of whatever origin (Table 26–14) is associated with lack of libido and consequent erectile dysfunction. These can also be the first clinical manifestations of a hyperprolactinemic disorder (Table 26–5). Other endocrine causes include hyperthyroidism, Addison's disease, and acromegaly. Impotence in diabetes may be related to inadequate penile blood flow or autonomic neuropathy. Vascular disease is a frequent factor in impotence in elderly men. Vascular claudication of the legs along with related impotence is known as **Leriche's syndrome.**

Many pharmacologic agents are known to cause varying degrees of impotence (Table 26–2). Selective serotonin reuptake inhibitors (SSRIs, eg, fluoxetine) cause reduced libido. SSRIs and clomipramine cause delayed ejaculation.

For idiopathic or neurogenic impotence, intraurethral alprostadil has been fairly effective. Evaluation and treatment of erectile dysfunction are covered in Chapter 23.

Table 26–2. Drugs causing impotence.

Alcohol	Marijuana
Amphetamines	Methadone
Antihistamines	Methyldopa
Barbiturates	Metoclopramide
Beta-blockers	Monoamine oxidase
Butyrophenones	inhibitors
Carbamazepine	Narcotics
Cimetidine	Phenothiazines
Clonidine	Sedatives
Cocaine	Spironolactone
Guanethidine	Thiazides
Ketoconazole	Tricyclic antidepres-
Leuprolide	sants

Padma-Nathan H et al: Treatment of men with erectile dysfunction with transurethral alprostadil. Medicated Urethral System for Erection (MUSE) Study Group. N Engl J Med 1997;336:1.

Cryptorchism

One or both testes may be absent from the scrotum at birth in about 20% of premature males and in 3–6% at full term. Cryptorchism is found in 1–2% of males after 1 year of age but must be distinguished from retractile testes, which require no treatment. Administration of hCG may promote testicular descent. Cryptorchism should be corrected before age 18–24 months in an attempt to reduce the risk of infertility, which occurs in up to 75% of men with bilateral cryptorchism and in 50% with unilateral cryptorchism. It is not clear, however, whether early orchiopexy improves ultimate fertility. Many patients have underlying hypogonadism.

The ultimate incidence of testicular neoplasia is about 0.002% in normal males, 0.06% in cryptorchid males, and up to 5% in patients with intra-abdominal testes.

Orchiopexy decreases the risk of neoplasia when performed before 10 years of age. Orchiopexy does not enhance the detection rate or contribute to the treatment of neoplasia, so adults are usually not treated. Orchiectomy after puberty is an option for intra-abdominal testes.

Gutierrez CS: Cryptorchidism. West J Med 1995;163:67.
King LR: Undescended testis. JAMA 1996;276:856.
Rozanski TA, Blood DA: The undescended testis: Theory and management. Urol Clin North Am 1995;222:107.

Bone Pain & Pathologic Fractures

Onset of pathologic fractures at an early age is seen in osteogenesis imperfecta (blue scleras may be present). Painful bowing of the bones and pseudofractures suggest rickets or osteomalacia. Hyperparathyroidism or malignancy is suspected in patients with bone pain and hypercalcemia. Back pain or pathologic fractures in hypogonadal men and women implicate osteoporosis; such pain may be relieved with calcitonin. Sex hormone replacement and alendronate are given to help prevent further fractures. In cases of osteopenia of unknown cause, hyperthyroidism and Cushing's syndrome should also be considered. Bone pain may occur also as a result of primary or metastatic tumors, multiple myeloma, and Paget's disease; such pain may be relieved with bisphosphonates such as pamidronate or alendronate. Treatment is that of the underlying disorder.

Hortobagyi GN et al: Efficacy of pamidronate in reducing skeletal complications in patients with breast cancer and lytic bone metastases. Protocol 19 Aredia Breast Cancer Study Group. N Engl J Med 1996;335:1785. (There was significantly less increase in bone pain and deterioration of performance status in the pamidronate group than in the placebo group.)

Muscle Cramps & Tetany

Muscle cramps are usually caused by sports or occupational muscle injury. Nocturnal leg cramps are commonly idiopathic but are seen in diabetes mellitus, Parkinson's disease, central nervous system or spinal cord lesions, a variety of neuromuscular conditions, hemodialysis, and in those receiving cisplatin or vincristine chemotherapy. Various other drugs can cause myalgias that patients describe as cramps (eg, cimetidine, cholestyramine). Alkalosis due to any cause (eg, severe vomiting or hyperventilation) may decrease ionized calcium and cause muscle cramping and paresthesias. Leg cramps during walking may be due to vascular insufficiency, hyperthyroidism, or hypothyroidism.

Diffuse, recurrent, or severe muscle cramping requires evaluation for hypocalcemia (Table 21–7). Treatment of hypocalcemia is discussed in Chapter 21. Magnesium deficiency must be considered in tetany unresponsive to calcium. Nocturnal recumbency leg cramps may be prevented by oral quinine sulfate, 200–500 mg in the evening. After 1–2 weeks of nights without leg cramps, the quinine may be discontinued to determine if continued therapy is necessary. Quinine is usually well tolerated but may occasionally cause hypersensitivity reactions, thrombocytopenia, or adverse central nervous system and gastrointestinal reactions. Quinine tends to increase plasma digoxin levels and may enhance the effect of warfarin.

Recurrent cervicofacial and laryngeal dystonias, as well as hand cramps, have been successfully treated with injections of botulinum toxin.

Leclerc K, Landry FJ: Benign nocturnal leg cramps. Current controversies over use of quinine. Postgrad Med 1996;99:177.
Mandal AK et al: Is quinine effective and safe in leg cramps? J Clin Pharmacol 1995;35:588.
Man-Song-Hing M, Wells G: Meta-analysis of efficacy of quinine for treatment of nocturnal leg cramps in elderly people. BMJ 1995;10:13.

Mental Changes

Disturbances of mentation may be important indications of underlying endocrine disorders. Nervousness and excitability are characteristic of the menopause and hyperthyroidism. Adult cretinism is the result of prolonged hypothyroidism in infancy. In adults, hypothyroidism is accompanied by mental slowness, depression, and lethargy. Occasionally it may be manifested by delusional psychosis ("myxedema madness"). Pheochromocytoma may cause anxiety, confusion, or psychosis. Prolonged hypocalcemia from untreated hypoparathyroidism may be associated with intellectual deterioration. Hypoglycemia of any origin may cause confusion, abnormal speech, and behavioral or personality changes as well as sudden loss of consciousness, somnolence and prolonged lethargy, or coma. Frank psychosis can occur but is rare. Mild hypercalcemia causes fatigue and emotional irritability. Severe hypercalcemia can cause confusion, psychosis, and coma. Confusion may occur in hypopituitarism or Addison's disease. Confusion, lethargy, and nausea may be the presenting symptoms of hyponatremia. Insomnia, mood changes, anxiety, and psychosis can be associated with Cushing's syndrome. Rapid changes in glucocorticoid status (either a sudden increase or a sudden decrease) may be associated with acute psychosis. Porphyria may cause affective and thought disorders, particularly during acute attacks.

Mental changes may result from vitamin deficiencies caused by malnutrition, malabsorption, and other conditions. Deficiency in vitamin B_1 (thiamin) is usually seen in alcoholism and can cause Korsakoff's syndrome with typical memory loss and confabulation. Deficiency in vitamin B_2 (riboflavin) may cause personality deterioration and occurs commonly with psychotropic and antimalarial drugs and with diabetes and other diseases. Vitamin B_3 (niacin) deficiency is seen with poor nutrition, alcoholism, mercaptopurine toxicity, and malignant carcinoid syndrome and can cause irritability, dementia, dermatitis, and diarrhea. Vitamin B_6 (pyridoxine) deficiency is frequently seen in alcoholics or during treatment with isoniazid or levodopa and can cause irritability, depression, and neuropathy. Deficiency of vitamin B_{12} (cobalamin) is caused by deficiency in gastric intrinsic factor and may be seen at any age; however, it is more common in the elderly, affecting about 10% of people over age 70 years. Vitamin B_{12} deficiency may cause depression, irritability, paranoia, confusion, and dementia. It is usually associated with other neurologic symptoms such as paresthesias and leg weakness. Mental changes may occur in the absence of megaloblastic anemia.

DISEASES OF THE HYPOTHALAMUS & PITUITARY GLAND

Anterior pituitary gland function is controlled by regulating hormones produced by the hypothalamus and by direct feedback inhibition. The **posterior pituitary** receives antidiuretic hormone and oxytocin from the hypothalamus, secreting them under central nervous system control (Table 26–3). Hypothalamic hormones generally stimulate the anterior pituitary except for dopamine, which inhibits the pituitary from spontaneously secreting prolactin.

Table 26–3. Pituitary hormones.

Anterior pituitary
 Growth hormone (GH)[1]
 Prolactin (PRL)
 Adrenocorticotropic hormone (ACTH)
 Thyroid-stimulating hormone (TSH)
 Luteinizing hormone (LH)[2]
 Follicle-stimulating hormone (FSH)
Posterior pituitary
 Arginine vasopressin (AVP)[3]
 Oxytocin

[1]GH closely resembles human placental lactogen (hPL).
[2]LH closely resembles human chorionic gonadotropin (hCG).
[3]AVP is identical with antidiuretic hormone (ADH).

HYPOPITUITARISM

Essentials of Diagnosis

- Sexual dysfunction; weakness; easy fatigability; lack of resistance to stress, cold, and fasting; axillary and pubic hair loss.
- Low blood pressure; may have visual field defects.
- Low free thyroxine; deficient cortisol response to cosyntropin.
- Low serum testosterone (men); amenorrhea; serum prolactin may be elevated; FSH and LH are low or low normal.
- MRI may reveal a pituitary or hypothalamic lesion.

General Considerations

Patients with hypopituitarism may have single or multiple hormonal deficiencies. When one hormonal deficiency is discovered, others must be sought.

Causes include mass lesions such as pituitary adenomas, brain tumors or aneurysms, apoplexy, metastatic carcinoma, granulomas, multifocal Langerhans cell granulomatosis, and pituitary abscess. Autoimmune hypophysitis and postpartum pituitary necrosis (Sheehan's syndrome) are rare causes. Causes of hypopituitarism without mass lesions include trauma, radiation or surgery, encephalitis, hemochromatosis, and stroke. Pituitary hormone deficiencies may be congenital and caused by a *Pit-1* gene mutation.

A pituitary tumor may be part of the syndrome of multiple endocrine neoplasia (type I), with concomitant tumors of the parathyroid glands and pancreatic islets.

Clinical Findings

Manifestations of hypopituitarism vary depending upon which specific hormones are lacking and whether their deficiency is partial or complete.

A. Symptoms and Signs: Gonadotropin deficiency includes loss of luteinizing hormone (LH) and follicle-stimulating hormone (FSH), which causes hypogonadism and infertility. Patients with isolated gonadotropin deficiency may present as delayed adolescence. (See also discussion of primary amenorrhea.) Congenital gonadotropin deficiency may be associated with a decreased sense of smell (from hypoplasia of the olfactory bulbs) in Kallman's syndrome. In acquired gonadotropin deficiency, both men and women lose axillary, pubic, and body hair gradually, particularly if they are also hypoadrenal. Men may note diminished beard growth. Libido is diminished. Women have amenorrhea; men note decreased erections. Infertility is the rule. (See section on secondary amenorrhea.)

Thyroid-stimulating hormone (TSH) deficiency causes hypothyroidism with manifestations such as fatigue, weakness, weight change, and hyperlipidemia. (See Hypothyroidism and Myxedema, below.)

Adrenocorticotropic hormone (ACTH) deficiency results in diminished cortisol secretion (see below). Symptoms include weakness, fatigue, weight loss, and hypotension. Adrenal mineralocorticoid secretion continues, so manifestations of adrenal insufficiency in hypopituitarism are usually less striking than in bilateral adrenal gland destruction (Addison's disease).

Growth hormone (GH) deficiency in adulthood tends to cause mild to moderate obesity, asthenia, and reduced cardiac output.

Panhypopituitarism is the absence of all anterior pituitary hormones. Besides the manifestations noted above, patients with long-standing hypopituitarism tend to have dry, pale, finely textured skin. The face has fine wrinkles and an apathetic countenance.

B. Laboratory Findings: The fasting blood glucose may be low. Hyponatremia is often present. Hyperkalemia usually does not occur, since aldosterone production is not affected.

The T_4 level is low, and TSH is not elevated. Plasma levels of sex steroids (testosterone and estradiol) are low or low normal, as are the serum gonadotropins as well. Elevated prolactin levels are found in patients with prolactinomas, acromegaly, or hypothalamic disease.

In secondary hypoadrenalism, administration of cosyntropin (synthetic ACTH 1–24), 0.25 mg (intramuscularly or intravenously) usually causes serum cortisol to rise to less than 20 µg/dL by 30–60 minutes after the injection. A low-dose cosyntropin test (0.001 mg intravenously) is slightly more sensitive in detecting subtle ACTH-cortisol insufficiency. A baseline ACTH level is low or normal in secondary hypoadrenalism, distinguishing it from primary adrenal disease.

Patients with a normal cosyntropin test but with clinically suspected pituitary-adrenal insufficiency may have a metyrapone stimulation test: Metyrapone 1.5 g is administered at 11 PM; serum is collected at 8 AM for 11-deoxycortisol and cortisol determinations.

Patients with hypoadrenalism usually have an 11-deoxycortisol concentration under 7 µg/dL in the presence of a cortisol suppressed to less than 5 µg/dL. The metyrapone test must be performed in the absence of replacement glucocorticoid. Side effects include frequent nausea and occasional vomiting.

C. Imaging: MRI provides the best visualization of parasellar lesions. The posterior pituitary usually has a high-intensity signal on sagittal MRI that is lacking in central diabetes insipidus.

Differential Diagnosis

Anorexia nervosa may occasionally simulate hypopituitarism. In fact, severe malnutrition may give rise to functional hypopituitarism. Cachexia is rare in hypopituitarism. In anorexia nervosa, loss of axillary and pubic hair is unusual; plasma cortisol is normal or high and may respond rapidly to cosyntropin stimulation; the gonadotropins are usually present at low levels. Thyroid function tests are not abnormal in anorexia nervosa except for low T_3. Pituitary growth hormone assays show high levels in anorexia nervosa and very low levels in hypopituitarism.

Primary adrenal or thyroid insufficiency is easily differentiated from pituitary insufficiency, since serum ACTH or TSH is invariably elevated in the former conditions.

Severe illness causes functional suppression of TSH and thyroxine as well as gonadotropins and sex steroids. Glucocorticoids or megestrol treatment suppresses ACTH-cortisol secretion. Hyperthyroxinemia suppresses TSH.

Complications

In addition to those of the primary lesion (eg, tumor), complications may develop at any time as a result of the patient's inability to cope with stressful illness. This may lead to high fever, shock, coma, and death. Sensitivity to thyroid may rarely precipitate adrenal crisis if thyroid hormone is administered without glucocorticoid treatment. Rarely, acute hemorrhage may occur in large pituitary tumors, manifested by rapid loss of vision, headache, and evidence of acute pituitary failure (pituitary apoplexy) requiring emergency decompression of the sella.

Treatment

Medical therapy for prolactinomas is bromocriptine, which is often the only treatment required (see section on hyperprolactinemia). Unresponsive prolactinomas and other lesions may be resected or biopsied via a transsphenoidal approach, which in expert hands is an effective and safe surgical procedure. Craniotomy is rarely necessary. Endocrine substitution therapy must be used before, during, and often permanently after such procedures.

GH-secreting tumors may respond to octreotide (see section on acromegaly). Radiation therapy with x-ray, gamma knife, or heavy particles may be necessary but increases the likelihood of hypopituitarism.

The mainstay of substitution therapy for pituitary insufficiency remains the lifetime replacement of the end-organ deficiencies (adrenal, thyroid, and gonad).

A. Corticosteroids: Give hydrocortisone tablets, 15–25 mg/d orally in divided doses. Most patients do well with 15 mg in the morning and 5–10 mg in the late afternoon. Some patients feel better taking prednisone, 5–7.5 mg/d, or dexamethasone, 0.25 mg/d. A mineralocorticoid is rarely needed. Additional hydrocortisone must be given during states of stress, eg, during infection, trauma, or surgical procedures. For mild illness, corticosteroid doses are doubled or tripled. For severe trauma or surgical stress, hydrocortisone is given in doses of 50 mg intramuscularly or intravenously every 6 hours and then reduced to normal doses as the stress subsides.

Patients with secondary adrenal insufficiency due to treatment with glucocorticoids at supraphysiologic doses require their usually daily dose of glucocorticoid during surgery and acute illness; supplemental hydrocortisone is not usually required.

B. Thyroid: Levothyroxine is given to correct hypothyroidism only after the patient is assessed for cortisol deficiency or is already receiving glucocorticoids. The usual maintenance dose is 0.125 mg daily (range, 0.05–0.3 mg daily).

C. Sex Hormones:

1. Androgen replacement is discussed in the section on male hypogonadism.

2. Estrogen replacement is discussed in the section on female hypogonadism.

3. To improve spermatogenesis, chorionic gonadotropin is given at a dosage of 2000–3000 units intramuscularly three times weekly and testosterone replacement is discontinued. The dose of hCG is adjusted to normalize serum testosterone levels. After 1 year of hCG treatment, human menopausal gonadotropins (hMG) may be given as menotropins (mixture of FSH and LH) or as hCG along with urofollitropins (FSH alone). Leuprolide (GnRH analog) by intermittent subcutaneous infusion may be substituted for the hMG in patients with a normal pituitary gland.

4. For fertility induction in females, ovulation may be induced with clomiphene, 50 mg daily for 5 days every 2 months. Urofollitropins and chorionic gonadotropin can induce multiple births and should be used only by those experienced with their administration. (See Chapter 17.)

D. Human Growth Hormone: hGH is synthesized by recombinant DNA techniques. Adults with hypopituitarism and severe growth hormone deficiency treated with GH—at doses of 0.04 units/kg (0.015 mg/kg) injected subcutaneously 3 days weekly—have experienced an improvement in muscle mass, work capacity, sense of well-being, and bone density.

GH levels normally decline with aging. Healthy elderly men treated with GH (at double the above dose) for 6 months were found to have an increase in muscle mass and bone density and a 13% drop in fat mass, but functional abilities were unchanged. Available data do not support the use of hGH to reverse normal aging effects.

Side effects of GH treatment are frequent and dosage-dependent and include hand stiffness, diffuse arthralgias, and pitting edema of the legs.

E. Other Drugs: Bromocriptine may reverse the hypogonadism seen in hyperprolactinomas. (See Disorders of Prolactin Secretion.)

Prognosis

The prognosis depends on the primary cause. Hypopituitarism resulting from a pituitary tumor may be reversible with careful selective resection of the tumor. Functional hypopituitarism due to starvation, suppression by hypercortisolism, or hyperthyroidism is also correctable.

Hypopituitarism is usually permanent. However, with appropriate therapy, a patient with hypopituitarism can expect a normal life span.

Bates AS et al: The effect of hypopituitarism on life expectancy. J Clin Endocrinol Metab 1996;81:1169.

Glowniak JV, Loriaux DL: A double-blind study of perioperative steroid requirements in secondary adrenal insufficiency. Surgery 1997;121:123.

Johansson G et al: Two years of growth hormone (GH) treatment increases bone mineral content and density in hypopituitary patients with adult-onset GH deficiency. J Clin Endocrinol Metab 1996;81:2865.

Meling TR, Nylen ES: Growth hormone deficiency in adults: A review. Am J Med Sci 1996;311:153.

Papadakis MA et al: Growth hormone replacement in healthy older men improves body composition but not functional ability. Ann Intern Med 1996;124:708.

Rasmussen S et al: A low dose ACTH test to assess the function of the hypothalamic-pituitary-adrenal axis. Clin Endocrinol 1996;44:151.

DIABETES INSIPIDUS

Essentials of Diagnosis

- Polyuria (2–20 L/d); polydipsia.
- Urine specific gravity usually < 1.006 during ad libitum fluid intake.
- Vasopressin reduces urine output (except in nephrogenic diabetes insipidus).

General Considerations

Diabetes insipidus is an uncommon disease characterized by an increase in thirst and the passage of large quantities of urine of low specific gravity. The urine is otherwise normal. It is caused by a deficiency of or resistance to vasopressin.

The causes may be classified as follows:

A. Deficiency of Vasopressin:

1. Primary diabetes insipidus (without an identifiable organic lesion noted on MRI of the pituitary and hypothalamus) may be familial, occurring as a dominant trait, or sporadic ("idiopathic"). It also occurs in Wolfram's syndrome, a rare autosomal recessive condition with diabetes insipidus, diabetes mellitus, optic atrophy, and deafness (DIDMOAD).

2. Secondary diabetes insipidus is due to damage to the hypothalamus or pituitary stalk by anoxic encephalopathy, surgical or accidental trauma, infection (eg, encephalitis, tuberculosis, syphilis), sarcoidosis, or multifocal Langerhans cell (eosinophilic) granulomatosis ("histiocytosis X"). Metastases to the pituitary are more likely to cause diabetes insipidus (33%) than are pituitary adenomas (1%).

3. Vasopressinase-induced diabetes insipidus may be seen in the last trimester of pregnancy and in the puerperium; it is often associated with preeclampsia or hepatic dysfunction. A circulating enzyme destroys native vasopressin; however, synthetic desmopressin is unaffected. The condition usually responds to desmopressin therapy (see below) and subsides spontaneously.

B. "Nephrogenic" Diabetes Insipidus: This disorder is due to a defect in the kidney tubules that interferes with water reabsorption. The polyuria is unresponsive to vasopressin. These patients have normal secretion of vasopressin. It occurs as a familial X-linked trait; adults often have hyperuricemia as well. Acquired forms of vasopressin-resistant diabetes insipidus are seen in pyelonephritis, renal amyloidosis, myeloma, potassium depletion, Sjögren's syndrome, sickle cell anemia, or chronic hypercalcemia. The disorder may occur also as a glucocorticoid effect or as an acute side effect of diuretics. Certain drugs (eg, demeclocycline, lithium, foscarnet, or methicillin) may induce nephrogenic diabetes insipidus. The recovery from acute tubular necrosis may also be associated with transient nephrogenic diabetes insipidus.

Clinical Findings

A. Symptoms and Signs: The symptoms of the disease are intense thirst, especially with a craving for ice water, and polyuria, the volume of ingested fluid varying from 2 L to 20 L daily, with correspondingly large urine volumes. Partial diabetes insipidus presents with less intense symptoms and should be suspected in patients with unremitting enuresis. Diabetes insipidus may present with hypernatremia and dehydration, especially after hypothalamic damage due to shock or anoxia.

B. Laboratory Findings: Evaluation for diabetes insipidus should include a 24-hour urine collection for volume, glucose, and creatinine and serum for glucose, urea nitrogen, calcium, potassium, and sodium.

The diagnosis of diabetes insipidus as a cause of polyuria or hypernatremia requires mostly clinical judgment. There is no single diagnostic laboratory test. If the clinical situation implicates central diabetes insipidus (and no other causes for polyuria are present; see Differential Diagnosis, below), a supervised "vasopressin challenge test" may be given: Desmopressin acetate is given in an initial dose of 0.05–0.1 mL intranasally (or 1 μg subcutaneously or intravenously), with measurement of prior and subsequent urine volumes. Serum sodium must be obtained immediately in the event of symptoms of hyponatremia. The dosage of desmopressin is doubled if the response is marginal. Patients with true central diabetes insipidus will notice a distinct reduction in their thirst and polyuria; serum sodium usually stays normal except in some salt-losing conditions (Table 26–4).

When nephrogenic diabetes insipidus is a diagnostic consideration, measurement of serum vasopressin

Table 26–4. Differential diagnosis of hyponatremia.[1,2]

Artifactual: hyperglycemia, hypertriglyceridemia
Syndrome of inappropriate ADH release or action (SIADH)
  Central nervous system lesions; reset osmostat
  Pulmonary lesions
  Other: acute intermittent porphyria, positive-pressure breathing
  Ectopic ADH production: especially small-cell carcinoma of the lung
  Drug-induced SIADH (see Table 21–3).
Hyponatremia with hypervolemia
  Decreased water excretion
    Congestive heart failure
    Cirrhosis
    Renal failure
  Excessive water intake
    Restriction of dietary salt without water restriction
    Compulsive water drinking
    Intravenous water
Hyponatremia due to sodium depletion
  Renal losses
    Diuretics
    Addison's disease; salt-wasting 21-hydroxylase deficiency; selective hypoaldosteronism
    Renal diseases: tubulointerstitial disease, renal tubular acidosis
    Central nervous system-induced natriuresis (associated with central nervous system injury, especially subarachnoid hemorrhage; also pituitary surgery)
    Nonsteroidal anti-inflammatory agents
  Gastrointestinal losses
    Vomiting
    Diarrhea
    Fistulas
  Third space losses
    Burns
    Pancreatitis
    Crush injuries
    Major surgery
Hypothyroidism
Severe illness

[1]Modified, with permission, from Fitzgerald PA: *Handbook of Clinical Endocrinology*, 2nd ed. Appleton & Lange, 1992.
[2]Two or more conditions may coexist.

is done during modest fluid restriction; typically, the vasopressin level is high.

In nonfamilial central diabetes insipidus, MRI of the pituitary and hypothalamus and of the skull is done to look for mass lesions. Absence of a posterior pituitary "bright spot" on T1-weighted MRI is suggestive of central diabetes insipidus.

Differential Diagnosis of Polyuria

Central diabetes insipidus must be distinguished from polyuria caused by Cushing's syndrome or glucocorticoid treatment, lithium, and the nocturnal polyuria of Parkinson's disease. It must also be distinguished from the excessive fluid intake seen in psychogenic polydipsia, central nervous system sarcoidosis, and intravenous fluid administration.

Central diabetes insipidus is distinguished from diabetes mellitus by checking the urine for glucose. It must also be distinguished from nephrogenic diabetes insipidus (see above).

Complications

If water is not readily available, the excessive output of urine will lead to severe dehydration. Patients with an impaired thirst mechanism are very prone to hypernatremia. All the complications of the primary disease may eventually become evident. In patients who are receiving antidiuretic therapy, there is a danger of induced water intoxication.

Treatment

A. Desmopressin: Desmopressin acetate is the treatment of choice for central diabetes insipidus. It is also useful in diabetes insipidus associated with pregnancy or the puerperium, since desmopressin is resistant to degradation by the circulating vasopressinase. It is usually given intranasally (100 μg/mL solution) every 12–24 hours as needed for thirst and polyuria. It may be administered via metered-dose inhaler containing 0.1 mL/spray or via a plastic calibrated tube rhinyle. Patients are started with 0.05–0.1 mL every 12–24 hours, and the dose is then individualized according to response.

Desmopressin is also available as a parenteral preparation containing 4 μg/mL. For central diabetes insipidus, it is given intravenously, intramuscularly, or subcutaneously in doses of 1–4 μg every 12–24 hours as needed to treat thirst or hypernatremia.

Desmopressin is also available as an oral preparation (0.1 or 0.2 mg tablets) which are given in a starting dose of 0.1 mg daily and increased to a maximum of 0.2 mg every 8 hours, if required. Mild increases in hepatic enzymes are common, so the drug is not given to patients with liver disease. Gastrointestinal symptoms and asthenia may occur.

Adverse reactions to desmopressin have included nasal irritation, occasional agitation, and erythromelalgia. Hyponatremia is uncommon if minimum effective doses are used and the patient allows thirst to occur periodically.

Aqueous vasopressin is an alternative for patients unable to take desmopressin. It is short-acting and causes vasoconstriction with reports of cardiac arrest. It must never be given intravenously.

B. Other Measures: Mild cases require no treatment other than adequate fluid intake. Reduction of aggravating factors (eg, glucocorticoids, which increase renal free water clearance) will improve polyuria. Both central and nephrogenic diabetes insipidus respond partially to hydrochlorothiazide, 50–100 mg/d (with potassium supplement or amiloride). Chlorpropamide is sometimes effective for central diabetes insipidus and can improve thirst sensation in patients with recurrent hypernatremia; however, chlorpropamide is usually reserved for special cases due to the danger of hypoglycemia. Nephrogenic diabetes insipidus may respond to combined treatments of indomethacin-hydrochlorothiazide, indomethacin-desmopressin, or indomethacin-amiloride. Indomethacin, 50 mg every 8 hours, is effective acutely.

Psychotherapy is required for most patients with compulsive water drinking. Thioridazine and lithium are best avoided if drug therapy is needed, since they cause polyuria.

Prognosis

Central diabetes insipidus appearing after pituitary surgery usually remits after days to weeks but may be permanent if the superior pituitary stalk is cut.

Central diabetes insipidus is made transiently worse by glucocorticoids in the high doses frequently given perioperatively.

Chronic diabetes insipidus is more an inconvenience than a dire medical condition. Treatment with desmopressin allows normal sleep and activity. Hypernatremia can occur, especially when the thirst center is damaged, but diabetes insipidus itself does not reduce life expectancy, and the prognosis is that of the underlying disorder.

Bianco CM: Diabetes insipidus. Am J Nurs 1996;96:30.

Holtzman EJ, Ausiello DA: Nephrogenic diabetes insipidus: Causes revealed. Hosp Pract (Off Ed) 1994 Mar;29:89.

Laredo S et al: Coexistence of central diabetes insipidus and salt wasting: The difficulties in diagnosis, changes in natremia, and treatment. J Am Soc Nephrol 1996;7:2527.

ACROMEGALY & GIGANTISM

Essentials of Diagnosis

- Excessive growth of hands (increased glove and ring size), feet (increased shoe width), jaw (protrusion of lower jaw), and internal organs; or gigantism before closure of epiphyses.
- Coarsening facial features; deeper voice.

- Amenorrhea, headaches, visual field loss, sweating, weakness.
- Soft, doughy, sweaty handshake.
- Serum GH not suppressed following oral glucose.
- Elevated insulin-like growth factor I (IGF-I).
- Imaging: Terminal phalangeal "tufting" on radiographs. CT or MRI demonstration of pituitary tumor in 90%.

General Considerations

Growth hormone exerts much of its growth-promoting effects through the release of IGF-I produced in the liver and other tissues.

An excessive amount of growth hormone is most often produced by a benign pituitary adenoma. Acromegaly is usually sporadic in distribution but may rarely be familial. The disease may be associated with adenomas elsewhere, such as in the parathyroids or pancreas (multiple endocrine neoplasia type I). Acromegaly may also be seen in McCune-Albright syndrome and as part of Carney's complex (atrial myxoma, acoustic neuroma, and spotty skin pigmentation). Acromegaly is rarely caused by ectopic GHRH or GH secreted by hypothalamic or bronchial carcinoid or pancreatic tumors. If the onset precedes closure of the epiphyses, gigantism will result. If the epiphyses have already closed at onset, only overgrowth of soft tissues and terminal skeletal structures (acromegaly) results. Rarely, the disease is transient and followed by partial pituitary insufficiency.

Clinical Findings

A. Symptoms and Signs: Concurrent secretion of prolactin and crowding of other hormone-producing cells causes hypogonadism. Production of excessive growth hormone causes doughy enlargement of the hands, with spade-like fingers; large feet, face, tongue, and internal organs; wide spacing of the teeth; and an oily, tough, "furrowed" skin and scalp. There is frequently enlargement of the jaw, with prognathism and malocclusion. Hoarseness is common. Obstructive sleep apnea may occur. Acanthosis nigricans may be present. Pituitary tumor enlargement may cause headache, bitemporal hemianopia, and diplopia. Other changes may include hypertension (50%), diabetes mellitus (30%), goiter, and galactorrhea. Less commonly, these may be the presenting picture in acromegaly. Excessive sweating may be the most reliable clinical sign of activity of the disease. Carpal tunnel syndrome and spinal stenosis may cause neurologic symptoms.

B. Laboratory Findings: After an overnight fast, a fasting serum specimen is obtained and assayed for prolactin (cosecreted by many GH-secreting tumors); IGF-I (increased to over five times normal in most acromegalics); glucose (diabetes is common in acromegaly); liver function tests and BUN; serum inorganic phosphorus (frequently elevated); serum free thyroxine; and TSH (secondary hypothyroidism is common in acromegaly; primary hypothyroidism may increase prolactin).

Glucose syrup (100 g) is then administered orally, and serum GH is measured 60 minutes afterward. A GH level higher than 2 ng/mL (males) or 5 ng/mL (females) is evidence of acromegaly. High serum GH levels can be caused by exercise or eating just prior to the test, acute illness or agitation, hepatic or renal failure, malnourishment, diabetes mellitus or concurrent treatment with estrogens, beta-blockers, or clonidine. Some patients with acromegaly have normal serum GH concentrations.

C. Imaging: MRI shows a pituitary tumor in 90% of acromegalics. MRI is generally superior to CT scanning, especially in the postoperative setting. X-rays of the skull may show an enlarged sella and thickened skull. X-rays may also show tufting of the terminal phalanges of the fingers and toes. A lateral view of the foot shows increased thickness of the heel pad.

Differential Diagnosis

Active acromegaly must be distinguished from familial coarse features, large hands and feet, and isolated prognathism. It must also be distinguished from inactive ("burned-out") acromegaly in which there has been a spontaneous remission due to infarction of the pituitary adenoma. Acromegaly is distinguished from these conditions by testing (see above) and by ongoing enlargement in ring or shoe size and by progressive coarsening of facial features, which can be seen in serial photographs.

Complications

Complications include hypopituitarism, hypertension, glucose intolerance or frank diabetes mellitus, cardiac enlargement, and cardiac failure. The carpal tunnel syndrome, due to compression of the median nerve at the wrist, may cause disability of the hand. Arthritis of hips, knees, and spine can be troublesome. Cord compression may be seen. Visual field defects may be severe and progressive. Acute loss of vision or cranial nerve palsy may occur if the tumor undergoes spontaneous hemorrhage and necrosis (pituitary apoplexy).

Treatment

Transsphenoidal pituitary microsurgery removes the adenoma while preserving anterior pituitary function in most patients. Growth hormone levels fall immediately, but IGF-I levels fall gradually over days to weeks. Diaphoresis and carpal tunnel syndrome often improve within a day after surgery. Pituitary irradiation is useful if operative therapy fails. Patients in remission tend to gain some weight. Periodic reassessment of pituitary function after these procedures is advisable. Large doses of bromocriptine (eg, 20 mg/d) may control GH secretion in a minority of patients, usually those with concomitant prolactin secretion.

Octreotide, a somatostatin analog, can be useful in

treating acromegaly. It may be used as first therapy in locales where transsphenoidal surgery is not available. Octreotide must be administered by injection at doses averaging 100 µg subcutaneously three times daily. A longer-acting preparation has been developed and appears effective. Most patients experience at least a partial response. Headache often improves, but tumor shrinkage is usually marginal. Octreotide may also be effective in ectopic acromegaly. Side effects are experienced by about one-third of patients and include injection site pain, loose acholic stools, abdominal discomfort, or cholelithiasis. Combined therapy with bromocriptine (also cabergoline or pergolide) and octreotide may have an additive effect.

Prognosis

Patients with untreated acromegaly tend to have premature cardiovascular disease and progressive acromegalic symptoms. Transsphenoidal pituitary surgery is successful in 90% of patients with tumors less than 2 cm in diameter and GH levels less than 50 ng/mL. Postoperatively, normal pituitary function is usually preserved. Conventional radiation therapy (alone) produces a remission in about 38% by 2 years and 73% by 5 years after treatment. Gamma knife radiation is also an option. Heavy particle pituitary radiation produces a remission in about 70% by 2 years and 80% by 5 years. Radiation therapy eventually produces some degree of hypopituitarism in most patients. Conventional radiation therapy may cause some degree of organic brain syndrome and predisposes to small strokes.

Caron P et al: Three year follow-up of acromegalic patients treated with intramuscular slow-release lanreotide. J Clin Endocrinol Metab 1997;82:18.

Flogstad AK et al: Sandostatin LAR in acromegalic patients: Long-term treatment. J Clin Endocrinol Metab 1997;82:23.

Frohman LA: Acromegaly: What constitutes optimal therapy? J Clin Endocrinol Metab 1996;81:443.

Maugans TA, Coates ML: Diagnosis and treatment of acromegaly. Am Fam Physician 1995;52:207.

Melmed S et al: Clinical review 75: Recent advances in pathogenesis, diagnosis, and management of acromegaly. J Clin Endocrinol Metab 1995;80:3395.

HYPERPROLACTINEMIA

Essentials of Diagnosis

- Women: Menstrual cycle disturbances (oligomenorrhea, amenorrhea); galactorrhea; infertility.
- Men: Hypogonadism; decreased libido and erectile dysfunction; infertility.
- Elevated serum prolactin.
- CT scan or MRI often demonstrates pituitary adenoma.

Normal Physiology

Prolactin's main role is to induce lactation. Serum prolactin levels increase during pregnancy from a normal (follicular phase) level of less than 20 ng/mL to as high as 600 ng/mL by the time of delivery. Under the combined effect of prolactin, increased estrogen, and progesterone, breast development takes place, with eventual formation of milk in the acini. Estrogens inhibit the actual secretion of milk. After parturition, the sudden withdrawal of estrogen caused by expulsion of the placenta results in the onset of lactation. During the puerperal period, suckling constitutes a powerful stimulus for the continued production of prolactin as well as oxytocin. Lactation will cease if prolactin secretion is interrupted by prolactin-lowering drugs or by pituitary destruction. Prolactin is an unusual hormone in terms of control of secretion in that it is under mainly inhibitory control. Thus, section of the pituitary stalk will result in marked increases in prolactin secretion. Prolactin inhibitory factor (PIF) is dopamine.

Elevated serum prolactin can be caused by numerous conditions (Table 26–5).

Table 26–5. Causes of hyperprolactinemia.

Physiologic Causes	Pharmacologic Causes	Pathologic Causes
Exercise	Amoxapine	Acromegaly
Idiopathic	Amphetamines	Chronic chest wall stimulation (post-thoracotomy, postmastectomy, herpes zoster, breast problems, etc)
Pregnancy	Anesthetic agents	
Puerperium	Butyrophenones	
Sleep (REM phase)	Cimetidine	Cirrhosis
Stress (trauma, surgery)	Estrogens	Hypothalamic disease
Suckling	Hydroxyzine	Hypothyroidism
	Methyldopa	Pituitary stalk section
	Metoclopramide	Prolactin-secreting tumors
	Narcotics	Pseudocyesis (false pregnancy)
	Nicotine	Renal failure (especially with zinc deficiency)
	Phenothiazines	Spinal cord lesions
	Progestins	
	Reserpine	
	Tricyclic antidepressants	
	Verapamil	

Clinical Consequences of Prolactin Excess

In women, prolactin excess produces disturbances of pituitary ovarian function with anovulatory cycles, oligomenorrhea, or (frequently) amenorrhea and (less commonly) galactorrhea. In men, excess prolactin is associated with erectile dysfunction and decreased libido (very common), hypogonadism (common), and gynecomastia (unusual).

Of all women with nongestational secondary amenorrhea, about 30% have hyperprolactinemia. Of women with nonpuerperal secondary amenorrhea and galactorrhea, about 70% have elevated serum prolactin levels. In men, increased prolactin concentrations are usually not associated with galactorrhea because the male breast tissue has not been primed by estrogens and progesterone.

Most women with hyperprolactinemia have amenorrhea, oligomenorrhea, or infertility. Hyperprolactinemic women tend to have decreased bone density and are therefore ultimately at increased risk to develop clinical osteoporosis if left untreated.

The most important cause of high serum prolactin is a pituitary tumor. As many as 65% of all pituitary tumors may be associated with hyperprolactinemia. The tumors may be small (microadenomas) or may produce clear-cut enlargement of the sella (macroadenomas). Hormone stimulation tests to distinguish a prolactin-secreting tumor from other causes of hyperprolactinemia are unreliable. The actual level of serum prolactin is useful, however. In the absence of renal failure or late pregnancy, levels greater than 250 ng/mL are almost diagnostic of prolactinoma. Macroadenomas tend to cause higher levels of serum prolactin than microadenomas and are more frequently associated with decreased secretion of gonadotropins (LH and FSH). MRI or CT scan of the pituitary often demonstrates small prolactinomas, but differentiation from normal variants is not always possible.

Other causes of nontumorous hyperprolactinemia (Table 26–5) must be considered; tests for hypothyroidism and unsuspected pregnancy are usually indicated.

Treatment

The treatment of hyperprolactinemia depends upon the cause. Medications known to increase prolactin are stopped, if possible. Hyperprolactinemia due to hypothyroidism is corrected by thyroxine. Patients with hyperprolactinemia not induced by drugs, hypothyroidism, or pregnancy should be examined by pituitary MRI. Patients with persistent hyperprolactinemia who have amenorrhea or other significant symptoms are usually treated with dopamine agonists (eg, bromocriptine, cabergoline, pergolide). These drugs bind to the pituitary dopamine receptor and thus inhibit prolactin secretion from the gland.

Bromocriptine and pergolide are about equally effective in improving symptoms and reducing serum prolactin levels when given at therapeutically comparable doses, ie, bromocriptine, 2.5–20 mg/d, or pergolide, 0.25–2 mg/d. Bromocriptine is substantially more expensive than pergolide.

Therapy should be started with a small dose (eg, bromocriptine, 1.25 mg/d) given at bedtime to minimize side effects of nausea, dizziness, and orthostatic hypotension. Fatigue commonly occurs, as do a variety of psychiatric side effects; these are not dose-related and may take many weeks to resolve once the dopamine agonist is discontinued. A patient who has been unable to tolerate one dopamine agonist may sometimes be able to tolerate another. *Note:* Most adverse symptoms may be reduced in women by *intravaginal administration* of the bromocriptine tablet. The dose is then gradually increased as necessary to bring prolactin levels down to normal.

With bromocriptine treatment, 90% of patients with prolactinomas experience a fall in serum prolactin to 10% or less of pretreatment levels; 67% of treated patients achieve a normal serum prolactin level. Shrinkage of a pituitary adenoma occurs early, but maximum effect may take up to 6 months. Nearly half shrink more than 50%. Discontinuing therapy even after many years usually results in reappearance of hyperprolactinemia and galactorrhea-amenorrhea. Since fertility is usually promptly restored with bromocriptine, many pregnancies have resulted—with no clear evidence that the drug is teratogenic. Patients with microadenomas may have bromocriptine safely withdrawn during pregnancy. Macroadenomas may enlarge significantly during pregnancy; if bromocriptine is withdrawn, patients should be followed most carefully clinically and with computer-assisted visual field perimetry.

Patients with prolactinomas resistant to bromocriptine may respond to cabergoline, a long-acting dopamine agonist; dosage begins at 0.25 mg orally once weekly for 1 week, then 0.25 mg twice weekly for the next week, then 0.5 mg twice weekly. Further dosage increases may be required monthly, based upon serum prolactin levels, up to a maximum of 1.5 mg twice weekly. Cabergoline may also be administered intravaginally if a woman has side effects from oral administration.

Transsphenoidal surgery may be urgently required for large tumors causing visual compromise or apoplexy. It is also used electively for patients who do not tolerate or respond to bromocriptine.

Colao A et al: Prolactinomas resistant to standard dopamine agonists respond to chronic cabergoline treatment. J Clin Endocrinol Metab 1997;82:876.

Kaye TB: Hyperprolactinemia: Causes, consequences, and treatment options. Postgrad Med 1996;99:265.

Moliten ME, Thorner MO, Wilson C: Management of prolactinomas. J Clin Endocrinol Metab 1997;82:996.

Motta T et al: Vaginal cabergoline in the treatment of hyperprolactinemic patients intolerant to oral dopaminergics. Fertil Steril 1996;65:440.

Stewart PM et al: Pituitary imaging is essential for women with moderate hyperprolactinaemia. BMJ 1993;306:507.

DISEASES OF THE THYROID GLAND

An adult's thyroid gland normally weighs about 15–20 g. Embryologic defects may result in a rare lingual thyroid, retrosternal thyroid, or agenesis of one or both lobes.

Thyroid-stimulating hormone (TSH, thyrotropin) is secreted by the pituitary and stimulates several steps of thyroid hormone production: trapping of iodine, peroxidase linking of iodine to tyrosine, coupling of monoiodotyrosine or diiodotyrosine to form T_3 (triiodothyronine) or T_4 (thyroxine), and release of T_3 and T_4. The thyroid secretes mostly T_4 and very little T_3. About 90% of circulating T_3, the most active thyroid hormone, is derived from peripheral deiodination of T_4. Circulating thyroid hormones have a direct feedback inhibition effect upon the pituitary thyrotroph cells, desensitizing them from the stimulatory effect of hypothalamic thyrotropin-releasing hormone (TRH).

Over 99% of circulating thyroid hormones are bound to serum proteins, mostly thyroid-binding globulin (TBG). Only free hormone enters cells, binding to nuclear hormone receptors, which regulate DNA control of oxidative processes throughout the body.

The thyroid tests discussed in the following section are ordinarily very helpful in the evaluation of thyroid disorders. However, many conditions and drugs alter serum thyroxine levels without affecting clinical status (Table 26–6). Furthermore, a serum thyroxine determination is not sufficiently sensitive to detect mild degrees of hypo- or hyperthyroidism. Therefore, other tests may be used, but all are imperfect.

TESTS OF THYROID FUNCTION
(Table 26–7)

The tests most widely used in clinical practice are serum immunoassays for TSH and "free" thyroxine (FT_4). Assays for FT_4 have largely supplanted measurements of total thyroxine (T_4), resin T_3 uptake (RT_3U), and free thyroxine index (FT_4I).

1. SERUM THYROID TESTS

Free Thyroxine Immunoassay (FT_4)

FT_4 is a direct measurement of the serum concentration of free (unbound) thyroxine. FT_4 represents

Table 26–6. Factors falsely altering serum thyroxine measurements without affecting clinical status.[1,2]

Factors Increasing T_4	Factors Decreasing T_4
Laboratory error	Laboratory error
Autoimmunity	Severe illness (eg, chronic renal failure, major surgery, caloric deprivation)
Acute illness (eg, viral hepatitis, chronic active hepatitis; primary biliary cirrhosis; acute intermittent porphyria; AIDS)	Acute psychiatric problems
	Cirrhosis
High-estrogen states (may also increase T_3)	Nephrotic syndrome
Oral estrogen-containing contraceptives	Hereditary TBG deficiency
Pregnancy	Drugs
Estrogen replacement therapy	Phenobarbital
Neonatal period	Phenytoin (T_4 may be as low as 2 µg/dL)
Acute psychiatric problems	Carbamazepine
Hyperemesis gravidarum and morning sickness (may also increase T_3)	Triiodothyronine (T_3) therapy
Familial thyroid hormone binding abnormalities	Androgens
Generalized resistance to thyroid hormone	Fluorouracil
Drugs	Halofenate (lowers triglycerides and uric acid; not marketed in USA)
Amiodarone	Mitotane
Amphetamines	Phenylbutazone
Clofibrate	Fenclofenac (nonsteroidal anti-inflammatory agent; not marketed in USA)
Heparin (dialysis method)	Salicylates (large doses)
Heroin	Chloral hydrate
Levothyroxine (T_4) replacement therapy	Asparaginase
Methadone (may also increase T_3)	
Perphenazine	

[1]Modified, with permission from Fitzgerald PA: *Handbook of Clinical Endocrinology*, 2nd ed. Appleton & Lange, 1992.
[2]Symptomatic hyperthyroidism or hypothyroidism may also be present incidentally.

Table 26–7. Appropriate use of thyroid tests.

Purpose	Test	Comment
Screening	Serum TSH (sensitive assay)	Most sensitive test for primary hypothyroidism and hyperthyroidism
	Free T_4	Excellent test
	T_4 (RIA)	Varies directly with TBG
	T_3 resin uptake (T_3RU)	Varies inversely with TBG
	Free thyroxine index	Useful combination of T_4 and T_3U
For hypothyroidism	Serum TSH	High in primary and low in secondary hypothyroidism
	Antithyroglobulin and antithyroperoxidase antibodies	Elevated in Hashimoto's thyroiditis
For hyperthyroidism	Serum TSH (sensitive assay)	Suppressed except in TSH-secreting pituitary tumor or hyperplasia (rare)
	T_3 (RIA)	Elevated
	^{123}I uptake and scan	Increased diffuse versus "hot" areas
	Antithyroglobulin and antimicrosomal antibodies	Elevated in Graves' disease
	TSH receptor antibody (TSH-R Ab [stim])	Usually positive in Graves' disease
For nodules	Fine-needle aspiration (FNA)	Best diagnostic method for thyroid cancer
	^{123}I uptake and scan	Cancer is usually "cold." Less reliable than FNA.
	^{99m}Tc scan	Vascular versus avascular
	Ultrasonography	Solid versus cystic. Pure cysts are usually not malignant.

only about 0.025% of the serum concentration of the total T_4. It is the only metabolically active fraction of T_4 that freely enters cells to produce its effects.

When performed properly, this assay is superior to the total T_4 assay and free thyroxine index, since it is not affected by variations in protein binding. It is the procedure of choice for following the thyroid's changing secretion of T_4 during treatment for hyperthyroidism. Unfortunately, even the FT_4 assay has some shortcomings; serum FT_4 levels may be suppressed in patients with severe nonthyroid illness. In patients receiving heparin, measured levels of FT_4 may be falsely high, particularly when a dialysis assay is used. Serum FT_4 levels may rise transiently in acute nonthyroidal illness, when thyroid-binding protein frequently falls.

T_4 Immunoassay

This test measures the total serum concentration of thyroxine (bound and free). An increased serum T_4 confirms a clinical diagnosis of hyperthyroidism, while a decreased serum T_4 confirms a clinical diagnosis of hypothyroidism. It is affected by altered states of thyroxine binding (see Table 26–6). Therefore, this test is usually run with a resin T_3 uptake to provide a free thyroxine index (see below).

Resin T_3 (or T_4) Uptake

This is an indirect inverse test of serum thyroid-binding proteins (TBP)—ie, it is high when thyroid-binding proteins are low. The assay involves adding labeled T_3 or T_4 to the serum sample; it competes with the patient's thyroxine for binding to TBP. This mixture is then added to a thyroid hormone-binding resin. The resin is then assayed for its uptake of the label. A high resin uptake indicates that the patient's serum contains relatively low amounts of TBP or high levels of thyroxine.

This test is used as a "fudge factor" to correct a total serum thyroxine measurement for the effect of increased or decreased binding, creating a free thyroxine index (see below). A low resin uptake (high TBP) is seen with estrogen therapy, pregnancy, acute hepatitis, genetic TBP increase, and hypothyroidism. A low resin uptake with low TBP may be seen in severe illness. A high resin uptake is seen with hyperthyroidism and with chronic liver disease, nephrotic syndrome, anabolic steroid administration, and high-dose glucocorticoid administration (low TBP).

Free Thyroxine Index (FTI)

The product of T_4 and resin T_3 uptake ($T_4 \times T_3$ uptake) helps correct for abnormalities of thyroxine binding. A good free T_4 assay is more accurate.

The FTI, when calculated using the RT_3U, may be elevated in euthyroid patients with familial dysalbuminemic hyperthyroxinemia. This is a benign autosomal dominant trait in which an abnormal albumin molecule binds T_4 with much greater affinity than T_3. The RT_3U is not decreased (failing to compensate for the increased binding, as it would for TBG excess), because the T_3 used in the RT_3U assay is not significantly affected. Serum levels of free thyroxine and TSH are normal.

T₃

This test is of value in the diagnosis of thyrotoxicosis with normal T_4 values (T_3 thyrotoxicosis). It is not useful for the diagnosis of hypothyroidism.

Free T₃

This test measures the very tiny amount of T_3 that circulates unbound. It is sometimes useful in looking for hyperthyroidism in women taking oral estrogen and thyroxine replacement.

2. THYROID RADIOACTIVE IODINE UPTAKE & SCAN

Radioiodine (¹²³I) Uptake of Thyroid Gland

A. Elevated: Graves' disease, dietary iodine deficiency, toxic nodular goiter, pregnancy, early Hashimoto's thyroiditis, some thyroid enzyme deficiencies, nephrotic syndrome, recovery from subacute thyroiditis, recovery from thyroid hormone suppression.

B. Low: Administration of iodides or iodine in any form (drugs, radiology contrast dyes, etc), antithyroid drugs, subacute thyroiditis, thyroid hormone administration, thyroid gland damage (from thyroiditis, surgery, or radioiodine), hypopituitarism, ectopic functioning thyroid tissue, azotemia, severe (high-turnover) Graves' disease, heart failure, and some thyroid enzyme abnormalities.

Radioiodine (¹²³I) Scan of Thyroid Gland

A rectilinear scan over the thyroid may be obtained after ^{123}I administration, thereby obtaining a life-sized picture of thyroid uptake.

3. OTHER THYROID TESTS

Thyroid-Stimulating Hormone (TSH) Immunoassay

"Third-generation" assays can detect TSH levels as low as 0.01 mU/L. **TSH levels are decreased** in patients with primary hyperthyroidism (eg, Graves' disease, toxic multinodular goiter, toxic nodule, subacute thyroiditis, or release of stored hormone in Hashimoto's thyroiditis). TSH levels may also be suppressed in some clinically euthyroid individuals with autonomous thyroid secretion (eg, euthyroid Graves' ophthalmopathy). TSH can also be suppressed by thyroid hormone administration in either excessive or adequate replacement amounts. TSH is also frequently low during severe nonthyroidal ill-

ness; distinction from hypopituitarism can usually be made clinically.

Dopamine can cause suppression of TSH and may cause true secondary hypothyroidism during prolonged administration. Other conditions associated with decreased TSH include pregnancy (especially with morning sickness), hCG-secreting trophoblastic tumors, acute psychiatric illness (1% incidence), and acute administration of glucocorticoids. Certain drugs cause mild suppression of TSH without clinical hyperthyroidism; these include nonsteroidal anti-inflammatory agents, narcotics, and certain calcium channel blockers (especially nifedipine; also verapamil, but not diltiazem).

In clinically euthyroid persons age 60 or older, the TSH is very low (≤ 0.1 mU/L) in 3% and mildly low (0.1–0.4 mU/L) in 9%. The chance of developing atrial fibrillation is higher with very low TSH (2.8% yearly) than with normal TSH (1.1% yearly). Asymptomatic patients with very low TSH are followed closely but not treated unless they develop atrial fibrillation or other manifestations of hyperthyroidism.

TSH levels are elevated in primary hypothyroidism, either clinical or subclinical. TSH may also be elevated or inappropriately normal in the very rare cases of hyperthyroidism due to pituitary neoplastic or nonneoplastic inappropriate secretion of thyrotropin. Autoimmune disease may also falsely elevate serum TSH levels by interfering with the assay. TSH may be transiently elevated during recovery from nonthyroidal illness and in about 14% of patients with acute psychiatric admissions; the TSH returns to normal in the great majority of these patients. TSH may be mildly elevated as a normal variant in some individuals, especially the elderly (over 2% incidence). Such euthyroid patients with normal T_4 levels must be followed carefully, since about 18% later become hypothyroid.

Thyroid Antibodies

Antibodies against several thyroid constituents (thyroglobulin and thyroperoxidase) are most commonly found in Hashimoto's thyroiditis and Graves' disease. Antithyroid antibodies are found in about 5–10% of normal subjects. There is an increasing incidence with age. About 20% of hospitalized patients have detectable antithyroid antibodies. In the latter, the titers tend to be low, and they increase with age. TSH receptor antibody (TSH-R Ab [stim]) titers are elevated in approximately 80% of patients with Graves' disease. These titers—and those of antithyroglobulin and antithyroperoxidase antibodies—often decrease during pregnancy and during treatment of Graves' disease with antithyroid drugs. TSH-R Ab [stim] titers have been used with variable results to predict the rate of relapse of Graves' disease after chronic thiourea therapy.

Serum Thyroglobulin

The level of serum thyroglobulin rises in autoimmune thyroid disease, thyroid injury or inflammation, and thyroid cancer. Levels are of little value in diagnosing or distinguishing among these conditions, but they provide a useful marker in thyroid cancer to indicate recurrence of disease and the need for further studies and therapy. Do not confuse serum thyroglobulin with serum thyroid binding globulin (see above).

Ultrasound

This simple technique has been used to determine if thyroid lesions are solid or cystic. Cysts are less likely to be malignant, since thyroid carcinomas rarely undergo cystic degeneration. However, most solid lesions are also benign.

Fine-Needle Thyroid Biopsy

Aspiration of thyroid tissue with a fine needle (25-gauge) is helpful in the diagnosis of thyroid disorders, especially nodular lesions. This technique has become the preferred approach to the diagnosis of thyroid masses.

Calcitonin Assay

This test is elevated in medullary thyroid carcinoma, azotemia, hypercalcemia, pernicious anemia, thyroiditis, and pregnancy. High levels are also seen in many other malignancies such as carcinomas of the lung (45%), pancreas, breast (38%), and colon (24%).

4. EFFECT OF NONTHYROIDAL ILLNESS & DRUGS UPON THYROID FUNCTION TESTS

Many factors affect thyroid function tests, causing misleading laboratory evidence of hypothyroidism or hyperthyroidism in patients who are clinically euthyroid. See Table 26–6.

Patients with severe illness, caloric deprivation, or major surgery have a shift in the peripheral conversion of serum T_4 to more inactive reverse T_3 (rT_3). In most patients who are critically ill, there is a circulating inhibitor of thyroid hormone binding to serum thyroid binding proteins. This causes the resin uptake of thyroid hormone (rT_3U) to be misleadingly low, causing the computed free thyroxine index to be very low. The presence of a very low serum T_4 in severe nonthyroidal illness indicates a poor prognosis. In one series of such patients with serum T_4 levels under 3 µg/dL, there was a mortality rate of 84%.

Direct assays of free thyroxine often show low levels of FT_4 in severe illness. Since studies of giving replacement thyroxine to such patients have shown no improvement in survival, they are considered "euthyroid." Serum TSH tends to be suppressed in severe nonthyroidal illness, making the diagnosis of primary hypothyroidism quite difficult, although the presence of a goiter suggests the diagnosis.

The clinician must decide whether such severely ill patients (with a low serum T_4 but nonelevated TSH) might have hypothyroidism due to pituitary insufficiency. Patients without symptoms of prior brain lesion or hypopituitarism are very unlikely to suddenly develop hypopituitarism during an unrelated illness. Patients with diabetes insipidus, hypopituitarism, or other signs of a central nervous system lesion may have thyroxine given empirically. Patients receiving prolonged dopamine infusions may develop true secondary hypothyroidism due to direct dopamine suppression of TSH-secreting cells.

Bauer DC, Brown AN: Sensitive thyrotropin and free thyroxine testing in outpatients: Are both necessary? Arch Intern Med 1996;156:2333.

Danese MD et al: Screening for mild thyroid failure at the periodic health examination: A decision and cost-effectiveness analysis. JAMA 1996;276:285.

Krahn AD et al: How useful is thyroid function testing in patients with recent-onset atrial fibrillation? The Canadian Registry of Atrial Fibrillation Investigators. Arch Intern Med 1996;156:2221.

THE NODULAR THYROID

Essentials of Diagnosis

- Single or multiple thyroid nodules are commonly found with careful thyroid examinations.
- Thyroid function tests mandatory.
- Thyroid biopsy for single or dominant nodules or for a history of prior head-neck radiation.
- Ultrasound examination sometimes useful for biopsy and follow-up.
- Clinical follow-up required.

General Considerations

Enlargement of the thyroid (goiter) may be diffuse or irregular (nodular) and may often be discovered on physical examination. Nodular goiters are very common in regions of dietary iodine deficiency (see Iodine Deficiency Disorders, below). Patients with a history of past head-neck radiation have about a 25% chance of developing thyroid disease years later, including a high rate of thyroid carcinoma. In others, a solitary nodule by palpation is most often a benign adenoma or colloid nodule. Thyroid adenomas may occasionally function enough to produce thyrotoxicosis. Other thyroid pathology may include cysts, thyroiditis (see below), infections, and primary or metastatic neoplasms.

Clinical Findings & Management

A. Symptoms and Signs: The thyroid is best examined in a well-lighted room. The seated patient is given water to drink and the anterior neck is observed during swallowing. The thyroid moves upward during swallowing and may be visible in a thin neck; enlargement or asymmetry of the thyroid may be noted. Palpation of the thyroid is best done from behind a seated patient using the second and third fingers of both hands. As the patient swallows water, thyroid nodules may be perceived moving beneath the fingers. The location of any nodules should be noted, along with their size, firmness, and tenderness. The neck should be examined for lymphadenopathy. Enlarged thyroids should be auscultated for bruits.

Patients with thyroid enlargement should be questioned and examined for symptoms and signs of thyroid eye disease, hyperthyroidism, or hypothyroidism (see below).

Patients discovered to have thyroid enlargement are questioned further about any family history of thyroid disorders, prior medical history of thyroid problems, and prior radiation therapy to the head or neck or other exposure to radiation.

B. Laboratory Findings: Thyroid nodules are an indication for thyroid function testing. Serum determinations for TSH (sensitive assay) and free thyroxine (FT_4) are preferred. Tests for antithyroid peroxidase antibodies and antithyroglobulin antibodies may also be helpful. Very high antibody levels are found in Hashimoto's thyroiditis. However, thyroiditis frequently coexists with malignancy, so a suspicious nodule should be biopsied.

Fine-needle aspiration (FNA) biopsy is the best way to assess a nodule for malignancy. A 25-gauge needle is used to biopsy suspicious nodules. The needle is attached to a syringe and special syringe holder. The biopsy is done without local anesthesia. Care must be taken to avoid bloody dilution of the specimens. Material obtained is placed on a slide; a thin smear is obtained by laying a second slide over the material and then drawing the slides apart. One slide is air-dried while the other is preserved in 95% alcohol. Two or more biopsies may be obtained. Reading by an experienced cytopathologist is mandatory.

In one review of thyroid biopsies, about 70% were benign, 10% follicular neoplasm (suspicious), 5% malignant, and 15% nondiagnostic. About 30% of patients with suspicious cytology harbor a malignancy. Patients with suspicious cytology usually undergo immediate thyroid surgery; however, those electing not to have surgery appear to have a benign course for at least several years.

C. Imaging Studies: Since the advent of needle biopsy, radioactive iodine (RAI; ^{123}I or ^{131}I) scans are of less use in evaluating thyroid nodules because both hypofunctioning (cold) and hyperfunctioning (hot) nodules may sometimes be malignant. RAI scanning and uptake is helpful if a patient is found to have evidence of hyperthyroidism. (See Hyperthyroidism, below.) Ultrasound evaluation of thyroid nodules may be of benefit to determine whether a palpable nodule is really just one of many nodules, thus having less chance of being malignant. It may also be helpful in following thyroid nodules and in difficult biopsies. Ultrasound is generally preferred over CT and MRI because of its accuracy, ease of use, and lower cost.

Treatment

A. Solitary Thyroid Nodules: Solitary thyroid nodules call for fine-needle aspiration biopsy (see above). Nodules with benign cytologic features need to be followed by periodic palpation and rebiopsied if further growth occurs. Thyroxine "suppression" therapy is ineffective in shrinking nodules unless the patient has primary hypothyroidism with an elevated TSH. A solitary thyroid nodule in a patient with a remote history of radiation therapy to the head or neck is considered at high risk of malignancy, calling for resection. Cystic nodules can be managed by removal of fluid for cytologic examination, which may deflate the cyst. However, cysts tend to recur, requiring repeated aspirations. Solitary nodules in a patient with hyperthyroidism are an indication for radioactive iodine scan, which generally distinguishes toxic adenoma from Graves' disease. However, Graves' disease may occasionally be unilateral owing to agenesis of the contralateral lobe, so additional studies with antithyroid antibodies may be helpful. A "hot" nodule is usually benign but is resected to cure the hyperthyroidism.

B. Multinodular Goiters: A thyroid containing multiple nodules is likely to be a benign multinodular goiter. Nevertheless, fine-needle aspiration biopsy is performed on any nodule that is growing or is particularly dominant or hard. Large retrosternal goiters rarely harbor a malignancy but can be followed by CT scan or MRI. Continued growth or compressive symptoms are reasons for surgical excision. Thyroxine "suppression" therapy (thyroxine, 0.05–0.1 mg daily) is useful for patients with elevated serum TSH but much less so for those with normal TSH levels. Thyroxine should not be prescribed for patients with suppressed TSH since this may add to autonomous secretion and cause thyrotoxicosis. Patients found to be hyperthyroid may have a radioactive iodine scan and uptake for additional evaluation, especially if ^{131}I is a therapeutic consideration.

C. Incidental Small Thyroid Nodules: Nonpalpable small thyroid nodules are detected in about 50% of scans of the neck (MRI, CT, ultrasound) done for other reasons. In one series, only 2% of such thyroids were found to have significant malignancy after surgical resection. Microscopic "micropapillary" carcinoma is a variant of normal, being found in 24% of thyroidectomies performed for benign thyroid disease when 2 mm sections were carefully examined. It thus appears that the overwhelming majority of these microscopic foci never become clinically significant. The surgical pathology report of such a tiny papillary carcinoma that is otherwise benign does not justify aggressive follow-up or treatment because a cancer diagnosis is unwarranted and harmful. All that may be required is yearly follow-up with palpation of the neck and mild TSH suppression by thyroxine. Therefore, ultrasound-guided FNA biopsy is reserved for patients with nonpalpable nodules over 1.5 cm in diameter and for those with a history of head-neck irradiation.

Prognosis

The great majority of thyroid nodules are benign. Benign thyroid nodules tend to persist or grow slowly, but they may involute. Only about 1% of benign nodules increase in diameter with follow-up. Conversion to a malignant nodule is rare. The prognosis for patients with thyroid nodules that prove to be malignant is that of the histologic type and other factors (see below). Overall, differentiated thyroid carcinoma has an excellent prognosis, but metastases do occur. Multinodular goiters tend to persist or grow slowly, even in iodine-deficient areas where iodine repletion frequently does not shrink established goiters. Patients with small incidentally discovered nonpalpable thyroid nodules are at very low risk for malignancy, and even those that are malignant have a minor effect on morbidity and mortality.

Cerosimo E et al: "Suspicious" thyroid cytologic findings: Outcomes in patients without immediate surgical treatment. Mayo Clin Proc 1993;68:343.

Fink A et al: Occult micropapillary carcinoma associated with benign follicular thyroid disease and unrelated thyroid neoplasms. Mod Pathol 1996;9:816.

Gharib B: Fine-needle aspiration biopsy of thyroid nodules: Advantages, limitations, and effect. Mayo Clinic Proc 1994;69:44. (Fine-needle aspiration biopsy is a safe, simple, reliable, and cost-effective means of detecting benign nodules and therefore should be the initial diagnostic test.)

Hurley DL, Gharib H: Evaluation and management of multinodular goiter. Otolaryngol Clin North Am 1996; 29:527.

Maxwell JG et al: Fine-needle aspiration cytology and thyroid surgery in the community hospital. Am J Surg 1996;172:529.

IODINE DEFICIENCY DISORDERS

Essentials of Diagnosis

- Common in regions of the world with low-iodine diets.
- High rate of congenital hypothyroidism and cretinism.
- Goiters may become multinodular and grow to great size.
- Most adults with endemic goiter are found to be euthyroid; however, some are hypothyroid or hyperthyroid.
- Impaired cognition and hearing may be subtle or severe.

General Considerations

Approximately 5% of the world's population have goiters. Of these, about 75% are in persons dwelling in geographic regions characterized by significant iodine deficiency. Areas of iodine deficiency are found in 115 countries, mostly in developing areas but also in areas of Europe. In certain highly endemic areas, up to 50% of the population may have goiters. Up to 0.5% of such populations may have full-blown cretinism, with less severe manifestations of congenital hypothyroidism being even more common (eg, isolated deafness, short stature, or impaired mentation). Intelligence quotients in iodine-deficient adults are an average of 13 points lower than expected. Although iodine deficiency is the most common cause of endemic goiter, certain foods (eg, sorghum, millet, maize, cassava) and water pollutants can themselves cause goiter or aggravate a goiter proclivity caused by iodine deficiency. Some individuals are particularly susceptible to goiter owing to congenital partial defects in thyroid enzyme activity.

Clinical Findings

A. Symptoms and Signs: Endemic goiters may become multinodular and very large; enlargement during pregnancy may cause compressive symptoms. Some patients with endemic goiter may become hypothyroid. Others may become thyrotoxic as the goiter grows and becomes more autonomous, especially if iodine is added to the diet.

B. Laboratory Findings: The serum thyroxine is usually normal. Serum TSH is generally normal or slightly elevated. TSH falls in the presence of hyperthyroidism if a multinodular goiter has become autonomous in the presence of sufficient amounts of iodine for thyroid hormone synthesis. Thyroid radioactive iodine uptake is usually elevated, but it may be normal if iodine intake has improved. Serum levels of antithyroid antibodies are usually either undetectable or in low titers. Serum thyroglobulin is often elevated.

Differential Diagnosis

Endemic goiter must be distinguished from all other forms of nodular goiter that may coexist in an endemic region (see above).

Prevention

Before the days of dietary iodine supplementation, the Great Lakes region of the USA was known as a "goiter belt." In certain cantons of Switzerland, 30% of young men were declared unfit for military service because of their large goiters. Iodine supplementation was started in Switzerland in 1922, initially by adding 5 mg of potassium iodide per kilogram of salt, with later increases to the current level of 20 mg/kg salt. This practice virtually eliminates endemic iodine-deficient goiter and cretinism. Unfortunately, many iodine-deficient countries have inadequate programs for iodine supplementation. The minimum dietary requirement for iodine is about 50 μg daily, with optimal iodine intake being 150–300 μg daily. Iodine sufficiency is assessed by measurement of urinary iodide excretion, the target being more than 100 μg of iodide per gram of creatinine.

Initiating iodine supplementation in a geographic area causes an increased frequency of hyperthyroidism in the first year, followed by greatly reduced rates of toxic nodular goiter and Graves' disease thereafter.

Treatment

Dietary supplementation with iodine successfully prevents iodine-deficient goiter and cretinism but is less successful in shrinking established goiter in such regions. Attempts to shrink such goiters with thyroxine are generally unsuccessful and may cause thyrotoxicosis, since nodular goiters tend to become autonomous over time. Adults with large multinodular goiter may require thyroidectomy for cosmesis, compressive symptoms, or thyrotoxicosis; but following partial thyroidectomy in iodine-deficient geographic areas, there is a high goiter recurrence rate.

Baltisberger BL et al: Decrease of incidence of toxic nodular goiter in a region of Switzerland after full correction of mild iodine deficiency. Eur J Endocrinol 1995; 132:546.

Dunn JT: Seven deadly sins in confronting endemic iodine deficiency, and how to avoid them. J Clin Endocrinol Metab 1996;81:1332.

HYPOTHYROIDISM & MYXEDEMA

Essentials of Diagnosis

- Weakness, fatigue, cold intolerance, constipation, weight change, depression, menorrhagia, hoarseness.
- Dry skin, bradycardia, delayed return of deep tendon reflexes.
- Anemia, hyponatremia.
- T_4 and radioiodine uptake usually low.
- TSH elevated in primary hypothyroidism.

General Considerations

Thyroid hormone deficiency may affect virtually all body functions. The degree of severity ranges from mild and unrecognized hypothyroid states to striking myxedema.

Hypothyroidism may be due to primary disease of the thyroid gland itself or lack of pituitary TSH. Although gross forms of hypothyroidism, ie, myxedema and cretinism, are readily recognized on clinical grounds alone, the far more common mild forms often escape detection without adequate laboratory testing.

Goiter is frequently noted when hypothyroidism is due to Hashimoto's thyroiditis, iodide deficiency, genetic thyroid enzyme defects, drug goitrogens (lithium, iodide, propylthiouracil or methimazole, phenylbutazone, sulfonamides, amiodarone), food goitrogens in iodide-deficient areas (eg, turnips, cassavas), or, rarely, peripheral resistance to thyroid hormone or infiltrating diseases (eg, cancer, sarcoidosis). A hypothyroid phase occurs in subacute (de Quervain's) viral thyroiditis following initial hyperthyroidism.

Goiter is usually absent when hypothyroidism is due to: deficient pituitary TSH secretion, or destruction of the gland by surgery, external radiation, or ^{131}I. Primary hypothyroidism may also be idiopathic.

Amiodarone, because of its high iodine content, causes clinically significant hypothyroidism in about 8% of patients. The T_4 level is normal or low, and the TSH is elevated, usually over 20 ng/dL. Another 17% of patients develop milder elevations of TSH and are asymptomatic. Low-dose amiodarone is less likely to cause hypothyroidism. Cardiac patients with amiodarone-induced symptomatic hypothyroidism are treated with just enough thyroxine to relieve symptoms.

Clinical Findings

These may vary from the rather rare full-blown myxedema to mild states of hypothyroidism, which are far more common.

A. Symptoms and Signs:

1. Early–Frequent symptoms are fatigue, lethargy, weakness, arthralgias or myalgias, muscle cramps, cold intolerance, constipation, dry skin, headache, and menorrhagia. Physical findings may be few or absent. Features may include thin, brittle nails, thinning of hair, and pallor, with poor turgor of the mucosa. Delayed return of deep tendon reflexes is often noted.

2. Late–The principal symptoms are slow speech, absence of sweating, constipation, peripheral edema, pallor, hoarseness, decreased sense of taste and smell, muscle cramps, aches and pains, dyspnea, weight changes (usually gain, but weight loss is not rare), and diminished auditory acuity. Some women have amenorrhea; others have menorrhagia. Galactorrhea may also be present. Physical findings include puffiness of the face and eyelids, typical carotenemic skin color, thinning of the outer halves of the eyebrows, thickening of the tongue, hard pitting edema, and effusions into the pleural, peritoneal, and pericardial cavities, as well as into joints. Cardiac enlargement ("myxedema heart") is often due to pericardial effusion. The heart rate is slow; the blood pressure is more often normal than low, and reversible diastolic hypertension may be found. Hypothermia may be present. Pituitary enlargement due to hyperplasia of TSH-secreting cells, which is reversible following thyroid therapy, may be seen in long-standing hypothyroidism. Hypothyroidism rarely causes true obesity.

B. Laboratory Findings: The T_4 may be low or low normal. TSH is increased with primary hypothyroidism but is low or normal with pituitary insufficiency. Other laboratory abnormalities may often be seen: increased serum cholesterol, liver enzymes, and creatine kinase; increased serum prolactin; hyponatremia, hypoglycemia, and anemia (with normal or increased mean corpuscular volume). Titers of antibodies against thyroperoxidase and thyroglobulin are high in patients with Hashimoto's thyroiditis. Serum T_3 is not a good test for hypothyroidism.

A number of factors can lower serum T_4 levels without causing true hypothyroidism (Table 26–6).

Differential Diagnosis

Hypothyroidism must be considered in states of asthenia, unexplained menstrual disorders, myalgias, constipation, weight change, hyperlipidemia, and anemia. Myxedema enters into the differential diagnosis of unexplained heart failure that does not respond to digitalis or diuretics, and unexplained ascites. The protein content of myxedematous effusions is high. The thick tongue may be confused with that seen in primary amyloidosis. Pernicious anemia may be suggested by the pallor and the macrocytic anemia sometimes seen in myxedema; the two disorders may even coexist. Some cases of depression, primary psychosis and structural diseases of the brain have been confused with myxedema. The pituitary is often quite enlarged in primary hypothyroidism due to reversible hyperplasia of TSH-secreting cells; the concomitant hyperprolactinemia seen in hypothyroidism can lead to the mistaken diagnosis of a pituitary adenoma.

Complications

Complications are mostly cardiac in nature, occurring as a result of advanced coronary artery disease and congestive failure, which may be precipitated by too vigorous thyroid therapy. There is an increased susceptibility to infection. Megacolon has been described in long-standing hypothyroidism. Organic psychoses with paranoid delusions may occur ("myxedema madness"). Rarely, adrenal crisis may be precipitated by thyroid therapy. Hypothyroidism is a rare cause of infertility, which may respond to thyroid medication. Pregnancy in a woman with untreated hypothyroidism often results in miscarriage. On the other hand, if the hypothyroidism is due to autoimmune disease, it may improve during pregnancy. Sellar enlargement and even well-defined TSH-secreting tumors may develop in untreated cases. These tumors decrease in size after replacement therapy is instituted.

A rare complication of severe hypothyroidism is deep stupor, at times progressing to **myxedema coma,** with severe hypothermia, hypoventilation, hy-

ponatremia, hypoxia, hypercapnia, and hypotension. Convulsions and abnormal central nervous system signs may occur. Myxedema coma is often induced by an underlying infection; cardiac, respiratory, or central nervous system illness; cold exposure; or drug use. It is most often seen in elderly women. The mortality rate is high. Myxedematous patients are unusually sensitive to opiates and may die from average doses.

Refractory hyponatremia is often seen in severe myxedema. Inappropriate secretion of antidiuretic hormone has been observed in some patients, but a defect in distal tubular reabsorption of sodium and water has been demonstrated in many others.

Treatment

A. Specific Therapy: Levothyroxine is the drug of choice. Levothyroxine is readily available, inexpensive, and well standardized. It is converted in the body to T_3, the most active thyroid hormone, in an enzymatically regulated manner that best meets the metabolic needs of the patient.

1. Patients who are elderly or have coronary insufficiency are treated with small doses of levothyroxine, 25–50 μg daily for 1 week, increasing the dose every 1–4 weeks by 25 μg daily up to a total of 75–150 μg daily. This dosage should be adjusted to optimally resolve symptoms while keeping TSH normal. Levothyroxine may also be administered once weekly, using a dose slightly higher than seven times the normal daily dose.

2. Patients who are younger and without coronary insufficiency may receive larger starting doses, 50–100 μg daily, increasing by 25 μg every 1–3 weeks until the TSH normalizes.

3. Maintenance—Each patient's dose must be adjusted to obtain the optimal effect. The proper dose should be decided mainly by careful clinical assessment. A serum TSH can be helpful, since persistently elevated levels usually indicate underreplacement with thyroxine, while very suppressed levels can indicate hyperthyroidism. Once a patient is feeling completely well, the dose is kept fairly constant. Frequent repeat determinations of serum thyroxine or TSH are unnecessary once the patient is feeling completely well and careful examinations show euthyroidism. In such patients, a sensitive TSH level may be obtained every 1–2 years. Serum thyroxine is usually high-normal or mildly elevated in patients receiving adequate doses of levothyroxine. Serum thyroxine levels in euthyroid patients may be quite high in patients also taking estrogen preparations. Serum TSH should be normal or slightly low. Most patients require 100–200 μg daily for maintenance.

Malabsorption of thyroxine may occur in short bowel syndrome; therapy with medium chain triglyceride oil may improve the diarrhea and absorption. Other diseases such as sprue, regional enteritis, pancreatitis, and liver disease may also cause reduced absorption of T_4. Certain substances interfere with the intestinal absorption of thyroxine, particularly sucralfate, aluminum hydroxide antacids, iron preparations, and phenytoin. Cholestyramine and other bile acid-binding resins can bind T_4; absorption of T_4 is reduced by 30% even when cholestyramine is given 5 hours before the thyroxine. Soybean infant formula also interferes with the absorption of thyroxine. Myxedema itself can interfere with its treatment by reducing thyroxine absorption, especially when severe. However, apparent malabsorption of thyroxine is often due to noncompliance.

Ironically, increased intestinal absorption of thyroxine has been reported with gastrojejunostomy and dumping syndrome.

4. Myxedema coma is a medical emergency with a high mortality rate. Levothyroxine sodium 400 μg is given intravenously and repeated daily in a dose of 100 μg intravenously. Hydrocortisone, 100 mg as an initial bolus, followed by 25–50 mg every 8 hours, should be given if adrenal insufficiency is suspected. The patient must not be warmed except by blanket. Infection is often present and must be aggressively treated. Assisted mechanical ventilation is almost always necessary to correct the hypercapnia.

5. There are special situations where the daily maintenance dose of thyroxine may have to be altered: Slightly higher doses may be necessary during pregnancy or in patients taking phenobarbital or bile acid-binding resins or changing their diet to one containing more fiber. Conversely, lower doses are often required in aging patients.

B. Needless Use of Thyroid: Thyroid medication should not be used as nonspecific stimulating therapy. Large doses given to euthyroid individuals to induce weight loss may induce cardiac arrhythmias, osteoporosis, muscle weakness, and anxiety.

The use of thyroid in cases of amenorrhea or infertility is indicated only if the patient is proved to be hypothyroid.

Prognosis

With early treatment, striking transformations take place both in appearance and mental function. Return to a normal state is usually the rule, but relapses will occur if treatment is interrupted. The patient may rarely die from the complications of myxedema coma. On the whole, response to thyroid treatment is most satisfactory. Chronic maintenance therapy with unduly large doses of thyroid hormone may lead to subtle but important side effects (eg, bone demineralization) and is to be avoided.

Grebe SKG et al: Treatment of hypothyroidism with once weekly thyroxine. J Clin Endocrinol Metab 1997; 82:870.

Harjai KJ, Licata AA: Effects of amiodarone on thyroid function. Ann Intern Med 1997;126:63.

Hurley DL, Gharib H: Detection and treatment of hypothyroidism and Graves' disease. Geriatrics 1995;50:41.

Klemperer JD et al: Thyroid hormone treatment after coronary-artery bypass surgery. N Engl J Med 1995; 333:1522.

Jordan RM: Myxedema coma. Pathophysiology, therapy and factors affecting prognosis. Med Clin North Am 1995;79:185.

HYPERTHYROIDISM (Thyrotoxicosis)

Essentials of Diagnosis

- Sweating, weight change, nervousness, loose stools, heat intolerance, irritability, fatigue, weakness, menstrual irregularity.
- Tachycardia; warm, moist skin; stare; tremor.
- In Graves' disease: goiter (often with bruit); ophthalmopathy.
- Suppressed TSH in primary hyperthyroidism; increased T_4, free T_4, and free T_4 index.

General Considerations

The term "thyrotoxicosis" denotes a series of clinical disorders associated with increased circulating levels of free thyroxine or triiodothyronine.

The various causes include the following:

(1) Graves' disease: By far the most common form of thyrotoxicosis is that associated with diffuse enlargement of the thyroid, hyperactivity of the gland, and the presence of antibodies against different fractions of the thyroid gland. This autoimmune thyroid disorder is called **Graves' disease** (Basedow's disease). It is much more common in women than in men (8:1), and its onset is usually between the ages of 20 and 40. It may be accompanied by infiltrative ophthalmopathy (Graves' exophthalmos) and, less commonly, by infiltrative dermopathy (pretibial myxedema). It may also be associated with other systemic autoimmune disorders such as pernicious anemia, myasthenia gravis, diabetes mellitus, etc. It has a familial tendency, and histocompatibility studies have shown an association with group HLA-B8 and HLA-DR3. The pathogenesis of the hyperthyroidism of Graves' disease involves the formation of autoantibodies that bind to the TSH receptor in thyroid cell membranes and stimulate the gland to hyperfunction. TSH receptor antibodies (TSH-R Ab [stim]) are demonstrable in the plasma of about 80% patients with Graves' disease. Other antibodies such as ANA are generated in Graves' disease, with antimicrosomal or antithyroglobulin antibodies being increased in most patients.

(2) Autonomous toxic adenomas of the thyroid may be single (Plummer's disease) or multiple (toxic multinodular goiter). These adenomas are not accompanied by infiltrative ophthalmopathy or dermopathy. Antithyroid antibodies are usually not present in the plasma, and tests for TSH-R Ab [stim] are negative.

(3) Subacute thyroiditis (thought to be due to viral infection) is characterized by a moderately enlarged, tender thyroid. If the gland is nontender, the disorder is called "silent thyroiditis." Hyperthyroidism is followed by hypothyroidism. During thyrotoxicosis, thyroid RAIU is low. A similar problem is seen with interleukin-2 therapy and after neck surgery for hyperparathyroidism. Treatment is with propranolol and analgesics until the condition subsides, usually over several months.

(4) Jodbasedow disease, or iodine-induced hyperthyroidism, may occur in patients with multinodular goiters after intake of large amounts of iodine in the diet or in the form of radiographic contrast materials or drugs, especially amiodarone.

(5) Thyrotoxicosis factitia is due to ingestion of excessive amounts of exogenous thyroid hormone. Isolated epidemics of thyrotoxicosis have been caused by consumption of ground beef contaminated with bovine thyroid gland.

(6) Struma ovarii: Thyroid tissue is contained in about 3% of ovarian dermoid tumors and teratomas. This thyroid tissue may autonomously secrete thyroid hormone due to a toxic nodule or in concert with the woman's thyroid gland in Graves' disease or toxic multinodular goiter.

(7) TSH hypersecretion by the pituitary may be caused by a tumor and is a rare cause of hyperthyroidism. Serum TSH is elevated or normal (determined by a sensitive TSH assay) in the presence of true thyrotoxicosis. No ophthalmopathy is present. Antithyroid antibodies and TSH-R Ab [stim] are usually normal. TSH hypersecretion may be caused by a pituitary adenoma, in which case it is known as "neoplastic inappropriate secretion of thyrotropin." The tumor may present as a mass lesion following treatment of hyperthyroidism. The pituitary adenoma is usually removed by transsphenoidal surgery; larger tumors may require radiation therapy. Tumors may sometimes respond to bromocriptine or octreotide. Hyperthyroidism is treated symptomatically with propranolol.

This condition may also be due to pituitary hyperplasia, in which case it is known as "nonneoplastic inappropriate secretion of thyrotropin." Pituitary hyperplasia may be detected on MRI scan as pituitary enlargement without a discrete adenoma being visible. This condition appears to be due to a diminished feedback effect of T_4 upon the pituitary. It may be familial, but it can also be caused by prolonged untreated hypothyroidism, especially in youth. Hyperthyroid symptoms are treated with propranolol. Definitive treatment is with radioactive iodine or thyroid surgery.

(8) Hashimoto's thyroiditis may cause transient hyperthyroidism during the initial destructive phase. It may occur transiently postpartum.

(9) Pregnancy and trophoblastic tumors–Although hCG generally has a low affinity for the thyroid's TSH receptors, very high serum levels of hCG may cause sufficient receptor activation to cause thyrotoxicosis. Mild gestational hyperthyroidism may occur during the first 4 months of pregnancy, when hCG levels are very high. Pregnant women are more likely to have thyrotoxicosis and hyperemesis gravidarum if they have high serum levels of sialo-hCG, a subfraction of hCG with greater affinity for TSH receptors.

Thyrotoxicosis may also be caused by the high serum levels of hCG seen in molar pregnancy, choriocarcinoma, and testicular malignancies.

(10) Metastatic functioning thyroid carcinoma is a rare cause of thyrotoxicosis.

(11) High-dose amiodarone causes symptomatic hyperthyroidism in about 2.5% of patients. The incidence in low-dose use is unknown. Since high levels of T_4 and free T_4 are normally seen in patients taking amiodarone, suppressed TSH (sensitive assay) must be present along with a greatly elevated T_4 (> 20 µg/dL) or T_3 (> 200 ng/dL). Treatment involves withdrawing the drug. Other options include thiourea drugs, potassium perchlorate, ipodate, thyroidectomy, and radioactive iodine if the radioiodine uptake is adequate for treatment.

Clinical Findings

A. Symptoms and Signs: Thyrotoxicosis due to any cause produces many different manifestations of variable intensity among different individuals. Patients may complain of nervousness, restlessness, heat intolerance, increased sweating, fatigue, weakness, muscle cramps, frequent bowel movements, or weight change (usually loss). There may be palpitations or angina pectoris. Women frequently report menstrual irregularities.

Hypokalemic periodic paralysis occurs in about 15% of Asian or Native American men with thyrotoxicosis. It usually presents abruptly with paralysis (and few thyrotoxic symptoms), often after intravenous dextrose, oral carbohydrate, or vigorous exercise. Attacks last 7–72 hours.

Signs of thyrotoxicosis may include stare and lid lag, tachycardia or atrial fibrillation, fine resting finger tremors, moist warm skin, hyperreflexia, fine hair, onycholysis, and (rarely) heart failure. Chronic thyrotoxicosis may cause osteoporosis. At times there may be clubbing and swelling of the fingers (acropachy). Graves' disease usually presents with additional findings of goiter (often with a bruit).

Graves' ophthalmopathy is clinically apparent in 20–40% and usually consists of chemosis, conjunctivitis, and mild proptosis. More severe lymphocytic infiltration of the eye muscles occurs in 5–10% and may produce exophthalmos and sometimes diplopia due to extraocular muscle entrapment. The optic nerve may be compressed in severe cases. Corneal drying may occur with inadequate lid closure. Eye changes may sometimes be asymmetric or unilateral. The severity of the eye disease is not closely correlated with the severity of the thyrotoxicosis. Some patients with Graves' ophthalmopathy are clinically euthyroid.

Skin "myxedema" occurs in about 3% of Graves' disease patients, usually in the pretibial region. Its texture resembles the skin of an orange.

B. Laboratory Diagnosis: Serum T_3, T_4, thyroid resin uptake, and free thyroxine are usually all increased. Sometimes the T_4 level may be normal but the serum T_3 is elevated. A reliable sensitive TSH assay is the best test for thyrotoxicosis; it is suppressed except in the very rare cases of pituitary inappropriate secretion of thyrotropin. Other laboratory abnormalities may include hypercalcemia, increased alkaline phosphatase, anemia, and decreased granulocytes.

TSH receptor antibody (TSH-R Ab [stim]) levels are usually high (80%), but TSH-R Ab [stim] measurement is not ordinarily required for diagnosis. Antithyroglobulin or antimicrosomal antibodies are usually elevated in Graves' disease. Serum ANA and anti-double-stranded DNA antibodies are also usually elevated without any evidence of lupus erythematosus or other collagen-vascular disease.

Patients with subacute thyroiditis often have an increased erythrocyte sedimentation rate.

Thyroid radioactive iodine uptake and scan is usually performed on patients with an established diagnosis of thyrotoxicosis. A high radioactive iodine uptake is seen in Graves' disease and toxic nodular goiter but can be seen in other conditions as well. A low radioactive iodine uptake is characteristic of subacute thyroiditis but can also be seen in other conditions. (For conditions affecting radioactive iodine uptake, see section on tests of thyroid function.)

C. Imaging: MRI of the orbits is the imaging method of choice to visualize Graves' ophthalmopathy affecting the extraocular muscles. CT scanning and ultrasound can also be used. Imaging is required only in severe cases or in euthyroid exophthalmos that must be distinguished from orbital tumors or other disorders.

Differential Diagnosis

True thyrotoxicosis must be distinguished from those conditions elevating serum thyroxine without affecting clinical status (Table 26–6).

Hyperthyroidism may be confused with anxiety neurosis or mania, but in the latter the thyroid is not enlarged and thyroid function tests are usually normal. Problems of diagnosis occur in patients with acute psychiatric disorders, about 30% of whom have hyperthyroxinemia without thyrotoxicosis. The TSH is not suppressed, distinguishing psychiatric disorder from true hyperthyroidism. T_4 levels return to normal gradually.

Exogenous thyroid administration will present the same laboratory features as thyroiditis. A rare pituitary tumor may produce the picture of thyrotoxicosis with high levels of TSH.

Some states of hypermetabolism without thyrotoxicosis—notably severe anemia, leukemia, polycythemia, and cancer—rarely cause confusion. Pheochromocytoma is often associated with hypermetabolism, tachycardia, weight loss, and profuse sweating. Acromegaly may also produce tachycardia, sweating, and thyroid enlargement. Appropriate laboratory tests will easily distinguish these entities.

Cardiac disease (eg, atrial fibrillation, angina) refractory to treatment suggests the possibility of underlying ("apathetic") hyperthyroidism. Other causes of ophthalmoplegia (eg, myasthenia gravis) and exophthalmos (eg, orbital tumor) must be considered. Graves' ophthalmopathy closely resembles pseudotumor of the orbit. Thyrotoxicosis must also be considered in the differential diagnosis of muscle weakness and osteoporosis. Diabetes mellitus and Addison's disease may coexist with thyrotoxicosis.

Complications

Cardiac complications of thyrotoxicosis include atrial fibrillation with a ventricular response that is difficult to control. Episodes of periodic paralysis induced by exercise or heavy carbohydrate ingestion and accompanied by hypokalemia may complicate thyrotoxicosis in Asian or Native American men. Hypercalcemia, osteoporosis, and nephrocalcinosis may occur. Decreased libido, impotence, decreased sperm count, and gynecomastia may be noted in men with hyperthyroidism.

Treatment

The methods used to treat thyrotoxicosis will vary according to the cause and severity of the hyperthyroidism, the patient's age, the clinical situation, and the desires of the patient.

A. Graves' Disease: The treatment of Graves' disease involves a choice of methods rather than a method of choice:

1. Propranolol–Propranolol is generally used for symptomatic relief until the hyperthyroidism is resolved. It effectively relieves the tachycardia, tremor, diaphoresis, and anxiety that occur with hyperthyroidism due to any cause. It is the initial treatment of choice for thyroid storm. The periodic paralysis seen in association with thyrotoxicosis is also effectively treated with beta blockade. It has no effect on thyroid hormone secretion. Treatment is usually begun with 10 mg orally and increased progressively until an adequate response is achieved, usually 20 mg four times daily. Doses as high as 80 mg four times daily are occasionally required.

2. Thiourea drugs–Methimazole or propylthiouracil is generally used for young adults or patients with mild thyrotoxicosis, small goiters, or fear of isotopes. Aged patients usually respond particularly well. These drugs are also useful for preparing hyperthyroid patients for surgery and elderly patients for radioactive iodide treatment. The drugs do not permanently damage the thyroid and are associated with a lower chance of posttreatment hypothyroidism (compared with radioactive iodide or surgery). Unfortunately, there is a high rate of recurrent hyperthyroidism (about 50%) after a year or more of therapy. A greater likelihood of long-term remission is seen in patients with small goiters or mild hyperthyroidism. Patients whose thyroperoxidase and thyroglobulin antibodies remain high after 2 years of therapy have been reported to have only a 10% rate of relapse.

A Japanese study reported that long-term remission rates were improved when thyroxine (about 0.1 mg daily) was added to the thiourea regimen once patients were euthyroid; however, a Scottish study failed to demonstrate such an effect.

a. Methimazole–Methimazole has the advantage of requiring less frequent dosing and fewer pills than propylthiouracil, making treatment more convenient. It is also associated with a lower incidence of acute hepatic necrosis. Rare complications peculiar to methimazole include serum sickness, cholestatic jaundice, loss of taste, alopecia, nephrotic syndrome, and hypoglycemia. Methimazole (10 mg tablets) is given orally in initial doses of 30–60 mg once daily. The dosage is usually reduced as manifestations of hyperthyroidism resolve and as the free thyroxine level becomes normal.

b. Propylthiouracil–Propylthiouracil has been considered the drug of choice during breast feeding or pregnancy, being less likely to cause aplasia cutis in the newborn. It blocks the peripheral conversion of T_4 to T_3 and is of some theoretic advantage over methimazole in thyroid storm, but this effect has not been demonstrated to be clinically significant. Rare complications peculiar to propylthiouracil include arthritis, lupus erythematosus, aplastic anemia, thrombocytopenia, and hypoprothrombinemia. Acute hepatitis occurs rarely and is treated with prednisone but may progress to liver failure. Propylthiouracil (available as 50 mg tablets) is given orally in initial doses of 300–600 mg daily in four divided doses. The dosage and frequency of administration is generally reduced as symptoms of hyperthyroidism resolve and the free thyroxine level becomes normal. During pregnancy, the dose is kept below 200 mg/d in order to avoid goitrous hypothyroidism in the infant.

c. Complications of thioureas–Agranulocytosis is an uncommon but serious complication of thiourea therapy, being reported in about 0.1% of patients taking methimazole and about 0.4% of patients taking propylthiouracil. Patients are warned that if they develop a sore throat or febrile illness, they should stop the drug while a white blood count is rechecked. The agranulocytosis is generally reversible and may be treated with filgrastim (G-CSF).

Periodic surveillance of the white blood count during treatment has been advocated by some clinicians, but onset is generally abrupt.

Other side effects common to thiourea drugs include pruritus, allergic dermatitis, nausea, and dyspepsia. Antihistamines may control mild pruritus without discontinuation of the drug. Since the two thiourea drugs are similar, patients who have had a major allergic reaction from one should not be given the other.

Primary hypothyroidism may occur. The patient may become clinically hypothyroid for 2 weeks or more before TSH levels rise, having been suppressed by the preceding hyperthyroidism. Therefore, the patient's changing thyroid status is best followed clinically and with serum levels of free thyroxine. Rapid growth of the goiter usually occurs if the patient is allowed to develop prolonged hypothyroidism; the goiter may sometimes become massive but usually regresses rapidly with thyroid hormone replacement.

3. Radioactive iodine (^{131}I)–The administration of radioiodine is an excellent method of destroying overactive thyroid tissue (either diffuse or toxic nodular goiter). The radioiodine damages the cells that concentrate it. Patients have no apparent risk of subsequent thyroid cancer, leukemia, or other malignancies. Children born to parents previously treated with ^{131}I show normal rates of congenital abnormalities. However, since fetal radiation is harmful, *radioactive iodine should not be given to pregnant women.*

Most patients may receive radioiodine while being symptomatically treated with just propranolol, which is then reduced in dosage as hyperthyroxinemia resolves. However, some patients (those with coronary diseases, elderly people, or those with severe hyperthyroidism) are usually rendered euthyroid with a thiouracil drug (see above) while the dosage of propranolol is reduced; once the patient is euthyroid, the thiourea is discontinued 3–5 days before ^{131}I treatment is given. There is a high incidence of hypothyroidism several years after ^{131}I even when small doses are given. However, hypothyroidism also occurs quite frequently years after surgical or medical treatment of Graves' disease, and eventual hypothyroidism may be part of the natural history of this condition. Prolonged follow-up, preferably with free T_4 and sensitive TSH measurements, is therefore mandatory.

4. Thyroid surgery–Thyroid surgery for Graves' disease and toxic nodular goiter has been performed less frequently as radioiodine treatment has become more widely accepted. Surgery is usually preferred for pregnant women whose thyrotoxicosis is not controlled with low doses of thioureas, for patients with particularly large goiters, and whenever there is a significant chance of malignancy.

Patients are ordinarily rendered euthyroid with a thiourea drug or ipodate preoperatively. Propranolol is given until the T_3 is normal preoperatively. Iodine is given (eg, Lugol's solution, 2–3 drops orally daily) for about 10 days preoperatively to reduce thyroid vascularity. If a patient undergoes surgery while thyrotoxic, larger doses of propranolol are given perioperatively to reduce the likelihood of thyroid crisis.

Morbidity includes possible damage to the recurrent laryngeal nerve that causes vocal cord paralysis. Hypoparathyroidism also occurs, which means that calcium levels must be checked postoperatively. These complications are unusual (< 1%) when the surgery is performed by a competent, experienced neck surgeon.

5. Iodinated contrast agents–Iopanoic acid and ipodate sodium are given orally (ipodate, 500 mg once daily) and quickly block peripheral conversion of T_4 to T_3 as well as T_4 release. Within 24 hours, serum T_3 levels fall an average of 62%. Treatment periods of 8 months or more are possible, but the effect tends to wane with time. These agents provide an important therapeutic option for patients in thyroid storm (see below), patients intolerant to thioureas, and newborns with thyrotoxicosis (due to maternal Graves' disease). Thyroid radioiodine uptake may be suppressed during treatment but returns to pretreatment uptake by 7 days after discontinuing the drug, allowing ^{131}I treatment.

B. Toxic Solitary Thyroid Nodules: Hyperthyroidism caused by a single hyperfunctioning thyroid nodule may be treated symptomatically with propranolol as in Graves' disease. Definitive treatment is with surgery or radioactive iodine. For patients under age 40, surgery is usually recommended; patients are made euthyroid with a thiourea preoperatively and given 10 days of iodine therapy before surgery as in Graves' disease (see above). Transient postoperative hypothyroidism resolves spontaneously. Permanent hypothyroidism occurs in about 14% of patients by 6 years after surgery. Patients over age 40 with a toxic solitary nodule are offered radioactive iodine. Permanent hypothyroidism occurs in about one-third of patients by 8 years after radioactive iodine. The nodule remains palpable in half and may grow in 10% of patients after radioactive iodine.

C. Toxic Multinodular Goiter: Hyperthyroidism caused by a toxic multinodular goiter may also be treated symptomatically with propranolol as in Graves' disease. This disorder usually affects older individuals, so radioactive iodine is ordinarily selected over surgery as definitive treatment. Thioureas do reverse hyperthyroidism, but there is a 95% recurrence rate after they are stopped. Older patients who are quite thyrotoxic are rendered nearly euthyroid with a thiourea, which is stopped about 3 days before radioactive iodine treatment. Meanwhile, the patient follows a low-iodine diet; this is done to enhance the thyroid gland's uptake of radioactive iodine, which may be relatively low in this condition

(compared to Graves' disease). Relatively high doses of radioactive iodine are usually required; recurrent thyrotoxicosis and hypothyroidism are common, so patients must be followed closely. Surgery is generally reserved for pressure symptoms or cosmetic indications. Patients are prepared for surgery as in Graves' disease (see above).

D. Subacute Thyroiditis: Patients with subacute thyroiditis are best treated symptomatically with propranolol. The condition subsides spontaneously within weeks to months. Thioureas are ineffective, since thyroid hormone production is actually low in this condition. Radioactive iodine is ineffective, since the thyroid's iodine uptake is low. Since periods of hypothyroidism may occur following the initial inflammatory episode, patients should have close clinical follow-up, with serum free thyroxine measurement when necessary. Prompt treatment of the transient hypothyroidism may reduce the incidence of recurrent thyroiditis. Pain can usually be managed with aspirin or other nonsteroidal anti-inflammatory agents.

E. Hashimoto's Thyroiditis: Rarely, patients develop hyperthyroidism as a result of release of stored thyroid hormone during severe Hashimoto's thyroiditis. The thyroperoxidase or thyroglobulin antibodies are usually high, but radioiodine uptake is low, thus distinguishing it from Graves' disease. This is especially common in postpartum women, in whom it may be transient. Treatment is with propranolol. Patients are followed carefully for the development of hypothyroidism and treated according to their thyroid status.

F. Treatment of Complications:

1. Graves' ophthalmopathy–Patients with ophthalmopathy may "flare" after radioactive iodide treatment, so they are prophylactically treated with prednisone for 4–6 weeks after treatment. For progressive exophthalmos, prednisone is given in doses of 40–60 mg/d, with dosage reduction over several weeks. Higher initial prednisone doses of 80–120 mg/d are used when there is optic nerve compression. Hypothyroidism and hyperthyroidism must be treated promptly. Other treatment options include low-dose radiation therapy to the extraocular muscles, avoiding the cornea and lens. Intravenous immunoglobulins may also be effective in doses of 1 g/kg for 2 consecutive days and repeated every 3 weeks for 3–4 months. For severe cases, orbital decompression surgery may save vision, though diplopia often persists postoperatively. General eye protective measures include wearing glasses to protect the protruding eye and taping the lids shut during sleep if corneal drying is a problem. Methylcellulose drops and gels ("artificial tears") may also help. Tarsorrhaphy or canthoplasty can frequently help protect the cornea and provide improved appearance.

2. Cardiac complications–

a. Sinus tachycardia or heart pounding is usually

present in thyrotoxicosis. Treatment consists of treating the thyrotoxicosis. A beta-blocker (as described above) such as propranolol is used in the interim unless there is an associated cardiomyopathy.

b. Atrial fibrillation is commonly seen in thyrotoxicosis and may be the presenting manifestation. Spontaneous conversion to normal sinus rhythm tends to occur with achievement of euthyroidism, but that likelihood decreases with age. Hyperthyroidism must be treated (see above). Other drugs may be required:

(1) Digoxin is used to slow a fast ventricular response; it must be used in larger than normal doses because of increased clearance and an increased number of cardiac sodium transport units requiring inhibition. Digoxin doses are reduced as hyperthyroidism is corrected.

(2) Beta-blockers may also reduce the ventricular rate, but they must be used with caution—particularly in patients with cardiomegaly or signs of heart failure—since their negative inotropic effect may precipitate congestive heart failure. Therefore, an initial trial of a short-duration beta-blocker should be considered, such as esmolol intravenously. If a beta-blocker is used, doses of digoxin must be reduced.

(3) Calcium channel blockers (or electrical cardioversion) are unlikely to convert atrial fibrillation to normal sinus rhythm while a patient is thyrotoxic. Their negative inotropic effect may precipitate congestive heart failure.

(4) Anticoagulation should be considered in order to prevent arterial thromboembolism in the following situations: left atrial enlargement on echocardiogram, global left ventricular dysfunction, recent congestive heart failure, hypertension, recurrent atrial fibrillation, or a history of previous thromboembolism. The doses of warfarin required in thyrotoxicosis are smaller than normal because of an accelerated plasma clearance of vitamin K-dependent clotting factors. Higher warfarin doses are usually required as hyperthyroidism subsides.

c. Heart failure due to thyrotoxicosis may be caused by extreme tachycardia, cardiomyopathy, or both. Very aggressive treatment of the hyperthyroidism is required in either case (see Thyroid Crisis, below). The tachycardia from atrial fibrillation is treated with digoxin as above. Intravenous furosemide is typically required. If tachycardia appears to be the main cause of the failure, beta-blockers are administered cautiously as described above.

Thyrotoxic dilated cardiomyopathy is caused by a direct toxic effect of prolonged excess thyroid hormone upon the heart and may occur at any age. Beta-blockers and calcium channel blockers are avoided. Emergency treatment may include afterload reduction, diuretics, digoxin, and other inotropic agents while the patient is being rendered euthyroid.

d. Apathetic hyperthyroidism may present with angina pectoris. Treatment is directed at reversing the hyperthyroidism as well as providing standard antianginal therapy. Coronary angioplasty or bypass grafting can often be avoided by prompt diagnosis and treatment.

3. Thyroid crisis or "storm"–This disorder, rarely seen today, is an extreme form of thyrotoxicosis that may occur with stressful illness, thyroid surgery, or radioactive iodine administration and is manifested by marked delirium, severe tachycardia, vomiting, diarrhea, dehydration, and, in many cases, very high fever. The mortality rate is high.

A thiourea drug is given (eg, propylthiouracil, 150–250 mg every 6 hours; or methimazole, 15–25 mg every 6 hours). Iodide is given 1 hour later as Lugol's solution (10 drops three times daily orally) or as sodium iodide (1 g intravenously slowly). Ipodate sodium (500 mg/d orally) can be helpful if begun 1 hour after the first dose of thiourea. Propranolol is given (cautiously in the presence of heart failure; see above) in a dosage of 0.5–2 mg intravenously every 4 hours or 20–120 mg orally every 6 hours. Hydrocortisone is usually given in doses of 50 mg every 6 hours, with rapid dosage reduction as the clinical situation improves. Aspirin is avoided since it displaces T_4 from thyroid-binding globulin, raising free T_4 serum levels. Definitive treatment with ^{131}I or surgery is delayed until the patient is euthyroid.

4. Hyperthyroidism and pregnancy–Diagnosis may be difficult, since normal pregnancy may be accompanied by tachycardia, warm skin, heat intolerance, increased sweating, and a palpable thyroid. Laboratory tests are helpful: Although the total T_4 is elevated in most pregnant women, values over 20 µg/dL are encountered only in hyperthyroidism. TSH is suppressed. The T_3 resin uptake, which is low in normal pregnancy because of high TBG concentration, is normal or high in thyrotoxic subjects. The free T_4 is clearly elevated. Pregnancy often has a beneficial effect upon the thyrotoxicosis of Graves' disease, with decreasing antibody titers and decreasing free T_4 levels as the pregnancy advances. Pregnant women with hyperthyroidism are treated with propylthiouracil in the smallest dose possible, permitting mild hyperthyroidism to occur since it is usually well tolerated. The drug does cross the placenta and rarely may induce TSH hypersecretion and thyroid enlargement in the fetus. Thyroid hormone administration to the mother does not prevent hypothyroidism in the fetus, since T_4 and T_3 do not freely cross the placenta. Fetal hypothyroidism is rare, since the mother's hyperthyroidism is often controlled with small daily doses of propylthiouracil (50–150 mg/d). If hyperthyroidism is severe, surgery may be necessary—best done during the second trimester.

Only minimal amounts of propylthiouracil are transferred to the maternal milk, so breast feeding is apt to be safe. This is less true for methimazole, which appears in higher concentrations in the milk.

5. Dermopathy–An uncommon complication

of Graves' disease, dermopathy is an abnormal thickening of the skin due to deposition of glycosaminoglycans. It is known as "pretibial myxedema" since it usually occurs in the anterior lower leg, sometimes also including the dorsum of the foot. Treatment involves application of a topical glucocorticoid (eg, fluocinolone) with nocturnal plastic occlusive dressings.

Prognosis

Graves' disease may subside spontaneously and may even result in spontaneous hypothyroidism. More commonly, however, it progresses. The ocular, cardiac, and psychologic complications often are more serious than the chronic wasting of tissues and may become irreversible even after treatment. Permanent hypoparathyroidism and vocal cord palsy are risks of surgical thyroidectomy. Recurrences are common following thiourea therapy but also occur after low-dose ^{131}I therapy or subtotal thyroidectomy. With adequate treatment and long-term follow-up, the results are good. Posttreatment hypothyroidism is common. It may occur within a few months or up to several years after radioactive iodine therapy or subtotal thyroidectomy. Malignant exophthalmos has a poor prognosis unless treated aggressively.

Kahaly G et al: Intravenous immunoglobulins vs. steroids in Graves' ophthalmopathy. Clin Exp Immunol 1996; 106:197.

Kennedy JW, Caro IF: The ABCs of managing hyperthyroidism in the older patient. Geriatrics 1996;51:22.

McIver B et al: Lack of effect of thyroxine in patients with Graves' hyperthyroidism who are treated with an antithyroid drug. N Engl J Med 1996;334:220.

Roti E, Minelli R, Salvi M: Clinical review 80: Management of hyperthyroidism and hypothyroidism in the pregnant woman. J Clin Endocrinol Metab 1996; 81:1679.

Singer PA et al: Treatment guidelines for patients with hyperthyroidism and hypothyroidism. Standards of Care Committee, American Thyroid Association. JAMA 1995;273:808.

Tietgens ST, Leinung MC: Thyroid storm. Med Clin North Am 1995;79:169.

Wartofsky L: Treatment options for hyperthyroidism. Hosp Pract 1996;31:69.

Yeatts RP: Graves' ophthalmopathy. Med Clin North Am 1996;79:195.

THYROID CANCER

Essentials of Diagnosis

- Painless swelling in region of thyroid.
- Thyroid function tests usually normal.
- Past history of irradiation to head and neck region may be present.
- Positive thyroid needle aspiration.

General Considerations (Table 26–8)

Although carcinoma of the thyroid is rarely associated with functional abnormalities, it enters into the differential diagnosis of all thyroid lesions. It is common in all age groups but especially in patients who have received any radiation therapy to the face, neck, or upper chest.

Papillary carcinoma is the most common and least aggressive thyroid malignancy. Pure papillary or mixed papillary-follicular carcinoma represents about 70% of all thyroid cancers. **Follicular carcinoma** represents about 15% of thyroid malignancies but is more likely to have distant metastases. Papillary and follicular thyroid carcinomas are classified as differentiated thyroid carcinoma. **Medullary thyroid carcinoma** represents less than 5% of thyroid cancers and tends to metastasize locally. Of all cases of medullary thyroid cancer, about one-third are sporadic, one-third are familial occurrences, and another third are associated with multiple endocrine neoplasia type II. **Anaplastic thyroid carcinoma** represents only about 1% of thyroid malignancies. Other malignancies involving the thyroid include lymphomas and metastases (especially melanoma, breast, renal, and bronchogenic carcinomas).

Table 26–8. Some characteristics of thyroid cancer.

	Papillary	Follicular	Medullary	Anaplastic
Incidence	Most common	Common	Uncommon	Rare
Average age	42	50	50	57
Females	70%	72%	56%	56%
Deaths due to thyroid cancer	6%	24%	33%	98%
Invasion: Juxtanodal	+++++	+	++++++	+++
Blood vessels	+	+++	+++	+++++
Distant sites	+	+++	++	++++
Resemblance to normal thyroid	+	+++	+	±
^{123}I uptake	+	++++	0	0
Degree of malignancy	+	++ to +++	+ to ++++	++++++++

Clinical Findings

A. Symptoms and Signs: The principal sign of thyroid carcinoma is a palpable, firm and nontender nodule in the thyroid area. Anterior cervical lymph nodes may be enlarged. Metastatic functioning differentiated thyroid carcinoma can sometimes secrete enough thyroid hormone to produce thyrotoxicosis. Medullary thyroid carcinoma frequently causes diarrhea, fatigue, and other symptoms. Signs of pressure or invasion of surrounding tissues are present in anaplastic or long-standing tumors with recurrent laryngeal nerve palsy or fixation of nodule to neighboring structures.

B. Laboratory Findings: With very few exceptions, all thyroid function tests are normal unless the cancer is associated with thyroiditis. Serum thyroid autoantibodies are sometimes found. Thyroglobulin levels are high in most metastatic papillary and follicular tumors.

In medullary carcinoma, calcitonin levels may be elevated, especially after stimulation by pentagastrin infusion. Since two-thirds of medullary carcinoma cases are familial or MEN 2, siblings and children of patients with medullary carcinoma are advised to have genetic testing to detect *RET* proto-oncogene mutations (see MEN 2a).

D. Imaging: Extensive bone and soft tissue metastases (some of which may take up radioiodine) may be demonstrable on radiographs or radioisotope scans. Medullary carcinoma tends to calcify; metastases may be detected with positron emission tomography (PET) scanning and MRI.

Differential Diagnosis (Table 26–9)

Lymphocytic thyroiditis, multinodular goiter, and colloid nodules can be distinguished from malignancies by FNA biopsy. However, FNA cannot distinguish benign follicular adenoma from follicular carcinoma.

Complications

The complications vary with the type of carcinoma. Papillary tumors invade local structures, such as lymph nodes; follicular tumors metastasize through the bloodstream; anaplastic carcinomas are highly aggressive, both locally and systemically. One-third of medullary carcinomas may secrete serotonin and prostaglandins, producing flushing and diarrhea, and may be complicated by the coexistence of pheochromocytomas or hyperparathyroidism. The complications of radical neck surgery often include permanent hypoparathyroidism and, less commonly, vocal cord palsy; permanent hypothyroidism is expected and should always be treated adequately.

Treatment

Surgical removal is the treatment of choice for thyroid carcinomas. Highly skilled surgeons can perform near-total thyroidectomies with a less than 1% rate of serious complications (hypoparathyroidism or recurrent laryngeal nerve damage). Other series have reported up to an 11% incidence of permanent hypoparathyroidism after total thyroidectomy. The incidence of hypoparathyroidism may be reduced if accidentally resected parathyroids are immediately autotransplanted into the neck muscles. The advantage of near-total thyroidectomy for differentiated thyroid carcinoma is that multicentric foci of carcinoma are more apt to be resected and there is then less normal thyroid tissue to compete with cancer for ^{131}I administered later for scans or treatment. Other surgeons prefer to do more conservative procedures. Neck muscle dissections are avoided for differentiated thyroid carcinoma. Thyroxine is prescribed in doses of 0.1–0.15 mg/d postoperatively. The dosage

Table 26–9. Clinical evaluation of thyroid nodules.[1]

Clinical Evidence	Low Index of Suspicion	High Index of Suspicion
History	Family history of goiter; residence in area of endemic goiter	Previous therapeutic radiation of head, neck, or chest; hoarseness
Physical characteristics	Older women; soft nodule; multinodular goiter	Young adults, men; solitary, firm nodule; vocal cord paralysis; enlarged lymph nodes; distant metastatic lesions
Serum factors	High titer of antithyroid antibody; hypothyroidism; hyperthyroidism	
Fine-needle aspiration biopsy	Colloid nodule or adenoma	Papillary carcinoma, follicular neoplasm, medullary or anaplastic carcinoma
Scanning techniques Uptake of ^{123}I Ultrasonogram Roentgenogram	"Hot" nodule Cystic lesion Shell-like calcification	"Cold" nodule Solid lesion Punctate calcification
Thyroxine therapy	Regression after 0.05–0.1 mg/d for 6 months or more	Increase in size

[1]Clinically suspicious nodules should be evaluated with fine-needle aspiration biopsy.

is adjusted to keep the serum TSH slightly suppressed during long-term follow-up of differentiated thyroid carcinoma.

About 2–4 months after surgery, a whole-body ^{131}I scan is performed: Iodide uptake is enhanced by stopping thyroxine for 6 weeks prior to the scan, thereby causing hypothyroidism; TSH then rises and stimulates iodide uptake. Iodine-containing foods and contrast media are avoided. Patients with "normal thyroid" remnants should receive 30–50 mCi of ^{131}I if their cancer was 1.5 cm or more in diameter. Patients with extrathyroidal uptake from metastatic disease are given larger doses of 100–150 mCi in the hospital. Another whole-body scan several days after ^{131}I treatment will sometimes detect metastases not visible on pretreatment scans.

False-positive ^{131}I scans are common with normal residual thyroid tissue and have been reported with Zenker's diverticulum, ovary, pleuropericardial cyst, gastric pull-up, and ^{131}I-contaminated bodily secretions. False-negative ^{131}I scans are common in early metastatic differentiated thyroid carcinoma but occur also in more advanced disease, including 14% of bone metastases.

Patients with differentiated thyroid carcinoma are followed clinically with neck palpation, physical examination, and chest x-ray and observed for thyrotoxicosis that might indicate functioning metastases. About 6–12 months after their postoperative scan, patients usually receive another ^{131}I whole body scan and serum thyroglobulin measurement while hypothyroid; these have a combined sensitivity of 95% for metastases. Serum thyroglobulin in a patient receiving thyroxine has a lower sensitivity of 62%.

Thallium-201 (^{201}Tl) scans may be useful for detecting metastatic differentiated thyroid carcinoma when ^{131}I scan is normal but serum thyroglobulin is elevated. MRI is useful in distinguishing recurrent thyroid tumor from postoperative changes.

Patients with papillary carcinoma should have at least two consecutively negative scans before they are considered in remission. Further scans may be required for patients with more aggressive follicular carcinomas, prior metastases, rising serum thyroglobulin, or other evidence of metastases. Patients with anaplastic thyroid carcinoma are treated with local resection and radiation. Thyroid lymphomas are best treated with external radiation therapy.

Patients with medullary thyroid carcinoma are treated surgically; medullary carcinoma does not take up ^{131}I.

Prognosis

The prognosis for differentiated thyroid carcinoma is directly related to the cell type and the age at diagnosis. Papillary carcinomas, when treated, are associated with a very low mortality rate, and life expectancy is nearly normal. Follicular carcinomas are generally more aggressive but still have a good prognosis, with a 1-year survival rate of nearly 100% and a 5-year survival rate of over 90%. Patients with lymph node and distant metastases have a lower survival rate. Patients with papillary and follicular carcinoma may be followed with serum thyroglobulin levels, which serve as a tumor marker after thyroidectomy. Hürthle cell carcinoma, a variant of follicular carcinoma, is more aggressive than papillary or follicular carcinoma. The prognosis is less favorable in patients presenting after age 45. Anaplastic carcinoma is locally aggressive; the 1-year survival rate is about 10%, and the 5-year rate is about 5%.

Medullary thyroid carcinoma has a variable prognosis. Patients with sporadic disease usually have lymph node involvement at the time of diagnosis, whereas distal metastases may not be noted for years; the 5-year survival is 82% and the 10-year survival rate is 69%. Familial cases or those associated with MEN 2a tend to be less aggressive; the 10-year survival rate is higher, in part due to earlier detection. Women with medullary thyroid carcinoma who are under age 40 also have a better prognosis.

Medullary thyroid carcinoma carries a worse prognosis if tumor tissue stains heavily for calcitonin or myelomonocytic antigen Leu-M1.

Serum calcitonin levels may be used as a tumor marker for medullary thyroid carcinoma. Serum CEA is also elevated in 70% of cases. Since these levels may remain elevated in patients with apparent complete resections and long-term remissions, it is a rising level of these markers (rather than the absolute level) that best indicates progression of the malignancy.

Clark OH: Predictors of thyroid tumor aggressiveness. West J Med 1996;165:131.

Moley JF: Medullary thyroid cancer. Surg Clin North Am 1995;75:405.

Singer PA et al: Treatment guidelines for patients with thyroid nodules and well-differentiated thyroid cancer. American Thyroid Association. Arch Intern Med 1996;156:2165.

Solomon BL, Wartofsky L, Burman KD: Current trends in the management of well differentiated papillary thyroid carcinoma. J Clin Endocrinol Metab 1996;81:333.

THYROIDITIS

Essentials of Diagnosis

- Swelling of thyroid gland, often causing pressure symptoms in acute and subacute forms; painless enlargement in chronic form.
- Thyroid function tests variable.
- Serum antithyroid antibody tests often positive.

General Considerations

Thyroiditis may be classified as follows: (1) chronic lymphocytic ("Hashimoto's") thyroiditis due to autoimmunity, (2) subacute thyroiditis, (3) suppurative thyroiditis, and (4) Riedel's thyroiditis.

Clinical Findings

A. Symptoms and Signs:

1. Hashimoto's thyroiditis—Hashimoto's thyroiditis—also called chronic lymphocytic thyroiditis—is the most common form of thyroiditis and probably the most common thyroid disorder in the USA. It tends to be familial and is six times more common in women than in men. Its frequency is increased by dietary iodine supplementation. Certain drugs (amiodarone, alpha interferon, interleukin-2, granulocyte-colony stimulating factor) frequently induce thyroid autoantibodies.

The thyroid gland is usually diffusely enlarged, firm, and finely nodular. One thyroid lobe may be asymmetrically enlarged, raising concerns about neoplasm. Although patients may complain of neck tightness, pain and tenderness are not usually present. About 10% of cases are atrophic, the gland being fibrotic, particularly in elderly women.

Patients with clinically evident disease usually have increased circulating levels of antithyroid peroxidase (95%) or antithyroglobulin (60%) antibodies.

Subclinical thyroiditis is very common, and in autopsy series about 40% of women and 20% of men exhibit focal thyroiditis. Low serum titers of antithyroid antibodies are found in 13% of women and 3% of men. However, only 1% of the population has antibody titers greater than 1:6400.

Postpartum thyroiditis is a form of autoimmune thyroiditis occurring soon after parturition and accompanied by transient hyperthyroidism followed by hypothyroidism; recovery of normal function occurs in most cases.

2. Subacute thyroiditis—This fairly common disorder—also called de Quervain's thyroiditis, granulomatous thyroiditis, giant cell thyroiditis—is an acute, usually painful enlargement of the thyroid gland, with dysphagia. The pain may radiate to the ears. If there is no pain, it is called "silent thyroiditis." The manifestations may persist for weeks or months and may be associated with signs of thyrotoxicosis and malaise. Young and middle-aged women are most commonly affected. Viral infection has been suggested as the cause. The erythrocyte sedimentation rate is markedly elevated, and antithyroid antibodies are low, which helps differentiate this form of thyroiditis from others. Radioactive iodine uptake is low, distinguishing this disorder from Graves' disease. Aspiration biopsy is usually not required but shows characteristic giant multinucleated cells.

3. Suppurative thyroiditis—Suppurative thyroiditis is a rare disorder causing severe pain, tenderness, redness, and fluctuation in the region of the thyroid gland. It is caused by pyogenic organisms, usually in the course of systemic infection.

4. Riedel's thyroiditis—Riedel's thyroiditis is also called chronic fibrous thyroiditis, Riedel's struma, woody thyroiditis, ligneous thyroiditis, and invasive thyroiditis. It usually causes hypothyroidism and may cause hypoparathyroidism as well. It is the rarest form of thyroiditis and is found most frequently in middle-aged or elderly women. Enlargement is often asymmetric; the gland is stony hard and adherent to the neck structures, causing signs of compression and invasion, including dysphagia, dyspnea, and hoarseness. It is usually a manifestation of a multifocal systemic fibrosis syndrome with retroperitoneal, mediastinal, and biliary tract sclerosis.

B. Laboratory Findings:
The T_4 and T_3 resin uptake are usually markedly elevated in acute and subacute thyroiditis and normal or low in the chronic forms. Radioiodine uptake is characteristically very low in the initial, hyperthyroid phase of subacute thyroiditis; it may be high with an uneven scan in chronic thyroiditis, with enlargement of the gland, and low in Riedel's struma. Thyroid autoantibodies are most commonly demonstrable in Hashimoto's thyroiditis but are also found in the other types. The serum TSH level is elevated if thyroid hormone is not elaborated in adequate amounts by the thyroid gland.

Complications

In the suppurative forms of thyroiditis, any of the complications of infection may occur; the subacute and chronic forms of the disease are complicated by the effects of pressure on the neck structures: dyspnea and, in Riedel's struma, vocal cord palsy. Hashimoto's thyroiditis may lead to hypothyroidism or transient thyrotoxicosis. Graves' disease may sometimes develop. Carcinoma or lymphoma may be associated with chronic thyroiditis and must be considered in the diagnosis of uneven painless enlargements that continue in spite of treatment. Hashimoto's thyroiditis may be associated with Addison's disease, hypoparathyroidism, diabetes, pernicious anemia, biliary cirrhosis, vitiligo, and other autoimmune conditions.

Differential Diagnosis

Thyroiditis must be considered in the differential diagnosis of all types of goiters, especially if enlargement is rapid. The very low radioiodine uptake in subacute thyroiditis with elevated T_4 and T_3 are helpful. Chronic thyroiditis, especially if the enlargement is uneven and if there is pressure on surrounding structures, may resemble carcinoma, and both disorders may be present in the same gland. The subacute and suppurative forms of thyroiditis may resemble any infectious process in or near the neck structures. Thyroid autoantibody tests have been of help in the diagnosis of chronic lymphocytic (Hashimoto's) thyroiditis, but the tests are not specific and may also be positive in patients with goiters, carcinoma, and thyrotoxicosis—though the titers are usually higher in Hashimoto's thyroiditis. Biopsy may be required for diagnosis.

Treatment

A. Suppurative Thyroiditis: Treatment is with antibiotics and with surgical drainage when fluctuation is marked.

B. Subacute Thyroiditis: All treatment is empiric and must be continued for several weeks. Recurrence is common. The drug of choice is aspirin, which relieves pain and inflammation. Thyrotoxic symptoms are treated with propranolol, 10–40 mg every 6 hours. Transient hypothyroidism is treated with thyroxine (0.05–0.1 mg/d) if symptomatic.

C. Hashimoto's Thyroiditis: Levothyroxine should be given in the usual doses (0.05–0.2 mg daily) if hypothyroidism or large goiter is present. If the thyroid gland is only minimally enlarged and the patient is euthyroid (with normal TSH levels), regular observation is in order, since hypothyroidism may develop subsequently—often years later. (See Hypothyroidism section.)

D. Riedel's Struma: Partial thyroidectomy is often required to relieve pressure; adhesions to surrounding structures make this a difficult operation.

Prognosis

The course of this group of diseases is quite variable. Spontaneous remissions and exacerbations are common in the subacute form, and therapy is nonspecific. The disease process may smolder for months. Hashimoto's thyroiditis is occasionally associated with other autoimmune disorders (diabetes mellitus, Addison's disease, pernicious anemia, etc). In general, however, patients with Hashimoto's thyroiditis have an excellent prognosis, since the condition either remains stable for years or progresses slowly to hypothyroidism, which is easily treated. Women with postpartum thyroiditis usually regain normal thyroid function.

Dayan CM, Daniels GH: Chronic autoimmune thyroiditis. N Engl J Med 1996;335:99.
Schubert MF, Kountz DS: Thyroiditis: A disease with many faces. Postgrad Med 1995;98:101.

THE PARATHYROIDS

The main physiologic effects of parathyroid hormone are as follows: (1) It increases the osteoclastic activity in bone, with increased delivery of calcium and phosphorus to the circulation; (2) it increases the renal tubular reabsorption of calcium in the glomerular filtrate; (3) it inhibits the net absorption of phosphate and bicarbonate by the renal tubule; and (4) it stimulates the synthesis of 1,25-dihydroxycholecalciferol by the kidney. All of these steps result in a net increase in the amount of ionized calcium circulating in plasma.

Vitamin D is a hormone with a complex set of actions and mechanism of synthesis. Cholecalciferol (vitamin D_3) is synthesized in the skin, under the influence of ultraviolet radiation, from 7-dehydrocholesterol. Two sequential hydroxylations are necessary for full biologic activity: The first one takes place in the liver—to 25-hydroxycholecalciferol ($25[OH]D_3$)—and the second one in the kidney, resulting in the formation of the most potent biologic metabolite of vitamin D, 1,25-dihydroxycholecalciferol ($1,25[OH]_2D_3$). The main action of vitamin D is the acceleration of calcium and phosphate absorption in the intestine.

HYPOPARATHYROIDISM & PSEUDOHYPOPARATHYROIDISM

Essentials of Diagnosis

- Tetany, carpopedal spasms, tingling of lips and hands, muscle and abdominal cramps, psychologic changes.
- Positive Chvostek's sign and Trousseau's phenomenon; defective nails and teeth; cataracts.
- Serum calcium low; serum phosphate high; alkaline phosphatase normal; urine calcium excretion reduced.
- Serum magnesium may be low.

General Considerations

Hypoparathyroidism is most commonly seen following thyroidectomy, when it is usually transient but may be permanent. It may also occur after surgical removal of a parathyroid adenoma for primary hyperparathyroidism due to suppression of the remaining normal parathyroids and accelerated remineralization of the skeleton (hungry bone syndrome).

Hypoparathyroidism may be autoimmune (rarely) and occur sporadically or as part of polyglandular autoimmune syndrome (PGA type I). This is also known as autoimmune polyendocrinopathy-candidiasis-ectodermal dystrophy (APECED). PGA type I presents in childhood with at least two of the following: candidiasis, hypoparathyroidism, and Addison's disease. Patients may also develop cataracts, uveitis, alopecia, vitiligo, or immune thyroid disease.

Parathyroid deficiency can also occur from dysembryogenesis (DiGeorge's syndrome) or as a result of damage from heavy metals (Wilson's disease, transfusion hemosiderosis, hemochromatosis), granulomas, metastatic tumors, or infection.

Functional hypoparathyroidism may also occur as

a result of magnesium deficiency (malabsorption, chronic alcoholism), which prevents the secretion of PTH. Correction of hypomagnesemia results in rapid disappearance of the condition. Hypoparathyroidism may rarely occur after neck irradiation.

Pseudohypoparathyroidism is a genetic defect of tissue resistance to PTH associated with short stature, round face, obesity, short fourth metacarpals and metatarsals, ectopic bone formation, and mental retardation. Patients without hypocalcemia but sharing the phenotypic abnormalities are said to have "pseudopseudohypoparathyroidism."

Clinical Findings

A. Symptoms and Signs: Acute hypoparathyroidism causes tetany, with muscle cramps, irritability, carpopedal spasm, and convulsions; tingling of the circumoral area, hands, and feet is almost always present. Symptoms of the chronic disease are lethargy, personality changes, anxiety state, blurring of vision due to cataracts, and mental retardation.

Chvostek's sign (facial muscle contraction on tapping the facial nerve in front of the ear) is positive, and Trousseau's phenomenon (carpal spasm after application of a cuff) is present. Cataracts may occur; the nails may be thin and brittle; the skin is dry and scaly, at times with fungus infection (candidiasis), and there may be loss of hair (eyebrows); deep tendon reflexes may be hyperactive. Papilledema and elevated cerebrospinal fluid pressure are occasionally seen. Teeth may be defective if the onset of the disease occurs in childhood.

B. Laboratory Findings: Serum calcium is largely bound to albumin. Therefore, ionized calcium should be determined, or the serum calcium level should be corrected for serum albumin level as follows:

$$\text{"Corrected" serum Ca}^{2+} = \text{Serum Ca}^{2+} \text{ mg/dL} + (0.8 \times [4.0 - \text{Albumin g/dL}])$$

Serum calcium is low, serum phosphate high, urinary calcium low, and alkaline phosphatase normal. Parathyroid hormone levels are low. Serum magnesium should be determined since hypomagnesemia frequently accompanies hypocalcemia and may exacerbate symptoms and decrease parathyroid function.

C. Imaging: Radiographs or CT scans of the skull may show basal ganglia calcifications; the bones may be denser than normal.

D. Other Examinations: Slit-lamp examination may show early posterior lenticular cataract formation. The ECG shows prolonged QT intervals and T wave abnormalities.

Complications

Acute tetany with stridor, especially if associated with vocal cord palsy, may lead to respiratory obstruction requiring tracheostomy. The complications of chronic hypoparathyroidism depend largely upon the duration of the disease. There may be associated autoimmunity causing sprue syndrome, pernicious anemia, or Addison's disease. In long-standing cases, cataract formation and calcification of the basal ganglia are seen. Occasionally, parkinsonian symptoms develop. Ossification of the paravertebral ligaments may occur with nerve root compression; surgical decompression may be required. Seizures are common in untreated patients. Overtreatment with vitamin D and calcium may produce nephrocalcinosis and impairment of renal function.

Differential Diagnosis

The symptoms of hypocalcemic tetany may be confused with paresthesias, muscle cramps, or tetany due to respiratory alkalosis, in which the serum calcium is normal. In fact, hyperventilation tends to accentuate hypocalcemic symptoms.

Hypocalcemia is frequently seen in patients with hypoalbuminemia; serum levels of ionized calcium are normal.

Hypocalcemia may also be due to malabsorption of calcium, magnesium, or vitamin D; patients do not always have diarrhea. It may also be caused by certain drugs such as loop diuretics, plicamycin, phenytoin, alendronate, and foscarnet. In addition, hypocalcemia may be seen in cases of rapid intravascular volume expansion or due to chelation from transfusions of large volumes of citrated blood. Transient hypocalcemia is also frequently seen following parathyroidectomy for hyperparathyroidism. It is also observed in patients with acute pancreatitis. Some patients with certain osteoblastic metastatic carcinomas (especially breast, prostate) may develop hypocalcemia instead of the expected hypercalcemia. Hypocalcemia with hyperphosphatemia (simulating hypoparathyroidism) is seen in azotemia but may also be caused by large doses of intravenous, oral, or rectal phosphate preparations and by chemotherapy of responsive lymphomas or leukemias.

Hypocalcemia with hypercalciuria may be due to a familial syndrome involving a mutation in the calcium-sensing receptor; such patients have levels of serum PTH that are in the normal range, distinguishing it from hypoparathyroidism. It is transmitted as an autosomal dominant. Such patients are hypercalciuric; treatment with calcium and vitamin D may cause nephrocalcinosis.

At times hypoparathyroidism is misdiagnosed as idiopathic epilepsy, choreoathetosis, or brain tumor (on the basis of brain calcifications, convulsions, choked disks) or, more rarely, as "asthma" (on the basis of stridor and dyspnea).

Treatment

A. Emergency Treatment for Acute Attack

(Hypoparathyroid Tetany): This usually occurs after surgery and requires immediate treatment.

1. Be sure an adequate airway is present.

2. Calcium gluconate, 10–20 mL of 10% solution intravenously, may be given *slowly* until tetany ceases. Ten to 50 mL of 10% calcium gluconate may be added to 1 L of 5% glucose in water or saline and administered by slow intravenous drip. The rate should be so adjusted that the serum calcium is maintained between 8 and 9 mg/dL.

3. Oral calcium–Calcium salts should be given orally as soon as possible to supply 1–2 g of calcium daily. Calcium carbonate (40% calcium) is effective and is the calcium salt of choice. Tablets containing 250 mg or 500 mg of calcium are well tolerated. Liquid calcium carbonate (Titralac), 400 mg/5 mL, may be especially useful. The dosage is 1–3 g calcium daily. Calcium citrate contains 21% calcium, but a higher proportion is absorbed with less gastrointestinal intolerance.

4. Vitamin D preparations–(Table 26–10.) Therapy should be started as soon as oral calcium is begun. The treatment of choice for chronic hypoparathyroidism is vitamin D_2 (ergocalciferol), which has been used successfully for many years. The usual dose ranges from 25,000 to 150,000 units/d. It is a slow-acting preparation, and if toxicity develops, hypercalcemia—treatable with hydration and prednisone—may persist for weeks after it is discontinued. Ergocalciferol gives a more stable serum calcium level than do the shorter-acting preparations.

Dihydrotachysterol is faster in onset of action and is three times more potent than ergocalciferol. The usual daily maintenance dose is 0.125–1 mg/d. It is more expensive than vitamin D_2.

The active metabolite of vitamin D, 1,25-dihydroxycholecalciferol (calcitriol), has a very rapid onset of action, and if toxicity develops it is not long-lasting. Because of its very high cost, it has been used primarily in the treatment of acute hypocalcemia in doses ranging from 0.25 to 4 µg/d rather than for chronic therapy.

Calcifediol (25-hydroxyvitamin D_3) is another option for treatment which has an intermediate onset and duration of action; the usual starting dose is 20 µg/d orally.

5. Magnesium–If hypomagnesemia is present (chronic alcoholism, malnutrition, renal loss, drugs such as cisplatin, etc), it must be corrected in order to treat the resulting hypocalcemia. Acutely, $MgSO_4$ is given intravenously, 1–2 g every 6 hours. Chronic magnesium replacement may be given as magnesium oxide tablets (600 mg), one or two per day, or as a combined magnesium and calcium preparation (Dolomite, others).

B. Maintenance Treatment: The goal should be to maintain the serum calcium in a slightly low but asymptomatic range (8–8.6 mg/dL). This will minimize the hypercalciuria that would otherwise occur and provides a margin of safety against overdosage and hypercalcemia, which may produce permanent damage to renal function. Calcium supplementation (1–2 g/d) is continued, and a vitamin D preparation (see above) is given. Monitoring of serum calcium at regular intervals (at least every 3 months) is mandatory. One should also monitor urine calcium with "spot" urine determinations and keep the level below 30 mg/dL if possible.

Caution: Phenothiazine drugs should be administered with caution to hypocalcemic patients, since they may precipitate extrapyramidal symptoms. Furosemide should be avoided, since it may enhance hypocalcemia.

Prognosis

The outlook is good if the diagnosis is made promptly and treatment instituted. Any dental changes, cataracts, and brain calcifications are permanent. Periodic blood chemical evaluation is required, since changes in calcium levels may call for modification of the treatment schedule. Hypercalcemia that develops in patients with seemingly stable, treated hypoparathyroidism may be a presenting sign of Addison's disease.

Table 26–10. Vitamin D preparations used in the treatment of hypoparathyroidism.[1]

	Potency	How Supplied	Daily Dose (Range)	Time Required for Toxic Effects to Subside
Ergocalciferol (ergosterol, vitamin D_2)	40,000 USP units/mg	Capsules of 25,000 and 50,000 units; solution, 8,000 units/mL	25,000–200,000 units	6–18 weeks
Dihydrotachysterol (Hytakerol)	120,000 USP units/mg	Tablets of 0.125, 0.2, and 0.4 mg	0.2–1 mg	1–3 weeks
Calcifediol (Calderol)	. . .	Capsules of 20 and 50 µg	20–200 µg	3–6 weeks
Calcitriol (Rocaltrol)	. . .	Capsules of 0.25 and 0.5 µg	0.25–4 µg	$1/2$–2 weeks

[1]Reproduced, with permission, from Greenspan FS, Baxter JD (editors): *Basic & Clinical Endocrinology*, 4th ed. Appleton & Lange, 1994.

Guise TA, Mundy GR: Clinical review 69: Evaluation of hypocalcemia in children and adults. J Clin Endocrinol Metab 1995;80:1473.

Olson JA Jr et al: Parathyroid autotransplantation during thyroidectomy. Results of long-term follow-up. Ann Surg 1996;223:472.

Pearce SH et al: A familial syndrome of hypocalcemia with hypercalciuria due to mutations in the calcium-sensing receptor. N Engl J Med 1996;335:1115. (Mutations in the calcium-sensing receptor are associated with a familial syndrome of hypocalcemia with hypercalciuria that needs to be distinguished from hypoparathyroidism.)

Tohme JF, Blezikian JP: Hypocalcemic emergencies. Endocrinol Metab Clin North Am 1993;22:363.

HYPERPARATHYROIDISM

Essentials of Diagnosis

- Patients frequently asymptomatic, detected by screening.
- Renal stones, polyuria, hypertension, constipation, fatigue, mental changes.
- Bone pain; rarely, cystic lesions and pathologic fractures.
- Serum and urine calcium elevated; urine phosphate high with low to normal serum phosphate; alkaline phosphatase normal to elevated.
- Elevated parathyroid hormone.

General Considerations

Primary hyperparathyroidism is an increasingly recognized disorder, present in up to 0.1% of adult patients examined. It can be seen at any age but is more frequent in persons over the age of 50 and is three times more common in women than in men.

The disease is caused by hypersecretion of parathyroid hormone, usually by a parathyroid adenoma, and less commonly by hyperplasia or carcinoma (rare). The pathologic classification of parathyroid adenoma versus hyperplasia is difficult when examining an isolated gland.

Parathyroid adenomas or hyperplasia can be familial (about 5%) and may be part of multiple endocrine neoplasia types 1, 2a, and 2b. (See Table 26–16.)

Hyperparathyroidism causes excessive excretion of calcium and phosphate by the kidneys; this can result in calculus formation within the urinary tract. At least 5% of renal stones are associated with this disease. Diffuse parenchymal calcification (nephrocalcinosis) is seen less commonly. Chronic bone resorption induced by excessive PTH in the circulation may produce diffuse demineralization, pathologic fractures, or cystic bone lesions throughout the skeleton ("osteitis fibrosa cystica").

In chronic renal failure, hyperphosphatemia and decreased renal production of $1,25(OH)_2D_3$ initially produce a decrease in ionized calcium. The parathyroid glands are stimulated (secondary hyperparathyroidism) and may enlarge, becoming autonomous (tertiary hyperparathyroidism). The bone disease seen in this setting is known as "renal osteodystrophy." Diabetics seem somewhat less prone to develop this syndrome. Hypercalcemia often occurs after renal transplant but usually subsides spontaneously.

Parathyroid carcinoma is an unusual cause of hyperparathyroidism but is more common in patients with severe hypercalcemia.

Clinical Findings

A. Symptoms and Signs: Hypercalcemia is usually discovered accidentally by blood "biochempanel" screening. Most patients are asymptomatic. Parathyroid adenomas are usually so small and deeply located in the neck that they are almost never palpable; when a mass is palpated, it usually turns out to be an incidental thyroid nodule.

Symptomatic patients are said to have problems with "bones, stones, abdominal groans, psychic moans, with fatigue overtones." The manifestations are more formally categorized as follows:

1. Skeletal manifestations–Significant bone disease is found in about 1.4% of patients with hyperparathyroidism; osteitis fibrosa cystica may cause "brown tumors" and cysts of the jaw or pathologic fractures. More commonly, patients have bone pain, arthralgias, and diminished bone density, particularly of cortical bone (eg, distal radius or hip).

2. Urinary tract manifestations–Polyuria and polydipsia may be present and are due to hypercalcemia. Calcium-containing kidney stones are reported in about 18% of those with newly discovered primary hyperparathyroidism. Nephrocalcinosis and renal failure can occur.

3. Manifestations of hypercalcemia–Mild hypercalcemia is often asymptomatic. In more severe cases, thirst, anorexia, nausea, and vomiting are present. Constipation, asthenia, anemia, weight loss, and hypertension are commonly found. Some patients present primarily with neuromuscular disorders such as muscle weakness, easy fatigability, or paresthesias. Depression, intellectual weariness, and increased sleep requirement are common. Pruritus and psychosis or even coma may accompany severe hypercalcemia. Calcium may precipitate in the corneas ("band keratopathy") or soft tissue (calciphylaxis).

B. Laboratory Findings: The hallmark of primary hyperparathyroidism is hypercalcemia (serum calcium > 10.5 mg/dL when corrected for serum albumin; see above). In hyperproteinemic states, the total serum calcium may be elevated but the ionized fraction is normal, whereas in primary hyperparathyroidism the ionized calcium is almost always elevated. The serum phosphate is often low (< 2.5 mg/dL). The urine calcium excretion may be high or normal (averaging 250 mg/g creatinine) but it is usually low for the degree of hypercalcemia. There is an excessive loss of phosphate in the urine in the presence of low (25% of cases) to low normal serum phosphate. (In secondary hyperparathyroidism due to renal failure, the serum phosphate is high.) The alkaline phosphatase is elevated only if bone disease is present. The plasma chloride and uric acid levels may be elevated. Elevated levels of parathyroid hormone confirm the diagnosis. The best immunoassay recognizes the intact molecule at two different sites—the amino terminal and the carboxyl terminal ends—with two different antibodies. This assay, known as *immunoradiometric assay* (IRMA), is specific and sensitive, making it easier to distinguish primary hyperparathyroidism from other causes of hypercalcemia.

C. Imaging: Unguided neck exploration by an experienced parathyroid surgeon is about equally successful at identifying a parathyroid adenoma as the best localization procedures. Localizing preoperative imaging may be reserved for patients with prior neck surgery. In such cases, performing two different types of studies reduces the chance of false positives. Since the gland or glands affected are rarely larger than 1.5 cm in diameter (and usually *much* smaller), preoperative imaging techniques are often unsuccessful. Imaging techniques include ultrasonography, CT, MRI, Tc-99m sestamibi, and thallium/technetium subtraction studies. The accuracy of a given technique depends upon the available equipment and technical personnel. Angiography and selective venous sampling for PTH are rarely required. Unsuspected small intrathyroidal nodules are discovered incidentally in nearly half of patients with hyperparathyroidism who have imaging with ultrasound or MRI.

Bone x-rays are usually normal and not required to make the diagnosis of hyperparathyroidism. There may be demineralization, subperiosteal resorption of bone (especially in the radial aspects of the fingers), or loss of the lamina dura of the teeth. There may be cysts throughout the skeleton, mottling of the skull ("salt-and-pepper appearance"), or pathologic fractures. Articular cartilage calcification (chondrocalcinosis) is sometimes found.

Patients with renal osteodystrophy may have ectopic calcifications around joints or in soft tissue. Such patients may exhibit x-ray changes of osteopenia, osteitis fibrosa, or osteosclerosis, alone or in combination. Osteosclerosis of the vertebral bodies is known as "rugger jersey spine."

Complications

Pathologic fractures are more common, especially in women. Urinary tract infection due to stone and obstruction may lead to renal failure and uremia. If the serum calcium level rises rapidly, clouding of sensorium, renal failure, and rapid precipitation of calcium throughout the soft tissues may occur. Peptic ulcer and pancreatitis may be intractable before surgery. Insulinomas or gastrinomas may be associated, as well as pituitary tumors (multiple endocrine neoplasia type I). Pseudogout may complicate hyperparathyroidism both before and after surgical removal of tumors. Hypercalcemia during gestation produces neonatal hypocalcemia.

In secondary hyperparathyroidism due to renal failure, high serum calcium and phosphate levels may cause disseminated calcification in the skin, soft tissues, and arteries (calciphylaxis); this can result in painful ischemic necrosis of skin and gangrene, cardiac arrhythmias, and respiratory failure. The actual serum levels of calcium and phosphate have not correlated well with calciphylaxis, but a calcium (mg/dL) × phosphate (mg/dL) product over 70 is usually present.

Differential Diagnosis

(1) Artifact: A report of hypercalcemia may be due to laboratory error or excess tourniquet time and should always be repeated. Hypercalcemia may be due to high serum protein concentrations; serum calcium should be corrected for albumin (see above). It may also be seen with dehydration.

(2) Hypercalcemia of malignancy: Many malignant tumors (breast, lung, pancreas, uterus, hypernephroma, etc) can produce hypercalcemia. In some cases (breast carcinoma especially), bony metastases are present. In others, no metastases to bone can be demonstrated. Most of these tumors secrete parathyroid hormone-related protein, which has tertiary structural homologies to PTH and causes bone resorption and hypercalcemia similar to those of parathyroid hormone. The clinical features of the hypercalcemia of cancer can closely simulate hyperparathyroidism. Serum phosphate is often low, but the plasma level of PTH by IRMA is *low*.

Multiple myeloma is a common cause of hypercalcemia in the older population. Many other hematologic cancers such as monocytic leukemia, T cell leukemia and lymphoma, Burkitt's lymphoma, etc, have also been associated with hypercalcemia. Multiple myeloma causes renal dysfunction; resultant increased levels of C-terminal PTH may cause it to be confused with hyperparathyroidism if a C-terminal PTH assay is used. Serum protein and urine electrophoresis and bone marrow biopsy establish the diagnosis.

(3) Sarcoidosis and other granulomatous disorders: Macrophages and perhaps other cells present in granulomatous tissue have the ability to synthesize 1,25-dihydroxycholecalciferol. Hypercalcemia has been reported in patients with tuberculosis, sarcoidosis, berylliosis, histoplasmosis, coccidioidomycosis, leprosy, and even foreign-body granuloma. Increased intestinal calcium absorption and hypercalciuria are more common than hypercalcemia. Serum levels of 1,25-dihydroxycholecalciferol are elevated.

(4) Calcium or vitamin D ingestion: Ingestion

of large amounts of calcium (usually as an antacid) or vitamin D can cause hypercalcemia, which is reversible following its cessation. If it persists, the possibility of associated hyperparathyroidism should be strongly considered.

In vitamin D intoxication, patients may take large amounts of vitamin D for unclear reasons, so a check of all medications is important. Hypercalcemia may persist for several weeks. Serum levels of 25-hydroxycholecalciferol are helpful to confirm the diagnosis. A brief course of glucocorticoid therapy may be necessary if hypercalcemia is severe.

(5) Familial hypocalciuric hypercalcemia: This benign condition can be easily mistaken for mild hyperparathyroidism. It is an autosomal dominant inherited disorder characterized by hypocalciuria (usually < 50 mg/24 h), variable hypermagnesemia, and normal or minimally elevated levels of PTH. These patients do not normalize their hypercalcemia after subtotal parathyroid removal and should not be subjected to surgery. The condition has an excellent prognosis and is easily diagnosed with family history and urinary calcium clearance determination.

(6) Adrenal insufficiency: Hypercalcemia is common in untreated Addison's disease. The mechanism is unclear, but a partial explanation relates to the hyperproteinemia often found in a dehydrated, hemoconcentrated addisonian patient, so that it is the total rather than the ionized calcium that is elevated.

(7) Hyperthyroidism: Increased bone turnover is a feature of thyrotoxicosis. Mild hypercalcemia may also be present.

(8) Other causes: Other causes of hypercalcemia are shown in Table 21–9. Modest hypercalcemia is also occasionally seen in patients taking thiazide diuretics or lithium; such patients may have an inappropriately nonsuppressed PTH level in the face of hypercalcemia. Prolonged immobilization at bed rest may also cause hypercalcemia, especially in children, adolescents, and patients with extensive Paget's disease of bone. Mild hypercalcemia is also commonly seen in acutely ill patients being treated in intensive care units.

Treatment

A. Surgical Measures: Parathyroidectomy is recommended for patients with symptomatic hyperparathyroidism, kidney stones, or bone disease. Seemingly asymptomatic patients may be surgical candidates for other reasons such as (1) serum calcium 1 mg/dL above the upper limit of normal with urine calcium excretion > 50 mg/24 h; (2) urine calcium excretion over 400 mg/24 h; (3) cortical bone density ≥ 2 SD below normal; (4) relative youth (under age 50–60 years); or (5) difficulty ensuring medical follow-up. Removal of a parathyroid adenoma usually results in cure. Multiple tumors occur, so bilateral neck exploration is usually advisable. Parathyroid glands are not uncommonly supernumerary (five

or more) or ectopic (eg, intrathyroidal, carotid sheath, mediastinum).

Parathyroid hyperplasia, commonly seen with chronic renal failure, is best treated with subtotal parathyroidectomy, leaving a metallic clip to mark the location of residual parathyroid tissue.

After surgery, the patient may develop paresthesias or even tetany (usually transient) as a result of rapid fall of blood calcium even though the calcium level may fall only to the normal range. Therefore, frequent postoperative monitoring of serum calcium and albumin is recommended. Serum PTH levels drawn immediately postoperatively are not as useful and may be misleading. Transient thyrotoxicosis may also occur postoperatively.

Caution: Postoperative hypocalcemia may require large amounts of calcium and short-acting vitamin D. Additional magnesium salts may be required postoperatively.

B. Medical Measures: Hypercalcemia is treated with a large fluid intake unless contraindicated. Severe hypercalcemia requires hospitalization and intensive hydration with intravenous saline. (See Chapter 21.)

Bisphosphonates such as pamidronate and alendronate are potent inhibitors of bone resorption and can temporarily treat the hypercalcemia of hyperparathyroidism, malignancy, or immobilization. They may relieve bone pain as with patients with metastatic breast or prostate cancer. Pamidronate in doses of 30–90 mg (in 0.9% saline) is administered intravenously over 4–12 hours. Pamidronate causes a gradual decline in serum calcium over several days that may last for weeks to months. Other bisphosphonates such as alendronate may be effective orally, but their long-term use for chronic hyperparathyroidism has not been studied. Such bisphosphonates are used generally for patients with severe hyperparathyroidism in preparation for surgery.

Patients with mild, asymptomatic hyperparathyroidism are often followed closely medically. Such patients are advised to keep active, avoid immobilization, and drink adequate fluids. They need to avoid thiazide diuretics, large doses of vitamins D and A, and calcium-containing antacids or supplements. Serum calcium and albumin are checked about twice yearly, renal function and urine calcium once yearly, and bone density every 1–2 years.

Estrogen replacement is given to postmenopausal women. Digitalis preparations are avoided, since patients with hypercalcemia are sensitive to its toxic effects. Propranolol may be useful for preventing the adverse cardiac effects of hypercalcemia. Glucocorticoid therapy is ineffective for treating hypercalcemia.

Renal osteodystrophy is caused by secondary hyperthyroidism during renal failure; it may be prevented by avoiding hyperphosphatemia. Calcium acetate is given with meals to bind phosphate. Calcitriol, given orally or intravenously after dialysis, also suppresses parathyroid hyperplasia of renal failure (see Chapter 22).

Prognosis

Completely asymptomatic patients with mild hypercalcemia may be treated medically as outlined above. The disease is usually a chronic progressive one unless surgically cured. There are at times unexplained exacerbations and partial remissions.

Spontaneous cure due to necrosis of the tumor has been reported but is exceedingly rare. The prognosis is directly related to the degree of renal impairment. The bones, in spite of severe cyst formation, deformity, and fracture, will heal if a parathyroid tumor is successfully removed. The presence of pancreatitis increases the mortality rate. Significant renal damage may progress even after removal of an adenoma. Parathyroid carcinoma tends to invade local structures and may sometimes metastasize; repeat surgical resections can prolong life. Aggressive surgical and medical management of parathyroid carcinoma can result in an 85% 5-year survival rate and a 57% 10-year survival rate.

Deftos LJ: Hypercalcemia: Mechanisms, differential diagnosis, and remedies. Postgrad Med 1996;100:119.

Hakaim AG, Esselsyn CB Jr: Parathyroid carcinoma: Fifty-year experience at the Cleveland Clinic Foundation. Cleve Clin J Med 1993;60:331.

Mitchell BK et al: Localization studies in patients with hyperparathyroidism. Surg Clin North Am 1995;75:483.

Silverberg SJ, Bilezikian JP: Evaluation and management of primary hyperparathyroidism. J Clin Endocrinol Metab 1996;81:2036.

Strewler GJ: Indications for surgery in patients with minimally symptomatic primary hyperparathyroidism. Surg Clin North Am 1995;75:439.

METABOLIC BONE DISEASE

The term "metabolic bone disease" denotes those conditions producing diffusely decreased bone density (osteopenia) and diminished bone strength. It is categorized by histologic appearance: osteoporosis (common; bone matrix and mineral both decreased) and osteomalacia (unusual; bone matrix intact, mineral decreased).

OSTEOPOROSIS

Essentials of Diagnosis

- Asymptomatic to severe backache.
- Spontaneous fractures often discovered incidentally on radiography; loss of height.

- Serum parathyroid hormone, $25(OH)D_2$, calcium, phosphorus, and alkaline phosphatase usually normal.
- Demineralization, especially of spine, hip, and pelvis.

General Considerations

Osteoporosis is the most common metabolic bone disease in the USA and the cause of hundreds of thousands of fractures every year. The morbidity and indirect mortality rates are very high. Since the usual form of the disease is clinically evident in middle life and beyond and since women are more frequently affected than men, it may be referred to as "postmenopausal" osteoporosis. It is characterized by a decrease in the amount of bone present to a level below which it is capable of maintaining the structural integrity of the skeleton. The rate of bone formation is often normal, whereas the rate of bone resorption is increased. There is a greater loss of trabecular bone than compact bone, accounting for the primary features of the disease, ie, crush fractures of vertebrae, fractures of the neck of the femur, and fractures of the distal end of the radius. Whatever bone is present is normally mineralized.

Osteogenesis imperfecta (see Chapter 20) is caused by a major mutation in the gene encoding for type I collagen, the major collagen constituent of bone. This causes severe osteoporosis. Spontaneous fractures occur in utero or during childhood. Less severe mutations in the type I collagen gene are common, resulting in collagen disarray and predisposing to hypogonadal (eg, menopausal), or idiopathic osteoporosis.

Etiology

The causes of osteoporosis are listed in Table 26–11.

Clinical Findings

A. Symptoms and Signs: Osteoporosis is usually asymptomatic until fractures occur. It may present as backache of varying degrees of severity or as a spontaneous fracture or collapse of a vertebra. Loss of height is common.

B. Laboratory Findings: Serum calcium, phosphate, and PTH are normal. The alkaline phosphatase is usually normal but may be slightly elevated, especially following a fracture.

C. Imaging: The principal areas of demineralization are the spine and pelvis, especially in the femoral neck and head; demineralization is less marked in the skull and extremities. Compression of vertebrae is common. Bone densitometry permits screening for osteopenia in high-risk individuals and allows assessment of response to therapy. CT densitometry of vertebrae is highly accurate and reproducible. Dual energy x-ray absorptiometry (DEXA)

Table 26–11. Etiologic classification of osteoporosis.[1,2]

Hormone deficiency	**Genetic disorders**
Estrogen (women)	Type I collagen mutations
Androgen (men)	Osteogenesis imperfecta
Hormone excess	Adult osteoporosis
Cushing's syndrome or glucocorticoid	Ehlers-Danlos syndrome
administration	Marfan's syndrome
Thyrotoxicosis	Homocystinuria
Hyperparathyroidism	**Miscellaneous**
Excessive vitamin D administration	Diabetes mellitus
Immobilization	Protein-calorie malnutrition
Tobacco	Liver disease
Malignancy, especially multiple myeloma	Rheumatoid arthritis
Idiopathic or geriatric	Heparin therapy
	Vitamin C deficiency
	Copper deficiency
	Juvenile osteoporosis
	Systemic mastocytosis
	Alcoholism-induced

[1]Modified, with permission, from Fitzgerald PA: *Handbook of Clinical Endocrinology*, 2nd ed. Appleton & Lange, 1992.
[2]See Table 26–12 for causes of osteomalacia.

can determine the density of any bone, is quite accurate, and delivers negligible radiation.

Differential Diagnosis

Osteoporosis has many causes (Table 26–11). Additionally, osteopenia and fractures can be caused by osteomalacia (see below) and bone marrow neoplasia such as myeloma or metastatic bone disease. Bone scintiscans, MRI, and biopsy may be required, since these conditions may coexist.

Treatment

A. Specific Measures: Several treatment options are available, so a regimen is tailored to each patient.

1. Sex hormones–Women with hypogonadism should be considered for replacement estrogen (see Hormone Replacement Therapy).

2. Bisphosphonates–These agents inhibit osteoclast-induced bone resorption. They should be given with 6–8 oz of water at least one-half hour before breakfast; calcium, coffee, and orange juice reduce absorption. Alendronate, one 10 mg tablet daily, effectively increases bone density and reduces fracture rates by about 50%. Alendronate can cause esophagitis. It is contraindicated for patients with esophageal strictures or achalasia and must be used with caution in those with a history of hiatal hernia, dysphagia, gastritis, or peptic ulcers. Etidronate (200 mg tablets) appears to be somewhat less effective but is less expensive when given cyclically in a dose of 400 mg daily for 2 weeks every 3 months. For patients receiving long-term pharmacologic doses of glucocorticoids, prophylactic treatment with alendronate or cycled etidronate may reduce osteoporosis.

3. Calcitonin–A nasal spray (Miacalcin) is available that contains 2200 units/mL in 2 mL me-

tered-dose bottles. The usual dose is one puff (0.09 mL, 200 IU) once daily, alternating nostrils. Nasal administration causes significantly less nausea and flushing than the parenteral route. However, nasal symptoms such as rhinitis and epistaxis occur commonly; other less common adverse reactions include flu-like symptoms, allergy, arthralgias, back pain, and headache. Five years of therapy increases bone 2–3% and reduces the number of new vertebral fractures.

The parenteral formulation of calcitonin (400 IU per 2 mL ampule) is administered in doses of 100 units/d subcutaneously. A few severe allergic reactions have occurred. Therefore, it is advisable to initiate parenteral therapy with a small test dose and stand-by epinephrine. Both nasal and parenteral calcitonin have analgesic effects on bone pain; reduction of pain may be noted within 2–4 weeks after commencing therapy.

B. General Measures: The diet should be adequate in protein, calcium, and vitamin D. Increased calcium intake by use of supplementary calcium salts (eg, calcium carbonate), up to 1–1.5 g calcium per day, is advisable. Adequate vitamin D (400 units/d) must be ensured, and additional vitamin D (2000–5000 units/d) may be needed if there is suspected deficiency in sun exposure or dietary vitamin D, malabsorption, or osteomalacia. Pharmacologic glucocorticoid doses should be reduced or discontinued if possible. Thiazides may be useful if hypercalciuria is present. Regular exercise is recommended. Patients should be kept active; bedridden patients should be given active or passive exercises. The spine may be adequately supported (though braces or corsets are usually not well tolerated), but rigid or excessive immobilization must be avoided. Patients must be protected from falling. Alcohol and smoking should be avoided.

Prognosis

The prognosis is good for preventing post-menopausal osteoporosis if estrogen therapy is started early and maintained for years. There may be improvement in osteoporosis once treatment is begun and any glucocorticoid (in supraphysiologic doses) is stopped. Measures to prevent progressive loss of bone mass are more effective than treatment of the clinical disease.

Black DM et al: Randomised trial of effect of alendronate on risk of fracture in women with existing vertebral fractures. Fracture Intervention Trial Research Group. Lancet 1996;348:1535. (Among women with low bone mass and existing vertebral fractures, alendronate substantially reduces the frequency of fractures.)

Bone HG et al: Dose-response relationships for alendronate treatment in osteoporotic elderly women. Alendronate Elderly Osteoporosis Study Centers. J Clin Endocrinol Metab 1997;82:265.

De Groen PC et al: Esophagitis associated with the use of alendronate. N Engl J Med 1996;335:1016.

Postmenopausal Estrogen/Progestin Interventions (PEPI) Trial Group: Effects of hormone therapy on bone mineral density. JAMA 1996;276:1389. (See related topics in same issue.)

Recommendations for the prevention and treatment of glucocorticoid-induced osteoporosis. American College of Rheumatology Task Force on Osteoporosis Guidelines. Arthritis Rheum 1996;39:1791.

Ross PD: Osteoporosis. Frequency, consequences, and risk factors. Arch Intern Med 1996;156:1399.

OSTEOMALACIA

Essentials of Diagnosis

- Painful proximal muscle weakness (especially pelvic girdle); bone pain and tenderness.
- Decreased bone density from diminished mineralization of osteoid.
- Unlike osteoporosis, common laboratory abnormalities may include increases in alkaline phosphatase, decreased 25-hydroxyvitamin D, or hypocalcemia, hypocalciuria, hypophosphatemia, secondary hyperparathyroidism.
- Classic radiologic features may be present.

General Considerations

Defective mineralization of the growing skeleton in childhood causes permanent bone deformities (rickets). The same defects occurring in adults cause osteomalacia.

Etiology
(Table 26–12)

Osteomalacia can be caused by any condition that results in inadequate calcium or phosphate mineralization of bone osteoid.

A. Calcium Deficiency: Calcium deficiency can be caused by inadequate vitamin D from insuffi-

---

Table 26–12. Causes of osteomalacia.[1,2]

Vitamin disorders
Decreased availability of vitamin D
  Insufficient sunlight exposure
  Nutritional deficiency of vitamin D
  Malabsorption
  Nephrotic syndrome
Vitamin D-dependent rickets type I
Liver disease
Chronic renal failure
Phenytoin, carbamazepine, or barbiturate therapy
Calcium deficiency
Phosphate deficiency
Decreased intestinal absorption
  Nutritional deficiency of phosphorus
  Malabsorption
  Phosphate-binding antacid therapy
Increased renal loss
  X-linked hypophosphatemic rickets
  Tumoral hypophosphatemic osteomalacia
  Association with other disorders, including paraproteinemias, glycogen storage diseases, neurofibromatosis, Wilson's disease, and Fanconi's syndrome
Disorders of bone matrix
Hypophosphatasia
Fibrogenesis imperfecta
Axial osteomalacia
Inhibitors of mineralization
Aluminum
Bisphosphonates

---

[1]Modified, with permission, from Fitzgerald PA: *Handbook of Clinical Endocrinology*, 2nd ed. Appleton & Lange, 1992.
[2]See Table 26–11 for causes of osteoporosis.

---

cient sun exposure, malnutrition, or malabsorption (pancreatic insufficiency, gluten-sensitive enteropathy, etc). The minimal vitamin D requirement is 2.5 μg (100 IU) daily; the recommended daily allowance is at least 10 μg (400 IU) daily.

Adults in the USA generally receive nutritional supplements of plant vitamin D (ergocalciferol, vitamin D_2) in milk or other processed foods, so that serious vitamin D deficiency is now quite rare. Nutritional vitamin D deficiency is common in less developed areas of the world.

Patients may have other defects of vitamin D synthesis or resistance. Renal disease causes deficient 1-hydroxylation of 25-hydroxyvitamin D.

Osteomalacia may also be caused by anticonvulsant medication, especially phenytoin and phenobarbital, probably by causing resistance to 1,25-hydroxyvitamin D. Familial 1,25-hydroxyvitamin D resistance syndromes have also been described.

B. Phosphate Deficiency: Congenital phosphate deficiency is caused most commonly by a familial X-linked renal tubular defect of phosphate resorption (vitamin D-resistant rickets). Acquired hypophosphatemia can be caused by malabsorption of phosphate due to gut-binding by aluminum hydroxide antacids, poor nutrition, and alcoholism. Hypophosphatemia can also be caused by soft tissue tumors that secrete a substance which causes phosphaturia and total body phosphate depletion. About 87% of such tumors are benign; serum $1,25(OH)_2D_3$ levels are low in oncogenic hypophosphatemia.

Clinical Findings

The clinical manifestations of defective bone mineralization depend on the age at onset and the severity. In adults, osteomalacia is typically asymptomatic at first. Eventually, muscle weakness, bone pain, and tenderness occur. Fractures may occur with little or no trauma.

Diagnostic Tests

Serum is obtained for calcium, albumin, phosphate, alkaline phosphatase, parathyroid hormone. and 25-hydroxyvitamin D $(25[OH]D_3)$ determinations. Bone densitometry helps document the degree of osteopenia. X-rays may show diagnostic features.

In one series of biopsy-proved osteomalacia, alkaline phosphatase was elevated in 94%; the calcium or phosphorus was low in 47%; $25(OH)D_3$ was low in 29%; pseudofractures were seen in 18%; and urinary calcium was low in 18%. $1,25(OH)_2D_3$ may be low even when $25(OH)D_2$ levels are normal.

Bone biopsy is not usually necessary but is diagnostic of osteomalacia if there is significant unmineralized osteoid.

Differential Diagnosis

Osteomalacia usually can be distinguished from osteoporosis by the relative absence of biochemical abnormalities in the latter.

Treatment

Treatment of osteomalacia depends upon the cause. Nutritional vitamin D deficiency is treated with ergocalciferol, 50,000 units orally once or twice weekly for 6–12 months, followed by at least 400 units daily. Larger and more frequent doses are sometimes required in malabsorption syndromes. Phenytoin-induced osteomalacia may be prevented with vitamin D, 50,000 units orally every 2 weeks.

Phosphate deficiency from renal phosphate wasting (vitamin D-resistant rickets) responds to lifetime phosphate supplementation; vitamin D must be given also to improve the impaired calcium absorption caused by the phosphate.

Isolated nutritional calcium deficiency (< 150 mg/d) does occur and is treated with oral calcium.

Bingham CT, Fitzpatrick LA: Noninvasive testing in the diagnosis of osteomalacia. Am J Med 1993;95:519.

Nellen JF et al: Hypovitaminosis D in immigrant women: Slow to be diagnosed. BMJ 1996;312:570.

Russel JA: Osteomalacic myopathy. Muscle Nerve 1994; 17:578.

Wilkins GE et al: Oncogenic osteomalacia: Evidence for a humoral phosphaturic factor. J Clin Endocrinol Metab 1995;80:1628.

PAGET'S DISEASE OF BONE (Osteitis Deformans)

Essentials of Diagnosis

- Often asymptomatic.
- Bone pain may be the first symptom.
- Kyphosis, bowed tibias, large head, deafness, and frequent fractures that vary with location of process.
- Serum calcium and phosphate normal; alkaline phosphatase elevated; urinary hydroxyproline elevated.
- Dense, expanded bones on x-ray.

General Considerations

Paget's disease is a bone disease that may be related to a paramyxovirus (canine distemper) infection. It causes excessive bone destruction and repair—with associated deformities, since the repair takes place in an unorganized fashion. Up to 3% of persons over age 50 have isolated lesions, but clinically important disease is much less common. There is a strong familial incidence of Paget's disease. A rare form occurs in young people.

Clinical Findings

A. Symptoms and Signs: Paget's disease is often mild or asymptomatic. Deep "bone pain" is usually the first symptom. The bones become soft, leading to bowed tibias, kyphosis, and frequent fractures with slight trauma. If the skull is involved, the patient may report headaches and an increased hat size. Deafness may occur. Increased vascularity over the involved bones causes increased warmth.

B. Laboratory Findings: Serum calcium and phosphorus are normal, but serum alkaline phosphatase is markedly elevated. Urinary hydroxyproline is also elevated in active disease. Serum calcium may be elevated, particularly if the patient is at bed rest.

C. Imaging: On radiographs the involved bones are expanded and denser than normal. Multiple fissure fractures may be seen in the long bones. The initial lesion may be destructive and radiolucent, especially in the skull ("osteoporosis circumscripta"). Technetium pyrophosphate bone scans are helpful in delineating activity of bone lesions even before any radiologic changes are apparent.

Differential Diagnosis

Paget's disease must be differentiated from primary bone lesions such as osteogenic sarcoma and multiple myeloma, and fibrous dysplasia and from secondary bone lesions such as metastatic carcinoma and osteitis fibrosa cystica. Fibrogenesis imperfecta ossium is a rare symmetric disorder that can mimic the features of Paget's disease; alkaline phosphate is likewise elevated. If serum calcium is elevated, hyperparathyroidism may be present in some patients as well.

Complications

Fractures are frequent and occur with minimal trauma. If immobilization takes place and there is an excessive calcium intake, hypercalcemia and kidney stones may develop. Vertebral collapse may lead to spinal cord compression. Osteosarcoma may develop in long-standing lesions. Sarcomatous change is suggested by marked increase in bone pain, sudden rise in alkaline phosphatase, and appearance of a new lytic lesion. The increased vascularity may give rise to high-output cardiac failure. Arthritis frequently develops in joints adjacent to involved bone.

Extensive skull involvement may cause cranial nerve palsies from impingement of the neural foramina. Ischemic neurologic events may occur as a result of a vascular "steal" phenomenon. Involvement of the auditory region frequently causes hearing loss (mixed sensorineural and conductive) and occasionally tinnitus or vertigo.

Treatment

Asymptomatic patients require no treatment except for those with extensive skull involvement, in whom prophylactic treatment may prevent deafness and stroke.

The bisphosphonate **alendronate** (10 mg tablets) inhibits osteoclast-mediated bone resorption and has become the drug of choice at a dosage of up to 40 mg daily. Tiludronate (200 mg tablets), 400 mg daily for 3 months, is also effective. Etidronate disodium is available in 200 mg and 400 mg tablets. The safest dose is 5 mg/kg daily for 90–180 days. In severe disease, 10 mg/kg/d may be used for 90 days, with rest periods before another course is given. Etidronate may have adverse effects on bone mineralization and can aggravate bone pain. One dose of pamidronate, 60–120 mg intravenously over 2–4 hours, may produce improvement lasting several months. Alkaline phosphatase continues to drop for 6 months after treatment. (See Treatment of Hypercalcemia.)

The calcitonins act by reducing osteoclastic activity. **Synthetic salmon calcitonin** (Calcimar, 400 units/2 mL ampule) is given in doses of 50–100 IU subcutaneously daily or three times weekly for months to years. Aside from local hypersensitivity reactions, systemic side effects—eg, flushing, nausea—are common but usually quite mild. Nasal calcitonin (200 IU daily, alternating nostrils) is as effective as the parenteral preparation and is associated with much less side effects.

Prognosis

The prognosis in general is good, but sarcomatous changes (in 1–3%) can alter the prognosis unfavorably. In general, the prognosis is worse the earlier in life the disease starts. Fractures usually heal well. In the severe forms, marked deformity, intractable pain, and cardiac failure are found. These complications should become rare with prompt treatment with the bisphosphonates now available or under development.

Ooi CG, Fraser WD: Paget's disease of bone. Postgrad Med J 1997;73:69.

Reid IR et al: Biochemical and radiologic improvement in Paget's disease of bone treated with alendronate: A randomized, placebo-controlled trial. Am J Med 1996; 101:341.

Siris E et al: Comparative study of alendronate versus etidronate for the treatment of Paget's disease of bone. J Clin Endocrinol Metab 1996;81:961. (The alendronate-treated group tolerated treatment well and had significantly greater decreases in both serum alkaline phosphatase [79% versus 44%] and urinary deoxypyridinoline [75% versus 51%] than the etidronate-treated group.)

DISEASES OF THE ADRENAL CORTEX

ADRENAL CORTEX PHYSIOLOGY

Aldosterone is the major mineralocorticoid secreted by the zona glomerulosa, the outer layer of the adrenal cortex. It stimulates the renal tubule to reabsorb sodium and excrete potassium, thereby protecting against hypovolemia and hyperkalemia.

Aldosterone secretion is stimulated by hypovolemia in an indirect way. Hypovolemia causes the renal juxtaglomerular cells to secrete renin; renin stimulates the peripheral conversion of angiotensin I to angiotensin II; angiotensin II then causes aldosterone secretion. Hyperkalemia directly stimulates aldosterone secretion. Secretion is inhibited by atrial natriuretic factor and by dopamine.

Cortisol is the major glucocorticoid secreted by the middle zona fasciculata and the inner zona reticularis of the adrenal cortex.

Cortisol counters insulin effects, tending to cause hyperglycemia by inhibiting insulin secretion and by increasing hepatic gluconeogenesis, substrate being provided by the increased amino acids made available by cortisol's inhibition of protein synthesis in muscles.

Cortisol is secreted in a diurnal pattern, being highest upon awakening and lowest at bedtime. Cortisol production normally increases during exercise, making more glucose and fatty acids available for energy. Cortisol is also secreted in response to acute trauma, infection, and other stresses; it dampens defense mechanisms, helping prevent their dangerous overactivity. It inhibits the production or action of many mediators of inflammation and immunity such as interleukin-6 (IL-6), lymphokines, prostaglandins, and histamine. Cortisol is required for production of angiotensin II, thereby helping maintain adequate vascular tone.

Glucocorticoids increase renal free water clearance. They lower serum calcium by inhibiting calcium uptake by the renal tubule and gut and by redistributing calcium intracellularly.

Androgens are produced in the adrenal cortex, mostly by the inner zona fasciculata. The adrenal cortex's fetal zone atrophies after birth, but the adrenal continues to make large amounts of dehydroepiandrosterone sulfate (DHEAS) and dehydroepiandrosterone (DHEA), which have no known significance during adult life, having minimal androgenic activity; but they continue to be the adrenals' most abundantly secreted steroids. DHEAS secretion declines steadily with age. There are individual differences in secretion, and—for unknown reasons—there is a positive correlation between DHEAS levels and longevity.

Testosterone and androstenedione are the major functional androgens secreted by the adrenal. Their secretion causes adrenarche, which precedes gonadal androgen secretion and stimulates the first sexual hair of puberty.

ADRENOCORTICAL HYPOFUNCTION (Adrenocortical Insufficiency)

1. ACUTE ADRENAL INSUFFICIENCY (Adrenal Crisis)

Essentials of Diagnosis

- Weakness, abdominal pain, fever, confusion, nausea, vomiting, and diarrhea.
- Low blood pressure, dehydration; skin pigmentation may be increased.
- Serum potassium high, sodium low, blood urea nitrogen high.
- Cosyntropin ($ACTH_{1-24}$) unable to stimulate a normal increase in serum cortisol.

General Considerations

Acute adrenal insufficiency is an emergency caused by insufficient cortisol. Crisis may occur in the course of chronic treated insufficiency, or it may be the presenting manifestation of adrenal insufficiency. Acute adrenal crisis is more commonly seen in primary adrenal insufficiency (Addison's disease) than in disorders of the pituitary gland causing secondary adrenocortical hypofunction.

Adrenal crisis may occur in the following situations: (1) Following stress, eg, trauma, surgery, infection, or prolonged fasting in a patient with latent insufficiency. (2) Following sudden withdrawal of adrenocortical hormone in a patient with chronic insufficiency or in a patient with temporary insufficiency due to suppression by exogenous glucocorticoids. (3) Following bilateral adrenalectomy or removal of a functioning adrenal tumor that had suppressed the other adrenal. (4) Following sudden destruction of the pituitary gland (pituitary necrosis), or when thyroid is given to a patient with hypoadrenalism. (5) Following injury to both adrenals by trauma, hemorrhage, anticoagulant therapy, thrombosis, infection, or, rarely, metastatic carcinoma.

Clinical Findings

A. Symptoms and Signs: The patient complains of headache, lassitude, nausea and vomiting, abdominal pain, and often diarrhea. Confusion or coma may be present. Fever may be 40 °C or more. The blood pressure is low. Other signs may include cyanosis, dehydration, skin hyperpigmentation, and sparse axillary hair (if hypogonadism is also present). Meningococcemia may be associated with purpura and adrenal insufficiency secondary to adrenal infarction (Waterhouse-Friderichsen syndrome).

B. Laboratory Findings: The eosinophil count may be high. Hyponatremia or hyperkalemia (or both) are usually present. Hypoglycemia is frequent. Hypercalcemia may be present. Blood, sputum, or urine culture may be positive if bacterial infection is the precipitating cause of the crisis.

The diagnosis is made by a simplified cosyntropin stimulation test, which is performed as follows: (1) Synthetic $ACTH_{1-24}$ (cosyntropin), 0.25 mg, is given parenterally. (2) Serum is obtained for cortisol between 30 and 60 minutes after cosyntropin is administered. Normally, serum cortisol rises to at least 20 μg/dL. For patients receiving glucocorticoid treatment, hydrocortisone must not be given for at least 8 hours before the test. Other glucocorticoids do not interfere with specific assays for cortisol.

Plasma ACTH is markedly elevated if the patient has primary adrenal disease (generally > 200 pg/mL).

Differential Diagnosis

Acute adrenal insufficiency must be distinguished from other causes of shock (eg, septic, hemorrhagic, cardiogenic). Hyperkalemia is also seen with gastrointestinal bleeding, rhabdomyolysis, hyperkalemic paralysis, and certain drugs (eg, ACE inhibitors, spironolactone). Hyponatremia is seen in many other conditions (eg, hypothyroidism, diuretic use, heart failure, cirrhosis, vomiting, diarrhea, severe illness, or major surgery). It must also be distinguished from an acute abdomen where neutrophilia is the rule, whereas eosinophilia and lymphocytosis are characteristic of adrenal insufficiency.

Treatment

A. Acute Phase: If the diagnosis is suspected, draw a blood sample for cortisol determination and treat with hydrocortisone, 100–300 mg intravenously, and saline *immediately*, without waiting for the results. Thereafter, give hydrocortisone phosphate or hydrocortisone sodium succinate, 100 mg intravenously immediately, and continue intravenous infusions of 50–100 mg every 6 hours for the first day. Give the same amount every 8 hours on the second day and then adjust the dosage in view of the clinical picture.

Since bacterial infection frequently precipitates acute adrenal crisis, broad-spectrum antibiotics should be administered empirically while waiting for the results of initial cultures. Hypoglycemia should be vigorously treated while serum electrolytes, blood urea nitrogen, and creatinine are monitored.

B. Convalescent Phase: When the patient is able to take food by mouth, give oral hydrocortisone, 10–20 mg every 6 hours, and reduce dosage to maintenance levels as needed. Most patients ultimately require hydrocortisone twice daily (AM, 10–20 mg; PM, 5–10 mg). Mineralocorticoid therapy is not needed when large amounts of hydrocortisone are being given, but as the dose is reduced it is usually necessary to add fludrocortisone acetate, 0.05–0.2 mg daily. Some patients never require fludrocortisone or become edematous at doses of more than 0.05 mg once or twice weekly. Once the crisis has passed, the patient must be investigated to assess the degree of permanent adrenal insufficiency and to establish the cause if possible.

Prognosis

Rapid treatment will usually be life-saving. However, acute adrenal insufficiency is frequently unrecognized and untreated since its manifestations mimic more common conditions; lack of treatment leads to shock that is unresponsive to volume replacement and vasopressors, resulting in death.

Barquist E, Kirton O: Adrenal insufficiency in the surgical intensive care unit patient. J Trauma 1997;42:27.

Oelkers W: Adrenal insufficiency. N Engl J Med 1996; 335:1206.

Soni A et al: Adrenal insufficiency occurring during septic shock: Incidence, outcome, and relationship to peripheral cytokine levels. Am J Med 1995;98:266. (Five of 21 patients with septic shock had adrenal insufficiency.)

2. CHRONIC ADRENOCORTICAL INSUFFICIENCY (Addison's Disease)

Essentials of Diagnosis

- Weakness, easy fatigability, anorexia, weight loss; nausea and vomiting, diarrhea; abdominal pain, muscle and joint pains; amenorrhea.
- Sparse axillary hair; increased skin pigmentation, especially of creases, pressure areas, and nipples.
- Hypotension, small heart.
- Serum sodium may be low; potassium, calcium, and urea nitrogen may be elevated; neutropenia, mild anemia, eosinophilia, and relative lymphocytosis may be present.
- Plasma cortisol levels are low or fail to rise after administration of corticotropin.
- Plasma ACTH level elevated.

General Considerations

Addison's disease is an uncommon disorder caused by destruction of the adrenal cortices. It is characterized by chronic deficiency of cortisol, aldosterone, and adrenal androgens and causes skin pigmentation that can be strikingly dark or subtle. Volume and sodium depletion and potassium excess eventually occur in primary adrenal failure. In contrast, if chronic adrenal insufficiency is secondary to pituitary failure (atrophy, necrosis, tumor), mineralocorticoid production (controlled by the renin-angiotensin system) persists and hyperkalemia is not present. Furthermore, if ACTH is not elevated, skin pigmentary changes are not encountered.

The term "Addison's disease" should be reserved for adrenal insufficiency due to adrenocortical disease. Autoimmune destruction of the adrenals is the most common cause of Addison's disease in the USA (accounting for about 80% of spontaneous cases). It may be isolated or may occur as part of a polyglandular autoimmune syndrome (PGA). **Type I PGA** begins in early childhood with chronic mucocutaneous candidiasis followed by hypoparathyroidism and Addison's disease by age 10–12 years. **Type II PGA** consists of Addison's disease, thyroid disease (hyperthyroidism 5%; hypothyroidism 10%) or insulin-dependent diabetes (10%). This syndrome is also known as "autoimmune polyendocrinopathy-candidiasis-ectodermal dysplasia (APECED)." The combination of Addison's disease and hypothyroidism is known as Schmidt's syndrome.

Other problems seen with autoimmune Addison's disease include vitiligo, premature primary ovarian failure (40% of women before age 50), testicular failure (5%), and pernicious anemia (4%).

Tuberculosis was formerly a leading cause of Addison's disease. The association is now relatively rare in the USA but common where tuberculosis is more prevalent.

Bilateral adrenal hemorrhage may occur in patients taking anticoagulants, during open heart surgery, and during other major trauma. It may also occur about 1 week postoperatively, presenting with pain, fever, and shock. Some cases are associated with antiphospholipid antibody syndrome.

Rare causes include metastatic carcinoma, coccidioidomycosis, histoplasmosis, cytomegalovirus infection (more frequent in patients with AIDS), syphilitic gummas, scleroderma, amyloid disease, and hemochromatosis. Adrenoleukodystrophy is an X-linked genetic disorder affecting about one in 20,000 males. Addison's disease may occur years prior to the onset of neurologic symptoms.

Adults with hereditary cortisol deficiency due to adrenal insensitivity to ACTH may develop achalasia, alacrima, and neurologic disease (Allgrove's syndrome); cortisol deficiency usually presents in childhood but may not occur until the third decade. Adults with congenital adrenal hypoplasia may have hypogonadotropic hypogonadism, myopathy, and high-frequency hearing loss.

Patients with hereditary defects in adrenal enzymes for cortisol synthesis develop "congenital adrenal hyperplasia" due to ACTH stimulation. The most common enzyme defect is P450c21 (21-hydroxylase). Patients with severely defective P450c21 enzymes manifest deficiency of mineralocorticoids (salt wasting) in addition to deficient cortisol and excessive androgens. Women with milder enzyme defects have adequate cortisol but develop hirsutism in adolescence or adulthood and are said to have "late-onset" congenital adrenal hyperplasia. (See Hirsutism section.)

Clinical Findings

A. Symptoms and Signs: The symptoms may include weakness and fatigability, weight loss, myalgias, arthralgias, fever, anorexia, nausea and vomiting, anxiety, and mental irritability. Some of these symptoms may be due to high serum levels of IL-6. Pigmentary changes consist of diffuse tanning over nonexposed as well as exposed parts or multiple freckles; hyperpigmentation is especially prominent over the knuckles, elbows, knees, and posterior neck and in palmar creases and nail beds. Nipples and areolas tend to darken. The skin in pressure areas such as the belt or brassiere lines and the buttocks also darkens. New scars are pigmented. Some patients have associated vitiligo (10%). Emotional changes are common. Hypoglycemia, when present, may worsen the patient's weakness and mental functioning, rarely leading to coma. Manifestations of other autoimmune disease (see above) may be present. Patients tend to be hypotensive and orthostatic; about 90% have systolic blood pressures under 110 mm Hg; blood pressure over 130 mm Hg is rare. Other findings may include a small heart, hyperplasia of lymphoid tissues, and scant axillary and pubic hair (especially in women).

B. Laboratory Findings: The white count usually shows moderate neutropenia, lymphocytosis, and a total eosinophil count over 300/µL. Among patients with *chronic* Addison's disease, the serum sodium is usually low (90%) while the potassium is elevated (65%). Patients with diarrhea may not be hyperkalemic. Fasting blood glucose may be low. Hypercalcemia may be present. Young men with idiopathic Addison's disease may be screened for adrenoleukodystrophy by determining plasma VLCFA

(very long chain fatty acid); affected patients have high levels of VLCFAs.

Low plasma cortisol (< 5 mg/dL) at 8 AM is diagnostic, especially if accompanied by simultaneous elevation of the plasma ACTH level (usually > 200 pg/mL). The cosyntropin stimulation test is performed as described above. Antiadrenal antibodies are found in the serum in about 50% of cases of autoimmune Addison's disease. Antibodies to thyroid (45%) and other tissues may be present.

C. Imaging: When Addison's disease is not clearly autoimmune, a chest x-ray is obtained to look for tuberculosis, fungal infection, or cancer as possible causes. CT scan of the abdomen will show small noncalcified adrenals in autoimmune Addison's disease. The adrenals are enlarged in about 85% of cases due to metastatic or granulomatous disease. Calcification is noted in about 50% of cases of tuberculous Addison's disease but is also seen with hemorrhage, fungal infection, pheochromocytoma, and melanoma.

Differential Diagnosis

Addison's disease should be considered in any patient with hypotension or hyperkalemia. Unexplained weight loss, weakness, and anorexia may be mistaken for occult cancer. Nausea, vomiting, diarrhea, and abdominal pain may be misdiagnosed as intrinsic gastrointestinal disease. The hyperpigmentation may be confused with that due to ethnic or racial factors. Weight loss may simulate anorexia nervosa. Hemochromatosis also enters the differential diagnosis of skin hyperpigmentation, but it should be remembered that it may truly be a cause of Addison's disease as well as diabetes mellitus and hypoparathyroidism. Serum ferritin is increased in most cases of hemochromatosis and is a useful screening test. About 17% of patients with AIDS have symptoms of cortisol resistance.

Complications

Any of the complications of the underlying disease (eg, tuberculosis) are more likely to occur, and the patient is susceptible to intercurrent infections that may precipitate crisis. Associated autoimmune diseases are common (see above).

Treatment

A. Specific Therapy: Replacement therapy should include a combination of glucocorticoids and mineralocorticoids. In mild cases, hydrocortisone alone may be adequate.

1. Hydrocortisone is the drug of choice. Most addisonian patients are well maintained on 15–25 mg of hydrocortisone orally daily in two divided doses, two-thirds in the morning and one-third in the late afternoon or early evening. Some patients respond better to prednisone in a dosage of about 3 mg in the morning and 2 mg in the evening. Many patients, however, do not obtain sufficient salt-retaining effect and require fludrocortisone supplementation or extra dietary salt.

2. Fludrocortisone acetate has a potent sodium-retaining effect. The dosage is 0.05–0.3 mg orally daily or every other day. If postural hypotension, hyperkalemia, or weight loss occurs, raise the dose. If edema, hypokalemia, or hypertension ensues, lower the dose.

B. General Measures: Treat all infections immediately and vigorously, and raise the dose of hydrocortisone appropriately. The dose of glucocorticoid should also be raised in case of trauma, surgery, stressful diagnostic procedures, or other forms of stress. The maximum hydrocortisone dose for severe stress is 50 mg intravenously or intramuscularly every 6 hours. Lower doses, oral or parenteral, are used for lesser stress. The dose is reduced back to normal as the stress subsides. Patients are advised to wear a medical alert bracelet or medal reading, "Adrenal insufficiency—takes hydrocortisone."

Patients with adrenoleukodystrophy receive dietary treatment and bone marrow transplantation.

Prognosis

With adequate replacement therapy, the life expectancy of patients with Addison's disease is markedly prolonged. Active tuberculosis responds to specific treatment. Withdrawal of treatment or increased demands due to infection, trauma, surgery, or other types of stress may precipitate crisis with a sudden fatal outcome unless large doses of parenteral corticosteroids are employed. With appropriate therapy, however, a fully active life is possible for most patients.

Brosnan CM, Gowing NF: Addison's disease. BMJ 1996;312:1085.

Freda PU et al: Primary adrenal insufficiency in patients with the acquired immunodeficiency syndrome: A report of five cases. J Clin Endocrinol Metab 1994;79:1540.

Grinspoon SK, Biller BM: Clinical review 62: Laboratory assessment of adrenal insufficiency. J Clin Endocrinol Metab 1994;79:923.

Keljo DJ, Squires RH Jr: Clinical problem-solving. Just in time. N Engl J Med 1996;334:46. (A clinical exercise highlighting the challenges of diagnosing Addison's disease.)

Laureti S et al: X-Linked adrenoleukodystrophy is a frequent cause of idiopathic Addison's disease in young adult male patients. J Clin Endocrinol Metab 1996;81:470.

Oelkers W: Adrenal insufficiency. N Engl J Med 1996; 335:1206.

CUSHING'S SYNDROME (Hypercortisolism)

Essentials of Diagnosis

- Central obesity, muscle wasting, thin skin, easy bruisability, psychologic changes, hirsutism, purple striae.
- Osteoporosis, hypertension, poor wound healing.
- Hyperglycemia, glycosuria, leukocytosis, lymphocytopenia, hypokalemia.
- Elevated serum cortisol and urinary free cortisol. Lack of normal suppression by dexamethasone.

General Considerations

The term Cushing's "syndrome" refers to the manifestations of excessive corticosteroids, commonly due to supraphysiologic doses of glucocorticoid drugs and rarely due to spontaneous production of excessive corticosteroids by the adrenal cortex. Adult cases of spontaneous Cushing's syndrome have several possible causes:

(1) About 70% are due to Cushing's "disease," which refers to the manifestations of hypercortisolism due to ACTH hypersecretion by the pituitary. It is usually caused by a benign pituitary adenoma that is typically very small (< 5 mm). It is at least five times more frequent in women than men.

(2) About 15% are due to nonpituitary neoplasms (eg, small-cell lung carcinoma), which produce excessive amounts of ectopic ACTH. Hypokalemia and hyperpigmentation are commonly found in this group.

(3) About 15% are unrelated to ACTH and are caused by excessive cortisol secretion by an adrenal tumor (adenoma or carcinoma) or rarely by bilateral adrenal nodular hyperplasia. Adrenal adenomas are generally small and produce mostly cortisol, whereas adrenal carcinomas are usually large when discovered and can also produce excessive amounts of androgens with resultant hirsutism and virilization.

Clinical Findings

A. Symptoms and Signs: Patients with Cushing's syndrome usually have central obesity with a plethoric "moon face," "buffalo hump," supraclavicular fat pads, protuberant abdomen, and thin extremities; oligomenorrhea or amenorrhea (or impotence in the male); weakness, backache, headache; hypertension; and acne and superficial skin infections. Patients may have thirst and polyuria (with or without glycosuria), renal calculi, glaucoma, purple striae (especially around the thighs, breasts, and abdomen), and easy bruisability. Wound healing is impaired. Mental symptoms may range from increased lability of mood to frank psychosis. Patients are subject to infections.

B. Laboratory Findings: Glucose tolerance is impaired as a result of insulin resistance. Polyuria is present as a result of increased free water clearance; diabetes mellitus with glycosuria may worsen it. Patients with Cushing's syndrome often have leukocytosis with relative granulocytosis and lymphopenia. Hypokalemia (but not hypernatremia) may be present, particularly in cases of ectopic ACTH secretion.

Tests for Hypercortisolism

The easiest screening test for hypercortisolism involves giving dexamethasone, 1 mg, at 11 PM and collecting serum for cortisol determination at about 8 AM the next morning; a cortisol level under 5 μg/dL excludes Cushing's syndrome with 98% certainty. Other patients require further investigation, which includes a 24-hour urine collection for cortisol and creatinine. An abnormally high 24-hour urine free cortisol (or free cortisol to creatinine ratio of > 95 μg cortisol/g creatinine) helps confirm hypercortisolism.

In cases of blatant Cushing's syndrome, no further confirmation of hypercortisolism is necessary. In less certain cases, a suppression test can also be done by giving dexamethasone, 0.5 mg orally every 6 hours for 48 hours; urine is collected on the second day. Urine free cortisol over 20 μg/d or urine 17-hydroxycorticosteroid over 4.5 mg/d also helps confirm hypercortisolism.

Samples for serum cortisol determinations may be obtained at 8 AM and 11 PM; an 11 PM cortisol over 50% of the 8 AM level indicates lack of diurnal variation that is characteristic of Cushing's syndrome in adults. Conditions that cause false-positive testing (see below) should be considered.

Finding the Cause of Hypercortisolism

Once hypercortisolism is confirmed, a baseline plasma ACTH is obtained. It must be collected properly on ice and processed quickly by a laboratory with a reliable, sensitive assay. A level of ACTH below the normal range (about 20 pg/mL) indicates a probable adrenal tumor, whereas higher levels are produced by pituitary or ectopic tumors.

Localizing Techniques

In ACTH-dependent Cushing's syndrome, MRI of the pituitary can demonstrate a pituitary adenoma in about 50% of cases. When the pituitary MRI is normal or shows a tiny irregularity that may be incidental, selective inferior petrosal venous sampling for ACTH is performed (with CRH stimulation) where available to confirm a pituitary ACTH source, distinguishing it from an occult nonpituitary tumor secreting ACTH.

Location of ectopic sources of ACTH is done with CT scan of the chest and abdomen, with special attention to the lungs (for carcinoid or small-cell carcinomas), the thymus, the pancreas, and the adrenals. Chest masses are frequently due to opportunistic infections, so biopsy is done to confirm the pathologic diagnosis prior to resection.

In non-ACTH-dependent Cushing's syndrome, a CT scan of the adrenals can localize the adrenal tumor in most cases.

Differential Diagnosis

Alcoholic patients can have hypercortisolism and many clinical manifestations of Cushing's syndrome. Depressed patients also have hypercortisolism that can be nearly impossible to distinguish biochemically from Cushing's syndrome. Patients with severe obesity frequently have an abnormal dexamethasone suppression test, but the urine free cortisol is usually normal, as is diurnal variation of serum cortisol. Patients with familial cortisol resistance have hyperandrogenism, hypertension, and hypercortisolism without actual Cushing's syndrome. Certain drugs such as phenytoin, phenobarbital, and primidone accelerate the metabolism of dexamethasone, thereby causing a "false-positive" dexamethasone suppression test. Estrogens—during pregnancy or as oral contraceptives—may also cause lack of dexamethasone suppressibility. In pregnancy, urine free cortisol is increased, while 17-hydroxycorticosteroids remain normal and diurnal variability of serum cortisol is normal.

Complications

Cushing's syndrome, if untreated, produces serious morbidity and even death. The patient may suffer from any of the complications of hypertension or of diabetes. Susceptibility to infections is increased. Compression fractures of the osteoporotic spine and aseptic necrosis of the femoral head may cause marked disability. Nephrolithiasis and psychosis may occur. Following bilateral adrenalectomy for Cushing's disease, a pituitary adenoma may enlarge progressively, causing local destruction (eg, visual field impairment) and hyperpigmentation; this complication is known as Nelson's syndrome.

Treatment

Cushing's disease is best treated by selective transsphenoidal resection of the pituitary adenoma, after which the rest of the pituitary usually returns to normal function; however, the normal corticotrophs are suppressed and require 6–36 months to recover normal function. Hydrocortisone replacement therapy is necessary in the meantime. Patients who fail to have a remission should undergo bilateral laparoscopic adrenalectomy. Patients may also receive pituitary irradiation, but only about 23% of patients are cured, and remissions require up to 6 months. Patients who are not surgical candidates may be given a trial of ketoconazole in doses of about 200 mg every 6 hours; liver enzymes must be monitored for progressive elevation.

Adrenal neoplasms secreting cortisol are resected laparoscopically. The contralateral adrenal is suppressed, so postoperative hydrocortisone replacement is required until recovery occurs. Metastatic adrenal carcinomas may be treated with mitotane; ketoconazole or metyrapone can help suppress hypercortisolism in unresectable adrenal carcinoma.

Ectopic ACTH-secreting tumors should be surgically resected. If that cannot be done, medical treatment with ketoconazole or metyrapone (or both) may at least suppress the hypercortisolism; however, metyrapone may exacerbate female virilization. Somatostatin analog (octreotide) given parenterally several times daily suppresses ACTH secretion in about one-third of such cases.

Prognosis

The best prognosis for total recovery is for patients in whom a benign adrenal adenoma has been removed and who have survived the postadrenalectomy state of adrenal insufficiency. Patients with Cushing's disease can be cured by transsphenoidal surgery, but there is a failure rate of about 10–20%. Those patients who have a complete remission after transsphenoidal surgery have about a 15–20% chance of recurrence over the next 10 years. Even patients who undergo bilateral adrenalectomy may have a recurrence of hypercortisolism due to growth of an adrenal remnant, stimulated by the high levels of ACTH found after adrenalectomy. The prognosis for ectopic ACTH-producing tumors is dependent upon the aggressiveness and metastatic status of the particular tumor type.

Estrada J et al: The long-term outcome of pituitary irradiation after unsuccessful transsphenoidal surgery in Cushing's disease. N Engl J Med 1997;336:172.

Findling JW, Doppman JL: Biochemical and radiologic diagnosis of Cushing's syndrome. Endocrinol Metab Clin North Am 1994;23:511. (Entire volume dedicated to Cushing's syndrome.)

Orth DN: Cushing's syndrome. (Medical Progress.) N Engl J Med 1995;332:791.

Sonino N et al: Risk factors and long-term outcome in pituitary-dependent Cushing's disease. J Clin Endocrinol Metab 1996;81:2647.

HIRSUTISM & VIRILIZATION

Essentials of Diagnosis

- Menstrual disorders, hirsutism, acne.
- Virilization may occur: increased muscularity, balding, deepening of the voice, enlargement of the clitoris.
- Occasionally a palpable pelvic tumor.
- Urinary 17-ketosteroids and serum DHEAS and androstenedione elevated in adrenal disorders, variable in others.
- Serum testosterone often elevated.

General Considerations

Major androgens include testosterone, androstenedione, and dehydroepiandrosterone sulfate (DHEAS). In women, circulating testosterone is derived from direct ovarian secretion (60%) and from peripheral conversion from androstenedione (40%). Androstenedione is secreted in about equal amounts by the adrenals and ovaries. DHEAS is secreted exclusively by the adrenals.

Testosterone is the most potent androgen, but 98% circulates in a bound state: About 65% is strongly bound to sex hormone-binding globulin (SHBG), while 33% is weakly bound to albumin. Only free testosterone and a portion of the weakly bound testosterone can enter target cells to exert androgenic effect. Assays have therefore been devised to measure "total," "free," or "free and weakly bound" testosterone.

Testosterone is converted in the skin to dihydrotestosterone (DHT), which actually stimulates the hair follicle. DHT is metabolized to androstanediol glucuronide, which can be measured and is elevated in most cases of hirsutism.

Etiology

Hirsutism may be caused by the following disorders:

(1) Idiopathic or familial: Many patients with hirsutism have no detectable hyperandrogenism. Patients often have a strong familial predisposition to hirsutism that may be considered normal in the context of their genetic background. Such patients may have elevated serum levels of androstanediol glucuronide, a metabolite of dihydrotestosterone that is produced by skin in cosmetically unacceptable amounts.

(2) Polycystic ovary syndrome (hyperthecosis, Stein-Leventhal syndrome): This is a common functional disorder of the ovaries which accounts for at least half the cases of clinical hirsutism. Patients frequently have amenorrhea or oligomenorrhea with anovulation and obesity. The serum LH:FSH ratio is often greater than 2.0. Both adrenal and ovarian androgen hypersecretion are commonly present.

(3) Adrenal enzyme defects: Baby girls with "classic" 21-hydroxylase deficiency have ambiguous genitalia and may become virilized unless treated with corticosteroid replacement; about half of such patients have clinically evident mineralocorticoid deficiency (salt-wasting) as well.

About 2% of patients with adult-onset hirsutism have been found to have a partial defect in adrenal 21-hydroxylase, whose phenotypic expression is delayed until adolescence or adulthood; such patients do not have salt wasting.

Some rare patients with hyperandrogenism and hypertension have 11-hydroxylase deficiency. This is distinguished from cortisol resistance by high cortisol levels in the latter and by high 11-deoxycortisol levels in the former.

(4) Ovarian tumors are very uncommon causes of hirsutism (0.8%) and include arrhenoblastomas, Sertoli-Leydig cell tumors, dysgerminomas, and hilar cell tumors.

(5) Adrenal carcinoma is a rare cause of hyperandrogenism that can be quite virilizing.

(6) Other rare causes of hirsutism include ACTH-induced Cushing's syndrome, acromegaly, and ovarian luteoma of pregnancy. Pharmacologic causes include minoxidil, cyclosporine, phenytoin, anabolic steroids, diazoxide, and certain progestins.

Clinical Findings

A. Symptoms and Signs: Modest androgen excess from any source increases sexual hair (chin, upper lip, abdomen, and chest) and increases sebaceous gland activity, producing acne. Menstrual irregularities, anovulation, and amenorrhea are common. If androgen excess is pronounced, defeminization (decrease in breast size, loss of feminine adipose tissue) and virilization (frontal balding, muscularity, clitoromegaly, and deepening of the voice) occurs. Virilization implicates the presence of an androgen-producing neoplasm.

Hypertension may be seen in rare patients with Cushing's syndrome, adrenal 11-hydroxylase deficiency, or cortisol resistance syndrome.

A pelvic examination may disclose clitoromegaly or ovarian enlargement that may be cystic or neoplastic.

B. Laboratory Testing and Imaging: Serum androgen testing is mainly useful to screen for rare occult adrenal or ovarian neoplasms. Some general guidelines are presented here, though exceptions are common:

A serum testosterone level greater than 200 ng/dL or free testosterone greater than 40 ng/dL indicates the need for pelvic examination and ultrasound. If that is negative, an adrenal CT scan is performed.

A serum androstenedione greater than 1000 ng/dL also implicates an ovarian or adrenal neoplasm. Patients with milder elevations of serum testosterone or androstenedione usually are treated with an oral contraceptive.

Patients with very elevated serum DHEAS (> 700 μg/dL) have an adrenal source of androgen. This usually is due to adrenal hyperplasia and rarely to adrenal carcinoma. An adrenal CT scan is performed.

No firm guidelines exist as to which patients (if any) with hyperandrogenism should be screened for "late-onset" 21-hydroxylase deficiency. The evaluation requires levels of serum 17-hydroxyprogesterone to be drawn at baseline and at 30–60 minutes after the intramuscular injection of 0.25 mg of cosyntropin ($ACTH_{1-24}$). Patients with congenital adrenal hyperplasia will usually have a baseline 17-hydroxyprogesterone over 300 ng/dL or a stimulated level over 1000 ng/dL. The diagnosis, once made, is interesting academically but not helpful to the patient since glucocorticoid treatment is not particularly more effective in this condition than are other treatment modalities (see below).

Patients with any clinical signs of Cushing's syndrome should receive a screening test. (See Cushing's Syndrome.)

Serum levels of FSH and LH are elevated if amenorrhea is due to ovarian failure. An LH:FSH ratio greater than 2.0 is common in patients with polycystic ovaries; pelvic ultrasound reveals enlarged or cystic ovaries in most cases.

Treatment

Any underlying cause of hyperandrogenism must be detected and treated if possible. Postmenopausal women with severe hyperandrogenism should undergo laparoscopic bilateral oophorectomy, even if the adrenal CT is normal, since small hilar cell tumors of the ovary may not be visible on scans. Any drugs causing hirsutism are stopped. Treatment options for other cases include the following:

(1) Spironolactone may be taken in doses of 50–100 mg twice daily on days 5–25 of the menstrual cycle or daily if used concomitantly with an oral contraceptive. Hyperkalemia or hyponatremia is uncommon.

(2) Cyproterone acetate is a potent antiandrogen with progestational activity. It is not available in the USA. It is available elsewhere as the progestin element in an oral contraceptive (Diane-35: ethinyl estradiol 35 μg with cyproterone acetate 2 mg). The dose of 2 mg is effective. An oral contraceptive is usually prescribed also. Side effects may include fatigue, nausea, or depression.

(3) Finasteride inhibits 5α-reductase, the enzyme that converts testosterone to active dihydrotestosterone in the skin. Given as 5 mg doses orally daily, it provides modest reduction in hirsutism over 6 months—comparable to results achieved with spironolactone. Side effects are rare.

(4) Flutamide, 250–375 mg/d, inhibits androgen receptor uptake and also suppresses serum androgen. Used with an oral contraceptive, it appears to be more effective than spironolactone in improving hirsutism, acne, and male pattern baldness. Hepatotoxicity has been reported but is rare.

(5) Oral contraceptives stimulate menses, if desired, but are less effective for hirsutism. Contraceptives with low-androgenic progestins (desogestrel, gestodene) may be tried.

(6) Local treatment by shaving or depilatories, waxing, electrolysis, or bleaching should be encouraged.

Note: Antiandrogen treatments must be given only to nonpregnant women. Women must be counseled to take oral contraceptives, when indicated, and avoid pregnancy, since use during pregnancy causes malformations and pseudohermaphroditism in male infants.

Kalve E, Klein IF: Evaluation of women with hirsutism. Am Fam Physician 1996;54:117.

MacKenna TJ: Screening for sinister causes of hirsutism. N Engl J Med 1994;331:1015.

Marshburn PB, Carr BR: Hirsutism and virilization: A systematic approach to benign and potentially serious causes. Postgrad Med 1995;97:99 and 105.

Rittmaster RS: Clinical review 73: Medical treatment of androgen-dependent hirsutism. J Clin Endocrinol Metab 1995;80:2559.

PRIMARY HYPERALDOSTERONISM

Essentials of Diagnosis

- Hypertension, polyuria, polydipsia, muscular weakness.
- Hypokalemia, alkalosis.
- Elevated plasma and urine aldosterone levels and low plasma renin level.

General Considerations

Classic hyperaldosteronism (with hypokalemia) accounts for about 0.7% of cases of hypertension; milder hyperaldosteronism is more frequent. The disorder is more common in females. Primary hyperaldosteronism may be due to unilateral adrenocortical adenoma (Conn's syndrome, 73%) or bilateral cortical hyperplasia (27%), which may be glucocorticoid-suppressible due to an autosomal dominant genetic defect allowing ACTH stimulation of aldosterone production.

Clinical Findings

A. Symptoms and Signs: Hypertension, muscular weakness (at times with paralysis simulating periodic paralysis), paresthesias with frank tetany, headache, polyuria, and polydipsia are the main complaints. Hypertension is typically moderate. Some patients have only diastolic hypertension, without other symptoms and signs. Malignant hypertension is rare. Edema is rarely seen in primary hyperaldosteronism.

B. Laboratory Findings: The patient must have a high sodium intake (> 120 meq/d) during the entire evaluation period; serum potassium is low. A 24-hour urine collection is assayed for aldosterone, free cortisol, and creatinine. A low plasma renin activity (< 5 µg/dL) with 24-hour urine aldosterone over 20 µg indicates hyperaldosteronism. A urine aldosterone of less than 20 µg/24 h is seen with rare adrenal or gonadal enzyme defects in the activity of 17α-hydroxylase (associated with ambiguous genitalia or primary amenorrhea) or 11β-hydroxylase (associated with virilization).

Once hyperaldosteronism is diagnosed, plasma is assayed for 18-hydroxycorticosterone; a level over 85 µg/dL is seen with adrenal neoplasms, whereas levels under 85 µg/dL are nondiagnostic. Additionally, plasma can be assayed for aldosterone at 8 AM while the patient is supine after overnight recumbency and again after 4 hours upright. Patients with an adrenal adenoma usually have a baseline plasma aldosterone greater than 20 µg/dL which does not rise. Patients with hyperplasia typically have a baseline plasma aldosterone less than 20 µg/dL which rises during upright posture. Exceptions occur.

If an adrenal adenoma is diagnosed by the above testing, a CT scan of the adrenals can lateralize it with 80% success. If not visualized by CT, the adenoma may be localized by adrenal vein catheterization for aldosterone or by a dexamethasone-suppressed iodocholesterol adrenal scan.

Differential Diagnosis

The differential diagnosis of hyperaldosteronism includes other causes of hypokalemia (see Chapter 21) in patients with essential hypertension. For example, many hypertensive patients taking diuretics develop hypokalemia even while taking potassium-sparing diuretics or potassium supplements. Chronic depletion of intravascular volume stimulates renin secretion and secondary hyperaldosteronism. Thus, it is important to discontinue diuretics and ensure adequate hydration and sodium intake when assessing a patient for primary hyperaldosteronism (see above).

Excessive ingestion of real licorice (black and derived from anise) may produce hypertension and hypokalemia caused by a derivative of its glycyrrhizinic acid inhibiting 11β-hydroxysteroid dehydrogenase, thereby enhancing cortisol's mineralocorticoid effect. Oral contraceptives may increase aldosterone secretion in some patients. Renal vascular disease can cause severe hypertension with hypokalemia; plasma renin activity is high, distinguishing it from primary hyperaldosteronism.

Excessive adrenal secretion of other corticosteroids (besides aldosterone) may also cause hypertension with hypokalemia. This occurs with certain congenital adrenal enzyme disorders such as P450c11 deficiency (increased deoxycorticosterone with virilization and deficient cortisol) or P450c17 deficiency (increased deoxycorticosterone, corticosterone, and progesterone but deficient estradiol and testosterone). Hyperaldosteronism may rarely be due to a malignant ovarian tumor.

Complications

All of the complications of chronic hypertension are encountered in primary hyperaldosteronism. Progressive renal damage is less reversible than hypertension.

Treatment

Conn's syndrome (unilateral adrenal adenoma secreting aldosterone) is treated by laparoscopic adrenalectomy, though lifelong spironolactone therapy is an option. Bilateral adrenal hyperplasia is best treated with spironolactone; bilateral adrenalectomy corrects the hypokalemia but not the hypertension and should *not* be performed. Antihypertensive agents may also be necessary. Hyperplasia sometimes responds well to dexamethasone suppression.

Prognosis

The hypertension is reversible in about two-thirds of cases but persists or returns in spite of surgery in the remainder. The prognosis is much improved by early diagnosis and treatment. Only 2% of aldosterone-secreting adrenal tumors are malignant.

The low renin levels found in this condition (and in about 25% of cases of essential hypertension) also confer a relatively good prognosis.

Blumenfeld JD et al: Diagnosis and treatment of primary hyperaldosteronism. Ann Intern Med 1994;121:877.

Litchfield WR, Dluhy RG: Primary aldosteronism. Endocrinol Metab Clin North Am 1995;24:593.

Lo CY et al: Primary aldosteronism. Results of surgical treatment. Ann Surg 1996;224:125.

Young WF Jr et al: Primary aldosteronism: Adrenal venous sampling. Surgery 1996;120:913.

DISEASES OF THE ADRENAL MEDULLA

PHEOCHROMOCYTOMA

Essentials of Diagnosis

- "Attacks" of headache, perspiration, palpitations.
- Hypertension, frequently sustained but often paroxysmal, especially during surgery or delivery.
- Attacks of nausea, pain, weakness, dyspnea, visual disturbance.
- Anxiety, tremor, weight loss, or heat intolerance.
- Elevated urinary catecholamines or their metabolites. Normal serum T_4 and TSH.

General Considerations

Pheochromocytomas are rare, being found in less than 0.1% of hypertensive individuals. Patients have disease characterized by paroxysmal or sustained hypertension due to a tumor located in either or both adrenals or anywhere along the sympathetic nervous chain, and rarely in such aberrant locations as the thorax, bladder, or brain. Primary extra-adrenal pheochromocytomas are known as "paragangliomas." Pheochromocytomas are characterized by a rough "rule of tens": About 10% of cases are not associated with hypertension; 10% are extra-adrenal, and of those about 10% are extra-abdominal; 10% occur in children; most tumors are sporadic, with only 10–15% familial; in about 10%, the tumor involves both adrenal glands (bilateral adrenal tumors tend to occur more frequently in familial cases); and about 10% of tumors are malignant.

Familial pheochromocytoma may be associated with the following: calcitonin-secreting medullary carcinoma of the thyroid and hyperparathyroidism (multiple endocrine neoplasia type II); medullary carcinoma of the thyroid and the syndrome of multiple mucosal neuromas (multiple endocrine neoplasia type IIb); neurofibromatosis (Recklinghausen's disease); von Hippel-Lindau disease (hemangioblastomas of retina, cerebellum, and other parts of the nervous system); and islet cell tumors (rare).

Clinical Findings

A. Symptoms and Signs: Pheochromocytoma typically causes attacks of severe headache (85%), palpitations (65%), and profuse sweating (65%). The absence of all three symptoms excluded pheochromocytoma with 99% certainty in one series. Vasomotor changes (including facial pallor) may occur, along with tachycardia, precordial or abdominal pain, increasing nervousness and irritability, increased appetite, and loss of weight. Anginal attacks may occur. Physical findings usually include hypertension (95%), which may be sustained (20%), sustained with paroxysms (50%), or paroxysmal only (25%). There may be cardiac enlargement; postural tachycardia (change of more than 20 beats/min) and postural hypotension; and mild elevation of basal body temperature. Retinal hemorrhage or cerebrovascular hemorrhage occurs occasionally.

The manifestations of pheochromocytoma are quite varied. Besides the above symptoms, some patients can present with psychosis or confusion, seizures, hyperglycemia, bradycardia, hypotension, paresthesias, or Raynaud's phenomenon. Other patients may have pulmonary edema and heart failure due to cardiomyopathy. Still other patients may be entirely asymptomatic or may have abdominal discomfort due to a pheochromocytoma presenting as a large abdominal mass.

B. Laboratory Findings: Hypermetabolism is present; thyroid function tests are normal, including serum T_4, free T_4, T_3, and TSH; and glycosuria or hyperglycemia (or both) may be present.

C. Special Tests:

1. Assay of urinary catecholamines (total and fractionated), metanephrines, vanilmandelic acid (VMA), and creatinine detects most pheochromocytomas, especially when samples are obtained during or immediately following an episodic attack. A 24-hour urine specimen is usually obtained, although an overnight or shorter collection may be used; patients with pheochromocytomas generally have more that 2.2 µg of metanephrine per milligram of creatinine and more than 5.5 µg of VMA per milligram of creatinine.

Many drugs and chemicals and some foods can affect the tests for pheochromocytoma (Table 26–13). Testing for catecholamines should be done using high-performance liquid chromatography with electrochemical detection (HPLC-ECD); this minimizes false test results.

Table 26–13. Drugs, foods, and conditions affecting chemical tests for pheochromocytoma.[1]

Test	Increase	Decrease
Universally affecting catecholamines, metanephrines, and vanilmandelic acid (VMA)	Sympathomimetics (amphetamines, ephedrine, nasal decongestants, bronchodilators, cocaine) Levodopa Rapid clonidine withdrawal Excess ingestion of bananas Vasodilators (nitroprusside, nitroglycerin) Methylxanthines (aminophylline) Severe stress (emotion, exercise, pain, myocardial infarction) Diseases: intracranial lesions, acute psychosis, Guillain-Barré syndrome, lead poisoning, eclampsia, hypoglycemia, carcinoid, acute porphyria, quadriplegia, amyotrophic lateral sclerosis Fluorescent substances:[2] quinidine, chloral hydrate, tetracyclines, methenamine, methocarbamol, nicotinic acid, erythromycin, quinine, riboflavin, bretylium	Large doses of ganglionic blockers: guanethidine, reserpine (with chronic administration; acute administration causes initial increases) Fenfluramine (anorectic) Renal insufficiency Diseases: malnutrition, dysautonomia, quadriplegia (quiescent)
Catecholamines	Ethanol, isoproterenol, methyldopa, monoamine oxidase inhibitors, phenothiazines, α-methyl-p-tyrosine, methenamine, urine bilirubin, labetalol	
Metanephrines	Ethanol, methyldopa, monoamine oxidase inhibitors, benzodiazepines, phenothiazines	Radiopaque media (methylglucamine): Renografin, Hypaque-M,[3] Renovist, Cardiografin, Urografin, Conray
Vanilmandelic acid (VMA)	Lithium, nalidixic acid, methocarbamol, glyceryl guaiacolate, p-aminosalicylic acid, salicylates, mephenesin, sulfonamides, excess ingestion[2] of chocolate, citrus, tea, vanilla, coffee	Ethanol, monoamine oxidase inhibitors, disulfiram, clofibrate, mandelamine, salicylates (Pisano method)

[1]Modified, with permission, from Fitzgerald PA: *Handbook of Clinical Endocrinology*, 2nd ed. Appleton & Lange, 1992.
[2]Fluorimetric assay methods are subject to most types of interference. The most specific assays use chromatographic, HPLC, and spectrophotometric methods. Drugs should be stopped for 1 week before testing.
[3]Hypaque as diatrizoate sodium is all right.

2. Direct assay of epinephrine and norepinephrine in blood and urine during or following an attack is the most sensitive test for pheochromocytoma associated with paroxysmal hypertension. High epinephrine levels favor tumor localization within the adrenal gland. Proper, quiet collection of plasma specimens is essential.

3. Imaging–CT scan and MRI have been very helpful in the confirmation and localization of pheochromocytoma. They should not ordinarily replace urinary catecholamine assays since incidental adrenal adenomas are not uncommon (over 2%) and may cause misdiagnosis. [123]I MIBG scan helps localize tumors with a sensitivity of about 85% and specificity of 99%.

4. Pharmacologic provocative and suppressive tests that evaluate the rise or fall in blood pressure are usually not required or recommended.

Differential Diagnosis

Tachycardia, tremor, palpitation, and hypermetabolism may give rise to confusion with thyrotoxicosis. Pheochromocytoma may also be misdiagnosed as essential hypertension, myocarditis, glomerulonephritis or other renal lesions, toxemia of pregnancy, eclampsia, and psychoneurosis (anxiety attack). It can sometimes be mistaken for an acute abdomen.

Other conditions that have manifestations similar to those of pheochromocytoma include acute intermittent porphyria, hypogonadal vascular instability (hot flushes), cocaine or amphetamine use, clonidine withdrawal, hypertensive crisis caused by foods containing tyramine (eg, cheeses) in patients taking MAO inhibitor antidepressants, labile hypertension, and unstable angina.

False-positive testing for catecholamines and

metabolites occurs in about 10% of hypertensives, but levels are usually less than 50% above normal and typically normalize with repeat testing.

Complications

All of the complications of severe hypertension may be encountered. Hypertensive crises with sudden blindness or cerebrovascular accidents are not uncommon. These may be precipitated by sudden movement, by manipulation during or after pregnancy, by emotional stress or trauma, or during surgical removal of the tumor. Cardiomyopathy may develop. Occasionally, the initial manifestation of pheochromocytoma may be hypotension or even shock.

After removal of the tumor, a state of severe hypotension and shock (resistant to epinephrine and norepinephrine) may ensue with precipitation of renal failure or myocardial infarction. Hypotension and shock may occur from spontaneous infarction or hemorrhage of the tumor; emergency surgical removal of the tumor is necessary in these cases.

On rare occasions, a patient dies as a result of the complications of diagnostic tests or during surgery. No patient with suspected pheochromocytoma should be subjected either to an invasive diagnostic procedure or to surgery unless there has been adequate alpha blockade with phenoxybenzamine.

Treatment

Laparoscopic removal of the tumor or tumors is the treatment of choice. Preoperative administration of α-adrenergic blocking drugs has made pheochromocytoma surgery a great deal safer in recent years. Give phenoxybenzamine, 10 mg orally every 12 hours, and increase the dose gradually—about every 3 days—until hypertension is controlled. The usual maintenance dose is 40–120 mg daily. Optimal alpha blockade is achieved when supine arterial pressure is below 160/90 mm Hg and standing arterial pressure is above 80/45 mm Hg.

After appropriate α-adrenergic receptor blockade with phenoxybenzamine, the beta-blocker propranolol or the combined alpha- and beta-blocker labetalol can be employed to control tachycardia and other arrhythmias. Maintain adrenergic blockade for a minimum of 10 days or until optimal cardiac status is established. Monitor the ECG until it becomes stable. (It may take a week or even months to correct electrocardiographic changes in patients with catecholamine myocarditis, and it is prudent to defer surgery until then in such cases.) Patients must be very closely monitored during surgery in order to promptly detect sudden changes in blood pressure or cardiac arrhythmias.

Hypertensive crisis can initially be managed with sublingual administration of nifedipine 10 mg (pierced capsule). Intraoperative severe hypertension is managed with continuous intravenous nitroprus-

side, 0.5–10 μg/kg/min. Tachyarrhythmia is treated with esmolol or lidocaine.

Autotransfusion of 1–2 units of blood per 12 hours preoperatively plus generous intraoperative volume replacement reduces the risk of postresection hypotension caused by persisting α-adrenergic blockade.

Plasma glucose is monitored for 2 days postoperatively to detect hypoglycemia.

Since there may be multiple or metastatic tumors, it is essential to recheck urinary catecholamine levels postoperatively (1–2 weeks after surgery).

For inoperable or metastatic tumors, oral phenoxybenzamine has been successfully used as chronic symptomatic treatment. Metyrosine is a competitive blocker in the synthesis of catecholamines that is also useful; the initial dosage is 250 mg four times daily, increased daily by increments of 250–500 mg to a maximum of 4 g/d. Metastatic pheochromocytomas may be treated with combination chemotherapy or with high doses of ^{131}I MIBG, which is available at some medical centers.

Prognosis

The prognosis depends upon how early the diagnosis is made. The malignancy of a pheochromocytoma cannot be determined by histologic examination. A tumor is considered malignant if metastases are present; this may take many years to become clinically evident. If the tumor is successfully removed before irreparable damage to the cardiovascular system has occurred, a complete cure is usually achieved. Complete cure (or improvement) may follow removal of a tumor that has been present for many years. In some cases, hypertension persists or returns in spite of successful surgery. Although this may be essential hypertension, biochemical reevaluation is then required, looking for a second or metastatic pheochromocytoma.

Before the advent of blocking agents, the surgical mortality rate was as high as 30%, but this has rapidly decreased. The importance of a team approach—endocrinologist, anesthesiologist, and surgeon—cannot be overemphasized. With optimal management, the surgical mortality rate is less than 3%.

Patients with metastatic pheochromocytoma have a median survival of about 4.5 years; however, prolonged survivals do occur.

Bravo EL: Evolving concepts in the pathophysiology, diagnosis, and treatment of pheochromocytoma. Endocr Rev 1994;15:356.

Heron E et al: The urinary metanephrine-to-creatinine ratio for the diagnosis of pheochromocytoma. Ann Intern Med 1996;125:300. (Measurement of the metanephrine-to-creatinine ratio is a sensitive and specific test for pheochromocytoma.)

Loh KC et al: Pheochromocytoma: A ten-year survey. Q J Med 1997;90:51.

Peaston RT, Lennard TW, Lai LC: Overnight excretion of urinary catecholamines and metabolites in the detection of pheochromocytoma. J Clin Endocrinol Metab 1996; 81:1378. (Compared to 24-hour results, overnight urinary norepinephrine levels provided a better diagnostic sensitivity [100%] and specificity [98%].)

Werbel SS, Ober KP: Pheochromocytoma: Update on diagnosis, localization, and management. Med Clin North Am 1995;779:131.

DISEASES OF THE PANCREATIC ISLET CELLS*

ISLET CELL FUNCTIONING PANCREATIC TUMORS

The pancreatic islets are composed of several types of cells, each with distinct chemical and microscopic features: the A cells (20%) secrete glucagon, the B cells (70%) secrete insulin, and the D cells (5%) secrete somatostatin or gastrin. F cells secrete "pancreatic polypeptide." Each type of cell may give rise to benign or malignant neoplasms that may be multiple and usually present with a clinical syndrome related to hypersecretion of a native or ectopic hormonal product. The diagnosis of a particular pancreatic islet neoplasm depends upon first suspecting it from its clinical manifestations. The serum concentration of that particular hormone may then be assayed.

Insulinomas are usually (about 85%) benign and secrete excessive amounts of insulin (as well as proinsulin and C-peptide), which causes hypoglycemia. The tumors may be multiple, especially in familial cases of MEN type 1.

Gastrinomas are generally benign and secrete excessive gastrin (as well as "big" gastrin), which stimulates the stomach to hypersecrete acid, thereby causing peptic ulceration (Zollinger-Ellison syndrome). About 25% are ultimately found to have multiple endocrine neoplasia, with hyperparathyroidism occurring from 14 years preceding the Zollinger-Ellison diagnosis to 38 years after. Surgical cure is unusual. The 5-, 10- and 20-year survival rates with MEN 1 are 94%, 75%, and 58%, respectively, while the survival rates for sporadic Zollinger-Ellison syndrome are 62%, 50%, and 31%, respectively. (See Chapter 14.)

Glucagonomas secrete excessive glucagon and may cause a peculiar dermatitis called **necrolytic migratory erythema.** Such patients also usually have diabetes mellitus, weight loss, and liver metastases by the time of diagnosis.

Somatostatinomas are very rare and are associated with weight loss, diabetes mellitus, malabsorption, and hypochlorhydria.

Other rare tumors secrete excessive amounts of **vasoactive intestinal polypeptide (VIP),** a substance that causes profuse watery diarrhea (Verner-Morrison syndrome). Treatment with octreotide improves the symptoms but does not halt tumor growth. Symptomatic improvement with calcitonin treatment has also been reported.

In addition to the native hormones, aberrant or ectopic hormones are often secreted by islet cell tumors, including ACTH, melanocyte-stimulating hormone, serotonin, and chorionic gonadotropin, with a variety of clinical syndromes. Islet cell tumors may be part of the syndrome of multiple endocrine adenomatosis type I (with pituitary and parathyroid adenomas).

Localization of pancreatic islet cell tumors and their metastases is best done with somatostatin receptor scintigraphy (SRS) for all but insulinomas; SRS detects about 75% of noninsulinomas. CT and MRI are also useful.

Direct resection of the tumor (or tumors), which often spreads locally, is the primary form of therapy for all types of islet cell neoplasm except Zollinger-Ellison syndrome, where use of a proton pump inhibitor, eg, omeprazole or lansoprazole, is the therapy of choice. Insulinomas are resected but in MEN 1 are rarely cured, so surgery is reserved for dominant masses in such cases. Palliation of functioning malignant disease often requires both antihormonal and anticancer chemotherapy. The use of streptozocin, doxorubicin, and asparaginase, especially for malignant insulinoma, has produced some encouraging results, though these drugs are quite toxic. Octreotide, a somatostatin analog, is now used in the therapy of islet cell tumor. The hypoglycemia of insulinoma may be counteracted by verapamil or diazoxide.

The prognosis in these neoplasms is variable. Long-term survival in spite of widespread metastases has been reported.

Bieligk S, Jaffe BM: Islet cell tumors of the pancreas. Surg Clin North Am 1995;75:1025.

Gibril F et al: Somatostatin receptor scintigraphy: Its sensitivity compared with that of other imaging methods in detecting primary and metastatic gastrinomas. A prospective study. Ann Intern Med 1996;125:26.

Meko JB et al: Evaluation of somatostatin-receptor scintigraphy for detecting neuroendocrine tumors. Surgery 1996;120:975.

Orloff SL, Debas HT: Advances in the management of patients with Zollinger-Ellison syndrome. Surg Clin North Am 1995;75:511.

Perry RR, Vinik AI: Clinical review 72: Diagnosis and

---

*Diabetes mellitus and the hypoglycemic states are discussed in Chapter 27.

management of functioning islet cell tumors. J Clin Endocrinol Metab 1995;80:2273.

Wermers RA et al: The glucagonoma syndrome. Clinical and pathologic features in 21 patients. Medicine 1996;75:53.

DISEASES OF THE TESTES

MALE HYPOGONADISM

Essentials of Diagnosis

- Diminished libido and erections.
- Decreased growth of body hair.
- Testes may be small or normal in size. Serum testosterone is usually decreased.
- Serum gonadotropins (LH and FSH) are decreased in hypogonadotropic hypogonadism; they are increased in testicular failure (hypergonadotropic hypogonadism).

General Considerations

Male hypogonadism is caused by deficient testosterone secretion by the testes. It may be classified according to whether it is due to (1) insufficient gonadotropin secretion by the pituitary (hypogonadotropic) or (2) pathology in the testes themselves (hypergonadotropic) (see Table 26–14). The evaluation for hypogonadism begins with a serum testosterone or free testosterone measurement. A low serum testosterone is evaluated with serum LH and FSH levels. Patients with low gonadotropins are further evaluated for other pituitary abnormalities, including hyperprolactinemia.

Etiology

A. Hypogonadotropic Hypogonadism: A deficiency in FSH and LH may be isolated or associated with other pituitary hormonal abnormalities. Patients must be evaluated for signs of Cushing's syndrome or adrenal insufficiency, growth hormone excess or deficiency, and thyroid hormone excess or deficiency.

Congenital hypogonadotropic hypogonadism presents as "delayed" puberty. Such boys may have already presented with childhood short stature owing to an associated deficiency in GH caused by a *Pit-1* gene mutation. Isolated FSH and LH deficiency may be associated with a diminished sense of smell (Kallman's syndrome) and certain other syndromes (see Hypopituitarism, above).

Acquired hypogonadotropic hypogonadism may be due to a pituitary or hypothalamic lesion but may be idiopathic. Hyperprolactinemia (Table 26–5) may also induce hypogonadism.

B. Hypergonadotropic Hypogonadism: A failure in testicular secretion of testosterone causes a rise in LH. If testicular Sertoli cell function is deficient, FSH will be elevated. Conditions that can cause testicular failure include viral infection (eg, mumps), irradiation, cancer chemotherapy, autoimmunity, XY gonadal dysgenesis, and Klinefelter's syndrome.

Klinefelter's syndrome (seminiferous tubule dysgenesis) is a common cause of male hypogonadism that is due to the expression of an abnormal karyotype, classically 47,XXY. Other forms are common, eg, 46,XY/47,XXY mosaicism, 48,XXYY, 48,XXXY, or 46,XX males.

The manifestations of Klinefelter's syndrome are variable. Testes feel normal during childhood, but during adolescence they usually become firm, fibrotic, small, and nontender to palpation. Although puberty occurs at the normal time, the degree of virilization is variable. About 85% have some gynecomastia at puberty.

Other common findings include tall stature and abnormal body proportions (height greater than arm span; crown-pubis length greater than pubis-floor). Patients with multiple X or Y chromosomes are more apt to have mental deficiency and other abnormalities such as clinodactyly or synostosis. They may also exhibit problems with coordination and social skills. Other problems include a higher incidence of breast cancer, chronic pulmonary disease, varicosities of the legs, and diabetes mellitus (8%); impaired glucose tolerance occurs in an additional 19%.

Most men (about 95%) have azoospermia, but

Table 26–14. Causes of male hypogonadism.

Hypogonadotropic (Low or Normal LH)	Hypergonadotropic (High LH)
Constitutional delay	Klinefelter's syndrome
Chronic illness	Bilateral anorchia
Malnourishment	Sertoli cell-only syndrome
Cushing's syndrome	Noonan's syndrome
Hypothyroidism	Bilateral anorchia
Hypopituitarism	Testicular trauma
Pituitary tumors	Orchitis
Hypothalamic lesions	Mumps
Hemochromatosis	Leprosy
Drugs	Tuberculosis
Alcohol	Lymphoma
Marijuana	Myotonic dystrophy
Spironolactone	Antitumor chemotherapy
Ketoconazole	Radiation therapy
GnRH agonist (leuprolide)	Male climacteric
Prior androgens (eg, nandrolone)	Idiopathic
Estrogen-secreting tumors (testicular, adrenal)	
Congenital syndromes	
Kallmann	
Prader-Willi	
Alström	
Idiopathic	

men with 46,XY/47,XXY mosaicism may be fertile. The diagnosis is confirmed by karyotyping or by determining the presence of RNA for X-inactive-specific transcriptase (XIST) in peripheral blood leukocytes by PCR.

The serum testosterone is low, and FSH and LH are elevated. Sometimes the serum testosterone is normal, but serum free testosterone is usually low.

All causes of gynecomastia (Table 26–1) must be differentiated from Klinefelter's syndrome. Testicular size, plasma LH, FSH, and prolactin and, if necessary, karyotyping or XIST will settle the diagnosis.

C. Androgen Insensitivity: Partial resistance to testosterone is a rare condition in which phenotypic males have variable degrees of apparent hypogonadism, gynecomastia, hypospadias, cryptorchism, and gynecomastia.

Clinical Findings

A. Symptoms and Signs: Hypogonadism that is congenital or acquired during childhood presents as delayed puberty. Men with acquired hypogonadism have variable manifestations. Most men experience decreased libido. Others complain of erectile dysfunction, hot sweats, asthenia, or depression. Their presenting complaint may also be infertility, gynecomastia, headache, fracture, or other symptoms related to the cause or result of the hypogonadism. The patient's history often gives a clue to the cause (Table 26–14).

Physical signs associated with hypogonadism may include decreased body, axillary, beard, or pubic hair; such diminished sexual hair growth is not reliably present except after years of severe hypogonadism. Examination should include measurements of arm span and height. Testicular size should be assessed with an orchidometer (normal volume is about 10–25 mL; normal length is usually over 6 cm). Testicular size may decrease but usually remains within the normal range in men with postpubertal hypogonadotropic hypogonadism, but it may be diminished with testicular injury or Klinefelter's syndrome. The testes must also be carefully palpated for masses, since Leydig cell tumors may secrete estrogen and present with hypogonadism.

B. Laboratory Findings: The hemoglobin and hematocrit may be slightly below the male range due to hypogonadism. Laboratory evaluation for male hypogonadism should always include measurement of serum testosterone. There are different sorts of testosterone assays. An assay for serum free testosterone is more sensitive than that for total testosterone. Testosterone levels fluctuate, generally being higher in the morning, so that more than one assay may be necessary for careful evaluation. In patients with low or borderline-low serum testosterone levels, serum LH and FSH should be measured. LH and FSH tend to be high in patients with primary hypogonadism but low or inappropriately normal in men with hypogonadotropic hypogonadism. Bone densitometry may be reduced in long-standing male hypogonadism.

1. Acquired hypogonadotropic hypogonadism–Men with hypogonadotropic hypogonadism have low serum testosterone levels without a compensatory increase in gonadotropins. Such men require careful evaluation for other manifestations of hypopituitarism, Cushing's syndrome, hemochromatosis, pituitary tumor, or brain tumor. Olfactory testing is performed even though Kallmann's syndrome ordinarily presents with delayed puberty. A serum prolactin determination is obtained but may be elevated for many reasons (Table 26–5). The serum estradiol level may be elevated in patients with cirrhosis and in rare cases of estrogen-secreting tumors (testicular Leydig cell tumor or adrenal carcinoma). Men with no discernible definite cause for hypogonadotropic hypogonadism should have an MRI of the pituitary and hypothalamic region to look for a tumor or other lesion. (See Hypopituitarism.)

2. Acquired hypergonadotropic hypogonadism–Men with hypergonadotropic hypogonadism have low serum testosterone levels with a compensatory increase in gonadotropins. It is most commonly seen in elderly men, in whom the cause is usually idiopathic (male climacteric). Younger men require a particularly careful evaluation. Patients should be examined for features of Klinefelter's syndrome, since signs of mosaic Klinefelter's syndrome may first appear in adulthood. Hypogonadism and gynecomastia may also present in adulthood as a late phenotypic expression of partial deficiency of testicular 17-ketosteroid reductase.

Uremic patients may have suppressed serum testosterone with an elevated LH level but may also have a suppressed LH level due to hyperprolactinemia. Patients with myotonic dystrophy also tend to have primary hypogonadism. The testicles must be carefully examined for evidence of trauma, infiltrative lesions (eg, lymphoma), or ongoing infection (eg, leprosy, tuberculosis). Testicular biopsy is usually reserved for younger patients in whom the reason for primary hypogonadism is unclear.

Treatment

Hypogonadism is usually treated with parenteral testosterone (enanthate or cypionate). The usual dose is about 300 mg intramuscularly every 3 weeks or 200 mg every 2 weeks. The preparation is oil-based and is usually given in the gluteal area. The dose is adjusted according to the patient's response. Oral androgen preparations include methyltestosterone and fluoxymesterone. These oral preparations have rarely caused liver tumors or peliosis hepatis with long-term use. Cholestatic jaundice occurs in 1–2% but usually remits after the medication is discontinued. The oral androgens are not as effective as parenteral testosterone.

Testosterone transdermal systems are applied as skin patches. One such system (Androderm) is applied as two new patches nightly on different areas of the thighs, upper arms, abdomen, or back; each patch's gel contains 12.5 mg of testosterone and delivers about 2.5 mg/d into the circulation.

Another system (eg, Testoderm) is a patch (10 mg/40 cm^2 or 15 mg/60 cm^2) which is placed on a shaved area of the scrotum for 22 hours daily.

Disadvantages of both patch systems include skin irritation, inconvenience, and expense. Side effects of testosterone therapy may include acne, gynecomastia, and reduced HDL cholesterol.

Prognosis of Hypogonadism

If hypogonadism is due to a pituitary lesion, the prognosis is that of the primary disease (eg, tumor, necrosis). The prognosis for restoration of virility is good if testosterone is given.

Bagatell CJ, Bremner WJ: Androgens in men: Uses and abuses. N Engl J Med 1996;334:707.

Katznelson L et al: Increase in bone density and lean body mass during testosterone administration in men with acquired hypogonadism. J Clin Endocrinol Metab 1996; 81:4358.

Kleinheinz A, Schutze W: Klinefelter's syndrome: New and rapid diagnosis by PCR analysis of XIST gene expression. Andrologia 1994;26:127.

Nachtigall LB et al: Adult-onset idiopathic hypogonadotropic hypogonadism: A treatable form of male infertility. N Engl J Med 1997;336:410.

Testosterone patches for hypogonadism. Med Lett Drugs Ther 1996;38:49.

TESTICULAR TUMORS IN ADULTS
(See also Chapter 23.)

About 95% of testicular tumors are germ cell tumors (seminomas or nonseminomas). They may produce (as serum markers) hCG and alpha-fetoprotein. Seminomas do not produce alpha-fetoprotein, but about 5–10% produce some hCG; nonseminomas, on the other hand, produce increased serum levels of one or both of these markers in about 90% of cases. Men with liver disease may have misleadingly high levels of alpha-fetoprotein.

About 5% of testicular tumors are Leydig or Sertoli cell tumors. Leydig cell tumors tend to produce estrogen (75%) and cause gynecomastia and impotence on that basis; they may sometimes produce androgens that can cause pseudoprecocious puberty in boys. Sertoli cell tumors may also produce estrogen (30%) with feminization; gynecomastia may be due to hCG secretion (25%).

Some testicular tumors may be small and nonpalpable yet may secrete sufficient amounts of hCG or estrogen to cause gynecomastia or impotence. Testicular ultrasound may help reveal small tumors.

After unilateral orchiectomy for testicular cancer, an elevated FSH level prior to further treatment indicates a patient at higher risk for cancer in the remaining testis.

Einhorn LH: Clinical trials in testicular cancer. Cancer 1993;71:3182.

Gilliland FD, Key CR: Male genital cancers. Cancer 1995;95:295.

Hentrich MU et al: Testicular germ cell tumors in patients with human immunodeficiency virus infection. Cancer 1996;77:2109. (Of 192 men with germ cell tumors, six were HIV-positive. Prognosis and treatment were unchanged.)

Presti JC et al: Fertility and testis cancer. Urol Clin North Am 1993;20:17.

DISEASES OF THE OVARIES
(See also Chapter 17.)

PRIMARY AMENORRHEA

Primary amenorrhea is defined as failure of appearance of any menses by age 16. It may be due to ovarian failure or other conditions.

Etiology

The causes of primary amenorrhea include the following:

A. Hypothalamic-Pituitary Causes (With Low-Normal FSH): A genetic deficiency of GnRH and gonadotropins may be isolated or associated with other pituitary deficiencies or diminished olfaction (Kallman's syndrome). Hypothalamic lesions, particularly craniopharyngioma, may be present. Pituitary tumors may be nonsecreting or may secrete prolactin or growth hormone. Cushing's syndrome may be caused by glucocorticoid treatment, a cortisol-secreting adrenal tumor, or an ACTH-secreting pituitary tumor. Hypothyroidism can delay adolescence. Head trauma or encephalitis can cause gonadotropin deficiency. Primary amenorrhea may also be caused by constitutional delay of adolescence, organic illness, vigorous exercise (eg, ballet dancing, running), stressful life events, dieting, or anorexia nervosa; however, these conditions should not be assumed to account for amenorrhea without a full physical and endocrinologic evaluation. (See section on hypopituitarism.)

B. Hyperandrogenism (With Low-Normal FSH): Excess testosterone may be secreted by adrenal tumors or by adrenal hyperplasia caused by steroidogenic enzyme defects such as P450c21 deficiency (salt-wasting) or P450c11 deficiency (hypertension). Ovarian tumors or polycystic ovaries may also secrete excess testosterone. Serum testosterone is above the normal female range. Androgenic steroids may also cause this syndrome.

C. Ovarian Causes (With High FSH): Gonadal dysgenesis (Turner's syndrome and variants; see below) is a frequent cause of primary amenorrhea. Ovarian failure due to autoimmunity is a common cause. Various rare steroidogenic enzyme deficiencies may block ovarian production of estrogen. A deficiency in P450c17 steroidogenic enzyme activity causes hypogonadism (associated with hypertension and hypokalemia), as may a whole-body deficiency in P450arom activity (associated with polycystic ovaries, tall stature, osteoporosis, and virilization).

D. Pseudohermaphroditism (With High LH): An enzymatic defect in testosterone synthesis may present as a sexually immature phenotypic girl with primary amenorrhea. Complete androgen resistance (testicular feminization) presents as a phenotypic young woman without sexual hair but with normal breast development and primary amenorrhea. In both cases, the uterus is absent and testes are intra-abdominal or cryptorchid. Intra-abdominal testes are surgically resected. Such patients are treated as normal but infertile, hypogonadal women.

E. Uterine Causes (With Normal FSH): Congenital absence or malformation of the uterus may be responsible for primary amenorrhea, as may an unresponsive or atrophic endometrium. An imperforate hymen is occasionally the reason for the absence of visible menses.

F. Pregnancy (With High hCG): Pregnancy may be the cause of primary amenorrhea even when the patient denies ever having had sexual intercourse.

Clinical Findings

A. Symptoms and Signs: Patients with primary amenorrhea require a thorough history and physical examination to look for signs of the conditions noted above. Headaches or visual field abnormalities implicate a hypothalamic or pituitary tumor. Signs of pregnancy may be present. Blood pressure abnormalities, acne, and hirsutism should be noted. Short stature may be seen with an associated growth hormone or thyroid hormone deficiency. Short stature with manifestations of gonadal dysgenesis indicates Turner's syndrome (see below). Olfaction testing screens for Kallman's syndrome. Obesity and short stature may be signs of Cushing's syndrome. Tall stature may be due to eunuchoidism or gigantism. Hirsutism or virilization suggests excessive testosterone.

An external pelvic examination plus a rectal examination should be performed to assess hymenal patency and the presence of a uterus.

B. Laboratory Findings: The initial endocrine evaluation should include serum determinations of FSH, LH, PRL, testosterone, TSH, free T_4, and hCG (pregnancy test). Patients who are virilized or hypertensive require serum electrolyte determinations and further hormonal evaluation. Girls with low-normal FSH and LH—especially those with high PRL levels—are evaluated by MRI of the hypothalamus and pituitary. Girls who have a normal uterus and high FSH without the classic features of Turner's syndrome may require a karyotype to diagnose X chromosome mosaicism.

Treatment

Treatment of primary amenorrhea is directed at the underlying cause. Girls with permanent hypogonadism are treated with estrogen replacement therapy (see below).

SECONDARY AMENORRHEA

Secondary amenorrhea is defined as absence of menses for 3 consecutive months in women who have passed menarche.

Etiology

The causes of secondary amenorrhea include the following:

A. Hypothalamic-Pituitary Causes (With Low-Normal FSH): Prolactin elevation due to any cause (see section on hyperprolactinemia) may cause amenorrhea. Pituitary tumors or other lesions may cause hypopituitarism. Patients with signs of adrenal insufficiency require a cosyntropin stimulation test (see section on adrenal insufficiency).

Secondary "hypothalamic" amenorrhea may be caused by stressful life events such as school examinations or leaving home. Such women usually have a history of normal sexual development and irregular menses since menarche. Amenorrhea may also be the result of strict dieting, vigorous exercise, organic illness, or anorexia nervosa. These conditions should not be assumed to account for amenorrhea without a full physical and endocrinologic evaluation. Young women in whom the results of evaluation and progestin withdrawal test are normal have noncyclic secretion of gonadotropins resulting in anovulation. Such women typically recover spontaneously but should have regular evaluations and a progestin withdrawal test about every 3 months to detect loss of estrogen effect.

B. Hyperandrogenism (With Low-Normal FSH): Elevated serum levels of testosterone can cause hirsutism, virilization, and amenorrhea. The cause may be a rare adrenal or ovarian neoplasm. Other causes are polycystic ovary syndrome and adrenal P450c21 deficiency. Anabolic steroids also cause amenorrhea.

C. Uterine Causes (With Normal FSH): Infection of the uterus commonly occurs following delivery or D&C but may occur spontaneously. Endometritis due to tuberculosis or schistosomiasis should be suspected in endemic areas. Endometrial scarring may result, causing amenorrhea (Asherman's syndrome). Such women typically continue to have monthly premenstrual symptoms. The vaginal estrogen effect is normal. Diagnosis and treatment is best done by direct hysteroscopic inspection of the endometrium and lysis of adhesions. A small Foley catheter is left in the uterus for 1 week while antibiotics are given. The catheter is then replaced by an IUD for about 2 months. Cyclic estrogen and progestin is given to build up the endometrial lining. After such treatment, menses usually resume and fertility is possible, but spontaneous abortions and other pregnancy complications occur commonly.

D. Pregnancy (High hCG): Pregnancy is the most common cause for secondary amenorrhea in women of childbearing age. The differential diagnosis includes rare ectopic secretion of hCG by a choriocarcinoma or bronchogenic carcinoma.

E. Premature Ovarian Failure (High FSH): This refers to primary hypogonadism that occurs before age 40. About 30% of such cases are due to autoimmunity against the ovary. About 8% of cases are due to X chromosome mosaicism. Other causes include surgical bilateral oophorectomy, radiation therapy for pelvic malignancy, and chemotherapy. Women who have undergone hysterectomy are prone to premature ovarian failure even though the ovaries were left intact. Other cases may be familial or idiopathic. Ovarian failure is usually irreversible. Treatment consists of estrogen replacement therapy plus a progestin if the uterus is present.

F. Menopause (High FSH): "Climacteric" is defined as the period of natural physiologic decline in ovarian function, generally occurring over about 10 years. By about age 40, the remaining ovarian follicles are those that are the least sensitive to gonadotropins. Increasing titers of FSH are required to stimulate estradiol secretion. Lower levels of estradiol and more frequent anovulation tend to cause menometrorrhagia (dysfunctional uterine bleeding). Fertility declines progressively. Psychologic symptoms may include depression and irritability. Women may experience fatigue, insomnia, headache, diminished libido, or rheumatologic symptoms. Vasomotor instability (hot flushes) are experienced by 80% of women, lasting seconds to many minutes. Hot flushes may be most severe at night or may be triggered by emotional stress. Some women continue to menstruate for many months despite symptoms of estrogen deficiency. Estrogen supplementation provides symptomatic relief.

"Menopause" is defined as the terminal episode of naturally occurring menses. It is a retrospective diagnosis, usually made after 6 months of amenorrhea. The normal age for menopause in the USA ranges between 48 and 55 years, with an average of about 51.5 years. Serum estradiol levels fall and the remaining estrogen after menopause is estrone, derived mainly from peripheral aromatization of adrenal androstenedione. Such peripheral production of estrone is enhanced by obesity and liver disease. Individual differences in estrone levels partly explain why the symptoms noted above may be minimal in some women but severe in others. The acute symptoms of estrogen deficiency noted above tend to decline in severity within several years after menopause. However, about 35% of women have symptoms for more than 5 years. The late manifestations of estrogen deficiency include urogenital atrophy with vaginal dryness and dyspareunia; dysuria, frequency, and incontinence may occur. Increased bone osteoclastic activity increases the risk for osteoporosis and fractures. The skin becomes more wrinkled. Increases in the LDL:HDL cholesterol ratio cause an increased risk for arteriosclerosis.

Clinical Findings

A. Symptoms and Signs: All women with amenorrhea require a complete history and physical examination. Nausea and breast engorgement are typical signs of early pregnancy. Hot flushes are common in ovarian failure. Headache or visual field abnormalities are seen with pituitary or hypothalamic tumors. Complaints of thirst and polyuria require evaluation; diabetes insipidus implicates a hypothalamic lesion. Goiter may be due to hyperthyroidism. Weight loss, diarrhea, or skin darkening may indicate adrenal insufficiency. Weight loss with a distorted body image implicates anorexia nervosa. The breasts are examined carefully for galactorrhea, a common sign of hyperprolactinemia. Hirsutism or virilization may be a sign of hyperandrogenism. Manifestations of hypercortisolism (eg, weakness, psychiatric changes, hypertension, central obesity, hirsutism, thin skin, ecchymoses) may indicate alcoholism or Cushing's syndrome. Signs of acromegaly or gigantism may also indicate a pituitary tumor. Signs of systemic illness (eg, cirrhosis, renal failure) should be appreciated. Various drugs may elevate prolactin and cause amenorrhea (see section on hyperprolactinemia). Needle tracks may indicate heroin or amphetamine abuse.

A careful pelvic examination is always required to check for uterine or adnexal enlargement and to obtain a Papanicolaou smear and a vaginal smear for assessment of estrogen effect. Various life stresses, vigorous exercise, and "crash" dieting all predispose to amenorrhea; however, such factors should not be assumed to account for amenorrhea without a complete workup to screen for other causes.

B. Laboratory Findings: Since pregnancy is the most common cause of amenorrhea, women of childbearing age are immediately screened with a serum or urine hCG (pregnancy test). An elevated hCG overwhelmingly indicates pregnancy; false-positive testing may occur very rarely with ectopic hCG secretion (eg, choriocarcinoma or bronchogenic carcinoma). Women without an elevated hCG receive further laboratory evaluation including serum PRL, FSH, LH, TSH, and plasma potassium. Hyperprolactinemia or hypopituitarism (without obvious cause; see section on hypopituitarism) should prompt an MRI study of the pituitary region. Routine testing for renal and hepatic function (eg, BUN, serum creatinine, bilirubin, alkaline phosphatase, and ALT) is also performed. A serum testosterone level is obtained in hirsute or virilized women. Patients with manifestations of hypercortisolism receive a 1 mg overnight dexamethasone suppression test for initial screening (see section on Cushing's syndrome). Nonpregnant women without any laboratory abnormality may receive a 10-day course of a progestin (eg, medroxyprogesterone acetate, 10 mg/d); absence of withdrawal menses typically indicates a lack of estrogen or a uterine abnormality.

Treatment

Treatment of secondary amenorrhea is directed at the cause. Therapy of hypogonadism generally consists of estrogen replacement therapy (see below). The doses of estrogen required for symptomatic relief from vasomotor symptoms are sometimes higher than typical physiologic replacement doses. If estrogen replacement therapy is declined or contraindicated, partial symptomatic relief from hot flushes may sometimes be afforded by medroxyprogesterone acetate or clonidine. Tamoxifen, an antiestrogen used in breast cancer management, gives some bone protection but no relief from hot flushes. Treatment or prevention of postmenopausal osteoporosis with bisphosphonates such as alendronate (see section on osteoporosis) is another therapeutic option.

Estrogen Replacement Therapy

The goals of estrogen replacement therapy are several:

(1) Replace adequate estrogen to prevent osteoporosis.

(2) Restore menses when the patient wants this for psychologic reasons.

(3) Reduce manifestations of estrogen deficiency such as hot flushes, mood changes, vaginal dryness, urinary incontinence, and skin wrinkling.

(4) Improve serum lipid profile, possibly reducing the risk of cardiovascular disease.

(5) Reduce the risks of Alzheimer's disease and perhaps of colon and lung cancer.

Estrogen replacement therapy should begin with the onset of hypogonadism. However, it is not necessary to treat all cases, especially temporary amenorrhea or irregular menses. Patients who have normal menses after a short course of medroxyprogesterone acetate (see above) may have menses induced every 1–3 months in this manner.

Women who have had a hysterectomy are given conjugated estrogens, usually 0.625–1.25 mg, either daily or cycled on days 1–25 of the calendar month. Alternative oral estrogen preparations include ethinyl estradiol (20 or 50 µg) and estradiol (0.5, 1, or 2 mg). Estradiol may be delivered by skin patch (0.05 or 0.1 mg) reapplied twice weekly. Parenteral (intramuscular) preparations of estrogen include estradiol cypionate in oil (5 mg/mL; 1–5 mg every 3–4 weeks) and estradiol valerate (10, 20, or 40 mg/mL; 10–20 mg every 3–4 weeks).

Women with an intact uterus may be treated with estrogen (as above) but must also receive a progestin in order to decrease the risk of estrogen-induced endometrial carcinoma. Women receiving unopposed estrogen have a risk of endometrial carcinoma that is ten times greater than the risk in untreated patients. The addition of a progestin reduces the risk below that of untreated women. The progestin of choice is medroxyprogesterone acetate. Medroxyprogesterone acetate (5–10 mg) is given on days 16–25 of the calendar month; conjugated estrogens, 0.625–1.25 mg, is given daily on days 1–25 of the month. Alternatively, medroxyprogesterone may be given as 2.5 to 5 mg daily with the estrogen; this tends to cause irregular spotting for about 4 months, but bleeding then usually stops by 1 year, and women are not bothered by menstruation. Continued abnormal bleeding necessitates a pelvic examination; endometrial biopsy may be done using a Vibra aspiration technique. These regimens can be tailored to the individual's requirements and response.

Long-term estrogen replacement therapy produces a very significant reduction in the overall mortality of postmenopausal women, mainly by reducing the number of deaths due to cardiovascular disease. Improvement in serum HDL cholesterol is greatest with unopposed estrogen but is also seen with the addition of a progestin. Cycled progestin regimens seem to allow an increase in HDL greater than that seen with daily progestins. Medroxyprogesterone acetate is favored over most other progestins as having the least adverse effect on HDL cholesterol, though micronized progesterone may be better than medroxyprogesterone acetate in this regard.

The effect of long-term estrogen replacement therapy upon the risk of breast cancer is controversial. The Nurses' Health Study indicated an increased risk, but only for women who consumed alcohol. The Iowa Women's Health Study reported an increase in breast cancer with estrogen replacement in women consuming more than 5 g of alcohol daily. Several other large-cohort studies have shown no increased risk of breast cancer with estrogen replacement therapy. No markedly accelerated risk of breast cancer has been seen in users of estrogen replacement therapy who have benign breast disease or a family history of breast cancer. Any increased risk of breast cancer is small compared with the greatly reduced mortality and morbidity from cardiovascular disease and hip fracture seen with estrogen replacement therapy. Certain studies suggest that women receiving estrogen replacement therapy have a reduced incidence of Alzheimer's disease and a lower mortality rate from lung and colon cancers.

Relative contraindications to estrogen replacement therapy include breast cancer, melanoma, seizure disorders, and large pituitary prolactinomas.

Side effects of estrogen replacement may also include weight gain, edema, and breast tenderness. A very slightly increased risk of venous thrombosis is seen with oral estrogen. Estrogen therapy may cause hypertriglyceridemia, particularly in patients with preexistent hyperlipidemia, which may rarely result in pancreatitis.

Hypogonadal women usually have diminished ovarian androgen secretion. This contributes to hot flushes, loss of libido and sexual hair, muscle atrophy, and osteoporosis. Selected women may be treated with low-dose methyltestosterone, which is available in combination with conjugated estrogens (eg, Estratest). Tablets contain either 1.25 mg conjugated estrogens with 2.5 mg methyltestosterone or 0.625 mg conjugated estrogens with 1.25 mg methyltestosterone. Estratest is usually started at the lowest strength every 2 days, alternating days with standard estrogen replacement (see above). It should be given cyclically at the lowest dose that controls symptoms. At such small doses, side effects are usually minimal but may include nausea, polycythemia, emotional changes, paresthesias, electrolyte disturbances, and potentiation of anticoagulant therapy. Reduction in HDL cholesterol may negate the beneficial effect on cardiovascular mortality conferred by estrogen replacement therapy. Cholestatic jaundice and elevation of liver enzymes occur rarely. Hepatocellular neoplasms and peliosis hepatis, rare complications of oral androgens at higher doses, have not been reported with lower doses. Side effects of excess androgen treatment include hirsutism and virilization. Androgens should not be given to women with liver disease or during pregnancy or breast feeding.

Colditz GA et al: The use of estrogens and progestins and the risk of breast cancer in postmenopausal women. N Engl J Med 1995;332:1589. (A follow-up of the Nurses' Health Study reports an increased incidence of breast cancer among postmenopausal women treated with estrogen, with or without a progestin.)

Daly E et al: Risk of venous thromboembolism in users of hormone replacement therapy. Lancet 1996;348:977. (Current hormone replacement therapy use is associated with risk of venous thromboembolism. The number of extra cases appears to be only about one in 5000 users per year. These findings need to be weighed against the benefits of long-term treatment.)

Ettinger B et al: Reduced mortality associated with long-term postmenopausal estrogen therapy. Obstet Gynecol 1996;87:6.

Grodstein F et al: Postmenopausal estrogen and progestin

use and the risk of cardiovascular disease. N Engl J Med 1996;335:453.

Mayeaux EJ Jr, Johnson C: Current concepts in postmenopausal hormone replacement therapy. J Fam Pract 1996;43:69.

Newcomb PA et al: Long-term hormone replacement therapy and risk of breast cancer in postmenopausal women. Am J Epidemiol 1995;142:788. (This population-based case-control study in the USA evaluated 3130 breast cancer cases. Estrogen replacement was not associated with higher rates of breast cancer).

Postmenopausal Estrogen/Progestin Intervention (PEPI) Trial: Effects of hormone therapy on bone mineral density. JAMA 1996;276:1389.

Stanford JL et al: Combined estrogen and progestin hormone replacement therapy in relation to risk of breast cancer in middle-aged women. JAMA 1995;274:137. (The use of estrogen with progestin does not appear to be associated with an increased risk of breast cancer in middle-aged women. See editorial on p 179 of same issue.)

Sullivan JM: Estrogen replacement therapy. Am J Med 1996;101(Suppl 4A):56S.

Zumoff B: The critical role of alcohol consumption in determining the risk of breast cancer with postmenopausal estrogen administration. J Clin Endocrinol Metab 1997;82:1656.

TURNER'S SYNDROME
(Gonadal Dysgenesis)

Turner's syndrome is a chromosomal disorder associated with primary hypogonadism, short stature, and other phenotypic anomalies. It is a common cause of primary amenorrhea. Patients with the classic syndrome lack one of the two X chromosomes and have a 45,XO karyotype.

Typical Turner's Syndrome (45,XO Gonadal Dysgenesis)

Features of Turner's syndrome (Table 26–15) are variable and may be subtle in girls with mosaicism. Typical manifestations in adulthood include short stature, hypogonadism, webbed neck, high-arched palate, wide-spaced nipples, hypertension, and renal abnormalities. 45,XO zygotes account for about 0.8% of all conceptuses, making this the most common major chromosomal abnormality in humans. Less than 3% of these zygotes survive to term, with the incidence of Turner's syndrome being about 1:10,000 female newborns.

Girls with Turner's syndrome may be diagnosed at birth, since they tend to be small and may exhibit severe lymphedema. Evaluation for childhood short stature often leads to the diagnosis. Growth hormone and somatomedin levels are normal. Hypogonadism presents as "delayed adolescence"; FSH and LH are high, making a diagnosis of primary hypogonadism. A blood karyotype showing 46,XO (or X chromo-

Table 26–15. Manifestations of Turner's syndrome.

Distinctive facial features:
  Ptosis
  Micrognathia
  Low-set ears
  Epicanthal folds
Short stature
Sexual infantilism due to gonadal dysgenesis
Webbed neck (40%)
Low hairline
High-arched palate
Cubitus valgus
Short fourth metacarpals (50%)
Lymphedema of hands and feet (30%)
Hypoplastic widely spaced nipples
Hyperconvex nails
Pigmented nevi
Keloid formation
Recurrent ear infections
Renal abnormalities (60%)
  Horseshoe kidney
  Hydronephrosis
Hypertension (idiopathic or due to coarctation or renal
  disease)
Gastrointestinal bleeding from intestinal telangiectases (rare)
Impaired space-form recognition, direction sense, and
  mathematical reasoning
Cardiovasular anomalies
  Coarctation of the aorta (10–20%)
  Aortic stenosis
  Bicuspid aortic valve
  Aortic dissection due to coarctation and cystic medial
    necrosis of aorta (rare)
Associated conditions
  Obesity
  Diabetes mellitus
  Hashimoto's thyroiditis
  Achlorhydria
  Cataracts: lenticular or corneal
  Rheumatoid arthritis
  Inflammatory bowel disease

some abnormalities or mosaicism) establishes the diagnosis.

Treatment of girls with Turner's syndrome is largely supportive. Treatment of girls over age 9 with daily injections of growth hormone (0.1 units/kg/d) plus an androgen for 4 years increases final height by a mean of about 8.5 cm over the mean predicted height of 145.7 cm. Estrogen replacement is begun as growth stops with low doses of conjugated estrogens (0.3 mg) or ethinyl estradiol (5 μg) given on days 1–25 per month; the dose is gradually increased over 2–3 years to 0.625–1.25 mg of conjugated estrogens or 10–20 μg of ethinyl estradiol. Medroxyprogesterone acetate, 5 mg, is added on days 16–25 of the month to induce menses.

Turner's Syndrome Variants

A. 46,X (Abnormal X) Karyotype: An abnormality or deletion of certain genes on the short arm of the X chromosome causes short stature and other signs of Turner's syndrome; some gonadal function and even fertility is possible. Abnormalities or dele-

tions of other genes located on both the long and short arms of the X chromosome can produce gonadal dysgenesis with few other somatic features.

B. 45,XO/46,XX Mosaicism: This karyotype results in a modified form of Turner's syndrome. Such girls tend to be taller and may have more gonadal function and fewer other manifestations of Turner's syndrome.

C. Other Variants: 45,XO/46,XY mosaicism can produce some manifestations of Turner's syndrome. Patients may have ambiguous genitalia or male infertility with an otherwise normal phenotype.

Gravholt CH et al: Prenatal and postnatal prevalence of Turner's syndrome: a registry study. BMJ 1996;312:16.

Nilsson KO et al: Improved final height in girls with Turner's syndrome treated with growth hormone and oxandrolone. J Clin Endocrinol Metab 1996;81:635.

Saenger P: Turner's syndrome. N Engl J Med 1996; 335:1749.

MULTIPLE ENDOCRINE NEOPLASIA

Several syndromes with multiple gland involvement have been described (Table 26–16).

MEN 1
(Wermer's Syndrome)

The most common multiglandular syndrome is multiple endocrine neoplasia type 1 (MEN 1). Biochemical testing identifies affected individuals by age 14–18 years, but the syndrome usually becomes clinically manifest in the fourth decade. **Hyperparathyroidism** occurs in over 80% of patients; it presents with hypercalcemia and usually involves hyperplasia or adenomas of several parathyroid glands. **Pancreatic islet cell tumors** occur in about 75% of patients; gastrinomas are the most common tumor and can result in gastric hyperacidity (Zollinger-Ellison syndrome) with peptic ulcer disease or diarrhea. Islet cell tumors may also secrete insulin, somatostatin, or glucagon. **Pituitary adenomas** occur in about 60% and may secrete prolactin, growth hormone, or ACTH but are usually nonfunctional; such tumors may produce local pressure effects and hypopituitarism. About 37% of these patients have adrenal cortical adenomas or hyperplasia—bilateral in about half. They are generally benign and nonfunctional. In one series, one out of 12 such patients developed a feminizing adrenal carcinoma. These adrenal lesions are pituitary-independent.

Tumors of the pituitary gland, the parathyroid gland, and the pancreatic islets may occur in the same patient, though not necessarily at the same

Table 26–16. Multiple endocrine neoplasia (MEN) syndromes.[1]

	MEN 1	MEN 2A	MEN 2B
Synonym	Wermer's syndrome	Sipple's syndrome	
Genetic transmission	Autosomal dominant	Autosomal dominant	Autosomal dominant
Tumor types (incidence)			
Parathyroid	> 80%	50%	Rare
Pancreatic	75%		
Pituitary	60%		
Medullary thyroid carcinoma		> 90%	80%
Pheochromocytoma		20%	60%
Mucosal and gastrointestinal ganglioneuromas		Rare	> 90%
Lipoma	Occasional		
Adrenocortical adenoma	Occasional		
Carcinoid	Occasional		
Thyroid adenoma	Occasional		

[1]From Fitzgerald PA (editor): *Handbook of Clinical Endocrinology*, 2nd ed. Appleton & Lange, 1992.

time. Some individuals in the same family express the abnormality as children, whereas in others the clinical manifestations may not appear until late in adult life. The clinical manifestations of MEN 1 are extremely variable, since the glandular tumors may secrete a variety of different hormones.

The kindreds expressing MEN 1 have been shown to harbor a gene mutation on the long arm of chromosome 11, which causes phenotypic expression as a dominant trait. Genetic linkage analysis can be used to determine which other family members will express this syndrome, permitting informed genetic counseling and avoiding unnecessary testing for unaffected individuals.

The differential diagnosis of MEN 1 includes sporadic or familial tumors of the pituitary, parathyroids, or pancreatic islets. Hypercalcemia (from any cause) may cause gastrointestinal symptoms and increased gastrin levels, simulating a gastrinoma. Treatment of gastrointestinal symptoms with H_2 blockers or metoclopramide causes hyperprolactinemia, simulating a pituitary prolactinoma.

MEN 2a (Sipple's Syndrome)

A separate disorder of multiglandular hypersecretion of hormones is multiple endocrine neoplasia type 2a. It too is inherited as an autosomal dominant trait. In MEN 2a, patients may have **medullary thyroid carcinoma** (> 90%); hyperparathyroidism (20–50%), due to hyperplasia or multiple adenomas in over 70% of cases; or **pheochromocytomas** (20–35%), which are often bilateral. The medullary thyroid carcinoma is of mild to moderate aggressiveness and generally occurs in the third or fourth decade in the familial syndrome and in the sixth decade in sporadic cases.

Siblings or children of patients with MEN 2a can have genetic testing to determine if they have a muta-

tion of the *RET* proto-oncogene, which identifies about 98% of such individuals. There is incomplete penetrance and about 30% of those with such mutations never manifest endocrine tumors. Alternatively, patients may have periodic serum calcitonin measurements after pentagastrin stimulation to screen for early medullary thyroid carcinoma: pentagastrin, 0.5 μg/kg, is given intravenously over 15 seconds; serum samples for calcitonin are obtained at 1½-, 5-, and 10-minute intervals; a peak level over 190 pg/mL in males or over 80 pg/mL in females implicates an occult medullary thyroid carcinoma. Alternatively, patients may be screened with a serum calcitonin drawn after 3 days of omeprazole, 20 mg orally twice daily; calcitonin levels rise in the presence of medullary thyroid carcinoma to levels seen with the pentagastrin test. Patients with *RET* mutations or abnormal stimulation testing are advised to have a total thyroidectomy after screening for latent pheochromocytoma.

MEN 2b

Patients with MEN 2b have a syndrome characterized by mucosal neuromas (> 90% with bumpy lips, enlarged tongue, Marfan-like habitus), pheochromocytomas (60%), and medullary thyroid carcinoma (80%), which can be quite aggressive. Patients also have intestinal abnormalities (75%), skeletal abnormalities (87%), and delayed puberty (43%). The medullary thyroid carcinoma is aggressive and tends to present in the third to fourth decades. Prophylactic thyroidectomy is advisable for patients with mucosal neuromas and family members with the syndrome or *RET* proto-oncogene mutations after screening for pheochromocytoma.

Buckley LM et al: Calcium and vitamin D_3 supplementation prevents bone loss in the spine secondary to low-dose corticosteroids in patients with rheumatoid arthri-

Table 26–17. Systemic versus topical activity
of corticosteroids.
(Hydrocortisone = 1 in potency.)

	Systemic Activity	Topical Activity
Prednisone	4–5	1–2
Fluprednisolone	8–10	10
Triamcinolone	5	1
Triamcinolone acetonide	5	40
Dexamethasone	30–120	10
Betamethasone	30	5–10
Betamethasone valerate	. . .	50–150
Methylprednisolone	5	5
Fluocinolone acetonide	. . .	40–100
Flurandrenolone acetonide	. . .	20–50
Fluorometholone	1–2	40
Deflazacort	3–4	. . .

tis: A randomized, double-blind, placebo-controlled trial. Ann Intern Med 1996;125:961.

Diamond T et al: Cyclical etidronate plus ergocalciferol prevents glucocorticoid-induced bone loss in post-menopausal women. Am J Med 1995;98:459.

Eng C; Seminars in medicine of the Beth Israel Hospital, Boston. The RET proto-oncogene in multiple endocrine neoplasia type 2 and Hirschsprung's disease. N Engl J Med 1996;335:943.

Erdőgan MF et al: Omeprazole:calcitonin stimulation test for the diagnosis, follow-up, and family screening in medullary thyroid carcinoma. J Clin Endocrinol Metab 1997;82:897.

Ledger GA et al: Genetic testing in the diagnosis and management of multiple endocrine neoplasia type II. Ann Intern Med 1995;122:118.

Mulligan LM, Ponder BA: Genetic basis of endocrine disease: Multiple endocrine neoplasia type 2. J Clin Endocrinol Metab 1995;80:1989.

Neumann HP et al: Pheochromocytomas, multiple endocrine neoplasia type 2, and von Hippel-Lindau disease. N Engl J Med 1993;329:1531. (All patients with pheochromocytomas should be screened for MEN 2 and von Hippel-Lindau disease to avert further morbidity and mortality in the patients and their families. Conversely, all patients in families with MEN 2 or von Hippel-Lindau disease should be screened for pheochromocytoma, even if they are asymptomatic.)

Table 26–18. Management of patients receiving systemic glucocorticoids.[1]

1. Do not administer glucocorticoids unless absolutely indicated and more conservative measures have failed.
2. Keep dosage and duration of administration to the minimum required for adequate treatment.
3. Screen for tuberculosis before treatment with a PPD or chest x-ray.
4. Screen for diabetes mellitus before treatment and at each physician visit. Train the patient to test urine weekly for glucose.
5. Screen for hypertension before treatment and at each physician visit.
6. Screen for glaucoma and cataracts before treatment, 3 months into treatment, and then at least yearly.
7. Prepare the patient and family for possible adverse effects on mood, memory, and cognitive function. Inform them about other possible side effects, particularly weight gain, osteoporosis, and aseptic necrosis of bone.
8. Institute a vigorous physical exercise and isometric regimen tailored to each patient's disabilities.
9. Administer calcium (1 g elemental calcium) and vitamin D_3, 400–800 IU orally daily. Check spot morning urines, and alter dosage to keep urine calcium concentration below 30 mg/dL. If the patient is receiving thiazide diuretics, check for hypercalcemia, and administer only 500 mg elemental calcium daily. Consider a bisphosphonate such as alendronate or cycled etidronate for prophylaxis against osteoporosis.
10. Avoid prolonged bed rest that will accelerate muscle weakness and bone mineral loss. Ambulate early after fractures.
11. Treat hypogonadism in women or men.
12. Avoid elective surgery, if possible. Vitamin A in a daily dose of 20,000 units orally for 1 week may improve wound healing.
13. Avoid activities that could cause falls or other trauma.
14. Watch for fungal or yeast infections of skin, nails, mouth, vagina, and rectum, and treat appropriately.
15. Ulcer prophylaxis: Administer oral glucocorticoids with meals. Glucocorticoids alone do not need prophylaxis with H_2 blockers or omeprazole. If administered with nonsteroidals, consider prophylaxis with omeprazole, 20–40 mg/d. Avoid large doses of antacids containing aluminum hydroxide (many popular brands); aluminum hydroxide binds phosphate and may cause a hypophosphatemic osteomalacia that can compound glucocorticoid osteoporosis.
16. Treat any infections aggressively. Consider unusual pathogens.
17. Weigh daily. Use dietary measures to avoid obesity and optimize nutrition.
18. Measure height frequently. This serves to document the degree of axial spine demineralization and compression.
19. Treat edema as indicated.
20. Monitor plasma potassium for hypokalemia. Treat as indicated.
21. Obtain bone densitometry before treatment and then periodically. Treat osteoporosis.
22. Avoid smoking and excessive ethanol consumption.
23. With dosage reduction, watch for signs of adrenal insufficiency or glucocorticoid withdrawal syndrome.

[1]Modified and reproduced, with permission, from Fitzgerald PA: *Handbook of Clinical Endocrinology*, 2nd ed. Appleton & Lange, 1992.

CLINICAL USE OF GLUCOCORTICOIDS

Mechanisms of Action

Cortisol is a steroid hormone that is normally secreted by the adrenal cortex in response to ACTH. It exerts its action by binding to nuclear receptors that then act upon chromatin to regulate gene expression, producing effects throughout the body.

Relative Potencies

Hydrocortisone and cortisone acetate, like cortisol, have mineralocorticoid effects that become excessive at higher doses. Other synthetic glucocorticoids such prednisone, dexamethasone, and deflazacort (an oxazoline derivative of prednisolone) have minimal mineralocorticoid activity. The relative potencies relative to hydrocortisone are listed in Table 26–17. Anticonvulsant drugs (eg, phenytoin, carbamazepine, phenobarbital) accelerate the metabolism of glucocorticoids other than hydrocortisone, making them significantly less potent. Megestrol, a synthetic progestin, has slight glucocorticoid activity that becomes significant when administered in high doses for appetite stimulation.

Adverse Effects

Prolonged treatment with systemic glucocorticoids causes a variety of adverse effects that can be life-threatening. Patients should be thoroughly informed of the major possible side effects of treatment such as insomnia, personality change, weight gain, muscle weakness, polyuria, kidney stones, diabetes mellitus, sex hormone suppression, occasional amenorrhea in women, candidiasis and opportunistic infections, osteoporosis with fractures, or aseptic necrosis of bones, particularly of the hips, which may become manifest many months after even brief treatment (see section on Cushing's syndrome). Therefore, it is wise to follow an organized treatment plan such as the one outlined in Table 26–18.

Buckley LM et al: Calcium and vitamin D_3 supplementation prevents bone loss in the spine secondary to low-dose corticosteroids in patients with rheumatoid arthritis. A randomized, double-blind, placebo-controlled trial. Ann Intern Med 1996;125:961.

Diamond T et al: Cyclical etidronate plus ergocalciferol prevents glucocorticoid-induced bone loss in postmenopausal women. Am J Med 1995;98:459.

Hahn BH, Mazzaferri EL: Glucocorticoid-induced osteoporosis. Hosp Pract (Off Ed) 1995 Aug;30:45.

Millard PS: Corticosteroid-induced bone loss. J Fam Pract 1996;42:347.

Picado C, Luengo M: Corticosteroid-induced bone loss: Prevention and management. Drug Saf 1996;15:347.

Steer KA et al: Megestrol-induced Cushing's syndrome. Clin Endocrinol 1995;42:91.

Diabetes Mellitus & Hypoglycemia   27

John H. Karam, MD

DIABETES MELLITUS

Essentials of Diagnosis

Type I diabetes, or insulin-dependent diabetes mellitus (IDDM):
- Polyuria, polydipsia, and rapid weight loss associated with unequivocal hyperglycemia.
- Plasma glucose of 140 mg/dL or higher after an overnight fast, documented on more than one occasion.
- Ketonemia, ketonuria, or both.

Type II diabetes, or non-insulin-dependent diabetes mellitus (NIDDM):
- Most patients are over 40 years of age and obese.
- Polyuria and polydipsia. Ketonuria and weight loss generally are uncommon at time of diagnosis. Candidal vaginitis in women may be an initial manifestation. Many patients have few or no symptoms.
- Plasma glucose of 140 mg/dL or higher after an overnight fast on more than one occasion. After 75 g oral glucose, diagnostic values are 200 mg/dL or more 2 hours after the oral glucose and at least once between 0 and 2 hours.
- Hypertension, hyperlipidemia, and atherosclerosis are often associated.

Classification & Pathogenesis

Diabetes mellitus represents a syndrome with disordered metabolism and inappropriate hyperglycemia due to either an absolute deficiency of insulin secretion or a reduction in its biologic effectiveness or both. It is classified into two major types in which age at onset is not a criterion (Table 27–1).

A. Type I: Insulin-Dependent Diabetes Mellitus (IDDM): This severe form is associated with ketosis in the untreated state. It occurs most commonly in juveniles but occasionally in adults, especially the nonobese and those who are elderly when hyperglycemia first appears. It is a catabolic disorder in which circulating insulin is virtually absent, plasma glucagon is elevated, and the pancreatic B cells fail to respond to all insulinogenic stimuli. Exogenous insulin is therefore required to reverse the catabolic state, prevent ketosis, reduce the hyperglucagonemia, and bring the elevated blood glucose level down.

The highest prevalence of type I diabetes is in Scandinavia, where it comprises as many as 20% of the total number of patients with diabetes. This decreases in prevalence to 13% in southern Europe and 8% in the USA, while in Japan and China less than 1% of patients with diabetes have type I diabetes.

Certain human leukocyte antigens (HLA) are strongly associated with the development of type I diabetes. About 95% of type I patients possess either HLA-DR3 or HLA-DR4, compared to 45–50% of Caucasian controls. HLA-DQ genes are even more specific markers of type I susceptibility, since a particular variety (HLA-DQw3.2) is generally found in the DR4 patients with type I, while a "protective" gene (HLA-DQw3.1) is often present in the DR4 controls. In addition, circulating islet cell antibodies have been detected in as many as 85% of patients tested in the first few weeks of their diabetes, and when sensitive immunoassays are used, the majority of these patients also have detectable anti-insulin antibodies prior to receiving insulin therapy. It has recently been documented that most islet cell antibodies are directed against glutamic acid decarboxylase, a 64,000-MW enzyme localized within pancreatic B cells. Immunoassay kits for this sensitive antibody marker of type I diabetes are now available (Kronus, San Clemente, California). These kits facilitate screening of siblings of affected children as well as adults with atypical features of type II for the presence of an autoimmune cause for their diabetes.

Because of these immune characteristics, type I diabetes is felt to result from an infectious or toxic environmental insult to persons whose immune system is genetically predisposed to develop a vigorous autoimmune response either against altered pancreatic B cell antigens or against molecules of the B cell resembling the viral protein (molecular mimicry). Extrinsic factors that affect B cell function include dam-

Table 27–1. Clinical classification of idiopathic diabetes mellitus syndromes.

Type	Ketosis	Islet Cell Antibodies	HLA Association	Treatment
(I) Insulin-dependent (IDDM)	Present	Present at onset	Positive	Insulin (mixtures of rapid- and intermediate-acting, at least twice daily) and diet
(II) Non-insulin-dependent (NIDDM) (a) Nonobese	Absent	Absent	Negative	(1) Eucaloric diet alone (2) Diet plus insulin or oral agents
(b) Obese				(1) Weight reduction (2) Hypocaloric diet, plus oral agents or insulin for symptomatic control only

age caused by viruses such as mumps or coxsackie B4 virus, by toxic chemical agents, or by destructive cytotoxins and antibodies released from sensitized immunocytes. Specific HLA genes may increase susceptibility to a diabetogenic virus or be linked to certain immune response genes that predispose patients to a destructive autoimmune response against their own islet cells (autoaggression). Amelioration of hyperglycemia in patients given cyclosporine shortly after onset of type I diabetes lends further support to the pathogenetic role of autoimmunity.

B. Type II: Non-Insulin-Dependent Diabetes Mellitus (NIDDM): This represents a heterogeneous group comprising milder forms of diabetes that occur predominantly in adults but occasionally in juveniles. More than 90% of all diabetics in the USA are included under this classification. Circulating endogenous insulin is sufficient to prevent ketoacidosis but is inadequate in the face of increased needs owing to tissue insensitivity. Type II diabetes is defined in essentially negative terms: It is a *non*ketotic form of diabetes that is *not* linked to HLA markers on the sixth chromosome; it has *no* islet cell antibodies or any other immune component; and it is *not* dependent on exogenous insulin therapy to sustain life, thereby being termed "*non*-insulin-dependent diabetes mellitus" (NIDDM). In most cases of this type of diabetes, the cause is unknown.

An element of tissue insensitivity to insulin has been noted in most type II patients irrespective of weight and has been attributed to several interrelated factors. These include a primary (and as yet undefined) genetic factor, which is aggravated in time by additional enhancers of insulin resistance such as aging and abdominal-visceral obesity. In addition, there is an accompanying deficiency in the response of pancreatic B cells to glucose. Both the tissue resistance to insulin and the impaired B cell response to glucose appear to be further aggravated by increased hyperglycemia, and both defects are ameliorated by treatment that reduces the hyperglycemia toward normal. Attempts to identify a genetic marker for type II have as yet been unsuccessful. However, most epidemiologic data indicate strong genetic influences, since in monozygotic twins over 40 years of age,

concordance is uniform within a year whenever one twin develops type II.

Two subgroups of patients with type II diabetes are currently distinguished by the absence or presence of obesity. The degree and prevalence of obesity varies among different racial groups. While obesity occurs in less than 30% of Chinese and Japanese patients with type II, it is found in 75–80% of North Americans, Europeans, or Africans with type II and approaches 100% of patients with type II among Pima Indians or Pacific Islanders from Nauru or Samoa.

1. Nonobese type II patients–These patients generally show an absent or blunted early phase of insulin release in response to glucose; however, it may often be elicited in response to other insulinogenic stimuli such as acute intravenous administration of sulfonylureas, glucagon, or secretin.

Although residual insulin resistance may be detected after therapeutic correction of the hyperglycemia in some cases, it does not seem to be clinically relevant to the treatment of most nonobese type II patients, who generally respond to appropriate therapeutic supplements of insulin in the absence of rare associated conditions such as lipoatrophy or acanthosis nigricans.

Among this heterogeneous subgroup of patients with nonobese type II diabetes, the vast majority are idiopathic. However, with increasing frequency, a variety of etiologic genetic abnormalities have been documented in these phenotypic type II diabetics. These include the following: (See Table 27–2.)

a. Maturity-onset diabetes of the young (MODY)–This subgroup is a relatively rare disorder characterized by non-insulin-dependent diabetes with autosomal dominant inheritance and an age at onset of 25 years or younger. Patients are nonobese, and their hyperglycemia is due to impaired glucose-induced secretion of insulin. Three types of MODY have been described, with single gene defects localized to chromosomes 20, 7, and 12—designated MODY 1, MODY 2 ,and MODY 3, respectively.

(1) MODY 1 includes 74 members of a pedigree known as the R-W family, who are descendants of a German couple who immigrated to Detroit, Michi-

Table 27–2. Nonobese "type II" diabetes with genetic markers.

SINGLE GENE MUTATIONS		
Syndrome	Mutation	Chromosome
MODY 1	Hepatocyte nuclear factor-4α	20q
MODY 2	Glucokinase gene	7p
MODY 3	Hepatocyte nuclear factor-1α	12q
Mutant insulin	Insulin gene	11p
Mutant insulin receptor	Insulin receptor gene	19p
Mitochondrial mutation	Transfer RNAs (leucine or lysine tRNA)	Mitochondrial DNA

POLYGENIC TRANSMISSION		
Syndrome	High-Risk Genotypes	Chromosome
Incomplete form of type I IDDM1	HLA DR3 or HLA DR4 (or both)	6p
IDDM2	Insulin gene region	11p

gan, in 1861. They have been studied prospectively since 1958, and in 1996 the genetic defect was shown to be a nonsense mutation of a nuclear transcription factor found in liver as well as in pancreatic B cells. This gene has been termed hepatocyte nuclear factor-4α (HNF-4α) and is found on chromosome 20. Just how it reduces glucose-induced insulin secretion has not yet been clarified, but it may contribute to impaired gene expression.

(2) MODY 2 has been described in all parts of the world, and at least 26 different mutations of the glucokinase gene on chromosome 7 have been identified. Reduced sensitivity of pancreatic B cell glucokinase to plasma glucose causes impaired insulin secretion, resulting in fasting hyperglycemia and mild diabetes.

(3) MODY 3 is caused by mutations of the hepatocyte nuclear factor-1α (HNF-1α), whose gene is located on chromosome 12. As many as seven different mutations of this gene have been identified in seven families. This transcription factor is expressed in pancreatic B cells as well as in liver and is a weak transactivator of the insulin gene. This may explain how mutations of HNF-1α impair glucose-induced insulin secretion.

b. Diabetes due to mutant insulins–This is a very rare subtype of nonobese type II diabetes, with no more than nine individuals and their families having been described. Since all affected individuals were heterozygous and possessed one normal insulin gene, diabetes was usually quite mild, did not appear until middle age, and showed autosomal dominant genetic transmission. These patients generally have

no evidence of clinical insulin resistance and respond well to standard therapy.

c. Diabetes due to mutant insulin receptors–Defects in the insulin receptor gene have been found in more than 40 people with diabetes, but most of them are patients with rare syndromes of extreme insulin resistance associated with acanthosis nigricans. Patients with classic forms of type II diabetes have not shown insulin receptor mutations and seem to have a postreceptor defect of unknown cause.

d. Diabetes mellitus associated with a mutation of mitochondrial DNA–Since sperm do not contain mitochondria, only the mother transmits mitochondrial genes to her offspring. Diabetes due to a mutation of mitochondrial DNA that impairs the transfer of leucine into mitochondrial proteins has been described in 22 Japanese families involving 52 individuals as well as in isolated case reports in Caucasians. Most patients have a mild form of maternally transmitted diabetes that responds to oral hypoglycemic agents, though four persons had a nonimmune form of IDDM. As many as 63% of patients with this subtype of diabetes have a hearing loss, and a smaller proportion (15%) had a syndrome of myopathy, encephalopathy, lactic acidosis, and stroke-like episodes (MELAS). A lysine transfer defect has also recently been found in a family with maternally transmitted diabetes.

e. Mild forms of type I diabetes–Certain unrecognized patients with a milder expression of type I diabetes initially retain enough B cell function to avoid ketosis but later in life develop increasing dependency on insulin therapy as their B cell mass diminishes.

2. Obese type II patients–This form of diabetes is secondary to extrapancreatic factors that produce insensitivity to endogenous insulin. It is characterized by nonketotic mild diabetes, mainly in adults but occasionally also in children. The primary problem is a "target organ" disorder resulting in ineffective insulin action (Table 27–3) that can secondarily influence pancreatic B cell function. Hyperplasia of

Table 27–3. Factors reducing response to insulin.

Prereceptor inhibitors: Anti-insulin antibodies
Receptor inhibitors:
  Insulin receptor antibodies
  "Down-regulation" of receptors by hyperinsulinism:
    Primary hyperinsulinism (B cell adenoma)
    Hyperinsulinism secondary to a postreceptor defect
      (obesity, Cushing's syndrome, acromegaly,
      pregnancy) or prolonged glycemia (diabetes mellitus,
      post-glucose tolerance test)
Postreceptor influences:
  Poor responsiveness of principal target organs; obesity;
    hepatic disease; muscle inactivity; sustained
    hyperglycemia
  Hormonal excess: glucocorticoids, growth hormone, oral
    contraceptive agents, progesterone, human chorionic
    somatomammotropin, catecholamines, thyroxine

pancreatic B cells is often present and probably accounts for the fasting hyperinsulinism and exaggerated insulin and proinsulin responses to glucose and other stimuli seen in the milder forms of this disorder. In more severe cases, secondary (but potentially reversible) failure of B cell secretion may result after exposure to prolonged fasting hyperglycemia. This phenomenon has been called "desensitization" of the pancreatic B cell. It is selective for glucose, and the B cell recovers sensitivity to glucose stimulation once the sustained hyperglycemia is corrected by any form of therapy, including diet, oral hypoglycemic agents, or insulin. Obesity is common in this type of diabetes and is generally associated with abdominal distribution of fat, producing an abnormally high waist-to-hip ratio. Refined radiographic techniques of assessing abdominal fat distribution with CT scans have documented that a "visceral" obesity, due to accumulation of fat in the omental and mesenteric regions, correlates with insulin resistance, whereas fat predominantly in subcutaneous tissues of the abdomen has little if any association with insulin insensitivity. Lipolysis of visceral fat directly into the portal circulation alters liver metabolism and increases hepatic glucose output much more than when peripheral fat is mobilized into systemic veins. Exercise may affect the deposition of visceral fat as suggested by CT scans of Japanese Sumo wrestlers, whose extreme obesity is predominantly subcutaneous. Their daily vigorous exercise program seems to prevent accumulation of visceral fat, and they have normal serum lipids and normoglycemia despite daily intakes of 5000–7000 kcal and development of massive subcutaneous obesity.

A major cause of the observed resistance to insulin in target tissues of obese patients is believed to be a postreceptor defect in insulin action. This is associated with overdistended storage depots, and there is a reduced ability to clear nutrients from the circulation after meals. A resulting hyperinsulinism can further enhance insulin resistance by down-regulation of insulin receptors. Moreover, when hyperglycemia develops, a specific glucose transporter protein within insulin target tissue also becomes down-regulated after continuous activation. This contributes to further defects in postreceptor insulin action, thereby aggravating the hyperglycemia.

When exercise increases blood flow to muscle as well as increasing muscle mass, and when overfeeding is corrected so that storage depots become less saturated, the cycle is interrupted. There is improvement in insulin sensitivity, which is further restored toward normal by a reduction of both the hyperinsulinism and the hyperglycemia.

Epidemiologic Considerations

An estimated 16 million people in the USA are known to have diabetes, of which 1.4 million have the insulin-dependent type. Use of the current "therapeutic" classification has been widely accepted throughout the world, but its deficiencies are apparent in many individual cases. For example, a 23-year-old nonobese woman whose mild diabetes is presently responding adequately to diet alone and who shows a low-normal C-peptide response to stimuli had presented with severe diabetes with ketosis and required insulin for several weeks following diagnosis. In addition, she has an associated autoimmune disorder, myasthenia gravis. From an etiologic standpoint, she probably has type I diabetes, but her present clinical status is "non-insulin-dependent." Similarly, many diabetics classified as "non-insulin-dependent" require insulin therapy. Now that assays to screen for islet cell antibodies as well as for antibodies against glutamic acid decarboxylase are more available (see above), a new classification will be forthcoming relating to cause and independent of therapy. To retain the acronyms, type I could aptly be termed "immune-dependent diabetes mellitus" (IDDM), and type II "non-immune-dependent diabetes mellitus" (NIDDM).

Insulin resistance syndrome (syndrome X, CHAOS). Investigators have speculated that the well-known association of **hyperglycemia, hyperinsulinemia, dyslipidemia,** and **hypertension,** which leads to coronary artery disease and stroke, may result from a genetic defect producing insulin resistance, particularly when obesity aggravates the degree of insulin resistance. They suggest that insulin resistance predisposes to hyperglycemia, which results in hyperinsulinemia, which may or may not be of sufficient magnitude to correct the hyperglycemia; and that this excessive insulin level then contributes to increased VLDL production in the liver, leading to hyperlipidemia and to increased sodium retention by renal tubules, thus inducing hypertension. Moreover, they propose that high insulin levels can stimulate endothelial proliferation—by virtue of insulin's action on growth factor receptors—to initiate atherosclerosis. Australian epidemiologists have called this association of disorders "CHAOS" (acronym for coronary artery disease, hypertension, atherosclerosis, obesity, and stroke). While these associations have been well known, the mechanism for their interrelationship remains speculative and an invitation to experimental investigation. Some investigators question the etiologic role of hyperinsulinism on hypertension, since these two manifestations, which often coexist in Caucasians, are not highly associated in blacks or Pima Indians. Moreover, patients with hyperinsulinism due to insulinoma are generally not hypertensive, and there is no fall in blood pressure after surgical removal of the insulinoma restores normal insulin levels. The main value of grouping these disorders as a syndrome, however, is to remind physicians that the therapeutic goals are not only to correct hyperglycemia but also to manage the elevated blood pressure and dyslipidemia that result in increased cerebrovascular and cardiac morbidity and mortality in these patients. Physicians aware of this syndrome are less likely to prescribe therapies that correct hypertension but raise lipids (diuretics, beta-blockers) or that correct hyperlipidemia but increase insulin resistance, with aggravation of diabetes (niacin). Finally, the use of long-acting insulins and sulfonylureas that promote sustained hyperinsulinism may have to be moderated, with insulin-sparing drugs such as metformin being preferable, if the hypothesis behind the insulin-resistance syndrome is ever substantiated.

Clinical Findings

The principal clinical features of the two major types of diabetes mellitus are listed for comparison in Table 27–4.

Patients with type I diabetes (IDDM) present with a characteristic symptom complex, as outlined below. An absolute deficiency of insulin results in excessive accumulation of circulating glucose and fatty acids, with consequent hyperosmolality and hyperketonemia. The severity of the insulin deficiency and the acuteness with which the catabolic state develops determine the intensity of the osmotic and ketotic excess.

Patients with type II diabetes (NIDDM) may or may not present with characteristic symptoms and signs. The presence of obesity or a strongly positive family history for mild diabetes suggests a high risk for the development of type II diabetes.

A. Symptoms and Signs:

1. Type I diabetes (IDDM)–Increased urination is a consequence of osmotic diuresis secondary to sustained hyperglycemia. This results in a loss of glucose as well as free water and electrolytes in the urine. Thirst is a consequence of the hyperosmolar state, as is blurred vision, which often develops as the lenses and retinas are exposed to hyperosmolar fluids.

Weight loss despite normal or increased appetite is

Table 27–4. Clinical features of diabetes at diagnosis.

	Type I Diabetes (IDDM)	Type II Diabetes (NIDDM)
Polyuria and thirst	++	+
Weakness or fatigue	++	+
Polyphagia with weight loss	++	–
Recurrent blurred vision	+	++
Vulvovaginitis or pruritus	+	++
Peripheral neuropathy	+	++
Nocturnal enuresis	++	–
Often asymptomatic	–	++

a common feature of type I when it develops subacutely over a period of weeks. The weight loss is initially due to depletion of water, glycogen, and triglyceride stores; thereafter, reduced muscle mass occurs as amino acids are diverted to form glucose and ketone bodies.

Lowered plasma volume produces dizziness and weakness due to postural hypotension when sitting or standing. Total body potassium loss and the general catabolism of muscle protein contribute to the weakness.

Paresthesias may be present at the time of diagnosis of type I diabetes, particularly when the onset is subacute. They reflect a temporary dysfunction of peripheral sensory nerves, which clears as insulin replacement restores glycemic levels closer to normal, suggesting neurotoxicity from sustained hyperglycemia.

When insulin deficiency is absolute and of acute onset, the above symptoms progress in an accelerated manner. Ketoacidosis exacerbates the dehydration and hyperosmolality by producing anorexia and nausea and vomiting, thus interfering with oral fluid replacement.

The patient's level of consciousness can vary depending on the degree of hyperosmolality. When insulin deficiency develops relatively slowly and sufficient water intake is maintained, patients remain relatively alert and physical findings may be minimal. When vomiting occurs in response to worsening ketoacidosis, dehydration progresses and compensatory mechanisms become inadequate to keep serum osmolality below 320–330 mosm/L. Under these circumstances, stupor or even coma may occur. The fruity breath odor of acetone further suggests the diagnosis of diabetic ketoacidosis.

Hypotension in the recumbent position is a serious prognostic sign. Loss of subcutaneous fat and muscle wasting are features of more slowly developing insulin deficiency. In occasional patients with slow, insidious onset of insulin deficiency, subcutaneous fat may be considerably depleted. An enlarged liver, eruptive xanthomas on the flexor surface of the limbs and on the buttocks, and lipemia retinalis indicate that chronic insulin deficiency has resulted in chylomicronemia, with circulating triglycerides elevated usually to over 2000 mg/dL.

2. Type II diabetes (NIDDM)–While many patients with type II diabetes present with increased urination and thirst, many others have an insidious onset of hyperglycemia and may be relatively asymptomatic initially. This is particularly true in obese patients, whose diabetes may be detected only after glycosuria or hyperglycemia is noted during routine laboratory studies. Occasionally, type II patients may present with evidence of neuropathic or cardiovascular complications because of underlying occult disease present for some time prior to diagnosis. Chronic skin infections are common. Generalized pruritus and symptoms of vaginitis are frequently the initial complaints of women with type II. Diabetes should be suspected in women with chronic candidal vulvovaginitis as well as in those who have delivered large babies (> 9 lb, or 4.1 kg) or have had polyhydramnios, preeclampsia, or unexplained fetal losses.

Obese diabetics may have any variety of fat distribution; however, diabetes seems to be more often associated in both men and women with localization of fat deposits on the upper segment of the body (particularly the abdomen, chest, neck, and face) and relatively less fat on the appendages, which may be quite muscular. Standardized tables of waist-to-hip ratio indicate that ratios of "greater than 0.9" in men and "greater than 0.8" in women are associated with an increased risk of diabetes in obese subjects. Mild hypertension is often present in obese diabetics.

B. Laboratory Findings:

1. Urinalysis–

a. Glucosuria–A specific and convenient method to detect glucosuria is the paper strip impregnated with glucose oxidase and a chromogen system (Clinistix, Diastix), which is sensitive to as little as 0.1% glucose in urine. Diastix can be directly applied to the urinary stream, and differing color responses of the indicator strip reflect glucose concentration.

Certain common therapeutic agents interfere with this determination. When taken in large doses, ascorbic acid, salicylates, methyldopa, and levodopa can give false-negative results, since these powerful reducing agents interfere with the color reaction and thus prevent accurate estimation of glucose in the urine of diabetics. A normal renal threshold for glucose as well as reliable bladder emptying is essential for interpretation.

b. Ketonuria–Qualitative detection of ketone bodies can be accomplished by nitroprusside tests (Acetest or Ketostix). Although these tests do not detect β-hydroxybutyric acid, which lacks a ketone group, the semiquantitative estimation of ketonuria thus obtained is nonetheless usually adequate for clinical purposes.

2. Blood testing procedures–

a. Glucose tolerance test–

(1) Methodology and normal fasting glucose–Plasma or serum from venous blood samples may be used and has the advantage over whole blood of providing values for glucose that are independent of hematocrit and that reflect the glucose concentration to which body tissues are exposed. For these reasons, and because plasma and serum are more readily measured on automated equipment, plasma and serum glucose measurements are rapidly replacing the whole blood glucose determinations used heretofore in most laboratories. If serum is used, samples should be refrigerated and separated within 1 hour after collection.

(2) Criteria for laboratory confirmation of diabetes mellitus–If the fasting plasma glucose level is over 140 mg/dL on more than one occasion, further evaluation of the patient with a glucose challenge is unnecessary. However, when fasting plasma glucose is less than 140 mg/dL in suspected cases, a standardized oral glucose tolerance test may be done (Table 27–5).

For proper evaluation of the test, the subjects should be normally active and free from acute illness. Medications that may impair glucose tolerance include diuretics, contraceptive drugs, glucocorticoids, niacin, and phenytoin.

Because of difficulties in interpreting oral glucose tolerance tests and the lack of standards related to aging, these tests are generally being replaced by documentation of fasting hyperglycemia as a means of diagnosing diabetes mellitus.

Since fasting plasma glucose is known to increase with aging, physicians should be more tolerant of slight abnormalities of fasting glucose values in elderly people (over 70 years of age) and not deprive patients of occasional sugar-containing snacks when symptoms are not evident. However, an occasional elderly patient may benefit from the diagnosis of mild diabetes in that macular edema may be detected earlier and laser treatment initiated before vision deteriorates permanently.

b. Glycosylated hemoglobin (hemoglobin A_1) measurements–Glycosylated hemoglobin is abnormally high in diabetics with chronic hyperglycemia and reflects their metabolic control. It is produced by nonenzymatic condensation of glucose molecules with free amino groups on the globin component of hemoglobin. The higher the prevailing ambient levels of blood glucose, the higher will be the level of glycosylated hemoglobin. The major form of glycohemoglobin is termed hemoglobin A_{1c}, which

Table 27–5. National Diabetes Data Group criteria for evaluating standard oral glucose tolerance test.[1]

	Normal Glucose Tolerance	Impaired Glucose Tolerance	Diabetes Mellitus[2]
Fasting plasma glucose (mg/dL)	< 115	116–139	> 140
Points between 0 and 120 minutes (mg/dL)	< 200	< 200	200 at least once
Two hours after glucose load (mg/dL)	< 140	> 140 but < 200	> 200

[1]Give 75 g of glucose dissolved in 300 mL of water after an overnight fast in subjects who have been receiving at least 150–200 g of carbohydrate daily for 3 days before the test.
[2]A fasting plasma glucose greater than 140 mg/dL is diagnostic of diabetes. However, if the plasma glucose is less than 140 mg/dL, both of the lower columns must be fulfilled to make the diagnosis of diabetes mellitus.

normally comprises only 4–6% of the total hemoglobin. The remaining glycohemoglobins (2–4% of the total) consist of phosphorylated glucose or fructose and are termed hemoglobin A_{1a} and hemoglobin A_{1b}. Many laboratories measure the sum of these three glycohemoglobins and report it as hemoglobin A_1, but more laboratories are converting to the more intricate but highly specific HbA_{1c} assay.

Since glycohemoglobins circulate within red blood cells whose life span lasts up to 120 days, they generally reflect the state of glycemia over the preceding 8–12 weeks, thereby providing an improved method of assessing diabetic control. When glycohemoglobins are measured in a reliable laboratory, they are extremely useful in monitoring the progress of patients. Measurements should be made in patients with either type of diabetes mellitus at 3- to 4-month intervals so that adjustments in therapy can be made if glycohemoglobin is either subnormal or if it is more than 2% above the upper limits of normal for a particular laboratory. In patients monitoring their own blood glucose levels, glycohemoglobin values provide a valuable check on the accuracy of monitoring. In patients who do not monitor their own blood glucose levels, glycohemoglobin values are essential for adjusting therapy. Attempts to use glycohemoglobin methods for diabetes screening have been controversial. Sensitivity in detecting known diabetes cases by hemoglobin A_{1c} measurements is only 85%, indicating that diabetes cannot be excluded by a normal value. On the other hand, elevated hemoglobin A_{1c} assays are quite specific (91%) in identifying the presence of diabetes mellitus.

Occasionally, fluctuations in hemoglobin A_1 are due to an acutely generated, reversible, intermediary (aldimine-linked) product that can falsely elevate glycohemoglobins when measured with "short-cut" chromatographic methods. This can be eliminated by using specific HPLC methods that detect HbA_{1c} or by dialysis of the hemolysate before chromatography. When hemoglobin variants are present, such as negatively charged hemoglobin F, acetylated hemoglobin from high-dose aspirin therapy, or carbamoylated hemoglobin produced by the complexing of urea with hemoglobin in uremia, falsely *high* "hemoglobin A_1" values are obtained with commonly used chromatographic methods. In the presence of positively charged hemoglobin variants such as hemoglobin S or C, or when the life span of red blood cells is reduced by increased hemolysis or hemorrhage, falsely *low* values for "hemoglobin A_1" result.

Serum fructosamine is formed by nonenzymatic glycosylation of serum proteins (predominantly albumin). Since serum albumin has a much shorter half-life than hemoglobin, serum fructosamine generally reflects the state of glycemic control for only the preceding 2 weeks. When abnormal hemoglobins or hemolytic states affect the interpretation of glycohemoglobin or when a narrower time frame is required, such as for ascertaining glycemic control at the time of conception in a diabetic woman who has recently become pregnant, serum fructosamine assays offer some advantage. Normal values are 1.5–2.4 mmol/L when the serum albumin level is 5 g/dL.

c. Self-monitoring of blood glucose–Capillary blood glucose measurements performed by patients themselves, as outpatients, are extremely useful, particularly in type I patients in whom "tight" metabolic control is attempted. A portable battery-operated glucometer provides a digital readout of the intensity of color developed when glucose oxidase paper strips are exposed to a drop of capillary blood for up to 45 seconds. Similar diagnostic strips made by Bio-Dynamics Corp. (Chemstrip-bG) have two chromogen indicators that permit *visual* estimation of the glucose concentration when compared to a series of color standards after timed exposure to a drop of blood. The Chemstrip-bG can also be read by a reflectance meter (Accu-Chek II). Second-generation glucometers—One Touch II (Lifescan, Inc), Glucometer II (Ames Co.), or ExacTech (Baxter Corp)—automatically time the reaction as soon as a drop of blood is applied to the previously inserted test strip. This relieves patients of the need to wipe off the strip after an exact interval of time and eliminates technical errors from improper blotting or timing. The timing for glucometer readouts varies from 12 to 45 seconds, with the most rapid result obtained from the Accu-Chek "Instant," which requires only 12 seconds. The memory in this device only holds nine entries, whereas other glucometers can retain memories of as many as 500 tests. As little as 2–5 µL of blood are needed for analysis by most meters, though the Accu-Chek "Instant" requires 12–50 µL. Various glucometers appeal to a particular consumer need and are relatively inexpensive, ranging from $50.00 to $100.00 each. However, test strips remain a major expense, costing 50–75 cents apiece. In self-monitoring of blood glucose, patients must prick their finger with a small lancet (Monolet, Ames Co.), which can be facilitated by a small plastic trigger device such as an Autolet (Ames Co.), Autoclix (Bio-Dynamics), or Penlet (Lifescan, Inc.). When used for multiple patients, as in a clinic, physician's office, or hospital ward, *disposable* finger-rest platforms are required to avoid inadvertent transmission of blood-borne viral diseases. Recent refinements provide a much smaller 28-gauge lancet to reduce the discomfort caused by the larger, standard-sized 21-gauge lancet.

The accuracy of data obtained by glucose monitoring requires careful education and training of the patient in sampling and measuring procedures as well as in proper calibration of the instruments. Bedside glucose monitoring in a hospital setting requires rigorous quality control programs and certification of personnel to avoid serious errors. When this is not feasible, glucose testing at the bedside is best done by technicians from the central laboratory.

Noninvasive glucose monitoring is a subject of active current research interest.

3. Lipoprotein abnormalities in diabetes– Levels of circulating lipoproteins are just as dependent on normal levels and action of insulin as is the plasma glucose. In type I diabetes, moderately deficient control of hyperglycemia is associated with only a slight elevation of LDL cholesterol and serum triglycerides and little if any change in HDL cholesterol. Once the hyperglycemia is corrected, lipoprotein levels are generally normal. However, in obese patients with type II diabetes, a distinct "diabetic dyslipidemia" is characteristic of the insulin resistance syndrome. Its features are a high serum triglyceride level (300–400 mg/dL), a low HDL-cholesterol (less than 30 mg/dL), and a qualitative change in LDL particles, producing a smaller dense LDL whose membrane carries supranormal amounts of free cholesterol. Since a *low* HDL-cholesterol is a major feature predisposing to macrovascular disease, the term "dyslipidemia" has preempted the term "hyperlipidemia," which mainly denoted the elevated triglycerides. Measures designed to correct the obesity and hyperglycemia, such as exercise, diet, and hypoglycemic therapy, are the treatment of choice for diabetic dyslipidemia, and in occasional patients in whom normal weight was achieved, all features of the lipoprotein abnormalities cleared. Since primary disorders of lipid metabolism may coexist with diabetes, persistence of lipid abnormalities after restoration of normal weight and blood glucose should prompt a diagnostic workup and possible pharmacotherapy of the lipid disorder. Chapter 28 discusses these matters in detail.

Differential Diagnosis

A. Hyperglycemia Secondary to Other Causes: (Table 27–6.) Secondary hyperglycemia has been associated with various disorders of insulin target tissues (liver, muscle, and adipose tissue).

Other secondary causes of carbohydrate intolerance include endocrine disorders—often specific endocrine tumors—associated with excess production of growth hormone, glucocorticoids, catecholamines, glucagon, or somatostatin. In the first four situations, peripheral responsiveness to insulin is impaired. With excess of glucocorticoids, catecholamines, or glucagon, increased hepatic output of glucose is a contributory factor; in the case of catecholamines, decreased insulin release is an additional factor in producing carbohydrate intolerance, and with excess somatostatin production it is the major factor.

A rare syndrome of extreme insulin resistance associated with acanthosis nigricans afflicts either young women with androgenic features as well as insulin receptor mutations or older people, mostly women, in whom a circulating immunoglobulin binds to insulin receptors and reduces their affinity to insulin.

Medications such as thiazide diuretics, phenytoin, niacin, and high-dose glucocorticoids can produce hyperglycemia that is reversible once the drugs are discontinued. Chronic pancreatitis reduces the number of functioning B cells and can result in a metabolic derangement very similar to that of genetic type I diabetes except that a concomitant reduction in pancreatic A cells may reduce glucagon secretion so that relatively lower doses of insulin replacement are needed. Insulin-dependent diabetes is occasionally associated with Addison's disease and autoimmune thyroiditis (**Schmidt's syndrome,** or **polyglandular failure syndrome**). This occurs more commonly in women and represents an autoimmune disorder in which there are circulating antibodies to adrenocortical and thyroid tissue, thyroglobulin, and gastric parietal cells.

B. Nondiabetic Glycosuria: Nondiabetic glycosuria (renal glycosuria) is a benign, asymptomatic condition wherein glucose appears in the urine despite a normal amount of glucose in the blood, either basally or during a glucose tolerance test. Its cause may vary from an autosomally transmitted genetic disorder to one associated with dysfunction of the proximal renal tubule (Fanconi's syndrome, chronic renal failure), or it may merely be a consequence of the increased load of glucose presented to the tubules by the elevated glomerular filtration rate during pregnancy. As many as 50% of pregnant women normally have demonstrable sugar in the urine, especially during the third and fourth months. This sugar is practically always glucose except during the late weeks of pregnancy, when lactose may be present.

Treatment

A. Goals of Treatment of Diabetes: Diabetes mellitus is a chronic disease that requires ongoing medical care as well as patient and family education both to prevent acute illness and to reduce the risk of long-term complications. Therapy directed toward these goals should not be too restrictive to the pa-

---

Table 27–6. Secondary causes of hyperglycemia.

Hyperglycemia due to tissue insensitivity to insulin
  Hormonal tumors (acromegaly, Cushing's syndrome, glucagonoma, pheochromocytoma)
  Pharmacologic agents (glucocorticoids, sympathomimetic drugs, niacin)
  Liver disease (cirrhosis, hemochromatosis)
  Muscle disorders (myotonic dystrophy)
  Adipose tissue disorders (lipoatrophy, lipodystrophy, truncal obesity)
  Insulin receptor disorders (acanthosis nigricans syndromes, leprechaunism)
Hyperglycemia due to reduced insulin secretion
  Hormonal tumors (somatostatinoma, pheochromocytoma)
  Pancreatic disorders (pancreatitis, hemosiderosis from excess transfusions, idiopathic hemochromatosis)
  Pharmacologic agents (thiazide diuretics, phenytoin, pentamidine, Vacor rodenticide)

tient's quality of life. The recent dramatic results of the Diabetes Control and Complications Trial (see below) indicate that the therapeutic objective is to restore known metabolic derangements toward normal in order to prevent and delay progression of diabetic complications. This objective should be approached while making every effort to avoid severe hypoglycemia.

B. Treatment Regimens:

1. Diet–A well-balanced, nutritious diet remains a fundamental element of therapy. However, in more than half of cases, diabetic patients fail to follow their diet. Consultation with a registered dietician is recommended. In prescribing a diet, it is important to relate dietary objectives to the type of diabetes. In obese patients with mild hyperglycemia, the major goal of diet therapy is weight reduction by caloric restriction. Thus, there is less need for exchange lists, emphasis on timing of meals, or periodic snacks, all of which are so essential in the treatment of insulin-requiring nonobese diabetics. This type of patient represents the most frequent challenge for the physician. Weight reduction is an elusive goal that can only be achieved by close supervision and education of the obese patient. See Chapter 29 for dietary management of obesity.

a. Revised ADA recommendations–In 1994, the American Diabetes Association released a position statement on medical nutrition therapy that replaced the calculated ADA diet formula of the past with suggestions for an individually tailored dietary prescription based on metabolic, nutritional, and lifestyle requirements. They contend that the concept of one diet for "diabetes" and the prescription of an "ADA diet" no longer can apply to both major types of diabetes. In their medical nutrition therapy recommendations for persons with type II diabetes, the 55–60% carbohydrate content of previous diets has been reduced considerably because of the tendency of high carbohydrate intake to cause hyperglycemia, triglyceridemia, and a lowered HDL-cholesterol. In obese type II patients, glucose and lipid goals join weight loss as the focus of therapy. These patients are advised to limit their carbohydrate content by substituting noncholesterologenic monounsaturated oils such as olive oil, rapeseed (canola) oil, or the oils in nuts and avocados. This maneuver is also indicated in type I patients on intensive insulin regimens in whom near-normoglycemic control is less achievable on higher carbohydrate diets. They should be taught "carbohydrate counting" so they can administer 1 unit of regular insulin for each 10 or 15 g of carbohydrate eaten at a meal. In these patients, the ratio of carbohydrate to fat will vary among individuals in relation to their glycemic responses, insulin regimens, and exercise pattern.

The new recommendations for both types of diabetes continue to limit cholesterol to 300 mg daily and advise a daily protein intake of 10–20% of total calories. They suggest that saturated fat be no higher than 8–9% of total calories with a similar proportion of polyunsaturated fat and that the remainder of caloric needs be made up of an individualized ratio of monounsaturated fat and of carbohydrate containing 20–35 g of dietary fiber. Poultry, veal, and fish continue to be recommended as a substitute for red meats for keeping saturated fat content low. In contrast to previous recommendations, the present ADA position statement proffers no evidence that reducing protein intake below 10% of total caloric intake (about 0.8 g/kg/d) is of any benefit in patients with nephropathy and renal impairment, and in fact it is felt that doing so may be detrimental.

Exchange lists for meal planning can be obtained from the American Diabetes Association and its affiliate associations or from the American Dietetic Association, 216 W. Jackson Blvd., Chicago, IL 60606 (312-899-0040). Their internet address is http://www.eatright.org.

b. Dietary fiber–Plant components such as cellulose, gum, and pectin are indigestible by humans and are termed dietary "fiber." Insoluble fibers such as cellulose or hemicellulose, as found in bran, tend to increase intestinal transit and may have beneficial effects on colonic function. In contrast, soluble fibers such as gums and pectins, as found in beans, oatmeal, or apple skin, tend to retard nutrient absorption rates so that glucose absorption is slower and hyperglycemia may be slightly diminished. Although its recommendations do not include insoluble fiber supplements such as added bran, the ADA recommends food such as oatmeal, cereals, and beans with relatively high soluble fiber content as staple components of the diet in diabetics. High soluble fiber content in the diet may also have a favorable effect on blood cholesterol levels.

c. Artificial sweeteners–Aspartame (Nutra-Sweet) has proved to be a popular sweetener for diabetic patients. It consists of two amino acids (aspartic acid and phenylalanine) that combine to produce a nutritive sweetener 180 times as sweet as sucrose. A major limitation is that it cannot be used in baking or cooking because of its lability to heat.

The nonnutritive sweetener saccharin continues to be available in certain foods and beverages despite warnings by the FDA about its potential long-term carcinogenicity to the bladder. The 1994 position statement of the ADA concludes that all nonnutritive sweeteners that have been approved by the FDA (such as aspartame and saccharin) are safe for consumption by all people with diabetes.

Nutritive sweeteners such as sorbitol and fructose have recently increased in popularity. Except for acute diarrhea induced by ingestion of large amounts of sorbitol-containing foods, their relative risk has yet to be established. Fructose represents a "natural" sugar substance that is a highly effective sweetener which induces only slight increases in plasma glucose levels. However, because of potential adverse effects of large amounts of fructose (up to 20% of total calories) on raising serum cholesterol and LDL-cholesterol, the ADA feels it may have no overall advantage as a sweetening agent in the diabetic diet. This does not preclude, however, ingestion of fructose-containing fruits and vegetables or fructose-sweetened foods in moderation.

2. Oral drugs for treating hyperglycemia– Sulfonylureas remain the most widely prescribed oral drugs for treating hyperglycemia. However, in December 1994 the FDA gave approval to a member of the biguanide family, metformin, for clinical use. In contrast to sulfonylureas, which work by stimulating the pancreas to secrete more insulin, metformin lowers hyperglycemia by other mechanisms and is an "insulin-sparing" drug that does not cause weight gain in treated diabetic patients. For these reasons, it has been advocated as a first-line drug for obese diabetics with the insulin resistance syndrome as well as for combination with a sulfonylurea in patients responding poorly to a sulfonylurea alone. The FDA feels that metformin has met satisfactory standards of safety after several years of clinical trials in the United States and over 20 years of use in more than 70 countries worldwide. Its tendency to cause lactic acidosis is only one-tenth that of phenformin, another biguanide, which was taken off the market in 1977 in the USA as well as in many other countries.

A third class of oral antihyperglycemic drugs are the competitive inhibitors of intestinal brush-border alpha-glucosidases. A representative of this class, acarbose, received FDA approval in 1995. It tends to reduce postprandial hyperglycemia by reducing the rate of absorption of most carbohydrates such as starches, dextrins, maltose, and sucrose (but not lactose, which has a beta linkage).

A fourth class of oral antihyperglycemic drugs are the potentiators of insulin action, the thiazolidinediones. Troglitazone was approved for use by the FDA in 1997 after clinical trials found it safe and effective in type II patients with insulin resistance syndrome. While lowering hyperglycemia and hypertriglyceridemia, it is not associated with weight gain or drug-induced hypoglycemia.

a. Sulfonylureas–(Table 27–7.) Slight modifications of the basic structure produce agents that have similar qualitative actions but differ widely in potency. The mechanism of action of the sulfonylureas when they are acutely administered is due to their insulinotropic effect on pancreatic B cells. Sulfonylureas apparently specifically bind to an ATP-sensitive potassium channel of the pancreatic B cell and close it, thereby depolarizing the cell membrane. This results in an influx of extracellular calcium through voltage-gated calcium channels, which causes insulin granules to move toward the cell surface, facilitating exocytosis. However, it remains unclear whether this well-documented *acute* action re-

quires additional extrapancreatic effects such as enhanced peripheral glucose utilization, hepatic glucose output suppression, and increased binding of insulin at insulin receptors to better explain the hypoglycemic effect of sulfonylureas during chronic administration.

Sulfonylureas are presently not indicated in the juvenile type ketosis-prone insulin-dependent diabetic, since these drugs seem to depend on functioning pancreatic B cells. There is little, if any, potentiation of insulin effectiveness on long-term glycemic control when sulfonylureas are added in type I patients, which argues against any substantial extrapancreatic effect of sulfonylureas.

The sulfonylureas seem most appropriate for use in the nonobese insulinopenic mild maturity-onset diabetic in whom acute administration improves the early phase of insulin release that is refractory to acute glucose stimulation. In obese mild diabetics and others with peripheral insensitivity to levels of circulating insulin, primary emphasis should be on weight reduction. When hyperglycemia in obese diabetics has been more severe, with consequent impairment of pancreatic B cell function, sulfonylureas may improve glycemic control until concurrent measures such as diet, exercise, and weight reduction can sustain the improvement without the need for oral drugs. Sulfonylureas are generally contraindicated in patients with hepatic or renal impairment.

(1) Tolbutamide is supplied in tablets of 250 and 500 mg. It is rapidly oxidized in the liver to inactive metabolites, and its approximate duration of effect is relatively short (6–10 hours). Tolbutamide is probably best administered in divided doses (eg, 500 mg before each meal and at bedtime); however, some patients require only one or two tablets daily with a maximum dose of 2000 mg/d. Because of its short duration of action, which is independent of renal function, tolbutamide is probably the safest sulfonylurea to use in elderly patients, in whom hypoglycemia would be a particularly serious risk. Prolonged hypoglycemia has been reported rarely with tolbutamide, mostly in patients receiving certain antibacterial sulfonamides (sulfisoxazole), or phenylbutazone for arthralgias. These drugs apparently compete with tolbutamide for plasma protein binding sites and for oxidative enzyme systems in the liver, resulting in maintenance of high levels of unmetabolized, active sulfonylurea in the circulation.

(2) Tolazamide is supplied in tablets of 100, 250, and 500 mg. It is comparable to chlorpropamide in potency but has a shorter duration of action and does not cause water retention. Tolazamide is more slowly absorbed than the other sulfonylureas, with effects on blood glucose not appearing for several hours. Its duration of action may last up to 20 hours, with maximal hypoglycemic effect occurring between the fourth and fourteenth hours. It is more potent than tolbutamide and is often effective, as are

Table 27–7. Oral antidiabetic drugs.

Drug	Tablet Size	Daily Dose	Duration of Action	Cost per Unit	Cost for 30 Days' Treatment Based on Maximum Dosage[1]
Tolbutamide (Orinase)	250 and 500 mg	0.5–2 g in 2 or 3 divided doses	6–12 hours	$0.10/500 mg	$12.00
Tolazamide* (Tolinase)	100, 250, and 500 mg	0.1–1 g as single dose or in 2 divided doses	Up to 24 hours	$0.12/100 mg $0.22/250 mg	$26.00
Acetohexamide* (Dymelor)[2]	250 and 500 mg	0.25–1.5 g as single dose or in 2 divided doses	8–24 hours	$0.23/250 mg $0.38/500 mg	$34.00
Chlorpropamide* (Diabinese)[2]	100 and 250 mg	0.1–0.5 g as single dose	24–72 hours	$0.07/100 mg $0.12/250 mg	$7.20
Glyburide (Diaβeta, Micronase)	1.25, 2.5, and 5 mg	1.25–20 mg as single dose or in 2 divided doses	Up to 24 hours	G: $0.50/5 mg B: $0.63/5 mg	G: $60.00 B: $75.60
(Glynase)	1.5, 3, and 6 mg	1.5–18 mg as single dose or in 2 divided doses	Up to 24 hours	$0.92/6 mg	$83.70
Glipizide (Glucotrol)	5 and 10 mg	2.5–40 mg as single dose or in 2 divided doses on an empty stomach	6–12 hours	G: $0.32/5 mg G: $0.60/10 mg B: $0.70/10 mg	G: $72.00 B: $84.00
(Glucotrol XL)	5 and 10 mg	Up to 20 or 30 mg daily as a single dose	Up to 24 hours	$0.33/5 mg $0.65/10 mg	$58.50
Glimeperide (Amaryl)	1, 2, and 4 mg	1–4 mg as single dose	Up to 24 hours	$0.69/4 mg	$20.70
Metformin (Glucophage)	500 and 850 mg	1–2.55 g. One tablet with meals 2 or 3 times daily	7–12 hours	$0.50/500 mg $0.85/850 mg	$76.00
Acarbose (Precose)	50 and 100 mg	75–300 mg in 3 divided doses with first bite of food	4 hours	$0.45/50 mg $0.59/100 mg	$53.00
Troglitazone (Rezulin)	200 and 400 mg	200–600 mg as single dose	24–30 hours	$3.47/200 mg $5.33/400 mg	$264.00

*Generic available.
[1]Cost to pharmacist (average wholesale price) for 30 days' treatment based on maximum dosage (generic when possible). Source: First Data Bank, Price Alert, April 1997.
[2]There has been a decline in use of these formulations. In the case of chlorpropamide, the decline is due to its numerous side effects (see text).

other longer-acting sulfonylureas, when tolbutamide fails to correct prebreakfast hyperglycemia. Tolazamide is metabolized to several compounds that retain hypoglycemic effects. If more than 500 mg/d is required, the dose should be divided and given twice daily. Doses larger than 1000 mg daily do not improve the degree of glycemic control.

(3) Acetohexamide is supplied in tablets of 250 and 500 mg. Its duration of action is about 10–16 hours, being intermediate in action between tolbutamide and chlorpropamide. A dose of 0.25–1.5 g is given daily in one or two doses. Liver metabolism is rapid, but the metabolite produced remains active.

(4) Chlorpropamide is supplied in tablets of 100 and 250 mg. This drug, with a half-life of 32 hours, is slowly metabolized, with approximately 20–30% excreted unchanged in the urine. Since the metabolites

retain hypoglycemic activity, elimination of the biologic effect is almost completely dependent on renal excretion. Its use is therefore contraindicated in patients with renal insufficiency because of its increased duration of action and prolonged half-life. The average maintenance dose is 250 mg daily, given as a single dose in the morning. Chlorpropamide is a potent agent, and prolonged hypoglycemic reactions are more common than with tolbutamide, particularly in elderly patients, in whom chlorpropamide therapy is contraindicated. Doses in excess of 500 mg daily increase the risk of cholestatic jaundice. A flush may occur when alcohol is ingested by patients taking chlorpropamide, appearing within 8 minutes of ingesting the alcohol and lasting for 10–12 minutes; it is believed to be dose-related and similar to a disulfiram reaction, though much milder.

Hyponatremia is a complication of chlorpropamide therapy in some patients, especially those taking diuretics. Chlorpropamide both stimulates vasopressin secretion and potentiates its action at the renal tubule, resulting in dilutional hyponatremia. This antidiuretic effect of chlorpropamide is relatively unique, and since other sulfonylureas have now become available with comparable potency but without the disadvantage of causing water retention or alcohol-induced flushing, there is less need to prescribe chlorpropamide in managing patients with type II.

(5) Second-generation sulfonylureas (glyburide, glipizide, and glimeperide)–Glyburide, glipizide, and glimeperide are from 100 to 200 times more potent than tolbutamide. These drugs should be used with caution in patients with cardiovascular disease or in elderly patients, in whom prolonged hypoglycemia would be especially dangerous.

Diabetic patients who have not responded to tolbutamide or even tolazamide may respond to the more potent first-generation sulfonylurea chlorpropamide or to any of the second-generation sulfonylureas. Unfortunately, substantial glycemic benefit has not always resulted when a maximum therapeutic dose of chlorpropamide has been replaced with that of a second-generation drug in type II patients whose glucose control has been unsatisfactory. Second-generation sulfonylureas tend to be more expensive than the first-generation agents.

(a) Glyburide–Glyburide is available in 1.25, 2.5, and 5 mg tablets. The usual starting dose is 2.5 mg/d, and the average maintenance dose is 5–10 mg/d given as a single morning dose; maintenance doses higher than 20 mg/d are not recommended. Some reports suggest that 10 mg is a maximum daily therapeutic dose, with 15–20 mg having no additional benefit in poor responders and doses over 20 mg actually worsening hyperglycemia. Glyburide is metabolized in the liver into products with such low hypoglycemic activity that they are considered clinically unimportant. Although assays specific for the unmetabolized compound suggest a plasma half-life of only 1–2 hours, the biologic effects of glyburide are clearly persistent 24 hours after a single morning dose in diabetic patients. Glyburide is unique among sulfonylureas in that it not only binds to a pancreatic B cell membrane receptor but also becomes sequestered within the B cell. This may explain its prolonged biologic effect despite its relatively short circulating half-life. A recently marketed "Press Tab" formulation of "micronized" glyburide—easy to divide in half with slight pressure if necessary—is currently available in tablet sizes of 1.5 mg, 3 mg, and 6 mg.

Glyburide has few adverse effects other than its potential for causing hypoglycemia. Flushing has rarely been reported after ethanol ingestion. It does not cause water retention, as chlorpropamide does, but rather slightly enhances free water clearance. Glyburide is absolutely contraindicated in the presence of hepatic impairment and probably should not be used in patients with renal insufficiency, in elderly patients, or in those who would be put at serious risk from an episode of hypoglycemia.

(b) Glipizide–Glipizide is available in 5 and 10 mg tablets. For maximum effect in reducing postprandial hyperglycemia, this agent should be ingested 30 minutes before meals, since rapid absorption is delayed when the drug is taken with food. The recommended starting dose is 5 mg/d with up to 15 mg/d given as a single daily dose before breakfast. When higher daily doses are required, they should be divided and given before meals. The maximum recommended dose is 40 mg/d, though doses above 10–20 mg probably provide little additional benefit in poor responders.

At least 90% of glipizide is metabolized in the liver to inactive products, and 10% is excreted unchanged in the urine. Glipizide therapy is therefore contraindicated in patients with hepatic or renal impairment, who would be at high risk for hypoglycemia, but because of its lower potency and shorter duration of action it is preferable to glyburide in elderly patients. Recently, a new formulation of glipizide has been marketed as Glucotrol-XL in 5 mg and 10 mg tablets. It provides extended release during transit through the gastrointestinal tract with greater effectiveness in lowering prebreakfast hyperglycemia than the shorter-duration immediate-release standard glipizide tablets. However, this formulation appears to have sacrificed its lower propensity for severe hypoglycemia compared with longer-acting glyburide without showing any demonstrable therapeutic advantages over glyburide.

(c) Glimeperide–This sulfonylurea has recently completed clinical trials and was approved in 1996 by the FDA for once-daily use as monotherapy or in combination with insulin to lower blood glucose in diabetes patients who cannot control their glucose level through diet and exercise. Glimeperide achieves blood glucose lowering with the lowest dose of any sulfonylurea compound and this tends to increase its cost-effectiveness. A single daily dose of 1 mg/d has been shown to be effective, and the maximal recommended dose is 8 mg. It has a long duration of effect with a pharmacodynamic half-life of 5 hours, allowing once-daily administration, which improves compliance. It is completely metabolized by the liver to relatively inactive metabolic products.

b. Metformin and other biguanides–The biguanides were introduced in the 1950s for the management of non-insulin-dependent diabetes mellitus. Phenformin was available in the USA until 1977, when it was discontinued because of its association with lactic acidosis. While it is still prescribed in some other countries to a limited extent, it has generally been replaced by other biguanides such as buformin and particularly metformin. Only metformin is discussed here.

Metformin (1,1-dimethylbiguanide hydrochloride) was introduced in France in 1957 as an oral agent for therapy of type II diabetes, either alone or in conjunction with sulfonylureas. It is marketed under the brand name Glucophage.

(1) Clinical pharmacology–The exact mechanism of action of metformin remains unclear. It reduces both the fasting level of blood glucose and the degree of postprandial hyperglycemia in patients with type II diabetes but has no effect on fasting blood glucose in normal subjects. Metformin does not stimulate insulin action, yet is particularly effective in reducing hepatic gluconeogenesis. Other proposed mechanisms include a slowing down of gastrointestinal absorption of glucose and increased glucose uptake by skeletal muscle, which have been reported in some but not all clinical studies. Because of its very high concentration in intestinal cells after oral administration, metformin increases glucose to lactate turnover, which may account for a reduction in hyperglycemia.

Metformin has a half-life of 1½–3 hours, is not bound to plasma proteins, and is not metabolized in humans, being excreted unchanged by the kidneys.

(2) Indications and dosage–Metformin may be used as an adjunct to diet for the control of hyperglycemia and its associated symptomatology in patients with type II diabetes, particularly those who are obese or are not responding optimally to maximal doses of sulfonylureas. A side benefit of metformin therapy is its tendency to improve both fasting and postprandial hyperglycemia and hypertriglyceridemia in obese diabetics without the weight gain associated with insulin or sulfonylurea therapy. Metformin is not indicated for patients with type I diabetes and is contraindicated in diabetics with renal or hepatic insufficiency, alcoholism, or a propensity to develop hypoxia (eg, disease associated with cardiorespiratory insufficiency, with its propensity to raise serum lactate).

Metformin is dispensed as 500 mg or 850 mg tablets, and the dosage range is from 500 mg to a maximum of 2.55 g daily, with the lowest possible effective dose being recommended. It is important that metformin be taken in divided doses—and with meals—to reduce minor gastrointestinal upsets. A common schedule would be one 500 mg tablet three times a day with meals or one 850 mg tablet twice daily at breakfast and dinner.

(3) Adverse reactions–The most frequent side effects of metformin are gastrointestinal symptoms (anorexia, nausea, vomiting, abdominal discomfort, diarrhea), which occur in up to 20% of patients. These effects are dose-related, tend to occur at onset of therapy, and often are transient. However, in 3–5% of patients, therapy may have to be discontinued because of persistent diarrheal discomfort.

Hypoglycemia does not occur with therapeutic doses of metformin, which permits its description as a "euglycemic" or "antihyperglycemic" drug rather than an oral hypoglycemic agent. Dermatologic or hematologic toxicity is rare.

Lactic acidosis (see below) has been reported as a side effect but is uncommon with metformin in contrast to phenformin, and almost all reported cases have involved subjects with associated risk factors that should have contraindicated its use (renal, hepatic, or cardiorespiratory insufficiency, alcoholism, advanced age). Acute renal failure can occur rarely in certain patients receiving radiocontrast agents. Metformin therapy should therefore be temporarily halted for 2 days prior to injection of radiocontrast agents to avoid potential lactic acidosis if renal failure occurs.

c. Alpha-glucosidase inhibitors–Acarbose is an oligosaccharide analog that binds 1000 times more avidly to the intestinal disaccharidases than do products of carbohydrate digestion or sucrose. This competitive inhibition of alpha-glucosidase limits postprandial rise of glucose and results in an insulin-sparing action. When used to treat hyperglycemic patients, its overall effect is slight, with a reduction of hemoglobin A_{1c} of only 0.5–1%, and a reduction of postprandial hyperglycemia by 30–50%. The principal adverse effect, seen in 20–30% of patients, is flatulence. This is caused by undigested carbohydrate reaching the lower bowel, where gases are produced by bacterial flora. In 3% of cases, troublesome diarrhea occurs. This gastrointestinal discomfort tends to discourage excessive carbohydrate consumption and promotes improved compliance of NIDDM patients with their diet prescriptions. The recommended starting dose of acarbose is 50 mg twice daily, gradually increasing to 100 mg three times a day. For maximal benefit on postprandial hyperglycemia, acarbose should be given with the first mouthful of food ingested. When acarbose is given alone, there is no risk of hypoglycemia. However if combined with insulin or sulfonylureas, it might increase the risk of hypoglycemia from these agents. A slight rise in hepatic aminotransferases has been noted in clinical trials (5% versus 2% in placebo controls, and particularly with doses > 300 mg/d). The levels generally return to normal on stopping the drug.

d. Insulin sensitizers (thiazolidinediones)–Troglitazone, a member of this new class of oral antidiabetic drugs, has recently been approved for use by the FDA for insulin-resistant patients who are responding poorly to insulin therapy. Clinical trials with doses of 400 mg/d have been shown to be effective in managing patients with type II diabetes, particularly when they manifest the insulin resistance syndrome; it has shown no adverse reactions as compared with placebo. Troglitazone appears to potentiate insulin action and is effective in improving glucose disposal and reducing hepatic glucose output only when circulating insulin levels are adequate. It reduces hyperglycemia, hypertriglyceridemia, and hyperinsulinemia and tends to slightly elevate both HDL and LDL cholesterol in insulin-resistant patients without causing weight gain or drug-induced hypoglycemia. It has no glucose-lowering effect in normal subjects.

The mechanism of action of troglitazone is unknown but requires the presence of circulating insulin and the metabolic state of insulin resistance for its effectiveness in humans. There is suggestive evidence that it acts on a family of nuclear transcription factors, particularly peroxisome proliferator-activated receptor-gamma (PPARγ) to potentiate insulin-induced expression of genes important for carbohydrate and lipid metabolism.

e. Safety of the oral hypoglycemic agents– The University Group Diabetes Program (UGDP) reported that the number of deaths due to cardiovascular disease in diabetic patients treated with tolbutamide or the no longer used phenformin was excessive compared to either insulin-treated patients or those receiving placebos. Controversy persists about the validity of the conclusions reached by the UGDP because of concerns about the heterogeneity of the population studied, with its preponderance of obese subjects, and because of certain features of the experimental design such as the use of a fixed dose of oral drug. At present, a warning label concerning potential cardiac deaths is inserted in each package of sulfonylureas and metformin, but there is no restriction upon recommending their use by the American Diabetes Association.

Idiosyncratic reactions to sulfonylureas are rare, with skin rashes or hematologic toxicity (transient leukopenia, thrombocytopenia) occurring in less than 0.1% of patients.

3. Insulin–Insulin is indicated for type I (IDDM) diabetics as well as for nonobese type II diabetics with insulinopenia whose hyperglycemia does not respond to diet therapy either alone or combined with oral hypoglycemic drugs.

With the development of highly purified human insulin preparations, immunogenicity has been markedly reduced, thereby decreasing the incidence of therapeutic complications such as insulin allergy, immune insulin resistance, and localized lipoatrophy at the injection site. However, the problem of achieving optimal insulin delivery remains unsolved with the present state of technology. It has not been possible to reproduce the physiologic patterns of intraportal insulin secretion with subcutaneous injections of soluble or longer-acting insulin suspensions. Even so, with the help of appropriate modifications of diet and exercise and careful monitoring of capillary blood glucose levels at home, it has often been possible to achieve acceptable control of blood glucose by using various mixtures of short- and longer-acting insulins injected at least twice daily or portable insulin infusion pumps.

a. Characteristics of available insulin preparations–Commercial insulin preparations differ with respect to the animal species from which they are obtained, their purity and solubility, and the time of onset and duration of their biologic action. As many as 23 different formulations of insulin are available in the USA.

(1) Species of insulin–Human insulin is now produced by recombinant DNA techniques (biosynthetic human insulin). It has been introduced for clinical use as Humulin (Eli Lilly) and as Novolin (Novo Nordisk) and dispensed as either Regular (R), NPH (N), Lente (L), or Ultralente (U) formulations (see Table 27–8). Recently, a very rapidly-acting analog of human insulin with reversal of the 28 and 29 amino acids of the B chain has become available for human use (see Insulin lispro, below). In addition to human insulin, insulin from pork and beef sources continues to be widely used throughout the world.

Because the supply of pork insulin has been too limited to satisfy the insulin requirements of all diabetic patients, most commercial insulins contain the slightly more antigenic beef insulin, which differs by three amino acids from human insulin (in contrast to the single amino acid distinguishing pork and human insulins). Standard preparations of Iletin I (Eli Lilly) are mixtures containing 70% beef and 30% pork insulin. However, a limited supply of monospecies pork insulin (Iletin II) is available for use in certain patients who seem to benefit from the slightly more prolonged and sustained effect of animal insulin, compared with human insulin. The cost of human insulin is approximately 1¼ times the cost of standard beef and pork insulin but slightly less than the cost of purified pork insulin. Because of declining production costs for biosynthesis of human insulin, it is expected that by 1998 human insulin will greatly exceed animal insulin in sales throughout most of the industrial countries.

(2) Purity of insulin–Recent improvements in purification techniques for insulins extracted from animal pancreas have reduced or eliminated contaminating insulin precursors which were capable of inducing anti-insulin antibodies. The degree of purification in which proinsulin contamination is greater than 10 but less than 25 ppm characterizes the main form of insulin produced commercially in the USA by Eli Lilly as Iletin I. When proinsulin content is reduced to less than 10 ppm, manufacturers are entitled by FDA regulations to label the insulin as "purified." Such highly purified insulins are presently marketed in the USA by Eli Lilly and Novo Nordisk. The Eli Lilly product is called Iletin II to identify this highly purified insulin, and it presently is available only as a monospecies pork insulin. All human insulins are also highly purified.

Purified insulins seem to preserve their potency quite well, so that refrigeration is recommended but not crucial. During travel, reserve supplies of insulin

Table 27–8. Some insulin preparations available in the USA.[1,2]

Preparation	Species Source	Concentration	Cost[2]
Ultra-short -acting insulins			
Insulin lispro (Humalog, Lilly)	Human analog (recombinant)	U100	$24.98
Short-acting insulins			
Standard[3]			
Regular Iletin I (Lilly)	Beef and pork	U100	$17.68
"Purified"[4]			
Regular (Novo Nordisk)[5]	Pork or human	U100	Pork: $28.88
Regular Humulin (Lilly)	Human	U100, U500	$19.89, $42.73
Regular Iletin II (Lilly)	Pork	U100, U500	$28.88, $149.52
Velosulin (Novo Nordisk)[6]	Human	U100	$22.00
Intermediate-acting insulins			
Standard[3]			
Lente Iletin I (Lilly)	Beef and pork	U100	$17.68
NPH Iletin I (Lilly)	Beef and pork	U100	$17.68
"Purified"[4]			
Lente Humulin (Lilly)	Human	U100	$19.84
Lente Iletin II (Lilly)	Pork	U100	$28.88
Lente (Novo Nordisk)	Pork or human	U100	$24.24
NPH Humulin (Lilly)	Human	U100	$19.84
NPH Iletin II (Lilly)	Pork	U100	$28.88
NPH (Novo Nordisk)	Pork or human	U100	$19.84
Premixed insulins (% NPH, % regular)			
Novolin 70/30 (Novo Nordisk)	Human	U100	$19.84
Humulin 70/30 and 50/50 (Lilly)	Human	U100	$19.84
Long-acting insulins			
"Purified"[4]			
Ultralente Humulin (Lilly)	Human	U100	$19.84

[1]Modified and reproduced, with permission, from Katzung BG (editor): *Basic and Clinical Pharmacology,* 7th ed. Appleton & Lange, 1997.
[2]All of these agents (except insulin lispro and U500) are available without a prescription. Costs to pharmacist (average wholesale price) per 10 mL bottle. Source: First Data Bank, Price Alert, April 1997. Wholesale prices for all preparations (except insulin lispro and U500) are similar.
[3]Greater than 10 but less than 25 ppm proinsulin.
[4]Less than 10 ppm proinsulin.
[5]Novo Nordisk human insulins are termed Novolin R, L, and N.
[6]Velosulin contains phosphate buffer, which favors its use to prevent insulin aggregation in pump tubing but precludes its being mixed with lente insulin.

can thus be readily transported for weeks without losing potency if protected from extremes of heat or cold.

(3) Concentration of insulin–At present, most insulins are available in a concentration of 100 units/mL (U100), and all are dispensed in 10 mL vials. With the popularity of "low-dose" (0.5 or 0.3 mL) disposable insulin syringes, U100 can be measured with acceptable accuracy in doses as low as 1–2 units, and the manufacture of all U40 concentrations has therefore been discontinued in the United States. For use in rare cases of severe insulin resistance in which large quantities of insulin are required, U500 regular porcine insulin (Iletin II) as well as U500 regular human insulin (Humulin R) are available from Eli Lilly.

b. Insulin preparations–(Table 27–8.) Four principal types of insulins are available: (1) ultrashort-acting, with very rapid onset and short duration; (2) short-acting, with rapid onset of action; (3) intermediate-acting; and (4) long-acting, with slow onset of action (Table 27–8 and Figure 27–1).

Ultra-short-acting and short-acting insulins are dispensed as clear solutions at neutral pH and contain small amounts of zinc to improve their stability and shelf life. All other commercial insulins have been modified to provide prolonged action and are dispensed as turbid suspensions at neutral pH with either protamine in phosphate buffer (NPH insulin) or varying concentrations of zinc in acetate buffer (ultralente and lente insulins). These suspensions of insulin are designed for subcutaneous administration only, while the short-acting and ultra-short-acting insulins can also be given intravenously.

(1) **Ultra-short-acting insulin**–Insulin lispro (Humalog) is a new insulin analog, produced by recombinant technology, wherein two amino acids near the terminal end of the B chain have been reversed in position: proline at position B28 has been moved to B29 and lysine has been moved from B29 to B28. Reversing these two amino acids results in a much lower propensity to form hexamers in contrast to human insulin. When injected subcutaneously, insulin lispro quickly dissociates into monomers and is absorbed very rapidly, reaching peak serum values in as early as 1 hour—in contrast to regular human insulin, whose hexamers require considerably more time to dissociate and become absorbed. Moreover, reversing these two amino acids does not interfere with insulin lispro's binding to the insulin receptor, its circulating half-life, or its immunogenicity, which are all identical with that of human regular insulin. Clinical trials have demonstrated that optimal time of preprandial subcutaneous injection of comparable doses of insulin lispro and of regular human insulin are 20 minutes and 60 minutes before the meal, respectively, in insulin-dependent diabetics requiring intensive insulin therapy. While this ultra-rapid onset of action of insulin lispro has been welcomed as a great convenience by diabetic patients who object to waiting as long as 60 minutes after injecting regular human insulin before they can begin their meal, patients must be taught to ingest adequate absorbable carbohydrate early in the meal to avoid hypoglycemia during the meal. Moreover, a property of insulin lispro which tends to reduce the frequency of late hypoglycemia following meals is that its duration of action, in contrast to regular human insulin, is not prolonged by increasing the dosage of the insulin. Regardless of the dose of insulin lispro injected subcutaneously, its duration is no more than 3–4 hours, whereas regular human insulin in moderate doses (15–40 units) lasts much longer, with its duration of action being proportionate to the dose. When the FDA approved insulin lispro, it indicated that—in contrast to other over-the-counter insulin formulations—insulin lispro will require a physician's prescription and medical supervision of its use until more experience with its novel pharmacokinetics is available.

(2) **Short-acting insulin**–Regular insulin is a short-acting soluble crystalline zinc insulin whose effect appears within 30 minutes after subcutaneous injection and lasts 5–7 hours when usual quantities are administered. Intravenous infusions of regular insulin are particularly useful in the treatment of diabetic ketoacidosis and during the perioperative management of insulin-requiring diabetics. When intravenous insulin is needed for hyperglycemic emergencies, insulin lispro has no advantage over regular human insulin, which is instantly converted to the monomeric form when given intravenously and which is 30–40% less costly than insulin lispro. Regular insulin is also preferred when the subcutaneous insulin requirement is changing rapidly, such as after surgery or during acute infections, although insulin lispro may be preferable in these situations.

Aggregation of insulin solutions which cause clogging of tubing in insulin infusion pumps appears to be reduced by use of phosphate-buffered insulins. Novo Nordisk's Velosulin human insulin is the only buffered regular insulin available for pump users. Although infusion sets made of newer materials such as polyfin seem to reduce aggregation tendencies of unbuffered regular insulin, it probably remains advisable to recommend buffered Velosulin for use with insulin pumps. The FDA has approved insulin lispro for injection only and not for use in insulin pumps. Concern has been expressed that because of insulin lispro's more rapid absorption it may entail greater risks of severe hyperglycemia and ketosis in the event of pump failure than those which occur with human insulin. Clinical trials are in progress to resolve this concern.

(3) **Intermediate- and long-acting insulins**– Lente insulin is a mixture of 30% semilente (an amorphous precipitate of insulin with zinc ions) with 70% ultralente insulin (an insoluble crystal of zinc and insulin). Its onset of action is delayed for up to 2 hours (Figure 27–1), and because its duration of action often is less than 24 hours (with a range of 18–24 hours), most patients require at least two injections daily to maintain a sustained insulin effect. Lente insulin has its peak effect in most patients between 8 and 12 hours, but individual variations in peak response time must be considered when interpreting unusual or unexpected patterns of glycemic responses in individual patients. While lente insulin is the most widely used of the lente series, particularly in conjunction with regular insulin, there has recently been a resurgence of use of ultralente in combination with multiple injections of rapid-acting insulin (regular insulin or insulin lispro) as a means of attempting optimal control in type I patients. Ultralente when made from beef insulin had had a very slow onset of action with a prolonged duration (Figure 27–1), and its administration once or twice daily had been advocated to provide a basal level of insulin comparable to that achieved by basal endogenous secretion or the overnight infusion rate programmed

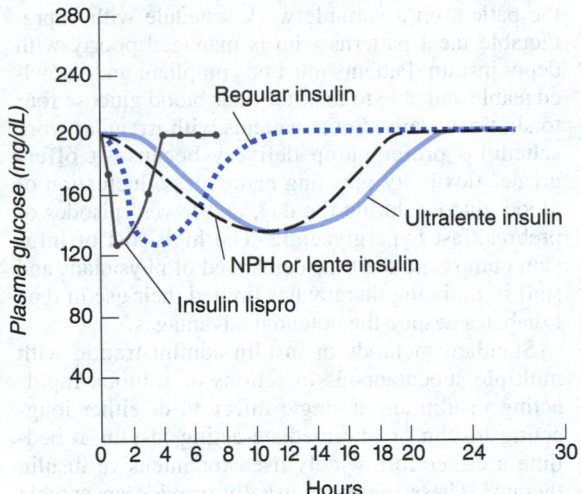

Figure 27–1. Extent and duration of action of various insulins (in a fasting diabetic). Duration is extended considerably when the dose of a given formulation increases above the average therapeutic doses depicted here (except for insulin lispro).

into insulin pumps. Unfortunately, manufacturers have discontinued production of beef ultralente insulin, and only the less sustained and much shorter-acting ultralente made from human insulin is currently available (Table 27–8). Because of its less sustained action compared with beef ultralente (which often achieved satisfactory basal insulin levels with only one injection daily), it is generally recommended that the daily dose of Humulin Ultralente be split into two equal doses given every 12 hours.

NPH (neutral protamine Hagedorn or isophane) insulin is an intermediate-acting insulin whose onset of action is delayed by combining two parts soluble crystalline zinc with 1 part protamine zinc insulin. This produces equivalent amounts of insulin and protamine, so that neither is present in an uncomplexed form ("isophane").

The onset and duration of action of NPH insulin are comparable to those of lente insulin (Figure 27–1); it is usually mixed with regular insulin and given at least twice daily for insulin replacement in type I patients. Occasional vials of NPH insulin have tended to show unusual clumping of their contents or "frosting" of the container, with considerable loss of bioactivity. This instability is a rare phenomenon and might occur less frequently if NPH human insulin were refrigerated when not in use and if bottles were discarded after 1 month of use.

(4) Mixtures of insulin–Since intermediate insulins require several hours to reach adequate therapeutic levels, their use in type I patients requires supplements of regular insulin preprandially. It is well established that insulin mixtures containing increased

proportions of lente to regular insulins may retard the rapid action of admixed regular insulin. The excess zinc in lente insulin binds the soluble insulin and partially blunts its action, particularly when a relatively small proportion of regular insulin is mixed with lente (eg, 1 part regular to 1½ or more parts lente). NPH preparations do not contain excess protamine and so do not delay absorption of admixed regular insulin. They are therefore preferable to lente when mixtures of intermediate and regular insulins are prescribed. For convenience, regular or NPH insulin may be mixed together in the same syringe and injected subcutaneously in split dosage before breakfast and supper. It is recommended that the regular insulin be withdrawn first, then the NPH insulin. No attempt should be made to mix the insulins in the syringe, and the injection is preferably given immediately after loading the syringe. Stable premixed insulins (70% NPH and 30% regular or 50% of each) are available as a convenience to patients who have difficulty mixing insulin because of visual problems or impairment of manual dexterity.

With increasing use of ultra-short-acting insulin lispro as a popular and convenient preprandial insulin, it has become evident that combination with a more sustained insulin is essential to maintain postabsorptive glycemic control. It has been demonstrated that insulin lispro can be acutely mixed with either NPH or ultralente insulin without affecting its rapid absorption. However, premixed preparations have been unstable since attempts to maintain a 70% NPH and 30% insulin lispro results in a variable loss of soluble insulin lispro as the human insulin in the protamine complex is partially displaced by the insulin lispro. Consequently, the soluble component becomes over time a mixture of human insulin and insulin lispro at varying ratios. In an attempt to remedy this, instead of using human insulin to produce NPH insulin, clinical trials in Europe are being performed with an intermediate insulin composed of isophane complexes of protamine with insulin lispro. This intermediate insulin has been designated as "NPL" (neutral protamine lispro) and has the same duration of action as NPH insulin. It has the advantage of being dispensable as premixed combinations of NPL and insulin lispro and has been tested in various concentrations of premixed vials, eg, 75% NPL/25% insulin lispro, 50% NPL/50% insulin lispro, and 25% NPL/75% insulin lispro. Preliminary results of clinical trials suggest that the latter given before each meal has served as a valuable premeal insulin to optimize glycemic excursions postprandially while maintaining postabsorptive basal insulin levels. At bedtime, an injection of NPL alone is being tested to maintain overnight basal insulin levels.

Since insulin lispro resists hexamer formation at pharmacologic concentrations, it appears to resist precipitation by high concentrations of zinc and thus cannot be used to make a lente or ultralente formulation. However, this lack of precipitation by zinc allows it to be mixed with any of the lente series—in contrast to regular insulin, which tends to be precipitated by the excess zinc in the lente series when mixed prior to injection.

c. Methods of insulin administration–

(1) Insulin syringes and needles–Plastic disposable syringes with half-inch ultrafine needles attached are available in 1 mL, 0.5 mL, 0.3 mL, and 0.25 mL sizes. In cases where very low insulin doses are prescribed, the specially calibrated 0.3 mL and 0.25 mL disposable syringes facilitate accurate measurement of U100 insulin in doses up to 30 or 25 units, respectively. The "low-dose" syringes have become increasingly popular, because diabetics generally should not take more than 25–30 units of insulin in a single injection, except in rare instances of extreme insulin resistance. Several recent reports have indicated that "disposable" syringes may be reused until blunting of the needle occurs (usually after three to five injections). Sterility adequate to avoid infection with reuse appears to be maintained by recapping syringes between uses. Cleansing the needle with alcohol may not be desirable since it can dissolve the silicon coating and can increase the pain of skin puncturing.

(2) Site of injection–Any part of the body covered by loose skin can be used, such as the abdomen, thighs, upper arms, flanks, and upper buttocks. Rotation of sites continues to be recommended to avoid delayed absorption when fibrosis or lipohypertrophy occurs from repeated use of a single site. However, considerable variability of absorption rates from different sites, particularly with exercise, may contribute to the instability of glycemic control in certain type I patients if injection sites are rotated too frequently in different areas of the body. Consequently, it is best to limit injection sites to a single region of the body and rotate sites within that region. The abdomen is recommended for subcutaneous injections, since regular insulin has been shown to absorb more rapidly from that site than from other subcutaneous sites.

(3) Insulin delivery systems–Efforts to administer soluble insulin by "closed-loop" systems (glucose-controlled insulin infusion system) have been successful for acute situations such as diabetic ketoacidosis or for administering insulin to diabetics during surgery. However, chronic use is prevented by the need for continually aspirating blood to reach an external glucose sensor and the large size of the computerized pump system.

In the United States, both the MiniMed and the Disetronic insulin infusion pumps are available for subcutaneous delivery of insulin. Clinical trials are under way to test the effectiveness of an implantable MiniMed pump for peritoneal delivery. A prime candidate for the insulin pump method of delivering subcutaneous insulin is the pregnant diabetic woman or the patient on a variable work schedule with unpredictable meal patterns who is managed poorly with depot insulin. Patients must be compliant and knowledgeable and able to monitor their blood glucose four to six times daily. Some patients with irregular work schedules prefer pump delivery because it offers greater flexibility in eating habits, less fluctuation of blood glucose during the day, and fewer episodes of prebreakfast hyperglycemia. The high cost of infusion pumps and the time demanded of physicians and staff in initiating therapy has limited their use in type I diabetes despite the potential advantages.

Standard methods of insulin administration with multiple subcutaneous injections of soluble, rapid-acting insulin and a single injection of either long-acting insulin or intermediate-acting insulin at bedtime are therefore widely used for intensive insulin therapy. These regimens usually provide acceptable glycemic control if frequent self-monitoring of blood glucose is practiced.

To facilitate these multiple injection regimens, portable pen-sized injectors have been introduced which contain cartridges of U100 regular human insulin and retractable needles (NovoPen, NovolinPen, Insuject). Cartridges of insulin lispro (Humalog) have also been made available by the Lilly Company. These injectors eliminate the need for carrying an insulin bottle and syringes during the day to provide multiple injections of rapid-acting insulin supplementary to one or two injections of long-acting insulin to maintain basal insulin levels.

4. Insulin-like growth factor-1 (IGF-1) therapy–In patients with severe insulin resistance who respond poorly to insulin, the use of IGF-1 has been advocated. IGF-1 is a 70-amino-acid peptide which is homologous to human proinsulin. An intravenous bolus of 13 nmol produces hypoglycemia in humans similar to a bolus of 1 nmol of insulin. Several patients with severe insulin resistance due to insulin receptor mutations have responded to IGF-1 but not to insulin, suggesting that the hypoglycemic action of IGF-1 is via its own receptor and not by cross-reacting with the receptor for insulin. While more studies are needed to verify this concept, its use in some cases of severe insulin resistance has been advocated. However, since IGF-1 may promote tumor growth, there are serious questions about its safety in other than short-term use.

C. General Considerations in Treatment of Diabetes: Patients with diabetes can have a full and satisfying life. However, "free" diets and unrestricted activity are still not advised for insulin-requiring diabetics. Until new methods of insulin replacement are developed that provide more normal patterns of insulin delivery in response to metabolic demands, multiple feedings will continue to be recommended, and certain occupations potentially hazardous to the patient or others will continue to be prohibited because of risks due to hypoglycemia. The American

Diabetic Association can act as a patient advocate in case of employment questions.

Exercise increases the effectiveness of insulin, and moderate exercise is an excellent means of improving utilization of fat and carbohydrate in diabetic patients. A judicious balance of the size and frequency of meals with moderate regular exercise can often stabilize the insulin dosage in diabetics who tend to slip out of control easily. Strenuous exercise could precipitate hypoglycemia in an unprepared patient, and diabetics must therefore be taught to reduce their insulin dosage in anticipation of strenuous activity or to take supplemental carbohydrate. Injection of insulin into a site farthest away from the muscles most involved in exercise may help ameliorate exercise-induced hypoglycemia, since insulin injected in the proximity of exercising muscle may be more rapidly mobilized.

All diabetic patients must receive adequate instruction on personal hygiene, especially with regard to care of the feet (see below), skin, and teeth. All infections—but especially pyogenic infections with fever and toxemia—provoke the release of high levels of insulin antagonists such as catecholamines or glucagon and thus bring about a marked increase in insulin requirements. Supplemental regular insulin is often required to correct hyperglycemia during infection.

Psychologic factors are of great importance in the control of diabetes, particularly when the disease is difficult to stabilize. One reason the diabetic may be particularly sensitive to emotional upset is that pancreatic A cells of diabetics are hyperresponsive to physiologic levels of epinephrine, producing excessive levels of glucagon with consequent hyperglycemia.

Counseling should be directed at avoiding extremes of compulsive rigidity or self-destructive neglect and is especially important for adolescents.

D. The Diabetes Control and Complications Trial (DCCT): In 1993, a long-term randomized prospective study involving 1441 type I patients in 29 medical centers reported that "near" normalization of blood glucose resulted in a delay in the onset and a major slowing of the progression of established microvascular and neuropathic complications of diabetes during an up to 10-year follow-up.

Multiple insulin injections (66%) or insulin pumps (34%) were used in the intensively treated group who were trained to modify their therapy depending on frequent glucose monitoring. The conventionally treated groups used no more than two insulin injections, and clinical well-being was the goal with no attempt to modify management based on HbA_{1c} or their glucose results.

In one-half of the subjects, a mean hemoglobin A_{1c} of 7.2% (normal: < 6%) and a mean blood glucose of 155 mg/dL was achieved using intensive therapy, while in the conventionally treated group, HbA_{1c} averaged 8.9% with an average blood glucose of 225 mg/dL. Over the study period, which averaged 7 years, there was an approximately 60% reduction in risk between the two groups in regard to diabetic retinopathy, nephropathy, and neuropathy.

Intensively treated patients had a threefold greater risk of serious hypoglycemia as well as a greater tendency toward weight gain. However, there were no deaths definitely attributable to hypoglycemia in any subjects in the DCCT study, and no evidence of posthypoglycemic cognitive damage was detected.

Reinterpretation of the published data from the DCCT trial suggests that "moderate" glycemic control (HbA_{1c} no higher than 2% above the upper limits of normal) rather than "tight" control was just as beneficial in reducing complications while producing fewer episodes of severe hypoglycemia. This implies that adjusting therapeutic glycemic goals a bit higher than those of the DCCT should retain the benefits of intensive insulin therapy at a somewhat lower risk.

The general consensus of the American Diabetes Association is that intensive insulin therapy associated with comprehensive self-management training should become standard therapy in type I patients after the age of puberty. Exceptions include those with advanced renal disease and the elderly, since, in these groups, the detrimental risks of hypoglycemia outweigh the benefits of tight glycemic control. This is especially true in small children, in whom the developing brain is particularly susceptible to hypoglycemic injury and in whom the benefits of control are limited since diabetic complications do not seem to occur until some years after the onset of puberty.

While patients with type II were not studied in the DCCT, there is no reason to believe that the effects of better control of blood glucose levels would not also apply to type II. The eye, kidney, and nerve abnormalities are quite similar in both types of diabetes, and it is likely that similar underlying mechanisms apply. Several important differences, however, must be considered. Since these patients are generally from an older population with a high incidence of macrovascular disease, an episode of severe hypoglycemia entails much greater risk than it would in younger type I patients of the DCCT. Moreover, weight gain may be much greater in obese type II patients in whom intensive insulin therapy is attempted. These risks take on greater relevance in older type II patients who have a relatively lower prevalence of microangiopathy than type I patients and in whom prevention of microvascular disease over the long term is much less likely to influence morbidity and mortality because of the much more ominous consequences of their macrovascular disease.

A preliminary study, the Veterans Affairs cooperative study on glycemic control and complications in type II diabetes, has raised some concern that major cardiovascular events occurred more frequently in NIDDM patients treated intensively with insulin as

INSTRUCTIONS IN THE CARE OF THE FEET
FOR PERSONS WITH DIABETES MELLITUS OR VASCULAR DISTURBANCES

Hygiene of the Feet

(1) Wash feet daily with mild soap and luke-warm water. Dry thoroughly between the toes by pressure. Do not rub vigorously, as this is apt to break the delicate skin.

(2) When feet are thoroughly dry, rub well with vegetable oil to keep them soft, prevent excess friction, remove scales, and prevent dryness. Care must be taken to prevent foot tenderness.

(3) If the feet become too soft and tender, rub them with alcohol about once a week.

(4) When rubbing the feet, always rub upward from the tips of the toes. If varicose veins are present, massage the feet very gently; never massage the legs.

(5) If the toenails are brittle and dry, soften them by soaking for one-half hour each night in lukewarm water containing 1 tbsp of powdered sodium borate (borax) per quart. Follow this by rubbing around the nails with vegetable oil. Clean around the nails with an orangewood stick. If the nails become too long, file them with an emery board. File them straight across and no shorter than the underlying soft tissues of the toe. Never cut the corners of the nails. (The podiatrist should be informed if a patient has diabetes.)

(6) Wear low-heeled shoes of soft leather that fit the shape of the feet correctly. The shoes should have wide toes that will cause no pressure, fit close in the arch, and grip the heels snugly. Wear new shoes one-half hour only on the first day and increase by 1 hour each day following. Wear thick, warm, loose stockings.

Treatment of Corns & Calluses

(1) Corns and calluses are due to friction and pressure, most often from improperly fitted shoes and stockings. Wear shoes that fit properly and cause no friction or pressure.

(2) To remove excess calluses or corns, soak the feet in lukewarm (not hot) water, using a mild soap, for about 10 minutes and then rub off the excess tissue with a towel or file. Do not tear it off. Under no circumstances must the skin become irritated.

(3) Do not cut corns or calluses. If they need attention it is safer to see a podiatrist.

(4) Prevent callus formation under the ball of the foot (a) by exercise, such as curling and stretching the toes several times a day; (b) by finishing each step on the toes and not on the ball of the foot; and (c) by wearing shoes that are not too short and that do not have high heels.

Aids in Treatment of Impaired Circulation (Cold Feet)

(1) Never use tobacco in any form. Tobacco contracts blood vessels and so reduces circulation.

(2) Keep warm. Wear warm stockings and other clothing. Cold contracts blood vessels and reduces circulation.

(3) Do not wear circular garters, which compress blood vessels and reduce blood flow.

(4) Do not sit with the legs crossed. This may compress the leg arteries and shut off the blood supply to the feet.

(5) If the weight of the bedclothes is uncomfortable, place a pillow under the covers at the foot of the bed.

(6) Do not apply any medication to the feet without directions from a physician. Some medicines are too strong for feet with poor circulation.

(7) Do not apply heat in the form of hot water, hot water bottles, or heating pads without a physician's consent. Even moderate heat can injure the skin if circulation is poor.

(8) If the feet are moist or the patient has a tendency to develop athlete's foot, a prophylactic dusting powder should be used on the feet and in shoes and stockings daily. Change shoes and stockings at least daily or oftener.

Treatment of Abrasions of the Skin

(1) Proper first-aid treatment is of the utmost importance even in apparently minor injuries. Consult a physician immediately for any redness, blistering, pain, or swelling. Any break in the skin may become ulcerous or gangrenous unless properly treated by a physician.

(2) Dermatophytosis (athlete's foot), which begins with peeling and itching between the toes or discoloration or thickening of the toenails, should be treated immediately by a physician or podiatrist.

(3) Avoid strong irritating antiseptics such as tincture of iodine.

(4) As soon as possible after any injury, cover the area with sterile gauze, which may be purchased at drugstores. Only fine paper tape or cellulose tape (Scotch Tape) should be used on the skin if adhesive retention of the gauze is required.

(5) Elevate and, as much as possible until recovery, avoid using the foot.

compared with those receiving standard insulin therapy. Hemoglobin A_{1c} was 7.2% in the intensively treated group compared with 9.5% in the group receiving standard therapy. Because this study was of relatively short duration (27 months) and because the sample size was small (n = 153), the investigators requested a long-term expanded trial before concluding that a detrimental effect results from intensive insulin therapy in NIDDM. An ongoing multicenter prospective clinical trial in the United Kingdom investigating the risks and benefits of intensive therapy of type II diabetic patients over an 8-year period will be completed in 1998 and should provide some data that will help resolve these questions. At present, the American Diabetes Association feels that common sense and clinical judgment on an individual basis should determine just what degree of glycemic control is appropriate in type II diabetes.

Steps in the Management of the Diabetic Patient

A. Diagnostic Examination: Any features of the clinical picture that suggest end-organ insensitivity to insulin, such as obesity, must be identified. The family history should document not only the incidence of diabetes in other members of the family but also the age at onset, whether it was associated with obesity, and whether insulin was required. Other factors that increase cardiac risk, such as smoking history, presence of hypertension or hyperlipidemia, or oral contraceptive pill use, should be recorded.

Laboratory diagnosis should document fasting plasma glucose levels above 140 mg/dL or postprandial values consistently above 200 mg/dL and whether ketonuria accompanies the glycosuria. A glycohemoglobin measurement is useful for assessing the effectiveness of future therapy. Some flexibility of clinical judgment is appropriate when diagnosing diabetes mellitus in the elderly patient with borderline hyperglycemia.

Baseline values include fasting plasma triglycerides, total cholesterol and HDL cholesterol, electrocardiography, renal function studies, peripheral pulses, and neurologic, podiatric, and ophthalmologic examinations to help guide future assessments.

B. Patient Education (Self-Management Training): Since diabetes is a lifelong disorder, education of the patient and the family is probably the most important obligation of the physician who provides initial care. The best persons to manage a disease that is affected so markedly by daily fluctuations in environmental stress, exercise, diet, and infections are the patients themselves and their families. The "teaching curriculum" should include explanations by the physician or nurse of the nature of diabetes and its potential acute and chronic hazards and how they can be recognized early and prevented or treated. The importance of regular tests for glucose on capillary blood specimens should be stressed and instructions on proper testing and recording of data provided. Moreover, patients should be provided with algorithms they can use to adjust the timing and quantity of their insulin dose, food, and exercise in response to recorded blood glucose values for optimal blood glucose control. The targets for blood glucose control should be elevated appropriately in elderly patients since they have the greatest risk if subjected to hypoglycemia and the least long-term benefit from more rigid glycemic control. Advice on personal hygiene, including detailed instructions on foot care, as well as individual instruction on diet and specific hypoglycemic therapy, should be provided. Patients should be told about community agencies, such as Diabetes Association chapters, that can serve as a continuing source of instruction. Finally, vigorous efforts should be made to persuade new diabetics who smoke to give up the habit, since large vessel peripheral vascular disease and debilitating retinopathy are less common in nonsmoking diabetic patients.

C. Self-Monitoring of Blood Glucose: Monitoring of blood glucose by patients has allowed greater flexibility in management while achieving improved glycemic control.

Self-monitoring of blood glucose is particularly useful in brittle diabetics, those attempting "ideal" glycemic control such as during pregnancy, patients who have little or no early warning of hypoglycemic attacks, and those with dysfunctional bladders from diabetic neuropathy or altered renal thresholds for glucose. Self-monitoring of blood glucose is recommended for all insulin-treated diabetic patients. The expert consensus on self-monitoring is that its proper use is to develop a database as an aid in making day-to-day informal decisions about therapy as well as to determine when emergency situations arise. It is particularly valuable as an educational and training tool to enhance understanding of diabetes by patients and their families. The usefulness of self-monitoring depends on the accuracy of the results obtained. Patients must be taught proper techniques, cautioned to calibrate instruments each day despite the expense of strips, to keep proper records, and, particularly, how to respond to unacceptably high or low blood glucose levels with appropriate therapeutic maneuvers. Self-monitoring has proved to be an effective and safe clinical tool that can improve glycemic control in compliant patients.

D. Initial Therapy: Treatment must be individualized on the basis of the type of diabetes and specific needs of each patient. However, certain general principles of management can be outlined for hyperglycemic states of different types.

1. The obese type II patient—The most common type of diabetic patient is obese, is non-insulin-dependent, and has hyperglycemia because of insensitivity to normal or elevated circulating levels of insulin.

a. Weight reduction–Treatment is directed toward achieving weight reduction, and prescribing a diet is only one means to this end. Behavior modification to achieve adherence to the diet, as well as increased physical activity to expend energy, is also required. Cure can be achieved by reducing adipose stores, with consequent restoration of tissue sensitivity to insulin, but weight reduction is hard to achieve and even more difficult to maintain with our current therapies. The presence of diabetes with its added risk factors may motivate the obese diabetic to greater efforts to lose weight. (See also Chapter 29.)

b. Hypoglycemic agents–Neither insulin nor sulfonylureas are indicated for long-term use in the obese patient with mild diabetes. The weight reduction program can be upset by real or imagined hypoglycemic reactions when insulin therapy or sulfonylureas are used and weight gain is a frequent complication. Monotherapy with acarbose, metformin, or troglitazone may be useful in the obese patient with mild diabetes if pharmacotherapy is required since they are not associated with weight gain or drug-induced hypoglycemia.

Oral agents such as metformin, troglitazone, and sulfonylureas have a role in the management of obese patients with moderately severe diabetes causing nocturia, blurred vision, or candidal vulvovaginitis. Insulin injections may be required if a trial of sulfonylurea therapy combined with troglitazone or metformin does not ameliorate symptoms. In such cases, short-term therapy (weeks or months) with either oral agents or insulin may be indicated to abate symptoms until simultaneous caloric restriction leading to weight reduction can occur.

Combining sulfonylureas with insulin replacement has not been effective in reducing insulin requirements or improving glycemic control in type I patients who have no residual pancreatic B cell function. On the other hand, type II patients do show modest glycemic improvement with a combined sulfonylurea-insulin regimen, but one that generally can be achieved with insulin therapy alone. At present, there is no overall consensus for using combined sulfonylurea therapy with insulin in type II. A recent double-blind trial in a group of obese type II patients who failed sulfonylureas demonstrated that a regimen of bedtime NPH insulin (mean dose of 40–50 units) plus a maximum dose of glipizide (20 mg twice daily) was able to produce near normoglycemia during a 1-year study. However, until more data are available to validate this approach, many diabetologists recommend stopping the sulfonylureas when patients are responding poorly to maximal doses and changing over to insulin therapy alone. In the case of type II patients requiring excessive amounts of insulin—exceeding 100 units/d—it is considered a reasonable option to *add* troglitazone at doses of 400–600 mg/d to improve glycemic control rather than to prescribe higher insulin doses.

2. The nonobese patient–In the nonobese diabetic, mild to severe hyperglycemia is usually due to refractoriness of B cells to glucose stimulation. Treatment depends on whether insulinopenia is mild (type II or mild type I in partial remission) or severe, with ketoacidosis (IDDM).

a. Diet therapy–If hyperglycemia is mild, normal metabolic control can occasionally be restored by means of multiple feedings of a diet limited in simple sugars and with a caloric content sufficient to maintain ideal weight. Restriction of saturated fats and cholesterol is also strongly advised.

b. Oral hypoglycemic agents–When diet therapy is not sufficient to correct hyperglycemia, a trial of sulfonylureas is often successful in reducing the glycohemoglobin concentration below 9.5%. Once the dosage of one of the more potent sulfonylureas reaches the upper recommended limit in a compliant patient without maintaining fasting blood glucose below 140 mg/dL during the day, combination therapy with metformin (up to 850 mg two or three times daily) and sulfonylureas should be tried. This has been effective in up to 50% of sulfonylurea failures. If fasting hyperglycemia above 140 mg/dL persists, insulin therapy is recommended by the ADA.

c. Treatment of type I with insulin–(Table 27–9.) The patient requiring insulin therapy should be initially regulated under conditions of optimal diet and normal daily activities. In patients with type I, information and counseling based on the findings of the DCCT (see above) should be provided about the advantages and disadvantages of taking multiple injections of insulin in conjunction with self blood glucose monitoring. If near-normalization of blood glucose is attempted, urine glucose measurements are not sufficient, and at least three measurements of capillary blood glucose are required daily to avoid frequent hypoglycemic reactions. Table 27–9 sets forth the advantages and disadvantages of various insulin regimens in this type of diabetes.

(1) Conventional split-dose insulin mixtures–A typical initial dose schedule in a 70-kg patient taking 2200 kcal divided into six or seven feedings might be 10 units of regular and 15 units of NPH insulin in the morning and 5 units of regular and 5 units of NPH insulin in the evening. The morning capillary blood glucose gives a measure of the effectiveness of NPH insulin administered the previous evening; the noon blood glucose reflects the effects of the morning regular insulin; and the 5:00 PM and 9:00 PM sugars represent the effects of the morning NPH and evening regular insulins, respectively. A properly educated patient should be taught to adjust insulin dosage by observing the pattern of glycemia and correlating it with the approximate duration of action and the time of peak effect after injection of the various insulin preparations (Figure 27–1). Adjustments to correct patterns of hyperglycemia

Table 27–9. Advantages and disadvantages of various insulin regimens in treatment of type I diabetes.

Two Injections (Conventional Split Doses of Regular and NPH Insulin Twice Daily)	Three Injections (Mixtures of Regular and NPH in AM; Regular at Dinner; NPH at Bedtime)	Four Injections (Regular or Insulin Lispro Before Meals and Long-Acting Insulin to Maintain Basal Insulin Levels)
ADVANTAGES		
Relatively convenient. Controls postprandial glycemia at breakfast and dinner.	Controls postprandial glycemia at breakfast and dinner. Can prevent prebreakfast hyperglycemia with less risk of nocturnal hypoglycemia. Less variability of absorption of NPH, since lower doses are injected to last overnight.	Controls postprandial glycemia. Allows flexibility of meal schedules and quantity. Less variability of absorption of small doses of insulins given more frequently. Tight glycemic control is possible with least risk of hypoglycemia.
DISADVANTAGES		
Prebreakfast hyperglycemia is common. Increased risk of nocturnal hypoglycemia in attempt to control prebreakfast hyperglycemia. Variability of absorption due to relatively large NPH doses to last overnight.	Less convenient. Lunch schedule is relatively inflexible as to time and quantity to avoid hypoglycemia from morning NPH. Dinner schedule cannot be delayed without extra feedings.	Relatively inconvenient. Pumps are expensive and are generally less convenient than multiple injections and add risk of skin infections and pump failures.

should include the following options, either alone or in combination: modification of diet and exercise programs and changes in the insulin dose or its preprandial timing.

(2) Intensive insulin therapy—In cases where conventional split doses of insulin mixtures cannot maintain near normalization of blood glucose without hypoglycemia, particularly at night, multiple injections of insulin may be required. An increasingly popular regimen consists of reducing or omitting the evening dose of intermediate insulin and adding a portion of it at bedtime. For example, 10 units of regular insulin mixed with 10 units of NPH insulin in the morning, 8–10 units of regular insulin before the evening meal, and 6 units of NPH insulin at bedtime is often more efficacious than the conventional split-dose regimen mentioned above. The dose of regular insulin prior to a meal should be selected so that each 10–15 g of carbohydrate is covered by 1 unit of regular insulin. With current availability of nutritional labeling, the counting of nutrient carbohydrates should be taught to all patients receiving intensive insulin therapy.

In cases where hypoglycemia occurs unexpectedly and at inconsistent times day or night, variable or delayed insulin absorption from large subcutaneous depots containing both regular and NPH insulin may be a contributing factor. Reducing the size and changing the character of the depots by administering small doses of regular insulin more frequently (eg, three times a day before meals), with one injection of a long-acting insulin (eg, ultralente insulin) at bedtime has often been most helpful in reducing the frequency and severity of hypoglycemia in patients attempting near normalization of blood glucose. This

regimen has become more convenient with the advent of pen-injectors and gives greater flexibility regarding meal patterns and diet than conventional therapy with split-dose insulin mixtures.

Insulin lispro has been advocated as a safer and more convenient alternative to regular human insulin for preprandial use in regimens of intensive insulin therapy. However, because of its relatively short duration (no more than 3–4 hours), it requires two injections of ultralente insulin at 12-hour intervals or concomitant small doses of intermediate-acting insulin with each preprandial injection to avoid hyperglycemia prior to the subsequent meal or bedtime snack. In addition to carbohydrate content of the meal, the effect of simultaneous fat ingestion must also be considered a factor in determining the insulin lispro dosage required to control the glycemic increment during and just after the meal. With low-carbohydrate content and high-fat intake there is an increased risk of hypoglycemia from insulin lispro within 2 hours after the meal. In a 65 kg person with type I diabetes eating meals of standard carbohydrate content and a moderate to low fat content, a possible regimen of insulin lispro might be started, with the following doses injected only 20 minutes before meals and adjusted depending on target blood glucose levels (Table 27–10).

Since insulin lispro reaches a peak serum level so quickly after subcutaneous administration, smaller doses are generally required compared with regular human insulin. Multiple injections of NPH insulin (or twice-daily ultralente insulin) can be mixed in the same syringe as the insulin lispro.

Occasional patients do not accept multiple injections of insulin and prefer continuous subcutaneous

Table 27–10. Example of an intensive insulin regimen using insulin lispro and ultralente insulin.

	Pre-Breakfast	Pre-Lunch	Pre-Dinner	At Bedtime
Insulin lispro	5 units	5 units	4 units	—
Ultralente insulin	12 units	—	12 units	—

infusions with portable open-loop insulin pumps, which require subcutaneous needle insertion only every 48 hours.

(3) Management of early morning hyperglycemia in type I–(Table 27–11.) One of the more difficult therapeutic problems in managing patients with type I is determining the proper adjustment of insulin dose when the prebreakfast blood glucose level is high.

(a) Somogyi effect–Patients with type I may develop nocturnal hypoglycemia, which may in turn stimulate a surge of counterregulatory hormones (Somogyi effect) to produce high blood glucose levels by 7:00 AM.

Clinicians have often observed that by reducing inappropriately high doses of administered insulin, hyperglycemia on the following morning may improve substantially. This "Somogyi effect" remains a factor to be considered as contributing to early morning hyperglycemia in patients treated with relatively high doses of insulin. Prescribing a lower dose of intermediate-acting insulin before dinner or at bedtime is a reasonable therapeutic option, particularly when nocturnal hypoglycemia is suspected.

(b) Dawn phenomenon–The dawn phenomenon is present in as many as 75% of type I patients and occurs in most type II and normal subjects as well. It is characterized by reduced tissue sensitivity to insulin developing between 5:00 AM and 8:00 AM. Recent evidence suggests that this phenomenon is evoked by spikes of growth hormone released hours before, at the onset of sleep. When the dawn phenomenon occurs alone, it may produce only mild hyperglycemia in the early morning, but when it is associated with the Somogyi effect or the waning phenomenon (or both), the hyperglycemia may be more severe.

(c) Waning of circulating insulin levels–The most common cause of prebreakfast hyperglycemia is probably the waning of circulating insulin levels. This would suggest that *more* rather than less intermediate-acting insulin should be given in the evening.

The Somogyi effect, the dawn phenomenon, and the waning of insulin levels are not mutually exclusive; if they occur together, more severe hyperglycemia develops.

Table 27–11 shows that diagnosis of the cause of prebreakfast hyperglycemia can be facilitated by self-monitoring of blood glucose at 3:00 AM in addition to the usual bedtime and 7:00 AM measurements. This is required for only a few nights until the diagnosis is established and appropriate adjustment of bedtime insulin dose or nighttime feeding is achieved.

(d) Therapy of prebreakfast hyperglycemia–When a particular pattern emerges from monitoring blood glucose levels overnight, appropriate therapeutic measures can be taken. The Somogyi effect can be treated by eliminating the dose of intermediate insulin at dinnertime and giving it at a lower dosage at bedtime or by supplying more food at bedtime. When the dawn phenomenon alone is present, the dosage of intermediate insulin can be divided between dinnertime and bedtime, or when insulin pumps are used, the basal infusion rate can be increased (eg, from 0.8 unit/h to 1 unit/h from 6:00 AM until breakfast). With waning insulin levels, either increasing the evening dose or shifting it from dinnertime to bedtime, or both, can be effective. A bedtime dose of NPH made from animal insulin provides more sustained overnight insulin levels than human NPH and may be effective in managing refractory prebreakfast hyperglycemia.

Table 27–11. Prebreakfast hyperglycemia: Classification by blood glucose and insulin levels.

	Blood Glucose (mg/dL)			Free Immunoreactive Insulin (μU/mL)		
	10:00 PM	3:00 AM	7:00 AM	10:00 PM	3:00 AM	7:00 AM
Somogyi effect	90	40	200	High	Slightly high	Normal
Dawn phenomenon	110	110	150	Normal	Normal	Normal
Waning of insulin dose plus dawn phenomenon	110	190	220	Normal	Low	Low
Waning of insulin dose plus dawn phenomenon plus Somogyi effect	110	40	380	High	Normal	Low

d. Treatment of type II with insulin–When sulfonylureas fail and type II patients require insulin to control their hyperglycemia, various insulin regimens may be effective. Although a single morning injection of insulin is not recommended in type I diabetes (see Table 27–9), in some patients with type II diabetes enough residual insulin secretion persists to allow a single morning injection of 25–30 units of NPH or lente insulin to replace their deficient insulin secretion. If prebreakfast hyperglycemia persists on this regimen, a number of alternatives are available. A convenient regimen includes split doses of a fixed 70:30 mixture of NPH:regular insulin, which can be started as 20 units before breakfast and 15 units before dinner and increased appropriately depending on target blood glucoses at 7:00 AM and 5:00 PM. When more than 50 units a day are required without achieving proper control, these patients may benefit from three or four injection regimens as described for type I in Table 27–9.

e. Acceptable levels of glycemic control: See above for a discussion of the Diabetes Control and Complications Trial and its implications for type II therapy. A reasonable aim of therapy is to approach normal glycemic excursions without provoking severe or frequent hypoglycemia. What has been considered "acceptable" control includes blood glucose levels of 80–130 mg/dL before meals and after an overnight fast and levels no higher than 180 mg/dL 1 hour after meals and 150 mg/dL 2 hours after meals. Glycohemoglobin levels should be no higher than 2% above the upper limit of the normal range for any particular laboratory. Among the intensively treated patients in the DCCT, very little progression of retinopathy occurred among the 90% of those whose hemoglobin A_{1c} was within 2% of the upper limit of normal, in contrast to the accelerated progression in the 10% who had higher values of glycohemoglobin. In elderly patients, criteria for optimal control should be adjusted upward, with glycohemoglobins 2–3% above the upper limits of normal and preprandial blood glucose levels below 200 mg/dL being acceptable.

Indications for Purified Insulins

Human insulin or purified pork insulins are indicated when insulin of conventional purity and containing beef species has been associated with allergy, immune resistance, or lipoatrophy. Also, they are preferable in any patient undergoing insulin therapy for the first time, since they reduce or eliminate the risk of occurrence of these rare immune complications. Moreover, absent or very low levels of anti-insulin antibodies enhance recovery from insulin-induced hypoglycemia and facilitate the measurement of therapeutic levels of circulating insulin as a guide for optimal management. In patients with type II whose therapy with insulin is to be for a limited time (eg, in gestational diabetes or during acute infections or surgery), human insulin or purified insulin reduces the risks of immunologic sensitization to future exposures to insulin.

Complications of Insulin Therapy

A. Hypoglycemia: Hypoglycemic reactions, the most common complication of insulin therapy, may result from delay in taking a meal or unusual physical exertion. With more type I patients attempting "tight" control, this complication has become even more frequent. In older diabetics, in those taking only longer-acting insulins, and often in those attempting to maintain euglycemia on infusion pumps, autonomic counterregulatory responses are less readily elicited during hypoglycemia, and the manifestations are mainly from impaired function of the central nervous system, ie, mental confusion, bizarre behavior, and ultimately coma. Even focal neurologic deficits mimicking stroke may be observed. More rapid development of hypoglycemia from the effects of regular insulin causes signs of autonomic hyperactivity, both sympathetic (tachycardia, palpitations, sweating, tremulousness) and parasympathetic (nausea, hunger), that may progress to coma and convulsions. Except for sweating, most of the sympathetic symptoms of hypoglycemia are blunted in patients receiving beta-blocking agents for angina or hypertension. Though not absolutely contraindicated, these drugs must be used with great caution in insulin-requiring diabetics, and, whenever possible, β_1-selective blocking agents should be used.

1. Altered awareness of hypoglycemia– Since autonomic responses correlate strongly with "awareness" of hypoglycemia, many poorly controlled diabetics—whose nervous systems have adapted to chronic hyperglycemia—may trigger adrenergic alarms at levels of blood glucose above the usual hypoglycemic range. Conversely, type I patients overtreated with insulin may be unaware of critically low levels of blood glucose because of an adaptive blunting of their alarm systems owing to repeated episodes of hypoglycemia. This has been shown to be reversible if higher average blood glucose levels are maintained in these patients to avoid recurrent hypoglycemia over a period of several weeks.

Controversy exists over whether there is a link between switching from animal insulin to human insulin and development of reduced awareness for hypoglycemia. However, in the absence of large-scale prospective studies, the consensus of most diabetologists is that the data questioning the safety of human insulin are insufficient to justify a restriction of its use at this time. They feel that loss of awareness can be induced by repeated episodes of hypoglycemia. The latter may occur in as many as half of patients switched from animal to human insulin if the switch is made at equivalent or nearly equivalent dosages, without taking the precaution of beginning with a

20–25% lower human insulin dose to compensate for the reduced neutralization of the injected insulin by preexisting anti-beef or anti-pork insulin antibodies. Another cause of frequent hypoglycemia could be the inclination of patients and their physicians to attempt tighter glycemic control at the time of switching from animal to human insulin as part of a general upgrading of their diabetes care. As evidenced by results of the DCCT, the risk of frequent severe hypoglycemic episodes is greatly increased when "normalization" of the blood glucose is attempted with presently available methods of insulin delivery, and this is independent of the species of insulin used.

2. Lack of glucagon response in type I–For unexplained reasons, patients with type I lose their glucagon responses to hypoglycemia (but not to amino acids in protein-containing meals) within a year or so after developing diabetes. These patients then rely predominantly on the sympathetic nervous system to counterregulate hypoglycemia and are at special risk in later years when aging, autonomic neuropathy, or frequent hypoglycemic episodes blunt their sympathetic responses.

3. Prevention and treatment of hypoglycemia–Because of the potential danger of insulin reactions, the diabetic patient should carry packets of table sugar or a candy roll at all times for use at the onset of hypoglycemic symptoms. *Tablets containing 3 g of glucose are available* (dextrosol). The educated patient soon learns to take the amount of glucose needed and avoids the excess that may occur with eating candy or drinking orange juice, causing very high hyperglycemia. An ampule of glucagon (1 mg) should be provided to every diabetic receiving insulin therapy, and family or friends should be instructed how to inject it intramuscularly in the event that the patient is unconscious or refuses food. *An identification MedicAlert bracelet, necklace, or card in the wallet or purse should be carried by every diabetic receiving hypoglycemic drug therapy.* The telephone number for the MedicAlert Foundation International in Turlock, California, is 800-ID-ALERT.

All of the manifestations of hypoglycemia are rapidly relieved by glucose administration. If more severe hypoglycemia has produced unconsciousness or stupor, the treatment is 50 mL of 50% glucose solution by rapid intravenous infusion. If intravenous therapy is not available, 1 mg of glucagon injected intramuscularly will usually restore the patient to consciousness within 15 minutes to permit ingestion of sugar. If the patient is stuporous and glucagon is not available, small amounts of honey or syrup can be inserted within the buccal pouch, but, in general, oral feeding is contraindicated in unconscious patients. Rectal administration of syrup or honey (30 mL per 500 mL of warm water) has been effective.

B. Immunopathology of Insulin Therapy: At least five molecular classes of insulin antibodies are produced during the course of insulin therapy in dia-

betes, including IgA, IgD, IgE, IgG, and IgM. With the increased therapeutic use of purified pork and human insulin in Western countries, the various immunopathologic syndromes such as insulin allergy, immune insulin resistance, and lipoatrophy have become quite rare. However, wherever less purified forms of beef insulin are still used, these disorders remain a clinical concern among some insulin-treated patients.

1. Insulin allergy–Insulin allergy, or immediate-type hypersensitivity, is a rare condition in which local or systemic urticaria is due to histamine release from tissue mast cells sensitized by adherence of anti-insulin IgE antibodies. In severe cases, anaphylaxis results. When only human insulin has been used from the onset of insulin therapy, insulin allergy is exceedingly rare. When allergy to beef or, more rarely, pork insulin is present, a species change (eg, to human insulin) may correct the problem, although in many cases cross-reaction between human and animal insulins results in persistent allergic responses. Antihistamines, corticosteroids, and even desensitization may be required, especially for systemic hypersensitivity.

2. Immune insulin resistance–All insulin-treated patients develop a low titer of circulating IgG anti-insulin antibodies that neutralize to a small extent the action of insulin. However, under rare circumstances, in some diabetic patients, principally those with some degree of tissue insensitivity to insulin (such as in the obese) and with a history of interrupted exposure to therapy with beef insulin, a high titer of circulating IgG anti-insulin antibodies may develop. This results in extremely high insulin requirements—often more than 200 units daily. This is often a self-limited condition and may clear spontaneously after several months. However, in cases where the circulating antibody is specifically more reactive with beef insulin—a more potent immunogen in humans than pork insulin—changing the patient to a less antigenic insulin (pork or human) may make possible a dramatic reduction in insulin dosage or at least may shorten the duration of immune resistance. Owing to the usual effectiveness of human insulin in treating this syndrome, immunosuppressive therapy with high doses of glucocorticoids is no longer required.

C. Lipodystrophy at Injection Sites: Atrophy of subcutaneous fatty tissue leading to disfiguring excavations and depressed areas may rarely occur at the site of injection. This complication results from an immune reaction, and it has become rarer with the development of pure insulin preparations. Injection of these preparations directly into the atrophic area often results in restoration of normal contours. Lipohypertrophy, on the other hand, is a consequence of the pharmacologic effects of insulin being deposited in the same location repeatedly. It can occur with purified insulins and is best treated with localized liposuction of the hypertrophic areas by an experienced plastic surgeon. Rotation of injection sites will prevent lipohypertrophy.

Chronic Complications of Diabetes

Late clinical manifestations of diabetes mellitus include a number of pathologic changes that involve small and large blood vessels, cranial and peripheral nerves, the skin, and the lens of the eye. These lesions lead to hypertension, renal failure, blindness, autonomic and peripheral neuropathy, amputations of the lower extremities, myocardial infarction, and cerebrovascular accidents. These late manifestations correlate with the duration of the diabetic state subsequent to the onset of puberty. In type I diabetes, up to 40% of patients develop end-stage renal disease, compared with less than 20% of patients with type II diabetes. As regards proliferative retinopathy, it ultimately develops in both types of diabetes but has a slightly higher prevalence in type I patients (25% after 15 years' duration). In patients with type I diabetes, complications from end-stage renal disease are a major cause of death, whereas patients with type II diabetes are more likely to have macrovascular diseases leading to myocardial infarction and stroke as the main causes of death.

A. Ocular Complications:

1. Diabetic cataracts–Premature cataracts occur in diabetic patients. These opacities resemble those found in elderly patients with "senile" cataracts but occur at a younger age and seem to correlate with both the duration of diabetes and the severity of chronic hyperglycemia. Nonenzymatic glycosylation of lens protein is twice as high in diabetic patients as in age-matched nondiabetic persons and may contribute to the premature occurrence of cataracts.

2. Diabetic retinopathy–Three main categories exist: background, or "simple," retinopathy, consisting of microaneurysms, hemorrhages, exudates, and retinal edema; preproliferative retinopathy with arteriolar ischemia manifested as cotton-wool spots (small infarcted areas of retina); and proliferative, or "malignant," retinopathy, consisting of newly formed vessels. Proliferative retinopathy is a leading cause of blindness in the USA, particularly since it increases the risk of retinal detachment. After 10 years of diabetes, half of all patients have retinopathy, and this proportion increases to more than 80% after 15 years of diabetes. Annual consultation with an ophthalmologist should be arranged for patients who have had type I diabetes for more than 5 years and for *all* patients with type II diabetes, because they were probably diabetic for an extensive period of time before diagnosis. Extensive "scatter" xenon or argon photocoagulation and focal treatment of new vessels reduce severe visual loss in those cases in which proliferative retinopathy is associated with *recent* vitreous hemorrhages or in which extensive new vessels are located on or near

the optic disk. Macular edema, which is more common than proliferative retinopathy in patients with type II diabetes (up to 18% prevalence), has also responded to this therapy with improvement in visual acuity. Avoiding tobacco use and correction of associated hypertension are important therapeutic measures in the management of diabetic retinopathy.

3. Glaucoma–Glaucoma occurs in approximately 6% of persons with diabetes. It is generally responsive to the usual therapy for open-angle disease. Neovascularization of the iris in diabetics can predispose to closed-angle glaucoma, but this is relatively uncommon except after cataract extraction, when growth of new vessels has been known to progress rapidly, involving the angle of the iris and obstructing outflow.

B. Diabetic Nephropathy:
As many as 4000 cases of end-stage renal disease occur each year among diabetic people in the United States. This is about one-fourth of all patients being treated for end-stage renal disease and represents a considerable national health expense.

The cumulative incidence of nephropathy differs between the two major types of diabetes. Patients with type I diabetes have a 30–40% chance of having nephropathy after 20 years—in contrast to the much lower frequency in type II diabetes patients, in whom only about 15–20% develop clinical renal disease. However, since there are many more individuals affected with type II diabetes, end-stage renal disease is much more prevalent in type II than in type I diabetes in the United States and especially throughout the rest of the world. Recent studies have documented that with improved glycemic control and more effective therapeutic measures to correct hypertension—and with the beneficial effects of angiotensin-converting enzyme inhibitors—there can be a substantial reduction in the development of end-stage renal disease among diabetics.

Diabetic nephropathy is initially manifested by proteinuria; subsequently, as kidney function declines, urea and creatinine accumulate in the blood.

1. Microalbuminuria–Sensitive radioimmunoassay methods of detecting small amounts of urinary albumin have permitted detection of microgram concentrations—in contrast to the less sensitive dipstick strips, whose minimal detection limit is 0.3–0.5%. Conventional 24-hour urine collections, in addition to being inconvenient for patients, also show wide variability of albumin excretion, since several factors such as sustained erect posture, dietary protein, and exercise tend to increase albumin excretion rates. For these reasons, most laboratories prefer to measure a timed overnight urine collection beginning at bedtime, when the urine is discarded and the time noted. Normal subjects excrete less than 15 μg/min during overnight urine collections; values of 20 μg/min or higher are considered to represent abnormal microalbuminuria. A convenient screening method involves analysis of the albumin-creatinine ratio in an early morning spot urine brought in by the patient. A ratio of albumin (mg/L) to creatinine (nmol/L) of 3.5 or less is normal, and a ratio of 10 or more indicates abnormal microalbuminuria. Values between 3.6 and 9.9 are borderline and should be repeated.

Subsequent renal failure can be predicted by persistent urinary albumin excretion rates exceeding 30 μg/min. Increased microalbuminuria correlates with increased levels of blood pressure and increased LDL cholesterol, and this may explain why increased proteinuria in diabetic patients is associated with an increase in cardiovascular deaths even in the absence of renal failure. Careful glycemic control as well as a low-protein diet (0.8 g/kg/d) may reduce both the hyperfiltration and the elevated microalbuminuria in patients in the early stages of diabetes and those with incipient diabetic nephropathy. Antihypertensive therapy also decreases microalbuminuria, and there is some evidence that angiotensin I converting enzyme (ACE) inhibitors may have a specific role in reducing intraglomerular pressure in addition to their lowering of systemic hypertension. A recent 2-year double-blind placebo-controlled clinical trial in type I diabetic patients who had persistent microalbuminuria but were normotensive showed that an ACE inhibitor (captopril, 50 mg twice daily) impeded progression to clinical proteinuria and prevented the increase in albumin excretion rate.

2. Progressive diabetic nephropathy–Progressive diabetic nephropathy consists of proteinuria of varying severity occasionally leading to nephrotic syndrome with hypoalbuminemia, edema, and an increase in circulating betalipoproteins as well as progressive azotemia. In contrast to all other renal disorders, the proteinuria associated with diabetic nephropathy does not diminish with progressive renal failure (patients continue to excrete 10–11 g daily as creatinine clearance diminishes). As renal failure progresses, there is an elevation in the renal threshold at which glycosuria appears.

Hypertension develops with progressive renal involvement, and coronary and cerebral atherosclerosis seems to be accelerated. Approximately two-thirds of adult patients with diabetes have hypertension. Once diabetic nephropathy has progressed to the stage of hypertension, proteinuria, or early renal failure, glycemic control is not beneficial in influencing its course. In this circumstance, antihypertensive medications, including ACE inhibitors, and restriction of dietary protein to 0.6 g/kg body weight per day are recommended. ACE inhibitors have been shown to protect against deterioration in renal function in IDDM patients with clinical nephropathy. This beneficial effect appears to be due to improved glomerular hemodynamics that cannot be explained only by the antihypertensive action of these drugs. One long term study using captopril (25 mg three times daily)

showed a 50% reduction in the risk of the combined end points of death, dialysis and transplantation in IDDM subjects with diabetic nephropathy and clinical proteinuria. During initiation of ACE-inhibitor therapy, the rare occurrence of persistent hyperkalemia (above 6 meq/L) is an indication to stop this medication.

When the serum creatinine reaches 3 mg/dL, consultation with a nephrologist or a diabetologist experienced in the treatment of diabetic nephropathy is recommended. When the serum creatinine reaches 5 mg/dL, consultation with personnel at a center where renal transplantation is performed is indicated.

Dialysis has been of limited value in the treatment of renal failure due to diabetic nephropathy. At present, experience in renal transplantation—especially from related donors—is more promising and is the treatment of choice in cases where there are no contraindications such as severe cardiovascular disease.

C. Gangrene of the Feet: The incidence of gangrene of the feet in diabetics is 20 times the incidence in matched controls. The factors responsible for its development are ischemia, peripheral neuropathy, and secondary infection. Occlusive vascular disease involves both microangiopathy and atherosclerosis of large and medium-sized arteries. Cigarette smoking should be avoided, and prevention of foot disease should be emphasized, since treatment is difficult once ulceration and gangrene have developed. Patients should be instructed to inspect their feet daily for reddened areas, blisters, abrasions, or lacerations, particularly when the foot is insensitive (see Instructions in the Care of the Feet). Physicians should inspect the feet of diabetic patients at each visit and instruct patients as necessary on filing calluses with an emery board, cutting toenails straight across, not walking barefoot, and avoiding tight shoes. When an uncomplicated neuropathic ulcer is present and blood flow is not impaired, consultation with a podiatrist or orthopedist is recommended. Cholesterol-lowering agents are useful as adjunctive therapy when early ischemic signs are detected. If blood supply is diminished or absent, patients with foot ulcers should be referred to an appropriate specialist (vascular or orthopedic surgeon). Special custom-built shoes are usually required to redistribute weight evenly over an insensitive foot, particularly when it has been deformed by surgery or asymptomatic fractures (Charcot's joint). Amputation of the lower extremities is sometimes required.

Nonselective beta-blockers are relatively contraindicated in patients with ischemic foot ulcers, because these drugs reduce peripheral blood flow.

D. Diabetic Neuropathy: Peripheral and autonomic neuropathy, the two most common chronic complications of diabetes, are poorly understood.

1. Peripheral neuropathy–

a. Distal symmetric polyneuropathy–This is the most common form of diabetic peripheral neuropathy where loss of function appears in a stocking-glove pattern and is due to an axonal neuropathic process. Sensory involvement usually occurs first and is generally bilateral, symmetric, and associated with dulled perception of vibration, pain, and temperature, particularly in the lower extremities. At times, discomfort of the lower extremities can be incapacitating. Both motor and sensory nerve conduction are delayed in peripheral nerves, and ankle jerks may be absent. In most cases, motor weakness is mild and confined to the most distal intrinsic muscles of the hands and feet. Long-term complications of diabetic polyneuropathy include insensitivity of the feet, leading to repeated "silent" trauma that predisposes to neuropathic plantar ulcers or deformities of the feet secondary to multiple "silent" fractures (Charcot's joint).

b. Isolated peripheral neuropathy—Involvement of the distribution of only one nerve ("mononeuropathy"), or of several nerves ("mononeuropathy multiplex") is characterized by sudden onset with subsequent recovery of all or most of the function. This neuropathology has been attributed to vascular ischemia or traumatic damage. Femoral and cranial nerves are commonly involved, and motor abnormalities predominate. These can result in sudden onset of diplopia due to ophthalmoplegia or in acute pain and weakness of thigh muscles (diabetic amyotrophy). Spontaneous resolution of these ischemic neuropathies generally occurs in 6–12 weeks. In more severe cases with extensive atrophy of limb musculature, this disorder has been termed "malignant cachexia" and mimics the end stages of advanced neoplasia, particularly when depression produces anorexia and weight loss. With this more severe manifestation of diabetic amyotrophy, recovery of muscle function may only be partial.

c. Painful diabetic neuropathy—Hypersensitivity to light touch and occasionally severe "burning" pain, particularly at night, can become physically and emotionally disabling. Amitriptyline, 25–75 mg at bedtime, has been recommended for pain associated with diabetic neuropathy. Dramatic relief has often resulted within 48–72 hours. This rapid response is in contrast to the 2 or 3 weeks required for an antidepressive effect. Patients often attribute benefit to their having a full night's sleep after amitriptyline compared to many previously sleepless nights occasioned by neuropathic pain. Mild to moderate morning drowsiness is a side effect that generally improves with time or can be lessened by giving the medication several hours before bedtime. This drug should not be continued if improvement has not occurred after 5 days of therapy. Desipramine in doses of 25–150 mg/d seems to have the same efficacy as amitriptyline. Other drugs used include carbamazepine and phenytoin, both of questionable benefit for leg pain. There has also been interest in use of the antiarrhythmic drug mexiletine for this pur-

pose in doses of up to 10 mg/kg/d. Capsaicin, a topical irritant, has recently been advocated for local nerve pain; it is dispensed as a cream (Zostrix 0.025%, Zostrix-HP 0.075%) to be rubbed into the skin over the painful region two to four times daily. A multicenter 8-week double-blind study (see Capsaicin Study Group reference) has recently reported that topical 0.075% capsaicin is effective in reducing pain among a population of 277 diabetic patients with painful diabetic neuropathy.

2. Autonomic neuropathy—With autonomic neuropathy, there is evidence of postural hypotension, decreased cardiovascular response to Valsalva's maneuver, gastroparesis, alternating bouts of diarrhea (particularly nocturnal) and constipation, inability to empty the bladder, and impotence. Gastroparesis should be considered in insulin-dependent diabetic patients who develop unexpected fluctuations and variability in their blood glucose levels after meals. Impotence due to neuropathy differs from psychogenic impotence in that the latter may be intermittent (erections occur under special circumstances), whereas diabetic impotence is usually persistent; aortoiliac occlusive disease may contribute to this problem.

a. Management of autonomic neuropathy—There is no consistently effective treatment for diabetic autonomic neuropathy. Metoclopramide has been of some help in treating diabetic gastroparesis over the short term, but its effectiveness seems to diminish over time. It is a dopamine antagonist that has central antiemetic effects as well as a cholinergic action to facilitate gastric emptying. It can be given intravenously (10 mg three or four times a day, 30 minutes before meals and at bedtime) or orally (20 mg of liquid metoclopramide) before breakfast and dinner. Drowsiness, restlessness, fatigue, and lassitude are common adverse effects. Tardive dyskinesia and extrapyramidal effects also occur. Cisapride (10 mg three or four times daily) is a newer agent that can improve the rate of gastric emptying of both liquids and solids by virtue of its cholinergic and antiserotonergic actions. It appears to be better tolerated and to cause fewer central nervous system side effects than metoclopramide, but it may cause troublesome increased stool frequency in some patients. Erythromycin appears to bind to motilin receptors in the stomach and has been found to improve gastric emptying in doses of 250 mg three times daily. Diarrhea associated with autonomic neuropathy has occasionally responded to broad-spectrum antibiotic therapy, though it often undergoes spontaneous remission. Refractory diabetic diarrhea is often associated with impaired sphincter control and fecal incontinence. Therapy with loperamide, 4–8 mg daily, or diphenoxylate with atropine, two tablets up to four times a day, may provide relief. In more severe cases, tincture of paregoric or codeine (60 mg tablets) may be required to reduce the frequency of diarrhea and improve the consistency of the stools. Clonidine has been reported to lessen diabetic diarrhea, but its tendency to lower blood pressure in these patients who already have autonomic neuropathy and some orthostatic hypotension often limits its usefulness. Bethanechol in doses of 10–50 mg three times a day has occasionally improved emptying of the atonic urinary bladder. Catheter decompression of the distended bladder has been reported to improve its function, and considerable benefit has been reported after surgical severing of the internal vesicle sphincter. Mineralocorticoid therapy with fludrocortisone, 0.2–0.3 mg/d, and elastic stockings or pressure suits have reportedly been of some help in patients with orthostatic hypotension occurring as a result of loss of postural reflexes.

b. Management of impotence–Local injection of papaverine or alprostadil (PGE₁) into the corpus cavernosum produces a penile erection if blood supply is competent. This helps differentiate erectile disabilities due to neuropathic causes from those that do not respond to papaverine because of vasculopathy. Impotence is usually permanent, and a penile prosthesis should be considered as a therapeutic option in appropriate cases. External vacuum therapy (Erec-Aid System) is a nonsurgical treatment consisting of a suction chamber operated by a hand pump that creates a vacuum around the penis. This draws blood into the penis to produce an erection which is maintained by a specially designed tension ring inserted around the base of the penis and which can be kept in place for up to 20–30 minutes. This approach has met with acceptance by a majority of patients with impotence, while others have opted for surgical implant of a penile prosthesis.

E. Skin and Mucous Membrane Complications: Chronic pyogenic infections of the skin may occur, especially in poorly controlled diabetic patients. Eruptive xanthomas can result from hypertriglyceridemia, associated with poor glycemic control. An unusual lesion termed **necrobiosis lipoidica diabeticorum** is usually located over the anterior surfaces of the legs or the dorsal surfaces of the ankles. They are oval or irregularly shaped plaques with demarcated borders and a glistening yellow surface and occur in women two to four times more frequently than in men.

"Shin spots" are not uncommon in adult diabetics. They are brownish, rounded, painless atrophic lesions of the skin in the pretibial area. Candidal infection can produce erythema and edema of intertriginous areas below the breasts, in the axillas, and between the fingers. It causes vulvovaginitis in most chronically uncontrolled diabetic women with persistent glucosuria and is a frequent cause of pruritus.

While antifungal creams containing miconazole or clotrimazole offer immediate relief of vulvovaginitis, recurrence is frequent unless glucosuria is reduced.

F. Special Situations:

1. Insulin replacement during surgery–It is likely that target glucose levels between 100 and 250 mg/dL are adequate in most patients to avoid postoperative infections or wound dehiscence, though this view is based on clinical observations rather than conclusive evidence. All diabetic patients should have serum electrolytes measured preoperatively so that abnormalities can be corrected prior to surgery. During major surgery and in the immediate recovery period in patients with insulin-requiring diabetes, 5% dextrose in physiologic saline should be infused intravenously at a rate of 100–200 mL/h with regular human insulin (25 units/250 mL 0.9% saline) infused into the intravenous tubing at a rate of 1–3 units/h. The patient's blood glucose should be monitored every hour initially and the rates of insulin or dextrose adjusted to maintain blood glucose values between 120 and 190 mg/dL (although levels up to 250 mg/dL may be acceptable).

Most patients with type II diabetes, whether or not they are receiving insulin therapy, should be treated with insulin during major surgery. In these patients, 10 units of regular human insulin added to 1000 mL of a D₅W solution containing 20 meq of potassium chloride and infused at a rate of 100 mL/h (1 unit/h) is generally adequate to regulate glycemia during surgery. The patient's glucose should be monitored hourly to prevent extremes of hyper- or hypoglycemia. If blood glucose values remain above 250 mg/dL at 1–2 hours, an infusion concentration of 15 units/L can be substituted.

NIDDM patients facing minor surgical procedures not requiring general anesthesia who have previously been controlled on oral agents or diet alone do not generally require insulin infusions. Glucose-containing solutions should be avoided during surgery in these patients, and blood glucose levels should be monitored every 4 hours. Regular human insulin or insulin lispro should be administered subcutaneously if needed to maintain blood glucose below 250 mg/dL (see Chapter 2).

2. Pregnancy and the diabetic patient–Several features distinguish the management of diabetics during pregnancy from the general therapy of diabetes. These include the following: (1) Oral hypoglycemic agents are contraindicated. (2) Weight reduction is not advised, since fetal nutrition can be adversely affected. (3) Intensive insulin therapy with frequent self-monitoring of blood glucose is generally recommended to improve the likelihood of having healthy normal babies. Every effort should be made, utilizing multiple injections of insulin or a continuous infusion of insulin by pump, to maintain near-normalization of fasting and preprandial blood glucose values while avoiding hypoglycemia. Glycohemoglobin should be maintained in the normal range.

Since many diabetic pregnancies persist beyond the expected term—or because the infants are usually large and hydramnios may be present—it has been suggested that pregnancy be terminated early (at

37–38 weeks), especially if glycemic control during pregnancy has been inadequate (eg, glycohemoglobin > 10%). There is a present trend away from elective cesarean section and toward induction of labor.

See Chapter 18 for further details.

Prognosis

Despite the present inadequacy of subcutaneous insulin delivery systems for physiologic insulin replacement, over 60% of patients with type I do reasonably well over the long term. The remainder develop severe disability leading to blindness, end-stage renal failure, and early demise.

The period between 10 and 20 years after onset of type I diabetes seems to be a critical one. If the patient survives this period without fulminating complications, there is a strong likelihood that reasonably good health will continue. In addition to poorly understood genetic factors relating to differences in individual susceptibility to development of long-term complications of hyperglycemia, it is clear that in both types of diabetes, the diabetic patient's intelligence, motivation, and awareness of the potential complications of the disease contribute significantly to the ultimate outcome.

Internet Addresses

[American Association of Diabetes Educators]
  http:// www.AADEnet.org
[American Diabetes Association]
  http://www.diabetesnet. com/ada.html
[American Dietetic Association]
http://www.eatright.org
[Juvenile Diabetes Foundation]
  http://www.jdfcure.com

Classification, Pathophysiology, & Diagnosis of Diabetes Mellitus

Atkinson MA, Maclaren NK: The pathogenesis of insulin-dependent diabetes mellitus. N Engl J Med 1996;331:1428. (Review of genetic and environmental aspects of the autoimmune etiology of type I diabetes and their implications for its prediction and prevention.)

Cheatham B, Kahn CR: Insulin action and the insulin signaling network. Endocr Rev 1995;16:117. (A review of recent progress in identifying targets of insulin action and pathways affecting metabolic substrate transport, energy storage, and cell growth.)

Kadowaki T et al: A subtype of diabetes mellitus associated with a mutation of mitochondrial DNA. N Engl J Med 1994;330:962. (A rare form of diabetes transmitted by an affected mother's mitochondrial genes and often associated with nerve deafness. While it generally presents as a type II diabetes, occasional cases show ketoacidosis and insulin dependence on a nonautoimmune basis.)

Kahn CR, Vicent D, Doria A: Genetics of non-insulin-dependent (type II) diabetes mellitus. Ann Rev Med 1996;47:509. (Genetic markers for this most prevalent form of diabetes remain elusive.)

Polonsky KS, Sturis J, Bell GI: Non-insulin dependent diabetes mellitus: A genetically programmed failure of the beta cell to compensate for insulin resistance. N Engl J Med 1996;334:777. (The pathogenesis of classic late-onset NIDDM remains an enigma. This authoritative review emphasizes the likelihood that genes affecting both the secretion and the action of insulin act in concert with nongenetic factors such as diet and the level of physical activity to cause the hyperglycemia of NIDDM.)

Yamagata K et al: Mutations in the hepatocyte nuclear factor-1α gene in maturity-onset diabetes of the young (MODY 3). Nature 1996;384:455.

Yamagata K et al: Mutations in the hepatocyte nuclear factor-4α gene in maturity-onset diabetes of the young (MODY 1). Nature 1996;384:458. (With these two reports identifying genetic mutations among nuclear transcription factors expressed in pancreatic B cells, the gene defects in all three known MODY syndromes have now been detected.)

Yamashita S et al: Insulin resistance and body fat distribution: Contribution of visceral fat accumulation to the development of insulin resistance and atherosclerosis. Diabetes Care 1996;19:287. (Using CT scans, the ratio of visceral fat area to subcutaneous fat area [V/S ratio] was used to define certain obese patients with the "visceral fat syndrome." This highly atherogenic state includes visceral fat accumulation, glucose intolerance [insulin resistance], hyperlipidemia, and hypertension.)

Therapy of Diabetes Mellitus

[Diet and exercise in NIDDM]
  gopher://gopher.nih.gov/00/clin/cdcs/individual/60. diabet

American Diabetes Association: Nutrition recommendations and principles for people with diabetes mellitus. (Position statement.) Diabetes Care 1997;20 (Suppl):S14. (Major changes in nutritional therapy of diabetes include the elimination of "ADA diet prescriptions," allowing freer substitution of sucrose in the meals and recommending tailored prescriptions for each diabetic patient based on individual goals.)

Anderson JH Jr et al: Reduction of postprandial hyperglycemia and frequency of hypoglycemia in IDDM patients on insulin-analog treatment. Diabetes 1997;46:265. (This multinational and multicenter randomized clinical trial in 1008 patients with IDDM documents that insulin lispro improves postprandial glycemic control, reduces hypoglycemic episodes, and improves patient convenience as compared with regular insulin.)

Burge MR, Castillo KR, Schade DS: Meal composition is a determinant of lispro-induced hypoglycemia in IDDM. Diabetes Care 1997;20:152. (When meals are relatively low in carbohydrate content, insulin lispro, because of its ultra-rapid absorption, predisposes to early postprandial hypoglycemia much more so than does regular insulin. The authors caution patients and their health care providers about this potential hazard of insulin lispro therapy.)

Colwell JA: The feasibility of intensive insulin management in non-insulin-dependent diabetes mellitus: Implications of the Veterans Affairs Cooperative Study on Glycemic Control and Complications in NIDDM. Ann Intern Med 1996;124(1 Part 2):131. (This preliminary study at five VAMCs in 153 NIDDM men in whom standard pharmacologic therapy had failed raised concern that intensive insulin therapy over 27 months was accompanied by more major cardiovascular events than did standard insulin therapy. Because of the small sample size and the relatively short duration of the study, the authors feel that a longer expanded trial is needed before this unexpected conclusion can be accepted.)

Coniff RF et al: Reduction of glycosylated hemoglobin and postprandial hyperglycemia by acarbose in patients with NIDDM. Diabetes Care 1995;18:817. (Acarbose, a complex oligosaccharide that inhibits digestion of ingested starch and most disaccharides, was moderately effective in lowering hemoglobin A_{1c} levels by 0.5–1% in a group of patients with NIDDM.)

Cryer PE, Fisher JN, Shamoon H: Hypoglycemia. Diabetes Care 1994;17:734. (The focus of this review is clinical hypoglycemia in insulin-treated diabetic patients. It describes syndromes of compromised glucose counterregulation and measures to prevent or reverse them when they are caused by frequent episodes of hypoglycemia.)

Davidson MB, Peters AL: An overview of metformin in the treatment of type II diabetes mellitus. Am J Med 1997;102:99. (A clinical review emphasizing the efficacy of metformin in patients with type II diabetes and its safety if avoided in those with contraindications to its use.)

DCCT Research Group: The effect of intensive treatment of diabetes on the development and progression of long-term complications in insulin-dependent diabetes mellitus. N Engl J Med 1993;329:977. (This 10-year randomized trial of 1441 IDDM patients in 29 centers, documented that intensive therapy was superior to conventional treatment in preventing or delaying the progress of chronic diabetic complications.)

DCCT Research Group: Hypoglycemia in the diabetes control and complications trial. Diabetes 1997; 46:271. (This report emphasizes the threefold higher risk of severe hypoglycemia among type I diabetic patients receiving intensive insulin therapy and analyzes the factors that were the strongest predictors of the risk of future episodes of hypoglycemia in these patients.)

Fanelli C et al: Long-term recovery from unawareness, deficient counterregulation and lack of cognitive dysfunction during hypoglycaemia, following institution of rational, intensive insulin therapy in IDDM. Diabetologia 1994;37:1265. (An important study in 21 IDDM patients whose hypoglycemic unawareness was reversed by meticulous attention to preventing hypoglycemia despite near-normal glycemic control for 1 year.)

Goldberg RB et al: A dose-response study of glimepiride in patients with NIDDM who have previously received sulfonylurea agents. Diabetes Care 1996;19:849. (A multicenter trial in 304 NIDDM patients which demonstrated that single daily doses of 4 or 8 mg of glimepiride, a newly approved sulfonylurea, were effective and well tolerated.)

Karam JH: Reversible insulin resistance in non-insulin-dependent diabetes mellitus. Horm Metab Res 1996;28:440. (This review focuses on mechanisms whereby glucotoxicity and lipotoxicity induce insulin resistance and discusses therapeutic measures to reverse these acquired factors in patients with type II diabetes.)

Saltiel AR, Olefsky JM: Thiazolidinediones in the treatment of insulin resistance and type II diabetes. Diabetes 1996;45:1661. (Troglitazone, an insulin enhancer, lowers coronary risk factors such as hyperglycemia, hypertriglyceridemia, and hyperinsulinemia in insulin-resistant NIDDM patients without causing weight gain or drug-induced hypoglycemia.)

Chronic Complications of Diabetes Mellitus

Caputo GM et al: Assessment and management of foot disease in patients with diabetes. N Engl J Med 1994;331:854. (The authors review the pathogenesis of diabetic foot disorders and provide practical suggestions for their prevention and treatment. They outline a comprehensive approach which they feel will meet the United States Department of Health goals of a 40% reduction in amputation rates in diabetic patients by the year 2000.)

Clark CM, Lee DA: Drug therapy: Prevention and treatment of the complications of diabetes mellitus. N Engl J Med 1995;332:1210. (A comprehensive review of medications available for the chronic complications of diabetes, including peripheral and autonomic neuropathy, retinopathy, and nephropathy.)

Davis MD: Diabetic retinopathy. Diabetes Care 1992; 15:1884. (This excellent clinical overview describes the pathogenesis and epidemiology of diabetic retinopathy and its current treatment.)

Pfeifer MA, Schumer MP: Clinical trials of diabetic neuropathy: Past, present and future. Diabetes 1995; 44:1355. (Current pharmacotherapy for diabetic neuropathy is unsuccessful in convincingly alleviating symptoms or leading to recovery of established neuropathy. Glycemic control remains the best method of slowing progression of diabetic neuropathy.)

Sowers JR, Epstein M: Diabetes mellitus and associated hypertension, vascular disease and nephropathy: An update. Hypertension 1995;26(Part 1):869. (This comprehensive review outlines current concepts of the pathogenesis of progressive diabetic nephropathy and details new and promising pharmacologic interventions that specifically address these pathophysiologic mechanisms.)

DIABETIC COMA

Coma may be due to a variety of causes not directly related to diabetes. Certain causes directly related to diabetes require differentiation: (1) Hypoglycemic coma resulting from excessive doses of insulin or oral hypoglycemic agents. (2) Hyperglycemic coma associated with either severe insulin deficiency (diabetic ketoacidosis) or mild to moderate insulin deficiency (hyperglycemic nonketotic hyperosmolar coma). (3) Lactic acidosis associated with diabetes, particularly in diabetics stricken with severe infections or with cardiovascular collapse.

DIABETIC KETOACIDOSIS

Essentials of Diagnosis

- Hyperglycemia > 250 mg/dL.
- Acidosis with blood pH < 7.3.
- Serum bicarbonate < 15 meq/L.
- Serum positive for ketones.

General Considerations

Diabetic ketoacidosis may be the initial manifestation of type I diabetes or may result from increased insulin requirements in type I diabetes patients during the course of infection, trauma, myocardial infarction, or surgery. It is a life-threatening medical emergency with a mortality rate just under 5%. Type II diabetics may develop ketoacidosis under severe stress such as sepsis. Recently, diabetic ketoacidosis has been found to be one of the more common serious complications of insulin pump therapy, occurring in approximately one per 80 patient-months of treatment. Many patients who monitor capillary blood glucose regularly ignore urine ketone measurements, which would signal the possibility of insulin leakage or pump failure before serious illness develops. Poor compliance is one of the most common causes of diabetic ketoacidosis, particularly when episodes are recurrent.

Clinical Findings

A. Symptoms and Signs: The appearance of diabetic ketoacidotic coma is usually preceded by a day or more of polyuria and polydipsia associated with marked fatigue, nausea and vomiting, and, finally, mental stupor that can progress to coma. On physical examination, evidence of dehydration in a stuporous patient with rapid deep breathing and a "fruity" breath odor of acetone would strongly suggest the diagnosis. Hypotension with tachycardia indicates profound fluid and electrolyte depletion, and mild hypothermia is usually present. Abdominal pain and even tenderness may be present in the absence of abdominal disease. Conversely, cholecystitis or pancreatitis may occur with minimal symptoms and signs.

B. Laboratory Findings: (Table 27–12.) Glycosuria of 4+ and strong ketonuria with hyperglycemia, ketonemia, low arterial blood pH, and low plasma bicarbonate are typical of diabetic ketoacidosis. Serum potassium is often elevated despite total body potassium depletion resulting from protracted polyuria or vomiting. Elevation of serum amylase is common but often represents salivary as well as pancreatic amylase. Thus, in this setting, serum amylase is not a good marker for acute pancreatitis. Azotemia may be a better indicator of renal status than serum creatinine, since multichannel chemical analysis of serum creatinine (SMA-6) is falsely elevated by nonspecific chromogenicity of keto acids and glucose. Most laboratories can correct for these interfering substances on request, and newer analyzers are being introduced that routinely eliminate this interference. Leukocytosis as high as 25,000/μL with a left shift may occur with or without associated infection. The presence of an elevated or even a normal temperature would suggest the presence of an infection, since patients with diabetic ketoacidosis are generally hypothermic if uninfected.

Complications

The two major metabolic aberrations of diabetic ketoacidosis are hyperglycemia and ketoacidemia, both due to insulin lack associated with hyperglucagonemia.

A. Hyperglycemia: Hyperglycemia results from increased hepatic production of glucose as well as diminished glucose uptake by peripheral tissues. Hepatic glucose output is a consequence of increased gluconeogenesis resulting from insulinopenia as well

Table 27–12. Laboratory diagnosis of coma in diabetic patients.

	Urine		Plasma		
	Glucose	**Acetone**	**Glucose**	**Bicarbonate**	**Acetone**
Related to diabetes					
Hypoglycemia	0[1]	0 or +	Low	Normal	0
Diabetic ketoacidosis	++++	++++	High	Low	++++
Nonketotic hyperglycemic coma	++++	0	High	Normal or slightly low	0
Lactic acidosis	0 or +	0 or +	Normal or low or high	Low	0 or +
Unrelated to diabetes					
Alcohol or other toxic drugs	0 or +	0 or +	May be low	Normal or low[2]	0 or +
Cerebrovascular accident or head trauma	+ or 0	0	Often high	Normal	0
Uremia	0 or +	0	High or normal	Low	0 or +

[1]Leftover urine in bladder might still contain glucose from earlier hyperglycemia.
[2]Alcohol can elevate plasma lactate as well as keto acids to reduce pH.

as from an associated hyperglucagonemia. When serum hyperosmolality exceeds 320–330 mosm/L, central nervous system depression or coma may ensue. Coma in a diabetic patient with a lower osmolality should prompt a search for cause of coma other than hyperosmolality.

B. Ketoacidemia: Ketoacidemia represents the effect of insulin lack at multiple enzyme loci. Insulin lack associated with elevated levels of growth hormone and glucagon contributes to an increase in lipolysis from adipose tissue and in hepatic ketogenesis. In addition, there is evidence that reduced ketolysis by insulin-deficient peripheral tissues contributes to the ketoacidemia. The only true "keto" acid present is acetoacetic acid, which, along with its by-product acetone, is measured by nitroprusside reagents (Acetest and Ketostix). The sensitivity for acetone, however, is poor, requiring over 10 mmol, which is seldom reached in the plasma of ketoacidotic subjects—although this detectable concentration is readily achieved in urine. Thus, in the plasma of ketotic patients, only acetoacetate is measured by these reagents. The more prevalent β-hydroxybutyric acid has no ketone group and is therefore not detected by conventional nitroprusside tests. This takes on special importance in the presence of circulatory collapse during diabetic ketoacidosis, wherein an increase in lactic acid can shift the redox state to increase β-hydroxybutyric acid at the expense of the readily detectable acetoacetic acid. Bedside diagnostic reagents would then be unreliable, suggesting no ketonemia in cases where β-hydroxybutyric acid is a major factor in producing the acidosis.

Treatment

A. Prevention: Education of diabetic patients to recognize the early symptoms and signs of ketoacidosis has done a great deal to prevent severe acidosis. Urine ketones should be measured in patients with signs of infection or in insulin pump-treated patients when capillary blood glucose is unexpectedly and persistently high. When heavy ketonuria and glycosuria persist on several successive examinations, supplemental regular insulin should be administered and liquid foods such as lightly salted tomato juice and broth should be ingested to replenish fluids and electrolytes. The patient should be instructed to contact the physician if ketonuria persists, and especially if vomiting develops or if appropriate adjustment of the infusion rate on an insulin pump does not correct the hyperglycemia and ketonuria. In juvenile-onset diabetics, particularly in the teen years, recurrent episodes of severe ketoacidosis often indicate poor compliance with the insulin regimen, and these patients will require intensive family counseling.

B. Emergency Measures: If ketosis is severe, the patient should be placed in the hospital for correction of the hyperosmolality as well as the ketoacidemia. An intensive care unit or, at the least, a step-down unit is preferable for more severe cases.

1. Therapeutic flow sheet—One of the most important steps in initiating therapy is to start a flow sheet listing vital signs and the time sequence of diagnostic laboratory values in relation to therapeutic maneuvers. Indices of the metabolic defects include urine glucose and ketones as well as arterial pH, plasma glucose, acetone, bicarbonate, serum urea nitrogen, and electrolytes. Serum osmolality should be measured or estimated and tabulated during the course of therapy.

A convenient method of estimating *effective* serum osmolality is as follows (normal values in humans are 280–300 mosm/L):

$$mosm/L = 2 [Na^+ (meq/L) + K^+ (meq/L)] + \frac{Glucose (mg/dL)}{18}$$

These calculated estimates are usually 10–20 mosm/L lower than values measured by standard cryoscopic techniques in patients with diabetic coma. While urea exerts an effect on freezing point depression as measured in the laboratory, it is freely permeable across cell membranes and therefore not included in calculations of effective serum osmolality. One physician should be responsible for maintaining this therapeutic flow sheet and prescribing therapy. An indwelling urinary catheter is required in all comatose patients but should be avoided if possible in a fully cooperative diabetic because of the risk of introducing bladder infection. Fluid intake and output should be recorded. Gastric intubation is recommended in the comatose patient to correct the commonly associated gastric dilatation that may lead to vomiting and aspiration. The patient should not receive sedatives or narcotics.

2. Insulin replacement—Only regular insulin should be used initially in all cases of severe ketoacidosis, and it should be given immediately after the diagnosis is established. Regular insulin can be given in a loading dose of 0.1 unit/kg as an intravenous bolus followed by 0.1 unit/kg/h, continuously infused or given hourly as an intramuscular injection; this is sufficient to replace the insulin deficit in most patients. Replacement of insulin deficiency helps correct the acidosis by reducing the flux of fatty acids to the liver, reducing ketone production by the liver, and also improving removal of ketones from the blood. Insulin treatment reduces the hyperosmolality by reducing the hyperglycemia. It accomplishes this by increasing removal of glucose through peripheral utilization as well as by decreasing production of glucose by the liver. This latter effect is accomplished by direct inhibition of gluconeogenesis and glycogenolysis, as well as by lowered amino acid flux from muscle to liver and reduced hyperglucagonemia.

The insulin dose should be "piggy-backed" into the fluid line so the rate of fluid replacement can be changed without altering the insulin delivery rate. For optimal effects, continuous low-dose insulin infusions should always be preceded by a rapid intravenous loading dose of regular insulin, 0.1 unit/kg, to prime the tissue insulin receptors. If the plasma glucose level fails to fall at least 10% in the first hour, a repeat loading dose is recommended. The availability of bedside glucometers and of laboratory instruments for rapid and accurate glucose analysis (Beckman or Yellow Springs glucose analyzer) has contributed much to achieving optimal insulin replacement. Rarely, a patient with immune insulin resistance is encountered, and this requires doubling the insulin dose every 2–4 hours if hyperglycemia does not improve after the first two doses of insulin.

3. Fluid and electrolyte replacement–In most patients, the fluid deficit is 4–5 L. Initially, 0.9% saline solution is the solution of choice to help reexpand the contracted vascular volume and should be started in the emergency room as soon as the diagnosis is established. The use of sodium bicarbonate has been questioned since clinical benefit was not demonstrated in one prospective randomized trial and because of the following potentially harmful consequences: (1) hypokalemia from rapid potassium shifts into cells; (2) tissue anoxia from reduced dissociation of oxygen from hemoglobin when acidosis is rapidly reversed; (3) cerebral acidosis resulting from a reduction of cerebrospinal fluid pH; and (4) a worsening of hyperosmolality. However, these concerns are relatively less important in certain clinical settings, and 1–2 ampules of sodium bicarbonate (44 meq per 50 mL ampule) added to a bottle of *hypotonic* saline solution may be administered whenever the blood pH is 7.0 or less or blood bicarbonate is below 9 meq/L. Once the pH reaches 7.1, no further bicarbonate should be given, since it aggravates rebound metabolic alkalosis as ketones are metabolized. Alkalosis causes potassium shifts that increase the risk of cardiac arrhythmias. In the first hour, at least 1 L of 0.9% saline should be infused, and fluid should be given thereafter at a rate of 300–500 mL/h with careful monitoring of serum potassium. If the blood glucose is above 500 mg/dL, 0.45% saline solution may be used after the first hour, since the water deficit exceeds the sodium loss in uncontrolled diabetes with osmotic diuresis. Failure to give enough volume replacement (at least 3–4 L in 8 hours) to restore normal perfusion is one of the most serious therapeutic shortcomings affecting satisfactory recovery. Likewise, excessive fluid replacement (more than 5 L in 8 hours) may contribute to acute respiratory distress syndrome or cerebral edema. When blood glucose falls to 250 mg/dL or less, 5% glucose solutions should be used to maintain blood glucose between 200 and 300 mg/dL while insulin therapy is continued in order to clear the ketonemia. Glucose administration has the dual advantage of preventing hypoglycemia and furthermore of reducing the likelihood of cerebral edema, which could result from too rapid a decline in hyperglycemia.

During therapy, hyperchloremic acidosis develops because of the considerable loss of keto acids in the urine during the initial phase of treatment. A portion of the bicarbonate deficit is replaced with chloride ions infused in large amounts as saline to correct the dehydration. Thus, in most patients, as the ketoacidosis clears during insulin replacement, they show a hyperchloremic, low bicarbonate pattern with a normal anion gap. This is a relatively benign condition that reverses itself over the subsequent 12–24 hours once intravenous saline is no longer being administered.

4. Potassium and phosphate replacement– Total body potassium loss from polyuria as well as from vomiting may be as high as several hundred milliequivalents. However, because of shifts from cells due to the acidosis, serum potassium is usually normal or high until after the first few hours of treatment, when acidosis improves and serum potassium returns into cells. Potassium in doses of 20–30 meq/h should be infused within 2–3 hours after beginning therapy, or sooner if initial serum potassium is inappropriately low. Potassium replacement should be deferred if serum potassium fails to respond to initial therapy and remains above 5 meq/L, as in cases of renal insufficiency. An ECG can be of help in monitoring the patient and reflecting the state of potassium balance at the time, but it should not replace accurate laboratory measurements.

Foods high in potassium content can be prescribed when the patient has recovered sufficiently to take food orally. (Tomato juice and grapefruit juice contain 14 meq of potassium per 240 mL and a medium-sized banana 10 meq.) See Chapter 21 for potassium content of foods.

Phosphate replacement is seldom required in treating diabetic ketoacidosis. However, if severe hypophosphatemia of less than 0.35 mmol/L (< 1 mg/dL) develops during insulin therapy, a small amount of phosphate can be replaced as the potassium salt. Hypophosphatemia of this severity is detrimental to membranes of skeletal muscle and may lyse red blood cells. The potassium need is several times that of phosphate and should be replaced separately, since replacing phosphorus ions too rapidly (while meeting potassium requirements) can precipitate serum calcium in the tissues and induce tetany.

A significant therapeutic benefit of routine phosphate replacement has not been documented in several randomized trials. However, certain potential advantages have been suggested. Treatment of hypophosphatemia helps to restore the buffering capacity of the plasma, thereby facilitating renal excretion of hydrogen; and it corrects the impaired oxygen dissociation from hemoglobin by regenerating 2,3-diphosphoglycerate. To minimize the risk of inducing tetany from an overload of phosphate replacement, an average deficit of 40–50 mmol phosphate in adults with diabetic ketoacidosis should be replaced by intravenous infusion *at a rate not to exceed 3 mmol/h.*

A stock solution available from Abbott Laboratories provides a mixture of 1.12 g KH_2PO_4 and 1.18 g K_2HPO_4 in a 5 mL single-dose vial representing 22 meq potassium and 15 mmol phosphate (27 meq). Five milliliters of this stock solution in 2 L of either 0.45% saline or 5% dextrose in water, infused at 400 mL/h, will replace the phosphate at the optimal rate of 3 mmol/h and will provide 4.4 meq of potassium per hour. If serum phosphate remains below 0.35 mmol/L (1 mg/dL), a repeat 5-hour infusion of potassium phosphate at a rate of 3 mmol/h would be reasonable.

5. Treatment of associated infection–Antibiotics are prescribed as indicated. Cholecystitis and pyelonephritis may be particularly severe in these patients.

Prognosis

The frequency of deaths due to diabetic ketoacidosis has been dramatically reduced by improved therapy of young diabetics, but this complication remains a significant risk in the aged and in patients in profound coma in whom treatment has been delayed. Acute myocardial infarction and infarction of the bowel following prolonged hypotension worsen the outlook. A serious prognostic sign is renal failure, and prior kidney dysfunction worsens the prognosis considerably because the kidney plays a key role in compensating for massive pH and electrolyte abnormalities. Cerebral edema has been reported to occur rarely as metabolic deficits return to normal. This is best prevented by avoiding sudden reversal of marked hyperglycemia. Maintaining glycemic levels of 200–300 mg/dL for the initial 24 hours after correction of severe hyperglycemia reduces this risk.

Fleckman AM: Diabetic ketoacidosis. Endocrinol Metab Clin North Am 1993;22:181. (A lucid description of the pathogenesis of diabetic ketoacidosis and a well-documented review of therapy, including a useful section on treatment during the recovery period in the hospital and after discharge.)

Okuda Y et al: Counterproductive effects of sodium bicarbonate in diabetic ketoacidosis. J Clin Endocrinol Metab 1996;81:314. (Sodium bicarbonate administration in patients with diabetic ketoacidosis increases ketonemia and delays its correction by insulin.)

Umpierrez GE, Khajavi M, Kitabchi AE: Review: diabetic ketoacidosis and hyperglycemic hyperosmolar nonketotic syndrome. Am J Med Sci 1996;311:225. (The pathophysiology and therapy of both of these hyperglycemic emergencies are reviewed in an authoritative

manner based on extensive clinical experience and participation in numerous clinical trials in this area. Controversial issues are discussed and a concise management protocol is presented.)

NONKETOTIC HYPERGLYCEMIC HYPEROSMOLAR COMA

Essentials of Diagnosis

- Hyperglycemia > 600 mg/dL.
- Serum osmolality > 310 mosm/kg.
- No acidosis; blood pH above 7.3.
- Serum bicarbonate > 15 meq/L.
- Normal anion gap (< 14 meq/L).

General Considerations

This second most common form of hyperglycemic coma is characterized by severe hyperglycemia in the absence of significant ketosis, with hyperosmolality and dehydration. It occurs in patients with mild or occult diabetes, and most patients are at least middle-aged to elderly. Lethargy and confusion develop as serum osmolality exceeds 310 mosm/kg, and coma can occur if osmolality exceeds 320–330 mosm/kg. Underlying renal insufficiency or congestive heart failure is common, and the presence of either worsens the prognosis. A precipitating event such as infection, myocardial infarction, stroke, or recent operation is often present. Certain drugs such as phenytoin, diazoxide, glucocorticoids, and diuretics have been implicated in its pathogenesis, as have procedures associated with glucose loading such as peritoneal dialysis.

Pathogenesis

A partial or relative insulin deficiency may initiate the syndrome by reducing glucose utilization of muscle, fat, and liver while inducing hyperglucagonemia and increasing hepatic glucose output. With massive glycosuria, obligatory water loss ensues. If a patient is unable to maintain adequate fluid intake because of an associated acute or chronic illness or has suffered excessive fluid loss, marked dehydration results. As plasma volume contracts, renal insufficiency develops, and the resultant limitation of renal glucose loss leads to increasingly higher blood glucose concentrations. Severe hyperosmolality develops that causes mental confusion and finally coma. It is not clear why ketosis is virtually absent under these conditions of insulin insufficiency, although reduced levels of growth hormone may be a factor, along with portal vein insulin concentrations sufficient to restrain ketogenesis.

Clinical Findings

A. Symptoms and Signs: Onset may be insidious over a period of days or weeks, with weakness, polyuria, and polydipsia. The lack of features of ketoacidosis may retard recognition of the syndrome and delay therapy until dehydration becomes more profound than in ketoacidosis. Reduced intake of fluid is not an uncommon historical feature, due to either inappropriate lack of thirst, nausea, or inaccessibility of fluids to elderly, bedridden patients. Lethargy and confusion develop, progressing to convulsions and deep coma. Physical examination confirms the presence of profound dehydration in a lethargic or comatose patient without Kussmaul respirations.

B. Laboratory Findings: Severe hyperglycemia is present, with blood glucose values ranging from 600 to 2400 mg/dL. In mild cases, where dehydration is less severe, dilutional hyponatremia as well as urinary sodium losses may reduce serum sodium to 120–125 meq/L, which protects to some extent against extreme hyperosmolality. However, as dehydration progresses, serum sodium can exceed 140 meq/L, producing serum osmolality readings of 330–440 mosm/kg. Ketosis and acidosis are usually absent or mild. Prerenal azotemia is the rule, with serum urea nitrogen elevations over 100 mg/dL being typical.

Treatment

A. Saline: Fluid replacement is of paramount importance in treating nonketotic hyperglycemic coma. The onset of hyperosmolarity is more insidious in elderly people without ketosis than in younger individuals with high serum ketone levels, which provide earlier indicators of severe illness (vomiting, rapid deep breathing, acetone odor, etc). Consequently, diagnosis and treatment are often delayed until fluid deficit has reached levels of 6–10 L.

If hypovolemia is present, fluid therapy should be initiated with isotonic saline. In all other cases, hypotonic (0.45%) saline appears to be preferable as the initial replacement solution because the body fluids of these patients are markedly hyperosmolar. As much as 4–6 L of fluid may be required in the first 8–10 hours. Careful monitoring of the patient is required for proper sodium and water replacement. Once blood glucose reaches 250 mg/dL, fluid replacement should include 5% dextrose in either water, 0.45% saline solution, or 0.9% saline solution. The rate of dextrose infusion should be adjusted to maintain glycemic levels of 250–300 mg/dL in order to reduce the risk of cerebral edema. An important end point of fluid therapy is to restore urine output to 50 mL/h or more.

B. Insulin: Less insulin may be required to reduce the hyperglycemia in nonketotic patients as compared to those with diabetic ketoacidotic coma. In fact, fluid replacement alone can reduce hyperglycemia considerably by correcting the hypovolemia, which then increases both glomerular filtration and renal excretion of glucose. An initial dose of only 15 units intravenously and 15 units subcutaneously of regular insulin is usually quite effective, and in most cases subsequent doses need not be greater than 10–20 units subcutaneously every 4 hours.

C. Potassium: With the absence of acidosis, there may be no initial hyperkalemia unless associated renal failure is present. This results in less severe total potassium depletion than in diabetic ketoacidosis, and less potassium replacement is therefore needed. However, because initial serum potassium is usually not elevated and because it declines rapidly as a result of insulin's effect on driving potassium intracellularly, it has been recommended that potassium replacement be initiated earlier than in ketotic patients, assuming that no renal insufficiency or oliguria is present. Potassium chloride (10 meq/L) can be added to the initial bottle of fluids administered if the patient's serum potassium is not elevated.

D. Phosphate: If severe hypophosphatemia (serum phosphate < 1 mg/dL [< 0.35 mmol/L]) develops during insulin therapy, phosphate replacement can be given as described for ketoacidotic patients (at 3 mmol/h).

Prognosis

The overall mortality rate of hyperglycemic, hyperosmolar, nonketotic coma is more than ten times that of diabetic ketoacidosis, chiefly because of its higher incidence in older patients, who may have compromised cardiovascular systems or associated major illnesses and whose dehydration is often excessive because of delays in recognition and treatment. (When patients are matched for age, the prognoses of these two hyperglycemic emergencies are reasonably comparable.) When prompt therapy is instituted, the mortality rate can be reduced from nearly 50% to that related to the severity of coexistent disorders.

Ennis ED, Stahl EJ, Kreisberg RA: The hyperosmolar hyperglycemic syndrome. Diabetes Reviews 1994;2:115. (An update relating to pathogenesis, and recommended therapy.)

Lorber D: Nonketotic hypertonicity in diabetes mellitus. Med Clin North Am 1995;79:39. (A review of clinical presentation, pathogenesis, and management of this disorder, with useful suggestions on education of patients and their caregivers regarding its prevention.)

LACTIC ACIDOSIS (See also Metformin & Other Biguanides.)

Essentials of Diagnosis

- Severe acidosis with hyperventilation.
- Blood pH below 7.30.
- Serum bicarbonate < 15 meq/L.
- Anion gap > 15 meq/L.
- Absent serum ketones.
- Serum lactate > 5 mmol/L.

General Considerations

Lactic acidosis is characterized by accumulation of excess lactic acid in the blood. Normally, the principal sources of this acid are the erythrocytes (which lack enzymes for aerobic oxidation), skeletal muscle, skin, and brain. Conversion of lactic acid to glucose and its oxidation principally by the liver but also by the kidneys represent the chief pathways for its removal. Overproduction of lactic acid (tissue hypoxia), deficient removal (hepatic failure), or both (circulatory collapse) can cause accumulation. Lactic acidosis is not uncommon in any severely ill patient suffering from cardiac decompensation, respiratory or hepatic failure, septicemia, or infarction of bowel or extremities. With the discontinuance of phenformin therapy in the USA, lactic acidosis in patients with diabetes mellitus has become uncommon but occasionally occurs in metformin-treated patients and it still must be considered in the acidotic diabetic, especially if the patient is seriously ill.

Clinical Findings

A. Symptoms and Signs: The main clinical feature of lactic acidosis is marked hyperventilation. When lactic acidosis is secondary to tissue hypoxia or vascular collapse, the clinical presentation is variable, being that of the prevailing catastrophic illness. However, in the idiopathic, or spontaneous, variety, the onset is rapid (usually over a few hours), blood pressure is normal, peripheral circulation is good, and there is no cyanosis.

B. Laboratory Findings: Plasma bicarbonate and blood pH are quite low, indicating the presence of severe metabolic acidosis. Ketones are usually absent from plasma and urine or at least not prominent. The first clue may be a high anion gap (serum sodium minus the sum of chloride and bicarbonate anions [in meq/L] should be no greater than 15). A higher value indicates the existence of an abnormal compartment of anions. If this cannot be clinically explained by an excess of keto acids (diabetes), inorganic acids (uremia), or anions from drug overdosage (salicylates, methyl alcohol, ethylene glycol), then lactic acidosis is probably the correct diagnosis. (See Chapter 21 also.) In the absence of azotemia, hyperphosphatemia may be a clue to the presence of lactic acidosis. The diagnosis is confirmed by demonstrating, in a sample of blood that is promptly chilled and separated, a plasma lactic acid concentration of 5 mmol/L or higher (values as high as 30 mmol/L have been reported). Normal plasma values average 1 mmol/L, with a normal lactate/pyruvate ratio of 10:1. This ratio is greatly exceeded in lactic acidosis.*

---

*In collecting samples, it is essential to rapidly chill and separate the blood in order to remove red cells, whose continued glycolysis at room temperature is a common source of error in reports of high plasma lactate. Frozen plasma remains stable for subsequent assay.

Treatment

Aggressive treatment of the precipitating cause of lactic acidosis is the main component of therapy. Empiric antibiotic coverage for sepsis should be given after culture samples are obtained in any patient in whom the cause of the lactic acidosis is not apparent.

Alkalinization with intravenous sodium bicarbonate to keep the pH above 7.2 has been recommended in the emergency treatment of severe lactic acidosis. Massive doses may be required (as much as 2000 meq in 24 hours has been used); however, there is no evidence that the mortality rate is favorably affected by administering bicarbonate, and the matter is at present controversial. Hemodialysis may be useful in cases where large sodium loads are poorly tolerated. Dichloroacetate, an anion that facilitates pyruvate removal by activating pyruvate dehydrogenase, reverses certain types of lactic acidosis in animals but is of no clinical utility in humans. In a prospective controlled clinical trial involving 252 cases of lactic acidosis, dichloroacetate failed to alter either hemodynamics or survival, despite its proved effectiveness in lowering lactate levels and raising arterial pH significantly.

Prognosis

The mortality rate of spontaneous lactic acidosis approaches 80%. The prognosis in most cases is that of the primary disorder that produced the lactic acidosis.

Cohen RD: Lactic acidosis: New perspectives on origins and treatment. Diabetes Reviews 1994;2:86. (A review of the controversy regarding whether or not bicarbonate therapy is beneficial or detrimental in the management of metabolic acidosis.)

Lalau JD et al: Role of metformin accumulation in metformin-associated lactic acidosis. Diabetes Care 1995;18:779. (In 14 NIDDM patients with metformin-associated lactic acidosis, five had very high levels of plasma metformin, five had moderately high levels, and four had no accumulation of metformin. While accumulation of metformin was the most common association, severe lactic acidosis occurs with normal levels in the face of severe sepsis, cardiac failure, or hepatic failure.)

Stacpoole PW et al: Natural history and course of acquired lactic acidosis in adults. Am J Med 1994;97:47. (A placebo-controlled randomized clinical trial of intravenous dichloroacetate in 252 patients with lactic acidosis. This therapy failed to alter either hemodynamics or survival.)

THE HYPOGLYCEMIC STATES

Spontaneous hypoglycemia in adults is of two principal types: fasting and postprandial. Fasting hypoglycemia is often subacute or chronic and usually presents with neuroglycopenia as its principal manifestation; postprandial hypoglycemia is relatively acute and is often heralded by symptoms of neurogenic autonomic discharge (sweating, palpitations, anxiety, tremulousness).

Differential Diagnosis (Table 27–13)

Fasting hypoglycemia may occur in certain endocrine disorders, such as hypopituitarism, Addison's disease, or myxedema; in disorders related to liver malfunction, such as acute alcoholism or liver failure; and in instances of renal failure, particularly in patients requiring dialysis. These conditions are usually obvious, with hypoglycemia being only a secondary feature. When fasting hypoglycemia is a primary manifestation developing in adults without apparent endocrine disorders or inborn metabolic diseases from childhood, the principal diagnostic possibilities include (1) hyperinsulinism, due to either pancreatic B cell tumors or surreptitious administration of insulin (or sulfonylureas); and (2) hypoglycemia due to non-insulin-producing extrapancreatic tumors.

Postprandial (reactive) hypoglycemia may be classified as early (within 2–3 hours after a meal) or late (3–5 hours after eating). Early, or alimentary, hypoglycemia occurs when there is a rapid discharge of ingested carbohydrate into the small bowel followed by rapid glucose absorption and hyperinsulinism. It may be seen after gastrointestinal surgery and is particularly associated with the dumping syndrome after gastrectomy. In some cases, it is functional and may represent overactivity of the parasympathetic nervous system mediated via the vagus nerve. Rarely, it results from defective counterregulatory responses such as deficiencies of growth hormone, glucagon, cortisol, or autonomic responses.

Alcohol-related hypoglycemia is due to hepatic glycogen depletion combined with alcohol-mediated inhibition of gluconeogenesis. It is most common in malnourished alcohol abusers but can occur in anyone who is unable to ingest food after an acute alcoholic episode followed by gastritis and vomiting. At presentation, blood ethanol may be below levels usually associated with legal standards relating to being "under the influence."

Immunopathologic hypoglycemia is an extremely rare condition in which anti-insulin antibodies or antibodies to insulin receptors develop spontaneously. In the former case, the mechanism is unclear, but it may relate to increasing dissociation of insulin from circulating pools of bound insulin. When antibodies to insulin receptors are found, most patients do not have hypoglycemia but rather severe insulin-resistant diabetes and acanthosis nigricans. However, during the course of the disease in these patients, certain anti-insulin receptor antibodies with agonist activity mimicking insulin action may develop, producing severe hypoglycemia.

Factitious hypoglycemia is self-induced hypoglycemia due to surreptitious administration of insulin or sulfonylureas.

HYPOGLYCEMIA DUE TO PANCREATIC B CELL TUMORS

Fasting hypoglycemia in an otherwise healthy, well-nourished adult is rare, and is most commonly due to an adenoma of the islets of Langerhans. Ninety percent of such tumors are single and benign, but multiple adenomas can occur as well as malignant tumors with functional metastases. B cell hyperplasia as a cause of fasting hypoglycemia is rare and not well documented in adults. Adenomas may be familial, and multiple adenomas have been found in conjunction with tumors of the parathyroids and pituitary (Wermer's syndrome; multiple endocrine neoplasia type I).

Clinical Findings

A. Symptoms and Signs: The symptoms and signs are those of subacute or chronic hypoglycemia, which may progress to permanent and irreversible brain damage. Delayed diagnosis has often resulted in prolonged psychiatric care or treatment for psychomotor epilepsy before the true diagnosis was established. In long-standing cases, obesity can result as a consequence of overeating to relieve symptoms.

Whipple's triad is characteristic of hypoglycemia regardless of the cause. It consists of (1) a history of hypoglycemic symptoms, (2) an associated fasting blood glucose of 40 mg/dL or less, and (3) immedi-

Table 27–13. Common causes of hypoglycemia.[1]

Fasting hypoglycemia
  Hyperinsulinism
    Pancreatic B cell tumor
    Surreptitious administration of insulin or sulfonylureas
    Extrapancreatic tumors
Postprandial (reactive) hypoglycemia
  Early hypoglycemia (alimentary)
Postgastrectomy
Functional (increased vagal tone)
  Late hypoglycemia (occult diabetes)
Delayed insulin release due to B cell dysfunction
  Counterregulatory deficiency
  Idiopathic
Alcohol-related hypoglycemia
Immunopathologic hypoglycemia
  Idiopathic anti-insulin antibodies (which release their
    bound insulin)
  Antibodies to insulin receptors (which act as agonists)
Pentamidine-induced hypoglycemia

[1]In the absence of clinically obvious endocrine, renal, or hepatic disorders and exclusive of diabetes treated with hypoglycemic agents.

ate recovery upon administration of glucose. The hypoglycemic symptoms in insulinoma often develop in the early morning or after missing a meal. Occasionally, they occur after exercise. They typically begin with evidence of central nervous system glucose lack and can include blurred vision or diplopia, headache, feelings of detachment, slurred speech, and weakness. Personality and mental changes vary from anxiety to psychotic behavior, and neurologic deterioration can result in convulsions or coma. Sweating and palpitations may not occur.

Hypoglycemic unawareness is very common in patients with insulinoma. They adapt to chronic hypoglycemia by increasing their efficiency in transporting glucose across the blood-brain barrier. Counterregulatory hormonal responses as well as neurogenic symptoms such as tremor, sweating, and palpitations are therefore blunted during hypoglycemia. However, symptoms and normal hormone responses during experimental insulin-induced hypoglycemia have been shown to be restored after successful surgical removal of the insulinoma. Presumably with return of euglycemia, adaptive effects on glucose transport into the brain are corrected and thresholds of counterregulatory responses and neurogenic autonomic symptoms are therefore restored to normal.

B. Laboratory Findings: B cell adenomas do not reduce secretion in the presence of hypoglycemia, and the critical diagnostic test is to demonstrate inappropriately elevated serum insulin levels at a time when hypoglycemia is present. A reliable serum insulin level of 8 µU/mL or more in the presence of blood glucose values below 40 mg/dL is diagnostic of inappropriate hyperinsulinism. Other causes of hyperinsulinemic hypoglycemia must be considered, including factitious administration of insulin or sulfonylureas. An elevated circulating proinsulin level is characteristic of most B cell adenomas and does not occur in factitious hyperinsulinism.

C. Diagnostic Tests:

1. Prolonged fasting under hospital supervision until hypoglycemia is documented is probably the most dependable means of establishing the diagnosis, especially in men. In patients with insulinoma, the blood glucose levels often drop below 40 mg/dL after an overnight fast. In normal male subjects, the blood glucose does not fall below 55–60 mg/dL during a 3-day fast. In contrast, in premenopausal women who have fasted for only 24 hours, the plasma glucose may fall normally to such an extent that it can reach values as low as 35 mg/dL. After 36 hours of fasting, premenopausal normal women occasionally achieve such low levels of glucose that clinical evaluation of this test for insulinoma becomes quite difficult. In these cases, however, the women are not symptomatic, presumably owing to the development of sufficient ketonemia to supply energy needs to the brain. Insulinoma patients, on the other hand, become symptomatic when plasma glucose drops to subnormal levels, since inappropriate insulin secretion restricts ketone formation. Moreover, the demonstration of a nonsuppressed insulin level (≥ 8 µU/mL) in the presence of hypoglycemia and of an *increasing* ratio of insulin to glucose (ie, glucose falls more rapidly than does insulin) suggests the diagnosis of insulinoma, since normal females show a falling insulin-to-glucose ratio during a fast. If hypoglycemia does not develop in a male patient after fasting for up to 72 hours—and particularly when this prolonged fast is terminated with a period of moderate exercise—insulinoma must be considered an unlikely diagnosis.

2. Proinsulin determinations–In contrast to normal subjects, whose proinsulin concentration is less than 20% of the total immunoreactive insulin, patients with insulinoma have elevated levels of proinsulin representing 30–90% of total immunoreactive insulin.

3. Stimulation tests with pancreatic B cell secretagogues such as tolbutamide, glucagon, or leucine are generally not needed in most cases if basal insulin is found to be nonsuppressible and therefore inappropriately elevated during fasting hypoglycemia. However, in occasional patients with a relatively fixed level of circulating insulin that is only barely inappropriate, stimulation may be helpful, bearing in mind that false-negative results can occur if the tumor is poorly differentiated and agranular.

Intravenous glucagon (1 mg over 1 minute) can be useful in patients with "borderline" fasting inappropriate hyperinsulinism. A serum insulin rise above baseline of 200 µU/mL or more at 5 and 10 minutes strongly suggests insulinoma, although poorly differentiated tumors may not respond. Glucagon has the advantage over tolbutamide of correcting rather than provoking hypoglycemia during stimulation testing and is diagnostic in 60–70% of patients with insulinoma.

D. Preoperative Localization of B Cell Tumors: Pancreatic arteriography has been disappointing, with an accuracy rate of only 20% and a false-positive rate of about 5%. A promising modification correlates imaging from selective arteriography of segments of the pancreas with simultaneous hepatic vein sampling for insulin during a bolus of intra-arterial calcium delivered selectively to these same pancreatic segments. Calcium has been found to be a secretagogue only for insulinomas and not for normal islet tissue, so that a rise in hepatic insulin concentration indicates segmental localization of the insulinomas. CT scan and standard MRI are not helpful in the preoperative localization of insulinoma because they do not distinguish small tumors within the pancreas. A kinetic MRI with multiple images during contrast injection offers the best current preoperative localization method, and intraoperative ultrasound should be available at the time of surgery as a means of localizing small tumors within the pancreas not palpable at laparotomy.

Percutaneous transhepatic pancreatic vein catheterization with insulin assay is also useful for localizing small insulinomas; it is particularly helpful when multiple insulinomas are suspected, as in patients with coexisting pituitary or parathyroid adenomas. However, this technique is not widely available and is associated with considerable discomfort.

Treatment

A. Surgical Measures: Resection by a surgeon with experience in removing islet cell tumors is the treatment of choice. Diazoxide, 300–400 mg/d orally, inhibits insulin release from tumors and is useful in the interval prior to surgery for prevention of hypoglycemic episodes. Hydrochlorothiazide, 25–50 mg daily, should also be prescribed to counteract the edema and hyperkalemia secondary to diazoxide therapy as well as to potentiate its hyperglycemic effect. However, because effective doses are tolerated poorly over the long term—particularly because of its tendency to produce hirsutism in women—diazoxide is not considered a desirable alternative to surgical excision. Blood glucose should be monitored throughout surgery, and 10% dextrose in water should be infused at a rate of 100 mL/h or faster. In cases where the diagnosis has been established but no adenoma is located after careful palpation and use of intraoperative ultrasound, subtotal pancreatectomy is usually indicated, including the entire body and tail of the pancreas. Total pancreatectomy is seldom required now in view of the efficacy of long-term medical therapy with diazoxide in most patients with insulinomas.

B. Diet and Medical Therapy: In patients with inoperable functioning islet cell carcinoma or in patients in whom subtotal removal of the pancreas has failed to produce cure, reliance on frequent feedings is necessary. Since most tumors are not responsive to glucose, carbohydrate feedings every 2–3 hours are usually effective in preventing hypoglycemia, although obesity may become a problem. Glucagon should be available for emergency use as indicated in the discussion of treatment of diabetes. Diazoxide, 300–600 mg daily orally, has been useful with concomitant thiazide diuretic therapy to control sodium retention. When patients are unable to tolerate diazoxide because of gastrointestinal upset, hirsutism, or edema, the calcium channel blocker verapamil may be beneficial in view of its inhibitory effect on insulin release from insulinoma cells. Octreotide, a potent long-acting synthetic octapeptide analog of somatostatin, has been used to inhibit release of hormones from a number of endocrine tumors, including inoperable insulinomas. When hypoglycemia persists after attempted surgical removal of the insulinoma and if diazoxide or verapamil is poorly tolerated or ineffective, a trial of 50 µg of octreotide acetate injected subcutaneously twice daily may control the hypoglycemic episodes in conjunction with multiple small feedings. Streptozocin is useful in decreasing insulin secretion in islet cell carcinomas, and effective doses have been achieved without the undue renal toxicity that characterized early experience.

Prognosis

When insulinoma is diagnosed early and cured surgically, complete recovery is likely, although brain damage following severe hypoglycemia is not reversible. A significant increase in survival rate has been shown in streptozocin-treated patients with islet cell carcinoma, with reduction in tumor mass as well as decreased hyperinsulinism.

Perry RR, Vinik AI: Diagnosis and management of functioning islet cell tumors. J Clin Endocrin Metab 1995; 80:2273. (Practical recommendations for the diagnosis and management of insulinomas by authors with considerable clinical experience.)

vanHeerden JA et al: Occult functioning insulinomas: which localizing studies are indicated? Surgery 1992; 112:1010. (In the extensive experience of surgeons at the Mayo Clinic, extensive preoperative radiologic investigation was neither indicated nor cost-effective. Intraoperative palpation in conjunction with an available ultrasound transducer was successful in locating 20 of 20 cases of insulinoma whose anatomic site was indeterminate preoperatively.)

HYPOGLYCEMIA DUE TO EXTRAPANCREATIC TUMORS

These rare causes of hypoglycemia include mesenchymal tumors such as retroperitoneal sarcomas, hepatocellular carcinomas, adrenocortical carcinomas, and miscellaneous epithelial type tumors. The tumors are frequently large and readily palpated or visualized on CT scans or MRI.

Laboratory diagnosis depends upon fasting hypoglycemia associated with serum insulin levels that are generally below 8 µU/mL. The mechanism of these tumors' hypoglycemic effect remains obscure. Although they do not release immunoreactive insulin, it has been suggested that they may produce certain insulin-like substances similar to the somatomedins or growth factors that may bind to the insulin receptor. A high-molecular-weight form of IGF-II has recently been implicated as a cause of hypoglycemia in patients with hepatocellular tumors.

The prognosis for these tumors is generally poor, and surgical removal should be attempted when feasible. Dietary management of the hypoglycemia is the mainstay of medical treatment, since diazoxide is usually ineffective.

Chung J, Henry RR: Mechanisms of tumor-induced hypoglycemia with intraabdominal hemangiopericytoma. J Clin Endocrinol Metab 1996;81:919. (An abnormal insulin-like growth factor-2 [IGF-2], with a high molecular weight, appears to explain many, but not all, cases of hypoglycemia secondary to extrapancreatic tumors.)

POSTPRANDIAL HYPOGLYCEMIA
(Reactive Hypoglycemia)

Postgastrectomy Alimentary Hypoglycemia

Reactive hypoglycemia following gastrectomy is a consequence of hyperinsulinism resulting from rapid gastric emptying of ingested food. Symptoms result from adrenergic hyperactivity in response to the hypoglycemia. Treatment consists of more frequent feedings with smaller portions of less rapidly assimilated carbohydrate and more slowly absorbed fat and protein.

Functional Alimentary Hypoglycemia

This syndrome is classified as functional when no postsurgical explanation exists for the presence of early alimentary type reactive hypoglycemia. It is most often associated with chronic fatigue, anxiety, irritability, weakness, poor concentration, decreased libido, headaches, hunger after meals, and tremulousness. However, most patients with these symptoms do not have hypoglycemia. (See Chronic Fatigue Syndrome in Chapter 1.)

Indiscriminate use and overinterpretation of glucose tolerance tests have led to an unfortunate tendency to overdiagnose functional hypoglycemia. *As many as one-third or more of normal subjects have hypoglycemia reaching nadirs as low as 40–50 mg/dL with or without symptoms during a 4-hour glucose tolerance test.* Accordingly, to increase diagnostic reliability, hypoglycemia should preferably be documented during a spontaneous symptomatic episode accompanying routine daily activity, with clinical improvement following feeding. Oral glucose tolerance tests are overly sensitive and mixed meals are relatively insensitive in detecting postprandial reactive hypoglycemia. Recently it has been shown that a high-carbohydrate breakfast has proved useful in differentiating persons with postprandial reactive hypoglycemia from normal controls. The test resulted in reactive hypoglycemia to levels below 59 mg/dL in 47% of 38 subjects, in contrast to only 2.2% of the 43 controls. This test was found to be much more sensitive than a standard mixed meal, which was also given to these two groups.

In patients with documented postprandial hypoglycemia on a functional basis, there is no harm and occasional benefit in reducing the proportion of carbohydrate in the diet while increasing the frequency and reducing the size of meals. Support and mild sedation should be the mainstays of therapy, with dietary manipulation only an adjunct.

Late Hypoglycemia (Occult Diabetes)

This condition is characterized by a delay in early insulin release from pancreatic B cells, resulting in initial exaggeration of hyperglycemia during a glucose tolerance test. In response to this hyperglycemia, an exaggerated insulin release produces a late hypoglycemia 4–5 hours after ingestion of glucose. These patients are usually quite different from those with early hypoglycemia, often being obese and frequently having a family history of diabetes mellitus.

In obese patients, treatment is directed at weight reduction to achieve ideal weight. Like all patients with postprandial hypoglycemia, regardless of cause, these patients often respond to reduced carbohydrate intake with multiple, spaced, small feedings high in protein. They should be considered potential diabetics and advised to have periodic medical evaluations.

Brun JF et al: Evaluation of a standardized hyperglucidic breakfast test in postprandial reactive hypoglycemia. Diabetologia 1995;38:494. (A high-carbohydrate breakfast was found to differentiate patients referred for symptomatic postprandial hypoglycemia [n = 38] from a control population [n = 43] much better than did a standard mixed meal. Blood glucose levels less than 59 mg/dL were found in 47% of the referred subjects after the hyperglucidic breakfast but in only 2.2% of the controls, implying that this may be a useful test in identifying postprandial reactive hypoglycemia.)

ALCOHOL-RELATED HYPOGLYCEMIA

Fasting Hypoglycemia After Ethanol

During the postabsorptive state, normal plasma glucose is maintained by hepatic glucose output derived from both glycogenolysis and gluconeogenesis. With prolonged starvation, glycogen reserves become depleted within 18–24 hours and hepatic glucose output becomes totally dependent on gluconeogenesis. Under these circumstances, a blood concentration of ethanol as low as 45 mg/dL (considerably below the California legal "under the influence" level for drivers of 80 mg/dL) can induce profound hypoglycemia by blocking gluconeogenesis. Neuroglycopenia in a patient whose breath smells of alcohol may be mistaken for alcoholic stupor. Prevention consists of adequate food intake during ethanol ingestion. Therapy consists of glucose administration to replenish glycogen stores until gluconeogenesis resumes.

Postethanol Reactive Hypoglycemia

When sugar-containing soft drinks are used as mixers to dilute alcohol in beverages (gin and tonic, rum and cola), there seems to be a greater insulin release than when the soft drink alone is ingested and a tendency for more of a late hypoglycemic overswing to occur 3–4 hours later. Prevention would consist of avoiding sugar mixers while ingesting alcohol and ensuring supplementary food intake to provide sustained absorption.

FACTITIOUS HYPOGLYCEMIA

Factitious hypoglycemia may be difficult to document. A suspicion of self-induced hypoglycemia is supported when the patient is associated with the health professions or has access to insulin or sulfonylurea drugs taken by a diabetic member of the family. The triad of hypoglycemia, high immunoreactive insulin, and suppressed plasma C peptide immunoreactivity is pathognomonic of exogenous insulin administration. Demonstration of circulating antibodies supports this diagnosis in suspected cases. When sulfonylureas are suspected as a cause of factitious hypoglycemia, a chemical test of the plasma to detect the presence of these drugs may be required to distinguish laboratory findings from those of insulinoma.

IMMUNOPATHOLOGIC HYPOGLYCEMIA

This rare cause of hypoglycemia, documented in isolated case reports, may occur as two distinct disorders: one associated with spontaneous development of circulating anti-insulin antibodies and another associated with antibodies to insulin receptors, in which the antibodies apparently have agonist capabilities. This latter disorder is extremely rare, having been documented in no more than five cases. However, development of anti-insulin antibodies has been reported in over 200 patients most of whom were being treated with methimazole for thyrotoxicosis. Occasional case reports in the United States include patients with a lupus-like syndrome or with various paraproteinemias.

Uchigata Y et al: Insulin autoimmune syndrome (Hirata disease): Clinical features and epidemiology in Japan. Diabetes Res Clin Prac 1994;22:89. (Over 200 cases have been reported with spontaneous hypoglycemia associated with circulating antibodies to insulin. Most cases were reported from Japan and were associated with administration of sulfhydryl drugs such as methimazole for Graves' disease. The syndrome is transient and responds to withdrawal of sulfhydryl drugs.)

PENTAMIDINE-INDUCED HYPOGLYCEMIA

With the increased prevalence of pulmonary infection by *Pneumocystis carinii* in patients with acquired immune deficiency syndrome, pentamidine given intravenously or by aerosol is being used more frequently and in 10–20% of patients produces symptomatic hypoglycemia. This apparently is due to lytic destruction of pancreatic B cells, causing acute hyperinsulinemia and hypoglycemia, followed later by insulinopenia and hyperglycemia that occasionally is persistent. Intravenous glucose should be administered during pentamidine administration and for the period immediately following to prevent or ameliorate hypoglycemic symptoms. Following a complete course of therapy with pentamidine, fasting blood glucose or a subsequent glycohemoglobin should be monitored to assess the extent of pancreatic B cell recovery or residual damage.

Assan R et al: Pentamidine-induced derangements of glucose homeostasis: Determinant roles of renal failure and drug accumulation—a study of 128 patients. Diabetes Care 1995;18:47. (Hypoglycemia associated with elevated insulin levels in plasma occurred in 25 of 128 pentamidine-treated patients due to pancreatic B cell toxicity. Drug accumulation due to excessive doses or renal impairment is the determining risk factor.)

Polansky KS: A practical approach to fasting hypoglycemia. N Engl J Med 1992;326:1020. (A succinct overview of the diagnostic criteria and clinical management of fasting hypoglycemia in adults.)

Service FJ: Hypoglycemia. Med Clin North Am 1995;79:1. (Reviews the endocrine emergency of hypoglycemia—its clinical presentation, acute treatment, and potential sequelae.)

28

Lipid Abnormalities

Robert B. Baron, MD, MS, & Warren S. Browner, MD, MPH

Lipid abnormalities are of importance to the clinician primarily because of their relation to atherosclerotic vascular disease, especially coronary heart disease. Clinical trials showing that lowering high blood cholesterol reduces the incidence of coronary heart disease have given impetus to nationwide campaigns to reduce serum cholesterol levels. For patients with known cardiovascular disease (secondary prevention), there are clear benefits from cholesterol lowering, including a reduction in total mortality in both men and women and in both middle-aged patients and older patients. Among patients without cardiovascular disease (primary prevention), however, there is more controversy about the overall benefit of aggressive cholesterol lowering. Although one study from Scotland suggests a beneficial effect on both heart disease mortality and total mortality in middle-aged men, the effects of cholesterol lowering on total mortality in women, young men, and the elderly are less clear. Nonetheless, several treatment algorithms have been developed to assist clinicians in selecting patients for this intervention.

LIPIDS & LIPOPROTEINS

The two main lipids in blood are cholesterol and triglyceride. They are carried in lipoproteins, which are globular packages that also contain proteins known as apoproteins. Cholesterol is an essential element of all animal cell membranes and forms the backbone of steroid hormones and bile acids; triglycerides are important in transferring energy from food into cells. Why lipids are deposited into the walls of large and medium-sized arteries—an event with potentially lethal consequences—is not known.

Lipoproteins are usually classified on the basis of how dense they are. Density is determined by the amounts of triglyceride (which makes them less dense) and apoproteins (which have the opposite effect). The least dense particles, known as chylomicrons, are normally found in the blood only after fat-containing foods have been eaten. Chylomicrons rise as a creamy layer when nonfasting serum is allowed

to stand. The other lipoproteins are suspended in serum and must be separated using a centrifuge. The densest (and smallest) family of particles consists mainly of apoproteins and cholesterol and are called high-density lipoproteins (HDL). Somewhat less dense are the low-density lipoproteins (LDL). Least dense are the large, very-low-density lipoproteins (VLDL), consisting mainly of triglyceride. In fasting serum, most of the cholesterol is carried on LDL particles and is therefore referred to as LDL cholesterol; most of the triglyceride is found in VLDL particles. Specific apoproteins are associated with each lipoprotein class.

Chylomicrons are made in the gut and travel via the portal vein into the liver and via the thoracic duct into the circulation. They are normally completely metabolized, transferring energy from food into muscle and fat cells. The liver manufactures VLDL particles from its own stores of fat and carbohydrate. VLDL particles transfer triglyceride to cells; after losing enough, they eventually become LDL particles, which provide cholesterol for cellular needs. Excess LDL particles are taken up by the liver, and the cholesterol they contain is then excreted into the bile. HDL particles are made in the liver and intestine and appear to facilitate the transfer of apoproteins among lipoproteins. They also participate in reverse cholesterol transport, either by transferring cholesterol into other lipoproteins or directly into the liver.

LIPOPROTEINS & ATHEROGENESIS

The plaques found in the arterial walls of patients with atherosclerosis contain large amounts of cholesterol, providing an early clue that serum cholesterol might be an important factor in their development. Epidemiologic studies have clearly established that the higher the level of LDL cholesterol, the greater the risk of atherosclerotic heart disease; conversely, the higher the level of HDL cholesterol, the lower the risk of coronary heart disease. This is true in men and women, in different racial and ethnic groups, and at all adult ages. Because most cholesterol in serum is LDL cholesterol, high total cholesterol levels are also associated with an increased risk of coronary heart disease. Middle-aged men whose serum cholesterol levels are in the highest quintile for age (above about 230 mg/dL) have a risk of coronary death before age 65 of about 11%; men in the lowest quintile (below about 170 mg/dL) have a 3% risk. Death from coronary heart disease before age 65 is less common in women, with equivalent risks about one-third those of men. As a general approximation in men, each 10 mg/dL increase in cholesterol (or LDL cholesterol) increases the risk of coronary heart disease by about 10%; each 5 mg/dL increase in HDL reduces the risk by about 10%. The effect of HDL cholesterol is greater in women, whereas the effects of total and LDL cholesterol are smaller. All of these relationships tend to diminish with age.

The exact mechanism by which LDL particles result in the formation of atherosclerotic plaques—or the means whereby HDL particles protect against their formation—is not known. The simple model of LDL carrying cholesterol into the walls of arteries, with HDL removing it, is more useful as a mnemonic than as a representation of what is known. Recent work suggests that LDL particles which have become oxidized (a process that occurs naturally) may be particularly atherogenic. Receptors on the surface of macrophages within atherosclerotic plaques bind and accumulate oxidized LDL. The formation of antibodies to oxidized LDL may also be important in plaque formation. Thus, there is growing interest in the role of antioxidants, such as vitamins C and E and beta-carotene, in the prevention and treatment of atherosclerotic disease. The size of the LDL molecule itself may also influence its atherogenesis; at the same LDL concentrations, those persons with large numbers of smaller particles appear to be at higher risk for coronary heart disease.

The relationship of VLDL cholesterol to atherogenesis is less certain. Perhaps the number, or size, or subtype of VLDL particles—rather than the total amount in serum—is important. In addition, HDL and VLDL levels are inversely related. Patients with a high VLDL level are likely to have a low HDL level and thus be at increased risk for coronary heart disease for that reason alone.

There are several genetic disorders that provide insight into the pathogenesis of lipid-related diseases. Most important—but fortunately rare in the homozygous state (about one per million)—is a condition in which the cell-surface receptors for the LDL molecule are absent or defective. This disorder is also known as **familial hypercholesterolemia.** These patients have reduced ability to metabolize LDL particles, resulting in high LDL levels and premature atherosclerosis. Patients with two abnormal genes (homozygotes) have extremely high LDL levels—up to eight times normal—and may present with athero-

sclerotic disease in childhood. Homozygotes may require liver transplantation to correct their severe lipid abnormalities. Those with one defective gene (heterozygotes) have LDL concentrations that are approximately twice normal; persons with this condition often present with coronary heart disease in their 30s or 40s.

Another rare condition is characterized by an abnormality of lipoprotein lipase, the enzyme that enables peripheral tissues (muscle and adipose cells, for example) to take up triglyceride from chylomicrons and VLDL particles. Patients with this condition (which is one of the causes of **familial hyperchylomicronemia**) have a marked increase in triglyceride concentrations and usually present with recurrent pancreatitis and hepatosplenomegaly in childhood.

There are several other genetic abnormalities of lipid metabolism, usually named for the abnormality that appears when serum is electrophoresed (eg, **dysbetalipoproteinemia**) or from the particular combinations of lipid abnormalities that appear in families (eg, **familial combined hyperlipidemia**). These entities are important to the clinician because they emphasize the need to screen family members of patients with severe lipid disorders. Some of these patients have abnormalities in the production of various apoproteins, such as increased levels of apoprotein B and its affiliated lipoproteins, LDL and VLDL, or reduced production of apoprotein AII and its affiliated particle, HDL.

Havel RJ, Rapaport E: Management of primary hyperlipidemia. N Engl J Med 1995;332:1491.

Levine GN, Keaney JF Jr, Vita JA: Cholesterol reduction in cardiovascular disease: Clinical benefits and possible mechanisms. N Engl J Med 1995;332:512.

NCEP Adult Treatment Panel II: Summary of the Second Report of the National Cholesterol Education Program Expert Panel on detection, evaluation, and treatment of high blood cholesterol in adults. JAMA 1993;269:3015.

Schwartz C et al: A modern view of atherogenesis. Am J Cardiol 1993;71:9B. (Role of oxidized LDL particles.)

Treasure CB et al: Beneficial effects of cholesterol-lowering therapy on the coronary endothelium in patients with coronary artery disease. N Engl J Med 1995;332:481.

LIPID FRACTIONS & THE RISK OF CORONARY HEART DISEASE

In fasting serum, cholesterol is carried primarily on three different lipoproteins—the VLDL, LDL, and HDL molecules. Total cholesterol equals the sum of these three components:

Total cholesterol = HDL cholesterol +

VLDL cholesterol + LDL cholesterol

Most clinical laboratories measure the total cholesterol, the total triglycerides, and the amount of cholesterol found in the HDL fraction, which is easily precipitated from serum. The vast majority of triglyceride is found in VLDL particles, which contain about five times as much triglyceride by weight as cholesterol. Thus, the amount of cholesterol found in the VLDL fraction can be estimated by dividing the triglyceride by 5:

$$\text{VLDL cholesterol} = \frac{\text{Triglycerides}}{5}$$

Because the triglyceride level is used as a proxy for the amount of VLDL, this formula only works in fasting samples. Furthermore, it only works when the triglyceride level is less than 400–500 mg/dL. At higher triglyceride levels (as is the case when serum appears lipemic), LDL and VLDL cholesterol levels can be determined after ultracentrifugation.

The total cholesterol is reasonably stable over time; however, measurements of HDL and especially triglycerides may vary considerably because of analytic error in the laboratory and because of biologic variation in a patient's triglyceride level. Thus, the LDL should always be estimated as the mean of at least two determinations; if those two estimates differ by more than 10%, a third lipid profile should be obtained. It is estimated as follows:

$$\text{LDL cholesterol} = \text{Total cholesterol} - \text{HDL cholesterol} - \frac{\text{Triglycerides}}{5}$$

When using SI units (which measure lipids by moles rather than weight), the formula becomes:

$$\text{LDL cholesterol} = \text{Total cholesterol (mmol/L)} - \text{HDL cholesterol (mmol/L)} - \frac{\text{Triglycerides (mmol/L)}}{2.2}$$

Understanding the relationships of the different lipid fractions leads to a more sophisticated and clinically accurate understanding of a patient's lipid-related coronary risk than simply knowing the total cholesterol level. Two persons with the same total cholesterol of 275 mg/dL may have very different lipid profiles. One may have an HDL cholesterol of 110 mg/dL with a triglyceride of 150 mg/dL, with an estimated LDL cholesterol of 135 mg/dL; the other may have an HDL cholesterol of 25 mg/dL with a triglyceride of 200 mg/dL and an LDL cholesterol of 210 mg/dL. All other risk factors being equal, the second patient would have more than a tenfold higher coronary heart disease risk than the first. Because high HDL cholesterol levels are common in

women, many women with apparently high total cholesterol levels actually have favorable lipid profiles. Thus, evaluation of the lipid fractions is essential before therapy for high blood cholesterol in individual patients is initiated.

Some authorities use the ratio of the total cholesterol to HDL cholesterol as an indicator of lipid-related coronary risk: the lower this ratio is, the better. (In the example from the previous paragraph, the first person would have a ratio of $275 \div 110 = 2.5$, while the second would have a much less favorable ratio of $275 \div 25 = 11$.) While intuitively convenient as a summary measure, the ratio may obscure potentially important information (a total cholesterol of 300 mg/dL and an HDL of 60 mg/dL results in the same ratio of 5 as a total cholesterol of 150 mg/dL with an HDL of 30 mg/dL). Moreover, errors in the measurement of HDL cholesterol are common in many laboratories, and the total cholesterol-to-HDL cholesterol ratio magnifies their importance.

There is no "normal" range for serum lipids. In Western populations, cholesterol values are about 20% higher than in Asian populations and exceed 300 mg/dL in nearly 5% of adults. About 10% of adults have LDL cholesterol levels above 200 mg/dL. In general, total and LDL cholesterol levels rise with age.

Declines in cholesterol levels are seen when a patient is acutely ill. Thus, it is rarely appropriate to measure lipid levels in an ill or hospitalized patient, with the notable exception of the serum triglyceride level in a patient with pancreatitis. Cholesterol levels (even when expressed as an age-matched percentile rank, such as the highest 20%) do not remain constant over time, especially from childhood through adolescence and young adulthood. Thus, children and young adults with relatively high cholesterol levels may have lower levels later in life, whereas those with low cholesterol levels may later have higher levels.

THERAPEUTIC EFFECTS OF LOWERING CHOLESTEROL

Most studies of the effect of cholesterol lowering have distinguished between primary prevention (treating high blood cholesterol in persons free of coronary heart disease) and secondary prevention (treating persons with manifest coronary heart disease). The important distinction is that primary prevention trials enroll healthy subjects who have relatively low rates of coronary disease but in whom other causes of morbidity and mortality are proportionately more common. Secondary prevention trials, on the other hand, follow patients who have a high rate of subsequent coronary disease; other causes of mortality are relatively less important.

Several clinical trials have established that reducing cholesterol levels in healthy middle-aged men without coronary heart disease (primary prevention) reduces their risk and that the reduction in risk is proportionate to the reduction in LDL cholesterol and the increase in HDL cholesterol. Patients in the treatment groups have had statistically significant and clinically important reductions in the rates of myocardial infarctions, new cases of angina, and need for coronary artery bypass procedures. The West of Scotland Study, for example, showed a 31% decrease in myocardial infarctions in middle-aged men treated with pravastatin compared with placebo. As with most primary prevention interventions, however, large numbers of healthy patients need to be treated to prevent a single event; for cholesterol lowering, it may be necessary to treat more than 600 patients for several years to prevent a single coronary death or five or six nonfatal coronary events.

Primary prevention studies have found a less consistent effect on mortality. Although the West of Scotland Study found a 22% decrease in total mortality that was almost statistically significant ($P = 0.051$), pooled results of prior primary prevention studies found a statistically significant *increase* in deaths from cancer (by 43%) and from injuries and violence (by 76%) and a 7% increase (not statistically significant) on total mortality.

In patients—mainly middle-aged men—who already have coronary heart disease, the net benefits of cholesterol lowering are clearer, with reductions in the progression of coronary atherosclerosis, fewer subsequent coronary events, less mortality from coronary heart disease, and a reduction in mortality from all causes. A clinical trial from Scandinavia using simvastatin found a 30% reduction in total mortality (and a 42% reduction in coronary heart disease mortality) in the treated group of men and women with known coronary heart disease. The important exceptions among currently available therapies are the fibric acid derivatives (clofibrate and gemfibrozil), which have not shown benefits in the secondary prevention of coronary heart disease, and probucol, which has not been studied with clinical end points. Several studies have also shown that cholesterol lowering actually causes regression of atherosclerotic plaques in some patients, including women. This effect appears to occur throughout the range of LDL cholesterol levels; the lower the LDL, the greater the regression. Evidence also suggests that cholesterol lowering can slow or even reverse carotid artery atherosclerosis, though no net effect on stroke risk has been shown.

These apparent disparities highlight several important points. The benefits and adverse effects of cholesterol lowering appear to be specific to each type of drug; the clinician cannot assume that the effects will generalize to other classes of medication. Second, the net benefits from cholesterol lowering depend upon the underlying risk of coronary heart disease and of

other disease. In patients with manifest atherosclerosis, morbidity and mortality rates associated with coronary heart disease are high, and measures that reduce coronary heart disease are more likely to be beneficial even if they have no effect—or even slightly harmful effects—on other diseases. Third, we do not know the full effects of cholesterol lowering in women and among older and younger men.

Cummings P, Psaty BM: The association between cholesterol and death from injury. Ann Intern Med 1994; 120:848. (Meta-analysis of primary prevention studies.)

Gaziano JM, Hebert PR, Hennekens CH: Cholesterol reduction: Weighing the benefits and risks. Ann Intern Med 1996;124:914. (Balanced review.)

Hebert P, Gaziano J, Hennekens C: An overview of trials of cholesterol lowering and risk of stroke. Arch Intern Med 1995;155:50. (No net benefit seen.)

Pedersen TR: Lowering cholesterol with drugs and diet. (Editorial.) N Engl J Med 1995;333:1350.

Scandinavian Simvastatin Survival Study Group: Randomized trial of cholesterol lowering in 4444 patients with coronary heart disease: the Scandinavian Simvastatin Survival Study (4S). Lancet 1994;344:1383. (Reductions in total and coronary heart disease mortality.)

Shepherd J et al: Prevention of coronary heart disease with pravastatin in men with hypercholesterolemia. West of Scotland Coronary Prevention Study Group. N Engl J Med 1995;333:1301. (First study to show a reduction in total mortality in the primary prevention setting.)

LOW CHOLESTEROL & OTHER DISEASES

While high cholesterol levels are clearly associated with an increased risk of coronary heart disease, low cholesterol levels (especially < 160 mg/dL) are associated with an increased risk of mortality from other causes, including cancer, respiratory disease, injuries and accidents, and liver disease. The biologic explanation for this excess mortality is not known, though it may be confined to certain subgroups (eg, smokers). Some studies have suggested that low cholesterol represents a preclinical manifestation of the underlying disease, eg, an undiagnosed malignancy. Other analyses have found that the increase in risk persists for at least several years. Thus, the net effect of the overall relationship between cholesterol and mortality is somewhat U-shaped, with mortality rates being highest in those with either low or high cholesterol levels.

Iribarren C et al: Serum total cholesterol and mortality. Confounding factors and risk modification in Japanese-American men. JAMA 1995;273:1926. (Suggests that U-shaped curve is seen only in men who smoke, drink, or have hypertension. The relationship between cholesterol and mortality is flat in other men.)

Law MR et al: Assessing possible hazards of reducing serum cholesterol. BMJ 1994;308:373. (One of three articles plus an editorial in this issue concluding that potential hazards are outweighed by benefits.)

SECONDARY CONDITIONS THAT AFFECT LIPID METABOLISM

Several factors, including drugs, can influence serum lipids (Table 28–1). These are of importance for two reasons: abnormal lipid levels (or changes in lipid levels) may be the presenting sign of some of these conditions, and correction of the underlying condition may obviate the need to treat an apparent lipid disorder. Diabetes and alcohol use, in particular, are commonly associated with high triglyceride levels that decline with improvements in glycemic control or reduction in alcohol use, respectively. Thus, secondary causes of high blood lipids should be considered in each patient with a lipid disorder before lipid-lowering therapy is started. In most instances, special testing is not needed: a history and physical

Table 28–1. Secondary causes of lipid abnormalities.

Cause	Associated Lipid Abnormality
Obesity	Increased triglycerides, decreased HDL cholesterol
Sedentary lifestyle	Decreased HDL cholesterol
Diabetes mellitus	Increased triglycerides, increased total cholesterol
Alcohol use	Increased triglycerides, increased HDL cholesterol
Hypothyroidism	Increased total cholesterol
Hyperthyroidism	Decreased total cholesterol
Nephrotic syndrome	Increased total cholesterol
Chronic renal insufficiency	Increased total cholesterol, increased triglycerides
Hepatic disease (cirrhosis)	Decreased total cholesterol
Obstructive liver disease	Increased total cholesterol
Malignancy	Decreased total cholesterol
Cushing's disease (or steroid use)	Increased total cholesterol
Oral contraceptives	Increased triglycerides, increased total cholesterol
Diuretics[1]	Increased total cholesterol, increased triglycerides
Beta-blockers[1,2]	Increased total cholesterol, decreased HDL

[1]Short-term effects only
[2]Beta-blockers with intrinsic sympathomimetic activity, such as pindolol and acebutolol, do not affect lipid levels.

examination are sufficient. One study, however, found that screening for hypothyroidism in patients with hyperlipidemia is cost-effective.

CLINICAL PRESENTATIONS

Most patients with high cholesterol levels have no specific symptoms or signs. The vast majority of patients with lipid abnormalities are detected by the laboratory, either as part of the workup of a patient with cardiovascular disease, as part of a preventive screening strategy, or on a "routine" chemistry panel. Extremely high levels of chylomicrons or VLDL particles (triglyceride level above 1000 mg/dL) result in the formation of **eruptive xanthomas** (red-yellow papules, especially on the buttocks). High LDL levels result in tendinous xanthomas on certain tendons (Achilles, patella, back of the hand). Such xanthomas usually indicate one of the underlying genetic hyperlipidemias. **Lipemia retinalis** (cream-colored blood vessels in the fundus) is seen with extremely high triglyceride levels (above 2000 mg/dL).

SCREENING FOR HIGH BLOOD CHOLESTEROL

All patients with cardiovascular disease—whether manifest (eg, angina, claudication) or asymptomatic (eg, Q waves, femoral bruit)—should be screened for elevated lipids (Figure 28–1); the only exceptions would be patients in whom lipid lowering is not indicated or desirable for other reasons. Patients who already have evidence of atherosclerosis are the group at highest risk of suffering additional manifestations in the near term and thus have the most to gain from reduction of blood lipids. Additional risk reduction measures for atherosclerosis are discussed in Chapter 10; lipid lowering should be just one aspect of a program to reduce the progression and effects of the disease.

Given the high prevalence of underlying lipid abnormalities in patients with cardiovascular disease, a complete lipid profile (total cholesterol, HDL cholesterol, and triglyceride levels) after an overnight fast should be obtained as a screening test. Those whose estimated LDL cholesterol level is high should have at least one repeat measurement. Specific treatments for high LDL cholesterol levels are discussed below. The goal of therapy should be to reduce the LDL cholesterol to below 100 mg/dL. If this goal cannot be reached, the clinician should recognize that any reduction in LDL is better than no reduction. Even treatment of only mildly elevated LDL cholesterol is clinically useful. The Cholesterol and Recurrent Events (CARE) study found that even individuals with "normal" LDL cholesterol levels had a statistically significant 24% reduction in fatal coronary

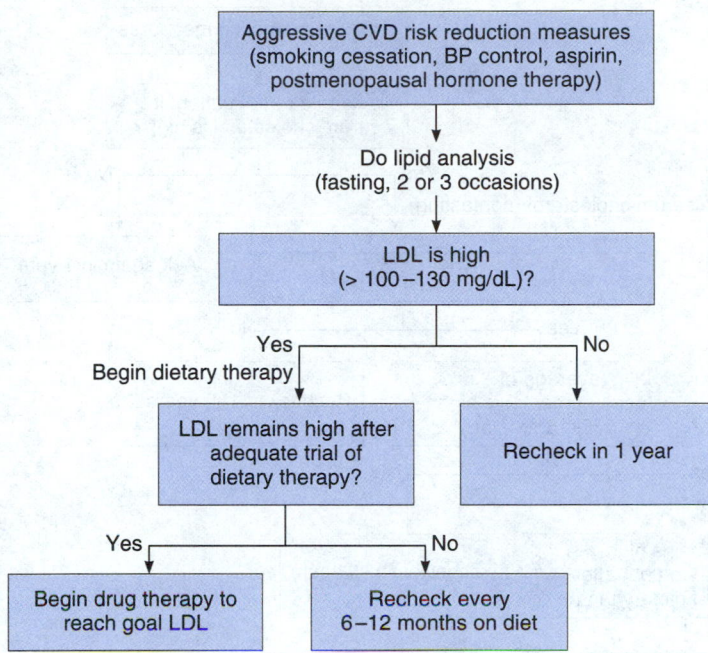

Figure 28–1. Suggested algorithm for screening and management of patients with known cardiovascular disease. Treatment cutpoints and goals discussed in text.

heart disease and recurrent myocardial infarctions when the LDL was lowered to 100 mg/dL.

The best screening and treatment strategy for the remainder of the adult population who do not have atherosclerotic cardiovascular disease is not clear. Several algorithms have been developed to guide the clinician in treatment decisions. Clinicians, however, must individualize management decisions for each patient to determine the potential benefits, risks, costs, and the patient's preferences with respect to cholesterol-lowering therapy.

Although the National Cholesterol Education program (NCEP) continues to recommend screening of all adults aged 20 or older for high blood cholesterol, both the American College of Physicians and the United States Preventive Services Task Force suggest beginning at age 35 in men and age 45 in women unless there is a striking family history or physical findings to suggest a genetic disorder. This strategy focuses cholesterol screening on those at most immediate risk of coronary artery disease and increases the cost effectiveness of cholesterol screening.

Individuals without cardiovascular disease can then be stratified according to risk factors as defined by the NCEP (Figure 28–2). Those with two or more risk factors are considered to be at intermediate risk of coronary artery disease, and those with less than two are at low risk. Risk factors include age and gender (men aged 45 or older, women aged 55 or older); a family history of premature coronary heart disease (myocardial infarction or sudden cardiac death before age 55 in a first-degree male relative or before age 65 in a first-degree female relative); hypertension (whether treated or not); current cigarette smoking (ten or more cigarettes per day); diabetes mellitus (whether treated or not); and low HDL cholesterol (< 35 mg/dL). Because HDL cholesterol is protective against coronary heart disease, a risk factor is subtracted if the level is greater than 60 mg/dL.

Several strategies for obtaining the initial cholesterol measurement have been proposed, including (1) measuring total cholesterol alone, (2) measuring total cholesterol and HDL cholesterol, or (3) measuring only LDL and HDL cholesterol. Each is acceptable as long as all treatment decisions are based on the LDL and HDL cholesterol levels. Measurement of the total cholesterol alone is the least expensive strategy and is adequate for low-risk individuals; those with total cholesterol greater than 200 mg/dL should then be reevaluated with a fasting LDL and HDL cholesterol measurement. Measurement of the total cholesterol and HDL cholesterol allows for better characterization of the risk factor profile but also requires reevaluation if the total cholesterol is greater than 200 mg/dL. Initial measurement of the LDL and HDL cholesterol is least likely to lead to patient misinformation and misclassification and is the strategy preferred by many clinicians.

Treatment decisions are based upon the LDL cholesterol and the patient's risk factor profile (including the HDL cholesterol level). Patients in the intermediate risk group (two or more risk factors) are selected for diet therapy if LDL cholesterol is greater than 130 mg/dL and for drug therapy if it is greater than 160 mg/dL. Low-risk individuals are selected for diet

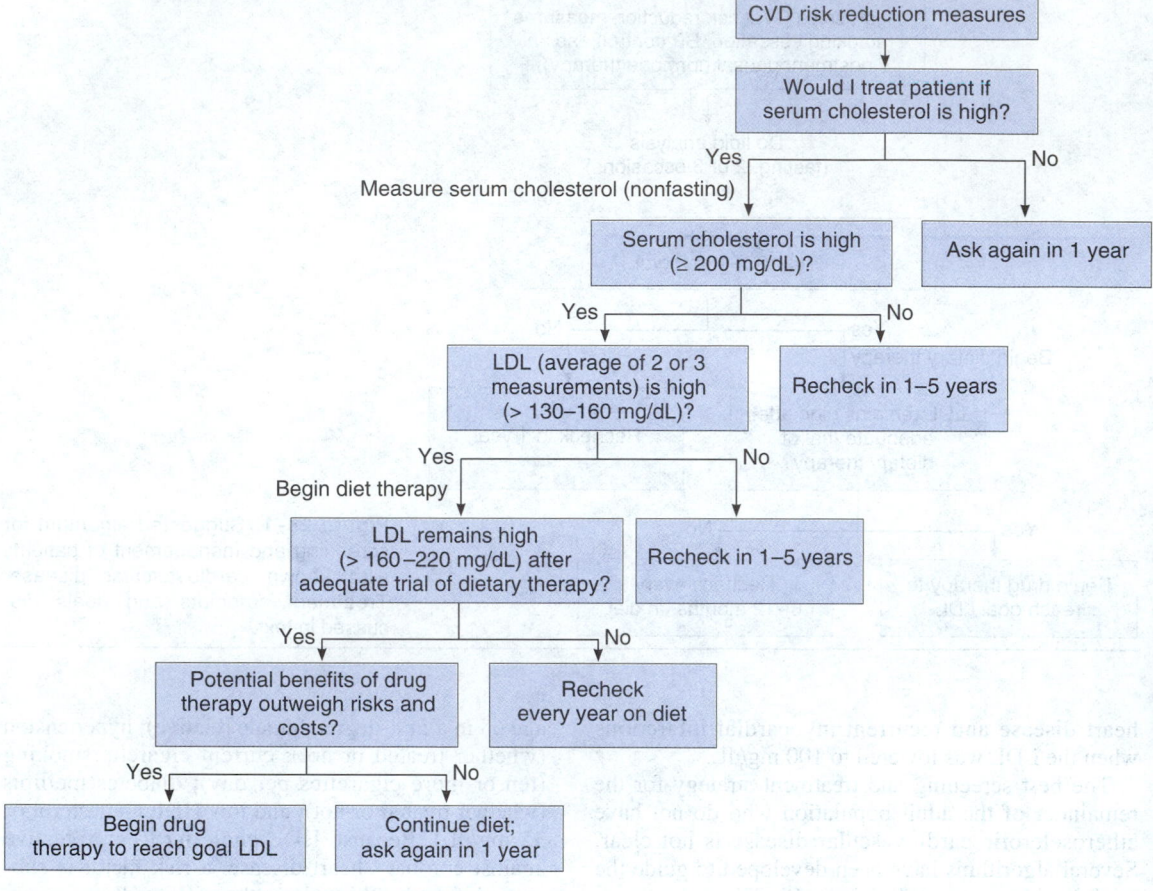

Figure 28–2. Algorithm for screening and management of patients free of cardiovascular disease. Treatment cutpoints, goals, and variations are discussed in the text.

therapy if LDL cholesterol is greater than 160 mg/dL and for drug therapy if it is greater than 190 mg/dL. Young individuals (men under age 35 and women under age 45) require an LDL cholesterol of 220 mg/dL or more before drug therapy is warranted.

Screening in Women

The foregoing screening and treatment guidelines, based largely on LDL cholesterol levels, are designed for both male and female patients. Yet observational studies suggest that HDL cholesterol is a more important risk factor for coronary heart disease in women than a high LDL cholesterol. Meta-analysis of clinical trials that have included women with known heart disease, however, has found that medications that primarily lower LDL cholesterol do prevent recurrent myocardial infarctions in women. There is insufficient clinical trial evidence to be certain of a similar effect from LDL-lowering therapy in women without evidence of coronary heart disease. Although most experts recommend application of the

same NCEP primary prevention guidelines for women as for men, clinicians should be aware of the uncertainty in this area.

Screening in Older Patients

Meta-analysis of observational evidence relating cholesterol to coronary heart disease in the elderly suggests that cholesterol is no longer a risk factor for coronary heart disease for persons over age 75. Clinical trials have rarely included such individuals. Although the NCEP recommends continuing treatment in the elderly, many clinicians will prefer to stop screening and treatment in patients age 75 or older who do not have coronary heart disease. In patients age 75 or older who have coronary heart disease, LDL-lowering therapy can be continued as recommended for younger patients with the disease. Decisions to discontinue therapy should be based on overall functional status and life expectancy, comorbidities, and patient preference and should be made in context with overall therapeutic goals and end-of-life decisions.

American College of Physicians: Guidelines for using serum cholesterol, high-density lipoprotein cholesterol, and triglyceride levels as screening tests for preventing coronary heart disease in adults. Part 1. Ann Intern Med 1996;124:515. (Recommendation to begin screening in men at age 35 and in women at age 45.)

Garber AM, Browner WS, Hulley SB: Cholesterol screening in asymptomatic adults, revisited. Part 2. Ann Intern Med 1996;124:518. (Literature review forming the basis of ACP recommendations.)

Krumholz HM et al: Lack of association between cholesterol and coronary heart disease mortality and morbidity and all-cause mortality in persons older than 70 years. JAMA 1994;272:1335. (Cholesterol is no longer a risk factor after age 75.)

U.S. Preventive Services Task Force: *Guide to Clinical Preventive Services,* 2nd ed. International Medical Publishing, 1996. (Another recommendation to begin screening at age 35 in men and age 45 in women.)

Walsh JM, Grady D: Treatment of hyperlipidemia in women. JAMA 1995;274:1152. (Meta-analysis of clinical trials that include women supports secondary prevention strategies but underscores lack of data for primary prevention.)

TREATMENT OF HIGH LDL CHOLESTEROL

Reduction of LDL cholesterol is just one part of a program to reduce the risk of cardiovascular disease. Other measures—including smoking cessation, hypertension control, chronic aspirin intake, and postmenopausal hormonal replacement therapy—are also of central importance. Less well studied but potentially of great value is raising the HDL cholesterol level. Several "healthy habits" have more than one benefit. Quitting smoking, for example, reduces the effect of other cardiovascular risk factors (such as a high cholesterol level); it may also increase the HDL cholesterol level. Exercise (and weight loss) may reduce the LDL cholesterol level and increase the HDL cholesterol level. Modest alcohol use (1–2 ounces a day) also raises HDL levels and appears to have a salutary effect on coronary heart disease rates. While the clinician may not wish to recommend alcohol use to patients, its safe use in moderation need not be discouraged.

Diet Therapy

Most treatment algorithms recommend diet therapy as the initial step for all patients with high blood cholesterol. Unfortunately, studies of nonhospitalized adults have reported only modest cholesterol-lowering benefits from such therapy, typically in the range of a 5–10% decrease in LDL cholesterol. The results of studies with longer periods of follow-up suggest that the long-term impact of diet therapy is even less. The effect of diet therapy, however, varies considerably among individuals. Although most patients will have a quite modest effect with dietary changes, some patients will have striking reductions in LDL cholesterol—up to a 25–30% decrease—while others will have clinically important increases. Thus, the results of diet therapy should be carefully monitored, typically about 4 weeks after initiation.

Cholesterol-lowering diets may also have a variable effect on lipid fractions. For example, diets that are very low in total fat or very low in saturated fat may lower HDL cholesterol as much as LDL cholesterol. It is not known how these diet-induced changes affect coronary risk.

Several nutritional approaches to diet therapy are available (Table 28–2). Most Americans currently eat 35–40% of calories as fat. Approximately 15% is saturated fat. Dietary cholesterol intake averages 400 mg/d. A standard "Step 1" cholesterol-lowering diet recommends reducing total fat to 30% and saturated fat to 10% of calories. Dietary cholesterol is limited to 300 mg/d. The "Step 2" diet further restricts saturated fat to 7% of calories and dietary cholesterol to 200 mg/d. These diets replace fat, particularly saturated fat, with carbohydrate. In most instances, this approach will also result in fewer total calories consumed and will facilitate weight loss in overweight patients. Other diet plans, including the Dean Ornish Diet, the Pritikin Diet, and most vegetarian diets, restrict fat even further. Low-fat, high-carbohydrate diets may, however, result in reductions in HDL cholesterol.

An alternative strategy is the "Mediterranean diet," which maintains total fat at approximately 35–40% of total calories but replaces saturated fat with monounsaturated fat such as that found in canola oil and in olives, peanuts, avocados, and their oils. This diet is equally effective at lowering LDL cholesterol but is less likely to lead to reductions in HDL cholesterol. Because of the substantial intake of dietary fat, this diet is less likely to lead to weight loss. Thus, a traditional low-fat approach is still preferred for patients with lipid disorders who are overweight. In thin patients, however, a Mediterranean diet can be considered.

Other dietary changes may also result in beneficial changes in blood lipids. Soluble fiber, such as that found in oat bran or psyllium, may reduce LDL cholesterol by 5–10%. Garlic, soy protein, vitamin C, and certain plant sterols may also result in reduction of LDL cholesterol. Because of current interest in oxidation of LDL cholesterol as an initiating event in atherogenesis, diets should also be rich in antioxidant vitamins, found primarily in fruits and vegetables (see Chapter 29).

Anderson JW, Johnstone BM, Cook-Newell ME: Meta-analysis of the effects of soy protein intake on serum lipids. N Engl J Med 1995;333:276. (High intakes of soy

Table 28–2. Macronutrient composition of three lipid-modifying diets.

Nutrient	Recommended Intake		
	Step 1 Diet	Step 2 Diet	Mediterranean Diet
Total fat	< 30% of calories	< 30% of calories	< 40% of calories
Saturated fat	< 10% of calories	< 7% of calories	< 10% of calories
Polyunsaturated fat	< 10% of calories	< 10% of calories	< 10% of calories
Monounsaturated fat	< 10% of calories	< 10% of calories	< 20% of calories
Carbohydrate	50–60% of calories	50–60% of calories	40–50% of calories
Protein	10–20% of calories	10–20% of calories	10–20% of calories
Cholesterol	< 300 mg/d	< 200 mg/d	< 300 mg/d
Total calories	For desirable weight	For desirable weight	For desirable weight

protein—five servings per day—results in a 9% decrease in cholesterol.)

Denke MA: Cholesterol-lowering diets: A review of the evidence. Arch Intern Med 1995;155:17. (Cholesterol-lowering diets are feasible in the outpatient setting, but response is quite variable.)

Gaziano JM et al: Moderate alcohol intake, increased levels of high density lipoprotein and its subfractions, and decreased risk of myocardial infarction. N Engl J Med 1993;329:1829. (Moderate alcohol intake is associated with increases in HDL cholesterol.)

Hunninghake DB et al: The efficacy of intensive dietary therapy alone or combined with lovastatin in outpatients with hypercholesterolemia. N Engl J Med 1993;328:1213. (A diet containing 28% of calories as fat was relatively ineffective, lowering LDL cholesterol by 5% but also lowering HDL cholesterol by 6%.)

Miettinen TA et al: Reduction of serum cholesterol with sitostanol-ester margarine in a mildly hypercholes-terolemic population. N Engl J Med 1995;333:1308. (Reduced LDL cholesterol by 14%.)

Neil H et al: Randomised trial of lipid lowering advice in general practice: The effects on serum lipids, lipoproteins, and antioxidants. BMJ 1995;310:569. (Modest effects in practice.)

Pharmacologic Therapy (Table 28–3)

All patients whose risk from coronary heart disease is considered high enough to warrant pharmacologic therapy of an elevated LDL cholesterol should be given aspirin prophylaxis at a dose of about 325 mg every other day unless there are contraindications such as aspirin sensitivity, bleeding diatheses, or active peptic ulcer disease. Current data suggest that the effect of aspirin in reducing the risk of coronary

Table 28–3. Effects of selected lipid-modifying drugs.

Drug	Lipid-Modifying Effects			Initial Daily Dose	Maximum Daily Dose	Cost for 30 Days' Treatment, With Dose Listed[1]
	LDL	HDL	Triglyceride			
Niacin	−15 to −25%	+25 to −35%	↓↓	100 mg once	3–4.5 g divided	$5.28 (1.5 g bid)
Lovastatin	−25 to −40%	+5 to −10%	↓	10 mg once	80 mg divided	$67.50 (20 mg once)
Simvastatin	−25 to −40%	+5 to −10%	↓	5 mg once	40 mg once	$60.00 (10 mg once)
Pravastatin	−25 to −40%	+5 to −10%	↓	20 mg once	40 mg once	$61.66 (20 mg once)
Fluvastatin	−20 to −30%	+5 to −10%	↓	20 mg once	40 mg once	$36.60 (20 mg once)
Atorvastatin	−25 to −40%	+5 to −10%	↓↓	10 mg once	80 mg once	$84.60 (20 mg once)
Cholestyramine	−15 to −25%	+5%	±	4 g bid	24 g divided	$80.00 (8 g divided)
Colestipol	−15 to −25%	+5%	±	5 g bid	30 g divided	$80.00 (10 g divided)
Gemfibrozil	−10 to −15%	+15 to −20%	↓↓	600 mg once	1200 mg divided	$58.00 (600 mg bid)
Estrogens (conjugated)	−15 to −20%	+15 to −20%	↑	0.625 mg once	0.625 mg once	$13.53 (0.625 mg once)

[1]Cost to pharmacist for 30 days' treatment based on daily dosage listed (generic when possible). Source: First Data Bank, Price Alert, April 1997.
± = variable, if any

heart disease is equal to or even greater than that of cholesterol lowering. Other coronary heart disease risk factors, such as hypertension and smoking, should also be controlled.

Treatment of postmenopausal women with oral estrogen replacement therapy is associated with a reduction in LDL levels and an increase in HDL levels. These lipid effects appear to be responsible for about half of the possible benefit of postmenopausal estrogens on reducing the incidence of coronary heart disease. Estrogen also may be an antioxidant and has direct effects on vascular endothelium. The addition of a progesterone to the hormone regimen does not substantially diminish the beneficial effect on lipids.

If the decision to treat a patient with an LDL-lowering drug is made, the clinician must select an appropriate agent based on the safety, efficacy, cost, and effects on lipid levels (Tables 28–3 and 28–4) and set a goal for treatment. Current recommendations do not include drug therapy for low HDL levels in patients who do not also have high LDL levels. As with all therapies for chronic conditions, the therapeutic goal is best approached slowly and steadily, watching carefully for side effects and encouraging continued compliance with nonpharmacologic measures. Combinations of drugs may be necessary. Once the goal is reached, the lipid profile should be monitored periodically (every 6–12 months), with consideration given to periodic reductions in drug dose. With the exception of niacin (available generically for a few dollars per month), lipid-lowering agents are expensive and may need to be given for decades. Thus, their cost-effectiveness is generally low. Therapy with lovastatin, for example, has been estimated to cost more than $1 million per year of life saved if it is used to treat a 35-year-woman with a cholesterol level of 300 mg/dL who has no other coronary risk factors (and this estimate assumes that there are no adverse effects of therapy). A recent analysis, based on animal data, has suggested that lipid-lowering agents may be carcinogenic. This possibility should remind clinicians of the importance of carefully balancing the risks and benefits of any therapy, especially one that may be lifelong.

Table 28–4. Selection of lipid-modifying medications.[1]

Primary prevention
Premenopausal women (rare):
    Resins, niacin, "statins"
Men (35–75 years):
    Niacin, "statins," resins
Postmenopausal women (50–75 years):
    Estrogens, niacin, "statins"
Secondary prevention
Men:
    "Statins," niacin, combinations
Women:
    Estrogen, "statins," niacin, combinations

[1]See text for indications and Table 28–3 for dosages.

A. Niacin (Nicotinic Acid): Niacin was the first lipid-lowering agent that was associated with a reduction in total mortality. Long-term follow-up of a secondary prevention trial of middle-aged men with previous myocardial infarction disclosed that about 52% of those who had been previously treated with niacin had died, compared with 58% in the placebo group. This favorable effect on mortality was not seen during the trial itself, though there was a reduction in the incidence of coronary heart disease.

Niacin reduces the production of VLDL particles, with secondary reduction in LDL and increases in HDL cholesterol levels. The average effect of full-dose niacin therapy, 3–4.5 g/d, is a 15–25% reduction in LDL cholesterol and a 25–35% increase in HDL cholesterol. Full doses of niacin are required to obtain the LDL effect, but the HDL effect may be observed at lower doses, eg, 1 g/d. Niacin will also reduce triglycerides by half and will lower lipoprotein(a) (Lp[a]) levels. Thus, its effect on blood lipids is nearly optimal. Unfortunately, intolerance to niacin is common; only 50–60% of subjects in clinical trials tolerate full doses. Niacin causes a prostaglandin-mediated flushing that patients may describe as hot flashes or pruritus. This problem can be decreased by pretreatment with aspirin (81–325 mg/d) or other nonsteroidal anti-inflammatory agents. Flushing may also be decreased by initiating niacin therapy with a very small dose, eg, 50–100 mg with the evening meal. The dose can be doubled each week until 1.5 g/d is tolerated. After rechecking blood lipids, the dose is divided and increased until the goal of 3–4.5 g/d is reached. Only immediate-release niacin is recommended for lipid modification. Sustained-release preparations are more expensive and have less effect on raising HDL cholesterol. Both immediate-release and sustained-release niacin are associated with hepatitis, but the most severe cases have been reported with the sustained-release preparations. It is not known whether routine monitoring of liver enzymes results in early detection and thus reduced severity of this side effect. Niacin can also exacerbate gout and peptic ulcer disease and may worsen hyperglycemia in patients with diabetes mellitus.

B. Bile Acid-Binding Resins (Cholestyramine, Colestipol): Treatment with these agents has been shown to reduce the incidence of coronary events (such as myocardial infarction) in middle-aged men by about 20%, with no significant effect on total mortality. The resins work by binding bile acids in the intestine. The resultant reduction in the enterohepatic circulation causes the liver to increase its production of bile acids, using hepatic cholesterol to do so. Thus, hepatic LDL receptor activity increases, with a decline in plasma LDL levels. The triglyceride level tends to increase slightly in some patients treated with bile acid-binding resins; they should be used with caution in those with elevated triglycerides and probably not at all in patients who have triglyceride levels above about 500 mg/dL. The clinician can anticipate a reduction of 15–25% in the LDL cholesterol level, with minor (if any) increases in the HDL level.

The usual dose of cholestyramine is 12–36 g of resin per day in divided doses with meals, mixed in water or, more palatably, juice. The prepackaged 4 g doses are more expensive than the bulk form; the "candy bars" are even more expensive. Doses of colestipol are 20% higher (the packets each contain 5 g of resin).

These agents often cause gastrointestinal symptoms, such as constipation and gas. They may interfere with the absorption of fat-soluble vitamins (thereby complicating the management of patients receiving warfarin) and may bind other drugs in the intestine. Concurrent use of psyllium may ameliorate the gastrointestinal side effects.

C. HMG-CoA Reductase Inhibitors (Lovastatin, Pravastatin, Simvastatin, Fluvastatin, Atorvastatin): These agents work by inhibiting the rate-limiting enzyme in the formation of cholesterol. They have been shown to reduce coronary heart disease and total mortality in secondary prevention settings, as well as in middle-aged men free of coronary heart disease. Cholesterol synthesis in the liver is reduced, with a compensatory increase in hepatic LDL receptors (presumably so that the liver can take more of the cholesterol that it needs from the blood), and a reduction in the circulating LDL cholesterol level by up to 35%. There are also modest increases in HDL levels and decreases in triglyceride levels.

Doses are as follows: lovastatin, 10–80 mg/d; pravastatin, 10–40 mg/d; simvastatin, 5–40 mg/d; fluvastatin, 20–40 mg/d; and atorvastatin, 10–80 mg/d. These agents are usually given once a day in the evening (most cholesterol synthesis takes place overnight); at the high end of the dose ranges, twice-a-day dosing may be used. Side effects include myositis, whose incidence may be higher in patients concurrently taking fibrates or niacin. Manufacturers recommend monitoring liver and muscle enzymes. Several agents (notably erythromycin and cyclosporine) reduce the metabolism of these agents.

D. Fibric Acid Derivatives (Gemfibrozil, Clofibrate): In the largest clinical trial that used clofibrate, there were significantly more deaths—especially due to cancer—in the treatment group than in the control group. Although still available, clofibrate is rarely used. Gemfibrozil reduced coronary heart disease rates in hypercholesterolemic middle-aged men free of coronary disease in the Helsinki Heart Study. The effect was only observed among those who also had lower HDL cholesterol levels and high triglyceride levels. Among men with previous myocardial infarction, however, gemfibrozil increased overall mortality as well as that due to coronary heart disease. Clinicians should also be aware of the trend toward increased numbers of cancer deaths among subjects treated with gemfibrozil in the Helsinki Heart Study.

The fibrates reduce the synthesis and increase the breakdown of VLDL particles, with secondary effects on LDL and HDL levels. They reduce LDL levels by about 10–15% and triglyceride levels by about 40% and raise HDL levels by about 15–20%. The usual dose of gemfibrozil is 600 mg once or twice a day. Side effects include cholelithiasis, hepatitis, and myositis. The incidence of the latter two conditions may be higher among patients also taking other lipid-lowering agents. Given that clofibrate caused a statistically significant increase in cancer mortality, it should not be used.

E. Probucol: The effects of probucol on coronary heart disease—and its long-term safety—are not known. It does reduce the deposition of LDL into xanthomas in humans (and into atherosclerotic plaques in rabbits). The mechanism of action of probucol is not clear. It apparently reduces the amount of oxidized LDL (it was originally used as an industrial antioxidant). Probucol reduces LDL levels by 10–15% but has the potentially important adverse effect of lowering HDL levels by up to 10%. It also may be cardiotoxic. Probucol, if used at all, should be reserved for patients with a clear genetic disorder who have failed other therapies.

Initial Selection of Medication

At present there are no absolute guidelines for selection of available lipid-modifying medications in particular patients. Nonetheless, the results of clinical trials can provide some guidance (Table 28–4). For men with known coronary heart disease who require a lipid-modifying medication, an HMG-CoA reductase inhibitor is preferred. For women with known coronary heart disease, hormone replacement therapy (Chapter 26) should be considered and an HMG-CoA reductase inhibitor prescribed if the goal LDL level is not achieved. Although niacin will also have beneficial effects on lipids in both men and women with coronary heart disease, there is less evidence from clinical trials demonstrating the desired effects on coronary heart disease and all-cause mortality.

For patients without known coronary heart disease, the choice of medications (and proof of a beneficial effect) is less clear. For men 45–64 years of age, an HMG-CoA reductase inhibitor is preferred. For men aged 35–44 and for men aged 65–75, either niacin or an HMG-CoA reductase inhibitor can be equally considered. For postmenopausal women up to age 75, hormone replacement therapy should be considered first, followed by niacin or an HMG-CoA reductase inhibitor. Premenopausal women rarely require lipid-modifying therapy. Resins are the only lipid-modifying medication considered safe in pregnancy. If pregnancy is not a concern, niacin or an HMG-CoA reductase inhibitor can be considered.

Combinations of lipid-modifying medications can also be used. Combinations may be more cost-effective than high doses of a single medication (usually an HMG-CoA reductase inhibitor) and may have beneficial effects on lipids. Low-dose niacin (0.5–1 g/d), for example, will substantially increase the HDL cholesterol when added to an HMG-CoA reductase inhibitor. Combinations, however, may increase the risk of severe complications of drug therapy. The combination of gemfibrozil and HMG-CoA reductase inhibitors increases the risk of myositis more than either drug alone.

Choice of cholesterol-lowering drugs. Med Lett Drugs Ther 1996;38:67.

Frick M et al: Efficacy of gemfibrozil in dyslipidaemic subjects with suspected heart disease: An ancillary study in the Helsinki heart study frame population. Ann Med 1993;25:41. (Disappointing results in the secondary prevention setting.)

Illingworth DR et al: Comparative effects of lovastatin and niacin in primary hypercholesterolemia: A prospective trial. Arch Intern Med 1994;154:1586. (More patients tolerate lovastatin, but the lipid-modifying effects of niacin are better.)

McKenney JM et al: A comparison of the efficacy and toxic effects of sustained- vs. immediate-release niacin in hypercholesterolemic patients. JAMA 1994;271:672. (Most severe hepatitis is seen with sustained-action niacin preparations.)

Newman TB, Hulley SB: Carcinogenicity of lipid-lowering drugs. JAMA 1996;275:55. (Presents animal data from the *PDR,* FDA, and published studies; an accompanying editorial suggests that the drugs are safe.)

Probstfield JL, Hunninghake DB: Nicotinic acid as a lipoprotein-altering agent: Therapy directed by the primary physician. Arch Intern Med 1994;154:1557. (Niacin is still useful as a lipid-modifying medication.)

Writing Group for the PEPI Trial: Effects of estrogen or estrogen/progestin regimens on heart disease risk factors in postmenopausal women. The Postmenopausal Estrogen/Progestin Intervention (PEPI) Trial. JAMA 1995; 273:199. (Favorable effects on lipids.)

HIGH BLOOD TRIGLYCERIDES

Patients with very high levels of serum triglycerides are at risk of pancreatitis. The pathophysiology is not certain, since there are some patients with very high triglyceride levels who never develop pancreatitis. Most patients with congenital abnormalities in triglyceride metabolism present in childhood; hypertriglyceridemia-induced pancreatitis that first presents in adults is more commonly due to an acquired problem in lipid metabolism.

Although there are no clear triglyceride levels that always result in pancreatitis, most clinicians are uncomfortable with levels above 1000 mg/dL. The risk of pancreatitis may be more related to the triglyceride level following consumption of a fatty meal. Because postcibal increases in triglyceride are inevitable if fat-containing foods are eaten, fasting triglyceride levels in persons prone to pancreatitis should be kept well below that level.

The primary therapy for high triglyceride levels is dietary, avoiding alcohol and fatty foods and restricting calories. Control of secondary causes of high triglyceride levels (see Table 28–1) may also be helpful. In patients with persistent elevations in the pancreatitis range despite adequate dietary compliance—and certainly in those with a previous episode of pancreatitis—therapy with a triglyceride-lowering drug (eg, niacin, in doses as described above) is indicated.

Whether patients with elevated triglycerides (> 250 mg/dL) and no other lipoprotein abnormalities are at increased risk of atherosclerotic disease is not known. Some of these patients may belong to families with a genetic disorder known as **familial combined hyperlipidemia.** This disorder is characterized by a variety of lipid abnormalities in different family members: Some have high cholesterol levels, some high triglyceride levels, and some both. It now appears that the common link is an abnormality in one of the LDL-associated apoproteins (B-100), and that this may be a coronary risk factor. However, the effect on coronary heart disease risk of treating an isolated high triglyceride level in these patients is not known.

Current indications for treatment of high blood triglycerides to prevent coronary heart disease are controversial. In patients with known coronary heart disease, it is reasonable to treat isolated increases in triglycerides to 400 mg/dL or greater with an HMG-CoA reductase inhibitor. Most of these patients will have elevated LDL cholesterol (≥ 130 mg/dL) and will benefit from drug therapy even though estimation of the LDL cholesterol level will not be possible until the triglyceride is below 400 mg/dL. In patients without known coronary heart disease, the optimal strategy is not known. Triglyceride levels above 400 mg/dL can be treated first with nonpharmacologic approaches, including weight loss, low-fat diet, avoidance of excess alcohol, and regular aerobic exercise. If serum triglyceride levels remain greater than 400 mg/dL (but < 1000 mg/dL), LDL cholesterol can be measured directly by ultracentrifugation. Treatment decisions can then be based on the LDL cholesterol level.

Backer-Irksome R et al: Efficacy and safety of a new HMG-CoA reductase inhibitor, atorvastatin, in patients with hypertriglyceridemia. JAMA 1996;275:128. (Atorvastatin reduces triglycerides more than other "statins" while also reducing LDL cholesterol.)

Criqui MH et al: Plasma triglyceride level and mortality from coronary heart disease. N Engl J Med 1993; 328:1220. (There was no evidence that an elevated triglyceride level was an independent predictor of death from coronary disease.)

NIH Consensus Development Panel on Triglyceride, High-Density Lipoprotein, and Coronary Heart Disease: Triglyceride, high-density lipoprotein, and coronary heart disease. JAMA 1993;269:505. ("Many important questions remain unanswered.")

29

Nutrition

Robert B. Baron, MD, MS

NUTRITIONAL REQUIREMENTS

Approximately 40 nutrients are required by the human body. Nutrients are considered essential if they cannot be synthesized by the body and if a deficiency causes recognizable abnormalities that disappear when the deficit is corrected. Required nutrients include the essential amino acids, water-soluble vitamins, fat-soluble vitamins, minerals, and the essential fatty acids. The body also requires an adequate energy substrate, a small amount of metabolizable carbohydrate, indigestible carbohydrate (fiber), additional nitrogen, and water.

Most of the required nutrients are harmful when consumed in excessive amounts. Thus, a range of acceptable intake levels can be established for most of them.

Nutritional requirements are most commonly expressed as the average daily amounts of nutrients a population group should consume. In the USA, the most widely used estimates of nutritional requirements are the Recommended Dietary Allowances (RDAs) developed by a subcommittee of the Food and Nutrition Board of the National Academy of Sciences. RDAs have been established for energy and protein; the water-soluble vitamins thiamin, riboflavin, niacin, vitamin B_6, folic acid, vitamin B_{12}, and vitamin C; the fat-soluble vitamins A, D, and K; and the minerals calcium, phosphorus, magnesium, iron, zinc, iodine, and selenium (Table 29–1).

The RDAs exceed the actual requirements of most individuals in the population because they are stated as 2 SD above the estimated mean requirement. Therefore, a dietary intake of less than the RDA of a specific nutrient is not necessarily inadequate for a given individual—it increases the *risk* of an inadequate intake. For most clinical situations, two-thirds of the RDA is considered an adequate nutritional intake.

The RDAs for energy are treated in a different manner. Because energy needs vary so greatly among individuals, the RDA Committee sets forth estimates of the average needs of the population rather than recommended intakes for individuals. About half of the population will require more energy than the RDA and half will require less.

Nutritional requirements vary not only from one individual to the next but from one day to the next in any given subject. They differ also with age, sex, and body size and during pregnancy and lactation. Different RDAs have been developed for different age and sex groups. Requirements vary also with such clinical circumstances as premature birth, aging, metabolic disorders, infections, chronic illness, medications, extremes of climate and physical activity, and the route of ingestion. The RDAs do not cover such situations—they are intended only for healthy populations.

ENERGY

The human body requires energy to support normal functions and physical activity, growth, and repair of damaged tissues. Energy is provided by oxidation of dietary protein, fat, carbohydrate, and alcohol. Oxidation of 1 g of each provides 4 kcal of energy from protein and carbohydrate, 9 kcal from fat, and 7 kcal from alcohol.

In healthy adults, energy expenditure is primarily determined by three factors: basal energy expenditure (BEE), thermic effect of food (TEF), and physical activity.

The BEE is the amount of energy required to maintain basic physiologic functions. It is measured while the subject is resting in a warm room, not having eaten for 12 hours. In healthy persons, the BEE (in kcal/24 h) can be estimated by the Harris-Benedict equation, which will correctly predict measured BEE in 90% ± 10% of healthy subjects (see Nutritional Requirements, below). In clinical practice, patients rarely meet the strict criteria for basal measurement. Energy expenditure measured in individuals at rest without food for 2 hours is the resting metabolic

Table 29-1. Recommended daily dietary allowances for adults (revised 1989).[1]

Category	Age (years) or Condition	Weight (kg)	(lb)	Height (cm)	(in)	Protein (g)	Fat-Soluble Vitamins				Water-Soluble Vitamins							Minerals						
							Vitamin A (mg RE)	Vitamin D (mg)	Vitamin E (mg α-TE)	Vitamin K (mg)	Vitamin C (mg)	Thiamine (mg)	Riboflavin (mg)	Niacin (mg NE)	Vitamin B6 (mg)	Folate (μg)	Vitamin B12 (μg)	Calcium (mg)	Phosphorus (mg)	Magnesium (mg)	Iron (mg)	Zinc (mg)	Iodine (μg)	Selenium (μg)
Males	15–18	66	145	176	69	59	1,000	10	10	65	60	1.5	1.8	20	2.0	200	2.0	1,200	1,200	400	12	15	150	50
	19–24	72	160	177	70	58	1,000	10	10	70	60	1.5	1.7	19	2.0	200	2.0	1,200	1,200	350	10	15	150	70
	25–50	79	174	176	70	63	1,000	5	10	80	60	1.5	1.7	19	2.0	200	2.0	800	800	350	10	15	150	70
	51+	77	170	173	68	63	1,000	5	10	80	60	1.2	1.4	15	2.0	200	2.0	800	800	350	10	15	150	70
Females	15–18	55	120	163	64	44	800	10	8	55	60	1.1	1.3	15	1.5	180	2.0	1,200	1,200	300	15	12	150	50
	19–24	58	128	164	65	46	800	10	8	60	60	1.1	1.3	15	1.6	180	2.0	1,200	1,200	280	15	12	150	55
	25–50	63	138	163	64	50	800	5	8	65	60	1.1	1.3	15	1.6	180	2.0	800	800	280	15	12	150	55
	51+	65	143	160	63	50	800	5	8	65	60	1.0	1.2	13	1.6	180	2.0	800	800	280	10	12	150	55
Pregnant						60	800	10	10	65	70	1.5	1.6	17	2.2	400	2.2	1,200	1,200	320	30	15	175	65
Lactating	1st 6 months					65	1,300	10	12	65	95	1.6	1.8	20	2.1	280	2.6	1,200	1,200	355	15	19	200	75
	2nd 6 months					62	1,200	10	11	65	90	1.6	1.7	20	2.1	260	2.6	1,200	1,200	340	15	16	200	75

[1]From: National Research Council: *Recommended Dietary Allowances*, 10th ed. National Academy of Sciences, 1989.

expenditure (RME) and is about 10% greater than BEE.

TEF is the amount of energy expended during and following the ingestion of food. TEF averages approximately 10% of the BEE.

Physical activity has a major impact on energy expenditure. The average energy expenditure per hour by adults engaged in typical activities is shown in Table 29–2.

Daily recommended energy intakes for healthy individuals are shown in Table 29–3.

PROTEIN

Protein is required for growth and for maintenance of body structure and function. Although the nutritional requirement is commonly stated in grams of protein, the true requirement is for nine **essential amino acids** plus additional nitrogen for protein synthesis. The essential amino acids are leucine, isoleucine, lysine, methionine, phenylalanine, threonine, tryptophan, valine, and histidine.

Adequate protein must be consumed each day to replace essential amino acids lost through protein turnover. On a protein-free diet, the average male loses 3.8 g of nitrogen per day—equivalent to 24 g of protein. Allowing for differences in protein quality and utilization and for individual variability, the RDA for protein is 56 g/d for men and 45 g/d for women.

Protein and energy requirements are closely related. Diets that provide insufficient energy will require additional protein to maintain nitrogen equilibrium.

CARBOHYDRATE

As long as adequate energy and protein are provided in the diet, there is no specific requirement for dietary carbohydrate. A small amount of carbohydrate—approximately 100 g/d—is necessary to prevent ketosis. In practice, however, most dietary energy should be provided by carbohydrate. In the USA, the average diet contains 45% of calories as carbohydrate. Current recommendations are to increase carbohydrate intakes to 55–60% of total calories in the diet.

Dietary carbohydrates include simple sugars, complex carbohydrates (starches), and indigestible carbohydrates (dietary fiber). Although simple sugars and complex carbohydrates provide equal amounts of calories, the bulk of dietary carbohydrates should be derived from starches. Sugars—particularly sucrose—are concentrated sources of calories without other sources of essential nutrients. Sucrose consumption is also thought to be an important factor in the development of tooth decay. Complex carbohydrates, when unrefined, provide carbohydrate calories and vitamins, minerals, and dietary fiber.

Dietary fiber is that portion of plant foods that cannot be digested by the human intestine. Fiber increases the bulk of the stool and facilitates excretion. Epidemiologic evidence suggests that diets high in dietary fiber are associated with a lower incidence of digestive and cardiovascular diseases. The more insoluble fibers, such as those found in wheat bran, have the greatest impact on colonic function. Soluble fibers such as those found in legumes, oats, and fruit result in lower blood sugar levels in diabetics and lower blood cholesterol.

FAT

Dietary fat is the most concentrated source of food energy. Like energy from dietary carbohydrate, energy derived from fat can support protein synthesis. Dietary fat also provides the essential fatty acid linoleic acid. Other than the need for adequate quantities of linoleic acid, there is no specific requirement for dietary fat as long as the diet provides adequate nutrients oxidizable for energy. Although the average American diet contains 35–40% of calories as fat,

Table 29–2. Average energy kilocalories expended per hour by adults at selected weights engaged in various activities.[1]

Activity	54 kg (120 lb)	64 kg (140 lb)	73 kg (160 lb)	82 kg (180 lb)	91 kg (200 lb)	100 kg (220 lb)
Sleeping: Reclining	50	58	69	78	86	99
Very light: Sitting	73	83	103	115	127	150
Light: Walking on level, shopping, light housekeeping	143	166	200	225	250	290
Moderate: Cycling, dancing, skiing, tennis	226	262	307	345	382	430
Heavy: Walking uphill, shoveling, swimming, playing basketball or football	440	512	598	670	746	840

Note: Range of rate of expenditure of calories per minute of activity (for a 70-kg man or a 58-kg woman): Sleeping, 0.9–1.2; very light, 1.5–2.5; light, 2–4.9; moderate, 5–7.4; heavy, 6–12.
[1]Data from: *Recommended Dietary Allowances*, 9th ed. National Academy of Sciences–National Research Council, 1980. Adapted from McArdle WD, Katch FI, Katch VL: *Exercise Physiology: Energy, Nutrition and Human Performance*. Lea & Febiger, 1981.

Table 29–3. Median heights and weights and recommended energy intake (REE) for nonpregnant adults.[1]

Category	Age (years)	Weight (kg)	Weight (lb)	Height (cm)	Height (in)	REE (kcal/d)	Average Energy Allowance[2] (kcal) Multiples of REE	Average Energy Allowance[2] (kcal) Per kg	Average Energy Allowance[2] (kcal) Per Day[3]
Males	19–24	72	160	177	70	1780	1.67	40	2900
	25–50	79	174	176	70	1800	1.60	37	2900
	51+	77	170	173	68	1530	1.50	30	2300
Females	19–24	58	128	164	65	1350	1.60	38	2200
	25–50	63	138	163	64	1380	1.55	36	2200
	51+	65	143	160	63	1280	1.50	30	1900

[1]Modified from: National Research Council: *Recommended Dietary Allowances*, 10th ed. National Academy of Sciences, 1989.
[2]In the range of light to moderate activity, the coefficient of variation is ± 20%.
[3]Figure is rounded.

most current recommendations are to limit dietary fat to 30% or less of total calories. Diets containing as little as 5–10% of total calories as fat appear to be safe and well tolerated.

Dietary fats are composed chiefly of fatty acids and dietary cholesterol. Fatty acids contain either no double bonds (saturated), one double bond (monounsaturated), or more than one double bond (polyunsaturated). Current dietary recommendations are to decrease total fat and replace saturated fats with monounsaturated fatty acids and complex carbohydrates. Saturated fatty acids are associated with increased serum cholesterol, while polyunsaturated and monounsaturated fatty acids lower serum cholesterol. Saturated fats are solid at room temperature and in general are derived from animal foods; unsaturated fats are liquid at room temperature and in general are derived from plant foods.

The polyunsaturated fatty acid **linoleic acid** is an essential nutrient, required by the body for the synthesis of arachidonic acid, the major precursor of prostaglandins. Deficiencies of linoleic acid result in dermatitis, hair loss, and impaired wound healing. For individuals with average energy requirements, approximately 5 g of linoleic acid per day—1–2% of total calories—is required to prevent essential fatty acid deficiency.

Cholesterol is a major constituent of cell membranes. It is synthesized easily by the body and is not an essential nutrient. Diets that contain large amounts of cholesterol partially inhibit endogenous cholesterol synthesis but result in a net increase in serum cholesterol concentrations because of suppression of synthesis of low-density lipoprotein receptors. Average American diets contain approximately 450 mg/d of cholesterol. Current recommendations are to limit dietary cholesterol to 300 mg or less per day.

VITAMINS

Vitamins are a heterogeneous group of organic molecules required by the body for a variety of es-

sential metabolic functions. They are grouped as **water-soluble vitamins:** thiamin, riboflavin, niacin, vitamin B_6 (pyridoxine), vitamin B_{12} (cobalamin), folate, pantothenic acid, biotin, and vitamin C (ascorbic acid); and **fat-soluble vitamins:** A, D, E, and K. Disorders of vitamin metabolism are discussed below.

MINERALS

The body also requires a number of inorganic minerals, commonly grouped as the **major minerals** calcium, magnesium, and phosphorus; the **electrolytes** sodium, potassium, and chloride; and the **trace elements** iron, zinc, copper, manganese, molybdenum, fluoride, iodine, cobalt, chromium, and selenium. Important characteristics of major minerals and electrolytes are summarized in Table 29–4.

DRUG-NUTRIENT INTERACTIONS

Many commonly used medications can have important effects on nutritional requirements. Chronic therapy with a variety of drugs can induce nutrient deficiencies by appetite suppression, intestinal malabsorption, and alterations in nutrient metabolism or excretion. The effects of selected drugs on nutrient absorption and metabolism are summarized in Table 29–5.

DIETARY RECOMMENDATIONS

Prior to the 1980s, the emphasis in nutrition education and diet planning was to ensure that the RDAs were met by diets that contained a wide variety of foods. The most important dietary education tool used for this purpose was *The Four Food Groups,* published by the United States Department of Agriculture (USDA). According to this model, two servings per day from both the milk group and the meat group and four servings per day from both the fruit

Table 29–4. Essential macrominerals: Summary of major characteristics.[1]

Elements	Functions	Deficiency Disease or Symptoms	Toxicity Disease or Symptoms[2]
Calcium	Constituent of bones, teeth; regulation of nerve, muscle function.	Children: rickets. Adults: osteomalacia. May contribute to osteoporosis.	Occurs with excess absorption due to hypervitaminosis D or hypercalcemia due to hyperparathyroidism, or other causes of hypercalcemia.
Phosphorus	Constituent of bones, teeth, ATP, phosphorylated metabolic intermediates. Nucleic acids.	Children: rickets. Adults: osteomalacia.	Low serum Ca^{2+}:P_i ratio stimulates secondary hyperparathyroidism; may lead to bone loss.
Sodium	Principal cation in extracellular fluid. Regulates plasma volume, acid-base balance, nerve and muscle function, Na^+-K^+ ATPase.	Unknown on normal diet, secondary to injury or illness.	Hypertension (in susceptible individuals).
Potassium	Principal cation in intracellular fluid; nerve and muscle function, Na^+-K^+ ATPase.	Occurs secondary to illness, injury, or diuretic therapy; muscular weakness, paralysis, mental confusion.	Cardiac arrest, small bowel ulcers.
Chloride	Fluid and electrolyte balance; gastric fluid.	Infants fed salt-free formula. Secondary to vomiting, diuretic therapy, renal disease.	Cardiac arrest, small bowel ulcers.
Magnesium	Constituent of bones, teeth; enzyme cofactor (kinases, etc).	Secondary to malabsorption or diarrhea, alcoholism.	Depressed deep tendon reflexes and respiration.

[1]Reproduced, with permission, from Murray RK et al: *Harper's Biochemistry,* 21st ed. Appleton & Lange, 1988.
[2]Excess mineral intake produces toxic symptoms. Unless otherwise specified, symptoms include nonspecific nausea, diarrhea, and irritability.

and vegetable group and the cereal group would meet the minimal nutritional requirements for most individuals.

Although this model ensured that the RDAs were met by a variety of foods, it did not guarantee that selected foods were of high quality. The effects of food processing on the nutrient density of food, the balance of macronutrients (percentages of fat, carbohydrate, and protein), and the character of macronutrients (simple versus complex carbohydrate; saturated versus unsaturated fat) are omitted.

In the last 2 decades, numerous governmental, professional, and public health agencies and associations have regularly published dietary recommendations that address these issues. Although attention has been directed to the differences between these reports, most agree on the basic principles of eating a wide variety of foods; increasing the consumption of foods containing complex carbohydrates; restricting the intake of sugar, fat (particularly saturated fat), cholesterol, salt, and alcohol; and maintaining an ideal body weight.

A new nutrition education guide, the "Food Guide Pyramid" (Figure 29–1), has been recently published by the USDA, replacing the "Four Food Groups." The Pyramid places greatest emphasis on consumption of bread, cereal, rice, and pasta (six to eleven servings); vegetables (three to five servings); and fruit (two to four servings); lesser emphasis on milk, yogurt, and cheese (two or three servings) and meat, poultry, fish, dry beans, eggs, and nuts (two or three servings); and recommends that fats, oils, and sweets be used sparingly.

ASSESSMENT OF NUTRITIONAL STATUS

The prevention and treatment of nutritional problems require the identification of patients at risk for the development of malnutrition and the identification of patients who already show symptoms and signs of malnutrition. Unfortunately, no single biochemical test or clinical technique is sufficiently accurate to serve as a reliable test for malnutrition. Current techniques of nutritional assessment utilize a combination of methods, including evaluation of dietary intake, anthropometric measurements, clinical examination, and laboratory tests. Some patients require serial measurements and close observation to confirm the diagnosis of malnutrition.

DIETARY HISTORY

Virtually all patients undergoing a complete history and physical examination should be asked screening dietary questions to help identify those high-risk patients who require further evaluation. Of particular importance are the regularity and availability of meals; who does the shopping and food preparation; recent changes in appetite, intake, or body weight; use of special diets or dietary supplements; use of alcohol, drugs, or medications; food prefer-

Table 29–5. Effect of drugs on nutrient absorption and metabolism.

Drug	Effect
Analgesics and anti-inflammatories	
Salicylates	Decrease serum ascorbic acid; increase urinary loss of ascorbic acid, potassium, and amino acids.
Sulfasalazine	Impairs folate absorption and antagonizes folate supplementation.
Antacids	
Aluminum antacids	Decrease absorption of phosphate and vitamin A.
H$_2$ blockers	Decrease iron and vitamin B$_{12}$ absorption.
Octreotide acetate	Hypo- and hyperglycemia; decreases fat and carotene absorption.
Anticonvulsants	
Phenobarbital	Decreases serum folate; increases vitamin D and vitamin K turnover and may cause deficiency.
Phenytoin	Decreases serum folate; increases vitamin D and vitamin K turnover and may cause deficiency.
Primidone	Decreases serum folate and vitamins B$_6$, B$_{12}$; decreases calcium absorption; increases vitamin D and vitamin K turnover and may cause deficiency.
Antimicrobials	
Neomycin	Binds bile acids and decreases absorption of fat, carotene; of vitamins A, D, K, and B$_{12}$; and of potassium, sodium, calcium, nitrogen.
Amphotericin B	Decreases serum magnesium and potassium.
Aminosalicylic acid	Increases absorption of folate, vitamin B$_{12}$, iron, cholesterol, fat.
Chloramphenicol	Increases need for vitamins B$_2$, B$_6$, B$_{12}$; increases serum iron.
Penicillin	Hypokalemia; renal potassium wasting.
Tetracycline	Calcium, iron, magnesium inhibit drug absorption; decreases vitamin K synthesis.
Cycloserine	May decrease absorption of calcium, magnesium; may decrease serum folate and vitamins B$_6$, B$_{12}$; decreases protein synthesis.
Isoniazid	Vitamin B$_6$ antagonist; may cause deficiency.
Sulfonamides	Decrease absorption of folate; decrease serum folate, iron.
Nitrofurantoin	Decreases serum folate.
Pyrimethamine	Decreases serum B$_{12}$ and folate.
Antimitotics	
Methotrexate	Decreases activation of folate.
Colchicine	Decreases absorption of vitamin B$_{12}$, carotene, fat, sodium, potassium, cholesterol, lactose, nitrogen.
Cathartics	
Phenolphthalein	Malabsorption, hypokalemia; deficiency of vitamin D, calcium.
Mineral oil	Malabsorption; decreased absorption of vitamins A, D, K.
Diuretics	Some cause hypokalemia, hypomagnesemia; may increase urinary excretion of vitamins B$_1$, B$_6$; calcium, magnesium, potassium.
Hypocholesterolemics	
Cholestyramine	Binds bile acids; decreases absorption of fat, carotene; vitamins A, D, K, B$_{12}$; folate, iron.
Clofibrate	Decreases absorption of carotene, vitamin B$_{12}$, iron, glucose.
Hypotensives	
Hydralazine	Vitamin B$_6$ deficiency.
Captopril	May cause hyponatremia, hyperkalemia; decreases taste acuity.
Oral contraceptives	Vitamin B$_6$, folate deficiency; may increase the need for other nutrients.

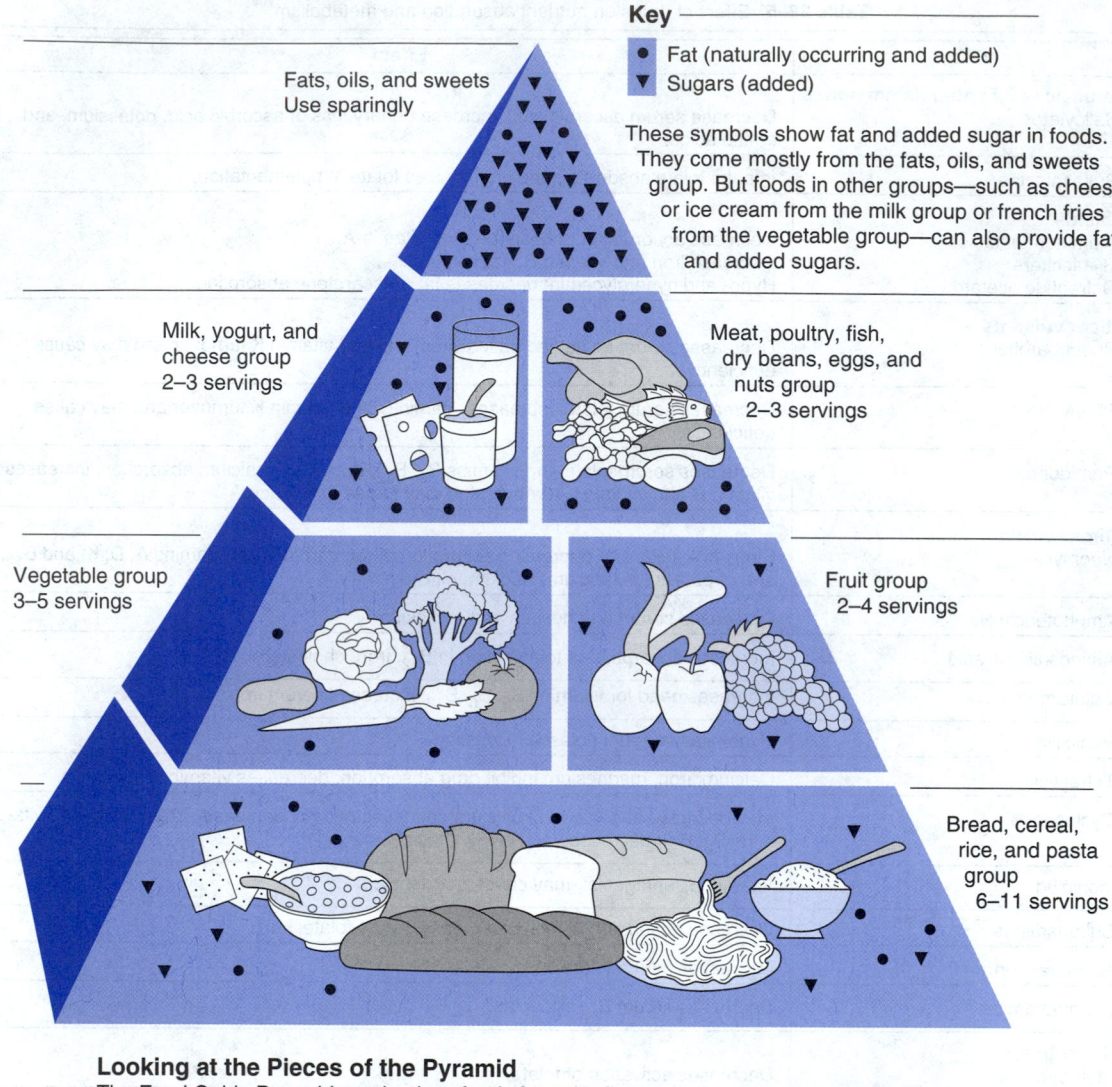

Key
- ● Fat (naturally occurring and added)
- ▼ Sugars (added)

These symbols show fat and added sugar in foods. They come mostly from the fats, oils, and sweets group. But foods in other groups—such as cheese or ice cream from the milk group or french fries from the vegetable group—can also provide fat and added sugars.

Fats, oils, and sweets
Use sparingly

Milk, yogurt, and cheese group
2–3 servings

Meat, poultry, fish, dry beans, eggs, and nuts group
2–3 servings

Vegetable group
3–5 servings

Fruit group
2–4 servings

Bread, cereal, rice, and pasta group
6–11 servings

Looking at the Pieces of the Pyramid
The Food Guide Pyramid emphasizes foods from the five major food groups shown in the three lower sections of the Pyramid. Each of these food groups provides some, but not all, of the nutrients you need. Foods in one group can't replace those in another. No one of these major food groups is more important than another—for good health, you need them all.

Figure 29–1. The Food Guide Pyramid. A guide to daily food choices.

ences and food allergies; and the presence of illnesses that affect nutritional intakes, losses, or requirements. Elderly and adolescent patients, pregnant or lactating women, and the poor and socially isolated are at particular risk for nutritional problems.

Further quantification of dietary intake can be performed using a variety of techniques. **Twenty-four-hour diet recalls** can be performed quickly and easily and provide rough estimates of nutrient intakes. Patients are asked to describe their dietary intake over the preceding 24 hours, including snacks, beverages, and alcohol. Problems with this technique include inaccurate reporting by patients, difficulties in estimating serving sizes, and the usual problems of generalizing from inadequate data: in this case, a single day's intake. More accurate quantitative information can be obtained by asking patients to complete a **3- to 5-day diet record.** Nutrient composition can then be analyzed with the aid of standard handbooks or computer software. Although this technique is prospective and less likely to be invalidated by memory lapses, omissions are still common as well as the usual difficulties in estimating serving sizes.

What Counts as One Serving?

The amount of food that counts as one serving is listed below. If you eat a larger portion, count it as more than one serving. For example, a dinner portion of spaghetti would count as two or three servings of pasta.

Be sure to eat at least the lowest number of servings from the five major food groups listed below. You need them for the vitamins, minerals, carbohydrates, and protein they provide. Just try to pick the lowest fat choices from the food groups. No specific serving size is given for the fats, oils, and sweets group because the message is USE SPARINGLY.

Food groups

Milk, yogurt, and cheese

| 1 cup of milk or yogurt | 1 1/2 ounces of natural cheese | 2 ounces of processed cheese |

Meat, poultry, fish, dry beans, eggs, and nuts

| 2–3 ounces of cooked lean meat, poultry, or fish | 1/2 cup of cooked dry beans, 1 egg, or 2 tablespoons of peanut butter count as 1 ounce of lean meat |

Vegetable

| 1 cup of raw leafy vegetables | 1/2 cup of other vegetables, cooked or chopped raw | 3/4 cup of vegetable juice |

Fruit

| 1 medium apple, banana, orange | 1/2 cup of chopped, cooked, or canned fruit | 3/4 cup of fruit juice |

Bread, cereal, rice, and pasta

| 1 slice of bread | 1 ounce of ready-to-eat cereal | 1/2 cup of cooked cereal, rice, or pasta |

How many servings do you need each day?

	Many women, older adults	Children, teenage girls, active women, most men	Teen-age boys, active men
Calorie level[1]	About 1600	About 2200	About 2800
Bread group servings	6	9	11
Vegetable group servings	3	4	5
Fruit group servings	2	3	4
Milk group servings	2–3[2]	2–3[2]	2–3[2]
Meat group servings	2, for a total of 5 ounces	2, for a total of 6 ounces	3, for a total of 7 ounces
Total fat (grams)	53	73	93

[1] These are the calorie levels if you choose low-fat, lean foods from the five major groups and use foods from the fats, oils, and sweets group sparingly.

[2] Women who are pregnant or breastfeeding, teenagers, and young adults to age 24 need three servings.

Figure 29–1. (Continued)

CLINICAL EXAMINATION

A nutritionally focused physical examination should be performed on each patient at risk for nutritional problems. The examination emphasizes muscle wasting, fat stores, volume status, and signs of micronutrient deficiencies (Table 29–6).

Evaluation of body weight is particularly useful. Body weight in relationship to height should be checked against reference tables of desirable weight (Table 29–7) and expressed as **relative weight:** current weight/desirable weight × 100. A recent change in body weight is a better index of undernutrition than a low relative weight. Changes in body weight are best expressed as a percentage of usual weight lost per unit of time. A loss of 10% or more of usual weight within a period of 1–2 months is generally considered to be predictive of a poor clinical outcome.

Evaluation of body composition—particularly fat stores and skeletal muscle—can be performed by visual inspection or, more quantitatively, by using **anthropometric measurements.** The most commonly used are the triceps skin fold, and mid arm muscle circumference. Because of significant individual variations and technical variations in measurement, however, anthropometry has limited clinical utility.

A number of more sophisticated techniques are

Table 29–6. Clinical signs that may be due to nutrient deficiency.

Clinical Sign	Nutrient Deficiency	Clinical Sign	Nutrient Deficiency
Hair		**Mouth** (cont'd)	
Transverse depigmentation	Protein, copper	Atrophic lingual papillae	Niacin, iron, riboflavin, folate, vitamin B_{12}
Easily pluckable	Protein		
Sparse and thin	Protein, zinc, biotin	Hypogeusia	Zinc, vitamin A
Skin		Tongue fissuring	Niacin
Dry, scaling	Zinc, vitamin A, essential fatty acids	**Neck**	
		Goiter	Iodine
Flaky paint dermatitis	Protein, niacin, riboflavin	**Chest**	
Follicular hyperkeratosis	Vitamins A and C	Thoracic rosary	Vitamin D
Perifollicular petechiae	Vitamin C	**Heart**	
Petechiae, purpura	Vitamins C and K	High-output failure	Thiamin
Pigmentation, desquamation	Niacin	Decreased output	Protein-calorie
		Abdomen	
Nasolabial seborrhea	Niacin, riboflavin, pyridoxine	Hepatosplenomegaly	Protein-calorie
Pallor	Iron, folate, vitamin B_{12}, copper	Distention	Protein-calorie
		Diarrhea	Niacin, folate, vitamin B_{12}
Scrotal/vulvar dermatoses	Riboflavin	**Extremities**	
Subcutaneous fat loss	Calorie	Muscle tenderness, pain	Thiamin, vitamin C
Nails		Muscle wasting	Protein-calorie
Spooning	Iron	Edema	Protein, thiamin
Transverse lines, ridging	Protein-calorie	Bone tenderness	Vitamin D, vitamin C, calcium, phosphorus
Head			
Temporal muscle wasting	Protein-calorie	**Neurologic**	
Parotid enlargement	Protein	Hyporeflexia	Thiamin
Eyes		Decreased position and vibratory sense	Vitamin B_{12}, thiamin
Night blindness	Vitamin A, zinc		
Corneal vascularization	Riboflavin	Paresthesias	Vitamin B_{12}, thiamin, niacin
Xerosis, Bitot spots, keratomalacia	Vitamin A	Confabulation, disorientation	Thiamin
Conjunctival inflammation	Riboflavin	Dementia	Niacin
Mouth		Ophthalmoplegia	Thiamin, phosphorus
Glossitis (scarlet, raw)	Niacin, pyridoxine, riboflavin, vitamin B_{12}, folate	Tetany	Calcium, magnesium
		Other	
Bleeding gums	Vitamin C, riboflavin	Delayed wound healing	Zinc, protein-calorie, vitamin C
Cheilosis	Riboflavin		
Angular stomatitis	Riboflavin, iron		

available for more precise assessment of body composition. Most, however, have little role in patient care. These include bioimpedance analysis, total body electrical conductivity, dual energy x-ray absorptiometry, underwater weighing, total body water and potassium, neutron activation analysis, and MRI.

LABORATORY TESTS

Serum albumin is the most important laboratory test for the diagnosis of protein-calorie undernutrition. Most patients with severe protein depletion will have abnormally low serum albumin levels. Unfortunately, many nonnutritional conditions can also cause low levels of serum albumin—particularly liver disease and severe illness in general. Other serum proteins with shorter half-lives (transferrin, prealbumin, etc) may more accurately reflect short-term changes in nutritional status but suffer from similar shortcomings.

Qualitative and quantitative tests of cellular immunity are also abnormal in many patients with protein-calorie undernutrition. Measurements of the **total lymphocyte count** and **delayed hypersensitivity reactions** to common skin test antigens are commonly used but are also nonspecific; ie, abnormalities may be due to nonnutritional factors.

Despite their uncertain diagnostic utility, these tests are useful prognostic indicators. Patients with abnormal nutritional assessment parameters have a markedly increased risk of poor clinical outcomes.

Despite the use of a nutritionally focused history and physical examination and judicious use of laboratory tests, it is often difficult to confirm a diagnosis of malnutrition. Continued close observation is often necessary. Monitoring dietary intakes during hospitalization can be quite helpful. **Calorie counts** by registered dietitians can be used to estimate energy and protein intakes for comparison with estimated requirements. Serial measurements of body weight and serial clinical assessments should also be performed.

Detsky AS, Smalley PS, Chang J: Is this patient malnourished? JAMA 1994;271:54. (A systematic approach to nutritional assessment emphasizing the history and physical examination.)

Table 29–7. Acceptable weights (in pounds, without shoes and clothes) for men and women, 1996.1

Height	Weight
5'0"	97–128
5'1"	101–132
5'2"	104–137
5'3"	107–141
5'4"	111–146
5'5"	114–150
5'6"	118–155
5'7"	121–160
5'8"	125–164
5'9"	129–169
5'10"	132–174
5'11"	136–179
6'0"	140–184
6'1"	144–189
6'2"	148–195
6'3"	152–200
6'4"	156–205
6'5"	160–211
6'6"	164–216

[1]United States Department of Health and Human Resources, 1996.

Dwyer JT, Gallo JJ, Reichel W: Assessing nutritional status in elderly patients. Am Fam Physician 1993;47:613. (Special considerations in nutritional assessment of the elderly.)

Gianotti L et al: Lack of improvement of prognostic performance of weight loss when combined with other parameters. Nutrition 1995;11:12. (Weight loss of 10% was the best predictor of prognosis in 398 surgical patients. Additional measures of nutritional assessment, including serum albumin and total lymphocyte count, had no additional predictive validity.)

NUTRITIONAL DISORDERS

PROTEIN-ENERGY MALNUTRITION

Essentials of Diagnosis

- Manifestations range from weight loss and growth failure to distinct syndromes, kwashiorkor, and marasmus.
- In severe cases, virtually all organ systems affected.
- History of decreased intake of energy or protein, increased nutrient losses, or increased nutrient requirements.

General Considerations

Protein-energy malnutrition occurs as a result of a relative or absolute deficiency of energy and protein. It may be primary, due to inadequate food intake, or secondary, as a result of other illness. For most developing nations, primary protein-energy malnutrition remains the most important nutritional problem and among the most significant of all health problems. Classically, protein-energy malnutrition has been described as two distinct syndromes. **Kwashiorkor,** caused by a deficiency of protein in the presence of adequate energy, is typically seen in weaning infants at the birth of a sibling in areas where foods containing protein are insufficiently abundant. **Marasmus,** caused by combined protein and energy deficiency, is most commonly seen where adequate quantities of food are not available.

In industrialized societies, protein-energy malnutrition is most often secondary to other diseases. As many as 20% of all patients admitted to the hospital have significant protein-energy malnutrition. In these patients, protein-energy malnutrition is caused either by decreased intake of energy and protein, increased nutrient losses, or increased nutrient requirements dictated by the underlying illness. For example, diminished oral intake may result from poor dentition or various gastrointestinal disorders. Loss of nutrients results from malabsorption and diarrhea as well as from glycosuria. Requirements are increased by fever, surgery, neoplasia, and burns. Few patients are sick enough to require acute hospitalization without manifesting some of these risk factors.

Pathophysiology

Protein-energy malnutrition results in important pathophysiologic changes that can affect virtually every organ system. The most obvious results are loss of body weight, adipose stores, and skeletal muscle mass. Weight losses of 5–10% are usually tolerated without significant loss of physiologic function; losses of 35–40% of body weight usually result in death. Loss of protein from skeletal muscle and internal organs is usually proportionate to weight loss. Protein mass is lost from the liver, gastrointestinal tract, kidneys, and heart.

As protein-energy malnutrition progresses, organ dysfunction may develop. Hepatic synthesis of serum proteins decreases, and depressed levels of circulating proteins may be observed. Cardiac output and contractility are decreased, and the ECG may show decreased voltage and a rightward axis shift. Autopsies of patients who die with severe undernutrition show myofibrillar atrophy and interstitial edema of the heart.

The lungs are affected primarily by weakness and atrophy of the muscles of respiration. Vital capacity and tidal volume are depressed, and mucociliary clearance is abnormal. The gastrointestinal tract is most importantly affected by mucosal atrophy and loss of villi of small intestine, resulting in a decrease in absorptive capacity. Intestinal disaccharidase deficiency and mild pancreatic insufficiency can also develop and result in malabsorption.

Changes in immunologic function are among the most important changes seen in protein-calorie undernutrition. The total lymphocyte count is commonly decreased, primarily because of a reduction in circulating T cells. T cell function is also depressed. Changes in B cell function are more variable. Other aspects of immunologic function are also affected, including total complement activity, granulocyte function, and anatomic barriers to infection. Virtually every phase of wound healing is also affected.

Clinical Findings

The clinical manifestations of protein-energy malnutrition are diverse, ranging from mild growth failure and weight loss to a number of distinct clinical syndromes. Children in the developing world, for example, may manifest the classic syndromes of marasmus and kwashiorkor. In secondary protein-energy malnutrition as seen in industrialized nations, clinical manifestations are affected by the degree of protein and energy deficiency, the underlying illness that resulted in the deficiency, and the patient's nutritional status prior to illness.

In mild cases of secondary protein-energy malnutrition, weight loss may be the only manifestation. In more severe cases, manifestations include depletion of fat stores in the face and extremities and loss of skeletal muscle, best seen in the interosseous and temporal muscles. The skin is often dry and the hair thin. If serum albumin is decreased, dependent edema or anasarca may be present.

The clinical manifestations of protein-energy malnutrition may be obscured in two other circumstances. Patients with significant obesity often appear to be overnourished because of their excess adipose stores. Rapid weight loss, however—particularly when due to illness—commonly results in depletion of skeletal and visceral protein and can lead to the pathophysiologic abnormalities described above despite the external appearance of obesity. In such patients, significant weight loss and depletion of serum proteins may be the only clues to protein depletion. Acutely ill patients—particularly those who are "hypermetabolic" and unable to eat—may develop visceral protein depletion rapidly without manifesting significant weight loss or other signs of undernutrition. In these patients, signs of hypermetabolism and decreased levels of serum protein may be the only clues to the diagnosis of undernutrition.

Treatment

The treatment of severe protein-energy malnutrition is a slow process requiring great care. Initial efforts should be directed at correcting fluid and electrolyte abnormalities and any significant acute infections. Of particular concern is depletion of potassium, magnesium, and calcium and acid-base abnormalities. The second phase of treatment is directed at repletion of protein, energy, and micronutrients. Treatment should be started with modest quantities of protein and calories calculated according to the patient's actual body weight. Adult patients can initially be given 0.8 g of protein and 30 kcal per kilogram. Concomitant administration of vitamins and minerals is necessary. Either the enteral or parenteral route can be used, although the former is preferable. Enteral fat and lactose are usually withheld initially. Patients with less severe protein-calorie undernutrition can be given calories and protein simultaneously with the correction of fluid and electrolyte abnormalities. Similar quantities of protein and calories are recommended for initial treatment.

All patients initially treated for protein-energy malnutrition require close follow-up. Both calories and protein can be advanced as tolerated. Adult patients can be advanced to 1.5 g/kg/d of protein and 40 kcal/kg/d of calories.

Patients who are refed too rapidly can develop a number of untoward clinical sequelae. During refeeding, circulating potassium, magnesium, phosphorus, and glucose move intracellularly and can result in low serum levels of each. The administration of water and sodium in combination with carbohydrate refeeding can overload hearts with depressed cardiac function and result in congestive heart failure. Enteral refeeding can result in malabsorption and diarrhea due to abnormalities in the gastrointestinal tract.

Refeeding edema is a benign condition that must be differentiated from congestive heart failure. Changes in renal sodium reabsorption and poor skin and blood vessel integrity result in the development of edema in dependent areas without other signs of congestive heart failure. Treatment is with reassurance, elevation of the dependent area, and modest sodium restriction. Diuretics are usually ineffective in this situation, may aggravate electrolyte deficiencies, and should not be used.

The prevention and early detection of protein-energy malnutrition in hospitalized patients require constant awareness of that possibility by the physicians and others responsible for their care. Each patient admitted to the hospital should be screened for risk factors. Patients at risk require formal assessment of nutritional status and close observation of dietary intake, body weight, and nutritional requirements during the hospital stay.

Baron RB: Protein-energy malnutrition. In: Bennet JC, Plum F (editors): *Cecil Textbook of Medicine,* 20th ed. Saunders, 1996.

Guirao X et al: Extracellular volume, nutritional status and refeeding changes. Nutrition 1994;10:558. (Strategies for identifying and preventing rapid increases in extracellular water during treatment of protein-energy malnutrition.)

Hardin TC: Cytokine mediators of malnutrition: Clinical implications. Nutr Clin Pract 1993;8:55. (Understanding the complex interactions of cytokines as mediators of intermediary metabolism may be increasingly important in the care of critically ill patients.)

Laviano A, Campos AC: The skeleton in the hospital closet 20 years later: Malnutrition in patients with GI disease, cancer and AIDS. Nutrition 1994;10:569. (Summary of 1995 conference reviewing the current prevalence of protein-energy malnutrition in hospitalized patients and current strategies for prevention and treatment.)

OBESITY

Essentials of Diagnosis

- Excess adipose tissue, resulting in body weight 20% or more in excess of expected ("desirable") weight.
- Upper body obesity (abdomen and flank) of greater health consequence than lower body obesity (buttocks and thighs).
- Associated with multiple metabolic and structural disorders.

General Considerations

Obesity is one of the most common disorders in medical practice and among the most frustrating and difficult to manage. Little progress has been made in obesity treatment in the last 25 years, yet major changes have occurred in our understanding of its causes and its implications for health.

Definition & Measurement

Obesity is defined as an excess of adipose tissue. The exact criterion for how much is too much is controversial. Accurate quantification of body fat requires sophisticated techniques not usually available in clinical practice. In most situations, physical examination is sufficient to detect excess body fat. Two methods commonly used for more quantitative evaluation are relative weight (RW) and body mass index (BMI).

Relative weight (RW) is the measured body weight divided by the "desirable weight" × 100. Desirable weight is defined as the midpoint value recommended for a given height in the weight tables published by the United States government (Table 29–7). Unfortunately, there is considerable controversy over which weight table best reflects the relationship between body weight and health. Weight tables published in 1990 allowed for a substantial increase in weight for height compared with earlier tables. Recent data, particularly from the Nurses' Health Study, suggest that earlier weight tables, such as the one published in 1985, are more accurate.

Because the RW does not differentiate between excess fat or "excess" muscle, the body mass index (BMI) can be used to more accurately reflect the presence of excess adipose tissue. The BMI is calculated by dividing measured body weight in kilograms by the height in meters squared. The "normal" BMI is 20–25 kg/m².

The National Institutes of Health currently define obesity as a relative weight over 120% (BMI > 27.5 kg/m²): Mild obesity is a relative weight of 120–140% (BMI 27.5–30 kg/m²); moderate obesity is a relative weight of 140–200% (BMI 30–40 kg/m²); and severe or "morbid" obesity is a relative weight over 200% (BMI > 40 kg/m²). Other factors besides total weight, however, are also important. Recent data suggest that upper body obesity (excess fat around the waist and flank) is a greater health hazard than lower body obesity (fat in the thighs and buttocks). Obese patients with high waist-hip ratios (> 1.0 in men; > 0.8 in women) have a significantly greater risk of diabetes mellitus, stroke, coronary artery disease, and early death than equally obese patients with lower ratios. Further differentiation of the location of excess fat suggests that visceral fat within the abdominal cavity is more hazardous to health than subcutaneous fat around the abdomen.

About 34% of people in the USA have relative weights in excess of 120%. Blacks—particularly black women—are more apt to be obese than whites, and the poor are more obese than the rich regardless of race.

Health Consequences of Obesity

Obesity is associated with significant increases in both morbidity and mortality. A great many disorders occur with greater frequency in obese people. The most important and common of these are hypertension, type II diabetes mellitus, hyperlipidemia, coronary artery disease, degenerative joint disease, and psychosocial disability; but certain cancers (colon, rectum, and prostate in men; uterus, biliary tract, breast, and ovary in women), thromboembolic disorders, digestive tract diseases (gallstones, reflux esophagitis), and skin disorders are also more prevalent in the obese. Surgical and obstetric risks are greater as well. Obese patients also have a greater risk of pulmonary functional impairment, endocrine abnormalities, proteinuria, and increased hemoglobin concentration.

The death rate increases in proportion to the degree of obesity: Relative weights of 130% are associated with an excess mortality rate of 35% and relative weights of 150% a greater than two-fold excess death rate. Patients with "morbid" obesity (relative weight > 200%) have as much as a ten-fold increase in death rate.

Etiology

Until recently, obesity was considered to be the direct result of a sedentary lifestyle plus chronic ingestion of excess calories. Obese people were *blamed* for being obese—by their friends and families, their employers, their physicians, and even by themselves. Although these factors are undoubtedly the principal cause of obesity in some cases, there is now evidence for strong genetic influences on the development of obesity. A recent study of 540 adopted children demonstrated a close relationship between their body mass index and that of their biologic parents. No such relationship was found between the children and their adoptive parents. Twin studies have also demonstrated substantial genetic influences on body mass index and little influence from the childhood environment. Although studies vary, as much as 50–75% of obesity can be explained by genetic influences.

Recent molecular genetic studies have confirmed important genetic determinants of some types of obesity. Studies in animals have identified a gene that when made useless by mutation causes obesity. The normal gene produces a protein called "leptin" that controls appetite. When leptin is defective, mice grow profoundly fat; when leptin is supplemented, the mice lose weight. Human studies have recently confirmed the existence of an almost identical human gene. Although mutations in this gene are rare, it is hypothesized that extra doses of leptin may be effective in reducing human obesity. Recently, a high-affinity receptor for leptin has been identified in the mouse hypothalamus and a possible leptin-induced satiety factor, glucagon-like peptide-1 (GLP-1), has been identified. Human studies have also identified a mutation in the gene for the β_3 receptor in adipose tissue, involved in lipolysis and thermogenesis, that markedly increases the risk of obesity.

These studies suggest that genetic factors may result in changes in both energy intake and energy expenditure. Further research will probably permit classification of obese patients into subgroups according to different etiologic features. Given our imperfect understanding of the causes of obesity, it is essential not to hold the patients personally responsible for their condition.

Medical Evaluation of the Obese Patient

The history and physical examination are the most important parts of the evaluation of obese patients. Historical information should be obtained about age at onset, recent weight changes, family history of obesity, occupational history, eating and exercise behavior, cigarette and alcohol use, previous weight loss experience, and psychosocial factors. Particular attention should be directed at use of laxatives, diuretics, hormones, nutritional supplements, and over-the-counter medications.

Physical examination should assess the degree and distribution of body fat, overall nutritional status, and signs of secondary causes of obesity.

Less than 1% of obese patients have an identifiable secondary cause of obesity. Hypothyroidism and Cushing's syndrome are important examples that can usually be diagnosed by physical examination in patients with unexplained recent weight gain. Such patients with physical findings suggesting hypothyroidism or Cushing's syndrome may require further endocrinologic evaluation, including serum TSH determination and dexamethasone suppression testing (see Chapter 26).

All obese patients should be evaluated for medical consequences of their obesity. Fasting levels of glucose, cholesterol, and triglycerides should be measured.

Treatment

There is no single effective method of treatment for obesity. Using conventional techniques, only 20% of patients will lose 20 lb and maintain the loss for over 2 years; 5% will maintain a 40-lb loss. Continued close provider-patient contact appears to be more important for success of treatment than the specific features of any given treatment regimen. Careful patient selection will improve success rates and lessen frustration of both patients and therapists. Only sufficiently motivated patients should enter treatment programs. Specific attempts to identify motivated patients—eg, requesting a 3-day diet record—are often useful.

Most successful programs employ a multidisciplinary approach to weight loss, with hypocaloric diets, behavior modification or other strategies to change eating behavior, aerobic exercise, and social support. Emphasis must be on *maintenance* of weight loss.

Dietary instructions should incorporate the same principles that apply to healthy people who are not obese, ie, a low-fat, high-complex carbohydrate, high-fiber diet. This is achieved by emphasizing intake of a wide variety of predominantly "unprocessed" foods. Special attention is usually paid to limiting foods that provide large amounts of calories without other nutrients, ie, fat, sucrose, and alcohol. There is no special advantage to diets that restrict carbohydrates, advocate large amounts of protein or fats, or recommend ingestion of foods one at a time.

Long-term changes in eating behavior are required to maintain weight loss. Although formal **behavior modification** programs are available to which patients can be referred, the clinician caring for obese patients can teach a number of useful behavioral techniques. The most important technique is to emphasize planning and record keeping. Patients can be taught to plan menus and exercise sessions and to record their actual behavior. Record keeping not only aids in behavioral change; the availability of records also helps the health care provider to make specific suggestions for problem solving. Patients can be taught to recognize "eating cues" (emotional, situational, etc) and how to avoid or control them. Reward systems and refundable financial contracts are also useful for many patients.

Exercise offers a number of advantages to patients

trying to lose weight and keep it off. Aerobic exercise directly increases the daily energy expenditure and is particularly useful for long-term weight maintenance. Exercise will also preserve lean body mass and partially prevent the decrease in basal energy expenditure seen with semistarvation.

Social support is essential for a successful weight loss program. Continued close contact with the therapist, family and peer group involvement, etc, are useful techniques for reinforcing behavioral change and preventing social isolation.

Patients with severe obesity may require more aggressive treatment regimens. **Very low calorie diets** (400–800 kcal/d) result in rapid weight loss and marked improvement in obesity-related metabolic complications. Side effects such as fatigue, orthostatic hypotension, cold intolerance, and fluid and electrolyte disorders are common and require regular supervision by a physician. Other less common complications include gout, gallbladder disease, and cardiac arrhythmias. Patients are commonly maintained on such programs for 4–6 months and lose an average of 2–4 lb a week. Long-term weight maintenance is less predictable and requires concurrent behavior modification and exercise. Recent studies suggest that 800 kcal diets are as effective as lower-calorie programs and are better tolerated.

Medications for the treatment of obesity include the amphetamines (with high abuse potential—DEA Schedule II); the nonamphetamine schedule IV appetite suppressants phentermine, diethylpropion, and mazindol; phenylpropanolamine; and the antidepressants fluoxetine and sertraline.

Controversy exists about the efficacy of these agents and the proper indications for their prescription. Confounding features of the dialogue include a widespread perception that obesity is caused simply by overeating, expectations that medications alone might be able to adequately treat obesity, limited research on long-term efficacy, and the abuse potential of some of the drugs.

Numerous studies of appetite suppressant drugs have been conducted. Although efficacy in producing weight loss has been documented for several agents, there have been alarming reports of toxicity, leading to withdrawal of FDA approval of dexfenfluramine and fenfluramine. Specifically, the combination of fenfluramine and phentermine has resulted in serious cardiac valvular abnormalities in a number of patients and one fatal case of pulmonary hypertension. Duration of therapy was short in many of the individuals with valvular disease—and less than a month in the patient with pulmonary hypertension.

Discontinuation of appetite suppressant drugs most commonly results in weight gain. Advocates of their use point out that stopping any successful medication results in recurrence of the condition being treated.

Proponents of these drugs also argue that long-term use of some of the approved medications is safe and efficacious, especially when they are used as adjuncts to a comprehensive weight loss program. Serious side effects, however, are a matter of continuing concern. In addition to the observations noted above, still another recent case-control study from Europe suggested an increased relative risk of pulmonary hypertension in patients using anorexiant drugs. In this study, the risks appeared to increase with longer duration of therapy.

Appetite suppressant drugs are contraindicated during pregnancy and lactation and in patients with renal, hepatic, or cardiac failure, severe systemic hypertension, pulmonary hypertension, glaucoma, or substance abuse. The serotonergic medications are contraindicated in patients using other pharmacologically similar agents such as antidepressants and drugs given for migraine.

Pharmacotherapy should be restricted to patients with a BMI $\geq$ 30 kg/m^2—or $\geq$ 27 kg/m^2 if there is obesity-related co-morbidity. Best results are observed in patients who enter a structured exercise program and adhere to dietary therapy. Those who meet these initial goals of diet and exercise are given 4 weeks of medication on the second visit. A third visit is scheduled 4 weeks later to monitor progress. Weight loss during the first 4 weeks on medications is the best predictor of success at 1 year. The optimal duration of therapy is not known, but patients should be monitored periodically for compliance and side effects. Medications are most rational for use in patients with chronic medical conditions (diabetes, hypertension, lipid disorders), in whom successful weight loss may lead to dosage reductions. Few data, however, support this hypothesis. When the relative merits and risks of diet versus pharmacologic management are explained, many patients will select a very low calorie diet rather than the drugs.

Although it is generally considered to be the last resort for the treatment of obesity, more than 100,000 obese patients have had **surgical therapy.** Few controlled trials exist, and the development of rational indications for surgery has been difficult. Most surgeons require relative weights greater than 200% before they will proceed. Gastric operations, such as the vertical-banded gastroplasty and gastric bypass procedures, are now the operations of choice. Although both types of procedures result in significant weight loss, direct comparisons tend to favor gastric bypass. The perioperative mortality rate averages less than 1% but ranges from nil to 4% at different centers. When reversals, revisions, and patients lost to follow-up are considered, failure rates approach 50%. Jejunoileal bypass operations have been abandoned by most surgeons owing to unacceptable long-term complications.

A recent concern has been the possible deleterious health effects of fluctuations of body weight produced by repeated cycles of weight loss and gain ("yo-yo dieting"). Numerous studies have evaluated the effect of weight fluctuations on coronary heart disease and all-cause mortality with mixed results. These concerns reinforce the common-sense approach to avoiding casual or short-lived attempts to lose weight. On the other hand, motivated individuals at risk for obesity-related illness should still be encouraged to lose weight, with particular emphasis on long-term weight maintenance.

Abenhaim L et al: Appetite-suppressant drugs and the risk of primary pulmonary hypertension. N Engl J Med 1996;335:609. (Case control study from Europe found a substantial increase in risk of primary pulmonary hypertension in individuals using appetite suppressant drugs.)

Brownell KD, Rodin J: The dieting maelstrom: Is it possible and advisable to lose weight? Am Psychol 1994;49:781. (An excellent recent review of dieting and weight loss.)

Carek PJ, Shere JT, Carson DS: Management of obesity: Medical treatment options. Am Fam Physician 1997; 55:551. (Behavior modification, including regular exercise and the development of healthy eating habits, remains the best hope for long-term weight loss. Surgery or medication should be reserved for special circumstances.)

Curfman GD: Diet pills redux. (Editorial.) N Engl J Med 1997;337:629. (Excellent summary of toxic effects of appetite suppressants, especially in combination. Two orginal articles appear on pages 581 and 602 of the same issue.)

Clément K et al: Genetic variation in β_3-adrenergic receptor and an increased capacity to gain weight in patients with morbid obesity. N Engl J Med 1995;333:352. (Genetics affect energy expenditure as well as energy intake.)

Leibel RL, Rosenbaum M, Hirsch J: Changes in energy expenditure resulting from altered body weight. N Engl J Med 1995;332:621. (Changes in body weight are associated with compensatory changes in energy expenditure that oppose the maintenance of the new weight.)

Lindpainter K: Finding an obesity gene: A tale of mice and men. N Engl J Med 1995;332:679. (A candidate gene for human obesity has been identified.)

Scott J: New chapter for the fat controller. Nature 1996;379:113. (Brief summary of the status of genetic investigation into the cause of obesity.)

Stahl KA, Imperiale TF: An overview of the efficacy and safety of fenfluramine and mazindol in the treatment of obesity. Arch Fam Med 1993;2:1033. (Medications result in modest short-term weight loss.)

EATING DISORDERS

ANOREXIA NERVOSA

Essentials of Diagnosis

- Disturbance of body image and intense fear of becoming fat.
- Weight loss leading to body weight 15% below expected.
- In females, absence of three consecutive menstrual cycles.

General Considerations

Anorexia nervosa characteristically begins in the years between adolescence and young adulthood. Approximately 90% of patients are females, most commonly from the middle and upper socioeconomic strata. The diagnosis is based on weight loss leading to body weight 15% below expected, a distorted body image, fear of weight gain or of loss of control over food intake, and, in females, the absence of at least three consecutive menstrual cycles. Other medical or psychiatric illnesses that can account for anorexia and weight loss must be excluded.

Recent studies suggest that the prevalence of anorexia nervosa is greater than previously suggested. In Rochester, Minnesota, for example, the prevalence of anorexia nervosa per 100,000 population is estimated to be about 270 for females and 22 for males. In Caucasian adolescent girls from middle- and upper-class families, anorexia nervosa is an even more common illness. Many other adolescent girls have features of the disorder without the severe weight loss.

The cause of anorexia nervosa is not known. Although multiple endocrinologic abnormalities exist in these patients, most authorities believe they are secondary to malnutrition and not primary disorders. Most authors favor a primary psychiatric origin, but no single psychiatric hypothesis satisfactorily explains all cases. The patient characteristically comes from a family whose members are highly goal- and achievement-oriented. Interpersonal relationships may be inadequate or destructive. The parents are usually overly directive and concerned with slimness and physical fitness, and much of the family conversation centers around dietary matters. One theory holds that the patient's refusal to eat is an attempt to regain control of her body in defiance of parental control. The patient's unwillingness to inhabit an "adult body" may also represent a rejection of adult responsibilities and the implications of adult interpersonal relationships. Patients are commonly perfectionistic in behavior and exhibit obsessional personality characteristics. Marked depression or anxiety may be present.

Clinical Findings

A. Symptoms and Signs: Clinically, patients with anorexia nervosa may exhibit severe emaciation and may complain of cold intolerance or constipation. Amenorrhea is almost always present. Bradycardia, hypotension, and hypothermia may be present in severe cases. Examination demonstrates loss of body fat, dry and scaly skin, and increased lanugo body hair. Parotid enlargement and edema may also be present.

B. Laboratory Findings: Laboratory findings are variable but may include anemia, leukopenia, electrolyte abnormalities, and elevations of BUN and serum creatinine. Serum cholesterol levels are often increased. Endocrine abnormalities include depressed levels of luteinizing and follicle-stimulating hormones and impaired response of LH to luteinizing hormone-releasing hormone.

Diagnosis & Differential Diagnosis

The diagnosis of anorexia nervosa can be difficult, since many common social and cultural factors promote and maintain anorexic behavior. Diagnosis depends upon identification of the common behavioral features and exclusion of medical disorders that would account for weight loss.

Behavioral features required for the diagnosis include intense fear of becoming obese, disturbance of body image, weight loss of at least 25%, and refusal to maintain body weight over a minimal normal weight.

The differential diagnosis includes endocrine and metabolic disorders such as panhypopituitarism, Addison's disease, hyperthyroidism, and diabetes mellitus; gastrointestinal disorders such as Crohn's disease and celiac sprue; chronic infections and cancers such as tuberculosis and lymphoma; and rare central nervous system disorders such as hypothalamic tumors.

Treatment

The goal of treatment is restoration of normal body weight and resolution of psychologic difficulties. Hospitalization is usually necessary for frank anorexia nervosa. Treatment programs conducted by experienced teams are successful in about two-thirds of cases, restoring normal weight and menstruation. One-half continue to experience difficulties with eating behavior and psychiatric problems. Occasional patients with anorexia develop obesity after treatment. Two to 6% of patients die from the complications of the disorder or commit suicide.

Various treatment methods have been used without clear evidence of superiority of one over another. Supportive care by physicians and nurses is probably the most important feature of therapy. Structured behavioral therapy, intensive psychotherapy, and family therapy may be tried. A variety of medications including tricyclic antidepressants, selective serotonin reuptake inhibitors, and lithium carbonate are effective in some cases. Patients with severe malnutrition must be hemodynamically stabilized and may require enteral or parenteral feeding. Forced feedings should be reserved for life-threatening situations, since the goal of treatment is to reestablish normal eating behavior.

Leach AM: The psychopharmacotherapy of eating disorders. Psychiatric Ann 1995;25:628. (Excellent review of medication options.)

Mehler PS: Eating disorders: 1. Anorexia nervosa. Hosp Pract (Off Ed) 1996 Jan;31:109. (Review from a general internist's perspective.)

Position of the American Dietetic Association: Nutrition intervention in the treatment of anorexia nervosa, bulimia nervosa, and binge eating. J Am Diet Assoc 1994; 94:902.

Practice guidelines for eating disorders: American Psychiatric Association. Am J Psychiatry 1993;150:212. (Current APA guidelines.)

Thiel A et al: Obsessive-compulsive disorder among patients with anorexia nervosa and bulimia nervosa. Am J Psychiatry 1995;152:72. (A high prevalence of obsessive-compulsive disorder was observed and correlated with severity of the eating disorder.)

Walters EE, Kendler KS: Anorexia nervosa and anorexic-like syndromes in a population-based female twin sample. Am J Psychiatry 1995;152:64. (A population-based descriptive analysis demonstrating a spectrum of anorexia-like syndromes and a familial pattern.)

BULIMIA NERVOSA

Essentials of Diagnosis

- Uncontrolled episodes of binge eating.
- Recurrent inappropriate compensation to prevent weight gain such as self-induced vomiting, laxatives, diuretics, fasting, or excessive exercise.
- A minimum average of two binge eating episodes a week for at least 3 months.
- Overconcern with weight and body shape.

General Considerations

Bulimia nervosa is the episodic uncontrolled ingestion of large quantities of food followed by recurrent inappropriate compensatory behavior in order to prevent weight gain such as self-induced vomiting, diuretics or cathartics, or strict dieting or vigorous exercise.

Like anorexia nervosa, bulimia nervosa is predominantly a disorder of young, white middle- and upper-class women. It is more difficult to detect than anorexia, and some studies have estimated the prevalence to be as high as 19% in college-age women.

Patients with bulimia nervosa typically consume large quantities of easily ingested high-calorie foods, usually in secrecy. Some patients may have several such episodes a day for a few days; others report regular and persistent patterns of binge eating. Binging is usually followed by vomiting, cathartics, or diuretics and is usually accompanied by feelings of guilt or depression. Periods of binging may be followed by intervals of self-imposed starvation. Body weights may fluctuate but generally are within 20% of desirable weights.

Some patients with bulimia nervosa also have a cryptic form of anorexia nervosa with significant weight losses and amenorrhea. Family and psychologic issues are generally similar to those encountered among patients with anorexia nervosa. Bulimics, however, have a higher incidence of premorbid obesity, greater use of cathartics and diuretics, and more impulsive or antisocial behaviors. Weights are closer to normal, and menstruation is usually preserved.

Depending on the type and severity of abnormal behavior, a variety of medical complications can occur. Gastric dilatation and pancreatitis have been reported after binges. Vomiting can result in poor dentition, pharyngitis, esophagitis, aspiration, and electrolyte abnormalities. Cathartic and diuretic abuse also commonly result in electrolyte abnormalities or dehydration. Constipation and hemorrhoids are common.

Treatment of bulimia and bulimarexia requires supportive care and psychotherapy. Individual, group, family, and behavioral therapy have all been utilized with modest success. Antidepressants may be helpful in some patients. The best published results to date have been with fluoxetine hydrochloride and other selective serotonin reuptake inhibitors. Although death from bulimia is rare, the long-term psychiatric prognosis in severe bulimia is worse than the prognosis in anorexia nervosa, which suggests that the underlying psychiatric disorder may be more severe.

Drewnowski A et al: Eating pathology and *DSM-III-R* bulimia nervosa: A continuum of behavior. Am J Psychiatry 1994;151:1217. (As with anorexia, a spectrum of bulimia was observed.)

Hetherington MM et al: Eating behavior in bulimia nervosa multiple meal analyses. Am J Clin Nutr 1994;60:864. (Bulimic patients exhibited chaotic eating patterns and high energy and fat intakes. Mood improved after both binging and purging, most significantly after purging.)

See also references under Anorexia Nervosa, above.

DISORDERS OF VITAMIN METABOLISM

Deficiencies of single vitamins are rarely encountered in current clinical practice, even in developing countries. Deficiencies of multiple vitamins are more commonly seen along with protein-calorie undernutrition. Although any cause of protein-calorie undernutrition can result in concurrent vitamin deficiency, most such instances are associated with malabsorption, alcoholism, medications, hemodialysis, total parenteral nutrition, food faddism, or inborn errors of metabolism.

Vitamin deficiency syndromes develop gradually.

Symptoms are commonly nonspecific, and the physical examination is rarely helpful in early diagnosis. Most characteristic physical findings, such as the perifollicular hemorrhages associated with vitamin C deficiency, are seen late in the course of the syndrome. Other characteristic physical findings, such as glossitis and cheilosis, are seen with deficiencies of many B vitamins. Such abnormalities strongly suggest the presence of a nutritional deficiency but do not indicate which nutrient is deficient.

Despite the relative ease of meeting the recommended daily allowances with a mixed diet, many adults in the USA take vitamin supplements. In fact, syndromes of vitamin excess may be more common than deficiency syndromes, particularly those due to excess of vitamins A, D, and B_6. Most claims for significant health benefits of such supplements, particularly those taken in megadoses, remain unsubstantiated.

Some vitamins can be used efficaciously as drugs. Derivatives of vitamin A are used to treat cystic acne and, more recently, skin wrinkles. Niacin is an effective medication for hyperlipidemia. Vitamin-responsive inborn errors of metabolism also commonly require pharmacologic doses of vitamins.

Greenberg ER, Sporn MB: Antioxidant vitamins, cancer and cardiovascular disease. N Engl J Med 1996; 334:1189.

Mertz W: A balanced approach to nutrition for health: The need for biologically essential minerals and vitamins. J Am Diet Assoc 1994;94:1259.

Russell RM, Suter PM: Vitamin requirements of elderly people: An update. Am J Clin Nutr 1993;58:4.

Sardesai VM: Role of antioxidants in health maintenance. Nutr Clin Pract 1995;10:19.

WATER-SOLUBLE VITAMINS

1. THIAMIN (B_1)

The primary role of thiamin is as precursor of thiamin pyrophosphate, a coenzyme required for several important biochemical reactions necessary for carbohydrate oxidation. Thiamin is also thought to have an independent role in nerve conduction in peripheral nerves. The recommended daily allowances of thiamin are listed in Table 29–1.

Thiamin Deficiency
   A. Clinical Findings: Most thiamin deficiency in the USA is due to alcoholism. Chronic alcoholics may have poor dietary intakes of thiamin and impaired thiamin absorption, metabolism, and storage. Thiamin deficiency is also associated with malabsorption, dialysis, and other causes of chronic protein-calorie undernutrition. Thiamin deficiency can be precipitated in patients with marginal thiamin status with intravenous dextrose solutions.

Early manifestations of thiamin deficiency include anorexia, muscle cramps, paresthesias, and irritability. Advanced deficiency affects chiefly the cardiovascular system ("wet beriberi") or the nervous system ("dry beriberi"). Wet beriberi occurs if severe physical exertion and high carbohydrate intakes accompany thiamin deficiency, whereas dry beriberi is seen with inactivity and low-calorie intake.

Beriberi heart disease is characterized by marked peripheral vasodilation resulting in classic high-output heart failure with dyspnea, tachycardia, cardiomegaly, and pulmonary and peripheral edema, with warm extremities mimicking cellulitis.

Involvement of the nervous system can include both the peripheral and the central nervous systems. Peripheral nerve involvement is typically a symmetric motor and sensory neuropathy with pain, paresthesias, and loss of reflexes. The legs are usually affected more than the arms. Central nervous system involvement results in Wernicke-Korsakoff syndrome. Wernicke's encephalopathy consists of nystagmus progressing to ophthalmoplegia, truncal ataxia, and confusion. Korsakoff's syndrome is characterized by amnesia, confabulation, and impaired learning.

B. Diagnosis: A variety of biochemical tests are available to assess thiamin deficiency. In most instances, however, the clinical response to empirical thiamine therapy is used to support a diagnosis of thiamin deficiency. The most commonly used and widely available biochemical tests are measurement of erythrocyte transketolase activity and urinary thiamin excretion. A transketolase activity coefficient greater than 15–20% suggests thiamin deficiency.

C. Treatment: Suspected thiamin deficiency should be treated promptly with large parenteral doses of thiamine. Fifty to 100 mg/d is typically administered for the first few days, followed by daily oral doses of 5–10 mg/d. All patients should simultaneously receive therapeutic doses of other water-soluble vitamins. Although treatment results in complete resolution in one-half of patients (one-fourth immediately and another one-fourth over days), the other half obtain only partial resolution or no benefit.

2. RIBOFLAVIN (B₂)

Riboflavin—as the coenzymes flavin mononucleotide and flavin adenine dinucleotide—participates in a variety of important oxidation-reduction reactions and is an essential component of a number of other enzymes. The recommended daily allowances of riboflavin are listed in Table 29–1.

Riboflavin Deficiency

A. Clinical Findings: Riboflavin deficiency almost always occurs in combination with deficiencies of other vitamins. Dietary inadequacy, interactions with a variety of medications, alcoholism, and other causes of protein-calorie undernutrition are the most common causes of riboflavin deficiency.

Manifestations of riboflavin deficiency include mouth soreness, cheilosis, angular stomatitis, glossitis, seborrheic dermatitis, weakness, corneal vascularization, and anemia.

B. Diagnosis: Riboflavin deficiency is usually treated empirically when the diagnosis is clinically suspected. Deficiency can be confirmed by measuring the riboflavin-dependent enzyme erythrocyte glutathione reductase. Activity coefficients greater than 1.2–1.3 are suggestive of riboflavin deficiency. Urinary riboflavin excretion and serum levels of plasma and red cell flavins can also be measured.

C. Treatment: Riboflavin deficiency is easily treated with riboflavin-containing foods such as meat, fish, and dairy products or with oral preparations of the vitamin. Administration of 5–15 mg/d until clinical findings are resolved is usually adequate. Riboflavin can also be given parenterally, but it is poorly soluble in aqueous solutions.

Riboflavin Toxicity

There is no known toxicity of riboflavin.

3. NIACIN

Niacin is a generic term for nicotinic acid and other derivatives with similar nutritional activity. Unlike most other vitamins, niacin can be synthesized by the human body from the essential amino acid tryptophan. Niacin is an essential component of the coenzymes nicotinamide adenine dinucleotide (NAD) and nicotinamide adenine dinucleotide phosphate (NADP), which are involved in many oxidation-reduction reactions. The recommended daily allowances of niacin are listed in Table 29–1; major food sources are protein foods containing tryptophan and numerous cereals, vegetables, and dairy products.

Niacin can also be used therapeutically for the treatment of hypercholesterolemia and hypertriglyceridemia. Daily doses of 3–6 g can result in significant reductions in levels of low-density lipoproteins (LDL) and very-low-density lipoproteins (VLDL) and in elevation of high-density lipoproteins (HDL). Niacinamide does not exhibit the lipid-lowering effects of nicotinic acid.

Niacin Deficiency

A. Clinical Findings: Historically, niacin deficiency occurred when corn, which is relatively deficient in both tryptophan and niacin, was the major source of calories. Currently, niacin deficiency is more commonly due to alcoholism and nutrient-drug interactions. Niacin deficiency can also occur in inborn errors of metabolism.

As with other B vitamins, the early manifestations of niacin deficiency are nonspecific. Common complaints include anorexia, weakness, irritability, mouth soreness, glossitis, stomatitis, and weight loss. More advanced deficiency results in the classic triad of pellagra: dermatitis, diarrhea, and dementia. The characteristic dermatitis is symmetric, involving sun-exposed areas. Skin lesions are dark, dry, and scaling. The dementia begins with insomnia, irritability, and apathy and progresses to confusion, memory loss, hallucinations, and psychosis. The diarrhea can be severe and may result in malabsorption due to atrophy of the intestinal villi. Advanced pellagra can result in death.

B. Diagnosis: In advanced cases, the diagnosis of pellagra can be made on clinical grounds. In early cases, diagnosis requires a high index of suspicion and attempts at confirmation of niacin deficiency. Niacin metabolites, particularly *N*-methylnicotinamide, can be measured in the urine. Low levels suggest niacin deficiency but may also be found in patients with generalized undernutrition. Serum and red cell levels of NAD and NADP are also low but are similarly nonspecific.

C. Treatment: Pellagra can be effectively treated with oral niacin, usually given as nicotinamide. Doses ranging from 10 to 150 mg/d have been used without difficulty.

Niacin Toxicity

At the high doses of niacin used to treat hyperlipidemia, side effects are common. These include cutaneous flushing (partially prevented by pretreatment with aspirin, 325 mg/d) and gastric irritation. Elevation of liver enzymes, hyperglycemia, and gout are less common untoward effects. Although sustained-release preparations of niacin cause less flushing, they are associated with a greater risk of fulminant hepatitis than immediate release and are rarely recommended.

Illingworth DR et al: Comparative effects of lovastatin and niacin in primary hypercholesterolemia: A prospective trial. Arch Intern Med 1994;154:1586. (Although lovastatin was better tolerated, niacin resulted in better overall lipid reduction.)

Lasagna L: Over-the-counter niacin. JAMA 1994;271:709. (An argument against OTC use of niacin.)

McKenney JM et al: A comparison of the efficacy and toxic effects of sustained- versus immediate-release niacin in hypercholesterolemic patients. JAMA 1994; 271:672. (The sustained-release forms of niacin are more hepatotoxic.)

4. VITAMIN B₆ (Pyridoxine)

Vitamin B_6 ("pyridoxine") is actually a group of closely related substances involved in intermediary metabolism. These include pyridoxine itself, pyridoxal, pyridoxamine, and their 5-phosphate esters. As the major coenzyme involved in the metabolism of amino acids, pyridoxal 5-phosphate is the most important. Pyridoxal phosphate is also required for the synthesis of heme. The recommended daily allowances of vitamin B_6 are listed in Table 29–1.

Vitamin B₆ Deficiency

A. Clinical Findings: Vitamin B_6 deficiency most commonly occurs as a result of interactions with medications—especially isoniazid, cycloserine, penicillamine, and oral contraceptives—or of alcoholism. A number of inborn errors of metabolism and other pyridoxine-responsive syndromes, particularly pyridoxine-responsive anemia, are not clearly due to vitamin deficiency but commonly respond to high doses of the vitamin.

Manifestations of vitamin B_6 deficiency result in a clinical syndrome similar to that seen with deficiencies of other B vitamins, including mouth soreness, glossitis, cheilosis, weakness, and irritability. Severe deficiency can result in peripheral neuropathy, anemia, and seizures.

B. Diagnosis: The diagnosis of vitamin B_6 deficiency can be confirmed by measurement of pyridoxal phosphate in blood. Normal levels are greater than 50 ng/mL.

C. Treatment: Vitamin B_6 deficiency can be effectively treated with oral vitamin B_6 supplements. Doses of 10–20 mg/d are usually adequate, though some patients taking medications that interfere with pyridoxine metabolism may need doses as high as 100 mg/d. Inborn errors of metabolism and the pyridoxine-responsive syndromes often require up to 600 mg/d.

Vitamin B_6 should be routinely prescribed for patients receiving medications (such as isoniazid) that interfere with pyridoxine metabolism to prevent vitamin B_6 deficiency. This is particularly true for elderly patients, the urban poor, and alcoholics, who are more likely to have diets marginally adequate in vitamin B_6.

Large doses of vitamin B_6 have also been advocated for treatment of premenstrual syndrome and carpal tunnel syndrome. No significant clinical benefits have been consistently demonstrated.

Vitamin B₆ Toxicity

A sensory neuropathy, at times irreversible, occurs in patients receiving large doses of vitamin B_6. Although most patients have taken 2 g or more per day, some patients have taken only 200 mg/d.

5. VITAMIN B₁₂ & FOLATE

Vitamin B_{12} (cobalamin) and folate are discussed in Chapter 13. The recommended daily allowances of vitamin B_{12} and folate are listed in Table 29–1. Vitamin B_{12} is abundant in meat and dairy products; fresh fruits and vegetables supply ample folic acid.

6. VITAMIN C (Ascorbic Acid)

Vitamin C is a potent antioxidant involved in many oxidation-reduction reactions and is also required for the synthesis of collagen. It increases the absorption of nonheme iron and is involved in tyrosine metabolism, wound healing, and drug metabolism. With the exception of collagen synthesis, the exact mechanism of action for most of these functions is poorly understood. The recommended daily allowances of vitamin C are listed in Table 29–1; major food sources are fresh fruits and vegetables.

Vitamin C Deficiency

A. Clinical Findings: Most cases of vitamin C deficiency seen in the USA are due to dietary inadequacy, most commonly in the urban poor, the elderly, and chronic alcoholics. Patients with chronic illnesses such as cancer and chronic renal failure and individuals who smoke cigarettes are also at risk for vitamin C deficiency. Infants 6–12 months of age whose diets are not supplemented with vitamin C or vitamin C-containing foods are also at high risk.

Early manifestations of vitamin C deficiency are nonspecific and include malaise and weakness. In more advanced stages, the typical features of scurvy develop. Manifestations may include perifollicular hemorrhages, perifollicular hyperkeratotic papules, petechiae and purpura, splinter hemorrhages, bleeding gums, joint hemorrhages, and subperiosteal hemorrhages. Anemia is common, and wound healing is impaired. The late stages of scurvy are characterized by edema, oliguria, neuropathy, intracerebral hemorrhage, and death.

B. Diagnosis: The diagnosis of advanced scurvy can be made clinically on the basis of the characteristic skin lesions and other manifestations. The diagnosis can be confirmed with decreased plasma ascorbic acid levels, typically below 0.1 mg/dL. Platelet levels can also be measured.

C. Treatment: Adult scurvy can be treated with 300–1000 mg of ascorbic acid per day. Improvement typically occurs, even in advanced cases, within days. Numerous epidemiologic studies have suggested that high intakes of vitamin C are associated with a decreased risk of cancer. Vitamin C may also protect against coronary heart disease by modifying blood cholesterol levels and preventing LDL-cholesterol from oxidation. A recent large study showed a significant decrease in all-cause and coronary heart disease mortality in individuals with high intakes (approximately 300–400 mg/d).

Vitamin C Toxicity

Although generally extremely safe, very large doses of vitamin C can have side effects. Most common are gastric irritation, flatulence, or diarrhea. Oxalate kidney stones are of theoretic concern because ascorbic acid is metabolized to oxalate, but stone formation has not been frequently reported. Vitamin C can also confuse common diagnostic tests by causing false-negative tests for fecal occult blood and both false-negative and false-positive tests for urine glucose.

FAT-SOLUBLE VITAMINS

1. VITAMIN A

Vitamin A (retinol) is a high-molecular-weight alcohol either ingested preformed or synthesized from plant carotenoids, particularly β-carotene. Isomers and derivatives of retinol are commonly called retinoids. Vitamin A is essential for normal retinal function and plays an important but still not fully understood role in cell growth and differentiation, particularly of epithelial cells. Vitamin A is also necessary for normal wound healing. The recommended daily allowances of vitamin A are listed in Table 29–1; the principal food sources are highly pigmented vegetables.

Because of its role in cell differentiation, vitamin A has been postulated to have a role in cancer prevention. The role of retinoids for chemoprevention of cancer is under intense investigation. The provitamin β-carotene may play an even more important role in prevention of cancer and heart disease by virtue of its antioxidant activity.

Vitamin A Deficiency

A. Clinical Findings: Vitamin A deficiency is one of the most common vitamin deficiency syndromes, particularly in developing countries. In many such regions, vitamin A deficiency is the most common cause of blindness. In the USA, vitamin A deficiency is usually due to fat malabsorption syndromes, alcoholism, or laxative abuse with mineral oil and occurs most commonly in the elderly and the urban poor.

Night blindness is the earliest symptom of vitamin A deficiency. Dryness of the conjunctiva (xerosis) and the development of small white patches on the conjunctiva (Bitot's spots) are early signs. Ulceration and necrosis of the cornea (keratomalacia), perforation, endophthalmitis, and blindness are late manifestations. Xerosis and hyperkeratinization of the skin and loss of taste may also occur.

B. Diagnosis: Abnormalities of dark adaptation are strongly suggestive of vitamin A deficiency. Serum levels below the normal range of 30–65 mg/dL are commonly seen in advanced deficiency.

C. Treatment: Night blindness, poor wound healing, and other signs of early deficiency can be effectively treated with 30,000 IU of vitamin A daily for 1 week. Advanced deficiency with corneal damage calls for administration of 20,000 units/kg for at least 5 days. The potential antioxidant effects of β-carotene can be achieved with supplements of 25,000–50,000 IU of β-carotene.

Vitamin A Toxicity

Excess intake of β-carotenes (hypercarotenosis) results in staining of the skin a yellow-orange color but is otherwise benign. Skin changes are most marked on the palms and soles, while the scleras remain white, clearly distinguishing hypercarotenosis from jaundice. Large doses of β-carotene are otherwise safe.

Excessive vitamin A (hypervitaminosis A), on the other hand, can be quite toxic. Chronic toxicity usually occurs after ingestion of daily doses of over 50,000 units/d for more than 3 months. Early manifestations include dry, scaly skin, hair loss, mouth sores, painful hyperostoses, anorexia, and vomiting. More serious findings include increased intracranial pressure, with papilledema, headaches, and decreased cognition; and hepatomegaly, occasionally progressing to cirrhosis. Acute toxicity can result from ingestion of massive doses of vitamin A, such as in drug overdoses or consumption of polar bear liver. Manifestations include nausea, vomiting, abdominal pain, headache, papilledema, and lethargy.

The diagnosis can be confirmed by elevations of serum vitamin A levels. The only treatment is withdrawal of vitamin A from the diet. Most symptoms and signs improve rapidly.

Bates CJ: Vitamin A. Lancet 1995;345:31.

2. VITAMIN D

Vitamin D is discussed in Chapter 26. The recommended daily allowances of vitamin D are listed in Table 29–1; a major food source is fortified milk, but sunlight on the skin is a prime resource as well.

3. VITAMIN E

Vitamin E activity is derived from at least eight naturally occurring tocopherols, the most potent of which is α-tocopherol. Although the exact function and mechanism of action of vitamin E in humans are unclear, it is commonly thought to function as an antioxidant, protecting membranes and other cellular structures from attack by free radicals. Dietary selenium and other antioxidants work in conjunction with vitamin E and may partially spare its requirement and reverse signs of vitamin E deficiency in animals. The recommended daily allowances of vitamin E are listed in Table 29–1; the major food source is vegetable seed oil.

Vitamin E, like β-carotene and vitamin C, may also play a role in protection against cancer, coronary heart disease, and cataracts through its antioxidant function.

Vitamin E Deficiency

A. Clinical Findings: Clinical deficiency of vitamin E is most commonly due to severe malabsorption, the genetic disorder abetalipoproteinemia, or, in children with chronic cholestatic liver disease, biliary atresia or cystic fibrosis. Manifestations of deficiency include areflexia, disturbances of gait, decreased proprioception and vibration, and ophthalmoplegia.

B. Diagnosis: Plasma vitamin E levels can be measured; normal levels are 0.5–0.7 mg/dL or higher. Since vitamin E is normally transported in lipoproteins, the serum level should be interpreted in relation to circulating lipids.

C. Treatment: The optimum therapeutic dose of vitamin E has not been clearly defined. Large doses, often administered parenterally, can be used to improve the neurologic complications seen in abetalipoproteinemia and cholestatic liver disease. The potential antioxidant benefits of vitamin E can be achieved with supplements of 100–400 units/d.

Vitamin E Toxicity

Vitamin E is the least toxic of the fat-soluble vitamins. Large doses, 20–80 times the recommended daily requirement, have been taken for extended periods of time without apparent harm, although nausea, flatulence, and diarrhea have been reported. Large doses of vitamin E can increase the vitamin K requirement and can result in bleeding in patients taking oral anticoagulants.

Kushi LH et al: Dietary antioxidant vitamins and death from coronary heart disease in postmenopausal women. N Engl J Med 1996;334:1156. (Large observational study suggesting reduction in coronary heart disease with increased vitamin E in foods.)
Meydani M: Vitamin E. Lancet 1995;345:170.
Rapola JM et al: Effect of vitamin E and beta carotene on the incidence of angina pectoris: A randomized, double blind controlled trial. JAMA 1996;275:693. (Vitamin E was associated with a minor decrease in incidence of angina. Beta-carotene was associated with a slight increase.)
Stephens NG: Randomised controlled trial of vitamin E in patients with coronary heart disease: Cambridge Heart Antioxidant Study (CHAOS). Lancet 1996;347:781. (Vitamin supplementation reduced the risk of nonfatal myocardial infarctions.)

4. VITAMIN K

Vitamin K is discussed in Chapter 13. The recommended daily allowances of vitamin K are listed in Table 29–1. It is synthesized by intestinal bacteria.

DIET THERAPY

Specific therapeutic diets can be designed to facilitate the medical management of most common illnesses. In most cases, consultation with a registered dietitian is necessary in order to design and implement major dietary changes. Physicians should be familiar with the indications for special diets and their basic composition to facilitate patient referrals and to maximize patient compliance.

Diet therapy is a difficult process, and not all patients are able to cooperate fully. Before starting specific dietary changes, one should assess the patient's motivation for change in eating habits. Patients who are not adequately motivated or who for other reasons are unable to change their diets should not be started on diet therapy, since embarking on a course that can only fail will interfere with other aspects of the therapeutic relationship between doctor and patient. Requesting the patient to record dietary intake for 3–5 days may provide useful insight into the patient's motivation.

Prescribed diets should take into account personal food preferences, cultural habits, and eating behavior. Changes should be introduced gradually. Close follow-up and a close patient-therapist relationship are necessary for sustained dietary change.

Therapeutic diets can be divided into three groups: (1) diets that alter the consistency of food; (2) diets that restrict or otherwise modify dietary components; and (3) diets that supplement dietary components.

DIETS THAT ALTER CONSISTENCY

Clear Liquid Diet

This diet provides adequate water, 500–1000 kcal as simple sugar, and some electrolytes. It is fiber-free and requires minimal digestion or intestinal motility.

A clear liquid diet is useful for patients with resolving postoperative ileus, acute gastroenteritis, partial intestinal obstruction, and as preparation for diagnostic gastrointestinal procedures. It is commonly used as the first diet for patients who have been taking nothing by mouth for long periods. Because of the low calorie and minimal protein content of the clear liquid diet, it should be used only for short periods.

Full Liquid Diet

The full liquid diet provides adequate water and can be designed to provide adequate calories and protein. Vitamins and minerals—especially folic acid, iron, and vitamin B_6—may be inadequate and should be provided in the form of supplements. Dairy products, soups, eggs, and soft cereals are used to supplement clear liquids. Commercial oral supplements can also be incorporated into the diet or used alone.

This diet is low in residue and can be used in many instances instead of the clear liquid diet described above—especially in patients with difficulty in chewing or swallowing, with partial obstructions, or in preparation for some diagnostic procedures. Full liquid diets are commonly used following clear liquid diets to "advance" diets in patients who have been taking nothing by mouth for long periods.

Soft Diets

Soft diets are designed for patients unable to chew or swallow hard or coarse food. Tender foods are used, and most raw fruits and vegetables and coarse breads and cereals are eliminated. Soft diets are commonly used to assist in progression from full liquid diets to regular diets in postoperative patients and patients who are too weak or those whose dentition is too poor to handle a general diet.

Mechanical soft diets include chopped, ground, and pureed foods as well as any foods patients are able to masticate. These diets are used for head and neck surgical patients, those with dental problems and esophageal strictures, and other patients who have difficulty with chewing or swallowing.

The soft diet can be designed to meet all nutritional requirements.

DIETS THAT RESTRICT NUTRIENTS

Diets can be designed to restrict (or eliminate) virtually any nutrient or food component. The most commonly used restricted diets are those that limit sodium, fat, and protein. Other restrictive diets include gluten restriction in sprue, potassium and phosphate reduction in renal insufficiency, and various elimination diets for food allergies.

Sodium-Restricted Diets

Low-sodium diets are useful in the management of hypertension and in conditions in which sodium retention and edema are prominent features, particularly congestive heart failure, chronic liver disease, and chronic renal failure. Sodium restriction is beneficial with or without diuretic therapy. When used in conjunction with diuretics, sodium restriction allows lower dosage of the diuretic medication and may prevent side effects. Potassium excretion, in particular, is directly related to distal renal tubule sodium delivery, and sodium restriction will decrease diuretic-related potassium losses.

Typical American diets contain about 4–6 g (175–260 meq) of sodium per day. A no-added-salt diet contains approximately 3 g of sodium (132 meq) per day. Further restriction can be achieved with sodium diets 2 g or 1 g per day. Diets with more severe restriction are poorly accepted by patients and are rarely used.

Dietary sodium includes sodium naturally occurring in foods, sodium added during food processing, and sodium added by the consumer during cooking and at the table. About a third of current dietary intake is derived from each. Diets that allow 2000 mg of sodium daily are easiest to design and implement. Such diets generally eliminate added salt, most processed foods, and selected foods with particularly high sodium content. Patients who follow such diets for 2–3 months lose their craving for salty foods and can often continue to restrict their sodium intake indefinitely. Many patients with mild hypertension will achieve significant reductions in blood pressure (approximately 5 mm Hg diastolic) with this degree of sodium restriction. Other patients require more severe sodium restriction (approximately 1000 mg of sodium per day) for reduction in blood pressure, and others may actually have increased blood pressure with sodium restriction.

Diets allowing 1000 mg of sodium require further restriction of commonly eaten foods. Special "low-sodium" products are now available to facilitate such diets. These diets are difficult for most people to follow and are generally reserved for hospitalized patients and highly motivated outpatients—most commonly those with severe liver disease and ascites.

Fat-Restricted Diets

Traditional fat-restricted diets are useful in the treatment of fat malabsorption syndromes. Such diets will improve the symptoms of diarrhea with steatorrhea independently of the primary physiologic abnormality by limiting the quantity of fatty acids that reach the colon. The degree of fat restriction necessary to control symptoms must be individualized. Patients with severe malabsorption can be limited to 40–60 g of fat per day. Diets containing 60–80 g of fat per day can be designed for patients with less severe abnormalities.

In general, fat-restricted diets require broiling, baking, or boiling meat and fish; discarding the skin of poultry and fish and using those foods as the main protein source; using nonfat dairy products; and avoiding desserts, sauces, and gravies.

Low-Cholesterol, Low-Saturated-Fat Diets

Fat-restricted diets that specifically restrict saturated fats and dietary cholesterol are the mainstay of dietary treatment of hyperlipidemia (see Chapter 28). Similar diets are recommended also for diabetes (Chapter 27) and for the prevention of coronary artery disease (Chapter 10). Current recommendations for the prevention of cancer by dietary modification also include fat restriction.

The aim of these diets is to restrict total fat to 30% of calories and to achieve a normal body weight by caloric restriction. Saturated fat and dietary cholesterol are further restricted. In the first phase of treatment ("step 1"), saturated fat is restricted to 10% of total calories and dietary cholesterol to 300 mg/d. "Step 2" consists of further reduction of saturated fat to 7% of total calories and dietary cholesterol to 200 mg/d. In both cases, up to 10% of calories is derived from polyunsaturated fats and 10–15% is monounsaturated. In both diets also, 50–60% of calories is from carbohydrates, particularly complex carbohydrates high in dietary fiber. Ideally, the "step 1" diet can lead to a decrease in serum cholesterol of 15–20% and the "step 2" diet a further 5% reduction.

Protein-Restricted Diets

Protein-restricted diets are most commonly used in patients with hepatic encephalopathy due to chronic liver disease and in patients with renal failure to ameliorate the progression of early disease and to decrease symptoms of uremia in more severe disease. Patients with selected inborn errors of amino acid metabolism and other abnormalities resulting in hyperammonemia also require restriction of protein or of specific amino acids.

Protein restriction is intended to limit the production of nitrogenous waste products. Energy intake must be adequate to facilitate the efficient use of dietary protein. Proteins must be of high biologic value and be provided in sufficient quantity to meet minimal requirements. For most patients, the diet should contain at least 0.6 g/kg/d of protein. Patients with encephalopathy who fail to respond to this degree of restriction are unlikely to respond to more severe restriction.

DIETS THAT SUPPLEMENT NUTRIENTS

High-Fiber Diet

Dietary fiber is a diverse group of plant constituents that are resistant to digestion by the human digestive tract. Typical American diets contain about 5–10 g of dietary fiber per day. Epidemiologic evidence has suggested that populations consuming greater quantities of fiber have a lower incidence of certain gastrointestinal disorders, including diverticulitis and colon cancer. Most authorities currently recommend higher intakes of dietary fiber for health maintenance.

Diets high in dietary fiber (20–35 g/d) are also commonly used in management of a variety of gastrointestinal disorders, particularly the irritable bowel syndrome and recurrent diverticulitis. Diets high in fiber may also be useful to reduce blood sugar in patients with diabetes and to reduce cholesterol levels in patients with hypercholesterolemia. Such diets include greater intakes of fresh fruits and vegetables, whole grains, legumes and seeds, and bran products. For some patients, the addition of psyllium seed (2 tsp per day) or natural bran (½ cup per day) may be preferable.

High-Potassium Diets

Potassium-supplemented diets are used most commonly to compensate for potassium losses caused by diuretics. Although potassium losses can be partially prevented by using lower doses of diuretics, concurrent sodium restriction, and potassium-sparing diuretics, some patients require additional potassium to prevent hypokalemia. Epidemiologic and experimental evidence suggests that high-potassium diets may also have a direct antihypertensive effect. Typical American diets contain about 3 g (80 meq) of potassium per day. High-potassium diets commonly contain 4.5–7 g (120–180 meq) of potassium per day.

Most fruits, vegetables, and their juices contain high concentrations of potassium (see Chapter 21). Supplemental potassium can also be provided with potassium-containing salt substitutes (up to 20 meq in ¼ tsp) or as potassium chloride in solution or capsules, but this is rarely necessary if the above measures are followed to prevent potassium losses and supplement dietary potassium.

High-Calcium Diets

Additional intakes of dietary calcium have recently been recommended for the prevention of postmenopausal osteoporosis, the prevention and treatment of hypertension, and the prevention of colon cancer. Although the evidence in each case is preliminary, most authorities currently recommend intakes of 1 g of calcium per day for most adults and 1.5 g/d for postmenopausal women. Current USA intakes are approximately 700 mg/d.

Low-fat and nonfat dairy products are the mainstay of supplemental calcium intakes. Patients with lactose intolerance who cannot tolerate liquid dairy products may be able to tolerate nonliquid products such as cheese and yogurt. Leafy green vegetables and canned fish with bones also contain high concentrations of calcium, although the latter is also very high in sodium.

[Optimal calcium intake.] gopher://gopher.nih.gov/11/clin/cdcs/individual/97.calcm

Denke MA, Grundy SM: Individual responses to a cholesterol-lowering diet in 50 men with moderate hypercholesterolemia. Arch Intern Med 1994;154:317. (Cholesterol-lowering diets in men resulted in a 15 mg/dL reduction in LDL-cholesterol and no change in HDL-cholesterol. The range of responses was quite large, however, including substantial increases in LDL-cholesterol in some subjects.)

Denke MA: Individual responsiveness to a cholesterol-lowering diet in postmenopausal women with moderate hypercholesterolemia. Arch Intern Med 1994;154:1977. (Cholesterol-lowering diets in women resulted in an 11 mg/dL reduction in LDL-cholesterol and a concurrent 3 mg/dL reduction in HDL-cholesterol. As with men, the range of responses was large, including substantial increases in LDL-cholesterol in some subjects.)

Expert Panel: Summary of the second report of the National Cholesterol Education Program (NCEP): Expert panel on detection, evaluation, and treatment of high blood cholesterol in adults. JAMA 1993;269:3015. (A thorough discussion of diet therapy for high blood cholesterol.)

National High Blood Pressure Education Working Group Report on primary prevention of hypertension. Arch Intern Med 1993;153:186. (Comprehensive review of diet and blood pressure.)

Pearson TA, Patel RV: The great quest for a cholesterol-decreasing diet: Should we subtract, substitute, or supplement? Ann Intern Med 1993;119:627. (Alternative strategies for cholesterol lowering.)

Position Statement: Nutrition recommendations and principles for people with diabetes mellitus. Diabetes Care 1994;17:519.

Tinker LF, Heins JM, Holler HJ: Commentary and translation: 1994 nutrition recommendations for diabetes. J Am Diet Assoc 1994;94:507. (1994 recommendations of the American Diabetes Association and American Dietetic Association emphasize much greater individualization of nutrition therapy for diabetics, particularly regarding carbohydrate and fat intake.)

NUTRITIONAL SUPPORT

Nutritional support is the provision of nutrients to patients who cannot meet their nutritional requirements by eating standard diets. Nutrients may be delivered enterally, using oral nutritional supplements, nasogastric and nasoduodenal feeding tubes, and tube enterostomies; or parenterally, using lines or catheters placed in peripheral or central veins, respectively. Current nutritional support techniques permit adequate nutrient delivery to virtually any patient. Nutrition support should only be utilized, however, if it is likely to improve the patient's clinical outcome. The financial costs and risks of side effects must be balanced against the potential advantages of improved nutritional status in each clinical situation.

INDICATIONS FOR NUTRITIONAL SUPPORT

The precise indications for nutritional support remain controversial. Most authorities agree that nutritional support is indicated for at least four groups of adult patients: (1) those with inadequate bowel syndromes; (2) those with severe prolonged hypercatabolic states (eg, due to extensive burns, multiple trauma, mechanical ventilation); (3) those requiring prolonged therapeutic bowel rest; and (4) those with severe protein-calorie undernutrition with a treatable disease who have sustained a loss of over 25% of body weight.

It has been difficult to prove the efficacy of nutritional support in the treatment of most other conditions. Over 100 randomized controlled clinical trials have been conducted in an attempt to address this question. In most cases it has not been possible to show a clear advantage of treatment by means of nutritional support over treatment without such support. Unfortunately, most of these studies have design flaws and do not disprove the effectiveness of nutritional support.

The American Society for Parenteral and Enteral Nutrition (ASPEN) has published recommendations for the rational use of nutritional support. The recommendations emphasize the need to individualize the decision to begin nutritional support, carefully weighing the risks and costs against the benefit to each patient. They also demonstrate the need to identify high-risk malnourished patients by nutritional assessment.

NUTRITIONAL SUPPORT METHODS

Selection of the most appropriate nutritional support method involves consideration of gastrointestinal function, the anticipated duration of nutritional support, and the ability of each method to meet the patient's nutritional requirements. The method chosen should meet the patient's nutritional needs with the lowest risk and lowest cost possible. For most patients, enteral feeding is safer and cheaper and offers significant physiologic advantages. An algorithm for

selection of the most appropriate nutritional support method is presented in Figure 29–2.

Prior to initiating specialized enteral nutritional support, efforts should be made to supplement food intake. Careful attention to patient preferences, timing of meals, diagnostic procedures and use of medications, and the use of foods brought to the hospital by family and friends can often significantly increase oral intake. Patients unable to eat enough at regular mealtimes to meet their nutritional requirements can be given **oral supplements** as snacks or to replace low-calorie beverages. Supplements of differing nutritional composition are available for the purpose of individualizing the diet in accordance with specific clinical requirements. Fiber and lactose content, caloric density, protein level, and amino acid profiles can all be modified as necessary.

Patients unable to take adequate oral nutrients who have functioning gastrointestinal tracts and who meet the criteria for nutritional support are candidates for **tube feedings.** Small-bore feeding tubes are placed via the nose into the stomach or duodenum. Patients able to sit up in bed who can protect their airways can be fed into the stomach. Because of the increased risk of aspiration, patients who cannot adequately protect their airways should be fed nasoduodenally. Feeding tubes can be passed into the duodenum by leaving an extra length of tubing and placing the patient in the right decubitus position. Metoclopramide, 10 mg intravenously, can be given 20 minutes prior to insertion and continued every 6 hours thereafter to facilitate passage through the pylorus. Occasionally patients will require fluoroscopy or endoscopic guidance to insert the tube distal to the pylorus. Placement of nasogastric and, particularly, nasoduodenal tubes should be confirmed radiographically before delivery of feeding solutions.

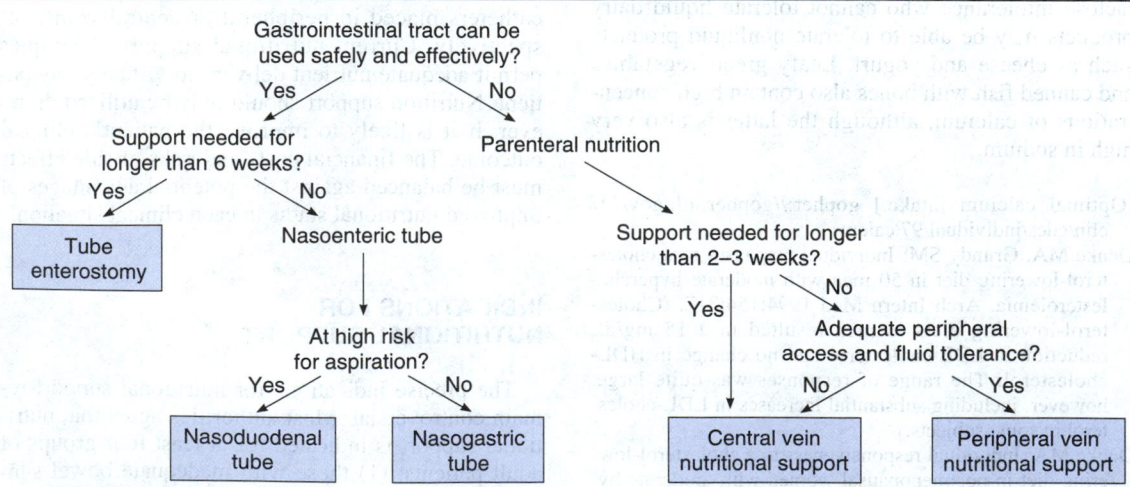

Figure 29–2. Nutritional support method decision tree.

Feeding tubes can also be placed directly into the gastrointestinal tract using **tube enterostomies.** Most tube enterostomies are placed in patients who require long-term enteral nutritional support. The most common application is the surgical placement of gastrostomies and jejunostomies. Gastrostomies have the advantage of allowing bolus feedings, while jejunostomies require continuous infusions. Gastrostomies—like nasogastric feeding—should only be used in patients at low risk for aspiration. Gastrostomies can also be placed percutaneously with the aid of endoscopy. These tubes can then be advanced to jejunostomies. Tube enterostomies can also be used in patients with unrelievable obstructions.

Patients who require nutritional support but whose gastrointestinal tracts are nonfunctional should receive **parenteral nutritional support.** Most patients receive parenteral feedings via a central vein—most commonly the subclavian vein. Peripheral veins can be used in some patients, but because of the high osmolality of parenteral solutions this is rarely tolerated for long periods.

Peripheral vein nutritional support is most commonly used in patients with nonfunctioning gastrointestinal tracts who require immediate support but whose clinical status is expected to improve within 1–2 weeks, allowing enteral feeding. Peripheral vein nutritional support is administered via standard intravenous lines. Solutions should always include lipid and dextrose in combination with amino acids to provide adequate nonprotein calories. Serious side effects are infrequent, but there is a high incidence of phlebitis and infiltration of intravenous lines.

Central vein nutritional support is most commonly delivered via intravenous catheters placed percutaneously using aseptic technique. Proper placement in the superior vena cava is documented radiographically before the solution is allowed to start running. Catheters must be carefully maintained by experienced nursing personnel and not used for anything other than nutritional support.

NUTRITIONAL REQUIREMENTS

Each patient's nutritional requirements should be determined independently of the method chosen. In most situations, solutions of equal nutrient value can be designed for delivery via enteral and parenteral routes, but differences in absorption must be considered. A complete nutritional support solution must contain water, energy, amino acids, electrolytes, vitamins, minerals, and essential fatty acids.

Water

For most patients, water requirements can be calculated by allowing 1500 mL for the first 20 kg of body weight plus 20 mL for every kilogram over 20.

Additional losses should be replaced as they occur. For average-sized adult patients, fluid needs are about 30–35 mL/kg, or approximately 1 mL/kcal of energy required (see below).

Energy

Energy requirements can be estimated by one of three methods: (1) by using standard equations to calculate resting energy expenditure (REE) plus additional calories for activity and illness; (2) by applying a simple calculation based on calories per kilogram of body weight; or (3) by measuring energy expenditure with indirect calorimetry.

Resting energy expenditure (REE) can be calculated by the **Harris-Benedict equation:** for men, REE = 66 + (13.7 × weight in kg) + (5 × height in cm) − (6.8 × age in years). For women, REE = 655 + (9.5 × weight in kg) + (1.7 × height in cm) − (4.7 × age). For undernourished patients, actual body weight should be used; and for obese patients, ideal body weight should be used. For most patients, an additional 20–50% of REE is administered as nonprotein calories to accommodate energy expenditures during activity or relating to the illness. Occasional patients are noted to have energy expenditures greater than 150% of REE.

Energy requirements can be estimated also by multiplying actual body weight in kilograms (for obese patients, ideal body weight) by 30–35 kcal.

Both of these methods provide imprecise estimates of actual energy expenditures, especially for the markedly underweight, overweight, and critically ill patient. Studies using indirect calorimetry have demonstrated that as many as 30–40% of patients will have measured expenditures 10% above or below estimated values. For accurate determination of energy expenditure, indirect calorimetry should be used.

Protein

Protein and energy requirements are closely related. If adequate calories are provided, most patients can be given 0.8–1.2 g of protein per kilogram per day. Patients undergoing moderate to severe stress should receive up to 1.5 g/kg/d. As in the case of energy requirements, actual weights should be used for normal and underweight patients and ideal weights for patients with significant obesity.

Patients who are receiving protein without adequate calories will catabolize protein for energy rather than utilizing it for protein synthesis. Thus, when energy intake is low, excess protein is needed for nitrogen balance. If both energy and protein intakes are low, extra energy will have a more significant positive effect on nitrogen balance than extra protein.

Electrolytes & Minerals

Requirements for sodium, potassium, and chloride vary widely. Most patients require 45–145 meq/d of each. The actual requirement in individual patients will depend on the patient's cardiovascular, renal, endocrine, and gastrointestinal status as well as measurements of serum concentration.

Patients receiving enteral nutritional support should receive adequate vitamins and minerals according to the recommended daily allowances (Table 29–1). Most premixed enteral solutions provide adequate vitamins and minerals as long as adequate calories are administered.

Patients receiving parenteral nutritional support require smaller amounts of minerals: calcium, 10–15 meq/d; phosphorus, 15–20 meq per 1000 nonprotein calories; and magnesium, 16–24 meq/d. Most patients receiving nutritional support do not require supplemental iron because body stores are adequate. Iron nutrition should be monitored closely by following the hemoglobin concentration, MCV, and iron studies. Parenteral administration of iron is associated with a number of adverse effects and should be reserved for iron-deficient patients unable to take oral iron.

Patients receiving parenteral nutritional support should be given the trace elements zinc (about 5 mg/d) and copper (about 2 mg/d). Patients with diarrhea will require additional zinc to replace fecal losses. Additional trace elements—especially chromium, manganese, and selenium—are provided to patients receiving long-term parenteral nutrition.

Parenteral vitamins are provided daily. Standardized multivitamin solutions are currently available to provide adequate quantities of vitamins A, B_{12}, C, D, E, thiamin, riboflavin, niacin, pantothenic acid, pyridoxine, folic acid, and biotin. Vitamin K is not given routinely but administered when the prothrombin time becomes abnormal.

Essential Fatty Acids

Patients receiving nutritional support should be given 2–4% of their total calories as linoleic acid to prevent essential fatty acid deficiency. Most prepared enteral solutions contain adequate linoleic acid. Patients receiving parenteral nutrition should be given at least 250 mL of a 20% intravenous fat (emulsified soybean or safflower oil) about two or three times a week. Intravenous fat can also be used as an energy source in place of dextrose.

ENTERAL NUTRITIONAL SUPPORT SOLUTIONS

Most patients who require enteral nutritional support can be given commercially prepared enteral solutions (Table 29–8). Nutritionally complete solutions have been designed to provide adequate proportions of water, energy, protein, and micronutrients. Nutritionally incomplete solutions are also available to provide specific macronutrients (eg, protein, carbohydrate, and fat) to supplement complete

Table 29–8. Enteral solutions.

Complete

Blenderized (eg, Compleat Regular, Compleat Modified,[1] Vitaneed[1])

Whole protein, lactose-containing (eg, Meritene, Carnation and Delmark Instant Breakfast, Forta Shake)

Whole protein, lactose-free, low-residue:
- 1 kcal/mL (eg, Ensure, Isocal, Osmolite, Nutren 1.0,[1] Nutrilan, Isolan,[1] Sustacal, Resource)
- 1.5 kcal/mL (eg, Ensure Plus, Sustacal HC, Comply, Nutren 1.5, Resource Plus)
- 2 kcal/mL (eg, Isocal HCN, Magnacal, TwoCal HN)
- High-nitrogen: > 15% total calories from protein (eg, Ensure HN, Attain,[1] Osmolite HN,[1] Replete, Entrition HN,[1] Isolan,[1] Isocal HN,[1] Sustacal HC, Isosource HN,[1] Ultralan)

Whole protein, lactose-free, high-residue:
- 1 kcal/mL (eg, Jevity,[1] Profiber,[1] Nutren 1.0 with fiber,[1] Fiberlan,[1] Sustacal with fiber, Ultracal,[1] Ensure with fiber, Fibersource)

Chemically defined peptide- or amino acid-based (eg, Accupep HPF, Criticare HN, Peptamen,[1] Reablin, Vital HN, AlitraQ, Tolerex, Vivonex TEN)

"Disease-specific" formulas:
- Renal failure: with essential amino acids (eg, Amin-Aid, Travasorb Renal, Aminess)
- Malabsorption: with medium-chain triglycerides (eg, Portagen,[1] Travasorb MCT)
- Respiratory failure: with > 50% calories from fat (eg, Pulmocare, NutriVent)
- Hepatic encephalopathy: with high amounts of branched-chain amino acids (eg, Hepatic-Acid II, Travasorb Hepatic)

Incomplete (modular)

Protein (eg, Nutrisource Protein, Promed, Propac)

Carbohydrate (eg, Nutrisource Carbohydrate, Polycose, Sumacal)

Fat (eg, MCT Oil, Microlipid, Nutrisource Lipid)

Vitamins (eg, Nutrisource Vitamins)

Minerals (eg, Nutrisource Minerals)

[1]Isotonic.

solutions for patients with unusual requirements or to design solutions that are not available commercially.

Nutritionally complete solutions are characterized as follows: (1) by osmolality (isotonic or hypertonic), (2) by lactose content (present or absent), (3) by the molecular form of the protein component (intact proteins; peptides or amino acids), (4) by the quantity of protein and calories provided, and (5) by fiber content (present or absent). For most patients, isotonic solutions containing no lactose or fiber are preferable. Such solutions generally contain moderate amounts of fat and intact protein. Most commercial isotonic solutions contain 1000 kcal and about 37–45 g of protein per liter.

Solutions containing hydrolyzed proteins or crystalline amino acids and with no significant fat content are called elemental solutions, since macronutrients are provided in their most "elemental" form. These solutions have been designed for patients with malabsorption, particularly pancreatic insufficiency and limited fat absorption. Elemental diets are extremely hypertonic and often result in more severe diarrhea. Their use should be limited to patients who cannot tolerate isotonic solutions.

Although formulas have been designed for specific clinical situations—solutions containing primarily essential amino acids (for renal failure), medium-chain triglycerides (for fat malabsorption), more fat (for respiratory failure and CO_2 retention), and more branched-chain amino acids (for hepatic encephalopathy and severe trauma)—they have not been shown to be superior to standard formulas for most patients.

Enteral solutions should be administered via continuous infusion, preferably with an infusion pump. Isotonic feedings should be started at full strength at about 25–33% of the estimated final infusion rate. Feedings can be advanced by similar amounts every 12 hours as tolerated. Hypertonic feedings should be started at half strength. The strength and the rate can then be advanced every 6 hours as tolerated.

COMPLICATIONS OF ENTERAL NUTRITIONAL SUPPORT

Minor complications of tube feedings occur in 10–15% of patients. Gastrointestinal complications include diarrhea (most common), inadequate gastric emptying, emesis, esophagitis, and occasionally gastrointestinal bleeding. Diarrhea associated with tube feeding may be due to intolerance to the osmotic load or to one of the macronutrients (eg, fat, lactose) in the solution. Patients being fed in this way may also have diarrhea from other causes (as side effect of antibiotics or other drugs; associated with infection, etc), and these possibilities should always be investigated in appropriate circumstances.

Mechanical complications of tube feedings are potentially the most serious. Of particular importance is aspiration. All patients receiving nasogastric tube feedings are at risk for this life-threatening complication. Limiting nasogastric feedings to those patients who can adequately protect their airway and careful monitoring of patients being fed by tube should limit these serious complications to 1–2% of cases. Minor mechanical complications are common and include tube obstruction and dislodgment.

Metabolic complications during enteral nutritional support are common but in most cases easily managed. The most important problem is hypernatremic dehydration, most commonly seen in elderly patients given excessive protein intake who are unable to respond to thirst. Abnormalities of potassium, glucose, and acid-base balance may also occur.

PARENTERAL NUTRITIONAL SUPPORT SOLUTIONS

Parenteral nutritional support solutions can be designed to deliver adequate nutrients to virtually any patient. The basic parenteral solution is composed of dextrose, amino acids, and water. Electrolytes, minerals, trace elements, vitamins, and medications can also be added. Most commercial solutions contain the monohydrate form of dextrose that provides 3.4 kcal/g. Crystalline amino acids are available in a variety of concentrations, so that a broad range of solutions can be made up that will contain specific amounts of dextrose and amino acids as required.

Typical solutions for central vein nutritional support contain 25–35% dextrose and 2.75–6% amino acids depending upon the patient's estimated nutrient and water requirements. These solutions typically have osmolalities in excess of 1800 mosm/L and require infusion into a central vein. A typical formula for patients without organ failure is shown in Table 29–9.

Solutions with lower osmolalities can also be designed for infusion into peripheral veins. Typical solutions for peripheral infusion contain 5–10% dextrose and 2.75–4.25% amino acids. These solutions have osmolalities between 800 and 1200 mosm/L and result in a high incidence of thrombophlebitis and line infiltration. These solutions will provide adequate protein for most patients but inadequate energy. Additional energy must be provided in the form of emulsified soybean or safflower oil. Such intravenous fat solutions are currently available in 10% and 25% solutions providing 1.1 and 2.2 kcal/mL, respectively. Intravenous fat solutions are isosmotic and well tolerated by peripheral veins. Typical patients are given 200–500 mL of a 20% solution each day. As much as 60% of total calories can be administered in this manner.

Intravenous fat can also be provided to patients receiving central vein nutritional support. In this instance, dextrose concentrations should be decreased to provide a fixed concentration of energy. Intra-

Table 29–9. Typical TPN solution (for stable patients without organ failure).

Dextrose (3.4 kcal/g)	25%
Amino acids (4 kcal/g)	6%
Na$^+$	50 meq/L
K$^+$	40 meq/L
Ca^{2+}	5 meq/L
Mg^{2+}	8 meq/L
Cl$^-$	60 meq/L
P	12 mmol/L
Acetate	Balance
MVI-12 (vitamins)	10 mL/d
MTE (trace elements)	5 mL/d
Fat emulsion 20%	250 mL five times a week
Typical rate	Day 1: 30 mL/h
	Day 2: 60 mL/h
By day 2, solution provides	Calories 1925 kcal total
	Protein 86 g
	Fat 19% of total kcal
	Fluid 1690 mL

venous fat has been shown to be equivalent to intravenous dextrose in providing energy to "spare protein." Intravenous fat is associated with less glucose intolerance, less production of carbon dioxide, and less fatty infiltration of the liver and has been increasingly utilized in patients with hyperglycemia, respiratory failure, and liver disease. Intravenous fat has also been increasingly used in patients with large estimated energy requirements. Recent studies suggest that the maximum glucose utilization rate is approximately 5–7 mg/min/kg. Patients who require additional calories can be given them as fat to prevent excess administration of dextrose. Intravenous fat can also be used to prevent essential fatty acid deficiency. The optimal ratio of carbohydrate and fat in parenteral nutritional support has not been determined.

Infusion of parenteral solutions should be started slowly to prevent hyperglycemia and other metabolic complications. Typical solutions are given initially at a rate of 50 mL/h and advanced by about the same amount every 24 hours until the desired final rate is reached.

COMPLICATIONS OF PARENTERAL NUTRITIONAL SUPPORT

Complications of central vein nutritional support occur in up to 50% of patients. Although most are minor and easily managed, about 5% of patients will develop significant complications. Complications of central vein nutritional support can be divided into catheter-related complications and metabolic complications.

Catheter-related complications can occur during insertion or while the catheter is in place. Pneumothorax, hemothorax, arterial laceration, air emboli, and brachial plexus injury can occur during catheter placement. The incidence of these complications is inversely related to the experience of the physician performing the procedure but will occur in at least 1–2% of cases even in major medical centers. Each catheter placement should be documented by chest radiograph prior to initiation of nutritional support.

Catheter thrombosis and catheter-related sepsis are the most important complications of indwelling catheters. Patients with indwelling central vein catheters who develop signs of sepsis without an apparent source should have their lines removed immediately, the tip cultured, and antibiotics begun empirically. Patients with less significant fevers without an apparent source should have their lines removed and be observed without antibiotics. Catheter-related sepsis occurs in 2–3% of patients even if maximal efforts are made to prevent infection.

Metabolic complications of central vein nutritional support occur in over 50% of patients (Table 29–10).

Table 29–10. Metabolic complications of parenteral nutritional support.

Complication	Common Causes	Possible Solutions
Hyperglycemia	Too-rapid infusion of dextrose, "stress," glucocorticoids.	Decrease glucose infusion. Insulin. Replacement of dextrose with fat.
Hyperosmolar nonketotic dehydration	Severe, undetected hyperglycemia.	Insulin, hydration, potassium.
Hyperchloremic metabolic acidosis	High chloride administration.	Decrease chloride.
Azotemia	Excessive protein administration.	Decrease amino acid concentration.
Hyperphosphatemia, hypokalemia, hypomagnesemia	Extracellular to intracellular shifting with refeeding.	Increase solution concentration.
Liver enzyme abnormalities	Lipid trapping in hepatocytes, fatty liver.	Decrease dextrose.
Acalculous cholecystitis	Biliary stasis.	Oral fat.
Zinc deficiency	Diarrhea, small bowel fistulas.	Increase concentration.
Copper deficiency	Biliary fistulas.	Increase concentration.

Most are minor and easily managed, and termination of support is seldom necessary.

PATIENT MONITORING DURING NUTRITIONAL SUPPORT

Every patient receiving enteral or parenteral nutritional support should be followed closely. Formal nutritional support teams composed of a physician, a nurse, a dietitian, and a pharmacist have been shown to decrease the rate of complications.

Patients should be monitored both for the adequacy of treatment and to prevent complications or detect them early when they occur. Because estimates of nutritional requirements are imprecise, frequent reassessment is necessary. Daily intakes should be recorded and compared with estimated requirements. Body weight, hydration status, and overall clinical status should be followed. Patients who do not appear to be responding as anticipated can be evaluated for nitrogen balance by means of the following equation:

$$\text{Nitrogen balance} = \frac{\text{24-hour protein intake (g)}}{6.25} - \left(\frac{\text{24-hour urinary nitrogen (g)}}{} + 4\right)$$

Patients with positive nitrogen balances can be continued on their current regimens; patients with negative balances should receive moderate increases in calorie and protein intake and then be reassessed.

Feeding tubes and catheters should be examined often to avoid mechanical and infectious complications.

Monitoring for metabolic complications should include urine glucose determination every 6 hours and daily measurements of electrolytes; serum glucose, phosphorus, magnesium, calcium, and creatinine; and BUN until the patient is stabilized. Once the patient is stabilized, electrolytes, phosphorus, calcium, magnesium, and glucose should be checked at least twice weekly. Red blood cell folate, zinc, and copper should be checked at least once a month.

ASPEN Board of Directors: Guidelines for the use of parenteral and enteral nutrition in adult and pediatric patients. JPEN J Parenter Enteral Nutr 1993;17:15A. (Current guidelines from the American Society of Parenteral and Enteral Nutrition.)

Buchman AL et al: Catheter-related infections associated with home parenteral nutrition and predictive factors for the need for catheter removal in their treatment. JPEN J Parenter Enteral Nutr 1994;18:297. (Catheter infection is relatively uncommon in home TPN patients.)

Burge JC et al: Efficacy of hypocaloric total parenteral nutrition in hospitalized obese patients: A prospective, double-blind randomized trial. JPEN J Parenter Enteral Nutr 1994;18:203. (Hypocaloric feedings can be used in obese patients with mild to moderate stress and still result in positive nitrogen balance.)

Eisenberg JM et al: Does perioperative total parenteral nutrition reduce medical care costs? JPEN J Parenter Enteral Nutr 1993;17;201. (Analysis of the large VA cooperative perioperative total parenteral nutrition trial showed no reduction in costs for any subgroup of patients receiving preoperative TPN.)

Everitt NJ, McMahon MJ: Peripheral intravenous nutrition. Nutrition 1994;10:49. (Review of indications and complications of peripheral vein nutritional support, suggesting that it is safe, effective, and underutilized.)

Klein S, Koretz RL: Nutrition support in patients with cancer: What do the data really show? Nutr Clin Pract 1994;9:91. (Review of studies suggesting that for most patients nutritional support does not improve clinical outcomes.)

Mueller C, Nestle M: Regulation of medical foods: Toward a rational policy. Nutr Clin Pract 1995;10:8. (An argument for the more careful federal regulation of enteral formulas.)

Phinney SD, Siepler J, Bach HT: Is there a role for parenteral feeding in clinical medicine? West J Med 1996;164:130. (Critical review of the effectiveness of parenteral nutrition.)

30

General Problems in Infectious Diseases

Richard A. Jacobs, MD, PhD

Most infections are confined to specific organ systems. In a book such as this—arranged principally by organ system—many of the important infectious disease entities are discussed in chapters dealing with specific anatomic areas. In this chapter are discussed some important general problems related to infectious diseases that are not covered elsewhere.

FEVER OF UNKNOWN ORIGIN (FUO)

To fulfill the criteria of FUO, a patient must have an illness of at least 3 weeks' duration, fever over 38.3 °C on several occasions, and must remain undiagnosed after 1 week of study in the hospital. The intervals specified are arbitrary ones intended to exclude patients with protracted but self-limited viral illnesses and to allow time for the usual radiographic, serologic, and cultural studies to be performed. Because of concerns over costs of hospitalization and the availability of most screening tests on an outpatient basis, the criterion requiring 1 week of hospitalization is often ignored. (For a general discussion of fever, see the section on fever and hyperthermia in Chapter 1.)

Etiologic Considerations

Certain general principles about FUO should be kept in mind in the diagnostic approach to these patients.

A. Common Causes: Most cases represent unusual manifestations of common diseases and not rare or exotic diseases—ie, tuberculosis, endocarditis, gallbladder disease, and HIV (primary infection or opportunistic infection) are more common causes of FUO than Whipple's disease or familial Mediterranean fever.

B. Age of Patient: In adults, infections (30–40% of cases) and cancer (20–35% of cases) account for the majority of FUOs. In children, infections are the most common cause of FUO (30–50% of cases) and cancer a rare cause (5–10% of cases). Autoimmune disorders occur with equal frequency in

adults and children (10–20% of cases), but the diseases differ. Juvenile rheumatoid arthritis is particularly common in children, whereas systemic lupus erythematosus, Wegener's granulomatosis, and polyarteritis nodosa are more common in adults. Adult Still's disease, giant cell arteritis, and polymyalgia rheumatica occur exclusively in adults.

C. Duration of Fever: The cause of FUO changes dramatically in patients who have been febrile for a prolonged period of time—ie, 6 months or longer. Infection, cancer, and autoimmune disorders combined account for only 20% of FUOs in these patients. Instead, other entities such as granulomatous diseases (granulomatous hepatitis, Crohn's disease, ulcerative colitis) and factitious fever become important causes. Up to 27% of patients who say they have been febrile for 6 months or longer actually have no true fever or underlying disease. Instead, the usual normal circadian variation in temperature (temperature 1–2 °C higher in the afternoon than in the morning) is interpreted as abnormal. Patients with episodic or recurrent fever (ie, those who meet the classic criteria for FUO but have fever-free periods of 2 weeks or longer) are similar to patients with prolonged fever. Infection, malignancy, and autoimmune disorders account for only 20–25% of such fevers, whereas various miscellaneous diseases (Crohn's disease, familial Mediterranean fever, allergic alveolitis) account for another 25%. Approximately 50% remain undiagnosed but have a benign course with eventual resolution of symptoms.

D. Immunologic Status: In the neutropenic patient, fungal infections and occult bacterial infection are important and common causes of FUO. In the patient taking immunosuppressive medications (particularly organ transplant patients), cytomegalovirus infections are a frequent cause of fever, as are fungal infections, nocardiosis, *Pneumocystis carinii* pneumonia, and mycobacterial infections.

E. Classification of Causes of FUO: Most patients with FUO will fit into one of five categories.

1. Infection–Both systemic and localized infections can cause FUO. Tuberculosis and endocarditis are the most common systemic infections, but mycoses, viral diseases (particularly infection with Epstein-Barr virus and cytomegalovirus), toxoplasmosis, brucellosis, Q fever, cat-scratch disease, salmonellosis, malaria, and many other less common infections have been implicated. Primary infection with human immunodeficiency virus (HIV) or opportunistic infections associated with the acquired immunodeficiency syndrome (AIDS)—particularly mycobacterial infections—can also present as FUO. The most common form of localized infection causing FUO is an occult abscess. Liver, spleen, kidney, brain, and bone are organs in which abscess may be difficult to find. A collection of pus may form in the peritoneal cavity or in the subdiaphragmatic, subhepatic, paracolic, or other areas. Cholangitis, osteomyelitis, urinary tract infection, dental abscess, or a collection of pus in a paranasal sinus may cause prolonged fever.

2. Neoplasms–Many cancers can present as FUO. The most common are lymphoma (both Hodgkin's and non-Hodgkin's) and leukemia. Other diseases of lymph nodes, such as angioimmunoblastic lymphoma, Kikuchi's syndrome, and Castleman's disease, can also cause FUO. Primary and metastatic tumors of the liver also are frequently associated with fever, as are renal cell carcinomas. Atrial myxoma is an often forgotten neoplasm that can result in fever. Chronic lymphocytic leukemia and multiple myeloma are rarely associated with fever, and the presence of fever in patients with these diseases should prompt a careful search for infection.

3. Autoimmune disorders–Still's disease, systemic lupus erythematosus, and polyarteritis nodosa are the most common autoimmune causes of FUO. Giant cell arteritis and polymyalgia rheumatica are seen almost exclusively in patients over 50 years of age and are nearly always associated with an elevated erythrocyte sedimentation rate (> 40 mm/h).

4. Miscellaneous causes–Many other diseases have been associated with FUO but less commonly than the foregoing types of illness. Examples include hyperthyroidism, thyroiditis, sarcoidosis, Whipple's disease, familial Mediterranean fever, recurrent pulmonary emboli, alcoholic hepatitis, drug fever, factitious fever, and others.

5. Undiagnosed FUO–Despite extensive evaluation, in 10–15% of patients the diagnosis remains elusive. In about three-fourths of these patients, the fever abates spontaneously and the clinician never knows the cause; in the remainder, more classic manifestations of the underlying disease appear over time, and the diagnosis then becomes obvious.

Approach to Diagnosis of FUO

Because the evaluation of a patient with FUO is so costly and time-consuming, it is imperative to document the presence of fever. This is done most reliably by observing the patient while the temperature is being taken to make certain that fever is not factitious (self-induced). Associated findings that usually accompany fever include tachycardia, chills, and piloerection. A thorough history—including family, occupational, social (sexual practices, use of intravenous drugs), dietary (unpasteurized products, raw meat), exposures (animals, chemicals), and travel histories—may give clues to the underlying diagnosis. Detailed and repeated physical examination may reveal subtle, evanescent clinical findings that are the key to diagnosis.

In addition to routine laboratory studies, blood cultures should always be obtained, preferably when the patient is off antibiotics. Serologic studies may be diagnostic for certain immunologic diseases but are less useful in diagnosing infectious causes of FUO. A single elevated titer rarely allows one to make a diagnosis of infection; instead, one must demonstrate a fourfold rise or fall in titer to confirm a specific infectious cause. Because infection is the most common cause of FUO, other body fluids are usually cultured, ie, urine, sputum, stool, cerebrospinal fluid, and morning gastric aspirates (if one suspects tuberculosis). Direct examination of blood smears may establish a diagnosis of malaria or relapsing fever *(Borrelia)*.

Almost all patients with FUO should have a chest radiograph, sinus films, upper gastrointestinal series with small bowel follow-through, barium enema, proctosigmoidoscopy, and evaluation of gallbladder function. CT scan of the abdomen and pelvis is also frequently performed and can be quite useful in evaluating patients with FUO. It is particularly useful for looking at the liver, spleen, and retroperitoneum. When the CT scan is positive, the findings are usually confirmed and often lead to a specific diagnosis. It is important to realize that a negative CT scan is not quite as useful; even with a negative CT scan, more invasive procedures such as biopsy or exploratory laparotomy may lead to the diagnosis. The role of MRI in the investigation of FUO has not been evaluated. In general, however, MRI is better than CT for detecting lesions of the nervous system. Ultrasound is very sensitive for detecting lesions of the kidney, pancreas, and biliary tree. Echocardiography should be used if one is considering endocarditis or atrial myxoma. Transesophageal echocardiography is more sensitive than surface echocardiography for detecting valvular lesions, but even a negative transesophageal study does not exclude endocarditis (10% false-negative rate). The usefulness of radionuclide studies has not been extensively studied in FUO. Theoretically, a gallium scan would be more helpful than an indium-labeled white blood cell scan, because gallium is useful for detecting infection and neoplasm whereas the indium scan is useful only for detecting infection. Both studies are limited by high rates of false-positive and false-negative results. Indium-labeled immunoglobulin is another radionuclide study that may prove to be useful in detecting infection and neoplasm and can be used in the neutropenic patient. It is not sensitive for lesions of the liver, kidney, and heart because of high background activity. Overall sensitivity is 80%, and specificity is 70%.

Invasive procedures are often required for diagnosis. Any abnormal finding should be aggressively evaluated: headache calls for lumbar puncture to rule out meningitis; skin from an area of rash should be biopsied to look for cutaneous manifestations of collagen vascular disease or infection; and enlarged lymph nodes should be aspirated or biopsied and examined for cytologic features to rule out neoplasm and sent for culture. Bone marrow aspiration with biopsy is a relatively low-yield procedure (except in HIV-positive patients, in whom mycobacterial infection is a common cause of FUO and bone marrow biopsy a high-yield procedure), but the risk is low and the procedure should be done if other less invasive tests have not yielded a diagnosis. Liver biopsy will yield a specific diagnosis in 10–15% of patients with FUO. One should consider this procedure in any patient with abnormal liver function tests even if the liver is normal in size on physical examination. The role of exploratory laparotomy is debatable. Studies on the usefulness of laparatomy in the diagnosis of FUO have not been done since the advent of CT scanning and MRI. One should consider laparotomy in the deteriorating patient if the diagnosis is elusive despite extensive evaluation.

Therapeutic Trials

Therapeutic trials are indicated if a diagnosis is strongly suspected—eg, it is reasonable to give antituberculous drugs if one suspects tuberculosis, or tetracycline if brucellosis is suspected. However, if there is no clinical response in several weeks, it is imperative to stop therapy and reevaluate the situation.

Empiric use of corticosteroids should be discouraged; these agents can suppress fever if given in high enough doses, but they can also exacerbate many infections, and infection remains a leading cause of FUO. Suppression of fever with low doses of nonsteroidal anti-inflammatory agents (eg, naproxen, 250 mg twice daily) has been reported to be specific for fever associated with malignancy, but published data are limited.

Cunha BA: Fever of unknown origin. Infect Dis Clin North Am 1996;10:111. (A general review of causes, diagnostic evaluation, and treatment.)

Hirschmann JV: Fever of unknown origin in adults. Clin Infect Dis 1997;24:291. (A comprehensive review.)

Miralles P et al: Fever of uncertain origin in patients infected with the human immunodeficiency virus. Clin Infect Dis 1995;20:872. (Evaluation of 50 patients. Mycobacterial disease the most common cause.)

INFECTIONS IN THE IMMUNOCOMPROMISED PATIENT

A description of the cellular basis of immune response, the role of various host responses in maintaining health, and the methods used for detection of deficiencies in the immune system can be found in Chapter 19.

Compromised hosts are individuals who have one or more defects in their natural defense mechanisms that put them at an increased risk of developing infections. Not only is the risk of infection greater in these individuals, but once infection develops it is often severe, rapidly progressive, and can be life-threatening. In addition, microorganisms that are not usually pathogens in the noncompromised patient may cause serious disease in the compromised patient. Individuals are most commonly compromised because of dysfunction of their immune system (granulocytopenia, T and B cell deficiency, hypogammaglobulinemia), but the presence of coexisting illness can also predispose to infection.

Granulocytopenia is common following bone marrow transplantation—as a result of myelosuppressive chemotherapy—and in acute leukemias. The risk of infection begins to increase when the absolute granulocyte count falls below 500/μL, with a dramatic increase in frequency and severity when the granulocyte count falls below 100/μL. The granulocytopenic patient is particularly susceptible to infections with gram-negative enteric organisms, *Pseudomonas,* gram-positive cocci (particularly *Staphylococcus aureus* and *Staphylococcus epidermidis*), *Candida, Aspergillus,* and other fungi that have recently emerged as pathogens such as *Trichosporon, Scedosporium, Fusarium,* and *Pseudallescheria.*

Defects in humoral immunity are often congenital, though hypogammaglobulinemia can occur in multiple myeloma and chronic lymphocytic leukemia. Patients with defects in humoral immunity lack opsonizing antibodies and are at particular risk of infection with encapsulated organisms such as *Haemophilus influenzae* and *Streptococcus pneumoniae.*

Patients with cellular immune deficiency encompass a large and rather heterogeneous group that includes patients with HIV infection (see Chapter 31), those with lymphoreticular malignancies such as Hodgkin's disease (which is associated with dysfunction of cellular immunity), and patients receiving immunosuppressive medications such as corticosteroids, cyclosporine, azathioprine, and other cytotoxic drugs. This latter group—immunosuppressed as a result of medications—includes transplant patients, many solid tumor patients receiving therapy, and patients receiving prolonged high-dose corticosteroid treatment (for asthma, temporal arteritis, systemic lupus, etc). Patients with cellular immune dysfunction are susceptible to infections by a large number of organisms, particularly ones that replicate intracellularly. Examples include bacteria such as *Listeria, Legionella, Salmonella,* and *Mycobacterium;* viruses such as herpes simplex, varicella, and cytomegalovirus; fungi such as *Cryptococcus, Coccidioides, Histoplasma,* and *Pneumocystis;* and protozoa such as *Toxoplasma.*

Patients who are functionally or anatomically asplenic fail to clear organisms from the bloodstream and are at an increased risk of overwhelming bacteremia with encapsulated bacteria (primarily *Streptococcus pneumoniae* but also *H influenzae* and *Neisseria meningitidis*).

Finally, a large group of patients who are not classically immunodeficient are at increased risk of infection because of debilitating injury (eg, burns or severe trauma), invasive procedures (eg, hyperalimentation lines, Foley catheters, dialysis catheters), central nervous system dysfunction (which predisposes to aspiration pneumonia and decubitus ulcers), the presence of obstructing lesions (eg, pneumonia due to an obstructed bronchus, pyelonephritis due to nephrolithiasis, cholangitis secondary to cholelithiasis), and use of broad-spectrum antibiotics.

Despite the generalizations made above about the relationship between type of immunosuppression and likely pathogen, it is important to remember that any pathogen can occur in any immunosuppressed patient at any time. Thus, a systematic evaluation to identify a specific organism is required.

Organisms not usually considered pathogens in the noncompromised patient may cause serious life-threatening infection in the compromised patient (eg, *S epidermidis, Corynebacterium jeikeium, Propionobacterium acnes, Bacillus* spp). Therefore, one must interpret culture results with caution and not disregard isolates as mere contaminants. A contaminating organism in the immunocompetent patient may be a pathogen in the immunocompromised one.

Approach to Diagnosis

Not all fevers are due to infection. Transplant rejection, organ ischemia and necrosis, thrombophlebitis, and lymphoma may all present as fever and must be considered in the differential diagnosis.

Because infections in the immunocompromised patient can be rapidly progressive and life-threatening, diagnostic procedures must be done promptly, and empiric therapy is often instituted before a specific diagnostic agent has been isolated:

(1) Routine evaluation includes complete blood count with differential, chest x-ray, and blood cultures; urine and sputum cultures should be obtained if indicated clinically or radiographically. Any focal complaints (localized pain, headache, rash) should prompt a thorough evaluation and cultures appropriate to the site.

(2) Because the types of organisms causing infec-

tion are so varied in the immunosuppressed patient, if a source of infection is identified every effort should be made to obtain specimens that may lead to a specific microbial diagnosis.

(3) Patients who remain febrile without an obvious source should be evaluated for viral infection (cytomegalovirus blood cultures or antigen test), abscesses (which usually occur near previous operative sites), systemic candidiasis that involves the liver or spleen, or aspergillosis. Serologic evaluation may be helpful if toxoplasmosis is a possible pathogen.

(4) Consider special diagnostic procedures. The cause of pulmonary infiltrates can be easily determined with simple techniques in some situations— eg, induced sputum yields a diagnosis of *P carinii* pneumonia in 50–80% of AIDS patients with this infection. In other situations, more invasive procedures may be required (bronchoalveolar lavage, transbronchial biopsy, or even open lung biopsy). Other procedures such as skin, liver, or bone marrow biopsy may be helpful in establishing a diagnosis.

(5) In patients who have undergone solid organ transplants, immediate postoperative infections often involve the transplanted organ. Following lung transplantation, pneumonia and mediastinitis are particularly common; following liver transplantation, intra-abdominal abscess, cholangiolitis, and peritonitis are common; following renal transplantation, urinary tract infections, perinephric abscesses, and infected lymphoceles can occur. In contrast to solid organ transplants, in bone marrow transplant patients the source of fever cannot be found in 60–70% of patients.

(6) The time of occurrence of infection, particularly following solid organ transplantation, can be helpful in determining the infectious origin. Most infections that occur in the first month posttransplant are related to the operative procedure and to hospitalization itself (wound infection, intravenous catheter infection, urinary tract infection from a Foley catheter) or are related to the transplanted organ (see paragraph [5], above). Infections that occur between the second and sixth months are often related to immunosuppression. During this period, reactivation of viruses occurs, and herpes simplex, varicella-zoster, and CMV infections are quite common. Opportunistic infections with fungi (*Candida, Aspergillus, Pneumocystis carinii,* and others), *Listeria monocytogenes, Nocardia,* and *Toxoplasma* are also common. After 6 months, when immunosuppression has been reduced to maintenance levels, common infections that are found in any population occur.

Prevention of Infection

There is great interest in preventing infection with prophylactic antimicrobial regimens, but there is no uniformity of opinion about what the optimal drugs or dosage regimens should be.

Trimethoprim-sulfamethoxazole, one double-strength tablet three times a week, one double-strength tablet twice daily on weekends, or one single-strength tablet daily for 3–6 months, is frequently used to prevent *P carinii* infections in transplant patients. It may also decrease the incidence of bacterial pneumonia, urinary tract infections, nocardia infections, and toxoplasmosis.

In patients allergic to trimethoprim-sulfamethoxazole, aerosolized pentamidine is used in a dosage of 300 mg once a month. Dapsone, 50 mg daily or 100 mg three times weekly, can also be used. Acyclovir has been shown to be effective in preventing herpes simplex and varicella infections in transplant recipients.

Prevention of CMV is more difficult, and no uniformly accepted approach has been adopted. Prevention strategies often depend on the serologic status of the donor and recipient and the organ transplanted, which determines the level of immunosuppression after transplant. In renal transplant patients, the risk of CMV disease is relatively low except in seronegative patients who receive kidneys from seropositive donors. These high-risk patients usually receive ganciclovir, 2.5–5 mg/kg intravenously twice daily during hospitalization (usually 10–14 days), and then are placed on a regimen of 800 mg of acyclovir orally daily for 3 months. Because immunosuppression is increased during periods of rejection, patients treated for rejection usually receive intravenous ganciclovir during rejection therapy.

Liver transplant recipients have a greater risk of developing CMV disease, and most patients are given intravenous ganciclovir during hospitalization followed by high-dose oral acyclovir for 3 months. For seronegative patients who receive livers from seropositive donors, a more aggressive approach is taken, giving intravenous ganciclovir in the hospital followed after discharge by intravenous ganciclovir 5 days a week for 3 months. Although oral ganciclovir in the outpatient setting is an attractive option and may be effective, large-scale clinical trials of its efficacy have not been conducted. In general, heart and lung recipients are treated in somewhat the same way as recipients of liver transplants.

Recipients of bone marrow transplants are more severely immunosuppressed than recipients of solid organ transplants, are at greater risk for developing serious CMV infection, and thus usually receive more aggressive prophylaxis. Two approaches have been used: universal prophylaxis or preemptive therapy. In the former, all CMV-seropositive patients receive 7.5–10 mg/kg/d of ganciclovir for 1 week prior to transplantation and a lower dose of 5 mg/kg/d after engraftment (which usually occurs on about day 30) for 5–7 days of each week for 3–4 months. This method is effective in preventing infection and disease but is limited by its high cost and toxicity. Alternatively, patients can be followed without specific therapy and have blood sampled weekly for the presence of CMV.

If CMV is detected by an antigenemia assay, preemptive therapy with ganciclovir is given (5 mg/kg intravenously twice daily for 7 days, followed by 5 mg/kg daily for the first 100–120 days after transplantation). This approach is also effective but does miss a small number of patients who subsequently develop CMV disease. In allogeneic marrow transplant patients, intravenous immune globulin, 500–1000 mg/kg, is given every 1–2 weeks for the first 3 months after transplantation as CMV prophylaxis. Following autologous bone marrow transplantation, immune globulin is not recommended and may be associated with increased toxicity.

In the neutropenic patient, the gastrointestinal tract is the source of many infections. Oral nonabsorbable antibiotics and quinolones have been used for gastrointestinal decontamination in an attempt to decrease bacteremia from this site. Because of poor compliance with nonabsorbable agents and concern about selection of resistant organisms with quinolones, neither approach has gained widespread acceptance. Small bowel decontamination with polymyxin E, gentamicin, and nystatin when given at least 3 days prior to liver transplantation is effective in reducing the incidence of postoperative infections. The role of prophylactic antifungal agents in neutropenic patients remains controversial. Fluconazole has been shown to decrease the incidence of superficial and invasive fungal infections in one study but has been associated with selection of resistant organisms (*Candida krusei*). In addition, fluconazole is not active against *Candida glabrata,* aspergillosis, or mucormycosis, common infections in neutropenic patients. Preliminary data on low-dose amphotericin B (0.1 mg/kg/d) for prophylaxis suggest efficacy in preventing invasive disease, but further data are required. Studies evaluating itraconazole are in progress. Prophylaxis in HIV-positive patients is summarized in Chapter 31.

Handwashing is the simplest and most effective means of decreasing nosocomial infections in *all* patients, especially the compromised host. Invasive devices such as central and peripheral lines and Foley catheters are a potential source of infection. The need for these devices should be continually assessed and their use discontinued at the earliest possible time.

Approach to Treatment

In addition to providing antimicrobial therapy, it is important to improve host defenses whenever possible, correct electrolyte imbalances, and maintain adequate nutrition. Because immunosuppression is often the reason for infection, it is important to decrease immunosuppressive medications even in organ transplant patients. Reduction or discontinuation of immunosuppressive medication may jeopardize the viability of the transplanted organ, but in life-threatening infections it is necessary as an adjunct to effective antimicrobial therapy. Hematopoietic growth factors (granulocyte and granulocyte-macrophage colony-stimulating factors) stimulate proliferation of bone marrow stem cells, resulting in an increase in peripheral leukocytes. These agents shorten the period of neutropenia and have been associated with fewer infections. Use of growth factors in patients with prolonged neutropenia (> 7 days) is an effective means of reversing immunosuppression.

Antimicrobial drug therapy should be rationally based on culture results (see Chapter 37). Therapy should be specific for isolated pathogens, and bactericidal agents should be used. Combinations of antimicrobials are often required to provide synergy, to prevent resistance, or to serve as broad-spectrum coverage of multiple pathogens (since infections in these patients are often polymicrobial).

Empiric therapy is often instituted at the earliest sign of infection in the immunosuppressed patient because prompt therapy favorably affects outcome. The antibiotic or combination of antibiotics used depends on the type of immunocompromise and the site of infection. For example, in the febrile neutropenic patient, one is concerned primarily about bacterial and fungal infections. A number of different antibiotics have been used to treat this patient population. (See discussion in Chapter 37.) If the patient fails to respond to antibiotics in 3–5 days, amphotericin B, 0.5–1 mg/kg/d, is added to treat a presumed fungal infection. Regardless of whether the patient becomes afebrile, therapy is continued until resolution of neutropenia. Failure to continue antibiotics through the period of neutropenia is associated with a high incidence of relapse that can be associated with septic shock. In the organ transplant patient with interstitial infiltrates, one is concerned mainly about *P carinii* or *Legionella* spp, so that empiric treatment with intravenous erythromycin and trimethoprim-sulfamethoxazole would be reasonable. If the patient fails to respond to empiric treatment, one must often decide between empiric addition of more antimicrobial agents or undertaking invasive procedures (see above) to make a specific diagnosis. By making a specific diagnosis, therapy can be specific and polypharmacy with multiple potentially toxic agents avoided.

Giamarellou H: Empiric therapy for infections in the febrile neutropenic compromised host. Med Clin North Am 1995;79:559. (Review of approaches used.)

Greene JN, Hipmenz JW (editors): Infectious complications of cancer therapy. Infect Dis Clin North Am 1996;10(2). (Entire issue contains articles on infections associated with antitumor chemotherapy.)

Rowe JM et al: Recommended guidelines for the management of autologous and allogeneic bone marrow transplantation: A report from the Eastern Cooperative Oncology Group (ECOG). Ann Intern Med 1994;129:143. (Review of all aspects, including prophylaxis and therapy of infection.)

Rubin RH (editor): Infection in transplantation. Infect Dis Clin North Am 1995;9(4):1. (Entire issue.)

NOSOCOMIAL INFECTIONS

Nosocomial infections are by definition those acquired in the course of hospitalization. At present in the USA, 5% of patients who enter the hospital free from infection acquire a nosocomial infection. Generally, patients acquire hospital infections with common organisms because of their own increased susceptibility to infection or because of procedures performed in the hospital.

Nosocomial infections can be attributed principally to the following aspects of contemporary medical care:

(1) Many hospitalized patients (especially in tertiary care hospitals, which have the highest nosocomial infection rate) are compromised because of deficiencies in their immunologic responses or impaired host defenses (skin ulcers, aspiration tendencies, etc). These may be congenital but commonly are acquired as a result of the administration of drugs for the treatment of cancer, for the maintenance of transplants, or for the suppression of autoimmune processes. The very young and the elderly are particularly susceptible to infection.

(2) Many aspects of medical care now require the use of invasive techniques for diagnosis, monitoring, and therapy. Examples are the indwelling urinary catheter; intravascular lines used for measurements, infusions of fluids or drugs, or parenteral alimentation; drainage tubes; and shunts.

(3) Materials administered in the intensive care unit may themselves be vectors of infection. Common examples are contaminated intravenous solutions or their containers; respirators and humidifiers that may introduce microorganisms into particularly susceptible lungs; and plastic tubing that may carry infectious agents into the body.

(4) The widespread use of antimicrobial drugs contributes to the selection of drug-resistant microorganisms both in the individual patient and in the hospital environment. Thus, nosocomial infections are often attributable to members of the endogenous human microflora or free-living microorganisms that happen to be particularly resistant to antimicrobial drugs, presenting difficult management problems. Such organisms often are not established human pathogens but can be classed as opportunists.

The principal anatomic sites of hospital-acquired infection are the urinary tract, surgical wounds, the respiratory tract, and skin sites where indwelling needles or tubes penetrate. Most notorious among nosocomial infections are those due to gram-negative enteric bacteria, staphylococci, or mycotic organisms that develop in patients with granulocyte counts below 500/µL as a result of cancer chemotherapy or organ transplant. In such patients, bloodstream invasion often occurs without a well-defined portal of entry. Patients with markedly depressed cell-mediated immunity may also develop viral infections in the hospital, eg, varicella-zoster, cytomegalovirus, and hepatitis. They are likewise open to opportunists such as *Legionella, Nocardia,* and *P carinii.*

In general, organisms that cause nosocomial infections tend to be multidrug-resistant and are often not sensitive to antibiotics used to treat community-acquired infections. For example, *Staphylococcus aureus* strains that cause hospital infections may be resistant to nafcillin and cephalosporins; *S epidermidis*—a frequent pathogen in patients with foreign bodies (shunts, hyperalimentation catheters, prosthetic heart valves, etc)—similarly may be resistant to nafcillin and sensitive only to vancomycin; *Enterococcus faecium* may be resistant to ampicillin and vancomycin and sensitive only to investigational drugs; and gram-negative organisms that cause nosocomial infections may be unusual subspecies of *Enterobacter, Acinetobacter,* and *Pseudomonas* and sensitive only to aminoglycosides, quinolones, or imipenem. For these reasons, it is often necessary to institute empiric therapy with drugs such as vancomycin and tobramycin (or a quinolone or imipenem) until a specific agent is isolated and sensitivities are known, at which time the least toxic and least costly active drug can be used. The bacteriology and sensitivity patterns of nosocomial infections are quite variable, and one must be aware of local patterns to best treat these patients.

Prevention is of paramount importance in controlling nosocomial infections. The concept of universal precautions emphasizes that all patients should be treated as though they have a potential blood-borne transmissible disease, and thus all body secretions should be handled with care to prevent spread of disease. Almost all hospitals have implemented body substance isolation, which requires use of gloves whenever a health care worker anticipates contact with blood or other body secretions. The use of gloves is intended to prevent contamination of the hands of health care workers with infected secretions and subsequent spread of infection to other patients by direct contact. The concept of body substance isolation is grounded in recognition of the fact that many nosocomial infections are transmitted on the hands of health care workers and the assumption that spread of infection can be reduced by using gloves as a protective barrier. However, even when gloves are used, hand contamination occurs 13% of the time (largely due to glove leaks), emphasizing the importance of hand washing. Hand washing is the easiest and most effective means of preventing nosocomial infections and should be done routinely even when gloves are utilized. Foley catheters, intravenous lines, hemodynamic monitoring devices, hyperalimentation lines, and similar invasive devices should be used only when critical to patient care and, when used, should be discontinued at the earliest possible time. Peripheral intravenous lines should be replaced every 3 days and arterial lines every 4 days. Lines in the central venous circulation (including those placed peripherally) can be left in indefinitely and are changed or removed when they are clinically suspected of being infected, when they are nonfunctional, or when they are no longer needed. Selective decontamination of the digestive tract with nonabsorbable antibiotics to prevent nosocomial pneumonia is widely used in Europe, but the therapeutic efficacy of this expensive intervention is controversial. Attentive nursing care (positioning to prevent decubitus ulcers, wound care, elevating the head during tube feedings to prevent aspiration) is critical in preventing nosocomial infections. In addition, careful monitoring of high-risk areas (intensive care units, neonatal units, surgical floors, hemodialysis and transplant units, etc) by skilled personnel—hospital epidemiologists—to detect increases in infection rates early is a key factor in prevention of these types of infections.

Pittet D, Wenzel RP: Nosocomial bloodstream infections: Secular trends in rates, mortality, and contribution to total hospital deaths. Arch Intern Med 1995;155:1177. (Summarizes changes in etiology and mortality over a 12-year period.)

Verhoef J, Verhage EAE, Visser MR: A decade of experience with selective decontamination of the digestive tract as prophylaxis for infections in patients in the intensive care unit: What have we learned? Clin Infect Dis 1993;17:1047. (Review of published studies.)

INFECTIONS OF THE CENTRAL NERVOUS SYSTEM

Infections of the central nervous system can be caused by almost any infectious agent, including bacteria, mycobacteria, fungi, spirochetes, protozoa, helminths, and viruses. Certain symptoms and signs are common to all types of central nervous system infection: headache, fever, sensorial disturbances, neck and back stiffness, positive Kernig and Brudzinski signs, and cerebrospinal fluid abnormalities. Although it is rare for all of these manifestations to be present in any one individual, the presence of even one of them should suggest the possibility of a central nervous system infection.

Central nervous system infection constitutes a *medical emergency.* Immediate diagnostic steps must be instituted to establish the specific cause. Normally, these include the history, physical examination, blood count, blood culture, lumbar puncture followed by careful study and culture of the cerebrospinal fluid, and a chest film. The fluid must be examined for cell count, glucose, and protein, and a smear must be stained for bacteria (and acid-fast organisms when appropriate) and cultured for pyogenic organisms and for mycobacteria and fungi when indicated. Counterimmunoelectrophoresis and latex agglutination tests can detect antigens of encapsulated organisms (*Streptococcus pneumoniae,*

Haemophilus influenzae, Neisseria meningitidis, and *Cryptococcus neoformans).* These tests are particularly helpful when the patient has already received antibiotics, so that cultures are likely to be negative. Although it is difficult to prove with existing clinical data that early antibiotic therapy improves outcome in bacterial meningitis, prompt therapy is still recommended.

Since performing a lumbar puncture in the presence of a space-occupying lesion (brain abscess, subdural hematoma, subdural abscess) can result in brain stem herniation and death, a CT scan is performed prior to lumbar puncture if a space-occupying lesion is suspected on the basis of papilledema, coma, seizures, or focal neurologic findings. If delays are encountered in obtaining a CT scan and bacterial meningitis is suspected, blood cultures should be drawn and antibiotics should be administered even before cerebrospinal fluid is obtained for culture to avoid unnecessary delays in treatment (Table 30–1). Animal studies suggest that antibiotics given within 4 hours before obtaining cerebrospinal fluid will not affect culture results.

Etiologic Classification

Central nervous system infections can be divided into several categories that usually can be readily distinguished from each other by cerebrospinal fluid examination as the first step toward etiologic diagnosis (Table 30–2).

A. Purulent Meningitis: Patients with bacterial meningitis usually present acutely within hours or 1–2 days after onset of symptoms. The organisms responsible depend primarily on the age of the patient as summarized in Table 30–1. The diagnosis is usually based on the gram-stained smear (positive in 60–80%) or culture (positive in over 90%).

B. Chronic Meningitis: Patients with chronic meningitis present less acutely with a history of symptoms lasting weeks to months. The most common pathogens are *Mycobacterium tuberculosis,* atypical mycobacteria, fungi (*Cryptococcus, Coccidioides, Histoplasma),* and spirochetes (*Treponema pallidum,* meningovascular syphilis; and *Borrelia burgdorferi,* Lyme disease). The diagnosis is made by culture or in some cases by serologic tests (cryptococcosis, coccidioidomycosis, syphilis, Lyme disease).

C. Aseptic Meningitis: Aseptic meningitis—a much more benign and self-limited syndrome—is caused principally by viruses, especially mumps virus, the enterovirus group (including coxsackieviruses and echoviruses), and herpesviruses. Infectious mononucleosis may be accompanied by aseptic meningitis. Leptospiral infection is usually placed in the aseptic group because of the lymphocytic cellular response and its relatively benign course. This type of meningitis also occurs during secondary syphilis and stage 2 Lyme disease.

D. Encephalitis: Encephalitis (due to herpesviruses, arboviruses, and many other viruses) produces disturbances of the sensorium, seizures, and many other manifestations. Cerebrospinal fluid may be entirely normal or may show some lymphocytes.

E. Partially Treated Bacterial Meningitis: Previous effective antibiotic therapy given for 12–24 hours will decrease the rate of positive Gram stain results by 20% and culture by 30–40% but will have little effect on cell count, protein, or glucose. Occasionally, previous antibiotic therapy will change a predominantly polymorphonuclear response to a lymphocytic pleocytosis, and some of the cerebrospinal fluid findings may be similar to those seen in aseptic meningitis.

Table 30–1. Initial antimicrobial therapy for purulent meningitis of unknown cause.

Age Group	Common Microorganisms	Standard Therapy
3 months to 18 years	*H influenzae, N meningitidis, S pneumoniae*[1]	Cefotaxime or ceftriaxone[2]
18–50 years	*S pneumoniae,*[1] *N meningitidis*	Cefotaxime or ceftriaxone[3]
Over 50 years	*S pneumoniae,*[1] *N meningitidis, L monocytogenes,* gram-negative bacilli	Ampicillin, cefotaxime, or ceftriaxone[3]
Impaired cellular immunity	*L monocytogenes* or gram-negative bacilli	Ampicillin[4] plus ceftazidime[5]
Postsurgical or posttraumatic	*S aureus, S pneumoniae,*[1] gram-negative bacilli	Vancomycin[6] plus ceftazidime[5]

[1]In areas where penicillin-resistant pneumococcus is prevalent, vancomycin, 15 mg/kg every 8 hours, should be included in the regimen.
[2]The dose of cefotaxime is 50 mg/kg every 6 hours; of ceftriaxone, 50–100 mg/kg every 12 hours.
[3]The usual dose of cefotaxime is 2 g every 6 hours and that of ceftriaxone is 2 g every 12 hours. If the organism is sensitive to penicillin, 3–4 million units IV every 4 hours is given.
[4]The dose of ampicillin is usually 2 g IV every 4 hours.
[5]Ceftazidime is given in a dose of 50–100 mg/kg every 8 hours up to 2 g every 8 hours.
[6]The dose of vancomycin is 15 mg/kg every 8 hours.

Table 30–2. Typical cerebrospinal fluid findings in various central nervous system diseases.

Diagnosis	Cells/μL	Glucose (mg/dL)	Protein (mg/dL)	Opening Pressure
Normal	0–5 lymphocytes	45–85[1]	15–45	70–180 mm H$_2$0
Purulent meningitis (bacterial)[2] (community-acquired)	200–20,000 polymorphonuclear neutrophils	Low (< 45)	High (> 50)	Markedly elevated
Granulomatous meningitis (mycobacterial, fungal)[2]	100–1000, mostly lymphocytes[3]	Low (< 45)	High (> 50)	Moderately elevated
Aseptic meningitis, viral or meningoencephalitis[4]	100–1000, mostly lymphocytes[3]	Normal	Moderately high (> 50)	Normal to slightly elevated
Spirochetal meningitis	25–2000, mostly lymphocytes[3]	Normal or low	High (> 50)	Slightly elevated
"Neighborhood" reaction[5]	Variably increased	Normal	Normal or high	Variable

[1]Cerebrospinal fluid glucose must be considered in relation to blood glucose level. Normally, cerebrospinal fluid glucose is 20–30 mg/dL lower than blood glucose, or 50–70% of the normal value of blood glucose.
[2]Organisms in smear or culture of cerebrospinal fluid; counterimmunoelectrophoresis or latex agglutination may be diagnostic.
[3]Polymorphonuclear neutrophils may predominate early.
[4]Viral isolation from cerebrospinal fluid early; antibody titer rise in paired specimens of serum.
[5]May occur in mastoiditis, brain abscess, epidural abscess, sinusitis, septic thrombus, brain tumor. Cerebrospinal fluid culture results usually negative.

F. Neighborhood Reaction: As noted in Table 30–2, this term denotes a purulent infectious process in close proximity to the central nervous system that spills some of the products of the inflammatory process— white blood cells or protein—into the cerebrospinal fluid. Such an infection might be a brain abscess, osteomyelitis of the vertebrae, epidural abscess, subdural empyema, or bacterial sinusitis or mastoiditis.

G. Noninfectious Meningeal Irritation: Meningismus, presenting with the classic signs of meningeal irritation with totally normal cerebrospinal fluid findings, may occur in the presence of other infections such as pneumonia and shigellosis. Carcinomatous meningitis, sarcoidosis, systemic lupus erythematosus, chemical meningitis, and certain drugs (NSAIDs, OKT3, trimethoprim-sulfamethoxazole, and others) can also produce symptoms and signs of meningeal irritation with associated cerebrospinal fluid pleocytosis, increased protein, and low or normal glucose.

H. Brain Abscess: Brain abscess presents as a space-occupying lesion; symptoms may include vomiting, fever, change of mental status, or focal neurologic manifestations. If brain abscess is suspected, a CT scan should precede lumbar puncture. The bacteriology of brain abscess is usually polymicrobial and includes *S aureus,* gram-negative bacilli, streptococci, and anaerobes (including anaerobic streptococci and *Prevotella* species).

I. Amebic Meningoencephalitis: These infections are caused by free-living amebas and present as two distinct syndromes. The diagnosis is confirmed by culture or identification of the organism in cerebrospinal fluid or on biopsy specimens. No effective therapy is available.

1. Primary amebic meningoencephalitis is caused by *Naegleria fowleri* and is an acute fulminant disease characterized by signs of meningeal irritation that rapidly progresses to encephalitis and death. Anecdotal reports of cure of primary amebic meningoencephalitis have been reported with intravenous and intraventricular administration of amphotericin B.

2. Granulomatous amebic encephalitis is caused by *Acanthamoeba* species. It is an indolent disease characterized by headache, nausea, vomiting, cranial neuropathies, seizures, and hemiparesis.

Treatment

Treatment consists of supporting circulation, ventilation, the airway, and other vital functions that may be compromised by infection and resulting disturbance of the central nervous system. Increased intracranial pressure due to brain edema often requires therapeutic attention. Hyperventilation, mannitol (25–50 g as a bolus intravenous infusion), and even drainage of cerebrospinal fluid through placement of ventricular catheters have been employed to control cerebral edema and increased intracranial pressure. Dexamethasone (4 mg every 4–6 hours) may also decrease cerebral edema. In the case of purulent meningitis, proper antimicrobial treatment is imperative. Since the identity of the causative microorganism may remain unknown or doubtful for a few days, initial antibiotic treatment as set forth in Table 30–1 should be directed against the microorganisms most common for each age group.

The duration of therapy for bacterial meningitis varies depending upon the etiologic agent: *Haemophilus influenzae* 7 days; *Neisseria meningitidis* 7 days; *Streptococcus pneumoniae* 10–14 days; *Listeria monocytogenes* 14–21 days; gram-negative bacilli 21 days.

Dexamethasone therapy (0.15 mg/kg every 6 hours for 4 days) for bacterial meningitis in infants and children may be beneficial in preventing hearing loss and decreasing the incidence of neurologic sequelae (ataxia and seizures) but has no effect on the survival rate. Most studies showing efficacy of corticosteroids in infants and children were done on patients infected with *H influenzae,* an uncommon pathogen since immunization against this organism has become commonplace. In infants infected with *S pneumoniae,* corticosteroids have not been shown to confer a statistically significant benefit. The role of corticosteroids in adults is even less clear. In addition, corticosteroids can decrease the penetration of vancomycin into the cerebrospinal fluid in adults—an observation of importance in areas where penicillin-resistant pneumococci are prevalent. Despite the uncertainties, dexamethasone is usually given to infants and children and has been recommended in adults with high bacteria loads (ie, positive Gram stain) and those with increased intracranial pressures. Therapy of brain abscess consists of drainage (excision or aspiration) in addition to 3–4 weeks of systemic antibiotics directed against organisms isolated. A regimen often used includes metronidazole, 500 mg intravenously every 8 hours, plus ceftizoxime, 2 g intravenously every 8 hours. In cases where abscesses are less than 2 cm in size, whenever there are multiple abscesses that cannot be drained, or if an abscess is located in an area where significant neurologic sequelae would result from drainage, antibiotics for 6–8 weeks without drainage can be employed.

Therapy of other types of meningitis is discussed elsewhere in this book (fungal meningitis, Chapter 36; syphilis and Lyme borreliosis, Chapter 34; tuberculous meningitis, Chapter 33; herpes encephalitis, Chapter 32).

Johnson RT: Acute encephalitis. Clin Infect Dis 1996;23:219. (Comprehensive review.)

Quaglierello VJ, Scheld WM: Treatment of bacterial meningitis. N Engl J Med 1997;336:708. (Review of etiology and therapy, including use of corticosteroids and treatment of infection with penicillin-resistant pneumococci.)

ANIMAL & HUMAN BITE WOUNDS

About 1% of emergency room visits in urban areas are for treatment of animal and human bites. Dog bites occur most commonly in the summer months, and most occur in children. Biting animals are usually known by their victims, and most biting incidents are provoked (ie, bites occur while playing with the animal or after surprising the animal or waking it abruptly from sleep). Failure to elicit a history of provocation is important, because an unprovoked attack raises the possibility that the animal is rabid. Human bites are usually inflicted by children while playing or fighting; in adults, bites are associated with alcohol use and closed-fist injuries that occur during fights.

The animal inflicting the bite, the location of the bite, and the type of injury inflicted are all important determinants of whether these injuries become infected. Cat bites are more likely to become infected than human bites—between 30% and 50% of all cat bites subsequently become infected. Infections following human bites are variable: Those inflicted by children rarely become infected, because they are superficial; and bites by adults become infected in 15–30% of cases, with a particularly high rate of infection in closed-fist injuries. Dog bites, for unclear reasons, become infected only 5% of the time. Bites of the head, face, and neck are less likely to become infected than bites on the extremities. Puncture wounds become infected more frequently than lacerations, probably because the latter are easier to irrigate and debride.

The bacteriology of bite infections depends upon the biting animal and when the infection occurs after the biting incident. Early infections (within 24 hours after the bite) following dog and cat bites are most frequently caused by *Pasteurella multocida.* These infections are characterized by rapid onset and progression, fevers, chills, cellulitis, and local adenopathy. Early infections following human bites are usually caused by mixed aerobic and anaerobic mouth flora and can produce a rapidly progressive necrotizing infection. Late infections (longer than 24 hours after the bite) are caused mainly by staphylococci and streptococci, but innumerable organisms have been implicated in these infections. *Capnocytophaga canimorsus* (formerly called a DF2 organism), a gram-negative organism that is part of canine oral flora; *Eikenella corrodens,* another gram-negative organism that can be part of human mouth flora; *Haemophilus* spp, *Pseudomonas* spp, and other gram-negative organisms—all have been implicated in bite infections.

There have been no documented cases of HIV transmission by human bites.

Treatment

A. Local Care: Vigorous cleansing and irrigation of the wound as well as debridement of necrotic material are the most important factors in decreasing the incidence of infections. X-rays should be obtained to look for fractures and the presence of foreign bodies. Careful examination to assess the extent of the injury (tendon laceration, joint space penetration) is critical to appropriate care.

B. Suturing: If wounds require closure for cosmetic or mechanical reasons, suturing can be done.

However, one should never suture a wound that is already infected, and wounds of the hand should generally not be sutured since a closed-space infection of the hand can result in loss of function.

C. Prophylactic Antibiotics: Prophylaxis is indicated in high-risk bites, eg, cat bites in any location (dicloxacillin, 0.5 g orally four times a day for 3–5 days) and hand bites by any animal or by humans (penicillin V, 0.5 g orally four times a day for 3–5 days). Although dicloxacillin and penicillin have been most extensively studied for prophylaxis, there is concern about their use because of their narrow spectrum of activity. Based on the microbiology of bite wounds noted above, other agents that have not been adequately studied but that have broader spectrums of activity may be even more effective as prophylactic agents. Examples include cefuroxime and amoxicillin-clavulanic acid. Immunocompromised patients and especially individuals without functional spleens are at risk for developing overwhelming bacteremia and sepsis following animal bites and thus should also receive prophylaxis.

D. Antibiotics: For wounds that are infected, antibiotics are clearly indicated. How they are given (orally or intravenously) and the need for hospitalization are individualized clinical decisions. In general, *P multocida* is best treated with penicillin or a tetracycline. Response to therapy is slow, and therapy should be continued for at least 2–3 weeks. Human bites frequently require admission to the hospital and intravenous therapy with a third-generation cephalosporin such as ceftizoxime. Because the bacteriology of these infections is so variable, one should always culture infected wounds and adjust therapy appropriately, especially if the patient is not responding to initial empiric treatment.

E. Tetanus and Rabies: All patients must be evaluated for the need for tetanus (see Chapter 33) and rabies (see Chapter 32) prophylaxis.

Cummings P: Antibiotics to prevent infection in patients with dog bite wounds: A meta-analysis of randomized trials. Ann Emerg Med 1994;23:535. (Reasonable for "high-risk" wounds.)

Griego RD et al: Dog, cat, and human bites. A review. J Am Acad Dermatol 1995;33:1019. (Microbiology, prophylaxis, therapy.)

Wiggins ME, Akelman E, Weiss A-PC: The management of dog bites and dog bite infections to the hand. Orthopedics 1994;17:617. (A review of recommendations for local care, prophylaxis, and antibiotic treatment.)

SEXUALLY TRANSMITTED DISEASES

Some infectious diseases are transmitted most commonly—or most efficiently—by sexual contact. Most of the infectious agents that cause sexually transmitted diseases are fairly easily inactivated when exposed to a harsh environment. They are thus particularly suited to transmission by contact with mucous membranes. They may be bacteria (eg, gonococci), spirochetes (syphilis), chlamydiae (nongonococcal urethritis, cervicitis), viruses (eg, herpes simplex, hepatitis B virus, cytomegalovirus, HIV), or protozoa (eg, *Trichomonas*). In most infections caused by these agents, early lesions occur on genitalia or other sexually exposed mucous membranes; however, wide dissemination may occur, and involvement of nongenital tissues and organs may mimic many noninfectious disorders. All sexually transmitted diseases have subclinical or latent phases that play an important role in long-term persistence of the infection or in its transmission from infected (but largely asymptomatic) persons to other contacts. Laboratory examinations are of particular importance in the diagnosis of such asymptomatic patients. Simultaneous infection by several different agents is common, and any person with a sexually transmitted disease should be tested for syphilis. If the test is negative, a repeat study should be done in 3 months, since seroconversion can be delayed.

For each patient, there are one or more sexual contacts who require diagnosis and treatment. As a rule, sexual partners should be treated simultaneously to avoid prompt reinfection. Finding a sexually transmitted disease in a child strongly suggests sexual abuse, and such cases must be reported to the authorities. The commonest sexually transmitted diseases are gonorrhea,* syphilis,* condyloma acuminatum, chlamydial genital infections, herpesvirus genital infections, *Trichomonas* vaginitis, chancroid,* granuloma inguinale,* scabies, louse infestation, and bacterial vaginosis (among lesbians). However, shigellosis,* hepatitis A, B, and C,* amebiasis,* giardiasis, cryptosporidiasis, salmonellosis,* and campylobacteriosis may also be transmitted by sexual (oralanal) contact, especially in homosexual males. Homosexual contact is the most prevalent method of transmission of HIV and AIDS,* though bidirectional heterosexual transmission can also occur (see Chapter 31).

The risk of developing a sexually transmitted disease following a sexual assault has not been extensively studied. Victims of assault have a high baseline rate of infection (*Neisseria gonorrhoeae* 6%, *Chlamydia trachomatis* 10%, *Trichomonas vaginalis* 15%, and bacterial vaginosis 34%), and the risk of acquiring infection as a result of the assault is significant but is lower than the preexisting rate (*N gonorrhoeae* 6–12%, *C trachomatis* 4–17%, *T vaginalis* 12%, syphilis 0.5–3%, and bacterial vaginosis 19%). Victims should be evaluated within 24 hours after the assault, and cultures for *N gonorrhoeae*, *C trachomatis,* and herpes simplex virus should be obtained and

---

*Reportable to public health authorities.

vaginal secretions examined for *Trichomonas* and bacterial vaginosis. In addition, a blood sample should be obtained for serologic testing for syphilis. (An additional sample should be stored for future testing for HIV and hepatitis B if needed.) Follow-up examination for sexually transmitted disease should be repeated at 2 weeks, since concentrations of infecting organisms may not have been sufficient to produce a positive culture at the time of initial examination. Follow-up serologic testing for syphilis and HIV should be performed in 3 months. Prophylactic antibiotics should be given if the assailant is known to be infected. The usefulness of presumptive therapy is controversial, some workers feeling that all patients should receive it and others that it should be limited to those in whom follow-up cannot be ensured or that it should be given only to those who request it. If therapy is given, a reasonable regimen would be one dose of ceftriaxone, 125 mg intramuscularly, plus metronidazole, 2 g orally as a single dose, plus doxycycline, 100 mg orally twice daily for 7 days. If the patient is pregnant, azithromycin, 1 g as a single dose, should be used instead of doxycycline, and metronidazole should be given only after the first trimester.

Although seroconversion to HIV has been reported following sexual assault when this was the only known risk, the risk of developing HIV is felt to be minimal. Because prophylactic antiretroviral therapy is not of proved benefit, it is generally not recommended in this setting.

Hampton HL: Care of the woman who has been raped. N Engl J Med 1995;332:234. (Review of medical, forensic, and psychologic issues associated with assault.)

1993 Sexually Transmitted Diseases Treatment Guidelines. MMWR Morb Mortal Wkly Rep 1993;42(RR-14):97. (CDC guidelines for management of victims of sexual assault.)

INFECTIONS IN DRUG USERS

The abuse of parenterally administered narcotic drugs has increased enormously in recent years. There are now an estimated 300,000 or more intravenous drug users in the USA, mostly in or near large urban centers. Consequently, physicians and hospitals serving such urban and suburban populations must deal with many problems—including infections—related to drug abuse.

Common Infections That Occur With Greater Frequency in Drug Users

(1) **Skin infections** are associated with poor hygiene and use of nonsterile technique when injecting drugs. *S aureus* is the most common organism involved, but streptococci, enteric gram-negative organisms, and anaerobes can also cause skin infections. Cellulitis and subcutaneous abscesses occur most commonly. Myositis and necrotizing fasciitis occur infrequently but are life-threatening.

(2) **Hepatitis** is very common among habitual drug users and is transmissible both by the parenteral (hepatitis B, C, and D virus) and by the fecal-oral route (hepatitis A). Multiple episodes of hepatitis with different agents can occur.

(3) **Aspiration pneumonia** and its complications (lung abscess, empyema, brain abscess) result from altered consciousness associated with drug abuse. Mixed aerobic and anaerobic mouth flora are usually involved.

(4) **Tuberculosis** also occurs in drug users, and infection with HIV has fostered the spread of tuberculosis in this population. Morbidity and mortality rates are increased in HIV-infected individuals with tuberculosis. Tuberculosis should be suspected in those who have classic radiographic findings and in those with infiltrates who do not respond to antibiotics.

(5) **Pulmonary septic emboli** may originate from venous thrombi or right-sided endocarditis.

(6) **Sexually transmitted diseases** are not directly related to drug abuse, but the practice of exchanging sex for drugs has resulted in an increased frequency of sexually transmitted diseases. Syphilis, gonorrhea, and chancroid are the most common.

(7) **AIDS** has a high incidence among intravenous drug abusers and their sexual contacts and the offspring of infected women (see Chapter 31).

(8) **Infective endocarditis** (see below). The coexistence of HIV infection with endocarditis is associated with a poor outcome in patients with CD4 counts less than 200/μL.

Infections Rare in USA

A. Tetanus: In the 1950s and 1960s, tetanus was commonly seen in drug users, especially in unimmunized women who injected drugs subcutaneously ("skin-popping"). Increased tetanus immunization among drug users has resulted in a decline in this disease, though cases are still reported.

B. Malaria: Needle transmission occurs from intravenous drug users who acquired the infection in malaria-endemic areas outside the USA.

C. Melioidosis: This chronic pulmonary infection caused by *Pseudomonas pseudomallei* is occasionally seen in debilitated drug users.

Osteomyelitis & Septic Arthritis

Osteomyelitis involving vertebral bodies, sternoclavicular joints, and other sites usually results from hematogenous distribution of injected organisms or septic venous thrombi. Pain and fever precede radiographic changes by several weeks. While staphylococci—often methicillin-resistant—are common organisms, *Serratia, Pseudomonas,* and other pathogens rarely encountered in spontaneous bone or joint disease are found in addicts who use drugs intravenously.

Infective Endocarditis

The organisms that cause infective endocarditis in those who use drugs intravenously are most commonly *S aureus, Candida* (especially *Candida parapsilosis*), *Enterococcus faecalis,* other streptococci, and gram-negative bacteria (especially *Pseudomonas* and *Serratia marcescens*).

Involvement of the right side of the heart is somewhat more frequent than involvement of the left side, and infection of more than one valve is not infrequent. Right-sided involvement, especially in the absence of murmurs, is often suggested by the presence of septic pulmonary emboli. The diagnosis must be established by blood culture. Therapy, including empiric treatment, is discussed in Chapter 33.

Approach to the Patient

A common and difficult clinical problem is management of the parenteral drug user who presents with fever. In general, after obtaining appropriate cultures (blood, urine, and sputum if the chest x-ray is abnormal), empiric therapy is begun. If the chest x-ray is suggestive of a community-acquired pneumonia (consolidation), therapy for outpatient pneumonia is begun with a second- or third-generation cephalosporin (many would add erythromycin to this regimen). If the chest x-ray is suggestive of septic emboli (nodular infiltrates), therapy for presumed endocarditis is initiated, usually with a combination of nafcillin and gentamicin. Ampicillin should be added if enterococci are a consideration. If the chest x-ray is normal and no focal site of infection can be found, endocarditis is presumed. While awaiting the results of blood cultures, empiric treatment with nafcillin and gentamicin (with or without ampicillin) is started. If blood cultures are positive for organisms that frequently cause endocarditis in drug users (see above), endocarditis is presumed to be present and treated accordingly. If blood cultures are positive for an organism that is an unusual cause of endocarditis, evaluation for an occult source of infection should go forward. In this setting, a transesophageal echocardiogram may be quite helpful since it is 90% sensitive in detecting vegetations and a negative study is strong evidence against endocarditis. If blood cultures are negative and the patient responds to antibiotics, therapy should be continued for 7–14 days (oral therapy can be given once an initial response has occurred). In every patient, careful examination for an occult source of infection (genitourinary, dental, sinus, gallbladder, etc) should be done.

Levine DP, Sobel JD: Infections in intravenous drug abusers. In: *Principles and Practice of Infectious Diseases,* 4th ed. Mandell GL, Bennett JE, Dolin R (editors). Churchill Livingstone, 1995.

Matthew J et al: Clinical features, sites of involvement, bacteriologic findings, and outcome of infective endocarditis in intravenous drug users. Arch Intern Med 1995;155:1641. (Review of 125 cases with emphasis on site of involvement, bacteriology, treatment, and complications.)

O'Conner PG, Selwyn PA, Schottenfield RS: Medical care for injection drug users with human immunodeficiency virus infection. N Engl J Med 1994;331:450. (Discussion of medical and social issues.)

FOOD POISONING & ACUTE GASTROENTERITIS

Food poisoning is a nonspecific term often applied to the syndrome of acute anorexia, nausea, vomiting, or diarrhea that is attributed to food intake, particularly if it afflicts groups of people and is not accompanied by fever. The actual cause of such acute gastrointestinal upsets might be emotional stress, viral or bacterial infections, food intolerance, inorganic (eg, sodium nitrite) or organic (eg, mushroom, shellfish) poisons, or drugs (eg, antimicrobials). More specifically, the term "food poisoning" denotes disorders caused by toxins produced by bacteria growing in food (staphylococci, clostridia, *Bacillus cereus*), or acute food infections with short incubation periods and a mild course (*Salmonella enterocolitis* [see above]), or infection with enterotoxigenic *Escherichia coli,* shigellae, or vibrios (*Vibrio cholerae,* El Tor vibrios, marine vibrios including *Vibrio parahaemolyticus, Vibrio vulnificus*). *Campylobacter jejuni* and *Yersinia enterocolitica* may produce similar clinical enterocolitis and can be identified only by special stool culture methods. *E coli* O157:H7 is an infrequent cause of hemorrhagic colitis. Adenoviruses, rotaviruses, astroviruses, and Norwalk-type viruses may produce a similar syndrome. Various protozoa (*Entamoeba histolytica, Giardia,* microsporidia, *Isospora,* cryptosporidia, and others) can also cause acute or chronic diarrhea. (See Chapter 35.) Some prominent features of some of these food poisonings are listed in Table 30–3. In general, the diagnosis must be suspected when groups of people who have shared a meal develop acute vomiting or diarrhea. Food and stools must be obtained for bacteriologic and toxicologic examination. In febrile patients, blood cultures are indicated.

Treatment usually consists of replacement of fluids and electrolytes and, very rarely, management of hypovolemic shock and respiratory embarrassment. In general, most cases of acute gastroenteritis are self-limited and do not require therapy other than supportive measures. When symptoms persist beyond 3–4 days, initial presentation is accompanied by fever or bloody diarrhea, or the patient is immunocompromised, cultures of stool are usually obtained. Symptoms have often resolved by the time

Table 30–3. Acute bacterial diarrheas and "food poisoning."

Organism	Incubation Period (hours)	Vomiting	Diarrhea	Fever	Microbiology	Pathogenesis	Clinical Features
Staphylococcus	1–8, rarely up to 18	+++	+	–	Staphylococci grow in meats, dairy, bakery products and produce enterotoxin.	Enterotoxin acts on receptors in gut that transmit impulses to medullary centers.	Abrupt onset, intense vomiting for up to 24 hours, regular recovery in 24–48 hours. Occurs in persons eating the same food. No treatment usually necessary except to restore fluids and electrolytes.
Bacillus cereus	1–8, rarely up to 18	+++	+	–	Reheated fried rice causes vomiting or diarrhea.	Enterotoxins formed in food or in gut from growth of *B cereus*.	After 1–6 hours, mainly vomiting. After 8–16 hours, mainly diarrhea. Both self-limited to less than 1 day.
Clostridium perfringens	8–16	±	+++	–	Clostridia grow in rewarmed meat dishes and produce enterotoxin.	Enterotoxin produced in food and in gut causes hypersecretion in small intestine.	Abrupt onset of profuse diarrhea; vomiting occasionally. Recovery usual without treatment in 1–4 days. Many clostridia in cultures of food and feces of patients.
Clostridium botulinum	24–96	±	Rare	–	Clostridia grow in anaerobic foods and produce toxin.	Toxin absorbed from gut blocks acetylcholine at neuromuscular junction.	Diplopia, dysphagia, dysphonia, respiratory embarrassment. Treatment requires clear airway, ventilation, and intravenous polyvalent antitoxin (see text). Toxin present in food and serum. Mortality rate high.
Clostridium difficile	?	–	+++	+	Associated with antimicrobial drugs, eg, clindamycin.	Enterotoxin causes epithelial necrosis in colon; pseudomembranous colitis.	Especially after abdominal surgery, abrupt bloody diarrhea, and fever. Toxin in stool. Oral vancomycin or metronidazole useful in therapy.
Escherichia coli (some strains)	24–72	±	+	–	Organisms grow in gut and produce toxin. May also invade superficial epithelium.	Enterotoxin causes hypersecretion in small intestine.	Usually abrupt onset of diarrhea; vomiting rare. A serious infection in neonates. In adults, "traveler's diarrhea" is usually self-limited to 1–3 days. Use diphenoxylate with atropine but no antimicrobials.

(continued)

Table 30–3. Acute bacterial diarrheas and "food poisoning." (continued)

Organism	Incubation Period (hours)	Vomiting	Diarrhea	Fever	Microbiology	Pathogenesis	Clinical Features
Vibrio parahaemo-lyticus	6–96	+	+	±	Organisms grow in seafood and in gut and produce toxin, or invade.	Hypersecretion in small intestine; stools may be bloody.	Abrupt onset of diarrhea in groups consuming the same food, especially crabs and other seafood. Recovery is usually complete in 1–3 days. Food and stool cultures are positive.
Vibrio cholerae (mild cases)	24–72	+	+++	–	Organisms grow in gut and produce toxin.	Enterotoxin causes hypersecretion in small intestine. Infective dose: 10^7–10^9 organisms.	Abrupt onset of liquid diarrhea in endemic area. Needs prompt replacement of fluids and electrolytes IV or orally. Tetracyclines shorten excretion of vibrios. Stool cultures positive.
Campylobacter jejuni	2–10 days	–	+++	+	Organisms grow in jejunum and ileum.	Invasion and enterotoxin production uncertain.	Fever, diarrhea; PMNs and fresh blood in stool, especially in children. Usually self-limited. Special media needed for culture at 43 °C. Erythromycin in severe cases with invasion. Usual recovery in 5–8 days.
Shigella spp (mild cases)	24–72	±	+	+	Organisms grow in superficial gut epithelium and gut lumen and produce toxin.	Organisms invade epithelial cells; blood, mucus, and PMNs in stools. Infective dose: 10^2–10^3 organisms.	Abrupt onset of diarrhea, often with blood and pus in stools, cramps, tenesmus, and lethargy. Stool cultures are positive. In severe cases, give trimethoprim-sulfamethoxazole, ampicillin, or chloramphenicol. Do not give opiates. Often mild and self-limited.
Salmonella spp	8–48	±	+	+	Organisms grow in gut. Do not produce toxin.	Superficial infection of gut, little invasion. Infective dose: 10^5 organisms.	Gradual or abrupt onset of diarrhea and low-grade fever. No antimicrobials unless systemic dissemination is suspected. Stool cultures are positive. Prolonged carriage is frequent.
Yersinia enterocolitica	?	±	+	+	Fecal-oral transmission (occasionally). Foodborne. In pets.	Gastroenteritis or mesenteric adenitis. Occasional bacteremia. Enterotoxin produced.	Severe abdominal pain, diarrhea, fever; PMNs and blood in stool; polyarthritis, erythema nodosum in children. If severe, give tetracycline or gentamicin. Keep stool at 4 °C before culture.

cultures are completed. In this case, even if a pathogen is isolated, therapy is not needed (except for *Shigella,* since the infecting dose is so small that therapy to eradicate organisms from the stool is indicated for epidemiologic reasons). If symptoms persist and a pathogen is isolated, it is reasonable to institute specific treatment even though therapy has not been conclusively shown to alter the natural history of disease for most pathogens. Exceptions include gastroenteritis due to *Salmonella* (where therapy may prolong the carrier state and increase the relapse rate) and *Campylobacter* (early therapy shortens the course of disease). Several studies examining the effect of antibiotic therapy on domestically acquired diarrhea have suggested that ciprofloxacin, 500 mg every 12 hours for 5 days, is effective in shortening the course of illness compared with placebo. Because of concerns about selecting for resistant organisms coupled with the fact that most infectious diarrhea is self-limited, routine use of antibiotics for all patients with diarrhea is not recommended. Antibiotics should be considered in patients with evidence of invasive disease (white cells in stool, dysentery), with symptoms 3–4 days or more in duration, with multiple stools (eight to ten or more per day) and in those with impaired immune responses. Antimotility drugs may relieve cramping and decrease diarrhea in mild cases. Their use should be limited to patients without fever and without dysentery (bloody stools), and they should be used in low doses.

Therapeutic recommendations for specific agents can be found elsewhere in this book.

Park SI, Giannella RA: Approach to the adult patient with acute diarrhea. Gastroenterol Clin North Am 1993; 22:483. (Review discussing etiology, diagnosis, and therapy.)

TRAVELER'S DIARRHEA

Whenever a person travels from one country to another—particularly if the change involves a marked difference in climate, social conditions, or sanitation standards and facilities—diarrhea is likely to develop within 2–10 days. There may be up to ten or even more loose stools per day, often accompanied by abdominal cramps, nausea, occasionally vomiting, and rarely fever. The stools do not usually contain mucus or blood, and aside from weakness, dehydration, and occasionally acidosis, there are no systemic manifestations of infection. The illness usually subsides spontaneously within 1–5 days, although 10% remain symptomatic for a week or longer, and in 2% symptoms persist for longer than a month.

Bacteria cause 80% of cases of traveler's diarrhea, with enterotoxigenic *E coli, Shigella* species, and *Campylobacter jejuni* being the most common pathogens. Less common causative agents include *Aeromonas, Salmonella,* noncholera vibrios, *Entamoeba histolytica,* and *Giardia lamblia.* Contributory causes may at times include unusual food and drink, change in living habits, occasional viral infections (adenoviruses or rotaviruses), and change in bowel flora. In patients with fever and bloody diarrhea, stool culture may be indicated, but in most cases cultures are reserved for those who do not respond to antibiotics. Chronic watery diarrhea may be due to amebiasis or giardiasis or, rarely, tropical sprue.

For most individuals, the affliction is short-lived, and symptomatic therapy with opiates or diphenoxylate with atropine is all that is required provided the patient is not systemically ill (fever $\geq$ 39 °C) and does not have dysentery (bloody stools), in which case antimotility agents should be avoided. Packages of oral rehydration salts to treat dehydration are available over the counter in the USA and in many foreign countries. Avoidance of fresh foods and water sources that are likely to be contaminated is recommended for travelers to developing countries, where infectious diarrheal illnesses are endemic. Prophylaxis is recommended for those with significant underlying disease (inflammatory bowel disease, AIDS, diabetes, heart disease in the elderly, conditions requiring immunosuppressive medications) and for those whose full activity status during the trip is so essential that even short periods of diarrhea would be unacceptable. Prophylaxis is started upon entry into the destination country and is continued for 1 or 2 days after leaving. For stays of more than 3 weeks, prophylaxis is not recommended because of the cost and increased toxicity. For prophylaxis, bismuth subsalicylate is effective but turns the tongue and the stools blue and can interfere with doxycycline absorption, which may be needed for malaria prophylaxis. Numerous antimicrobial regimens for once-daily prophylaxis also are effective, such as norfloxacin 400 mg, ciprofloxacin 500 mg, ofloxacin 300 mg, or trimethoprim-sulfamethoxazole 160/800 mg. Because not all travelers will have diarrhea and because most episodes are brief and self-limited, an alternative approach that is currently recommended is to provide the traveler with a 3- to 5-day supply of antimicrobials to be taken if significant diarrhea occurs during the trip. Commonly used regimens include ciprofloxacin 500 mg twice daily, ofloxacin 300 mg twice daily, or norfloxacin 400 mg twice daily. Trimethoprim-sulfamethoxazole 160/800 mg twice daily can be used as an alternative (especially in children), but resistance is common in many areas. Aztreonam, a poorly absorbed monobactam with activity against most bacterial enteropathogens, also is efficacious when given orally in a dose of 100 mg three times daily for 5 days.

DuPont HL, Capsuto EG: Persistent diarrhea in travelers. Clin Infect Dis 1996;22:124. (Discussion of etiology, diagnosis, and therapy.)

DuPont HL, Ericsson CD: Prevention and treatment of traveler's diarrhea. N Engl J Med 1993;328:1821. (Pros and cons of prophylaxis.)

ACTIVE IMMUNIZATION AGAINST INFECTIOUS DISEASES

RECOMMENDED IMMUNIZATION OF INFANTS, CHILDREN, & ADOLESCENTS

Every individual—child or adult—should maintain an adequate defense against infectious disease by immunization. The recommended schedules and dosages change often, so that one should always consult the manufacturer's package inserts.

The schedule for active immunizations in children is presented in Table 30–4. Of note is the recommendation that all adolescents should see a health care provider at age 11–12. The objective is to ensure vaccination of those who have not received varicella or hepatitis B vaccine; to make certain that a second dose of measles-mumps-rubella (MMR) has been given as well as a booster for tetanus and diphtheria (Td); and to provide immunizations (influenza and pneumococcal vaccines) that may be indicated for certain high-risk individuals.

RECOMMENDED IMMUNIZATION OF ADULTS

Several vaccines are recommended for adults depending upon the individual's previous vaccination status and the risks of exposure to certain diseases.

Tetanus-Diphtheria Toxoid

Everyone should receive a primary series of immunizations against tetanus and diphtheria once (Table 30–4). Adults who have not previously been immunized should receive two doses of Td 1–2 months apart, followed by a booster dose 6–12 months later. Adults partially immunized in childhood with DTP need only a total of three doses of tetanus and diphtheria toxoid (ie, if one dose was given in childhood, give two doses of Td; if two doses were given, only one dose of Td is needed to complete primary immunization). The traditional recommendation has been to give booster doses of Td every 10 years throughout life. An alternative approach emphasizes ensuring that all adults receive primary immunization and recommending a single midlife (age 50 years) booster dose of Td to those who have received the full pediatric immunization, including the booster in the teenage years. If booster doses are given too frequently, an Arthus reaction as well as severe local pain and swelling can occur. Pertussis vaccine, which is combined with tetanus-diphtheria toxoid for use in children (DTP), should not be used in adults because of the frequency of adverse reactions to the whole-cell pertussis component. The recently released acellular pertussis vaccine (DTaP) appears to be immunogenic and well-tolerated in adults but is not yet recommended for adult immunization.

Measles

Adults born before 1957 are considered immune to measles. Adults born in 1957 or later who lack documentation of immunization after age 1 or who do not have a physician-documented history or laboratory evidence of previous infection should receive at least one dose of vaccine. Persons born between 1963 and 1967—a period when inactivated measles vaccine was the only product available—should also receive one dose of live attenuated vaccine. Persons vaccinated before their first birthday should also receive a single dose of vaccine. Because most adults do not have detailed information about childhood immunization or illnesses, a practical approach is to administer a single dose of MMR to all healthy adults born after 1956. Because outbreaks of measles have occurred in young adults who have received a single dose of measles vaccine, revaccination is recommended, particularly before going to college, entering a health care profession, or embarking on foreign travel to areas where measles is endemic. Entrants to colleges and universities and employees of health care institutions who have not previously been vaccinated should receive two doses of vaccine at least 1 month apart. Revaccination of an immune person is not associated with adverse effects—if the vaccination status is unknown and an indication for vaccination exists, it can be safely done. Vaccination of susceptible adults within 72 hours after exposure to an active case of measles is protective.

About 5–15% of unimmunized individuals will develop fever and about 5% a mild rash 5–12 days after vaccination. Fever and rash are self-limiting, lasting only 2–3 days. Local swelling and induration are particularly common in individuals previously vaccinated with inactivated vaccine. Pregnant women and immunosuppressed persons should not be vaccinated (with the exception of asymptomatic HIV-infected individuals, who should be vaccinated if susceptible). Recent data suggest that MMR vaccine can be safely given to patients with a history of egg allergy even when severe. A single 0.5 mL dose can be given without prior skin testing or desensitization as long as postvaccination observation for 90 minutes is possible.

Rubella

The major purpose of rubella vaccination is to pre-

Table 30–4. Recommended childhood vaccinations—United States, January–June 1996.[1,2]

Vaccine	Age										
	Birth	1 mo	2 mos	4 mos	6 mos	12 mos	15 mos	18 mos	4–6 yrs	11–12 yrs	14–16 yrs
Hepatitis B[3]	Hep B-1										
		Hep B-2			Hep B-3					Hep B[4]	
Diphtheria and tetanus toxoids and pertussis vaccine[5]			DTP	DTP	DTP	DTP (DTaP at ≥ 15 mo)			DTP or DTaP	Td	
Haemophilus influenzae type b[6]			Hib	Hib	Hib	Hib					
Poliovirus[7]			OPV (IPV)	OPV (IPV)	OPV				OPV		
Measles-mumps-rubella[8]						MMR			MMR or MMR		
Varicella-zoster virus[9]						Var				Var[10]	

■ Range of Acceptable Ages for Vaccination

▨ "Catch-Up" Vaccination[4,10]

[1]Source: Advisory Committee on Immunization Practices, American Academy of Pediatrics, and American Academy of Family Physicians. Use of trade names and commercial sources is for identification only and does not imply endorsement by the Public Health Service or the U.S. Department of Health and Human Services.
[2]Vaccines are listed under the routinely recommended ages.
[3]Infants born to hepatitis B surface antigen (HBsAg)-negative mothers should receive 2.5 μg of Recombivax HB (Merck & Co.) or 10 μg of Engerix-B (SmithKline Beecham). The second dose should be administered ≥ 1 month after the first dose. Infants born to HBsAg-positive mothers should receive 0.5 mL hepatitis B immune globulin (HBIG) within 12 hours of birth, and either 5 μg of Recombivax HB or 10 μg of Engerix-B at a separate site. The second dose is recommended at age 1–2 months and the third dose at age 6 months. Infants born to mothers whose HBsAg status is unknown should receive either 5 μg of Recombivax HB or 10 μg of Engerix-B within 12 hours of birth. The second dose of vaccine is recommended at age 1 month and the third dose at age 6 months.
[4]Adolescents who have not received three doses of hepatitis B vaccine should initiate or complete the series at age 11–12 years. The second dose should be administered at least 1 month after the first dose, and the third dose should be administered at least 4 months after the first dose and at least 2 months after the second dose.
[5]The fourth dose of diphtheria and tetanus toxoids and pertussis vaccine (DTP) may be administered at age 12 months, if at least 6 months have elapsed since the third dose of DTP. Diphtheria and tetanus toxoids and acellular pertussis vaccine (DTaP) is licensed for the fourth and/or fifth vaccine dose(s) for children aged ≥ 15 months and may be preferred for these doses in this age group. Tetanus and diphtheria toxoids, adsorbed, for adult use (Td) is recommended at age 11–12 years if at least 5 years have elapsed since the last dose of DTP, DTaP, or diphtheria and tetanus toxoids, absorbed, for pediatric use (DT).
[6]Three *Haemophilus influenzae* type b (Hib) conjugate vaccines are licensed for infant use. If PedvaxHIB (Merck & Co.) *Haemophilus* b conjugate vaccine (Meningococcal Protein Conjugate) (PRP-OMP) is administered at ages 2 and 4 months, a dose at 6 months is not required. After completing the primary series, any Hib conjugate vaccine may be used as a booster. Comvax, a combination vaccine using antigenic components from Pedvax HIB and Recombivax HB, can be used to immunize against hepatitis B and *Haemophilus.* Doses are given at ages 2, 4, and 12–15 months.
[7]Oral poliovirus vaccine (OPV) is recommended for routine infant vaccination. Because of the small but definite risk of vaccine-associated polio, which most commonly follows the first or second dose of vaccine, IPV can be substituted for the first two doses of OPV. Inactivated poliovirus vaccine (IPV) is recommended for persons—or household contacts of persons—with a congenital or acquired immune deficiency disease or an altered immune status resulting from disease or immunosuppressive therapy, and is an acceptable alternative for other persons. The primary three-dose series for IPV should be given with a minimum interval of 4 weeks between the first and second doses and 6 months between the second and third doses.
[8]The second dose of measles-mumps-rubella vaccine (MMR) is routinely recommended at age 4–6 years or at age 11–12 years but may be administered at any visit provided at least 1 month has elapsed since receipt of the first dose.
[9]Varicella-zoster virus vaccine (Var) can be administered to susceptible children any time after age 12 months.
[10]Unvaccinated children who lack a reliable history of chickenpox should be vaccinated at age 11–12 years.

vent transmission to the fetus. Immunization is recommended for all adults but particularly for women of childbearing age who have not previously been immunized. In addition, both male and female hospital workers who may be exposed to patients with rubella or who might have contact with pregnant patients should be immunized. A single immunization is given. Because of the expense of serologic testing to identify susceptible individuals and because revaccination of immune individuals is not associated with adverse effects, routine serologic testing is not required prior to vaccination.

Adverse effects are usually mild. Up to 40% of unvaccinated adults (usually women) experience joint pain. Joint symptoms begin 1–3 weeks after vaccination and are self-limited, lasting 3–10 days. Frank arthritis is rare. Although vaccination of pregnant women is *not* recommended, available data suggest that with the RA27/3 vaccine strain (the one presently available), the congenital rubella syndrome does not occur in the offspring of those inadvertently vaccinated during pregnancy or within 3 months before conception. Persons immunosuppressed by virtue of disease or medication should not receive vaccine. HIV infection is an exception—vaccine should be given to asymptomatic individuals and may be considered in symptomatic patients. Since the vaccine contains trace amounts of neomycin, a history of anaphylaxis to this agent is a contraindication to vaccine use.

Mumps

Mumps vaccine is recommended for all adults thought to be susceptible. Persons born before 1957 are considered to be naturally immune and do not require vaccination. Those born in 1957 or later should be considered susceptible unless they can document infection, prove vaccination, or have laboratory evidence of immunity. Vaccination in those already immune is not associated with an increased incidence of adverse effects.

Mumps vaccine is generally safe. It should not be given to those who are immunosuppressed (except HIV-infected individuals) or who have a history of anaphylaxis to neomycin.

Influenza

Influenza vaccination is recommended yearly. Those at greatest risk for severe complications of influenza should have priority in vaccination programs: (1) Adults and children with chronic cardiopulmonary disease, including children with asthma. (2) Residents of nursing homes and other chronic care facilities. (3) Healthy adults 65 years of age or older. (4) Adults and children who have required either regular medical follow-up or hospitalization in the last year for chronic metabolic disorders (including diabetes) or renal disease, those with hemoglobinopathies, and those receiving immunosuppressive

drugs. (5) Children and teenagers (age 6 months to 18 years) who are on long-term aspirin therapy and would be at increased risk for developing Reye's syndrome following influenza. Certain high-risk groups of patients (the elderly, persons with AIDS, transplant patients) may have a poor antibody response to vaccine, but there is no reason not to vaccinate them. Recent studies have suggested that following vaccination of HIV-positive patients there is a brief (2- to 4-week) period of increased HIV viremia and viral replication. The clinical significance of this is not known, and progression of disease after vaccination has not been observed. Thus, the potential benefit of vaccination of HIV-positive individuals outweighs any theoretic risks. In an attempt to prevent disease in high-risk patients, vaccination of household members and health care providers who have contact with these high-risk patients should also be vaccinated. Vaccination is recommended also for otherwise healthy adults who provide essential community services.

Local reactions (erythema and tenderness) at the site of injection are common, but fevers, chills, and malaise (which last in any case only 2–3 days) are rare. Like measles, mumps, and yellow fever vaccines, influenza vaccine is prepared using embryonated chicken eggs, and persons with a history of anaphylaxis to eggs should not be vaccinated. Influenza vaccination may be associated with multiple false-positive serologic tests to HIV, HTLV-1, and hepatitis C. Seropositivity is self-limited, lasting 2–5 months.

Pneumococcal Pneumonia

Pneumococcal vaccine contains purified polysaccharide from 23 of the most common strains of *Streptococcus pneumoniae,* which cause 90% of bacteremic episodes in the USA. Antibody response following vaccination is dependent upon the patient's immune status and the presence of concomitant disease. Healthy adults have an excellent antibody response, as do patients who are postsplenectomy and those with sickle cell disease. Elderly individuals and those with chronic diseases (diabetes mellitus, alcoholic cirrhosis, chronic obstructive pulmonary disease) have increased antibody levels following vaccination but to a lesser extent than young healthy adults. Patients with Hodgkin's disease respond to vaccination if it is given before splenectomy, radiation, or chemotherapy, whereas patients with leukemia, lymphoma, and HIV infection respond poorly.

Although the efficacy of pneumococcal vaccine has been questioned, most postlicensure studies indicate that vaccination is about 60–70% effective in preventing bacteremic disease in immunocompetent persons. It is 50% effective in patients with underlying diseases (not severely immunocompromised) and even less effective in immunocompromised patients (only 10% effective) largely because of inability to mount an antibody response in this population of patients. It is presently recommended for patients at increased risk for developing severe pneumococcal disease, especially asplenic patients and those with sickle cell disease. It is also recommended for adults who are at increased risk of developing pneumococcal disease, including those with chronic illnesses (eg, cardiopulmonary disease, alcoholism, cirrhosis, cerebrospinal fluid leaks), those who are immunocompromised (eg, patients with Hodgkin's disease, lymphoma, chronic lymphocytic leukemia, multiple myeloma, chronic renal failure, nephrotic syndrome, organ transplant recipients, and asymptomatic or symptomatic HIV infection), and those taking immunosuppressive medications. In addition, it is recommended for all individuals over 65 years of age. Whether 65 is the appropriate age to vaccinate healthy adults is unclear. Antibody response declines with age, and some have suggested routine immunization at age 50 similar to the recommendation for tetanus (see above). A single dose of vaccine usually confers lifelong immunity. Revaccination every 6 years should be considered only in those at highest risk of fatal pneumococcal infection (eg, asplenic patients), those known to have a rapid decline in antibody titers (eg, those with nephrotic syndrome or renal failure, transplant recipients), and those 65 years of age who were previously immunized because of risk factors and have not been immunized in the last 6 years. Revaccination should also be considered for high-risk individuals previously immunized with the older 14-valent vaccine. Since immunocompetent patients respond best to the vaccine, it should be given 1 month before splenectomy or before starting chemotherapy if that can be anticipated.

Mild reactions (erythema and tenderness) occur in up to 50% of recipients, but systemic reactions are uncommon. The incidence of adverse reactions with revaccination is unknown but is probably related to the interval between vaccinations. Early reports suggested frequent adverse reactions when revaccination occurred within 1–2 years. Subsequent reports have indicated few adverse reactions when revaccination occurs 5 or more years later.

Hepatitis B

Recombinant hepatitis B vaccine is given intramuscularly in the deltoid—gluteal injection often results in deposition of vaccine in fat rather than muscle, with fewer serologic conversions—on three separate occasions: the first two doses 1 month apart and the last dose 5 months after the second one. It is recommended for all individuals at increased risk of developing hepatitis B for social reasons (intravenous drug users, male homosexuals), family reasons (household and sexual contacts of hepatitis B carriers), or occupational reasons (those with frequent exposure to blood and blood products, hemodialysis patients and staff, house officers, medical students, morticians). For immunosuppressed patients and those being maintained on hemodialysis, seroresponse to standard doses of vaccine is low, and for that reason preparations delivering a higher vaccine dose (40 µg/mL) have become available. In addition to higher vaccine doses, these patients may require more frequent immunizations, and some experts have recommended annual screening to determine whether booster doses are needed. Although most often used for preexposure prophylaxis, the vaccine is also given as postexposure prophylaxis along with hepatitis B immunoglobulin following needle stick injury or mucous membrane exposure to blood from an individual who is HBsAg-positive. It is also given along with hepatitis B immunoglobulin to infants of mothers who are HBsAg-positive. Immunity wanes with time, but recommendations for routine revaccination have not been established. Adverse reactions are minor and limited to local soreness.

Following vaccination, 90–95% of healthy young individuals develop protective antibodies. A number of factors decrease serologic response, including increasing age over 30, renal failure, HIV infection, diabetes, chronic liver disease, obesity, and smoking. Postvaccination serologic testing is not routinely done. It is reserved for those whose clinical management would be influenced by their immune status (eg, health care workers, infants born to HBsAg-positive mothers, dialysis patients), and those who may have an impaired response. Those who do not respond can receive up to three additional doses at 1- to 2-month intervals with serologic testing after each dose.

Varicella

A live attenuated varicella virus vaccine is currently recommended as part of routine childhood immunization (Table 30–4). Although only 10% of adults remain susceptible, varicella in adolescents and adults is a more severe disease. Only about 2% of all cases of varicella occur in adults, but almost 50% of all deaths are in the adult population. Thus, susceptible adolescents and adults should be immunized, with special emphasis on certain high-risk groups, ie, health care workers, susceptible household contacts of immunosuppressed individuals, persons in high-risk environments such as those who work in day care centers or elementary schools, nonpregnant women of childbearing age, individuals in closed populations such as prisons or the armed forces, and international travelers. The role of the present vaccine in postexposure prophylaxis is not known, though previous formulations tested in Japan were 90% effective when given within 3 days after exposure. The vaccine is very immunogenic. Seroconversion occurs in 95% of children after a single dose. In adolescents (older than 12 years of age) and adults, seroconversion is seen in 78% after one dose and 99% after two doses. For this reason, two doses given 4–8 weeks apart are recommended in persons 12 years of age and older. The duration of immunity is not known but is probably 10 years. Although the vaccine is very effective in preventing disease, breakthrough infections do occur—but are much milder than in unvaccinated individuals (usually less than 50 lesions, with milder systemic symptoms). Although the vaccine is very safe, adverse reactions can occur as late as 4–6 weeks after vaccination. Tenderness and erythema at the injection site are seen in 25%, fever in 10–15%, a localized maculopapular or vesicular rash in 5%, and a smaller percentage develop a diffuse rash, usually with five or fewer vesicular lesions. Spread of virus from vaccinees to susceptible individuals is possible, but the risk of such transmission even to immunocompromised patients is small and disease, when it develops, is mild and treatable with acyclovir. Nonetheless, the vaccine, being a live attenuated virus, should not be given to immunocompromised individuals or pregnant women. The vaccine is contraindicated in persons allergic to neomycin. For theoretic reasons, it is recommended that following vaccination salicylates should be avoided for 6 weeks (to prevent Reye's syndrome). Several unresolved issues remain, including the need for booster doses, whether universal childhood vaccination will shift the incidence of disease to adolescence or adulthood with the possibility of more severe disease, and whether vaccination might prevent development of herpes zoster.

Hepatitis A

Two inactivated hepatitis A vaccines (Havrix, VAQTA) are approved for use in the USA. They are indicated for individuals 2 years of age or older who are at an increased risk of developing hepatitis A. Potential vaccinees include travelers (including military personnel) to areas where hepatitis is endemic (Africa, Asia, Central and South America, Mexico, parts of the Caribbean); certain populations that experience episodic hepatitis A outbreaks (such as indigenous Alaskans, certain American Indian reservations, certain religious communities); certain high-risk groups such as employees of day care centers, caretakers for developmentally impaired institutionalized individuals, and laboratory workers who handle live hepatitis A virus; homosexual men; illicit drug users; and those with chronic liver disease. Vaccine has been used as a means of controlling spread of disease during outbreaks in communities with high rates of infection. The role of hepatitis A vaccine in controlling outbreaks in day care centers, hospitals, and institutions for the disabled has not been investigated, and immune globulin is used in those settings. A single intramuscular injection in adults elicits antibodies in 80–90% of individuals at 2 weeks and 96% by 1 month. The different formulations come in different strengths, and dosage depends on the age of the vaccinee and the preparation used (see package insert). In general, two doses are required, the second given 6–18 months after the first. The duration of immunity is not known but may be lifelong, and at present repeat vaccination is not recommended. Adverse effects are minimal and consist mainly of soreness at the injection site. If vaccine is not available, temporary passive immunity may be induced by the intramuscular injection of immune globulin, 0.02 mL/kg every 2–3 months or 0.1 mL/kg every 6 months. Protection with immune globulin is recommended for persons traveling to all parts of the world where sanitation is poor and the risk of exposure to hepatitis A is high because of contaminated food and water supplies and contact with infected persons. Preparation of immunoglobulin from plasma involves steps that inactivate HIV, thus making immunoglobulin preparations incapable of transmitting HIV infection.

RECOMMENDED IMMUNIZATIONS FOR TRAVELERS

Individuals traveling to other countries frequently require immunizations in addition to those listed above and may benefit from chemoprophylaxis against various diseases. Every traveler must fulfill the immunization requirements of the health authorities of different countries. These are listed in *Health Information for International Travel,* published by the Centers for Disease Control. An updated version is published yearly and is available from the Superintendent of Documents, United States Government Printing Office, Washington, DC 20402.

When individuals request information and vaccinations for travel from a physician, their entire immunization history should be reviewed and updated, including those immunizations listed above that are not specifically required for travel.

Various vaccines can be given simultaneously at different sites. Some, such as cholera, plague, and typhoid vaccine, which cause significant discomfort, are best given at different times. In general, live attenuated vaccines (measles, mumps, rubella, yellow fever, oral typhoid vaccine, and oral poliovaccine) should not be given to immunosuppressed individuals or household members of immunosuppressed people or to pregnant women. Immunoglobulin should not be given for 3 months before or at least 2 weeks after live virus vaccines, because it may attenuate the antibody response.

Chemoprophylaxis of malaria is discussed in Chapter 35.

Cholera

Because the incidence of cholera among travelers is very low and because the vaccine is only marginally effective, the World Health Organization does not routinely require immunization even for persons traveling to and from endemic areas. Although no country officially requires cholera vaccination, some local authorities may still require documentation of vaccination.

Cholera vaccine contains a suspension of killed vibrios, including prevalent antigenic types. Two injections are given intramuscularly 2–6 weeks apart, followed by booster injections every 6 months during periods of possible exposure. Protection depends largely on booster doses. An inactivated oral vaccine appears to be more effective than the parenteral vaccine but is not available in the USA. A live attenuated oral vaccine is being investigated. The WHO certificate is valid for 6 months only.

Hepatitis B

Persons traveling to and spending more than 6 months in endemic areas of HBV infection who will have close contact with the local population should be considered for vaccination. Short-term travelers to areas of moderate or high endemic infection (Southeast Asia and sub-Saharan Africa) who will be in contact with potentially infected body secretions of residents should be vaccinated. Vaccination should begin at least 6 months before travel to allow for completion of the series.

Meningococcal Meningitis

If travel is contemplated to an area where meningococcal meningitis is epidemic (Nepal, sub-Saharan Africa, New Delhi) or highly endemic, polysaccharide vaccines from types A, C, W-135, and Y may be indicated. Follow the manufacturer's dosage recommendations. The vaccine is also recommended for persons with anatomic or functional asplenia and those with terminal complement deficiencies.

Plague

Plague vaccine is a suspension of killed plague bacilli that is given intramuscularly. Three injections are given—the second, 4 weeks after the initial injection; and the third, 5 months after the second. The risk of acquiring plague is so low that routine vaccination is not recommended. Vaccination is reserved for travelers who will have exposure to rodents or rabbits in rural areas where plague is endemic (some areas in South America, Southeast Asia, occasionally others). For continuing exposures, booster doses at intervals of 1–2 years are recommended.

Poliomyelitis

Adult travelers to tropical or developing countries who have not previously been immunized against poliomyelitis should receive a primary series of three doses of inactivated enhanced-potency poliovaccine (IPV), as follows: two doses of 0.5 mL subcutaneously 4–8 weeks apart and then a third dose at least 4 weeks and preferably 6–12 months after the

second dose. Because of the risk of vaccine-associated paralytic poliomyelitis, live attenuated oral poliovaccine (OPV) should not be routinely used for primary vaccination of adults. It may be used if protection is needed within 4 weeks of travel, in which case a single dose of OPV or IPV is given and primary immunization is then completed with either IPV or OPV. (Primary immunization with OPV includes two doses given 6–8 weeks apart and a third dose given at least 6 weeks and preferably 8–12 months after the second dose.) Travelers who have previously been fully immunized with OPV or IPV should receive a one-time booster dose with either OPV or IPV.

Rabies

For travelers to areas where rabies is common in domestic animals (eg, India, Asia, Mexico), preexposure prophylaxis with human diploid cell vaccine or rabies vaccine adsorbed should be considered. It usually consists of two intramuscular (deltoid area) injections of 1 mL of human diploid cell vaccine or rabies vaccine adsorbed given 1 week apart with a booster dose 2–3 weeks later. Alternatively, two intradermal injections of 0.1 mL of human diploid cell vaccine are given 1 week apart, with a booster dose given 2–3 weeks later. Chloroquine can blunt the immunologic response to rabies vaccine. If malaria prophylaxis with this agent is required, vaccination should be given intramuscularly (*not* intradermally) to ensure adequate antibody response. There are no data on the interaction between mefloquine and rabies vaccine. It would seem reasonable to administer rabies vaccine intramuscularly if mefloquine is to be given until further studies are done.

Typhoid

Typhoid vaccination is recommended for travelers to developing countries (especially Latin America, Africa, and Asia) who will have prolonged exposure to contaminated food and water. Three preparations of approximately equal efficacy (50–75% effective) are available: (1) a heat-phenol-inactivated vaccine for parenteral use; (2) an oral live-attenuated Ty21a vaccine supplied as enteric-coated capsules; and (3) a Vi capsular polysaccharide (Vi CPS) vaccine for parenteral use. The phenol-inactivated preparation that has been historically used is associated with the most side effects and is not recommended unless the other preparations are not available. The Ty2la vaccine is given as one capsule every other day for four doses. The capsules must be refrigerated and taken with cool liquids (37 °C or less) at least 1 hour before meals. All four doses must be taken for maximum protection. Adverse effects are minimal and consist primarily of gastrointestinal upset. It is not recommended for children less than 6 years of age. The Vi CPS vaccine is given as a single intramuscular injection. Adverse effects consist mainly of local irritation at the site of injection, but fever and headache have been reported. The vaccine is not recommended for children under 2 years of age. If continued or repeated exposures are anticipated, booster doses are recommended. A booster dose of the heat-inactivated vaccine is recommended every 3 years. Boosters of the Vi CPS are given every 2 years. The optimal booster dose of the Ty2la is not known, but the manufacturer recommends repeating the four-dose series every 5 years. The live attenuated vaccine should not be used in immunosuppressed patients, including those with HIV infection.

Yellow Fever

The live attenuated yellow fever virus vaccine is administered once subcutaneously. Although the risk of yellow fever is low for most conventional travelers, a number of countries require vaccination for all visitors and others require it for travelers to or from endemic areas (mainly equatorial Africa and parts of South and Central America). The WHO certificate requires registration of the manufacturer and the batch number of the vaccine. Vaccination is available in the USA only at approved centers. (Contact the local health department for available resources.) Reimmunization is recommended at 10-year intervals if continued risk exists.

Because it is a live attenuated vaccine prepared in embryonated eggs, the yellow fever vaccine should not be given to immunosuppressed individuals or those with a history of anaphylaxis to eggs. Pregnancy is a relative contraindication to vaccination.

Japanese B Encephalitis

This is a mosquito-borne viral encephalitis that affects primarily children and older adults (65 years and older) and occurs primarily from May to September. It is the leading cause of encephalitis in Asia. Because the risk of infection is low and because adverse effects of the vaccine can be serious, not all travelers to Asia should be vaccinated. Vaccine should be given to travelers to endemic areas who will be staying at least 30 days and who are traveling during the transmission season, particularly if they are visiting rural areas. Travelers who spend less than 30 days in the region should be considered for vaccination if they intend to visit areas of epidemic transmission or if extensive outdoor activities are planned in rural rice-growing areas. The recommended primary immunization schedule is 1 mL of vaccine administered subcutaneously on days 0, 7, and 30. If time constraints are compelling, the last dose can be given on day 14. The last dose should be given at least 10 days before embarkation because adverse effects in the form of urticaria and angioedema have been described, occurring from minutes up to 10 days after vaccination. Following vaccination, patients should be observed for 30 minutes and advised of the possibility of delayed reactions of angioedema

and urticaria. In addition, local reactions have been reported in 20% of vaccinees and systemic reactions (fever, chills, malaise, headache) in 10%.

[Immunization information.]
  http://www.cdc.gov/nip/home.html
Gardner P, Eckhoff T: Immunization in adults in the 1990's. Curr Clin Top Infect Dis 1995;15:271. (Textbook style review.)
Gardner P et al: Adult immunizations. Ann Intern Med 1996;124:35. (Updates new vaccines since publication of previous reference.)
Guide for Adult Immunization, 3rd ed. American College of Physicians, 1994. (Comprehensive review in textbook format.)
Recommended childhood immunization schedule, United States, January–June 1996. MMWR Morb Mortal Wkly Rep 1996;44:940. (A consensus statement from the Advisory Committee on Immunization Practices and the American Academy of Pediatrics.)
Update: Vaccine side effects, adverse reactions, contraindications, and precautions: Recommendations of the Advisory Committee on Immunization Practices (ACIP). MMWR Morb Mortal Wkly Rep 1996;45(RR-12). (Comprehensive review of adverse effects, with recommendations for vaccine use.)

HYPERSENSITIVITY TESTS & DESENSITIZATION

One should test for hypersensitivity before injecting antitoxin, materials derived from animal sources, or drugs (eg, penicillin) to which a patient has had a severe reaction in the past. If the test described below is negative, desensitization is not necessary, and a full dose of the material may be given. If the test is positive, alternative drugs should be strongly considered. If that is not feasible, desensitization is necessary.

Intradermal Test for Hypersensitivity

Penicillin is the drug that most frequently serves as an indication for sensitivity testing and desensitization. Skin testing requires two preparations: PPL (penicilloyl-polylysine) and a minor determinant mixture. Several points should be emphasized in performing and interpreting these tests. Whenever possible, both PPL and a minor determinant should be used, since 85% of skin test reactors are positive to PPL but 15% react only to the minor determinant mixture. In addition, if penicillin G is used instead of the minor determinant mixture, some allergic patients will be missed. About 25% of individuals who react to minor determinant mixture may not react to penicillin G, and such patients may still have an anaphylactic or accelerated reaction to penicillin. A pinprick test is performed with each solution at different sites by placing a small drop of solution on the skin and making small indentations of the skin with a needle.

If there is no reaction within 10 minutes, 0.01–0.02 mL is injected intradermally, raising a small bleb. Development of a wheal greater than 5 mm in diameter is considered a positive test and an indication for desensitization. If the test is negative, the drug can be administered with the precautions listed below. Even if the test is negative, about 1% of patients will have an immediate or accelerated reaction. Thus, the drug can be administered with relative safety, but the precautions below should be followed.

Desensitization

A. Precautions:

1. The desensitization procedure is not innocuous—deaths from anaphylaxis have been reported. If extreme hypersensitivity is suspected, it is advisable to use an alternative structurally unrelated drug and to reserve desensitization for situations when treatment cannot be withheld and no alternative drug is available.

2. An antihistaminic drug (25–50 mg of hydroxyzine or diphenhydramine intramuscularly or orally) should be administered before desensitization is begun in order to lessen any reaction that occurs.

3. Desensitization should be conducted in an intensive care unit where cardiac monitoring and emergency endotracheal intubation can be performed.

4. Epinephrine, 1 mL of 1:1000 solution, must be ready for immediate administration.

B. Desensitization Method:

Several methods of desensitization have been described for penicillin, including use of both oral and intravenous preparations. All methods start with very small doses of drug and gradually increase the dose until therapeutic doses are achieved. For penicillin, 1 unit of drug is given intravenously and the patient observed for 15–30 minutes. If there is no reaction, some recommend doubling the dose while others recommend increasing it tenfold every 15–30 minutes until a dosage of 2 million units is reached; then give the remainder of the desired dose.

For recommendations on skin testing and desensitization for other preparations (botulism antitoxin, diphtheria antitoxin, etc), one should consult the manufacturer's package inserts.

Treatment of Reactions

A. Mild Reactions: If a mild reaction occurs, drop back to the next lower dose and continue with desensitization. If a severe reaction occurs, administer epinephrine (see below) and discontinue the drug unless treatment is urgently needed. If desensitization is imperative, continue slowly, increasing the dosage of the drug more gradually.

B. Severe Reactions: If bronchospasm occurs, epinephrine, 0.3–0.5 mL of 1:1000 dilution, should be given subcutaneously every 10–20 minutes. The following can also be given if symptoms persist: inhaled metaproterenol (0.3 mL of a 5% solution in 2.5 mL of saline), intravenous aminophylline (0.3–0.9 mL/kg/h maintenance after a 6 mg/kg loading dose over 30 minutes), or corticosteroids (250 mg of hydrocortisone or 50 mg of methylprednisolone intravenously every 6 hours for two to four doses). Hypotension should be treated with intravenous fluids (saline or colloid), epinephrine (1 mL of 1:1000 dilution in 500 mL of D_5W intravenously at a rate of 0.5–5 µg/min), and antihistamines (25–50 mg of hydroxyzine or diphenhydramine intramuscularly or orally every 6–8 hours as needed). Cutaneous reactions, manifested as urticaria or angioedema, respond to epinephrine subcutaneously and antihistamines in the doses set forth above.

Weiss ME: Evaluation and treatment of patients with prior reactions to β-lactam antibiotics. Curr Clin Top Infect Dis 1993;13:131. (Review of pathogenesis and diagnosis with regimens of desensitization.)

31

HIV Infection

Mitchell H. Katz, MD, & Harry Hollander, MD

Essentials of Diagnosis

- Risk factors: sexual contact with an infected person, parenteral exposure to infected blood by transfusion or needle sharing, perinatal exposure.
- Prominent systemic complaints such as sweats, diarrhea, weight loss, and wasting.
- Opportunistic infections due to diminished cellular immunity—often life-threatening.
- Aggressive cancers, particularly Kaposi's sarcoma and extranodal lymphoma.
- Neurologic manifestations, including dementia, aseptic meningitis, and neuropathy.

General Considerations

When AIDS was first recognized in the USA in 1981, cases were identified by finding severe opportunistic infections such as *Pneumocystis carinii* pneumonia that indicated profound defects in cellular immunity in the absence of other causes of immunodeficiency. When the syndrome was found to be caused by the human immunodeficiency virus (HIV), it became obvious that severe opportunistic infections and unusual neoplasms were at one end of a spectrum of disease, while healthy seropositive individuals were at the other end.

In 1993, the Centers for Disease Control and Prevention expanded the AIDS definition (Table 31–1). The 1993 definition includes all 23 opportunistic infections (eg, pneumocystis pneumonia) and neoplasms (eg, Kaposi's sarcoma) that were included in the 1987 definition. As with the 1987 definition, it also includes as AIDS cases persons with documented weight loss, diarrhea, or dementia and a positive HIV serology. There remain criteria for both definitive and presumptive diagnoses. The expansion is that persons with a positive HIV serology and who have ever had a CD4 lymphocyte count below 200 cells/μL or a CD4 lymphocyte percentage below 14% are considered to have AIDS. Inclusion of persons with low CD4 counts as AIDS cases reflects the recognition that immunodeficiency is the defining characteristic of AIDS. The choice of a cutoff point at 200 cells/μL is supported by several cohort studies showing that over 80% of persons with counts below

this level will develop AIDS within 3 years. The 1993 definition was also expanded to include persons with positive HIV serology and pulmonary tuberculosis, recurrent pneumonia, and invasive cervical cancer. One consequence of the expanded definition has been that HIV-infected persons are diagnosed with AIDS an average of 1.6 years earlier in the course of the disease. The definition doubled to tripled the number of new cases of AIDS in 1993. However, the impact of the new definition on the number of new cases has been less since then.

The goal of the current definition is to enhance efforts at surveillance of HIV disease. It does not affect eligibility for most social services benefits, since the Social Security Administration has decided not to use the CDC definition as presumptive eligibility of disability. Instead, SSA has developed a functional assessment for determining eligibility for benefits for HIV-infected persons. In the past, the term "AIDS-related complex" (ARC) was used to denote those HIV-infected patients who were symptomatic but did not fit the CDC definition of AIDS. This group of patients is heterogeneous, with varying clinical problems and prognoses. Therefore, the use of the term "ARC" should be avoided. While the majority of general internists, family physicians, and general practitioners do treat HIV-infected patients, many feel uncomfortable doing so. The discomfort stems from attitudes toward gay men and intravenous drug users, lack of sufficient knowledge to treat the disease, and inadequate reimbursement for the time-consuming care required by AIDS patients. Resources are available to help clinicians care for HIV-infected persons. Clinicians should call their state medical associations for a list of local resources.

For HIV-infected patients, primary care providers should perform periodic physical examinations, monitor prognostic markers (eg, CD4 lymphocyte counts), prescribe initial antiviral and prophylactic therapy, initiate diagnostic evaluation and therapy for HIV-related complications, provide supportive counseling, and offer assistance with terminal care (eg, pain control and durable power of attorney for health care). Specialists should be consulted for patients in-

Table 31–1. CDC AIDS case definition for surveillance of adults and adolescents.

Definitive AIDS diagnoses (with or without laboratory evidence of HIV infection)
1. Candidiasis of the esophagus, trachea, bronchi, or lungs.
2. Cryptococcosis, extrapulmonary.
3. Cryptosporidiosis with diarrhea persisting > 1 month.
4. Cytomegalovirus disease of an organ other than liver, spleen, or lymph nodes.
5. Herpes simplex virus infection causing a mucocutaneous ulcer that persists longer than 1 month, or bronchitis, pneumonitis, or esophagitis of any duration.
6. Kaposi's sarcoma in a patient < 60 years of age.
7. Lymphoma of the brain (primary) in a patient < 60 years of age.
8. *Mycobacterium avium* complex or *Mycobacterium kansasii* disease, disseminated (at a site other than or in addition to lungs, skin, or cervical or hilar lymph nodes).
9. *Pneumocystis carinii* pneumonia.
10. Progressive multifocal leukoencephalopathy.
11. Toxoplasmosis of the brain.

Definitive AIDS diagnoses (with laboratory evidence of HIV infection)
1. Coccidioidomycosis, disseminated (at a site other than or in addition to lungs or cervical or hilar lymph nodes).
2. HIV encephalopathy.
3. Histoplasmosis, disseminated (at a site other than or in addition to lungs or cervical or hilar lymph nodes).
4. Isosporiasis with diarrhea persisting > 1 month.
5. Kaposi's sarcoma at any age.
6. Lymphoma of the brain (primary) at any age.
7. Other non-Hodgkin's lymphoma of B cell or unknown immunologic phenotype.
8. Any mycobacterial disease caused by mycobacteria other than *Mycobacterium tuberculosis*, disseminated (at a site other than or in addition to lungs, skin, or cervical or hilar lymph nodes).
9. Disease caused by extrapulmonary *M tuberculosis*.
10. *Salmonella* (nontyphoid) septicemia, recurrent.
11. HIV wasting syndrome.
12. CD4 lymphocyte count below 200 cells/μL or a CD4 lymphocyte percentage below 14%.
13. Pulmonary tuberculosis.
14. Recurrent pneumonia.
15. Invasive cervical cancer.

Presumptive AIDS diagnoses (with laboratory evidence of HIV infection)
1. Candidiasis of esophagus: (a) recent onset of retrosternal pain on swallowing; and (b) oral candidiasis.
2. Cytomegalovirus retinitis. A characteristic appearance on serial ophthalmoscopic examinations.
3. Mycobacteriosis. Specimen from stool or normally sterile body fluids or tissue from a site other than lungs, skin, or cervical or hilar lymph nodes, showing acid-fast bacilli of a species not identified by culture.
4. Kaposi's sarcoma. Erythematous or violaceous plaque-like lesion on skin or mucous membrane.
5. *Pneumocystis carinii* pneumonia: (a) a history of dyspnea on exertion or nonproductive cough of recent onset (within the past 3 months); and (b) chest x-ray evidence of diffuse bilateral interstitial infiltrates or gallium scan evidence of diffuse bilateral pulmonary disease; and (c) arterial blood gas analysis showing an arterial oxygen partial pressure of < 70 mm Hg or a low respiratory diffusing capacity of < 80% of predicted values or an increase in the alveolar-arterial oxygen tension gradient; and (d) no evidence of a bacterial pneumonia.
6. Toxoplasmosis of the brain: (a) recent onset of a focal neurologic abnormality consistent with intracranial disease or a reduced level of consciousness; and (b) brain imaging evidence of a lesion having a mass effect or the radiographic appearance of which is enhanced by injection of contrast medium; and (c) serum antibody to toxoplasmosis or successful response to therapy for toxoplasmosis.
7. Recurrent pneumonia: (a) more than one episode in a 1-year period; and (b) acute pneumonia (new symptoms, signs, or radiologic evidence not present earlier) diagnosed on clinical or radiologic grounds by the patient's physician.
8. Pulmonary tuberculosis: (a) apical or miliary infiltrates and (b) radiographic and clinical response to antituberculosis therapy.

tolerant of standard antiviral drugs, those in need of systemic chemotherapy, and those with complicated opportunistic infections, particularly when invasive procedures or experimental therapies are needed. In many cases, a single consultation with follow-up to the primary care physician will provide the needed expertise while ensuring continuity in care. With 1 million HIV-infected Americans, it is impossible for all care to be delivered by infectious disease and oncology specialists.

Epidemiology

The modes of transmission of HIV are similar to those of hepatitis B, in particular with respect to sexual, parenteral, and vertical transmission. The risk of sexual transmission varies with particular sexual practices; receptive anal intercourse is the riskiest. The risk of sustaining HIV infection from a needle stick with infected blood is approximately 1:300, which is significantly less than the risk of contracting hepatitis B from a contaminated needle stick. Between 13% and 40% of children born to HIV-infected mothers contract HIV infection. The HIV has not been shown to be transmitted by respiratory droplet spread, by vectors such as mosquitoes, or by casual nonsexual contact.

Current estimates are that about 1 million Americans are infected with HIV. Estimates of the number of people who have developed AIDS in the 1990s have been scaled down from prior estimates, based on recent AIDS incidence data. In 1996, there were 223,000 Americans living with AIDS. Projections beyond that year are not yet available. In the USA, 44% of AIDS cases are reported in gay or bisexual men, and 26% are heterosexual intravenous drug users, the majority of whom live in major metropolitan areas. The remainder of cases occur in infants of infected mothers, heterosexual contacts of infected individuals, and recipients of contaminated blood or blood products. Among risk groups, the most rapid percentage increases are anticipated among young gay and bisexual men, women, and inner city intravenous drug users, especially blacks and Latinos.

The rapid increase of AIDS cases among women is of great concern. Whereas women represented only 7% of cases prior to 1985, they represented 18% of prevalent AIDS cases in 1996. Intravenous drug use and heterosexual contact with an infected partner are the two major risk factors for women. With the rapid increase of HIV infection among women, there has been a corresponding rise in the number of perinatally infected children.

A recent multicenter trial showed that when AZT is administered to women during pregnancy, labor, and delivery and to their newborns, the rate to transmission of HIV is decreased by two-thirds. This finding increases the importance of offering HIV counseling and testing to all women who are pregnant or are considering pregnancy.

The natural history of HIV infection is different in men than in women, though it has been difficult to determine whether the differences are due to biologic or to social factors. In general, women appear later for medical care than men. Therefore, those studies that compared men with women with reference to rates of progression to AIDS found that women progressed more rapidly. Most studies that have adequately adjusted for disease stage have reported no differences in rates of progression. However, one large study reported that women have shorter survival times than men and that many have died without an AIDS diagnosis. Violence toward women, drugs, pregnancy, and poverty may all play a role in this higher rate of death. In addition, women are at risk for gynecologic complications of HIV infection, including recurrent candidal vaginitis, pelvic inflammatory disease, and cervical dysplasia.

HIV infection will continue to spread outward from major metropolitan areas to suburban and rural parts of the country. Because blood donor screening using the HIV-enzyme-linked immunosorbent assay (ELISA) is universally practiced in the USA, the number of new AIDS cases due to transfusion has already peaked and is expected to decline further. The current risk of contracting HIV from a screened unit of blood is 1:100,000. Since 1983, transmission of HIV to at-risk gay men in San Francisco has dramatically fallen to about 1% per year. Recent surveys have indicated a relapse from "safe sex" practices among certain populations of gay men, raising concern that there will be an increase in the number of new seroconverters. This finding underlines the need for continued counseling and education of at-risk individuals.

There are an estimated 10 million persons infected worldwide. In Central and East Africa in some urban areas, as many as a third of sexually active adults are infected. HIV infection began to spread in Asia in the late 1980s, and it is expected that new infections in Asia will exceed new infections in Africa by the late 1990s. The most common mode of transmission is bidirectional heterosexual spread. The reason for the greater risk for transmission with heterosexual intercourse in Africa and Asia than in the United States may relate to cofactors such as general health status, the presence of genital ulcers, and the number of sexual partners.

Connor EM et al: Reduction of maternal-infant transmission of human immunodeficiency virus type 1 with zidovudine treatment. N Engl J Med 1994;331:1173. (Results of a multicenter placebo-controlled trial of AZT during pregnancy.)

Legg JJ: Women and HIV. J Am Board Fam Pract 1993; 6:367. (Reviews epidemiology, gynecologic manifestations, and natural history of HIV among women.)

1993 revised classification system for HIV infection and expanded surveillance case definition for AIDS among adolescents and adults. MMWR Morb Mortal Wkly Rep 1992;41(RR-17):1. (Explains the most prevalent AIDS case definition.)

US Public Health Service recommendations for human immunodeficiency virus counseling and voluntary testing for pregnant women. MMWR Morb Mortal Wkly Rep 1995;44(RR-7):1. (Reviews recommendations for voluntary HIV testing for pregnant women.)

Etiology

The syndromes described below are due to infection with human retroviruses known as human immunodeficiency viruses (HIV or HIV-1, formerly HTLV-III or LAV). Retroviruses depend upon a unique enzyme, reverse transcriptase (RNA-directed DNA-polymerase), to replicate within host cells. The other major pathogenic human retrovirus, HTLV-I, is associated with lymphoma, while HIV is not directly oncogenic. The HIV genomes contain genes for three basic structural proteins and at least five other regulatory proteins; *gag* codes for group antigen proteins, *pol* codes for polymerase, and *env* codes for the external envelope protein. The greatest variability in strains of HIV occurs in the viral envelope. Since neutralizing activity is found in antibodies directed against the envelope, this variability presents problems for vaccine development.

In addition to the classic AIDS virus (HIV-1), a group of related viruses, HIV-2, have been isolated in West African patients. HIV-2 has the same genetic organization as HIV-1, but there are significant differences in the envelope glycoproteins. Some infected individuals exhibit AIDS-like illnesses, but most West Africans infected with HIV-2 are currently asymptomatic. HIV-2 has been found in several people in the USA. Thus, this variant may be less pathogenic or have a longer period of latency preceding disease. Cases have been documented in which AIDS-like illnesses have occurred in the absence of HIV infection. The syndrome of idiopathic CD4 lymphocytopenia appears to represent a heterogeneous form of immunodeficiency. No convincing infectious or other cause has been identified.

Pathogenesis

The hallmark of symptomatic HIV infection is immunodeficiency. The virus can infect all cells expressing the T4 (CD4) antigen, which serves as a receptor for HIV. Once it enters a cell, HIV can replicate and cause cell fusion or death by unknown mechanisms. In many cases, a latent state is established, with integration of the HIV genome into the cell's genome. The cell principally infected is the CD4 (helper-inducer) lymphocyte, which directs many other cells in the immune network. With increasing duration of infection, the number of CD4 lymphocytes falls. Some of the immunologic defects, however, are explained not by *quantitative* abnormalities of lymphocyte subsets but by *qualitative* defects in CD4 responsiveness induced by HIV.

Other cells in the immune network that are infected by HIV include B lymphocytes and macrophages. The defect in B cells is partly due to disordered CD4 lymphocyte function. However, HIV can also alter B cell function directly. These direct and indirect effects can lead to generalized hypergammaglobulinemia and can also depress B cell responses to new antigen challenges. Because of these defects, the immunodeficiency of HIV is mixed. Elements of humoral and cellular immunodeficiency are present, especially in children.

The role of macrophage-monocyte infection in immunodeficiency is not as clear. It is possible that macrophage dysfunction plays a role in some of the clinical manifestations of the disease, such as pneumocystis pneumonia. Macrophages also act as a reservoir for HIV and serve to disseminate it to other organ systems (eg, the central nervous system).

Apart from the immunologic effects of HIV, the virus can also directly cause a variety of neurologic effects. Rare glial cells and oligodendrocytes express CD4 antigen and thus may be permissive of infection by HIV. However, these cells are rarely infected, whereas multinucleated giant cells of macrophage origin are more commonly seen in brain specimens of infected individuals. The envelope of HIV is ho-

mologous with neuroleukins; the neuropathologic features may be partly dependent upon inhibition of neurologic growth factors by the virus. Other factors such as coexistent CMV infection may also be important. Perturbations of excitatory neurotransmitters and calcium flux may contribute to neurologic dysfunction.

Pathophysiology

Clinically, the syndromes caused by HIV infection are usually explicable by one of three known mechanisms. Some HIV-associated manifestations, however, are not explained by any of these proposed mechanisms.

A. Immunodeficiency: Immunodeficiency is a direct result of the effects of HIV upon immune cells. A spectrum of infections and neoplasms is seen, as in other congenital or acquired immunodeficiency states. Two remarkable features of HIV immunodeficiency are the low incidence of certain infections such as listeriosis and aspergillosis and the frequent occurrence of certain neoplasms such as lymphoma or Kaposi's sarcoma. This latter complication has been seen primarily in gay or bisexual men, and its incidence has steadily declined through the first 10 years of the epidemic. Evidence now strongly suggests that a new herpesvirus is the cause of Kaposi's sarcoma.

B. Autoimmunity: Autoimmunity can occur as a result of disordered cellular immune function or B lymphocyte dysfunction. Examples of both lymphocytic infiltration of organs (eg, lymphocytic interstitial pneumonitis) and autoantibody production (eg, immunologic thrombocytopenia) occur. These phenomena may be the only clinically apparent disease or may coexist with obvious immunodeficiency.

C. Neurologic Dysfunction: Little is known about the mechanisms of neurologic dysfunction, since relatively few neural cells are infected and the inflammatory response is minimal. Possibilities include homology with and blockade of neurologic growth factors, other toxic effects of viral products, or release of neurotoxic compounds from infected macrophages.

Clinical Findings

The complications of HIV-related infections and neoplasms affect virtually every organ. The general approach to the HIV-infected person with symptoms is to evaluate the organ systems involved, aiming to diagnose treatable conditions rapidly. As can be seen in Figure 31–1, the CD4 lymphocyte count provides very important prognostic information. Certain infections may occur at any CD4 count, while others rarely occur unless the CD4 lymphocyte count has dropped below a certain level. For example, a patient with a CD4 count of 600 cells/µL, cough, and fever may have a bacterial pneumonia but would be very unlikely to have pneumocystis pneumonia.

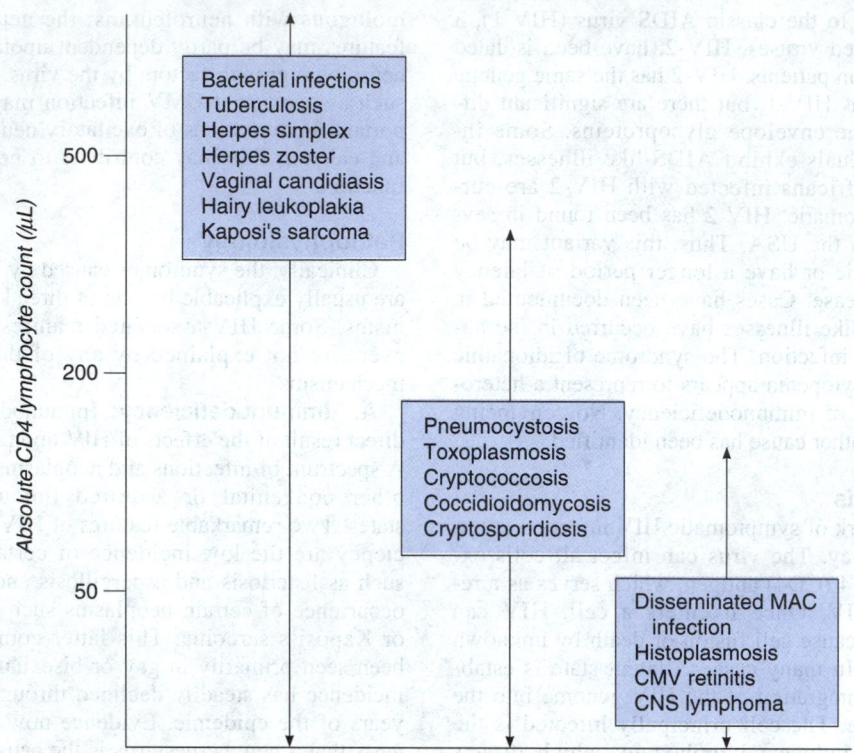

Figure 31–1. Relationship of CD4 count to development of opportunistic infections.

A. Symptoms and Signs: Many individuals with HIV infection remain asymptomatic for years, with a mean time of approximately 10 years between exposure and development of AIDS. When symptoms occur, they may be remarkably protean and nonspecific. Since virtually all the findings may be seen with other diseases, a combination of complaints is more suggestive of HIV infection than any one symptom.

Physical examination may be entirely normal. Abnormal findings range from completely nonspecific to highly specific for HIV infection. Those that are predictive of HIV infection include hairy leukoplakia of the tongue and disseminated Kaposi's sarcoma.

1. Systemic complaints–Fever, night sweats, and weight loss are common symptoms in HIV-infected patients and may occur without a complicating opportunistic infection. Patients with persistent **fever** and no localizing symptoms should nonetheless be carefully examined, and evaluated with a chest radiograph (pneumocystis pneumonia can present without respiratory symptoms), bacterial blood cultures if the fever is greater than 38.5 °C, serum cryptococcal antigen, and mycobacterial cultures of the blood. Sinus radiographs or sinus CT scans should be considered to evaluate occult sinusitis. If these studies are normal, patients should be observed closely. Antipyretics are useful because HIV-infected patients

have a propensity for high fevers and subsequent dehydration. Generally, nonsteroidal anti-inflammatory agents are more effective than aspirin or acetaminophen in the relief of fever.

Weight loss is a particularly distressing complication of long-standing HIV infection. Patients typically have disproportionate loss of muscle mass, with maintenance or less substantial loss of fat stores. The mechanism of HIV-related weight loss is not completely understood but appears to be multifactorial.

Tumor necrosis factor (TNF; cachectin) is known to be elevated in AIDS patients with secondary infections such as pneumocystis pneumonia. TNF decreases lipoprotein lipase activity, decreases the synthesis of fatty acids, and promotes the breakdown of fat. AIDS patients also have high alpha interferon levels, which may result in decreased clearance of triglycerides. However, the exact roles of tumor necrosis factor, alpha interferon, and other cytokines, as well as their combined effect on weight loss, are still unknown.

AIDS patients frequently suffer from anorexia, nausea, and vomiting, all of which contribute to weight loss by decreasing caloric intake. In some cases, these symptoms are secondary to a specific infection, such as viral hepatitis. In other cases, however, evaluation of the symptoms yields no specific pathogen, and it is assumed to be due to a primary effect of HIV. Malabsorption also plays a role in decreased caloric intake. Patients may suffer diarrhea from infections with bacterial, viral, or parasitic agents.

Exacerbating the decrease in caloric intake, many AIDS patients have an increased metabolic rate. This increased rate has been shown to exist even among asymptomatic HIV-infected persons, but it accelerates with disease progression and secondary infection. AIDS patients with secondary infections also have decreased protein synthesis, which makes maintaining muscle mass difficult.

Several strategies have been developed to slow AIDS wasting. Patients should be counseled to maintain high caloric diets. Food supplementation with high-calorie drinks may enable patients with not much appetite to maintain their intake. Selected patients with otherwise good functional status and weight loss due to unrelenting nausea, vomiting, or diarrhea may benefit from total parenteral nutrition. It should be noted, however, that TPN is more likely to increase fat stores than to reverse the muscle wasting process.

Two pharmacologic approaches for increasing appetite and weight gain are the progestational agent megestrol acetate (80 mg four times a day) and the antiemetic agent dronabinol (2.5–5 mg three times a day). Side effects from megestrol acetate are rare. Thromboembolic phenomena, edema, nausea, vomiting, and rash have been reported. Euphoria, dizziness, paranoia, and somnolence and even nausea and vomiting have been reported in 3–10% of patients using dronabinol.

Growth hormone at a dose of 0.1 mg/kg/d subcutaneously for 12 weeks has resulted in modest increases in lean body mass; its cost is approximately $150 per day. Although there are no studies proving that anabolic steroids increase lean body mass among HIV-infected patients, clinical experience suggests that these agents do enable many patients to gain muscle mass. Anabolic steroids seem to work best for patients who are able to do weight training. The most commonly used regimens are testosterone enanthate or testosterone cypionate (100–200 mg intramuscularly every 2–4 weeks). Testosterone patches (4–6 mg/d) applied to the shaved scrotum can also be used. A transdermal delivery system (2.5 mg/d) is also available that can be applied to nonhairy parts of the body.

Nausea leading to weight loss is sometimes due to esophageal candidiasis. Patients with oral candidiasis and nausea should be empirically treated with an oral antifungal agent. Patients with weight loss due to nausea of unclear origin may benefit from use of antiemetics prior to meals (prochlorperazine, 10 mg three times daily, or metoclopramide, 10 mg three times daily). Effective fever control decreases the metabolic rate and may slow the pace of weight loss. Dronabinol (5 mg three times daily) can also be used

to increase appetite. Depression and adrenal insufficiency are two potentially treatable causes of weight loss.

2. Sinopulmonary disease–

a. Pneumocystis pneumonia–(See also discussions in Chapter 36.) The lungs are a frequently involved site of disease. Pneumocystis pneumonia is the most common opportunistic infection, affecting 75% of patients. Pneumocystis pneumonia may be difficult to diagnose because the symptoms— fever, cough, and shortness of breath—are nonspecific. Furthermore, the severity of symptoms ranges from fever and no respiratory symptoms through mild cough or dyspnea to frank respiratory distress.

Hypoxemia may be severe, with a P_{O_2} less than 60 mm Hg. The cornerstone of diagnosis is the chest radiograph. Diffuse or perihilar infiltrates are most characteristic, but only two-thirds of patients with pneumocystis pneumonia have this finding. Normal chest radiographs are seen in 5–10% of patients with pneumocystis pneumonia, while the remainder have atypical infiltrates. Apical infiltrates are commonly seen among patients with pneumocystis pneumonia who have been receiving aerosolized pentamidine prophylaxis. Large pleural effusions are uncommon with pneumocystis pneumonia; their presence suggests bacterial pneumonia, other infections such as tuberculosis, or pleural Kaposi's sarcoma. Isolated elevations of serum lactate dehydrogenase concentrations are consistent with a diagnosis of pneumocystis pneumonia, as well as lymphoma, disseminated histoplasmosis, and long-term treatment with zidovudine.

Definitive diagnosis can be obtained by Wright-Giemsa stain of induced sputum in 50–80% of cases. Sputum induction is performed by having patients inhale an aerosolized solution of 3% saline produced by an ultrasonic nebulizer. Patients should not eat for at least 8 hours and should not use toothpaste or mouthwash prior to the procedure since they can interfere with test interpretation. The next step for patients with negative sputum examinations still suspected of having pneumocystis pneumonia should be bronchoalveolar lavage. This technique establishes the diagnosis in over 95% of cases.

In patients with symptoms suggestive of pneumocystis pneumonia but with negative or atypical chest radiographs and negative sputum examinations, other diagnostic tests may provide additional information in deciding whether to proceed to bronchoalveolar lavage. Elevation of serum lactate dehydrogenase occurs in 95% of cases of pneumocystis pneumonia, but the specificity of this finding is at best 75%. Patients with serum lactate dehydrogenase levels of 220 units/L or less and erythrocyte sedimentation rates less than 50 mm/h are unlikely to have pneumocystis pneumonia and may be clinically followed. In addition, a CD4 count above 250 cells/μL within 2 months prior to evaluation of respiratory symptoms makes a diagnosis of pneumocystis pneumonia unlikely; only 1–5% of cases occur at this CD4 count level (Figure 31–1).

Pneumothoraces are common in HIV-infected patients with a history of pneumocystis pneumonia, especially if they have received aerosolized pentamidine treatment. Because patients may have a pneumothorax as their presenting symptom of recurrent pneumocystis pneumonia, such patients who have not had therapy for pneumocystis pneumonia in the preceding 3 months may need evaluation for pneumocystis. Pneumothoraces in HIV-infected individuals should be treated initially in the same fashion as in other patients. Unfortunately, they frequently recur with clamping or removal of the chest tube. Sclerosis with bleomycin or talc is the treatment of choice for recurrent pneumothoraces, but it is not uniformly successful even when multiple treatments are performed. If sclerosis fails, thoracoscopic stapling or thoracotomy may be required.

b. Other infectious pulmonary diseases– Other infectious causes of pulmonary disease in AIDS patients include bacterial, mycobacterial, and viral pneumonias. An increased incidence of pneumococcal pneumonia with septicemia and *Haemophilus influenzae* pneumonia has been reported. The incidence of infection with *Mycobacterium tuberculosis* has markedly increased in metropolitan areas because of HIV infection as well as homelessness. Tuberculosis occurs in an estimated 4% of persons who have AIDS. It is thought to result mainly from reactivation of prior infection; atypical infiltrates and disseminated disease occur more commonly than among immunocompetent hosts. Multidrug-resistant tuberculosis has emerged as a major problem in several metropolitan areas. Noncompliance with prescribed antituberculous drugs is a major risk factor. Several of the reported outbreaks appear to implicate nosocomial spread. The emergence of drug resistance makes it essential that antibiotic sensitivities be performed on all positive cultures. Drug therapy should be individualized. Patients with multidrug-resistant *Mycobacterium tuberculosis* infection should receive at least three drugs to which their organism is sensitive. Atypical mycobacteria can cause pulmonary disease in AIDS patients with or without preexisting lung disease and responds variably to treatment. Making a distinction between *Mycobacterium tuberculosis* and atypical mycobacteria requires culture of sputum specimens. If culture of the sputum produces acid-fast bacilli, definitive identification may take several weeks. DNA probes allow for presumptive identification usually within days of a positive culture. While awaiting definitive diagnosis, clinicians should err on the side of treating patients as if they have *M tuberculosis* infection. In cases where the risk of atypical mycobacteria is very high (eg, a person without risk for tuberculosis expo-

sure with a CD4 count under 50 cells/μL—see Figure 31–1), clinicians may wait for definitive diagnosis if the person is smear-negative for acid-fast bacilli and not living in a communal setting. Isolation of cytomegalovirus from bronchoalveolar lavage fluid occurs commonly in AIDS patients but does not establish a definitive diagnosis. Diagnosis of cytomegalovirus pneumonia requires biopsy; response to treatment is poor.

c. Noninfectious pulmonary diseases–Noninfectious causes of lung disease include Kaposi's sarcoma, non-Hodgkin's lymphoma, and interstitial pneumonitis. In patients with known Kaposi's sarcoma, pulmonary involvement complicates the course in approximately one-third of cases. Non-Hodgkin's lymphoma may involve the lung as the sole site of disease but more commonly involves other organs as well, especially the brain, liver, and gastrointestinal tract. Both of these processes may show nodular or diffuse parenchymal involvement, pleural effusions, and mediastinal adenopathy on chest radiographs.

Nonspecific interstitial pneumonitis may mimic pneumocystis pneumonia. Pulmonary involvement by HIV may result in a lymphocytic interstitial pneumonitis seen in lung biopsies. Whether this pathologic pattern represents direct HIV infection or is an autoimmune response to infection is unclear. This pathologic pattern is common in childhood HIV infection and is being recognized more commonly in adults. It has a variable clinical course. Typically, these patients present with several months of mild cough and dyspnea; chest radiographs show interstitial infiltrates. Many patients with this entity undergo transbronchial biopsies in an attempt to diagnose pneumocystis pneumonia. Instead, the tissue shows interstitial inflammation ranging from an intense lymphocytic infiltration (consistent with lymphoid interstitial pneumonitis) to a mild mononuclear inflammation. Corticosteroids may be helpful in some cases.

d. Sinusitis–Chronic sinusitis can be a frustrating problem for HIV-infected patients. Symptoms include sinus congestion and discharge, headache, and fever. Some patients may have radiographic evidence on sinus x-ray or sinus CT scan of sinus disease in the absence of significant symptoms. Nonsmoking patients with purulent drainage should be treated with amoxicillin (500 mg orally three times a day). Patients who smoke should be treated with amoxicillin-potassium clavulanate (500 mg orally three times a day) to cover *Haemophilus influenzae*. Prolonged treatment (3–6 weeks) with an antibiotic and guaifenesin (600 mg orally twice daily) to decrease sinus congestion may be required. For patients not responding to amoxicillin-potassium clavulanate, ciprofloxacin should be tried (500 mg orally twice a day). Some patients may require referral to an otolaryngologist for sinus drainage.

3. Central nervous system disease—Central nervous system disease in HIV-infected patients can be divided into intracerebral space-occupying lesions, encephalopathy, meningitis, and spinal cord processes.

a. Toxoplasmosis—Toxoplasmosis is the most common space-occupying lesion in HIV-infected patients. Patients may present with headache, focal neurologic deficits, seizures, or altered mental status. The diagnosis is usually made presumptively based on the characteristic appearance of cerebral imaging studies. Typically, toxoplasmosis appears as multiple lesions, contrast-enhancing on CT scan, with a predilection for the basal ganglia.

Single lesions are atypical of toxoplasmosis. When a single lesion has been detected by CT scanning, MRI scanning—because of its greater sensitivity—may reveal multiple lesions. If a patient has a single lesion on MRI and is neurologically stable, clinicians may pursue a 2-week empiric trial of toxoplasmosis therapy. A repeat scan should be performed at 2 weeks. If the lesion has not diminished in size, biopsy of the lesion should be performed. Since many HIV-infected patients will have detectable titers, a positive *Toxoplasma* serologic test does not confirm the diagnosis. Conversely, as many as 15% of patients with toxoplasmosis have negative titers by enzyme immunoassay or immunofluorescence assays.

b. Central nervous system lymphoma—Non-Hodgkin's lymphoma is the second most common space-occupying lesion in HIV-infected patients. Symptoms are similar to those with toxoplasmosis. While imaging techniques cannot distinguish these two diseases with certainty, lymphoma more often is solitary. Other less common lesions should be suspected if there is preceding bacteremia, positive tuberculin test, fungemia, or intravenous drug use. These include bacterial abscesses, cryptococcomas, tuberculomas, and *Nocardia* lesions.

Because techniques for stereotactic brain biopsy have improved, this procedure plays an increasing role in diagnosing cerebral lesions. Biopsy should be strongly considered if lesions are solitary or do not respond to toxoplasmosis treatment, especially if they are easily accessible. Diagnosis of lymphoma is important because patients who have not had a prior opportunistic infection are likely to benefit from treatment (radiation therapy).

c. AIDS dementia complex—AIDS dementia complex (HIV-associated cognitive/motor complex) is the most common cause of mental status changes in HIV-infected patients. The diagnosis is one of exclusion based on a brain imaging study and spinal fluid analysis that exclude other pathogens. Neuropsychiatric testing is helpful in distinguishing patients with dementia from those with depression. Patients with AIDS dementia complex typically have difficulty with cognitive tasks and exhibit diminished motor speed. Patients may first notice a deterioration in their handwriting. The manifestations of dementia may wax and wane, with persons exhibiting periods of lucidity and confusion over the course of a day. Although the mechanism by which HIV causes neurologic dysfunction is not completely understood, many patients improve with zidovudine. The calcium channel blocker nimodipine has been shown to be well tolerated but is of uncertain efficacy. Metabolic abnormalities may also cause changes in mental status: hypoglycemia, hyponatremia, hypoxia, and drug overdose are important considerations in this population. Other less common infectious causes of encephalopathy include progressive multifocal leukoencephalopathy, cytomegalovirus, syphilis, and herpes simplex encephalitis.

d. Cryptococcal meningitis—Cryptococcal meningitis typically presents with fever and headache. Less than 20% of patients have meningismus. Diagnosis is based on a positive latex agglutination test or positive culture of spinal fluid for *Cryptococcus*. Seventy to ninety percent of patients with cryptococcal meningitis have a positive serum agglutination test for *Cryptococcus* (CRAG). Thus, a negative serum CRAG test makes a diagnosis of cryptococcal meningitis unlikely and can be useful in the initial evaluation of a patient with headache, fever, and normal mental status. HIV meningitis, characterized by lymphocytic pleocytosis of the spinal fluid with negative culture, is common early in HIV infection and may mimic cryptococcal meningitis in its clinical presentation.

e. HIV myelopathy—Spinal cord function may also be impaired in HIV-infected individuals. HIV myelopathy presents with leg weakness and incontinence. Spastic paraparesis and sensory ataxia are seen on neurologic examination. Myelopathy is usually a late manifestation of HIV disease, and most patients will have concomitant HIV encephalopathy. Pathologic evaluation of the spinal cord reveals vacuolation of white matter. Because HIV myelopathy is a diagnosis of exclusion, symptoms suggestive of myelopathy should be evaluated by lumbar puncture to rule out cytomegalovirus polyradiculopathy (described below) and an MRI or CT scan to exclude epidural lymphoma.

4. Peripheral nervous system—Peripheral nervous system syndromes include inflammatory polyneuropathies, sensory neuropathies, and mononeuropathies.

An inflammatory demyelinating polyneuropathy similar to Guillain-Barré syndrome occurs in HIV-infected patients, usually prior to frank immunodeficiency. The syndrome in many cases improves with plasmapheresis, supporting an autoimmune basis of the disease. Cytomegalovirus can cause an ascending polyradiculopathy characterized by lower extremity weakness and a neutrophilic pleocytosis on spinal fluid analysis with a negative bacterial culture.

Transverse myelitis can be seen with herpes zoster or cytomegalovirus.

About 30% of patients with advanced HIV disease develop sensory neuropathies. Affected patients typically complain of numbness, tingling, and pain in their lower extremities. Symptoms are disproportionate to findings on gross sensory and motor evaluation. In contrast to inflammatory demyelinating polyneuropathy, sensory neuropathies occur late in HIV-disease progression and are due to axonal loss. Evaluation should rule out other causes of sensory neuropathy such as alcoholism, thyroid disease, vitamin B_{12} deficiency, and syphilis. Severe sensory neuropathy is a contraindication to initiation of three antiretroviral drugs, the dideoxynucleosides didanosine (ddI), zalcitabine (ddC), and stavudine (d4T). Occasionally, sensory neuropathies improve with zidovudine therapy, but more commonly treatment is symptomatic with amitriptyline.

5. Rheumatologic manifestations–Arthritis, involving single or multiple joints, with or without effusion, has been commonly noted in HIV-infected patients. Involvement of large joints is most common. While the cause of HIV-related arthritis is unknown, most patients will respond to nonsteroidal anti-inflammatory agents. Patients with a sizable effusion, especially if the joint is warm or erythematous, should have the joint tapped, followed by culture of the fluid to rule out suppurative arthritis as well as fungal and mycobacterial disease.

Several rheumatologic syndromes, including Reiter's syndrome, psoriatic arthritis, sicca syndrome, and systemic lupus erythematosus, have been reported in HIV-infected patients (Chapter 19). However, it is unclear if the prevalence is greater than in the general population.

6. Myopathy–Myopathies are increasingly noted in HIV-infected patients. Proximal muscle weakness is typical, and patients may have varying degrees of muscle tenderness. The most important clinical distinction is between myopathy due to the primary effect of HIV and that due to zidovudine. Patients with symptomatic myopathy, especially with creatine kinase levels greater than 1000 units/L, should have their dose of zidovudine decreased or stopped and be considered for alternative antiviral therapy (didanosine or zalcitabine). A muscle biopsy can distinguish HIV myopathy from zidovudine myopathy and should be considered in patients for whom continuation of zidovudine is essential.

7. Retinitis–Complaints of visual changes must be evaluated immediately in HIV-infected patients. Cytomegalovirus retinitis, characterized by perivascular hemorrhages and fluffy exudates, is the most common retinal infection in AIDS patients and can be rapidly progressive. In contrast, cotton wool spots, which are also common in HIV-infected people, are benign, remit spontaneously, and appear as small indistinct white spots without exudation or hemorrhage. This distinction may be difficult at times for the nonspecialist, and patients with visual changes should be seen by an ophthalmologist. Other rare retinal processes include other herpesvirus infections or toxoplasmosis.

8. Oral lesions–The findings of oral candidiasis and hairy leukoplakia are significant for several reasons. First, these lesions are almost pathognomonic for HIV infection. Second, several studies have indicated that patients with these lesions have a high rate of progression to AIDS, though it is not known whether this increased risk within 3 years is independent of other parameters of immune function, such as the CD4 count.

Hairy leukoplakia is caused by the Epstein-Barr virus. The lesion is not usually troubling to patients and sometimes regresses spontaneously. Hairy leukoplakia is commonly seen as a white lesion on the lateral aspect of the tongue. It may be flat or slightly raised, is usually corrugated, and has vertical parallel lines with fine or thick ("hairy") projections. Patients who are bothered by hairy leukoplakia can be treated with acyclovir, 800 mg orally four times a day. Oral candidiasis can be bothersome to patients, many of whom report an unpleasant taste or mouth dryness. There are two types of oral candidiasis: pseudomembranous (removable white plaques) and erythematous (red friable plaques). Treatment is with topical agents such as clotrimazole 10 mg troches (one four or five times a day). Patients with candidiasis that does not respond to topical antifungals can be treated with fluconazole (50–100 mg orally once a day for 3–7 days). Chronic suppression of oral candidiasis with fluconazole has been associated with development of candidiasis resistant to all available azoles and thus should be avoided except in frequently recurring cases.

Angular cheilitis—fissures at the sides of the mouth—is usually due to *Candida* as well and can be treated topically with ketoconazole cream (2%) twice a day.

Gingival disease is common in HIV-infected patients and is thought to be due to an overgrowth of microorganisms. It usually responds to professional dental cleaning and chlorhexidine rinses. Some HIV-infected patients will develop a particularly aggressive gingivitis or periodontitis; these patients should be started on antibiotics that cover anaerobic oral flora (eg, metronidazole, 250 mg four times a day for 4 or 5 days) and referred to oral surgeons with experience with these entities.

Aphthous ulcers are painful and may interfere with eating. They can be treated with fluocinonide (0.05% ointment mixed 1:1 with plain Orabase and applied six times a day to the ulcer). For lesions that are difficult to reach, patients should use dexamethasone swishes (0.5 mg in 5 mL elixir three times a day). The pain of the ulcers can be relieved with use of an anesthetic spray (10% lidocaine). Other lesions seen in the mouths of

HIV-infected patients include Kaposi's sarcoma (usually on the hard palate), and warts.

9. Gastrointestinal manifestations–

a. Candidal esophagitis–(See also discussion in Chapter 14.) Esophageal candidiasis is a common AIDS infection. In a patient with characteristic symptoms, empiric antifungal treatment is begun with fluconazole (200 mg daily). Further evaluation to identify other causes of esophagitis (herpes simplex, cytomegalovirus) is reserved for patients who do not improve with treatment.

b. Hepatic disease–Autopsy studies have demonstrated that the liver is a frequent site of infections and neoplasms in HIV-infected patients. However, many of these infections are not clinically symptomatic. Clinicians may note elevations of alkaline phosphatase and aminotransferases on routine chemistry panels. Mycobacterial disease, cytomegalovirus, hepatitis B virus, and lymphoma cause liver disease and can present with varying degrees of nausea, vomiting, and right upper quadrant abdominal pain. Sulfonamides, imidazole drugs, antituberculous medications, pentamidine, clarithromycin, and didanosine (ddI) have also been associated with hepatitis. HIV-infected patients with chronic active hepatitis may have less severe bouts of hepatitis because of the concomitant immunodeficiency. Percutaneous liver biopsy may be helpful in diagnosing liver disease, but frequently the cause can be determined by other tests (eg, blood culture, biopsy of a more accessible site). Moreover, because the majority of hepatic infections do not respond well to treatment (eg, *M avium* complex), liver biopsy should be reserved for people with persistent symptoms and laboratory abnormalities in whom no other cause for illness can be determined.

c. Biliary disease–Biliary disease is common in AIDS patients. Cholecystitis presents with similar manifestations as seen in immunocompetent hosts but is more likely to be acalculous. Sclerosing cholangitis and papillary stenosis have also been increasingly reported in HIV-infected patients. Typically, the syndrome presents with severe nausea, vomiting, and right upper quadrant pain. Liver function tests generally show alkaline phosphatase elevations disproportionate to elevation of the aminotransferases. Although dilated ducts can be seen on ultrasound, the diagnosis is made by endoscopic retrograde cholangiopancreatography, which reveals intraluminal irregularities of the proximal intrahepatic ducts with "pruning" of the terminal ductal branches. Stenosis of the distal common bile duct at the papilla is commonly seen with this syndrome. Cytomegalovirus and *Cryptosporidium* are thought to play inciting roles in this syndrome. Initial reports of symptomatic improvement with performance of sphincterotomies were encouraging, but enthusiasm for the procedure has waned because many patients had recurrence of symptoms.

d. Enterocolitis–Enterocolitis is a common problem in HIV-infected individuals. Organisms known to cause enterocolitis include bacteria (*Campylobacter, Salmonella, Shigella*), viruses (cytomegalovirus, adenovirus), and protozoans (*Cryptosporidium, E histolytica, Giardia, Isospora,* Microsporida). HIV itself may cause enterocolitis. Several of the organisms causing enterocolitis in HIV-infected individuals also cause diarrhea in immunocompetent hosts. However, HIV-infected patients tend to have more severe and more chronic symptoms, including high fevers and severe abdominal pain that can mimic acute abdominal catastrophes. Bacteremia and concomitant biliary involvement are also more common with enterocolitis in HIV-infected patients. Relapses of enterocolitis following adequate therapy have been reported with both *Salmonella* and *Shigella* infections.

Because of the wide range of agents known to cause enterocolitis, a stool culture and multiple stool examinations for ova and parasites (including modified acid-fast staining for *Cryptosporidium*) should be performed. Those patients who have *Cryptosporidium* on one stool with improvement in symptoms in less than 1 month should not be considered to have AIDS, as *Cryptosporidium* is a cause of self-limited diarrhea in HIV-negative hosts. More commonly, HIV-infected patients with *Cryptosporidium* have persistent enterocolitis with profuse watery diarrhea.

To date, no consistently effective treatments have been developed for *Cryptosporidium* infection. There are anecdotal reports of good responses to paromomycin, 25 mg/kg/d orally, although it appears that patients with high CD4 counts are more likely to respond to this regimen. Patients who do not respond to paromomycin alone should be given a trial of azithromycin (1000 mg orally daily). Because azithromycin contains lactose, some clinicians recommend use of lactose-free azithromycin, which is available through a compassionate use protocol (Pfizer: 215-972-0420, XT 2424). Nitazoxanide (NTZ) is producing promising results as a treatment for cryptosporidiosis and is also available through a compassionate use protocol (Unimed: 800-864-6330 XT 3032). Immune bovine colostrum, the newer macrolide antibiotics, and diclazuril are being evaluated as oral therapy. Patients should be given diphenoxylate with atropine (one or two tablets orally three or four times a day). Those who do not respond may be given paregoric with bismuth (5–10 mL orally three or four times a day). Octreotide in escalating doses (starting at 0.05 mg subcutaneously every 8 hours for 48 hours) has been found to ameliorate symptoms in approximately 40% of patients with cryptosporidial or idiopathic HIV-associated diarrhea.

Patients with a negative stool examination and persistent symptoms should be evaluated with colonoscopy and biopsy. Patients whose symptoms last longer than 1 month with no identified cause of diarrhea are considered to have a presumptive diagnosis of AIDS enteropathy. A primary effect of the HIV on the colonic epithelium may be the cause. Upper endoscopy with small bowel biopsy is not recommended as a routine part of the evaluation. Many patients who undergo upper endoscopy have nonspecific abnormalities, but these rarely reflect treatable diseases.

e. Other disorders–Two other important gastrointestinal abnormalities in HIV-infected patients are gastropathy and malabsorption. It has been documented that some HIV-infected patients do not produce normal levels of stomach acid and therefore are unable to absorb drugs such as ketoconazole that require an acid medium. This decreased acid production may explain, in part, the susceptibility of HIV-infected patients to *Campylobacter, Salmonella,* and *Shigella,* all of which are sensitive to acid concentration. There is no evidence to suggest that *Helicobacter pylori* is more common in HIV-infected persons.

A malabsorption syndrome occurs commonly in HIV-infected patients. It can be due to infection of the small bowel with *M avium* complex or *Cryptosporidium.* In other cases, biopsy of the small bowel reveals no pathogens but histologic changes consistent with Whipple's disease.

10. Endocrinologic manifestations–The adrenal gland is the most commonly afflicted endocrine gland in patients with AIDS. Abnormalities demonstrated on autopsy include infection (especially with cytomegalovirus and *M avium-intracellulare*), infiltration with Kaposi's sarcoma, and injury from hemorrhage and presumed autoimmunity. The prevalence of clinically significant adrenal insufficiency is unknown. Patients with suggestive symptoms should undergo a cosyntropin stimulation test. Those who do not achieve a cortisol level of 20 µg/dL (552 nmol/L) 30–60 minutes following cosyntropin administration should undergo a 3-day ACTH stimulation test.

While frank deficiency of cortisol is rare, an isolated defect in mineralocorticoid metabolism may lead to salt wasting and hyperkalemia. Such patients should be treated with fludrocortisone (0.1–0.2 mg daily).

AIDS patients appear to have abnormalities of thyroid function tests different from those of patients with other chronic diseases. AIDS patients have been shown to have high levels of triiodothyronine (T_3), thyroxine (T_4), and thyroid-binding globulin and low levels of reverse triiodothyronine (rT_3). The causes and clinical significance of these abnormalities are unknown.

11. Skin manifestations–HIV-infected patients commonly develop skin manifestations that can be grouped into viral, bacterial, fungal, neoplastic, and nonspecific dermatitides.

Herpes simplex infections occur more frequently, tend to be more severe, and are more likely to disseminate in AIDS patients than in immunocompetent hosts. Because of the risk of progressive local disease, all herpes simplex attacks should be treated with acyclovir (200 mg orally five times a day), or famciclovir (500 mg orally three times a day) for 7 days. To avoid the complications of attacks, many clinicians recommend chronic acyclovir administration (400 mg orally twice a day) for HIV-infected patients with a history of recurrent herpes. However, the finding of acyclovir resistance among some herpes strains cultured from HIV-infected patients raises concern about this practice.

Herpes zoster is a common manifestation of HIV infection. As with herpes simplex infections, patients with zoster should be treated with acyclovir to prevent dissemination (800 mg orally four or five times per day). Vesicular lesions should be cultured if there is any question about their origin, since herpes simplex responds to much lower doses of acyclovir. Disseminated zoster and cases with ocular involvement should be treated with intravenous (10 mg/kg every 8 hours) rather than oral acyclovir.

Molluscum contagiosum is seen in HIV-infected patients, as in other immunocompromised patients. Lesions have a propensity for spreading widely over the patient's skin and should be treated with topical liquid nitrogen.

Staphylococcus is the most common bacterial cause of skin disease in HIV-infected patients; it usually presents as folliculitis, superficial abscesses (furuncles), or bullous impetigo. Because dissemination with sepsis has been reported, attempts should be made to treat these lesions aggressively. Folliculitis is initially treated with topical clindamycin or mupirocin, and patients may benefit from regular washing with an antibacterial soap such as chlorhexidine. Intranasal mupirocin has been used successfully for staphylococcal decolonization in other settings. In HIV-infected patients with recurrent staphylococcal infections, weekly intranasal mupirocin should be considered in addition to topical care and systemic antibiotics. Abscesses often require incision and drainage. Patients may need antistaphylococcal antibiotics such as dicloxacillin, 250–500 mg orally four times daily, or erythromycin, 250 mg orally four times daily (with rifampin, 600 mg orally daily for 10 days for nasal staphylococcal decolonization), for severe folliculitis.

Bacillary angiomatosis is a well-described entity in HIV-infected patients. It is caused by two closely related organisms: *Bartonella* (formerly *Rochalimaea*) *henselae* and *Bartonella quintana.* The epidemiology of *B henselae* infection suggests zoonotic transmission from young cats. The most common manifestation is raised, reddish, highly vascular skin lesions that can mimic the lesions of Kaposi's sarcoma. Fever is a common manifestation of this infection; involvement of bone, lymph nodes, and liver has also been reported. Responses to doxycycline, 100 mg orally twice daily, and erythromycin, 250 mg orally four times daily, have been reported. Therapy is continued for at least 14 days, and patients who are seriously ill with visceral involvement may require months of therapy.

The majority of fungal rashes afflicting AIDS patients are due to dermatophytes and *Candida*. These are particularly common in the inguinal region but may occur anywhere on the body. Fungal rashes generally respond well to topical clotrimazole (1% twice a day) or ketoconazole (2% twice a day).

Kaposi's sarcoma lesions are red or purple, flat or raised papules that generally do not blanch. Cutaneous lesions can be treated with radiation or with intralesional injection of vinblastine, 0.01–0.02 mg in 0.1 mL of saline. Other dermatologic malignancies seen disproportionately among HIV-infected persons include basal cell and squamous cell carcinomas.

Seborrheic dermatitis is more common in HIV-infected patients. Scrapings of seborrhea have revealed *Malasezzia furfur (Pityrosporum ovale),* implying that the seborrhea is caused by this fungus. Consistent with the isolation of this fungus is the clinical finding that seborrhea responds well to topical clotrimazole (1% cream) as well as hydrocortisone (1% cream).

Xerosis presents in HIV-infected patients with severe pruritus. The patient may have no rash, or nonspecific excoriations from scratching. Treatment is with emollients (eg, absorption base cream) and antipruritic lotions (eg, camphor 9.5% and menthol 0.5%).

Psoriasis can be very severe in HIV-infected patients. Phototherapy and etretinate (0.25–9.75 mg/kg/d orally in divided doses) may be used for recalcitrant cases in consultation with a dermatologist. Because of the underlying immunodeficiency, methotrexate should be avoided.

12. HIV-related malignancies–Four cancers are currently included in the CDC classification of AIDS: Kaposi's sarcoma, non-Hodgkin's lymphoma, primary lymphoma of the brain, and invasive cervical carcinoma. Epidemiologic studies have shown that between 1973 and 1987 among single men in San Francisco, the risk of Kaposi's sarcoma increased more than 5000-fold and the risk of non-Hodgkin's lymphoma more than tenfold. Although Hodgkin's disease is not an AIDS-defining malignancy, epidemiologic studies indicate that it is about three times more common among HIV-infected gay men than among uninfected gay men. The increase in incidence of malignancies is probably a function of impaired cell-mediated immunity.

Kaposi's sarcoma is still the most common HIV-related malignancy. Kaposi's lesions may appear anywhere; careful examination of the eyelids, conjunctiva, pinnae, palate, and toe webs is mandatory to locate potentially occult lesions. In light-skinned individuals, Kaposi's lesions usually appear as purplish, nonblanching lesions that can be papular or nodular. In dark-skinned individuals, the lesions may appear more brown. In the mouth, lesions are most often palatal papules, though exophytic lesions of the tongue and gingivae may also be seen. Kaposi's lesions may be confused with other vascular lesions such as angiomas and pyogenic granulomas. About 40% of patients with dermatologic Kaposi's sarcoma will develop visceral disease (eg, gastrointestinal, pulmonary). Rapidly progressive dermatologic or visceral disease is best treated with systemic chemotherapy. Commonly used regimens include alternating weekly vincristine and vinblastine or combination doxorubicin, bleomycin, and vincristine. Alpha interferon has activity against Kaposi's sarcoma and may result in remission of lesions in minimally symptomatic patients with high CD4 counts and no history of opportunistic infection. However, even in this subgroup, subjective symptoms (eg, malaise, anorexia) limit the utility of this therapy. Bulky lesions of the lower extremities accompanied by lymphedema are a common presentation of Kaposi's sarcoma. Radiation and conservative measures (eg, leg elevation, elastic stockings) may be helpful.

Non-Hodgkin's lymphoma in HIV-infected persons tends to be very aggressive. The malignancies are usually of B cell origin and characterized as diffuse large-cell tumors. Over 90% of the malignancies are extranodal, with the central nervous system being a common site.

Patients with central nervous system disease are treated with radiation therapy. Systemic disease is treated with chemotherapy. Common regimens are CHOP (cyclophosphamide, doxorubicin, vincristine, and prednisone) and modified M-BACOD (methotrexate, bleomycin, doxorubicin, cyclophosphamide, vincristine, and dexamethasone). Granulocyte colony-stimulating factor (G-CSF; filgrastim) is used to maintain white blood counts with this latter regimen.

Although Hodgkin's disease is not included as part of the CDC definition of AIDS, studies have found that HIV infection is associated with a fivefold increase in the incidence of Hodgkin's disease. HIV-infected persons with Hodgkin's disease are more likely to have mixed cellularity and lymphocyte depletion subtypes of Hodgkin's disease and to present at an advanced stage of disease.

Anal dysplasia and squamous cell carcinoma have been noted in HIV-infected homosexual men. These lesions have been strongly correlated with previous infection by human papillomavirus (HPV). While many of the infected men report a history of anal warts or have visible warts, a significant percentage have silent papillomavirus infection. Cytologic (using Papanicolaou smears) and papillomavirus DNA studies can easily be performed on specimens obtained by anal swab. Although many questions remain unanswered, the growing frequency of these problems and the risk of progression from dysplasia to cancer in immunocompromised patients suggest that annual anal swabs for cytologic examination should be done in all HIV-infected persons who have engaged in anal intercourse.

HPV also appears to play a causative role in cervical dysplasia and neoplasia. The incidence and clinical course of cervical disease in HIV-infected women are discussed below.

13. Gynecologic manifestations–Vaginal candidiasis, cervical dysplasia and neoplasia, and pelvic inflammatory disease are more common in HIV-infected women than in uninfected women. These manifestations also tend to be more severe when they occur in association with HIV infection. Therefore, HIV-infected women need frequent gynecologic care. Vaginal candidiasis may be treated with topical agents (see Chapter 36). However, HIV-infected women with recurrent or severe vaginal candidiasis may need systemic therapy.

The incidence of cervical dysplasia in HIV-infected women is 40%. Because of this finding, HIV-infected women should have Papanicolaou smears every 6 months (as opposed to the AHCPR Guideline recommendation for every 12 months). Some clinicians recommend routine colposcopy or cervicography because cervical intraepithelial neoplasia has occurred in women with negative Papanicolaou smears. Cone biopsy is indicated in cases of serious cervical dysplasia.

Cervical neoplasia appears to be more aggressive among HIV-infected women. Most HIV-infected women with cervical cancer die of that disease rather than of AIDS. Because of its frequency and severity, cervical neoplasia was added to the CDC definition of AIDS in 1993.

While pelvic inflammatory disease appears to be more common in HIV-infected women, the bacteriology of this condition appears to be the same as among HIV-uninfected women. At present, HIV-infected women with pelvic inflammatory disease should be treated with the same regimens as uninfected women (see Chapter 17). However, inpatient therapy is generally recommended.

B. Laboratory Findings: Specific tests for HIV include antibody and antigen detection (Table 31–2). Screening serology is done by enzyme-linked immunosorbent assay (ELISA). Positive specimens are then confirmed by a different method (eg, Western blot). The sensitivity of screening serologic tests is greater than 99.5%. The specificity of positive results by two different techniques approaches 100% even in low-risk populations. False-positive screening tests may occur as normal biologic variants or in association with other disease states, such as connective tissue disease. These are usually detected by negative confirmatory tests. Molecular biology techniques (polymerase chain reaction) show a small incidence of individuals (< 1%) who are infected with HIV for up to 36 months without generating an antibody response. However, the vast majority will develop antibodies detectable by screening serologic tests within several months of infection. Core protein antigen (p24) may be detectable before a serologic response occurs, and antigenemia may also reappear in the course of the disease as immunosuppression progresses.

Nonspecific laboratory findings with HIV infection may include anemia, leukopenia (particularly lymphopenia) and thrombocytopenia in any combination, polyclonal hypergammaglobulinemia, and hypocholesterolemia. Cutaneous anergy is frequent early in the course and becomes universal as the disease progresses.

Table 31–2. Laboratory findings with HIV infection.

Test	Significance
HIV enzyme-linked immunosorbent assay (ELISA)	Screening test for HIV infection. Sensitivity > 99.9%; to avoid false-positive results, repeatedly reactive results must be confirmed with Western blot.
Western blot	Confirmatory test for HIV. Specificity when combined with ELISA > 99.9%. Indeterminate results with early HIV infection, HIV-2 infection, autoimmune disease, pregnancy, and recent tetanus toxoid administration.
CBC	Anemia, neutropenia, and thrombocytopenia common with advanced HIV infection.
Absolute CD4 lymphocyte count	Most widely used predictor of HIV progression. Risk of progression to an AIDS opportunistic infection or malignancy is high with CD4 < 200 cells/μL.
CD4 lymphocyte percentage	Percentage may be more reliable than the CD4 count. Risk of progression to on AIDS opportunistic infection or malignancy is high with percentage < 20%.
HIV viral load tests	These tests measure the amount of actively replicating HIV virus. Correlate with disease progression and response to antiretroviral drugs. Levels > 5000–10,000 copies/mL indicate the need for treatment.
β_2-Microglobulin	Cell surface protein indicative of macrophage-monocyte stimulation. Levels > 3.5 mg/dL associated with rapid progression of disease. Not useful with intravenous drug users.
p24 antigen	Indicates active HIV replication. Tends to be positive prior to seroconversion and with advanced disease.

Several laboratory markers are available to provide prognostic information and guide therapy decisions (Table 31–2). The most widely used marker is the absolute CD4 lymphocyte count. As counts decrease, the risk of serious opportunistic infection increases (Figure 31–1).

With the increased use of the CD4 count, the limitations of the test have become more apparent. There is substantial diurnal variation (counts are generally lower in the morning), and counts may be depressed by any intercurrent illness. Therefore, the trend in counts is more important than any single value. Because of laboratory variation, serial counts should be performed in the same laboratory. The frequency of performance of counts depends on the patient's health status. Patients whose CD4 counts are substantially above the threshold for initiation of antiviral therapy (500 cells/μL) should have counts performed every 6 months. Those who have counts near or below 500 cells/μL should have counts performed every 3 months. This is necessary for evaluating the efficacy of antiviral therapy and for initiating *P carinii* prophylactic therapy when the CD4 count drops below 200 cells/μL. Some studies suggest that the percentage of CD4 lymphocytes is a more reliable indicator of prognosis than the absolute counts because the percentage does not depend on calculating a manual differential. While the CD4 count measures immune dysfunction, it does not provide a measure of how actively HIV is replicating in the body. This large gap in our ability to assess HIV replication has been filled by "viral load" tests. These are PCR-based quantitative measures of the number of copies of HIV RNA or branched DNA. Changes in viral load from one test to another in the same patient are evaluated on a logarithmic scale, base 10.

Tests that determine evidence of macrophage-monocyte stimulation may provide additional useful prognostic information in infected individuals. Beta$_2$-microglobulin, for example, is a cell surface protein that increases at the time of HIV seroconversion and continues to rise with progression of disease. Asymptomatic individuals with elevated serum β_2-microglobulin concentrations may have a twofold to threefold increased incidence of disease progression. Epidemiologic studies have shown that even after stratification by CD4 count, β_2-microglobulin is an independent risk factor for the progression of disease. Because many intravenous drug users have chronically elevated β_2-microglobulin levels, this test is not generally helpful for patients in this group. Patients with malignant tumors, autoimmune processes, and other infections may also have elevated levels. Clinically, the test may not be very useful because current treatment guidelines are tied to CD4 count levels. Therefore, in most settings, the results are helpful prognostically but do not actually change therapeutic decisions.

The presence of detectable p24 antigen in serum indicates a higher risk of progression of disease even after adjusting for the level of CD4 lymphocyte count. An immune-complex-dissociated p24 assay is more sensitive and appears useful for demonstrating antiviral activity of drugs.

Early HIV Guideline Panel: Evaluation and management of early HIV infection: Clinical practice guideline. AHCPR Publication No. 94–0572. Rockville, MD: Agency for Health Care Policy and Research, Public Health Service, U.S. Department of Health and Human Services, 1994.

Fischl MA et al: An outbreak of tuberculosis caused by multiple-drug-resistant tubercle bacilli among patients with HIV infection. Ann Intern Med 1992;117:177. (Classic description of the disease profile and documentation of nosocomial spread.)

Saksela K et al: HIV-1 messenger RNA in peripheral blood mononuclear cells as an early marker of risk for progression to AIDS. Ann Intern Med 1995;123:641. (Prognostic value of plasma HIV-1 RNA levels.)

Schambelan M et al: Recombinant human growth hormone in patients with HIV-associated wasting: A randomized, placebo-controlled trial. (Treatment with growth hormone increased body weight, lean body mass, and exercise tolerance.)

Simpson DM et al: Neurologic manifestations of HIV infection. Ann Intern Med 1994;121:769. (Defines current understanding of central and peripheral neurologic problems.)

Tompkins DC et al: *Rochalimaea*'s role in cat scratch disease and bacillary angiomatosis. Ann Intern Med 1993;118:388. (Current state of knowledge about these newly identified organisms.)

Weber R, Bryan RT: Microsporidial infections in immunodeficient and immunocompetent patients. Clin Infect Dis 1994;19:517.

Differential Diagnosis

HIV infection may mimic a variety of other medical illnesses. Specific differential diagnosis depends upon the mode of presentation. In patients presenting with constitutional symptoms such as weight loss and fevers, differential considerations include cancer, chronic infections such as tuberculosis and endocarditis, and endocrinologic diseases such as hyperthyroidism. When pulmonary processes dominate the presentation, acute and chronic lung infections must be considered as well as other causes of diffuse interstitial pulmonary infiltrates. When neurologic disease is the mode of presentation, conditions that cause mental status changes or neuropathy—eg, alcoholism, liver disease, renal dysfunction, thyroid disease, and vitamin deficiency—should be considered. If a patient presents with headache and a cerebrospinal fluid pleocytosis, other causes of chronic meningitis enter the differential. When diarrhea is a prominent complaint, infectious enterocolitis, antibiotic-associated colitis, inflammatory bowel disease, and malabsorptive symptoms must be considered.

Prevention

A. Primary Prevention: Until vaccination is a reality, prevention of HIV infection will depend upon effective precautions regarding sexual practices and intravenous drug use, screening of blood products, and infection control practices in the health care setting. Primary care physicians should routinely obtain a sexual history and provide risk factor assessment of their patients and, when appropriate, screening for HIV infection with pre- and posttest counseling. Pretest counseling should include review of risk factors for HIV infection, discussion of safe sex, and the meaning of a positive test. Posttest counseling should include a review of the importance of safe sex practices. For persons who test positive, information on available medical and mental health services should be provided as well as guidance for contacting sexual or needle-sharing partners. It is the duty of physicians to counsel HIV-negative patients on how to avoid exposure to HIV. Patients should be counseled not to exchange bodily fluids unless they are in a long-term mutually monogamous relationship with someone who has tested HIV antibody-negative and has not engaged in unsafe sex for at least 6 months prior to or at any time since the negative test.

Only latex condoms should be used, along with a water-soluble lubricant. Although nonoxynol-9, a spermicide, kills HIV, it cannot be enthusiastically recommended as an ingredient in lubricants because of the possibility that it may cause genital ulcers which could facilitate HIV transmission. Patients should be counseled that condoms are not 100% effective. They should be made familiar with the use of condoms, including, specifically, the advice that condoms must be used every time; that space should be left at the tip of the condom as a receptacle for semen; that intercourse with a condom should not be attempted if the penis is only partially erect; that men should hold on to the base of the condom when withdrawing the penis to prevent slippage; and that condoms should not be reused. Although anal intercourse remains the sexual practice at highest risk of transmitting HIV, seroconversions have been documented with vaginal and oral intercourse as well. Therefore, condoms should be used when engaging in these activities. Women as well as men should understand how to use condoms so as to be sure that their partners are using them correctly.

Persons using intravenous drugs should be cautioned never to exchange needles or other drug paraphernalia. When sterile needles are not available, bleach does appear to inactivate HIV and should be used to clean needles.

Current efforts to screen blood and blood products have lowered the risk of HIV transmission with transfusion to 1:100,000.

In the hospital, concerns about nosocomial infection have led to the recommendation for universal body fluid precautions. This involves the rigorous use of gloves when handling any body fluid and the addition of gown, mask, and goggles for procedures that may result in splash or droplet spread. Reports of transmission of drug-resistant tuberculosis in health care settings also have had infection control implications. All patients with cough in outpatient settings should be encouraged to wear masks. Hospitalized HIV-infected patients with cough should be placed in respiratory isolation until tuberculosis can be excluded by chest x-ray and sputum smear examination. Primate model data have suggested that development of a protective vaccine may be possible. Clinical trials in humans using gp120 or its precursor gp160 have shown development of neutralizing antibodies to laboratory but not field isolates of HIV and may not be protective of infection. Phase II trials are under way using a vaccine that combines gp120 with a canarypox vector. In phase I trials, this combination appeared to be more successful in stimulating both antibody production and cell-mediated immunity than simpler subunit vaccines.

A second aspect of vaccine development focuses on boosting the immunologic responses of individuals who are already HIV-infected. One study suggested the possibility of eliciting new humoral and cellular immune responses in seropositive individuals with CD4 counts of over 500 cells/µL, but there is no evidence that clinical outcome is improved.

B. Secondary Prevention: The percentage of HIV-infected persons who will ultimately progress to AIDS is not known. However, cohort studies of individuals with documented dates of seroconversion demonstrate that approximately 50% of untreated seropositive persons develop AIDS within 10 years. The risk of developing AIDS is inversely correlated with the CD4 count; over 80% of patients with a CD4 count below 200 cells/µL develop AIDS within 3 years. A CD4 count of less than 50 cells/µL is also an important natural history landmark, since most deaths occur once the count has fallen below this level.

There is substantial evidence that medical intervention with antiretroviral and prophylactic regimens can prevent opportunistic infections and improve survival. Treatment prevents several infectious diseases, including tuberculosis and syphilis, which are transmissible to others. Recommendations are listed in Table 31–3.

Because of the increased occurrence of tuberculosis among HIV-infected patients, all such individuals should undergo PPD testing. Although anergy is common among AIDS patients, the likelihood of a false-negative result is much lower when the test is done early in infection. Those with positive tests (defined for HIV-infected patients as > 5 mm of induration) need a chest x-ray. Patients with an infiltrate in any location, especially if accompanied by mediastinal adenopathy, should have sputum sent for acid-fast staining. Those patients with a positive PPD but

Table 31–3. Health care maintenance
of HIV-infected individuals.

For all HIV-infected individuals
  CD4 counts every 3–6 months
  Viral load tests every 3–6 months and 1 month following a
    change in therapy
  PPD with anergy controls
  INH for those with positive PPD and normal chest x-ray
  RPR or VDRL
  Toxoplasma IgG serology
  Cytomegalovirus IgG serology
  Pneumococcal vaccine
  Influenza vaccine in season
  Hepatitis vaccine for those who are HBsAb-negative
  Haemophilus influenzae b vaccination
  Papanicolaou smears every 6 months for women
  Consider anal swabs for cytologic evaluation yearly for
    men with history of receptive anal intercourse
For HIV-infected individuals with CD4 < 500 cells/μL
  Zidovudine (AZT) or other antiretroviral drug as indicated
    (see Table 31–5)
For HIV-infected individuals with CD4 < 200 cells/μL
  P carinii prophylaxis (see Table 31–6)
For HIV-infected individuals with CD4 < 100 cells/μL
  M avium complex prophylaxis

negative evaluations for active disease should receive isoniazid (300 mg daily) for 9 months to a year regardless of their age. Recent analysis suggests also that HIV-infected individuals at high risk for tuberculosis should receive a course of isoniazid prophylaxis regardless of PPD status. This would include homeless individuals and injection drug users.

HIV-infected patients are at increased risk of reactivation of syphilis and progression to tertiary syphilis despite standard treatment. Because the only widely available tests for syphilis are serologic and because HIV-infected individuals are known to have disordered antibody production, there is concern about the interpretation of these titers. This concern has been fueled by a report of an HIV-infected patient with secondary syphilis and negative syphilis serologic testing. Furthermore, HIV-infected individuals may lose FTA-ABS reactivity after treatment for syphilis, particularly if they have low CD4 counts. Thus, in this population, a nonreactive treponemal test does not rule out a past history of syphilis. In addition, persistence of treponemes in the spinal fluid after one dose of benzathine penicillin has been demonstrated in HIV-infected patients with primary and secondary syphilis. Therefore, the CDC has recommended an aggressive diagnostic approach to HIV-infected patients with reactive RPR or VDRL tests of greater than 1 year or unknown duration. All such patients should have a lumbar puncture with cerebrospinal fluid cell count and CSF-VDRL. Those with a normal cerebrospinal fluid evaluation are treated as having late latent syphilis (benzathine penicillin G, 2.4 million units intramuscularly weekly for 3 weeks) with follow-up titers. Those with a pleocytosis or a positive CSF-VDRL test are

treated as having neurosyphilis (aqueous penicillin G, 2–4 million units intravenously every 4 hours; or procaine penicillin G, 2.4 million units intramuscularly daily, with probenecid, 500 mg four times daily, for 10 days). Some clinicians take a less aggressive approach to patients who have low titers (less than 1:8), a history of having been treated for syphilis, and a normal neurologic examination. Close follow-up of titers is mandatory if such a course is taken. For a more detailed discussion of this topic, see Chapter 34.

The efficacy of pneumococcal, *Haemophilus influenzae* b, and influenza vaccines is debated, but since they are safe, HIV-infected individuals should receive them. Patients without evidence of hepatitis B antigen or surface antibody should receive hepatitis B vaccination. Live vaccines, such as yellow fever vaccine, should be avoided. Measles vaccination, while a live virus vaccine, appears relatively safe when administered to HIV-infected individuals and should be given if the patient has never had measles or been adequately vaccinated.

HIV-infected individuals should be counseled with regard to safe sex. Because of the risk of transmission, they should be warned to use condoms with sexual intercourse, including oral intercourse. HIV-infected women should use latex barriers such as dental dams (available at dental supply stores) to prevent their partners from having direct oral contact with vaginal secretions. Substance abuse treatment should be recommended for persons who are using recreational drugs. They should be warned to avoid consuming raw meat or eggs to avoid infections with *Toxoplasma, Campylobacter,* and *Salmonella.* Because of the emotional impact of HIV infection and subsequent illness, many patients will benefit from supportive counseling.

C. HIV Risk for Health Care Professionals:
Epidemiologic studies show that needle sticks occur commonly among health care professionals, especially among surgeons performing invasive procedures and inexperienced hospital house staff. Efforts to reduce needle sticks should focus on avoiding recapping needles and, whenever possible, doing invasive procedures under controlled circumstances. The risk of HIV transmission from a needle stick with blood from an HIV-infected patient is about 1:250. The risk from mucous membrane contact is too low to quantitate.

Health care professionals who sustain needle sticks should be counseled and offered HIV testing as soon as possible. HIV testing is done to establish a negative baseline for worker's compensation claims in case there is a subsequent conversion. Follow-up testing is usually performed at 6 weeks, 3 months, and 6 months.

A case control study by the Centers for Disease Control and Prevention indicates that administration of AZT following a needle stick decreases the rate of

HIV seroconversion by 79%. Furthermore, data from animal models suggest potential efficacy of zidovudine when given soon after exposure. Therefore, providers should be offered therapy with zidovudine (200 mg orally three times daily) and lamivudine (150 mg orally twice daily). Providers who have high-risk exposures (eg, deep punctures), exposures to source patients with advanced disease or with high viral loads (eg, > 50,000 copies per milliliter), or exposures to source patients who may have virus resistant to standard antiretroviral therapy should be offered a protease inhibitor in addition to the above regimen (eg, indinavir, 800 mg orally three times daily). Therapy should be started as soon as possible after exposure and continued for 4 weeks. Unfortunately, there have been documented cases of seroconversion following parenteral exposure to HIV despite prompt use of zidovudine prophylaxis. Counseling of the provider should include "safe sex" guidelines.

D. Preventing Perinatal Transmission of HIV: A multicenter trial showed that when zidovudine is administered to women during pregnancy, labor, and delivery and then to their newborns, the rate of transmission of HIV is decreased by two-thirds. For this reason, all women who are pregnant or considering pregnancy should be offered an HIV antibody test. Ideally, pregnant HIV-infected women should be started on zidovudine during the second trimester. Because about half of fetal infections in non-breast-feeding women occur shortly before or during the birth process, zidovudine should be administered whenever a woman initiates perinatal care even if she did not begin therapy in the second trimester. Breast feeding is thought to increase the rate of transmission by 10–20% and should be avoided.

Case-control study of HIV seroconversion in health-care workers after percutaneous exposure to HIV-infected blood—France, United Kingdom, and United States, January 1988–August 1994. MMWR Morb Mortal Wkly Rep 1995;44:929. (AZT reduces the risk of seroconversion after percutaneous exposure by approximately 79%.)

Gallant JE, Moore RD, Chaisson RE: Prophylaxis for opportunistic infections in patients with HIV infections. Ann Intern Med 1994;120:932. (Reviews efficacy of prophylaxis for a variety of opportunistic infections.)

Gerberding JL: Prophylaxis for occupational exposure to HIV. Ann Intern Med 1996;125:497. (Thorough discussion of issues of occupational exposures, including treatment.)

Jewett JF, Hecht FM: Preventive health care for adults with HIV infection. JAMA 1993;269:1144. (Review of evidence supporting preventive medical interventions for HIV-infected persons.)

Letvin NL: Vaccines against human immunodeficiency virus: Progress and prospects. N Engl J Med 1993; 329:1400. (State of the art review of basic science and practical problems.)

Makadon HJ, Selin JG: Prevention of HIV infection in primary care: Current practice, future possibilities. Ann Intern Med 1995;123:715. (Discusses strategies for improving the HIV-prevention strategies of primary care physicians.)

Update: Provisional Public Health Service recommendations for chemoprophylaxis after occupational exposure to HIV. MMWR Morb Mortal Wkly Rep 1996;45:468. (Consensus recommendations for treatment of occupational exposure.)

Zidovudine for the prevention of HIV transmission from mother to infant. MMWR Morb Mortal Wkly Rep 1994;43:285. (Efficacy of zidovudine in reducing perinatal transmission.)

Treatment

Treatment for HIV infection can be divided into four categories: therapy for opportunistic infections and malignancies, antiretroviral treatment, hematopoietic stimulating factors, and prophylaxis of opportunistic infections.

Experimental treatment regimens for HIV infection are constantly changing. Clinicians may obtain up-to-date information on experimental treatments by calling the AIDS Clinical Trials Information Service (ACTIS), 800-TRIALS-A (English and Spanish); and the National AIDS Hot Line, 800-342-AIDS (English), 800-344-SIDA (Spanish), and 800-AIDS-TTY (hearing impaired).

A. Therapy for Opportunistic Infections and Malignancies: Treatment of common HIV infections and malignancies is detailed in Table 31–4. In general, AIDS patients require protracted therapy, including lifelong therapy for toxoplasmosis, cryptococcosis, and cytomegalovirus retinitis. The emergence of resistance is more common for some infections of HIV-infected people (eg, acyclovir-resistant herpes simplex) than among immunocompetent individuals. In addition, HIV-infected patients have an increased incidence of side effects to standard drugs such as trimethoprim-sulfamethoxazole.

Treating patients with repeated episodes of the same opportunistic infection can pose difficult therapeutic challenges. For example, patients with second or third episodes of pneumocystis pneumonia may have developed allergic reactions to standard treatments with a prior episode. Fortunately, there are several alternatives available for the treatment of *P carinii* infection. Trimethoprim with dapsone—and primaquine and clindamycin—are two combinations that often are tolerated in patients with a prior allergic reaction to trimethoprim-sulfamethoxazole and intravenous pentamidine. On the positive side, patients who develop second episodes of pneumocystis pneumonia while taking prophylaxis tend to have milder courses.

Well-established alternative regimens now also exist for most AIDS-related opportunistic infections: amphotericin B or fluconazole for cryptococcal meningitis; ganciclovir or foscarnet for cytomeg-

Table 31–4. Treatment of AIDS-related opportunistic infections and malignancies.[1]

Infection or Malignancy	Treatment	Complications
P carinii infection[2]	Trimethoprim-sulfamethoxazole, 15 mg/kg/d (based on trimethoprim component) orally or IV for 14–21 days.	Nausea, neutropenia, anemia, hepatitis, drug rash, Stevens-Johnson syndrome.
	Pentamidine, 3–4 mg/kg/d IV for 14–21 days.	Hypotension, hypoglycemia, anemia, neutropenia, pancreatitis, hepatitis.
	Trimethoprim, 15 mg/kg/d orally, with dapsone, 100 mg/d orally, for 14–21 days.	Nausea, rash, hemolytic anemia in G6PD-deficient patients. Methemoglobinemia (weekly levels should be < 10% of total hemoglobin).
	Primaquine, 15–30 mg/d orally, and clindamycin, 600 mg every 8 hours orally, for 14–21 days.	Hemolytic anemia in G6PD-deficient patients. Methemoglobinemia, neutropenia, colitis.
	Atovaquone, 750 mg orally 3 times daily for 14–21 days.	Rash, elevated aminotransferases, anemia, neutropenia.
	Trimetrexate, 45 mg/m² IV for 21 days (given with leucovorin calcium) if intolerant of all other regimens.	Leukopenia, rash, mucositis.
M avium complex infection	Clarithromycin, 500 mg orally twice daily, with ethambutol, 15 mg/kg/d orally (maximum, 1 g). May also add: Rifabutin, 300 mg orally daily.	Clarithromycin: hepatitis, nausea, diarrhea; ethambutol: hepatitis, optic neuritis. Rash, hepatitis, uveitis.
Toxoplasmosis	Pyrimethamine, 100–200 mg orally as loading dose, followed by 50–75 mg/d, combined with sulfadiazine, 4–6 g orally daily in 4 divided doses, and folinic acid, 10 mg daily for 4–8 weeks; then pyrimethamine, 25–50 mg/d, with clindamycin, 2 g/d, and folinic acid, 5 mg/d.	Leukopenia, rash.
Lymphoma	Combination chemotherapy (eg, modified CHOP, M-BACOD,[3] with or without G-CSF or GM-CSF).[4] Central nervous system disease: radiation treatment with dexamethasone for edema.	Nausea, vomiting, anemia, leukopenia, cardiac toxicity (with doxorubicin).
Cryptococcal meningitis	Amphotericin B, 0.6 mg/kg/d IV, to a total dose of about 1.5 g.	Fever, anemia, hypokalemia, azotemia.
	Fluconazole, 400 mg orally daily for 6 weeks, then 200 mg orally daily.	Hepatitis.
Cytomegalovirus infection	Ganciclovir, 10 mg/kg/d IV in 2 divided doses for 10 days, followed by 6 mg/kg 5 days a week indefinitely. (Decrease dose for renal impairment.) May use ganciclovir as maintenance therapy (1 g orally with fatty foods three times a day).	Neutropenia (especially when used concurrently with zidovudine).
	Foscarnet, 60 mg/kg IV every 8 hours for 10–14 days (induction), followed by 90 mg/kg once daily. (Adjust for changes in renal function.)	Nausea, hypokalemia, hypocalcemia, hyperphosphatemia, azotemia.
Esophageal candidiasis or recurrent vaginal candidiasis	Fluconazole, 100–200 mg daily for 10–14 days.	Hepatitis, development of imidazole resistance.
	Ketoconazole, 200 mg orally twice daily for 10–14 days.	Hepatitis, adrenal insufficiency, ventricular tachycardia when given with terfenadine or astemizole.
Herpes simplex infection	Acyclovir, 200 mg 5 times daily for 7–10 days; or acyclovir, 5 mg/kg IV every 8 hours for severe cases.	Resistant herpes simplex with chronic therapy.
	Foscarnet, 40 mg/kg IV every 8 hours, for acyclovir-resistant cases. (Adjust for changes in renal function.)	See above.

(continued)

Table 31–4. Treatment of AIDS-related opportunistic infections and malignancies.[1] (continued)

Infection or Malignancy	Treatment	Complications
Herpes zoster	Acyclovir, 800 mg orally 4 or 5 times daily for 7–10 days. Intravenous therapy at 10 mg/kg every 8 hours for ocular involvement, disseminated disease.	See above.
	Famciclovir, 50 mg orally 3 times daily.	Headache, nausea.
	Foscarnet, 40 mg/kg IV every 8 hours for acyclovir-resistant cases. (Adjust for changes in renal function.)	See above.
Kaposi's sarcoma Limited cutaneous disease	Observation, intralesional vinblastine.	Inflammation, pain at site of injection.
Extensive or aggressive cutaneous disease	Systemic chemotherapy (eg, alternating weekly vinca alkaloids). Alpha interferon (for patients with CD4 > 200 cells/μL and no constitutional symptoms). Radiation (amelioration of edema).	Bone marrow suppression, peripheral neuritis, flu-like syndrome.
Visceral disease (eg, pulmonary)	Combination chemotherapy (eg, daunorubicin, bleomycin, vinblastine).	Bone marrow suppression, cardiac toxicity, fever.

[1]For treatment of *Mycobacterium tuberculosis* infection, see Chapter 8.
[2]For moderate to severe *P carinii* infection (oxygen saturation < 90%), corticosteroids should be given with specific treatment. The dose of prednisone is 40 mg twice daily for 5 days, then 40 mg daily for 5 days, and then 20 mg daily until therapy is complete.
[3]CHOP = cyclophosphamide, doxorubicin, vincristine (Oncovin), and prednisone. Modified M-BACOD = methotrexate, bleomycin, doxorubicin, cyclophosphamide, vincristine (Oncovin), and dexamethasone.
[4]G-CSF = granulocyte colony-stimulating factor (filgrastim); GM-CSF = granulocyte-macrophage colony-stimulating factor (sargramostim).

alovirus infection; and sulfadiazine or clindamycin with pyrimethamine for toxoplasmosis.

Corticosteroids. Although conceptually it would seem that corticosteroid therapy should be avoided in HIV-infected patients, steroid use has been shown to improve the course of patients with moderate to severe pneumocystosis (oxygen saturation < 90%, PO_2 < 65 mm Hg) when administered within 72 hours after diagnosis. The mechanism of action is presumed to be a decrease in alveolar inflammation.

B. Antiretroviral Treatment: The development of drugs that suppress the HIV infection itself rather than its complications has been an important development (Table 31–5). In general, patients who have never been treated for HIV are given first-line treatment as shown in Figure 31–2. However, for patients with advanced disease (eg, CD4 lymphocyte counts < 200 cells/μL) or a high viral load (eg, greater than 50,000 copies per milliliter), it may be preferable to begin with second-line treatment, which includes a protease inhibitor.

Treatment recommendations for HIV-infected patients are in flux. Nonetheless, there are a few principles for which there is consensus. Treatment decisions should be guided primarily by HIV viral load test results. Persons with viral loads greater than 5000–10,000 copies per milliliter should be offered treatment to reduce the load. If the treatment does not lower the viral load by at least 0.5 log (at 4 weeks following initiation of a new therapy), the treatment should be changed. Similarly, treatment should be changed if the patient has an increase of viral load of 0.5 log while on therapy. The theory is that by reduc-

ing virus replication, antiretroviral therapy can prevent destruction of the immune system. Also, if the virus is not actively reproducing, it is less likely that mutations will occur that confer resistance to the antiretroviral agents. As therapy in patients with high viral loads but normal CD4 counts has not yet been proved, some clinicians do not initiate antiretroviral therapy until the patient's CD4 count drops below 500 cells/μL. In contrast, some researchers argue that HIV is best treated "early and hard" and advocate treating as early as possible following HIV infection with two nucleoside analogs plus a protease inhibitor.

Monotherapy should be avoided. For a patient who does not want to take more than one drug, didanosine is preferred to zidovudine. When patients show evidence of progression on therapy, two new drugs should be introduced at the same time if possible. The goal is to reduce the chance that the virus will become resistant.

The ideal combination of drugs to use is better understood after a review of the available agents. These agents can be grouped into three major categories: nucleoside analogs, protease inhibitors, and nonnucleoside reverse transcriptase inhibitors.

1. Nucleoside analogs–

a. Zidovudine–Zidovudine (azidothymidine; AZT) was the first approved antiviral drug for HIV infection. It has been proved to decrease symptoms and prolong the life of patients with AIDS or severe symptomatic disease. Zidovudine has also been shown to slow the progression to severe disease among patients with mild symptoms as well as asymptomatic patients with CD4 counts below

Table 31–5. Antiretroviral therapy.

Drug	Indication	Dose	Common Side Effects	Monitoring	Cost[1]
Nucleoside analogs					
Zidovudine (AZT) (Retrovir)	First-line treatment in combination with ddl, ddC, or 3TC	500–600 mg orally daily in three divided doses	Anemia, neutropenia, nausea, malaise, headache, insomnia, myopathy	Complete blood count and differential (every 3 months once stable)	$1.59/100 mg
Didanosine (ddl) (Videx)	First-line treatment alone or in combination with AZT	125–300 mg orally twice daily (for pill formulation)	Peripheral neuropathy, pancreatitis, dry mouth, hepatitis	CBC and differential, aminotransferases, K$^+$, amylase, triglycerides, monthly neurologic examination	$2.40/150 mg $4.00/250 mg powder
Zalcitabine (ddC) (Hivid)	First-line treatment in combination with AZT	0.375–0.75 mg orally 3 times a day	Peripheral neuropathy, aphthous ulcers, hepatitis	Monthly neurologic examination, aminotransferases	$2.29/0.75 mg
Stavudine (d4T) (Zerit)	In combination with 3TC in patients intolerant to zidovudine	20 mg orally twice daily	Peripheral neuropathy, hepatitis, pancreatitis	Monthly neurologic examination, aminotransferases, amylase	$2.53/40 mg
Lamivudine (3TC) (Epivir)	CD4 ≤ 500 cells/μL or symptomatic disease; first-line treatment in combination with AZT	150 mg orally twice daily	Rash, peripheral neuropathy	Monthly neurologic examination	$3.85/150 mg
Protease inhibitors					
Saquinavir (Invirase)	Progression of disease on first-line treatment; use in combination with nucleoside analogs	600 mg orally three times daily	Gastrointestinal distress, headache	No additional monitoring	$2.12/200 mg
Ritonavir (Norvir)	Progression of disease on first-line treatment; use in combination with nucleoside analogs	600 mg orally twice daily	Gastrointestinal distress, peripheral paresthesias	Monthly aminotransferases, CK, uric acid, triglycerides	$1.85/100 mg
Indinavir (Crixivan)	Progression of disease on first-line treatment; use in combination with nucleoside analogs	800 mg orally three times daily	Kidney stones	Monthly aminotransferases, bilirubin level	$1.25/200 mg $1.67/400 mg
Nelfinavir (Veracept)	Failure of or intolerance to other protease inhibitors	750 mg orally three times daily	Diarrhea	To be determined	To be determined
Nonnucleoside reverse transcriptase inhibitors (NNRTIs)					
Nevirapine (Viramune)	To be determined in combination with nucleoside analogs	200 mg orally daily for 2 weeks, then 200 mg orally twice daily	Rash	No additional monitoring	$4.13/200 mg
Delavirdine	To be determined in combination with nucleoside analogs	400 mg orally three times daily	Rash	To be determined	To be determined

[1]Cost to pharmacist (average wholesale price) for unit dose indicated. Source: First Data Bank, Price Alert, April 1997.

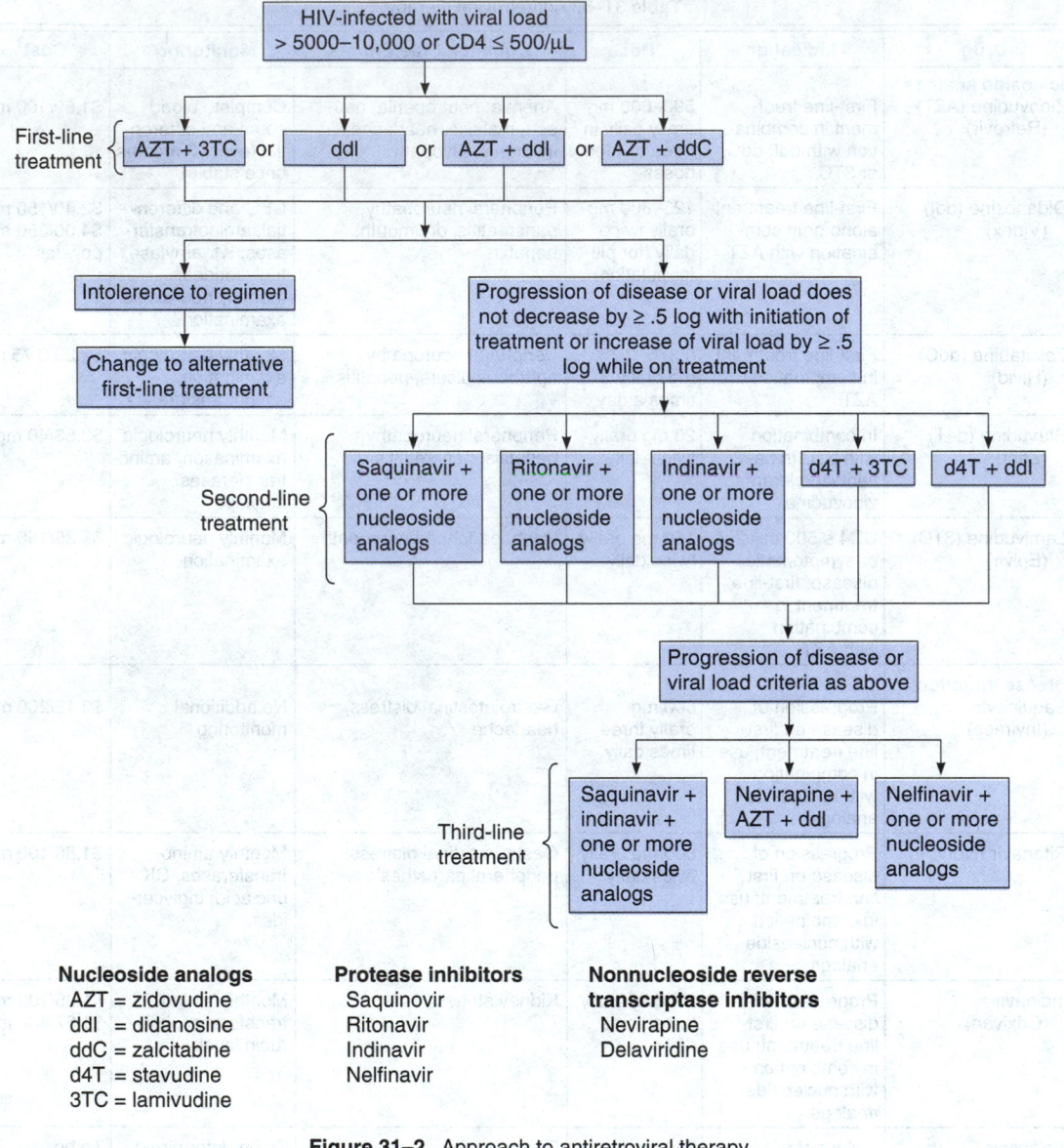

Figure 31–2. Approach to antiretroviral therapy.

500 cells/μL. Based on this finding, zidovudine was approved by the Food and Drug Administration for patients with CD4 counts below 500 cells/μL. However, two large studies, the Veterans Affairs Cooperative Study and the Concorde Study, have raised questions about whether zidovudine should automatically be recommended for patients with CD4 counts below that number. Both studies found that starting zidovudine early slows progression of disease but does not increase survival time compared with patients started on zidovudine later in the course of illness. Interpretation of these studies is complicated because they were performed prior to the availability of other antiretroviral agents. Zidovudine monotherapy is no longer recommended, especially for patients who have progressed on zidovudine.

While the dosing of zidovudine had been controversial, a total daily dose of 600 mg (200 mg orally three times daily) for an individual of average weight (50–74 kg) is now standard based upon studies in both early and late disease. While some antiviral effect is preserved at a total daily dose of 300 mg, this is a suboptimal dose. Conversely, the only setting in which a higher dose (1000–2000 mg/d) might be considered would be in the patient who develops dementia despite receiving the standard dose. One study suggested dose-related amelioration of neurologic symptoms.

Although all of the major trials of zidovudine have used every 4 hour dosing, clinicians are increasingly using three times a day dosing to improve patient compliance. The rationale for less frequent dosing is the long half-life of zidovudine once phosphorylated inside of infected cells (in contrast to the short half-life of zidovudine in the serum). The cost of zidovudine (at a dose of 600 mg/d) is approximately $270 a month.

Side effects seen with zidovudine are listed in Table 31–5. Approximately 40% of patients will experience subjective side effects that generally remit within 6 weeks. The common dose-limiting side effects of zidovudine are anemia and neutropenia. Although the anemia is usually macrocytic, it does not respond to vitamin B_{12} or folic acid supplementation. Both the anemia and the neutropenia generally respond to dose reductions and interruptions. Erythropoietin (epoetin alfa) and G-CSF (filgrastim) may also be used to ameliorate these side effects if the use of other antiretroviral agents is not possible. Zidovudine also causes myopathy, characterized by proximal muscle weakness. However, since this can also occur with advanced AIDS, it can be difficult to determine whether zidovudine is the inciting cause.

In monitoring patients receiving zidovudine, complete blood counts—with platelet and differential counts—should be done monthly for the first 2 months of therapy and then every 1–3 months depending on the clinical situation. Liver function tests and creatine phosphokinase levels should be checked every 3 months. Zidovudine can be taken concomitantly with other medicines except probenecid, which prolongs the serum half-life of zidovudine. Because of the synergistic bone marrow toxicity with some antibiotics, it may be prudent to withhold zidovudine while treating patients for serious opportunistic infections such as pneumocystis pneumonia. Long-term administration of zidovudine with ganciclovir can pose a difficult problem. Only 15% of patients tolerate this combination without significant hematologic toxicity. One approach to neutropenia is to add G-CSF (filgrastim) to the regimen; another is to substitute another agent for zidovudine. Finally, foscarnet has been shown to be well tolerated with concomitant zidovudine therapy. Since longer survival has been demonstrated in patients with CMV retinitis given foscarnet than in those given ganciclovir—perhaps because they were better able to tolerate simultaneous zidovudine—foscarnet probably represents the optimal antiviral approach. However, foscarnet therapy is more time-consuming and technically difficult for the patient than ganciclovir therapy since maintenance infusions last 2 hours instead of 1 hour and require a home infusion pump. Some patients may therefore prefer ganciclovir.

b. Didanosine–Both didanosine (dideoxyinosine; ddI) and zalcitabine (dideoxycytidine; ddC) have been approved by the FDA. Didanosine and zalcitabine are recommended for patients who are intolerant to zidovudine or have progressive HIV disease (eg, a significant drop of the CD4 lymphocyte count despite zidovudine treatment). Both drugs have been shown to increase CD4 lymphocyte counts and lower p24 antigen levels in a manner similar to zidovudine.

Didanosine alone has been shown to be superior to zidovudine alone in some patients who have taken zidovudine for at least 8–16 weeks. Several studies have extended this finding and shown that in previously untreated individuals with CD4 counts in the 200–500 cells/μL range, didanosine, alone or in combination with zidovudine, provides a survival benefit compared with zidovudine alone. This has resulted in a shift to earlier use of this agent.

Administration of didanosine is inconvenient. Because the drug is degraded by stomach acid, patients must take the medication on an empty stomach (1 hour before or 2–3 hours after meals). It is supplied in two forms: pills and packets of powder. To receive adequate buffering agent, the pills should be taken two at a time and thoroughly chewed or dissolved in water. The tablet formulation was improved in 1996 to make it easier to chew. Diarrhea (due to the buffering agent used) is more common with the powder.

Dosing of these two formulations is by weight. For adults weighing 35–49 kg, dosing is 125 mg (tablets) or 167 mg (powder) twice a day; for adults weighing 50–74 kg, 200 mg (tablets) or 250 mg (powder) twice a day; and for adults weighing over 75 kg, 300 mg (tablets) or 375 mg (powder) twice a day. Unlike zidovudine, didanosine does not cause anemia but may cause neutropenia. It has also been associated with pancreatitis. The incidence of pancreatitis with didanosine is 5–10%—of fatal pancreatitis, less than 0.4%. Patients with a history of pancreatitis, as well as those taking other medications associated with pancreatitis (including trimethoprim-sulfamethoxazole and intravenous pentamidine) are at higher risk of this complication. Patients should be warned not to use alcohol while taking didanosine. Clinicians should also teach patients to watch for the symptoms of pancreatitis and to stop treatment if they develop abdominal pain, nausea, or vomiting while taking didanosine until it can be determined if they have pancreatitis. Other common side effects with didanosine include a dose-related, reversible, painful peripheral neuropathy which occurs in about a third of patients, and dry mouth. Fulminant hepatic failure and electrolyte abnormalities, including hypokalemia, hypocalcemia, and hypomagnesemia, have been reported in patients taking didanosine.

c. Zalcitabine–Zalcitabine has several advantages as a potential antiviral agent. It is inexpensive, easy to administer, and has no known hematologic side effects. The usual dosage of zalcitabine is approximately 0.005–0.01 mg/kg orally every 8 hours. This drug is formulated in 0.375 mg and 0.75 mg tablets. A comparative trial of zidovudine and zalcitabine as single antiretroviral agents in patients without prior therapy showed superiority of zidovudine. However, zalcitabine has shown promise in combination with zidovudine (see below) and appears to be as efficacious as didanosine when used as monotherapy in persons who have previously received zidovudine.

Zalcitabine, like didanosine, may cause peripheral neuropathy. It is also associated with aphthous ulcers, rash, and rare cases of pancreatitis.

d. Stavudine–Stavudine (d4T) has shown promise as an antiretroviral drug. It has been found to increase CD4 counts and decrease p24 antigenemia. It is currently available for patients with CD4 counts below 500 cells/μL who are intolerant to didanosine and zidovudine or who have shown progression of disease. Side effects noted are peripheral neuropathy and hepatitis. Pancreatitis has been reported in patients taking stavudine, but it is unclear if the drug was the cause of the pancreatitis. The dose is 20 mg orally twice daily.

e. Lamivudine–Lamivudine is the newest available reverse transcriptase inhibitor. It appears to be a safe and well-tolerated agent that has shown great promise when used in combination with zidovudine. This combination results in more sustained suppression of viral replication and increase in CD4 cell counts than other combinations of nucleoside drugs studied to date. Zidovudine and lamivudine have a unique interaction whereby lamivudine suppresses the development and effect of zidovudine resistance mutations. Thus, it is not known whether this drug will show the same promising results in combination with other nucleoside agents. The dose of lamivudine is 150 mg orally twice daily.

2. Protease inhibitors–Four protease inhibitors—saquinavir, ritonavir, indinavir, and nelfinavir—have been approved for use. Protease inhibitors have been shown to potently suppress HIV replication in vitro and in vivo, particularly when combined with nucleoside analogs.

Saquinavir, given at a dose of 600 mg orally three times a day, causes some gastrointestinal side effects but has been generally well tolerated. One problem with its current formulation is poor bioavailability, which may favor the rapid development of drug resistance. Absorption may be improved by taking it with a high-fat meal.

Ritonavir and indinavir are two other potent protease inhibitors which have just been released and which appear to be better absorbed than saquinavir. Probably for this reason, they appear to be more effective in clinical practice. The usual dose for ritonavir is 600 mg orally twice a day. The dose for indinavir is 800 mg orally three times a day, and it is recommended that it be administered without food but with water 1 hour before or 2 hours after a meal. The most common side effects are gastrointestinal distress and peripheral paresthesias with ritonavir and kidney stones with indinavir; patients taking the latter drug should drink at least 48 ounces of liquids a day to ensure adequate hydration.

Nelfinavir was approved in 1997, and there is relatively little clinical experience with this agent. There does not appear to be significant cross-resistance with indinavir and ritonavir. The dose is 750 mg (three 250 mg tablets) three times daily with food. The most common side effect is diarrhea, which generally can be controlled with over-the-counter antidiarrheal agents.

Since the metabolism of these drugs is dependent upon the cytochrome P450 system, drugs such as rifabutin that induce this system should be avoided in favor of alternative agents where such choices exist. Because of the large number of drugs that should be avoided with these agents, clinicians should consult the product inserts before prescribing ritonavir, indinavir, or nelfinavir with other medications.

When any protease inhibitor is used incorrectly, drug resistance develops rapidly. For this reason, it is important to stress to patients the importance of complying with the prescribed treatment regimen. Patients should be counseled that if they feel they will miss doses or days of treatment, it would be better for them to not take a protease inhibitor. Protease inhibitors should not be used alone. In general, they should not be dose-escalated. The one exception is ritonavir, which should be initiated with a dose escalation schedule. The reason is that the body metabolizes the drug more slowly at the start of therapy, so that full dosing results in overdosing in the initial period. The manufacturer recommends a schedule of 300 mg twice daily for 1 day, 400 mg twice daily for 2 days, 500 mg twice daily for 1 day, and then 600 mg twice daily thereafter. Some clinicians have slowed this dose escalation even further over a period of 10 days to 3 weeks, starting with doses of 200 mg orally twice daily for two days.

3. Nonnucleoside reverse transcriptase inhibitors–Nevirapine is the first of a third class of antiretroviral drugs to be approved. While initial studies of this agent as monotherapy were discouraging owing to the rapid development of drug resistance, more recent clinical trials suggest beneficial effects and delayed development of resistance when nevirapine is combined with nucleoside analogs. The dose is 200 mg orally daily for 2 weeks, then 200 mg orally twice daily. The major toxicity of nevirapine is rash, the incidence of which can be reduced by starting with half the dose for the first 2 weeks. Delavirdine (400 mg orally three times daily) is a second drug in this class that is currently undergoing trials and is available on a compassionate use basis.

4. Combination therapy–While there is consensus that combination therapy is best for HIV infection, it is not clear which combinations are best. Zidovudine plus lamivudine has clearly demonstrated superior viral suppression and CD4 response compared with zidovudine monotherapy. For this reason, zidovudine plus lamivudine is a widely prescribed combination of nucleoside analogs. Zidovudine plus either didanosine or zalcitabine increased survival in antiretroviral-naive patients compared with zidovudine alone, but neither combination performed better than didanosine alone. For this reason, zidovudine plus didanosine and zidovudine plus zalcitabine are common combinations. For patients who cannot or do not want to take more than one antiretroviral agent, didanosine is a good choice.

In general, zidovudine and stavudine should not be used together since there is laboratory evidence of antagonism and because both can cause anemia. Similarly, didanosine, zalcitabine, and lamivudine are rarely used together because they all cause peripheral neuropathy.

Use of a protease inhibitor with two nucleoside analogs is a particularly potent combination because the drugs inhibit HIV at different points in the virus's life cycle. Addition of ritonavir to existing regimens of nucleoside analogs has been shown to increase survival for patients with advanced disease. Patients treated with zidovudine, lamivudine, and indinavir have been shown to have undetectable HIV viral load results. Saquinavir with zalcitabine was shown to be superior to either agent alone. Saquinavir can be used with indinavir. When used together with saquinavir, ritonavir increases the bioavailability of the latter drug. The dose of saquinavir with this combination is reduced to 400–600 mg twice daily. It may be possible to reduce the dose of ritonavir as well to 400 mg twice daily. However, data on the efficacy of this combination, as well as the ideal dosing schedule, are not yet available.

Much remains to be learned about the use of non-nucleoside reverse transcriptase inhibitors with other antiretroviral agents. Preliminary studies show that nevirapine may significantly reduce serum levels of the protease inhibitors; thus, optimal combinations of these agents cannot be established.

Clinicians and patients face difficult choices in this era of expanding therapeutic options. Aggressive combination therapy can certainly be justified in individuals who initially present with low CD4 cell counts or high viral loads, both of which indicate an unfavorable prognosis and early development of drug resistance; and in patients who have had disease progression despite antiretroviral monotherapy. More difficult is the decision about the regimen for people with earlier disease and lower risk of rapid progression. Starting combination therapy in this setting may burden patients with complicated medication regimens, high medical costs, long-term toxicities, and the significant risk of development of resistance.

C. Hematopoietic Stimulating Factors: Epo-

etin alfa (erythropoietin) has been approved for use in HIV-infected patients with anemia, including those with anemia secondary to zidovudine use. It has been shown to decrease the need for blood transfusions. The drug is expensive, and a low endogenous erythropoietin level (less than 500 mU/mL) should be demonstrated before starting therapy. The starting dose is 8000 units subcutaneously three times a week. The target hematocrit is 35–40%. The dose may be increased by 12,000 units every 4–6 weeks as needed to a maximum dose of 48,000 units per week. Hypertension is the most common side effect.

Human granulocyte colony-stimulating factor (G-CSF [filgrastim]) and granulocyte-macrophage colony-stimulating factor (GM-CSF [sargramostim]) have been shown to increase the neutrophil counts of HIV-infected patients. G-CSF is preferred because of the theoretical concern of GM-CSF-stimulating HIV replication in infected monocytes. In patients receiving cytotoxic chemotherapy for lymphoma or Kaposi's sarcoma, daily subcutaneous doses of G-CSF at approximately 5 μg/kg (a 300 μg or 480 μg vial, depending upon weight) are given beginning 5–7 days after chemotherapy until the neutrophil count has rebounded to above 1000/μL. G-CSF may also have a role in ameliorating neutropenia caused by other drugs such as zidovudine or ganciclovir, when other therapeutic alternatives are not possible. Since the cost of this therapy is approximately $150 per vial, dosage should be closely monitored and minimized, aiming for a neutrophil count of 1000/μL. When the drug is used for indications other than cytotoxic chemotherapy, one or two doses at 5 μg/kg per week is usually sufficient.

D. Prophylaxis of Opportunistic Infections: Patients with a history of pneumocystis pneumonia should receive secondary prophylaxis for that disease. Primary prophylaxis should be offered to patients with CD4 counts below 200 cells/μL, or less than 14% CD4 lymphocyte counts, or weight loss or oral candidiasis.

Three regimens for prophylaxis are trimethoprim-sulfamethoxazole, aerosolized pentamidine, and dapsone (see Table 31–6). Trimethoprim-sulfamethoxazole is inexpensive and widely available. In two recent studies comparing once-daily double-strength trimethoprim-sulfamethoxazole with aerosolized pentamidine for primary and secondary prophylaxis of pneumocystis pneumonia, patients randomized to trimethoprim-sulfamethoxazole were significantly less likely to develop pneumocystis pneumonia. In the study of secondary prophylaxis, there was a threefold decrease in the risk of recurrence with trimethoprim-sulfamethoxazole. This study also found that patients randomized to trimethoprim-sulfamethoxazole were less likely to develop bacterial infections (eg, pneumonia, sinusitis) than persons in the aerosolized pentamidine group—another reason

Table 31–6. *Pneumocystis carinii* prophylaxis.

Drug	Dose	Side Effects	Limitations
Trimethoprim-sulfamethoxazole	One double-strength tablet three times a week to one tablet daily	Rash, neutropenia, hepatitis, Stevens-Johnson syndrome	Hypersensitivity reaction is common, but, if mild, one may be able to treat through.
Dapsone	50–100 mg daily or 100 mg two or three times per week	Anemia, nausea, methemoglobinemia, hemolytic anemia	Efficacy not established. G6PD level should be checked prior to therapy. Check methemoglobin level at 1 month.
Aerosolized pentamidine	300 mg monthly	Bronchospasm (pretreat with bronchodilators); rare reports of pancreatitis	Apical *P carinii* pneumonia, extrapulmonary *P carinii* infections, pneumothorax.

to use trimethoprim-sulfamethoxazole instead of aerosolized pentamidine. There is a higher incidence of side effects with trimethoprim-sulfamethoxazole (primarily fever, rash, and nausea and vomiting) than with aerosolized pentamidine. Nonetheless, trimethoprim-sulfamethoxazole (one double-strength tablet three times a week to once daily) should be considered the prophylactic agent of choice if tolerated. Patients who develop mild rashes on this regimen may be treated with diphenhydramine (25–50 mg every 4 hours). However, clinicians and patients must watch carefully for signs of Stevens-Johnson syndrome. Some clinicians are also using desensitization regimens to overcome allergic reactions. Reports suggest that desensitization may be successful in 40% of cases.

Aerosolized pentamidine has the advantage of minimal systemic side effects. Its disadvantages are expense (approximately $160.00 per monthly treatment) and decreased effectiveness in the apical and peripheral areas of the lung. Cases of extrapulmonary *P carinii* infections in patients receiving aerosolized pentamidine have also been reported.

Aerosolized pentamidine may also increase the incidence of pneumothorax in patients with a history of *Pneumocystis* infection.

Although dapsone has not been widely studied, it appears to be an effective prophylactic agent with minimal side effects. As with trimethoprim-sulfamethoxazole, it is inexpensive and widely available and may be used in patients with an allergic reaction to trimethoprim-sulfamethoxazole. Before prescribing dapsone, clinicians should document that the patient is not G6PD-deficient. Such patients are at high risk of developing hemolytic anemia with dapsone therapy. Patients taking dapsone concomitantly with didanosine should take the dapsone at least 2 hours prior to the didanosine. Dapsone is not absorbed well in the neutral pH stomach environment created by the didanosine buffering agent.

Patients who develop *P carinii* infection on a particular prophylactic regimen should be switched to a different one or should receive a combination regimen (eg, aerosolized pentamidine plus trimethoprim-sulfamethoxazole).

M avium complex infection occurs in at least one-third of AIDS patients. Once the CD4 count falls below 75–100 cells/μL, prophylaxis should be started with a macrolide agent. Clarithromycin (500 mg orally twice daily) and azithromycin (1200 mg orally weekly) have both been shown to decrease the incidence of disseminated disease by approximately 75%, with a low rate of breakthrough of resistant disease. The latter regimen is generally preferred on the basis of ease of compliance and cost. Adding rifabutin increases the toxicity of the regimen but does not significantly increase its efficacy and is therefore not recommended. As sole therapy, rifabutin (300 mg orally daily) is less effective and more toxic than clarithromycin or azithromycin. Clinicians should make certain that patients do not have active *M tuberculosis* infection by examination of a chest radiograph prior to starting rifabutin because of concern about the development of resistance to rifabutin with cross-resistance to rifampin. Similarly, clinicians should establish with a blood culture that the patient does not have disseminated *M avium* complex infection. Common side effects of both azithromycin and clarithromycin are nausea and diarrhea. Two common side effects with rifabutin are rash and hepatic dysfunction. Rifabutin may induce hepatic enzymes, thereby decreasing the activity of some drugs metabolized by the liver.

Prophylaxis for *M tuberculosis*—isoniazid, 300 mg daily for 9 months to a year—should be given to all HIV-infected patients with positive PPD reactions (defined for HIV-infected patients as > 5 mm of induration).

Toxoplasmosis prophylaxis is desirable in patients with positive IgG *Toxoplasma* serology. Trimethoprim-sulfamethoxazole (one double-strength tablet daily) offers good protection against toxoplasmosis, as does a combination of pyrimethamine, 25 mg orally once a week, plus dapsone, 100 mg orally daily.

Cytomegalovirus infection is also common in late

HIV disease. Oral ganciclovir has been approved for CMV prophylaxis among HIV-infected persons with CD4 counts below 50 cells/µL. However, because the drug causes neutropenia, it is not widely used. Clinicians should consider performing serum CMV IgG antibody testing. Persons who are CMV IgG-negative are not at risk for development of CMV disease. Importantly, patients who are CMV IgG-negative should receive CMV-negative blood if they require a transfusion. Because over 99% of gay men are positive for CMV IgG, it is appropriate to reserve testing for heterosexuals with HIV.

Cryptococcosis and endemic fungal diseases are also candidates for prophylaxis. One prophylactic trial showed a decreased incidence of cryptococcal disease with the use of fluconazole, 200 mg orally daily, but the treated group had no benefit in terms of mortality. In areas of the world where histoplasmosis and coccidioidomycosis are endemic and are frequent complications of HIV infection, prophylactic use of fluconazole or itraconazole may prove to be useful prophylactic strategies. However, the problem of identifying individuals at highest risk makes the targeting of prophylaxis difficult.

Since individuals with advanced HIV infection are susceptible to a number of opportunistic pathogens, the use of agents with activity against more than one pathogen is envisioned. It has been shown, for example, that trimethoprim-sulfamethoxazole confers some protection against toxoplasmosis in individuals receiving this drug for *P carinii* prophylaxis. The newer macrolide antibiotics such as clarithromycin offer promise in this regard, since they have activity against bacterial, mycobacterial, and parasitic pathogens.

Course & Prognosis

The rate of progression to symptomatic disease is reviewed above. Once clinical findings develop, outcome varies. With improvements in therapy, some cohorts of patients are living longer after the diagnosis of AIDS. In San Francisco, mean survival after a first bout of pneumocystis pneumonia is 18–24 months. This is increased from approximately 12 months at the start of the epidemic. However, survival after diagnosis of HIV-related lymphomas still averages less than 8 months.

[Linked pages from community-based organizations in NYC]
   http://www.aidsnyc.org
[National AIDS Treatment Information Project (Kaiser) phone: 800-656-4KFF]
   http://www.kff.org/kff/topiclist.html?topic=AIDS%FHI
   V&submit.x=16&submit.y=9
[SFGH AIDS program website]
   http://HIVInSite.UCSF.edu
Armitage K et al: Treatment of cryptosporidiosis with paromomycin. Arch Intern Med 1992;152:2497. (Five cases with apparent response to this agent.)

Carpenter CCJ et al: Antiretroviral therapy for HIV infection in 1996: Recommendations of an International Panel. JAMA 1996;276:146. (Useful approaches to antiretroviral treatment in different clinical scenarios.)
Collier AC et al: Combination therapy with zidovudine and didanosine compared with zidovudine alone in HIV-1 infection. Ann Intern Med 1993;119:786. (Zidovudine plus didanosine resulted in a more sustained CD4 response than zidovudine alone.)
Collier AC et al: Treatment of human immunodeficiency virus infection with saquinavir, zidovudine, and zalcitabine. N Engl J Med 1996;34:1011. (Treatment with saquinavir, zidovudine, and ddC was superior to treatment with zidovudine and ddC or saquinavir and zidovudine.)
Dannemann B et al: Treatment of toxoplasmic encephalitis in patients with AIDS. Ann Intern Med 1992;116:33. (Multicenter study suggesting the equivalence of clindamycin and sulfadiazine in addition to pyrimethamine therapy.)
D'Aquila RT et al: Nevirapine, zidovudine, and didanosine compared with zidovudine and didanosine in patients with HIV-1 infection. A randomized, double-blind, placebo-controlled trial. Ann Intern Med 1996; 124:1019. (Addition of nevirapine to zidovudine and ddI improved immunologic and virologic response but was associated with severe rashes in 9% of patients receiving nevirapine.)
Deeks SG et al: HIV-1 protease inhibitors: A review for clinicians. JAMA 1997;277:145. (Reviews available data on the use of protease inhibitors.)
Eron JJ et al: Treatment with lamivudine, zidovudine, or both in HIV-positive patients with 200 to 500 CD4+ cells per cubic millimeter. N Engl J Med 1995; 333:1662. (Treatment with a combination of lamivudine and zidovudine is found to be superior to either treatment alone.)
Havlir DV et al: Prophylaxis against disseminated *Mycobacterium avium* complex with weekly azithromycin, daily rifabutin, or both. N Engl J Med 1996;335:392. (As monotherapy azithromycin is superior to rifabutin. Adding rifabutin increases side effects without significantly increasing efficacy.)
Horsburgh CR: Advances in the prevention and treatment of *Mycobacterium avium* disease. N Engl J Med 1996; 335:428. (Review of prevention and treatment of this common opportunistic infection.)
Kahn J et al: A controlled trial comparing continued zidovudine with didanosine in human immunodeficiency virus infection. N Engl J Med 1992;327:581. (Patients switched from zidovudine to didanosine had a lower rate of disease progression than those maintained on zidovudine.)
Lane HC et al: Recent advances in the management of AIDS-related opportunistic infections. Ann Intern Med 1994;120:945. (Reviews pneumocystis pneumonia, toxoplasmosis, *M tuberculosis*, *M avium* complex, and cytomegalovirus.)
Masur H: Drug therapy: Prevention and treatment of *Pneumocystis* pneumonia. N Engl J Med 1992;327:1853. (Summary of available treatments for prophylaxis and treatment.)
Montaner JSG et al: Didanosine compared with continued zidovudine therapy for HIV-infected patients with 200 to 500 CD4 cells/mm^3. Ann Intern Med 1995;123:561.

(Randomized, double-blind controlled study showing a change to didanosine to be superior to continuing with zidovudine in patients treated with zidovudine for at least 6 months.)

O'Brien WA et al: Changes in plasma HIV-1 RNA and CD4+ lymphocyte counts and the risk of progression to AIDS. N Engl J Med 1996;334:426. (Response of plasma HIV-1 RNA levels to treatment predicted progression of disease.)

Pierce M et al: A randomized trial of clarithromycin as prophylaxis against disseminated *Mycobacterium avium* complex infection in patients with advanced acquired immunodeficiency syndrome. N Engl J Med 1996; 335:384. (Clarithromycin compared with placebo significantly decreases the incidence of *M avium* complex infection.)

Powderly WG et al: A controlled trial of fluconazole or amphotericin-B to prevent relapse of cryptococcal meningitis in patients with the acquired immunodeficiency syndrome. N Engl J Med 1992;326:793. (Fluconazole was clearly superior and less toxic.)

Richman DD: Resistance, drug failure, and disease progression. AIDS Res Human Retro 1994;10:901. (A balanced overview of this controversial topic.)

Saag MS et al: Comparison of amphotericin B with fluconazole in the treatment of acute AIDS-associated cryptococcal meningitis. N Engl J Med 1992;326:83. (Fluconazole and amphotericin B are equivalent in neurologically intact patients with cryptococcal meningitis.)

Studies of Ocular Complications of AIDS Research Group: Mortality in patients with the acquired immunodeficiency syndrome treated with either foscarnet or ganciclovir for cytomegalovirus retinitis. N Engl J Med 1992;326:213. (Foscarnet-treated patients had a survival advantage, but the ganciclovir-treated group received less antiretroviral therapy.)

USPHS/IDSA Working Group: USPHS/IDSA guidelines for the prevention of opportunistic infections in persons infected with human immunodeficiency virus: A summary. Ann Intern Med 1996;124:348.

Infectious Diseases: Viral & Rickettsial

32

Wayne X. Shandera, MD, & Maria E. Carlini, MD

I. VIRAL DISEASES

In this section we will review herpesviruses, viruses associated with vaccine-preventable diseases, viruses whose major pathologic feature is neurotropic, systemic, respiratory, exanthematous, and gastrointestinal, and a final unclassifiable group. The hepatotropic viruses and the human immunodeficiency virus (HIV) are discussed in Chapters 15 and 31, respectively.

Clinical Diagnostic Considerations

Some viral illnesses present with clear clinical syndromes (measles, mumps, chickenpox). In many instances, however, the clinical picture is suggestive of viral infection but the causative agent could be any of a number of viruses. For example, aseptic meningitis can be caused by mumps virus, lymphocytic choriomeningitis virus, or any of several enteroviruses. Symptoms of respiratory disease with many viruses are typically indistinguishable, being characterized by erythema, nasal secretions, minimal purulence, and interstitial disease when pneumonia is present. Specific diagnosis requires laboratory assistance, which may be costly and may not influence therapy for an individual patient.

Identification of a virus is usually required only for confirmation of atypical cases, help with outbreak investigation, or elucidation of confusing syndromes. The frequency with which certain pathogens cause certain diseases allows for educated guesses, eg, respiratory syncytial virus (RSV) for bronchiolitis or parainfluenza virus for croup. Instances where rapid diagnosis assists in patient management are outlined in this chapter.

Laboratory Diagnostic Considerations

Three basic laboratory techniques are used for diagnosis of viral infections:

A. Isolation and Identification of Virus: Identification may be by a stain (eg, the nonspecific Tzanck smear for herpesviruses), cell culture (eg, coxsackievirus in suckling mice), or antibody detection (eg, rabies virus on skin biopsy). Isolation of virus from a normally sterile site (cerebrospinal fluid, lung) or from a lesion (vesicles) in an immunocompetent individual is diagnostically significant. From nonsterile sites (nasopharynx, stool), finding virus may denote only carriage, and seroconversion and pathologic change are needed for diagnosis.

B. Microscopic Methods: Microscopic techniques are used to examine cells, body fluids, biopsy material, or aspirates in search of virus or cytopathic changes specific for one or a group of viruses (eg, multinucleated giant cells at the base of herpes lesions, rotavirus structures on electron micrographs of diarrheal stools).

Immunofluorescent methods, often with monoclonal antibodies, can rapidly identify some antigens (rabies, varicella, herpes simplex, respiratory syncytial virus) in desquamated or scraped cells.

C. Immunologic Studies of Sera: Specific antibodies to viruses rise during the course of illness, though the rise and persistence of titer depend on the virus. A fourfold or greater rise in antibody titer during illness is considered evidence of disease.

Single titers are seldom helpful, and laboratories may require paired sera (acute and convalescent, 2–3 weeks apart). Serologic panels against many viruses are not practical in individual patients, since serologic studies require suspicion of the involved virus. Antigenic detection is used for certain viruses (HBsAg, HCV, HIV) and detects viral presence independently of disease duration or host response.

Therapeutic Considerations

The armamentarium of antiviral therapy has expanded greatly with the advent of the HIV outbreak (currently at least 22 antivirals are available in the United States), though for many common viruses (rhinoviruses, adenoviruses) and many serious but less common ones (arboviruses, hantaviruses) there is no definitive antiviral therapy.

The mainstay of preventing viral diseases is vaccination. Currently available live vaccines include those against the agents responsible for measles, mumps, rubella, poliovirus (Sabin vaccine), yellow fever, varicella, Japanese B encephalitis, and, in the near future, rotaviruses. The inactivated vaccines protect against the agents implicated in poliovirus (Salk vaccine), hepatitis A, hepatitis B, and respiratory syncytial virus (RSV). Passive immunoprophylaxis remains a vanguard of prevention against rabies, hepatitis A and B, RSV infection, and, among the immunosuppressed, varicella.

HUMAN HERPESVIRUSES

These viruses share features important in human disease. Eight identified human herpesviruses include herpes simplex virus (HSV) type 1, HSV type 2, varicella-zoster virus (type 3), Epstein-Barr (EB)-infectious mononucleosis virus (type 4), and cytomegalovirus (CMV) (type 5). A sixth type (HHV-6) has been identified as a causative agent of roseola (exanthema subitum), and a seventh (HHV-7) has been serologically associated with the disease. Another herpesvirus (HHV-8) may be associated with Kaposi's sarcoma (see Chapter 31).

Subclinical primary infection with the herpesviruses is more common than clinically manifest illness. Each persists in a latent state for the remainder of the host's life. Reactivation producing clinical recurrence of disease may follow known or unknown triggering mechanisms. With HSV and VZV, virus remains latent in sensory ganglia, and upon reactivation lesions appear in the distal sensory nerve distribution. As a result of disease-, drug-, or radiation-induced immunosuppression, virus reactivation may lead to widespread lesions in affected organs such as the viscera or the central nervous system. Severe or fatal illness may occur in infants and the immunodeficient. Herpesviruses can transform cells in tissue culture, though only EBV has been clearly associated with malignancy (see EBV section).

DeClercq E: Antivirals for the treatment of herpesvirus infections. J Antimicrob Chemother 1993;32(Suppl):121. (Includes a discussion of newer agents, such as famciclovir and cidofovir.)

1. HERPESVIRUSES 1 & 2

Essentials of Diagnosis

- Spectrum of illness from stomatitis to facial nerve paralysis (Bell's palsy) and encephalitis.
- Incubation period indeterminate since virus remains latent in ganglia and reactivates.
- Successful management usually with acyclovir.

General Considerations

Herpesviruses 1 and 2 affect primarily the oral and genital areas, respectively. Seroprevalence to both agents increases with age and, for HSV-2, with sexual activity. Disease is typically a manifestation of reactivation, and the triggers for clinical reactivation are multifactorial and not well understood.

Clinical Findings

A. Mucocutaneous Disease: Herpes simplex type 1 mucocutaneous disease largely involves the mouth and oral cavity ("herpes labialis") but also includes whitlows and a minority of urogenital infections. Vesicles typically form moist ulcers after several days and if untreated epithelialize over 2–3 weeks. Primary infection may be asymptomatic. Recurrences are usually milder and involve fewer lesions and faster healing.

Herpes simplex type 2 lesions largely involve the genital tract. Latency in presacral ganglia with reactivation in response to unknown stimuli is responsible for recurrent disease. A manifestation of primary infection in women may be aseptic meningitis. Asymptomatic shedding is common, especially following primary type 2 infection or symptomatic recurrences, and appears to be responsible for transmission.

Diagnosis is usually made clinically. Viral cultures of vesicular fluid or direct fluorescent antibody staining of scraped lesions may confirm the diagnosis.

B. Ocular Disease: HSV can cause keratitis, blepharitis, and keratoconjunctivitis. Keratitis is usually unilateral and is diagnosed by branching (dendritic) ulcers that stain with fluorescein. Visual acuity may be impaired from adjacent corneal involvement.

C. Neonatal Infection: Both herpesviruses can infect the fetus and induce congenital malformations (organomegaly, bleeding, central nervous system abnormalities). Neonatal herpes may also occur from unrecognized shedding in the mother's genital tract at time of delivery (even without a history of symptomatic genital herpes). Vesicular lesions, conjunctivitis, and neurologic symptoms from seizures to coma may be present beginning days to weeks postpartum.

D. Encephalitis, Recurrent Meningitis: Herpes simplex encephalitis presents with nonspecific symptoms: a flu-like prodrome, followed by headache, fever, behavioral and speech disturbances, and seizures that may be focal or generalized. A distinguishing feature is a propensity to involve the temporal lobe ("mass-like" lesions on scans, temporal lobe seizure foci on EEGs).

HSV DNA polymerase chain reaction (PCR) in the cerebrospinal fluid is a rapid and sensitive tool for early detection of HSV encephalitis and should probably replace brain biopsy when available. Untreated disease and presentation with coma carry a high mortality rate, with many survivors suffering neurologic sequelae. HSV-2 has been implicated as a major cause of benign recurrent lymphocytic meningitis.

E. Disseminated Infection: Disseminated HSV infection typically occurs in the setting of immunosuppression, either primary or iatrogenic, including steroid usage or, rarely with pregnancy. Skin lesions are not always present.

F. Bell's Palsy: An association between HSV-1 and Bell's palsy has been established.

G. Esophagitis: Esophagitis occurs with HSV-1 in AIDS patients and is diagnosed by endoscopic biopsy and cultures; the chief differential in the diagnosis of CMV esophagitis distinguished by the size and depth of the lesion (smaller and deeper for HSV).

Treatment & Prevention:

Drugs that inhibit replication of herpesvirus 1 and 2 include idoxuridine and trifluridine (for keratitis), acyclovir and vidarabine (for encephalitis or disseminated disease), and foscarnet (for resistant mucocutaneous disease in the immunocompromised) (see Table 32–1).

A. Mucocutaneous Disease: Oral and topical (5%) acyclovir are useful in treating mucocutaneous disease in immunosuppressed patients. Oral acyclovir is also useful in symptomatic primary genital infections, especially in women. A dosage of 200 mg five times a day can reduce the frequency and severity of recurrent oral or genital disease. When applied six times a day, topical 5% acyclovir solutions can reduce viral shedding, alleviate pain, and shorten the interval to healing, although the effect on recurrence or rate of recurrences is less substantial.

Acyclovir-resistant isolates associated with mucocutaneous lesions in the HIV-positive population should be treated with foscarnet (phosphonoformic acid), 40–60 mg/kg intravenously every 8 hours, adjusting for renal dysfunction. Rare cases resistant to foscarnet may require both foscarnet and acyclovir. The acyclic nucleoside analog cidofovir shows promise for treating both resistant HSV and CMV infections.

Acyclovir is effective in primary and secondary prevention. Patients with recurrent genital infections should be placed on maintenance acyclovir at a dosage of 600–800 mg/d in two or three divided doses. Prophylaxis may be especially useful for patients exposed to ultraviolet radiation such as during skiing or sailing trips. Famciclovir (250 mg twice daily) and valacyclovir (500 mg twice daily) are promising alternatives for recurrent disease because of their less frequent administration. AIDS patients with a history of mucocutaneous disease should receive lifelong acyclovir suppression.

B. Keratitis: Ophthalmic trifluridine or acyclovir, given as drops for 10 days (without corticosteroids), is the agent of choice.

C. Neonatal Disease: Acyclovir intravenously is effective for disseminated lesions in neonatal disease (5 mg/kg intravenously every 8 hours for 5 days).

D. Encephalitis: Because of the need for rapid treatment and the difficulties associated with brain biopsy, patients with suspected HSV encephalitis are typically given intravenous acyclovir (10 mg/kg every 8 hours for 10 days or more, adjusting for renal impairment), starting upon suspicion of diagnosis, and stopping if the biopsy is negative or another diagnosis is established. If the PCR is negative and clinical suspicion remains high in the absence of a biopsy, treatment should be continued for 10 days because it is relatively nontoxic.

E. Disseminated Disease: Disseminated disease responds best to parenteral acyclovir (see the preceding paragraph for dosages) when treatment is initiated early.

F. Bell's Palsy: Treatment with acyclovir does not change the clinical course of Bell's palsy.

G. Esophagitis: Patients with esophagitis should receive intravenous acyclovir at a dosage of 5–10 mg/kg every 8 hours; AIDS patients should be maintained on acyclovir at a dosage of 400 mg three to five times daily.

Prevention

Recurrent mucocutaneous disease is most effectively treated with acyclovir as outlined above; recurrent genital disease also requires use of barrier precautions during sexual activity. Preventing spread to hospital staff and other patients from cases with mucocutaneous, disseminated, or genital disease requires isolation and the use of handwashing and gloving-gowning precautions. Staff with active lesions (eg, whitlows) should not have contact with patients.

Benedetti J et al: Recurrence rates in genital herpes after symptomatic first-episode infection. Ann Intern Med 1994;121:847. (Acyclovir does not decrease recurrence rates; higher recurrence rates are reported in men—this explains higher transmission rates from men to women—and those with extended first infections.)

Frenkel LM et al: Clinical reactivation of herpes simplex virus type 2 infection in seropositive pregnant women with no history of genital herpes. Ann Intern Med 1993;118:414. (Serologic evidence of HSV-2 infection was common in pregnant women without a history of genital herpes.)

Lakeman FD et al: Application of PCR to CSF from brain-biopsied patients and correlation with disease. J Infect Dis 1995;171:857. (PCR is replacing brain biopsy as the standard of diagnosis.)

Mertz GJ: Management of genital herpes. Adv Exp Med Biol 1996;394:1.

Young EJ et al: Disseminated herpesvirus infection during pregnancy. Clin Infect Dis 1996;22:51. (Hepatic involvement portends a poor prognosis; review of 27 cases in the literature.)

Table 32–1. Agents for viral infections.

Drug	Dosing	Spectrum	Renal Clearance/ Hemodialysis	CSF Penetration	Toxicities
Acyclovir	200–800 mg orally five times daily; 250–500 mg/m² IV every 8 hours for 7 days	HSV	Yes/Yes	Yes	Neurotoxic reactions, reversible renal dysfunction, local reactions
Amantadine	100 mg orally twice daily (100 mg/d in elderly) for 10 days	Influenza A	Yes/No	Yes	Confusion, gastrointestinal symptoms
Cidofovir	5 mg/kg IV weekly for 2 weeks, then every other week	CMV	Yes/NA	NA	Neutropenia, renal failure, ocular hypotonia
Didanosine (ddl)	125–300 mg orally twice daily based on weight	HIV-1, HIV-2	Yes (moderate)/ Poorly dialyzed	Yes	Pancreatitis, neuropathy; magnesium toxicity in renal failure
Famciclovir	500 mg orally three times daily	VZV, ?HSV	Yes/NA	NA	NA
Foscarnet	20 mg/kg IV bolus, then 120 mg/kg IV every 8 hours for 2 weeks; maintain with 60 mg/kg/d IV for 5 days each week	CMV, HSV resistant to acyclovir, VZV, HIV-1	Yes/Yes	Variable	Nephrotoxicity, genital ulcerations, calcium disturbances
Ganciclovir	5 mg/kg IV bolus every 12 hours for 14–21 days; maintain with 3.75 mg/kg/d IV for 5 days each week	CMV	Yes/Yes	Yes	Neutropenia, thrombocytopenia, CNS side effects
Idoxuridine	Topical, 0.1% every 1–2 hours for 3–5 days	HSV keratitis	—	—	Local reactions
Indinavir	800 mg orally three times daily	HIV-1, ?HIV-2	MInimal/NA	See note 1	Nephrolithiasis, ↑ bilirubin, nausea, vomiting, flank pain
Interferon alfa-2b	SC: 3–5 million IU three times weekly to daily. Intralesionally: 1 million IU per 0.1 mL in up to five warts three times weekly for 3 weeks	HBV, HCV, papillomavirus (HPV)	Yes/Yes	—	Influenza-like syndrome, myelosuppression, neurotoxicity
Interferon alfa-n3	0.05 mL/wart biweekly up to 8 weeks	HPV	NA/NA	NA	Local reactions
Lamivudine (3TC)	12 mg/kg/d	HIV-1, ?HIV-2, HBV	Yes/NA	Yes	Skin rash, headache, insomnia
Nevirapine	200 orally daily or twice daily	HIV-1	NA/NA	Yes	Rash, including Stevens-Johnson reactions, thrombocytopenia, ↑ aminotransferases
Ribavirin	Aerosol: 1.1 g/d as 20 mg/mL dilution over 12–18 hours for 3–7 days (See text for Lassa fever doses.)	RSV, severe influenza A or B, Lassa fever	Yes/No	Yes	Wheezing
Rimantadine	100 mg orally twice daily	Influenza A	Yes/No	Yes	Same as amantadine, but less severe
Ritonavir	Dose escalates from 300 mg orally twice daily to 600 mg orally three times daily (requires refrigeration)	HIV-1, ?HIV-2	No/No	See note 1	Paresthesias, nausea, vomiting, diarrhea, ↑ triglycerides, ↑ aminotransferases
Saquinavir	600 mg orally three times daily with food	HIV-1, HIV-2	No/No	See note 1	Nausea, diarrhea
Stavudine (d4T)	40 mg twice daily	HIV-1, ?HIV-2	Yes (moderate)/ NA	Yes	Neuropathy, increased liver function tests, pancreatitis

Table 32–1. Agents for viral infections. (continued)

Drug	Dosing	Spectrum	Renal Clearance?/ Hemodialysis	CSF Penetration	Toxicities
Trifluridine	Topical, 1% drops every 2 hours to 9 drops/d	HSV keratitis	—	—	Local reactions
Valacyclovir	1 g orally three times daily for 7 days for VZV; 500 mg twice daily for HSV	VZV, ?HSV	Yes/Poorly	NA	Thrombotic thrombocyto-penic purpura or hemoly-tic uremic syndrome in AIDS
Vidarabine	15 mg/kg/d IV for 10 days	HSV, VZV	Yes/Yes	Yes	Teratogenic, megaloblastosis, neurotoxicity
Zalcitabine (ddC)	0.75 mg three times daily	HIV-1, HIV-2	Yes/—	Yes	Rash, fevers, aphthous stomatitis, neurotoxicity; rarely, pancreatitis and myelosuppression
Zidovudine (AZT)	200 mg three times daily (capsules for 300 mg twice daily are available) Total daily dose: 400–600 mg	HIV-1, HIV-2	Yes (moderate)/ Yes (moderate)	Yes	Bone marrow sup-pression, neurotoxic-ity

Note 1: Generally, the protease inhibitors are tightly protein-bound and do not penetrate the cerebrospinal fluid well.

2. VARICELLA (Chickenpox) & HERPES ZOSTER (Shingles)

Essentials of Diagnosis

- Exposure 14–21 days before onset.
- Fever and malaise just before or with eruption.
- Rash: pruritic, centripetal, papular, changing to vesicular ("dewdrops on a rose petal"), pustular, and finally crusting.

General Considerations

Varicella-zoster virus is human herpesvirus 3. Disease manifestations are either chickenpox (varicella) or shingles (herpes zoster, a reactivation of varicella). Chickenpox is highly contagious and is generally a disease of childhood, with spread by inhalation of infective droplets or contact with lesions after 10–20 days (average, 14–15 days).

Clinical Findings

A. Varicella:

1. Symptoms and signs–(Table 32–2.) Fever and malaise are usually mild in children and more severe in adults. Vesicular lesions, quickly rupturing to form small ulcers, may appear first in the oropharynx. The pruritic rash is centripetal and most prominent on the face, scalp, and trunk, but to a lesser extent it commonly involves the extremities. Maculopapules change in a few hours to vesicles that become pustular and eventually form crusts. New lesions may erupt for 1–5 days, so that all stages of the eruption are generally present simultaneously. The crusts usually slough in 7–14 days. The vesicles and pustules are superficial and elliptic, with slightly serrated borders.

Many infections are subclinical. In immunosuppressed patients, visceral VZV infection can occur in the absence of cutaneous lesions. The generalized nondermatomal distribution and the evolution of lesions (all stages simultaneously) distinguish primary varicella from herpes zoster.

2. Laboratory findings–Leukopenia is common. Multinucleated giant cells are evident on Tzanck smears of scrapings of vesicle bases. Diagnosis is usually made on the basis of clinical findings, though virus is isolable from vesicles and by detection of antigens in vesicle fluid.

B. Herpes Zoster: Pain is often severe and may precede the appearance of rash. Lesions follow any nerve root distribution, with thoracic and lumbar roots commonest, and cervical or trigeminal involvement is typical. In most cases a single unilateral dermatome is involved. The occurrence of zoster does not correlate with progression to AIDS in HIV-infected patients, but recurrent zoster indicates a poorer prognosis in established AIDS.

Skin lesions resemble those of chickenpox, developing as maculopapules and evolving into vesicles and pustules. Lesions on the tip of the nose indicate involvement of the nasociliary nerve, a branch of the ophthalmic division of the trigeminal nerve; this nerve also serves the cornea. Facial palsy, lesions of the external ear with or without tympanic membrane involvement, vertigo and tinnitus, and deafness signify geniculate ganglion involvement (Ramsay Hunt syndrome). In either, treatment is indicated (see below).

Table 32–2. Diagnostic features of some acute exanthems.

Disease	Prodromal Signs and Symptoms	Nature of Eruption	Other Diagnostic Features	Laboratory Tests
Eczema herpeticum	None.	Vesiculopustular lesions in area of eczema.		Herpes simplex virus isolated in cell culture. Multinucleate giant cells in smear of lesion.
Varicella (chicken-pox)	0–1 day of fever, anorexia, headache.	Rapid evolution of macules to papules, vesicles, crusts; all stages simultaneously present; lesions superficial, distribution centripetal.	Lesions on scalp and mucous membranes.	Specialized complement fixation and virus neutralization in cell culture. Fluorescent antibody test of smear of lesions.
Infectious mono-nucleosis (EBV)	Fever, adenopathy, sore throat.	Maculopapular rash resembling rubella, rarely papulovesicular.	Splenomegaly, tonsillar exudate.	Atypical lymphocytes in blood smears; heterophil agglutination. Monospot test.
Exanthema subitum (HHV-6,7; roseola)	3–4 days of high fever.	As fever falls by crisis, pink maculopapules appear on chest and trunk; fade in 1–3 days.		White blood count low.
Measles (rubeola)	3–4 days of fever, coryza, conjunctivitis, and cough.	Maculopapular, brick-red; begins on head and neck; spreads downward and outward, in 5–6 days rash brownish, desquamating. See atypical measles.	Koplik's spots on buccal mucosa.	White blood count low. Virus isolation in cell culture. Antibody tests by hemagglutination inhibition or neutralization.
Atypical measles	Same as measles.	Maculopapular centripetal rash, becoming confluent.	History of measles vaccination.	Measles antibody present in past, with titer rise during illness.
Rubella	Little or no prodrome.	Maculopapular, pink; begins on head and neck, spreads downward, fades in 3 days. No desquamation.	Lymphadenopathy, postauricular or occipital.	White blood count normal or low. Serologic tests for immunity and definitive diagnosis (hemagglutination inhibition).
Erythema infectiosum (parvovirus B19)	None. Usually in epidemics.	Red, flushed cheeks; circumoral pallor; maculopapules on extremities.	"Slapped face" appearance.	White blood count normal.
Enterovirus infections	1–2 days of fever, malaise.	Maculopapular rash resembling rubella, rarely papulovesicular or petechial.	Aseptic meningitis.	Virus isolation from stool or cerebrospinal fluid; complement fixation titer rise.
Typhus	3–4 days of fever, chills, severe headaches.	Maculopapules, petechiae, initial distribution centrifugal (trunk to extremities).	Endemic area, lice.	Complement fixation.
Rocky Mountain spotted fever	3–4 days of fever, vomiting.	Maculopapules, petechiae, initial distribution centripetal (extremities to trunk, including palms).	History of tick bite.	Complement fixation.
Ehrlichiosis	Headache, malaise.	Rash in one-third, similiar to Rocky Mountain spotted fever.	Pancytopenia, elevated liver function tests.	Polymerase chain reaction, immunofluorescent antibody.
Scarlet fever	One-half to 2 days of malaise, sore throat, fever, vomiting.	Generalized, punctate, red; prominent on neck, in axillae, groin, skinfolds; circumoral pallor; fine desquamation involves hands and feet.	Strawberry tongue, exudative tonsillitis.	Group A hemolytic streptococci in cultures from throat; antistreptolysin O titer rise.
Meningo-coccemia	Hours of fever, vomiting.	Maculopapules, petechiae, purpura.	Meningeal signs, toxicity, shock.	Cultures of blood, cerebrospinal fluid. High white blood count.
Kawasaki disease	Fever, adenopathy, conjunctivitis.	Cracked lips, strawberry tongue, maculopapular polymorphous rash, peeling skin on fingers and toes.	Edema of extremities. Angiitis of coronary arteries.	Thrombocytosis, electrocardiographic changes.

Complications

A. Varicella: Secondary bacterial infections, particularly with group A beta-hemolytic streptococci, are common; cellulitis, erysipelas, epiglottitis, osteomyelitis, scarlet fever, and, rarely, meningitis have been observed. Pitted scars are frequent sequelae. Interstitial pneumonia is more common in adults than in children and may result in ARDS or death. Encephalitis is infrequent (1:1000), is characterized by ataxia and nystagmus, and usually results in complete recovery.

Reye's syndrome also complicates varicella (and other viral infections, especially influenza B), usually in childhood, and has been associated with aspirin therapy (see Influenza, below). Varicella in immunosuppressed patients is often severe and may be fatal. Many manifestations of VZV infection occur in HIV infection.

When contracted during the first or second trimesters of pregnancy, varicella carries a risk of congenital malformations, including cicatricial lesions of an extremity, growth retardation, microphthalmia, cataracts, chorioretinitis, deafness, and cerebrocortical atrophy. If a mother develops varicella within 5 days after delivery, the newborn is at great risk of severe disease and should receive varicella-zoster immune globulin (VZIG). (See below for dosage.)

B. Herpes Zoster: In immunosuppressed patients, herpes zoster may disseminate, producing skin lesions beyond the dermatome, visceral lesions, and encephalitis. Postherpetic neuralgias occur in 50% of zoster patients over age 60.

Prevention

The care of patients with active varicella or zoster requires isolation and infection control precautions (handwashing, gowns, gloves). Respiratory isolation is needed when managing a case of varicella pneumonia. Susceptible employees should not care for active varicella cases. Exposed susceptible individuals should refrain from patient care until after the incubation period.

A. Varicella: A live attenuated vaccine is recommended for administration to all children over 12 months of age who have not had clinical chickenpox. Susceptible household contacts of children with documented varicella should also be vaccinated, assuming they are neither immunocompromised nor have had previous varicella. In this latter instance, the vaccine is 85% effective in preventing illness. Children receiving the vaccine should not take aspirin for at least 6 weeks, because of the possibility Reye's syndrome.

Varicella-zoster immune globulin (VZIG) is effective in preventing chickenpox in exposed susceptible, particularly immunosuppressed, individuals. It is given by deep intramuscular injection in a dosage of 12.5 units/kg up to a maximum of 625 units, with a repeat dose in 3 weeks if a high-risk patient remains exposed. VZIG has no place in acute therapy. It may be obtained by calling any Red Cross Blood Center or the Centers for Disease Control and Prevention (404-639-1870). Because VZIG appears to bind the varicella vaccine, it should not be given concomitantly with it.

B. Zoster: There are no known means of effectively preventing zoster eruptions.

Treatment

A. General Measures: Patient should be isolated until primary crusts have disappeared and kept at bed rest until afebrile. Hospitalized patients with VZV infections should be isolated, and caregivers should wear gowns, gloves, and masks when in contact with them. The skin needs to be kept clean. Pruritus can be relieved with oral antihistamines, topical calamine lotion, and colloidal oatmeal baths. As an antipyretic, acetaminophen is used.

B. Antiviral Therapy: For the infrequent varicella infections when antiviral therapy is indicated, the mainstay of therapy is acyclovir, which is effective in reducing the severity and shortening the duration of chickenpox and zoster both in adults and in children. However, acyclovir has little effect on postherpetic pain. Corticosteroids have been used to reduce the incidence of postherpetic neuralgia in the elderly but the drugs are usually ineffective; a short course will probably not have deleterious effects.

In immunocompromised patients, antiviral therapy with high-dose acyclovir (30 mg/kg/d in three divided doses intravenously for at least 7 days) should be started once the diagnosis is suspected. It should also be instituted for pneumonitis or corneal or trigeminal ganglion involvement in immunocompetent persons. Acyclovir-resistant varicella has been observed in AIDS patients receiving chronic acyclovir therapy. Foscarnet may be used for acyclovir-resistant virus; however, resistance to foscarnet has also been observed.

Newer agents (famciclovir, valacyclovir) are available for varicella-zoster infection (Table 32–1).

Eye involvement in zoster demands ophthalmologic referral and mydriatics, topical steroids, and, as noted, antivirals (oral acyclovir, topical vidarabine or acyclovir).

C. Treatment of Complications: Secondary bacterial infections of lesions are managed with bacitracin-neomycin, mupirocin (2% ointment), or oral antistaphylococcal antibiotics if lesions are extensive (eg, dicloxacillin, 250 mg four times daily for 10 days).

Prognosis

The total duration of varicella from onset of symptoms to disappearance of crusts rarely exceeds 2 weeks. Fatalities are rare except in immunosuppressed patients.

Zoster resolves in 2–6 weeks. Antibodies persist longer and at higher levels than with primary varicella.

Baren JM et al: Primary varicella in adults: Pneumonia, pregnancy, and hospital admission. Ann Emerg Med 1996;28:165. (While 10% of 130 patients presenting to an ER with varicella had pneumonia, there was no increased risk of pneumonia among the pregnant patients.)

Gray F et al: Varicella-zoster virus infection of the central nervous system in the acquired immune deficiency syndrome. Brain 1994;117:987. (Syndromes associated with VZV in AIDS include multifocal encephalitis, ventriculitis, acute hemorrhagic meningomyeloradiculitis, a focal necrotizing myelitis, and vasculopathy of leptomeningeal arteries.)

Strauss SE: Shingles: Sorrows, salves, and solutions. JAMA 1993;269:1836. (Brief review of antivirals, steroids, topical treatment, and vaccines for VZV infection.)

Watson BM et al: Safety and immunogenicity of a combined live attenuated measles, mumps, rubella, and varicella vaccine (MMR[II]V) in healthy children. J Infect Dis 1996;173:731.

3. INFECTIOUS MONONUCLEOSIS

Essentials of Diagnosis

- Fever, sore throat, malaise, lymphadenopathy.
- Splenomegaly and occasionally a maculopapular rash.
- Positive heterophil agglutination test (Monospot).
- "Atypical" large lymphocytes in blood smear; lymphocytosis.
- Hepatitis; occasionally myocarditis, neuritis, encephalitis.

General Considerations

Infectious mononucleosis is an acute infectious disease due to the Epstein-Barr (EB) virus (human herpesvirus 4). It is universal in distribution and may occur at any age but usually occurs between the ages of 10 and 35, either in an epidemic form or as sporadic cases. Rare cases have been reported in the elderly, usually without the full complex of symptoms. Its mode of transmission is probably by saliva. The incubation period is probably 5–15 days or longer.

Clinical Findings

A. Symptoms and Signs: Symptoms are varied but typically include fever, lymphadenopathy (discrete, nonsuppurative, slightly painful, especially along the posterior cervical chain), and splenomegaly (in about one-half). Sore throat is usually present, and toxic symptoms (malaise, anorexia, and myalgia) occur frequently in the early phase of the illness. A maculopapular or occasionally petechial rash occurs in fewer than 15% of cases unless ampicillin has been given (when rash may be seen in > 90%). Exudative pharyngitis, tonsillitis, or gingivitis may occur.

Other manifestations of infectious mononucleosis are hepatitis, nausea, anorexia, and jaundice; central nervous system involvement with headache, neck stiffness, photophobia, painful mononeuropathies (including Bell's palsy), and occasionally aseptic meningitis, encephalitis, or Guillain-Barré syndrome; pulmonary involvement with chest pain, dyspnea, and cough; and myocardial involvement with tachycardia and arrhythmias.

The varying symptoms of infectious mononucleosis—especially sore throat, hepatitis, rash, and lymphadenopathy—raise difficult problems in differential diagnosis.

B. Laboratory Findings: Initially, there is a granulocytopenia followed within 1 week by a lymphocytic leukocytosis. Many lymphocytes are atypical, ie, are larger than normal mature lymphocytes, stain more darkly, and frequently show vacuolated, foamy cytoplasm and dark chromatin in the nucleus. Hemolytic anemia secondary to anti-i antibodies is occasionally encountered, as is thrombocytopenia (at times severe).

Heterophil (sheep cell agglutination) antibody tests and the correlated mononucleosis spot (Monospot) test usually become positive in infectious mononucleosis before the fourth week after onset of illness. Heterophil-negative tests are not uncommon in children. Titer rises in antibodies directed at several EB virus antigens can be detected. During acute illness there is a rise and fall in IgM antibody to EB virus capsid antigen (VCA) and a rise in IgG antibody to VCA, which persists for life. Antibodies to EB virus nuclear antigen (EBNA) appear at 3–4 weeks after onset and also persist. A false-positive VDRL or RPR test occurs in 10% of cases. Culture of viruses is not routinely available.

Hepatic aminotransferases and bilirubin are commonly elevated. Cryoglobulins are present in up to 90% of patients. In central nervous system involvement, the cerebrospinal fluid may show increase of pressure, abnormal lymphocytes, and protein.

Differential Diagnosis

Causes of exudative pharyngitis include diphtheria, gonococcal and streptococcal infections, and infections with adenovirus and herpes simplex; potentially severe head and neck infections (pharyngeal and tonsillar abscesses) may occasionally be mistaken for the lymphadenopathy of mononucleosis. CMV infection, toxoplasmosis, and rubella may be indistinguishable from infectious mononucleosis due to EB virus, but the heterophil antibody and Monospot tests are negative and pharyngitis is usually absent. Mycoplasmal infection may also present primarily with pharyngitis, though lower respiratory symptoms usually predominate. A hypersensitivity syndrome induced by carbamazepine may mimic infectious mononucleosis.

Complications

Secondary bacterial throat infection can occur and is often streptococcal. Autoimmune hemolytic anemia occurs in up to 3% of cases. Splenic rupture is a rare but dramatic complication, and a history of preceding trauma can be elicited in half of the cases. Pericarditis and myocarditis are also rare complications, although nonspecific electrocardiographic changes are seen in about 5% of patients. Neurologic involvement—including transverse myelitis—is infrequent.

Treatment

A. General Measures: No specific treatment is available, and acyclic antiviral compounds (acyclovir, ganciclovir) are not helpful, although newer agents such as penciclovir (the prodrug for famciclovir) appear to have anti-EBV properties. The patient requires support and reassurance because of the frequent feeling of lassitude and the duration of symptoms. Symptomatic relief can be afforded by the administration of aspirin or another nonsteroidal anti-inflammatory agent, and warm saline throat irrigations or gargles three or four times daily. In severely ill patients, when enlarged lymphoid tissue threatens to obstruct the airway, a 5-day course of corticosteroids (eg, prednisolone, 50 mg/d for 3 days, with tapering) may be beneficial; severe thrombocytopenia and autoimmune hemolytic anemia also may respond to corticosteroids; pericarditis and impending splenic rupture are not clear-cut indications for corticosteroid therapy. Corticosteroids are not indicated for uncomplicated acute infectious mononucleosis.

B. Treatment of Complications: Hepatitis, myocarditis, and encephalitis are treated symptomatically. Rupture of the spleen requires emergency splenectomy. In order to avoid this complication, it is best to avoid frequent deep palpation of the spleen or vigorous activity for at least 1 month or until splenomegaly has regressed.

Prognosis

In uncomplicated cases, fever disappears in 10 days and lymphadenopathy and splenomegaly in 4 weeks. The debility sometimes lingers for 2–3 months.

Death is uncommon; when it does occur it is usually due to splenic rupture, hypersplenic phenomena (severe hemolytic anemia, thrombocytopenic purpura), or encephalitis.

Bacon TH, Boyd HR: Activity of penciclovir against Epstein-Barr virus. Antimicrob Ag Chemother 1995;39:1559.

Connelly KP, DeWitt LD: Neurologic complications of infectious mononucleosis. Pediatr Neurol 1994;101:181.

Kieff E: EBV: Increasing evidence of a link to carcinoma. N Engl J Med 1995;333:724. (Editorial on p 693 of the same issue.)

Strauss SE (moderator) et al: Epstein-Barr virus infections: Biology, pathogenesis, and management. Ann Intern Med 1993;118:45. (NIH conference.)

See also references at end of next section.

4. OTHER EBV SYNDROMES

EBV viral antigens have been found in over 90% of patients with African Burkitt's lymphoma or nasopharyngeal carcinoma. A causative role for EBV has been postulated with both neoplasms. An inability to eliminate EBV has a well-established association with X-linked lymphoproliferative syndrome (Duncan's disease). EBV-induced uncontrolled lymphoproliferation appears to give rise to B cell lymphomas in the setting of immunodeficiency. Immunologically privileged areas such as the central nervous system are particularly susceptible. EBV has also been associated with leiomyomas in children with AIDS and with nasal T cell lymphomas. There is no credible evidence that chronic fatigue syndrome is caused by chronic EBV infection. Oral hairy leukoplakia is discussed in Chapter 8.

Lekstrom-Hines JA et al: Periodic illness associated with Epstein-Barr virus infection. Clin Infect Dis 1996;22:22. (See also the editorial on p 28. A chronic lymphoproliferative, nonmalignant state appears to also be associated with EBV by serologic and virologic data.)

Liebowitz D: Epstein-Barr virus: An old dog with new tricks. N Engl J Med 1995;332:55.

Swanink CMA et al: EBV and the chronic fatigue syndrome. Clin Infect Dis 1995;20:1390. (No difference in viral antigen load between patients and controls.)

5. CYTOMEGALOVIRUS DISEASE

Most cytomegalovirus (CMV) infections in healthy individuals are asymptomatic, with the virus remaining latent (exact cells of latency are not known). However, the virus is isolable from up to 25% of salivary glands, 10% of uterine cervices, and 1% of neonatal urine samples. Seroprevalence increases with age and with the number of sexual partners. Detectable antibody is present in the serum of most homosexual men. Transmission is sexual, congenital, through blood products or transplantation, and person-to-person (eg, day care centers). Severe disease occurs primarily in the immunocompromised, especially those with AIDS and transplant patients.

Clinical Findings

A. Classification: There are three recognizable clinical syndromes.

1. Perinatal disease and CMV inclusion disease–Intrauterine infection of infants whose mothers had a primary infection during pregnancy results in a neonatal syndrome of jaundice, hepatosplenomegaly, thrombocytopenia, periventricular central nervous system calcifications, mental retardation, motor disability, and purpura. Neonatally acquired disease may resemble mononucleosis and therefore is often asymptomatic; neurologic deficits may ensue later in life.

2. Acute acquired CMV infection–This syndrome, akin to EBV-associated infectious mononucleosis, is characterized by fever, malaise, myalgias and arthralgias (but not pharyngitis or respiratory symptoms), atypical lymphocytes, and abnormal liver function tests. Heterophil antibody is absent. Transmission occurs by sexual contact, in milk, via respiratory droplets among nursery or day care center attendants, and by transfusions of blood.

3. Disease in immunocompromised hosts– Tissue and bone marrow transplant patients are at increased risk for CMV infection, especially in the first 100 days after allograft transplantation. HIV-infected patients may have a variety of CMV manifestations. CMV is itself immunosuppressive and may worsen manifestations of HIV infection, including *Pneumocystis carinii* pneumonia.

a. CMV retinitis–Retinitis due to CMV infection occurs primarily in AIDS patients. Screening for visual symptoms may be helpful, but ophthalmologic documentation of neovascular, proliferative lesions ("pizza-pie" retinopathy) is required for diagnosis.

b. Gastrointestinal and hepatobiliary CMV– Serious gastrointestinal CMV disease occurs in AIDS and after organ transplantation, cancer chemotherapy, or steroid therapy. Esophagitis presents with odynophagia; small bowel disease may mimic inflammatory bowel disease or may present as ulceration or perforation. Colonic CMV disease causes diarrhea, hematochezia, abdominal pain, fever, and weight loss. CMV has been identified, often with other pathogens, in up to 15% of patients with AIDS cholangiopathy. Diagnosis is by mucosal biopsy showing characteristic CMV histopathologic findings of intranuclear ("owl's eye") and intracytoplasmic inclusions.

c. Pulmonary CMV–Pulmonary CMV infection occurs in about 15% of bone marrow transplant recipients; the mortality rate is 80–90% in this group. CMV seronegative blood products should be used in seronegative recipients of seronegative transplants. High-titer CMV immunoglobulins may be effective in preventing CMV pneumonia in the seronegative recipients.

d. Neurologic CMV–Polyradiculopathy and encephalitis have been reported but are uncommon. The latter has a subacute onset in patients with advanced AIDS and is usually associated with disseminated CMV infections. The isolation of CMV in the cerebrospinal fluid is indicative usually of disseminated CMV infection. Prolonged ganciclovir may be helpful, and treatment should be continued indefinitely.

4. Other disease associations–CMV has been linked serologically to non-HIV-associated Kaposi's sarcoma and more recently to coronary artery disease. The significance of these associations remains under investigation.

B. Laboratory Findings: CMV is isolable from urine, cervical secretions, semen, saliva, blood, and other tissues, but virus isolation is most useful when combined with the pathologic findings described. Cultures alone are of little use in diagnosing AIDS-related CMV infections. The acute mononucleosis syndrome is associated with lymphocytosis, often 2 weeks after the fever, but absolute leukoplakia may also be noted. Serologic tests are useful primarily in seroepidemiologic studies. Antigen detection by virus technology (including the polymerase chain reaction technique) must be interpreted in the context of clinical and pathologic findings.

Prevention

No vaccine is currently available. CMV hyperimmune globulin given to seronegative bone marrow or renal transplant recipients may be prophylactic. Limiting transfusions, using products filtered to remove leukocytes, and selecting CMV-seronegative donors are all important in reducing the rate of CMV transmission. Ganciclovir at a dosage of 5 mg/kg intravenously twice daily for 5 days, beginning when the absolute neutrophil count is 750 cells/μL, then daily until day 100 posttransplant, reduces CMV infection and disease, leaving mortality unchanged.

Treatment

Two antiviral agents with efficacy against CMV infections are ganciclovir, 5 mg/kg intravenously every 12 hours for 14–21 days; and foscarnet, loading with 20 mg/kg intravenously, followed by 60 mg/kg every 8 hours over weeks. A daily maintenance regimen using both ganciclovir (3.75 mg/kg intravenously) and foscarnet (60 mg/kg intravenously), each over 1 hour, has been shown to be safe and effective in inhibiting CMV replication. Both medications require dosage adjustments for renal impairment.

The induction phase is required for AIDS patients with CMV disease involving critical parts of the retina; for less critical areas, maintenance therapy can be used from the outset. Both agents are effective in preventing progression of retinitis, and oral ganciclovir is an effective but expensive alternative for maintenance therapy. Complications include neutropenia with ganciclovir (preventing concomitant zidovudine therapy) and renal impairment with foscarnet (often manageable with hydration) (Table 32–1). The nucleoside analog cidofovir is given intravenously every 2 weeks and represents a promising new alternative therapy for CMV retinitis.

DeRodriguez W, Fuhrer J: Cytomegalovirus colitis in patients with acquired immunodeficiency syndrome. J R Soc Med 1994;87:203. (While diarrhea is common, bloody diarrhea is not.)

Drew WL et al: Oral ganciclovir as maintenance treatment for CMV retinitis in patients with AIDS. N Engl J Med 1995;333:615. (Oral and intravenous ganciclovir had similar mean times to progression of retinitis, but the oral form had fewer side effects.)

Goodgame RW: Gastrointestinal cytomegalovirus disease. Ann Intern Med 1993;119:924. (Review of gastrointestinal manifestations in immunocompromised and immunocompetent patients.)

Goodrich JM et al: Ganciclovir prophylaxis to prevent cytomegalovirus disease after allogeneic marrow transplant. Ann Intern Med 1993;118:173. (Reduced morbidity but not mortality. Another protocol for bone marrow transplant patients also reduced the probability of CMV disease in the first 120 days. See Winston JD et al: Ann Intern Med 1993;118:179.)

Masur H et al: Advances in the management of AIDS-related cytomegalovirus retinitis. Ann Intern Med 1996;125;126.

6. HUMAN HERPESVIRUSES 6, 7, & 8

Human herpesvirus 6 (HHV-6) is a B cell lymphotropic virus that is the principal cause of exanthema subitum (roseola infantum, sixth disease). Primary HHV-6 infection occurs most commonly in children under 2 years of age and may cause one-third of infantile febrile seizures. HHV-6 is infrequently a pathogen of older children and adults, though it has been associated with several illnesses including hepatitis, infectious mononucleosis-like syndromes, interstitial pneumonitis, and lymphoproliferative disease in immunocompromised patients and histiocytic necrotizing lymphadenitis and idiopathic bone marrow suppression in bone marrow transplant recipients.

Two variants (A and B) of HHV-6 have been identified. The latter is sensitive to ganciclovir, and both are sensitive to foscarnet, which should be given for serious HHV-6 infections (see cytomegalovirus section for dosages). HHV-6 has been isolated from blood in lymphoma patients and may play a role in angioimmunoblastic lymphadenopathy with dysproteinemia and Hodgkin's disease.

HHV-7 is a T cell lymphotropic virus that has also been serologically associated with roseola. The membrane glycoprotein CD4 is involved in HHV-7 recognition, and an antagonistic interaction between HHV-7 and HIV has been shown.

A herpesvirus (HHV-8) is now known to be responsible for AIDS-associated Kaposi's sarcoma. See Chapter 31 for pathogenesis and management.

Luppi M, Torelli G: The new lymphotropic herpesviruses and hepatitis C virus in human lymphoproliferative diseases: An overview. Haematologica 1996;81:265.

Robinson WS: HHV-6. Curr Clin Top Infect Dis 1994;14:159.

MAJOR VACCINE-PREVENTABLE VIRAL INFECTIONS

1. MEASLES

Essentials of Diagnosis

- Exposure 10–14 days before onset in an unvaccinated patient.
- Prodrome of fever, coryza, cough, conjunctivitis, photophobia, Koplik's spots.
- Rash: brick-red, irregular, maculopapular; onset 3–4 days after onset of prodrome; begins on the face and proceeds "downward and outward," affecting the palms and soles last.
- Leukopenia.

General Considerations

Measles is an acute systemic viral (paramyxovirus) infection transmitted by inhalation of infective droplets. The virus preferentially infects monocytes. It is the cause of death for 1 million children worldwide yearly. Its highest incidence is in young children. Illness confers permanent immunity. Communicability is greatest during the preeruptive and catarrhal stages but continues as long as the rash remains. Sporadic recent outbreaks of the disease in adults, adolescents, and unvaccinated preschool children in dense urban areas have led to changes in recommendations concerning prevention (see below).

Clinical Findings

A. Symptoms and Signs: (Table 32–2.) Fever is often as high as 40–40.6 °C. It persists through the prodrome and early rash (about 5–7 days). Malaise may be marked. Coryza (nasal obstruction, sneezing, and sore throat) resembles that seen with upper respiratory infections. Cough is persistent and nonproductive. Conjunctivitis manifests as redness, swelling, photophobia, and discharge.

Koplik's spots are pathognomonic of measles. They appear about 2 days before the rash and last 1–4 days as tiny "table salt crystals" on the dull red mucous membranes of the cheeks and often on inner conjunctival folds and vaginal mucous membranes. Other findings include pharyngeal erythema, a yellowish exudate on the tonsils, coating of the tongue in the center with a red tip and margins, moderate generalized lymphadenopathy, and, in occasional cases, splenomegaly.

The rash usually appears first on the face and behind the ears 4 days after the onset of symptoms. The initial lesions are pinhead-sized papules which coalesce to form a brick-red, irregular, blotchy maculopapular rash. In severe cases, the rash may coalesce to form a nearly uniform erythema on some body areas. The rash next appears on the trunk, followed by the extremities, including the palms and soles. It fades in order of appearance. Hyperpigmentation remains in fair-skinned individuals and severe cases. Slight desquamation may follow.

Atypical measles is a syndrome occurring in adults who received inactivated measles vaccine (available 1963–1967) or who received live measles vaccine before age 12 months and as a result developed hypersensitivity rather than protective immunity. When infected later with wild measles virus, such individuals may develop a potentially fatal illness with high fever, unusual rashes (papular, hemorrhagic) without Koplik's spots, headache, arthralgias, hepatitis, and interstitial or nodular infiltrates, occasionally with pleural effusions.

B. Laboratory Findings: Leukopenia is usually present unless secondary bacterial complications exist. Proteinuria is often present. Although technically difficult, virus can be cultured from nasopharyngeal washings and from blood. A fourfold rise in serum hemagglutination inhibition antibody supports the diagnosis.

Complications

A. Central Nervous System Complications: Encephalitis occurs in approximately 0.05–0.1% of cases. Its onset is usually 3–7 days after the rash. Vomiting, convulsions, coma, and a variety of severe neurologic signs and symptoms develop. Treatment is symptomatic and supportive. Demyelination is prominent. Virus is usually not found in the central nervous system, though demyelination is prominent. There is an appreciable mortality rate (10–20%), and many patients are left with neurologic morbidity.

Subacute sclerosing panencephalitis (SSPE) is a very late central nervous system complication, the measles virus acting as a "slow virus" to produce degenerative central nervous system disease years after the initial infection. SSPE is rare (1:100,000 cases of measles) and occurs more often when measles develops early in life, among males, and in persons living in rural environments.

An acute progressive encephalitis (subacute measles encephalitis), characterized by seizures, neurologic deficits, and often progressive stupor and death, can occur among immunosuppressed patients; measles virus opportunistically invades the central nervous system. Treatment is supportive, withholding immunosuppressive chemotherapy when feasible. Interferon and ribavirin have been variably successful.

B. Respiratory Tract Disease: Early in the course of the disease, bronchopneumonia or bronchiolitis due to the measles virus may occur in 1–7% and result in serious respiratory difficulties. Pneumonia occurring with or without an evanescent rash is seen in atypical measles.

C. Secondary Bacterial Infections: Immediately following measles, secondary bacterial infection—particularly cervical adenitis, otitis media, and pneumonia—occurs in about 15% of patients.

D. Tuberculosis: Measles produces temporary anergy to the tuberculin skin test. There may be exacerbations in tuberculosis patients.

Prevention

In the United States, it is recommended that children receive their first vaccine dose at 12–15 months and a second at age 4–6 years prior to entry into school (see Table 30–4). Students beyond high school and medical staff starting employment must have the above vaccination schedule documented or must have serologic evidence of immunity if they were born after 1956. For individuals born before 1957, herd immunity can be assumed. Health care workers should be screened and vaccinated if necessary regardless of date of birth.

Outbreak control is similar. If outbreaks are occurring in preschool children under 1 year of age, initial vaccination may be given at 6 months, with repeat at 15 months. When outbreaks take place in day care centers, K–12 institutions, or colleges and universities, revaccination is probably indicated for all, in particular for students and their siblings born after 1956 who do not have documentation of immunity as defined above. Susceptible personnel who have been exposed should be isolated from patient contact from the fifth to the 21st day after exposure irrespective of whether they have been vaccinated or have received immune globulin. If they develop measles, they should be isolated from patient contact until 7 days after the rash develops.

When susceptible individuals are exposed to measles, the live virus vaccine can prevent disease if given within 5 days of exposure. This is rarely feasible in a household. Later, gamma globulin (0.25 mL/kg [0.11 mL/lb] body weight) can be injected for prevention of clinical illness. This must be followed by active immunization with live measles vaccine 3 months later. Vaccination of all immunocompetent persons born after 1956 who travel to the developing world is essential.

Pregnant women and the immunosuppressed in general should *not* receive this or other live virus vaccines. There are two exceptions: asymptomatic HIV-infected patients, who have typically not shown adverse effects from measles vaccination; and HIV-infected children, in whom exposure to vaccines improves survival after measles. In the developing world, the use of "high-titer" vaccine is associated with a higher delayed mortality rate in several series. Immune globulin should be considered for postexposure prophylaxis in any HIV-infected person exposed to measles.

Treatment

A. General Measures: The patient should be isolated for the week following onset of rash and keep at bed rest until afebrile. Treatment is symptomatic as needed. Vitamin A, 400,000 units/d orally (the beneficial effects of which include maintenance of gastrointestinal and respiratory epithelial mucosa and probably immune enhancement), has been shown to reduce pediatric morbidity and mortality rates in hospitalized measles patients.

B. Treatment of Complications: Secondary bacterial infections are treated with appropriate antimicrobial drugs. Postmeasles encephalitis, including SSPE, can only be treated symptomatically.

Prognosis

The mortality rate of measles in infants was 0.6% in a recent outbreak in California; the mortality rate may be as high as 10% in developing nations. Deaths in the USA are due principally to encephalitis (15% mortality rate) and secondary bacterial pneumonia. Deaths in the developing world are mainly related to diarrhea and protein-losing enteropathy.

Anders JF et al: Secondary failure rates of measles vaccines: A metaanalysis of published studies. Pediatr Infect Dis J 1996;15:62. (Secondary failure rates appear to be < 0.2%.)

General recommendations on immunization. Recommendations of the Advisory Committee on Immunization Practices (ACIP). MMWR Morb Mortal Wkly Rep 1994; 43(RR-1):1.

Hutchins S et al: Measles outbreaks in the United States, 1987 through 1990. Pediatr Infect Dis J 1996;15:31.

James JM et al: Safe administration of the measles vaccine to children allergic to eggs. N Engl J Med 1995;332: 1262. (No anaphylaxis was observed after vaccine administration in children with proved egg allergy.)

Measles control—resetting the agenda: A report of the Children's Vaccine Initiative Ad Hoc Committee on an Investment Strategy for Measles Control. J Infect Dis 1994; 170(Suppl 1):1. (Excellent discussions on pathogenesis, cytokines, hyperimmune globulins, and new vaccines.)

Recommended childhood immunization schedule—United States, 1997. MMWR Morb Mortal Wkly Rep 1997; 46:35. (Published also in JAMA 1997;277:371.)

Trotter AC et al: MMR vaccine administration in egg-sensitive children: Systemic reactions during vaccine desensitization. Ann Allergy 1994;72:25. (An accompanying editorial reminds readers that reactions to MMR can occur in vaccinees not allergic to eggs; no skin test predicts such reactions.)

Watson BM et al: Safety and immunogenicity of a combined live attenuated measles, mumps, rubella, and varicella vaccine (MMR[II]V) in healthy children. J Infect Dis 1996;173:731.

2. MUMPS

Essentials of Diagnosis

- Exposure 14–21 days before onset.
- Painful, swollen salivary glands, usually parotid.

- Frequent involvement of other tissues, including testes, pancreas, and meninges, in unvaccinated individuals.

General Considerations

Mumps is a viral (paramyxovirus) disease spread by respiratory droplets that usually produces inflammation of the salivary glands and, less commonly, orchitis, aseptic meningitis, pancreatitis, and oophoritis. Most patients are children. The incubation period is 14–21 days (average, 18 days). Infectivity precedes the symptoms by about 1 day and is maximal for 3 days but may last a week.

Clinical Findings

A. Symptoms and Signs: Parotid tenderness and overlying facial edema are the most common physical findings. Occasionally, swelling in one gland subsides completely before the other parotid or salivary glands become involved. Swelling and tenderness of the submaxillary and sublingual glands are variable. The orifice of Stensen's duct may be red and swollen.

Fever and malaise are variable and are often minimal in young children. High fever usually accompanies meningitis or orchitis. Neck stiffness, headache, and lethargy suggest meningitis. Testicular swelling and tenderness (unilateral in 75%) denote orchitis. Orchitis occurs in about 25% of postpubertal men. Upper abdominal pain, nausea, and vomiting suggests pancreatitis. Mumps is the leading cause of pancreatitis in children. Lower abdominal pain and ovarian enlargement suggest oophoritis and occur in 25% of postpubertal women, but the diagnosis may be difficult. Pain and swelling of one or both (75%) of the parotid or other salivary glands occur, usually in succession 1–3 days apart. Occasionally, one gland subsides completely (usually in 7 days or less) before others become involved.

B. Laboratory Findings: Relative lymphocytosis may be present. Serum amylase is commonly elevated with or without pancreatitis. Lymphocytic pleocytosis (and normal to low glucose) of the cerebrospinal fluid is present in meningitis, which may be asymptomatic. The diagnosis is confirmed by isolating mumps virus from saliva or cerebrospinal fluid or demonstrating a fourfold rise in complement-fixing antibodies in paired sera.

Differential Diagnosis

Swelling of the parotid gland may be due to calculi in the parotid ducts or to a reaction to iodides. Other causes include starch ingestion, sarcoidosis, cirrhosis, diabetes, bulimia, and Sjögren's syndrome. Parotitis may also be produced by pyogenic organisms (eg, *Staphylococcus aureus*), particularly in debilitated individuals, drug reaction (phenothiazines, propylthiouracil), and other viruses (influenza A, parainfluenza, EBV infection, coxsackieviruses).

Swelling of the parotid gland must be differentiated from inflammation of the lymph nodes located more posteriorly and inferiorly than the parotid gland.

Complications

The "complications" of mumps are other manifestations of the disease less common than inflammation of the salivary glands. These usually follow the parotitis but may precede it or occur without salivary gland involvement: meningitis (30%), orchitis (occurs mainly after puberty in 25% of infected men, and on rare occasion leads to priapism or testicular infarction), pancreatitis, oophoritis, thyroiditis, neuritis, myocarditis, thrombocytopenia, migratory arthralgias, and nephritis.

Aseptic meningitis is common during the course of mumps and may occur without salivary gland involvement. This is a very benign self-limited illness. Rare neurologic complications include encephalitis, Guillain-Barré syndrome, and transverse myelitis. Encephalitis is associated with cerebral edema, serious neurologic manifestations, and sometimes death. Deafness develops rarely from eighth nerve neuritis.

Prevention

Mumps live virus vaccine is safe and highly effective. It is recommended for routine immunization for children over age 1 year, either alone or in combination with other virus vaccines (eg, with measles and rubella—in MMR vaccine). It should not be given to pregnant women or to immunocompromised individuals, though the vaccine has been given to asymptomatic HIV-infected individuals without adverse sequelae. Its use has markedly decreased the incidence of mumps in the USA; an outbreak in Tennessee was attributable to primary vaccine failure, perhaps associated with waning immunity. The mumps skin test is less reliable in determining immunity than are serum neutralization titers.

Treatment

A. General Measures: The patient should be isolated until swelling subsides and kept at bed rest during the febrile period. Treatment is symptomatic as needed.

B. Management of Complications:

1. Meningitis–The treatment of aseptic meningitis is purely symptomatic. The management of encephalitis requires attention to cerebral edema, the airway, and vital functions.

2. Orchitis–The scrotum should be suspended in a suspensory or toweling "bridge" and ice bags applied. Incision of the tunica may be necessary in severe cases. Codeine or meperidine may be given as necessary for pain. Pain can also be relieved by injection of the spermatic cord at the external inguinal ring with 10–20 mL of 1% procaine solution. Hydrocortisone sodium succinate (100 mg intravenously, followed by 20 mg orally every 6 hours for 2 or

3 days) to reduce the inflammatory reaction is of questionable benefit.

3. Pancreatitis–Symptomatic treatment should be provided and parenteral fluids if necessary.

4. Oophoritis–Symptomatic treatment should be given as needed.

Prognosis

The entire course of mumps rarely exceeds 2 weeks. Fatalities (from encephalitis) are rare.

Orchitis often makes the patient very uncomfortable but rarely results in sterility. Mumps is not known to be associated with stillbirths or teratogenicity.

Briss PA et al: Sustained transmission of mumps in a highly vaccinated population: Assessment of primary vaccine failure and waning vaccine-induced immunity. J Infect Dis 1994;169:77.

Gershon AA: Present and future challenges of immunizations on the health of our patients. Pediatr Infect Dis J 1995;14:445.

Recommended childhood immunization schedule—United States, 1997. MMWR Morb Mortal Wkly Rep 1997;46:35. (Published also in JAMA 1997;277:371.)

Watson BM et al: Safety and immunogenicity of a combined live attenuated measles, mumps, rubella, and varicella vaccine (MMR[II]V) in healthy children. J Infect Dis 1996;173:731.

3. POLIOMYELITIS

Essentials of Diagnosis

- Muscle weakness, headache, stiff neck, fever, nausea and vomiting, sore throat.
- Lower motor neuron lesion (flaccid paralysis) with decreased deep tendon reflexes and muscle wasting.
- Cerebrospinal fluid shows excess leukocytes. Lymphocytes predominate; rarely more than 500/μL.

General Considerations

Poliomyelitis virus, an enterovirus, is present in throat washings and stools. Infection is most commonly acquired by the fecal-oral route. Since the introduction of effective vaccine, poliomyelitis has become a rare disease in developed areas of the world. Among 133 cases reported in the United States between 1980 and 1994, six were imported and 125 (94%) were vaccine-associated (two were indeterminate). Wild poliovirus disease has been eradicated from the Western hemisphere. Three antigenically distinct types of poliomyelitis virus (I, II, and III) are recognized, with no cross-immunity between them. The incubation period is 5–35 days (usually 7–14 days). Infectivity is maximal during the first week, but virus is excreted in stools for several weeks.

Clinical Findings

A. Symptoms and Signs: At least 95% of infections are asymptomatic, but in those who become ill the following manifestations are seen.

1. Minor illness (abortive poliomyelitis)–The symptoms are fever, headache, vomiting, diarrhea, constipation, and sore throat.

2. Nonparalytic poliomyelitis–In addition to the above symptoms, signs of meningeal irritation and muscle spasm occur.

3. Paralytic poliomyelitis–Paralytic poliomyelitis represents 0.1% of all poliomyelitis cases. Paralysis may occur at any time during the febrile period. Tremors, muscle weakness, constipation, and ileus may appear. Paralytic poliomyelitis may be divided into two forms, which may coexist: **(1) spinal poliomyelitis,** with weakness of the muscles supplied by the spinal nerves; and **(2) bulbar poliomyelitis,** with weakness of the muscles supplied by the cranial nerves (especially nerves IX and X), involvement of the respiratory and vasomotor centers, and variable "encephalitis" symptoms.

In spinal poliomyelitis, paralysis of the shoulder girdle often precedes intercostal and diaphragmatic paralysis, which leads to diminished chest expansion and decreased vital capacity.

In bulbar poliomyelitis, symptoms include diplopia (uncommonly), facial weakness, dysphagia, dysphonia, nasal voice, weakness of the sternocleidomastoid and trapezius muscles, difficulty in chewing, inability to swallow or expel saliva, and regurgitation of fluids through the nose. The most life-threatening aspect of bulbar poliomyelitis is respiratory paralysis. Lethargy or coma may be due to hypoxia, most often from hypoventilation. Hypertension, hypotension, and tachycardia may occur. Convulsions are rare.

B. Laboratory Findings: The peripheral white blood cell count may be normal or mildly elevated. Cerebrospinal fluid pressure and protein are normal or slightly increased; glucose is not decreased; cells usually number fewer than $500/\mu L$ (predominantly lymphocytes; polymorphonuclear cells may be elevated at first). Cerebrospinal fluid is normal in 5% of patients. The virus may be recovered from throat washings (early) and stools (early and late). Neutralizing and complement-fixing antibodies appear during the first or second week of illness.

Differential Diagnosis

Nonparalytic poliomyelitis is similar to other forms of enteroviral meningitis; the distinction is made serologically. Acute infectious polyneuritis (Guillain-Barré) and tick paralysis may initially resemble poliomyelitis. In Guillain-Barré syndrome (see Chapter 24), the weakness is more symmetric and ascending in most cases, but the Fischer variant is quite similar to bulbar polio. Cerebrospinal fluid usually has a high protein content but normal cell count.

Complications

Urinary tract infection, atelectasis, pneumonia, myocarditis, and pulmonary edema may occur. Respiratory failure may be a result of paralysis of respiratory muscles, airway obstruction from involvement of cranial nerve nuclei, or lesions of the respiratory center.

Prevention

Recommendations for prevention of poliomyelitis have been modified as a result of changing epidemiology, eradication of polio in the Western Hemisphere, and continued concern about vaccine-associated disease with the oral live vaccine. Current recommendations are to provide the inactive (Salk) vaccination for the first two doses (in infancy, at 2 and 4 months) followed by the oral (Sabin) vaccination for the third dose (at 6 months) if there are no immunologically incompetent individuals in the household or among close contacts. The third dose is not needed in the developing world.

The oral live trivalent virus vaccine (Sabin) is easily administered, safe, and very effective in providing local gastrointestinal immunity as well as circulating antibody. Routine immunization of adults in the USA is not recommended because of the low incidence of the disease. However, adults who are exposed to poliomyelitis or plan to travel to endemic areas and who have not received polio immunization within the past decade should be given inactivated poliomyelitis vaccine (Salk). This vaccine should also be given when immunization of immunodeficient or immunosuppressed individuals and members of their households is required.

In the developing world, the interval between OPV doses should probably be longer than 1 month (because of interference from enteric pathogens). Intramuscular injections should be routinely avoided during the month following oral poliomyelitis vaccination to prevent provocation paralysis.

Treatment

Strict bed rest in the first few days of illness reduces the rate of paralysis. Cranial nerve involvement must be detected promptly. Comfortable but rotating positions should be maintained in a "polio bed" (firm mattress, footboard, sponge rubber pads or rolls, sandbags, and light splints). Fecal impaction and urinary retention (especially with paraplegia) are managed appropriately. In cases of respiratory weakness or paralysis, intensive care is needed.

Prognosis

During the febrile period, paralysis may develop or progress. Mild weakness of small muscles is more likely to regress than severe weakness of large muscles. Bulbar poliomyelitis carries a mortality rate of up to 50%. New muscle weakness may develop and progress slowly years after recovery from acute paralytic poliomyelitis. This entity, postpoliomyelitis syndrome, presents with signs of chronic and new denervation, is not infectious in origin, and is associated with increasing dysfunction of surviving motor neurons.

Miller MA et al: Cost-effectiveness of incorporating inactivated poliovirus vaccine into the routine childhood immunization schedule. JAMA 1996;276:967. (Cost analyses suggest that prevention of vaccine-associated polio, by changing to inactive poliovirus vaccination, will cost over $3 million per case prevented.)

Strebel PM et al: Epidemiology of poliomyelitis in the United States after the last reported case of indigenous wild virus-associated disease. J Infect Dis 1992;14:568.

Strebel PM et al: Intramuscular infections within 30 days of immunization with oral poliovirus vaccine: A risk factor for vaccine-associated paralytic poliomyelitis. N Engl J Med 1995;332:500.

4. RUBELLA

Essentials of Diagnosis

- Exposure 14–21 days before onset.
- Arthralgia, particularly in young women.
- No prodrome in children (mild in adults); mild symptoms (fever, malaise, coryza) coinciding with eruption.
- Posterior cervical and postauricular lymphadenopathy 5–10 days before rash.
- Fine maculopapular rash of 3 days' duration; face to trunk to extremities.
- Leukopenia, thrombocytopenia.

General Considerations

Rubella is a systemic disease caused by a togavirus transmitted by inhalation of infective droplets. It is only moderately communicable. One attack usually confers permanent immunity. The incubation period is 14–21 days (average, 16 days). The disease is transmissible from 1 week before the rash appears until 15 days afterward.

The clinical picture of rubella is difficult to distinguish from other viral illnesses such as infectious mononucleosis, echovirus infections, and coxsackievirus infections. Definitive diagnosis can be made only by isolating the virus or serologically.

The principal importance of rubella lies in its devastating effects on the fetus in utero, producing teratogenic effects and a continuing congenital infection. A cluster of cases of congenital rubella syndrome was reported from Southern California in 1990–1991.

Clinical Findings

A. Symptoms and Signs: (Table 32–2.) Fever and malaise, usually mild, accompanied by tender suboccipital adenitis, may precede the eruption by 1 week. Mild coryza may be present. Polyarthritis oc-

curs in about 25% of adult cases. These symptoms usually subside within 7 days but may persist for weeks.

Posterior cervical and postauricular lymphadenopathy is very common. Erythema of the palate and throat, sometimes patchy, may be noted. A fine, pink maculopapular rash appears on the face, trunk, and extremities in rapid progression (2–3 days) and fades quickly, usually lasting 1 day in each area. Rubella without rash may be at least as common as the exanthematous disease. Diagnosis can be suspected when there is epidemiologic evidence of the disease in the community but requires laboratory confirmation.

B. Laboratory Findings: Leukopenia may be present early and may be followed by an increase in plasma cells. Virus isolation and serologic tests of immunity (rubella virus hemagglutination inhibition and fluorescent antibody tests) are available. Definitive diagnosis is based on a fourfold rise in the antibody titer.

Complications

A. Exposure During Pregnancy: It is important to know whether rubella antibodies are present at the beginning of pregnancy, since fetal infection during the first trimester may lead to congenital rubella in at least 80% of fetuses.

When a pregnant woman is exposed to a possible case of rubella, an immediate hemagglutination-inhibiting rubella antibody level should be obtained; there is no reason for concern in positive tests. If no antibodies are found, clinical and serologic follow-up is essential. Confirmation of rubella in the expectant mother raises the question of therapeutic abortion, an alternative to be considered in the light of personal, religious, legal, and other factors. The risk to the fetus is highest for maternal infection in the first trimester but continues into the second trimester.

B. Congenital Rubella: An infant acquiring the infection in utero may be normal at birth but more likely will have a wide variety of manifestations, including early-onset cataracts, glaucoma and microphthalmia, hearing deficits, psychomotor retardation, congenital heart defects, organomegaly, and maculopapular rash. Viral excretion in the throat and urine persists for many months despite high antibody levels. The diagnosis is confirmed by isolation of the virus. A specific test for IgM rubella antibody is useful for diagnosis in the newborn. Treatment is directed to the many anomalies.

C. Postinfectious Encephalopathy: In 1:6000 cases, postinfectious encephalopathy develops 1–6 days after the rash; the virus is not always isolable. The mortality rate is 20%, but residual deficits are rare among the recovered. The mechanism is unknown.

Prevention

Live attenuated rubella virus vaccine should be

given to all infants and to susceptible girls before the menarche. When women are immunized, they must not be pregnant, and the absence of antibodies should be established. (In the USA, about 80% of 20-year-old women are immune to rubella.) Birth control should be practiced for at least 3 months after vaccine administration, though there are no reports of congenital rubella syndrome after rubella immunization and inadvertent immunization of a pregnant woman is not considered an indication for therapeutic abortion. Arthritis, often more prominent than in native rubella, may follow vaccination, is more common in women, and may relate to hormonal and genetic influences of the immune response to rubella proteins. It is often more severe than that which occurs with disease. MMR may be given in conjunction with DPT boosters; adequate serologic response has been shown.

Treatment

Acetaminophen provides symptomatic relief. Encephalitis and non-life-threatening thrombocytopenia should be treated symptomatically.

Prognosis

Rubella (other than the congenital form) is a mild illness and rarely lasts more than 3–4 days. Congenital rubella, on the other hand, has a high mortality rate, and the associated congenital defects are largely permanent. The association between chronic arthritis and rubella vaccination is currently under study.

Mellinger AK et al: High incidence of congenital rubella syndrome after a rubella outbreak. Pediatr Infect Dis J 1995;14:573. (A high rate [2.1%] was noted among infants born to unimmunized Amish women infected during a recent outbreak.)

Peltola H et al: The elimination of indigenous measles, mumps, and rubella from Finland by a 12-year, two-dose vaccination program. New Engl J Med 1994; 331:1397. (The two doses were given at 14–18 months of age and again at 6 years of age.)

Rubella and congenital rubella syndrome: United States, January 1, 1991–May 7, 1994. MMWR Morb Mortal Wkly Rep 1994;3:397.

Vetter RT, Johnson GM: Vaccination update: Diphtheria, tetanus, pertussis, mumps, rubella, measles. Postgrad Med 1995;98:133.

OTHER NEUROTROPIC VIRUSES

1. RABIES

Essentials of Diagnosis

- History of animal bite.
- Paresthesia, hydrophobia, rage alternating with calm.
- Convulsions, paralysis, thick tenacious saliva.

General Considerations

Rabies is a viral (rhabdovirus) encephalitis transmitted by infected saliva that gains entry into the body by an animal bite or an open wound. Bats, skunks, foxes, and raccoons are widely infected. Biting species that cause rabies in the United States tend to be geographically determined: raccoons in the East and New England; skunks in the Midwest, Southwest, and California; coyotes in Texas; and foxes in the Southwest, New England, and Alaska. Dogs and cats are infected in developing countries (including the Mexican border), and 10 of 20 Americans with rabies acquired the disease abroad during the 1980s. Rodents and lagomorphs (eg, rabbits) are unlikely to have rabies. The virus gains entry into the salivary glands of dogs 5–7 days before their death from rabies, thus limiting their period of infectivity. The incubation period may range from 10 days to many years but is usually 3–7 weeks. The interval is dependent in part on distance of the wound from the central nervous system. The virus travels in the nerves to the brain, multiplies there, and then migrates along the efferent nerves to the salivary glands.

Rabies is almost uniformly fatal, with surviving cases likely due to rabies-related viruses. The most common clinical problem confronting the physician is the management of a patient bitten by an animal (see Prevention).

Clinical Findings

A. Symptoms and Signs: There is usually a history of animal bite. Patients with scratches from rabid animals are about 50 times less likely than those with bites to develop rabies. Pain appears at the site of the bite, followed by paresthesias. The skin is quite sensitive to changes of temperature, especially air currents. Attempts at drinking cause extremely painful laryngeal spasm (hydrophobia). Restlessness, muscle spasm, extreme excitability and bizarre behavior, convulsions, and paralysis occur. Large amounts of thick tenacious saliva are present.

B. Laboratory Findings: Biting animals who are apparently well should be kept under observation for 7–10 days. Sick or dead animals should be examined for rabies. A wild animal, if captured, should be sacrificed and the head shipped on ice to the nearest laboratory qualified to examine the brain for evidence of rabies virus; the diagnosis is made by the fluorescent antibody technique. When the animal cannot be examined, skunks, bats, coyotes, foxes, and raccoons should be presumed to be rabid.

Fluorescent antibody testing of skin biopsy material from the posterior neck or a corneal impression may be positive early in the disease. The test may become negative after antibodies develop.

Prevention

Since rabies is almost always fatal, prevention is the only reasonable approach, and all exposures must be evaluated individually. Immunization of household dogs and cats and active immunization of persons with significant animal exposure (eg, veterinarians) are important. However, the most important common decisions concern animal bites.

A. Local Treatment of Animal Bites and Scratches: Thorough cleansing, debridement, and repeated flushing of wounds with soap and water are important. If rabies immune globulin or antiserum is to be used, a portion should be infiltrated locally around the wound (see below) and the remainder given intramuscularly. Wounds caused by animal bites should not be sutured.

B. Postexposure Immunization: Therapy is indicated when the disease is seriously under consideration. Medical decisions should be based on recommendations of the USPHS Advisory Committee but also be on circumstances of the bite, including the extent and location of the wound, the biting animal, and the local endemicity of rabies. Consultation is available from state and local health departments. Postexposure treatment includes both passive antibody and vaccination.

The optimal form of passive immunization is rabies immune globulin (40 units/kg). Up to 50% of the globulin is infiltrated around the wound; the rest is administered intramuscularly. If immune globulin (human) is not available, equine rabies antiserum (20 units/kg) can be used after appropriate tests for horse serum sensitivity. An inactivated human diploid cell rabies vaccine (HDCV) is given as five injections of 1 mL intramuscularly (in the deltoid rather than the gluteal muscle) on days 0, 3, 7, 14, and 28 after exposure.

Rabies immune globulin and rabies vaccine (human diploid cell vaccine) should never be given in the same syringe or at the same site. Allergic reactions to the vaccine are rare, though local reactions (pruritus, erythema, tenderness) occur in about 25% and mild systemic reactions (headaches, myalgias, nausea) in about 20% of recipients. The vaccine is commercially available or can be obtained through health departments. For patients who previously received pre- or postexposure vaccine, rabies immune globulin should not be given; vaccine, 1 mL in the deltoid, should be given twice (on days 0 and 3).

In other countries, inactivated duck embryo vaccine or mouse brain vaccine may be available, but the method of administration is more complex, the rate of allergic reactions—including particularly ascending paralysis—is higher, and the efficacy is less.

Preexposure prophylaxis with three injections of diploid cell vaccine is recommended for persons at high risk of exposure (veterinarians, animal handlers, etc). Simultaneous chloroquine prophylaxis for malaria may diminish the antibody response.

Treatment

This very severe illness with an almost universally fatal outcome requires skillful intensive care with attention to the airway, maintenance of oxygenation, and control of seizures. Universal blood and body fluid precautions are essential.

Prognosis

Once the symptoms have appeared, death almost inevitably occurs after 7 days, usually from respiratory failure.

Cantor SB et al: A decision-analytic approach to post-exposure rabies prophylaxis. Am J Public Health 1994;84:1144. (Treatment was optimized when the probability of the biting animal being rabid was at least 1:2000.)

Compendium of animal rabies control, 1996. National Association of State Public Health Veterinarians, Inc. MMWR Morb Mortal Wkly Rep 1996;45(RR-3):1.

Fishbein DB, Robinson LE: Rabies. N Engl J Med 1993;329:1632. (A map outlines the species predominant in the USA.)

2. ARBOVIRUS ENCEPHALITIDES

Essentials of Diagnosis

- Fever, malaise, stiff neck, sore throat, and nausea and vomiting, progressing to stupor, coma, and convulsions.
- Signs of an upper motor neuron lesion (exaggerated deep tendon reflexes, absent superficial reflexes, pathologic reflexes, spastic paralysis).
- Cerebrospinal fluid protein and pressure often increased, with lymphocytic pleocytosis.

General Considerations

The arboviruses are mosquito- and tick-borne agents that produce clinical manifestations in humans. They include three alphaviruses (causing Western, Eastern, and Venezuelan equine encephalitis), four flaviviruses (causing St. Louis and Japanese B encephalitis, dengue, and yellow fever), and bunyaviruses (causing California [the LaCrosse agent] encephalitis and a series of viral hemorrhagic fevers [Rift Valley fever; hemorrhagic fever with renal syndrome from the Hantaan agent]). Only those agents causing primarily encephalitis will be discussed here (Table 32–3).

The leading causes of arbovirus encephalitis are St. Louis and California encephalitis. Agent-specific reservoirs (typically small mammals or birds) are responsible for maintaining the encephalitis-producing viruses in nature; horses serve as sentinels for infection with the equine agents, though birds maintain the life cycle. Eleven North Americans died of Japanese B encephalitis between 1981 and 1992—most of them military personnel stationed in Asia.

Clinical Findings

A. Symptoms and Signs: The symptoms are fever, malaise, sore throat, nausea and vomiting, lethargy, stupor, coma, and convulsions. Signs in-

Table 32–3. Arbovirus (arthropod-borne) encephalitis.[1]

Disease	Geographic Distribution	Vector; Reservoir	Comment
California encephalitis	Throughout USA, especially Midwest	Mosquitoes; small mammals	Mainly in children
Eastern (equine) encephalitis	Eastern part of North, Central, and South America (coastal areas)	Mosquitoes; birds	Often occurs in horses in the area. High mortality rate (50–75%); frequent sequelae (seizures, paresis), especially in children.
St. Louis encephalitis	Western and central USA, Florida	Mosquitoes; birds (including domestic fowl)	Frequent cranial nerve findings; prolonged convalescence.
Venezuelan encephalitis	South America; Florida (rarely), Texas (rarely)	Mosquitoes; rodents	Rare in USA; low mortality rate; rare sequelae.
Western (equine) encephalitis	Throughout Western Hemisphere	Mosquitoes; birds	Often occurs in horses in the area; particularly affects infants and older adults.
Japanese B encephalitis	Temperate East Asia, southern and southeastern Asia	Mosquitoes; pigs and birds	Vaccine available. High mortality rate (25%) and morbidity rate (50% with neuropsychiatric sequelae).

[1]Seasonal incidence varies with the mosquito season in different areas. It is mainly summer and fall (May through October) in the Northern Hemisphere.

clude stiff neck, signs of meningeal irritation, tremors, convulsions, cranial nerve palsies, paralysis of extremities, exaggerated deep tendon reflexes, absent superficial reflexes, and pathologic reflexes.

B. Laboratory Findings: The white blood cell count is variable. Cerebrospinal fluid pressure and protein content are often increased; glucose is normal; lymphocytic pleocytosis may be present (polymorphonuclears may predominate early). The virus may sometimes be isolated from blood or, rarely, from cerebrospinal fluid. Serologic tests of blood or cerebrospinal fluid may be diagnostic in specific types of encephalitis (by demonstrating virus-specific IgM or a fourfold change in complement-fixing or neutralizing antibodies). CT or MRI of the brain may be useful in excluding the temporal lobe lesions indicative of herpesvirus or mass lesions.

Differential Diagnosis

Mild forms of encephalitis must be differentiated from aseptic meningitis, lymphocytic choriomeningitis, and nonparalytic poliomyelitis; severe forms from cerebrovascular accidents, brain tumors, brain abscess, and intoxications.

Arbovirus encephalitides (Table 32–3) must be differentiated from other causes of viral encephalitis (herpes simplex virus, mumps virus, poliovirus or other enteroviruses, HIV), encephalitis accompanying exanthematous diseases of childhood (measles, varicella, infectious mononucleosis, rubella), encephalitis following vaccination (a demyelinating type following rabies, measles, and pertussis vaccination), toxic encephalitis (from drugs, poisons, or bacterial toxins such as *Shigella dysenteriae* type 1), and Reye's syndrome.

Complications

Bronchial pneumonia, urinary retention and infection, and decubitus ulcers may occur. Late sequelae are mental deterioration, parkinsonism, and epilepsy.

Prevention

Effective measures include mosquito control (repellents, protective clothing, insecticides). A vaccine against Japanese B encephalitis has been licensed for use in the United States. A dose of 1 mL is given subcutaneously on days 0, 3, and 20, with a booster 2 years later; it is recommended for summer travelers to rural areas of East Asia.

Treatment

Although specific antiviral therapy is not available for most causative entities, vigorous supportive measures can be helpful. Such measures include reduction of intracranial pressure (mannitol), monitoring of intraventricular pressure, the control of convulsions, maintenance of the airway, administration of oxygen, and attention to adequate nutrition during periods of prolonged coma. The efficacy of corticosteroids in these infections is not established.

Prevention or early treatment of decubitus ulcers, pneumonia, and urinary tract infections is important. Anticonvulsants should be given as needed.

Prognosis

The prognosis is always guarded, especially in younger children. Sequelae may become apparent late in the course of what appears to be a successful recovery.

Calisher CH: Medically important arboviruses of the United States and Canada. Clin Microbiol Rev 1994; 7:89.

Dobler G: Arboviruses causing neurological disorders in the central nervous system. Arch Virol Suppl 1996; 11:33.

Patz JA et al: Global climate change and emerging infectious diseases. JAMA 1996;276:372. (Dengue and other viral encephalitides are expected to increase in prevalence if global climate change theories are correct.)

3. LYMPHOCYTIC CHORIOMENINGITIS

Essentials of Diagnosis

- "Influenza-like" prodrome of fever, chills, malaise, and cough, followed by meningitis with associated stiff neck.
- Aseptic meningitis with positive Kernig sign, headache, nausea, vomiting, and lethargy.
- Cerebrospinal fluid: slight increase of protein, lymphocytic pleocytosis (500–3000/µL); low glucose (≥ 25%).
- Complement-fixing antibodies within 2 weeks.

General Considerations

Lymphocytic choriomeningitis is a viral (arenavirus) infection of the central nervous system. The reservoir of infection is the infected house mouse, although naturally infected guinea pigs, monkeys, dogs, and swine have been observed. Pet hamsters may be a source of infection. The virus is shed by the infected animal via oronasal secretions, urine, and feces, with transmission to humans probably through contaminated food and dust. The incubation period is 8–13 days to the appearance of systemic manifestations and 15–21 days to the appearance of meningeal symptoms. CD4 cells may be involved in pathogenesis. The virus is not spread person-to-person. Outbreaks have occurred among laboratory workers from rodent exposure. Complications are rare.

This disease is principally confined to the eastern seaboard and northeastern states of the USA.

Clinical Findings

A. Symptoms and Signs: Symptoms are biphasic. The prodromal illness is characterized by fever, chills, headache, myalgia, cough, and vomiting, the meningeal phase by headache, nausea and vomiting, and lethargy. Signs of pneumonia are occasionally present during the prodromal phase. During the meningeal phase there may be neck and back stiffness with a positive Kernig sign. Obstructive hydrocephalus is a rare complication. Arthralgias can develop late.

The prodrome may terminate in complete recovery, or meningeal symptoms may appear after a few days of remission.

B. Laboratory Findings: Leukocytosis or leukopenia and thrombocytopenia may be present. Cerebrospinal fluid lymphocytic pleocytosis (total count is often 500–3000/µL) may occur, with slight increase in protein and normal to low glucose in at least 25%. Complement-fixing antibodies appear during or after the second week. The virus may be recovered from the blood and cerebrospinal fluid by mouse inoculation.

Differential Diagnosis

The influenza-like prodrome and latent period help distinguish this from other aseptic meningitides, and bacterial and granulomatous meningitis. A history of exposure to mice or other potential vector is an important diagnostic clue.

Treatment

Treatment is supportive as for encephalitis or aseptic meningitis.

Prognosis

Fatalities are rare. The illness usually lasts 1–2 weeks, although convalescence may be prolonged.

Jahrling PB, Peters CJ: Lymphocytic choriomeningitis virus: A neglected pathogen of man. Arch Pathol Lab Med 1992;116:486. (Editorial review.)

4. VIRUS-LIKE AGENTS WITH LONG LATENCY (Including Prion Disease)

Several animal diseases (visna, scrapie) are caused by communicable agents with slow replication and long latent intervals in the host. Such agents have been called *pro*teinaceous *in*fectious particles resistant to most procedures that modify nucleic acid and are increasingly being referred to as "prions." Four such agents or related agents that cause human disease are discussed here.

Kuru and **Creutzfeldt-Jakob disease** are called spongiform encephalopathies, referring to the appearance of central nervous system tissue on pathologic examination. The agents are transmissible in brain or eye tissue to primates, including humans. On reactivation from the latent state after months to years, diseases ensue that are characterized by an inexorably progressive downhill course. Kuru—once prevalent in central New Guinea but no longer seen since the abandonment of cannibalism—was characterized by cerebellar ataxia, tremors, dysarthria, and emotional lability.

Creutzfeldt-Jakob disease presents usually in late middle age with rapidly progressive dementia, myoclonic fasciculations, ataxia, and somnolence and has an electroencephalographic pattern characterized by paroxysms with high voltages and slow waves. There is a rapid decline to akinetic mutism. There are no definitive risk factors for Creutzfeldt-Jakob disease, though in 15% of cases there is a family history of the disorder. MRI typically shows bilateral areas of increased signal intensity, predominantly in the caudate and putamen. There is no specific treatment, and the only known means of prevention is avoidance of contamination by affected brain tissue, electrodes, or neurosurgical tools or by transplants of cornea, dura, or cadaveric growth hormone from infected donors. Disinfection of equipment requires autoclaving at 15 psi for 1 hour, and disinfection of contaminated surfaces requires 5% hypochlorite or 0.1 N sodium hydroxide solution.

A variant of Creutzfeldt-Jakob disease has been reported recently in a small outbreak from Britain. The patients were younger adults, the duration of disease was longer, the clinical symptomatology was less severe, and the electroencephalographic findings were not typical of classic Creutzfeldt-Jakob disease. The disease is believed to result from ingestion of beefsteak from livestock infected with "mad cow disease." Statistical analysis appears to support a causative relationship.

Subacute sclerosing panencephalitis is also a slowly progressive disorder, but pathologic examination shows demyelination rather than spongiform lesions. The disease clinically presents in children (mean age at onset is 7 years) with seizures and dementia and is uniformly fatal. It has been associated with a defective measles virus or possibly vaccination. Measles antibodies are elevated in the cerebrospinal fluid. Inexplicably, the disease is more common among rural boys.

Progressive multifocal leukoencephalopathy is another progressive demyelinating central nervous system disorder with a propensity for immunosuppressed adults, including AIDS patients. The cause is probably JC virus (JCV), a papovavirus whose main central nervous system target is myelinating oligodendrocytes. JCV has also been cultured and identified by PCR—though not necessarily associated with disease—in central nervous system tissue from HIV-infected and other individuals.

Hsich G et al: The 14-3-3 brain protein in cerebrospinal fluid as a marker for transmissible spongiform encephalopathy. N Engl J Med 1996;335:924.

Johnson RT: Prion disease. N Engl J Med 1992;326:486.

Major EO, Ault GS: Progressive multifocal leukoencephalopathy: Clinical and laboratory observations in a viral induced demyelinating disease in the immunodeficient patient. Curr Opin Neurol 1995;8:184.

Will RG et al: A new variant of Creutzfeldt-Jakob disease in the UK. Lancet 1996;347:921.

5. HUMAN T CELL LYMPHOTROPIC VIRUS (HTLV)

Retroviruses include both the lympholytic HIV agents and the lymphotropic oncoviruses, human T cell leukemia viruses types 1 and 2 (HTLV-1 and -2). The isolation of HTLV-1 from a young male with T cell lymphoma established an association of the virus with adult T cell lymphoma/leukemia (ATL) that has been confirmed from highly endemic areas (the Caribbean, southern Japan) and from other areas, including sub-Saharan Africa and the southeastern United States. Common clinical features of ATL include diffuse lymphadenopathy, maculopapular skin lesions that may evolve into an erythroderma, organomegaly, lytic bone lesions, and sometimes hypercalcemia. A predisposition to dermatophytoses, strongyloidiasis, and the usual AIDS-associated opportunistic infections (pneumocystis pneumonia, CMV infection, cryptococcosis) has been reported. Diagnosis requires identification of HTLV antibodies. Confirmatory demonstration of monoclonal proviral DNA integration in tumor cells is helpful.

A variety of neurologic syndromes characterized by slow progression and onset in middle age, with weakness and spasticity, typically of the legs, have been associated with HTLV. Such entities are referred to as either tropical spastic paraparesis or HTLV-associated myelopathy. Other symptoms and findings include sensory disturbances, hyperactive reflexes, and cerebrospinal fluid lymphopleocytosis.

HTLV-2 is less strongly associated with ATL, HTLV-2, and hairy cell leukemia, but not strongly; associations with a syndrome resembling tropical spastic paraparesis have also been reported. Native American populations appear to be at particular risk for HTLV-2 infection.

Management of ATL is similar to that for non-Hodgkin's lymphoma and includes combination chemotherapy and radiation of particular sites (weight-bearing bony lesions, paraspinal masses, intracerebral lesions). The myelopathy of human T cell leukemia virus is discussed in Chapter 24; care is supportive but may include the use of corticosteroids. Screening of the blood supply for HTLV-1 is required in the United States, since transfusion is a recognized mode of transmission, along with sexual activity, vertical transmission, and perhaps other methods (seroprevalence increases with age). Ten to 40 percent of HTLV-2 carriers are not cross-reactive to HTLV-1 screening assays, and new methods for improving blood screening are under development.

Rios M et al: Transmission of human T cell lymphotropic virus (HTLV) type II by transfusion of HTLV-I-screened blood products. J Infect Dis 1994;170:206.

Rosenblatt JD: Human T-lymphotropic virus types I and II. West J Med 1993;158:379. (Molecular analogies to HIV explained.)

OTHER SYSTEMIC VIRAL DISEASES

1. DENGUE

Essentials of Diagnosis

- Exposure 7–10 days before onset.
- Sudden onset of high fever, chills, severe aching, headache, sore throat, prostration, and depression.
- Biphasic fever curve: initial phase, 3–7 days; remission, few hours to 2 days; second phase, 1–2 days.
- The rash is biphasic: first evanescent, followed by maculopapular, scarlatiniform, morbilliform, or petechial changes from extremities to torso.
- Leukopenia.

General Considerations

Dengue is a viral (togavirus, flavivirus) disease transmitted by the bite of the *Aedes* mosquito. It may be caused by one of several serotypes widely distributed between latitudes 25 °N and 25 °S (eg, Thailand, India, Philippines; Caribbean, including Puerto Rico and Cuba; Central America; Africa). It occurs only in the active mosquito season (warm weather). The incubation period is 3–15 days (usually 7–10 days). Endemic transmission has occurred in the USA (the last such case was in southern Texas in 1986). A recent outbreak has been reported from the Mexican border city of Reynosa.

Clinical Findings

A. Symptoms and Signs: Dengue is usually a nonspecific, self-limited, febrile illness, but its presentation may range from asymptomatic infection to severe hemorrhage and sudden fatal shock. Severe dengue begins with a sudden onset of high fever, chilliness, and severe aching ("breakbone") of the head, back, and extremities, accompanied by sore throat, prostration, and depression. There may be conjunctival redness and flushing or blotching of the skin. The initial febrile phase lasts 3–7 days, typically but not inevitably followed by a remission of a few hours to 2 days.

The rash appears in 80% of cases during the remission or during the second febrile phase, which lasts 1–2 days and is accompanied by similar but usually milder symptoms than in the first phase. The rash may be scarlatiniform, morbilliform, maculopapular, or petechial. It appears first on the dorsum of the hands and feet and spreads to the arms, legs, trunk, and neck but rarely to the face. The rash lasts 2 hours to several days and may be followed by desquamation.

Petechial rashes and gastrointestinal hemorrhages occur with **dengue hemorrhagic fever,** caused possibly by strains of any subtype in Asia and increasingly in the Caribbean, Mexico, and Central America. Some dengue virus envelope glycoproteins are homologous with segments of clotting factors, in-

cluding plasminogen, and thus the hemorrhagic fever may represent an autoimmune reaction.

Before the rash appears, it is difficult to distinguish dengue from malaria, yellow fever, or influenza; the rash makes dengue far more likely.

B. Laboratory Findings: Leukopenia is characteristic. Thrombocytopenia occurs in the hemorrhagic form of the disease. Virus may be recovered from the blood during the acute phase.

Complications

Depression, pneumonia, bone marrow failure, iritis, orchitis, and oophoritis are unusual complications. Shock occurs in hemorrhagic dengue.

Prevention

Available prophylactic measures include control of mosquitoes by screening and insect repellents, particularly during early morning and late afternoon exposures. An effective vaccine has been developed but has not been produced commercially.

Treatment

Treatment entails the appropriate use of volume and pressors, acetaminophen rather than aspirin for analgesia, and the gradual restoration of activity during prolonged convalescence.

Prognosis

Fatalities are rare, though convalescence tends to be slow.

Ramirez-Ronda CH: Dengue in the Western Hemisphere. Infect Dis Clin North Am 1994;8:107. (Includes an algorithm for assessing severity of infection based on spectrum of disease.)

Rodriguez-Figueroa L et al: Risk factors for dengue infection during an outbreak in Puerto Rico in 1991. Am J Trop Med Hyg 1995;52:496. (Mosquito control is essential.)

2. COLORADO TICK FEVER

Essentials of Diagnosis

- Onset 1–19 days (average, 4 days) following tick bite.
- Fever, chills, myalgia, headache, prostration.
- Leukopenia.
- Second attack of fever after remission lasting 2–3 days.

General Considerations

Colorado tick fever is an acute viral (recently reclassified as a coltivirus) infection transmitted by *Dermacentor andersoni* bites. The disease is limited to the western USA and Canada and is most prevalent during the tick season (March to August). The incubation period is 3–6 days.

Clinical Findings

A. Symptoms and Signs: The onset of fever (to 38.9–40.6 °C) is abrupt, sometimes with chills. Severe myalgia, headache, photophobia, anorexia, nausea and vomiting, and generalized weakness are prominent symptoms. Abnormal physical findings are limited to an occasional faint rash. Fever continues for 3 days, followed by a remission of 1–3 days and then by a full recrudescence lasting 2–4 days. In an occasional case there may be three bouts of fever.

Influenza, Rocky Mountain spotted fever, and other acute leukopenic fevers must be differentiated.

B. Laboratory Findings: Leukopenia (2000–3000/μL) with a shift to the left occurs. Viremia may be demonstrated by inoculation of blood into mice or by fluorescent antibody staining of the patient's red cells (with adsorbed virus). Complement-fixing antibodies appear during the third week of disease.

Complications

Aseptic meningitis, encephalitis, and hemorrhagic fever occur rarely. Asthenia may follow, but fatalities are very rare.

Treatment

No specific treatment is available. Aspirin or another nonsteroidal anti-inflammatory agent—or codeine or hydrocodone—may be given for pain.

Prognosis

The disease is usually self-limited and benign.

Calisher CH: Medically important arboviruses of the United States and Canada. Clin Microbiol Rev 1994; 7:89.

3. HEMORRHAGIC FEVERS

This is a diverse group of illnesses resulting from viral infections and perhaps immunologic responses to them. The common clinical features include high fever; hemorrhagic diathesis with petechiae or purpura; and bleeding from the nose, gastrointestinal tract, and genitourinary tract, with thrombocytopenia, leukopenia, and marked toxicity, often leading to shock and death. The viruses may be tick-borne (eg, Omsk hemorrhagic fever, Russia; Kyasanur Forest hemorrhagic fever, India), mosquito-borne (eg, Chikungunya hemorrhagic fever, yellow fever, dengue), or zoonotic (often derived from rodents, eg, hemorrhagic fever with renal syndrome secondary to Hantaan virus infection, Junin hemorrhagic fever, Argentina; Machupo hemorrhagic fever, Bolivia; Lassa hemorrhagic fever, West Africa; the Puumala virus, Scandinavia; Belgrade virus, Yugoslavia; and Dobrava virus, the Balkans). The zoonotic group also includes Marburg hemorrhagic fever (from contact with African vervet monkeys) and Ebola hemor-

rhagic fever in central Africa. Lassa fever has been associated with rodent consumption.

Persons who present with symptoms compatible with those of hemorrhagic fever and who have traveled from a possible endemic area should be strictly isolated for diagnosis and symptomatic treatment. Conclusive diagnosis may be made by growing the virus from blood obtained early in the disease or by showing a significant specific antibody titer rise. Isolation is particularly important, because some of these infections are highly transmissible to close contacts, including medical personnel, and carry a mortality rate of 50–70%.

For most of these entities, no specific treatment is available. Lassa fever and hemorrhagic fever with renal failure can be effectively treated—if started early—with intravenous ribavirin (33 mg/kg as loading dose, followed by 16 mg/kg every 6 hours for 4 days and then 8 mg/kg every 8 hours for 3 days) (see Chapter 37). It is important to differentiate hemorrhagic fever from such easily treated entities as meningococcemia and Rocky Mountain spotted fever.

Christopher J et al: Ebola hemorrhagic fever in Zaire, 1995; a perspective. Curr Opin Infect Dis 1995;8:225.

Ruo SL et al: Retrospective and prospective studies of hemorrhagic fever with renal syndrome in rural China. J Infect Dis 1994;170:527. (Twelve percent antibody prevalence, with rural activities a risk factor.)

Sodhi A: Ebola virus disease: Recognizing the face of a rare killer. Postgrad Med 1996;99:75.

4. HANTAVIRUSES

Hantaviruses are rodent-borne RNA viruses with at least five distinct serotypes. These differ in rodent hosts, geographic distribution, and degree of pathogenicity for humans. The Hantaan serotype viruses cause severe hemorrhagic fever with renal syndrome and are found primarily in Korea, China, and eastern Russia. The Seoul viruses produce a less severe form and are found primarily in Korea and China. The Puumala viruses are found in Scandinavia and Europe and are associated with a relatively mild form of the syndrome. A fifth serotype, the newly discovered Muerto Canyon virus, is responsible for the **hantavirus pulmonary syndrome,** most cases of which have been reported in the southwestern United States. Hantavirus pulmonary syndrome begins as a nonspecific febrile illness followed by rapid progression to a shock-like state, associated with increased pulmonary vascular permeability and ARDS. Hematologic features include thrombocytopenia, hemoconcentration, and leukocytosis.

Diagnosis can be made serologically, by immunohistochemical staining, or by PCR amplification of viral tissue DNA.

Prevention

Since infection is thought to occur by inhalation of rodent wastes, prevention is aimed toward eradication of rodents in houses and avoidance of exposure to rodent excreta in rural settings.

Treatment

No treatment has been established as definitely effective. Intravenous ribavirin has been used, since it is effective in treating severe cases of Hantaan virus infection.

Hantavirus pulmonary syndrome—United States, 1995–1996. MMWR Morb Mortal Wkly Rep 1996;45:291.

Simonsen L et al: Evaluation of the magnitude of the 1993 hantavirus outbreak in the southwestern United States. J Infect Dis 1995;172:729.

Warner GS: Hantavirus illness in humans: Review and update. South Med J 1996;89:264. (A reminder that the mortality rate of hantavirus pulmonary syndrome is ten times that of its Eurasian counterparts.)

Zeitz PS et al: A case-control study of hantavirus pulmonary syndrome during an outbreak in the southwestern United States. J Infect Dis 1995;171:864. (The syndrome is associated with peridomestic cleaning and agricultural activity in rodent-infested areas.)

5. YELLOW FEVER

Essentials of Diagnosis

- Endemic area exposure (tropical South and Central America, Africa, but not Asia).
- Sudden onset of severe headache, aching in legs, and tachycardia.
- Brief (1 day) remission, followed by bradycardia, hypotension, jaundice, hemorrhagic tendency.
- Proteinuria, leukopenia, bilirubinemia, bilirubinuria.

General Considerations

Yellow fever is a viral (group B arbovirus, togavirus) infection transmitted by the *Aedes* and jungle mosquitoes. It is endemic only in Africa and South America (tropical or subtropical), but epidemics have extended far into the temperate zone during warm seasons. The mosquito transmits the infection by first biting an individual having the disease and then biting a susceptible individual after the virus has multiplied within the mosquito's body. The incubation period in humans is 3–6 days. Adults and children are equally susceptible, though attack rates are highest among adult males because of their work habits.

Clinical Findings

A. Symptoms and Signs:

1. Mild form—Symptoms are malaise, headache, fever, retro-orbital pain, nausea, vomiting, and photophobia. Bradycardia may be present.

2. Severe form—Symptoms are the same as in the mild form, with sudden onset and then severe pains throughout the body, extreme prostration, bleeding into the skin and from the mucous membranes, oliguria, and jaundice. Signs include tachycardia, erythematous face, and conjunctival redness during the congestive phase, followed by a period of calm (on about the third day) with a normal temperature and then a return of fever, bradycardia, hypotension, jaundice, hemorrhages (gastrointestinal tract, bladder, nose, mouth, subcutaneous), and later delirium.

B. Laboratory Findings: Leukopenia occurs, although it may not be present at the onset. Proteinuria is present, sometimes as high as 5–6 g/L, and disappears completely with recovery. With jaundice there are bilirubinuria and bilirubinemia. Serologic diagnosis may be established by showing fourfold or greater increases in hemagglutination inhibition, complement fixation, or neutralizing antibodies. An IgM capture enzyme immunoassay (EIA) is a rapid, specific diagnostic aid.

Differential Diagnosis

It may be difficult to distinguish yellow fever from hepatitis, malaria, leptospirosis, dengue, and other hemorrhagic fevers, and other forms of jaundice on clinical evidence alone.

Prevention

Transmission is prevented through mosquito control. Live virus vaccine is highly effective, safe, and should be provided for immunocompetent adults living in or traveling to endemic areas. Pregnant women should not be immunized. (See Chapter 30.)

Treatment

No specific antiviral therapy is available. Treatment is directed toward symptomatic relief and management of complications.

Prognosis

The mortality rate is high in the severe form, with death occurring most commonly between the sixth and the tenth days. In survivors, the temperature returns to normal by the seventh or eighth day. The prognosis in any individual case is guarded at the onset, since sudden changes for the worse are common. Intractable hiccup, copious black vomitus, melena, and anuria are unfavorable signs. Convalescence is prolonged, including 1–2 weeks of asthenia.

Monath TP, Nasidi A: Should yellow fever vaccine be included in the expanded program of immunization in Africa? A cost-effectiveness analysis for Nigeria. Am J Trop Med Hyg 1993;48:274. (Inclusion in ongoing immunization programs rather than in only emergency epidemic containment may be a more effective prevention strategy for the developing world.)

Tsai TF et al: Congenital yellow fever virus infection after immunization in pregnancy. J Infect Dis 1993:168:1520.
Yellow fever vaccine. Recommendations of the Immunization Practices Advisory Committee (ACIP). MMWR Morb Mortal Wkly Rep 1990;39(RR-6):1.

COMMON VIRAL RESPIRATORY INFECTIONS

Infections of the respiratory tract are perhaps the most common human ailments. Specific associations of certain groups of viruses with certain disease syndromes have been established. In young infants and in the elderly, or in persons with impaired respiratory tract reserve, bacterial superinfection increases morbidity and mortality.

Croup, epiglottitis, and the common cold are discussed in Chapter 8.

Mossad SB: Zinc gluconate lozenges for treating the common cold: A randomized, double-blind placebo controlled study. Ann Intern Med 1996;125:81. (Zinc reduces the duration of cold symptoms.)

1. RESPIRATORY SYNCYTIAL VIRUS

Respiratory syncytial virus (RSV) causes annual outbreaks of pneumonia, bronchiolitis, and tracheobronchitis in the very young. Reinfection is common and manifests itself typically as a mild upper respiratory tract infection and tracheobronchitis in older children or adults. Serious pulmonary RSV infections have been described in elderly and immunocompromised adults, including outbreaks with a high mortality rate in bone marrow transplant and pediatric liver transplant patients. Infants with congenital heart disease are at high risk for severe RSV infection.

Annual epidemics occur in winter and spring. The average incubation period is 5 days. Inoculation may occur through the nose or the eyes.

In bronchiolitis, proliferation and necrosis of bronchiolar epithelium develop, producing obstruction from sloughed epithelium and increased mucus secretion. Signs include low-grade fever, tachypnea, and wheezes. Hyperinflated lungs, decreased gas exchange, and increased work of breathing are present. Otitis media is a frequent complication.

RSV is the only respiratory pathogen that produces its most serious illness at a time when specific maternal antibody is invariably present, though high titers can modify or prevent infection.

Rapid diagnosis may be made by viral antigen identification of nasal washings using an ELISA or immunofluorescent assay. Culture of nasopharyngeal secretions remains the standard of diagnosis.

Treatment consists of hydration, humidification of inspired air, and ventilatory support as needed. In in-fants, aerosolized ribavirin may help (1.1 g/d, diluted to 20 mg/mL, delivered as a particulate with oxygen over 12–18 hours per day for 3–7 days—although high-dose, short-duration therapy may be as effective). Pregnant women should avoid ribavirin exposure—and indeed, patients with upper respiratory RSV infections probably do not need ribavirin. Hyperimmune RSV immunoglobulin G is not effective in the management of these infections among infants, though it may be tried in combination with ribavirin for RSV infections among immunocompromised adults. Hyperimmune RSV immunoglobulin G prophylaxis is, however, safe and effective in preventing lower respiratory tract infection in infants and young children at high risk because of prematurity or pulmonary or cardiac disease. A subunit vaccine given to pregnant women may provide passive protection against respiratory syncytial virus in neonates. Because nosocomial RSV infections disseminate rapidly, prevention in hospitals entails rapid diagnosis, cohorting cases, handwashing, and perhaps passive immunization.

Englund JA et al: Passive protection against RSV disease in infants; the role of maternal antibody. Ped Infect Dis J 1994;13:449. (Antibody of purified F [fusion] protein correlates with immunity, and trials are under way to vaccinate pregnant women with RSV glycoproteins.)
Falsey AR et al: RSV and influenza A infections in the hospitalized elderly. J Infect Dis 1995;172:389. (In this large series from Rochester, 10% had RSV infections and RSV was often associated with bronchospasm.)
Ruuskanen O: RSV—is it preventable? J Hosp Infect 1995;30S:494.

2. INFLUENZA

Essentials of Diagnosis

- Cases usually in epidemic pattern, not sporadic.
- Abrupt onset with fever, chills, malaise, cough, coryza, and muscle aches.
- Aching, fever, and prostration out of proportion to catarrhal symptoms.
- Leukopenia.

General Considerations

Influenza (an orthomyxovirus) is transmitted by the respiratory route. In contrast to RSV and rhinoviruses, transmission occurs by droplet nuclei rather than fomites or large particle aerosols. Although sporadic cases occur, epidemics and pandemics appear at varying intervals, usually in the fall or winter. Antigenic types A and B produce clinically indistinguishable infections, whereas type C is usually a minor illness. The incubation period is 1–4 days.

It is difficult to diagnose influenza in the absence of an epidemic. The disease resembles many other mild febrile illnesses but is almost always accompanied by a cough.

Clinical Findings

A. Symptoms and Signs: The onset is usually abrupt, with fever, chills, malaise, muscular aching, substernal soreness, headache, nasal stuffiness, and occasionally nausea. Fever lasts 1–7 days (usually 3–5). Coryza, nonproductive cough, and sore throat are present. Signs include mild pharyngeal injection, flushed face, and conjunctival redness.

B. Laboratory Findings: Leukopenia is common. Proteinuria may be present. The virus may be isolated from the throat washings by inoculation of embryonated eggs or cell cultures. Complement-fixing and hemagglutination-inhibiting antibodies appear during the second week.

Complications

Influenza causes necrosis of the respiratory epithelium, which predisposes to secondary bacterial infections. The interactions between bacteria and influenza are bidirectional, with bacterial enzymes (eg, proteases, trypsin-like compounds, streptokinase, plasminogen) activating influenza viruses. Frequent complications are acute sinusitis, otitis media, purulent bronchitis, and pneumonia; the elderly and the chronically ill are at high risk for complications.

Pneumonia is commonly due to bacterial infection with pneumococci or staphylococci and on occasion to the influenza virus itself. The circulatory system is not usually involved, but pericarditis, myocarditis, and thrombophlebitis sometimes occur.

Reye's syndrome is a rare and severe complication of influenza and other viral diseases (eg, varicella), particularly in young children. It consists of rapidly progressive hepatic failure and encephalopathy, and there is a 30% fatality rate. The pathogenesis is unknown, but the syndrome is associated with aspirin use. Hypoglycemia, elevation of serum transaminases and blood ammonia, prolonged prothrombin time, and change in mental status all occur within 2–3 weeks after onset of the viral infection. Histologically, the periphery of liver lobules shows striking fatty infiltration and glycogen depletion. Treatment is supportive and directed to the management of cerebral edema.

Prevention

Trivalent influenza virus vaccine provides partial immunity (about 85% efficacy) for a few months to 1 year. The vaccine's antigenic configuration changes yearly and is based on prevalent strains of the preceding year. Vaccination (0.5 mL intramuscularly once in October or November each year) is recommended annually for persons over 65, children and teenagers receiving chronic aspirin therapy, nursing home residents, those with chronic lung or heart disease or other debilitating illnesses, and health care workers. The vaccine is contraindicated in persons with hypersensitivity to chicken eggs or other components of the vaccine, persons with an acute febrile illness, or thrombocytopenia. Concomitant warfarin or steroid therapy is not a contraindication. Side effects are infrequent and include tenderness, redness, or induration at the site of the injection and, rarely, myalgias or fever. Adequate immunity is achieved about 2 weeks after vaccination. The vaccination effectively reduces both morbidity (preventing 35–60% of hospital admissions in the elderly) and mortality (preventing 35–80% of hospital deaths). A live attenuated vaccine has been widely used among Russian adults.

HIV-infected persons can be safely vaccinated, and concerns about activating replication of the HIV virus by the immunogen are probably exaggerated. However, immune responses are impaired in severely CD4-lymphopenic individuals, so vaccination is recommended only when the CD4 counts are greater than 100/μL. False-positive assays with HIV, HTLV-I, and HCV have been reported for weeks in the wake of influenza vaccination.

Chemoprophylaxis for epidemiologically or virologically confirmed influenza A with amantadine hydrochloride, 200 mg/d orally in two divided doses (100 mg/d in the elderly, who may develop central nervous system side effects), or rimantadine (200 mg/d in two divided doses) will markedly reduce the attack rate among exposed unvaccinated individuals if begun immediately and continued for 10 days. Amantadine or rimantadine may also be used during an outbreak while waiting for immunity to develop following vaccination.

Treatment

Many patients with influenza prefer to rest in bed. Analgesics and a cough mixture may be used. Amantadine or rimantadine, in the same doses as are used for prophylaxis, appreciably decrease the duration of signs and symptoms. Rimantadine is preferred in patients with renal failure. The clinical significance of resistance to antiviral agents is controversial. Ribavirin (1.1 g/d, diluted to 20 mg/mL and delivered as particulate aerosol with oxygen over 12–18 hours a day for 3–7 days [Table 32–1]) has helped severely ill patients with influenza A or B. Newer agents such as nasally applied zanamivir, an antineuraminidase, are under development.

Antibacterial antibiotics should be reserved for treatment of bacterial complications. Acetaminophen rather than aspirin should be used for fever in children.

Prognosis

The duration of the uncomplicated illness is 1–7 days, and the prognosis is excellent. Purulent bronchitis and bronchiectasis may result in chronic pulmonary disease and fibrosis that persist throughout life. Most fatalities are due to bacterial pneumonia. Influenzal pneumonia has a high mortality rate among pregnant women and persons with a history of rheumatic heart disease. In recent epidemics, the mortality rate has been low except in debilitated individuals.

If the fever persists for more than 4 days with productive cough and white cell count over 10,000/μL, secondary bacterial infection should be suspected. Pneumococcal pneumonia is most common and staphylococcal pneumonia most serious.

Gross PA et al: The efficacy of influenza vaccine in elderly persons; a metaanalysis and review of the literature. Ann Intern Med 1995;123:518. (Immunization reduces the risk of pneumonia, hospitalization, and death.)

Honkanen PO: Reactions following administration of influenza vaccine alone or with pneumococcal vaccine to the elderly. Arch Intern Med 1996;156:205. (The two vaccines can be safely coadministered.)

Khan AS et al: Comparison of US inactivated split-virus and Russian live attenuated, cold-adapted trivalent influenza vaccines in Russian schoolchildren. J Infect Dis 1996;173:453. (The ease of administration of the live, attenuated vaccine may compensate for its slightly lower efficacy.)

Kroon FP et al: Antibody response to influenza, tetanus, and pneumococcal vaccines in HIV-seropositive individuals in relations to the number of CD4+ lymphocytes. AIDS 1994;8:469. (Influenza vaccination is not recommended for HIV-infected individuals whose CD4 value is less than 100×10^6/L.)

Nichol KL et al: Side effects associated with influenza vaccination in healthy working adults: A randomized, placebo-controlled trial. Arch Intern Med 1996; 156:1546. (Systemic symptoms are not increased among influenza vaccinees.)

ADENOVIRUS INFECTIONS

Adenoviruses (there are more than 40 antigenic types) produce a variety of clinical syndromes. These infections are self-limited or clinically inapparent and most common among infants, young children, and military recruits. Outbreaks in liver, bone marrow, and renal transplant recipients have been reported, and dissemination may occur. The incubation period is 4–9 days.

Clinical syndromes of adenovirus infection, often overlapping, include the following: (1) The **common cold** (see Chapter 8) is characterized by rhinitis, pharyngitis, and mild malaise without fever. (2) **Non-streptococcal exudative pharyngitis** is characterized by fever lasting 2–12 days accompanied by malaise and myalgia. Sore throat is often manifested by diffuse injection, a patchy exudate, and cervical lymphadenopathy. Cough is sometimes accompanied by rales and x-ray evidence of pneumonitis. Conjunctivitis is often present. (3) **Pharyngoconjunctival fever** is manifested by fever and malaise, conjunctivitis (often unilateral), and mild pharyngitis. (4) **Epidemic keratoconjunctivitis** (transmissible person-to-person) oc-

curs in adults and is manifested by unilateral conjunctival redness, pain, tearing, and an enlarged preauricular lymph node. Keratitis leads to subepithelial opacities (especially with types 8, 19, or 37). (5) **Acute hemorrhagic cystitis** is a disorder of children often associated with adenovirus type 11. (6) Sexually transmitted **genitourinary ulcers** and **urethritis** may be caused by types 2, 8, and 37 in particular. (7) Adenoviruses also cause acute **gastroenteritis** (types 40, 41) and **intussusception** and have been rarely associated with **encephalitis** and **pericarditis**.

Infected liver transplant recipients tend to develop hepatitis (type 5 adenovirus), whereas bone marrow and renal transplant recipients tend to develop pneumonia or hemorrhagic cystitis. Ribavirin has been used to treat adenovirus infections among HIV-infected individuals.

Vaccines are not available for general use. Live oral vaccines containing attenuated type 4 and type 7 have been used in military personnel.

Treatment is symptomatic.

Klapper PE: Adenovirus cross-infection: A continuing problem. J Hosp Infect 1995;30(Suppl):S262. (Evidence for nosocomial transmission.)

Wilson JM et al: Adenoviruses as gene delivery vehicles. N Engl J Med 1996;334:1185. (Adenoviruses, although a common cause of human disease, have received particular recent recognition through their role in gene therapy.)

OTHER EXANTHEMATOUS VIRAL INFECTIONS

1. PARVOVIRUS INFECTIONS

Parvovirus B19 causes several syndromes. In children, an exanthematous illness is characterized by fiery red "slapped cheeks," circumoral pallor, and a subsequent lacy, maculopapular, evanescent truncal rash. Malaise, headache, and pruritus occur, but little fever. In immunosuppressed patients, especially those with HIV infection and sickle cell disease, anemia due to red cell hypoplasia occurs. Middle-aged persons (especially women) develop polyarthralgias that mimic lupus erythematosus and preferentially involve the proximal interphalangeal joints of the hands and the wrists and knees. In pregnancy, fetal loss and hydrops fetalis have been reported.

The diagnosis is clinical (Table 32–2) but may be confirmed by an elevated titer of IgM anti-parvovirus antibodies in serum. Scarlet fever is the most similar disorder. The prognosis is excellent. Besides arthritis with hypocomplementemia, which is common in some outbreaks, encephalitis, chronic hemolytic anemia, and hepatitis are rare complications.

Treatment is symptomatic. Screening of donated blood could potentially prevent transfusion-related infection and is under investigation. Several nosocomial outbreaks have been documented, and hospital infection control personnel should administer standard containment guidelines (handwashing after patient exposure, avoiding contact with pregnant women).

Gratacos E et al: The incidence of human parvovirus B19 infection during pregnancy and its impact on perinatal outcome. J Infect Dis 1995;171:1360. (In a series of 1610 pregnant females from Barcelona, vertical transmission occurred in 25% and fetal loss in 1.6%.)

Heegaard ED, Hornsleth A: Parvovirus: The expanding spectrum of disease. Acta Paediatr 1995;84:109.

Qari M, Qadri SM: Parvovirus B19 infection: Associated diseases, common and uncommon. Postgrad Med 1996;100:239.

2. POXVIRUS INFECTIONS

Among the nine poxviruses causing disease in humans, five are clinically important: (1) **Variola:** Smallpox was a highly contagious disease characterized by severe headache, fever, and prostration and accompanied by a centrifugal rash developing in order of progression from macules to papules to vesicles to pustules. Immunization with vaccinia virus, culminating in a worldwide effort by WHO, apparently succeeded in eradicating smallpox from the world as of 1979. After much debate among public health personnel and virologists, a decision was made to destroy the virus. (2) **Molluscum contagiosum** may be transmitted sexually or by other close contact. It is manifested by pearly, raised, umbilicated skin nodules sparing the palms and soles. It tends to persist in AIDS patients. Treatment is by local chemoabrasion, cryotherapy, or surgical removal. (3) **Vaccinia:** The efficacy of vaccination with vaccinia was responsible in part for smallpox eradication. Since the world is free of smallpox, civilian vaccination is indicated only for laboratory workers who must handle virus related to variola. Vaccination is still practiced among some military forces. Smallpox vaccination is not required for any international travel. Any form of immunosuppression is an absolute contraindication to smallpox vaccination. Eczema (or a history of it) in a patient or family member, other forms of dermatitis, and burns also contraindicate vaccination. There is no indication for therapeutic use of smallpox vaccine. (4) **Orf** (contagious pustular dermatitis or ecthyma contagiosa) and (5) **paravaccinia** (milkers' nodules) are occupationally acquired diseases acquired by contact with sheep and cattle, respectively.

VIRUSES & GASTROENTERITIS

Viruses are responsible for probably 30–40% of cases of infectious diarrhea in the USA, and ro-

taviruses are a leading worldwide cause of dehydrating gastroenteritis in young children. The agents that can cause disease include group B rotaviruses (responsible for outbreaks in China), Norwalk agent (which causes epidemics of vomiting and diarrhea and is often transmitted by food—especially shellfish—and water), astroviruses, and enteric adenoviruses.

Rotaviruses (four major serotypes) can also cause infections in adults exposed to infected infants and are ubiquitous in the environment of an outbreak. (Secondary rates are between 16% and 30%.) The disease is usually mild, but cases have also occurred among travelers, in epidemic fashion, and after waterborne exposure. Sensitive and specific immunoassays to detect viral RNA in fecal specimens are available. Treatment is symptomatic, with fluid and electrolyte replacement. Immunity does not appear to be serotype-specific, and lymphoproliferative responses are important.

The **Norwalk agent** and **Norwalk-like agents** are responsible for about 40% of cases of group-related or institutional diarrhea, transmission usually being the fecal-oral route, though airborne transmission may also occur. Nausea and vomiting are especially common with Norwalk agent. An ELISA can detect the agent in stool samples. Treatment again is symptomatic.

Orenstein WA et al: Rotavirus vaccines—from licensure to disease reduction. J Infect Dis 1996(Suppl);174:S118.

Sherman PM et al: Infectious gastroenterocolitides in children: An update on emerging pathogens. Pediatr Clin North Am 1996;43:391.

VIRUSES THAT PRODUCE SEVERAL SYNDROMES

1. COXSACKIEVIRUS INFECTIONS

Coxsackievirus infections cause several clinical syndromes. As with other enteroviruses, infections are most common during the summer. Two groups, A and B, are defined either serologically or by mouse bioassay. There are more than 50 serotypes.

Clinical Findings

A. Symptoms and Signs: The clinical syndromes associated with coxsackievirus infection may be described briefly as follows:

1. Summer grippe (A and B)–A febrile illness, principally of children, lasting 1–4 days; minor symptoms and respiratory tract infection are often present.

2. Herpangina (A2–6, 10)–Sudden onset of fever, which may be as high as 40.6 °C, sometimes with febrile convulsions; headache, myalgia, vomiting; and sore throat characterized early by petechiae or papules on the soft palate that become shallow ulcers in about 3 days and then heal.

3. Epidemic pleurodynia (B1–5)–Sudden onset of recurrent pain in the area of diaphragmatic attachment (lower chest or upper abdomen). Fever is often present during attacks of pain. Other findings are headache, sore throat, malaise, nausea; tenderness, hyperesthesia, and muscle swelling of the involved area; orchitis, pleurisy, and aseptic meningitis. Serum creatine kinase may be elevated. Relapse may occur after recovery.

4. Aseptic meningitis (A and B)–Fever, headache, nausea, vomiting, stiff neck, drowsiness, and cerebrospinal fluid lymphocytosis without chemical abnormalities. A focal encephalitis and a transverse myelitis have been reported with coxsackievirus group A and a disseminated encephalitis after group B infection.

5. Acute nonspecific pericarditis (B types)–Sudden onset of anterior chest pain, often worse with inspiration and in the supine position; fever, myalgia, headache; pericardial friction rub appear early; pericardial effusion with paradoxic pulse, increased venous pressure, and increase in heart size are noted. Electrocardiographic and x-ray evidence of pericarditis is often present. Relapses may occur.

6. Myocarditis (B1–5)–Heart failure in the neonatal period secondary to in utero myocarditis. Adult dilated cardiomyopathy has been correlated with group B infections (especially B2, B5).

7. Hand, foot, and mouth disease (A5, 10, 16)–Sometimes epidemic and characterized by stomatitis and a vesicular rash on hands and feet.

8. Hepatitis (B1)–Fulminant neonatal hepatitis with thrombocytopenia has been reported.

9. Insulin-dependent diabetes mellitus (B types)–An association has been made with the onset of diabetes mellitus shortly after Coxsackie B infection.

B. Laboratory Findings: Routine laboratory studies show no characteristic abnormalities. Neutralizing antibodies appear during convalescence. The virus may be isolated from throat washings or stools inoculated into suckling mice.

Treatment & Prognosis

Treatment is symptomatic. With the exception of myocarditis, pericarditis, perhaps diabetes, and rare illnesses such as pancreatitis or polio-like syndrome, the syndromes caused by coxsackieviruses are benign and self-limited. There are anecdotal reports of success with immunoglobulin in severe disease.

Fohlman J: Is juvenile diabetes a viral disease? Ann Med 1993;25:569.

2. ECHOVIRUS INFECTIONS

Echoviruses are enteroviruses that produce several clinical syndromes, particularly in children. Infection is most common during summer.

Over 30 serotypes have been demonstrated. Most cause aseptic meningitis, which may be associated with a rubelliform rash. Type 16 causes Boston exanthem, characterized by sudden onset of fever, nausea, and sore throat and a roseola-like rash over the face and trunk that persists 1–10 days. Diseases associated with echoviruses range from common respiratory diseases and epidemic diarrhea to myocarditis, encephalitis, and septic shock.

As with other enterovirus infections, diagnosis is best established by correlation of clinical, epidemiologic, and laboratory evidence. Cytopathic effects are produced in tissue culture after recovery of virus from throat washings, blood, or cerebrospinal fluid. Fourfold or greater rises in antibody titer signify systemic infection.

Treatment is symptomatic. The prognosis is excellent, though there are reports of mild paralysis after central nervous system infection. Handwashing is an effective control measure in outbreaks of aseptic meningitis.

Helfand RF et al: Echovirus 30 infection and aseptic meningitis in parents of children attending a child care center. J Infect Dis 1994;169:1133.

II. RICKETTSIAL DISEASES

The rickettsioses are febrile exanthematous diseases caused by rickettsiae, small gram-negative obligate intracellular bacterial parasites of arthropods. In arthropods, rickettsiae grow in the gut lining, often without harming the host. Human infection results from either an arthropod bite or contamination with its feces. In humans, rickettsiae grow principally in endothelial cells of small blood vessels, producing vasculitis, cell necrosis, thrombosis of vessels, skin rashes, and organ dysfunctions.

Different rickettsiae and their vectors are endemic in different parts of the world, but two or more types may coexist in the same geographic area. A summary of epidemiologic features is given in Table 32–4. The clinical picture is variable but usually includes a prodromal stage followed by fever, rash, and prostration. Isolation of rickettsiae from the patient is cumbersome and difficult and is best left to specialized laboratories. A promising new means of isolation is the centrifugation shell-vial technique. Diagnosis is usually based on clinical examination and epidemiologic

Table 32–4. Rickettsial diseases.[1]

Disease	Rickettsial Pathogen	Geographic Areas of Prevalence	Insect Vector	Mammalian Reservoir	Weil-Felix Agglutination[2]		
					OX19	OX2	OXK
Typhus group							
Epidemic (louse-borne) typhus	*Rickettsia prowazekii*	South America, Africa, Asia, North America	Louse	Humans, flying squirrels	+	±	—
Endemic (murine) typhus	*Rickettsia typhi*	Worldwide; small foci (USA: southeastern Gulf Coast)	Flea	Rodents	+	—	—
Scrub typhus	*Rickettsia tsutsugamushi*	Southeast Asia, Japan, Australia	Mite[3]	Rodents	—	—	+
Spotted fever group							
Rocky Mountain spotted fever	*Rickettsia rickettsii*	Western Hemisphere; USA (especially mid-Atlantic coastal region)	Tick[3]	Rodents, dogs	+	+	—
Boutonneuse fever, Kenya tick typhus, South African tick fever, Indian tick typhus	*Rickettsia conorii*	Africa, India, Mediterranean regions	Tick[3]	Rodents, dogs	+	+	—
Queensland tick typhus	*Rickettsia australis*	Australia	Tick[3]	Rodents, marsupials	+	+	—
North Asian tick typhus	*Rickettsia sibirica*	Siberia, Mongolia	Tick[3]	Rodents	+	+	—
Rickettsialpox	*Rickettsia akari*	USA, Korea, former USSR	Mite[3]	Mice	—	—	—
RMSF-like	*Rickettsia canada*	North America	Tick[3]	Rodents	?	?	—
Other							
Ehrlichiosis	*Ehrlichia chaffeensis*	Southeastern North America	Tick[3]	Dogs	?	?	?
Q fever	*Coxiella burnetii*	Worldwide	None[4]	Cattle, sheep, goats	—	—	—

[1]Modified from Brooks GF, Butel JS, Ornston LN: Jawetz, Melnick & Adelberg's Medical Microbiology, 19th ed. Appleton & Lange, 1991.
[2]Weil-Felix titers lack sensitivity and specificity and should not be used when other, more reliable tests are available.
[3]Also serve as arthropod reservoir by maintaining rickettsiae through transovarian transmission.
[4]Human infection results from inhalation of dust.

evidence. Laboratory diagnosis relies on the development of specific antibodies detected by complement fixation (for diagnosis), immunofluorescence, or hemagglutination (for species identification) tests. The Weil-Felix reaction lacks sufficient sensitivity and specificity to be used as a sole diagnostic test.

Prevention & Treatment

Preventive measures are directed at control of the vector, and avoidance of exposure by use of repellents and protective clothing. A thorough search of body surfaces should be conducted after potential exposure and the vector (louse, tick, or mite) gently removed.

All rickettsiae can be inhibited by tetracyclines or chloramphenicol. All early clinical infections respond in some degree to treatment with these drugs. Treatment usually consists of giving either tetracycline or chloramphenicol in the dosage schedules listed below.

Kostman JR: Laboratory diagnosis of rickettsial diseases. Clin Dermatol 1996;14:301. (Entire dedicated to rickettsial issues.)

Middleton DB: Tick-borne infections: What starts as a tiny bite may have a serious outcome. Postgrad Med 1994;95(5):131.

Walker DH, Dumler SJ: Emerging and reemerging rickettsial disease. N Engl J Med 1994;331:1651.

TYPHUS GROUP

1. EPIDEMIC LOUSE-BORNE TYPHUS

Essentials of Diagnosis

- Prodrome of headache, then chills and fever.
- Severe, intractable headaches, prostration, persisting high fever.
- Macular rash appearing on the fourth to seventh days on the trunk and in the axillae, spreading to

the rest of the body but sparing the face, palms, and soles.

• Diagnosis confirmed by specific antibodies using complement fixation, microagglutination, or immunofluorescence.

General Considerations

Epidemic louse-borne typhus is due to infection with *Rickettsia prowazekii,* a parasite of the body louse that ultimately kills the louse. Transmission is favored by crowded living conditions, famine, war, or any circumstances that predispose to heavy infestation with lice. When the louse sucks the blood of a person infected with *R prowazekii,* the organism becomes established in the gut of the louse and grows there. When the louse is transmitted to another person (through contact or clothing) and has a blood meal, it defecates simultaneously, and the infected feces are rubbed into the itching bite wound. Dry, infectious louse feces may also enter the respiratory tract.

In a person who recovers from clinical or subclinical typhus infection, *R prowazekii* may survive in lymphoid tissues. Years later, there may be a recrudescence of disease (Brill's disease) without exposure to infected lice.

Mild and atypical cases of *R prowazekii* have rarely occurred in the USA after contact with flying squirrels or their ectoparasites or decades following exposure (eg, among concentration camp victims of World War II). Cases can be acquired by travel to pockets of infection (eg, central and northeastern Africa, including Somalia).

Clinical Findings

A. Symptoms and Signs: (Table 32–4.) Prodromal malaise, cough, headache, backache, arthralgia, and chest pain begin after an incubation period of 10–14 days, followed by an abrupt onset of chills, high fever, and prostration, with flu-like symptoms progressing to delirium and stupor. The headache is severe, the fever prolonged.

Other findings consist of conjunctivitis, flushed facies, rales at the lung bases, and often splenomegaly. A macular rash (that may become confluent) appears first in the axillas and then over the trunk, spreading to the extremities but rarely involving the face, palms, or soles. In severely ill patients, the rash becomes hemorrhagic, and hypotension becomes marked. There may be renal insufficiency, stupor, and delirium. In spontaneous recovery, improvement begins 13–16 days after onset with rapid drop of fever.

B. Laboratory Findings: The white blood cell count is variable. Proteinuria and hematuria commonly occur. Serum obtained 5–12 days after onset of symptoms usually shows specific antibodies for *R prowazekii* antigens as demonstrated by complement fixation, microagglutination, or immunofluorescence. In primary rickettsial infection, early antibodies are

IgM; in recrudescence (Brill's disease), early antibodies are predominantly IgG.

C. Imaging: Radiographs of the chest may show patchy consolidation.

Differential Diagnosis

The prodromal symptoms and the early febrile stage are not specific enough to permit diagnosis in nonepidemic situations. The rash is usually sufficiently distinctive for diagnosis, but it may be absent in up to 10% of cases or may be difficult to observe in dark-skinned persons. A variety of other acute febrile diseases may have to be considered.

Brill's disease (recrudescent epidemic typhus) has a more gradual onset than primary *R prowazekii* infection, fever and rash are of shorter duration, and the disease is milder and rarely fatal.

Complications

Pneumonia, thromboses, vasculitis with major vessel obstruction and gangrene, circulatory collapse, myocarditis, and uremia may occur.

Prevention

Prevention consists of louse control with insecticides, particularly by applying chemicals to clothing or treating it with heat, and frequent bathing. A deloused and bathed typhus patient is not infectious.

Immunization with vaccines consisting of inactivated egg-grown *R prowazekii* gives some protection to laboratory personnel, physicians, or field workers who are exposed to the parasite. This vaccine is not currently commercially available in the USA or Canada. An improved cell culture vaccine is being developed.

Treatment

Treatment consists of either tetracycline (25 mg/kg/d in four divided doses) or chloramphenicol (50–100 mg/kg/d in four divided doses) for 4–10 days.

Prognosis

The prognosis depends greatly upon age and immunization status. In children under age 10, the disease is usually mild. The mortality rate is 10% in the second and third decades but in the past reached 60% in the sixth decade. Effective vaccination can convert a potentially serious disease into a mild one.

Perine PL et al: A clinico-epidemiological study of epidemic typhus in Africa. Clin Infect Dis 1992;14:1149. (Combines a discussion of global epidemiology with clinical experience in Addis Ababa.)

2. ENDEMIC FLEA-BORNE TYPHUS (Murine Typhus)

Rickettsia typhi is transmitted from rat to rat through the rat flea. Humans acquire the infection when bitten by an infected flea, which releases infected feces while sucking blood. A second etiologic agent, which closely resembles *R typhi*, has been linked to the cat flea and opossum exposures. Most cases in the USA are found in southern Texas and California. Rare cases follow travel, usually to Southeast Asia. Recent cases in Los Angeles have been linked to cat or opossum exposure and transmission via the cat flea.

Endemic typhus resembles recrudescent epidemic typhus in that it has a gradual onset and the fever and rash are of shorter duration (6–13 days). The symptoms are less severe than in epidemic typhus and may mimic measles, rubella, or roseola. The rash is maculopapular and concentrated on the trunk and fades fairly rapidly. Pneumonia and gangrene are rare. Fatalities are rare and limited to the elderly.

Clinical differentiation from Rocky Mountain spotted fever is established by the season of onset (earlier in the year for Rocky Mountain spotted fever), the character of the rash, and geography (urban or rural, versus rural for Rocky Mountain spotted fever). Complement-fixing or immunofluorescent antibodies can be detected in the patient's serum with specific *R typhi* antigens.

Preventive measures are directed at control of rats and ectoparasites (rat fleas) with insecticides, rat poisons, and rat-proofing of buildings. Antibiotic treatment with tetracycline (25–50 mg/kg/d in four divided doses) or chloramphenicol (50–75 mg/kg/d in four divided doses) is indicated through 3 full days of defervescence.

Esperanza L et al: Murine typhus: Forgotten but not gone. Southern Med J 1992;85:754.

Sorvillo FJ et al: A suburban focus of endemic typhus in Los Angeles County: Association with seropositive domestic cats and opossums. Am J Trop Med Hyg 1993; 48:269.

3. SCRUB TYPHUS (Tsutsugamushi Disease)

Essentials of Diagnosis

- Exposure to mites in endemic area of Southeast Asia, the western Pacific (including Korea), and Australia.
- Black eschar at site of bite, with regional and generalized lymphadenopathy.
- Conjunctivitis and a short-lived macular rash.
- Frequent pneumonitis, encephalitis, and cardiac failure.
- Laboratory confirmation with agglutinins to *Proteus* OXK and specific antibodies by immunofluorescence.

General Considerations

Scrub typhus is caused by *Rickettsia tsutsuga-mushi (R orientalis)*, which is principally a parasite of rodents transmitted by mites in the endemic areas listed above. The mites live on vegetation but complete their maturation cycle by biting humans who come in contact with infested vegetation. Serosurveys of suburban Bangkok blood donors show over 20% seroprevalence.

Clinical Findings

A. Symptoms and Signs: After a 1- to 3-week incubation period, malaise, chills, severe headache, and backache develop. At the site of the bite, a papule evolves into a flat black eschar. The regional lymph nodes are enlarged and tender, and there may be generalized adenopathy. Fever rises gradually, and a macular rash appears primarily on the trunk after a week of fever and may be fleeting or may last a week. The patient may become obtunded. During the second or third week, pneumonitis, myocarditis and cardiac failure, and, rarely, encephalitis, acute abdominal pain, granulomatous hepatitis, or acute renal failure may develop.

B. Laboratory Findings: Blood obtained during the first few days of illness may permit isolation of the rickettsial organism by mouse inoculation. Fluorescein-labeled antirickettsial assays are preferred to complement fixation tests. PCR may be the most sensitive means of diagnosis.

Differential Diagnosis

Leptospirosis, typhoid, dengue, malaria, and other rickettsial infections should be considered. Scrub typhus is a recognized cause of obscure tropical fevers, especially in children. When the rash is fleeting and the eschar not evident, laboratory results are the best guide to diagnosis.

Prevention

Repeated application of long-acting miticides can make endemic areas safe. When this is not possible, insect repellents on clothing and skin provide some protection. For short exposure, chemoprophylaxis with doxycycline (200 mg weekly) can prevent the disease but permits infection. No effective vaccines are available at present.

Treatment & Prognosis

Without treatment, fever may subside spontaneously after 2 weeks, but the mortality rate may be 10–30%. Treatment for 3 days with doxycycline, 100 mg twice daily, or for 7 days with chloramphenicol, 25 mg/kg/d in four divided doses, virtually eliminates deaths and relapses, though chloramphenicol- and tetracycline-resistant strains have been reported from Southeast Asia, and azithromycin may become the drug of choice for children, pregnant women, and patients with refractory disease.

Song J-H et al: Short-course doxycycline treatment versus conventional tetracycline therapy for scrub typhus: A multicenter trial. Clin Infect Dis 1995;21:506. (Three days is sufficient therapy when using doxycycline.)

SPOTTED FEVERS

1. ROCKY MOUNTAIN SPOTTED FEVER

Essentials of Diagnosis

- Exposure to tick bite in endemic area.
- "Influenzal" prodrome followed by chills, fever, severe headache, widespread aches and pains, restlessness, and prostration; occasionally, delirium and coma.
- Red macular rash appears between the second and sixth days of fever, first on the wrists and ankles and then spreading centrally; it may become petechial.
- Laboratory confirmation by agglutination of *Proteus* OX19 and OX2 and by specific antibodies with complement fixation and immunofluorescence.

General Considerations

The causative agent, *R rickettsii*, is transmitted to humans by the bite of ticks, including the wood tick, *Dermacentor andersoni,* in the western USA and by the bite of the dog tick, *Dermacentor variabilis,* in the eastern USA. Other hard ticks transmit the organism in the southern USA and in Central and South America and are responsible for transmitting it among rodents, dogs, porcupines, and other animals. Most human cases occur in late spring and summer. In the USA, most cases occur in the eastern third of the country, with nearly 1000 reported per year.

Clinical Findings

A. Symptoms and Signs: Three to 10 days after the bite of an infectious tick, symptoms begin with fever, chills, headache, nausea and vomiting, myalgias, restlessness, insomnia, and irritability. Cough and pneumonitis may develop. Delirium, lethargy, seizures, stupor, and coma may appear. The face is flushed and the conjunctiva injected. The rash (faint macules that progress to maculopapules and then petechiae) appears between days 2 and 6 of fever, first on the wrists and ankles, spreading centrally to the arms, legs, and trunk for 2–3 days; involvement of the palms and soles is characteristic. About 10% of cases occur without rash or with minimal rash. In some cases there is splenomegaly, hepatomegaly, jaundice, gangrene, myocarditis, or uremia.

B. Laboratory Findings: Leukocytosis, thrombocytopenia, hyponatremia, proteinuria, and hematuria are common. Cerebrospinal fluid may show hypoglycorrhachia and mild pleocytosis. Owing to endothelial damage, there is activation of platelets, coagulation pathways, and fibrinolysis. Diagnosis during the acute phase of the illness can be made by immunohistologic demonstration of *R rickettsiae* in skin biopsy specimens. Isolation of the organism using the shell vial technique is available in some laboratories. A rise in antibody titer during the second week of illness can be detected by specific complement fixation, immunofluorescence, and microagglutination tests. Laboratory confirmation can be made by immunofluorescent antibody (IFA), latex agglutination, or complement fixation.

Differential Diagnosis

The early signs and symptoms of Rocky Mountain spotted fever are shared with many other infections. The rash may be confused with that of measles, typhoid, ehrlichiosis, or meningococcemia. The suspicion of the latter requires blood cultures and cerebrospinal fluid examination.

Prevention

Protective clothing, tick-repellent chemicals, and the removal of ticks at frequent intervals are helpful measures.

Treatment & Prognosis

In mild, untreated cases, fever subsides at the end of the second week. The response to chloramphenicol (25–50 mg/kg/d orally or intravenously in four divided doses) or doxycycline (200 mg daily intravenously or orally) is prompt if the drugs are started early. Treatment is given for 7 days or through the third day of defervescence.

The mortality rate for Rocky Mountain spotted fever varies strikingly with age. In the untreated elderly, the mortality rate may be 70%, but it is usually less than 20% in children. The usual cause of death is pneumonitis with respiratory or cardiac failure. Sequelae, more common than formerly recognized, may include seizures, encephalopathy, peripheral neuropathy, paraparesis, bowel and bladder incontinence, cerebellar and vestibular dysfunction, hearing loss, and motor deficits.

Archibald LK, Sexton DJ: Long-term sequelae of Rocky Mountain spotted fever. Clin Infect Dis 1995;20:1155.
Quintal D: Rocky Mountain spotted fever. Clin Dermatol 1996;14:3. (Entire issue devoted to rickettsial diseases.)

2. RICKETTSIALPOX

Rickettsia akari is a parasite of mice, transmitted by mites *(Allodermanyssus sanguineus).* Rickettsialpox occurs in humans where crowded conditions and mouse-infested housing allow transmission of the pathogen to humans. Pathologic findings include dermal edema, subepidermal vesicles, and at times a lymphocytic vasculitis. The incubation period is 7–12 days. Onset is sudden, with chills, fever, headache, photophobia, and disseminated aches and pains. The primary lesion is a painless red papule that vesicates and forms a black eschar. Two to 4 days after onset of symptoms, a widespread papular eruption appears that becomes vesicular and forms crusts that are shed in about 10 days. Early lesions may resemble those of chickenpox (typically vesicular versus papulovesicular in rickettsialpox).

Leukopenia and a rise in antibody titer to rickettsial antigen with complement fixation or indirect fluorescent assays using a conjugated antirickettsial globulin can identify antigen in punch biopsies of skin lesions.

Treatment includes tetracycline, 15 mg/kg/d orally in four divided doses for 3–5 days.

Even without treatment, the disease is fairly mild and self-limited, treatment only hastening resolution. Control requires the elimination of mice from human habitations after insecticide has been applied to suppress the mite vectors.

Boyd AS: Rickettsialpox. Dermatol Clin 1997;15:313. (Review article.)

Heymann WR: Rickettsialpox. Clin Dermatol 1996;14:279.

Kass EM et al: Rickettsialpox in a New York City Hospital, 1980–1989. N Engl J Med 1994;331:1612. (Discusses diagnosis by direct immunofluorescence and describes histopathologic findings of lesional skin.)

3. TICK TYPHUS

The term "tick typhus" denotes a variety of spotted rickettsial fevers (often named by geography: eg, Israel tick fever, Kenya tick fever, Mediterranean spotted fever, Queensland tick typhus, Flinders Island spotted fever) transmitted by ticks (under introduction above) by the rickettsial agents *R conorii, R australis, R japonica, R africae,* and *R sibirica.* Dogs and wild animals may serve as reservoirs. The pathogens usually produce a black spot (tâche noire) at the site of the tick bite that may be useful in diagnosis, though spotless boutonneuse fever has been reported. Rarely, papulovesicular lesions may resemble rickettsialpox. Endothelial injury produces perivascular edema (this may be the presenting symptom) and dermal necrosis; regional adenopathy, disseminated lesions, focal hepatic necrosis, and encephalitis may occur. The disease has occurred among travelers, and in the USA, 67 cases were recorded over a 10-year interval, largely among returnees from Africa, including Somalia. Diagnosis is clinical, with serologic or PCR confirmation. Prevention entails protective clothing, repellents, and inspection for and removal of ticks. Treatment is with the following drugs given for 7–10 days: tetracycline (25–50 mg/kg/d in four divided doses), chloramphenicol (50–75 mg/kg/d in four divided doses), or ciprofloxacin (500 mg twice daily).

Morschang A et al: Imported rickettsiosis in German travelers. Infection 1995;23:94. (Eighty-two percent [18 of 22 cases] were boutonneuse fever.)

OTHER RICKETTSIAL & RICKETTSIAL-LIKE DISEASES

1. EHRLICHIOSIS

Ehrlichiosis is due to *Ehrlichia chaffeensis,* an obligatory intracellular parasite of leukocytes that forms intracellular inclusions bodies. It is a tick-borne pathogen most consistently identified with the tick vector *Amblyomma americanum.* Human ehrlichiosis has been diagnosed mainly in the Southeastern and South Central USA in patients exposed to ticks. Clinical disease ranges from mild to life-threatening. Typically, after about a 9-day incubation period and a prodrome consisting of malaise, rigors, and nausea, patients develop worsening fever and headache; a pleomorphic rash may occur. Leukopenia and absolute lymphopenia as well as thrombocytopenia occur often. Serious reported sequelae include acute respiratory failure, encephalopathy, and acute renal failure. An indirect fluorescent antibody assay is available through CDC and requires acute and convalescent sera. A PCR assay applied to whole blood samples has been reported as a rapid diagnostic tool.

A form of ehrlichiosis in which neutrophils are infected has recently been recognized in the northern United States; it is referred to as human granulocytic ehrlichiosis, and the causal agent is closely related to *Ehrlichia equi* or *Ehrlichia phagocytophila.*

Doxycycline is effective given as 200 mg orally or IV for at least 7 days or until 3 days of defervescence.

Dawson JE: Human ehrlichiosis in the United States. Curr Clin Top Infect Dis 1996;16:164.

Dumler JS, Bakken JS: Ehrlichial diseases of humans: Emerging tick-borne infections. Clin Infect Dis 1995; 20:1102.

Fishbein DB, Dennis DT: Tick-borne diseases—a growing risk. N Engl J Med 1995;333:452. (Three of the ten tick-borne diseases recognized in the USA have been recognized only in the last decade: Lyme disease and the two forms of ehrlichiosis.)

Walker DH: Emerging bacterial and zoonotic and vector borne diseases; ecological and epidemiological factors. JAMA 1996;275:463.

2. Q FEVER

Essentials of Diagnosis

- Exposure to sheep, goats, cattle, or their products is common; some infections are laboratory-acquired.

- An acute or chronic febrile illness with severe headache, cough, prostration, and abdominal pain.
- Extensive pneumonitis, hepatitis, or encephalopathy; rarely endocarditis.

General Considerations

Coxiella burnetii is unique among rickettsiae in that it is usually transmitted to humans not by arthropods but by inhalation or ingestion. It primarily infects cattle, sheep, and goats, in which it produces mild or subclinical infection. It is transmitted by cows and goats principally through the milk and placenta and by sheep through feces, placenta, and milk. Dry feces and milk, dust contaminated with them, and the tissues of these animals contain large numbers of infectious organisms that are spread by the airborne route. Inhalation of contaminated dust and of droplets from infected animal tissues is the main source of human infection. Outbreaks have been described in association with parturient cats. There is an occupational risk for animal handlers, slaughterhouse workers, veterinarians, and laboratory workers.

The route of acquisition appears to determine the main clinical syndrome; in Eastern Canada, pneumonia is the usual manifestation, whereas in France granulomatous hepatitis is more common. The French have also noted an association with HIV positivity, a finding not confirmed in Spain. Endocarditis is an uncommon but serious form of *Coxiella* infection and has been linked with immunocompromising conditions, urban residence, and raw milk ingestion. *Coxiella* is resistant to heat and drying, perhaps because the organism forms endospore-like structures. Thus, it survives in dust, on the fleece of infected animals, or in inadequately pasteurized milk. Spread from one human to another does not seem to occur even in the presence of florid pneumonitis, but maternal-fetal infection can occur.

Clinical Findings

A. Symptoms and Signs: After an incubation period of 1–3 weeks, a febrile illness develops with headache, prostration, and muscle pains, occasionally with a nonproductive cough. Physical signs of pneumonitis are slight; hepatitis is often present and may be severe. Endocarditis of the aortic valve is rare and occurs almost exclusively in the setting of preexisting valve disease or immunosuppression. Other uncommon manifestations include encephalitis, hemolytic anemia, orchitis, acute renal failure, and mediastinal lymphadenopathy. The clinical course may be acute or chronic and relapsing.

B. Laboratory Findings: Laboratory examination shows elevated liver function tests, occasionally leukocytosis, and a diagnostic rise in complement-fixing antibodies. Antibodies to phospholipids have been reported.

In Q fever endocarditis, there is an IgG titer of 1:200 or more by complement fixation or indirect immunofluorescence with IgA antibodies against phase 1 antigen of *C burnetii*. Isolation of *C burnetii* is possible using the shell-vial technique. A serum ELISA is also available.

C. Imaging: Radiographs of the chest show patchy pulmonary infiltrates.

Differential Diagnosis

Viral, mycoplasmal, and bacterial pneumonias; viral hepatitis; brucellosis; tuberculosis; psittacosis; and other animal-borne diseases must be considered. The history of exposure to animals or animal dusts or tissues (eg, in slaughterhouses) should lead to appropriate specific serologic tests. Unexplained fevers with negative blood cultures in association with vascular or cardiac disease should make one consider Q fever, especially in immunocompromised patients.

Prevention

Prevention is based on detection of the infection in livestock, reduction of contact with infected animals or dusts contaminated by them, special care when working with animal tissues, and effective pasteurization of milk. A vaccine of formalin-inactivated phase 1 *Coxiella* is being developed for persons at high risk of infection and appears to be protective. A vaccine is available in some countries for persons with high-risk exposures.

Treatment & Prognosis

Treatment with tetracyclines (25 mg/kg/d in four divided doses) can suppress symptoms and shorten the clinical course but does not always eradicate the infection. Treatment should continue through 3 full days of defervescence. Even in untreated patients, the mortality rate is usually low, except with endocarditis.

Treatment of endocarditis consists of protracted—often for years—antibiotic therapy with doxycycline (200 mg/d) and either trimethoprim-sulfamethoxazole (320/1600 mg/d) or rifampin (900 mg/d, though this drug may interact adversely with anticoagulants if they should be required), or quinolones (ofloxacin, 400 mg/d, or equivalent). Heart valves often need replacement, since the mainstays of antibiotic therapy (chloramphenicol, tetracycline) for rickettsial organisms are bacteriostatic. The combination of hydroxychloroquine and doxycycline is bactericidal in vitro, and human studies are under way.

Fournier PE et al: Modification of the diagnostic criteria proposed by the Duke Endocarditis Service to permit improved diagnosis of Q fever endocarditis. Am J Med 1996;100:629. (The sensitivity of the criteria were significantly increased by including serologic results and single blood culture as major diagnostic criteria.)

Marrie TJ et al: Route of infection determines the clinical manifestations of acute Q fever. J Infect Dis 1996; 173:484.

Montes M et al: *Coxiella burnetii* infection in subjects with HIV infection and HIV infection in patients with Q fever. Scand J Infect Dis 1995;27:344.

Raoult D, Marrie T: Q fever. Clin Infect Dis 1995;20:489.

KAWASAKI SYNDROME

Kawasaki syndrome is a worldwide multisystemic disease also known as mucocutaneous lymph node syndrome. It occurs mainly in children but occasionally in adults, at times in epidemic fashion. The epidemiology suggests an infectious origin, though no agent has been identified. Disease is probably not mediated by a bacterial toxin, though a staphylococcal toxin may serve as a "superantigen" that interacts with T cells. The disease is characterized by fever and four of the following: bilateral nonexudative conjunctivitis; mucous membrane changes of at least one type (injected pharynx, cracked lips, strawberry tongue); extremity changes of at least one type (edema, desquamation, erythema, a polymorphous rash); and cervical lymphadenopathy greater than 1.5 cm.

A major complication is arteritis of the coronary vessels, occurring in 20% of untreated cases. Factors associated with the development of coronary artery aneurysms are leukocytosis and elevated C-reactive protein. Arteritis of extremity vessels and peripheral gangrene have been reported also. The cause of these complications is likewise unknown.

Management is with aspirin (80–100 mg/kg/d in divided doses with subsequent tapering) and intravenous immune globulin in high doses. Plasmapheresis may be useful in cases unresponsive to immune globulin. Corticosteroids are thought to increase the likelihood of development of coronary aneurysms.

Shulman ST et al: Kawasaki disease. Pediatr Clin North Am 1995;42:1205. (A reminder that this is a very common cause of acquired pediatric heart disease in America.)

Terai M et al: The absence of evidence of a staphylococcal toxin involved in the pathogenesis of Kawasaki disease. J Infect Dis 1995;172:558.

Infectious Diseases: Bacterial & Chlamydial

33

Henry F. Chambers, MD

INFECTIONS CAUSED BY GRAM-POSITIVE BACTERIA

STREPTOCOCCAL INFECTIONS

1. PHARYNGITIS

Essentials of Diagnosis

- Abrupt onset of sore throat, fever, malaise, nausea, and headache.
- Throat red and edematous, with or without exudate; cervical nodes tender.
- Diagnosis confirmed by culture of throat.

General Considerations

Beta-hemolytic streptococci, classically group A, are the most common bacterial cause of exudative pharyngitis. Transmission is by droplets of infected secretions. Group A streptococci producing erythrogenic toxin may cause scarlet fever rashes in susceptible persons.

Clinical Findings

A. Symptoms and Signs: "Strep throat" is characterized by a sudden onset of fever, sore throat, pain on swallowing, tender cervical adenopathy, malaise, and nausea. The pharynx, soft palate, and tonsils are red and edematous, and there may be a purulent exudate. The rash of scarlet fever is diffusely erythematous, resembling a sunburn, with superimposed fine red papules, and is most intense in the groin and axillas. It blanches on pressure, may become petechial, and fades in 2–5 days, leaving a fine desquamation. In scarlet fever, the face is flushed, with circumoral pallor; and the tongue is coated, with enlarged red papillae (strawberry tongue).

B. Laboratory Findings: Leukocytosis with an increase in polymorphonuclear neutrophils is common. Throat culture onto a single blood agar plate has a sensitivity of 70–80%. Currently available rapid diagnostic tests, which are based on detection of streptococcal antigen, are generally less sensitive than culture.

Complications

The suppurative complications of streptococcal sore throat include sinusitis, otitis media, mastoiditis, peritonsillar abscess, and suppuration of cervical lymph nodes, among others.

Nonsuppurative complications are rheumatic fever and glomerulonephritis. Rheumatic fever may follow recurrent episodes of pharyngitis beginning 1–4 weeks after the onset of symptoms. Glomerulonephritis follows a single infection with a nephritogenic strain of *Streptococcus* group A (eg, types 4, 12, 2, 49, and 60), more commonly on the skin than in the throat, and begins 1–3 weeks after the onset of the infection.

Differential Diagnosis

Streptococcal sore throat resembles (and cannot be reliably distinguished clinically from) pharyngitis caused by adenoviruses, Epstein-Barr virus, and other agents. Pharyngitis and lymphadenopathy are common findings in primary HIV infection. Generalized lymphadenopathy, splenomegaly, atypical lymphocytosis, and a positive serologic test (eg, Monospot) distinguish mononucleosis from streptococcal pharyngitis. Diphtheria is characterized by a pseudomembrane; candidiasis shows white patches of exudate and less erythema; and necrotizing ulcerative gingivostomatitis (Vincent's fusospirochetal disease) presents with shallow ulcers in the mouth. Bacterial epiglottitis with odynophagia and difficulty handling secretions should be considered when severity of symptoms is disproportionate to findings on examination of the pharynx.

Treatment

Antimicrobial therapy has a minimal effect on resolution of symptoms. Because its main purpose is prevention of complications, therapy may be withheld pending results of culture. Because throat culture (especially if a single plate is used) and rapid detection methods may be falsely negative in 30% or more of cases, when clinical suspicion is high (eg, presence of exudative pharyngitis, tender adenopathy, high fever, and absence of cough and rhinorrhea) and the risk of therapy is low (eg, no drug allergy), antimicrobial therapy may be given without laboratory evaluation.

A. Benzathine penicillin G, 1.2 million units intramuscularly as a single dose, is optimal therapy.

B. Penicillin V potassium, 500 mg orally four times a day (or amoxicillin, 150–500 mg orally three times a day) for 10 days, is effective, but compliance may be poor after the patient becomes asymptomatic in 2–4 days.

C. Patients allergic to penicillin may be treated with erythromycin, 0.5 g four times daily (40 mg/kg/d) for 10 days.

D. Azithromycin, 500 mg (10 mg/kg in children) once daily for 3 days, is an alternative. This regimen is less effective than penicillin in eradication of organisms from the pharynx, but the clinical response probably is similar—though Pacifico et al (1996) found azithromycin to be clinically less effective than penicillin.

Prevention of Recurrent Rheumatic Fever

Effectively controlling rheumatic fever depends upon identification and treatment of primary streptococcal infection and secondary prevention of recurrences. Patients who have had rheumatic fever should be treated with a continuous course of antimicrobial prophylaxis for at least 5 years. Effective alternative regimens are erythromycin, 250 mg orally twice daily, and penicillin G, 500 mg orally daily.

Bisno AL: Acute rheumatic fever: A present day perspective. Medicine 1993;72:278. (The history of rheumatic fever, its diagnosis, and its recent resurgence.)

Carroll K, Reimer L: Microbiology and laboratory diagnosis of upper respiratory tract infections. Clin Infect Dis 1996;23:442. (Microbial causes of pharyngitis and accuracy of various diagnostic tests.)

Pacifico L et al: Comparative efficacy and safety of 3-day azithromycin and 10-day penicillin V treatment of group A beta-hemolytic streptococcal pharyngitis in children. Antimicrob Agents Chemother 1996;40:1005. (Bacteriologic cure rate [54%] and clinical response rate [75%] for azithromycin are inferior compared with penicillin [86% and 91%, respectively].)

Perkins A: An approach to diagnosing the acute sore throat. Am Fam Physician 1997;55:131, 141.

Schaad UB, Heynen G: Evaluation of the efficacy, safety and toleration of azithromycin vs. penicillin V in the treatment of acute streptococcal pharyngitis in children: Results of a multicenter, open comparative study. Pediatr Infect Dis J 1996;15:791. (Multicenter trial in 343 children comparing 10 days of penicillin to 3 days of azithromycin; clinical response rates were similar, but 35–45% of azithromycin-treated patients were culture-positive after treatment compared with 18–20% of penicillin-treated patients.)

2. STREPTOCOCCAL SKIN INFECTIONS

Streptococci are not part of normal skin flora. Streptococcal skin infections usually result from colonization of normal skin by contact with other infected individuals or by preceding streptococcal respiratory infection.

Clinical Findings

A. Symptoms and Signs: Impetigo is a focal, vesicular, pustular lesion with a thick, amber-colored crust that has a "stuck-on" appearance.

Erysipelas is a painful superficial cellulitis that frequently involves the face. It is well demarcated from the surrounding normal skin. Erysipelas also affects skin with impaired lymphatic drainage, such as edematous lower extremities or wounds.

B. Laboratory Findings: Cultures obtained from a wound or pustule are likely to grow group A streptococci. Other cultures of the skin (eg, direct cultures or tissue fluid aspirated from an area of cellulitis or erysipelas) may be positive if the specimen is obtained from the leading edge of the lesion. Blood cultures are occasionally positive.

Treatment

Parenteral antibiotics are indicated for patients with facial erysipelas or evidence of systemic infection. Penicillin, 2 million units intravenously every 4 hours, is the drug of choice.

Cutaneous infections caused by staphylococci may at times be difficult to differentiate from streptococcal infections. Coinfection with staphylococci also occurs. Therefore, initial therapy for severely ill patients or those who have risk factors for staphylococcal infection (eg, intravenous drug use, wound infection, diabetes) should include an agent—such as nafcillin, 1.5 g intravenously every 6 hours—that also is active against *Staphylococcus aureus*. In the patient with minor penicillin allergy, cefazolin, 500 mg intravenously or intramuscularly every 8 hours, may be used. In the patient with a serious penicillin allergy (ie, anaphylaxis), vancomycin, 1000 mg intravenously every 12 hours, should be used.

Patients who do not require parenteral therapy may be treated with penicillin V potassium, 500 mg orally, or erythromycin, 500 mg orally, four times daily for 7–10 days.

Bisno AL, Stevens DL: Streptococcal infections of skin and soft tissue. N Engl J Med 1996;334:240.

3. OTHER GROUP A STREPTOCOCCAL INFECTIONS

Arthritis, pneumonia, empyema, endocarditis, and necrotizing fasciitis are relatively uncommon infections that may be caused by group A streptococci. A toxic shock-like syndrome also occurs.

Arthritis generally occurs in association with cellulitis. In addition to intravenous therapy with penicillin G, 2 million units every 4 hours (or cefazolin or vancomycin in doses recommended above for penicillin-allergic patients), frequent percutaneous needle aspiration should be performed to remove joint effusions. Open surgical drainage usually is not necessary unless the hip or shoulder is infected, because these are less amenable to percutaneous drainage.

Pneumonia and **empyema** often are characterized by extensive tissue destruction and an aggressive, rapidly progressive clinical course associated with significant morbidity and mortality rates. High-dose penicillin and chest tube drainage are indicated for treatment of empyema. Vancomycin is an acceptable substitute in penicillin-allergic patients.

Group A streptococci can cause **endocarditis.** This complication should be suspected when bacteremia accompanies pneumonia, particularly if the patient abuses parenteral drugs. The tricuspid valve is most commonly involved. A patient with suspected endocarditis should be treated with 4 million units of penicillin G every 4 hours for 4 weeks. Vancomycin, 1000 mg every 12 hours, is recommended for persons allergic to penicillin.

Necrotizing fasciitis is a rapidly spreading infection involving the fascia of deep muscle. The clinical findings at presentation may be those of severe cellulitis, but the presence of systemic toxicity and severe pain, which may be followed by anesthesia of the involved area due to destruction of nerves as infection advances through the fascial planes, are important clues to the diagnosis. Surgical exploration is mandatory when the diagnosis is suspected. Early and extensive debridement is essential for survival.

Any streptococcal infection—and necrotizing fasciitis in particular—can be associated with **streptococcal toxic shock-like syndrome,** characterized by invasion of skin or soft tissues, acute respiratory distress syndrome, and renal failure. The very young, the elderly, and those with underlying medical conditions are at particularly high risk for invasive disease. Bacteremia, which is uncommon in staphylococcal toxic shock syndrome, occurs in the majority of cases. Skin rash and desquamation may not be present. Mortality rates up to 80% have been reported for patients with the full-blown syndrome. The syndrome is due to elaboration of pyrogenic erythrotoxin (which also causes **scarlet fever**), a superantigen that stimulates massive release of inflammatory cytokines felt to mediate the shock. Clindamycin—but not penicillin—inhibits toxin production.

Penicillin remains the drug of choice for treatment of serious streptococcal infections, but some authorities recommend adding clindamycin (600 mg every 8 hours intravenously) to the regimen. Outbreaks of invasive disease have been associated with colonization by invasive clones that can be transmitted to close contacts who, though asymptomatic, may be a reservoir for disease. Tracing contacts of patients with invasive disease is controversial.

Bisno AL, Stevens DL: Streptococcal infections of skin and soft tissue. N Engl J Med 1996;334:240.

Brook I, Frazier EH: Clinical and microbiological features of necrotizing fasciitis. J Clin Microbiol 1995;33:2382.

Cockerill FR 3rd et al: An outbreak of invasive group A streptococcal disease associated with high carriage rates of the invasive clone among school-aged children. JAMA 1997;277:38. (A clonal outbreak and the role of colonization is described.)

Davies HD et al: Invasive group A streptococcal infections in Ontario, Canada. Ontario Group A Streptococcal Study Group. N Engl J Med 1996;335:547. (Risk factors, including risk to household contacts of cases, and mortality rates for toxic shock-like syndrome and other invasive streptococcal infections are reported.)

Forni AL et al: Clinical and microbiological characteristics of severe group A streptococcus infections and streptococcal toxic shock syndrome. Clin Infect Dis 1995; 21:333.

4. NON-GROUP A STREPTOCOCCAL INFECTIONS

Non-group A streptococci produce a spectrum of disease similar to that of group A streptococci. Some non-group A streptococci are β-hemolytic (eg, groups B, C, and G). The treatment of infections caused by these strains is the same as for group A streptococci.

Group B streptococci are an important cause of sepsis, bacteremia, and meningitis in the neonate. This organism, which is part of the normal vaginal flora, may cause septic abortion, endometritis, or peripartum infections and, less commonly, cellulitis, bacteremia, and endocarditis in adults. Treatment of infections caused by group B streptococci is with either penicillin or vancomycin in doses recommended for group A streptococci. Because of in vitro synergism, some authorities recommend the addition of low-dose gentamicin, 1 mg/kg every 8 hours.

Viridans streptococci, which are nonhemolytic or α-hemolytic (ie, producing a green zone of hemolysis on blood agar), are part of the normal oral flora. Although these strains may produce focal pyogenic infection, they are most notable as the leading cause of native valve endocarditis (see below).

Group D streptococci include *Streptococcus bovis* and the enterococci. *S bovis* is a cause of endocarditis in association with bowel neoplasia or cirrhosis. Endocarditis caused by *S bovis* is treated like viridans streptococci.

ENTEROCOCCAL INFECTIONS

Enterococci have been classified into a genus separate from other streptococci. Two species, *Enterococcus faecalis* and *Enterococcus faecium,* are responsible for most human enterococcal infections. Enterococci cause wound infections, urinary tract infections, and endocarditis. Except for serious infections such as meningitis, endocarditis, bacteremia in the immunocompromised host, and osteomyelitis, most enterococcal infections can still be treated with penicillin, 3 million units every 4 hours; ampicillin (which is slightly more active than penicillin in vitro), 2 g every 6 hours; or vancomycin, 1 g every 12 hours. Because these antibiotics are not bactericidal for enterococci, gentamicin in a dose of 1 mg/kg every 8 hours is added for treatment of endocarditis or other serious infection.

Enterococci, which are intrinsically resistant to multiple antibiotics, have until recently been susceptible to penicillin, vancomycin, and gentamicin. Strains that are resistant to all known antibiotics are now being encountered, and nosocomial outbreaks of infection caused by strains resistant to gentamicin or vancomycin are increasingly common. It is essential to determine antimicrobial susceptibility of clinical isolates in order to detect these resistant organisms. Infection control measures that may be indicated to limit their spread include isolation, strict adherence to barrier precautions, and avoidance of overuse of vancomycin and gentamicin. Optimal therapy for infection caused by vancomycin- and gentamicin-resistant strains is not known, but some are susceptible in vitro to fluoroquinolones, rifampin, or teicoplanin. Synercid, an investigational streptogramin combination agent, may be effective against vancomycin-resistant enterococci.

Dever LL et al: Treatment of vancomycin-resistant *Enterococcus faecium* infections with an investigational streptogramin antibiotic (quinupristin/dalfopristin); a report of fifteen cases. Microb Drug Resist 1996;2:407.

Preventing the spread of vancomycin resistance: Report from the Hospital Infection Control Practices Advisory Committee. Federal Register 1994;59:25758. (Recommendations for surveillance, susceptibility testing, screening, and infection control measures.)

PNEUMOCOCCAL INFECTIONS

1. PNEUMOCOCCAL PNEUMONIA

Essentials of Diagnosis

- Productive cough, fever, rigors, dyspnea, early pleuritic chest pain.
- Consolidating lobar pneumonia on chest x-ray.
- Lancet-shaped gram-positive diplococci on Gram stain of sputum.

General Considerations

The pneumococcus is the most common cause of community-acquired pyogenic bacterial pneumonia. Alcoholism, infection by HIV, sickle cell disease, splenectomy, and hematologic disorders are predisposing factors. The mortality rate remains high in the setting of advanced age, multilobar disease, severe hypoxemia, extrapulmonary complications, and bacteremia.

Clinical Findings

A. Symptoms and Signs: The illness typically evolves over a period of a few days. The patient presents with high fever, productive cough, occasionally hemoptysis, and pleuritic chest pain, features that distinguish it from mycoplasmal or pneumocystis pneumonia. Rigors occur within the first few hours of infection but are uncommon thereafter. Bronchial breathing is an early sign.

B. Laboratory Findings: Classically, pneumococcal pneumonia is a lobar pneumonia with radiographic signs of consolidation and occasionally effusion. Infiltrates may also be patchy.

Gram's stain of sputum always should be examined. Adequately collected samples (with < 10 epithelial cells and > 25 polymorphonuclear leukocytes per high-power field) show gram-positive diplococci 80–90% of the time. Sputum culture alone is less sensitive than Gram's stain, and false positives are common as well. Blood cultures are positive in up to 25% of selected cases and much more commonly so in HIV-positive patients.

Complications

Parapneumonic (sympathetic) effusion is common and may cause recurrence or persistence of fever. These sterile fluid accumulations need no specific therapy. Empyema occurs in 5% or less of cases and is differentiated from sympathetic effusion by the presence of organisms on Gram-stained fluid or positive pleural fluid cultures.

Pneumococcal pericarditis is a rare complication that can cause tamponade. Pneumococcal arthritis also is uncommon. Pneumococcal endocarditis usually involves the aortic valve and often occurs in association with meningitis and pneumonia. Early heart failure and multiple embolic events are typical.

Treatment

A. Specific Measures: Uncomplicated pneumococcal pneumonia (ie, arterial Po_2 > 60 mm Hg, no coexisting medical problems, and single-lobe disease without signs of extrapulmonary infection) may be treated on an outpatient basis with penicillin V potassium, 500 mg orally four times a day for 7–10 days. For penicillin-allergic patients, any of the following regimens may be used: erythromycin, 500 mg orally four times a day; trimethoprim-sulfamethoxazole, one double-strength tablet (320 mg trimethoprim and 1600 mg sulfamethoxazole) orally twice a day; or azithromycin, one 500 mg dose on the first day and 250 mg once a day for the next 4 days. Patients should be followed for clinical response (eg, less cough, defervescence within 2–3 days) because pneumococci may be resistant to penicillin or any of the second-line agents. Lack of clinical response may indicate infection with a resistant strain, and hospitalization should be considered.

More seriously ill patients or those with other medical problems should be admitted and treated parenterally with aqueous penicillin G, 2 million units intravenously every 4 hours. A low-dose regimen of procaine penicillin, 600,000 units intramuscularly every 12 hours, is effective for pneumonia caused by penicillin-susceptible strains; however, because 10% or more of pneumococcal isolates are of intermediate or high-level resistance, higher doses of penicillin are recommended until susceptibility of the isolate is known. For penicillin-allergic patients without anaphylaxis or other serious reactions, cefazolin, 500 mg either intravenously or intramuscularly every 8 hours, is effective. For serious penicillin or cephalosporin allergy or infection caused by a highly penicillin-resistant strain (MIC > 1 μg/mL), vancomycin, 30 mg/kg/d, up to 2000 mg total, in two divided doses, can be used. Trimethoprim-sulfamethoxazole given intravenously in amounts providing 10 mg/kg/d of the trimethoprim component divided into three doses also is effective.

B. Treatment of Complications: Pleural effusions developing after initiation of antimicrobial therapy usually are sterile, and thoracentesis need not be performed if the patient is otherwise improving. Thoracentesis is indicated for an effusion that is present prior to initiation of therapy and in the patient who has significant fever or who otherwise has not responded to antibiotics after 3–4 days. Chest tube drainage may be required if pneumococci are identified by culture or Gram stain.

Echocardiography should be done if pericardial effusion is suspected. Patients with pericardial effusion who are responding to therapy and have no signs of tamponade may be followed and treated with indomethacin, 50 mg three times daily, for pain. In patients with increasing effusion, unsatisfactory clinical response, or evidence of tamponade, pericardiocentesis will determine if the pericardial space is infected. Infected fluid must be drained either percutaneously (by tube placement or needle aspiration), by placement of a pericardial window, or by pericardiectomy. Pericardiectomy eventually may be required to prevent or treat constrictive pericarditis, a common sequela of bacterial pericarditis.

Endocarditis should be treated with 24 million units of penicillin G (or vancomycin for penicillin-allergic patients) daily for 3–4 weeks. Mild heart failure may respond to medical therapy alone, such as digoxin and diuretics, but moderate to severe heart failure is an indication for prosthetic valve implantation, as are systemic emboli or large friable vegetations as determined by echocardiography.

C. Penicillin-Resistant Pneumococci: The prevalence of penicillin-resistant pneumococci (MIC > 0.1 μg/mL) in the United States is increasing, accounting for 10–15% of bloodstream isolates in some regions. All blood and cerebrospinal fluid isolates should be tested for resistance to penicillin. The 1 μg oxacillin disk diffusion assay is an easily performed, reliable screen for resistance. Pneumonia caused by intermediately resistant strains (penicillin MIC > 0.1 μg/mL but ≤ 1 μg/mL) generally will respond to high-dose penicillin therapy. High-dose penicillin also may be effective for infections other than meningitis caused by highly penicillin-resistant strains (MIC > 1 μg/mL). However, some authorities recommend that ceftriaxone, 2 g once daily, cefotaxime 3 g every 6 hours, or vancomycin, 1 g every 12 hours be used instead, especially for immunocompromised patients, because of superior in vitro activity and a more favorable ratio between serum drug concentration and MIC. Penicillin-resistant strains of pneumococci may be resistant to multiple antibiotics, including erythromycin, azithromycin, clarithromycin, trimethoprim-sulfamethoxazole, and chloramphenicol, and susceptibility to these agents must be documented prior to their use.

Friedland IR, McCracken GH Jr: Management of infections caused by antibiotic-resistant *Streptococcus pneumoniae.* N Engl J Med 1994;331:377. (Excellent review of the literature concerning treatment of infections caused by penicillin-resistant pneumococci with specific recommendations for therapy.)

Gilks CF et al: Invasive pneumococcal disease in a cohort of predominantly HIV-1 infected female sex-workers in Nairobi, Kenya. Lancet 1996;347:718. (The clinical features of pneumococcal disease, including the unusual finding of bacteremia without a source.)

Niederman MS et al: Guidelines for the initial management of adults with community-acquired pneumonia: Diagnosis, assessment of severity, and initial antimicrobial therapy. Am Rev Respir Dis 1993;148:1418. (Recommendations of American Thoracic Society for diagnosis, management, and therapy of patients with community-acquired pneumonia; includes an excellent discussion of etiology.)

2. PNEUMOCOCCAL MENINGITIS

Essentials of Diagnosis

- Fever, headache, altered mental status.
- Meningismus.
- Gram-positive diplococci on Gram stain of cerebrospinal fluid; counterimmunoelectrophoresis may be positive in partially treated cases.

General Considerations

Streptococcus pneumoniae is the most common

cause of meningitis in adults and the second most common cause of meningitis in children over the age of 6 years. Head trauma, cerebrospinal fluid leaks, and sinusitis may precede pneumococcal meningitis.

Clinical Findings

A. Symptoms and Signs: The onset is rapid, with fever, headache, and altered mentation. Pneumonia may be present. Compared with meningitis caused by the meningococcus, pneumococcal meningitis lacks a rash, and focal neurologic deficits, cranial nerve palsies, and obtundation are more prominent features.

B. Laboratory Findings: The cerebrospinal fluid typically has more than 1000 white blood cells per microliter, over 60% of which are polymorphonuclear leukocytes; the glucose concentration is less than 40 mg/dL, or less than 50% of the simultaneous serum concentration; the protein usually exceeds 150 mg/dL. Not all cases of meningitis will have these typical findings, and alterations in cerebrospinal fluid cell counts and chemistries may be surprisingly minimal, overlapping with those of aseptic meningitis.

Gram stain of cerebrospinal fluid shows gram-positive cocci in 80–90% of cases, and in untreated cases blood or cerebrospinal fluid cultures are almost always positive. Tests such as counterimmunoelectrophoresis or latex agglutination to detect pneumococcal antigens in cerebrospinal fluid are less sensitive than culture and Gram stain. Antigen detection tests may occasionally be helpful in establishing the diagnosis in the patient who has been partially treated and in whom cultures and stains are negative.

Treatment

Antibiotics should be given as soon as the diagnosis of meningitis is suspected. If lumbar puncture must be delayed (eg, while awaiting results of an imaging study to exclude a mass lesion), ceftriaxone, 4 g, is given intravenously after blood cultures (positive in 50% of cases) have been obtained. Ceftriaxone is preferred as initial therapy instead of penicillin pending determination of in vitro susceptibility because of the recent increased prevalence of penicillin-resistant strains of pneumococci. In the penicillin-allergic patient, chloramphenicol, 1.5 g every 6 hours, may be used, but some penicillin-resistant strains are also resistant to this antibiotic. Once susceptibility has been confirmed, penicillin, 24 million units daily in six divided doses, ceftriaxone, 4 g/d, or chloramphenicol, 6 g/d in four divided doses, is continued for 10–14 days in documented cases.

The best therapy for penicillin-resistant strains is not known. Penicillin-resistant strains often are cross-resistant to the third-generation cephalosporins as well as other antibiotics. Susceptibility testing is essential to proper management of this infection.

Treatment failures have been reported with ceftriaxone or cefotaxime for meningitis caused by strains with penicillin MICs ≥ 2 μg/mL. If the MIC of ceftriaxone or cefotaxime is ≤ 0.5 μg/mL, single-drug therapy with either of these cephalosporins is likely to be effective. If the MIC is ≥ 1 μg/mL, treatment with a combination of ceftriaxone, 2 g every 12 hours, plus either rifampin, 10 mg/kg/d (up to 600 mg/d) intravenously, or vancomycin, 30 mg/kg/d (up to 2 g/d) in two to four divided doses, is recommended. Experimental data from animal models also suggest that a ceftriaxone-rifampin or ceftriaxone-vancomycin combination is effective. If a patient with a penicillin-resistant organism has not responded clinically to therapy with a third-generation cephalosporin, repeat lumbar puncture is indicated to assess the bacteriologic response.

The role of steroids in adjunctive therapy of meningitis in the adult remains controversial. Dexamethasone, 0.15 mg/kg intravenously every 6 hours, may be given when coma, focal deficits, and other signs of increased intracranial pressure are present. Dexamethasone may interfere with the penetration of vancomycin (in adults but not in children) and, to a lesser extent, ceftriaxone into cerebrospinal fluid, which could adversely affect the efficacy of these drugs in meningitis caused by penicillin-resistant strains.

Durand ML et al: Acute bacterial meningitis in adults: A review of 493 episodes. N Engl J Med 1993;328:21. (Analysis of microbiology, morbidity, mortality, and risk factors.)

John C: Treatment failure with use of a third-generation cephalosporin for penicillin-resistant pneumococcal meningitis: Case report and review. Clin Infect Dis 1994;18:188. (Review of the experience with cefotaxime and ceftriaxone for treatment of meningitis caused by penicillin-resistant pneumococci.)

Quagiliarello V, Scheld WM: Treatment of bacterial meningitis. N Engl J Med 1997;336:708.

STAPHYLOCOCCUS AUREUS INFECTIONS

1. SKIN & SOFT TISSUE INFECTIONS

Essentials of Diagnosis

- Localized erythema with induration.
- Tendency toward abscess formation.
- Folliculitis commonly observed.
- Gram stain of pus with gram-positive cocci in clusters; cultures usually positive.

General Considerations

Most staphylococci found on cultures of normal skin belong to the *Staphylococcus epidermidis* group. *Staphylococcus aureus* is not normal skin flora. *S au-*

reus tends to cause more localized skin infections than streptococci, and abscess formation is common.

Clinical Findings

A. Symptoms and Signs: *S aureus* skin infections may begin around one or more hair follicles, causing folliculitis. These infections may localize to form boils (or furuncles) or spread to adjacent skin and deeper subcutaneous tissue (ie, a carbuncle). Myositis or fasciitis may occur, often in association with a deep wound or other inoculation or injection.

B. Laboratory Findings: Cultures of the wound or abscess material will almost always yield the organism. In patients with other systemic signs of infection, blood cultures should be obtained because of potential endocarditis, osteomyelitis, or metastatic seeding of other sites.

Treatment

Proper drainage of abscess fluid or other focal infections is the mainstay of therapy. Drainage may be all that is needed for cutaneous abscess. Antibiotic therapy alone is unlikely to be effective if collections of infected material are undrained.

For uncomplicated skin infections, oral therapy is satisfactory. An oral penicillinase-resistant penicillin or cephalosporin, such as dicloxacillin or cephalexin, 500 mg four times a day for 7–10 days, is the drug of choice. Erythromycin, 500 mg four times a day, may be used in the penicillin-allergic patient, although the prevalence of erythromycin-resistant strains makes this regimen less attractive empirically.

For more complicated infections with extensive cutaneous or deep tissue involvement or fever, parenteral therapy is indicated initially. A penicillinase-resistant penicillin such as nafcillin or oxacillin in a dosage of 1.5 g every 6 hours intravenously is the drug of choice. In allergic patients without a serious reaction, cefazolin, 0.5–1 g intravenously or intramuscularly every 8 hours, can be used. In patients with a serious allergy to β-lactam antibiotics or if the strain is methicillin-resistant, vancomycin, 1000 mg intravenously every 12 hours, is the drug of choice.

2. OSTEOMYELITIS

S aureus is the cause of approximately 60% of all cases of osteomyelitis. Osteomyelitis may be caused by direct inoculation, eg, from an open fracture or as a result of surgery; by extension from a contiguous focus of infection or open wound; or, more commonly, by hematogenous spread. Long bones and vertebrae are the usual sites. Epidural abscess with or without bone involvement is a common complication of vertebral osteomyelitis and should be suspected if fever and back pain are accompanied by radicular pain or neurologic signs or symptoms indicative of spinal cord compression (eg, incontinence).

Clinical Findings

A. Symptoms and Signs: The infection may be acute, with abrupt development of local symptoms and systemic toxicity; or indolent, with insidious onset of vague pain over the site of infection, progressing to local tenderness. Fever is absent in one-third or more of cases. Abscess formation is a late and unusual manifestation. Draining sinus tracts occur in chronic infections or infections of foreign body implants.

B. Laboratory Findings: The diagnosis is established by isolation of *S aureus* from the blood or bone of a patient with signs and symptoms of focal bone infection. Blood culture will be positive in approximately 60% of untreated cases of staphylococcal osteomyelitis. Bone biopsy and culture should be considered if blood cultures are sterile.

C. Imaging: Bone scan and gallium scan, each with a sensitivity of approximately 95% and a specificity of 60–70%, are useful in identifying or confirming the site of bone infection. Plain bone films early in the course of infection are often normal but will become abnormal in most cases even with effective therapy. Spinal infection (unlike malignancy) traverses the disk space to involve the contiguous vertebral body. CT is more sensitive than plain films and can be useful in localizing associated abscesses. MRI is somewhat less sensitive than bone scan but has a specificity of 90%. MRI is indicated when epidural abscess is suspected in association with vertebral osteomyelitis.

Treatment

Prolonged therapy is required to cure staphylococcal osteomyelitis. Durations of 4–6 weeks or longer are recommended. Although oral regimens can be effective, parenteral regimens are advised during the acute phase of the infection for patients with systemic toxicity. Nafcillin or oxacillin, 9–12 g/d in six divided doses, is the drug of choice. Cefazolin, 1 g every 8 hours, also is effective. Vancomycin, 1 g every 12 hours, may be used for the penicillin-allergic patient.

Oral regimens are dicloxacillin or cephalexin, 1 g every 6 hours. Ciprofloxacin, 750 mg twice a day, may be an effective alternative. Some authorities recommend that rifampin be added to the regimen for treatment of staphylococcal osteomyelitis. The dose is 300 mg twice a day.

Aliabaldi P, Nikpoor N: Imaging osteomyelitis. Arthritis Rheum 1994;37:617.

Dirschl DR, Almekinders LC: Osteomyelitis: Common causes and treatment recommendations. Drugs 1993; 45:29.

Torda AJ, Gottlieb T, Bradbury R: Pyogenic vertebral osteomyelitis: Analysis of 20 cases and review. Clin Infect Dis 1995;20:320. (Nosocomial infection and *S aureus* etiology are predominant features. Utility of various imaging modalities is reviewed.)

3. STAPHYLOCOCCAL BACTEREMIA

S aureus readily invades the bloodstream and infects sites distant from the primary site of infection, which may be relatively minor or even inapparent. Though commonly arising from skin lesions or intravenous lines, whenever *S aureus* is recovered from blood cultures, the possibility of endocarditis, osteomyelitis, or other metastatic deep infection must be considered. The appropriate duration of therapy for uncomplicated bacteremia arising from a removable source (eg, intravenous device) or drainable focus (eg, skin abscess) has not been well defined, but at least 10–14 days of parenteral therapy appear to be the minimum. However, approximately 5% or more of patients still relapse, usually with endocarditis or osteomyelitis, even if treated for 2 weeks.

Because of this tendency—and based on the impression that longer courses of therapy reduce the relapse rate—10–14 days of nafcillin or oxacillin, 1.5 g intravenously every four to six hours, cefazolin, 500–1000 mg every 8 hours, or vancomycin, 1000 mg every 12 hours, is recommended for uncomplicated staphylococcal bacteremia. Vancomycin should be reserved for patients with serious penicillin allergy or with infections caused by methicillin-resistant strains because of data suggesting that it is less active than β-lactam antibiotics. Longer courses of either parenteral or oral therapy may be considered for patients (eg, those with diabetes, immunocompromised persons) at risk for late complications from bacteremia and for those in whom endocarditis is suspected.

Jernigan JA, Farr BM: Short-course therapy of catheter-related *Staphylococcus aureus* bacteremia: A meta-analysis. Ann Intern Med 1993;119:304. (The optimal duration of therapy remains unknown.)

Malanoski GJ et al: *Staphylococcus aureus* catheter-associated bacteremia. Arch Intern Med 1995;155:1161.

4. TOXIC SHOCK SYNDROME

Some strains of staphylococci elaborate toxins that can cause three important entities: "scalded skin syndrome" in children, toxic shock syndrome in adults, and enterotoxin food poisoning. Toxic shock syndrome is characterized by abrupt onset of high fever, vomiting, and watery diarrhea. Sore throat, myalgias, and headache are common. Hypotension with renal and cardiac failure is an ominous manifestation in severe cases. A diffuse macular erythematous rash and nonpurulent conjunctivitis are common, and desquamation, especially of palms and soles, is typical during recovery. Fatality rates may be as high as 15%. Although toxic shock syndrome has occurred in children and in males, most cases (90% or more) have been reported in women of childbearing age. Of these, symptoms begin in nearly all patients within 5 days of the onset of a menstrual period in women who have used tampons. The syndrome is possible in any patient with a focus of toxin-producing *S aureus.* Nonmenstrual cases of toxic shock syndrome are now about as common as menstrual cases. Organisms from various sites, including the nasopharynx, vagina, or rectum or from wounds, have all been associated with the illness. Toxic shock syndrome is most often caused by toxic shock syndrome toxin-1 (TSST-1). Nonmenstrual cases of toxic shock syndrome are frequently caused by strains that do not produce TSST-1. Blood cultures are negative, because symptoms are due to the effects of the toxin and not to the invasive properties of the organism.

Important aspects of treatment include rapid rehydration, antistaphylococcal drugs, management of renal or cardiac insufficiency, and removal of sources of toxin, eg, removal of tampon, drainage of abscess.

Strausbaugh LJ: Toxic shock syndrome. Are you recognizing its changing presentations? Postgrad Med 1993;94:107. (Review of clinical presentation of nonmenstrual toxic shock syndrome.)

5. INFECTIONS CAUSED BY COAGULASE-NEGATIVE STAPHYLOCOCCI

Coagulase-negative staphylococci are an important cause of infections of intravascular and prosthetic devices and of wound infection following cardiothoracic surgery. On rare occasions, these organisms can cause infections such as osteomyelitis and endocarditis in the absence of a prosthesis. More than 20 species have been identified, but most human infections are caused by *Staphylococcus epidermidis, S haemolyticus, S hominis, S warnerii, S saprophyticus, S saccharolyticus,* and *S cohnii.* These common nosocomial pathogens are less virulent than *S aureus,* and infections caused by them tend to be more indolent.

Because coagulase-negative staphylococci are normal inhabitants of human skin, it can be difficult to determine whether their isolation is caused by infection or contamination, the latter perhaps accounting for three-fourths of blood culture isolates. Infection is more likely if the patient has a foreign body (eg, sternal wires, prosthetic joint, prosthetic cardiac valve, intracranial pressure monitor, cerebrospinal fluid shunt, peritoneal dialysis catheter) or an intravascular device in place. Purulent or serosanguineous drainage, erythema, pain, or tenderness at the site of the foreign body or device suggests infection. Instability and pain are signs of prosthetic joint infection. Fever, a new murmur, instability of the prosthesis, or signs of systemic embolization are evidence of prosthetic valve infection. Immunosuppression and recent antimicrobial therapy also are risk factors for infection.

Infection is also more likely if the same strain is consistently isolated from two or more blood cultures (particularly if samples were obtained at different times) and from the foreign body site. Contamination rather than infection is favored by a single positive blood culture or if more than one strain is isolated from blood cultures. The antimicrobial susceptibility pattern and speciation—also called biotyping—is commonly used to determine whether one or more strains have been isolated. More sophisticated typing methods, such as plasmid pattern analysis or restriction endonuclease pattern analysis, may be required to identify distinct strains.

Whenever possible, the intravascular device or foreign body suspected of being infected by coagulase-negative staphylococci should be removed. However, removal and replacement of some devices (eg, prosthetic joint, prosthetic valve, cerebrospinal fluid shunt) can be a difficult or risky procedure, and it may sometimes be preferable to treat with antibiotics alone with the understanding that the probability of cure is low and that surgical management may eventually be necessary.

Coagulase-negative staphylococci are commonly resistant to methicillin and multiple other antibiotics. For patients with normal renal function, vancomycin, 1 g intravenously every 12 hours, is the treatment of choice for suspected or confirmed infection caused by these organisms until susceptibility to penicillinase-resistant penicillins or other agents has been confirmed. Duration of therapy has not been established for relatively uncomplicated infections, such as those secondary to intravenous devices, which may be eliminated by simply removing the infected device. Infection involving bone or a prosthetic valve should be treated for 6 weeks. A combination regimen of vancomycin plus rifampin, 300 mg orally twice daily, and gentamicin, 1 mg/kg intravenously every 8 hours, is recommended for treatment of prosthetic valve endocarditis caused by methicillin-resistant strains.

Herwaldt LA et al: The positive predictive value of isolating coagulase-negative staphylococci from blood cultures. Clin Infect Dis 1996;22:14. (Twenty-six percent of 227 episodes of blood cultures growing coagulase-negative staphylococci represented true bacteremia. Risk factors associated with true infection are discussed.)

L'Ecuyer PB et al: The epidemiology of chest and leg wound infections following cardiothoracic surgery. Clin Infect Dis 1996;22:424. (Coagulase-negative staphylococci account for approximately one-fourth of chest wound infections, second only to *S aureus*.)

Rupp MA, Archer GL: Coagulase-negative staphylococci: Pathogens associated with medical progress. Clin Infect Dis 1994;19:231.

CLOSTRIDIAL DISEASES

1. CLOSTRIDIAL MYONECROSIS (Gas Gangrene)

Essentials of Diagnosis

- Sudden onset of pain and edema in an area of wound contamination.
- Prostration and systemic toxicity.
- Brown to blood-tinged watery exudate, with skin discoloration of surrounding area.
- Gas in the tissue by palpation or x-ray.
- Gram-positive rods in culture or smear of exudate.

General Considerations

Gas gangrene or clostridial myonecrosis is produced by entry of one of several clostridia (*Clostridium perfringens, Clostridium ramosum, Clostridium bifermentans, Clostridium histolyticum, Clostridium novyi,* etc) into devitalized tissues. Toxins produced under anaerobic conditions result in shock, hemolysis, and myonecrosis.

Clinical Findings

A. Symptoms and Signs: The onset of gas gangrene is usually sudden, with rapidly increasing pain in the affected area, fall in blood pressure, and tachycardia. Fever is present but is not proportionate to the severity of the infection. In the last stages of the disease, severe prostration, stupor, delirium, and coma occur.

The wound becomes swollen, and the surrounding skin is pale. There is a foul-smelling brown, blood-tinged serous discharge. As the disease advances, the surrounding tissue changes from pale to dusky and finally becomes deeply discolored, with coalescent, red, fluid-filled vesicles. Gas may be palpable in the tissues.

B. Laboratory Findings: Gas gangrene is a clinical diagnosis, and empirical therapy is indicated whenever the diagnosis is suspected. Radiographic studies may show gas within the soft tissues, but this is not sufficient to make the diagnosis because other organisms may produce gas. The smear typically shows a remarkable absence of neutrophils and the presence of gram-positive rods. Anaerobic culture confirms the diagnosis.

Differential Diagnosis

Other types of infection can cause gas formation in the tissue, eg, *Enterobacter, Escherichia,* and mixed anaerobic infections including *Bacteroides* and peptostreptococci. Clostridia may produce serious puerperal infection with hemolysis.

Treatment

Penicillin, 2 million units every 3 hours intravenously, is effective. Although other agents (eg, tetracycline, clindamycin, metronidazole, chloramphenicol, cefoxitin) are active against *Clostridium* species in vitro and probably in vivo as well, their clinical efficacy has not been demonstrated. Adequate surgical debridement and exposure of infected areas is essential, with radical surgical excision often necessary. Hyperbaric oxygen therapy has been used, but clinical data demonstrating its efficacy are lacking.

Brown DR et al: A multicenter review of the treatment of major truncal necrotizing infections with and without hyperbaric oxygen therapy. Am J Surg 1994;167:485. (Retrospective analysis of hyperbaric oxygen therapy in 54 patients showing no significant benefit, though mortality was slightly lower [30% verses 42%] in those treated with hyperbaric oxygen.)

Stephens MB: Gas gangrene: Potential for hyperbaric oxygen therapy. Postgrad Med 1996;99:217, 224. (Treatment of gas gangrene and potential role of hyperbaric oxygen therapy.)

TETANUS

Essentials of Diagnosis

- History of wound and possible contamination.
- Jaw stiffness followed by spasms of jaw muscles (trismus).
- Stiffness of the neck and other muscles, dysphagia, irritability, hyperreflexia.
- Finally, painful convulsions precipitated by minimal stimuli.

General Considerations

Tetanus is caused by the neurotoxin elaborated by *Clostridium tetani*. Spores of this organism are ubiquitous in soil. When introduced into a wound, spores may germinate. The vegetative bacteria produce a toxin, tetanospasmin, which is a zinc metalloprotease that cleaves synaptobrevin, a protein essential for neurotransmitter release. Tetanospasmin interferes with neurotransmission at spinal synapses of inhibitory neurons. As a result, minor stimuli result in uncontrolled spasms, and reflexes are exaggerated. The incubation period is 5 days to 15 weeks, with the average being 8–12 days.

In the United States, most cases occur in unvaccinated individuals. Persons at risk are the elderly, migrant workers, newborns, and injection drug users, who may acquire the disease through subcutaneous injections. While puncture wounds are recognized as particularly prone to causing tetanus, any wound, including decubiti, where dead tissue and anaerobic conditions are present may become colonized and infected by *C tetani*.

Clinical Findings

A. Symptoms and Signs: The first symptom may be pain and tingling at the site of inoculation, followed by spasticity of the muscles nearby. More frequently, however, the presenting symptoms are stiffness of the jaw, neck stiffness, dysphagia, and irritability. Hyperreflexia develops later, with spasms of the jaw muscles (trismus) or facial muscles and rigidity and spasm of the muscles of the abdomen, neck, and back. Painful tonic convulsions precipitated by minor stimuli are common. Spasms of the glottis and respiratory muscles may cause acute asphyxia. The patient is awake and alert throughout the illness. The sensory examination is normal. The temperature is normal or only slightly elevated.

B. Laboratory Findings: The diagnosis of tetanus is made clinically.

Differential Diagnosis

Tetanus must be differentiated from various acute central nervous system infections. Trismus may occasionally develop with the use of phenothiazines. Strychnine poisoning should also be considered.

Complications

Airway obstruction is common. Urinary retention and constipation may result from spasm of the sphincters. Respiratory arrest and cardiac failure are late, life-threatening events.

Prevention

Tetanus is completely preventable by active immunization. Immunizations for children include tetanus toxoid, usually as DTP (see Table 30–4 for schedule). For primary immunization of adults, tetanus toxoid is administered as two doses 4–6 weeks apart, with a third dose 6–12 months later. Booster doses are given every 10 years or at the time of major injury if it occurs more than 5 years after a dose.

Passive immunization should be used in nonimmunized individuals and those whose immunization status is uncertain whenever a wound is contaminated or likely to have devitalized tissue. Tetanus immune globulin, 250 units, is given intramuscularly. Active immunization with tetanus toxoid should be started concurrently. Table 33–1 provides a guide to prophylactic management.

Treatment

A. Specific Measures: Give tetanus immune globulin, 5000 units intramuscularly. Tetanus does not produce natural immunity, and a full course of immunization with tetanus toxoid should be administered once the patient has recovered.

B. General Measures: Minimal stimuli can provoke spasms, so the patient should be placed at bed rest and monitored under the quietest conditions possible. Sedation, paralysis with curare-like agents, and mechanical ventilation are often necessary to control tetanic spasms. Penicillin, 20 million units daily, is administered to all patients—even those with mild illness—to eradicate toxin-producing organisms.

Prognosis

High mortality rates are associated with a short incubation period, early onset of convulsions, and delay in treatment. Contaminated lesions about the head and face are more dangerous than wounds on other parts of the body. The overall mortality rate historically is about 40%, but this can be considerably reduced with ventilator management as described.

Sun KO et al: Management of tetanus: A review of 18 cases. J R Soc Med 1994;87:135.

BOTULISM

Essentials of Diagnosis

- History of recent ingestion of home-canned or smoked foods or of injection drug use and demonstration of toxin in serum or food.
- Sudden onset of diplopia, dry mouth, dysphagia, dysphonia, and muscle weakness progressing to respiratory paralysis.
- Pupils are fixed and dilated.

General Considerations

Botulism is food poisoning usually caused by ingestion of preformed toxin (usually type A, B, or E) of *Clostridium botulinum*, a ubiquitous, strictly anaerobic, spore-forming bacillus found in soil. Canned, smoked, or vacuum-packed anaerobic foods are involved—particularly home-canned vegetables, smoked meats, and vacuum-packed fish—but commercial foods have also been associated with outbreaks of botulism. Infant botulism and wound botu-

Table 33–1. Guide to tetanus prophylaxis in wound management. (Modified from MMWR Morb Mortal Wkly Rep 1991;40:70.)

History of Absorbed Tetanus Toxoid	Clean, Minor Wounds		All Other Wounds[1]	
	Td[2]	TIG[3]	Td[2]	TIG[3]
Unknown or < 3 doses	Yes	No	Yes	Yes
3 or more doses	No[4]	No	No[5]	No

[1]Such as, but not limited to, wounds contaminated with dirt, feces, soil, saliva, etc; puncture wounds; avulsions; and wounds resulting from missiles, crushing, burns, and frostbite.
[2]Tetanus toxoid and diphtheria toxoid, adult form. Use only this preparation (Td-adult) in children older than 6 years.
[3]Tetanus immune globulin.
[4]Yes if more than 10 years have elapsed since last dose.
[5]Yes if more than 5 years have elapsed since last dose. (More frequent boosters are not needed and can enhance side effects.)

lism, which occurs in injection drug users, differ in that organisms present in the gut or wound, respectively, elaborate toxin in vivo. Botulinum toxins, like tetanus toxin, are zinc metalloproteases that cleave specific components of the synaptic vesicle membrane docking and fusion complex. Botulinum toxin inhibits release of acetylcholine at the neuromuscular junction. Clinically, early nervous system involvement leads to respiratory paralysis. The mortality rate in untreated cases is high.

Clinical Findings

A. Symptoms and Signs: Twelve to 36 hours after ingestion of the toxin, visual disturbances appear, particularly diplopia and loss of accommodation. Ptosis, cranial nerve palsies with impairment of extraocular muscles, and fixed dilated pupils are characteristic signs. The sensory examination is normal. Other symptoms are dry mouth, dysphagia, and dysphonia. Nausea and vomiting may be present, particularly with type E toxin. The sensorium remains clear and the temperature normal. Respiratory paralysis may lead to death unless mechanical assistance is provided.

B. Laboratory Findings: Toxin in patients' serum and in suspected foods may be shown by mouse inoculation and identified with specific antiserum.

Differential Diagnosis

Cranial nerve involvement suggests vertebrobasilar insufficiency, the C. Miller Fisher variant of Guillain-Barré syndrome, myasthenia gravis, or any basilar meningitis, infectious or carcinomatous. Intestinal obstruction or other types of food poisoning are considered when nausea and vomiting are present.

Treatment

If botulism is suspected, the physician should contact the state health authorities or the Centers for Disease Control and Prevention for advice and help with procurement of botulinus antitoxin and for assistance in obtaining assays for toxin in serum, stool, or food. During off hours, the CDC provides assistance via a recorded message at 404-639-2206.

Respiratory failure is managed with intubation and mechanical ventilation. Parenteral fluids or alimentation should be given while swallowing difficulty persists.

The removal of unabsorbed toxin from the gut may be attempted. Any remnants of suspected foods should be assayed for toxin. Persons who might have eaten the suspected food must be located and observed.

Burningham MD et al: Wound botulism. Ann Emerg Med 1994;24:1184.
Townes JM et al: An outbreak of type A botulism associ-

ated with a commercial cheese sauce. Ann Intern Med 1996;125:558.

ANTHRAX

Anthrax is a disease of sheep, cattle, horses, goats, and swine caused by *Bacillus anthracis,* a gram-positive spore-forming aerobic rod. The organism is transmitted to humans by inoculation of broken skin or mucous membranes or by inhalation, causing either cutaneous or pulmonary infection. Anthrax is a rare occupational disease of farmers, veterinarians, and tannery and wool workers; prospective military use of the organism may result in future cases.

In cutaneous anthrax, an erythematous papule appears on an exposed area of skin and becomes vesicular, with a purple to black center. The surrounding area is edematous and vesicular. The center of the lesion finally forms a necrotic eschar and sloughs. Regional adenopathy, fever, malaise, headache, and nausea and vomiting may be present. After the eschar sloughs, hematogenous spread and sepsis may occur, resulting in shock, cyanosis, sweating, and collapse. Hemorrhagic meningitis may also occur.

Pulmonary anthrax follows inhalation of spores from hides, bristles, or wool. It is characterized by fever, malaise, headache, dyspnea, and cough; congestion of the nose, throat, and larynx; and evidence of pneumonia or mediastinitis.

Culture of sputum, blood, or a skin lesion may be positive for *B anthracis.* Smears of skin lesions show gram-positive encapsulated rods.

The mortality rate is high despite proper therapy, especially in pulmonary disease. Penicillin G, 2 million units intravenously every 4 hours, is the therapy of choice. Tetracycline, 500 mg orally every 6 hours, may be used for mild, localized cutaneous infection.

Force FM: Anthrax. Clin Infect Dis 1994;19:1009.

DIPHTHERIA

Essentials of Diagnosis

- Tenacious gray membrane at portal of entry in pharynx.
- Sore throat, nasal discharge, hoarseness, malaise, fever.
- Myocarditis, neuropathy.
- Culture confirms the diagnosis.

General Considerations

Diphtheria is an acute infection, caused by *Corynebacterium diphtheriae,* that usually attacks the respiratory tract but may involve any mucous membrane or skin wound. The organism is spread chiefly by respiratory secretions. Exotoxin produced by the organism is responsible for myocarditis and neuropathy. This exotoxin inhibits elongation factor, which is required for protein synthesis.

Clinical Findings

A. Symptoms and Signs: Nasal, laryngeal, pharyngeal, and cutaneous forms of diphtheria occur. Nasal infection produces few symptoms other than a nasal discharge. Laryngeal infection may lead to upper airway and bronchial obstruction. In pharyngeal diphtheria, the most common form, a tenacious gray membrane covers the tonsils and pharynx. Mild sore throat, fever, and malaise are followed by toxemia and prostration.

Myocarditis and neuropathy are the most common and most serious complications. Myocarditis causes cardiac arrhythmias, heart block, and heart failure. The neuropathy usually involves the cranial nerves first, producing diplopia, slurred speech, and difficulty in swallowing.

B. Laboratory Findings: The diagnosis is made clinically but can be confirmed by culture of the organism.

Differential Diagnosis

Diphtheria must be differentiated from streptococcal pharyngitis, infectious mononucleosis, adenovirus or herpes simplex infection, Vincent's angina, and candidiasis. A presumptive diagnosis of diphtheria must be made on clinical grounds without waiting for laboratory verification, since emergency treatment is needed.

Prevention

Active immunization with diphtheria toxoid is part of routine childhood immunization (usually as DTP) with appropriate booster injections. The immunization schedule for adults is the same as for tetanus. In order to avoid major allergic reactions, only the "adult type" toxoid (Td) should be used.

Susceptible persons exposed to diphtheria should receive a booster dose of toxoid plus active immunization if not previously immunized, as well as a course of penicillin.

Treatment

Antitoxin, which is prepared from horse serum, must be given in all cases when diphtheria is suspected. For mild early pharyngeal or laryngeal disease, the dose is 20,000–40,000 units; for moderate nasopharyngeal disease, 40,000–60,000 units; for severe, extensive, or late (3 days or more) disease, 80,000–100,000 units. Diphtheria equine antitoxin can be obtained from the Centers for Disease Control and Prevention.

Antibiotics are a useful adjunct to antitoxin. Both penicillin and erythromycin are effective. The dosage of erythromycin is 500 mg orally four times daily for 7–10 days. Removal of membrane by direct laryngoscopy or bronchoscopy may be necessary to prevent or alleviate airway obstruction.

LISTERIOSIS

Listeria monocytogenes is a motile, gram-positive rod that is a facultative intracellular organism capable of invading several cell types. Most cases of infection caused by *L monocytogenes* are sporadic, but outbreaks have been traced to eating contaminated food, especially unpasteurized dairy products. Five types of infection are recognized:

(1) Infection during pregnancy, usually in the last trimester, is a mild febrile illness without an apparent primary focus. This is a relatively benign disease for both mother and fetus that may resolve without specific therapy.

(2) Granulomatosis infantisepticum is a neonatal infection acquired in utero and characterized by disseminated abscesses and granulomas and by a high mortality rate.

(3) Bacteremia with or without sepsis syndrome is an infection of neonates or immunocompromised adults. The presentation is that of a febrile illness without a recognized source.

(4) Meningitis caused by *L monocytogenes* affects infants under 2 months of age and adults, ranking third and fourth, respectively, among the common causes of bacterial meningitis. Adults with meningitis are usually immunocompromised, and cases have been associated with HIV infection. Cerebrospinal fluid shows a *neutrophilic* pleocytosis.

(5) Finally, focal infections, including adenitis, brain abscess, endocarditis, osteomyelitis, and arthritis, occur rarely.

Therapy of infections caused by *Listeria* is controversial with respect both to the most effective agent and the duration of treatment. The drug of choice is probably ampicillin, 8–12 g/d intravenously in four to six divided doses (the higher dose being recommended in cases of meningitis). It has relatively good penetration into cerebrospinal fluid, and, although there are few data, the response to ampicillin seems to be better than that to penicillin, erythromycin, or chloramphenicol. Gentamicin is synergistic with ampicillin against *Listeria* in vitro and in animal models, and the use of combination therapy may for that reason be considered during the first few days of treatment to enhance eradication of organisms. Mortality and morbidity rates still are high, and relapse does occur, perhaps related to poor penetration of ampicillin into cells where organisms reside. Anecdotal clinical data indicating efficacy of trimethoprim-sulfamethoxazole and its excellent penetration into cells and into the cerebrospinal fluid support its use for therapy of listeriosis. The dose is 10–20 mg/kg/d of the trimethoprim component. Therapy should be administered for at least 2–3 weeks.

Longer durations—between 3 and 6 weeks—have been recommended for treatment of meningitis, especially in severely immunocompromised patients.

Chang J et al: Listeriosis in bone marrow transplant recipients: Incidence, clinical features, and treatment. Clin Infect Dis 1995;21:1289.

Dalton CB et al: An outbreak of gastroenteritis and fever due to *Listeria monocytogenes* in milk. N Engl J Med 1997;336:100. (Chocolate milk was identified as the source of this food-borne outbreak.)

INFECTIONS CAUSED BY GRAM-NEGATIVE BACTERIA

BORDETELLA PERTUSSIS INFECTION (Whooping Cough)

Essentials of Diagnosis

- Predominantly in infants under age 2 years. Adults may be an important reservoir of infection for children.
- Two-week prodromal catarrhal stage of malaise, cough, coryza, and anorexia.
- Paroxysmal cough ending in a high-pitched inspiratory "whoop."
- Absolute lymphocytosis, often striking; culture confirms diagnosis.

General Considerations

Pertussis is an acute infection of the respiratory tract caused by *Bordetella pertussis* that is transmitted by respiratory droplets. The incubation period is 7–17 days. Infants are most commonly infected; half of all cases occur before age 2 years. Neither immunization nor disease confers lasting immunity to pertussis. Consequently, adults are an important reservoir of the disease.

Clinical Findings

The symptoms of classic pertussis last about 6 weeks and are divided into three consecutive stages. The catarrhal stage is characterized by its insidious onset, with lacrimation, sneezing, and coryza, anorexia and malaise, and a hacking night cough that tends to become diurnal. The paroxysmal stage is characterized by bursts of rapid, consecutive coughs followed by a deep, high-pitched inspiration (whoop). The convalescent stage usually begins 4 weeks after onset of the illness with a decrease in the frequency and severity of paroxysms of cough. The diagnosis often is not considered in adults, who may not have a typical presentation. Cough persisting more than 2 weeks is suggestive of pertussis. Infection may also be asymptomatic.

The white blood cell count is usually 15,000–20,000/μL (rarely, as high as 50,000/μL or more), 60–80% of which are lymphocytes. The diagnosis is established by isolating the organism from nasopharyngeal culture. A special medium (eg, Bordet-Gengou agar) must be requested.

Prevention

Active immunization with pertussis vaccine is recommended for all infants, usually combined with diphtheria and tetanus toxoids (DTP). Infants and susceptible adults with significant exposure to pertussis should receive prophylaxis with erythromycin (40 mg/kg/d, up to 2 g/d, for 10 days). Booster doses of pertussis vaccine have not been recommended after age 6 except to control outbreaks. Recognition of adults as an important reservoir of infection and development of an effective acellular vaccine with fewer side effects than the whole cell vaccine undoubtedly will prompt a reevaluation of the current recommendations for vaccination of adults.

Treatment

Erythromycin, 500 mg four times a day orally for 10 days, shortens the duration of carriage. It also may diminish the severity of coughing paroxysms.

Cherry JD. Historical review of pertussis and the classical vaccine. J Infect Dis 1996;174(Suppl 3):S259.
Postels-Multani S et al: Symptoms and complications of pertussis in adults. Infection 1995;23:139.

MENINGOCOCCAL MENINGITIS

Essentials of Diagnosis

- Fever, headache, vomiting, confusion, delirium, convulsions.
- Petechial rash of skin and mucous membranes in many.
- Neck and back stiffness with positive Kernig and Brudzinski signs is characteristic.
- Purulent spinal fluid with gram-negative intracellular and extracellular diplococci.
- Culture of cerebrospinal fluid, blood, or petechial aspiration confirms the diagnosis.

General Considerations

Meningococcal meningitis is caused by *Neisseria meningitidis* of groups A, B, C, Y, W-135, and others. Meningitis due to serogroup A is uncommon in the United States. Serogroup B generally causes sporadic cases. The frequency of outbreaks of meningitis caused by group C meningococcus has increased in recent years, and this serotype is the most common cause of epidemic disease in the United States. Up to 40% of persons are nasopharyngeal carriers of meningococci, but relatively few develop disease. Infection is transmitted by droplets. The clinical illness may take the form of meningococcemia (a fulminant form of septicemia without meningitis), meningococcemia with meningitis, or predominantly meningitis. Chronic recurrent meningococcemia with fever, rash, and arthritis can occur, particular in those with terminal complement deficiencies (C7–C9).

Clinical Findings

A. Symptoms and Signs: High fever, chills, and headache; back, abdominal, and extremity pains; and nausea and vomiting are present. In severe cases, rapidly developing confusion, delirium, seizures, and coma occur.

On examination, nuchal and back rigidity are typical, with positive Kernig and Brudzinski signs. A petechial rash often first appearing in the lower extremities and at pressure points is found in most cases. Petechiae may vary from pinhead-sized to large ecchymoses or even areas of skin gangrene that may later slough if the patient survives.

B. Laboratory Findings: Lumbar puncture typically reveals a cloudy or purulent cerebrospinal fluid, with elevated pressure, increased protein, and decreased glucose content. The fluid usually contains more than 1000 cells/μL, with polymorphonuclear cells predominating and containing gram-negative intracellular diplococci. The absence of organisms in a Gram-stained smear of the cerebrospinal fluid sediment does not rule out the diagnosis. The capsular polysaccharide can often be demonstrated in cerebrospinal fluid or urine by latex agglutination; this is especially useful in partially treated patients, though sensitivity is only 60–80%. The organism is usually demonstrated by smear or culture of the cerebrospinal fluid, oropharynx, blood, or aspirated petechiae.

Disseminated intravascular coagulation is an important complication of meningococcal infection. Prothrombin time and partial thromboplastin time are prolonged, fibrin dimers are elevated, fibrinogen is low, and the platelet count is depressed.

Differential Diagnosis

Meningococcal meningitis must be differentiated from other bacterial and viral meningitides. In small infants and in the elderly, the presentation may be atypical, without fever or stiff neck.

Rickettsial or echovirus infection and, rarely, other bacterial infections (eg, staphylococcal infections, scarlet fever) may also produce a petechial rash.

Prevention

Effective polysaccharide vaccines for groups A, C, Y, and W-135 are available. A and C vaccine has reduced the incidence of infections with these meningococcus groups in military recruits. The vaccines are effective for control of epidemics in civilian populations.

Outbreaks in closed populations are best controlled by eliminating nasopharyngeal carriage of meningococci. Rifampin is the drug of choice in dosages as follows: 600 mg twice a day for 2 days for adults; 10 mg/kg twice a day for 2 days for children 1 month to 12 years; 5 mg/kg twice a day for 2 days for infants.

Household members exposed to a person with meningococcal meningitis are at increased risk and should be given rifampin prophylaxis. Day care center contacts are treated in the same manner. School and work contacts need not be treated. Hospital contacts need not be treated unless intense exposure has occurred (eg, mouth-to-mouth resuscitation).

Accidentally discovered carriers without known close contact with meningococcal disease do not require prophylactic antimicrobials.

Treatment

Blood cultures must be obtained and intravenous antimicrobial therapy started immediately. This may be done prior to lumbar puncture in patients in whom the diagnosis is not straightforward and who therefore require CT scanning to exclude mass lesions. Aqueous penicillin G is the antibiotic of choice (24 million units/24 h) in divided doses every 4 hours. In penicillin-allergic patients or those in whom *Haemophilus influenzae* or gram-negative meningitis is a consideration, ceftriaxone, 4 g intravenously once a day, should be used. Chloramphenicol, 1 g every 6 hours, is an alternative in the severely penicillin- or cephalosporin-allergic patient.

Treatment should be continued in full doses by the intravenous route until the patient is afebrile for 5 days. In the past, the recommended duration of therapy has been 7–10 days. More recent studies suggest that shorter courses—as few as 4 days if ceftriaxone is used—are also effective.

Obtundation or deterioration in mental status may result from cerebral edema and increased intracranial pressure. In critically ill patients with evidence of increased intracranial pressure, administration of dexamethasone (0.6 mg/kg/d in four divided doses) should be considered.

Heparinization is of theoretic value in disseminated intravascular coagulation and bleeding, but it does not influence prognosis.

INFECTIONS CAUSED BY *HAEMOPHILUS* SPECIES

Haemophilus influenzae type b is primarily a pathogen of children less than 5 years old. Meningitis and epiglottitis, which are almost always caused by type B strains, occur most often in this group. *H influenzae* and other *Haemophilus* species may cause sinusitis, otitis, bronchitis, epiglottis, pneumonitis, cellulitis, arthritis, meningitis, and endocarditis in adults at any age, however.

In adults, **pneumonia** is one of the more common infections caused by *H influenzae* type b. Nontypable strains of *H influenzae* actually are more common as a cause of pneumonia in HIV-infected patients, however. The presentation is that of a typical bacterial pneumonia, with purulent sputum containing a predominance of gram-negative, pleomorphic rods. Alcoholism, smoking, chronic lung disease, advanced age, and HIV infection are important risk factors.

Although *Haemophilus* species and nontypable strains of *H influenzae* may cause pneumonia, they more frequently colonize the upper respiratory tract. Consequently, in the absence of positive pleural fluid or blood cultures, distinguishing pneumonia from colonization is difficult. Pneumonia from *Haemophilus* species probably is overdiagnosed for this reason.

Nontypable strains of *H influenzae* and other *Haemophilus* species cause **sinusitis, otitis,** and **respiratory tract infections.** Alcoholics, smokers, HIV-infected individuals, and patients with chronic lung disease are particularly at risk for respiratory infections with these organisms. *Haemophilus* species other than *H influenzae* (eg, *H parainfluenzae, H aphrophilus*) infrequently cause **endocarditis.**

Beta-lactamase-producing strains are less common in adults than in children. For most adult patients with sinusitis, otitis, or respiratory tract infection, oral amoxicillin, 500 mg every 8 hours for 10–14 days is adequate. For the penicillin-allergic patient, trimethoprim-sulfamethoxazole, 800 mg/160 mg, orally twice daily for 10–14 days, or azithromycin, 500 mg orally as a first dose and then 250 mg once a day for four days, is also effective.

In the more seriously ill patient (eg, the toxic patient with multilobar pneumonia), use of a second- or third-generation cephalosporin—cefuroxime, 750 mg every 8 hours, or ceftriaxone, 1 g/d—is advisable pending determination of whether the infecting strain is a β-lactamase producer. Trimethoprim-sulfamethoxazole, administered based on a dose of 10 mg/kg/d of trimethoprim, can be used for the penicillin-allergic patient. A 10- to 14-day course of therapy is adequate for most cases.

Epiglottitis, which occasionally occurs in adults, is characterized by an abrupt onset of high fever, drooling, and inability to handle secretions. A foreign body sensation in the pharynx may precede these symptoms by several hours. Stridor and respiratory distress result from laryngeal obstruction. Early, elective intubation is recommended because airway obstruction may progress unpredictably and rapidly. The diagnosis is best made by direct visualization of the cherry-red, swollen epiglottis at laryngoscopy. Because laryngoscopy may provoke laryngospasm and obstruction, it should be performed in an intensive care unit or similar setting, and only at the time of intubation. Cefuroxime, 1.5 g every 8 hours for 7–10 days, or ceftriaxone, 1 g every 24 hours for 7–10 days, is the drug of choice. Trimethoprim-sulfamethoxazole (see above for dosage) or chloramphenicol, 4 g/d, may be used in the patient with serious penicillin allergy.

Meningitis—also rare but still a possibility in adults—becomes a consideration in the patient who has meningitis associated with sinusitis or otitis. The presentation is the same as that of other bacterial meningitides. Initial therapy of suspected *H influenzae* meningitis should be with ceftriaxone, 4 g/d in one or two divided doses, until the strain is proved not to produce β-lactamase. Chloramphenicol, 100 mg/kg/d in four divided doses, can be used if the patient has a serious, life-threatening allergy to β-lactam antibiotics. Traditionally, meningitis has been treated for 10–14 days, but a 7-day regimen of ceftriaxone has been shown to be safe and effective in infants and children. Dexamethasone, 0.15 mg/kg intravenously every 6 hours, has been shown to be a valuable adjunctive agent in treatment of meningitis in infants and children, resulting in reduction in long-term sequelae, principally hearing loss. The role of corticosteroids in management of adult meningitis is controversial.

INFECTIONS CAUSED BY MORAXELLA CATARRHALIS

Moraxella catarrhalis is a gram-negative aerobic coccus that is morphologically and biochemically similar to *Neisseria*. This organism has recently been recognized as a cause of sinusitis, bronchitis, and pneumonia. Bacteremia and meningitis have also been reported in immunocompromised patients. The organism frequently colonizes the respiratory tract, and differentiation of colonization from infection can be difficult. If *M catarrhalis* is the predominant isolate, therapy should be directed against it. *M catarrhalis* typically produces β-lactamase and therefore is usually resistant to ampicillin and amoxicillin. It is susceptible to amoxicillin-clavulanate, ampicillin-sulbactam, trimethoprim-sulfamethoxazole, ciprofloxacin, and second- and third-generation cephalosporins. Treatment is similar to that for *Haemophilus* infections.

LEGIONNAIRE'S DISEASE

Essentials of Diagnosis

- Patients are often immunocompromised, smokers, or have chronic lung disease.
- Scant sputum production, pleuritic chest pain, toxic appearance.
- Chest x-ray shows focal patchy infiltrates or consolidation.

- Gram's stain of sputum shows polymorphonuclear leukocytes and no organisms.

General Considerations

Legionella infection ranks among the three or four most common causes of community-acquired pneumonia. The diagnosis must be considered whenever the etiology of a pneumonia is in question. Legionnaire's disease is more common in immunocompromised persons, in smokers, and in those with chronic lung disease. Outbreaks of legionellosis have been associated with contaminated water sources, such as shower heads and faucets in patient rooms and air conditioning cooling towers.

Clinical Findings

A. Symptoms and Signs: Legionnaire's disease is one of the atypical pneumonias, so called because a Gram-stained smear of sputum does not show organisms. However, many features of Legionnaire's disease are more like typical pneumonia, with high fevers, a "toxic" appearance of the patient, pleurisy, and purulent sputum (without predominant or identifiable organisms). Classically, this pneumonia is caused by *Legionella pneumophila*, though other species can cause disease that is clinically indistinguishable.

B. Laboratory Findings: Culture onto charcoal-yeast extract agar or similar enriched medium is the most sensitive method (80–90% sensitivity) for diagnosis of legionellosis and permits identification of infections caused by species and serotypes other than *L pneumophila* serotype 1. Dieterle's silver staining of tissue, pleural fluid, or other infected material is also a reliable method for detecting *Legionella* species. Direct fluorescent antibody stains and serologic testing are less sensitive because these will detect only infection caused by *L pneumophila* serotype 1.

Treatment

The drug of choice for treatment of legionellosis is erythromycin administered at a dose of 1 g intravenously every 6 hours initially, then 500 mg every 6 hours orally once the patient has responded, for a total of 14–21 days. Azithromycin, 500 mg orally every 24 hours, or clarithromycin, 500 mg orally every 12 hours, is also active against *Legionella*, and these drugs are suitable (but expensive) alternatives for patients unable to tolerate erythromycin. Rifampin, 300 mg twice a day in combination with erythromycin, may be synergistic and may be considered for those with severe illness and in immunocompromised hosts, who tend to have more aggressive disease.

Tetracyclines and trimethoprim-sulfamethoxazole occasionally have been used to treat legionellosis, and ciprofloxacin is active in vitro. These agents are of unproved efficacy and should be considered for use only if erythromycin or the other macrolides are contraindicated or cannot be tolerated.

Edelstein PH: Legionnaires' disease. Clin Infect Dis 1993; 16:741. (Epidemiology and clinical manifestations.)

Roig J, Carreres A, Domingo C: Treatment of Legionnaires' disease. Current recommendations. Drugs 1993; 46:63.

Yu V: Legionnaires' disease: New understanding of community-acquired pneumonia. Hosp Pract (Off Ed) 1993;28(1):63. (Epidemiology, diagnosis, and management.)

GRAM-NEGATIVE BACTEREMIA & SEPSIS

There are several hundred thousand episodes of gram-negative sepsis annually. Patients with rapidly fatal underlying diseases (neutropenic patients or those immunosuppressed by virtue of an underlying disease or medication) have a mortality rate of 40–60%; patients with ultimately fatal underlying diseases (diseases likely to be fatal in 5 years, such as solid tumors, severe liver disease, and aplastic anemia) have a mortality rate of 15–20%; and patients with no underlying disease have a low mortality rate—5% or less. Gram-negative bacteremia can originate in a number of sites, the most common being the genitourinary system, hepatobiliary tract, gastrointestinal tract, and lungs. Less common sources include intravenous lines, infusion fluids, surgical wounds, surgical drains, and decubitus ulcers.

Clinical Findings

A. Symptoms and Signs: Most patients have fevers and chills, often with an abrupt onset. However, 15% of patients are hypothermic (temperature ≤ 36.4 °C) at the onset of sepsis, and 5% of patients never develop a temperature above 37.5 °C. Hyperventilation with respiratory alkalosis and changes in mental status are important early manifestations. Hypotension and shock, which occur in 20–50% of patients, are unfavorable prognostic signs.

B. Laboratory Findings: Neutropenia or neutrophilia, often with increased numbers of immature forms of polymorphonuclear leukocytes, is the most common laboratory abnormality in septic patients. Thrombocytopenia occurs in 50% of patients, laboratory evidence of coagulation abnormalities in 10%, and frank DIC in 2–3%. Both clinical manifestations and the laboratory abnormalities are nonspecific and insensitive, which accounts for the relatively low rate of blood culture positivity (approximately 20–40%) in patients with suspected gram-negative sepsis. If possible, three blood cultures should be obtained in rapid succession before starting antimicrobial therapy. The chance of recovering the organism from the blood of the septic patient with bacteremia in at least one of the three blood cultures is greater than 95%.

The false-negative rate for a single culture of 5–10 mL of blood is 30%. This may be reduced to a 5–10% false-negative rate (albeit with a slight false-positive rate due to isolation of contaminants) if a single volume of 30 mL is inoculated into several blood culture bottles. Because blood cultures may be falsely negative, if the patient with presumed septic shock, negative blood cultures, and no other good explanation for the clinical course responds to antimicrobials, therapy should be continued for 10–14 days.

Treatment

Several factors are important in the management of patients with sepsis.

A. Removal of Predisposing Factors: This usually means decreasing or stopping immunosuppressive medications and in certain circumstances (eg, documented positive blood cultures) giving granulocyte colony-stimulating factor (filgrastim; G-CSF) to the neutropenic patient.

B. Identifying the Source of Bacteremia: A search for the source of bacteremia should be made. By simply finding the source and either removing it (intravenous line) or draining it (abscess), it is possible to transform what might be a fatal disease into one that is easily treatable.

C. Supportive Measures: The use of fluids and pressors for maintaining blood pressure is discussed in Chapter 11; management of disseminated intravascular coagulation is discussed in Chapter 13.

D. Antibiotics: Antibiotics should be given as soon as the diagnosis of sepsis is seriously considered, since delays in therapy have been associated with increased mortality rates. In general, bactericidal antibiotics should be used and should be given intravenously to ensure therapeutic serum levels. Penetration of antibiotics into the site of primary infection is critical for successful therapy—ie, if the infection originates in the central nervous system, antibiotics that penetrate the blood-brain barrier should be used—eg, penicillin, ampicillin, chloramphenicol, and third-generation cephalosporins—but not first-generation cephalosporins or aminoglycosides, which penetrate poorly. Sepsis caused by gram-positive organisms cannot be differentiated on clinical grounds from that due to gram-negative bacteria. Therefore, initial therapy should include antibiotics active against both types of organisms.

The number of antibiotics necessary to treat sepsis remains controversial and depends upon the underlying disease. Table 37–2 provides a guide for empirical therapy. Most authorities believe that for patients with rapidly fatal underlying diseases, a synergistic combination of antibiotics, including an aminoglycoside, should be used. For patients with nonfatal and ultimately fatal underlying diseases and who are not in shock, a single-drug regimen with any of several broad-spectrum antibiotics (eg, a third-generation cephalosporin, ticarcillin-clavulanate, imipenem) is adequate. Therapy can be altered once results of culture and sensitivity are known.

E. Corticosteroids: There is no role for corticosteroids in the therapy of sepsis or septic shock.

F. Adjunctive Therapy: Expanded knowledge of the pathophysiology of sepsis and septic shock and recognition that cytokines play a critical role have led to novel approaches to reduce morbidity and mortality associated with sepsis. Strategies include blocking the effects of endotoxin with anti-endotoxin monoclonal antibodies; blockade of TNFα, a potent cytokine mediator of septic shock, with anti-TNF monoclonal antibody or soluble TNF receptor; and use of IL-1 receptor antagonists to inhibit the proinflammatory effects of IL-1 binding to its receptor. Results of clinical trials with these agents so far have been largely disappointing, with no significant improvement in overall survival. The ultimate role and long-term benefits of adjunctive therapy have yet to be defined.

Bone RC: Gram-positive organisms and sepsis. Arch Intern Med 1994;154:26. (Pathophysiology and increasing incidence.)

Natanson C: Selected treatment strategies for septic shock based on proposed mechanisms of pathogenesis. Ann Intern Med 1994;120:771. (The current state of research to find effective adjunctive therapies for septic shock.)

Parrillo JE: Mechanisms of disease: Pathogenetic mechanisms of septic shock. N Engl J Med 1993;328:1471. (Pathogenesis and management.)

Rangel-Frausto MS et al: The natural history of the systemic inflammatory response syndrome (SIRS): A prospective study. JAMA 1995;273:117. (Natural history study documenting epidemiology and progression of disease from the earlier phase of systemic inflammatory response syndrome to septic shock.)

SALMONELLOSIS

Salmonellosis includes infection by any of approximately 2000 serotypes of salmonellae. The taxonomy of *Salmonella* species has been confusing. All *Salmonella* serotypes are considered members of a single species, *S enterica*. Human infections are caused almost exclusively by *S enterica* subsp *enterica,* of which three serotypes—typhi, typhimurium, and choleraesuis—are predominantly isolated. Three clinical patterns of infection are recognized: (1) enteric fever, the best example of which is typhoid fever, due to serotype typhi; (2) acute enterocolitis, caused by serotype typhimurium, among others; and (3) the "septicemic" type, characterized by bacteremia and focal lesions, exemplified by infection with serotype choleraesuis. All types are transmitted by ingestion of the organism, usually from contaminated food or drink.

1. ENTERIC FEVER (Typhoid Fever)

Essentials of Diagnosis

- Gradual onset of malaise, headache, sore throat, cough, and finally "pea soup" diarrhea, though constipation is more typical.
- Rose spots, relative bradycardia, splenomegaly, and abdominal distention and tenderness.
- Slow (stepladder) rise of fever to maximum and then slow return to normal.
- Leukopenia; blood, stool, and urine culture positive for *S enterica* serotype typhi.

General Considerations

Enteric fever is a clinical syndrome characterized by constitutional and gastrointestinal symptoms and by headache. It can be caused by any *Salmonella* species. The term "typhoid fever" applies when serotype typhi is the cause of enteric fever accompanied by bacteremia. Infection is transmitted by consumption of contaminated food or drink. The incubation period is 5–14 days. Infection begins when organisms penetrate the intestinal wall and invade mesenteric lymph nodes and the spleen. Serotypes other than typhi usually do not cause invasive disease, presumably because they lack the necessary human-specific virulence factors. Bacteremia occurs, and the infection then localizes principally in the lymphoid tissue of the small intestine (particularly within 60 cm of the ileocecal valve). Peyer's patches become inflamed and may ulcerate, with involvement greatest during the third week of disease. The organism may disseminate to the lungs, gallbladder, kidneys, or central nervous system.

Clinical Findings

A. Symptoms and Signs: The onset is usually insidious but in children may be abrupt, with chills and high fever. During the prodromal stage, there is increasing malaise, headache, cough, and sore throat, often with abdominal pain and constipation, while the fever ascends in a stepwise fashion. After about 7–10 days, the fever reaches a plateau and the patient is much more ill, appearing exhausted and often prostrated. There may be marked constipation, or "pea soup" diarrhea; marked abdominal distention occurs as well. If there are no complications, the patient's condition will gradually improve over 7–10 days. However, relapse may occur for up to 2 weeks after defervescence.

During the early prodrome, physical findings are few. Later, splenomegaly, abdominal distention and tenderness, relative bradycardia, dicrotic pulse, and occasionally meningismus appear. The rash (rose spots) commonly appears during the second week of disease. The individual spot, found principally on the trunk, is a pink papule 2–3 mm in diameter that fades on pressure. It disappears in 3–4 days.

B. Laboratory Findings: Typhoid fever is best diagnosed by isolation of the organism from blood culture, which is positive in the first week of illness in 80% of patients who have not taken antimicrobials. The rate of blood culture positivity declines thereafter, but one-fourth or more of patients still have positive blood cultures in the third week. Cultures of bone marrow occasionally are positive when blood cultures are not. Stool culture is not reliable because it may be positive in gastroenteritis without typhoid fever.

Differential Diagnosis

Enteric fever must be distinguished from other gastrointestinal illnesses and from other infections that have few localizing findings. Examples include tuberculosis, infective endocarditis, brucellosis, lymphoma, and Q fever. Often there is a history of recent travel to endemic areas, and viral hepatitis, malaria, or amebiasis may be in the differential diagnosis as well.

Complications

Complications occur in about 30% of untreated cases and account for 75% of all deaths. Intestinal hemorrhage, manifested by a sudden drop in temperature and signs of shock followed by dark or fresh blood in the stool, or intestinal perforation, accompanied by abdominal pain and tenderness, is most likely to occur during the third week. Less frequent complications are urinary retention, pneumonia, thrombophlebitis, myocarditis, psychosis, cholecystitis, nephritis, osteomyelitis, and meningitis.

Prevention

Immunization is not always effective but should be provided for household contacts of a typhoid carrier, for travelers to endemic areas, and during epidemic outbreaks. A multiple-dose oral vaccine and a single-dose parenteral vaccine are available. Their efficacies are similar, but oral vaccine causes fewer side effects. Boosters, when indicated, should be given every 5 years and 3 years for oral and parenteral preparations, respectively.

Adequate waste disposal and protection of food and water supplies from contamination are important public health measures to prevent salmonellosis. Carriers must not be permitted to work as food handlers.

Treatment

A. Specific Measures: Ampicillin, chloramphenicol, and trimethoprim-sulfamethoxazole may be effective. All can be given orally or intravenously depending on the patient's condition. Because resistance to ampicillin and chloramphenicol is common, trimethoprim-sulfamethoxazole, administered as 10 mg/kg/d of trimethoprim, is probably the first choice. Ceftriaxone, 2 g once a day, also is effective. Fluoroquinolones such as ciprofloxacin, 750 mg twice a day, also are effective, but their use is contraindicated in children and pregnant women. The recommended duration of therapy is 2 weeks, though limited data suggest that shorter courses are also effective.

B. Treatment of Carriers: Chemotherapy often is unsuccessful in eradicating the carrier state. While treatment of carriage with ampicillin, trimethoprim-sulfamethoxazole, or chloramphenicol may be successful, one recent study suggests that ciprofloxacin, 750 mg twice a day for 4 weeks, is highly effective. Cholecystectomy may also achieve this goal.

Prognosis

The mortality rate of typhoid fever is about 2% in treated cases. Elderly or debilitated persons are likely to do poorly. The course is milder in children.

With complications, the prognosis is poor. Relapses occur in up to 15% of cases. A residual carrier state frequently persists in spite of chemotherapy.

Plotkin SA, Bouveret-Le Cam N: A new typhoid vaccine composed of the Vi capsular polysaccharide. Arch Intern Med 1995;155:2293. (Efficacies of 55–75% can be achieved with a single parenteral dose of vaccine.)

Smith MD et al: Comparison of ofloxacin and ceftriaxone for short-course treatment of enteric fever. Antimicrob Agents Chemother 1994;38:1716.

2. *SALMONELLA* GASTROENTERITIS

By far the most common form of salmonellosis is acute enterocolitis. Numerous *Salmonella* serotypes may cause enterocolitis. The incubation period is 8–48 hours after ingestion of contaminated food or liquid.

Symptoms and signs consist of fever (often with chills), nausea and vomiting, cramping abdominal pain, and diarrhea, which may be grossly bloody, lasting 3–5 days. Differentiation must be made from viral gastroenteritis, food poisoning, shigellosis, amebic dysentery, acute ulcerative colitis, and acute surgical abdominal conditions. The diagnosis is made by culturing the organism from the stool.

The disease is usually self-limited, but bacteremia with localization in joints or bones may occur, especially in patients with sickle cell disease.

Treatment of uncomplicated enterocolitis is symptomatic only. Malnourished or severely ill patients, those with sickle cell disease, and those with suspected bacteremia should be treated for 3–5 days with trimethoprim-sulfamethoxazole (one double-strength tablet twice a day), ampicillin (100 mg/kg intravenously or orally), or ciprofloxacin (750 mg twice a day).

3. *SALMONELLA* BACTEREMIA

Rarely, *Salmonella* infection may be manifested by prolonged or recurrent fevers accompanied by bacteremia and local infection in bone, joints, pleura, pericardium, lungs, or other sites. Mycotic abdominal aortic aneurysms may also cause this problem. Serotypes other than typhi usually are isolated. This complication tends to occur in immunocompromised persons and is seen in HIV-infected individuals, who frequently have bacteremia without an obvious source. Treatment is the same as for typhoid fever, plus drainage of any abscesses. In HIV-infected patients, relapse is common, and lifelong suppressive therapy may be needed. Ciprofloxacin, 750 mg twice a day, is effective both for therapy of acute infection and for suppression of recurrence.

SHIGELLOSIS

Essentials of Diagnosis

- Diarrhea, often with blood and mucus.
- Crampy abdominal pain and systemic toxicity.
- White blood cells in stools; organism isolated on stool culture.

General Considerations

Shigella dysentery is a common disease, often self-limited and mild but occasionally serious. *Shigella sonnei* is the leading cause in the USA, followed by *Shigella flexneri*. *Shigella dysenteriae* causes the most serious form of the illness. Shigellae are invasive organisms: The infective dose is 10^2–10^3 organisms. Recently, there has been a rise in strains resistant to multiple antibiotics.

Clinical Findings

A. Symptoms and Signs: The illness usually starts abruptly, with diarrhea, lower abdominal cramps, and tenesmus. The diarrheal stool often is mixed with blood and mucus. Systemic symptoms are fever, chills, anorexia and malaise, and headache. The patient becomes progressively weaker and more dehydrated. The abdomen is tender. Sigmoidoscopic examination reveals an inflamed, engorged mucosa with punctate, sometimes large areas of ulceration.

B. Laboratory Findings: The stool shows many leukocytes and red cells. Stool culture is positive for shigellae in most cases, but blood cultures grow the organism in less than 5% of cases.

Differential Diagnosis

Bacillary dysentery must be distinguished from *Salmonella* enterocolitis and from disease due to enterotoxigenic *E coli*, *Campylobacter*, and *Y enterocolitica*. Amebic dysentery may be similar clinically and is diagnosed by finding amebas in the fresh stool specimen. Ulcerative colitis in the adolescent and adult is an important cause of bloody diarrhea.

Complications

Temporary disaccharidase deficiency may follow the diarrhea. Reiter's syndrome is an uncommon complication, usually occurring in HLA-B27 individuals infected by *Shigella*.

Treatment

Treatment of dehydration and hypotension is lifesaving in severe cases. The current antimicrobial treatment of choice is trimethoprim-sulfamethoxazole, one double-strength tablet twice a day for 7–10 days, or ciprofloxacin (contraindicated in pregnancy), 750 mg twice daily for 7–10 days. Shigellae resistant to ampicillin are common, but if the isolate is susceptible, a dose of 500 mg four times a day is also effective. Amoxicillin, which is less effective, should not be used. A single dose of a quinolone (eg, norfloxacin, 400 mg, or ciprofloxacin, 750 mg) may be as effective as a 5-day course of therapy with other drugs.

GASTROENTERITIS CAUSED BY *ESCHERICHIA COLI*

Escherichia coli causes gastroenteritis by a variety of mechanisms. Enterotoxigenic *E coli* (ETEC) elaborates either a heat-stable or heat-labile toxin that mediates the disease. ETEC is an important cause of traveler's diarrhea. Enteroinvasive *E coli* (EIEC) differs from other *E coli* bowel pathogens in that these strains invade cells, causing bloody diarrhea and dysentery similar to infection with *Shigella* species. EIEC is uncommon in the United States. Neither ETEC nor EIEC strains are routinely isolated and identified from stool cultures because there is no selective medium. Antimicrobial therapy directed against *Salmonella* and *Shigella* shortens the clinical course, but the disease is self-limited.

Enterohemorrhagic *E coli* (EHEC) produces two *Shiga*-like toxins that mediate the clinical manifestations, which include an asymptomatic carriage stage, nonbloody diarrhea, hemorrhagic colitis, hemolytic-uremic syndrome, and thrombotic thrombocytopenic purpura. Although there are several serotypes of EHEC, serotype O157:H7 is responsible for most cases in the United States. *E coli* O157:H7 has been responsible for several outbreaks of diarrhea and hemolytic-uremic syndrome related to consumption of undercooked hamburger and unpasteurized apple juice. Elderly individuals and young children are most severely affected, with hemolytic-uremic syndrome being a common and often fatal complication in the latter group. *E coli* O157:H7 is not identified by routine stool cultures. Isolation requires identification of sorbitol-negative colonies of *E coli* on sorbitol-MacConkey agar followed by serologic testing to confirm the serotype. Antimicrobial therapy does not alter the course of the disease, and treatment is primarily supportive. Hemolytic-uremic syndrome or thrombotic thrombocytopenic purpura occurring in association with a diarrheal illness suggests the diagnosis and should prompt evaluation for EHEC. Confirmed infections should be reported immediately to public health officials.

Su C, Brandt LJ: *Escherichia coli* O157:H7 infection in humans. Ann Intern Med 1995;123:698. (Review of recent outbreaks, epidemiology, pathogenesis, and clinical manifestations.)

CHOLERA

Essentials of Diagnosis

- Voluminous diarrhea.
- Stool is liquid, gray, turbid, and without fecal odor, blood, or pus ("rice water stool").
- Rapid development of marked dehydration.
- History of travel in endemic area or contact with infected person.
- Positive stool cultures and agglutination of vibrios with specific sera.

General Considerations

Cholera is an acute diarrheal illness caused by certain serotypes of *Vibrio cholerae*. The disease is toxin-mediated, and fever is unusual. The toxin activates adenylyl cyclase in intestinal epithelial cells of the small intestines, producing hypersecretion of water and chloride ion and a massive diarrhea of up to 15 L per day. Death results from profound hypovolemia.

Cholera occurs in epidemics under conditions of crowding, war, and famine (eg, in refugee camps) and where sanitation is inadequate. Infection is acquired by ingestion of contaminated food or water. Cholera was rarely seen in the United States until 1991, when epidemic cholera returned to the Western Hemisphere, originating as an outbreak in coastal cities of Peru. The epidemic spread to involve several countries in South and Central America as well as Mexico, and cases have been imported into the United States. Cholera should be considered in the differential diagnosis of severe watery diarrhea, especially in those who have traveled to affected countries.

Clinical Findings

A. Symptoms and Signs: Cholera is characterized by a sudden onset of severe, frequent watery diarrhea (up to 1 L per hour). The liquid stool is gray, turbid, and without fecal odor, blood, or pus ("rice water stool"). Dehydration and hypotension develop rapidly.

B. Laboratory Findings: Stool cultures are positive, and agglutination of vibrios with specific sera can be demonstrated.

Prevention

A vaccine is available that confers short-lived, limited protection and may be required for entry into or reentry after travel to some countries. It is administered in two doses 1–4 weeks apart. A booster dose every 6 months is recommended for persons remaining in areas where cholera is a hazard.

Vaccination programs are expensive and not particularly effective in managing outbreaks of cholera. When outbreaks occur, efforts should be directed toward establishing clean water and food sources and proper waste disposal.

Treatment

Treatment is by replacement of fluids. In mild or moderate illness, oral rehydration usually is adequate and has dramatically decreased the mortality rate in developing countries. A simple oral replacement fluid can be made from 1 teaspoon of table salt and 4 heaping teaspoons of sugar added to 1 L of water. Intravenous fluids are indicated for persons in shock or those with other signs of severe hypovolemia and those who cannot take adequate fluids orally. Either lactated Ringer's infusion or an intravenous fluid containing 4 g (approximately 70 meq) of NaCl, 1 g (10 meq) of KCl, 5.4 g (50 mmol) of sodium lactate, and 8 g (45 mmol) of glucose per liter is satisfactory.

Antimicrobial therapy will shorten the course of illness. Several antimicrobials are active against *V cholerae*, including tetracycline, ampicillin, chloramphenicol, trimethoprim-sulfamethoxazole, and fluoroquinolones. Multiple antibiotic resistance does occur, so susceptibility testing, if available, is advisable.

Seas C et al: Practical guidelines for the treatment of cholera. Drugs 1996;51:966.

INFECTIONS CAUSED BY OTHER *VIBRIO* SPECIES

Vibrios other than *Vibrio cholerae* that cause human disease are *Vibrio parahaemolyticus, Vibrio vulnificus,* and *Vibrio alginolyticus*. All are halophilic marine organisms. Infection is acquired by exposure to organisms in contaminated, undercooked, or raw crustaceans or shellfish and warm (> 20 °C) ocean waters and estuaries. Infections are more common during the summer months from regions along the Atlantic coast and the Gulf of Mexico in the United States and from tropical waters around the world. Oysters are implicated in up to 90% of food-related cases. *V parahaemolyticus* causes an acute watery diarrhea with crampy abdominal pain and fever, typically occurring within 24 hours after ingestion of contaminated shellfish. The disease is self-limited, and antimicrobial therapy is usually not necessary. *V parahaemolyticus* may also cause cellulitis and sepsis, though these findings are more characteristic of *V vulnificus* infection.

V vulnificus and *V alginolyticus*—neither of which is associated with diarrheal illness—are important causes of cellulitis and primary bacteremia, which may follow ingestion of contaminated shellfish or exposure to sea water. Cellulitis with or without sepsis may be accompanied by bulla formation and necrosis with extensive soft tissue destruction, at times requiring debridement and amputation. The infection can be rapidly progressive and is particularly severe in immunocompromised individuals—especially those with cirrhosis—with death rates as high as 50%. Patients with chronic liver disease and those who are immunocompromised should be cautioned to avoid eating raw oysters.

Tetracycline at a dose of 500 mg four times a day is the drug of choice for treatment of suspected or documented primary bacteremia or cellulitis caused by *Vibrio* species. *V vulnificus* is susceptible in vitro to penicillin, ampicillin, cephalosporins, chloramphenicol, aminoglycosides, and fluoroquinolones, and these agents may also be effective. *V parahaemolyticus* and *V alginolyticus* produce β-lactamase and therefore are resistant to penicillin and ampicillin, but susceptibilities otherwise are similar to those listed for *V vulnificus*.

INFECTIONS CAUSED BY *CAMPYLOBACTER* SPECIES

Campylobacters are microaerophilic, motile, gram-negative rods. Two species infect humans: *Campylobacter jejuni,* an important cause of diarrheal disease; and *Campylobacter fetus* subsp *fetus*, which typically causes systemic infection and not diarrhea. Dairy cattle are an important reservoir for campylobacters. Outbreaks of enteritis have been associated with consumption of raw milk. *Campylobacter* gastroenteritis is associated with fever, abdominal pain, and diarrhea characterized by loose, watery, or bloody stools. The differential diagnosis includes shigellosis, salmonella gastroenteritis, and enteritis caused by *Yersinia enterocolitica* or invasive *Escherichia coli*. The disease is self-limited, but its duration can be shortened with antimicrobial therapy. Both erythromycin, 250–500 mg four times daily for 5–7 days, and ciprofloxacin, 500 mg twice daily for 5–7 days, are effective regimens. Pending identification of the causative agent of suspected bacterial gastroenteritis, ciprofloxacin is a rational choice for empirical therapy because all of the common bacterial pathogens are susceptible.

C fetus causes systemic infections that can be fatal, including primary bacteremia, endocarditis, meningitis, and focal abscesses. It infrequently causes gastroenteritis. Patients infected with *C fetus* are often elderly, debilitated, or immunocompromised. Closely related species, collectively termed *Campylobacter*-like organisms, cause bacteremia in HIV-infected individuals. Systemic infections respond to therapy with gentamicin, chloramphenicol, or ceftriaxone. These organisms are also susceptible in vitro to ciprofloxacin. Ceftriaxone or chloramphenicol should be used to treat infections of the central nervous system because of their ability to penetrate the blood-brain barrier.

BRUCELLOSIS

Essentials of Diagnosis

- Insidious onset: easy fatigability, headache, arthralgia, anorexia, sweating, irritability.
- Intermittent fever, especially at night, which may become chronic and undulant.
- Cervical and axillary lymphadenopathy; hepatosplenomegaly.
- Lymphocytosis, positive blood culture, elevated agglutination titer.

General Considerations

The infection is transmitted from animals to humans. *Brucella abortus* (cattle), *Brucella suis* (hogs), and *Brucella melitensis* (goats) are the main agents. Transmission to humans occurs by contact with infected meat (slaughterhouse workers), placentae of infected animals (farmers, veterinarians), or ingestion of infected unpasteurized milk or cheese. The incubation period varies from a few days to several weeks. The disorder may become chronic. In the USA, brucellosis is very rare except in the midwestern states (from *B suis*) and in visitors or immigrants from countries where brucellosis is endemic (eg, Mexico, Spain, South American countries).

Clinical Findings

A. Symptoms and Signs: The onset may be acute, with fever, chills, and sweats, but typically is insidious. It may be weeks before the patient seeks medical care for weakness, weight loss, low-grade fevers, sweats, and exhaustion upon minimal activity. Symptoms also include headache, abdominal or back pains with anorexia and constipation, and arthralgia. Epididymitis occurs in 10% of cases in men. The chronic form may assume an undulant nature, with periods of normal temperature between acute attacks; symptoms may persist for years, either continuously or intermittently.

Physical findings are minimal. Half of cases have peripheral lymph node enlargement and splenomegaly; hepatomegaly is less common.

B. Laboratory Findings: Early in the course

of infection, the organism can be recovered from the blood, cerebrospinal fluid, urine, and bone marrow. Because the organism is slow-growing, cultures should be incubated for 21 days before being read as negative. Cultures are more likely to be negative in chronic cases. The diagnosis often is made by serologic testing. Rising serologic titers or an absolute agglutination titer of greater than 1:100 supports the diagnosis. Occasionally, falsely negative agglutination studies are reported when antibodies are present in extremely high titer (prozone phenomenon). In such cases, it is necessary to ask the laboratory to repeat the study on a diluted serum specimen.

Differential Diagnosis

Brucellosis must be differentiated from any other acute febrile disease, especially influenza, tularemia, Q fever, mononucleosis, and enteric fever. In its chronic form it resembles Hodgkin's disease, tuberculosis, HIV infection, malaria, and disseminated fungal infections such as histoplasmosis and coccidioidomycosis.

Complications

The most frequent complications are bone and joint lesions such as spondylitis and suppurative arthritis (usually of a single joint), endocarditis, and meningoencephalitis. Less common complications are pneumonitis with pleural effusion, hepatitis, and cholecystitis.

Treatment

Single-drug regimens are not recommended because the relapse rate may be as high as 50%. Combination regimens of two or three drugs are more effective. Either (1) doxycycline plus rifampin or streptomycin (or both) *or* (2) trimethoprim-sulfamethoxazole plus rifampin or streptomycin (or both) is effective in doses as follows for 21 days: doxycycline, 100–200 mg/d in divided doses; trimethoprim 320 mg/d plus sulfamethoxazole 1600 mg/d in divided doses; rifampin, 600–1200 mg/d; and streptomycin, 500 mg intramuscularly twice a day. Longer courses of therapy (eg, several months) may be required to cure relapses, osteomyelitis, or meningitis.

TULAREMIA

Essentials of Diagnosis

- Fever, headache, nausea, and prostration.
- Papule progressing to ulcer at site of inoculation.
- Enlarged regional lymph nodes.
- History of contact with rabbits, other rodents, and biting arthropods (eg, ticks in summer) in endemic area.
- Serologic tests or culture of ulcer, lymph node aspirate, or blood confirm the diagnosis.

General Considerations

Tularemia is an infection of wild rodents—particularly rabbits and muskrats—with *Francisella (Pasteurella) tularensis*. Humans usually acquire the infection by contact with animal tissues (eg, trapping muskrats, skinning rabbits) or from ticks. Infection in humans often produces a local lesion and widespread organ involvement but may be entirely asymptomatic. The incubation period is 2–10 days.

Clinical Findings

A. Symptoms and Signs: Fever, headache, and nausea begin suddenly, and a local lesion—a papule at the site of inoculation—develops and soon ulcerates. Regional lymph nodes may become enlarged and tender and may suppurate. The local lesion may be on the skin of an extremity or in the eye. Pneumonia may develop from hematogenous spread of the organism or may be primary after inhalation of infected aerosols, which are responsible for human-to-human transmission. Following ingestion of infected meat or water, an enteric form may be manifested by gastrointestinal symptoms, stupor, and delirium. In any type of involvement, the spleen may be enlarged and tender and there may be nonspecific rashes, myalgias, and prostration.

B. Laboratory Findings: Culturing the organism from blood or infected tissue requires special media. For this reason and because cultures of *F tularensis* may be hazardous to laboratory personnel, the diagnosis is usually made serologically. A positive agglutination test (> 1:80) develops in the second week after infection and may persist for several years.

Differential Diagnosis

Tularemia must be differentiated from rickettsial and meningococcal infections, cat-scratch disease, infectious mononucleosis, and various bacterial and fungal diseases.

Complications

Hematogenous spread may produce meningitis, perisplenitis, pericarditis, pneumonia, and osteomyelitis.

Treatment

Streptomycin, 0.5 g intramuscularly every 6–8 hours, together with tetracycline 0.5 g orally every 6 hours, is administered until 4–5 days after the patient becomes afebrile. Chloramphenicol may be substituted for tetracycline in the same dosage.

PLAGUE

Essentials of Diagnosis

- History of exposure to rodents in endemic area.

- Sudden onset of high fever, malaise, muscular pains, and prostration.
- Axillary or inguinal lymphadenitis (bubo).
- Bacteremia, sepsis, and pneumonitis may occur.
- Positive smear and culture from bubo and positive blood culture.

General Considerations

Plague is an infection of wild rodents with *Yersinia pestis,* a small bipolar-staining gram-negative rod. Plague is endemic in California, Arizona, Nevada, and New Mexico. It is transmitted among rodents and to humans by the bites of fleas or from contact with infected animals. If a plague victim develops pneumonia, the infection can be transmitted by droplets to other individuals. The incubation period is 2–10 days.

Following the flea bite, the organisms spread through the lymphatics to the lymph nodes, which become greatly enlarged (bubo). They may then reach the bloodstream to involve all organs. When pneumonia or meningitis develops, the outcome is often fatal.

Clinical Findings

A. Symptoms and Signs: The onset is sudden, with high fever, malaise, tachycardia, intense headache, and severe myalgias. The patient appears profoundly ill. Delirium may ensue. If pneumonia develops, tachypnea, productive cough, blood-tinged sputum, and cyanosis also occur. Signs of meningitis may develop. A pustule or ulcer at the site of inoculation and signs of lymphangitis may be observed. Axillary, inguinal, or cervical lymph nodes become enlarged and tender and may eventually suppurate and drain. With hematogenous spread, the patient may rapidly become toxic and comatose, with purpuric spots (black plague) appearing on the skin.

Primary plague pneumonia is a fulminant pneumonitis with bloody, frothy sputum and sepsis. It is usually fatal unless treatment is started within a few hours after onset.

B. Laboratory Findings: The plague bacillus may be found in smears from aspirates of buboes examined with Gram's stain. Cultures from bubo aspirate or pus and blood are positive but may grow slowly. In convalescing patients, an antibody titer rise may be demonstrated by agglutination tests.

Differential Diagnosis

The lymphadenitis of plague is most commonly mistaken for the lymphadenitis accompanying staphylococcal or streptococcal infections of an extremity, sexually transmitted diseases such as lymphogranuloma venereum or syphilis, and tularemia. The systemic manifestations resemble those of enteric or rickettsial fevers, malaria, or influenza. The pneumonia resembles other bacterial pneumonias, and the meningitis is similar to those caused by other bacteria.

Prevention

Drug prophylaxis may provide temporary protection for persons exposed to the risk of plague infection, particularly by the respiratory route. Tetracycline hydrochloride, 500 mg orally once or twice daily for 5 days, can accomplish this.

Plague vaccines—both live and killed—have been used for many years, but their efficacy is not clearly established.

Treatment

Therapy must be started promptly when plague is suspected. Streptomycin, 1 g intramuscularly, is administered immediately, and 0.5 g intramuscularly is then given every 6–8 hours. Tetracycline, 2 g daily orally (or parenterally if necessary), is given at the same time. Intravenous fluids, pressor drugs, oxygen, and intubation and mechanical ventilation are used as required. Patients with plague pneumonia should be strictly isolated.

GONOCOCCAL INFECTIONS

Essentials of Diagnosis

- Purulent and profuse urethral discharge, especially in men, with dysuria, yielding positive smear.
- Epididymitis, prostatitis, periurethral inflammation, proctitis in men.
- Cervicitis in women with purulent discharge, or asymptomatic, yielding positive culture; vaginitis, salpingitis, proctitis also occur.
- Fever, rash, tenosynovitis, and arthritis with disseminated disease.
- Gram-negative intracellular diplococci seen in a smear or cultured from any site, particularly the urethra, cervix, pharynx, and rectum.

General Considerations

Gonorrhea is the most prevalent reportable communicable disease in the USA, with an estimated 2.5 million or more cases annually. It is caused by *Neisseria gonorrhoeae,* a gram-negative diplococcus typically found inside polymorphonuclear cells. It is most commonly transmitted during sexual activity and has its greatest incidence in the 15- to 29-year-old age group. The incubation period is usually 2–8 days.

Anatomic Classification

A. Urethritis and Cervicitis: In men, there is initially burning on urination and a serous or milky discharge. One to 3 days later, the urethral pain is more pronounced and the discharge becomes yellow, creamy, and profuse, sometimes blood-tinged. The disorder may regress and become chronic or progress to involve the prostate, epididymis, and periurethral glands with acute, painful inflammation. Chronic infection leads to prostatitis and urethral strictures.

Rectal infection is common in homosexual men. Atypical sites of primary infection (eg, the pharynx) must always be considered. Asymptomatic infection is common and occurs in both sexes.

Gonococcal infection in women often becomes symptomatic during menses. Women may have dysuria, urinary frequency, and urgency, with a purulent urethral discharge. Vaginitis and cervicitis with inflammation of Bartholin's glands are common. Infection may be asymptomatic, with only slightly increased vaginal discharge and moderate cervicitis on examination. Infection may remain as a chronic cervicitis—an important reservoir of gonococci. It may progress to involve the uterus and tubes with acute and chronic salpingitis and with ultimate scarring of tubes and sterility. In pelvic inflammatory disease, anaerobes and chlamydiae often accompany gonococci. Rectal infection may result from spread of the organism from the genital tract or from anal coitus.

Smears of urethral discharge in men, especially during the first week after onset, typically show gram-negative diplococci in polymorphonuclear leukocytes. Smears are less often positive in women. Cultures are essential in all cases where gonorrhea is suspected and gonococci cannot be shown in gram-stained smears. This applies particularly to cervical, rectal, pharyngeal, and joint specimens. Specimens of pus or secretions are streaked on a selective medium such as Thayer-Martin or Transgrow. The latter is suitable for transport if a laboratory is not immediately available.

B. Disseminated Disease: Systemic complications follow the dissemination of gonococci from the primary site via the bloodstream. Gonococcal bacteremia is associated with intermittent fever, arthralgia, and skin lesions ranging from maculopapular to pustular or hemorrhagic, which tend to be few in number and peripherally located. Rarely, gonococcal endocarditis or meningitis develops. Arthritis and tenosynovitis are common complications, particularly involving the knees, ankles, and wrists. One or occasionally a few joints usually are involved. Gonococci can be isolated from less than half of patients with gonococcal arthritis.

C. Conjunctivitis: The most common form of eye involvement is direct inoculation of gonococci into the conjunctival sac. In adults, this occurs by autoinoculation of a person with genital infection. The purulent conjunctivitis may rapidly progress to panophthalmitis and loss of the eye unless treated promptly. A single 1-g dose of ceftriaxone is effective.

Differential Diagnosis

Gonococcal urethritis or cervicitis must be differentiated from nongonococcal urethritis; cervicitis or vaginitis due to *Chlamydia trachomatis, Gardnerella vaginalis, Trichomonas, Candida,* and many other agents associated with sexually transmitted diseases; pelvic inflammatory disease, arthritis, proctitis, and skin lesions. Often, several such agents coexist in the same patient. Reiter's disease (urethritis, conjunctivitis, arthritis) may mimic gonorrhea or coexist with it.

Prevention

Prevention is based on education, mechanical or chemical prophylaxis, and early diagnosis and treatment. The condom, if properly used, can reduce the risk of infection. Effective drugs taken in therapeutic doses within 24 hours of exposure can abort an infection.

Treatment

Therapy typically is administered before antimicrobial susceptibilities are known. The choice of which regimen to use should be based on the prevalence of penicillin-resistant organisms. Recent data indicate a nationwide distribution of penicillin- and tetracycline-resistant gonococci. Consequently, penicillin should no longer be considered first-line therapy. All sexual partners should be treated.

A. Uncomplicated Gonorrhea: For urethritis or cervicitis, ceftriaxone, 125 mg intramuscularly, is the treatment of choice. Effective single-dose oral regimens are also available, such as cefixime, 400 mg, or one of the fluoroquinolones—ciprofloxacin, 500 mg, or ofloxacin, 400 mg. Spectinomycin, 1 g intramuscularly once, may be used for the penicillin-allergic patient. Amoxicillin is no longer recommended owing to the prevalence of penicillin-resistant strains of gonococci. Anal gonorrhea in women responds to the same drugs, but in males ceftriaxone is most effective. Pharyngeal gonorrhea responds to ceftriaxone in the same dosage or to trimethoprim-sulfamethoxazole, nine regular-strength tablets orally daily for 5 days.

Since coexistent chlamydial infection is common, the above courses should be followed by erythromycin, 500 mg four times daily orally, or doxycycline, 100 mg twice daily orally, for 7 days. A single 1 g oral dose of azithromycin, given concurrently, is also effective and an attractive option when treating a patient population in which compliance is often an issue.

B. Treatment of Other Infections: Salpingitis, prostatitis, bacteremia, arthritis, and other complications due to susceptible strains in adults should be treated with penicillin G, 10 million units intravenously daily, for 5 days. Ceftriaxone, 2 g intravenously daily for 5 days, also is effective. Endocarditis should be treated with ceftriaxone, 1 g every 12 hours intravenously, for at least 3 weeks. Postgonococcal urethritis and cervicitis, which is usually caused by *Chlamydia,* is treated with a regimen of erythromycin, doxycycline, or azithromycin as described above. Serologic tests for syphilis should also be obtained.

Pelvic inflammatory disease requires cefoxitin, 2 g parenterally every 6 hours, or cefotetan, 2 g intravenously every 12 hours. Clindamycin, 900 mg intravenously every 8 hours, plus gentamicin, administered as a 2 mg/kg loading dose followed by 1.5 mg/kg every 8 hours, is also effective. Cefoxitin, 2 g intramuscularly, plus probenecid, 1 g orally as a single dose, followed by a 14-day oral regimen of doxycycline, 100 mg twice a day, is an effective outpatient regimen. Concurrent treatment for chlamydial infection also is indicated. Alternative drug choices exist.

Moran JS, Levine WC: Drugs of choice for the treatment of uncomplicated gonococcal infections. Clin Infect Dis 1995;20(Suppl 1):S47.

CHANCROID

Chancroid is a sexually transmitted disease caused by the short gram-negative bacillus *Haemophilus ducreyi*. Nonvenereal inoculation has occurred in medical personnel through contact with chancroid patients. The incubation period is 3–5 days.

The initial lesion at the site of inoculation is a vesicopustule that breaks down to form a painful, soft ulcer with a necrotic base, surrounding erythema, and undermined edges. Multiple lesions—started by autoinoculation—and inguinal adenitis often develop. The adenitis is usually unilateral and consists of tender, matted nodes of moderate size with overlying erythema. These may become fluctuant and rupture spontaneously. With lymph node involvement, fever, chills, and malaise may develop. Women may have no external signs of infection.

Swabs from lesions are best cultured on chocolate agar with 1% Isovitalex and vancomycin, 3 mg/mL, to yield *H ducreyi*. Mixed sexually transmitted disease is very common (including syphilis, herpes simplex, and HIV infection), as is infection of the ulcer with fusiforms, spirochetes, and other organisms.

Balanitis and phimosis are frequent complications.

Chancroid must be differentiated from other genital ulcers. The chancre of syphilis, by contrast, is clean and painless, with a hard base.

A single dose of either azithromycin, 1 g orally, or ceftriaxone, 250 mg intramuscularly, is effective treatment. Effective multiple-dose regimens are amoxicillin-potassium clavulanate (500/125) three times a day orally for 7 days; erythromycin, 500 mg orally four times a day for 7 days; or ciprofloxacin, 500 mg orally twice a day for 3 days.

Martin DH et al: Comparison of azithromycin and ceftriaxone for the treatment of chancroid. Clin Infect Dis 1995;21:409. (A single 1 g dose of azithromycin was as effective as a single 250 mg dose of ceftriaxone.)

GRANULOMA INGUINALE

Granuloma inguinale is a chronic, relapsing granulomatous anogenital infection due to *Calymmatobacterium (Donovania) granulomatis*. The pathognomonic cell, found in tissue scrapings or secretions, is large (25–90 μm) and contains intracytoplasmic cysts filled with bodies (Donovan bodies) that stain deeply with Wright's stain.

The incubation period is 8 days to 12 weeks. The onset is insidious. The lesions occur on the skin or mucous membranes of the genitalia or perineal area. They are relatively painless infiltrated nodules that soon slough. A shallow, sharply demarcated ulcer forms, with a beefy-red friable base of granulation tissue. The lesion spreads by contiguity. The advancing border has a characteristic rolled edge of granulation tissue. Large ulcerations may advance onto the lower abdomen and thighs. Scar formation and healing may occur along one border while the opposite border advances.

Superinfection with spirochete-fusiform organisms is common. The ulcer then becomes purulent, painful, foul-smelling, and extremely difficult to treat.

Several therapies are available. Because of the indolent nature of the disease, duration of therapy tends to be relatively long. Erythromycin or tetracycline, 500 mg four times a day for 21 days, is effective. Ampicillin, 500 mg four times a day, also is effective, but up to 12 weeks of therapy may be necessary.

Since other sexually transmitted diseases frequently coexist, cultures for these and a serologic test for syphilis must be performed.

BARTONELLA SPECIES

A revised classification of the α_2 subdivision of proteobacteria has grouped the species previously known as *Rochalimaea* as members of the genus *Bartonella* based on ribosomal RNA. These organisms (which include *B quintana, B henselae, B vinsonii,* and *B elizabethae*) are responsible for a wide variety of clinical syndromes. **Bacillary angiomatosis,** an important manifestation of bartonellosis, is discussed in Chapter 31.

Trench fever is a self-limited, louse-borne relapsing febrile disease caused by *B quintana*. The disease has occurred epidemically in louse-infested troops and civilians during wars and endemically in residents of scattered geographic areas (eg, Central America). Humans acquire infection when infected lice feces enter sites of skin breakdown. Onset of symptoms is abrupt and fever lasts 3–5 days, with relapses. The patient complains of weakness and severe pain behind the eyes and typically in the back and legs. Lymphadenopathy, splenomegaly, and a transient maculopapular rash may appear. Subclinical infection is frequent, and a carrier state is recognized. The differential diagnosis includes other febrile, self-limited states such as dengue, leptospirosis, malaria, relapsing fever, and typhus. Recovery occurs regularly even in the absence of treatment.

Karim A et al: Cat scratch disease, bacillary angiomatosis and other infections due to *Rochalimaea*. N Engl J Med 1994;330:1509.

CAT-SCRATCH DISEASE

Essentials of Diagnosis

- A primary infected ulcer or papule-pustule at site of inoculation (30% of cases).
- Regional lymphadenopathy that often suppurates.
- History of scratch by cat at involved area.
- Positive intradermal test.

General Considerations

This is an acute infection that occurs worldwide and is more common in children and young adults in contact with cats. It may be transmitted by a scratch or other injury, but some cases lack such a history. Cat-scratch disease is caused by the gram-negative bacillus *Bartonella* (formerly *Rochalimaea*) *henselae.*

Clinical Findings

A. Symptoms and Signs: A few days after the scratch, about one-third of patients develop a primary lesion at the site of inoculation. This primary lesion appears as an infected, scabbed ulcer or a papule with a central vesicle or pustule. One to 3 weeks later, symptoms of generalized infection appear (fever, malaise, headache), and the regional lymph nodes become enlarged without evidence of lymphangitis. The nodes may be tender and fixed, with overlying inflammation; or nontender, discrete, and without evidence of surrounding inflammation. Suppuration may occur, with the discharge of sterile pus. While the course is usually benign, some adults have fever and severe systemic symptoms for weeks.

Lymph node enlargement must be differentiated from that of lymphoma or other malignancy, tuberculosis, lymphogranuloma venereum, and acute bacterial infection.

B. Laboratory Findings: The sedimentation rate is elevated, the white blood cell count is usually normal, and the pus from the nodes is sterile. Lymph node morphology is fairly characteristic; excisional biopsy, usually performed to exclude lymphoma, confirms the diagnosis.

Complications

Encephalitis occurs rarely. Macular or papular rashes and erythema nodosum are occasionally seen. A disseminated form of cat-scratch disease, recently renamed **bacillary angiomatosis,** has been reported in HIV-infected persons and other immunocompromised individuals. Clinically, the lesions—which can be cutaneous, lymphatic, or visceral—are vasculoproliferative and histopathologically distinct from the granulomatous lesions of cat-scratch disease. A closely related organism, *Bartonella* (formerly *Rochalimaea*) *quintana,* the agent of trench fever (see above), also can cause bacillary angiomatosis, but its mode of transmission is uncertain. Bacillary angiomatosis responds to treatment with erythromycin (the drug of choice) or tetracycline.

Treatment

The role of antimicrobials in the therapy of uncomplicated cat-scratch disease is not established. Symptoms usually resolve without specific therapy in 1–2 weeks.

Koehler JE et al: *Rochalimaea henselae* infection. A new zoonosis with the domestic cat as reservoir. JAMA 1994;271:531. (Definitive study that establishes the link between *Rochalimaea* [since renamed *Bartonella*] *henselae* infection of cats and their role as the reservoir for infection of humans.)

ANAEROBIC INFECTIONS

Anaerobic bacteria make up the majority of normal human flora. Prominent members of the normal microbial flora of the mouth (anaerobic spirochetes, *Prevotella,* fusobacteria), the skin (anaerobic diphtheroids), the large bowel (*Bacteroides,* anaerobic streptococci, clostridia), and the female tract (*Bacteroides,* anaerobic streptococci, fusobacteria) may produce disease when displaced from their normal sites into tissues or closed body spaces.

Certain characteristics are suggestive of anaerobic infections: (1) They are polymicrobial. (2) Abscess formation is the rule. (3) Pus and infected tissue often are malodorous. (4) Septic thrombophlebitis and metastatic infection are frequent and may require incision and drainage. (Most of the important anaerobes except *Bacteroides fragilis* are highly sensitive to penicillin G. Diminished blood supply that favors proliferation of anaerobes because of reduced tissue oxygenation interferes with the delivery of antimicrobials to the site of anaerobic infection.) (5) Bacteriologic examination may yield negative results or only inconsequential aerobes unless rigorous culture conditions are used.

Important types of infections that are most commonly caused by anaerobic organisms are listed below. Treatment of all these infections consists of surgical exploration and judicious excision in conjunction with administration of antimicrobial drugs.

Upper Respiratory Tract

Prevotella melaninogenica (formerly *Bacteroides melaninogenicus*) together with anaerobic spirochetes is commonly involved in periodontal infections. These organisms, fusobacteria, and peptostreptococci are responsible for a substantial percentage of cases of chronic sinusitis and probably of peritonsillar abscess, chronic otitis media, and mastoiditis. Hygiene and drainage are as important in treatment as antimicrobials. Oral anaerobic organisms have been uniformly susceptible to penicillin, but there has been a recent trend of increasing penicillin resistance, usually due to β-lactamase production. Penicillin remains the drug of choice: 1–2 million units intravenously every 4 hours if parenteral therapy is required or 0.5 g orally four times daily for less severe infections. In the penicillin-allergic patient, clindamycin can be used (600 mg intravenously every 8 hours or 300 mg orally every 6 hours).

Chest Infections

Usually in the setting of poor oral hygiene and periodontal disease, aspiration of saliva (which contains 10^8 anaerobic organisms per milliliter in addition to aerobes) may lead to necrotizing pneumonia, lung abscess, and empyema. While polymicrobial infection is the rule, anaerobes—particularly *P melaninogenica,* fusobacteria, and peptostreptococci—are common etiologic agents. Most pulmonary infections respond to antimicrobial therapy alone. Percutaneous chest tube or surgical drainage is indicated for empyema.

Penicillin has long been considered the drug of choice for treatment of anaerobic lung infections, but penicillin-resistant *B fragilis* and *P melaninogenica* are isolated in up to 25% of cases. Clindamycin is more effective than penicillin for treatment of anaerobic lung infections. Penicillin failures have been associated with the presence of penicillin-resistant organisms. Clindamycin, 600 mg intravenously once, followed by 300 mg orally every 6–8 hours, is the treatment of choice for these infections. Penicillin, 2 million units intravenously every 4 hours, followed by amoxicillin, 500 mg every 8 hours orally, is a reasonable alternative. The second-generation cephalosporins cefoxitin, cefotetan, and cefmetazole are active in vitro against anaerobes, including those that are penicillin-resistant. Chloramphenicol is also effective, but it is used uncommonly given the numerous alternatives.

Central Nervous System

Anaerobes are a common cause of brain abscess, subdural empyema, or septic central nervous system thrombophlebitis. The organisms reach the central nervous system by direct extension from sinusitis, otitis, or mastoiditis or by hematogenous spread from chronic lung infections. Antimicrobial therapy—eg, penicillin, 20 million units intravenously, in combination with metronidazole, 750 mg intravenously, every 8 hours—is an important adjunct to surgical drainage. Some small multiple brain abscesses can be treated with antibiotics alone for 6–8 weeks and may heal without surgical drainage.

Intra-abdominal Infections

In the colon there are up to 10^{11} anaerobes per gram of content—predominantly *B fragilis,* clostridia, and peptostreptococci. These organisms play a central etiologic role in most intra-abdominal abscesses following trauma to the colon, diverticulitis, appendicitis, or perirectal abscess and may also participate in hepatic abscess and cholecystitis, often in association with aerobic coliform bacteria. The gallbladder wall may be infected with clostridia as well. The bacteriology includes anaerobes as well as enteric gram-negative rods and on occasion enterococci. Therapy should be directed both against anaerobes and gram-negative aerobes. Multiple antibiotics may be required. Antibiotics reliably active against *B fragilis* include metronidazole, chloramphenicol, imipenem, ampicillin-sulbactam, and ticarcillin-clavulanic acid. Cefoxitin, cefotetan, and clindamycin are active against 80–90% of strains, but most third-generation cephalosporins have poor activity, inhibiting only 50% of isolates. Non-*fragilis* species of *Bacteroides* may be less susceptible to the cephalosporins.

Table 33–2 summarizes the antibiotic regimens for management of moderate to moderately severe infections (eg, patient hemodynamically stable, good surgical drainage possible or established, low APACHE score, no multiple organ failure) and severe infections (eg, major peritoneal soilage, large or multiple abscesses, patient hemodynamically unstable), particularly if drug-resistant organisms are suspected. An effective oral regimen for patients able to take oral medications is presented also.

Female Genital Tract & Pelvic Infections

The normal flora of the vagina and cervix includes several species of *Bacteroides,* peptostreptococci, group B streptococci, lactobacilli, coliform bacteria, and, occasionally, spirochetes and clostridia. These organisms commonly cause genital tract infections and may disseminate from there.

While salpingitis is commonly caused by gonococci and chlamydiae, tubo-ovarian and pelvic abscesses are associated with anaerobes in a majority of cases. Postpartum infections may be caused by aerobic streptococci or staphylococci, but anaerobes are often found, and the most severe cases of postpartum or postabortion sepsis are associated with clostridia and *Bacteroides.* These have a high mortality rate, and treatment requires both antimicrobials directed against anaerobes and coliforms (see above) and abscess drainage or early hysterectomy.

Table 33–2. Treatment of anaerobic intra-abdominal infections.

Oral therapy

Ciprofloxacin, 750 mg twice daily, plus metronidazole, 500 mg three times daily

Intravenous therapy

Moderate to moderately severe infections:

Ticarcillin/clavulanate, 3 g/0.1 g every 6 hours

or—

Cefotetan, 2 g every 12 hours

or—

Clindamycin, 600 mg every 8 hours, or metronidazole, 500 mg every 8 hours, plus gentamicin, 5 mg/kg/d

Severe infections:

Imipenem, 0.5 g every 6–8 hours, or ceftriaxone, 1 g every 24 hours, plus either clindamycin, 600 mg every 8 hours, or metronidazole, 500 mg every 8 hours

Bacteremia & Endocarditis

Anaerobic bacteremia usually originates from the gastrointestinal tract, the oropharynx, decubitus ulcers, or the female genital tract. Endocarditis due to anaerobic and microaerophilic streptococci and *Bacteroides* originates from the same sites. Most cases of anaerobic or microaerophilic streptococcal endocarditis can be effectively treated with 12–20 million units of penicillin G daily, but optimal therapy of other types of anaerobic bacterial endocarditis must rely on laboratory guidance. Anaerobic corynebacteria *(Propionibacterium)*, clostridia, and *Bacteroides* occasionally cause endocarditis.

Skin & Soft Tissue Infections

Anaerobic infections in the skin and soft tissue usually follow trauma, inadequate blood supply, or surgery and are commonest in areas that are contaminated by oral or fecal flora. There may be progressive tissue necrosis and a putrid odor.

Several terms, such as bacterial synergistic gangrene, synergistic necrotizing cellulitis, necrotizing fasciitis, and nonclostridial crepitant cellulitis, have been used to classify these infections. Although there are some differences in microbiology among them, their differentiation on clinical grounds alone is difficult. All are mixed infections caused by aerobic and anaerobic organisms and require aggressive surgical debridement of necrotic tissue for cure. Surgical consultation is obligatory to assist in diagnosis and treatment.

Broad-spectrum antibiotics active against both anaerobes and gram-positive and gram-negative aerobes (eg, vancomycin plus metronidazole plus gentamicin or tobramycin) should be instituted empirically and modified by culture results (Table 37–2). They are given for about a week after progressive tissue destruction has been controlled and the margins of the wound remain free of inflammation.

Solomkin JS et al: Results of a randomized trial comparing sequential intravenous/oral treatment with ciprofloxacin plus metronidazole to imipenem/cilastatin for intra-abdominal infections. The Intra-Abdominal Infection Study Group. Ann Surg 1996;223:303.

ACTINOMYCOSIS

Essentials of Diagnosis

- History of recent dental infection or abdominal trauma.
- Chronic pneumonia or indolent intra-abdominal or cervicofacial abscess.
- Sinus tract formation.

General Considerations

Actinomyces israelii and other species of *Actinomyces* occur in the normal flora of the mouth and tonsillar crypts. They are anaerobic, gram-positive, branching filamentous bacteria (1 μm in diameter) that may fragment into bacillary forms. When introduced into traumatized tissue and associated with other anaerobic bacteria, these actinomycetes become pathogens.

The most common site of infection is the cervicofacial area (about 60% of cases). Infection typically follows extraction of a tooth or other trauma. Lesions may develop in the gastrointestinal tract or lungs following ingestion or aspiration of the organism from its endogenous source in the mouth.

Clinical Findings

A. Symptoms and Signs:

1. Cervicofacial actinomycosis–Cervicofacial actinomycosis develops slowly. The area becomes markedly indurated, and the overlying skin becomes reddish or cyanotic. Abscesses eventually draining to the surface persist for long periods. Sulfur granules—masses of filamentous organisms—may be found in the pus. There is usually little pain unless there is secondary infection. Trismus indicates that the muscles of mastication are involved. Radiography may reveal bony involvement.

2. Thoracic actinomycosis–Thoracic involvement begins with fever, cough, and sputum production with night sweats and weight loss. Pleuritic pain may be present. Multiple sinuses may extend through the chest wall, to the heart, or into the abdominal cavity. Ribs may be involved. Radiography shows areas of consolidation and in many cases pleural effusion. Cervicofacial or thoracic disease may occasionally result in central nervous system complications, most commonly brain abscess or meningitis.

3. Abdominal actinomycosis–Abdominal

actinomycosis usually causes pain in the ileocecal region, spiking fever and chills, vomiting, and weight loss and may be confused with Crohn's disease. Irregular abdominal masses may be palpated. Pelvic inflammatory disease caused by actinomycetes has been associated with prolonged use of an intrauterine contraceptive device. Sinuses draining to the exterior may develop. CT scanning reveals an inflammatory mass that may extend to involve bone.

B. Laboratory Findings: The anaerobic, gram-positive organism may be demonstrated as a granule or as scattered branching gram-positive filaments in the pus. Anaerobic culture is necessary to distinguish *Actinomyces* from *Nocardia*, because specific therapy differs for the two infections.

Treatment

Penicillin G is the drug of choice. Ten to 20 million units are given via a parenteral route for 2–4 weeks, followed by oral penicillin V, 500 mg four times daily.

Sulfonamides such as sulfamethoxazole may be an alternative regimen at a total daily dosage of 2–4 g. Response to therapy is slow. Therapy should be continued for weeks to months after clinical manifestations have disappeared in order to ensure cure. Surgical procedures such as drainage and resection may be beneficial.

With penicillin and surgery, the prognosis is good. The difficulties of diagnosis, however, may permit extensive destruction of tissue before the diagnosis is identified and therapy is started.

NOCARDIOSIS

Nocardia asteroides and *Nocardia brasiliensis,* aerobic filamentous soil bacteria, cause pulmonary and systemic nocardiosis. Bronchopulmonary abnormalities (eg, alveolar proteinosis) predispose to colonization, but infection is unusual unless the patient is also receiving systemic corticosteroids or is otherwise immunosuppressed.

Pulmonary involvement usually begins with malaise, loss of weight, fever, and night sweats. Cough and production of purulent sputum are the chief complaints. Radiography may show infiltrates accompanied by pleural effusion. The lesions may penetrate to the exterior through the chest wall, invading the ribs.

Dissemination may involve any organ. Brain abscesses and subcutaneous nodules are most frequent. Dissemination is seen exclusively in immunocompromised patients.

N asteroides is usually found as delicate, branching, gram-positive filaments. It may be weakly acid-fast, occasionally causing diagnostic confusion with tuberculosis. Identification is made by culture.

Therapy is initiated with intravenous trimethoprim-sulfamethoxazole and continued with oral trimethoprim-sulfamethoxazole, one double-strength tablet twice a day. Surgical procedures such as drainage and resection may be needed as adjunctive therapy.

Response may be slow, and therapy must be continued for at least 6 months. The prognosis in systemic nocardiosis is poor when diagnosis and therapy are delayed.

INFECTIONS CAUSED BY MYCOBACTERIA

NONTUBERCULOUS ATYPICAL MYCOBACTERIAL DISEASES

About 10% of mycobacterial infections seen in clinical practice are caused not by *Mycobacterium tuberculosis* but by atypical mycobacteria. Atypical mycobacterial infections are among the most common opportunistic infections in advanced HIV disease. These organisms have distinctive laboratory characteristics, occur ubiquitously in the environment, are not communicable from person to person, and are often strikingly resistant to antituberculous drugs.

Disseminated *Mycobacterium avium* Infection

Mycobacterium avium complex (MAC) produces asymptomatic colonization or a wide spectrum of diseases, including coin lesions, bronchitis in patients with chronic lung disease, and invasive pulmonary disease that is often cavitary and occurs in patients with underlying lung disease. MAC is a common cause of disseminated disease in the late stages of HIV infection, when the CD4 cell count is less than 50–100/μL. Persistent fever and weight loss are the most common symptoms. The organism can usually be cultured from multiple sites, including blood, liver, lymph node, or bone marrow. Blood culture is the preferred means of establishing the diagnosis and has a sensitivity of 98%.

Agents with proved activity against MAC in humans are rifabutin, azithromycin, clarithromycin, and ethambutol. Amikacin and ciprofloxacin have activity in vitro, but clinical data are lacking. Single-agent therapy should not be used because of rapid emergence of secondary resistance. Clarithromycin, 500 mg orally twice daily, plus ethambutol, 15 mg/kg/d as a single dose, with or without rifabutin, 300 mg/d, is the treatment of choice. Azithromycin, 500 mg once daily, may be used instead of clarithromycin. Too few data are available to permit specific recommendations about second-line regimens for patients intolerant of macrolides or those who have disease caused by macrolide-resistant organisms. However, a combination of two or more active agents should be used.

Several clinical trials have now shown that antimicrobial prophylaxis of MAC prevents disseminated disease and prolongs survival. It is the standard of care to offer prophylaxis against MAC to all HIV-infected patients with CD4 counts ≤ 50/μL. Single-drug regimens of clarithromycin, 500 mg twice daily, azithromycin, 1200 mg once weekly, or rifabutin, 300 mg once daily, have been shown to be effective. Clarithromycin and azithromycin are more effective and better tolerated than rifabutin, and for that reason a macrolide is preferred over rifabutin. Patients who develop disseminated disease while receiving macrolide prophylaxis may have macrolide-resistant organisms, a factor to consider when pondering treatment options. Which regimen to use is not established, but most authorities recommend addition of rifabutin and ethambutol. Whether to continue the macrolide if the isolate is resistant in vitro is controversial.

Pulmonary Infections

MAC causes a chronic, slowly progressive pulmonary infection resembling tuberculosis in immunocompetent patients, who typically have underlying pulmonary disease.

Treatment of immunocompetent patients with pulmonary infection is almost completely empirical and based almost entirely on anecdotal data. A combination of agents should be used. Rifampin, 600 mg once daily, plus ethambutol, 15–25 mg/kg/d, plus streptomycin, 1 g intramuscularly three to five times a week for the first 4–6 months, have been used. The role of rifabutin, fluoroquinolones, and the macrolides is not known, but based upon their excellent efficacy in immunocompromised AIDS patients, they may actually be more effective than the relatively weak agents traditionally used in immunocompetent patients. Clarithromycin is a very potent drug in the treatment of MAC in AIDS patients. Based on this, inclusion of clarithromycin in the initial treatment regimen of immunocompetent patients should be strongly considered.

Mycobacterium kansasii can produce clinical disease resembling tuberculosis, but the illness progresses more slowly. Most such infections occur in patients with preexisting lung disease, though 40% of patients have no known pulmonary disease. Microbiologically, *M kansasii* is similar to *M tuberculosis* and is sensitive to the same drugs. Therapy with isoniazid, ethambutol, and rifampin for 2 years (or

1 year after sputum conversion) has been highly successful.

Less common causes of pulmonary disease include *Mycobacterium xenopi, Mycobacterium szulgai,* and *Mycobacterium gordonae.* These organisms have variable sensitivities, and treatment is based on results of sensitivity tests. *Mycobacterium fortuitum* and *Mycobacterium chelonei* also can cause pneumonia.

Lymphadenitis

Most cases of lymphadenitis (scrofula) in adults are caused by *Mycobacterium tuberculosis* and can be a manifestation of disseminated disease. In children, the majority of cases are due to nontuberculous mycobacterial species, with *Mycobacterium scrofulaceum* and MAC being the most common. *Mycobacterium kansasii, Mycobacterium bovis, Mycobacterium chelonei,* and *Mycobacterium fortuitum* are less commonly observed. Unlike disease caused by *M tuberculosis,* which requires systemic therapy for 9 months, infection with nontuberculous mycobacteria can be successfully treated by surgical excision without antituberculous therapy.

Skin & Soft Tissue Infections

Skin and soft tissue infections such as abscesses, septic arthritis, and osteomyelitis can result from direct inoculation or hematogenous dissemination or may occur as a complication of surgery.

M chelonei and *M fortuitum* are frequent causes of this type of infection. Most cases occur in the extremities and initially present as nodules. Ulceration with abscess formation often follows. The organisms are resistant to the usual antituberculous drugs but may be sensitive to a variety of antibiotics, including erythromycin, doxycycline, amikacin, cefoxitin, sulfonamides, imipenem, and ciprofloxacin. Therapy includes surgical debridement along with drug therapy. Initially, parenteral drugs are given for several weeks, and this is followed by an oral regimen to which the organism is sensitive. The duration of therapy is variable but usually continues for several months after the soft tissue lesions have healed.

Mycobacterium marinum infection ("swimming pool granuloma") presents as a nodular skin lesion following exposure to nonchlorinated water. The lesions respond to therapy with doxycycline, minocycline, or trimethoprim-sulfamethoxazole.

Mycobacterium ulcerans infection (Buruli ulcer) is seen mainly in Africa and Australia and produces a large ulcerative lesion. Therapy consists of surgical excision and skin grafting.

Sullam PM: Rifabutin therapy for disseminated *Mycobacterium avium* complex infection. Clin Infect Dis 1996;22(Suppl 1):S37. (Review of the role of rifabutin in therapy of MAC infection.)

Shafran SD et al: A comparison of two regimens for the

treatment of *Mycobacterium avium* complex bacteremia in AIDS: Rifabutin, ethambutol, and clarithromycin versus rifampin, ethambutol, clofazimine, and ciprofloxacin. Canadian HIV Trials Network Protocol 010 Study Group. N Engl J Med 1996;335:377. (A three-drug regimen of rifabutin, ethambutol, and clarithromycin was superior, with resolution of bacteremia in approximately 70% of cases.)

MYCOBACTERIUM TUBERCULOSIS INFECTIONS

The case rate of tuberculosis in the United States has been increasing since 1986, largely due to a dramatic increase in cases among HIV-infected individuals. Compared to a lifetime risk of developing active tuberculosis of approximately 10% in an infected immunocompetent person, the risk is up to 7% per year for the HIV-infected individual who is also infected with *M tuberculosis*. This greatly increased risk of developing active disease—as well as the recent occurrence in HIV-infected individuals of outbreaks of tuberculosis caused by strains of *M tuberculosis* resistant to multiple drugs—underscore the importance of early case identification and administration of effective antituberculous therapy. Accordingly, the principles of antituberculous therapy, the preferred treatment regimens, and the currently available antimicrobial agents are reviewed.

Except for the special case of tuberculous meningitis, which is discussed below, the clinical manifestations of tuberculous infection are discussed in the chapters pertaining to the organ system involved.

Treatment Considerations

A. Initial Therapy: Patients with suspected or documented active tuberculosis should be treated with at least two drugs to which the strain is susceptible. Single-drug regimens are notoriously ineffective, with failure rates of 70% or more due to emergence of resistant mutants, which occurs at a frequency of one bacillus in 10^6. Because 10^7 to 10^9 acid-fast bacilli typically are present at the site of active infection, resistant mutants are invariably present when therapy is initiated. Therapy with two drugs, each possessing a different mechanism of action, is effective because the odds that a bacillus is resistant to both are $10^{-6} \times 10^{-6}$, or one in 10^{12}, which is at least three orders of magnitude less than the number of infecting organisms.

The results of susceptibility tests usually are not known when therapy is initiated. Therefore, drugs are chosen based on their relative potency and on prior susceptibility data obtained from within the community or within the relevant patient population. Isoniazid and rifampin are the two most potent antituberculous agents, and because clinical isolates from newly diagnosed cases were predictably susceptible

to both (98% or more of strains), initial therapy with these two drugs was until recently considered appropriate for most cases. Three or four drug regimens were reserved for patients who had one or more risk factors for drug-resistant tuberculosis. Patients at risk for infection with resistant strains were those who had been previously treated for tuberculosis; those who failed to complete a prescribed course of therapy or were otherwise noncompliant; and patients or their close contacts who were from regions (eg, the Philippines, China, Southeast Asia, and Haiti) where the prevalence of primary drug-resistant strains is above 5%.

Recent outbreaks of multidrug-resistant tuberculosis in HIV-infected patients from Miami and New York have led to new recommendations for initial therapy of suspected tuberculosis. Initial therapy with an oral four-drug regimen consisting of isoniazid (INH), 300 mg, rifampin, 600 mg, pyrazinamide, 25 mg/kg, and ethambutol, 15 mg/kg, each administered as a single daily dose, is recommended pending results of culture and susceptibility tests. It may be reasonable to add or substitute other drugs (Table 33–3) depending on the epidemiologic data. For example, if a patient has had a relapse or has not responded to a particular regimen, two other drugs not used previously should be included in the regimen. If a strain is known to be resistant to a particular drug, another drug to which the strain is likely to be susceptible should be substituted. As a rule of thumb, at least two new drugs are added to a failing regimen. Which drug or drugs eventually are selected will also depend upon their toxicities and the ability of the patient to tolerate them.

B. Definitive Therapy: Assuming that the four-drug regimen recommended above is used and that the strain is susceptible, ethambutol can be discontinued and the three-drug regimen of isoniazid, ri-

Table 33–3. Antituberculous agents, ranked in order of preference, and usual daily doses.

Drug	Daily Dose and Route
First-line agents	
Isoniazid	300 mg orally or IM
Rifampin	600 mg orally or IV
Ethambutol	15–25 mg/kg orally
Pyrazinamide	25 mg/kg orally
Streptomycin	15 mg/kg IM
Second-line agents	
Amikacin	15 mg/kg IM
Capreomycin	15 mg/kg IM
Ethionamide	0.5–1 g orally
Cycloserine	0.5–1 g orally
Ofloxacin	600–800 mg/d orally
Ciprofloxacin	750 mg twice daily orally

fampin, and pyrazinamide administered for a total of 2 months. The pyrazinamide is then stopped, and isoniazid and rifampin are administered for at least four more months (total of 6 months). If pyrazinamide is not used during the first 2 months of therapy, isoniazid and rifampin should be administered for a minimum of 9 months. If other drug combinations must be used because of toxicity or drug resistance, longer durations of therapy are required (Table 33–4).

The regimens used for treatment of active pulmonary tuberculosis are effective also against extrapulmonary disease. However, some authorities recommend longer durations (eg, 12 months of isoniazid plus rifampin instead of 6–9 months) for extrapulmonary disease such as meningitis or bone and joint infections, where drug penetration is an issue, and for disseminated infection. The relapse rate in HIV-infected patients treated with a 6-month regimen of isoniazid-rifampin-pyrazinamide is higher than in HIV-seronegative patients. Relapse has been associated with low CD4 counts. Because extending therapy does not improve survival, current recommendations for treatment of active tuberculosis in HIV-infected patients are the same as for other patients.

Prognosis & Follow-Up

Response to therapy is monitored clinically and, if possible, bacteriologically. A qualitative decrease in numbers of acid-fast bacilli seen on sputum smears over the course of therapy is a reliable indicator of response. Most patients who are treated with the recommended four-drug regimen are culture-negative by 3 months. If sputum smears remain persistently positive, noncompliance should be suspected and institution of supervised daily therapy strongly considered. If noncompliance is unlikely, the possibility of drug resistance should be entertained and the regimen altered accordingly.

The period of infectivity after initiation of chemotherapy is poorly defined. Three consecutive sputum smears negative for acid-fast bacilli using samples obtained on separate days are a reliable indication that the patient is no longer infectious to others.

Table 33–4. Minimum recommended duration of antituberculous therapy.

Regimen	Duration (mo)
Isoniazid + rifampin + pyrazinamide[1]	6
Isoniazid + rifampin	9
Rifampin + ethambutol	12
Isoniazid + ethambutol	18–24

[1]Pyrazinamide for the first 2 months only.

Preventive Therapy

Administration of isoniazid, 300 mg once daily for 6 months (12 months for HIV-infected or other immunocompromised patients), is approximately 80% effective in preventing active disease in persons with a positive tuberculin (PPD) skin test. The test is considered positive when there is ≥ 10 mm of induration at 48–72 hours after intradermal injection of 0.1 mL of tuberculin antigen. The cut-off is ≥ 5 mm for HIV-infected individuals and close contacts of active cases of pulmonary tuberculosis. Isoniazid prophylaxis is recommended for tuberculin skin test-positive individuals aged 35 or younger and for all close contacts of active cases, HIV-infected or otherwise immunocompromised individuals, and the skin test converters (defined as individuals with a prior documented negative test within 2 years of a newly positive one) regardless of age. The recommendations of the American Thoracic Society (Bass et al, 1994) should be consulted for more detailed information and advice concerning tuberculin skin testing and preventive therapy.

Bass JB et al: Treatment of tuberculosis and tuberculous infection in adults and children. Am J Respir Crit Care Med 1994;149:1359.

Iseman MD: Treatment of multidrug-resistant tuberculosis. N Engl J Med 1993;329:784.

Perrièens JH et al: Pulmonary tuberculosis in HIV-infected patients in Zaire: A controlled trial of treatment for either 6 or 12 months. N Engl J Med 1995;332:779. (The relapse rate was 9% for HIV-infected patients receiving the 6-month regimen compared with 5.3% for HIV-seronegative patients and 2% for HIV-infected patients treated for 12 months. Survival rates of HIV-infected cases were not increased by extending therapy to 12 months.)

Pulido F et al: Relapse of tuberculosis after treatment in human immunodeficiency virus-infected patients. Arch Intern Med 1997;157:227. (Shorter duration of treatment and a low CD4 cell count were associated with a greater probability of relapse, which occurred in 10 [24%] of 41 patients who were treated for less than 9 months.)

Raviglione MC, Snider DE, Kochi A: Global epidemiology of tuberculosis: Morbidity and mortality of a worldwide epidemic. JAMA 1995;273:220.

TUBERCULOUS MENINGITIS

Essentials of Diagnosis

- Gradual onset of listlessness, irritability, and anorexia.
- Headache, vomiting, and seizures common.
- Cranial nerve abnormalities typical.
- Tuberculosis focus may be evident elsewhere.
- Cerebrospinal fluid shows several hundred lymphocytes, low glucose, and high protein.

General Considerations

Tuberculous meningitis is caused by rupture of a

meningeal tuberculoma resulting from earlier hematogenous seeding of tubercle bacillus from a pulmonary focus, or it may be a consequence of miliary spread.

Clinical Findings

A. Symptoms and Signs: The onset is usually gradual, with listlessness, irritability, anorexia, and fever, followed by headache, vomiting, convulsions, and coma. In older patients, headache and behavioral changes are prominent early symptoms. Nuchal rigidity and cranial nerve palsies occur as the meningitis progresses. Evidence of active tuberculosis elsewhere or a history of prior tuberculosis is present in up to 75% of patients.

B. Laboratory Findings: The spinal fluid is frequently yellowish, with increased pressure, 100–500 cells/μL (early, polymorphonuclear neutrophils; later, lymphocytes), increased protein, and decreased glucose. Acid-fast stains of cerebrospinal fluid usually are negative, and cultures also may be negative in 15–25% of cases. Chest x-ray often reveals abnormalities compatible with tuberculosis but may be normal.

Differential Diagnosis

Tuberculous meningitis may be confused with any other type of meningitis, but the gradual onset, the predominantly lymphocytic pleocytosis of the spinal fluid, and evidence of tuberculosis elsewhere often point to the diagnosis. The tuberculin skin test is usually positive, though in a significant proportion of patients it is negative.

Fungal and other granulomatous meningitides, syphilis, and carcinomatous meningitis are in the differential diagnosis.

Complications

Complications of tuberculous meningitis include chronic brain syndrome, seizure disorders, cranial nerve palsies, stroke, and obstructive hydrocephalus. These result from inflammatory exudate primarily involving the basilar meninges and arteries.

Treatment

Presumptive diagnosis followed by early, empiric antituberculous therapy is essential for survival and to minimize sequelae. Even if cultures are not positive, a full course of therapy is warranted if the clinical setting is suggestive of tuberculous meningitis.

Regimens that are effective for pulmonary tuberculosis are effective also for tuberculous meningitis (Table 33–3). Rifampin, isoniazid, and pyrazinamide all penetrate into cerebrospinal fluid well. The penetration of ethambutol is more variable, but therapeutic concentrations can be achieved, and the drug has been successfully used for meningitis. Aminoglycosides penetrate less well. Regimens that do not include both isoniazid and rifampin may be effective but are less reliable and generally must be given for longer periods. Other regimens may also be effective, but they are less reliable and generally must be given for longer periods.

Some authorities recommend the addition of corticosteroids for patients with focal deficits or altered mental status. Dexamethasone, 0.15 mg/kg four times daily for 1–2 weeks, then discontinued in a tapering regimen over 4 weeks, may be used.

LEPROSY

Essentials of Diagnosis

- Pale, anesthetic macular—or nodular and erythematous—skin lesions.
- Superficial nerve thickening with associated anesthesia.
- History of residence in endemic area in childhood.
- Acid-fast bacilli in skin lesions or nasal scrapings, or characteristic histologic nerve changes.

General Considerations

Leprosy is a chronic infectious disease caused by the acid-fast rod *Mycobacterium leprae*. The mode of transmission probably is respiratory and involves prolonged exposure in childhood. The disease is endemic in tropical and subtropical Asia, Africa, Central and South America and the Pacific regions, and southern USA.

Clinical Findings

A. Symptoms and Signs: The onset is insidious. The lesions involve the cooler body tissues: skin, superficial nerves, nose, pharynx, larynx, eyes, and testicles. Skin lesions may occur as pale, anesthetic macular lesions 1–10 cm in diameter; discrete erythematous, infiltrated nodules 1–5 cm in diameter; or a diffuse skin infiltration. Neurologic disturbances are manifested by nerve infiltration and thickening, with resultant anesthesia, neuritis, and paresthesia. Bilateral ulnar neuropathy is highly suggestive. In untreated cases, disfigurement due to the skin infiltration and nerve involvement may be extreme, leading to trophic ulcers, bone resorption, and loss of digits.

The disease is divided clinically and by laboratory tests into two distinct types: lepromatous and tuberculoid. The lepromatous type occurs in persons with defective cellular immunity. The course is progressive and malignant, with nodular skin lesions; slow, symmetric nerve involvement; abundant acid-fast bacilli in the skin lesions; and a negative lepromin skin test. In the tuberculoid type, cellular immunity is intact and the course is more benign and less progressive, with macular skin lesions, severe asymmetric nerve involvement of sudden onset with few bacilli present in the lesions, and a positive lepromin skin test. Intermediate ("borderline") cases are frequent.

Eye involvement (keratitis and iridocyclitis), nasal ulcers, epistaxis, anemia, and lymphadenopathy may occur.

B. Laboratory Findings: Laboratory confirmation of leprosy requires the demonstration of acid-fast bacilli in a skin biopsy. Biopsy of skin or of a thickened involved nerve also gives a typical histologic picture. *M leprae* does not grow in artificial media.

Differential Diagnosis

The skin lesions of leprosy often resemble those of lupus erythematosus, sarcoidosis, syphilis, erythema nodosum, erythema multiforme, cutaneous tuberculosis, and vitiligo.

Complications

Renal failure and hepatomegaly from secondary amyloidosis may occur with long-standing disease.

Treatment

Combination therapy is recommended for treatment of all types of leprosy. Single-drug treatment is accompanied by emergence of resistance, and primary resistance to dapsone also occurs. For borderline and lepromatous cases, a three-drug regimen such as dapsone, 50–100 mg/d, clofazimine, 50 mg/d, and rifampin, 10 mg/kg/d (up to 600 mg/d), all given orally, should be used. The triple-drug combination should be administered for a minimum of 2–3 years and, ideally, until all biopsies are negative for acid-fast bacilli. For indeterminate and tuberculoid leprosy, the dapsone-rifampin combination is recommended for 6–12 months, often followed by a course of dapsone alone for 2 or more years.

Two reactional states—erythema nodosum leprosum and reversal reactions—may occur as a consequence of therapy. The reversal reaction, typical of borderline lepromatous leprosy, probably results from enhanced host immunity. Skin lesions and nerves become swollen and tender, but systemic manifestations are not seen. Erythema nodosum leprosum, typical of lepromatous leprosy, is a consequence of immune injury from antigen-antibody complex deposition in skin and other tissues; in addition to skin and nerve manifestations, fever and systemic involvement may be seen. Prednisone, 60 mg/d, or thalidomide, 300 mg/d (in the nonpregnant patient only), is effective for erythema nodosum leprosum. Improvement is expected within a few days after initiating prednisone, and thereafter the dose may be tapered over several weeks to avoid recurrence. Thalidomide is also tapered over several weeks to a 100 mg bedtime dose. Erythema nodosum leprosum is usually confined to the first year of therapy, and prednisone or thalidomide can be discontinued. Thalidomide is ineffective for reversal reactions, and prednisone, 60 mg/d, is indicated. Reversal reactions tend to recur, and the dose of prednisone should be slowly tapered over weeks to months. Therapy for leprosy should not be discontinued during treatment of reactional states.

INFECTIONS CAUSED BY CHLAMYDIAE

Chlamydiae are a large group of obligate intracellular parasites closely related to gram-negative bacteria. They are assigned to three species—*Chlamydia trachomatis, Chlamydia psittaci,* and *Chlamydia pneumoniae*—on the basis of intracellular inclusions, sulfonamide susceptibility, antigenic composition, and disease production. *C trachomatis* causes many different human infections involving the eye (trachoma, inclusion conjunctivitis), the genital tract (lymphogranuloma venereum, nongonococcal urethritis, cervicitis, salpingitis), or the respiratory tract (pneumonitis). *C psittaci* causes psittacosis in humans and many animal diseases. *Chlamydia pneumoniae,* TWAR strain, is a newly identified species that causes respiratory tract infections. A few specific diseases are described.

CHLAMYDIA TRACHOMATIS INFECTIONS

1. LYMPHOGRANULOMA VENEREUM

Essentials of Diagnosis

- Evanescent primary genital lesion.
- Lymph node enlargement, softening, and suppuration, with draining sinuses.
- Proctitis and rectal stricture in women or homosexual men.
- Positive complement fixation test.

General Considerations

Lymphogranuloma venereum is an acute and chronic sexually transmitted disease caused by *Chlamydia trachomatis* types L1–L3. After the genital lesion disappears, the infection spreads to lymph channels and lymph nodes of the genital and rectal areas. The disease is acquired during intercourse or through contact with contaminated exudate from active lesions. The incubation period is 5–21 days. Inapparent infections and latent disease are not uncommon.

Clinical Findings

A. Symptoms and Signs: In men, the initial vesicular or ulcerative lesion (on the external genitalia) is evanescent and often goes unnoticed. Inguinal buboes appear 1–4 weeks after exposure, are often bilateral, and have a tendency to fuse, soften, and break down to form multiple draining sinuses, with extensive scarring. In women, the genital lymph drainage is to the perirectal glands. Early anorectal manifestations are proctitis with tenesmus and bloody purulent discharge; late manifestations are chronic cicatrizing inflammation of the rectal and perirectal tissue. These changes lead to obstipation and rectal stricture and, occasionally, rectovaginal and perianal fistulas. They are also seen in homosexual men.

B. Laboratory Findings: The complement fixation test may be positive, but cross-reaction with other chlamydiae occurs. Although a positive reaction may reflect remote infection, high titers usually indicate active disease. Specific immunofluorescence tests for IgM are more specific for acute infection.

Differential Diagnosis

The early lesion of lymphogranuloma venereum must be differentiated from the lesions of syphilis, genital herpes, and chancroid; lymph node involvement must be distinguished from that due to tularemia, tuberculosis, plague, neoplasm, or pyogenic infection; rectal stricture must be distinguished from that due to neoplasm and ulcerative colitis.

Treatment

The antibiotic of choice is tetracycline (contraindicated in pregnancy), 0.25–0.5 g orally four times daily, or doxycycline, 0.1 g twice daily for 21 days. Erythromycin, 500 mg four times a day, or trimethoprim-sulfamethoxazole, 160/800 mg twice a day for 21 days, also is effective.

2. CHLAMYDIAL URETHRITIS & CERVICITIS

Chlamydia trachomatis immunotypes D–K are isolated in about 50% of cases of nongonococcal urethritis and cervicitis by appropriate techniques. In other cases, *Ureaplasma urealyticum* can be grown as a possible etiologic agent. *C trachomatis* is an important cause of postgonococcal urethritis. Co-infection with gonococci and chlamydiae is common, and postgonococcal (ie, chlamydial) urethritis may persist after successful treatment of the gonococcal component. Occasionally, epididymitis, prostatitis, or proctitis is caused by chlamydial infection.

Females infected with *Chlamydia* may be asymptomatic or may have signs and symptoms of cervicitis, salpingitis, or pelvic inflammatory disease. *Chlamydia* is probably the leading cause of infertility in females in the United States.

Culture is reliable but difficult and expensive because of the requirement for growth in cell culture. Three indirect methods for diagnosis are direct immunofluorescence assay, enzyme-linked immunoassay, and DNA probing of cervical samples, none of which are as sensitive as culture. Sensitivities and specificities of the indirect methods are similar—about 75–90% and 95%, respectively. For these reasons, the diagnosis often is made clinically and by exclusion, ie, failure to identify gonococci in a patient with urethritis or cervicitis. The urethral or cervical discharge tends to be less painful, less purulent, and more watery in chlamydial versus gonococcal infection. Absence of gram-negative intracellular diplococci in urethral discharge from a male is very suggestive of chlamydial infection.

Therapy often must be given presumptively. Sexual partners of infected patients should also be treated. Effective treatment regimens are tetracycline or erythromycin, 500 mg four times a day, or doxycycline, 100 mg twice daily, for 7 days. Trimethoprim-sulfamethoxazole, 160/800 mg twice a day, is acceptable but may be less effective than tetracyclines or erythromycin. Erythromycin is the drug of choice in the pregnant patient. A single 1 g dose of azithromycin is effective for uncomplicated urethritis and cervicitis and has the advantage of improved patient compliance and minimal toxicity.

Stamm WE et al: Azithromycin for empirical treatment of the nongonococcal urethritis syndrome in men: A randomized double-blind study. JAMA 1995;274:545. (Azithromycin as a single dose is as effective as a 7-day course of doxycycline.)

CHLAMYDIA PSITTACI & PSITTACOSIS (Ornithosis)

Essentials of Diagnosis

- Fever, chills, and cough; headache common.
- Atypical pneumonia with slightly delayed appearance of signs of pneumonitis.
- Contact with infected bird (psittacine, pigeons, many others) 7–15 days previously.
- Isolation of chlamydiae or rising titer of complement-fixing antibodies.

General Considerations

Psittacosis is acquired from contact with birds (parrots, parakeets, pigeons, chickens, ducks, and many others), which may or may not be ill. The history may be difficult to obtain if the patient acquired infection from an illegally imported bird.

Clinical Findings

The onset is usually rapid, with fever, chills, myalgia, dry cough, and headache. Signs include temperature-pulse dissociation, dullness to percussion, and rales. Pulmonary findings may be absent early. Dyspnea and cyanosis may occur later. Endocarditis, which is culture-negative, may occur. The radiographic findings in typical psittacosis are those of atypical pneumonia, which tends to be interstitial and diffuse in appearance, though consolidation can occur. Psittacosis is indistinguishable from other bacterial or viral pneumonias by radiography.

The organism is rarely isolated from cultures. The diagnosis is usually made serologically; antibodies appear during the second week and can be demonstrated by complement fixation or immunofluorescence. Antibody response may be suppressed by early chemotherapy.

Differential Diagnosis

The illness is indistinguishable from viral, mycoplasmal, or other atypical pneumonias except for the history of contact with birds. Psittacosis is in the differential diagnosis of culture-negative endocarditis.

Treatment

Treatment consists of giving tetracycline, 0.5 g orally every 6 hours or 0.5 g intravenously every 12 hours, for 14–21 days. Erythromycin may be effective as well.

Verweij PE et al: Severe human psittacosis requiring artificial ventilation: A case report and review. Clin Infect Dis 1995;20:440.

CHLAMYDIA PNEUMONIAE, TWAR STRAIN

Chlamydia pneumoniae causes pneumonia and bronchitis and has been associated seroepidemiologically with coronary artery disease. The clinical presentation of pneumonia is that of an atypical pneumonia. The organism accounts for approximately 10% of community-acquired pneumonias, ranking second to *Mycoplasma* as an agent of atypical pneumonia. Its role in coronary artery disease remains to be defined, but *C pneumoniae* has been detected in up to 50% of coronary atheromatous lesions.

Like *C psittaci,* TWAR strains are resistant to sulfonamides. Erythromycin or tetracycline, 500 mg four times a day for 10–14 days, appears to be effective therapy.

Campbell LA et al: Detection of *Chlamydia pneumoniae* TWAR in human coronary atherotomy tissue. J Infect Dis 1995;172:585.

Marrie TJ et al: Ambulatory patients with community-acquired pneumonia: Frequency of atypical agents and clinical course. Am J Med 1996;101:508.

Infectious Diseases: Spirochetal

Richard A. Jacobs, MD, PhD

SYPHILIS

NATURAL HISTORY & PRINCIPLES OF DIAGNOSIS & TREATMENT

Syphilis is a complex infectious disease caused by *Treponema pallidum,* a spirochete capable of infecting almost any organ or tissue in the body and causing protean clinical manifestations (Table 34–1). Transmission occurs most frequently during sexual contact, through minor skin or mucosal lesions; sites of inoculation are usually genital but may be extragenital. The risk of developing syphilis after unprotected sex with an individual with early syphilis is approximately 30–50%. The organism is extremely sensitive to heat and drying but can survive for days in fluids; therefore, it can be transmitted in blood from infected persons. Syphilis can be transferred via the placenta from mother to fetus after the tenth week of pregnancy (congenital syphilis).

The immunologic response to infection is complex, but it provides the basis for most clinical diagnoses. The infection induces the synthesis of a number of antibodies, some of which react specifically with pathogenic treponemes and some with components of normal tissues (see below). If the disease is untreated, sufficient defenses develop to produce a relative resistance to reinfection; however, in most cases these immune reactions fail to eradicate existing infection and may contribute to tissue destruction in the late stages. Patients treated early in the disease are fully susceptible to reinfection.

The natural history of acquired syphilis is generally divided into two major clinical stages: early (infectious) syphilis and late syphilis. The two stages are separated by a symptom-free latent phase during the first part of which (early latency) the infectious stage is liable to recur. Infectious syphilis includes the primary lesions (chancre and regional lymphadenopathy); the secondary lesions (commonly in-volving skin and mucous membranes, occasionally bone, central nervous system, or liver); relapsing lesions during early latency; and congenital lesions. The hallmark of these lesions is an abundance of spirochetes; tissue reaction is usually minimal. Late syphilis consists of so-called benign (gummatous) lesions involving skin, bones, and viscera; cardiovascular disease (principally aortitis); and a variety of central nervous system and ocular syndromes. These forms of syphilis are not contagious. The lesions contain few demonstrable spirochetes, but tissue reactivity (vasculitis, necrosis) is severe and suggestive of hypersensitivity phenomena.

As a result of intensive public health efforts during and after World War II, there was a reduction in the incidence of infectious syphilis. With the marked increase in all sexually transmitted diseases since the 1970s, there has been a rise in the number of reported cases of syphilis. In the early 1980s, the incidence of infectious syphilis increased, with a particularly high rate among homosexual men. In the mid 1980s, there was a slight decrease in the incidence of syphilis, chiefly as a result of changes in sexual practices in response to the AIDS epidemic. Between 1985 and 1990, there was again a dramatic increase in infectious syphilis, with 50,223 cases of primary and secondary syphilis reported in 1990. This increase was broad-based, affecting both men and women in inner city urban and rural areas, particularly in the southern regions of the United States. Although adolescent and young adult blacks were primarily affected, increases were seen in other ethnic groups also, as well as adults over 60. Limited access to health care, decreases in health department clinical services, increased use of illicit drugs (especially "crack cocaine"), the exchange of sex for drugs or money to buy drugs, and the difficulty of contact tracing when multiple sexual partners are involved all contributed to the dramatic increase. Concomitantly with the increase in acquired syphilis, there has also been an increase in congenital syphilis, particularly in urban areas. In response to this increase in infectious syphilis, intensive syphilis control programs targeting high-risk populations—women of childbearing age, sexu-

Table 34–1. Stages of syphilis and common clinical manifestations.

Primary syphilis
Genital ulcer: painless ulcer with clean base and firm indurated borders
Regional lymphadenopathy
Secondary syphilis
Skin and mucous membranes
Rash: diffuse (including palms and soles), macular, papular, pustular, and combinations
Condylomata lata
Mucous patches: painless, silvery ulcerations of mucous membrane with surrounding erythema
Generalized lymphadenopathy
Constitutional symptoms
Fever, usually low-grade
Malaise
Anorexia
Arthralgias and myalgias
Central nervous system
Asymptomatic
Symptomatic
Headache
Meningitis
Cranial neuropathies (II–VIII)
Ocular
Iritis
Iridocyclitis
Other
Renal: glomerulonephritis, nephrotic syndrome
Liver: hepatitis
Bone and joint: arthritis, periostitis
Late syphilis
Late benign (gummatous): granulomatous lesion usually involving skin, mucous membranes and bones, but any organ can be involved
Cardiovascular
Aortic insufficiency
Coronary ostial stenosis
Aortic aneurysm
Neurosyphilis
Asymptomatic
Meningovascular
Seizures
Hemiparesis or hemiplegia
Tabes dorsalis
Impaired proprioception and vibratory sensation
Argyll Robertson pupil
Shooting pains
Ataxia
Romberg's sign
Urinary and fecal incontinence
Charcot joint
Cranial nerve involvement (II–VIII)
General paresis
Personality changes
Hyperactive reflexes
Argyll Robertson pupil
Decreased memory
Slurred speech
Optic atrophy

ally active teens, drug users, inmates of penal institutions, persons with multiple sexual partners or those who have sex with prostitutes—and emphasizing screening, early treatment, contact tracing, and condom use were instituted and have been successful in limiting the spread of this disease—as evidenced by

the decrease in reported cases of primary and secondary syphilis to 16,500 in 1995.

Laboratory Diagnosis

Since the infectious agent of syphilis cannot be cultured in vitro, diagnostic measures must rely mainly on serologic testing, microscopic detection of *T pallidum* in lesions, and other examinations (biopsies, lumbar puncture, x-rays) for evidence of tissue damage.

A. Serologic Tests for Syphilis: (Table 34–2.) There are two general categories of serologic tests for syphilis: (1) Nontreponemal tests detect antibodies to lipoidal antigens present in either the host or *T pallidum*. The original antigens used to measure these nonspecific antibodies (reagin) were crude extracts of beef heart or liver and resulted in significant false-positive reactions. The cardiolipin-cholesterol-lecithin preparation presently used is much purer and gives fewer false-positive reactions. (2) Treponemal tests employ live or killed *T pallidum* as antigen to detect antibodies specific for pathogenic treponemes.

1. Nontreponemal antigen tests–The most commonly used nontreponemal antigen tests are the VDRL and RPR, which measure the ability of heated serum to flocculate a suspension of cardiolipin-cholesterol-lecithin. The flocculation tests are easy, rapid, and inexpensive to perform and are therefore used primarily for routine (often automated) screening for syphilis. Quantitative expression of the reactivity of the serum, based upon titration of dilutions of serum, may be valuable in establishing the diagnosis and in evaluating the efficacy of treatment.

The VDRL test (the nontreponemal test in widest use) generally becomes positive 4–6 weeks after infection, or 1–3 weeks after the appearance of a primary lesion; it is almost invariably positive in the secondary stage. The VDRL titer is usually high (> 1:32) in secondary syphilis and tends to be lower (< 1:4) or even negative in late forms of syphilis. These serologic tests are not highly specific and must be closely correlated with other clinical and laboratory findings. The tests are positive in patients with non-sexually transmitted treponematoses (see below). More importantly, "false-positive" serologic re-

Table 34–2. Percentage of patients with positive serologic tests for syphilis.[1]

Test	Stage		
	Primary	**Secondary**	**Tertiary**
VDRL[2]	70–75%	99%	75%
FTA-ABS[3]	85–95%	100%	98%

[1]Based on untreated cases.
[2]VDRL = Venereal Disease Research Laboratory test.
[3]FTA-ABS = Fluorescent treponemal antibody-absorption test.

actions are frequently encountered in a wide variety of nontreponemal states, including connective tissue diseases, infectious mononucleosis, malaria, febrile diseases, leprosy, intravenous drug use, infective endocarditis, old age, hepatitis C viral infection, and pregnancy. False-positive tests also occur more commonly in HIV-seropositive patients (4%) than in HIV-seronegative patients (0.8%). False-positive reactions are usually of low titer and transient and may be distinguished from true positives by specific treponemal antibody tests. False-negative results can be seen when very high antibody titers are present (the prozone phenomenon). If syphilis is strongly suspected and the nontreponemal test is negative, the laboratory should be instructed to dilute the specimen to detect a positive reaction. The rapid plasma reagin (RPR) test is a simple, rapid, and reliable substitute for the traditional VDRL test. RPR titers are often higher than VDRL titers and thus are not comparable. The RPR test is suitable for automated screening.

Nontreponemal antibody titers are used to assess adequacy of therapy. The time required for the VDRL or RPR to become negative depends on the stage of the disease, the height of the initial titer, and whether the infection is an initial or repeat episode. In general, individuals with repeat infections, higher initial titers, and more advanced stages of disease at the time of treatment have a slower seroconversion rate and are more likely to remain serofast (ie, titers do not become negative). Older data on which recommendations for re-treatment are based and which employed more intensive treatment regimens than are presently used (see below) indicate that in primary and secondary syphilis, the VDRL usually decreases fourfold by 3 months and eightfold by 6 months. Furthermore, seronegativity was seen in 97% of those with primary syphilis and 76% of those with secondary syphilis at 2 years. More recent data based on currently recommended treatment regimens (see below) suggest that decreases in titer may be slower, ie, in primary and secondary syphilis it may take 6 months to see a fourfold decrease in titer and 12 months to see an eightfold drop. In patients with early latent syphilis, response is even slower, with a fourfold drop in titer taking 12–24 months. Seronegativity was seen in 72% of patients with primary syphilis and only 56% of those with secondary syphilis after 3 years. Whether these recent data more accurately reflect response of nontreponemal serologies to current treatment regimens needs confirmation.

2. Treponemal antibody tests–The fluorescent treponemal antibody absorption (FTA-ABS) test is the most widely employed treponemal test. It measures antibodies capable of reacting with killed *T pallidum* after absorption of the patient's serum with extracts of nonpathogenic treponemes. The FTA-ABS test is of value principally in determining whether a positive nontreponemal antigen test is "false-positive" or is indicative of syphilis. Because of its great sensitivity, particularly in the late stages of the disease, the FTA-ABS test is also of value when there is clinical evidence of syphilis but the nontreponemal serologic test for syphilis is negative. The test is positive in most patients with primary syphilis and in virtually all with secondary syphilis. Like nontreponemal antigen tests, the specific treponemal antibody test may revert to negative with adequate therapy. This is seen almost exclusively in initial infections in individuals with primary syphilis. In one study, 11% of individuals with a first episode of primary syphilis were seronegative by the FTA-ABS test at 1 year posttreatment, and 24% were negative by 3 years. Immunologic status may also affect antibody titers. Seven percent of asymptomatic HIV-infected patients became seronegative after treatment, as opposed to 38% of symptomatic HIV-infected individuals. The long-held belief that a positive FTA-ABS persists indefinitely is clearly not valid, and this test therefore cannot be used as a reliable marker of previous infection. False-positive FTA-ABS tests occur rarely in systemic lupus erythematosus and in other disorders associated with increased levels of gamma globulins. It is noteworthy that Lyme disease may cause a false-positive FTA-ABS test but rarely causes a false-positive reaginic test. A *T pallidum* hemagglutination (TPHA) test and microhemagglutination test for antibody to *T pallidum* (MHA-TP) are comparable in specificity and sensitivity to the FTA-ABS test but may become positive somewhat later in infection.

Investigational tests such as direct antigen detection, Western immunoblot, ELISA (CAPTIA Syph G, CAPTIA Syph M), and PCR are under study as diagnostic tools. They have shown promise in clinical trials, especially for diseases difficult to diagnose such as neurosyphilis and congenital syphilis. The increased sensitivity (ELISA) and specificity (Western blot) of these tests make them attractive, but because of lack of clinical evaluation in field trials they have not yet supplanted the more traditional methods of diagnosis.

Final decisions about the significance of the results of serologic tests for syphilis must be based upon a total clinical appraisal.

B. Microscopic Examination: In infectious syphilis, *T pallidum* may be shown by darkfield microscopic examination of fresh exudate from lesions or material aspirated from regional lymph nodes. The darkfield examination requires considerable experience and care in the proper collection of specimens and in the identification of pathogenic spirochetes by observing characteristic features of morphology and motility. Repeated examinations may be necessary. Spirochetes usually are not found in late syphilitic lesions by this technique.

An immunofluorescent staining technique for

demonstrating *T pallidum* in dried smears of fluid taken from early syphilitic lesions is available. Slides are fixed and treated with fluorescein-labeled antitreponemal antibody that has been preabsorbed with nonpathogenic treponemes. The slides are then examined for fluorescing spirochetes in an ultraviolet microscope. Because of its simplicity and convenience to physicians (slides can be mailed), this technique has replaced darkfield microscopy in most health departments and medical center laboratories.

C. Spinal Fluid Examination: Cerebrospinal fluid findings in neurosyphilis are variable. In "classic" cases there is an elevation of total protein, lymphocytic pleocytosis, and a positive cerebrospinal fluid reagin test (VDRL). However, cerebrospinal fluid may be completely normal in neurosyphilis, and the VDRL may be negative. In one study, 25% of patients with primary or secondary syphilis in whom *T pallidum* was isolated from cerebrospinal fluid had a normal cerebrospinal fluid examination. In later stages of syphilis, normal cerebrospinal fluid analysis in the presence of infection can occur, but it is unusual. Because false-positive reagin tests rarely occur in the cerebrospinal fluid, a positive test confirms the presence of neurosyphilis. Because the cerebrospinal fluid VDRL may be negative in 30–70% of cases of neurosyphilis, *a negative test does not exclude neurosyphilis.* The use of FTA-ABS in the diagnosis of neurosyphilis is controversial. Some feel that it is more sensitive than the VDRL, but this is not accepted uniformly, and a high serum titer of FTA-ABS may result in a positive cerebrospinal fluid titer in the absence of neurosyphilis. A negative cerebrospinal fluid FTA-ABS is strong evidence against the diagnosis of neurosyphilis. Other treponemal antibody tests, such as the MHA-TP and the TPHA index, likewise are not reliable in making the diagnosis of neurosyphilis, although a negative test is helpful in excluding the diagnosis.

Cerebrospinal fluid examination is recommended depending on clinical manifestations and stage of disease, as discussed below. Asymptomatic neurosyphilis (ie, positive cerebrospinal fluid findings without symptoms) requires prolonged penicillin treatment as given for symptomatic neurosyphilis. Adequate treatment is indicated by gradual decrease in cerebrospinal fluid cell count, protein concentration, and VDRL titer. Rarely, serologic tests of cerebrospinal fluid may remain positive for years after adequate treatment of neurosyphilis even though all other parameters have returned to normal.

Treatment

A. Specific Measures:

1. Penicillin, as benzathine penicillin G or aqueous procaine penicillin G, is the drug of choice for all forms of syphilis and other spirochetal infections. Effective tissue levels must be maintained for several days or weeks because of the spirochete's long generation time (about 30 hours). Penicillin is highly effective in early infections and variably effective in the late stages. The principal contraindication is hypersensitivity to the penicillins. The recommended treatment schedules are included below in the discussion of the various forms of syphilis.

2. Other antibiotic therapy–Oral tetracyclines are effective in the treatment of syphilis for patients who are sensitive to penicillin. Tetracycline, 500 mg orally four times daily for 14 days, or doxycycline, 100 mg orally twice daily for 14 days, is given for infectious syphilis. In syphilis of more than 1 year's duration or of unknown duration, treatment is continued for 28 days in the same doses. Azithromycin, 500 mg daily for 10 days (total dose 5 g) or 500 mg on alternate days for 11 days (total dose 3 g), is also effective for infectious syphilis.

Human clinical trials using ceftriaxone for infectious syphilis are limited, and this agent is therefore not officially recommended at present. However, based on animal data and pharmacologic predictions, some have suggested ceftriaxone in multiple-dose regimens to treat infectious syphilis (250 mg intravenously or intramuscularly once a day for 5 days) and latent neurosyphilis (1 g intravenously or intramuscularly once a day for 14 days). Multiple doses of ceftriaxone are more costly than a single dose of benzathine penicillin and more inconvenient for the patient.

B. Local Measures (Mucocutaneous Lesions): Local treatment is usually not necessary. No local antiseptics or other chemicals should be applied to a suspected syphilitic lesion until specimens for microscopy have been obtained.

C. Public Health Measures: Patients with infectious syphilis must abstain from sexual activity until rendered noninfectious by antibiotic therapy. All cases of syphilis must be reported to the appropriate public health agency for assistance in identifying and treating contacts. In addition, all patients with syphilis should have an HIV test at the time of diagnosis.

D. Epidemiologic Treatment: Patients who have been exposed to infectious syphilis within the preceding 3 months may be infected but seronegative and thus should be treated as for early syphilis. Others at high risk either for infection (ie, those with other sexually transmitted diseases and those infected with HIV) or its consequences (ie, pregnant women) should undergo serologic tests for syphilis. The present recommended therapy for gonorrhea (ceftriaxone and doxycycline) is only partially effective in treating incubating syphilis. Therefore, patients with gonorrhea and a known exposure to syphilis should be treated with separate regimens effective against both diseases.

Complications of Specific Therapy

The Jarisch-Herxheimer reaction is ascribed to the

sudden massive destruction of spirochetes by drugs and release of toxic products and is manifested by fever and aggravation of the existing clinical picture. It is most likely to occur in early syphilis. Treatment should not be discontinued unless the symptoms become severe or threaten to be fatal or unless syphilitic laryngitis, auditory neuritis, or labyrinthitis is present, where the reaction may cause irreversible damage.

The reaction may be prevented or modified by simultaneous administration of antipyretics or corticosteroids. It usually begins within the first 24 hours and subsides spontaneously within the next 24 hours of penicillin treatment.

Follow-Up Care

Because treatment failures can occur and reinfection is always a possibility, patients treated for syphilis should be followed clinically and serologically. Response to therapy is difficult to assess, and no definite criteria exist for cure in patients with primary or secondary syphilis. Failure of nontreponemal antibody titers to decrease fourfold by 3 months may identify a group at high risk of treatment failure. Optimal management of these patients is unclear, but close clinical and serologic follow-up is indicated. If titers fail to decrease fourfold by 6 months or if recurrent symptoms develop, an HIV test should be repeated (all patients with syphilis should have an HIV test at the time of diagnosis), a lumbar puncture performed, and retreatment given. In patients with latent syphilis, nontreponemal serologic tests should be repeated at 6 and 12 months. If titers increase fourfold or initially high titers ($\geq$ 1:32) fail to decrease fourfold by 12–24 months, an HIV test and lumbar puncture should be performed and re-treatment given according to the stage of the disease.

Prevention

Avoidance of sexual contact is the only completely reliable method of prophylaxis but is an impractical public health measure for obvious reasons.

A. Mechanical: The standard latex condom is effective but protects covered parts only. The exposed parts should be washed with soap and water as soon after contact as possible. This applies to both sexes.

B. Antibiotic: If there is known exposure to infectious syphilis, abortive penicillin therapy may be used. Give 2.4 million units of procaine penicillin G intramuscularly. Treatment of gonococcal infection with penicillins, tetracyclines, and ceftriaxone is probably effective against incubating syphilis in most cases. However, other antimicrobial agents (eg, spectinomycin) may be ineffective in aborting preclinical syphilis. In view of the increasing use of antibiotics other than penicillin for gonococcal disease, patients treated for gonorrhea should have a serologic test for syphilis 3–6 months after treatment.

Course & Prognosis
(See Table 34–3.)

The lesions associated with primary and secondary syphilis are self-limiting and resolve with few or no residua. Late syphilis may be highly destructive and permanently disabling and may lead to death. In broad terms, if no treatment is given, about one-third of people infected with syphilis will undergo spontaneous cure, about one-third will remain in the latent phase throughout life, and about one-third will develop serious late lesions.

CLINICAL STAGES OF SYPHILIS

1. PRIMARY SYPHILIS

Essentials of Diagnosis
- History of sexual contact (often unreliable).
- Painless ulcer on genitalia, perianal area, rectum, pharynx, tongue, lip, or elsewhere 2–6 weeks after exposure.
- Nontender enlargement of regional lymph nodes.

Table 34–3. Natural course of untreated syphilis.

Stage of Disease	Likelihood of Developing Clinical Manifestations (%)	Comment
Latent	24%	90% of relapses occur in first year after infection.
Late Benign (gummatous)	15%	Many patients have more than one late manifestation.
Cardiovascular	10%	Seen only in those who develop syphilis after 15 years of age. Pathologic findings more common, ie, 50–80%.
Neurosyphilis	6.5%	Asymptomatic neurosyphilis has been reported in 8–40%.

- Fluid expressed from lesion contains *T pallidum* by immunofluorescence or darkfield microscopy.
- Serologic test for syphilis often positive.

General Considerations

This is the stage of invasion and may pass unrecognized. The typical lesion is the chancre at the site or sites of inoculation, most frequently located on the penis, labia, cervix, or anorectal region. Anorectal lesions are especially common among male homosexuals. The primary lesion occurs occasionally in the oropharynx (lip, tongue, or tonsil) and rarely on the breast or finger. The chancre starts as a small erosion 10–90 days (average, 3–4 weeks) after inoculation that rapidly develops into a painless superficial ulcer with a clean base and firm, indurated margins, associated with enlargement of regional lymph nodes, which are rubbery, discrete, and nontender. Bacterial infection of the chancre may occur and may lead to pain. Healing occurs without treatment, but a scar may form, especially with secondary bacterial infection.

Laboratory Findings

The serologic test for syphilis is usually positive 1–2 weeks after the primary lesion is noted; rising titers are especially significant when there is a history of previous infection. Immunofluorescence or darkfield microscopy shows treponemes in at least 95% of chancres. Cerebrospinal fluid pleocytosis has been reported in 10–20% of patients with primary syphilis.

Differential Diagnosis

The syphilitic chancre may be confused with chancroid, lymphogranuloma venereum, genital herpes, or neoplasm. Any lesion on the genitalia should be considered a possible primary syphilitic lesion.

Treatment

Benzathine penicillin G, 2.4 million units intramuscularly in the gluteal area, is given once. For the penicillin-allergic patient (who is not pregnant), doxycycline, 100 mg orally twice daily for 2 weeks, tetracycline, 500 mg orally four times a day for 2 weeks, or azithromycin, 500 mg daily for 10 days or 500 mg on alternate days for 11 days, can be used.

2. SECONDARY SYPHILIS

Essentials of Diagnosis

- Generalized maculopapular skin rash.
- Mucous membrane lesions, including patches and ulcers.
- Weeping papules (condylomas) in moist skin areas.
- Generalized nontender lymphadenopathy.
- Fever.
- Meningitis, hepatitis, osteitis, arthritis, iritis.

- Many treponemes in scrapings of mucous membrane or skin lesions by immunofluorescence or darkfield microscopy.
- Serologic tests for syphilis always positive.

General Considerations & Treatment

The secondary stage of syphilis usually appears a few weeks (or up to 6 months) after development of the chancre, when sufficient dissemination of *T pallidum* has occurred to produce systemic signs (fever, lymphadenopathy) or infectious lesions at sites distant from the site of inoculation. The most common manifestations are skin and mucosal lesions. The skin lesions are nonpruritic, macular, papular, pustular, or follicular (or combinations of any of these types), though the maculopapular rash is the most common. The skin lesions usually are generalized; involvement of the palms and soles is especially suspicious. Annular lesions simulating ringworm are observed in blacks. Mucous membrane lesions range from ulcers and papules of the lips, mouth, throat, genitalia, and anus ("mucous patches") to a diffuse redness of the pharynx. Both skin and mucous membrane lesions are highly infectious at this stage. Specific lesions—**condylomata lata**—are fused, weeping papules on the moist areas of the skin and mucous membranes.

Meningeal (aseptic meningitis or acute basilar meningitis), hepatic, renal, bone, and joint invasion may occur, with resulting cranial nerve palsies, jaundice, nephrotic syndrome, and periostitis. Alopecia (moth-eaten appearance) and uveitis may also occur.

All serologic tests for syphilis are positive in almost all cases. The cutaneous and mucous membrane lesions often show *T pallidum* on darkfield microscopic examination. A transient cerebrospinal fluid pleocytosis is seen in 30–70% of patients with secondary syphilis, though only 5% have positive serologic cerebrospinal fluid reactions. There may be evidence of hepatitis or nephritis (immune complex type). Circulating immune complexes exist in the blood and are deposited in blood vessel walls.

Skin lesions may be confused with the infectious exanthems, pityriasis rosea, and drug eruptions. Visceral lesions may suggest nephritis or hepatitis due to other causes. The diffusely red throat may mimic other forms of pharyngitis.

Treatment is as for primary syphilis unless central nervous system or ocular disease is present, in which case treatment is as for neurosyphilis (see below). Isolation of the patient is important.

3. RELAPSING SYPHILIS (Early Latent Syphilis)

The essentials of diagnosis are the same as in secondary syphilis.

The lesions of secondary syphilis heal spontaneously, but secondary syphilis may relapse if undiagnosed or inadequately treated. These relapses may include any of the findings noted under secondary syphilis: skin and mucous membrane, neurologic, ocular, bone, or visceral. Unlike the usual asymptomatic neurologic involvement of secondary syphilis, neurologic relapses may be fulminating, leading to death. Relapse is almost always accompanied by a rising titer in quantitative serologic tests; indeed, a rising titer may be the first or only evidence of relapse. About 90% of relapses occur during the first year after infection.

Treatment is as for primary syphilis unless central nervous system disease is present.

4. LATE LATENT ("HIDDEN") SYPHILIS

Essentials of Diagnosis

- No physical signs.
- History of syphilis with inadequate treatment.
- Positive serologic tests for syphilis.

General Considerations & Treatment

Latent syphilis is the clinically quiescent phase during the interval after disappearance of secondary lesions and before the appearance of tertiary symptoms. Early latency is defined as the first year after infection, during which time most infectious lesions recur ("relapsing syphilis"); after the first year, the patient is said to be in the late latent phase. Transmission to the fetus, however, can probably occur in any phase. There are (by definition) no clinical manifestations during the latent phase, and the only significant laboratory findings are positive serologic tests. A diagnosis of latent syphilis is justified only when the cerebrospinal fluid is entirely negative, x-ray and physical examination shows no evidence of cardiovascular involvement, and false-positive tests for syphilis have been ruled out. The latent phase may last from months to a lifetime.

It is important to differentiate latent syphilis from a false-positive serologic test for syphilis, which can be due to the many causes listed above.

Treatment is with benzathine penicillin G, 2.4 million units three times at 7-day intervals (total dose, 7.2 million units). In the penicillin-allergic patient, give tetracycline, 0.5 g orally four times a day for 28 days, or doxycycline, 100 mg orally twice daily for 28 days. If there is evidence of cerebrospinal fluid involvement, treat as for neurosyphilis. Only a small percentage of serologic tests will be appreciably altered by treatment with penicillin. The treatment of this stage of the disease is intended to prevent the late sequelae.

5. LATE (TERTIARY) SYPHILIS

Essentials of Diagnosis

- Infiltrative tumors of skin, bones, liver (gummas).
- Aortitis, aneurysms, aortic regurgitation.
- Central nervous system disorders, including meningovascular and degenerative changes, paresthesias, shooting pains, abnormal reflexes, dementia, or psychosis.

General Considerations

This stage may occur at any time after secondary syphilis, even after years of latency, and is seen in about one-third of untreated patients (Table 34–3). Late lesions probably represent, at least in part, a delayed hypersensitivity reaction of the tissue to the organism and are usually divided into two types: (1) a localized gummatous reaction, with a relatively rapid onset and generally prompt response to therapy ("benign late syphilis"); and (2) diffuse inflammation of a more insidious onset that characteristically involves the central nervous system and large arteries, is often fatal if untreated, and is at best arrested by treatment. Gummas may involve any area or organ of the body but most often the skin or long bones. Cardiovascular disease is usually manifested by aortic aneurysm, aortic regurgitation, or aortitis. Various forms of diffuse or localized central nervous system involvement may occur.

Late syphilis must be differentiated from neoplasms of the skin, liver, lung, stomach, or brain; other forms of meningitis; and primary neurologic lesions.

Although almost any tissue and organ may be involved in late syphilis, the following are the most common types of involvement.

Skin

Cutaneous lesions of late syphilis are of two varieties: (1) multiple nodular lesions that eventually ulcerate (lues maligna) or resolve by forming atrophic, pigmented scars; and (2) solitary gummas that start as painless subcutaneous nodules, then enlarge, attach to the overlying skin, and eventually ulcerate.

Mucous Membranes

Late lesions of the mucous membranes are nodular gummas or leukoplakia, highly destructive to the involved tissue.

Skeletal

Bone lesions are destructive, causing periostitis, osteitis, and arthritis with little or no associated redness or swelling but often marked myalgia and myositis of the neighboring muscles. The pain is especially severe at night.

Eyes

Late ocular lesions are gummatous iritis, chorioretinitis, optic atrophy, and cranial nerve palsies, in addition to the lesions of central nervous system syphilis.

Respiratory System

Respiratory involvement by late syphilis is caused by gummatous infiltrates into the larynx, trachea, and pulmonary parenchyma, producing discrete pulmonary densities. There may be hoarseness, respiratory distress, and wheezing secondary to the gummatous lesion itself or to subsequent stenosis occurring with healing.

Gastrointestinal System

Gummas involving the liver produce the usually benign, asymptomatic hepar lobatum. Occasionally a picture resembling Laennec's cirrhosis is produced by liver involvement. Gastric involvement can consist of diffuse infiltration into the stomach wall or focal lesions that endoscopically and microscopically can be confused with lymphoma or carcinoma. Epigastric pain, early satiety, regurgitation, belching, and weight loss are common symptoms.

Cardiovascular System

Cardiovascular lesions (10–15% of late syphilitic lesions) are often progressive, disabling, and life-threatening. Central nervous system lesions are often present also. Involvement usually starts as an arteritis in the supracardiac portion of the aorta and progresses to cause one or more of the following: (1) Narrowing of the coronary ostia with resulting decreased coronary circulation, angina, and acute myocardial infarction. (2) Scarring of the aortic valves, producing aortic regurgitation with its water-hammer pulse, aortic diastolic murmur, frequent aortic systolic murmur, cardiac hypertrophy, and eventually congestive heart failure. (3) Weakness of the wall of the aorta, with saccular aneurysm formation and associated pressure symptoms of dysphagia, hoarseness, brassy cough, back pain (vertebral erosion), and occasionally rupture of the aneurysm. Recurrent respiratory infections are common as a result of pressure on the trachea and bronchi.

Treatment of tertiary syphilis (excluding neurosyphilis; see below) is as for latent syphilis. Reversal of positive serologic tests does not usually occur. A second course of penicillin therapy may be given if necessary. There is no known method for reliable eradication of the treponeme from humans in the late stages of syphilis. Viable spirochetes are occasionally found in the eyes, in cerebrospinal fluid, and elsewhere in patients with "adequately" treated syphilis, but claims for their capacity to cause progressive disease are speculative.

Neurosyphilis

Neurosyphilis (15–20% of late syphilitic lesions; often present with cardiovascular syphilis) is also a progressive, disabling, and life-threatening complication. It develops more commonly in men than in women and in whites than in blacks.

A. Classification: There are four clinical types.

1. Asymptomatic neurosyphilis–This form is characterized by spinal fluid abnormalities (positive spinal fluid serology, increased cell count, occasionally increased protein) without symptoms or signs of neurologic involvement.

2. Meningovascular syphilis–This form is characterized by meningeal involvement or changes in the vascular structures of the brain (or both), producing symptoms of low-grade meningitis (headache, irritability); cranial nerve palsies (basilar meningitis); unequal reflexes; irregular pupils with poor light and accommodation reflexes; and, when large vessels are involved, cerebrovascular accidents. The cerebrospinal fluid shows increased cells (100–1000/μL), elevated protein, and usually a positive serologic test for syphilis. The symptoms of acute meningitis are rare in late syphilis.

3. Tabes dorsalis–This form is a chronic progressive degeneration of the parenchyma of the posterior columns of the spinal cord and of the posterior sensory ganglia and nerve roots. The symptoms and signs are impairment of proprioception and vibration sense, Argyll Robertson pupils (which react poorly to light but well to accommodation), and muscular hypotonia and hyporeflexia. Impairment of proprioception results in a wide-based gait and inability to walk in the dark. Paresthesias, analgesia, or sharp recurrent pains in the muscles of the leg ("shooting" or "lightning" pains) may occur. Crises are also common in tabes: gastric crises, consisting of sharp abdominal pains with nausea and vomiting (simulating an acute abdomen); laryngeal crises, with paroxysmal cough and dyspnea; urethral crises, with painful bladder spasms; and rectal and anal crises. Crises may begin suddenly, last for hours to days, and cease abruptly. Neurogenic bladder with overflow incontinence is also seen. Painless trophic ulcers may develop over pressure points on the feet. Joint damage may occur as a result of lack of sensory innervation (Charcot joint). The cerebrospinal fluid may have a normal or increased cell count (3–200/μL), elevated protein, and variable results of serologic tests.

4. General paresis–This is generalized involvement of the cerebral cortex with insidious onset of symptoms. There is usually a decrease in concentrating power, memory loss, dysarthria, tremor of the fingers and lips, irritability, and mild headaches. Most striking is the change of personality; the patient becomes slovenly, irresponsible, confused, and psychotic. Combinations of the various forms of neurosyphilis (especially tabes and paresis) are not uncommon. The cerebrospinal fluid findings resemble those of tabes dorsalis.

B. Special Considerations in Treatment of Neurosyphilis: It is most important to prevent neurosyphilis by prompt diagnosis, adequate treatment, and follow-up of early syphilis. Indications for lumbar puncture vary depending upon the stage of the disease and the host's immune status. In early syphilis (primary and secondary syphilis and early latent syphilis of less than 1 year's duration), cerebrospinal fluid abnormalities occur commonly, but neurosyphilis rarely develops in patients who have received the standard therapy outlined above. Thus, unless clinical symptoms and signs of neurosyphilis are present, a lumbar puncture in early syphilis is not recommended as part of the routine evaluation. In theory, all patients with syphilis of more than 1 year's duration should have a lumbar puncture. This is rarely strictly adhered to, and each case is usually individualized. In one study of hospitalized patients with latent syphilis detected by routine screening, cerebrospinal fluid abnormalities occurred frequently (in 32% of HIV-negative patients and 67% of HIV-positive patients) but were nonspecific, not indicative of active neurosyphilis, and rarely influenced therapeutic decisions—emphasizing the low yield of routine lumbar puncture in this setting. Cerebrospinal fluid evaluation is, however, strongly suggested in the later stages of syphilis if neurologic symptoms and signs are present; therapy other than with penicillin is to be given; if the patient is HIV-positive (see next section); if serum nontreponemal antibody titers are 1:32 or higher; or if there is evidence of active syphilis at other sites (aortitis, iritis, optic atrophy, etc). In the presence of definite cerebrospinal fluid or neurologic abnormalities, treat for neurosyphilis. The pretreatment clinical and laboratory evaluation should include neurologic, ocular, psychiatric, and cerebrospinal fluid examinations.

The regimen of 2.4 million units of benzathine penicillin intramuscularly weekly for three consecutive weeks results in low to undetectable cerebrospinal fluid levels of penicillin, and treatment failures have been described when this regimen has been used to treat neurosyphilis. For these reasons, present recommendations for the therapy of neurosyphilis employ higher doses of short-acting penicillin in order to achieve better penetration and higher levels of drug in the cerebrospinal fluid. Recommended regimens include 2–4 million units of aqueous crystalline penicillin G intravenously every 4 hours for 10–14 days. Alternatively, 2–4 million units of procaine penicillin can be given intramuscularly once daily along with 500 mg of probenecid orally four times daily, both for 10–14 days. Because of concerns about slowly dividing organisms that may persist, many experts recommend subsequent administration of 2.4 million units of benzathine penicillin intramuscularly once weekly for 3 weeks as additional therapy. Alternative therapy to penicillin has not been established for treatment of neurosyphilis. Chloramphenicol (2 g daily for 30 days), doxycycline (200 mg twice daily for 21 days), and ceftriaxone (1 g daily for 14 days) have all been shown to achieve treponemicidal levels in the cerebrospinal fluid, but clinical experience is limited, and failures have been reported. Thus, patients with a history of penicillin allergy should be skin-tested, desensitized, and treated with penicillin.

All patients should have spinal fluid examinations at 6-month intervals until the cell count is normal. Response may be gauged by clinical improvement and reversal of cerebrospinal fluid changes. A second course of penicillin therapy may be given if the cell count has not decreased at 6 months or is not normal at 2 years. Not infrequently, there is progression of neurologic symptoms and signs despite high and prolonged doses of penicillin. It has been postulated that these treatment failures are related to the unexplained persistence of viable *T pallidum* in central nervous system or ocular lesions in at least some cases.

6. SYPHILIS IN HIV-INFECTED PATIENTS

Because syphilis has variable clinical manifestations and an unpredictable course, evaluation of case reports of unusual clinical or laboratory manifestations of syphilis in HIV-infected patients is difficult. Nonetheless, recent reports have suggested that certain clinical manifestations of syphilis in HIV-infected individuals may differ from those seen in noninfected individuals. Persons infected with HIV are more likely to present with secondary syphilis and have chancres than patients who are HIV-negative. Ulceronodular cutaneous disease (lues maligna), a manifestation of secondary syphilis, may be more common in HIV-infected individuals. Accelerated clinical courses have been described, with neurosyphilis occurring within months after the diagnosis of early syphilis. Similarly, the serologic response to infection may be blunted or delayed, and an increasing number of reports has emphasized that standard regimens of benzathine penicillin used to treat noninfected patients may be inadequate to treat the HIV-infected patient. As a result, the approach to the HIV-infected patient with syphilis has changed over the years as information has evolved. Because of concern about false-negative serologic tests or a delayed immunologic response, if the diagnosis of syphilis is suggested on clinical grounds but reagin tests are negative, alternative tests should be performed. These tests include darkfield examination of lesions and direct fluorescent antibody staining for *T pallidum* of lesion exudate or biopsy specimens.

The diagnosis of neurosyphilis in HIV-infected patients is complicated by the fact that cerebrospinal fluid abnormalities are frequently seen and may be due to neurosyphilis or HIV infection itself. The exact prevalence of neurosyphilis in HIV-infected patients with positive serum nontreponemal tests is not precisely known. Retrospective studies have suggested that as many as 10–50% of asymptomatic patients with positive serum tests who have consented to lumbar puncture have neurosyphilis defined by a positive cerebrospinal fluid VDRL test. The use of cerebrospinal fluid treponemal antibody titers (MHA-TP or FTA-ABS) in making the diagnosis of neurosyphilis is controversial. Because of the high rate of false-positive reactions, the specificity of this test is low. Conversely, a negative test has been considered by some to be strong evidence against neurosyphilis. Because of the high potential for neurosyphilis and because neurosyphilis requires more aggressive therapy, all HIV-infected patients who have syphilis (regardless of stage of disease) should be encouraged to have a lumbar puncture.

Treatment failures with presently recommended regimens of benzathine penicillin have been documented in HIV-infected patients. In one study, three of four patients treated with 2.4 million units of benzathine penicillin for secondary syphilis failed therapy, and all three were HIV-positive. Up to 45% of HIV-infected patients with neurosyphilis have been previously treated for early syphilis with benzathine penicillin, usually a single dose of 2.4 million units, but some with as much as 7.2 million units. In addition, currently recommended therapy for neurosyphilis (see above) may not be curative in the HIV-infected patient. In one study, serologic or clinical failure was documented in 4 of 11 patients treated intravenously with 18–24 million units of penicillin G daily for 10 days. Because there is no way to identify beforehand those at high risk for relapse and because alternative treatment regimens have not been studied, officially there has been no change in recommendations for treating syphilis in patients coinfected with HIV, and emphasis has been placed on close follow-up (see below). However, because of increasing numbers of failures using standard regimens, some have advocated a more aggressive approach such as treating early syphilis with multiple-dose regimens of penicillin (2.4 million units weekly for 3 weeks), longer courses of intravenous therapy for neurosyphilis, or periodic re-treatment of patients with persistently abnormal cerebrospinal fluid analyses.

Whether HIV-infected patients with syphilis have a different serologic response to penicillin therapy than noninfected individuals is unsettled. Nontreponemal titers tend to be higher in HIV-infected persons, and some studies have suggested a slower decline in these titers following treatment whereas others have not. Similarly, some studies have found that specific treponemal antibody tests (eg, FTA-ABS) revert to negative more frequently in HIV-infected patients, while others have found no difference in serologic response to therapy between HIV-positive and HIV-negative individuals. Despite the difficulties in interpretation of serologic test results, current recommendations are that in patients infected with HIV, nontreponemal quantitative tests should be repeated at 1, 2, 3, 6, 9, and 12 months after therapy. Treatment failure (as defined above for non-HIV-infected patients) should prompt a lumbar puncture and re-treatment. Most would re-treat primary and secondary syphilis with 2.4 million units of benzathine penicillin weekly for 3 weeks if the cerebrospinal fluid is normal. HIV-infected patients with neurosyphilis should be followed as described above for non-HIV-infected patients.

7. SYPHILIS IN PREGNANCY

All pregnant women should have a nontreponemal serologic test for syphilis at the time of the first prenatal visit. In women suspected of being at increased risk for syphilis, another nontreponemal test should be performed during the third trimester and again at delivery. The serologic status of all women who have delivered should be known before discharge from the hospital. Seropositive women should be considered infected and should be treated unless prior treatment with fall in antibody titer is medically documented.

The preferred treatment is with penicillin in dosage schedules appropriate for the stage of syphilis (see above). Penicillin prevents congenital syphilis in 90% of cases, even when treatment is given late in pregnancy. Tetracycline and doxycycline are contraindicated in pregnancy, and erythromycin is associated with a high risk of failure in the fetus. Women with a history of penicillin allergy should be skin-tested and desensitized if necessary.

The infant should be evaluated immediately, as noted below, and at 6–8 weeks of age.

8. CONGENITAL SYPHILIS

Congenital syphilis is a transplacentally transmitted infection that occurs in infants of untreated or inadequately treated mothers. The physical findings at birth are quite variable: The infant may have many or only minimal signs or even no signs until 6–8 weeks of life (delayed form). The most common findings are on the skin and mucous membranes—maculopapular rash, condylomas, mucous membrane patches, and serous nasal discharge (snuffles). These lesions are infectious; *T pallidum* can easily be found microscopically, and the infant must be isolated. Other common findings are hepatosplenomegaly, anemia, or osteochondritis. These early active lesions subsequently heal, and if the disease is left untreated it produces the characteristic stigmas of syphilis—interstitial keratitis, Hutchinson's teeth, saddle nose, saber shins, deafness, and central nervous system involvement.

The presence of negative serologic tests at birth in both the mother and the infant usually means that the newborn is free of infection. However, recent infection near the time of delivery may result in negative tests because there has been insufficient time to develop a serologic response. Thus, one must maintain a high index of suspicion in infants who present with delayed onset of symptoms despite negative serologic tests at birth, especially in infants born to high-risk mothers (HIV-positive, illicit drug users). Infants should be evaluated for congenital syphilis if the mother is seropositive and has not been treated or was treated with a nonpenicillin regimen, was treated within 1 month of delivery, or was treated before pregnancy but was not followed serologically to ensure response. The serologic evaluation for syphilis in newborn infants is complicated by the transplacental acquisition of maternal antibody (IgG). Evaluation of a newborn suspected of having congenital syphilis includes the history of maternal therapy, a careful physical examination, hematocrit (for possible anemia), a nontreponemal serologic test performed on serum, a cerebrospinal fluid examination, and x-rays of long bones. Examination of the placenta for histologic changes associated with congenital syphilis, special stains for spirochetes, and even PCR for treponemal DNA may provide supportive data for the diagnosis of congenital syphilis.

Infants should be treated at birth if maternal treatment was inadequate, unknown, or done with drugs other than penicillin or if adequate follow-up cannot be ensured. In addition, infants should be treated if there is clinical or radiologic evidence of active disease; if there is evidence of neurosyphilis (positive CSF-VDRL or pleocytosis); or if a serum nontreponemal titer is four times the mother's titer or higher.

Seropositive infants not treated at birth should be followed carefully at 1, 2, 3, 6, and 12 months of age. Nontreponemal antibody titers that are passively transferred should decline by 3 months and be gone by 6 months. If titers are stable or rising, a lumbar puncture should be obtained and therapy given. Treponemal antibody titers that are passively transferred can persist for a year. If they persist longer, the child should be evaluated for neurosyphilis and treated.

Treated infants should be followed clinically and serologically every 2–3 months. Nontreponemal antibody titers should be negative by 6 months of age, and if they are not the infant should be evaluated for neurosyphilis and re-treated. Infants with neurosyphilis should undergo lumbar puncture every 6 months or until pleocytosis has resolved. Re-treatment is indicated if the CSF-VDRL is positive at 6 months, if there is not a downward trend in cell count at each examination, or if there is still pleocytosis at 2 years.

Therapy for congenital syphilis is 100,000–150,000 units/kg of aqueous crystalline penicillin G daily given in two or three divided doses intravenously, or 50,000 units/kg of procaine penicillin daily given as a single intramuscular injection, both for 10–14 days.

Jonas S et al: Postneonatal screening for congenital syphilis. J Fam Pract 1995;41:286. (Congenital syphilis in infants with negative serology.)

Larsen SA, Steiner BM, Rudolph AH: Laboratory diagnosis and interpretation of tests for syphilis. Clin Microbiol Rev 1995;8:1. (Comprehensive review of diagnostic tests.)

1993 Sexually transmitted diseases treatment guidelines. MMWR Morb Mortal Wkly Rep 1993;42 (No. RR-14):1.

Scheck DN, Hook EW III: Neurosyphilis. Infect Dis Clin North Am 1994;8:769. (Review of neurosyphilis, including impact of HIV infection on diagnosis and treatment.)

Tramont EC: Syphilis in adults: From Christopher Columbus to Sir Alexander Fleming to AIDS. Clin Infect Dis 1995;21:1361. (Review of manifestations, diagnosis, and current therapeutic recommendations.)

NON-SEXUALLY TRANSMITTED TREPONEMATOSES

A variety of treponemal diseases other than syphilis occur endemically in many tropical areas of the world. They are distinguished from disease caused by *T pallidum* by their nonsexual transmission, their relatively high incidence in certain geographic areas and among children, and their tendency to produce less severe visceral manifestations. As in syphilis, organisms can be demonstrated in infectious lesions with darkfield microscopy or immunofluorescence but cannot be cultured in artificial media; the serologic tests for syphilis are positive, including the newer tests such as CAPTIA Syph G; the diseases have primary, secondary, and sometimes tertiary stages; and penicillin is the drug of choice. There is evidence that infection with these agents may provide partial resistance to syphilis and vice versa. Treatment with penicillin in doses appropriate to primary syphilis (eg, 2.4 million units of benzathine penicillin G intramuscularly) is generally curative in any stage of the non-sexually transmitted treponematoses. In cases of penicillin hypersensitivity, tetracycline is usually the recommended alternative.

YAWS
(Frambesia)

Yaws is a contagious disease largely limited to tropical regions that is caused by *Treponema pallidum* subsp *pertenue*. It is characterized by granulomatous lesions of the skin, mucous membranes, and bone. Yaws is rarely fatal, though if untreated it may lead to chronic disability and disfigurement. Yaws is acquired by direct nonsexual contact, usually in childhood, although it may occur at any age. The "mother yaw," a painless papule that later ulcerates, appears 3–4 weeks after exposure. There is usually associated regional lymphadenopathy. Six to 12 weeks later, similar secondary lesions appear and last for several months or years. Painful ulcerated lesions on the soles are frequent and are called "crab yaws." Late gummatous lesions may occur, with associated tissue destruction involving large areas of skin and subcutaneous tissues. The late effects of yaws, with bone change, shortening of digits, and contractions, may be confused with similar changes occurring in leprosy. Central nervous system, cardiac, or other visceral involvement is rare.

PINTA

Pinta is a non-sexually transmitted spirochetal infection caused by *Treponema carateum*. It occurs endemically in rural areas of Latin America, especially in Mexico, Colombia, and Cuba, and in some areas of the Pacific. A nonulcerative, erythematous primary papule spreads slowly into a papulosquamous plaque showing a variety of color changes (slate, lilac, black). Secondary lesions resemble the primary one and appear within a year after it. These appear successively, new lesions together with older ones; are commonest on the extremities; and later show atrophy and depigmentation. Some cases show pigmentary changes and atrophic patches on the soles and palms, with or without hyperkeratosis, that are indistinguishable from "crab yaws." Very rarely, central nervous system or cardiovascular disease is observed late in the course of infection.

ENDEMIC SYPHILIS

Endemic syphilis is an acute or chronic infection caused by an organism indistinguishable from *T pallidum* subsp *endemicum*. It has been reported in a number of countries, particularly in the eastern Mediterranean area, often with local names: bejel in Syria, Saudi Arabia, and Iraq; and dichuchwa, njovera, and siti in Africa. It also occurs in Southeast Asia. The local forms have distinctive features. Moist ulcerated lesions of the skin or oral or nasopharyngeal mucosa are the most common manifestations. Generalized lymphadenopathy and secondary and tertiary bone and skin lesions are also common. Deep leg pain points to periostitis or osteomyelitis. Cardiovascular and central nervous system involvement is rare.

Chulay JD: *Treponema* species (yaws, pinta, bejel). In: *Principles and Practice of Infectious Diseases*, 4th ed.

Mandell GL, Bennett JE, Dolin R (editors). Churchill Livingstone, 1995. (A textbook review of non-sexually transmitted treponemal diseases.)

MISCELLANEOUS SPIROCHETAL DISEASES

RELAPSING FEVER

Relapsing fever is endemic in many parts of the world. The main reservoir is rodents, which serve as the source of infection for ticks (eg, *Ornithodoros*). The distribution and seasonal incidence of the disease are determined by the ecology of the ticks in different areas. In the USA, infected ticks are found throughout the West, especially in mountainous areas, but clinical cases are uncommon in humans.

The infectious organism is a spirochete, *Borrelia recurrentis*, though other poorly characterized borrelia-like organisms can cause similar disease. It may be transmitted transovarially from one generation of ticks to the next. The spirochetes occur in all tissues of the tick, and humans can be infected by tick bites or by rubbing crushed tick tissues or feces into the bite wound. Tick-borne relapsing fever is endemic but is not transmitted from person to person. Different species (or strain) names have been given to *Borrelia* in different parts of the world where the organisms are transmitted by different ticks.

When an infected person harbors lice, the lice become infected with *Borrelia* by sucking blood. A few days later, the lice serve as a source of infection for other persons. Large epidemics may occur in louse-infested populations, and transmission is favored by crowding, malnutrition, and cold climate.

Clinical Findings

A. Symptoms and Signs: There is an abrupt onset of fever, chills, tachycardia, nausea and vomiting, arthralgia, and severe headache. Hepatomegaly and splenomegaly may develop, as well as various types of rashes. Delirium occurs with high fever, and there may be various neurologic and psychic abnormalities. The attack terminates, usually abruptly, after 3–10 days. After an interval of 1–2 weeks, relapse occurs, but often it is somewhat milder. Three to ten relapses may occur before recovery.

B. Laboratory Findings: During episodes of fever, large spirochetes are seen in blood smears stained with Wright's or Giemsa's stain. The organisms can be cultured in special media but rapidly lose pathogenicity. The spirochetes can multiply in injected rats or mice and can be seen in their blood. A variety of anti-*Borrelia* antibodies develop during the illness; sometimes the Weil-Felix test for rickettsioses and nontreponemal serologic tests for syphilis may also be falsely positive. Cerebrospinal fluid abnormalities occur in patients with meningeal involvement. Mild anemia and thrombocytopenia are common, but the white blood cell count tends to be normal.

Differential Diagnosis

The manifestations of relapsing fever may be confused with malaria, leptospirosis, meningococcemia, yellow fever, typhus, or rat-bite fever.

Prevention

Prevention of tick bites (as described for rickettsial diseases) and delousing procedures applicable to large groups can prevent illness. Arthropod vectors should be controlled if possible.

An effective means of chemoprophylaxis has not been developed.

Treatment

A single dose of tetracycline or erythromycin, 0.5 g orally, or a single dose of procaine penicillin G, 400,000–600,000 units intramuscularly, probably constitutes adequate treatment for louse-borne relapsing fevers. Because of higher relapse rates, tickborne disease is treated with 0.5 g of tetracycline or erythromycin given four times daily for 5–10 days. Jarisch-Herxheimer reactions occur commonly following treatment and may be life-threatening. Treatment with aspirin—but not hydrocortisone—may ameliorate this reaction. The Jarisch-Herxheimer reaction is mediated in part by tumor necrosis factor, and administration of antibody to this cytokine prior to antibiotic therapy is effective in preventing the reaction.

Prognosis

The overall mortality rate is usually about 5%. Fatalities are most common in old, debilitated, or very young patients. With treatment, the initial attack is shortened and relapses are largely prevented.

Johnson WD Jr: *Borrelia* species: Relapsing fever. In: *Principles and Practice of Infectious Diseases,* 4th ed. Mandell GL, Bennett JE, Dolin R (editors). Churchill Livingston, 1995.
Rawlings JA: An overview of tick-borne relapsing fever with emphasis on outbreaks in Texas. Tex Med 1995;91:56. (A review of epidemiology and clinical manifestations.)

RAT-BITE FEVER
(Spirillary Rat-Bite Fever, Sodoku)

Rat-bite fever is an uncommon acute infectious disease caused by *Spirillum minus*. It is transmitted to humans by the bite of a rat. Inhabitants of rat-infested slum dwellings and laboratory workers are at greatest risk.

Clinical Findings

A. Symptoms and Signs: The original rat bite, unless secondarily infected, heals promptly, but 1 to several weeks later the site becomes swollen, indurated, and painful; assumes a dusky purplish hue; and may ulcerate. Regional lymphangitis and lymphadenitis, fever, chills, malaise, myalgia, arthralgia, and headache are present. Splenomegaly may occur. A sparse, dusky-red maculopapular rash appears on the trunk and extremities in many cases, and there may be frank arthritis.

After a few days, both the local and systemic symptoms subside, only to reappear again in a few more days. This relapsing pattern of fever for 3–4 days alternating with afebrile periods lasting 3–9 days may persist for weeks. The other features, however, usually recur only during the first few relapses.

B. Laboratory Findings: Leukocytosis is often present, and the nontreponemal test for syphilis is often falsely positive. The organism may be identified in darkfield examination of the ulcer exudate or aspirated lymph node material; more commonly, it is observed after inoculation of a laboratory animal with the patient's exudate or blood. It has not been cultured in artificial media.

Differential Diagnosis

Rat-bite fever must be distinguished from the rat bite-induced lymphadenitis and rash of streptobacillary fever. Clinically, the severe arthritis and myalgias seen in streptobacillary disease is rarely seen in disease caused by *S minus*. Reliable differentiation requires an increasing titer of agglutinins against *Streptobacillus moniliformis* or identification of the causative organism. Rat-bite fever must also be distinguished from tularemia, rickettsial disease, *Pasteurella multocida* infections, and relapsing fever by identification of the causative organism.

Treatment

Treat with procaine penicillin G, 600,000 units intramuscularly every 12 hours; or tetracycline hydrochloride, 0.5 g every 6 hours for 10–14 days. Give supportive and symptomatic measures as indicated.

Prognosis

The reported mortality rate of about 10% should be markedly reduced by prompt diagnosis and antimicrobial treatment.

Washburn RG: *Spirillum minus* (rat-bite fever). In: *Principles and Practice of Infectious Diseases,* 4th ed. Mandell GL, Bennett JE, Dolin R (editors). Churchill Livingstone, 1995.

LEPTOSPIROSIS

Leptospirosis is an acute and often severe infection that frequently affects the liver or other organs and is caused by serovars of *Leptospira interrogans.* The three most common serovars of infection are *Leptospira icterohaemorrhagiae* of rats, *Leptospira canicola* of dogs, and *Leptospira pomona* of cattle and swine. Several other varieties can also cause the disease, but *L icterohaemorrhagiae* causes the most severe illness. The disease is worldwide in distribution, and the incidence is higher than usually supposed. The leptospires are often transmitted to humans by the ingestion of food and drink contaminated by the urine of the reservoir animal. The organism may also enter through minor skin lesions and probably via the conjunctiva. Recreational cases have followed swimming in contaminated water, and occupational cases occur among sewer workers, rice planters, abattoir workers, and farmers. Sporadic urban cases have been seen in the homeless exposed to rat urine. The incubation period is 2–20 days.

Clinical Findings

A. Symptoms and Signs: Anicteric leptospirosis is the more common and milder form of the disease and is often biphasic. The initial or "septicemic" phase begins with abrupt fever to 39–40 °C, chills, abdominal pain, severe headache, and myalgias, especially of the calf muscles. There is marked conjunctival suffusion. Leptospires can be isolated from blood, cerebrospinal fluid, and tissues. Following a 1- to 3-day period of improvement in symptoms and absence of fever, the second or "immune" phase begins. Leptospires are absent from blood and cerebrospinal fluid but are still present in the kidney, and specific antibodies appear. A recurrence of symptoms is seen as in the first phase of disease with the onset of meningitis. Uveitis, rash, and adenopathy may occur. The illness is usually self-limited, lasting 4–30 days, and complete recovery is the rule.

Icteric leptospirosis (Weil's syndrome) (usually caused by *L icterohaemorrhagiae*) is the most severe form of the disease, characterized by impaired renal and hepatic function, abnormal mental status, hypotension, and a 5–10% mortality rate. Symptoms and signs are continuous and not biphasic.

Pretibial fever, a mild form of leptospirosis caused by *Leptospira autumnalis,* occurred during World War II at Fort Bragg, USA. In pretibial fever, there is patchy erythema on the skin of the lower legs or generalized rash occurring with fever.

Leptospirosis with jaundice must be distinguished from hepatitis, yellow fever, and relapsing fever.

B. Laboratory Findings: The leukocyte count may be normal or as high as 50,000/μL, with neutrophils predominating. The urine may contain bile, protein, casts, and red cells. Oliguria is not uncommon, and in severe cases uremia may occur. In cases with meningeal involvement, organisms may be found in the cerebrospinal fluid during the first 10 days of illness. Early in the disease, the organism may be identified by darkfield examination of the patient's blood or by culture on a semisolid medium (eg, Fletcher's EMJH). Cultures take 1–6 weeks to become positive. The organism may also be grown from the urine from the tenth day to the sixth week. Diagnosis is usually made by means of serologic tests, of which several are available. Agglutination tests (microscopic, using live organisms; and macroscopic, using killed antigen) become positive after 7–10 days of illness, peak at 3–4 weeks, and may persist at high levels for many years. Thus, to make a diagnosis, a fourfold or greater rise in titer must be documented. Indirect hemagglutination, immunofluorescent antibody, and ELISA tests are also available. The IgM ELISA is particularly useful in making an early diagnosis, as it is positive as early as 2 days into illness, a time when the clinical manifestations may be nonspecific. PCR methods (presently investigational) appear to be sensitive, specific, positive early in disease, and able to detect leptospiral DNA in blood, urine, cerebrospinal fluid, and aqueous humor. Serum CK is usually elevated in leptospirosis patients and normal in hepatitis patients.

Complications

Myocarditis, aseptic meningitis, renal failure, and massive hemorrhage are not common but are the usual causes of death. Iridocyclitis may occur.

Treatment

Various antimicrobial drugs, including penicillin and tetracyclines, show antileptospiral activity. Penicillin (eg, 6 million units daily intravenously) is said to be beneficial in severe leptospirosis, especially if started within the first 4 days of illness. Jarisch-Herxheimer reactions may occur. Observe for evidence of renal failure, and treat as necessary. Effective prophylaxis consists of doxycycline, 200 mg orally once weekly during the risk of exposure. Doxycycline, 100 mg twice daily for 7 days, can also reduce the severity and duration of symptoms if given within 3 days after onset of disease.

Prognosis

Without jaundice, the disease is almost never fatal. With jaundice, the mortality rate is 5% for those under age 30 and 30% for those over age 60.

Farr RW: Leptospirosis. Clin Infect Dis 1995;21:1. (Clinical review.)

Vinetz JM et al: Sporadic urban leptospirosis. Ann Intern Med 1996;125:794. (Epidemiology of an urban outbreak.)

LYME DISEASE
(Lyme Borreliosis)

Essentials of Diagnosis

- Erythema migrans, a flat or slightly raised red lesion that expands with central clearing.
- Headache or stiff neck.
- Arthralgias, arthritis, and myalgias; arthritis is often chronic and recurrent.
- Wide geographic distribution, with most United States cases in the Northeast, mid-Atlantic, Upper Midwest, and Pacific coastal regions.

General Considerations

This illness, named after the town of Old Lyme, Connecticut, is caused by the spirochete *Borrelia burgdorferi* and is transmitted to humans by ixodid ticks that are part of the *Ixodes ricinus* complex. Three genomic groups of the *B burgdorferi sensu lato* group have been identified: *B burgdorferi sensu stricto,* which causes disease in North America and less commonly in Europe and Asia; *B garinii,* and *B afzelii,* the latter two of which are the predominant etiologic agents of Lyme disease in Europe and Asia. Lyme disease is the most common vector-borne disease in the United States and is being reported with increasing frequency, but the true incidence is not known. Overreporting of Lyme disease remains a problem. In 1995, there were 11,603 cases (down from 13,083 cases in 1994), in 43 states of the USA, but enzootic cycles of *B burgdorferi* could be documented in only 19 states. Overdiagnosis of Lyme disease is also a major problem. In a Lyme disease clinic at a major teaching hospital in an endemic area, 788 patients were referred over a 4.5-year period. Only 23% were found to have active disease. The remaining patients had adequately treated disease in the past and another concurrent illness (20%) or did not have Lyme disease at all (57%). The overreporting and overdiagnosis of Lyme disease is in part explained by the recent discovery of a nonculturable spirochete in the lone star tick *(Amblyomma americanum).* This organism produces a Lyme disease-like illness with a skin lesion very similar to that of erythema migrans. As the lone star tick is found in the Midwest and Southern areas where enzootic cycles for *B burgdorferi* have not been reported, cases of Lyme disease reported from these areas are probably due to this newly discovered organism. Most cases of Lyme disease occur in the Northeast, Upper Midwest, and along the Pacific Coast. The vector is *Ixodes scapularis* (also known as *I dammini*) in the northeastern, midwestern, and southeastern United States, *Ixodes pacificus* on the West Coast, *Ixodes ricinus* in Europe, and *Ixodes persulcatus* in Asia. The disease also occurs in Australia (vector unknown). Mice and deer make up the major animal reservoir of *B burgdorferi,* but other rodents and birds may also be infected. Domestic animals such as dogs, cattle, and horses can also develop clinical illness, usually manifested as arthritis.

Ticks feed once during each of their three stages of life. Larval ticks feed in late summer, nymphs in the following spring and early summer, and adults during the fall. The preferred host for the nymphs and larvae is the white-footed mouse in the USA (the black-striped mouse in Europe). This animal is tolerant of infection—a fact that is critical in maintaining infection, since the mouse can remain spirochetemic and transmit the agent to the larvae the following spring after being infected by the nymphal form in early summer. Adult ticks prefer the white-tailed deer as host. Although only 20–25% of nymphs harbor spirochetes compared with 50–65% of adults, most infections occur in the spring and summer (when nymphs are active), and fewer cases occur in the cooler months (October to April), when adults feed. This is probably due to the greater abundance of nymphs; greater human outdoor activity in spring and summer, when nymphs feed; and the fact that adult ticks are larger, easier to detect by the human host, and thus can be removed before disease is transmitted. Less than 1% of larvae are infected with spirochetes, and transmission of the disease through contact with larvae is unlikely.

The increased incidence of Lyme disease is due in part to the resurgence of the once-decimated deer population, the spread of tick vectors to new areas (infected *Ixodes* ticks have been isolated from migratory birds), and the encroachment of suburbs on once rural areas, bringing humans and ticks into closer proximity. Control of Lyme disease is best accomplished by avoiding tick-infested areas, wearing protective clothing, using repellents, and inspecting for ticks after possible exposures. Controlling ticks on residential property and in parks may also be helpful, but limiting the spread of ticks and deer control are not currently feasible.

Under experimental conditions, ticks must feed for 24 hours or longer to transmit infections, though human epidemiologic data suggest that disease transmission is possible in some patients with shorter tick attachment times. In addition, the percentage of ticks infected varies on a regional basis. In the Northeast and Midwest, 15–65% of *I scapularis* ticks are infected with the spirochete; in the Western United States, only 2% of *I pacificus* are infected. These are important epidemiologic features in assessing the likelihood that tick exposure will result in disease. Exposure to *I pacificus* is unlikely to result in disease, since so few ticks are infected, but this is not true of exposure to *I scapularis.* Eliciting a history of brushing a tick off the skin (ie, the tick was not feeding) or removing a tick on the same day as exposure (ie, the tick did not feed long enough) decreases the likelihood that infection will develop, since the vast majority of cases occur when ticks feed for at least 24 hours.

Ixodes ticks are smaller than the more common dog ticks *(Dermacentor variabilis)*. Larvae are less than 1 mm in size, and the adult female is 2–3 mm in size, with a red body and black legs. After a blood meal, ticks can reach two to three times their unengorged size. Because the tick is so small, the bite is usually painless and goes unnoticed. After feeding, the tick drops off in 2–4 days. If a tick is found, it should be removed immediately. The best way to accomplish this is to grab the mouth part—not the body—where it enters the skin with a fine-tipped tweezers and pull firmly and repeatedly until the tick releases its hold. Saving the tick in a bottle of alcohol for future identification may be useful, especially if symptoms develop.

Congenital infection has been documented, but the exact frequency and manifestations have not been clearly defined. Similarly, because the organism can be latent, it is not known if women infected prior to becoming pregnant can activate the disease and transmit infection to the fetus. In one retrospective study, 5 of 19 pregnancies complicated by Lyme disease resulted in an adverse outcome, but all of the outcomes were different and could not be conclusively linked to infection. Several serosurveys involving over 2000 pregnant women in endemic areas have not found any association between seropositivity in prospective mothers and the prevalence of congenital malformations, fetal death, and prematurity. Thus, if *B burgdorferi* causes a congenital syndrome like some other spirochetal illnesses, it must be extremely uncommon.

Clinical Findings

The typical clinical description of Lyme disease divides the illness into three stages: stage 1, flu-like symptoms and a typical skin rash **(erythema migrans)**; stage 2, weeks to months later, Bell's palsy or meningitis; and stage 3, months to years later, arthritis. The problem with this simplified scheme is that there is a great deal of overlap, and the skin, central nervous system, and musculoskeletal system can be involved early or late. A more accurate classification divides disease into early and late manifestations and specifies whether disease is localized or disseminated.

A. Symptoms and Signs:

1. Stage 1, early localized infection–Stage 1 infection is characterized by erythema migrans. About 1 week after the tick bite (range, 3–30 days; median 7–10 days), a flat or slightly raised red lesion appears at the site, which is commonly seen in areas of tight clothing such as the groin, thigh, or axilla. This lesion expands over several days, with central clearing. About 20% of patients either do not have typical skin lesions or the lesions go unnoticed. A flu-like illness with fever, chills, and myalgia occurs in about half of patients. Even without treatment, the symptoms and signs of erythema migrans resolve in

3–4 weeks. Although the classic lesion of erythema migrans is not difficult to recognize, atypical forms can occur that may lead to misdiagnosis. Vesicular, urticarial, and evanescent erythema migrans have been reported, as have lesions that develop central intensification instead of clearing. Similarly, chemical reactions to tick and spider bites, drug eruptions, urticaria, and staphylococcal and streptococcal cellulitis have been mistaken for erythema migrans.

2. Stage 2, early disseminated infection–In stage 2, the spirochete may spread in the patient's blood or lymph to cause a wide variety of symptoms and signs. This usually occurs within days to weeks after inoculation of the organism. The most common manifestations involve the skin, central nervous system, and musculoskeletal system. In about half of patients, secondary lesions develop that are not associated with a tick bite. These lesions are similar in appearance to the primary lesion but are usually smaller. A rare skin lesion (1% of patients) seen primarily in Europe is *Borrelia* lymphocytoma. This presents as a small reddish nodule or plaque on the ear in children and on the nipple in adults. Headache and stiff neck can occur, as well as migratory pains in joints, muscles, and tendons. Fatigue and malaise are common. Generally, the neurologic and musculoskeletal symptoms are intermittent and last only hours to a few days, whereas fatigue is persistent. After hematogenous spread, the organism sequesters itself in certain areas and produces focal symptoms. Some patients experience cardiac (4–10% of patients) or neurologic (10–20% of patients) manifestations. Involvement of the heart includes myopericarditis, with atrial or ventricular arrhythmias and heart block. Neurologic disease is most commonly manifested as aseptic meningitis with mild headache and neck stiffness, Bell's palsy, or encephalitis with irritability, personality change, and forgetfulness that can wax and wane. Even in the absence of symptoms, seeding of the central nervous system can occur. Peripheral neuropathy (sensory or motor), transverse myelitis, and mononeuritis multiplex have also been described. Conjunctivitis, keratitis, and, rarely, panophthalmitis can occur.

3. Stage 3, late persistent infection–Stage 3 infection occurs months to years after the initial infection and again primarily manifests itself as musculoskeletal, neurologic, and skin disease. Up to 60% of patients develop musculoskeletal complaints. Clinical manifestations are quite variable and include (1) joint and periarticular pain without objective findings (perhaps a manifestation of fibromyalgia that may be triggered by Lyme disease); (2) frank arthritis, mainly of large joints, that is chronic or recurrent over years (recurrences become less severe, less frequent, and shorter with time); and (3) chronic synovitis, which may result in permanent disability. The pathogenesis of chronic Lyme arthritis may be an immunologic phenomenon rather than persistence of infection. The observations that individuals with chronic arthritis have an increased frequency of HLA-DR4 gene expression, antibodies to OspA and OspB protein in joint fluid (major outer surface proteins of *B burgdorferi*), lack *B burgdorferi* DNA in synovial fluid as detected by polymerase chain reaction (PCR), and often fail to respond to antibiotics—all support the inference of an immunologic mechanism.

Both the central and the peripheral nervous systems may be involved. Subacute encephalopathy, characterized by memory loss, mood changes, and sleep disturbance, is the most common chronic neurologic manifestation. An axonal polyneuropathy, manifested as distal sensory paresthesias or radicular pain, can occur either alone or, more commonly, in association with encephalopathy. Most of these patients have objective signs of disease when tested by electromyography. A rare form of chronic neurologic dysfunction—leukoencephalitis—presents with cognitive dysfunction, spastic paraparesis, ataxia, and bladder dysfunction. This form of the disease is seen more commonly in Europe than in the United States.

The cutaneous manifestation of late infection, which can occur up to 10 years after infection, is **acrodermatitis chronicum atrophicans.** It has been described mainly in Europe and is due to infection with *Borrelia afzelii,* a species that commonly causes disease in Europe but not the United States. There is usually bluish-red discoloration of a distal extremity with associated swelling. These lesions become atrophic and sclerotic with time and eventually resemble localized scleroderma. At least two cases of diffuse fasciitis with eosinophilia, a rare entity that resembles scleroderma, have been associated with infection with *B burgdorferi.*

B. Laboratory Findings: The diagnosis of Lyme disease is based on both clinical manifestations and laboratory findings. The National Surveillance Case Definition specifies a person with exposure to a potential tick habitat (within the 30 days just prior to developing erythema migrans) with (1) erythema migrans diagnosed by a physician or (2) at least one late manifestation of the disease and (3) laboratory confirmation as fulfilling the criteria for Lyme disease. Laboratory confirmation requires detection of specific antibodies to *B burgdorferi* in serum, either by indirect immunofluorescence assay (IFA) or enzyme-linked immunosorbent assay (ELISA); the latter is now preferred, because it is more sensitive and specific. A Western blot assay that can detect both IgM and IgG antibodies is used as a confirmatory test. IgM antibody appears first 2–4 weeks after onset of erythema migrans, peaks at 6–8 weeks, and then declines to low levels after 4–6 months of illness. Persistence of IgM or reappearance of IgM late in the disease may be indicative of recurrent disease. IgG occurs later (6–8 weeks after onset of disease), peaks at 4–6 months, and may remain elevated at low lev-

els indefinitely despite appropriate therapy and resolution of symptoms. A two-test approach is now recommended for the diagnosis of active Lyme disease. All specimens positive or equivocal by ELISA or IFA should be tested by Western immunoblot. When Western immunoblot is done during the first 4 weeks of illness, both IgM and IgG should be tested. If a patient with suspected early Lyme disease has negative serologic studies, acute and convalescent titers should be obtained since up to 50% of patients with early disease can be antibody-negative in the first several weeks of illness. A fourfold rise (or fall) in antibody titer would be diagnostic of recent infection. In patients with later stages of disease, almost all are antibody-positive. False-positive reactions in the ELISA and IFA have been reported in juvenile rheumatoid arthritis, rheumatoid arthritis, systemic lupus erythematosus, infectious mononucleosis, subacute infective endocarditis, syphilis, relapsing fever, leptospirosis, enteroviral and other viral illnesses, and patients with gingival disease (presumably because of cross-reactivity with oral treponemes). False-negative serologic reactions occur early in illness, and antibiotic therapy early in disease can abort subsequent seroconversion. Other investigational tests include an antibody-capture ELISA, which appears to be more specific and sensitive than the routine ELISA or IFA, especially in early disease. It is positive in up to 90% of patients with stage 1 disease. It is difficult to perform and is presently available only in reference and research laboratories. Use of flagellar antigen, which produces an early immune response, to detect antibodies by both ELISA and immunoblotting may improve the ability to detect early disease and is under investigation.

Caution should be exercised in basing the diagnosis of Lyme disease on serologic testing. In addition to the lack of sensitivity of the available tests as noted above, interlaboratory variation in test results is a major problem. In one study, aliquots of serum were sent to different laboratories, and there was a marked difference in reported test results, with known positive serum being identified in less than half of cases. When a second specimen of the same serum was sent 2 weeks later, 8 of 18 laboratories reported a fourfold difference in titers. These data demonstrate the difficulty in making the diagnosis of Lyme disease by serologic testing and emphasize the need for national standards. Lack of specificity is also a problem, and several diseases can cause false-positive reactions as noted above.

B burgdorferi has rarely been cultured from blood or cerebrospinal fluid. Aspiration of erythema migrans lesions has yielded positive cultures in up to 29% of cases, and cultures of biopsy specimens have been reported positive in 60–70%. The ability to culture organisms from skin lesions is greatly influenced by antibiotic therapy. Even a brief course of several days will result in negative cultures. Special silver staining of chronically inflamed synovial tissue demonstrates spirochetes in one-third of patients.

Detection of bacterial DNA by PCR may become a useful diagnostic tool in view of difficulties in culturing the organism and interpreting serologic tests. Although quite specific, the sensitivity of the test varies and depends upon which body fluid is tested and the stage of disease. In patients with arthritis, 85% of synovial fluid samples are positive for *B burgdorferi* DNA by PCR. Sensitivity in blood and cerebrospinal fluid is not as good. PCR is more sensitive than culture for detecting spirochetemia in early disease (18% versus 5%), but serology (IgG or IgM) detects over 50% of cases. Similarly, PCR can detect *B burgdorferi* DNA in cerebrospinal fluid of 25% of chronic cases of neuroborelliosis and 38% of acute cases, but sensitivity is obviously a limiting factor. The significance of a positive reaction is unclear. Whether a positive PCR indicates persistence of viable organisms that will respond to further treatment or is a marker for residual DNA (not active infection) has not been clarified and depends on the clinical specimen and the stage of disease. In chronic Lyme arthritis, some have suggested that a positive PCR indicates active infection that requires further therapy, while others have found a positive reaction despite months of therapy. At present, this test remains investigational.

The diagnosis of neuroborelliosis is often difficult since clinical manifestations, such as memory impairment, may be difficult to document. Most patients with neuroborelliosis have a history of previous mono- or polyarticular arthritis, and the vast majority have antibody present in serum. When cerebrospinal fluid is sampled, there is usually a pleocytosis or elevated protein (or both) and evidence of localized antibody production, ie, a ratio of cerebrospinal fluid to serum antibody of > 1.0. The role of other tests such as PCR in detection of DNA or ELISA in detecting the presence of OspA antigen is unclear, but in difficult cases these tests can be performed and, if positive, help establish the diagnosis. In addition, many patients with neuroborelliosis will have a peripheral neuropathy that may be detected by electromyography. In the absence of any of the above findings, it is difficult to make the diagnosis of central nervous system borrelia infection.

Nonspecific laboratory abnormalities can be seen, particularly in early disease. The most common are an elevated sedimentation rate of > 20 mm/h seen in 50% of cases and mildly abnormal liver function tests present in 30%. The abnormal liver function tests are transient and return to normal within a few weeks of treatment. A mild anemia, leukocytosis (11,000–18,000/µL), and microscopic hematuria have been reported in 10% or less of patients.

Prevention

Simple preventive measures such as covering exposed areas with long-sleeved shirts and wearing long trousers tucked into socks, using repellents, and inspecting for ticks after exposure will greatly reduce the number of tick bites. Environmental controls directed at limiting ticks on residential property would be helpful, but trying to limit the deer, tick, or white-footed mouse populations over large areas is not feasible.

The role of prophylactic antibiotics following tick bites is controversial. Analysis of the cost-effectiveness of prophylactic therapy suggests that antibiotics administered for 2 weeks would be beneficial in preventing illness in endemic areas, where the risk of acquiring disease following a tick bite is 3.6% or greater. However, studies designed to examine the effect of prophylaxis have not shown any significant benefit. In one study of almost 400 patients in a highly endemic area, amoxicillin, 250 mg three times daily for 10 days, was no better than placebo in preventing disease in patients who had been bitten by a deer tick within the previous 72 hours. Since most patients who develop Lyme disease are symptomatic and since treatment of early disease prevents late sequelae, it is reasonable to reserve treatment for patients who develop symptoms rather than to routinely administer prophylactic antibiotics. Exceptions might include situations where the follow-up is uncertain, the patient is extremely anxious, the patient is a pregnant woman, or the tick was engorged when removed.

Vaccination with a recombinant outer surface protein (OspA) has been protective in a mouse model of disease. Preliminary data in humans suggest that the vaccine is well tolerated and highly immunogenic.

Treatment

Antibiotic sensitivity of *B burgdorferi* has been established in vitro. Tetracycline is effective against the spirochete, but penicillin is only moderately so. Erythromycin is effective in vitro but has been disappointing in clinical trials. Ampicillin, ceftriaxone, azithromycin, cefuroxime, and imipenem are also effective in vitro, but aminoglycosides, ciprofloxacin, and rifampin are not.

Present recommendations for therapy are outlined in Table 34–4. In general, infection confined to skin is treated for 10 days while disseminated disease requires longer therapy (20–30 days). For central nervous system disease (with the exception of Bell's palsy), systemic therapy is used. Other organ system involvement usually responds to oral medication. For early disease, oral antibiotic therapy shortens the duration of rash and usually prevents late sequelae. Either doxycycline, 100 mg twice daily, or tetracycline, 250–500 mg four times daily, is most commonly used. Amoxicillin is also effective and is recommended for children, for pregnant or lactating women, and for those who cannot tolerate doxycycline or tetracycline. Cefuroxime axetil, 500 mg

Table 34–4. Treatment of Lyme disease.

Manifestation	Drug and Dosage	Pediatric Dosage
Erythema migrans	Doxycycline, 100 mg twice daily for 10 days; or tetracycline, 500 mg 4 times daily for 10 days; or amoxicillin, 250–500 mg 3 times daily for 10 days; or cefuroxime axetil, 500 mg twice daily for 10 days; or erythromycin, 250 mg 4 times daily for 10 days.	Amoxicillin, 20–40 mg/kg/d for 10 days; or erythromycin, 30 mg/kg/d for 10 days; or cefuroxime axetil, 250 mg twice daily for 10 days.
Neurologic disease Bell's palsy	Doxycycline, tetracycline, or amoxicillin as above for 1 month.	Amoxicillin, 20–40 mg/kg/d for 1 month.

Other central
    nervous system
    disease
	Ceftriaxone, 2 g IV once daily for 3–4 weeks; or penicillin G, 20 million units daily IV in 6 divided doses for 3–4 weeks; or cefotaxime, 2 g IV every 8 hours for 3–4 weeks.	Ceftriaxone, 50–80 m/kg IV once daily for 3–4 weeks; or penicillin, 250–400 units/kg/d IV in divided doses for 3–4 weeks.

Cardiac disease
  First-degree block
    (PR < 0.3 s)
	Doxycycline, tetracycline, or amoxicillin as above for 10–30 days.	Amoxicillin as above for 10–30 days.

High-degree
    atrioventricular
    block
	Ceftriaxone or penicillin G as above for 14 days.	Penicillin G or ceftriaxone as above for 14 days.

Arthritis Oral dosage	Doxycycline, tetracycline, or amoxicillin as above for 1 month.	Amoxicillin as above for 1 month.
Parenteral dosage	Ceftriaxone or penicillin G as above for 14 days.	Penicillin G as above for 14 days.

Acrodermatitis
  chronicum
  atrophicans
	Doxycycline, tetracycline, or amoxicillin as above for 1 month.	Amoxicillin as above for 1 month.

twice daily for 20 days, is as effective as doxycycline, 100 mg twice daily for 20 days. Erythromycin is less effective. Azithromycin, 500 mg/d for 7 days, was not as effective as amoxicillin, 500 mg three times a day for 20 days, for erythema migrans. Complete resolution of symptoms was less common in the azithromycin group, and relapses occurred more commonly. For disseminated stage 2 disease, oral medication—doxycycline or amoxicillin—can be used for Bell's palsy. If other central nervous system manifestations are present (meningitis), ceftriaxone is given intravenously. Intravenous penicillin is also effective for central nervous system disease, but ceftriaxone penetrates into the cerebrospinal fluid better and can be given once daily. Mild cardiac disease (PR < 0.3 s) can be treated with oral agents, but high-degree atrioventricular block should be treated with either intravenous ceftriaxone or penicillin. Therapy of arthritis is difficult because some patients fail to respond to any therapy and others who do respond do so slowly. Initial studies suggested that intravenous penicillin was superior to benzathine penicillin. In one small study, ceftriaxone appeared to be superior to intravenous penicillin. In a recent study, however, oral agents (doxycycline or amoxicillin) were just as effective as intravenous regimens (penicillin or ceftriaxone). A reasonable approach to the patient with Lyme arthritis is to start with oral therapy and if this fails to switch to an intravenous agent. Data for treatment in pregnancy are limited. Tetracycline and doxycycline should not be used in pregnancy (be-

cause of subsequent tooth staining of infant). Because of the failure of oral agents to prevent fetal infection in one case, some have recommended parenteral therapy. In one study, 53 women in various trimesters with erythema migrans were treated with ceftriaxone for 2 weeks. The drug was tolerated well, no clinical disease developed in infants, and preterm births and congenital anomalies occurred no more frequently than in the general population.

Physicians are often confronted with patients with nonspecific symptoms (such as fatigue and myalgias) and positive serologic tests for Lyme disease who request (or demand) therapy for their illness. It is important in managing these patients to remember (1) that the diagnosis of Lyme disease is primarily a clinical one, and nonspecific symptoms alone are not diagnostic; (2) that serologic tests are fraught with difficulty (as noted above), and in areas where disease prevalence is low, false-positive serologic tests are much more common than true-positive tests; and (3) that parenteral therapy with ceftriaxone for 2–4 weeks is costly (approximately $5000) and has been associated with significant adverse effects (cholelithiasis). Parenteral therapy should be reserved for those most likely to benefit, ie, those with cutaneous, neurologic, cardiac, or rheumatic manifestations that are characteristic of Lyme disease.

Prognosis

Most patients respond to appropriate therapy with prompt resolution of symptoms. In a study of 201 children—most with early disease—treated with oral medications, complete resolution of symptoms was seen in 94% at 4 weeks, and none developed long-term complications when followed for an average of 2 years. With adequate therapy, only a small percentage of patients will fail to respond or will develop a late relapse. True treatment failures are thus uncommon, and in most cases re-treatment or prolonged treatment of Lyme disease is instituted because of misdiagnosis or misinterpretation of serologic results rather than inadequate therapy. It is important to remember that most areas endemic for Lyme disease are also endemic for babesiosis and ehrlichiosis. Coinfection with the etiologic agents of these diseases may be associated with more severe symptoms than infection with either agent alone and is another possible explanation for failure to respond to therapy directed at Lyme disease.

The long-term outcome of adult patients with Lyme disease is not clear. A recent study involving 38 patients found that one-third of patients followed for 6 years had musculoskeletal, neurologic, or cognitive problems. Although all patients received therapy, it was often delayed for months to years, and antibiotic regimens used were not the ones currently recommended. It is not known whether similar results would be found in patients treated early in the course of disease with more aggressive regimens.

Gerber MA et al: Lyme disease in children in southeastern Connecticut. N Engl J Med 1996;335:1270. (Natural history with therapy of early disease.)

Halperin JJ et al: Practice parameters for the diagnosis of patients with nervous system Lyme borreliosis (Lyme disease). Neurology 1996;46:619. (Superb review of manifestations of neurologic disease, diagnostic criteria, and therapy.)

Luft BJ et al: Appropriateness of parenteral antibiotic treatment for patients with presumed Lyme disease. Ann Intern Med 1993;119:518. (A position paper of the American College of Rheumatology and the Council of the Infectious Diseases Society of America.)

Sigal LH (editor): A symposium: National Clinical Conference on Lyme Disease. Am J Med 1995;98(Suppl 4A):[Entire issue.] (Eleven articles on various topics including epidemiology, clinical manifestations, and therapy.)

Spach DH et al: Tick-borne diseases in the United States. N Engl J Med 1993;329:936. (Review includes Lyme disease. Good color photos of ticks.)

Steere AC et al: The overdiagnosis of Lyme disease. JAMA 1993;269:1812. (Review of experience in a Lyme disease clinic in an endemic area.)

Walker DH et al: Emerging bacterial zoonotic and vector-borne diseases: Ecological and epidemiologic factors. JAMA 1996;275:463. (Review of emerging tick-borne diseases.)

Infectious Diseases: Protozoal & Helminthic

Robert S. Goldsmith, MD, MPH, DTM&H

I. PROTOZOAL INFECTIONS

AFRICAN TRYPANOSOMIASIS
(Sleeping Sickness)

Essentials of Diagnosis

- History of exposure to tsetse flies. Bite lesion.

Hemolymphatic stage (usually absent or unnoticed in *T b gambiense* infections):

- Irregular fevers, headaches, joint pains, malaise, pruritus, papular skin rash, edemas.
- Posterior cervical or generalized lymphadenopathy; hepatosplenomegaly.
- Anemia, weight loss.
- Trypanosomes in blood or lymph node aspirates; positive serology.

Meningoencephalitic stage:

- Insomnia, motor and sensory disorders, abnormal reflexes, somnolence to coma.
- Trypanosomes and increased white cells and protein in cerebrospinal fluid.

General Considerations

African trypanosomiasis is caused by *Trypanosoma brucei rhodesiense* and *Trypanosoma brucei gambiense,* both hemoflagellates. The organisms are transmitted by bites of tsetse flies (*Glossina* species), which inhabit shaded areas along streams and rivers. Human disease occurs locally throughout tropical Africa from south of the Sahara to about 20° south latitude. *T b gambiense* infections are in the moist sub-Saharan savannah and riverine forests of West and Central Africa up to the eastern Rift Valley. *T b rhodesiense* occurs to the east of the Rift Valley in the savannah of East and Southeast Africa and along the shores of Lake Victoria. There are an estimated 10,000–20,000 new cases annually and 5000 deaths.

T b rhodesiense infection is primarily a zoonosis of game animals; humans are infected sporadically. Humans are the principal mammalian host for *T b*

gambiense, but recent information suggests an animal reservoir as well.

Clinical Findings

A. Symptoms and Signs: *T b rhodesiense* infections go through the following three stages, are much more virulent, and untreated patients die within weeks to a year. In *T b gambiense* infections, however, chancres do not appear and the hemolymphatic stage is usually absent or goes unnoticed; when symptoms do become manifest after weeks to years, they are initially so mild that they are often ignored by the patient.

1. The trypanosomal chancre–This is a local pruritic, painful inflammatory reaction (3–10 cm) with regional lymphadenopathy that appears about 48 hours after the tsetse fly bite and lasts 2–4 weeks.

2. The hemolymphatic stage–This stage usually begins 3–10 days later with invasion of the bloodstream and reticuloendothelial system. High fever, severe headache, joint pains, and malaise recur at irregular intervals corresponding to waves of parasitemia. Between febrile episodes there are symptom-free periods that last up to 2 weeks. Transient rashes may appear, often pruritic and papular or circinate. Examination reveals mild enlargement of the liver and spleen, and edema (peripheral, pleural, ascites, etc). Enlarged, rubbery, and painless lymph nodes occur in 75% of patients. In *T b gambiense,* only the posterior cervical group (Winterbottom's sign) may be enlarged. With progression of the disease, there is increasing weight loss and debilitation. Signs of myocardial involvement may appear early in Rhodesian infection, and the patient may succumb to myocarditis before signs of central nervous system invasion appear.

3. The meningoencephalitic stage–This stage appears within a few weeks or months of onset of Rhodesian infection but in Gambian sleeping sickness develops more insidiously, starting 6 months to several years after onset. Insomnia, anorexia, personality changes, apathy, and headaches are among the early findings. A variety of motor or tonus disorders may develop, including tremors and disturbances of speech, gait, and reflexes; somnolence appears late. The patient becomes severely emaciated and, finally, comatose. Death often results from secondary infection.

B. Laboratory Findings: Definitive diagnosis requires identifying motile organisms in wet films and after Giemsa staining in specimens from the bite lesion (rare), lymph node aspirates, bone marrow, or cerebrospinal fluid. Because the number of trypanosomes in blood fluctuates and often is undetectable 3 out of 5 days, specimens should be examined daily for about 15 days, including after concentration by microhematocrit centrifugation of 10–15 mL of heparinized blood (trypanosomes are concentrated in the buffy coat). Other diagnostic tests with blood are the quantitative buffy coat technique, intraperitoneal inoculation into laboratory rodents (most sensitive approach, but only effective for *T b rhodesiense*), culture, Millipore filtration, and DEAE-cellulose anion exchange. Only soft lymph nodes (not fibrosed) should be selected for aspiration; they should be gently kneaded. Cerebrospinal fluid shows an increase in lymphocytes and protein; centrifugation to detect the parasite should be done both rapidly and twice (at least twice as sensitive as single centrifugation). The fluid should also be inoculated into an experimental animal and culture medium.

Serologic tests are available for IgM and IgG antibody. Circulating IgM levels become positive about 12 days after onset of infection and may reach 10–20 times normal. Normal or low levels, however, do not rule out the infection, for titers may fluctuate when brief periods of excess antigens may depress the titers, even to below detectable levels. In late central nervous system disease, though both circulating antibody and parasitemia may fall below detectable levels, serologic tests of the cerebrospinal fluid may yet prove useful. In central nervous system at any stage of the disease, an elevated IgM in the cerebrospinal fluid is pathognomonic for central nervous system infection except that false-negative results have been reported. Additional immunodiagnostic tests include ELISA and immunofluorescent assays.

Other findings include anemia, increased sedimentation rate, thrombocytopenia, reduced total serum protein, and increased serum globulin.

Differential Diagnosis

Trypanosomiasis may be mistaken for a variety of other diseases, including malaria, influenza, pneumonia, infectious mononucleosis, leukemia, lymphoma, the arbovirus encephalitides, cerebral tumor, and various psychoses. Serologic tests for syphilis may be falsely positive in trypanosomiasis.

Treatment

Because most of the drugs used are highly toxic (mortality during drug treatment can reach 5–10%),

immunoassays are insufficient to make the diagnosis; detection of the organism is required. (See references for dosages, adverse reactions, and modes of administration.)

A. Hemolymphatic Stage: Drugs of choice are suramin for both parasites or eflornithine (DMFO) for *T b gambiense*. The alternative drug for *T b gambiense* is pentamidine. Suramin and pentamidine frequently cause severe adverse reactions. A third alternative for both parasites—but not to be used as a first choice because of severe toxicity—is melarsoprol.

B. Late Disease With Central Nervous System Involvement: The drugs of choice are melarsoprol for both parasites or eflornithine for *T b gambiense*. Alternative treatments for *T b gambiense* are eflornithine or tryparsamide plus suramin.

Suramin and pentamidine, which do not penetrate the blood-brain barrier, cannot be used when the central nervous system is involved. Melarsoprol causes a reactive encephalopathy in up to 5% of patients; corticosteroids have been used by some workers to prevent this. Eflornithine, approved for use in the USA but available only from the manufacturer, is highly effective and associated with only mild toxicity in early and late *T b gambiense* infections, but its efficacy in *T b rhodesiense* infection is inconsistent. In the USA, suramin and melarsoprol are available only from the CDC Drug Service, Centers for Disease Control and Prevention, Atlanta, GA 30333. Telephone: 404-639-3670; 404-639-2888 evenings, weekends, and holidays. See references for dosages.

Proper follow-up to ensure detection of the encephalitic stage requires initial cerebrospinal fluid examination, repeat studies at intervals during treatment, 3 months after treatment, and then at 6-month intervals for 2 years.

Prevention

Individual prevention in endemic areas should include wearing long sleeves and trousers, avoiding dark-colored clothing, and using mosquito nets while sleeping. Repellents have no effect. Pentamidine is used in chemoprophylaxis (controversial) only against the Gambian type. In *T b rhodesiense* infection, pentamidine may suppress early symptoms, resulting in recognition of the disease too late in its course for effective treatment. Excretion of pentamidine is slow; therefore, one intramuscular injection (4 mg/kg, maximum 300 mg) protects for 3–6 months. The drug is potentially toxic and should only be used for persons at high risk (ie, those with constant, heavy exposure to tsetse flies in areas with known transmission of Gambian disease). Performing serologic tests every 6 months during exposure and for 3 years afterward is the safest method for detecting the disease at an early stage.

Prognosis

Most patients—even those with advanced disease—recover following treatment. Relapses are common (about 2%). When therapy is started late, irreversible brain damage or death is common. Most persons with African trypanosomiasis will die if untreated.

Brun RL: Advances in chemotherapy of African trypanosomiasis. (Editorial.) Acta Trop 1993;54:3.

Drugs for parasitic infections: Med Lett Drugs Ther 1995;37:99. (Important resource for dosages.)

Kuzoe FAS: Current situation of African trypanosomiasis. Acta Trop 1993;54:153.

Milord F et al: Eflornithine concentrations in serum and cerebrospinal fluid of 63 patients treated for *Trypanosoma brucei gambiense* sleeping sickness. Trans R Soc Trop Med Hyg 1993;87:473.

Pepin J et al: Risk factors for encephalopathy and mortality during melarsoprol therapy of *Trypanosoma brucei gambiense* sleeping sickness. Trans R Soc Trop Med Hyg 1995;89:92.

AMERICAN TRYPANOSOMIASIS
(Chagas' Disease)

Essentials of Diagnosis

Acute stage:

• Inflammatory lesion at site of inoculation; prolonged fever, tachycardia, hepatosplenomegaly, lymphadenopathy, signs of myocarditis.

• Parasites in peripheral blood, positive serologic tests.

Chronic stage:

• Heart failure with cardiac arrhythmias; decreased intensity of heart sounds; episodes of thromboembolism.

• In some geographic regions, dysphagia, severe constipation, and radiologic evidence of megaesophagus or megacolon.

• Positive xenodiagnosis or hemoculture, positive serologic tests; abnormal ECG.

General Considerations

Chagas' disease is caused by *Trypanosoma cruzi,* a protozoan parasite of humans and wild and domestic animals. *T cruzi* occurs only in the Americas; it is found in wild animals and to a lesser extent in humans from southern South America to southern USA. An estimated 16 million people are infected, mostly in rural areas, resulting in about 45,000 deaths yearly. In many countries of South America, Chagas' disease is the most important cause of heart disease. In southern USA, although the organism has been found in triatomine bugs and wild and domestic animals, only three confirmed indigenous cases have been reported. However, a large number of immigrants from Latin America (particularly Central America) are infected (estimated to be more than 50,000).

T cruzi is transmitted by many species of triatomine (reduviid) bugs that become infected by ingesting blood from infected animals or humans who have circulating trypanosomes. Multiplication occurs in the digestive tract of the bug; infective forms are eliminated in feces. Infection in humans is through "contamination" with bug feces; the parasite penetrates the skin (generally through the bite wound), mucus membranes, or the conjunctiva. Transmission can also occur by blood transfusion or in utero.

The trypanosomes first multiply close to the point of entry. They then enter the bloodstream as trypanosomes and later invade the heart and other tissues, where they assume a leishmanial form. Multiplication causes cellular destruction, inflammation, and fibrosis. Infection continues for many years, probably for life.

Clinical Findings

A. Symptoms and Signs: Most infected persons are asymptomatic. The **acute stage,** seen principally in children, lasts 2–4 months and leads to death in up to 10% of cases. The earliest findings are at the site of inoculation either in the eye—Romaña's sign (unilateral bipalpebral edema, conjunctivitis, local lymphadenopathy)—or in the skin—a chagoma (furuncle-like lesion with local lymphadenopathy). Subsequent findings include fever, malaise, headache, hepatomegaly, mild splenomegaly, and generalized lymphadenopathy. Acute myocarditis may lead to biventricular failure, but arrhythmias are rare. Meningoencephalitis is limited to young children and is often fatal.

A **latent period** may last from 10 to 30 years in which the patient is asymptomatic but in which serologic tests and sometimes parasitologic examination confirm the presence of the infection. Reactivation of Chagas' disease in AIDS has been reported.

The **chronic stage** is usually manifested by cardiac disease in the third and fourth decades of life, characterized by arrhythmias, congestive heart failure (often with prominent right-sided findings), and systemic or pulmonary embolization originating from mural thrombi. Sudden cardiac arrest in young persons may occur and is attributed to ventricular fibrillation. Megacolon and megaesophagus, caused by damage to nerve plexuses in the bowel or esophageal wall, occur in some areas of Chile, Argentina, and Brazil; symptoms include dysphagia, regurgitation, and constipation.

B. Laboratory Findings: Appropriate selection of tests allows a definitive parasitologic diagnosis in most acute cases and in up to 40% of chronic ones. In the acute stage, trypanosomes should be looked for by examination of anticoagulated fresh blood for motile organisms and by examination of the following stained preparations: thick blood films, buffy coat, and the sediment after centrifuging (600 Hz) the supernatant of clotted blood. In the chronic stage, the parasite can only be detected by culture or xenodiagnosis. The latter consists of permitting uninfected laboratory-reared bugs of the local major vector to feed on the patients and then examining their intestinal contents for trypanosomes. In both acute and chronic infection, blood should also be cultured using Nicolle-Novy-MacNeal medium and inoculated into laboratory mice or rats 3–10 days old. *Trypanosoma rangeli,* a nonpathogenic blood trypanosome also found in humans in Central America and northern South America, must not be mistaken for *T cruzi.* Several serologic tests are routinely used and are of presumptive value when positive; when possible, two or three tests should be used. Antibodies of the IgM class are usually elevated early in the acute stage but are replaced by IgG antibodies as the disease progresses. Maximum titers are reached in 3–4 months; thereafter, titers can remain positive at a low level for life. False-positive reactions can occur in the presence of leishmaniasis or *T rangeli* infection or because of autoantibodies. In chronic infections, when circulating organisms are difficult to find, the polymerase chain reaction procedure shows promise as a sensitive detection method. Serologic tests generally fail to assess the effectiveness of chemotherapy. The most important electrocardiographic abnormalities are right bundle branch block, other conduction defects, and arrhythmias. In certain regions of South America, radiologic examination may show megaesophagus, megacolon, or cardiac enlargement with characteristic apical aneurysms.

Treatment

Therapy is unsatisfactory. Treatment is indicated in acute but not latent infection and is controversial in the chronic stage. Two drugs are used: nifurtimox and benznidazole—both must be used for long periods and are potentially toxic. In acute disease, the drugs are effective in reducing the duration and severity of infection, but cure is achieved in only about 50% of patients. In the chronic phase, most reports indicate that although parasitemia and xenodiagnosis may become negative, treatment does not alter the serologic reaction, cardiac function, or progression of the disease. Some evidence indicates that pathogenesis may have an autoimmune basis not dependent on persistence of infection.

Nifurtimox is given orally in daily doses of 10 mg/kg in four divided doses after meals for 120 days. It generally produces anorexia, weight loss, tremors, and peripheral neuropathy. Hallucinations, pulmonary infiltrates, and convulsions are rare. In the USA, nifurtimox is available only from the Parasitic Disease Drug Service, Centers for Disease Control, Atlanta, GA 30333 (call 404-639-3670). Benznidazole, where available (not in the USA), is the alternative drug of choice at a dosage of 5–10 mg/kg/d for 30–60 days; it has side effects similar to those of nifurtimox.

In the chronic stage, diuretics are usually effective in cardiac failure, but digoxin is commonly not well tolerated. The most effective antiarrhythmic drug is amiodarone, but pulmonary and cardiac toxicity can be problems with its use. Arrhythmias are treated in the usual way; cardiac pacemakers are used for atrioventricular blocks. In endemic areas, blood should not be used for transfusion unless at least two serologic tests are negative; otherwise, blood can be treated with gentian violet to kill the parasites.

Prognosis

Acute infections in infants and young children are often fatal, particularly when the central nervous system is involved. Adults with chronic cardiac infections also may ultimately succumb to the disease.

De Castro SL: The challenge of Chagas' disease chemotherapy: An update of drugs assayed against *Trypanosoma cruzi.* Acta Trop (Basel) 1993;53:83.

Hagar JM, Rahimtoola SH: Chagas' heart disease. Curr Probl Cardiol 1995;20:825.

Kirchhoff LV: Chagas disease: American trypanosomiasis. Infect Dis Clin North Am 1993;7:487.

Prata A: Chagas' disease. Infect Dis Clin North Am 1994; 8:61.

Rossi MA, Bestetti RB: The challenge of chagasic cardiomyopathy: The pathologic roles of autonomic abnormalities, autoimmune mechanisms and microvascular changes, and therapeutic implications. Cardiology 1995;86:1.

AMEBIASIS

Essentials of Diagnosis

- Mild to moderate colitis: recurrent diarrhea and abdominal cramps, sometimes alternating with constipation; mucus may be present; blood is usually absent.
- Severe colitis: semiformed to liquid stools streaked with blood and mucus, fever, colic, prostration. In fulminant cases, ileus, perforation, peritonitis, and hemorrhage occur.
- Hepatic amebiasis: fever, hepatomegaly, pain, localized tenderness.
- Laboratory findings: amebas in stools or in abscess aspirate; serologic tests positive with severe colitis or hepatic abscess, which is readily imaged by ultrasonography or CT scan.

General Considerations

Amebiasis is infection of the large colon, liver, and other tissues by the protozoan parasite *Entamoeba histolytica.* Formerly considered one organism with varying virulence, the current general view is that there are two distinct though morphologically identical species in the *Entamoeba* complex: (1) *E dispar,* which remains in the colon as a stable commensal that is avirulent and produces an asymptomatic carrier state; and (2) *E histolytica* (about 10% of the complex), which shows varying degrees of virulence ranging from a commensal state in the colon—in which it does not cause disease, yet is potentially invasive—to being invasive of the intestinal wall and resulting in acute diarrhea or dysentery or chronic diarrhea. *E histolytica* may also be carried by the blood to the liver, where they may produce hepatic abscesses. Rarely, they are carried to the lungs, brain, or other organs or invade the perianal skin.

The infection is present worldwide but is most prevalent and severe in subtropical and tropical areas, where rates may exceed 40% under conditions of crowding, poor sanitation, and poor nutrition. It is estimated that there are about 50–100 million cases of invasive amebiasis and up to 100,000 deaths annually worldwide. In temperate areas, however, amebiasis tends to be asymptomatic or a mild, chronic infection that often remains undiagnosed. In the USA, seropositive rates up to 2–5% have been reported in some populations.

E histolytica exists as two forms in the lumen and mucosal crypts of the large bowel: cysts (10–14 μm) and motile trophozoites (12–50 μm). In the absence of diarrhea, trophozoites encyst in the large bowel. Trophozoites passed into the environment die rapidly, but cysts remain viable in soil and water for several weeks to months at appropriate temperature and humidity.

Humans are the only established host and are universally susceptible. Only cysts are infectious, since after ingestion they survive gastric acidity whereas trophozoites are destroyed. Transmission generally occurs through ingestion of cysts from fecally contaminated food or water. Flies and other arthropods also serve as mechanical vectors; to an undetermined degree, transmission results from contamination of food by the hands of food handlers. Where human excrement is used as fertilizer, it is often a source of food and water contamination. Person-to-person contact is also important in transmission; therefore, all household members as well as an infected person's sexual partner should have their stools examined. Sexual transmission of *E histolytica* among male homosexuals in some temperate urban areas is predominantly of nonpathogenic strains. In communal settings such as mental hospitals (but not child day care centers), prevalence rates as high as 50% have been reported. Amebiasis is rarely epidemic, but urban outbreaks have occurred because of common-source water contamination. Amebiasis is not an opportunistic infection in AIDS.

E histolytica and *E dispar* appear to be stable with regard to pathogenicity. As this is further confirmed and when simplified laboratory methods are developed to differentiate them, *E dispar* infections will not need to be treated. At present, isoenzyme analysis, typing with monoclonal antibodies to surface antigens, and restriction fragment length polymorphisms—not convenient laboratory procedures—differentiate the two organisms.

Malnutrition and alcoholism probably predispose to enhanced virulence. Fulminant infections may occur in pregnancy and in young children. Corticosteroids and other immunosuppressive drugs often convert a commensal infection to an invasive one.

The characteristic intestinal lesion is the amebic ulcer, which can occur anywhere in the large bowel (including the appendix) and sometimes in the terminal ileum but predominates in the cecum, descending colon, and the rectosigmoid colon—areas of greatest fecal stasis. Trophozoites invade the colonic mucosa by means of their ameboid movement and proteolytic secretions and induce necrosis to form the characteristic flask-shaped ulcers. Ulcers are usually limited to the muscularis, but if penetration to the serous layer occurs, bowel perforation, local abscess, or generalized peritonitis may result. In fulminating cases, ulceration may be extensive, and the bowel becomes thin and friable. Hepatic abscesses range from a few millimeters to 15 cm or larger, usually are single, occur more often in the right lobe (particularly the upper portion), and are more common in men.

Clinical Findings

A. Symptoms and Signs: Amebiasis can be classified into intestinal and extraintestinal disease and further subdivided into the clinical syndromes described below. Some patients have an acute onset of severe diarrhea as early as 8 days (commonly 2–4 weeks) after infection. Others may have an asymptomatic or mild intestinal infection for months to several years before either intestinal symptoms or liver abscess appears. Transition may occur from one type of intestinal infection to another, and each may give rise to hepatic abscess, or the intestinal infection may clear spontaneously.

1. Intestinal amebiasis–

a. Asymptomatic infection–In most infected persons, the organism lives as a commensal, and the patient is without symptoms.

b. Mild to moderate colitis (nondysenteric colitis)–A few stools a day are passed that are semiformed and have mucus but no blood. There may be abdominal cramps, flatulence, fatigue, and weight loss. Periods of remission and recurrence may last days to weeks or longer; during remissions, the patient may have constipation. Abdominal examination may show distention, hyperperistalsis, and tenderness. In some patients with chronic infection, the colon is thick and palpable, particularly over the cecum and descending colon. Toxic products released as a result of the bowel infection may induce periportal inflammation, mild hepatomegaly, and low-grade liver enzyme abnormalities, but without demonstrable trophozoites in the liver.

c. Severe colitis (dysenteric colitis)–As the severity of intestinal infection increases, the number of stools increases, and they change from semiformed to liquid with streaks of blood beginning to appear. With larger numbers of stools, 10–20 or more, little fecal material is present, but blood (fresh or dark) and bits of necrotic tissue become increasingly evident. With increasing severity, the patient may become prostrate and toxic, with fever up to 40.5 °C, and have colic, tenesmus, vomiting, generalized abdominal tenderness, and nonspecific hepatic enlargement and tenderness. Rare complications include appendicitis, bowel perforation (followed by peritonitis, pericolonic abscess, retroperitoneal fecal cellulitis, fistula to the abdominal surface), and fulminating colitis (with paralytic ileus, hypotension, massive mucosal sloughing, and hemorrhage). Death may follow.

d. Localized ulcerative lesions of the colon–Bowel ulcerations limited to the rectal area may result in passage of formed stools with bloody exudate. Ulcerations limited to the cecum may induce mild diarrhea and simulate acute appendicitis. Amebic appendicitis, in which the appendix is extensively involved but not the remainder of the large bowel, is rare.

e. Localized granulomatous lesions of the colon (ameboma)–This occurs as a result of excessive production of granulation tissue in response to amebic infection, either in the course of dysentery or slowly in chronic intestinal infection. These masses may present as an irregular tumor (single or multiple) that projects into the bowel or as an annular constricting mass up to several centimeters in length. Clinical findings (pain, obstructive symptoms, and hemorrhage) and x-ray findings may simulate bowel carcinoma, inflammatory bowel disease, tuberculosis, or lymphogranuloma venereum. At endoscopy, the mass is deep red and bleeds easily, and biopsy specimens show granulation tissue and *E histolytica,* though the number of organisms may be relatively few. Antiamebic drugs are usually adequate in treatment; surgical removal of the lesion without prior or immediate postoperative drug therapy is likely to result in death.

2. Extraintestinal amebiasis–

a. Hepatic amebiasis–Amebic liver abscess, although a relatively infrequent consequence of intestinal amebiasis, is not uncommon given the large number of intestinal infections. A large proportion of patients with liver abscess do not have concurrent intestinal symptoms, nor can they recall having had chronic intestinal symptoms. The onset of symptoms can be sudden or gradual, ranging from a few days to many months. Cardinal manifestations are fever (often high), pain (continuous, stabbing, or pleuritic, and sometimes severe), and an enlarged and tender liver. Patients may also experience malaise or prostration, sweating, chills, anorexia, and weight loss. The liver enlargement may present subcostally, in the epigastrium, as a localized bulging of the rib cage, or, as a result of enlargement against the dome of the diaphragm, it may produce coughing and findings at the right lung base (dullness to percussion, rales, and diminished breath sounds). Intercostal tenderness is common. Localizing signs on the skin may be an area of edema or a point of maximum tenderness. Without prompt treatment, the hepatic abscess may rupture into the pleural, peritoneal, or pericardial space or other contiguous organs, and death may follow.

b. Other extraintestinal infections–Skin infections may develop in the perianal area. Metastatic infection may rarely occur throughout the body, particularly the lungs, brain, and genitalia.

B. Laboratory Findings:

1. Intestinal amebiasis–Three specimens obtained under optimal conditions will generally detect only 80% of amebic infections, and three additional tests will raise the diagnostic rate to about 90%. Trophozoites predominate in liquid stools, cysts in formed stools.

A standard procedure is to collect three specimens at 2-day intervals or longer, with one of the three obtained after a laxative such as (1) sodium sulfate or phosphate (Fleet's Phospho-Soda), 30–60 g in a glass of water; or (2) bisacodyl 5–15 mL. Oil laxatives such as mineral oil should not be used. Specimens should be collected in a clean container. Because trophozoites rapidly autolyze, specimens should be examined within about 30 minutes or should immediately be mixed with a preservative.

If the patient has received specific therapy, antibiotics, antimalarials, antidiarrheal preparations (containing bismuth, kaolin, or magnesium hydroxide), barium, or mineral oil, specimen collection should be delayed 10–14 days.

On sigmoidoscopic examination, no findings are typical in mild intestinal disease; in severe disease, ulcers may be found that are 1 mm to 2 cm across, with intact intervening mucosa. If present, exudate should be collected with a glass pipette (not with cotton, to which trophozoites may adhere) or by scraping with a metal curette and examined immediately. The colon should not be cleansed before sigmoidoscopy, since this washes exudate from ulcers and destroys trophozoites. In some centers, rectal biopsy has enhanced diagnosis; the specimens are best examined by immunofluorescence methods. Where possible, in vitro culture of amebas can be attempted.

Most patients with amebic colitis test positive for occult blood, whereas findings for fecal leukocytes are noncontributory. Detection of trophozoites that contain ingested red blood cells is diagnostic for invasive *E histolytica* (they are not found in *E dispar* infections), but they may be confused with the occasional macrophage that also contains red blood cells. *E histolytica* cysts and trophozoites must be differentiated from the other pathogenic and nonpathogenic intestinal protozoa.

In dysentery, the white blood cell count can reach 20,000 or higher, but it is not elevated in mild colitis. A low-grade eosinophilia is occasionally present.

Serologic testing for *E histolytica* infection is specific (*E dispar* has not been shown to elicit serum antibodies) and usually positive if there has been substantial tissue invasion (as occurs in severe intestinal infection). In mild or asymptomatic intestinal infection, few patients are positive; it has been shown, however, that in asymptomatic infection with pathogenic *E histolytica* a positive serum antibody and antigenemia can result. The indirect hemagglutination test is sensitive and apparently produces no false-positive reactions. Titers become positive within a week after onset of symptoms and persist for up to 10 years after successful treatment; therefore, the test does not distinguish present from past infection. The agar gel methods, though less sensitive, are rapidly conducted laboratory tests that measure current invasion; the tests become negative within about 3–6 months after eradication of infection. Other tests for antibody include the ELISA and immunofluorescent tests. The polymerase chain reaction and other methods, which continue under evaluation for detection of antigen in stool or liver abscess aspirate, show promise of differentiating *E dispar* from *E histolytica*.

2. Hepatic abscess—Elevation of the right dome of the diaphragm and the size and location of abscess can be determined by ultrasonography (usually round or oval nonhomogeneous lesions, abrupt transition from normal liver to the lesion, hypoechoic center with diffuse echoes throughout the abscess), CT (well-defined, round, low-density lesions with an internal, nonhomogeneous structure), MRI, and radioisotope scanning. After intravenous injection of contrast material, CT may show a hyperdense halo around the periphery of the abscess. Gallium scans, only infrequently useful, show a cold spot (sometimes with a bright rim) as opposed to the increased gallium uptake in the center of pyogenic abscesses. Serologic tests are usually positive, but stools often no longer contain the parasite. The white count ranges from 15,000 to 25,000/μL. Eosinophilia is not present. Liver function test abnormalities, when present, are usually minimal. Indications and risks of percutaneous aspiration of abscesses when used in diagnosis and treatment are described below.

Differential Diagnosis

Amebiasis should be considered in patients with acute or chronic diarrhea (including cases associated with only mild changes in bowel habits in patients who have an exposure history, including travel or household or sexual exposure), liver abscess, and annular lesions of the colon. All patients with presumed inflammatory bowel disease should be tested serologically, by multiple stool examinations, and by colonoscopy with biopsy because of the risk of overwhelming amebic disease if corticosteroid therapy were to be given in the presence of amebiasis. The differential diagnosis of amebic liver abscess includes pyogenic abscess, echinococcal cyst, and hepatocellular carcinoma.

Treatment

The choice of drug depends on the type of clinical presentation and the site of drug action. Treatment may require the concurrent or sequential use of several drugs. Table 35–1 outlines a preferred and an alternative method of treatment for each clinical type of amebiasis.

The **tissue amebicides** dehydroemetine and emetine act on organisms in the bowel wall and in other tissues but not on amebas in the bowel lumen. Chloroquine is active principally against amebas in the liver. The **luminal amebicides** diloxanide furoate, iodoquinol, and paromomycin act on organisms in the bowel lumen but are ineffective against amebas in the bowel wall or other tissues. Oral tetracycline inhibits the bacterial associates of *E histolytica* and thus has an indirect effect on amebas in the bowel lumen and bowel wall but not in other tissues. Given parenterally, antibiotics have little antiamebic activity at any site. Metronidazole is unique in that it is effective both in the bowel lumen and in the bowel wall and other tissues. However, metronidazole when used alone for bowel infections is not sufficient as a luminal amebicide, for it fails to cure up to 50% of infections. Metronidazole also reaches the central nervous system.

A. Asymptomatic Intestinal Infection: Cure rates with a single course of diloxanide furoate or iodoquinol are 80–85%. Usually in asymptomatic infection, a tissue amebicidal drug is not given to prevent liver infection. Alternatives for treatment or retreatment are paromomycin or metronidazole plus iodoquinol or diloxanide furoate. Within endemic areas, asymptomatic carriers generally are not treated because of the frequency of reinfection. In nonendemic areas, a viewpoint of many authorities is that until *E dispar* and *E histolytica* can be conveniently differentiated, asymptomatic carriers should be treated with a luminal amebicide.

B. Mild to Moderate Intestinal Infection: Metronidazole plus a luminal amebicide is the treatment of choice. Alternative treatments are set forth in Table 35–1. The minimum dose of chloroquine needed to destroy trophozoites carried to the liver or to eradicate an undetected early-stage liver abscess is not established.

C. Severe Intestinal Infection: Fluid and electrolyte therapy and opiates to control bowel motility are necessary adjuncts to specific therapy. Though opiates relieve symptoms, they should be used cautiously because of the potential risk of toxic megacolon.

D. Hepatic Abscess: Hospitalization and bed rest are necessary. Opinions differ on whether a course of chloroquine should follow metronidazole to avoid rare long-term failures. Regarding rare

Table 35–1. Treatment of amebiasis.

	Drug(s) of Choice	Alternative Drug(s)
Asymptomatic intestinal infection	Diloxanide furoate[1,2]	Iodoquinol (diiodohydroxyquin)[3] or paromomycin[4]
Mild to moderate intestinal infection (nondysenteric colitis)	(1) Metronidazole[5] **plus** (2) Diloxanide furoate,[2] iodoquinol,[3] or paromomycin[4]	(1) Diloxanide furoate[2] or iodoquinol[3] **plus** (2) A tetracycline[6] **followed by** (3) Chloroquine[7] **or** (1) Paromomycin[4] **followed by** (2) Chloroquine[7]
Severe intestinal infection (dysentery)	(1) Metronidazole[8] **plus** (2) Diloxanide furoate[2] or iodoquinol[3] **or, if parenteral therapy is needed initially:** (1) Intravenous metronidazole[9] until oral therapy can be started; (2) Then give oral metronidazole[8] plus diloxanide furoate[2] or iodoquinol[3]	(1) A tetracycline[6] **plus** (2) Diloxanide furoate[2] or iodoquinol[3] **followed by** (3) Chloroquine[10] **or, if parenteral therapy is needed initially:** (1) Dehydroemetine[1,11] or emetine[11] **followed by** (2) A tetracycline[6] plus diloxanide furoate[2] or iodoquinol[3] **followed by** (3) Chloroquine[10]
Hepatic abscess	(1) Metronidazole[8,9] **plus** (2) Diloxanide furoate[2] or iodoquinol[3] **followed by** (3) Chloroquine[10]	(1) Dehydroemetine[1,12] or emetine[12] **followed by** (2) Chloroquine[13] **plus** (3) Diloxanide furoate[2] or iodoquinol[3]
Ameboma or extra-intestinal infection	As for hepatic abscess, but not including chloroquine	As for hepatic abscess, but not including chloroquine

[1]Available in the USA only from the Parasitic Disease Drug Service, Centers for Disease Control and Prevention, Atlanta, GA 30333. Telephone requests may be made by calling the central number: 404-639-3670.

[2]Diloxanide furoate, 500 mg three times daily with meals for 10 days.

[3]Iodoquinol (diiodohydroxyquin), 650 mg three times daily for 21 days.

[4]Paromomycin, 25–30 mg/kg (base) (maximum 3 g) in three divided doses after meals daily for 7 days.

[5]Metronidazole, 750 mg three times daily for 10 days. In countries where it is available (not in the USA), tinidazole is preferred over metronidazole as the nitroimidazole component in treatment; although the two drugs are equally effective, tinidazole is given in a shorter course of treatment and is better tolerated. The tinidazole dosage is 800 mg three times daily for 3 days; in severe intestinal disease and hepatic abscess, continue for 5 days.

[6]Tetracycline, 250 mg four times daily for 10 days; in severe dysentery, give 500 mg four times daily for the first 5 days, then 250 mg four times daily for 5 days. Tetracycline should not be used during pregnancy.

[7]Chloroquine, 500 mg (salt) daily for 7 days.

[8]Metronidazole, 750 mg three times daily for 10 days.

[9]An intravenous metronidazole formulation is available; change to oral medication as soon as possible. See manufacturer's recommendation for dosage.

[10]Chloroquine, 500 mg (salt) daily for 14 days.

[11]Dehydroemetine or emetine, 1 mg/kg subcutaneously (preferred) or intramuscularly daily for the least number of days necessary to control severe symptoms (usually 3–5 days) (maximum daily dose for dehydroemetine is 90 mg; for emetine, 65 mg).

[12]Use dosage recommended in footnote 11 for 8–10 days.

[13]Chloroquine, 500 mg (salt) orally twice daily for 2 days and then 500 mg orally daily for 19 days.

short-term metronidazole failures, if during the course of metronidazole treatment a satisfactory clinical response does not occur in about 3 days, the abscess should be drained for therapeutic purposes and to evaluate for pyogenic abscess. Continued failure to achieve an adequate clinical response of a suspected amebic abscess requires changing to the potentially toxic alternative drug dehydroemetine (or emetine) plus chloroquine. Treatment also requires a luminal amebicide (diloxanide furoate or iodoquinol), whether or not the organism is found in the stool. Antibiotics are added only when there is concomitant bacterial liver abscess, which is rare. However, metronidazole itself is highly effective against anaerobic bacteria, a major cause of bacterial liver abscesses. After successful treatment, imaging defects in the liver disappear slowly (range: 3–130 months); some calcify.

Most patients treated with metronidazole for an amebic liver abscess do not require percutaneous aspiration for diagnostic or therapeutic purposes. The indications for aspiration are (1) a large abscess, threatening rupture; (2) a left lobe abscess, which is associated with a higher rate of severe complications; (3) lack of medical response after about 3 days of metronidazole; and (4) a need to evaluate for pyogenic abscess. The risks of aspiration are bacterial superinfection, bleeding, peritoneal spillage, and inadvertent puncture of an infected hydatid cyst. The aspirate is divided into serial 30- to 50-mL aliquots, but only the last sample is examined, as organisms are found only at the edge of the abscess.

E. Adverse Drug Reactions: Metronidazole often induces transient nausea or vomiting; if alcohol is taken during or shortly after treatment, a disulfiram-like reaction may occur. Metronidazole increases the rate of naturally occurring tumors in mice but not in nonrodent species. However, some authorities consider the drug to be essentially free of cancer risk in humans. Nevertheless, prudence requires that metronidazole be given to pregnant or nursing mothers only if other drugs cannot be used.

Dehydroemetine and emetine cause nausea, vomiting, and pain at the injection site. They are general protoplasmic poisons that have adverse effects on many tissues (particularly the heart) and a narrow range between therapeutic and toxic effects; dehydroemetine may be the safer of the two drugs. The tetracyclines should not be used for pregnant women; use erythromycin stearate or paromomycin instead. Iodoquinol may cause mild, transient diarrhea; neurotoxicity has not been reported at standard doses. Flatulence is common with diloxanide furoate. Paromomycin may cause mild gastrointestinal symptoms, infrequently intense diarrhea, and rarely overgrowth of nonsusceptible organisms.

Follow-Up Care

In follow-up, examine at least three stools at 2- to 3-day intervals, starting 2–4 weeks after the end of treatment. For some patients, sigmoidoscopy and re-examination of stools within 3 months may be indicated.

Postdysenteric colitis is an uncommon sequela of severe amebic colitis. Following adequate treatment, diarrhea continues and the mucosa may be reddened and edematous, but no ulcers or organisms are found. Most such cases are self-limited, with permanent remission in weeks to months. Uncommonly, the diarrhea may be profound and unremitting and in some instances probably represents ulcerative colitis triggered by the amebic infection.

Prevention & Control

Prevention requires safe water supplies, sanitary disposal of human feces, adequate cooking of foods, protection of foods from fly contamination, washing hands after defecation and before preparing or eating foods, and, in endemic areas, avoidance of foods that cannot be cooked or peeled. Water supplies can be boiled (briefly) or treated with iodine (0.5 mL tincture of iodine per liter for 20 minutes, or longer if the water is cold). Filters are also available to purify drinking water. Disinfection dips for fruits and vegetables are not advised, and no drug is safe or effective in prophylaxis.

Prognosis

The mortality rate from untreated amebic dysentery, hepatic abscess, or ameboma may be high. With chemotherapy instituted early in the course of the disease, the prognosis is good.

Gonzalez-Ruiz A et al: Diagnosis of amebic dysentery by detection of *Entamoeba histolytica* fecal antigen by an invasive strain-specific, monoclonal antibody-based enzyme-linked immunosorbent assay. J Clin Microbiol 1994;32:964.

Haque R et al: Rapid diagnosis of *Entamoeba* infection by using *Entamoeba* and *Entamoeba histolytica* stool antigen detection kits. J Clin Microbiol 1995;33:2558.

Islam S, Kundi AK, Akhter J: Retrospective study of treatment of amoebic liver abscess with and without aspiration. Trop Doct 1995;25:40.

Ravdin JI: Amebiasis. Clin Infect Dis 1995;20:1453.

Reed SL: New concepts regarding the pathogenesis of amebiasis. Clin Infect Dis 1995;21:S182.

INFECTIONS WITH PATHOGENIC FREE-LIVING AMEBAS

Primary Amebic Meningoencephalitis

Primary amebic meningoencephalitis is a fulminating, purulent meningoencephalitis that resembles bacterial meningitis and is rapidly fatal. Most infections have been in children and young adults. The usual cause is the free-living ameboflagellate *Nae-*

gleria fowleri. Other agents, the *Acanthamoeba* species (see below) and the leptomyxid ameba, cause a multifocal granulomatous encephalitis in immunosuppressed persons, including those with AIDS. *Balamuthia mandrillaris* has recently been isolated from AIDS patients.

N fowleri is a thermophilic organism found in fresh and polluted warm lake water, domestic water supplies, swimming pools, thermal water, and sewers. Most patients give a history of exposure to fresh water; dust is also a possible source of infection. Nasal and throat swabs have shown a human carrier state, and serologic surveys suggest that inapparent infections occur.

The organism apparently invades the central nervous system through the cribriform plate. The incubation period varies from 2 to 7 days. Early symptoms include headache, fever, and lethargy, often associated with rhinitis and pharyngitis. Vomiting, disorientation, and other signs of meningoencephalitis develop within 1 or 2 days, followed by coma and then death on the fifth or sixth day. At autopsy, some victims have a nonspecific myocarditis.

Lumbar or ventricular cerebrospinal fluid contains several hundred to 25,000 leukocytes/µL (50–100% neutrophils) and erythrocytes (up to several thousand/µL). Protein is usually somewhat elevated, and glucose is normal or moderately reduced. If conventional examinations for bacteria and fungi are negative, the fluid must then be examined for free-living amebas to make the specific diagnosis. A wet mount examined by an ordinary optical microscope with the aperture restricted or condenser down will enhance contrast and refractility; a warm stage is not needed. The fluid should not be centrifuged or refrigerated, as this tends to immobilize the amebas. Their brisk motility distinguishes them from leukocytes of various types, which they closely resemble. Staining, culture, and mouse inoculation should be performed. Serologic testing for antibody and circulating antigen is experimental.

Precise species identification is based on morphology, demonstration of flagellate transformation (*Naegleria* only), and various immunologic methods.

Only four well-documented survivors have been reported. One was treated with intravenous and intrathecal amphotericin B and another with a combination of amphotericin B, miconazole, and rifampin. Experimental studies have shown a marked synergistic effect between amphotericin B and either tetracycline or rifampin.

Acanthamoeba Infections

Free-living amebas of the genus *Acanthamoeba* are found in soil and in fresh, brackish, and thermal water as trophozoites (15–45 µm) or cysts (10–25 µm). Several species have been recognized only recently as human pathogens that cause a number of poorly defined syndromes: (1) a subacute and chronic focal granulomatous necrotizing encephalitis that invariably has led to death in weeks to months, (2) skin lesions that resemble deep fungal infections, (3) granulomatous dissemination to many tissues, and (4) uveitis or chronic keratitis that may lead to blindness. Portals of entry may include the skin, eyes, or respiratory tract. A commensal nasal carrier state is established. Immunocompromised patients, including HIV-infected persons, may have increased susceptibility.

In the encephalitis syndrome, cerebrospinal fluid lymphocytosis has been described. Antemortem diagnosis has been made via biopsy specimens. Specific identification is based on the immunofluorescence reactivities of the amebas in tissue sections. No treatment has been effective, but ketoconazole, miconazole, sulfonamides, clotrimazole, pentamidine, paromomycin, propamidine, neomycin, amphotericin B, or flucytosine can be tried.

Hundreds of cases of *Acanthamoeba* keratitis have been documented, most associated with wearing contact lenses; some cases are due to penetrating corneal trauma or exposure to contaminated water. The advent of the imaging power of new confocal microscopy increases sensitivity and provides rapid and easy definition of cysts and trophozoites. The clinical features suggestive of *Acanthamoeba* keratitis are (1) severe ocular pain, (2) partial or 360-degree paracentral stromal ring infiltrate on ophthalmologic examination, (3) recurrent corneal epithelial breakdown, and (4) a corneal lesion refractory to the usual medications. Typically, the keratitis progresses slowly over months. The diagnosis can be confirmed by vigorously scraping the cornea with a swab or platinum-tipped scapula. The material is microscopically examined after staining with Giemsa's or trichrome stain or by immunofluorescent techniques and is also placed in culture on nonnutrient agar seeded with *Escherichia coli.*

Medical treatment has improved for *Acanthamoeba* keratitis; a large proportion of patients can expect a good visual result and cure with treatment that follows early medical diagnosis. Topical chlorhexidine digluconate 0.02% with propamidine is more effective than polyhexamethylene biguanide plus propamidine. Oral itraconazole can be added for deep keratitis. Use of corticosteroid therapy is controversial. In spite of medical treatment, penetrating keratoplasty is often necessary to excise diseased tissue; corneal grafting can be used for noninflamed eyes.

Prevention requires immersion of contact lenses in disinfectant solutions for at least 6 hours.

Clavel A et al: Primary amebic meningoencephalitis in a patient with AIDS: Unusual protozoological findings. Clin Infect Dis 1996;23:1314.

Illingworth CD et al: *Acanthamoeba* keratitis: Risk factors and outcome. Br J Ophthalmol 1995;79:1078.

Sison JP et al: Disseminated *Acanthamoeba* infection in patients with AIDS: Case reports and review. Clin Infect Dis 1995;20:1207.

Walker CM: *Acanthamoeba:* Ecology, pathogenicity and laboratory detection. Br J Biomed 1996;53:146.

BABESIOSIS
(Piroplasmosis)

Babesia are tick-borne protozoal parasites of wild and domestic animals worldwide. Babesiosis in humans is a rare intraerythrocytic infection caused by two *Babesia* species. Heretofore, the infection has been recognized only in Europe *(Babesia divergens)* (rare) and North America *(Babesia microti);* it has recently been reported from Taiwan and Mexico. In the USA, more than 200 cases of *B microti* infection have been reported from coastal and island areas of northeastern and mid-Atlantic states as well as from Wisconsin, Minnesota, Missouri, Washington, and California. A new *Babesia* species (WA1) has recently been described in humans in Washington, Georgia, and California. Natural hosts for *B microti* are various wild and domestic animals, particularly the white-footed mouse and white-tailed deer. With extension of the deer's habitat, the range of human infection appears to be increasing as well.

Humans are infected as a result of *Ixodes dammini* tick bites, but transmission from blood transfusion has also been reported. Coinfections with Lyme disease may occur. Without passing through an exoerythrocytic stage, *B microti* enters the red blood cell and multiplies, resulting in cell rupture followed by infection of other cells.

Surveys have shown an antibody prevalence of up to 2% in humans, which indicates a high level of subclinical infections. The incubation period is 1–4 weeks, but patients usually do not recall the tick bite. The illness is characterized by irregular fever, chills, headache, diaphoresis, myalgia, and fatigue but is without malaria-like periodicity of symptoms. Most patients have a moderate hemolytic anemia, and some have hemoglobinuria or hepatosplenomegaly. Although parasitemia may continue for months, with or without symptoms, the disease is self-limited and, after several weeks or months, most patients recover without sequelae. Splenectomized, elderly, or immunosuppressed persons are the most likely to have severe manifestations.

Only a few *B divergens* infections have been reported, all in splenectomized patients. These infections progress rapidly with high fever, severe hemolytic anemia, jaundice, hemoglobinuria, and renal failure; death usually follows.

Diagnosis is by identification of the intraerythrocytic parasite (2–3 μm) on Wright- or Giemsa-stained thick or thin blood smears; no gametocytes and no intracellular pigment are seen. A single red cell may contain different stages of the parasite, and parasitemia can exceed 10%. Repeated smears may be necessary; parasitemia is usually evident in 2–4 weeks. The organism must be differentiated from malarial parasites, particularly *Plasmodium falciparum.* Isolation can be attempted by inoculating patient blood into hamsters or gerbils. Serum antibody by indirect immunofluorescent test appears within 2–4 weeks and persists for 6–12 months; cross-reactions occur between *Babesia* species and malaria parasites, but antibody titers are generally highest to the infecting organism. The polymerase chain reaction method, where available, is more sensitive but of equal specificity.

No drug treatment is satisfactory. Since *B microti* infections in patients with an intact spleen are usually self-limiting, most infections can be treated symptomatically. In some patients, particularly those who have undergone splenectomy, limited experience suggests that 7–10 days of quinine (650 mg three times a day) plus clindamycin (2.4 g in three or four divided doses daily parenterally or 600 mg three times a day orally) may be useful; exchange transfusion has also been successful in several ill patients with parasitemia greater than 10%. New reports suggest effectiveness for atovaquone or combined pentamidine and trimethoprim-sulfamethoxazole. Management of *B divergens* infection can be attempted with exchange transfusion and clindamycin-quinine therapy.

Boustani MR, Gelfand JA: Babesiosis. Clin Infect Dis 1966;22:611.

Persing DH et al: Infection with a *Babesia*-like organism in northern California. N Engl J Med 1995;332:298.

Pruthi RK et al: Human babesiosis. Mayo Clin Proc 1995;70:853.

Wittner M et al: Atovaquone in the treatment of *Babesia microti* infections in hamsters. Am J Trop Med Hyg 1996;55:219.

BALANTIDIASIS

Balantidium coli is a large ciliated intestinal protozoan found worldwide, but particularly in the tropics. Infection results from ingestion of cysts passed in stools of humans or swine, the reservoir hosts. In the new host, the cyst wall dissolves and the trophozoite may invade the mucosa and submucosa of the terminal ileum and large bowel, causing abscesses and irregularly rounded ulcerations. Many infections are asymptomatic and probably need not be treated. Chronic recurrent diarrhea, alternating with constipation, is most common, but severe dysentery with bloody mucoid stools, tenesmus, and colic may occur intermittently. The organisms do not spread hematogenously to other organs.

Diagnosis is established by finding trophozoites in liquid stools, cysts in formed stools, or the trophozoite in scrapings or biopsy of ulcers of the large bowel. Specimens must be examined rapidly or placed in preservative.

The treatment of choice is tetracycline hydrochloride, 500 mg four times daily for 10 days. The alternative drug is iodoquinol (diiodohydroxyquin), 650 mg three times daily for 21 days. Occasional success has also been reported with metronidazole (750 mg three times daily for 5 days) or paromomycin (25–30 mg/kg [base] in three divided doses for 5–10 days).

In properly treated mild to moderate symptomatic cases, the prognosis is good, but in spite of treatment, fatalities have occurred in severe infections as a result of intestinal perforation or hemorrhage.

Dodd LG: *Balantidium coli* infestation as a cause of acute appendicitis. J Infect Dis 1991;163:1392.

COCCIDIAL & MICROSPORIDIAL INFECTIONS: CRYPTOSPORIDIOSIS, ISOSPORIASIS, CYCLOSPORIASIS, & SARCOCYSTOSIS

Coccidiosis and microsporidiosis are intestinal infections usually accompanied by diarrhea and abdominal discomfort. The infections, which occur worldwide but particularly in tropical climates, are increasingly recognized because of their frequent occurrence in HIV infections. Currently identified causes of coccidiosis are *Cryptosporidium parvum, Isospora belli, Cyclospora cayetanensis,* and *Sarcocystis bovihominis* and *S suihominis. Encephalitozoon* species are the etiologic agents for microsporidiosis (see below). The diseases are rarely life-threatening except in patients with AIDS, in whom isosporiasis, cryptosporidiosis, and microsporidiosis are opportunistic infections. In diagnosis, three stool specimens should be obtained fresh and in preservative over 5–7 days, and, because special diagnostic methods beyond standard testing methods are required, the laboratory should be notified that coccidia and microsporidia are being sought.

General Considerations

A. Cryptosporidiosis: *Cryptosporidium parvum* is found in humans and many animals species. Human infection ranges from a sporadic mild diarrhea in all ages, acute childhood diarrhea (particularly malnourished children in developing countries), traveler's diarrhea, and severe diarrhea in immunocompromised persons.

Infection occurs as a result of ingestion of oocysts excreted in feces of infected humans or animals. The source of infection is contaminated drinking water, food, recreational water, or environmental surfaces. Direct person-to-person transmission can occur, resulting in clustering in households, in day care centers, and among homosexuals. Of concern is repetition of such waterborne outbreaks as that in Milwaukee in 1993, in which 400,000 persons became ill. Since chlorine disinfection of water is not effective, adequate filtration is required. The incubation period appears to be 5–21 days. Oocysts (4–5 μm) passed in stools are fully sporulated and infectious; therefore, hospitalized patients should be isolated and stool precautions strictly observed. Oocysts can persist in the environment for up to 6 months under moist conditions. The prevalence of asymptomatic human carriers in the USA is estimated to be about 1%.

The full life cycle of *Cryptosporidium* occurs within a single host—asexual and sexual proliferation and parasite amplification. The organisms attach to the microvillous borders of enterocytes of the small bowel and also are found free in mucosal crypts. The host cell membrane deteriorates, leaving the parasitic membrane in direct contact with epithelial cell cytoplasm. The organisms do not, however, invade the tissues. Voluminous secretory or malabsorptive diarrhea results, but the mechanism has not been elucidated.

In AIDS, infection may involve any part of the gastrointestinal tract, including the biliary tract (sclerosing cholangitis has been described); respiratory tract infection, lymphadenopathy, and hepatosplenomegaly may occur, as well as multisystem involvement.

Diagnosis is by detection of oocysts in fresh or fixed stool specimens by a variety of flotation or concentration methods or by finding developmental stages in small bowel mucosal biopsies. Three stools submitted fresh or in preservative should be examined over 5–7 days, and—as for *Isospora*—the laboratory should be notified that *Cryptosporidium* is being sought. Routine fecal staining methods do not detect the organisms; instead, a modified acid-fast staining method must be used—which, however, is relatively low in sensitivity and specificity. Where available, fluorescent microscopy using auramine staining or a monoclonal antibody enhances diagnosis. Several new, commercially available ELISA tests that detect cryptosporidial antigen in feces appear to have high sensitivity and specificity and provide for ease of use. Stools are free of white or red blood cells. Blood leukocytosis and eosinophilia are uncommon. Serodiagnostic tests have been developed, including ELISA and immunofluorescent tests that detect IgG and IgM antibody, but they are not yet useful in diagnosing acute disease. Radiologic changes have been reported in the stomach, intestines, and bile ducts in severe disease. In AIDS patients with unexplained diarrhea, the organism should also be looked for in sputum and bronchoalveolar lavage fluid; specimens obtained from lung tissue have sometimes been positive in patients with negative stool specimens.

B. Isosporiasis: Isosporiasis, caused by *Iso-*

spora belli, is considered host-specific for humans. Infection is by the fecal-oral route following ingestion of oocysts. Sporozoites excyst and invade jejunal and duodenal epithelial cells, in which they undergo both a sexual and an asexual cycle in the same host, resulting in the liberation of unsporulated ellipsoidal oocysts ($20–30 \times 10–20$ μm) into the feces. Opinion differs about whether the oocyst can be transmitted directly from person to person by anal-oral sexual contact or if it must pass into the environment and mature to its infectious stage. Outbreaks have occurred in day care centers and mental institutions. The incubation period is 7–11 days.

Diagnosis by stool examination is often difficult, for the organisms may be scanty even in the presence of significant symptoms. The laboratory should be notified of the need to search for the organisms, so that special concentration techniques and acid-fast staining will be used. Because of their buoyancy, oocysts must be looked for just beneath the coverslip of the preparation. The peroral duodenal string test and duodenal aspiration may also assist in diagnosis; frequently, however, diagnosis can be made only after duodenal biopsy and search of multiple serial sections. Serologic tests are not available.

C. Cyclosporiasis: Cyclosporiasis, caused by *C cayetanensis,* is a recently recognized intestinal coccidian oocyst (8–9 μm) infection responsible for a diarrheal illness that is not clinically distinguishable from cryptosporidiosis or isosporiasis, including chronicity in HIV-infected persons with instances of biliary disease. The infection has been reported in many parts of the world, including in travelers, and as a causative agent for water-borne outbreaks. The incubation period appears to be 1–7 days. Transmission is presumed to be fecal-oral; the life cycle and host range are unknown. Oocysts (the sporulated stage shows two sporocysts, each enclosing two sporozoites) can be identified in stool by examination of wet mounts under phase microscopy, by use of modified acid-fast stains (oocysts are variably acid-fast), or by autofluorescence with ultraviolet epifluorescence microscopy. These procedures are not routine for most clinical laboratories.

D. Sarcocystosis: *Sarcocystis* is a two-host coccidian. Human disease occurs as two syndromes, both rare: (1) an enteric infection in which humans are the definitive host and (2) a muscle infection in which humans are an intermediate host. In the enteric form, sporocysts passed in human feces are not infective for humans but must be ingested by cattle or pigs. Humans become infected by eating poorly cooked beef or pork containing oocysts of *Sarcocystis bovihominis* or *Sarcocystis suihominis,* respectively. (Formerly, the causative agent was known as *Isospora hominis.*) Organisms enter intestinal epithelial cells and are transformed into oocysts that release sporocysts into the feces. Clinically, the intestinal infection is often asymptomatic or causes mild but protracted diarrhea. Diagnosis is by stool examination using a flotation method.

The muscle form of sarcocystosis results when humans ingest sporocysts in feces from an infected carnivore that has eaten prey which harbored sarcocysts. The sporocysts liberate sporozoites that invade the intestinal wall and are disseminated to skeletal muscle. This results in subcutaneous and muscular inflammation lasting several days to 2 weeks and the finding of swellings at these sites, sometimes associated with eosinophilia. Sarcocysts are often asymptomatic, however, such as those found incidentally at autopsy in cardiac muscle.

E. Microsporidiosis: Microsporidia are obligate intracellular protozoans that are pathogens of arthropods, fish, and vertebrates. First recognized about 25 years ago, infections in humans are due mainly to *Encephalitozoon* species and occur for the most part in HIV-infected persons. On ingestion of infectious spores, multiplication within enterocytes results in formation of sporoblasts that metamorphose into spores passed in feces. On release into the environment, the spores can persist for several months. *E bieneusi* primarily infects small intestinal enterocytes and causes chronic diarrhea not unlike that in cryptosporidiosis; a sclerosing cholangitis-like syndrome has also been described. *E cuniculi* has been associated with neurologic disorders, hepatitis, peritonitis, and keratoconjunctivitis. *E hellum* infects the corneal epithelium and also disseminates to the lungs and kidneys. *Septata intestinalis* disseminates widely after an initial intestinal enterocyte infection. Microsporidia are probably the leading cause of diarrhea in AIDS patients; *E hellum* and *E cuniculi* are found in both AIDS and non-AIDS patients. Microsporidia in humans are gram-positive organisms with mature spores ($0.5–2 \times 1–4$ μm). Definitive diagnosis initially was by detecting organisms in biopsies by electron and light microscopy; the organisms can now be recognized in feces, body fluids, and conjunctival scrapings by light microscopy using various staining methods.

Symptoms & Signs of Coccidial & Microsporidial Infections

Generally, the forms of diarrhea caused by the coccidial and microsporidial agents are clinically indistinguishable from each other.

A. In Immunocompetent Persons: Infection varies from no symptoms to a mild diarrhea with flatulence and bloating to severe, frequent watery diarrhea; the onset may be explosive. Mucus may be present in stools, but no microscopic or gross blood. Other findings may include low-grade fever, malaise, anorexia, abdominal cramps, vomiting, and myalgia. These symptoms are generally self-limited and last a few days up to several weeks (sometimes longer for isosporiasis). Weight loss can be marked. Parasitologic clearance may take several months.

B. Immunologically Deficient Patients: The diarrhea can be profuse (up to 15 L daily has been reported), with cholera-like watery movements, accompanied by severe malabsorption, electrolyte imbalance, and marked weight loss; fever is uncommon. Mucus is seen in the stools, but blood and leukocytes are seldom present. The diarrhea may recur or persist, and passage of organisms continues for months to indefinitely.

Treatment of Coccidial & Microsporidial Infections

Supportive treatment for diarrhea includes fluid and electrolyte replacement and, in chronic cases, parenteral nutrition.

In **isosporiasis,** effective treatment has been described using (1) trimethoprim (160 mg) and sulfamethoxazole (800 mg) (TMP-SMZ) four times daily for 10 days and then twice daily for 3 weeks; or (2) sulfadiazine, 4 g, and pyrimethamine, 35–75 mg, in four divided doses daily, plus leucovorin calcium, 10–25 mg daily, for 3–7 weeks. In immunocompromised patients, it may be necessary to continue a maintenance dose indefinitely with TMP-SMZ three times weekly or Fansidar once weekly. Efficacy in primary infection has also been reported for furazolidone (400 mg/d for 10 days), nitrofurantoin, metronidazole, quinacrine, and diclazuril. In the treatment of **cyclosporiasis,** TMP-SMZ twice daily for 7 days should be tried; in HIV infections, higher dosages and long-term maintenance may be needed. In **microsporidiosis,** there is no established treatment. For intestinal infections, albendazole (400 mg twice daily) may be useful and may require extended treatment. Octreotide has sometimes provided symptomatic relief.

No treatment has been successful for **sarcocystosis** or **cryptosporidiosis.** Cryptosporidiosis in immunologically competent persons is a self-limiting disease, though nonspecific supportive measures may be needed. In cryptosporidiosis in immunologically incompetent persons, spiramycin (1 g three times daily for 2 weeks or longer), zidovudine (AZT), azithromycin, paromomycin, octreotide, eflornithine, letrazuril, and hyperimmune bovine colostrum have occasionally been reported to be of value.

Bryan RT: Microsporidiosis as an AIDS-related opportunistic infection. Clin Infect Dis 1995;21:S62.

Fayer R: *Cryptosporidium* and *Cryptosporidiosis*. CRC Press, 1997.

Goodgame RW: Understanding intestinal spore-forming protozoa: Cryptosporidia, microsporidia, isospora, and cyclospora. Ann Intern Med 1996;124:429.

Mannheimer SB, Soave R: Protozoal infections in patients with AIDS: Cryptosporidiosis, isosporiasis, cyclosporiasis, and microsporidiosis. Infect Dis Clin North Am 1994;8:483.

Soave R, Johnson WD: *Cyclospora:* Conquest of an emerging pathogen. Lancet 1995;345:667.

GIARDIASIS

Essentials of Diagnosis

- Most infections are asymptomatic.
- In some cases, acute or chronic diarrhea, mild to severe, with bulky, greasy, frothy, malodorous stools, free of blood and pus.
- Upper abdominal discomfort, cramps, distention, excessive flatus, and lassitude.
- Cysts and occasionally trophozoites in stools.
- Trophozoites in duodenal fluid.

General Considerations

Giardiasis is a protozoal infection of the upper small intestine caused by the flagellate *Giardia lamblia* (also called *G intestinalis* and *G duodenalis*). The parasite occurs worldwide, and in children in developing countries can reach 20% and even higher. In the USA and Europe, the infection is considered the most common intestinal protozoal pathogen. Persons of all ages are affected, but occurrence is particularly high among children.

The organism occurs in feces as a symmetric, heart-shaped flagellated trophozoite measuring $10–25 \times 6–12$ μm and as a cyst measuring $8–13 \times 6–11$ μm. Only the cyst form is infectious by the oral route; trophozoites are destroyed by gastric acidity. Humans are the reservoir for *Giardia,* but dogs, cats, and beavers have been implicated—but not confirmed—as zoonotic sources of infection. Under suitable moist conditions, cysts can survive in the environment for weeks to months.

A large proportion of infections are sporadic, resulting from cysts transmitted as a result of fecal contamination of water or food, by person-to-person contact, or by anal-oral sexual contact. Multiple infections are common in households, children's day care centers (often the nidus for spread of organisms to the community), and mental institutions. Outbreaks occur as a result of contamination of water supplies. Giardiasis is a well-recognized problem in special groups including travelers abroad, campers who drink water from USA streams, male homosexuals, and persons with impaired immune states. Giardiasis has not been an opportunistic infection in AIDS.

After the cysts are ingested, trophozoites emerge in the duodenum and jejunum. They can cause epithelial damage, atrophy of villi, hypertrophic crypts, and extensive cellular infiltration of the lamina propria. It is likely that hypogammaglobulinemia, low secretory IgA levels in the gut, achlorhydria, and malnutrition favor the development of infection. *Giardia* has recently been detected in the stomach; to be determined is whether this represents reflux from the duodenum or localized infection.

Clinical Findings

A. Symptoms and Signs: A large proportion of infected persons remain asymptomatic cyst carriers, and their infection clears spontaneously. The clinical forms of giardiasis are (1) acute diarrhea, (2) chronic diarrhea, and (3) malabsorption syndrome. The incubation period is usually 1–3 weeks but may be longer. The illness may begin gradually or suddenly. The acute phase may last days or weeks, but it is usually self-limited, although cyst excretion may be prolonged. In a few patients, the disorder may become chronic and last for years, but it does not appear to last indefinitely.

In both the acute and chronic forms, diarrhea ranges from mild to severe; most often it is mild. There may be no complaints other than of one bulky, loose bowel movement a day, often after breakfast. With larger numbers of movements, the stools become increasingly watery and may contain mucus but are usually free of blood and pus; they are copious, frothy, malodorous, and greasy. The diarrhea may be daily or recurrent; if recurrent, stools may be normal to mushy during intervening days, or the patient may be constipated. Weight loss and weakness may occur. Less common are anorexia, nausea and vomiting, midepigastric discomfort and cramps (often after meals), belching, flatulence, borborygmi, and abdominal distention. Low-grade fever is infrequent, and headache, urticaria, and myalgia are rare.

A malabsorption syndrome occasionally develops in the acute or chronic stage that may result in marked weight loss and debility. Findings may include fat- and protein-losing enteropathy and vitamin B_{12} and disaccharidase deficiencies. The latter may persist for a long time in persons apparently cured after specific treatment.

B. Laboratory Tests: Diagnosis is by identifying cysts or trophozoites in feces or duodenal fluid. Detection can be difficult, because the number of cysts passed varies considerably from day to day, and at the onset of infection, patients may have symptoms for about a week before organisms can be detected.

If clinically warranted, diagnostic accuracy can be increased by proceeding as follows: (1) routine stool examinations → (2) examination of upper intestinal fluid by the duodenal string test (Entero-Test) or by duodenal aspiration followed by concentration (500 Hz for 5 minutes) → (3) duodenal biopsy examined after permanent staining. Three stool specimens should be examined; they should be collected at intervals of 2 days or longer. Of patients with giardiasis, one specimen will detect 50–75% of cases and three specimens about 90%. Unless the specimens can be submitted within an hour, they should be preserved immediately in a fixative. Purges do not increase the likelihood of finding the organism. Use of barium, antibiotics, antacids, kaolin products, or oily laxatives may temporarily (about 10 days) reduce the number of parasites or interfere with detection. Duodenal biopsy specimens should first be pressed onto a slide to obtain a mucosal imprint for staining and

then be sectioned for histologic examination. Biopsy is rarely done, however; most workers prefer instead an empiric course of treatment after presumptive diagnosis.

Coproantigen test results by ELISA and IFA are sensitive (85–98%) and specific (90–100%). Commercial kits are available but as yet should be reserved for situations where stool specimens are negative for *Giardia* and other pathogens or in circumstances where only the presence of *Giardia* need be determined, as in diarrhea among day care children or campers. An ELISA developed for serum IgG antibody does not distinguish present from past infection; however, an IgM test now under evaluation may do so. Radiologic examination of the small bowel is usually normal in mildly ill persons but may show nonspecific findings of increased transit time, altered motility, thickened mucosal folds, and barium column segmentation in patients with marked symptoms.

Treatment

Symptomatic patients should be treated. Although controversial, treatment of asymptomatic patients should be considered since they can transmit the infection to others and may occasionally become symptomatic themselves. In selected instances of asymptomatic infection, it may be best to wait a few weeks before starting treatment, as some infections will clear spontaneously in the absence of treatment.

Treatment is effective with tinidazole, metronidazole, quinacrine, or furazolidone. However, rare drug resistance (failure has also been induced experimentally) has resulted occasionally in treatment failures that require re-treatment with an alternative drug. Tinidazole, where available, is the drug of choice, based on reports that it is effective as a single dose. In follow-up, wait about 2 weeks before rechecking two or more stools at weekly intervals.

All of these drugs occasionally have unpleasant side effects. The potential carcinogenicity of furazolidone, metronidazole, and tinidazole appears to be negligible based on 2 decades of use. None of the agents cure more than about 90% of cases (80% for furazolidone).

A. Metronidazole: The dose is 250 mg three times daily for 7–10 days. Metronidazole may cause gastrointestinal symptoms, headache, dizziness, a metallic taste, and candidal overgrowth. Patients must be warned that alcohol may cause a disulfiram-like reaction.

B. Furazolidone: The dose is 100 mg (in suspension) four times daily for 7–10 days. Gastrointestinal symptoms, fever, headache, rash, and a disulfiram-like reaction with alcohol occur. Furazolidone can cause mild hemolysis in glucose-6-phosphate dehydrogenase-deficient persons and rarely causes hypersensitivity reactions.

C. Quinacrine (Mepacrine): (Not available in

the USA.) The dose is 100 mg three times daily after meals for 5–7 days. The drug has a bitter taste. Gastrointestinal symptoms, headache, and dizziness are common; harmless yellowing of the skin is infrequent. Toxic psychosis and exfoliative dermatitis, which are rare, may be severe and long-lasting. Quinacrine is contraindicated in psoriasis or in persons with a history of psychosis.

D. Tinidazole: (Not available in the USA.) A dose of 2 g given once has had reported cure rates of 90–100%. Adverse reactions consist of mild gastrointestinal side effects in about 10% of patients; headache and vertigo are less common.

E. Others: Albendazole (400 mg daily for 5 days) has shown cure rates that range from 10% to 95%. Reports with **paromomycin** also have been mixed.

Prevention

There is no effective chemoprophylaxis for giardiasis. Prevention is as for amebiasis (above).

Prognosis

With treatment and successful eradication of the infection, there are no sequelae. Without treatment, severe malabsorption may rarely contribute to death from other causes.

Aldeen WE et al: Evaluation of a commercially available ELISA assay for detection of *Giardia lamblia* in fecal specimens. Diagn Microbiol Infect Dis 1995;21:77.

Hill DR: Giardiasis. Issues in diagnosis and management. Infect Dis Clin North Am 1993;7:503.

Lengerich EJ, Addiss DG, Juranek DD: Severe giardiasis in the United States. Clin Infect Dis 1994;18:760.

Thompson RCA, Reynoldson JA, Lymbery AJ (editors): *Giardia, from Molecules to Disease.* CAB International, 1994.

Walterspiel JN, Pickering LK: *Giardia* and giardiasis. Prog Clin Parasitol 1994;4:1.

LEISHMANIASIS

Leishmaniasis is infection by species of the genus *Leishmania.* The disease is a zoonosis transmitted by bites of sandflies (*Phlebotomus* [Old World leishmaniasis] and *Lutzomyia* [New World leishmaniasis] species) from the wild animal reservoir (eg, rodents, Canidae, sloths, marsupials) and domestic dogs (they can die from *L infantum* infections) to humans; however, kala azar is transmitted directly from humans to humans. Leishmaniae have two distinct forms in their life cycle: (1) In mammalian hosts, the parasite is found in its amastigote form (Leishman-Donovan bodies, 2×5 μm) within mononuclear phagocytes. When sandflies feed on an infected host, the parasitized cells are ingested with a blood meal. (2) In the sandfly vector, the parasite converts to, multiplies,

and is then transmitted during feeding as a flagellated extracellular promastigote (10–15 μm).

Four clinical syndromes occur. The speciation of leishmaniasis is complex (about 20 species are known to infect humans) and unsettled, and some species can cause more than one syndrome, not all of which are noted below.

(1) **Visceral leishmaniasis** (kala azar), characterized by hepatosplenomegaly and anemia, is caused mainly by the *L donovani* group of agents: *L d donovani, L infantum, L chagasi,* and *L archbaldi.*

(2) **Old World cutaneous leishmaniasis**—moist or dry leishmaniasis—is caused mainly by *L tropica, L major,* and *L aethiopica.* **New World cutaneous leishmaniasis** is caused by the *L mexicana* complex.

(3) **Mucocutaneous leishmaniasis** (espundia), characterized by an initial cutaneous ulcer that is followed in months to years by destructive nasopharyngeal lesions, is caused by the *Leishmania (Viannia)* group of agents, principally by *L (V) braziliensis* and rarely by *L (V) panamensis.*

(4) **Diffuse cutaneous leishmaniasis** is a state of deficient cell-mediated immunity, in which the widespread, leprosy-like skin lesions are generally progressive and refractory to treatment. The causative organisms are the *L mexicana* complex in the New World and *L aethiopica* in the Old World.

In tropical and temperate zones, an estimated 12 million persons are infected, and 1–2 million new cases and 5000 deaths occur yearly. Severity of infection ranges from subclinical or minimally pathogenic (self-healing or easily treated) to severely incapacitating, metastasizing, mutilating, and fatal.

Leishmaniae are capable of latent infection and can become opportunistic pathogens in immunoincompetent persons; more than 700 coinfections with HIV-visceral leishmaniasis have been reported from 22 countries, but the problem is worse in southern Europe. Antibodies are readily detected in these cases, but the skin test is negative.

Diagnosis

Definitive diagnosis is by finding the intracellular, nonflagellated amastigote in stained scrapings, aspirates, or biopsies or the flagellated promastigote stage in culture (requires up to 28 days, using specialized media held at 22–28 °C). Hamster or Balb/c mouse inoculation of the nose, footpad, or tail base may also be useful (requires 2–12 weeks). Specimens should be obtained at a raised ulcer margin through an area of intact skin cleansed with 70% alcohol. For scrapings, press the site with the fingers (to obtain tissue fluid, not blood) and incise a 3-mm slit. For needle aspiration, sterile preservative-free saline is inserted with a 23- to 27-gauge needle; the aspirate is then cytospun at 800 g for 5 minutes. Biopsies (4–6 mm) are used for impression smears, histologic examination, and culture. The sensitivities of direct staining and smears are 60–65%. Serologic tests and a skin (Montenegro) test are also available (see under each syndrome below). The polymerase chain reaction is promising for its high sensitivity in diagnosis, particularly in early infections, as well as its ability to discriminate parasite species.

Treatment

Treatment is less than adequate because of drug toxicity, long courses required, and frequent need for hospitalization. The drug of choice is sodium stibogluconate; however, resistance to the agent is increasing in frequency in many countries. Alternative drugs for some forms of infection—but more toxic—are amphotericin B and pentamidine. See specialized sources for additional details on toxicity and mode of treatment with these drugs.

A. Sodium Stibogluconate: Sodium stibogluconate is provided as a solution that contains 100 mg of antimony (Sb) per milliliter; only fresh solutions should be used. Treatment is started with a 200-mg Sb test dose followed by 20 mg Sb/kg/d, but there is no upper limit on the maximum daily dose. Although the drug can be administered as a 5% solution intramuscularly (may be locally painful), intravenous administration is preferred (cough may occur) when the volume is high, as is the case for most adults. Meglumine antimoniate (85 mg Sb/mL) is equal in efficacy and toxicity when used in equivalent Sb doses. The appropriate volume of drug is mixed with 50 mL of 5% dextrose in water and infused over at least a 10-minute interval. The drug is given on consecutive days: 28 days for visceral and mucocutaneous leishmaniasis and 20 days for cutaneous leishmaniasis. In certain regions of the world, because of resistance, longer courses are indicated. Although few side effects occur initially, they are more likely to appear with cumulative doses. Most common are gastrointestinal symptoms, fever, myalgia, arthralgia, phlebitis, and rash; hemolytic anemia and liver, renal, and heart damage and pancreatitis are rare. Patients should be monitored weekly for the first 3 weeks and twice weekly thereafter by serum chemistries, complete blood counts, and electrocardiography. Discontinue therapy if the following occur: aminotransferases three to four times normal levels or significant arrhythmias, corrected QT intervals greater than 0.50 s, or concave ST segments. Relapses should be treated at the same dosage level for at least twice the previous duration. In the USA, the drug is available only from the Parasitic Drug Service, Centers for Disease Control and Prevention, Atlanta, GA 30333 (404-639-3670).

B. Amphotericin B: Amphotericin B is dissolved in 500 mL of 5% dextrose and injected slowly intravenously over 6 hours on alternate days. The initial dose of 0.25 mg/kg/d is gradually increased to 1 mg/kg/d ($0.25 \rightarrow 0.5 \rightarrow 1$) until a total of about 30 mg/kg is given. Under evaluation is the use of lipid formulations of amphotericin B, particles of which enter infected mononuclear phagocytic cells; this preparation achieves higher concentrations in the liver and spleen and is much less toxic.

C. Pentamidine Isethionate: Pentamidine isethionate, 2–4 mg/kg intramuscularly (preferable) or intravenously, is given daily or on alternate days (up to 15 injections). For some forms of visceral leishmaniasis, it may be necessary to treat for a longer period or to repeat treatment.

D. Paromomycin: Paromomycin (aminosidine) has been used topically for cutaneous leishmaniasis with varying success. The drug is showing promise in parenteral treatment (potentially severely toxic) of refractory visceral leishmaniasis in India and cutaneous disease in Central America.

Prevention & Control

Infection occurs when humans encroach on sandfly habitats—warm, humid microclimates, including rodent burrows, rock piles, or tree holes; these are often in sylvatic areas near forests or semiarid ecosystems. Biting is generally at twilight or at night but may occur in shaded areas during the day. Personal protection may fail but is partially accomplished by clothing (pants, long sleeves) that covers exposed skin, deet repellent (see under Malaria), avoidance of endemic areas (especially at night), use of mosquito coils, and use of fine-mesh sandfly netting for sleeping (may be too warm in tropical areas). Although sandflies can traverse the mesh of standard mosquito nets, insecticide-impregnated nets may prevent this. Often useful in control are destruction of animal reservoir hosts, mass treatment of humans in kala azar-prevalent areas, residual insecticide spraying in domestic and peridomestic areas, and keeping dogs and other domesticated animals out of the house, particularly at night.

Albrecht H et al: Visceral leishmaniasis emerging as an important opportunistic infection in HIV-infected persons living in areas nonendemic for *Leishmania donovani*. Arch Pathol Lab Med 1996;120:189.

Azulay RD, Azulay Junior DR: Immune-clinical-pathologic spectrum of leishmaniasis. Int J Dermatol 1995;34:303.

Grevelink SA, Lerner EA: Leishmaniasis. J Am Acad Dermatol 1996;34:257.

Herwaldt BL, Berman JD: Recommendations for treating leishmaniasis with sodium stibogluconate (Pentostam) and review of pertinent clinical studies. Am J Trop Med Hyg 1992;46:296.

Kalter DC: Laboratory tests for the diagnosis and evaluation of leishmaniasis. Dermatol Clin 1994;12:37.

Kar K: Serodiagnosis of leishmaniasis. Crit Rev Microbiol 1995;21:123. (Reviews serology, etiology of syndromes, diagnostic methods, differential diagnosis, diagnostic culture media.)

Magill AJ: Epidemiology of the leishmaniases. Dermatol Clin 1995;13:505.

1. VISCERAL LEISHMANIASIS (Kala Azar)

Visceral leishmaniasis is caused mainly by the *Leishmania donovani* complex: (1) *L d donovani* (eastern India, Bangladesh, Southeast Asia, Sudan, Ethiopia, Kenya, scattered foci in central Africa, Soviet Central Asia, and China), (2) *L d infantum* (Mediterranean littoral, Middle East, Iran, Saudi Arabia, Afghanistan, Pakistan), and (3) *L d chagasi* (South America, Central America, Mexico). In each locale, the disease has its own peculiar clinical and epidemiologic features; India, China, and East Africa have had epidemics. Both *L tropica* in the Middle East, the Mediterranean littoral, Kenya, India, and western Asia and *L mexicana amazonensis* in the Amazon Basin have also been shown to cause visceral leishmaniasis in a few patients, generally in a milder form. Although humans are the major reservoir, animal reservoirs such as the dog, other canids, and rodents are important. The incubation period is usually 4–6 months (range: 10 days to 24 months).

A local nonulcerating nodule at the site of the bite may precede systemic manifestations but usually is inapparent. The onset may be acute (as early as 2 weeks after infection) or insidious. Fever often peaks twice daily, with chills and sweats, weakness, weight loss, cough, and diarrhea. The spleen progressively becomes huge, hard, and nontender. The liver is somewhat enlarged, and generalized lymphadenopathy is common. Hyperpigmentation of skin, especially on the hands, feet, abdomen, and forehead, is marked in light-skinned patients. In blacks, there may be warty eruptions or skin ulcers. Petechiae, bleeding from the nose and gums, jaundice, edema, and ascites may occur. Wasting is progressive; death, often due to intercurrent infection, occurs within months to 1–2 years. In some regions, oral and nasopharyngeal or cutaneous manifestations occur with or without visceral involvement.

Post-kala azar dermal leishmaniasis may appear 1–2 years after apparent cure (up to 10 years in India and China). It may simulate leprosy, as multiple hypopigmented macules or nodules develop on preexisting lesions. Erythematous patches may appear on the face. Leishmaniae are present in the skin. Antimony treatment should be tried but is often ineffective.

In HIV-infected persons—with or without AIDS—visceral leishmaniasis can be an opportunistic infection. Numerous cases have been reported from the Mediterranean area and some from South America. These patients may have a shorter duration of symptoms, no fever or splenomegaly, and a poor response to treatment.

The diagnosis is made by demonstrating the organism in buffy coat preparations of blood; on stained smears of aspirates of sternal marrow or iliac crest, liver, enlarged lymph nodes, or spleen; and by culture. Because of the hazard of splenic aspiration, it should only be performed by experienced persons; contraindications are a soft spleen in the acute phase, a prolonged prothrombin time, and platelet counts under 40,000/μL. The direct agglutination IgM test and ELISAs are positive early in the disease. In most patients, the immunofluorescent IgG antibody test is positive at titers of 1:256 or higher. The leishmanin skin test is always negative during active disease and becomes positive months to years after recovery. Other characteristic findings are progressive leukopenia (seldom over 3000/μL after the first 1–2 months), with lymphocytosis and monocytosis, normochromic anemia, and thrombocytopenia. There is a marked increase in total protein up to or greater than 10 g/dL owing to an elevated IgG fraction; serum albumin is 3 g/dL or less. Liver function tests show hepatocellular damage. Proteinuria may be present.

The differential diagnosis includes leukemia, lymphoma, tuberculosis, brucellosis, malaria, typhoid, schistosomiasis, African trypanosomiasis, infective endocarditis, cirrhosis, and other entities.

Sodium stibogluconate (20 mg/kg/d for 30 days) is the drug of choice. Whereas Mediterranean kala azar responds to 10–15 daily doses, the disease in Kenya, Sudan, and India requires at least 30 days of treatment. With incomplete response or relapse, the treatment should be repeated for up to 60 days. Failure should lead to use of pentamidine or amphotericin B. Other drugs under evaluation individually or in combination with antimony, pentamidine, amphotericin B, or liposomal encapsulated amphotericin B are allopurinol, human gamma interferon, and parenteral paromomycin.

Without treatment, the case-fatality rate can reach 90%. Early diagnosis and treatment reduces the mortality rate to 2–5%. Relapses (up to 10% in India and 30% in Kenya) are most likely to occur within 6 months after completion of treatment.

Dietze R et al: Treatment of kala-azar in Brazil with Amphocil (amphotericin B cholesterol dispersion) for 5 days. Trans R Soc Trop Med Hyg 1995;89:309.

Tanner CE: Immunobiology of visceral leishmaniasis. Clin Immunol Immunopathol 1996;78:105.

Thakur CP et al: Aminosidine plus sodium stibogluconate for the treatment of Indian kala-azar: A randomized dose-finding clinical trial. Trans R Soc Trop Med Hyg 1995;89:219.

Thakur CP et al: Comparison of three treatment regimens with liposomal amphotericin B (AmBisome) for visceral leishmaniasis in India: A randomized dose-finding study. Trans R Soc Trop Med Hyg 1996;90:319.

2. CUTANEOUS LEISHMANIASIS

Cutaneous swellings appear 2 weeks to several months after sandfly bites and can be single or multiple. Depending on the leishmanial species and host immune response, lesions begin as small papules and develop into nonulcerated dry plaques or large encrusted ulcers with well-demarcated raised and indurated margins. Satellite lesions may be present. The lesions are painless unless secondarily infected. Local lymph nodes may be enlarged. Systemic symptoms are rare, but a low-grade fever of short duration may be present at the onset. For most species, healing usually occurs spontaneously in months to 1–3 years, starting with central granulation tissue that spreads peripherally. Pyogenic complications may be followed by lymphangitis or erysipelas. Contraction of scars can cause deformities and disfigurement, especially if lesions are on the face.

Diffuse cutaneous leishmaniasis is caused by the *L mexicana* complex and *L aethiopica*. Nonulcerating lesions (that resemble lepromatous leprosy) occur over the entire body. The condition is associated with anergy, in which the skin test is negative but amastigotes are abundant. In spite of repeated doses of antimony, pentamidine, or amphotericin, cures are rare.

Definitive diagnosis is by identification of the organisms (see above). Where available, species identification should be done by molecular methods. The serologic and leishmanin skin tests become positive in 4–6 weeks but are unreliable; most assays cannot distinguish between leishmaniasis and *Trypanosoma cruzi* infections and may cross-react at low titers in malaria, toxoplasmosis, and amebiasis.

Old World Cutaneous Leishmaniasis

Agents of Old World cutaneous leishmaniasis are as follows:

(1) *L tropica* is the agent responsible for an urban infection of dogs and humans. It is found in the Middle East, northwestern India, East Africa, central Asian area of the former Soviet Union, Afghanistan, Pakistan, Turkey, Armenia, Greece, and southern France and Italy. The incubation period is 2 months or longer, and healing is complete in 1–2 years. The lesions of *L tropica* infection tend to be single and dry, to ulcerate slowly or not at all, and to persist for a year or longer. **Leishmaniasis recidivans** is a relapsing form of *L tropica* infection in which the primary lesion nearly heals, lateral spread follows, and scarring can be extensive; it is associated with hypersensitivity and a strongly positive skin test but scarce amastigotes. Visceral involvement by *L tropica* has been reported rarely and is relatively resistant to antimony treatment.

(2) *L major* infection causes lesions in dry or desert rural areas and is primarily a disease of desert rodents. Human disease occurs in the Middle East, central Asian area of the former Soviet Union, Arabian peninsula, Afghanistan, and Africa (North, East, and sub-Saharan Africa from Senegal to Sudan and Kenya). The lesions are characterized by multiple,

wet, rapidly ulcerating sores with crusting. Spontaneous healing is generally complete in 6–12 months.

(3) *L aethiopica* infection occurs in the Ethiopian and Kenyan highlands. Ulceration is rare; spontaneous healing is slow over several years. An uncommon complication is diffuse cutaneous leishmaniasis.

(4) *L donovani* sometimes causes cutaneous disease with visceral manifestations.

Old World leishmaniasis, especially in the Middle East, is generally self-healing in about 6 months and does not metastasize to the mucosa. Thus, it may be justified to withhold treatment if the lesions are small, in an unobtrusive place, and appear to be healing. Pentavalent antimony (20 days) should be used to treat patients with large or multiple lesions or if the lesions are on cosmetically or functionally important areas (eg, the wrist). Complete healing may not be evident until weeks after the course of treatment has been completed. Pentamidine or amphotericin B is used for failures. Other treatments for less severe disease are physical measures (local cryotherapy or heat therapy, electrocoagulation, surgical removal) and intralesional injection of sodium stibogluconate. Paromomycin ointment may also be effective. Lesions should be kept clean and antibiotics used if secondary infection occurs.

New World Cutaneous Leishmaniasis

Agents of New World cutaneous leishmaniasis are as follows:

(1) The *L mexicana* group: *L m mexicana* (Texas, Mexico, Central America); *L m amazonensis* (Amazonian basin, Venezuela, Panama, Trinidad); other species (Venezuela and Dominican Republic).

(2) The *Leishmania (Viannia)* group: *L (V) braziliensis* (Central and South America); *L (V) panamensis* (Central and northeastern South America; and *L (V) guyanensis* (South America).

L mexicana and *L braziliensis* infections generally result from forest-related activities or from dwellings situated near forests. *L panamensis* foci are found both in rain forest and drier habitats.

Most New World cutaneous lesions are ulcers, but vegetative, verrucous, or nodular lesions may occur also. *L m mexicana* ("chiclero's ulcer") in the Yucatan and Central America produces destructive lesions on the ear cartilage. Up to 80% of *L b braziliensis* cutaneous lesions progress to espundia (see below); some *L braziliensis* complex strains also show a chain of palpable local lymph nodes and some *L m mexicana* and South American strains can cause diffuse cutaneous leishmaniasis.

In New World *L mexicana* infections from Mexico and Central America, solitary nodules or ulcers in inconspicuous sites generally will heal spontaneously, but metronidazole, 750 mg three times daily for 10 days, can be tried. Lesions on the ear, face, or hands should be treated with sodium antimony gluconate but usually require only a 12- to 14-day course. Under evaluation are ketoconazole, itraconazole, liposome-encapsulated compounds, combined sodium stibogluconate and allopurinol, and topically applied paromomycin. Cutaneous lesions acquired in regions of mucocutaneous leishmaniasis may be due to *L braziliensis* or *L panamensis* and should be treated with a full course of sodium stibogluconate.

Hepburn NC, Tidman MJ, Hunter JAA: Aminosidine (paromomycin) versus sodium stibogluconate for the treatment of American cutaneous leishmaniasis. Trans R Soc Trop Med Hyg 1994;88:700.

Martinez S, Gonzalez M, Vernaza ME: Treatment of cutaneous leishmaniasis with allopurinol and stibogluconate. Clin Infect Dis 1997;24:165.

McHugh CP, Melby PC, LaFon SG: Leishmaniasis in Texas: Epidemiology and clinical aspects of human cases. Am J Trop Med Hyg 1996;55:547.

Momeni AZ, Aminjavaheri M: Treatment of recurrent cutaneous leishmaniasis. Int J Dermatol 1995;34:129.

Momeni AZ et al: Treatment of cutaneous leishmaniasis with itraconazole. Arch Dermatol 1996;132:784.

3. MUCOCUTANEOUS LEISHMANIASIS (Espundia)

Mucocutaneous leishmaniasis occurs in lowland forest areas and is caused by the *Leishmania (Viannia)* group of organisms, usually by *L (V) braziliensis* (Central and South America) and rarely by *L (V) panamensis* (Central and northeastern South America). The initial lesion, single or multiple, is on exposed skin; at first it is papular (can be pruriginous or painful), then nodular, and later may ulcerate or become wart-like or papillomatous. Local healing follows, with scarring within several months to a year. Subsequent naso-oral involvement occurs in a small proportion of patients either by direct extension or, more often, metastatically to the mucosa. It may appear concurrently with the initial lesion, shortly after healing, or after many years. The mucosa of the anterior part of the nasal septum is generally the first area to be involved. Extensive destruction of the soft tissues and cartilage of the nose, oral cavity, and lips may follow and may extend to the larynx and pharynx. Gross and hideous destruction and marked suffering can result. Secondary bacterial infection is common. Regional lymphangitis, lymphadenitis, fever, weight loss, keratitis, and anemia may be present.

Diagnosis is by finding amastigotes in scrapings, biopsy impressions or histologic sections, or aspirated tissue fluid. The organism grows with difficulty in culture or after inoculation of hamsters; if positive, speciation should be attempted. The leishmanin skin test is useful if it produces a fully developed papule in 2–3 days that disappears after a week. The direct agglutination test for IgM antibodies becomes positive in 4–6 weeks. IgG antibodies are detectable in most cases and disappear with cure. The main considerations in the differential diagnosis are paracoccidioidomycosis, polymorphic reticulosis, Wegener's granulomatosis, lymphoma, and nasopharyngeal carcinoma, which are distinguishable by biopsy.

Treatment of this condition is difficult; failure rates are high in severe disease even when a full course of sodium stibogluconate treatment is used. Some workers recommend extended treatment for 6–8 weeks. Under evaluation are combined antimony and gamma interferon treatment. Corticosteroids may be needed to control local inflammation due to release of antigens. If repeated and extended antimony treatment fails, amphotericin B is used. Antibiotics are usually needed to treat associated bacterial or fungal infection.

Franke ED et al: Efficacy of 28-day and 40-day regimens of sodium stibogluconate (Pentostam) in the treatment of mucosal leishmaniasis. Am J Trop Med Hyg 1994; 51:77.

Samandy JA, Janniger CK, Schwartz RA: Cutaneous and mucocutaneous leishmaniasis. Cutis 1996;57:13.

MALARIA

Essentials of Diagnosis

- History of exposure in a malaria-endemic area.
- Periodic attacks of sequential chills, fever, and sweating.
- Headache, myalgia, splenomegaly; anemia, leukopenia.
- Characteristic parasites in erythrocytes, identified in thick or thin blood films.
- Complications of falciparum malaria: Cerebral findings (mental disturbances, neurologic signs, convulsions), hemolytic anemia, hyperpyrexia, dysenteric or cholera-like stools, dark urine, anuria.

General Considerations

Four species of the genus *Plasmodium* are responsible for human malaria: *P vivax, P malariae, P ovale,* and *P falciparum.* Although the disease has been eradicated from most temperate zone countries, it continues to be endemic in many parts of the tropics and subtropics, and imported cases occur in the USA and other countries free of transmission. Malaria is present in parts of Mexico, Haiti, Dominican Republic, Central and South America, Africa, the Middle East, the Indian subcontinent, Southeast Asia, China, and Oceania. *P vivax* and *P falciparum* are responsible for most infections and are found throughout the malarious regions. *P malariae* is also widely distributed but is less common. *P ovale,* although generally rare, seems to replace *P vivax* in West Africa. *P vivax* infection is uncommon among blacks because their red blood cells do not have the Duffy factor surface antigen. Annually worldwide, malaria causes clinical illness in 300–500 million people and results in 1.5–2.7 million deaths; its greatest impact is on young children, particularly in sub-Saharan Africa. The USA experiences each year an average of 1000 imported infections with different species; a few cases of locally acquired, mosquito-transmitted infection from an imported case; and an average of four deaths from falciparum malaria. Most of the imported infections are acquired in tropical Africa.

Malaria is transmitted from human to human by the bite of infected female *Anopheles* mosquitoes. **Induced malaria**—congenital transmission and transmission by blood transfusion—also occurs. Other than the mosquito, there are no animal reservoirs for human malaria.

The mosquito becomes infected by ingesting blood containing the sexual forms of the parasite (micro- and macrogametocytes). After a developmental phase in the mosquito, sporozoites in the salivary glands are inoculated into humans when the mosquito next feeds. The first stage of development in humans, the exoerythrocytic stage, takes place in the liver. In all four infections, the sporozoites invade hepatocytes to mature as tissue schizonts. However, in *P vivax* and *P ovale* infections only—but not in induced infections with these parasites—some sporozoites enter hepatocytes to become dormant hypnozoites; activation of the hypnozoites 6–8 months later results in a primary infection or in relapse. Subsequently, when liver schizonts escape from the liver into the bloodstream, they invade red blood cells, multiply, and 48 hours later (or 72 with *P malariae*) cause the red cells to rupture, releasing a new crop of parasites (merozoites). Within the bloodstream, this cycle of invasion, multiplication, and red cell rupture may be repeated many times.

In *P falciparum* and *P malariae* malaria, the liver infection ceases spontaneously in less than 4 weeks; thereafter, multiplication is confined to the red cells. Thus, 4 weeks after departure from an endemic area, treatment that eliminates these species from the red cells will cure the infection. Cure of *P vivax* and *P ovale* malaria, however, requires treatment to eradicate infection from both red cells and liver hypnozoites.

The incubation period after exposure or after stopping chemoprophylaxis is, for *P falciparum,* approximately 12 days (range: 9–60 days); for *P vivax* and *P ovale,* 14 days (range: 8–27 days [initial attacks for some temperate strains may not occur for up to 8 months]); and for *P malariae,* 30 days (range: 16–60 days). If untreated, *P falciparum* infections usually terminate spontaneously in 6–8 months but can persist for up to 1.5 years; *P vivax* and *P ovale* infections can persist without treatment for as long as 5 years; and *P malariae* infections have lasted for as long as 50 years.

Clinical Findings

A. Symptoms and Signs: Typical malarial attacks show sequentially, over 4–6 hours, shaking chills (the cold stage); fever (the hot stage) to 41 °C or higher; and marked diaphoresis (the sweating stage). Associated symptoms may include fatigue, headache, dizziness, gastrointestinal symptoms (anorexia, nausea, slight diarrhea, vomiting, abdominal cramps), myalgia, arthralgia, backache, and dry cough. These symptoms appear to be due in large part to release of tissue necrosis factor and other cytokines during schizogony.

Either from the onset or with progression of the disease, the attacks may show an every-other-day (tertian) periodicity in vivax, ovale, or falciparum malaria or an every-third-day (quartan) periodicity in malariae malaria. Splenomegaly usually appears when acute symptoms have continued for 4 or more days; the liver is frequently mildly enlarged. The patient may be tired between attacks but otherwise feels well. After this primary episode, recurrences are common, each separated by a latent period.

Because of its frequent and severe complications, *P falciparum* is the more serious infection and causes the most deaths, sometimes within 24 hours. In severe falciparum infections, red blood cell parasitemia is higher than 3–5%. Severe disease results in part from intense sequestration and cytoadherence of parasitized red cells in capillaries and postcapillary venules. Complications include (1) cerebral malaria with edema (headache, mental disturbances, neurologic signs, retinal hemorrhages, convulsions, delirium, coma); (2) hyperpyrexia; (3) hemolytic anemia; (4) noncardiogenic pulmonary edema; (5) acute tubular necrosis and renal failure, rarely with production of dark urine (blackwater fever); (6) acute hepatopathy, with centrilobular necrosis and marked jaundice but no liver failure; (7) hypoglycemia; (8) an adrenal insufficiency-like syndrome; (9) cardiac dysrhythmias; (10) gastrointestinal syndromes (including secretory diarrhea and dysentery); (11) lactic acidosis and hypoglycemia; (12) coexisting pneumonia; and (13) water and electrolyte imbalance. The prognosis is bad when there are multiple complications or if more than 20% of infected red cells contain mature parasites or more than 5% of neutrophils contain pigment. Gram-negative bacteremia may contribute to death.

Immunologic disorders resulting from chronic infection are tropical splenomegaly and nephrotic syndrome (the latter due to *P malariae* only). Malaria infections do not appear to act as an opportunistic infection in AIDS patients.

B. Laboratory Findings: The thick and thin blood film, dehemoglobinized and Giemsa-stained, is the mainstay of diagnosis. The much less sensitive thin film is used primarily for species differentiation after the presence of an infection is detected on a thick film. Because the level of parasitemia varies from hour to hour—especially for *P falciparum* infections, in which parasites may be difficult to find—blood should be examined at 8-hour intervals for 3 days, during and between febrile spikes. The newly described quantitative buffy coat method to detect parasitemia is slightly more sensitive than thick smears, but it is expensive and requires fluorescent microscopy.

The number of red cells infected seldom exceeds 2% of the total cells. During paroxysms, there may be transient leukocytosis; leukopenia develops subsequently, with a relative increase in large mononuclear cells. In severe falciparum malaria, parasitemia may reach 30% or higher; mature asexual forms disappear (sequestered in the microcirculation); hepatic function tests often become abnormal; and hemolytic jaundice, thrombocytopenia, and marked anemia with reticulocytosis may develop.

Serologic tests are not commonly used in the diagnosis of acute attacks, but an ELISA for *P falciparum* infection is now commercially available. Antibody persists for 10 or more years; testing does not distinguish between present and past infection. A rapid and simply accomplished dipstick antigen capture assay appears promising for field diagnosis, with a specificity and sensitivity of about 90% for *P falciparum*.

Differential Diagnosis

Uncomplicated malaria must be distinguished from a variety of other causes of fever, splenomegaly, anemia, or hepatomegaly. Often considered are influenza, urinary tract infections, typhoid fever, infectious hepatitis, dengue, kala azar, amebic liver abscess, leptospirosis, and relapsing fever. Malaria complications can mimic many diseases.

Prevention

Prevention is based on evaluating the risk of exposure to infection, preventing mosquito bites, and chemoprophylaxis. Advice should also be given regarding medical care if malaria-like symptoms occur while traveling. All persons who will be exposed should receive chemoprophylaxis; however, because of rare but potentially serious side effects, chemoprophylaxis should not be prescribed in the absence of malaria risk. Travelers should be advised that in spite of all precautions, no prophylactic regimen gives complete protection. Fever or other symptoms can develop in malaria as early as 8 days (range: 8–60 days) after exposure or stopping prophylaxis; for *P vivax* infections in temperate areas, the delay may be up to 8 months.

A. Consultative Resources Regarding Risks, Chemoprophylaxis, and Treatment: Consultation with a center working on malaria may be necessary to obtain up-to-date information on malaria risks and prophylaxis (by country) and treatment. A source on information and advice in the

USA is the Malarial Branch, Centers for Disease Control, Atlanta, GA. For recorded information on prophylaxis, phone: 404-332-4559; fax: 404-332-4565; Internet: http://www.cdc.gov (choose the Travelers' Health category). For management of acute attacks, phone 770-488-7760. See also the references below.

B. Risk of Exposure: The risk of exposure to mosquitoes may be difficult to estimate since it varies by climate, rainy season, altitude, degree of mosquito control in urban versus rural areas, and according to whether exposure will occur during the time malaria mosquitoes are biting (chiefly between dusk and dawn). Travel to urban areas of Central and South America and Southeast Asia entails minimal risk.

C. Preventing Mosquito Bites: When out of doors between dusk and dawn, protective measures should be used: Clothing should cover most of the body, and deet (N,N-diethyl-3-methylbenzamide) mosquito repellent should be applied to exposed areas every 3–4 hours. To minimize the slight risk of toxic encephalopathy from deet, it should be applied sparingly and only to exposed skin and outer clothing; avoid high concentrations (over 35%) of the repellent; avoid inhalation and contamination of eyes, mouth, wounds, or irritated skin; and wash skin after coming indoors. The Ultrathon formulation provides a reduced concentration of deet (33%) with extended protection (12 hours). Living quarters should be screened; if screening is not available, mosquito bed nets should be used at night, preferably ones impregnated every 6 months with permethrin (0.2 g/m^2) (Permonone). To kill mosquitoes in living quarters, use an antimosquito pyrethrum-containing spray or a powdered insecticide dispenser of pyrethroid tablets or burn pyrethroid mosquito coils. Garments can also be impregnated (sprayed or soaked) with permethrin, which repels for several weeks.

D. Advice Regarding Treatment if Malaria-Like Febrile Symptoms Occur While Traveling: Medical care should be sought immediately. The traveler should insist that blood smears be done and, if negative, repeated at intervals. If malaria is suspected but blood smears cannot be done, malaria treatment should be started.

Emergency self-treatment (standby treatment): Individuals who may be exposed to malaria and for whom medical attention will not be readily available are advised to carry medication for self-treatment if they develop fever or flu-like symptoms. However, *it is imperative that medical follow-up be sought promptly.* Patients should be given written instructions. The choice among available drugs depends on the anticipated type of exposure to drug-resistant *P falciparum* (see above for areas of resistance and Table 35–3 for dosages): (1) chloroquine (for 2 days) for persons taking no prophylaxis in chloroquine-sensitive areas; (2) Fansidar (three

Table 35–2. Prevention of malaria in travelers.[1]

**TO PREVENT ATTACKS OF ALL FORMS OF MALARIA
AND TO ERADICATE *P FALCIPARUM* AND *P MALARIAE* INFECTIONS**[2,3,4,5]

REGIONS WITH CHLOROQUINE-SENSITIVE *P FALCIPARUM* MALARIA: Central America north and west of the Panama Canal, the Caribbean, North Africa, and parts of the Middle East, including Egypt

Chloroquine
Dose: Chloroquine phosphate, 500 mg salt (300 mg base). Give a single dose of chloroquine weekly starting 1 week before entering the endemic area, while there, and for 4 weeks after leaving.

REGIONS WITH CHLOROQUINE-RESISTANT *P FALCIPARUM* MALARIA: All other regions of the world; the frequency and intensity of resistance vary by region.

Mefloquine (preferred method)[6]
Dose: one 250-mg tablet salt (228 mg base). Give a single dose of mefloquine weekly starting 1 week before entering the endemic area, while there, and for 4 weeks after leaving.

Doxycycline (alternative method)[7]
Dose: 100 mg daily. Give the daily dose for 2 days before entering the endemic area, while there, and for 4 weeks after leaving.

Chloroquine combined with proguanil[8] **(second alternative method)**
Dose:
Chloroquine, weekly at the above schedule.
Proguanil, 200 mg daily while in the endemic area and for 4 weeks after leaving.

TO ERADICATE *P VIVAX* AND *P OVALE* INFECTIONS[2]

Primaquine[9]
Primaquine is indicated only for persons who have had a high probability of exposure to *P vivax* or *P ovale* (see text). Start primaquine only after returning home, during the last 2 weeks of chemoprophylaxis. Dose: 26.3 mg salt (15 mg base) daily for 14 days.

---

[1]See text for additional information on drug cautions, contraindications, and side effects. For additional information on prophylaxis for specific countries, see the references or call the Centers for Disease Control and Prevention (CDC), Atlanta, GA (404-332-4559; fax 404-332-4565). The information is also available on the Internet at http://www.cdc.gov (choose the Travel Health category).

[2]The blood schizonticides (chloroquine, mefloquine, and doxycycline), when taken for 4 weeks after leaving the endemic area, are curative for sensitive *P falciparum* and *P malariae* infections; primaquine, however, is needed to eradicate the persistent liver stages of *P vivax* and *P ovale*. Give the drug after a meal.

[3]Test doses of chloroquine and doxycycline (single doses) and of mefloquine (one dose weekly for 3 weeks) allows for changing to an alternative drug in the event of significant side effects.

[4]See text for standby drugs for emergency self-treatment of presumptive malaria; such drugs should be used only when a physician is not immediately available. It is imperative, however, that medical follow-up be sought promptly.

[5]Chloroquine and proguanil can be used in pregnancy; in chloroquine-resistant areas, mefloquine can also be used, but preferably not in the first trimester.

[6]Because of the high frequency of resistance, mefloquine should not be used in Thailand or adjacent countries; it is now the preferred drug for sub-Saharan Africa.

[7]Doxycycline is used in Thailand and adjacent countries and in other regions by persons who cannot tolerate mefloquine. It is contraindicated in pregnant women. Take with evening meals. See text for side effects.

[8]The combination can be used in countries with a low frequency of chloroquine-resistant falciparum malaria such as southern Asia (not Bangladesh) and parts of the Middle East. Proguanil is not available in the USA but can be purchased in other countries.

[9]Before taking primaquine, patients should be screened to detect glucose-6-phosphate dehydrogenase deficiency. Primaquine is contraindicated in pregnancy. An alternative regimen in regions where chloroquine is effective in prophylaxis is chloroquine phosphate, 500 mg (salt), plus primaquine phosphate, 78.9 mg (salt), weekly for 8 weeks.

---

tablets once only); and (3) quinine for 3–7 days plus tetracycline for 7 days (7 days of quinine is toxic for some patients). Mefloquine and halofantrine are not recommended because of their potential for severe toxicity.

Drugs Used in Chemoprophylaxis & Treatment
(Tables 35–2 and 35–3)

A. Drug Classification: By chemical groups, some of the major antimalarial drugs are as follows: **4-aminoquinolines**—chloroquine, hydroxychloro- quine, amodiaquine;* **diaminopyrimidines**— pyrimethamine, trimethoprim; **biguanides**— proguanil* (chlorguanide,* chlorproguanil*); **8-aminoquinolines**—primaquine; **cinchona alkaloids**—quinine, quinidine; **sulfonamides**—sulfadoxine, sulfadiazine, sulfamethoxazole; **sulfones**—dapsone; **4-quinoline-carbinolamines**—mefloquine; and **antibiotics**—tetracycline, doxycycline, clin-

---

*Not available in the USA but available in some countries.

Table 35–3. Treatment of malaria in nonimmune adult populations.

Treatment[1] of Infection With All Species (Except Chloroquine-Resistant *P falciparum*)	Treatment[1] of Infection With Chloroquine-Resistant *P falciparum* Strains
Oral treatment of *P falciparum*[2] or *P malariae* infection Chloroquine phosphate, 1 g (salt)[3,4] as initial dose, then 0.5 g at 6, 24, and 48 hours.	**Oral treatment** Quinine sulfate, 10 mg/kg (salt) 3 times daily for 3–7 days,[8] plus one of the following: (1) doxycycline,[9] 100 mg twice daily for 7 days, or clindamycin,[9] 900 mg 3 times daily for 3 days; (2) pyrimethamine, 25 mg twice daily for 3 days, and sulfadiazine, 500 mg 4 times daily for 5 days; (3) tetracycline,[9] 250–500 mg 4 times daily for 7 days; (4) once only, pyrimethamine, 75 mg, and sulfadoxine, 1500 mg (= 3 tablets of Fansidar[10]).
Oral treatment of *P vivax* or *P ovale* infection Chloroquine[3,4] as above followed by 0.5 g on days 10 and 17 plus primaquine phosphate, 26.3 mg (salt)[5] daily for 14 days starting about day 4.	
Parenteral treatment of severe attacks Quinine dihydrochloride[6] or quinidine gluconate.[7] Start oral chloroquine therapy as soon as possible; follow with primaquine if the infection is due to *P vivax* or *P ovale*.	*or* Mefloquine,[11] 1250 mg (salt) once or 750 mg followed after 6–8 hours by 500 mg.
or	*or*
Chloroquine hydrochloride IM;[13] repeat every 6 hours. Start oral therapy as soon as possible; follow with primaquine if infection is due to *P vivax* or *P ovale*.	Halofantrine[12]
	or
or	Artemisinin derivatives[14]
Artemisinin derivatives[14]	**Parenteral treatment of severe attacks** Quinine dihydrochloride[6] or quinidine gluconate[7] plus intravenous doxycycline or clindamycin. Start oral therapy with quinine sulfate plus the second drug above as soon as possible to complete 7 days of treatment.

[1]See text for cautions, contraindications, and side effects of each drug. For advice on management, call the Centers for Disease Control and Prevention (CDC), Atlanta, GA (770-488-7760).

[2]In falciparum malaria, if the patient has not shown a clinical response to chloroquine (48–72 hours for mild infections, 24 hours for severe ones), parasitic resistance to chloroquine should be considered. Chloroquine should be stopped and oral quinine plus doxycycline, or mefloquine, or halofantrine started.

[3]500 mg chloroquine phosphate = 300 mg base.

[4]Chloroquine alone is curative for infection with sensitive strains of *P falciparum* and for *P malariae,* but primaquine is needed to eradicate the persistent liver stages of *P vivax* and *P ovale.* Start primaquine after the patient has recovered from the acute illness; continue chloroquine weekly during primaquine therapy. Patients should be screened for glucose-6-phosphate dehydrogenase deficiency before use of primaquine. An alternative mode for primaquine therapy is combined primaquine, 78.9 mg (salt), and chloroquine, 0.5 g (salt), weekly for 8 weeks.

[5]26.3 mg of primaquine phosphate = 15 mg primaquine base.

[6]Quinine dihydrochloride. Give 10 mg/kg (salt) in 500 mL of 5% glucose solution IV slowly over 4 hours; repeat every 8 hours until oral therapy is possible (maximum, 1800 mg/d). Blood pressure and ECG should be monitored constantly to detect arrhythmias or hypotension. As severe hypoglycemia may occur, blood glucose levels should be monitored. A higher initial loading dose of quinine is given (20 mg/kg) to patients who acquired infections in Southeast Asia if it is known with certainty that they have not already taken the medication. Extreme caution is required in treating patients with quinine who previously have been taking mefloquine in prophylaxis. In the USA, quinine dihydrochloride is no longer available.

[7]When parenteral quinine is unavailable (as in the USA), quinidine gluconate can be used, administered as a continuous infusion. A loading dose of 10 mg/kg (salt) (maximum, 600 mg) is diluted in 300 mL of normal saline and administered over 1–2 hours, followed by 0.02 mg/kg/min (salt) (maximum, 10 mg/kg every 8 hours) by continuous infusion until oral quinine therapy is possible. If more than 48 hours of parenteral treatment is required, some authorities reduce the quinidine dose by one-third to one-half. Fluid status, blood glucose levels, blood pressure, and ECG should be closely monitored; widening of the QRS interval or lengthening of the QT interval requires discontinuation.

[8]Although quinine sulfate is usually given for 3 days, it should be continued for 7 days in patients who acquired infections in Southeast Asia and South America, where diminished responsiveness to quinine has been noted.

[9]Contraindicated in pregnant women.

[10]Fansidar should not be used for infections acquired in Southeast Asia, the Indian subcontinent, or parts of the Amazon Basin.

[11]Serious side effects are rare. See text for cautions and contraindications.

[12]The dosage is 500 mg (salt) every 6 hours for three doses and repeat in 1 week. See text for cautions and contraindications. Although halofantrine is approved for use in the USA, it has not been marketed.

[13]To avoid potential severe toxicity, give parenteral chloroquine by low-dose intramuscular injection (maximum, 3.5 mg/kg [salt] every 6 hours).

[14]Artemisinin and its derivatives are not available in the USA but are available in some countries. For dosages, see White NJ: The treatment of malaria. N Engl J Med 1996;335:800.

damycin; and **others**—halofantrine,* and artemisinin (qinghaosu)* and its derivatives. Pyrimethamine and proguanil are known as **antifolates,** since they inhibit dihydrofolate reductase of plasmodia. Drug combinations used to treat *P falciparum* malaria resistant to chloroquine include Fansidar (pyrimethamine plus sulfadoxine) and Maloprim (pyrimethamine plus dapsone).

The effectiveness of antimalarial drugs differs with different species of the parasite and with different stages of the life cycle. Drugs that act in the liver to eliminate developing exoerythrocytic schizonts or latent hypnozoites are called **tissue schizonticides** (primaquine). Those that act on blood schizonts are **blood schizonticides** or **suppressive agents** (eg, chloroquine, amodiaquine, proguanil, pyrimethamine, mefloquine, quinine, quinidine, halofantrine, and qinghaosu and its derivatives). **Gametocides** are drugs that prevent infection of mosquitoes by destroying gametocytes in the blood (eg, primaquine for *P falciparum* and chloroquine for *P vivax*, *P malariae*, and *P ovale*). **Sporonticidal** agents are drugs that render gametocytes noninfective in the mosquito (eg, pyrimethamine, proguanil).

None of the drugs prevent infection (ie, are true **causal prophylactic drugs**). However, proguanil and chlorproguanil—and to some extent the antibiotics and primaquine—prevent maturation of the early *P falciparum* and *P vivax* hepatic schizonts. Blood schizonticides destroy circulating plasmodia and thus prevent malarial attacks (**suppressive prophylaxis**) and, when given weekly for 4 weeks after departure from the endemic area, result in cure of *P falciparum* and *P malariae* infections. Only primaquine destroys the hypnozoites of *P vivax* and *P ovale* and, when given with a blood schizonticide, prevents relapse from infection with these parasites and thus effects **radical cure (terminal prophylaxis).**

B. Parasite Resistance to Drugs:

1. *P falciparum* resistance–

a. Chloroquine-resistant strains of *P falciparum* have been confirmed or are probably present in all malarious areas except in the Caribbean, Central America north and west of the Panama Canal, North Africa, and parts of the Middle East, including Egypt. In regions of resistance, some strains of *P falciparum* are only partially resistant to the drug, as manifested by temporary subsidence of symptoms and transient decrease or disappearance in asexual parasitemia, followed by return of both after several days to weeks.

b. Resistance to pyrimethamine-sulfadoxine (Fansidar) is present at high levels in Southeast Asia, the Indian subcontinent, and parts of the Amazon basin. The drug is still useful (controversial) in sub-Saharan Africa because of still infrequent but increasingly occurring resistance. Fansidar shows no cross-resistance with other antimalarial drugs.

c. Resistance to pyrimethamine or proguanil when used alone is common in most endemic areas, but the degree and distribution are not accurately known.

d. Mefloquine–Sporadic or low levels of mefloquine resistance have been reported from Southeast and southern Asia and parts of Africa, South America, the Middle East, and Oceania. Along the Thai-Burmese and Thai-Cambodian borders, however, the frequency reaches 30–60%.

e. Quinine and quinidine–Variable degrees of decreased responsiveness have been reported, though rarely, in Southeast Asia and Oceania and apparently in sub-Saharan Africa and Brazil.

f. Halofantrine–A high degree of resistance has been reported in eastern Thailand. Strains resistant to halofantrine are commonly resistant to mefloquine also.

2. *P vivax* resistance–

a. Antifolates–Resistance of *P vivax* blood schizonts to pyrimethamine and proguanil, including the pyrimethamine-containing drugs Fansidar and Maloprim, has been reported in many areas of the world, particularly Southeast Asia.

b. Primaquine–Partial resistance of some strains of *P vivax* hepatic schizonts to primaquine in areas of Southeast Asia, Oceania, and the Amazon basin may necessitate a larger dose for cure (15 mg of base per day for 21 days).

c. Chloroquine–Recent reports from Indonesia (Irian Jaya, Sumatra) and Papua New Guinea indicate high levels of *P vivax* schizonts resistant to chloroquine. Decreased susceptibility may also be appearing in the Solomon Islands, Myanmar, India, Brazil, and Colombia. Mefloquine appears to be effective in prophylaxis and treatment of *P vivax* in these areas.

3. *P ovale* and *P malariae*–These forms have not shown resistance.

C. Selected Drugs: Indications, Limitations, and Adverse Side Effects:

1. Chloroquine phosphate–Chloroquine is the drug of choice in chemoprophylaxis and in treatment for all forms of malaria except for infections due to resistant strains of *P falciparum* (see also ¶2c, above). However, in *P vivax* and *P ovale* infections, primaquine is needed to eradicate the persistent liver phases and thus prevent relapse.

Oral chloroquine is usually well tolerated when used for malaria prophylaxis or treatment and is safe to use in pregnancy. Gastrointestinal symptoms, mild headache, pruritus (especially in blacks), dizziness, blurred vision, anorexia, malaise, and urticaria may occur; taking the drug after meals or in divided twice-weekly doses may reduce these side effects.

In parenteral treatment of severely ill patients, qui-

---

*Not available in the USA but available in some countries.

nine or quinidine is the preferred drug. If neither is available, chloroquine can be given intramuscularly or intravenously. However, chloroquine can be severely toxic unless it is given in small amounts (3.5 mg [salt]/kg) intramuscularly every 6 hours or by slow intravenous infusion.

Rare reactions from oral chloroquine include impaired hearing, psychosis, convulsions, blood dyscrasias, skin reactions, and hypotension. When given in large doses for prolonged periods as an anti-inflammatory agent in autoimmune diseases, chloroquine has caused ocular damage. Theoretically, a total cumulative dosage of 100 g (base) may be critical in the development of ocular, ototoxic, and myopathic effects. However, with weekly long-term administration of chloroquine, serious eye damage has not been confirmed; therefore, periodic eye examinations may no longer be indicated. Chloroquine should be used with caution in patients who have histories of liver damage, alcoholism, or neurologic or hematologic disorders. It is contraindicated in patients with psoriasis. Chloroquine suppresses the immune response to the rabies vaccine.

Certain antacids and antidiarrheal agents (kaolin, calcium carbonate, and magnesium trisilicate) should not be taken within about 4 hours before or after chloroquine administration, since they interfere with its absorption.

2. Mefloquine hydrochloride–Mefloquine, a quinoline methanol derivative, is used for oral prophylaxis and treatment of chloroquine-resistant and multidrug-resistant *P falciparum* malaria. In treatment, it is used only for mildly to moderately ill patients; severely ill patients require parenteral (quinine or quinidine) treatment. Mefloquine has strong schizonticidal activity against *P falciparum* (except for resistant strains) and *P vivax*—and presumably against *P ovale* and *P malariae*—but it is not active against *P falciparum* gametocytes or the hepatic stages of *P vivax* or *P ovale,* which require a course of primaquine.

With the lower doses used in prophylaxis, frequent minor and transient side effects (apparently no more frequent than those associated with chloroquine) include nausea, vomiting, epigastric pain, diarrhea, headache, dizziness, syncope, and extrasystoles. Severe neuropsychiatric symptoms are rare (estimated 1:10,000). If prophylaxis is continued for more than a year, periodic liver function and ophthalmologic tests should be done. With treatment doses—particularly over 1000 mg—gastrointestinal symptoms and fatigue are more likely to occur, and the frequency of neuropsychiatric symptoms (dizziness, headache, visual disturbances, vertigo, tinnitus, insomnia, restlessness, anxiety, depression, confusion, disorientation, acute psychosis, or seizures) may be of the order of 1:1200–1:200. In experimental animals, the drug affects fertility and is teratogenic; it also causes degenerative changes in the epididymis in rats and in

the lens and retina of some species. In human males, however, no deleterious effects on spermatozoa were found, and no effects have been noted in the human retina or lens.

Mefloquine is contraindicated in the presence of a cardiac conduction abnormality, liver impairment, or a history of a psychiatric or neurologic disorder, perhaps including epilepsy. Also contraindicated is concurrent administration of mefloquine with quinine, quinidine, or halofantrine. If these drugs precede use of mefloquine, 12 hours should elapse before mefloquine is started; however, because of the long elimination half-life of mefloquine (13–26 days), extreme caution is required if one of these drugs is used to treat malaria after mefloquine has been taken. Concurrent administration with tetracyclines or ampicillin results in increased mefloquine blood levels.

The development of neuropsychiatric symptoms during prophylaxis is an indication for stopping the drug. Patients should be instructed to use caution when driving or operating machinery, and some persons whose work requires fine coordination and spatial discrimination should not take the drug. Patients taking anticonvulsant drugs (particularly valproic acid and divalproex sodium) may have breakthrough seizures. CDC has recently advised that mefloquine can be used throughout pregnancy; nevertheless, its use during the first trimester should be based on risk-benefit assessment. Women of childbearing potential who take mefloquine for antimalarial prophylaxis should preferably avoid conception for the duration of mefloquine usage and for 2 months after the last dose.

Note: The tablet formulation in the USA contains 250 mg of the salt (= 228 mg of base). However, in Canada and many other countries, the tablets contain 274 mg of the salt (= 250 mg of base). Mefloquine should not be taken on an empty stomach and should be taken with 8 oz of water.

3. Primaquine phosphate–Primaquine is used to prevent relapse by eliminating persistent liver forms of *P vivax* or *P ovale* in patients who have had an acute attack and for individuals returning from an endemic area who have probably been exposed to malaria. However, in persons with a low probability of exposure, it is preferable to avoid primaquine's potential toxicity by not giving the drug. Instead, such patients are advised to seek medical evaluation in the event of malaria-like symptoms, which usually occur within 2 years after infection but can occur up to 4 years after. Primaquine is sometimes given as a single 45 mg (base) dose to eliminate *P falciparum* gametocytes.

Primaquine is generally well tolerated. Occasional side effects of the drug are gastrointestinal disturbances, headache, dizziness, or neutropenia. Primaquine should not be used in pregnancy (risks of hemolytic disease in the fetus), in autoimmune disorders, or concurrently with quinine.

All patients should be tested for glucose-6-phosphate dehydrogenase (G6PD) deficiency before therapy is begun and followed carefully during treatment; this is because primaquine may cause mild, self-limited hemolysis or marked hemolysis (pallor, weakness, abdominal pain, dark urine) or methemoglobinemia. G6PD deficiency is most common among persons of Mediterranean, African, or certain East Asian extractions. Patients with severe G6PD deficiency (< 10% residual enzyme activity) should not receive primaquine. For individuals with 10–60% residual activity, it is generally safe to give combined primaquine phosphate, 78.9 mg (45 mg base), and chloroquine phosphate, 0.5 g (0.3 g base), weekly for 8 weeks. However, for persons suspected of having the Mediterranean or Canton forms of G6PD deficiency, it may be preferable not to give primaquine but to treat attacks of malaria with chloroquine as they occur.

4. Quinine–Oral quinine sulfate is used to treat malaria due to multidrug-resistant strains of *P falciparum* that do not respond to chloroquine, Fansidar, or mefloquine. Although quinine alone will control acute attacks, in many infections—particularly with strains from Southeast Asia—it fails to prevent recurrence. Addition of one of several drugs (Table 35–3) lowers the rate of recurrence. For treatment of acute attacks of *P vivax, P ovale,* and *P malariae* malaria, however, chloroquine is more effective than quinine and is the drug of choice.

Because quinine is an irritant to the gastric mucosa, it should be taken with food. Mild to moderate quinine toxicity (cinchonism) is manifested by headache, nausea, slight visual disturbances, dizziness, and mild tinnitus. These symptoms may abate as treatment continues and usually do not require discontinuation of treatment. Where available, quinine blood levels can be monitored; desired plasma levels are 5–10 µg/mL. Severe cinchonism requiring temporary or permanent discontinuation of therapy is rare and begins to appear at plasma levels greater than 7 µg/mL; findings include fever, skin eruptions, deafness, marked visual abnormalities (scotomas, diplopia, contracted visual fields, retinal vessel spasticity, optic atrophy, blindness), other central nervous system abnormalities (vertigo, somnolence, confusion, seizures), disturbances in cardiac rhythm or conduction, massive intravascular hemolysis with renal failure (blackwater fever), agranulocytosis, and thrombocytopenia.

Parenteral quinine dihydrochloride is used in the treatment of severe attacks of malaria due to *P falciparum* strains sensitive or resistant to chloroquine. The drug is given only intravenously at a slow rate (Table 35–3); rapid infusions may be severely toxic. The drug should be used with extreme caution and only for patients who cannot take the medication orally; appropriate oral therapy should be started as soon as possible. Infusions may cause thrombophlebitis. In the USA, parenteral quinine is no longer available and parenteral quinidine gluconate is used instead.

See references and manufacturers' recommendations for drug interactions (including aluminum-containing antacids, digoxin, anticoagulants, and cimetidine). Quinine is safe to use in pregnancy; relative contraindications are a history of tinnitus or of optic atrophy. Systemic clearance of quinine slows in proportion to the severity of the disease.

5. Quinidine gluconate–Quinidine is the dextrorotatory diasterioisomer of quinine. The two drugs are equally efficacious in parenteral treatment of severe malaria (Table 35–3). The two drugs are also similar with regard to toxicity and drug interactions, but quinidine has a greater cardiosuppressant effect.

6. Halofantrine–Halofantrine is a schizonticide for all four malaria species, including multidrug-resistant *P falciparum.* The drug is used only in oral treatment at a dosage of 500 mg (salt) given three times at 6-hour intervals and repeated in 1 week. Infrequent to rare, minor side effects are abdominal pain, diarrhea, cough, rash, and pruritus. The drug should not be given from 1 hour before to 3 hours after a meal, because fatty food enhances and results in irregular absorption. Halofantrine is not used for prophylaxis or standby treatment because of this variable bioavailability; because the standard dose prolongs the QT_c interval; and because there have been rare reports of ventricular arrhythmias, sometimes fatal. The drug should not be used in the presence of preexisting cardiac disease, or recent usage (3 weeks) or concomitant treatment with mefloquine, or with other drugs that prolong the QT_c interval. Because halofantrine is embryotoxic in animals, it should not be given to pregnant women. Halofantrine is widely available abroad; in the USA, however, although approved by the FDA, it has not been marketed.

7. Pyrimethamine-sulfadoxine (Fansidar)– Fansidar is supplied as tablets that contain pyrimethamine (25 mg) and sulfadoxine (500 mg). Fansidar's limitations are that it is effective only against susceptible strains of *P falciparum* (see above); its low efficacy against *P vivax, P ovale,* or *P malariae* and that it is slow-acting. Fansidar is no longer used for weekly prophylaxis because of rare reports of severe cutaneous toxicity and death. However, in single-dose treatment, Fansidar is generally well tolerated. Cutaneous reactions are more common in persons who are HIV-positive.

Current indications for Fansidar are (1) as a single dose (slow-acting) in conjunction with quinine (rapid-acting) in treatment of sensitive strains of acute chloroquine-resistant falciparum malaria and (2) in presumptive self-treatment of malaria (see above).

Fansidar is contraindicated for individuals with known sulfonamide sensitivity and those in the last month of pregnancy (the sulfadoxine component, which has a long half-life, can cause kernicterus in the newborn). The drug should be used with caution in the presence of impaired renal or hepatic function, in patients with G6PD deficiency (hemolysis occurs in some), and in those with severe allergic disorders or bronchial asthma. If folic acid is needed, ingestion should be delayed 1 week to avoid an inhibitory effect on the antimalarial action of Fansidar.

8. Doxycycline–Doxycycline is effective against chloroquine-sensitive and chloroquine-resistant *P falciparum, P vivax,* and (apparently) against *P ovale* and *P malariae.* It is used prophylactically against chloroquine-resistant and mefloquine-resistant falciparum malaria in Thailand and adjacent countries and elsewhere for patients who cannot tolerate mefloquine (Table 35–2). Doxycycline is also used as an adjunct drug with quinine for the treatment of resistant falciparum malaria (Table 35–3). Side effects include infrequent gastrointestinal symptoms (take with meals plus copious amounts of water to avoid esophageal irritation; avoid milk, which reduces absorption); candidal vaginitis (advise carrying a self-treatment antifungal regimen, either vaginal suppositories or cream); and rare photosensitivity (prevention may be achieved by use of sunscreens that absorb ultraviolet radiation and by avoidance of exposure to direct sunlight as much as possible). The drug is contraindicated in pregnancy, in nursing mothers, and in persons with hepatic dysfunction.

9. Artemisinin (qinghaosu) derivatives–Artemisinin and related drugs, which continue under evaluation, are available in some countries but not in the USA. They are rapidly acting schizonticides against all malaria parasites, including falciparum malaria resistant to chloroquine, mefloquine, and quinine. Recrudescences are common but may be prevented by follow-up treatment with mefloquine or an antibiotic. Artemisinin and its derivatives are not effective against the parasite's liver stages, and, because of their short half-lives, are of no use for prophylaxis. Adverse events, which include gastrointestinal symptoms, pruritus, and fever, are mild. Animal studies suggest a potential for embryo and central nervous system toxicity; the latter, however, has not been documented in more than 2 million drug usages in humans.

10. Proguanil–Proguanil (chlorguanide, paludrine; not available in the USA), 200 mg/d, is a schizonticide against three of the malaria parasites (unknown degree against *P malariae*) and has some causal prophylactic action. It is used in prophylaxis in combination with chloroquine (0.5 g/wk) in areas with no or low-intensity chloroquine-resistant *P falciparum.* It is not used in treatment, either alone or in combination. Rarely reported side effects are nausea, vomiting, hair loss, and mouth ulcers. The drug is safe to use in pregnancy; it should not be used in persons with hepatic or renal dysfunction. Clinical trials of proguanil plus atovaquone suggest high cure rates

in multidrug-resistant *P falciparum* malaria and that the combination is well tolerated.

Chemoprophylaxis for Nonimmune Populations (See Table 35–2 for methods and dosages.)

Selected drugs should be taken with water at mealtime. It is preferable that they be tested in advance of departure for malarious regions—weekly for 1–2 weeks for chloroquine, daily for 3 days for doxycycline, weekly for 2–3 weeks for mefloquine—to evaluate for side effects and to allow time for selection of an alternative drug if needed. Subsequently, to achieve satisfactory blood levels, chloroquine or mefloquine should be started 1 week before initial exposure or, in the case of doxycycline, 2 days before exposure. Thereafter, chemoprophylaxis is taken weekly (daily for doxycycline) while in the endemic area *and for 4 weeks afterward.* On returning home, primaquine is given to eradicate persistent liver stages of *P vivax* or *P ovale* if there has been significant exposure to these parasites (see above under Primaquine). For additional details on the following drugs, see Table 35–2 and under the individual drugs (above).

A. Chemoprophylaxis in Regions Where *P falciparum* Is Sensitive to Chloroquine:

1. Drug of choice–Chloroquine prevents attacks for all forms of malaria and is curative for *P falciparum* and *P malariae* when taken for 4 weeks after leaving the endemic area.

2. Alternative drugs–For persons who cannot take chloroquine, hydroxychloroquine sulfate (400 mg [salt]) can be tried.

Schizonticides *not used for chemoprophylaxis* are halofantrine (erratic absorption and variable bioavailability), Fansidar (hypersensitivity reactions with rare deaths), amodiaquine (agranulocytosis and toxic hepatitis), pyrimethamine (widespread resistance of both *P falciparum* and *P vivax*), artemisinin and related drugs (short duration of action), proguanil (except in combination with chloroquine), and generally quinine (toxicity).

B. Chemoprophylaxis in Regions Where *P falciparum* Is Resistant to Chloroquine:

1. Drug of choice–Mefloquine is the drug of choice. Note its cautions and contraindications (see above).

2. First alternative–Doxycycline's side effects can be a problem for some persons (see above).

3. Second alternative–When daily proguanil (200 mg) is added to weekly chloroquine (0.5 g), more protection is obtained than when chloroquine is used alone. The combination is recommended by some authorities (Bradley and Warhurst, 1995) for some countries where chloroquine resistance is uncommon. The combination is not effective in Thailand or Papua New Guinea; for sub-Saharan Africa, mefloquine appears to be more reliable. In selected circumstances, medication should be provided for self-treatment of breakthrough attacks (see above).

C. Chemoprophylaxis in Southeast Asia: Multidrug *P falciparum* resistance is extensive in Southeast Asia. Chloroquine cannot be used throughout the region. Fansidar is not effective in Thailand, Cambodia, and Myanmar and probably in other areas. Additionally, because of the increasing frequency of mefloquine resistance, doxycycline (100 mg daily) is recommended instead in Thailand, Cambodia, Myanmar, and Papua New Guinea.

D. Prophylaxis for Pregnant Women: Pregnant women should be protected; malaria infection during pregnancy may be particularly severe. Drugs contraindicated in pregnancy are doxycycline and primaquine. Therefore, the best course is weekly chloroquine (or hydroxychloroquine) with or without proguanil. In areas of chloroquine-resistant malaria, mefloquine can be used except in the first trimester.

Treatment of Acute Attacks
(See under individual drugs and Table 35–3 for dosages.)

A. General Considerations: It is important to determine whether a patient has been treated with antimalarials in the previous 1–2 days (3 weeks for mefloquine because of its slow excretion) to avoid the risk of overdose or adverse drug interactions. In the event of mefloquine prophylaxis or treatment failure, it is hazardous—although it may be essential—to use quinine, quinidine, or halofantrine (Table 35–3); under these circumstances, apparently the safest drug to use is artemisinin or one of its derivatives, which are available in some countries.

In falciparum malaria, indications for parenteral treatment are (1) failure to retain ingested drugs, (2) cerebral malaria, (3) multiple complications, and (4) a peripheral asexual parasitemia of 5% (250,000/μL) or higher. Patients with falciparum malaria should be hospitalized to observe for therapeutic response. It is essential to determine the density of parasites on the blood smear (as a measure of severity of infection) and to recheck at least daily. Within 48–72 hours, patients usually become afebrile and improve clinically; within 48 hours, parasitemia is generally reduced by about 75% (though there may be an initial increase during the first 6–12 hours). If there is no improvement within 48–72 hours for mild infections or 24 hours for severe ones or if there is increasing asexual parasitemia after 1–2 days (in the presence of adequate drug ingestion and retention), parasite resistance to the drug must be assumed and treatment changed.

B. Treatment of All Forms of Malaria Except *P falciparum* Strains Resistant to Chloroquine:

1. Elimination of asexual erythrocytic parasites–Infection by all four species of malaria is generally treated with oral chloroquine (Table 35–3). Al-

ternative oral drugs if chloroquine cannot be tolerated are mefloquine, quinine sulfate, halofantrine (approved but not available in the USA), and artemisinin or its derivatives.

If the patient is severely ill, treat with intravenous quinine dihydrochloride (not available in the USA) or quinidine gluconate (Table 35–3); a third alternative drug is chloroquine hydrochloride, given intramuscularly. Start oral therapy with chloroquine as soon as possible.

2. Eradication of *P vivax* or *P ovale* infections–This is accomplished with a standard course of primaquine (Table 35–3).

3. Elimination of persistent gametocytemia–Gametocytes of *P vivax*, *P ovale*, and *P malariae* can be eliminated by chloroquine. Gametocytes of *P falciparum* are eliminated by a single dose of 26.3 mg of primaquine salt.

4. Treatment of semi-immunes–Treatment of attacks in semi-immune patients generally requires shorter courses of drug treatment.

C. Treatment of Falciparum Malaria Acquired in Areas Where *P falciparum* Is Resistant to Chloroquine: Start treatment with oral quinine sulfate and a second drug (Table 35–3) (but not Fansidar if the infection was acquired in an area with Fansidar resistance). Alternative drugs are mefloquine, halofantrine (approved but not yet available in the USA), and artemisinin or its derivatives; in Southeast Asia, multidrug resistance extends to Fansidar, mefloquine, and halofantrine.

If the patient is severely ill, treat with intravenous quinine or quinidine (Table 35–3). A second drug (doxycycline or clindamycin) should also be given parenterally. Oral treatment with quinine plus the antibiotic should be started as soon as possible.

D. Special Measures for Treatment of Severe *P falciparum* Malaria: (See references for further details.) Severe and complicated falciparum malaria is a medical emergency that requires hospitalization, intensive care and the initiation of intravenous chemotherapy as rapidly as possible. In patients requiring more than 48 hours of parenteral therapy, reduce the quinine or quinidine dose by one-third to one-half. Rehydration of the patient should be done with great caution, particularly in the first 24 hours, since overhydration may precipitate noncardiogenic pulmonary edema. Fluid, electrolyte, and acid-base balance must be monitored. In general, 2–3 L of fluid is required the first day, followed by 10–20 mL/kg/d; intake and output should be carefully recorded. Early dialysis may be necessary for renal failure, particularly in the presence of multiple complications. Blood glucose levels should be monitored every 6 hours during the acute and early convalescent period, since hypoglycemia may be severe, either as a result of the malaria infection or the use of quinine or quinidine; treatment is with 50% dextrose (1–2 mL/kg) followed by a 4-hour infusion of 10%

dextrose. Patients with clinically significant disseminated intravascular coagulation should be treated with fresh whole blood. Anticonvulsants (eg, phenobarbital, diazepam) are used for seizures; the temperature is maintained below 38.5 °C. Exchange transfusion (5–10 L for adults) is in use on an experimental basis when more than 15% of red blood cells are parasitized (5% if severe dysfunction of other organs is present). Corticosteroids, heparin, and aspirin have been shown to be deleterious in cerebral malaria and should not be used.

Follow-Up for *P falciparum* Malaria

Blood films should be checked daily until parasitemia clears; check weekly thereafter for 4 weeks to observe for recrudescence of infection.

Prognosis

The uncomplicated and untreated primary attack of *P vivax, P ovale,* or *P falciparum* malaria usually lasts 2–4 weeks; that of *P malariae* about twice as long. Attacks of each type of infection may subsequently recur (once or many times) before the infection terminates spontaneously. With prompt antimalarial therapy, the prognosis is generally good, but in *P falciparum* infections, when severe complications such as cerebral malaria develop, the prognosis is poor even with treatment. It is now recognized that after cerebral malaria, residual neurologic deficits can occur.

Bhavnani SN, Preston SL: Monitoring of intravenous quinidine infusion in the treatment of *Plasmodium falciparum* malaria. Ann Pharmacother 1995;29:33.

Bradley DJ, Warhurst DC: Malaria prophylaxis: Guidelines for travelers from Britain. BMJ 1995;310:709.

Centers for Disease Control and Prevention: Health information for international travel. 1995. HHS Publication No. CDC 95-8280. For sale from the Superintendent of Documents, U.S. Government Printing Office, Washington, DC 20402. Telephone: 202-783-3238.

Collins WE, Jeffery GM: Primaquine resistance in *Plasmodium vivax.* Am J Trop Med Hyg 1996;55:243.

Cook GC: Malarial prophylaxis. Mefloquine toxicity should limit its use to treatment alone. BMJ 1995;311:190.

Eisenman A et al: Blood exchange [correction of exchange]—A rescue procedure for complicated falciparum malaria. Vox Sang 1995;68:19.

Hoffman SL: Artemether in severe malaria—still too many deaths. (Editorial.) N Engl J Med 1996;335:124.

Kuile FOK et al: Mefloquine treatment of acute falciparum malaria: A prospective study of non-serious adverse effects in 3673 patients. Bull WHO 1995;73:631.

Masinde GL, Krogstad DJ: Biologic and geographic factors in prevention and treatment of malaria. Curr Clin Top Infect Dis 1994;14:80.

Matson PA et al: Cardiac effects of standard-dose halofantrine therapy. Am J Trop Med Hyg 1996;54:229.

Svenson JE et al: Imported malaria. Clinical presentation and examination of symptomatic travelers. Arch Intern Med 1995;155:861.

White NJ: The treatment of malaria. N Engl J Med 1996;335:800.

TOXOPLASMOSIS

Essentials of Diagnosis

Acute primary infection:

• Fever, malaise, headache, lymphadenopathy (especially cervical), myalgia, arthralgia, stiff neck, sore throat; occasionally, rash, hepatosplenomegaly, retinochoroiditis, confusion; in various combinations.

• Positive serologic tests with high and rising IgG and IgM.

• Isolation of *Toxoplasma gondii* from blood or body fluids; tachyzoites in histologic sections of tissue or cytologic preparations of body fluids.

Acute primary or recrudescent infection in immunocompromised patients:

• Central nervous system mass lesions; retinochoroiditis, pneumonitis, myocarditis less common; sometimes other findings as above.

• Positive IgG titers moderately high; IgM antibody usually absent. Tissue diagnosis as above.

General Considerations

T gondii, an obligate intracellular protozoan, is found worldwide in humans and in many species of animals and birds. The parasite is a coccidian of cats, the definitive host, and exists in three forms: The *trophozoite* (tachyzoite) (3×7 μm) is the rapidly proliferating form seen in the tissues and body fluids in the acute stage. The trophozoites can enter and multiply in most mammalian nucleated cells. The *cyst* (bradyzoite), containing viable trophozoites, is the latent form that can persist indefinitely as a chronic infection and is found particularly in muscle and nerve tissue. The *oocyst* is the form passed only in the feces of the cat family. In the intestinal epithelium of cats, a sexual cycle occurs, with subsequent release of oocysts for 3–14 days; cats may, however, become reinfected and excrete oocysts multiple times. Human infection results from ingestion of cysts in raw or undercooked meat; from ingestion of oocysts on contaminated vegetables or other foods, following careless handling of cat litter, or from soil by soil-eating children; from transplacental transmission; or, rarely, from direct inoculation of trophozoites, as in blood transfusion. Dogs, insects, and public water supplies may contribute to mechanical transmission. Antibody prevalence rates range from less than 5% in some parts of the world (absence of cats, minimal ingestion of meat) to about 55% in the USA and over 80% in France.

Clinical Findings

A. Symptoms and Signs: Over 80% of primary infections are asymptomatic. The incubation period for symptomatic persons is 1–2 weeks. Generally, on recovery, both asymptomatic and symptomatic infections persist as chronic latent (cyst) infections. Reactivation occurs almost exclusively in severely immunocompromised patients.

The clinical manifestations of toxoplasmosis may be grouped into four syndromes:

1. Primary infection in the immunocompetent host–Most infections are acute, mild, febrile multisystem illnesses that resemble infectious mononucleosis. Lymphadenopathy, usually nontender, particularly of the head and neck, is the most common finding. Other features in various combinations are malaise, myalgia, arthralgia, headache, sore throat, and maculopapular or urticarial rash. Hepatosplenomegaly may occur. Rarely, severe cases are complicated by pneumonitis, meningoencephalitis, hepatitis, myocarditis, and retinochoroiditis. Symptoms may fluctuate, but most patients recover spontaneously within a few months.

2. Congenital infection–Congenital transmission occurs only as a result of infection (generally asymptomatic) in a nonimmune woman during pregnancy. Infection has been detected in up to 1% of women during pregnancy; 15–60% of such infections, varying by trimester, are transmitted to the fetus, but only a small percentage result in abortions or stillbirths or in active disease in premature or full-term, live-born infants. Though fetal infection may occur in any trimester, it is more severe early in pregnancy. Treatment of the mother reduces the congenital infection rate by about 60%. See specialized sources for clinical manifestations and approach to diagnosis.

3. Retinochoroiditis–This develops gradually weeks to years after congenital infection (the preponderant form, which is generally bilateral) or rarely after an acquired infection in a young child (generally unilateral). Acquired infections in older children and adults rarely progress to retinochoroiditis. The inflammatory process persists for weeks to months as focally necrotic retinal lesions with blurred margins. Visual defects include blurring, central defects, and scotomas. Rarely, progression may result in glaucoma and blindness. With healing, white or dark-pigmented scars may result. Panuveitis may accompany retinochoroiditis.

4. Reactivated disease in the immunologically compromised host–Reactivated toxoplasmosis occurs in patients with AIDS, cancer, or those given immunosuppressive drugs. The infection may present in specific organs (brain, lungs, and eye most commonly, but also heart, skin, gastrointestinal tract, and liver) or as disseminated disease. In AIDS, depletion of CD4 T cell lymphocytes and macrophage dysfunction predispose to reactivation of latent *Toxoplasma* infection. Between 30% and 50% of AIDS patients seropositive for past *Toxoplasma* infection will develop focal or (less often) diffuse intracerebral toxoplasma lesions, associated with clinical findings of fever, headache, altered mental status, seizures, and focal (or, infrequently, nonfocal) neurologic deficits (see also Chapter 31).

B. Laboratory Findings: Diagnosis depends principally on serologic tests, which are sensitive and reliable. However, diagnosis is occasionally made from tissue (blood, bone marrow aspirates, cerebrospinal fluid sediment, sputum, and other tissues or body fluids or placental tissue) either histologically (demonstration of trophozoites or characteristic histology) or by isolation of the organism in mice or tissue culture.

1. Histology–Cysts or trophozoites may be directly identified by staining blood (buffy coat from centrifuged heparinized blood) or other tissues or body fluids. Demonstration of cysts does not establish a causal relationship to clinical illness, since cysts may be found in both acute and chronic infections. However, finding tachyzoites confirms active infection. In the placenta, fetus, or newborn, the presence of cysts indicates congenital infection.

2. Serologic tests–The Sabin-Feldman dye test and the indirect hemagglutination, indirect immunofluorescence (IFA), ELISA, and other tests—can be done on blood, cerebrospinal fluid, aqueous humor, and other body fluids. The dye test, which is extremely sensitive and specific, is the standard, but it is rarely used because of laboratory safety factors. The ELISA, immunosorbent, and IFA tests permit separation of IgM and IgG antibody. In the IFA test for IgM, antibody appears 1–2 weeks after start of infection, reaches a peak at 6–8 weeks, and then gradually declines; low titers may persist for more than 12 months. IgG antibody persists for life in most patients. False-positive and false-negative tests can occur with the IFA test; the former can be avoided by use of IgM capture tests. Other tests that may be useful for patients who, after 3 months, continue to have low-positive, equivocal, or negative IgM titers are the IgA-ELISA and IgE tests by ELISA and immunosorbent agglutination assay. Using various body fluids, diagnosis by polymerase chain reaction or by detection of antigen or of nucleic acid sequences specific for *T gondii* is highly promising, especially for early diagnosis and to avoid invasive procedures.

The following are selected serologic and other findings in specific toxoplasmosis syndromes:

a. Acute infection in immunocompetent persons–The diagnosis is established by seroconversion from negative to positive, by a fourfold rise in serologic titers by any test, or by a single high titer (1:160) of IgM antibody. A presumptive diagnosis is based on a single IgM titer of over 1:64 and a very high IgG titer (> 1:1000). The diagnosis of acute toxoplasmosis is excluded if the dye test and an IgM test are negative for 3 months after onset of symptoms.

b. Recrudescent infection in immunosup-

pressed patients—In AIDS patients, *Toxoplasma* can sometimes be isolated from the blood. Alternatively, definitive diagnosis is only by finding *Toxoplasma* organisms in cerebrospinal fluid (Wright-Giemsa stain) or by brain biopsy. To avoid the latter, empiric antibiotic treatment is generally started after presumptive evidence is obtained by MRI (the more sensitive test) or CT scan (typically: multiple, isodense or hypodense, ring-enhancing mass lesions). Antibody titers cannot be depended on, since most patients have IgG titers that reflect past infection, significant rises are infrequent, and IgM antibody is rare. However, absence of IgG is strong evidence against the diagnosis of central nervous system toxoplasmosis. The cerebrospinal fluid may show mild pleocytosis (predominantly lymphocytes and monocytes), elevated protein, and normal glucose; rarely seen is a rise in antibody titers. (See also Chapter 31.)

c. Toxoplasmic retinochoroiditis—This is usually associated with stable, usually low IgG titers and no IgM antibody. If IgG antibody in aqueous humor is higher than in the serum, the diagnosis is supported.

3. Other laboratory findings—Leukocyte counts are normal or reduced, often with lymphocytosis or monocytosis with rare atypical cells, but there is no heterophil antibody. Chest radiographs may show interstitial pneumonia.

Differential Diagnosis

In acute febrile disease, consider cytomegalovirus infection, infectious mononucleosis, and other causes of pneumonitis, myocarditis, myositis, hepatitis, and splenomegaly. With lymphadenopathy, possibilities include sarcoidosis, tuberculosis, tularemia, lymphoma, cat-scratch disease, and metastatic carcinoma. With brain lesions in the immunosuppressed host, herpes simplex, cytomegalovirus infection, other viral encephalitides, multifocal leukoencephalopathy, fungal encephalitis, vascular stroke, tuberculosis, psychosis, and, in particular, central nervous system lymphoma.

Treatment

A. Approach to Treatment: Asymptomatic **infections** in immuno competent hosts are not treated except in children under 5 years of age.

Symptomatic patients should be treated until manifestations of the illness have subsided and there is serologic evidence that immunity has been acquired.

Since most episodes of **retinochoroiditis** are self-limited, opinions vary on indications for and type of treatment. (See specialized texts.)

Immunocompromised patients with active infection (primary or recrudescent) must be treated. Therapy should continue for 4–6 weeks after cessation of symptoms—which may require up to a 6-month course, to be followed by drug prophylaxis as long as immunosuppression persists. In AIDS patients, treatment should be continued indefinitely. Chronic asymptomatic infection in these patients usually need not be treated, but prophylaxis may be started if significant increase in antibody titer is noted. (See also Chapter 31.)

During **pregnancy,** because early treatment reduces (but does not eliminate) the incidence of fetal infection, most workers feel that treatment is justified. For details on management of infections during pregnancy, see specialized texts.

B. Choice of Drugs: The treatment of choice in nonimmunocompromised patients is pyrimethamine, 25–50 mg daily, plus either trisulfapyrimidines (2–6 g/d in four divided doses) or sulfadiazine (100 mg/kg/d [maximum 6 g/d] in four divided doses); continue this treatment for 2–4 weeks. Note that the loading doses to initiate treatment are pyrimethamine (100 mg twice daily for 1 day) plus the chosen sulfonamide (75 mg/kg [maximum 4 g]). Patients should be screened for a history of sulfonamide sensitivity (skin rashes, gastrointestinal symptoms, hepatotoxicity); to prevent crystal-induced nephrotoxicity, good urine output should be maintained (alkalinization with sodium bicarbonate may also be useful). Pyrimethamine side effects include headache and gastrointestinal symptoms; folinic acid (calcium leucovorin), 10 mg/d in two to four divided doses, is given to avoid the hematologic effects of pyrimethamine-induced folate deficiency. Platelet and white blood cell counts should be performed at least twice weekly. Clindamycin (600 mg four times daily) may be a useful alternative drug; because it concentrates in the choroid, it is also used in the treatment of ocular disease. Immunotherapy and newer drugs such as azithromycin and atovaquone (which may be active against the cyst form) are under evaluation.

In toxoplasmosis in pregnancy, spiramycin is given at a dosage of 3 g in four divided doses; the drug is not effective in other forms of the infection. In the USA, the drug is available from the manufacturer.

Prevention

Freezing of meat to –20 °C for 2 days or heating to 60 °C for 4 minutes kills cysts in tissues. Under appropriate environmental conditions, oocysts passed in cat feces can remain infective for a year or more. Thus, children's play areas, including sandboxes, should be protected from cat (and dog) feces; hand washing is indicated after contact with soil potentially contaminated by animal feces. Indoor cats should be fed only dry, canned, or cooked meat. Litter boxes should be changed daily, as freshly deposited oocysts are not infective for 48 hours.

Pregnant women should have their serum examined for *Toxoplasma* antibody. If the IgM test is negative but an IgG titer is present and less than 1:1000, no further evaluation is necessary. Those with negative titers should take measures to prevent infection—preferably by having no further contact with cats, by thoroughly cooking meat, and by hand washing after handling raw meat and before eating or touching the face. For seronegative women who continue to have significant environmental exposure, serologic screening should be conducted several times during pregnancy.

Prognosis

The outlook for acute toxoplasmosis in adults is excellent as long as the patient is immunocompetent. In immunosuppressed patients, the disease is usually fatal if untreated; improvement results if treatment is started early, but recrudescence is common. Chronic asymptomatic infection, as indicated by a persistent antibody titer, is usually benign.

Extermann P: Screening for toxoplasmosis in pregnancy. Arch Gynecol Obstet 1995;256:S170.

Georgiev VS: Management of toxoplasmosis. Drugs 1994;48:179.

Hay J, Dutton GN: Toxoplasma and the eye. (Editorial.) BMJ 1995;310:1021.

Israelski DM, Remington J: Toxoplasmosis in the non-AIDS immunocompromised host. Curr Clin Top Infect Dis 1993;13:57.

New LC, Holliman RE: Toxoplasmosis and human immunodeficiency virus (HIV) disease. J Antimicrob Chemother 1994;33:1079.

II. HELMINTHIC INFECTIONS

TREMATODE (FLUKE) INFECTIONS

SCHISTOSOMIASIS
(Bilharziasis)

Essentials of Diagnosis

- Acute phase: Abrupt onset (2–6 weeks postexposure) of abdominal pain, weight loss, headache, malaise, chills, fever, myalgia, diarrhea (sometimes bloody), dry cough, hepatomegaly, and eosinophilia.
- Chronic phase: Either (1) diarrhea, abdominal pain, blood in stool, hepatomegaly or hepatosplenomegaly, and bleeding from esophageal varices (*Schistosoma mansoni* or *Schistosoma japonicum* infection); or (2) terminal hematuria, urinary frequency, and urethral and bladder pain (*Schistosoma haematobium* infection).
- Depending on species, characteristic eggs in feces, urine, or scrapings or biopsy of rectal or bladder mucosa.

General Considerations

Schistosomiasis, which infects more than 200 million persons worldwide, induces severe consequences in 20 million persons annually, resulting in up to 200,000 deaths. The disease is caused mainly by three blood flukes (trematodes). *S mansoni*, which causes intestinal schistosomiasis, is widespread in Africa and occurs in the Arabian peninsula, South America (Brazil, Venezuela, Suriname), and the Caribbean (including Puerto Rico but not Cuba). Vesical (urinary) schistosomiasis, caused by *S haematobium*, is found throughout the Middle East and Africa. Asiatic intestinal schistosomiasis, due to *S japonicum,* is important in China and the Philippines, and a small focus is present in Sulawesi, Indonesia, but transmission in Japan has been interrupted. A number of schistosome species of animals sometimes infect humans, including *Schistosoma intercalatum* in central Africa and *Schistosoma mekongi* in the Mekong delta in Thailand, Cambodia, and Laos. In the USA, an estimated 400,000 immigrants are infected, but transmission does not occur.

Mammals are important reservoirs for *S japonicum.* Humans are the main reservoir for *S mansoni* and *S haematobium;* the few animal species infected with *S mansoni* are not epidemiologically important.

In the life cycle involving humans, the adult worms live in terminal venules of the bowel (*S mansoni, S japonicum*) or bladder (*S haematobium*). When eggs passed in feces or urine reach fresh water, a larval form is released that subsequently infects snails, the intermediate host. After development, infective larvae (cercariae) leave the snails, enter water, and infect exposed persons through the skin or mucous membranes. After penetration, the cercariae become schistosomula larvae that reach the portal circulation in the liver, where they rapidly mature. After a few weeks, adult worms pair, mate, and migrate mainly to terminal venules of specific veins, where females deposit their eggs. By means of lytic secretions, some eggs reach the lumen of the bowel or bladder and are passed with feces or urine. Others are retained in the bowel or bladder wall, while still others are carried in the circulation to the liver, lung, and (less often) to other tissues.

Except for the allergic response in the acute syndrome (see below), disease is primarily due to delayed hypersensitivity. Antigens released by the eggs stimulate a local T cell-dependent granulomatous response, followed by a strong fibrotic reaction. Live worms produce no lesions and rarely cause symptoms. The type or degree of tissue damage and symptoms varies with the intensity of infection (worm burden), host genetic factors, site of egg deposition, concurrent infection (eg, hepatitis B), and duration of infection.

S mansoni adults migrate to the inferior mesenteric veins of the large bowel and *S japonicum* to the superior and inferior mesenteric veins in the large and small bowel. Ulcers and polyps (common only in Egypt) result from granuloma formation and fibrosis in the bowel wall. Egg accumulation in the liver may result in periportal fibrosis and portal hypertension of the presinusoidal type, but liver function typically remains intact even in advanced disease. Portal-systemic collateralization due to portal hypertension can result in embolization of eggs to the lungs, with subsequent endarteritis, pulmonary hypertension, and cor pulmonale. Because greater numbers of eggs are produced by *S japonicum,* the resulting disease is often more severe.

Adult *S haematobium* mature in the venous plexus of the bladder, ureters, rectum, prostate, and uterus. Ulcers and polyps result from granuloma formation and fibrosis in the bladder wall, and eggshell remnants may calcify. Stricture or distortion of the ureteral orifices or terminal ureters may result in hydroureter, hydronephrosis, and ascending infection. Lesions in the pelvic organs rarely progress to extensive fibrosis and infection. Eggs are carried to the liver or lungs, but severe pathologic changes in these organs are less frequent than in *S mansoni* and *S japonicum* infections.

In size, adult *S mansoni* are 6–13 × 1 mm. The prepatent period—from cercarial penetration until appearance of eggs in feces—is about 50 days. The life span of the worms ranges from 5 to 30 years or more.

Clinical Findings

A. Symptoms and Signs: Although a large proportion of infected persons have light infections and are asymptomatic, an estimated 50–60% have symptoms and 5–10% advanced organ damage. In children, schistosomal infections may contribute to decreased nutritional status and growth retardation.

1. Cercarial dermatitis–Following cercarial penetration, clinical findings progress from a localized itchy erythematous or petechial rash to macules and papules that last up to 5 days. Most cases occur in fresh or marine water (worldwide) and are due to skin invasion by bird schistosome cercariae, parasites that do not mature in humans and do not cause systemic symptoms. The syndrome is uncommon with human schistosome infections.

2. Acute schistosomiasis (Katayama fever)–This syndrome, primarily an allergic response to the developing schistosomes, may occur with the three schistosomes (rare with *S haematobium*) and usually is not seen in natives. The incubation period is 2–7 weeks; the severity of illness ranges from mild to (rarely) life-threatening. In addi-

tion to fever, malaise, urticaria, diarrhea (sometimes bloody), myalgia, dry cough, leukocytosis, and marked eosinophilia, the liver and spleen may be temporarily enlarged. The patient again becomes asymptomatic in 2–8 weeks. Early in the infection, stool examination may be negative (examinations should be repeated for at least 6 months) but serologic tests positive. Controversy continues about whether praziquantel and corticosteroids are safe and effective in treatment of acute disease.

3. Chronic schistosomiasis–This stage begins 6 months to several years after infection. In *S mansoni* and *S japonicum* infections, findings include diarrhea, abdominal pain, irregular bowel movements, blood in the stool, a hard enlarged liver, and splenomegaly. With subsequent slow progression over 5–15 years or longer, the following may appear: anorexia, weight loss, weakness, polypoid intestinal tumors, and features of portal and pulmonary hypertension. Immune complex glomerulonephritis may also occur.

In *S haematobium* infection, early symptoms of urinary tract disease are frequency and dysuria, followed by terminal hematuria and proteinuria. Frank hematuria may be recurrent. Sequelae may include bladder polyp formation, cystitis, chronic *Salmonella* infection, pyelitis, pyelonephritis, urolithiasis, hydronephrosis due to ureteral obstruction, renal failure, and death. Severe liver, lung, genital, or neurologic disease is rare. Bladder cancer has been associated with vesicular schistosomiasis.

4. Other complications–In heavily infected children, growth can be markedly retarded. Portal hypertension may result in a contracted liver, splenomegaly, pancytopenia, esophageal varices, and variceal bleeding. Abnormal liver function, jaundice, ascites, and hepatic coma are end-stage findings. Pulmonary hypertension with cor pulmonale is characterized by a parasternal lift and loud S_2; neck vein distention and edema due to right heart failure may supervene. Other large bowel complications include stricture, granulomatous masses, and persistent *Salmonella* infection; colonic polyposis is manifested by bloody diarrhea, anemia, hypoalbuminemia, and clubbing. Transverse myelitis, epilepsy, or optic neuritis may result from collateral circulation of eggs or ectopic worms.

B. Laboratory Findings: Screening is by testing for eggs (repeated testing may be necessary) and occult blood in urine and feces, examination for proteinuria and leukocyturia, and serologic testing.

1. Eggs–Definitive diagnosis is made by finding characteristic live eggs in excreta or by mucosal biopsy. Ultrasound examination of the liver, which shows the pathognomonic pattern of periportal fibrosis, replaces wedge liver biopsy to detect hepatic eggs.

In *S haematobium* infection, eggs may be found in the urine or, less frequently, in the stools. Eggs are sought in urine specimens collected between 9 AM and 2 PM or in 24-hour collections. They are processed either by examination of the sediment or preferably by membrane filtration. Occasionally, eggs are sought by vesical mucosa biopsy.

In *S mansoni* and *S japonicum* infections, eggs may be found in stool specimens by direct examination, but some form of concentration is usually necessary; most commonly, the Kato-Katz quantitative method is used. Repeated examinations and sampling of large quantities of stool are often needed to find eggs in light infections. If results are negative, rectal mucosal biopsy of suspicious lesions or random biopsy specimens at two or three sites of normal mucosa may yield the diagnosis. Biopsy specimens should be examined as crush preparations between two glass slides.

2. Serologic tests–ELISA, immunoblot, and other tests are used in screening and may detect rare egg-negative or ectopic infections, but the tests do not distinguish active from past infection. The Centers for Disease Control and Prevention uses a "fast ELISA" for screening (sensitivity and specificity = 99%) and a Western blot (specificity = 100%) for confirmation and speciation. Detection of circulating antigen and antigen in urine is promising. Skin testing is to be discouraged.

3. Other tests–Anemia is common. Eosinophilia, common during the acute stage, usually is absent in the chronic stage. In *S mansoni* and *S japonicum* infections, barium swallow, esophagoscopy, barium enema or colonoscopy, chest x-ray, or an ECG may be indicated. Ultrasound examination of the liver may show the pathognomonic pattern of periportal fibrosis and replaces the need for liver biopsy.

In *S haematobium* infection, occult hematuria can often be detected either microscopically or by reagent strip test, particularly if the first portion of the urine specimen is evaluated. In advanced disease, cystoscopy may show "sandy patches," ulcers, and areas of squamous metaplasia; lower abdominal plain films may show calcification of the bladder wall or ureters. Sonography is considered the imaging technique of choice but may fail to show the calcification. CT—which may demonstrate pathognomonic "turtleback" calcifications—intravenous pyelography and retrograde cystography and pyelography may be useful.

Differential Diagnosis

Early intestinal schistosomiasis may be mistaken for amebiasis, bacillary dysentery, or other causes of diarrhea and dysentery. Later, the various causes of portal hypertension or of bowel polyps must be considered. In endemic areas, vesical schistosomiasis must be differentiated from other causes of urinary symptoms such as genitourinary tract cancer, bacterial infections of the urinary tract, nephrolithiasis, and the like.

Treatment

A. Medical Treatment: Treatment should be given only if live ova are identified. The safety and effectiveness of current drugs make it possible to treat all infections orally, including advanced disease, and without concern for serious side effects. Praziquantel can be used to treat all species; alternative drugs of choice are oxamniquine for *S mansoni* and metrifonate for *S haematobium*.

After treatment, periodic laboratory follow-up for continued passage of eggs is essential, starting at 3 months and continuing at intervals for 1 year; if found, viability should be determined, since dead eggs are passed for some months.

1. Praziquantel–Cure rates at 6 months for *S haematobium, S mansoni,* and *S japonicum* infections are 87%, 80%, and 84%, respectively, with marked reduction in egg counts in those not cured.

The dosage for treatment of all forms of schistosomiasis is 20 mg/kg three times for 1 day at 4- to 6-hour intervals. Lower dosages (20 mg/kg twice in 1 day) have been reported to be highly effective in some parts of the world for *S haematobium* and *S mansoni.* Tablets are taken with water after a meal and should not be chewed.

Mild and transient side effects persisting for hours to 1 day are common and include malaise, headache, dizziness, and anorexia. Less frequent are fatigue, drowsiness, nausea, vomiting, generalized abdominal pain, loose stools, pruritus, urticaria, arthralgia and myalgia, and low-grade fever. Minimal elevations of liver enzymes have occasionally been reported. The drug should not be used in pregnancy, and because of drug-induced dizziness, patients should not drive and should be cautioned if their work requires physical coordination or alertness. In areas where cysticercosis may coexist with a schistosomal infection being treated with praziquantel, treatment is best conducted in a hospital to monitor for death of cysticerci, which may be followed by neurologic complications.

2. Metrifonate–Metrifonate is a highly effective alternative drug for the treatment of *S haematobium* infections only. The dosage is 7.5–10 mg/kg (maximum 600 mg) once and then repeated twice at 2-week intervals. Cure rates range from 44% to 93%. Those not cured show marked reduction in egg counts. Side effects range from none to mild and transient findings, including gastrointestinal symptoms, headache, bronchospasm, weakness, and vertigo. Metrifonate is not available in the USA.

3. Oxamniquine is highly effective in *S mansoni* infections. For strains in the western hemisphere and western Africa, a dose of 12–15 mg/kg is given once. In Africa and the Arabian peninsula, give 15 mg/kg twice daily for 2 days. The drug is administered with food; when divided doses are needed, they are separated by 6–8 hours. Cure rates are 70–95%, with marked reduction in egg counts in those not cured. Side effects occur within hours: dizziness is most common; less frequent are drowsiness, nausea and vomiting, diarrhea, abdominal pain, and headache. An orange or red discoloration of the urine may occur. Rarely reported is central nervous system stimulation with behavioral changes, hallucinations, or seizures; patients should be observed for 2 hours after ingestion of the drug for appearance of these findings. Since the drug makes some patients dizzy or drowsy, it should be used with caution in patients whose work or activity requires mental alertness. The drug has shown mutagenic and embryocidal effects and is contraindicated in pregnancy.

B. Surgical Measures: In selected instances, surgery may be indicated for removal of polyps and for obstructive uropathy. For bleeding esophageal varices, sclerotherapy is the treatment of choice. As a last resort in patients who have repeated bleeding, shunting procedures (esophagogastric devascularization with splenectomy or distal—but not proximal—splenorenal shunt) are used, though their effectiveness and relative usefulness are not well established. Severe pancytopenia is an indication for splenectomy.

Prognosis

With treatment, the prognosis is excellent in early and light infections. There may be shrinkage or elimination of bladder and bowel ulcerations, granulomas, and polyps and reduction in detectable fibrosis by sonography. In advanced disease with extensive involvement of the intestines, liver, bladder, or other organs, the outlook is poor even with treatment. In endemic areas, mass treatment of children diminishes the risk of developing severely diseased organs, even though reinfection may occur.

al Karawi MA et al: Long term outcome of endoscopic sclerotherapy of variceal bleeding; comparative study between schistosomiasis and others. Hepatogastroenterology 1966;43:287.

Jordan P (editor): *Human Schistosomiasis.* CAB International, 1993.

Lucey DR, Maguire JH: Schistosomiasis. Infect Dis Clin North Am 1993;7:635.

McKerrow JH, Sun E: Hepatic schistosomiasis. Prog Liv Dis 1994;12:121.

Nooman ZM et al: The use and limitations of ultrasonography in the diagnosis of liver morbidity attributable to *Schistosoma mansoni* infection in community-based surveys. Mem Inst Oswaldo Cruz 1995;90:147.

Rocha MO et al: Pathogenic factors of acute schistosomiasis mansoni: Correlation of worm burden, IgE, blood eosinophilia and intensity of clinical manifestations. Trop Med Int Health 1996;1:213.

Strickland GT: Gastrointestinal manifestations of schistosomiasis. Gut 1994;35:1334.

FASCIOLOPSIASIS

The large intestinal fluke, *Fasciolopsis buski,* is a common parasite of humans and pigs in central and Southern China, Taiwan, Southeast Asia, Indonesia, eastern India, and Bangladesh. When eggs shed in stools reach water, they hatch to produce free-swimming larvae that penetrate and develop in the flesh of snails. Cercariae subsequently escape from the snails and encyst on various water plants. Humans are infected by eating these plants uncooked (usually water chestnuts, bamboo shoots, or caltrops). Adult flukes (length 2–7.5 cm) mature in about 3 months and live in the small intestine attached to the mucosa or buried in mucous secretions. The number of parasites ranges from a few to several thousand.

After an incubation period of 2–3 months, manifestations of gastrointestinal irritation appear in all but light infections. Symptoms in severe infections include nausea, anorexia, upper abdominal pain, and diarrhea, sometimes alternating with constipation. Ascites and edema of the face and lower extremities may occur later; the physiologic mechanism is not understood. Intestinal obstruction, ileus, cachexia, and extreme prostration have been described.

Diagnosis depends on finding characteristic eggs or, occasionally, flukes in the stools. Leukocytosis with moderate eosinophilia is common. No serologic test is available. Because the adult worms live for only 6 months, absence from the endemic area for a longer period makes the diagnosis unlikely.

The drug of first choice is praziquantel, given as a 25 mg/kg dose three times a day for 1 day. The alternative drug is niclosamide, administered as for taeniasis but given every other day for three doses.

In light infections—even without treatment—the prognosis is good; generally, spontaneous cure occurs within 1 year. In rare cases—particularly in children—heavy infections with severe toxemia have resulted in death from cachexia or intercurrent infection.

Liu LX, Harinasuta KT: Liver and intestinal flukes. Gastroenterol Clin North Am 1996;25:627.

FASCIOLIASIS

Infection by *Fasciola hepatica,* the sheep liver fluke, results from ingestion of encysted metacercariae on watercress or other aquatic vegetables or in water. A wide range of herbivorous mammals are reservoir hosts. The disease in humans probably occurs worldwide but is most prevalent in sheep-raising countries, particularly where raw salads are eaten. The infection has been reported from Europe, mainland USA, Hawaii, the West Indies, the Middle East, China, Siberia, and North, East and South Africa. Eggs of the worm, passed in host feces into fresh water, release a miracidium that infects snails; the snails subsequently release cercariae that in turn encyst as metacercariae on vegetation (some cercariae become metacercariae directly in the water) to complete their life cycle. The leaf-shaped adult flukes measure 3 × 1.5 cm.

In humans, metacercariae excyst, penetrate and migrate through the liver, and mature in the bile ducts, where they cause local parenchymal necrosis and abscess formation. Although the infection is usually mild, three clinical syndromes can develop: acute, chronic latent, and chronic obstructive. The acute illness, associated with migration of immature larvae through the liver, shows an enlarged and tender liver, high fever, leukocytosis, and marked eosinophilia (to 90%). Pain may be present in the epigastrium or right upper quadrant, and the patient may experience headache, anorexia, and vomiting. Myalgia, urticaria, and other allergic reactions. Jaundice, cachexia, and prostration may appear in severe illness. Anemia and hypergammaglobulinemia are common; other liver function tests may be abnormal. Early diagnosis is difficult in the acute phase, because eggs are not found in the feces for 3–4 months. The chronic latent phase may be asymptomatic or characterized by hepatomegaly and other acute findings. The chronic obstructive phase takes place if the extrahepatic bile ducts are occluded, producing a clinical picture similar to that of sclerosing cholangitis, biliary cirrhosis, or choledocholithiasis. Occasionally, adult flukes migrate and produce lesions and symptoms in ectopic sites.

Diagnosis is established by detecting characteristic eggs in the feces; repeated examinations may be necessary. Sometimes the diagnosis can only be made by finding eggs in biliary drainage and, in rare instances, only after liver biopsy or at surgical exploration. Exogenous transient fecal carriage can occur as a result of ingestion of egg-containing cow or sheep liver. Eosinophilia is characteristic. Liver imaging and cholangiography may be useful. Serologic tests are often useful in presumptive diagnosis, particularly in the acute phase. The ELISA is highly sensitive and specific in detection of both antibody and antigen, but cross-reactions have occurred with schistosomiasis. Successful treatment appears to correlate with a decline in antibody titer. A fecal ELISA is promising.

Evidence is increasing that triclabendazole, a veterinary fasciolicide, is the drug of choice. At present, it is used in humans only on an experimental basis; further confirmation is needed of its effectiveness, dosage, and safety. In a recent report, a single 10 mg/kg dose achieved an 80% cure rate with an absence of side effects. Bithionol is the alternative drug of choice; its deficiencies are its long course (given as for paragonimiasis), failure rates of up to 50%, and frequent adverse reactions. Albendazole trials continue, but that drug also has shown high failure rates.

Reports on praziquantel have been variable; generally, it is ineffective even when used for up to 7 days at a dose of 25 mg/kg three times daily with a 4- to 6- hour interval between doses. If triclabendazole, bithionol, or praziquantel is not effective, dehydroemetine or emetine hydrochloride in dosages used for amebic liver abscess may help; both drugs are potentially toxic, but dehydroemetine may be less so. For any of the drugs, the destruction of parasites followed by release of antigen in sensitized patients may evoke symptoms.

Bithionol and dehydroemetine are available in the USA only from the Parasitic Disease Drug Service, Centers for Disease Control, Atlanta, GA 30333.

In endemic areas, aquatic plants should not be eaten raw; washing does not destroy the metacercariae, but cooking will. Drinking water must be boiled or purified.

Apt W et al: Treatment of human chronic fascioliasis with triclabendazole: Drug efficacy and serologic response. Am J Trop Med Hyg 1995;52:532.

Bacq Y et al: Successful treatment of acute fascioliasis with bithionol. Hepatology 1991;14:1066.

Dias LM et al: Biliary fascioliasis: Diagnosis, treatment, and follow-up by ERCP. Gastrointest Endosc 1996; 43:616.

Price TA, Tuazon CU, Simon GL: Fascioliasis: Case Reports and Review. Clin Infect Dis 1993;17:426.

CLONORCHIASIS & OPISTHORCHIASIS

Infection by *Clonorchis sinensis,* the Chinese liver fluke, is endemic in areas of Japan, Korea, China, Taiwan, and Southeast Asia. Over 20 million people are affected. Opisthorchiasis is caused by worms of the genus *Opisthorchis,* generally either *O felineus* (central, eastern, and southern Europe, eastern Asia, Southeast Asia, India) or *O viverrini* (Thailand, Laos, Vietnam). Clinically and epidemiologically, opisthorchiasis and clonorchiasis are identical.

Certain snails are infected when they ingest eggs shed into water in human or animal feces. Larval forms escape from the snails, penetrate the flesh of various freshwater fish, and encyst as metacercariae. Fish-eating mammals, including dogs and cats, are of great importance in maintaining the natural cycle. Human infection results from eating such fish, either raw or undercooked. Pickling, smoking, or drying may not suffice to kill the metacercariae. In humans, the ingested parasites excyst in the duodenum and ascend the bile ducts into the medium and small biliary radicals, but also into the larger ducts and the gallbladder, where they mature and remain throughout their lives (15–25 years), shedding eggs in the bile. In size, the worms are 7–20 × 1.5–3 mm. In the chronic stage of infection, there is progressive bile duct thickening, periductal fibrosis, dilation, biliary stasis, and secondary infection. Little fibrosis occurs in the portal tracts.

Most patients harbor few parasites and are asymptomatic. Among symptomatic patients, an acute and chronic syndrome occurs. Acute symptoms follow entry of immature worms into the biliary ducts and may persist for several weeks. Findings include malaise, low-grade fever, an enlarged, tender liver, pain in the hepatic area or epigastrium, urticaria, arthralgia, leukocytosis, eosinophilia, and an elevated serum alanine aminotransferase. The acute syndrome is difficult to diagnose, since ova may not appear in the feces until 3–4 weeks after onset of symptoms.

In chronic infections, findings include weakness, anorexia, epigastric pain, diarrhea, prolonged low-grade fever, intermittent episodes of right upper quadrant pain, localized hepatic area tenderness, and progressive hepatomegaly; liver function tests are normal.

Complications include intrahepatic bile duct calculi that may lead to recurrent pyogenic cholangitis, biliary abscess, or endophlebitis of the portal-venous branches. Although focal initially, this may gradually result in destruction of the liver parenchyma, fibrosis, and, in a few patients, cirrhosis with jaundice and ascites. Chronic cholecystitis, cholelithiasis, and a non-functional, enlarged gallbladder may occur. Flukes may also enter the pancreatic duct, causing acute pancreatitis or cholelithiasis. Cholangiocarcinoma has been causally linked with prolonged *Clonorchis* and *Opisthorchis* infection.

Diagnosis is made by finding characteristic eggs in stools (repeated tests may be necessary) or duodenal aspirate (sensitivity approaches 100%). During the chronic stage, leukocytosis varies according to the intensity of infection; eosinophilia may be present. In severe infection, the number of eggs per gram of feces may not reflect the heavy worm burden. In the advanced chronic disease, (1) liver function tests will indicate parenchymal damage; (2) CT and sonography may show diffuse dilation of small intrahepatic bile ducts with no or minimal dilation of the large intra- and extrahepatic ducts; and (3) transhepatic cholangiograms may show alternating stricture and dilation of the biliary tree, with worms visualized as filling defects. Of the several evaluated serologic tests, the ELISA is preferred (sensitivity, 77%); however, unless a specific monoclonal antibody is used, cross-reactions are common with other trematode and cestode infections, tuberculosis, and liver cancer.

The drug of choice is praziquantel. With a dosage of 25 mg/kg three times daily for 2 days (with a 4- to 6-hour interval between doses), cure rates over 95% can be anticipated for *Clonorchis* infections. One day of treatment may be sufficient for *Opisthorchis* infections. (For side effects, see Schistosomiasis, above.) Albendazole, at a dosage of 10 mg/kg twice daily for 7 days, appears to be less effective and requires a longer course of treatment. Mebendazole, at a dosage of 30 mg/kg for 20–30 days, has sometimes been effective.

The disease is rarely fatal, but patients with advanced infections and impaired liver function may succumb more readily to other diseases. The prognosis is good for light to moderate infections.

Ip M, Leung N, Cheng AF: Acute clonorchiasis. Scand J Infect Dis 1995;27:645.

Liu LX, Harinasuta KT: Liver and intestinal flukes. Gastroenterol Clin North Am 1996;25:627.

Mairiang E et al: Reversal of biliary tract abnormalities associated with *Opisthorchis viverrini* infection following praziquantel treatment. Trans R Soc Trop Med Hyg 1993;87:194.

PARAGONIMIASIS

Paragonimus westermani, the lung fluke, commonly infects humans (estimated 20 million) throughout the Far East; foci are also present in West Africa, South and Southeast Asia, the Pacific Islands, Indonesia, and New Guinea. Many carnivores and omnivores in addition to humans serve as reservoir hosts for the adult fluke (8–16 × 4–8 × 3–5 mm). A number of other *Paragonimus* species also infect humans in China, Japan, and Central and South America.

Eggs reaching water, either in sputum or feces, hatch in 3–6 weeks. Released miracidia penetrate and develop in snails. Emergent cercariae encyst as metacercariae in the tissues of crabs and crayfish. Human infection results if metacercariae are ingested when the crustaceans are eaten raw or pickled or are crushed and food, vessels, drinking water or fingers become contaminated. The metacercariae excyst in the small intestine and penetrate the peritoneal cavity. Most migrate through the diaphragm and enter the peripheral lung parenchyma; some may lodge in the brain (about 1% of all cases) or at other ectopic sites. In the lungs, the parasite becomes encapsulated by granulomatous fibrous tissue, reaching up to 2 cm in diameter. The lesion, which usually opens into a bronchiole, may subsequently rupture, resulting in expectoration of eggs, blood, and inflammatory cells. Rarely, the eggs may also enter the general circulation and produce ectopic in any tissue. The prepatent period until appearance of expectorated eggs is about 6 weeks.

In pulmonary infections, most persons have light to moderate worm burdens and are asymptomatic. In symptomatic cases, low-grade fever and dry cough are present initially; subsequently, pleuritic pain is common, and a rusty, blood-flecked, viscous sputum or frank hemoptysis may occur. Following slow progression, complications of bronchitis, bronchiectasis, bronchopneumonia, lung abscess, fibrosis, and pleural thickening or effusion may appear.

Only a minority of patients with cerebral infections present with acute disease, usually manifested by meningitis. In chronic central nervous system disease, seizures, cranial neuropathies, or meningoencephalitis may occur; death can follow. Parasites in the peritoneal cavity or the intestinal wall may cause abdominal pain, diarrhea or dysentery, and a palpable tumor mass. Migratory subcutaneous nodules (a few millimeters to 1 cm in diameter) occur with about 10% of *P westermani* infections and up to 60% of *Paragonimus skrjabini* infections.

Pulmonary disease is diagnosed by finding (1) characteristic eggs in sputum (rusty sputum is nearly pathognomonic), feces, bronchoscopic washings, biopsy specimens, or pleural fluid; or (2) adult flukes in subcutaneous nodules or other surgical specimens. If eggs are not found after multiple direct sputum examinations, they may be detectable in a 24-hour sputum collection processed by alkaline sodium hypochlorite concentration. Serum and cerebrospinal fluid serologic tests (ELISA, 92% sensitivity; and immunoblot, 96% sensitivity and 99% specificity) are available but do not differentiate active from prior infection. An antigen detection assay is promising. Eosinophilia and low-grade leukocytosis are common. Chest films may show infiltrates, fibrosis, nodules, cavitary lesions, pleural thickening or effusion, or calcifications. By CT, round, low-attenuation cystic lesions (5–15 mm) filled with fluid or gas are seen within the consolidation. In acute cerebral disease, CT shows multilocular, ring-like enhancement with surrounding low-density areas. In chronic cerebral disease, plain skull films often show round or oval-shaped calcifications, sometimes surrounded by low-density areas. Cerebrospinal fluid may be turgid or bloody, with numerous eosinophils. The EEG is almost always abnormal.

Paragonimiasis and tuberculosis must be differentiated, though chest x-ray appearance alone does not make the distinction. Since *Paragonimus* ova are destroyed by Ziehl-Neelsen stain for acid-fast bacilli, the sputum should first be examined for the eggs. The presence of a large number of eosinophils or Charcot-Leyden crystals in sputum suggests paragonimiasis.

In pulmonary paragonimiasis, praziquantel is the drug of choice (25 mg/kg after meals three times daily for 3 days, with a 4- to 6-hour interval between doses). (For side effects, see above under Schistosomiasis.) Bithionol is the alternative drug (30–50 mg/kg, given on alternate days for 10–15 doses [20–30 days]; the daily dose should be divided into a morning and evening dose). Side effects are frequent but generally mild and transient. Gastrointestinal side effects, particularly diarrhea, occur in most patients. Liver function should be tested serially. Bithionol is available in the USA only from the Parasitic Disease Drug Service, Centers for Disease Control, Atlanta, GA 30333. Antibiotics may be necessary for secondary pulmonary infection. Cure rates of over 90% can be anticipated for both praziquantel and bithionol.

In the acute stage of cerebral paragonimiasis, particularly meningitis, praziquantel or bithionol may be effective. With death of parasites, severe local reactions may occur; corticosteroids should therefore be given as in cerebral cysticercosis. In the chronic stage, both surgical removal of the parasites and drug usage are likely to be ineffective in diminishing neurologic symptoms.

Cha SH et al: Cerebral paragonimiasis in early active stage: CT and MR features. AJR Am J Roentgenol 1994; 162:141.

Kusner DJ, King CH: Cerebral paragonimiasis. Semin Neurol 1993;13:201.

Ripert C et al: Therapeutic effect of triclabendazole in patients with paragonimiasis in Cameroon: A pilot study. Trans R Soc Trop Med Hyg 1992;86:417.

Zihao Z et al: Antigen detection assay to monitor the efficacy of praziquantel for treatment of *Paragonimus westermani* infections. Trans R Soc Trop Med Hyg 1996; 90:43.

CESTODE INFECTIONS

TAPEWORM INFECTIONS
(See also Cysticercosis and Echinococcosis, below.)

Classification

Six tapeworms infect humans frequently. The large tapeworms are *Taenia saginata* (the beef tapeworm, up to 25 m in length), *Taenia solium* (the pork tapeworm, 7 m), and *Diphyllobothrium latum* (the fish tapeworm, 10 m). The small tapeworms are *Hymenolepis nana* (the dwarf tapeworm, 25–40 mm), *Hymenolepis diminuta* (the rodent tapeworm, 20–60 cm), and *Dipylidium caninum* (the dog tapeworm, 10–70 cm). Four of the six tapeworms occur worldwide; the pork and fish tapeworms have more limited distribution. Humans are the only definitive host of *T saginata and T solium*.

An adult tapeworm consists of a head (scolex), a neck, and a chain of individual segments (proglottids) in which eggs form in mature segments. The scolex is the attachment organ and generally lodges in the upper part of the small intestine.

Multiple infections are the rule for small tapeworms and may occur for *D latum;* however, it is rare for a person to harbor more than one or two of the taeniae.

A. Beef Tapeworm: The infection occurs in most countries with beef husbandry but is highly endemic in parts of the Far East, central and eastern Africa, and the central Asian area of the former Soviet Union. Gravid segments of *T saginata* in the human intestine detach themselves from the chain and are passed in feces to soil. When proglottids or eggs are ingested by grazing cattle or other domesticated bovines, the eggs hatch to release embryos that encyst in muscle as cysticerci. Humans are infected by eating raw or undercooked beef containing viable cysticerci, *Cysticercus bovis*. In the human intestines, the cysticercus develops into an adult worm.

B. Pork Tapeworm: This tapeworm is particularly prevalent in Mexico, Latin America, the Iberian Peninsula, the Slavic countries, Africa, Southeast Asia, India, and China. In the USA and Canada, human infection is rare, usually encountered in persons infected abroad; cysticercosis in hogs is uncommon. The infection is no longer found in northwestern Europe. The life cycle of *T solium* is similar to that of *T saginata* except that pigs ingest human feces containing proglottids and eggs to become the host of the larval stage. Humans become infected when they eat undercooked pork containing viable *C cellulosae*. Humans are also the intermediate host when they become infected with the larval stage (see Cysticercosis, below) by accidentally ingesting eggs in human feces; the eggs are immediately infectious. Transmission of eggs may occur as a result of autoinfection (hand to mouth), direct person-to-person transfer, ingestion of food or drink contaminated by eggs, or (rarely) regurgitation of proglottids into the stomach.

C. Fish Tapeworm: *D latum* is found in temperate and subarctic lake regions in many areas of the world, including northern Europe, Canada, Alaska, the Pacific Coast of the USA (the infection may no longer be present in the Great Lakes areas), Japan, Taiwan, Siberia, Manchuria, Australia, and southern South America and southern Africa. Eggs passed in human feces that reach fresh water are taken up first by crustaceans that in turn are eaten by fish, both of which are intermediate hosts. Human infection results from eating raw or inadequately cooked brackish or freshwater fish, including salmon. Nonhuman reservoir hosts include dogs, bears, and other fish-eating mammals.

D. Dwarf Tapeworm: *H nana* is the most common cestode. It can reach high prevalence, particularly in children, in regions of the world with poor fecal hygiene and in closed institutions worldwide. Humans are the definitive host of the human strain of the parasite; rodent-adapted strains occur in rodents. The life cycle is unusual in that both larval and adult stages are found in the human intestine, internal autoinfection can occur, and generally there is no intermediate host. Transmission usually results from eggs transferred directly from human to human (the eggs are immediately infective) but sometimes involves fomites, water, or food or the swallowing of fleas or beetles infected with the larval stage. *H nana* infections in children are usually lost spontaneously in adolescence.

E. Rodent Tapeworm: *H diminuta* is a common parasite of rodents. Many arthropods (eg, rat fleas, beetles, and cockroaches) serve as intermediate

hosts. Humans—most commonly young children—are infected by accidentally swallowing the infected arthropods, usually in cereals or stored products.

F. Dog Tapeworm: *D caninum* infection generally occurs in young children in close association with infected dogs or cats. Transmission results from swallowing the infected intermediate hosts, ie, fleas or lice.

Clinical Findings

A. Signs and Symptoms:

1. Large tapeworms–Large tapeworm infections are generally asymptomatic. Occasionally, vague gastrointestinal symptoms (eg, nausea, diarrhea, abdominal pain) and systemic symptoms (eg, fatigue, hunger, dizziness) have been attributed to the infections. Vomiting of proglottid segments or obstruction of the bile duct, pancreatic duct, or appendix is rare.

Some persons (mostly Scandinavian residents) who harbor the fish tapeworm develop a macrocytic megaloblastic anemia accompanied by thrombocytopenia and mild leukopenia. Gastric acidity is normal. The anemia is a result of the worm's competing with the host for vitamin B_{12}. Clinical findings are indistinguishable from those of pernicious anemia and include glossitis, dyspnea, tachycardia, and neurologic findings (numbness, paresthesias, disturbances of coordination, impairment of vibration and position sense, and dementia).

2. Small tapeworms–Light infections are generally asymptomatic. Heavy infections, particularly with *H nana,* may cause diarrhea, abdominal pain, anorexia, vomiting, weight loss, and irritability.

B. Laboratory Findings: Infection by a beef or pork tapeworm is often discovered by the patient finding segments in stool, clothing, or bedding. To determine the species, proglottid segments are either flattened between glass slides and examined microscopically for anatomic detail or differentiated by enzyme electrophoresis of glucose phosphate isomerase. Eggs are only infrequently present in stools, but the perianal cellophane tape test, as used to diagnose pinworm, is sometimes useful in detecting *T saginata* eggs. However, *Taenia* eggs look alike and do not permit species differentiation except by specialized methods. Detection of *Taenia*-specific antigens in stool, currently a research method, may become the most sensitive method for detecting infection.

Fish tapeworm is diagnosed by finding characteristic operculated eggs in stool; repeat examinations may be necessary. Proglottids are passed occasionally, and their internal morphology is also diagnostic. The presence of hydrochloric acid in the stomach differentiates the anemia from pernicious anemia; in both conditions, the Schilling test is abnormal.

H nana and *H diminuta* infections are diagnosed by finding characteristic eggs in feces; proglottids are usually not seen. *D caninum* infection is diagnosed by detection of proglottids (the size of melon seeds) in feces or after their active migration through the anus.

Serologic tests are not available for tapeworm infections; an ELISA for detection of coproantigens is under evaluation.

Treatment

A. Specific Measures: Although niclosamide and praziquantel are both drugs of choice for most tapeworm infections, praziquantel is more effective in hymenolepiasis, and some workers consider it to be somewhat more effective in taeniasis. In areas endemic for neurocysticercosis, a dose of praziquantel of 5 mg/kg or higher carries a small risk of activating the lesions.

1. *T saginata* and *D latum*—Praziquantel in a single dose of 10 mg/kg achieves cure rates of about 99%. At this dose, side effects (see under Schistosomiasis, above) are minimal. With a single dose of four tablets (2 g) of niclosamide, cure rates over 90% can be anticipated. The drug is given in the morning before the patient has eaten. The tablets *must be chewed thoroughly* and swallowed with water. Eating may be resumed in 2 hours. Niclosamide usually produces no side effects.

Pre- and posttreatment purges are not used for either drug. The anemia and neurologic manifestations of *D latum* respond to vitamin B_{12} as used in treatment of pernicious anemia.

2. *T solium*—The choice of drugs and methods of treatment are as above. For both drugs, it may be useful to give a moderate purgative 2–3 hours after treatment to rapidly eliminate segments from the bowel. The patient must be instructed about the need after defecation for careful washing of the hands and perianal area and for safe disposal of feces for 4 days following therapy.

3. *H nana*—Praziquantel, the drug of choice, produces 95% cure rates with a single 25 mg/kg dose. Niclosamide, the alternative drug, produces cure rates of 75% when given at the above dosage for 5–7 days; some workers repeat the course 5 days later.

4. *H diminuta* and *D caninum*—Treatment is with niclosamide or praziquantel in dosages as for *H nana*. Cure rates are not established.

B. Follow-Up Care: In treatment of large tapeworm infections, a disintegrating worm is usually passed within 24–48 hours of treatment. Since efforts are not generally made to recover and identify the scolex, cure can be presumed only if regenerated segments have not reappeared 3–5 months later. If it is preferred that parasitic cure be established immediately, the head (scolex) must be found in posttreatment stools; a laxative is given 2 hours after treatment, and stools must be collected in a preservative for 24 hours. To facilitate examination, toilet paper must be disposed of separately.

Prevention & Prognosis

C cellulosae is killed by cooking at 65 °C or freezing at –20 °C for 12 hours; *C bovis* at 56 °C or –10 °C for 5 days. Pickling is not adequate. Because the prognosis is often poor in cerebral cysticercosis (see below), *T solium* infections must be immediately eradicated.

Botero D et al: Taeniasis and cysticercosis. Infect Dis Clin North Am 1993;7:683.

Flisser A: Taeniasis and cysticercosis due to *Taenia solium*. Prog Clin Parasitol 1994;4:77.

Geerts S: The efficacy of praziquantel for the treatment of cestode and metacestode infections. Int J Antimicrob Ag 1994;4:321.

Shantz P: Tapeworms (cestodiasis). Gastroenterol Clin North Am 1996;25:637.

CYSTICERCOSIS

Essentials of Diagnosis

- History of exposure to *Taenia solium* in an endemic region; concomitant or past intestinal infection.
- Seizures and other symptoms and signs of a focal space-occupying central nervous system lesion.
- Subcutaneous or muscular nodules (5–10 mm); calcified lesions on x-rays of soft tissues.
- Calcified or uncalcified cysts by CT scan or MRI; positive serologic tests.

General Considerations

Human cysticercosis is infection by the larval (cysticercus) stage of the tapeworm *T solium* (see above). Prevalence rates to 10% are recognized in some endemic areas.

The natural history of the infection is incompletely known. Cysticerci complete their development within 2–4 months after larval entry and live for months to years. Several factors give rise to symptomatology: Initially, the live larva within a thin-walled cyst (vesicular cyst) is minimally antigenic. When the host immune response or chemotherapy results in gradual death of the cyst, there may be cyst enlargement (colloidal cyst) with mechanical compression, inflammation with pericyst edema, and (sometimes) vasculitis that can result in small cerebral infarcts; increased intracranial pressure and cerebrospinal fluid changes may follow. Subsequently, as the cyst degenerates over 2–7 years, it may disappear or be replaced by a granuloma, calcification, or residual fibrosis. Cysts at different life cycle stages—active (live), transitional, and inactive (dead)—may be present in the same organ. Although some patients develop an intense immune response to the parasite, others show a remarkable tolerance.

Locations of cysts in order of frequency are the central nervous system, subcutaneous tissues and striated muscle, globe of the eye, and, rarely, other tissues. Cysts reach 5–10 mm in soft tissues but may be larger (up to 5 cm) in the central nervous system. Attached to the inner wall of the cyst is an invaginated protoscolex with four suckers and a crown of hooks.

Clinical Findings

A. Signs and Symptoms:

1. Neurocysticercosis–In many patients, cysts remain asymptomatic. When symptomatic, the incubation period is highly variable (usually from 1 to 5 years but sometimes shorter). Manifestations are due to mass effect, inflammatory response, or obstruction of the brain foramina and ventricular systems. Neurologic findings are varied and nonspecific, in large part determined by the number and location of the cysts.

a. Acute invasive stage–This rare event, occurring shortly after invasion, results from extensive acute spread of cysticerci to the brain parenchyma. Fever, headache, myalgia, marked eosinophilia, and coma may occur.

b. Parenchymal cysts–Cysticerci can present singly or multiply and may be scattered or in clumps. Findings include epilepsy (focal or generalized), focal neurologic deficits, intracranial hypertension (intense headache, vomiting, papilledema, visual loss), and altered mental status. Seizures usually do not occur until the cyst or cysts have begun to die.

c. Subarachnoid space cysts and meningeal cysts–Small to large cysts are generally located in the cortical sulci or basal cisterns. The arachnoid is the principal basal membrane affected. Adhesive arachnoiditis may result in obstructive hydrocephalus, intracranial hypertension, arterial thrombosis leading to transient ischemia or stroke, and cranial nerve dysfunction (most often of the optic nerve).

d. Ventricular cysts may float freely (usually singly) within the ventricles or cerebral aqueduct or may be attached to the ventricular wall. They are usually asymptomatic but can cause increased intracranial pressure as a result of intermittent or total blockage.

e. Racemose cysts are rare aberrant forms that are multiple-branched, nonencysted, and lack a scolex; they present as grape-like irregular clusters and may reach over 10 cm in diameter. They generally are found in the ventricular and basal subarachnoid spaces, where they cause marked adhesive arachnoiditis and often obstructive hydrocephalus.

f. Spinal cord cysts can be extraspinal or intraspinal and cause arachnoiditis (meningitis, radiculopathy) or pressure symptoms.

2. Ophthalmocysticercosis–Usually there is a single cyst, free-floating in the vitreous or under the retina. Presenting symptoms include periorbital pain, scotomas, and progressive deterioration of visual acuity. Findings may include disk hemorrhage and edema, retinal detachment, iridocyclitis, and chorioretinitis. MRI but not CT may assist in diagnosis; immunologic tests are negative.

3. Subcutaneous and striated muscle cysticercosis–Subcutaneous cysts present as nodules that tend to appear, collapse and disappear, and then reappear in other sites after variable periods of time. They are usually asymptomatic.

B. Laboratory Tests:
Definitive diagnosis of neurocysticercosis requires finding the parasite on histologic section of specimens removed by excisional biopsy of skin or subcutaneous tissues (not of brain tissue). Patients should be thoroughly examined by palpation for pea-sized nodules. Presumptive diagnosis may be made by the following tests.

1. Imaging–Plain radiographs of muscle may detect oval or linear calcified lesions (4–10×2–5 mm). The lesions are usually multiple, sometimes in the hundreds, and the long axes of the cysts are nearly always in the plane of the surrounding muscle fibers. Plain skull films may demonstrate one or more cerebral calcifications (generally 5–10 mm; sometimes 1–2 mm when only the scolex is calcified).

The most useful procedures for examining the skull are imaging by CT and MRI. CT patterns for parenchymal cysts include (1) vesicular cysts (viable cysts with no host immune reaction), which are rounded areas of low density with little or no enhancement after contrast medium; (2) colloidal cysts (dead or dying cysts with host immune reaction), which are hypodense or isodense lesions surrounded by edema associated with ring-like or nodular enhancement; and (3) granuloma or calcifications (dead cysts), which are often several millimeters in diameter but variable in size. Signs of increased intracranial pressure and diffuse brain edema may also be seen. A combination of images is often found, owing to different developmental stages. As compared with CT, MRI has superior resolution for vesicular cysts (isodense, similar to cerebrospinal fluid) and for colloidal cysts (hyperdense). However, CT is superior for granulomas and calcifications, the most frequent presentations of cysticercosis, which MRI may miss. The MRI sometimes detects pathognomonic 2- to 4-mm nodules (protoscoleces) within cyst fluid. Intraventricular cysts (isodense) are not seen on routine CT but require intraventricular contrast medium. Spinal cysticercosis is evaluated by CT myelography or MRI.

2. Immunologic tests–With serum, the new immunoelectrotransfer blot test appears to reach nearly 100% specificity and 95% sensitivity (sensitivity appears to decline if only one or two cysts are present), whereas the ELISA showed, respectively, 63% and 65%. Hydatid disease and *H nana* infections cross-react in the ELISA. Sensitivity using cerebrospinal fluid was 86% by immunoblot and 62% by ELISA. Patients presenting with only calcified lesions or granulomas are generally serologically negative.

3. Other tests–The cerebrospinal fluid in neurocysticercosis should be evaluated for IgM (by ELISA) and IgG antibody; the fluid typically shows increased protein, decreased glucose, and a cellular reaction of mainly lymphocytes and eosinophils; eosinophilia over 20% is diagnostically important. Lumbar puncture is contraindicated in case of increased intracerebral pressure. The EEG may be abnormal. Though the patient usually no longer harbors a tapeworm, stools from both the patient and family members should be examined over several days by each individual for the passage of proglottids and by the laboratory for proglottids and eggs.

Differential Diagnosis

The differential diagnosis includes tuberculoma, tumor, hydatid disease, vasculitis, chronic fungal disorders, toxoplasmosis and other parasitic diseases, and neurosyphilis.

Treatment

Medical treatment is with albendazole (preferred) or praziquantel. Albendazole is more effective, and when corticosteroids are given concurrently, the plasma level of albendazole increases but that of praziquantel decreases. Anthelmintic treatment is most effective for parenchymal cysts; less effective for intraventricular, subarachnoid, or racemose cysts; and has no effect on and is not needed for granulomatous or calcified cysts. It remains to be fully established that medical treatment is preferable to symptomatic treatment followed by normal death of the parasites. Some clinicians wait 3 months, with selected patients, to see if cysts will spontaneously disappear without treatment. Drug treatment is withheld during the acute phase of cysticercotic encephalitis if intracranial hypertension is present.

Treatment should be conducted in hospital. In less than a week after starting treatment, inflammatory reactions around dying parasites may be manifested by meningismus, headache (analgesics may be sufficient for mild symptoms), vomiting, hyperthermia, mental changes, and convulsions; decompensation with death is very rare. It remains controversial whether to give steroids concomitantly to avoid or diminish this reaction or to use them only if marked symptoms appear or increase. Even when steroids are given prospectively, the inflammatory reaction may occur. Prednisone, 30 mg/d in two or three divided doses, starting 1–2 days before use of the drug and continuing at diminishing doses for about 14 days afterward, is one regimen. The reaction usually subsides in 48–72 hours, but continuing severity may require steroids in higher dosage and mannitol. Anticonvulsants must be continued during drug treatment and probably for an indefinite time afterward.

Following treatment, 50% cure rates (disappearance of cysts and clearing of symptoms) have been reported both for albendazole and praziquantel. Of the remaining patients, many have amelioration of symptoms, including intracranial hypertension and seizures.

In ocular cysticercosis, treatment with albendazole plus corticosteroids kills the cysts, reducing subretinal cysts to a small scar and allowing for easy extraction of vitreous cysts.

A. Specific Measures:

1. Albendazole–A dosage of 15 mg/kg/d in divided doses with meals for 8 days is as effective as the former 30-day course. Albendazole should be taken with a fatty meal to increase absorption. The drug is now available in the USA.

2. Praziquantel–Give 50 mg/kg/d for 15 days in three divided doses. Phenytoin, phenobarbital, and corticosteroids, when administered with praziquantel, reduce serum levels of the latter; high doses of praziquantel have been tried in these circumstances.

3. Surgery–Surgery has successfully removed orbital, cisternal, and ventricular cysts and, if accessible, cerebral, meningeal, or spinal cord cysts. When hydrocephalus is present, surgical shunt is required even when the parasites have been destroyed.

B. General Measures: Symptomatic treatment of neurocysticercosis is based on the use of steroids and mannitol for cerebral edema and anticonvulsants for seizures.

Prognosis

The fatality rate for untreated neurocysticercosis is about 50%; survival time from onset of symptoms ranges from days to many years. Drug treatment has reduced the mortality rate to about 5–15%. Surgical procedures to relieve intracranial hypertension along with use of steroids to reduce edema improve the prognosis for those not effectively treated with the drugs.

Carpio A et al: Is the course of neurocysticercosis modified by treatment with anthelmintic agents? Arch Intern Med 1995;155:1982.

Sotelo J, Del Brutto OH, Roman GC: Cysticercosis. Curr Clin Top Infect Dis 1996;16:240.

Webbe G: Human cysticercosis: Parasitology, pathology, clinical manifestations and available treatment. Pharmacol Ther 1994;64:175.

White AC: Neurocysticercosis: A major cause of neurologic disease worldwide. Clin Infect Dis 1997;24:101.

ECHINOCOCCOSIS
(Hydatid Disease, Hydatidosis)

Human echinococcosis results from parasitism by the larval stage of four *Echinococcus* species of which *Echinococcus granulosus* (cystic hydatid disease) and *Echinococcus multilocularis* (alveolar hydatid disease) are the most important. Minor species are *Echinococcus vogeli* (polycystic hydatid disease) from northern South America and Panama and *Echinococcus oligarthrus*. Echinococcosis is a zoonosis in which humans are an intermediate host of the larval stage of the parasite. The definitive host is a carnivore (all of which, except for the lion, are Canidae) that harbors the adult tapeworm in the small intestine; the carnivore becomes infected by ingesting the larval form in tissue of the intermediate host. The intermediate hosts, chiefly herbivorous mammals but also humans, become infected by ingesting tapeworm eggs passed in carnivore feces. The larval stage is referred to as a hydatid cyst.

1. CYSTIC HYDATID DISEASE (Unilocular Hydatid Disease)

Essentials of Diagnosis

- History of exposure to dogs associated with livestock in a hydatid-endemic region.
- Avascular cystic tumor of liver, lung, or, infrequently, bone, brain, or other organs as detected by imaging procedures.
- Symptoms and signs of a space-occupying mass.
- Positive serologic tests.

General Considerations

Human infection with *E granulosus* is common throughout southern South America, the Mediterranean littoral and the Middle East, central Asia, and East Africa. Endemic foci are in eastern Europe, Russia, Australia, New Zealand, India, and the United Kingdom; in North America, foci have been reported from the western USA, the lower Mississippi valley, Alaska, and northwestern Canada.

The pastoral strain—which is more pathogenic to humans—has a transmission cycle in which dogs are the definitive host, and sheep (usually) but also cattle and other domestic livestock are intermediate hosts. However, the strain in horses, pigs, and camels may be of low or no infectivity for humans. The sylvatic, or northern, strain is maintained in wolves and wild ungulates (moose and reindeer) in northern Alaska, Canada, Scandinavia, and Eurasia.

Human infection occurs when eggs passed in dog feces are accidentally swallowed. Liberated embryos penetrate the intestinal mucosa, enter the portal bloodstream, and are carried to the liver where they become hydatid cysts (65% of all cysts). Some larvae reach the lung (25%) and develop into pulmonary hydatids. Infrequently, cysts form in the brain, bones, skeletal muscles, kidneys, spleen, or other tissues. Cysts of the sylvatic strain tend to localize in the lungs.

The cyst wall has three layers: an inner germinal layer that gives rise within the cyst to germinal elements, a supporting intermediate layer, and an outer layer produced by the host. In the liver, cysts may in-

crease in size 1–30 mm in diameter per year and become enormous, but symptoms generally do not develop until they reach about 10 cm. Some cysts die spontaneously; others may persist unchanged for years. Part or all of the inner layer of hepatic and splenic cysts may calcify, which does not necessarily mean cyst death.

Clinical Findings

A. Symptoms and Signs: A liver cyst may remain silent for 10–20 or more years until it becomes large enough to be palpable, to be visible as an abdominal swelling, to produce pressure effects, or (rarely) to produce symptoms due to leakage or rupture. There may be right upper quadrant pain, nausea, and vomiting. The effects of pressure may result in biliary obstruction, with secondary bacterial cholangitis, cirrhosis, and portal hypertension. If a cyst ruptures suddenly, anaphylaxis and death may occur. If fluid and hydatid particles escape slowly, allergic manifestations may result, including a rise in the eosinophil count. Rupture can occur into the pleural, pericardial, or peritoneal space or into the duodenum, colon, or renal pelvis. Dissemination of germinal elements may be followed by the development of multiple secondary cysts. A characteristic clinical syndrome may follow intrabiliary extrusion of cyst contents—jaundice, biliary colic, and urticaria.

Pulmonary cysts cause no symptoms until they leak; become large enough to obstruct a bronchus, causing segmental collapse; or erode into a bronchus and rupture. Brain cysts produce symptoms earlier and may cause seizures or symptoms of increased intracranial pressure. Cysts in the bone marrow or spongiosa do not have a host layer, are irregular in shape, erode osseous tissue, and may present as pain or as spontaneous fracture. The bones most often affected are the vertebrae; many of these patients develop epidural extension with compression of the spinal cord and paraplegia. Because 20% of patients have multiple cysts, upon diagnosis each patient should be screened for cysts in the liver, spleen, kidneys, lungs, brain, bones, skin, tongue, vitreous, and other tissues.

B. Imaging: Sonography and CT scan are most commonly used to detect a cystic mass in the liver. Nearly pathognomonic is the presence within a hydatid cyst of daughter cysts; they must be distinguished, however, from blood clots within the cavity of simple cysts. The mass can also be defined by MR imaging, scintillation scan, or by angiography (rarely used). Spotty calcified densities or a calcified cyst wall may be seen in the liver or spleen. Chest films and thoracic CT scans may show a pulmonary lesion, but calcification of the wall does not occur. An intravenous urogram or bone scan may detect cysts at other sites.

C. Laboratory Findings: The immunoblot test, where available, is the test of choice (98% specific and 91% sensitive). The arc 5 test is also diagnostic except for cross-reactions with *T solium* cysticercosis infections. Several other serologic tests (ELISA and indirect hemagglutination and immunofluorescence) are useful for screening. Persons from whom cysts have been completely removed and carriers of dead cysts may become seronegative. The Casoni intracutaneous skin test has been abandoned because of poor specificity.

Eosinophilia is uncommon except after cyst rupture. Liver function tests are usually normal. Confirmation of the diagnosis is possible only by examination of cyst contents after surgical removal.

Percutaneous aspiration of hydatid cysts for diagnostic and therapeutic (injection of a scolicidal agent) purposes until recently has been contraindicated because of risk of leakage at the aspiration site (viable cysts are usually under pressure), with potential for anaphylaxis and dissemination of infection. Several workers have recently reported safe results achieved with the aid of sonographic monitoring, but the number of patients so treated is small and the duration of follow-up is short.

Differential Diagnosis

Noninfected hydatid cysts of the liver need to be differentiated from simple epithelial cysts; infected cysts, from bacterial and amebic abscesses. Hydatid cysts in any site may be mistaken for a variety of malignant and nonmalignant tumors and cysts. In the lung, a cyst may be confused with cavitary tuberculosis. Allergic symptoms arising from cyst leakage may resemble those associated with many other diseases.

Treatment & Prevention

Definitive treatment of hydatid cysts still consists of surgical removal. Although the role of drug treatment remains to be defined, information on the long-term safety and effectiveness of albendazole is accumulating. Decision making in the choice between the two modes of treatment must take into account (1) historical surgical mortality rates (1–4%), postoperative complications (10–25%), and recurrence rates after surgery (10% or higher); and (2) cure rates after albendazole treatment of 30–40%. One approach is to give a course of treatment to selected asymptomatic patients whose cysts are small and not in danger of rupture. If, after 6–9 months, the cyst has not disappeared or clearly died, it can then be removed surgically.

A. Surgical Treatment: Operative treatment of liver cysts involves several problems: total removal of all infective components of the cyst, avoiding cyst content spillage, selection of a scolicidal agent to be placed within the cyst, management of communications between the cyst and biliary tract (if present), management of the residual cavity, and minimizing the risk of operation. Scolicidal solutions, which include cetrimide (5%), hypertonic saline (20%), silver nitrate (0.5%), ethanol (70–95%), and sodium hypochlorite (3.75%), have come under criticism because of their potential for direct and indirect toxicity (an estimated 20% of cysts are thought to communicate with the biliary tract). To reduce the risk of recurrence due to spillage, albendazole is used preoperatively (at least 4 days) and postoperatively (1 month); the postoperative use of praziquantel is under evaluation. The treatment of bone cysts is by combined curettage, lavage, instillation of sterilization substances, and chemotherapy.

B. Drug Treatment:

1. Albendazole–Albendazole is more readily absorbed than mebendazole; this permits a lower dosage of albendazole to be used, yet its active metabolite, the sulfoxide, reaches effective concentrations in cyst wall and fluid. A current regimen is four tablets (800 mg) daily in divided doses with meals for 3 months. Among 253 patients treated in multiple studies, the outcomes for liver and lung cysts were, respectively, as follows: cured (33%, 40%), improved (44%, 37%), no change (21%, 22%), and worse (2%, 1%). In another study, findings for 59 patients with liver cysts (< 10 cm) followed for 3–7 years were as follows: cured (41%), improved (41%), no change (15%), worsened (none), and recurrences (two cases, or 3%). Bone cysts are more refractory and may require a year of treatment. In the 3-month courses, drug side effects include reversible low-grade aminotransferase elevations (17%), leukopenia to 2900/μL (2%), rare gastrointestinal symptoms (including pain at cyst sites), dizziness or headache, alopecia, rash, and pruritus. Anaphylaxis has been reported once and eosinophilia rarely, probably related to cyst fluid leakage.

2. Mebendazole–When mebendazole was used at high doses for several months, marked regression and apparent death of cysts occurred in some patients. In others, cysts were either stable or continued to grow and if removed were viable. The dosage is 50 mg/kg/d in three divided doses for 3 months, with many patients requiring repeated courses. The drug is taken with fatty meals. When possible, mebendazole levels should be monitored; serum levels in excess of 74 ng/mL 1–2 hours after an oral dose may be necessary for parasite killing. Occasional side effects with treatment include pruritus, rash, alopecia, reversible leukopenia, gastric irritation, musculoskeletal pain, fever, and acute pain in the cyst area; six cases of glomerulonephritis and three of agranulocytosis (with one death) have been reported.

3. Praziquantel–Praziquantel kills protoscoleces within hydatid cysts but does not affect the germinal membrane. The drug is being evaluated as adjunctive therapy with albendazole both pre- and postsurgery to protect against cyst spillage.

C. Prevention: In endemic areas, prevention is by prophylactic treatment of pet dogs with 5 mg/kg of praziquantel at monthly intervals to remove adult tapeworms and by health education to prevent feeding of offal to dogs.

Prognosis

Most liver and lung cysts can be removed surgically without great difficulty, but in patients with cysts in less accessible sites the prognosis is less favorable. The prognosis is always grave when there has been spillage and the development of secondary cysts. About 15% of untreated patients eventually die because of the disease or its complications.

2. ALVEOLAR HYDATID DISEASE (Multilocular Hydatid Disease)

Alveolar hydatid disease results from infection by the larval form of *Echinococcus multilocularis*. The life cycle involves foxes as definitive host and microtine rodents as intermediate host. Domestic dogs and cats can also become infected with the adult tapeworm when they eat infected wild rodents. Human infection is by accidental ingestion of tapeworm eggs passed in fox or dog feces. The disease in humans has been reported in parts of central Europe, much of Siberia, northern Japan, northwestern Canada, and western Alaska. Recent information has extended the Old World range southward to Iran and northern India and China. Increasing numbers of cases have been reported from central North America (eleven USA states and four Canadian provinces). The primary localization of alveolar cysts is in the liver, where they may extend locally or metastasize to other tissues. The larval mass has poorly defined borders and behaves like a neoplasm; it infiltrates and proliferates indefinitely by exogenous budding of the germinative membrane, producing an alveolus-like pattern of microvesicles. X-rays show hepatomegaly and characteristic scattered areas of radiolucency often outlined by 2- to 4-mm calcific rings. Serologic tests are the same as for cystic hydatid disease and cannot distinguish between the species. Treatment is by surgical removal of the entire larval mass when possible, accompanied by drug treatment. Ninety percent of patients with nonresectable masses die within 10 years. Long-term drug therapy (5 years to life) is with albendazole (preferred) (800 mg/d in divided doses) or with mebendazole (40 mg/kg/d in divided doses with fatty meals); the drugs inhibit growth of the parasite and have extended patient survival, but larval tissue is not completely destroyed.

Azar C, Bastid C: Echinococcus of the liver. Gut 1995;36:947.

Fenton-Lee D, Mossis DL: The management of hydatid disease of the liver. Part 1. Trop Doct 1996;26:173. (Review of surgical management.)

Nahmias J et al: Three- to 7-year follow-up after albendazole treatment of 68 patients with cystic echinococcosis (hydatid disease). Ann Trop Med Parasitol 1994;88:295.

WHO informal working group on echinococcosis in humans. Bull World Health Organ 1996;74:231.

Wilson JF, Rausch RL, Wilson FR: Alveolar hydatid disease. Review of the surgical experience in 42 cases of active disease among Alaskan Eskimos. Ann Surg 1995;221:315.

NEMATODE (ROUNDWORM) INFECTIONS

ANISAKIASIS

Anisakiasis is larval invasion of the stomach or intestinal wall by anisakid nematodes. In the acute form, the infection may mimic surgical abdomen; in the chronic form, mild symptoms may persist for weeks to years.

Definitive hosts are marine mammals, including whales, seals, and dolphins. Eggs discharged with feces are ingested by crustaceans, in which larvae develop that are infective for squids, mackerel, herring, cod, halibut, rockfish, salmon, tuna, and other marine fish. In the fish, the larvae pass to the musculature and are able to transfer from fish to fish along the food chain, eventually reaching a marine mammal, where they mature into the adult stage.

Humans are infected when they ingest larvae in marine fish or squid eaten raw, undercooked, salted, or lightly pickled. Larvae liberated in the stomach attach to or partially penetrate the gastric or intestinal mucosa (small bowel is more common; colon is rare), resulting in localized ulceration, edema, and eosinophilic granuloma formation; eventually, the parasite dies. Rarely, worms are coughed up and expectorated or penetrate the gut wall, enter the peritoneal cavity, and migrate. Most larvae, however, probably fail to cause infection and are passed in feces. Although the larvae sometimes develop to the adult stages, gravid females are not found in humans.

The infection occurs worldwide, but most cases have been reported in Japan and the Netherlands, with a few in the United States, Scandinavia, Chile, and other fish-eating countries. Regional foods eaten raw such as sashimi in Japan, pickled herring in the Netherlands, and ceviche (seviche) in Latin America are common vehicles of infection.

Clinical Findings

A. Symptoms and Signs: The majority of acute cases present as gastric anisakiasis. Occasionally, acute infection is followed by a chronic course.

1. Acute gastric anisakiasis—Within hours after larval ingestion, the patient experiences nausea, vomiting, and epigastric pain that progressively becomes more severe. Urticaria has been reported; hematemesis is rare.

2. Acute intestinal anisakiasis—Within 1–7

days, colicky pain appears in the lower abdomen, often localized at the ileocecal region, accompanied by diarrhea, nausea, vomiting, diffuse abdominal tenderness, and mild fever.

3. Chronic disease–For weeks to several years, symptoms may continue that mimic gastric ulcer, gastritis, gastric tumor, bowel obstruction, or inflammatory bowel disease.

B. Laboratory Findings: Stools may show occult blood, but eggs are not produced. Mild leukocytosis and eosinophilia may be present. ELISA and RAST serologic tests may be tried but are not reliable in chronic disease.

C. Imaging and Endoscopy: In acute infection, endoscopy is preferred because the larvae sometimes can be seen and removed from the stomach. X-rays of the stomach may show a localized edematous, ulcerated area with an irregularly thickened wall, decreased peristalsis, and rigidity. Double contrast technique may show the threadlike larvae. Small bowel x-rays may show thickened mucosa and segments of stenosis with proximal dilation. Ultrasound examination of gastric and intestinal lesions may also be useful.

In the chronic stage, x-rays and endoscopy of the stomach—but not of the bowel—may be helpful. The diagnosis is often made only at laparotomy with surgical removal of the parasite.

Prevention & Treatment

Prevention is by avoidance of ingestion of raw or incompletely cooked squid or marine fish, especially salmon, rockfish, herring, and mackerel; early evisceration of fish is recommended. Larvae within fish may with difficulty be seen as colorless, tightly coiled or spiraled worms in 3-mm whorls or as reddish or pigmented larvae lying open in muscles or viscera. The larvae are killed by temperatures about 60 °C or by freezing at –20 °C for 24 hours (7 days is advised by some workers). Smoking procedures that do not bring the temperature to 60 °C, marinating in vinegar, and salt-curing are not reliable.

There is no drug treatment. Except where larvae can be removed by fiberoptic gastroscopy or colonoscopy, treatment of acute and chronic lesions is limited to symptomatic measures; symptoms generally improve in 1–2 weeks. Surgical excision of the worm may be necessary in severe cases.

Bouree P, Paugam A, Petithory JC: Anisakidosis: Report of 25 cases and review of the literature. Comp Immunol Microbiol 1995;18:75.

Ishikura H et al: Anisakidae and anisakidosis. Prog Clin Parasitol 1993;3:43.

Kakizoe S et al: Endoscopic findings and clinical manifestations of gastric anisakiasis. Am J Gastroenterol 1995;90:761.

Muraoka A et al: Acute gastric anisakiasis: 28 cases during the past 10 years. Dig Dis Sci 1996;41:2362.

ANGIOSTRONGYLIASIS

1. ANGIOSTRONGYLIASIS CANTONENSIS (Eosinophilic Meningoencephalitis)

A nematode of rats, *Angiostrongylus cantonensis,* is the causative agent of a form of eosinophilic meningoencephalitis. It has been reported from Hawaii and other Pacific islands, Southeast Asia, Japan, China, Taiwan, Hong Kong, Australia, Egypt, Madagascar, Nigeria, Bombay, Cuba, Puerto Rico, Bahamas, Brazil, and New Orleans.

Human infection results from the ingestion of infective larvae contained in uncooked food—either the intermediate mollusk hosts (snails, slugs, planarians) or transport hosts that have ingested mollusks (crabs, shrimp, fish). Leafy vegetables contaminated by small mollusks or by mollusk slime may also be the source of infection, as can fingers during collection and preparation of snails for cooking. The mollusks become infected by ingesting larvae excreted in feces of infected rodents, the definitive host.

The incubation period in humans is 1–3 weeks. Ingested larvae (0.5 × 0.025 mm) invade the central nervous system, where, during migration, they may cause extensive tissue damage; at their death, a local inflammatory reaction ensues. The usual clinical findings are those of meningoencephalitis, including severe headache, fever, neck stiffness, nausea and vomiting, and multiple neurologic findings, particularly asymmetric transient cranial neuropathies. Worms in the spinal cord may result in sensory abnormalities in the trunk or extremities; worms have also been seen in the eye.

The spinal fluid characteristically shows elevated protein, eosinophilic pleocytosis, and normal glucose. Occasionally, the parasite can be recovered from spinal fluid. Peripheral eosinophilia with a low-grade leukocytosis is common. A serologic test is available from the Centers for Disease Control and Prevention; its sensitivity and specificity are not established. CT and MRI may show a central nervous system lesion.

The differential diagnosis includes tuberculosis, coccidioidal or aseptic meningitis, syphilis, lymphoma, gnathostomiasis, cysticercosis, paragonimiasis, echinococcosis, and schistosomiasis japonicum.

No specific treatment is available; however, levamisole, albendazole, thiabendazole (25 mg/kg three times daily for 3 days), mebendazole (100 mg twice daily for 5 days), or ivermectin can be tried. Theoretically, parasite deaths may exacerbate central nervous system inflammatory lesions. Symptomatic treatment with analgesics or corticosteroids may be necessary. The illness usually persists for weeks to months, the parasite dies, and the patient then recovers spontaneously, usually without sequelae. However, fatalities have been recorded.

Prevention is by rat control; by cooking of snails, prawns, fish, and crabs for 3–5 minutes or by freezing them (–15 °C for 24 hours); and by examining vegetables for mollusks before eating. Washing contaminated vegetables to eliminate larvae contained in mollusk mucus is not always successful.

Noskin GA, McMenamin MB, Grohmann SM: Eosinophilic meningitis due to *Angiostrongylus cantonensis.* Neurology 1992;42:1423.

2. ANGIOSTRONGYLIASIS COSTARICENSIS

Angiostrongylus costaricensis, which causes an eosinophilic ileocolitis, has been identified in humans (predominantly children) in Mexico, Central America, Venezuela, Brazil, and the USA (Texas). The known geographic range of the parasite in rodents (the definitive host) extends from northern South America to Texas. Infection occurs from ingestion of the larvae in the intermediate host (slugs, snails) or from food contaminated by larvae in slug or snail mucus. In humans, the larvae mature in the mesenteric vessels, where they cause thrombosis and ischemic necrosis of the intestine. Eggs lodging in capillaries give rise to eosinophilic granulomas, most commonly in the appendix but also in the terminal ileum, the cecum, the first part of the ascending colon, and the regional lymph nodes. Findings include fever, right lower quadrant abdominal pain and a mass, leukocytosis, and eosinophilia. Bowel complications consist of incomplete or complete obstruction and infarction. No serologic test is available; neither eggs nor larvae are passed in stool. The disease usually simulates acute appendicitis, which can in fact be caused by the parasite. Intra-abdominal mass can mimic tumor. There is no specific treatment; albendazole, thiabendazole, or mebendazole can be tried. Operative treatment is frequently necessary.

Hulbert TV, Larsen RA, Chandrasoma PT: Abdominal angiostrongyliasis mimicking acute appendicitis and Meckel's diverticulum: Report of a case in the United States and review. Clin Infect Dis 1992;14:836.

Vazquez JJ, Sola JJ, Boils AL: Hepatic lesions induced by *Angiostrongylus costaricensis.* Histopathology 1994; 25:489.

ASCARIASIS

Essentials of Diagnosis

- Pulmonary phase: Transient cough, dyspnea, wheezing, urticaria, with eosinophilia and transient pulmonary infiltrates.
- Intestinal phase: Vague upper abdominal discomfort; occasional vomiting, abdominal distention.
- Eggs in stools; worms passed per rectum, nose, or mouth.

General Considerations

Ascaris lumbricoides is the most common of the intestinal helminths; an estimated 1 billion people are infected worldwide. It is cosmopolitan in distribution and is found in high prevalence wherever there are low standards of hygiene and sanitation (including focally in southeastern USA) or where human feces are used as fertilizer. The infection is specific for humans and occurs in all age groups. Heavy worm burdens, however, are usually seen only in children, in whom there may be reduced nitrogen, fat, and D-xylose absorption and reduced mucosal lactate activity resulting in decreased growth rates.

Adult worms live in the upper small intestine. After fertilization, the female produces enormous numbers of eggs that pass in feces. Direct transmission between humans does not occur, as the eggs must remain on the soil for 2–3 weeks before they become infective. Thereafter, they can survive for years. Infection occurs through ingestion of mature eggs in fecally contaminated food and drink. The eggs hatch in the small intestine, releasing motile larvae that penetrate the wall of the small intestine and reach the right heart via the mesenteric venules and lymphatics. From the heart they move to the lung, burrow through the alveolar walls, and migrate up the bronchial tree into the pharynx, down the esophagus, and back to the small intestine. Egg production begins 60–75 days after ingestion of infective eggs. Adult worms (20–40 cm × 3–6 mm) live for 1 year or more.

Clinical Findings

A. Symptoms and Signs: As a result of their migration and induction of hypersensitivity, larvae in the lung cause capillary and alveolar damage, which may result in low-grade fever, nonproductive cough, blood-tinged sputum, wheezing, dyspnea, and substernal pain. There may be urticaria and localized rales. Rarely, larvae lodge ectopically in the brain, kidney, eye, spinal cord, etc, and may cause symptoms referable to those organs.

Small numbers of adult worms in the intestine usually produce no symptoms. With heavy infection, peptic ulcer-like symptoms or vague pre- or postprandial abdominal discomfort may be seen. Adult worms may also migrate with heavy infections; they may be coughed up, vomited, or emerge through the nose or anus. They may also force themselves into the common bile duct, pancreatic duct, appendix, diverticula, and other sites, which may lead to cholangitis, cholecystitis, pyogenic liver abscess, or pancreatitis. With very heavy infestations, masses of worms may cause intestinal obstruction, volvulus, or intussusception. During typhoid fever, worms may penetrate the weakened bowel wall. Rare cases of lung abscess or laryngeal obstruction with suffocation have been described. Moderate to high worm loads have been associated with stunting of growth in children. Periodic treatment of children with albendazole for multiple intestinal parasitism has resulted in improved nutrition.

B. Imaging: During the larval migratory phase, chest radiographs may show transitory, patchy, ill-defined asymmetric infiltrations (Löffler's syndrome). Intestinal infection is sometimes established by chance, when radiologic examination of the abdomen (with or without barium) shows the presence of worms. The diagnosis of biliary ascariasis can be made by endoscopic retrograde cholangiopancreatography, which has the therapeutic potential of removing the worms, and by ultrasonography. In intestinal obstruction, plain abdominal films show air-filled levels and multiple linear images of ascarides in dilated bowel loops; ultrasonography can also demonstrate the dilated bowel and worm mass.

C. Laboratory Findings: During the pulmonary phase, eosinophils may reach 30–50% and remain high for about a month; larvae are occasionally found in sputum. During the intestinal phase, diagnosis usually depends upon finding the characteristic eggs in feces. Occasionally, an adult worm spontaneously passed per rectum or orally reveals an unsuspected infection. Serologic tests are not useful, and there is no eosinophilia.

Differential Diagnosis

Pulmonary ascariasis with eosinophilia must be differentiated from nonparasitic causes (asthma, Löffler's syndrome, eosinophilic pneumonia, allergic bronchopulmonary aspergillosis), and parasitic causes (tropical pulmonary eosinophilia, toxocariasis, strongyloidiasis, hookworm, paragonimiasis). *Ascaris*-induced pancreatitis, appendicitis, diverticulitis, etc, must be differentiated from other causes of inflammation of these tissues. Postprandial dyspepsia may simulate duodenal ulcer, hiatal hernia, gallbladder disease, or pancreatic disease.

Treatment

Albendazole and pyrantel pamoate are the treatments of choice. None of the drugs listed below require pre- or posttreatment purges. Stools should be rechecked at 2 weeks and patients re-treated until all ascarids are removed. Ascariasis, hookworm, and trichuriasis infections, which often occur together, may be treated simultaneously by albendazole, mebendazole, or oxantel-pyrantel pamoate.

Because anesthesia stimulates the worms to become hypermotile, they should be removed in advance in infected patients undergoing elective surgery. In pregnancy, ascariasis should be treated after the first trimester.

Drug treatment should not be used in the migratory phase. In intestinal obstruction or biliary ascariasis, surgery may be avoided by nasogastric suction followed by a standard dose of an anthelmintic given via the tube. In biliary ascariasis, endoscopic removal of the worm under ultrasonographic guidance is often successful.

A. Albendazole: In light infections, a single dose of albendazole (400 mg) results in cure rates over 95%; in heavy infections, however, a 2- to 3-day course is indicated. Side effects, including migration of *Ascaris* through the nose or mouth, are rare. Albendazole is available in the USA though not approved for this indication. The drug is contraindicated in pregnancy.

B. Pyrantel Pamoate: Pyrantel pamoate as a single oral dose of 10 mg base/kg (maximum, 1 g) results in 85–100% cure rates. It may be given before or after meals. Infrequent and mild side effects include vomiting, diarrhea, headache, dizziness, and drowsiness.

C. Mebendazole: Mebendazole is highly effective when given in a dosage of 100 mg twice daily before or after meals for 3 days. Gastrointestinal side effects are infrequent. The drug is contraindicated in pregnancy.

D. Piperazine: The dosage for piperazine (as the hexahydrate) is 75 mg/kg body weight (maximum, 3.5 g) for 2 days in succession, giving the drug orally before or after breakfast. For heavy infestations, treatment should be continued for 4 days in succession or the 2-day course should be repeated after 1 week.

Gastrointestinal symptoms and headache occur occasionally; central nervous system symptoms (temporary ataxia and exacerbation of seizures) are rare. Allergic symptoms have been attributed to piperazine. The drug should not be used for patients with hepatic or renal insufficiency or in those with a history of seizures or chronic neurologic disease.

E. Levamisole: Levamisole, available in the USA but not approved for this indication, is highly effective as a single oral dose of 150 mg. Occasional mild and transient side effects are nausea, vomiting, abdominal pain, headache, and dizziness.

Prognosis

The complications caused by wandering adult worms require that all *Ascaris* infections be treated and eradicated.

Akgun Y: Intestinal obstruction caused by *Ascaris lumbricoides.* Dis Colon Rectum 1996;39:1159.

Albonico M et al: A randomized controlled trial comparing mebendazole and albendazole against *Ascaris, Trichuris* and hookworm infections. Trans R Soc Trop Med Hyg 1994;88:585.

Khuroo MS: Ascariasis. Gastroenterol Clin North Am 1996;25:553. (Review, including surgical diagnosis and treatment.)

Madiba TE, Hadley GP: Surgical management of worm volvulus. S Afr J Surg 1996;34:33.

CUTANEOUS LARVA MIGRANS
(Creeping Eruption)

Cutaneous larva migrans, prevalent throughout the tropics and subtropics, including southeastern USA, is caused by larvae of the dog and cat hookworms, *Ancylostoma braziliense* and *Ancylostoma caninum*. A number of other animal hookworms, gnathostomiasis, and strongyloidiasis are rarely also causative agents. Moist sandy soil (eg, beaches, children's sand piles) contaminated by dog or cat feces is a common site of infection. The infection is also reported in travelers to the tropics, among whom delayed onset beyond several weeks has been described.

At the site of larval entry, particularly on the hands or feet, up to several hundred minute, intensely pruritic erythematous papules appear. Two to 3 days later, serpiginous eruptions appear as the larvae migrate at a rate of several millimeters a day; the parasite lies slightly ahead of the advancing border. The process may continue for weeks; the lesions may become severely pruritic, vesiculate, encrusted, or secondarily infected. Without treatment, the larvae eventually die and are absorbed.

The diagnosis is based on the characteristic appearance of the lesions and the frequent presence of eosinophilia. Biopsy is usually not indicated.

Mild transient cases may not require treatment. For mild cases, thiabendazole cream (15% in a hygroscopic base) applied topically daily for 5 or more days is usually effective. In more severe cases, albendazole (now available in the USA), is the drug of choice at a dosage of 400 mg daily or twice daily for 3–5 days. It is nearly free of side effects. Albendazole applied as a paste to the skin is being evaluated. Based on increasing evidence, it is likely that a single oral dose of ivermectin (12 mg) will be a highly effective alternative drug. A third alternative, thiabendazole given orally as for strongyloidiasis, has significant side effects in about one-third of patients. Progression of the lesions and itching are usually stopped within 48 hours. Antihistamines are helpful in controlling pruritus; antibiotic ointments may be necessary to treat secondary infections.

Davies HD, Sakuls P, Keystone JS: Creeping eruption: A review of clinical presentation and management of 60 cases presenting to a tropical disease unit. Arch Dermatol 1993;129:588.

Jelinek T et al: Cutaneous larva migrans in travelers: Synopsis of histories, symptoms, and treatment of 98 patients. Clin Infect Dis 1994;19:1062.

Rodilla F, Colomia J, Magraner J: Current treatment recommendations for cutaneous larva migrans. Ann Pharmacother 1994;28:672.

Zaiman H: Cutaneous larva migrans. Trop Doct 1995; 25:136.

DRACUNCULIASIS
(Guinea Worm Infection, Dracunculosis, Dracontiasis)

Dracunculiasis is an infection of connective and subcutaneous tissues by the nematode *Dracunculus medinensis*. It occurs only in humans and is a major cause of disability. Since the start of the WHO eradication program, the number of infected persons has declined about 97% from over 3 million to 100,000. Endemic areas have been the Indian subcontinent; West and Central Africa north of the equator (Cameroon to Mauritania, Uganda, and southern Sudan); and Saudi Arabia, Iran, and Yemen. Almost all remaining cases are reported from Africa—75% from Sudan. All ages are affected, and prevalence may reach 60%.

Infection occurs by swallowing water containing the infected intermediate host, the crustacean *Cyclops* (copepods, water fleas). In the stomach, larvae escape from the crustacean and mature in subcutaneous connective tissue. After mating, the male worm dies and the gravid female (60–80 cm × 1.7–2.0 mm) moves to the surface of the body, where its head reaches the dermis and provokes a blister that ruptures on contact with water. Intermittently over 2–3 weeks, whenever the ulcer comes in contact with water, the uterus discharges great numbers of larvae, which are ingested by copepods. Most adult worms are gradually extruded; some worms retract and reemerge; and others die in the tissues, disintegrate, and may provoke a severe inflammatory reaction. Infection does not induce protective immunity.

Clinical Findings

A. Symptoms and Signs: The incubation period is 9–14 months. Infection may be at one or several sites. Several hours before the head appears at the skin surface, local erythema, burning, pruritus, and tenderness often develop at the site of emergence. There may also be a 24-hour systemic allergic reaction (pruritus, fever, nausea and vomiting, dyspnea, periorbital edema, and urticaria). After rupture, the tissues surrounding the ulceration frequently become indurated, reddened, and tender. Because most lesions appear on the leg or foot, patients often must give up walking and working for days to several months. Uninfected ulcers heal in 4–6 weeks. The worm rarely reaches ectopic sites.

Secondary infections, including tetanus, are common. Deep "cold" abscesses may result at the sites of dying, nonemergent worms. Ankle and knee joint infections with resultant deformity are common complications.

B. Laboratory Findings: When an emerging adult worm is not visible in the ulcer or under the skin, the diagnosis may be made by detection of larvae in smears from discharging sinuses. Immersion of an ulcer in cold water stimulates larval expulsion.

Eosinophilia is usually present. Skin and serologic tests are not useful. Calcified worms can be recognized on radiographs.

Treatment

All persons in an endemic area should be actively immunized against tetanus.

A. General Measures: The patient should be at bed rest with the affected part elevated. Cleanse the lesion, control secondary infection with topical antibiotics, and change dressings twice daily.

B. Manual Extraction: Traditional extraction of emerging worms by gradually rolling them out a few centimeters each day on a small stick is still useful, especially when done along with chemotherapy and use of aseptic dressings. The process appears to be facilitated by placing the affected part in water several times a day. If the worm is broken during removal, however, secondary infection almost always results, leading to cellulitis, abscess formation, or septicemia.

C. Anthelmintic Therapy: Metronidazole and thiabendazole are sometimes useful in alleviating symptoms and in reducing the duration of infection (by expediting spontaneous extrusion of worms or facilitating their manual extraction). The drugs have an anti-inflammatory effect but do not kill the adult or larvae.

1. Metronidazole, 250 mg three times daily for 10 days, causes only minimal toxicity. (See under Amebiasis).

2. Thiabendazole, 25 mg/kg twice daily for 2–3 days after meals, frequently causes side effects, sometimes severe (see under Strongyloidiasis, below).

3. Mebendazole, 400–800 mg daily for 6 days, can be tried.

D. Surgical Removal: Preemergent female worms can be surgically removed intact under local anesthesia if not firmly embedded in deep fascia or around tendons.

Prevention & Control

The disease is readily prevented by use of only noncontaminated drinking water. This can be accomplished either (1) by preventing contamination of community water supplies through use of tube wells, hand pumps, or cisterns or treating water sources with temephos; or (2) by filtering water through nets (eg, nylon nets of 100 μm pore size) or by boiling water. Eradication of the disease appears to be imminent. The last cases may now be appearing in Pakistan and India, with eradication remaining to be achieved in Yemen and parts of Africa. Since the WHO-sponsored eradication program began, estimated world annual incidence has dropped from 10 million to 2 million, and the disease has nearly been eradicated from Asia.

Hours M, Cairncross S: Long-term disability due to guinea worm. Trans R Soc Trop Med Hyg 1994;88:559.

Magnussen P, Yakubu A, Bloch P: The effect of antibiotic- and hydrocortisone-containing ointments in preventing secondary infections in guinea worm disease. Am J Trop Med Hyg 1994;51:797.

Progress toward global eradication of dracunculiasis. MMWR Morb Mortal Wkly Rep 1995;44:875.

Rohde JE et al: Surgical extraction of guinea worm: Disability reduction and contribution to disease control. Am J Trop Med Hyg 1993;48:71.

ENTEROBIASIS
(Pinworm Infection)

Essentials of Diagnosis

- Nocturnal perianal and vulvar pruritus, insomnia, irritability, restlessness.
- Vague gastrointestinal symptoms.
- Eggs demonstrable by cellulose tape test; worms visible on perianal skin or in stool.

General Considerations

Enterobius vermicularis (8–13 × 0.5 mm) is common worldwide. Humans, the only host, can harbor a few to hundreds of worms. Young children are affected more often than adults, and multiple infections occur in households and institutions with young children. High rates have been recorded in homosexual men, but the infection does not become opportunistic in HIV. A second species, *Enterobius gregorii,* has been described in England.

The adult worms inhabit the cecum and adjacent bowel areas, lying loosely attached to the mucosa. Gravid females migrate through the anus to the perianal skin and deposit eggs in large numbers. The eggs become infective in a few hours and may then infect others or be autoinfective if transferred to the mouth by contaminated food, drink, fomites, or hands. After being swallowed, the eggs hatch in the duodenum, and the larvae migrate down to the cecum. Retroinfection occasionally occurs when the eggs hatch on the perianal skin and the larvae migrate through the anus into the large intestine. The development of a mature ovipositing female from an ingested egg requires about 3–4 weeks. Eggs remain viable for 2–3 weeks outside the host. The life span of the worm is 30–45 days.

Clinical Findings

A. Symptoms and Signs: Many patients are asymptomatic. The most common and important symptom is perianal pruritus (particularly at night), due to the presence of the female worms or deposited eggs. Insomnia, restlessness, enuresis, and irritability are common symptoms, particularly in children. Many mild gastrointestinal symptoms have also been attributed to enterobiasis, but the association is difficult to prove. At night, worms may occasionally be seen near the anus. Perianal scratching may result in excoriation and impetigo. Adults sometimes report a "crawling" sensation in the anal area. Rarely, worm migration—including migration through the female genital tract or into the urethra—results in ectopic inflammation (vulvovaginitis, diverticulitis, appendicitis, cystitis) or granulomatous reactions (colon, genital tract, peritoneum, and elsewhere). Colonic ulceration and eosinophilic colitis have been reported.

B. Laboratory Findings: Diagnosis is made by finding eggs on the perianal skin (eggs are seldom found on stool examination). The most reliable method is by applying a short strip of sealing cellulose pressure-sensitive tape (eg, Scotch Tape) to the perianal skin and then spreading the tape on a slide for low-power microscopic study; toluene is used to clear the preparation. Three such preparations made on consecutive mornings before bathing or defecation will establish the diagnosis in about 90% of cases. Before the diagnosis can be ruled out, five to seven such examinations are necessary. Nocturnal examination of the perianal area or gross examination of stools may reveal adult worms, which should be placed in preservative, alcohol, or saline for laboratory examination. The worms can sometimes be seen on anoscopy. Eosinophilia is rare.

Differential Diagnosis

Pinworm pruritus must be distinguished from similar pruritus due to mycotic infections, allergies, hemorrhoids, proctitis, fissures, strongyloidiasis, and other conditions.

Treatment

A. General Measures: Symptomatic patients should be treated, and in some situations all members of the patient's household should be treated concurrently, since for each overt case there are usually several inapparent cases. Generally, however, treatment of all nonsymptomatic cases is not necessary. Careful washing of hands with soap and water after defecation and again before meals is important. Fingernails should be kept trimmed close and clean and scratching of the perianal area avoided. Ordinary washing of bedding will usually kill pinworm eggs; some workers recommend daily washing.

B. Specific Measures: Treatment with the following drugs should be repeated at 2 and 4 weeks. Albendazole, mebendazole, and pyrantel pamoate are the drugs of choice and can be given with or without food. Albendazole and mebendazole should not be used in pregnancy.

1. Albendazole is available in the USA though not approved for this indication. It may reach a 100% cure rate when given as a single 400 mg dose. Abdominal pain and diarrhea are rare.

2. Mebendazole as a single 100 mg dose is also

highly effective. It should be chewed for best effect. Gastrointestinal side effects are infrequent.

3. Pyrantel pamoate is highly effective, with cure rates of over 95%. It is administered as a 10 mg (base)/kg (maximum, 1 g) dose. Infrequent side effects include vomiting, diarrhea, headache, dizziness, and drowsiness. In the USA, pyrantel is available as self-medication for pinworm infection.

4. Other drugs–Piperazine, although effective, is not recommended because treatment requires 1 week. Thiabendazole is not recommended, because it causes frequent side effects which rarely are severe and life-threatening.

Prognosis

Although annoying, the infection is benign. Cure is readily attainable with one of several effective drugs. Reinfection is common, especially in children, because of continued exposure outside the home.

Cook GC: *Enterobius vermicularis* infection. Gut 1994; 35:1159.

Dahlstrom JA, Macarthur EB: *Enterobius vermicularis:* A possible cause of symptoms resembling appendicitis. Aust N Z J Surg 1994;64:692.

Grencis RK, Cooper ES: Enterobius, trichuris, capillaria, and hookworm including ancylostoma caninum. Gastroenterol Clin North Am 1996;25:579.

Lie LX et al: Eosinophilic colitis associated with larvae of the pinworm *Enterobius vermicularis*. Lancet 1995; 346:410.

FILARIASIS

More than 80 million people are infected with lymphatic filariasis, which is caused by three filiarial nematodes: *Wuchereria bancrofti, Brugia malayi,* or *Brugia timori.* W bancrofti is widely distributed in the tropics and subtropics of both hemispheres and on Pacific islands and is transmitted by *Culex, Aedes,* and *Anopheles* mosquitoes. *B malayi* is transmitted by *Mansonia* and *Anopheles* mosquitoes of South India, Sri Lanka, Southeast Asia, South China, the northern coastal areas of China, and South Korea. *B timori* is found on the southeastern islands of Indonesia.

No animal reservoir hosts are known for *W bancrofti* or *B timori*; cats, monkeys, and other animals may harbor *B malayi*. Mosquitoes become infected by ingesting microfilariae with a blood meal; at subsequent feedings, they can infect new susceptible hosts. Over months, adult worms (females, 8–9 cm × 0.2–0.3 mm) mature and live in or near superficial and deep lymphatics and lymph nodes and produce large numbers of viviparous circulating microfilariae, which may be seen in the blood starting 6–12 months after infection.

Pathologic changes in lymph vessels are due to host immunologic reactions to developing and mature worms. Living microfilariae generally cause no lesions, with the exception of tropical pulmonary eosinophilia. Rapid death of microfilariae, however, does produce findings, and an abscess may form at the site of a dying adult worm.

Dirofilariasis, infection by *Dirofilaria immitis,* the dog heartworm, has been reported in the USA, Japan, and Australia. Nodules have been found in the skin or as solitary 1–2 cm "coin" lesions in the periphery of the lungs. The serologic test for filariasis is positive, but there is no microfilaremia.

Other filiarial worms. Several other species infect humans—*Mansonella perstans, Mansonella streptocerca,* and *Mansonella ozzardi*—but usually without causing important findings.

Clinical Findings

A. Symptoms and Signs: The incubation period is generally 8–16 months in expatriates but may be longer in indigenous persons. Many infections remain asymptomatic, with or without microfilariae.

1. Acute disease–Episodes of fever (filarial fever), with or without inflammation of lymphatics and nodes, occur at irregular intervals and last for several days. Characteristically, the adenolymphangitis presents as retrograde extension from the affected node. With disease progression, epididymitis and orchitis as well as involvement of pelvic, abdominal, or retroperitoneal lymphatics may also occur intermittently. Lymph node enlargement may persist. In travelers, allergic-like findings (hives, rashes, eosinophilia) and lymphangitis and lymphadenitis are more likely to be present.

2. Chronic disease–Obstructive phenomena occur as a result of interference with normal lymphatic flow; this includes hydrocele, scrotal lymphedema, lymphatic varices and elephantiasis, particularly of the extremities, genitals, and breasts. Chyluria may result from rupture of distended lymphatics into the urinary tract. Extrapulmonary manifestations seen in some patients include lymphadenopathy or moderate hepatomegaly or splenomegaly.

3. Occult disease–A small proportion of infected persons develop occult disease, in which the classic clinical manifestations and microfilaremia are not present but microfilariae are present in the tissues.

In **tropical pulmonary eosinophilia,** microfilariae of *W bancrofti* or *B malayi* are sequestered in the lungs but not found in the blood. The condition is characterized by episodic nocturnal coughing or wheezing, hypereosinophilia, high filarial antibody titers and IgE levels, diffuse miliary lesions or increased bronchovascular markings on chest films, fever (sometimes), and a response to diethylcarbamazine treatment (6 mg/kg daily for 21 days). Relapses (in 20%) require re-treatment with up to 12 mg/kg

daily for up to 30 days. If untreated, the condition can progress to chronic pulmonary fibrosis.

B. Laboratory Findings: Diagnosis is established by finding microfilariae in the blood. In indigenous persons, they are rare in the first 2–3 years, abundant as the disease progresses, and again rare in the obstructive stage. In persons from nonendemic areas, inflammatory reactions may be prominent in the absence of microfilariae. Microfiliariae of *W bancrofti* are found in the blood chiefly at night (nocturnal periodicity 10 PM to 2 AM), except for a nonperiodic variety in the South Pacific. *B malayi* microfilariae are usually nocturnally periodic but in Southeast Asia may be present at all times, with a slight nocturnal rise. Anticoagulated blood specimens are collected at times related to the periodicity of the local strain. Specimens may be stored at ambient temperatures until examined in the morning by wet film for motile larvae and by Giemsa-stained smears—thick for sensitivity and thin for specific morphology. A formalin-anionic detergent preservative can also be used. If these are negative, the blood specimens should be concentrated by the Knott concentration or membrane filtration technique. If all are negative, oral administration of 50 mg of diethylcarbamazine often results in positive blood specimens (within minutes to an hour) or a systemic reaction (itching, papular rash, myalgia). If negative, repeat with 200 mg. When onchocerciasis or loiasis may be present, this test must be done with extreme caution.

Serologic tests may be helpful in diagnostic screening, but false-positive (other filarial and helminthic infections) and false-negative reactions occur. An indirect hemagglutination titer of 1:128 and a bentonite flocculation titer of 1:5 in combination are considered minimum significant titers. ELISA-IgG and IgE tests are available. Eosinophil counts may be elevated. Testing for antigenemia, now experimental, may prove useful in diagnosis (examining daytime blood specimens and detecting some amicrofilaremic infections) and in monitoring efficacy of treatment. In differential diagnosis, lymphangiography (potentially damaging to the lymphatics) and radionuclide lymphoscintigraphy may be useful lymphatic imaging methods. As live adult worms can be detected by ultrasonography, the method can be useful in detecting adult worms in amicrofilaremic persons.

Treatment, Prevention, & Prognosis

Diethylcarbamazine, the drug of choice, rapidly kills blood microfilariae but only slowly kills or injures adult worms. Cure may require multiple 3-week courses (2 mg/kg three times a day after meals, starting with small doses, and gradually increasing over 3–4 days). At this dose, the drug rarely produces direct toxicity. However, adverse immunologic reactions to dying microfilariae and adult worms are common—more so with brugian than with bancroftian filariasis. Reactions are local (lymphadenitis, abscess, ulceration) and systemic (fever, headache, myalgia, dizziness, malaise, and other allergic responses). Antipyretics and analgesics may be helpful. In areas where onchocerciasis or loiasis is also prevalent, special care must be taken not to provoke reactions to dying microfilariae of these parasites. Diethylcarbamazine has also been extensively used in mass treatment programs and is being evaluated for prophylaxis. In the USA, the drug is available only from the manufacturer, Lederle Laboratories, 914-735-5000.

During acute inflammatory episodes, it is controversial whether to treat and whether drug usage will shorten the attack. General measures include bed rest, antibiotics for secondary infections, use of elastic stockings and pressure bandages for leg edema, and suspensory bandaging for orchitis and epididymitis.

Small hydroceles may benefit from a locally injected sclerosing agent, or surgery may be indicated. To manage elephantiasis, lymphovenous shunt procedures may be useful, combined with removal of excess subcutaneous fatty and fibrous tissue, postural drainage, and physiotherapy.

Ivermectin, a microfilaricide, continues under evaluation as a single 400 µg/kg dose, which is repeated in 6 months. Diethylcarbamazine is still needed to kill the adult worms. Both drugs appear to be equally efficacious in reducing microfilarial burdens; mild side effects (myalgia, headache, fever) are similar in some studies but less so for ivermectin in others.

The prognosis is good with treatment of early and mild cases (including low-grade lymphedema, chyluria, small hydrocele), but in advanced infection the prognosis is poor.

Andrade LD et al: Comparative efficacy of three different diethylcarbamazine regimens in lymphatic filariasis. Trans R Soc Trop Med Hyg 1995;89:319.

Moore TA et al: Diethylcarbamazine-induced reversal of early lymphatic dysfunction in a patient with bancroftian filariasis: Assessment with use of lymphoscintigraphy. Clin Infect Dis 1996;23:1007.

Moulia-Pelat JP et al: Combination ivermectin plus diethylcarbamazine, a new effective tool for control of lymphatic filariasis. Trop Med Parasitol 1995;46:9.

Ottesen EA: Filarial infections. Infect Dis Clin North Am 1993;7:619.

Sharma S: Drugs for filariasis: Adv Drug Res 1993;24:200.

GNATHOSTOMIASIS

Gnathostomiasis, due for the most part to infection by the larval stage of the nematode *Gnathostoma spinigerum,* is rarely caused by other *Gnathostoma* species. Infection is most common in Thailand and Japan but is also reported from Southeast Asia, China, India, Mexico, Ecuador, Israel, and East Africa. In the USA, though *G spinigerum* has rarely been seen in minks, it has not been reported in humans. Eggs passed in feces of the definitive hosts, wild and domestic dogs and cats, are infective for copepods (water fleas). Ingestion of copepods by secondary hosts results in encysted larvae in their tissues; humans are infected when these larvae are ingested in raw, marinated, or inadequately cooked freshwater fish, chicken or other fowl, frogs, or pork. Infection has also been attributed to ingestion of infected copepods in water.

Within 24–48 hours, larval migration through the intestinal wall can cause acute epigastric pain, vomiting, urticaria, and eosinophilia. The worm then migrates to subcutaneous and other tissues but is unable to mature. Most common is a pruritic subcutaneous swelling up to 25 cm across, occasionally accompanied by stabbing pain. Over weeks to years, the swelling may remain in one area for days or weeks, or move continuously. Occasionally the worm becomes visible under the skin.

Internal organs and the eye may also be invaded. Spontaneous pneumothorax, leukorrhea, hematemesis, hematuria, hemoptysis, paroxysmal coughing, and edema of the pharynx with dyspnea have been reported as complications. Invasion of the brain can result in an eosinophilic meningoencephalitis or subarachnoid hemorrhage. Spinal cord invasion can lead to myelitis or radiculopathy.

Definitive diagnosis is sometime possible by surgical removal of the worm when it appears close to the skin. Marked eosinophilia is common, except for parasites in the central nervous system. Serodiagnosis by immunoblot assay or ELISA is promising. Skin and other serologic tests are unsatisfactory.

Treatment with albendazole may be effective. Among presumptively diagnosed cases, 94 of 100 persons were apparently cured after a dosage of 400 mg or 800 mg (in divided doses) of the drug daily for 21 days. Larval death appeared to occur slowly over 1–2 weeks. Ivermectin has been reported to be effective in animals. Courses of prednisolone have provided temporary relief of symptoms.

Crowley JJ, Kim YH: Cutaneous gnathostomiasis. J Am Acad Dermatol 1995;33:825.

Houston S: Gnathostomiasis: Report of a case and brief review. Can J Infect Dis 1994;5:125.

Kraivichian P et al: Albendazole in the treatment of human gnathostomiasis. Trans R Soc Trop Med Hyg 1992;86:418.

Rusnak JM, Lucey DR: Clinical gnathostomiasis: Case report and review of the English language literature. Clin Infect Dis 1993;16:33.

HOOKWORM DISEASE

Essentials of Diagnosis

Early findings (not commonly recognized):
- Dermatitis: pruritic, erythematous, papulovesicular eruption at site of larval invasion.

- Pulmonary migration of larvae: transient episodes of coughing, asthma, fever, blood-tinged sputum, marked eosinophilia.

Later findings:

- Intestinal symptoms: anorexia, diarrhea, abdominal discomfort.
- Anemia (iron deficiency): fatigue, pallor, dyspnea on exertion, poikilonychia, heart failure.
- Characteristic eggs and occult blood in the stool.

General Considerations

Hookworm disease, widespread in the moist tropics and subtropics and sporadically in southeastern USA, is caused by *Ancylostoma duodenale* and *Necator americanus.* Probably a quarter of the world's population is infected, and in many areas the infection is a major cause of general debility, retardation of growth and development of children, and increased susceptibility to infections. About 50,000 deaths of young children yearly are attributed directly to hookworm infection; other deaths of young infected children occur from various infections that could normally be tolerated, such as malaria, measles, and those that cause diarrhea.

In the Western Hemisphere and tropical Africa, *Necator* was the prevailing species, and in the Far East, India, China, and the Mediterranean area, *Ancylostoma* was prevalent, but both species have now become widely distributed. Infection is rare in regions with less than 40 inches of rainfall annually. Humans are the only host for both species.

The adult worms are approximately 1 cm long. Eggs produced by females are passed in the stool and must fall on warm, moist soil if hatching followed by larval development is to take place. Larvae remain infective for hours to about a week, depending on environmental conditions. Following skin penetration, the larvae migrate in the bloodstream to the pulmonary capillaries, break into alveoli, and then are carried by ciliary action upward to the bronchi, trachea, and mouth. After being swallowed, they reach and attach to the mucosa of the upper small bowel; maturation and release of egg occurs in 6–8 weeks. *Ancylostoma* infection can also be acquired by ingestion of the larvae in food or water. Adult *Ancylostoma* survive about a year; *Necator,* about 3–5 years.

The worms suck blood at their attachment sites. The estimated hookworm load for 1000 eggs per gram of feces (light infection) is 11 for *Ancylostoma* and 32 for *Necator;* the daily blood loss per worm is estimated, respectively, to be 0.2 mL and 0.04 mL. Over a period of years, even small worm burdens can significantly deplete iron reserves: Depending on the host's dietary intake of iron, severe anemia may result if 30 or more *Ancylostoma* or 100 or more *Necator* worms are present. A moderate worm load is 2000–8000 eggs per gram of feces.

Clinical Findings

A. Symptoms and Signs: Ground itch, the first manifestation of infection, is a pruritic erythematous dermatitis, either maculopapular or vesicular, that follows skin penetration of the infective larvae. Severity is a function of the number of invading larvae and the sensitivity of the host. Scratching may result in secondary infection. Strongyloidiasis and cutaneous larva migrans must be considered in the differential diagnosis at this stage.

The pulmonary stage, in which there is larval migration through the lungs, may show dry cough, wheezing, blood-tinged sputum, and low-grade fever. The pulmonary migration of *Ascaris* and *Strongyloides* larvae can produce similar findings.

After two or more weeks, maturing worms attach to the mucosa of the duodenum and upper jejunum. In heavy infections, worms may reach the ileum. Patients who have light infections and adequate iron intake often remain asymptomatic. In heavy infections, however, there may be anorexia, diarrhea, vague abdominal pain, and ulcer-like epigastric symptoms. Severe anemia may result in pallor, deformed nails, pica, and cardiac decompensation. Marked protein loss may also occur, resulting in hypoalbuminemia, with edema and ascites. There are conflicting reports of malabsorption in some severe infections.

Reduction in worm loads and symptoms after the first decade of life suggests that a moderate degree of immunity develops.

B. Laboratory Findings: Diagnosis depends upon demonstration of characteristic eggs in feces; a concentration method may be needed. The two species cannot be differentiated by the appearance of their eggs. The stool usually contains occult blood. Hypochromic microcytic anemia can be severe, with hemoglobin levels as low as 2 g/dL, a low serum iron and a high iron-binding capacity, and low serum ferritin. Eosinophilia (as high as 30–60% of a total white blood count reaching 17,000/μL) is usually present in the pulmonary migratory stage of infection but is not marked in the chronic intestinal stage.

Treatment

A. General Measures: The availability of safe anthelmintics makes it possible to treat all patients initially, irrespective of the intensity of infection; nevertheless, it may not be necessary or beneficial to treat light infections. Re-treatment may be necessary at 2-week intervals until the worm burden is reduced to a low level as estimated by semiquantitative egg counts. Eradication of infection is not essential, since light infections do not injure the well-nourished patient and iron loss is replaced if the patient is receiving adequate dietary iron.

If anemia is present, oral ferrous sulfate and a diet high in protein and vitamins are required for at least 3 months after the anemia has been corrected in order to replace iron stores. A dosage schedule for ferrous sulfate tablets (200 mg) is one tablet three times daily for 2 months followed by one tablet daily for 4 months. Parenteral iron is rarely indicated. Blood transfusion may be necessary if anemia is severe.

B. Specific Measures: Mebendazole, pyrantel, and albendazole are highly effective drugs for treatment of both hookworm species; mebendazole or albendazole can be used to treat concurrent trichuriasis, and all three drugs can be used to treat concurrent ascariasis. The drugs are given before or after meals, without purges. For the three drugs, mild gastrointestinal side effects are rare; none should be used in pregnancy. Albendazole and mebendazole should not be given to children under about 1 year of age.

1. Pyrantel pamoate–In *A duodenale* infections, pyrantel given as a single dose, 10 mg (base)/kg (maximum 1 g), produces cures in 76–98% of cases and a marked reduction in the worm burden in the remainder. For *N americanus* infections, a single dose may give a satisfactory cure rate in light infection, but for moderate or heavy infection a 3-day course is necessary. If the species is unknown, treat as for necatoriasis. Mild and transient drowsiness and headache may occur.

2. Mebendazole–When mebendazole is given at a dosage of 100 mg twice daily for 3 days, reported cure rates for both hookworm species range from 35% to 95%.

3. Albendazole, given orally once only at a dosage of 400 mg, results in the cure of 85–95% of patients with *Ancylostoma* infection and markedly reduces the worm burden in those not cured. Because cure rates for single-dose treatments of *Necator* infection were 33–90%, treatment should be continued for 2–3 days, especially in heavy infections. Albendazole is available in the USA, though it is not FDA-approved for this indication.

Prognosis

If the disease is recognized before serious secondary complications appear, complete recovery is the rule following treatment.

Eosinophilic Enteritis

In Australia, *Ancylostoma caninum,* the dog hookworm, has been found to cause abdominal pain, diarrhea, and peripheral eosinophilia.

Croese J et al: Human enteric infection with canine hookworms. Ann Intern Med 1994;120:369.

Gilles HM, Ball PAJ: *Hookworm Infections.* Elsevier Science, 1991.

Grencis RK, Cooper ES: Enterobius, trichuris, capillaria, and hookworm including ancylostoma caninum. Gastroenterol Clin North Am 1996;25:579.

Hotez PJ, Pritchard DI: Hookworm infection. Sci Am 1995 Jun;272:68.

LOIASIS

Loiasis is a chronic filarial disease caused by infection with *Loa loa.* The infection occurs in humans and monkeys in rain and swamp forest areas of West Africa from Nigeria to Angola and throughout the Congo river watershed of central Africa eastward to southwest Sudan and western Uganda. An estimated 3–13 million persons are infected.

The adult worms live in the subcutaneous tissues for up to 12 years. Gravid females release microfilariae into the bloodstream which subsequently are ingested in a blood meal by the vector-intermediate host, female *Chrysops* species, day-biting flies. When the fly feeds again, the larval stage can infect a new host or cause superinfection. The time to worm maturity and detection of new microfilariae is 6 months to several years.

Clinical Findings

A. Symptoms and Signs: Many infected persons are asymptomatic. In symptomatic persons, the worms (females, 4–7 cm × 0.5 mm) are evidenced by their temporary appearance beneath the skin or conjunctiva, by unilateral edema of an extremity, or by Calabar swellings. The latter are subcutaneous edematous reactions, 3–10 cm in diameter, nonpitting and nonerythematous, and at times associated with low-grade fever, local pain, and pruritus. The swellings may migrate a few centimeters for 2–3 days or stay in place before they subside. At irregular intervals, they recur at the same or different sites, but only one appears at a time. When near joints, they may be temporarily disabling. Migration across the eye may be asymptomatic or may produce pain, intense conjunctivitis, and eyelid edema. Dying adult worms may elicit small nodules or local sterile abscesses, and dead worms may result in radiologically detectable calcification.

Microfilariae in the blood do not induce symptoms. Rarely, however, they enter the central nervous system and may cause encephalitis, myelitis, or jacksonian seizures; the larvae can also induce lesions and complications in the retina, heart, lungs, and other tissues.

Natives generally have a mild form of the infection or are asymptomatic but are microfilaremic and serologically positive. The disease among visitors, however, is often characterized by more pronounced immunologically mediated symptoms (frequent and debilitating Calabar swellings, elevated leukocyte and eosinophil counts, hypergammaglobulinemia, increased polyclonal IgE) and frequently a positive serologic test but nondetectable microfilaremia.

B. Laboratory Findings: Specific diagnosis is made by finding characteristic microfilariae in daytime (10 AM to 4 PM) blood specimens by concentration methods; in order of increasing sensitivity, they are (1) thick films, (2) Knott's concentration, and

(3) Nuclepore filtration. Presumptive diagnosis that permits treatment is based on Calabar swellings or eye migration, a history of residence in an endemic area, and marked eosinophilia (40% or greater). Serologic tests may be positive, but cross-reactions occur with other filarial diseases and sometimes with nematode infections.

Treatment & Prognosis

See references for details on proper use of diethyl-carbamazine (drug of choice both as a micro- and macrofilaricide), since side effects to dying microfilariae may be severe, and life-threatening encephalitis can occur rarely. The dosage is 50 mg once (day 1), 50 mg three times daily (day 2), 100 mg three times daily (day 3), and 3 mg/kg three times daily (days 4–21). One course of treatment cures about 50% of patients; three courses, 90%. Reactions are more likely with pretreatment microfilaria counts greater than 25/μL. Cytapheresis has been used to reduce parasite loads before starting diethycarbamazine. Prednisone is sometimes indicated to minimize reactions. Ivermectin is being evaluated for initial treatment of patients with high microfilaria loads; however, even among amicrofilaremic patients, a few have a severe reaction and require hospitalization. Surgical removal of adult worms from the eye or skin is not recommended.

Individual protection is facilitated by daytime use of insect repellent and by wearing light-colored clothing with long sleeves and trousers. Diethylcarbamazine prophylaxis, 300 mg weekly, may be useful if the risk of exposure is high. It is not indicated, however, for the casual traveler or for persons who might previously have acquired any of the filarial infections.

Most infections run a benign course, but some are accompanied by severe and temporarily disabling symptoms. The prognosis is excellent with treatment.

Churchill DR et al: Clinical and laboratory features of patients with loiasis (*Loa loa* filariasis) in the U.K. J Infect 1996;33:103.

Hovette P et al: Efficacy of ivermectin treatment of *Loa loa* filariasis patients without microfilaraemias. Ann Trop Med Parasitol 1994;88:93.

Klion AD, Otteson EA, Nutman TB: Effectiveness of diethylcarbamazine in treating loiasis acquired by expatriate visitors to endemic regions: Long-term follow-up. J Infect Dis 1994;169:604.

Wahl G, Georges AJ: Current knowledge on the epidemiology, diagnosis, immunology, and treatment of loiasis. Trop Med Parasitol 1995;46:287.

ONCHOCERCIASIS

Onchocerciasis is a chronic filarial disease caused by *Onchocerca volvulus*. The advent of the safe and effective drug ivermectin has led to effective treatment and control of the disease. Primary findings are subcutaneous nodules that contain adult worms and skin and eye changes that result from dead or dying microfilariae. Heavy infection leads to chronic pruritus, disfiguring skin lesions, visual impairment, and debility. An estimated 18 million persons are infected, of whom 0.3 million are blinded by the condition and 0.5 million severely visually impaired. In hyperendemic areas, more than 40% of inhabitants over 40 years of age are blind. The infection, predominant in West Africa, also occurs in many other parts of tropical Africa and in localized areas of the southwestern Arabian peninsula, southern Mexico, Guatemala, Venezuela, Colombia, and northwestern Brazil. The West African savanna strain is especially associated with severe blinding eye lesions.

Humans are the only important host. The vector and intermediate host are *Simulium* flies, day biters that breed in rivers and fast-flowing streams and become infected by ingesting microfilariae with a human blood meal; at subsequent feedings, they can infect new susceptible hosts.

Clinical Findings

A. Symptoms and Signs: Adult worms, which can live for up to 14 years, typically are in fibrous subcutaneous nodules that are painless, freely movable, and 0.5–1 cm in diameter. Many nodules, however, are deep in the connective and muscular tissues and nonpalpable. The interval from exposure to onset of symptoms can be as long as 1–3 years. Female worms release motile microfilariae into the skin, subcutaneous tissues, lymphatics, and eyes; microfilariae are occasionally seen in the urine but rarely in blood or cerebrospinal fluid. Skin manifestations are localized or cover large areas. Pruritus may be severe, leading to skin excoriation and lichenification; other findings include pigmentary changes, papules, scaling, atrophy, pendulous skin, and acute inflammation. Pruritus may occur in the absence of skin lesions. There may be marked enlargement of femoral and inguinal nodes and generalized lymph node enlargement. Microfilariae in the eye may lead to visual impairment and blindness; findings include itching, photophobia, anterior segment changes (limbitis, punctuate and sclerosing keratitis, iritis, secondary glaucoma, cataract), and posterior segment changes (optic neuritis, optic atrophy, chorioretinitis, and other retinal and choroidal findings). Infected visitors, as compared with indigenous persons, may show a more prominent dermatitis despite a low to nondetectable microfiladerma or eosinophilia and an absence of nodules and eye disease.

B. Laboratory Findings: Diagnosis is by demonstrating microfilariae in skin snips (usually obtained with a punch biopsy instrument), identifying them in the cornea or anterior chamber by slitlamp examination, or by nodule aspiration or excision.

Skin snips are placed in saline and incubated overnight before examination. Adult worms may be recovered in excised nodules, whereas ultrasound has been used to detect nonpalpable onchocercomas and to distinguish them from other lesions (lipomas, fibromas, lymph nodes, foreign body granulomas). Skin and serologic tests are usually positive, but cross-reactions occur with other forms of filariasis. Immunoblot analysis of IgG4 antibodies appears to be more sensitive than skin snips earlier in infection, but cross-reactions also occur with other filarial infections. Diagnosis by polymerase chain reaction on skin snips may prove to be the most sensitive test for diagnosis and for assessing posttreatment status. Eosinophilia (15–50%), polyclonal hypergammaglobulinemia, and elevated IgE levels are common.

Treatment & Prognosis

Nodules on or near the head should be removed surgically. Drug treatment is with ivermectin (a microfilaricide) as a single oral dose of 150 µg/kg given with water on an empty stomach. The number of microfilariae in the skin diminishes markedly within 2–3 days, remains low for months, and then gradually increases; microfilariae in the anterior chamber of the eye decrease slowly in number over months, eventually disappear, and then gradually return. The optimum frequency of treatment to control symptoms and prevent disease progression remains to be determined. In one schedule, the dose is repeated at 3-month intervals for 12 months; in another, the dose is repeated monthly three times. Thereafter, treatment is repeated at 12-month intervals until the adult worms die, which may take 10 years or longer. With the first treatment only, patients with microfilariae in the cornea or anterior chamber may benefit from several days of prednisone treatment (1 mg/kg/d) to avoid inflammatory eye reactions. Although single-dose ivermectin does not kill the adult worms, with repeated doses at 3-month or yearly intervals, increasing evidence suggests that the drug has a low-level macrofilaricidal action. Ivermectin is now marketed in the USA. See specialized sources for further details concerning its use.

In comparison studies, ivermectin was as effective as diethylcarbamazine in reducing the number of microfilariae but did so with significantly fewer systemic and ocular adverse reactions. Diethylcarbamazine is no longer recommended by WHO in onchocerciasis therapy. For selected patients in whom repeated ivermectin treatments do not control symptoms, suramin can be given for its macrofilaricidal action; however, because of suramin's toxicity and complex administration, it should only be administered by experts. Amocarzine is under evaluation for its macro- and microfilaricidal actions.

With treatment, some skin and ocular lesions improve and ocular progression is prevented, except for some instances of further deterioration of chorioret-

initis. The prognosis is unfavorable only for those patients who are seen for the first time with already far-advanced ocular onchocerciasis.

Burnham G: Ivermectin treatment of onchocercal skin lesions: Observations from a placebo-controlled, double-blind trial in Malawi. Am J Trop Med Hyg 1995;52:270.

Onchocerciasis and its control. Report of a WHO Expert Committee on Onchocerciasis Control. WHO Tech Rep Ser 1995;852:1.

Ottesen EA: Immune responsiveness and the pathogenesis of human onchocerciasis. J Infect Dis 1995;171:659.

Whitworth JAG, Maude GH, Downham MD: Clinical and parasitological responses after up to 6.5 years of ivermectin treatment for onchocerciasis. Trop Med Int Health 1996;1:786.

STRONGYLOIDIASIS

Essentials of Diagnosis

- Pruritic dermatitis at sites of larval penetration.
- Diarrhea, epigastric pain, nausea, malaise, weight loss.
- Cough, rales, transient pulmonary infiltrates.
- Eosinophilia; characteristic larvae in stool specimens, duodenal aspirate, or sputum.
- Hyperinfection syndrome: Severe diarrhea, bronchopneumonia, ileus.

General Considerations

Strongyloidiasis is caused by infection with *Strongyloides stercoralis* (2–2.5 × 30–50 mm). Major symptoms result from adult parasitism, principally in the duodenum and jejunum, or from larval migration through pulmonary and cutaneous tissues. The primary host is humans, but dogs, cats, and primates have been found infected with strains indistinguishable from those of humans.

The disease is endemic in tropical and subtropical regions; although the prevalence is generally low, in some areas disease rates exceed 25%. In temperate areas, the disease occurs sporadically. In the USA, highest infection rates are found in immigrants from endemic areas, in parts of Appalachia, and in southeastern areas. Multiple infections in households are common, and prevalence in institutions, particularly mental institutions, may be high.

The parasite is uniquely capable of maintaining its life cycle both within the human host and in soil. Infection occurs when filariform larvae in soil penetrate the skin, enter the bloodstream, and are carried to the lungs, where they escape from capillaries into alveoli and ascend the bronchial tree to the glottis. The larvae are then swallowed and carried to the duodenum and upper jejunum, where maturation to the adult stage takes place. The parasitic female, generally held to be parthenogenetic, matures and lives embedded in the mucosa, where its eggs are laid and hatch. Rhabditiform larvae, which are noninfective, emerge, and migrate into the intestinal lumen to leave the host via the feces. The life span of the adult worm may be as long as 5 years.

In the soil, the rhabditiform larvae metamorphose into the infective (filariform) larvae. However, the parasite also has a free-living cycle in soil, in which some rhabditiform larvae develop into adults that produce eggs from which rhabditiform larvae emerge to continue the life cycle.

Autoinfection in humans, which probably occurs at a low rate in most infections, is an important factor in determining worm burden and is responsible for the persistence of infections. Internal autoinfection takes place in the lower bowel when some rhabditiform larvae develop into filariform larvae that penetrate the intestinal mucosa, enter the intestinal lymphatic and portal circulation, are carried to the lungs, and return to the small bowel to complete the cycle. This process is accelerated by achlorhydria, constipation, diverticula, and other conditions that reduce bowel motility. In addition, an external autoinfection cycle can occur as a result of fecal contamination of the perianal area.

In the hyperinfection syndrome, autoinfection is greatly increased, resulting in a marked increase in the intestinal worm burden and in massive dissemination of filariform larvae to the lungs and most other tissues, where they can cause local inflammatory reactions and granuloma formation. Occasionally, in the lungs and elsewhere, larvae metamorphose into adults. Hyperinfection is generally initiated under conditions of depressed host cellular immunity, especially in debilitated, malnourished persons and in patients receiving immunosuppressive therapy, particularly corticosteroids. Only a few cases of strongyloidiasis have been reported in AIDS patients. Penetration of the bowel wall by filariform larvae can result in bacterial or fungal sepsis.

Clinical Findings

A. Symptoms and Signs: The time from larval penetration of the skin by filariform larvae until their appearance in the feces is 3–4 weeks. An acute syndrome can sometimes be recognized in which cutaneous symptoms are followed by pulmonary and then intestinal symptoms. Patients usually present, however, with chronic symptoms (continuous or with irregular exacerbations) that can persist for years or for life.

1. Cutaneous manifestations–Skin invasion is usually of the feet. In sensitized patients, there may be focal edema, inflammation, petechiae, serpiginous or urticarial tracts, and intense itching. In chronic infections, there may be both stationary urticaria and larva currens, the latter characterized by transient eruptions that migrate in serpiginous tracts.

2. Intestinal manifestations–Symptoms range from mild to severe, the most common being diarrhea, abdominal pain, and flatulence. Anorexia, nausea, vomiting, epigastric tenderness, and pruritus ani may be present; with increasing severity, fever and malaise may appear. Diarrhea may alternate with constipation, and in severe cases the feces contain mucus and blood. The pain is often epigastric in location and may mimic duodenal ulcer. Malabsorption or a protein-losing enteropathy can result from a large intestinal worm burden.

3. Pulmonary manifestations–With migration of larvae through the lungs, bronchi, and trachea, symptoms may be limited to a dry cough and throat irritation or low-grade fever, dyspnea, wheezing, and hemoptysis may occur. Bronchopneumonia, bronchitis, pleural effusion, progressive dyspnea, and miliary abscesses can develop; the cough may become productive of an odorless, mucopurulent sputum.

4. Hyperinfection syndrome–Intense dissemination of larvae to the lungs and other tissues can result in additional complications, including pleural effusion, pericarditis and myocarditis, hepatic granulomas, cholecystitis, purpura, ulcerating lesions at all levels of the gastrointestinal tract, central nervous system involvement, paralytic ileus, perforation and peritonitis, gram-negative septicemia, meningitis, cachexia, shock, and death.

B. Laboratory Findings:

1. Detection of eggs and larvae–Eggs are seldom found in feces. Diagnosis, which may be difficult, requires finding the larval stages in feces or duodenal fluid. Rhabditiform larvae may be found in recently passed stool specimens; filariform larvae will be present in specimens held in the laboratory for some hours. Four to six specimens, preserved or unpreserved, should be collected at 2-day intervals or longer, since the number of larvae in feces may vary considerably from day to day. Each specimen should be examined by direct microscopy, and several should be processed by the Baermann concentration or agar plate culture method to increase sensitivity of testing; stool specimens must be received unpreserved.

Although larvae cannot be found in the stools of 25% or more of infected patients, the diagnosis can often be made by finding rhabditiform larvae or ova in mucus obtained by means of the duodenal string test or by duodenal intubation and aspiration. Duodenal biopsy is seldom indicated but will confirm the diagnosis in most patients. Occasionally, filariform or rhabditiform larvae can be detected in sputum or bronchial washings during the pulmonary phase of the disease.

2. Serologic and hematologic findings–In chronic low-grade intestinal strongyloidiasis, the white blood cell count is often normal, with a slightly elevated percentage of eosinophils. However, with increasing larval migration, eosinophilia may reach 50% and leukocytosis 20,000/μL. Mild anemia may be present. Serum IgE immunoglobulins may be elevated. An ELISA is sensitive (85%), but cross-reactions can occur with filariasis and other helminthic infections.

3. Imaging–Small bowel x-rays may show inflammation, irritability, and prominent mucosal folds; there may also be bowel dilation, delayed emptying, and ulcerative duodenitis. In chronic infections, the findings can resemble those in nontropical and tropical sprue, or there may be narrowing, rigidity, and diminished peristalsis. During pulmonary migration of larvae, fine miliary nodules or irregular changing patches of pneumonitis may be seen.

4. Hyperinfection–In the hyperinfection syndrome, there may also be findings of hypoproteinemia, malabsorption, abnormal liver function, and extensive pulmonary opacities. Filariform larvae may appear in the urine. Eosinopenia, when present, is thought to be an unfavorable prognostic sign.

Differential Diagnosis

Because of varied signs and symptoms, the diagnosis of strongyloidiasis is often difficult. Eosinophilia plus one or more of the following factors should further enhance consideration of the diagnosis: endemic area exposure, duodenal ulcer-like pain, persistent or recurrent diarrhea, or malabsorption, recurrent coughing or wheezing, and transient pulmonary infiltrates. The duodenitis and jejunitis of strongyloidiasis can also mimic giardiasis, cholecystitis, and pancreatitis. Transient pulmonary infiltrates must be differentiated from tropical pulmonary eosinophilia and Löffler's syndrome. The diagnosis should be considered among the many causes of malabsorption in the tropics and in immunocompromised persons, including HIV-infected patients.

Treatment

Since *Strongyloides* can multiply in humans, treatment should continue until the parasite is eradicated. Patients receiving immunosuppressive therapy should be examined for the presence of the infection before and probably at intervals during treatment. In concurrent infection with *Strongyloides* and *Ascaris* or hookworm (which is common), eradicate *Ascaris* and hookworms first and *Strongyloides* subsequently. In selected patients negative for *Strongyloides* larvae, an empiric course of ivermectin may be indicated.

A. Ivermectin: Ivermectin, available in the USA, is the drug of choice. It appears to be equal in effectiveness to thiabendazole but has far fewer side effects. In a study of patients without the hyperinfection syndrome, all of 34 persons treated with 200 μg/kg for 1–2 days were cured; in another study, 83% of 29 persons treated with 150–200 μg/kg were cured. In the hyperinfection syndrome in AIDS patients, all seven patients who received 200 μg/kg on days 1, 2, 15, and 16 were cured. Failures have also occurred in AIDS.

B. Thiabendazole: An oral dose of 25 mg/kg (maximum, 1.5 g per dose) is given after meals twice daily for 2–3 days. A 5- to 7-day course is needed for disseminated infections. Tablet and liquid formulations are available; tablets should be chewed. Side effects, including headache, weakness, vomiting, vertigo, and decreased mental alertness, occur in as many as 30% of patients and may be severe. These symptoms are lessened if the drug is taken after meals. Other potentially serious side effects occur rarely. Erythema multiforme and the Stevens-Johnson syndrome have been associated with thiabendazole therapy; several fatalities have occurred in children.

C. Albendazole: Albendazole is given at a dosage of 400 mg twice daily for 3–7 days and repeated in 1 week; cure rates in several studies ranged from 38% to 80%. In comparative studies, albendazole is less effective than ivermectin.

Prognosis

The prognosis is favorable except in the hyperinfection syndrome and in infections associated with emaciation, advanced liver disease, cancer, immunologic disorders, or the use of immunosuppressive drugs. In selected instances, a 2-day course of treatment with thiabendazole once monthly can be tried to control infections that cannot be eradicated.

Dreyer G et al: Patterns of detection of *Strongyloides stercoralis* in stool specimens: Implications for diagnosis and clinical trials. J Clin Microbiol 1996;34:2569.

Gann PJ, Neva FA, Gam AA: A randomized trial of single- and two-dose ivermectin versus thiabendazole for treatment of strongyloidiasis. J Infect Dis 1994;169:1076.

Grove DI: Human strongyloidiasis. Adv Parasitol 1996;38:251.

Mahmoud AAF: Strongyloidiasis. Clin Infect Dis 1996;23:949.

Marti H et al: A comparative trial of a single-dose ivermectin versus three days of albendazole for the treatment of *Strongyloides stercoralis* and other soil-transmitted helminth infections in children. Am J Trop Med Hyg 1996;55:477.

TRICHINOSIS
(Trichinelliosis, Trichinellosis)

Essentials of Diagnosis

- History of ingestion of raw or inadequately cooked pork, boar, or bear.
- First week: diarrhea, cramps, malaise.
- Second week to 1–2 months: muscle pain and tenderness, fever, periorbital and facial edema, conjunctivitis.
- Eosinophilia and elevated serum enzymes; positive serologic tests; larvae in muscle biopsy.

General Considerations

Trichinosis is caused worldwide by *Trichinella spiralis*. The disease is present wherever pork is eaten but is a greater problem in many temperate areas than in the tropics. In the USA, there has been a marked reduction in prevalence in pigs (rates in commercial pork are nil to 0.7%) and humans (fewer than 100 cases are reported yearly). Three other species of *Trichinella* have been recognized in humans: *T nativa* appears to be restricted to Arctic and sub-Arctic regions and *T nelsoni* to tropical Africa. *T pseudospiralis,* reported rarely worldwide, occurs as a persistent infection accompanied by a chronic fatigue syndrome.

Human infections occur sporadically or in outbreaks. Infection is usually acquired by eating viable encysted larvae in raw or uncooked pork or pork products. Ground beef has also been a source of infection when adulterated with pork or inadvertently contaminated in a common meat grinder. In some cases, the source of infection is the flesh of dog (East Asia), horse (France), or wild animals, particularly bear, walrus, or bush pigs.

Gastric juices liberate the encysted larvae. They rapidly mature and mate, and the adult female then burrows into the mucosa of the small intestine. Within 4–5 days, the female begins to discharge viviparous larvae (100 × 6 µm) that are disseminated via the lymphatics and bloodstream to most body tissues. Larvae that reach striated muscle encyst and remain viable for months to years; those that reach other tissues are rapidly destroyed. The adult worms (2–3.6 mm × 75–90 µm) survive for up to about 6 weeks.

In the natural cycle, larvae develop into adult worms in the intestines when a carnivore or omnivore ingests parasitized muscle. Pigs generally become infected by feeding on uncooked food scraps or, less often, by eating infected rats. Other reservoir hosts include swine, dogs, cats, rats, and many wild animals, including the wolf, bear, and boar; marine animals in the Arctic; and the hyena, jackal, and lion in the tropics.

Clinical Findings

A. Symptoms and Signs: The incubation period is 2–7 days (range: 12 hours to 28 days). Severity depends upon intensity of infection, tissues invaded, immune status and age of the host (children have less severe infections), and perhaps the strain of the parasite. Findings range from asymptomatic to a mild febrile illness with short-lasting symptoms to a severe progressive illness with multiple system involvement that in rare cases is fatal.

1. Intestinal stage—When present, intestinal symptoms persist for 1–7 days: diarrhea, abdominal cramps, and malaise are the major findings; nausea and vomiting occur less frequently; and constipation is uncommon. Fever, eosinophilia, and leukocytosis are rare during the first week.

2. Muscle invasion stage—This begins at the end of the first week and lasts about 6 weeks. Parasitized muscles show an intense inflammatory reaction. Findings include fever (low-grade to marked); muscle pain and tenderness, edema, and spasm; periorbital and facial edema; sweating; photophobia and conjunctivitis; weakness or prostration; pain on swallowing; dyspnea, coughing, and hoarseness; subconjunctival, retinal, and nail splinter hemorrhages; and rashes and formication. The most frequently parasitized muscles and sites of findings are the masseters, the tongue, the diaphragm, the intercostal muscles, and the extraocular, laryngeal, paravertebral, nuchal, deltoid, pectoral, gluteus, biceps, and gastrocnemius muscles. Inflammatory reactions around larvae that reach tissues other than muscle may result in a broad range of findings, including the development of meningitis, encephalitis, myocarditis, bronchopneumonia, nephritis, and peripheral and cranial nerve disorders.

3. Convalescent stage—This generally begins in the second month but in severe infections may not begin before 3 months or longer. Vague muscle pains and malaise may persist for several more months. Permanent muscular atrophy has been reported.

B. Laboratory Findings: The diagnosis is supported by findings of eosinophilia, elevated serum muscle enzymes, and positive serologic tests. There may be a marked hypergammaglobulinemia with reversal of the albumin-globulin ratio. Absence of an elevated sedimentation rate is a useful diagnostic clue. Confirmation of the diagnosis is by detection of larvae in muscle biopsy specimens.

Leukocytosis and eosinophilia appear during the second week. The proportion of eosinophils rises to a maximum of 20–90% in the third or fourth week and then slowly declines to normal over the next few months.

Serologic tests can detect most clinically manifest cases but are not sufficiently sensitive to detect low-level infections (ie, a few larvae per gram of ingested muscle). More than one test should be used and then repeated to observe for seroconversion or for a rising titer. A qualitative latex agglutination test is available for screening. The bentonite flocculation (BF) test (positive titer, ≥ 1:5) is highly sensitive and is considered nearly 100% specific. It becomes positive in the third or fourth week, and reaches a maximum titer at about 2 months, and generally reverts to negative in 2–3 years. The immunofluorescence test (positive titer > 16) is also highly sensitive, though less specific than the BF test; it may become positive in the second week. The IgM and IgG ELISAs are also showing high sensitivity and specificity for antibody and detection of circulating antigens. The intradermal test is no longer recommended, as it may remain positive for years and batches of antigen vary in potency.

Adult worms may be looked for in feces, though they are seldom found. In the second week, there are occasional larvae in blood, duodenal washings, and, rarely, in centrifuged spinal fluid. In the third to fourth weeks, biopsy of skeletal muscle may be definitive (particularly gastrocnemius and pectoralis), preferably at a site of swelling or tenderness or near tendinous insertions. Portions of the specimen should be examined microscopically by compression between glass slides, by digestion, and by preparation of multiple histologic sections. If the biopsy is done too early, larvae may not be detectable. Myositis even in the absence of larvae is a significant finding.

C. Imaging: Chest films during the acute phase may show disseminated or localized infiltrates. Late calcification of muscle cysts cannot be detected radiologically.

Complications

The more important complications are granulomatous pneumonitis, encephalitis, and cardiac failure.

Differential Diagnosis

Because of its protean manifestations, trichinosis may resemble many other diseases. Eosinophilia, muscle pain and tenderness, and fever should lead the physician to consider collagen vascular disorders such as dermatomyositis or polyarteritis nodosa.

Prevention

The frequency and intensity of infection in the USA and other countries have been significantly reduced by public health measures to prevent feeding of uncooked garbage to hogs and by animal inspection (not in the USA). The chief safeguard against trichinosis is adequate cooking of pork at 77 °C or by freezing meat at –15 °C for 30 days (longer if meat is over 15 cm thick). *T spiralis* in game is often relatively resistant to freezing. Low doses of gamma irradiation are also effective in killing larvae.

Treatment

Treatment is principally supportive, since in most cases recovery is spontaneous without sequelae.

A. Intestinal Phase: Though supporting evidence for efficacy is limited, albendazole, because of its relatively high absorption and freedom from adverse reactions, is proposed as the drug of choice in a dosage of 400 mg twice daily for up to 60 days. Mebendazole is an alternative drug at a dosage of 200–400 mg three times daily for 3 days, followed by 400–500 mg three times daily for 10 days. A second alternative drug is thiabendazole at a dosage of 25 mg/kg (maximum, 1.5 g per dose) twice daily after meals for 3–7 days; side effects, sometimes severe, are common (see Strongyloidiasis, above). Corticosteroids are contraindicated in the intestinal phase.

B. Muscle Invasion Phase: In this stage, severe infections require hospitalization and high doses of corticosteroids for 24–48 hours, followed by lower doses for several days or weeks to control symptoms.

However, because corticosteroids may suppress the inflammatory response to adult worms, they should be used only when symptoms are severe. Thiabendazole has been tried in the muscle stage with equivocal relief of muscle pain or tenderness or lysis of fever; further trials are recommended. Mebendazole and albendazole may also be tried.

Prognosis

Death is rare—sometimes within 2–3 weeks in overwhelming infections, more often in 4–8 weeks from a major complication such as cardiac failure or pneumonia.

Andrews JRH, Ainsworth R, Abernethy D: *Trichinella pseudospiralis* in humans: Description of a case and its treatment. Trans R Soc Trop Med Hyg 1994;88:200.

Cabie A et al: Albendazole versus thiabendazole as therapy for trichinosis: A retrospective study. Clin Infect Dis 1996;22:1033.

Capo V, Despommier DD: Clinical aspects of infection with *Trichinella* spp. Clin Microbiol Rev 1996;9:47.

Clausen MR et al: *Trichinella* infection and clinical disease. Q J Med 1996;89:631.

TRICHURIASIS
(Trichocephaliasis, Whipworm)

Trichuris trichiura is a common intestinal parasite of humans throughout the world, particularly in the subtropics and tropics. Persons of all ages are affected, but infection is heaviest and most frequent in children. The slender worms, 30–50 mm in length, attach by means of their anterior whip-like end to the mucosa of the large intestine, particularly to the cecum. Eggs are passed in the feces but require 2–4 weeks for larval development after reaching the soil before becoming infective; thus, person-to-person transmission is not possible. Infections are acquired by ingestion of the infective egg. The larvae hatch in the small intestine and mature in the large bowel but do not migrate through the tissues.

Clinical Findings

A. Symptoms and Signs: Light (fewer than 10,000 eggs per gram of feces) to moderate infections rarely cause symptoms. Heavy infections (30,000 or more eggs per gram of feces) may be accompanied by abdominal cramps, tenesmus, diarrhea, distention, flatulence, nausea, vomiting, and weight loss. Rectal prolapse and hematochezia or chronic occult blood loss may also occur, most often in malnourished young children. Sometimes, adult worms are seen in stools. Invasion of the appendix, with resulting appendicitis, is rare.

B. Laboratory Findings: Diagnosis is by identification of characteristic eggs and, sometimes, adult worms in stools. Eosinophilia (5–20%) is common with all but light infections. Severe iron deficiency anemia may be present with heavy infections.

Treatment

Patients with asymptomatic light infections do not require treatment. For those with heavier or symptomatic infections, give mebendazole, albendazole, or oxantel. Thiabendazole should *not* be used, because it is not effective and is potentially toxic.

A. Mebendazole: The dosage is 100 mg twice daily before or after meals for 3 days. It may be therapeutically advantageous for the tablets to be chewed before swallowing. Cure rates of 60–80% and higher are reported after one course of treatment, with marked reduction in ova counts in the remaining patients. For severe trichuriasis, a longer course of treatment (up to 6 days) or a repeat course will often be necessary. Gastrointestinal side effects from the drug are rare. The drug is contraindicated in pregnancy.

B. Albendazole: Albendazole, given orally at a single dose of 400 mg, has resulted in cure rates of 33–90%, with marked reduction in egg counts in those not cured. An appropriate dosage to achieve higher cure rates in moderate to heavy infections remains to be determined, but daily treatment for 2–3 days can be tried. Albendazole (now available in the USA) should not be used in pregnancy.

C. Oxantel Pamoate: Oxantel pamoate is an analogue of pyrantel pamoate and acts only on *T trichiura.* Cure rates of 57–100% have been reported in various trials. One treatment schedule is 15 mg/kg (base) daily for 2 days for patients with mild to moderate intensity of infection. For patients with severe infection, give 10 mg/kg (base) daily for 5 days. Oxantel is not available in the USA. Safety in pregnancy is not established.

Callender JE et al: Treatment effects in *Trichuris* dysentery syndrome. Acta Paediatr 1994;83:1182.

Cooper ES et al: "Catch-up" growth velocities after treatment for *Trichuris* dysentery syndrome. Trans R Soc Trop Med Hyg 1995;89:653.

Ramdath DD et al: Iron status of schoolchildren with varying intensities of *Trichuris trichiura* infection. Parasitology. 1995;110:347.

VISCERAL LARVA MIGRANS (Toxocariasis)

Most visceral larva migrans cases are due to *Toxocara canis,* an ascarid of dogs and other canids; in a few cases, *Toxocara cati* in domestic cats has been implicated and rarely *Belascaris procyonis* of raccoons. The adult worms live in the intestinal tracts of their respective hosts and release large numbers of eggs in the stool.

The reservoir mechanism for *T canis* is latent infection in female dogs which is reactivated during pregnancy. Transmission from mother to puppies is via the placenta and milk. Most eggs passed to the environment are from puppies (2 weeks to 6 months) and lactating bitches (up to 6 months after parturition). The life cycle of *T cati* is similar, but transplacental transmission does not occur.

Human infections are sporadic and probably occur worldwide. In the USA, antibody seroprevalence is 5–7%. Infection is generally in dirt-eating young children who ingest *T canis* or *T cati* eggs from soil or sand contaminated with animal feces, most often from puppies. Direct contact with infected animals does not produce infection, as the eggs require a 3- to 4-week extrinsic incubation period to become infective; thereafter, eggs in soil remain infective for months to years.

In humans, hatched larvae are unable to mature but continue to migrate through the tissues for up to 6 months. Eventually they lodge in various organs, particularly the lungs and liver and less often the brain, eyes, and other tissues, where they produce eosinophilic granulomas up to 1 cm in diameter.

Clinical & Laboratory Findings

A. Acute Infection: Migrating larvae may induce fever, cough, wheezing, hepatosplenomegaly, and lymphadenopathy. A variety of other findings may occur when other organs are invaded, including myelitis, encephalitis, and carditis. The acute phase may last 2–3 weeks, but resolution of all physical and laboratory findings may take up to 18 months.

Leukocytosis is marked (may exceed 100,000/µL), with 30–80% due to eosinophils. Hyperglobulinemia occurs when the liver is extensively invaded and is a useful clue in diagnosis. An ELISA test is the most specific (92%) and sensitive (78%) serologic test and may permit a presumptive diagnosis, although it does not distinguish acute from prior infection. Nonspecific isohemagglutinin titers (anti-A and anti-B) are usually greater than 1:1024. Chest radiographs may show infiltrates. With central nervous system involvement, the cerebrospinal fluid may show eosinophils. No parasitic forms can be found by stool examination.

Ultrasonography has been used to detect 1-cm hypoechoic lesions in the liver, each with a thread-like hyperechoic line. Specific diagnosis can only be made by percutaneous liver biopsy or by direct biopsy of a granuloma at laparoscopy, but these procedures are seldom justified.

B. Ocular Toxocariasis: Most cases occur in children, most commonly 5–10 years old, who present with visual impairment in one eye and sometimes leukocoria, squint, and red eye. The principal pathologic entity is eosinophilic granuloma of the retina that resembles retinoblastoma. Until the recent development of the ELISA test, this resulted in the enucleation of many eyes. Other common clinical findings are a diffuse, painless endophthalmitis; posterior pole granuloma; and a peripheral inflammatory mass. Uncommonly seen are an iris nodule, optic nerve granuloma, uniocular pars planitis, and a migrating retinal nematode. Ocular toxocariasis, which is generally recognized years after the acute infection, is generally not associated with peripheral eosinophilia, hypergammaglobulinemia, or isohemagglutinin elevation. Serum ELISA tests may be positive, but a negative test does not rule out the diagnosis. If doubt exists about whether a patient with a positive serum ELISA test has retinoblastoma, examination of the vitreous humor for ELISA antibody and eosinophils can be helpful. High-resolution CT scanning of the orbit should be done.

Prevention, Treatment, & Prognosis

Disease in humans is best prevented by periodic treatment of puppies, kittens, and nursing dog and cat mothers, starting at 2 weeks postpartum, repeating at weekly intervals for 3 weeks and then every 6 months.

A. Acute Infection: There is no proved specific treatment, but thiabendazole (as used in strongyloidiasis), mebendazole (200–400 mg in divided doses for 10–15 days), albendazole (400 mg twice daily for 21 days), diethylcarbamazine (6 mg/kg in divided doses for 21 days), or ivermectin should be tried. Theoretically, release of antigens from dying parasites may exacerbate clinical findings. Corticosteroids, antibiotics, antihistamines, and analgesics may be needed to provide symptomatic relief. Symptoms may persist for months but generally clear within 1–2 years. The ultimate outcome is usually good, but permanent neuropsychologic deficits have been seen.

B. Ocular Toxocariasis: Treatment includes corticosteroids (subconjunctival applications may be preferable to oral usage), vitrectomy for vitreous traction, laser photocoagulation, and an anthelmintic drug. Partial or total permanent visual impairment is rare.

Bhatia V, Sarin SK: Hepatic visceral larva migrans: Evolution of the lesion, diagnosis, and role of high-dose albendazole therapy. Am J Gastroenterol 1994;89:624.

Kerr-Muir MG: *Toxocara canis* and human health. BMJ 1994;309:5.

Magnaval J: Comparative efficacy of diethylcarbamazine and mebendazole for the treatment of toxocariasis. Parasitology 1995;119:529.

Sommer C et al: Adult *Toxocara canis* encephalitis. J Neurol Neurosurg Psychiatry 1994;57:229.

Richard J. Hamill, MD

Fungal infections have assumed an increasingly important role as use of broad-spectrum antimicrobial agents has increased and the number of immunodeficient patients has risen. Some pathogens (eg, *Cryptococcus, Candida, Pneumocystis, Fusarium*) virtually never cause serious disease in normal hosts. Other endemic fungi (eg, *Histoplasma, Coccidioides, Paracoccidioides*) commonly cause disease in normal hosts but tend to be more aggressive in immunocompromised ones.

CANDIDIASIS

Essentials of Diagnosis

- Common normal flora but opportunistic pathogen.
- Gastrointestinal mucosal disease, particularly esophagitis, most common; catheter-associated fungemia occurs in hospitals.
- Diagnosis of invasive systemic disease requires tissue biopsy or evidence of retinal disease.

General Considerations

Candida albicans can be cultured from the mouth, vagina, and feces of most people. Cutaneous and oral lesions are discussed in Chapters 6 and 8, respectively. The risk factors for invasive candidiasis include prolonged neutropenia, recent surgery, broad-spectrum antibiotic therapy, the presence of intravascular catheters (especially when providing total parenteral nutrition), and intravenous drug use. Cellular immunodeficiency predisposes to mucocutaneous disease. When no other underlying cause is found, persistent oral or vaginal candidiasis should arouse a suspicion of HIV infection; over the course of their disease, AIDS patients will almost without exception have candidiasis as a complication.

Clinical Findings & Treatment

A. Mucosal Candidiasis: Esophageal involvement is the most frequent type of invasive mucosal

disease. Individuals present with substernal odynophagia, gastroesophageal reflux, or nausea without substernal pain. Oral candidiasis, though often associated, is not invariably present. Diagnosis is best confirmed by endoscopy with biopsy and culture, since radiographically the condition may be difficult to distinguish from esophagitis caused by infection with cytomegalovirus or herpes simplex virus. Therapy depends upon the severity of disease. If patients are able to swallow and take adequate amounts of fluid orally, fluconazole, 100 mg/d for 10–14 days will usually suffice. In the individual who is more ill or has developed esophagitis while taking fluconazole, a 10- to 14-day course of amphotericin B at a dose of 0.3 mg/kg/d intravenously usually results in resolution. Relapse is common when there is underlying HIV infection.

Vulvovaginal candidiasis occurs in an estimated 75% of women during their lifetime. Risk factors include pregnancy, uncontrolled diabetes mellitus, broad-spectrum antimicrobial treatment, corticosteroid use, and AIDS. In women with AIDS, vaginal candidiasis is usually the first and most frequent opportunistic infection. Common symptoms include acute vulvar pruritus, burning vaginal discharge, and dyspareunia. Various topical azole preparations (eg, clotrimazole, 100 mg vaginal tablet for 7 days, or miconazole, 200 mg vaginal suppository for 3 days) are effective. One 150 mg oral dose of fluconazole has been shown to have equivalent efficacy with better patient acceptance.

B. Candidal Funguria: Candidal funguria usually resolves with discontinuance of antibiotics or removal of bladder catheters. When symptomatic funguria persists, oral fluconazole, 50 mg/d for 7–10 days, can be used if renal function is normal. If creatinine clearance is less than 10 mL/min, irrigation for 5 days with 50 mg/d of amphotericin B mixed in 1 L of D_5W may be necessary. Rare complications of candidal funguria are ureteral obstruction and dissemination.

C. Candidal Fungemia: Candidal fungemia may represent a benign, self-limited process, but until proved otherwise it should be considered a sign of

---

*Superficial mycoses are discussed in Chapter 6.

serious disseminated disease. If fungemia resolves with removal of intravascular catheters, there are often no further complications. The incidence of endophthalmitis may be higher than previously recognized, and a short course of intravenous amphotericin B to a total dose of 200 mg appears to lower this incidence. Such an approach is strongly recommended for patients with candidal fungemia. (See Amphotericin B, Chapter 37.)

If fungemia is documented repeatedly, if retinal lesions are identified, or if *Candida* is isolated from other sites, the patient is considered to have disseminated disease. Important clinical findings in disseminated candidiasis are fluffy white retinal infiltrates that extend into the vitreous and raised, erythematous skin lesions that may be painful. However, though characteristic, these are seen in less than 50% of cases. Other organ system involvement in disseminated disease may include the brain, meninges, and myocardium. Amphotericin B to a total dose of 1 g is the agent of choice. Flucytosine, 150 mg/kg/d orally in four divided doses, is added if central nervous system involvement occurs until clinical improvement results. Individuals who do not tolerate amphotericin B may be given fluconazole, 200–400 mg/d intravenously, with equivalent efficacy. Serologic tests for *Candida* have not proved helpful in differentiating transient fungemia from disseminated disease.

Another form of disseminated disease is hepatosplenic candidiasis. This results from aggressive chemotherapy and prolonged neutropenia in patients with underlying hematologic cancers. Patients typically present with fever and variable abdominal pain weeks after chemotherapy, when neutrophil counts have recovered. Blood cultures are generally negative. Hepatic enzymes reveal an alkaline phosphatase elevation that may be marked. CT scanning of the abdomen shows hepatosplenomegaly, most often with multiple low-density defects in the liver. Diagnosis is established by liver biopsy, histopathology, and culture. Amphotericin B is given to a total dose of 1 g intravenously but often works poorly; fluconazole, 400 mg daily, or liposomal preparations of amphotericin B may be better. Therapy is continued until clinical and radiographic improvement occurs.

D. Candidal Endocarditis: Candidal endocarditis rarely is a complication of transient fungemia. It usually results from direct inoculation at the time of open heart surgery or repeated inoculation with intravenous drug use. Candidal endocarditis occurs with increased frequency on prosthetic valves in the first few months following surgery. Splenomegaly and petechiae are common, and there is a predilection for large-vessel embolization. Non-*albicans* species such as *Candida parapsilosis* and *Candida tropicalis* are more often important etiologic agents in endocarditis than in fungemia, when *C albicans* is usual. The diagnosis is established definitively by culturing *Candida* from emboli or from

large vegetations at the time of valve replacement. Valve destruction (usually aortic or mitral) is common, and surgical therapy is necessary in addition to a prolonged course of amphotericin therapy, usually to a total dose of 1–1.5 g intravenously.

It is important to note that non-*albicans* species of *Candida* are often resistant to imidazole antibiotics such as fluconazole. The widespread use of these agents for prophylaxis in immunocompromised patients can lead to the emergence of pathogens such as *Candida krusei*. Dissemination of this organism has been reported in patients undergoing bone marrow transplantation for leukemia. Imidazole-resistant *C albicans* has increased in frequency in immunocompromised patients, particularly in patients with late-stage AIDS receiving chronic suppressive fluconazole.

In all forms of invasive candidiasis, an important element of therapy is reversal of the underlying predisposing factor when possible.

Ozun O et al: Problems and controversies in the management of hematogenous candidiasis. Clin Infect Dis 1996;22(Suppl 2):S95. (Provides algorithm for approach to therapy in patients with candidemia.)

Reef SE et al: Treatment options for vulvovaginal candidiasis, 1993. Clin Infect Dis 1995;20(Suppl 1):S80.

Rex JH et al: A randomized trial comparing fluconazole with amphotericin B for the treatment of candidemia in patients without neutropenia. N Engl J Med 1994; 331:1325. (Fluconazole was equivalent to amphotericin B for treatment of candidemia. Intravenous catheters were the source of candidemia in the majority of patients.)

HISTOPLASMOSIS

Essentials of Diagnosis

- Epidemiologically linked to bird droppings and bat exposure; common along river valleys.
- Most patients asymptomatic; respiratory illness most common clinical problem.
- Rare patients with normal immune function develop dissemination, with hepatosplenomegaly, lymphadenopathy, and oral ulcers.
- Widespread disease especially common in AIDS or other immunosuppressed states, with poor prognosis.
- Skin test and serology seldom diagnostic; biopsy of affected organs with culture, urinary polysaccharide antigen most useful.

General Considerations

Histoplasmosis is caused by *Histoplasma capsulatum,* a dimorphic fungus that has been isolated from soil in endemic areas (central and eastern USA, eastern Canada, Mexico, Central America, South America, Africa, and southeast Asia). Infection presumably takes place by inhalation of conidia. These convert into small budding cells that are engulfed by phagocytic cells in the lungs. The organism proliferates and is carried hematogenously to other organs.

Clinical Findings

A. Symptoms and Signs: Most cases of histoplasmosis are asymptomatic or mild and so are unrecognized. Past infection is recognized by the development of a positive histoplasmin skin test and occasionally by pulmonary and splenic calcification noted on incidental x-rays. Symptoms and signs of pulmonary involvement are usually absent even in patients who subsequently show areas of calcification on chest x-ray. Symptomatic infection may present with mild influenza-like illness, often lasting 1–4 days. Moderately severe infections are frequently diagnosed as atypical pneumonia. These patients have fever, cough, and mild chest pain lasting 5–15 days. Physical examination is usually negative. Radiographic findings during acute illness are variable and nonspecific.

Clinically evident infections occur also in several other forms: (1) **Acute histoplasmosis** frequently occurs in epidemics. It is a severe disease manifested by marked prostration, fever, and relatively few pulmonary complaints even when x-rays show pneumonia. The illness may last from 1 week to 6 months but is almost never fatal. (2) **Progressive disseminated histoplasmosis** is usually fatal within 6 weeks or less. Symptoms usually consist of fever, dyspnea, cough, loss of weight, and prostration. Diarrhea is usually present in children. Ulcers of the mucous membranes of the oropharynx may be present. The liver and spleen are nearly always enlarged, and all the organs of the body are involved, particularly the adrenal glands. (3) **Chronic progressive pulmonary histoplasmosis** is usually seen in older patients with chronic obstructive lung disease and in mildly immunocompromised patients. The lungs show chronic progressive changes, often with apical cavities. (4) **Disseminated disease in the profoundly immunocompromised host** often represents reactivation of prior infectious foci or may reflect acute infection. This form is commonly seen in patients with underlying HIV infection and is characterized by fever and multiple organ system involvement. Chest x-rays may show a miliary pattern. Presentation may be fulminant, with death ensuing rapidly unless treatment is provided.

B. Laboratory Findings: Most patients with progressive pulmonary disease show anemia of chronic disease. Bone marrow involvement may be prominent in disseminated forms with occurrence of pancytopenia. Alkaline phosphatase and marked LDH and ferritin elevations are also common.

In pulmonary disease, sputum culture is rarely positive except in chronic disease; in contrast, blood or bone marrow cultures from immunocompromised patients with acute disseminated disease are positive more than 80% of the time. A urine antigen assay has a sensitivity of greater than 90% for disseminated disease in AIDS patients and can be used to diagnose relapse. The sensitivity of screening immunodiffusion is 50% in acute pulmonary histoplasmosis, and complement fixation titers are positive in about 80% of cases. Combined results in immunodeficient patients approach 80%. Since skin test reactivity may persist for years following infection, it is generally not useful for establishing the diagnosis. Skin testing may also interfere with subsequent serologic diagnosis.

Treatment

For progressive localized disease and for mild to moderately severe nonmeningeal disseminated disease in immunocompetent or immunocompromised patients, itraconazole, 200–400 mg/d orally is the treatment of choice with an overall response rate of approximately 80%. Duration of therapy ranges from weeks to several months depending upon the severity of illness. Amphotericin B is reserved for individuals who cannot take oral medications, failure of itraconazole therapy, meningitis, or severe disseminated disease in an immunocompromised host. Up to 2.5 g total may need to be given in the latter two situations. (See Amphotericin B, Chapter 37.) Patients with AIDS-related histoplasmosis require lifelong suppressive therapy with itraconazole, 200–400 mg/d orally.

Wheat J et al: Itraconazole treatment of disseminated histoplasmosis in patients with the acquired immunodeficiency syndrome. Am J Med 1995;98:336. (Itraconazole is safe and effective induction therapy for mild disseminated histoplasmosis in AIDS patients.)

Wheat J et al: Prevention of relapse of histoplasmosis with itraconazole in patients with the acquired immunodeficiency syndrome. Ann Intern Med 1993;118:610. (Itraconazole was 95% effective.)

COCCIDIOIDOMYCOSIS

Essentials of Diagnosis

- Influenza-like illness with malaise, fever, backache, headache, and cough.
- Arthralgia and periarticular swelling of knees and ankles.
- Erythema nodosum common.
- Dissemination may result in meningitis, bony lesions, or skin and soft tissue abscesses.
- X-ray findings vary widely from pneumonitis to cavitation.
- Serologic tests useful; spherules containing endospores demonstrable in sputum or tissues.

General Considerations

Coccidioidomycosis should be considered in the

diagnosis of any obscure illness in a patient who has lived in or visited an endemic area.

Infection results from the inhalation of arthroconidia of *Coccidioides immitis,* a mold that grows in soil in certain arid regions of the southwestern USA, in Mexico, and in Central and South America.

About 60% of infections are subclinical and unrecognized other than by the subsequent development of a positive coccidioidin skin test. In the remaining cases, symptoms may be of severity warranting medical attention. Fewer than 1% of immunocompetent hosts show dissemination, but among these patients the mortality rate is high.

In HIV-infected people in endemic areas, coccidioidomycosis is now a common opportunistic infection, occurring in approximately 25% of patients over the course of HIV disease.

Clinical Findings

A. Symptoms and Signs: Symptoms of primary coccidioidomycosis occur in about 40% of infections. The onset (after an incubation period of 10–30 days) is usually that of a respiratory tract illness with fever and occasionally chills. Pleuritic pain is common. Nasopharyngitis may be followed by bronchitis accompanied by a dry or slightly productive cough.

Arthralgia accompanied by periarticular swellings, often of the knees and ankles, is common. Erythema nodosum may appear 2–20 days after onset of symptoms. Erythema multiforme may also occur rarely. Persistent pulmonary lesions, varying from cavities and abscesses to parenchymal nodular densities or bronchiectasis, occur in about 5% of diagnosed cases.

About 0.1% of white and 1% of nonwhite patients are unable to localize or control infection caused by *C immitis.* Filipinos and blacks are especially susceptible, as are pregnant women. Symptoms in progressive coccidioidomycosis depend upon the site of dissemination. Any organ may be involved. Pulmonary findings usually become more pronounced, with mediastinal lymph node enlargement, cough, and increased sputum production. Lung abscesses may rupture into the pleural space, producing an empyema. Extension to bones and skin may take place, and pericardial and myocardial extension has been occasionally observed. Dissemination may be associated with fungemia, characterized clinically by a diffuse miliary pattern on chest x-ray and by early death. The course may be particularly rapid in immunosuppressed patients. HIV-infected persons with disseminated disease have a higher incidence of miliary infiltrates, lymphadenopathy, and meningitis, but skin lesions are uncommon.

Bone lesions most often occur at bony prominences. Meningitis occurs in 30–50% of cases of dissemination. Subcutaneous abscesses and verrucous skin lesions are especially common in fulminating cases. Lymphadenitis may occur and may progress to suppuration. Mediastinal and retroperitoneal abscesses are not uncommon.

B. Laboratory Findings: In primary coccidioidomycosis, there may be moderate leukocytosis and eosinophilia and an elevated sedimentation rate. A persisting elevated or increasing sedimentation rate is a sign of progressive disease. The coccidioidin skin test becomes positive early after localized infection and may remain positive for years; however, it is typically negative with disseminated disease. Serologic testing is useful for both diagnosis and prognosis. The immunodiffusion test (CIE) and the tube precipitin test are useful for screening, and IgG and IgM by immunodiffusion are also adequate for diagnosis. Historically, a persistent rising complement fixation titer ($\geq$ 1:16) has been considered suggestive of disseminated disease. Serum complement fixation titer may be low when there is meningitis but no other disseminated disease. A false-negative rate up to 30% is seen in patients with HIV-related coccidioidomycosis. Demonstrable antibodies in spinal fluid are diagnostic of coccidioidal meningitis. These are found in over 90% of cases. Spinal fluid findings include increased cell count with lymphocytosis and reduced glucose. Spherules filled with endospores may be found in biopsy specimens; though they are not infectious, they convert to the highly contagious arthroconidia when grown in culture media. Exoantigen testing is in widespread use and substantially reduces the risk to laboratory personnel. Blood cultures in appropriate media are only uncommonly positive in disseminated disease. Spinal fluid culture is positive in approximately 30% of meningitis cases.

C. Imaging: Radiographic findings vary, but patchy, nodular pulmonary infiltrates and thin-walled cavities are most common. Hilar lymphadenopathy may be visible and is seen in localized disease; mediastinal lymphadenopathy suggests dissemination. There may be pleural effusions and lytic lesions in bone.

Treatment

General symptomatic therapy is given as needed for disease limited to the chest with no evidence of progression. For progressive pulmonary or extrapulmonary disease, amphotericin B intravenously has proved effective in some patients (see Chapter 37). Therapy should be continued to a total dose of 2.5–3 g. For meningitis, treatment consists of the intrathecal administration of amphotericin B daily in increasing doses up to 1–5 mg/d until the patient is clinically stable. The drug can then be tapered to once every 6 weeks for several years thereafter. Systemic therapy with amphotericin B, 0.6 mg/kg/d intravenously, is generally given concurrently with the initial therapy. Once the patient is clinically stable, oral therapy with an azole for an indefinite period, in dosages as discussed below, is an alternative to intrathecal therapy.

Results with fluconazole at a dose of 400 mg/d suggest that it may be possible to treat approximately 75% of selected patients with mild coccidioidal meningitis with oral fluconazole. Such therapy is suppressive only and must be continued indefinitely.

Ketoconazole, 200–800 mg orally daily 1–2 hours before breakfast, fluconazole, 200–400 mg orally daily, and itraconazole, 400 mg orally daily, are alternative regimens for disease limited to the chest; however, therapy must be continued for 6 months or longer after the disease is inactive in order to prevent relapse.

Thoracic surgery is occasionally indicated for giant, infected, or ruptured cavities. Surgical drainage is also useful for soft tissue abscesses. Amphotericin B, 1 mg/kg/d intravenously, is advisable following extensive surgical manipulation of infected tissue until the disease is inactive, whereupon therapy may be continued with an azole.

Prognosis

The prognosis in the case of limited disease is good, but persistent pulmonary cavities may cause complications. Nodules, cavities, and fibrotic residuals may rarely progress after long periods of stability or regression. Disseminated and meningeal forms still have mortality rates exceeding 50%.

Dewsnup DH et al: Is it ever safe to stop azole therapy for *Coccidioides immitis* meningitis? Ann Intern Med 1996;124:305. (Discontinuing therapy in patients who have achieved clinical remission while maintained on azoles results in an inordinately high relapse rate.)

Singh VR et al: Coccidioidomycosis in patients infected with human immunodeficiency virus: Review of 91 cases at a single institution. Clin Infect Dis 1996;25:563. (Most patients are treated initially with an azole; however, the mortality rate was 60%.)

Stevens DA: Coccidioidomycosis. N Engl J Med 1995; 332:1077. (Good review with discussions of treatment regimens for the various complications of coccidioidomycosis.)

PNEUMOCYSTOSIS
(*Pneumocystis carinii* Pneumonia)

Essentials of Diagnosis

- Fever, dyspnea, nonproductive cough.
- Bilateral diffuse interstitial disease without hilar adenopathy by chest x-ray.
- Bibasilar crackles on auscultation in many cases; others have no findings.
- Reduced partial pressure of oxygen.
- *P carinii* in lung tissue, sputum, or bronchoalveolar lavage fluid.

General Considerations

Phylogenetic analysis suggests that *P carinii* is a fungus. The organism has been found in the lungs of a variety of domesticated and wild mammals and is distributed worldwide in humans. Although *P carinii* infection is rare in the general population, serologic evidence indicates that asymptomatic infections have occurred in most persons by a young age. The overt infection (pneumocystosis) is an acute interstitial plasma cell pneumonia that occurs with high frequency among two groups: (1) as epidemics of primary infections among prematures or debilitated or marasmic infants on hospital wards, and (2) as sporadic cases among older children and adults who have an abnormal or altered immune status. Cases occur generally in patients with cancer or severe malnutrition and debility, in patients treated with immunosuppressive or cytotoxic drugs or irradiation for the management of organ transplants and cancer, and, most commonly, in patients with AIDS (see Chapter 31).

The mode of transmission in primary infection is unknown, but the evidence suggests airborne transmission. Following asymptomatic primary infection, latent and presumably inactive organisms are sparsely distributed in the alveoli. Unsettled, however, is whether acute infection in older children and adults results from de novo infection or from reactivation of latent infection.

In AIDS, without specific prophylaxis, pneumocystis pneumonia occurs in up to 80% of patients and is a major cause of death. Its incidence increases in direct proportion to the fall in CD4 cells, with most cases occurring when the cells are below 200/μL. Dissemination of the infection to tissues other than the lung is rare, except in those who have received prophylactic aerosolized pentamidine. In non-AIDS patients receiving immunosuppressive therapy, symptoms frequently begin after corticosteroids have been tapered or discontinued.

Clinical Findings

A. Symptoms and Signs: Findings are generally limited to the pulmonary parenchyma, but extrapulmonary disease is being reported with increasing frequency. In the sporadic form of the disease associated with deficient cell-mediated immunity, the onset is abrupt, with fever, tachypnea, shortness of breath, and usually nonproductive cough. Pulmonary physical findings may be slight and disproportionate to the degree of illness and to the radiologic findings; many patients have bibasilar crackles, but others do not. Without treatment, the course is usually one of rapid deterioration and death. In adult disease, patients may present with spontaneous pneumothorax, usually in patients with previous episodes or those receiving aerosolized pentamidine prophylaxis. In the infantile form of the disease, the patient is generally free of fever and may show eosinophilia. Patients with AIDS will usually have other evidence of HIV-associated disease, including fever, fatigue, and weight loss, for weeks or months preceding the illness.

B. Laboratory Findings: Chest radiographs most often show diffuse "interstitial" infiltration, which may be heterogeneous or miliary or patchy early in infection. There may also be diffuse or focal consolidation, cystic changes, nodules, or cavitation within nodules; 5–10% of patients with pneumocystis pneumonia have normal chest films. Chest films are more often atypical in patients who have received prophylaxis with aerosolized pentamidine, demonstrating upper lobe infiltrates.

Typically, there is reduction in vital and total lung capacity, and the single-breath diffusing capacity for carbon monoxide shows impaired diffusion. The blood gases usually show hypoxemia with hypocapnia. Gallium lung scanning (sensitivity > 95%, specificity 20–40%) shows diffuse uptake; the test should be reserved for those with normal chest films and normal pulmonary function in whom the disease is suspected. Isolated elevation or rising levels of serum LDH are characteristic. Lymphopenia with depleted CD4 lymphocytes is common. Serologic tests, including tests to detect antigenemia, are not helpful in diagnosis.

Specific diagnosis depends on morphologic demonstration of the organisms in clinical specimens using specific stains. The organism cannot be reliably cultured. Although patients rarely spontaneously produce sufficient sputum for examination, adequate specimens can usually be obtained with induced sputum by having patients inhale an aerosol of hypertonic saline (3%) produced by an ultrasonic nebulizer. Specimens are then stained with Giemsa's stain or methenamine silver, either of which allows detection of cysts. The use of monoclonal antibody with immunofluorescence has increased the sensitivity of diagnosis. Additional techniques for obtaining specimens include bronchoalveolar lavage (sensitivity 86–97%) followed if necessary by transbronchial lung biopsy (85–97%). Open lung biopsy and needle lung biopsy are infrequently done. Although conclusions are still preliminary, the polymerase chain reaction (PCR) test for the detection of *P carinii* appears to be sensitive but does not provide more rapid diagnosis.

Treatment
(See Table 31–4.)

Treatment should be based on a proved diagnosis because of the toxicity of therapy and the possible coexistence of other infections. Trimethoprim-sulfamethoxazole (TMP-SMZ) and pentamidine isethionate are equally effective, but severe adverse reactions can occur in up to 50% of patients receiving either drug. In non-AIDS patients, the former drug is preferred because of its lower incidence of side effects. In AIDS patients, the choice of agent therefore depends on other factors (eg, in mild to

moderately severe infection, TMP-SMZ but not pentamidine can be given orally; TMP-SMZ is used in preexisting renal disease; pentamidine is used if fluid must be restricted or if there is a history of sulfonamide drug sensitivity). Therapy should be continued with the selected drug for at least 5–10 days before one considers changing agents, as fever, tachypnea, and pulmonary infiltrates persist for 4–6 days after starting treatment; some patients have a transient worsening of their disease during the first 3–5 days, which may be related to an inflammatory response secondary to the presence of dead or dying organisms. See below and Chapter 31 for a discussion of the role of corticosteroids in treatment. Some clinicians prefer to treat episodes of AIDS-associated pneumocystis pneumonia for 21 days rather than the usual 14 days recommended for non-AIDS cases.

A. Trimethoprim-Sulfamethoxazole: The dosage is TMP 20 mg/kg (12–15 mg/kg may decrease side effects without decreasing efficacy) and SMZ 100 mg/kg given orally or intravenously daily in three or four divided doses for 14–21 days. Adverse reactions are generally those of the sulfonamide component. Patients with AIDS have a high frequency of hypersensitivity reactions—fever, rashes (sometimes severe), malaise, neutropenia, hepatitis, nephritis, thrombocytopenia, and hyperbilirubinemia.

B. Pentamidine Isethionate: This drug is administered intravenously (preferred) or intramuscularly as a single dose of 3 mg (salt) per kilogram per day for 14–21 days. To avoid injection site pain or sterile abscesses, most workers administer the drug only intravenously by diluting it in 250 mL of 5% dextrose in water and giving it slowly over 1 hour. Pentamidine causes side effects in nearly 50% of patients. Occasional reactions include rash, neutropenia, abnormal liver function tests, serum folate depression, hyperkalemia, and hypocalcemia. Hypoglycemia (often clinically inapparent), hyperglycemia, hyponatremia, and delayed nephrotoxicity with azotemia may occur. Rarely, a variety of other severe adverse reactions may occur, including anemia, thrombocytopenia, ventricular arrhythmias, and fatal pancreatitis. Blood glucose levels should be monitored. Inadvertent rapid intravenous infusion may cause precipitous hypotension.

C. Atovaquone: Atovaquone is a hydroxynaphthoquinone that has been FDA-approved for patients with mild to moderate disease who cannot tolerate TMP-SMZ or pentamidine, but failure is reported in 15–30% of cases. Mild side effects are common, but no serious reactions have been reported. The dosage is 750 mg three times daily for 21 days. Because absorption can be a problem leading to low serum concentrations and treatment failure, the drug should be taken with food, especially a fatty meal.

D. Other Drugs: Clindamycin, 600 mg three

times daily, plus primaquine, 15 mg/d; and dapsone, 100 mg/d, plus trimethoprim 15 mg/kg/d, in three divided doses daily, are alternative oral regimens for mild to moderate disease or for continuation of therapy after intravenous therapy is initiated. Trimetrexate, 45 mg/m^2/d intravenously, plus high-dose leucovorin has been approved for salvage use in patients not responding to other therapies, but the success rate is less than 25%.

E. Prednisone: In conjunction with antimicrobials, prednisone is given when PaO$_2$ on admission is < 70 mm Hg; its use improves the prognosis in severe pneumocystis pneumonia. For dosages and durations of therapy, see the section on corticosteroids in Chapter 31 and the footnote in Table 31–4.

F. Supportive Care: Because of the hypoxia usually associated with this disease, oxygen therapy is indicated to maintain the oxygen saturation over 90% by pulse oximeter.

Prevention

See Chapter 31 and Table 31–6.

Prognosis

In the absence of early and adequate treatment, the fatality rate for the endemic infantile form of pneumocystosis is 20–50%; for the sporadic form in immunodeficient persons, the fatality rate is nearly 100%. Early treatment reduces the mortality rate to about 3% in the former and 25% in the latter forms of infection. In immunodeficient patients who do not receive prophylaxis, recurrences are common (30% in AIDS).

Black JR et al: Clindamycin and primaquine therapy for mild-to-moderate episodes of *Pneumocystis carinii* pneumonia in patients with AIDS: AIDS Clinical Trials Group 044. Clin Infect Dis 1994;18:905. (This regimen is comparable to trimethoprim-sulfamethoxazole for mild disease.)

Hughes WT: The role of atovaquone tablets in treating *Pneumocystis carinii* pneumonia. J Acquir Immune Defic Syndr Hum Retrovirol 1995;8:247. (Atovaquone has similar clinical success as trimethoprim-sulfamethoxazole and pentamidine and is associated with fewer side effects.)

Sepkowitz KA: *Pneumocystis carinii* pneumonia without acquired immunodeficiency syndrome. More patients, same risk. Arch Intern Med 1995;155:1125.

CRYPTOCOCCOSIS

Essentials of Diagnosis

- Most common cause of fungal meningitis.
- Predisposing factors: Hodgkin's disease, corticosteroids, HIV infection.
- Symptoms of headache, abnormal mental states; meningismus seen occasionally, though rarely in HIV-infected patients.
- Demonstration of capsular antigen in cerebrospinal fluid diagnostic; 95% of HIV-infected patients also show it in serum.

General Considerations

Cryptococcosis is caused by *Cryptococcus neoformans*, an encapsulated budding yeast that has been found worldwide in soil and on dried pigeon dung.

Infections are acquired by inhalation. In the lung, the infection may remain localized, heal, or disseminate. Immunocompetent hosts rarely develop clinically apparent cryptococcal pneumonia. Progressive lung disease and dissemination most often occur in the setting of cellular immunodeficiency, including underlying hematologic cancer under treatment, Hodgkin's disease, long-term corticosteroid therapy, or HIV infection.

Clinical Findings

A. Symptoms and Signs: Disseminated disease may involve any organ, but central nervous system disease usually predominates. Headache is usually the first symptom of meningitis. Confusion and other mental status changes as well as cranial nerve abnormalities, nausea, and vomiting may be seen as the disease progresses. Nuchal rigidity and meningeal signs occur about 50% of the time but are uncommon in HIV-infected patients with this complication. Intracerebral mass lesions (cryptococcomas) are rarely seen. Obstructive hydrocephalus may complicate the course.

B. Laboratory Findings: Spinal fluid findings include increased pressure, variable pleocytosis, budding encapsulated fungus cells, increased protein, and decreased glucose, though as many as 50% of AIDS patients have no pleocytosis. Cryptococcal antigen in cerebrospinal fluid and culture establish the diagnosis 90% of the time. Patients with AIDS often have the antigen in both cerebrospinal fluid and serum, and extrameningeal disease is common.

Treatment

In AIDS-related cryptococcal meningitis, oral fluconazole, 400 mg/d for a minimum of 10 weeks, has reasonable efficacy for acute therapy in patients with mild disease. The best candidates for initial fluconazole therapy are patients with an intact level of consciousness and a spinal fluid cryptococcal antigen titer of less than 1:128. Higher-risk patients should receive amphotericin B initially, but it may be possible to shorten the course and change to fluconazole once clinical stability has been achieved.

There has been a trend away from regimens based on prolonged amphotericin B therapy, particularly in HIV-infected patients. However, this agent remains important, especially in severe disease. Amphotericin B, 0.7–1 mg/kg/d intravenously for 14 days, followed by an additional 8 weeks of fluconazole, 400 mg/d orally, have been quite effective, achieving clinical responses and cerebrospinal fluid sterilization. It does not appear that the addition of flucytosine substantially contributes to improved cure rates; patients who are very ill but can still take oral medications may benefit from flucytosine, 150 mg/kg/d orally, divided into four equal doses and given every 6 hours. The addition of flucytosine at this early stage does appear to prevent late relapses. Repeated lumbar punctures or ventricular shunting may be important to relieve high cerebrospinal fluid pressures or if hydrocephalus is a complication. The end points for amphotericin B therapy are clinical response and culture negativity of the cerebrospinal fluid.

A similar approach is reasonable for patients with cryptococcal meningitis in the absence of AIDS, though the mortality rate is considerably higher. Because of serious underlying illnesses and generally greater age, this group of patients does not tolerate the higher doses of amphotericin B as well as patients with AIDS. Therapy is generally continued if cerebrospinal fluid cultures remain positive or cerebrospinal fluid antigen titers remain greater than 1:8.

A preliminary study in patients with AIDS suggests that fluconazole plus flucytosine is efficacious for mild cases, but this regimen has not been compared with fluconazole alone.

Maintenance antifungal therapy is important after treatment of an acute episode in HIV-related cases, since otherwise the rate of relapse is greater than 50%. Fluconazole, 200 mg/d, is the maintenance therapy of choice, decreasing the relapse rate approximately tenfold compared with placebo and threefold compared with weekly amphotericin B in patients whose cerebrospinal fluid has been sterilized by the induction therapy.

Prognosis

Factors that indicate a poor prognosis include the activity of the predisposing conditions, lack of spinal fluid pleocytosis, high initial antigen titer in either serum or cerebrospinal fluid, decreased mental status, and the presence of disease outside the nervous system.

de Lalla F et al: Amphotericin B as primary therapy for cryptococcosis in patients with AIDS: Reliability of relatively high doses administered over a relatively short period. Clin Infect Dis 1995;20:263. (Relatively high doses of amphotericin B for the first 2 weeks of therapy result in a high rate of microbiologic and clinical success.)

Haubrich RH et al: High-dose fluconazole for treatment of cryptococcal disease in patients with human immunodeficiency virus infection. The California Collaborative Treatment Group. J Infect Dis 1994;170:238. (Small study suggesting benefit of raising daily dose of fluconazole to 800 mg.)

Powderly WG et al: A randomized trial comparing fluconazole with clotrimazole troches for the prevention of fungal infections in patients with advanced human immuno-
deficiency virus infection. N Engl J Med 1995;332:700. (Fluconazole taken prophylactically reduces the frequency of cryptococcosis as well as esophageal candidiasis and superficial fungal infections in HIV-infected patients, especially those with < 50 CD4 lymphocytes/μL, but the drug does not reduce overall mortality. Questions regarding costs, drug interactions, and development of resistant *Candida* remain.)

ASPERGILLOSIS

Aspergillus fumigatus is the usual cause of aspergillosis, though many species of *Aspergillus* may cause a wide spectrum of disease. Burn eschar and detritus in the external ear canal are often colonized by these fungi. Clinical illness results either from an aberrant immunologic response or tissue invasion.

Allergic bronchopulmonary aspergillosis occurs in patients with preexisting asthma who develop worsening bronchospasm and fleeting pulmonary infiltrates accompanied by eosinophilia, high levels of IgE, and *Aspergillus* precipitins in the blood. It also may complicate cystic fibrosis. The disease characteristically pursues a waxing and waning course with gradual improvement over time, but it may result in saccular bronchiectasis and end-stage fibrotic lung disease. For acute exacerbations, oral prednisone is begun at a dose of 1 mg/kg/d and then tapered slowly over several months. Antifungal agents do not have a role in the management of allergic aspergillosis, since the disease is due to an immunologic reaction to the fungus and not related to tissue invasion.

Invasive manifestations may be seen in immunocompetent adults. These include chronic sinusitis and colonization of preexisting pulmonary cavities (**aspergilloma**). Sinus disease may require long courses of antibiotics (itraconazole, 200 mg twice daily, for weeks to months) as well as surgical debridement. Aspergillomas of the lung may be found by incidental radiographic studies but may also present with significant hemoptysis. Intracavitary instillation of amphotericin B and bronchoscopic removal have been tried with little success; several uncontrolled trials have suggested some benefit from itraconazole. The most effective therapy for symptomatic aspergilloma remains surgical resection.

Life-threatening **invasive aspergillosis** most commonly occurs in profoundly immunodeficient patients, particularly those with prolonged severe neutropenia. Patients with very advanced HIV disease may also be at risk for invasive aspergillosis, particularly if they have other risk factors for the disease. Pulmonary disease is most common, with patchy infiltration leading to a severe necrotizing pneumonia. There is often tissue infarction as the organism grows into blood vessels; clues to this are the development of pleuritic chest pain and elevation of serum LDH. AIDS patients are also predisposed to a unique ulcerative tracheobronchitis that may coexist with parenchymal pulmonary disease. At any time, there may be hematogenous dissemination to the central nervous system, skin, and other organs. Early diagnosis and reversal of any correctable immunosuppression are essential. Blood cultures have very low yield. In contrast to allergic aspergillosis, serologic tests and antigen detection have low sensitivities for invasive disease. Isolation of *Aspergillus* from pulmonary secretions does not necessarily imply invasive disease. Therefore, the mainstay of diagnosis is demonstration of *Aspergillus* in tissue. Histologically, one sees branched septate hyphae. Biopsy specimens will not invariably grow the organism.

When severe invasive aspergillosis is considered clinically likely or is demonstrable by biopsy, rapid institution of high doses of amphotericin B may be life-saving (see Chapter 37). The total daily dose is rapidly increased to 0.8–1.5 mg/kg/d intravenously as tolerated for the first several weeks of therapy. Thereafter, more traditional doses of 0.6 mg/kg/d are continued until a total dose of at least 2 g has been reached. The addition of flucytosine is of unclear benefit. Itraconazole orally at a dose of 200–400 mg/d has activity against *Aspergillus,* and initial clinical experience is favorable for less severe disease. Until more data accumulate, amphotericin B should remain the first-line drug for invasive disease. The mortality rate of pulmonary or disseminated disease in the immunocompromised patient remains well above 50%, however.

Andriole VT: *Aspergillus* infections: Problems in diagnosis and treatment. Infect Agents Dis 1996;5:47. (Serologic methods for diagnosis of invasive aspergillosis.)

Denning DW: Therapeutic outcome in invasive aspergillosis. Clin Infect Dis 1996;23:608. (Therapy of invasive aspergillosis continues to be suboptimal. It is not yet clear what role the newer liposomal amphotericin preparations or itraconazole have in management.)

MUCORMYCOSIS

The term "mucormycosis" (zygomycosis, phycomycosis) is applied to opportunistic infections caused by members of the genera *Rhizopus, Mucor, Absidia,* and *Cunninghamella.* Predisposing conditions include diabetic ketoacidosis, chronic renal failure, and treatment with steroids or cytotoxic drugs. These organisms appear in tissues as broad, branching nonseptate hyphae. Biopsy is almost always required for diagnosis. Invasive disease of the sinuses, orbits, and the lungs may be noted. Widely disseminated disease has been more commonly seen recently in patients who have received aggressive chemotherapy. The diagnosis should be considered in acidotic diabetic patients with black necrotic lesions of the nose or sinuses or with new cranial nerve abnormali-

ties. Without treatment, meningeal invasion may ensue. A prolonged course of high-dosage amphotericin B (1–1.5 mg/kg/d intravenously) should be started early. Control of diabetes and other underlying conditions, along with extensive repeated surgical removal of necrotic, nonperfused tissue, are essential. Even when these measures are introduced in a timely fashion, the prognosis is poor, with a 30–50% mortality rate for localized disease and higher rates in disseminated cases.

Nussbaum ES et al: Rhinocerebral mucormycosis: Changing patterns of disease. Surg Neurol 1994;41:152. (Rhinocerebral mucormycosis is increasingly affecting populations of patients with other risk factors besides diabetes mellitus. Early aggressive therapy provides the best chance for a favorable outcome.)

BLASTOMYCOSIS

Blastomycosis occurs more often in men and in a geographically delimited area of the south central and midwestern USA and Canada. A few cases have been found in Mexico and Africa.

Pulmonary infection may be asymptomatic. When dissemination takes place, lesions are most frequently seen on the skin, in bones, and in the urogenital system.

Cough, moderate fever, dyspnea, and chest pain are evident in symptomatic patients. These may resolve or progress, with bloody and purulent sputum production, pleurisy, fever, chills, loss of weight, and prostration. Radiologic studies usually reveal infiltrates and enlarged regional lymph nodes, though less commonly than in histoplasmosis or coccidioidomycosis. Raised, verrucous cutaneous lesions that have an abrupt downward sloping border are usually present in disseminated blastomycosis. The border extends slowly, leaving a central atrophic scar. These lesions persist untreated for long periods, mimicking skin cancer. Bones—often the ribs and vertebrae—are frequently involved. Lesions appear to be both destructive and proliferative on radiography. Epididymitis, prostatitis, and other involvement of the male urogenital system may occur. Central nervous system involvement is uncommon. Cases in HIV-infected persons may progress rapidly, with dissemination common.

Laboratory findings usually include leukocytosis and anemia, though these are not specific. The organism is found in clinical specimens as a thick-walled cell 5–20 mm in diameter that may have a single broad-based bud. It grows readily on culture. Serologic tests are not well standardized.

Itraconazole, 100–200 mg/d orally for at least 2–3 months, is now the therapy of choice for nonmeningeal disease, with a response rate of over 80%. Amphotericin B, 0.3–0.6 mg/kg/d intravenously for a total dose of 1.5–2.5 g, is given for treatment failures or cases with central nervous system involvement.

Follow-up for relapse should be regularly made for several years so that therapy may be resumed or another drug instituted.

Pappas PG et al: Treatment of blastomycosis with fluconazole: A pilot study. Clin Infect Dis 1995;20:267. (Fluconazole was moderately effective for blastomycosis but appears inferior to similar doses of itraconazole.)

PARACOCCIDIOIDOMYCOSIS
(South American Blastomycosis)

Paracoccidioides brasiliensis infections have been found only in patients who have resided in South or Central America or Mexico. Long asymptomatic periods enable patients to travel far from the endemic areas before developing clinical problems. Ulceration of the naso- and oropharynx is usually the first symptom. Papules ulcerate and enlarge both peripherally and deeper into the subcutaneous tissue. Differential diagnosis includes mucocutaneous leishmaniasis and syphilis. Extensive coalescent ulcerations may eventually result in destruction of the epiglottis, vocal cords, and uvula. Extension to the lips and face may occur. Eating and drinking are extremely painful. Skin lesions may occur, usually on the face. Variable in appearance, they may have a necrotic central crater with a hard hyperkeratotic border. Lymph node enlargement may follow mucocutaneous lesions, eventually ulcerating and forming draining sinuses; in some patients, it is the presenting symptom. Hepatosplenomegaly may be present as well. Cough, sometimes with sputum, indicates pulmonary involvement, but the symptoms and signs are often mild, even though radiographic findings indicate severe parenchymatous changes in the lungs. The extensive ulceration of the upper gastrointestinal tract may prevent caloric intake and result in cachexia.

Laboratory findings are nonspecific. Serology by immunodiffusion is positive in 98% of cases. Complement fixation titers correlate with progressive disease and fall with effective therapy. The fungus is found in clinical specimens as a spherical cell that may have many buds arising from it. If direct examination does not reveal the organism, biopsy with Gomori staining may be helpful.

Itraconazole, 100–200 mg orally daily, is the treatment of choice and generally results in a clinical response within 1 month and effective control after 2–6 months.

Brummer E et al: Paracoccidioidomycosis: An update. Clin Microbiol Rev 1993;6:89. (Microbiology, diagnosis, and therapy.)

Restrepo A: Treatment of tropical mycoses. J Am Acad Dermatol 1994;31:S91. (Emphasizes short-course therapy with itraconazole.)

SPOROTRICHOSIS

Sporotrichosis is a chronic fungal infection caused by *Sporothrix schenckii*. It is worldwide in distribution; most patients have had contact with soil, plants, or decaying wood. Infection takes place when the organism is inoculated into the skin—usually on the hand, arm, or foot.

The most common form of sporotrichosis begins with a hard, nontender subcutaneous nodule. This later becomes adherent to the overlying skin and ulcerates. Within a few days to weeks, similar nodules usually develop along the lymphatics draining this area, and these may ulcerate as well. The lymphatic vessels become indurated and are easily palpable. Blood-borne dissemination is rare, and the general health of the patient is not affected.

Disseminated sporotrichosis is rare in the immunocompetent host but may present with lung, bone, joint, and central nervous system involvement in immunocompromised patients.

Cultures are needed to establish diagnosis. Antibody tests may be useful for diagnosis of disseminated disease, especially meningitis.

Itraconazole, 200–400 mg orally daily for several months, is now the treatment of choice for localized disease and some cases of disseminated disease. Amphotericin B intravenously, 1.5–2 g (see Chapter 37), is tried in severe systemic infection. Surgery is usually contraindicated except for simple aspiration of secondary nodules.

The prognosis is good for all forms of sporotrichosis except the disseminated type.

Kauffman CA: Old and new therapies for sporotrichosis. Clin Infect Dis 1995;21:981. (Itraconazole is the drug of choice for most forms of sporotrichosis.)

PENICILLIUM MARNEFFEI INFECTIONS

Penicillium marneffei is a dimorphic fungus, endemic in southeast Asia, that causes systemic infection in both healthy and compromised hosts. There have been increasing reports of patients with advanced AIDS presenting with disseminated infections, including travelers returning from southeast Asia. Clinical manifestations include fever, generalized papular rash, lymphadenopathy, cough, and diarrhea. The best sites for isolation of the fungus include the skin, blood, bone marrow, respiratory tract, and lymph nodes. Patients with mild to moderate infection can be treated with itraconazole, 400 mg daily for 8 weeks. Amphotericin B, 0.5–0.7 mg/kg/d, is the drug of choice for severe disease. Because the relapse rate after successful treatment is 30%, maintenance therapy with itraconazole, 200–400 mg daily, is indicated.

Duong TA: Infection due to *Penicillium marneffei,* an emerging pathogen: Review of 155 reported cases. Clin Infect Dis 1996;23:125.

CHROMOMYCOSIS

Chromomycosis is a chronic, principally tropical cutaneous infection caused by several species of closely related black molds (*Fonsecaea* species and *Phialophora* species).

Lesions are slowly progressive and occur most frequently on a lower extremity. The lesion begins as a papule or ulcer. Over months to years, papules enlarge to become vegetating, papillomatous, verrucous elevated nodules. Satellite lesions may appear along the lymphatics. There may be secondary bacterial infection. Elephantiasis may result.

The fungus is seen as brown, thick-walled, spherical, sometimes septate cells in pus. The type of reproduction found in culture determines the species.

Itraconazole, 100–400 mg/d orally for 6–18 months, has also resulted in a response rate of 65%.

MYCETOMA
(Maduromycosis & Actinomycetoma)

Maduromycosis is the term used to describe mycetoma caused by the true fungi. Actinomycotic mycetoma is caused by *Nocardia* and *Actinomadura* spp. The disease begins as a papule, nodule, or abscess that over months to years progresses slowly to form multiple abscesses and sinus tracts ramifying deep into the tissue. Secondary bacterial infection may result in large open ulcers. Radiographs may show destructive changes in the underlying bone. The agents occur as white, yellow, red, or black granules in tissue or pus. Microscopic examination assists in the diagnosis.

The prognosis is good for patients with actinomycetoma, since they usually respond well to sulfonamides and sulfones, especially if treated early. Trimethoprim-sulfamethoxazole, 160/800 mg orally twice a day, or dapsone, 100 mg twice daily after meals, has also been reported to be effective. Streptomycin, 14 mg/kg/d intramuscularly, may be useful during the first month of therapy. All other medications must be taken for months and continued for several months after clinical cure to prevent relapse. Debridement assists healing.

The prognosis for maduromycosis is poor, though prolonged itraconazole therapy may result in a response rate of 70%. Amputation is necessary in far-advanced cases.

Restrepo A: Treatment of tropical mycoses. J Am Acad Dermatol 1994;31:S91. (Emphasizes short-course therapy with itraconazole.)

OTHER OPPORTUNISTIC MOLD INFECTIONS

Fungi previously considered to be harmless colonizers (eg, *Pseudallescheria boydii, Fusarium, Paecilomyces, Penicillium*) are emerging as significant pathogens in immunocompromised patients. This occurs most often in patients being treated for hematopoietic malignancies. Infection may be localized in the skin, lungs, or sinuses, or widespread disease may appear with lesions in multiple organs. Colonization of old cavitary disease may cause minimal symptoms or may precede dissemination with meningitis or brain abscesses. Endocarditis occurs more commonly in intravenous drug abusers. Sinus infection may cause bony erosion. Infection in subcutaneous tissues following traumatic implantation may develop as a well-circumscribed cyst or as an ulcer.

Nonpigmented septate hyphae are seen in tissue and are indistinguishable from those of *Aspergillus* when infections are due to *Pseudallescheria boydii* or species of *Fusarium, Paecilomyces, Penicillium,* or other hyaline molds. Spores or mycetoma-like granules are rarely present in tissue.

Infection by any of a number of black molds is designated as **phaeohyphomycosis.** These black molds are common in the environment, especially on decaying vegetation, and do not cause infection in the normal host, although some black molds, as well as some hyaline molds, are allergens. In tissues of patients with phaeohyphomycosis, the mold is seen as black or faintly brown hyphae, yeast cells, or both. Culture on appropriate medium is needed to identify the agent. Histologic demonstration of these organisms is definitive evidence of invasive infection; positive cultures must be interpreted cautiously and not assumed to be contaminants in immunocompromised hosts. Some isolates are sensitive to antifungal antibiotics. The differentiation of *Pseudallescheria boydii* and *Aspergillus* is particularly important, since the former is uniformly resistant to amphotericin B but may be sensitive to imidazole antibiotics.

Perfect JR et al: The new fungal opportunists are coming. Clin Infect Dis 1996;22(Suppl 2):S112. (Review of recently recognized fungal opportunists and suggestions for therapy.)

ANTIFUNGAL THERAPY

Table 36–1 summarizes the major properties of currently available antifungal agents. In addition to the newer antimicrobial agents that have been introduced over the past several years, there are several other important developments in the treatment of invasive fungal disease. A number of lipid-based amphotericin B formulations have recently become available. In early noncomparative studies, these

Table 36–1. Agents for systemic mycoses.

Drug	Dosing	Renal Clearance?	CSF Penetration?	Toxicities	Spectrum of Activity
Amphotericin B	0.3–1.5 mg/kg/d IV	No	Poor	Rigors, fever, azotemia, hypokalemia, hypomagnesemia, renal tubular acidosis, anemia	All major pathogens except *Pseudallescheria*
Amphotericin B lipid complex	5 mg/kg/d IV	No	Poor	Fever, rigors, nausea, hypotension, anemia, azotemia, tachypnea	Same as amphotericin B, above
Amphotericin B colloidal suspension	3–6 mg/kg/d IV	No	Poor	Fever, rigors, nausea, hypotension, azotemia, hypomagnesemia, anemia, tachypnea	Same as amphotericin B, above
Liposomal amphotericin B	3–6 mg/kg/d IV	No	Poor	Fever, rigors, nausea, hypotension, azotemia, anemia, tachypnea, chest tightness	Same as amphotericin B, above
Flucytosine (5-FC)	150 mg/kg/d orally in 4 divided doses	Yes	Yes	Leukopenia,[1] rash, diarrhea, hepatitis, nausea, vomiting	Cryptococcosis,[2] candidiasis,[2] chromomycosis
Ketoconazole	200–800 mg/d orally in 1 or 2 doses	No	Poor	Anorexia, nausea, suppression of testosterone and cortisol, rash, hepatitis[3]	Nonmeningeal histoplasmosis and coccidioidomycosis, blastomycosis, paracoccidioidomycosis, mucosal candidiasis (except urinary)
Fluconazole	100–400 mg/d in 1 or 2 doses IV or orally	Yes	Yes	Nausea, rash, alopecia[4]	Mucosal candidiasis (including urinary tract), cryptococcosis, histoplasmosis, perhaps coccidioidomycosis
Itraconazole	100–400 mg/d orally as single dose	No	Variable	Nausea, hypokalemia, edema, hypertension[3]	Same as ketoconazole plus sporotrichosis, aspergillosis, chromomycosis

[1]Use should be monitored with blood levels to prevent this or the dose adjusted according to creatinine clearance.
[2]In combination with amphotericin B.
[3]Drug interaction with terfenadine, astemizole, or cisapride may produce prolongation of the QT interval, ventricular arrhythmias, and torsades de pointes.
[4]Drug interaction with cisapride may produce prolongation of the QT interval, ventricular arrhythmias, and torsades de pointes.

agents have shown promise in the treatment of systemic candidiasis, invasive aspergillosis, and cryptococcal meningitis. Their principal advantage appears to be substantially reduced nephrotoxicity, allowing administration of much higher doses. Because of their expense, use of these agents should be reserved for individuals who develop significant nephrotoxicity during amphotericin B therapy. Cytokine therapy and use of growth factors such as GM-CSF (sargramostim or molgramostim) have been shown in animal models to increase clearance of fungi and result in better clinical outcomes.

Coma JA et al: Oral azole drugs as systemic antifungal therapy. N Engl J Med 1994;330:263.
Hiemenz JW et al: Lipid formulations of amphotericin B: Recent progress and future directions. Clin Infect Dis 1996;22(Suppl 2):S133.
Sarosi GA et al: Therapy for fungal infections. Mayo Clin Proc 1994;69:1111. (Provides suggested antifungal regimens for the major mycoses.)

37

Anti-infective Chemotherapeutic & Antibiotic Agents

Richard A. Jacobs, MD, PhD, & B. Joseph Guglielmo, PharmD

Some Principles of Antimicrobial Therapy

Antimicrobial drugs are used on a very large scale, and their proper use gives striking therapeutic results. On the other hand, they can create serious untoward reactions and should therefore be administered only upon proper indication.

Drugs of first choice and alternative drugs are presented in Table 37–1.

The following steps are required in each patient considered for antibiotic therapy.

A. Etiologic Diagnosis: Formulate an etiologic diagnosis based on clinical observations. Microbial infections are best treated early. The physician must decide on clinical grounds (1) whether the patient has a microbial infection that can be favorably influenced by antimicrobial drugs and (2) the kind of pathogen most probably causing such infection. Based on the organ system involved, the bacteria causing infection can usually be predicted ("best guess"). See Tables 37–2 and 37–3.

B. "Best Guess": Select a specific antimicrobial drug on the basis of past experience for empirical therapy. Based on a "best guess," the physician should choose a drug or combination of drugs that is likely to be effective against the suspected pathogens.

C. Laboratory Control: In most cases, specimens for laboratory examination are obtained before antimicrobial therapy is started to determine the causative infectious organism and, if desirable, susceptibility to antimicrobial drugs.

D. Clinical Response: Based on the clinical response of the patient, evaluate the laboratory reports and consider the desirability of changing the antimicrobial drug regimen. Laboratory results should not overrule clinical judgment. Isolation of an organism that confirms the initial clinical impression is useful. Conversely, laboratory results may contradict the initial clinical impression and compel its reconsideration. If the specimen was obtained from a site that is normally devoid of bacterial flora and not exposed to the external environment (eg, blood, cerebrospinal fluid, pleural fluid, joint fluid), the recovery of a microorganism is a significant finding even if the organism recovered is different from the clinically suspected etiologic agent, and this may force a change in treatment. On the other hand, isolation of unexpected microorganisms from the respiratory tract, gastrointestinal tract, or surface lesions (sites that have a complex flora) must be critically evaluated before drugs are abandoned that were judiciously selected on the basis of an initial "best guess" for empirical treatment.

E. Drug Susceptibility Tests: Some microorganisms are fairly uniformly susceptible to certain drugs; if such organisms are isolated, they need not be tested for drug susceptibility. For example, most group A hemolytic streptococci and clostridia respond predictably well to penicillin. On the other hand, some organisms (eg, enteric gram-negative rods) are variably susceptible to antimicrobial agents and require drug susceptibility testing whenever they are isolated from a significant specimen. Recently, organisms that have had predictable antibiotic susceptibility patterns have become resistant and now require susceptibility testing. Examples include the pneumococcus, which may be resistant to multiple agents, including penicillin, and the enterococci, which may be resistant to penicillin, aminoglycosides, and vancomycin.

Antimicrobial drug susceptibility tests may be performed on solid media as "disk tests," in broth in tubes, or in wells of microdilution plates. The latter two methods yield results expressed as MIC (minimal inhibitory concentration), and the technique can be modified to give MBC (minimal bactericidal concentration) results. In some infections, the MIC or MBC permits a better estimate of the amount of drug required for therapeutic effect in vivo.

Disk tests usually indicate whether an isolate is susceptible or resistant to serum concentrations of drug achieved in vivo with conventional dosage regimens, thus providing valuable guidance in selecting therapy. When there appear to be marked discrepancies between test results and clinical response of the patient, the following possibilities must be considered:

Table 37–1. Drugs of choice for suspected or proved microbial pathogens, 1998.[1] (± = alone or combined with)

Suspected or Proved Etiologic Agent	Drug(s) of First Choice	Alternative Drug(s)
Gram-negative cocci		
Moraxella catarrhalis	TMP-SMZ[2]	Cefuroxime, cefotaxime, ceftizoxime, ceftriaxone, cefepime, cefuroxime axetil, an erythromycin,[3] a tetracycline,[4] azithromycin, amoxicillin-clavulanic acid, clarithromycin, a fluoroquinolone[5]
Neisseria gonorrhoeae (gonococcus)	Ceftriaxone or cefixime	Ciprofloxacin, spectinomycin, ofloxacin, cefpodoxime proxetil
Neisseria meningitidis (meningococcus)	Penicillin[6]	Cefotaxime, ceftizoxime, ceftriaxone, ampicillin, chloramphenicol
Gram-positive cocci		
Streptococcus pneumoniae[7] (pneumococcus)	Penicillin[6]	An erythromycin,[3] a cephalosporin,[8] vancomycin, TMP-SMZ, chloramphenicol, clindamycin, azithromycin, clarithromycin
Streptococcus, hemolytic, groups A, B, C, G	Penicillin[6]	An erythromycin,[3] a cephalosporin,[8] vancomycin, clindamycin, azithromycin, clarithromycin
Viridans streptococci	Penicillin[6] ± gentamicin	Cephalosporin,[8] vancomycin
Staphylococcus, methicillin-resistant	Vancomycin ± gentamicin ± rifampin	TMP-SMZ,[2] minocycline
Staphylococcus, non-pencillinase-producing	Penicillin[6]	A cephalosporin,[8] vancomycin, imipenem, clindamycin
Staphylococcus, penicillinase-producing	Penicillinase-resistant penicillin[9]	Vancomycin, a cephalosporin,[8] clindamycin, amoxicillin-clavulanic acid, ticarcillin-clavulanic acid, ampicillin-sulbactam, piperacillin-tazobactam, imipenem, TMP-SMZ[2]
Enterococcus faecalis	Ampicillin + gentamicin	Vancomycin + gentamicin
Enterococcus faecium	Vancomycin + gentamicin	Quinupristin-dalfopristin (Synercid)[10]
Gram-negative rods		
Acinetobacter	Imipenem	Minocycline, TMP-SMZ,[2] doxycycline, aminoglycosides,[11] pipericillin, ceftazidime, a fluoroquinolone[5]
Prevotella, oropharyngeal strains	Clindamycin	Penicillin,[6] metronidazole, cefoxitin, cefotetan
Bacteroides, gastrointestinal strains	Metronidazole	Cefoxitin, chloramphenicol, clindamycin, cefotetan, cefmetazole, imipenem, ticarcillin-clavulanic acid, ampicillin-sulbactam, piperacillin-tazobactam
Brucella	Tetracycline[4] + gentamicin	TMP-SMZ[2] ± gentamicin; chloramphenicol ± gentamicin
Campylobacter	A fluoroquinolone[5]	Tetracycline,[4] erythromycin[3]
Enterobacter	TMP-SMZ,[2] imipenem	Aminoglycoside,[11] aztreonam, a fluoroquinolone,[5] cefepime
Escherichia coli (sepsis)	Cefotaxime, ceftizoxime, ceftriaxone, ceftazidime, cefepime	Ampicillin, TMP-SMZ,[2] imipenem, aminoglycosides, a fluoroquinolone[5]
Escherichia coli (first urinary infection)	Sulfonamide,[12] TMP-SMZ[2]	Ampicillin, cephalosporin,[8] ciprofloxacin, ofloxacin
Haemophilus (meningitis and other serious infections)	Cefotaxime, ceftizoxime, ceftriaxone, ceftazidime	Chloramphenicol
Haemophilus (respiratory infections, otitis)	TMP-SMZ[2]	Ampicillin, amoxicillin, doxycycline, azithromycin, clarithromycin, cefotaxime, ceftizoxime, ceftriaxone, cefepime, cefuroxime, cefuroxime axetil
Helicobacter pylori	Tetracycline + metronidazole + bismuth subsalicylate	Amoxicillin + metronidazole + bismuth subsalicylate; tetracycline + clarithromycin + bismuth subsalicylate
Klebsiella	Cefotaxime, ceftizoxime, ceftriaxone, ceftazidime, cefepime	TMP-SMZ,[2] aminoglycoside,[11] imipenem, a fluoroquinolone,[5] piperacillin, mezlocillin
Legionella species (pneumonia)	Erythromycin[2] ± rifampin	TMP-SMZ,[2] clarithromycin, azithromycin, ciprofloxacin
Pasteurella (Yersinia) (plague, tularemia)	Streptomycin	Chloramphenicol, a tetracycline,[4] gentamicin
Proteus mirabilis	Ampicillin	An aminoglycoside,[11] TMP-SMZ,[2] ciprofloxacin, ofloxacin
Proteus vulgaris and other species (_Morganella, Providencia_)	Cefotaxime, ceftizoxime, ceftriaxone, ceftazidime, cefepime	Aminoglycoside,[11] imipenem, TMP-SMZ,[2] a fluoroquinolone[5]
Pseudomonas aeruginosa	Aminoglycoside[11] + antipseudomonal penicillin[13]	Ceftazidime ± aminoglycoside; imipenem ± aminoglycoside; aztreonam ± aminoglycoside; ciprofloxacin ± piperacillin; ciprofloxacin ± ceftazidime

(continued)

Table 37–1. Drugs of choice for suspected or proved microbial pathogens, 1998.[1] (± = alone or combined with) (continued)

Suspected or Proved Etiologic Agent	Drug(s) of First Choice	Alternative Drug(s)
Pseudomonas pseudomallei (melioidosis)	Ceftazidime	Chloramphenicol, tetracycline,[4] TMP-SMZ,[2] amoxicillin-clavulanic acid, imipenem
Pseudomonas mallei (glanders)	Streptomycin + tetracycline[4]	Chloramphenicol + streptomycin
Salmonella (bacteremia)	Ceftriaxone, a fluoroquinolone[5]	TMP-SMZ,[2] ampicillin, chlorampenicol
Serratia	Cefotaxime, ceftizoxime, ceftriaxone, ceftazidime, cefepime	TMP-SMZ,[2] aminoglycosides,[11] imipenem, a fluoroquinolone[5]
Shigella	A fluoroquinolone[5]	Ampicillin, TMP-SMZ,[2] ceftriaxone
Vibrio (cholera, sepsis)	Tetracycline[4]	TMP-SMZ,[2] a fluoroquinolone[5]
Gram-positive rods		
Actinomyces	Penicillin[6]	Tetracycline,[4] clindamycin
Bacillus (eg, anthrax)	Penicillin[6]	Erythromycin,[3] tetracycline[4]
Clostridium (eg, gas gangrene, tetanus)	Penicillin[6]	Metronidazole, chloramphenicol, clindamycin, imipenem
Corynebacterium diphtheriae	Erythromycin[3]	Penicillin[6]
Corynebacterium jeikeium	Vancomycin	Ciprofloxacin, penicillin + gentamicin
Listeria	TMP-SMZ[2]	Ampicillin ± aminoglycoside[11]
Acid-fast rods		
Mycobacterium tuberculosis[14]	INH + rifampin + pyrazinamide ± ethambutol or streptomycin	Other antituberculous drugs
Mycobacterium leprae	Dapsone + rifampin ± clofazimine	Minocycline, ofloxacin, clarithromycin
Mycobacterium kansasii	INH + rifampin ± ethambutol	Ethionamide, cycloserine
Mycobacterium avium complex	Clarithromycin or azithromycin + one or more of the following: ethambutol, clofazimine, ciprofloxacin, amikacin	Other antituberculous drugs
Mycobacterium fortuitum-chelonei	Amikacin + doxycycline	Cefoxitin, erythromycin, sulfonamide
Nocardia	TMP-SMZ[2]	Minocycline, imipenem, sulfisoxazole[12]
Spirochetes		
Borrelia burgdorferi (Lyme disease)	Tetracycline[4]	Amoxicillin, ceftriaxone, cefuroxime axetil, azithromycin, clarithromycin, penicillin
Borrelia recurrentis (relapsing fever)	Tetracycline[4]	Penicillin[6]
Leptospira	Penicillin[6]	Tetracycline[4]
Treponema pallidum (syphilis)	Penicillin[6]	Tetracycline,[4] ceftriaxone
Treponema pertenue (yaws)	Penicillin[6]	Tetracycline[4]
Mycoplasmas	Erythromycin[3] or tetracycline[4]	Clarithromycin, azithromycin
Chlamydiae		
C psittaci	Tetracycline[4]	Chloramphenicol
C trachomatis (urethritis or pelvic inflammatory disease)	Doxycycline or azithromycin	Ofloxacin or sulfisoxazole
C pneumoniae	Tetracycline[4]	Erythromycin,[3] clarithromycin
Rickettsiae	Tetracycline[4]	Chloramphenicol, ciprofloxacin, ofloxacin

[1]Adapted from Med Lett Drugs Ther 1996;38:25.

[2]TMP-SMZ is a mixture of 1 part trimethoprim and 5 parts sulfamethoxazole.

[3]Erythromycin estolate is best absorbed orally but carries the highest risk of hepatitis; erythromycin stearate and erythromycin ethylsuccinate are also available.

[4]All tetracyclines have similar activity against microorganisms. Dosage is determined by rates of absorption and excretion of various preparations.

[5]Fluoroquinolones include ciprofloxacin, ofloxacin, levofloxacin, sparfloxacin, and others (see text).

[6]Penicillin G is preferred for parenteral injection; penicillin V for oral administration—to be used only in treating infections due to highly sensitive organisms.

[7]Most cephalosporins (with the exception of ceftazidime) have good activity against gram-positive cocci.

[8]Intermediate and high-level resistance to penicillin has been described. Infections caused by strains with intermediate resistance may respond to high doses of penicillin, cefotaxime, or ceftriaxone. Infections caused by highly resistant strains should be treated with vancomycin ± rifampin. Some strains of penicillin-resistant pneumococci are resistant to erythromycin, macrolides, TMP-SMZ, and chloramphenicol.

[9]Parenteral nafcillin or oxacillin; oral dicloxacillin, cloxacillin, or oxacillin.

[10]Synercid is an investigational drug available through Rhône-Poulenc Rorer.

[11]Aminoglycosides—gentamicin, tobramycin, amikacin, netilmicin—should be chosen on the basis of local patterns of susceptibility.

[12]Oral sulfisoxazole is highly soluble in urine; parenteral TMP-SMZ can be injected intravenously in treating severely ill patients.

[13]Antipseudomonal penicillins: ticarcillin, mezlocillin, pipericillin.

[14]Resistance may be a problem, and susceptibility testing should be done.

Table 37–2. Examples of initial antimicrobial therapy for acutely ill adults pending identification of causative organism.

	Suspected Clinical Diagnosis	Likely Etiologic Diagnosis	Drugs of Choice
(A)	Meningitis, bacterial	Pneumococcus,[1] meningococcus	Cefotaxime,[2] 2–3 g IV every 6 hours, or ceftriaxone, 2 g IV every 12 hours
(B)	Meningitis, bacterial, age > 50	Pneumococcus, meningococcus, *Listeria monocytogenes,*[3] gram-negative bacilli	Ampicillin, 2 g IV every 4 hours, plus cefotaxime or ceftriaxone as in (A)
(C)	Meningitis, postoperative (or posttraumatic)	*S aureus,* gram-negative bacilli (pneumococcus, posttraumatic)	Vancomycin, 10 mg/kg every 8 hours, plus ceftazidime, 3 g IV every 8 hours
(D)	Brain abscess	Mixed anaerobes, pneumococci, streptococci	Penicillin G, 4 million units IV every 4 hours, or metronidazole, 500 mg IV every 8 hours, plus cefotaxime or ceftriaxone as in (A)
(E)	Pneumonia, acute, community-acquired, severe	Pneumococci, *M pneumoniae,* Legionella, *C pneumoniae*	Erythromycin,[4] 0.5 g orally or IV four times daily, or doxycycline, 100 mg IV or orally every 12 hours, plus cefotaxime, 1–2 g IV every 12 hours (or ceftriaxone, 1 g IV every 24 hours)
(F)	Pneumonia, postoperative or nosocomial	*S aureus,* mixed anaerobes, gram-negative bacilli	Cefotaxime (or ceftriaxone) with or without tobramycin
(G)	Endocarditis, acute (including IV drug user)	*S aureus, E faecalis,* gram-negative aerobic bacteria, viridans streptococci	Penicillin G, 2–3 million units IV every 4 hours, plus nafcillin, 2 g IV every 4 hours, plus gentamicin, 2 mg/kg every 8 hours
(H)	Septic thrombophlebitis (eg, IV tubing, IV shunts)	*S aureus,* gram-negative aerobic bacteria	Nafcillin, 2 g IV every 4 hours, plus gentamicin,[5] 2 mg/kg every 8 hours
(I)	Osteomyelitis	*S aureus*	Nafcillin, 2 g IV every 4 hours
(J)	Septic arthritis	*S aureus, N gonorrhoeae*	Ceftriaxone, 1–2 g IV every 4 hours
(K)	Pyelonephritis with flank pain and fever (recurrent UTI)	*E coli, Klebsiella, Enterobacter, Pseudomonas*	Ciprofloxacin, 400 mg IV every 12 hours, or levofloxacin, 500 mg IV once daily
(L)	Suspected sepsis in neutropenic patient receiving cancer chemotherapy	*S aureus, Pseudomonas, Klebsiella, E coli*	Ceftazidime, 2 g IV every 8 hours, or piperacillin-tazobactam, 4.5 g IV every 6 hours
(M)	Intra-abdominal sepsis (eg, post-operative, peritonitis, cholecystitis)	Gram-negative bacteria, *Bacteroides,* anaerobic bacteria, streptococci, clostridia	Ampicillin, 1–2 g every 6 hours, or gentamicin, 2 mg/kg every 8 hours, plus metronidazole, 500 mg IV every 8 hours

[1]Some strains may be resistant to penicillin, in which case vancomycin, 30–40 mg/kg/d in two or three divided doses, should be used with or without rifampin.
[2]Cefotaxime, ceftriaxone, ceftazidime, or ceftizoxime can be used. Most studies on meningitis have been done with cefotaxime or ceftriaxone (see text).
[3]TMP-SMZ can be used to treat *Listeria monocytogenes* in patients allergic to penicillin in a dosage of 15–20 mg/kg of TMP in three or four divided doses.
[4]Other macrolides such as azithromycin or clarithromycin can be used.
[5]Depending on local drug susceptibility pattern, use tobramycin, 5–7 mg/kg/d, or amikacin, 15 mg/kg/d, in place of gentamicin.

1. Selection of an inappropriate drug, dosage, or route of administration.

2. Failure to drain a collection of pus or to remove a foreign body.

3. Failure of a poorly diffusing drug to reach the site of infection (eg, central nervous system) or to reach intracellular phagocytosed bacteria.

4. Superinfection in the course of prolonged chemotherapy. After suppression of the original infection or of normal flora, a second type of microorganism may establish itself against which the originally selected drug is ineffective.

5. Emergence of drug-resistant or tolerant organisms.

6. Participation of two or more microorganisms in the infectious process, of which only one was originally detected and used for drug selection.

7. Inadequate host defenses, including immunodeficiencies and diabetes.

8. Noninfectious causes, including drug fever, malignancy, and autoimmune disease.

F. Adequate Dosage: Adequacy of therapy is usually assessed by a favorable clinical response. The rapidity of response depends on a number of factors, including the host (immunocompromised patients respond slower than immunocompetent patients), the site of infection (deep-seated infections such as osteomyelitis and endocarditis respond more slowly than superficial infections such as cystitis or cellulitis), the pathogen (virulent organisms such as *Staphylococcus aureus* respond more slowly than viridans streptococci; mycobacterial and fungal infections respond slower than bacterial infections), and the duration of illness (in general, the longer the

Table 37–3. Examples of empirical choices of antimicrobials for adult outpatient infections.

Suspected Clinical Diagnosis	Likely Etiologic Agents	Drugs of Choice	Alternative Drugs
Erysipelas, impetigo, cellulitis, ascending lymphangitis	Group A *streptococcus*	Phenoxymethyl penicillin, 0.5 g orally four times daily.	Erythromycin, 0.5 g orally four times daily, or cephalexin, 0.5 g orally four times daily for 7–10 days; azithromycin, 500 mg on day 1, and 250 mg on days 2–5.
Furuncle with surrounding cellulitis	*Staphylococcus aureus*	Dicloxacillin, 0.5 g orally four times daily for 7–10 days.	Cephalexin, 0.5 g orally four times daily for 7–10 days.
Pharyngitis	Group A *streptococcus*	Phenoxymethyl penicillin, 0.5 g orally four times daily for 10 days.	Erythromycin, 0.5 g orally four times daily for 10 days; azithromycin, 500 mg on day 1 and 250 mg on days 2–5, or clindamycin, 200 mg orally two to four times daily, or clarithromycin, 800 mg four times daily for 10 days.
Otitis media	*Streptococcus pneumoniae, Haemophilus influenzae, Moraxella catarrhalis*	Amoxicillin, 0.5 g orally three times daily; or TMP-SMZ, one double-strength tablet twice daily for 10 days.	Augmentin,[2] 0.5 g orally 3 times daily; cefuroxime, 0.5 g orally twice daily; or cefoxime, 0.2–0.4 g daily for 10 days.
Acute sinusitis	*S pneumoniae, H influenzae, M catarrhalis*	Amoxicillin, 0.5 g orally three times daily; or TMP-SMZ, one double-strength tablet twice daily for 10 days.	Augmentin,[2] 0.5 g orally three times daily; cefuroxime, 0.5 g orally twice daily; or cefoxime, 0.2–0.4 g daily for 10 days.
Aspiration pneumonia	Mixed oropharyngeal flora, including anaerobes	Clindamycin, 0.3 g orally four times daily for 10–14 days.	Phenoxymethyl penicillin, 0.5 g orally four times daily for 10–14 days.
Pneumonia	*S pneumoniae, Mycoplasma pneumoniae, Legionella pneumophila, Chlamydia pneumoniae*	Erythromycin 0.5 g orally four times daily for 10–14 days, or doxycycline, 100 mg orally every 12 hours.	Phenoxymethyl penicillin, 0.5 g orally four times daily for 10 days, or azithromycin as above or clarithromycin as above.
Cystitis	*Escherichia coli, Klebsiella pneumoniae, Proteus* species, *Staphylococcus saprophyticus*	TMP-SMZ,[1] one double-strength tablet twice daily for 3 days.	Fluoroquinolones[4]
Pyelonephritis	*E coli, K pneumoniae, Proteus* species, *S saprophyticus*	Fluoroquinolones[4].	TMP-SMZ,[1] one double-strength tablet twice daily.
Gastroenteritis	*Salmonella, Shigella, Campylobacter, Entamoeba histolytica*	See Note 3.	
Urethritis, epididymitis	*Neisseria gonorrhoeae, Chlamydia trachomatis*	Ceftriaxone, 250 mg IM once for *N gonorrhoeae*; doxycycline, 100 mg twice daily for 10 days for *C trachomatis*.	Ofloxacin, 400 mg once, or ciprofloxacin, 500 mg once, for *N gonorrhoeae*; doxycycline, 100 mg twice daily for 10 days, or ofloxacin, 300 mg orally twice daily for 10 days for *C trachomatis*.
Pelvic inflammatory disease	*N gonorrhoeae, C trachomatis*, anaerobes, gram-negative rods	Ceftriaxone, 250 mg IM once, followed by doxycycline, 100 mg orally twice daily for 10–14 days.	Cefoxitin, 2 g IM, with probenecid, 1 g orally, followed by doxycycline, 100 mg orally twice daily for 10–14 days, or ofloxacin, 400 mg orally twice daily for 14 days, plus clindamycin, 450 mg orally four times daily, or metronidazole, 500 mg orally twice daily for 14 days.
Syphilis Early syphilis (primary, secondary, or latent) of < 1 year's duration	*Treponema pallidum*	Benzathine penicillin G, 2.4 million units IM once.	Doxycycline, 100 mg orally twice daily or tetracycline, 0.5 g orally four times daily for 2 weeks.
Latent syphilis of > 1 year's duration or cardiovascular syphilis		Benzathine penicillin G, 2.4 million units/d IV for 10 days.	Tetracycline, 0.5 g orally four times daily; or doxycycline, 100 mg orally twice daily for 4 weeks.

(continued)

Table 37–3. Examples of empirical choices of antimicrobials for adult outpatient infections. (continued)

Suspected Clinical Diagnosis	Likely Etiologic Agents	Drugs of Choice	Alternative Drugs
Neurosyphilis		Aqueous penicillin G, 12–24 million units/d IV for 10 days.	Procaine penicillin G, 2–4 million units/d IM, plus probenecid, 500 mg orally four times daily, both for 10 days.

[1]TMP-SMZ is a fixed combination of 1 part trimethoprim and 5 parts sulfamethoxazole. Single-strength tablets: 80 mg TMP, 400 mg SMZ; double-strength tablets: 160 mg TMP, 800 mg SMZ.
[2]Augmentin is a combination of amoxicillin, 250 mg or 500 mg, plus 125 mg of clavulanic acid.
[3]The diagnosis should be confirmed by culture before therapy. *Salmonella* gastroenteritis does not require therapy. For *Shigella*, give TMP-SMZ double-strength tablets twice daily for 5 days; or ampicillin, 0.5 g orally four times daily for 5 days; or ciprofloxacin, 0.5 g orally four times daily for 5 days. For *Campylobacter*, give erythromycin, 0.5 g orally four times daily for 5 days; or ciprofloxacin, 0.5 g orally four times daily for 5 days. For *E histolytica*, give metronidazole, 750 mg orally three times daily for 5–10 days, followed by diiodohydroxyquin, 600 mg three times daily for 3 weeks.
[4]Fluoroquinolines and dosages include ciprofloxacin, 500 mg orally twice daily; ofloxacin, 400 mg orally twice daily; levofloxacin, 500 mg daily; and sparfloxacin, 500 mg as loading dose and then 200 mg once daily. For others see text.

symptoms are present, the longer it takes to respond). Thus, depending on the clinical situation, persistent fever and leukocytosis several days after initiation of therapy may not indicate improper choice of antibiotics but may be due to the natural history of the disease being treated. In most infections, either a bacteriostatic or a bactericidal agent can be used. In some infections (eg, infective endocarditis and meningitis), one must kill the infecting organism to achieve a cure. When potentially toxic drugs (eg, aminoglycosides, flucytosine) are used, the serum levels of the drug should be measured to avoid toxicity and ensure appropriate dosage. In patients with altered clearance of drugs, the dosage or frequency of administration must be adjusted. Especially in elderly, morbidly obese patients or those with altered renal function, it is best to measure levels directly and adjust therapy accordingly.

In renal or hepatic failure, the dosage must be adjusted as shown in Table 37–4.

G. Duration of Antimicrobial Therapy: Generally, effective antimicrobial treatment results in reversal of the clinical and laboratory parameters of active infection and marked clinical improvement. However, varying periods of treatment may be required for cure. Key factors include (1) the type of infecting organism (bacterial infections can be cured more rapidly than fungal or mycobacterial ones), (2) the location of the process (eg, endocarditis and osteomyelitis require prolonged therapy), and (3) the immunocompetence of the patient. It is noteworthy that very few studies have examined appropriate length of treatment to effect a cure, and duration of therapy is often arbitrary.

H. Adverse Reactions: All antimicrobials can cause adverse effects. Most commonly these are (1) hypersensitivity reactions (eg, fever, rashes, anaphylaxis), (2) direct toxicity (eg, diarrhea, vomiting, impairment of renal or hepatic function, neurotoxicity), (3) superinfection by drug-resistant microorganisms, or (4) drug interactions such as the increased

INR associated with trimethoprim-sulfamethoxazole added to warfarin.

If the infection is life-threatening and treatment cannot be stopped, the reactions may be managed symptomatically (especially if mild) or another drug may be chosen that does not cross-react with the offending one (Table 37–1). If the infection is less severe, it may be possible to stop all antimicrobials and follow the patient carefully.

I. Route of Administration: Parenteral therapy is preferred for acutely ill patients with serious infections (eg, endocarditis, meningitis, sepsis, severe pneumonia) when high levels of antibiotics are required for successful therapy. Certain drugs (eg, fluconazole, rifampin, metronidazole, and fluoroquinolones) are so well absorbed that they can be administered orally even in seriously ill patients.

Food does not significantly influence the bioavailability of most oral antimicrobial agents. Exceptions include the tetracyclines and the quinolones, which are chelated by heavy metals. Azithromycin capsules are associated with decreased bioavailability when taken with food and should be given 1 hour before or 2 hours after meals.

A major complication of intravenous antibiotic therapy is catheter infections. To minimize infections, peripheral Teflon catheters are routinely changed every 48–72 hours to prevent phlebitis. Most catheter-related infections present with local signs of infection (erythema, tenderness) at the insertion site; in some, there is a normal-appearing insertion site. In the evaluation of a patient with fever who is receiving intravenous therapy, the catheter must always be considered as a potential source. Some small-gauge (20–23F) peripherally inserted silicone or polyurethane catheters (Per Q Cath, A-Cath, Ven-A-Cath, and others) are associated with a very low infection rate and can be maintained for 3–6 months without replacement. Such catheters are ideal for long-term outpatient antibiotic therapy.

J. Cost of Antibiotics: Because of the wide-

Table 37–4. Use of antimicrobials in patients with renal failure[1] and hepatic failure.

	Principal Mode of Excretion or Detoxification	Approximate Half-Life in Serum		Proposed Dosage Regimen in End-Stage Renal Failure		Removal of Drug by Hemodialysis	Dose After Hemodialysis	Dosage in Hepatic Failure
		Normal	Renal Failure[2]	Initial Dose[3]	Maintenance Dose			
Acyclovir	Renal	2.5–3.5 hours	20 hours	2.5 mg/kg	2.5 mg/kg q24h	Yes	2.5 mg/kg	No change
Ampicillin–subactam	Renal	0.5–1 hour	8–12 hours	3 g	1.5 g q8–12h	Yes	1.5 g	No change
Amphotericin B	Unknown	360 hours	360 hours	No change	No change	No	None	No change
Ampicillin	Tubular secretion	0.5–1 hour	8–12 hours	1 g	1 g q8–12h	Yes	1 g	No change
Azithromycin	Renal 20%; hepatic 35%	3–4 hours	Not known	500 mg	250 mg q24h	No	None	Not known[4]
Aztreonam	Renal	1.7 hours	6 hours	1–2 g	0.5–1 g q6–8h	Yes	0.5–1 g	No change
Chloramphenicol	Mainly liver	3 hours	4 hours	0.5 g	0.5 g q6h	Yes	0.5 g	0.25–0.5 g q12h
Ciprofloxacin	Renal and liver	4 hours	8.5 hours	0.5 g	0.25–0.75 g q24h	No	None	No change
Clarithromycin	Renal 30%; hepatic >50%	3–4 hours	15 hours	500 mg	250 mg q12h	No	None	Not known[4]
Clindamycin	Liver	2–4 hours	2–4 hours	0.6 g IV	0.6 g q8h	No	None	0.3–0.6 g q8h
Doxycycline	Renal	15–24 hours	15–24 hours	100 mg	100 mg q12h	No	None	Not known[4]
Erythromycin	Mainly liver	1.5 hours	1.5 hours	0.5–1 g	0.5–1 g q6h	No	None	0.25–0.5 g q6h
Famciclovir[5]	Renal	2.5 hours	13–20 hours	500 mg	500 mg q24h	Yes	500 mg	No change
Fluconazole	Renal	30 hours	98 hours	0.2 g	0.1 g q24h	Yes	Give q24h dose	No change
Flucytosine	Renal	3–6 hours	30–250 hours	37.5 mg/kg	25 mg/kg q24h	Yes	25 mg/kg	No change
Foscarnet	Renal	3–8 hours	Not known	90–120 mg	Not known[6]	No	None	No change
Fosfomycin	Renal	6 hours	11–50 hours	NA	NA	NA	NA	No change
Ganciclovir[7]	Renal	3 hours	11–28 hours	1.25 mg/kg	1.25 mg/kg q24h	Yes	Give q24h dose	No change
Imipenem	Glomerular filtration	1 hour	3 hours	0.5 g	0.25–0.5 g q12h	Yes	0.25–0.5 g	No change
Isoniazid	Renal	1–5 hours	2.5 hours	300 mg	300 mg q24h	Yes	300 mg	Not known[4]
Itraconazole	Hepatic	21 hours	25 hours	50–200 mg	50–200 mg q24h	No	None	Not known[4]
Ketoconazole	Hepatic	8 hours	8 hours	200 mg	200–400 mg q24h	No	None	Not known[4]
Lomefloxacin	Renal	10–12 hours	25 hours	400 mg	200 mg q24h	No	None	No change
Meropenem	Renal	1 hour	5–10 hours	1 g	0.5–1 g q24h	Yes	0.5 g	No change
Metronidazole	Liver	6–10 hours	6–10 hours	0.5 g IV	0.5 g q8h	Yes	0.25 g	0.25 g q12h
Mezlocillin	Renal 50–70%; biliary 20–30%	1 hour	3–6 hours	3 g	2 g q6–8h	Yes	1 g	1–2 g q8h
Nafcillin	Liver 80%; kidney 20%	0.75 hours	1.5 hours	1.5 g	1.5 g q4h	No	None	2–3 g q12h
Ofloxacin	Renal	6–8 hours	36 hours	400 mg	200 mg q24h	Not known	Not known	No change
Penicillin G	Tubular secretion	0.5–1 hours	7–10 hours	1–2 million units	1 million units q8h	Yes	500,000 units	No change
Pentamidine	Not known	6–9 hours	6–9 hours	4 mg/kg	4 mg/kg q24h	No	None needed	No change

								1–2 g q8h
Piperacillin and piperacillin + tazobactam	Renal 50–70%; biliary 20–30%	1 hour	3–6 hours	3 g	2 g q6–8h	Yes	1 g	
Rifampin	Hepatic	2–3 hours	3–5 hours	600 mg	600 mg q24h	No	None	Not known[4]
Ticarcillin	Tubular secretion	1.1 hour	15–20 hours	3 g	2 g q6–8h	Yes	1 g	No change
Trimethoprim-sulfamethoxazole	Some liver	TMP 10–12 hours; SMZ 8–10 hours	TMP 24–48 hours; SMZ 18–24 hours	320 mg TMP + 1600 mg SMZ	80 mg TMP + 400 mg SMZ every 12 hours	Yes	80 mg TMP + 400 mg SMZ	No change
Trimetrexate	Hepatic	15 hours	Not known	45 mg/m²	40 mg/m² q24h	No	None	Not known
Vancomycin	Glomerular filtration	6 hours	6–10 days	1 g	1 g q6–10d based on serum levels[8]	No	None	No change

[1] For cephalosporins, see text and Table 37–7; for aminoglycosides, see Table 37–7; for tetracyclines, see Table 37–8.

[2] Considered here to be marked by creatinine clearance of 10 mL/min or less.

[3] For a 70-kg adult with a serious systemic infection.

[4] Dose adjustment in hepatic failure has not been studied, but because clearance of the drug is principally hepatic, dose reduction may be required.

[5] Pharmacokinetics and dosing are in reference to the active agent, penciclovir.

[6] When creatinine clearance is 30 mL/min, a dose of 60 mg/kg is given once daily. For clearances less than 30 mL/min, the dose has not been established.

[7] Oral ganciclovir is same as IV ganciclovir except that the initial dose is 1000 mg, maintenance dose is 500 mg daily, and dose after hemolysis is 500 mg.

[8] When serum levels reach 5–10 µg/mL, another dose should be given.

spread use of antibiotics, the cost of these agents can be substantial both to institutions and to individuals. In addition to the direct cost of purchasing a drug, one must consider the costs of monitoring for toxicity (drug levels, liver function tests, electrolytes, etc), the cost of treating adverse reactions, the cost of treatment failure, and the costs associated with the time required for administering drugs that are given at frequent intervals. Although cost should not be the only determinant in choosing antibiotics, if several drugs with equal efficacy and toxicity are available, one should choose the least expensive. Table 37–5 lists the costs of commonly used antibiotics.

The Choice of Antimicrobial Drugs. Med Lett Drugs Ther 1996;38:25. (Current recommendations.)
Barriere SL, Jacobs RA: Clinical use of antimicrobials. In: *Basic & Clinical Pharmacology,* 6th ed. Katzung BG (editor). Appleton & Lange, 1995.

PENICILLINS

The penicillins are a large group of antimicrobial substances, all of which share a common chemical nucleus (6-aminopenicillanic acid) that contains a β-lactam ring essential to their biologic activity. All β-lactam antibiotics inhibit formation of microbial cell walls.

Penicillins fall into four major categories, discussed below.

Antimicrobial Action & Resistance

The initial step in penicillin action is the binding of the drug to receptors—penicillin-binding proteins—some of which are transpeptidation enzymes. The penicillin-binding proteins of different organisms differ in number and in affinity for a given drug. After penicillins have attached to receptors, peptidoglycan synthesis is inhibited because the activity of transpeptidation enzymes is blocked. The final bactericidal action is the removal of an inhibitor of the autolytic enzymes in the cell wall, which activates the enzymes and results in cell lysis. Organisms that are defective in autolysin function are inhibited but not killed by β-lactam antibiotics ("tolerance"). Organisms that produce β-lactamases (penicillinases) are resistant to some penicillins because the β-lactam ring is broken and the drug is inactivated. Only organisms that are actively synthesizing peptidoglycan (in the process of multiplication) are susceptible to β-lactam antibiotics. Nonmultiplying organisms or those lacking cell walls (L forms) are not susceptible but may act as "persisters."

Microbial resistance to penicillins is caused by four factors:

(1) Production of β-lactamases, eg, by staphylococci, gonococci, *Haemophilus* species, and coliform organisms.

(2) Lack of penicillin-binding proteins or decreased affinity of penicillin-binding protein for β-lactam antibiotic receptors (eg, resistant pneumococci, methicillin-resistant staphylococci, enterococci) or impermeability of cell envelope, so that penicillins cannot reach receptors (eg, metabolically inactive bacteria).

(3) Failure of activation of autolytic enzymes in the cell wall; "tolerance," eg, in staphylococci, group B streptococci.

(4) The presence of cell wall-deficient (L) forms or mycoplasmas, which do not synthesize peptidoglycans.

1. NATURAL PENICILLINS

The natural penicillins include forms of penicillin G for parenteral administration (aqueous crystalline, procaine, and benzathine penicillin G) or for oral administration (penicillin G and phenoxymethyl penicillin [penicillin V]). They are most active against gram-positive organisms, less active against gram-negatives, and susceptible to hydrolysis by β-lactamases. They are used for infections caused by susceptible pneumococci (however, up to 25% of strains now demonstrate intermediate- or high-level resistance to penicillin), streptococci, meningococci, non-β-lactamase-producing staphylococci and gonococci, *Treponema pallidum* and other spirochetes, *Bacillus anthracis* and other gram-positive rods, clostridia, *Actinomyces,* and most anaerobes except β-lactamase-producing strains, eg, *Bacteroides fragilis* (Table 37–1).

Pharmacokinetics & Administration

While aqueous crystalline penicillin G can be given intramuscularly, the intravenous route, by intermittent bolus injection or continuous infusion, is often preferred to avoid local pain. After parenteral administration, penicillin is widely distributed in tissues. An intravenous dose of 1 million units of penicillin G produces a peak serum level of 10 μg/mL. (One million units of penicillin G equals 0.6 g.) Levels equal to those in serum occur in many tissues, but lower levels prevail in the eye, prostate, and central nervous system. However, with acute inflammation of the meninges (eg, in bacterial meningitis), penicillin G levels in the cerebrospinal fluid exceed 0.2 μg/mL with a daily parenteral dose of 20 million units. This level is more than is required to kill sensitive pneumococci and meningococci. Consequently, systemically administered penicillin G is adequate to treat meningitis caused by exquisitely susceptible organisms.

Special dosage forms of penicillin permit delayed absorption to yield low blood and tissue levels for long periods, eg, benzathine penicillin G. After a sin-

Table 37–5. Approximate costs of antimicrobials.

Drug	Dose per Day[1]	Cost per Unit[2]	Daily Cost of Therapy[3]
INTRAVENOUS PREPARATIONS			
Acyclovir	15 mg/kg (mucocutaneous herpes)	$56.00/0.5 g	$168.00
Acyclovir	30 mg/kg (CNS herpes)	$113.00/1 g	$339.00
Amikacin	15 mg/kg	$68.00/0.5 g	$136.00
Ampicillin	100 mg/kg	$4.00/2 g	$16.00
Ampicillin plus sulbactam	3 g q8h	$13.00/3 g (IV)	$39.00
Aztreonam	50 mg/kg	$16.00/1 g	$48.00
Cefazolin	50 mg/kg	$7.00/1 g (IV)	$21.00
Cefoxitin	80 mg/kg	$10.00/1 g	$30.00
Ceftazidime	50 mg/kg	$14.50/1 g	$43.50
Ceftizoxime	50 mg/kg	$12.00/1 g	$36.00
Ceftriaxone	30 mg/kg	$37.00/1 g	$74.00
Cefuroxime	60 mg/kg	$12.00/1.5 g	$36.00
Ciprofloxacin	0.8 g	$15.60/0.2 g	$62.40
Clindamycin	2400 mg	$5.00/0.6 g	$20.00
Fluconazole	0.2–0.4 g	$81.00/0.2 g $119.00/0.4 g	$81.00–119.00
Foscarnet	180 mg/kg (induction) 90–120 mg/kg (maintenance)	$73.00 (24 mg/mL × 250 mL = 6000 mg)	$146.00 $73.00–102.00
Ganciclovir	10 mg/kg	$35.00/0.5 g	$70.00
Gentamicin	5 mg/kg	$1.50/80 mg	$7.50
Imipenem	50 mg/kg	$25.00/0.5 g	$100.00
Metronidazole	1500 mg	$9.00/0.5 g (B), $7.00/0.5 g (G)	$27.00 (B), $21.00 (G)
Mezlocillin	250 mg/kg	$13.00/3 g	$52.00
Nafcillin	100 mg/kg	$8.00/2 g, $5.00/2 g (SB)	$32.00 or $20.00
Ofloxacin	400 mg twice daily	$26.40/0.4 g	$52.80
Penicillin	12 million units	$1.30/1 million units	$15.60
Piperacillin	250 mg/kg	$17.00/3 g	$68.00
Piperacillin plus tazobactam	3.75 g q6–8h	$15.00/3.75 g	$60.00
Ticarcillin	250 mg/kg	$10.00/3 g	$40.00
Ticarcillin-potassium clavulanic acid	3.1 g q6h	$14.00/3.1 g	$56.00
Tobramycin	5 mg/kg	$7.00/80 mg	$35.00
Trimethoprim-sulfamethoxazole	15 mg/kg TMP	$45.00 (0.48 g TMP in 30 mL) (B)	$90.00
Trimetrexate	45 mg/m^2	$50.00/25 mg	(Depends on surface area.)
Vancomycin	20–30 mg/kg	$7.00/0.5 g	$28.00
ORAL PREPARATIONS			
Acyclovir	1000 mg (therapy of herpes)	$1.00/0.2 g	$5.00
Acyclovir	800 mg three times daily (herpes suppression for immunocompromised patient)	$4.00/0.8 g	$12.00
Amoxicillin	20–30 mg/kg	$0.60/0.5 g	$1.80
Ampicillin	20–30 mg/kg	$0.20/0.5 g	$0.80
Augmentin (0.5 g amoxicillin plus 0.125 g clavulanic acid)	30 mg/kg	$3.00/0.5 g	$9.00
Azithromycin	500 mg as loading dose, then 250 mg/d for 4 days	$6.00/0.25 g	$12.00 load, then $6.00
Azithromycin	1 g as single dose for *C trachomatis* infection	$19.20/1 g packet	$19.20/1 g packet
Cefaclor	20–30 mg/kg	$4.00/0.5 g	$12.00

(continued)

Table 37–5. Approximate costs of antimicrobials. (continued)

Drug	Dose per Day[1]	Cost per Unit[2]	Daily Cost of Therapy[3]
ORAL PREPARATIONS			
Cefixime	400 mg	$6.30/0.4 g	$6.30
Cefpodoxime proxetil	400 mg	$4.00/0.2 g	$8.00
Cefprozil (0.5 g)	15 mg/kg	$5.50/0.5 g	$11.00
Cefuroxime (0.5 g)	0.5 g twice daily	$6.65/0.5 g	$13.30
Cephalexin (0.5 g)	30 mg/kg	$0.60/0.5 g	$2.40
Ciprofloxacin (0.5 g)	0.5–0.75 g twice daily	$4.14/0.5 g	$8.28
Ciprofloxacin (0.75 g)		$5.78/0.75 g	$11.56
Clarithromycin (0.25 or 0.5 g)	250–500 mg twice daily	$3.26/0.5 g	$6.52
Clindamycin (0.3 g)	15 mg/kg	$2.40/0.3 g	$9.60
Doxycycline (0.1 g)	3 mg/kg	$0.40/0.1 g	$0.80
Erythromycin (0.5 g)	30 mg/kg	$0.20/0.5 g	$0.60
Famciclovir (0.5 g)	500 mg three times daily	$7.00/0.5 g	$21.00
Fluconazole (0.1 g)	0.1–0.2 g daily	$6.90/0.1 g	$6.90
Fluconazole (0.2 g)		$11.25/0.2 g	$11.25
Flucytosine (0.5 g)	150 mg/kg	$2.00/0.5 g	$40.00
Ganciclovir (0.25 g)	1 g three times daily	$3.90/0.25 g	$46.80
Itraconazole (0.1 g)	200–400 mg	$6.00/0.1 g	$12.00–24.00
Ketoconazole (0.2 g)	0.2–0.4 g	$3.00/0.2 g	$3.00–6.00
Levofloxacin (0.5 g)	0.5 g daily	$7.00/0.5 g	$7.00
Lomefloxacin (0.4 g)	400 mg	$6.35/0.4 g	$6.35
Loracarbef (0.4 mg)	800 mg	$4.00/0.4 mg	$8.00
Metronidazole (0.5 g)	2 g (*Trichomonas*) 20 mg/kg	$0.30/0.5 g (G), $2.50/0.5 g (B)	$1.20 (G), $10.00 (B), $0.85 (G), $7.00 (B)
Ofloxacin (0.4 g)	400 mg twice daily	$4.00/0.4 g	$8.00
Phenoxymethyl penicillin (0.5 g)	30 mg/kg	$0.12/0.5 g (G)	$0.48
Sparfloxacin (0.2 g)	0.2 g daily	$6.97/0.2 g	$13.94 day 1, then $6.97/d
Tetracycline (0.5 g)	30 mg/kg	$0.09/0.5 g	$0.36
Trimethoprim-sulfamethoxazole	5 mg/kg TMP	$0.20/80 mg TMP and 400 mg SMZ	$0.80
Valacyclovir (0.5 g)	0.5–1 g three times daily	$2.75/0.5 g	$8.25–16.50
Vancomycin	125 mg three times daily	$5.00/125 mg	$15.00

[1]Doses based on a 70-kg individual with normal renal function.
[2]Cost to pharmacist (average wholesale price). B = brand name; G = generic. Source: First Data Bank, Price Alert, April, 1997.
[3]Daily cost for intravenous antibiotics includes acquistion cost only and not preparation and administrations costs.

gle intramuscular injection of 1.2 million units (0.9 g), serum levels in excess of 0.02 µg/mL are maintained for 10 days and levels in excess of 0.004 µg/mL for 3 weeks. The latter level is sufficient to protect against β-hemolytic streptococcal infection; the former, to treat an established infection with these organisms. Procaine penicillin also has delayed absorption. After intramuscular injection of 1–2 million units (1–2 g), serum levels of 0.1 µg/mL persist for 18–24 hours.

Phenoxymethyl penicillin (penicillin V) is the oral penicillin of choice. It is more acid-stable than oral penicillin G, is better absorbed, and gives higher serum levels. A 250 mg dose results in serum levels of 2–3 µg/mL.

Most of the absorbed penicillin is rapidly excreted by the kidneys into the urine; small amounts are excreted by other routes. About 10% of renal excretion is by glomerular filtration and 90% by tubular secretion. Tubular secretion can be partially blocked by probenecid, 0.5 g (10 mg/kg) every 6 hours orally, to achieve higher systemic levels. Individuals with impaired renal function likewise tend to maintain higher penicillin levels longer, and the dose should be reduced in moderate to severe renal failure. One commonly used formula for calculating the maximum daily dose of penicillin in millions of units in patients with a creatinine clearance of less than 40 mL/min is as follows (see also Table 37–4):

$$\text{Dosage} = 3.2 + \frac{\text{Creatinine clearance}}{7}$$

Clinical Uses

Most infections caused by organisms sensitive to penicillin will respond to aqueous penicillin G in daily doses of 0.6–5 million units (0.36–3 g) administered intravenously in divided doses every 4–6 hours. For severe or life-threatening infections (meningitis, endocarditis), much larger daily doses (10–24 million units) should be given by intermittent intravenous infusion every 2–4 hours in equally divided doses.

Penicillin V is indicated only in minor disorders such as mild respiratory infections, pharyngitis, and skin and soft tissue infections. The usual dose is 1–2 g/d in four equally divided doses.

A single injection of 1.2 million units of benzathine penicillin intramuscularly is satisfactory for treatment of β-hemolytic streptococcal pharyngitis. An injection of 1.2–2.4 million units every 3–4 weeks provides satisfactory prophylaxis for rheumatics against reinfection with group A streptococci. Syphilis can be treated with benzathine penicillin, 2.4 million units intramuscularly weekly for 1–3 weeks, depending on the stage of the disease (see Table 37–3).

Procaine penicillin is used primarily for treatment of uncomplicated pneumococcal pneumonia in a dose of 600,000 units twice a day and for treatment of neurosyphilis (Table 37–3).

2. EXTENDED-SPECTRUM PENICILLINS

The extended-spectrum group of penicillins includes the aminopenicillins: ampicillin and amoxicillin; the carboxypenicillins: ticarcillin; and the ureidopenicillins: piperacillin and mezlocillin. These drugs are all susceptible to destruction by staphylococcal (and other) β-lactamases. They tend to be active against many gram-negative rods and have the same activity as natural penicillins against gram-positive bacteria.

Antimicrobial Activity

Ampicillin and amoxicillin are active against most strains of *Proteus mirabilis, Listeria,* and non-β-lactamase-producing strains of *Haemophilus influenzae* but inactive against most strains of *Klebsiella, Pseudomonas, Serratia, Enterobacter,* and indole-positive *Proteus.* Activity against *Salmonella* species and *Shigella* species is variable. While these drugs are less active than penicillin in vitro against pneumococci and streptococci, they are clinically effective in treating infections caused by susceptible strains of these organisms. They are more active than penicillin G against enterococci.

Ticarcillin extends the activity of ampicillin to include many strains of *Pseudomonas, Serratia,* and indole-positive *Proteus,* but it has poor activity against most strains of *Klebsiella* and enterococci.

The ureidopenicillins are similar to ticarcillin but exhibit slight differences in activity against gram-negative organisms. Piperacillin is more active than ticarcillin against *Pseudomonas aeruginosa* and *Klebsiella,* but otherwise its spectrum of activity is similar to that of ticarcillin. Mezlocillin is similar in activity to piperacillin but slightly less active against *P aeruginosa.* Both mezlocillin and piperacillin are active against enterococci. The extended-spectrum penicillins are active against most anaerobes. Ampicillin and amoxicillin are not active against β-lactamase-producing strains of *B fragilis*—in contrast to the other drugs in this class which are active at high concentrations.

Pharmacokinetics & Administration

Ampicillin can be given orally or parenterally. The usual oral dose is 1–2 g/d (15–50 mg/kg/d), resulting in serum levels of 4–6 μg/mL. Intravenous dosages range from 20 to 200 mg/kg/d (the higher dosages required in meningitis), resulting in serum levels of up to 40 μg/mL. Amoxicillin is given orally only, in dosages of 25–100 mg/kg/d, usually as 250 or 500 mg tablets three times daily, and is absorbed better than ampicillin, resulting in serum levels twice as high as those achieved with ampicillin. Amoxicillin is the oral drug of choice in the treatment of intermediately penicillin-susceptible pneumococci.

The carboxy- and ureidopenicillins are given intravenously (200–300 mg/kg/d) in dosages of 3–4 g every 4–6 hours, resulting in serum levels of 250–300 μg/mL.

Dosage adjustments in renal failure are required for the extended-spectrum penicillins and are summarized in Table 37–4.

Clinical Uses

Ampicillin and amoxicillin are given orally for minor infections, such as bronchitis, sinusitis, otitis, or urinary tract infections. Ampicillin is given intravenously for pneumonia, meningitis, bacteremia, or endocarditis. In meningitis in the neonate or elderly, ampicillin is given concurrently with a third-generation cephalosporin to cover *Listeria.*

Amoxicillin is frequently used for urinary tract infections, sinusitis, otitis, and bronchitis and as antibacterial prophylaxis to prevent endocarditis (see section on Antimicrobial Chemoprophylaxis). It has also been used in combination with metronidazole and bismuth subsalicylate to treat recurrent gastric and duodenal ulcers caused by *Helicobacter pylori.* Although ticarcillin, mezlocillin, and piperacillin have been used as single drugs, they are commonly administered in combination with an aminoglycoside or a quinolone to treat serious *Pseudomonas* infections and as empirical therapy in the febrile neutropenic patient.

3. PENICILLINS COMBINED WITH β-LACTAMASE INHIBITORS

The addition of β-lactamase inhibitors (clavulanic acid, sulbactam, tazobactam) can prevent inactivation of the parent penicillin by bacterial β-lactamases. Augmentin (amoxicillin, 250 mg, 500 mg, or 875 mg, plus 125 mg of clavulanic acid), Timentin (ticarcillin, 3 g, plus 100 mg of clavulanic acid), Unasyn (ampicillin 1 g plus sulbactam 0.5 g, and ampicillin 3 g plus sulbactam 1.5 g), and Zosyn (piperacillin 3 g plus tazobactam 0.375 g, and piperacillin 4 g plus tazobactam 0.5 g) are available. Augmentin is given orally and the others intravenously. In general, the β-lactamase inhibitors effectively inactivate β-lactamases produced by anaerobes, *Staphylococcus aureus, H influenzae, Moraxella catarrhalis,* and *Bacteroides fragilis,* thus making Augmentin, Timentin, Unasyn, and Zosyn effective agents for infections with these organisms. In contrast, the β-lactamase inhibitors are variably and unpredictably effective against certain β-lactamases produced by aerobic enteric gram-negative rods, enterobacters, and pseudomonads and thus cannot be relied upon to treat these organisms unless specific sensitivity testing is done. Of the available parenteral drugs, Zosyn has the broadest spectrum of activity. Like Unasyn (but not Timentin) it is active against ampicillin-susceptible enterococci. It has greater in vitro activity against *Pseudomonas aeruginosa* than Timentin and is more active than either Timentin or Unasyn against *Serratia* and *Klebsiella* species.

Augmentin, because of its high cost and gastrointestinal intolerance, is limited to the treatment of refractory cases of sinusitis and otitis that have not responded to less costly agents and is used for therapy and prophylaxis of infections resulting from animal and human bites. The roles of Timentin, Unasyn, and Zosyn are not well defined at present. One possible application of these agents would be to use them alone or in combination with an aminoglycoside to treat polymicrobial infections such as peritonitis from a ruptured viscus, osteomyelitis in a diabetic patient, or traumatic osteomyelitis.

The dosage regimens of these drugs are the same as those of the parent drugs. When Timentin or Zosyn is used to treat *Pseudomonas* infections, higher doses (200–300 mg/kg/d) are used.

4. PENICILLINASE-RESISTANT PENICILLINS

Methicillin, oxacillin, cloxacillin, dicloxacillin, nafcillin, and others are relatively resistant to destruction by β-lactamases produced by staphylococci and are limited to the treatment of infections with such organisms. They are less active than natural penicillins against gram-positives; however, they are still adequately effective against streptococcal infections.

Oxacillin, cloxacillin, and dicloxacillin are given orally in dosages of 0.25–0.5 g every 6 hours in mild or localized staphylococcal infections (50–100 mg/kg/d for children).

For serious systemic staphylococcal infections, nafcillin, 6–12 g/d, is given intravenously in four to six divided doses (50–100 mg/kg/d for children). Eighty percent of administered nafcillin is excreted into the biliary tract and only 20% by renal tubular secretion.

5. ADVERSE EFFECTS OF PENICILLINS

Allergy

All penicillins are cross-sensitizing and cross-reacting. Any preparation containing penicillin may induce sensitization, including foods or cosmetics. In general, sensitization occurs in proportion to the duration and total dose of penicillin received in the past. The responsible antigenic determinants appear to be degradation products of penicillins, particularly penicilloic acid and products of alkaline hydrolysis (minor antigenic determinants) bound to host protein. Skin tests with penicilloyl-polylysine, with minor antigenic determinants, and with undegraded penicillin can identify most hypersensitive individuals. Among positive reactors to skin tests, the incidence of subsequent immediate severe penicillin reactions is high. Although many persons develop IgG antibodies to antigenic determinants of penicillin, the presence of such antibodies is not correlated with allergic reactivity (except for rare instances of hemolytic anemia), and serologic tests have little predictive value. A history of a penicillin reaction in the past is not reliable. Only one-fourth of patients with a history of penicillin allergy have an adverse reaction when challenged with the drug. The decision to administer penicillin or related drugs (other β-lactams) to patients with an allergic history depends upon the severity of the reported reaction, the severity of the infection being treated, and the availability of alternative drugs. For patients with a history of severe reaction (anaphylaxis), alternative drugs should be used. In the rare situations when there is a strong indication for using penicillin (eg, syphilis in pregnancy) despite a history of severe reaction, desensitization can be performed. If the history is unclear or the reaction mild (rash), the patient may be rechallenged with penicillin or may be given another β-lactam antibiotic. (See Chapter 30 for discussion and methods of desensitization.)

Allergic reactions include anaphylaxis, serum sickness (urticaria, fever, joint swelling, angioneurotic edema 7–12 days after exposure), and a variety of skin rashes, oral lesions, fever, interstitial nephritis, eosinophilia, hemolytic anemia, other hematologic disturbances, and vasculitis. The incidence of hypersensitivity to penicillin is estimated to be 1–5% among adults in the USA. Life-threatening anaphylactic reactions are very rare (0.05%). Ampicillin produces maculopapular skin rashes more frequently than other penicillins, but some ampicillin rashes are not allergic in origin. The nonallergic ampicillin rash usually occurs after 3–4 days of therapy, is maculopapular, is more common in patients with coexisting viral illness (especially Epstein-Barr infection), and resolves with continued therapy. Penicillins can induce nephritis with primary tubular lesions association with anti-basement membrane antibodies.

Individuals known to be hypersensitive to penicillin can at times tolerate the drug during corticosteroid administration.

Toxicity

Since the action of penicillin is directed against a unique bacterial structure, the cell wall, it is virtually without effect on animal cells. The toxic effects of penicillin G are due to the direct irritation caused by intramuscular or intravenous injection of exceedingly high concentrations (eg, 1 g/mL). Such concentrations may cause local pain, induration, thrombophlebitis, or degeneration of an accidentally injected nerve. All penicillins are irritating to the central nervous system and can cause seizures. There is no indication for intrathecal administration since they sufficiently cross the blood-brain barrier with inflamed meninges. In rare cases, a patient with renal insufficiency receiving large doses may exhibit signs of cerebrocortical irritation as a result of passage of unusually large amounts of penicillin into the central nervous system. With doses of this magnitude, direct cation toxicity (Na^+, K^+) can also occur.

Large doses of penicillins given orally may lead to gastrointestinal upset, particularly nausea and diarrhea. This is most pronounced with the broad-spectrum penicillins—ampicillin or amoxicillin—and Augmentin and may be due to overgrowth of staphylococci, *Pseudomonas,* clostridia, or yeasts or to toxin production by *Clostridium difficile.* Superinfections in other organ systems may occur with penicillins as with any other antibiotic. Nafcillin administered at high doses is associated with a modest leukopenia. High doses of ticarcillin, mezlocillin, or pipericillin can produce hypokalemic alkalosis and elevation of serum aminotransferases and can inhibit platelet aggregation.

Bush LM, Calmon J, Johnson CC: Newer penicillins and beta-lactamase inhibitors. Infect Dis Clin North Am 1995;9:653. (Pharmacology, spectrum of activity, clinical indications, toxicity.)

CEPHALOSPORINS
(Tables 37–6 and 37–7)

The cephalosporins are structurally related to the penicillins. They consist of a β-lactam ring attached to a dihydrothiazoline ring. Substitutions of chemical groups at various positions on the basic structure have resulted in a proliferation of drugs with varying pharmacologic properties and antimicrobial activities.

The mechanism of action of cephalosporins is analogous to that of the penicillins: (1) binding to specific penicillin-binding proteins that serve as drug receptors on bacteria, (2) inhibition of cell wall synthesis, and (3) activation of autolytic enzymes in the cell wall that result in bacterial death. Resistance to cephalosporins may be due to poor permeability of the drug into bacteria, lack of penicillin-binding proteins, or degradation by β-lactamases.

Cephalosporins have been divided into four major groups or "generations" (Table 37–6) based mainly on their antibacterial activity: First-generation cephalosporins have good activity against aerobic gram-positive organisms and some community-acquired gram-negative organisms (*P mirabilis, E coli, Klebsiella* species); second-generation drugs have a slightly extended spectrum against gram-negative bacteria, and some are active against anaerobes; and third-generation cephalosporins have less activity against gram-positives but are extremely active against most gram-negative bacteria (except *Enterobacter* and *Citrobacter*). Not all cephalosporins fit neatly into this grouping, and there are exceptions to the general characterization of the drugs in the individual classes; however, the generational classification of cephalosporins is useful for discussion purposes. Cefepime, a fourth-generation cephalosporin, has recently been approved. The drug is considered a fourth-generation agent because it is stable against plasmid-mediated β-lactamase and has little or no β-lactamase-inducing capacity. Cefepime compares favorably with ceftazidime with respect to its gram-negative activity; however, its stability versus plasmid-mediated β-lactamase results in improved coverage against *Enterobacter* and *Citrobacter* species. The gram-positive coverage of cefepime approaches that of cefotaxime or ceftriaxone.

Table 37–6. Major groups of cephalosporins.

First Generation	Second Generation	Third Generation	Fourth Generation
Cephalothin	Cefamandole	Cefotaxime	Cefepime
Cephapirin	Cefuroxime	Ceftizoxime	
Cefazolin	Cefonicid	Ceftriaxone	
Cephalexin[1]	Ceforanide	Ceftazidime	
Cephadrine[1]	Cefaclor[1]	Cefoperazone	
Cefadroxil[1]	Cefoxitin	Moxalactam	
	Cefotetan	Cefixime[1]	
	Cefprozil[1]	Cefpodoxime proxetil[1]	
	Cefuroxime axetil[1]	Ceftibuten[1]	
	Cefmetazole		

[1]Oral agents.

Both parenteral and oral cephalosporins—especially second- and third-generation agents—are quite costly (Table 37–5). Because of their broad spectrum of activity and low toxicity, these drugs are used to treat many infections. Because of their cost, their broad spectrum of activity, and concerns about selecting for resistant organisms, the use of cephalosporins should be limited to those situations in which clear-cut superiority over less expensive drugs with narrower spectrums of activity has been demonstrated.

1. FIRST-GENERATION CEPHALOSPORINS

Antimicrobial Activity

These drugs are very active against gram-positive cocci, including most pneumococci, viridans streptococci, group A hemolytic streptococci, and *S aureus.* Like all cephalosporins, they are inactive against enterococci and methicillin-resistant staphylococci. Among gram-negative bacteria, *E coli, Klebsiella pneumoniae,* and *P mirabilis* are usually sensitive except for some hospital-acquired strains. There is very little activity against such gram-negatives as *P aeruginosa,* indole-positive *Proteus, Enterobacter, Haemophilus influenzae, Serratia marcescens, Citrobacter,* and *Acinetobacter.* Anaerobic cocci are usually sensitive, but *B fragilis* is not.

Pharmacokinetics & Administration

A. Oral: Cephalexin, cephradine, and cefadroxil are variably absorbed. Urine levels of these drugs are several hundred times higher than serum levels, but concentrations in other tissues are variable and usually lower than in the serum. Cefadroxil, because of its longer half-life, can be given twice daily. Dosage adjustment is required in renal insufficiency.

B. Intravenous: Cefazolin is preferred over cephalothin and cephapirin because it has a longer half-life, requires less frequent dosing, and achieves higher serum levels. In renal insufficiency, all of these agents require dosage adjustments.

C. Intramuscular: Both cephapirin and cefazolin can be given intramuscularly, but pain on injection is less with cefazolin.

Clinical Uses

Although the first-generation cephalosporins have a broad spectrum of activity and are relatively nontoxic, they are rarely the drugs of choice. Oral drugs are indicated for treatment of urinary tract infections in patients who are allergic to sulfonamides, and they can be used for minor staphylococcal infections. Oral cephalosporins may also be preferred for minor polymicrobial infections (eg, cellulitis, soft tissue abscess). Oral cephalosporins should not be relied on in serious systemic infections.

Intravenous first-generation cephalosporins penetrate most tissues well and are the drugs of choice for surgical prophylaxis in many cases. More expensive second- and third-generation cephalosporins offer no advantage over the first-generation drugs for surgical prophylaxis except where anaerobes play an important role, such as for colorectal surgery or for hysterectomy.

Other major uses of intravenous first-generation cephalosporins include infections for which they are the least toxic drugs (eg, *Klebsiella* infections) and infections in persons with a history of *mild* penicillin allergy (not anaphylaxis).

First-generation cephalosporins do not penetrate the cerebrospinal fluid and cannot be used to treat meningitis.

2. SECOND-GENERATION CEPHALOSPORINS

Second-generation cephalosporins are a heterogeneous group with marked individual differences in activity, pharmacokinetics, and toxicity. In general, all are active against organisms also covered by first-generation drugs, but they have an extended gram-negative coverage. Indole-positive *Proteus,* and *Klebsiella* (including cephalothin-resistant strains) are usually sensitive. Cefamandole, cefuroxime, cefonicid, ceforanide, cefuroxime axetil, and cefprozil are active against *H influenzae,* including β-lactamase-producing strains, but have little activity against *Serratia* and *B fragilis.* In contrast, cefoxitin and cefotetan are active against 80–90% of strains of *B fragilis* and some strains of *Serratia.* Cefmetazole is similar in activity to cefoxitin and cefotetan but has more activity against *H influenzae.* Against gram-positive organisms, these drugs are generally less active than the first-generation cephalosporins (cefuroxime and cefuroxime axetil are exceptions). Like the latter, second-generation drugs have no activity against *P aeruginosa* or enterococci.

Pharmacokinetics & Administration

A. Oral: Only cefaclor, cefuroxime axetil, and cefprozil can be given orally. All are available as capsules (0.25 or 0.5 g) and in suspension (0.125 or 0.25 g/5 mL). Cefuroxime axetil releases cefuroxime after absorption. Its longer half-life permits twice-daily dosing, and absorption is enhanced when it is taken with food (as is not the case with many other oral antibiotics).

B. Intravenous and Intramuscular: Because of differences in drug half-life and protein binding, peak serum levels achieved and dosing intervals vary greatly for this group of drugs (Table 37–7). Drugs

Table 37–7. Pharmacology of the cephalosporins.

Drug	Peak Serum Level (μg/mL) After 1 g IV	Serum Half-Life (min)	Total Daily Dose (mg/kg)	Dosage Interval (hours)	Dosage Adjustments in Renal Failure		
					Moderate (Cl_{cr} 10–50) mL/min)	Severe (Cl_{cr} <10 mL/min)	Post-hemodialysis Dose
Cephalothin, cephapirin	40–60	40	50–200	4–6	1–2 g every 6–12 hours	1 g every 12 hours	1 g
Cefazolin	90–120	90	25–100	8	0.5–1 every 12 hours	0.5 g daily	0.5 g
Cephalexin, cephradine[1]	15–20	50–60	15–30	6	0.25–0.5 g every 8–12 hours	0.25–0.5 g daily	0.5 g
Cefadroxil[1]	15	75	15–30	12–24	1 g daily	0.5 g daily	0.5 g
Cefamandole	60–80	45	75–200	6–8	1 g every 12 hours	1–2 g daily	0.5 g
Cefepime	60–70	120	50–75	8–12	1 g every 12 hours	1 g every 24 hours	1 g
Ceftibuten[1]	20	120	9	12–24	0.4 g daily	0.1–0.2 g daily	0.7 g
Cefuroxime	80–100	80	50	6–12	1 g every 12 hours	1–2 g daily	0.5 g
Cefuroxime axetil[1]	6–8	75	5–15	12	0.5 g every 24 hours	0.25 g daily	0.25 g
Cefonicid	200–250	240	15–30	24	0.5 g daily	1 g every 72 hours	0.25 g
Ceforanide	125	180	15–30	12	1 g daily	1 g every 48 hours	0.25 g
Cefaclor[1]	15–20	50	20–40 children, 10–15 adults	6–8	0.5 g every 8–12 hours	0.25–0.5 g every 12–24 hours	0.25–0.5 g
Cefixime[1]	3–5	180–240	8 (with maximum of 0.4 g/d total)	12–24	0.4 g daily	0.1 g daily	None
Cefpodoxime proxetil[1]	2	150	5	12	0.2 g every 24 hours	0.2 g 3 times per week after dialysis	0.2 g
Cefprozil[1]	10	90	10–15	12	0.5 g every 12–24 hours	0.25–0.5 g every 12–24 hours	0.5 g
Cefotetan	60–80	150	50–100	8–12	1 g every 8–12 hours	0.5–1 g daily	0.5 g
Cefotaxime	40–60	60	50–75	6–8	1–2 g every 6–8 hours	1–2 g every hours	1–2 g
Cefoxitin	60–80	60	50–100	6–8	1 g every 12 hours	1–2 g daily	0.5 g
Cefmetazole	70–100	60–80	50–100	6–8	1 g every 12–24 hours	1–2 g every 24–48 hours	1 g
Ceftizoxime	80–100	100	50–75	8–12	0.5–1 g every 8–12 hours	0.25–0.5 g every 12–24 hours	0.5 g
Ceftriaxone	150	480	30–50	12–24	1–2 g daily	1–2 g daily	None
Ceftazidime	100–120	120	50–75	8–12	1 g every 12 hours	0.5–1 g daily	0.5 g
Cefoperazone	150	120	30–200	8–12	1–2 g every 12 hours	1–2 g every 12 hours	None
Loracarbef[1]	10	60	10–15	12	0.2 g every 24 hours	0.2 g 3 times per week after dialysis	0.2 g
Moxalactam	60–100	120	50–200	6–12	0.5–1 g every 12 hours	0.25–0.5 g every 12 hours	0.5 g

[1]Oral agents. Serum levels based on 0.5 g oral dose.

with shorter half-lives (cefoxitin, cefamandole) require higher doses and more frequent dosing than drugs with longer half-lives (cefuroxime, cefonicid, ceforanide, cefotetan). Dosage adjustments are required with renal impairment.

Clinical Uses

Because of their activity against β-lactamase-producing *H influenzae* and *M catarrhalis,* cefprozil and cefuroxime axetil can be used to treat sinusitis and otitis media in patients who are allergic to ampicillin or amoxicillin or have not responded to treatment with those drugs.

Because of their activity against *B fragilis,* cefoxitin, cefmetazole, and cefotetan can be used to treat mixed anaerobic infections, eg, peritonitis and diverticulitis. However, since 10–15% of *B fragilis* and many enteric gram-negative organisms are resistant to these drugs, for severe life-threatening intra-abdominal infections metronidazole plus an aminoglycoside or a third-generation cephalosporin is preferred. Cefoxitin and cefotetan have been used as prophylaxis in colorectal surgery, vaginal or abdominal hysterectomy, and appendectomy because of their activity against *Bacteroides fragilis.* Cefonicid and ceforanide have also been promoted for surgical prophylaxis, but there is no evidence that they are more effective than first-generation cephalosporins, and they tend to be more expensive. Cefamandole, like cefuroxime, may be useful for the treatment of community-acquired pneumonia, but it has few other uses.

3. THIRD- & FOURTH-GENERATION CEPHALOSPORINS

Antimicrobial Activity

These drugs are active against staphylococci (not methicillin-resistant strains) but less so than first-generation cephalosporins. They have no activity against enterococci but do inhibit most nonenterococcal streptococci. A major advantage of these cephalosporins is their expanded gram-negative coverage. In addition to organisms inhibited by other cephalosporins, they are consistently active against *S marcescens, Providencia, Haemophilus,* and *Neisseria,* including β-lactamase-producing strains. Two drugs—ceftazidime and cefoperazone—have good activity against *P aeruginosa. Acinetobacter, Citrobacter, Enterobacter,* and non-*aeruginosa* strains of *Pseudomonas* are variably sensitive to third-generation cephalosporins, and *Listeria* is resistant. Activity against *B fragilis* is variable, and these agents should not be relied upon to treat serious infections with this organism. In contrast to the third-generation agents, cefepime, the only currently available fourth-generation cephalosporin, is active against *Enterobacter* and *Citrobacter.*

Cefixime, cefpodoxime proxetil, and ceftibuten, the only oral agents in this group, are more active than cefuroxime axetil but are not as active as parenteral third-generation cephalosporins against gram-negative organisms such as *Pseudomonas, Enterobacter, Morganella,* and *S marcescens.* The major differences in these drugs are activity against gram-positive bacteria. All are active against *Streptococcus pyogenes* (group A streptococcus). Cefpodoxime proxetil is active against methicillin-sensitive *S aureus,* whereas cefixime and ceftibuten have little activity (neither is active against methicillin-resistant strains). Both cefixime and cefpodoxime proxetil are active against penicillin-sensitive strains of *Streptococcus pneumoniae* (the pneumococcus). Like other members of this class, these drugs are inactive against enterococci and *Listeria monocytogenes.*

Pharmacokinetics & Administration

The intravenous agents penetrate well into body fluids and tissues and—except for cefoperazone—reach levels in the cerebrospinal fluid that exceed those needed to inhibit most pathogens, including gram-negative rods. The half-lives of these drugs are variable, which accounts for the differences in dosing intervals (Table 37–7). Cefoperazone and ceftriaxone are eliminated primarily by biliary excretion, and no dosage adjustment is required in renal insufficiency. The other drugs are eliminated by the kidney and thus require dosage adjustments in renal insufficiency.

Clinical Uses

Because of their penetration into the cerebrospinal fluid, third-generation cephalosporins—except cefoperazone—can be used to treat meningitis. Meningitis due to susceptible pneumococci (strains that are moderately resistant or highly resistant to penicillin may have high MICs to third-generation cephalosporins, and these agents should not be used to treat meningitis caused by penicillin-resistant pneumococci), meningococci, *H influenzae,* and susceptible enteric gram-negative rods has been successfully treated. In meningitis in the elderly, third-generation cephalosporins should be combined with ampicillin until *L monocytogenes* has been excluded as the etiologic agent. Ceftazidime has been used to treat *Pseudomonas* meningitis. The dosage for meningitis should be at the upper limits of the recommended range, because cerebrospinal fluid levels of these drugs are only 10–20% of serum levels. Ceftazidime is frequently administered empirically in the febrile neutropenic patient. Ceftriaxone is indicated for gonorrhea, chancroid, and certain more serious forms of Lyme disease (see Chapter 34). Because of its long half-life and once-daily dosing requirement, ceftriaxone is also an ideal drug for outpatient parenteral therapy of infections due to susceptible organisms.

Cefepime is useful for indications similar to those of ceftazidime, including treatment of the febrile neutropenic patient.

Cefixime, because of its long half-life, can be given once daily. For improved compliance, this may be advantageous in treating sinusitis and otitis in children. Ceftibuten also can be given once daily, 400 mg. Although approved for use in otitis media and acute exacerbations of chronic bronchitis, its limited activity against *Moraxella catarrhalis* and *Streptococcus pneumoniae,* frequent pathogens in these entities, makes it a poor choice for these infections. Cefixime (400 mg as a single dose) and cefpodoxime proxetil (200 mg as a single dose) are as effective as ceftriaxone (125 mg intramuscularly) for the therapy of genital, rectal, and pharyngeal gonorrhea.

Because of the high cost and broad spectrum of activity of third- and fourth-generation cephalosporins, their use should be limited. When they are used empirically, therapy can be changed to the most efficacious, least toxic, and least expensive drug once the etiologic agent has been identified.

4. ADVERSE EFFECTS OF CEPHALOSPORINS

Allergy

Cephalosporins are sensitizing, and a variety of hypersensitivity reactions occur, including anaphylaxis, fever, skin rashes, nephritis, granulocytopenia, and hemolytic anemia. The frequency of cross-allergy between cephalosporins and penicillins is not known but is estimated to be about 6–10%. Persons with a history of anaphylaxis to penicillins should not receive cephalosporins.

Toxicity

Local pain can occur after intramuscular injection, or thrombophlebitis after intravenous injection. Hypoprothrombinemia is a frequent adverse effect (40–68%) of cephalosporins that have a methylthiotetrazole group (eg, cefamandole, cefmetazole, cefoperazone, cefotetan). Prophylactic administration of vitamin K, 10 mg twice weekly, can prevent this complication. Drugs containing the methylthiotetrazole ring can also cause severe disulfiram-like reactions, and use of alcohol or medications containing alcohol (eg, theophylline elixir) must be avoided. Ceftriaxone has been associated with cholelithiasis due to precipitation of drug when its solubility in bile is exceeded. All β-lactams have been associated with leukopenia, and this adverse effect may occur more frequently in those who have severe hepatic dysfunction.

Superinfection

Third- and fourth-generation cephalosporins have little activity against gram-positive organisms, particularly methicillin-resistant staphylococci and enterococci. Superinfection with these organisms—as well as with fungi—may occur.

Klein NC, Cunha BA: Third-generation cephalosporins. Med Clin North Am 1995;79:705. (Pharmacology, spectrum of activity, indications, toxicities.)

OTHER β-LACTAM DRUGS

Monobactams

These are drugs with a monocyclic β-lactam ring that are resistant to β-lactamases and active against gram-negative organisms (including *Pseudomonas*) but have no activity against gram-positive organisms or anaerobes. Aztreonam resembles ceftazidime in its gram-negative activity. The usual dosage is 1–2 g intravenously every 6–8 hours, providing peak serum levels of 100 μg/mL. Clinical uses of aztreonam are limited because of the availability of third-generation cephalosporins with a broader spectrum of activity and minimal toxicity. Despite the structural similarity of aztreonam to penicillin, cross-reactivity is limited, and it can therefore be used in most patients with penicillin allergy.

Carbapenems

This class of drugs is structurally related to β-lactam antibiotics. Imipenem, the first drug of this type, has a wide spectrum of activity that includes most gram-negative rods (including *P aeruginosa*) and gram-positive organisms and anaerobes, with the exception of *Pseudomonas cepacia, Stenotrophomonas* (formerly *Xanthomonas*) *maltophilia, Enterococcus faecium,* and most methicillin-resistant *S aureus* and *S epidermidis*. It is resistant to β-lactamases but is inactivated by dipeptidases in renal tubules. Consequently, it must be combined with cilastatin, a dipeptidase inhibitor, for clinical use.

The half-life of imipenem is 1 hour. Penetration into body tissues and fluids, including the cerebrospinal fluid, is good. The usual dosage is 0.5–1 g intravenously every 6 hours (maximum dose 50 mg/kg/d). Dosage adjustment is required in renal insufficiency. For patients with creatinine clearances of 10–30 mL/min, one-half the usual dose is given; for those with clearances of 10 mL/min, 0.5 g is given every 12 hours. An additional dose is given after hemodialysis.

Meropenem is similar to imipenem in spectrum of activity and pharmacology. It is not inactivated by dipeptidase. It is less likely to cause seizures than imipenem, though the risk of seizures is actually quite low with imipenem if dosage is appropriately adjusted for renal insufficiency.

Imipenem and meropenem should not be routinely used as first-line therapy unless the organism causing infection is multidrug-resistant and is known to be sensitive to these agents. In patients hospitalized for a prolonged period who may have infection with a multidrug-resistant organism, empirical use of imipenem or meropenem while awaiting culture results is reasonable. *Pseudomonas* may rapidly develop resistance to these drugs. The use of imipenem or meropenem alone appears to be as effective as combination therapy in the febrile neutropenic patient and as effective as combination therapy in certain polymicrobial infections such as peritonitis and obstetric pelvic infections.

The most common adverse effects of imipenem and meropenem are nausea, vomiting, diarrhea, reactions at the infusion site, and skin rashes. Seizures can occur, especially in patients with impaired renal function. Patients allergic to penicillins may be allergic to imipenem and meropenem as well.

Carbacephems

Loracarbef is a β-lactam antibiotic that is structurally similar to cefaclor except that a methylene group has replaced the sulfur in the dihydrothiazine ring. This structural change adds chemical stability to the drug but does not greatly enhance its antibacterial activity, which is essentially the same as that of cefaclor, cefuroxime axetil, and cefprozil. The high cost of loracarbef precludes its use as a first-line agent, and it should be reserved for the therapy of sinusitis, otitis media, bronchitis, and urinary tract infections in patients who have failed therapy with less expensive agents (eg, ampicillin, amoxicillin, trimethoprim-sulfamethoxazole). The usual dosage is 200–400 mg orally every 12 hours.

Ennis DM, Cobbs CG: The newer cephalosporins, aztreonam and impinemem. Infect Dis Clin North Am 1995; 9:687.

Norrby SR: Carbapenems. Med Clin North Am 1995; 79:745. (Pharmacology, spectrum of activity, indications, toxicity.)

ERYTHROMYCIN GROUP (Macrolides)

The erythromycins are a group of closely related compounds characterized by a macrocyclic lactone ring to which various sugars are attached.

Antimicrobial Activity

Erythromycins inhibit protein synthesis by binding to the 50S subunit of bacterial ribosomes. They are bacteriostatic or bactericidal for gram-positive organisms, including most pneumococci, streptococci, and corynebacteria in a concentration of 0.02–2 μg/mL. Similar to penicillin, macrolide-resistant *S pneumoniae* is being reported with increased frequency (15%). Erythromycin-resistant pneumococci are azalide-resistant as well (azithromycin, clarithromycin). Chlamydiae, mycoplasmas, *Legionella,* and *Campylobacter* are also susceptible.

Pharmacokinetics & Administration

Preparations for oral use include erythromycin base, erythromycin stearate, estolate, and ethyl succinate. The base is most acid-stable, and the estolate is the best-absorbed of the oral forms. Clinically, however, none of the oral preparations have any advantage over others. The usual adult oral dose is 250–500 mg four times daily, resulting in serum levels of 1–2 μg/mL. Erythromycins are excreted largely in the bile; only 5% is excreted in the urine, and no adjustment is therefore required in renal failure.

Erythromycin lactobionate and gluceptate are available for intravenous use. The usual dosage is 250–500 mg every 6 hours, but higher dosages (1 g every 6 hours) are used initially in the treatment of Legionnaires' disease.

Clinical Uses

Erythromycins are drugs of choice for infections caused by *Legionella, Mycoplasma, Corynebacterium* (including diphtheria and bacteremia), and *Chlamydia* (including ocular and respiratory infections). They are effective in streptococcal and pneumococcal disease and for endocarditis prophylaxis in dental procedures in penicillin-allergic patients. They can also be used in combination with sulfisoxazole for acute otitis media and with neomycin in prophylaxis for bowel surgery. When administered early, erythromycin may shorten the course of *Campylobacter* enteritis.

Adverse Effects

Nausea, vomiting, and diarrhea may occur after oral intake. Erythromycins—particularly the estolate—can produce acute cholestatic hepatitis (fever, jaundice, impaired liver function), probably as a hypersensitivity reaction. Most patients recover, but hepatitis recurs if the drug is readministered. Reversible auditory impairment can occur when large doses (4 g/d or more) are given to patients with impaired renal or hepatic function. Erythromycins can increase the effects of oral anticoagulants, digoxin, theophylline, nonsedating antihistamines, and cyclosporine by inhibiting cytochrome P450. Patients taking these medications who are treated with erythromycin should have levels monitored and dosages adjusted appropriately.

AZALIDES

Azalides (azithromycin, clarithromycin, dirythromycin, and others) are a group of antibiotics closely related structurally to the macrolides. Like erythromycin, they are active against *Streptococcus pneumoniae,* group A streptococcus, viridans streptococci, *M catarrhalis, Legionella, Mycoplasma pneumoniae,* and *Chlamydia pneumoniae* and are slightly more active in vitro than erythromycin against *H influenzae* (with azithromycin having better activity than clarithromycin and dirythromycin having activity equivalent to that of erythromycin). They are also active against *Chlamydia trachomatis, N gonorrhoeae, Ureaplasma urealyticum,* and *Haemophilus ducreyi.* In addition, these drugs have in vitro activity against a number of unusual pathogens. including atypical mycobacteria *(Mycobacterium avium-intracellulare, Mycobacterium chelonei, Mycobacterium fortuitum, Mycobacterium marinum), Toxoplasma gondii, Campylobacter jejuni, Helicobacter pylori,* and *Borrelia burgdorferi.*

The azalides are more acid-stable than erythromycin, penetrate tissues well, and have a long terminal half-life, with high tissue concentrations that persist for days. Azithromycin, clarithromycin, and dirythromycin are approved for treatment of streptococcal pharyngitis, uncomplicated skin infections, and acute bacterial exacerbations of chronic bronchitis. Because of the long half-life, treatment with azithromycin is with once-daily dosing for a total of 5 days (500 mg on day 1 and then 250 mg on days 2–5). Clarithromycin is usually administered in a dosage of 250–500 mg twice daily, and dirythromycin is given as a single daily dose of 500 mg.

The azalides are more expensive than erythromycin. Whether the decreased gastrointestinal distress that occurs and the less frequent dosing that is required outweigh the increased cost is not yet determined.

Azithromycin has also been approved as single-dose therapy (1 g) for chlamydial genital infections. This is much more expensive than 7 days of treatment with doxycycline (Table 37–5), but the assurance of adequate supervised therapy for this infection makes azithromycin preferred therapy in some patients. Azithromycin can also be used as single-dose therapy (1 g) for chancroid, and a single-dose of 1 g is as efficacious as 7 days of doxycycline for nongonococcal urethritis in men. The spectrum of activity of erythromycin suggests that it might be useful for community-acquired pneumonia and can be used for mild to moderate cases that are appropriate for oral therapy. Weekly 1200 mg doses of azithromycin are effective in preventing *Mycobacterium avium* complex infections in HIV-positive patients and in doses of 600 mg daily may be effective in *M avium* complex pulmonary infections in non-HIV-positive patients. Clarithromycin has been used for the therapy of *M avium* complex infections, usually in combination with other drugs (eg, rifabutin and ethambutol). Clarithromycin (500 mg twice daily for 6 months) is very effective therapy for disseminated *Mycobacterium chelonei* infections and may be the drug of choice for use against this pathogen. Cla-

rithromycin has also been used in combination regimens for the therapy of *Helicobacter pylori* infections. When clarithromycin is given with omeprazole, cure rates in excess of 80% have been achieved. The role of these agents in the therapy of toxoplasmal encephalitis is under investigation.

Adverse effects of these agents are similar to those of erythromycin, but gastrointestinal upset, the major side effect, occurs about 50% less often with the azalides. Hepatic enzyme elevations, interstitial nephritis, headache, dizziness, and ototoxicity at high doses have rarely been reported.

Kanatani MS, Guglielmo BJ: The new macrolides azithromycin and clarithromycin. West J Med 1994; 160:31. (Activity, clinical trials, and adverse effects.)

TETRACYCLINE GROUP

The tetracyclines are a large group of drugs with common basic chemical structures, antimicrobial activity, and pharmacologic properties. Microorganisms resistant to this group show extensive cross-resistance to all tetracyclines.

Antimicrobial Activity

Tetracyclines are inhibitors of protein synthesis and are bacteriostatic for many gram-positive and gram-negative bacteria. They are strongly inhibitory for the growth of mycoplasmas, rickettsiae, chlamydiae, spirochetes, and some protozoa (eg, amebas). Over 90% of pneumococci remain susceptible to these agents, as are 99% of *H influenzae* as well. Tetracyclines also have moderate activity against some vancomycin-resistant enterococci. There are great differences in the susceptibility of different strains of a given species of microorganism. Because of the emergence of resistant strains, tetracyclines have lost some of their former usefulness. *Proteus* and *Pseudomonas* are regularly resistant; *Bacteroides,* streptococci, shigellae, and vibrios are increasingly so.

Pharmacokinetics & Administration

Tetracyclines are absorbed irregularly from the gastrointestinal tract. Absorption is impaired by dairy products, aluminum hydroxide gels (antacids), and chelation with divalent cations, eg, Ca^{2+} or Fe^{2+}. Absorption is least with chlortetracycline (30%); intermediate with tetracycline, oxytetracycline, and demeclocycline (60–80%); and highest with doxycycline and minocycline (95% or more). An oral dose of 250 mg of tetracycline hydrochloride gives serum levels of 2–3 $\mu g/mL$, and 100 mg of doxycycline gives serum levels of 1–2 $\mu g/mL$. Tetracyclines are widely distributed, and low levels can be found in many tissues. Lipid solubility of minocycline and doxycycline probably accounts for their penetration into the cerebrospinal fluid, tears, and saliva.

The usual dosage of tetracyclines is 250–500 mg four times daily. Doxycycline and minocycline are given as 100 mg twice daily and demeclocycline and methacycline as 150 mg four times daily or 300 mg twice daily.

Tetracyclines are metabolized in the liver and concentrated in bile. Excretion is mainly through bile and urine. All tetracyclines—except doxycycline—accumulate in renal insufficiency and are antianabolic in high doses. Doxycycline requires no dosage adjustment in renal failure; the other tetracyclines should be avoided or given in reduced dosage.

For patients unable to take oral medication, some tetracyclines (doxycycline, minocycline) are formulated for parenteral administration in doses similar to the oral ones. A 1% topical tetracycline ointment is available for conjunctival infections.

Clinical Uses

Tetracyclines are the drugs of choice for chlamydial, rickettsial, and *Vibrio* infections and some spirochetal infections. Sexually transmitted diseases in which chlamydiae often play a role—endocervicitis, urethritis, proctitis, and epididymitis—should be treated with a tetracycline for 7–14 days. Pelvic inflammatory disease is often treated with doxycycline plus cefoxitin or cefotetan. Other chlamydial infections (psittacosis, lymphogranuloma venereum, trachoma) and sexually transmitted diseases (granuloma inguinale) also respond to tetracyclines. Other uses include treatment of acne, respiratory infections, Lyme disease and relapsing fever, brucellosis, glanders, and tularemia (often in combination with streptomycin), cholera, mycoplasmal pneumonia, and infections caused by *M marinum* and *Pasteurella multocida* (often after an animal bite). Tetracycline has also been used in combination with other drugs for amebiasis, falciparum malaria, and recurrent ulcers due to *H pylori*. Because of generally good activity against pneumococci, *Haemophilus influenzae, Chlamydia, Legionella,* and *Mycoplasma,* doxycycline should be considered as empiric therapy for outpatient pneumonia.

Minocycline achieves a high concentration in the saliva and can be used for eradication of meningococci in carriers who cannot tolerate rifampin. Minocycline is equally as efficacious as doxycycline for the therapy of nongonococcal urethritis and cervicitis.

Adverse Effects

A. Allergy: Hypersensitivity reactions with fever or skin rashes are uncommon.

B. Gastrointestinal Side Effects: Gastrointestinal side effects, especially diarrhea, nausea, and anorexia, are common. These can be diminished by reducing the dose, but sometimes they force discontinuance of the drug.

C. Bones and Teeth: Tetracyclines are bound to calcium deposited in growing bones and teeth, causing fluorescence, discoloration, enamel dysplasia, deformity, or growth inhibition. Therefore, tetracyclines should not be given to pregnant women or children under 6 years of age.

D. Liver Damage: Tetracyclines can impair hepatic function or even cause liver necrosis, particularly during pregnancy or in the presence of preexisting liver damage.

E. Kidney Effects: Demeclocycline can cause nephrogenic diabetes insipidus and has been used therapeutically to treat inappropriate antidiuretic hormone secretion. Tetracyclines may increase blood urea nitrogen when diuretics are administered.

F. Other: Vaginal candidiasis is a common complication of tetracycline therapy. Tetracyclines—principally demeclocycline—may induce photosensitization, especially in fair-skinned individuals. Minocycline induces vestibular reactions (dizziness, vertigo, nausea, vomiting), with a frequency of 35–70% after doses of 200 mg daily and has also been implicated as a cause of hypersensitivity pneumonitis. Demeclocycline inhibits antidiuretic hormone.

Klein NC, Cunha BA: Tetracyclines. Med Clin North Am 1995;79:789. (Pharmacology, spectrum of activity, indications, toxicities.)

CHLORAMPHENICOL

Antimicrobial Activity

Chloramphenicol is active against many gram-positive and gram-negative bacteria and rickettsiae. It binds to the 50S subunit of ribosomes and inhibits protein synthesis. It is bacteriostatic for most organisms but bactericidal for *S pneumoniae, H influenzae,* and *Neisseria meningitidis.* This bactericidal activity accounts for the efficacy of chloramphenicol in the treatment of meningitis caused by these organisms. Of currently available agents, it is one of the few with any activity against some vancomycin-resistant enterococci.

Pharmacokinetics & Administration

For most systemic infections, chloramphenicol, 30 mg/kg/d, is given intravenously, but meningitis in adults may require 50 mg/kg/d in four divided doses. With a dose of 1 g intravenously, serum levels reach 15–20 µg/mL. Since the intravenous preparation—chloramphenicol sodium succinate—must be hydrolyzed to active drug by nonspecific plasma esterases, it yields somewhat lower levels than the oral form. A 1 g oral dose gives serum levels of 20–25 µg/mL.

Chloramphenicol is widely distributed in tissues, including the eye and central nervous system. Cerebrospinal fluid levels are 70–80% of peak serum levels, and the levels in brain tissue may even exceed those in serum.

Chloramphenicol is metabolized in the liver, and less than 10% is excreted unchanged in the urine. Thus, no dosage adjustment is needed in renal insufficiency. Patients with liver disease may accumulate the drug, and levels should be monitored.

Clinical Uses

Chloramphenicol is a possible choice in the following circumstances: (1) Meningococcal, *H influenzae,* or pneumococcal infections of the central nervous system in patients with a history of anaphylaxis to β-lactam drugs. (2) Anaerobic or mixed infections in the central nervous system, eg, brain abscess. (3) As an alternative to tetracyclines in rickettsial infections, especially in pregnant women, in whom tetracycline is contraindicated. (4) For treatment of vancomycin-resistant enterococcal infections if susceptibility has been demonstrated.

Adverse Effects

Nausea, vomiting, and diarrhea occur infrequently. The most serious adverse effects pertain to the hematopoietic system. Adults taking chloramphenicol in excess of 50 mg/kg/d regularly exhibit disturbances in red cell maturation within 1–2 weeks. There is anemia, hyperferremia, reticulocytopenia, and the appearance of vacuolated nucleated red cells in the bone marrow. These changes regress when the drug is stopped and are not related to aplastic anemia. The latter is an irreversible consequence of chloramphenicol administration and represents a specific, probably genetically determined individual defect. It occurs in 1:40,000–1:25,000 courses of chloramphenicol treatment.

Chloramphenicol inhibits the metabolism of certain drugs. Thus, it may prolong the action and raise the blood concentration of tolbutamide, phenytoin, chlorpropamide, and warfarin sodium.

Chloramphenicol is specifically toxic for newborns, particularly premature infants. Because these patients lack the mechanism for detoxification of chloramphenicol in the liver, the drug may accumulate, producing the highly fatal "gray baby syndrome," with vomiting, flaccidity, hypothermia, and hypotension.

AMINOGLYCOSIDES

Aminoglycosides are a group of bactericidal drugs sharing chemical, antimicrobial, pharmacologic, and toxic characteristics. At present, the group includes streptomycin, neomycin, kanamycin, amikacin, gentamicin, tobramycin, sisomicin, netilmicin, paromomycin, and spectinomycin. All these agents inhibit protein synthesis in bacteria by attaching to and inhibiting the function of the 30S subunit of the bacterial ribosome. Resistance is based on (1) a deficiency of the ribosomal receptor (chromosomal mutant); (2) the enzymatic destruction of the drug (plasmid-mediated transmissible resistance of clinical importance) by acetylation, phosphorylation, or adenylylation; or (3) a lack of permeability to the drug molecule or failure of active transport across cell membranes. (This can be chromosomal, eg, streptococci are relatively impermeable to aminoglycosides; or plasmid-mediated, eg, in gram-negative enteric bacteria.) Anaerobic bacteria are resistant to aminoglycosides because transport across the cell membrane is an oxygen-dependent energy-requiring process.

All aminoglycosides are more active at alkaline than at acid pH. All are potentially ototoxic and nephrotoxic, though to different degrees. All can accumulate in renal insufficiency; therefore, dosage adjustments must be made in patients with renal dysfunction (see Table 37–8).

Because of their considerable toxicity and the availability of other antibiotics with broad spectrums of activity and fewer adverse effects (eg, third-generation cephalosporins, quinolones, imipenem, meropenem), aminoglycosides have been used less often in recent years. They are most commonly used to treat resistant gram-negative organisms that are sensitive only to aminoglycosides, or in low doses in combination with β-lactam drugs for their synergistic effect (eg, enterococci, penicillin-resistant viridans streptococci, right-sided *S aureus* endocarditis, *S aureus* and *S epidermidis* prosthetic valve infection). Although aminoglycosides demonstrate in vitro activity against many gram-positive bacteria, they should never be used alone to treat infections caused by these organisms—both because there is no clinical experience with the treatment of such infections and because less toxic alternatives are available.

General Properties of Aminoglycosides

Because of the similarities of the aminoglycosides, a summary of properties is presented briefly.

A. Absorption, Distribution, Metabolism, and Excretion: Aminoglycosides are well absorbed after intramuscular or intravenous injection, but they are not absorbed from the gastrointestinal tract. They are distributed widely in tissues and penetrate into pleural, peritoneal, or joint fluid in the presence of inflammation. They diffuse poorly into the eye, prostate, bile, central nervous system, or spinal fluid after parenteral injection.

There is no significant metabolic breakdown of aminoglycosides. The serum half-life is 2–3 hours in

Table 37–8. Dosing of aminoglycosides.[1]

	Creatinine Clearance (mL/min)				
	> 80	**60–80**	**40–60**	**20–40**	**< 20**
Gentamicin, tobramycin, netilmycin	5 mg/kg q24h	1.5–2.5 mg/kg q12h	1.2–1.5 mg/kg q24h	1.2–1.5 mg/kg q12–24h	2 mg/kg as loading dose and then 1–1.5 mg/kg q24–48h
Amikacin	15 mg/kg q24h	4.5–7.5 mg/kg q12h	3.5–4.5 mg/kg q12h	3.5–4.5 mg/kg q12–24h	7.5 mg/kg as loading dose and then 3–4.5 mg/kg q24–48h

[1]Dosing should be guided by serum level measurements (peaks 30 minutes after the end of intravenous infusion and troughs ≤ 30 minutes before the next dose). When a single large daily dose is given, peak levels are not required. The dosage ranges given in the table are those used to treat gram-negative infections and are intended to achieve, for gentamicin, tobramycin, and netilmicin, peak levels of 6–10 mg/L and trough levels of ≤ 2 mg/L; for amikacin, peak levels of 20–30 mg/L and trough levels of ≤ 5 mg/L.

patients with normal renal function. Excretion is almost entirely by glomerular filtration. Urine levels usually are 10–50 times higher than serum levels. Aminoglycosides are removed fairly effectively by hemodialysis but irregularly by peritoneal dialysis.

B. Dosage and Effect of Impaired Renal Function: In persons with normal renal function, the dosage of amikacin is 15 mg/kg/d in a single daily dose; that for gentamicin, tobramycin, or netilmicin is 5 mg/kg injected once daily. A single large daily dose of gentamicin, tobramycin, netilmicin, or amikacin is just as efficacious as—and no more toxic than—traditional dosing every 8–12 hours. In patients with renal insufficiency, some investigators recommend administering the same dose but extending the interval to every 48–72 hours, while others have suggested maintaining the dosage interval but decreasing the dose. Patients with renal failure, volume overload, or obesity have altered antibiotic clearance or volume of distribution. While nomograms have been useful in dosing, they are less accurate in volume overload or obesity. Furthermore, none of these nomograms adequately incorporate the use of once-daily dosing of aminoglycosides in the treatment of infection. In patients with abnormal renal function or body composition, aminoglycoside levels are recommended to guide dosing. In general, peak levels greater than 6 μg/mL are necessary for optimal outcome in the treatment of serious gram-negative infection, including pneumonia. Trough levels of more than 2 μg/mL have been associated with an increased incidence of nephrotoxicity. In patients with normal body composition, dosing regimens as set forth in Table 37–8 should be followed. Reduced gentamicin doses (1 mg/kg every 8 hours) are recommended when used synergistically with β-lactams or vancomycin in the treatment of serious gram-positive infection (eg, enterococcal endocarditis).

C. Adverse Effects: All aminoglycosides can cause ototoxicity and nephrotoxicity. Ototoxicity, though rare, is worrisome because it can be irreversible and is cumulative. Ototoxicity presents as

hearing loss (cochlear damage), noted first with high-frequency tones, or as vestibular damage, manifested by vertigo and ataxia. Amikacin appears to be more ototoxic than gentamicin, tobramycin, or netilmicin. Nephrotoxicity, which is more frequent than ototoxicity, is accompanied by rising serum creatinine levels or reduced creatinine clearance. Nephrotoxicity is usually reversible and occurs with similar frequency with gentamicin, tobramycin, amikacin, and netilmycin.

In very high doses, particularly with irrigation of an inflamed peritoneum, aminoglycosides can be neurotoxic, producing a curare-like effect with neuromuscular blockade that results in respiratory paralysis. Calcium gluconate or neostigmine can serve as an antidote to this reaction.

1. STREPTOMYCIN

Streptomycin is bactericidal for both gram-positive and gram-negative bacteria. The usual dosage is 15–25 mg/kg/d (about 1 g/d) injected in one or two divided doses intramuscularly. Streptomycin exhibits all the adverse effects typically associated with the aminoglycosides; however, it has greater vestibular toxicity and less nephrotoxicity when compared with gentamicin.

Resistance emerges so rapidly and has become so widespread that only a few specific indications for this drug remain:

(1) Plague and tularemia.

(2) Endocarditis caused by *Enterococcus faecalis* or viridans streptococci (use in conjunction with penicillin or vancomycin) in strains that are susceptible to high levels of streptomycin (ie, ≤ 2000 μg/mL). Gentamicin is often substituted for streptomycin in this setting.

(3) Serious active tuberculosis.

(4) Acute brucellosis (use with tetracycline).

2. NEOMYCIN & KANAMYCIN

These aminoglycosides are closely related, with similar activity and complete cross-resistance. Systemic use has been abandoned because of oto- and nephrotoxicity.

Ointments containing 1–5 mg/g of neomycin, often combined with bacitracin and polymyxin, can be applied to infected superficial skin lesions. The drug mixture covers most staphylococci and gram-negative bacteria likely to be present, but the efficacy is questionable. Solutions of neomycin, 2.5–5 mg/mL, have been used for irrigation of infected joints or wounds. The total amount of drug must be kept below 15 mg/kg/d, since absorption leads to systemic toxicity.

In preparation for elective bowel surgery, 1 g of neomycin is given orally every 6–8 hours for 1–2 days (often combined with erythromycin, 1 g) to reduce aerobic bowel flora. Action on gram-negative anaerobes is negligible. In hepatic coma, the coliform bacteria can be suppressed for prolonged periods by oral neomycin or kanamycin, 1 g every 6–8 hours, during reduced protein intake, resulting in diminished ammonia production.

Kanamycin is less toxic than neomycin and is used for the same indications and in the same doses as neomycin for topical application and oral intake.

In addition to oto- and nephrotoxicity, which can result from systemic absorption, neomycin or kanamycin can give rise to allergic reactions when applied topically to skin or eye. Respiratory arrest has followed the instillation of 3–5 g of kanamycin into the peritoneal cavity after colonic surgery; this is treated with neostigmine.

Paromomycin, closely related to neomycin and kanamycin, is poorly absorbed after oral administration and has been used mainly to treat asymptomatic intestinal amebiasis. A dosage of 500 mg orally three or four times daily is effective for cryptosporidiosis in AIDS.

3. AMIKACIN

Amikacin is a semisynthetic derivative of kanamycin. It is relatively resistant to several of the enzymes that inactivate gentamicin and tobramycin, and bacterial resistance is increasing only slowly. Many gram-negative enteric bacteria—including many strains of *Proteus, Pseudomonas, Enterobacter,* and *Serratia*—are inhibited by 1–20 μg/mL of amikacin in vitro. After injection of 500 mg of amikacin intramuscularly every 12 hours (15 mg/kg/d), peak levels in serum are 10–30 μg/mL. Some infections caused by Enterobacteriaceae resistant to gentamicin respond to amikacin. Central nervous system infections require intrathecal or intraventricular injection of 5–10 mg daily. In addition to therapy for serious gram-negative infections, amikacin is often included with other drugs for therapy of *M avium* complex and *Mycobacterium fortuitum* complex.

Like all aminoglycosides, amikacin is nephrotoxic and ototoxic (particularly for the auditory portion of the eighth nerve). Its levels should be monitored in patients with renal failure.

4. GENTAMICIN

With doses of 5 mg/kg/d of this aminoglycoside, serum levels are sufficient for bactericidal effect against many strains of staphylococci, coliforms, and other gram-negative organisms. Enterococci are resistant unless a penicillin or vancomycin is also given. Gentamicin may be synergistic with penicillins active against *Pseudomonas, Proteus, Enterobacter, Klebsiella,* and other gram-negatives. Sisomicin resembles the C1a component of gentamicin.

Indications, Dosages, & Routes of Administration

Gentamicin is used in severe infections caused by gram-negative bacteria. Included are sepsis, infected burns, pneumonia, pyelonephritis, and other serious infections. The usual dosage is 5 mg/kg/d intravenously administered once daily. In endocarditis due to viridans streptococci or *E faecalis,* gentamicin in lower doses (3 mg/kg/d in two or three divided doses) is combined with penicillin or ampicillin. In renal insufficiency, the dose should be adjusted as noted above. For infected burns or skin lesions, creams containing 0.1% gentamicin are used. Such topical use should be restricted to avoid favoring the development of resistant bacteria in hospitals. In meningitis due to gram-negative bacteria, 5–10 mg of gentamicin has been injected daily intraventricularly in adults.

5. TOBRAMYCIN

Tobramycin closely resembles gentamicin in antibacterial activity, toxicity, and pharmacologic properties and exhibits partial cross-resistance. Tobramycin may be effective against some gentamicin-resistant pseudomonads. Dosing is the same as for gentamicin. Tobramycin has also been given by aerosol (600 mg in three divided doses) to patients with cystic fibrosis. It was effective in improving pulmonary function and decreasing colonization with *Pseudomonas* without toxicity and without selecting for resistant strains. This therapy may prove beneficial in decreasing the need for hospitalization in these patients.

Netilmicin shares many characteristics with gentamicin and tobramycin and can be given in a dosage of 5–7 mg/kg/d. It may be less ototoxic and less nephrotoxic than the other aminoglycosides.

6. SPECTINOMYCIN

Spectinomycin is an aminocyclitol antibiotic (related to aminoglycosides) for intramuscular administration. Its sole application is in the treatment of gonococci producing β-lactamase in persons with gonorrhea who are hypersensitive to penicillin. It is not effective for pharyngeal gonorrhea. One injection of 2 g (40 mg/kg) is given. About 5–10% of gonococci are probably resistant. There is usually pain at the injection site, and there may be nausea and fever.

Lortholary O et al: Aminoglycosides. Med Clin North Am 1995;79:761.

POLYMYXINS

The polymyxins are basic polypeptides that are bactericidal for most gram-negative aerobic rods, including *Pseudomonas*. Because of poor distribution into tissues and substantial toxicity (primarily nephrotoxicity and ototoxicity), systemic use of these agents is limited to infections caused by multidrug-resistant gram-negative organisms that are sensitive only to the polymyxins. Polymyxins B and E (colistin) are the only parenteral agents available. Polymyxin B can be given intravenously in a dose of 1.5–2.5 mg/kg/d in four divided doses or intramuscularly in a dose of 2.5–3 mg/kg/d. Colistin is given intramuscularly or intravenously in a dosage of 2.5–5 mg/kg/d in two divided doses. Dosage adjustments are required with renal insufficiency.

Topical preparations are used more commonly but with unproved efficacy. Solutions of polymyxin B sulfate, 1 mg/mL, can be applied to infected surfaces; injected into joint spaces, the pleural cavity, or subconjunctivally; or inhaled as aerosols. Ointments containing 0.5 mg/g of polymyxin B sulfate in a mixture with neomycin or bacitracin (or both) are often applied to superficial infected skin lesions. Polymyxins are inactivated by purulent exudates. They rarely cause local sensitization.

ANTITUBERCULOUS DRUGS

Singular problems exist in the treatment of tuberculosis and other mycobacterial infections, which are chronic but may give rise to hyperacute lethal complications. The organisms are intracellular, have long periods of metabolic inactivity, and tend to develop resistance to any one drug. Therefore, combined drug therapy is employed to delay the emergence of this resistance. First-line drugs, increasingly used together in all tuberculosis, are isoniazid, ethambutol, rifampin, and pyrazinamide. A series of second-line drugs will be mentioned only briefly.

1. ISONIAZID

Isoniazid is the hydrazide of isonicotinic acid (INH), the most active antituberculosis drug. Isoniazid in a concentration of 0.2 μg/mL or less inhibits and kills most tubercle bacilli. However, some atypical mycobacteria as well as some strains of *M tuberculosis* are resistant. In susceptible large populations of *M tuberculosis*, isoniazid-resistant mutants occur. Their emergence is delayed in the presence of a second drug. There is no cross-resistance between isoniazid and other antituberculosis drugs.

Isoniazid is well absorbed from the gastrointestinal tract and diffuses readily into all tissues, including the central nervous system. The inactivation of isoniazid—particularly its acetylation—is under genetic control. However, the speed of isoniazid acetylation has little influence over the selection of drug regimens. Isoniazid and its conjugates are excreted mainly in the urine.

Indications, Dosages, & Routes of Administration

Isoniazid is the most widely used drug in tuberculosis. It should not be given as the sole drug in active tuberculosis. This favors emergence of resistance (up to 30% in some countries). In active, clinically manifest disease, it is given in conjunction with one or more drugs. The usual oral adult dose is 300 mg/d. In noncompliant patients, it can be given twice weekly in a dose of 15 mg/kg/dose (maximum, 900 mg/dose). In anephric patients, the dose is reduced to 200 mg/d.

Toxic reactions to isoniazid include insomnia, restlessness, fever, myalgia, hyperreflexia, and even convulsions and psychotic episodes. Some of these are attributable to a relative pyridoxine deficiency and along with peripheral neuritis can be prevented by the administration of pyridoxine, 25–50 mg/d. Isoniazid can induce hepatitis. Progressive liver damage occurs rarely in patients under age 20; in 1.5% of persons between 30 and 50 years of age; and in 2.5% of older individuals. The risk of hepatitis is greater in alcoholics. Mild elevations (two to three times normal) of aminotransferases are common, occurring in 10–20% of patients taking isoniazid. If they are elevated more than three to five times normal, the drug should be discontinued. The drug is also stopped if clinical hepatitis occurs. Isoniazid can reduce the metabolism of phenytoin, increasing its blood level and toxicity.

2. ETHAMBUTOL

Ethambutol is a synthetic, water-soluble, heat-stable compound, dispensed as the hydrochloride.

Many strains of *M tuberculosis* and of "atypical"

mycobacteria are inhibited in vitro by ethambutol, 1–5 μg/mL. The mechanism of action is not known.

Ethambutol is well absorbed from the gastrointestinal tract. About 20% of the drug is excreted in feces and 50% in the urine, in unchanged form. Excretion is delayed and dosage adjustment is required in renal insufficiency; with creatinine clearance of 10–30 mL/min, one-half the usual dose is given, and with clearance of less than 10 mL/min, 35% of the usual dose. In meningitis, ethambutol appears in the cerebrospinal fluid in relatively low levels (1–2 μg/mL).

Resistance to ethambutol emerges fairly rapidly among mycobacteria when the drug is used alone. Therefore, ethambutol, 15 mg/kg, is given as a single daily dose in combination with other antituberculosis drugs.

Hypersensitivity to ethambutol is uncommon. It may cause a rise in the serum uric acid. The commonest side effects are visual disturbances: Reduction in visual acuity, optic neuritis, and perhaps retinal damage occur in some patients receiving ethambutol, 25 mg/kg/d for several months. Most changes are reversible, but periodic visual acuity testing is mandatory when doses above 15 mg/kg/d are used. At lower doses, side effects are rare.

3. RIFAMPIN & RIFABUTIN

Rifampin is a semisynthetic derivative of rifamycin. Rifampin, 1 μg/mL or less, inhibits many gram-positive cocci, meningococci, and mycobacteria in vitro. Gram-negative organisms are often more resistant. Highly resistant mutants occur frequently in susceptible microbial populations (one in 10^6–10^8 bacteria).

Rifampin binds strongly to DNA-dependent bacterial RNA polymerase and thus inhibits RNA synthesis in bacteria. Rifampin penetrates well into phagocytic cells and can kill intracellular organisms.

Rifampin given orally is well absorbed and widely distributed in tissues, including the central nervous system. Levels in cerebrospinal fluid are 50% of those in serum. The drug is excreted mainly through the liver and to a lesser extent in the urine. With oral doses of 600 mg, serum levels exceed 5 μg/mL for 4–6 hours, and urine levels may be 3–20 times higher. No adjustment is needed in renal insufficiency.

In the treatment of tuberculosis, a single oral dose of 600 mg (10–20 mg/kg) is given daily or, in noncompliant patients, 600 mg twice weekly. In order to delay the rapid emergence of resistant microorganisms, combined treatment with other antituberculous drugs is required. Rifampin is effective for treatment of leprosy (see below), and 600 mg twice daily for 2 days can terminate the meningococcal carrier state; rifampin-resistant strains emerge in 10% of subjects.

Close contacts of children with manifest *H influenzae* infection (eg, in the family or in day care centers) can receive rifampin, 20 mg/kg/d for 4 days, as prophylaxis. Rifampin combined with trimethoprim-sulfamethoxazole can eradicate staphylococcal carriage in the nasopharynx. Combination of rifampin with either penicillin or clindamycin is effective in eradication of group A β-hemolytic streptococci from the pharynx of chronic carriers. Synergistic action of rifampin with nafcillin and vancomycin against staphylococci in vitro is of uncertain clinical significance. However, in patients with *S aureus* or *S epidermidis* prosthetic valve endocarditis, rifampin at a dose of 300 mg every 8 hours for 6 weeks is recommended along with nafcillin or vancomycin for 6 weeks and gentamicin for 2 weeks. With the exception of prophylaxis, rifampin should never be used alone.

Rifampin imparts an orange color to urine, sweat, and contact lenses. Occasional adverse effects include rashes, thrombocytopenia, impaired liver function, light-chain proteinuria, and some impairment of immune response. In intermittent administration, rifampin must be given at least twice weekly to avoid a "flu syndrome" and anemia. Rifampin increases the metabolism of oral anticoagulants and contraceptives and lowers serum levels of methadone, ketoconazole, chloramphenicol, oral hypoglycemic drugs, some antiarrhythmic agents, and cyclosporine.

Rifabutin is structurally similar to rifampin but is 10–20 times more active against *M avium* complex. In a dose of 0.3 g/d, it is effective for prophylaxis against *M avium* complex in HIV-infected patients with CD4 counts less than 100/μL. When rifabutin is used as part of a multidrug regimen to treat *M avium* complex pulmonary infections, adverse effects (leukopenia, nausea, vomiting, polyarthralgia, uveitis) occur commonly—particular when clarithromycin is in the regimen; in such circumstances, doses of rifabutin should not exceed 300 mg/d. Adverse effects and drug interactions are the same as those associated with rifampin. Uveitis can also occur with rifabutin.

4. STREPTOMYCIN

The general pharmacologic features and toxicity of streptomycin are described above in the section on aminoglycosides. Streptomycin, 1–10 μg/mL, is inhibitory and bactericidal for most tubercle bacilli, whereas most atypical mycobacteria are resistant. All large populations of tubercle bacilli contain some streptomycin-resistant mutants. Therefore, streptomycin is employed only in combination with other antituberculosis drugs.

Streptomycin penetrates poorly into cells and exerts its action mainly on extracellular organisms. Since at any moment 90% of tubercle bacilli are intracellular and thus unaffected by streptomycin, treatment for many months is required.

For combination therapy in tuberculous meningitis, miliary dissemination, and severe organ tuberculosis, streptomycin is given intramuscularly, 0.5–1 g daily (30 mg/kg/d for children) for weeks or months. This is followed by streptomycin, 1 g intramuscularly two or three times a week for months.

Prolonged streptomycin treatment may impair eighth nerve function. A total cumulative dose of 120 g should not be exceeded, and the drug should be used with caution in persons over 60 years of age since they are more prone to oto- and nephrotoxicity.

5. PYRAZINAMIDE

Pyrazinamide is bactericidal for most *M tuberculosis* strains and also for many "atypical" mycobacteria. It is well absorbed after oral administration and is widely distributed in tissues. It penetrates well into the cerebrospinal fluid and achieves levels equal to those in serum. The usual oral dose is 20–30 mg/kg (1.5–2 g) given once daily, and this results in serum levels of 30–50 μg/mL. In noncompliant patients, 50–70 mg/kg can be given twice weekly. Pyrazinamide is commonly used in the therapy of tuberculosis because of its demonstrated efficacy in short-course therapy regimens (see below).

The major adverse effect is hepatotoxicity. When pyrazinamide is used at recommended doses of 20–30 mg/kg/d, hepatotoxicity is relatively uncommon. When higher doses are given, toxicity can be seen in up to 5% of patients. Nausea, vomiting, drug fever, and hyperuricemia can occur.

6. FIXED-DOSE COMBINATIONS

Two fixed-dose combinations are available in the United States. **Rifamate** contains rifampin 300 mg and isoniazid 150 mg. The usual adult dose is two tablets each day. **Rifater** contains a combination of rifampin 120 mg, isoniazid 50 mg, and pyrazinamide 300 mg. Dosage varies by weight (ie, four tablets for those weighing < 44 kg, five tablets for those weighing 45–54 kg, and six tablets for those weighing > 55 kg). These combinations prevent selecting for resistance, which may occur with monotherapy. Such combinations are rational and should be encouraged.

7. ALTERNATIVE DRUGS IN TUBERCULOSIS TREATMENT

The drugs listed alphabetically below are usually considered only in cases of drug resistance (clinical or laboratory) to first-line drugs.

Aminosalicylic acid (PAS), closely related to

p-aminobenzoic acid, inhibits most tubercle bacilli in concentrations of 1–5 μg/mL but has no effect on other bacteria.

Aminosalicylic acid is readily absorbed from the gastrointestinal tract. Doses of 8–12 g/d orally give peak blood levels of 50–70 μg/mL. The drug is widely distributed in tissues (except the central nervous system) and rapidly excreted into the urine.

Common side effects include anorexia, nausea, diarrhea, and epigastric pain. Sodium aminosalicylate may be given parenterally. Hypersensitivity reactions include fever, skin rashes, granulocytopenia, lymphadenopathy, and arthralgias.

Clofazimine is a phenazine dye used in the treatment of leprosy and is active in vitro against *M avium* complex and *M tuberculosis*. It is given orally as a single daily dose of 100 mg for treatment of *M avium* complex disease. Its clinical efficacy for the therapy of tuberculosis has not been established. Adverse effects include nausea, vomiting, abdominal pain, and skin discoloration from red-brown to black.

Capreomycin is an injectable agent given intramuscularly in doses of 15–30 mg/kg/d (maximal dose 1 g). Major toxicities include ototoxicity (both vestibular and cochlear) and nephrotoxicity. If the drug must be used in older patients, the dose should not exceed 750 mg.

Cycloserine, a bacteriostatic agent, is given in doses of 15–20 mg/kg (not to exceed 1 g) orally and has been used in re-treatment regimens and for primary therapy of highly resistant *M tuberculosis*. It can induce a variety of central nervous system dysfunctions and psychotic reactions. These may be controlled by phenytoin, 100 mg/d orally, or pyridoxine, 50–100 mg daily.

Ethionamide, like cycloserine, is bacteriostatic and is given orally in a dose of 15–20 mg/kg (maximal dose 1 g). It has been used in combination therapy but produces marked gastric irritation and is the least well tolerated antimycobacterial agent.

The **fluoroquinolones** ofloxacin and ciprofloxacin are active in vitro against *M tuberculosis,* with MICs of 0.25–2 μg/mL. Limited data suggest that these drugs are efficacious in therapy of tuberculosis, particularly in re-treatment regimens. In re-treatment schedules or for infection with resistant organisms, high doses should be used (ciprofloxacin, 750 mg orally twice daily; ofloxacin, 400 mg orally twice daily).

Barnes PF, Barrows SA: Tuberculosis in the 1990's. Ann Intern Med 1993;119:400. (Epidemiology, diagnosis, therapy, and prophylaxis.)

Ellner JJ et al: Tuberculosis symposium: Emerging problems and promises. J Infect Dis 1993;168:537. (Epidemiology, new diagnostic techniques, resistance, and therapy.)

Iseman MD: Treatment of multidrug-resistant tuberculosis. N Engl J Med 1993;329:784. (Useful drugs, treatment regimens, and prophylaxis.)

SULFONAMIDES & ANTIFOLATE DRUGS

More than 150 different sulfonamides have been marketed at one time or another, the modifications being designed principally to achieve greater antibacterial activity, a wider antibacterial spectrum, greater solubility, or more prolonged action. Because of their low cost and relative efficacy in many infections, sulfonamides are still used widely.

Antimicrobial Activity

Sulfonamides are structural analogues of *p*-aminobenzoic acid (PABA) and compete with PABA to block its conversion to dihydrofolic acid. Organisms that require exogenous PABA in the synthesis of folates and pyrimidines are inhibited. Animal cells and some resistant microorganisms use exogenous folate and thus are not affected by sulfonamides.

Trimethoprim, pyrimethamine, and trimetrexate are compounds that inhibit the conversion of dihydrofolic acid to tetrahydrofolic acid by blocking the enzyme dihydrofolate reductase. These agents have been used alone or (more commonly) in combination with other drugs (usually sulfonamides) to prevent or treat a number of bacterial and parasitic infections. Trimetrexate is the most potent agent and is about 1500 times more active than trimethoprim. At high doses, all can inhibit mammalian dihydrofolate reductase, but clinically this is a problem only with pyrimethamine and trimetrexate. Folinic acid (leucovorin) is given concurrently with pyrimethamine and trimetrexate to prevent bone marrow suppression.

Sulfonamides inhibit many gram-positive (including *Nocardia*) and gram-negative organisms. Emerging resistance, particularly among streptococci, gonococci, meningococci, and enteric gram-negative organisms, has limited their use. Sulfonamides are also active against some strains of *Chlamydia* and such organisms as *Toxoplasma, Plasmodium,* and *Pneumocystis carinii.*

The combination of trimethoprim (TMP) (one part) plus sulfamethoxazole (SMZ) (five parts) is bactericidal for such gram-negative organisms as *E coli, Klebsiella, Enterobacter, Salmonella,* and *Shigella,* though resistance is beginning to emerge. It is also active against many strains of *Serratia, Providencia, Stenotrophomonas maltophilia, P cepacia, Pseudomonas pseudomallei,* and *Pseudomonas mallei* but not against *P aeruginosa.* It is inactive against anaerobes and enterococci but inhibits *S aureus* and about 50% *S epidermidis. M catarrhalis, H influenzae, H ducreyi, L monocytogenes,* and some atypical mycobacteria, eg, *M marinum, M kansasii,* and *M scrofulaceum,* are also inhibited by this combination.

Pharmacokinetics & Administration

Sulfisoxazole, like other soluble sulfonamides (sulfadiazine, sulfamethoxazole), is well absorbed from the gastrointestinal tract and widely distributed in tissues. For mild infections due to susceptible organisms (eg, urinary tract infections), the usual dose is 0.5–1 g four times daily (30–60 mg/kg/d), while for systemic infections, 100 mg/kg/d is appropriate. A 1 g oral dose of sulfisoxazole yields serum levels of 50–100 µg/mL.

One-half the dose of sulfisoxazole is excreted unchanged in the urine. In mild renal insufficiency, no dosage adjustment is needed; in severe renal failure (creatinine clearance < 5 mL/min), one-third to one-half the usual dose is given.

Insoluble sulfonamides, eg, phthalylsulfathiazole and salicylazosulfapyridine (sulfasalazine), are poorly absorbed from the gastrointestinal tract and are largely excreted in the feces. Phthalylsulfathiazole has been used for preparation of the bowel for surgery (8–15 g/d for 5–7 days), sulfasalazine for ulcerative colitis (6 g/d in four doses); it is broken down to sulfapyridine and the anti-inflammatory salicylate in the bowel.

For patients who are unable to take oral drugs, some intravenous sulfonamide preparations are available. Most widely used is trimethoprim-sulfamethoxazole. Each vial contains 80 mg TMP + 400 mg SMZ in a volume of 5 mL, which must be diluted in 125 mL of 5% dextrose in water. For many bacterial infections, the dose is 10 mg TMP + 50 mg SMZ/kg/d in two doses; for pneumocystis infections, 15–20 mg TMP + 75–100 mg SMZ/kg/d is given in four doses. This dosage is suitable for patients with creatinine clearances above 50 mL/min. Half to three-fourths of that dosage is suitable for patients with creatinine clearances of 10–50 mL/min and one-quarter of the dosage for clearances under 5 mL/min.

Topical uses of sulfonamides include the application of sodium sulfacetamide solution (30%) or ointment (10%) to the conjunctiva and mafenide acetate cream or silver sulfadiazine to burn wounds.

Clinical Uses

Present indications for sulfonamides include the following.

A. Urinary Tract Infections: Coliform bacteria, the commonest cause of urinary tract infections, often remain susceptible to sulfonamides. Short-course therapy (3 days) with double-strength TMP-SMZ (160 mg TMP + 800 mg SMZ) given twice daily is effective therapy for lower urinary tract infections in women who are symptomatic for less than a week. Since TMP is concentrated in the prostate, TMP-SMZ, one double-strength tablet twice daily for 14–21 days, is effective in acute prostatitis. In chronic prostatitis, treatment for 6–12 weeks is indicated. *E coli,* the most common urinary pathogen, has become progressively more resistant to TMP-SMZ over the years, particularly in HIV-positive patients. If this trend continues, the routine use of

TMP-SMZ for empiric therapy of urinary tract infections will have to be reevaluated.

B. Parasitic Infections: TMP-SMZ is effective for prophylaxis and treatment of pneumocystis pneumonia and *Isospora belli* infection. For therapy of pneumocystis pneumonia, 15–20 mg/kg/d of trimethoprim and 75–100 mg/kg/d of sulfamethoxazole in four divided doses is administered intravenously or orally—depending upon the severity of disease—for 3 weeks. The dose for prophylaxis is 160 mg TMP + 800 mg SMZ daily or three times per week. (When given daily, it is also effective prophylaxis against toxoplasmal encephalitis.) *I belli* infection in AIDS has been successfully treated with 160 mg TMP + 800 mg SMZ orally four times daily for 10 days followed by twice-daily administration for 3 weeks. Treatment with 160 mg TMP + 800 mg SMZ three times a week or 500 mg sulfadoxine with 25 mg pyrimethamine once a week has prevented recurrences. Sulfadiazine with pyrimethamine is also used to treat and prevent recurrence of toxoplasmosis and sulfadoxine plus pyrimethamine is used to treat chloroquine-resistant falciparum malaria.

C. Bacterial Infections: Sulfonamides are the drugs of choice for *Nocardia* infections. TMP-SMZ is widely distributed in tissues, penetrates into the cerebrospinal fluid and has been used to treat meningitis caused by gram-negative rods, though third-generation cephalosporins are now preferred. TMP-SMZ is a frequent choice for management of acute sinusitis, otitis media, and shigellosis. The usual dose for adults is 160 mg TMP + 800 mg SMZ twice daily for 10 days.

TMP-SMZ is effective also for infections with *Pseudomonas pseudomallei* (melioidosis), *Stenotrophomonas maltophilia,* or *Burkholderia cepacia;* for treatment of chancroid; in combination with rifampin, for eradication of nasopharyngeal carriage of staphylococci; for prophylaxis against meningococcal disease when susceptible strains predominate; for antibacterial prophylaxis in organ transplant recipients or patients with chronic granulomatous disease; for therapy of legionellosis in patients who cannot tolerate or fail to respond to erythromycin; for treatment of *Listeria monocytogenes* meningitis; and perhaps also for management of Wegener's granulomatosis.

D. Chlamydial Infections: Sulfonamides effectively suppress trachoma, urethritis, inclusion conjunctivitis, and other manifestations, but erythromycin or tetracyclines are preferred.

E. Leprosy: Certain sulfones are widely used (see below).

Adverse Effects

Adverse reactions to sulfonamides occur in 10–15% of non-AIDS patients (usually a minor rash or gastrointestinal disturbance) and in up to 50% of patients with AIDS (predominantly rash, fever, neutropenia, and thrombocytopenia, often severe enough to require discontinuation of therapy). These drugs are capable of producing a wide variety of side effects—due partly to hypersensitivity, partly to direct toxicity—that must be considered whenever unexplained symptoms or signs occur in a patient who may have received these drugs.

A. Systemic Side Effects: Fever, skin rashes, urticaria; nausea, vomiting, or diarrhea; stomatitis, conjunctivitis, arthritis, aseptic meningitis, exfoliative dermatitis; bone marrow depression, thrombocytopenia, hemolytic (in G6PD deficiency) or aplastic anemia, granulocytopenia, leukemoid reactions; hepatitis, polyarteritis nodosa, vasculitis, Stevens-Johnson syndrome; psychosis; reversible hyperkalemia; and many others.

HIV-positive patients intolerant to TMP-SMZ can often be desensitized. A 70% success rate has been reported after giving 0.004 mg TMP/0.02 mg SMZ as oral suspension and increasing the dose tenfold each hour to achieve a final dose of 160 mg TMP/500 mg SMZ.

B. Urinary Tract Disturbances: Older sulfonamides were relatively insoluble and would precipitate in urine. The most commonly used sulfonamides presently (sulfisoxazole and sulfamethoxazole) are quite soluble, and the old admonition to force fluids is no longer warranted. Sulfonamides have been implicated in interstitial nephritis.

Gluckstein D, Ruskin J: Rapid oral desensitization to trimethoprim-sulfamethoxazole (TMP-SMZ): Use in prophylaxis for *Pneumocystis carinii* pneumonia in patients with AIDS who were previously intolerant to TMP-SMZ. Clin Infect Dis 1995;20:849. (Description of method.)

SULFONES USED IN THE TREATMENT OF LEPROSY

A number of drugs closely related to the sulfonamides (eg, dapsone; diaminodiphenylsulfone, DDS) have been used effectively in the long-term treatment of leprosy. The clinical manifestations of both lepromatous and tuberculoid leprosy can often be suppressed by treatment extending over several years. At least 5–30% of *Mycobacterium leprae* organisms are resistant to dapsone, so initial combined treatment with rifampin is advocated. Dapsone, 100 mg daily, is effective therapy for pneumocystis pneumonia in AIDS when combined with trimethoprim, 20 mg/kg/d in four divided doses. At a dose of 50–100 mg daily or 100 mg two or three times a week, it is effective prophylaxis for *P carinii* infection and, when combined with pyrimethamine, 50 mg per week, also prevents *Toxoplasma* encephalitis in HIV-infected patients.

Absorption, Metabolism, & Excretion

All sulfones are well absorbed from the intestinal tract, are distributed widely in all tissues, and tend to be retained in skin, muscle, liver, and kidney. Skin involved by leprosy contains ten times more drug than normal skin. Sulfones are excreted into the bile and reabsorbed by the intestine. Consequently, blood levels are prolonged. Excretion into the urine is variable, and the drug occurs in urine mostly as a glucuronic acid conjugate. Some persons acetylate sulfones slowly and others rapidly; this requires dosage adjustment.

Dosages & Routes of Administration

See Leprosy, Chapter 33, for recommendations.

Adverse Effects

The sulfones may cause any of the side effects listed above for sulfonamides. Anorexia, nausea, and vomiting are common. Hemolysis, methemoglobinemia, or agranulocytosis may occur. G6PD levels should be determined prior to initiation of dapsone therapy. If sulfones are not tolerated, clofazimine can be substituted.

SPECIALIZED DRUGS USED AGAINST BACTERIA

1. BACITRACIN

This polypeptide is selectively active against gram-positive bacteria. Because of severe nephrotoxicity upon systemic administration, its use has been limited to topical application on surface lesions, usually in combination with polymyxin or neomycin. Occasionally it is given orally for pseudomembranous colitis caused by toxin-producing *C difficile;* however, it is inferior to oral vancomycin or metronidazole.

2. MUPIROCIN

Mupirocin (formerly pseudomonic acid) is a naturally occurring antibiotic produced by *Pseudomonas fluorescens* that is active against most gram-positive cocci, including methicillin-sensitive and methicillin-resistant *S aureus.* It is used topically. It is effective in eliminating staphylococcal nasal carriage in the majority of patients for up to 3 months after application to the anterior nares twice daily for 5 days. However, recurrent colonization can occur (53% are recolonized at the end of 1 year) and when mupirocin is used chronically over months, resistant organisms can emerge. Monthly application for 5 days each month for up to a year decreases staphylococcal colonization, which in turn lowers the risk of recurrent staphylococcal skin infections. Whether it is more effective than trimethoprim-sulfamethoxazole or dicloxacillin plus rifampin for eradication of staphylococcal nasal carriage is unknown.

3. CLINDAMYCIN

Clindamycin resembles erythromycin (though different in structure) and is active against gram-positive organisms (except enterococci and most methicillin-resistant staphylococci). A dosage of 0.15–0.3 g orally every 6 hours yields serum concentrations of 2–5 µg/mL. It is widely distributed in tissues. Excretion is through the bile and urine. Clindamycin is an alternative to erythromycin as a substitute for penicillin. Clindamycin is currently recommended as the alternative drug for prophylaxis against endocarditis following oral procedures in patients allergic to amoxicillin. Clindamycin, 300 mg orally twice daily for 7 days, can be used as an alternative to metronidazole for the therapy of bacterial vaginosis. Topical application of a 2% vaginal cream once or twice daily for 7 days is also effective. Clindamycin is active against most anaerobes, including *Bacteroides.* It is frequently used to treat infections in which anaerobes are significant pathogens (eg, aspiration pneumonia, pelvic and abdominal infections), often in combination with other drugs (aminoglycosides, cephalosporins, aztreonam). In patients with necrotizing pneumonia or lung abscess following aspiration, clindamycin appears to be superior to penicillin. Seriously ill patients are given clindamycin, 600–900 mg (20–30 mg/kg/d) intravenously, during a 1-hour period every 8 hours. Success has also been reported in staphylococcal osteomyelitis. In the sulfonamide-allergic patient, high-dose clindamycin therapy (600–1200 mg intravenously every 6 hours or 600 mg orally every 6 hours) in conjunction with pyrimethamine has been used to treat toxoplasmosis of the central nervous system and appears to be as effective as pyrimethamine and sulfadiazine. Clindamycin in combination with primaquine has been reported to be effective in the therapy of pneumocystis pneumonia in patients with AIDS. These drugs are ineffective in meningitis.

Common side effects are diarrhea, nausea, and skin rashes. Impaired liver function and neutropenia have been noted. If 3–4 g is given rapidly intravenously, cardiorespiratory arrest may occur. Bloody diarrhea with pseudomembranous colitis has been associated with the administration of clindamycin and other antibiotics. This antibiotic-associated colitis is due to a necrotizing toxin produced by *C difficile.* The organism is resistant to the antimicrobial, is selected out by its presence, and is favored in its growth and toxin production. *C difficile* is usually susceptible to—and can be treated with—vancomycin, bacitracin, or metronidazole given orally, though metronidazole is the drug of choice (see below).

4. METRONIDAZOLE

Metronidazole is an antiprotozoal drug (see Chapter 35) that also has striking antibacterial effects against most anaerobes, including *Bacteroides*. It is well absorbed after oral administration, is widely distributed in tissues, and yields serum levels of 4–6 µg/mL after a 250 mg dose. It penetrates well into the cerebrospinal fluid, yielding levels similar to those in serum. The drug is metabolized in the liver, and dosage reduction is required in severe hepatic insufficiency. Metronidazole can be given intravenously.

Metronidazole is employed in amebiasis and giardiasis (see Chapter 35) and in the following circumstances:

(1) *Trichomonas* vaginitis responds to either a single dose (2 g) or to 250 mg orally three times daily for 7–10 days. Bacterial vaginosis responds to a single 2 g dose or to 500 mg twice daily for 7 days. Metronidazole vaginal cream (0.75%) applied twice daily for 5 days is also effective.

(2) In anaerobic infections, metronidazole can be given orally or intravenously, 500 mg three times daily (30 mg/kg/d). It is less expensive and more predictable against *B fragilis* than clindamycin or second-generation cephalosporins with anaerobic activity.

(3) Metronidazole is less expensive and equally as efficacious as oral vancomycin for the therapy of *C difficile* colitis and is the drug of choice for the disease. A dosage of 500 mg orally three times daily is recommended. If oral medication cannot be tolerated, intravenous metronidazole can be tried at the same dose; however, this route may be less effective than the oral one. Because of the emergence of vancomycin-resistant enterococci as a major pathogen and the role of oral vancomycin in selecting for these resistant organisms, metronidazole should always be used as first-line therapy for *C difficile* disease.

(4) Preparation of the colon before bowel surgery.

(5) Therapy of brain abscess, often in combination with penicillin or a third-generation cephalosporin.

(6) In combination with H_2-blockers and amoxicillin for therapy of some *H pylori* infections.

Adverse effects include stomatitis, nausea, and diarrhea. Ingestion of alcohol while taking metronidazole can result in flushing, hypotension, nausea, and vomiting. With prolonged use at high doses, reversible peripheral neuropathy can develop. Metronidazole can decrease the metabolism of warfarin and increase the prothrombin time, necessitating careful monitoring of the prothrombin time and dosage adjustment of warfarin when both drugs are used together. Metronidazole has been shown to be carcinogenic in certain animal models and mutagenic for certain bacteria. To date, human studies have not confirmed an increased incidence of malignancy.

Falagas ME, Gorbach SL: Clindamycin and metronidazole. Med Clin North Am 1995;79:845. (Pharmacology, spectrum of activity, indications, toxicity.)

5. VANCOMYCIN

This drug is bactericidal for most gram-positive organisms, particularly staphylococci and streptococci—and is bacteriostatic for most enterococci—in concentrations of 0.5–1 µg/mL. Although vancomycin has retained activity against staphylococci and streptococci, vancomycin-resistant strains of enterococci (particularly *Enterococcus faecium*) have become a major problem and account for 15–25% of isolates in some areas of the country. Vancomycin is not absorbed from the gastrointestinal tract. It is given orally only for the treatment of antibiotic-associated enterocolitis. For systemic effect the drug must be administered intravenously (20–30 mg/kg/d in two or three divided doses). An intravenous injection of 10 mg/kg over a period of 20 minutes yields blood levels of 20–30 µg/mL. Vancomycin is excreted mainly via the kidneys but may accumulate to some extent also in liver failure. In renal insufficiency, the half-life may be up to 8 days. Thus, only one dose of 0.5–1 g may be given every 4–8 days to a uremic individual undergoing chronic hemodialysis. Patients receiving high-flux hemodialysis or continuous arteriovenous hemofiltration (CAVH) require more frequent maintenance dosing. In patients with impaired renal function, the dosing interval is determined by measuring serum levels. When levels reach 5–15 µg/mL, repeat dosing is required to maintain therapeutic levels.

Indications for parenteral vancomycin include the following: (1) Severe staphylococcal infections in penicillin-allergic patients; it is the drug of choice for methicillin-resistant *S aureus* and *S epidermidis* infections. (2) Severe enterococcal infections in the penicillin-allergic patient, usually in combination with an aminoglycoside. (3) Other gram-positive infections in penicillin-allergic patients, eg, viridans streptococcal endocarditis. (4) Surgical prophylaxis in penicillin-allergic patients. (5) For gram-positive infections due to organisms that are multidrug-resistant, ie, *Corynebacterium jeikeium*. (6). Endocarditis prophylaxis in the penicillin-allergic patient undergoing certain genitourinary and gastrointestinal procedures (in combination with an aminoglycoside). (See Table 33–3.)

In antibiotic-associated enterocolitis, vancomycin, 0.125–0.5 g, is given orally four times daily.

Vancomycin is irritating to tissues; chills, fever,

and thrombophlebitis sometimes follow intravenous injection. The drug is infrequently ototoxic and potentially nephrotoxic when administered with aminoglycosides. Rapid infusion or high doses (1 g or more) may induce diffuse hyperemia ("red man syndrome") and can be avoided by extending infusions over 1–2 hours or by pretreating with a histamine antagonist such as hydroxyzine.

Cunha BA: Vancomycin. Med Clin North Am 1995; 79:817. (Pharmacology, spectrum of activity, indications, toxicity.)

STREPTOGRAMINS

Streptogramins are structurally similar to macrolides but do not share cross-resistance with that class. **Pristinamycin** is an oral streptogramin marketed in France for treatment of gram-positive infections. **Synercid** is a combination of two synthetic derivatives of pristinamycin—quinupristin and dalfopristin—in a 30:70 ratio that is administered intravenously. It is bacteriostatic and inhibits protein synthesis by binding to bacterial ribosomes. In vitro it has a wide spectrum of activity, including *Moraxella catarrhalis, Haemophilus influenzae, Clostridium* species, *Peptostreptococcus* species, *Mycoplasma, Legionella,* and *Chlamydia.* It has no activity against enteric gram-negative bacilli. However, its major clinical use is in the therapy of gram-positive infections, including those due to streptococci (including penicillin-resistant pneumococci) staphylococci (including methicillin-sensitive and methicillin-resistant *S aureus* and *S epidermidis*) and enterococci, including vancomycin-resistant *Enterococcus faecium.* It is currently an investigational drug available through Rhône-Poulenc Rorer for the therapy of vancomycin-resistant enterococcal infections.

QUINOLONES

The quinolones are synthetic analogues of nalidixic acid that have an exceedingly broad spectrum of activity against many bacteria. The mode of action of all quinolones involves inhibition of bacterial DNA synthesis by blocking the enzyme DNA gyrase.

The earlier quinolones (nalidixic acid, oxolinic acid, cinoxacin) did not achieve systemic antibacterial levels after oral intake and thus were useful only as urinary antiseptics. The newer fluorinated derivatives (norfloxacin, ciprofloxacin, enoxacin, pefloxacin, ofloxacin, lomefloxacin, levofloxacin, and sparfloxacin) have greater antibacterial activity, achieve clinically useful levels in blood and tissues, and have low toxicity.

Antimicrobial Activity

A number of fluoroquinolones are currently available. Most have quite similar spectrums of activity. In general, these drugs have superb activity against Enterobacteriaceae but are also active against other gram-negative bacteria such as *Haemophilus, Neisseria, Moraxella, Brucella, Legionella, Salmonella, Shigella, Campylobacter, Yersinia, Vibrio,* and *Aeromonas.* Ciprofloxacin has slightly better activity against *P aeruginosa* than the other fluoroquinolones, and none of these agents have reliable activity against *S maltophilia* or *P cepacia.* Against genital tract pathogens such as *Mycoplasma hominis, Ureaplasma urealyticum,* and *C pneumoniae,* ofloxacin possesses more activity than the others, and against *Gardnerella vaginalis* ciprofloxacin and ofloxacin are the most active. *M tuberculosis* is sensitive to the quinolones, as is *M fortuitum* and *Mycobacterium kansasii.* Although most *M avium* complex organisms are resistant to fluoroquinolones when combined with other agents (ethambutol, rifampin, and amikacin), ciprofloxacin appears to be effective in treating infections caused by this organism.

In general, the fluoroquinolones are less active against gram-positive than gram-negative organisms, with norfloxacin, enoxacin, and lomefloxacin having less activity than ciprofloxacin and ofloxacin. Ciprofloxacin and ofloxacin are active against most *S aureus* and *S epidermidis,* including about 50% of methicillin-resistant strains. However, recent reports of the emergence of ciprofloxacin-resistant strains of staphylococci developing during therapy may severely limit the use of quinolones to treat infections caused by these organisms. *M pneumoniae* and enterococci, including *E faecalis, S pneumoniae,* group A, B, and D streptococci, and viridans streptococci are only moderately sensitive to the quinolones. Anaerobic bacteria, *T pallidum,* and *Nocardia* are resistant to the fluoroquinolones.

Levofloxacin and sparfloxacin are very similar to the previously described fluoroquinolones with the notable exception of improved activity against streptococci, including penicillin-resistant pneumococci. Clinafloxacin and trovafloxacin will most likely be marketed in the near future. Clinafloxacin offers improved activity against anaerobes (including *Bacteroides* and *Prevotella* species) and gram-positive organisms, while trovafloxacin is the most potent quinolone against enterococcal infections.

Pharmacokinetics & Administration

After oral administration, the fluoroquinolones are well absorbed and widely distributed in body fluids and tissues and are concentrated intracellularly. Fluoroquinolones are bound by some heavy metals, and absorption is inhibited when they are given with iron, calcium, and other multivalent cations. Highest serum levels are achieved if they are given 1 hour before or 2 hours after meals. Ofloxacin and pefloxacin appear to penetrate into the cerebrospinal fluid better than other fluoroquinolones. The serum half-life ranges from 4 hours (ciprofloxacin) to 20 hours (sparfloxacin), with ofloxacin and enoxacin having a half-life of 6–8 hours. After ingestion of 500 mg, the peak serum level of ciprofloxacin is 2.5 μg/mL and is lower than that of the other quinolones (4–6 μg/mL), but this is offset by ciprofloxacin's slightly greater in vitro activity against most gram-negative organisms. A number of the fluoroquinolones can be administered intravenously, resulting in peak serum levels ranging from 4 to 9 μg/mL. The fluoroquinolones are excreted mainly through the kidney by tubular secretion (which can be blocked by probenecid) and by glomerular filtration. Up to 20% of the dose is metabolized by the liver. In renal insufficiency, half-lives are prolonged, but only slight dosage adjustment is needed with the exception of ofloxacin, in which the half-life increases from 8 to 35 hours. These drugs are not removed by hemodialysis or peritoneal dialysis.

Clinical Uses

Because of their high cost, broad spectrum of activity, and tendency for some organisms (eg, *P aeruginosa,* staphylococcal species) to develop resistance, these agents should not be routinely used as first-line therapy when less expensive agents with narrower spectrums are available.

Urinary tract infections caused by multidrug-resistant gram-negative organisms that are sensitive to quinolones can be treated with any of the available agents.

Because of good penetration into prostatic tissue, quinolones are effective in treating bacterial prostatitis and are alternatives to trimethoprim-sulfamethoxazole (doses for prostatitis are the same as for urinary tract infection, but the duration should be 6–12 weeks).

Quinolones have been approved for use in therapy of certain sexually transmitted diseases. Ofloxacin, 300 mg twice daily for 7 days, is as effective as doxycycline, 100 mg twice daily for 7 days, for the therapy of *C trachomatis* cervicitis, urethritis, and proctitis. It is also effective for nongonococcal urethritis caused by *U urealyticum.* Ciprofloxacin and norfloxacin are not effective for the therapy of chlamydial infections or nongonococcal urethritis. In general, the use of quinolones for the therapy of any sexually transmitted disease will be limited by their lack of efficacy in concomitant syphilis. Although ceftriaxone, 125–250 mg intramuscularly as a single injection, remains the treatment of choice for uncomplicated gonococcal urethritis, cervicitis, pharyngitis, and proctitis, these infections can also be treated with a single dose of 500 mg of ciprofloxacin, 400 mg of ofloxacin, or 400 mg of enoxacin. While not currently common in the United States, the increased prevalence of *N gonorrhoeae* resistant to fluoroquinolones may limit their usefulness for this infection in the future.

Pelvic inflammatory disease is usually caused by *Chlamydia trachomatis, N gonorrhoeae,* or anaerobes. Oral outpatient treatment with ofloxacin, 400 mg twice daily for 14 days, in addition to clindamycin, 450 mg orally four times daily for 14 days, or metronidazole, 500 mg orally twice daily for 14 days, can be used. Epididymitis in young men (< 35 years of age) is caused most commonly by *Chlamydia* and the gonococcus, and outpatient therapy with single-dose ciprofloxacin (500 mg) or ofloxacin (400 mg) followed by doxycycline, 100 mg twice daily for 10 days, is adequate therapy. Alternatively, ofloxacin, 300 mg twice daily for 10 days, can be used. *H ducreyi,* the agent that causes chancroid, is sensitive to quinolones, and ciprofloxacin, 500 mg twice daily, or enoxacin, 400 mg daily for 3 days, can be used as an alternative to erythromycin, azithromycin, or ceftriaxone as therapy for this disease.

Ciprofloxacin and ofloxacin have been successfully used to treat complicated skin and soft tissue infections and osteomyelitis caused by gram-negative organisms. Ciprofloxacin, 500–750 mg twice daily for at least 6 weeks, has been effective therapy for malignant otitis externa.

Because quinolones are the only available oral agents active against *Campylobacter* and the other major bacterial pathogens associated with diarrhea (*Salmonella, Shigella,* toxigenic *E coli),* they have been used for the therapy of traveler's diarrhea as well as domestically acquired acute diarrhea. Norfloxacin, ciprofloxacin, and ofloxacin may be effective in eradicating the chronic carrier state of *Salmonella* when therapy is continued for 4–6 weeks.

Ciprofloxacin has been used to eradicate meningococci from the nasopharynx of carriers.

Norfloxacin, ciprofloxacin, and ofloxacin are effective for prophylaxis against gram-negative infections in the neutropenic patient, and intravenous ciprofloxacin in combination with aminoglycosides or β-lactam antibiotics has been used successfully to treat the febrile neutropenic patient.

Although some clinical studies have suggested that ciprofloxacin and ofloxacin are efficacious in the therapy of lower respiratory tract infections, caution should be exercised since the drug has only marginal activity against *S pneumoniae* and *M pneumoniae,* and failures in treating pneumococcal pneumonia have been reported. It is possible that newer agents such as levofloxacin and sparfloxacin will be useful in community-acquired pneumonia, especially that due to penicillin-resistant pneumococci. One setting in which ciprofloxacin is indicated for the therapy of lower respiratory tract infections is in cystic fibrosis, where *P aeruginosa* is the predominant pathogen.

As noted above, ciprofloxacin in combination with other agents has been used to treat *M avium* complex infections, and ciprofloxacin and ofloxacin may be efficacious in the therapy of multidrug-resistant tuberculosis.

Adverse Effects

The most prominent adverse effects of the quinolones are nausea, vomiting, and diarrhea. Occasionally, headache, dizziness, seizures, insomnia, impaired liver function, and skin rashes have been observed as well as more serious reactions such as acute renal failure and anaphylaxis. Superinfections with enterococci and yeasts can develop. Clearance of theophylline may be inhibited by fluoroquinolones (especially enoxacin), and drug levels should be monitored in patients receiving both drugs. Prolongation of the prothrombin time has been observed in some patients receiving stable doses of warfarin after ciprofloxacin has been given, but this interaction is unpredictable and modest. Because fluoroquinolones cause joint damage in young animals, they are used with caution in children. Cartilage toxicity is rare in children with cystic fibrosis receiving ciprofloxacin, but tendonitis and tendon rupture, while infrequent, have been reported with several quinolone agents. Patients experiencing musculoskeletal symptoms should discontinue therapy.

Hendershot EF: Fluoroquinolones. Infect Dis Clin North Am 1995;9:715. (Pharmacology, spectrum of activity, indications, toxicity.)

Sparfloxacin and levofloxacin. Med Lett Drugs Ther 1997;41. (Activity, kinetics, toxicity, clinical use.)

PENTAMIDINE & ATOVAQUONE

Pentamidine and atovaquone are antiprotozoal agents that are primarily used to treat pneumocystis pneumonia. Pentamidine is discussed in Chapters 31 and 35. Atovaquone inhibits mitochondrial electron transport and probably also folate metabolism. It is poorly absorbed and should be given with food to maximize bioavailability. It has moderate activity against *P carinii*. In comparative trials with trimethoprim-sulfamethoxazole and pentamidine in the therapy of pneumocystis pneumonia in AIDS, atovaquone, 750 mg orally three times daily for 3 weeks, was less effective than both agents but better tolerated. Major adverse effects include rash, nausea, vomiting, diarrhea, fever, and abnormal liver function tests. The use of atovaquone is limited to patients with mild to moderate pneumocystis infections who have failed or cannot tolerate other therapies.

Hughes W et al: Comparison of atovaquone (566C80) with trimethoprim/sulfamethoxazole to treat *Pneumocystis carinii* pneumonia in patients with AIDS. N Engl J Med 1993;328:1521. (Results of study showing decreased efficacy but better tolerance than TMP-SMZ.)

URINARY ANTISEPTICS

These drugs exert antimicrobial activity in the urine but have little or no systemic antibacterial effect. Their usefulness is limited to urinary tract infections.

1. NITROFURANTOIN

Nitrofurantoin is bacteriostatic and bactericidal for both gram-positive (including enterococci and staphylococci) and many gram-negative bacteria (not *S marcescens* or *P aeruginosa*) in concentrations of 10–500 μg/mL. Microbial resistance does not emerge rapidly. The activity of nitrofurantoin is greatly enhanced at pH 6.5 or less.

Nitrofurantoin is rapidly absorbed from the gastrointestinal tract, but levels in serum and tissues are negligible. Thus, there is no systemic antibacterial effect. Use of the drug is limited to lower urinary tract infections. It is rapidly excreted in urine, where concentrations may be 200–400 μg/mL. In renal failure, there is virtually no excretion into the urine and no therapeutic effect.

The average daily dose in urinary tract infections is 100 mg orally four times daily, taken with food. A single daily dose of 50–100 mg can prevent recurrent urinary tract infections in women.

Oral nitrofurantoin often causes nausea and vomiting. Hemolytic anemia may occur in G6PD deficiency. Other side effects are skin rashes and pulmonary infiltration.

2. FOSFOMYCIN

Fosfomycin tromethamine is a phosphonic acid derivative useful in the treatment of uncomplicated urinary tract infection. The spectrum of activity includes *E coli, E faecalis,* and other gram-negative aerobic pathogens. Available as a 3 g sachet, fosfomycin may be useful for the single-dose treatment of the above organisms. Like nitrofurantoin, fosfomycin should not be used for systemic infection. However, the increased concentrations in urine allow for its use in uncomplicated bacteriuria. The most frequently reported adverse effects include diarrhea, headache, and nausea.

3. ACIDIFYING AGENTS

Urine with a pH below 5.5 tends to be antibacterial. Many substances have been used in an attempt to acidify urine, including ammonium chloride, ascorbic acid, methionine, and mandelic acid. In general, large doses are required and none are consistently effective. In view of the plethora of antibiotics that are available for therapy and prophylaxis of urinary tract infections, acidifying agents are of limited value.

SYSTEMICALLY ACTIVE DRUGS IN URINARY TRACT INFECTIONS

Many antimicrobial drugs are excreted in the urine in high concentrations. For this reason, low and relatively nontoxic dosages of penicillins, cephalosporins, aminoglycosides, quinolones, and trimethoprim-sulfamethoxazole can reach high urinary concentrations and are effective in urinary tract infections.

ANTIFUNGAL DRUGS

Empiric antifungal therapy is rarely instituted except for febrile neutropenic patients. Therapy is reserved for situations in which yeast or mold is seen on KOH preparation or when isolated organisms are thought to be pathogenic. Antifungal sensitivity testing has not yet been standardized and is not routinely recommended. Thus, therapy is based on experience and clinical trials and not on susceptibility tests.

1. AMPHOTERICIN B

Amphotericin B in vitro inhibits several organisms producing systemic mycotic disease in humans, including *Histoplasma, Cryptococcus, Coccidioides, Candida, Blastomyces, Sporothrix,* and others. This drug can be used for treatment of these systemic fungal infections. Intrathecal administration is necessary for the treatment of *Coccidioides* meningitis and may be required in meningitis caused by other fungi if systemic therapy fails (eg, *Cryptococcus, Candida*). *Pseudallescheria boydii* and *Fusarium* are often resistant to amphotericin B.

There is no consensus on how amphotericin B should be administered or on the dosage and the duration of therapy. The first few milliliters of the initial dose are administered over 10–20 minutes to test for anaphylaxis. The daily dose of amphotericin B for most fungal infections varies from 0.3 to 1 mg/kg, though infections caused by *Aspergillus* and *Mucor* are often treated with 1.5 mg/kg daily. Full doses are reached by increasing the dose incrementally over several days. The initial dose is usually 0.25 mg/kg given over 1–2 hours; on day 2, 0.5 mg/kg is given; and on day 3, 0.7–1/mg/kg is administered depending on the infection. The final dose is continued daily or every other day.

In fungal meningitis, amphotericin B, 0.5 mg, is injected intrathecally three times weekly; continuous treatment (many weeks) with an Ommaya reservoir is generally required. The dose is slowly increased over several weeks to improve tolerance (first week: 0.05 mg, 0.1 mg, 0.2 mg every other day; second week: 0.3 mg, 0.4 mg, 0.5 mg every other day). Relapses of fungal meningitis (especially *Coccidioides* meningitis) occur commonly and can be seen years after completion of therapy. Thus, when treating meningitis due to *Coccidioides immitis,* intrathecal therapy is given three times a week for 8–10 weeks initially, and the frequency is then decreased to once-weekly doses for 6 months. Subsequent therapy is dictated by cerebrospinal fluid titers. In meningitis due to other fungi, long-term therapy beyond the initial 8–10 weeks is rarely needed. Combined treatment with flucytosine is beneficial in cryptococcal meningitis and possibly systemic candidiasis. Amphotericin B may have some benefit in *Naegleria* meningoencephalitis.

Amphotericin B in low doses (0.1–0.25 mg/kg/d) has been used prophylactically to prevent invasive fungal infections in bone marrow transplant recipients and may be beneficial in this setting. Whether prophylactic administration is better than early empirical therapy in febrile patients who have not responded to broad-spectrum antibiotics has not been determined.

In patients with Foley catheters in place who have candiduria, amphotericin B bladder irrigations have been used to decrease colony counts. Twenty-five to 50 milligrams of drug is added to 500–1000 mL of sterile water. This solution is used for continuous (30–50 mL/h) or intermittent irrigation (200 mL four or five times daily with clamping of the catheter for ½–1 hour). Although the procedure is widely used, the efficacy of amphotericin B bladder irrigation has never been proved. Long-term eradication of candiduria following amphotericin B bladder irrigation rarely occurs.

In impaired renal function, the dose of amphotericin B need not be reduced initially. However, if the serum creatinine reaches 2.5–3 mg/dL, the dose is temporarily lowered (or even stopped for a few days) until renal function recovers. Amphotericin B is then resumed at about one-half the previous dosage and increased in increments as tolerated. The drug is not removed by hemodialysis, so that no additional drug is needed after dialysis.

The intravenous administration of amphotericin B usually produces chills, fever, vomiting, and headache. As a rule, infusions given over 1–2 hours are as well tolerated as those given over 4–6 hours. However, patients who experience infusion-related adverse effects may benefit from slowing the rate of administration. Tolerance may be enhanced by temporary lowering of the dose or premedication with aspirin (or acetaminophen) and diphenhydramine.

Addition of 25 mg of hydrocortisone to the infusion decreases the incidence of rigors, and meperidine, 25–50 mg, is effective in arresting rigors once they start. Amphotericin B can cause phlebitis when given peripherally, and this can be prevented by adding 500–1000 units of heparin to the infusion. Central intravenous administration eliminates the likelihood of this complication. Amphotericin B commonly impairs kidney function and produces anemia (impaired iron utilization by bone marrow). Electrolyte disturbances (hypokalemia, hypomagnesemia, distal renal tubular acidosis) also occur. Animal and limited human data suggest that the renal insufficiency commonly seen with amphotericin B administration can be prevented with salt supplementation. As a result, administration of 0.5–1 L of 0.9% saline prior to infusion of amphotericin B may prevent nephrotoxicity.

The nephrotoxicity of amphotericin has resulted in the development of lipid-based amphotericin B products. At the present time, two products—amphotericin B lipid complex (ABLC; Abelcet) and amphotericin B colloidal dispersion (ABCD; Amphotec)—are available, with a third product—liposomal amphotericin B (AmBisome)—likely to be released soon. Complexing amphotericin B with lipid allows larger doses to be administered (3–5 mg/kg, depending on the preparation and the fungal species. Infusion-related fevers and chills occur in about 15% of patients, but nephrotoxicity occurs less commonly (about 5% of patients) than with amphotericin B. The drug appears to be efficacious for therapy of invasive *Aspergillus* infections, invasive fungal infections in bone marrow transplant patients, cryptococcal meningitis in HIV-positive patients, and hepatosplenic candidiasis. The liquid-based products cost about ten times as much as amphotericin B, and at present their use is limited to those patients who have failed therapy with conventional amphotericin B or those who develop renal insufficiency (serum creatinine 2.5–3 mg/dL).

Kline S et al: Limited toxicity of prolonged therapy with high doses of amphotericin B lipid complex. Clin Infect Dis 1995;21:1154. (Describes six patients who received an average 1 year of therapy.)

Sharkey PK et al: Amphotericin B lipid complex compared with amphotericin B in the treatment of cryptococcal meningitis in patients with AIDS. Clin Infect Dis 1996;22:315. (Clinical response equivalent. Some questions about mycologic cure with lipid complex.)

2. GRISEOFULVIN

Griseofulvin is an agent that can inhibit the growth of some dermatophytes but has no effect on bacteria or on the fungi that cause deep mycoses. Absorption of griseofulvin microsize, 1 g/d, gives blood levels of 0.5–1.5 µg/mL. The absorbed drug has an affinity for skin and is deposited there, bound to keratin. Thus, it makes keratin resistant to fungal growth, and the new growth of hair or nails is free of infection. As keratinized structures are shed, they are replaced by uninfected ones. The bulk of ingested griseofulvin is excreted in the feces. Topical application of griseofulvin has little effect.

Oral doses of 0.5–1 g/d for 3–5 weeks are given if only the skin is involved and for 3–6 months or longer if the hair and nails are involved. Griseofulvin is most successful in severe dermatophytosis, particularly if caused by *Trichophyton rubrum,* though some strains are resistant.

An ultramicrosize particle formulation (Gris-PEG) is better absorbed. The dosage is 0.33–0.66 g orally daily.

Griseofulvin is relatively nontoxic and has a long history of clinical safety. Headache, nausea, vomiting, diarrhea, photosensitivity, and leukopenia have all been reported but are reversible and often will resolve without interruption of therapy. Routine monitoring for adverse effects is not required.

Major indications for use of this drug include tinea capitis, widespread tinea corporis, and tinea unguium (onychomycosis), though success rates in the latter are only 25–30%. Preserved agents in the treatment of onychomycosis include itraconazole and terbinafine. Preliminary data suggest that these drugs are at least as effective as griseofulvin; however, failures are reported in 30–50% of cases.

3. NYSTATIN

Nystatin has a wide spectrum of antifungal activity but is used almost exclusively to treat superficial candidal infections. It is too toxic for systemic administration, and the drug is not absorbed from mucous membranes or the gastrointestinal tract. Several preparations are available, including oral suspension (100,000 units/mL) and ointments, gels, and creams (100,000 units/g). For oral candidiasis, 500,000 units of suspension is used to rinse the mouth and is retained in the mouth as long as possible before it is swallowed. This is repeated four times a day for at least 2 days after resolution of the infection. Infections of skin are treated with cream or ointment, 100,000 units applied to the affected area twice daily until resolution of the infection. Nystatin is less effective than miconazole and clotrimazole for therapy of vaginal candidiasis.

4. FLUCYTOSINE

Flucytosine inhibits some strains of *Candida, Cryptococcus, Aspergillus, Torulopsis,* and other fungi. Dosages of 3–8 g daily (150 mg/kg/d) orally produce good levels in serum and cerebrospinal fluid. Clinical remissions of meningitis or sepsis due to yeasts have occurred. However, resistant organisms are selected out rapidly, and flucytosine is therefore not employed as a single drug except in urinary tract infections.

In renal insufficiency, flucytosine may accumulate to toxic levels, and dosage adjustments are needed. With normal renal function, the usual dosage is 37.5 mg/kg every 6 hours; for creatinine clearance of 26–50 mL/min, 37.5 mg/kg every 12 hours is given; for creatinine clearance of 10–25 mL/min, 37.5 mg/kg once daily is given; and for clearance less than 10 mL/min, 12–25 mg/kg once daily is given. Because patients with HIV infection and normal renal function do not tolerate the above-listed doses of flucytosine (150 mg/kg/d), 75–100 mg/kg/d is recommended. The drug is effectively removed by hemodialysis. Toxic effects include bone marrow depression, abnormal liver function, loss of hair, and others. Bone marrow suppression is caused by conversion of flucytosine to fluorouracil. Combined use of flucytosine and amphotericin B in systemic candidiasis and cryptococcal meningitis has been shown to be of value. Flucytosine is effective for therapy of urinary tract infections caused by sensitive organisms.

5. NATAMYCIN

Natamycin is a polyene antifungal drug effective against many different fungi in vitro. When it is combined with appropriate surgical measures, topical application of 5% ophthalmic suspension may be beneficial in the treatment of keratitis caused by *Fusarium, Cephalosporium,* or other fungi. The drug may also be effective in the treatment of oral or vaginal candidiasis. The toxicity after topical application appears to be low.

6. TERBINAFINE

Terbinafine, an allylamine, inhibits fungal cell membrane function by blocking ergosterol synthesis. Terbinafine is now available orally in 250 mg tablets. The recommended dosage is 250 mg daily for 12 weeks for toenail infections and 250 mg daily for 6 weeks for fingernail infections (success rate about 70%). Terbinafine is well tolerated. Most adverse effects are minor (diarrhea, dyspepsia) or transient (taste disturbance). Rare cases of hepatic injury have been reported.

7. ANTIFUNGAL IMIDAZOLES & TRIAZOLES

These antifungal drugs also inhibit synthesis of ergosterol, resulting in inhibition of membrane-associated enzyme activity, cell wall growth, and replication.

Clotrimazole, taken orally in the form of 10 mg troches five times daily, can prevent and treat oral candidiasis. Vaginal tablets (200 mg) inserted daily for 3 days are effective for vaginal candidiasis. Topical preparations for treatment of cutaneous dermatophytes are also available. Toxicity precludes systemic use.

Miconazole is active in vitro against *Coccidioides, Candida, Histoplasma, Cryptococcus, Paracoccidioides, Pseudallescheria, Sporothrix,* and other fungi. However, it has substantial toxicity and little clinical activity and is rarely used intravenously. It is a drug of choice only for *P boydii* infections in a dosage of 30 mg/kg/d in three divided doses. Its major use is as a 2% cream for dermatophytosis and as a 200 mg vaginal suppository for vaginal candidiasis.

Ketoconazole, an imidazole, can be given orally as a single daily dose of 200–600 mg, preferably with food. It is well absorbed and reaches serum levels of 2–4 µg/mL. The dosage remains the same in renal or hepatic failure. Absorption is impaired by antacid and H_2-blockers; coadministration of phenytoin, isoniazid, and rifampin can cause enhanced metabolism of ketoconazole and lower plasma levels.

Ketoconazole is primarily used to treat superficial infections caused by *Candida,* including oral, vaginal, and esophageal candidiasis. It dramatically improves lesions of chronic mucocutaneous candidiasis. Ketoconazole is also effective therapy for some deep-seated fungal infections such as blastomycosis, paracoccidioidomycosis, and nonmeningeal, localized histoplasmosis. However, this drug has been disappointing in the treatment of deep-seated candidal and coccidioidal infections (other than cutaneous lesions) and cryptococcal meningitis, where amphotericin B remains the drug of choice.

Adverse effects include nausea, vomiting, skin rashes, and occasional elevations in aminotransferase levels. Although most elevations of liver enzymes are asymptomatic, on rare occasions symptomatic and even fatal hepatitis can occur. All patients receiving azoles should be informed of the potential toxicity. Ketoconazole blocks the synthesis of adrenal steroids and testosterone and can cause gynecomastia and impotence. Ketoconazole can also cause increased levels of cyclosporine when administered with this drug, and careful monitoring of serum levels is needed to avoid toxicity. This interaction between ketoconazole and cyclosporine has been used successively in cardiac transplant patients to lower the dose of cyclosporine needed for immunosuppression by 60–80%. This resulted in significant cost savings as well as a decreased rate of rejection and infection. However, ketoconazole-resistant organisms may emerge using this strategy.

Fluconazole, a *bis*-triazole with activity similar to that of miconazole (the exception being *Blastomyces* *dermatitidis,* which is sensitive to fluconazole but not miconazole), is water-soluble and can be given both orally and intravenously. Absorption of the drug after oral administration is less pH-dependent than that of ketoconazole, and therapeutic serum levels are obtained even when H_2 receptor antagonists are given simultaneously. It penetrates well into the cerebrospinal fluid and eye and reaches therapeutically significant levels in the urine. The drug has been shown to be effective primarily in therapy of infections with *Candida, Cryptococcus,* and *Blastomyces. Candida albicans* is almost always sensitive to fluconazole, but other species of *Candida (C tropicalis, C krusei,* etc) are often resistant, as is *Torulopsis glabrata.* The drug is inactive against *Aspergillus, Mucor,* and *Pseudallescheria.* Fluconazole (50–100 mg) is as efficacious as ketoconazole (200 mg/d) and clotrimazole troches in the therapy of oropharyngeal candidiasis and is superior to ketoconazole for therapy of candidal esophagitis in immunosuppressed patients. It is also effective therapy for vaginal candidiasis, where a single oral dose of 150 mg is 80–90% effective, and chronic mucocutaneous candidiasis. Fluconazole (400 mg/d) may be as effective as amphotericin B (0.67 mg/kg/d) for therapy of invasive candidal infections (peritonitis, genitourinary infections, abdominal abscesses, wound infections) in both neutropenic and nonneutropenic patients. Response to fluconazole in leukemic patients with hepatosplenic candidiasis has also been observed. These patients either failed to respond to amphotericin B or had severe reactions to it. Fluconazole, 400 mg daily, has been shown to be effective as amphotericin B, 0.5–0.6 mg/kg/d, for candidemia in both neutropenic and nonneutropenic patients. Most of these infections were line-related, and removal of the line was critical to successful therapy. Candidal pyelonephritis would theoretically respond well to fluconazole, since the drug is concentrated in the urine and kidneys. Fluconazole (200 mg/d) is effective as chronic suppressive therapy of cryptococcal meningitis in patients with AIDS and is the drug of choice in this setting. Its use as initial therapy is not established. At a dose of 200 mg/d, response rates and overall mortality rates are the same in patients treated with oral fluconazole and with amphotericin B. However, the mortality rate in the first 2 weeks is higher in the fluconazole-treated group, and it takes longer to sterilize the cerebrospinal fluid in the group. Higher dosages (400–800 mg daily) may be more effective, but data are lacking. A reasonable approach would be to initiate therapy with amphotericin B for 2 weeks and then switch to oral fluconazole. A dosage of 400 mg of fluconazole daily is effective therapy for coccidioidal meningitis (80% response), but improvement was slow, taking as long as 4–8 months; efficacy was noted in both non-HIV-infected and HIV-infected individuals. Higher doses (800–1200 mg/d) may be even more efficacious. Fluconazole,

400 mg daily, has been shown to be effective as prophylaxis against superficial and invasive fungal infections in bone marrow transplant recipients, but concern has been raised about superinfection with resistant organisms *(Candida krusei).* The same dose of fluconazole has not reduced the incidence of invasive fungal disease in leukemic patients undergoing intensive chemotherapy; concomitant amphotericin B remained unchanged. Thus, the role of fluconazole in prophylaxis in the neutropenic patient has not been established. In advanced HIV disease, prophylactic fluconazole has been more convincingly shown to be effective in preventing invasive fungal disease. Fluconazole, 200 mg daily, is more effective than clotrimazole troches, 10 mg five times daily, in preventing cryptococcal disease, candidal esophagitis, and superficial fungal infections, especially in those with 50 or less CD4 lymphocytes. Because the overall incidence of invasive fungal disease is low, the value of universal prophylaxis to prevent disease in a few is questionable.

Fluconazole is well absorbed after oral administration (80% bioavailability), and serum levels approach those seen after administering the same dose intravenously. In addition, the intravenous preparation is about ten times more expensive than the oral medication. Thus, unless the patient cannot take medication by mouth or has an overwhelming infection, the preferred route of administration is orally.

Itraconazole is an oral triazole with antifungal and pharmacologic properties similar to those of ketoconazole. It is moderately well absorbed from the gastrointestinal tract (food increases absorption from 30% to 60%; antacids and H_2 receptor antagonists decrease absorption) and widely distributed in tissues with the notable exception of the central nervous system, where levels in spinal fluid are undetectable. Itraconazole solution is more predictably absorbed than the tablets. However, this preparation also is affected by elevated gastric pH. The drug is metabolized by the liver, and no dosage adjustment is needed in renal insufficiency. Itraconazole is very active against most strains of *Histoplasma capsulatum, Blastomyces dermatitidis, Cryptococcus neoformans, Sporotrichum schenkii,* and various dermatophytes. It is also active, though less so, against *Candida* (but may inhibit some fluconazole-resistant strains) and *Aspergillus* species but is inactive against *Fusarium* and zygomycetes. Itraconazole in doses of 200–400 mg/d is effective and approved therapy for localized or disseminated histoplasmosis and is more effective than ketoconazole in AIDS patients with histoplasmosis. It is also effective prophylaxis against recurrent histoplasmosis in these patients. Itraconazole is preferred over ketoconazole for therapy of blastomycosis because it is more efficacious and better tolerated. It is also effective in sporotrichosis, dermatophytic infections (including those of the nails), and oral and esophageal candidiasis. Noncomparative clinical trials indicate efficacy in therapy of invasive aspergillosis (55–80%) and coccidioidomycosis (57–94%). In the absence of comparative trials with other agents active against *C immitis* and *Aspergillus,* it is difficult to know if itraconazole should be used as a first-line drug against these organisms. Certainly the oral route of administration makes the drug attractive, particularly in patients who are not critically ill. Itraconazole has been approved for onychomycosis. Pulse therapy with 200 mg twice daily for 1 week each month, repeated for 4 consecutive months, is effective in 70% of cases.

Adverse effects are similar to those of ketoconazole and fluconazole, with anorexia, nausea, vomiting, and abdominal pain occurring most commonly. Skin rash has been reported in up to 8% of patients. Hepatitis and hypokalemia occur uncommonly. Drugs that increase hepatic drug-metabolizing enzymes (isoniazid, rifampin, phenytoin, phenobarbital) may increase itraconazole metabolism, and higher doses may be needed when these drugs are administered concurrently with itraconazole. Itraconazole also impairs the metabolism of cyclosporine and can result in toxic levels unless the dosage is adjusted. Like ketoconazole, itraconazole increases blood levels of digoxin, astemizole, and loratadine and can cause fatal arrhythmias.

The usual dosage is 200 mg once or twice daily with meals, the latter regimen being preferred in immunosuppressed patients and those with invasive aspergillosis. In patients with life-threatening infections, a 600 mg loading dose is given for 3 or 4 days.

Como JA, Dismukes WE: Oral azole drugs as systemic antifungal therapy. N Engl J Med 1994;330:263. (Pharmacology, activity, adverse effects, and clinical indications.)
Systemic antifungal drugs. Med Lett Drugs Ther 1996; 38:10. (Activity, adverse effects, and clinical trials.)

ANTIVIRAL CHEMOTHERAPY

Several compounds can influence viral replication and the development of viral disease.

Amantadine is active against influenza A (but not influenza B) and has efficacy both in prophylaxis and therapy of this infection. Yearly immunization against influenza is recommended (see Chapter 30) for disease prevention, but in certain select situations amantadine can be used for this purpose. Amantadine prophylaxis is 70–90% effective and is suggested for the influenza season (6–8 weeks) in patients who cannot be immunized who are at increased risk of developing complications of influenza (those with chronic pulmonary and cardiac diseases, persons over 65 years of age, persons with chronic metabolic diseases such as diabetes mellitus, and chronic renal

failure); in medical personnel who cannot receive vaccine but are capable of transmitting influenza to high-risk patients; if vaccine is not available; and if vaccine strains differ from the strain causing an epidemic. Short-term prophylaxis (2 weeks) is indicated if an outbreak occurs before vaccination has been given. In this setting, amantadine will protect against disease while antibody production is induced and will not interfere with antibody production. Because of its modest therapeutic benefit, high-risk patients and others with influenza A may benefit from treatment with amantadine if it is instituted within 48 hours after the onset of symptoms and continued for 1 week. The usual adult dosage is 200 mg orally per day (in persons over 65 years of age, 100 mg). The most marked untoward effects are insomnia, nightmares, and ataxia, especially in the elderly. Amantadine may accumulate and be more toxic in patients with renal insufficiency, and the dosage should be reduced.

Rimantadine, an analogue of amantadine, is as effective as amantadine and is associated with fewer central nervous system adverse effects. It is considerably more expensive than amantadine and thus should be considered only in the elderly, in whom central nervous system side effects occur more commonly.

Idoxuridine, 0.1% solution or 0.5% ointment, can be applied topically every 2 hours to the lesions of acute dendritic herpetic keratitis to enhance healing. It is also used, with corticosteroids, for stromal disciform lesions of the cornea to reduce the chance of acute epithelial herpes. Because of its toxicity for the cornea, it must not be used for more than 2–3 weeks.

Trifluridine ointment (1%) is more effective than idoxuridine in herpetic keratitis but also more expensive.

Vidarabine (adenine arabinoside), 3% administered topically, is very effective in herpetic keratitis. Vidarabine, 15 mg/kg/d intravenously, provides systemic treatment for some herpesvirus infections. It is effective in the therapy of herpes zoster infections in immunocompromised patients, for herpes encephalitis, and for neonatal herpes infections. Its use is limited, however, since acyclovir has equal or greater efficacy in these infections and is less toxic. Vidarabine is not effective for acyclovir-resistant mucocutaneous infections. (Foscarnet is the drug of choice; see below.) Topical vidarabine likewise has no effect on herpetic lesions of skin or mucous membranes.

The untoward effects of vidarabine include rashes, gastrointestinal disturbances, and neurologic abnormalities, including tremors, ataxia, abnormal electroencephalogram, paresthesias, and encephalopathy. All of these are enhanced in renal failure.

Acyclovir is the least toxic antiviral drug, with therapeutic effects in infections due to herpes simplex and in herpes zoster-varicella infections. In herpes-infected cells, it is selectively active against viral DNA polymerase and thus inhibits virus proliferation. Given intravenously (15 mg/kg/d in three divided doses), it can prevent and promote healing of mucocutaneous herpes simplex in immunocompromised patients. It can reduce pain, accelerate healing, and prevent dissemination of herpes zoster and varicella in immunocompromised patients. The usual dosage for varicella-zoster infections is 30 mg/kg/d intravenously in three equal doses. The drug has no effect on establishment of latency, frequency of recurrence, or incidence of postherpetic neuralgia. Acyclovir (30 mg/kg/d intravenously in three equal doses) is the drug of choice for herpes encephalitis. Intravenous or oral acyclovir is effective prophylaxis against recurrent mucocutaneous and visceral herpes infections in transplant and other severely immunosuppressed patients. Investigation of the role of intravenous acyclovir in the prevention of cytomegalovirus disease in transplant recipients has yielded conflicting data. Acyclovir appears to be effective in some transplant settings (renal and perhaps bone marrow) but not in others (liver).

Oral acyclovir, 200 mg five times daily, has therapeutic effects similar to those achieved with intravenous acyclovir, particularly in primary genital herpes simplex infections. Oral acyclovir for recurrent genital herpes reduces viral shedding but has marginal effects on symptoms and is generally not used in this setting. When taken prophylactically (200 mg three times daily or 400 mg twice daily) for 4–6 months, oral acyclovir can reduce the frequency and severity of recurrent genital herpetic lesions during this period. Acyclovir minimally affects symptoms or viral shedding in recurrent herpes labialis and is not generally used for this disease. However, in a dose of 400 mg twice daily, it is effective in preventing recurrent herpes labialis in those with frequent relapses and in preventing sun-induced relapses.

Other possible uses of oral acyclovir include (1) therapy of herpetic keratitis, (2) prevention and treatment of herpetic whitlow, (3) acceleration of healing of herpes zoster in immunocompetent patients if initiated within 48 hours after onset (800 mg five times daily for 7 days), (4) more rapid healing of rash and lessened clinical symptoms of primary varicella in adults and children if instituted within 24 hours after onset of rash and continued for 5–7 days, (5) therapy of herpes proctitis (400 mg five times daily for 10 days), (6) prevention of herpes simplex and cytomegalovirus infections in transplant recipients (in doses of 800 mg four or five times daily), (7) prevention of erythema multiforme that is herpes simplex-related, and (8) prophylaxis against varicella in susceptible household contacts.

Topical 5% acyclovir ointment can shorten the period of pain and viral shedding in herpes simplex mucocutaneous oral lesions in immunosuppressed patients but not in patients with normal immunity.

Topical acyclovir has largely been replaced by the oral form of the drug.

Serum levels of 2.5 μg/mL are achieved after a 200 mg oral dose, and levels of 35–50 μg/mL are seen after an intravenous infusion of 5 mg/kg. Newer agents (famciclovir, valacyclovir; see below) are significantly better absorbed than oral acyclovir. If costs are equal among these agents, they would be preferable to acyclovir. Dosage reduction in renal insufficiency is required. For most herpes simplex infections except encephalitis, the dose is 5 mg/kg every 8 hours. For patients with creatinine clearances of 25–50 mL/min, give 5 mg/kg every 12 hours; for clearances of 10–24 mL/min, give 5 mg/kg every 24 hours; and for clearances of 0–10 mL/min, give 2.5 mg/kg every 24 hours. Since hemodialysis reduces serum levels significantly, the daily dose should be given after hemodialysis.

Acyclovir is relatively nontoxic. Precipitation of drug in renal tubules has been described and can best be avoided by maintaining adequate hydration and urine flow. Central nervous system toxicity manifested by confusion, agitation, tremors, and hallucinations has been reported. Resistance has been described, usually in immunosuppressed patients who have received multiple courses of therapy.

Famciclovir is a prodrug of penciclovir. After oral administration, 75–80% of the famciclovir is absorbed and is deacetylated in the intestinal wall to the active drug, penciclovir. Penciclovir, like acyclovir, inhibits viral replication by interfering with viral DNA polymerase. Acyclovir-resistant strains of herpes simplex and varicella-zoster virus are also resistant to famciclovir. Famciclovir in a dose of 500 mg three times daily for 7 days has been approved for treatment of acute herpes zoster. It does not appear to have a major effect on the incidence or duration of postherpetic neuralgia. At a dose of 125 mg twice daily, famciclovir is effective prophylaxis for recurrent genital herpes. Its role in treating other herpesvirus infections awaits further study.

Valacyclovir is a prodrug of acyclovir that has better bioavailability than acyclovir. After absorption, it is converted to acyclovir and serum levels are three to five times higher than those achieved with acyclovir. Valacyclovir at a dose of 1 g three times a day is effective therapy for herpes zoster and at a dose of 1 g twice daily is effective prophylaxis for recurrent genital herpes.

Foscarnet (trisodium phosphonoformate) is a pyrophosphate analogue that inhibits viral DNA polymerase of human herpesviruses (CMV, herpes simplex, varicella-zoster) and the reverse transcriptase of human immunodeficiency virus. The drug is more expensive than ganciclovir, less well tolerated, and more difficult to administer. Therefore, its use is largely limited to patients who do not respond to ganciclovir or cannot tolerate it. Isolates of CMV resistant to ganciclovir and herpes simplex and varicella-zoster resistant to acyclovir are sensitive to foscarnet. Foscarnet appears to be effective for CMV retinitis and has been used successfully in patients who have failed to respond to ganciclovir. Once therapy is stopped, recurrences develop, and lifelong suppressive therapy is required. In one study comparing foscarnet with ganciclovir for CMV retinitis in AIDS, the mortality rate was significantly lower in the foscarnet-treated group (35% versus 50%). It is not clear whether this result was due to the antiretroviral activity of foscarnet or to the lower dosage of zidovudine in the ganciclovir-treated group because of bone marrow suppression. Combination therapy with ganciclovir and foscarnet has been associated with improved efficacy over monotherapy in the treatment of CMV retinitis. While combination therapy reduced progression of disease (eg, retinal changes), no improvement of visual acuity was observed over either drug used alone. Foscarnet has also been used to treat acyclovir-resistant mucocutaneous herpes simplex in AIDS patients (and is more effective than vidarabine in this setting) as well as varicella cutaneous lesions in AIDS patients who failed to respond to acyclovir. Uncontrolled trials suggest efficacy in CMV gastrointestinal disease, therapy of CMV infection following bone marrow and renal transplantation, and prevention of CMV disease when the drug is given prophylactically to seropositive bone marrow transplant recipients. Oral absorption is poor, and the drug must be given intravenously. The half-life is 3–5 hours, and this is prolonged with renal insufficiency. The usual induction dose is 60 mg/kg every 8 hours, and the dose for maintenance therapy is 120 mg/kg once daily. Adjustments are required for even minimal impairment in renal function (see package insert).

Toxicity is a major drawback to widespread use of foscarnet. The drug can cause severe phlebitis and must be diluted to a concentration of 12 mg/mL to be given peripherally. At higher concentrations, it must be given centrally. Nephrotoxicity, which is dose-dependent and reversible, is its major toxicity. Uncontrolled studies have suggested that prehydration with 2.5 L of 0.9% saline may protect against nephrotoxicity. Foscarnet binds divalent cations and hypocalcemia with peripheral neuropathy, seizures and arrhythmias, hypomagnesemia, and hypophosphatemia can occur. Monitoring of electrolytes and renal function is required during therapy. Anemia (20–50%) and nausea and vomiting (20–30%) are other common adverse effects.

Resistance of herpes simplex virus to foscarnet has been described. Resistance is usually seen in patients who are infected with HIV and either have received foscarnet previously or were receiving suppressive therapy. Isolates may be sensitive to acyclovir.

Cidofovir is a nucleotide analog that is active against all human herpesviruses. The drug has a prolonged pharmacokinetic intracellular half-life, allowing for administration every 1–2 weeks. Phosphorylation of cidofovir to its active form does not depend on viral enzymes. Thus, strains of cytomegalovirus, herpes simplex virus, and herpes zoster virus that are resistant to ganciclovir or acyclovir often are sensitive to cidofovir. Cidofovir delays progression of CMV retinitis in newly diagnosed disease (5 mg/kg weekly for 2 weeks, followed by maintenance of 3–5 mg/kg every other week) and is effective therapy in relapsed disease or in patients who are intolerant of traditional therapy (5 mg/kg every other day). Limited data suggest that direct intravitreal injection (20 μg every 5–6 weeks) of cidofovir is also effective for initial and maintenance therapy. To avoid nephrotoxicity, probenecid and intravenous saline must be administered with each dose.

Ribavirin aerosols sprayed into the respiratory tract early in influenza A and B infection of young adults or respiratory syncytial virus infections of small children resulted in a reduction of symptoms and more rapid recovery. Intravenous ribavirin can significantly lower the fatality rate of Lassa fever and is being studied as a potential therapeutic agent for Hanta virus pneumonia. The drug is teratogenic in animals, and pregnant women should not take care of patients receiving the aerosol.

Zidovudine (AZT), didanosine (dideoxyinosine, ddI), **zalcitabine** (dideoxycytidine, ddC), stavudine (d4T), and lamivudine (3TC) inhibit reverse transcriptase of the HIV virus. They are used exclusively in the therapy of HIV-infected individuals (except lamivudine, which may be effective therapy for chronic hepatitis B infection) and are discussed in detail in Chapter 31.

Inhibitors blocking HIV protease and active against strains resistant to reverse transcriptase antagonists are also discussed in Chapter 31. These include saquinavir, ritonavir, and indinavir.

Ganciclovir is an analogue of acyclovir that has broad antiviral activity, including activity against CMV. Most information about its potential usefulness for the therapy of CMV infections comes from uncontrolled open trials. The drug is efficacious in the therapy of CMV retinitis in AIDS patients, but once therapy is stopped, the relapse rate is high, and long-term maintenance suppressive therapy is required. Direct intravitreal injection of ganciclovir (400 mg) weekly is as efficacious as systemic therapy for maintenance. Ganciclovir has a modest effect on CMV colitis in AIDS patients. Ganciclovir at a dosage of 5 mg/kg every 12 hours for 14 days decreases the incidence of positive cultures and improves the appearance of the colon compared with placebo, but diarrhea, weight loss, and fever are unaffected. In bone marrow transplant recipients with CMV gastroenteritis (esophagitis, gastritis, duodenitis), ganciclovir is no better than placebo in relief of symptoms. Therapy of CMV pneumonitis with this agent has been disappointing. Studies of small numbers of patients have suggested that the addition of intravenous immunoglobulin or CMV immune globulin to ganciclovir may improve CMV pneumonitis. CMV viremia and hepatitis are often self-limited diseases, and the role of ganciclovir in treating these syndromes awaits clarification. However, because CMV viremia often predicts the presence of invasive disease, it is usually treated when it occurs. Ganciclovir is most efficacious as a prophylactic agent. Administration of ganciclovir for 100–120 days to seropositive bone marrow transplant recipients decreases the incidence of CMV disease. Similar results have been demonstrated in heart and liver transplant recipients treated for 28 days. In renal transplant patients, ganciclovir during periods of maximum immunosuppression (ie, when antilymphocyte antibody therapy is administered for rejection) prevents development of disease in seropositive individuals. Although ganciclovir alone is not effective in the therapy of CMV pneumonia, if the drug is initiated when asymptomatic viral excretion occurs (as determined by a positive culture in bronchoalveolar lavage), there is a marked reduction in the subsequent development of pneumonia. This again emphasizes ganciclovir's efficacy as a prophylactic agent. It should be emphasized that regimens employing high-dose intravenous and oral acyclovir have also been shown to be effective in preventing CMV disease following bone marrow, liver, and renal transplants. In practice, most high-risk solid organ transplant recipients receive ganciclovir intravenously for 10–14 days posttransplant followed by high-dose acyclovir therapy (800 mg four or five times daily adjusted for renal insufficiency) for 3–4 months or oral ganciclovir (1 g three times daily; see below). Because of the profound immunosuppression associated with bone marrow transplantation, following engraftment (usually at 1 month), intravenous ganciclovir, 5 mg/kg/d three times a week, is given for the first 100–120 days posttransplant, at which time high-dose acyclovir is given for an additional year. An alternative approach in the marrow transplant patient is to follow patients without therapy and to do surveillance cultures of blood (buffy coat) every 2–4 weeks or assay the blood for the presence of CMV-DNA by branched-chain DNA or PCR. If cultures are positive or CMV DNA is detected, therapy with ganciclovir, 5 mg/kg twice daily, is initiated.

The initial dose of ganciclovir is usually 5 mg/kg every 12 hours, resulting in peak serum levels of 18–24 μg/mL and cerebrospinal fluid levels of 2–2.7 μg/mL. The drug is cleared by the kidneys, and dosage adjustments are required for creatinine clearances less than 50 mL/min. For clearances of 30–50 mL/min, 2.5 mg/kg every 12 hours should be given; for clearances of 10–29 mL/min, 2.5 mg/kg once daily should be given; and for a clearance of less than 10 mL/min, 1.25 mg/kg is given as a single daily dose. Usual maintenance therapy in a patient with normal renal function is 5 mg/kg/d for 5 days a week.

The major adverse effect is neutropenia, which is reversible but requires dosage reduction. Thrombocytopenia, disorientation, nausea, rash, and phlebitis occur less commonly. **Oral ganciclovir** has poor bioavailability, with maximum absorption of only 6–9% when taken with food. After a dose of 1 g, peak serum levels are about 1 μg/mL (clinical isolates of CMV are inhibited by 0.02–3.5 μg/mL). Controlled clinical studies indicate that the oral drug in a dose of 1 g three times a day is slightly less effective than intravenous ganciclovir, 5 mg/kg daily as maintenance therapy for CMV retinitis (time to progression is 5–12 days shorter in those treated with the oral drug). Thus, in selected populations with peripheral non-sight-threatening lesions, oral ganciclovir maintenance may be convenient and effective therapy compared with long-term intravenous therapy. Because of its poor bioavailability, oral ganciclovir is unlikely to be effective as primary therapy for active CMV infection. The role of oral ganciclovir in prevention of CMV infection following bone marrow or solid organ transplantation has not been well studied, but preliminary data in liver transplant recipients suggest that oral ganciclovir, 1 g three times daily for 3 months, was efficacious in preventing CMV disease when compared with placebo (4% versus 17%).

Vitrasert is a polymer impregnated with 6 mg of ganciclovir that has been designed to allow for the slow release of 1 or 2 mg per hour. The 2.5 mm disk is implanted into the affected eye in a minor outpatient surgical procedure. Limited studies in HIV-positive individuals with CMV retinitis have indicated that the device is about 90% effective in preventing disease progression when used as initial therapy or when used in those who have previously failed intravenous therapy. Implants last about 4–8 months depending upon rate of release of drug. Complications can occur. The most common is blurred vision, which usually only lasts 2–4 weeks after implantation. Other less common complications include retinal detachment, vitreal hemorrhage, and endophthalmitis secondary to the surgical procedure. The obvious advantage of not requiring intravenous therapy may be offset by the local delivery of drug and the risk of developing disease in the contralateral eye, which occurred in 67% of patients in one study.

Human interferons. Interferons have been prepared from stimulated lymphocytes and more recently by DNA recombinant technology. These agents have antiviral, antitumor, and immunoregulatory properties. The most common uses of these agents include therapy of chronic hepatitis due to hepatitis B, C, and D (see Chapter 15), condyloma acuminatum, prophylaxis against infection in patients with chronic granulomatous disease, and therapy of a number of malignancies such as hairy cell leukemia,

Kaposi's sarcoma in AIDS, chronic myelogenous leukemia, multiple myeloma, renal cell carcinoma, and others, as well as therapy for relapsing multiple sclerosis. Other potential uses are for therapy of certain intracellular pathogens such as leprosy, atypical mycobacterial infection, toxoplasmosis, and leishmaniasis. Relapse of the underlying disease after cessation of therapy is common but usually responds to reinstitution of drug. Adverse effects are common and include an influenza-like illness with fever, chills, nausea, vomiting, headache, arthralgia, and myalgias. Bone marrow suppression, especially with high-dose therapy, has also been reported.

Crumpacker CS: Ganciclovir. N Engl J Med 1996;335:721. (Review of mechanisms of action, therapeutic indications, and adverse effects.)

Drugs for non-HIV viral infections. Med Lett Drugs Ther 1994;36:27.

Goodrich JM, Boeckh M, Bowden R: Strategies for prevention of cytomegalovirus disease after marrow transplantation. Clin Infect Dis 1994;19:287. (Review of published studies.)

Lea AP, Bryson NM: Cidofovir. Drugs 1996;52:225. (Review of activity, kinetics, toxicity, clinical use.)

Singh N et al: High-dose acyclovir compared with short-course preemptive ganciclovir therapy to prevent cytomegalovirus disease in liver transplant recipients: A randomized trial. Ann Intern Med 1994;120:375. (Efficacy of surveillance cultures and treatment only when cultures are positive.)

Wagstaff AJ, Bryson HM: Foscarnet: A reappraisal of its antiviral activity, pharmacokinetic properties and therapeutic use in immunocompromised patients with viral infections. Drugs 1994;48:199.

Disorders Due to Physical Agents 38

Richard Cohen, MD, MPH, & Brent R.W. Moelleken, MD

DISORDERS DUE TO COLD

Cold tolerance varies considerably among individuals. Factors that increase the likelihood of injury from exposure to cold include poor general physical conditioning, nonacclimatization, advanced age, systemic illness, poor tissue oxygenation, and the use of alcohol or other sedative drugs. High wind velocity ("wind-chill factor") increases the severity of cold injury at low temperatures.

Cold Urticaria

Some persons have a familial or acquired hypersensitivity to cold and may develop urticaria upon even limited exposure to a cold wind. The urticaria usually occurs only on exposed areas, but in markedly sensitive individuals the response can be generalized. Immersion in cold water may result in severe systemic symptoms, including shock. Recognition of the disorder is important because it has been responsible for deaths from swimming in cold water. Familial cold urticaria, manifested as a burning sensation of the skin occurring about 30 minutes after exposure to cold, does not seem to be a true urticarial disorder. In some patients with acquired cold urticaria, the disorder may be associated with the administration of drugs such as griseofulvin or with infections such as infectious mononucleosis. Cold urticaria may occur secondarily to cryoglobulinemia. Cold urticaria may be associated with cold hemoglobinuria as a complication of syphilis. In most cases of acquired cold urticaria, the cause is not known. For diagnosis, an ice cube is usually applied to the skin of the forearm for 4–5 minutes, then removed, and the area is observed for 10 minutes. As the skin rewarms, an urticarial wheal appears at the site and may be accompanied by itching. Histamine and other mediators released in the cold urticaria response are similar to those found in allergic reactions. Cyproheptadine, 16–32 mg/d in divided doses, is the drug of choice for cold urticaria. As an alternative, a combination of terbutaline, 5 mg three times daily, and aminophylline, 150 mg three times daily, has been recommended.

Raynaud's Phenomenon

See Chapter 12.

SYSTEMIC HYPOTHERMIA

Systemic hypothermia may result from exposure (atmospheric or immersion) to prolonged or extreme cold. The condition may arise in otherwise healthy individuals in the course of occupational or recreational exposure or in victims of accidents.

Systemic hypothermia may follow exposure even to cool but not cold temperatures when there is altered homeostasis due to debility or disease. In colder climates, elderly and inactive individuals living in inadequately heated housing are particularly susceptible. Acute alcoholism is commonly a predisposing cause. Patients with cardiovascular or cerebrovascular disease, mental retardation, malnutrition, myxedema, and hypopituitarism are more vulnerable to accidental hypothermia. The use of sedative and tranquilizing drugs may be a contributing factor. Prolonged postoperative hypothermia with increased mortality rates after surgery has been reported, especially in elderly patients. Administration of large amounts of refrigerated stored blood (without rewarming) can cause systemic hypothermia.

Pathogenesis

Systemic hypothermia is a reduction of core (rectal) body temperature below 35 °C. It causes reduced physiologic function—with decreased oxygen consumption and slowed myocardial repolarization, peripheral nerve conduction, gastrointestinal motility, and respirations—as well as hemoconcentration and pancreatitis. The body defends itself against cold exposure by superficial blood vessel constriction and increased metabolic heat production.

Clinical Findings

Early manifestations of hypothermia are not specific. There may be weakness, drowsiness, lethargy, irritability, confusion, and impaired coordination. A lowered body temperature may be the sole finding.

The internal (core) body temperature in accidental hypothermia may range from 25 to 35 °C. Oral temperatures are useless, so an esophageal or rectal probe that reads as low as 25 °C is required. At core temperatures below 35 °C, the patient may become delirious, drowsy, or comatose and may stop breathing. Indeed, the pulse and blood pressure may be unobtainable, leading clinicians to believe the patient is dead. Metabolic acidosis, hyperkalemia, pneumonia, pancreatitis, ventricular fibrillation, hypoglycemia or hyperglycemia, coagulopathy, and renal failure may occur. Abnormalities in cardiac rhythm are directly related to the lowering of core temperature; cardiac arrhythmias may occur, especially during the rewarming process. Progression of electrocardiographic abnormalities can also occur, including the pathognomonic J wave of Osborn—a second upward wave immediately following the S wave, which has been well described in lead II (Figure 38–1). Death in systemic hypothermia usually results from cardiac asystole or ventricular fibrillation.

Treatment
(Figure 38–2)

Patients with mild hypothermia (rectal temperature > 33 °C) who have been otherwise physically healthy usually respond well to a warm bed or to rapid passive rewarming with a warm bath or warm packs and blankets. A conservative approach is also usually employed in treating elderly or debilitated patients, using an electric blanket kept at 37 °C.

Patients with moderate or severe hypothermia (core temperatures of < 33 °C) do not have the thermoregulatory shivering mechanism and so require active rewarming with individualized supportive care. Adequate cardiovascular support, acid-base balance, arterial oxygenation, and adequate intravascular volume should be established prior to rewarming to minimize the risk of organ infarction and "afterdrop" (recurrent hypothermia). The methods and rate of active rewarming are controversial. Successful treatment usually includes a combination of active external and internal methods (see below). Aggressive rewarming should be attempted only by those experienced in the methods. *Once begun, CPR should continue until the patient has been rewarmed to at least 32 °C.* The need for oxygen therapy, endotracheal intubation, controlled ventilation, warmed intravenous fluids, and treatment of metabolic acidosis should be dictated by careful clinical and laboratory monitoring during the rapid rewarming process. Essential laboratory tests include complete blood count, prothrombin time, partial thromboplastin time, electrolytes, blood urea nitrogen, serum creatinine, liver function tests, amylase, glucose, pH, blood gases, urinalysis, and urine volume. Cardiac rhythm should be monitored, and cardiac, central vascular, or chest trauma or stimulation (catheter, cannulas, etc) should be avoided unless essential because of the risk

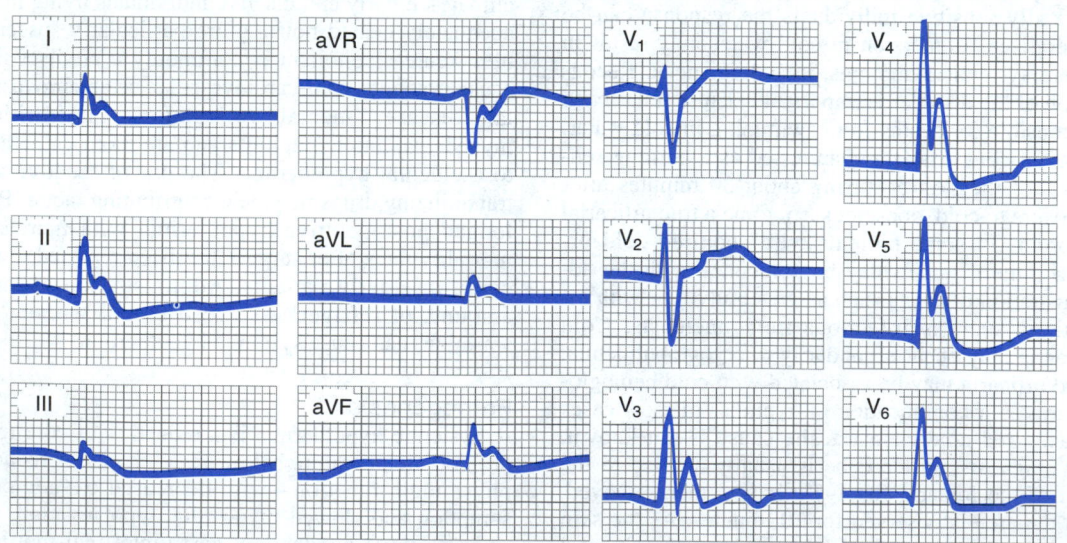

Figure 38–1. Hypothermia. The ventricular rate is 50/min. Atrial activity is not seen. The QRS complexes are narrow and are deformed at their terminal portions by a slurred wave occurring prior to the inscription of the ST–T waves; this is the J wave. The QT interval is prolonged. (Courtesy of R Brindis. Reproduced, with permission from Goldschlager N, Goldman MJ: *Principles of Clinical Electrocardiography,* 13th ed. Appleton & Lange, 1989.)

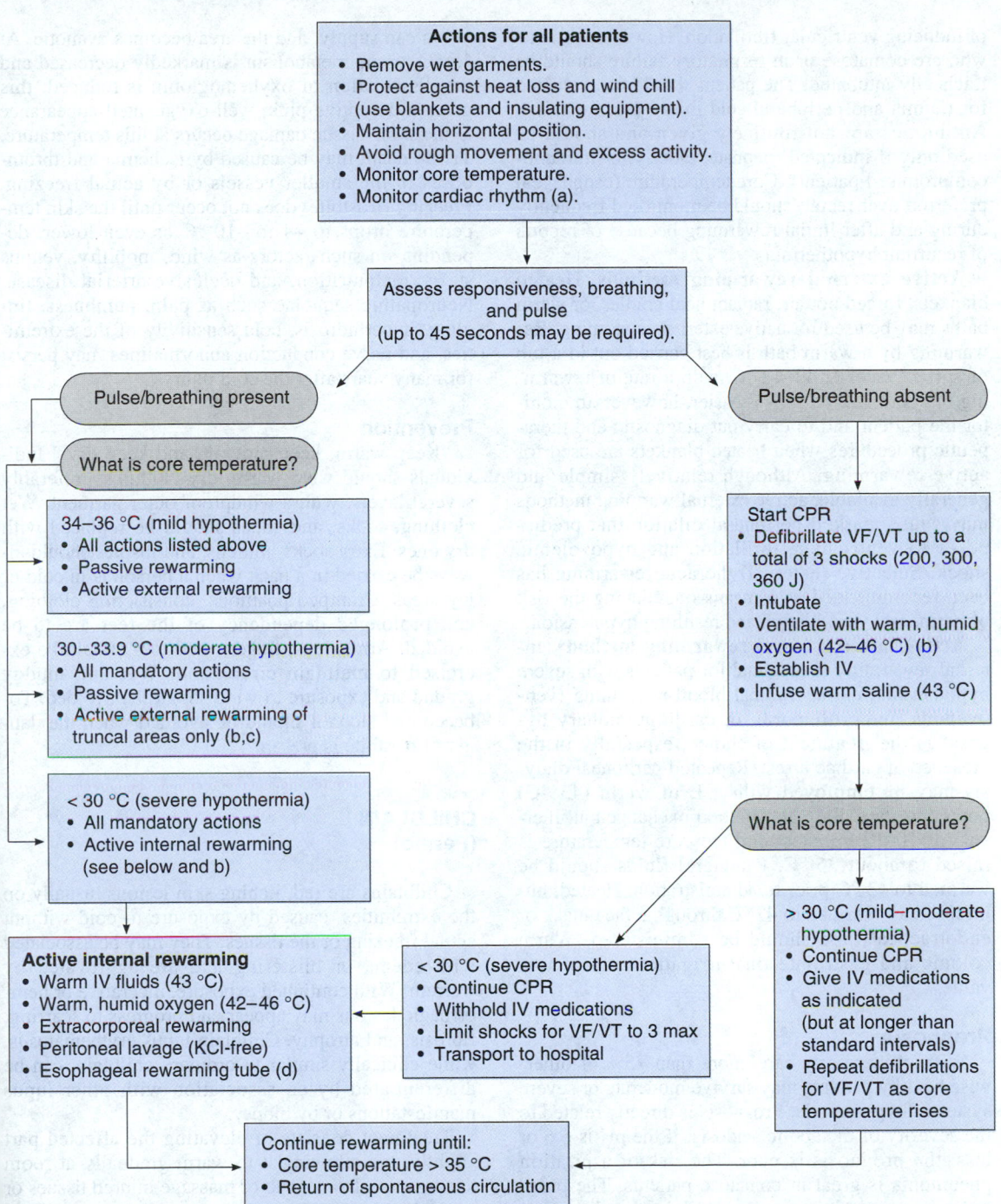

Actions for all patients
- Remove wet garments.
- Protect against heat loss and wind chill (use blankets and insulating equipment).
- Maintain horizontal position.
- Avoid rough movement and excess activity.
- Monitor core temperature.
- Monitor cardiac rhythm (a).

Assess responsiveness, breathing, and pulse
(up to 45 seconds may be required).

Pulse/breathing present

What is core temperature?

34–36 °C (mild hypothermia)
- All actions listed above
- Passive rewarming
- Active external rewarming

30–33.9 °C (moderate hypothermia)
- All mandatory actions
- Passive rewarming
- Active external rewarming of truncal areas only (b,c)

< 30 °C (severe hypothermia)
- All mandatory actions
- Active internal rewarming (see below and b)

Active internal rewarming
- Warm IV fluids (43 °C)
- Warm, humid oxygen (42–46 °C)
- Extracorporeal rewarming
- Peritoneal lavage (KCl-free)
- Esophageal rewarming tube (d)

Pulse/breathing absent

Start CPR
- Defibrillate VF/VT up to a total of 3 shocks (200, 300, 360 J)
- Intubate
- Ventilate with warm, humid oxygen (42–46 °C) (b)
- Establish IV
- Infuse warm saline (43 °C)

What is core temperature?

> 30 °C (mild–moderate hypothermia)
- Continue CPR
- Give IV medications as indicated (but at longer than standard intervals)
- Repeat defibrillations for VF/VT as core temperature rises

< 30 °C (severe hypothermia)
- Continue CPR
- Withhold IV medications
- Limit shocks for VF/VT to 3 max
- Transport to hospital

Continue rewarming until:
- Core temperature > 35 °C
- Return of spontaneous circulation

Figure 38–2. Hypothermia treatment algorithm. **(a):** May require needle electrodes through the skin. **(b):** Many experts think this should be done only in the hospital. **(c):** Methods include electric or charcoal warming devices, hot water bottles, heating pads, radiant heat sources, and warming bed. **(d):** Esophageal rewarming tubes are widely used in Europe. (VF, ventricular fibrillation; VT, ventricular tachycardia; J, joules.) (Reproduced, with permission, from Weinberg AD: Hypothermia. Ann Emerg Med 1993;22:370.)

of inducing ventricular fibrillation. However, patients who are comatose or in respiratory failure should be tracheally intubated. The patient should be evaluated for trauma and peripheral cold injury (eg, frostbite). Antibiotics are not routinely given and should be used only if indicated (neonate, elderly, or immuno-compromised patient). Core temperature (esophageal preferred over rectal) should be monitored frequently during and after initial rewarming because of reports of recurrent hypothermia.

Active external rewarming methods. Heated blankets, forced hot air, radiant heat cradles, or warm baths may be used for active external rewarming. Rewarming by a warm bath is best carried out in a tub of stirred water at 40–42 °C, with a rate of rewarming of about 1–2 °C/h. It is easier, however, to monitor the patient and to carry out diagnostic and therapeutic procedures when heated blankets are used for active rewarming. Although relatively simple and generally available, active external warming methods may cause marked peripheral dilation that predisposes to ventricular fibrillation and hypovolemic shock. Selective (external) thoracic rewarming has been recommended as a means of reducing the risk of peripheral vasodilation and resulting hypotension.

Active internal (core) rewarming methods. Internal rewarming is essential for patients with severe hypothermia; extracorporeal blood rewarming (venovenous, femorofemoral, or cardiopulmonary bypass) is the treatment of choice, especially in the presence of cardiac arrest. Repeated peritoneal dialysis may be employed with 2 L of warm (43 °C) potassium-free dialysate solution exchanged at intervals of 10–12 minutes until the core temperature is raised to about 35 °C. Parenteral fluids should be warmed to 43 °C prior to administration. Heated, humidified air warmed to 42 °C through a face mask or endotracheal tube should be administered. Warm colonic and gastrointestinal irrigations are of less value.

Prognosis

With proper early care, more than 75% of otherwise healthy patients may survive moderate or severe systemic hypothermia. Prognosis is directly related to the severity of metabolic acidosis; if the pH is 6.6 or less, the prognosis is poor. The risk of aspiration pneumonia is great in comatose patients. The prognosis is grave if there are underlying predisposing causes or treatment is delayed.

HYPOTHERMIA OF THE EXTREMITIES

Exposure of the extremities to cold produces immediate localized vasoconstriction followed by generalized vasoconstriction. When the skin temperature falls to 25 °C, tissue metabolism is slowed, but the demand for oxygen is greater than the slowed circulation can supply, and the area becomes cyanotic. At 15 °C, tissue metabolism is markedly decreased and the dissociation of oxyhemoglobin is reduced; this gives a deceptive pink, well-oxygenated appearance to the skin. Tissue damage occurs at this temperature. Tissue death may be caused by ischemia and thromboses in the smaller vessels or by actual freezing. Freezing (frostbite) does not occur until the skin temperature drops to −4 to −10 °C or even lower, depending on such factors as wind, mobility, venous stasis, malnutrition, and occlusive arterial disease. Neuropathic sequelae such as pain, numbness, tingling, hyperhidrosis, cold sensitivity of the extremities, and nerve conduction abnormalities may persist for many years after the cold injury.

Prevention

"Keep warm, keep moving, and keep dry." Individuals should wear warm, dry clothing, preferably several layers, with a windproof outer garment. Wet clothing, socks, and shoes should be replaced with dry ones. Extra socks, mittens, and insoles should always be carried in a pack when a person is in cold or icy areas. Cramped positions, constricting clothing, and prolonged dependency of the feet are to be avoided. Arms, legs, fingers, and toes should be exercised to maintain circulation. Wet and muddy ground and exposure to wind should be avoided. Tobacco and alcohol should be avoided when the danger of frostbite is present.

CHILBLAIN (Pernio)

Chilblains are red, itching skin lesions, usually on the extremities, caused by exposure to cold without actual freezing of the tissues. They may be associated with edema or blistering and are aggravated by warmth. With continued exposure, ulcerative or hemorrhagic lesions may appear and progress to scarring, fibrosis, and atrophy. Chilblain lupus erythematosus, while clinically similar to ordinary chilblain, can be differentiated by an association with other lupus manifestations or by biopsy.

Treatment consists of elevating the affected part slightly and allowing it to warm gradually at room temperature. Do not rub or massage injured tissues or apply ice or heat. Protect the area from trauma and secondary infection. Prazosin, 1 mg daily, has been recommended for treatment and prevention of recurrence.

FROSTBITE

Frostbite is injury of the tissues due to freezing. In mild cases, only the skin and subcutaneous tissues are involved; the symptoms are numbness, prickling, and itching. With increasing severity, deep frostbite involves deeper structures, and there may be paresthesia and stiffness. Thawing causes tenderness and burning pain. The skin is white or yellow, loses its elasticity, and becomes immobile. Edema, blisters, necrosis, and gangrene may appear. Scintigraphy has been used to assess the degree of involvement in severe frostbite and to distinguish viable from nonviable tissue.

Treatment

A. Immediate Treatment: Treat the patient for associated systemic hypothermia.

1. Rewarming–Superficial frostbite (frostnip) of extremities in the field can be treated by firm steady pressure with the warm hand (without rubbing), by placing fingers in the armpits, and, in the case of the toes or heels, by removing footwear, drying feet, rewarming, and covering with adequate dry socks or other protective footwear.

Rapid thawing at temperatures slightly above body heat may significantly decrease tissue necrosis. If there is any possibility of refreezing, the frostbitten part should not be thawed, even if this might mean prolonged walking on frozen feet. Refreezing results in increased tissue necrosis. Rewarming is best accomplished by immersing the frozen portion of the body for several minutes in a moving water bath heated to 40–42 °C until the distal tip of the part being thawed flushes. Water in this temperature range feels warm but not hot to the normal hand. Dry heat (eg, stove or open fire) is more difficult to regulate and is not recommended. After thawing has occurred and the part has returned to normal temperature (usually in about 30 minutes), discontinue external heat. Victims and rescue workers should be cautioned not to attempt rewarming by exercise or thawing of frozen tissues by rubbing with snow or ice water.

A protocol for treatment of frostbite is presented in Figure 38–3.

2. Protection of the part–Pressure or friction is avoided and physical therapy contraindicated in the early stage. The patient is kept at bed rest with

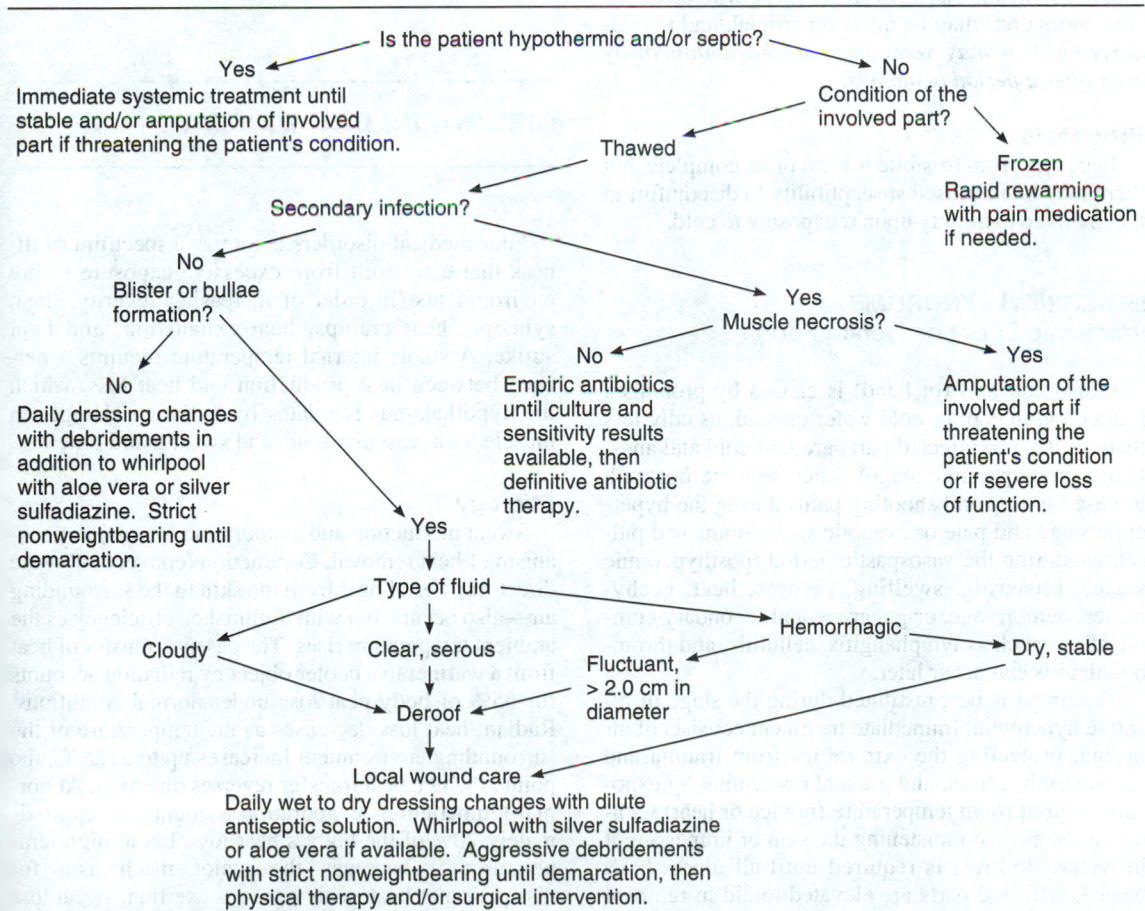

Figure 38–3. Treatment protocol for frostbite. (Modified and reproduced, with permission, from Pulla RJ et al: Frostbite: An overview with case presentations. J Foot Ankle Surg 1994;33:56.)

the affected parts elevated and uncovered at room temperature. Casts, dressings, or bandages are not applied. A combination of ibuprofen, 200 mg four times daily, and aloe vera has been used to prevent dermal ischemia.

3. Anti-infective measures–It is very important to prevent infection after the rewarming process. Protect skin blebs from physical contact. Local infections may be treated with mild soaks of soapy water or povidone-iodine. Whirlpool therapy at temperatures slightly below body temperature twice daily for 15–20 minutes for a period of 3 or more weeks helps cleanse the skin and debrides superficial sloughing tissue. Antibiotics may be required for deep infections.

B. Follow-Up Care: Gentle, progressive physical therapy to promote circulation should be instituted as soon as tolerated.

C. Surgery: Early regional sympathectomy (within 36–72 hours) has been reported to protect against the sequelae of frostbite, but the value of this measure is controversial. In general, other surgical intervention is to be avoided. *Amputation should not be considered until it is definitely established that the tissues are dead.* Tissue necrosis (even with black eschar formation) may be quite superficial, and *the underlying skin may sometimes heal spontaneously even after a period of months.*

Prognosis

Recovery from frostbite is most often complete, but there may be increased susceptibility to discomfort in the involved extremity upon reexposure to cold.

IMMERSION SYNDROME
(Immersion Foot or Trench Foot)

Immersion foot (or hand) is caused by prolonged immersion in cool or cold water or mud, usually less than 10 °C. The affected parts are first cold and anesthetic (prehyperemic stage). They become hot with intense burning and shooting pains during the hyperemic stage and pale or cyanotic with diminished pulsations during the vasospastic period (posthyperemic stage); blistering, swelling, redness, heat, ecchymoses, hemorrhage, or gangrene and secondary complications such as lymphangitis, cellulitis, and thrombophlebitis can occur later.

Treatment is best instituted during the stage of reactive hyperemia. Immediate treatment consists of air drying, protecting the extremities from trauma and secondary infection, and gradual rewarming by exposure to air at room temperature (not ice or heat) without massaging or moistening the skin or immersing it in water. Bed rest is required until all ulcers have healed. Affected parts are elevated to aid in removal of edema fluid, and pressure sites (eg, heels) are protected with pillows. Later treatment is as for Buerger's disease (see Chapter 12).

Gentilello LM: Advances in the management of hypothermia. Surg Clin North Am 1995;75:243. (Comparison of efficacy of rewarming methods.)

Larach MG: Accidental hypothermia. Lancet 1995;345:493. (Resuscitation and rewarming.)

Mills WJ Jr, O'Malley J, Kappes B: Cold and freezing: A historical chronology of laboratory investigations and clinical experience. Alaska Med 1993;35:89. (Pathophysiology and treatment experience and recommendations for hypothermia, frostbite, and immersion foot.)

Pulla RJ, Pickard IJ, Carnett TS: Frostbite: An overview with case presentations. J Foot Ankle Surg 1994;33:53. (Pathophysiology, diagnosis, treatment, and case reports of frostbite.)

Schrijver G, van der Maten J: Severe accidental hypothermia: Pathophysiology and therapeutic options for hospitals without cardiopulmonary bypass equipment. Neth J Med 1996;49:167. (Rewarming technique plus venovenous hemofiltration and dialysis.)

Spittell JA Jr, Spittell PC: Chronic pernio: Another cause of blue toes. Int Angiol 1992;11:46. (Diagnosis and treatment of chronic pernio and chilblains.)

Toth-Kasa I, Kiss M, Dobozy A: Treatment of cold urticaria. Int J Dermatol 1994;33:210. (Diagnosis of cold urticaria and evaluation of treatment protocol utilizing terbutaline and aminophylline.)

DISORDERS DUE TO HEAT

Four medical disorders comprise a spectrum of illness that can result from excessive exposure to hot environments (in order of increasing severity): heat syncope, heat cramps, heat exhaustion, and heat stroke. A stable internal temperature requires a balance between heat production and heat loss, which the hypothalamus regulates by initiating changes in muscle tone, vascular tone, and sweat gland function.

Etiology

Sweat production and evaporation is a major mechanism of heat removal. Conduction (convection)—the direct transfer of heat from the skin to the surrounding air—also occurs, but with diminished efficiency as the ambient temperature rises. The passive transfer of heat from a warmer to a cooler object by radiation accounts for 65% of body heat loss under normal conditions. Radiant heat loss decreases as the temperature of the surrounding environment increases up to 37.2 °C, the point at which heat transfer reverses direction. At normal temperatures, evaporation accounts for approximately 20% of the body's heat loss, but at high temperatures it becomes the major mechanism for dissipation of heat; with vigorous exertion, sweat loss can be as much as 2.5 L/h. This mechanism is also limited as humidity increases.

Health conditions that inhibit sweat production o

evaporation and increase susceptibility to heat disorders include obesity, generalized skin diseases (miliaria), diminished cutaneous blood flow, dehydration, malnutrition, hypotension, and reduced cardiac output. Medications that impair the sweating mechanism are the anticholinergics, antihistamines, phenothiazines, tricyclic antidepressants, monoamine oxidase inhibitors, and diuretics; reduced cutaneous blood flow results from use of vasoconstrictors and β-adrenergic blocking agents; and dehydration results from use of alcohol. Illicit drugs—eg, phencyclidine, LSD, amphetamines, and cocaine—can cause increased muscle activity and thus generate increased body heat. Drug withdrawal syndromes may have the same effect, as may prolonged seizures.

The risk of heat disorder also increases with age, impaired cognition, concurrent illness, reduced physical fitness, and insufficient acclimatization.

Prevention

Medical evaluation and monitoring should be used to identify individuals at increased risk of heat disorders. The exposed public should be made aware of the early symptoms and signs of heat disorders. It is not recommended to make salt tablets available for use without medical supervision; close monitoring of fluid and electrolyte intake may be necessary in situations necessitating activity in hot environments. Athletic events should be organized and managed with attention to thermoregulation: the WBGT (wet bulb globe temperature) Index should be monitored, fluid consumption should be encouraged, and medical support should be immediately accessible. Competition is not recommended when the WBGT exceeds 28 °C. Workers should not begin work in hot temperatures without proper acclimatization and should be encouraged to drink water frequently.

Protective air-cooled suits have been used successfully in the nuclear power industry for prolonged work in environments up to 60 °C.

Acclimatization is achieved by scheduled regulated exposure to hot environments and by gradually increasing the duration of exposure and the work load, until the body adjusts by starting to produce sweat of lower salt content in greater amounts at lower ambient temperatures. Acclimatization is accompanied by increased plasma volume, cardiac output, and cardiac stroke volume and a slower heart rate.

SPECIFIC SYNDROMES DUE TO HEAT EXPOSURE

1. HEAT SYNCOPE

Sudden unconsciousness can result from cutaneous vasodilation with consequent systemic and cerebral hypotension. Systolic blood pressure is usually less than 100 mm Hg, and there is typically a history of vigorous physical activity for 2 hours or more just preceding the episode. The skin is typically cool and moist, and the pulse is weak.

Treatment consists of rest and recumbency in a cool place, with fluids by mouth (or intravenously if necessary).

2. HEAT CRAMPS

Fluid and electrolyte depletion can result in slow, painful skeletal muscle contractions ("cramps") and even severe muscle spasms lasting 1–3 minutes, usually of the muscles most heavily used. Cramping results from salt depletion as sweat losses are replaced with water alone. The skin is moist and cool, and the muscles are tender. There may be muscle twitching. The victim is alert, with stable vital signs, but may be agitated and complaining of pain. The body temperature may be normal or slightly increased. Involved muscle groups are hard and lumpy. There is almost always a history of vigorous activity just preceding the onset of symptoms. Laboratory evaluation may show low serum sodium and hemoconcentration.

The patient should be moved to a cool environment and given oral saline solution (4 tsp of salt per gallon of water) to replace both salt and water. *Because of their slower absorption, salt tablets are not recommended.* The victim may have to rest for 1–3 days with continued dietary salt supplementation before returning to work or resuming heavy activity in the heat.

3. HEAT EXHAUSTION

Heat exhaustion results from prolonged heavy activity with inadequate salt intake in a hot environment and is characterized by dehydration, sodium depletion, or isotonic fluid loss with accompanying cardiovascular changes.

The diagnosis is based on prolonged symptoms and a rectal temperature over 37.8 °C, increased pulse rate—usually more than half again the patient's normal rate—and moist skin. Symptoms associated with heat syncope and heat cramps may also be present. The patient may be quite thirsty and weak, with central nervous system symptoms such as headache, fatigue, and, in cases due chiefly to water depletion, anxiety, paresthesias, impaired judgment, hysteria, and in some cases psychosis. Hyperventilation secondary to heat exhaustion can lead to respiratory alkalosis. Heat exhaustion may progress to heat stroke if sweating ceases.

Treatment consists of placing the patient in a shaded, cool environment and providing adequate hydration (1–2 L over 2–4 hours) and salt replenishment—orally, if possible. Physiologic saline or isotonic glucose solution can be administered intravenously in severe cases or when oral administration is not appropriate. Intravenous 3% (hypertonic) saline may be necessary if sodium depletion is severe. At least 24 hours of rest is recommended.

4. HEAT STROKE

Heat stroke is a life-threatening medical emergency resulting from failure of the thermoregulatory mechanism. Heat stroke is imminent when the core (rectal) temperature approaches 41 °C. It presents in one of two forms: classic heat stroke occurs in patients with compromised homeostatic mechanisms; exertional heat stroke occurs in previously healthy persons undergoing strenuous exertion in a thermally stressful environment. Morbidity or even death can result from cerebral, cardiovascular, hepatic, or renal damage.

The hallmarks of heat stroke are cerebral dysfunction with impaired consciousness, high fever, and absence of sweating. Persons at greatest risk are the very young, the elderly (> age 65) or chronically infirm, and patients receiving medications (eg, anticholinergics, antihistamines, phenothiazines) that interfere with heat-dissipating mechanisms.

Exertional heat stroke and exertion-related illnesses, including rhabdomyolysis, are appearing more frequently as complications of participation by unconditioned amateurs in strenuous athletic activities such as marathon running and triathlon competition.

Clinical Findings

A. Symptoms and Signs: Failure of the heat dissipation mechanism for any reason results in dizziness, weakness, emotional lability, nausea and vomiting, diarrhea, confusion, delirium, blurred vision, convulsions, collapse, and unconsciousness. The skin is hot and initially covered with perspiration. Later it dries. The pulse is strong initially. Blood pressure may be slightly elevated at first, but hypotension develops later. The core temperature is usually over 41 °C. As with heat exhaustion, hyperventilation can occur, leading to respiratory alkalosis. Metabolic (lactic) acidosis may also develop.

Exertional heat stroke may present with sudden collapse and loss of consciousness followed by irrational behavior. Anhidrosis may not be present. Twenty-five percent of heat stroke victims have prodromal symptoms for minutes to hours which may include dizziness, weakness, nausea, confusion, disorientation, drowsiness, and irrational behavior.

B. Laboratory Findings: Laboratory evaluation reveals dehydration, leukocytosis, elevated BUN, hyperuricemia, hemoconcentration, and decreased serum potassium, calcium, and phosphorus; urine is concentrated, with elevated protein, tubular casts, and myoglobinuria. Thrombocytopenia, in-

creased bleeding and clotting times, fibrinolysis, and consumption coagulopathy may also be present. Rhabdomyolysis and myocardial, hepatic, or renal damage may be identified by elevated creatine kinase, liver function tests, and BUN, and anuria, proteinuria, and hematuria. Electrocardiographic findings may include ST–T changes consistent with myocardial ischemia.

Treatment

Treatment is aimed at reducing the core temperature rapidly (within 1 hour) and controlling the secondary effects. Evaporative cooling is rapid and effective and is easily performed in most emergency settings. The patient's clothing should be removed and the entire body sprayed with water (15 °C) while cooled or ambient air is passed across the patient's body with large fans or other means at high velocity (100 ft/min). The patient should be in the lateral recumbent position or supported in a hands-and-knees position to expose as much skin surface as possible to the air. Other alternatives include use of cold wet sheets accompanied by fanning or isopropyl alcohol instead of water. Cardiopulmonary bypass provides rapid cooling but is often not practical.

Immersion in an ice-water bath as initial treatment is no longer preferred because of its greater potential for complications of hypotension and shivering. However, it should be considered if core temperature is not decreased rapidly in response to other treatment. Alternatives include ice packs (groin, axillas, neck) and iced gastric lavage, though these are much less effective than evaporative cooling.

Treatment should be continued until the rectal temperature drops to 39 °C. The temperature remains stable in most cases, but it should continue to be monitored for 24 hours. Chlorpromazine (25–50 mg intravenously) can be given initially and every 4 hours to control shivering and other muscular activity associated with increased heat load. Antipyretics (aspirin, acetaminophen) have no effect on environmentally induced hyperthermia and are contraindicated.

Hypovolemic and cardiogenic shock must be carefully distinguished, as either or both may occur. Central venous or pulmonary artery wedge pressure should be monitored. Five percent dextrose in saline (500–1000 mL) may be given without overloading the circulation if hypovolemic shock is present.

The patient should also be observed for renal failure due to rhabdomyolysis, hypokalemia, cardiac arrhythmias, disseminated intravascular coagulation, and hepatic failure. Hypokalemia frequently accompanies heat stroke but may not appear until rehydration. Maintenance of extracellular hydration and electrolyte balance should reduce the risk of renal failure due to rhabdomyolysis. Fluid administration to ensure a high urine output (> 50 mL/h), mannitol administration, and alkalinizing the urine (intravenous bicarbonate administration) are recom mended. Corticosteroids have not been shown to be of value.

Fluid output should be monitored through the use of an indwelling urinary catheter.

Because sensitivity to high environmental temperature continues in some patients for prolonged periods following an episode of heat stroke, immediate reexposure should be avoided.

Brody GM: Hyperthermia and hypothermia in the elderly. Clin Geriatric Med 1994;10:213. (Diagnosis and treatment of heat syndromes in the elderly.)

Bross NH, Binford TN Jr, Carlton FB Jr: Heat emergencies. Am Fam Physician 1994;50:389. (Diagnosis and treatment of heat disorders.)

Khogali M: Heat-related illness. Middle East J Anesthesiol 1994;12:531.

BURNS

The incidence and severity of burn injuries has been declining, with both deaths and acute hospitalizations attributable to burns down about 50%. More than 75% of burns involve less than 10% of total body surface area. Aggressive, early (between 24 and 72 hours postburn) excision of deeply burned tissues and skin grafting—and improved infection control—have contributed to significantly lower mortality rates and shorter hospitalizations. Nonetheless, an estimated 1.25 million burn injuries and 51,000 acute hospitalizations occur each year in the USA. Severe burns cause problems in the initial phase from hemodynamic compromise, related injuries such as smoke inhalation or fractures, and associated multiorgan failure and sepsis. Later, secondary scarring and constrictive wounds occur.

Clinically, a massive burn injury, usually over 15–20% of the body surface area, is characterized by hypovolemic shock due to dramatically increased whole-body capillary leak. Edema formation can be massive. Aggressive, monitored fluid resuscitation is necessary in severely burned patients, ideally in a dedicated burn unit. Children, the elderly, and those with underlying medical problems are at particular risk for untoward outcomes.

CLASSIFICATION

Burns are classified by extent, depth, patient age, and associated illness or injury.

Extent

The "rule of nines" (Figure 38–4) is useful for

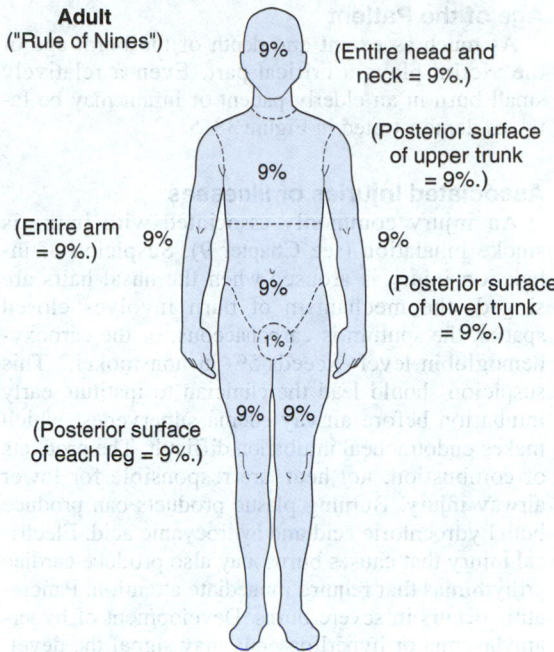

Figure 38–4. Estimation of body surface area in burns.

rapidly assessing the extent of a burn. More detailed charts based on age are available when the patient reaches the burn unit. Therefore, it is important to view the entire patient after cleaning soot to make an accurate assessment, both initially and on subsequent examinations. Only second- and third-degree burns are included in calculating the total burn surface area (TBSA), since first-degree burns usually do not represent significant injury in terms of prognosis or fluid and electrolyte management. However, first- or second-degree burns may convert to deeper burns, especially if treatment is delayed or bacterial colonization or superinfection occurs.

Depth

Judgment of depth of injury is difficult. The **first-degree burn** may be red or gray but will demonstrate excellent capillary refill. First-degree burns are not blistered initially. If the wound is blistered, this represents a partial-thickness injury to the dermis, or a **second-degree burn.** As the degree of burn is progressively deeper, there is a progressive loss of adnexal structures. Hairs can be easily extracted or are absent, sweat glands become less visible, and the skin appears smoother. The distinction between second- and third-degree burns is blurred and in a sense artificial. Deep second-degree burns are generally treated as full-thickness (third-degree) burns and excised and grafted earlier because of the long time necessary for reepithelialization and the thin, poor quality of the resultant skin.

Age of the Patient

As much as extent and depth of the burn, age of the victim plays a critical part. Even a relatively small burn in an elderly patient or infant may be fatal, as demonstrated in Figure 38–5.

Associated Injuries or Illnesses

An injury commonly associated with burns is smoke inhalation (see Chapter 9). Suspicion of inhalation injury is aroused when the nasal hairs are singed, the mechanism of burn involves closed spaces, the sputum is carbonaceous, or the carboxyhemoglobin level exceeds 5% in nonsmokers. This suspicion should lead the clinician to institute early intubation before airway edema supervenes, which makes endotracheal intubation difficult. The products of combustion, not heat, are responsible for lower airway injury. Burning plastic products can produce both hydrochloric acid and hydrocyanic acid. Electrical injury that causes burns may also produce cardiac arrhythmias that require immediate attention. Pancreatitis occurs in severe burns. Development of hyperamylasemia or hyperlipasemia may signal the development of pancreatic inflammation and subsequent pseudocyst or abscess formation.

Toxic epidermal necrolysis (TEN) occasionally occurs following sulfonamide or phenytoin administration (see Chapter 6). If TEN is severe, patients are best transferred to a burn unit and treated as having severe burn injury. Corticosteroid therapy should be avoided.

Premorbid physical and psychosocial disorders that complicate recovery from burn injury include cardiac or pulmonary disease, diabetes, alcoholism, drug abuse, and psychiatric illness.

SYSTEMIC REACTIONS TO BURN INJURY

The actual burn injury is only the incipient event in a cascade of deleterious local tissue and systemic inflammatory reactions leading to multiorgan system failure in the severely burned patient. Locally, substance P, serotonin, prostaglandins E_2 and $F_{2\alpha}$, histamine, platelet-activating factor, nitric oxide, bradykinin, and leukotrienes B_4 and D_4 play a role in the increased local capillary permeability and initiation of the systemic inflammatory cascade. Systemically, levels of interleukin-2 and interleukin-6 are elevated in proportion to the severity of the burn injury, perhaps as part of a generalized systemic release of inflammatory mediators. In addition, in the first 24 hours following a significant burn, there is production of tumor necrosis factor (TNF) and interferon-gamma (IFN-γ), which in turn stimulate production of the enzyme nitric oxide synthetase in hepatocytes. After 24 hours, lipopolysaccharide (LPS) plays a dominant role in its production. Nitric oxide has been proposed as a mediator of the acute inflammation. Clinical efforts at modification of these factors have had mixed success. Anti-LPS immunoglobulin G in freeze-dried plasma has resulted in

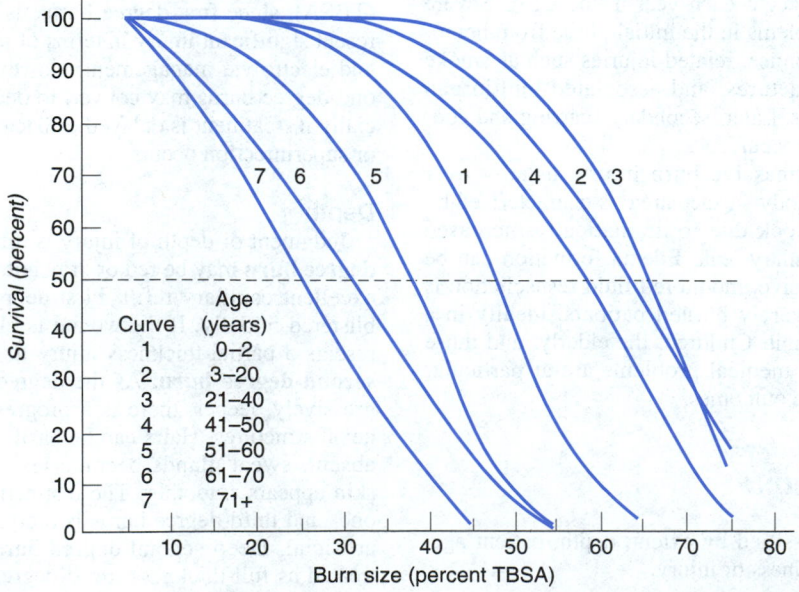

Figure 38–5. Patient survival and burn size according to patient age. (TBSA, total body surface area.) (Reproduced with permission, from Merrell SW et al: Increased survival after major thermal injury. Am J Surg 1987;154:623.)

significantly decreased endotoxin levels and a slight decrease in burn wound infections, though no reduction in mortality rates. Neutrophil-endothelial cell adhesion underlies many of the deleterious secondary effects of burn injury. Inhibition of this adhesion has decreased cellular injury, ischemia, and reperfusion injury and circulatory shock in both animals and humans.

INITIAL MANAGEMENT

Airway

The physician or emergency medical technician should proceed as with any other trauma using standard Advanced Trauma Life Support (ATLS) guidelines. The priorities are first to establish an airway, recognizing the frequent necessity to intubate a patient who may appear to be breathing normally but who has sustained an inhalation injury; next, to evaluate the cervical spine and head injuries; and finally, to stabilize fractures. *The burn wound itself has a lower priority*—nonetheless, fluid resuscitation by the Parkland formula (see below) may be instituted simultaneously with initial resuscitation. Endotracheal intubation should be considered for major burn cases, regardless of the area of the body involved, for as fluid resuscitation proceeds, generalized edema develops, including the soft tissues of the upper airway and perhaps the lungs as well. *Tracheostomy is rarely indicated for the burn victim* unless dictated by other circumstances such as delay in endotracheal intubation and subsequent upper airway edema, preventing vocal cord visualization. Chest radiographs are typically normal initially but may show an acute respiratory distress syndrome picture in 24–48 hours with severe inhalation injury. Supplemental oxygen should be administered. Inhalation injuries should be followed by serial blood gas determination and bronchoscopy. The use of corticosteroids is contraindicated because of the potential for immunosuppression.

History

Since mental disturbances, confusion resulting from the injury, or the presence of an endotracheal tube may later prevent the recording of an accurate history, one should as soon as possible obtain a detailed history of the circumstances of the injury, including locale, the possibility of closed-space injury, substances involved (including medications), and the duration of exposure as well as the past medical history (especially cardiopulmonary problems).

Vascular Access

All clothing and jewelry should be removed and an expedient physical examination performed to assess the extent of burn and associated injuries. Simultaneously with the above procedures, venous access must be sought, since the victim of a major burn may develop hypovolemic shock. A percutaneous large-bore (14 or 16 gauge) intravenous line through non-burned skin is preferred. Subclavian lines are avoided in the emergency setting because of the risk of pneumothorax and subclavian vein laceration when such a line is placed in a volume-depleted patient. Femoral lines provide good temporary access during resuscitation. *All lines—without exception— placed in the emergency department should be changed within 24 hours because of the high risk of nonsterile placement.* Distal saphenous cutdown is occasionally necessary. An arterial line is useful for monitoring mean arterial pressure and drawing blood.

FLUID RESUSCITATION

Crystalloids

Generalized capillary leak results from burn injury over more than 25% of the total body surface area. This often necessitates replacement of a large volume of fluid.

There are many guidelines for fluid resuscitation. The **Parkland formula** relies upon the use of lactated Ringer's injection. The fluid requirement in the first 24 hours is estimated as 4 mL/kg body weight per percent of body surface area burned. Deep electrical burns and inhalation injury increase the fluid requirement. Adequacy of resuscitation is determined by clinical parameters, including urine output and specific gravity, blood pressure, and central venous catheter or, if necessary, Swan-Ganz catheter readings.

Half the calculated fluid is given in the first 8-hour period. The remaining fluid, divided into two equal parts, is delivered over the next 16 hours. An extremely large volume of fluid may be required. For example, an injury over 40% of the total body surface area in a 70-kg victim may require 13 L *in the first 24 hours.* The first 8-hour period is calculated from the hour of injury.

Because it may contribute to renal failure and death, use of hypertonic sodium in resuscitation of burn patients, once thought to be reasonable, has been abandoned in favor of conventional Ringer's lactate.

Colloids

Overly aggressive crystalloid administration must be avoided in patients with pulmonary injury, since significant pulmonary edema can develop in patients with normal pulmonary capillary wedge and central venous pressures. In addition, routine colloid administration, commonplace 5 years ago, must now be considered suspect in routine burn resuscitation in view of its deleterious effect on glomerular filtration and its association with pulmonary edema.

Monitoring Fluid Resuscitation

A Foley catheter is essential for monitoring urinary output. *Diuretics have no role in this phase of patient management unless fluid overload has occurred or mannitol diuresis is performed in the case of rhabdomyolysis.*

Escharotomy

As edema fluid accumulates, ischemia may develop under any constricting eschar of an extremity, neck, or trunk if the full-thickness burn is circumferential. Escharotomy incisions through the anesthetic eschar can save life and limb and can be performed in the emergency department or operating room.

Fasciotomy in Electrical Burns & Associated Crush Injuries

When high-voltage electrical injury occurs, extensive deep tissue necrosis is almost invariably present. Deep tissue necrosis leads to profound tissue swelling. Because deep tissue compartments in the arms and legs are contained by unyielding fascia, these compartments must be opened by surgical fasciotomy to prevent further soft tissue, vascular, and nerve death.

Electrical burn injuries remain the most devastating and underrecognized burn injuries. A recent study reported musculoskeletal involvement in 44% of patients with electrical burns. Fully 79% of these patients required major amputations (often because of unrecognized compartment syndromes). Acute renal failure, resulting in part from rhabdomyolysis, occurred in 15% of these patients, and 59% of those developing acute renal failure died. Prompt recognition of the severity of electrical burns, with early fasciotomy and debridement, may reduce the incidence of such complications.

THE BURN WOUND

Treatment of the burn wound is based on several principles: (1) Protection from desiccation and further injury of those burned areas that will spontaneously reepithelialize in 7–10 days by application of topical antibiotic such as silver sulfadiazine or mafenide acetate. Prophylactic systemic antibiotics are not recommended. (2) Early excision and grafting of burned areas as soon as 24 hours after burn injury or when the patient will hemodynamically tolerate the excision and grafting procedure. Hyperbaric oxygen therapy has been shown to reduce the extent of burn injury, but reports are largely anecdotal, and this modality has not gained universal acceptance.

Topical Antibiotics

Silver sulfadiazine is currently the most popular topical agent. It is painless, easy to apply, and effective against most *Pseudomonas*. Mafenide acetate penetrates deeper and is indicated for burns over cartilage such as the ears and nose. Mafenide, when used as a 10% solution, inhibits carbonic anhydrase and results in metabolic acidosis. It also delays epithelization and may be painful. When it is diluted to a 5% solution, pain and metabolic side effects are lessened.

Povidone-iodine is especially useful against *Candida* and both gram-positive and gram-negative microorganisms. However, it penetrates eschar poorly, is very desiccating to the wound surface, and is painful. Also, significantly high blood iodine levels have been demonstrated in patients receiving this agent.

Regular and thorough cleansing of burned areas is a critically important intervention in burn units. Debridement of burn wounds may be aided by application of collagenase; such treatment may be as effective as—or more effective than—silver sulfadiazine treatment alone.

Wound Closure

The goal of therapy after fluid resuscitation is closure of the wound. Nature's own blister is the best cover to protect wounds that spontaneously epithelialize in 7–10 days (ie, superficial second-degree burns). Where the blister has been disrupted, silver sulfadiazine, porcine heterografts (preferably fresh, or frozen and meshed), or collagen composite dressings (Biobrane) can be used as skin substitutes. These expedients are temporary and not indicated in deep partial or full-thickness burns or in burns that are heavily colonized or infected. Cadaver homografts can also serve this purpose if available.

Wounds that will not heal spontaneously in 7–10 days (ie, deep second-degree or third-degree burns) are best treated by excision and autograft; otherwise, granulation and infection may develop, and the quality of the skin in regenerated deep partial thickness burns is marginal because of the very thin dermis that emerges. Cultured keratinocytes remain an experimental modality owing to the lack of dermis. Although research is continuing, clinical results have been largely disappointing owing to the poor quality of reconstructed skin. The main usefulness of keratinocytes may be as a temporary dressing.

PATIENT SUPPORT

Burn patients require extensive support. An attempt must be made to maintain normal core body temperature in patients with burns over more than 20% of total body surface area, since the hypermetabolic state of burns is exacerbated by subnormal temperatures. Respiratory injury, sepsis, and multiorgan failure are common. Enteral feedings may be started once the ileus of the resuscitation period has resolved, usually the day after the injury. If the patient does not tolerate low-residue tube feedings, TPN should be started without delay through a central venous catheter. As much as 4000–6000 kcal/d may be required in the postburn period. The metabolic demands are immense. A useful guide is to provide 25 kcal/kg body weight plus 40 kcal per percent of burn surface area. Fat emulsions (Intralipid) given intravenously are useful during the resuscitation period to span the period of ileus. This ileus may be due to mesenteric ischemia mediated by thromboxane A_2. Acidification of tube feedings may decrease bacterial translocation in critically ill patients and may decrease morbidity from infections.

Occasionally, burn patients may develop acute respiratory distress syndrome or respiratory failure unresponsive to maximal ventilatory support. Heroic resuscitative measures are sometimes successfully employed, with use of extracorporeal life support (ECLS), in children who would otherwise die of ARDS, inhalation injury, or pneumonia in the postburn period.

H_2 receptor blockers may be used to reduce acid production.

Early burn care and grafting, splinting, and hand therapy are the result of coordinated care by general, hand, and plastic surgeons, therapists, and nurses. Late burn reconstruction is best handled by a plastic and reconstructive surgeon. Recent advances in reconstructive burn surgery include the use of microsurgery to perform muscle and fasciocutaneous flaps and tissue expansion. However, complex reconstructive options such as free tissue transfer involve much higher than normal complication rates when performed in the acutely burned patient. In late reconstruction of burns involving the head and neck, tissue expansion is sometimes used instead of conventional skin grafting, since this technique provides skin most similar to that lost because of the burn. After severe burns to the hand, hand function may be aided by expedient hand splinting or axial pin fixation to prevent flexion contractures and facilitate prompt skin grafting and hand physical therapy.

Brigham PA, McLoughlin E: Burn incidence and medical care use in the United States: Estimate, trends, and data sources. J Burn Care Rehabil 1996;17:95.

Caldwell FT Jr, Wallace BH, Cone JB: Sequential excision and grafting of the burn injuries of 1507 patients treated between 1967 and 1986: End results and determinants of death. J Burn Care Rehabil 1996;17:137.

Cianci P, Sato R: Adjunctive hyperbaric oxygen therapy in the treatment of thermal burns: A review. Burns 1994;20:5.

D'Amato TA et al: High voltage electrical injury: A role for mandatory exploration of deep muscle compartments. J Natl Med Assoc 1994;86:535.

Darling GE et al: Pulmonary complications in inhalation injuries with associated cutaneous burn. J Trauma 1996; 40:83.

Fuller FW, Parrish M, Nance FG: A review of the dosimetry of 1% silver sulfadiazine cream in burn wound treatment. J Burn Care Rehab 1994;15:213.

Gore DC et al: Colloid infusions reduce glomerular filtration in resuscitated burn victims. J Trauma 1996;40:356.

Hansbrough JF et al: Wound healing in partial-thickness wounds treated with collagenase ointment versus silver sulfadiazine cream. J Burn Care Rehabil 1995;16:241.

Herndon DN, Zeigler ST: Bacterial translocation after thermal injury. Crit Care Med 1993;21(2 Suppl):S50.

Jenkins ME et al: Enteral feedings during operative procedures in thermal injuries. J Burn Care Rehabil 1994; 15:199.

Jones EB: Prophylactic anti-lipopolysaccharide freeze-dried plasma in major burns: A double blind controlled trial. Burns 1995;21:267.

Kelemen JJ 3rd et al: Effect of ambient temperature on metabolic rate after thermal injury. Ann Surg 1996; 223:406.

Kowal-Vern A et al: Interleukin-2 and interleukin-6 in relation to burn wound size in the acute phase of thermal injury. J Am Coll Surg 1995;178:357.

Nguyen TT et al: Current treatment of severely burned patients. Ann Surg 1996;223:14.

Platt AJ, McKiernan MV, McLean NR: Free tissue transfer in the management of burns. Burns 1996;22:474.

Saffle JR, Davis B, Williams P: American Burn Association Registry Participant Group. Recent outcomes in the treatment of burn injury in the United States: A report from the American Burn Association Patient Registry. J Burn Care Rehabil 1995;16(3 Part 1):219.

Sheridan RL et al: The acutely burned hand: Management and outcome based on a ten-year experience with 1047 burned hands. J Trauma 1995;38:406.

Wainwright DJ: Use of an acellular allograft dermal matrix (Alloderm) in the management of full thickness burns. Burns 1995;21:243.

Williamson JS et al: Cultured epithelial autograft: Five years of clinical experience with twenty-eight patients. J Trauma 1995;39:309.

ELECTRIC SHOCK

The possibility of life-threatening electrical injury exists wherever there is electric power or lightning. The amount and type of current, the duration and area of exposure, and the pathway of the current through the body determine the degree of damage. If the current passes through the heart or brain stem, death may occur immediately owing to ventricular fibrillation or apnea. Current passing through skeletal muscle can cause contractions severe enough to result in bone fracture. Current traversing peripheral nerves can cause acute or delayed neuropathy. Delayed effects can include damage to the spinal cord, peripheral nerves, bone, kidneys, and gastrointestinal tract as well as cataracts.

Direct current is much less dangerous than alternating current. Alternating current of high voltage with a very high number of cycles per second (hertz, Hz) may be less dangerous than a low voltage with fewer cycles per second. With alternating currents of 25–300 Hz, low voltages (< 220 Hz) tend to produce ventricular fibrillation; high voltages (> 1000 Hz), respiratory failure; intermediate voltages (220–1000 Hz), both. More than 100 mA of domestic house current (AC) of 110 volts at 60 Hz is, accordingly, dangerous to the heart, since it can cause ventricular fibrillation. DC current contact is more likely to cause asystole.

Lightning injuries differ from high-voltage electric shock injuries in that lightning usually involves higher voltage, briefer duration of contact, asystole rather than ventricular fibrillation, nervous system injury, a shock wave characteristic, and multisystem pathologic involvement.

Electrical burns are of three distinct types: flash (arcing) burns, flame (clothing) burns, and the direct heating effect of tissues by the electric current. The latter lesions are usually sharply demarcated, round or oval, painless yellow-brown areas (Joule burn) with inflammatory reaction. Significant subcutaneous damage can be accompanied by little skin injury, particularly with larger skin surface area electrical contact.

Electric shock may produce loss of consciousness. With recovery there may be muscular pain, fatigue, headache, and nervous irritability. The physical signs vary according to the action of the current. Ventricular fibrillation or respiratory failure (or both) can occur; the patient may be unconscious, pulseless, hypotensive, cold and cyanotic, and without respirations.

Electric shock may be a hazard in equipment that is usually considered to be harmless (eg, home appliances and medical equipment). Proper installation, utilization, and maintenance of equipment by qualified personnel should minimize this hazard.

Treatment

A. Emergency Measures: The victim may be freed from the current in many ways, but the rescuer must be protected. Turn off the power, sever the wire with a dry wooden-handled axe, make a proper ground to divert the current, or drag the victim carefully away by means of dry clothing or a leather belt.

CPR is instituted if breathing and pulses are absent and continued according to the usual AHA protocol.

Lightning injury. Victims of lightning injury, in whom coma may last for a few minutes to several days, should receive prompt and sustained artificial resuscitation. This should be continued as long as there is no clinical evidence of brain death.

B. Hospital Measures: Lightning or unstable electric shock victims should be hospitalized when revived and observed for shock, arrhythmia, thrombosis, infarction, sudden cardiac dilation, hemorrhage, and myoglobinuria. Electric shock injury cases should also be evaluated for blunt trauma, dehydration, skin burns, hypertension, posttraumatic stress, acid-base disturbances, and neurologic damage. Indications for hospitalization include significant arrhythmia or electrocardiographic changes, large burn, loss of consciousness, pulmonary or cardiac symptoms, or evidence of significant deep tissue or organ damage. Extra caution is indicated when the electroshock current has followed a transthoracic route (hand to hand or hand to foot).

For electric shock (not lightning) burns, aggressive hydration with Ringer's lactate should seek to achieve a urine output of 50–100 mL/h.

Prognosis

Complications may occur in almost any part of the body but most commonly include sepsis, gangrene requiring limb amputation, or neurologic, cardiac, or psychiatric dysfunction.

Carleton SC: Cardiac problems associated with electrical injury. Cardiol Clin 1995;13:263.

Cooper MA: Emergent care of lightning and electrical injuries. Semin Neurol 1995;15:268. (Physics, pathophysiology, assessment, and therapy).

Semin Neurol 1995;15(3–4):227–400. (September and December issues dedicated to neurologic, behavioral, ophthalmologic, and related aspects of lightning and electroshock injuries).

IONIZING RADIATION REACTIONS

The effects of ionizing radiation on the body have been observed in clinical use of x-rays and radioactive agents, after occupational or accidental exposure, and following the use of atomic weaponry. The extent of damage due to radiation exposure depends on the quantity of radiation delivered to the body, the dose rate, the organs exposed, the type of radiation (x-rays, neutrons, gamma rays, alpha or beta particles), the duration of exposure, and the energy transfer from the radioactive wave or particle to the exposed tissue. The Chernobyl experience suggests that the best biologic indicators of dose are the duration of the asymptomatic latent period (particularly for nausea or emesis), the severity of early symptoms, the rate of decline of the lymphocyte count, and the number and distribution of dicentric chromosomes in peripheral lymphocytes.

The National Committee on Radiation Protection has set the maximum permissible radiation exposure for occupationally exposed workers over age 18 a

0.1 rem* per week for the whole body (but not to exceed 5 rem per year) and 1.5 rem per week for the hands. (For purposes of comparison, routine chest x-rays deliver from 0.1–0.2 rem.)

Death after acute lethal radiation exposure is usually due to hematopoietic failure, gastrointestinal mucosal damage, central nervous system damage, widespread vascular injury, or secondary infection. The acute radiation syndrome may be dominated by central nervous system, gastrointestinal, or hematologic manifestations depending on dose and survival. Four hundred to 600 cGy of x-ray or gamma radiation applied to the entire body at one time may be fatal within 60 days; death is usually due to hemorrhage, anemia, and infection secondary to hematopoietic injury. Levels of 1000–3000 cGy to the entire body destroy gastrointestinal mucosa; this leads to toxemia and death within 2 weeks. Total body doses above 3000 cGy cause widespread vascular damage, cerebral anoxia, hypotensive shock, and death within 48 hours.

ACUTE (IMMEDIATE) IONIZING RADIATION EFFECTS ON NORMAL TISSUES

Clinical Findings

A. Injury to Skin and Mucous Membranes: Irradiation may cause erythema, epilation, destruction of fingernails, or epidermolysis.

B. Injury to Deep Structures:

1. Hematopoietic tissues–Injury to the bone marrow may cause diminished production of blood elements. Lymphocytes are most sensitive, polymorphonuclear leukocytes next most sensitive, and erythrocytes least sensitive. Damage to the blood-forming organs may vary from transient depression of one or more blood elements to complete destruction.

2. Cardiovascular system–Pericarditis with effusion or constrictive pericarditis may occur after a period of months or even years. Myocarditis is less common. Smaller vessels (the capillaries and arterioles) are more readily damaged than larger blood vessels.

3. Reproductive effects–In males, small single doses of radiation (200–300 cGy) cause temporary aspermatogenesis, and larger doses (600–800

cGy) may cause permanent sterility. In females, single doses of 200 cGy may cause temporary cessation of menses, and 500–800 cGy may cause permanent castration. Moderate to heavy irradiation of the embryo in utero results in injury to the fetus (eg, mental retardation) or in embryonic death and abortion.

4. Respiratory tract–High or repeated moderate doses of radiation may cause pneumonitis, often delayed for weeks or months.

5. Mouth, pharynx, esophagus, and stomach–Mucositis with edema and painful swallowing of food may occur within hours or days after onset of irradiation. Gastric secretion may be temporarily (occasionally permanently) inhibited by moderately high doses of radiation.

6. Intestines–Inflammation and ulceration may follow moderately large doses of radiation.

7. Endocrine glands and viscera–Hepatitis and nephritis may be delayed effects of therapeutic radiation. The normal thyroid, pituitary, pancreas, adrenals, and bladder are relatively resistant to low or moderate doses of radiation; parathyroid glands are especially resistant.

8. Nervous system–The brain and spinal cord are much more sensitive to acute exposures than the peripheral nerves.

C. Systemic Reaction (Radiation Sickness): The basic mechanisms of radiation sickness are not known. Anorexia, nausea, vomiting, weakness, exhaustion, lassitude, and in some cases prostration may occur, singly or in combination. Dehydration, anemia, and infection may follow. Radiation sickness associated with x-ray therapy is most likely to occur when the therapy is given in large dosage to large areas over the abdomen, less often when given over the thorax, and rarely when therapy is given over the extremities.

Prevention

Persons handling radiation sources can minimize exposure to radiation by recognizing the importance of time, distance, and shielding. Areas housing x-ray and nuclear materials must be properly shielded. X-ray equipment should be periodically checked for reliability of output, and proper filters should be employed. When feasible, it is advisable to shield the gonads, especially of young persons. Fluoroscopic examination should be performed as rapidly as possible, using an optimal combination of beam characteristics and filtration and the beam size should be kept to a minimum required by the examination. Special protective clothing may be necessary to protect against contamination with radioisotopes. In the event of accidental contamination, all clothing should be removed and the body vigorously bathed with soap and water. This should be followed by careful instrument (Geiger counter) check to localize the ionizing radiation.

In radiation terminology, a rad is the unit of absorbed dose and a rem is the unit of any radiation dose to body tissue in terms of its estimated biologic effect. Roentgen (R) refers to the amount of radiation dose delivered to the body. For x-ray or gamma ray radiation, rems, rads, and roentgens are virtually the same. For particulate radiation from radioactive materials, these terms may differ greatly (eg, for neutrons, 1 rad equals 10 rems). In the Système International (SI) nomenclature, the rad has been replaced by the gray (Gy), and 1 rad equals 0.01 Gy = 1 cGy. The SI replacement for the rem is the Sievert (Sv), and 1 rem equals 0.01 Sv.

Emergency Treatment for Radiation Accident Victims

The proliferation of radiation equipment and nuclear energy plants and the increased transportation of radioactive materials necessitate hospital plans for managing patients who are accidentally exposed to ionizing radiation or contaminated with radioisotopes. The plans should provide for effective emergency care and disposition of victims and materials with the least possible risk of spreading radioactive contamination to personnel and facilities.

Treatment

The success of treatment of local radiation effects depends upon the extent, degree, and location of tissue injury. Particulate or radioisotope exposures should be decontaminated in designated confined areas. For many radioisotopes, chelation, blocking, or dilution therapy is indicated (see NCRP No. 65 reference, below). Treatment of systemic reactions is symptomatic and supportive. Ondansetron, 8 mg orally twice or three times daily, has been recommended for nausea and vomiting. Alternatives include chlorpromazine, 25–50 mg given deeply intramuscularly every 4–6 hours as necessary or 10–25 mg orally every 4–6 hours as necessary; and dimenhydrinate, 50–100 mg, or perphenazine, 4–8 mg, 1 hour before and 1 and 4 hours after radiation therapy has been recommended. Simple, palatable foods and emotional support may help.

When radiation dosage levels are sufficient to cause damage to gastrointestinal mucosa, bone marrow, and other important tissues, good medical and nursing care may be lifesaving. Blood and platelet transfusions, bone marrow transplants, antibiotics, fluid and electrolyte maintenance, and other supportive measures may be useful. Recombinant hematopoietic growth factors (filgrastim and sargramostim or molgramostim) have been effective in accelerating hematopoietic recovery. Bone marrow transplantation should be considered following whole body exposures above 500–800 cGy.

CHRONIC (DELAYED) EFFECTS OF EXCESSIVE DOSES OF IONIZING RADIATION

Skin scarring, atrophy and telangiectasis, cataract, dry eye syndrome, retinopathy, neuropathy, myelopathy, cerebral injury, obliterative endarteritis, coronary artery disease, pericarditis, hypothyroidism, pulmonary fibrosis, hepatitis, intestinal stenosis, and nephritis are known to occur following high-dose exposure. Neoplastic disease, including leukemia, is increased in persons exposed to excessive radiation. Higher dose radon exposure is associated with increased risk of lung cancer. There is an increased incidence of thyroid cancer in patients who have received radiation exposure or therapy to the thymus, and the incidence of basal cell carcinoma of the skin is increased following radiotherapy. The latency period between radiation therapy and the development of cancer may be 30 years or longer. Prenatal irradiation may increase the risk of childhood cancer.

Microcephaly and other congenital abnormalities may occur in children exposed in utero, especially if the fetus was exposed during early pregnancy. Carcinogenesis from low-dose (< 10 rem) exposure to adults has not been demonstrated. However, because of age-related differences in sensitivity to radiation, carcinogenesis following childhood exposures has been observed (eg, Chernobyl and childhood thyroid cancer).

Axelson O: Cancer risks from exposure to radon in homes. Environ Health Perspect 1995;103(Suppl 2):37.

Cardis E et al: Effects of low doses and low dose rates of external ionizing radiation: Cancer mortality among nuclear industry workers in three countries. Radiat Res 1995;142:117.

Doll R: Hazards of ionizing radiation: 100 years of observation on man. Br J Cancer 1995;72:1339.

National Council on Radiation Protection and Measurement (NCRP): *Management of Persons Accidentally Contaminated With Radionuclides.* Report No. 65. NCRP, 1985. (Treatment recommendations for exposure to specific isotopes.)

Vyas DR et al: Management of radiation accidents and exposures. Pediatr Emerg Care 1994;10:232.

DROWNING

Drowning is the fifth leading cause of accidental death in the USA. The number of deaths due to drowning could undoubtedly be significantly reduced if adequate preventive and first aid instruction programs were instituted.

The asphyxia of drowning is usually due to aspiration of fluid, but it may result from airway obstruction caused by laryngeal spasm while the victim is gasping under water. About 10% of victims develop laryngospasms after the first gulp and never aspirate water ("dry drowning"). The rapid sequence of events after submersion—hypoxemia, laryngospasm, fluid aspiration, ineffective circulation, brain injury, and brain death—may take place within 5–10 minutes. This sequence may be delayed for longer periods if the victim, especially a child, has been submerged in very cold water or if the victim has ingested significant amounts of barbiturates. Immersion in cold water can also cause a rapid fall in the victim's core temperature, so that systemic hypothermia and death may occur before actual drowning.

The primary effect is hypoxia due to perfusion of poorly ventilated alveoli, intrapulmonary shunting, and decreased compliance. *The first requirement of rescue is immediate cardiopulmonary resuscitation.*

A number of circumstances or primary events may precede near drowning and must be taken into consideration in management: (1) use of alcohol or other drugs (a contributing factor in an estimated 25% of adult drownings), (2) extreme fatigue, (3) intentional hyperventilation, (4) sudden acute illness (eg, epilepsy, myocardial infarction), (5) head or spinal cord injury sustained in diving, (6) venomous stings by aquatic animals, and (7) decompression sickness in deep water diving.

When first seen, the near-drowning victim may present with a wide range of clinical manifestations. Spontaneous return of consciousness often occurs in otherwise healthy individuals when submersion is very brief. Many other patients respond promptly to immediate ventilation. Other patients, with more severe degrees of near drowning, may have frank respiratory failure, pulmonary edema, shock, anoxic encephalopathy, cerebral edema, and cardiac arrest. A few patients may be deceptively asymptomatic during the recovery period, only to deteriorate or die as a result of acute respiratory failure within the following 12–24 hours.

Clinical Findings

A. Symptoms and Signs: The patient may be unconscious, semiconscious, or awake but apprehensive, restless, and complaining of headaches or chest pain. Vomiting is common. Examination may reveal cyanosis, trismus, apnea, tachypnea, and wheezing. A pink froth from the mouth and nose indicates pulmonary edema. Cardiovascular manifestations may include tachycardia, arrhythmias, hypotension, cardiac arrest, and circulatory shock. Hypothermia may be present.

B. Laboratory Findings: Urinalysis shows proteinuria, hemoglobinuria, and acetonuria. There is usually a leukocytosis. The PaO_2 is usually decreased and the $PaCO_2$ increased or decreased. The blood pH is decreased as a result of metabolic acidosis. Chest x-rays may show pneumonitis or pulmonary edema.

Prevention

Avoidance of alcohol during recreational swimming or boating, close supervision of toddlers, swimming lessons early in life, and use of personal flotation devices when boating are recommended. All swimming pools should be fenced.

Treatment

A. First Aid: Immediate measures to combat hypoxemia at the scene of the incident—with sustained effective ventilation, oxygenation, and circulatory support—are critical to survival with complete recovery. Hypothermia and cervical spine injury should always be suspected.

1. Standard CPR is initiated if pulse and respirations are absent.

2. *Do not* waste time attempting to drain water from the victim's lungs, since this measure is most often of no value. The Heimlich maneuver (subdiaphragmatic pressure) should be used only if airway obstruction by a foreign body is suspected. The cervical spine should be immobilized if neck injury is possible.

3. *Do not* discontinue basic life support for seemingly "hopeless" patients until core temperature reaches 32 °C. Complete recovery has been reported after prolonged resuscitation of hypothermic patients.

B. Hospital Care: Careful observation of the patient; continuous monitoring of cardiorespiratory function; serial determination of arterial blood gases, pH, and electrolytes; and measurement of urinary output are required. Pulmonary edema may not appear for 24 hours.

1. Ensure optimal ventilation and oxygenation–The danger of hypoxemia exists even in the alert, conscious patient who appears to be breathing normally. Oxygen should be immediately administered at the highest available concentration. Endotracheal intubation and mechanical ventilation are necessary for patients unable to maintain an open airway or normal blood gases and pH. Nasogastric intubation will allow removal of swallowed water and prevention of aspiration. If the victim does not have spontaneous respirations, intubation is required. Oxygen saturation should be maintained at 90% or higher. Continuous positive airway pressure (CPAP) is the most effective means of reversing hypoxia in patients with spontaneous respirations and patent airways. Assisted ventilation may be necessary with pulmonary edema, respiratory failure, aspiration, pneumonia, or severe central nervous system injury. Serial physical examinations and chest x-rays should be carried out to detect possible pneumonitis, atelectasis, and pulmonary edema. Bronchospasm due to aspirated material may require use of bronchodilators. Antibiotics should be given only when there is clinical evidence of infection—not prophylactically.

2. Cardiovascular support–Central venous pressure (or, preferably, pulmonary artery wedge pressure) may be monitored as a guide to determining whether vascular fluid replacement and pressors or diuretics are needed. If low cardiac output persists after adequate intravascular volume is achieved, pressors should be given. Otherwise, standard therapy for pulmonary edema, cardiogenic or not, is administered.

3. Correction of blood pH and electrolyte abnormalities–Metabolic acidosis is present in 70% of near-drowning victims, but it is usually of minor importance and corrected through adequate ventilation and oxygenation. While controversial, bicarbonate administration (1 meq/kg) has been recommended for comatose patients (see Chapter 21).

4. Cerebral injury–Some near-drowning patients may progress to irreversible central nervous system damage despite apparently adequate treatment of hypoxia and shock. Mild hyperventilation to achieve a $PaCO_2$ between 25 and 30 mm Hg is recommended.

5. Hypothermia–Core temperature should be measured and managed as appropriate (see Systemic Hypothermia, above).

Course & Prognosis

Victims of near drowning who have had prolonged hypoxemia should remain under close hospital observation for 2–3 days after all supportive measures have been withdrawn and clinical and laboratory findings have been stable. Residual complications of near drowning may include intellectual impairment, convulsive disorders, and pulmonary or cardiac disease.

Bross MH, Clark JL: Near-drowning. Am Fam Physician 1995;51:1545. (Pathophysiology and treatment.)
Modell JH: Drowning. N Engl J Med 1993;328:253.

OTHER DISORDERS DUE TO PHYSICAL AGENTS

DECOMPRESSION SICKNESS & DYSBARIC ILLNESS

Decompression sickness and other disorders related to rapid changes in environmental pressure are occupational hazards for fliers and professional divers who are involved in deep-water exploration, rescue, salvage, or construction. In recent years, the sport of scuba diving has exposed amateurs to the hazards of decompression sickness.

At low depths the greatly increased pressure (eg, at 30 meters [100 ft] the pressure is four times greater than at the surface) compresses the respiratory gases into the blood and other tissues. During ascent from depths greater than 9 meters, gases dissolved in the blood and other tissues escape as the external pressure decreases. The appearance of symptoms depends on the depth and duration of submersion; the degree of physical exertion; the age, weight, and physical condition of the diver; and the rate of ascent. The size and number of gas bubbles (notably nitrogen) escaping from the tissues depend on the difference between the atmospheric pressure and the partial pressure of the gas dissolved in the

tissues. The release of gas bubbles and (particularly) the location of their release determine the symptoms.

Decompression sickness also occurs among fliers during rapid ascent from sea level to high altitudes when there is no adequate pressurizing protection. Deep-sea and scuba divers may be vulnerable to air embolism if airplane travel is attempted too soon (within a few hours) after diving.

The range of clinical manifestations includes gas bubble formation in the joints ("bends"), cerebral or pulmonary decompression sickness, arterial gas embolism (cerebral, pulmonary), ear and sinus barotrauma, and dysbaric osteonecrosis.

Predisposing factors include exercise, injury, obesity, dehydration, alcoholic excess, hypoxia, some medications (eg, narcotics, antihistamines), and cold. Reported sequelae include hemiparesis, neurologic dysfunction, and bone damage. Asthma, pneumothorax, low results on pulmonary function testing, lung cysts, or thoracic trauma may contraindicate diving.

The onset of acute decompression symptoms occurs within 30 minutes in half of cases and almost invariably within 6 hours. Symptoms, which are highly variable, include pain (largely in the joints), headache, confusion, pruritic rash, visual disturbances, nausea, vomiting, loss of hearing, weakness or paralysis, dizziness or vertigo, dyspnea, paresthesias, aphasia, and coma.

Pulmonary decompression sickness ("chokes") presents with burning, pleuritic substernal pain, cough, and dyspnea.

Early recognition and prompt treatment are extremely important. Continuous administration of oxygen is indicated as a first aid measure, whether or not cyanosis is present. Aspirin may be given for pain, but narcotics should be used very cautiously, since they may obscure the patient's response to recompression. Rapid transportation to a treatment facility for recompression, hyperbaric oxygen, hydration treatment of plasma deficits, and supportive measures is necessary not only to relieve symptoms but also to prevent permanent impairment. It has been recommended, however, that decompression symptoms be treated whenever they are seen—even up to 2 weeks postinjury—since it is still possible to completely alleviate symptoms. The physician should be familiar with the nearest compression center. The local public health department or nearest naval facility should be able to provide such information. The National Divers Alert Network (DAN) (919-684-8111) provides assistance in the management of underwater diving accidents.

Clenney TL, Lassen LF: Recreational scuba diving injuries Am Fam Physician 1996;53:1761. (Diagnosis, treatment, and prevention of scuba diving injuries.)
Jerrard DA: Diving medicine. Emerg Med Clin North Am 1992;10:329. (Diagnosis and treatment of dysbaric disorders.)

Madsen J et al: Diving physiology and pathophysiology. Clin Physiology 1994;14:597. (Pathophysiology of decompression illness.)

MOUNTAIN SICKNESS

Lack of sufficient time for acclimatization, increased physical activity, and varying degrees of health may be responsible for the acute, subacute, and chronic disturbances that result from hypoxia at altitudes greater than 2000 meters (6560 ft). Marked individual differences in tolerance to hypoxia exist. Patients with sickle cell disease are at high risk of painful crises from altitude-induced hypoxemia.

Acute Mountain Sickness

The severity of acute mountain sickness correlates with altitude and rate of ascent. Initial manifestations include headache (most severe and persistent symptom), lassitude, drowsiness, dizziness, chilliness, nausea and vomiting, facial pallor, dyspnea, and cyanosis. Later, there is facial flushing, irritability, difficulty in concentrating, vertigo, tinnitus, visual disturbances, auditory disturbances, anorexia, insomnia, increased dyspnea and weakness on exertion, increased headaches (due to cerebral edema), palpitations, tachycardia, Cheyne-Stokes breathing, and weight loss. More severe manifestations include pulmonary edema and encephalopathy (see below). Voluntary, periodic hyperventilation may relieve symptoms. In most individuals, symptoms clear within 24–48 hours, but in some instances, if the symptoms are sufficiently persistent or severe, the patient must be returned to lower altitudes. Definitive treatment is immediate descent, which must be managed if reduced consciousness, ataxia, or pulmonary edema is present. Administration of oxygen, 2–3 L/min, will often relieve acute symptoms. Acetazolamide, 250 mg every 8 hours, or dexamethasone, 8 mg initially followed by 4 mg every 6 hours, for as long as symptoms persist, is recommended therapy; they may be used together in severe cases. Portable hyperbaric chambers can provide limited short-term symptom relief.

Preventive measures include slow ascent—300 meters (984 feet) per day—adequate rest and sleep the day before travel, reduced food intake, and avoidance of alcohol, tobacco, and unnecessary physical activity during travel. Acetazolamide, 250 mg every 8–12 hours, beginning the day before ascent and continuing for 48–72 hours at altitude, may be used as prophylaxis. Dexamethasone, 2–4 mg every 6 hours beginning on the day of ascent, continuing for 3 days at the higher altitude, and then tapering over 5 days, is an alternative.

Acute High-Altitude Pulmonary Edema

This serious complication usually occurs at levels above 3000 meters (9840 ft). Early symptoms of pulmonary edema may appear within 6–36 hours after arrival at a high-altitude area—dry, incessant cough, shortness of breath disproportionate to exertion, headache, decreased exercise performance, fatigue, dyspnea at rest, and substernal oppression. Later, wheezing, orthopnea, and hemoptysis may occur. Recognition of the early symptoms may enable the patient to descend before incapacitating pulmonary edema develops, but strenuous exertion should be avoided. An early descent of even 500 or 1000 meters may result in improvement of symptoms. Physical findings include rales, tachycardia, mild fever, tachypnea, cyanosis, prolonged respiration, and rales and rhonchi. The patient may become confused or even comatose, and the entire clinical picture may resemble severe pneumonia. The white count is often slightly elevated, but the blood sedimentation rate is usually normal. Chest x-ray findings vary from irregular patchy infiltration in one lung to nodular densities bilaterally or with transient prominence of the central pulmonary arteries. Transient, nonspecific electrocardiographic changes, occasionally showing right ventricular strain, may occur. Pulmonary arterial blood pressure is elevated, whereas pulmonary wedge pressure is normal.

Treatment, which must often be given under field conditions, consists of rest in the semi-Fowler position (head raised) and administration of 100% oxygen by mask at a rate of 6–8 L/min for 15–30 minutes. *Immediate descent is essential.* Recompression in a portable hyperbaric bag will temporarily reduce symptoms if rapid or immediate descent is not possible. To conserve oxygen, lower flow rates may be used for the next 24–48 hours until the victim recovers or can be evacuated to a lower altitude. Treatment for acute respiratory distress syndrome (see Chapter 9) may be required for some patients who have a prolonged course of pulmonary edema. Nifedipine, 10 mg sublingually and 20 mg by slow release orally immediately, followed by 20 mg long-acting every 6 hours, may provide symptomatic relief. Dexamethasone, 4 mg every 6 hours, has been recommended if central nervous system symptoms are present. Acetazolamide, 250 mg every 8 hours, should be administered if acute mountain sickness is suspected. If bacterial pneumonia exists, appropriate antibiotic therapy should be given.

Preventive measures include education of prospective mountaineers regarding the possibility of serious pulmonary edema, optimal physical conditioning before travel, gradual ascent to permit acclimatization, and a period of rest and inactivity for 1–2 days after arrival at high altitudes. Prompt medical attention with rest and high-flow oxygen if respiratory symptoms develop may prevent progression to frank pulmonary edema. Persons with a history of high-altitude pulmonary edema should be hospitalized for further observation if possible. Pulmonary embolism and high-altitude bronchitis can also occur. Mountaineering parties at levels of 3000 meters (9843 ft) or higher should carry a supply of oxygen and equipment sufficient for several days. Persons with symptomatic cardiac or pulmonary disease should avoid high altitudes.

Acute High-Altitude Encephalopathy

High-altitude encephalopathy appears to be an extension of the central nervous symptoms of acute mountain sickness (see above). It usually occurs at elevations above 2500 meters (8250 ft) and is more common in unacclimatized individuals. Clinical findings are due largely to hypoxemia and cerebral edema. Severe headaches, confusion, truncal ataxia, staggering gait, focal deficits, nausea and vomiting, and seizures may progress to obtundation and coma. Papilledema and retinal hemorrhages may be observed in about 50% of patients.

Early recognition of the encephalopathic symptoms is essential. Oxygen should be administered by mask. Dexamethasone, 4–8 mg every 6 hours, is recommended thereafter. If descent is accomplished as quickly as possible, recovery is usually rapid and complete.

Subacute Mountain Sickness

This occurs most frequently in unacclimatized individuals and at altitudes above 4500 meters (14,764 ft). Symptoms, which are probably due to central nervous system anoxia without associated alveolar hyperventilation, are similar to but more persistent and severe than those of acute mountain sickness. There are additional problems of dehydration, skin dryness, and pruritus. The hematocrit may be elevated, and there may be electrocardiographic and chest x-ray evidence of right ventricular hypertrophy. Treatment consists of rest, oxygen administration, and return to lower altitudes.

Chronic Mountain Sickness (Monge's Disease)

This uncommon condition of chronic hypoxia, which is encountered in residents of high-altitude communities who have lost their acclimatization to such an environment, is difficult to differentiate clinically from chronic pulmonary disease. The disorder is characterized by somnolence, mental depression, hypoxemia, cyanosis, clubbing of fingers, polycythemia (hematocrit often > 75%, hemoglobin > 22 g/dL), signs of right ventricular failure, electrocardiographic evidence of right axis deviation and right atrial and ventricular hypertrophy, and x-ray evidence of right heart enlargement and central pulmonary vessel prominence. There is no x-ray evidence of structural pulmonary disease. Pulmonary function tests usually disclose alveolar hypoventila-

tion and elevated PCO_2 but fail to reveal defective oxygen transport. There is a diminished respiratory response to CO_2. Almost complete disappearance of all abnormalities eventually occurs when the patient returns to sea level.

A'Court CHD et al: Doctor on a mountaineering expedition. BMJ 1995;310:1248. (Preparation for climbing expeditions and prevention.)

McMurray SJ: High altitude medicine for family physicians. Can Fam Physician 1994;40:711. (Pathophysiology, diagnosis, and treatment of acute high-altitude disorders.)

Richalet JP: High altitude pulmonary oedema: Still a place for controversy? Thorax 1995;50:923. (Pathophysiology and treatment of high-altitude pulmonary edema.)

MEDICAL EFFECTS OF AIR TRAVEL & SELECTION OF PATIENTS FOR AIR TRAVEL

The decision about whether or not it is advisable for a patient to travel by air depends not only upon the nature and severity of the illness but also upon such factors as the duration of flight, the altitude to be flown, pressurization, the availability of supplementary oxygen and other medical supplies, the presence of attending physicians and trained nursing attendants, and other special considerations. Air carriers in the USA cannot legally allow the use of personal (passenger-supplied) oxygen containers, but most major airlines will supply oxygen upon advance written request from the passenger's physician. Airline policies, charges, and other details must be checked with each carrier. Medical hazards or complications of modern air travel are remarkably uncommon; unless there is some specific contraindication (Table 38–1), air transportation may actually be the best means of moving patients. The medical hazard most likely to be realized is hypoxia. The most common in-flight emergencies are cardiovascular, syncopal, neuropsychiatric, and abdominal. The Air Transport Association of America defines an incapacitated passenger as "one who is suffering from a physical or mental disability and who, because of such disability or the effect of the flight on the disability, is incapable of self-care; would endanger the health or safety of such person or other passengers or airline employees; or would cause discomfort or annoyance of other passengers."

All commercial airlines retain medical consultants to assist their personnel in making decisions regarding the transportation of passengers with noticeable symptoms of sickness or injury. Physicians may contact these medical consultants by calling or writing the medical departments of major airlines.

Cardiovascular Disease

A. Cardiac Decompensation: Patients in con-

Table 38–1. Contraindications to commercial air travel.[1]

Cardiovascular
  Active thrombophlebitis
  Recent deep vein thrombosis (within 4 weeks)
  Recent myocardial infarction (within 6 weeks)[2]
  Recent cerebrovascular accident (within 2 weeks)
  Severe hypertension
  Decompensated (or unstable) cardiovascular disease or
    restricted cardiac reserve[3]
  Recent thoracic surgery (within 3 weeks)
Bronchopulmonary
  Pneumothorax
  Congenital or noncommunicating pulmonary cysts
  Acute bronchospasm
  Cyanosis
  Dyspnea at rest
  Pulmonary hypertension
  Pneumonia
  Inadequate pulmonary function, including
    1. Vital capacity <50% of predicted
    2. Hypercapnia ($PaCO_2$ >50 mm Hg)
    3. Hypoxemia (PaO_2 <50 mm Hg predicted in flight)
    4. Diffusing capacity <50% of predicted
Eye, ear, nose, and throat
  Recent eye or middle ear surgery
  Acute sinusitis or otitis media
  Surgical mandibular fixation (permanent wiring of jaw)
Gastrointestinal tract
  Recent abdominal surgery (within 14 days)
  Acute diverticulitis or ulcerative colitis
  Acute esophageal varices
  Acute gastroenteritis
Neuropsychiatric
  Epilepsy (unless well controlled medically and cabin
    altitude does not exceed 2500 meters [8000 ft])
  Previous violent or unpredictable behavior
  Recent skull fracture
  Brain tumor
Hematologic
  Anemia (Hb <8.5 g/dL or RBC < 3 million/μL in an adult)
  Sickle cell disease (unless cabin altitude does not exceed
    6800 meters [22,500 ft])
  Blood dyscrasias with active bleeding (hemophilia,
    leukemia)
Pregnancy
  Beyond 240 days or with threatened miscarriage
Miscellaneous
  Need for intravenous fluids or special medical apparatus[2]

[1]Modified and reproduced, with permission, from Mod Med
(June) 1982;50:196. Based on recommendations of the
American Medical Association in JAMA 1982;247:1009.
[2]Consultation with an airline flight surgeon is suggested.
[3]In some cases, low-altitude flights can be made without supplemental oxygen in accordance with recommendations of
the American College of Chest Physicians.

gestive failure should not fly until they are compensated by appropriate treatment, or unless they are in a
pressurized plane with 100% oxygen therapy available during the entire flight.

**B. Compensated Valvular or Other Heart
Disease:** Patients should not fly above 2400–2800
meters (7874–9187 ft) unless the aircraft is pressurized and oxygen is administered at altitudes of 2400
meters (7874 ft) or higher.

**C. Acute Myocardial Infarction, Convales-
cent and Asymptomatic:** At least 6 weeks of convalescence is recommended even for asymptomatic
patients if flying is contemplated. Coronary disease
patients with severe or poorly controlled hypertension or ventricular ectopy should not fly. Ambulatory, stabilized, and compensated patients tolerate air
travel well. Oxygen should be available.

D. Angina Pectoris: Air travel is inadvisable
for patients with new-onset severe or unstable
angina. In mild to moderate cases of angina, air
travel may be permitted, especially in pressurized
planes. Oxygen should be available.

E. Deep Venous Thrombosis: Patients with
deep venous thrombosis should not fly until their anticoagulant therapy is stable and they have no evidence of pulmonary complications. Long flights increase the risk of deep vein thrombosis and resulting
embolic disease. Prevention includes avoidance of
smoking and alcohol, low-dose aspirin, support hose,
and leg exercises and walking during the flight.

Respiratory Disease

A. Nasopharyngeal Disorders: Nasal allergies and infections predispose to development of
aerotitis. Chewing gum, nasal decongestants (pseudoephedrine timed-release, one 120 mg capsule 30
minutes before departure), appropriate anti-infective
treatment, and avoiding sleep on descent may prevent barotitis. (See Barotrauma, Chapter 8.)

B. Asthma: Patients with mild asthma can
travel without difficulty. Patients with status asthmaticus should not be permitted to fly.

C. Congenital Pulmonary Cysts: Patients
should not travel unless cleared by a physician.

D. Tuberculosis: Patients with active, communicable tuberculosis or pneumothorax should not be
permitted to travel by air.

E. Other Pulmonary Disorders: Breathlessness at rest is a contraindication to air travel. The degree of hypoxemia and hypercapnia should be assessed, and vital capacity should be evaluated (Table
38–1).

Anemia

Patients with severe anemia (hemoglobin < 8.5
g/dL or red cell count < 3 million/μL) should not
travel by air until hemoglobin has been raised to a
reasonable level. If hemoglobin is less than 8–9 g/dL,
oxygen should be available. Patients with sickle cell
disease appear to be particularly vulnerable.

Diabetes Mellitus

Diabetics who do not need insulin or who can administer their own insulin during flight may fly
safely. "Brittle" diabetics who are subject to frequent
episodes of hypoglycemia should be in optimal control before flying and should carry sugar or candy in
case hypoglycemic reactions occur. Adjustment of
insulin administration schedule should be discussed
prior to travel across time zones.

Patients With Surgical Problems

Patients convalescing from thoracic or abdominal surgery should not fly until 10 days (abdominal) to 21 days (thoracic) after surgery, and then only if the wound is healed and there is no drainage.

Colostomy patients may be permitted to travel by air providing they are nonodorous and colostomy bags are emptied before flight.

Patients with large hernias unsupported by a truss or binder should not be permitted to fly in nonpressurized aircraft because of an increased danger of strangulation of the herniated bowel.

Postsurgical or posttraumatic eye cases require pressurized cabins and oxygen therapy to avoid retinal damage due to hypoxia and intraocular gas bubbles.

Psychiatric Disorders

Severely psychotic, agitated, or disturbed patients should not be permitted to fly on scheduled airlines even when accompanied by a medical attendant.

Extremely nervous or apprehensive patients may travel by air if they receive adequate sedatives or tranquilizers before and during flight.

Motion Sickness

Patients subject to motion sickness can be given sedatives or antihistamines (eg, dimenhydrinate, 50 mg every 4–6 hours; promethazine, 25 mg every 6 hours; or meclizine, 25–50 mg every 24 hours) before and during the flight. Small meals of easily digested food before and during the flight may reduce the tendency to nausea and vomiting.

Pregnancy

Pregnant women may be permitted to fly during the first 8 months of pregnancy unless there is a history of habitual abortion or premature birth. During the ninth month of pregnancy, air travel is not recommended; if travel is essential, a physician's authorization is required. Infants less than 1 week old should not be flown at high altitudes or for long distances.

Advising patients about air travel. Drug Ther Bull 1996;34:30.

Alexander JK: Coronary problems associated with altitude and air travel. Cardiol Clin 1995;13:271. (Pathogenesis, prevention.)

Poisoning

Kent R. Olson, MD

INITIAL EVALUATION OF THE PATIENT WITH POISONING OR DRUG OVERDOSE

Patients with drug overdoses or poisoning may initially present with no symptoms or with varying degrees of overt intoxication. The asymptomatic patient may have been exposed to or may have ingested a lethal dose of a poison but not yet have any manifestations of toxicity. It is always important to (1) quickly assess the potential danger, (2) perform gut decontamination to prevent absorption, and (3) observe the patient for an appropriate interval.

Assess the Danger

If the toxin is known, the danger can be assessed by consulting a text or computerized information resource (eg, POISINDEX) or by calling a regional poison control center (Table 39–1). Assessment will usually take into account the dose ingested (in milligrams per kilogram of body weight), the time interval since ingestion, the presence of any clinical signs, preexisting cardiac, respiratory, renal, or liver disease, and, occasionally, specific serum drug or toxin levels. Be aware that the history given by the patient or family may be incomplete or unreliable.

The manufacturer or its local representative may be able to provide information over the phone concerning the toxic ingredients in question and can be contacted directly or via the regional poison control center (Table 39–1).

Gut Decontamination

The choice of gut decontamination procedure depends on the toxin and the circumstances. (See below for more discussion of methods.)

Observation of the Patient

Asymptomatic or mildly symptomatic patients should be observed for at least 4–6 hours. Longer observation is indicated if the ingested substance is a sustained-release preparation or is known to slow gastrointestinal motility or if there may have been exposure to a poison with delayed onset of symptoms (such as acetaminophen, colchicine, or hepatotoxic mushrooms). After that time, the patient may be discharged if no symptoms have developed and adequate gastric decontamination has been provided. Before discharge, psychiatric evaluation should be performed to assess suicidal risk. Intentional ingestions in adolescents should raise the possibility of unwanted pregnancy or sexual abuse.

THE SYMPTOMATIC PATIENT

In symptomatic patients, treatment of life-threatening complications takes precedence over in-depth diagnostic evaluation. Patients with mild symptoms may deteriorate rapidly, which is why all potentially significant exposures should be observed in an acute care facility. The following complications may occur, depending on the type of poisoning.

COMA

Assessment & Complications

Coma is commonly associated with ingestion of large doses of antihistamines, barbiturates, benzodiazepines, ethanol, opioids, phenothiazines, or tricyclic antidepressants. The most common cause of death in comatose patients is respiratory failure, which may occur abruptly. Aspiration of gastric contents may also occur, especially in victims who are deeply obtunded or convulsing. Hypoxia and hypoventilation may cause or aggravate arrhythmias and seizures. Thus, protection of the airway and assisted ventilation are the most important treatment measures for any poisoned patient.

Table 39–1. AAPCC-certified regional poison control centers.[1]

The American Association of Regional Poison Control Centers has certified the following regional poison control centers as meeting their minimum operating criteria. Regional poison control centers operate 24 hours a day, utilizing specially trained and dedicated staff with access to a variety of texts, files, and computerized poison information resources. They can also provide immediate telephone consultation with a physician specializing in medical toxicology.

ALABAMA
  Alabama Poison Center, Tuscaloosa: 800-462-0800 (Alabama only), 205-345-0600
  Regional Poison Control Center, The Children's Hospital of Alabama, Birmingham: 205-939-9201, 800-292-6678 (Alabama only), 205-933-4050
ARIZONA
  Arizona Poison and Drug Information Center, Tucson: 800-362-0101 (Arizona only), 602-626-6016
  Arizona Poison and Drug Information Center, Tucson: 800-362-0101, 602-626-6016
  Samaritan Regional Poison Center, Phoenix: 602-253-3334
CALIFORNIA
  California Poison Control System: 800-876-4766 (public); 800-411-8080 (health professionals)
COLORADO
  Rocky Mountain Poison and Drug Center, Denver: 303-629-1123
DISTRICT OF COLUMBIA
  National Capital Poison Center, Washington: 202-625-3333, 202-362-8563 (TTY)
FLORIDA
  Florida Poison Information Center, Jacksonville: 904-549-4480, 800-282-3171 (Florida only)
  Florida Poison Information Center and Toxicology Resource Center, Tampa: 813-253-4444, 800-282-3171 (Florida only)
GEORGIA
  Georgia Poison Center, Atlanta: 800-282-5846 (Georgia only), 404-616-9000
INDIANA
  Indiana Poison Center, Indianapolis: 800-382-9097 (Indiana only); 317-929-2323
KENTUCKY
  Kentucky Regional Poison Center of Kosair Children's Hospital, Louisville: 502-629-7275, 800-722-5725 (Kentucky only)
MARYLAND
  Maryland Poison Center, Baltimore: 800-492-2414 (Maryland only), 410-528-7701
MASSACHUSETTS
  Massachusetts Poison Control System, Boston: 800-682-9211, 617-232-2120
MICHIGAN
  Poison Control Center, Children's Hospital, Detroit: 313-745-5711
MINNESOTA
  Hennepin Regional Poison Center, Minneapolis: 612-347-3141, Petline: 612-337-7387, 612-337-7474 (TDD)
  Minnesota Regional Poison Center, St. Paul: 612-221-2113
MISSOURI
  Cardinal Glennon Children's Hospital Regional Poison Center, St. Louis: 314-772-5200, 800-366-8888
MONTANA
  Rocky Mountain Poison and Drug Center, Denver: 303-629-1123
NEBRASKA
  The Poison Center: 402-390-5555 (Omaha), 800-955-9119 (Nebraska and Wyoming)
NEW JERSEY
  New Jersey Poison Information and Education System, Newark: 800-962-1253
NEW MEXICO
  New Mexico Poison and Drug Information Center, Albuquerque: 800-432-6866 (New Mexico only), 505-843-2551
NEW YORK
  Hudson Valley Regional Poison Center, North Tarrytown: 800-336-6997, 914-366-3030
  Long Island Regional Poison Control Center, Mineola: 516-542-2323, -2324, -2325, -3813
  New York City Poison Control Center, New York City: 212-340-4494, 212-POISONS, 212-689-9014 (TDD)
OHIO
  Central Ohio Poison Center, Columbus: 614-228-1323, 800-682-7625, 614-228-2272 (TTY), 614-461-2012
  Cincinnati Drug and Poison Information Center, Cincinnati: 800-872-5111 (Ohio only), 513-558-5111
OREGON
  Oregon Poison Center, Portland: 800-452-7165 (Oregon only), 503-494-8968
PENNSYLVANIA
  Central Pennsylvania Poison Center, Hershey: 800-521-6110
  The Poison Control Center Serving the Greater Philadelphia Metropolitan Area, Philadelphia: 215-386-2100
  Pittsburgh Poison Center, Pittsburgh: 412-681-6669
RHODE ISLAND POISON CENTER
  Rhode Island Poison Center, Providence: 401-277-5727

(continued)

Table 39–1. AAPCC-certified regional poison control centers.[1] (continued)

The American Association of Regional Poison Control Centers has certified the following regional poison control centers as meeting their minimum operating criteria. Regional poison control centers operate 24 hours a day, utilizing specially trained and dedicated staff with access to a variety of texts, files, and computerized poison information resources. They can also provide immediate telephone consultation with a physician specializing in medical toxicology.

TEXAS
North Texas Poison Center, Dallas: 214-590-5000; Texas WATS 800-441-0040
Southeast Texas Poison Center: 409-765-1420 (Galveston); 713-654-1701 (Houston)
South Texas Poison Center, San Antonio: 800-POISON-1
UTAH
Utah Poison Control Center, Salt Lake City: 801-581-2151, 800-456-7707 (Utah only)
VIRGINIA
Blue Ridge Poison Center, Charlottesville: 804-924-5543, 800-451-1428
National Capital Poison Center (Northern Virginia only): 202-625-3333, 202-362-8563 (TTY)
WEST VIRGINIA
West Virginia Poison Center, Charleston: 800-642-3625 (West Virginia only); 304-348-4211
WYOMING
The Poison Center, Omaha: 800-955-9119 (Nebraska and Wyoming)

[1]American Association of Poison Control Centers, January, 1995.

Treatment

A. Emergency Management: The initial emergency management of coma can be remembered by the mnemonic *ABCD,* for Airway, Breathing, Circulation, and Drugs (dextrose, thiamine, and naloxone or flumazenil), respectively (Table 39–2).

1. Airway–Establish a patent airway by positioning, suction, or insertion of an artificial nasal or oropharyngeal airway. If the patient is deeply comatose or if there is no gag or cough reflex, perform endotracheal intubation. These airway interventions may not be necessary if the patient is intoxicated by an opioid or a benzodiazepine and responds rapidly to intravenous naloxone or flumazenil (see below).

2. Breathing–Clinically assess the quality and depth of respiration, and provide assistance if necessary with a bag-valve-mask device or mechanical ventilator. Provide supplemental oxygen. The arterial blood CO_2 tension is useful in determining the adequacy of ventilation. The arterial blood PO_2 determination may reveal hypoxemia, which may be caused by respiratory arrest, bronchospasm, pulmonary aspiration, or noncardiogenic pulmonary edema. Pulse oximetry is not reliable in patients with methemoglobinemia or carbon monoxide poisoning.

Table 39–2. Initial management of coma.

A	Airway control
B	Breathing
C	Circulation
D	Drugs (give all three) Dextrose 50%, 50–100 mL IV Thiamine, 100 mg IM or IV Naloxone, 0.45–2 mg IV And consider flumazenil, 0.2–0.5 mg IV[1,2]

[1]Repeated doses, up to 5–10 mg, may be required.
[2]Do not give if patient has co-ingested a tricyclic antidepressant or cocaine or has a seizure disorder.

3. Circulation–Measure the pulse and blood pressure, and estimate tissue perfusion (eg, by measurement of urinary output, skin signs, arterial blood pH). Insert an intravenous line, and draw blood for complete blood count, glucose, electrolytes, serum creatinine and liver tests, and possible toxicologic testing.

4. Drugs–

a. Dextrose and thiamine–Unless promptly treated, severe hypoglycemia can cause irreversible brain damage. Therefore, in all comatose or convulsing patients, give 50% dextrose, 50–100 mL by intravenous bolus, unless a rapid bedside blood sugar test is available and rules out hypoglycemia. In alcoholic or very malnourished patients who may have marginal thiamine stores, give thiamine, 100 mg intramuscularly or over 2–3 minutes intravenously.

b. Narcotic antagonists–Naloxone, 0.4–2 mg intravenously, may reverse opioid-induced respiratory depression and coma. If opioid overdose is strongly suspected, give additional doses of naloxone (up to 5–10 mg may be required to reverse potent opioids). *Caution:* Naloxone has a much shorter duration of action (2–3 hours) than most common opioids; repeated doses may be required, and continuous observation for at least 3–4 hours after the last dose is mandatory.

c. Flumazenil–Flumazenil, 0.2–0.5 mg intravenously, repeated every 30 seconds as needed up to a maximum of 3 mg, may reverse benzodiazepine-induced coma. *Caution:* Flumazenil has a short duration of effect (2–3 hours), and resedation requiring additional doses is common. Furthermore, flumazenil should not be given if the patient has co-ingested a tricyclic antidepressant or has a seizure disorder.

HYPOTHERMIA

Assessment & Complications

Hypothermia commonly accompanies coma due to opioids, ethanol, hypoglycemic agents, phenothiazines, barbiturates, benzodiazepines, and other sedative-hypnotics and depressants. Hypothermic patients may have a barely perceptible pulse and blood pressure and often appear to be dead. Hypothermia may cause or aggravate hypotension, which will not reverse until the temperature is normalized.

Treatment

Hypothermia treatment is discussed in Chapter 38. Gradual rewarming is preferred unless the patient is in cardiac arrest.

HYPOTENSION

Assessment & Complications

Hypotension may be due to poisoning by many different drugs and poisons. The most common drugs causing hypotension are antihypertensive drugs, beta-blockers, calcium channel blocking agents, iron, theophylline, phenothiazines, barbiturates, and tricyclic antidepressants. Poisons causing hypotension include cyanide, carbon monoxide, hydrogen sulfide, arsenic, and certain mushrooms.

Hypotension in the poisoned or drug-overdosed patient may be caused by venous or arteriolar vasodilation, hypovolemia, depressed cardiac contractility, or a combination of these effects. The only certain way to determine the cause of hypotension in any individual patient is to insert a pulmonary artery catheter and measure the left ventricular filling pressure and then calculate the cardiac output and peripheral vascular resistance. Alternatively, a central venous pressure (CVP) monitor may indicate a need for further fluid therapy.

Treatment

Most patients respond to empiric treatment (200 mL intravenous boluses of 0.9% saline or other isotonic crystalloid up to total of 1–2 L). If fluid therapy is not successful, give dopamine, 5–15 µg/kg/min by intravenous infusion in a large peripheral or central line. Consider pulmonary artery catheterization if hypotension persists.

Hypotension caused by certain toxins may respond to specific treatment. For hypotension caused by overdoses of tricyclic antidepressants or related drugs, administer sodium bicarbonate, 1–2 meq/kg by intravenous bolus injection. For beta-blocker overdose, glucagon intravenously may be of value. For calcium antagonist overdose, administer calcium chloride, 15–20 mg/kg intravenously (repeated doses may be necessary).

HYPERTENSION

Assessment & Complications

Hypertension may be due to poisoning with amphetamines, anticholinergics, cocaine, phenyl-propanolamine, or monoamine oxidase inhibitors (mainly as a result of a concomitantly administered drug).

Severe hypertension (eg, diastolic blood pressure > 105–110 mm Hg in a person who does not have chronic hypertension) can result in acute intracranial hemorrhage, myocardial infarction, or aortic dissection. Patients often present with headache, chest pain, or encephalopathy.

Treatment

Treat hypertension (see Chapter 11) if the patient is symptomatic or if the diastolic pressure is greater than 105–110 mm Hg—especially if there is no prior history of hypertension.

Administer phentolamine, 2–5 mg intravenously, or nitroprusside sodium, 0.25–8 µg/kg/min intravenously. If excessive tachycardia is present, add propranolol, 1–5 mg intravenously, or esmolol 25–100 µg/kg/min intravenously. *Caution:* Do not give beta-blockers alone, since doing so may paradoxically worsen hypertension.

ARRHYTHMIAS

Assessment & Complications

Arrhythmias may occur with a variety of drugs or toxins (Table 39–3). They may also occur as a result of hypoxia, metabolic acidosis, or electrolyte imbalance (eg, hyper- or hypokalemia, hypocalcemia), or following exposure to chlorinated solvents or chloral hydrate overdose.

Treatment

Arrhythmias are often caused by hypoxia or electrolyte imbalance, and these conditions should be sought and treated. If ventricular arrhythmias persist, administer lidocaine at usual antiarrhythmic doses.

Table 39–3. Common toxins or drugs causing arrhythmias.

Arrhythmia	Common Causes
Sinus bradycardia	Beta-blockers, verapamil, organophosphates, digitalis glycosides, opioids, clonidine, sedative-hypnotics.
Atrioventricular block	Beta-blockers, digitalis glycosides, calcium antagonists, tricyclic antidepressants, lithium.
Sinus tachycardia	Theophylline, caffeine, cocaine, amphetamines, phencyclidine, beta-agonists (eg, albuterol), iron, anticholinergics, tricyclic antidepressants, antihistamines.
Wide QRS complex	Tricyclic antidepressants, quinidine and class 1a antiarrhythmics, class 1c antiarrhythmics, phenothiazines, potassium (hyperkalemia).

Caution: Avoid class Ia agents (quinidine, procainamide, disopyramide), which may aggravate arrhythmias caused by tricyclic antidepressants, calcium antagonists, or beta-blockers. Wide QRS complex tachycardia in the setting of tricyclic antidepressant overdose (or quinidine and other class Ia drugs) should be treated with sodium bicarbonate, 50–100 meq intravenously by bolus injection. (See discussion of tricyclic antidepressant poisoning.)

For tachyarrhythmias induced by chlorinated solvents, chloral hydrate, or sympathomimetic agents, use propranolol or esmolol (see doses given above in hypertension section).

CONVULSIONS

Assessment & Complications

Convulsions may be due to poisoning with many drugs and poisons, including amphetamines, antihistamines, camphor, cocaine, isoniazid, lindane, phencyclidine (PCP), phenothiazines, theophylline, and tricyclic antidepressants.

Convulsions may also be caused by hypoxia, hypoglycemia, hypocalcemia, hyponatremia, withdrawal from alcohol or sedative-hypnotics, head trauma, central nervous system infection, or idiopathic epilepsy.

Prolonged or repeated convulsions commonly lead to hypoxia, metabolic acidosis, hyperthermia, and rhabdomyolysis.

Treatment

Administer diazepam, 5–10 mg intravenously over 2–3 minutes, or lorazepam, 2–3 mg intravenously, or—if intravenous access is not immediately available—midazolam, 5–10 mg intramuscularly. If convulsions continue, administer phenobarbital, 15–20 mg/kg slowly intravenously over no less than 30 minutes; or phenytoin, 15 mg/kg intravenously over no less than 30 minutes (maximum infusion rate, 50 mg/min). The drugs may be used together if necessary. Maintenance doses may be required if drug toxicity is expected to last more than 18–24 hours.

Convulsions due to a few drugs and toxins may require antidotes or other specific therapies (as listed in Table 39–4).

HYPERTHERMIA

Assessment & Complications

Hyperthermia may be associated with poisoning by amphetamines, atropine and other anticholinergic drugs, cocaine, dinitrophenol and pentachlorophenol, phencyclidine (PCP), salicylates, strychnine, tricyclic antidepressants, and various other medications. Use of drugs which may increase serotonin concentrations or enhance its effects (eg, fluoxetine, paroxe-

Table 39–4. Convulsions requiring special consideration (see text for doses).

Toxin or Drug	Comments
Isoniazid (INH)	Administer pyridoxine.
Lithium	May indicate need for hemodialysis.
Organophosphates	Administer pralidoxime (2-PAM) and atropine.
Strychnine	"Convulsions" are actually spinally mediated muscle spasms and usually require neuromuscular paralysis.
Theophylline	Convulsions indicate need for hemodialysis or charcoal hemoperfusion.
Tricyclic antidepressants	Hyperthermia and cardiotoxicity are common complications of repeated convulsions; paralyze early with neuromuscular blockers to reduce muscular hyperactivity.

tine, and other selective serotonin reuptake inhibitors; meperidine; dextromethorphan; others) in a patient taking a monoamine oxidase inhibitor may cause agitation, hyperactivity, and hyperthermia. Haloperidol and other antipsychotic agents can cause rigidity and hyperthermia (neuroleptic malignant syndrome [NMS]).

Hyperthermia is a rapidly life-threatening complication. Severe hyperthermia (temperature > 40–41 °C) may rapidly cause brain damage and multiorgan failure, including rhabdomyolysis, renal failure, and coagulopathy (see Chapter 38).

Treatment

Treat hyperthermia aggressively by removing all clothing, spraying with tepid water, and fanning the patient. If this is not rapidly effective, as shown by a normal rectal temperature within 30–60 minutes, or if there is significant muscle rigidity or hyperactivity, induce neuromuscular paralysis with pancuronium, 0.1 mg/kg intravenously, or another nondepolarizing neuromuscular blocker. Once paralyzed, the patient must be intubated and mechanically ventilated. Absence of visible muscular convulsive movements may give the false impression that brain seizure activity has ceased; however, this must be confirmed by electroencephalography.

Dantrolene (2–5 mg/kg intravenously) may be effective for hyperthermia associated with muscle rigidity that does not respond to neuromuscular blockade (ie, malignant hyperthermia). Bromocriptine, 2.5–7.5 mg orally daily, has been recommended for neuroleptic malignant syndrome.

ANTIDOTES & OTHER TREATMENT

ANTIDOTES

Give an antidote (if available) when there is reasonable certainty of a specific diagnosis (Table 39–5). Antidotes themselves may have serious side effects. The indications and dosages for specific antidotes are discussed in the respective sections for specific toxins. See also Table 39–6.

DECONTAMINATION OF THE SKIN

Corrosive agents rapidly injure the skin and eyes and must be removed immediately. In addition, many toxins are readily absorbed through the skin, and systemic absorption can be prevented only by rapid action.

Wash the affected areas with copious quantities of lukewarm water or saline. Wash carefully behind the ears, under the nails, and in skin folds. For oily substances (eg, pesticides), wash the skin at least twice with plain soap and shampoo the hair. Specific decontaminating solutions or solvents (eg, alcohol) are rarely indicated and in some cases may enhance absorption.

Table 39–5. Some toxic agents for which there are specific antidotes.

Toxic Agent	Specific Antidote
Acetaminophen	Acetylcysteine
Anticholinergics (eg, atropine)	Physostigmine
Anticholinesterases (eg, organophosphate pesticides)	Atropine and pralidoxime (2-PAM)
Benzodiazepines	Flumazenil
Carbon monoxide	Oxygen
Cyanide	Sodium nitrite, sodium thiosulfate
Digitalis glycosides	Digoxin-specific Fab antibodies
Heavy metals (eg, lead, mercury, iron) and arsenic	Specific chelating agents
Isoniazid	Pyridoxine (vitamin B_6)
Methanol, ethylene glycol	Ethanol (ethyl alcohol)
Opioids	Naloxone
Snake venom	Specific venom antisera

Table 39–6. Examples of ineffective or dangerous "antidotes."[1]

"Antidote"	Application	Problems
Amphetamines, caffeine, or doxapram	Nonspecific arousal, eg, sedative overdose	Cardiac arrhythmias, seizures
Mineral oil	Petroleum distilate ingestion	Lipoid pneumonia
Physostigmine	Nonspecific arousal, eg, diazepam overdose, tricyclic antidepressants	Bradycardia, asystole, seizures
"Universal antidote" (burnt toast, tea)	Adsorbent in gut	Ineffective; aspiration; wastes time
Vinegar, other weak acids	Neutralization of alkali burns	Ineffective; may worsen injury

[1]Reproduced, with permission, from Saunders CE, Ho MT (editors): *Current Emergency Diagnosis & Treatment*, 4th ed. Appleton & Lange, 1992.

DECONTAMINATION OF THE EYES

Act quickly to prevent serious damage. Flush the eyes with copious amounts of saline (preferred) or water. (If available, instill local anesthetic drops in the eye before beginning irrigation.) Remove contact lenses if present. Direct the irrigating stream so that it will flow across both eyes after running off the nasal bridge. Lift the tarsal conjunctiva to look for undissolved particles and to facilitate irrigation. Continue irrigation for 15 minutes by the clock or until each eye has been irrigated with at least 1 L of solution. If the toxin is an acid or a base, check the pH of the tears after irrigation, and continue irrigation until the pH is between 6.5 and 7.5.

After irrigation is complete, perform fluorescein examination of the eye, using a slitlamp or Wood's lamp to identify areas of corneal injury. Patients with serious conjunctival or corneal injury should be immediately referred to an ophthalmologist.

GASTROINTESTINAL DECONTAMINATION

Removal of ingested poisons is an essential part of emergency treatment. However, studies indicate that if more than 60 minutes has passed, induced emesis and gastric lavage are relatively ineffective. For small or moderate ingestions of most substances, toxicologists generally recommend activated charcoal alone without prior gastric emptying. Exceptions are large ingestions of anticholinergic compounds and salicylates, which often delay gastric emptying, and ingestion of sustained-release or enteric-coated tablets, which may remain intact for several hours.

Gastric emptying is not generally used for ingestion of corrosive agents or petroleum distillates, because further esophageal injury or pulmonary aspiration may result. However, in certain cases, removal of the toxin may be more important than concern over possible complications. Consult a medical toxicologist or regional poison control center (Table 39–1) for advice.

Emesis

Emesis using syrup of ipecac is a convenient and fairly effective way to evacuate gastric contents if given very soon after ingestion (eg, at work or at home). However, it may delay or prevent use of oral activated charcoal and is not generally used in the hospital management of ingestions.

A. Indications: For removal of poison in conscious, cooperative patients and for promptness, ipecac can be given in the home or at work in the first few minutes after poisoning.

B. Contraindications: Induced emesis is contraindicated for drowsy, unconscious, or convulsing patients and for patients who have ingested kerosene or other hydrocarbons (danger of aspiration of stomach contents), corrosive poisons, or rapidly acting convulsants (eg, tricyclic antidepressants, strychnine, nicotine, camphor).

C. Technique: Give syrup of ipecac, 30 mL (15 mL in children), followed by an 8-oz glass of water. Repeat in 20 minutes if necessary.

Gastric Lavage

Gastric lavage is more effective for liquid poisons or small pill fragments than for intact tablets or pieces of mushroom. It is most effective when started within 60 minutes after ingestion. The lavage procedure may delay administration of activated charcoal and may hasten passage of pills and other toxic material into the small intestine.

A. Indications: Gastric lavage is indicated for removal of ingested poisons when emesis is refused, contraindicated, or unsuccessful; for collection and examination of gastric contents for identification of poison; and for convenient administration of charcoal and antidotes.

B. Contraindications: Do *not* use lavage for stuporous or comatose patients with absent gag reflexes unless they are endotracheally intubated beforehand. Some authorities advise against lavage when caustic material has been ingested; others regard it as essential to remove liquid corrosives from the stomach.

C. Technique: In obtunded or comatose patients, the danger of aspiration pneumonia is reduced by placing the patient in a head down, left lateral decubitus position and, if necessary, protecting the airway with endotracheal intubation. Gently insert a lubricated, soft but noncollapsible stomach tube (at least 37–40F) through the mouth or nose into the stomach. Aspirate and save the contents, and then lavage repeatedly with 50–100 mL of fluid until the return fluid is clear. Use lukewarm tap water or saline.

Activated Charcoal

Activated charcoal effectively adsorbs almost all drugs and poisons. Poorly absorbed substances include iron, lithium, potassium, sodium, cyanide, mineral acids, and alcohols.

A. Indications: Activated charcoal should be used for prompt adsorption of drugs or toxins in the stomach and intestine. Studies show that activated charcoal given alone may be as effective as or more effective than ipecac-induced emesis or gastric lavage.

B. Contraindications: Activated charcoal should not be used for stuporous, comatose, or convulsing patients unless it can be given by gastric tube and the airway is first protected by cuffed endotracheal tube. This substance is contraindicated also for patients with ileus or intestinal obstruction or those who have ingested corrosives for whom endoscopy is planned.

C. Technique: Administer activated charcoal, 60–100 g orally or via gastric tube, mixed in aqueous slurry. Repeated doses may be given to ensure gastrointestinal adsorption or to enhance elimination of some drugs (see below).

Catharsis

A. Indications: For stimulation of peristalsis to hasten the elimination of unabsorbed drugs and poisons and the activated charcoal slurry.

B. Contraindications and Cautions: Do not use mineral oil or other oil-based cathartics. Avoid sodium-based cathartics in patients with hypertension, renal failure, and congestive heart failure and magnesium-based cathartics in those with renal failure.

C. Technique: Magnesium sulfate 10%, 2–3 mL/kg; or sorbitol 70%, 1–2 mL/kg. Sorbitol is commonly used in prepackaged charcoal slurry products.

Whole Bowel Irrigation

Whole bowel irrigation utilizes large volumes of balanced polyethylene glycol-electrolyte solution to mechanically cleanse the entire intestinal tract. There is no net gain or loss of systemic fluids or electrolytes.

A. Indications: Whole bowel irrigation is particularly effective for massive iron ingestion in which intact tablets are visible on abdominal x-ray. It has also been used for ingestions of sustained-release and enteric-coated tablets as well as drug-filled packets.

B. Contraindications: Same as for cathartics.

C. Technique: Administer the balanced polyethylene glycol-electrolyte solution (CoLyte,

GoLYTELY) into the stomach via gastric tube at a rate of 1–2 L/h until the rectal effluent is clear.

Increased Drug Removal

A. Forced Diuresis: Forced diuresis is hazardous; the risk of complications (pulmonary edema, electrolyte imbalance) usually outweighs its benefits. Acidic drugs (eg, salicylates, phenobarbital) are more rapidly excreted with an alkaline urine. Acidification (sometimes promoted for amphetamines, phencyclidine) is *not* very effective and is contraindicated in the presence of rhabdomyolysis or myoglobinuria.

B. Dialysis (Hemodialysis or Hemoperfusion): The indications for dialysis are as follows: (1) Known or suspected potentially lethal amounts of a dialyzable drug (Table 39–7). (2) Poisoning with deep coma, apnea, severe hypotension, fluid and electrolyte or acid-base disturbance, or extreme body temperature changes that cannot be corrected by conventional measures. (3) Poisoning in patients with severe renal, cardiac, pulmonary, or hepatic disease who will not be able to eliminate the toxin by usual mechanisms.

Many of the substances that cannot be removed effectively by aqueous dialysis can be removed by he-moperfusion through specially designed coated charcoal columns. Indications are the same as for dialysis. Peritoneal dialysis may occasionally be employed for acute poisonings when hemodialysis is not available, but it is very inefficient. Dialysis should usually augment rather than replace well-established emergency and supportive measures. Continuous arteriovenous and venovenous hemodiafiltration is of uncertain benefit for elimination of poisons.

C. Repeat-Dose Charcoal: Repeated doses of activated charcoal, 20–30 g every 3–4 hours, may hasten elimination of some drugs (eg, digitoxin, theophylline, phenobarbital) by adsorbing drug excreted into the gut lumen ("gut dialysis"). Sorbitol or other cathartics should *not* be used with each dose, or resulting large stool volumes may lead to dehydration or hypernatremia.

Bosse GM et al: Comparison of three methods of gut decontamination in tricyclic antidepressant overdose. J Emerg Med 1995;13:203. (Prospective randomized study suggests benefit of charcoal combined with lavage, but sample size was small.)

DIAGNOSIS OF POISONING

The identity of the ingested substance is usually known, but occasionally a comatose patient is found with an unlabeled container or refuses or otherwise fails to give a coherent history. By performing a directed physical examination and ordering common clinical laboratory tests, the clinician can often make a tentative diagnosis that may allow empiric interventions or may suggest specific toxicologic tests.

PHYSICAL EXAMINATION

Important diagnostic variables in the physical examination include blood pressure, pulse rate, temperature, pupil size, sweating, and the presence or absence of peristaltic activity. Poisonings with many drugs fit into one of four common syndromes.

Sympathomimetic Syndrome

The blood pressure and pulse rate are elevated, though with severe hypertension reflex bradycardia may occur. The temperature is often elevated, pupils are dilated, and the skin is sweaty, though mucous membranes are dry. Patients are usually agitated, anxious, or frankly psychotic.

Examples: Amphetamines, cocaine, ephedrine and pseudoephedrine, phencyclidine (pupils normal or small), phenylpropanolamine (bradycardia common).

Table 39–7. Recommended use of hemodialysis (HD) and hemoperfusion (HP) in poisoning.

Poison	Procedure	Indications[1]
Carbamazepine	HP	Seizures, severe cardiotoxicity.
Digitoxin[2]	HP	Severe toxicity, Fab not available.
Ethylene glycol	HD	Acidosis, serum level > 100 mg/dL.
Lithium	HD	Severe symptoms.
Methanol	HD	Acidosis, serum level > 50 mg/dL.
Phenobarbital	HP	Intractable hypotension, acidosis despite maximal supportive care.
Salicylate	HD	Severe acidosis, CNS symptoms, level > 100 mg/dL (100 mg/L).
Theophylline	HP or HD	Serum level > 90–100 mg/L (acute) or seizures and serum level > 40–60 mg/L (chronic).
Valproic acid	HD	Serum level > 900–1000 mg/L or deep coma, severe acidosis.

[1]Contact a regional poison control center or a clinical toxicologist before undertaking these procedures. See text for further discussion of indications.
[2]Digoxin and other cardiac glycosides are not removed by hemoperfusion.

Sympatholytic Syndrome

The blood pressure and pulse rate are decreased and body temperature is low. The pupils are small or even pinpoint. Peristalsis is usually decreased. Patients are usually obtunded or comatose.

Examples: Barbiturates, benzodiazepines and other sedative hypnotics, clonidine and related antihypertensives, ethanol, opioids.

Cholinergic Syndrome

Stimulation of muscarinic receptors causes bradycardia, miosis, sweating, and hyperperistalsis as well as bronchorrhea, wheezing, excessive salivation, and urinary incontinence. Nicotinic receptor stimulation may produce initial hypertension and tachycardia as well as fasciculations and muscle weakness. Patients are usually agitated and anxious.

Examples: Carbamates, nicotine, organophosphates, physostigmine.

Anticholinergic Syndrome

Tachycardia with mild hypertension is common, and the body temperature is often elevated. Pupils are widely dilated. The skin is flushed, hot and dry. Peristalsis is decreased, and urinary retention is common. Patients may have myoclonic jerking or choreoathetoid movements. Agitated delirium is frequently seen, and severe hyperthermia may occur.

Examples: Atropine, scopolamine, other naturally occurring and pharmaceutical anticholinergics, amantadine, antihistamines, phenothiazines (hypotension, small pupils), tricyclic antidepressants.

CLINICAL LABORATORY TESTS IN MANAGEMENT OF POISONING

The following clinical laboratory tests are recommended for screening of the overdosed patient: measured serum osmolality and osmolar gap, electrolytes, glucose, creatinine, BUN, urinalysis (eg, oxalate crystals with ethylene glycol poisoning, myoglobinuria with rhabdomyolysis), and electrocardiography. Serum acetaminophen and ethanol levels should be determined in all patients with drug overdoses.

OSMOLAR GAP

The osmolar gap is defined and calculation of the gap is described in Table 39–8. It is increased in the presence of large quantities of low-molecular-weight substances, most commonly ethanol. Common poisons associated with increased osmolar gap are ace-

Table 39–8. Use of the osmolar gap in toxicology.[1]

The osmolar gap (Δosm) is determined by subtracting the calculated serum osmolality from the measured serum osmolality.

$$\text{Calculated osmolality (osm)} = 2[Na+ \text{(meq/L)}] + \frac{\text{Glucose (mg/dL)}}{18} + \frac{\text{BUN (mg/dL)}}{2.8}$$

$$\Delta\text{osm} = \text{Measured osmolality} - \text{Calculated osmolality}$$

Serum osmolality may be increased by contributions of circulating alcohols and other low-molecular-weight substances. Since these substances are not included in the calculated osmolality, there will be a gap proportionate to their serum concentration and inversely proportionate to their molecular weight:

$$\frac{\text{Serum concentration (mg/dL)}}{} = \Delta\text{osm} \times \frac{\text{Molecular weight}}{10}$$

For ethanol (the commonest cause of Δosm), a gap of 30 mosm/L indicates an ethanol level of approximately

$$30 \times \frac{46}{10} = 138 \text{ mg/dL}$$

	Molecular Weight	Toxic Concentration	Approximate Corresponding Δosm (mosm/L)
Ethanol	46	300	65
Methanol	32	50	16
Ethylene glycol	60	150	25
Isopropanol	60	150	25

[1]Modified from Saunders CE, Ho MT (editors): *Current Emergency Diagnosis & Treatment,* 4th ed. Appleton & Lange, 1992.
Note: Most laboratories use the freezing point method for calculating osmolality. If the vaporization point method is used, alcohols are driven off and their contribution to osmolality is lost.

tone, ethanol, ethylene glycol, isopropyl alcohol, methanol, and propylene glycol.

ANION GAP

Metabolic acidosis associated with an elevated anion gap is usually due to an accumulation of lactic acid or other acids (see Chapter 21). Common causes of elevated anion gap in poisoning include carbon monoxide, cyanide, ethylene glycol, medicinal iron, isoniazid, methanol, phenformin, and salicylates.

One should also check the osmolar gap; combined elevated anion and osmolar gap suggests poisoning by methanol or ethylene glycol, though this may also occur in patients with diabetic ketoacidosis and alcoholic ketoacidosis.

TOXICOLOGY LABORATORY EXAMINATION

The routine toxicology screen (Table 39–9) is of little value in the initial care of the poisoned patient—on the contrary, it is time-consuming, expensive, and frequently erroneous. Specific quantitative levels of certain drugs may be extremely helpful (Table 39–10), however, especially if specific antidotes or interventions (eg, dialysis, antidotes) would be indicated based upon the results.

If a toxicology screen is required, urine is the best specimen for broad qualitative screening. Blood samples may be saved for possible quantitative testing, but blood is not appropriate for screening purposes since it is relatively insensitive for many common drugs, including psychotropic agents, opioids, and stimulants.

ABDOMINAL X-RAYS

A plain film of the abdomen may reveal radiopaque iron tablets, drug-filled condoms, or other toxic material. Studies suggest that few tablets are predictably visible (eg, ferrous sulfate, sodium chloride, calcium carbonate, and potassium chloride). Thus, the x-ray is useful only if positive.

TREATMENT OF COMMON SPECIFIC POISONINGS (Alphabetical Order)

ACETAMINOPHEN

Acetaminophen is a common analgesic found in many nonprescription and prescription products. After absorption, it is metabolized mainly by glu-

Table 39–9. Common drugs screened for in blood and urine in the toxicology laboratory.[1]

Blood
Acetaminophen, alcohols, barbiturates, benzodiazepines, carisoprodol, ethchlorvynol, glutethimide, meprobamate, phenytoin, salicylates.

Urine
Acetaminophen, alcohols, amphetamines, barbiturates, chlorpheniramine, cocaine, codeine, dextromethorphan, diphenhydramine, ethchlorvynol, lidocaine, meperidine, meprobamate, methadone, methyprylon, morphine, pentazocine, phencyclidine, phenothiazines, propoxyphene, salicylates, tricyclic antidepressants.

[1]**Note:** The urine screen is generally more comprehensive, detecting drugs of abuse (opiates, stimulants), antihistamines, and, in many cases, drugs also found in serum.

Table 39–10. Specific quantitative levels and potential therapeutic interventions.[1]

Drug or Toxin	Treatment
Acetaminophen	Use of specific antidote (acetylcysteine) based on serum level.
Carbon monoxide	High carboxyhemoglobin level indicates need for 100% oxygen.
Digitalis (digoxin or digitoxin)	On basis of serum digitalis and potassium levels, treatment with Fab antibody fragments may be indicated.
Ethanol	Low serum level may suggest nonalcoholic cause for coma (eg, trauma, other drugs, other alcohols). May also be used in monitoring ethanol therapy for methanol or ethylene glycol poisoning.
Iron	Level may indicate need for chelation with deferoxamine.
Lithium	Serum levels and calculated half-life can guide decision to hemodialyze.
Methanol	Acidosis, high methanol level indicate need for hemodialysis, ethanol therapy.
Methemoglobin	Methemoglobinemia can be treated with methylene blue intravenously.
Salicylates	High level may indicate need for hemodialysis, alkaline diuresis.
Theophylline	Immediate hemodialysis or hemoperfusion may be indicated based on serum level.
Valproic acid	Elevated levels may indicate need to consider hemodialysis.

[1]Some drugs or toxins may have profound and irreversible toxicity unless rapid and specific management is provided outside of routine supportive care. For these agents, laboratory testing may provide the serum level or other evidence required for administering a specific antidote or arranging for hemodialysis.

curonidation and sulfation, with a small fraction metabolized via the P450 mixed-function oxidase system to a highly toxic reactive intermediate. This toxic intermediate is normally detoxified by cellular glutathione. With acute acetaminophen overdose (> 140 mg/kg, or 7 g in an average adult), hepatocellular glutathione is rapidly depleted and the reactive intermediate attacks other cell proteins, causing necrosis. Patients with enhanced P450 activity, such as chronic alcoholics and patients taking anticonvulsants, are at increased risk of developing hepatotoxicity. Hepatic toxicity may also occur after chronic accidental overuse of acetaminophen—eg, as little as 1 g of acetaminophen every 4–6 hours for 1–2 days in a patient with chronic alcohol abuse.

Clinical Findings

Shortly after ingestion, patients may have nausea

or vomiting, but there are usually no other signs of toxicity until 24–48 hours after ingestion, when hepatic aminotransferase levels begin to increase. With severe poisoning, massive hepatic necrosis may occur, resulting in jaundice, hepatic encephalopathy, renal failure, and death.

The diagnosis of severe poisoning after acute overdose is based on measurement of the serum acetaminophen level. Plot the serum level versus the time since ingestion on the acetaminophen nomogram shown in Figure 39–1. Ingestion of sustained-release products, such as Tylenol Extended Relief, may cause delayed elevation of serum levels.

Treatment

A. Emergency and Supportive Measures:
Empty the stomach by emesis (at home) or gastric lavage (within 1 hour after ingestion). (If more than 1–2 hours have passed since ingestion, do not attempt gut emptying procedures.) Administer activated charcoal. Although charcoal may bind the oral antidote acetylcysteine, this is not considered clinically significant.

B. Specific Treatment:
If the serum acetaminophen level is higher than the toxic line on the nomogram (Figure 39–1), begin treatment with a loading dose of acetylcysteine, 140 mg/kg orally, fol-

lowed by 70 mg/kg every 4 hours. The FDA-approved protocol in the USA continues treatment for 72 hours. However, other protocols have demonstrated equivalent success with 20–48 hours of treatment. Treatment with acetylcysteine is most effective if started within 8–10 hours after ingestion.

Acetylcysteine may also be given intravenously; this is the preferred method in Europe and Canada, but there is no approved parenteral formulation or dosing schedule in the United States. If the patient cannot tolerate acetylcysteine despite antiemetics and administration via a gastric tube, the drug may be given intravenously. Call the regional poison control center for assistance.

Anker AL, Smilkstein MJ: Acetaminophen: Concepts and controversies. Emerg Med Clin North Am 1994;12:335. (Review of mechanism of toxicity, treatment, and recent controversies regarding length of treatment and late use of acetylcysteine.)

Vale JA, Proud AT: Paracetamol (acetaminophen) poisoning. Lancet 1995;346:547. (An excellent review of the pathophysiology, diagnosis, and treatment of acetaminophen poisoning.)

ACIDS, CORROSIVE
(Table 39–11)

The strong mineral acids exert primarily a local corrosive effect on the skin and mucous membranes. In severe burns, circulatory collapse may result. Symptoms include severe pain in the throat and upper gastrointestinal tract, marked thirst, bloody vomitus; difficulty in swallowing, breathing, and speak-

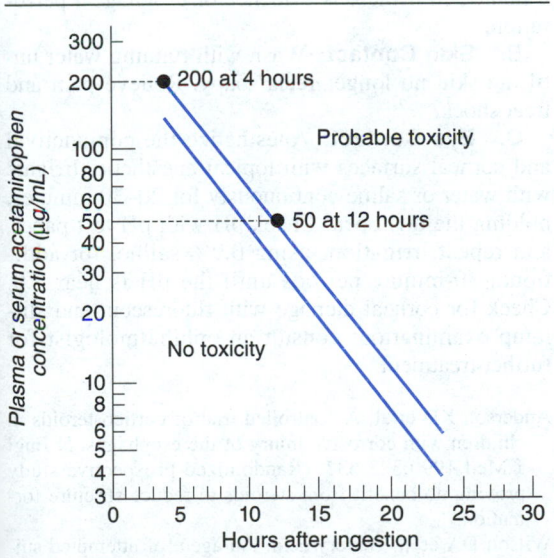

Figure 39–1. Nomogram for prediction of acetaminophen hepatotoxicity following acute overdosage. The upper line defines serum acetaminophen concentrations known to be associated with hepatotoxicity; the lower line defines serum levels 25% below those expected to cause hepatotoxicity. To give a margin for error, the lower line should be used as a guide to treatment. (Modified and reproduced, with permission, from Rumack BH, Matthew H: Acetaminophen poisoning and toxicity. Pediatrics 1975;55:871.)

Table 39–11. Common corrosive agents.[1]

Category and Examples	Injury Caused
Concentrated alkalies Clinitest tablets Drain cleaners Industrial-strength ammonia Lye Oven cleaners	Penetrating liquefaction necrosis
Concentrated acids Pool disinfectants Toilet bowl cleaners	Coagulation necrosis
Weaker cleaning agents Cationic detergents (dishwasher detergents) Household ammonia Household bleach	Superficial burns and irritation; deep burns (rare)
Other Hydrofluoric acid	Penetrating, delayed, destructive injury

[1]Reproduced, with permission, from Saunders CE, Ho MT (editors): *Current Emergency Diagnosis & Treatment,* 4th ed. Appleton & Lange, 1992.

ing; discoloration and destruction of skin and mucous membranes in and around the mouth; and shock. Severe systemic metabolic acidosis may occur.

Severe deep destructive tissue damage may occur after exposure to hydrofluoric acid because of the penetrating and highly toxic fluoride ion. Systemic hypocalcemia and hyperkalemia may occur.

Inhalation of volatile acids, fumes, or gases such as chlorine, fluorine, bromine, or iodine causes severe irritation of the throat and larynx and may cause upper airway obstruction and noncardiogenic pulmonary edema.

Treatment

A. Ingestion: Do *not* induce emesis. Dilute immediately by giving a glass (4–8 oz) of milk or water to drink. Do *not* give bicarbonate or other neutralizing agents. Some experts recommend immediate gastric lavage.

Perform flexible endoscopic esophagoscopy promptly to determine the presence and extent of injury. X-rays of the chest and abdomen may reveal the presence of free air in patients with esophageal or gastric perforation. Perforation, peritonitis, and major bleeding are indications for surgery.

B. Skin Contact: Flood with water for 15 minutes. Use no chemical antidotes; the heat of the reaction may cause additional injury.

For hydrofluoric acid burns, soak the affected area in magnesium sulfate solution or apply 2.5% calcium gluconate gel (prepared by adding 3.5 g calcium gluconate to 5 oz of water-soluble surgical lubricant, eg, K-Y Jelly); then arrange immediate consultation with a plastic surgeon or other specialist. Binding of the fluoride ion may be achieved by injecting 0.5 mL of 5% calcium gluconate per square centimeter under the burned area. (*Caution: Do not use calcium chloride.*)

C. Eye Contact: Anesthetize the conjunctiva and corneal surfaces with topical local anesthetic drops. Flood with water for 15 minutes, holding the eyelids open. Check pH with pH 6.0–8.0 test paper, and repeat irrigation, using 0.9% saline, until pH is near 7.0. Check for corneal damage with fluorescein and slitlamp examination; consult an ophthalmologist about further treatment.

D. Inhalation: Remove from further exposure to fumes or gas. Check skin and clothing. Treat pulmonary edema.

Chan TC, Williams SR, Clark RF: Formic acid skin burns resulting in systemic toxicity. Ann Emerg Med 1995;26:383. (Case report illustrating the potential for serious systemic poisoning after corrosive skin exposure.)

Gumaste W, Dave PB: Ingestion of corrosive substances by adults. Am J Gastroenterol 1992;87:1. (A review of gastrointestinal injuries from corrosive acids and alkali.)

ALKALIES
(Table 39–11)

The strong alkalies are common ingredients of some household cleaning compounds and may be suspected by their "soapy" texture. Those with alkalinity above pH 12.0 are particularly corrosive. Clinitest tablets and disk batteries are also a source. Alkalies cause liquefactive necrosis, which is deeply penetrating. Symptoms include burning pain in the upper gastrointestinal tract, nausea, vomiting, and difficulty in swallowing and breathing. Examination reveals destruction and edema of the affected skin and mucous membranes and bloody vomitus and stools. X-ray may reveal the presence of disk batteries in the esophagus or lower gastrointestinal tract.

Treatment

A. Ingestion: Do *not* induce emesis. Dilute immediately with a glass of water. Some gastroenterologists recommend immediate gastric lavage after ingestion of liquid caustic substances to remove residual material.

Immediate endoscopy is recommended to evaluate the extent of damage. If x-ray reveals the location of ingested disk batteries in the esophagus, immediate endoscopic removal is mandatory.

The use of corticosteroids to prevent stricture formation is of no proved benefit and is definitely contraindicated if there is evidence of esophageal perforation.

B. Skin Contact: Wash with running water until the skin no longer feels soapy. Relieve pain and treat shock.

C. Eye Contact: Anesthetize the conjunctival and corneal surfaces with topical anesthetic. Irrigate with water or saline continuously for 20–30 minutes, holding the lids open. Check pH with pH test paper, and repeat irrigation, using 0.9% saline, for additional 30-minute periods until the pH is near 7.0. Check for corneal damage with fluorescein and slitlamp examination; consult an ophthalmologist for further treatment.

Anderson KD et al: A controlled trial of corticosteroids in children with corrosive injury of the esophagus. N Engl J Med 1990;323:637. (Randomized prospective study proving no benefit from steroids to reduce stricture formation.)

Wilson DA et al: Battery acid: An agent of attempted suicide in black South Africans. S Afr Med J 1995;85:529. (Case series of 27 patients; four required surgical intervention.)

AMPHETAMINES & COCAINE

Amphetamines and cocaine are widely abused for their euphorigenic and stimulant properties. Both drugs may be smoked, snorted, ingested, or injected.

The forms most commonly used for smoking are "ice" (amphetamine base) and "crack" or "freebase" (cocaine base). Amphetamines and cocaine produce central nervous system stimulation and a generalized increase in central and peripheral sympathetic activity. The toxic dose of each drug is highly variable and depends on the route of administration and individual tolerance. The onset of effects is most rapid after intravenous injection or smoking. Amphetamine derivatives and related drugs include methylenedioxymethamphetamine (MOMA, "ecstasy"), ephedrine ("herbal ecstasy"), and methcathinone ("cat").

Clinical Findings

Patients may present with anxiety, tremulousness, tachycardia, hypertension, diaphoresis, dilated pupils, agitation, muscular hyperactivity, and psychosis. Metabolic acidosis may occur. In severe intoxication, seizures and hyperthermia may occur. Sustained or severe hypertension may result in intracranial hemorrhage, aortic dissection, or myocardial infarction.

The diagnosis is supported by finding amphetamines, cocaine, or the cocaine metabolite benzoylecgonine in the urine. Blood screening is not sensitive enough to detect these drugs.

Treatment

A. Emergency and Supportive Measures: Maintain a patent airway and assist ventilation, if necessary. Treat coma or seizures as described at the beginning of this chapter. Rapidly lower the body temperature (see p 1469) in patients who are hyperthermic (40 °C). Treat agitation or psychosis with a benzodiazepine such as diazepam, 5–10 mg intravenously (repeated as needed up to 20 mg), or midazolam, 0.1–0.2 mg/kg intramuscularly.

For poisoning by ingestion, perform gastric lavage and administer activated charcoal, or administer activated charcoal alone without prior gut emptying (see p 1445). Do *not* induce emesis, because of the risk of seizures.

B. Specific Treatment: Treat hypertension with a vasodilator drug such as phentolamine (1–5 mg intravenously) or nifedipine (10–20 mg orally) or a combined α- and β-adrenergic blocker such as labetalol (10–20 mg intravenously). Do *not* administer a pure beta-blocker such as propranolol alone, as this may result in paradoxic worsening of the hypertension as a result of unopposed α-adrenergic effects.

Treat tachycardia or tachyarrhythmias with a short-acting beta-blocker such as esmolol (25–100 μg/kg/min by intravenous infusion).

Callawa CW, Clark RF: Hyperthermia in psychostimulant overdose. Ann Emerg Med 1994;24:68. (Hyperthermia is a life-threatening complication of psychostimulant overdose and may be related to intense central nervous system dopamine activity.)

Stevens DC et al: Acid-base abnormalities associated with cocaine toxicity in emergency department patients. J Toxicol Clin Toxicol 1994;32:31. (Severe metabolic acidosis, with serum pH as low as 6.4, occasionally occurs in patients with severe cocaine toxicity.)

ANTICOAGULANTS

Warfarin and related compounds (including ingredients of many commercial rodenticides) inhibit the clotting mechanism by blocking hepatic synthesis of vitamin K-dependent clotting factors.

Anticoagulants may cause hemoptysis, gross hematuria, bloody stools, hemorrhages into organs, widespread bruising, and bleeding into joint spaces. The prothrombin time is increased within 12–24 hours (peak 36–48 hours) after a single overdose. After ingestion of brodifacoum and indanedione rodenticides (so-called superwarfarins), inhibition of clotting factor synthesis may persist for several weeks or even months after a single dose.

Treatment

A. Emergency and Supportive Measures: Discontinue the drug at the first sign of gross bleeding, and determine the prothrombin time. If the patient has ingested an acute overdose, empty the stomach by emesis (at home) or lavage and administer activated charcoal (see p 1471).

B. Specific Treatment: Do not treat prophylactically—wait for the evidence of anticoagulation (elevated prothrombin time). If the prothrombin time is elevated, give phytonadione (vitamin K), 5–10 mg subcutaneously, and give fresh-frozen plasma as needed to rapidly correct the coagulation factor deficit if there is serious bleeding. If the patient is chronically anticoagulated and has strong medical indications for being maintained in that status (eg, prosthetic heart valve), give much smaller doses of vitamin K (1 mg) and fresh-frozen plasma (or both) to titrate to the desired prothrombin time.

If the patient has ingested brodifacoum or related super-rodenticides, prolonged observation (over weeks) and repeated administration of vitamin K may be required.

Sheen SR, Spiller HA: Symptomatic brodifacoum ingestion requiring high-dose phytonadione therapy. Vet Hum Toxicol 1994;36:216. (Case report describes vitamin K dose of up to 200 mg/d for 152 days.)

ANTICONVULSANTS
(Carbamazepine, Phenytoin, Valproic Acid)

These drugs are widely used in the management of seizure disorders. In addition, carbamazepine and valproic acid are increasingly used for treatment of mood disorders.

Phenytoin can be given orally or intravenously. Rapid intravenous injection of phenytoin can cause acute myocardial depression and cardiac arrest owing to the solvent propylene glycol; a newer form of phenytoin (fosphenytoin) is available that does not contain this diluent. Phenytoin intoxication can occur with only slightly increased doses because of the small toxic-therapeutic window. Phenytoin intoxication can also occur following acute intentional or accidental overdose. The overdose syndrome is usually mild even with high serum levels. The most common manifestations are ataxia, nystagmus, and drowsiness. Choreoathetoid movements have been described.

Carbamazepine was first used for the treatment of trigeminal neuralgia. It has since become a first-line agent for temporal lobe epilepsy and other seizure disorders. Intoxication causes drowsiness, stupor, and, with high levels, coma and seizures. Dilated pupils and tachycardia are common. Toxicity may be seen with serum levels greater than 20 mg/L, though severe poisoning is usually associated with concentrations greater than 30–40 mg/L. Because of erratic and slow absorption, intoxication may progress over several hours to days.

Valproic acid intoxication produces a unique syndrome consisting of hypernatremia (from the sodium component of the salt), metabolic acidosis, hypocalcemia, elevated serum ammonia, and mild liver aminotransferase elevation. Hypoglycemia may occur as a result of hepatic metabolic dysfunction. Coma with small pupils may be seen and can mimic opioid poisoning. Delayed sequelae include encephalopathy and cerebral edema.

Treatment

A. Emergency and Supportive Measures: For recent ingestions, give activated charcoal orally or by gastric tube. For large ingestions of carbamazepine or valproic acid—especially of sustained-release formulations—consider whole bowel irrigation (see p 1471). Multiple-dose activated charcoal may be beneficial in ensuring gut decontamination for large ingestions and may enhance elimination of absorbed drugs.

B. Specific Treatment: There are no antidotes. Naloxone was reported to have reversed valproic acid overdose in one anecdotal case. Consider hemodialysis (valproic acid) or hemoperfusion (carbamazepine) for massive intoxication (eg, carbamazepine levels > 100 mg/L or valproic acid poisoning with levels > 1000 mg/L).

Anderson GO et al: Life threatening intoxication with valproic acid. J Toxicol Clin Toxicol 1995;33:279.

Schmidt S et al: Signs and symptoms of carbamazepine overdose. J Neurol 1995;242:169.

ARSENIC

Arsenic is found in pesticides and industrial chemicals. Symptoms of poisoning usually appear within 1 hour after ingestion but may be delayed as long as 12 hours. They include abdominal pain, vomiting, watery diarrhea, and skeletal muscle cramps. Profound dehydration and shock may occur. In chronic poisoning, symptoms can be vague but often include those of peripheral sensory neuropathy. Urinary arsenic levels may be misleading and are falsely elevated after certain meals (eg, seafood) that contain large quantities of relatively nontoxic organic arsenic.

Treatment

A. Emergency Measures: Induce vomiting or perform gastric lavage, and administer 60–100 g of activated charcoal (see p 1471).

B. Antidote: For symptomatic patients or those with massive overdose, give dimercaprol injection (BAL), 10% solution in oil, 3–5 mg/kg dimercaprol intramuscularly every 4–6 hours for 2 days. The side effects include nausea, vomiting, headache, and hypertension. Follow dimercaprol with oral penicillamine, 100 mg/kg/d in four divided doses (maximum, 2 g/d), or succimer (DMSA), 10 mg/kg every 8 hours, for 1 week. Consult a medical toxicologist or regional poison control center (Table 39–1) for advice regarding chelation.

Kasarskis EJ et al: Arsenic poisoning in central Kentucky: A case report. Am J Ind Med 1993;24:723. (Case report and review of 21 cases over 20 years.)

Moore DF et al: Acute arsenic poisoning: Absence of polyneuropathy after treatment with 2,3-dimercaptopropanesulphonates. J Neurol Neurosurg Psychiatry 1994;57:1133. (Case report of two men treated successfully with DMPS, a compound similar to DMSA, after accidental arsenic trioxide ingestion.)

ATROPINE & ANTICHOLINERGICS

Atropine, scopolamine, belladonna, diphenoxylate with atropine, *Datura stramonium, Hyoscyamus niger,* some mushrooms, tricyclic antidepressants, and antihistamines are antimuscarinic agents with variable central nervous system effects. The patient complains of dryness of the mouth, thirst, difficulty in swallowing, and blurring of vision. The physical signs include dilated pupils, flushed skin, tachycardia, fever (although hypothermia has been reported), delirium, myoclonus, ileus, and flushed appearance. Antidepressants and antihistamines may induce convulsions.

Antihistamines are commonly available with or without prescription. Diphenhydramine commonly causes delirium, tachycardia, and seizures. Massive overdose may mimic tricyclic antidepressant poisoning. The newer nonsedating antihistamines terfenadine and astemizole have caused QT interval prolongation and torsades de pointes (atypical ventricular tachycardia).

Treatment

A. Emergency and Supportive Measures: Induce vomiting or perform gastric lavage, and administer activated charcoal (see p 1471). Do *not* induce emesis in patients who have ingested antidepressants, because seizures may occur abruptly. Tepid sponge baths and sedation are indicated to control high temperatures (see p 1469).

B. Specific Treatment: For pure atropine or related anticholinergic syndrome, if symptoms are severe (eg, hyperthermia or excessively rapid tachycardia), give physostigmine salicylate, 0.5–1 mg slowly intravenously over 5 minutes, with electrocardiographic monitoring, until symptoms are controlled. Bradyarrhythmias and convulsions are a hazard with physostigmine administration, and it should not be used in patients with tricyclic antidepressant overdose.

Christensen RC: Misdiagnosis of anticholinergic delirium as schizophrenic psychosis. Am J Emerg Med 1995; 13:117. (Case report of a 38-year-old man with episodes of agitation auditory and visual hallucinations following abuse of diphenhydramine.)

Coremans P et al: Anticholinergic intoxication with commercially available thorn apple tea. J Toxicol Clin Toxicol 1994;32:589. (Case report of two adolescents with acute psychosis and peripheral signs of anticholinergic intoxication after drinking tea made from *Datura stramonium*.)

BETA-ADRENERGIC BLOCKERS

There are a wide variety of β-adrenergic blocking drugs, with varying pharmacologic and pharmacokinetic properties (see Table 11–4). The most commonly used and most toxic beta-blocker is propranolol. Propranolol competitively blocks β_1 and β_2 adrenoceptors and also has direct membrane-depressant and central nervous system effects.

Clinical Findings

The most common findings with mild or moderate intoxication are hypotension and bradycardia. Cardiac depression from more severe poisoning is often unresponsive to conventional therapy with β-adrenergic stimulants such as dopamine and norepinephrine. In addition, with propranolol and other lipid-soluble drugs, seizures and coma may occur.

The diagnosis is based on typical clinical findings. Routine toxicology screening does not usually include beta-blockers.

Treatment

A. Emergency and Supportive Measures: Initially, treat bradycardia or heart block with at-

ropine (0.5–2 mg intravenously), isoproterenol (2–20 µg/min by intravenous infusion, titrated to the desired heart rate), or an external transcutaneous cardiac pacemaker. Specific antidotal treatment may be necessary (see below).

For ingested drugs, empty the stomach by gastric lavage and administer activated charcoal (see p 1471). Do *not* induce emesis because of the risk of seizures.

B. Specific Treatment: If the above measures are not successful in reversing bradycardia and hypotension, give glucagon, 5–10 mg intravenously, followed by an infusion of 1–5 mg/h. Glucagon is an inotropic agent that acts at a different receptor site and is therefore not affected by beta-blockade.

Kerns W 2nd, Kline J, Ford MD: Beta-blocker and calcium channel blocker toxicity. Emerg Med Clin North Am 1994;12:365. (Mechanism, diagnosis, and treatment, including use of glucagon.)

Kollef MH: Labetolol overdose successfully treated with amrinone and alpha-adrenergic receptor agonists. Chest 1994;105:626. (Case report of successful use of amrinone after failure of glucagon.)

CALCIUM ANTAGONISTS

Calcium antagonists used in the United States include verapamil, diltiazem, nifedipine, nicardipine, and nimodipine. These drugs share the ability to cause arteriolar vasodilation and depression of cardiac contractility, especially after acute overdose. Patients may present with bradycardia, AV nodal block, hypotension, or a combination of these effects. With severe poisoning, cardiac arrest may occur. The diagnosis is made clinically; these drugs are not included in routine toxicology screening.

Treatment

A. Emergency and Supportive Measures: Maintain a patent airway and assist ventilation, if necessary. Treat coma, hypotension, and seizures as described at the beginning of this chapter. Treat bradycardia with atropine (0.5–2 mg intravenously), isoproterenol (2–20 µg/min by intravenous infusion), or a transcutaneous or internal cardiac pacemaker.

For ingested drugs, administer activated charcoal (see p 1471). Because of the risk of hypotension and seizures, *do not* induce emesis.

B. Specific Treatment: If bradycardia and hypotension are not reversed with these measures, administer calcium chloride 10%, 10 mL intravenously, or calcium gluconate 10%, 20 mL intravenously. Calcium is most useful in reversing negative inotropic effects and is less effective for AV nodal blockade and bradycardia. The serum calcium should be raised by at least 2–3 mg/dL for maximum benefit. Epinephrine infusion (1–4 meq/min initially) and glucagon, 5–10 mg intravenously, have also been recommended.

Howarth DM et al: Calcium channel blocking drug overdose: An Australian series. Hum Exp Toxicol 1994;13:161. (Case series of 15 patients emphasizes early gastric decontamination, use of high-dose calcium, and inotropic support.)

CARBON MONOXIDE

Carbon monoxide is a colorless, odorless gas produced by the combustion of carbon-containing materials. Poisoning may occur as a result of suicidal or accidental exposure to automobile exhaust, smoke inhalation in a fire, or accidental exposure to an improperly vented gas heater or other appliance. Carbon monoxide avidly binds to hemoglobin, with an affinity approximately 250 times that of oxygen. This results in reduced oxygen-carrying capacity and altered delivery of oxygen to cells (see also Smoke Inhalation in Chapter 9).

Clinical Findings

At low carbon monoxide levels (carboxyhemoglobin saturation 10–20%), victims may have headache, dizziness, abdominal pain, and nausea. With higher levels, confusion, dyspnea, and syncope may occur. Hypotension, coma, and seizures are common with levels greater than 50–60%. Survivors of acute severe poisoning may develop permanent neurologic deficits. The fetus and newborn may be more susceptible because of high carbon monoxide affinity for fetal hemoglobin.

Carbon monoxide poisoning should be suspected in any person with severe headache or acutely altered mental status, especially in cold weather, when improper heating systems may have already been used. Diagnosis depends on specific measurement of the arterial or venous carboxyhemoglobin saturation, although the level may have declined if high-flow oxygen therapy has been administered. Routine arterial blood gas testing and pulse oximetry are not useful because they give falsely normal calculated oxyhemoglobin saturation determinations.

Treatment

A. Emergency and Supportive Measures: Maintain a patent airway and assist ventilation, if necessary. Remove the victim from exposure. Treat patients with coma, hypotension, or seizures, as described at the beginning of this chapter.

B. Specific Treatment: The half-life of the carboxyhemoglobin complex is about 4–5 hours in room air but is reduced dramatically by high concentrations of oxygen. Administer 100% oxygen by tight-fitting high-flow reservoir face mask or endotracheal tube. Hyperbaric oxygen (HBO) can provide 100% oxygen under higher than atmospheric pressures, further shortening the half-life; it may be useful if immediately available for patients with coma or seizures and in pregnant women, though controlled studies have failed to prove that HBO is superior to high-flow oxygen at normal pressure.

Seger D, Welch L: Carbon monoxide controversies: Neuropsychologic testing, mechanism of toxicity, and hyperbaric oxygen. Ann Emerg Med 1994;24:242. (Proposed mechanisms of carbon monoxide poisoning and pitfalls in the use of neuropsychiatric testing to evaluate outcome.)

Tribbles PM, Perrotta PL: Treatment of carbon monoxide poisoning: A critical review of human outcome studies comparing normobaric oxygen with hyperbaric oxygen. Ann Emerg Med 1994;24:269. (The authors review currently published studies and call for a properly designed, prospective, randomized, double-blind study to evaluate the effectiveness of hyperbaric oxygen therapy.)

CHEMICAL WARFARE AGENTS

Nerve agents used in chemical warfare work by cholinesterase inhibition and are most commonly organophosphates. Agents such as **tabun** (dimethylphosphoramidocyanidic acid ethyl ether) and **sarin** (methylphosphonofluoridic acid 1-methylethyl ester) are similar to insecticides such as malathion but are vastly more potent. They may be inhaled or absorbed through the skin. Systemic effects due to unopposed action of acetylcholine include miosis, salivation, abdominal cramps, diarrhea, and muscle paralysis producing respiratory arrest. Inhalation also produces severe bronchoconstriction and copious nasal and tracheobronchial secretions.

Treatment

A. Emergency and Supportive Measures: Perform thorough decontamination of exposed areas with repeated soap and shampoo washing. Personnel caring for such patients must wear protective clothing and gloves, since cutaneous absorption may occur through normal skin.

B. Specific Treatment: Give atropine in an initial dose of 2 mg intravenously, and repeat as needed to reverse signs of acetylcholine excess. (Some victims have required several hundred milligrams.) Treat also with the cholinesterase-reactivating agent pralidoxime, 1–2 g intravenously initially followed by 200–400 mg/h. United States military personnel in the Persian Gulf war were equipped with autoinjectable units containing 2 mg of atropine plus 600 mg of the cholinesterase-reactivating agent pralidoxime.

Okumura T et al: Report on 640 victims of the Tokyo subway sarin attack. Ann Emerg Med 1996;28:223.

CHLORINATED INSECTICIDES
(Chlorophenothane [DDT], Lindane, Toxaphene, Chlordane, Aldrin, Endrin)

Lindane (Kwell) and other chlorinated insecticides are central nervous system stimulants that can cause poisoning by ingestion, inhalation, or direct contact. The estimated lethal dose is about 20 g for DDT, 3 g for lindane, 2 g for toxaphene, 1 g for chlordane, and less than 1 g for endrin and aldrin. The manifestations of poisoning are nervous irritability, muscle twitching, convulsions, and coma. Arrhythmias may occur. Hepatic and renal damage are reported.

Treatment

Do *not* induce emesis, since seizures may occur abruptly. Perform lavage, and give activated charcoal (see p 1471). Repeat-dose activated charcoal may be effective for large ingestions. For convulsions, give diazepam, 5–10 mg slowly intravenously, or other anticonvulsants.

Perform thorough decontamination of exposed areas with repeated soap and shampoo washing. Personnel caring for such patients must be wear protective clothing and gloves, since cutaneous absorption may occur through normal skin.

Waller K et al: Seizures after eating a snack food contaminated with the pesticide endrin. West J Med 1992; 157:648. (Five patients who developed seizures after eating taquitos contaminated with this highly toxic insecticide. The source of contamination was not found.)

CLONIDINE & OTHER SYMPATHOLYTIC ANTIHYPERTENSIVES
(Clonidine, Methyldopa, Prazosin)

Overdosage with these agents causes bradycardia, hypotension, miosis, respiratory depression, and coma. (Hypertension occasionally occurs after clonidine overdosage, a result of peripheral alpha-adrenergic effects of this drug in high doses.) Symptoms are usually resolved in less than 24 hours, and deaths are rare. Similar symptoms may occur after ingestion of topical nasal decongestants chemically similar to clonidine (oxymetazoline, tetrahydrozoline, naphazoline).

Treatment
A. Emergency and Supportive Measures: Give activated charcoal and a cathartic (see p 1445). Maintain the airway and support respiration if necessary. Symptomatic treatment is usually sufficient even in massive overdose. Maintain blood pressure with intravenous fluids. Dopamine can also be used. Atropine is usually effective for bradycardia.
B. Specific Treatment: There is no specific antidote. Although tolazoline has been recommended

for clonidine overdose, its effect are unpredictable and it should not be used. Naloxone has been reported to be successful in a few anecdotal and poorly substantiated cases.

Vitezic D et al: Naphazoline nasal drops intoxication in children. Arh Hig Rada Toksikol 1994;45:25. (Case series of 11 children hospitalized with somnolence following nasal drop ingestion.)

COCAINE

See Amphetamines and Cocaine, above.

CYANIDE

Cyanide is a highly toxic chemical used widely in research and commercial laboratories and many industries. Its gaseous form, hydrogen cyanide, is an important component of smoke in fires. Cyanide-generating glycosides are also found in the pits of apricots and other related plants. Cyanide is generated by the breakdown of nitroprusside, and poisoning can result from rapid high-dose infusions. Cyanide is also formed by metabolism of acetonitrile, found in some over-the-counter fingernail glue removers. Cyanide is rapidly absorbed by inhalation, skin absorption, or ingestion. It disrupts cellular function by inhibiting cytochrome oxidase and preventing cellular oxygen utilization.

Clinical Findings

The onset of toxicity is nearly instantaneous after inhalation of hydrogen cyanide gas but may be delayed for minutes to hours after ingestion of cyanide salts or cyanogenic plants or chemicals. Symptoms of intoxication include headache, dizziness, nausea, abdominal pain, and anxiety, followed by confusion, syncope, shock, seizures, coma, and death. The odor of "bitter almonds" may be detected on the victim's breath or in vomitus, though this is not a reliable finding. The venous oxygen saturation may be elevated (> 90%) in severe poisonings because tissues have failed to take up arterial oxygen. There are no reliable rapid bedside laboratory tests for cyanide.

Treatment
A. Emergency and Supportive Measures: Remove the victim from exposure, taking care to avoid exposure to rescuers. For suspected cyanide poisoning due to nitroprusside infusion, stop or slow the rate of infusion. (Metabolic acidosis and other signs of cyanide poisoning usually clear rapidly.)

For cyanide ingestion, empty the stomach by gastric lavage with charcoal, or immediate oral administration of charcoal, or immediate emesis (if lavage or charcoal is not available) (see p 1471). Although charcoal has a low affinity for cyanide, the usual doses of 60–100 g are adequate to bind typically ingested lethal doses (100–200 mg).

B. Specific Treatment: In the United States, the cyanide antidote kit (Table 39–12) contains nitrites (to induce methemoglobinemia, which binds free cyanide) and thiosulfate (to promote conversion of cyanide to the less toxic thiocyanate). Administer amyl nitrite by crushing an ampule under the victim's nose or at the end of the endotracheal tube; and administer 3% sodium nitrite solution, 10 mL intravenously. *Caution:* Nitrites may induce hypotension and dangerous levels of methemoglobin. Also administer 25% sodium thiosulfate solution, 50 mL intravenously (12.5 g).

Yen D et al: The clinical experience of acute cyanide poisoning. Am J Emerg Med 1995;13:524. (Case series of 21 victims over a 10-year period.)

DIGITALIS & OTHER CARDIAC GLYCOSIDES

Cardiac glycosides are derived from a variety of plants and are widely used to treat heart failure and supraventricular arrhythmias. These drugs paralyze the Na^+-K^+ ATPase pump and have potent vagotonic effects. Intracellular effects include enhancement of calcium-dependent contractility and shortening of the action potential duration. Digoxin and ouabain are highly tissue-bound, but digitoxin has a volume of distribution of just 0.6 L/kg, making it the only cardiac glycoside accessible to enhanced removal procedures such as hemoperfusion or repeated doses of activated charcoal.

Clinical Findings

Intoxication may result from acute single exposure or chronic accidental overmedication. After acute overdosage, patients frequently develop nausea and vomiting, bradycardia, hyperkalemia, and atrioventricular block. Patients who develop toxicity gradu-

ally during chronic therapy are often hypokalemic and hypomagnesemic owing to concurrent diuretic treatment and more commonly present with ventricular arrhythmias (eg, ectopy, bidirectional ventricular tachycardia, or ventricular fibrillation).

Treatment

A. Emergency and Supportive Measures: Maintain a patent airway and assist ventilation, if necessary. Monitor potassium levels and cardiac rhythm closely. Treat ventricular arrhythmias initially with lidocaine (2–3 mg/kg intravenously) or phenytoin (10–15 mg/kg intravenously slowly over 30 minutes) and treat bradycardia initially with atropine (0.5–2 mg intravenously), isoproterenol (1–5 µg/min initially), or a transcutaneous external cardiac pacemaker.

After acute ingestion, perform gastric lavage and administer activated charcoal (see p 1445). Emesis is not recommended because it may enhance vagotonic effects such as bradycardia and AV block.

B. Specific Treatment: For patients with severe intoxication (eg, marked bradycardia or AV block unresponsive to atropine, or ventricular arrhythmias unresponsive to lidocaine or phenytoin), administer digoxin-specific antibodies (digoxin immune Fab [ovine]; Digibind). Estimation of the Digibind dose is based on the body burden of digoxin calculated from the ingested dose or the steady-state serum digoxin concentration:

1. From the ingested dose–Number of vials = approximately 1.5 × ingested dose (mg).

2. From the serum concentration–Number of vials = approximately serum digoxin (ng/mL) × body weight (kg) × 10^{-2}. After acute overdose, serum levels are falsely high before tissue distribution is complete, and overestimation of the Digibind dose is likely.

3. Empiric dosing of Digibind may be utilized if the patient's condition is relatively stable and an underlying condition (eg, atrial fibrillation) suggests a residual level of digitalis activity. Start with one or two vials and reassess the clinical condition after 20–30 minutes.

Note: After administration of Digibind, serum digoxin levels are falsely elevated.

Table 39–12. Currently available (prepackaged) cyanide antidotes.[1,2]

Antidote	How Supplied	Dose
Amyl nitrite	0.3 mL (aspirol inhalant)	Break 1–2 aspirols under patient's nose.
Sodium nitrite	3 g/dL (300 mg in 10 mL [vials])	6 mg/kg intravenously (0.2 mL/kg)
Sodium thiosulfate	25 g/dL (12.5 g in 50 mL [vials])	250 mg/kg intravenously (1 mL/kg)

[1]Reproduced, with permission, from Saunders CE, Ho MT (editors): *Current Emergency Diagnosis & Treatment*, 4th ed. Appleton & Lange, 1992.
[2]In USA, manufactured by Eli Lilly & Co.

Bosse GM, Pope TM: Recurrent digoxin overdose and treatment with digoxin-specific Fab antibody fragments. J Emerg Med 1994;12:179. (Case report of use of Fab in the same patient on three separate occasions without adverse effects.)

Deaths associated with a purported aphrodisiac: New York City February 1993–May 1995. MMWR Morb Mortal Wkly Rep 1995;44:853, 861. (Ingestion of a substance derived from the toad *Bufo bufo gargarizaus* and sold as a topical aphrodisiac caused deaths in four young men. Measurable levels of digoxin were found at autopsy.)

ETHANOL, BARBITURATES, BENZODIAZEPINES, & OTHER SEDATIVE-HYPNOTIC AGENTS

The group of agents known as sedative-hypnotic drugs includes a variety of products used for the treatment of anxiety, depression, insomnia, and epilepsy. Ethanol and other selected agents are also popular recreational drugs. All of these drugs depress the central nervous system reticular activating system, cerebral cortex, and cerebellum.

Clinical Findings

Mild intoxication produces euphoria, slurred speech, and ataxia. Ethanol intoxication may produce hypoglycemia, even at relatively low concentrations. With more severe intoxication, stupor, coma, and respiratory arrest may occur. Death or serious morbidity is usually the result of pulmonary aspiration of gastric contents. Bradycardia, hypotension, and hypothermia are common. Patients with massive intoxication may appear to be dead, with no reflex responses and even absent electroencephalographic activity. Diagnosis and assessment of severity of intoxication are usually based on clinical findings. Ethanol serum levels greater than 300 mg/dL (0.3 g/dL; 65 mmol/L) usually produce coma in persons who are not chronically abusing the drug, but regular users may remain awake at much higher levels. Phenobarbital levels greater than 80–100 mg/L usually cause coma.

Treatment

A. Emergency and Supportive Measures: Empty the stomach by emesis or gastric lavage and administer activated charcoal (see p 1471). Repeat-dose charcoal may enhance elimination of phenobarbital, and hemoperfusion may be necessary for patients with severe phenobarbital intoxication, but these procedures are not effective for most other drugs in this group.

B. Specific Treatment: Flumazenil is a benzodiazepine receptor-specific antagonist; it has no effect on ethanol, barbiturates, or other sedative-hypnotic agents. Flumazenil is given slowly intravenously, 0.2 mg over 30–60 seconds, repeated in 0.5 mg increments as needed up to a total dose of 3–5 mg. *Caution:* Flumazenil may induce seizures in patients with preexisting seizure disorder, benzodiazepine addiction, or concomitant tricyclic antidepressant overdose. If seizures occur, diazepam and other benzodiazepine anticonvulsants will not be effective. As with naloxone, the duration of action of flumazenil is short (2–3 hours) and resedation may occur, requiring repeated doses.

Hoffman RS et al: The poisoned patient with altered consciousness. Controversies in the use of a "coma cock-tail." JAMA 1995;274:562. (The authors downplay the use of flumazenil.)

GAMMA HYDROXYBUTYRATE

Gamma hydroxybutyrate has become a popular drug of abuse. It originated as a short-acting general anesthetic and is occasionally used in the treatment of narcolepsy. It gained popularity among bodybuilders for its alleged growth hormone stimulation and found its way into social settings, where it is consumed as a liquid. Its rapid onset leads to incapacitation and coma. Symptoms after ingestion include drowsiness and lethargy followed by coma with respiratory depression. Muscle twitching and seizures are sometimes observed. Recovery is usually rapid, with patients awakening within a few hours.

Treatment

For recent ingestions, give activated charcoal orally or by gastric tube. There is no specific treatment. Most patients recover rapidly with supportive care.

Ferrara SD et al: Fatality due to gamma-hydroxybutyric acid (GHB) and heroin intoxication. J Forensic Sci 1995;40:501. (Case report.)

Thomas G et al: Coma induced by abuse of gamma-hydroxybutyrate (GHB or liquid ecstasy). BMJ 1997; 314:35. (Case report.)

IRON

Iron is widely used therapeutically for the treatment of anemia and as a daily supplement in multiple vitamin preparations. Most children's preparations contain about 12–15 mg of elemental iron (as sulfate, gluconate, or fumarate salt) per dose, compared with 60–90 mg in most adult-strength preparations. Severe iron intoxications occur most often in children who ingest adult-strength preparations. Iron is corrosive to the gastrointestinal tract and, once absorbed, has depressant effects on the myocardium and on peripheral vascular resistance. Intracellular toxic effects of iron include disruption of Krebs cycle enzymes.

Clinical Findings

Ingestion of less than 30 mg/kg of elemental iron usually produces only mild gastrointestinal upset. Ingestion of more than 40–60 mg/kg may cause vomiting (sometimes with hematemesis), diarrhea, hypotension, and acidosis. Death may occur as a result of profound hypotension due to massive fluid losses and bleeding, metabolic acidosis, peritonitis from intestinal perforation, or sepsis. Fulminant hepatic failure may occur. Survivors of the acute ingestion may suffer permanent gastrointestinal scarring.

Serum iron levels greater than 350–500 µg/dL are considered toxic, and levels over 1000 µg/dL are usually associated with severe poisoning. A plain abdominal x-ray may reveal radiopaque tablets.

Treatment

A. Emergency and Supportive Measures: Maintain a patent airway and assist ventilation if necessary. Treat hypotension aggressively with intravenous crystalloid solutions (0.9% saline or lactated Ringer's solution). Fluid losses may be massive owing to vomiting and diarrhea as well as third-spacing into injured intestine.

Perform whole bowel irrigation to remove unabsorbed pills from the intestinal tract (see p 1471). Activated charcoal is not effective but may be used if other ingestants are suspected.

B. Specific Treatment: Deferoxamine is a selective iron chelator. It may be given intramuscularly or intravenously but is not useful as an oral binding agent. For patients with established manifestations of toxicity—and particularly those with markedly elevated serum iron levels (eg, greater than 500–600 µg/dL)—administer 10–15 mg/kg/h by constant intravenous infusion; higher doses (up to 40–50 mg/kg/h) have been used in massive poisonings. Hypotension may occur. The presence of iron-deferoxamine complex in the urine may give it a "vin rosé" appearance. Deferoxamine is safe for use in pregnant women with acute iron overdose. Prolonged infusion of deferoxamine (> 36–48 hours) has been associated with development of ARDS—the mechanism is not known.

Jackson TW et al: The effect of oral deferoxamine on iron absorption in humans. J Toxicol Clin Toxicol 1995;33:325. (Oral deferoxamine was not effective in reducing iron absorption after a simulated overdose in volunteers.)

Mills KE, Curry SC: Acute iron poisoning. Emerg Med Clin North Am 1994;12:397. (Pathophysiology and treatment.)

ISONIAZID

Isoniazid (INH) is an antibacterial drug used mainly in the treatment and prevention of tuberculosis. It may cause hepatitis in certain patients with chronic use. It produces acute toxic effects by competing with pyridoxal 5-phosphate, resulting in lowered brain γ-aminobutyric acid (GABA) levels. Acute ingestion of as little as 1.5–2 g of isoniazid can cause toxicity, and severe poisoning is likely to occur after ingestion of more than 80–100 mg/kg.

Clinical Findings

Confusion, slurred speech, and seizures may occur abruptly after acute overdose. Severe lactic acidosis—out of proportion to the severity of seizures—is probably due to inhibited metabolism of lactate.

Diagnosis is based on a history of ingestion and the presence of severe acidosis associated with seizures. Isoniazid is not usually included in routine toxicologic screening, and serum levels are not readily available.

Treatment

A. Emergency and Supportive Measures: Seizures may require higher doses of diazepam (15–20 mg intravenously) or administration of pyridoxine as antidote (see below).

Empty the stomach by gastric lavage and administer activated charcoal (see p 1471). Do *not* induce emesis, because of the risk of abrupt onset of seizures.

B. Specific Treatment: Pyridoxine (vitamin B_6) is a specific antagonist of the acute toxic effects of isoniazid and is usually successful in controlling convulsions that do not respond to diazepam. Give 5 g intravenously over 1–2 minutes or, if the amount ingested is known, give a gram-for-gram equivalent amount of pyridoxine.

Alvarez FG et al: Isoniazid overdose: Four case reports and a review of the literature. Intens Care Med 1995;21:641. (Isoniazid overdose should be suspected in any patient presenting with seizures and metabolic acidosis.)

LEAD

Lead is used in a variety of industrial and commercial products, such as storage batteries, solders, paints, pottery, plumbing, and gasoline and is found in some traditional ethnic medicines. Lead toxicity usually results from chronic repeated exposure and is rare after a single ingestion. Lead produces a variety of adverse effects on cellular function and primarily affects the nervous system, gastrointestinal tract, and hematopoietic system.

Clinical Findings

Lead poisoning often goes undiagnosed initially because presenting symptoms and signs are nonspecific and exposure is not suspected. Common symptoms include colicky abdominal pain, constipation, headache, and irritability. Severe poisoning may cause coma and convulsions. Chronic intoxication can cause learning disorders (in children) and motor neuropathy (eg, wrist drop).

Diagnosis is based on measurement of the blood lead level. Whole blood lead levels less than 10 µg/dL are usually considered nontoxic. Levels between 10 and 25 µg/dL have been associated with impaired neurobehavioral development in children. Levels of 25–50 µg/dL may be associated with headache, irritability, and subclinical neuropathy. Levels of 50–70 µg/dL are associated with moderate toxicity, and levels greater than 70–100 µg/dL are often associated with severe poisoning. Other laboratory findings of lead poisoning include microcytic anemia with basophilic stippling and elevated free erythrocyte protoporphyrin.

Treatment

A. Emergency and Supportive Measures:

For patients with encephalopathy, maintain a patent airway and treat coma and convulsions as described at the beginning of this chapter.

For recent acute ingestion, give activated charcoal and a cathartic (see p 1471). If a large lead-containing object (eg, fishing weight) is still visible in the stomach on abdominal x-ray, repeated cathartics, whole bowel irrigation, endoscopy, or even surgical removal may be necessary to prevent subacute lead poisoning. (The acidic gastric contents may corrode the metal surface, enhancing lead absorption. Once the object passes into the small intestine, the risk of toxicity declines.)

Conduct an investigation into the source of the lead exposure. Workers with a single lead level greater than 60 μg/dL (or three successive monthly levels greater than 50 μg/dL) must by federal law be removed from the site of exposure. Contact the regional office of the United States Occupational Safety and Health Administration (OSHA). Several states mandate reporting of cases of confirmed lead poisoning.

B. Specific Treatment:
The indications for chelation depend on the blood lead level and the patient's clinical state. A medical toxicologist or regional poison control center (Table 39–1) should be consulted for advice about selection and use of these antidotes.

1. Severe toxicity–Patients with severe intoxication (encephalopathy or levels greater than 70–100 μg/dL) should receive edetate calcium disodium (EDTA), 1500 mg/m^2/kg/d (approximately 50 mg/kg/d) in four to six divided doses or as a continuous intravenous infusion. Some clinicians also add dimercaprol (BAL), 4–5 mg/kg intramuscularly every 4 hours for 5 days.

2. Less severe toxicity–Patients with less severe symptoms and asymptomatic patients with blood lead levels between 55 and 69 μg/dL may be treated with edetate calcium disodium alone in dosages as above. A new chelator, succimer (dimercaptosuccinic acid, DMSA), is now available for oral use in patients with mild to moderate intoxication. The usual dose is 10 mg/kg orally every 8 hours for 5 days, then every 12 hours for 2 weeks.

Note: It is impermissible under the law to treat asymptomatic workers with elevated levels in order to keep their levels under 50 μg/dL rather than remove them from the exposure.

Landrigan PJ, Todd AC: Lead poisoning. West J Med 1994;161:153. (Review.)

Lohiya GS, Lohiya S: Lead poisoning in a radiator repairer.

West J Med 1995;162:160. (Case report illustrates continued lack of compliance with workplace exposure prevention efforts.)

LSD & OTHER HALLUCINOGENS

A variety of substances—ranging from naturally occurring plants and mushrooms to synthetic substances such as phencyclidine (PCP), toluene and other solvents, and LSD—are abused for their hallucinogenic properties. The mechanism of toxicity and the clinical effects vary for each substance.

Many hallucinogenic plants and mushrooms produce anticholinergic delirium (see p 1452), with flushed skin, dry mucous membranes, dilated pupils, tachycardia, and urinary retention. Some plants and mushrooms may contain hallucinogenic indoles such as mescaline and lysergic acid diethylamide (LSD), which typically cause marked visual hallucinations and perceptual distortion, widely dilated pupils, and mild tachycardia. Phencyclidine (PCP), a dissociative anesthetic agent similar to ketamine, can produce fluctuating delirium and coma, often associated with vertical and horizontal nystagmus. Toluene and other hydrocarbon solvents (butane, trichloroethylene, "chemo," etc) cause euphoria and delirium and may sensitize the myocardium to the effects of catecholamines, leading to fatal dysrhythmias.

Treatment

A. Emergency and Supportive Measures:
Maintain a patent airway and assist respirations if necessary. Treat coma, hyperthermia, and seizures as outlined at the beginning of this chapter. For recent ingestions, give activated charcoal orally or by gastric tube.

B. Specific Treatment:
Patients with anticholinergic delirium may benefit from a dose of physostigmine (see p 1479). However, this drug should not be used if poisoning by tricyclic antidepressants is suspected. Dysphoria, agitation, and psychosis associated with LSD or mescaline intoxication may respond to benzodiazepines or haloperidol. Monitor patients who have sniffed solvents for cardiac dysrhythmias (most commonly premature ventricular contractions, ventricular tachycardia, ventricular fibrillation); treatment with beta-blockers such as propranolol or esmolol may be more effective than lidocaine.

Christensen RC: Misdiagnosis of anticholinergic delirium as schizophrenic psychosis. Am J Emerg Med 1995; 13:117. (Case report.)

MERCURY

Acute mercury poisoning usually occurs by ingestion of inorganic mercuric salts or inhalation of metallic mercury vapor. Ingestion of the mercuric salts causes a metallic taste, salivation, thirst, a burning sensation in the throat, discoloration and edema of oral mucous membranes, abdominal pain, vomiting, bloody diarrhea, and shock. Direct nephrotoxicity causes acute renal failure. Inhalation of high concentrations of metallic mercury vapor may cause acute fulminant chemical pneumonia. Chronic mercury poisoning causes weakness, ataxia, intention tremors, irritability, and depression. Exposure to alkyl (organic) mercury derivatives from contaminated fish or fungicides used on seeds has caused ataxia, tremors, convulsions, and catastrophic birth defects.

Treatment

A. Acute Poisoning: There is no effective specific treatment for mercury vapor pneumonitis. Remove ingested mercuric salts by emesis and lavage, and administer activated charcoal and a cathartic (see p 1471). For acute ingestion of mercuric salts, give dimercaprol (BAL) at once, as for arsenic poisoning. Unless the patient has severe gastroenteritis, consider succimer (DMSA), 10 mg/kg orally every 8 hours for 5 days and then every 12 hours for 2 weeks. Maintain urine output. Treat oliguria and anuria if they occur.

B. Chronic Poisoning: Remove from exposure. Neurologic toxicity is not considered reversible with chelation, though some authors recommend a trial of succimer.

Malecki JM, Hopkins R: Mercury exposure in a residential community. MMWR Morb Mortal Wkly Rep 1995; 44:436. (Report of a large-scale elemental mercury exposure resulting in evacuation of 86 persons.)
Schwartz JG, Snider TE, Moniel MM: Toxicity of a family from vacuumed mercury. Am J Emerg Med 1992;10: 258. (Poisoning resulted from inhalation of vaporized liquid mercury due to vacuuming.)

METHANOL & ETHYLENE GLYCOL

Methanol (wood alcohol) is commonly found in a variety of products, including solvents, duplicating fluids, record cleaning solutions, and paint removers. It is sometimes ingested intentionally by alcoholics as a substitute for ethanol and may also be found as a contaminant in bootleg whiskey. Ethylene glycol is the major constituent in most antifreeze compounds. The toxicity of both agents is caused by metabolism to highly toxic organic acids—methanol to formic acid; ethylene glycol to glycolic and oxalic acids.

Clinical Findings

Shortly after ingestion of either of these agents, patients usually appear "drunk." The serum osmolality (measured with the freezing point device) is usually elevated, but acidosis is often absent early. After several hours, metabolism to toxic organic acids leads to a severe anion gap metabolic acidosis, tachypnea, confusion, convulsions, and coma. Methanol intoxication frequently causes visual disturbances, while ethylene glycol often produces oxalate crystalluria and renal failure.

Treatment

A. Emergency and Supportive Measures: For patients presenting within 30–60 minutes after ingestion, empty the stomach by emesis or gastric lavage and administer activated charcoal (see p 1471). (*Note:* Charcoal is not very effective.)

B. Specific Treatment: Patients with significant toxicity (manifested by severe acidosis, altered mental status, serum methanol or ethylene glycol level > 50 mg/dL, or significant osmolar gap) should undergo hemodialysis as soon as possible to remove the parent compound and the toxic metabolites.

Ethanol blocks metabolism of the parent compounds by competing for the enzyme alcohol dehydrogenase. The desired serum ethanol concentration is 100 mg/dL. To achieve this, administer a loading dose of approximately 750 mg/kg orally or in a dilute intravenous solution (available from the pharmacy in 5% and 10% solution), and then provide a maintenance infusion of 100–150 mg/kg/h. The infusion will have to be increased to about 175–250 mg/kg/h during hemodialysis to replace dialysis elimination of ethanol.

Hanif M et al: Fatal renal failure caused by diethylene glycol in paracetamol elixir: The Bangladesh epidemic. BMJ 1995;311:88. (Use of this glycol in a pediatric acetaminophen elixir resulted in an epidemic of renal failure.)
Palatwick W et al: Methanol half-life during ethanol administration. Ann Emerg Med 1995;25:202. (The average elimination half-life of methanol during ethanol administration was 43 hours, with a range of 30–52 hours. The authors advise hemodialysis to enhance methanol elimination.)

METHEMOGLOBINEMIA-INDUCING AGENTS

A large number of chemical agents are capable of oxidizing ferrous hemoglobin to its ferric state (methemoglobin), a form that cannot carry oxygen. Drugs and chemicals known to cause methemoglobinemia include benzocaine (a local anesthetic), aniline, nitrites, nitrogen oxide gases, nitrobenzene, dapsone, pyridium, and many others. Dapsone has a long elimination half-life and may produce prolonged or recurrent methemoglobinemia after initial treatment.

Clinical Findings

Methemoglobinemia reduces oxygen-carrying capacity and may cause dizziness, nausea, headache dyspnea, confusion, seizures, and coma. The severity of symptoms depends on the percentage of hemoglobin oxidized to methemoglobin; severe poisoning is usually present with methemoglobin fractions of greater than 40–50%. Even at low levels (15–20%), victims appear cyanotic because of the "chocolate brown" color of methemoglobin, but they have normal PO_2 results on arterial blood gas determinations. Pulse oximetry gives inaccurate oxygen saturation measurements. Severe metabolic acidosis may be present. Hemolysis may occur, especially in patients susceptible to oxidant stress (ie, those with glucose-6-phosphate dehydrogenase deficiency).

Treatment

A. Emergency and Supportive Measures: High-flow oxygen is given. If the causative agent was recently ingested, empty the stomach by gastric lavage and administer activated charcoal (see p 1471). For dapsone ingestion, give repeat-dose activated charcoal to enhance dapsone elimination (see p 1472).

B. Specific Treatment: Methylene blue enhances the conversion of methemoglobin to hemoglobin by increasing the activity of the enzyme methemoglobin reductase. For symptomatic patients, administer 1–2 mg/kg (0.1–0.2 mL/kg of 1% solution) intravenously. The dose may be repeated once in 15–20 minutes if necessary. Patients with hereditary methemoglobin reductase deficiency or glucose-6-phosphate dehydrogenase deficiency may not respond to methylene blue treatment.

McGoldrick MD, Bailie GR: Severe accidental dapsone overdose. Am J Emerg Med 1995;13:414. (Case report.)

Truman TL, Dallessio JJ, Weibley RE: Life-threatening Pyridium-Plus intoxication: A case report. Pediatr Emerg Care 1995;11:103.

MONOAMINE OXIDASE INHIBITORS (Isocarboxazid, Phenelzine)

Overdoses cause ataxia, excitement, hypertension, and tachycardia, followed several hours later by hypotension, convulsions, and hyperthermia.

Ingestion of tyramine-containing foods may cause a severe hypertensive reaction. These foods include aged cheese and red wines. Hypertensive reactions may also occur with any sympathomimetic drug. Severe or fatal hyperthermia (serotonin syndrome) may occur if patients receiving monoamine oxidase inhibitors are given meperidine, fluoxetine, paroxetine, fluvoxamine, venlafaxine, tryptophan, dextromethorphan, or other serotonin-enhancing drugs. This reaction can also occur with the newer selective MAO inhibitor moclobemide.

Treatment

Remove ingested drug by gastric lavage, and administer activated charcoal and a cathartic (see p 1471). Treat severe hypertension with nitroprusside, phentolamine, or other rapid-acting vasodilators (see p 1468). Treat hypotension with fluids and positioning, but avoid use of pressor agents. Observe patients for at least 24 hours, since hyperthermic reactions may be delayed. Treat hyperthermia with aggressive cooling; neuromuscular paralysis may be required (see p 1469).

Power BM et al: Fatal serotonin syndrome following a combined overdose of moclobemide, clomipramine, and fluoxetine. Anaesth Intensive Care 1995;23:499. (Case report.)

Sporer KA: The serotonin syndrome: Implicated drugs, pathophysiology, and management. Drug Safety 1995;13:94. (Review.)

MUSHROOMS

There are thousands of mushroom species that cause a variety of toxic effects. The most dangerous species of mushrooms are *Amanita phalloides, Amanita verna, Amanita virosa, Gyromitra esculenta,* and the *Galerina* species, all of which contain amatoxin, a potent cytotoxin. Ingestion of part of one mushroom of a dangerous species may be sufficient to cause death.

The pathologic finding in fatalities from amatoxin-containing mushroom poisoning is acute massive necrosis of the liver, kidneys, and skeletal muscles.

Clinical Findings
(Table 39–13)

A. Symptoms and Signs:

1. Amatoxin-type cyclopeptides–(*Amanita phalloides, Amanita verna, Amanita virosa,* and *Galerina* species.) After a latent interval of 8–12 hours, severe abdominal cramps and vomiting begin and progress to profuse diarrhea, followed by hepatic necrosis, hepatic encephalopathy, and frequently renal failure. The fatality rate is about 20%. Cooking the mushrooms does not prevent poisoning.

2. Gyromitrin type–(*Gyromitra* and *Helvella* species.) Toxicity is more common following ingestion of uncooked mushrooms. Vomiting, diarrhea, hepatic necrosis, convulsions, coma, and hemolysis may occur after a latent period of 8–12 hours. The fatality rate is probably less than 10%.

3. Muscarinic type–(*Inocybe* and *Clitocybe* species.) Vomiting, diarrhea, bradycardia, hypotension, salivation, miosis, bronchospasm, and lacrimation occur shortly after ingestion. Cardiac arrhythmias may occur. Fatalities are rare.

4. Anticholinergic type–(Eg, *Amanita muscaria, Amanita pantherina.*) This type causes a variety of symptoms that may be atropine-like, including excitement, delirium, flushed skin, dilated pupils,

Table 39–13. Poisonous mushrooms.

Toxin	Genus	Symptoms and Signs	Onset	Treatment
Amanitin	Amanita (A phalloides, A verna, A virosa)	Severe gastroenteritis, followed by delayed hepatic and renal failure after 48–72 hours	6–24 hours	Supportive. Correct dehydration. Give repeated doses of activated charcoal orally. Penicillin, thioctic acid, and silibinin are unproved antidotes.
Muscarine	Inocybe, Clitocybe	Muscarinic (salivation, miosis, bradycardia, diarrhea)	30–60 minutes	Supportive. Give atropine, 0.5–2 mg intravenously, for severe cholinergic symptoms and signs.
Ibotenic acid, muscimol	Amanita muscaria ("fly agaric")	Anticholinergic (mydriasis, tachycardia, hyperpyrexia, delirium)	30–60 minutes	Supportive. Give physostigmine, 0.5–2 mg intravenously, for severe anticholinergic symptoms and signs.
Coprine	Coprinus	Disulfiram-like effect occurs with ingestion of ethanol	30–60 minutes	Supportive. Abstain from ethanol for 3–4 days.
Monomethyl-hydrazine	Gyromitra	Gastroenteritis; occasionally hemolysis, hepatic and renal failure	6–12 hours	Supportive. Correct dehydration. Pyridoxine, 2.5 mg/kg intravenously, may be helpful.
Orellanine	Cortinarius	Nausea, vomiting; renal failure after 1–3 weeks	2–14 days	Supportive.
Psilocybin	Psilocybe	Hallucinations	15–30 minutes	Supportive.
Gastrointestinal irritants	Many species	Nausea and vomiting, diarrhea	½–2 hours	Supportive. Correct dehydration.

and muscular jerking tremors, beginning 1–2 hours after ingestion. Fatalities are rare.

5. Gastrointestinal irritant type–(Eg, *Boletus, Cantharellus.*) Nausea, vomiting, and diarrhea occur shortly after ingestion. Fatalities are rare.

6. Disulfiram–(*Coprinus* species.) Disulfiram-like sensitivity to alcohol may persist for several days. Toxicity is characterized by flushing, hypotension, and vomiting after coingestion of alcohol.

7. Hallucinogenic–(*Psilocybe* and *Panaeolus* species.) Mydriasis, nausea and vomiting, and intense visual hallucinations occur 1–2 hours after ingestion. Fatalities are rare.

8. *Cortinarius orellanus*–This mushroom may cause acute renal failure due to tubulointerstitial nephritis.

Treatment

A. Emergency Measures: After the onset of symptoms, efforts to remove the toxic agent are probably useless, especially in cases of amatoxin or gyromitrin poisoning, where there is usually a delay of 12 hours or more before symptoms occur and patients seek medical attention. However, induction of vomiting is recommended for any recent ingestion of an unidentified or potentially toxic mushroom. Activated charcoal and a cathartic should also be given (see p 1471).

B. General Measures:

1. Amatoxin-type cyclopeptides–A variety of unproved antidotes (eg, thioctic acid, silibinin, penicillin, corticosteroids) have been suggested for amatoxin-type mushroom poisoning, but experimental results are equivocal. Aggressive fluid replacement for diarrhea and intensive supportive care for hepatic failure are the mainstays of treatment.

Interruption of enterohepatic circulation of the amatoxin by the administration of activated charcoal and laxatives may be of value. However, by the time this method is employed, most of the amatoxin has already caused cellular damage and has already been excreted. Charcoal hemoperfusion has been recommended but is of unproved value.

Liver transplant may be the only hope for survival in gravely ill patients—contact a liver transplant center early.

2. Gyromitrin type–For gyromitrin poisoning, give pyridoxine, 25 mg/kg intravenously.

3. Muscarinic type–For mushrooms producing predominantly muscarinic-cholinergic symptoms, give atropine, 0.005–0.01 mg/kg intravenously, and repeat as needed.

4. Anticholinergic type–For anticholinergic type, physostigmine, 0.5–1 mg intravenously, may calm extremely agitated patients and reverse peripheral anticholinergic manifestations, but it may also cause bradycardia, asystole, and seizures.

5. Gastrointestinal irritant type–Treat with antiemetics and intravenous or oral fluids.

6. Disulfiram type–For *Coprinus* ingestion

avoid alcohol. Treat alcohol reaction with fluids and supine position.

7. Hallucinogenic type–Provide a quiet, supportive atmosphere. Diazepam or haloperidol may be used for sedation.

8. *Cortinarius*–Provide supportive care and hemodialysis as needed for renal failure.

Feinfeld DA et al: Poisoning by amatoxin-containing mushrooms in suburban New York: Report of four cases. J Toxicol Clin Toxicol 1994;32:715. (Case series. The authors advise charcoal hemoperfusion, though this treatment is not of proved benefit.)

Scheulerein C et al: *Amanita phalloides* intoxications in a family of Russian immigrants. Gastroenterol 1994; 32:399. (Three patients developed liver failure—one of them required liver transplantation on day 4; the others recovered.)

OPIOIDS
(Morphine, Heroin, Codeine, Propoxyphene, etc)

Prescription and illicit opioids are popular drugs of abuse and the cause of frequent hospitalizations for overdose. These drugs have widely varying potencies and durations of action; for example, some of the illicit fentanyl derivatives are up to 2000 times more potent than morphine. All of these agents decrease central nervous system activity and sympathetic outflow by acting on opiate receptors in the brain.

Clinical Findings

Mild intoxication is characterized by euphoria, drowsiness, and constricted pupils. More severe intoxication may cause hypotension, bradycardia, hypothermia, coma, and respiratory arrest. Pulmonary edema may occur. Death is usually due to apnea or pulmonary aspiration of gastric contents. Propoxyphene may cause seizures and prolongation of the QRS interval. While the duration of effect for heroin is usually 3–5 hours, methadone intoxication may last for 48–72 hours or longer. Most opioids, with the exception of illicit newer fentanyl derivatives, are detectable on urine toxicology screening.

Treatment

A. Emergency and Supportive Measures: If the patient arrives for medical care shortly after ingestion, empty the stomach by emesis or gastric lavage and administer activated charcoal (see p 1471).

B. Specific Treatment: Naloxone is a specific opioid antagonist that can rapidly reverse signs of narcotic intoxication. Although it is structurally related to the opioids, it has no agonist effects of its own. Administer 0.4–2 mg intravenously, and repeat as needed to awaken the patient and maintain airway protective reflexes and spontaneous breathing. Very large doses (10–20 mg) may be required for patients intoxicated by some opioids (eg, propoxyphene, codeine, fentanyl derivatives). **Caution:** The duration of effect of naloxone is only about 2–3 hours; repeated doses may be necessary for patients intoxicated by long-acting drugs such as methadone. Continuous observation for at least 3 hours after the last naloxone dose is mandatory.

Leo PJ et al: Heroin body packing. J Accid Emerg Med 1995;12:43. (Ingestion of heroin-filled condoms for purposes of smuggling can lead to intoxication—sometimes fatal—if one or more of the containers ruptures.)

Stork CM et al: Propoxyphene-induced wide QRS complex dysrhythmia responsive to sodium bicarbonate: A case report. J Toxicol Clin Toxicol 1995;33:179. (Suggests propoxyphene may have membrane-stabilizing effects similar to those of tricyclic antidepressants.)

PARAQUAT

Paraquat is used as an herbicide. Concentrated solutions of paraquat are highly corrosive to the oropharynx, esophagus, and stomach. The fatal dose after absorption may be as small as 4 mg/kg. If ingestion of paraquat is not rapidly fatal because of its corrosive effects, the herbicide may cause progressive pulmonary fibrosis, with death ensuing after 2–3 weeks. Patients with plasma paraquat levels above 2 mg/L at 6 hours or 0.2 mg/L at 24 hours are likely to die.

Treatment

Remove ingested paraquat by immediate induced emesis, or by gastric lavage if the patient is already in a health care facility. Clay (bentonite or fuller's earth) and activated charcoal are effective adsorbents. Administer repeated doses of 60 g of activated charcoal by gastric tube every 2 hours for at least three or four doses. Charcoal hemoperfusion, 8 hours per day for 2–3 weeks, has been anecdotally reported to be lifesaving. Supplemental oxygen should be withheld unless the P_{O_2} is less than 70 mm Hg because oxygen may contribute to the pulmonary damage, which is mediated through lipid peroxidation. For further information and for rapid determination of paraquat levels, call the nearest regional poison center or ICI America Inc (800-327-8633).

Suzuki K et al: Effect of aggressive hemoperfusion on the clinical course of patients with paraquat poisoning. Hum Exp Toxicol 1993;12:323. (Aggressive hemoperfusion—10 hours or more during the first 24 hours—has been advocated to remove the maximum possible amount of paraquat. However, the authors found no improvement in overall mortality data compared with conventional hemoperfusion.)

PESTICIDES: CHOLINESTERASE INHIBITORS (Organophosphates: Parathion, Malathion, etc; Carbamates: Carbaryl, Aldicarb, etc)

Organophosphate and carbamate insecticides are widely used in commercial agriculture and home gardening and have largely replaced older, more environmentally persistent organochlorine compounds such as DDT and chlordane. The organophosphates and carbamates—also called anticholinesterases because they inhibit the enzyme acetylcholinesterase—cause an increase in acetylcholine activity at nicotinic and muscarinic receptors and in the central nervous system. There are a variety of chemical agents in this group, with widely varying potencies. Most of them are poorly water-soluble and are formulated with an aromatic hydrocarbon solvent such as xylene. Most of them are well absorbed through intact skin. Most chemical warfare "nerve agents" (see p 1454) are organophosphates.

Clinical Findings

Inhibition of cholinesterase results in abdominal cramps, diarrhea, vomiting, excessive salivation, sweating, lacrimation, miosis (constricted pupils), wheezing and bronchorrhea, seizures, and skeletal muscle weakness. Initial tachycardia is usually followed by bradycardia. Profound skeletal muscle weakness, aggravated by excessive bronchial secretions and wheezing, may result in respiratory arrest and death. Signs and symptoms of poisoning may persist or recur over several days, especially with highly lipid-soluble agents such as fenthion.

The diagnosis is suspected in patients who present with miosis, sweating, and hyperperistalsis. Serum and red blood cell cholinesterase activity can be measured in the laboratory and is usually depressed at least 50% below baseline in those victims who have severe intoxication.

Treatment

A. Emergency and Supportive Measures: If the agent was recently ingested, empty the stomach by gastric lavage and administer activated charcoal (see p 1471). Do not induce emesis because of the risk of abrupt onset of seizures. If the agent is on the victim's skin or hair, wash repeatedly with soap or shampoo and water. Providers must take care to avoid skin exposure by wearing gloves and waterproof aprons.

B. Specific Treatment: Atropine reverses excessive muscarinic stimulation and is effective for treatment of salivation, wheezing, abdominal cramping, and sweating. However, it does not interact with nicotinic receptors at autonomic ganglia and at the neuromuscular junction and has no effect on muscle weakness. Administer 2 mg intravenously, and give repeated doses as needed to dry bronchial secretions and decrease wheezing; as much as several hundred milligrams of atropine have been given to treat severe poisoning.

Pralidoxime (2-PAM, Protopam) is a specific antidote that reverses organophosphate binding to the cholinesterase enzyme; therefore, it is effective at the neuromuscular junction as well as other nicotinic and muscarinic sites. It should be started as soon as possible, to prevent permanent binding of the organophosphate to cholinesterase. Administer 1–2 g intravenously, and begin a continuous infusion (200–400 mg/h). Constant infusion is more effective because of the short duration of action of single doses. Continue to give pralidoxime as long as there is any evidence of acetylcholine excess. Pralidoxime is of questionable benefit for carbamate poisoning, because carbamates have only a transitory effect on the cholinesterase enzyme.

Bardin PG et al: Organophosphate and carbamate poisoning. Arch Intern Med 1994;154:1433.

PETROLEUM DISTILLATES & SOLVENTS

Petroleum distillate toxicity may occur from inhalation or as a result of pulmonary aspiration during or after ingestion. Acute manifestations of aspiration pneumonitis are vomiting, coughing, and bronchopneumonia. Some hydrocarbons—ie, those with aromatic or halogenated subunits—can also cause severe systemic poisoning after oral ingestion (Table 39–14). Hydrocarbons can also cause systemic intoxication by inhalation. Vertigo, muscular incoordination, irregular pulse, myoclonus, and convulsions occur with serious poisoning and may be due to hypoxemia or the systemic effects of the agents. Chlorinated and fluorinated hydrocarbons (trichloroethylene, freons, etc) and many other hydrocarbons can cause ventricular arrhythmias by a mechanism of myocardial sensitization after inhalation.

Treatment
(Table 39–14)

Remove the patient to fresh air. Since aspiration is the primary danger with many common products, use of lavage or emesis is controversial. Removal of ingested hydrocarbon is usually suggested only if the preparation contains toxic solutes (eg, an insecticide) or is an aromatic or halogenated product. Watch the victim closely for 6–8 hours for signs of aspiration pneumonitis (cough, localized rales or rhonchi, tachypnea, and infiltrates on chest radiograph). The use of corticosteroids to treat pneumonitis is controversial. If fever occurs, give a specific antibiotic after identification of pathogens by laboratory studies. Because of the risk of arrhythmias, use bronchodilators

Table 39–14. Clinical features of hydrocarbon poisoning.[1]

Type	Examples	Risk of Pneumonia	Risk of Systemic Toxicity	Treatment
High-viscosity	Vaseline[2] Motor oil	Low	Low	None.
Low-viscosity, nontoxic	Furniture polish Mineral seal oil Kerosene Lighter fluid	High	Low	Observe for pneumonia. *Do not* induce emesis.
Low-viscosity, unknown systemic toxicity	Turpentine Pine oil	High	Variable	Observe for pneumonia. Give activated charcoal.
Low-viscosity, known systemic toxicity	Camphor Phenol Chlorinated insecticides Aromatic hydrocarbons (benzene, toluene, etc)	High	High	Give activated charcoal.

[1]Reproduced, with permission, from Saunders CE, Ho MT (editors): *Current Emergency Diagnosis & Treatment,* 4th ed. Appleton & Lange, 1992.
[2]"Vaseline" is one of several proprietary names for petrolatum (petroleum jelly, paraffin jelly).

only with caution in patients with chlorinated or fluorinated solvent intoxication.

Ford ES et al: Deaths from exposure to trichloroethylene. J Occup Environ Med 1995;37:749. (Case series of deaths in young men working with this solvent in confined spaces without adequate ventilation.)
Pande TK et al: Turpentine poisoning: A case report. Forensic Sci Int 1994;65:47. (Case report, including status epilepticus.)

PHENOTHIAZINES & OTHER ANTIPSYCHOTIC AGENTS
(Chlorpromazine, Promazine, Haloperidol, Prochlorperazine, Risperidone, Clozapine, etc)

Chlorpromazine and related drugs are used as antiemetics and antipsychotic agents and as potentiators of analgesic and hypnotic drugs.

Minimum doses of phenothiazines induce drowsiness and mild orthostatic hypotension in as many as 50% of patients. Larger doses can cause obtundation, miosis, severe hypotension, tachycardia, convulsions, and coma. Abnormal cardiac conduction may occur (particularly with thioridazine), resulting in prolongation of QRS or QT intervals (or both) and ventricular arrhythmias.

With therapeutic doses, some patients develop an acute extrapyramidal reaction similar to Parkinson's disease, with spasmodic contractions of the face and neck muscles, extensor rigidity of the back muscles, carpopedal spasm, and motor restlessness. Severe rigidity accompanied by hyperthermia and metabolic acidosis ("neuroleptic malignant syndrome") may occasionally occur and is life-threatening (see Chapters 1 and 25).

Treatment
A. Emergency and Supportive Measures:
Administer activated charcoal. Consider gastric lavage for massive ingestions. For severe hypotension, treatment with fluids and pressor agents may be necessary. Treat hyperthermia as outlined on p 1469. Maintain cardiac monitoring.

B. Specific Treatment:
Hypotension and cardiac arrhythmias associated with widened QRS intervals on the ECG may respond to intravenous sodium bicarbonate as used for tricyclic antidepressants.

For extrapyramidal signs, give diphenhydramine, 0.5–1 mg/kg intravenously, or benztropine mesylate, 1–2 mg intramuscularly. Treatment with oral doses of these agents should be continued for 24–48 hours.

Bromocriptine (2.5–7.5 mg orally daily) may be effective for mild or moderate neuroleptic malignant syndrome. Dantrolene (2–5 mg/kg intravenously) has also been used.

Buckley NA, Whyte IM, Dawson AH: Cardiotoxicity is more common in thioridazine overdose than with other neuroleptics. J Toxicol Clin Toxicol 1995;33:199. (Of 299 consecutive patients with antipsychotic agent overdose, thioridazine was most commonly associated with prolonged QT and QRS intervals.)
Ganelin L et al: Suspected neuroleptic malignant syndrome in a patient receiving clozapine. Ann Pharmacother 1996;30:248. (A patient with a previous history of neuroleptic malignant syndrome associated with haloperidol

developed the syndrome after 9 days of clozapine therapy.)

QUINIDINE & RELATED ANTIARRHYTHMICS

Quinidine, procainamide, and disopyramide are class Ia antiarrhythmic agents, and flecainide is a class Ic agent. These drugs have membrane-depressant effects on the sodium-dependent channel responsible for cardiac cell depolarization. Manifestations of cardiotoxicity include arrhythmias, syncope, and hypotension. The ECG may show widening of the QRS complex, a lengthened QT and PR interval, and atypical or polymorphous ventricular tachycardia (torsades de pointes).

Treatment

A. Emergency and Supportive Measures: Remove ingested drug by gastric lavage followed by activated charcoal and catharsis (see p 1471).

B. Specific Treatment: Treat cardiotoxicity (atrioventricular block, hypotension, QRS interval widening) with intravenous boluses of sodium bicarbonate, 50–100 meq. Ventricular tachycardia of the torsades de pointes variety may be treated with intravenous magnesium (1–2 g), isoproterenol (1–5 μg/min), or overdrive pacing.

Kim SY, Benowitz NL: Poisoning due to class IA antiarrhythmic drugs. Quinidine, procainamide, and disopyramide. Drug Saf 1990;5:393. (Pharmacology, pathophysiology of overdose, and treatment options, including use of bicarbonate and dialysis procedures.)

Leblanc M et al: N-Acetylprocainamide intoxication with torsades de pointes treated by high dialysate flow rate continuous arteriovenous hemodiafiltration. Crit Care Med 1995;23:589. (Case report.)

SALICYLATES

Salicylates (aspirin, methyl salicylate, etc) are found in a variety of over-the-counter and prescription medications. Salicylates uncouple cellular oxidative phosphorylation, resulting in anaerobic metabolism and excessive production of lactic acid and heat, and they also interfere with several Krebs cycle enzymes. A single ingestion of more than 200 mg/kg of salicylate is likely to produce significant acute intoxication. Poisoning may also occur as a result of chronic excessive dosing over several days. Although the half-life of salicylate is 2–3 hours after small doses, it may increase to 20 hours or more with intoxication.

Clinical Findings

Acute ingestion often causes nausea and vomiting, occasionally with gastritis. Moderate intoxication is characterized by hyperpnea (deep and rapid breathing), tachycardia, tinnitus, and elevated anion gap metabolic acidosis. Serious intoxication may result in agitation, confusion, coma, seizures, cardiovascular collapse, pulmonary edema, hyperthermia, and death. The prothrombin time is often elevated owing to salicylate-induced hypoprothrombinemia.

Diagnosis is suspected in any patient with metabolic acidosis and is confirmed by measuring the serum salicylate level. Patients with levels greater than 100 mg/dL (1000 mg/L) after an acute overdose are more likely to have severe poisoning. On the other hand, patients with chronic intoxication may suffer severe symptoms with levels of only 60–70 mg/dL. The arterial blood gas typically reveals a respiratory alkalosis with an underlying metabolic acidosis.

Treatment

A. Emergency and Supportive Measures: After acute suicidal or accidental ingestion of more than 150–200 mg/kg salicylate, empty the stomach by gastric lavage and administer activated charcoal (see p 1471). Extra doses of activated charcoal may be needed in patients who ingest more than 10 g of aspirin. The desired ratio of charcoal to aspirin is about 10:1 by weight; while this cannot always be given as a single dose, it may be administered in divided doses every 2–4 hours. Treat metabolic acidosis with intravenous sodium bicarbonate.

B. Specific Treatment: Alkalinization of the urine enhances renal salicylate excretion by trapping the salicylate anion in the urine. Add 100 meq (two ampules) of sodium bicarbonate to 1 L of 5% dextrose in 0.2% saline, and infuse this solution intravenously at a rate of about 150–200 mL/h. Unless the patient is oliguric, add 20–30 meq of potassium to each liter of intravenous fluid.

Hemodialysis may be lifesaving and is indicated for patients with severe metabolic acidosis, markedly altered mental status, or significantly elevated salicylate levels (eg, > 100–120 mg/dL [1000–1200 mg/L] after acute overdose or > 60–70 mg/dL [600–700 mg/L] with chronic intoxication).

Chan TY: The risk of severe salicylate poisoning following the ingestion of topical medicaments or aspirin. Postgrad Med J 1996;72:109. (In a retrospective case review, the two highest serum salicylate levels occurred in patients who had ingested topical medicines containing oil of wintergreen [methyl salicylate].)

Yip L, Dart RC, Gabow PA: Concepts and controversies in salicylate toxicity. Emerg Med Clin North Am 1994; 12:351.

SEAFOOD POISONINGS

A variety of intoxications may occur after eating certain types of fish or other seafood. These include scombroid, ciguatera, paralytic shellfish, and puffer fish poisoning. The mechanisms of toxicity and clinical presentations are described in Table 39–15. In the majority of cases, the seafood has a normal appearance and taste (scombroid may have a peppery taste).

Treatment

A. Emergency and Supportive Measures: *Caution:* Abrupt respiratory arrest may occur with paralytic shellfish and puffer fish poisoning. Observe symptomatic patients for at least 4–6 hours. Replace fluid and electrolyte losses from gastroenteritis with intravenous saline or other crystalloid solution.

For recent ingestions, it may be possible to adsorb residual toxin in the gut with activated charcoal, 50–60 g orally.

B. Specific Treatment: There is no specific antidote for paralytic shellfish or puffer fish poisoning.

1. Ciguatera–There are anecdotal reports of successful treatment of severe neurologic symptoms with mannitol, 1 g/kg intravenously.

2. Scombroid–Antihistamines such as diphenhydramine, 25–50 mg intravenously, and the H_2 blocker cimetidine, 300 mg intravenously, are usually effective. For severe reactions, give also epinephrine, 0.3–0.5 mL of a 1:1000 solution subcutaneously.

Barton ED et al: Ciguatera fish poisoning: A southern California epidemic. West J Med 1995;163:31. (Epidemic of 25 cases traced to fish caught off the coast of Baja, California.)

Lau FL et al: Puffer fish poisoning. J Accid Emerg Med 1995;12:214. (Seven Vietnamese refugees in a Hong Kong detention center ate a puffer fish and developed typical symptoms; one patient died.)

SNAKE BITES

The venom of poisonous snakes and lizards may be predominantly neurotoxic (coral snake) or predominantly cytolytic (rattlesnakes, other pit vipers). Neurotoxins cause respiratory paralysis; cytolytic venoms cause tissue destruction by digestion and hemorrhage due to hemolysis and destruction of the endothelial lining of the blood vessels. The manifestations of rattlesnake envenomation are mostly local pain, redness, swelling, and extravasation of blood. Perioral tingling, metallic taste, nausea and vomiting, hypotension, and coagulopathy may also occur. Neurotoxic envenomation may cause ptosis, dysphagia, diplopia, and respiratory arrest.

Treatment

A. Emergency Measures: Immobilize the patient and the bitten part in a horizontal position. Avoid manipulation of the bitten area. Transport the patient to a medical facility for definitive treatment. Do *not* give alcoholic beverages or stimulants; do *not* apply ice; do *not* apply a tourniquet. The trauma to

Table 39–15. Common seafood poisonings.

Type of Poisoning	Mechanism	Clinical Presentation
Ciguatera	Reef fish ingest toxic dinoflagellates, whose toxins accumulate in fish meat. Commonly implicated fish in the USA are barracuda, jack, snapper, and grouper.	1–6 hours after ingestion, victims develop abdominal pain, vomiting, and diarrhea accompanied by a variety of neurologic symptoms, including paresthesias, reversal of hot and cold sensation, vertigo, headache, and intense itching. Autonomic disturbances, including hypotension and bradycardia, may occur.
Scombroid	Improper preservation of large fish results in bacterial degradation of histidine to histamine. Commonly implicated fish include tuna, mahimahi, bonita, mackerel, and kingfish.	Allergic-like (anaphylactoid) symptoms are due to histamine, usually begin within 15–90 minutes, and include skin flushing, itching, urticaria, angioedema, bronchospasm, and hypotension as well as abdominal pain, vomiting, and diarrhea.
Paralytic shellfish poisoning	Dinoflagellates produce saxitoxin, which is concentrated by filter-feeding mussels and clams. Saxitoxin blocks sodium conductance and neuronal transmission in skeletal muscles.	Onset is usually within 30–60 minutes. Initial symptoms include perioral and intraoral paresthesias. Other symptoms include nausea and vomiting, headache, dizziness, dysphagia, dysarthria, ataxia, and rapidly progressive muscle weakness that may result in respiratory arrest.
Puffer fish poisoning	Tetrodotoxin is concentrated in liver, gonads, intestine, and skin. Toxic effects are similar to those of saxitoxin. Tetrodotoxin is also found in some North American newts and Central American frogs.	Onset is usually within 30–40 minutes but may be as short as 10 minutes. Inital perioral paresthesias are followed by headache, diaphoresis, nausea, vomiting, ataxia, and rapidly progressive muscle weakness that may result in respiratory arrest.

underlying structures resulting from incision and suction performed by unskilled people is probably not justified in view of the small amount of venom that can be recovered.

B. Specific Antidote and General Measures:

1. Pit viper (eg, rattlesnake) envenomation–With local signs such as swelling, pain, and ecchymosis but no systemic symptoms, give four or five vials of polyvalent crotalid antivenin by intravenous drip in 250–500 mL saline. (This should be preceded by skin testing for horse serum sensitivity with the kit supplied.) For more serious envenomation with marked local effects and systemic toxicity (eg, hypotension, coagulopathy), 10–20 vials may be required. Epinephrine should be available for immediate use in the event of an allergic reaction. Specific antiserum therapy is more effective if given soon after the bite. Monitor vital signs and the blood coagulation profile. Type and cross-match blood. The adequacy of venom neutralization is indicated by improvement in signs and symptoms, and the rate of swelling slows. Serum sickness reactions are common after antivenin use, usually occur 5–10 days after antivenin administration, and may be treated with prednisone, 45–60 mg daily with tapering doses.

2. Elapid (coral snake) envenomation–Give 1–2 vials of specific antivenom as soon as possible. To locate antisera for exotic snakes, call the local poison control center.

Guisto JA: Severe toxicity from crotalid envenomation after early resolution of symptoms. Ann Emerg Med 1995;26:387. (Case report illustrating importance of continued observation.)

SPIDER BITES & SCORPION STINGS

The toxin of most species of spiders in the USA causes only local pain, redness, and swelling. That of the more venomous black widow spiders (*Latrodectus mactans*) causes generalized muscular pains, muscle spasms, and rigidity. The brown recluse spider (*Loxosceles reclusa*) causes progressive local necrosis as well as hemolytic reactions (rare). Stings by most scorpions in the USA cause only local pain. Stings by the more toxic *Centruroides* species (found in the southwestern USA) may cause muscle cramps, twitching and jerking, and occasionally hypertension, convulsions, and pulmonary edema.

Treatment

A. Black Widow Spider Bites: Pain may be relieved with parenteral narcotics or muscle relaxants (eg, methocarbamol, 15 mg/kg). Calcium gluconate 10%, 0.1–0.2 mL/kg intravenously, may relieve muscle rigidity, though its effectiveness is questionable. Antivenin is rarely indicated, usually only for very young or elderly patients who do not respond to the above measures. Horse serum sensitivity testing is required. (Instruction and testing materials are included in the antivenin kit.)

B. Brown Recluse Spider Bites: Because bites occasionally progress to extensive local necrosis, some authorities recommend early excision of the bite site, whereas others use oral corticosteroids. Recently, interest has focused on the use of dapsone and colchicine. An antivenin is being developed. All of these treatments remain of unproved value.

C. Scorpion Stings: No specific treatment is available. For *Centruroides* stings, some toxicologists use a specific antivenom developed in Arizona, but this is neither FDA-approved nor widely available.

Clark RF et al: Clinical presentation and treatment of black widow spider envenomation: A review of 163 cases. Ann Emerg Med 1992;21:782. (The authors found calcium relatively ineffective compared with intravenous opioids and benzodiazepines.)

THEOPHYLLINE

Theophylline is commonly used in the treatment of bronchospasm due to asthma, chronic lung disease, and congestive heart failure. Its toxicity may be caused by several of its pharmacologic effects, including inhibition of phosphodiesterase and adenosine and release of catecholamines. Theophylline may cause intoxication after an acute single overdose or as a result of chronic accidental repeated overmedication or reduced elimination caused by hepatic dysfunction or interacting drug (eg, cimetidine, erythromycin). The usual serum half-life of theophylline is 4–6 hours, but this may increase to more than 20 hours after overdose.

Clinical Findings

Mild intoxication causes nausea, vomiting, tachycardia, and tremulousness. Severe intoxication is characterized by ventricular and supraventricular tachyarrhythmias, hypotension, and seizures. Status epilepticus is common and often intractable to usual anticonvulsants. After acute overdose (but not chronic intoxication), hypokalemia, hyperglycemia, and metabolic acidosis are common. Seizures and other manifestations of toxicity may be delayed for several hours after acute ingestion, especially if a sustained-release preparation such as Theo-Dur was taken.

Diagnosis is based on measurement of the serum theophylline concentration. Acute overdose patients with serum levels greater than 100 mg/L are likely to develop seizures and hypotension. Patients with chronic intoxication may develop serious toxicity at lower levels (ie, 60 mg/L).

Treatment

A. Emergency and Supportive Measures:

After acute ingestion, administer activated charcoal and a cathartic (see p 1445). Repeated doses of activated charcoal may enhance theophylline elimination by "gut dialysis" (see p 1446).

Hemoperfusion and hemodialysis are effective in removing theophylline and are indicated for patients with status epilepticus or markedly elevated serum theophylline levels (eg, > 100 mg/L after acute overdose or > 60 mg/L with chronic intoxication). Whole bowel irrigation may help eliminate intact sustained-release pills after massive ingestion.

B. Specific Treatment:

There is no antidote for seizures, but hypotension and tachycardia—which are mediated through excessive β_2-adrenergic stimulation—may respond to beta-blocker therapy. Administer esmolol, 25–50 μg/kg/min by intravenous infusion, or propranolol, 0.5–1 mg intravenously.

Shannon M: Hypokalemia, hyperglycemia and plasma catecholamine activity after severe theophylline intoxication. J Toxicol Clin Toxicol 1994;32:41. (Hypokalemia and hyperglycemia are more common with acute overdose than chronic intoxication.)

TRICYCLIC ANTIDEPRESSANTS

Tricyclic and related cyclic antidepressants are among the most commonly implicated products in suicidal overdose. These drugs have anticholinergic and cardiac depressant properties. Tricyclic antidepressants produce more marked membrane-depressant cardiotoxic effects than the phenothiazines. All of these drugs are highly tissue-bound and are not effectively removed by hemodialysis procedures.

Newer antidepressants such as trazodone, fluoxetine, paroxetine, sertraline, bupropion, venlafaxine, and fluvoxamine are not chemically related to the tricyclic antidepressant agents and do not generally produce cardiotoxic effects. However, bupropion, venlafaxine, and fluvoxamine may cause seizures in overdoses.

Clinical Findings

Signs of severe intoxication may occur abruptly and without warning within 30–60 minutes after acute overdose. Anticholinergic effects include dilated pupils, tachycardia, dry mouth, flushed skin, muscle twitching, and decreased peristalsis. Cardiotoxic effects include QRS interval widening (> 0.12 s; see Figure 39–2), ventricular arrhythmias, atrioventricular block, and hypotension. Seizures and coma are common with severe intoxication. Life-threatening hyperthermia may result from status epilepticus and anticholinergic-induced impairment of sweating.

The diagnosis should be suspected in any overdose

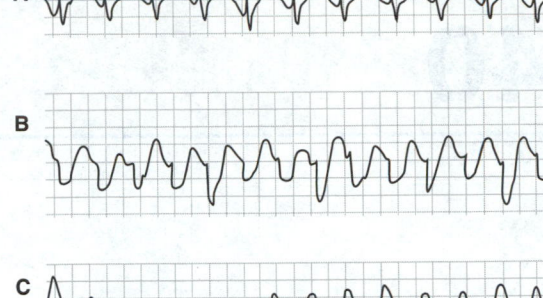

Figure 39–2. Cardiac arrhythmias resulting from tricyclic antidepressant overdose. **A:** Delayed intraventricular conduction results in prolonged QRS interval (0.18 s). **B and C:** Supraventricular tachycardia with progressive widening of QRS complexes mimics ventricular tachycardia. (Reproduced, with permission, from Benowitz NL, Goldschlager N: Cardiac disturbances in the toxicologic patient. In: *Clinical Management of Poisoning and Drug Overdose,* 2nd ed. Haddad LM, Winchester JF [editors]. Saunders, 1990.)

patient with anticholinergic side effects, especially if there is widening of the QRS interval or seizures. For intoxication by most tricyclics, the QRS interval correlates with the severity of intoxication more reliably than the serum drug level.

Treatment

A. Emergency and Supportive Measures:

Observe patients for at least 6 hours, and admit all patients with evidence of anticholinergic effects (eg, delirium, dilated pupils, tachycardia) or signs of cardiotoxicity.

Perform gastric lavage and administer activated charcoal (see p 1471). Do *not* induce emesis because of the risk of seizures.

B. Specific Treatment:

Cardiotoxic membrane-depressant effects may respond to boluses of sodium bicarbonate (50–100 meq intravenously). Sodium bicarbonate provides a large sodium load that alleviates depression of the sodium-dependent channel. Reversal of acidosis may also have beneficial effects at this site. Maintain the pH between 7.45 and 7.50.

Liebelt EL, Francis PD, Woolf AD: ECG lead aVR versus QRS interval in predicting seizures and arrhythmias in acute tricyclic antidepressant toxicity. Ann Emerg Med 1995;26:175. (Prospective study of 79 patients with tricyclic antidepressant overdose found that increased amplitude of the R wave in aVR was more predictive of seizures and arrhythmias than the QRS interval.)

Newton EH, Shih RD, Hoffman RS: Cyclic antidepressant overdose: A review of current management strategies. Am J Emerg Med 1994;12:376. (Comprehensive review.)

40

Medical Genetics

Reed E. Pyeritz, MD, PhD

The rapid and in some cases spectacular advances in human genetics during the past decade have had important implications for clinical medicine. Familiarity with the fundamental principles of both basic and clinical genetics is now necessary if the physician is to provide a high standard of care. Within the professional lifetimes of most physicians practicing today, all 3 billion nucleotides of the human genome will have been sequenced. The great hope, of course, is that with this exponential growth in information will come new insights into the causes and pathogenetic mechanisms of human disease, more accurate diagnosis, and effective treatment for many disorders now considered beyond the practitioner's therapeutic reach. Along with this optimistic prospect, however, have come some urgent concerns about (1) the ethical, legal, and sociologic implications of what has been termed "genetic engineering" but is better and more broadly called "molecular medicine"; (2) the problem for medical educators of how best to transmit such an enormous body of information to their students and to primary care practitioners; and (3) the seemingly esoteric nature of much of that information paired with the realization that any one of the obscure facts of medical genetics might achieve clinical relevance at any time.

Goldstein JL, Brown MS: Genetic aspects of disease. In: *Harrison's Principles of Internal Medicine,* 13th ed. Isselbacher KJ et al (editors). McGraw-Hill, 1994. (A succinct review of basic principles.)

Jorde LB et al: *Medical Genetics.* Mosby, 1995. (An up-to-date and comprehensive textbook for the medical student.)

Pyeritz RE: A revolution in medicine like no other. FASEB J 1992;6:2761. (Current and future importance of genetics in clinical medicine.)

Rimoin DL, Connor JM, Pyeritz RE (editors): *Principles and Practice of Medical Genetics,* 3rd ed. Churchill Livingstone, 1997. (Multiauthored compendium covering the basic principles of human genetics, the importance of genetics in medicine, and the diagnosis and management of many genetic disorders.)

Seashore WR, Wappner RS: *Genetics in Primary Care & Clinical Medicine.* Appleton & Lange, 1996. (A succinct
review of syndromes and diseases of chromosomal, multifactorial, and single-gene causation.)

INTRODUCTION TO MEDICAL GENETICS

Physicians at one time concerned themselves only with what they could discover by bedside interrogation and inspection and laboratory investigation. In the parlance of genetics, the patient's symptoms and signs constitute his or her **phenotype.** Now the means are at hand for defining a person's **genotype,** the actual information content inscribed in the 2 meters of coiled DNA present in each cell of the body—or half that amount in every mature ovum or sperm. Virtually all phenotypic characteristics—and this includes diseases as well as human traits such as personality, height, and intelligence—are to some extent determined by the genes. The importance of the genetic contribution varies widely among human phenotypes, and methods are only now being developed to identify the gene involved in complex traits and most common diseases. Moreover, the importance of the environment and of interactions between environment and genotype in producing phenotypes cannot be overstated despite the obscurity of the actual mechanisms.

The billions of nucleotides in the nucleus of a cell are organized linearly along the DNA double helix in functional units called **genes,** and each of the 50,000–100,000 human genes is accompanied by various regulatory elements that control when it is active in producing **messenger RNA (mRNA)** by a process called **transcription.** In most situations, mRNA is transported from the nucleus to the cytoplasm, where its genetic information is **translated** into **proteins,** which perform the functions that ultimately determine phenotype. For example, proteins serve as enzymes that facilitate metabolism and cell synthesis; as DNA binding elements that regulate transcription of other genes; as structural elements of cells and the extracellular matrix; and as receptor molecules for intra- and intercellular communication.

Chromosomes are the vehicles in which the genes are carried from generation to generation. Each chromosome is a complex of protein and nucleic acid in which an unbroken double helix of DNA is coiled and supercoiled into a space many orders of magnitude less than the extended length of the DNA. Within the chromosome there occur highly complicated and integrated processes, including DNA replication, recombination, and transcription. Humans normally have 46 chromosomes, which are arranged in 23 pairs. One of these pairs, the **sex chromosomes** X and Y, determines the sex of the individual; females have the pair XX and males the pair XY. The remaining 22 pairs are called **autosomes** (Figure 40–1).

In all somatic cells, the 44 autosomes and one of the X chromosomes are transcriptionally active. In males, the active X is the only X; portions of the Y chromosome are also active. In females, the requirement for **dosage compensation** (to be equivalent to the situation in males) is satisfied by inactivation of most of one X chromosome early in embryogenesis. This process of X chromosomal inactivation, while not understood biochemically, is known to be random, so that on average, in 50% of a female's cells, one of the X chromosomes will be active, and in the other 50% the **homologous** member of the pair will be active. The phenotype of the cell is determined by which genes on the chromosomes are active in producing mRNA at any given time.

GENES & CHROMOSOMES

In all genes, information is contained in parcels called **exons,** which are interspersed with stretches of DNA called **introns** that do not encode any information about the protein sequence. However, introns may contain genetic regulatory sequences, and some introns are so large that they encode an entirely distinct gene.

The exact location of a gene on a chromosome is its **locus,** and the array of loci constitutes the **human gene map.** Currently, the chromosomal site of more than 4500 genes is known, often to a high degree of resolution. A variation of this map, identifying se-

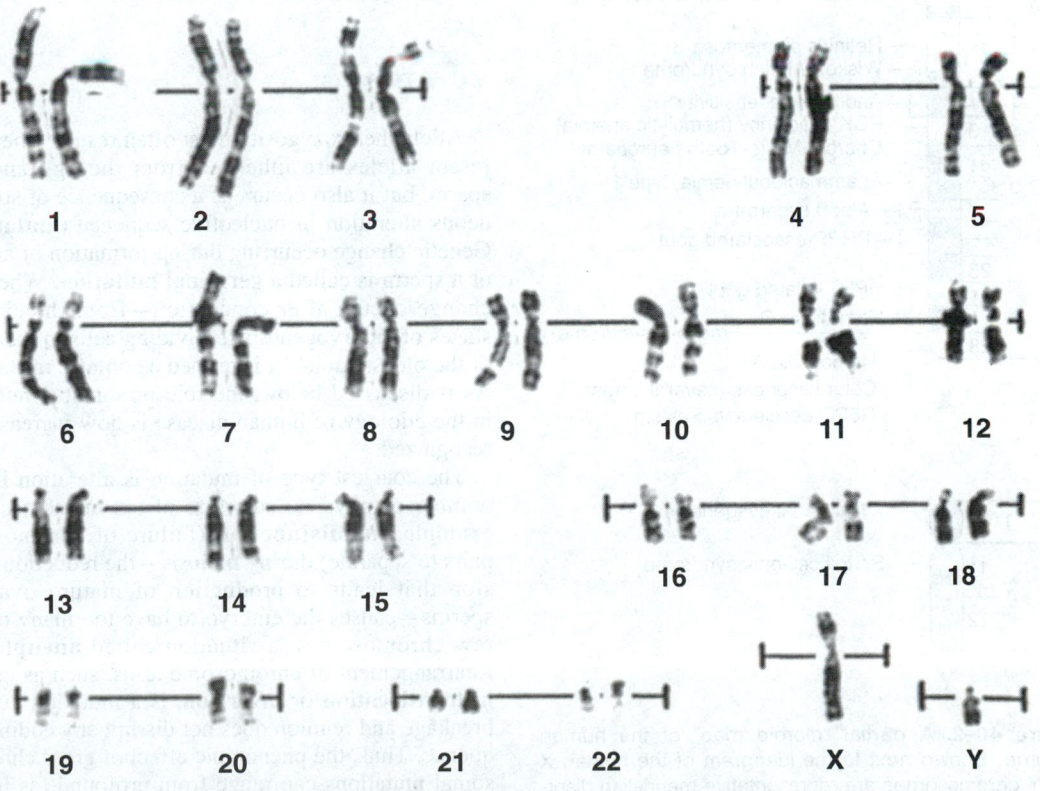

Figure 40–1. Normal karyotype of a human male. Prepared from cultured amniotic cells and stained with Giemsa's stain. About 400 bands are detectable per haploid set of chromosomes.

lected loci known to be involved in human disease, is shown in Figure 40–2. The difference in resolution of the ordering of genes achievable by molecular techniques (such as linkage analysis) compared to cytogenetic techniques (such as visualization of small defects) is substantial, though the gap is narrowing. The chromosomes in the "standard" karyotype shown in Figure 40–1 have about 450 visible bands; under the best of cytologic and microscopic conditions, a total of about 1600 bands can be seen. But even in this extended configuration, each band contains dozens— sometimes hundreds—of individual genes. Thus, loss (**deletion**) of a small band, which is the smallest type of defect identifiable under the microscope, will involve loss of many coding sequences and will have diverse effects on the phenotype.

The number and arrangement of genes on homologous chromosomes are identical even though the actual coding sequences of homologous genes may not be. Homologous copies of a gene are termed **alleles.** In comparing alleles, it must be specified at what level of analysis the comparison is being made. When alleles are truly identical—in that their coding

sequences are invariant—the individual is **homozygous** at that locus. At a coarser level, the alleles may be functionally identical despite subtle variations in nucleotide sequence—with the result either that the proteins produced from the two alleles are identical or that whatever differences there may be in amino acid sequence will have no bearing on the function of the protein. If the individual is being analyzed at the level of the protein phenotype, allelic homozygosity would again be an apt descriptor. However, if the analysis were at the level of the DNA—as occurs in restriction enzyme examination or nucleotide sequencing—then, despite functional identity, the alleles would be viewed as different and the individual would be **heterozygous** for that locus. Heterozygosity based on differences in the protein products of alleles has been detectable for decades and was the first hard evidence concerning the high degree of human biologic variability. In the past decade, analysis of DNA sequences has shown this variability to be much more remarkable—differences in nucleotide sequence between individuals occur about once every 400 nucleotides.

Hoffman EP: The evolving genomic project: Current and future impact. Am J Hum Genet 1994;54:129.

Strachan T, Read AP: *Human Molecular Genetics.* Wiley-Liss, 1996. (A comprehensive text on molecular biology and its interface with human genetics.)

MUTATION

Allelic heterozygosity most often results when different alleles are inherited from the egg and the sperm, but it also occurs as a consequence of spontaneous alteration in nucleotide sequence (**mutation**). Genetic change occurring during formation of an egg or a sperm is called a **germinal mutation.** When the change occurs after conception—from the earliest stages of embryogenesis to dividing cells in the body of the oldest adult—it is termed a **somatic mutation.** As is discussed below, the role of somatic mutation in the etiology of human disease is now increasingly recognized.

The coarsest type of mutation is alteration in the number or physical structure of chromosomes. For example, **nondisjunction** (failure of chromosome pairs to separate) during **meiosis**—the reduction division that leads to production of mature ova and sperms—causes the embryo to have too many or too few chromosomes, a situation called **aneuploidy.** Rearrangement of chromosome arms, such as occurs in **translocation** or **inversion,** is a mutation even if breakage and reunion does not disrupt any coding sequence. Thus, the phenotypic effect of gross chromosomal mutations can range from profound (as in aneuploidy) to nil.

A bit less coarse, but still detectable cytologically,

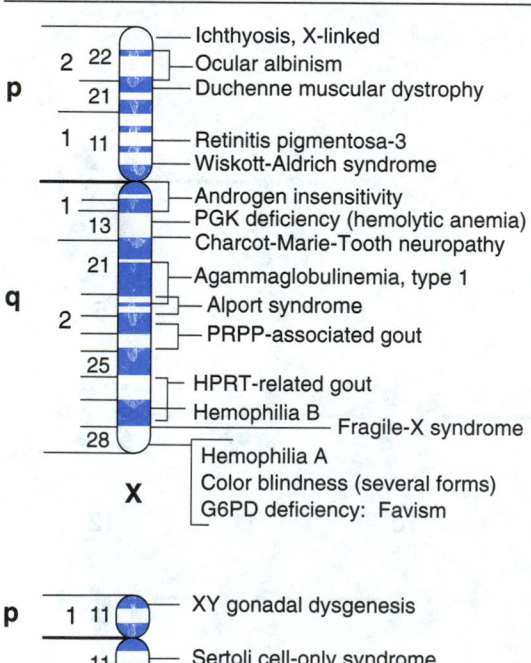

Figure 40–2. A partial "morbid map" of the human genome. Shown next to the ideogram of the human X and Y chromosomes are representative mendelian disorders caused by mutations at that locus. (Courtesy of McKusick and Strayer.)

are **deletions** of part of a chromosome. Such mutations almost always alter phenotype, because a number of genes are lost; however, a deletion *may* involve only a single nucleotide, whereas about 1–2 million nucleotides (1–2 megabases) must be lost before the defect can be visualized by the most sensitive cytogenetic methods short of in situ hybridization. Molecular biologic techniques are needed to detect smaller losses.

Mutations of one or a few nucleotides in exons have several potential consequences. Changes in one nucleotide can alter which amino acid is encoded; if the amino acid is in a critical region of the protein, function might in this way be severely deranged. On the other hand, some amino acid substitutions have no detectable effect on function, and the phenotype is therefore unaltered by the mutation. Similarly, because the genetic code is **degenerate** (two or more different three-nucleotide sequences called **codons** encode some amino acids), nucleotide substitution does not necessarily alter the amino acid sequence of the protein. Three specific codons signal termination of translation; thus, a nucleotide substitution in an exon that generates one of the stop-codons usually causes a truncated protein, which is nearly always dysfunctional. Other nucleotide substitutions can disrupt the signals that direct splicing of the mRNA molecule and grossly alter the protein product. Finally, insertions and deletions of one or more nucleotides can have dramatic effects—any change that is not a multiple of three nucleotides disrupts the reading frame of the remainder of the exon—or potentially minimal effects (if the protein can tolerate the insertion or loss of an amino acid).

Mutations in introns may disrupt mRNA splicing signals or may be entirely silent with respect to the phenotype. A great deal of variation in nucleotide sequences among individuals (averaging one difference every few hundred nucleotides) resides within introns. Mutations in the DNA between adjacent genes may also be silent or may have a profound effect on phenotype if regulatory sequences are disrupted. A novel mechanism for mutation, which also helps explain clinical variation among relatives, has recently been discovered in myotonic dystrophy, Huntington's disease, fragile-X mental retardation syndrome, Friedreich's ataxia, and other disorders. A region of repeated sequences within a gene can be unstable in some families; expansion of the number of repeated units within this segment is associated with a more severe phenotype.

Mutations may occur spontaneously or may be induced by such environmental factors as radiation, medication, or viral infections. Both advanced maternal and paternal age favor mutation, but of different types. In women, meiosis is completed only when an egg ovulates, and chromosomal nondisjunction is more common the older the egg. The risk that an aneuploid egg will result increases exponentially and becomes a major clinical worry for women older than their early 30s. In men, mutations of a subtler sort—affecting nucleotide sequences—increase with age. Offspring of men over 40 are at an increased risk of having mendelian conditions, primarily autosomal dominant ones.

Antonarakis SE: Mutations in human disease. in: *Principles and Practice of Medical Genetics,* 3rd ed. Rimoin DL, Conner JM, Pyeritz RE (editors). Churchill Livingstone, 1997. (How mutations occur and their effect on gene function.)

Barsh G: Genetic disease. In: *Pathophysiology of Disease: An Introduction to Clinical Medicine,* 2nd ed. McPhee SJ et al (editors): Appleton & Lange, 1997. (Discusses pathogenesis of fragile X-associated mental retardation.)

Warren ST, Nelson DL: Advances in molecular analysis of fragile X syndrome. JAMA 1994;271:536. (A review of trinucleotide repeat mutations and their diagnosis, using this common cause of mental retardation as an example.)

GENES IN INDIVIDUALS

For some quantitative traits such as height or serum glucose concentration in normal individuals, it is virtually impossible to distinguish the contributions of individual genes; this is because in general, phenotypes are the products of multiple genes acting in concert. However, if one of the genes in the system is aberrant, a major departure from the "normal" or expected phenotype might arise. Whether the aberrant phenotype is serious (ie, a disease) or even recognized will depend on the nature of the defective gene product and how resilient the system is to disruption. The latter point emphasizes the importance of homeostasis in both physiology and development—many mutations go unrecognized because the system can cope, even though tolerances for further perturbation might be narrowed.

In other words, virtually all human characteristics are **polygenic,** while many of the disordered phenotypes thought of as "genetic" are **monogenic** but still influenced by other loci in a person's genome.

Phenotypes due to alterations at a single gene are also characterized as **mendelian,** after the monk and part-time biologist who studied the reproducibility and recurrence of variation in garden peas. Gregor Mendel showed that some traits were **dominant** to others, which he called **recessive.** The dominant traits required only one copy of a "factor" to be expressed, regardless of what the other copy was, whereas the recessive traits required two copies before expression occurred. In modern terms, the mendelian factors are genes, and the alternative copies of the gene are alleles. Let A be the common (normal) allele and let a be a mutant allele at a locus: If the same phenotype is present no matter whether the genotype is A/a or a/a, the phenotype is dominant, whereas if the phenotype is present only when the genotype is a/a, it is recessive.

In medicine, it is important to keep two considerations in mind: First, dominance and recessiveness are attributes of the phenotype, not the gene; and second, the concepts of dominance and recessiveness depend on how one defines the phenotype. To illustrate both points, consider sickle cell disease. This condition occurs when a person inherits two alleles for β^S-globin, in which the normal glutamate at position 6 of the protein has been replaced by valine; the genotype for the β-globin locus is *HbS/HbS*, compared to the normal *HbA/HbA*. When the genotype is *HbS/HbA*, the individual does not have sickle cell disease, so this condition satisfies the criteria for being a recessive phenotype. But now consider the phenotype of sickled erythrocytes. Red cells with the genotype *HbS/HbS* clearly sickle—but, if the oxygen tension is reduced, so do cells with the genotype *HbS/HbA*. Therefore, sickling is a dominant trait.

A mendelian phenotype is characterized not only in terms of dominance and recessiveness but also according to whether the determining gene is on the X chromosome or on one of the 22 pairs of autosomes. Traits or diseases are therefore called autosomal dominant, autosomal recessive, X-linked recessive, and X-linked dominant.

Leder P, Clayton DA, Rubenstein E (editors): *Scientific American Introduction to Molecular Medicine.* Scientific American Medicine, 1994. (A series of lucid accounts of general topics in human and molecular genetics, the human genome project, cancer, and hereditary disorders.)

Mueller R, Cook J: Mendelian inheritance. In: *Principles and Practice of Medical Genetics,* 3rd ed. Rimoin DL, Connor JM, Pyeritz RE (editors): Churchill Livingstone, 1997.

Roses AD: From genes to mechanisms to therapies: Lessons to be learned from neurological disorders. Nat Med 1996;2:267. (A brief, lucid statement of what it will take to reap the benefits of the Human Genome Project.)

GENES IN FAMILIES

Since the first decade of this century, the patterns of recurrence of specific human phenotypes have been explained in terms of principles first described by Mendel in the garden pea plant. Mendel's second principle—usually referred to as his first*—is called

---

*Mendel's first law stated that—from the perspective of the phenotype—it mattered not from which parent a particular allele was inherited. For years this principle was thought to be too obvious to be codified as anybody's "law" and was therefore ignored. In fact, however, recent evidence from studies of human disorders suggests that certain genes are "processed" **(imprinted)** as they move through the gonad and that processing in the testis is different from that in the ovary. Thus, not only is this first mendelian principle important, it was incorrect as originally formulated from observations in peas.

the **law of segregation** and states that a pair of factors (alleles) that determines some trait separates (segregates) during formation of gametes. In simple terms, a heterozygous *(A/a)* person will produce two types of gametes with respect to this locus—one containing only *A* and one containing only *a*, in equal proportions. Offspring of this person will have a 50–50 chance of inheriting the *A* allele and a similar chance of inheriting the *a* allele.

The concepts of genes in individuals and in families can be combined to specify how mendelian traits will be inherited.

Autosomal Dominant Inheritance

The characteristics of autosomal dominant inheritance in humans can be summarized as follows:

(1) There is a vertical pattern in the pedigree, with multiple generations affected (Figure 40–3).

(2) Heterozygotes for the mutant allele show an abnormal phenotype.

(3) Males and females are affected with equal frequency and severity.

(4) Only one parent must be affected for an offspring to be at risk for developing the phenotype.

(5) When an affected person mates with an unaffected one, each offspring has a 50% chance of inheriting the affected phenotype. This is true regardless of the sex of the affected parent—specifically, male-to-male transmission occurs.

(6) The frequency of sporadic cases is positively associated with the severity of the phenotype. More precisely, the greater the **reproductive fitness** of affected persons, the less likely it is that any given case resulted from a new mutation.

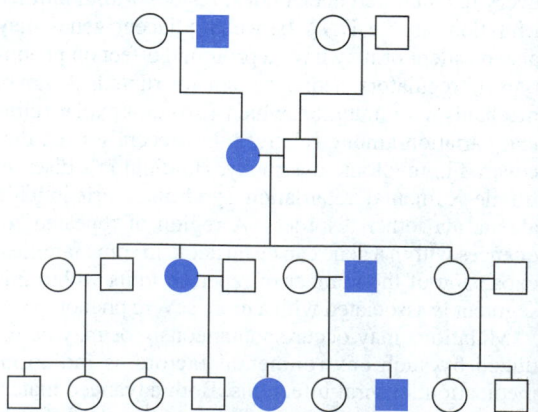

Figure 40–3. A pedigree illustrating autosomal dominant inheritance. Square symbols indicate males and circles females; open symbols indicate that the person is phenotypically unaffected, and filled symbols indicate that the phenotype is present to some extent.

(7) The average age of fathers is advanced in the case of isolated (sporadic or new mutation) cases.

Autosomal dominant phenotypes are often age-dependent, less severe than autosomal recessive ones, and associated with malformations or other physical features. They are **pleiotropic** in that multiple, even seemingly unrelated clinical manifestations derive from the same mutation; and **variable** in that expression of the same mutation among people will differ.

Penetrance is a concept often associated with mendelian conditions—especially dominant ones—and the term is often misused. It should be defined as an expression of the frequency of appearance of a phenotype (dominant or recessive) when one or more mutant alleles are present. For individuals, penetrance is an all-or-none phenomenon—the phenotype is either present (penetrant) or not (nonpenetrant). The term **variability**—not "incomplete penetrance"—should be used to denote differences in expression of an allele.

The most frequent cause of apparent nonpenetrance is insensitivity of the methods for detecting the phenotype. If an apparently normal parent of a child with a dominant condition were in fact heterozygous for the mutation, the parent would have a 50% chance at each subsequent conception of having another affected child. A common cause of nonpenetrance in adult-onset mendelian diseases is death of the affected person before the phenotype becomes evident but after transmission of the mutant allele to offspring. Thus, accurate genetic counseling demands careful attention to the family medical history and high-resolution scrutiny of both parents of a child with a condition known to be a mendelian dominant trait.

When both alleles are expressed in the heterozygote, as in blood group AB, in sickle trait (HbS/HbA), in the major histocompatibility antigens (eg, A2B5/A3B17), or in sickle-C disease (HbS/HbC), the phenotype is called **codominant.**

In human dominant phenotypes, the homozygous state for the mutant allele is almost always more severe than in heterozygotes.

Autosomal Recessive Inheritance

The characteristics of autosomal recessive inheritance in humans can be summarized as follows:

(1) There is a horizontal pattern in the pedigree, with a single generation affected (Figure 40–4).

(2) Males and females are affected with equal frequency and severity.

(3) Inheritance is from both parents, each a heterozygote (carrier) and each usually clinically unaffected.

(4) Each offspring of two carriers has a 25% chance of being affected, a 50% chance of being a carrier, and a 25% chance of inheriting neither mu-

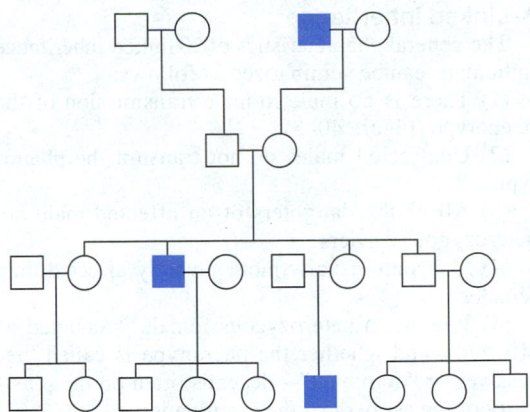

Figure 40–4. A pedigree illustrating X-linked inheritance. (Symbols as in Figure 40–3.)

tant allele. Thus, two-thirds of all clinically unaffected offspring are carriers.

(5) In matings between individuals, each with the same recessive phenotype, all offspring will be affected.

(6) Affected individuals who mate with unaffected individuals who are not carriers have only unaffected offspring.

(7) The rarer the recessive phenotype, the more likely it is that the parents are **consanguineous** (related).

Autosomal recessive phenotypes are often associated with deficient activity of enzymes and are thus termed **inborn errors of metabolism.** Such disorders include phenylketonuria, Tay-Sachs disease, and the various glycogen storage diseases and tend to be more severe, less variable, and less age-dependent than dominant conditions.

When an autosomal recessive condition is quite rare, the chance that the parents of affected offspring are consanguineous is increased. As a result, the prevalence of rare recessive conditions is high among inbred groups such as the Old Order Amish. On the other hand, when the autosomal recessive condition is common, the chance of consanguinity between parents of cases is no higher than in the general population (about 0.5%).

Two different *mutant* alleles at the same locus, as in HbS/HbC, form a **genetic compound.** The phenotype usually lies between those produced by either allele present in the homozygous state. Because of the large number of mutations possible in a given gene, many autosomal recessive phenotypes are probably due to genetic compounds. Sickle cell disease is an exception. Consanguinity is strong presumptive evidence for true homozygosity of mutant alleles and against a genetic compound.

X-Linked Inheritance

The general characteristics of X-linked inheritance in humans can be summarized as follows:

(1) There is no male-to-male transmission of the phenotype (Figure 40–5).

(2) Unaffected males do not transmit the phenotype.

(3) All of the daughters of an affected male are heterozygous carriers.

(4) Males are usually more severely affected than females.

(5) Whether a heterozygous female is counted as affected—and whether the phenotype is called "recessive" or "dominant"—depends often on the sensitivity of the assay or of the examination.

(6) Some mothers of affected males will not themselves be heterozygotes (ie, they will be homozygous normal) but will have a germinal mutation. The proportion of heterozygous (carrier) mothers is negatively associated with the severity of the condition.

(7) Heterozygous women transmit the mutant gene to one-half of sons, who are affected, and to one-half of daughters, who are heterozygotes.

(8) If an affected male mates with a heterozygous female, half of the male offspring will be affected, giving the false impression of male-to-male transmission. One-half of the female offspring of such matings will be affected as severely as the average hemizygous male; in small pedigrees, this pattern may simulate autosomal dominant inheritance.

The characteristics of X-linked inheritance depend on phenotypic severity. For some disorders, affected males do not survive to reproduce. In such cases, about two-thirds of affected males have a carrier mother; in the remaining third, the disorder arises by new germinal mutation in an X chromosome of the mother. When the disorder is nearly always manifest in heterozygous females (X-linked dominant inheritance), females tend to be affected about twice as often as males; and on average an affected female transmits the phenotype to half of her sons and half of her daughters.

X-linked phenotypes are often clinically variable—particularly in heterozygous females—and suspected of being autosomal dominant with nonpenetrance. For example, Fabry's disease (α-galactosidase A deficiency) may be clinically silent in carrier women or may cause stroke, renal failure, or myocardial infarction by middle age.

Germinal mosaicism occurs in mothers of boys with X-linked conditions. The chance of such a mother having a second affected son or a heterozygous daughter depends on the fraction of her oocytes that carries the mutation. Currently, this fraction is impossible to determine. However, the presence of germinal mosaicism can be detected in some conditions (eg, Duchenne's muscular dystrophy) in a family by analysis of DNA, and this knowledge becomes crucial for genetic counseling.

Nearly 7000 human genes have been identified through their phenotypes and inheritance patterns in families. This total represents 5–10% of all genes thought to be encoded by the 22 autosomes and 2 sex chromosomes. Victor McKusick coordinates an international effort to catalogue human mendelian variation.

McKusick VA: *Mendelian Inheritance in Man,* 11th ed. Johns Hopkins Univ Press, 1994. (A catalogue consisting, for each phenotype, of a six-digit identification number—used extensively in the medical literature—a summary statement, and a list of pertinent references. Editions are published biennially, but the catalogue is updated continuously and is computer-accessible as Online Mendelian Inheritance in Man [OMIM], accessible through the National Center for Biotechnology Information [http://www.nchi.nlm.nih.gov/emim]. For information, contact OMIM User Support, FAX 410-955-4999.)

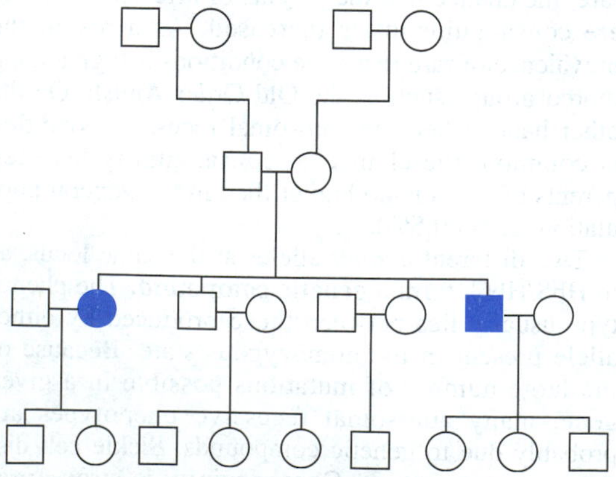

DISORDERS OF MULTIFACTORIAL CAUSATION

Many disorders cluster in families but are not associated with evident chromosomal aberrations or mendelian inheritance patterns. Examples include congenital malformations such as cleft lip, pyloric stenosis, and spina bifida; coronary artery disease; adult-onset diabetes mellitus; and various forms of neoplasia. They are often characterized by varying frequencies in different racial or ethnic groups, disparity in sexual predilection, and greater frequency (but less than full concordance) in monozygotic than in dizygotic twins. This inheritance pattern is called "multifactorial" to signify that multiple genes interact with various environmental agents to produce the phenotype. The familial clustering is assumed to be due to sharing of both alleles and environment.

Figure 40–5. A pedigree illustrating autosomal recessive inheritance. (Symbols as in Figure 40–3.)

For most multifactorial conditions, there is little understanding of which particular genes are involved, how they and their products interact, and in what way different nongenetic factors contribute to the phenotype. For some disorders, biochemical and genetic studies have identified mendelian conditions within the coarse phenotype: Defects of the low-density lipoprotein receptor account for a small fraction of cases of ischemic heart disease (a larger fraction if only patients under age 50 are considered); familial polyposis of the colon predisposes to adenocarcinoma; and some patients with emphysema have inherited deficiency of α_1-proteinase inhibitor. Despite these notable examples, this reductionistic preoccupation with mendelian phenotypes is unlikely to explain the great majority of human disease; but even so, in the last analysis, much of human pathology will prove to be associated with genetic factors in cause, pathogenesis, or both.

Our ignorance about fundamental genetic mechanisms in development and physiology has not completely restricted practical approaches to the genetics of multifactorial disorders. For example, recurrence risks are based on empiric data derived from observation of many families. The risk of recurrence of multifactorial disorders is increased in several instances: (1) to close relatives (sibs, offspring, and parents) of an affected individual; (2) when two or more members of a family have the same condition; (3) when the first case in a family is in the less commonly affected sex (eg, pyloric stenosis is five times more common in boys; an affected woman has a three- to fourfold greater risk of having a child with pyloric stenosis); and (4) in ethnic groups in which there is a high incidence of a particular condition (eg, spina bifida is 40 times more common in Caucasians—and even more frequent among the Irish—than in Asians).

For many apparently multifactorial disorders, enough families have not been examined to have established empiric risk data. A useful approximation of recurrence risk in close relatives is the square root of the incidence. For example, many common congenital malformations have an incidence of 1:2000 to 1:500 live births; the calculated recurrence risks are thus in the 2–5% range—values that correspond closely to experience.

Childs B: A logic of disease. In: *The Metabolic and Molecular Bases of Inherited Disease,* 7th ed. Scriver CR et al (editors). McGraw-Hill, 1995. (A cogent and comprehensive approach to how genes are involved in pathophysiology.)

CHROMOSOMAL ABERRATIONS

Any deviation from the structure and number of chromosomes as displayed in Figure 40–1 is, techni-

cally, a chromosomal aberration. Not all aberrations cause problems in the affected individual, but some that do not may lead to problems in offspring. About 1:200 live-born infants have a chromosomal aberration that is detected because of some effect on phenotype. This frequency increases markedly the earlier in fetal life the chromosomes are examined. By the end of the first trimester of gestation, most fetuses with abnormal numbers of chromosomes have been lost through spontaneous abortion. For example, Turner's syndrome—due to absence of one sex chromosome and the presence of a single X chromosome—is a relatively common condition, but it is estimated that only 2% of fetuses with this form of aneuploidy survive to term. Even more striking in live-born children is the complete absence of most autosomal trisomies and monosomies despite their frequent occurrence in young fetuses.

Types of Chromosomal Abnormalities

Major structural changes occur in either **balanced** or **unbalanced** form. In the latter, there is a gain or loss of genetic material; in the former, there is no change in the amount of genetic material but only a rearrangement of it. At the sites of breaks and new attachments of chromosome fragments, there may be permanent structural or functional damage to one gene or to only a few genes. Despite no visible loss of material, the aberration may nonetheless be recognized as unbalanced through an abnormal phenotype and the chromosomal defect confirmed by molecular analysis of the DNA.

Aneuploidy results from nondisjunction—the failure of a chromatid pair to separate in a dividing cell. Nondisjunction in either the first or second division of meiosis results in gametes with abnormal chromosomal constitutions. In aneuploidy, more or fewer than 46 chromosomes are present (Table 40–1). The following are all forms of aneuploidy: (1) **monosomy,** in which only one member of a pair of chromosomes is present; (2) **trisomy,** in which three chromosomes are present instead of two; and (3) **polysomy,** in which one chromosome is represented four or more times.

If nondisjunction occurs in mitosis, **mosaic** patterns occur in somatic tissue, with some cells having one karyotype and other cells of the same organism another karyotype. Patients with a mosaic genetic constitution often have manifestations of each of the genetic syndromes associated with the various abnormal karyotypes.

Translocation results from an exchange of parts of two chromosomes.

Deletion is loss of chromosomal material.

Duplication is the presence of two or more copies of the same region of a given chromosome. The redundancy may occur in the same chromosome or in a

Table 40–1. Clinical phenotypes resulting from aneuploidy.

Condition	Karyotype	Incidence at Birth
Trisomy 13	47,XX or XY,+13	1:15,000
Trisomy 18	47,XX or XY,+18	1:11,000
Trisomy 21 (Down's syndrome)	47,XX or XY,+21	1:900
Klinefelter's syndrome	47,XXY	1:1000 males
XYY	47,XYY	1:1000 males
Turner's syndrome	45,X	1:7500 females
XXX syndrome	47,XXX	1:1000 females

nonhomologous chromosome. In the latter case, a translocation will also have occurred.

An **isochromosome** is one in which the arms on either side of the centromere have the same genetic material in the same order—ie, the chromosome has at some time divided in such a way that it has a double dose of one arm and absence of the other.

In an **inversion,** a chromosomal region becomes reoriented 180 degrees out of ordinary phase. The same genetic material is present, but in a different order.

Ferguson-Smith MA, Andrews T: Cytogenetic analysis. In: *Principles and Practice of Medical Genetics,* 3rd ed. Rimoin DL, Connor JM, Pyeritz RE (editors). Churchill Livingstone, 1997. (A review of the indications for and techniques of clinical cytogenetics.)

THE TECHNIQUES OF MEDICAL GENETICS

The diagnosis and management of hereditary disorders should bring to bear the skills and knowledge of a general physician. The disorders affect multiple organ systems and people of all ages. Many disorders are chronic ones, but often there are acute crises. The concerns of patients and families span a wide range of medical, psychologic, social, and economic issues. These characteristics emphasize the need for pediatricians, internists, obstetricians, and family practitioners to provide medical genetics services for their patients. Those physicians therefore need to know what laboratory and consultative services are available from clinical geneticists and the indications for their use. This section reviews these matters.

CYTOGENETICS

Cytogenetics is the study of chromosomes by light microscopy. The chromosomal constitution of a single cell or an entire individual is specified by a standardized notation. The total chromosome count is determined first, followed by the sex chromosome complement and then by any abnormalities. The autosomes are all designated by numbers from 1 to 22. A plus (+) or minus (–) sign indicates, respectively, a gain or loss of chromosomal material. For example, a normal male is 46,XY, while a girl with Down's syndrome caused by trisomy 21 is 47,XX,+21.

Chromosomal analyses are done by growing human cells in tissue culture, chemically inhibiting mitosis, and then staining, observing, photographing, sorting, and counting the chromosomes. The display of all of the chromosomes is termed the **karyotype** (Figure 40–1) and is the end result of the technical aspect of cytogenetics.

Specimens for cytogenetic analysis can be obtained for routine analysis from the peripheral blood, in which case T lymphocytes are examined; from amniotic fluid for culture of amniocytes; from trophoblastic cells from the chorionic villus; from bone marrow; and from cultured fibroblasts, usually obtained from a skin biopsy. Enough cells must be examined so that the chance of missing a cytogenetically distinct cell line (a situation of mosaicism) is statistically low. For most clinical indications, 20 mitoses are examined and counted under direct microscopic visualization, and two are photographed and karyotypes prepared. Observation of aberrations usually prompts more extended scrutiny and in many cases further analysis of the original culture.

A variety of methods can be used to reveal banding patterns—unique to each pair of chromosomes—in the analysis of aberrations. The number of bands that can be visualized is a function of how "extended" the chromosomes are, which in turn depends chiefly on how early in metaphase (or even in prophase for the most extensive banding) mitosis was arrested. The "standard" karyotype reveals about 400 bands per haploid set of chromosomes, whereas a prophase karyotype might reveal four times that number. As invaluable as extended karyotypes are in certain clinical circumstances, their interpretation is often difficult—in terms of the time and effort required and of ambiguity about what is abnormal, what is a normal variation, and what is a technical artifact. In situ hybridization with DNA probes for specific chromosomes or regions of chromosomes can be labeled and used to identify subtle aberrations. Given proper technique, fluorescent in situ hybridization (FISH) yields sensitivities and specificities of virtually 100%. Some applications are being used routinely and marketed commercially, though the FDA has been slow to approve any probes for clinical use.

Indications for Cytogenetic Analysis

The current indications are listed in Table 40–2. A wide array of clinical syndromes have been found to be associated with chromosomal aberrations, and analysis of the karyotype is useful any time a patient is discovered to have the manifestations of one of these syndromes. When a chromosomal aberration is revealed, not only does the patient's physician obtain valuable information about prognosis, but the parents gain insight into the cause of their child's problems and the family can be counseled accurately—and usually reassured—about the risks of recurrence.

Mental retardation is a frequent component of congenital malformation syndromes because of coincident defective development of the central nervous system. However, one of the most frequent causes of mental retardation is associated with few systemic effects. The fragile-X syndrome—so called because of the gap, or **fragile site,** evident at the end of the long arm of the X chromosome—occurs in one of every 2000 males and is second only to Down's syndrome as a cause of retardation in males. This aberration is inherited from mothers who are heterozygous for the fragile-X site; many carrier women have apparently normal intellect, but some are retarded. Thus, any person with unexplained mental retardation should be studied by chromosomal analysis, with particular attention paid to this aberration. Since special techniques are required, the laboratory request must clearly indicate that a search for fragile sites is needed.

Abnormalities of sexual differentiation can only be understood once the patient's **genetic sex** is clarified. Hormonal therapy and plastic surgery can to some extent determine **phenotypic sex,** but genetic sex is dictated by the complement of sex chromosomes. The best-known example of dichotomy between the genetic sex and phenotypic sex is the testicular feminization syndrome, in which the chromosomal constitution is 46,XY but, because of a defect in the testosterone receptor protein (specified by a gene on the Y chromosome), the external phenotype is completely female.

Failure or delay in developing secondary sexual characteristics occurs in Turner's syndrome (the most common cause being a form of aneuploidy, ie, monosomy for the X chromosome, 45,X), in Klinefelter's syndrome (the most common karyotype is 47,XXY), and in other much rarer chromosomal aberrations.

Tall stature is perhaps the only consistent phenotypic feature associated with having an extra Y chromosome (karyotype 47,XYY); most men with this chromosomal aberration lead normal lives, and thus tall stature in a male is itself no indication for chromosomal analysis. However, some evidence suggests that an increased prevalence of learning difficulties may be associated with this aberration. Furthermore, Klinefelter's syndrome often causes tall stature, albeit with a eunuchoid habitus, and learning and behavioral problems. Thus, the combination of learning or behavioral difficulties and unexpectedly increased height in a male should prompt consideration of cytogenetic analysis.

As discussed below, most tumors are associated with chromosomal aberrations, some of which are highly specific for certain malignancies. Cytogenetic analysis of tumor tissue may assist in diagnosis, prognosis, and management.

Whenever a person is shown to have a chromosome translocation—whether it be balanced and asymptomatic or unbalanced, causing a syndrome—the physician should consider the importance of identifying the source of the translocation. If the proband is a child and the parents are interested in having more children, both parents should be studied cytogenetically. How far the primary physician or consultant should go in tracking a translocation through a family is an unsettled question with legal and ethical as well as medical implications. Certainly the proband (if an adult) or the parents of the proband need to be counseled and the potential risks to relatives discussed. The physician should document, both in the medical record and by correspondence, that the burden of disclosing relevant data to the extended family has been assumed by specific named individuals.

Inability to produce offspring, either through failure to conceive or as a result of repeated miscarriages, is a frustrating and discouraging problem for affected couples and their physicians. Considerable progress in the urologic and gynecologic understanding of infertility has benefited many couples. However, chromosomal aberrations remain an important

---

Table 40–2. Indications for cytogenetic analysis.

1. Patients with malformations suggestive of one of the recognized syndromes associated with a specific chromosome aberration.
2. Patients of any age who are grossly retarded physically or mentally, especially if there are associated anomalies.
3. Any patient with ambiguous internal or external genitalia or suspected hermaphroditism.
4. Girls with primary amenorrhea and boys with delayed pubertal development. Up to 25% of patients with primary amenorrhea have a chromosomal abnormality.
5. Males with learning or behavioral disorders who are taller than expected (based on parental height).
6. Certain malignant and premalignant diseases (see Tables 40–8 and 40–9).
7. Parents of a patient with chromosome translocation.
8. Parents of a patient with a suspected chromosomal syndrome if there is a family history of similarly affected children.
9. Couples with a history of multiple spontaneous abortions of unknown cause.
10. Couples who are infertile after more common obstetric and urologic causes have been excluded.
11. Prenatal diagnosis (see Table 40–7).

problem in reproductive medicine, and cytogenetic analysis should be utilized at some stage in extended evaluation. Infertility can be caused by Klinefelter's and Turner's syndromes; the external phenotype may be subtle, particularly if the chromosomal aberration is mosaic. Any early spontaneous abortion may be due to fetal aneuploidy. Recurrence may be due to parental translocation predisposing to an unbalanced fetal karyotype.

Borgaonkar D: *Chromosomal Variation in Man,* 7th ed. Wiley, 1994. (A comprehensive catalogue; the companion of McKusick's *Mendelian Inheritance in Man.*)

Flint J et al: The detection of subtelomeric chromosomal rearrangements in idiopathic mental retardation. Nat Genet 1995;9:132. (A demonstration of the power of molecular detection of subtle chromosome defects, with application to diagnosing causes of retardation.)

Mitelman F: *Catalog of Chromosome Aberrations in Cancer,* 5th ed. Wiley, 1994. (Common and rare cytogenetic aberrations in tumors of all types.)

Mitelman F (editor): *An International System for Human Cytogenetic Nomenclature (1995).* Karger, 1995. (The most recent revision to the standard approach for designating normal and abnormal chromosomes.)

Schröck E et al: Multicolor spectral karyotyping of human chromosomes. Science 1996;273:499. (By using FISH and computerized classification of emission spectra, each human chromosome acquires a unique color. Enables detection of subtle rearrangements.)

BIOCHEMICAL GENETICS

Biochemical genetics deals not only with enzymatic defects but also with proteins of all functions, including cytoskeletal and extracellular structure, regulation, and receptors. The principal functions of the biochemical genetics laboratory are to determine the presence or absence of proteins, to assess the qualitative characteristics of proteins, and to verify the effectiveness of proteins in vitro. The key elements from the referring physician's perspective are (1) to indicate what the suspected clinical diagnoses are and (2) to make certain that the proper specimen is obtained and transported to the laboratory in a timely manner.

Indications for Biochemical Investigations

Some inborn errors are relatively common in the general population, eg, hemochromatosis, defects of the low-density lipoprotein receptor, and cystic fibrosis (Table 40–3). Others, while rare across the entire population, are common in certain ethnic groups, such as Tay-Sachs disease in Ashkenazic Jews, sickle cell disease in African-Americans, and thalassemias in populations from around the Mediterranean basin and Asia. Many of these disorders are autosomal recessive, and the frequency of heterozygotes is many times that of the fully expressed disease. Screening for carrier status can be effective if certain requirements are satisfied (Table 40–4). For example, all of the United States and the District of Columbia require screening of newborns for one or more metabolic diseases. Such programs are cost-effective even for rare conditions such as phenylketonuria, which occurs in only one of every 11,000 births. Unfortunately, not all disorders that meet the requirements in Table 40–4 are screened for in every state. Furthermore, compliance is highly variable among programs, and follow-up diagnostic tests, management, and counseling are in some cases inadequate. Babies most likely to be missed are those born at home and those discharged before they have digested much milk or formula. In some states, parents can refuse to have their infants studied.

Use of the biochemical genetics laboratory for other than screening purposes must be justified by

Table 40–3. Representative inborn errors of metabolism.

General Class of Defect	Example	Biochemical Defect	Inheritance[1]
Aminoacidopathy	Phenylketonuria	Phenylalanine hydroxylase	AR
Connective tissue	Osteogenesis imperfecta type II	$\alpha1(I)$ and $\alpha2(I)$ procollagen	AD
Gangliosidosis	Tay-Sachs disease	Hexosaminidase A	AR
Glycogen storage disease	Type I	Glucose-6-phosphatase	AR
Immune function	Chronic granulomatous disease	Cytochrome b, β chain	XL
Lipid metabolism	Familial hypercholesterolemia	LDL receptor	AD
Mucopolysaccharidosis	MPS II (Hunter's syndrome)	Iduronate sulfatase	XL
Porphyria	Acute intermittent	Porphobilinogen deaminase	AD
Transport	Cystic fibrosis	CF transmembrane conductance regulator	AR

[1]AR = autosomal recessive; AD = autosomal dominant; XL = X-linked recessive.

Table 40–4. Requirements for effective screening for inborn errors of metabolism.

1. The disease should be clinically severe or have potentially severe consequences.
2. The natural history of the disease should be understood.
3. Effective treatment should be generally available and depend on early diagnosis for optimal results.
4. The disease incidence should be high enough to warrant screening.
5. The screening test should have favorable specificity (low false-positive rate) and sensitivity (low false-negative rate).
6. The screening test should be available for and used by the entire population at risk.
7. An adequate system for follow-up of positive results should be provided.
8. The economic cost-benefit analysis should favor screening and treatment.

the need for data on which to base a diagnosis of specific disorders or classes of related disorders. The possibilities are limited only by the extent of knowledge, the enthusiasm of the primary physician or consultant, the willingness of the patient or family to pursue the diagnosis and specimens to be taken, and the availability of a laboratory to examine the specimens.

Though many inborn defects are so subtle they escape detection, there are a number of clinical situations in which an inborn error should be part of the differential diagnosis. The urgency with which the investigation is undertaken will vary depending on the severity of the disorder and the availability of treatment. Table 40–5 lists various clinical presentations.

The possibility of acute metabolic disease of the neonate is the most important indication, because prompt diagnosis and treatment may often make the difference between life and death. The clinical features are nonspecific because the newborn has a limited repertoire of responses to severe metabolic insults. The physician must be both inclusive and systematic in evaluating such ill babies.

Scriver CR et al (editors): *The Metabolic and Molecular Bases of Inherited Disease,* 7th ed. McGraw-Hill, 1995. (The standard reference work and source of information about most hereditary disorders.)
Seashore WR, Wappner RS: *Genetics in Primary Care & Clinical Medicine.* Appleton & Lange, 1996. (Contains a general approach to the child with a suspected metabolic disorder.)

DNA ANALYSIS

Direct inspection of nucleic acids—often called "molecular genetics" or "DNA diagnosis"—is achieving an increasingly prominent role in a number of clinical areas, including oncology, infectious disease, forensic medicine, and the general study of pathophysiology. A major impact has been in the diagnosis of mendelian disorders. Once a particular gene is shown to be defective in a given condition, the nature of the mutation itself can be determined, often by sequencing the nucleotides and comparing the array with that of a normal allele. One of a variety of techniques can then be used to determine whether that same mutation is present in other patients with the same disorder. Genetic heterogeneity is so extensive that most mendelian conditions are associated with numerous mutations at one locus—or occasionally multiple loci—that produce the same phenotype. Mutations at no less than 13 different genes cause retinitis pigmentosa, and changes in at least six genes cause familial hypertrophic cardiomyopathy. This fact complicates DNA diagnosis of patients and screening for carriers of defects in specific genes.

A few conditions are associated with relatively few mutations or with only one highly prevalent mutation. For example, all sickle cell disease is caused by exactly the same change of glutamate to valine at position 6 of β-globin, and that substitution in turn is due to a change of one nucleotide at the sixth codon in the β-globin gene. But such uniformity is the exception. In cystic fibrosis, about 70% of heterozy-

Table 40–5. Manner of presentation of inborn errors of metabolism.

Presentation and Course	Examples
Acute metabolic disease of the neonate	Galactosemia, urea cycle disorders
Chronic disorders with little progression	Phenylketonuria, hypothyroidism
Chronic disorders with insidious, incessant progression	Tay-Sachs disease
Disorders causing abnormalities of structure	Skeletal dysplasias, Marfan's syndrome
Disorders of transport	Cystinuria, lactase deficiency
Disorders that determine susceptibilities	LDL receptor deficiency, agammaglobulinemia
Episodic disorders	Most porphyrias, G6PD deficiency
Disorders causing anemia	Pyruvate kinase deficiency, hereditary spherocytosis
Disorders interfering with hemostasis	Hemophilia A and B, von Willebrand disease
Congenital disorders with no possibility of reversal	Testicular feminization
Disorders with protean manifestations	Pseudohypoparathyroidism, hereditary amyloidoses
Inborn errors with no clinical effects	Pentosuria, histidinemia

gotes have an identical deletion of three nucleotides that causes loss of a phenylalanine residue from a chloride transport protein; however, the remaining 30% of mutations of that protein are diverse (over 300 have been discovered), so that no simple screening test will detect *all* carriers of cystic fibrosis.

Reviews of the current technical status of DNA analysis appear regularly in the medical literature. Polymerase chain reaction (PCR) studies have revolutionized many aspects of molecular biology, and DNA diagnosis has come to involve this technique in many instances. If the sequences of the 10–20 nucleotides at the ends of a region of DNA of interest (such as a portion of a gene) are known, then "primers" complementary to these sequences can be synthesized. When even a minute amount of DNA from a patient (eg, from a few leukocytes, buccal mucosal cells, or hair bulbs) is combined with the primers in a reaction mixture that replicates DNA—and after several dozen cycles are then performed—the region of DNA between the primers will be amplified exponentially. For example, the presence of early HIV infection can be detected after PCR amplification of a portion of the viral genome.

Indications for DNA Diagnosis

The basic requirement for the use of nucleic acids in the diagnosis of hereditary conditions is that a **probe** be available for the gene in question. The probe may be a piece of the actual gene, a sequence close to the gene, or just a few nucleotides at the actual mutation. The closer the probe is to the actual mutation, the more accurate and the more useful will be the information derived. DNA diagnosis involves one of two general approaches: (1) direct detection of the mutation and (2) linkage analysis, whereby the presence of a mutation is inferred from the nature of a probe DNA sequence remote from the mutation. In the latter approach, as the probe moves farther from the mutation, the chances increase that recombination will have separated the two sequences and confused the interpretation of the data.

Some of the conditions for which direct detection is possible are listed in Table 40–6. Conditions that can be diagnosed only indirectly are also listed; while their number also is increasing, there is a gratifying shift to diagnosis by direct detection as the molecular nature of mutations is defined.

DNA diagnosis is finding frequent application in presymptomatic detection of individuals with age-dependent disorders such as Huntington's disease and adult polycystic kidney disease, screening for carriers of autosomal recessive conditions such as cystic fibrosis and thalassemias, screening for female heterozygotes of X-linked conditions such as Duchenne's muscular dystrophy and hemophilia A and B, and prenatal diagnosis (see below). The full range of indications is undefined at this time. However, primary care providers and specialists alike must be mindful that substantive ethical, psychologic, legal, and social issues remain unresolved. For example, some conditions for which hereditary susceptibility can be readily defined (such as Alzheimer's disease, hemochromatosis, Huntington's disease, and many cancers) have no effective therapy at this time. For these same conditions, health insurance and life insurance providers may be especially interested in learning who among their current or prospective customers is at higher risk. Some states have enacted legislation to protect people identified as having one

Table 40–6. Selected DNA probes with current diagnostic applications.

Gene Probe	Disorder	Diagnostic Application
β-Globin	Sickle cell disease Beta thalassemia	Prenatal screening Prenatal screening
α-Globin	Alpha thalassemia Polycystic kidney disease	Prenatal screening Presymptomatic, prenatal screening
Factor VIII	Hemophilia A	Prenatal screening, carrier detection
Dystrophin	Duchenne's muscular dystrophy	Presymptomatic, prenatal screening, carrier detection
α_1-AP	α_1-Antiprotease deficiency	Prenatal screening
Phe hydroxylase	Phenylketonuria	Prenatal screening
CFTR	Cystic fibrosis	Prenatal, presymptomatic screening, carrier detection
Trinucleotide repeat (CAG) in huntingtin	Huntington's disease	Presymptomatic, prenatal screening
Growth hormone	Growth hormone deficiency	Prenatal screening, carrier detection, early diagnosis
HLA	Hemochromatosis Congenital adrenal hyperplasia	Presymptomatic, prenatal screening Prenatal screening

or another genetic risk. (When all is said and done, all of us fall in this category.)

Logistics of DNA Diagnosis

Lymphocytes are a ready source of DNA; 10 mL of whole blood yields up to 0.5 mg of DNA, enough for dozens of analyses based on hybridization, each of which requires only 5 μg. If the analysis is quite narrowly focused on a specific mutation (such as in a family study, in which only one specific nucleotide change is addressed), PCR analysis can often be used and the amount of DNA needed is truly infinitesimal—a few hair bulbs or sperm are adequate. Once isolated, the DNA sample can be divided into aliquots and frozen. Alternatively, lymphocytes can be transformed with viruses into lymphoblasts; these cells are immortal, can be frozen, and—whenever DNA is required—can be thawed, propagated, and their DNA isolated. These stored specimens provide access to a person's genome long after the individual dies. This is such an important advantage that many clinical genetics centers and commercial laboratories "bank" DNA from patients and informative relatives even if the samples cannot be put to use immediately. The specimens may later prove invaluable to relatives or to other patients being evaluated. DNA in some instances has become more reliable than the medical record and even more readily retrievable!

Blood for DNA isolation should be drawn in EDTA anticoagulant (purple-top tubes); blood for lymphoblast culture should be drawn in heparin (green-top tubes). Neither should be frozen. Specimens for DNA isolation can be stored or shipped at room temperature over a period of a few days. Lymphoblast cultures should be established within 48 hours, so prompt shipment is essential.

Fetal DNA can be isolated from amniotic cells, from trophoblastic cells taken by chorionic villus sampling, or from either cell type grown in culture. Samples need to be processed promptly but can be shipped by overnight mail and *must not be frozen*.

Elias S, Annas GJ: Generic consent for genetic screening. N Engl J Med 1994;330:1611. (The importance of discussing the indications for and implications of a wide variety of genetic screening tests.)

Karnes PS: Ordering and interpreting DNA tests. Mayo Clinic Proc 1996;71:1192.

Korf B: Molecular medicine: Molecular diagnosis. N Engl J Med 1995;332:1218, 1499. (A brief review of the principles and applications of DNA analysis to clinical medicine.)

Krawczak M, Schmidtke J: *DNA Fingerprinting*. BIOS Scientific, 1994. (A survey of methods and applications of DNA analysis for human identification.)

Wertz DC et al: Genetic testing for children and adolescents: Who decides? JAMA 1994;272:875. (Young people raise special concerns when presymptomatic disorders may be detected by DNA testing.)

PRENATAL DIAGNOSIS

It is possible to diagnose in utero, before the middle of the second trimester, several hundred mendelian disorders, all chromosome aberrations, and a number of congenital malformations that are not mendelian. The first step toward prenatal diagnosis is taken when the expecting couple, the primary physician, or the obstetrician thinks of the need for it. Recent surveys suggest that even for the most common indication for such service—advanced maternal age—less than half of all women 35 years and older are offered prenatal testing.

Techniques Used in Prenatal Diagnosis

Prenatal diagnosis depends on the ability to assay the fetus directly (fetal blood sampling, fetoscopy), indirectly (analysis of amniotic fluid, amniocytes or trophoblastic cells, ultrasound), or remotely (analysis of maternal serum). Some of these techniques satisfy the requirements for screening (Table 40–4) and should be offered to all pregnant women; others carry considerable risk and should be reserved for specific circumstances. A few centers are developing preimplantation diagnosis of the embryo; a single cell is plucked from the six- to eight-cell blastocyst, which has been cultured after in vitro fertilization, without harming future development. The chromosomes of the cell can be studied by FISH or the genes by PCR. Another new approach, with considerable potential, is isolation of fetal cells that are circulating in minute numbers in the maternal circulation.

Ultrasound scanning of the fetus is a safe, noninvasive procedure that can diagnose gross skeletal malformations as well as nonbony malformations known to be associated with specific diseases. Some obstetricians routinely perform fetal ultrasound at least once between 12 and 20 weeks of gestation, though this practice does not yet represent the standard of care.

Other prenatal diagnostic procedures—fetoscopy, fetography, and amniography—are more invasive and a definite risk to the mother and fetus. They are indicated only if the risk of the suspected abnormality is high and the information cannot be obtained by other means.

All of the cytogenetic, biochemical, and DNA analytic techniques discussed above can be applied to specimens from the fetus. Aside from screening for α-fetoprotein in maternal serum, analysis of fetal chromosomes is the most frequently performed test. Chromosomal analysis can be performed on amniotic cells and on trophoblastic cells grown in culture and directly on any trophoblastic cells that happen to be undergoing mitosis. Amniotic fluid cells are derived chiefly from the fetal urinary system. Amniocentesis can be performed between gestational weeks 16 and 18 to permit unhurried sample analysis, transmission of results, and reproductive decisions. The time from obtaining the sample to a final reading of the karyotype has now been shortened to an average of 10–14 days, and automated methods may reduce the time a bit further. Sampling the chorionic villus (CVS) for trophoblastic cells (derived embryologically from the same fertilized egg as the fetus) is usually done between gestational weeks 10 and 11. If the tissue can be analyzed directly, cytogenetic results can be obtained within a few hours; however, the quality of the karyotypes is inferior to that from cultured cells, and most laboratories routinely culture cells and reexamine any suspected abnormalities. The advantage of CVS is that the results are available early in pregnancy, so that termination, if elected, can occur earlier in the pregnancy and the obstetric complications of termination are fewer.

The risk of CVS is somewhat higher than that of amniocentesis, though both are relatively safe. Between 0.5% and 1% of pregnancies are lost as a complication of CVS, whereas less than one in 300 amniocenteses result in fetal loss. These figures are lower than—but are in addition to—the 2–3% spontaneous abortion rate after the first trimester ends.

Indications for Prenatal Diagnosis

The indications for prenatal diagnosis are listed in Table 40–7. A few deserve comment.

Most studies done for advanced maternal age will detect no chromosomal aberration, and the couple will be reassured by this news. However, it is always appropriate to emphasize that the average risk of producing a child with a defect evident at birth, such as a physical malformation or some inborn error of metabolism, is about 3%, and that the risk increases with the age of either parent. Simply examining the chromosomes reduces this risk minimally. On the other hand, unless one of the other indications is present, it is simply not possible to "screen" a pregnancy for most birth defects (neural tube defects being an exception).

A history for cytogenetic aberrations emphasizes a chromosomal defect in a parent, a family history of a chromosomal defect, or a previous child or conceptus with a defined or undefined chromosomal defect. The factors that render some couples susceptible to repeated episodes of aneuploidy are unclear, and routine prenatal testing is warranted once a defect has occurred.

Cytogenetic analysis of the fetus will of course give information about the sex chromosomes. Some couples do not desire advance knowledge of the sex of their child, and the person transmitting the results to the couple should always address this issue first. On the other hand, some couples *only* want to know the sex of the fetus and plan to terminate the pregnancy if the undesired sex is detected. Virtually no centers in the United States consider sex selection to be an appropriate indication for prenatal diagnosis.

The level of α-fetoprotein in maternal serum changes with gestational age, with the mother's medical status, and with abnormalities of the fetus. If the first two factors can be well controlled, the assay can be used to provide information about the fetus. Levels are expressed as multiples of the median value for a particular gestational age. Higher than normal levels are associated with open neural tube defects (the conditions for which the test was developed), recent or impending fetal demise, gastroschisis, and fetal renal disease. Extremely high levels are highly specific for fetal anomalies—a level three times the median increases 20-fold the risk of meningomyelocele or anencephaly. Low α-fetoprotein levels in maternal serum are associated with fetal trisomy, especially Down's syndrome; the reason for this association remains unclear. The addition of two other analytes in maternal serum—human chorionic gonadotropin (hCG) and unconjugated estriol (uE3)—to the assay for α-fetoprotein (to produce the "triple screen") enhances by several times the ability to detect a fetus with trisomy 21 and trisomy 18. While the triple screen in the second—and probably the first—trimester improves both the sensitivity and specificity of detection of trisomic pregnancies, all positive results need to be followed by amniocentesis for confirmation.

Table 40–7. Indications for prenatal diagnosis.

Indications	Methods
Age of mother ≥ 35 years at expected delivery, previous child with chromosome aberration, intrauterine growth delay	Cytogenetics (amniocentesis, chorionic villus sampling)
Biochemical disorder	Protein assay, DNA diagnosis
Congenital anomaly	Sonography, fetoscopy
Screening for neural tube defects and trisomy	Maternal serum α-fetoprotein and chorionic gonadotropin

Biagiotti R et al: Maternal serum screening for Down's syndrome in the first trimester of pregnancy. Br J Obstet Gynaecol 1995;102:660. (Concise review of the potential for screening earlier in pregnancy.)

D'Alton ME, DeCherney AH: Prenatal diagnosis. N Engl Med 1993;328:114. (Concise review of current possibilities.)

Delhanty JDA: Preimplantation diagnosis. Prenatal Dia 1995;14:1217. (A concise review of this new approach to diagnosing chromosomal and genetic problems after in vitro fertilization.)

Milunsky A (editor): *Genetic Disorders and the Fetus*, 3r ed. Johns Hopkins Univ Press, 1992. (Multiauthored text that covers methods and specific fetal and maternal disorders.)

Simoni G, Sirchia SM: Confined placental mosaicism. Pr

natal Diag 1995;14:1185. (A discussion of a cause of false-positive results in chorionic villus sampling.)

Simpson JL, Elias S: Isolating fetal cells in maternal circulation for prenatal diagnosis. Prenatal Diag 1995;14:1229. (Two of the principal investigators in developing this technique review progress.)

NEOPLASIA: CHROMOSOMAL & DNA ANALYSIS

Studies of both chromosomes and nucleic acids support Boveri's 1914 hypothesis that cancer is caused by a change in genetic material at the cellular level. Two classes of genes have been discovered that function in neoplastic transformation.

Oncogenes arise from preexisting normal genes (proto-oncogenes) that have been altered by both viral and nonviral factors. As a result, the cells synthesize either normal proteins in inappropriate amounts or proteins that are aberrant in structure and function. Many of these proteins are cellular growth factors, controllers of messenger RNA, and initiators and regulators of RNA; others are receptors for growth factors. The net result of oncogene activation is unregulated cell division. Mutations that activate oncogenes virtually always arise in somatic cells and are not usually inherited. Although some oncogenes are more likely to be activated in certain tumors, in general the same mutations may be found in neoplasia arising in different cells and tissues.

Tumor suppressor genes can be viewed as the antithesis of oncogenes. Their normal function is to suppress transformation; mutation in both alleles is necessary to obliterate this important function. The first mutant allele at any tumor suppressor gene might arise spontaneously or might be inherited; mutation in the other allele (the "second hit") virtually always arises spontaneously, but by any of a number of molecular mechanisms. These genes show considerably more tumor specificity than do oncogenes; however, while some specific mutations are necessary for certain tumors to arise, no loss of single tumor suppressor function is sufficient. Clearly, a person who inherits one copy of a mutant tumor suppressor gene is at increased risk that in some susceptible cell, at some time during life, the function of that gene will be lost. This susceptibility is inherited as an autosomal dominant trait. For example, mutation in one allele of the p53 locus results in the Li-Fraumeni syndrome, in which susceptibility before age 45 years to sarcomas and other tumors occurs in males and females in successive generations. Inherited mutations in this locus also increase the risk that a second tumor will develop following radiation or chemotherapy for the first tumor, suggesting that the initial treatment may induce a "second hit" in a p53 locus in another tissue. However, inheriting a p53 mutation is not a guarantee that cancer will develop at an early age; much more needs to be learned about the pathogenesis of neoplasia before the genetic counseling of families with a molecular predisposition to cancer is clarified. *BRCA1,* a gene that predisposes women to breast and ovarian cancer, is another example of a tumor suppressor gene. Women who inherit one mutant allele of *BRCA1* have an 85% lifetime risk of developing breast cancer, and the average age of tumor detection is in the fifth decade.

In selected cases, a patient's DNA can be analyzed for the presence of a mutated gene and thereby assess that individual's risk for developing a tumor. Examples are retinoblastoma, certain forms of Wilms' tumor, breast cancer, and familial colon cancer. To illustrate how noninvasive and sensitive the methodology has become, it is possible to analyze stool for the presence of mutations in tumor suppressor genes that might indicate the presence of a clinically undetected adenocarcinoma of the colon. The analysis—not yet in general use—depends on the ability of the polymerase chain reaction to amplify minute quantities of the mutant DNA present in epithelial cells shed from the tumor.

A third class of genes that predispose to malignancy has been discovered in the past few years. So-called **mutator genes** have joined oncogenes and tumor suppressor genes as risk factors. Mutator genes normally function to repair damage to DNA that occurs from environmental insults such as exposure to carcinogens and ultraviolet irradiation. When a mutator gene is mutated itself, DNA damage accumulates and eventually affects oncogenes and tumor suppressor genes, thereby making cancer more likely. Hereditary nonpolyposis colon cancer is one familial syndrome due to mutations in one of the four mutator genes identified thus far.

This exciting work on the molecular nature of oncogenesis was preceded by years of study of the cytogenetics of tumors. Indeed, the retinoblastoma tumor suppressor gene was ultimately isolated because a small number of patients with this tumor have a constitutive deletion of chromosome 13 where this gene maps. Other chromosomal aberrations have been found to be highly characteristic of—or even specific for—certain tumors (Table 40–8). Detection of one of these cytogenetic aberrations can thus aid in diagnosis.

Hematologic malignancies are especially amenable to study because of the relative ease of performing cytogenetic analysis. Such malignancies are associated with over 100 specific chromosomal rearrangements, chiefly translocations. Most of these rearrangements are restricted to a specific type of cancer (Table 40–9), and the remainder occur with many cancers.

In the leukemias, the chromosomal aberration is the basis of one of the subclassifications of the disease. When cytogenetic information is combined with the FAB classification, it is possible to define

Table 40–8. Chromosome aberrations associated with representative solid tumors.

Tumor	Chromosome Aberration
Meningioma	del(22)(q11)[1]
Neuroblastoma	del(1)(p36) or amplification
Renal cell carcinoma	del(3)(p14.2–p25) or translocation of this region
Retinoblastoma, osteosarcoma	del(13)(q14.1) or translocation of this region
Small-cell lung carcinoma	del(3)(p14–p23)
Wilms' tumor	del(11)(p15)

[1]Nomenclature means, "a deletion at band q11 of chromosome 22."

subsets of patients in which response to therapy, clinical course, and prognosis are predictable. If at the time of diagnosis there are no chromosomal changes in the bone marrow cells, the survival time is longer than if any or all of the bone marrow cells have abnormal cytogenetic characteristics. As secondary chromosomal changes occur, the leukemia becomes more aggressive, often associated with drug resistance and a reduced chance for complete or prolonged remission. The least ominous chromosomal change is numerical alteration without morphologic abnormality.

Less cytogenetic information is available for lymphomas and premalignant hematologic disorders than for leukemia. In Hodgkin's disease, studies have been limited by the low yield of dividing cells and the low number of clear-cut aneuploid clones, so that complete chromosomal analyses with banding are available for far fewer patients with Hodgkin's disease than for any other type of lymphoma. In Hodgkin's disease, the modal chromosomal number tends to be triploid or tetraploid. About one-third of the samples have a 14q+ chromosome. In non-Hodgkin's

Table 40–9. Chromosomal aberrations associated with representative hematologic malignancies.

Tumor	Chromosomal Aberration
Leukemias	
Acute myeloblastic	t(8;21)(q22;q11)[1]
Acute promyelocytic	t(15;17)(q22;q11–q12)
Acute monocytic	t(10;11)(p15–p11;q23)
Chronic myelogenous	t(9;22)(q23;q11)
Lymphomas	
Burkitt's	t(8;14)(q24.1;q32.3)
B cell	t(1;14)(q42;q43)
T cell	inv, del, and t of 1p13–p12
Premalignancy	
Polycythemia vera	del(20)(q11)

[1]Nomenclature means, "a translocation with the union at band q22 of chromosome 8 and q11 of chromosome 21."

lymphomas, high-resolution techniques of banding detect abnormalities in 95% of cases. Cytogenetic findings are now being correlated with the immunologic and histologic features and with prognosis.

In Burkitt's lymphoma, a solid tumor of B cell origin, 90% of patients have a translocation between the long arm of chromosome 8 and the long arm of chromosome 14, with chromosomal breakage sites being at or near immunoglobulin and oncogene loci.

Instability of chromosomes also predisposes to the development of some malignancies. In certain autosomal recessive diseases such as ataxia-telangiectasia, Bloom's syndrome, and Fanconi's anemia, the cells have a tendency to **genetic instability,** ie, to chromosomal breakage and rearrangement in vitro. These diseases are associated with a fairly high incidence of neoplasia, particularly leukemia and lymphoma.

Some chromosomal aberrations, better known for their effect on phenotype, also predispose to tumors. For example, patients with Down's syndrome (trisomy 21) have a 20-fold increase in the risk of leukemia; 47,XXY males (Klinefelter's syndrome) have a 30-fold increase in the risk of breast cancer; and XY phenotypic females have a heightened risk of developing ovarian cancer, primarily gonadoblastoma.

The indications for cytogenetic analysis of neoplasia continue to evolve. Not all tumors require study. However, in cases of tumors of unclear type (especially leukemias and lymphomas), with a strong family history of early neoplasia, or for certain tumors associated with potential generalized chromosomal defects (present in nonneoplastic cells), cytogenetic analysis should be strongly considered.

Cline MJ: The molecular basis of leukemia. N Engl J Med 1994;330:328. (Current understanding of the etiology and pathogenesis of leukemia in molecular terms.)

Fearon E, Cho KR: The molecular biology of cancer. In: *Principles and Practice of Medical Genetics,* 3rd ed. Rimoin DL, Connor JM, Pyeritz RE (editors): Churchill Livingstone, 1997.

Fishel R et al: The human mutator gene homolog *MSH2* and its association with hereditary nonpolyposis colon cancer. Cell 1993;75:1027. (Description of the first gene in a new class of loci that predispose to neoplasia.)

Hoskins KF et al: Assessment and counseling for women with a family history of breast cancer: A guide for clinicians. JAMA 1995;273:577. (A concise guide to current application of genetic insights to a common tumor.)

Lerman C, Croyle R: Psychological issues in genetic testing for breast cancer susceptibility. Arch Intern Med 1994;154:609. (Reviews the host of issues raised by DNA testing for germ-line mutations in genes that predispose to breast cancer.)

Olopade OI: Genetics in clinical cancer care—the future is now. N Engl J Med 1996;335:1455. (Brief review of use of *BRCA1* testing.)

Rabbitts TH: Chromosomal translocations in human cancer. Nature 1994;372:143. (Extends the range of clinic utility of detecting chromosomal aberrations in tumors from diagnosis by karyotype to diagnosis by immunologic reactivity to a mutant fusion protein to therapy by immunologic means.)

Szabo CI, King M-C: Inherited breast and ovarian cancer. Hum Mol Genet 1995;4:1819.

SELECTED GENETIC DISORDERS

ACUTE INTERMITTENT PORPHYRIA

Essentials of Diagnosis

- Unexplained abdominal crisis, generally in young women.
- Acute peripheral or central nervous system dysfunction.
- Recurrent psychiatric illnesses.
- Hyponatremia.
- Porphobilinogen in the urine during an attack.

General Considerations

Though there are several different types of porphyrias, the one with the most serious consequences and the one that usually presents in adulthood is acute intermittent porphyria, which is inherited as an autosomal dominant, though it remains clinically silent in the majority of patients who carry the trait. Those who develop clinical illness are usually women, with symptoms beginning in the teens or 20s, but in rare cases onset can begin after menopause. The disorder is caused by deficiency of porphobilinogen deaminase activity, leading to increased excretion of aminolevulinic acid and porphobilinogen in the urine. The diagnosis may be elusive if not specifically considered. The characteristic abdominal pain may be due to abnormalities in autonomic innervation in the gut. In contrast to other forms of porphyria, cutaneous photosensitivity is absent in acute intermittent porphyria. Attacks are precipitated by numerous factors, including drugs and intercurrent infections. Harmful and relatively safe drugs for use in treatment are listed in Table 40–10. Hyponatremia may be seen, due in part to inappropriate release of antidiuretic hormone, though gastrointestinal loss of sodium in some patients may contribute.

Clinical Findings

A. Symptoms and Signs: Patients show intermittent abdominal pain of varying severity, and in some instances it may so simulate acute abdomen as to lead to exploratory laparotomy. Since the origin of the abdominal pain is neurologic, there is absence of fever and leukocytosis. Complete recovery between

Table 40–10. Some "unsafe" and "probably safe" drugs for patients with acute porphyrias.

Unsafe	Probably Safe
Alkylating agents	Acetaminophen
Barbiturates	Amitriptyline
Carbamazepine	Aspirin
Chloroquine	Atropine
Chlorpropramide	Chloral hydrate
Clonidine	Chlordiazepoxide
Dapsone	Diazepam
Ergots	Digoxin
Erythromycin	Diphenhydramine
Estrogens, synthetic	Guanethidine
Food additives	Glucocorticoids
Griseofulvin	Hyoscine
Hydralazine	Ibuprofen
Ketamine	Imipramine
Meprobamate	Insulin
Methyldopa	Labetalol
Metoclopramide	Lithium
Nortriptyline	Naproxen
Pentazocine	Nitrofurantoin
Progestins	Opioid analgesics
Pyrazinamide	Penicillamine
Rifampin	Penicillin and derivatives
Spironolactone	Phenothiazines
Sulfonamides	Procaine
Theophylline	Propranolol
Tolazamide	Streptomycin
Tolbutamide	Succinylcholine
Valproic acid	Tetracycline
	Thiouracil
	Vitamins B and C

attacks is usual. Any part of the nervous system may be involved, with evidence for autonomic and peripheral neuropathy. Peripheral neuropathy may be symmetric or asymmetric and mild or profound; in the latter instance, it can even lead to quadriplegia with respiratory paralysis. Other central nervous system manifestations include seizures, psychosis, and abnormalities of the basal ganglia. Hyponatremia may further cause or exacerbate central nervous system manifestations.

B. Laboratory Findings: Often there is profound hyponatremia. The diagnosis can be confirmed by demonstrating an increased amount of porphobilinogen in the urine during an acute attack. Freshly voided urine is of normal color but may turn dark upon standing in light and air.

Most families have a different mutation in the porphobilinogen deaminase gene causing acute intermittent porphyria. With some effort in research laboratories, mutations can be discovered and used for presymptomatic and prenatal diagnosis.

Prevention

Avoidance of factors known to precipitate attacks of acute intermittent porphyria—especially drugs (sulfonamides and barbiturates, or drugs listed in Table 40–10)—can reduce morbidity. Starvation diets also cause attacks and so must be avoided.

Treatment

Treatment with a high-carbohydrate diet diminishes the number of attacks in some patients and is a reasonable empiric gesture considering its benignity. Acute attacks may be life-threatening and require prompt diagnosis, withdrawal of the inciting agent (if possible), and treatment with analgesics and intravenous glucose and hematin. A minimum of 300 g of carbohydrate per day should be provided orally or intravenously. Electrolyte balance requires close attention. Hematin therapy is still evolving and should be undertaken with full recognition of adverse consequences, especially phlebitis and coagulopathy. The intravenous dosage is up to 4 mg/kg once or twice daily.

Kappas A et al: The porphyrias. In: *The Metabolic Bases of Inherited Disease,* 7th ed. Scriver CR et al (editors). McGraw-Hill, 1995. (Review of all defects causing forms of porphyria, including the acute intermittent type.)
McGovern MM et al: Inherited porphyrias. In: *Principles and Practice of Medical Genetics,* 3rd ed. Rimoin DL, Conner JM, Pyeritz RE (editors). Churchill Livingstone, 1997. (Diagnosis and management are stressed.)

ALKAPTONURIA

Alkaptonuria is caused by a recessively inherited deficiency of the enzyme homogentisic acid oxidase. This acid derives from metabolism of both phenylalanine and tyrosine and is present in large amounts in the urine throughout the patient's life. An oxidation product accumulates slowly in cartilage throughout the body, leading to degenerative joint disease of the spine and peripheral joints. Indeed, examination of patients in the third and fourth decades shows a slight darkish blue color below the skin in areas overlying cartilage, such as in the ears, a phenomenon called "ochronosis." In some patients, a more severe hyperpigmentation can be seen in the sclera, conjunctiva, and cornea. Accumulation of metabolites in heart valves can lead to aortic or mitral stenosis. A predisposition to coronary artery disease may also be present. While the syndrome causes considerable morbidity, life expectancy is reduced only modestly. Symptoms are more often attributable to spondylitis with back pain, leading to a clinical picture difficult to distinguish from that of ankylosing spondylitis, though on radiographic assessment the sacroiliac joints are not fused in alkaptonuria.

The diagnosis is established by demonstrating homogentisic acid in the urine, which turns black spontaneously on exposure to the air; this reaction is particularly noteworthy if the urine is alkaline or when alkali is added to a specimen. Molecular analysis of the homogentisic acid oxidase gene, recently mapped to chromosome 3, is not necessary for diagnosis.

Treatment of the arthritis is similar to that for other arthropathies. Though in theory rigid dietary restriction might reduce accumulation of the pigment, this has not proved to be of practical benefit.

La Du BN: Alcaptonuria. In: *The Metabolic Bases of Inherited Disease,* 7th ed. Scriver CR et al (editors). McGraw-Hill, 1995. (Clinical and biochemical aspects of one of Garrod's original inborn errors of metabolism.)
Scriver CR: Alkaptonuria: Such a long journey. Nat Genet 1996;14:5. (An instructive editorial about the history of the disorder and the importance of mapping the causative gene.)

DOWN'S SYNDROME

Down's syndrome is usually diagnosed at birth on the basis of the typical facial features, hypotonia, and single palmar crease. Several serious problems that may be evident at birth or may develop early in childhood include duodenal atresia, congenital heart disease (especially atrioventricular canal defects), and leukemia. The intestinal and cardiac anomalies usually respond to surgery, and the leukemia generally responds to conservative management. Intelligence varies across a wide spectrum. Many people with Down's syndrome do well in sheltered workshops and group homes, but few achieve full independence in adulthood. An Alzheimer-like dementia usually becomes evident in the fourth or fifth decade and, for those who survive childhood, accounts for a reduced life expectancy. Studies addressing the risk and severity of dementia in relation to the apolipoprotein E *E4* genotype have had conflicting results. Cytogenetic analysis should always be performed—even though most patients will have simple trisomy for chromosome 21—to detect unbalanced translocations; such patients will usually have a parent with a balanced translocation, and there will be a recurrence risk of Down's syndrome in future offspring.

The risk of bearing a child with Down's syndrome increases exponentially with the age of the mother at conception and begins a marked rise after age 35. By age 45 years, a mother has one chance in 40 of having an affected child. The risk of other conditions associated with trisomy also increases, because of the increased predisposition of older oocytes to nondisjunction during meiosis. There is virtually no risk of trisomy associated with increased paternal age. However, older men do have an increased risk of fathering a child with a new autosomal dominant condition. But because there are so many distinct conditions, the chance of fathering an offspring with any given one is extremely small.

Barsh G: Genetic disease. In: *Pathophysiology of Disease. An Introduction to Clinical Medicine,* 2nd ed. McPhee SJ et al (editors): Appleton & Lange, 1997. (Discusses pathogenesis of Down's syndrome.)

Epstein CJ: The Down syndrome (trisomy 21). In: *The Metabolic and Molecular Bases of Inherited Disease,* 7th ed. Scriver CR et al (editors). McGraw-Hill, 1995. (Current perspectives on managing the diverse medical and social issues that arise in patients of all ages and their families.)

Tolmie JL: Down syndrome and other autosomal trisomies. In *Principles and Practice of Medical Genetics,* 3rd ed. Rimoin DL, Conner JM, Pyeritz RE (editors). Churchill Livingstone, 1997.

GAUCHER'S DISEASE

Gaucher's disease is inherited as an autosomal recessive. A deficiency of β-glucocerebrosidase causes an accumulation of sphingolipid within phagocytic cells throughout the body. Anemia and thrombocytopenia are common and may be symptomatic; both are due primarily to hypersplenism, but marrow infiltration with Gaucher cells may contribute. Cortical erosions of bones, especially the vertebrae and femur, are due to local infarctions, but the mechanism is unclear. Episodes of bone pain (termed "crises") are reminiscent of those in sickle cell disease. A hip fracture in a patient with a palpable spleen—especially in a Jewish person of Eastern European origin—suggests the possibility of Gaucher's disease. Bone marrow aspirates reveal typical Gaucher cells, which have an eccentric nucleus and PAS-positive inclusions, along with wrinkled cytoplasm and inclusion bodies of a fibrillar type. In addition, the serum acid phosphatase is elevated. Definitive diagnosis requires the demonstration of deficient glucocerebrosidase activity in leukocytes.

Until recently, treatment has been supportive and has included splenectomy for thrombocytopenia secondary to platelet sequestration. The purification of sufficient quantities of alglucerase (glucocerebrosidase-β-glucosidase) to permit intravenous administration on a regular basis now permits a reduction in total body stores of glycolipid and improvement in orthopedic and hematologic manifestations. The major drawback is the exceptional cost of alglucerase, which can exceed $350,000 per year, though recent studies suggest that more frequent administration of less enzyme (30 units/kg per month) is just as effective and reduces the cost to about $100,000 annually for an adult.

Beutler E, Grabowski GA: Gaucher disease. In: *The Metabolic and Molecular Bases of Inherited Disease,* 7th ed. Scriver CR et al (editors). McGraw-Hill, 1995. (A comprehensive review.)

Pollack CE et al: Individualised low-dose alglucerase therapy for type 1 Gaucher's disease. Lancet 1995;345: 1474. (Frequent administration of low doses of alglucerase is effective in terms of both outcome and cost.)

NIH Technology Assessment Panel: Gaucher disease: Current issues in diagnosis and treatment. JAMA 1996;275: 548. (An expert panel recommends appropriate use of biochemical and DNA analysis, the indications for treatment, and the guidelines for enzyme replacement therapy.)

HOMOCYSTINURIA

Homocystinuria in its classic form is caused by cystathionine β-synthase deficiency and exhibits an autosomal recessive pattern of inheritance. This results in extreme elevations of plasma and urinary homocystine levels, a basis for diagnosis of this disorder. Homocystinuria is similar in certain superficial aspects to Marfan's syndrome, since patients may show a similar body habitus and ectopia lentis is almost always present. However, mental retardation is often present, and the cardiovascular events are those of repeated venous and arterial thromboses whose precise cause remains obscure. Life expectancy is reduced, especially in untreated and pyridoxine-unresponsive patients; myocardial infarction, stroke, and pulmonary embolism are the most common causes of death. This condition is diagnosed in some states by newborn screening for hypermethioninemia; however, pyridoxine-responsive infants may not be detected. The diagnosis should be suspected in patients in the second and third decades of life who show evidence of arterial or venous thromboses and have no other risk factors. Although many mutations have been identified in the cystathionine β synthase gene, amino acid analysis of plasma remains the most appropriate diagnostic test. Patients should be studied after they have been off folate or pyridoxine supplementation for at least 1 week. The plasma should be separated promptly from the fresh venous blood specimen.

About one-half of patients have a form of cystathionine β-synthase deficiency that improves biochemically and clinically through pharmacologic doses of pyridoxine and folate. For these patients, treatment from infancy can prevent retardation and the other clinical problems. Patients who are pyridoxine-nonresponders must be treated with dietary reduction in methionine and supplementation of cysteine, also from infancy. The vitamin betaine is also useful in reducing plasma methionine levels by facilitating a metabolic pathway that bypasses the defective enzyme. Patients who have suffered venous thrombosis should be anticoagulated, but there are no studies to support prophylactic use of warfarin or antiplatelet agents.

Mudd H, Levy HL, Skovby F: Disorders of transsulfuration. In: *The Metabolic and Molecular Bases of Inherited Disease,* 7th ed. Scriver CR et al (editors). McGraw-Hill, 1995. (A comprehensive review of the genetics and clinical features of all of the disorders associated with elevated homocysteine, including the risk of vascular disease in heterozygotes.)

Pyeritz RE: Homocystinuria. In: *McKusick's Heritable Disorders of Connective Tissue,* 5th ed. Mosby, 1993. (Clinical, genetic, and biochemical aspects of an inborn error of metabolism with extensive effects on the extracellular matrix.)

HOMOCYSTEINE & ARTERIAL OCCLUSIVE DISEASE

Over the past 5 years, considerable evidence has accumulated to support the 20-year-old observation that patients with clinical and angiographic evidence of coronary artery disease tend to have higher levels of plasma homocysteine than controls without coronary artery disease. The relationship has been extended to cerebrovascular and peripheral vascular diseases. Although this effect was initially thought to be due at least in part to heterozygotes for cystathionine β-synthase deficiency (see above), in fact there is little evidence for this. Rather, the major factor leading to hyperhomocysteinemia is folate deficiency. Pyridoxine (vitamin B_6) and vitamin B_{12} are also important in the metabolism of methionine, and deficiency of any of these vitamins can lead to accumulation of homocysteine. A number of genes influence utilization of these vitamins and can predispose to deficiency. However, both nutritional and most genetic deficiencies of these vitamins can be corrected by dietary supplementation. Studies are ongoing to determine the long-term utility of routine vitamin supplementation in people at risk for arterial occlusive disease, but many workers in this field recommend, at a minimum, taking 1 mg of folic acid per day. Because patients with end-stage renal disease tend to have marked hyperhomocysteinemia and low serum folate, 5 mg of folic acid per day seems warranted.

Relatively few laboratories currently provide highly reliable assays for homocysteine. Processing of the specimen is crucial to obtain accurate results. The plasma must be separated within 30 minutes; otherwise, blood cells release the amino acid and the measurement will then be artificially elevated.

Boushey CJ et al: A quantitative assessment of plasma homocysteine as a risk factor for vascular disease: Probable benefits of increasing folic acid intakes. JAMA 1995;274:1049. (A review of all of the evidence supporting homocysteine as an independent risk factor and how dietary folic acid can be pivotal in modifying the risk.)

Kang SS, Wong PW: Genetic and nongenetic factors for moderate hyperhomocyst(e)inemia. Atherosclerosis 1996;119:135. (A brief review of the causes of elevated homocysteine.)

Motulsky AG: Nutritional ecogenetics: Homocysteine-related arteriosclerotic vascular disease, neural tube defects, and folic acid. Am J Hum Genet 1996;58:17. (A perspective that ties together congenital and adult-onset diseases through a common metabolic pathway.)

KLINEFELTER'S SYNDROME

Boys with an extra X chromosome are normal in appearance before puberty; thereafter, they have disproportionately long legs and arms, a female escutcheon, gynecomastia, and small testes. Infertility is due to azoospermia; the seminiferous tubules are hyalinized. The diagnosis is often not made until a couple is evaluated for inability to conceive. Mental retardation is somewhat more common than in the general population. Many men with Klinefelter's syndrome have learning problems. The risk of breast cancer is much higher in men with Klinefelter's syndrome than in 46,XY men, as is the risk of diabetes mellitus. Treatment with testosterone after puberty is advisable but will not restore fertility.

Paulsen CA, Plymate SR: Klinefelter's syndrome. In: *The Genetic Basis of Common Diseases.* King RA, Rotter JI, Motulsky AG (editors). University Press, 1992.

MARFAN'S SYNDROME

Essentials of Diagnosis
- Disproportionately tall stature, thoracic deformity, and joint laxity or contractures.
- Ectopia lentis and myopia.
- Aortic dilation and dissection.
- Mitral valve prolapse.

General Considerations
Marfan's syndrome, a systemic connective tissue disease, is inherited as an autosomal dominant. It is characterized by abnormalities of the skeletal system, ocular system, and cardiovascular system. Spontaneous pneumothorax, dural ectasia, and striae atrophicae can also occur. Of most concern is disease of the ascending aorta, which is associated with a dilated aortic root. Histology of the aorta shows diffuse medial abnormalities. Aortic and mitral valve leaflets are also abnormal and mitral regurgitation may be present as well, often with elongated chordae tendineae, which on occasion may rupture.

Clinical Findings
A. Symptoms and Signs: Affected patient are typically tall, with particularly long arms, legs and digits (arachnodactyly). However, there can be wide variability in the clinical presentation. Commonly, joint dislocations and pectus excavatum are found. Ectopia lentis may lead to severe myopia and retinal detachment. Mitral valve prolapse is seen in about 85% percent of patients. Aortic root dilation with aortic regurgitation or dissection with rupture can occur. To diagnose Marfan's syndrome, people with an affected relative need features in at least two systems. People with no family history need features in the skeletal system, two other systems, and one

the major criteria of ectopia lentis, dilation of the aortic root, or aortic dissection.

B. Laboratory Findings: Mutations in the fibrillin gene on chromosome 15 cause Marfan's syndrome. Nonetheless, no simple laboratory test is available to support the diagnosis in questionable cases because related conditions may also be due to defects in fibrillin.

Prevention

There is prenatal and presymptomatic diagnosis for patients in whom the molecular defect in fibrillin has been found and for large enough families in whom linkage analysis using polymorphic markers around the fibrillin gene can be performed.

Treatment

Children with Marfan's syndrome require regular ophthalmologic surveillance to correct visual acuity and thus prevent amblyopia, and annual orthopedic consultation for diagnosis of scoliosis at an early enough stage so that bracing might delay progression. Patients of all ages require echocardiography at least annually to monitor aortic diameter and mitral valve function. All patients should use standard endocarditis prophylaxis. Chronic beta-adrenergic blockade, titrated to individual tolerance but enough to produce a negative inotropic effect (atenolol, 1–2 mg/kg), retards the rate of aortic dilation. Restriction from vigorous physical exertion protects from aortic dissection. Prophylactic replacement of the aortic root with a composite graft when the diameter reaches 50–55 mm (normal: < 40 mm) prolongs life.

Prognosis

People with Marfan's syndrome who are untreated commonly die in the fourth or fifth decade from aortic dissection or congestive heart failure secondary to aortic regurgitation.

Deitz HC, Pyeritz RE: Mutations in the human gene for fibrillin-1 *(FBN1)* in the Marfan syndrome and related disorders. Hum Mol Genet 1995;4:1799. (A review of the molecular biology of microfibrils and an important group of connective tissue disorders.)

DePaepe A et al: Revised diagnostic criteria for the Marfan syndrome. Am J Med Genet 1996;62:417. (A new matrix for assigning the diagnosis based on clinical findings, family history, and molecular biology.)

Gott VL et al: Aortic root replacement: Risk factor analysis of a seventeen-year experience with 270 patients. J Thorac Cardiovasc Surg 1995;109:536. (The largest published series demonstrating excellent long-term results from prophylactic surgery.)

Pereira L et al: A molecular approach to the stratification of cardiovascular risk in families with Marfan's syndrome. N Engl J Med 1994;331:148. (The utility of linkage analysis in presymptomatic detection—and exclusion—of the Marfan diagnosis.)

Pyeritz RE: Marfan syndrome and other disorders of fibrillin. In: *Principles and Practice of Medical Genetics,* 3rd ed. Rimoin DL, Connor JM, Pyeritz RE (editors). Churchill Livingstone, 1997. (A comprehensive survey of Marfan's syndrome and related conditions.)

Rossiter JP et al: A prospective longitudinal evaluation of pregnancy in the Marfan syndrome. Am J Obstet Gynecol 1995;173:1599. (Pregnancy is not that dangerous for the Marfan woman with an aortic diameter less than 40 mm.)

Shores J et al: Progression of aortic dilatation and the benefit of long-term beta-adrenergic blockade in Marfan's syndrome. N Engl J Med 1994;330:1335.

41

Diagnostic Testing & Medical Decision Making

C. Diana Nicoll, MD, PhD, & William M. Detmer, MD

The clinician's main task is to make reasoned decisions about patient care despite imperfect clinical information and uncertainty about clinical outcomes. While data elicited from the history and physical examination are often sufficient for making a diagnosis or for guiding therapy, more information may be required. In these situations, clinicians often turn to diagnostic tests for help.

BENEFITS; COSTS & RISKS

When used appropriately, diagnostic tests can be of great assistance to the clinician. Tests can be helpful for **screening,** ie, to identify risk factors for disease and to detect occult disease in asymptomatic persons. Identification of risk factors may allow early intervention to prevent disease occurrence, and early detection of occult disease may reduce disease morbidity and mortality through early treatment. Optimal screening tests meet the criteria listed in Table 41–1.

Tests can also be helpful for **diagnosis,** ie, to help establish or exclude the presence of disease in symptomatic persons. Some tests assist in early diagnosis after onset of symptoms and signs; others assist in differential diagnosis of various possible diseases; others help determine the stage or activity of disease.

Finally, tests can be helpful in **patient management.** Tests can help (1) evaluate the severity of disease, (2) estimate prognosis, (3) monitor the course of disease (progression, stability, or resolution), (4) detect disease recurrence, and (5) select drugs and adjust therapy.

When ordering diagnostic tests, clinicians should weigh the potential benefits against the potential costs and disadvantages:

(1) An individual test such as MRI of the head can cost more than $1400.00, and diagnostic tests as a whole account for approximately one-fifth of health care expenditures in the USA.

(2) Some tests carry a risk of morbidity or mortality—eg, intravenous contrast material used in some CT scans leads to death from anaphylaxis in approximately 1:30,000 examinations.

(3) The discomfort associated with tests such as sigmoidoscopy or barium enema will deter some patients from completing a diagnostic work-up.

(4) The result of a diagnostic test often has implications for further care in that a test result may mandate further testing or frequent follow-up. This means that a patient with a falsely positive fecal occult blood test may incur significant cost, risk, and discomfort during follow-up sigmoidoscopy, barium enema, or colonoscopy.

(5) A false-positive test may lead to further unnecessary testing. Classifying a healthy patient as diseased based on a falsely positive diagnostic test can cause psychologic distress and may lead to risks from unnecessary therapy.

PERFORMANCE OF DIAGNOSTIC TESTS

TEST PREPARATION

Factors affecting both the patient and the specimen are important. The most crucial element in a properly conducted laboratory test is an appropriate specimen

Patient Preparation

The preparation of the patient is important for certain tests. For example, a fasting state is needed for optimal glucose and triglyceride measurements. Controlled conditions are frequently needed for endocrinology testing. For instance, posture and sodium intake must be strictly controlled when measuring renin and aldosterone levels. Strenuous exercise should be avoided before obtaining some tes

Table 41–1. Criteria for use of screening procedures.

Characteristics of population
1. Sufficiently high prevalence of disease.
2. Likely to be compliant with subsequent tests and treatments.

Characteristics of disease
1. Significant morbidity and mortality.
2. Effective and acceptable treatment available.
3. Presymptomatic period detectable.
4. Improved outcome from early treatment.

Characteristics of test
1. Good sensitivity and specificity.
2. Low cost and risk.
3. Confirmatory test available and practical.

Table 41–2. Properties of useful diagnostic tests.

1. Test methodology has been described in detail so that it can be accurately and reliably reproduced.
2. Test accuracy and precision have been determined.
3. The reference range has been established appropriately.
4. Sensitivity and specificity have been reliably established by comparison with a gold standard. The evaluation has used a range of patients, including those who have different but commonly confused disorders and those with a spectrum of mild and severe, treated and untreated disease. The patient selection process has been adequately described so that results will not be generalized inappropriately.
5. Independent contribution to overall performance of a test panel has been confirmed if a test is advocated as part of a panel of tests.

such as creatine kinase, since vigorous muscle activity can lead to falsely abnormal results.

Specimen Collection

Careful attention must be paid to patient identification and specimen labeling. Knowing when the specimen was collected may be important. For instance, aminoglycoside levels cannot be interpreted appropriately without knowing whether the specimen was drawn just before ("trough" level) or after ("peak" level) drug administration. Drug levels cannot be interpreted if they are drawn during the drug's distribution phase (eg, digoxin levels drawn during the first 6 hours after an oral dose). Substances that have a circadian variation (eg, cortisol) can be interpreted only in the context of the time of day the sample was drawn.

During specimen collection, other principles should be remembered. Specimens should not be drawn above an intravenous line, as this may contaminate the sample with intravenous fluid. Excessive tourniquet time will lead to hemoconcentration and increased concentration of protein-bound substances such as calcium. Lysis of cells during collection of a blood specimen will result in spuriously increased serum levels of substances concentrated in cells (eg, lactate dehydrogenase and potassium). Certain test specimens may require special handling or storage (eg, blood gas specimens). Delay in delivery of specimens to the laboratory can result in ongoing cellular metabolism and therefore spurious results for some studies (eg, low blood glucose).

TEST CHARACTERISTICS

Table 41–2 lists the characteristics of all useful diagnostic tests. Most of the principles detailed below can be applied not only to diagnostic tests but also to historical facts and physical examination findings.

Accuracy

The accuracy of a laboratory test is its correspondence with the true value. An inaccurate test is one that differs from the true value even though the results may be reproducible (Figures 41–1A and 1B). In the clinical laboratory, accuracy of tests is maximized by calibrating laboratory equipment with reference material and by participation in external quality control programs.

Precision

Test precision is a measure of a test's reproducibility when repeated on the same sample. An imprecise test is one that yields widely varying results on repeated measurements (Figure 41–1B). The precision of diagnostic tests, which is monitored in clinical laboratories by using control material, must be good enough to distinguish clinically relevant changes in a patient's status from the analytic variability of the test. For instance, the manual white blood cell differential count is not precise enough to detect important changes in the distribution of cell types, because it is calculated by subjective evaluation of a small sample (100 cells). Repeated measurements by different technicians on the same sample result in widely different results. Automated differential counts are more precise because they are obtained from machines that use objective physical characteristics to differentiate a much larger sample (10,000 cells).

Reference Range

Patient test results are interpreted by comparing them with published reference ranges. These ranges are method- and laboratory-specific. In practice, reference ranges often represent test results found in

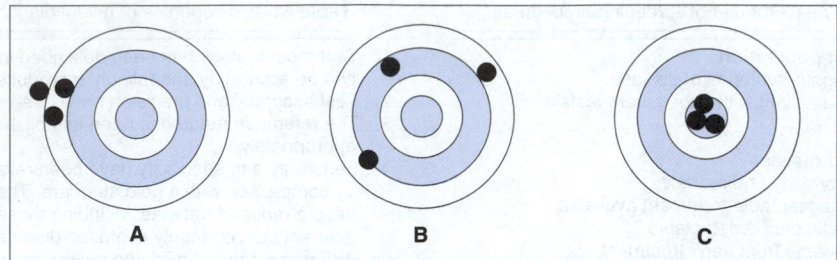

Figure 41–1. Relationship between accuracy and precision in diagnostic tests. The center of the target represents the true value of the substance being tested. Figure "A" represents a diagnostic test which is precise but inaccurate; on repeated measurement, the test yields very similar results, but all results are far from the true value. Figure "B" shows a test which is imprecise and inaccurate; repeated measurement yields widely different results, and the results are far from the true value. Figure "C" shows an ideal test, one that is both precise and accurate.

95% of a small population presumed to be healthy; by definition, 5% of healthy patients will have a positive (abnormal) test (Figure 41–2). As a result, slightly abnormal results should be interpreted in a critical fashion: they may be either truly abnormal or falsely abnormal. The practitioner should be aware also that the more tests ordered, the greater the chance for obtaining a falsely abnormal result. For instance, a healthy person subjected to 20 independent tests has a 64% probability of having at least one abnormal test result (Table 41–3).

It is important to consider also whether published reference ranges are appropriate for the patient being evaluated, since some ranges depend on age, sex, weight, diet, time of day, activity status, or posture. For instance, the reference ranges for hemoglobin concentration are age- and sex-dependent. The Appendix contains the reference ranges for commonly used chemistry and hematology tests.

Interfering Factors

The results of diagnostic tests can be altered by external factors, such as ingestion of drugs; and internal factors, such as abnormal physiologic states.

External interferences can affect test results in vivo or in vitro. In vivo, alcohol increases γ-glutamyl transpeptidase, and diuretics can affect sodium and potassium concentrations. Cigarette smoking can induce hepatic enzymes and thus reduce levels of substances such as theophylline that are metabolized by the liver. In vitro, cephalosporins may produce spurious serum creatinine levels due to interference with a common laboratory method.

Internal interferences result when an abnormal physiologic state interferes with the measurement of a test result. As an example, patients with gross lipemia may have spuriously low serum sodium levels if the test methodology used includes a step where serum is diluted before sodium is measured. Because of the potential for test interference, clinicians should be wary of unexpected test results and should investigate reasons other than disease that may explain abnormal results, including laboratory error.

Sensitivity & Specificity

Clinicians should use measures of test performance

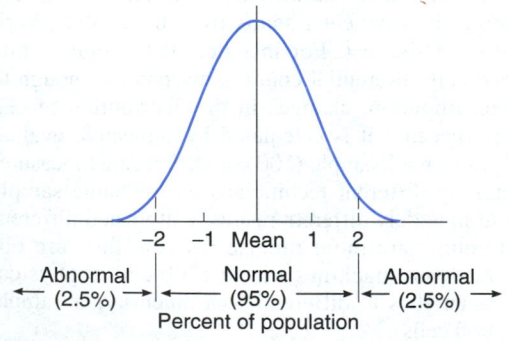

Figure 41–2. The reference range is usually defined as within 2 SD of the mean test result (shown as −2 and 2) in a small population of healthy volunteers. Note that in this example, test results are normally distributed; however, many biologic substances will have distributions that are skewed.

Table 41–3. Relationship between the number of tests and the probability that a healthy person will have one or more abnormal results.

Number of Tests	Probability That One or More Results Will Be Abnormal
1	5%
6	26%
12	46%
20	64%

such as sensitivity and specificity to judge the quality of a diagnostic test for a particular disease. Test **sensitivity** is the likelihood that a diseased patient has a positive test. If all patients with a given disease have a positive test (ie, no diseased patients have negative tests), then the test sensitivity is 100%. A test with high sensitivity is useful to exclude a diagnosis because a highly sensitive test will render few results that are falsely negative. To exclude infection with the AIDS virus, for instance, a clinician might choose a highly sensitive test such as the HIV antibody test.

A test's **specificity** is the likelihood that a healthy patient has a negative test. If all patients who do not have a given disease have negative tests (ie, no healthy patients have positive tests), then the test specificity is 100%. A test with high specificity is useful to confirm a diagnosis, because a highly specific test will have few results that are falsely positive. For instance, to make the diagnosis of gouty arthritis, a clinician might choose a highly specific test, such as the presence of negatively birefringent needle-shaped crystals within leukocytes on microscopic evaluation of joint fluid.

To determine test sensitivity and specificity for a particular disease, the test must be compared against a "gold standard," a procedure that defines the true disease state of the patient. For instance, the sensitivity and specificity of the ventilation/perfusion scan for pulmonary embolus are obtained by comparing the results of scans with the gold standard, pulmonary arteriography. However, for many disease states (eg, pancreatitis), such a gold standard either does not exist or is very difficult or expensive to apply. Therefore, reliable estimates of test sensitivity and specificity are sometimes difficult to obtain.

Sensitivity and specificity values can also be affected by the population from which these values are derived. For instance, many diagnostic tests are evaluated first using patients who have severe disease and control groups who are young and well. Compared with the general population, this study group will have more results that are truly positive (because patients have more advanced disease) and more results that are truly negative (because the control group is healthy). Thus, test sensitivity and specificity will be higher than would be expected in the general population, where more of a spectrum of health and disease are found. Clinicians should be aware of this **spectrum bias** when generalizing test results to their own practice.

Test sensitivity and specificity depend on the reference range used, ie, the cutoff point above which a test is interpreted as abnormal (Figure 41–3). If the cutoff is modified, sensitivity will be enhanced at the expense of specificity or vice versa.

Figure 41–4 shows how test sensitivity and specificity can be calculated using test results from patients previously classified by the gold standard as diseased or nondiseased.

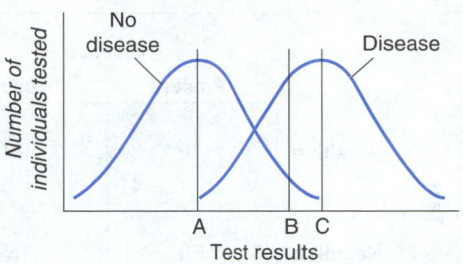

Figure 41–3. Hypothetical distribution of test results for healthy and diseased individuals. The position of the "cutoff point" between "normal" and "abnormal" (or "negative" and "positive") test results determines the test's sensitivity and specificity. If point "A" is the cutoff point, the test would have 100% sensitivity but low specificity. If point "C" is the cutoff point, the test would have 100% specificity but low sensitivity. For most tests, the cutoff point is determined by the reference range, ie, the range of test results that are within 2 SD of the mean (point "B"). In some situations, the cutoff is altered to enhance either sensitivity or specificity. (Modified and reproduced, with permission, from Griner PF et al: Selection and interpretation of diagnostic tests and procedures: Principles and applications. Ann Intern Med 1981;84[4 Part 2]:453.)

The performance of two different tests can be compared by plotting the sensitivity and (one minus the specificity) of each test at various reference range cutoff values. The resulting receiver operator characteristic (ROC) curve will often show which test is better; a clearly superior test will have an ROC curve that always lies above and to the left of the inferior test curve, and, in general, the better test will have a larger area under the ROC curve. For instance, Figure 41–5 shows the ROC curves for prostate-specific antigen (PSA) and prostatic acid phosphatase (PAP) in the diagnosis of prostate cancer. PSA is a superior test because it has higher sensitivity and specificity for all cutoff values.

USE OF TESTS IN DIAGNOSIS & MANAGEMENT

The value of a test in a particular clinical situation depends not only on the test's sensitivity and specificity but also on the probability that the patient has the disease before the test result is known (**pretest probability**). The results of a valuable test will substantially change the probability that the patient has the disease (**posttest probability**). Figure 41–4 shows how posttest probability can be calculated from the known sensitivity and specificity of the test

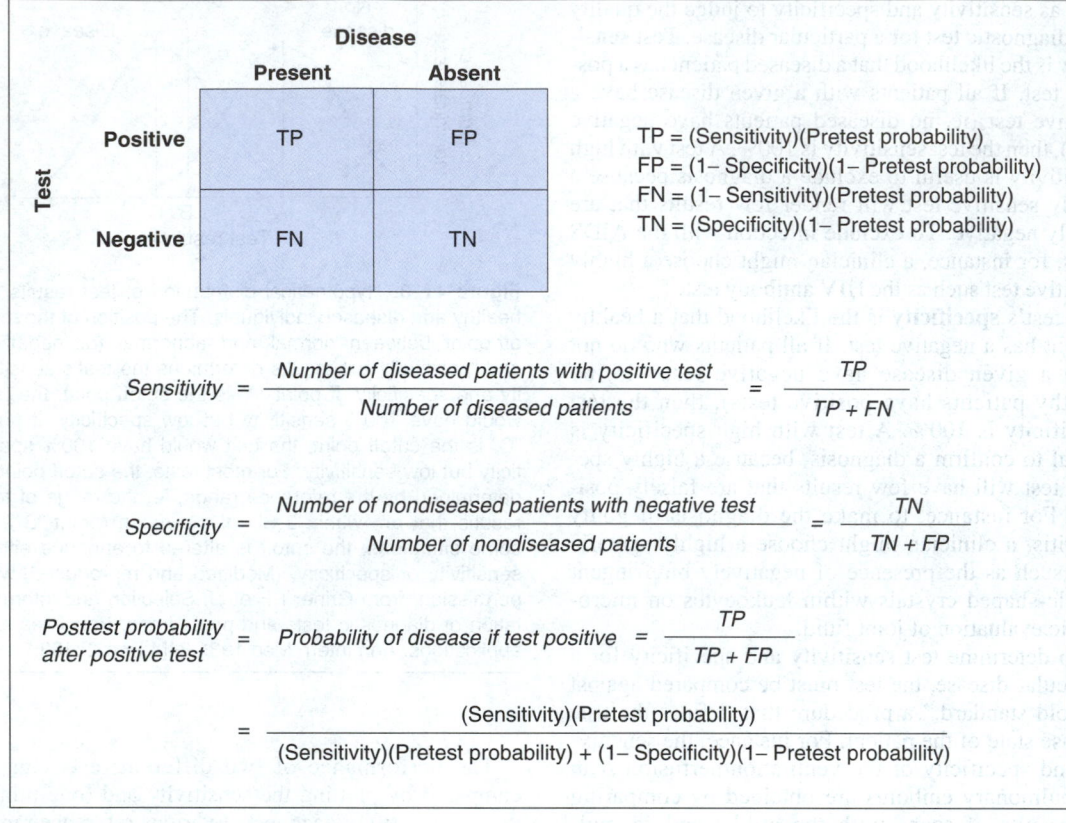

Figure 41–4. Calculation of sensitivity, specificity, and probability of disease after a positive test (posttest probability). (TP, true positive; FP, false positive; FN, false negative; TN, true negative.)

and the estimated pretest probability of disease (or disease prevalence).

The pretest probability of disease has a profound effect on the posttest probability of disease. As demonstrated in Table 41–4, when a test with 90% sensitivity and specificity is used, the posttest probability can vary from 1% to 99% depending on the pretest probability of disease. Furthermore, as the pretest probability of disease decreases, it becomes less likely that someone with a positive test actually has the disease and more likely that the result represents a false positive.

As an example, suppose the clinician wishes to calculate the posttest probability of prostate cancer using the PSA test and a cut-off value of 4 ng/mL. Using the data shown in Figure 41–5, sensitivity is 90% and specificity is 60%. The clinician estimates the pretest probability of disease given all evidence and then calculates the posttest probability using the approach shown in Figure 41–5. The pretest probability that an otherwise healthy 50-year-old man has prostate cancer is equal to the prevalence of prostate cancer in that age group (probability = 10%) and the

posttest probability is only 20%—ie, even though the test is positive, there is still an 80% chance that the patient does not have prostate cancer (Figure 41–6A). If the clinician finds a prostate nodule on rectal examination, the pretest probability of prostate cancer rises to 50% and the posttest probability using the same test is 69% (Figure 41–6B). Finally, if the clinician estimates the pretest probability to be 98% based on a prostate nodule, bone pain, and lytic lesions on spine x-rays, the posttest probability using PSA is 99% (Figure 41–6C). This example illustrates that pretest probability has a profound effect on posttest probability and that tests provide more information when the diagnosis is truly uncertain (pretest probability about 50%) than when the diagnosis is either unlikely or nearly certain.

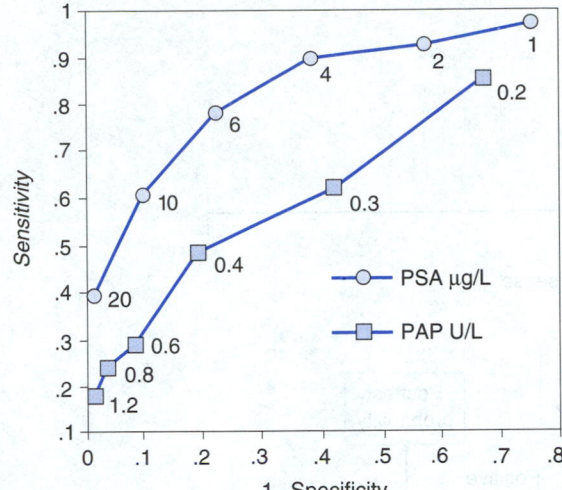

Figure 41–5. Receiver operator characteristic (ROC) curves for prostate-specific antigen (PSA) and prostatic acid phosphatase (PAP) in the diagnosis of prostate cancer. For all cutoff values, PSA has higher sensitivity and specificity; therefore, it is a better test based on these performance characteristics. (Modified and reproduced, with permission, from Nicoll D et al: Routine acid phosphatase testing for screening and monitoring prostate cancer no longer justified. Clin Chem 1993;39:2540.)

ODDS-LIKELIHOOD RATIOS

An easier way to calculate the posttest probability of disease is to use the odds-likelihood approach. Sensitivity and specificity are combined into one entity called the likelihood ratio (LR).

$$LR = \frac{\text{Probability of result in diseased persons}}{\text{Probability of result in nondiseased persons}}$$

Every test has two likelihood ratios, one corresponding to a positive test (LR^+) and one corresponding to a negative test (LR^-):

Table 41–4. Influence of pretest probability on the posttest probability of disease when a test with 90% sensitivity and 90% specificity is used.

Pretest Probability	Posttest Probability
0.01	0.08
0.50	0.90
0.99	0.999

$$LR^+ = \frac{\text{Probability that test is positive in diseased persons}}{\text{Probability that test is positive in nondiseased persons}}$$

$$= \frac{\text{Sensitivity}}{1 - \text{Specificity}}$$

$$LR^- = \frac{\text{Probability that test is negative in diseased persons}}{\text{Probability that test is negative in nondiseased persons}}$$

$$= \frac{1 - \text{Sensitivity}}{\text{Specificity}}$$

Lists of likelihood ratios can be found in some textbooks, journal articles, and computer programs (see Table 41–5 for sample values). Likelihood ratios can be used to make quick estimates of the usefulness of a contemplated diagnostic test in a particular situation. The simplest method for calculating posttest probability from pretest probability and likelihood ratios is to use a nomogram (Figure 41–7). The clinician places a straightedge through the points that represent the pretest probability and the likelihood ratio and then reads where the straightedge crosses the posttest probability line.

A more formal way of calculating posttest probabilities uses the likelihood ratio as follows:

Pretest odds × Likelihood ratio = Posttest odds

To use this formulation, probabilities must be converted to odds, where the odds of having a disease are expressed as the chance of having the disease divided by the chance of not having the disease. For instance, a probability of 0.75 is the same as 3:1 odds (Figure 41–8).

To estimate the potential benefit of a diagnostic test, the clinician first estimates the pretest odds of disease given all available clinical information and then multiplies the pretest odds by the positive and negative likelihood ratios. The results are the **posttest odds,** or the odds that the patient has the disease if the test is positive or negative. To obtain the posttest probability, the odds are converted to a probability (Figure 41–8).

For example, if the clinician believes that the patient has a 60% chance of having a myocardial infarction (pretest odds of 3:2) and the creatine kinase MB test is positive ($LR^+ = 32$), then the posttest odds of having a myocardial infarction are

$$\frac{3}{2} \times 32 = \frac{96}{2} \text{ or } 48:1 \text{ odds} \left(\frac{^{48}/_1}{^{48}/_1 + 1} = \frac{48}{48 + 1} = 98\% \text{ probability} \right)$$

If the CKMB test is negative ($LR^- = 0.05$), then the posttest odds of having a myocardial infarction are

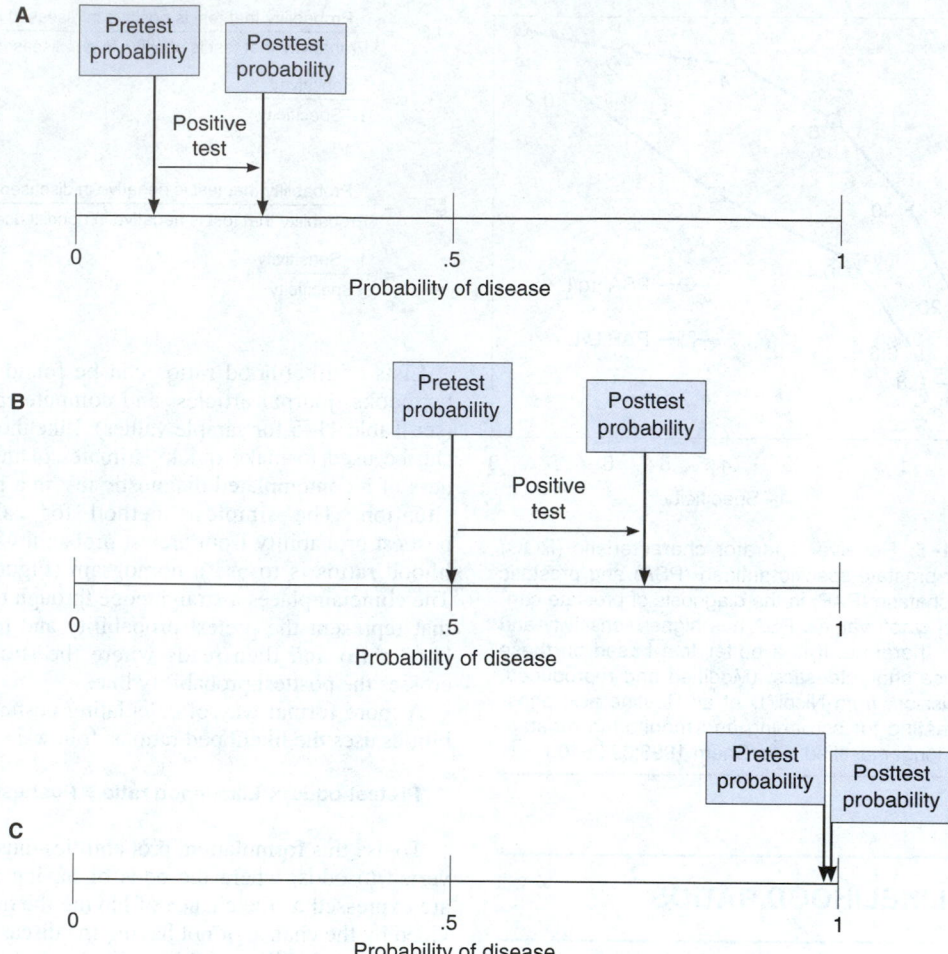

Figure 41–6. Effect of pretest probability and test sensitivity and specificity on the posttest probability of disease. (See text for explanation.)

$$\frac{3}{2} \times 0.05 = \frac{0.15}{2} \text{ odds} \left(\frac{^{0.15}/_2}{^{0.15}/_2 + 1} = \frac{0.15}{0.15 + 2} = 7\% \text{ probability} \right)$$

Sequential Testing

To this point, the impact of only one test on the probability of disease has been discussed, whereas during most diagnostic experiences, clinicians obtain clinical information in a sequential fashion. To calculate the posttest odds after three tests, for example, the clinician might estimate the pretest odds and use the appropriate likelihood ratio for each test:

Pretest odds × LR₁ × LR₂ × LR₃ = Posttest odds

When using this approach, however, the clinician should be aware of a major assumption: the chosen

Table 41–5. Likelihood ratios for a sample of diagnostic tests.

Test	Disease	LR⁺	LR⁻
Carcinoembryonic antigen	Dukes A colon cancer	1.6	0.87
Creatine kinase MB	Myocardial infarction	32	0.05
Free thyroxine index	Hyperthyroidism	6.8	0.06
Ferritin	Iron deficiency anemia	85	0.15
Antinuclear antibody	SLE	4.5	0.13

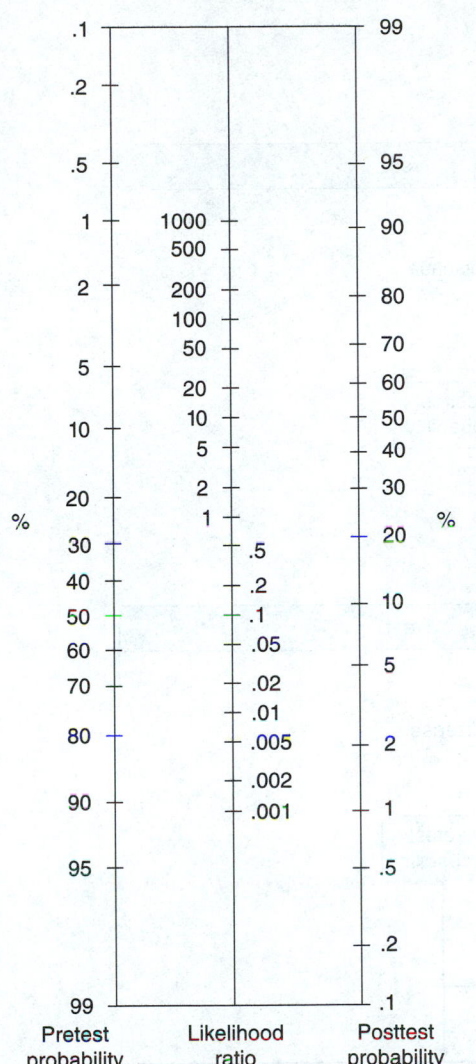

Figure 41–7. Nomogram for determining posttest probability from pretest probability and likelihood ratios. To figure the posttest probability, place a straightedge between the pretest probability and the likelihood ratio for the particular test. The posttest probability will be where the straightedge crosses the posttest probability line. (Adapted and reproduced, with permission, from Fagan TJ: Nomogram for Bayes's theorem. N Engl J Med 1975;293:257.)

$$Odds = \frac{Probability}{1 - Probability}$$

Example: If probability = 0.75, then

$$Odds = \frac{0.75}{1 - 0.75} = \frac{0.75}{0.25} = \frac{3}{1} = 3{:}1$$

$$Probability = \frac{Odds}{Odds + 1}$$

Example: If odds = 3:1, then

$$Probability = \frac{3/1}{3/1 + 1} = \frac{3}{3 + 1} = 0.75$$

Figure 41–8. Formulas for converting between probability and odds.

Threshold Approach to Decision Making

A key aspect of medical decision making is the selection of a treatment threshold, ie, the probability of disease at which treatment is indicated. Figure 41–9 shows a possible way of identifying a treatment threshold by considering the value (utility) of the four possible outcomes of the treat/don't treat decision.

A diagnostic test is useful only if it shifts the disease probability across the treatment threshold. For example, a clinician might decide to treat with antibiotics if the probability of streptococcal pharyngitis in a patient with a sore throat is greater than 25% (Fig-

tests or findings must be **conditionally independent.** For instance, with liver cell damage, the aspartate aminotransferase (AST) and alanine aminotransferase (ALT) enzymes may be released by the same process and are thus not conditionally independent. If conditionally dependent tests are used in this sequential approach, an overestimation of posttest probability will result.

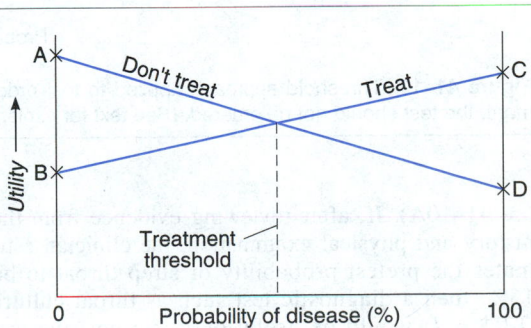

Figure 41–9. The "treat/don't treat" threshold. **A:** Patient does not have disease and is not treated (highest utility). **B:** Patient does not have disease and is treated (lower utility than A). **C:** Patient has disease and is treated (lower utility than A). **D:** Patient has disease and is not treated (lower utility than C).

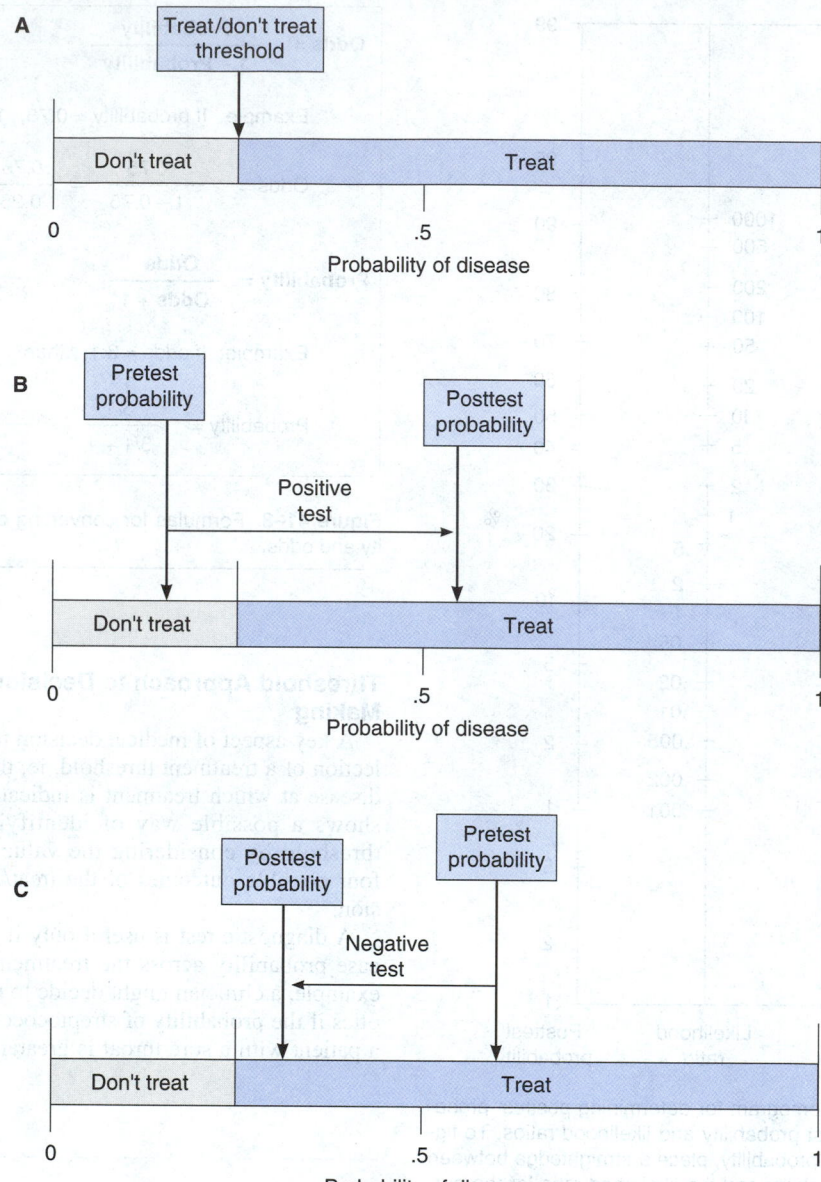

Figure 41–10. Threshold approach applied to test ordering. If the contemplated test will not change patient management, the test should not be ordered. (See text for explanation.)

ure 41–10A). If, after reviewing evidence from the history and physical examination, the clinician estimates the pretest probability of strep throat to be 15%, then a diagnostic test such as throat culture ($LR^+ = 7$) would be useful only if a positive test would shift the posttest probability above 25%. Use of the nomogram shown in Figure 41–7 indicates that the posttest probability would be 55% (Figure 41–10B); thus, ordering the test would be justified as it affects patient management. On the other hand, if the history and physical examination had suggested

that the pretest probability of strep throat was 60%, the throat culture ($LR^- = 0.33$) would be indicated only if a negative test would lower the posttest probability below 25%. Using the same nomogram, the posttest probability after a negative test would be 33% (Figure 10–C). Therefore, ordering the throat culture would not be justified.

Decision Analysis

Up to this point, the discussion of diagnostic testing has focused on test characteristics and methods

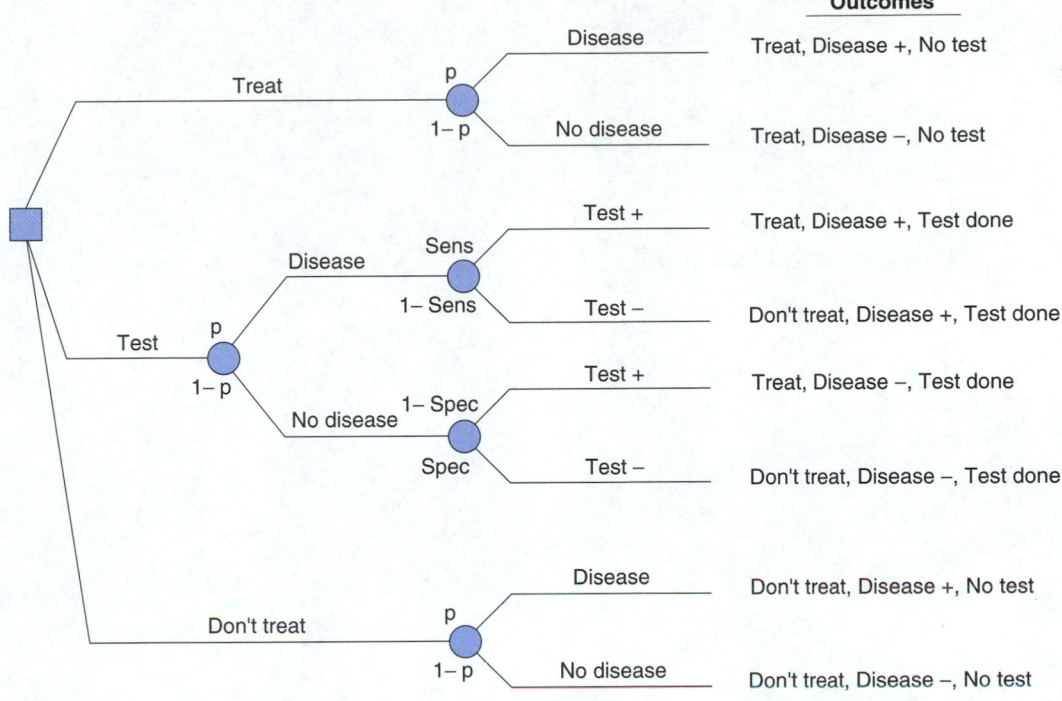

Outcomes

Treat, Disease +, No test

Treat, Disease −, No test

Treat, Disease +, Test done

Don't treat, Disease +, Test done

Treat, Disease −, Test done

Don't treat, Disease −, Test done

Don't treat, Disease +, No test

Don't treat, Disease −, No test

Figure 41–11. Generic tree for a clinical decision where the choices are (1) to treat the patient empirically, (2) to test and then treat if the test is positive, or (3) to withhold therapy. The square node is called a decision node, and the round nodes are called chance nodes. (p, pretest probability of disease; Sens, sensitivity; Spec, specificity.)

for using these characteristics to calculate the probability of disease in different clinical situations. Although useful, these methods are limited because they do not incorporate the many outcomes that may occur in clinical medicine or the values that patients and clinicians place on those outcomes. To incorporate outcomes and values with characteristics of tests, decision analysis can be used.

The basic idea of decision analysis is to model the options in a medical decision, assign probabilities to the alternative actions, assign values (utilities) to the various outcomes, and then calculate which decision gives the greatest value. To complete a decision analysis, the clinician would proceed as follows:

(1) Draw a decision tree showing the elements of the medical decision.
(2) Assign probabilities to the various branches.
(3) Assign values (utilities) to the outcomes.
(4) Determine the expected utility (the product of probability and utility) of each branch.
(5) Select the decision with the highest expected utility.

Figure 41–11 shows a decision tree where the decision to be made is whether to treat without testing, perform a test and then treat based on the test result, or perform no tests and give no treatment. The clinician begins the analysis by building a decision tree showing the important elements of the decision. Once the tree is built, the clinician assigns probabilities to all the branches. In this case, all the branch probabilities can be calculated from (1) the probability of disease before the test (pretest probability), (2) the chance of a positive test if the disease is present (sensitivity), and (3) the chance of a negative test if the disease is absent (specificity). Next, the clinician assigns utility values to each of the outcomes.

After the expected utility is calculated, the clinician may identify which alternative has the highest value by this analysis.

Although time-consuming, decision analysis can help to structure complex clinical problems and to make difficult clinical decisions.

Appendix: Therapeutic Drug Monitoring & Laboratory Reference Ranges

C. Diana Nicoll, MD, PhD

Table 1. Therapeutic drug monitoring.[1]

Drug	Effective Concentrations	Half-Life (hours)	Dosage Adjustment	Comments
Amikacin	Peak: 10–25 µg/mL; trough: <10 µg/mL	2–3 ↑ in uremia	↓ in renal dysfunction	Concomitant kanamycin or tobramycin therapy may give falsely elevated amikacin results by immunoassay.
Amitriptyline	160–240 ng/mL	9–46		Drug is highly protein-bound. Patient-specific decrease in protein binding may invalidate quoted range of effective concentration.
Carbamazepine	4–8 µg/mL	10–30		Induces its own metabolism. Metabolite 10,11-epoxide exhibits 13% cross-reactivity by immunoassay.
Cyclosporine	150–400 mg/mL (ng/L) whole blood	6–12	Need to know specimen and methodology used	Cyclosporine is lipid-soluble (20% bound to leukocytes; 40% to erythrocytes; 40% in plasma, highly bound to lipoproteins). Binding is temperature-dependent, so whole blood is preferred to plasma or serum as specimen. High-performance liquid chromatography (HPLC) or monoclonal fluorescence polarization measures cyclosporine reliably; polyclonal fluorescence polarization immunoassays cross-react with metabolites, so the therapeutic range used with those assays is higher. Anticonvulsants and rifampin increase metabolism. Erythromycin, ketoconazole, and calcium channel blockers decrease metabolism.
Desipramine	100–250 ng/mL	13–23		Drug is highly protein-bound. Patient-specific decrease in protein binding may invalidate quoted range of effective concentration.
Digoxin	0.8–2 ng/mL	42 ↑ in uremia, CHF, hypothyroidism; ↓ in hyperthyroidism	↓ in renal dysfunction, CHF	Bioavailability of digoxin tablets is 50–90%. Specimen must not be drawn within 6 hours of dose. Dialysis does not remove a significant amount. Hypokalemia potentiates toxicity. Digitalis toxicity is a clinical and *not* a laboratory diagnosis. Digibind (digoxin-specific antibody) therapy of digoxin overdose can interfere with measurement of digoxin levels depending on the digoxin assay. Elimination reduced by quinidine, verapamil, and amiodarone.
Ethosuximide	40–100 mg/L	Child: 30 Adult: 50		Levels used primarily to assess compliance. Toxicity is rare and does not correlate well with plasma concentrations.
Gentamicin	Peak: 4–8 µg/mL; trough: <2 µg/mL	2–5 ↑ in uremia (7.3 on dialysis)	↓ in renal dysfunction	Draw peak specimen 30 minutes after end of infusion. Draw trough just before next dose. In uremic patients, carbenicillin may decrease gentamicin half-life from 46 hours to 22 hours.

(continued)

Table 1. Therapeutic drug monitoring.[1] (continued)

Drug	Effective Concentrations	Half-Life (hours)	Dosage Adjustment	Comments
Imipramine	180–350 ng/mL	10–16		Drug is highly protein-bound. Patient-specific decrease in protein binding may invalidate quoted range of effective concentration.
Lidocaine	1–5 µg/mL	1.8 ↔ in uremia, CHF; ↑ in cirrhosis	↓ in CHF, liver disease	Levels increased with cimetidine therapy. CNS toxicity common in the elderly.
Lithium	0.7–1.5 meq/L	22 ↑ in uremia	↓ in renal dysfunction	Thiazides and loop diuretics may increase serum lithium levels.
Methotrexate		8.4 ↑ in uremia	↓ in renal dysfunction	7-Hydroxymethotrexate cross-reacts 1.5% in immunoassay. To minimize toxicity, leucovorin should be continued if methotrexate level is > 0.1 µmol/L at 48 hours after start of therapy. Methotrexate > 1 µmol/L at > 48 hours requires an increase in leucovorin rescue therapy.
Nortriptyline	50–140 ng/mL	18–44		Drug is highly protein-bound. Patient-specific decrease in protein binding may invalidate quoted range of effective concentration.
Phenobarbital	10–30 µg/mL	86 ↑ in cirrhosis	↓ in liver disease	Metabolized primarily by the hepatic microsomal enzyme system. Many drug-drug interactions.
Phenytoin	10–20 µg/mL; 5–10 µg/mL in uremia, hypoalbuminemia	Dose-dependent		Metabolite cross-reacts 10% in immunoassay. Metabolism is capacity-limited. Increase dose cautiously when level approaches therapeutic range, since new steady-state level may be disproportionately higher. Drug is very highly protein-bound; protein binding is decreased in uremia and hypoalbuminemia.
Primidone	5–10 µg/mL	8		Phenobarbital cross-reacts 0.5%. Metabolized to phenobarbital. Primidone/phenobarbital ratio > 1:2 suggests poor compliance.
Procainamide	4–8 µg/mL	3 ↑ in uremia	↓ in renal dysfunction	30% of patients with plasma levels of 12–16 µg/mL have electrocardiographic changes; 40% of patients with plasma levels of > 16 µg/mL have severe toxicity.
Quinidine	1–4 µg/mL	7 ↔ in CHF; ↑ in liver disease	↓ in liver disease, CHF	Effective concentration is lower in chronic liver disease and nephrosis, where binding is decreased.
Salicylate	15–300 µg/mL	Dose-dependent		
Theophylline	5–20 µg/mL	9	↓ in CHF, cirrhosis, and with cimetidine	Caffeine cross-reacts 10%. Elimination is increased 1½–2 times in smokers. 1,3-Dimethyl uric acid metabolite increased in uremia and, because of cross-reactivity, may cause an apparent slight increase in serum theophylline.
Tobramycin	Peak: 5–10 µg/mL; trough: <2 µg/mL	2–3; ↑ in uremia	↓ in renal dysfunction	Tobramycin, kanamycin, and amikacin may cross-react in immunoassay.
Valproic acid	55–100 µg/mL	13–19		95% protein-bound. Decreased binding in uremia and cirrhosis.
Vancomycin	Trough: 5–15 µg/mL	6 ↑ in uremia	↓ in renal dysfunction	Toxicity in uremic patients leads to irreversible deafness. Keep peak level < 30–40 µg/mL to avoid toxicity.

↔ = unchanged; ↑ = increase(d); ↓ = decrease(d); CHF = congestive heart failure.
[1]Modified and reproduced, with permission, from Nicoll D et al: *Pocket Guide to Diagnostic Tests,* 2nd ed. Appleton & Lange 1996.

Table 2. Reference ranges for commonly used tests.[1,2]
Current metric units × Conversion factor = SI units
SI units ÷ Conversion factor = Current metric units

Test	Specimen	Conventional Units	Conversion Factor	SI Units[2]	Collection
Acetaminophen	Serum	10–20 mg/L **Panic:** >50 mg/L	66.16	66–132 µmol/L	Marbled
Acetoacetate	Serum or urine	Negative		Negative	Marbled or urine container
Adrenocorticotropic hormone (ACTH)	Plasma	20–100 pg/mL (laboratory-specific)	0.22	4–22 pmol/L	Heparinized plastic container
Alanine aminotransferase (ALT, SGPT, GPT)	Serum	0–35 units/L (laboratory-specific)	0.02	0–0.58 µkat/L (laboratory-specific)	Marbled
Albumin	Serum	3.4–4.7 g/dL	10.00	34–47 g/L	Marbled
Aldosterone	Plasma	Salt-loaded (120 meq Na+/d): Supine: 3–10 ng/dL Upright: 5–30 ng/dL Salt-depleted (20 meq Na+/d): Supine: 12–36 ng/dL Upright: 17–137 ng/dL	27.74	83–277 pmol/L 139–831 pmol/L 332–997 pmol/L 471–3795 pmol/L	Lavender or green
Alkaline phosphatase	Serum	41–133 units/L (method- and age-dependent)	0.02	0.7–2.2 µkat/L (method- and age-dependent)	Marbled
Ammonia (NH_3)	Plasma	18–60 µg/dL	0.59	11–35 µmol/L	Green
Amylase	Serum	20–110 units/L (laboratory-specific)	0.02	0.33–1.83 µkat/L (laboratory-specific)	Marbled
Angiotensin-converting enzyme (ACE)	Serum	12–35 units/L (method-dependent)	16.67	<590 nkat/L (method-dependent)	Marbled
Antithrombin III (AT III)	Plasma	84–123% (qualitative) 22–39 mg/dL (quantitative)			Blue
α_1-Antitrypsin[3]	Serum	110–270 mg/dL	0.01	1.1–2.7 g/L	Marbled
Aspartate aminotransferase (AST, SGOT, GOT)	Serum	0–35 units/L (laboratory-specific)	0.02	0–0.58 µkat/L (laboratory-specific)	Marbled
Basophil count	Whole blood	$0.01–0.12 \times 10^9$/L			Lavender
Bilirubin	Serum	Total: 0.1–1.2 mg/dL Direct (conjugated to glucuronide): 0.1–0.4 mg/dL Indirect (unconjugated): 0.1–0.7 mg/dL	17.10	2–21 µmol/L <7 µmol/L <12 µmol/L	Marbled
Blood urea nitrogen (BUN)	Serum	8–20 mg/dL	0.36	2.9–7.1 mmol/L	Marbled
C-peptide	Serum	0.8–4.0 ng/mL	1.00	0.8–4.0 µg/L	Marbled (fasting)
Calcitonin	Plasma	Male: <90 pg/mL Female: <70 pg/mL	1.00	Male: <90 ng/L Female: <70 ng/L	Green
Calcium (Ca^{2+})	Serum	8.5–10.5 mg/dL **Panic:** <6.5 or >13.5 mg/dL	0.25	2.1–2.6 mmol/L	Marbled
Calcium (ionized)	Serum	4.6–5.3 mg/dL	0.25	1.15–1.32 mmol/L	Marbled
Calcium (U_{Ca})	Urine	100–300 mg/d	0.025	2.5–7.5 mmol/d	Urine bottle containing hydrochloric acid

(continued)

Table 2. Reference ranges for commonly used tests.[1,2] (continued)

Test	Specimen	Conventional Units	Conversion Factor	SI Units[2]	Collection
Carbon dioxide, partial pressure (P_{CO_2})	Whole blood	32–48 mm Hg	0.13	4.26–6.38 kPa	Heparinized syringe
Carbon dioxide (CO_2), total (bicarbonate)	Serum	22–28 meq/L **Panic:** <15 or >40 meq/L	1.00	22–28 mmol/L **Panic:** <15 or >40 mmol/L	Marbled
Carboxyhemoglobin (HbCO)	Whole blood	<9% of total hemoglobin (Hb)	0.01	<0.09 fraction of total hemoglobin	Lavender
Carcinoembryonic antigen (CEA)	Serum	0–2.5 ng/mL	1.00	0–2.5 μg/L	Marbled
Ceruloplasmin	Serum	20–35 mg/dL (laboratory-specific)	10.00	200–350 mg/L	Marbled
Chloride (Cl^-)	Serum	98–107 meq/L	1.00	98–107 mmol/L	Marbled
Cholesterol	Serum	Desirable: <200 mg/dL Borderline: 200–239 mg/dL High risk: >240 mg/dL	0.03	Desirable: <5.2 mmol/L Borderline: 5.2–6.1 mmol/L High risk: >6.2 mmol/L	Marbled
Chorionic gonadotropin, β-subunit (β-hCG), quantitative	Serum	Males and nonpregnant females: undetectable or <5 mU/mL	1.00	Males and nonpregnant females: undetectable or <5 IU/L	Marbled
Complement C3	Serum	64–166 mg/dL	10.00	640–1660 mg/L	Marbled
Complement C4	Serum	15–45 mg/dL	10.00	150–450 mg/L	Marbled
Complement CH50	Plasma or serum	22–40 units/mL (laboratory-specific)			Marbled
Cortisol	Plasma or serum	8:00 AM: 5–20 μg/dL	27.59	140–550 nmol/L	Marbled, lavender, or green
Cortisol (urinary free)	Urine	10–110 μg/24 h	2.76	30–300 nmol/d	Urine bottle containing boric acid
Creatine kinase (CK)	Serum	32–267 units/L (method-dependent)	0.02	0.53–4.45 μkat/L (method-dependent)	Marbled
Creatine kinase MB (CKMB)	Serum	<16 units/L or <4% of total CK (laboratory-specific)	0.04	<0.27 μkat/L	Marbled
Creatinine (Cr)	Serum	0.6–1.2 mg/dL	83.3	50–100 μmol/L	Marbled
Creatinine clearance (Cl_{Cr})	See Collection column.	Adults: 90–140 mL/min/1.73 m² BSA	0.017	1.5–2.3 mL/s/1.73 m² BSA	Carefully timed 24-hour urine and simultaneous serum or plasma creatinine sample
Cryoglobulins	Serum	<0.12 mg/dL			Marbled at 37 °C
Eosinophil count	Whole blood	0.4–0.5 × 10⁹/L			Lavender
Erythrocyte count (RBC count)	Whole blood	4.2–5.6 × 10⁶/μL	1.00	4.2–5.6 × 10¹²/L	Lavender
Erythrocyte sedimentation rate	Whole blood	Male: <10 mm/h Female: <15 mm/h (laboratory-specific)		Same	Lavender
Erythropoietin (EPO)	Serum	5–20 mU/mL	1.00	5–20 IU/L	Marbled
Ethanol	Serum	mg/dL Legal "driving under the influence" in many states is defined as >80 mg/dL (>17 mmol/L)	0.217	mmol/L	Marbled
Factor VIII assay	Plasma	40–150% of normal (varies with age)			Blue

Table 2. Reference ranges for commonly used tests.[1,2] (continued)

Test	Specimen	Conventional Units	Conversion Factor	SI Units[2]	Collection
Fecal fat	Stool	Random: <60 droplets of fat per high-power field 72-hour: <7 g/d			Qualitative: Random stool sample Quantitative: 72-hour collection following 2-day dietary fat regimen
Ferritin	Serum	Male: 16–300 ng/mL Female: 4–161 ng/mL	1.00	Male: 16–300 µg/L Female: 4–161 µg/L	Marbled
α-Fetoprotein (AFP)	Serum	0–15 ng/mL	1.00	0–15 µg/L	Marbled
Fibrin D-dimers	Plasma	Negative			Blue
Fibrinogen (functional)	Plasma	175–433 mg/dL **Panic:** <75 mg/dL	0.01	1.75–4.3 g/L	Blue
Folic acid (red cells)	Whole blood	165–760 ng/mL	2.27	370–1720 nmol/L	Lavender
Follicle-stimulating hormone (FSH)	Serum	Female: Follicular phase 4–13 mU/mL Luteal phase 2–13 mU/mL Midcycle 5–22 mU/mL Postmenopausal 30–138 mU/mL Male: 1–10 mU/mL (laboratory-specific)	1.00	Female: 4–13 IU/L 2–13 IU/L 5–22 IU/L 30–138 IU/L Male: 1–10 IU/L (laboratory-specific)	Marbled
Free erythrocyte protoporphyrin (FEP)	Whole blood	<35 µg/dL (method-dependent)			Lavender
Gamma-glutamyltranspeptidase (GGT)	Serum	9–85 units/L (laboratory-specific)	0.02	0.15–1.42 µkat/L (laboratory-specific)	Marbled
Gastrin	Serum	<100 pg/mL (laboratory-specific)	1.00	<100 ng/L	Marbled
Glucose	Serum	60–115 mg/dL **Panic:** <40 or >500 mg/dL	0.06	3.3–6.3 mmol/L	Marbled (fasting)
Glucose-6-phosphate dehydrogenase (G6PD) screen	Whole blood	5–14 units/g Hb	0.02	0.1–0.28 µkat/L	Green or blue
Glutamine	CSF	6–16 mg/dL **Panic:** >40 mg/dL	0.07	0.1–0.28 mmol/L	Collect CSF in a plastic tube
Glycated (glycosylated) hemoglobin (HbA_{1c})	Serum	3.9–6.9% (method-dependent)			Lavender
Growth hormone (GH)	Serum	0–5 ng/mL	1.00	0–5 µg/L	Marbled
Haptoglobin	Serum	46–316 mg/dL	0.01	0.5–3.2 g/L	Marbled
HDL cholesterol	Serum	Male: 27–67 mg/dL Female: 34–88 mg/dL	0.026	0.7–1.73 mmol/L 0.88–2.28 mmol/L	Marbled
Hematocrit (Hct)	Whole blood	Male: 39–49% Female: 35–45% (age-dependent)	0.01	Male: 0.39–0.49 Female: 0.35–0.45	Lavender
Hemoglobin A_2 (HbA_2)	Whole blood	1.5–3.5% of total hemoglobin	0.01	0.015–0.035	Lavender
Hemoglobin electrophoresis	Whole blood	HbA: >95% HbA_2: 1.5–3.5%			Lavender, blue, or green

(continued)

Table 2. Reference ranges for commonly used tests.[1,2] (continued)

Test	Specimen	Conventional Units	Conversion Factor	SI Units[2]	Collection
Hemoglobin, fetal (HbF)	Whole blood	Adult: <2% (varies with age)			Lavender, blue, or green
Hemoglobin, total (Hb)	Whole blood	Male: 13.6–17.5 g/dL Female: 12.0–15.5 g/dL **Panic:** ≤7 g/dL (age-dependent)	10.00	Male: 136–175 g/L Female: 120–155 g/L	Lavender
Hemosiderin	Urine	Negative			Urine container
5-Hydroxyindoleacetic acid (5-HIAA)	Urine	2–8 mg/24 h	5.23	10–40 µmol/d	Urine bottle containing hydrochloric acid
IgG index	Serum and CSF	0.29–0.59 ratio			Marbled and glass or plastic tube for CSF
Immunoglobulins (Ig)	Serum	IgA: 78–367 mg/dL IgG: 583–1761 mg/dL IgM: 52–335 mg/dL	0.01	IgA: 0.78–3.67 g/L IgG: 5.83–17.6 g/L IgM: 0.52–3.35 g/L	Marbled
Insulin, immuno-reactive	Serum	6–35 µU/mL	7.18	42–243 pmol/L	Marbled
Insulin-like growth factor-1	Plasma	123–463 ng/mL (age- and sex-dependent)	1.0	123–463 µg/L	Lavender
Iron (Fe^{2+})	Serum	50–175 µg/dL	0.18	9–31 µmol/L	Marbled
Iron-binding capacity, total (TIBC)	Serum	250–460 µg/dL	0.18	45–82 µmol/L	Marbled
Lactate dehydrogenase (LDH)	Serum	88–230 units/L (laboratory-specific)	0.02	1.46–3.82 µkat/L (laboratory-specific)	Marbled
Lactate dehydrogenase (LDH) isoenzymes	Serum	LDH_1/LDH_2: <0.85			Marbled
Lactic acid (lactate)	Venous blood	0.5–2.0 meq/L	1.00	0.5–2.0 mmol/L	Gray
LDL cholesterol	Serum	<130 mg/dL	0.026	<3.37 mmol/L	Marbled
Lead (Pb)	Whole blood	Child: <25 µg/dL Adult: <40 µg/dL	0.05	Child: <1.21 µmol/L Adult: <1.93 µmol/L	Navy
Lecithin/sphingomyelin (L/S) ratio	Amniotic fluid	>2.0 (method-dependent)			Collect in a plastic tube
Leukocyte alkaline phosphatase (LAP)	Whole blood	40–130 Based on 0 to 4+ rating of 100 PMNs stained for alkaline phosphatase			Green
Leukocyte (white blood cell) count, total (WBC count)	Whole blood	3.4–10 × 10³/µL **Panic:** <1.5 × 10³/µL	1.00	3.4–10 × 10⁹/L	Lavender
Lipase	Serum	0–160 units/L (laboratory-specific)	0.02	0–2.66 µkat/L (laboratory-specific)	Marbled

Luteinizing hormone (LH)	Serum	Female:
		  Follicular phase 1–18 mU/mL
		  Luteal phase 0.4–20 mU/mL
		  Midcycle 24–105 mU/mL
		  Postmenopausal 15–62 mU/mL
		Male: 1–10 mU/mL
		(laboratory-specific)
			1.00	1–18 units/L
				
				0.4–20 units/L
				
				24–105 units/L
				
				15–62 units/L
				Male: 1–10 units/L
				(laboratory-specific)
					Marbled

Lymphocyte count	Whole blood	0.8–3.5 × 10⁹/L			Lavender

(continued)

Table 2. Reference ranges for commonly used tests.[1,2] (continued)

Test	Specimen	Conventional Units	Conversion Factor	SI Units[2]	Collection
Magnesium (Mg^{2+})	Serum	1.8–3.0 mg/dL **Panic:** <0.5 or >4.5 mg/dL	0.41	0.75–1.25 mmol/L	Marbled
Mean corpuscular hemoglobin (MCH)	Whole blood	26–34 pg			Lavender
Mean corpuscular hemo-globin concentration (MCHC)	Whole blood	31–36 g/dL	10.00	310–360 g/L	Lavender
Mean corpuscular volume (MCV)	Whole blood	80–100 fL			Lavender
Metanephrines	Urine	0.3–0.9 mg/24 h	5.46	1.6–4.9 µmol/d	Urine bottle con-taining hydro-chloric acid
Methemoglobin (MetHb)	Whole blood	<1% of total hemoglobin	0.01	<0.01 fraction of total hemoglobin	Lavender
β$_2$-Microglobulin (β$_2$M)	Serum	<2.0 mg/dL	10.00	<2 mg/L	Marbled
Monocyte count	Whole blood	0.2–0.8 × 10^9/L			Lavender
Neutrophil count	Whole blood	2.2–8.6 × 10^9/L			Lavender
Osmolality	Serum	275–293 mosm/kg H$_2$O **Panic:** <240 or >320 mosm/kg H$_2$O	1.00	275–293 mmol/kg H$_2$O	Marbled
	Urine	Random: 100–900 mosm/kg H$_2$O	1.00	Random: 100–900 mmol/kg H$_2$O	Urine container
Oxygen, partial pressure (PO$_2$)	Whole blood	83–108 mm Hg	0.13	11.04–14.36 kPa	Heparinized syringe
Parathyroid hormone (PTH)	Serum	Intact PTH: 11–54 pg/mL (laboratory-specific)	0.11	Intact PTH: 1.2–5.7 pmol/L (laboratory-specific)	Marbled
Partial thromboplastin time, activated (PTT)	Plasma	25–35 seconds (range varies) **Panic:** ≥60 seconds			Blue
pH	Whole blood	Arterial: 7.35–7.45 Venous: 7.31–7.41			Heparinized syringe
Phosphorus	Serum	2.5–4.5 mg/dL **Panic:** <1.0 mg/dL	0.32	0.8–1.45 mmol/L	Marbled
Platelet count (Plt)	Whole blood	150–450 × 10^3/µL **Panic:** <25 × 10^3/µL	1.00	150–450 × 10^9/L **Panic:**<25 × 10^9/L	Lavender
Platelet-associated IgG	Whole blood	Negative			Yellow (17 mL of blood)
Porphobilinogen (PBG)	Urine	Negative			
Potassium (K$^+$)	Serum	3.5–5.0 meq/L **Panic:** <3.0 or >6.0 meq/L	1.00	3.5–5.0 mmol/L	Marbled
Prolactin (PRL)	Serum	<20 ng/mL	1.00	<20 µg/L	Marbled
Prostate-specific antigen (PSA)	Serum	0–4 ng/mL	1.00	0–4 µg/L	Marbled
Protein C	Plasma	71–176%			Blue

(continued)

Table 2. Reference ranges for commonly used tests.[1,2] (continued)

Test	Specimen	Conventional Units	Conversion Factor	SI Units[2]	Collection
Protein electrophoresis	Serum	Adults: Albumin: 3.3–4.7 g/dL α_1: 0.1–0.4 g/dL α_2: 0.3–0.9 g/dL β_2: 0.7–1.5 g/dL γ: 0.5–1.4 g/dL	10.00	33–47 g/L 1–4 g/L 3–9 g/L 7–15 g/L 5–14 g/L	Marbled
Protein S (antigen)	Plasma	76–178%			Blue
Protein, total	Plasma or serum	6.0–8.0 g/dL	10.00	60–80 g/L	Marbled
Prothrombin time (PT)	Whole blood	11–15 seconds **Panic:** ≥30 seconds (laboratory-specific) INR (international normalized ratio): 2–3.5 **Panic:** >6			Blue
Red blood cell count	Whole blood	4.7–6.1 × 10^9/mL			Lavender
Red cell volume	Whole blood	25–35 mL/kg			Green
Renin activity (PRA)	Plasma	High-sodium diet (75–150 meq Na+/d): Supine: 0.2–2.3 ng/mL/h Standing: 1.3–4.0 ng/mL/h Low-sodium diet (30–75 meq Na+/d): Standing: 4.0–7.7 ng/mL/h			Lavender
Reptilase clotting time	Plasma	13–19 seconds			Blue
Reticulocyte count	Whole blood	33–137 × 10^3/μL	1.00	33–137 × 10^9/L	Lavender
Russell's viper venom clotting time (dilute) (RVVT)	Plasma	24–37 seconds			Blue
Salicylate (aspirin, others)	Serum	20–30 mg/dL **Panic:** >35 mg/dL	10.00	200–300 mg/L	Marbled
Sodium (Na+)	Serum	135–145 meq/L **Panic:** <125 or >155 meq/L	1.00	135–145 mmol/L	Marbled
Testosterone	Serum	Male: 3.0–10.0 ng/mL Female: 0.3–0.7 ng/mL	3.47	Male: 10–35 nmol/L Female: 1.0–2.4 nmol/L	Marbled
Thrombin time	Plasma	24–35 seconds (laboratory-specific)			Blue
Thyroglobulin	Serum	3–42 ng/mL	1.00	3–42 μg/L	Marbled
Thyroid-stimulating hormone (TSH)	Serum	0.4–6 μU/mL	1.00	0.4–6 mU/L	Marbled
Thyroid-stimulating hormone receptor antibody (TSH-R Ab [stim])	Serum	<130% of basal activity. Based on cAMP generation in thyroid cell tissue culture.			
Thyroxine, free (FT$_4$)	Serum	9–24 pmol/L (varies with method)			Marbled
Thyroxine (T$_4$), total	Serum	5–11 μg/dL	12.80	64–142 nmol/L	Marbled
Thyroxine index, free (FT$_4$I)	Serum	6.5–12.5			Marbled
Transferrin	Serum	190–375 mg/dL	0.01	1.9–3.75 g/L	Marbled
Triglycerides	Serum	<165 mg/dL	0.01	<1.65 g/L	Marbled (fasting)

(continued

Table 2. Reference ranges for commonly used tests.[1,2] (continued)

Test	Specimen	Conventional Units	Conversion Factor	SI Units[2]	Collection
Triiodothyronine (T$_3$), total	Serum	95–190 ng/dL	0.015	1.5–2.9 nmol/L	Marbled
Troponin-I (cTnI)	Serum	<1.5 ng/mL			Marbled
Uric acid	Serum	Male: 2.4–7.4 mg/dL Female: 1.4–5.8 mg/dL	59.48	Male: 140–440 µmol/L Female: 80–350 µmol/L	Marbled
Vanillylmandelic acid (VMA)	Urine	2–7 mg/24 h	5.05	10–35 µmol/d	Urine bottle containing hydrochloric acid
Vitamin B$_{12}$	Serum	140–820 pg/mL	0.74	100–600 pmol/L	Marbled
Vitamin B$_{12}$ absorption test (Schilling test)	24-hour urine	Excretion of >8% of administered dose			Urine bottle
Vitamin D, 25-hydroxy (25[OH]D)	Serum or plasma	10–50 ng/mL	2.5	25–125 nmol/L	Marbled or green
Vitamin D, 1,25-dihydroxy (1,25[OH]$_2$D)	Serum or plasma	20–76 pg/mL		48–182 pmol/L	Marbled or green
White blood cell count	Whole blood	4.8–10.8 × 10^9/L			Lavender

[1]The reference ranges given here in conventional units and in SI units are from several large medical centers. Always use the reference ranges provided by your clinical laboratory, since ranges may be method-dependent.
[2]Reference: Young DS: Implementation of SI units for clinical laboratory data. Ann Intern Med 1987;106:114.
[3]Also called α_1-antiprotease in some clinical contexts.

Commonly Used Specimen Collection Tubes

Tube Color	Tube Contents	Typical Use
Lavender	EDTA	Complete blood count
Marbled	Serum separator	Serum chemistry tests
Red	None	Blood banking (serum)
Blue	Citrate	Coagulation studies
Gray	Inhibitor of glycolysis (sodium fluoride)	Lactic acid
Green	Heparin	Plasma studies
Yellow	Acid citrate	HLA typing
Navy	Trace metal free	Trace metals (eg, lead)

Index

NOTE: Page numbers in bold face type indicate a major discussion. A *t* following a page number indicates tabular material and an *i* following a page number indicates an illustration. Drugs are listed under their generic names. When a drug trade name is listed, the reader is referred to the generic name.

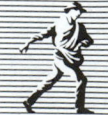